# INTERNATIONAL TEXTBOOK
# OF MEDICINE

**General Editors**

## A. H. Samiy, M.D.

Professor of Clinical Medicine, Attending Physician,
New York Hospital, Cornell Medical Center

## Lloyd H. Smith, Jr., M.D.

Professor and Chairman, Department of Medicine
University of California, San Francisco

## James B. Wyngaarden, M.D.

Frederic M. Hanes Professor and Chairman,
Department of Medicine, Duke University Medical Center

### Volume I
### PATHOPHYSIOLOGY
### The Biological Principles of Disease

### Volume II
### MEDICAL MICROBIOLOGY AND INFECTIOUS DISEASES

### Volume III
### CECIL TEXTBOOK OF MEDICINE

# MEDICAL MICROBIOLOGY
# and INFECTIOUS DISEASES

**ABRAHAM I. BRAUDE, M.D., Ph.D.**
Professor of Medicine and Pathology
University of California, San Diego

*Associate Editors*

**CHARLES E. DAVIS, M.D.**
Professor of Pathology
University of California, San Diego

**JOSHUA FIERER, M.D.**
Associate Professor of Medicine
University of California, San Diego

**W. B. SAUNDERS COMPANY** Philadelphia
London
Toronto
Mexico City
Sydney
Tokyo

W. B. Saunders Company:   West Washington Square
Philadelphia, PA   19105

1 St. Anne's Road
Eastbourne, East Sussex BN21 3UN, England

1 Goldthorne Avenue
Toronto, Ontario M8Z 5T9, Canada

Cedro 512
Mexico 4, D.F. Mexico

9 Waltham Street
Artarmon, N.S.W. 2064, Australia

Ichibancho, Central Bldg., 22-1
Chiyoda-ku, Tokyo 102, Japan

**Library of Congress Cataloging in Publication Data**

Braude, Abraham I.

Medical microbiology and infectious diseases.

(International textbook of medicine)

1. Medical microbiology.    2. Communicable diseases.
I. Title.    II. Series. [DNLM: 1. Microbiology.
2. Communicable diseases. QW4 B824m]

QR46.B68      616'.01      79–3986

ISBN 0–7216–1919–3

INTERNATIONAL TEXTBOOK OF MEDICINE
Medical Microbiology and Infectious
Diseases   Vol. II       ISBN   0-7216-1919-3

Last digit is the print number:   9  8  7  6  5  4  3  2

## Dedication

To medical students and physicians throughout the world, who strive with dedication and hard work to achieve better health for mankind.

# CONTRIBUTORS

YOUSEF AL-DOORY, Ph.D.
Associate Professor of Pathology, George Washington University School of Medicine; Chief, Sections of Mycology and Serology, Division of Laboratory Medicine, George Washington University Hospital, Washington, D.C.
DEMATIACEAE: AGENTS OF CHROMOMYCOSIS

AARON D. ALEXANDER, Ph.D.
Professor of Microbiology, Department of Microbiology, Chicago College of Osteopathic Medicine, Chicago, Illinois.
LEPTOSPIRA

A. O. ANYA, Ph.D.
Professor of Zoology and Director, School of Postgraduate Studies, University of Nigeria, Nsukka, Nigeria.
NEMATHELMINTHES

DONALD ARMSTRONG, M.D.
Professor of Medicine, Cornell University Medical College; Chief, Infectious Disease Service, Memorial Sloan-Kettering Cancer Center, New York, New York
CEREBRAL ASPERGILLOSIS; CEREBRAL MUCORMYCOSIS

HOWARD ROBERT ATTEBERY, D.D.S.
Research Microbiologist, Veterans Administration Medical Center, San Diego, California.
FUSOBACTERIA; GRAM-POSITIVE COCCI: PEPTOCOCCUS, PEPTOSTREPTOCOCCUS, STREPTOCOCCUS (ANAEROBIC), AND SARCINIA; VEILLONELLA

HERMAN BAER, M.D.
Associate Professor of Pathology and Medical Microbiology; Director, Clinical Microbiology Laboratories, Shands Teaching Hospital and Clinics, Miller Health Center, University of Florida, College of Medicine, Gainesville, Florida.
CLASSIFICATION OF BACTERIA; MORAXELLA AND ACINE-TOBACTER

ANN SULLIVAN BAKER, M.D.
Assistant Professor of Medicine, Harvard Medical School; Assistant in Medicine, Massachusetts General Hospital; Consultant in Infectious Diseases, Massachusetts Eye and Ear Infirmary, Boston, Massachusetts.
SPINAL EPIDURAL ABSCESS; SUBDURAL EMPYEMA

JEFFRY D. BAND, M.D.
Medical Epidemiologist, Center for Disease Control, Atlanta, Georgia.
LEGIONELLOSIS

ALAN G. BARBOUR, M.D.
Fellow, Division of Infectious Diseases, Department of Medicine, University of Utah, Salt Lake City, Utah.
COLORADO TICK FEVER

LANE BARKSDALE, M.D.
Professor of Microbiology, New York University School of Medicine and Medical Center, New York, New York.
DIPHTHERIA BACILLI AND OTHER CORYNEBACTERIA

ELIZABETH BARRETT-CONNOR, M.D.,
D.C.M.T. (London)
Associate Professor, Division of Epidemiology, Departments of Community Medicine and Medicine, University of California, San Diego, School of Medicine, San Diego, California.
AFRICAN SLEEPING SICKNESS; FLUKE INFECTIONS; INTESTINAL ROUNDWORMS

JOSEPH H. BATES, M.D.
Professor of Medicine and Microbiology, University of Arkansas for Medical Sciences; Chief, Medical Service, Little Rock Veterans Medical Center, Little Rock, Arkansas.
TULAREMIA

WILLIAM R. BEISEL, A.B., M.D., F.A.C.P.
Deputy for Science, US Army Medical Research

Institute of Infectious Diseases, Fort Dietrick, Maryland.
METABOLIC EFFECTS OF INFECTION

DONALD W. BELCHER, M.D.
Associate Professor of Medicine, University of Washington, School of Medicine; Staff Physician, MCCU, Veterans Administration Medical Center, Seattle, Washington.
DRACUNCULIASIS

FRANCISCO BIAGI, M.D.
Professor of Medical Parasitology, National University of Mexico, School of Medicine; American British Cowdray Hospital, Hospital Infantil Privado, Mexico City, Mexico.
AMEBIC DYSENTERY; CUTANEOUS AMEBIASIS

PERRY S. BINDER, M.D., F.A.C.S.
Associate Professor of Ophthalmology, University of California, San Diego; Chief of Ophthalmology, San Diego Veterans Administration Medical Center; Consultant, Naval Regional Medical Center, San Diego, California.
OCULAR BACTERIAL INFECTIONS; OCULAR FUNGAL, PARASITIC, CHLAMYDIAL, AND RICKETTSIAL INFECTIONS; OCULAR INFLAMMATORY DISEASE

RUTH BISHOP, D.Sc.
Principal Research Fellow (NHMRC), Department of Gastroenterology, Royal Children's Hospital, Melbourne, Australia.
VIRAL GASTROENTERITIS

ALAN L. BISNO, M.D.
Chief, Division of Infectious Diseases, and Professor of Internal Medicine, University of Tennessee Center for the Health Sciences; Attending Physician, City of Memphis Hospitals, Memphis, Tennessee.
ROCKY MOUNTAIN SPOTTED FEVER

DONALD L. BORNSTEIN, M.D.
Associate Professor of Medicine, Chief of Infectious Disease Section, Department of Medicine, State University of New York Upstate Medical Center; Attending Physician, State University Hospital, Syracuse Veterans Administration Hospital, Crouse-Irving Memorial Hospital, Syracuse, New York.
BACTEROIDES SEPTICEMIA; CLOSTRIDIAL MYONECROSIS; CLOSTRIDIAL SEPTICEMIA

PAULA BRANEFORS, M.D., Ph.D.
Assistant Professor, University of Goteborg, Institute of Medical Microbiology, Department of Bacteriology, Goteborg, Sweden.
EPIGLOTTITIS AND PSEUDOCROUP

ABRAHAM I. BRAUDE, M.D., Ph.D.
Professor of Medicine and Pathology, University of California, San Diego, California.
ACTINOMYCOSIS; THE ASPERGILLI; BACTERIAL ENDOTOXINS; BACTERIAL LUNG ABSCESS; BANCROFTIAN AND MALAYAN FILARIASIS; CANDIDA AND TORULOPSIS; COCCIDIOIDOMYCOSIS; DESCRIPTION OF ANTIMICROBIAL DRUGS; DENGUE AND OTHER HEMORRHAGIC FEVERS; LASSA FEVER; MECHANISMS OF ACQUIRED RESISTANCE TO INFECTION; MECHANISMS OF ACTION OF ANTIMICROBIALS; MECHANISMS OF IMMUNOLOGIC INJURY IN INFECTIOUS DISEASES; MECHANISMS OF NATURAL RESISTANCE TO INFECTION; MISCELLANEOUS FUNGI; THE AGENTS OF MYCETOMA AND RHINOSPORIDIUM; NORTH AMERICAN BLASTOMYCOSIS; POXVIRUSES; RESISTANCE TO ANTIMICROBIAL DRUGS; SPOROTRICHOSIS; THE ZYGOMYCETES.

RUDOLF BREZINA, M.D., Ph.D.
Head, Department of Rickettsiae, Institute of Virology, Slovak Academy of Sciences, Bratislava, Czechoslovakia.
ENDEMIC TYPHUS; EPIDEMIC TYPHUS; OTHER RICKETTSIAL SPOTTED FEVERS.

S. J. D. BROOKS, M.D.
Formerly Fellow in Infectious Diseases, Department of Medicine, University of California, San Diego, California.
BACTERIAL LUNG ABSCESS

RICHARD E. BRYANT, M.D.
Professor of Internal Medicine, Director of Infectious Diseases Division, University of Oregon Health Sciences Center, Portland, Oregon.
VIRAL PNEUMONIA

ANTHONY D. M. BRYCESON, M.D., F.R.C.P.E., D.T.M. & H.
Senior Lecturer, London School of Hygiene and Tropical Medicine; Consultant Physician, Hospital for Tropical Diseases, London, England.
CUTANEOUS AND MUCOCUTANEOUS LEISHMANIASIS; VISCERAL LEISHMANIASIS

JOHN J. S. BURTON, Ph.D.
University of California ICMR, Institute for Medical Research, Kuala Lumpur, Malaysia.
ARTHROPODS OF MEDICAL IMPORTANCE

LUBOR ČERVA, RNDr, Dr. Sc.
Senior Resident Scientist, Department of Protozoology, Czechoslovak Academy of Sciences, Dejvice, Czechoslovakia.
AMEBIC MENINGOENCEPHALITIS

BARUN DEB CHATTERJEE, M.B.B.S., Ph.D.
Professor and Head, Department of Bacteri-

ology and Serology, School of Tropical Medicine, Calcutta, India.
VIBRIOS

T. H. CHEN, M.D.
Research Microbiologist, Department of Biomedical and Environmental Health Sciences, School of Public Health, University of California, Berkeley, California.
YERSINIA, PASTEURELLA, AND FRANCISELLA

DAVID FRANCIS CLYDE, M.D., Ph.D., D.T.M. & H.
Senior Malaria Adviser, World Health Organization, Regional Office for Southeast Asia, New Delhi, India.
MALARIA

STEPHEN N. COHEN, M.D.
Clinical Professor of Laboratory Medicine, Medicine, and Microbiology, University of California, San Francisco, School of Medicine; Director of Clinical Laboratories and Attending Physician, University of California, San Francisco, Medical Center, San Francisco, California.
INFECTION WITH PNEUMOCYSTIS CARINII

RICHARD W. COMPANS, Ph.D.
Professor of Microbiology, University of Alabama Medical Center, Birmingham, Alabama.
MORPHOLOGY AND STRUCTURE OF VIRUSES

JAMES D. CONNOR, M.D.
Professor of Pediatrics, University of California, San Diego; Consultant, Mercy Hospital, Camp Pendleton, Naval Hospital (Balboa), Children's Hospital, San Diego, California.
HAND-FOOT-MOUTH DISEASE; HERPANGINA; PERTUSSIS

EUGENE H. COTA-ROBLES, Ph.D.
Professor of Biology, University of California, Santa Cruz, California.
THE STRUCTURE OF THE BACTERIAL CELL

MANUEL CUADRA, M.D.
Professor (Retired) of Infectious, Parasitic, and Tropical Diseases, Universidad Nacional Mayor de San Marcos, Facultad de Medicina, Lima, Peru; Staff Member, Robert Koch Institut, Associated with Virchow Krankenhaus, Berlin, West Germany.
BARTONELLA BACILLIFORMIS; BARTONELLOSIS

SCOTT F. DAVIES, M.D.
Assistant Professor of Medicine, University of

Minnesota Medical School; Chief, Pulmonary Section, Hennepin County Medical Center, Minneapolis, Minnesota.
HISTOPLASMOSIS

CHARLES E. DAVIS, M.D.
Professor of Pathology, University of California, San Diego, School of Medicine; Associate Director of Microbiology, University Hospital, San Diego, California.
BABESIOSIS; CLASSIFICATION AND IDENTIFICATION OF BACTERIA; CRYPTOCOCCUS; CUTANEOUS LARVA MIGRANS; ERYSIPELOTHRIX RHUSOPATHIAE; GLANDERS; PARAGONIMIASIS.

GÉRARD De CROUSAZ, M.D.
Associate Professor, Faculty of Medicine, University of Lausanne; Consultant Neurologist, Centre Hospitalier Universitaire Vaudois, Lausanne, Switzerland.
TUBERCULOUS MENINGITIS

GUNTHER DENNERT, Ph.D.
Department of Cancer Biology, The Salk Institute, San Diego, California.
SCHISTOSOMIASIS

DENNIS M. DIXON, Ph.D.
Assistant Professor, Department of Biology, Loyola College of Maryland, Baltimore, Maryland.
BLASTOMYCES AND PARACOCCIDIOIDES

ALEXANDER L. DOHANY, Ph.D., Maj, MSC.
Chief, Department of Acarology, US Army Medical Research Unit, Kuala Lumpur, Department of State, Washington, D.C.
ARTHROPODS OF MEDICAL IMPORTANCE

JEAN M. DOLBY, Ph.D.
Member of the Senior Scientific Staff of the Medical Research Council, Clinical Research Centre, Harrow, Middlesex, England.
BORDETELLA

SAM T. DONTA, M.D.
Professor of Medicine, University of Iowa, College of Medicine; Director, Infectious Disease Services, University of Iowa and Veterans Administration Medical Center, Iowa City, Iowa.
FOOD POISONING

R. GORDON DOUGLAS, Jr., M.D.
Professor of Medicine and Microbiology and Head of Infectious Disease Unit, University of Rochester, School of Medicine and Dentistry;

Physician, Strong Memorial Hospital, Rochester, New York.
INFLUENZA

HERBERT L. DuPONT, M.D.
Professor and Director, Program in Infectious Diseases and Clinical Microbiology, The University of Texas Medical School at Houston; Attending Internist, Hermann Hospital, Houston, Texas.
GRANULOMATOUS HEPATITIS

WERNER DUTZ, M.D., F.R.C. Path.
Professor of Pathology, Medical College of Virginia, Richmond, Virginia.
ANTHRAX

GEORGE A. EDWARDS, M.D.
Professor of Medicine, Chief of Staff, Veterans Administration Hospital, Dallas, Texas.
LEPTOSPIROSIS

JOHN E. EDWARDS, Jr., M.D.
Assistant Professor of Medicine, University of California at Los Angeles School of Medicine; Attending Physician, Department of Medicine, and Staff Physician, Division of Infectious Diseases, Los Angeles County, Harbor/UCLA Medical Center, Los Angeles, California.
FUNGEMIA; MONILIASIS OF THE SKIN; THRUSH OF THE MOUTH AND ESOPHAGUS

SANFORD S. ELBERG, Ph.D.
Professor of Microbiology and Immunology, Department of Biomedical and Environmental Health Sciences, School of Public Health, University of California, Berkeley, California.
YERSINIA, PASTEURELLA, AND FRANCISELLA

MAKOTO ENOMOTO, M.D.
Lecturer of Pathology, St. Marianna University, School of Medicine; Consulting Pathologist, Sagamihara Kyodo Hospital, Sagamihara, Japan.
FUNGAL TOXINS

WILLIAM R. FAIR, M.D.
Professor of Surgery and Chairman, Division of Urology, Washington University, School of Medicine, St. Louis, Missouri.
PROSTATITIS

VLADIMIR FARKAŠ, Ph.D.
Researcher, Institute of Chemistry, Department of Biochemistry of Saccharides, Slovak Academy of Sciences, Bratislava, Czechoslovakia.
MORPHOLOGY AND STRUCTURE OF FUNGI

JANOS FEHER, M.D., C.Sc.
Associate Professor of Internal Medicine, Semmelweis Medical University; Attending Hepatologist, Semmelweis Medical University, 3rd Department of Medicine, Budapest, Hungary.
SPIROCHETAL HEPATITIS

JOSHUA FIERER, M.D.
Associate Professor of Medicine, University of California, San Diego, School of Medicine; Chief, Microbiology Laboratory, Veterans Administration Medical Center; Attending Physician, University Hospital, San Diego, California.
GRAM-POSITIVE COCCI; HERPESVIRUS SIMIAE ENCEPHALITIS; STREPTOBACILLUS MONILIFORMIS

ROBERT H. FITZGERALD, Jr., M.D.
Assistant Professor of Orthopedic Surgery, Mayo Medical School; Consultant, Department of Orthopedics, Mayo Clinic and Mayo Foundation, Rochester, Minnesota.
BACTERIAL ARTHRITIS; BACTERIAL OSTEOMYELITIS

DAVID W. FRASER, M.D.
Medical Epidemiologist, Center for Disease Control, Atlanta, Georgia.
LEGIONELLOSIS

LAWRENCE R. FREEDMAN, M.D.
Professor and Chairman, Department of Medicine, Veterans Administration Wadsworth Medical Center, UCLA School of Medicine, Los Angeles, California.
INFECTIVE ENDOCARDITIS AND OTHER INTRAVASCULAR INFECTIONS

STANLEY D. FREEDMAN, M.D.
Head, Division of Infectious Diseases, Scripps Clinic, Associate Clinical Professor of Medicine, University of California, San Diego, California; Attending Staff, Green Hospital of Scripps Clinic, La Jolla, California.
PSITTACOSIS; WHIPPLE'S DISEASE

CHANTAL FRELAND
Doctor in Bio-chemistry, Former Teaching Assistant in Bacteriology at the Nantes University Medical School; Chef de Service, Laboratoire de Biologie Medicale, Hôpital Médico-Chirurgical Léon Bellier, Nantes-Cedex, France.
ERYSIPELOID

WESLEY FURSTE, M.D., F.A.C.S.
Clinical Professor of Surgery, Ohio State University; Senior Attending Surgeon, Riverside

Methodist and Mt. Carmel Hospitals, Columbus, Ohio.
TETANUS

ROBERT G. GARRISON, Ph.D.
Associate Professor of Microbiology, Department of Microbiology, University of Kansas Medical Center; Research Microbiologist, Veterans Administration Medical Center, Kansas City, Missouri.
SPOROTHRIX SCHENKII

O. J. A. GILMORE, M.S., F.R.C.S. (Eng.), F.R.C.S. (Ed.)
Consultant Surgeon, St. Bartholemew's Hospital, Hackney Hospital, London, England.
APPENDICITIS AND DIVERTICULITIS

ISAAC GINSBURG, M.Sc., Ph.D.
Professor of Microbiology, The Hebrew University Hadassah, Faculty of Dental Medicine Founded by the Alpha Omega Fraternity; Chairman, Department of Oral Biology, Faculty of Dental Medicine, Hebrew University; Member, Institute for Microbiology, Faculty of Medicine, Hebrew University Hadassah Medical Center, Jerusalem, Israel.
STREPTOCOCCUS

MICHAEL PIERRE GLAUSER, M.D.
Privat-Dolent and Aggregé, Faculty of Medicine, University of Lausanne; Médicin Adjoint, Division of Infectious Diseases, Centre Hospitalier Universitaire Vaudois, Lausanne, Switzerland.
URINARY TRACT INFECTION AND PYELONEPHRITIS

RUTH E. GORDON, Ph.D.
Professor of Microbiology, Waksman Institute of Microbiology, Rutgers, The State University of New Jersey, Piscataway, New Jersey.
NOCARDIA AND STREPTOMYCES

MICHAEL G. GROVES, D.V.M., Ph.D.
Commander, US Army Medical Research Unit, Institute for Medical Research, Kuala Lumpur, Malaysia.
BABESIOSIS

ASHLEY T. HAASE, M.D.
Associate Professor, Department of Medicine and Microbiology, School of Medicine, University of California, San Francisco; Chief, Infectious Disease, Veterans Administration Medical Center, San Francisco, California.
SLOW INFECTIONS

NANCY K. HALL, Ph.D.
Assistant Professor of Pathology, Health Science Center, University of Oklahoma, Oklahoma City, Oklahoma.
HISTOPLASMA CAPSULATUM

H. HUNTER HANDSFIELD, M.D.
Assistant Professor of Medicine, University of Washington, School of Medicine; Venereal Disease Control Officer, Seattle–King County Department of Public Health, Seattle, Washington.
LYMPHOGRANULOMA VENEREUM, CHANCROID, AND GRANULOMA INGUINALE

HERBERT S. HEINEMAN, M.D.
Clinical Professor of Medicine, Jefferson Medical College of Thomas Jefferson University; Attending Physician and Consultant in Infectious Diseases, Mercy Catholic Medical Center; Director, Public Health Laboratory, Department of Public Health, Philadelphia, Pennsylvania.
BACTERIAL BRAIN ABSCESS; SHOCK IN INFECTIOUS DISEASES

JUNJI H. HIGUCHI, M.D.
Instructor in Internal Medicine, The University of Texas Health Science Center at San Antonio; Attending Physician, Audie L. Murphy Memorial Veterans Hospital, San Antonio, Texas.
COMMON GRAM-NEGATIVE BACILLARY PNEUMONIAS; COMMON PNEUMONIAS DUE TO PYOGENIC COCCI

SHALOM Z. HIRSCHMAN, M.D.
Professor of Medicine and Director, Division of Infectious Diseases, The Mount Sinai School of Medicine of The University of New York; Attending Physician, The Mount Sinai Hospital, New York, New York.
HEPATITIS VIRUSES; VIRAL HEPATITIS

MONTO HO, M.D.
Professor of Medicine and Microbiology, University of Pittsburgh; Chief, Division of Infectious Diseases, Presbyterian-University Hospital, Pittsburgh, Pennsylvania.
CENTRAL NERVOUS SYSTEM INFECTIONS CAUSED BY TOGAVIRIDAE AND RELATED AGENTS; INTERFERON AND INTERFERENCE

BETTY C. HOBBS, D.Sc., Ph.D., Dip. Bact., F.R.C.Path., F.R.S.H.
Director (Retired), Food Hygiene Laboratory, Central Public Health Laboratory, London, England; Consultant Microbiologist, Christian Medical and Brown Memorial Hospital, Punjab, India.
THE CLOSTRIDIA

PATRICIA A. HOFFEE, Ph.D.
Professor of Microbiology, University of Pittsburgh, School of Medicine, Pittsburgh, Pennsylvania.
BACTERIAL GENETICS

THOMAS A. HOFFMAN, M.D.
Associate Professor of Medicine, University of Miami, School of Medicine; Chief, Division of Infectious Diseases, Jackson Memorial Hospital, Miami, Florida.
MENINGOCOCCEMIA; PURULENT BACTERIAL MENINGITIS

TOR HOFSTAD, M.D.
Associate Professor of Microbiology, Faculty of Medicine, University of Bergen; Chief Physician, Department of Microbiology, Haukeland Hospital, Bergen, Norway.
BACTEROIDES

HOOSHANG HOOSHMAND, M.D.
Neurological Associates, Vero Beach, Florida.
NEUROSYPHILIS

MARIAN C. HORZINEK, D.V.M., Ph.D.
Professor of Virology and Head, Department of Virology, Veterinary Faculty, State University, Utrecht, The Netherlands.
TOGAVIRUSES

CAROLYN COKER HUNTLEY, M.D.
Professor of Pediatrics, Bowman Gray School of Medicine; Attending Physician, North Carolina Baptist Hospital, Winston-Salem, North Carolina.
VISCERAL LARVA MIGRANS

ROBERT R. JACOBSON, Ph.D.
Clinical Instructor in Medicine, Louisiana State University Medical School, New Orleans, Louisiana; Chief of the Clinical Branch and Medical Department, US Public Health Service Hospital, Carville, Louisiana.
LEPROSY

W. G. JOHANSON, Jr., M.D.
Professor of Internal Medicine, The University of Texas Health Science Center at San Antonio; Chief, Pulmonary Disease Section, Audie L. Murphy Memorial Veterans Hospital, San Antonio, Texas.
COMMON GRAM-NEGATIVE BACILLARY PNEUMONIAS; COMMON PNEUMONIAS DUE TO PYOGENIC COCCI

ANSSI M. M. JOKIPII, M.D.
Docent in Clinical Microbiology and Immunology, University of Helsinki, Helsinki, Finland.
GIARDIASIS AND BALANTIDIASIS

LIISA JOKIPII, M.D.
Docent in Clinical Microbiology and Immunology, University of Helsinki, Helsinki, Finland.
GIARDIASIS AND BALANTIDIASIS

HARVEY S. KANTOR, M.D.
Associate Professor of Medicine and Pathology, and Director, Division of Infectious Diseases, Chicago Medical School; Chief, Infectious Diseases Section, Veterans Administration Medical Center, North Chicago, Illinois; Consultant in Infectious Diseases, Highland Park Hospital, Highland Park, Illinois; Consultant in Infectious Diseases, St. Mary of Nazareth Hospital, Chicago, Illinois.
BACTERIAL ENTERITIS

DENNIS L. KASPER, M.D.
Associate Professor of Medicine, Harvard Medical School; Chief, Division of Infectious Diseases, Beth Israel Hospital, Boston, Massachusetts.
PERITONITIS

HERBERT E. KAUFMAN, M.D.
Professor, Louisiana State Medical Center in New Orleans; Director, Louisiana State University Eye Center; Medical Director, Eye & Ear Institute of Louisiana, New Orleans, Louisiana.
VIRAL OCULAR INFECTIONS

PATRICK J. KELLY, M.D.
Professor of Orthopedic Surgery, Mayo Medical School; Consultant, Department of Orthopedics, Mayo Clinic and Mayo Foundation, Rochester, New York.
BACTERIAL ARTHRITIS; BACTERIAL OSTEOMYELITIS

GERALD T. KEUSCH, M.D.
Professor of Medicine, Tufts University School of Medicine; Attending Physician, New England Medical Center Hospitals, Boston, Massachusetts.
MALNUTRITION AND INFECTION; YERSINIA ENTERITIS

MOGENS KILIAN, D.D.S., Ph.D.
Associate Professor of Microbiology, Royal Dental College, Aarhus, Denmark.
HAEMOPHILUS

ALEXANDER L. KISCH, M.D.
Associate Professor of Internal Medicine, University of New Mexico, School of Medicine, Albuquerque, New Mexico.
PLAGUE

STEVE KOHL, M.D.
Associate Professor of Pediatrics, Program in Infectious Diseases and Clinical Microbiology, The University Medical School at Houston; Attending Pediatrician, Hermann Hospital; Pediatric Infectious Disease Consultant, M.D. Anderson Hospital and Tumor Research Institute, Houston, Texas.
GRANULOMATOUS HEPATITIS

REISAKU KONO, M.D., M.P.H., Dr. Med. Sci.
Lecturer in Virology in Tropical Medicine, Institute for Medical Science, University of Tokyo; Director, Central Virus Diagnostic Laboratory, National Institute of Health of Japan, Tokyo, Japan.
ENTEROVIRAL INFECTIONS OTHER THAN POLIOMYELITIS

HOWARD W. LARSH, Ph.D.
Research Professor of Microbiology, University of Oklahoma, Norman, Oklahoma; Director of Research and Laboratories, Missouri State Chest Hospital, Mt. Vernon, Missouri.
HISTOPLASMA CAPSULATUM

WILLIAM LAWSON, M.D., D.D.S.
Associate Professor of Otolaryngology, The Mount Sinai School of Medicine of the University of New York; Chief of Otolaryngology, The Bronx Veterans Administration Hospital; Attending Otolaryngologist, The Mount Sinai Hospital, New York, New York; Attending Otolaryngologist, City Hospital at Elmhurst, New York.
OTITIS MEDIA AND OTITIS EXTERNA

DONALD L. LEAKE, A.B., M.A., D.M.D., M.D.
Professor of Oral and Maxillofacial Surgery, UCLA School of Dentistry; Professor of Surgery, UCLA School of Medicine; Chairman, Department of Dentistry, Dental Director and Chief of Oral Surgery, Harbor-UCLA Medical Center, Torrance, California; Visiting Oral and Maxillofacial Surgeon, UCLA Hospital, Los Angeles, California.
BACTERIAL PAROTITIS

D. L. LEE, B.Sc., Ph.D.
Professor of Agricultural Zoology and Head of Department of Pure and Applied Zoology, University of Leeds, Leeds, England.
CLASSIFICATION AND ANATOMY OF PARASITES

AMORN LEELARASAMEE, M.D.
Assistant Professor, Infectious Unit, Department of Internal Medicine, Siriraj Hospital, Mahidol University, Thailand.
DENGUE AND OTHER HEMMORHAGIC FEVERS

FRITZ LEHMANN-GRUBE, M.D.
Professor of Virology, University of Hamburg, Hamburg, Germany.
ARENAVIRUSES; LYMPHOCYTIC CHORIOMENINGITIS

STANLEY M. LEMON, M.D.
Assistant Professor of Medicine, Department of Virus Diseases, Walter Reed Army Institute of Research, Walter Reed Army Medical Center; Staff Physician, Walter Reed General Hospital; Staff Physician, Walter Reed Army Medical Center, Washington, D.C.
THE HERPESVIRUSES

A. MARTIN LERNER, M.D.
Professor of Medicine and Director of Division of Infectious Diseases, Wayne State University, School of Medicine; Chief, Department of Medicine, Hutzel Hospital, Detroit, Michigan.
MYOCARDITIS AND PERICARDITIS

WILLIAM LESTER, M.D.
Professor of Medicine, University of Chicago, Pritzker School of Medicine; Attending Physician, University of Chicago Hospitals and Clinics, Chicago, Illinois.
NONTUBERCULOUS MYCOBACTERIAL INFECTIONS; TUBERCULOSIS

ALBERTO THOMAZ LONDERO, M.D.
Professor of Medical Mycology, Department of Microbiology and Parasitology, University of Santa Maria; Attending Medical Mycologist, University Hospital, Santa Maria, Brazil.
CHROMOBLASTOMYCOSIS; PARACOCCIDIOIDOMYCOSIS

W. H. RUSSELL LUMSDEN, D.Sc., M.D., F.R.C.P.E., F.R.S.E.
Retired Professor and Head of Department, Department of Medical Protozoology, London School of Hygiene and Tropical Medicine, London, England; Honorary Research Fellow, University of Dundee, Animal Services Unit, Ninewells Hospital and Medical School, Dundee, Scotland.
TRYPANOSOMIASIS

G. PHILIP MANIRE, Ph.D.
Kenan Professor of Bacteriology and Immunology, Vice Chancellor and Dean of Graduate School, University of North Carolina, Chapel Hill, North Carolina.
THE CHLAMYDIAE

FRANCOIS MARIAT, Dr. es Sciences (Paris)
Professor, Institut Pasteur, Paris, France.
SPOROTHRIX SCHENCKII

MELVIN I. MARKS, M.D.
  Director, Pediatric Infectious Diseases, Oklahoma Children's Memorial Hospital, Oklahoma City, Oklahoma.
MUMPS; PLEURODYNIA

HORACIO FIGUEROA MARROQUÍN, M.D.
  Emeritus Professor, University of San Carlos of Guatemala.
ONCHOCERCIASIS

FRANCIS D. MARTINSON, M.B., Ch.B. (ED), F.R.C.S. (ENG & ED).
  Professor of Oto-rhino-laryngology, University of Ibadan, College of Medicine; Consultant Otolaryngologist, University College Hospital, Ibadan, Nigeria.
PHYCOMYCOSIS

WILLIAM R. McCABE, M.D.
  Professor of Medicine and Microbiology, Boston University, School of Medicine; Director, Maxwell Finland Laboratory for Infectious Diseases, Boston City Hospital; Director, Division of Infectious Diseases, Boston University, School of Medicine; Consultant in Infectious Diseases, Farmingham Union Hospital; Consultant in Infectious Diseases, Carney Veterans Administration Hospital; Consultant in Infectious Diseases, Boston Veterans Administration Hospital, Boston, Massachusetts.
GRAM-NEGATIVE BACTEREMIA

RICHARD V. McCLOSKEY, M.D.
  Professor of Medicine, Jefferson Medical College; Chairman of Medicine and Head, Section of Infectious Diseases, Albert Einstein Medical Center, Daroff Division, Philadelphia, Pennsylvania.
DIPHTHERIA

J. ALLEN McCUTCHAN, M.D.
  Assistant Professor of Medicine, University of California, San Diego School of Medicine, Attending Physician, University Hospital, San Diego, California.
FACTITIOUS AND DELUSIONAL ILLNESSES SIMULATING INFECTION; GONOCOCCEMIA; GONORRHEA AND NONGONOCOCCAL URETHRITIS

ZELL A. McGEE, M.D.
  Professor of Medicine, Vanderbilt University, School of Medicine; Director, George Hunt Laboratory; Chief, Division of Infectious Diseases, Department of Medicine, Vanderbilt University Hospital, Vanderbilt, Tennessee.
CELL WALL–DEFECTIVE BACTERIA; MYCOPLASMAS

RIMA McLEOD, M.D.
  Fellow in Infectious Diseases, Department of Medicine, Division of Infectious Diseases, Stanford University, School of Medicine, Stanford, California; Fellow in Infectious Diseases, Division of Allergy, Immunology, and Infectious Diseases, Palo Alto Medical Research Foundation, Palo Alto, California.
TOXOPLASMOSIS

GERALD MEDOFF, M.D.
  Professor of Medicine, Microbiology, and Immunology and Chief of the Infectious Disease Division, Washington University, School of Medicine; Physician, Barnes Hospital, St. Louis, Missouri.
CRYPTOCOCCAL MENINGITIS; PULMONARY CRYPTOCOCCOSIS

MARIAN E. MELISH, M.D.
  Associate Professor of Pediatrics, Tropical Medicine, and Medical Microbiology, John A. Burns School of Medicine, University of Hawaii; Attending Pediatrician, Consultant in Infectious Disease, Kapiolani Children's Medical Center, Honolulu, Hawaii.
IMPETIGO; KAWASAKI SYNDROME; PYOGENIC SKIN INFECTIONS; STAPHYLOCOCCAL SCALDED SKIN SYNDROME

JOSEPH L. MELNICK, Ph.D.
  Distinguished Service Professor and Chairman, Department of Virology & Epidemiology, Baylor College of Medicine, Houston, Texas.
CLASSIFICATION OF VIRUSES

BURT R. MEYERS, M.D.
  Professor of Medicine, Mount Sinai School of Medicine of The University of New York; Attending Physician, Elmhurst General Hospital, Elmhurst, New York; Attending Physician, Mount Sinai Hospital, New York, New York.
ENDOPHTHALMITIS; LUDWIG'S ANGINA; OTITIS MEDIA AND OTITIS EXTERNA; PULMONARY MUCORMYCOSIS

WAYNE M. MEYERS, M.D., Ph.D.
  Chief, Division of Microbiology, Department of Infectious and Parasitic Diseases Pathology, Armed Forces Institute of Pathology, Washington, D.C.
MYCOBACTERIAL INFECTIONS OF THE SKIN

JOSEPH H. MILLER, M.S., Ph.D.
  Professor of Medical Parasitology, Louisiana State University Medical Center; Visiting Sci-

entist, The Charity Hospital in New Orleans, New Orleans, Louisiana.
THE PROTOZOA

DAVID L. MINKOFF, M.D.
Department of Pediatrics, University Hospital, San Diego, California.
HAND-FOOT-MOUTH DISEASE

JOSÉ LISBÔA MIRANDA, M.D.
Professor of Dermatology, Escola Médica do Rio de Janeiro, Universidade Gama Filho, Rio de Janeiro, Brazil.
LOBOMYCOSIS

SAROJ K. MISHRA, Ph.D.
Chief, Serodiagnostic Division, Robert Koch Institute, Berlin, Germany.
NOCARDIA AND STREPTOMYCES

SUSUMU MITSUHASHI, Ph.D., Dr. Med. Sci.
Professor, Department of Microbiology, and Director, Laboratory of Bacterial Resistance, Gunma University, School of Medicine, Maebishi City, Japan.
RESISTANCE TO ANTIMICROBIAL DRUGS

PETER M. MOODIE, M.D., B.S., D.T.M. & H.
Associate Professor of Tropical Medicine, Commonwealth Institute of Health, The University of Sydney, Sydney, Australia.
YAWS, PINTA, AND BEJEL

STEPHEN A. MORSE, Ph.D.
Asssociate Professor, Department of Microbiology and Immunology, University of Oregon Health Sciences Center, Portland, Oregon.
NEISSERIA

STEPHEN I. MORSE, M.D. (Deceased)
Professor and Chairman, Microbiology and Immunology, State University of New York, Downstate Medical Center, Brooklyn, New York.
STAPHYLOCOCCAL BACTEREMIA; STAPHYLOCOCCI

MAURICE A. MUFSON, M.D.
Professor and Chairman, Department of Medicine, Marshall University, School of Medicine; Associate Chief of Staff for Research and Development, Huntington Veterans Administration Medical Center; Active Attending Staff, Cabell Huntington Hospital and St. Mary's Hospital, Huntington, West Virginia.
MYCOPLASMA PNEUMONIA

DANIEL M. MUSHER, M.D.
Professor of Medicine, Professor of Microbiology and Immunology, Baylor College of Medicine; Chief, Infectious Disease Section, Veterans Administration Hospital, Houston, Texas.
SPIROCHETES; TREPONEMA AND BORRELIA; SYPHILIS OF THE GENITAL TRACT; SYPHILIS OF THE SKIN

HAROLD C. NEU
Professor of Medicine and Pharmacology, Columbia University, College of Physicians and Surgeons; Chief of Infectious Diseases Columbia-Presbyterian Medical Center, New York, New York.
PHARMACOLOGY AND TOXICOLOGY OF ANTIMICROBIAL AGENTS

FRITS ØRSKOV, M.D.
Collaborative Centre for Reference and Research on Escherichia (WHO), Statens Seruminstitut, Copenhagen, Denmark.
ENTEROBACTERIACEAE

IDA ØRSKOV, M.D.
Collaborative Centre for Reference and Research on Escherichia (WHO), Statens Seruminstitut, Copenhagen, Denmark.
ENTEROBACTERIACEAE

MICHAEL N. OXMAN, M.D.
Professor of Medicine and Pathology, University of California, San Diego School of Medicine; Chief, Infectious Diseases and Clinical Virology Sections, Veterans Administration Medical Center, San Diego, California.
GENITAL HERPES; HERPES SIMPLEX ENCEPHALITIS AND MENINGITIS; HERPES STOMATITIS; HERPES ZOSTER; PAPOVAVIRUSES; VARICELLA

JOSEPH S. PAGANO, M.D.
Director, Cancer Research Center, and Professor of Medicine and of Bacteriology and Immunology, University of North Carolina at Chapel Hill School of Medicine; Attending Physician in Medicine and Infectious Disease, North Carolina Memorial Hospital, Chapel Hill, North Carolina.
THE HERPESVIRUSES

ZBIGNIEW S. PAWLOWSKI, M.D., D.T.M. & H.
Professor of Medical Parasitology, Medical Faculty, Academy of Medicine, Poznań, Poland; Chief, Clinic of Parasitic and Tropical Diseases, Academy of Medicine, Poznań, Poland.
CESTODIASIS; PLATYHELMINTHES; TRICHINELLOSIS

LENNART PHILIPSON, M.D., Dr. Med. Sci.
Professor of Microbiology, Uppsala University, Uppsala, Sweden.
ADENOVIRUS

M. J. PICKETT, Ph.D.
Professor of Microbiology, University of California, Los Angeles, California.
GENUS PSEUDOMONAS

ALEXANDER W. PIERCE, Jr., M.D.
Professor of Family Practice, The University of Texas Medical School at San Antonio; Director, Family Health Center, Robert B. Green Hospital, San Antonio, Texas.
MYIASIS

LEO PINE, B.S., M.S., Ph.D.
Chief, Products Development Branch, Biological Products Division, Center for Disease Control, Atlanta, Georgia.
ACTINOMYCES AND MICROAEROPHILIC ACTINOMYCETES

FRANCISCO de PAULA PINHEIRO, M.D.
Director, Institute Evandro Chagas, Fundação Serviços de Saúda Pública, Ministry of Health, Belém, Pará, Brazil; Professor of Virology, Centro Ciências Biológicas, Federal University of Pará, Brazil.
YELLOW FEVER

BOSKO POSTIC, M.D.
Professor of Medicine, University of South Carolina, School of Medicine; Chief, Medical Service, William Jennings Bryan Dorn Veterans Hospital, Columbia, South Carolina.
RABIES; RHABDOVIRUS

ROY POSTLETHWAITE, B.Sc., M.D.
Professor of Virology, University of Aberdeen Medical School; Honorary Consultant Bacteriologist, Aberdeen Royal Infirmary and Associated Hospitals, Aberdeen, Scotland.
MOLLUSCUM CONTAGIOSUM

C. R. PRINGLE, B.Sc., Ph.D.
Honorary Lecturer, University of Glasgow; Member of the Medical Research Council, MRC Virology Unit, Glasgow, Scotland.
THE GENETICS OF VIRUSES

SEPPO PYRHÖNEN, M.D.
Docent in Virology, University of Helsinki; Oncologist, Department of Radiotherapy, University Central Hospital of Helsinki, Helsinki, Finland.
WARTS

T. RAMAKRISHNAN, M.Sc., Ph.D.
Professor, Microbiology and Cell Biology Laboratory, Indian Institute of Science, Bangalore, India.
BACTERIAL PHYSIOLOGY

A. RAMACHANDRA RAO, M.B., B.S., B.Sc.
Retired Health Officer, Corporation of Madras, Madras, India.
SMALLPOX, VACCINIA, AND COWPOX

G. RAMANANDA RAO, M. PHARM., Ph.D.
Assistant Professor, Microbiology and Cell Biology Laboratory, Indian Institute of Science, Bangalore, India.
BACTERIAL PHYSIOLOGY

GARRISON RAPMUND, M.D.
Brigadier General, MC, US Army; Assistant Surgeon General (Research and Development), Department of the Army, Washington, D.C.
RICKETTSIA; RICKETTSIALPOX; SCRUB TYPHUS; TRENCH FEVER

JACK S. REMINGTON, M.D.
Professor of Medicine, Division of Infectious Diseases, Stanford University, School of Medicine, Stanford, California; Chief, Division of Allergy, Immunology, and Infectious Diseases, Palo Alto Medical Research Foundation, Palo Alto, California.
TOXOPLASMOSIS

DOUGLAS D. RICHMAN, M.D.
Assistant Professor of Pathology and Medicine, University of California, San Diego, School of Medicine; Attending Physician, Veterans Administration Medical Center, San Diego, California.
ORTHOMYXOVIRUSES AND PARAMYXOVIRUSES; TUBERCULOMAS OF THE BRAIN

DAVID L. RINGO, Ph.D.
Assistant Research Biologist, University of California, Santa Cruz, California.
THE STRUCTURE OF THE BACTERIAL CELL

LEON ROSEN, M.D., Dr.P.H.
Head, Pacific Research Section, Laboratory of Parasitic Diseases, National Institute of Allergy and Infectious Diseases, Honolulu, Hawaii.
CEREBRAL ANGIOSTRONGYLIASIS

EDWARD BROOK ROTHERAM, Jr., M.D.
Clinical Associate Professor of Medicine, University of Pittsburgh, School of Medicine; Head, Division of Infectious Diseases, Allegheny General Hospital, Pittsburgh, Pennsylvania.
LIVER AND SUBPHRENIC ABSCESS; NONVENEREAL INFECTIONS OF THE FEMALE GENITALIA

J. L. RYAN, Ph.D., M.D.
Assistant Professor of Medicine, Yale University School of Medicine, New Haven, Connecticut; Chief, Infectious Disease Section, Veterans Administration Medical Center, West Haven, Connecticut.
BITES: P. MULTOCIDA, S. MONILIFORMIS, AND S. MINOR

ALBERT B. SABIN, M.D.
Distinguished Research Professor of Biomedicine, Medical University of South Carolina, Charleston, South Carolina.
POLIOMYELITIS

GEORGE A. SAROSI, M.D., F.A.C.P.
Professor of Medicine and Vice-Chairman, Department of Medicine, University of Minnesota; Chief, Medical Service, Veterans Administration Medical Center, Minneapolis, Minnesota.
ASPERGILLOSIS; HISTOPLASMOSIS

HOWARD J. SAZ, Ph.D.
Professor of Biology, University of Notre Dame, Notre Dame, Indiana.
BIOCHEMISTRY OF PARASITES: HELMINTHS

FENTON SCHAFFNER, M.D.
Professor of Medicine and Director, Division of Liver Diseases, The Mount Sinai School of Medicine of The University of New York; Attending Physician, The Mount Sinai Hospital, New York, New York.
VIRAL HEPATITIS

GILBERT M. SCHIFF, M.D.
Professor of Medicine, University of Cincinnati, College of Medicine; Director of Medicine, The Christ Hospital Institute of Medical Research; Attending Staff, Cincinnati General Hospital, Holmes Hospital, Cincinnati Veterans Administration Hospital, Christ Hospital; Consultant, Children's Hospital, Jewish Hospital, Cincinnati, Ohio.
MEASLES; RUBEOLA

H. P. R. SEELIGER, M.D.
Full Professor of Hygiene and Microbiology and Director of Institute of Hygiene, Bayerische Julius-Maximilians-Universität Wuerzburg, Federal Republic of Germany.
LISTERIA MONOCYTOGENES

SMITH SHADOMY, Ph.D.
Professor of Medicine and Microbiology, Medical College of Virginia, Virginia Commonwealth University, Richmond, Virginia.
BLASTOMYCES AND PARACOCCIDIOSIS

KAORU SHIMADA, M.D.
Attending Staff, Tokyo University Medical School; Chief, Infectious Disease Section, Tokyo Metropolitan Geriatric Hospital, Tokyo, Japan.
CHOLECYSTITIS AND CHOLANGITIS

RUDOLF SIEGERT, M.D.
Professor of Medical Microbiology, Institute of Hygiene, Philipps-Universität, Marburg, Federal Republic of Germany.
EBOLA VIRUS DISEASE; MARBURG VIRUS AND EBOLA VIRUS; MARBURG VIRUS DISEASE

SAMUEL C. SILVERSTEIN, M.D.
Associate Professor and Physician, Laboratory of Cellular Physiology and Immunology, Rockefeller University; Physician, Rockefeller University Hospital, New York, New York.
VIRAL REPLICATION

IRVING J. SLOTNICK, Ph.D.
Chief Microbiologist, Cedars Sinai Medical Center, Los Angeles, California.
ACTINOBACILLUS AND CARDIOBACTERIUM

DONALD W. SMITH, Ph.D.
Professor of Medical Microbiology, University of Wisconsin, Madison, Wisconsin.
MYCOBACTERIA

B. A. SOUTHGATE, M.B., B.S., F.F.C.M.
Senior Lecturer in Tropical Hygiene, University of London, London School of Hygiene and Tropical Medicine; Consultant Physician, North-West Thames Area Health Authority, London, England.
LOAIASIS

STEPHEN A. SPECTOR, M.D.
Assistant Professor of Pediatrics, University of California, San Diego, School of Medicine; Assistant Professor of Pediatrics, Division of Infectious Diseases, University of California, San Diego, University Hospital, San Diego, California.
IMMUNOPROPHYLAXIS AND IMMUNOTHERAPY

WESLEY W. SPINK, A.B., M.D.
Emeritus Regents' Professor of Medicine and Comparative Medicine, University of Minnesota Medical School; Staff Member, University of Minnesota Hospitals, Minneapolis, Minnesota.
BRUCELLA; BRUCELLOSIS

SPOTSWOOD L. SPRUANCE, M.D.
Associate Professor of Medicine, Department

of Internal Medicine, Division of Infectious Diseases, The University of Utah, Salt Lake City, Utah.
COLORADO TICK FEVER

NEVILLE F. STANLEY, B.Sc., D.Sc., F.R.A.C.P. (Hon.), M.A.S.M.
Professor and Chairman, Department of Microbiology, University of Western Australia; Director, Clinical Microbiology Services, Queen Elizabeth II Medical Centre, Perth, Western Australia.
REOVIRIDAE PATHOGENIC FOR MAN

DAVID A. STEVENS, M.D.
Associate Professor, Department of Medicine, Stanford University, School of Medicine, Stanford, California; Chief, Division of Infectious Diseases, Santa Clara Valley Medical Center, San Jose, California.
COCCIDIOIDAL MENINGITIS; INFECTIOUS MONONUCLEOSIS

H. HARLAN STONE, M.D.
Professor of Surgery, Emory University, School of Medicine; Chief of Trauma and Burn Services, Grady Memorial Hospital, Atlanta, Georgia.
NONCLOSTRIDIAL ANAEROBIC CELLULITIS

RICHARD B. STOUGHTON, M.D.
Professor and Director, Division of Dermatology, University of California, San Diego; Attending Physician, University of California, San Diego, University Hospital, San Diego, California.
DERMATOPHYTOSIS

WILLARD ALLEN TABER
Professor, Department of Biology, Texas A & M University, College of Sciences, College Station, Texas.
CLASSIFICATION OF FUNGI

DAVID TAYLOR-ROBINSON, M.D.
Division of Communicable Diseases, M.R.C. Clinical Research Centre; Hon. Consultant Microbiologist, Northwick Park Hospital, Harrow, Middlesex, England.
MYCOPLASMAS

ROBERT NICOL THIN, M.D., F.R.C.P.E.
Recognised Teacher, University of London; Honorary Senior Lecturer, Institute of Urology; Consultant in Charge, Department of Genital Medicine, St. Bartholemew's Hospital; Consultant, St. Peter's Hospitals, London, England.
MELIOIDOSIS

DORIS A. TRAUNER, M.S., M.D.
Assistant Professor of Neurosciences and Pediatrics, University of California, San Diego, School of Medicine; Chief of Pediatric Neurology, University Hospital Medical Center of San Diego County, San Diego, California.
REYE'S SYNDROME

WALTER P. G. TURCK, M.B., F.R.C.P.
Clinical Lecturer in Medicine, University of Hong Kong; Consultant Physician, Alice Ho Miu Ling Nethersole Hospital, Hong Kong.
CHRONIC Q FEVER, Q FEVER

D. A. J. TYRRELL, C.B.E., M.D., D.Sc., F.R.C.P., F.R.C.Path., F.R.S.
Head, Division of Communicable Diseases, Clinical Research Centre; Consultant Physician, Northwick Park Hospital, Harrow, Middlesex, London, England.
CORONAVIRUS

HANS A. VALKENBURG, M.D., Ph.D.
Professor of Epidemiology, Erasmus University Medical School, Rotterdam, Holland.
PHARYNGITIS AND TONSILLITIS

PAUL B. VAN CAUWENBERGE, M.D.
Lecturer, State University, Gent, Belgium; Consultant Otorhinolaryngologist, University Hospital, Gent, Belgium.
SINUSITIS

WILLIAM EDWARD VAN HEYNINGEN, Ph.D., Sc.D., D.Sc.
Emeritus Reader in Bacterial Chemistry, Sir William Dunn School of Pathology, University of Oxford, Oxford, England.
BACTERIAL EXOTOXINS

PANKAJALAKSHMI V. VENUGOPAL, M.D.
Associate Professor of Microbiology, Institute of Microbiology, Madras Medical College; Microbiologist, Government General Hospital, Madras, India.
MYCETOMA

TARALAKSHMI V. VENUGOPAL, M.D.
Associate Professor of Pathology, Department of Pathology, Madras Medical College; Pathologist, Government General Hospital, Madras, India.
MYCETOMA

HENRY A. WALCH, Ph.D.
Professor of Microbiology, San Diego State University, San Diego, California.
COCCIDIOIDES IMMITIS

esda, Maryland; Chief of Internal Medicine, Naval Regional Medical Center, Camp Pendleton, California.
CHOLERA

WARREN J. WARWICK, M.D.
Professor of Pediatrics, University of Minnesota; Attending Physician, University of Minnesota Hospitals, Minneapolis, Minnesota.
CAT SCRATCH DISEASE

TADEUSZ J. WIKTOR, D.V.M.
Member, The Wistar Institute, Philadelphia, Pennsylvania.
RABIES; RHABDOVIRUS

ROBERT P. WILLIAMS
Professor of Microbiology and Immunology, Baylor College of Medicine, Houston, Texas.
BACILLUS ANTHRACIS AND OTHER AEROBIC SPORE-FORMING BACILLI

SHELDON M. WOLFF, M.D.
Endicott Professor and Chairman, Department of Medicine, Tufts University, School of Medicine; Physician-in-Chief, New England Medical Center Hospital, Boston, Massachusetts.
FEVER

NATHANIEL A. YOUNG, M.D. (Deceased)
Head, Viral Oncology and Molecular Pathology Sections, Laboratory of Pathology, National Institutes of Health; Senior Attending Physician in Infectious Diseases, Clinical Center, National Institutes of Health, Bethesda, Maryland.
PICORNAVIRUSES

JULIUS S. YOUNGNER, Sc.D.
Professor and Chairman, Department of Microbiology, University of Pittsburgh, School of Medicine, Pittsburgh, Pennsylvania.
PERSISTENT VIRAL INFECTIONS

# FOREWORD

"Medicine is the only world-wide profession, following everywhere the same methods, activated by the same ambitions, and pursuing the same ends."

SIR WILLIAM OSLER

"From the earliest time, medicine has been a curious blend of superstition, empiricism, and that kind of sagacious observation, which is the stuff out of which ultimately science is made. Of these three strands — superstition, empiricism, and observation — medicine was constituted in the days of the priest-physicians of Egypt and Babylonia; of the same strands, it is still composed. The proportions have, however, varied significantly. An increasingly alert and determined effort, running through the ages, has endeavored to expel superstition, to narrow the range of empiricism, and to enlarge, refine, and systematize the scope of observation."

ABRAHAM FLEXNER

The traditions of medicine are as old as recorded history and are interwoven into all civilizations, both past and present. Avicenna, Galen, Hippocrates, Maimonides, Harvey, Pasteur, Koch, and many others, celebrated and obscure, have created that tradition, which is still being modified in our time. Clearly, superstition in medicine is not yet expelled nor empiricism sufficiently narrowed. They remain to adulterate and diminish the science and humanism of medical practice.

The science of medicine is universal in its origins and in its relevance. In fact, universality in time and place is the bedrock of scientific observation. Human biology is basically the same in Sri Lanka as in Sweden. It is true that biological variation exists. Gene pools have been modified by mutation and natural selection. Balanced polymorphism, for example, seems to have created a high incidence of sickle cell disease only where the associated increased resistance to falciparum malaria constitutes a significant biological advantage. Such examples of differing gene pools in ethnic groups abound. Much more impressive, however, is the constancy of human biology, representing a high conservation of the human genome and therefore close homology of gene products. Out of infinite possibilities, the same molecular species transport oxygen, capture energy from carbohydrates, and transmit nerve impulses in all humans without regard for national borders. It would be astonishing if it were otherwise in view of the recentness of the "ascent of man" from a common ancestry. It is reasonable, therefore, to present Volume I of this textbook as "international." Its discussions of cell biology, genetics, immunology, hematology, metabolism, endocrinology, cardiology, respiration, nephrology, gastroenterology, neurology, connective tissue, dermatology and clinical pharmacology are universally relevant. They are the disciplines that underlie the practice of medicine in whatever setting that practice may occur.

Although human biology is relatively constant, the environments in which men exist are extraordinarily diverse. Differences in nutrition, culture, education, economics, climate, crowding, application of the technologies of public health and preventive medicine, and many other environmental influences dictate the occurrence of disease and the maintenance of health far more than do differences in genomic nucleotide sequences. Disease presents in different patterns, therefore, throughout the world (geographic medicine) and in subsets within a given society (epidemiology). Differences exist in the incidence of all kinds of diseases (cancer, cardiovascular disorders, rheumatic diseases); in fact, it is difficult to find any disorder with equal geographical prevalence. Nutritional disorders, the infectious and parasitic diseases, and their deadly interactions are without question the medical problems with the most sharply defined geographical and economic foci—largely in the developing countries of the world.

All living things protect themselves as vigorously from invasion by smaller living things as they do from engulfment by larger ones; for it is as bad to rot from within as to be eaten from without—at least it is as decisive. Poor nutrition causes that protection to falter in ways not yet fully explained. Inadequate sanitation, poverty, and crowding have their own epidemiology and assist the invasion by smaller living things. Furthermore, some infectious diseases, once comfortably remote from western countries, are now alarmingly close in a shrinking world marked by increasing commerce in goods and people. Lassa fever, although still confined to Africa, warrants attention; kuru may be an analog for slow virus diseases yet to be detected. Volume II, edited by Doctors Braude, Davis, and Fierer, is truly international in its description of the parasitic and infectious diseases. Fifty-eight participants from 27 countries outside the United States have contributed to its completion with the authority of direct personal observation. More than any single book now available, it describes the world experience with the parasitic and infectious diseases.

The first two volumes of the *International Textbook of Medicine* were designed to articulate with the *Cecil Textbook of Medicine,* which has had an international audience in internal medicine for more than half a century, to complete this "system of medicine." The practice of clinical medicine requires a frame of reference, which for this series is the western world with its assumption of the availability of high technology and its recommended therapeutic programs.

The *International Textbook of Medicine,* then, has created two new books designed to be used with a third, a well known classic textbook of medicine. All three of these textbooks are capable of standing alone and each will have its specific audience. What is the motivation for presenting them in such a series or system of medicine? More than three-fourths of the earth's population live in the developing countries of the world. Achievement of better health is one of the highest aspirations of the people of these countries. "The health of all the people is really the foundation upon which all their happiness and all their powers as a state depend" (Disraeli). The prospects for better health in most of these countries, even in those that are wealthier and more fortunate, depend more directly upon the ultimate conquest of persistent poverty, malnutrition, illiteracy, and a multitude of other social problems than upon expansion of personal health services. These are problems that transcend the work of the physician, although the physician may be unusually influential in their alleviation. This is perhaps particularly true in countries where physicians constitute one of the few highly educated segments of society.

Despite the crushing burden of these external factors, most of which are beyond the traditional purview of medicine, the education of physicians and other health workers remains a top priority. The number of medical schools, medical students, and physicians continues to rise throughout the world. A severe limitation to both undergraduate and continuing medical education, however, has been a deficit of appropriate textbooks. Students living in the developing countries of Asia, Africa, or Latin America often have no easy access to libraries and can rarely afford to own the required textbooks. In most circumstances the student must rely on didactic lectures or notes distributed by teachers.

On the basis of these observations, as well as from many years of personal experience in medical education in developing countries, one of us (AHS) conceived this plan to publish a comprehensive textbook of medicine to meet the needs of students and physicians in the international medical community. Not unexpectedly, this turned out to be impossible to attain in a single volume. Volume I was therefore designed to give a comprehensive presentation of the most pertinent aspects of basic science and pathophysiology for medical practice. In view of the importance of infectious diseases as the leading cause of morbidity and mortality in the developing countries, it was considered essential to devote an entire volume to microbiology and to the clinical problems of infectious diseases. Of the many authoritative textbooks of clinical medicine, the *Cecil Textbook of Medicine* was judged to lend itself most readily to this series. At this time, the *International Textbook of Medicine* does not attempt to encompass all aspects of medical practice, such as pediatrics, surgery, or psychiatry. As such it is not totally comprehensive, but it is a start. It is also not a primer but rather presents medicine and its relevant pathophysiology at a level of rigor consistent with that taught at advanced medical schools throughout the world.

The practice of medicine is truly international in its scope. The editors hope that the *International Textbook of Medicine* will make a contribution to its common purposes.

ABDOL HOSSEIN SAMII, M.D.
LLOYD H. SMITH, JR., M.D.
JAMES B. WYNGAARDEN, M.D.

# PREFACE

This book tries to do two things that haven't been done before. First, it presents a full coverage of both microbiology and infectious diseases. Second, it takes advantage of the expert knowledge of authorities throughout the world by presenting contributions from nearly 30 different countries. About one-third of the authors are from outside the United States.

The reason for combining medical microbiology and infectious diseases is simply that they are inseparable. Recognizing that neither subject can be presented properly without the other, the authors of textbooks on medical microbiology have incorporated some material on infectious diseases as well, but the clinical coverage has not been enough to help the practicing physician. The reverse is true in texts dealing with clinical infectious diseases; these usually present a summary of the microbial agents causing each disease but not enough information to give the serious students of microbiology what they need. In order to avoid a superficial coverage of either subject, we have invited distinguished authorities to contribute thorough accounts of their subjects that would give even the specialist in those fields the information he is looking for. For the most part, this approach has brought together the two related disciplines so that they fully reinforce each other; each clinical problem is backed up by whatever relevant scientific data and ideas can be marshalled to help elucidate it.

The reason for an international approach is that different environments and ecologies throughout the world breed different germs, and different infections, so that the cause and nature of the diseases differ from one part of the world to another. In order to avoid the parochial approach of inviting American professors to write about infections they seldom see, we have called upon contributors who have had an unmatched experience in dealing with the disease they write about. If nothing else, we have in this way brought together an authoritative coverage of international infections by real experts with a vast first-hand encounter with their subject. In this way we can provide physicians and microbiologists throughout the world with reliable information on infections indigenous to their region, or infections carried there for the first time by international travellers, refugees, or migrants.

The picture of infectious diseases is greatly influenced by the enormous increase in such international mobility in the last 25 years. At least 4 waves of mobility to and from underdeveloped countries can be identified, and each of these is having its impact on the worldwide problem of infection. First, the rise in tourism, cultural exchange, and business travel to and from underdeveloped countries has created a remarkable growth in air travel. In 1977 alone, there were over 600 million passengers on international flights and a substantial portion of these people were visiting, coming from, or passing through underdeveloped countries. Second, the migration of laborers has accounted for another large element of movement from underdeveloped countries. Migrant workers from Mexico to the United States are increasing in number, and even greater shifts in worker populations are going on in Europe, especially from North Africa, Turkey, the middle eastern Arab countries, and India. The third mobile group of international significance is composed of pilgrims and is best illustrated by the 2 million people who go to Mecca from all over the world during the annual pilgrimage. Finally, there are the refugees from Southeast Asia who are pouring into centers in the United States and many other countries and who often pick up tropical infections in displaced person camps in Indochina and other way stations. The movement of these 4 large population groups carries two inevitable risks: one is to the person who gets the infection, and the other is to the community through which he passes or where he settles. Both problems were anticipated in planning this text and they are dealt with in the relevant chapters.

The international approach was not limited to selecting contributors on clinical chapters. Each country has its specialists in the basic sciences, as well, and a number of important scientists, known for the originality and scope of their research, have written chapters.

We hope that all this will add up to a useful work for anyone who has an interest in microbiology and infectious diseases. The medical student, for example, should be able to learn what he needs to know about microbiology in his preclinical studies, and then have a text on infectious diseases when he moves into his clinical years. By concentrating on microbiologic principles first, he should be equipped with the scientific background needed for undertaking an intelligent study of clinical infectious diseases. But even when he is concentrating on microbiology, he will have at hand a ready reference source with those clinical examples that clarify the basic science. Physicians, on the other hand, who use the book mainly for information about problems seen in their practice, will be able to find answers to theoretical or basic microbiologic questions that have a bearing on infectious diseases.

Finally, two explanatory notes are in order. First, medical microbiology is presented here in the strict sense so that related subjects, such as immunology, are presented only as they relate to microbiology (See Chapters 81 to 84). Whereas most immunologic concepts are taken into account with this approach, they are covered more fully and as a comprehensive unit in Volume I. Second, the clinical diseases are presented by system. This is partly because the etiologic approach was needed in the first half of this volume for dealing with specific microbial agents of disease, but mainly because most infections present themselves as a disease of a specific organ or system. We feel, therefore, that physicians can find an answer to their problem more quickly if the disease is described under the appropriate system. If he needs to know more about etiology he can refer to the chapters on specific microbial agents.

If anyone finds this work useful, he or she should know that Gita Braude, Sharon McFarlin, Elizabeth Thurlow, and Pat Campbell are the unsung heroines behind its production.

ABRAHAM I. BRAUDE

# CONTENTS

**B. Pleuropulmonary Infections**

## C. Abdominal Infections

**F. Vascular and Hematologic Infections**

**H.  Ocular Infections**

## I.  Musculoskeletal Infections

## J.  Infections Acquired From Animals

## K.  Illnesses Simulating Infections

# I  Microbiology

## A.  GENERAL MICROBIOLOGY

## Bacteriology

## *THE STRUCTURE OF THE* 1
## *BACTERIAL CELL*

*Eugene H. Cota-Robles, Ph.D.*
*and David L. Ringo, Ph.D.*

The structure of bacteria can be best understood by contrasting their cellular organization to that of the higher biologic forms — animals, plants, protozoa, algae, and fungi. In these life forms the cells are divided into internal compartments by membrane systems. These compartments (cellular *organelles)* have specific activities for the maintenance of the life functions of the cell. The nuclear compartment *(nucleus)* contains the cell's hereditary material, *deoxyribonucleic acid* (DNA). The nucleus is separated by a nuclear membrane from the rest of the cell, the *cytoplasm.* The DNA of higher cells is organized in two or more chromosomes.

Bacterial cells are not compartmentalized and therefore are considered to lack organelles. The hereditary material of bacteria consists of a single chromosome. This bacterial *nucleoid* is a single, tightly bundled, long strand of DNA that lies within the cytoplasm not surrounded by a nuclear membrane. For this reason bacteria are referred to as *prokaryotic,* that is, having a primitive nuclear structure; and higher cells are designated as *eukaryotic,* literally, having a true nucleus. All bacteria (as well as the blue-green algae) possess the prokaryotic form of organization.

In a broad sense, all types of cells function in the same manner. The information stored in the DNA is transcribed as *messenger ribonucleic acid* (mRNA), which moves from the nucleus into the cytoplasm. Here the messenger RNA attaches to ribosomes, where the genetic information is translated into specific proteins by the polymerization of amino acids. The synthesis of proteins is one of the most basic of cell processes, since virtually every metabolic activity of the cell is mediated by enzymes, the proteins that catalyze specific chemical reactions.

The basic function of a bacterial cell is to assimilate chemicals from its environment in order to grow and divide. Some bacteria perform these functions by using the simplest inorganic chemicals (carbon dioxide and minerals), and are termed *autotrophs.* Certain members of this group, photosynthetic bacteria and blue-green algae, rely on light as a source of energy and thus resemble plants in their photoautotrophic metabolism. Another and larger group of bacteria, the *heterotrophs,* use simple organic molecules from their environment as a source of energy and as building blocks for cellular material. Many of this latter group have adapted to growth within the animal body. Some are harmless symbionts, such as *Escherichia coli,* which normally inhabits the mammalian gut. Others are harmful and may cause human disease. These bacteria are termed *pathogens,* and their infection of body tissues results in a characteristic illness. Many of the features of bacterial cell structure are related, in one way or another, to their role as disease organisms and to the ways in which these diseases are treated and controlled.

1

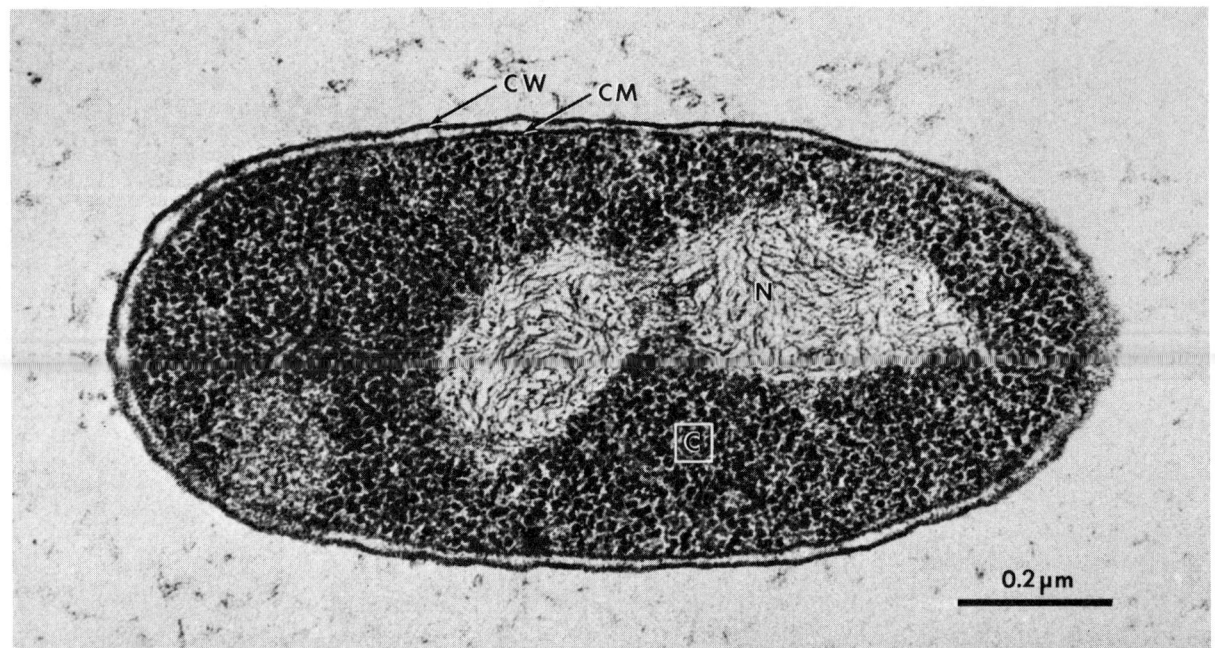

**FIGURE 1.** *This electron micrograph outlines the organization that is common to all bacterial cells. The nucleoid (N) occupies the central area of the cell; the cytoplasm (C) contains many ribosomes (individual dark granules); a cytoplasmic membrane (CM) and cell wall (CW) surround the cell. This bacterium,* Alteromonas espejiana, *is a marine pseudomonad that possesses a very simple wall structure.*

The generalized structure of a typical bacterial cell is shown in Figure 1. The prokaryotic cell consists of a cell wall, a cytoplasmic membrane surrounding a cytoplasm packed with ribosomes, and a more or less central nucleoid. The figure is an example of the image produced by the electron microscope of a very thin section cut through a chemically preserved (fixed) bacterium. It is possible to determine the overall shape and size of such a bacterial cell with the light microscope, but details that are smaller than about 0.2 $\mu$m cannot be resolved (Table 1). Thus, the internal structure of the bacterium can be deduced only through the use of the higher resolving power of the electron microscope, and all such detailed knowledge has been obtained only within the past 25 years.

**TABLE 1.    Units Used to Describe Bacteria and their Structures, and the Useful Limits of Resolution of the Human Eye, the Light Microscope, and the Electron Microscope**

Units:
  1 m $\times$ 10$^{-3}$  = 1 mm (millimeter)
  1 mm $\times$ 10$^{-3}$ = 1 $\mu$m (micrometer or micron)
  1 $\mu$m $\times$ 10$^{-3}$ = 1 nm (nanometer)
Limits of Resolving Power:
  Unaided human eye: 0.2 mm
  Compound light microscope: 0.2 $\mu$m
  Transmission electron microscope: 2 nm to 0.2 nm

## NUCLEOID

Embedded in the ribosome-rich cytoplasm is the bacterial genetic apparatus, the nucleoid. No boundary separates it from the rest of the cytoplasm; the nucleoid's physical segregation is maintained by the very nature of the DNA that is its make up. The DNA consists of one very long and narrow molecule — a double helix — which if stretched to its full length would measure more than 1.0 mm long and only 0.000002 mm (2 nm) wide. Genetic analysis has shown that most of the bacterial genes are linked to one another in an orderly fashion, and, moreover, that the linkage is continuous and circular. We therefore describe the bacterial nucleoid as a single, circular chromosome. Physical studies also demonstrate that the DNA strand of the chromosome is a circle that is tightly coiled into a bundle to produce the nucleoid image shown with the electron microscope. The chromosome replicates in the growing cell in preparation for cell division. Bacterial cells divide by binary fission into two daughter cells, each of which retains a copy of the chromosome. A small percentage of the cell's genetic information is present as much smaller DNA molecules, *plasmids*, which may be present in many copies and replicate independently. Bacterial plasmids often carry the genes involved in resistance to chemotherapeutic drugs. Plasmids cannot be observed within cells by the electron microscope because they are masked by the dense cytoplasm.

## CYTOPLASM

Although certain autotrophic bacteria contain internal membranes associated with photosynthesis and other special metabolic functions, the cytoplasm of most heterotrophic bacteria contains only ribosomes and storage granules. Ribosomes are the site of protein synthesis, and their large numbers reflect the importance of this synthetic role in the bacterial cell. Many enzymes are present in the cytoplasm, whereas others are bound to the cell membrane. It is impossible, however, to recognize individual protein molecules with the electron microscope, except when special preparative techniques are used.

Each ribosome is a complex structure about 20 nm in diameter, and is an aggregate of several RNA molecules and many protein molecules. The ribosome consists of two major subunits, one somewhat larger than the other. Although the ribosomes of all types of cells function in a similar manner in protein synthesis, it is possible to distinguish the ribosomes of prokaryotic cells from those of eukaryotic cells by their different sedimentation velocity in the ultracentrifuge. Bacte-

rial ribosomes have a sedimentation value of 70S (Svedberg units), whereas eukaryotic ribosomes are slightly larger and heavier with a sedimentation value of 80S. The antibiotics tetracycline, streptomycin, and chloramphenicol act by interfering with one stage or other of protein synthesis by bacterial (70S) ribosomes.

A second class of cytoplasmic particles, which are frequently but not always found, are storage granules (Fig. 2). The presence and amount of these particles vary with the type of bacterium and its level of metabolic activity. Storage granules represent a mechanism for temporary storage of excess metabolites. Three types of such granules are common: glycogen, a glucose polymer that serves as a carbohydrate reserve; poly-β-hydroxybutyric acid, a lipid reserve; and volutin, a polyphosphate compound. These granules are often large enough to be seen with the light microscope. Volutin granules are also known as metachromatic granules because of their staining behavior; that is, they appear red when stained with methylene blue dye.

## CELL MEMBRANE

The cytoplasmic membrane, a delicate structure that is only 6 nm thick, represents the true

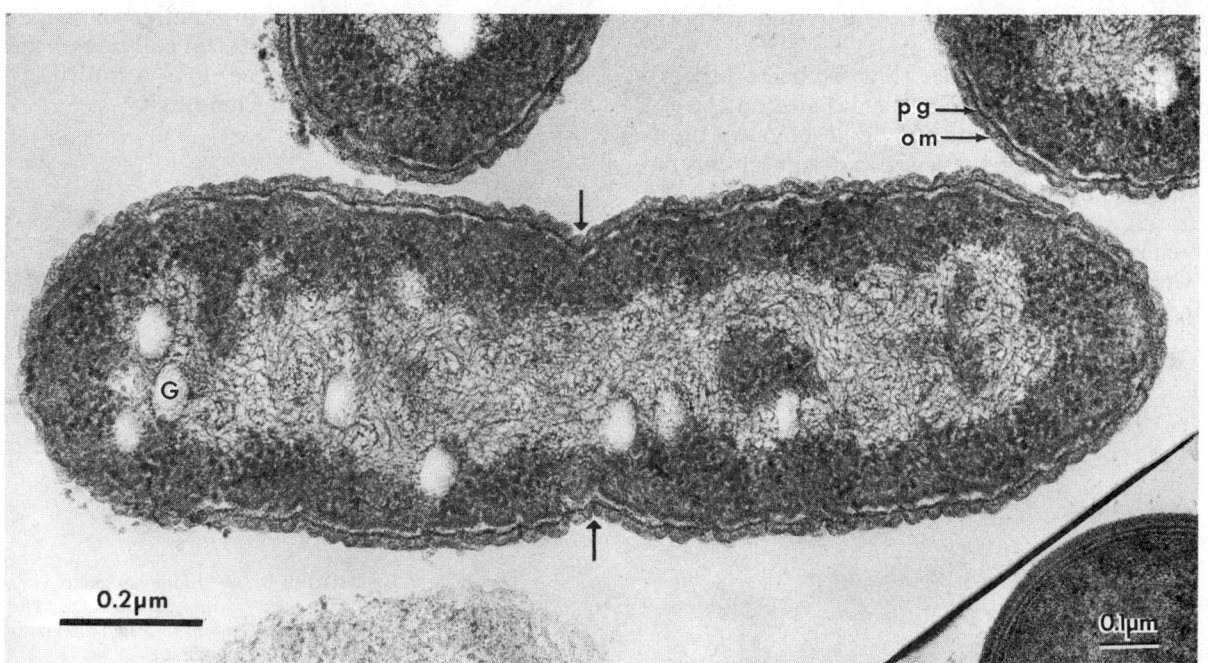

**FIGURE 2.**   *A typical rod-shaped gram-negative cell,* Chromobacterium violaceum, *is seen here in longitudinal and cross-section. It contains several storage granules (G), probably poly-β-hydroxybutyric acid. This cell is in the process of division, as indicated by the inward constriction of the cell wall around the middle of the cell (arrows). The outer membrane and peptidoglycan layers of the cell wall may be seen. The insert at the lower right shows the wall of a gram-positive cell,* Bacillus sphaericus, *for comparison. (Insert courtesy of Drs. Stanley Holt and Donald Tipper, University of Massachusetts.)*

barrier between the inside and the outside of the cell. In addition to a membrane, the bacterial cell requires the presence of a cell wall to permit it to withstand the cell's osmotic pressure and other forces encountered in nature. Removal of the cell wall normally results in the rupture of the cell membrane, causing *lysis,* the dissolution and death of the cell. In an osmotically protected environment the cell may remain intact and alive even after the cell wall is removed. A cell having no wall is called a *protoplast,* if the wall is completely removed, or a *spheroplast,* if some wall fragments remain.

The selective permeability of the cell membrane determines which molecules from the cell's environment can enter the cell and which are excluded. Some molecules diffuse passively into the cell; others require active transport across the membrane by specific enzymes. Enzymes involved in cell wall synthesis and synthesis of extracellular products are lodged in the cytoplasmic membrane. The antibiotic properties of polymyxin-B result from its interference with normal membrane permeability.

The electron transport system, the primary energy-generating system of the cell, is also located on the cell membrane. Thus, the membrane is the site where most chemical energy available through metabolism is converted into a form of energy (ATP) that can be used in the biosynthesis of cell materials or in other energy-requiring cellular reactions.

There is some evidence that the bacterial chromosome is attached to a special site on the cell membrane. This would provide a physical mechanism by which one of the two daughter chromosomes produced by DNA replication could be segregated into each of the daughter cells during cell division.

Generally, the bacterial membrane is found solely at the cell periphery. However, some bacterial cells exhibit complex infoldings or invaginations of the membrane into the cytoplasmic space (Fig. 3). These invaginations have been named *mesosomes* to distinguish them from the membrane proper and from the cytoplasm. This distinction may not be necessary, since mesosomes are not really separate bodies but rather extensions of the cell membrane. A number of efforts have been made to ascertain whether mesosomal invaginations have unique or specific functions. It has been suggested that they serve to increase the surface area of the cell membrane or that they represent specialized areas of the membrane; they are often seen in association with cell division or spore formation. However, to date no specialized functions have been conclusively demonstrated to be associated with the mesosomal membrane. Mesosomes have been observed only with the electron microscope, and some evidence suggests that the structures may be artifacts of the preparation of the cells for electron microscopy.

The appearance and chemical composition of the membrane of prokaryotic cells are quite similar to those of the cell membrane of eukaryotic cells. One notable chemical difference is that most bacterial membranes do not contain sterols (e.g., cholesterol) as do the membranes of higher life forms. In the bacterial cell, the cytoplasmic membrane performs many functions that are localized in the specialized organelles of higher cells. Thus, although the bacterial cell membrane may be simple in appearance, it is a multifunctional structure of extreme complexity.

## FLAGELLA

A number of bacterial cell types demonstrate a striking rapid motility that is the product of a specialized cell structure, the bacterial *flagellum.*

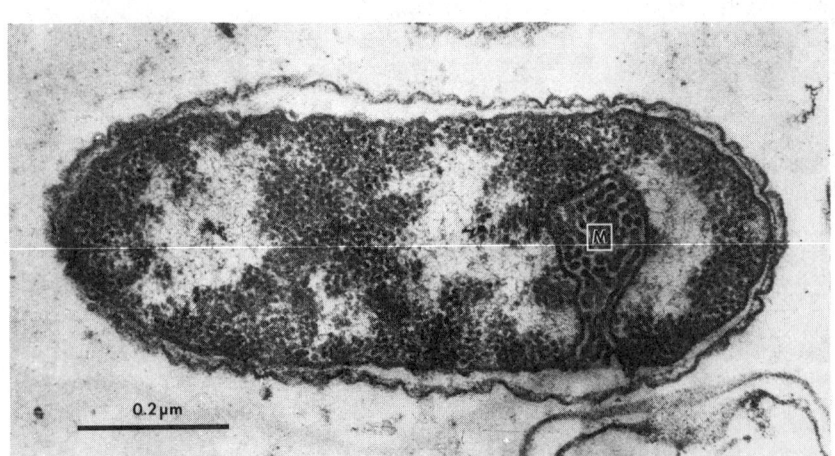

**FIGURE 3.** *A Chromobacterium violaceum cell, showing a single large mesosome (M), a complex invagination of the cytoplasmic membrane.*

Bacterial flagella are completely different in their structure and mechanism of function from the flagella and cilia of protozoa and other eukaryotic cells. In the higher cells a planar wave motion is generated within a membrane-bound flagellum by the sliding action of multiple protein filaments, the flagellar microtubules. In bacteria, a single proteinaceous filament, about 15 nm in diameter, projects from the cell. At its base a complex structure, which is highly integrated with the cell wall and membrane, produces a rotary motion in the flagellar filament. The cell is driven forward by the propeller-like motion of the flagellum. The mechanism of operation of this fascinating, chemically driven rotary motor is currently under investigation.

Motility is also linked to membrane-bound receptors that identify the presence of specific molecules in the cell's environment. This phenomenon of *chemotaxis* allows bacteria to move toward higher concentrations of nutrients and away from harmful substances.

Bacterial flagella may be arranged in a diverse manner in different cell types. Some bacteria possess many flagella distributed over the entire surface of the cell (*peritrichous* flagella), whereas others possess a single flagellum or a bundle of flagella located at one pole of the cell (*polar* flagella). Special flagellar stains are used to enlarge the dimensions of the flagella artificially so that they may be observed with the light microscope. Motility versus nonmotility and the arrangement of flagella are useful diagnostic characteristics for identifying bacteria.

## FIMBRIAE OR PILI

Electron microscopic examination of intact gram-negative cells frequently reveals the presence of long, slender projections extending from the surface of the cells. These projections, which originate at the cell membrane and extend through the cell wall, are of two types: the first are called *fimbriae*, or *common pili*, and the second are called *sex pili*.

The most common of these projections are the fimbriae, or common pili. Fimbriae are frequently found in large numbers (as many as several hundred per cell) projecting from the entire surface of freshly isolated gram-negative bacteria. They are made of a single protein, whose molecules are arranged in a helix to form a long filament. The function of fimbriae has not been completely clarified, but there is mounting evidence that these slender projections play a role in facilitating the adherence of bacterial cells to other surfaces. Fimbriae are rather stable and are not easily removed from the surface of the bacterial cell. The length and width of a common pilus vary greatly among different bacterial types but generally fall within the range of 3 to 15 nm in width and from 0.2 $\mu$m to a few micrometers in length.

Sex pili are less common than fimbriae; only a few gram-negative species are known to possess them. They act as specific bridges between bacterial cells during *conjugation,* a process in which unidirectional transfer of genetic information takes place between cells. The sex pilus has the form of a hollow tube, and it is believed that bacterial DNA migrates through the narrow central space of the pilus during conjugation. Sex pili are long (1 $\mu$m or more), relatively thick (about 25 nm), and very fragile. They can be broken by simple physical treatment. Very few (no more than ten) sex pili are found on bacteria that possess these fragile appendages.

## CELL WALL

The wall of the bacterium confers protective rigidity to the cell. The chemical composition and organization of the prokaryotic cell wall is a unique structure that is not found in eukaryotic cells. Its basic component is a mixed polymer called *peptidoglycan*. The peptidoglycan is made of two components: Linear polymers, called glycan strands, are made of two substituted hexose sugars — $N$-acetylglucosamine   and   $N$-acetylmuramic acid. These sugars are present in equal amounts and occupy alternate positions along the chains, which may contain dozens of sugar molecules. The second component is short peptides — identical chains of four amino acids — that attach to the glycan strand (but only to the $N$-acetylmuramic acid residues), thus forming side branches to the glycan strands. Some of these tetrapeptides are, in turn, linked to one another by other short peptides, forming cross-bridges between the glycan strands (Fig. 4). Peptidoglycan forms a single, bag-shaped macromolecule that surrounds the cytoplasmic membrane — conferring cell shape, countering the osmotic force exerted by the cell, and forming a physical barrier against the outside environment.

Besides the occurrence in peptidoglycan of the two unusual $N$-acetyl sugars, the peptide chains contain some amino acids that are found nowhere else except in bacterial cell walls. Among these are *meso*-diaminopimelic acid and the D-isomers of glutamic acid and alanine. (The amino acids found in all proteins are the L-isomers.)

Peptidoglycan is a component in the walls of almost all bacterial cells. Two notable exceptions are the cells of *Mycoplasma* and *Halobacteria*. *Mycoplasma* are very small bacteria that actually have no cell wall, being surrounded by a cytoplas-

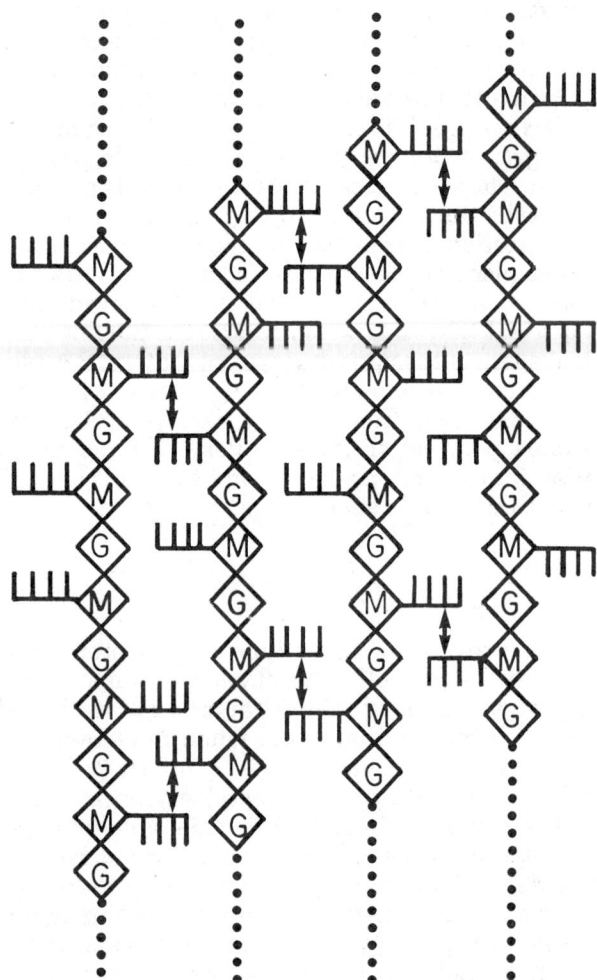

**FIGURE 4.** *This diagram schematically represents the structure of peptidoglycan. The glycan strands are composed of alternating units of N-acetylglucosamine (G) and N-acetylmuramic acid (M). Tetrapeptide side chains connect to the muramic acid residues. Some of the tetrapeptides are joined by other peptides (short arrows) to form cross-bridges between the glycan strands.*

peptidoglycan structure, consisting of many layers (although they are not visible as such with the electron microscope) of peptidoglycan, making a total cell wall thickness of 10 to 100 nm (Figs. 2 and 5). Peptidoglycan represents the major component of the gram-positive cell wall, although minor components known as teichoic acids are also present. Examples of gram-positive bacteria include *Bacillus, Streptococcus, Staphylococcus,* and *Clostridium.*

The original basis of division of bacteria into gram-negative and gram-positive forms was the staining procedure devised almost 100 years ago by the Danish physician Christian Gram. This stain, which is still in common clinical use for diagnostic purposes, involves four steps: Cells are 1) stained with crystal violet; 2) treated with iodine to form a crystal violet–iodine complex; 3) washed with an organic solvent such as alcohol; and 4) stained again with safranin. In gram-positive cells the purple dye complex is retained, whereas in gram-negative cells the dye complex is removed by the solvent. Thus gram-positive cells appear purple under the microscope; gram-negative cells are counterstained by the safranin and appear red. Although the exact mechanism of the staining reaction is not known, it appears that the staining occurs within the cell, not on the cell wall, and that the thicker peptidoglycan wall of the gram-positive cell protects the dye-iodine complex to a greater extent from the action of the solvent.

Since the cell wall of gram-positive bacteria consists of a layer of peptidoglycan that may be many times thicker than the peptidoglycan of the gram-negative cell wall, gram-positive cells tend to be sturdier and less susceptible to breakage by physical forces. In contrast, the presence in the gram-negative cell of other cell wall components in addition to peptidoglycan gives those bacteria certain advantages.

The gram-negative cell wall contains significant amounts of lipoprotein and lipopolysaccharide in association with the thin peptidoglycan layer. This layer of lipid material lies outside the peptidoglycan and is frequently called the *outer membrane.* Although it appears as a membrane in electron micrographs and has the property of excluding some large molecules, it appears to contain no enzymes, and its function and organization are much less complex than those of the cytoplasmic membrane.

An example of an advantage that gram-negative cells possess is a lower susceptibility to cell lysis by the naturally occurring hydrolytic enzyme *lysozyme.* Lysozyme is widespread in nature and specifically attacks peptidoglycan by cleaving the bonds of the glycan strand between *N*-acetylmuramic acid and *N*-acetylglucosamine.

mic membrane only. *Halobacteria,* which live in high-salt environments, have a wall that lacks peptidoglycan. The composition of peptidoglycan is not absolutely uniform among all types of bacteria; however, the variation is not in the carbohydrate backbone of the glycan strand but in the type of amino acids in the tetrapeptide and in the types and number of amino acids that cross-link the tetrapeptides to one another.

Bacteria can be divided into two major groups on the basis of their cell wall structure. The first, *gram-negative* organisms, have a thin peptidoglycan layer adjacent to the cytoplasmic membrane, plus other major cell wall components exterior to the peptidoglycan. Examples of gram-negative bacteria are *Escherichia, Salmonella, Pseudomonas, Treponema,* and *Chlamydia.* The second, *gram-positive* organisms, have a much thicker

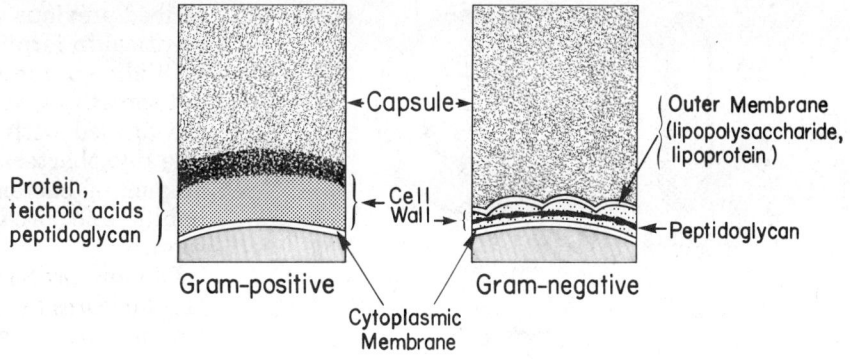

**FIGURE 5.** *These diagrams compare the structures of the gram-positive and the gram-negative bacterial cell walls, indicating the relative positions of the cytoplasmic membrane and the bacterial capsule.*

In the absence of the protective peptidoglycan layer, the bacterial cell swells excessively owing to osmotic forces. Eventually the cytoplasmic membrane ruptures from the internal pressure. The walls of gram-positive cells are generally quite sensitive to degradation by lysozyme. Gram-negative bacteria are less susceptible to such attack, since the outer membrane excludes lysozyme and prevents it from binding to its site of action on the cell wall's peptidoglycan.

The uniqueness of bacterial peptidoglycan has proved to be particularly useful in the treatment of many bacterial diseases. The biosynthesis of peptidoglycan can be disturbed by a number of antibiotics, including penicillin. The sensitive target of penicillin action is one of the final chemical reactions in peptidoglycan synthesis — the one that effects the linking of the peptide side chains. Thus, the drug prevents cross-bridges from being formed between the glycan strands. Without this bonding the integrity of the peptidoglycan is weakened, producing a fragile wall that cannot protect the cell adequately.

Since penicillin interferes with peptidoglycan synthesis, and since such synthesis does not occur in eukaryotic cells, cells of the animal body are resistant to the primary action of penicillin. Penicillin affects sensitive bacteria only when the cell wall is being synthesized, since it blocks synthesis rather than attacking existing peptidoglycan, as does lysozyme. Thus, if a penicillin-sensitive cell is not growing at the time the antibiotic is used, the cell wall will not be affected. Gram-negative bacteria are significantly less susceptible to the antibiotic action of penicillin than are gram-positive bacteria. This difference, as with lysozyme, is primarily the result of the protective effect of the outer membrane of the gram-negative cell wall, which makes it difficult for the penicillin molecule to reach its site of inhibition. However, forms of penicillin have been synthesized that can penetrate this barrier and attack gram-negative organisms.

## CAPSULE

A few bacterial types, including a number of disease-producing bacteria, manufacture an inert capsule that surrounds the entire cell. Capsular material is easily visualized with the light microscope by negative stains such as India ink. The role of the capsule in the life of bacteria has yet to be established; however, for some bacteria the capsule serves as a protective structure. Certain encapsulated cells are resistant to ingestion by animal phagocytes; thus, these bacteria cannot be destroyed by the phagocytic line of defense of animal blood.

Capsules have a defined chemical composition that is characteristic of the cell type that produces it. In most bacteria the capsule is composed of polysaccharides. A few bacteria produce capsules composed of polypeptides containing D amino acids. The structure of the bacterial capsule is not a highly ordered one as is the structure of the cell wall, thus a general form of capsule structure is not recognized.

## VARIATIONS IN BACTERIAL FORM

Within the large group of prokaryotic organisms, there is a great range in the size and shape of individual cells (Fig. 6). Some are at the limit of visibility of the light microscope; others are as large as some eukaryotic cells. Common cell shapes include spheres (cocci), rods (bacilli), comma shapes (vibrio), and spirals (spirillum, spirochete). Cell size and shape are valuable diagnostic characteristics and are readily seen with the light microscope.

Another diagnostic characteristic of bacteria is the way in which cells do or do not remain associated during growth. They may exist as solitary individuals, or they may remain attached in random clusters, in linear chains, or in ordered sheets or packets.

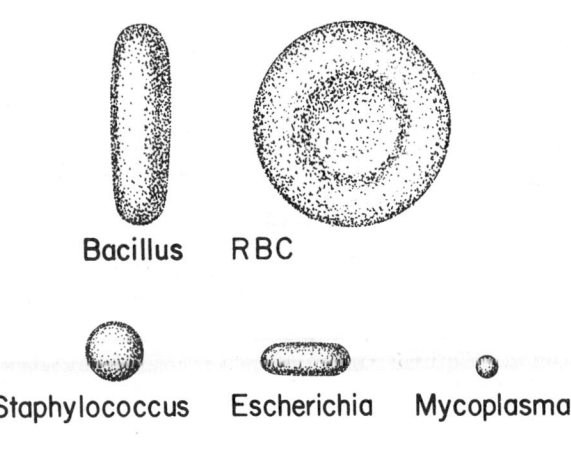

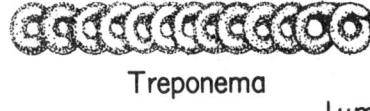

**FIGURE 6.** *Schematic drawings of common bacteria of different sizes and shapes are illustrated here with a human red blood cell to show their relative size.*

Although all the cells of an individual animal originate from a single fertilized egg cell, they show many forms in the adult, meaning that they have *differentiated* to perform certain specialized functions within the organism. When a single bacterial cell divides many times to form a colony of cells, the cells in that colony may be associated in characteristic spatial arrangements, as de-scribed previously, but all individuals are usually identical in form. Differentiation of cells as found in higher organisms does not occur in bacteria; but something akin to it occurs when special cells are formed with certain reproductive functions. The myxobacteria and the actinomycetes are examples of bacteria that have elaborate growth habits and produce fruiting bodies that bear spores.

Of more practical importance are the formation of *endospores* by certain gram-positive organisms. An endospore results when part of a cell, including the nucleoid and some cytoplasm, is walled off from the rest of the mother cell. A complex multilayered wall structure then forms around it (Fig. 7). The total process is called *sporulation.* The resulting endospore demonstrates no metabolic activity and is highly resistant to radiation, chemicals, dessication, and heat. This dormant stage represents a powerful mechanism for both dispersal and cell survival under adverse conditions. Since spores are relatively large refractile bodies, they may be seen with the light microscope. Their presence or absence and the position of the spore within the mother cell (median or terminal) are another set of useful diagnostic characteristics.

Under favorable circumstances the endospore is able to germinate rapidly. Metabolic activity resumes, and the spore swells and breaks open to release a cell identical to the one that originally produced the endospore. Such a cell, although again sensitive to heat and other adverse environmental conditions, can resume normal growth.

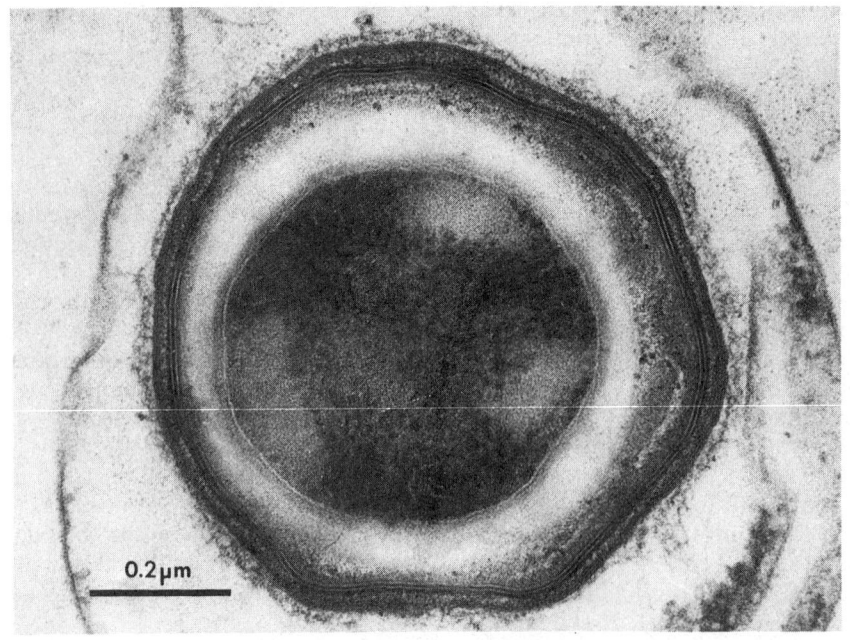

**FIGURE 7.** *This electron micrograph of a bacterial endospore of Bacillus sphaericus illustrates the complex layer structure of the spore wall. The spore is surrounded by remnants of the mother cell. (Courtesy of Drs. Stanley Holt and Donald Tipper, University of Massachusetts.)*

The organization of endospores differs substantially from that of vegetative (growing) cells. New structures are produced during sporulation as a result of the expression of specific bacterial genes. Among the new structures formed is a spore coat composed of a thin yet highly organized layer of extremely hydrophobic proteins. Also produced is the spore cortex, which lies between the spore coat and the significantly reduced cell protoplast. The cortex may be thick and is composed of a unique peptidoglycan; as such it may be analogous to the cell wall of the vegetative cell. As the spore is forming, large amounts of calcium are taken up, and corresponding quantities of dipicolinic acid are synthesized. This chemical combination appears to be responsible for the spore's heat resistance.

The production of endospores is limited to a small number of bacterial types, primarily *Bacillus, Clostridium,* and *Sporosarcina.* However, because of the extreme resistance of endospores to inactivation by physical and chemical means, endospore-forming bacteria are of major importance to human society. Most nonspore-forming bacteria are readily destroyed by boiling, but much higher temperatures are required to kill endospores (for example, autoclaving at 121° C for 20 minutes). Thus, sterilization procedures must acknowledge the high resistance of bacterial endospores even though the actual number of endospores in a given environment may be rather small.

## *SUMMARY*

Bacteria are enormously diverse in their form, habitat, and metabolic patterns. The outline of bacterial cell structure presented here represents a series of rather broad generalizations. They are based, of necessity, on those organisms that have been the subject of the most thorough investigation because of their importance in medicine, industry, or laboratory research. Consequently, gaps in our knowledge and exceptions to our generalizations will occur, particularly among the less common and more poorly studied groups of bacteria.

We can draw an overall conclusion, however: Although bacteria are generally smaller and appear simpler in their organization than the cells of animals and plants, this simplicity is only relative. Bacteria perform a variety of cellular functions common to all living systems and other functions that are peculiar to the prokaryotic kingdom; their biochemical and physiologic machinery is quite complex.

# CLASSIFICATION AND IDENTIFICATION OF BACTERIA    2

*Herman Baer, M.D.
and Charles E. Davis, M.D.*

Classification is the orderly arrangement of sets of organisms into a system; nomenclature deals with the naming or labeling of these organisms; and the recognition and allocation of an unknown organism is called identification. Classification, nomenclature, and identification are the three interdependent essentials of taxonomy.

## *BACTERIAL NOMENCLATURE*

The naming of bacteria is subject to the rules and recommendations of the Bacteriological Code; the need to comply with the Code has been responsible for many changes in bacterial nomenclature. As with the nomenclature of higher organisms, bacterial nomenclature is binomial: The designation of the genus is given first, with the first letter capitalized; the species designation, which is given a lower case first letter, follows the designation of the genus.

The shifting of an organism into a different genus will automatically change its generic name. Since there are no rules for classification, the rearrangement of organisms is more or less left to the whim of the taxonomist. Frequent changes of the generic designations of bacteria are the unfortunate consequence.

## BACTERIAL CLASSIFICATION

The classification of higher organisms is designed to reflect natural relatedness and phylogenetic relationships. The classification is hierarchic, proceeding from the large taxonomic groups to the species. In bacteria, studies of phylogenetic relationships are only beginning (see further on). In general, the hierarchic approach has met with limited success in bacterial classification, and its use has been sharply reduced in the latest edition of *Bergey's Manual of Determinative Bacteriology* (1974), the standard work on bacterial classification. The species is the fundamental unit of bacterial classification, and taxonomic ranks higher than the genus have limited importance, with the exception of the family Enterobacteriaceae (see Chapter 31).

In the conventional approach to bacterial classification, exemplified in *Bergey's Manual,* the genera of medically important bacteria are grouped together according to certain easily observable and relatively constant properties.

### Staining Reactions

The *gram reaction* is by far the most important of these properties. The Gram stain, which was devised by Christian Gram in 1884, divides bacteria into two fundamentally different categories, gram-positive and gram-negative. Infected material obtained directly from patients or from small portions of bacterial colonies or liquid cultures are allowed to dry in air and are heat fixed on glass slides before treatment with Gram's reagents. All conventional bacteria are stained purple by crystal violet, the primary dye of the Gram stain. After treatment with Gram's iodine (3 per cent $I_2$-KI at pH 8.0), which complexes with the crystal violet, only gram-positive bacteria resist decolorization with alcohol, ether, or acetone. Because they have retained the crystal violet, gram-positive bacteria do not color with safranin, the red counterstain used in the last step of the Gram stain. Gram-negative bacteria stain red from the safranin because they lose the crystal violet when treated with decolorizing agents. The gram-positive cell wall itself does not stain. Instead, it presents a permeability barrier to elution of the crystal violet–iodine complex from the interior of the cell by the decolorizing agent. Gram-negative walls contain lipopolysaccharide and thinner, less complex peptidoglycan (see Chapter 1) that do not resist penetration of the cell by the decolorizers.

Another staining reaction used in the classification of bacteria is the *Ziehl-Neelson (acid-fast) stain.* Mycobacteria (Chapter 40) are difficult to stain by ordinary techniques because of their high content of waxes and lipids. They are stained red, however, when they are flooded for five to seven minutes with carbol fuchsin that is kept steaming hot by placing the glass slide over a flame or on a hot plate during the staining. All bacteria are stained by this procedure, but only mycobacteria retain the carbol fuchsin when treated with 3 per cent HCl in alcohol (acid-fast). After decolorization, other bacteria are stained by a cold counterstain such as methylene blue to contrast with the red mycobacteria. Nocardia (Chapter 41) do not stain with the conventional Ziehl-Neelsen stain but remain red (acid-fast) if they are decolorized either by 1 per cent sulfuric acid or brief exposure to 3 per cent HCl. The "firmly bound" lipids of mycobacteria, which are resistant to extraction by organic solvents, are responsible for the acid-fastness of mycobacteria (see Chapter 40).

## MORPHOLOGY

Microscopically, bacterial cells can be identified as either spherical (cocci) or rod-shaped. Cocci may be arranged singly, or in pairs, clusters, or chains. Rod-shaped bacteria may be straight and regular or they may be club-shaped, curved, or spiral-shaped, or they may have pointed ends. Microscopic examination reveals the presence of spores. With the help of special staining procedures, the presence, number, and arrangement of flagella are noted. Flagella may be distributed over the entire surface of the cell (peritrichous flagellation), or they may be limited to the poles (polar flagellation).

### Metabolic Reactions

The reaction to atmospheric oxygen separates bacteria into aerobic, facultative (capable of either aerobic or anaerobic growth) and strictly anaerobic organisms. The study of nutritional requirements, or the ability to grow on certain kinds of culture media, provides useful information for classification. The mode of attack on carbohydrates, usually glucose, is of taxonomic significance: Glucose is degraded anaerobically in the absence of atmospheric oxygen by the so-called fermentative organisms. Oxidative organisms require atmospheric oxygen for the degradation of glucose. Other organisms fail to metabolize glucose at all. This fermentative (F) versus oxidative (O) metabolism of carbohydrates is determined in the so-called OF test in which part of the media is exposed to air and part is anaerobic. Other characteristics thought to be of fundamental taxonomic significance include the enzyme catalase, which decomposes $H_2O_2$, and oxidase, which transfers hydrogen directly from its substrate to oxygen.

The properties just described and others have

been used successfully by bacteriologists for many years to classify bacteria and have been accepted as fundamental and important; that is, they were weighted heavily in the classification. With the help of these properties, medically important bacteria can often be divided to the generic level, or placed into a group of genera. This is illustrated in the following list in an oversimplified fashion for the classification of some medically important gram-positive cocci:

Facultatively anaerobic, arranged in clusters, catalase-positive:
  fermentative: *Staphylococcus*
  oxidative: *Micrococcus*
Facultatively anaerobic, arranged in pairs or chains, catalase-negative: *Streptococcus*
Anaerobic, arranged in clusters, catalase-variable: *Peptococcus*
Arranged in pairs or chains, catalase-negative: *Peptostreptococcus*

The definition of the various species within a genus is based on a set of physiologic and biochemical characteristics, including the degradation of carbohydrates, amino acids, and a variety of other substrates. Certain characteristics are quite constant and highly discriminating — they separate otherwise very similar species. For example, among all species of staphylococci, the production of coagulase is unique to *Staphylococcus aureus* and has become part of the definition of the species.

Coagulase is an enzyme that causes clotting of citrated or oxalated plasma by reacting with the coagulase-reacting factor (prothrombin) to activate thrombin. Coagulase-positive staphylococci usually also produce clumping factor ("bound coagulase") that causes macroscopic agglutination of the staphylococci when they are mixed with plasma on a glass slide. More commonly, bacterial species are defined by means of a whole pattern of biochemical properties.

Many bacterial species have been subdivided further by a variety of techniques, including antigen analysis, biochemical reactions, and susceptibility to bacteriophages — viruses that penetrate and lyse bacteria. The resulting serotypes, biotypes, and phage types have considerable clinical and epidemiologic significance.

The fact that the conventional scheme of bacterial classification is artificial and based on arbitrarily chosen criteria has not detracted from its great practical usefulness. Although it has never been possible to define the concept of the bacterial species satisfactorily, the operational value of the concept of bacterial species to medicine and epidemiology has been immense.

In recent years, new approaches to bacterial classification have evolved in an effort to sup-
plant the conventional taxonomy by a more rational system. These include the Adansonian method of classification, or numerical classification, and the study of DNA-relatedness.

## Adansonian and Numerical Classification

The numerical classification was developed by Adanson and applied by him successfully to the taxonomy of groups of higher organisms. Instead of studying a relatively small number of properties considered to be important, a very large number of characteristics is examined, each of which is assigned equal weight. Taxonomic groups are established on the basis of the overall similarity of organisms. Similarity between two organisms can be expressed as the similarity coefficient, which is defined as the percentage of shared properties among all the properties tested. (Only those tests that give a positive result with at least one of the organisms are used for determination of the similarity coefficient.) If two organisms show a similarity coefficient of about 90, they are likely to belong to the same species.

The massive amounts of data generated by the study of a large number of properties of a great many strains is best handled by a computer. The greatest value of this so-called numerical taxonomy or numerical classification system lies in the re-evaluation of the conventional classification of groups of bacteria. Numerical classification has confirmed the appropriateness of the classification of many organisms and has suggested the reclassification of others.

## Classification by DNA-relatedness

The emerging field of genetic or molecular taxonomy is based on the analysis of bacterial DNA (Brenner and Falkow, 1971). In contrast to conventional taxonomy, this method can be expected to discover phylogenetic relationships among organisms and therefore provide a truly natural classification.

The degree to which organisms are related can be evaluated by the number of genes they have in common. Organisms of the same species would be expected to share most of their genes. As a consequence, the nucleotide composition and sequence of their DNA should be very similar. Techniques for determining the nucleotide sequence of nucleic acids are available, and the complete base sequence of several small viruses is known. It seems likely that this will have a major impact on the recognition of phylogenetic relationships among viruses. However, it is not practical to determine the base sequence of the much larger bacterial DNA at the present time. Other criteria to determine the DNA-relatedness of two bacteria include the comparison of the nucleotide base composition of their DNA, the degree to which their DNA will hybridize, and the ability of their DNA to undergo recombination.

The nucleotide base composition of DNA varies widely among different groups of bacteria and is characteristic for bacteria of the same genus. Since adenine (A) pairs with thymine (T), and guanine (G) pairs with cytosine (C), the percentage of each nucleotide in double-stranded DNA can be expressed by the formula AT + GC = 100 per cent. It is customary to express the base composition of DNA in terms of its GC content, which can vary from 22 per cent to 74 per cent for bacterial DNA. Bacteria with a different GC content have few base sequences in common and therefore have different genes and cannot be closely related. Conversely, organisms with a similar GC content may or may not be closely related, since a similarity in GC content does not necessarily mean that the base sequences are similar. For example, *E. coli,* a gram-negative bacillus of the family Enterobacteriaceae, and certain species of *Bacillus,* spore-forming gram-positive bacilli, have a GC content of 50 per cent, but are clearly unrelated. Determination of the nucleotide base composition is a powerful tool in reassessing the conventional classification of bacteria, and it is widely used for that purpose. For example, the genus *Micrococcus* appeared reasonably homogeneous by the usual bacteriologic criteria; however, some micrococci were found to have a GC content of 30 to 37 per cent, which corresponds to the GC content of staphylococci, instead of 66 to 75 per cent, which is typical of the other micrococci. Hence, these micrococci have recently been reclassified as staphylococci.

Hybridization is used to determine the degree to which base sequences of the DNA of two organisms are shared, or "homologous." The procedure for the hybridization experiment is performed as follows: The DNA of one organism is made radioactive biosynthetically, extracted from the bacteria, sheared into small fragments, and mixed with a large excess of nonradioactive DNA from the other organism. The mixture is heated to achieve separation of the DNA into single strands. After cooling, the complementary strands of DNA reanneal into double-stranded DNA. If the two organisms are related, they have many base sequences in common, and radioactive fragments will reanneal with nonradioactive complementary DNA. The percentage of radioactive DNA bound to nonradioactive DNA can be used to estimate the degree of complementarity and therefore the genetic relatedness between the organisms. Hybridization has been used extensively to study DNA homology between members of the family Enterobacteriaceae and has great potential for supplying new information on the taxonomy of other groups of organisms.

Under certain conditions, DNA can be transferred from one organism to another by the mechanisms of transformation, transduction, and conjugation (see Chapter 4). The transferred (donor) DNA can recombine with the resident (host) DNA to produce a genetic change that may manifest itself as a newly acquired property — for example, antibiotic resistance. It is assumed that two organisms are closely related if their DNA can recombine (Jones and Sneath, 1970). Recombination generally involves small pieces of DNA that are equivalent to only a few genes, and many factors other than gene similarity influence recombination rates. It must also be kept in mind that transfer of extrachromosomal genetic material (plasmids) can occur between organisms that are taxonomically unrelated.

Transformation and recombination have been used successfully for taxonomic studies of *Neisseria, Moraxella,* and related organisms, but recombination is less universally applicable than other methods of determining DNA-relatedness.

## *BACTERIAL IDENTIFICATION*

Bacterial classification is a basic science; in contrast, bacterial identification is an applied discipline of microbiology with great practical significance. The identification of a bacterium suspected of being the cause of an infection is one of the major tools for the objective diagnosis of infectious diseases. The approach to the identification of bacterial isolates in the diagnostic laboratory is quite different from that taken by the bacterial taxonomist in the classification of a new or unknown organism. The taxonomist will study as many characteristics as possible; time and cost are of little concern. In contrast, in order to be clinically useful and relevant, the identification of a clinical isolate must be provided as quickly as possible. Economics and practicality dictate the use of only a minimal number of diagnostic tests (Bartlett, 1974). Thus, by necessity, identification in the clinical laboratory will always represent a compromise between accuracy on the one hand, and speed and economy on the other. Just how this compromise is made will determine the quality of a laboratory.

The practical limitation on the number of properties that can be used for identification of bacteria makes the selection of the diagnostic tests very important. The same properties of bacteria that are used in the conventional classification are employed in the identification of clinical isolates. For this reason, identification is sometimes referred to as "classification in reverse."

A hierarchic set of tables permits the identification process to proceed in a rational, stepwise fashion. A logical, practical example of a hierarchic set of diagnostic tables for medically important bacteria is presented by Cowan and Steel (1974). In the first stage of identification, the unknown organism is assigned either to a single genus or to a group of genera with the help of a small number of characteristics. The groups of organisms established by the first set of tests are differentiated to the species level by one or two additional sets of biochemical or serologic tests. The obvious advantage of this stepwise approach to identification is that it requires fewer tests than the shotgun approach, in which a very large number of tests is performed initially.

A diagnostic key is indispensible for the objective identification of clinical isolates in the modern laboratory. Nevertheless, a key is useless without consideration of the time-honored methods of the Gram stain, colonial morphology, and growth characteristics.

Examples of diagnostic keys or flow sheets based on these stable characteristics are given in Tables 1 through 7. The first-stage tables (Tables 1 and 2) classify medically important bacteria according to their gram reactions and microscopic morphology. This type of classification system reflects the thinking of the experienced microbiologist when he analyzes Gram stains of primary material from patients and is often the only guide to treatment during the first 24 hours. The second-stage tables (Table 3 through 7) illustrate the identification of medically important bacteria according to growth characteristics, ability to grow in the presence of oxygen, colonial morphology, pigment production, motility, and the presence of certain stable enzymes such as catalase, oxidase, or coagulase. These simple observations permit the rapid determination of the genera of many bacteria and both the genera and species of a suprisingly large number of bacteria. More important, attention to these major, easily established properties prevents naive errors. Laboratories that use the Gram stain and pure single colony bacteriology as the cornerstones of bacterial identification will not misidentify a gram-negative bacillus as a gram-positive bacillus or a coccus just because the biochemical reactions are similar.

Third-stage tables that involve second or third subcultures into biochemical media are not included in this chapter. When a subculture into one or two simple, defined media permits identification of a bacterium to the species level, this step is included in the second-stage tables. The appendix to this chapter provides a glossary explaining some of these reactions. Additional information about the definitive identification of medically important species is provided in Part One of this book.

Gram-positive bacteria (Table 1) are easily divided into cocci and bacilli on the basis of microscopic morphology. Careful consideration of cell shape as well as the usual search for chains or tetrads virtually always separates streptococci from staphylococci. *Clostridium* and *Bacillus* cannot be differentiated from one another by Gram stain and microscopic morphology, but are readily differentiated from the other Gram-positive bacilli. The typical club-shaped, palisading *Corynebacterium* and the extensively branched, beaded, filamentous *Nocardia* or *Actinomyces israelii* are also distinctive, but the remainder of the gram-positive rods are more difficult to separate microscopically. *Propionobacterium, Listeria,* and *Erysipelothrix* are usually indistinguishable from diptheroids (corynebacteria). In contrast, *Propionobacterium* and *Erysipelothrix* may also be filamentous and indistinguishable from other filamentous bacteria with rudimentary branching. Although extensive branching is a uniform characteristic of *A. israelii* and *Nocardia,* the other *Actinomyces* species and *Arachnia* may exhibit only rudimentary branching. *Nocardia* may be separated from *Actinomyces* and *Streptomyces* by its tendency to retain carbol fuchsin in the acid-fast stain. The rapid-growing, atypical mycobacteria, which take the gram stain well, may be distinguished from other club-shaped bacteria by the Ziehl-Neelsen stain.

The gram-negative bacteria shown in Table 2 are more difficult to separate by microscopic morphology, but can readily be separated into cocci, the pleomorphic group, and the uniformly-shaped, larger Enterobacteriaceae-Pseudomonas group. In addition, the following bacteria can frequently be identified accurately by microscopy: *Neisseria* (kidney-shaped diplococci with flattened apposing edges), the *Acinetobacter-Moraxella* group (a mixture of *Neisseria*-like and bacillary forms), *Brucella* (tiny, faintly-staining bacilli), *Bacteroides* (small, uniformly encapsulated bacilli with occasional filamentous forms), *Haemophilus* (similar to *Bacteroides* but more pleomorphic with a larger population of filamentous forms), *Fusobacterium nucleatum* (severely pointed with a rigid, crystalline appearance), *Fusobacterium necrophorum* (spheroplastic), and *Vibrio* (when markedly comma-shaped). Generally, the Enterobacteriaceae cannot be separated microscopically from one another or from the other bacteria listed in the group with uniform shape. Although most of the coccobacillary, pleomorphic bacteria may be confused with one another, the source of the clinical specimen aids the microbiologist. A spinal fluid is more likely to contain *Haemophilus influenzae;* a surgical wound, *Bacteroides;* and a cat or dog bite, *Pasteurella multocida.*

**TABLE 1.  Classification of Medically Important Bacteria by Staining Reactions
and Microscopic Morphology***
**First-stage Table**

GRAM-POSITIVE

| Cocci | | Bacilli | |
|---|---|---|---|

| Round, in clusters & tetrads | Oval Shape, chains | Club-shaped palisading | Filamentous | | Spore-bearing large, uniform |
|---|---|---|---|---|---|

*Staphylococcus*    *Streptococcus*    Corynebacterium                 *Bacillus*

*Micrococcus*    *Peptostreptococcus*    *Listeria*    | Branching rudi-mentary or absent | | Extensive branching |    *Clostridium*

*Peptococcus*            *Erysipelothrix*    *Erysipelothrix*    *Actinomyces*

              *Mycobacterium* (rapid-growers)    *Lactobacillus*    *Arachnia*

              *Propionobacterium* (*Eubacterium*)    *Eubacterium*    *Nocardia*

                         (*Actinomyces*)    *Streptomyces*

             | Acid-fast |    (*Propionobacterium*)    | Partially acid-fast |

             Mycobacterium                   *Nocardia*

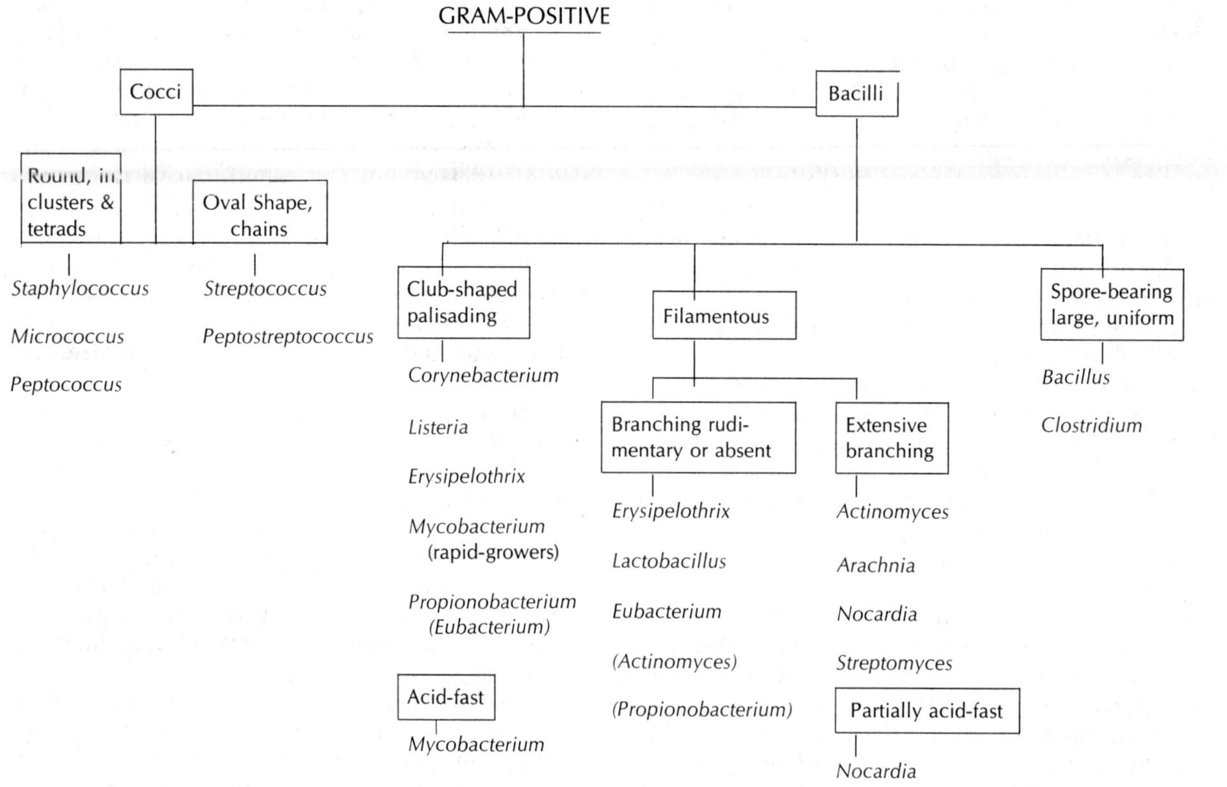

*Bacteria are listed in parenthesis when another shape or arrangement occurs more commonly.

**TABLE 2.  Classification of Medically Important Bacteria by Gram Stain and Microscopic Morphology**
**First-stage Table**

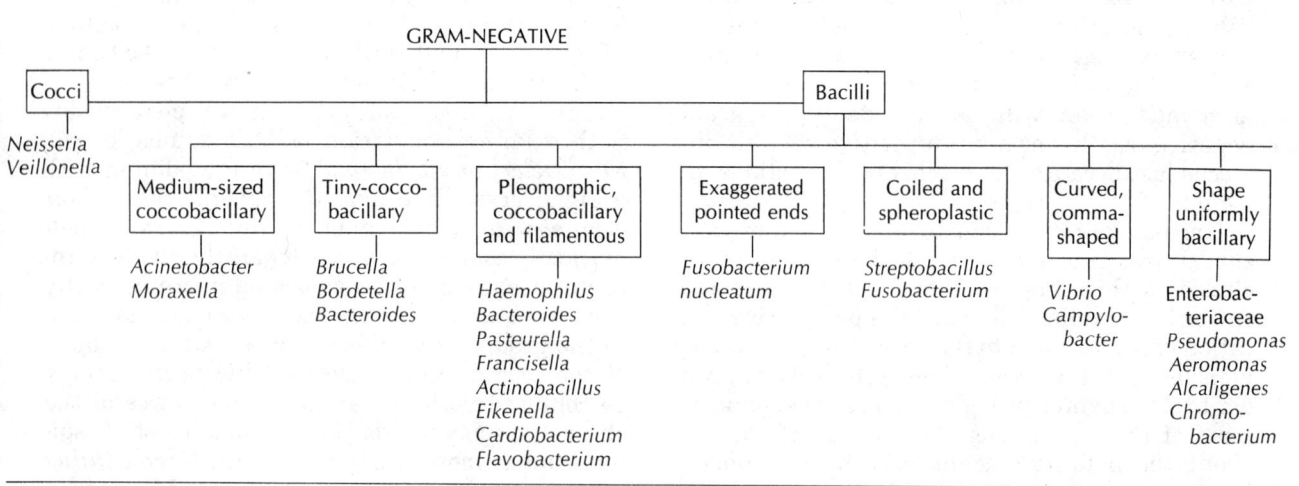

GRAM-NEGATIVE

| Cocci | | Bacilli | | | | | |
|---|---|---|---|---|---|---|---|

*Neisseria*
*Veillonella*

| Medium-sized coccobacillary | Tiny-cocco-bacillary | Pleomorphic, coccobacillary and filamentous | Exaggerated pointed ends | Coiled and spheroplastic | Curved, comma-shaped | Shape uniformly bacillary |
|---|---|---|---|---|---|---|

*Acinetobacter*   *Brucella*   *Haemophilus*   *Fusobacterium*   *Streptobacillus*   *Vibrio*   Enterobac-
*Moraxella*   *Bordetella*   *Bacteroides*   *nucleatum*   *Fusobacterium*   *Campylo-*   teriaceae
   *Bacteroides*   *Pasteurella*          *bacter*   *Pseudomonas*
     *Francisella*               *Aeromonas*
     *Actinobacillus*               *Alcaligenes*
     *Eikenella*                *Chromo-*
     *Cardiobacterium*              *bacterium*
     *Flavobacterium*

The second-stage table for identification of gram-positive cocci best illustrates the usefulness of microscopic and colonial morphology, selective media, and simple techniques for detection of enzymes. As shown in Table 3, virtually all gram-positive cocci can be identified from properly chosen primary or secondary cultures. Tables 4, 5, 6, and 7 — the second-stage tables for gram-positive bacilli, anaerobic gram-negative bacilli, and facultative gram-negative bacilli, respectively, demonstrate the other end of the spectrum. Identification of many of these bacteria require complete diagnostic tables listing fermentation and decarboxylation patterns, end products of glucose metabolism, nitrate reductase activity, urease activity, end products of tryptophane metabolism, and many other properties. Nevertheless, there are a large number of distinctive organisms among these groups that can be identified from primary or secondary cultures. Furthermore, this approach permits the intelligent selection of further tests for definitive identification. Bacteria that can be definitively identified from primary cul-

ture plates are indicated in Tables 4, 5, 6, and 7 either by giving the genus and species names or by listing a group of bacteria under the heading of Unique Characteristics.

The taxonomy of the anaerobic nonspore–forming gram-positive bacilli (Table 4) is currently in a most confused state. Many organisms such as the ramibacteria, the catenabacteria, and the bifidobacteria have been listed as separate genera, as *Actinomyces,* as *Lactobacillus,* and as *Eubacterium.* The eubacteria are given generic status with characteristics intermediate between the propionobacteria and the *Actinomyces.* Catenabacteria and ramibacteria have found a temporary home among the lactobacilli, and *Bifidobacterium* is regarded as a separate genus among the Actinomycetaceae family.

Taxonomists have recently divided the fusobacteria and the *Bacteroides* (Table 5) on the basis of end products of glucose metabolism. Fusobacteria produce predominantly butyric acid from glucose metabolism, whereas *Bacteroides* produce a mixed acid pattern. This rational approach to tax-

**TABLE 3.   Identification of Gram-Positive Cocci**
**Second-stage Table**

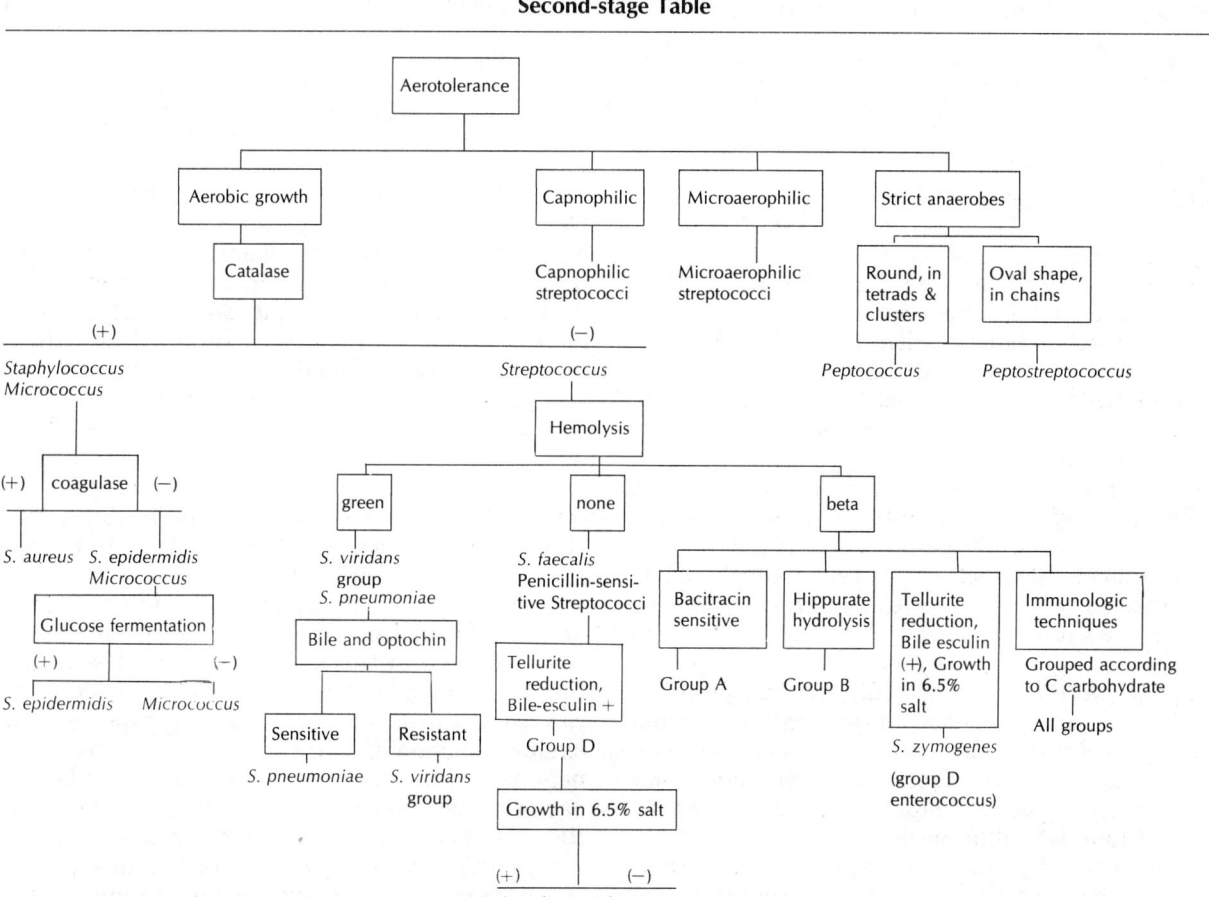

**TABLE 4.   Identification of Gram-positive Bacilli**
**Second-stage Table**

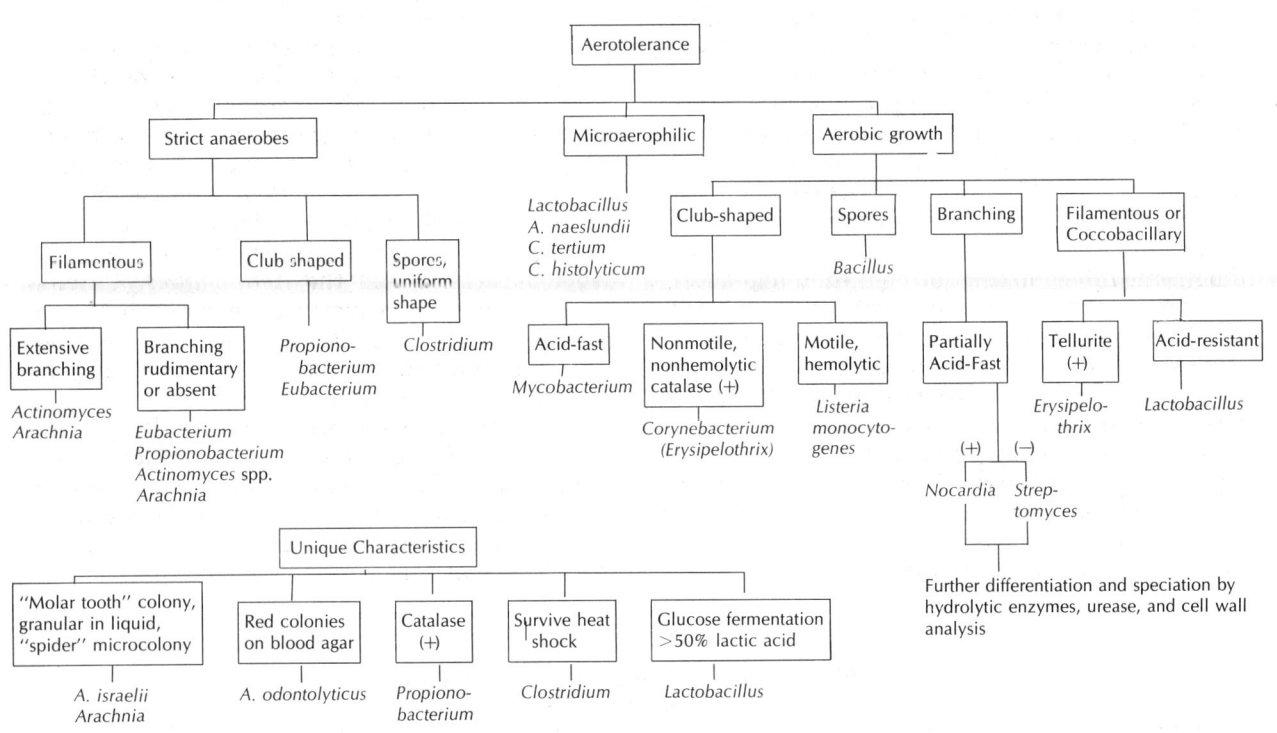

Further differentiation of anaerobic gram-positive bacilli by biochemical reactions and GLC of metabolic products

onomy with a precedent among the Enterobacteriaceae (butylene glycol versus mixed acid fermentation patterns — see Chapter 31) has not greatly disturbed the older, morphologic method of characterizing fusobacteria as the anaerobic gram-negative bacilli with pointed ends. The pleomorphic, spheroplastic bacterium that was best known to microbiologists as *Bacteroides funduliformis* has now been reclassified as *F. necrophorum* because it produces primarily butyric acid from glucose fermentation. The tendency to split *Bacteroides* into multiple species on the basis of minor differences in fermentation patterns and end products of glucose metabolism has resulted in confusion, however. For example, the bile-resistant (or enhanced) *Bacteroides* that were considered to be one species ten years ago *(B. fragilis)* were first divided into five subspecies of *B. fragilis*, and then each subspecies was granted full species status about three years ago. Despite this confusion, the majority of *Bacteroides* that are clearly capable of causing disease can be assigned to a definable species.

Tables 6 and 7 are the most extensive and complicated because there are more recognized species of facultative and aerobic gram-negative ba-

cilli than there are in the other groups. Nevertheless, this approach to identification works well. The fastidious bacteria listed in Table 6 generally produce smaller, more delicate colonies on blood agar than the Enterobacteriaceae, *Pseudomonas,* and vibrios (Table 7). Furthermore, they are inhibited or fail to grow on selective media such as eosin–methylene blue (EMB) or MacConkey agar. Although most of these bacteria cannot be differentiated from one another by gram stain, the group can be distinguished from the hardier members of the Gram-negative bacilli. Determination of the oxidase reaction, catalase production, enhancement by $CO_2$, and nutritional requirements permit the identification of most of these bacteria to the generic level and some of them to the level of species. The nutritionally versatile, hardier bacteria in Table 7 can be divided into two major groups by the oxidase reaction. Enterobacteriaceae are oxidase-negative, glucose-fermenting, nitrate-reducing bacteria that have peritrichous flagella when motile. The *Yersinia* species *(pestis, pseudotuberculosis,* and *enterocolitica)* and certain *Erwinia* species fit this definition and are now classified with the Enterobacteriaceae. The vibrios and *Campy-*

*lobacter* (formerly *V. fetus)* can sometimes be differentiated from the other oxidase-positive, hardy gram-negative bacilli by Gram stain. Otherwise, these nutritionally versatile bacteria are differentiated from one another as indicated in Table 7 by pigment production, oxidation and fermentation patterns, and other biochemical reactions.

## Bacterial Identification and Clinical Relevance

The function of the diagnostic bacteriology laboratory is to provide clinically useful information at a reasonable cost in the shortest length of time (Bartlett, 1974). It is clearly not the function of the laboratory to do sophisticated bacterial identification as an end in itself. For this reason, a question that each laboratory must constantly ask itself is how far to go with the identification of bacterial isolates obtained from clinical specimens. Ideally, each organism could be identified

fully to reflect the current status of bacterial classification, but this is not always feasible. The amount of work and the cost involved could be prohibitive. Furthermore, this approach would generate an enormous amount of clinically irrelevant data. Reporting the identity of all organisms regardless of potential pathogenic significance from a site normally inhabited by indigenous flora will confuse and frustrate most physicians. It is customary in most diagnostic laboratories to establish the identity of all organisms isolated from a specimen of a normally sterile anatomic site, but to identify and report only known pathogens from sites normally inhabited by indigenous flora. This approach is universally accepted for certain specimens (e.g., feces) but remains controversial for other specimens (e.g., throat and lower respiratory tract). This decision becomes especially important for specimens from immunocompromised patients who may be infected with opportunistic members of the normal flora.

**TABLE 5.   Identification of Strictly Anaerobic Gram-Negative Bacteria**
**Second-stage Table**

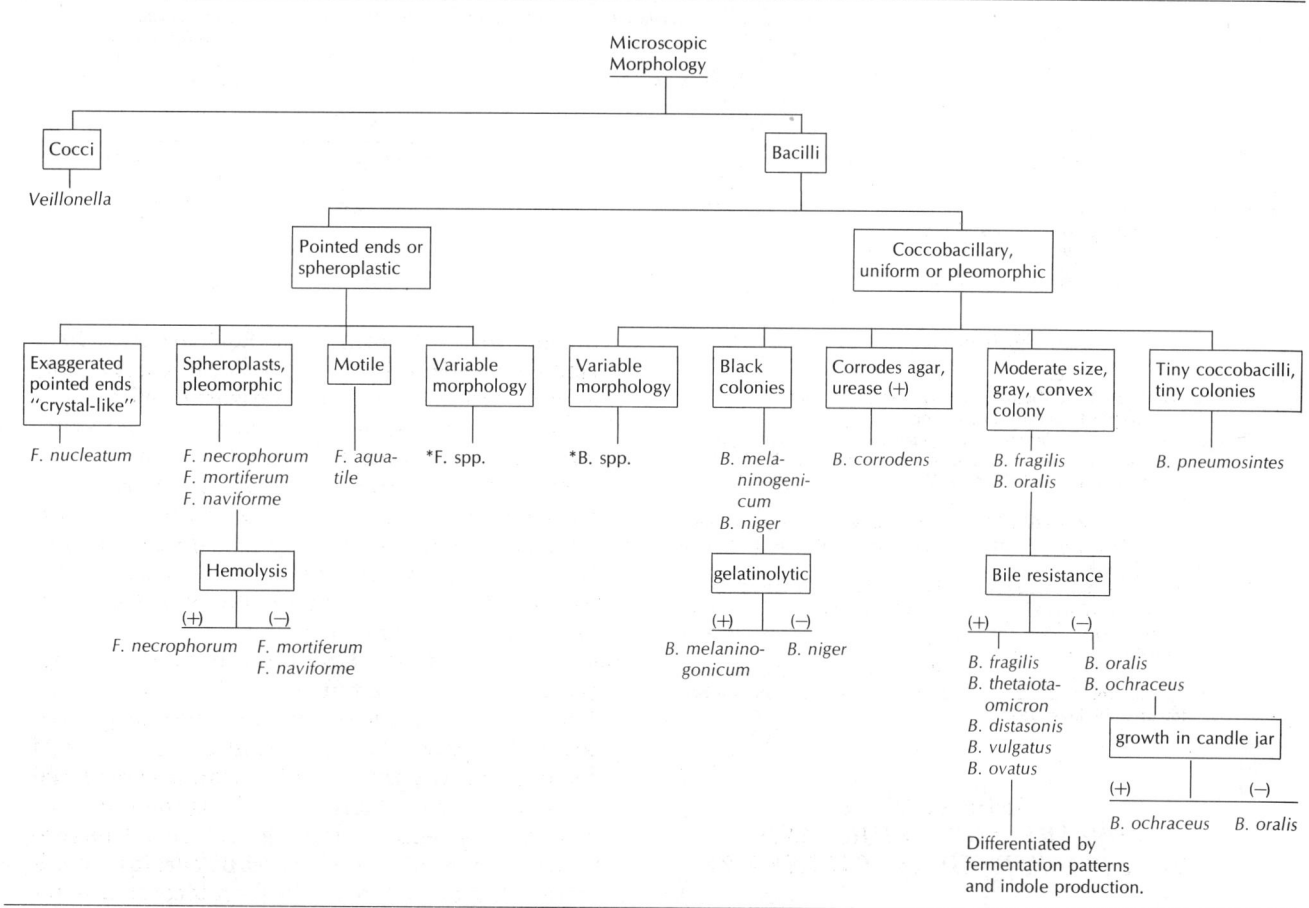

*F. species and B. species are differentiated by biochemical profiles and gas-liquid chromatography of metabolic products of spent cultures. Fusobacteria produce predominantly butyric acid from glucose fermentation. Bacteroides produce a mixed pattern of succinic, acetic, formic, and others.

**TABLE 6.   Identification of Facultative and Aerobic Gram-negative Bacteria
Second-stage Table for Fastidious Genera***

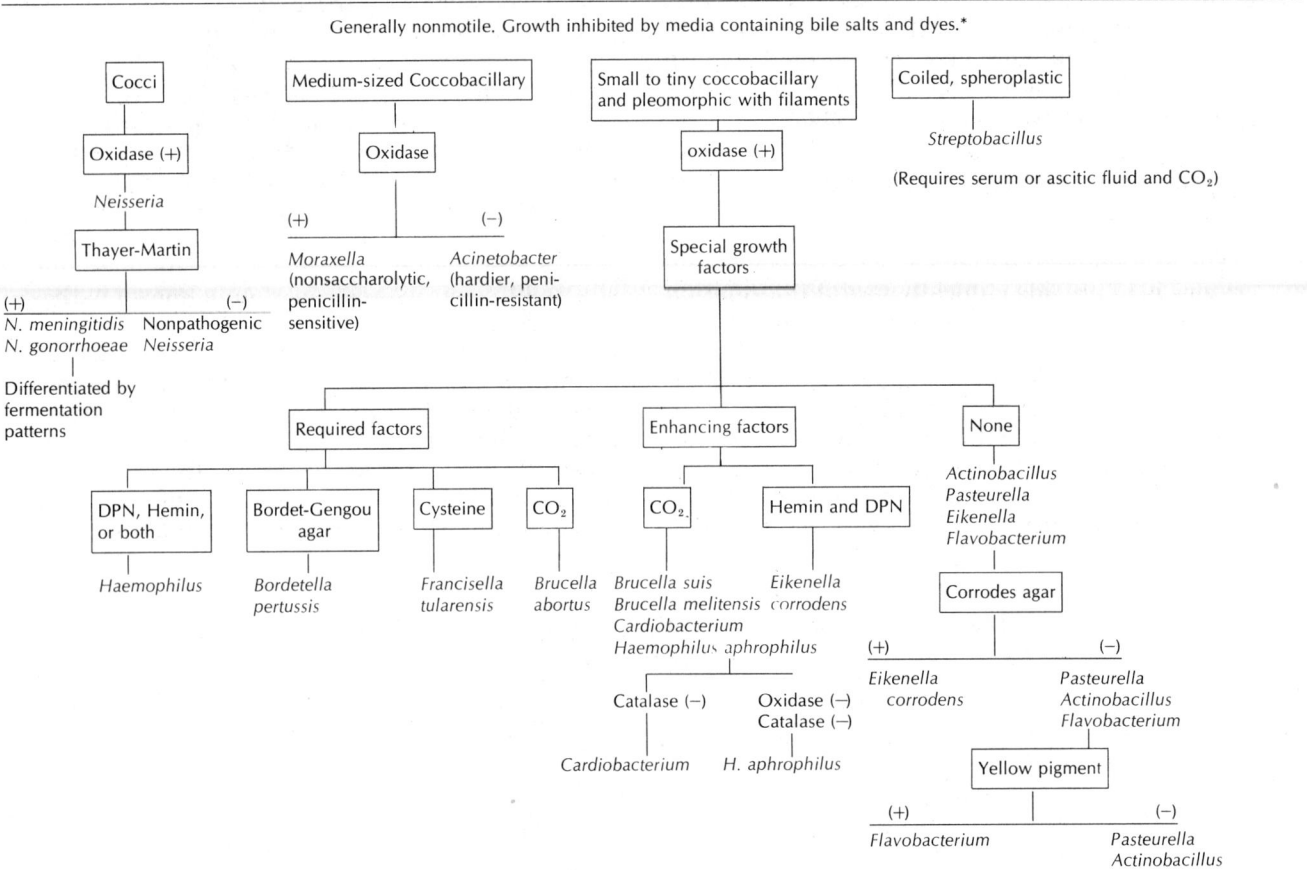

*See Table 7 for nutritionally versatile genera.

## References

Bartlett, R. C.: Medical Microbiology. Quality, Cost and Clinical Relevance. New York, John Wiley & Sons, 1974.

Brenner, D. J., and Falkow, S.: Molecular relationships among members of the enterobacteriaceae. In Caspari, E. W. (ed.): Advances in Genetics, Vol. 16. New York, Academic Press, 1971, pp. 81–118.

Buchanan, R. E., and Gibbons, N. E. (eds.): Bergey's Manual of Determinative Bacteriology. 8th ed. Baltimore, Williams & Wilkins Company, 1974.

Cowan, S. T., and Steel, K. J.: Manual for the Identification of Medical Bacteria. 2nd ed. Cambridge, Cambridge University Press, 1974.

Jones, D., and Sneath, P. H. A.: Genetic transfer and bacterial taxonomy. Bacteriol Rev. 34:40–81, 1970.

Lennette, E. H., Spaulding, E. H., and Truant, J. P. (eds.): Manual of Clinical Microbiology. 2nd ed. Washington, D.C., American Society for Microbiology, 1974.

## *APPENDIX*
## *GLOSSARY FOR TERMS AND*
## *REACTIONS USED IN TABLES 1–7*

*Acid-fast:* The property of mycobacteria to resist decolorization by 3 per cent HCl in 95 per cent alcohol after staining with hot carbol fuchsin (Ziehl-Neelsen stain). *Nocardia,* but not *Actinomyces species,* resist decolorization with 1 per cent $H_2SO_4$ in alcohol or with very brief exposures to 3 per cent HCl after treatment with carbol fuchsin. Since they are decolorized by the conventional Ziehl-Neelsen stain, *Nocardia* are referred to as *partially acid-fast.* "Firmly-bound" lipids, which are not extractable by organic solvents, are responsible for the acid-fastness of mycobacteria.

*Bacitracin sensitivity:* Group A β-hemolytic streptococci are differentiated from other β-hemolytic streptococci by inhibition of growth around a paper disc containing 0.04 units of bacitracin. Any zone of inhibition is considered a positive test. Many green streptococci (α-hemolytic streptococci) are sensitive to this concentration, so hemolysis must be carefully evaluated. Other β-hemolytic streptococci are inhibited only rarely by the bacitracin disc.

*Bile-"positive":* Capable of growth in bile. Group

D streptococci grow on agar containing 40 per cent oxgall bile. *Streptococcus faecalis* and *S. zymogenes* (the penicillin-resistant enterococci) can be differentiated from other group D streptococci (such as *S. bovis)* because the enterococci will also grow in broth containing 6.5 per cent NaCl. Growth of the intestinal *Bacteroides*, especially *B. fragilis,* is enhanced in the presence of 20 per cent oxgall bile. The growth of other *Bacteroides* is inhibited.

*Bile soluble:* The addition of an equal volume of 10 per cent oxgall bile or deoxycholate to turbid broth cultures or saline suspensions of *S. pneumoniae* (the pneumococcus), but not to *S. viridans* or other α-hemolytic streptococci, clears the cultures within 30 minutes because the pneumococci are lysed. Bile and optochin (see further on) activate an autolytic enzyme of pneumococci, L-alanine-muramyl amidase, which acts on the peptidoglycan and actually causes the lysis.

*Bile-esculin:* A medium that differentiates group D streptococci from all other streptococci because only group D grows on bile *and* hydrolyzes esculin. It does not differentiate the enterococci from the other group D streptococci. (See *Bile-"positive"*).

*Bordet-Gengou agar:* An enriched medium containing 20 per cent sheep blood for isolation and identification of *Bordetella pertussis,* the cause of whooping cough. Penicillin (0.25 μg/ml) is usually added to a portion of the media, and the patient's secretions are inoculated onto Bordet-Genjou agar, both with and without penicillin, to inhibit the normal bacterial flora. Plates are frequently inoculated by permitting patients to cough directly onto the medium.

*C carbohydrate* (group-specific C antigens): An antigenic layer of the cell wall of streptococci that lies just outside the peptidoglycan layer. β-hemolytic streptococci may be separated into groups A through O by precipitin reactions of acid extracts of the bacteria against group-specific antisera prepared in rabbits (Lancefield grouping scheme).

*Capnophilic:* Bacteria are called capnophilic when their growth either requires or is enhanced by $CO_2$.

*Catalase:* An enzyme that decomposes hydrogen peroxide to $H_2O$ and free oxygen. In the laboratory, catalase is usually tested for by adding 3 per cent $H_2O_2$ directly to colonies on solid agar or by transferring a colony directly to a drop of 30 per cent $H_2O_2$. Immediate bubbling consti-

**TABLE 7. Identification of Facultative and Aerobic Gram-negative Bacteria**
**Second-stage Table for Nutritionally Versatile Genera***

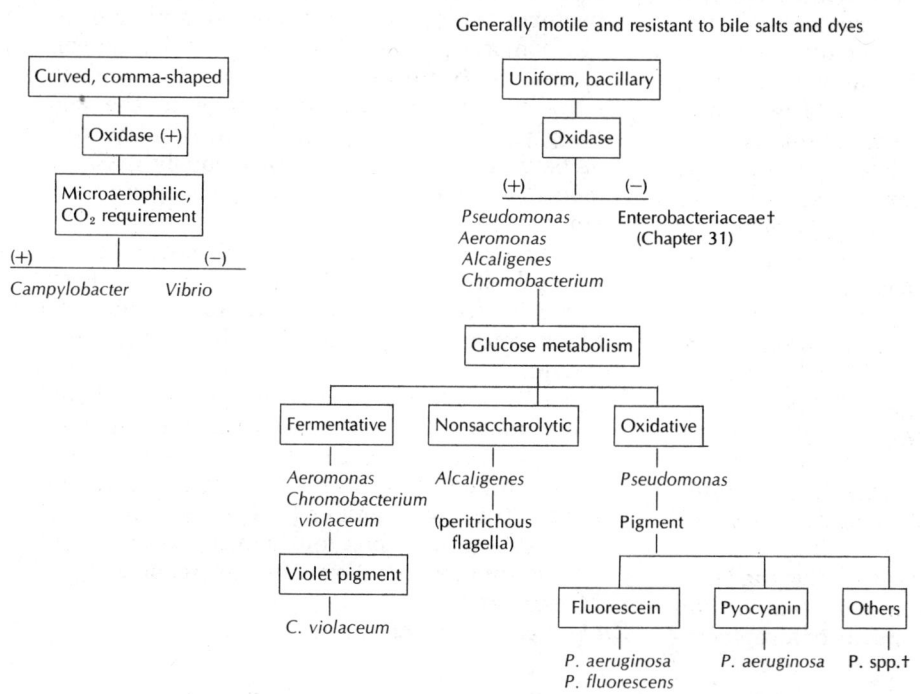

*See Table 6 for fastidious genera.
†Most organisms identified to species by fermentation patterns, oxidation patterns, production of nitrate reductase, urease, and occasionally by characteristic pigment.

tutes a positive test. Catalase should not be tested for on blood agar plates because red blood cells contain catalase.

*Coagulase:* An enzyme synthesized only by *Staphylococcus aureus* that clots plasma by reacting with the coagulase-reacting factor (prothrombin) to activate thrombin. Coagulase-positive staphylococci usually also produce clumping factor ("bound coagulase"), which causes macroscopic agglutination of the staphylococci when they are mixed with plasma on a glass slide.

*Cysteine:* An amino acid derived from cystine that enhances the growth of several bacteria. *Francisella tularensis* will grow only on media supplemented with either cysteine or cystine.

*Facultative* (facultative anaerobe): As used in bacteriology, facultative refers to bacteria that will grow either anerobically or in the presence of atmospheric concentrations of oxygen.

*Fluorescein:* A greenish yellow, water-diffusible pigment produced by *Pseudomonas aeruginosa* and *P. fluorescens.*

*Gelatinolytic:* Property of liquefying boiled gelatin; used in bacteriology as an identifying characteristic of some proteolytic bacteria.

*Gram stain:* Stain devised by Christian Gram in 1884 that divides bacteria into two fundamentally different categories, gram-positive and gram-negative. All bacteria are stained purple by crystal violet, the primary dye of the Gram stain. After treatment with 3 per cent $I_2$-KI, only gram-positive bacteria resist decolorization with alcohol, ether, or acetone. Gram-negative bacteria, which would otherwise be colorless, are stained by treatment with a red counterstain, usually safranin. The gram-positive cell wall acts as a permeability barrier to elution of the crystal violet–iodine complex by the decolorizing agent. Gram-negative walls, which are lipid-rich and glycopeptide-poor, do not prevent access of the decolorizing agents to the interior of the cell.

*Hippurate hydrolysis:* Cultures of group B streptococci, but not other streptococci, break down sodium hippurate to benzoic acid and glycine. A positive test is detected by the addition of ninhydrin, which is reduced by glycine to a purple color. Occasional strains of enterococci will hydrolyze hippurate but are easily differentiated from group B streptococci by other tests (see *Bile sculin).*

*Microaerophilic:* Generally used to designate organisms that grow better anerobically than aerobically, such as many strains of streptococci and lactobacilli. Some bacteria, such as *Campylobacter* (vibrio) *fetus* actually grow better at reduced concentrations of oxygen than they do either in atmospheric concentrations or in the absence of oxygen.

*Optochin:* Ethylhydrocupreine hydrochloride. The growth of *S. pneumoniae,* but not other α-hemolytic streptococci, are inhibited around a paper disc containing a 1:4000 concentration of optochin. The size of the zone of inhibition is larger when the pneumococcus is incubated in an environment without added $CO_2$. Zones of less than 12 to 15 mm should be confirmed by bile solubility (see earlier definition).

*Oxidase test:* When colonies of bacteria containing cytochrome C are flooded with methylphenylenediamine compounds, they turn black within seconds because of the production of a colored compound, indophenol oxide. *Neisseria* and *Pseudomonas species* are examples of oxidase-positive bacteria. Many bacteria with functional electron transport systems contain cytochromes other than cytochrome C and are oxidase-negative in spite of their ability to use oxidative phosphorylation as a major energy source.

*Pyocyanin:* A bluish green, diffusible phenazine pigment produced only by *Pseudomonas aeruginosa.*

*Spheroplasts* (spheroplastic): Bacteria that assume bizarre, swollen shapes because of a lack of integrity of the peptidoglycan. This rigid layer of the cell wall encases the cell contents of bacteria, which are always under higher internal osmotic pressure than body fluids or conventional bacteriologic media. Spheroplasts usually form because of damage to the peptidoglycan by cell wall–active antibiotics such as penicillin, but occur spontaneously in *Streptobacillus moniliformis* and *Fusobacterium necrophorum.*

*Tellurite* (sodium tellurite): Diphtheria bacilli, group D streptococci, *Erysipelothrix,* and a few other bacteria can reduce tellurite and form black colonies in media containing this compound.

*Thayer-Martin media:* Chocolate agar (laked blood agar or blood agar with enrichments) with the antibiotics colistin, vancomycin, and nystatin added to inhibit the normal bacterial flora of the mouth and vagina. Pathogenic *Neisseria* (the gonococcus and meningococcus), but not nonpathogenic *Neisseria,* grow on Thayer-Martin agar.

*Ziehl-Neelsen stain:* See *Acid-fast.*

# BACTERIAL PHYSIOLOGY 3

## T. Ramakrishnan, M.Sc., Ph.D.
## and G. Ramananda Rao, M. Pharm., Ph.D.

The origin of all free energy reaching this planet is the nuclear fusion reactions taking place in the sun. With the exception of chemoautotrophic bacteria, all living organisms draw energy from this source — either directly or indirectly. As in all other living organisms the requirement of energy for microorganisms is fundamental and essential. This need is explained by the fact that several processes involved in the biosynthesis of proteins, nucleic acids, and polysaccharides require the input of energy (endergonic), that is, having a positive change in free energy ($\Delta F'$ value). These thermodynamically unfavorable reactions are made possible under conditions in living organisms by coupling them with energy-yielding, or exergonic, reactions (negative change in $\Delta F'$ value).

The release of energy in exergonic reactions and the manner in which energy is trapped, stored, and utilized for endergonic reactions, are some of the fascinating aspects of bacterial metabolism. The central role of adenosine triphosphate (ATP) in energy exchanges in biologic systems was postulated by Fritz Lipmann and Hermann Kalckar in 1941 (Lipmann, 1941). It consists of three molecular species, adenine, D-ribose, and a triphosphate unit (Fig. 1).

The $\alpha$- and $\beta$-phosphates and the $\beta$- and $\gamma$-phosphates are connected by acid anhydride linkages called energy-rich bonds and are symbolized by a wriggle bond ($\sim$). The electrostatic repulsion between the negatively charged phosphate groups, which results from their close proximity, is reduced when ATP is hydrolyzed. The high potential energy of ATP is due to the fact that adenosine diphosphate (ADP) and $P_i$ enjoy greater resonance stabilization than ATP. The presence of this energy in ATP makes it the most functionally important compound in biologic systems.

In addition to ATP, a variety of other energy-rich compounds occur in biologic systems. They include 1) derivatives of phosphoric acid such as triphosphates of guanosine (GTP), cytidine (CTP), and uridine (UTP); and 2) derivatives of carboxylic acids, which include acyl thioesters such as acetyl coenzyme A. In fact, some of these compounds, such as phosphoenolpyruvate and creatine phosphate, have a higher potential energy than ATP.

ATP is formed by a number of reactions that are all of the general type ADP + X $\sim$ P $\to$ ATP + X, where X $\sim$ P is a high-energy intermediate. ATP is formed by two mechanisms in bacteria — substrate level phosphorylation and oxidative phosphorylation.

### Substrate Level Phosphorylation

In this mechanism the energy required for the conversion of ADP to ATP is supplied by high-energy metabolic intermediates such as phosphoenolpyruvate, succinyl coenzyme A, or creatine phosphate — a compound regarded as a store of high-energy phosphate.

$$\text{Phosphoenolpyruvate} + \text{ADP} \longrightarrow \text{Pyruvate} + \text{ATP}$$

$$\text{Succinyl coenzyme A} + \text{ADP} \xrightarrow{\text{GDP}} \text{Succinate} + \text{ATP} + \text{Coenzyme A}$$

$$\text{Creatine phosphate} + \text{ADP} \longrightarrow \text{Creatine} + \text{ATP}$$

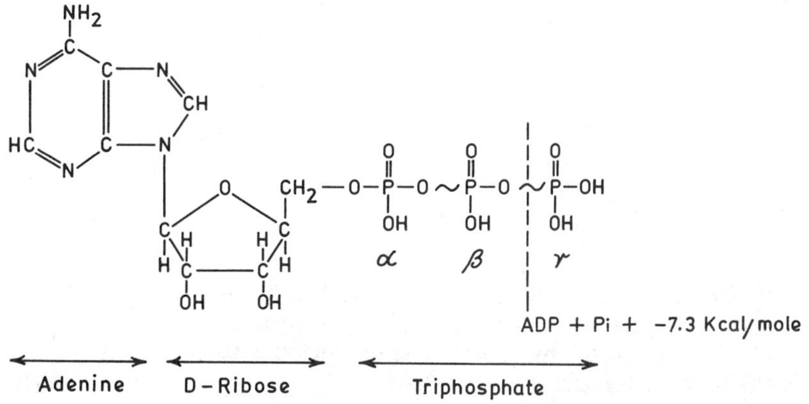

**FIGURE 1.** *Structure of ATP and energy release.*

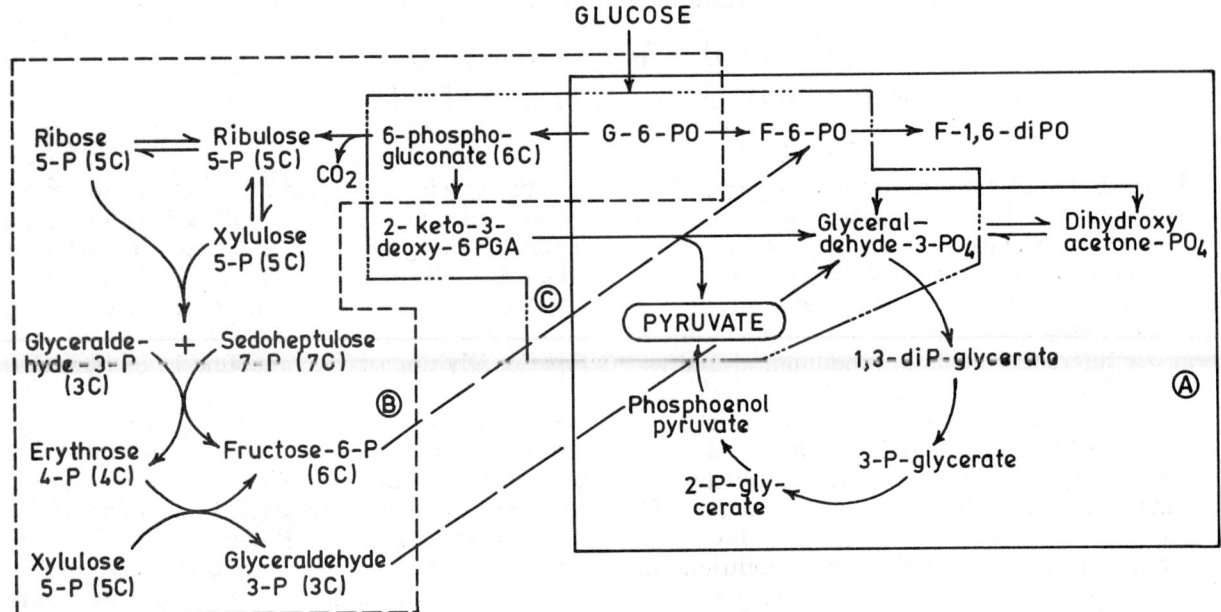

**FIGURE 2.** *Pathways involved in the metabolism of glucose to pyruvate A, Embden Myerhoff pathway (EMP); B, pentose-phosphate pathway; and C, Entner-Doudoroff pathway. In EMP, one molecule of fructose-1,6 diphosphate is split into two three-carbon compounds, glyceraldehyde 3-phosphate. Two molecules of ATP are needed to start the pathway, but four molecules of ATP are formed by the fermentation of glucose to pyruvic acid.*

The energy is released from the high-energy phosphate bonds in the substrate by means of substrate oxidation. This can be illustrated by reactions occurring in the glycolytic cycle (Fig. 2). The oxidation of glyceraldehyde 3-phosphate to 1,3 diphosphoglyceric acid by nicotinamide-adenine dinucleotide (NAD) produces a high-energy phosphate bond through the carboxy-linkage (as indicated by $\downarrow$) in the following manner:

$$\begin{array}{ccc}
\begin{array}{l} HC{=}O \\ | \\ HC{-}OH + P_i \\ | \\ CH_2OPO_3{=} \end{array} & \xrightarrow[\text{NAD} \qquad \text{NADH}]{} & \begin{array}{l} \overset{O}{\underset{||}{C}}{-}O\overset{\downarrow}{-}PO_3{=} \\ | \\ HC{-}OH \\ | \\ CH_2OPO_3{=} \end{array}
\end{array}$$

Glyceraldehyde-3-phosphate                  1,3-Diphosphoglyceric acid

This high-energy phosphate bond is then transferred to ADP to form a molecule of ATP, as follows:

$$\begin{array}{ccc}
\begin{array}{l} \overset{O}{\underset{||}{C}}{-}O{-}PO_3{=} \\ | \\ HCOH \\ | \\ CH_2OPO_3{=} \end{array} & \xrightarrow[\text{ADP} \qquad \text{ATP}]{} & \begin{array}{l} \overset{O}{\underset{||}{C}}{-}OH \\ | \\ HCOH \\ | \\ CH_2OPO_3{=} \end{array}
\end{array}$$

It should be noted that formation of the high-energy phosphate bond in 1,3-diphosphoglyceric acid is accompanied by the release of electrons to NAD to form NADH (reduced NAD).

**Oxidative Phosphorylation**

This phosphorylation is associated with electron transport. It is a coupled process wherein reduced substrates are oxidized with concomitant phosphorylation of ADP to ATP. During this process hydrogen atoms or electrons pass through oxidation-reduction reactions mediated by closely linked respiratory enzymes, especially flavoproteins and cytochromes, until the electrons reach a final acceptor, usually oxygen (see section on Aerobic Respiration). The energy present in reduced coenzymes is not released all at once but in a stepwise manner. This liberated energy is trapped in an unidentified form, X ~ P, which in turn, is utilized in the phosphorylation of ADP to ATP.

## How Do Bacteria Derive Energy?

Bacteria are classified into autotrophs and heterotrophs, depending on the mode in which they derive energy. Autotrophs (Greek *autos* = self, *trophe* = nutrition) such as *Nitrosomonas, Nitrobacter,* and *Thiobacillus* obtain energy by oxidizing $NH^+_4$, $HNO_2$, and S, respectively, and by utilizing molecular oxygen to do so (see section on Autotrophic Nutrition). In heterotrophs (Greek *heteros* = another), preformed organic compounds

such as polysaccharides, fats, and proteins are oxidized either aerobically (respiration) or anaerobically (fermentation), with release of energy. In respiration, molecular oxygen serves as the ultimate hydrogen acceptor, whereas in fermentation (which was defined by Pasteur as life without air) organic compounds serve as both electron donors and acceptors.

The brilliant contributions of Embden, Meyerhof, and Parnas led to the elucidation of the major pathway used by bacteria for the fermentation of glucose (Meyerhof, 1942). This pathway is termed the Embden-Meyerhof-Parnas (EMP) pathway, or glycolysis, and describes the conversion of glucose to pyruvic acid (Fig. 2A). This series of reactions also occurs in mammalian cells. Pyruvic acid is further metabolized to alcohol in yeast and to lactic acid in muscle. In the vast majority of bacteria, glucose is metabolized through the EMP pathway to pyruvate (Fig. 2A).

In obligate aerobic bacteria, which do not possess the EMP pathway, glucose is metabolized to pyruvate through the pentose phosphate pathway (hexose monophosphate shunt) (Fig. 2B). The

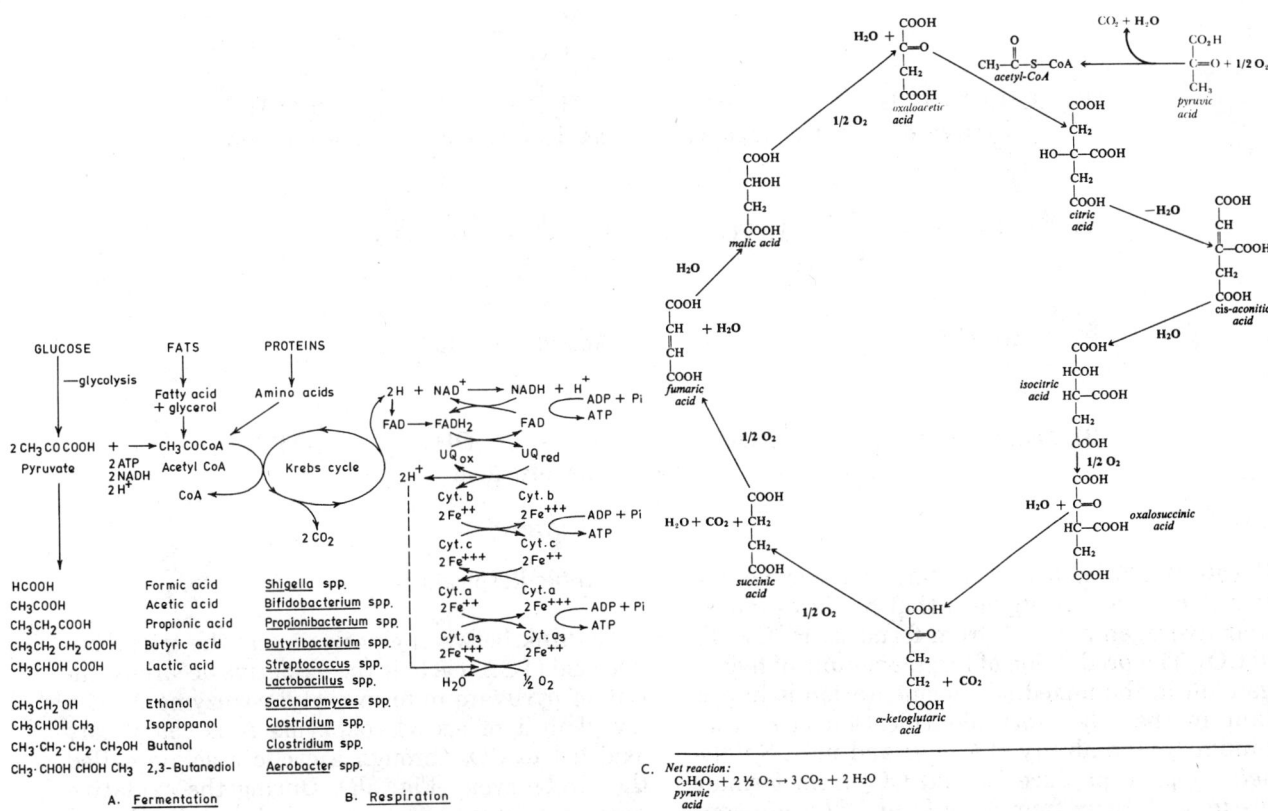

**FIGURE 3.** *A, Key role of pyruvate in the formation of fermentatation products and B, its oxidation through respiration, yielding ATP.*

reaction sequence of this pathway provides the ribose and erythrose-4-phosphate essential for the biosynthesis of nucleic acids and aromatic amino acids, respectively (Horecker, 1962). Another intermediate of this pathway — namely, ribulose-5-phosphate — is converted to ribulose-1,5-diP, the acceptor of $CO_2$ in autotrophic fixation of $CO_2$. The net yield of ATP is half that characteristic of the EMP pathway.

A facultative aerobic organism such as *Escherichia coli* has the ability to degrade glucose by either the EMP pathway or the pentose phosphate pathway. Whereas the EMP pathway gives more energy, the pentose phosphate pathway provides more reducing power in the form of NADPH (reduced nicotinamide adenine dinucleotide phosphate). However, a balance between these two pathways is controlled by phosphofructokinase, which phosphorylates fructose-6-P to fructose-1,6-diP. When the intracellular level of ATP increases, phosphofructokinase is strongly inhibited. As a result, phosphorylation of fructose-6-P is restricted, and the carbon flows via the pentose phosphate pathway. Increased levels of ATP similarly inhibit carbon flow through the EMP pathway under aerobic conditions and is termed the *Pasteur effect.*

In many species of aerobic bacteria glucose is metabolized by the Entner-Duodoroff pathway (Fig. 2C). In this pathway, 6-phosphogluconate of the pentose phosphate pathway is converted to 2-keto-3-deoxy-6-phosphogluconate (instead of ribulose 5-P as in the pentose phosphate pathway). The enzyme aldolase cleaves this into pyruvate and glyceraldehyde-3-P, intermediates in glycolysis. The latter is metabolized via the EMP pathway.

Pyruvate occupies a key position in carbohydrate fermentation. As a result of the conversion of glucose to pyruvate, NAD is reduced. Additional fermentations yield different products from pyruvate (Fig. 3A) and cause reoxidation of NADH, so that the oxidation-reduction balance of the cell is restored. In medical microbiology, one of the more important fermentations of pyruvate is the mixed acid fermentation by Enterobacteriaceae, such as *Escherichia coli* and *Shigella* spp. The reaction produces formic, lactic, and succinic acids, as well as a number of other products. The production of formate and acetate involves decarboxylation of pyruvate by the following series of reactions:

(1)   $CH_3COCO_2H$   +   CoASH   →   $H_3\overset{O}{\overset{\|}{C}}$ SCOA   +   $HCO_2H$
      Pyruvate     Coenzyme A   Acetyl Coenzyme A   Formic acid

(2)   $H_3CO$ SCOA   +   $H_3PO_4$   →   $CH_3-\overset{O}{\overset{\|}{C}}-O-\overset{O}{\overset{\|}{\underset{\underset{OH}{|}}{P}}}-OH$

     Acetyl COA             Acetyl Phosphate

(3) Acetyl-phosphate +   ADP   →   $CH_3-\overset{O}{\overset{\|}{C}}-OH$   +   ATP
                        Acetic acid

*E. coli* and *Salmonella spp.* have an enzyme system (formic hydrogenylase) that produces molecular hydrogen and $CO_2$ from formate: $HCO_2 \rightarrow H_2 + CO_2$. The production of large amounts of hydrogen ion in the mixed acid fermentation is important in the laboratory identification of *E. coli*. Similarly, the ability of *E. coli* and most *Salmonella* spp. to produce $H_2$ and $CO_2$ from formate distinguish them from *S. typhi* and *Shigella* spp., which cannot break down formate to these gases.

### Aerobic Respiration

The link between glycolysis and the tricarboxylic acid (TCA) cycle is the oxidative decarboxylation of pyruvate to form acetyl coenzyme A. The acetyl unit of acetyl coenzyme A is completely oxidized to $CO_2$ through a cyclic reaction called the Krebs cycle (Fig. 3B). During the oxidative process electrons flow from reduced NAD and FAD (Flavin adenine dinucleotide) to molecular oxygen through a chain of electron carriers with coupled synthesis of ATP at two or three sites, depending upon the substrate oxidized.

Glucose oxidation results in the production of 38 moles of ATP. These are derived from the net production of 2 ATP moles during the conversion of 1 mole of glucose to 2 moles of pyruvate and 36 moles of ATP during the conversion of 2 moles of pyruvate to 6 moles each of $CO_2$ and $H_2O$. The free energy change of glucose oxidation is 686,000 cal./mole. If 7000 calories are required in the synthesis of 1 mole of ATP, the efficiency of energy trapped is $\frac{7000 \times 38}{686,000} \times 100 = 39$ per cent. Since free energy of ATP synthesis may approach 12,000 cal./mole, depending on the concentrations of ADP, ATP, and phosphate at the actual site on the enzyme catalyzing the reactions, the efficiency could be as high as 60 per cent.

## The Glyoxylate Cycle

In addition to its role in terminal respiration, the TCA cycle is also important in providing the compounds required for biosyntheses. One of these is $\alpha$-oxoglutarate, which is the precursor of glutamic acid, a key compound in protein synthesis. During biosynthesis $\alpha$-oxoglutarate and other important intermediates, such as 4-carbon dicarboxylic acids, are continually removed from the TCA cycle and must be resynthesized from acetate. For this resynthesis of TCA intermediates, bacteria use a modified TCA cycle in which the reaction sequence between isocitric acid and malic acid (Fig. 3C) is changed through the glyoxalate bypass, which short-circuits the reactions that lead to the evolution of carbon dioxide. The bypass excludes the following reactions:

$$\text{Isocitrate} \rightarrow \alpha\text{-oxoglutarate} \rightarrow \text{succinate} + CO_2$$

This bypass consists of two enzymatic reactions:

1) $\text{Isocitrate} \xleftrightarrow{\text{isocitrate lyase}} \text{succinate} + \text{glyoxylate}$

2) $\text{Acetyl COA} + \text{glyoxalate} \xrightarrow{\text{malate synthase}} \text{malate} + \text{COA-SH}$

Thus, acetate is not used as a source of energy, but rather as a precursor of malic COOH and other 4-carbon dicarboxylic acids.

$$\begin{array}{l} CH_2 \\ CHOH \\ | \\ COOH \end{array}$$

### BIOSYNTHESIS

Microorganisms offer several advantages for biosynthetic studies, including rapid growth, the ability to synthesize all cell components, and the homogeneity of the cell population. Beadle and Tatum (1941) isolated mutants having a block in a metabolic pathway resulting from a lack of or defective activity of key enzymes. Such mutants (auxotrophic mutants) require for their growth the product of the blocked reaction, which the wild-type strain (prototroph) can synthesize de novo. The discovery that auxotrophic mutants accumulate previously undetectable compounds that were intermediates in the biosynthetic pathways for the formation of various macromolecules led to the elucidation of many of these pathways. These macromolecules that bacteria synthesize are classified as 1) repeating units (capsules and cell walls), 2) information molecules such as deoxyribonucleic acid (DNA) and ribonucleic acid (RNA), 3) proteins, and 4) structurally and functionally important lipids and polysaccharides.

### Repeating Polymers

The synthesis of peptidoglycan and lipopolysaccharide are similar in that the structural subunits of each are assembled on a lipid carrier in the cell membrane and are then transferred to growing ends of the polymer in the cell wall. The structural units, biosynthetic precursors, and polymerization sites of these polymers, as well as the capsular polysaccharides, are shown in Table 1. The biosynthesis of the lipopolysaccharide is discussed in Chapter 6.

The peptidoglycan is the most important of these polymers because it is an indispensable structural component of all bacteria. It is necessary for the structural integrity of the cell wall, it provides the characteristic shape of the bacterial cell, and it acts as a rigid corset that prevents the rupture of the cell. The internal osmotic pressure reaches 5 to 20 atmospheres in most bacteria as a result of active transport of solutes and would cause the cell to burst in water and other hypotonic environments if it were not for the strength

**TABLE 1. Capsular and Cell Wall Polysaccharides in Bacteria**

| 1 POLYSACCHARIDES | 2 REPEATING UNIT | 3 LINKAGE | 4 PRECURSORS | 5 SITE OF POLYMERIZATION | 6 ORGANISMS |
|---|---|---|---|---|---|
| *Capsular* | | | | | |
| Dextran | Glucose | $\alpha$-1,6 | Sugar-NDP (nucleoside diphosphates such as ADP, UDP, GDP, CDP) | Outer surface of the cell Syntheisized within the cell but excreted outside | *Leuconostoc* |
| Levan | Fructose | a-1,6 | | | *Acetobacter xylinum* |
| Cellulose | Glucose | $\beta$-1,4 | | | |
| Glycogen | Glucose | $\alpha$-1,4 | | | *Clostridium* spp. |
| Poly-L-glutamic acid | Glutamic acid | $\gamma$-peptide bond | Glutamate, ATP | Cytoplasm | *Bacillus anthracis* |
| Pneumococcus type III polysaccharide | Glucuronic acid, glucose | $\beta$-1,4 | UDP-glucuronic acid, UDP-glucose | | *Streptococcus pneumoniae* |
| *Cell wall* | | | | | |
| Glycopeptide | GlcNAc-MurNAc-pentapeptide | $\beta$-1,4 (between sugars). Tetrapeptide side chain is attached to the -COOH of the lactic group of MurNAc | UDP-MurNAc UDP-GlcNAc Glycyl tRNA | Cell membrane murein sub-unit is added to the growing chains in the cell wall through the participation of bactoprenol-P-P | Gram-positive bacteria such as *Staphylococcus aureus*, *Micrococcus lysodeikticus* (high content) |
| Lipopolysaccharide | *Core:* (KDO-heptose)-glu-gal-glu-GlcNAc *Specific side chains:* (-rha-man-gal-)$_n$ abequose | Side chain sugars are attached with their reducing groups toward the core $(1 \to 4, 1 \to 6$ and so forth) | *Core:* UDP-(glu-gal-GlcNAc) *Side chain:* GDP-(gal-man)-TDP-rha | Repeating side chain subunits are constructed by attachment to bactoprenol on membrane and then transferred to the "open" end of the growing polymer of the wall | Gram-negative true bacteria. Best studied in *Salmonella* spp. |
| Cell wall teichoic acids | Glycerol or ribitol substituted at OH groups with sugars or amino acids | Phosphodiester | Glycerol or ribitol, D-alanine, glucose succinate, oligo-saccharides | Covalently linked to peptido-glycan at C6-hydroxyl of N-acetylmuramic acid | Gram-positive bacteria such as staphylococci, strepto-cocci, *Lactobacillus*, and *Bacillus* |
| Lipoteichoic acids | Glycerol substituents | Phosphodiester | Fatty acid substituted glycerophosphate, & glycerol teichoic acid | Membrane | All gram-positive bacteria |

of the peptidoglycan. As the name implies, the peptidoglycan is composed of sugar and peptides.

The basic unit of the sugar is a disaccharide containing N-acetylglucosamine and muramic acid:

N-acetylglucosamine      N-acetylmuramic acid

$CH_2OH$      $CH_2OH$

$CH_3$

Muramic acid is a derivative of N-acetylglucosamine, to which lactic acid is incorporated at the 3-position. The two sugars in the disaccharide are linked at the $\beta$-1,4-position. The peptide is attached at the arrow through an amide linkage between L-alanine and the carboxyl group of muramic acid. The peptidoglycan is thus made up of polysaccharide chains linked together by peptides. The polysaccharide chains are composed of repeating units of the muramic acid N-acetylglucosamine disaccharide. In *E. coli* the cross-linking peptide strands consist of L-alanine, D-glutamic acid, $\alpha$-$\epsilon$ = diaminopimelic acid (DAP), and finally D-alanine to form a tetrapeptide (Fig. 4). The free carboxyl groups in the D-alanine residues are also attached to the NH$_2$ group of the diaminopimelic acid in adjacent tetrapeptides to produce a cross-linked structure (Fig. 4). In staph-

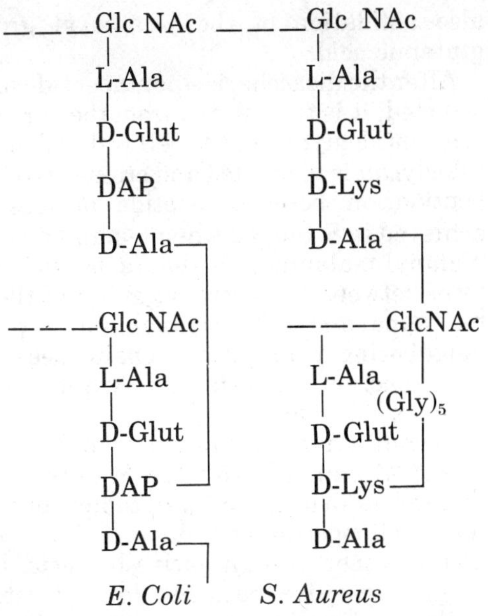

```
____Glc NAc  ____ ____Glc NAc
     |                 |
   L-Ala             L-Ala
     |                 |
   D-Glut            D-Glut
     |                 |
    DAP              D-Lys
     |                 |
   D-Ala┐            D-Ala┐
                          
____Glc NAc        ____ ____GlcNAc
     |                 |
   L-Ala             L-Ala
     |                 |  (Gly)₅
   D-Glut            D-Glut
     |                 |
    DAP ┘            D-Lys┘
     |                 |
   D-Ala┘            D-Ala

   E. Coli           S. Aureus
```

**FIGURE 4.** *Comparison of peptidoglycans in* S. aureus *and* E. coli. *Both bacteria contain linear sugar polymers (GlcNac + MurNAc) attached to pentapeptides through an amide linkage between N-acetylmuramic acid and* L-*alanine. In* E. coli *these sugar peptides are cross-linked by a peptide bond between the terminal* D-*alanine and diaminopimelic acid. In staphylococci, the cross-linkage between strands is achieved through a pentaglycine bridge that connects the terminal* D-*alanine of one peptide to the preterminal* L-*lysine of the neighboring peptide.*

ylococci a second chain composed of five glycine molecules — (Gly) 5 — is used to connect neighboring peptides.

Synthesis of the peptidoglycan begins in the cytoplasm with formation of $N$-acetyl glucosamine-6-phosphate (Glc Nac-6-P) from fructose-6-phosphate, glutamine, and acetyl COA.

Glc Nac-6-P is attached to a nucleoside diphosphate (as generally occurs when sugars are polymerized) to form uridine diphospho-$N$-acetylglucosamine (UDP Glc Nac). UDP-$N$-acetyl muramic acid (UDP-Mur Nac) is then produced by the following reaction involving phosphoenolpyruvate and 2H:

$$UDP \text{ Glc Nac} + CH_2 = C\text{-}CO_2H \xrightarrow{2(H)} UDP\text{-}Mur \text{ Nac}$$

phosphoenolpyruvate

The cross-linking pentapeptide is then attached, first by addition of L-alanine to the lactyl carboxyl group of UDP-Mur Nac, followed by serial addition of the remaining four amino acids. The formation of each peptide bond requires ATP and a specific enzyme.

The second step in peptidoglycan synthesis is the transfer of UDP Glc Nac and the muramyl pentapeptide to the carrier lipid, bactoprenol — a

$C_{55}$ polyisoprenoid alcohol with the formula $H_2O_3P - O (CH_2 = CH\text{-}CH_2)_{11} H$. This carrier lipid is the site of disaccharide formation, which results from the addition of acetylglucosamine (from UDP Glc Nac) to the $C_4$ hydroxyl group of muramic acid. At this stage the $\beta$-1,4-linked disaccharide forms the following complex with the pentapeptide and carrier lipid:

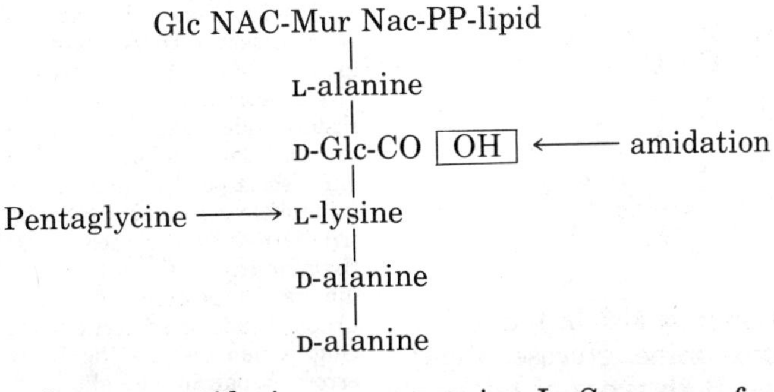

```
Glc NAC-Mur Nac-PP-lipid
            |
       L-alanine
            |
      D-Glc-CO OH  ←——— amidation
            |
Pentaglycine ——→ L-lysine
            |
       D-alanine
            |
       D-alanine
```

Note that the muramyl pentapeptide is connected to the lipid by a pyrophosphate bridge (PP). Further changes occur, depending on the

species. In *S. aureus,* for example, the pentaglycine bridge is attached to L-lysine by sequential addition of glycine from glycyl-tRNA. There is also amidation of the γ-carboxyl group of D-glutamic acid.

After the disaccharide-pentapeptide unit is constructed, it is transferred from the carrier lipid to the peptidoglycan in the cell wall, where the peptidoglycan is elongated and cross-linked by transpeptidation between peptide bridges. This is achieved in *S. aureus* when D-alanine is split from D-alanyl-D-alanine, so that a peptide bond can form between the carboxyl group of the residual D-alanine and the terminal amino group of a neighboring pentaglycine chain (see Figure 4). This reaction completes the synthesis of the cell wall peptidoglycan.

In addition to the differences in structure of the peptidoglycan of *E. coli* and *S. aureus,* there are differences in other cell wall components. Characteristic lipopolysaccharides are found in *E. coli* and all other gram-negative bacteria, but never in gram-positive bacteria. In contrast, teichoic acids are found only in gram-positive bacteria. Teichoic acids are cell wall polymers composed of long chains of either glycerol or ribitol. These chains are linked (to each other) by phosphodiester bonds and contain substitutions of both amino acids and monosaccharides. In some bacteria they are connected to the cell wall through muramic acid-6-phosphate. Glycerol teichoic acids have the general formula

The R group is often D-alanine. The formula for ribitol teichoic acid is generally

The R group substitution may also be D-alanine but is often *N*-acetylglucosamine, glucose, oligosaccharides, or succinate. Both types of teichoic acid are bound to the peptidoglycan and may be important surface antigens in streptococci, staphylococci, and other gram-positive bacteria. In ad-

dition, glycerol teichoic acid is bound to a glycolipid in the cytoplasmic membrane of all gram-positive bacteria and is known as lipoteichoic acid. In spite of their widespread occurrence, the physiologic role of lipoteichoic acids are not well understood. They may participate in the synthesis of peptidoglycan-associated teichoic acids, in binding $Mg^{++}$ ions at the cell surface, and in regulating cell division. In the pneumococci, the lipoteichoic acid, which contains choline, inhibits autolysis of the cell wall and prevents pneumococcal cells from separating, so that they form chains. This is brought about by inhibition of the autolytic enzyme mucopeptide amidohydrolase (Höltje and Tomasz, 1975).

### Information Molecules

DNA, RNA, and proteins are polymers composed of subunits (monomers). The subunits are linked to one another in a linear sequence by a phosphodiester bond (DNA and RNA) or a peptide bond (protein). The biosynthetic relationship between these macromolecules is shown in Figure 5. Three types of reactions are involved in the genetic flow from DNA→RNA→protein: replication, transcription, and translation.

In replication, free deoxyribonucleotides are assembled linearly to form an identical replica of the original DNA structure for hereditary transmission. The basis for the exact replication of a DNA strand is the base complementarity between adenine and thymine and between guanine and cytosine as proposed by the Watson and Crick model. DNA polymerase in extracts of *E. coli* has been found to catalyze the sequential addition of deoxyribonucleotides to the free 3'-OH ends using the opposite intact strand as template (Fig. 6*A*). There are three different DNA polymerases in *E. coli,* designated I, II, and III.*

DNA-dependent RNA polymerase brings about polymerization of ribonucleotide triphosphates to form a polynucleotide strand having complemen-

---

*The function of different polymerases is not clear, except with respect to DNA repair (repair of the patch) by polymerases and ligase. Polymerases II and III can repair more extensive genetic damage than polymerase I. Polymerases II and III restore wide areas of DNA injury (1000 to 3000 nucleotides), a process known as "long patch" repair. Polymerase I carries out only "short patch" repair limited to 10 to 30 nucleotides of an injured DNA molecule. Such injury can occur from ultraviolet irradiation that causes pyrimidine dimer formation (e.g., thymine-thymine, thymine-cytosine, or cytosine-cytosine dimers). These dimers form through the linkage of 5, 6 unsaturated bonds of adjacent pyrimidines to form a cyclobutane ring, which distorts the DNA helix and causes replication errors. Repair in the light involves separation of the dimers by photoligase in the presence of light (photoreactivation). Repair in the dark is more complex and requires excision of the dimer by endonucleases and re-establishment of the continuity of the DNA molecule.

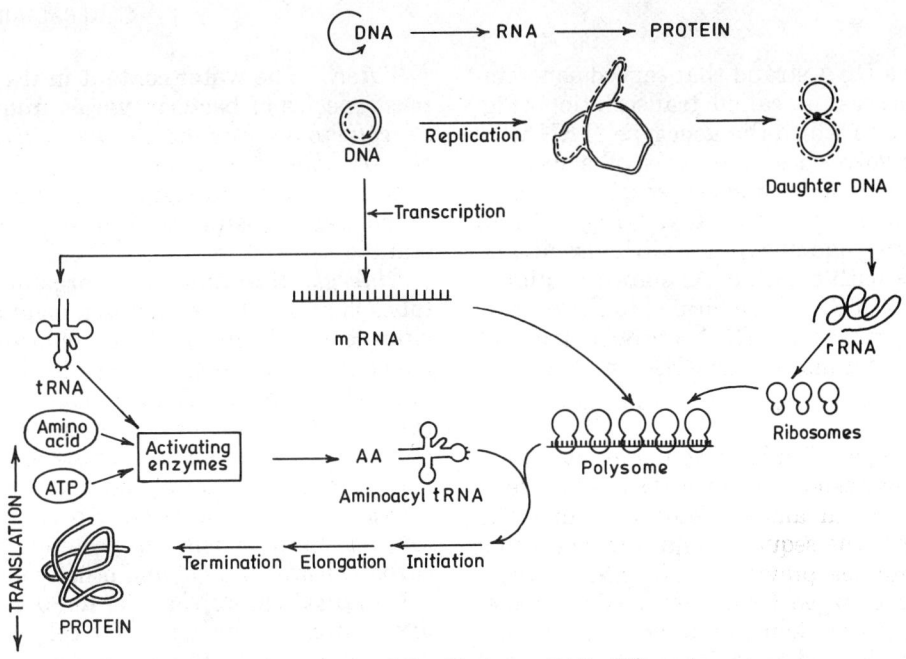

**FIGURE 5.** *Biosynthetic relationship among DNA, RNA, and proteins.*

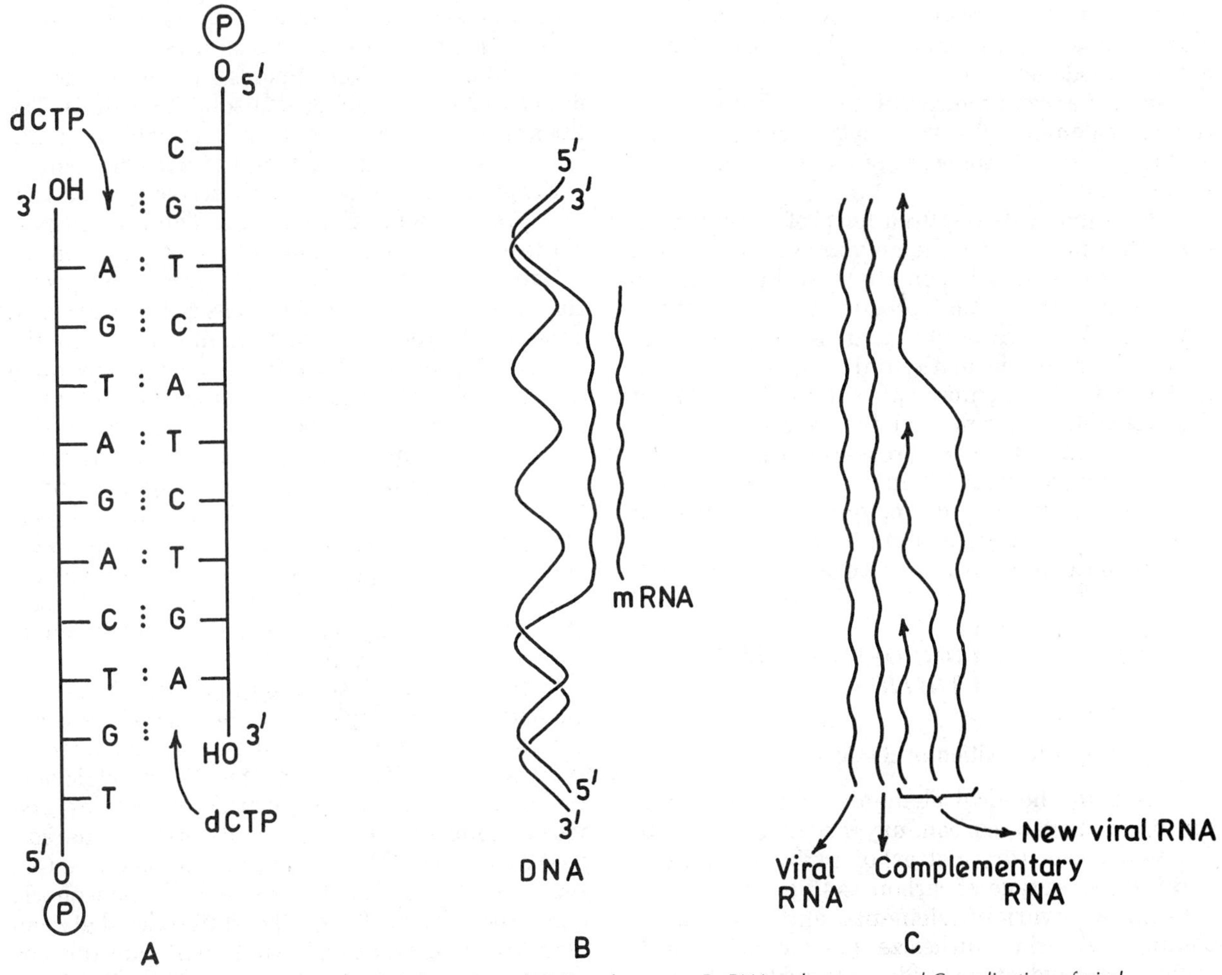

**FIGURE 6.** *Diagram showing A, the action of DNA polymerase, B, RNA polymerase, and C, replication of viral RNA.*

tarity with the DNA strand that served as a template. This process is called transcription (Fig. 6B). In viruses in which the genotype is RNA, its replication involves the synthesis of a complementary strand, which then serves as a template for production of new viral RNA (Fig. 6C). In RNA synthesis, adenine pairs with uracil and guanine pairs with cytosine. As shown in Figure 5, three classes of RNAs are formed in the cells by transcription: ribosomal RNA (rRNA), transfer RNA (tRNA), and messenger RNA (mRNA).

### Proteins

The phenotype of microorganisms is determined and manifested both directly and indirectly by its structural and enzymic proteins. The mRNA specifies the sequence of amino acids in a protein. Ribosomes provide nonspecific surfaces on which the charged (aminoacyl) tRNA molecules bind, transfer their amino acids to the nascent polypeptide, and are released as uncharged tRNAs (Fig. 5). The sequence of three nucleotide bases (triplet code) in mRNA specifies which amino acid is to be added onto the growing chain. Since there are 64 possible codons from A, U, G, and C, some of the 20 amino acids are specified by multiple codons.

The sequence of molecular events that occur in the lengthening of a polypeptide chain on the surface of 70S ribosome are summarized in Chapter 20.

The amino acids required for protein synthesis are either provided in the medium or synthesized from precursors. All open chain amino acids are synthesized from four precursors: oxalacetate, pyruvate, $\alpha$-oxoglutarate, and 3-phosphoglycerate. Among the aromatic amino acids, histidine is derived from pentose, phosphate, and others (for example, tyrosine and tryptophane) from a condensation of D-erythrose-4-phosphate and phosphoenolpyruvate. When amino acids are present in the growth medium, precursor synthesis is prevented through end-product inhibition (see section on Regulation of Growth at end of chapter).

## CHEMICAL COMPOSITION AND NUTRITION

### Chemical Composition of Bacteria

The main chemical elements in the bacterial cell are nitrogen, carbon, oxygen, and hydrogen. The percentage (dry matter) of nitrogen is 8 to 15 and the percentage of carbon is 45 to 55.

From the various elements and their compounds, bacteria synthesize nucleic acids, proteins, carbohydrates, lipids, glycoproteins, lipoproteins, nucleoproteins, enzymes, and vitamins.

*Water.* The water content in the cytoplasm of most species of bacteria varies from 75 per cent (*E. coli*) to 85 per cent (*Corynebacterium diphtheria, Mycobacterium tuberculosis, Vibrio cholerae*). Water is the main component of the cell and is found free or bound with other component substances.

*Mineral Substances.* Inorganic substances (phosphorus, sulphur, sodium, magnesium, potassium, calcium, iron, silicon, chlorine) and trace elements (molybdenum, cobalt, boron, manganese, zinc, copper) are also found in the bacterial cell. The total amount of mineral substances in bacteria grown on standard nutrient media varies from 2 to 14 per cent of the microbial mass.

*Dry Matter.* The organic part of the dry matter of bacteria consists of proteins, nucleic acids, carbohydrates, lipids, and other compounds.

*Proteins.* More than 50 to 80 per cent of the dry matter of the bacterial cell is made up of proteins found in the cytoplasm, nucleoid, cytoplasmic membrane, and other cell structures (Fig. 7).

In nucleoproteins, the prosthetic group is made up of nucleic acids. Similarly, in lipoproteins the prosthetic group is made up of either fats (lipids) or fat-like substances (lipoids). Lipoproteins are found within the cell as semisolid inclusions. The lipoproteins of the cytoplasmic membrane regulate the substances entering the bacterial cell.

Enzymes are proteins with active groups that catalyze biochemical reactions. The protein part of the enzyme is known as the apoenzyme and the active (prosthetic) group catalyzes the specific chemical reaction. In some cases the active, or prosthetic, groups are not bound firmly to the protein (apoenzyme) and are easily separated from it, whereas others can bind themselves to different proteins. These freely existing nonprotein catalysts involved in biochemical transformations are known as coenzymes. Another group of enzymes contain hemin compounds as the active group. Enzymes concerned with oxidation belong to this group. Enzymes act as oxidoreductases, transferases, hydrolases, lyases, isomerases, and ligases. Their functions in bacteria are summarized in Table 2.

*Nucleic Acids.* The amount of nucleic acids in the bacterial cell depends on the bacterial species and the nutrient medium, and it varies within 10 to 30 per cent of the dry matter. Ribonucleic acid (RNA) takes part in the synthesis of proteins, and deoxyribonucleic acid (DNA) determines hereditary properties. DNA is composed of adenine (A), guanine (G), cytosine (C), thymine (T), phosphoric acid, and ribose. Thus the difference between these two nucleic acids is that DNA contains the nitrogenous base, thymine, and deoxyribose, whereas RNA contains uracil and ribose.

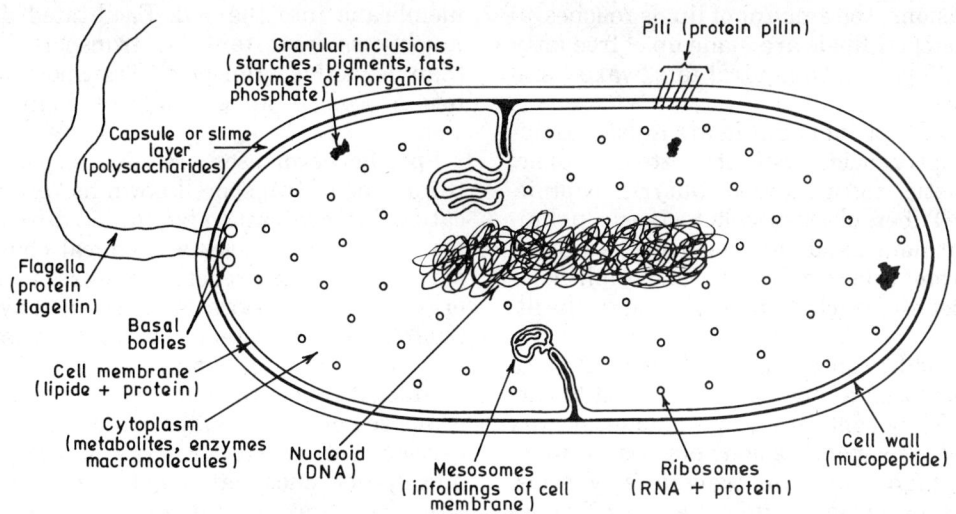

**FIGURE 7.** *Outline of generalized ultrastructure of a bacterial cell to indicate structural proteins (see Chapter 1).*

The structure of DNA was elucidated by Watson and Crick, who established that DNA is composed of two polynucleotide chains spirally wound and held together by hydrogen bonds between guanine and cytosine on one hand and adenine and thymine on the other. For every species of bacteria there is a definite ratio of paired bases $\dfrac{\text{guanine} + \text{cytosine}}{\text{adenine} + \text{thymine}}$. The guanine + cytosine (GC) content of bacteria varies from 28 per cent (some lactobacilli species) to 73 per cent (certain mycobacteria).

*Carbohydrates.* Carbohydrates and polyatomic alcohols compose 12 to 18 per cent of the dry matter in the bacterial cell. Most of the carbohydrate is a polysaccharide complex, sometimes bound to proteins and lipids, that is found in the cell wall and slime layer. The cytoplasm of many bacteria has a comparatively large amount of inclusions, chemically resembling glycogen or starch.

The polysaccharides of the capsules of types II,
III, and VIII pneumococcus belong to the group of compounds that do not contain nitrogen. They are polymers of aldobionic acids, and during complete hydrolysis break down into glucose and glucuronic acid. The polysaccharides of other microorganisms include dextrans, levans (fructosans), and cellulose (Table 1).

Some bacteria have hexosamines that on hydrolysis break down into monosaccharides, aminosaccharides, and amino acids (types I, IV, and XIV pneumococcus, *C. diphtheriae, M. tuberculosis*). Acid hydrolysis of polysaccharides releases galactose, glucose, fructose, and other monosaccharides.

The type specificity in *Salmonella* spp depends on the polysaccharide side chains of their lipopolysaccharides. This is of great significance in laboratory identification.

*Lipids.* In those bacteria that do not store fat in the form of inclusions, lipids constitute 10 per cent of the dry matter (in *C. diphtheriae* it is only 5 per cent). In those bacteria that store fats as

**TABLE 2.  Enzymes Found in Bacteria**

| TYPE | REACTION CATALYZED | EXAMPLES |
|---|---|---|
| Oxidoreductase | Oxidation and reduction | Dehydrogenase, oxidase, peroxidase |
| Transferase | Transfer of a group containing C, N, P, or S from one substrate to another | Transaminase, transferase, transmethylase, transketolase |
| Hydrolase | Hydrolytic cleavage | Esterase, amidase, peptidase, phosphatase |
| Lyase | Nonhydrolytic removal of chemical group, usually from a double bond | Decarboxylases, deaminase, aldolase |
| Isomerase | Intramolecular rearrangements as in the interconversion of one isomer into the other | Isomerase, racemase, epimerase, mutase |
| Ligase | Joining together of two different molecules, or of two ends in the same molecule. The reaction catalyzed by these enzymes involves the cleavage of a high-energy phosphate bond in ATP or another energy donor. | Synthetases |

special inclusions, the amount of lipids reaches 40 per cent. Bacterial lipids are made up of free fatty acids (26 to 28 per cent), neutral fats, waxes, and phospholipids.

The lipids of typhoid bacteria are almost exclusively free fatty acids (palmitic, stearic, oleic, lauric, myristic, tetracosanoic, butyric, caproic, and others). Tuberculostearic, ketostearic, palmitostearic, phthienic, and phthioic acids have been extracted from tubercle bacilli, and diphtheric acid have been extracted from diphtheria bacilli.

Tubercle bacilli contain bound lipids (12 to 15 per cent) composed of mycolic acid linked to carbohydrates. They contain a large amount of wax (wax D) that on saponification releases up to 84 per cent of high molecular weight fatty acids. These fatty acids possess a characteristically high resistance to the action of minerals, alcohols, and alkalies. A modicum of other specific components have been recognized in *M. tuberculosis:* phthiocerol dimycocerosate, and cardiolipin, which along with wax D may be important in pathogenicity.

The chemical composition of the microbial cells depends on the composition of the medium and the environmental conditions. In the case of pathogens isolated from their hosts, the extra-and intracellular milieu may determine the bacterial composition to a large extent.

### Nutrition

*Transport of Nutrients.* The phospholipid bilayer, which constitutes the bacterial cell membrane, is a barrier to the passage of most nutrients into the cytoplasm because nutrients are largely water soluble (polar). There are, however, proteins embedded in the membrane, with an average molecular weight of 30,000, that can actively transport into the cell a variety of molecules, including amino acids, lactose, glucose, galactose, and sulfate. This active transport allows the nutrient to reach a concentration within the cell that is thousands of times greater than on its exterior. In order to meet the work requirement for such transport against a concentration gradient, energy must be supplied by metabolic processes within the cell.

Another set of proteins, known as permeases, also facilitate transfer of nutrients into the cytoplasm, but this process requires no energy because the substrate moves from a higher concentration outside the cell to a lower concentration inside. The process is sometimes called "facilitated diffusion" and differs from simple diffusion in that the permease discriminates among substrates (Cohen and Monod, 1957). In other words, a specific permease selectively binds certain substrates, but not others, on the outside of the cell and catalyzes their movement across the cell membrane into the cell. Facilitated diffusion is much less important for transport in bacteria than is active transport. Transport of glycerol into *E. coli* is an example of facilitated diffusion.

Specific permeases are also responsible for a third type of transport known as "group translocation." In contrast to facilitated diffusion, group translocation involves a chemical change in the substrate, and the reaction requires metabolic energy. Group translocation is typified by the phosphotransferase system that can transfer fructose, glucose, mannose, mannitol, and other sugars against a concentration gradient. The system is composed of two enzymes and a small heat stable carrier protein, HPr. Energy is provided by the energy-rich phosphate bond of phosphoenolpyruvate. The first enzyme, enzyme I, catalyzes the transfer of phosphate (P) to the carrier protein HPr in the following reaction:

$$P\text{-enolpyruvate} + HPr \rightarrow pyruvate + P\text{-}HPr$$

The activated carrier protein, P-HPr, then reacts with free hexose so as to carry hexose across the membrane into the cell as hexose-6-phosphate. A second enzyme, enzyme II, catalyzes phosphorylation of the sugar as follows:

$$P\text{-}HPr + hexose \rightarrow hexose\text{-}6\text{-}P + HPr$$

There is a specific enzyme II for each hexose.

Species of bacteria vary in the method of transport used to carry nutrients into a cell. In addition, simple diffusion allows passage into the cell of substances present in high concentration outside the cell. Water is the most important substance that passes across the cell membrane by passive diffusion.

*Types of Nutrition.* *Autotrophic,* chemosynthetic, and photosynthetic bacteria are able to produce organic substances from inorganic compounds. They do not require organic carbon compounds and synthesize the component parts of their cell by absorbing carbon dioxide, in addition to water and simple nitrogen compounds (ammonia and its salts, nitrate, and others). Nitrifying bacteria and many sulphur bacteria belong to the autotrophic microbes. They synthesize complex substances at the expense of the energy they receive from the oxidation of ammonia to nitrites (*Nitrosomonas*) and nitrates (*Nitrobacter*) and the oxidation of sulphur, sulphides, and thiosulphates to sulphuric acid and its salts (*Thiobacillus thiooxidans*).

Some species of microorganisms — anaerobic purple and green sulphur bacteria (*Thiorhodaceae, Chlorobacteriaceae*) — contain chlorophyll and use radiant energy for photosynthesis.

The autotrophic bacteria use carbon dioxide as the sole source of carbon and are unable to absorb more complex carbon compounds. For this reason, such organisms cannot be pathogenic for humans and animals.

*Heterotrophic* bacteria require organic carbon (carbohydrates and keto, amino, and fatty acids), inorganic substances, trace elements, and vitamins. Heterotrophic bacteria can be subdivided into 1) saprophytes and 2) parasites.

1) *Saprophytes* (Greek *sapros* = decaying, *phyton* = plant) live at the expense of organic substances found in the surrounding environment. These include most species of bacteria inhabiting our planet.

2) *Parasites* make up a comparatively small number of species of bacteria that, in the process of evolution, have adapted themselves to a parasitic mode of life. However, this division of heterotrophic bacteria into saphrophytes and parasites is not absolute. Certain species of bacteria pathogenic to man can exist in the environment as saprophytes, and, conversely, some saprophytes under unfavorable conditions can cause disease in humans and animals.

*Nutrients Essential for Growth.*   The majority of bacteria develop only on complex media containing peptone (a product of enzymatic breakdown of meat and other protein substances), meat extract, and products of similar biologic origin, which contain all the nutrients in the form of high molecular weight compounds essential for growth.

NITROGEN.   According to the character of nitrogen nutrition, bacteria have been subdivided into a number of groups including those that function by 1) fixing atmospheric nitrogen; 2) absorbing mineral forms of nitrogen (ammonium sulphate); 3) assimilating ammonium salts, nitrates, or nitrates in the presence of amino acids or purines; 4) growing in the presence of individual amino acids or their mixtures; and 5) growing in protein nutrient media.

CARBON.   The sources of carbon for bacteria may be different carbohydrates, polyhydric alcohols, or organic acids. According to their ability to synthesize complex compounds, bacteria may be divided into four groups. 1) Those that obtain carbon from carbon dioxide and nitrogen from inorganic compounds. These organisms use radiant energy (light). Autotrophs that are capable of chemosynthesis obtain energy by the simple process of oxidation of inorganic compounds (nitrifying bacteria, sulphur bacteria, some iron bacteria). 2) Those that derive carbon and obtain energy from organic carbon compounds and nitrogen from its inorganic compounds (the majority of saprophytes). 3) Those that obtain carbon and energy from organic carbon compounds and nitrogen from amino acids (majority of commensals). 4) Those that absorb carbon and obtain energy from organic compounds, obtain nitrogen from a complex of many amino acids, and require one or more vitamins (pathogenic bacteria).

VITAMINS.   Besides peptones, carbohydrates, fatty acids, and inorganic elements, bacteria require special substances — vitamins or growth factors that function as coenzymes. As coenzymes, vitamins act as acceptors or donors of chemical groups or H atoms, which are transferred to or from the substrate by various enzymes. These are summarized in Table 3.

**TABLE 3.   Vitamins and Their Coenzyme Function in Bacteria**

| VITAMIN | COENZYME FORM | TRANSFER REACTION IN WHICH COENZYME COLLABORATES |
|---|---|---|
| Thiamine | Thiamine pyrophosphate (TPP) | Oxidative decarboxylation of $\alpha$-keto acids |
| Nicotinamide | Nicotinamide-adenine dinucleotide (NAD) | Hydrogen transfer in fermentation and respiration |
| | Nicotinamide-adenine dinucleotide phosphate (NADP) | NAD reversibly transfers electrons by coupling to different enzymes |
| Riboflavin | Flavin mononucleotide (FMN) Flavin adenine dinucleotide (FAD) | Hydrogen transfer in respiration. FAD is an electron acceptor for the oxidizing enzymes known as flavoproteins. FAD similar in action to NAD |
| Pyridoxine | Pyridoxal phosphate (PALP) | Catalyzes completely different reactions varying from amino-transfer and decarboxylation to racemization. It is the coenzyme of amino acid metabolism and the active group for amino transferases, decarboxylases, lyases, and synthetases. In all cases it acts by combination of its aldehyde group with the amino group of the substrate |
| Pantothenic acid | Coenzyme A (CoA) adenosine 3′5′ diphosphate + panthotheine phosphate | Transfer of acyl groups—All acyltransferases transfer acyl groups to or from CoA |
| Folic acid | Tetrahydrofolate (THFA) | Acts as a carrier of methyl, hydroxymethyl, formyl, or formimino groups |
| Biotin | Biotin | Carboxyl transfer; energy is derived from ATP |
| Cobalamine | $B_{12}$ coenzyme | Methyl transfer; isomerase reactions |

Some bacteria do not require a supplement of vitamins to the nutrient medium because they can synthesize these compounds. Others grow poorly on vitamin-free media, but their growth is enhanced upon the addition of vitamins. Bacteria such as pneumococcus and hemolytic streptococcus cannot be cultivated without vitamins. *Hemophilus influenzae* requires supplements of hemin and NAD for growth.

The amount of vitamins in the nutrient medium is expressed in micrograms, and they are required in concentrations varying from 0.001 to 10 mg/L. The concentrations of vitamins in bacterial cells (parts per million of dry weight) vary with different species but have the following ranges: nicotinic acid 210 to 250, riboflavin 44 to 67, thiamine 9 to 26, pyridoxine 6 or 7, pantothenic acid 90 to 140, and folic acid 3 to 15.

Intestinal microflora supply humans and animals directly with vitamins. Many bacteria participate in the vitamin metabolism of plants, in enriching food products with vitamins, and in producing vitamins.

INORGANIC SUBSTANCES. Potassium exerts a catalytic action and activates enzyme systems. Calcium participates in nitrification, in nitrogen fixation by soil microorganisms (*Azotobacter*), and in the production of gelatinase. Iron is found in the respiratory enzymes and functions as a catalyst in oxidation processes. Trace elements are incorporated into the structure of the active groups of some enzymes. Sulfur is a constituent of cysteine and methionine and of the coenzymes CoA and cocarboxylase. Phosphorus is a constituent of nucleic acids, phospholipids, ATP, and NADP. Magnesium is a cofactor for enzymes, and serves to bind enzymes to substrates. Cobalt is a constituent of vitamin $B_{12}$. Manganese, zinc, and copper are also essential for the activity of certain enzymes.

## BACTERIAL GROWTH

The growth of bacteria represents the increase in mass of bacterial cytoplasm as a result of the synthesis of cellular material.

Bacteria reproduce by simple transverse division, vegetative reproduction that occurs in different planes and produces many different cellular arrangements (clusters, chains, pairs). The transverse division of bacteria is not only a process of cell division of one mother cell into two equal daughter cells, but also represents a continuous separation of daughter cells from the mother cell so that the former in their turn become mother cells.

The rate of cell division differs among bacteria. It depends on the species of microorganism, age of culture, nutrient medium, temperature, concentration of carbon dioxide, and other factors.

The length of the generation of *E. coli, Clostridium perfringens,* and *Streptococcus faecalis* is 20 minutes in nutrient broth medium, whereas for the cells of a mammalian tissue culture it is 24 hours. Thus, bacteria reproduce about 100 times faster than a tissue in culture. The increase in the number of cells can be expressed in the following way:

1-2-4-8-16-32   N   (number of cells)

0-1-2-3-4-5      n   (number of generations)

The total amount of bacteria (N) after n generations will be equal to $2^n$ per cell of seeded material. If we take the original amount of bacteria inoculated into the nutrient medium as a single individual, and the time for one division as 30 minutes, theoretically, the total amount of bacteria produced per 24 hours would be $N = 2^{48}$. Given a division every 20 minutes, in 36 hours the microbial mass will be equal to 400 tons. Thermophilic microbes divide even more rapidly.

However, in natural as well as in artificial conditions the reproduction of bacteria is on a considerably smaller scale. It is limited by a number of internal and external factors described in the section on regulation of growth. Figure 8 illustrates schematically the rate of growth expressed as the number of cells per milliliter of the medium.

There are six principal phases of reproduction that are designated in Figure 8 by Roman numerals:

I. An initial *lag phase* represents a period of physiologic adjustment, during which the cells may need to synthesize new enzymes and reestablish minimal intracellular concentrations of substrates, enzymes, and inorganic ions.

II. A phase of *increasing growth* rate reflects the randomness of adjustment of individuals in the population and the increase in the rate of growth of each individual as the rates of its separate metabolic processes become maximum.

III. A phase of *logarithmic growth* is characterized by a maximal division rate and decrease in cell size. The "growth rate" of a culture is usually expressed in terms of cell doubling time, which is equated with generation time. This rate is influenced by temperature, the nature of the carbon source, the concentration of an essential nutrient if very low, the variety of nutrients available, and, for facultative anaerobes, the $O_2$ tension.

IV. A phase of *declining growth* rate represents the cessation of growth as a consequence of the exhaustion of the various nutrients in the medium.

V. A maximal *stationary phase* occurs when the number of newly produced bacteria is almost

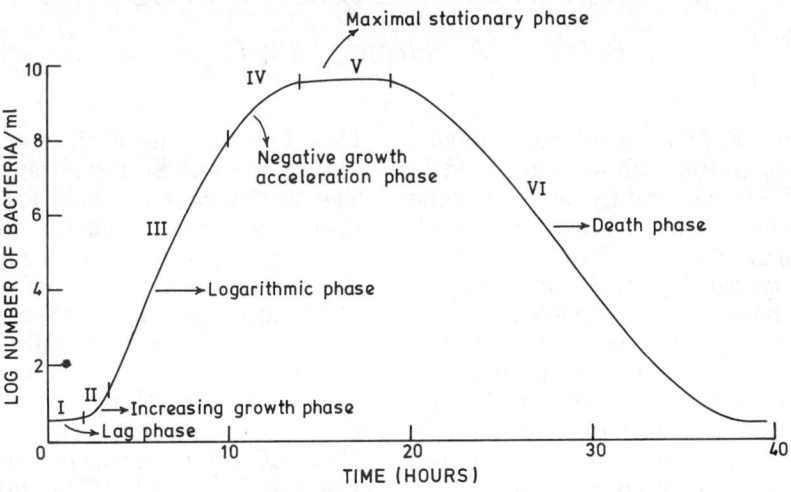

**FIGURE 8.** *Bacterial growth curve.*

equal to the number of organisms that die because of the lack of essential nutrients.

VI. The *death phase* is a consequence of the loss of selective permeability and of lysis — disintegration of cells.

The length of these phases is arbitrary, for it can vary depending on the species of bacteria and the conditions of cultivation. Thus, *E. coli* divide every 20 minutes, *Salmonella typhosa* divide every 25 minutes, *Streptococcus pyogenes* divide every 30 minutes, and *M. tuberculosis* divide every 18 hours under optimal growth conditions.

### Regulation of Growth

The biosynthetic pathways involved in growth are controlled by *feedback regulation.* The enzyme that mediates the first reaction in the pathway is inhibited by the end-product or end-products of the pathway, a process designated *end-product inhibition.* This process prevents an accumulation of the end-product or its intermediates. It assures the balanced operation of both catabolic and biosynthetic pathways.

The mechanism of end-product inhibition is not known, but it is thought that the binding of the end-product distorts the enzyme and creates a conformational change in the site for substrate attachment, so that the enzyme no longer binds properly to its substrate. An important example of this phenomenon is the inhibition of pyrimidine biosynthesis by cytidine triphosphate (CTP). The synthesis of cytidine begins when the enzyme aspartic transcarbamylase (ATCase) catalyzes

the condensation of carbamyl phosphate and aspartic acid with the production of carbamyl aspartic acid as follows:

$$\text{carbamyl phosphate} + \text{aspartic acid} \xrightarrow{\text{ATCase}} \text{carbamyl aspartic acid}$$

The end-product of this reaction is CTP, which inhibits aspartic transcarbamylase and prevents overproduction of the pyrimidine. This control of enzyme function is called *allosteric,* a term that refers to the fact that the enzyme inhibitor has a different shape, or structure, than the substrate, whose attachment to the enzyme is prevented (Monod et al., 1963). Another device for controlling metabolic pathways is known as *catabolite repression.* This phenomenon, described in Chapter 4, represses synthesis of the enzyme.

## References

Beadle, G.W., and Tatum, E.L.: Genetic control of biochemical reactions in Neurospora. Proc. Natl Acad Sci USA 27:499, 1941.

Cohen, G.N., and Monod, J.: Bacterial permeases. Bacteriol Rev 21:169, 1957.

Höltje, J.-V., and Tomasz, A.: Lipoteichoic acid: a specific inhibitor of autolysin activity in *Pneumococcus.* Proc Natl Acad Sci USA, 72:1690, 1975.

Horecker, B.L.: Pentose metabolism in bacteria. New York, John Wiley & Sons, 1962.

Lipmann, F.: Metabolic generation and utilization of phosphate bond energy. Adv Enzymol 1:99, 1941.

Meyerhof, O.: Intermediate carbohydrate metabolism. *In* A Symposium on Respiratory Enzymes. Vol. 3. Madison, University of Wisconsin Press, 1942.

Monod, J., Changeux, J., and Jacob, F.: Allosteric proteins and cellular control systems. J Mol Biol 6:306, 1963.

# 4 BACTERIAL GENETICS

*Patricia A. Hoffee, Ph.D.*

At first, bacteria were not considered to have a regular genetic apparatus such as that found in eukaryotic cells. This was mainly because of the lack of a well-defined nucleus and their small size. However, during the past 35 years extensive work has demonstrated that bacteria do have a form of genetic inheritance comparable to higher organisms, with the main exception that they contain a haploid genome in almost all instances. In fact, bacteria have been used as a model system to establish most of the basic concepts of molecular genetics that we have today (Hayes, 1968; Stanier et al., 1970; Watson, 1976).

## MOLECULAR ASPECTS

### The Bacterial Chromosome: Its Structure and Replication

In the intact bacterial cell there is a single, continuous molecule of deoxyribonucleic acid (DNA) that makes up the chromosome. This molecule has a molecular weight of about $3 \times 10^9$ and is a closed circle. The molecular structure of this chromosome was determined by the Nobel prize–winning work of Watson and Crick (Watson, 1976; Watson and Crick, 1953). It is composed of a double helix made of two complementary strands of polynucleotides that contain purine and pyrim-idine bases arranged along a backbone of alternating deoxyribose and phosphate groups (Fig. 1). The two strands are held together by hydrogen bonds that occur between a purine and a pyrimidine. This bonding is formed specifically between the pyrimidine thymine and the purine adenine (A-T base pair), or between the pyrimidine cytosine and the purine guanine (G-C base pair) (Fig. 2). Thus, the sequence of bases on one strand always has a complementary sequence of bases on the opposite strand; that is, the sequence AT-TATCCG will have a complementary sequence on the opposite strand of TAATAGGC. The presence of the complementary strands allows for faithful replication of the chromosome during division. The two strands separate at a particular origin of replication, each strand acting as its own template, and a new complementary strand is made by the enzymatic polymerization of the deoxyribonucleotide subunits — dATP, dTTP, dCTP, and dGTP. Because of the specificity of the bonding, the new strands will be the exact complement of the template strand, and the genetic information will be faithfully transmitted to the daughter cells. This mode of replication is referred to as *semiconservative* and is illustrated in Figure 3. By this mechanism the daughter cells in the first generation will have one strand of the double-stranded DNA molecule that originated from the

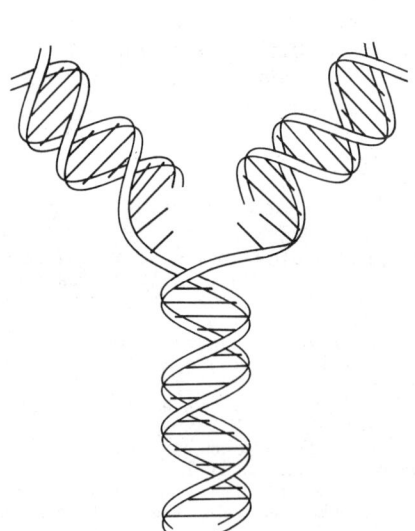

**FIGURE 1.** *The Watson-Crick model of DNA structure and replication. Two complementary strands are held together by the hydrogen bonding of adenine with thymine, and guanine with cytosine. The strands unwind during replication, and each strand acts as a template for the synthesis of the new daughter strands.*

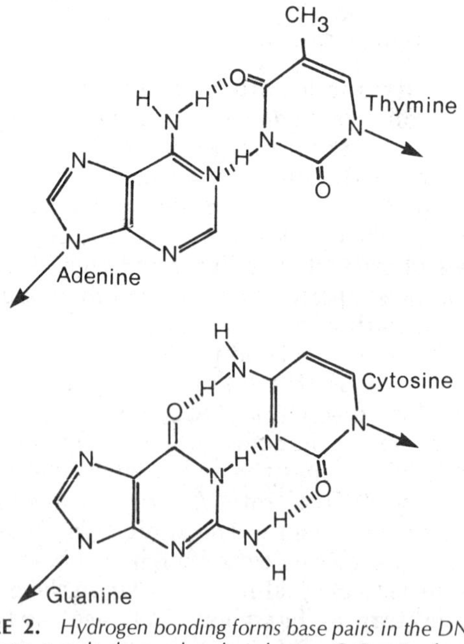

**FIGURE 2.** *Hydrogen bonding forms base pairs in the DNA. A-T pairs form two hydrogen bonds, whereas G-C pairs form three hydrogen bonds. The arrow indicates the position that binds to deoxyribose.*

DENSITY GRADIENT

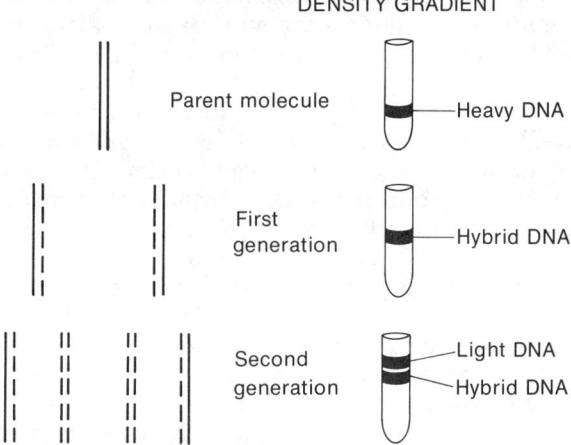

FIGURE 3. *Semiconservative replication of DNA in E. coli as demonstrated by the experiment of Meselson and Stahl (1958). The DNA of the parents is labeled with $^{15}N$, so that it appears heavy in a density gradient. After one generation in $^{14}N$ medium, the DNA from the first generation progeny is hybrid in density, since it has one strand of heavy DNA and one strand of light DNA. After the second generation, DNA or light density begins to appear along with the DNA of hybrid density. This pattern of density bands is consistent with semiconservative replication.*

parent cell and one new strand. In the second generation, two of the daughter cells will have no strand from the original parent cell. The mechanism of semiconservative replication was demonstrated by the experiment of Meselson and Stahl (1958) in which the parent cell DNA was labeled with heavy nitrogen and the pattern of distribution of the heavy label was then followed through several generations (Fig. 3).

In order for each daughter cell to receive a copy of the chromosome at cell division some control must be maintained over the replication of the chromosome. It is hypothesized that the bacterial chromosome has some attachment point on the cell membrane so that replication can be synchronized with cell division. A model proposed by Jacob and Brenner (1963), referred to as the *replicon model,* proposes that there is a specific point on the chromosome that is activated by an "initiator" protein. Replication begins at this point on the chromosome and then proceeds in a bidirectional manner until the whole chromosome has been replicated. Numerous proteins are involved in the replication process, and a number of them have been identified by the isolation of mutants of *Escherichia coli,* which are temperature sensitive for DNA replication (a temperature-sensitive mutant is one that can function normally at a permissive, or lower, temperature and is unable to do so at a nonpermissive, or higher, temperature; see section on Mutation). At least five specific genes have already been identified as being involved in the process of replica-

tion, and several other ones have been postulated but have yet to be identified.

### The Chromosome as a Functioning Unit

All the genetic potential of the bacterial cell is contained in the base sequence of the DNA molecule. (However, many bacteria contain extrachromosomal elements also of DNA that can confer additional genetic potential on a cell; see section on Gene Transfer in Bacteria). In order for this information to be expressed in the cellular behavior of the cell a number of complex processes must occur. The first process involves the transcription of the DNA base sequence into a ribonucleic acid molecule that will serve as a message — hence, the name messenger ribonucleic acid (mRNA). Segments of the DNA molecules are transcribed into mRNA by the action of an enzyme called RNA polymerase. This enzyme can polymerize ribonucleotides (ATP, GTP, CTP, and UTP) into a complementary strand of RNA, so that the presence of A in the DNA will result in U in the RNA, G in the DNA will give C in the RNA, T in the DNA will result in A in the RNA, and C in the DNA will give G in the RNA. Each discrete segment of DNA will specify an RNA message that will eventually be translated into a protein molecule. Such a segment or sequence of bases in the DNA is referred to as a *gene.* The mRNA molecule is translated into protein by the protein-synthesizing machinery of the cell, which is made up of activated amino acids, transfer RNA (tRNA), and ribosomes. The mRNA and the tRNA, which has a specific amino acid attached, come together on the surface of the ribosome. The tRNA molecule has a triplet of bases on one end that is complementary to a triplet of bases on the mRNA. Each tRNA molecule finds its complementary triplet on the mRNA, and the amino acid that it carries is put into a peptide linkage with the amino acid of the preceding tRNA molecule. As the ribosome moves along the mRNA, the peptide grows by the addition of each amino acid in a sequential manner until the complete mRNA has been translated into a sequence of amino acids. The sequence of bases in the DNA represents a code that was broken some 15 years ago. Each three bases in the DNA (a *codon*), and thus in the mRNA, specifies a particular amino acid. So whenever this codon appears in the DNA, a particular amino acid will be found in a particular position in the protein coded for by that segment of DNA. This genetic code is presented in Figure 4. Any possible sequence of three bases specifies an amino acid, thus AAU will specify asparagine, whereas AAG will specify lysine. The exceptions are the three codons UAG (amber), UAA (ochre), and UGA (opal). These codons do not specify an amino acid and are involved in the termination of

| First | Second | | | | Third |
|---|---|---|---|---|---|
|  | U | C | A | G |  |
| U | phe | ser | tyr | cys | U |
|  | phe | ser | tyr | cys | C |
|  | leu | ser | (ochre) | (opal) | A |
|  | leu | ser | (amber) | trp | G |
| C | leu | pro | his | arg | U |
|  | leu | pro | his | arg | C |
|  | leu | pro | gln | arg | A |
|  | leu | pro | gln | arg | G |
| A | ile | thr | asn | ser | U |
|  | ile | thr | asn | ser | C |
|  | ile | thr | lys | arg | A |
|  | met, fmet | thr | lys | arg | G |
| G | val | ala | asp | gly | U |
|  | val | ala | asp | gly | C |
|  | val | ala | glu | gly | A |
|  | val | ala | glu | gly | G |

**FIGURE 4.** *The genetic code. The combinations of the four bases gives 64 possible triple codons, which are listed with their amino acid assignments. Three codons, UAA (ochre), UAG (amber), and UGA (opal), do not code for any amino acid and are the nonsense codons that are used for termination signals.*

peptide synthesis. They are called *nonsense codons*. In order for the proper DNA sequences to be read at the appropriate times and in the right way, various mechanisms of control of transcription have evolved in bacterial cells. Some of these mechanisms will be discussed later in this chapter.

Although the detailed work on the genetic code and its translation and transcription led to a universal hypothesis of colinearity of the gene and its protein, recent work with viruses and mammalian cells suggests that other mechanisms of gene structure exist. It is now known that in some mammalian viruses such as SV-40 there exist overlapping genes in which codons are read in different phases, so that the same sequence of bases in the DNA may code for more than one protein. Another mechanism of interest is the recent finding of genes in pieces, or gene splicing, in which discontinuous sequences of bases in the DNA can code for a single polypeptide, such as in antibody synthesis. Thus, in addition to the "one-gene, one-polypeptide" hypothesis there is now a "one-gene, two-polypeptide" hypothesis as well as a "three-gene, one-polypeptide" hypothesis.

## MUTATION

### Molecular Basis of Mutation

A mutation is defined as a change in the base sequence of the DNA. In many cases such a base change will result in an altered amino acid sequence of a protein that will, in turn, alter the normal functioning of that protein. In addition, the base change will be propagated when the DNA is replicated. Thus, a mutation is characterized by its effect on cell growth or metabolism and by its stability in the progeny cells. The base change can occur in the DNA by one of two mechanisms: 1) substitution of one base pair by a different base pair, or 2) an addition or deletion of a base pair or a segment of DNA during breakage of the sugar-phosphate backbone of the DNA. Single base pair changes are referred to as point mutations. Such mutations can occur spontaneously during replication or repair of the DNA or can be increased in rate of appearance by chemicals or physical agents that can interact with the DNA molecule. Chemicals that can enhance the rate of mutation are called mutagens. The first group of mutagens includes base analogues, which are incorporated into the DNA in place of the natural base. These analogues have an increased tendency to pair with the wrong base during replication, which results in the replacement of one base pair by a different base pair. Such base analogues include compounds such as bromouracil, an analogue of thymine, and 2-aminopurine, an analogue of adenine. A second group is composed of compounds that chemically alter bases in the DNA and thus alter their pairing ability. These compounds include chemicals such as nitrous acid and alkylating reagents, of which the most powerful is *N*-methyl-*N*-nitroso-*N'*-nitroguanidine (nitrosoguanidine). The third group consists of still other chemicals, such as the acridine dyes, that cause mutation by intercalating between stacked base pairs in the DNA, which results in the insertion or deletion of base pairs during replication.

Substitution of one base pair by another may lead to a change in a codon that results in the replacement of the original amino acid in the protein by a new amino acid. For example, if there is a change from a A-T pair to a G-C pair, one might have a change in the anticodon (the name given to the codon in the mRNA) from UCG to CCG and thus a change in the amino acid sequence in which serine is replaced by proline. This type of change, in which one amino acid replaces another in the protein, is referred to as a *missense mutation*. If the base change results in one of the anticodons — UAA, UGA, or UAG — being produced, no amino acid is placed in the polypeptide chain, and termination of peptide synthesis occurs. This type of change, in which no amino acid is designated by the anticodon, is termed a *nonsense mutation*.

Whenever additions or deletions of single base pairs occur, such as with acridine dyes, there is a change in the reading frame of the mRNA so that all codons from the point of insertion or deletion are misread. For example, if the base sequence *UGG-UGG-UGG-UGG* occurs in the mRNA it will be translated in the protein as the amino acid sequence trp-trp-trp-trp. When a base addition occurs, such as the insertion of C, the base sequence becomes UGG-CUG-GUG-GUG, and each triplet is then misread from the point of insertion, giving the amino acid sequence trp-leu-val-val. Such mutants are termed *frameshift mutants* and are found when additions or deletions of one or two bases occur.

Another type of mutation is found when a large segment of DNA is either deleted or inserted. Mutations caused by large deletions are referred to as *deletion mutants* and those caused by large additions are termed *insertion mutants*. Insertion mutants are a relatively new concept, although such mutations have been described in the literature for some time. They are caused by the insertions of specific base sequences of about 800 to 1400 base pairs that are called *insertion sequences* (IS). These IS elements have now been found in the chromosome of *E. coli,* in various bacterial viruses, and in plasmids, and they act as a mechanism for joining pieces of DNA that occur in bacterial cells.

Just as mutations occur in the forward direction, as described previously, similar chemical changes occur that can result in getting back the original or a pseudooriginal phenotype. These changes, referred to as *reversions,* will be dependent in type on the kind of forward mutation that initially occurred. For example, in the case of base substitution, a reversion can simply be the change of the same base pair back to the one that was originally present. If the triplet UCG mutated to CCG, it could revert back to UCG by a change in the same base pair. Such revertants are termed *true revertants* and are genetically identi-

cal to the original parent. In addition, there are revertants that result not from changing the mutated initial base pair but from changing a base pair at another site in the DNA. Such a revertant, in which a second mutation compensates for the original mutation, is referred to as a *suppressor mutation*. They can occur within the same gene as the original mutation (*intragenic*) or they can occur in a gene outside the gene in which the initial mutation occurred *(extragenic)*. Intragenic suppression can correct both point mutations and frameshift mutations. Extragenic suppression is usually the result of a mutation occurring in a gene that codes for a product involved in translation, such as a tRNA molecule. The secondary mutation corrects the original defect by recognizing this defect as normal for translation. An important class of extragenic suppressors are those that correct a nonsense mutation. Some of these suppressors have been shown to be the result of a mutant tRNA that now recognizes the nonsense codon as one of the sense codons, and allows an amino acid to be inserted into the peptide chain and its synthesis to continue. Deletion mutants are not capable of reversion, but insertion mutants can revert to the original genotype of the parent cell by a simple loss of the inserted sequence.

### The Phenotypic Expression of Mutation

The preceding discussion gives one an understanding of what mutation is at the molecular level. However, such mutations, or changes in the base sequence of DNA, can be recognized only if they have an effect on the phenotype of the bacterial cell or virus that is being studied. Early in the study of bacteriology the apparent rapidity with which mutations occurred in bacteria and the selection of such mutants by the environment

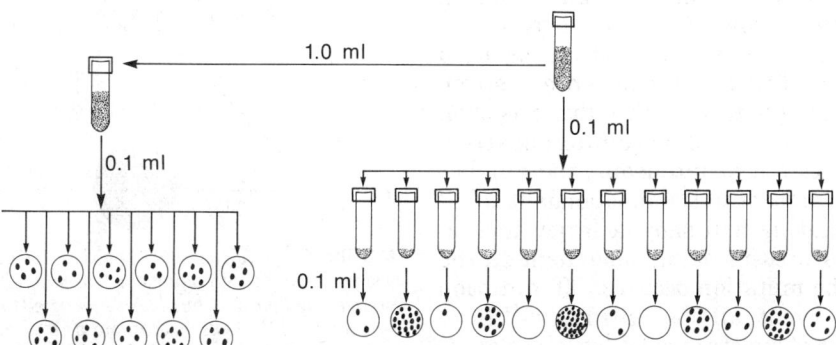

**FIGURE 5.**   *The fluctuation test of Luria and Delbrück (1943). A series of individual culture tubes containing 1 ml of nutrient medium are inoculated at low density with equal numbers of wild-type bacteria. After incubation overnight, a sample of each tube is plated on nutrient agar containing a selective agent such as streptomycin. Resistant cells will appear as colonies on the plates. A large fluctuation is seen in the numbers of resistant cells from different tubes, supporting the theory of spontaneous mutation. The control tube on the left is sampled multiple times to determine the fluctuation caused by random error.*

made it difficult to accept that bacteria had a genetic apparatus like that found in eukaryotic systems. It was as if the bacterial cell was altered as a direct response to environmental changes. The acceptance of bacterial cells as having a genetic makeup similar to other living organisms came with the classic experiment of Luria and Delbrück in 1943. This experiment, called the *fluctuation test,* is diagrammed in Figure 5. To understand the fluctuation test one must remember that a culture of bacteria grows exponentially, with each cell giving rise to two daughter cells until the culture reaches stationary phase. If, during growth, mutations arise spontaneously in bacteria, the point of time during the growth cycle at which the mutation occurs will determine how many cells will carry that mutation at the end of the growth cycle. For example, if we start with a dilute culture of *E. coli* that is sensitive to the presence of streptomycin ($str^s$ will not grow in the presence of streptomycin), and if the theory of spontaneous mutation is true, there is the probability a mutation that will make a cell resistant to the action of streptomycin ($str^r$) will occur at any point in the growth cycle. If this mutation occurs early during the growth of the culture, at the end of the growth phase there will be a large number of $str^r$ cells that will have been derived from the original mutant cell. If the mutation occurs late during the growth of the culture, at the end of the growth phase there will be only a few cells that are $str^r$. The number of $str^r$ cells present in the population at the end of the growth phase is determined by plating out an aliquot of the cells on a nutrient agar plate containing streptomycin. The $str^s$ cells will be killed, and only the $str^r$ cells will grow into colonies. If mutation in bacteria does not occur spontaneously, but instead is directed by the environment, the number of cells that become $str^r$ at the end of the growth phase will be independent of time. The fluctuation test sets up a large number of independent cultures, each started from a few $str^s$ cells, to test this hypothesis. The cultures are allowed to grow for a definitive amount of time in the absence of streptomycin, and a sample from each culture is then plated on a nutrient agar plate containing streptomycin. If mutation is spontaneous, the number of resistant cells present in the independent tubes at the time of plating will show a large fluctuation, the number present being dependent on the time at which the mutation occurred. If mutation is not a random event, all the cultures will have the same number of resistant colonies, since exposure to streptomycin occurs at the same time, and all cells have the same probability of becoming resistant. In all instances that were tested, a large fluctuation in the number of mutant cells occurred, providing evidence for the theory of

spontaneous mutation in bacteria. This type of analysis is important today as one of the best methods for providing evidence for the occurrence of mutation, particularly in the newly developing field of somatic cell genetics.

Although the results of the fluctuation test convinced most workers that bacteria undergo spontaneous mutation, there were a few workers who objected to the statistical nature of the data. These doubters were finally convinced by the development of the replica plating or indirect selection technique of Lederberg and Lederberg in 1952. The technique of replica plating is diagrammed in Figure 6. Although it was initially used to provide evidence that one could select a mutant cell without ever having that cell come into contact with the selecting agent, replica plating is now a valuable technique for the scoring of numerous genetic markers in a large number of colonies with a minimum amount of work. The technique involves using a square of velveteen, which has a raised surface, and placing it over the

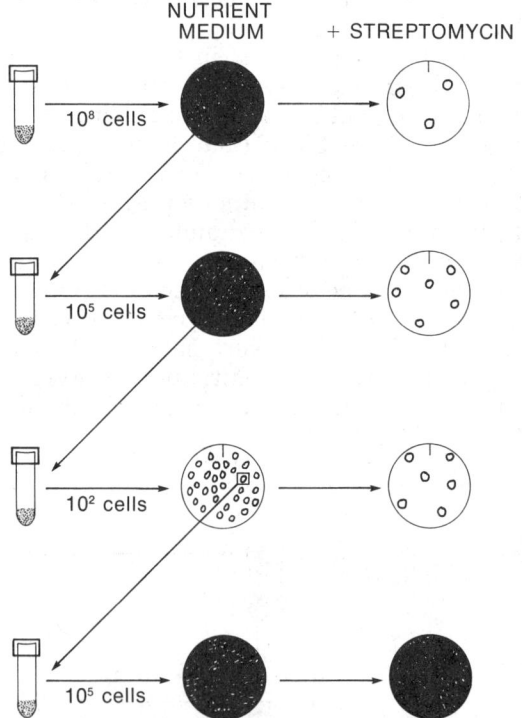

**FIGURE 6.** *Replica plating or indirect selection of Lederberg and Lederberg (1952). Streptomycin-sensitive cells, $10^8$, are spread on a nutrient medium and the plate is incubated to allow growth that will be confluent. The cells on the plate are then replicated using a sterile velveteen cloth to a sterile plate containing streptomycin. A few colonies develop after overnight incubation. The location on the original plate of resistant cells is determined by comparing the plates. The cells on this area are removed and transferred to fresh nutrient broth and allowed to grow. The procedure is repeated until an isolated clone is picked, the progeny of which are all streptomycin resistant.*

flattened surface of a wood block with a diameter slightly less than the size of a petri dish. A plate containing colonies of bacterial cells is pressed against the velveteen, and the cells are transferred to the cloth. Sterile plates containing various selective media are then inverted onto the fabric and replicas of the initial plate are transferred to the selective media. By sequential plating, picking, and growing of the cells, as shown in Figure 6, one can eventually isolate a colony of bacteria, the progeny of which are all resistant to the selective agent, even though they never came into contact with the agent. Thus, bacteria are constantly undergoing mutation, and any change in the environment can select a cell that has a growth advantage over the parent cells.

*Mutation Rate.*   The rate at which mutation occurs is expressed as a probability of the event occurring per cell generation, or each time one cell divides to form two new cells. To determine the mutation rate it is necessary to know within a specified time the increase that has occurred in the number of cells and in the number of mutations. The mutation rate (a) can be expressed as $a = \dfrac{M_t - M_o}{N_t - N_o}$, where $M_o$ is the number of mutations present at time zero and $M_t$ is the number present at time t, and $N_0$ is the number of cells present at time zero and $N_t$ is the number of cells present at time t. Another method for the determination of mutation rate is based on the use of the fluctuation test. If there are tubes found in the fluctuation test in which no mutations are present at the time of plating, the mutation rate can be determined from the Poisson distribution, where ln $P_o = -m$. Although it is difficult to get an absolute value for the mutation rate because of various problems in lag of expression of the phenotype, in general, values range from $10^{-6}$ to $10^{-9}$; that is, there is a probability that a given type of mutant will be present to the extent of 1 mutant cell per $10^6$ to $10^9$ cell divisions. Even though mutant cells may be present at a low frequency, if the environment of such a culture is altered to give these cells a growth advantage, eventually this cell type will take over the population. For example, if one cell that is resistant to streptomycin is present in a population of $10^8$ streptomycin-sensitive cells, this one cell will survive if the culture is exposed to the antibiotic. That one mutant cell will eventually develop into a population of streptomycin-resistant organisms.

*Selection Procedures.*   In the study of microbial genetics, selection of specific mutant phenotypes depends on the ability to alter the environment of bacterial cells. It is from the study of mutants with altered growth properties and altered control mechanisms that one can begin to understand the normal and infectious properties of microorganisms. Thus, the basis for the study of microbial genetics is the ability to select from a large population a few cells that have the genetic characteristics one wishes to study. To this end various standard selection procedures have been developed to enable one to isolate particular types of mutant cells. Most of these studies have been done with *E. coli* or *Salmonella typhimurium,* because of the ability of these gram-negative enteric bacteria to grow on a minimal medium consisting of only salts, trace metals, and a carbon and nitrogen source. Provided with one of a variety of carbohydrates these bacteria have all the necessary enzymes and proteins to make all their necessary growth requirements, including amino acids, purines, pyrimidines, vitamins, and other metabolic intermediates. The organisms (as isolated from nature) with these genetic capabilities are referred to as *wild type* cells. Cells isolated from the wild type that differ in one or more genes are designated as *mutants*. Mutant strains with additional growth requirements are termed *auxotrophs*. The nomenclature used to designate these strains is given in Table 1. The compound usually is listed by the first three letters of the name, hence *ara* for arabinose and *his* for histidine, followed by + or −. Resistance or sensitivity to a particular environment is designated as $^s$ or $^r$. The following procedures have been developed to isolate various classes of mutants.

RESISTANCE.   This is the easiest type of mutant to isolate. The procedure involves plating a large number of sensitive organisms in the presence of the selective agent. Surviving clones are purified and are resistant to that agent. This method can be used to isolate cells resistant to bacteriophages, antibiotics, chemicals, or physical agents such as ultraviolet light or x-rays.

AUXOTROPHS.   This type of mutant is difficult to isolate because the parent cells grow as well as

### TABLE 1.   Notation of Genetic Markers

+: Ability to utilize a carbohydrate or synthesize an intermediate, usually wild-type

−: Lack of ability to utilize a carbohydrate or synthesize an intermediate, usually mutant

*Examples:*

$ara^+$:  Ability to utilize arabinose as a carbon and energy source

$ara^-$:  Inability to utilize arabinose as a carbon and energy source but will utilize other sugars

$his^+$:  Ability to synthesize histidine

$his^-$:  Inability to synthesize histine, requires histidine for growth, histidine auxotroph

s:  Sensitivity to agent—chemical or antibiotic

r:  Resistance to agent—chemical or antibiotic

*Examples:*

$str^s$:  Sensitive and will not grow in the presence of streptomycin

$str^r$:  Resistant and will grow in the presence or absence of streptomycin

the mutant under all conditions. The method for the isolation of auxotrophs makes use of the fact that the parent will grow under conditions in which the mutant will not. The antibiotic penicillin, which kills only growing cells, is used. Wild-type cells are placed in a minimal glucose medium containing penicillin and are incubated for 18 to 20 hours. During this time wild-type cells grow and are killed by the action of penicillin. Any auxotrophs present are not able to grow because of the lack of a specific growth factor and so are not killed by penicillin. The surviving cells are plated on a supplemented medium in the absence of penicillin. To select for a particular mutant among the survivors, the clones can be tested by replica plating on a large number of media containing different supplements; that is, a *his*⁻ auxotroph will be selected for by looking for growth on a medium with histidine, but no growth will occur when histidine is omitted. Using the penicillin method of selecting auxotrophs, mutants in nearly all known biosynthetic pathways that are coded for by the bacterial chromosomes of *E. coli* and *S. typhimurium* are now available.

FERMENTATION-NEGATIVE MUTANTS. A fermentation-negative mutant is a strain that has lost the ability to use a particular carbohydrate as a carbon and energy source but can still use other carbohydrates for growth. These mutants generally are deficient in the specific enzymes necessary for the catabolism of the specific carbohydrate. For example, mutants unable to use the carbohydrate lactose are deficient either in a protein necessary for the transport of the sugar into the cell or in the enzyme β-galactosidase, which catalyzes the breakdown of lactose into galactose and glucose. Such mutants can be isolated by combining the penicillin selection procedure with the identification of the specific mutant on a differential medium such as eosin-methylene blue (EMB) lactose medium or McConkey's lactose medium, in which the lactose-fermenting colonies give a color reaction (due to acid production) and the lactose-negative cells (*lac*⁻) show a lack of color. For the penicillin selection, the sugar lactose is used in place of glucose in the minimal medium with penicillin. Lactose-negative cells that are not growing survive, whereas the growing lactose-positive cells are killed.

CONDITIONAL LETHAL MUTANTS. Conditional lethal mutants have a mutation that is expressed under one set of environmental conditions but not under others. The environmental conditions in which the mutation is expressed do not permit growth and are referred to as *nonpermissive conditions*. Similarly, when the mutation is not expressed, conditions permit growth and are called *permissive conditions*. A major class of such mutants are temperature-sensitive mutants (*ts*). Such *ts* mutants will grow at a lower temperature (25° C) but will not survive at a higher temperature (42° C), whereas the wild-type cells are capable of growing at both temperatures. These mutants usually have a missense mutation that results in the production of a protein that will function normally at a low temperature but not at the higher temperature. A second class of conditional lethal mutants result from a nonsense mutation. Such mutants can grow only in the presence of a secondary mutation or in a suppressor strain that allows for correction of the mutational defect at the translational level. Conditional lethal mutants are extremely valuable, since they allow the isolation, where no other selection procedure exists, of mutants defective in essential functions. A *ts* mutant can be isolated by plating cells at the permissive temperature and then, by replica plating, screening clones that will not grow at the nonpermissive temperature. The defective function must then be determined by biochemical analysis of the *ts* mutants.

## GENE TRANSFER IN BACTERIA

Bacteria can exchange genetic material; however, the mechanisms of exchange differ strikingly from genetic exchange in eukaryotes. The three methods of gene transfer that occur in bacteria — *transformation, conjugation,* and *transduction* — have several features in common: 1) Only fragments of the chromosome of one parent (called the donor cell) are usually transferred to a second cell (called the recipient cell). 2) Fragments of the donor chromosome are assumed to pair with the homologous regions of the recipient chromosome. 3) After pairing, the genetic material of the donor usually replaces its allelic material on the recipient chromosome to yield haploid recombinants. This is referred to as *replacement integration*. 4) In some special instances, certain genetic elements (plasmids or bacteriophages) can recombine in total with the bacterial chromosome to form a composite molecule containing all the genetic material from both DNA molecules. This type of recombination is referred to as *additive recombination*.

### Transformation

Transformation is gene transfer resulting from the uptake by a recipient cell of naked DNA released by a donor cell. For example, DNA released or purified in the laboratory from a donor strain that is *str*ʳ is mixed with cells that are *str*ˢ. An aliquot of the mixture is plated on a nutrient medium containing streptomycin, and approximately 1 in 100 cells plated are capable of growth.

Thus, resistance to streptomycin has appeared with a frequency of $10^{-2}$. These $str^r$ cells do not arise from mutations, since mutation to $str^r$ occurs with a frequency of only 1 in $10^8$ cells plated, but rather must result from the transfer of the $str^r$ DNA to the recipients. This type of gene transfer was originally described by Griffith in 1928 while working with the pneumococcus. This organism is virulent to mice only if the strains produce a polysaccharide capsule and hence have a smooth appearance during colony growth. If the capsule is absent, as in rough strains, virulence is also absent. Griffith showed that injection into a mouse of heat-killed smooth strains of pneumococci plus live rough strains killed the mouse and that live smooth pneumococci appeared in the dead mouse. He did not understand the mechanisms involved but suggested the name of "transforming factor" for the agent responsible for this phenomenon. In 1944, Avery, Macleod, and McCarty showed that the factor involved was DNA.

Transformation takes place in a large number of gram-negative and gram-positive bacteria, including *Pneumococcus, Hemophilus, Bacillus, Neisseria, Streptococcus, Xanthomonas,* and *Rhizobium.* Studies on transformation have been carried out in the laboratory, in most cases with *Pneumococcus, Hemophilus,* or *Bacillus.* More recently it has been found that *E. coli* also can undergo transformation if high concentrations of calcium ion are present.

In the interaction of transforming DNA with recipient cells, three determinants appear to be of major importance:

*The size of the DNA.* DNA that can transform cells has a minimum molecular weight of about 5 $\times 10^5$ but may be as large as $10^8$. Double-stranded DNA is many times more efficient for transformation than are single-stranded DNA structures.

*The concentration of the DNA.* Transformation is a function of DNA concentration. At a concentration of DNA below 100 m$\mu$g/ml, the number of transformants is proportional to the DNA concentration. This indicates that each transformant arises from the interaction of a recipient with a single molecule of transforming DNA. DNA that is foreign to the bacterial recipient DNA can also be taken up if it is double stranded. Thus, *Pneumococcus* can take up calf thymus DNA. Such foreign DNA, however, does not integrate into the recipient DNA and thus cannot transform.

*The physiologic state of the recipient cell.* In order for a recipient cell to take up DNA it must be in a physiologic state called *competence.* The period in the growth cycle when competence appears can vary with each bacterial species but generally appears near the end of the growth phase, just before the stationary phase (Fig. 7).

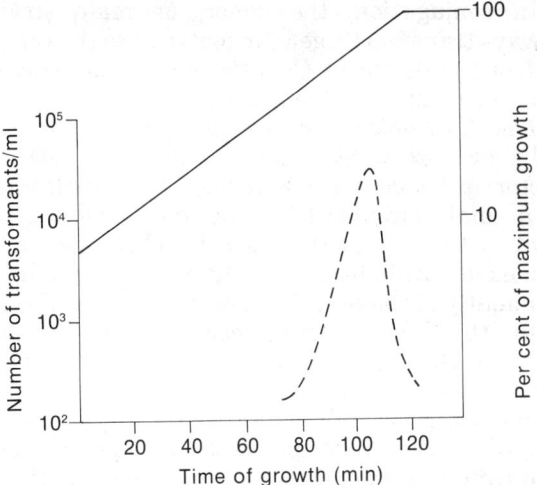

**FIGURE 7.** *The appearance of competence during cell growth. During cell growth (——) samples are removed from the culture and tested for their ability to be transformed (---). Competence peaks in late log phase.*

This is usually a transient state, but cells can be maintained in the competent state by freezing at $-40°$ C in 10 to 15 per cent glycerol. Competence is genetically controlled, and a protein can be extracted from competent cells that can make noncompetent cells competent. The mechanism of action of this protein, as well as the biochemical basis for competence, are unknown.

In the process of transformation, double-stranded DNA binds to the surface of the recipient cells. This DNA is cut by a membrane-bound endonuclease, and entry of the DNA is initiated. The uptake of the DNA occurs with digestion of one of the two complementary strands and the entrance into the cell of the other strand of DNA. This single-stranded piece of DNA is then integrated into the recipient cell at the homologous region of DNA replacing the recipient allele. The initial recombinant formed has a short region of the DNA that is part donor DNA and part recipient DNA. However, during the first replication cycle each strand of DNA is replicated faithfully and a new haploid cell emerges that now carries some new genetic information derived from the donor cell.

## Conjugation

Conjugation is gene transfer that occurs between sexually differentiated bacteria. It requires cell-to-cell contact between two viable cells, a donor, or male cell, and a recipient, or female cell. Conjugation was discovered in 1946 by Lederberg and Tatum and was shown to differ from transformation. The gene transfer they described was resistant to the action of DNAse and needed physical contact between two cells.

In conjugation, the donor, or male strain, always transfers its genetic material to the recipient, or female strain. Genetic material does not go from the female to the male cell.

***The Sex Factor.*** Male cells differ from female cells by possessing a factor called the fertility factor, or *F factor*. The F factor, a typical plasmid, is a small, circular DNA molecule, about 2 per cent of the size of the bacterial chromosome. It can exist within bacterial cells and replicate independently of the host chromosome. Male cells carrying the F factor can be recognized by the presence on the cell surface of a protein appendage referred to as an *F pilus* (see Chap. 1). The F pilus serves as a receptor site for the binding of various male-specific bacteriophages that can contain either DNA or RNA. The genetic information for the synthesis of the F pilus is contained in a series of genes located in the F factor. When the F factor is in the autonomous state, that is, not associated with the chromosome, the host cells are referred to as *$F^+$ cells*. $F^+$ cells are capable of transferring the F factor to recipient, or *$F^-$ cells,* upon cell-to-cell contact. Within a short time as many as 70 per cent of the $F^-$ cells can become $F^+$ cells. However, the $F^+$ cells remain $F^+$, suggesting that the factor must be replicated sometime during or before the transfer to the $F^-$ cells. In a cross between an $F^+$ and an $F^-$ cell one can detect a few recombinants for some bacterial markers with a frequency of about $10^{-5}$.

***Hfr Strains.*** In 1950, Cavelli isolated a male strain of bacteria that was unusual in that it had a 1000-fold increase in the frequency with which recombinants appeared, and it did not transfer the F factor to the recipients except in very rare instances. Such strains, and there are many now that have been isolated, are called *Hfr strains,* or high frequency of recombination strains. These strains arise in $F^+$ populations and are the result of the association of the F factor with the bacterial chromosome (see later discussion).

With the finding of Hfr strains that showed such high recombination values, the kinetics of the conjugation process could be investigated. Such studies were initiated in the late 1950s by Jacob and Wollman with the development of interrupted mating experiments. An interrupted mating experiment is performed by mixing together male and female cells in a ratio of 1 Hfr to 20 female cells. The female cells contain a series of genetic defects, for example: $thr^-$, auxotrophic for threonine; $leu^-$, auxotrophic for leucine; $lac^-$, unable to ferment lactose; $gal^-$, unable to ferment galactose; $azi^s$, sensitive to azide; $T_1^s$, sensitive to the phage T1; and $str^r$, resistant to streptomycin. In contrast, the male strain carries the opposite markers, that is, sensitive to streptomycin, resistant to azide and T1; prototrophic for threonine

and leucine, and ferments both lactose and galactose. The two cultures are mixed at high density for five minutes, and are then diluted to stop additional pair formation. At this point samples are removed at timed intervals. The samples are agitated violently to break up the mating pairs, then aliquots are plated on various selective media to determine what genetic information has been transferred from the Hfr strain to the recipient strain. The media are made so that neither parent strain is able to grow. For example, including streptomycin will eliminate growth of the Hfr; the absence of threonine or leucine will prevent growth of $F^-$ cells unless they have received the respective genes from the donor. Data from a typical mating experiment are shown in Figure 8. Several things are characteristic of these experiments: 1) The curves do not go through the origin. Thus, if the mating is interrupted at zero time no recombinants are formed. However, the longer the mating time, the more genetic material is transferred, so that at 30 minutes all the tested markers have appeared in the recipient — some to a greater and some to a lesser extent. 2) The time that a curve begins to rise represents the time of entry of the marker into the recipient. Thus, 18 minutes is the time that lactose enters the recipient. 3) The timed order of transfer reflects the order of genes on the chromosome and is characteristic of a particular Hfr strain. In the example in Figure 8, the first marker to enter the recipient is the azide gene, followed by T1, *lac*,

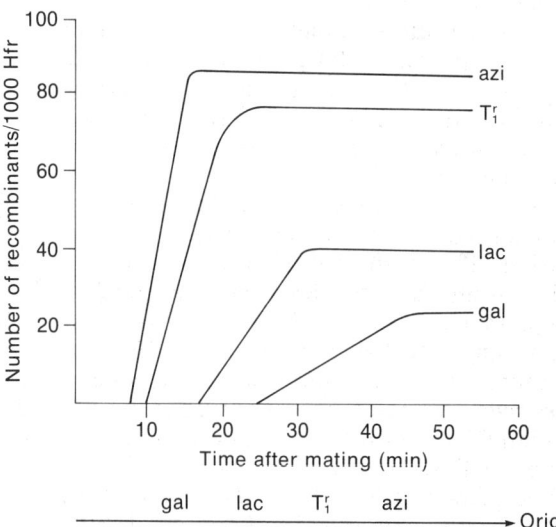

**FIGURE 8.** *Interrupted mating between Hfr and $F^-$ cells. An Hfr strain is mixed with a genetically marked $F^-$ strain (see text). At the specified time, samples are taken, the mating is stopped by vigorous agitation, and aliquots are plated on various selective media. The data are summarized in the bottom arrow and give the order of transfer of the markers from the Hfr to the $F^-$ cell.*

and *gal*, in that order. Since the time of entrance is dependent on their location on the chromosome, one can construct a chromosome map by timing the genes entering the F⁻ cell. Such mapping is usually only accurate within one minute.

Different Hfr strains vary in the time that certain markers enter the recipient and in their point of origin (defined as the part of the chromosome that is first to enter the recipient), but the order of genetic markers with respect to each other does not change. Let us assume that we have three different Hfr strains, and the genetic markers are represented as A, B, C, D, and E, with O representing the point of origin. Interrupted mating experiments between each Hfr and the same recipient give the following pattern of gene transfer. Hfr-1 transfers the markers as — O-D-C-B-A-E, Hfr-2 transfers the markers as — O-A-B-C-D-E, and Hfr-3 transfers the markers as — O-B-C-D-E-A. All the data, however, are consistent if we assume that the chromosome is a circular structure that can be broken at any point. The point of rupture becomes the point of origin of transfer, but the direction of transfer can be either clockwise or counterclockwise, as shown in Figure 9. Indeed, this is exactly what happens. The F factor, which exists in the cytoplasm, will sometimes associate itself with the bacterial chromosome. It does so as illustrated in Figure 10. The circular DNA structure that is the F factor will associate with specific areas on the chromosome. The two circular structures will break and recombine with one another, allowing complete integration of the F factor DNA into the chromo-

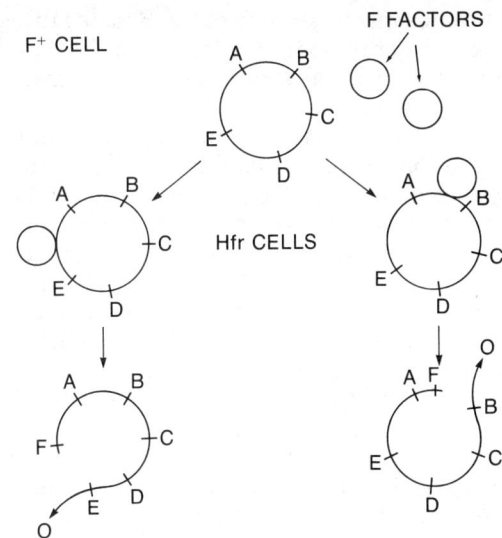

**FIGURE 10.**   *Association of the F factor with the bacterial chromosome. The F factor can integrate into the chromosome at various sites that have an area of base pair homology. The site of intergration will determine the point of origin for the Hfr during transfer of the DNA to an F⁻ cell.*

somal DNA. The point at which the F factor integrates will determine the point of origin of a particular Hfr strain as well as the direction of marker transfer. During the transfer, part of the F factor will be the last marker to enter the F⁻ cell. The entire chromosome is not usually transferred during the mating, since it is ruptured before the end is transferred explaining why the F⁻ recipient in a cross with an Hfr strain does not become male.

F-PRIME FACTORS.   Hfr strains are not always stable, and sometimes the F factor will be lost from the chromosome, once again giving an F⁺ cell. In most cases this reversal results in the original F factor as well as the complete bacterial chromosome. Occasionally, however, the F factor will bring with it part of the bacterial chromosome and is then called an F-prime (F′) factor. These F′-factors are designated by the bacterial genes they carry. For example, if an F factor carries the genes for lactose fermentation it is referred to as an F′-*lac* plasmid. These factors can transfer the attached bacterial genes with high frequency to recipient cells and have been used extensively to do complementation analyses in bacteria cells.

KINETICS OF TRANSFER.   When a culture of Hfr cells is mixed with an excess of F⁻ cells, the Hfr cell attaches to the F⁻ cell by way of the F-pilus. The tip of the pilus attaches to the gram-negative wall of the recipient, and the cells are brought into direct contact — presumably by retraction of the F pilus. When pair formation occurs there is some form of signal that initiates replication of

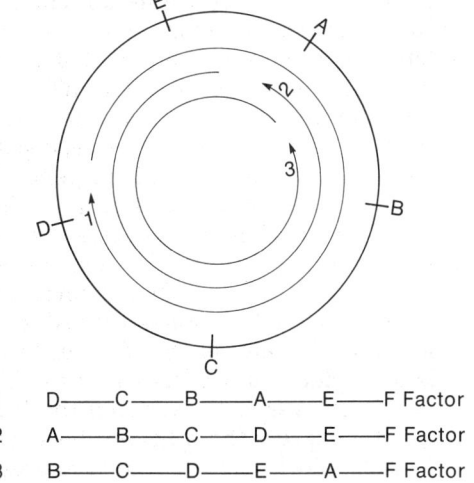

| 1 | D——C——B——A——E——F Factor |
| 2 | A——B——C——D——E——F Factor |
| 3 | B——C——D——E——A——F Factor |

**FIGURE 9.**   *Genetic evidence that the bacterial chromosome is a circular structure. Data from interrupted mating experiments with Hfr 1, Hfr 2, or Hfr 3 and the same F⁻ strain give the order of transfer of markers as shown, with the F factor the last marker to enter. These data are consistent with a circular chromosome, which can be broken at various points.*

the chromosome at the site of the F factor integration. As the chromosome is replicated in the Hfr strain, one parental strand of DNA passes into the recipient cell, and the other remains in the donor cell (see Figure 11). In both the donor and the recipient cells complementary strands are synthesized during the transfer. Rarely is the entire chromosome transferred, although plasmids not associated with the chromosome are transferred in total by the same mechanisms. The piece of chromosome that is transferred to the recipient is presumed to align itself with the homologous region on the recipient chromosome, followed by replacement of the recipient allele by the donor allele. The progeny of the initial recombinant event are thus haploid. In the case in which F′ factors are transferred to the recipient cells, the progeny of the recombination event become partially diploid for the genes carried on the F factor. This is true even if the F′ factor integrates into the chromosome, because it does so by additive recombination.

## Plasmids

The F factor discussed previously is a prototype of other small extrachromosomal genetic elements that exist in bacterial cells. These elements, termed *plasmids,* replicate autonomously and often confer new genetic properties on the bacterial host cell. The plasmids can be divided into two major classes: *transmissible plasmids,* which have the ability to initiate their own transfer by cell-to-cell contact; and *nontransmissible plasmids,* which lack the ability to promote their own transfer by cell-to-cell contact. Non-

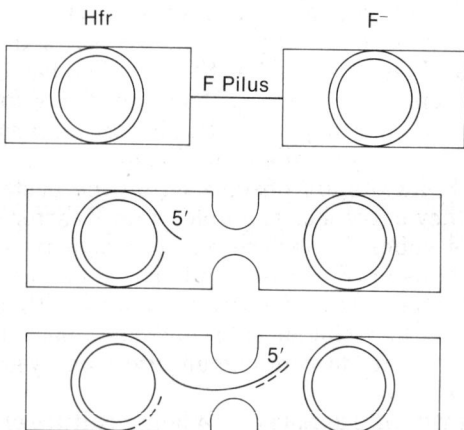

**FIGURE 11.** *Transfer of DNA from an Hfr cell to F⁻ cell. The cells become connected by way of the F pilus, which can act as a grappling hook to bring the two cells in contact. The chromosome in the donor breaks and begins replication with the transfer of one of the original donor DNA strands into the F⁻ cell. The DNA enters the F⁻ cells with a leading 5′ end and is replicated inside the F⁻ cell. Simultaneous replication of the donor DNA occurs in the Hfr cell.*

transmissible plasmids can be transferred from one bacterial cell to another by transduction, or transformation, or mobilization by a self-transmissible plasmid. Among the best characterized transmissible plasmids are F factors, antibiotic resistance factors (R factors), and some of the Colicinogenic factors (Col factors).

### Transmissible Plasmids

F FACTORS. The sex factor is best characterized for its mediation of conjugation and is a circular double-stranded DNA molecule with a molecular weight of $60 \times 10^6$. The F factor carries a number of genes, 13 of which are involved in the transmission of the plasmid (*tra* genes). The plasmid controls its own replication in the autonomous state allowing only one or two copies of the plasmid per cell. Transmission of the F factor is dependent on the presence of the F pilus. The pilus is expressed in all cells carrying the F factor and can be identified by the sensitivity of such cells to male-specific viruses that use the pilus as a receptor site. F factors cannot coexist in the same cell with some types of plasmids. Two plasmids that cannot coexist are said to be in the same incompatibility group. In addition, autonomous F factors cannot coexist in a cell that has an integrated F factor (Hfr strain). All transmissible plasmids studied to date appear to have analogous *tra* systems for the transfer of the plasmid from cell to cell.

R FACTORS. The R factors are plasmids that carry genes determining resistance to antibiotics. Some R plasmids consist of two components, the RTF, or resistance transfer factor (analogous to the F factor), and the r determinants. The r determinant portion of the R factor carries one or more genes that code for proteins that abolish the effectiveness of various antibiotics. The RTF component is similar in size to the F factor, but the r determinant component varies in size, depending on the number of genes carried. In general, the composite R factors have a molecular weight of about 60 to $70 \times 10^6$. The two components of the R factor are connected by insertion sequences (see further on) on both sides of the r determinant to give a single, closed double-stranded circular DNA molecule. Transfer of the R factor from cell to cell is dependent on a pilus structure. Unlike the F⁺ cells, however, cells carrying the R factor do not usually express the pilus on the surface of the cell. Only newly infected cells express the pilus, allowing for a rapid transfer of the R factor from R⁺ to R⁻ cells, followed by a repression of the pilus formation after several generations. The structure of the pilus of the R factor differs from that of the F pilus. One group of R factors, however, has an F-like pilus (that is, sensitive to

F-specific viruses), whereas other R factors code for other types of pili (that is, I-like pili). R factors can be grouped by incompatibility or compatibility with each other and with the F factor. (See Chapter 21 for further discussion of R factors.)

Other transmissible plasmids in *E. coli* have been associated with toxins that produce diarrhea in animals and in man. Certain *E. coli* produce two enterotoxins, a low molecular weight heat-stable toxin (ST) and a heat-labile toxin (LT), that have many properties similar to cholera toxin. The *E. coli* ST and LT are both coded for by plasmid genes and are often associated with the presence of drug-resistant factors and, in some porcine strains, the production of alpha hemolysin and the K88 antigen responsible for attachment to the bowel mucosa. It appears that LT and ST may be coded for by the same plasmid.

COL FACTORS.   Colicinogenic factors are plasmids that code for bactericidal substances called *colicins* or *bacteriocins*. These substances are proteins that kill closely related strains of bacteria that do not carry the same plasmid. As with the F factor and the R factor, the Col factors are closed, double-stranded circular DNA molecules. Col factors that are transmissible and classified as group II have a molecular weight of 60 to 110 $\times$ $10^6$. They carry a *tra* system analogous to the F factor, allowing transfer by cell-to-cell contact. The Col factors are designated by capital letters. Group II contains the factors B, I, and V. These factors show controlled replication and have one or two copies per cell. Like the F factor they code for a pilus structure that is involved in their transmission from cell to cell. Col factors can also transfer chromosomal genes and form strains analogous to Hfr strains. The colicins produced act by binding to receptors in the outer membrane of sensitive bacterial cells. After some rearrangement, they come into contact with the cytoplasmic membrane and exert their effect. The different colicins act in killing sensitive cells by a variety of mechanisms that include degradation of DNA and RNA, interference with the energy system of the cells, and inactivation of ribosome structure with inhibition of protein synthesis. It appears that only a few cells in a Col$^+$ population actually produce the colicin, whereas most of the cells are in a repressed state similar to that seen in lysogenic cells. Like lysogenic cells, the repression is destroyed by exposing the cells to agents such as mitomycin C. Although most of the studies on colicins have been in gram-negative organisms, recent work has focused on similar substances produced by gram-positive organisms. For example, in the group D streptococcus there has been described a streptocin that appears to be coded for by genes on a self-transmissible plasmid.

### Nontransmissible Plasmids

COL FACTORS.   The nontransmissible Col factors include the factors E$_1$, E$_2$, E$_3$, K, and D. These plasmids are much smaller than the transmissible plasmids and have molecular weights from 3 to 6 $\times$ $10^6$. This group of Col factors also differs from group II by having between 5 and 25 copies of the factor produced per chromosome-equivalent under a variety of growth conditions, suggesting a relaxed control of replication.

STAPHYLOCOCCAL PLASMIDS.   The best known plasmid occurring in *Staphylococcus* carries a gene for the determination of penicillinase, rendering the bacterial cell resistant to the action of penicillin. Other plasmids also occur in this organism, giving resistance to other antimicrobial agents. Self-transmissable plasmids have not been described in the staphylococcus, but transfer of plasmids by transduction has been shown to occur both in vitro and in vivo.

### Insertion Sequences and Recombination of Plasmids

Plasmids have the ability to recombine with each other as well as with the bacterial host chromosome. This ability is mainly due to the presence in the plasmids and in the bacterial chromosome of insertion sequences (IS). Insertion sequences are segments of DNA that have a specific base sequence and range in length from 800 to 1400 base pairs. They have been designated as IS1, IS2, IS3, IS4, and so on. The insertion sequences IS1, IS2, and IS3 are found at numerous points on the *E. coli* chromosome. Identical IS elements are found in various R factors, lambda phages, and F factors. The presence of these common base sequences allows for these various genomes to recombine and form new combinations of genes. Insertion sequences belong to a group of elements known as transposable elements, defined as segments of DNA that, as discrete genetic and physical entities, can move from one position in a genome to another position in the same or different genome. The IS elements are elements containing no known genes unrelated to the insertion function. More complex elements are the *Tn elements,* which contain IS segments usually as an inverted repeat on either end of the DNA fragment and additional genes unrelated to the insertion function. Many of the Tn elements are translocatable drug-resistance elements such as Tn10 (a tetracycline-resistant element) that can translocate from its position on an R factor to the bacterial chromosome and then to a bacteriophage. Other drug-resistance Tn elements have been described, such as Tn5 (kanamycin resistance) and Tn9 (chloramphenicol resistance), and are often referred to as *transposons.* More complex transposable elements are the plasmids or viruses that can contain both IS segments and Tn elements in addition to other genes needed for replication and transmission, that is, R factors. Thus, insertion sequence elements can act as sites for joining various DNA segments and allowing for new arrangements of genes in bacteria. This process results in optimal growth of the bacteria under a variety of changing environmental conditions and helps ensure survival.

### Transduction

Transduction is the transfer of genetic information from a donor cell to a recipient cell by way of a virus vector. For the most part transduction is carried out by temperate DNA-containing bacteriophages. A temperature phage is a virus that can either lyse or lysogenize a host cell upon infection. In the lysogenic response, the genes of the virus that are responsible for initiating the lytic response are repressed, and the viral DNA is integrated into the host DNA by a mechanism similar to the integration of the F factor. In the integrated, or *prophage,* state the virus genes replicate with the host cell genes and all daughter cells will have a viral gene integrated into their chromosome. Bacterial cells that have a viral genome integrated into their chromosome are called *lysogenic cells.* They differ from nonlysogenic cells in two respects: 1) they are immune to superinfection by the same type virus, and 2) they usually can be induced to produce virus particles without infection from the outside. A repressor gene product produced by the virus maintains the repressed and integrated state by preventing transcription of the lytic genes of the virus. Induction of a lysogenic cell to enter the lytic cycle occurs when this repressor protein is destroyed or prevented from functioning.

There are three major types of transduction: 1) *generalized transduction,* in which any genetic marker can be transduced, and the donor DNA is integrated by replacement of the recipient allele; 2) *specialized* or *restricted transduction,* in which only markers that are adjacent to the site where the viral DNA is integrated into the host DNA are transduced, and integration is usually by additive recombination; 3) *abortive transduction,* in which any marker can be transduced, but the DNA is not integrated into the recipient chromosome.

*Generalized Transduction.* To carry out generalized transduction, a bacterial culture is infected with a temperate virus under conditions of low multiplicity of infection (moi) of about .01 to 0.1 phage particles per cell. The culture is then allowed to grow through several cycles of phage development until most of the cells have been infected and lysed. During the maturation of the viral particles an occasional mistake is made and instead of packaging viral DNA, host DNA of the same size is put into the viral protein coat. These particles, which are now the *transducing particles,* are characterized by the fact that they contain only host DNA and no phage DNA. When an appropriately marked recipient strain is then mixed with this lysate at an moi of 5 phage particles to each cell, some cells will be infected by both a normal particle and a transducing, or defective, particle. By plating aliquots of the infected culture on appropriate selective media, one selects for transductants that now have donor DNA incorporated into the recipient DNA. Such generalized transductants can be selected for any genetic marker and arise at a frequency of about $10^{-5}$ or one transductant for every $10^5$ phage particles added. The transductants are characterized by being stable once they are formed, which is a result of the fact that the donor DNA has replaced the recipient DNA during the process. The size of the DNA that can be transduced is dependent on the size of the virus but is generally about 1 per cent of the size of the bacterial chromosome. Only closely linked genetic markers can be cotransduced on the same DNA particle, which enables transduction to be used for the genetic mapping of closely linked genes.

*Abortive Transduction.* During the process of generalized transduction, as described previously, there are instances when the donor DNA that is injected into the recipient cells does not integrate into the recipient DNA. These cells are referred to as *abortive transductants.* The piece of donor DNA exists in the recipient cell and is capable of functioning normally; however, it is not capable of being replicated. The result is that only one cell at any time in the population derived from the initially infected cell carries the DNA piece. The other daughter cells will receive, upon cell division, products coded for by the DNA and thus will be capable of carrying out several cell divisions until the protein product has become diluted out. As a result only minute colonies are formed by abortive transduction, although they may appear at 100 times the frequency of stable generalized transductants. Abortive transductants are seen only if two negative phenotypes happen to be defective in different genes, and thus, it is a useful method for carrying out complementation analyses.

*Specialized Transduction.* Specialized transduction is limited to genes that are adjacent to the site of prophage integration. This is clearly due to the mechanism by which specialized transducing particles are formed. Such particles can only be generated by starting with a bacteria culture that has been made lysogenic. Such a culture of cells when treated with short doses of ultraviolet light will lose the active viral repressor protein and begin to enter the lytic cycle. During this process the viral DNA is detached from the host DNA by a reversal of the mechanism by which it had been integrated. In the majority of cases this detachment is performed without any mistake, and a normal virus genome is released. However, in 1 in $10^6$ cells this excision will result in a mistake, and a particle will be released that now carries part of the viral DNA and part of the bacterial DNA (Fig. 12). In the case of lambda phage, the host DNA carried will be either the genes for galactose fermentation or the genes for biotin synthesis. These two loci occur on either side of the integrated virus. These particles are referred to as λ*dgal* or λ*dbio*, which stands for lambda-defective galactose or biotin. The particles are termed defective because they are missing part of the viral genes and cannot carry out a normal productive infection of a bacterial cell without the presence of a

normal viral particle. They will, however, inject their hybrid DNA into a recipient cell. The DNA will integrate at the homologous site on the recipient DNA by adding to the chromosome rather than by replacing the recipient allele. The transductants produced are therefore partially diploid for this region of the bacterial chromosome and are termed *heterogenotes*. In addition to carrying the defective particle, most of these transductants will also carry a normal phage genome and thus can be considered to be doubly lysogenic. The presence of the donor DNA is detected by infecting a *gal⁻* recipient with the lysate produced by ultraviolet irradiation of the lysogenic cells and then plating samples onto plates containing EMB-galactose medium. Cells that have received the galactose genes will give dark clones with a green sheen on this medium. If these galactose-positive clones are picked and restreaked, it is found that they are unstable. That is, in 1 in $10^3$ cell divisions, segregation of a galactose-negative clone will result. This is due to the loss of the λ*dgal* particle in some cells at division. The initial number of galactose-positive transductants found is about 1 in $10^5$ galactose-negative cells infected. If, however, one starts with a heterogenote clone and treats it with ultraviolet light to produce the lysate, a lysate is found that can now transduce the *gal* genes at a very high frequency. About 1 in 10 *gal⁻* cells infected can become galactose-positive. These lysates are referred to as *HFT,* or *high frequency transducing,* lysates. They occur because the lysate from the heterozygote has many particles carrying the *gal* genes, approximately one half of the viral particles produced. This is a result of the presence in the heterogenote of a normal virus particle that allows for replication of the defective particle in each cell in the culture.

## REGULATION OF GENE EXPRESSION

Bacteria have evolved rather intricate and elegant mechanisms to control the phenotypic expression of their genotype. In catabolic pathways, the enzymes needed for the breakdown of a substrate are expressed only if the substrate is available in the environment. In anabolic pathways, if the end-product is available in the environment the enzymes needed for the synthesis of that product are not expressed. When mutants became available that had lost their ability to control the synthesis of the enzymes involved in these pathways, an understanding of what was occurring at the molecular level began. The basic mechanism of control was elaborated by the work of Jacob and Monod in 1961 and is referred to as the *operon theory.* In this theory they describe two

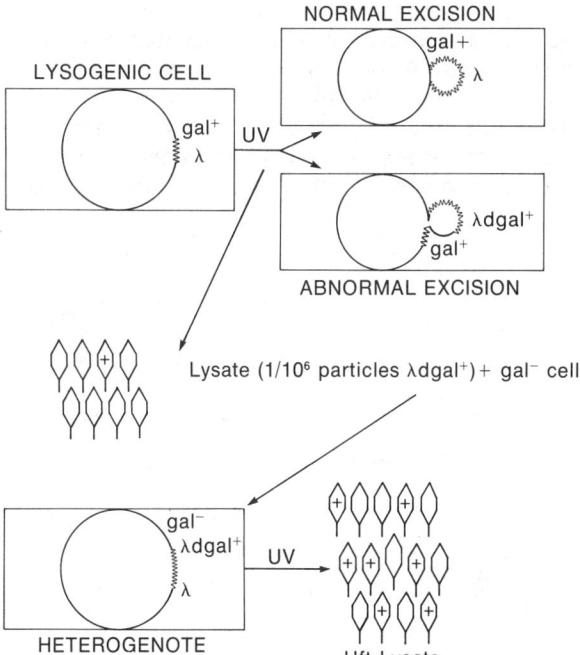

**FIGURE 12.** *Specialized transduction of the galactose genes in E. coli by lambda phage. A lysogenic cell is treated with UV light to cause cells to undergo the lytic cycle. In nearly all cells, excision of the virus is normal, and normal virus particles result. In one in 10⁶ cells, abnormal excision takes place giving a defective particle λdgal⁺. The presence of λdgal⁺ particles in the lysate can be shown by mixing the lysate with a gal⁻ strain and selecting for gal⁺ transductants. Many of these transductants will be heterogenotes and will carry both λdgal⁺ and normal λ. Ultraviolet irradiation of these cells yields a lysate that is half normal particle and half λdgal⁺ particles or an HFT lysate. These result because the normal λ particles will provide the functions missing in λdgal⁺ and allow its replication in each cell.*

major classes of genes: 1) *structural genes* — genes that specify the structure of a specific protein such as an enzyme, and 2) *regulatory genes, or sites* — genes, or sites, on the chromosome that control the rate of synthesis of the structural genes. The operon is defined as a group of contiguous structural genes showing coordinate expression, together with their closely linked controlling sites. The best understood operon, that concerned with the catabolism of lactose, is diagrammed in Figure 13. This type of control is referred to as *negative control,* since the presence of a repressor protein, which is bound to a site on the DNA called the operator site, prevents the synthesis of the mRNA from the structural genes. In the presence of the substrate or inducer, the structure of the repressor product is altered so that it no longer binds to the DNA, and mRNA production begins. The site at which mRNA synthesis is initiated by RNA polymerase is called the promoter site. This is also the site for the action of another regulator molecule, the cAMP activator protein − cAMP complex.

Mutations that occur in the structural genes usually result in the loss of enzyme activity caused by the alteration of the protein structure. Mutations that occur in the regulatory gene or controlling sites result either in strains that cannot be induced to produce enzymes *(noninducible)* or in strains that always produce the enzymes, even in the absence of the inducer *(constitutive).* To determine whether such mutations have occurred in the regulator gene or in the operator site, partial diploid studies are carried out using *F'lac* factors that carry different forms of the mutated genes (Fig. 14). In a diploid study, constitutivity is recessive to the wild-type inducible state if the regulator has been altered but is dominant

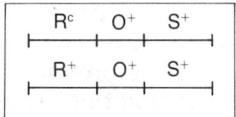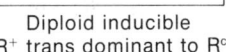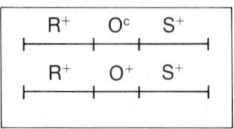

Diploid inducible     Diploid constitutive
$R^+$ trans dominant to $R^c$    $O^c$ cis dominant to $O^+$

**FIGURE 14.** *Differentiation of constitutive mutants as mutations in the regulator gene ($R^c$) or the operator site ($O^c$) in an operon under negative control. Partial diploids are constructed with F'-lac plasmids and then assayed for S enzyme activity after growth in the presence and absence of the inducer. Mutations in the R gene are constitutive because of the lack of repressor, and these are recessive and inducible in the presence of a wild-type repressor. Mutations in the O site are constitutive because they do not bind repressor and thus are dominant and still constitutive in the presence of the wild-type repressor.*

to the wild-type inducible state if the alteration has occurred in the operator site. If the regulator has been altered to give a noninducible state, this is dominant to both inducibility and constitutivity (Fig. 15).

A more complex but similar control pattern is seen in the pathway for the catabolism of arabinose. This operon is under *positive control.* Positive control differs from negative control in that it requires the presence of an activator protein to initiate mRNA transcription by RNA polymerase. Diploid studies in a positive control system give a different pattern than that seen in a negative control system. In this case alteration of the regulator to give the noninducible state is reces-

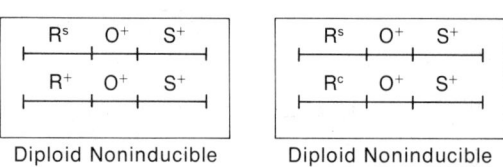

Diploid Noninducible     Diploid Noninducible

$R^s$ trans dominant to $R^+$ and $R^c$ in negative control

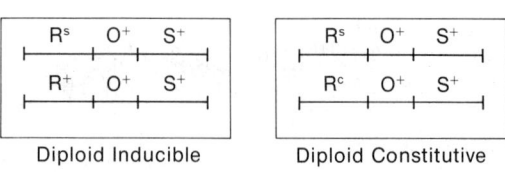

Diploid Inducible     Diploid Constitutive

$R^s$ recessive to $R^+$ and $R^c$ in positive control

**FIGURE 15.** *Differentiation of negative and positive control by partial diploid studies. $R^s$, or noninducible, strains in a negative control system result from the production of a mutated repressor that no longer binds the inducer and thus remains attached to the operative site. This $R^s$ repressor will also bind to the operative site on the opposite DNA strand and thus is dominant both to wild type and constitutivity. The $R^s$, or noninducible, state in positive control systems results from lack of production of an activator protein. Thus, the absence of the product makes the $R^s$ state recessive to either the presence of the wild-type activator or an altered $R^c$ constitutive activator.*

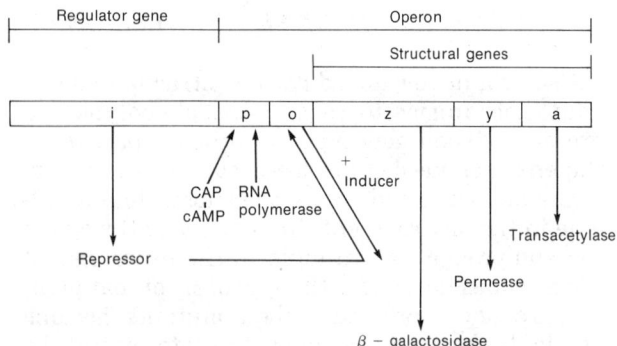

**FIGURE 13.** *The operon model for regulation of lactose fermentation. The repressor, the product of the regulator gene, prevents the synthesis of mRNA for the structural genes, z, y, and a, by binding to the operator site O. Addition of the inducer prevents the repressor from binding at O, and mRNA synthesis is initiated at the promoter, or p, site by RNA polymerase. The promotor site also has a binding site for the CAP-cAMP complex.*

sive to the wild-type inducible state. Likewise, constitutivity is dominant to noninducibility (Fig. 15). These results are consistent with a requirement for the presence of an activator protein to get expression of the operon.

Catabolite repression is an additional control mechanism that has evolved in bacterial cells and is superimposed on the operator-repressor interaction seen in both negative and positive control. It has been known for many years that bacterial cells growing in the presence of glucose will not use a carbon source that requires inducible enzyme synthesis until all of the glucose has been used. It is now known that in the presence of glucose, the level of cAMP in bacterial cells drops from $10^{-4}$ M to $10^{-7}$ M. cAMP is essential for the initiation of mRNA transcription. This compound binds to a protein called CAP or *catabolite gene activator product,* and this complex interacts with the DNA at the promotor site to stimulate transcription. This is a general control mechanism added to the very specific controls seen within each catabolic pathway.

## References

Avery, O. T., Macleod, C. M., and McCarty, M.: Studies on the chemical nature of the substance inducing transformation of pneumococcal types. J Exp Med 79:137, 1944.

Griffith, F.: The significance of pneumococcal types. J Hyg 27:113, 1928.

Hayes, W.: The Genetics of Bacteria and their Viruses. 2nd ed. New York, John Wiley & Sons, 1968.

Jacob, F., and Brenner, S.: Sur la régulation de la synthése du DNA chez les bacteries: 1'hypothèse du replicon. C R Acad Sci (Paris), 256:298, 1963.

Jacob, F., and Monod, J.: Genetic regulatory mechanisms in the synthesis of proteins. J Mol Biol 3:318, 1961.

Jacob, F., and Wollman, F.: Sur les processus de conjugaison et de recombination genetique chez *E. coli.* Ann Inst Pasteur 91:486, 1956.

Lederberg, J., and Lederberg, E. M.: Replica plating and indirect selection of bacterial mutants. J Bacteriol 63:399, 1952.

Lederberg, J., and Tatum, E.L.: Gene recombination in *E. coli.* Nature 158:582, 1946.

Luria, S.E., and Delbrück, M.: Mutations of bacteria from virus sensitivity to virus resistance. Genetics 28:491, 1943.

Meselson, M., and Stahl, F.: The replication of DNA in *Escherichia coli.* Proc Natl Acad Sci USA 44:671, 1958.

Stanier, R., Doudoroff, M., and Adelberg, E. A.: The Microbial World. 3rd ed. Englewood Cliffs, N.J., Prentice Hall, 1970.

Watson, J. D.: The Molecular Biology of the Gene. 3rd ed. New York, Benjamin Company, Inc., 1976.

Watson, J.D., and Crick, F.H.C.: Genetic implications of the structure of DNA. Nature 171:964, 1953.

# *BACTERIAL EXOTOXINS* **5**

## *William Edward van Heyningen, Ph.D., Sc.D.*

There are not more than three or four infectious diseases for which we have a reasonably clear understanding of the means by which the infecting organism brings about its harmful effects. The ability of the organism to grow in the body is not the same thing as its capacity to produce disease, for there is no intrinsic reason why the mere presence of a very small weight of infecting organisms in the body of the patient — from a few micrograms in tetanus to 100 mg at most in anthrax — should be harmful. The idea that pathogenic organisms produce poisons is an old and obvious one, and it is indeed a fact that many pathogenic bacteria do produce antigenic poisons,

TABLE 1.   Differences Between Bacterial Exotoxins and Endotoxins

|  | EXOTOXINS | ENDOTOXINS |
|---|---|---|
| Parent organisms | gram-positive and gram-negative | gram-negative |
| Within or without parent organism | within and without | within |
| Chemical nature | simple protein | protein-lipid-polysaccharide |
| Stability to heating (100°) | labile | stable |
| Detoxification by formaldehyde | detoxified | not detoxified |
| Neutralization by homologous antibody | complete | partial |
| Biologic activity | individual to toxin | same for all toxins |
| Toxicity compared with strychnine as 1 | 100 to 1,000,000 | 0.1 |

usually known as toxins. There are two types of toxins — the exotoxins, which are discussed in this chapter, and the endotoxins, which are discussed in Chapter 6. The differences between these two types of toxin are shown in Table 1. The harmful effects of endotoxins are perhaps due more to their immunologic properties than to their comparatively low toxicity, but their pathologic importance must not be underestimated.

Table 2 lists the better known bacterial exotoxins. The fact that a pathogenic organism produces a particular exotoxin does not necessarily mean that this toxin plays an important part in producing the harmful effects of the infectious disease.

**TABLE 2.   Exotoxins of Pathogenic Bacteria**

| BACTERIUM | DISEASE CAUSED IN MAN | TOXINS |
|---|---|---|
| *Bacillus anthracis* | anthrax | complex lethal edema-producing toxin |
| *Bordetella pertussis* | whooping cough | lethal, dermonecrotizing toxin |
| *Clostridium botulinum* | botulism | **6 type-specific lethal neurotoxins** |
| *Cl. oedematiens* | gas gangrene | 1. alpha, lethal, dermonecrotizing<br>2. beta, lethal, dermonecrotizing, hemolytic<br>3. gamma, lethal, dermonecrotizing, hemolytic<br>4. delta, hemolytic<br>5. epsilon, lethal, hemolytic<br>6. zeta, hemolytic |
| *Cl. perfringens* | gas gangrene and enteritis necroticans | 1. **alpha, lethal, dermonecrotizing, hemolytic**<br>2. beta, lethal<br>3. gamma, lethal<br>4. delta, lethal<br>5. epsilon, lethal, dermonecrotizing<br>6. eta, lethal (?)<br>7. iota, lethal, dermonecrotizing<br>8. theta, lethal, cardiotoxic, hemolytic<br>9. kappa, lethal, proteolytic<br>10. **enterotoxin** |
| *Cl. septicum* | gas gangrene | alpha, lethal, hemolytic |
| *Cl. sordellii* | gas gangrene | 1. edema-producing toxin<br>2. hemorrhagic toxin |
| *Cl. tetani* | tetanus | 1. **tetanospasmin, lethal, neurotoxic**<br>2. neurotoxin, nonspasmogenic<br>3. tetanolysin, lethal, cardiotoxic, hemolytic |
| *corynebacterium diphtheriae* | diphtheria | **diphtheria toxin, lethal, dermonecrotizing** |
| *Escherichia coli* | diarrhea | 1. **heat-labile enterotoxin**<br>(2. heat-stable enterotoxin) |
| *Pseudomonas aruginosa* | pyogenic infections | **exotoxin A** |
| *Staphylococcus aureus* | pyogenic infections, enterotoxaemia | 1. alpha, lethal, dermonecrotizing, hemolytic<br>2. beta, lethal, hemolytic<br>3. gamma, lethal, hemolytic<br>4. delta, hemolytic<br>5. **exfoliating toxin**<br>6. **enterotoxin** |
| *Streptococcus pyogenes* | pyogenic infections, scarlet fever, rheumatic fever | 1. Dick toxin, erythrogenic, nonlethal<br>2. streptolysin O, lethal, hemolytic, cardiotoxic<br>3. streptolysin S, lethal, hemolytic |
| *Vibrio cholerae Vibrio El Tor* | cholera | **cholera toxin, lethal, enterotoxic** |
| *Salmonella typhimurium* | enteritis | **enterotoxin?** |
| *Shigella shiga* | dysentery | **enterotoxin** |
| *Yersinia pestis* | plague | murine toxin |

**TABLE 3.   Criteria for Judging Whether Toxins are
Responsible for the Harmful Effects of an Infectious Disease**

1. The organism produces a toxin.
2. Virulent strains produce the toxin; avirulent do not.
3. The organism produces disease without multiplying profusely or spreading extensively.
4. The blood and lymph are sterile.
5. Organs and tissue at a distance from the site of infection are affected.
6. Introduction of sterile cell-free toxin into animals produces symptoms mimicking the disease.
7. The clinician sees toxic effects in the patient: peripheral vascular collapse; direct action on the heart muscle; central or peripheral nervous system affected (see Figure 1).
8. The disease can be prevented by immunization against the toxin.

In most cases there is no good reason for concluding whether it does or does not. The criteria that must be considered in coming to the conclusion that it does are listed in Table 3. These criteria need not all be fulfilled, and the toxins that fulfill at least some of them, or are relevant to those that do, are shown in bold type in Table 2. These are the toxins that we will discuss in this chapter, and in doing so we will be obliged to dismiss a number of well-known toxins, such as the staphylococcal and streptococcal hemolysins, that are of great scientific interest but as yet of no proven medical relevance.

Further reading (the references in this chapter should be consulted as much for their lists of references as for their texts): van Heyningen, 1970.

## NEUROTOXINS

### Tetanus Toxin (Tetanospasmin)

The harmful effects of tetanus are entirely due to this toxin, which fulfills all of the criteria in Table 3. Tetanus toxin is one of the most poisonous toxins known — purified preparations of the toxin may contain 100 million lethal doses (mouse) per milligram (i.e., 1 g kills two million tons of living matter). It is also one of the most

dangerous toxins known. Reliable statistics on tetanus do not exist, but it is possible that the toxin kills perhaps two million people every year, mainly newborn babies (*tetanus neonatorum,* or umbilical tetanus), in the underdeveloped countries of Asia, Africa, and South America.

The toxin acts only on the nervous system, without producing any morphologic changes. The disease is characterized by a spastic paralysis, which nearly always involves the jaw muscles (lockjaw) and the muscles of deglutition, and eventually leads to generalized convulsions (Fig. 1). The spasticity is due to the action of the toxin in blocking pre- and postsynaptic inhibition in the central nervous system, particularly in the spinal cord and cerebellum, which it reaches by ascending in the nerves by retrograde axonal transport, after uptake from the anaerobically replicating organisms near the wound of entry (which is often so small as to be undetectable *post mortem*). Apart from eradication of the organisms with penicillin to prevent formation of more toxin, treatment of tetanus is aimed at controlling convulsions by curarization. However, the toxin can also block neuromuscular transmission (like botulinum toxin; see below), and it also, perhaps indirectly, causes overactivity in the sympathetic nervous system. The latter effects involve drastic swings in blood pressure and heart rate, and a high mortality rate is associated with the

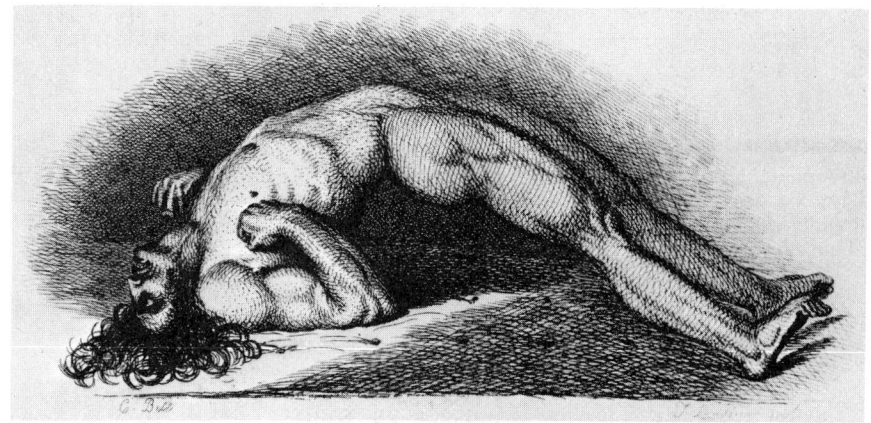

FIGURE 1. *Sir Charles Bell's drawing (1832) of a British soldier suffering from tetanus (lockjaw) as a result of wounds received at the Battle of Corunna. Note the spastic paralysis resulting from opposing muscles pulling against each other, owing to tetanus toxin blocking synaptic inhibition. This man will certainly die.*

appearance of these symptoms, unless they are controlled.

The toxin blocks both evoked and spontaneous transmitter release at the central and peripheral synapses on which it acts. The mechanism of action is not yet understood, and neither are the factors that determine its specificity with respect to particular synapses. Its effects are long lasting, and it appears that, at least at peripheral synapses, restoration of function requires sprouting of new nerve terminals.

What is known about the structure of the toxin is shown in Figure 2. The toxin is a simple protein, apparently consisting of two components, a "heavy" and a "light" polypeptide chain bound together by a peptide bond that is easily "nicked" by proteolytic enzymes in the culture filtrate, and a disulfide bond that is easily cleaved by reduction. The two chains are further held together by noncovalent forces that can be broken with urea or sodium dodecyl sulfate. These chains are inert

and antigenically distinct when separated, but can be recombined to form the fully toxic protein.

The mode of action of the toxin at the molecular level has not yet been determined, but it has been shown that the well-known specific binding of tetanus toxin to nervous tissue (Wassermann-Takaki phenomenon, 1898) is due to the binding of the toxin to certain gangliosides. The gangliosides are components of the cell membranes of most tissues, and are particularly concentrated in nervous tissue. Since they consist of a water-insoluble ceramide moiety and a water-soluble oligosaccharide moiety (Fig. 3), they are amphipathic — i.e., they are both water soluble and fat soluble, and are therefore well suited to play a role in cell membranes. Tetanus toxin shows a particular affinity for the sialidase-sensitive ganglioside GGnSSLC, which contains two sialosyl residues attached to the internal galactosyl residue, and can bind with it in a ratio of 3 to 4

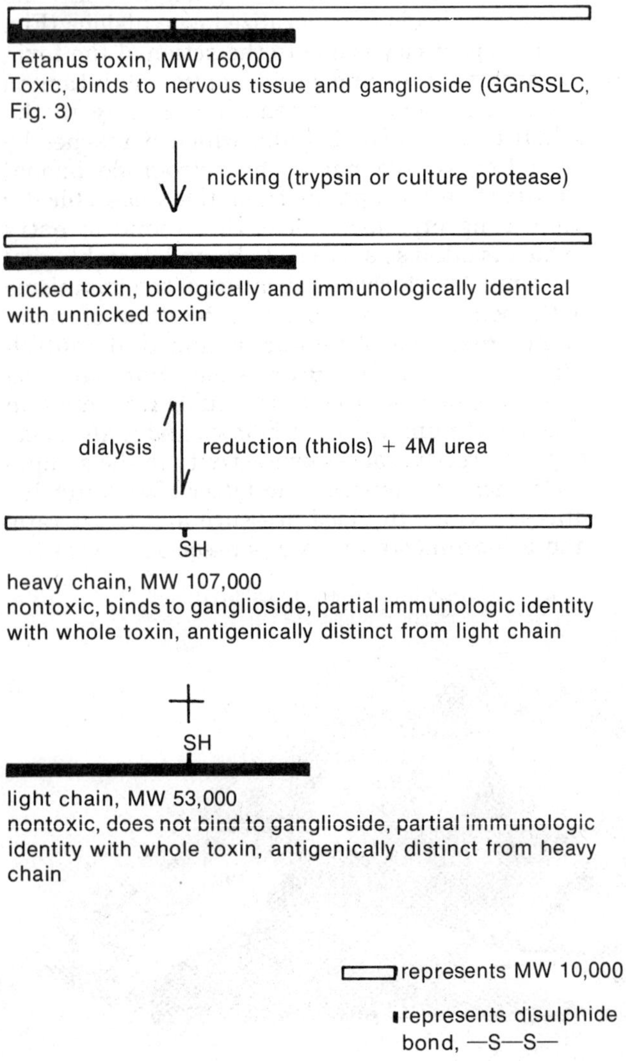

Tetanus toxin, MW 160,000
Toxic, binds to nervous tissue and ganglioside (GGnSSLC, Fig. 3)

nicking (trypsin or culture protease)

nicked toxin, biologically and immunologically identical with unnicked toxin

dialysis | reduction (thiols) + 4M urea

SH
heavy chain, MW 107,000
nontoxic, binds to ganglioside, partial immunologic identity with whole toxin, antigenically distinct from light chain

+
SH
light chain, MW 53,000
nontoxic, does not bind to ganglioside, partial immunologic identity with whole toxin, antigenically distinct from heavy chain

represents MW 10,000

represents disulphide bond, —S—S—

FIGURE 2. *Diagrammatic representation of the structure of tetanus toxin. As in Figures 4, 5, and 6, the black and white bands represent polypeptide chains. In each figure the lengths of these bands are proportional to their relative molecular weights, but note the different scales. Folding of chains by noncovalent bonds is not depicted and the only folding shown is that known to be due to disulfide bonds ( — S — S— ) from one part of a chain to another. These disulfide bonds can be broken by reduction with thiols (to convert —S —S to —SH═SH—), and restored by dialysing away the thiols. The fact that a protein denaturing agent (urea) is also necessary to separate the light and heavy chains of tetanus toxin suggests that they are held together by noncovalent bonds in addition to the covalent disulfide and peptide bond (see cholera toxin, Fig. 6).*

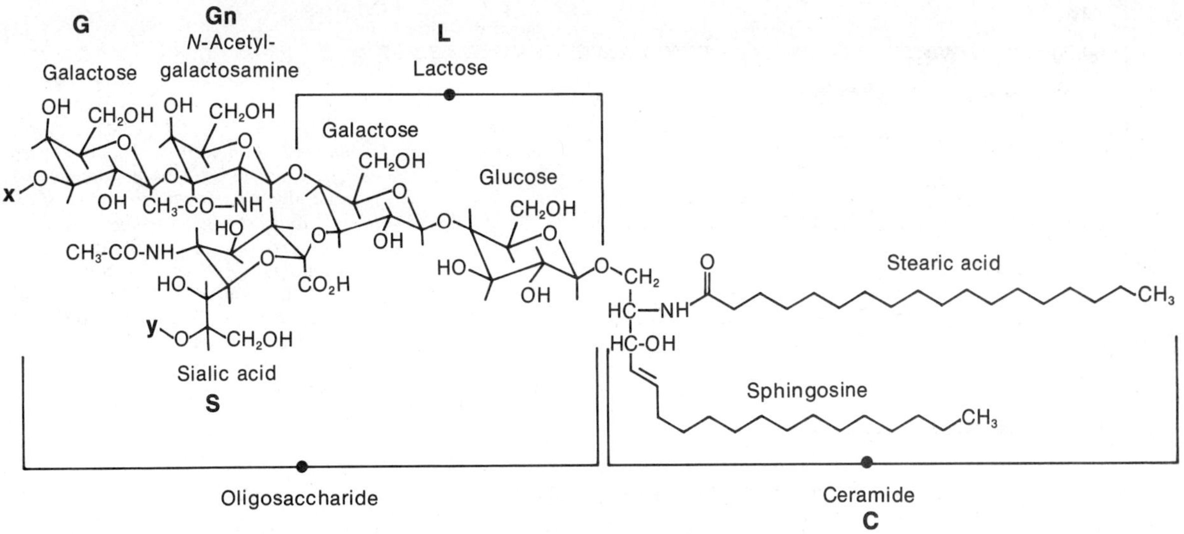

**FIGURE 3.** *Structures of some of the best-known gangliosides. The bond attaching the sialosyl (S) residue to the galactose moiety of the lactose (L) residue is sialidase- (that is, neuraminidase) insensitive. When sialosyl residues substitute for X or Y they are attached by sialidase-sensitive bonds.*
*GGn = H; y = H: Monosialosylganglioside SLC (GM3)*
*G = H; y = H: Monosialosylganglioside GnSLC (GM2)*
*x = H; y = H: Monosialosylganglioside GGnSLC (GM1)*
*x = S; y = H: Disialosylganglioside SGGnSLC (GD1a)*
*x = H; y = S: disialosylganglioside GGnSSCL (GD1b)*
*x = S; y = S: trisialosylganglioside SGGnSSLC (GT1)*
*(The shorthand names in brackets are more widely used but are not self-explanatory.)*

molecules ganglioside to 1 molecule toxin (Table 4). It is the only "heavy" component of the tetanus toxin molecule that combines with ganglioside.

Other bacterial toxins, notably cholera toxin, and certain other biologically active proteins, also bind to gangliosides (Table 4). The significance of this will be discussed below.

Further reading: Bizzini, 1977; Helting et al., 1977; S. van Heyningen, 1976; van Heyningen and Mellanby, 1971; Mellanby and Pope, 1976; and van Heyningen, 1963.

## Botulinum Toxins

Botulism generally assumes the form of food poisoning resulting from the ingestion of toxins preformed by *Clostridium botulinum* growing on food. There are six serologic types, A to F, of the organism, each producing an immunologically type-specific toxin. These toxins have different molecular weights, but they all have apparently the same neurotoxic activity. Only Types A, B, E, and F are known to affect man. Figure 4 shows

**TABLE 4.   Biologically Active Proteins Binding to Ganglioside Receptors**

| PROTEIN | RECEPTOR | TARGET |
|---|---|---|
| Tetanus toxin[1] | GGnSSLC>SGGnSSLC>SGGnSLC>GGnSLC | synaptic transmission |
| Botulinum toxin[2] | not identified—sialidase labile? | synaptic transmission |
| Cholera enterotoxin[3] | GGnSLC only | adenylate cyclase |
| E. coli enterotoxin[4] | GGnSLC only | adenylate cyclase |
| Staphylococcus alpha-toxin[5] | SGGlnLC[6] | cell membrane? |
| Vibrio parahaemolyticus toxin[7] | SGGnSSLC | ? |
| Thyrotropin hormone[8] | GGnSSLC>SGGnSSLC>GGnSLC>GnSLC=SLC>SGGnSLC | adenylate cyclase |
| Human chorionic gonadotropin[9] | SGGnSSLC>SGGnSLC>GGnSSLC>GnSLC>GGnSLC | adenylate cyclase |
| Interferon[10] | GnSLC | cell reaction to virus |
| Sendai virus[11] | not identified—sialidase labile? | ? |

1. van Heyningen (1963); 2. at pH 5, Mellanby and Pope (1976); 3. van Heyningen (1973); 4. Pierce (1973); 5. Kato and Naiki (1976); 6. Gln = N-acetyl-glucosamine (this ganglioside so far found only in red blood cells); 7. Takeda et al. (1976); 8. Mullin et al. (1976); 9. Lee et al. (1976); 10. Besancon et al. (1976); 11. Haywood (1974).

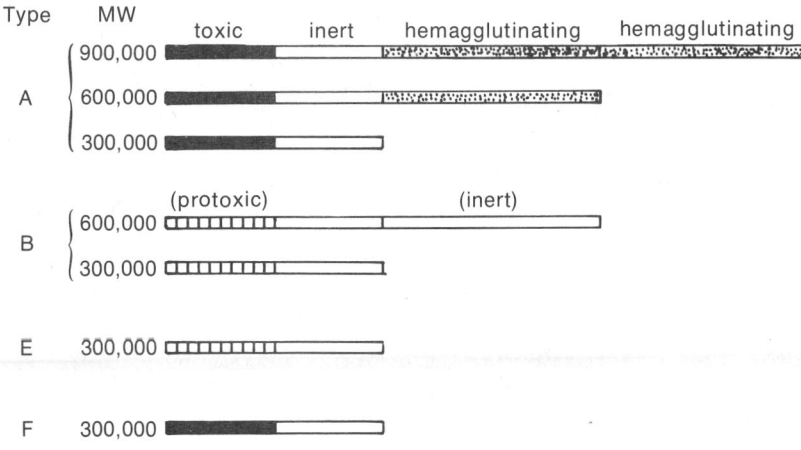

represents MW 75,000

**FIGURE 4.** *Diagrammatic representation of the composition of botulinum toxins (see legend to Fig. 2) as they appear to exist naturally. Under certain conditions of pH and ionic strength smaller toxic components (MW about 150,000) may be found in laboratory preparations. The toxins from Cl. botulinum types B and E appear as nontoxic protoxins that are converted to active toxins by proteolytic enzymes without appreciable change in molecular weight.*

that these toxins appear to be aggregates of two or three kinds of protein components — toxic, inert, and hemagglutinating. Only the Type A toxin contains the hemagglutinating component, and in the Types B and E toxins the toxic components are produced by the organism as inert protoxins that are converted by proteolytic enzymes into active toxins with no detectable change in molecular weight.

Botulinum toxin is as toxic as tetanus toxin; like tetanus toxin, it acts only on nervous tissue, and does not directly cause any detectable morphologic change in this tissue. It apparently has no central action, and seems to act only peripherally at the neuromuscular junctions, where (like tetanus toxin) it blocks both evoked and spontaneous release of acetylcholine from cholinergic motor nerve endings.

Nothing is yet known of the action of the toxin at the molecular level. The toxic component of the toxin (Fig. 4) has a molecular weight of about 150,000 (similar to that of tetanus toxin). It can be separated from the inert and hemagglutinating components without loss or change in character of the toxicity. Nothing is yet known of the structure of this toxic component.

It used to be thought that botulinum toxin does not bind to nervous tissue, or to gangliosides, but recent work has demonstrated that it is bound to synaptic membranes and to gangliosides under different physical conditions (pH, salt concentration) from those suitable for the binding of tetanus toxin. Perhaps these differences may be related to the different conditions under which these toxins block synaptic transmission in the laboratory. Thus, the in vitro effect of botulinum toxin on a phrenic nerve diaphragm preparation can be seen within 30 minutes of adding the toxin to the bathing medium, whereas the similar effect

of tetanus toxin can be reproduced only by injecting the toxin into the living animal and studying a nerve-muscle preparation isolated some hours later.

Recently it has been shown that the cause of the Sudden Infant Death Syndrome (crib death) can sometimes be due to botulism resulting from ingestion of *Cl. botulinum* spores, their survival of the passage through the infant stomach, followed by their vegetation and consequent toxin production in the gut. This means that, contrary to previously held opinion, botulism can be an infectious disease (in infants) and an exotoxinosis.

Further reading: Arnon *et al,* 1978; and Boroff and DasGupta, 1971.

## TOXINS BLOCKING PROTEIN SYNTHESIS

### Diphtheria Toxin

Diphtheria toxin is produced only by lysogenic strains of *Corynebacterium diphtheriae* infected with a bacteriophage carrying the *tox* gene, which carries the structural information for the synthesis of the toxin. The expression of this information is regulated, at least in part, by the bacterial host. The toxin must be considered responsible for the harmful effects of diphtheria since it fulfills all the criteria listed in Table 3. Unlike tetanus and botulinum toxins, diphtheria toxin appears to act on all tissues of susceptible animals. It has a necrotizing effect on cells, as may be seen when it is injected intracutaneously, as in the Schick test. In the diphtheria patient or the experimentally injected animal, the effect of the toxin is best seen in the heart muscles and the adrenal glands.

The mode of action of the toxin at the molecular level is well understood. It acts by blocking protein synthesis in susceptible cells by inhibiting polypeptide synthesis. The toxin inhibits the polypeptide synthesis by catalyzing the following reaction:

$$NAD^+ + EF\text{-}2 \rightleftharpoons ADPR\text{—}EF\text{-}2 + nicotinamide + H^+$$
$$\text{active} \qquad\qquad \text{inactive}$$

EF-2 is the Elongation Factor-2, which is required for translocating polypeptide-transfer RNA from the acceptor site to the donor site on the eukaryotic ribosome. It is inactivated by being coupled with the adenosine diphosphate ribose (ADPR) resulting from the cleavage of nicotinamide adenine diphosphate (NAD).

The structure of diphtheria toxin is shown in Figure 5. It consists of two peptide chains, A and B, linked together by easily cleavable peptide and disulfide bonds. Only the A (active) part of the diphtheria toxin molecule is responsible for the reaction above, resulting in the inactivation of Elongation Factor-2, and this active part must therefore be considered as an enzyme. The other part (B, binding) of the toxin molecule is responsible for binding the toxin to the membranes of

susceptible cells and facilitating the entry of A into the cytoplasm of the cell, where it catalyzes the reaction above. The whole toxin AB is toxic to susceptible animals or whole cells, whereas part A is not toxic to animals or whole cells, but will catalyze the reaction in cell extracts. On the other hand, the whole toxin AB is ineffective in cell extracts. Cells from species of animals that are relatively insusceptible to diphtheria toxin (e.g., mice) do not contain the receptor for the B-component and therefore do not bind toxin, but protein synthesis in extracts from these cells is blocked by A. This important concept of a bipartite (AB) toxin was first revealed with diphtheria toxin, and has led to similar concepts for other toxins and biologically active proteins (see below).

Although the target of diphtheria toxin — that is, the substrate for the enzymic A component — has been identified (NAD + EF-2), the receptor for the toxin — that is, the substance in the susceptible cell membrane to which the B component binds — has not yet been identified. It may be very difficult to do so, since the affinity constant of diphtheria toxin for susceptible cells is low

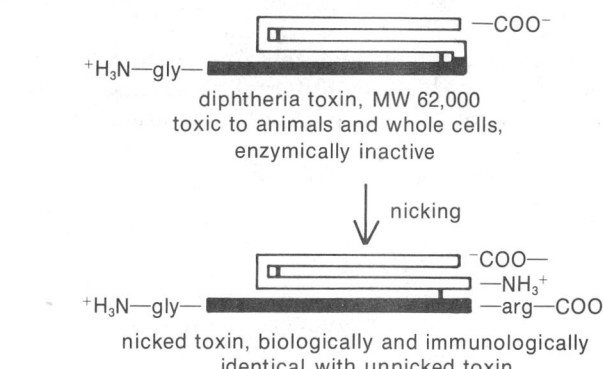

diphtheria toxin, MW 62,000
toxic to animals and whole cells,
enzymically inactive

**FIGURE 5.** *Diagrammatic representation of the structure of diphtheria toxin (see legend to Fig. 2).*

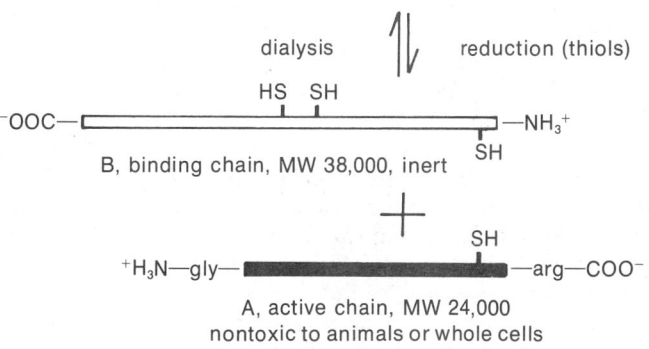

B, binding chain, MW 38,000, inert

A, active chain, MW 24,000
nontoxic to animals or whole cells
enzymically active in cell extracts

▭ = MW 5000
▮ = disulphide bond, —S—S—

compared with that of other toxins and since very few molecules of toxin are bound per cell.

Further reading: Boquet and Pappenheimer, 1976; Collier, 1975; Collier, 1977; Murphy, 1976; and Pappenheimer and Gill, 1973.

### Pseudomonas Aeruginosa Exotoxin A

Recently a lethal, necrotizing toxin (Exotoxin A) has been shown to be produced by most clinical isolates of *Pseudomonas aeruginosa,* which is a major source of hospital infection. The organism is an "opportunistic" pathogen that commonly infects patients whose defense mechanism is impaired because of genetic immunodeficiency, or because they are being treated with immunosuppressive drugs, or because of extensive burns. Exotoxin A is mentioned here because it is similar to diphtheria toxin insofar as it catalyzes the reaction of NAD with EF-2 to form ADPR — EF-2 and thereby blocks protein synthesis in animals, cells, and cell extracts. But there are differences. Unlike whole diphtheria toxin, the whole exotoxin A (MW about 66,000) is active in cell extracts as well as on whole cells; and although a smaller product of natural proteolysis (MW about 33,000) appears to be more active than the whole toxin in cell extracts, it is also active on whole cells. The toxins also differ in their relative toxicity to different species of animals and cell lines, which suggests that they bind to different receptors. There is no immunologic relationship between the two toxins.

Further reading: Collier, 1975.

## *ENTEROTOXINS*

An enterotoxin is a toxin produced in the intestinal tract by an infecting organism. This toxin causes diarrhea or vomiting. This effect generally results from the direct action of the toxin on the intestinal wall (e.g., cholera), but may also follow the absorption of the toxin into the bloodstream and its action elsewhere, as is thought to be the case with the staphylococcal enterotoxins. It is now recognized that acute gastroenteritis is a global medical problem, particularly severe in terms of morbidity, mortality, and economic impact in the less developed countries of the world. It is also being recognized that many of these enteropathies are enterotoxinoses.

Further reading: Banwell and Sherr, 1973; and Craig, 1972.

### Cholera Toxin

Cholera toxin, diphtheria toxin, and tetanus toxin are the three toxins that are quite certainly responsible for the harmful effects of the diseases caused by their parent organisms. Cholera is a disease of acute diarrhea, which may be so severe that a patient may lose up to 30 liters of watery stools in a day. Death follows the consequent dehydration. The toxic nature of cholera was recognized by John Snow in 1849, well before the germ theory of disease was established, and then reaffirmed 35 years later by Robert Koch who postulated a cholera toxin; but the existence of such a toxin was not proved until a further 75 years later, when S. N. De showed that cell-free culture filtrates of *Vibrio cholerae* promoted fluid accumulation when introduced directly into the gut. Since then the toxin has been isolated and subjected to a great deal of study all over the world. The toxin gene resides in the chromosomes of both biotypes, *V. cholerae* and *V. El Tor,* and both serotypes, Ogawa and Inaba. Cholera toxin causes diarrhea by stimulating a net output of chloride ions by the brush border cells of the small intestine. The stimulation of chloride secretion follows an increased output of adenosine-3′:5′-cyclic monophosphate (cyclic AMP), which results from stimulation of the enzyme adenylate cyclase by the toxin. The toxin acts on all eukaryotic cells containing this enzyme (and containing a particular ganglioside in the membrane; see below), besides those of the intestinal mucosa, and brings about a great diversity of effects, including increase in capillary permeability when injected into the skin, morphologic changes in Chinese hamster ovary (CHO) cells and in adrenal tumor cells (together with increased steroidogenesis), increased glycogenolysis in liver cells, and lipolysis in fat cells. The stimulation of adenylate cyclase by cholera toxin differs from that caused by hormones such as epinephrine and thyrotropin in that it involves a permanent change in the enzyme. For this reason recovery from cholera depends on the replacement of the affected cells of the intestinal wall, which takes place within hours.

Like diphtheria toxin, cholera toxin is a complex of two parts, A and B, but unlike diphtheria toxin these parts are held together by noncovalent bonds (hydrogen bonds, ionic bonds, hydrophobic interactions, and van der Waals forces, Fig. 6). Under fairly mild conditions the bonds linking A and B are broken, yielding one molecule of A and an aggregate of five molecules of subunits of B. This aggregate of subunits of B may occur along with the intact toxin during purification, and is known as "choleragenoid"; it is biologically inert, and immunologically almost (but not quite) identical with the whole toxin. Part A comprises two parts, held together by a peptide bond and a sulfhydryl bond. The peptide bond is usually nicked by natural proteolysis, and

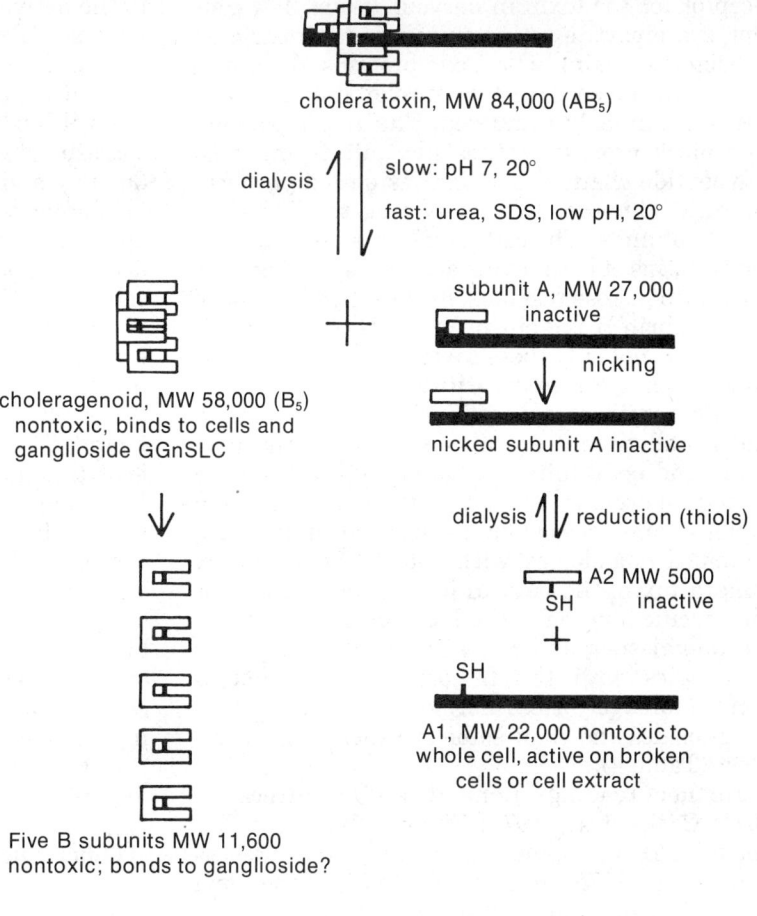

cholera toxin, MW 84,000 (AB₅)

dialysis

slow: pH 7, 20°

fast: urea, SDS, low pH, 20°

subunit A, MW 27,000
inactive

nicking

nicked subunit A inactive

choleragenoid, MW 58,000 (B₅)
nontoxic, binds to cells and
ganglioside GGnSLC

dialysis    reduction (thiols)

A2 MW 5000
inactive
SH

SH

A1, MW 22,000 nontoxic to
whole cell, active on broken
cells or cell extract

Five B subunits MW 11,600
nontoxic; bonds to ganglioside?

represents MW 5000

represents disulphide bond, —S—S—

**FIGURE 6.** *Diagrammatic representation of structure of cholera toxin (see legend to Fig. 2). The A component is held to the B (choleragenoid) component by noncovalent bonds (hydrogen bonds, van der Waals forces, etc.) as are the subunits of the B component. The A2 and A1 fragments of the A component are held together by a nickable peptide bond and a reducible disulfide bond.*

on reduction with a thiol the sulfhydryl bond is also broken to yield a smaller fragment A2 and a larger fragment A1. The biologic activity of cholera toxin resides in the fragment A1. The function of the "choleragenoid" aggregate, like that of the B component of diphtheria toxin, is to bind the toxin to the cell membrane and thus to facilitate the entry of the active component A1 into the cell.

The cell membrane receptor that recognizes and binds the choleragenoid part of cholera toxin has been identified as the sialidase- (or neuraminidase) stable ganglioside GGnSLC, generally known as GM1 (Table 4). Cells that do not contain this ganglioside are not susceptible to the action of the toxin, but if the ganglioside is simply added to the cells it becomes incorporated into their membranes and they become susceptible to this toxin.

The A1 fragment, like diphtheria toxin fragment A, is inactive on the whole cell but active on broken or lysed cells and on extract of the cells; it appears also to be an enzyme catalyzing the cleavage of NAD into ADPR and nicotinamide. The ADPR is bound not to EF2, but probably to some arginine-containing protein, possibly adenylate cyclase itself, and as a result of this the adenylate cyclase is permanently stimulated. The strong evidence that the action of the A1 component of cholera toxin is enzymic refutes the suggestion (Bennett and Cuatrecasas, 1977) that it stimulates adenylate cyclase by combining with it directly.

An important concept with wide implications is revealed by diphtheria and cholera toxins. This concept holds that biologically active proteins can have two distinct and separable parts, one part binding to the cell surface receptor and the other acting on a target within the cell. It is likely that the *Escherichia coli* enterotoxin is similarly constituted (see below); and it may be significant that tetanus toxin appears to consist of two separable components that are inactive singly but active again when rejoined, and that one of these components is responsible for the binding of tetanus toxin to the ganglioside that appears to be the receptor for the toxin in nervous tissue. The concept of a bipartite active protein is not restricted to bacterial toxins. The toxic proteins abrin and ricin from the seeds of two unrelated plant families are similarly composed. The A components both block protein synthesis by interfering with polypeptide chain elongation (as does diphtheria toxin), in this case by inactivating the 60S ribosomal subunits. The cell membrane receptors for the B chains of both toxins are similar and appear to contain lactose residues. Fully active hybrids of ricin A/abrin B and abrin A/ricin B can be constituted. It is not only these toxic bacterial and plant proteins that are so constituted — certain glycoprotein tropic hormones (including thyrotropin and gonadotropin) are also known to consist of alpha and beta units. The alpha units stimulate adenylate cyclase (but not permanently, the way cholera toxin does) and have some amino acid sequence homologies with the A component of cholera toxin; the beta units are responsible for the specific binding of the hormones to their susceptible tissues and have amino acid sequence homologies with the B component of cholera toxin. Moreover, these hormones bind to certain gangliosides and show some specificity in this respect (Table 4).

Further reading: Bennett and Cuatrecasas, 1977; Craig et al., 1976; Finkelstein, 1973; Finkelstein, 1976; Fishman and Brady, 1976; Flores and Sharp, 1975; Moss et al., 1976; Olsnes and Pihl, 1977; and van Heyningen, 1974.

### Escherichia Coli Enterotoxin

Enteropathogenicity and the ability to produce both a heat-stable small molecular and a heat-labile protein enterotoxin is conferred on *E. coli* by an enterotoxin plasmid (Ent$^+$). It is likely that these strains of *E. coli* contribute very heavily to enterotoxic enteropathies throughout the world. We will be concerned only with the heat-labile toxin that bears many resemblances to cholera toxin: (1) it stimulates adenylate cyclase, with the same consequences; (2) it cross-reacts immunologically with cholera toxin and choleragenoid, i.e., antisera to cholera toxin and choleragenoid neutralize both toxins, antisera to coli toxin neutralizes cholera toxin poorly; (3) both toxins bind to the ganglioside GGnSLC (but see below). There are, however, some differences. Coli toxin preparations vary considerably in molecular weight and have not yet been properly purified. This may be due to association of the toxin with other materials in the culture filtrate. It is also several orders of magnitude less toxic than cholera toxin, even taking into account the impurity of the preparations tested. Coli toxin appears to be synthesized as a protoxin, which is converted to the active form by proteolytic enzymes (thus it may be fully active in the gut, which contains trypsin-like enzymes, and inactive in the skin). Partially purified coli toxin preparations from several laboratories show faint bands in SDS gel corresponding to molecular weights of 23,000 to 30,000, and when *E. coli* is treated with the antibiotic polymyxin a protein of MW 23,000 is obtained that is very similar to cholera toxin A1 active component, but has some activity on whole cells.

As to the cell receptor for coli toxin, some workers have found that the ganglioside GGnSLC binds coli toxin as well as it binds cholera toxin; others find that coli toxin is far less readily bound. The results so far obtained seem to suggest that although coli and cholera toxins may have the same active component, and although the binding components may bind to the same receptor, they differ in their binding capacity. This might be connected with the variations found in the structure of coli toxin, and the possibility that the toxin might be associated with other components of culture filtrates. These other components may block binding capacity to varying degrees, and thus affect toxicity.

Further reading: Gill et al., 1976; and Craig et al., 1976.

### Other Enterotoxins

*Salmonella enteritidis* and *S. typhimurium* have been reported to produce enterotoxins possessing similarities to the *E. coli* enterotoxin, and *S. typhimurium* has been reported to produce a heat-labile factor inducing capillary permeability in rabbit skin, like *V. cholerae* and *E. coli* enterotoxins. These observations have not yet been confirmed, but they might prove to be important in the future in considerations of the intestinal effects of salmonella infections.

*Shigella dysenteriae* has been known for a long time to produce an exotoxin that appears to be as potent as botulinum toxin in producing flaccid paralysis in rabbits. The toxin is in fact not a neurotoxin but causes hemorrhages in the spinal cord of the rabbit, which leads to edema, and thus to pressure on nerves. Recently it has been shown that this toxin is a cytotoxic enterotoxin capable of causing fluid accumulation in ligated ileal loops of the rabbit. The role of this toxin in the pathogenesis of shigellosis has not yet been determined. There has been some evidence that toxin-producing strains of *S. dysenteriae* are no more pathogenic than invasive atoxic strains, but it has been proposed that both toxinogenesis and invasiveness play a role in the disease.

Food poisoning due to contamination by *Bacillus cereus, Clostridium perfringens, Staphylococ-*

*cus aureus,* and *Vibrio parahaemolyticus* is now recognized as a health hazard. *B. cereus* culture filtrate induces fluid accumulation in ligated rabbit ileal loops and an increase in capillary permeability in the skin. Apparently an enterotoxin is produced, but as yet little is known about its nature or its medical significance. Sporulating cultures of *Cl. perfringens* cause fluid accumulation in the gut, possibly owing to decreased absorption rather than increased secretion. A diarrheagenic and emetic toxin, different from the other known toxins of *Cl. perfringens,* has been isolated, with a molecular weight of 35,000. Little is known about the mode of action of the toxin, but it is likely that it is an important factor in *Cl. perfringens* food poisoning. The staphylococcus produces five enterotoxins, A to E, that can be differentiated serologically but have similar physicochemical properties (MW 26,000 to 30,000) and gastrointestinal effects, causing diarrhea and vomiting. The emetic effect is neurologically mediated. The site of the emetic action of these toxins has been shown to be in the abdominal viscera, and the sensory emetic stimulus reaches the vomiting center via the vagus and sympathetic nerves. The diarrheagenic mechanism has not yet been elucidated. The toxins seem most active on the middle segment of the small intestine where they enhance secretory activity without blocking absorption of sodium or water.

*Vibrio parahaemolyticus* is a major cause of seafood-borne gastroenteritis in Japan and elsewhere. The organism produces a heat-stable protein of MW 45,000 that is hemolytic, cardiotoxic, and capable of causing fluid accumulation in ligated rabbit ileal loops, causing degenerative changes at the same time (unlike cholera toxin). This toxin is blocked by a sialidase-sensitive ganglioside (Table 4).

Further reading: Finkelstein, 1976; Takeda et al., 1976; and van Heyningen, 1971.

## OTHER TOXINS

### Clostridium Perfringens Alpha Toxin

This toxin is discussed in order to show that a fatal disease resulting from an infection by an organism producing a lethal exotoxin need not necessarily be an exotoxinosis. *Clostridium perfringens* is the main causative organism of gas gangrene, a disease resulting from the infection of deep penetrating wounds, and characterized by tissue destruction and toxemia and shock. Several toxins are produced, including a proteolytic collagenase (kappa), a cardiotoxic oxygen-labile hemolysin (theta), and a tissue-necrotizing oxygen-stable hemolysin (alpha). The alpha toxin

is an enzyme, a phospholipase C, which catalyzes the cleavage of phosphyryl choline, phosphoryl ethanolamine, and other compounds from phospholipids. It has been shown that gas gangrene can be prevented in experimentally infected animals by prophylactic active or passive immunization against the alpha toxin, but not against the other toxins. In view of this, and of the undoubted fact that the injection of a lethal dose of alpha toxin can produce symptoms of shock, it is not unreasonable to suggest that *Cl. perfringens* gas gangrene is an exotoxinosis, like tetanus, diphtheria, and cholera, which were discussed earlier.

However, the situation in gas gangrene is much more complicated. Although alpha antitoxin gives good protection when infection is initiated in slightly damaged muscle, it gives little or no protection when infection is initiated in severely damaged muscle, or in slightly damaged muscle when the bacteriostatic action of serum proteins (transferrin) is lowered by pretreating the experimental animals with iron compounds. It would seem that the protective role of alpha antitoxin is not so much due to its neutralizing the lethality of the toxin, but rather to its neutralizing the ability of the toxin to cause tissue necrosis and so pave the way for further growth of the organism. In effect, the role of antitoxin is bacteriostatic. But if other factors prevail that favor bacterial growth, such as severe tissue damage, or if the bacteriostatic action of serum proteins is lowered, then massive growth of the organism results in a number of effects, such as removal of oxygen from the environment; fall in redox potential; marked changes in vascular permeability; loss of plasma protein; and severe hemoconcentration. It may be that these conditions are responsible for the fatal shock of gas gangrene.

Further reading: Bullen, 1970.

### Staphylococcal Exfoliative Toxin

Some phage group II strains of staphylococci are responsible for an exfoliative dermatitis (staphylococcal scalded skin syndrome, SSSS) in very young infants, and more rarely in older children and adults. The epidermis can be displaced at the slightest touch, like the skin of a ripe peach, and more than half the body may be denuded to give an appearance resembling severely scalded skin. It is distressing to endure, and to see, but it passes quickly and is rarely fatal, since the denuded areas dry up and the skin is rapidly replaced. The effect can be reproduced experimentally in newborn mice by infecting the skin with group II staphylococci or by injecting sterile culture filtrates. In children and adults exfoliation may also result from sensitivity to certain drugs, including sulfa compounds, phenylbutazone and barbiturates, but in these latter cases the splitting of the skin occurs at the dermoepidermal junction, whereas SSSS is characterized by intraepidermal splitting.

The exfoliative effect of group II staphylococcal skin infection is a clear case of a harmful effect of an infection being due to an exotoxin. This toxin (exfoliatin) has been freed of other active staphylococcal products and purified. It is a protein with reported molecular weights ranging from 24,000 to 33,000. Reports on its heat stability also vary, and it may be that there is more than one form of the toxin. Nothing is as yet known about the mode of action of the toxin at the molecular level.

Further reading: Taylor, 1976.

## IMMUNIZATION AGAINST EXOTOXINOSES

Since some or all of the harmful effects of some infections are entirely due to exotoxins, and since these exotoxins are antigenic, the question arises whether protection against the diseases can be obtained by passive or active immunization against the relevant exotoxins. Active immunization obviously has only prophylactic possibilities because the production of sufficiently high levels of antibodies can be attained only some weeks after injection of the antigen. Therapeutic passive immunization is of limited value because exotoxins are rapidly fixed to their susceptible cells, and once fixed they cannot be neutralized by antitoxin. In fact, the bound toxin may not remain on the surface of the cell, where it can be reached by antitoxin, for more than a few minutes. In the case of diphtheria and cholera toxins we know that the active components, A, of the toxins are rapidly "eclipsed," and pass into the interior of the cell where they are unavailable to antitoxin. In the case of cholera toxin we know that the cell-binding component, B, which also has most of the antitoxin binding capacity, remains on the surface of the cell while the A component acts inside; in the case of diphtheria toxin it is not yet known what happens to the B component; in either case the cell-damaging A component is sheltered from antitoxin.

Although antitoxin probably has little therapeutic value, there may be circumstances in which it might have some prophylactic value if it is administered soon enough, especially in suspected tetanus and diphtheria, before all the toxin has reached its susceptible tissue.

Active immunization can be achieved in advance of infection by injecting toxoid, that is toxin that has been rendered nontoxic without affecting its antigenicity, by treatment with agents such as formaldehyde or glutaraldehyde. Obviously it is feasible to consider actively immunizing only subjects that are at risk, such as children against diphtheria and tetanus, and soldiers against tetanus and gas gangrene. Pregnant women should also be immunized against tetanus to protect their babies from umbilical tetanus. It is not feasible to immunize infants against SSSS, for example, because the disease is very rare. It may be possible to immunize soldiers against gas gangrene toxin, but, as we have seen, it is likely that only those who receive wounds that do not bring about much tissue damage will be protected. This might still be worthwhile.

It might be instructive to compare the problems of active immunization against the three frank exotoxinoses we have already discussed: diphtheria, tetanus, and cholera.

People who have had diphtheria are probably immune to it, or at least to its worst effects, for the rest of their lives; they have been exposed to enough toxin to ensure this. The same state of affairs can be achieved by active immunization with purified toxoid. In developed countries where active immunization with diphtheria toxoid is carried out extensively, diphtheria has more or less disappeared. In countries where active immunization is not practiced, it is rife, and only survivors of the disease, or people who have had frequent contact with the organism without getting diseased, are immune.

People who have had tetanus and survived are no more immune to the disease than people who have not had it. The reason for this is that a sublethal (or lethal) dose of tetanus toxin is such a small amount of antigen (a few picograms or nanograms) that it is quite inadequate to elicit immunity. In Brazil and in India there is some evidence that some members of the indigenous populations may have protective levels of antitoxin in their sera, probably as a result of frequent experience of sublethal amounts of toxin. Active immunity to the disease is easily attained by immunization with the purified toxoid. In the early phase of World War I, when immunization was not practiced, the incidence of tetanus in the British Army was nearly 7 in every 1000 wounded; in World War II only 35 British soldiers died of tetanus and there are good reasons to doubt whether half of them had in fact been immunized.

How effective is antitoxic active immunization against cholera? The answer is still being sought. Although cholera is a frank exotoxinosis, it is otherwise a very different disease from either diphtheria or tetanus. For one thing, the toxin acts enterally not parenterally as in the other two diseases, and for another, the disease is very quick, with the time interval between onset and death being measured in hours rather than days.

The enteral nature of the disease suggests that for the actively produced antitoxin to be effective it must be present in the small intestine, secreted from the wall of the intestine in the form of IgA antibodies. Research is at present being conducted on the practical means of bringing about such enteral active immunity to the toxin. The rapid course of the disease means that there is not enough time for the anamnestic response of antibody production to secondary antigenic stimulus to play an important part. Protection therefore must probably depend on there being sufficient antibody present enterally at the time of infection.

If effective antitoxic immunity to cholera toxin can ever be achieved, it will have the very important added advantage that such immunity will also be effective against many *E. coli* diarrheas, since cholera antitoxin neutralizes *E. coli* toxin.

## References

Arnon, S. S., Midura, T. F., Damus, D., Wood, R. M., and Chin, J.: Intestinal infection and toxin production by *Clostridium botulinum* as one cause of sudden infant death syndrome. Lancet 1:1273, 1978.

Banwell, J. G., and Sherr, H.: The effect of bacterial enterotoxins on the gastrointestinal tract. Gastroenterology 65:467, 1973.

Bennett, F., and Cuatrecasas, P.: Cholera toxin: Membrane gangliosides and activation of adenylate cyclase. In Cuatrecasas, P. (ed.): The Specificity and Action of Animal, Bacterial and Plant Toxins. London, Chapman and Hall, 1977, p. 1.

Bizzini, B.: Tetanus toxin structure as a basis for elucidating its immunological and neuropharmacological activities. In Cuatrecasas, P. (ed.): The Specificity and Action of Animal, Bacterial and Plant Toxins. London, Chapman and Hall, 1977, p. 175.

Boroff, D. A., and DasGupta, B. R.: Botulinum toxin. In Kadis, S., Montie, T. C., and Ajl, S. J. (eds.): Microbial Toxins Volume IIA. New York and London, Academic Press, 1971, p. 1.

Boquet, P., and Pappenheimer, Jr., A. M.: Interaction of diphtheria toxin with mammalian cell membranes. J Biol Chem 251:5770, 1976.

Bullen, J. J.: Role of toxins in host-parasite relationships. In Ajl, S. J., Kadis, S., and Montie, T. C. (eds.): Microbial Toxins I. New York and London, Academic Press, 1970, p. 233.

Collier, R. J.: Diphtheria toxin: Mode of action and structure. Bacter Rev 39:54, 1975.

Collier, R. J.: Inhibition of protein synthesis by exotoxins from *Corynebacterium diphtheriae* and *Pseudomonas aeruginosa*. In Cuatrecasas, P. (ed.): The Specificity and Action of Animal, Bacterial and Plant Toxins. London, Chapman and Hall, 1977, p. 67.

Craig, J. P.: The enterotoxic enteropathies. In Symposia of the Society for General Microbiology XXII, Microbial Pathogenicity in Man and Animals. Cambridge, The University Press, 1972, p. 129.

Craig, J. P., Benenson, A. S., Hardegree, M. C., Pierce, N. F., and Richardson, S. H. (eds.): The Structure and Functions of Enterotoxins. J Infect Dis 133: March Supplement, 1976.

Finkelstein, R. A.: Cholera. CRC Critical Reviews in Microbiology 2:553, 1973.

Finkelstein, R. A.: Progress in the study of cholera and related enterotoxins. In Bernheimer, A. W. (ed.): Mechanisms in Bacterial Toxinology. New York, London, Sydney, Toronto, John Wiley and Sons, 1976, p. 53.

Fishman, P. H., and Brady, R. O.: Biosynthesis and function of gangliosides. Science 194:906, 1976.

Flores, J., and Sharp, W. G.: Effects of cholera toxin on adenylate cyclase. Studies with guanylimidodiphosphate. J Clin Invest 56:1345, 1975.

Gill, D. M., Evans, Jr., D. J., and Evans, D. G.: Mechanism of activation of adenylate cyclase in vitro by polymyxin-released heat-labile enterotoxin of *Escherichia coli*. J Infect Dis 33:S103, 1976.

Helting, T. B., Swizler, O., and Wiegandt, H.: Structure of Tetanus toxin. II Toxin binding to ganglioside. J Biol Chem 252:194, 1977.

Mellanby, J., and Pope, D.: The relationship between the action of tetanus toxin and its binding to membranes and gangliosides. In Porcellati, G., Ceccarelli, B., and Tettamanti, G. (eds.): Ganglioside Function. New York and London, Plenum Press, 1976, p. 215.

Moss, J., Manganiello, V. C., and Vaughan, M.: Hydrolysis of nicotinamide adenine dinucleotide by choleragen and its A protomer: Possible role in the activation of adenylate cyclase. Proc Nat Acad Sci U.S.A. 73:4424, 1976.

Murphy, J. R.: Structure activity relationships of diphtheria toxin. In Bernheimer, A. W. (ed.): Mechanisms in Bacterial Toxinology. New York, London, Sydney, Toronto, John Wiley and Sons, 1976, p. 31.

Olsnes, S., and Pihl, A.: Abrin, ricin, and their associated agglutinins. In Cuatrecasas, P. (ed.): The Specificity and Action of Animal, Bacterial and Plant Toxins. London, Chapman and Hall, 1977, p. 129.

Pappenheimer, Jr., A. M., and Gill, D. M.: Diphtheria. Science 182:353, 1973.

Takeda, Y., Takeda, T., Honda, T., and Miwatani, T.: Inactivation of the biological activities of the thermostable direct haemolysin of Vibrio parahaemolyticus by ganglioside GT1. Infect and Immun 14:1, 1976.

Taylor, A. G.: Toxins and the genesis of specific lesions: enterotoxin and exfoliatin. In Bernheimer, A. W. (ed.): Mechanisms in Bacterial Toxinology. New York, London, Sydney, Toronto, John Wiley and Sons, 1976, p. 195.

van Heyningen, S.: Binding of ganglioside by the chains of tetanus toxin. FEBS Letters 68:5, 1976.

van Heyningen, W. E.: The fixation of tetanus toxin, strychnine, serotonin and other substances by ganglioside. J Gen Microbiol 31:375, 1963.

van Heyningen, W. E.: General characteristics. In Ajl, S. J., Kadis, S., and Montie, T. C. (eds.): Microbial Toxins Volume I. New York and London, Academic Press, 1970, p. 1.

van Heyningen, W. E.: The exotoxin of *Shigella dysenteriae*. In Kadis, S., Montie, T. C., and Ajl, S. J. (eds.): Microbial Toxins Volume IIA. New York and London, Academic Press, 1971, p. 255.

van Heyningen, W. E.: Gangliosides as membrane receptors for tetanus toxin, cholera toxin and serotonin. Nature 249:415, 1974.

van Heyningen, W. E., and Mellanby, J.: Tetanus toxin. In Kadis, S., Montie, T. C., and Ajl, S. J. (eds.): Microbial Toxins Volume IIA. New York and London, Academic Press, 1971, p. 69.

# BACTERIAL ENDOTOXINS 6

## Abraham I. Braude, M.D.

The lipopolysaccharides (LPS) in the cell wall of gram-negative bacteria can cause hypotension, shock, fever, intravascular coagulation, and death. Because of this toxicity, and because they are incorporated within the bacterial cell wall, they are called endotoxins. Exotoxins, by contrast, are not structural components of the cell, and are released from the bacteria, so that their

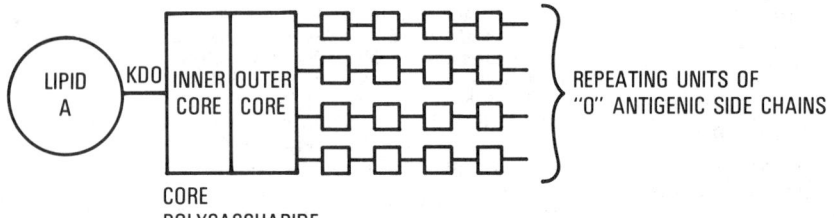

**FIGURE 1.** *Diagram of lipopolysaccharide showing three main regions: lipid A, core, and "O" antigens. Note key position of KDO as a link between lipid A and polysaccharides. KDO is attached via a ketoacidic linkage to glucosamine residues of lipid A.*

biologic activity is far greater in the culture filtrates than in the parent cell suspension. Although endotoxin may also escape into surrounding fluids, the whole cell of gram-negative bacteria retains the major portion of the endotoxic activity.

## CHEMICAL STRUCTURE OF ENDOTOXINS

The toxic LPS or endotoxins of smooth bacteria are macromolecules composed of three main regions: Lipid A, core polysaccharide, and "O" antigens (Fig. 1).

Each of these regions has a unique composition. The "O" antigens are made up of a series of repeating oligosaccharide units, each composed of three or four different hexoses. There may be as many as 10 such units in the smoothest gram-

negative bacteria. Although the lipid A and core polysaccharide of most gram-negative bacteria share a similar, if not identical, structure, the "O" antigens vary with each species and serologic type of organism. In rough bacteria, the "O" antigens are lost through a mutation that deprives the bacteria of enzymes required to synthesize the "O" antigen or attach them to the core. These rough bacteria thus lose hydrophilic surface properties provided by the abundant external sugars and no longer form smooth suspensions in liquid cultures (Fig. 2) or smooth colonies on solid media.

### Lipid A

The key to isolation of lipid A is KDO, a unique sugar with the formula 2-keto-3-deoxyoctonate (Heath and Ghalambor, 1963). A trisaccharide of KDO links lipid A to the core region, and mild acid hydrolysis will cleave the ketosidic linkage

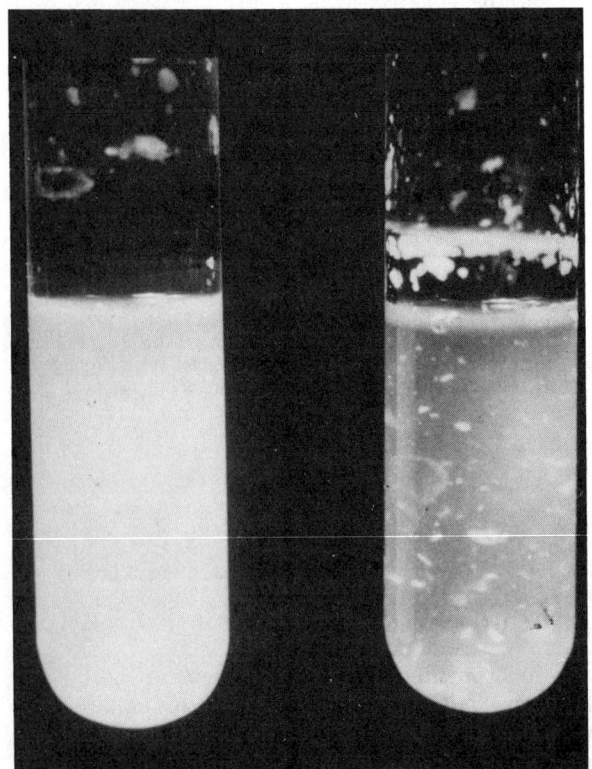

**FIGURE 2.** *Comparison of smooth parent culture of E. coli 0113 with rough mutant. The rough mutant is galactose deficient and cannot attach the "O" antigenic sugars to the core. The absence of "O" antigen deprives the LPS of abundant hydrophilic surface sugars and exposes the central hydrophobic lipids that are insoluble in water. (Rough mutant is on the right.)*

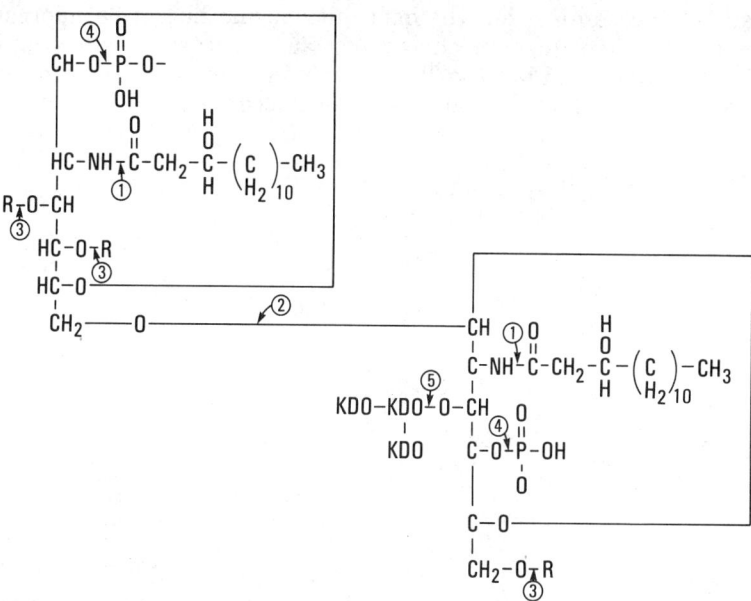

**FIGURE 3.** *Diagram of proposed structure of lipid A from* S. minnesota. *Note the following key structural features as indicated by arrows: 1) amide-linked β hydroxymyristic acid, 2) β-1,6 linkage of glucosamine disaccharide, 3) ester-linked long-chain fatty acids (R) at hydroxyl groups in positions 3,4, and 6 — these fatty acids are either lauric, palmitic, and 3-myristoxymystic, 4) phosphate groups at 1 and 4' may serve as bridges connecting the dissaccharide subunits, and 5) KDO trisaccharide.*

of KDO to lipid A, yielding water-insoluble preparations of lipid A with a molecular weight of approximately 2000. Another approach to the isolation of lipid A is through the use of mutants that synthesize a defective polysaccharide containing only lipid A and KDO. Mutants without lipid A have never been isolated, and therefore it appears indispensable for survival of bacteria.

Lipid A in most gram-negative bacilli of medical importance is composed of glucosamine-4-phosphate, long-chain fatty acids, and ethanolamine. [In certain saprophytes such as *Rhodopseudomonas,* glucosamine is absent from the lipid A (Hase and Rietschel, 1976)]. Thus, lipid A is an unusual phospholipid that uses D-glucosamine instead of glycerol as a skeleton. Disaccharides of glucosamine have β1,6 linkages in *Salmonella, Shigella, Escherichia coli, Yersinia, Fusobacterium, Pseudomonas,* and *Proteus.* The disaccharide subunits appear to be connected to each other through pyrophosphate or phosphodiester groups. The fatty acids are attached to the glucosamine subunit by ester or amide linkages (Fig. 3). In lipid A of *Salmonella minnesota,* for example, the hydroxyl groups in positions 6', 3, and 4 are esterified by lauric, palmitic, and 3-myristoxymyristic acid. The amino groups, on the other hand, are acylated with β-hydroxymyristic acid (3-hydroxytetradecanoic acid), a 14-carbon compound characteristically present in enterobacterial lipid A. Other β-hydroxy-fatty acids containing 10 to 17 carbon atoms are characteristic of different bacteria. In *Pseudomonas,* for example, the lipid A contains β-hydroxymyristic as in the enteric bacteria. These long-chain fatty acids give lipid A its lipoidal characteristics.

## Core Polysaccharide

This region contains not only KDO, the link to lipid A, but also heptose, phosphate, ethanolamine, and three hexoses. The hexoses, which consist of galactose, glucose and *N*-acetyl glucosamine, are designated the outer core, whereas the remainder is called the inner core. Much of the information on core sugars was obtained by examination of *Salmonella* mutants that were blocked in different steps in the biosynthesis of the core. These blocks resulted from defective activity of enzymes involved in transfer (transferase) or synthesis (synthetase; epimerase) of sugars. The sugars are transferred as sugar-nucleotides, usually as derivatives of uridine diphosphate (UDP) or guanosine diphosphate (GDP). The enzymes are associated with the cytoplasmic membrane where they catalyze the stepwise addition of the sugar-nucleotides to the nonreducing terminus of the growing core polymer. The inner core is constructed in the membrane by stepwise addition of KDO, heptose phosphate, and ethanolamine, followed by the hexose units of the outer core (Nikaido, 1973).

In rough mutants containing only KDO and heptose in the core, the LPS is designated chemotype Rd (Lüderitz et al., 1966). Such mutants lack the enzyme UDP-glucose synthetase so that synthesis of the core is not completed. In mutants with LPS designated Rc, the enzyme UDP galactose-4-epimerase is deficient so that glucose, but not galactose, is synthesized and incorporated into the core. The molecular weight of the Rc mutant is about 10,000. In chemotype Rb, the LPS contains all basal sugars except *N-*

acetylglucosamine, but the deficient enzyme has not been identified. In chemotype Ra, the core LPS is completed but the "O" side chains cannot be attached. The stepwise buildup of the core can be appreciated from its sugar sequences in the following diagrams showing each of the chemotypes of *Salmonella* LPS:

```
              Rd                                                  Rc

             KDO                                                 KDO
              |                                                   |
      heptose phosphate                               glucose—heptose phosphate
              |                                                   |
      heptose phosphate                                       heptose phosphate
              |                                                   |
      heptose phosphate                               glucose—heptose phosphate
              |                                                   |
      heptose phosphate                                       heptose phosphate
```

```
                                         Rb

                              galactose        KDO
                                  |             |
          glucose—galactose—glucose——heptose phosphate
                                          |
                              galactose—heptose phosphate
                                          |
          glucose—galactose—glucose——heptose phosphate
                                  |             |
                              galactose   heptose phosphate
```

```
                                             Ra

                                   galactose        KDO
                                       |             |
  N-acetyl glucosamine—glucose—galactose—glucose——heptose phosphate
                                                      |
                                   galactose—heptose phosphate
                                                      |
  N-acetyl glucosamine —glucose—galactose—glucose——heptose phosphate
                                       |
                                   galactose—heptose phosphate
```

### "O" Antigens

The outermost region of the LPS molecule consists of repeating oligosaccharide units containing usually three to five sugars each. Among these are certain unusual sugars that are rare except in gram-negative bacteria. Such rare sugars as 6-deoxyhexoses and 3,6-dideoxyhexoses are among the antigenic determinants that help classify the LPS and bacteria into serotypes through the use of specific antisera. Fucose and rhamnose are 6-deoxyhexoses commonly present in "O" side chains. Paratose, abequose, colitose, and tyvelose are important $\alpha$-3,6-dideoxyhexoses (Table 1). The synthesis of "O" side chains apparently begins on the inner surface of the cytoplasmic membrane where the oligosaccharide units are constructed (Nikaido, 1973). In *S. typhimurium,* for example, the unit is a tetrasaccharide built up by sequential addition of galactose, rhamnose, mannose, and the 3,6-dideoxyhexose abequose. The sugars are transported as nucleotides, and the tetrasaccharide is synthesized on a carrier lipid. The carrier lipid apparently transfers the tetrasaccharide across the cytoplasmic membrane where the units are polymerized into "O" side chains before attachment to the core region. The carrier lipid is a phosphorylated C55 polyisoprenoid alcohol (undecaprenol) with the following formula:

$$
\begin{array}{ccc}
\qquad CH_3 & & CH_3 \\
\qquad | & & | \\
CH_3-C=CH-CH_2-(CH_2-C=CH-CH-CH_2)_{10}- \\
\end{array}
$$

$$
\begin{array}{c}
OH \\
| \\
O-P-OH \\
\| \\
O
\end{array}
$$

This carrier lipid is probably identical to that which functions in the biosynthesis of cell wall peptidoglycan.

The chemical structure of many O-specific side chains has been determined by biosynthetic studies. The composition of the repeating oligosaccharide units in these side chains is given for certain pathogenic gram-negative bacilli in Table

**TABLE 1.  Composition of Repeating Oligosaccharide Units in Certain Pathogenic Gram-Negative Bacteria**

| BACTERIA | STRUCTURE | IMMUNE DOMINANT SUGAR | GROUP OR SEROGROUP |
|---|---|---|---|
| *Salmonella typhosa* | $\alpha$-Tyv                    $\alpha$-Glc<br>$\mid$                              $\mid$<br>2—($\alpha$)—Man—1,4—Rha—1,3 $\alpha$-Gal—1 | $\alpha$-Tyvelose | D |
| *Salmonella typhimurium* | $\alpha$-Abe                 $\alpha$-Glc$_{1,4}$<br>$\mid$                          $\mid$<br>2—d—Man—1,4—Rha $\rightarrow$ $\alpha$-Gal—1 | $\alpha$-Abequose | B |
| *Salmonella paratyphi* | $\alpha$-Par$_{1,3}$            $\alpha$-Glc$_{1,4}$<br>$\mid$                          $\mid$<br>2—$\alpha$-Man—1,4—Rha—1,3—$\alpha$-Gal—1 | Paratose | A |
| *Salmonella thompson* | Glc<br>$\mid$<br>Man—1,2—Man, 1,2—Man 1,2—Man—1 | Glucose | C$_1$ |
| *Salmonella anatum* | 6—B Man—1,4—Rha—1,3 $\alpha$-Gal—1 | Mannose | E$_1$ |
| *Shigella flexneri* | Ac<br>6—Glc Nac—1,2—Rha—1,4—Rha—1 | Rhamnose | 2a |

Glc = glucose; Gal = galactose; Rha = rhamnose; Man = mannose; Par = paratose; Glc Nac = *N*-acetyl glucosamine; Ab = abequose; Tyv = tyvelose; Ac = acetyl

1. It should be noted that for each repeating unit there is one or more immunodominant sugar that is most responsible for the serologic specificity of antiserum against each "O" antigen (Lüderitz et al., 1966). It is the sugar with the highest affinity for the reactive site of the "O" antibody, as determined by its ability to inhibit serologic reactions. From Table 1 it can be seen that the immunodominant sugar may be a terminal nonreducing sugar in the side chain ($\alpha$-tyvelose in *S. typhosa*) or main chain (rhamnose in *S. flexneri*). It may also be a nonterminal sugar in the main chain.

## BIOLOGIC ACTIVITY OF ENDOTOXINS

Injections of small doses of endotoxins into experimental animals bring about dramatic changes in blood pressure, clotting, body temperature, circulating blood cells, metabolism, humoral immunity, cellular immunity, and resistance to infection. A large dose is lethal. These changes can be elicited with LPS from gram-negative bacteria or the intact organisms. There are many ways to isolate LPS but the most widely used is the phenol-water method of Westphal et al. (1952). The organisms are extracted with 45 per cent aqueous phenol at 65 to 68° C. After cooling, the LPS is recovered in the aqueous phase, and must then be separated by ultracentrifugation from RNA, which also partitions into the aqueous layer. In rough organisms, the LPS is hydrophobic and is found mainly in the phenol phase; recovery from the aqueous phase is poor. Rough LPS is best extracted by a solvent containing phenol, petroleum ether, and chloroform and recovered by ultracentrifugation (Galanos et al., 1969).

### General Response to LPS

After intravenous injection of LPS the physiologic and biochemical changes depend on its dose and the animal species. In most animals (rabbits, dogs, monkeys, swine) injection of LPS in doses ranging from 0.1 to 100 $\mu$g will cause rapid onset of fever, neutropenia, and hypotension. The onset of neutropenia occurs almost immediately after injection of LPS, but fever and hypotension follow quickly, usually within 30 minutes. With large doses of LPS the hypotension may become irreversible and cause fatal shock. The pattern of fever, neutropenia, and hypotension has also been seen in patients given LPS or intravenous typhoid vaccine for fever therapy.

### Fever

The most detailed studies of fever after injection of LPS have been carried out in rabbits. After intravenous injection of 0.1 $\mu$g LPS from most smooth bacteria the temperature begins to rise after a latent period of 10 to 20 minutes and reaches a peak at about 70 minutes. After the first peak the temperature declines slightly but starts to rise again at 2 hours and reaches a second higher peak at about 3 hours. The second peak alone is dose dependent; it is absent with minimal pyogenic doses of LPS and gradually increases with rising doses until it reaches a ceiling that cannot be exceeded. According to current concepts the fever occurring after intravenous injection of endotoxin is mediated by a protein released from neutrophils or monocytes and designated endogenous pyrogen (EP) (Atkins and Bodel, 1972). No latent period precedes the rise in fever after injection of EP because it stimulates the fever centers in the hypothalamus directly without the intermediate reaction between pyrogen and leukocyte that occurs with LPS. It is possible, however, that endotoxin itself can stimulate the fever centers directly because the amount of LPS needed to cause fever after injection into the cerebrospinal fluid is only one-one thousandth that required by intravenous injection, and the latent period is less after intraspinal injection (Bennett et al., 1957). These findings would suggest that fever production requires EP in bacteremia but not in meningitis (e.g., meningococcemia vs meningococcal meningitis).

One of the classic features of endotoxin fever is tolerance (Fig. 4). The tolerance phenomenon occurs after repeated injections of the same dose of LPS and is characterized by a diminution in the height and duration of fever with successive injections. In rabbits this causes mainly a decline in the second peak. Two forms of tolerance are seen: (1) *early* tolerance, which is seen within 12 hours of the first injection; and (2) *late* tolerance, which appears gradually over several days. Early tolerance has been attributed to depletion of EP, or to a refractory response of the heat centers, which protects against sustained hypothermia. Late tolerance results from an immune reaction in which circulating antibody neutralizes LPS. Late tolerance can be transferred passively with serum, and causes accelerated disappearance of LPS into the reticuloendothelial system (Carey et al., 1958).

These febrile reactions are seen in nearly all mammals, including humans. In fact, man is far more sensitive to the pyrogenic action of LPS than any other animal, requiring 10 times less LPS than rabbits for the same febrile response (Wolff, 1973). Man also exhibits a longer latent period between injection of LPS and onset of fever and the fever curves are always monophasic. In tolerant human subjects the monophasic fever disappears completely, whereas tolerant rabbits maintain a monophasic response.

Rats and mice are exceptions to the rule that LPS injection causes fever in mammals. These

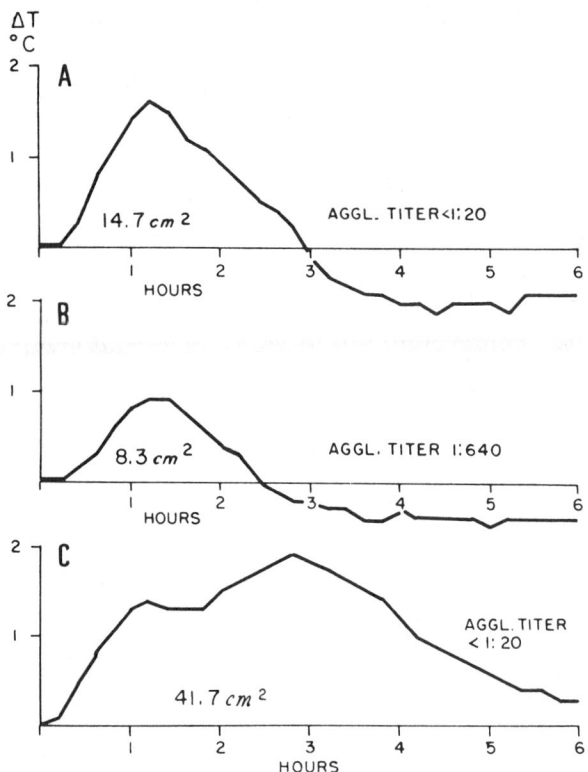

**FIGURE 4.** *A comparison in rabbits of A, early tolerance, B, late tolerance, and C, no tolerance to the pyrogenic activity of lipopolysaccharides. Note biphasic fever peaks in nontolerant rabbits and disappearance of second peak after tolerance develops. Curve "A" is produced in rabbits challenged 24 hours after one I.V. injection and curve "B" after the last of seven daily I.V. injections of 1.0 μg of endotoxin. Curve "C" was obtained in control rabbits with no prior injections (Milner, 1973.)*

two rodents respond to injection of LPS by a depression in body temperature.

### Hypotension

The blood pressure may fall in animals given the small doses of endotoxin required to produce fever, but sustained hypotension and shock usually require larger doses of LPS. For example, 100 μg *Escherichia coli* endotoxin will induce severe hemodynamic disturbances in 75 per cent of rabbits after intravenous injection.

Severe hypotension occurs about 30 minutes after injection of LPS and is the terminal manifestation of a series of preceding hypodynamic disturbances. The first of these in rabbits is a rise in pulmonary artery pressure due to an increase in acute resistance in the pulmonary veins. This obstruction to flow causes a drop in cardiac output with a secondary fall in arterial pressure as seen in Figure 5 (Neuhof, 1975). In dogs the first reaction is constriction of hepatic and small mesenteric veins so that blood is pooled in the mesenteric circulation. The resultant decrease in ve-

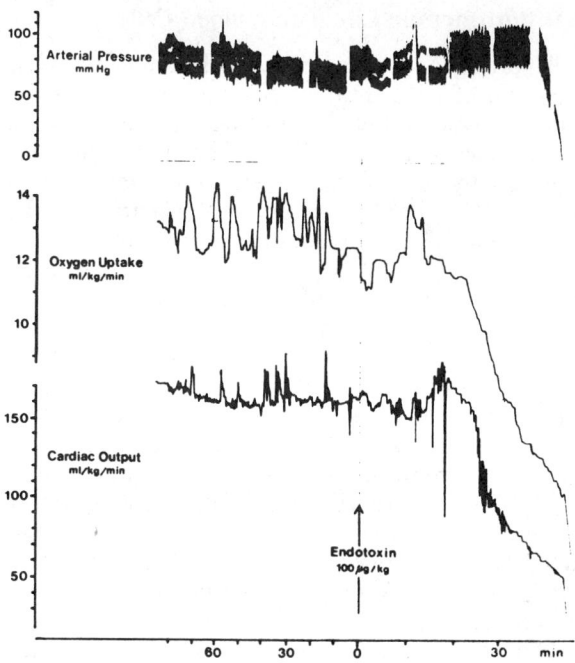

**FIGURE 5.** *Early phase of endotoxin shock in the rabbit. Fall in cardiac output precedes drop in blood pressure (Neuhof, 1975).*

nous return to the heart lowers the cardiac output but prevents pulmonary hypertension despite increased resistance in the pulmonary vascular system. The fall in cardiac output in all animals undergoing endotoxic shock results in reduced oxygen supply to the tissues. The low arterial pressure causes, in turn, reduced coronary perfusion.

In contrast to shock from fluid loss by hemorrhage, diarrhea, sweating, or vomiting, the hypotension in endotoxic shock cannot be corrected by administration of intravenous saline or blood. Fluid administration is likewise ineffective in overcoming shock in patients with heavy bacteremia due to gram-negative organisms.

## Intravascular Coagulation

The local and generalized Shwartzman reactions are the classic manifestations of abnormal clotting from endotoxin (Table 2). To produce either phenomenon animals are given two injections of endotoxin 12 to 18 hours apart. In the local Shwartzman reaction, the first dose is injected intradermally and the second intravenously. An area of hemorrhagic necrosis occurs at the site of intradermal injection within a few hours after the second injection. In the generalized Shwartzman reaction both injections of LPS are given intravenously and the animals develop bilateral cortical necrosis of the kidneys within a few hours after the second dose.

Both reactions are the result of intravascular coagulation and the selective occlusion of small vessels by fibrin. The mechanism proposed for the local reaction involves two steps: first, the intravenous dose initiates intravascular coagulation with production of fibrin polymers; second, these polymers are trapped in the skin vessels that had been injured by the inflammatory reaction around the intradermal dose of LPS. There is no renal cortical necrosis because most of the circulating fibrin is cleared by the reticuloendothelial system (RE). In the generalized Shwartzman reaction, the first intravenous dose of LPS initiates coagulation and the second blocks RE removal of fibrin. The excess circulating fibrin is then filtered by the glomerular capillaries, which become occluded so that the renal cortex is infarcted. Small vessels in other organs may also filter fibrin. Both local and generalized reactions can be prevented by anticoagulants such as heparin.

The mechanism by which endotoxin initiates coagulation is not clear but there is good evidence that both intrinsic (plasma) and extrinsic (tissue) factors are involved (Morrison and Ulevitch, 1978). Clotting via the *intrinsic* pathway appears to be initiated when endotoxin activates Hageman factor (XIII) through a reaction involving the negatively charged phosphate residues of

**TABLE 2.   Comparison of Local and Generalized Shwartzman Reactions**

| TYPE OF REACTION | FIRST DOSE | SECOND DOSE | INTERVAL BETWEEN DOSES (Hours) | DOSE OF ENDOTOXIN (mg), e.g., *E. coli* 0111 LPS First | Second | MANIFESTATIONS OF REACTION | CLINICAL EXAMPLE |
|---|---|---|---|---|---|---|---|
| Local Shwartzman | Intradermal | Intravenous | 21–24 | 0.25 | 0.03 | Hemorrhagic necrosis of skin | Meningococcal purpura |
| Generalized Shwartzman | Intravenous | Intravenous | 21–24 | 0.125 | 0.03 | Bilateral renal cortical necrosis | Bilateral renal cortical necrosis in *E. coli* septicemia of pregnancy |

lipid A. Hageman activation requires that a complex be formed between endotoxin and Hageman factor, probably by binding it to lipid A. Activation of Hageman factor eventuates in clotting because it initiates steps leading to the conversion of prothrombin to thrombin. The *extrinsic* pathway has been implicated because blood leukocytes are needed for both the local and generalized Shwartzman reactions, which are prevented by nitrogen mustard and other agents that cause leukopenia. Among the leukocytes, monocytes are currently regarded as the important circulating mediator cell for releasing the tissue factor (TF) that initiates clotting through the extrinsic pathway. TF is a lipoprotein in the plasma membrane of various cells, which complexes with factor VII and calcium ions to activate factor X. Activated factor X then converts prothrombin to thrombin.

The intravascular coagulation that leads to the generalized Shwartzman reaction depletes clotting factors such as fibrinogen, platelets, and prothrombin. During intravascular coagulation, fibrinolysis is activated so that fibrin-degradation fragments (or fibrin split-products) accumulate in the blood. These fragments become anticoagulants since they inhibit both proteolysis of fibrinogen by thrombin and the polymerization of fibrin monomer to form a clot. In addition, the split-products inhibit platelet aggregation. This combined effect of split-products on clotting and platelet function can cause serious bleeding in patients whose clotting factors are consumed by disseminated intravascular coagulation in meningococcemia and other severe infections caused by gram-negative bacteria (Davis and Arnold, 1974).

### In Vitro Coagulation

The addition of endotoxin to whole blood markedly shortens clotting time by activating Hageman factor and by stimulating leukocytes to release TF.

Endotoxin also clots the lysate prepared from the amebocytes of the horseshoe crab, *Limulus polyphemus* (Levin and Bang, 1964). This reaction has become important because clotting occurs in the presence of extremely small concentrations of endotoxin. The limulus lysate contains a clottable protein that forms a gel when exposed to as little as 0.0005 $\mu$g/ml of LPS. Endotoxin activates a high molecular weight (84,000) enzyme, which then reacts with a clottable protein to produce a gel. This reaction has been used to detect endotoxin in drugs, fluids, and other materials prepared for injection into patients. Limulus lysate has also been used to demonstrate endotoxin in the blood and spinal fluid of patients with gram-negative bacterial infections.

### Disturbances in Circulating Blood Cells

Severe neutropenia occurs within minutes after injection of LPS into rabbits and other animals and persists at levels less than 10 per cent of normal for 4 hours (Fig. 6). The neutropenia is followed by leukocytosis, with normoblasts and many other immature cells appearing in the circulation. The neutropenia results from sequestration of neutrophils in capillaries of the lung and other organs; and the leukocytosis results from the release of granulocytes from the bone marrow. Higher doses of LPS are required for neutropenia than for leukocytosis, probably because the numbers released from the marrow mask the mild sequestration of neutrophils produced by small doses. Because human beings cannot tolerate the relatively large doses given to rabbits and other animals, neutropenia has not always been observed in human studies but leukocytosis is constant and reproducible in them (Wolff, 1973).

The number of circulating platelets also falls rapidly after intravenous injection of LPS, and they are found in leukocyte-platelet thrombi or platelet-aggregates in small vessels of the lung and liver. As the platelets fall, there is a simultaneous release from them of platelet constituents such as serotonin and platelet factor 8. This rapid drop in platelets requires complement. From in vitro experiments it appears that endotoxin also causes platelet lysis through a reaction that requires the alternative pathway of complement. Primates, including man, appear to be much less susceptible to thrombocytopenia after endotoxin injection than are lower mammals, and primate platelets do not seem to react to endotoxin in vitro. In contrast to rabbit platelets, which undergo massive aggregation in platelet-rich plasma, human platelets do not aggregate when exposed to endotoxin (Morrison and Ulevitch, 1978).

Lymphocytes fall less precipitously than granulocytes and platelets and return more slowly to the circulation. They are also unaffected by tolerance. Daily injections of the same dose of endotoxin elicit a shorter period of neutrophil response. These tolerant animals develop only a brief period of neutropenia and a brisk rise in circulating neutrophils that begins between 1 and 2 hours after injection of endotoxin (Fig. 6). Lymphocytes, on the other hand, maintain their slow decline in tolerant animals.

### Immune Reactions: Cellular

*Lymphocytes.* Endotoxin stimulates proliferation of bone marrow-derived (B) lymphocytes (Peavy et al., 1973). This mitogenic effect of B lymphocytes results from the action of lipid A. It is demonstrated morphologically by transforma-

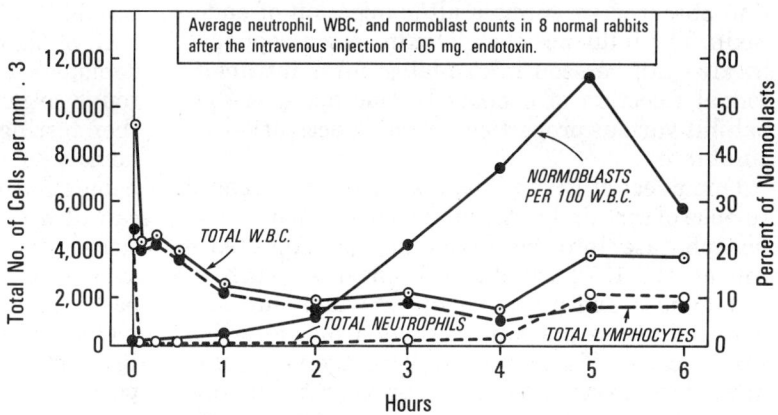

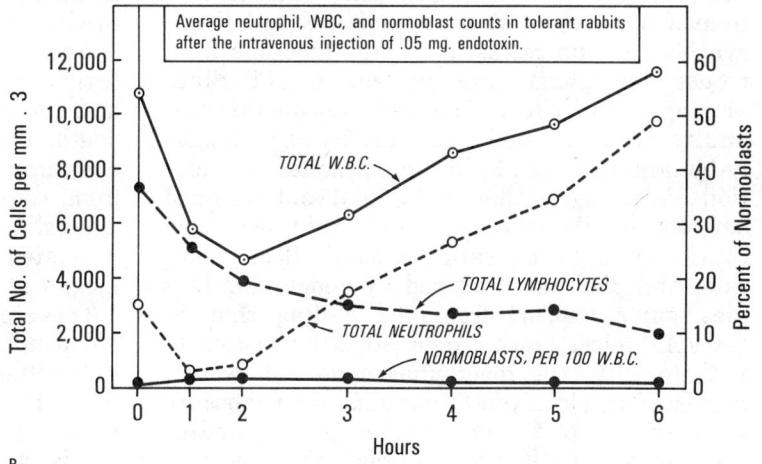

**FIGURE 6.** *Comparison of hematologic responses to intravenous lipopolysaccharide in A, normal (nontolerant) and B, tolerant rabbits.*

tion of B lymphocytes to blast cells and biochemically by increased synthesis of RNA, DNA, and protein. The phenomenon is seen in vitro with mouse lymphocytes, but not human or rabbit lymphocytes. It appears that stimulation by LPS of B cell mitosis results in division and differentiation into cells that secrete at a high rate the specific antibodies that are genetically determined for each cell. If such a reaction occurs in vivo, it could explain the increased nonspecific resistance to infection that occurs in mice shortly after an injection of endotoxin.

This idea is supported by the fact that mice (C3H/H$_e$J) whose B lymphocytes do not proliferate when exposed to LPS also fail to develop increased resistance to infection when injected with LPS. The defective response of B lymphocytes to LPS is genetic and is accompanied by increased resistance of the mice to LPS toxicity (Sulzer and Goodman, 1977).

*Macrophages.* LPS activates macrophages most likely by a direct effect of lipid A on the cell membrane and without the mediation of T lymphocytes (Rosenstreich et al., 1977). Activation of macrophages by LPS causes them to increase in size, become more adherent to glass, exhibit greater random migration, and carry out increased phagocytosis. There is increased phagocytosis of certain bacteria, complement- (C3b) coated particles, and IgG antibody-coated particles. Activated macrophages are metabolically more active, showing an increased consumption of glucose via the hexosemonophosphate shunt. They also increase their production of certain enzymes such as collagenase, lactic dehydrogenase (cytoplasmic), and acid phosphatase (lysosomal). Electron microscopy reveals hypertrophy of the Golgi region and an increase in the number and size of lysosomes. As little as 1 μg/ml of LPS will stimulate increased phagocytosis in vitro, and similar concentrations in vivo will cause activation of the reticuloendothelial system so that endotoxin and various colloidal particles are cleared more rapidly from the circulation. These properties of activated macrophages might also contribute to the nonspecific resistance to infection observed in animals after injection of endotoxin. The influence of endotoxin on macrophages in vivo can be seen in exudates; after intraperitoneal injection of endotoxin, macrophages that exhibit various properties typical of activation accumulate.

One effect of LPS on macrophages is increased release of certain lysosomal enzymes, such as acid phosphatase, into the surrounding medium (Allison et al., 1973). Proteolytic enzymes, such as collagenase and plasminogen activator, are also released. Since plasmin (activated plasminogen) would cause fibrinolysis and collagenase could disrupt connective tissue, it is easy to imagine how macrophages might mediate certain toxic effects of LPS. Prostaglandins, a group of biologically active aliphatic acids, have also been implicated as mediators of LPS toxicity upon release from macrophages. Prostaglandins E and F are synthesized and released in large amounts from mouse macrophages after exposure to LPS. Since prostaglandins cause increased vascular permeability, vasodilatation, vasoconstriction (especially by prostaglandin $F_2$ in the pulmonary circulation), decreased cardiac output, and contraction of smooth muscle (uterus, bowel, bronchi), they could account for the cardiovascular effects, abortion, and diarrhea produced by endotoxin. This idea gains support from the finding that in $C3H/H_eJ$ mice, which are genetically resistant to LPS toxicity, the macrophages do not secrete increased levels of prostaglandins upon exposure to endotoxin. Moreover, levels of prostaglandins are elevated in susceptible animals after injection of endotoxin, and indomethacin, which inhibits prostaglandin synthesis, also prevents certain toxic effects of endotoxin.

Endotoxin is taken up by macrophages by pinocytosis. The endotoxin is first adsorbed onto the cell membrane and then enters the cell through membrane invaginations. Peritoneal macrophages of guinea pigs are reported not to detoxify ingested endotoxin in vitro, but information on macrophages of other species in vitro and in vivo is too limited for general conclusions on cellular detoxification.

Large doses of endotoxin (e.g., 50 $\mu$g/ml *Escherichia coli* LPS) will kill macrophages in vitro.

### Immune Reactions: Humoral

*Antibody.* Injection of endotoxin or infection with gram-negative bacteria stimulates circulating antibody to LPS. Smooth endotoxins stimulate primarily antibody to the "O" antigenic side chains and endotoxin from rough bacteria, antibody to the core. Antibody to lipid A has also been described after injection of bacterial cells of *Salmonella minnesota* R595, which have the glycolipid KDO-lipid A on their surface. Antibody to each of these antigens ("O", core, lipid A) can be demonstrated by adsorbing LPS from smooth or rough organisms to the surface of red cells and then testing the antisera for their ability to cause hemolysis (in the presence of complement) or hemagglutination. Antibody to these antigens can also be demonstrated by precipitation reactions, precipitation-inhibition with individual sugars, enzyme-linked immunoabsorption, and bactericidal reactions in the presence of complement. Antibodies against LPS are both IgM and IgG. When lipid A is removed from the "O" polysaccharides by mild acid treatment, the "O" antigenic unit can no longer stimulate the formation of antibodies unless it is coupled to protein. The uncoupled, lipid-free O antigen is thus a nonantigenic hapten and can be identified only by in vitro reactions with specific antibody.

Antibody to "O" or "core" antigens can prevent toxicity of LPS, including the local Shwartzman and generalized Shwartzman reactions and death. The protection by "O" antibody is specific and limited to homologous LPS, whereas that from core antibody provides broad protection against LPS from a wide range of bacteria with unrelated "O" antigens (Braude et al., 1977; Ziegler et al., 1973).

The ability of LPS to stimulate antibody is independent of T lymphocytes. In this respect, LPS differs from most protein and cellular antigens that require a cooperation between T and B lymphocytes, in which the T lymphocytes activate the B lymphocytes to synthesize immunoglobulin.

*Complement.* Endotoxins can activate the complement system so that the various components are consumed and their activity disappears from serum (Mergenhagen et al., 1973). This activation can occur through either the classic or the alternative pathways, depending on the preparation of LPS. Activation of the classic pathway begins with activating of C1, which in turn catalyzes the assembly of C4,2 into the enzyme C3 convertase. C3 convertase activates C3 and the remaining components of complement. The first step in the reaction occurs in the presence of specific antibody against LPS, i.e., either IgG or IgM. After LPS combines with the Fab portion of the antibody, its Fc portion binds with C1 through its subunit C1q, and C1 becomes activated. There is also evidence that LPS from rough strains, as well as lipid A, can bind C1 directly and thereby activate the classic pathway without participation of antibody to LPS (Morrison and Ulevitch, 1978).

When the alternative pathway is activated by

LPS, the first two steps of the classic pathway are omitted. Instead, LPS causes the enzymatic activation of a protein that can cleave C3. The activated protein, designated C3 activator, splits C3 into C3A and C3B. The C3B activates the remaining complement components.

Activation of complement by either pathway can kill gram-negative (but not gram-positive) bacteria. Complement activated by the classic pathway kills bacteria more rapidly, and rough bacteria are generally more susceptible than smooth bacteria to this bactericidal action. It has been suggested that this difference in susceptibility to killing by the complement system is due to the greater ability of LPS from rough bacteria to activate the more efficient classic pathway.

Complement can also be activated by endotoxin in vivo (Spink et al., 1964; Gilbert and Braude, 1962). Endotoxins obtained by trichloroacetic extraction (Boivin preparation) are more effective in lowering complement levels in vivo. The initial hypotensive response to endotoxin is dependent on complement activation, and in patients with shock due to gram-negative bacteremia the levels of C3 are reduced (McCabe, 1973). These findings suggest that bacteremic shock may be mediated to some extent through a reaction between endotoxin and complement.

*Adjuvant Effect.* When endotoxin is injected intravenously along with a protein antigen, the subsequent antibody response to the protein antigen begins earlier, increases faster, and reaches a higher level than in controls given no endotoxin (Johnson, 1964). This enhancement of antibody response by endotoxin in known as its adjuvant effect, and explains the well known clinical observation that incorporation of typhoid vaccine with diphtheria or tetanus toxoid produces more antitoxin. Endotoxin does not need to be given by the same route as the protein antigen, but for maximal effect it should be given at the same time or within 6 hours of the antigen. Repeated injections of endotoxin, leading to tolerance to LPS toxicity, also abolish the adjuvant effect. The mechanism of the adjuvant effect of LPS is unknown. Since LPS can be detoxified by succinylation without losing its adjuvant activity, LPS toxicity does not seem essential for the adjuvant effect.

### Stimulation of Interferon Activity

When endotoxin is injected intravenously into experimental animals peak levels of interferon in the serum are reached within 2 to 3 hours (Youngner and Stinebring, 1966). Earlier data suggested that endotoxin caused the release of preformed interferon, but more recent evidence indicates that both endotoxin and viruses stimulate synthesis of interferon.

### Other Effects

*Abortion.* Injections of sublethal amounts of endotoxin can interrupt pregnancy in mice (Zahl and Bjerknes, 1943). The abortion is accompanied by placental hemorrhage and is apparently related to serotonin release. Endotoxins obtained from smooth or rough gram-negative bacteria, as well as lipid A, are abortifacient.

*Tumor Necrosis.* Endotoxin causes hemorrhagic necrosis of tumors in guinea pigs, rats, mice, and man. Most studies have been done with transplantable sarcomas of mice. The tumor becomes hemorrhagic 4 hours after the intravenous injection of crude or purified endotoxins and may undergo extensive necrosis and complete regression. The appearance of the necrotic tumor has suggested a similarity to the local Shwartzman reaction, but no thrombosis is observed in the hemorrhagic tumor.

*Metabolic Effects.* Intravenous injection of LPS causes changes in carbohydrates, lipids, iron, and sensitivity to epinephrine (Fiser et al., 1974). The level of blood glucose rises to a maximum within 2 hours after injection of LPS and then declines to severe hypoglycemic levels in shocked animals. This reaction is accompanied by rapid depletion of total body carbohydrate and impaired synthesis of glucose and glycogen (Berry, 1975). Administration of glucose or pyruvate fails to restore gluconeogenesis or glycogen synthesis to normal.

Hyperglyceridemia has been found in rabbits and rhesus monkeys after intravenous endotoxin (Lequire et al., 1959). It has also been seen in patients during septicemia due to gram-negative bacteria, but not gram-positive bacteria. It appears that endotoxin elevates serum triglyceride concentrations by interfering with the activation of lipid-clearing enzymes and the clearance of lipids by the reticuloendothelial system.

Hypoferremia occurs in mice and rats after injection of small doses (0.1 $\mu$g) of LPS and can be used as a bioassay for endotoxin.

The increased susceptibility to epinephrine is manifested by its ability to produce skin hemorrhages after intradermal injection in rabbits given intravenous LPS simultaneously, or after intradermal infections of mixtures of LPS and epinephrine (Thomas, 1956). As little as 5 $\mu$g of intradermal epinephrine and 1 $\mu$g of intravenous LPS can produce hemorrhagic necrosis resembling the local Shwartzman reaction. In contrast to the Shwartzman reaction, the epinephrine lesion is not blocked by heparin or nitrogen mustard, but is prevented by cortisone, dibenzaline, and chlorpromazine, which do not prevent the Shwartzman. This reaction to epinephrine may reflect either an increased sensitivity of the arterioles to adrenergic stimulation or an increased release of catecholamines at the peripheral nerve endings resulting from endotoxin activation of the sympathetic nervous system. The combined effects of local catecholamines and injected epinephrine might cause sufficient vasoconstriction to infarct the skin, whereas neither could do so alone.

## ALTERATION OF LPS TOXICITY

### Reduced Toxicity

The toxicity of LPS can be reduced in vivo with antiserum or by inducing tolerance, as described earlier. It can also be reduced by the administration of cortisone (Chedid and Boyer, 1955) or polymyxin B sulfate. Cortisone prevents death when given before lethal doses of endotoxin are injected. When polymyxin B is injected before or together with endotoxin it can neutralize the Shwartzman reactions and prevent death of mice from endotoxin (Rifkind and Hill, 1967). Polymyxin B acts by disrupting the structure of LPS.

Although relatively resistant to heat, the toxicity of endotoxin can be abolished in vitro by dry heat at 170° C for 3 hours. It is also detoxified by acid hydrolysis at elevated temperatures (0.1 N acid), by alkaline hydrolysis, and by oxidation with periodate, $H_2O_2$, or permanganate. It can be reversibly inactivated by a heat-labile factor in serum that appears to depolymerize LPS. Sodium dodecyl sulfate and sodium deoxycholate are also reputed to inactivate LPS by depolymerizing it; after removal of these agents the LPS reaggregates and toxicity is restored.

### Potentiation of Toxicity

A variety of procedures can potentiate LPS toxicity in experimental animals. One mechanism is reticuloendothelial blockage by thorium dioxide, which enhances the ability of endotoxin to kill animals and eliminates the increased resistance to the Shwartzman reaction and fever (tolerance) that follows repeated injections of endotoxins (Beeson, 1947). Colloidal iron saccharate, trypan blue, and lead acetate all enhance LPS toxicity when injected. A high molecular weight polygalactose, known as carrageenan, can increase the lethality of endotoxin by 100- to more than 3000-fold (Becker and Rudbach, 1978). Carrageenan is believed to function as a macrophage toxin by destabilizing the lysosomal membrane. All these agents probably enhance the toxicity of LPS by impairing macrophage function and blocking the reticuloendothelial system.

Other techniques for potentiating LPS toxicity are adrenalectomy (Parant and Chedid, 1971), mycobacterial infection, and high environmental temperatures. The mechanisms involved in lowering resistance to endotoxin by these procedures are unknown. Hypersensitivity to endotoxin, induced by repeated small intraperitoneal injections, increases the lethality of endotoxin for mice. These hypersensitivity deaths resemble anaphylaxis, occurring within 2 hours after challenge with endotoxin (Braude, 1975).

## References

Allison, A., Davies, P., and Page, R.: Effect of endotoxin on macrophages and other lymphoreticular cells. J Infect Dis 128(S):204, 1973.

Atkins, E., and Bodel, P.: Fever. N Engl J Med 286:27, 1972.

Becker, L., and Rudbach, J. A.: Potentiation of endotoxicity by carrageenan. Infect Immun 19:1099, 1978.

Beeson, P.: Effect of reticuloendothelial blockage on immunity to the Shwartzman phenomenon. Proc Soc Exp Biol Med 64:146, 1947.

Bennett, I. L., Jr., Petersdorf, R. G., and Keene, W. R.: Pathogenesis of fever: evidence for direct cerebral action of bacterial endotoxins. Trans Assoc Am Physicians 70:64, 1957.

Berry, L. J.: Metabolic effects of endotoxin. In Schlesinger, D. (ed.): Microbiology 1975. Washington D.C., American Society for Microbiology, 1975, p. 315.

Braude, A.: Opposing effects of immunity to endotoxin: hypersensitivity versus protection. In Urbaschek, B., Urbaschek, R., and Neter, E. (eds.): Gram-Negative Bacterial Infections. New York, Springer-Verlag, 1975, p. 69.

Braude, A., Ziegler, E., Douglas, H., and McCutchan, J.: Antibody to cell wall glycolipid of Gram-negative bacteria: induction of immunity to bacteremia and endotoxemia. J Infect Dis 136(S):167, 1977.

Carey, F., Zalesky, M., and Braude, A.: Studies with radioactive endotoxin. III. The effect of tolerance on the distribution of radioactivity after intravenous injection of Escherichia coli endotoxin labeled with $Cr^{51}$. J Clin Invest 37:441, 1958.

Chedid, L., and Boyer, F.: Étude comparative du pouvoir antitoxique de la cortisone et de la chlorpromazine. Ann Inst Pasteur 88:336, 1955.

Davis, C., and Arnold, K.: Role of meningococcal endotoxin in meningococcal purpura. J Exp Med 140:159, 1974.

Fiser, R., Denniston, J., and Beisel, W.: Endotoxemia in the rhesus monkey; alterations in host lipid and carbohydrate metabolism. Pediatr Res 8:13, 1974.

Galanos, C., Lüderitz, O., and Westphal, O.: A new method for the extraction of R lipopolysaccharides. Eur J Biochem 9:245, 1969.

Gilbert, V., and Braude, A.: Reduction in serum complement in rabbits after injection of endotoxin. J Exp Med 116:477, 1962.

Hase, S., and Rietschel, E. T.: Isolation and analysis of the lipid A backbone, lipid A structure of lipopolysaccharides from various bacterial groups. Eur J Biochem 63:101, 1976.

Heath, E. C., and Ghalambor, M. A.: 2-keto-3-deoxyoctonate, a constituent of cell wall lipopolysaccharide preparations obtained from E. coli. Biochem Biophys Res Commun 10:340, 1963.

Johnson, A.: Adjuvant action of bacterial endotoxin of the primary antibody response. In Landy, M., and Braun, W. (eds.): Bacterial Endotoxins. New Brunswick, N. J., Rutgers University Press, 1964, p. 252.

Lequire, V., Hutcherson, J., Hamilton, R., and Gray, M.: The effects of bacterial endotoxin on lipid metabolism. I. The responses of the serum lipids in rabbits to single and multiple injections of Shear's polysaccharide. J Exp Med 110:293, 1959.

Levin, J., and Bang, F.: The role of endotoxin in the extracellular coagulation of limulus blood. Bull Johns Hopkins Hosp 115:265, 1964.

Lüderitz, O., Staub, A. M., and Westphal, O.: Immunochemistry of O and R antigens of Salmonella and related Enterobacteriaceae. Bacteriol Rev 30:192, 1966.

McCabe, W.: Serum complement levels in bacteremia due to gram negative organisms. N Engl J Med 288:21, 1973.

Mergenhagen, S., Snyderman, R., and Phillips, K.: Activation of complement by endotoxin. J Infect Dis 128(S):78, 1973.

Milner, K.: Patterns of tolerance to endotoxin. J Infect Dis 128(S):229, 1973.

Morrison, D., and Ulevitch, R.: The effects of bacterial endotoxins on host mediation systems: A review. Am J Path 93:527, 1978.

Neuhof, H.: Changes in hemodynamics and gas metabolism after endotoxin injection. In Urbaschek, B., Urbaschek, R., and Neter, E. (eds.): Gram-Negative Bacterial Infections. New York, Springer-Verlag, 1975, p. 259.

Nikaido, H.: Biosynthesis and assembly of lipopolysaccharide and the outer membrane layer of Gram-negative cell wall. In Leive, L. (ed.): Bacterial Membranes and Walls. New York, Marcel Dekker, Inc., 1973, p. 131.

Parant, M., and Chedid, L.: Sensibilization de la souris aux endotoxines par la surrénalectomie ou par l'administration d'actinomycine D. C R Acad Sci (D) (Paris) 272:1308, 1971.

Peavy, D., Shands, J., Adler, W., and Smith, R.: Selective effects of bacterial endotoxins on various subpopulations of lymphoreticular cells. J Infect Dis 128(S):83, 1973.

Rifkind, D., and Hill, R.: Neutralization of the Shwartzman reactions by polymyxin B. J Immunol 99:564, 1967.

Rosenstreich, D., Glode, L., Wahl, L., Sandberg, A., and Mergenhagen, S.: Analysis of the cellular defects of endotoxin-unresponsive mice. In Schlesinger, D. (ed.): Microbiology 1977. Washington, D.C., American Society for Microbiology, 1977, p. 314.

Spink, W., Davis, R., Potter, R., and Chartrand, S.: The initial stage of canine endotoxin shock as an expression of anaphylactic shock: studies on complement titers and plasma histamine concentrations. J Clin Invest 43:696, 1964.

Sulzer, B., and Goodman, G.: Characteristics of Endotoxin. Resistant Low-Responder Mice. In Schlesinger, D. (ed.): Microbiology 1977. Washington D.C., American Society for Microbiology, 1977, p. 304.

Thomas, L.: The role of epinephrine in the reactions produced by the endotoxins of Gram-negative bacteria. I. Hemorrhagic necrosis produced by epinephrine in the skin of endotoxin-treated rabbits. J Exp Med 104:865, 1956.

Westphal, O., Lüderitz, O., and Bister, F.: Uber die extraktion von Bakterien mit Phenol/Wasser. Z Naturforsch 7b:148, 1952.

Wolff, S. M.: Biologic effects of bacterial endotoxins in man. J Infect Dis 128(S):251, 1973.

Youngner, J. S., and Stinebring, W. R.: Comparison of interferon production in mice by bacterial endotoxin and statolon. Virology 29:310, 1966.

Zahl, P., and Bjerknes, C.: Induction of decidua-placental hemorrhage in mice by the endotoxins of certain gram-negative bacteria. Proc Soc Exp Biol Med 54:329, 1943.

Ziegler, E., Douglas, H., and Braude, A.: Human antiserum for prevention of the local Shwartzman reaction and death from bacterial lipopolysaccharides. J Clin Invest 52:3236, 1973.

# Virology

# MORPHOLOGY AND STRUCTURE OF VIRUSES  7

## Richard W. Compans, Ph.D.

Viruses were first distinguished from other microorganisms on the basis of size, as determined by filtration techniques. Most infectious virus particles, or *virions,* are smaller than any bacteria, and are below the limit of resolution of the light microscope. The smallest virions are 20 to 30 nanometers in diameter (1 nanometer, nm, = $10^{-9}$ meter) and are the simplest agents known to cause infectious diseases of man.

In addition to their size, virions may be distinguished from other microorganisms by the fact that they contain only a single type of nucleic acid, either DNA or RNA. RNA-containing viruses are unique in possessing this type of nucleic acid as their genetic material.

Virions lack metabolic activity and do not possess ribosomes or many of the enzymes necessary for macromolecular synthesis, although they may contain certain specialized enzymes, as discussed in Chapter 9. As a consequence, viruses depend on cellular processes for their replication and are obligate intracellular parasites. Their replication process involves intracellular dissolution of virions into their macromolecular components, followed by synthesis of viral proteins and nucleic acids, whose structures are specified by the viral genome. The individual viral macromolecules are then assembled into progeny virions in yields as high as thousands of particles per infected cell. This type of replication cycle differs markedly from division by binary fission, which is the process by which bacteria multiply.

### METHODS FOR ANALYSIS OF VIRUS STRUCTURE

Filtration through membranes with graded pore sizes provided the earliest information on the size characteristics of different viruses. Similarly, ultracentrifugation studies enabled estimates of virus particle size before viruses could be visualized in the electron microscope. The ultracentrifuge is still essential for the concentration and purification of viruses, both of which are prerequisites for direct biochemical analyses. Differential centrifugation enables viruses to be concentrated and partially purified; alternatively, many viruses may be concentrated by precipitation with reagents such as ammonium sulfate or polyethylene glycol. Subsequently, most viruses may be purified by density gradient centrifugation in various media, the choice of which depends on the buoyant density as well as the stability of the virion. The most common are aqueous solutions of sucrose or potassium tartrate for the less dense and more fragile viruses, and cesium chloride solutions for the more stable viruses.

The structure of almost all animal viruses has now been examined directly by electron microscopy. If purified or concentrated virus suspensions are available, negative staining is usually the method of choice for specimen preparation. The procedure involves drying a suspension of virions in an aqueous solution of a heavy atom salt such as uranyl acetate or sodium phosphotungstate, which forms an electron-dense background. Virions, or other biologic structures, stand out as electron-lucent particles by this staining method, and it is possible to visualize the fine structure of the particles with high resolution (see Figs. 4 and 6). Virus-infected cells may also be examined in thin section by electron-microscopy after embedding in suitable polymers, and this approach has afforded much information on the intracellular aspects of virus replication.

The recent growth of *molecular virology* as an experimental science has yielded a wealth of information on the molecular structure and replication processes of viruses. Cell culture systems are available for propagation and assay of most animal viruses. Extensive use is made of radioisotopic labeling with specific precursors that are incorporated into viral macromolecules — for example, nucleosides into nucleic acids and amino acids into proteins. Viral macromolecules are analyzed by various procedures, of which density gradient centrifugation and gel electrophoresis are most popular. Since most virions contain only a few types of macromolecules, it has been possible to catalog the type and number of macromolecular components present and to study the events involved in their biosynthesis in infected cells.

## GENERAL STRUCTURAL ORGANIZATION OF VIRUSES

The simplest virions consist solely of nucleic acid enclosed in a protein coat. Early electron microscopic observations indicated that most virions were either rodlike or roughly spherical particles, and chemical analyses of plant viruses demonstrated that they contained only a small percentage of nucleic acid — for example, 5 per cent for tobacco mosaic virus (TMV). Crick and

Watson suggested that the viral coat consisted of multiple identical subunits, which would allow such a limited amount of nucleic acid to direct the synthesis of a large amount of coat protein. Subsequent biochemical analyses and x-ray diffraction studies of virus crystals have demonstrated such a subunit structure. Further, the protein subunits form a symmetric shell, termed the *capsid*. The capsid together with the nucleic acid is designated the *nucleocapsid*. Two types of capsid symmetry are observed in viruses: *helical* for the viruses that appeared rodlike, and *icosahedral* for the "spherical" viruses. Although the simplest virions consist solely of the naked nucleocapsid, many are more complex and possess an outer lipid-containing membrane, termed the *viral envelope*. Schematic diagrams of the structural components of the virion and their designations are shown in Figure 1.

The nucleic acid is contained within the nucleocapsid and is thus protected by the viral protein from degradation by nucleases. In addition to serving a protective function, the external proteins of the virion are important for specific interactions with receptors on host cells in the ini-

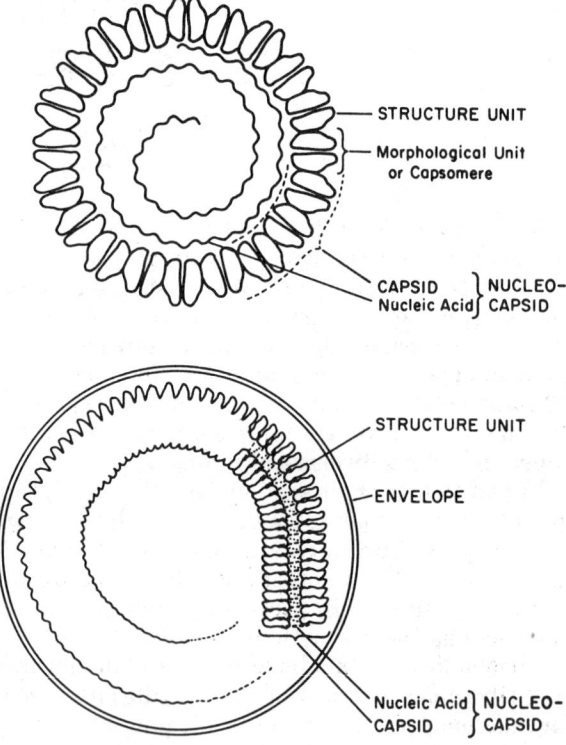

**FIGURE 1.** *Schematic cross sections through virus particles, illustrating the structural components and the terms used to describe them. Above: "spherical" virus with a naked icosahedral capsid. Below: enveloped virus with a helical nucleocapsid. (Modified from D. L. D. Caspar et al., Cold Spring Harbor Symp Quant Biol 27:49, 1962.)*

tial stages of the infection process and are the antigens that elicit an immune response following virus infection. Lipid-containing virions are much more heat labile than are virions consisting of naked nucleocapsids and are sensitive to lipid solvents or detergents.

Although there is no limit to the number of different sizes and shapes of viruses that could conceivably exist, only a few structural types have been observed. This finding forms the basis for a rational classification of animal viruses into families with common structural features, as discussed in Chapter 8. Classification is based on the size and structure of the viral nucleic acid, the size and symmetry of the capsid, and the presence or absence of an envelope. Fortunately, viruses that are classified together on the basis of structure also replicate by similar processes and frequently exhibit other similarities in their interactions with host cells. A total of 16 different families of animal viruses have been identified, five containing DNA genomes, and ten containing RNA genomes (Table 1). A more detailed description of the morphology and biologic properties of these agents is presented in Chapter 8.

## VIRAL NUCLEIC ACIDS

The molecular weight and configuration of the viral nucleic acid is an important characteristic of each virus family (Table 1). DNA viruses exhibit much greater variation in genome size than is observed with RNA-containing viruses. Most DNA-containing animal viruses contain double-stranded nucleic acid, whereas parvoviruses are exceptional in containing single-stranded DNA.

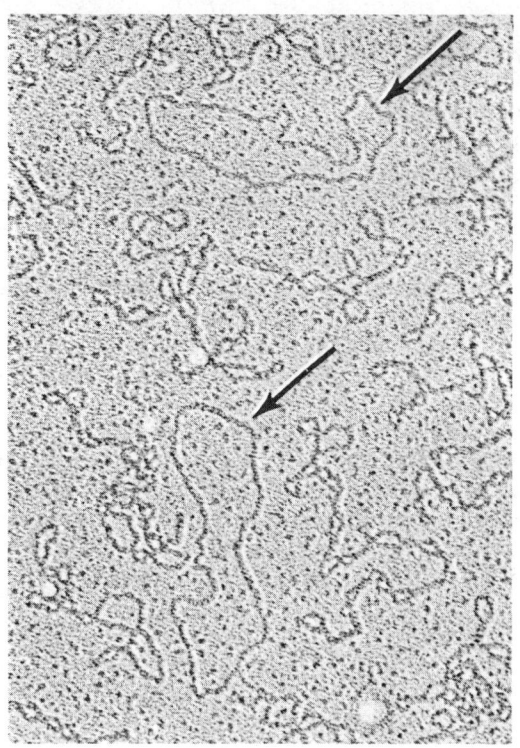

**FIGURE 2.** *Electron micrograph of the DNA genome of a papova-virus (simian virus 40). Most molecules are in a circular configuration containing several superhelical twists, although some molecules (arrows) are seen as open, untwisted circles. One strand of the DNA is broken in such molecules, which enables unwinding of the twists. Courtesy of Dr. Patricia Hale. Magnification: × 70,000.*

Viral DNA may occur as linear molecules, or as covalently closed circular molecules (for example, in papovaviruses, Fig. 2).

The RNA viruses exhibit great variation in the configuration of their nucleic acids. The possibilities include one linear molecule of single-strand-

**TABLE 1. Structural Properties of Animal Viruses**

| VIRUS FAMILY | MOLECULAR WEIGHT OF VIRAL NUCLEIC ACID × 10⁻⁶ | CAPSID SYMMETRY | PRESENCE OF ENVELOPE | DIAMETER OF VIRION (nm) |
|---|---|---|---|---|
| **DNA Viruses** | | | | |
| Parvoviridae | 1.5–2 | icosahedral | − | 20 |
| Papovaviridae | 3–5 | icosahedral | − | 45–55 |
| Adenoviridae | 20–25 | icosahedral | − | 75 |
| Herpesviridae | 100 | icosahedral | + | 150 |
| Poxviridae | 160–200 | complex | + | 240 × 300 |
| **RNA Viruses** | | | | |
| Picornaviridae | 2.6 | icosahedral | − | 25–30 |
| Togaviridae | 4 | icosahedral | + | 50–70 |
| Arenaviridae | 4–5 | helical (?) | + | 80–300 |
| Bunyaviridae | 4–5 | helical (?) | + | 80–100 |
| Orthomyxoviridae | 4–5 | helical | + | 90–120 |
| Paramyxoviridae | 6–7 | helical | + | 120–150 |
| Rhabdoviridae | 3.8 | helical | + | 70 × 170 |
| Coronaviridae | 5–6 | helical | + | 80–120 |
| Retroviridae | 6–7 | icosahedral | + | 100–120 |
| Reoviridae | 12–15 | icosahedral | − | 70–80 |

ed RNA (picorna-, toga-, paramyxo-, and rhab-doviruses), multiple segments of single-stranded RNA (arena-, bunya-, and orthomyxoviruses), multiple segments of double-stranded RNA (reovirus), and a complex of two identical copies of a single-stranded RNA (retroviruses). Thus far, no covalently closed circular molecules have been identified in RNA animal viruses. For several viruses with segmented RNA genomes, it has been shown that each segment functions as a gene that specifies a particular viral protein.

For some virus families, the nucleic acid alone is infectious. This provides the most convincing demonstration that the viral nucleic acid is the sole genetic information required for the formation of progeny virions. Infectious nucleic acids have been demonstrated only for those virus families in which the nucleic acid is present as a single molecule and in which no enzymatic activities essential for replication are present in the virion.

## STRUCTURE OF ICOSAHEDRAL NUCLEOCAPSIDS

An icosahedron consists of 20 equilateral triangular faces, and has 12 vertices at which five triangular faces meet (Fig. 3). It exhibits axes of fivefold symmetry through each vertex, threefold symmetry at the center of each triangular face, and twofold symmetry at the midpoints of the edges between two faces. The simplest icosahedral viruses possess 60 identical asymmetric protein subunits (structure units), three of which are positioned on each of the triangular faces of the

particle. The icosahedron is formed, and maintains its stability, by means of identical protein-protein bonds between adjacent subunits. Most icosahedral viruses, however, are larger and possess many more protein subunits. Frequently, such subunits are arranged in clusters, which form the *morphologic units,* or *capsomers,* that are the subunits visible by electron microscopy. The most common pattern of clustering results in formation of groups of five (pentamers) found at the vertices, and groups of six (hexamers) found on faces of the particle. The adenovirus capsid (Fig. 4) is an example of a complex icosahedral structure exhibiting this type of clustering.

The triangular facets of an icosahedron may be further subdivided into smaller equilateral triangles, and the term *triangulation number* is used to indicate the number of smaller units present on each face. Only certain triangulation numbers are possible, and they are given by the relationship $T = h^2 + hk + k^2$, where h and k are any integers. Thus, some of the possible triangulation numbers are 1, 3, 4, 7, 12, and so on. In terms of virus capsid structure, three structure units would be present on each of the smaller triangles. If these are clustered into pentamers and hexamers, the number of morphologic units in the capsid is equal to 10 T + 2. Thus, a capsid of triangulation number T will consist of 12 pentamers and 10 (T−1) hexamers.

Although simpler viruses may have only one type of structural subunit, more complex particles contain several types of protein as capsid components. Each protein, however, is specified by a particular viral gene; thus, virions contain the same set of capsid proteins irrespective of the host

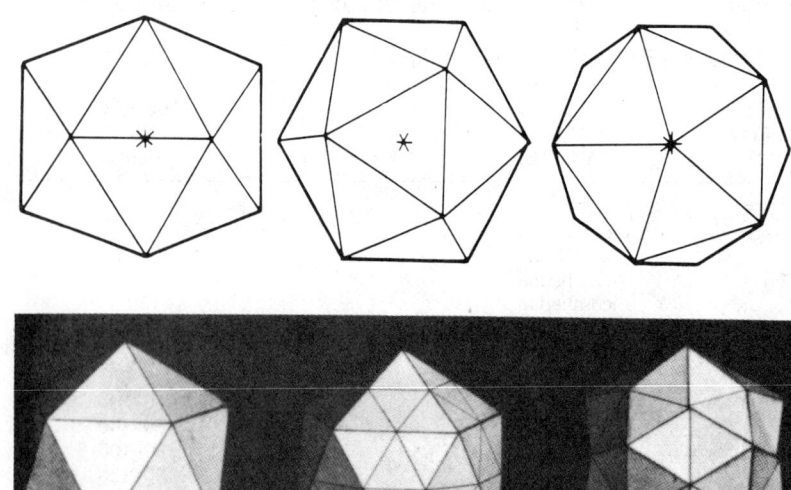

**FIGURE 3.** *Structural features of an icosahedron. Above, diagrams of an icosahedron viewed along different axes of symmetry ( *). From left to right, the structure is viewed along a twofold, threefold, and fivefold axis of symmetry. Below, examples of the subdivision of an icosahedron into surfaces of different triangulation numbers. From left to right, T = 1; T = 4; T = 3. (The lower portion is taken from Caspar and Klug, Cold Spring Harbor Symp Quant Biol 27:1, 1962.)*

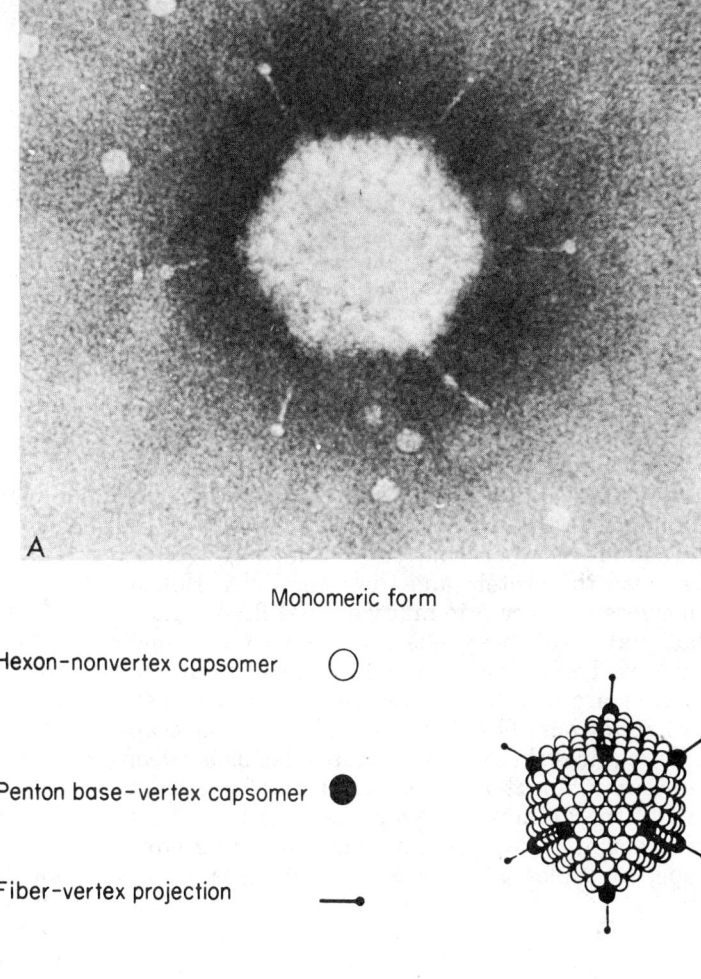

**FIGURE 4.** A, adenovirus particle negatively stained with sodium silicotungstate, illustrating the icosahedral capsid structure with fibers projecting from each of the vertices. (From Valentine and Pereira: J Mol Biol 13:13, 1965; supplied courtesy of Dr. N. G. Wrigley). B, schematic diagram of the structure of an adenovirus particle, illustrating the different capsid proteins and their arrangement, as well as the terms used to describe the individual structural components. (From E. Norrby: J Gen Virol 5:221, 1969.)

Monomeric form

Hexon-nonvertex capsomer

Penton base-vertex capsomer

Fiber-vertex projection

Penton-vertex capsomer
plus projection

Virion

B

cell of origin. Viruses with large genomes can direct the synthesis of more different proteins than can viruses with more limited genetic information, and for DNA viruses there is a good correlation between genetic information content and complexity of the capsid. For adenoviruses, the *hexon* subunit found on the faces of the particle consists of a different polypeptide species from that contained in the *penton* (vertex) subunit, and another distinct protein, the *fiber*, radiates outward from each vertex of the particle. Some icosahedral particles contain internal core proteins associated with the nucleic acid that differ from those of the capsid, whereas in other virus types, the nucleic acid is directly associated with the capsid proteins. At least one icosahedral virus, reovirus, contains two distinct capsid layers. Treatment of reovirus particles with proteases

removes the outer capsid layer and reveals an internal capsid that also appears to exhibit icosahedral symmetry.

For icosahedral viruses, the dimensions of each virion are uniform, as a result of identical protein-protein interactions that determine the structure of each particle. The process of assembly of an icosahedral virus is obviously designed to accommodate the viral genome in a capsid of suitable size; nucleic acids of a much larger size than a particular viral genome would probably not fit into its particular capsid. However, the presence of viral nucleic acid is not essential for the assembly of the capsid, and aberrant particles are produced by infected cells, including empty icosahedral capsids devoid of any nucleic acid. The size and organization of empty capsids is very similar to that of fully infectious virions; thus it is apparent that the capsid proteins possess the shapes and bonding characteristics that cause them to form a particular structure. Icosahedral capsids may also be produced that contain segments of cellular nucleic acid instead of the viral genome.

## HELICAL NUCLEOCAPSIDS

A helical arrangement of protein subunits has been demonstrated by crystallographic analysis of plant viruses such as TMV. As shown in Fig. 5, the RNA itself is in a helical arrangement in the TMV particle, and lies in a groove at a radius of 4 nm from the cylindric axis. The particle itself has a central hollow core 4 nm in diameter and an overall particle diameter of 18 nm. Virus particles consist of a single type of structural protein arranged in the form of repeating units, with interactions between adjacent subunits as well as between the protein and the viral RNA. Helical nucleocapsids occur in many animal RNA viruses but have not been observed in DNA animal viruses. The helical ribonucleoproteins in animal viruses are flexible, whereas many plant viruses are rigid rods. The flexibility of such nucleocapsids requires that there be no firm bonds between protein subunits in adjacent turns of the helix. All of the animal viruses containing helical nucleocapsids also possess a lipid-containing envelope; examples of some enveloped viruses with

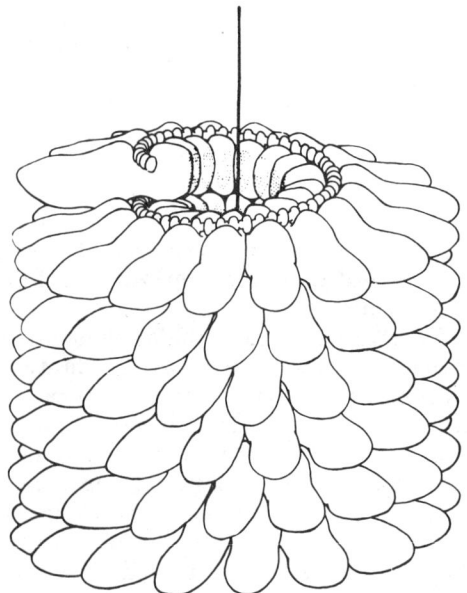

**FIGURE 5.** *Schematic diagram of the structure of tobacco mosaic virus based on x-ray diffraction studies. The RNA is coiled between the turns of the protein subunits; there are 49 nucleotides and about 16 1/3 protein subunits in each turn of the helix. The central hole is about 4 nm in diameter, and the overall diameter of the helix is 18 nm. (From Caspar and Klug: Cold Spring Harbor Symp Quant Biol 27:1, 1962.)*

helical nucleocapsids are shown in Figure 6. In such viruses, flexibility of the helix is important to enable folding of these nucleocapsids for enclosure within the viral membrane.

The length of the helical nucleocapsid is determined by the length of the viral RNA molecule itself; for TMV, a particle length of 300 nm is observed. The TMV protein can aggregate by itself to form rods of the same diameter as the virion, but such particles are of random length, due to the absence of the RNA as a length-determining factor. It is also possible for TMV protein to form helices with RNA from other sources, or with synthetic polynucleotides, indicating that the protein does not show strict specificity for a particular nucleic acid sequence for the interactions that lead to the assembly of the helical virus.

## VIRAL ENVELOPES

More than half of the established families of animal viruses contain lipids as major structural components, which are present in a limiting membrane, or *envelope*. The lipids are acquired during the maturation process, which usually occurs by budding at a cellular membrane. Thus the viral lipids are acquired from a membrane of the host cell and are similar to that membrane in composition; they are arranged in the form of a bilayer similar to that observed in other biologic membranes. The general arrangement of the other structural components of viral envelopes also closely resembles that observed in other biologic membranes in many respects. The viral envelope is asymmetric with respect to the distribution of carbohydrate components, as are cellular membranes: glycoproteins and glycolipids are found only on the external surface. The virion glycoproteins are virus-specific (that is, the polypeptide backbone is coded by the viral genome); however, the carbohydrate portion may vary with the host cell type and is synthesized by cellular enzymes. Viral glycoproteins form projections or spikes on the external surface of the virion. These glycoproteins are essential for viral infectivity and are responsible for adsorption of viruses to receptors on cell surfaces. They are also the antigens of importance in immunity to such viruses, in that antibody directed against the viral glycoproteins will neutralize virus infectivity. Host cell membrane proteins are effectively excluded from the viral membrane during the assembly of lipid-containing viruses.

Viral envelope glycoproteins appear to be amphipathic; that is, they have hydrophobic and hydrophilic domains. The isolated glycoproteins form rosette-like clusters (Fig. 6B) presumably because they aggregate by their hydrophobic ends. The hydrophobic end appears to be involved

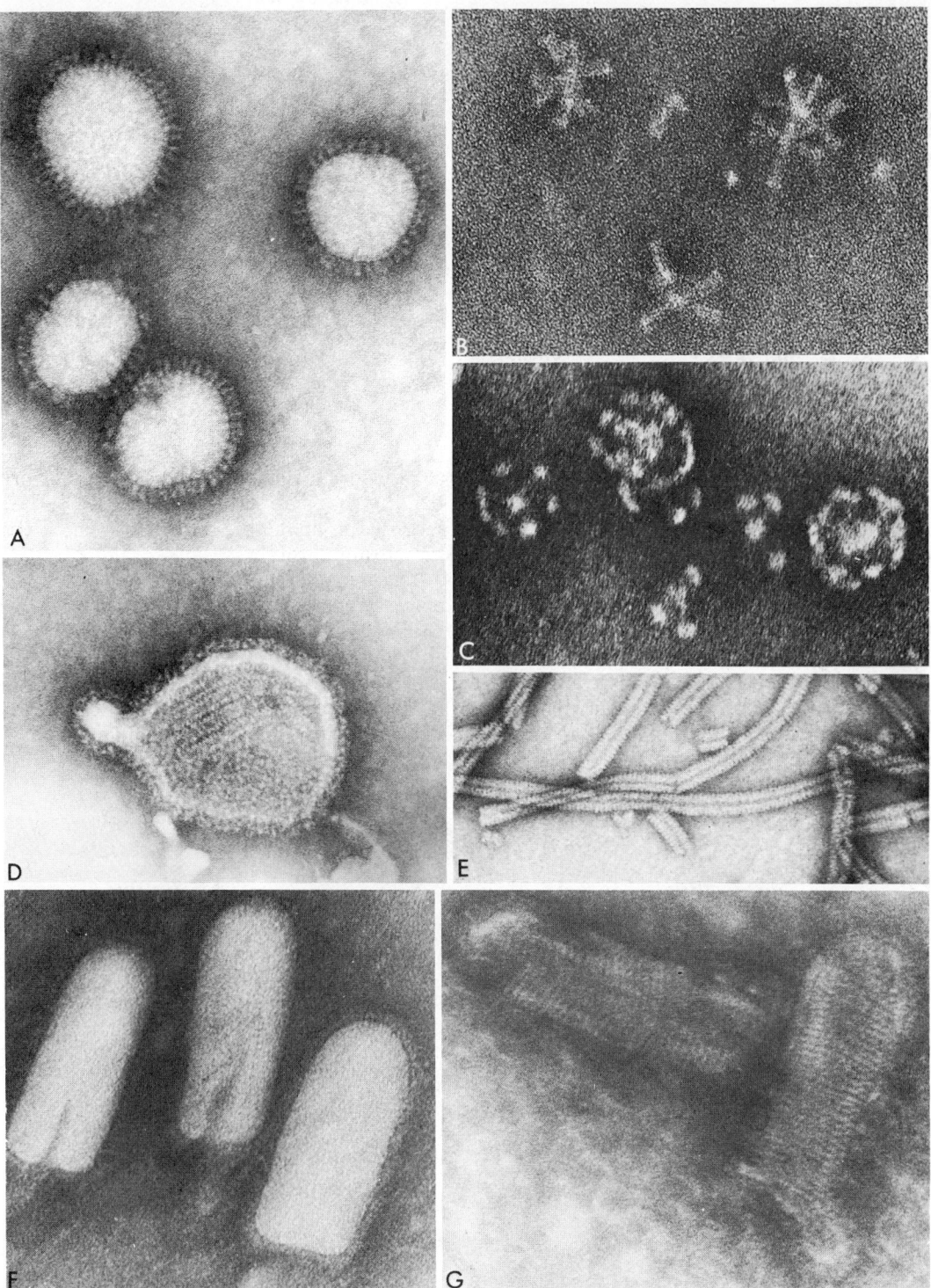

**FIGURE 6.** *Electron micrographs of some enveloped animal viruses and their structural components. A, Influenza virions, showing prominent surface spikes protruding from the viral membrane. The spikes consist of two types of glycoproteins, the hemagglutinin and neuraminidase. Isolated hemagglutinin spikes (B) consist of rodlike subunits that usually aggregate into rosette-like clusters because one end of the spike is hydrophobic; this end anchors the spike to the membrane. Isolated neuraminidase spikes (C) are mushroom-shaped, and also aggregate into characteristic clusters. D, Parainfluenza (SV5) particle penetrated by stain, revealing the internal helical nucleocapsid. E, Isolated SV5 nucleocapsids, some of which are broken into short fragments. The helical structure has a central hollow core, and the turns of the helix give the structure a herringbone-like appearance. F, Rhabdovirus (vesicular stomatitis) particles showing the bullet shape that is characteristic of this virus family. G, Partially disrupted vesicular stomatitis virions, in which the structure of the tightly coiled internal ribonucleoproteins can be observed. B and C are from Laver and Valentine, Virology 38:105, 1969 (Courtesy of Dr. W. G. Laver). D and E are from Compans and Nakamura, CRC Handbook Series in Clinical Laboratory Sciences, Section H, Volume 1, pp. 361–385, 1978. Magnifications: A, + 200,000; B and C, × 500,000; D, × 175,000; E, × 200,000; F and G, × 300,000.*

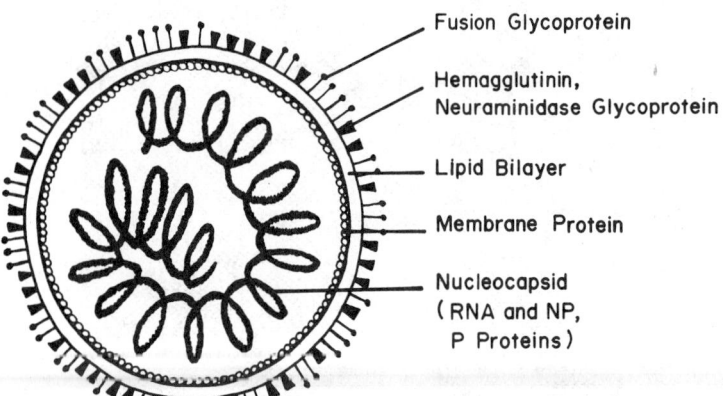

Fusion Glycoprotein

Hemagglutinin,
Neuraminidase Glycoprotein

Lipid Bilayer

Membrane Protein

Nucleocapsid
(RNA and NP,
P Proteins)

**FIGURE 7.** *Schematic diagram of the arrangement of structural proteins in a parainfluenza virion. Two types of glycoproteins form projections on the external surface of the lipid bilayer, and a membrane protein lines the inner surface of the bilayer. The helical nucleocapsid is coiled inside the envelope, and consists of the viral RNA and a nucleoprotein (NP) as well as other minor proteins (P) which may possess RNA polymerase activity. (From Compans and Nakamura, CRC Handbook Series in Clinical Laboratory Sciences, Section H, Volume 1, pp. 361–385, 1978).*

in binding of the glycoprotein to the viral membrane and may extend into or traverse the lipid bilayer to interact with proteins on the internal surface of the virion. Such interactions may be essential for the assembly process.

Virus-specific proteins are also components of the internal surface of the envelope. In the case of viruses with icosahedral nucleocapsids, the lipid membrane with its associated glycoproteins may be wrapped closely around the capsid itself, although intervening proteins may be present in some instances. For enveloped viruses with helical nucleocapsids, a particular type of protein is usually found in association with the inner surface of the envelope, and it is termed the M, or membrane, protein.

The morphology of some representative enveloped viruses is shown in Figure 6. The overall shapes and sizes of the virions are features characteristic of each virus family and are primarily determined by the arrangement of internal structural components. Some enveloped viruses are highly pleomorphic and may contain multiple nucleocapsids and genomes in a single

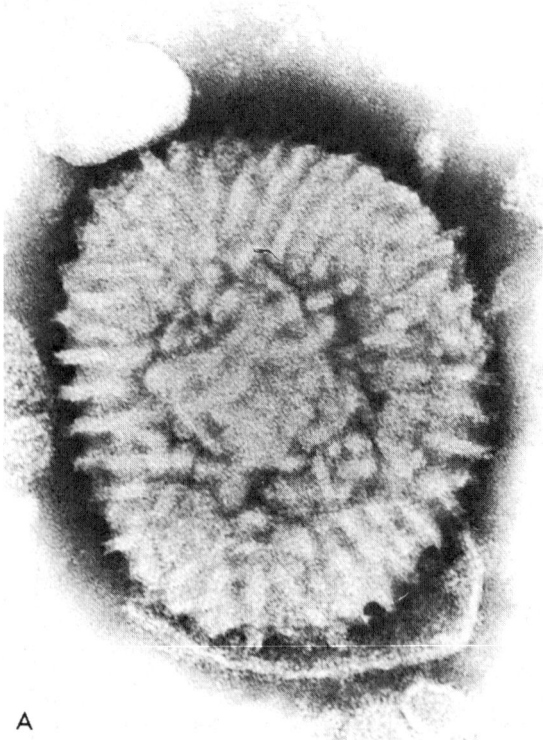

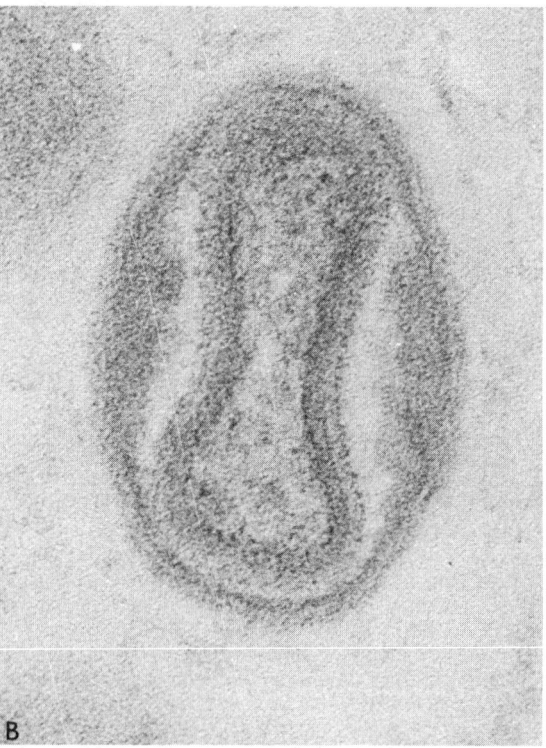

A

B

**FIGURE 8.** *Electron micrographs of vaccinia (poxvirus) virions. A, Negatively stained particle showing ridges or tubular elements covering the surface. B, Thin section of vaccinia virion showing a central biconcave core, two lateral bodies, and an outer membrane. A is from Dales, S.: J Cell Biol 18:51, 1963; B is from Pogo and Dales: Proc Natl Acad Sci U.S. 63:820, 1969. (Courtesy of Dr. Samuel Dales.) Magnification: A, × 228,000; B, × 220,000.*

envelope. All enveloped viruses possess glycoprotein spikes, but the shapes and lengths of these structures are also a distinctive property of each virus. The location of each structural protein has been elucidated in many enveloped viruses, as depicted for the parainfluenza virion in Figure 7.

### OTHER TYPES OF VIRUS STRUCTURE

Poxviruses are the largest and most complex of any of the viruses infecting man, containing about 30 or more different types of protein in the virion. They do not contain a capsid with either helical or icosahedral symmetry (Fig. 8). The virion contains DNA encased in a core structure, with two structures termed lateral bodies adjacent to the core. A lipid layer is also present in the interior of the particle. The resulting particle is oblong, and the surface is covered with distinct ridges. Poxviruses are more stable than most other lipid-containing viruses.

Certain plant diseases are caused by infectious nucleic acid molecules that lack any protein coat, and the term *viroid* has been given to such infectious agents. The known plant viroids are small, covalently closed, circular RNA molecules. It is possible that viroids may also occur in certain diseases of animals or man in which no conventional virus has been identified.

### References

*General*

Caspar, D. L. D., and Klug, A.: Physical principles in the construction of regular viruses. Cold Spring Harbor Symp Quant Biol 27: 1–24, 1962.
Crick, F. H. C., and Watson, J. D.: Structure of small viruses. Nature 177:473–475, 1956.

*Methods*

Brenner, S., and Horne, R. W.: A negative staining method for high resolution electron microscopy of viruses. Biochem Biophys Acta 34:103–110, 1959.
Brakke, M. K.: Density gradient centrifugation. In Maramorosch, R., and Koprowski, H. (eds.): Methods in Virology Vol. II. New York, Academic Press, pp. 93–117, 1967.
Elford, W. J.: The sizes of viruses and bacteriophages and methods for their determination. In Doerr, H., and Hallauer, C. (eds.): Handbuch der Virusforschung. Vienna, Springer.
Maizel, J. V.: Acrylamide gel electrophoresis of proteins and nucleic acids. In: Fundamental Techniques in Virology. Habel, K. and Salzman N. P. (eds.): New York, Academic Press, pp. 334–362, 1969.

*Viral Nucleic Acids*

Air, G. M.: DNA sequencing of viral genomes. In Fraenkel-Conrat. H., and Wagner, R. R. (eds.): Comprehensive Virology. New York, Plenum Press, Vol. 13, pp. 205–292, 1979.
Shatkin, A. J.: Animal RNA viruses: genome structure and function. Ann Rev Biochem 43:643–664, 1974.

*Icosahedral Nucleocapsids*

Finch, J. T., and Klug, A.: The structure of viruses of the papilloma-polyoma type. III. Structure of rabbit papilloma virus. J Mol Biol 13:1–12, 1965.
Valentine, R. C., and Pereira, H. G. Antigens and the structure of adenovirus. J Mol Biol 13:13–20, 1965.

*Helical Nucleocapsids*

Caspar, D. L. D.: Assembly and stability of the tobacco mosaic virus particle. Adv Prot Chem 18:37–121, 1963.
Compans, R. W., Mountcastle, W. E., and Choppin, P. W.: The sense of the helix of paramyxovirus nucleocapsids. J Mol Biol 65:167–169, 1971.
Finch, J. T., and Gibbs, A. J.: Observations on the structure of the nucleocapsids of some paramyxoviruses. J Gen Virol 6:141–150, 1970.

*Viral Envelopes*

Compans, R. W., and Klenk, H.-D.: Viral membranes. In Fraenkel-Conrat, H., and Wagner, R. R. (eds.): Comprehensive Virology. New York, Plenum Press, Vol. 13, pp. 293–407, 1979.
Harrison S. C., David, A., Jumblatt, J., and Darnell, J. E.: Lipid and protein organization in Sindbis virus. J Mol Biol 60:523–528, 1971.
Lenard, J., and Compans, R. W.: The membrane structure of lipid-containing viruses. Biochem Biophys Acta 344:51–94, 1974.

*Other Types of Virus Structure*

Dales, S.: The structure and replication of poxviruses as exemplified by vaccinia. In Dalton, A. J., and Haguenau, F. (eds.): Ultrastructure of Animal Viruses and Bacteriophages. New York, Academic Press, pp. 109–129, 1973.
Diener, T. O.: Viroids: The smallest known agent of infectious disease. Ann Rev Microbiol 28:23–40, 1974.

# CLASSIFICATION OF **8** VIRUSES

*Joseph L. Melnick, Ph.D.*

Until about 1950, so little was known about viruses other than their pathogenic effect in causing diseases that they were classified according to the diseases they caused rather than the properties of the virus particle. Now, we are approaching the end of an important phase of discovery and characterization of animal viruses. The knowledge thus gained concerning the viruses themselves has made it possible to establish broad groupings for these agents. It appears that most of the major groups of viruses of vertebrates — at least of man and the animals important to man — have been recognized and described. Many of these virus groupings, initially established on tentative and provisional bases, now appear to form real families and genera, in which the members are indeed related in fundamental ways. For example, the validity of the original grouping of the enteroviruses based on an enteric habitat and small size is being borne out by sophisticated techniques of molecular virology that compare the genetic makeup of different members of the group and their mode of replication.

The shift in emphasis — from sketching the broad outlines of the virus kingdom based on disease causation to filling in essential details about the viruses themselves — has been recognized by the change in the name of the International Committee on Nomenclature of Viruses (ICNV) to the International Committee on Taxonomy of Viruses (ICTV). The first report of the ICNV was published in 1971 (Wildy, 1971). Work of the Study Groups and Subcommittees of the ICTV is proceeding, and reports from these groups in their special areas of virology appear regularly in *Intervirology,* the journal of the Virology Section of the IAMS. Subsequent reports of the ICTV have been published (Fenner, 1976; Matthews, 1979).

Figures 1 and 2 serve as useful reference points for the following discussion of classification based upon properties of the virus particles. Comparison of these figures also shows how rapidly knowledge of virus composition and structure has advanced. Figure 1 is taken from a text published in 1967 (Davis et al., 1967); it remains fundamentally applicable in current virology. However, Figure 2, a diagram prepared about ten years

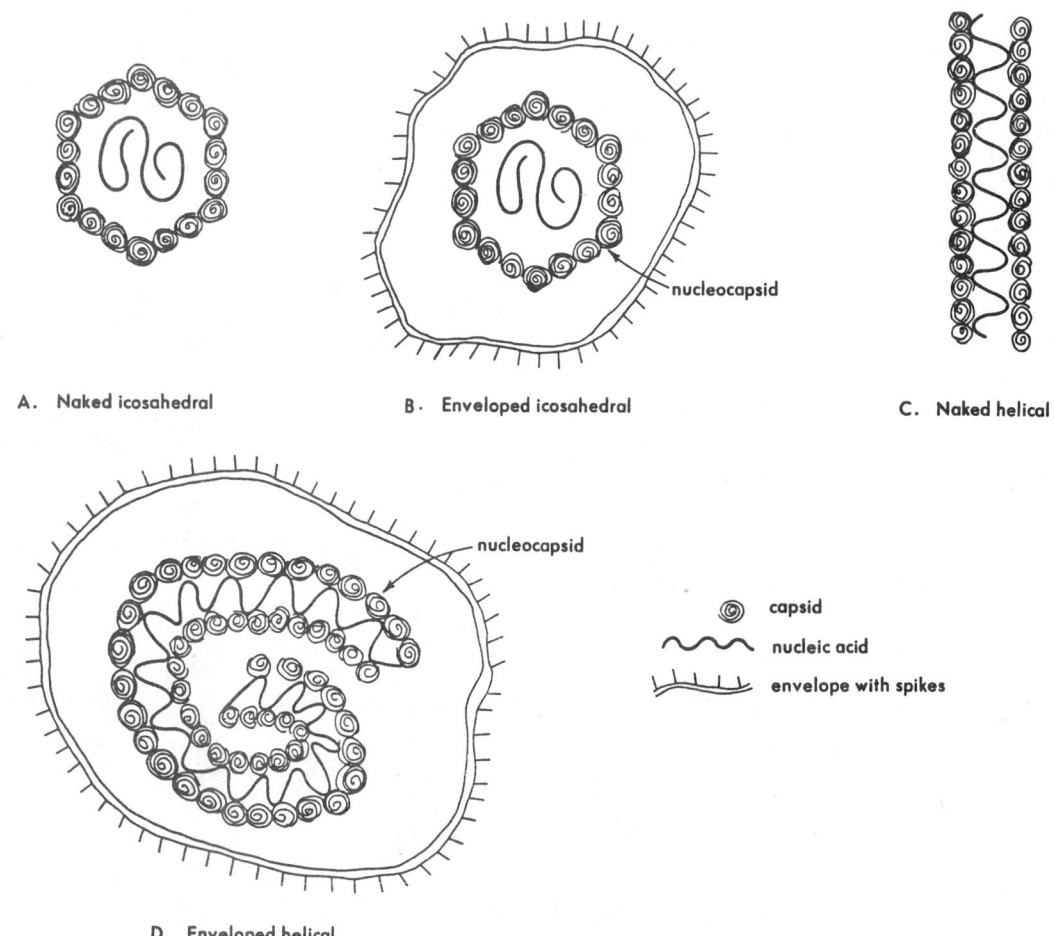

A.  Naked icosahedral

B.  Enveloped icosahedral

C.  Naked helical

D.  Enveloped helical

⊚  capsid

〰  nucleic acid

⊥⊥⊥  envelope with spikes

**FIGURE 1.**  *Schematic diagram of simple forms of virions and their components. The naked icosahedral virions resemble small crystals; the naked helical virions resemble rods with a fine regular helical pattern in their surface. The enveloped icosahedral virions are made up of icosahedral nucleocapsids surrounded by the envelope; the enveloped helical virions are helical nucleocapsids bent to form a coarse, often irregular coil, within the envelope. (From Davis, B. D., et al.: Microbiology. New York, Hoeber Medical Division, 1967.)*

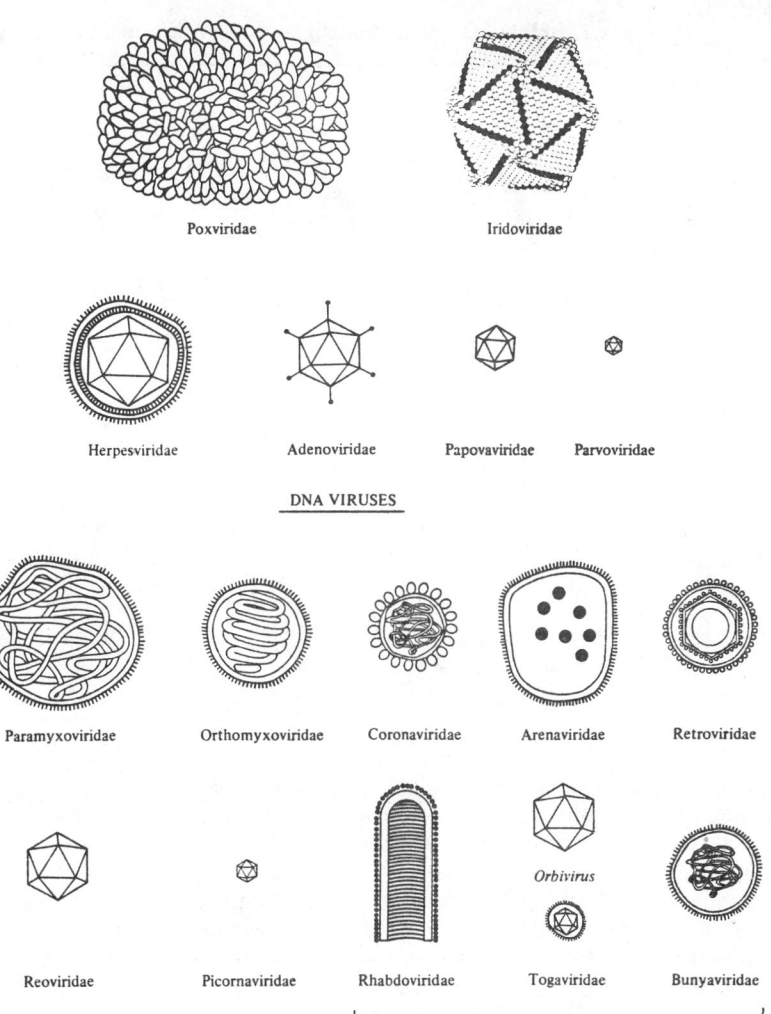

**FIGURE 2.** *Diagram illustrating the shapes and relative sizes of animal viruses of the major families (bar = 100 nm). From Fenner, F., and White, D. O.: Medical Virology. 2nd ed. New York, Academic Press, 1976.*

later (Fenner and White, 1976), not only draws upon additional information gained in the interim but also illustrates the wide variety of size and structure that is found among viruses of vertebrates.

Tables 1 to 5 are schematic diagrams showing separation of viruses of vertebrates into 16 families (Melnick, 1979). Table 1 describes viruses that have a DNA genome, cubic symmetry, and a naked nucleocapsid; Table 2 describes DNA-containing viruses with envelopes or complex coats. RNA-containing viruses are presented in three tables: Table 3, those with cubic capsid symmetry; Table 4, those with helical symmetry; and Table 5, those with capsid architecture either asymmetric or unknown. Commentaries follow on the viruses that have been definitely assigned to these groups. Also included are hepatitis viruses A and B, and some other agents whose classification is still tentative.

# DNA VIRUSES

### *PARVOVIRIDAE*
### (Bachmann et al., 1975)

Originally named picodnaviruses to reflect their small size and DNA-containing genome (Mayor and Melnick, 1966), the family Parvoviridae now includes three named genera, *Parvovirus, Densovirus,* and *Adeno-associated-virus.* A typical member is adeno-associated satellite virus, several serotypes of which are indigenous

**TABLE 1.   DNA-Containing Viruses With Cubic Symmetry and Naked Nucleocapsid**

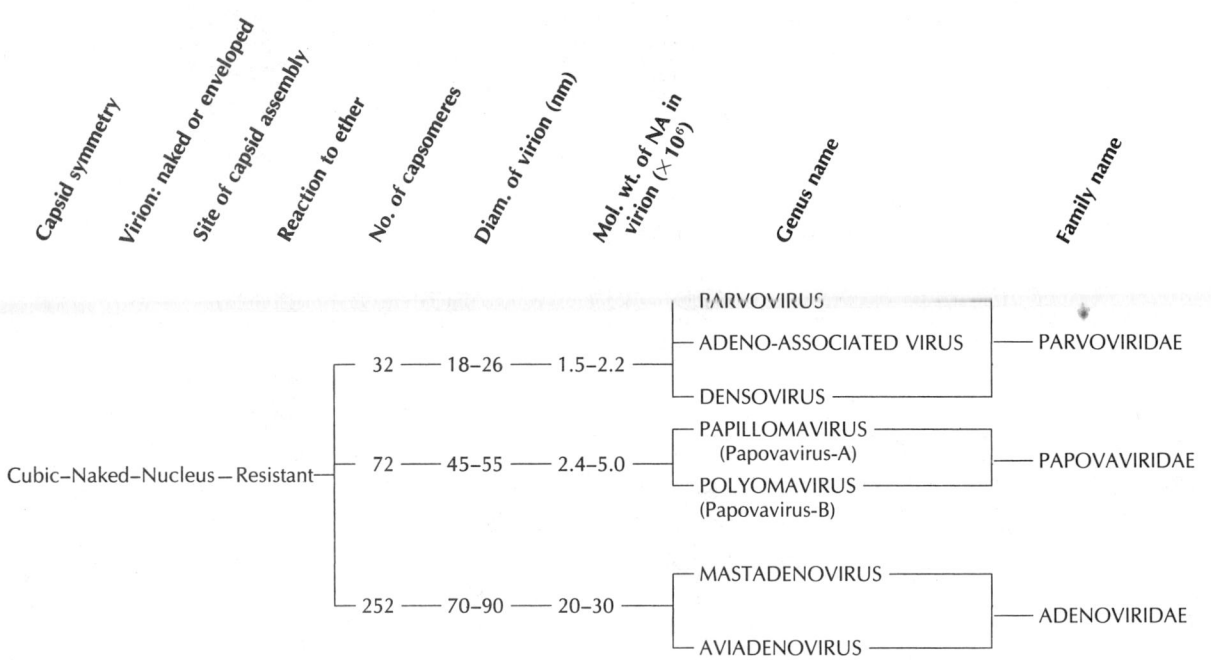

| Capsid symmetry | Virion: naked or enveloped | Site of capsid assembly | Reaction to ether | No. of capsomeres | Diam. of virion (nm) | Mol. wt. of NA in virion ($\times 10^6$) | Genus name | Family name |
|---|---|---|---|---|---|---|---|---|
| Cubic | Naked | Nucleus | Resistant | 32 | 18–26 | 1.5–2.2 | PARVOVIRUS / ADENO-ASSOCIATED VIRUS / DENSOVIRUS | PARVOVIRIDAE |
| | | | | 72 | 45–55 | 2.4–5.0 | PAPILLOMAVIRUS (Papovavirus-A) / POLYOMAVIRUS (Papovavirus-B) | PAPOVAVIRIDAE |
| | | | | 252 | 70–90 | 20–30 | MASTADENOVIRUS / AVIADENOVIRUS | ADENOVIRIDAE |

to man — but as yet with no known disease association in human beings. Reading from the left-hand side of Table 1, these are DNA-containing viruses that have cubic symmetry and a naked (unenveloped) nucleocapsid; during replication, capsid assembly takes place in the nucleus of the host cell. For the DNA viruses whose capsid assembly takes place in the nucleus (not only parvoviruses, but also papovaviruses, adenoviruses, and herpesviruses), a phase of replication — that is, viral protein synthesis — occurs in the cytoplasm. Messenger RNA of these viruses is associated with polyribosomes.

Infectivity is resistant not only to ether and other lipid solvents but also to heat (56° C for 60 minutes). The capsid has 32 capsomeres, the diameter of the virus particle is 18 to 26 nm, and the molecular weight of the nucleic acid is 1.5 to $2.2 \times 10^6$. The genus *Parvovirus* includes autonomously replicating viruses of several animal species (cat, cow, dog, goose, mink, mouse, pig, rabbit, rat). Members of the *Densovirus* genus also replicate autonomously; they are viruses of insects, but also can produce cytopathic effects in cultures of certain vertebrate cells (L cells). In contrast, adeno-satellite viruses are defective; that is, they cannot multiply in the absence of a replicating adenovirus, which serves as a "helper virus" — herpesvirus can act as a partial helper. Satellite viruses occur in cow, chicken, dog, horse, man, and monkey hosts.

Parvoviridae are the only DNA-containing viruses of vertebrates whose DNA genome is single-stranded within the virion; all the others (see Tables 1 and 2) have double-stranded DNA. In the case of adeno-satellite viruses and densoviruses, separate virions contain single strands of positive or negative DNA; these strands are complementary and when isolated from the virion shells they come together to form a double strand. In contrast, for members of the genus *Parvovirus,* the DNA in the virion is a positive strand only. However, the single-stranded DNA molecule has a hairpin-like structure at both the 5′ and the 3′ ends. In members of this genus, about 1 per cent of the virions form double strands similar to the self-complementary strands of the other two genera. Members of the *Parvovirus* genus show marked preference for actively dividing cells, have been shown to be transmissible transplacentally, and are receiving attention for their special disease potential in fetuses and neonates (Kilham and Margolis, 1975). One member has been associated with acute viral gastroenteritis of man.

In the light of accumulating data, it is becoming clear that hepatitis virus type B has a number of important properties similar to those of representative members of the parvovirus family. The 42-nm "Dane" particle (found in the serum of individuals infected with hepatitis B) is now recognized as the virus of this disease. The morphology, nucleic acid type, and nucleic acid strandedness of the Dane particles place them in a class by themselves, unrelated to any other known viruses. However, the 25 nm central core, which is assembled in the nucleus of the infected hepatocyte and which can be readily released from Dane particles, shares biochemical and biophysical properties with several members of the family Parvoviridae.

### *PAPOVAVIRIDAE*
(Melnick, 1962; Melnick et al., 1974a)

These relatively small, ether-resistant viruses contain double-stranded DNA in circular form. Many are unusually heat-stable, surviving temperatures that inactivate most viruses. The representatives that infect human beings are the papilloma or wart virus (of which at least two serotypes exist) and SV40-like viruses such as JC virus, which has been isolated from the brain tissue of patients with progressive multifocal leukoencephalopathy (PML), or BK virus, which has been isolated from the urine of immunosuppressed recipients of renal transplants. Other members include papilloma viruses of several vertebrate species, polyoma and K viruses of mice, and vacuolating viruses of monkeys (SV40)

and of rabbits. These viruses have relatively slow growth cycles characterized by replication within the nucleus. Papovaviruses produce latent and chronic infections in their natural hosts. Many produce tumors, particularly in experimentally infected rodents, serving as model systems to study viral carcinogenesis.

There are two genera whose names are in dispute: *Papillomavirus* (or *Papovavirus-A*) and *Polyomavirus* (or *Papovavirus-B*). Serious concern has been expressed at the use of "polyomavirus" for the human viruses, since the group B papoviruses of man have *not* been shown to be "polyoma" in character — that is, "produce many types of tumors in the host." For example, even though antibodies against BK virus are widespread in the population, human tumors and human malignant cell lines were negative when analyzed for BK virus-specific DNA sequences. Because the probes used could detect one copy of BK virus DNA if only 10 per cent of the cells were tumor cells, the results are very strong evidence that the tumors analyzed did not have a BK virus etiology. The tumors tested represent about 50 per cent of all types of cancers in the United States; thus there is no evidence that this member of papovavirus group B is involved in production of these tumors in the host.

**TABLE 2.   DNA-Containing Viruses With Envelopes or Complex Coats**

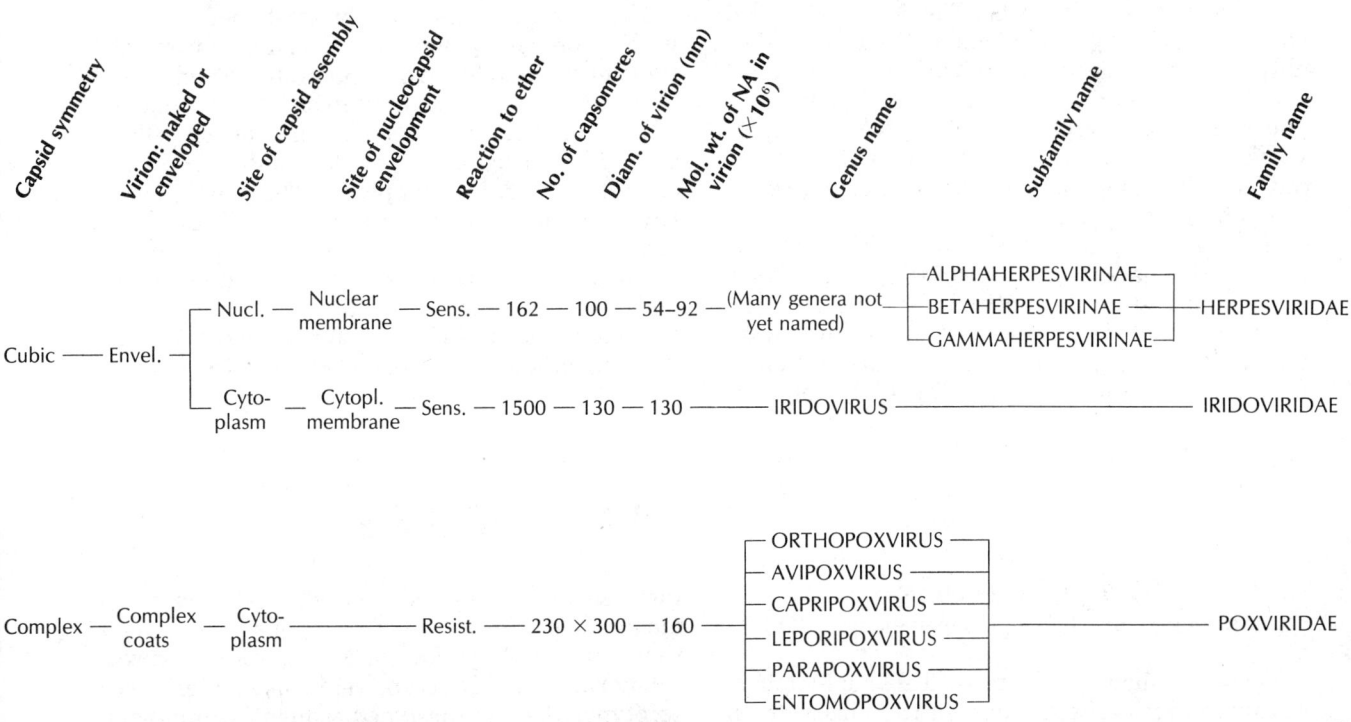

## ADENOVIRIDAE
### (Norrby et al., 1976)

The adenovirus virion is a nonenveloped isometric particle with 252 capsomeres, each 7 to 9 nm in diameter. Vertex capsomeres are antigenically distinct from the others and carry one or two filamentous projections. The adenovirus genome is a single linear molecule of double-stranded DNA. At least 33 serotypes infect man, and there are distinct serotypes for a number of other species. Adenoviruses have a predilection for mucous membranes and may persist for years in lymphoid tissue. Some cause acute respiratory diseases, febrile catarrhs, pharyngitis, and conjunctivitis. Human adenoviruses rarely cause disease in laboratory animals, but certain serotypes do produce tumors in newborn hamsters. Common antigens are shared by all mammalian adenoviruses (*Mastadenovirus* genus); these antigens are different from the corresponding antigens of members of the genus *Aviadenovirus*.

## HERPESVIRIDAE
### (O'Callaghan and Randall, 1976)

The herpesvirus family is a heterogeneous group of viruses identified by their structure. As shown in Table 2, the particle consists of a DNA-containing core enclosed by an icosahedral capsid with 162 hollow cylindric capsomeres. A lipid membrane containing virus-specific proteins surrounds the inner structures. The double-stranded DNA of various herpesviruses differs considerably in size ($92$ to $102 \times 10^6$ molecular weight), cytosine and guanine content (44 to 74 per cent), and structural complexity. The DNA of herpesviruses is sufficiently large to carry the genetic code for 80 to 100 proteins, of which about 50 have been observed.

Herpesviruses are noteworthy for their ability to establish latent and/or persistent infections, which may last for the lifetime of the host, even in the presence of circulating antibodies. Special interest has been generated by the association of EB herpesvirus with human Burkitt lymphomas and nasopharyngeal carcinomas and by the possible role of the genital herpesvirus, herpes simplex type 2, in cancer of the uterine cervix. Several simian herpesviruses have been shown to be oncogenic in experimentally infected animals. Herpesvirus infections of heterologous species are in many cases very serious; examples are the fatal infection of man by one of the simian herpesviruses, so-called B virus, and the infection of cattle by swine pseudorabies virus. Human diseases include oral and genital herpes; chickenpox and shingles due to varicella/zoster virus; cytomegalic inclusion disease; and infectious mononucleosis. Subfamilies have now been established to include most of the members of this large virus family (Matthews, 1979).

## IRIDOVIRIDAE

The best-known members of this family are the members of the insect iridescent virus group (for example, *Tipula* iridescent virus), now placed in the genus *Iridovirus*. However, other members of this family include important pathogens of vertebrates: African swine fever virus and many viruses of frogs and fish. No human iridovirus is known.

## POXVIRIDAE
### (Fenner, 1978)

These large viruses are brick-shaped or ovoid with a complex virion structure. The virion contains more than 30 structural proteins and several viral enzymes including a DNA-dependent RNA polymerase. This is the major DNA-containing virus family whose members replicate entirely within the cytoplasm. The genus *Orthopoxvirus* includes smallpox virus and the other poxviruses of man. Some of the animal poxviruses (for example, monkeypox) can infect humans, and with the eradication of smallpox from the world it has been speculated that human infections by these agents might be detected more frequently.

# RNA VIRUSES

## PICORNAVIRIDAE
### (Melnick et al., 1974b; Cooper et al., 1978)

These are shown at the top of Table 3. Members of this family — the smallest of the viruses with RNA genomes — are classed into four genera and into several hundred species. At least 70 members of the *Enterovirus* genus infect man; these include polioviruses, coxsackieviruses, echoviruses, and in recent years, new enterovirus serotypes that are assigned sequential numbers, such as enterovirus 68. Well over 100 viruses that

TABLE 3.    RNA-Containing Viruses With Cubic Capsid Symmetry

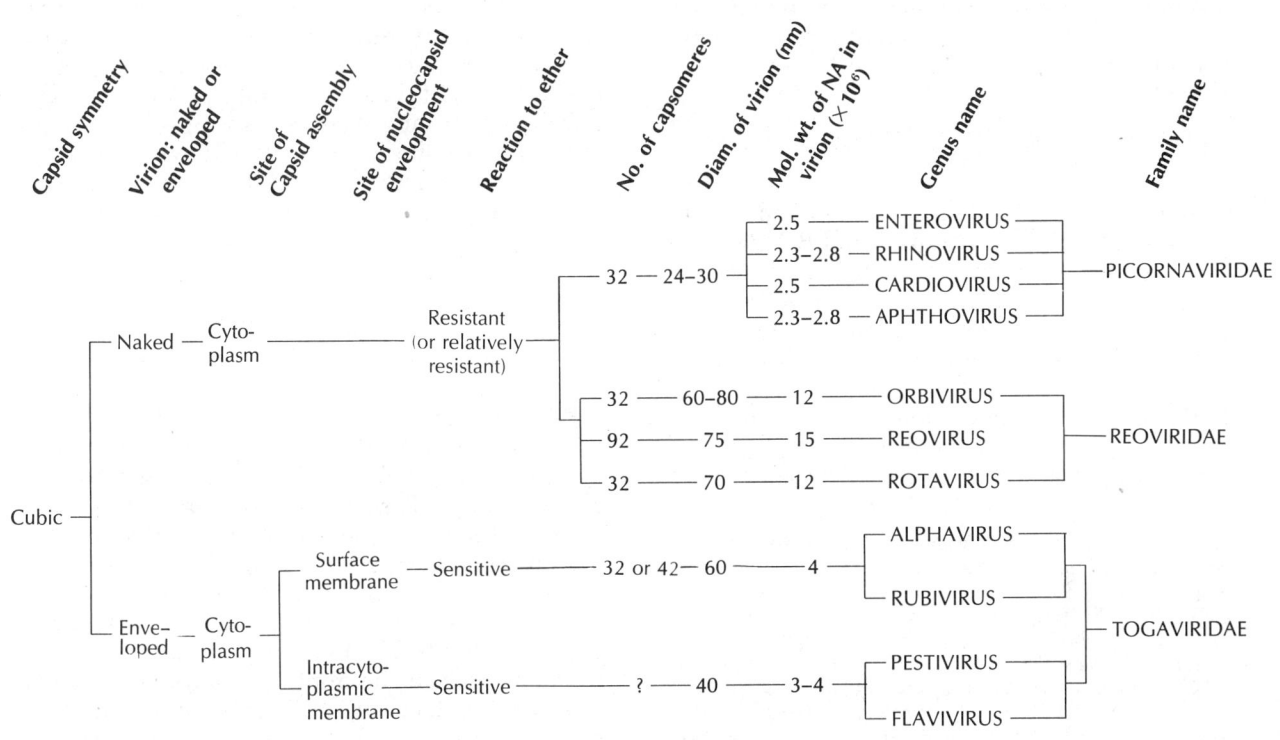

| Capsid symmetry | Virion: naked or enveloped | Site of Capsid assembly | Site of nucleocapsid envelopment | Reaction to ether | No. of capsomeres | Diam. of virion (nm) | Mol. wt. of NA in virion ($\times 10^6$) | Genus name | Family name |
|---|---|---|---|---|---|---|---|---|---|
| Cubic | Naked | Cytoplasm | | Resistant (or relatively resistant) | 32 | 24–30 | 2.5 | ENTEROVIRUS | PICORNAVIRIDAE |
| | | | | | | | 2.3–2.8 | RHINOVIRUS | |
| | | | | | | | 2.5 | CARDIOVIRUS | |
| | | | | | | | 2.3–2.8 | APHTHOVIRUS | |
| | | | | | 32 | 60–80 | 12 | ORBIVIRUS | REOVIRIDAE |
| | | | | | 92 | 75 | 15 | REOVIRUS | |
| | | | | | 32 | 70 | 12 | ROTAVIRUS | |
| | Enveloped | Cytoplasm | Surface membrane | Sensitive | 32 or 42 | 60 | 4 | ALPHAVIRUS | TOGAVIRIDAE |
| | | | | | | | | RUBIVIRUS | |
| | | | Intracytoplasmic membrane | Sensitive | ? | 40 | 3–4 | PESTIVIRUS | |
| | | | | | | | | FLAVIVIRUS | |

infect human beings belong to the genus *Rhinovirus.* Large numbers of agents from both of these genera are indigenous to other hosts. The two other genera are *Cardiovirus,* a rodent agent that may also infect man, and *Aphthovirus,* which includes the economically important foot-and-mouth disease viruses of cattle. The caliciviruses, once thought to belong to the Picornaviridae, have recently been shown to differ in both virus structure and method of replication.

The picornavirus genome is one piece of linear, single-stranded RNA of low molecular weight (about $2.5 \times 10^6$). The RNA is infectious and serves as its own messenger for protein translation. The enteroviruses and cardioviruses are acid-stable and have a buoyant density in CsCl of about 1.34 g/cm³; in contrast, the rhinoviruses and aphthoviruses are acid-labile and have a higher buoyant density, about 1.4 g/cm³.

The diseases caused by picornaviruses range from severe paralysis (paralytic poliomyelitis) to aseptic meningitis, pleurodynia, myocarditis, skin rashes, and common colds; inapparent infection is very common. Different viruses may produce the same syndrome; on the other hand, the same picornavirus may cause more than a single syndrome. After decades of investigation it now seems that hepatitis A virus is an enterovirus.

## REOVIRIDAE
### (Joklik et al., 1980)

Members of this virus family share a property unique among the RNA-containing viruses of vertebrates — the possession of a double-stranded, rather than single-stranded, RNA genome. The genome consists of several segments. The capsid has a double shell, and the structure of the outer capsid layer is indistinct, but icosahedral symmetry has been demonstrated in the inner capsid layers of all three recognized groups of reoviruses that infect vertebrates, the genera *Reovirus, Orbivirus,* and *Rotavirus.* The capsomeres of the orbiviruses are unusually large (10 to 15 nm wide) and appear ring-shaped. The human reoviruses are found in the bowel but their association with disease is not clear. Some orbiviruses have been considered to be arboviruses. The diseases caused by orbiviruses include Colorado tick fever of man, blue-tongue of sheep, African horsesickness, and epizootic hemorrhagic disease of deer. The members of the genus *Rotavirus* that infect human beings are increasingly recognized as major pathogens, responsible for a large share of nonbacterial infantile diarrhea. The gastroenteritis syndrome they cause is clinically very severe and is one of the commonest childhood illnesses throughout the world; in developing countries it is a leading cause of death. Much of the initial study of the rotaviruses was accomplished by electron microscopy and immune microscopy, and rotaviruses that infect man have not been isolated in cell cultures.

## TOGAVIRIDAE
### (Porterfield et al., 1978)

Members of this family include most arboviruses* of antigenic groups A and B, now classed in the genus *Alphavirus* (group A) and the genus *Flavivirus* (group B), and in newly designated genera, which include nonarbo togaviruses, rubella *(Rubivirus),* and the mucosal disease virus group *(Pestivirus).* The virions are spherical, 40 to 70 nm in diameter, and have a lipoprotein envelope with lipid and virus-specified glycopeptide tightly applied to an icosahedral nucleocap-

---

*One important and well-known virus group name that does not appear in the diagrams is a category based on ecologic properties, the *arbovirus group* (Berge, 1975). The more than 350 arthropod-borne viruses survive through a complex cycle involving vertebrate hosts and arthropods that serve as vectors, transmitting the viruses by their bites. This grouping, based on transmission, remains a useful one despite the wide diversity of its members in regard to properties of the virion. The vast majority of arboviruses now have been sufficiently well-characterized to permit their taxonomic placement. Their classic serologic interrelationships previously delineated by arbovirologists are paralleled by morphologic similarities, and have provided vital clues that can speed the taxonomic location of large numbers of viruses. Once some of the members of a classic serologic group have been characterized in terms of biophysical and biochemical properties, attention of taxonomists can be focused on their antigenic relatives. Arboviruses now are included in a number of families, chiefly Togaviridae, Bunyaviridae, Rhabdoviridae, Arenaviridae, and Reoviridae.

sid. The genome is a single molecule of single-stranded RNA. The alphaviruses and flaviviruses include many of the major human arboviral pathogens: the viruses of Venezuelan, eastern, and western equine encephalitis are alphaviruses, and the viruses of yellow fever, dengue, Japanese encephalitis, St. Louis encephalitis, Omsk hemorrhagic fever, and Russian spring-summer encephalitis are flaviviruses. Rubella virus thus far is the only member placed in the genus *Rubivirus.* Members of the *Pestivirus* genus include the viruses of hog cholera, bovine virus diarrhea, and other animal viruses.

## ORTHOMYXOVIRIDAE
### (Dowdle et al., 1975) (See Table 4)

All orthomyxoviruses recognized to date are influenza viruses. The virions may be spherical, elongated, or filamentous. For most members of the family, there are "spikes" projecting from the surface of the envelope; these are glycosylated protein peplomers 10 to 14 nm long and 4 nm in diameter, consisting of two types, the hemagglutinin and the neuraminidase. (In the nomenclature of variants of influenza type A, which arise frequently either as minor variants or as major new strains, the designation of these two antigens as $H_1N_1$, $H_3N_2$, and so on, supplies an important part of the information needed about new strains — their relatedness, if any, to strains that circulated previously — as a guide to the probable degree of immunity in the population.) During replication the helical nucleocapsid is first detected in the nucleus, whereas the hemagglutinin and neuraminidase are formed in the cytoplasm. The virus matures by budding at the cell surface

---

**TABLE 4.   RNA-Containing Viruses With Helical Symmetry**

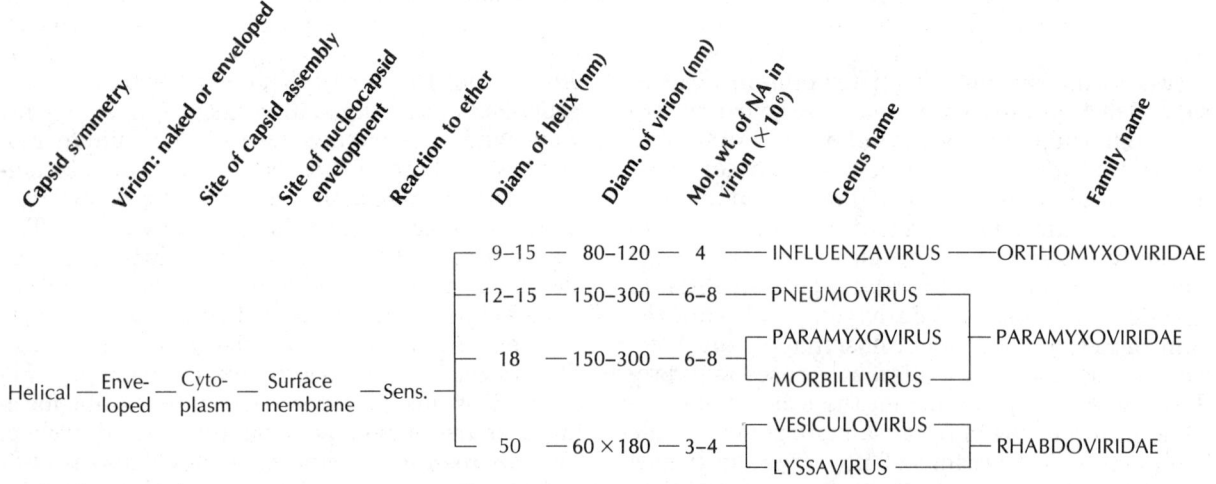

| Capsid symmetry | Virion: naked or enveloped | Site of capsid assembly | Site of nucleocapsid envelopment | Reaction to ether | Diam. of helix (nm) | Diam. of virion (nm) | Mol. wt. of NA in virion (× 10⁶) | Genus name | Family name |
|---|---|---|---|---|---|---|---|---|---|
| | | | | | 9–15 | 80–120 | 4 | INFLUENZAVIRUS | ORTHOMYXOVIRIDAE |
| | | | | | 12–15 | 150–300 | 6–8 | PNEUMOVIRUS | |
| | | | | | 18 | 150–300 | 6–8 | PARAMYXOVIRUS / MORBILLIVIRUS | PARAMYXOVIRIDAE |
| Helical | Enveloped | Cytoplasm | Surface membrane | Sens. | 50 | 60 × 180 | 3–4 | VESICULOVIRUS / LYSSAVIRUS | RHABDOVIRIDAE |

**TABLE 5.**    **RNA-Containing Viruses With Architecture Unsymmetric or Unknown**

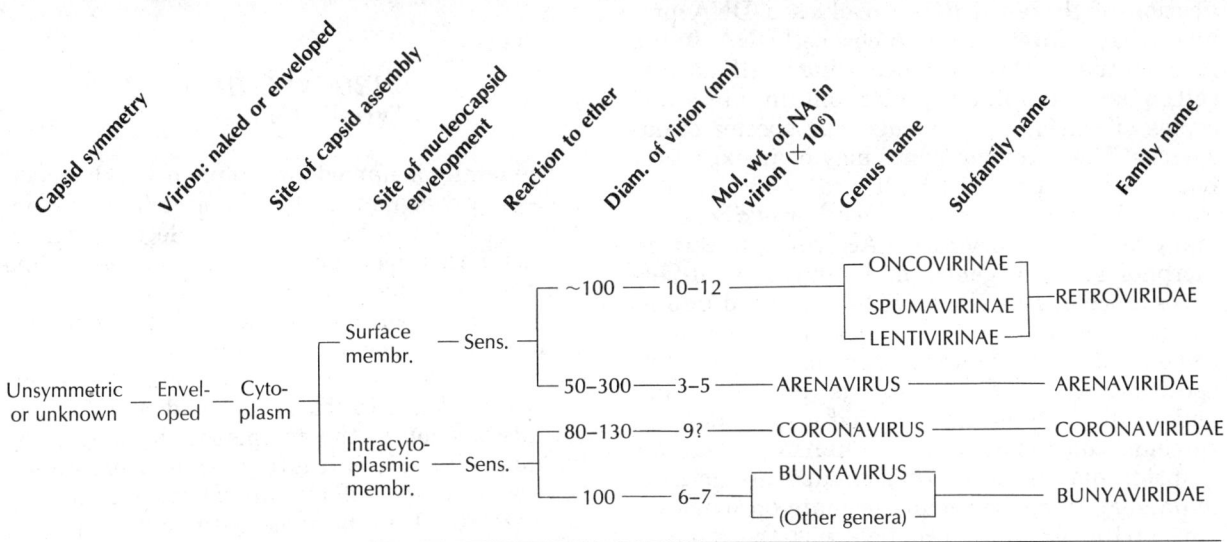

membrane. The genus *Influenzavirus* has been established and includes viruses of type A and type B; type C is considered a "probable genus." Antigenic variation is common, particularly among members of type A. Recombination occurs with high frequency within types but not between types or genera. Type A influenza viruses include agents of human, equine, and swine influenza and of fowl plague. Only human strains are known for types B and C.

### PARAMYXOVIRIDAE
(Kingsbury et al., 1978)

Usually spherical, these virions may also be pleomorphic; filamentous forms may be several micrometers long. On the lipid bilayer envelope are surface projections. Virions are formed in the cytoplasm by budding from the plasma membrane. Paramyxovirus infectivity is sensitive to ether, acid, and heat. The genera include the following: *Paramyxovirus* (parainfluenza viruses, mumps virus, Newcastle disease virus, Yucaipa and other avian paramyxoviruses); *Morbillivirus* (the viruses of measles, canine distemper, rinderpest, and peste de petite ruminant); and *Pneumovirus* (respiratory syncytial viruses of man and of cattle, and pneumonia virus of mice). Paramyxoviridae are genetically stable and genetic recombination does not occur.

### RHABDOVIRIDAE
(Fenner, 1976)

Members of this family have enveloped virions that are rod-shaped, resembling a bullet (with one end rounded and the other flattened) or bacilliform. Enclosed within the lipoprotein envelope and membrane protein is the long tubular nucleocapsid with helical symmetry. Members of some genera multiply in arthropods as well as in vertebrates or higher plants; others multiply only in insects. Infectivity is sensitive to ether, acid, and heat. The genera that infect vertebrates are *Lyssavirus* (including rabies virus, Duvenhage virus, and Mokola virus, all of which infect man; Lagos bat virus; and several agents isolated as yet only from insects), and *Vesiculovirus* (including vesicular stomatitis virus and a number of antigenically interrelated viruses from various animal species). Marburg virus, a simian virus highly pathogenic for man, is rhabdovirus-like in most properties but has very elongated forms.

### RETROVIRIDAE
(Dalton et al., 1974; Vogt, 1976)
(See Table 5)

Much remains to be settled concerning this family, but a good deal of progress has been made. The members include all of the RNA tumor viruses ("oncornaviruses"; "leukoviruses"), which are now assigned to a subfamily, Oncovirinae; other subfamilies are Lentivirinae (the slow viruses of the maedi/visna group) and Spumavirinae (the foamy virus group — agents that form syncytia in cell cultures). Members of the Retroviridae characteristically have a reverse transcriptase (RNA-dependent DNA polymerase) within the virion. For the most thoroughly studied members, the lipoprotein envelope encloses an inner shell with icosahedral symmetry and a central core or nucleocapsid with helical symmetry. Infectivity is ether, acid, and heat sensitive. Replication of the viral RNA involves a DNA provirus that is integrated into host cell DNA. In the case of the subfamily Oncovirinae, all normal cells of several animal species contain integrated copies of genes of the endogenous species of oncovirus. The oncovirus genes may be unexpressed but can be activated by physical and chemical agents, by superinfection with other oncoviruses, and even by herpesviruses. According to certain morphologic, antigenic, and enzymatic differences, oncoviruses also have been divided into A, B, and C (and possibly D) types of viruses. With some exceptions, oncoviruses fall into host-species–specific groups of agents inducing either leukemias or sarcomas — that is, leukemia-sarcoma complexes of avian, murine, feline, or hamster oncoviruses; other groups are murine mammary tumor virus and primate oncoviruses. One of the primate oncoviruses is the monkey mammary tumor virus (MoMTV).

### *ARENAVIRIDAE*
### (Pfau et al., 1974)

Members of this family have spherical or pleomorphic virions with a dense lipid bilayer membrane that bears surface projections; within the virion core are electron-dense RNA-containing granules about 20 to 30 nm in diameter that resemble ribosomes. Most member viruses have a single restricted rodent host in which persistent infection occurs; spread to other mammals and to man can take place, but is unusual. Members include lymphocytic choriomeningitis virus (LCM virus), which infects mice but may spread to man; Lassa virus; and members of the Tacaribe complex (Junin and Machupo viruses of South American hemorrhagic fevers, Pichinde virus, and several other viral agents that have been isolated as yet only from arthropods). Some arenaviruses (for example, Junin and Machupo, and Lassa) are

very serious pathogens when they do spread to man.

### *CORONAVIRIDAE*
### (Tyrrell et al., 1975)

The family is named for unique petal-shaped or club-shaped peplomers that project from the envelope; in negatively stained electron micrographs these projections form a fringe resembling the solar corona. The interior structure of the virion is believed to be a loosely-wound helically symmetric nucleocapsid. The genome consists of one large molecule of single-stranded RNA. Infectivity is sensitive to ether, acid, and heat. Nucleocapsids develop in the cytoplasm and mature by budding through intracytoplasmic membranes. Several serotypes of human coronaviruses have been isolated from patients with acute upper respiratory tract illnesses, primarily through the use of human embryonic tracheal and nasal organ cultures. There are distinct coronaviruses that infect a number of animal species.

### *BUNYAVIRIDAE*
### (Porterfield et al., 1975/76)

This family is the largest and most recently recognized taxonomic grouping assigned to an antigenically interrelated set of arboviruses. There are at least 200 members, more than 100 belonging to the Bunyamwera supergroup of arboviruses. The virions are spherical; they develop in the cytoplasm and mature by budding through intracytoplasmic membranes. Members of the family produce a number of important diseases of man and of domestic animals — for example, California encephalitis, Crimean hemorrhagic fever, sandfly fever, Rift Valley fever, and Nairobi sheep disease. Most Bunyaviridae members are mosquito-transmitted, but some are tickborne.

# EMERGING PROBLEMS IN VIRUS CLASSIFICATION

Some of the present and developing problems that viral taxonomists will have to meet are those posed by the recently discovered forms of life called viroids, and also by viral hybrids (between unrelated viruses), pseudovirions, and recombinant DNA.

*Viroids* constitute a recently discovered class of infectious agents smaller than viruses. They are

known to cause several diseases of plants (for example, potato spindle tuber disease), and may ultimately be found to cause disease in man and higher animals. (For example, the agent of scrapie disease of sheep — one of the puzzling "slow viruses" not yet placed taxonomically — may, according to recent findings, prove to be a viroid.) Viroids exhibit the characteristics of nucleic acids in crude extracts; that is, they are insensitive to heat and to organic solvents but are sensitive to nucleases. They do not appear to possess a protein coat. Viroids known at present consist solely of a short strand of RNA with a molecular weight of 75,000 to 100,000.

## VIRUS HYBRIDS

The fact that virus hybrids can exist in nature should be more widely recognized. If the simian papovavirus SV40 had not already been known as a virus before the discovery of SV40-adenovirus hybrid particles, these particles would have presented viral taxonomists with a very confusing puzzle. The hybrid particles, in which portions of SV40 genome material are covalently linked to adenovirus genetic material and encased within an adenovirus coat, would have seemed to be a new and very strange virus that reacted antigenically like an adenovirus (of the serotype from which its coat was derived) but whose progeny had many properties altogether different from other members of the adenovirus group.

## PSEUDOVIRION

This is another viral form that is difficult to classify. During viral replication the capsid sometimes encloses *host* nucleic acid rather than viral nucleic acid. Such particles look like ordinary virus particles when observed by electron microscopy, but they do not replicate. Pseudovirions contain the "wrong" nucleic acid. These particles present the taxonomist with problems based on natural events, but future laboratory manipulations will probably add to these problems of classification.

## RECOMBINANT DNA

Recently developed techniques allow DNA to be cleaved into specific pieces by using enzymes from bacteria called restriction endonucleases. These distinct fragments have importance in two areas: (1) the physical mapping of genes in large, complicated DNA genomes, and (2) genetic engineering. In addition to the overriding concern for safety precautions to ensure that new genetic combinations thus produced do not result in new organisms with dangerous properties, virologists must also give attention to how the new recombinant organisms should be classified. Classification of these new forms of life needs to be developed in ways that will reflect their origin and

relatedness to each other and to other living things.

## References

Bachmann, P. A., Hoggan, M. D., Melnick, J. L., Pereira, H. G., and Vago, C.: Parvoviridae. Intervirology 5:83, 1975.

Berge, T. O.: International Catalogue of Arboviruses Including Certain Other Viruses of Vertebrates. DHEW Publication No. (CDC) 75-8301, U. S. Dept. of Health, Education and Welfare, 1975.

Cooper, P. D., et al.: Picornaviridae: Second Report. Intervirology 10:165, 1978.

Dalton, A. J., Melnick, J. L., Bauer, H., Beaudreau, G., Bentvelzen, P., Bolognesi, D., Gallo, R., Graffi, A., Haguenau, F., Heston, W., Huebner, R., Todaro, G., and Heine, U. I.: The case for a family of reverse transcriptase viruses: Retraviridae. Intervirology 4:201, 1974.

Davis, B. D., Dulbecco, R., Eisen, H. N., Ginsberg, H. S., and Wood, W. B., Jr.: Microbiology. New York, Hoeber Medical Division, 1967.

Dowdle, W. R., Davenport, F. M., Fukumi, H., Schild, G. C., Tumova, B., Webster, R. G., and Zakstelskaja, L. Ya.: Orthomyxoviridae. Intervirology 5:245, 1975.

Fenner, F.: Classification and Nomenclature of Viruses: Second Report of the International Committee on Taxonomy of Viruses. Intervirology 7:1, 1976.

Fenner, F.: Portraits of viruses: The poxviruses. Intervirology 11:137, 1979.

Fenner, F., and White, D. O.: Medical Virology. 2nd ed. New York, Academic Press, 1976.

Joklik, W. K., et al.: Reoviridae. Intervirology, 1980.

Kilham, L., and Margolis, G.: Problems of human concern arising from animal models of intrauterine and neonatal infections due to viruses. Progr Med Virology 20:113, 1975.

Kingsbury, D. W., Bratt, M. A., Choppin, P. W., Hanson, R. P., Hosaka, Y., ter Meulen, T., Norrby, E., Plowright, W., Rott, R., and Wunner, W. H.: Paramyxoviridae. Intervirology 10:137, 1978.

Matthews, R. E. F.: Classification and Nomenclature of Viruses. Third Report of the International Committee on Taxonomy of Viruses. Intervirology 12:129, 1979.

Mayor, H. D., and Melnick, J. L.: Small deoxyribonucleic acid-containing viruses (picodnavirus group). Nature 210:331, 1966.

Melnick, J. L.: Papovavirus group. Science 135:1128, 1962.

Melnick, J. L.: Taxonomy of viruses, 1978. Progr Med Virology 25:160, 1979.

Melnick, J. L., Allison, A. C., Butel, J. S., Eckhart, W., Eddy, B. E., Kit, S., Levine, A. J., Miles, J. A. R., Pagano, J. S., Sachs, L., and Vonka, V.: Papovaviridae. Intervirology 3:106, 1974a.

Melnick, J. L., et al.: Picornaviridae. Intervirology 4:303, 1974b.

Norrby, E., Bartha, A., Boulanger, P., Dreizin, R. S., Ginsberg, H. S., Kalter, S. S., Kawamura, H., Rowe, W. P., Russell, W. C., Schlesinger, R. W., and Wigand, R.: Adenoviridae. Intervirology 7:117, 1976.

O'Callaghan, D. J., and Randall, C. C.: Molecular anatomy of herpesviruses: Recent studies. Progr Med Virology 22:152, 1976.

Pfau, C. J., Bergold, G. H., Casals, J., Johnson, K. M., Murphy, F. A., Pedersen, I. R., Rawls, W. E., Rowe, W. P., Webb, P. A., and Weissenbacher, M. C.: Arenaviruses. Intervirology 4:207, 1974.

Porterfield, J. S., Casals, J., Chumakov, M. P., Gaidamovich, S. Ya., Hannoun, C., Holmes, I. H., Horzinek, M. C., Mussgay, M., Oker-Blom, N., and Russell, P. K.: Bunyaviruses and Bunyaviridae. Intervirology 6:13, 1975/76.

Porterfield, J. S., Casals, J., Chumakov, M. P., Gaidamovich, S. Ya., Hannoun, C., Holmes, I. H., Horzinek, M. C., Mussgay, M., Oker-Blom, N., Russell, P. K., and Trent, D. W.: Togaviridae. Intervirology 9:129, 1978.

Tyrrell, D. A. J., Almeida, J. D., Cunningham, C. H., Dowdle, W. R., Hofstad, M. S., McIntosh, K., Tajima, M., Zakstelskaya, L. Ya., Easterday, B. C., Kapikian, A., and Bingham, R. W.: Coronaviridae. Intervirology 5:76, 1975.

Vogt, P. K.: The oncovirinae — a definition of the group. In First Report of the WHO Collaborating Centre for Collection and Evaluation of Data on Comparative Virology (Proceedings of the Official Opening of the Centre, in Munich). Published by the WHO Centre, Munich, 1976.

Wildy, P.: Classification and Nomenclature of Viruses: First Report of the International Committee on Nomenclature of Viruses. Monographs in Virology, Vol. 5, Basel, S. Karger, 1971.

# 9 VIRAL REPLICATION

*Samuel C. Silverstein, M.D.*

All viruses share a common problem: namely, to maintain and propagate their genetic information. To this end viruses parasitize the biosynthetic machinery of their host cells, availing themselves of one or more of the many subcellular compartments, synthetic capacities, processing pathways and substrates available in animal cells. Even the picornaviruses, which are among the smallest and apparently least complex of the animal viruses, require dozens of host-cell cytoplasmic functions and structures to replicate their genomes. The larger DNA-containing viruses, such as herpesviruses, require for their replication the biosynthetic capacities of both the nucleus and cytoplasm of their cellular hosts. Some tumor-forming viruses, such as the papova and oncornaviruses, integrate their genomes into their host cells' DNA. Locked together in this way, papovavirus or oncornavirus genes and host-cell genes replicate coordinately.

The number and variety of replicative strategies utilized by the different classes of RNA and DNA viruses suggest that they have left no potential replicative or biosynthetic pathway unexplored. Even the central dogma of molecular biology, "DNA makes RNA," must be qualified in the case of the oncornaviruses in which DNA is synthesized on an RNA template. Viewed in this context, each virus group occupies a specific ecologic niche among intracellular parasites and identifies one of the many pathways that have evolved for the faithful and efficient transfer of genes from cell to cell.

## INITIATION OF A VIRAL INFECTION

The initial problem facing any potential pathogen, be it bacterial, protozoan, or viral, is to enter the host. This is an especially demanding task for viruses since, unlike schistosomules or salmonellae, they cannot crawl through the skin or break open the junctions that join the cells of the intestinal epithelium. Viruses enter their hosts by infecting a susceptible cell.

Viral pathogens that enter without the assistance of an insect or animal vector do so by infecting cells of the respiratory, intestinal, and genital tracts. Although epithelial cells represent the major targets in these locations, viruses also appear to have access to the lymphoid tissues that surround the oropharynx. Once infected, the epithelial cells may release progeny virions into the bloodstream as occurs with smallpox and polioviruses, or the recirculating cells of the lymphoid tissues may themselves become infected and carry the virus to tissues elsewhere in the body. For viruses that utilize an insect (arboviruses), animal (rabies), or human (hepatitis B) vector, entry into the host is not synonymous with infection; these agents must still find and penetrate a susceptible cell to initiate the infectious process.

## CELL SURFACE RECEPTORS AND TISSUE TROPISM

The precise mechanism(s) that regulate the entry of viral nucleic acids or nucleoproteins into the cytoplasm or nucleus are poorly understood. It is clear that different viruses adsorb to unique "receptor" molecules on the host cells' surface and that these plasma membrane receptors determine the susceptibility of cells bearing them to infection with a given virus. For instance, both mouse and human cells produce poliovirus when they are infected with RNA extracted from poliovirus Type 1. That is, both human and mouse cells are biosynthetically capable of translating and replicating poliovirus RNA and encapsidating it into virions. However, human cells, unlike mouse cells, have plasma membrane receptors for poliovirus. As a consequence, only human cells bind and uncoat the intact virus, thereby allowing the viral RNA to gain access to the cell's cytoplasm and to initiate an infection.

Why have viral receptors been retained on the surface of cells? If the presence of these receptors served only to enhance the susceptibility of cells to a viral pathogen, then cells retaining these receptors would have a selective disadvantage in terms of survival. If, on the other hand, these surface receptors perform important roles in the maintenance of normal cellular function, then selective pressures for their elimination would be balanced by pressures for their retention. Although no data are available concerning the evolutionary history of cellular receptors for viruses, we do know that many cells have membrane receptors that mediate the binding and internalization of hormones, vitamins, immunoglobulins, and other physiologically important macromolecules. Viruses may utilize one or more of these receptor systems to penetrate their host cells.

Specific viral capsid proteins determine cell and tissue tropisms of closely related viruses. For instance, reovirus Type 1 infects ependymal cells in suckling mice and causes hydrocephalus; reovirus Type 3 infects neurons and causes a fatal encephalitis in these animals. The viral protein that controls these type-specific effects is the outer capsid protein responsible for the hemagglutinating properties of the virus. Each reovirion contains less than 30 copies of Type 1 or Type 3 hemagglutinin protein on its surface. Recombinant viruses containing all Type 3 genes, except for the single Type 1 gene encoding the hemagglutinin protein, behave like reovirus Type 1. That is, this recombinant virus infect ependymal cells, not neurons, and causes hydrocephalus, not encephalitis.

## PENETRATION OF THE VIRAL GENOME

Studies of avian RNA tumor viruses and of reoviruses suggest that the interaction of cell membrane receptors with viral capsid proteins regulates the penetration of a viral nucleoprotein into the cytoplasm, and not merely the attachment of the virus to the cell's surface. We currently recognize two mechanisms by which penetration occurs: fusion of the virus with the cell surface and endocytosis of the intact virion.

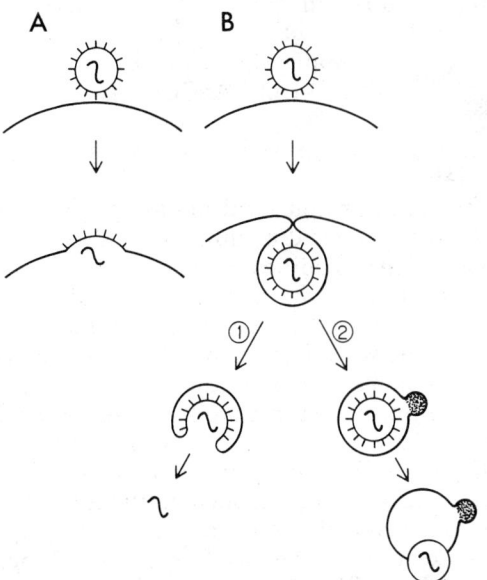

**FIGURE 1.** *Pathways of viral uncoating. A, The viral envelope fuses with the cell surface, resulting in release of viral nucleoprotein into the cytoplasmic matrix. B, The virus is endocytosed. Encircled 1, The interaction of the viral envelope with the membrane of the endocytic vacuole causes fusion or dissolution of the vacuolar membrane and partial or complete uncoating of the virus. Encircled 2, The virus-containing vacuole fuses with lysosomes. The outer viral capsids are degraded by lysosomal enzymes, and the viral nucleoprotein is released into the cytoplasm.*

### Fusion

Herpes, pox, and paramyxoviruses are agents whose outer envelope is composed of a lipid bilayer in which viral glycoproteins are embedded. These viruses appear to enter by fusion of this envelope with the host cell's plasma membrane (Fig. 1A). Fusion of a viral envelope with the cell membrane has been shown most convincingly for the paramyxoviruses. A glycoprotein named F (fusion factor) has been identified on the surface of paramyxoviruses, and activity of the F protein has been proved to be required for viral infectivity. As a consequence of its fusion with the cell's surface, viral envelope proteins are incorporated into the host cell's plasma membrane, and the viral nucleoprotein is released directly into the cytoplasm. It is of interest that most of the viruses that enter by fusion also have the capacity to fuse infected cells with their uninfected neighbors. Presumably the same viral glycoproteins that promote viral penetration are inserted into the plasma membranes of infected cells and are responsible for the fusion of these cells with neighboring cells.

### Endocytosis

Fusion factors have not been identified in several classes of enveloped viruses (myxo, toga, rhabdo, and oncorna), or in viruses (picorna, reo, papova, adeno) containing only proteins in their outer shells. These agents appear to be engulfed by the host cell in a phagocytic vacuole. The interaction of the viral capsids with the membrane of the phagocytic vacuole is presumed to result in the modification of the surface structure of the virus and the lysis of the phagocytic vacuole (Fig. 1B, pathway I). In this way the picorna, toga, myxo, rhabdo, and oncornaviruses are thought to release their infectious nucleic acids or nucleoproteins into the cytoplasm. Papova and adenoviruses require an additional uncoating step within the cytoplasm. These viruses are partially uncoated during their escape from the phagocytic vacuole. Subsequently, these partially uncoated virions are transported to the nuclear membrane at which site their infectious DNA is released and transported via the nuclear pores into the nucleoplasm.

Reoviruses illustrate a unique variation of this uncoating pathway. These viruses enter by phagocytosis but are transported within endocytic vacuoles to the host cell's lysosomes. Proteolytic enzymes within the lysosomal compartment degrade the outer viral capsids; the resulting nucleoprotein core is resistant to further proteolysis and appears to be released from the lysosomes into the cytoplasmic matrix (Fig. 1B, pathway 2).

## THE ROLE OF ANTIBODIES AND COMPLEMENT IN PREVENTING INFECTION

Antibodies directed against viral surface determinants inhibit viral infection by several mechanisms. First, antibodies block the interaction of viral capsids with cell-surface receptors and thereby markedly decrease the efficiency of viral adsorption to cells. Second, antibodies stimulate the fixation of serum complement to the virus. In the case of some enveloped viruses, complement causes lysis of the viral particle. Third, antibodies enhance the binding of viruses to the antibody and complement receptors of monocytes and macrophages and promote phagocytosis of neutralized viruses by these cells. Mononuclear phagocytes exhibit a reduced capacity to replicate a variety of viruses and thereby may slow the spread of an infection. Fourth, antibodies promote the segregation of antibody-coated virus into cellular lysosomes. Most viruses are destroyed by the degradative enzymes contained in this cellular compartment.

Although serum and/or secretory antibodies generally protect against infections with viruses, several exceptions have been noted. Infants with low antibody titers against dengue virus may develop an exceptionally severe disease on reexposure to the virus, presumably because at low levels the antibodies promote adsorption to and infection of mononuclear phagocytes. Individuals experiencing recurrent herpes infections have high titers of neutralizing antibody against herpes virus. Reactivation of the latent virus leads to virus spread by cell-cell fusion, a process that is controlled poorly by humoral immunity.

## REPLICATION

Having successfully gained access to the cell's biosynthetic machinery, viruses have the opportunity to subvert this machinery for their own purposes. Lytic animal viruses quickly shut off host-cell synthetic processes while temperate and transforming viruses rely on the integrity and longevity of the host cell for their own survival. Regardless of the replicative strategy to be employed, however, the initial problem facing all viruses is that of synthesizing messenger RNA (mRNA); it is only by forming new proteins that the virus can take command of the cell. In the sections that follow I summarize the steps leading to mRNA formation, genome replication, and synthesis of progeny virus for each of the major virus groups. Throughout, single-stranded polynucleotides of the same polarity as messenger RNA are termed plus (+) strands and single-stranded polynucleotides of complementary base sequence are termed minus (−) strands.

## SYNTHESIS AND STRUCTURE OF MESSENGER RNA

Polynucleotide chains are synthesized by the sequential addition of nucleotides. The direction of polymerization is $3' \rightarrow 5'$ with respect to the template and $5' \rightarrow 3'$ with respect to the newly formed polynucleotide. For example, an RNA template that has the sequence 3′ HO-UpGpApCp, etc.* at its 3′ end directs the formation of a complementary RNA strand with ATP at its 5′ terminus

$$5' \text{ pppA-OH } 3'$$
$$(3' \text{ HO-UpGpApCp---etc.}).$$

The next nucleotide, cytidylic acid, will join to the 3′ hydroxyl of ATP to give

$$5' \text{ pppApC-OH } 3'$$
$$3' \text{ HO-UpGpApCp---etc.}$$

Polymerization continues by the stepwise addition of nucleotides until the polynucleotide chain is completed. In the case of the RNA chain illustrated above, the next two nucleotides specified by the template RNA are uridylic and guanylic acids, giving the structure

$$5' \text{ pppApCpUpGp-OH } 3'$$
$$3' \text{ HO-UpGpApCp---etc.}$$

As the chain is synthesized, it is released from the template.

Most cellular and viral messenger RNAs have distinctive chemical modifications at their 5′ and 3′ ends. These modifications enhance the efficiency of messenger RNA translation by the ribosomes. The 5′ end is modified by a guanylic acid residue, the so-called "capping" nucleotide, joined by an unusual 5′ to 5′ linkage to the 5′ end of the RNA chain; both the capping guanylic acid residue and the nucleotide to which it is joined are methylated. Assuming the polynucleotide illustrated above is to be capped and methylated, the reactions proceed in the sequence pppApCpUpG-OH → GpppApCpUpG-OH → methyl-GpppAmethylpCpUpG-OH. The enzymes that carry out the capping and methylating reactions may be viral, as occurs in the formation of reovirus mRNAs, or

---

*p represents the phosphates that join the ribonucleosides in phosphodiester linkages. pppA-OH is adenosine triphosphate. The OH is the hydroxyl group at the 3′ position of the ribose of the nucleotide. Gppp is guanosine triphosphate.

cellular, as occurs in the formation of influenza virus mRNAs.

The 3' end of most messengers is modified by a sequence of 50 to 200 adenylic acid residues. By and large these adenylic acid residues are not determined by a sequence of complementary nucleotides in the template. Rather, they are added to the 3' end of the nascent mRNA chain by a viral or a cellular polyadenylic acid polymerase according to the reaction sequence - - -pU-OH $3' + (ATP) \rightarrow_n$ - - -pU(pA)$_n^-$OH 3'.

## POSITIVE-STRAND RNA VIRUSES

### Picornaviruses

The entero and rhinoviruses, the smallest of the RNA-containing animal viruses, contain a single molecule of single-stranded RNA of molecular weight $2.6 \times 10^6$ daltons. The genome RNA has the same size, base sequence, and polarity as mRNA. Upon entry into the cytoplasm, the genome RNA binds to ribosomes and initiates the synthesis of viral proteins (Fig. 2, pathway I). One or more of these proteins forms an RNA polymerase, and this enzyme catalyzes the synthesis of a negative RNA strand, using as its template the parental RNA plus (+) strand (Fig. 2, pathway II). The RNA minus strands act as templates for the synthesis of single-stranded RNA plus strands. Some of these progeny plus strands function as mRNA and direct the synthesis of viral proteins. Other plus strands are enclosed in viral capsids and thus become the genomes of the newly formed progeny virus.

The initial translation product of the viral

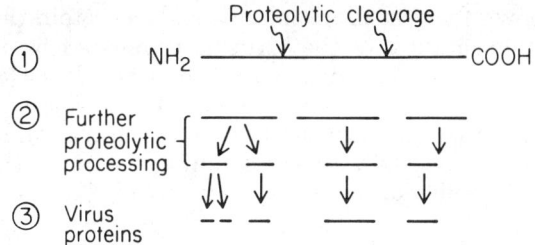

**FIGURE 3.** *Processing of the large precursor protein, encircled 1, that is the primary translation product of poliovirus messenger RNA. Proteolytic enzymes in the cytoplasm of the host cell perform the initial cleavage steps, encircled 2. Viral encoded enzymes may be involved in later cleavages. The proteins derived from the left (amino) half of the large protein form the viral coat proteins. The proteins derived from the right (carboxyl) half of the precursor protein form the viral RNA polymerases.*

mRNA is a large precursor protein (Fig. 3). Proteases present in the cytoplasm of the host cell catalyze the cleavage of this "polyprotein" into the smaller proteins that form the viral polymerase and capsid proteins. The capsid proteins self-assemble with one another, and with viral RNA, to form the completed virus. Progeny virus particles accumulate at an exponential rate within the cytoplasm until, for unknown reasons, the biosynthetic capacity of the cell is exhausted. The cell then lyses, releasing virus into the surrounding tissues.

### Togaviruses or Arthropod-borne Viruses

These agents have a slightly larger RNA genome ($4 \times 10^6$ daltons) than the picornaviruses, but replicate their genomes in essentially the same manner. However, in addition to genome-sized RNA, togavirus-infected cells contain an additional species of mRNA that is about one-third the length of viral genome RNA. This mRNA directs the synthesis of the viral core protein, and the three viral envelope glycoproteins $E_1$, $E_2$, and $E_3$. Viral genome RNA also serves as mRNA and is presumed to encode nonstructural proteins in addition to the envelope glycoproteins described above. Both genome-sized and shorter RNA plus strands are formed on genome length complementary RNA minus strands. Transcription of the less-than-genome length mRNA on the minus-strand RNA template is initiated independently of genome-length RNA.

Togaviruses are composed of an RNA-containing core wrapped within a lipoprotein envelope. The envelope is composed of host-cell lipids and viral glycoproteins. The core is assembled in the cytoplasmic matrix from RNA and soluble proteins while the envelope glycoproteins are synthesized in the rough endoplasmic reticulum and transported to the cell surface in membrane vesicles in a manner similar to that

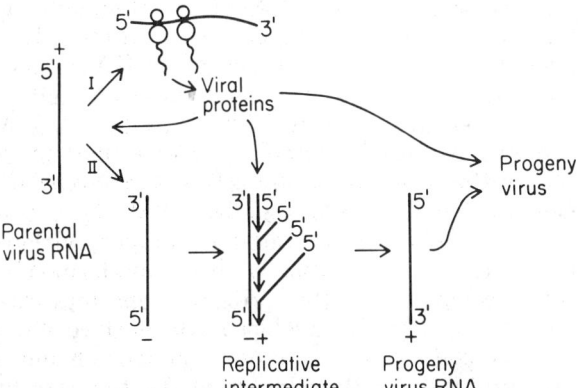

**FIGURE 2.** *Replication of picornavirus RNA. Pathway I. Parental virus RNA binds to host cell polyribosomes and serves as messenger RNA for the synthesis of viral proteins. Pathway II. Viral proteins form an RNA-dependent RNA polymerase that makes a negative-strand RNA copy of the parental positive-strand RNA. This negative-strand serves as a template for the synthesis of progeny positive strands.*

shown for vesicular stomatitis glycoprotein (Fig. 6). Formation of the virus is completed by the encapsidation of cores within their envelopes (see Fig. 6), and their release from the cell surface. Mature togaviruses do not accumulate in the cell but are released into the surrounding tissues as they are completed.

## Coronaviruses

In comparison with the picorna and togaviruses, our information about the molecular biology of coronavirus replication is less complete. Human coronaviruses contain single-stranded RNA of ~ $6 \times 10^6$ daltons molecular weight. This RNA, like picornavirus RNA and most messenger RNAs, contains a polyadenylic acid sequence at its 3' terminus. RNA extracted from coronaviruses is infectious. These findings, and the lack of a nucleic acid polymerase within the virus, suggest that coronaviruses are positive-strand viruses and that they replicate their RNA by a mechanism similar to the one described for picornaviruses.

Coronaviruses are named for the prominent spikes that radiate from their lipid envelopes. They replicate in the cytoplasm. Their helical viral ribonucleoprotein is encapsidated by budding into the cisternae of the endoplasmic reticulum. The virus is presumably released by lysis of infected cells; transport of coronaviruses from the rough endoplasmic reticulum to the cell surface in membrane vesicles may also occur.

## Oncornaviruses

These RNA-containing viruses have been identified as tumor-causing agents in a variety of vertebrates. Although they are not presently associated with disease in man, it seems unlikely that the species *Homo sapiens* has been excluded as a host for these ubiquitous viruses.

Oncornaviruses are diploid; they contain duplicate copies of single-stranded RNA of the same polarity as viral messenger RNA. In addition, they contain a specific transfer RNA (tryptophanyl tRNA in the case of avian oncornaviruses) hydrogen bonded to genome RNA, and an RNA-dependent DNA polymerase that synthesizes a double-stranded DNA copy of the viral RNA. The mechanism of synthesis of this double-stranded DNA copy is not completely understood, but the following steps have been identified (Fig. 4). Upon release of the virus core into the cytoplasm, synthesis of a DNA minus strand is initiated using viral RNA as template and the transfer RNA that is bound to viral RNA as primer (Fig. 4, *encircled 1*). Minus-strand synthesis is followed by plus-strand formation (Fig. 4, *encircled 2*), and the resulting linear DNA duplex is circularized

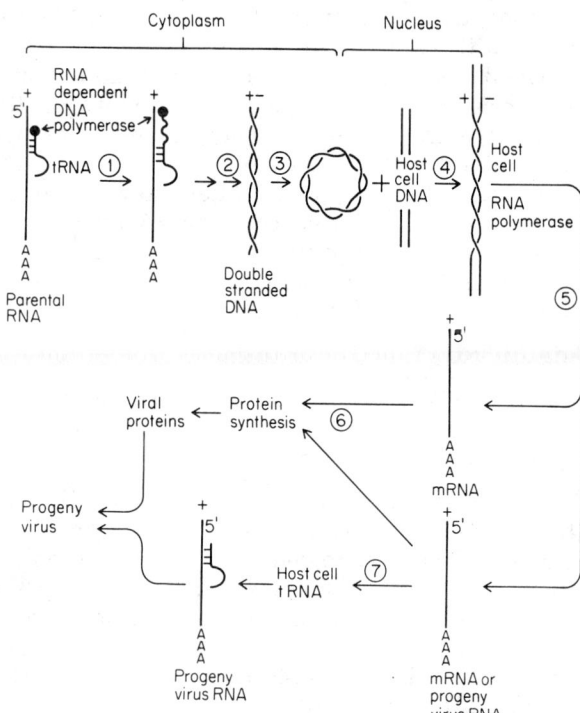

**FIGURE 4.** *Replication of oncornavirus RNA. Reactions shown on the left side of the diagram occur in the cytoplasm; those on the right side occur in the nucleus. Synthesis of a DNA copy of viral RNA begins (encircled 1) as soon as the viral ribonucleoprotein is released into the cytoplasm. Following its covalent integration into host cell DNA (encircled 4), the double-stranded DNA copy of the viral genome becomes a template for host cell RNA polymerases (encircled 5). These enzymes synthesize viral messenger RNAs (encircled 6) and progeny virus RNAs (encircled 7), using the integrated viral DNA as template. Proteins encoded by these messengers form the envelope and internal proteins of progeny virions. See text and Figure 6 for further details of oncornavirus morphogenesis.*

and integrated into host-cell DNA (Fig. 4, *encircled 3 and 4*). Host-cell RNA polymerases now synthesize messenger RNAs of less than genome length, and single-stranded RNA plus strands of genome length (Fig. 4, *encircled 5*). RNAs of both sizes are capped and polyadenylated at their 5' and 3' ends, respectively. They are exported from the nucleus into the cytoplasm where they direct the synthesis of viral proteins (Fig. 4, *encircled 6*). Genome-length RNA, together with host cell transfer RNA, is incorporated into progeny virions (Fig. 4, *encircled 7*). Progeny virions are formed by the envelopment of their ribonucleoprotein core within a lipoprotein envelope at the surface of the infected cell. Synthesis of oncornavirus envelope glycoproteins and their insertion into the nascent virus particle as it buds from the cell's surface occurs by a mechanism that is similar to the one described in Figure 6 for the formation of the envelope of vesicular stomatitis virus. The host cell is not destroyed by an oncornavirus infection; it continues to divide and to release virus. Thus oncornavirus-infected cells express viral envelope glycoproteins on their plasma membranes and viral proteins in their cytoplasm indefinitely.

A 60,000 molecular-weight protein that is encoded by the viral sarcomagenic ("sarc") gene has been identified as the molecule responsible for oncogenic transformation of cells infected with avian oncornaviruses. This protein has kinase activity; that is, using ATP as a cofactor, it catalyzes the phosphorylation of cellular and/or viral proteins. Whether this enzymatic activity is responsible for the malignant behavior of cells transformed by avian sarcoma viruses is unknown.

## NEGATIVE-STRAND RNA VIRUSES

These viruses contain RNA genomes that are complementary in nucleotide sequence to messenger RNA. Since messenger RNAs are by definition plus strands, complementary RNAs are termed minus or negative strands. Three virus groups of major significance are classified under this heading. In order of increasing genome complexity, they are rhabdoviruses (rabies, vesicular stomatitis virus); paramyxoviruses (measles, mumps, parainfluenza, and respiratory syncytial viruses); and orthomyxoviruses (influenza viruses). These viruses share several design features. They have envelopes whose lipids are derived from the surfaces of their host cells; they have helical nucleocapsids containing RNA of negative polarity; and they contain RNA-dependent RNA transcriptases, enzymes that make positive-strand mRNA using the viral genome as template.

The mechanisms of messenger RNA transcription by negative-strand viruses have been examined in great detail. Nevertheless, key issues regarding mRNA synthesis are unresolved. The intermediate steps in the replication of genome RNA are even less clearly defined. Thus the steps in mRNA synthesis and viral genome replication shown in Figures 5 and 7 should be taken as representative of the overall process of progeny-negative RNA strand formation but not as a precise description of mechanisms or of the intermediates involved.

### Rhabdoviruses

Rhabdoviruses are bullet-shaped; they contain five proteins and a single strand of RNA of molecular weight $4.5 \times 10^6$ daltons. The RNA is not by itself infectious. Within the virus, the RNA is associated throughout its length with multiple copies of the nucleocapsid protein. Also associated with the ribonucleoprotein are two proteins that form an RNA transcriptase. A matrix protein lies

on the under or internal surface of the lipid bilayer that forms the viral envelope. A single glycoprotein spans the lipid bilayer; this glycoprotein forms the spikes that project from the virus surface. Information concerning rhabdovirus replication is chiefly derived from studies of vesicular stomatitis viruses. These viruses replicate in the cytoplasm.

Entry of the viral nucleoprotein into the cytoplasm activates the nucleoprotein-associated RNA transcriptase and initiates the synthesis of viral messenger RNA (Fig. 5, pathway I). Messenger RNA molecules are synthesized sequentially from the 3' end of the viral genome. They are presumably cleaved from a large RNA transcript that is formed as the transcriptase proceeds down the genome from the 3' to the 5' end. These RNA messages are modified by the addition of methylated guanylic acid "caps" at their 5' ends and of polyadenylic acid at their 3' ends. Each messenger RNA directs the synthesis of one of the five viral proteins. Synthesis of viral proteins is required for the formation of full-length RNA plus strands and of progeny virus minus-strand RNA. Progeny minus strands serve as templates for amplification of messenger RNA synthesis and as the genomes of newly formed virions.

The viral proteins that form the internal components of the virus (in the case of vesicular stomatitis virus, these are the nucleocapsid, RNA transcriptase, and matrix proteins) are synthesized on polyribosomes that are free in the cy-

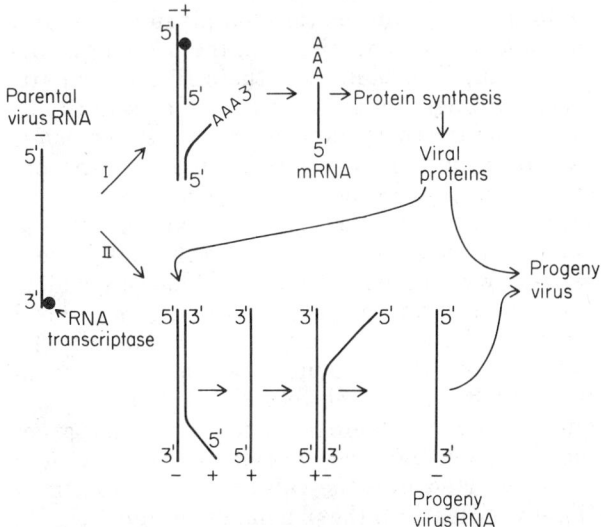

**FIGURE 5.** *Replication of rhabdovirus RNA. Pathway I. Complementary messenger RNAs are formed by the virus RNA transcriptase (•), using the parental negative-strand RNA as template. These viral messengers direct the synthesis of enzymes that make full length positive-strand RNA copies of the parental negative-strand RNAs (pathway II). The positive strands are the templates on which progeny virus negative-strand RNA is formed.*

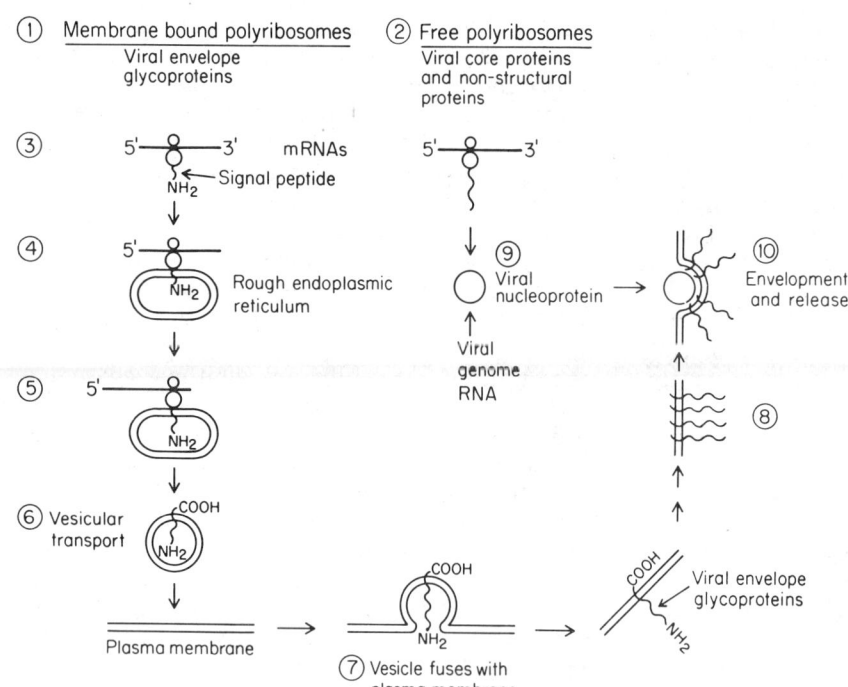

**FIGURE 6.** *Formation of viral envelope glycoproteins and the assembly of enveloped viruses. See text for details.*

toplasmic matrix (Fig. 6, *encircled 2*). The viral envelope glycoprotein (G) is formed on the ribosomes of the rough endoplasmic reticulum (Fig. 6, *encircled 1*). A "signal" peptide at the amino terminus of the nascent G protein promotes ribosome binding to the membranes of the rough endoplasmic reticulum and is responsible for the incorporation of the G protein into these membranes during its synthesis (Fig. 6, *encircled 3, 4, 5*). In this way, information contained in the viral messenger RNA specifies both the primary structure of the G protein and the cellular compartments through which it is to be processed. Glycosyl transferases within the rough endoplasmic reticulum add oligosaccharide chains to the nascent viral glycoprotein (Fig. 6, *encircled 5*). The viral glycoprotein is then transported via the smooth endoplasmic reticulum to the Golgi apparatus in which the final sugar residues are added. The composition and sequence of sugars in viral glycoproteins are determined by the host cell. The glycoproteins are thought to be transported from the smooth endoplasmic reticulum to the Golgi apparatus and from there to the cell surface as part of membrane-bound vesicles (Fig. 6, *encircled 6*), and to be inserted into the cell surface by fusion of these vesicles with the plasma membrane (Fig. 6, *encircled 6, 7, 8*).

The viral glycoprotein has the same orientation in the membranes of the rough endoplasmic reticulum as it has in the plasma membrane and in the completed virus. The glycoprotein spans the lipid bilayer. Its amino terminus and carbohy-

drate lie on the outside of the viral envelope while its carboxyl terminus projects into the interior of the virus. Viral glycoproteins in the plasma membrane can be thought of as the nucleation sites for the assembly of matrix proteins on the cytoplasmic side of the membrane. The interaction of the ribonucleoprotein with membrane-bound matrix protein leads to the formation of the completed virus and its release from the cell (Fig. 6, *encircled 9, 10*).

The mechanisms governing the synthesis, glycosylation, vesicular transport, and insertion of G protein into the cell surface are generally applicable to the formation of viral envelope glycoproteins. Thus, it seems likely that these pathways and principles are employed in the morphogenesis of most enveloped viruses.

### Paramyxoviruses

Paramyxoviruses are pleomorphic, filamentous, and spherical particles containing single-stranded RNA of molecular weight 5.5 to $6 \times 10^6$ daltons. They have two externally disposed glycoproteins, each of which forms spikes on the surface of the virion. One of these glycoproteins (termed HN) is both a hemagglutinin and a neuraminidase. It is responsible for attaching the virus to sialic acid residues on cell surfaces during penetration and for the virus's hemagglutinating activity. The neuraminidase removes sialic acid from cellular glycolipids and glycoproteins, thereby enhancing virus release from the surfaces of infected cells. The second viral glycoprotein (called F) promotes fusion of the viral envelope with cell surfaces, and fusion of infected cells with neighboring uninfected cells. Virus particles with an inactive fusion protein are not infectious.

Aside from these differences, paramyxoviruses resemble rhabdoviruses in overall replication strategy. Paramyxovirus ribonucleoprotein contains one major nucleocapsid protein and two other proteins that form the RNA transcriptase. A matrix protein lines the inner surface of the viral envelope. Release of the paramyxovirus ribonucleoprotein into the cytoplasm activates its RNA transcriptase and initiates the synthesis of viral messenger RNAs. Subsequently, viral proteins and progeny genome RNA are formed as outlined in Figure 5. Synthesis and insertion of viral glycoproteins HN and F into the cell surface occur in a manner similar to that described in Figure 6 for vesicular stomatitis G proteins. Matrix protein and ribonucleoprotein assemble at the cytoplasmic face of plasma membrane segments that contain HN and F proteins. Envelopment of the nucleoprotein and release of mature virions from the cell surface complete the replicative cycle.

### Orthomyxoviruses

Influenza virions occur in spheric and filamentous forms. Both forms have lipid envelopes containing two glycoproteins, a hemagglutinin and a neuraminidase. The hemagglutinin is responsible for virus attachment to sialic acid residues on the surface of the host cell, while the neuraminidase promotes release of progeny virus from infected cells. Unlike the paramyxoviruses, myxoviruses lack a fusion protein and do not cause cell fusion.

The influenza viruses contain eight segments of single-stranded RNA of negative polarity. Each RNA segment has a unique nucleotide sequence; each encodes a single messenger RNA and thereby a single protein. The genome contains 5.6 to 6 $\times 10^6$ daltons of RNA.

Each RNA segment forms a helical coil around the nucleocapsid proteins. Four other viral proteins are bound to the viral nucleoprotein; the entire complex has RNA transcriptase activity. The RNA transcriptase catalyzes the synthesis of single-stranded messenger RNA copies of all eight segments of the viral genome.

After penetration, the influenza ribonucleoproteins are transported into the host cell's nucleus. Formation of viral messenger RNA requires host-cell RNA synthesis. The capped and methylated 5' ends of host-cell messenger RNAs are used as "primers" for the viral RNA transcriptase. These primers are joined to RNA sequences encoded by the parental RNA templates. The host's polyadenylic acid polymerase adds adenylic acid residues to the 3' ends of viral RNA transcripts (Fig. 7, pathway I). These messenger RNAs are exported into the cytoplasm where they direct the synthesis of viral proteins (Fig. 7, pathway I) and serve as templates for genome (minus strand) RNA formation (Fig. 7, pathway II). Viral envelope glycoproteins (neuraminidase and hemagglutinin) are synthesized on membrane-bound ribosomes; viral nucleocapsid* and matrix proteins* are formed on free polysomes. The envelope glycoproteins are inserted into the plasma membrane by vesicular transport; the final steps of myxovirus assembly are similar in principle to those described for paramyxo- and rhabdoviruses (Fig. 6); that is, matrix protein is bound to the

---

*See Chapter 7 for a description of the location of these proteins in the virion.

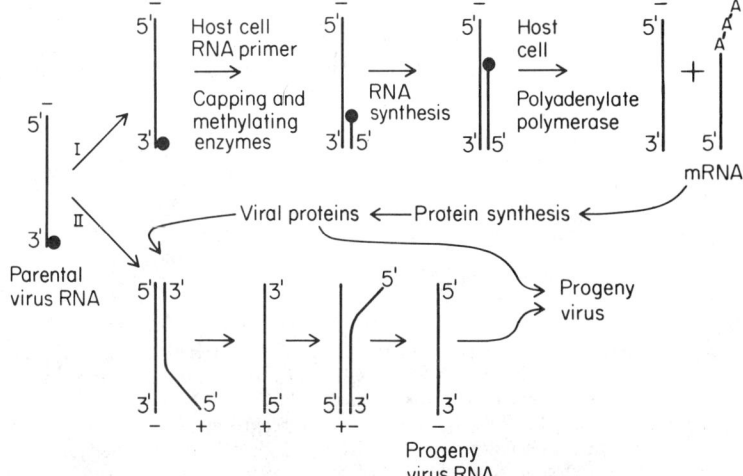

**FIGURE 7.** *Replication of influenza virus RNA. Pathway I. Viral messenger RNAs are synthesized by the virion-contained RNA transcriptase (•), using the parental genome RNAs as templates. Proteins encoded by these messengers form an RNA polymerase. This enzyme synthesizes positive-strand RNA copies of each of the segments of the parental genome (pathway II). These positive strands serve as templates for progeny negative-strand RNAs.*

cytoplasmic face of the plasma membrane. It is assumed, but not proved, that matrix protein binds preferentially to plasma membrane segments containing viral envelope glycoproteins. The eight pieces of viral ribonucleoprotein may bind to the matrix proteins; they are enveloped as the segment of membrane to which they are attached evaginates around them.

Sialic acid residues are removed from the host cell's surface by viral neuraminidase. Removal of those sialic acid groups prevents readsorption of progeny virions to the host cell and promotes the release of virus into the surrounding tissues. The negative-strand viruses are not stored within the cells they infect. They are released throughout the infectious cycle. Viral replication is terminated by death of the host cell.

The process by which viruses containing segmented genomes package one copy of each RNA segment is not known. It is possible, albeit unlikely, that packaging is a random event.

### VIRUSES CONTAINING DOUBLE-STRANDED RNA

Reo and rotaviruses contain 10 and 12 separate segments, respectively, of double-stranded RNA. A single messenger RNA encoding a single viral protein is transcribed from each segment of the double-stranded RNA genome. These viruses contain no lipid. They are composed of two concentric protein shells; the RNA is contained within the inner shell or core.

Reoviruses enter their host cells within endocytic vacuoles and are subsequently concentrated within lysosomes (Fig. 1B, pathway 2). Lysosomal proteases degrade the outer layer of viral proteins and thereby activate the RNA transcriptase contained within the core. This enzyme synthesizes single-stranded RNA plus strands using the complementary minus strands of the viral double-stranded RNAs as templates. The mechanism of RNA transcription on genome double-stranded RNA is analogous to the mechanism of RNA transcription on double-stranded DNA. That is, the parental double strands are conserved, and the newly synthesized single-stranded RNA transcripts are released (Fig. 8, *encircled 2*). In the case of reoviruses, the parental double-stranded RNAs are conserved within the virus's core. The parental virions synthesize multiple single-stranded RNA copies of each segment of genome double-stranded RNA. These newly formed RNA transcripts are exported from the particle (Fig. 8, *encircled 2*) and serve as messengers for the synthesis of viral proteins (Fig. 8, *encircled 3*) or as templates for the formation of progeny double-stranded RNA (Fig. 8, *encircled 4*). Synthesis of double-stranded RNA occurs within the cores of nascent progeny virions (Fig. 8, *encircled 5*). The mechanism(s) responsible for segregating one copy of each of the ten or twelve single-stranded RNA templates into each nascent core particle are unknown. Cores containing newly formed double-stranded RNA (Fig. 8, *encircled 6*) synthesize additional RNA single strands and thereby amplify the rate of messenger and genome template RNA formation. RNA synthesis is terminated by the assembly of the outer layer of capsid proteins on the viral core (Fig. 8, *encircled 7*). Progeny virus accumulates in the cytoplasm and is released by lysis of the host cell.

### VIRUSES CONTAINING DNA GENOMES

#### Papovaviruses

Papova is an acronym that stands for *papi*lloma, *pol*yoma, and simian *va*cuolating viruses. Of

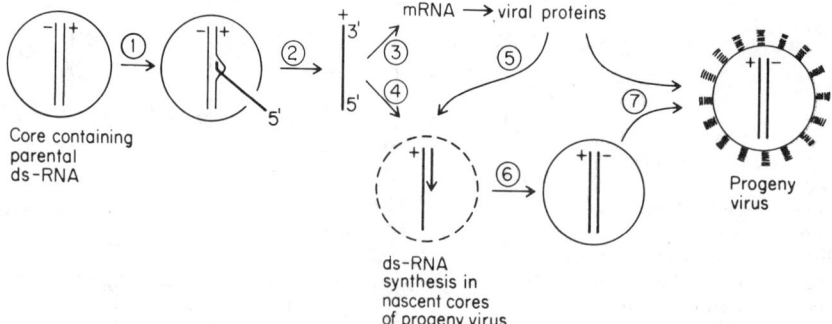

**FIGURE 8.** *Replication of reovirus double-stranded RNAs. Following lysosomal uncoating, the core, containing parental double-stranded (ds) RNA, is released into the the cytoplasmic matrix (encircled 1). Enzymes within the core synthesize and export single-stranded RNA plus strands (encircled 2). Progeny plus strands serve as messengers (encircled 3) for the synthesis of viral proteins (encircled 5), or as templates (encircled 4) for double-stranded RNA formation. Completed cores (encircled 6) containing all ten segments of double-stranded RNA combine with outer capsid proteins (encircled 7) to form progeny virions. See text for further details.*

these, wart virus (a papilloma virus) and JC virus (a vacuolating virus that is the putative causative agent of progressive multifocal leukoencephalopathy) are human pathogens. Interest in these viruses derives principally from the finding that simian virus 40 (a vacuolating virus) and polyoma virus cause oncogenic transformation of hamster and mouse cells, respectively. Cells transformed by SV40 or polyoma virus have one or more copies of the viral genome integrated into cellular DNA.

SV40 virions are small, icosahedral particles about 500 Å in diameter containing only protein and DNA. The genome is a circular molecule of double-stranded DNA of molecular weight $3 \times 10^6$ daltons. The DNA is infectious.

Bacterial restriction endonucleases, enzymes that cleave double-stranded DNA at sites containing specific nucleotide sequences, have been used to map the SV40 genome. One of these endonucleases, EcoRI, produces a single cut in the SV40 genome, converting it from a circular to a linear molecule. This EcoRI cleavage site provides a point of reference on SV40 DNA, and all functions of the DNA are mapped with respect to it. For instance, the origin of viral DNA replication begins roughly two-thirds of the way around the circle from the EcoRI cleavage site, and DNA replication occurs bidirectionally from this point of origin (Fig. 9).

After viral penetration into a permissive host cell, SV40 DNA is found in the nucleus. Host-cell RNA polymerase initiates transcription of "early" messenger RNAs using viral DNA as template. "Early" viral functions are messenger RNAs and their protein products that are synthesized prior to the replication of the viral genome. "Late" functions are messenger RNAs and proteins whose

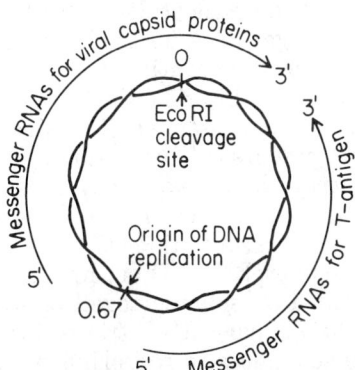

**FIGURE 9.** *Map of SV40 DNA. Early messenger RNAs are encoded by one strand of the DNA duplex. These messenger RNAs direct the synthesis of viral T-antigens. Late messengers are encoded by the complementary DNA strand on the opposite half of the circular molecule. These messengers direct the synthesis of viral capsid proteins. Messenger transcription begins near the origin of DNA replication (0.67) and proceeds in opposite directions on the two DNA strands.*

synthesis is initiated after replication of the viral genome. In general, early functions are enzymes required for genome replication, while late functions are viral capsid proteins. This is so for SV40-infected cells.

SV40 produces a single class of early messenger RNAs. These RNAs are exported to the cytoplasm where they direct the synthesis of tumor (T) antigens. T-antigens are a group of proteins, the largest of which has a molecular weight of 90,000. Animals with SV40-induced tumors have antibodies directed against T-antigens. These antibodies show that T-antigens are located principally in the nucleus of SV40-infected and transformed cells.

T-antigens stimulate the production of host-cell enzymes involved in DNA replication, and they induce host-cell DNA synthesis. T-antigens also regulate the replication of SV40 DNA. In cells that are transformed by SV40 the viral DNA is integrated into host-cell DNA early in the replicative cycle, and later viral genes encoding capsid proteins are not expressed. Monkey cells support a lytic infection with SV40. In these cells, the late genes that encode the three viral capsid proteins are transcribed and translated, and SV40 virions are formed within the nucleus. Virus is released when the cell lyses.

### Adenoviruses

Adenoviruses are icosahedral particles containing linear double-stranded DNA of about $25 \times 10^6$ daltons molecular weight. Like SV40, they replicate in the nucleus, use host-cell RNA polymerase to initiate their RNA transcription, produce a unique T-antigen, and cause transformation in some cell lines (rat) and lytic infections in others (human). Cells transformed by adenovirus contain a specific segment of adenovirus DNA integrated into cellular DNA. This "transforming" DNA comprises less than 10 per cent of the adenovirus genome.

Adenoviruses enter their host cells by endocytosis. Fibers projecting from the 12 vertices of these icosahedral particles bind to the cell surface and are required for successful penetration. These fibers are removed from the particle as it enters the cytoplasmic matrix. The particle is then transported to the nucleus. The final stage of adenovirus uncoating occurs at the pores of the nuclear envelope and results in the release of viral DNA into the nucleus. Within the nucleus, early adenovirus messenger RNAs are transcribed by host-cell RNA polymerase. These messengers direct the synthesis of viral proteins required for DNA replication and late RNA transcription. Late messenger RNAs direct the synthesis of adenovirus capsid proteins.

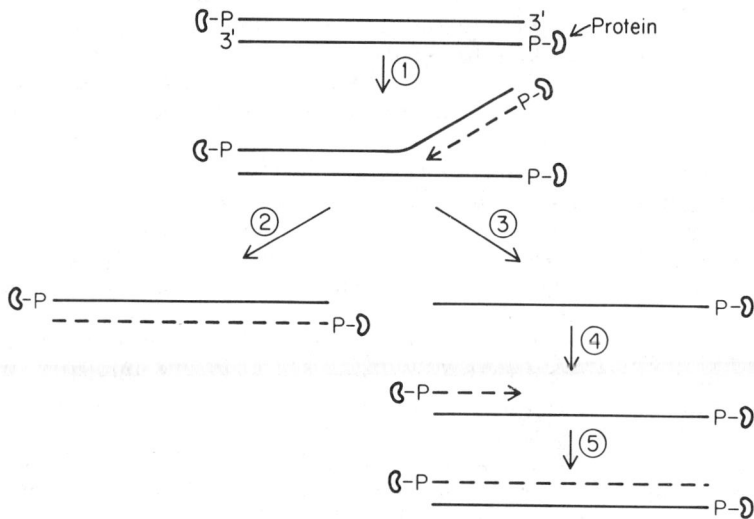

FIGURE 10. *Replication of adenovirus DNA. Solid lines (——) signify parental DNA strands. Dotted lines (---) indicate newly synthesized DNA. DNA synthesis is initiated at the 3' end of one strand of the double-stranded DNA molecule (encircled 1). An adenovirus protein-nucleotide complex may be required to initiate DNA replication. Completion of DNA elongation produces one double-stranded progeny DNA molecule (encircled 2) and one single-stranded parental DNA molecule (encircled 3). A complementary DNA strand is formed on the parental single strand (encircled 4), giving a second molecule of double-stranded DNA (encircled 5).*

Both strands of adenovirus DNA have a protein covalently linked to their 5' termini. Nucleotides linked to this protein may act as primers for progeny DNA synthesis. Adenovirus DNA is replicated by displacement of a parental DNA strand by a progeny DNA strand (Fig. 10). This yields one double-stranded progeny DNA molecule and one single-stranded DNA molecule. Synthesis of a complementary DNA strand using this single-stranded DNA as template yields a second molecule of double-stranded DNA (Fig. 11). Although the resultant DNA molecules contain one parental and one progeny DNA strand, this mechanism of DNA replication differs markedly from that observed for papovavirus or cellular DNA. In the latter cases, the DNA replication forks grow bidirectionally from a single initiation site.

Incubation of adenovirus DNA with a bacterial endonuclease, such as EcoRI, results in the formation of a small number of DNA fragments of limited size. The order of these fragments along

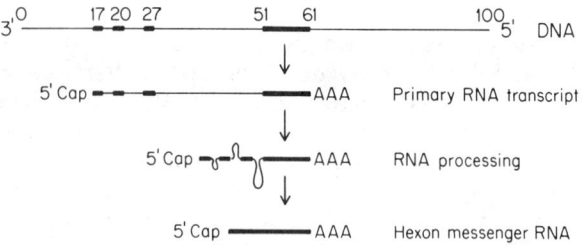

FIGURE 11. *Formation of adenovirus messenger RNA. Adenovirus DNA is shown at the top. Numbers along the DNA are map coordinates representing the percentage of the distance from the left to the right ends of the DNA of any specific nucleotide sequence. For instance, the bulk of the hexon messenger RNA is encoded by the segment of DNA that lies between 51 and 61 per cent of the distance from the 3' to the 5' ends of the DNA. Heavy lines (——) = DNA or RNA sequences that appear in the completed messenger RNA. Light lines (—) = intervening nucleotide sequences. See text for further explanation.*

the genome has been determined and the fragments have been used to map the position on the viral chromosome of specific messenger RNAs. In this way, the nucleotide sequences encoding a major viral capsid protein, the hexon, were shown to lie between 51 and 61 per cent of the distance from the left to the right ends of the viral DNA (Fig. 11).

By separating the two strands of viral DNA from one another, it has been possible to identify the strand encoding each messenger RNA. Experiments of this kind show that both DNA strands contain nucleotide sequences encoding the various early and late messenger RNAs. Thus, unlike SV40 (see Fig. 9, legend), the switch from early to late adenovirus messenger RNA synthesis is not a consequence of a switch in the DNA strand that is transcribed.

Studies of the regulation of adenovirus messenger RNA transcription led to the unexpected observation that the nucleotide sequences that specify the messenger RNA for the hexon protein are located in several noncontiguous segments of the viral chromosome (Fig. 11). Further studies have shown that hexon messenger RNA is derived from a large RNA precursor. This precursor, or primary RNA transcript, is an exact copy of all the DNA sequences lying in the interval between the sites of initiation and termination (17 to 61 per cent) of hexon messenger RNA. Thus, hexon messenger RNA is formed by splicing together specific segments of the primary RNA transcript (Fig. 11). Nucleotide sequences in the primary RNA transcript that are not required in the messenger RNA are cleaved from the primary transcript and degraded within the nucleus.

The presence of intervening DNA sequences and the formation of messenger RNAs by splicing of noncontiguous RNA segments are now recognized as general features of gene structure and function of all eukaryotic cells and of the DNA viruses that parasitize them. The discovery of RNA splicing has added a new dimension to our understanding of the genetics of eukaryotic cells.

### Herpes Viruses

Herpes viruses are relatively large (2000 Å in diameter), spherical particles composed of a lipoprotein envelope wrapped around a protein shell. The shell contains 162 regularly spaced capsomeres arranged in the shape of an icosahedron.* Within this shell lies the linear double-stranded DNA genome ($\sim 10^8$ daltons molecular weight) of the virus. The DNA appears to be wound around a central protein hublike thread on a spool.

Although they have similar anatomic features, the viruses of the herpes group are distinguishable from one another by the antigens they bear, by the structure of their DNA genomes, and by the diseases they cause. In terms of human pathology, herpes simplex virus (oral and genital herpes), Epstein-Barr (EB) virus (mononucleosis), cytomegalovirus (respiratory disease), and varicella-zoster virus ("chickenpox," "shingles") are the most frequently encountered members of this group. Of these viruses, herpes simplex is the prototypic strain. It is the easiest to grow to high titer in tissue culture. Its replicative cycle is summarized below and in Figure 13.

The structure of herpes simplex DNA is complex. Four DNA isomers have been identified in all virus stocks. Each arm has an inverted repeated nucleotide sequence at its ends. The two arms differ in their nucleotide sequences and in the proteins they encode. It is evident from their structures that the DNA sequences of the long and short arms can be joined together in four different orientations with respect to one another (Fig. 12). Presumably, randomization of the orientation of the long and short segments is a consequence of the mechanisms of herpes DNA replication, a process that is not well understood at present.

Penetration of herpes simplex virus into a suit-

---

*See Chapter 7 for a definition of icosahedral symmetry.

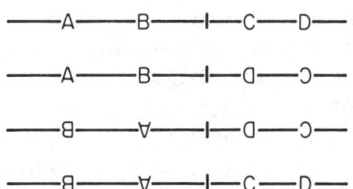

**FIGURE 12.**   *Orientations of the long (A–B) and short (C–D) arms of herpes simplex DNA. "Stick" figures represent double-stranded DNA molecules.*

able host cell occurs by the fusion of the lipoprotein envelope of the virus with the plasma membrane or with the membrane of an endocytic vacuole. In either case, the DNA-containing icosahedral shell of the virus is released into the cytoplasm; the viral DNA is subsequently concentrated in the nucleus (Fig. 13, *upper left*). Cellular RNA polymerases initiate transcription of RNA messengers on the herpes DNA. Like cellular messenger RNAs, these viral messengers are capped and polyadenylated and exported from the nucleus into the cytoplasm in which they direct the synthesis of herpes virus proteins. With the exception of viral glycoproteins, the newly synthesized herpes proteins return to the nucleus in which they regulate the synthesis of additional classes of viral messenger RNAs, shut off cellular RNA and DNA synthesis, initiate herpes DNA replication, and provide structural proteins for the assembly of virions.

Herpes-encoded glycoproteins are inserted into intracellular membranes (nuclear envelope, rough endoplasmic reticulum) and plasma membrane, presumably by a mechanism similar to that described for the insertion of vesicular stomatitis virus glycoprotein into the internal and surface membranes of vesicular stomatitis virus-infected cells (Fig. 6). Virus-encoded glycoproteins in the nuclear envelope form the outer envelope of progeny virions during the final stages of particle maturation (see below and Figure 13). Similar glycoproteins are inserted into the cell surface and may regulate spread of the virus by promoting fusion of infected cells with their uninfected neighbors.

Herpes DNA replicates in the nucleus. Newly replicated viral DNA occurs in concatemers, i.e., DNA molecules of greater than unit ($10^8$ MW) length. These multimeric genomes are then cleaved to molecules of unit length, condensed, and packaged within the icosahedral shell of the virus. Virus morphogenesis is completed when the DNA-containing icosahedron buds through the inner membrane of the nuclear envelope (Fig. 13). By this means the virus acquires its lipoprotein envelope and enters the cisternae of the endoplasmic reticulum. From this site it is transported to the extracellular environment, presumably by a process that is analogous to the transport of secretory proteins from the exocrine pancreas. That is, the virus is contained in smooth surfaced vesicles and carried within them to the plasma membrane. Fusion of these vesicles with the plasma membrane results in release of virus from the cell. In this way herpes virus-infected cells release virus throughout the replicative cycle. Ultimately, however, the cell is lysed as a result of the viral infection.

Several aspects of herpes virus-host cell in-

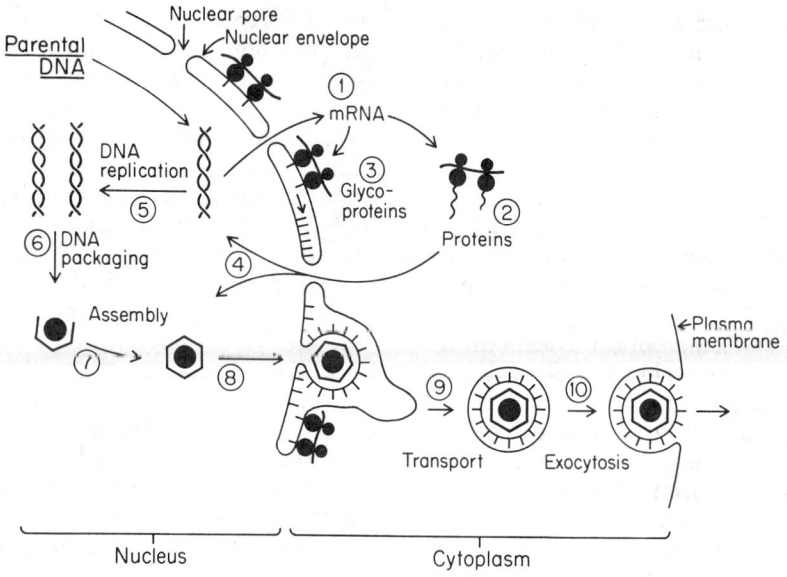

**FIGURE 13.** *Herpes simplex virus morphogenesis. Diagram begins with parental DNA (upper left) in nucleus of host cell. Encircled 1, Viral messenger RNAs are synthesized by host cell RNA polymerase on the viral DNA template. Messengers are exported from the nucleus and initiate the synthesis of viral proteins (free polyribosomes, encircled 2) and glycoproteins (membrane-bound polyribosomes, encircled 3). Viral proteins enter the nucleus (encircled 4), where they promote synthesis of additional classes of viral messenger RNAs. Viral DNA polymerase enters the nucleus and initiates viral DNA replication (encircled 5). DNA is cut into unit lengths, packaged into nucleoids (encircled 6) and encapsidated (encircled 7) within an icosahedral shell. The icosahedral shell buds through the nuclear membrane, acquiring a lipoprotein envelope containing viral glycoproteins (encircled 8). The mature virus is transported in vesicles to the plasma membrane (encircled 9). Fusion of the vesicle with the plasma membrane results in the release of the virus into the extracellular space (encircled 10).*

teractions have direct medical relevance and deserve further emphasis here.

### Cell Fusion

Cells infected with herpes simplex viruses fuse with their neighbors, forming multinucleated giant cells, presumably as a consequence of the insertion of viral glycoproteins into the cell surface. Fusion of infected with uninfected cells may allow spread of an infection even when virus-neutralizing antibodies are present in the extracellular fluids.

### Biosynthetic Requirements

Herpes viruses encode a thymidine kinase. The virus specified enzyme has a less stringent substrate specificity then the host enzyme and has been identified, together with the virus-induced DNA polymerase, as a target for nucleoside analogs exhibiting potent antiviral effects. For instance, 5′-iodo-5′-amino 2′,5′dideoxyuridine (AIdU), and 9-(2-hydroxyethoxymethyl) guanine (acyclo-guanine) are efficiently converted to their respective triphosphates by viral, but not by cellular, thymidine kinase. Both compounds efficiently inhibit DNA synthesis in herpes-infected cells but have little effect on DNA synthesis in uninfected cells.

Biosynthesis of viral glycoproteins is essential for formation of the viral envelope. Glucose and mannose analogs such as 2-deoxyglucose have proved to be effective inhibitors of viral glycoprotein biosynthesis in tissue culture. The potential therapeutic efficacy of these compounds is now being evaluated.

### Latent Infections

Herpes simplex, varicella-zoster, and EB virus cause latent infections in man. The recurrent nature of herpes infections, even in the presence of high titers of circulating antibodies, the recovery of infectious virus from ganglion cells of man and animals (simplex, zoster), and the identification of EB viral antigens and DNA in lymphoid cell lines from "normal" individuals indicate that the genomes of these viruses have the capacity to lie dormant for decades within the cells of the host. Efforts to prove that the entire genome of any one of these agents is integrated into host-cell DNA have as yet been unsuccessful. Multiple copies of EB virus DNA are found in human lymphoblasts and Burkitt's lymphoma cells. Although the DNA extracted from EB virus is linear, the EB DNA molecules found in transformed cells are closed circular duplex DNAs. These circular molecules resemble bacterial episomes; that is, they replicate in step with host-cell DNA without becoming part of it.

### Oncogenic Agents

A number of herpes-type viruses have been shown to be oncogenic agents in frogs, chickens, and monkeys, and herpes simplex and cytomegaloviruses, whose DNA has been damaged by ultraviolet light, have the capacity to transform cells in culture. Most important is the demonstration that EB virus causes lymphomas in monkeys and that EB virus can be recovered from the lymphoma cells of these primates. At present EB virus is the best candidate for a human tumor virus.

EB virus selectively infects and transforms human bone marrow-derived (B) lymphocytes. Its narrow host-cell range may be a consequence of the close association of EB virus receptors with the receptors for the cleaved third component of complement (C3d) on B-lymphocytes. The entire EB genome appears necessary for transformation. All EB transformed cells express an EB-specific nuclear antigen (EBNA). This antigen appears analogous to the T (tumor) antigens induced in the nuclei of animal cells transformed by papovaviruses or by adenoviruses. The vast majority of lymphocytes transformed by EB virus do not produce progeny virions. Viral capsid antigen (VCA) is found in the small proportion of cells that do synthesize infectious virus. These cells are destroyed as a result of the infection.

### Poxviruses

Poxviruses, the largest of all animal viruses, are brick shaped particles roughly 3500 by 2500 Å in size. They contain a single linear molecule of double-stranded DNA of about $1.3 \times 10^8$ molecular weight. Like cellular chromosomal DNA, the two strands of poxvirus DNA are covalently cross-linked at or near the ends of the DNA molecule.

In the virus, the DNA lies within a protein core. Also packed within this core are a DNA-dependent RNA transcriptase, a polyadenylic acid polymerase, a nucleotide phosphohydrolase, and RNA-capping and methylating enzymes. Flanking the core on two sides are protein-containing structures called lateral bodies; their functions are unknown. A lipoprotein envelope containing viral glycoproteins surrounds the entire particle.

Unlike other DNA-containing viruses, poxviruses replicate in the cytoplasm. However, host-cell nuclear functions are required late in the replicative cycle for the formation of infectious virus from immature virions (Fig. 14, *encircled 11*).

Entry of the viral core into the cytoplasm is accomplished by fusion of the viral envelope with the cell surface or by endocytosis of the virus and release of the core from the endocytic vacuole. Both processes have been shown to occur. Once liberated from its lipoprotein envelope and exposed to substrates in the cytoplasm, the core becomes biosynthetically active. Enzymes within the core synthesize and export single-stranded RNA messengers (Fig. 14, *encircled 2*) that direct the synthesis of proteins such as the thymidine kinase, DNA polymerase, and uncoating enzyme; these enzymes are used in subsequent biosynthet-

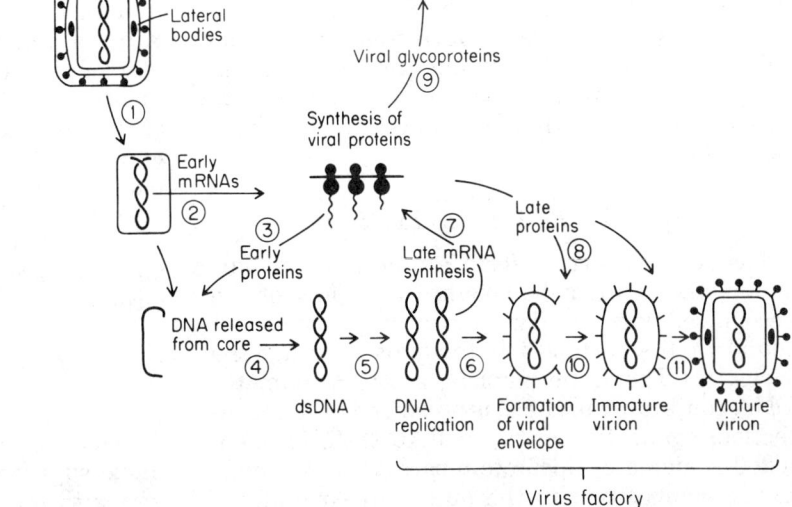

**FIGURE 14.** *Poxvirus replication. Infecting virus is shown at upper left. Progeny virus at lower right. See text for an explanation of the numbered intermediate steps.*

ic steps. Since these proteins are the products of the first RNA transcripts formed by the virus, they are termed "early" proteins.

Uncoating enzyme opens the viral core (Fig. 14, *encircled 4*), thereby releasing poxvirus DNA into the cytoplasmic matrix. Poxvirus DNA replicates semiconservatively; progeny double-stranded DNAs are composed of one parental and one progeny DNA strand. However, the precise mechanisms of DNA duplication and of breakage and synthesis of the bonds that cross-link the two DNA strands are not known.

Viral morphogenesis takes place in factories within the cytoplasm (Fig. 14, *encircled 5, 6, 10, 11*). These factories can be though of as "extranuclear nuclei." That is, viral DNA (Fig. 13, *encircled 5*) and viral messenger RNAs (Fig. 14, *encircled 7*), are synthesized within the factories. The DNA is retained in this location while the messenger RNAs are exported into the surrounding cytoplasm where they direct the synthesis of viral proteins (Fig. 14, *encircled 7 and 8*. Viral proteins return to the factories where they are assembled into virions.

In the factories the newly formed viral envelope appears to engulf a small portion of the matrix of the factory, thereby forming an immature particle (Fig. 14, *encircled 6 and 10*). The DNA-containing core and lateral bodies condense and assemble within these immature particles. Subsequently, other proteins are added to the envelope. Maturation of envelope and internal components completes the replicative cycle (Fig. 14, *encircled 11*). A small number of completed virions are released continuously from the infected cell throughout the replicative cycle. However, the major portion of virions is not released until the cell lyses.

Viral envelope glycoproteins are inserted into the host cell's plasma membrane. These glycoproteins alter the properties of the cell surface so that virus-infected cells fuse with nearby uninfected cells. In this way, poxviruses spread from cell to cell without entering the extracellular compartment. Mutant poxviruses that encode glycoproteins that inhibit cell-cell fusion have been identified.

## HEPATITIS VIRUS TYPE B

Hepatitis B viruses form a unique taxonomic group; they cannot be clasified with any of the recognized viruses. Two types of particles are found in the serum of individuals carrying the virus: (1) The Dane particle, a 420-Å diameter DNA-containing particle, is presumed to be the infectious agent of hepatitis B; (2) Australia antigen, a 200-Å diameter lipoprotein particle that is similar in composition to the outer envelope of the Dane particle. No nucleic acid has been found in Australia antigen, and it is presumed to be noninfectious.

The outer lipoprotein envelope of the Dane particle contains Australia or hepatitis B surface antigen. Within this envelope is core-containing circular DNA of molecular weight $1.6 \times 10^6$. Each DNA molecule is composed of a single-stranded covalently closed circular DNA and a complementary linear DNA strand that is about two-thirds the length of the circular DNA. Thus, the intact molecule is a circle that is double-stranded for two-thirds of its circumference and linear for the remaining one-third.

The Dane particle contains less genetic information than any known DNA or RNA virus. There is presently no cell culture system for in vitro growth of the virus. Thus the number of proteins encoded by the viral genome is not known. Since individuals infected with hepatitis B produce antibodies to Australia antigen, core antigen, and viral DNA polymerase, it is assumed that these proteins are viral gene products. Immunofluorescent studies indicate that the virus replicates in the hepatocyte nucleus.

### Viroids

Viroids are naked pieces of infectious circular single-stranded RNA of defined nucleotide sequence and weighing approximately 120,000 daltons. This is barely enough genetic information to code for a single protein of moderate molecular weight. However, no viroid-encoded protein has yet been found.

Viroids have been identified as the agents of plant diseases whose names range from the mundane (potato tuber spindle disease) to the exotic (Cadang-Cadang, a disease of coconut trees). They have not been identified as the agents of human disease, but they are candidate agents for Kuru, a progressive degenerative neurologic disease of New Guinea cannibals, transmissible dementias such as Creutzfeldt-Jakob disease, and scrapie, a progressive neurologic disease of sheep and goats. All three diseases have been transmitted to primates, and scrapie has been passaged in mice as well. The agents of these diseases appear to be smaller than any known virus and exhibit physical properties that suggest that they are viroids.

### DEFECTIVE INTERFERING PARTICLES

Defective interfering (DI) particles, as their name suggests, are defective viruses that interfere with the replication of their parent viruses.

DI particles contain insufficient genomic information to replicate themselves. In some cases, they contain less nucleic acid than standard virus. DI reo or influenza viruses lack the largest segment of viral RNA, while DI polio, vesicular stomatitis, and papovaviruses contain nucleic acids that are less than unit length. In other cases, DI particles contain gene duplications or segments of host DNA that have been substituted for viral DNA.

DI particles share four essential properties: (1) They are unable to propagate themselves. (2) They multiply only in the presence of a helper virus. (3) They interfere with the replication of homologous standard virus but not with the replication of viruses of another type (vesicular stomatitis DI particles interfere with VSV but not with poliovirus replication). (4) They have the capacity to compete with the standard virus and thereby to enrich their numbers at the expense of standard virus.

DI particles have been identified in stocks of virtually every virus type. They appear in increasing frequency when viruses are repeatedly passaged at high titer.

Persistent infections have been established in cell cultures with mixtures of DI particles and standard virus. Mice inoculated with a mixture of DI and standard vesicular stomatitis viruses develop a slowly progressive paralytic disease, while mice infected with standard vesicular stomatitis virus alone are rapidly killed. Whether DI particles promote chronic or persistent virus infections in man is not known.

DI particles may also provide protection against viral infection. Animals immunized with DI particles are protected against challenge with the homologous standard virus. Some strains of polio vaccine have been shown to contain DI particles.

## CONCLUSION

It is evident that the animal viruses have explored every possible combination of nucleic acids for the transfer of their genetic information. Negative strands encode complementary positive strands, positive strands encode complementary negative strands, and information shuttles back and forth between single and double strands and between RNA and DNA. The viruses have been no less adventurous in exploring cellular pathways for penetration of macromolecules into the cytoplasm, insertion of proteins into membranes, and assembly of complex structures than they have for information transfer. They highlight the major biosynthetic and morphogenetic pathways of eucaryotic cells. Where a pathway exists, a virus has evolved to exploit it.

## References

*General*

Luria, S. E., Darnell, J. E., Jr., Baltimore, D., and Campbell, A.: General Virology. New York, John Wiley and Sons, 1978.
Fraenkel-Conrat, H., and Wagner, R. R.: Comprehensive Virology. Vols. 1–10. New York, Plenum Press.

*Virus Penetration*

Dales, S.: Early events in cell-animal virus interactions. Bacteriol Rev 37:103, 1973.

*Picornaviruses*

Dasgupta, A., Baron, M. H., and Baltimore, D.: Poliovirus replicase. A soluble enzyme able to imitate copying of poliovirus RNA. Proc Natl Acad Sci USA 76:2679, 1979.
Nomoto, A., Kitemmura, N., Golini, F., and Wimmer, E.: The 5′ terminal structures of poliovirion RNA and poliovirus mRNA differ only in the genome-linked protein VPg. Proc Natl Acad Sci USA 74:5345, 1977.

*Oncornaviruses*

Bishop, J. M.: Retroviruses. Ann Rev Biochem 47:35, 1978.
Collett, M. S., and Erickson, R. L.: Protein kinase activity associated with the avian sarcoma virus Src gene product. Proc Natl Acad Sci USA 75:2021, 1978.

*Rhabdoviruses*

Banerjee, A. K., Abraham, G., and Colonno, R. J.: Vesicular stomatitis virus: Mode of transcription. J Gen Virol 34:1, 1977.

*Formation of Membranes of Enveloped Viruses*

Katz, F. N., Rothman, J. E., Knipe, D. M., and Lodish, H. F.: Membrane assembly: Synthesis and intracellular processing of the vesicular stomatitis viral glycoprotein. J Supramol Struct 7:353, 1977.
Blobel, G., and Lingappa, V. R.: Transfer of proteins across intracellular membranes. In Silverstein, S. C. (ed.): Transport of Macromolecules in Cellular Systems. Berlin, Abakon Verlagsgesellschaft, 1978, pp. 289–298.

*Paramyxoviruses*

Scheid, A., and Choppin, P. W.: Two disulfide-linked polypeptide chains consitute the active F protein of paramyxoviruses. Virology 80:54, 1977.

*Myxoviruses*

Palese, P., Plotch, S. J., Bouloy, M., and Krug, R. M.: The genes of influenza virus. Transfer of 5′-terminal cap of globin mRNA to influenza viral complementary RNA during transcription *in vitro*. Proc Natl Acad Sci USA 76:1618, 1979.

*Reoviruses*

Silverstein, S. C., Christman, J. C., and Acs, G.: The reovirus replicative cycle. Ann Rev Biochem 45:375, 1976.
Weiner, H. L., Drayna, D., Averil, D., Jr., and Fields, B. N.: Molecular basis of reovirus virulence: Role of the S1 gene. Proc Natl Acad Sci USA 74:5744, 1978.

*Papova and Adenoviruses*

Nathans, D.: Dissecting the genome of a small tumor virus (SV-40). (The Harvey Lectures, vol. 70.) New York, Academic Press, 1976, pp. 111–157.
Griffin, J. D., Spangler, G., and Livingston, D. M.: Protein kinase activity associated with SV40 T-antigen. Proc Natl Acad Sci USA 76:2610, 1979.

Sussenbach, J. S.: The mechanism of replication of adenovirus DNA. Virology 84:509, 1978.

*Restriction Endonucleases*

Nathans, D., and Smith, H. D.: Restriction endonucleases in the analysis and restructuring of DNA molecules. Ann Rev Biochem 44:273, 1975.

*Gene Splicing*

Abelson, J.: RNA processing and the intervening sequence problem. Ann Rev Biochem 48:1035, 1979.
Crick, F.: Split genes and RNA splicing. Science 204:264, 1979.

*Herpes Viruses*

Jacob, R. J., Morse, L. S., and Roizman, B.: Anatomy of herpes simplex virus DNA. J Virol 29:448, 1979.
Klein, R. J.: Pathogenetic mechanisms of recurrent herpes simplex virus infection. Arch Virol 51:1, 1976.
Henle, W., Henle, G., and Lennette, E. T.: The Epstein-Barr virus. Sci Am 241:48, 1979.

*Poxviruses*

Stern, W., and Dales, S.: Biogenesis of vaccinia. Virology 75:232, 1976.

Esteban, M., Flores, L., and Holowaczak, J. A.: Model for vaccinia virus DNA replication. Virology 83:467, 1977.

*Hepatitis B Virus*

Blumberg, B. S.: Australia antigen and the biology of hepatitis B. Science 197:17, 1977.
Charnay, R., Pourcel, C., Louise, A., Fritsch, A., and Tiollais, P.: Cloning in *E. coli* and physical structure of hepatitis B virion DNA. Proc Natl Acad Sci USA 76:2222, 1979.
Robinson, W. S.: The genome of hepatitis B virus. Ann Rev Microbiol 31:351, 1977.
Summer, J., Smolec, J. M., and Snyder, R.: A virus similar to human hepatitis B virus associated with hepatitis and hepatoma in woodchucks. Proc Natl Acad Sci USA 75:4533, 1978.

*Viroids*

Gajdusek, D. C.: Slow infections with unconventional viruses. (The Harvey Lectures.) New York Academic Press, 1978, pp. 283–353.
Randles, J. W., and Hatta, T.: Circularity of the ribonucleic acids associated with Cadang-Cadang disease. Virology 96:47, 1979.

*Defective Interfering Particle*

Huang, A. S., and Baltimore, D.: Defective Interfering Animal Viruses. New York, Planum Press, 1977, pp. 73–116.

# 10 THE GENETICS OF VIRUSES

## C. R. Pringle, B.Sc., Ph.D

## INTRODUCTION: THE SIGNIFICANCE OF VIRUS GENETICS

The science of virus genetics is concerned with the origin and mechanism of variation of viruses. The variability of viruses and the extent to which it is heritable have great importance for human medicine. The surface antigens of some viruses are inherently stable, and the diseases associated with these infectious agents can be controlled by vaccination (e.g., rubella, measles, rabies) or in exceptional circumstances even eradicated (e.g., smallpox). Other viruses exist as a range of antigenic types (e.g., the enteroviruses and rhinoviruses) or appear to change progressively in response to the development of immunity in their host (e.g., the antigenic drift of influenza virus). Control of these agents by vaccination is more difficult and ultimately may depend on accurate prediction of the potential evolution of the antigens of these viruses. Indeed, the design and development of appropriate influenza virus vaccines in anticipation of epidemics and even pandemics could become one of the principal applications of virus genetics in human medicine.

Viruses that cause diseases characterized by short incubation period, recurrent infection, and aviremia may be difficult to combat by vaccination and may be controllable only by chemotherapy. Suitable antiviral drugs have not been developed yet, and progress towards successful chemotherapy of virus infection depends on clear discrimination of virus-specific processes from those processes that are part of the biosynthetic apparatus of the host cell and essential for the viability of both the virus and its host. The isolation of virus mutants helps to identify these virus-specific processes, defining appropriate targets for pharmacologic attack and allowing a rational approach to antiviral chemotherapy.

Assessment of the oncogenic potential of a virus requires knowledge of the nature of its genome. To be oncogenic, the genome of the virus must exist as DNA at some stage to permit integration of viral information into the genome of the host cell and to produce a heritable change (transformation) in the growth properties of the cell. However, integration by itself does not invariably cause transformation and may not be obligatory in all cases. Determination of what is critical for virus-induced transformation and oncogenesis requires additional analysis of the organization and function of the viral genome.

## THE NATURE AND CODING CAPACITY OF VIRAL GENOMES

The viruses of man and animals exhibit great diversity of genome structure. From a genetic standpoint, viruses fall into three distinct categories: the *DNA-containing viruses*, the *RNA-containing viruses*, and the viruses endowed with reverse transcriptase (the *retroviruses*), whose genome alternates between RNA in the virion and proviral DNA in the host cell.

The DNA viruses, with the exception of the poxviruses, multiply in the nucleus of the host cell, and messenger RNA (mRNA) is transcribed by the host cell transcriptase. Hence, the naked genome of these viruses is infectious. The RNA viruses multiply predominantly in the cytoplasm, and since the host cell is unable to replicate RNA molecules, an RNA polymerase (or the information for its synthesis) must be introduced with the virus. It is an accepted convention to call a single-stranded RNA molecule the positive strand if it functions as the messenger for protein synthesis, and to call its complement the negative strand (or antimessage). The genome of RNA viruses may be represented by a positive or negative strand or both. The genome of positive-strand RNA viruses is infectious because it functions as mRNA for synthesis of the entire complement of viral proteins including the RNA replicase. The genome of negative-strand RNA viruses, on the other hand, is not infectious because it cannot replicate or be translated directly into protein. Consequently, the nucleocapsid of these viruses includes an RNA transcriptase to initiate synthesis of mRNA in the infected cell. The genome of retroviruses functions as mRNA and is therefore the positive strand; however, this RNA is not infectious, and the reverse transcriptase enzyme is a part of the structure of the virion. The proviral DNA form of these viruses is infectious, however.

The diverse nature of the viral genome can be rationalized by regarding the genome as a particular stage in the cycle of replication of nucleic acids sequestered in an extracellular particle. This concept is illustrated in Figure 1. The only

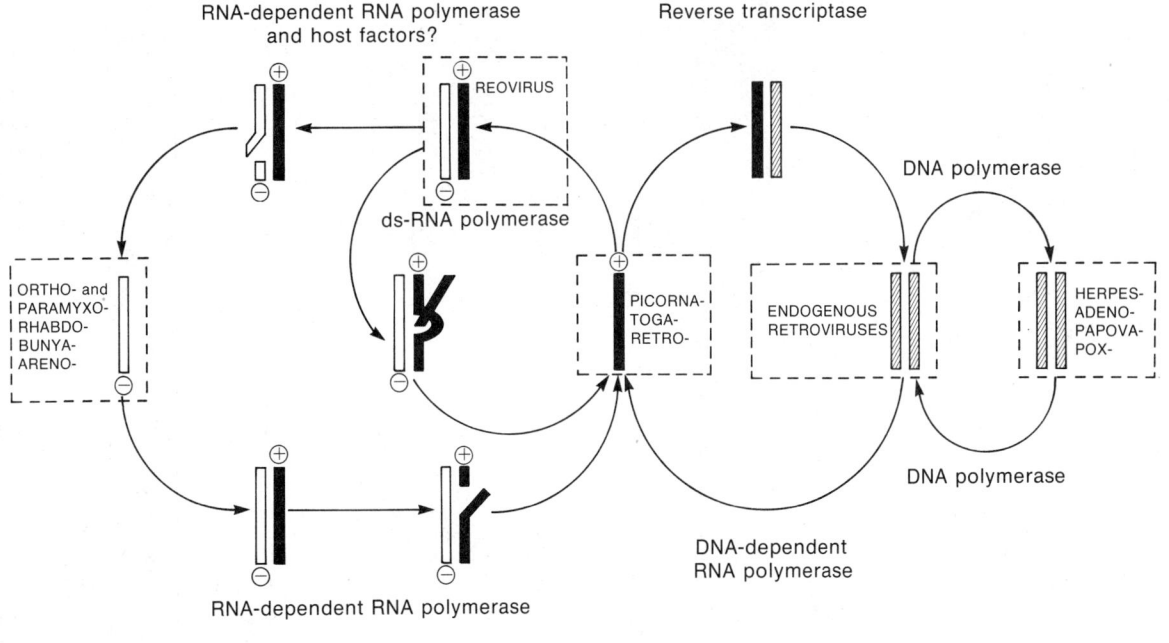

**FIGURE 1.** *Replication of nucleic acid and sequestration of the viral genome.*

*RNA replication follows the five-intermediate model proposed by Spiegelman. Reovirus replication follows a different path because there is no displacement of strands, and the parental duplex RNA is conserved. Positive strands are shown as black; negative strands are shown as white. DNA strands are indicated by cross-hatching. The stages of the nucleic acid replication cycles sequestered in extracellular virus particles are indicated by dashed lines.*

*The segmentation of the genome of some RNA viruses is not considered here, because subdivision of the genome is probably a form of transcriptional control. The single-strand DNA viruses have been omitted for simplicity. The only form among known viruses not represented is the RNA:DNA intermediate in the reverse transcription cycle.*

## TABLE 1. The Physical and Genetic Characteristics of the Genomes of Animal Viruses

| Group[a] | Example | Site of Replication | NUCLEIC ACID | | | | | GENETIC PROPERTIES | | | Special Features |
|---|---|---|---|---|---|---|---|---|---|---|---|
| | | | Type | Strand in Virion | Form | Infectivity | MW × 10⁶ | Relative Coding Capacity[b] | Complementation Groups | Recombination Frequency and Grouping | |
| Parvo | Murine minute | Nucleus | SS-DNA | − | Linear | ? | 1.7 | 3–4 | N.D. | N.D. | Replicates in unison with host; mitosis-dependent |
| | Adeno-associated | Nucleus | SS-DNA | −and+ | Linear | Yes | 1.8 | 3–4 | N.D. | N.D. | Helper and mitosis-dependent. Inverted terminal repeat |
| Papova | SV40 | Nucleus | DS-DNA | +/− | Super-coiled helix | Yes | 3.0 | 3 | 3 (or 5) | Low | Induces host DNA synthesis |
| Adeno | Adeno 5 | Nucleus | DS-DNA | +/− | Linear | Yes | 23.0 | 23 | 12 | Low-high linear map | Inverted terminal repetition. Covalently bonded protein at 5′ terminus |
| Herpes | HSV-2 | Nucleus | DS-DNA | +/− | Linear | Yes | 100.0 | 100 | 18 | Low-high linear map | Terminal and internal inverted repeats |
| Pox | Vaccinia | Cytoplasm | DS-DNA | +/− | Linear | No | 160.0 | 160 | N.D. | Low-high linear map | Cross-linked ends. DNA-dependent RNA polymerase and other virion enzymes |
| Picorna | Polio-1 | Cytoplasm | SS-RNA | + | Linear | Yes | 2.6 | 5 | Nil | Low linear map | One polycistronic message, post-translational cleavage; covalently bonded protein at 5′ terminus |
| Alpha | Sindbis | Cytoplasm | SS-RNA | + | Linear | Yes | 4.0 | 8 | 6 | None | Two polycistronic messages; post-translational cleavage |
| Flavi | Dengue | Cytoplasm | SS-RNA | + | Linear | N.D. | 4.0 | 8 | N.D. | None | Polycistronic (with internal initiation of translation?) |
| Bunya | Snowshoe hare | Cytoplasm | SS-RNA | − | 3 unique subunits | No | 6.4 | 13 | 2 | High 2 groups | Virion RNA-dependent RNA polymerase |
| Areno | Pichinde | Cytoplasm | SS-RNA | − | 3 unique subunits | No | 3.2 | 6 | N.D. | High 2 groups | Virion RNA-dependent RNA polymerase |
| Orthomyxo | Influenza | Cytoplasm (and nucleus?) | SS-RNA | − | 8 unique subunits | No | 5.0 | 10 | N.D. | High 8 groups | Virion RNA-dependent RNA polymerase |
| Paramyxo | Sendai | Cytoplasm | SS-RNA | − | Linear | No | 7.0 | 14 | 7 | None | Virion RNA-dependent RNA polymerase |
| Rhabdo | Vesicular stomatitis | Cytoplasm | SS-RNA | − | Linear | No | 4.0 | 8 | 6 | None | Virion RNA dependent RNA polymerase |
| Diplorna | Reo | Cytoplasm | DS-RNA | +/− | 10 unique subunits | No | 15.0 | 15 | N.D. | High 10 groups | Virion DS-RNA-dependent RNA polymerase |
| Retro | Rous sarcoma | Nucleus and cytoplasm | SS-RNA | + | 2 identical subunits | RNA no DNA Yes | 6.0 | 6 | N.D. | High | Virion RNA-dependent DNA polymerase |

[a] The papilloma, corona, irido, orbi, and metamyxovirus have been omitted because of lack of information.
[b] The number of possible gene products, assuming that an average sized protein contains 500 amino acids.

stage, excluding the replicative intermediates, not represented in known viruses, is the RNA:DNA intermediate in the reverse transcription pathway.

The *information capacity* of the genome is determined by the universal coding assignment of three nucleotides per amino acid. Therefore, 1500 nucleotides (or nucleotide pairs in the case of double-stranded nucleic acid) are required for an average-sized protein of 500 amino acids. The information content of different viruses is indicated in Table 1, together with other characteristics that define the properties of the genome. The genomes of DNA viruses differ by as much as fiftyfold in coding capacity, whereas the RNA viruses vary only within a threefold range (or fourfold if the retroviruses are included). A large proportion of the genome of the large DNA viruses, e.g., herpes simplex virus, is concerned with regulation of DNA synthesis, since nearly half of all *ts* mutants (see Mutation and Mutants) have DNA-negative phenotypes. This is probably reflected in the complex biology of herpes viruses and their tendency to cause latent infection.

These estimates of the information content of the viral genome are minimum values and do not take account of proteolytic cleavage and other modifications of primary gene products. Furthermore, recent analysis of the genome of the small single-stranded DNA bacteriophage ΦX174 has shown that polypeptides of entirely different amino acid sequence can be transcribed from the same polynucleotide by displacement of the triplet reading frame; thus gene E of ΦX174 lies entirely within gene D, and gene B within gene A. Similarly, functionally distinct gene products can be obtained by translation of mRNA from a fixed point with occasional read-through of a specific stop signal resulting in two polypeptides with overlapping sequences (e.g., the A and A' proteins of bacteriophage Qβ). Also, among the mammalian viruses, polyomavirus conserves the coding potential of its genome by utilizing host proteins as structural compounds of the virion (Table 1).

## MUTATION AND MUTANTS

Mutation can be defined as a discontinuous event that results in a change in information content. Virus mutants arise spontaneously or can be induced by chemical or physical agents (mutagens). *Mutagens* that have proven effective with human and animal viruses include base analogues (5-fluorouracil and 5-azacytidine for RNA viruses and 5-bromode oxyuridine for DNA viruses), alkylating agents (ethyl methane sulfonate, among others), intercalating agents (pro-

flavine and NTG), deaminating agents (nitrous acid), hydroxylamine and ionizing irradiation (ultraviolet light). The base analogues are incorporated into the genome, and mutations are produced by miscoding during replication. The other mutagens induce mutation by direct chemical change of the nucleic acid. Frameshift and nonsense (polypeptide chain-terminating) mutants of human or animal viruses have not been unequivocally identified, and most induced mutants appear to be missense mutants in which substitution of an amino acid modifies the functional activity of a gene product.

*Mutants* may have specific phenotypes such as resistance to heat inactivation or an inhibitory drug; for instance, mutants of poliovirus resistant to guanidine hydrochloride have played an important role in mapping the poliovirus genome. In general, however, mutants with specific phenotypes are less useful than conditional lethal mutants, in which a single common phenotype (e.g., inability to multiply at high temperature) is sufficient to provide mutants with lesions in any gene that is indispensable for normal replication. This is because a change in amino acid sequence of any polypeptide can produce a conformational change that affects the stability of a protein at high temperature. *Conditional lethal mutants* of animal viruses are exclusively temperature-sensitive (*ts*) mutants. Host-restricted mutants, analogous to the amber-ochre mutants of prokaryotes, are unknown probably because mammalian cells with the characteristics of the suppressor strains of prokaryotes have not yet been identified.

Extensive changes in polynucleotide sequence of the genome can occur by rearrangement, duplication, and deletion. Spontaneous *deletion mutants* of viruses are common and occur in all virus groups. Particles with defective genomes frequently interfere specifically with the replication of the undeleted genome and are known as DI (defective interfering) particles. It has been suggested that the generation of DI particles is responsible for the self-limitation of many virus diseases by moderating the course of infection until an immune response is developed. Figure 2 illustrates the extent of the deletions observed in DI particles of the rhabdovirus vesicular stomatitis virus (VSV). Deletion mutants can only multiply with the assistance of a helper virus. This complex relationship is exemplified best in the leukemia-sarcoma viruses, in which the mammalian sarcoma viruses lack genetic information for envelope protein (and internal proteins according to the strain), and these viruses are entirely dependent on the "helper" leukemia virus for normal maturation.

The deletion of sequences in DI particles of

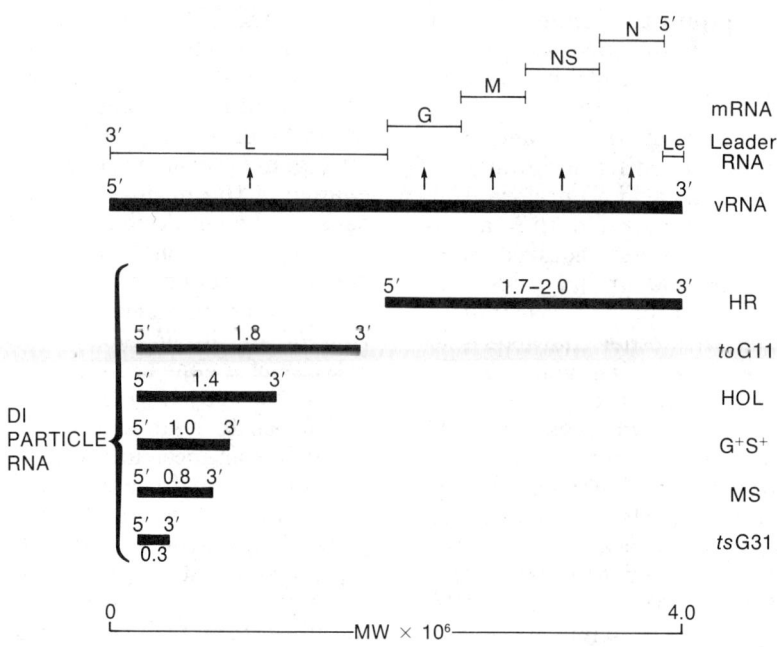

**FIGURE 2.** *Physical maps of DI particle RNA of vesicular stomatitis virus (VSV).*
*The DI particles of VSV are deletion mutants. The physical location of the RNA from six different DI particles (HR, tsG11, HOL, Gts⁺, MS and tsT31) are illustrated. All these DI particles have interfering activity with homotypic virus. The HR DI particle is unique in its ability to interfere heterotypically. It is also the only DI particle that contains complete viral genes.*

papovaviruses, on the other hand, may be accompanied by rearrangements, reiteration of sequences, and substitutions of extraneous host DNA. Indeed, *duplications* and rearrangements are characteristic features of the normal genome of the herpes viruses and presumably have arisen by mutational events during the evolution of these viruses. The location and orientation of the redundant (duplicated) sequences in the herpes simplex virus genome are illustrated in Figure 3. The four forms of the genome are present simultaneously in any population of molecules and are thought to be continually generated by recombinational events within the redundant sequences.

## GENETIC INTERACTIONS BETWEEN VIRUSES

### Recombination in RNA Viruses and Subunit Reassortment

Since informational RNA is unique to viruses, so also is recombination between RNA molecules. The genome of several RNA viruses (influenza, reo, bunya, and arenoviruses) is segmented, and high frequency recombination is a characteristic feature of all these viruses. Recombination occurs by *reassortment* of the subunits of the genome. The mechanism that ensures that the correct complement of subunits is assembled in the mature virion is still unknown. Each of the eight subunits of the influenza virus genome codes for a single protein, and hybrid viruses can be selected from the progeny of mixed infections. For example, if the PR8 and Hong Kong strains are crossed, a recombinant with the Hong Kong hemagglutinin and the PR8 neuraminidase can be selected by exposure to antiPR8 hemagglutinin and anti–Hong Kong neuraminidase sera. The genomic subunits of different strains of influenza virus (and similarly their gene products) have different electrophoretic mobilities in polyacrylamide gel, and by analysis of the subunits present in specific recombinants, it has been possible to map completely the influenza virus genome. The coding assignment of the subunits of the genome of the PR8 and Hong Kong strains, and a recombinant with the hemagglutinin of Hong Kong (HK) and the neuraminidase of PR8 are illustrated in Figure 4. From the relative mobilities of the subunits, it is apparent that only the hemagglutinin subunit has been exchanged in this particular recombinant. In any cross of two influenza viruses, 254 different recombinants (i.e., $[1/2]^8 - 2$) are possible by subunit rearrangement. This particular recombinant was obtained because one of the parents had been irradiated by ultraviolet light, so that most viable progeny viruses would derive all their genomic segments from the unirradiated parent with the exception of the hemagglutinin

A

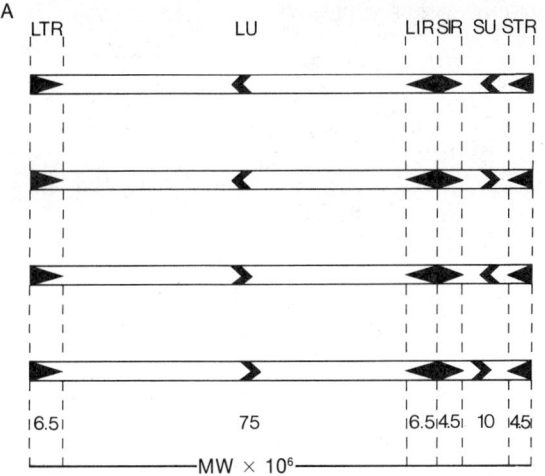

B

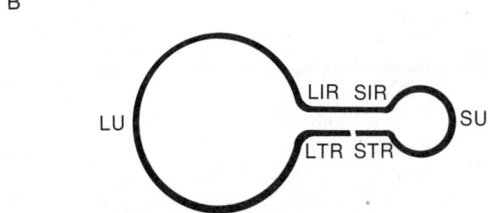

**FIGURE 3.** *The herpes simplex virus genome. A, The four arrangements of the genome of herpes simplex virus. LTR = long terminal repeat; LU = long unique region; LIR = long internal repeat; SIR = short internal repeat; SU = short unique region; STR = short terminal repeat. Inversion of the long and short regions is indicated by arrows and could occur as a result of internal recombination within the redundant sequences. B, The homology of the internal and terminal repeat regions. This double ring structure is observed in electronmicrographs of single-strand DNA following self-annealing.*

*This arrangement of the genome is characteristic for herpes simplex virusesType 1 and Type 2 but not for other members of the herpes group. The least complex herpesvirus genome is that of channel catfish virus, which lacks a short unique region and has no internal redundancy.*

gene, which was selected against by exposure to antiPR8 hemagglutinin.

The retroviruses also exhibit high frequency recombination. However, although the genome exists as two subunits, the mechanism is not independent reassortment because the two components of the genome are identical, and therefore the particles are genetically *diploid*. The subunits of the retrovirus genome are linked by base pairing at their 5′ end as an inverted dimer, and transcription is initiated from primers (tryptophan tRNA in Rous sarcoma virus) located close to the 5′ ends. Synthesis of a complete progeny strand necessitates a jump from the 5′ end of one strand to the 3′ end of the same or the other strand of the dimer. Hence, each round of transcription provides an opportunity for intermolecular recombination, which could account for the high frequency of recombination.

Recombination has not been detected in any negative-strand RNA virus with an unsegmented genome, but it does occur at low frequency with at least some positive-strand RNA viruses (see Table 1). *Genetic maps* of poliovirus and foot-and-mouth disease virus (FMDV) have been constructed from crosses of *ts* mutants. In both cases, the mutants were oriented relative to the locus for resistance to the inhibitor guanidine and then arranged in a linear order on the basis of the recombination frequencies observed in crosses of pairs of mutants. The genetic map of poliovirus is illustrated in Figure 5. Analysis of the properties of the constituent *ts* mutants defines the different coding regions. The organization of the genome of FMDV is probably similar to that of poliovirus, but the gene order in other RNA viruses differs from the picornavirus pattern. For example, in Sindbis virus and VSV the coat protein genes are located centrally or towards but not at the 5′ end. These differences probably reflect different modes of transcription and translation. In fact, the genome of picornaviruses is polycistronic and not partitioned into genes, since the entire genome is translated directly into a single giant polypeptide, which is subsequently cleaved into smaller polypeptides, which are the functional gene products. *Post-translation cleavage* is probably a feature of all positive-strand viruses, because in eukaryotic cells, initiation of translation occurs at only a single site in all mRNA. (A recent study of Kunjin virus suggests, however, that the flavi-

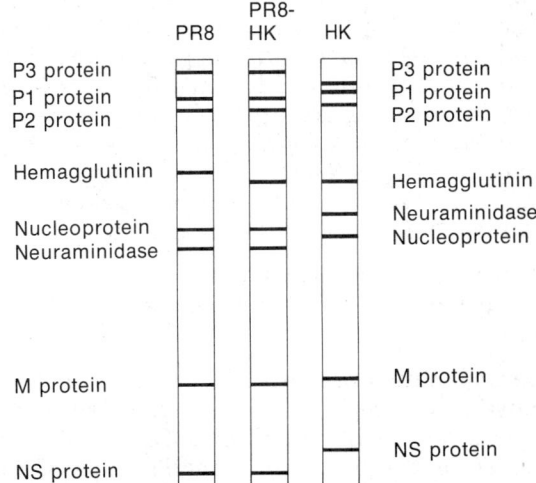

**FIGURE 4.** *The influenza virus genome.*

*The eight subunits of the influenza virus genome can be separated by polyacrylamide gel electrophoresis. The relative mobilities of the RNA subunits of the PR8 (A/PR/8/34) and HK(A/HK/8/68) strains of influenza virus, and the assignments of gene function are illustrated in the left and right tracks, respectively. The center track is a recombinant clone, and it can be seen by inspection that it contains the hemagglutinin gene of the HK strain together with seven subunits from the PR8 strain.*

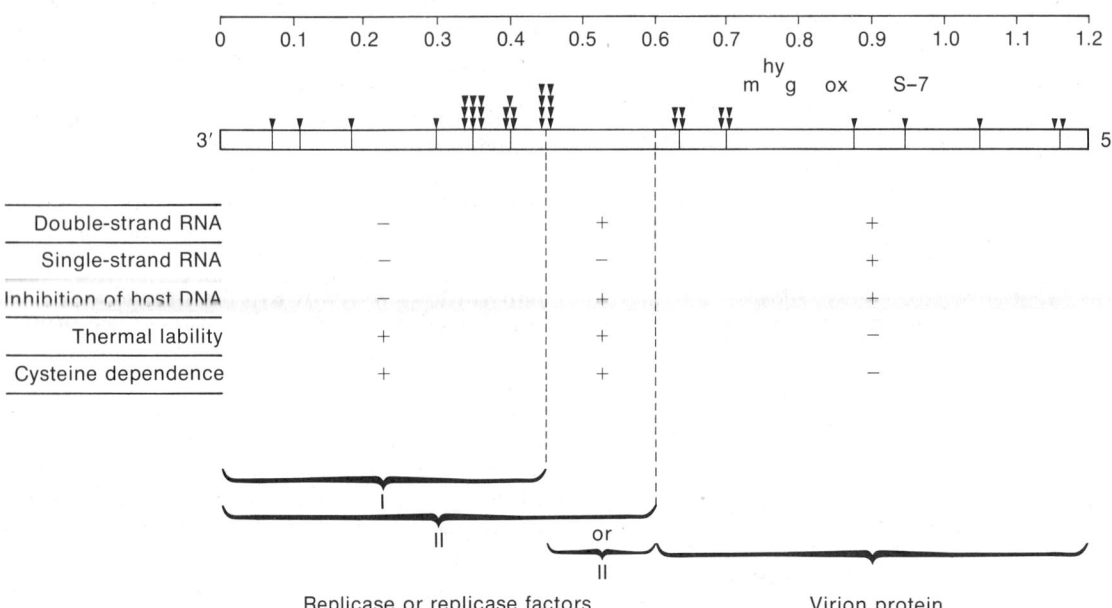

**FIGURE 5.** *The picornavirus genome.*

*Recombination map of 39 ts mutants of poliovirus Type 1 and the assignment of gene function. The symbol indicates the map position of a ts mutant. Identification of gene function is summarized in the lower part of the figure. The loci of four inhibitors of multiplication all fall within the coat protein region. The inhibitors are guanidine (g), dextran sulfate (m), and derivatives of hydantoin (hy), oxadiazole (ox), and pyrimidine carboxylate (S–7).*

*The genetic map of foot-and-mouth disease virus, an unrelated picornavirus, closely resembles that of poliovirus. Thirty-five mutants have been arranged in a linear sequence extending over 0.7 map units. Again, the locus of the guanidine inhibitor falls in the presumptive coat protein region.*

viruses may prove exceptions to this generalization.)

The gene order of avian sarcoma virus has been established by a combination of genetic and physical methods to be the following: 5'-*gag-pol-env-src*-3', in which *gag* is the gene for the precursor of the internal proteins, *pol* is the gene for viral polymerase, *env* is the gene for the surface glycoproteins, and *src* is the sarcomagenic sequence. In avian leukemia viruses, the *src* gene is deleted.

### Recombination in DNA Viruses and Correlation of Physical and Genetic Maps

Recombination between DNA viruses does not require any exceptional mechanisms, since the enzymes capable of recombining DNA molecules preexist in the host cell. Genetic maps of the genomes of polyomavirus, SV40 virus, adenovirus, and herpes simplex virus have been derived from crosses of *ts* mutants and correlated with physical maps of the genome. In adenovirus, for example, the *physical mapping* of cross-over events was achieved by isolating recombinants between *ts* mutants of two serologically distinct strains of adenovirus, whose DNA differed in

their pattern of cleavage by restriction endonucleases. (Restriction endonucleases are bacterial enzymes that recognize particular nucleotide sequences in double-stranded DNA and cleave specific phosphodiester bonds within these sites to produce unique DNA fragments that can be separated by electrophoresis in polyacrylamide gel). Since the genome of the recombinant contains sequences from each parent, the position of the cross-over event can be determined by comparison of the types of DNA fragment produced. The location of mutants to particular regions of DNA can also be determined by *marker rescue* experiments in which *ts* mutant-infected cells are coinfected with individual fragments of the DNA of wild-type virus obtained by restriction endonuclease treatment. The genetic and physical maps of the genome of adenovirus and the two papovaviruses, SV40 and polyoma, have been aligned by these methods, and mapping of the more complex herpes simplex virus is progressing rapidly. Genetic mapping is an important step towards the goal of defining the specific features of viral biosynthesis. Analysis of the properties of the different mutants locates the regions of the molecule that code for particular proteins. Figure

6 illustrates the alignment of the genetic and physical maps of adenovirus. Perhaps one of the most significant features of this map is that the viral genes that are responsible for transformation of the growth properties of cells are confined to one region of the molecule (the 5' end).

### Hybrid Viruses

Genetic recombination between two completely unrelated DNA viruses can occur in certain special circumstances. Adenovirus Type 7 has been adapted to grow in nonpermissive monkey-kidney cells by serial passage. This modified adenovirus was found to induce SV40-type tumors in hamsters, however, and it was evident that the adaptation was due to the "helper" effect of contaminating SV40 virus. Attempts to eliminate the SV40 component by antiserum treatment led instead to isolation of a true hybrid of adenovirus and SV40, in which 10 per cent of the adenovirus genome had been deleted and replaced by 75 per cent of the SV40 genome. The hybrid was defective and only able to replicate in the presence of "helper" adenovirus, presumably because essential genes had been deleted. The inserted fragment of the SV40 genome included the early region (with a small repetition) and part of the late region, and consequently the hybrid virus expressed SV40 T-antigen in infected cells and induced SV40-type tumors in hamsters. *Defective adenovirus Type 2-SV40 hybrids* have been isolated that have up to one half of the adenovirus genome deleted and more than one genome equivalent of SV40 inserted.

*Nondefective adenovirus Type 2-SV40 hybrids* have also been isolated with 4.5 to 7.1 per cent of the adenovirus genome deleted and substituted by 7 to 59 per cent of the SV40 genome. Again, it is the early region of the SV40 genome that is inserted. Evidently the region of the adenovirus genome between map positions 0.79 and 0.86 (see Fig. 6), where all the deletions occur, is not essential for replication. The generation of these nondefective hybrids was a unique event, since it has not been possible to produce this hybrid again. Nevertheless, it illustrates that under rare circumstances DNA viruses at least have the potential to acquire genes from other DNA viruses, and how a nononcogenic virus might become oncogenic.

## NONGENETIC INTERACTIONS

### Complementation and Genetic Analysis in the Absence of Recombination

When cells are simultaneously infected by two *ts* mutants and incubated at high temperature, an enhanced yield may result if the mutations are in different viral genes. This is because the normal gene product of one virus compensates for the defective gene product of the other virus and vice versa. This phenomenon is termed *complementation*. Complementation defines the functional units of the genome and involves interaction of gene products only. Progeny virus produced by complementation retains the *ts* phenotype of the parents. In some cases, complementation may be unidirectional or even result in a depressed yield if a defective protein is produced in excess and incorporated into the majority of virions. The operational distinction of complementation and recombination is illustrated in Figure 7. Mutants can be grouped according to their ability to complement other mutants, and the number of complementation groups gives a minimum estimate of the number of genes in the genome of any virus (Table 1). In addition, complementation facili-

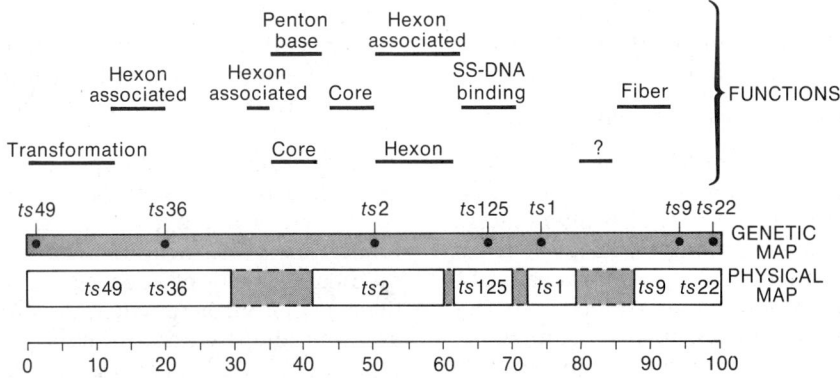

**FIGURE 6.**  *The adenovirus genome.*
*The genetic map of seven* ts *mutants of adenovirus Type 5 obtained by crosses of* ts *mutants is compared with the location of the same seven mutants obtained by physical mapping where fragments of adenovirus DNA generated by restriction endonuclease treatment are used to rescue* ts *mutants. There is no discrepancy between the two maps. The presumptive gene functions of the various regions are also illustrated.*

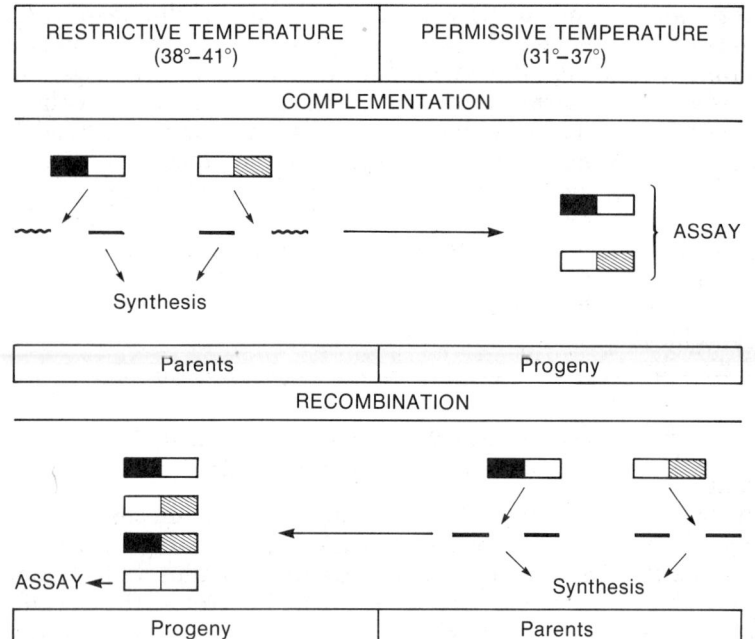

**FIGURE 7.** *The operational distinction between complementation and recombination using temperature-sensitive mutants.*

*In complementation the mixed infection is conducted at restrictive temperature, and the yield is assayed at permissive temperature. The progeny are temperature-sensitive like the parents. In recombination the mixed infection is conducted at permissive temperature, and the yield is assayed at restrictive temperature. Thus, only one of the recombinants (the nonmutant) is assayed, since the parents and the double mutant recombinant are restricted.* ☐ *= normal gene;* ■ *= independent;* ▨ *= ts mutants;* —— *= normal gene product;* ⋁⋀ *= defective gene product.*

tates analysis of the organization of the genome of viruses (such as the unsegmented negative-strand RNA viruses) that do not undergo recombination. The example of the rhabdovirus VSV illustrates the value of this approach. Five proteins are present in the virion of VSV, and no other virus-specified proteins have been detected in infected cells. The existence of six groups of complementing mutants points to the existence of another VSV protein, as yet undetected. Further study of the properties of *ts* mutants may lead to identification of this putative VSV protein and its function. So far four of the complementation groups of VSV Indiana have been correlated with viral proteins. Identification of gene functions in this way has confirmed that the RNA-dependent RNA polymerases of negative-strand viruses and the RNA-dependent DNA polymerase (reverse transcriptase) of retroviruses are virus-specified enzymes.

### Phenotypic Mixing and Pseudotypes

Two different viruses multiplying in the same cell may produce progeny with the phenotypic characteristics of both parents. This phenomenon is particularly evident among enveloped viruses that mature by budding from membranes, but it is also prevalent among nonenveloped viruses. For instance, influenza virus can acquire antigens from serologically related strains and also from quite unrelated parainfluenza viruses and rhabdoviruses. The majority of phenotypically mixed particles contain antigens from both parents and can be neutralized by antisera to both viruses. A minority may be entirely invested by the envelope of the heterologous virus. This can have important epidemiologic consequences, since it would allow a virus to survive and persist in an apparently immune population.

The defective avian and mammalian sarcoma viruses exist only as *pseudotypes*, i.e., as phenotypically mixed particles whose envelope proteins are donated by the nondefective helper leukemia virus. Pseudotypes are also produced when cytolytic viruses (VSV is often used experimentally) multiply in cells chronically infected with oncornaviruses (the oncogenic retroviruses). Virions with the envelope antigens of avian leukosis virus and the nucleocapsid of VSV, designated VSV (ALV), and the reciprocal pseudotype ALV (VSV), have been identified among the progeny following VSV infection of chick embryo cells carrying avian leukosis virus. Pseudotype formation is also known to occur between DNA viruses (herpes simplex) and RNA viruses (VSV).

Production of pseudotypes of VSV can be used as a sensitive probe for detection of cryptic RNA tumor virus agents, as an aid in the study of membranes and host restriction, or as a rapid method of assay of such agents as mouse mammary tumor virus in which the alternative in vivo assay is lengthy and difficult. However, pseudotypes of the ALV (VSV) type constitute a potential biohazard. The leukemogenic and sarcoma genic viruses of animals are characteristically host-restricted, and envelopment in a membrane provided by an unrestricted virus like VSV could enable the oncogenic virus to reach cells that are normally inaccessible, with unpredictable consequences.

Phenotypic mixing is not confined to envelope proteins. The $\alpha$ mutants of Rous sarcoma virus, for example, have part of the polymerase gene deleted (as well as the entire envelope gene), and they can only be propagated in the presence of a helper virus that contributes the polymerase and envelope functions.

### Host-Induced Modification

Host-induced modification, i.e., nonheritable phenotypic variation, can occur in certain circumstances. The lipid and the carbohydrate portions of the glycolipids and glycoproteins of the viral envelope are contributed by the host cell and therefore vary according to the cell of origin. For instance, the glycoproteins of arthropod-borne viruses released from insect cells lack sialic acid, while the same virus propagated in mammalian cells may possess sialic acid. However, in general this variability does not appear to have important biologic consequences.

## DETERMINATION OF VIRULENCE, DISEASE POTENTIAL, AND ONCOGENICITY

The factors that determine the pathogenic potential of viruses can be defined by study of the effects of mutations in specific genes. For instance, study of temperature-sensitive mutants of reovirus revealed that mutation in a late function of the viral genome resulted in a change of disease pattern. Wild-type reovirus is lethal for newborn rats, whereas *ts* mutants exhibit greatly reduced virulence. In the case of one mutant (*ts* B1), although the majority of animals survived infection with high doses of virus, later in life progressive neurologic disease developed, which culminated in death. The assembly of the outer capsid is defective in *ts* B1-infected cells, and it was proposed that intracellular accumulation of viral nucleocapsid is responsible for the altered disease pattern.

Mutations affecting *neurovirulence* have been described frequently. One mutant of measles virus is less neurovirulent than wild-type measles in suckling hamsters. Hydrocephalus, a response to infection normally masked by the dominant neurologic signs, is a consequence of infection with this mutant. On the other hand, *ts* mutants of VSV often exhibit enhanced neurovirulence for newborn hamsters. However, there is no specific association of neurovirulence with a particular gene. The alteration in disease pattern is related more to the increased survival time of infected animals.

The virulence of avian influenza (fowl plague) virus appears to be influenced by many factors; so far no one gene has been implicated as a major determinant of virulence, and probably the same is true for human influenza virus. However, the virulence of the avian parainfluenza virus (Newcastle disease virus) for chickens is dependent on extracellular cleavage of an envelope glycoprotein (the F or fusion protein). Mutation affecting the sensitivity of this protein to proteolytic cleavage influences host range in vitro and virulence in vivo. Furthermore, there are known mutants of a murine parainfluenza virus that differ in the sensitivity of the F protein to cleavage by specific proteases and, as a consequence, their ability to infect different cells.

The role of viruses in *oncogenesis* can also be approached by study of the properties of mutants. Transformation defective (*td*) mutants of Rous sarcoma virus occur spontaneously and are predominantly deletion mutants in which part or all of the sarcoma determinant (the *src* gene) is missing. These mutants are still oncogenic, however, because they retain the ability to induce leukosis. The genome of *td* deletion mutants and the naturally occurring avian leukosis viruses are similar in size. The *src* gene sequences of different avian sarcoma viruses are homologous, indicating that they have been conserved in evolution. *Src* sequences can be detected also in the normal cells of several avian species, including Japanese quail (which has no inducible endogenous retrovirus). The prevalence of these *src*-related sequences suggests that the *src* gene of avian sarcoma viruses, which is a function not required for virus multiplication, was acquired from the cell at some time in the past.

The origin of the *src* gene in mammalian sarcoma viruses is more complex. The Harvey and Kirsten strains of murine sarcoma virus appear to have acquired rat genome sequences and transforming ability during passage in rats. The Moloney strain of murine sarcoma virus, on the other hand, acquired transforming ability during passage in mice, and there is no sequence homology between the *src* gene of the Moloney virus and the *src* genes of the Harvey or Kirsten viruses.

Almost all *ts* mutants of avian sarcoma virus that affect transformation are late mutants. Temperature-shift experiments with *ts* mutants have shown that transformation is dependent on the continuous activity of a viral gene. However, the nature of the *src* gene product is still unknown.

Cells transformed by SV40 virus carry viral

DNA sequences integrated into their chromosomes. All or only part of the SV40 genome may be present. Study of cells transformed by *ts* mutants of SV40 virus showed that expression of an early gene function of SV40 only was necessary for initiation and maintenance of the transformed state. However, there seems to be no single chromosomal site of integration of SV40 (in rat cells at least), and the number of insertions of the SV40 genome or its early genes is variable in different cell lines.

Similarly, the isolation of *ts* mutants of adenovirus that failed to transform rodent cells at nonpermissive temperature showed that a viral gene product was required at least for initiation of transformation by adenovirus. These mutants map at one end of the adenovirus genome, and only those fragments of the adenovirus genome obtained by restriction endonuclease digestion that contain the left-hand end are able to transform cells; no more than 8 per cent of the genome is required to cause transformation.

## EVOLUTION IN ACTION

Human influenza A virus undergoes dramatic changes in its surface antigens (*antigenic shift*) at intervals, causing severe pandemics. Between pandemics, the virus is constantly changing in a more progressive manner (*antigenic drift*). The available evidence supports the hypothesis that antigenic drift occurs by accumulation of small mutational changes, whereas antigenic shift is the result of hybridization between a human influenza and a virus maintained in a reservoir species. The pandemic of 1918 was caused by a strain that may have acquired an antigenically novel hemagglutinin by recombination with a swine influenza virus. Reconstruction experiments in animals have confirmed that hybridization between different influenza virus strains can occur in vivo. For example, reciprocal recombinants of swine influenza and fowl plague virus (FPV) have been obtained from pigs, despite the inability of FPV to multiply efficiently in this host animal.

The history of the introduction of *myxomatosis* into Australia illustrates that evolutionary changes may occur in both the virus and its host. Myxomavirus was extremely lethal for European rabbits when it was liberated in Australia in 1950 as a pest control measure: mortality rates were in excess of 99 per cent. However, attenuated variants soon made their appearance and within 3 to 4 years they became dominant, because reduced virulence favored survival of animals from one season to the next and allowed a susceptible population to be reestablished each year. Following appearance of the initial attenuated variants, there was a corresponding increase in the genetic resistance of the host animal, so that the mortality induced by a standard virulent strain fell from over 90 per cent to 25 per cent in 5 years. Thus, a milder disease and stable endemicity were evolved by changes in the disease potential of the virus and the genetic resistance of the host animals. It is possible that similar factors have had a similar influence in the evolution of endemic virus disease in man.

## References

*The Nature and Coding Capacity of Viral Genomes*

Baltimore, D.: Expression of animal virus genomes. Bacteriol Rev 35:235, 1971.
Watson, J. D.: Molecular Biology of the Gene, 2nd ed. New York and Amsterdam, W. A. Benjamin Inc., 1970.
Weisbeek, P. J., Borrias, W. E., Langeveld, S. A., Baas, P. D., and van Arkel, G. A.: Bacteriophage ΦX174: gene A overlaps gene B. Proc Natl Acad Sci USA 74:2504, 1977.

*Mutation and Mutants*

Fenner, F.: Conditional lethal mutants of animal viruses. Curr Topics Microbiol Immunol 48:1, 1969.
Fraenkel-Conrat, H., and Wagner, R. R.(eds.): Comprehensive Virology, Vol. 9: Regulation and Genetics, The Genetics of Animal Viruses. New York and London, Plenum Press, 1977.
Huang, A. S., and Baltimore, D.: Defective viral particles and viral disease processes. Nature (London) 226:325, 1973.
Pringle, C. R.: Conditional lethal mutants of vesicular stomatitis virus. Curr Topics Microbiol Immunol 68:85, 1975.

*Genetic Interactions Between Viruses*

Fenner, F., McAuslan, B. R., Mims, C. A., Sambrook, J., and White, D. O.: The Biology of Animal Viruses, 2nd ed. New York and London, Academic Press, 1974.
Kelly, T. J., Jr., and Nathans, D.: The genome of simian virus 40. Adv Virus Res 21:86, 1977.
Palese, P.: The genes of influenza virus. Cell 10:1, 1977.
Tooze, J. (ed.): The Molecular Biology of Tumour Viruses. Cold Spring Harbor Laboratory, 1973.
Westway, E. G.: Strategy of the flavivirus genome; evidence for multiple internal initiation of translation of proteins specified by Kunjin virus in mammalian cells. Virology 80:320, 1977.
Williams, J., Grodzicker, T., Sharp, P., and Sambrook, J.: Adenovirus recombination: physical mapping of cross-over events. Cell 4:113, 1975.

*Nongenetic Interactions*

Fields, B. N.: Genetic manipulation of reovirus — a model for modification of disease? N Engl J Med 287:1026, 1972.
Stehelin, D., Guntaka, R. C., Varmus, H. E., and Bishop, J. M.: Purification of DNA complementary to nucleotide sequences required for neoplastic transformation of fibroblasts by avian sarcoma viruses. J Mol Biol 101:349, 1976.

*Determination of Virulence, Disease Potential, and Oncogenicity*

Fenner, F., and Ratcliffe, F. N.: Myxomatosis. London and New York, Cambridge University Press, 1965.
Kilbourne, E. D. (ed.): The Influenza Viruses and Influenza. New York, Academic Press, 1975.

# PERSISTENT VIRAL INFECTIONS 11

*Julius S. Youngner, Sc.D.*

The attention of medical virologists has been focused primarily on acute febrile diseases. Acute infections, such as influenza, smallpox, and measles, have incubation periods of days to weeks, well-defined symptoms, and closely associated pathologic manifestations. In individuals who recover from acute viral infections, both cellular and humoral mechanisms operate during the incubation period and the virus usually disappears from the body within several weeks after the first symptoms appear. The period in which virus can be isolated from clinical specimens is very limited; in most cases virus is demonstrable only briefly before and after the onset of clinical disease. In virus infections, such as poliomyelitis and mumps, the pattern of acute disease and recovery is often more difficult to study, since the infection may be subclinical and produce no clear-ly recognizable or characteristic symptomatology.

Increasing attention is being devoted to persistent viral infections in which the infectious agent is present for long periods of time. Infections of this type are diverse and difficult to classify with precision. A great variety of viruses, patterns of pathogenesis, and clinical entities contribute to the complexity of this group of infections (Table 1).

## CLASSIFICATION OF PERSISTENT VIRAL INFECTIONS IN HUMANS AND ANIMALS

Persistent viral infections can be classified into three general categories: (1) latent infections, (2)

**TABLE 1. Persistent Viral Infections of Humans**

| VIRUS Genome | CLASSIFICATION Group | AGENT | DISEASE | VIRUS PRESENCE* | MECHANISM OF PATHOGENESIS† |
|---|---|---|---|---|---|
| DNA | Herpesvirus | Herpes simplex virus (Types 1 and 2) | Herpes | Latent | Cytolysis |
| | | Varicella-Zoster virus | Zoster | Latent | Cytolysis |
| | | Cytomegalovirus | Cytomegalo-inclusion disease | Latent | Cytolysis |
| | | | Mononucleosis | Latent | Transformation |
| | | EB virus | Mononucleosis | Latent | Transformation |
| | | | Lymphoma | Latent | Transformation |
| DNA | Papovavirus | JC virus | Progressive multifocal leuko-encephalopathy (PML) | Minimal | Cytolysis |
| | | BK virus | ? | Latent | ? |
| | | Human papilloma virus | Warts | Overt | Transformation |
| DNA | Adenovirus | Adenovirus (many types) | ? | Latent | ? |
| DNA | Unclassified | Hepatitis B virus | Hepatitis | Overt | Immunopathology(?) |
| ? | | Non A/B hepatitis virus | Hepatitis | Overt | Immunopathology(?) |
| RNA | Paramyxovirus | Measles | Subacute sclerosing panencephalitis (SSPE) | Minimal | Cytolysis |
| RNA | Togavirus | Rubella | Fetal anomalies | Overt | Inhibition of cell division(?) |
| | | | Panencephalitis | | Cytolysis(?) |
| ? | ? | Creutzfeldt-Jakob agent | Spongiform encephalopathy | Overt | Cytolysis |
| | | Kuru agent | Spongiform encephalopathy | Overt | Cytolysis |

*Latent = infective virus cannot be demonstrated, except during active or recrudescent symptoms of disease.
 Minimal = infective virus difficult to demonstrate; may be absent or present in exceedingly small numbers.
 Overt = infective virus usually demonstrable with or without presence of symptoms.

†Cytolysis = lesions result from cell destruction by virus.
 Transformation = lesions due to cell proliferative response to infection in the absence of cytolysis.
 Immunopathology = lesions due to specific virus antigen-antibody complex reactions in affected tissues.

chronic infections, and (3) slow infections (Fenner and White, 1976).

### Latent Infections

In this type of persistence, the virus disappears after acute primary disease and reappears during recurrences of disease. There may be one or more such recurrences after long intervals. The best understood diseases in this class are caused by members of the herpesvirus group, herpes simplex, and varicella-zoster viruses.

The most common manifestations of herpes simplex is a recurrent vesicular eruption ("cold sores"), which appears most commonly at the mucocutaneous junctions around the lips or nostrils. These eruptions progress to pustules and crust formation and then disappear. The virus remains latent in the sensory cells of the trigeminal nerve ganglion between attacks (Stevens, 1975). The mechanism that is responsible for reactivation of virus is not fully understood. Nonspecific stimuli, such as respiratory infection, fever, or sunlight cause the virus to spread from the trigeminal ganglion via the sensory nerves to the areas of the skin supplied by the nerves. The relapses of herpes simplex occur despite the presence of circulating antibody in patients with recurring disease. The virus probably passes directly from cell to cell without release; this protects the virus from exposure to antibody in the body fluids.

A similar pattern of latency is seen in herpes zoster, a disease due to reactivation of virus latent in dorsal root or cranial nerve ganglia, many years after childhood varicella. In herpes zoster, which mainly affects adults, painful vesicles erupt in an area of skin supplied by a sensory nerve fiber from a single dorsal root. Most commonly affected are the thoracic nerves; less frequently the ophthalmic nerve of the trigeminal ganglion may be involved.

Disseminated infection with cytomegalovirus, a ubiquitous member of the herpesvirus group, is seen when immunosuppressive therapy, neoplasms, or other debilitating diseases lower resistance of the patient. Reactivation of latent cytomegalovirus is frequently seen in renal transplant recipients; these reactivations are often not associated with any overt signs or symptoms of disease. The site of latency of cytomegalovirus is not clearly established. In some cases, cytomegalovirus infection may be transmitted during the transfusion of large volumes of fresh blood, and reflects the widespread occurrence of healthy carriers of cytomegalovirus.

### Chronic Infections

Persistent infections in this class have a common characteristic: virus is always demonstrable and often is shed. Disease symptoms may be absent or associated with immunopathologic manifestations. A good example of chronic human infection is hepatitis B, a disease associated with varying degrees of hepatic necrosis, and usually contracted by transmission of virus in blood from a chronic carrier (Committee on Viral Hepatitis, 1975). A large amount of a virus-associated antigen (HB-Ag) is commonly present in the serum. This antigen usually disappears rapidly after an acute clinical or subclinical infection. However, in about 5 per cent of infected individuals, HB-Ag may persist in serum in high concentration for years. Although the concentration of infective virus is lower than the HB-Ag, sera from such carriers are highly infectious for recipients of blood transfusion, staff of renal dialysis units, and drug addicts who use unsterilized syringes.

Sera from patients acutely or chronically ill with hepatitis B infection contain antigen-antibody complexes that may play a role in the pathogenesis of acute and chronic hepatic disease. In addition, there is evidence that the glomerulonephritis and polyarteritis nodosa seen in some HB-Ag carriers may be caused by antigen-antibody complexes.

Another example of a chronic infection in humans is the rubella syndrome seen in infants infected in utero with rubella virus during the first 16 weeks of pregnancy. Such infants have various disorders and defects due to generalized infection with rubella virus, and it is usually possible to isolate virus from almost any of their organs. Maternal antibody may inhibit the spread of virus but does not eliminate virus-producing cells. These cells divide at a slower rate than normal uninfected cells, probably giving rise to some of the developmental abnormalities common in infants with rubella syndrome.

### Slow Infections

Diseases in this group have many of the characteristics of the chronic infections described in the previous section. However, they differ from chronic infections in several important characteristics. Slow infections have very long incubation periods ranging from months to years; the disease has a long, chronic, and progressive course, and the outcome is usually fatal (Kimberlin, 1976).

The viruses that cause slow infections are heterogeneous. Nononcogenic retroviruses cause visna, maedi, and progressive pneumonia, which are slowly progressive infections of sheep. Another group of agents is poorly defined and difficult to isolate and assay — namely, the agents that produce subacute spongiform encephalopathies in sheep (scrapie), in mink (mink encephalopathy), and in humans (kuru and Creutzfeldt-Jakob disease). The agents of these diseases resemble viruses in that they pass filters with small pore diameters and can be transmitted to experimental animals. The resistance of these agents to irradiation, chemicals, and heat, and the failure of the agents to elicit a detectable antibody response in infected hosts indicate that they are not typical viruses. A third group of agents is made up of conventional viruses that produce slow, degenerative diseases of the central nervous system in humans: subacute sclerosing panencephalitis (measles and rubella viruses) and progressive multifocal leukoencephalopathy (JC virus, a papovavirus). Table 2 summarizes the characteristics of slow virus infections of humans.

*Spongiform Encephalopathies.* Kuru was the first chronic degenerative disease of the central nervous system of humans proved to have a viral etiology. This disease occurred only among a group of about 50,000 highland New Guineans. The classic studies of Gajdusek (1977) revealed that the kuru agent was spread by ritualistic cannibalism and had an incubation period of from four to 20 years. The incidence of the disease has declined since the early 1960s, when the practice of cannibalism was discouraged. All attempts to cultivate the agent of kuru in cell cultures have been unsuccessful. However, transmission experiments have shown that intracerebral inoculation of brain tissue from kuru victims into chimpanzees and monkeys causes the animals to develop symptoms of kuru after an incubation period of about two years.

The importance of the studies of kuru has been illuminated by the demonstration that a rare, progressive, fatal neurologic disease of humans, Creutzfeldt-Jacob disease, is due to an agent with many of the characteristics of the kuru virus. Creutzfeldt-Jakob disease is characterized by presenile dementia with symptoms due to lesions in the cerebral cortex (status spongiosus) and lesions in the spinal cord. The disease is reproduced in chimpanzees and other monkeys by intracere-bral inoculation of brain tissue from victims of the disease; the incubation period in experimental animals is about one year. The natural route of infection is not known, but the disease has been accidentally transmitted via a cornea graft (Duffy et al., 1974). Transmission has also been reported via electrodes used for electroencephalography from a patient with the disease to other patients in whom the electrodes were subsequently implanted (Bernoulli et al., 1977).

*Subacute Sclerosing Panencephalitis (SSPE).* This severe chronic neurologic disease is seen in children and young adults several years after primary, and usually uncomplicated, measles (ter Meulen et al., 1972). Affected children have high titers of measles antibody in their serum and spinal fluid. The earliest signs of illness are personality and behavioral changes with intellectual impairment. The disease progresses to convulsions, myoclonal spasms, and increasing neurologic deterioration leading to coma and death. At postmortem there is electron microscopic evidence of measles virus infection, but measles virus cannot be recovered directly. Only by cocultivation of brain tissue with permissive indicator cells can infective measles virus be recovered. Despite the presence of high levels of specific antibody in serum and cerebrospinal fluid, the progress of the disease is not arrested. The factors involved in determining the occurrence of this slow complication of measles in rare individuals are not known. Chronic infection with rubella virus infrequently produces a progressive neurologic disease resembling SSPE (Weil et al., 1975).

*Progressive Multifocal Leukoencephalopathy (PML).* This is a rare disease that occurs only in patients whose immunologic responsiveness has been severely compromised by such preexisting conditions as leukemia, reticulosis, or immunosuppressive therapy. There are varied neurologic signs, such as dementia, incoordination, and impaired vision; the disease is usually fatal in three or four months. On autopsy, multiple foci of demyelination are found in the cerebral hemi-

**TABLE 2.  Slow Virus Infections of Humans**

| DISEASE | SITE | PATHOLOGY | VIRUSES |
|---|---|---|---|
| Kuru | Brain | Spongiform encephalopathy, especially in cerebellum | Filterable agent transmissible to chimpanzees and monkeys |
| Creutzfeldt-Jakob disease | Brain and spinal cord | Spongiform encephalopathy | Filterable agent transmissible to chimpanzees and monkeys |
| Subacute sclerosing panencephalitis (SSPE) | Brain | Neuronal degeneration | Measles and rubella viruses |
| Progressive multifocal leukoencephalopathy (PML) | Brain | Multiple foci of demyelination in cerebral hemispheres and cerebellum | Human papovavirus (JC virus) |

spheres and cerebellum; the brain stem and basal ganglia may also be affected. Most cases are due to a papovavirus (JC virus) but some are caused by a virus almost identical to SV40, another papovavirus. These viruses can be grown in human fetal glial cell cultures. Another serotype of papovavirus (BK virus) has been recovered from the urine and genitourinary tract of patients undergoing immunosuppression to prevent rejection of transplanted kidneys. BK virus has not yet been associated with any specific clinical disease (Padgett and Walker, 1976).

Infections with both JC and BK viruses appear to be widespread, since serologic surveys show that many people have antibody to these agents. However, the type of disease caused by primary infection with these viruses during childhood or early adolescence has not been identified. The site of viral latency in the body before reactivation is also not known.

In spite of the increased understanding of the etiology of the slow virus diseases described above, the causes of the most important demyelinating diseases of the central nervous system — that is, multiple sclerosis, the common presenile dementias, and Parkinson's disease — are all still obscure. In the case of multiple sclerosis, common viruses such as measles and parainfluenza type 1 have been suggested as the causative agent in the recent past. However, these associations have so far not stood up to thorough and critical investigation.

## PERSISTENT VIRAL INFECTION AT THE CELLULAR LEVEL

The complexities involved in studying persistent infections in humans and the difficulties in establishing model systems in animals have led to intensive efforts to use cell culture models of persistent viral infection. Infection of permissive cells with lytic viruses in culture usually leads to productive infection, the release of large numbers of progeny viruses, and cell death. However, many animal viruses that are considered to be highly cytocidal can establish infections of cell cultures that result in long-term multiplication of the virus while at the same time the cells continue to grow and divide. These stable virus-host cell relationships can be classified into several general categories.

### Cell Culture Models of Persistent Viral Infections

The classification that follows is oversimplified because, in many systems, cells may be protected by several mechanisms that may function simultaneously or sequentially. Despite these complexities, the following classification is useful in understanding the model systems that have been established in cell cultures (Walker, 1968). The salient characteristics of these model systems are summarized in Table 3.

*Class I. Carrier State in Genetically Resistant Cells.* In this type of infection a majority of the cells is genetically resistant. However, permissive (susceptible) cells continually appear and these cells, when infected by free virus in the medium, permit a normal cycle of virus replication and the release of progeny. Characteristically, viral specific antibody or other antiviral factors, such as interferon, are not required to maintain the stable carrier state. Only a small proportion of the cells is infected; when persistently infected cells are cloned, infected cells are destroyed and the clones obtained are free of virus. The clearest examples of this type of carrier culture are infections of a human cell line (HeLa) by poliovirus and Coxsackie virus, members of the picornavirus group.

*Class II. Carrier State in Permissive Cells Protected by Antibody in the Medium.* In this type of carrier culture only a small fraction of the genetically susceptible cells is infected; most cells are protected from infection by the presence of antiviral factors, usually antibody, in the me-

TABLE 3.  Classification of Persistently Infected Carrier Cultures

| Class of Carrier Culture | Antiviral Antibody Required | All or Most Cells Infected | Infected Cells Can Divide and Form Colonies | Infection Cured by Antiviral Antibody | Interfering Factors Produced in Medium |
|---|---|---|---|---|---|
| I. Genetically resistant cells | No | No | No | Yes | Yes or No |
| II. Permissive cells protected by antibody in medium | Yes | No | No | Yes | Yes or No |
| III. Permissive cells protected by interference or interferon | No | No | No | Yes | Yes |
| IV. Regulated infections | No | Yes | Yes | No | Yes or No |
| V. Virus DNA integrated into the host cell genome | No | Yes | Yes | No | No |

dium. Removal of the antibody from the medium results in the spread of the infection and destruction of the cell culture. Infected cells do not divide and grow into colonies except in the presence of antibody in the medium. In the absence of antibody, the cell clones obtained are virus-free. The best documented example of this type of carrier state is the persistent infection of various human cell lines by herpes simplex virus.

*Class III. Carrier Cultures of Permissive Cells Protected by Interference or Interferon.* The general characteristics of this class of persistently infected cells are the following: only a small fraction of the cell population is infected at any time; infected cells do not divide and cannot be cloned; cell clones, when obtained, are free of virus; endogenously produced interfering factors are always present in the culture medium; therefore, antibody or other antiviral factors do not have to be provided for establishment or maintenance of the carrier state. The relative importance of different endogenously produced interfering factors, such as defective-interfering virus particles and interferon, will be considered below.

An outstanding feature of cultures of this type is that the cells are resistant to superinfection by the carried virus or by heterologous viruses, even though only a small fraction of the cells is infected and producing virus at any given time. However, when the infections are cured by prolonged exposure to antibody, the cured cells are just as susceptible to the homologous and heterologous viruses as the original cell line, indicating that genetically resistant cells do not arise during the carrier phase. There are many examples of Class III carrier cultures involving paramyxoviruses and togaviruses.

*Class IV. Carrier Cultures in Which the Infections Are "Regulated."* The first three classes of persistently infected cells that were described above have important common characteristics. Only a small fraction of the cell population is infected at any given time, infected cells do not divide and grow into colonies but are killed by virus, and clones of cells that are obtained form the carrier culture are free of virus. In contrast, the "regulated" infections of Class IV have the following properties: (1) a high proportion, sometimes all, of the cells in the culture are infected; (2) infected cells can divide and grow into clones that consist of infected cells; (3) antibody or other antiviral factors are not required to establish or maintain the persistently infected state and the culture is not cured of virus by the addition of antibody to the medium; (4) although carrier cultures of this type are fully resistant to superinfection by the homologous virus, they exhibit no resistance to unrelated viruses.

Little is known about the mechanisms by which the "regulated" infections prevent the virus from going through the usual replicative events and cell destruction characteristic of cytocidal infections. The designation "regulated" infection seems appropriate because there seems to be some sort of intracellular regulation or control not yet understood. A large variety of enveloped, budding, RNA viruses can establish this type of persistence — for example, the paramyxoviruses (mumps, measles, parainfluenza viruses 1 and 3, Sendai), rubella, and rabies viruses.

*Class V. Carrier State Due to Virus DNA Integration into the Host Cell Genome.* Another model for persistent infections involves the integration of the viral genome into the DNA genome of the host cell, an event that would permit the long-term maintenance of viral genetic information in infected cells. There is strong evidence in cell culture systems that persistence by some members of the papovavirus, adenovirus, and herpesvirus groups is maintained by this mechanism. However, in most instances rigorous proof is lacking that genomes of these DNA viruses are integrated into the host cell chromosome in humans or animals. Even in cell culture models, the mechanisms by which the viral genomes are regulated and the phenomena associated with activation are mostly unknown.

There is convincing evidence that visna virus, an RNA C-type retrovirus, which causes a persistent inflammatory demyelinating disease of the central nervous system of sheep, replicates via a DNA intermediate that is integrated into the host cell genome (Haase, 1977). The reverse transcriptase present in the visna virion is responsible for the transcription of a DNA copy of the RNA genome, and it is this DNA intermediate that is inserted into the host DNA.

The possibility has been raised that some enveloped cytolytic RNA viruses, such as paramyxoviruses and togaviruses, which do not contain reverse transcriptase, have the choice of alternate pathways of nucleic acid synthesis and can employ an integrated DNA intermediate for maintaining long-term persistence in infected cells. This mechanism, which is yet to be proved, will be considered in more detail below.

### Virus-Specific Factors That May Be Involved in the Establishment and Maintenance of Persistent Infections

*Mechanisms of Persistence of DNA Viruses.* Herpes simplex, varicella-zoster, and cytomegaloviruses, all members of the herpes-virus group, probably establish persistence in which the virus remains latent; the DNA genomes are present as cytoplasmic or nuclear plasmid forms in either a completely regulated or a nonreplicating state. Also likely is the possibility that in some instances a less tightly controlled, very slowly replicating state may be involved. In either case there is no a priori need to postulate integration as a means of perpetuating the infection.

In regard to the papovaviruses, the best-studied example is SV40, a virus of simian origin that is related to human papovavirus (JC virus) associated with progressive multifocal leukoencephalopathy. SV40 virus maintains a latent state in cell cultures by integration of the viral DNA into the host genome; such cells may contain up to 10 copies of SV40 DNA per cell (Doerfler, 1975). In the case of human papilloma virus, a papovavirus that causes warts, the mechanism by which the viral DNA persists is not yet known.

There is strong circumstantial evidence that persistence of adenovirus in certain cell systems is maintained by the integration of the viral genome into the host cell DNA (Doerfler, 1975). There is, however, no rigorous proof of this mechanism, and the manner in which adenoviruses persist in adenoids and tonsils of humans is unknown. Also unknown is the mechanisms of persistence of the SV40-related viruses, JC and BK, which are isolated from patients with progressive multifocal leukoencephalopathy or from immunosuppressed patients shedding these viruses in their urine.

The only definitive information concerning integration of viral DNA of herpesviruses comes from studies of the Epstein-Barr (EB) virus that is associated with infectious mononucleosis, Burkitt's lymphoma, and nasopharyngeal carcinoma (Klein, 1973). There is evidence that both in lymphoblastoid cell lines and in the tumors, the EB virus DNA is maintained in two physical states; a linear form integrated into cellular DNA, and a circular, extrachromosomal plasmid.

In summary, although there is some understanding of the state of the viral DNA in cell culture systems latently infected with some papovaviruses (except papilloma virus), adenoviruses, and EB virus, there is little definitive information concerning other herpesviruses. With the exception of EB virus, little is known about the mechanisms of DNA virus latency in man or animals. The mechanism by which the viral genomes are controlled and regulated during latent infection, and more particularly, the phenomena associated with reactivation are, at this time, poorly understood.

*Mechanisms of Persistence of RNA Viruses.* A number of different mechanisms, which are not necessarily mutually exclusive, have been proposed to explain the persistence of ordinarily cytolytic RNA viruses in cell cultures. Although there is some evidence that these mechanisms may oper-

ate in animal models, there is no direct support at this time for their involvement in human disease (Rima and Martin, 1976).

ROLE OF DEFECTIVE-INTERFERING (DI) PARTICLES. Evidence is accumulating that defective particles capable of interfering with the replication of homologous standard virus occur spontaneously in almost every virus system that has been studied (Huang, 1973). Serial passage of viruses at high multiplicities of infection (high virus per cell ratios in the inoculum) results in the production of DI particles that have the following general characteristics: (1) they contain normal structural capsid proteins; (2) a portion of the viral genome is missing (in reality they are deletion mutants); (3) they can replicate only in cells coinfected with the homologous virus helper; and (4) they can interfere specifically with the replication of homologous standard virus.

It has been postulated that the production of DI particles may regulate the synthesis of virus in persistent infections by specifically inhibiting production of the homologous standard virus, thereby damping down infection (Huang and Baltimore, 1970). There is some evidence that this concept is plausible even for a highly cytolytic virus. When vesicular stomatitis virus (VSV), a rhabdovirus, is passaged serially at high multiplicity in susceptible Chinese hamster ovary cells, and the relative concentrations of standard VSV and DI particles are determined at each passage, there is a cyclical overlapping pattern of production of complete virus and production of DI particles. This pattern, based on serial high multiplicity passages, serves as a theoretical model for persistent infection.

Evidence concerning the possible role of DI particles in persistent infection is provided by a model system involving a line of hamster cells (BHK-21) persistently infected with VSV (Holland and Villarreal, 1974). A mixture of infective standard virus and large numbers of DI particles is required to establish the initial persistent infection. During the course of the infection, more DI particles are generated.

Synthesis of DI particles has been implicated in maintenance of measles virus persistence in human cell lines, and in cultured cells persistently infected with such diverse viruses as reovirus, rabies, several togaviruses, and lymphocytic choriomeningitis virus. The precise relationship of DI particles to autointerference and to persistence is not well understood. Although it is evident that DI particles play an important role in many carrier cell cultures, much more work is needed to prove a role for DI particles in persistent infections in animals and humans.

ROLE OF TEMPERATURE-SENSITIVE (TS) MUTANTS. A body of information has accumulated that shows that viruses recovered from persistent infections often differ in biologic properties from the standard virus used to initiate the infection. Quite commonly, when compared to wild-type viruses, the agents recovered from persistently infected cells produce smaller plaques in cell cultures and are less able to infect experimental animals. In many model systems, there is a natural selection of ts mutants* that replace the standard virus population during the evolution of the persistently infected state (Preble and Youngner, 1975). Such ts viruses occur in a variety of host cells persistently infected with agents such as mumps, measles, rubella, Sendai, Newcastle disease, Sindbis, Western equine encephalomyelitis, and vesicular stomatitis viruses. Selection of ts mutants in persistent infections is not limited to any particular class of virus or type of cultured cell. In fact, one report (Valentine et al., 1969) describes a commonly occurring spontaneous ts mutant of bacteriophage Qβ that causes a persistent infection of its bacterial host, *Escherichia coli.*

The reasons why ts mutants are selected under conditions of persistent infection are not fully understood, but the following is known. In the cases of such viruses as VSV, Newcastle disease virus, and Sindbis, ts mutants interfere strongly with the replication of standard virus at both permissive and nonpermissive temperatures, interference occurring before or at the level of RNA transcription. Second, ts mutants of VSV are rescued by standard virus at nonpermissive temperatures; in effect, ts mutants act as conditionally defective interfering (DI) viruses at the nonpermissive temperature. As a result, the replication of ts virus tends to be dominant at the nonpermissive or partially restrictive temperature, thereby explaining why ts mutants are selected. Also, since under these conditions ts mutants tend to be less cytocidal and the replication of standard virus is suppressed, an explanation is provided of why ts mutants tend to be elected and why this selection leads to the maintenance of persistent infections.

Despite these observations, the presence of multiple genetic alterations in viruses isolated from persistently infected cells mandates caution in attributing to any one defect a key role in the establishment and maintenance of a persistent infection. Any genetic alteration that converts a lytic virus-cell interaction to a noncytocidal one has the potential to cause a persistent infection.

There is much evidence that ts mutation plays a role in the establishment and maintenance of many persistent infections in cell cultures. However, in animals and humans the relationship of these observations to persistence is not yet established.

ROLE FOR DEFECTS IN HOST CONTRIBUTIONS TO VIRUS REPLICATION. It is likely that increasing evidence will appear dealing with the importance of defects or alterations in virus assembly and release in persistent infections, particularly those involving enveloped viruses. The yield of these viruses from persistently infected cells is often less than in cytocidal infections, and frequently no infective virus is produced. Several mechanisms could operate in such a system.

Specific protein cleavages, especially of viral envelope glycoproteins, are important steps in virus maturation (Scheid and Choppin, 1976). In some paramyxoviruses, cleavage is accomplished by a host enzyme and activates virus activities such as cell fusion, hemolysis, and viral penetration of host cells. The host range and tissue tropisms in large measure depend on the presence in host tissue of the appropriate activating protease. Since virus mutants have been isolated in the laboratory that require different proteases for activation, the possibility exists that infection of a tissue not normally susceptible to a given virus may result from the appearance of a mutant that can be activated by a protease present in that tissue. In addition, infection by a cytocidal virus of a cell that cannot cleave the progeny viral glycoprotein could result in persistent infection without the production infective virus. If proper cleavage reactions fail in paramyxoviruses, mature but noninfective virus is produced, whereas failure of cleavage in togaviruses prevents virus assembly. It is possible that specific proteolysis of viral proteins by host enzymes is important in many persistent infections.

POSSIBLE ROLE OF INTEGRATED VIRAL GENOMES. DNA copies of RNA virus genomes are integrated into chromosomes of cells persistently infected by tumorigenic retroviruses and by visna virus, a retrovirus that causes persistent central nervous system disease in sheep. There have been several reports that DNA copies of usually cytocidal single-stranded RNA viruses have been integrated into the genome of persistently infected host cells (Simpson and Iinuma, 1975; Zhdanov, 1975). The viruses involved include respiratory syncytial virus, SV5, measles, Sindbis, and tickborne encephalitis virus. A mechanism proposing an integrated DNA intermediate of usually cytolytic RNA viruses raises questions concerning (1) the source of the RNA-dependent DNA polymerase

---

*Temperature-sensitive (ts) conditional lethal mutants have been described for many different viruses (Fenner, 1969). These ts viruses occur in low frequency spontaneously and in higher frequency after exposing standard virus to mutagens. Ts viruses replicate well at low temperatures (31 to 33° C) and poorly at higher temperatures (38 to 40° C); in contrast, standard wild-type viruses replicate almost equally as well at both permissive and nonpermissive (restrictive) temperatures.

that initially transcribes the RNA of the infecting virus into a DNA copy, (2) the nature of the integration of this DNA copy into the host cell DNA, and (3) the regulation of the expression of the integrated DNA copy of the viral RNA. Some workers have not found DNA intermediates in cells persistently infected with several cytolytic RNA viruses (Haase et al., 1977). The implications and potential of this mechanism are so important that the original observations concerning integrated DNA copies of RNA virus genomes should be confirmed.

There is abundant evidence, however, that a DNA integration mechanism is not necessary for persistence of RNA viruses. In many instances the viral genome persists as RNA, replicates independently of the host cell genome, and passes from one daughter cell to another for generations, with viral products demonstrable at any stage.

OTHER MECHANISMS. The intact animal probably has more mechanisms for establishing and maintaining persistent infections than cultured cells possess. Both nonspecific resistance factors (fever; interferon production) and specific immunity complicate the situation. Much more information is needed to understand the mechanisms by which virus-infected cells are eliminated in the body. The role of antibody modulation of viral antigens from the cell surface in persistent infection in the animal must also be clarified (Joseph and Oldstone, 1975).

## References

Bernoulii, C., Siegfried, J., Baumgartner, G., Regli, F., Rabinowtiz, T., Gajdusek, D. C., and Gibbs, C. J.: Danger of accidental person-to-person transmission of Creutzfeldt-Jakob disease by surgery. Lancet 1:478, 1977.

Committee on Viral Hepatitis: Symposium on Viral Hepatitis. Am J Med Sci 270:2, 1975.

Doerfler, W.: Integration of viral DNA into the host genome. Curr Top Microbiol Immunol 71:1, 1975.

Duffy, P., Wolf, J., Collins, G., De Voe, A. G., Streeten, B., and Cowen,

D.: Possible person-to-person transmission of Creutzfeldt-Jakob disease. N Engl J Med 290:692,1974.

Fenner, F.: Conditional lethal mutants of animal viruses. Curr Top Microbiol Immunol 48:1, 1969.

Fenner, F., and White, D. O.: Medical Virology, 2nd ed. New York, Academic Press, Inc., 1976.

Gajdusek, D. C.: Unconventional viruses and the origin and disappearance of kuru. Science 197:943, 1977.

Haase, A. T., Stowring, L., Ventura, P., Traynor, B., Johnson, K., Swoveland, P., Smith, M., Britten-Darnall, M., Faras, A., and Morayan, O.: Role of DNA intermediates in persistent infections caused by RNA viruses. In Schlessinger, D. (ed.): Microbiology— 1977, Washington, American Society for Microbiology, 1977, p. 478.

Holland, J. J., and Villarreal, L. P.: Persistent noncytocidal vesicular stomatitis virus infections mediated by defective T particles that suppress virion transcriptase. Proc Natl Acad Sci USA 71:2956, 1974.

Huang, A. S.: Defective interfering viruses. Ann Rev Microbiol 27:101, 1973.

Huang, A. S., and Baltimore, D.: Defective viral particles and viral disease processes. Nature 226:325, 1970.

Joseph, B. S., and Oldstone, M. B. A.: Immunologic injury in measles virus infection. II. Suppression of immune injury through antigenic modulation. J Exp Med 142:864, 1975.

Kimberlin, R. H. (ed.): Slow virus diseases of animals and man. Frontiers in Biology. Amsterdam, North-Holland Publishing Co., 1976.

Klein, G.: The Epstein-Barr virus. In Kaplan, A. S. (ed.): The herpesviruses. New York, Academic Press, 1973, p. 521.

Padgett, B. L., and Walker, D. L.: New human papovaviruses. Prog Med Virol 22:1, 1976.

Preble, O. T., and Youngner, J. S.: Temperature-sensitive viruses and the etiology of chronic and inapparent infections. J. Infect Dis 131:467, 1975.

Rima, B. K., and Martin, S. J.: Persistent infection of tissue culture cells by RNA viruses. Med Microbiol Immunol 162:89, 1976.

Scheid, A., and Choppin, P: Protease activation mutants of Sendai virus. Activation of biologic properties by specific proteases. Virology 69:265, 1976.

Simpson, R. W., and Iinuma, M.: Recovery of infectious proviral DNA from mammalian cells infected with respiration syncytial virus. Proc Natl Acad Sci USA 72:3230, 1975.

Stevens, J. G.: Latent herpes simplex virus and the nervous system. Curr Top Microbiol Immunol. 70:31, 1975.

ter Meulen, V., Katz, M., and Müller, D.: Subacute sclerosing panencephalitis: a review. Curr Top Immunol 57:1, 1972.

Valentine, R. C., Ward, R., and Strand, M.: The replication cycle of RNA bacteriophages. Adv Virus Res 15:1, 1969.

Walker, D. L.: Persistent viral infection in cell cultures. In Sanders, M., and Lennette, E. H. (eds.) Medical and Applied Virology. St. Louis, Missouri, Warren H. Green, Inc., 1968, p. 99

Weil, M. L., Itabashi, H. H., Cremer, N. E., Oshers, L. S., Lennette, E. H., and Carnay, L.: Chronic progressive panencephalitis due to rubella virus simulating subacute sclerosing panencephalitis. N Engl J Med 19:994, 1975.

Zhdanov, V. M.: Integration of viral genomes. Nature 256:471, 1975.

# 12 INTERFERON AND INTERFERENCE

## Monto Ho, M.D.

The story of interferon illustrates how an obscure phenomenon originally of interest only to laboratory scientists can become important for the whole field of biomedical and clinical sciences (Finter,

1973; Ho and Armstrong, 1975; Metz, 1975). In the 1930s and 1940s, virologists were already familiar with "viral interference." They found that, for example, if virus A was injected into an experimental animal at the same time or shortly before virus B, the replication of virus B would be inhibited. Virus A, the "interfering virus," frequently interfered even if it was inactivated or made noninfectious by heat or ultraviolet irradiation. No satisfactory explanation for this phenomenon was provided until 1957 when Isaacs and Lindenmann did a classic experiment, described in Figure 1.

The experiment formed the basis of a simple but important discovery. This was that viruses can induce in cells an antiviral substance, interferon, which in turn inhibited the replication of the challenge virus. In many ways, interferon is an ideal antiviral substance. It is relatively nontoxic, and it is broadly effective against a large number of RNA and DNA viruses. Further, since interferon is produced by cells under "natural" conditions of viral infections in animals, it was thought that a novel antiviral defense system was discovered.

## INDUCTION AND INDUCERS

Interferon is a cellular protein. In this respect it is like hormones, enzymes, antibodies, and other cellular proteins. Such proteins are usually made by specialized cells, but as far as we know all cells can make interferon if given the appropriate stimulus ("induced"). The interferon-making capacity of cells is ordinarily not expressed; it is "repressed." It is widely believed that when cells are "induced" to make interferon, this capacity is "derepressed." However, there is a curious aspect of "derepression" of interferon production. Usually in induced or derepressed protein synthesis, the presence of the inducer or derepressor guarantees continued production. In the case of interferon production, it is a "one-shot affair" no matter how much inducer is applied or for how long the inducer is present, as shown in Figure 2 (Finter, 1973).

This suggests that another regulatory mechan-

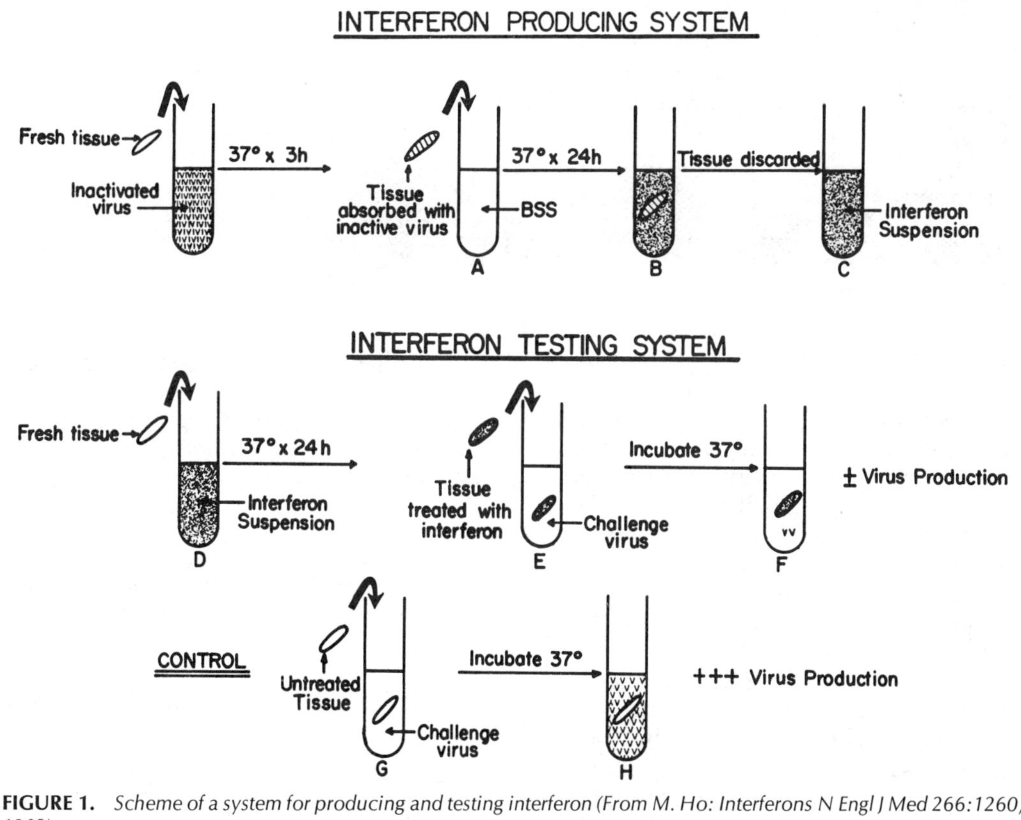

**FIGURE 1.** *Scheme of a system for producing and testing interferon (From M. Ho: Interferons N Engl J Med 266:1260, 1962).*

*Fragments of chick chorioallantoic tissue are bathed in a suspension of inactivated Type A influenza virus (interfering virus). The tissue absorbed with the inactivated virus was incubated for 24 hours (A, B). A substance called "interferon" was released (C). Its presence was demonstrated in the "Interferon Testing System." Fresh tissue fragments are treated in the suspension containing interferon (D). The treated tissue (E) along with untreated controls (G) is inoculated with a "challenge virus." Virus production in treated and control tissue is measured. The degree of reduction in (F) as compared with (H) represents the potency of interferon. This testing system is still the conceptual basis for all methods of interferon assay.*

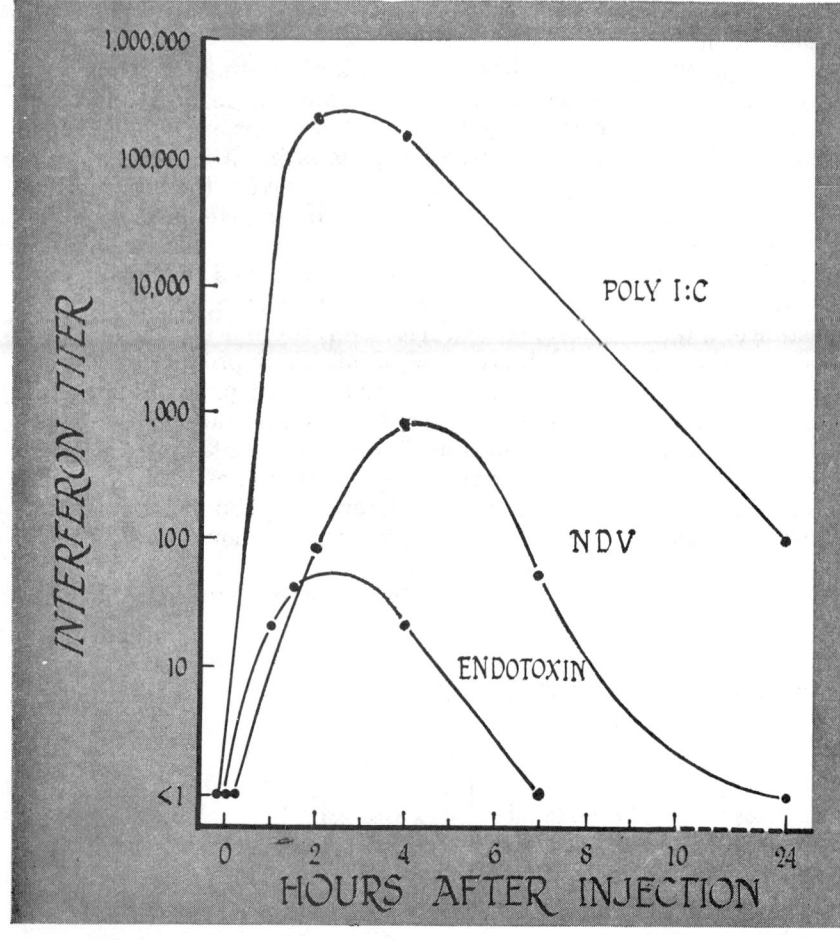

**FIGURE 2.** *The appearance of interferon in the serum of a rabbit after injection of E. coli lipopolysaccharide (endotoxin), Newcastle disease virus (NDV), or a complexed synthetic double-stranded ribonucleic acid, polyriboinosinic-polyribocytidylic acid (poly I:C). Note the marked variation in the effectiveness of these three inducers, and that maximum interferon levels are only transiently maintained. (From Ho, M.: Factors influencing the interferon response. Arch Int Med 126:136, 1970.)*

ism in cells that inhibits interferon synthesis is triggered off by the inducer. Cells in culture as well as animals cannot respond to an interferon inducer for varying intervals after being induced. This "hyporeactive" or "refractory" period varies from hours to days. In animals it may be as long as one week and is a serious deterrent to repeated administrations of inducers to achieve steady interferon concentrations in tissues.

There are many substances that induce interferon. They are classified in Table 1 (Ho and Armstrong, 1975). Two types of interferon production may be distinguished. Type 1 follows stimulation with specific, known inducers. These inducers are divided into two classes, A and B.

Class A inducers are good inducers that induce the production of 1000 units/ml or more of interferon in cell culture or in the bloodstream of animals. They contain double-stranded RNA, or may form such RNA in the course of cell infection. Newcastle disease virus and poly I:C (see Fig. 2) are examples.

Class B inducers are moderate to poor inducers that may act only when injected in animals. They

are a motley group of macromolecular substances often without effect in fibroblast or epithelial cell cultures. Some are microorganisms that infect intracellularly. It is assumed that uptake by macrophages is necessary in induction by many of

**TABLE 1.   Types of Interferon Production and Inducers**

I. Type I Interferon Production: Stimulated by Inducers
   A. Class A Inducers (good inducers, double-stranded RNA):
      1. RNA animal viruses
      2. DNA animal viruses
      3. Plant, insect fungus and bacterial viruses
      4. Natural and synthetic double-stranded RNA's
   B. Class B Inducers (moderate to poor inducers):
      1. Intracellular organisms (bacteria, rickettsia, protozoa)
      2. Bacterial products (lipopolysaccharides, polysaccharides)
      3. Polymers (polycarboxylic, polysulfates, polyphosphates)
      4. Low molecular weight substances (tilorone, cycloheximide, etc.)

II. Type II Interferon Production: Specific and Nonspecific Immune Induction
   A. Immune Specific Induction
   B. Nonspecific Stimulation of T or B Lymphocytes by Mitogens

these substances. Some members of this class may eventually relate to class A inducers or to Type II production.

Type II is the production of interferon by specific and nonspecific immunologic activation of lymphocytes and macrophages. Although this important phenomenon produces only moderate amounts of interferon, it may be an effector limb of cell-mediated immunity.

During immune specific induction, interferon is produced by sensitized lymphocytes upon exposure to specific antigen. The sensitizing antigen may be a viral antigen, or nonviral antigens such as PPD, diphtheria, or tetanus toxoid. Immune induction may occur in vitro or in the animal. A most effective method is to stimulate circulating interferon in mice infected with BCG by an intravenous injection of BCG or PPD.

Interferon is also produced when lymphocytes are stimulated by nonspecific mitogens such as phytohemagglutinin, pokeweed antigen, and concanavalin A. The responding lymphocyte is the one specifically stimulated by the mitogen.

## PROPERTIES OF INTERFERON

Interferon is a heterogeneous class of proteins with unique biologic properties. Biochemically it is still inadequately characterized.

Its definitive biologic effect is its ability to inhibit intracellular replication of viruses. In addition it has a host of other less apparent but rather bewildering biologic properties. Interferon can inhibit the multiplication of normal and cancerous cells, act as an immunologic adjuvant or depressant, enhance or inhibit the production of interferon itself, enhance the toxicity of polyribonucleotides for cells, and enhance the phagocytic effect of phagocytes. The significance of these heterogeneous effects is still unclear, but at this time they appear insufficient to render interferon toxic. In any case, interferon can no longer be assumed to be a pristine antiviral substance. Eventually, its other effects may explain its efficacy or toxicity, depending on whichever action one may be observing. The antitumor effect of interferon is potentially of great therapeutic interest.

Another cardinal property of interferon is its so-called "species," or actually genus, specificity. That is, its antiviral effect is observed only in cells of the same species or genus as the cells from which the interferon was made. For example, chick cell interferon acts only on chick cells or other fowl cells but not human cells. To obtain interferon effective for human cells or for human beings, it is necessary to produce interferon in human or primate cells. This implies interferons from different species vary biochemically, but

such chemical differences have not been worked out.

The purification of interferon has been an elusive objective. Almost every physicochemical method used to study interferon has revealed a new dimension of heterogeneity. Interferon, even from one species, is heterogeneous with respect to molecular weight, isoelectric point, carbohydrate content, physical stability, and polyacrylamide gel electrophoresis. That is, more than one type of molecule is always obtained.

Immunologic analyses have recently revealed another dimension of the heterogeneity of interferon. Antibody affinity column chromatography has also been a powerful tool in interferon purification. For example, it has been shown that antibody made against human fibroblast interferon neutralizes the homologous interferon but it has no effect on leukocyte interferon. Conversely, antibody made against leukocyte interferon neutralizes both fibroblast and leukocyte interferon. This suggests that human leukocyte interferon possesses both "L" and "F" antigens, whereas fibroblast interferon possesses only "F" antigen. Apparently the type of cell producing interferon is one of the determinants of the characteristics of the interferon produced. Other work suggests that the mode of induction also plays a role. Interferon produced by the Type I method (Table 1) is antigenically different from interferon production by Type II, or "immune," induction. At this time we still do not understand why there are so many different interferons, or how it is explained genetically or developmentally. Apparently, in the case of human interferon, at least two chromosomes, 2 and 5, are involved in interferon production. But we have no idea whether the different interferons are variations of one basic gene product or of many.

## MECHANISM OF ACTION OF INTERFERON

Very little is understood about the actions of interferon, except its antiviral effect. It was realized soon after its discovery that interferon does not directly inactivate viruses, nor does it affect their adsorption on cells. The antiviral property of interferon was found to be eliminated if cell RNA or protein synthesis was inhibited. The interpretation was that interferon, in order to be active, must induce in the cell another protein that is the active antiviral substance. This explains why interferon must first incubate with the cell to create an "antiviral state." Once this state is created, the presence of interferon is no longer required, in striking contrast to other antimicrobial substances, whose activity usually requires their constant presence. It is also possible that the full expression of the antiviral state induced by interferon requires a virus infection.

Another piece of indirect evidence suggesting that interferon itself is not antiviral, and that an intermediary substance is needed comes from somatic hybrid studies. In cultures of fused hybrid human and mouse cells, in which specific human chromosomes are lost, the sensitivity to interferon (or the ability of interferon to induce the antiviral state) is lost in cells without chromosome G 21. Presumably this chromosome has a gene that facilitates the expression of interferon, perhaps by coding for the antiviral protein.

Little is known about the "actual" antiviral substance or how it acts. Indeed, its existence is still largely inferential, although some studies suggest its isolation in cell-free systems. Interferon has been thought to act at the transcriptional or translational level, and there are experiments to support each thesis. These two views are not necessarily exclusive. It is possible that with further advances in the state of the art both in molecular virology and in the study of interferons, these two views may be reconciled or subsumed by a more basic mechanism of action.

Inhibition of transcription was demonstrated by two types of experiments. First, interferon was found to inhibit the synthesis of early RNA in SV 40–infected cells. Such early RNA includes transcripts of the SV 40 genome, which code for T antigen and other early viral proteins, also found to be inhibited by interferon. Second, a number of RNA viruses (such as vesicular stomatitis virus) contain, as part of the virus, an RNA polymerase. After infection, transcription of the viral RNA by the polymerase occurs. This transcript, a product complementary to the viral RNA, has also been reported to be inhibited in interferon-treated cells.

A number of experiments suggest that translation of viral messenger RNA is inhibited in interferon-treated cells. In cell-free systems containing ribosomes, transfer RNA's, elongation factors, messenger RNA, and labeled amino acids extracted from interferon-treated cells, translation of viral messenger is not supported as well as it is in extracts from untreated cells (Fig. 3). In some studies, certain nonviral messengers, such as rabbit globin messenger RNA, may not be translated either. The question arises as to how specific is the antiviral effect of interferon. Perhaps interferon, in view of its other effects, such as inhibition of normal cell multiplication, is a metabolic regulator of broader significance.

## ROLE OF INTERFERON IN HOST DEFENSE

Interferon is a novel antiviral substance produced in the course of natural virus infections, but its relative importance among specific and nonspecific antiviral defenses is uncertain. The missing link in our understanding is that there is no "experiment in nature" in which a viral infection may be observed in an animal whose capacity to make interferon or react to it is genetically deficient. Analogous congenital deficiencies in humoral and cellular immunity are well known and highly instructive. The best evidence that interferon probably plays some role in host defense is that viral infections in mice run a more lethal course if interferon formed is neutralized by specific antiserum against interferon (Gresser et al., 1976).

The discovery that lymphocytes activated by mitogens and sensitized lymphocytes exposed to specific antigens produce interferon adds another, although uncertain, dimension to the role of interferon in host defense. Interferon may be regarded as one of the many lymphokines, such as migration inhibition factor, which help explain how cellular immunity works. A number of viruses, particularly the Herpetoviridae, produce more frequent and more severe infections when

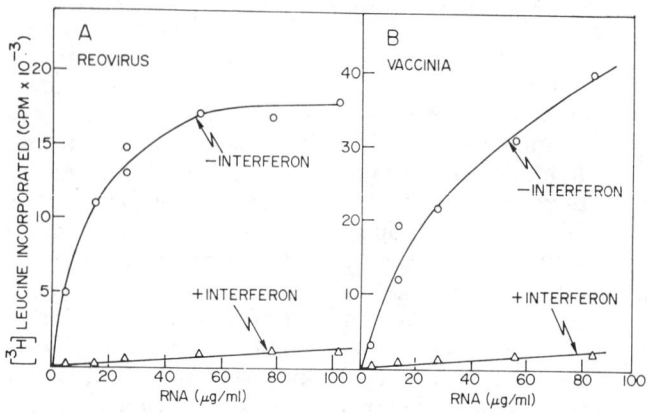

**FIGURE 3.** *The translation of reovirus and vaccinia virus messenger RNA by cell-free fraction (S10) of Krebs II ascites tumor cells (a form of suspended mouse tumor cell) pretreated or untreated with interferon. Interferon pretreatment inhibits translation of these two viral proteins, but not of normal cell mRNA. (From Samuel, C. E., and Joklik, W. K., Virology 58: 483, 1974.)*

cellular immunity is suppressed. One method by which cellular immunity is assumed to work is by release of interferon from sensitized T lymphocytes that come in contact with viral antigen. This mechanism should be particularly effective in the lesions, such as the vesicles of herpes simplex or herpes zoster, where there is an abundance of viral antigens and inflammatory lymphocytes. Interferon is produced in such lesions, but what would happen if interferon were not produced is less clear. Herpes zoster is reported to disseminate more frequently when the interferon content of vesicles is low in patients who have lymphomas and are on chemotherapy. But immunosuppression by disease or chemotherapy has not been shown to reduce interferon formation.

## THERAPEUTIC ROLE AS AN ANTIVIRAL SUBSTANCE

There are two ways to use the interferon system therapeutically. One may administer either an inducer of interferon or interferon itself. In animals the administration of "inducer" may be effective against viral infections. "Hyporeactivity" to repeated induction is an intrinsic problem of this method. It limits the efficacy of repeated administration of inducer and places a limit on the amount of interferon that can be induced, but it is not insurmountable. A more serious problem has been the toxicity of practically every inducer that has been carefully studied. Some of the best and chemically purest inducers, such as synthetic double-stranded polyribonucleotides, are prohibitively toxic. The search for nontoxic inducers, either by molecular manipulation of polyribonucleotides or by search for new types of inducers, continues.

Although interferon has properties of an ideal antiviral substance, it is still not available in the physician's armamentarium, more than 20 years after its discovery, for two main reasons. First, interferon does not eradicate viral infections. It is unusually potent, since as little as 0.001 $\mu$g possesses detectable antiviral activity, but its antiviral activity at any dose is incomplete so that it cannot cure or prevent a viral infection even with relatively large amounts. Any clinical effect requires large amounts of interferon. Second, interferon is species specific and difficult to prepare in large amounts, especially human interferon, but this technical problem can be solved.

Studies in experimental animals suggest that interferon should be more effective as a prophylactic than a curative agent. In humans it has been shown that when relatively large amounts are sprayed in the nose, subsequent infection by a rhinovirus may be ameliorated. The severity of established herpes zoster in Hodgkin's disease can also be lessened by interferon. Eventually, interferon may be useful in prevention of a widespread epidemic viral disease, or in treatment of severe infections.

Two observations suggest other unexpected possibilities for the use of interferon. One is the report that interferon reduced hepatitis B virus activity in patients with chronic aggressive hepatitis (Greenberg et al., 1976). Thus, interferon may even have a place in the therapy of chronic viral infection. Second, interferon has been reported to retard the progression of osteogenic sarcoma in humans. It is unclear whether this effect is due to the antiviral or some other effect of interferon. It is also possible that the antitumor effect is due to some impurity from the white cells from which the interferon was made. These questions can be answered only by further studies.

## OTHER TYPES OF VIRAL INTERFERENCE

There are three types of viral interference that are not mediated by interferon.

### Receptor Interference

One type of interference is based on competition for specific viral receptors. Infection by a myxovirus, such as Newcastle disease virus, may be interfered with if cell receptors are occupied or blocked by a prior infection. Another example of this type of interference may be found in the avian leukoviruses. It is used to study the relatedness of these agents and their titration. For example, inapparent infection of chick cells by one leukovirus will abrogate cellular receptors for this and related agents, so that a superinfection by a related transforming or cytocidal agent will be interfered with.

### Intracellular Homologous Interference

Another type of interference involves competition for limiting factor *within cells* among homologous or homotypic viruses. Examples are known among many viruses, such as influenza virus, vesicular stomatitis virus, and poliovirus. The best studied example is the ability of defective particles to interfere. These defective interfering particles (DIP) explain "autointerference" and may have a modifying role on viral infections. They are discussed in Chapter 11.

### Interference by Heterologous Agents

This is also intracellular and may be based on repression of transcription or translation. One example is so-called "intrinsic interference," which depends on a protein (not interferon) specified by the interfering virus. A number of viruses, such as rubella virus or measles virus, may interfere in chick embryo fibroblast cultures with the replication of Newcastle disease virus. This type of interference may be used to titer noncytopathic or nonreplicating virus.

## References

Finter, N. B.: Interferons and Interferon Inducers. New York, American Elsevier Pub. Co., Inc., 1973, p. 598.

Greenberg, H. B., Pollard, R. B., Lutwick, L. I., Gregory, P. B., Robinson, W. S., and Merigan, T. C.: Effect of human leukocyte interferon on hepatitis B virus infection in patients with chronic active hepatitis. N Engl J Med 295:517, 1976.

Gresser, I., Tovey, M. G., et al.: Role of interferon in the pathogenesis of virus diseases in mice as demonstrated by the use of anti-interferon serum. I. Rapid evolution of encephalomyocarditis virus infection. J Exper Med 144:1305, 1976.

Ho, M., and Armstrong, J. A.: Interferon. Ann Rev Micro 29:131, 1975.

Isaacs, A., and Lindenmann, J.: Virus interference. I Interferon Proc Roy Soc B, 147:258, 1957.

Metz, D. H.: Interferon and interferon inducers. Adv Drug Res 10:101, 1975.

Samuel, C. E., and Joklik, W. K.: A protein synthesizing system from interferon-treated cells that discriminates between cellular and viral messenger RNAs. Virology 58:476, 1974.

# Mycology

# 13 MORPHOLOGY AND STRUCTURE OF FUNGI

*Vladimir Farkaš, Ph.D.*

The fungi (Latin: *fungus,* mushroom) can be defined as eukaryotic, thallus-forming organisms *(Thallobiota)* that lack both chlorophyll and chemolithotrophic machinery. Consequently, they can produce structural elements neither from carbon dioxide via photosynthesis nor from inorganic matter. For this reason they depend on external sources of organic carbon. The fungi can live as saprophytes on dead organic matter or as parasites on other organisms, mainly plants, but also animals and man. (For the taxonomic position of fungi, see Chapter 14).

The vegetative body of the fungus, the *thallus,* is never differentiated into roots, stem, and leaves, and the fungi have no specialized vessels for transport of water and nutrients as in vascular plants. The fungi can form only a plectenchymatic type of "tissue" consisting of aggregates of cells largely retaining their individuality. In certain cases, as in sexual processes, the cells can communicate by means of hormone-like compounds.

In the vegetative phase the fungal population grows essentially as an undifferentiated group of similar cells. The differentiation occurs in the second developmental phase, known as the reproductive or fruiting phase. The hyphae that penetrate into the growth medium or spread over its surface absorbing the nutrients are called *vegetative mycelium*. The vegetative mycelium projects above the surface of the medium as *aerial mycelium* bearing reproductive structures. Some parasitic fungi produce special branches of the vegetative mycelium called *haustoria* (s. haustorium), which penetrate into the cytoplasm of host cells and absorb the necessary nutrients.

## *REPRODUCTION*

The fungi usually reproduce by means of motile or nonmotile *spores;* however, in many cases even small fragments of viable mycelium are sufficient to initiate growth of a new individual. The spores can be one-celled, two-celled, or many-celled. They are derived from the parent thallus and contain all the genetic information necessary for the development of a new thallus. The shapes of spores and the mode of sporulation are important characteristics in classification and identification of fungi (Fig. 1).

The spores can arise either asexually by differentiation of the thallus or sexually as a result of fusion of parent haploid nuclei. This is followed by formation of a sexual zygote and by restoration of the haploid state by meiosis. The sexual process is initiated by fusion of pairs of motile or nonmotile sexual cells *(gametes)* of opposite sexes or by somatic copulation of undifferentiated vegetative hyphae (Fig. 2).

## *MORPHOLOGY*

Morphologically, the fungi represent a very heterogeneous group of microorganisms. Some fungi grow as single cells *(yeasts),* others as multinuclear filaments *(molds).* Certain fungi, including many human pathogens, exhibit dimorphism — that is, they can grow as yeast or as mold (Fig. 3). In deep infections the yeast form predominates, whereas in superficial infections of keratinized skin layers the mycelial form of fungi is more common. The biochemical nature of dimorphism is poorly understood. The yeast–mold transitions of the fungal phenotype can be influenced by temperature, nutrition, redox potential, partial pressure of carbon dioxide, and other environmental factors. The two morphologic types of the same organism are distinctly different in the chemical composition of their cell walls.

### Yeasts

Yeasts are unicellular fungi that reproduce by budding or fission; the latter can be considered as a broad-base type of budding. Yeast cells are spherical or ellipsoidal, usually about 3 to 10 $\mu$m in diameter and 5 to 30 $\mu$m in length. Different species of yeast differ in their mode of budding (apical, lateral, bipolar, multipolar) and in other details. Yeast cells grow by a somewhat uniform extension of the cellular surface of the growing bud. During budding the nucleus of the mother cell divides, and one daughter nucleus passes into the bud. The two cells are then separated by a crosswall, called a *septum,* and after a certain period the bud breaks away. A birth scar is visible on the daughter cell, and a prominent bud scar remains on the mother cell's wall surface. The chemical composition of the bud scar with the septum usually differs from that of the rest of the cell wall. The bud scars remain as permanent

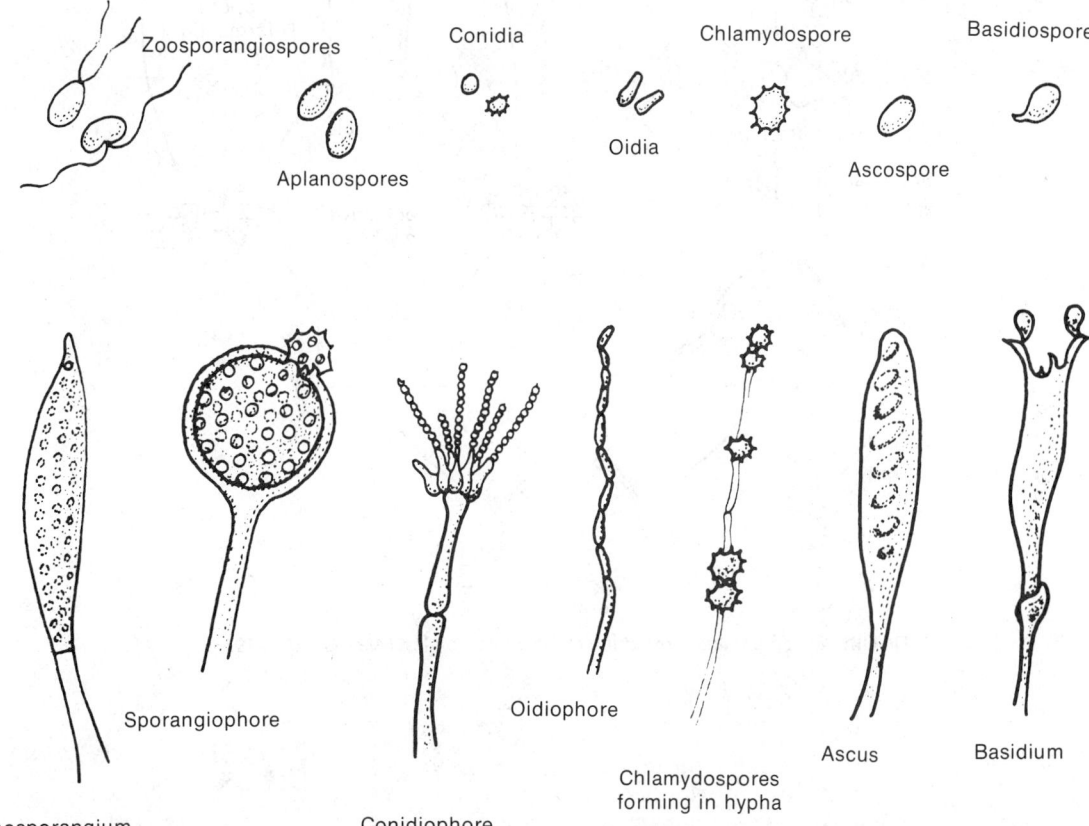

**FIGURE 1.** *Different types of reproductive structures and spores in fungi. (After Encyclopedia of Science and Technology. Vol. 5. New York, McGraw-Hill Book Company, 1971, p. 117.)*

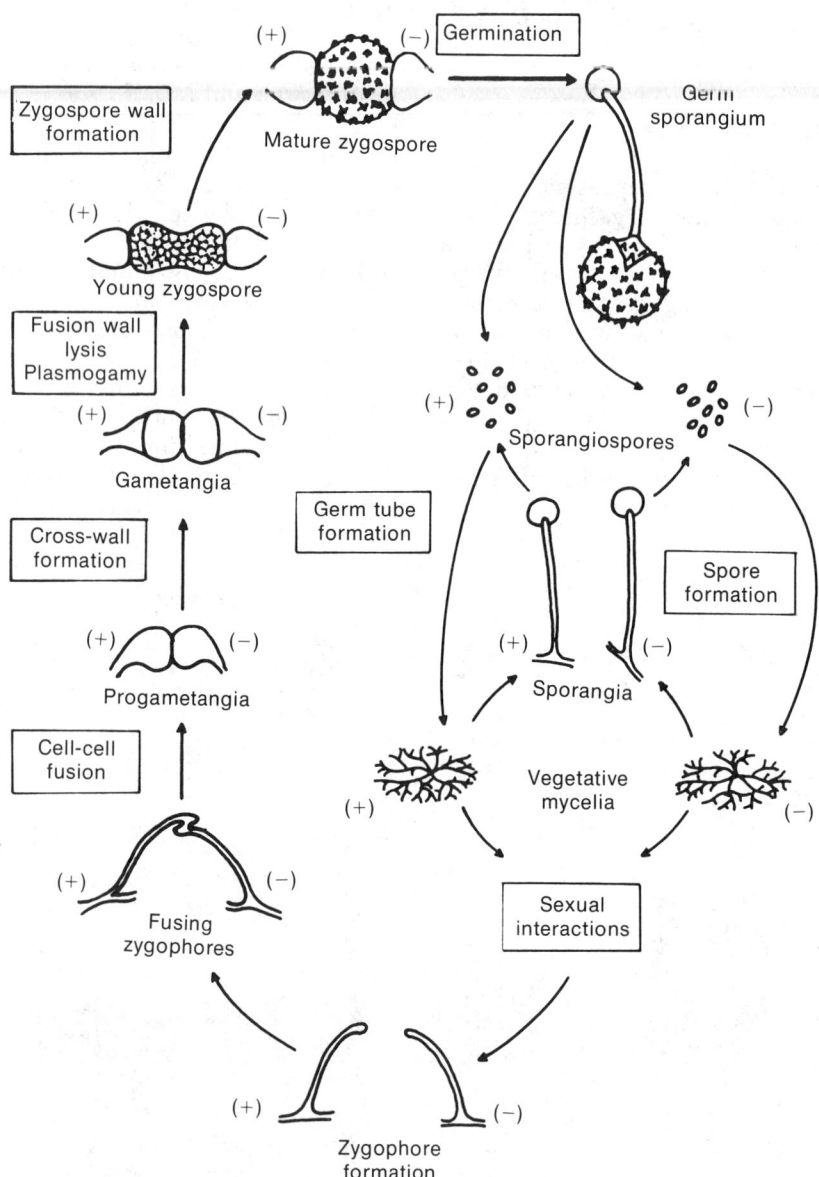

**FIGURE 2.** *Sexual and asexual life cycles of Mucorales. (After Gooday, 1973.)*

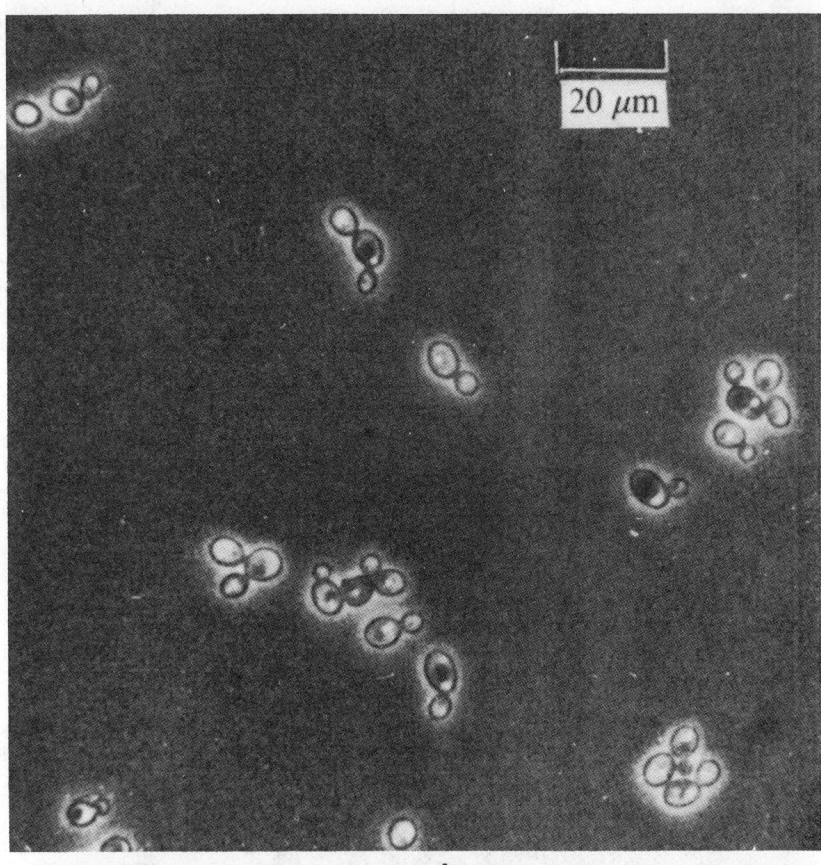

**A**

**FIGURE 3.** *Yeast* (A) *and mycelial* (B) *forms of* Candida albicans. *(From Mariott, M. S.: J Gen Microbiol 86:115, 1975.)*

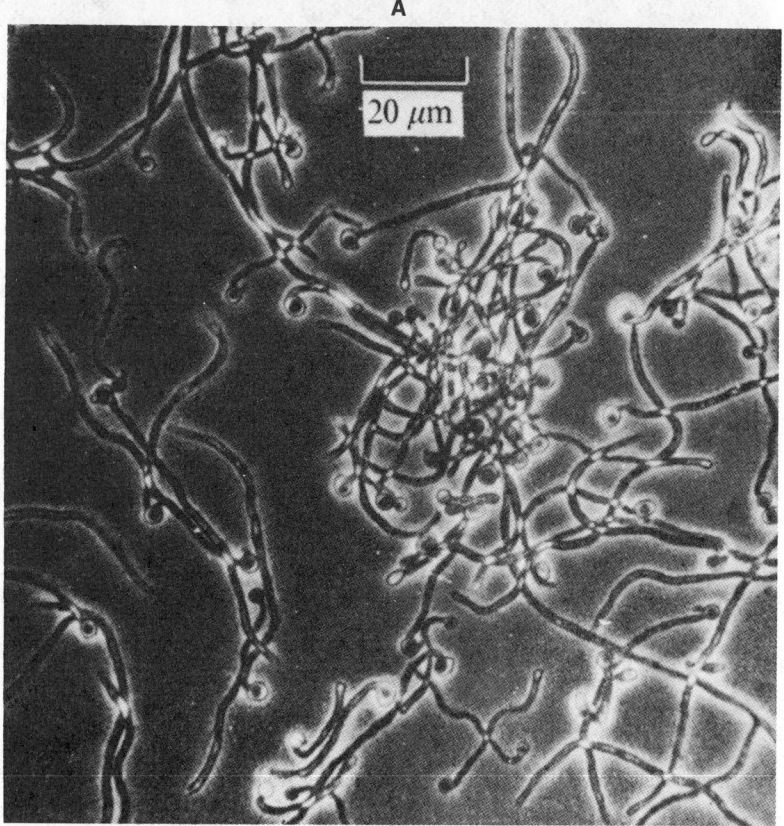

**B**

structures on the surface of the walls, and their number indicates the age of the cells (Fig. 4).

## Molds

The principal living unit of a mold is a *hypha.* Hyphae are about 3 to 12 μm diameter and can reach several centimeters in length. The hyphae grow by elongation at the tip *(apex).* In older portions of the hypha lateral branches arise that then develop like the main hypha. The densely

packed, interwoven hyphae constitute web-like *mycelia,* which are visible as macroscopic fungal *colonies* (Fig. 5).

In lower fungi the hyphae are usually not divided by septa into individual cells, but rather the whole mycelium is coenocytic — that is, it contains many nuclei in nonseparated cytoplasm. Regular septation observed in higher fungi does not change the coenocytic character of the hyphae because the septa have fine pores that ensure the continuity of the cytoplasm.

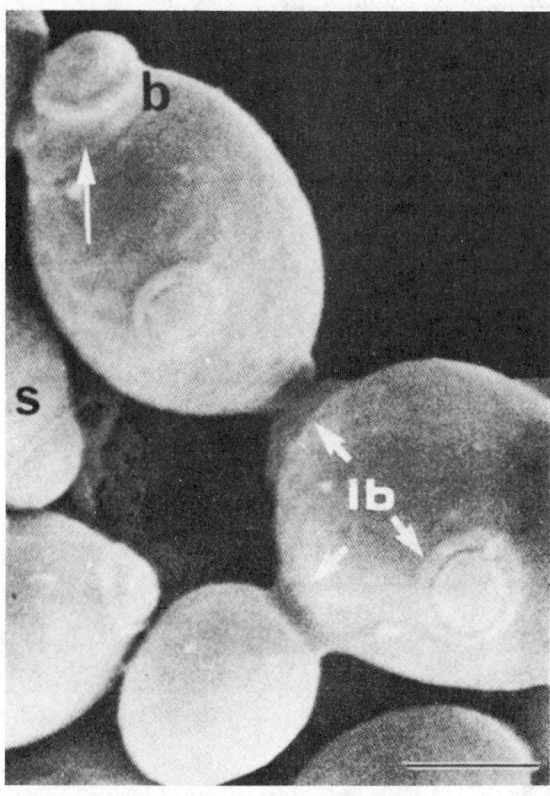

**FIGURE 4.** A, *Scanning electronmicrograph of the cells of* Candida slooffii *showing lateral budding (1b), bud scar (bs) and a birth scar (s). Bar indicates 1 μm. (From Watson, K., and Arthur, H.: J Bacteriol 130:312, 1976.)*

B, *Electronmicrograph of an ultrathin section through the cell of* Cryptococcus neoformans. C, capsule; CW, cell wall; M, mitochondria; N, nucleus; V, vacuole; B, bud. Bar indicates 1 μm. (From Peterson, E. M., Hawley, R. J., and Calderone, R. A.: Can J Microbiol 22:1518, 1976.)*

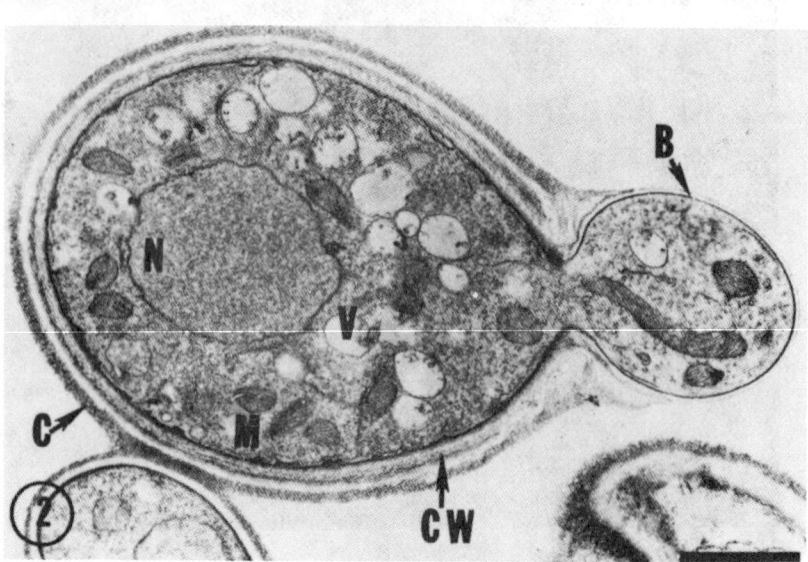

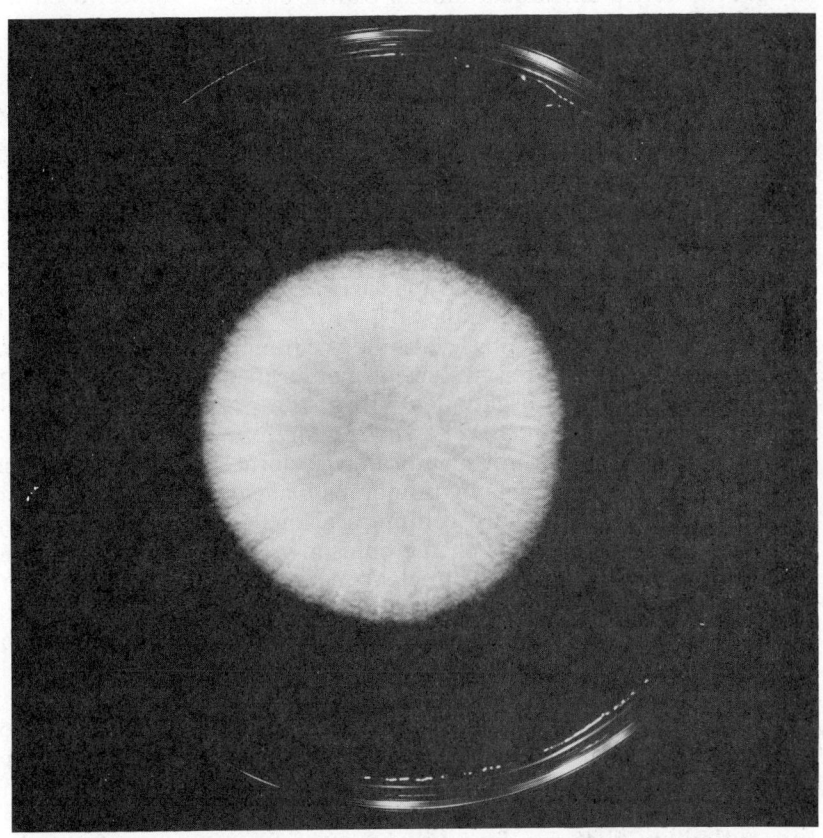

**FIGURE 5.** A, *Colony of the mold* Aspergillus niger. B, *Microphotograph from the margin of the same colon showing individual hyphae. Bar represents 50 μm.*

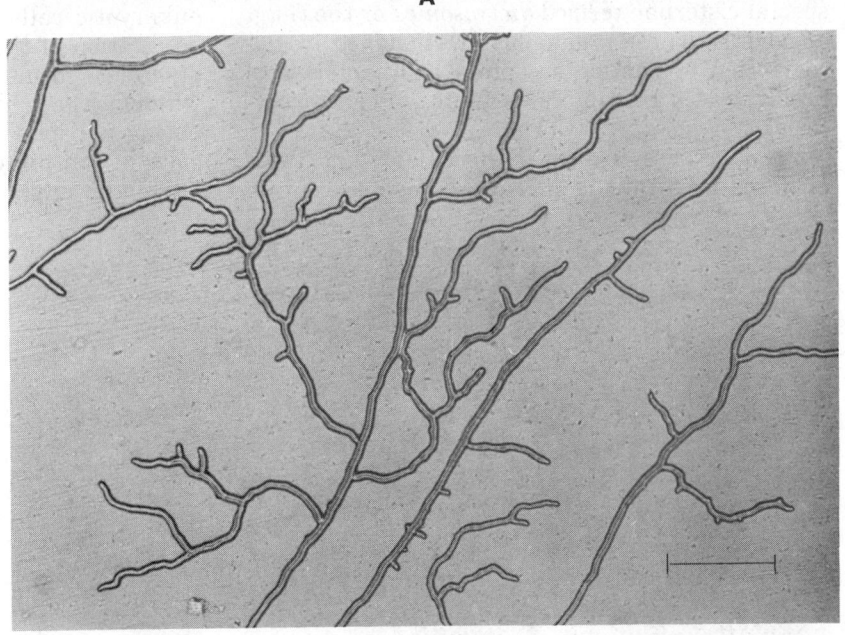

## ULTRASTRUCTURE

In the anatomic complexity of their cells the fungi resemble plants and animals. Unlike bacteria, the fungi possess a "true" nucleus that is typical of eukaryotic cells; it contains different chromosomes separated from the cytoplasm by a nuclear envelope and a mitotic apparatus within the nucleus that ensures the separation of duplicated chromosomes into two identical parts during mitosis. The quantity of DNA per cell varies from four to ten times the amount present in bacterial cells. This figure can be compared with the 1000 to 10,000-fold increase of DNA content observed in plants and animals.

Electron microscopic observations on fungal cells reveal a complicated system of membranes and membrane-bound organelles within the cytoplasm (see Figs. 4B and 6). The *nuclear envelope* consists of two parallel unit membranes perforated at their mutual contacts by numerous *nuclear pores*. Nuclear pores assure communication between the nucleoplasm and the cytoplasm.

Closely associated with the nuclear membrane is the complicated system of membranes called the *endoplasmic reticulum*. The membranes of the endoplasmic reticulum serve as the attachment sites for *ribosomes* that are involved in protein synthesis. The endoplasmic reticulum also channels different components within the cytoplasm and divides the cytoplasm into compartments. The closely packed membranes of the endoplasmic reticulum that are free of ribosomes form special cisternae termed *dictyosomes* or the *Golgi apparatus*. These organelles are involved in glycosylation of peptide acceptors and excretion of prefabricated glycoproteins from the cell (exocytosis).

*Vacuoles* are spherical vesiculoid structures enclosed by a unit membrane. They can contain water with dissolved solutes, gases, polymetaphosphate granules (volutine), waste products of cellular metabolism, and various hydrolytic enzymes used for breakdown of polymeric substances. Small vacuolar bodies derived from the membranes of the endoplasmic reticulum or from the cisternae of the Golgi apparatus can convey prefabricated glycoproteins to the cell exterior.

Metabolic energy is produced in *mitochondria* in the form of adenosine 5'-triphosphate (ATP) through respiration-mediated oxidative phosphorylation of adenosine 5'-diphosphate (ADP). The mitochondria, about 1 $\mu$m in diameter and several micrometers in length, are ubiquitous organelles of all eukaryotic cells.

Besides the principal organelles described above, the fungal cytoplasm can contain granules of reserve materials (lipids and glycogen) and various other inclusions.

The cytoplasm is surrounded by a single unit membrane, about 8 to 9 nm thick, called the *cytoplasmic membrane* or *plasmalemma*. The cytoplasmic membrane fulfills many functions in mediating communication between the cytoplasm and the cell exterior. Among these functions are the diffusion of solutes and nutrients and the passive and active carrier transport of amino acids and sugars. It is also an attachment site of enzymes involved in the biosynthesis of the cell wall. The cytoplasmic membrane, like other cellular membranes, is composed of phospholipids, proteins (or glycoproteins) and sterols. The presence of sterols distinguishes the membranes of eukaryotic cells from bacterial membranes. By association of their lipophilic portions, the phospholipids form a lipid bilayer or sandwich, whereby the hydrophilic portions of the participating phospholipid molecules face out on both sides of the bilayer. The phospholipid bilayer is broken up in places by globular protein (or glyco-

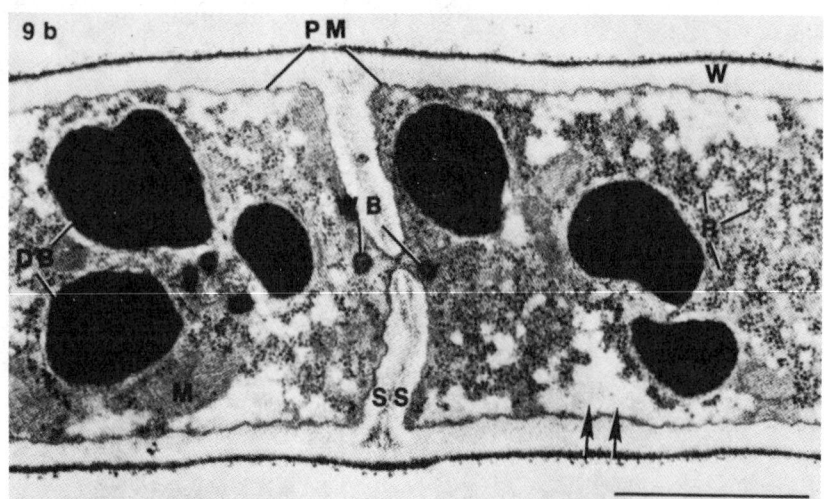

**FIGURE 6.** *Electronmicrograph of sectioned hyphal cell of* Phialophora dermatitis. *W, cell wall; R, ribosomes; DB, dense bodies; WB, Woronin bodies; M, mitochondria; SS, single septum. Double arrows indicate polysaccharide storage areas. Bar indicates 1 $\mu$m. (From Oujezdsky, K. B., Grove, S. N., and Szaniszlo, P. J.: J Bacteriol 113:468, 1973.)*

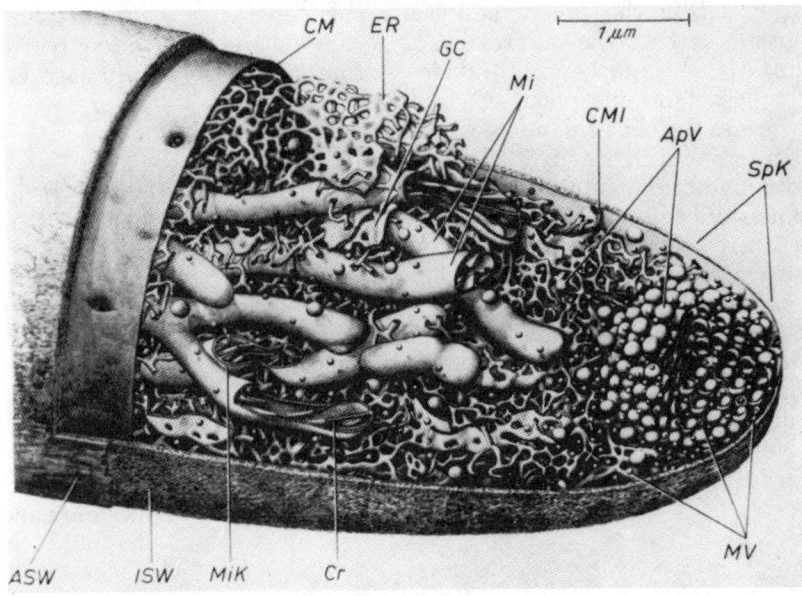

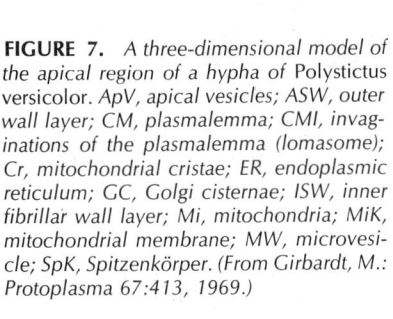

**FIGURE 7.**   *A three-dimensional model of the apical region of a hypha of Polystictus versicolor. ApV, apical vesicles; ASW, outer wall layer; CM, plasmalemma; CMI, invaginations of the plasmalemma (lomasome); Cr, mitochondrial cristae; ER, endoplasmic reticulum; GC, Golgi cisternae; ISW, inner fibrillar wall layer; Mi, mitochondria; MiK, mitochondrial membrane; MW, microvesicle; SpK, Spitzenkörper. (From Girbardt, M.: Protoplasma 67:413, 1969.)*

protein) molecules, which are completely or partially immersed in the lipids. The "fluid mosaic" model of the cytoplasmic membrane (Singer and Nicolson, 1972) presumes in extreme cases a free lateral movement of the protein globules in the lipid bilayer.

The space between the cytoplasmic membrane and the cell wall, called the *periplasmic space,* contains soluble macromolecular precursors of the cell wall and various extracellular hydrolases that cleave the oligomeric substrates to monomers before their transport into the cell. A three-dimensional model of a fungal cell is shown in Figure 7.

## CELL WALLS

In the great majority of fungi the outer surface of the cytoplasmic membrane is covered by a rigid cell wall. The primary role of the cell wall is to determine and to maintain cellular morphology. Dissolution of the cell walls by special lytic enzymes liberates osmotically fragile protoplasts that are shaped spherically by hydrostatic forces. Under suitable conditions (osmotic stabilizers, nutrition) the protoplasts can regenerate the cell wall on their surface. Lowering the osmolarity of the medium causes lysis of the protoplasts and kills them.

Besides their morphogenetic role, the cell walls mediate the interactions of the fungus cells with their environment, other cells, and the infected host.

### Chemical Composition

The fungal walls are composed of polysaccharides, protein-polysaccharide complexes, variable amounts of lipids, and lesser quantities of other components.

Polysaccharides, which represent about 80 to 90 per cent of the dry matter of the cell walls, are composed of amino sugars, hexoses, hexuronic acids, methylpentoses, and pentoses (Bartnicki-Garcia, 1970). Owing to their distinctive physicochemical properties, the different polymers fulfill specific functions in the cell walls. The crystalline, insoluble polysaccharides, such as cellulose, chitin, and beta-glucans, form the wall skeleton that is responsible for the mechanical strength and morphology of the walls. The amorphous homo- and heteropolysaccharides, often in association with proteins, act as cementing substances, constitute the carbohydrate moieties of extracellular enzymes, and form the immunodeterminant groups of wall antigens.

### Wall Architecture

The organization of individual components within the wall can be different in various genera of fungi and can vary with the age of the cells. The older parts of the walls are usually thicker, more rigid, and more resistant to hydrolytic enzymes.

Refined electron microscopic techniques coupled with cytochemical staining and selective action of purified polysaccharide-hydrolases have revealed that several layers of building material exist within the fungal cell wall. The general picture is that the outer surface of the wall is smooth or slightly granular in texture and is composed of amorphous glycoprotein material, whereas the skeletal, microcrystalline component is prominent in the layer adjacent to the cytoplasmic membrane (Fig. 8). The spaces between the fibrils of the microcrystalline layer, the *wall matrix,* are filled with an amorphous component that also penetrates the periplasmic space. Some yeasts (e.g., *Cryptococcus* sp.) produce viscous polysaccharide capsules on the outer surface of the cell wall. The chemical nature of the capsular slime closely resembles that of the protein-polysaccharides from the cell walls. A great portion of the capsular material is released into the medium during growth.

## STRUCTURE AND BIOSYNTHESIS OF CELL-WALL COMPONENTS

The polysaccharides of the fungal cell walls are polymerized from their activated monomers, nucleoside 5'-diphosphate sugars (NDP-sugars; Fig. 9) under the catalytic action of corresponding glycosyl transferases. The general equation for this process is:

$$\underset{\text{donor}}{\text{NDP–sugar}} + \underset{\text{acceptor}}{\text{(sugar)}_n} \xrightarrow{\text{glycosyl transferase}} \underset{\text{product}}{\text{(sugar)}_{n+1} + \text{NDP}}$$

The result of the transglycosylic reaction is the lengthening of the saccharidic chain of the acceptor molecule by one glycosyl unit. A single carbohydrate unit as well as the product from the preceding reaction can serve as the acceptor. The multiple repetition of this process leads to formation of long chains of glycosyl units linked by glycosidic bonds.

In the biosynthesis either of heteropolysaccharides containing different carbohydrate units, or of polymers containing different glycosidic bonds, any of several glycosyl transferases may catalyze the transfer of a specific sugar and the formation of a specific glycosidic bond. The following are examples of biosynthesis of some principal cell-wall constituents in fungi.

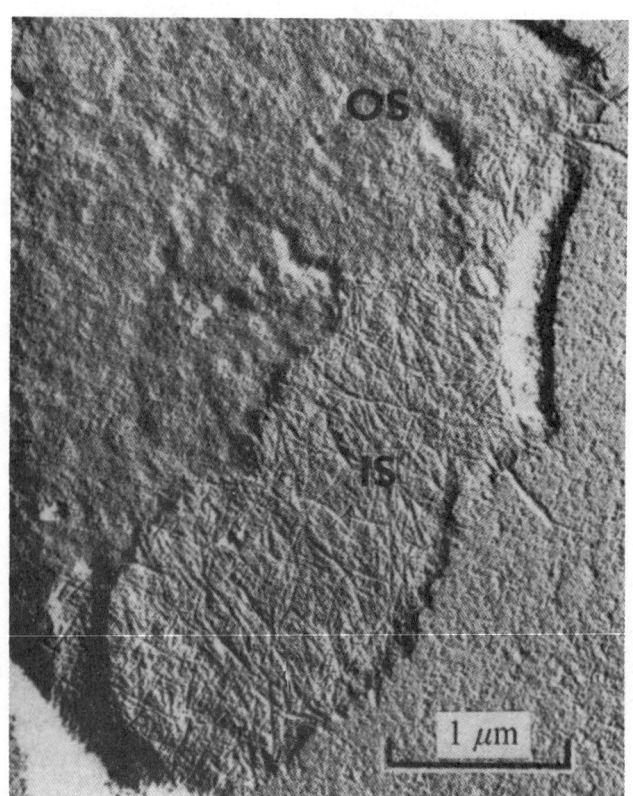

**FIGURE 8.** *Electronmicrograph of an isolated empty hyphal wall of* Pythium accanthicum *showing granular outer surface (OS) and microfibrillar inner surface (IS) of the cell wall. (From Siestma, J. H., Child, J. J., Nesbitt, L. R., and Haskins, R. H.: J Gen Microbiol 86:29, 1975.)*

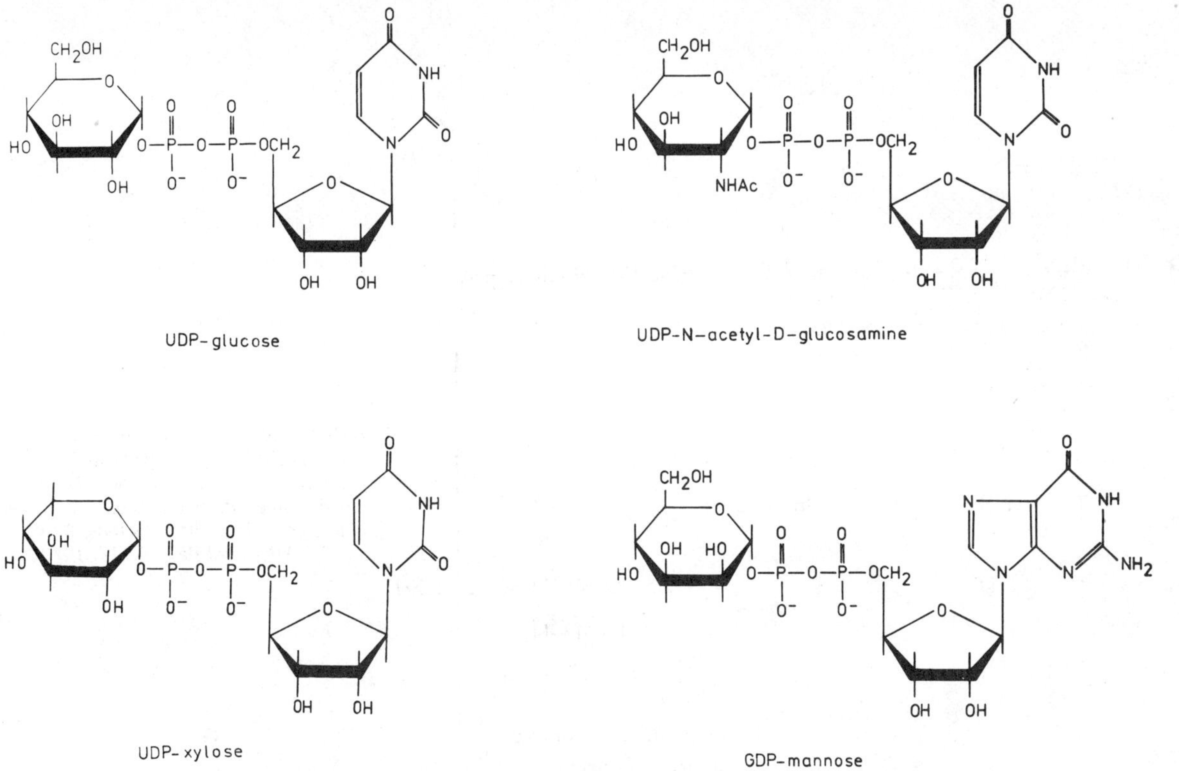

**FIGURE 9.**   *Structural formulae of some nucleoside 5'-diphosphate sugars serving as precursors in biosynthesis of fungal wall polysaccharides.*

## Chitin

Chitin is a linear polysaccharide composed exclusively of *N*-acetyl-D-glucosamine units linked by beta-1,4 glycosidic bonds. Owing to low solubility the linear chitin molecules tend to form microcrystalline aggregates in water. Chitin is polymerized from UDP-*N*-acetyl-D-glucosamine under the catalytic action of the enzyme chitin synthetase. The enzyme is located in the cytoplasmic membrane, where it can exist in two interconvertible forms, as active enzyme or as temporarily inactive zymogen. The interconversion of the two forms of chitin synthetase is supposed to play a decisive role in regulation of biosynthesis of the cell wall and, consequently, of fungal morphogenesis.

## Glucans

Various polymers of glucose represent important cell-wall constituents in many fungi. The insoluble cellulose and beta-glucans (i.e., those containing only beta-glycosidic bonds) form, together with chitin, the skeletal portion of the walls, whereas the alpha-glucans are usually amorphous and are located in the wall matrix.

Most glucans are polymerized by transglycosylic reactions from UDP-glucose. The exact cellular location of the reactions is, so far, not known. It is supposed that the skeletal wall glucans are synthesized by enzymes closely associated with the plasmalemma.

## Protein-Polysaccharide Complexes

Protein-polysaccharides, or glycoproteins, are the center of much interest because they are both structural components of the cell walls and determinants of biologic specificity on cell surfaces. Structurally, the fungal wall glycoproteins exhibit many similarities with surface protein-polysaccharide complexes from higher organisms. For this reason the glycoproteins of fungi are used as models to study various aspects of glycoprotein structure, function, and biosynthesis.

So far, the most systematic studies on fungal glycoproteins have been performed with yeast mannan (Ballou, 1976). The polysaccharide moiety of yeast mannan consists of an alpha-1,6-linked polymannose backbone to which short side chains of mannosyl units linked by alpha-1,2 and alpha-1,3 glycosidic bonds are attached. The whole polysaccharide is linked via a diacetylchi-

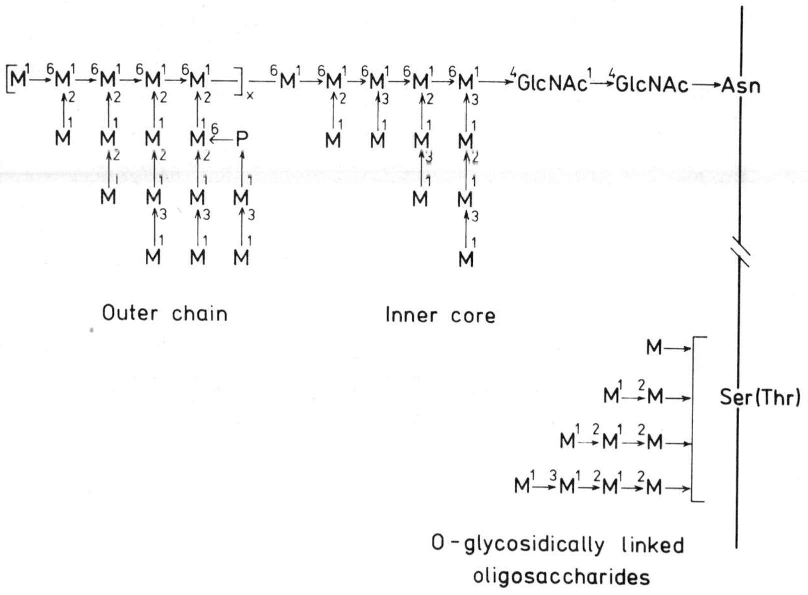
GlcNAc
GlcNAc
Asn
P
Outer chain
Inner core
Ser(Thr)
O-glycosidically linked
oligosaccharides

**FIGURE 10.** *Structure of mannan from the yeast* Saccharomyces cerevisiae. *M, mannopyranose residue; GlcNAc, N-acetyl-D-glucosamine; P, phosphate; Asn, asparagine; Ser, serine; Thr, threonine. (From Farkaš, V.: Microbiol Rev 43:117, 1979.)*

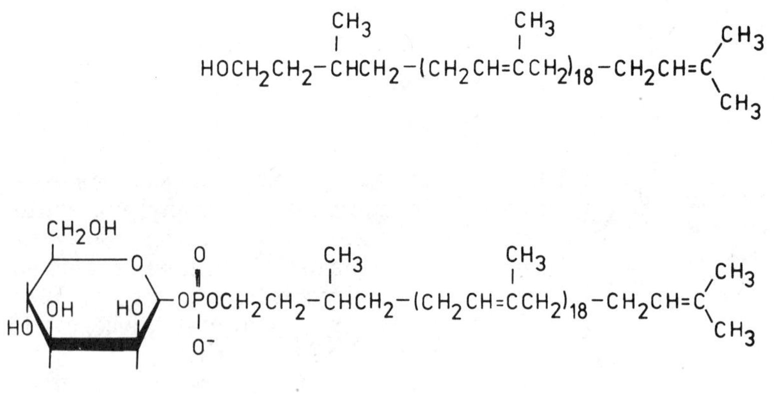

**FIGURE 11.** *Structural formula of dolichol monophosphate-mannose.*

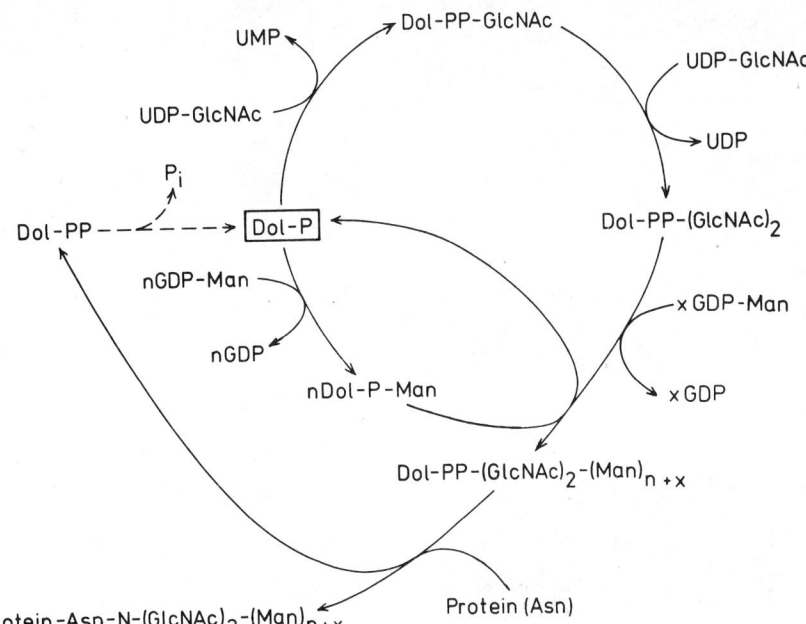

**FIGURE 12.** *Schematic representation of possible steps in biosynthesis of the "inner core" of yeast mannan. Dol-P, dolichol phosphate; Dol-PP, dolichol pyrophosphate; $P_i$, inorganic phosphate. $x + n = 0$ to 17. (From Farkaš, V.: Microbiol Rev 43:117, 1979.)*

tobiose bridge to an asparaginyl residue in the protein part of the molecule. Besides that, short manno-oligosaccharides containing alpha-1,2 and alpha-1,3 glycosidic links are attached directly to the hydroxyaminoacids serine and threonine by O-glycosidic bonds (Fig. 10).

Biosynthesis of the relatively complex structure of yeast mannan requires participation of a whole set of mannosyltransferases, each of them catalyzing the formation of a specific linkage. The precursor of mannosyl units in the biosynthesis of yeast mannan is guanosine 5'-diphospho mannose (GDP-Man). The transfer of mannosyl units from their donor to the acceptor can proceed either in a single step or through lipophilic intermediates such as dolichol-monophosphate mannose (Fig. 11). It is assumed that the involvement of dolichols is necessary in those reactions that take place in a lipophilic environment, as for example on the surface or inside the membranes of the endoplasmic reticulum. The binding of hydrophilic sugar residues to a lipophilic carrier facilitates

their solubility in the membrane and, consequently, their translocation within the cell. The biosynthesis of the whole "inner core" of yeast mannan probably proceeds while the product is attached to the dolichol carrier (Fig. 12).

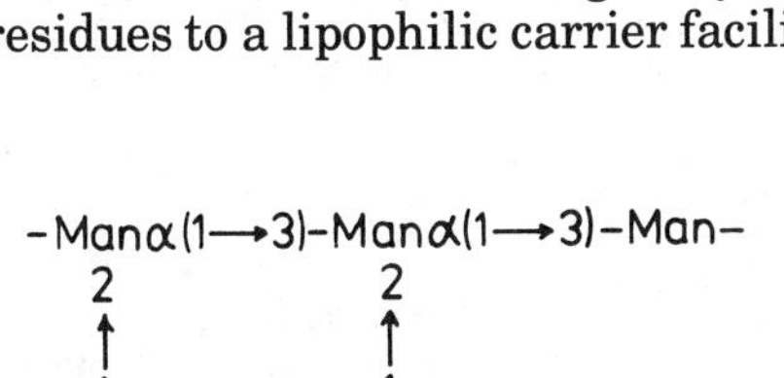

The mannan of *Candida albicans* has a structure very similar to that depicted in Figure 10. The difference is that the mannan from *Candida albicans* contains a much higher proportion of unsubstituted mannosyl units in the polymannose backbone and, in addition, contains longer side branches that reach the size of a heptasaccharide. The side chains containing terminal alpha-1,3 linked mannosyl units are immunodeterminant groups in the mannan antigens, and the intensity of the precipitin reaction with antibodies induced by whole cells increases with the length of the side chains in the mannan.

Surface antigens from other fungi have usually more complex structures than the yeast mannans. The polysaccharide portions of these antigens can be chemically characterized as neutral or acidic heteropolysaccharides, composed of hexoses, pentoses, methylpentoses, and, in acidic heteropolysaccharides, uronic acids. For example, the capsular glucurono-xylo-mannan from *Cryptococcus neoformans* has a branched structure in which a linear alpha-1,3 linked polymannose chain is substituted at positions C-2 by beta-glycosidically linked glucuronic acid or xylose, with the xylose predominating (Fig. 13).

Glycosylation of nascent proteins takes place in

$$-\text{Man}\alpha(1{\longrightarrow}3)-\text{Man}\alpha(1{\longrightarrow}3)-\text{Man}-$$

**FIGURE 13.** *Structure of acidic polysaccharide from capsules of Cryptococcus neoformans. Man, mannopyranose residue; Xyl, xylopyranose residue; GlcA, glucuronic acid residue.*

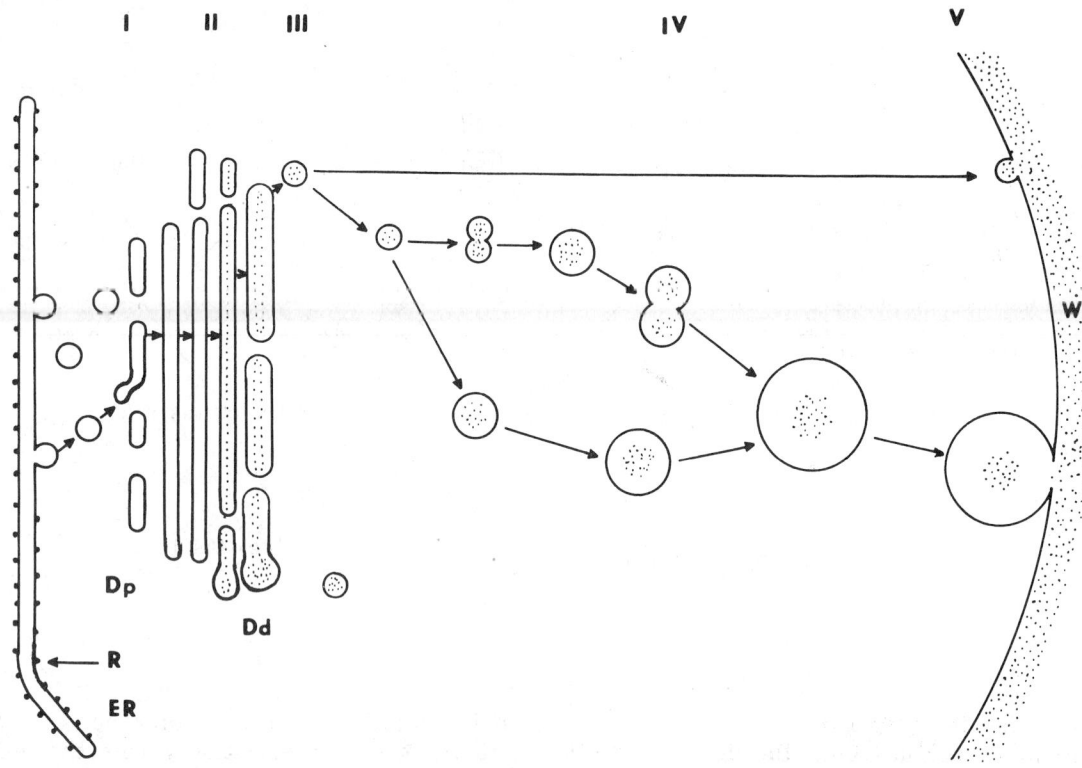

**FIGURE 14.** *Diagrammatic representation of biosynthesis and excretion of cell wall glycoproteins. Stage I: Formed proteins are transferred from ER to dictyosome by blebbing of ER and refusion of vesicles to form a cisterna at the proximal pole of the dictyosome (Dp). Stage II: Cisternal contents and the membranes are transformed as the cisterna is displaced to the distal pole (Dd) by the continued formation of new cisternae. Stage III: Cisternae vesiculate to form secretory vesicles as they approach and reach the distal pole. Stage IV: Secretory vesicles migrate to the cell wall. Some may increase in size or fuse with other vesicles to form large secretory vesicles, while others are carried directly to the cell surface. Stage V: Vesicles accumulate at the growth region of the wall and fuse with the cytoplasmic membrane, liberating their contents into the wall region (W). (After Grove et al., 1970.)*

dictyosomes and in the smooth endoplasmic reticulum. In the course of this process the formed glycoproteins are packed into vesicles derived from the original membrane systems and carried toward the cytoplasmic membrane. The carrier vesicles fuse with the membrane and discharge their contents into the cell exterior (Fig. 14). A portion of the supplied glycoproteins remains entrapped in the periplasm or anchored to the cell wall, and the other part diffuses into the surrounding medium. Some of the extracellular glycoproteins exhibit enzymatic activity; they act as hydrolases of various kinds. The hydrolytic action of these enzymes facilitates the growth and penetration of the fungus into the solid substrate or the invaded tissue.

## References

Ballou, C. E.: Structure and biosynthesis of the mannan component of the yeast cell envelope. Adv Microbiol Physiol 14:93, 1976.

Bartnicki-Garcia, S.: Cell wall composition and other biochemical markers in fungal phylogeny. In Hasborne, J. B. (ed.): Phytochemical Phylogeny. New York and London, Academic Press, 1970, p. 81.

Farkaš, V.: Biosynthesis of cell walls of fungi. Microbiol Rev 43:117, 1979.

Girbardt, M.: Die Ultrastruktur der Apikalregion von Pilzhyphen. Protoplasma 67:413, 1969.

Gooday, G. W.: Differentiation in *Mucorales*. Symp Soc Gen Microbiol 23:269, 1973.

Grove, S. N., Bracker, C. E., and Morré, D. J.: An ultrastructural basis for hyphal tip growth in *Pythium ultimum*. Am J Botany 57:245, 1970.

Mariott, M. S.: Isolation and chemical characterization of plasma membranes from the yeast and mycelial forms of *Candida albicans*. J Gen Microbiol 86:115, 1975.

Oujezdsky, K. B., Grove, S. N., and Szaniszlo, P. J.: Morphological and structural changes during the yeast-to-mold conversion of *Phialophora dermatitis*. J Bacteriol 113:468, 1973.

Peterson, E. M., Hawley, R. J., and Calderone, R. A.: An ultrastructural analysis of protoplast-spheroplast induction in *Cryptococcus neoformans*. Can J Microbiol 22:1518, 1976.

Siestma, J. H., Child, J. J., Nesbitt, L. R., and Haskins, R. H.: Chemistry and ultrastructure of the hyphal walls of *Pythium accanthicum*. J Gen Microbiol 86:29, 1975.

Singer, S. J., and Nicolson, G. L.: The fluid mosaic model of the structure of cell membranes. Science 175:720, 1972.

Watson, K., and Arthur, H.: Cell surface topography of *Candida* and *Leucosporidium* yeasts as revealed by scanning electron microscopy. J Bacteriol 130:312, 1976.

# CLASSIFICATION OF FUNGI 14

## Willard A. Taber, Ph.D.

Fungi live in soil, on plants, in water, and occasionally on man. Most plant diseases are caused by fungi; most diseases of animals are caused by bacteria and viruses. For this reason fungi are usually associated with botany, whereas bacteria are associated with zoology. For an overview of fungi and their impact on man, see Taber and Taber, 1967.

The term fungus refers to nonphotosynthetic plant-like forms that resemble plants in possessing cell walls and the glyoxylate bypass of the Krebs cycle. Fungi resemble both plants and animals in being eukaryons — that is, they possess nuclei, mitochondria, endoplasmic reticula, more than one chromosome, protoplasmic streaming, and the capacity to synthesize steroids. They differ from bacteria, which are prokaryons, and which lack the above structures and activities. Whether microscopic or macroscopic in size (Fig. 1), fungi are united by the possession of hyphae (Fig. 2) or hypha-like structures. Fungi vary greatly in structural detail, and consequently a single all-inclusive definition is difficult to formulate. Fungi are nonphotosynthetic forms that consist of multinucleated cytoplasm within a much-branched system of tubes (the hyphae of filamentous fungi), of naked multinucleated cytoplasm (the plasmodium of Myxomycota), or of single vegetative cells that multiply either by formation of buds (the yeasts) or of motile spores (certain primitive aquatic phycomycetes).

There are a minimum of 50,000 species of fungi (Ainsworth, 1968b) distributed in approximately 4000 genera. Enumeration of fungal taxa is made difficult because some species have two generic names. This results from the fact that fungal taxa are based on sexual structures even though many fungi exist that produce only asexual spore structures. They are given a form-type name. If such a fungus is found to produce a sexual stage, it is given a second name to relate it to similar fungi of

the classification. As an example, recent crossings of various strains of the deadly asexual fungus *Cryptococcus neoformans* showed it to be capable of producing a sexual stage characteristic of the Basidiomycetes and according to the provisions of the International Code of Botanical Nomenclature was given a second name, *Filobasidiella neoformans*. The species name is always retained although the ending may have to be changed to conform to the new generic name. Either name can be used, but the name based on the sexual state takes preference taxonomically. For definition of mycological terms, see the *Dictionary of Fungi* (Ainsworth, 1971).

## SOME CHARACTERISTICS OF REPRESENTATIVE FUNGI

### Myxomycota

The Myxomycota as represented by the common myxomycetes, or slime molds, possess a vegetative or assimilative phase that consists of a naked mass of multinucleated cytoplasm, the plasmodium. This plasmodium increases in size as it crawls over the substrate consuming small forms of life and soluble nutrients (Fig. 3). When food or water supply becomes limited, the plasmodium is transformed into sporangia-bearing spores. Meiosis precedes either formation or germination of these spores. A spore breaks open and approximately four amoeboid or flagellated cells escape and feed on surrounding nutrients. Pairs of such cells functioning as gametes fuse (Fig. 3) and develop into the 2N plasmodium. Myxomycete plasmodia or sporangia can be found on logs, fallen leaves, or grass after rains. None is known to be pathogenic to animals although the related Plasmodiophoromycetes are pathogens of certain

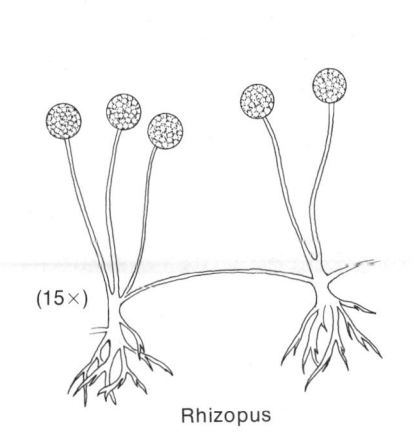

(15×)

Rhizopus

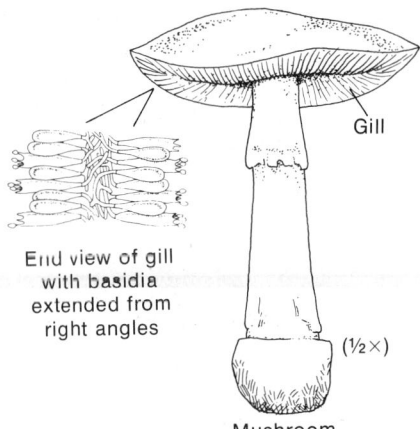

Gill

End view of gill
with basidia
extended from
right angles

(½×)

Mushroom

**FIGURE 1.** *Asexual sporangiospores are borne in sporangia that are supported on sporangiophores. Rhizopus also possesses rhizoids at the base of the sporangiophore. (Left) Basidiocarp of Amanita sp. Basidiospores are borne on basidia. (Right)*

**FIGURE 2.** *Vegetative or assimilative forms of growth of Fungi. (Left) Hyphal form with branches. (Center) Yeast form of growth in which proliferation occurs by budding. (Right) Unicellular growth characteristic of certain simple Phycomycetes. Approximate size of a bacterium is shown for comparison. Bacteria are always very narrow.*

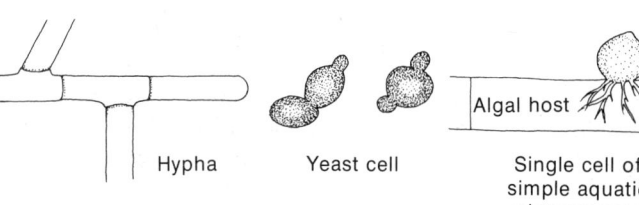

Hypha

Yeast cell

Algal host

Single cell of
simple aquatic
phycomycete

Bacteria
for size
comparison

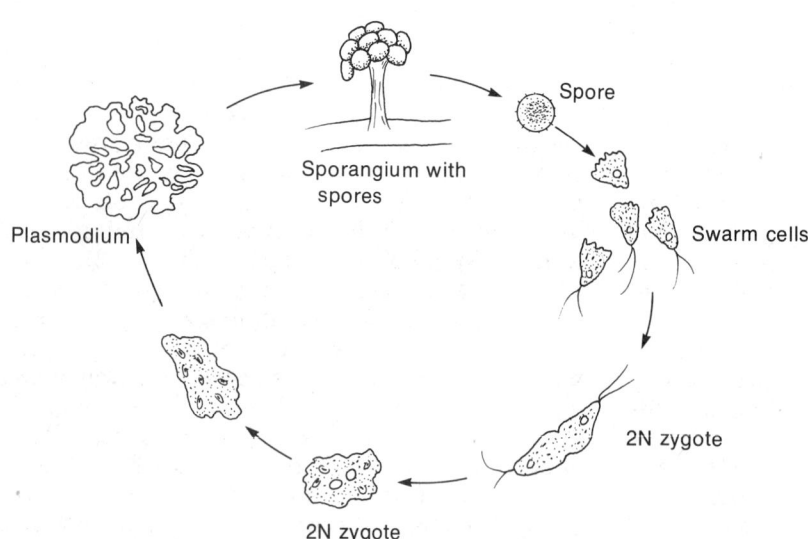

Spore

Sporangium with
spores

Swarm cells

Plasmodium

2N zygote

2N zygote

**FIGURE 3.** *Life cycle of myxomycete.*

plants. For descriptions of species, see Martin and Alexopoulos, 1969.

## Eumycota

### Mastigomycotina

Mastigomycotina are nonplasmodial fungi that produce motile cells. Motility is by flagella of the eukaryotic type. Many species, such as some of the Chytridiomycetes, consist of a single cell with rhizoids (Fig. 2), which becomes transformed into a sporangium containing motile spores. Chytridiomycetes possess one posterior flagellum, Hypochytridiomycetes possess one anterior flagellum, and the Oomycetes possess two flagella and in addition are usually mycelial (Table 1). Oomycetes also possess a female oogonium and a male antheridium (Table 1). The fertilized oosphere in the oogonium becomes an oospore. The oospore germinates by germ tube, which develops into mycelium or hyphae. Some species of Saprolegnia can parasitize aquatic animals, producing a woolly halo of mycelium around the host. The Oomycetes consist of four orders, Saprolegniales, Leptomitales, Lagenidiales, and Peronosporales. The Peronosporales embrace many plant pathogens, such as the downy mildews, which cause severe crop losses (Fig. 4). The asexual spores of some can produce germ tubes as well as flagella, and this group represents a transition to nonmotile terrestrial forms of fungi.

### Zygomycotina

Zygomycetes are nonmotile phycomycetes that possess coenocytic hyphae, thick-walled sexual spores called zygospores (Table 1), and sporangia containing asexual spores (Hesseltine, 1973). Most species produce woolly aerial mycelium when grown on spoiled foods or agar in a Petri plate. The aerial hyphae may fill the air space of a Petri plate culture; other fungi do not. Some species are homothallic. That is, hyphae developing from one spore can produce the sexual spore. Others are heterothallic, and hyphae of different mating types must fuse before sexual spores can be produced. Hormones are involved in hyphal attraction. Several species are pathogenic to man (Table 2) and their invasiveness is associated with diabetes. These fungi grow rapidly on sugars and are frequently referred to as sugar fungi. Members of the Entomophthorales attack insects, grow in association with amphibians, or grow in ground litter. Dead flies fixed to window panes and surrounded by a halo have been killed by *Entomophthora muscae*. The halo consists of sporangia shot off from the fungus growing on the fly.

### Ascomycotina

There are approximately 15,000 species of ascomycetes distributed in 1950 genera. Ascomycetes are those fungi that produce the sexual spore, the ascospore, in an ascus (Table 1, Fig. 5). The vegatative or assimilative phase can consist either of coenocytic hyphae compartmentalized by regularly placed simple perforated septa (crosswalls) or yeast cells. An ascus usually contains eight ascospores but certain species can produce four and others more than eight ascospores.

Ascomycetes are divided into three major categories: Euascomycetes, which possess a unitunicate ascus and usually an ascocarp (Table 1) that forms around the developing asci; Loculoascomycetes, which possess a bitunicate ascus (Fig. 5) that is formed within a cavity or locule hollowed out of a stroma that may superficially resemble an ascocarp; and Laboulbeniomycetes, which are minute nonmycelial ascomycetes living exclusively on the exoskeletons of insects and mites (Benjamin, 1973). Certain species of Euascomycetes can also possess a stroma, but if so, the ascocarp develops in or on top of it. The stroma is composed of pseudoparenchymatous tissue (see Taber and Taber 1973 for a review of structures). Unexplainably, the concept Euascomycete is not employed taxonomically.

#### Euascomycetes

**Hemiascomycetes.**  Yeast and yeast-like fungi that produce unitunicate asci but not in an ascocarp are placed in this class. At least one, *Pichia guilliermondii*, is pathogenic to man.

**Plectomycetes.**  Plectomycetes are normally filamentous ascomycetes that produce a simple closed ascocarp, the cleistothecium, containing globose dissolving asci at various heights in the ascocarp (Table 1). Many of the human pathogenic fungi are members of this class and most are in the Family Gymnoascaceae. *Histoplasm capsulatum, Blastomyces dermatitidis, Paracoccidioides brasiliensis*, and the unrelated *Sporothrix schenkii* grow as true yeasts in human tissue and as hyphae elsewhere in nature. Note that the first three names represent the asexual forms of these fungi, the forms generally observed. Names of the sexual and asexual forms are listed in Table 2. Many of the dermatophytes are members of this group. Note that dermatophytes are housed in three asexual genera: Trichophyton, Microsporum, and Epidermophyton; and note that those producing a sexual state are also members of either Arthroderma or Nannizzia (Table 2). Microascus produces a perithecium (Table 2) but here is placed in the Plectomycetes because the

**TABLE 1.   Overview of the Fungi**

| OLD | NEW | CHARACTERISTICS |
|---|---|---|
| Myxomycetes (Class) | MYXOMYCOTA (Division)<br>Myxomycetes (Class) "Slime molds"<br>Plasmodiophoromycetes Plant Pathogens<br>Acrasiomycetes<br>"Labyrinthulales" | Vegetative phase is a plasmodium that consists of fused or single amoeba. Creeps over surface of substrate. Some produce dry spore-bearing structures that resemble fungal structures. |
| | EUMYCOTA (Division)<br>All other fungi. | Do not creep over substrate. Spread by growing. Vegetative phase a hypha, yeast cell, or single cell. |
| Phycomycete-Oomycete<br>Aquatic phycomycetes, many are plant pathogens | Mastigomycotina (Subdivision)<br>Chytridiomycetes (Class)<br>Hyphochytridiomycetes<br>Oomycetes | Asexual Spores are motile owing to flagella. Hyphae, when present, multinucleate (coenocytic) without regular cross walls (septa). |

Sexual phase                           Asexual phase

| | | |
|---|---|---|
| Phycomycete-Zygomycete | Zygomycotina (Subdivision)<br>Zygomycetes (Class)<br>Sexual spore is a zygospore and asexual spore is usually a sporangiospore (borne within a sporangium). Human pathogens are found among: Rhizopus, Absidia, Mucor, and Basidiobolus.<br>Trichomycetes (on or in arthropods) | Coenocytic hyphae without regular perforated septa but no motile spores. |

Sexual spore                           Asexual spore

| | | |
|---|---|---|
| Ascomycete<br>Ascocarp is a structure housing or supporting asci. It forms around the developing asci of the Euascomycetes. Loculoascomycetes possess a hollowed-out stroma in which asci develop. | Ascomycotina (Subdivision)<br>1. Euascomycetes. Unitunicate ascus (no classification)<br>Hemiascomycetes. (Class). Yeast or yeast-like. No ascocarp; no ascogenous hyphae. Yeasts usually have no hyphae.<br>Plectomycete. Round asci scattered throughout cleistothecium type ascocarp; asci dissolving. (Human pathogens: dermatophytes, Histoplasma, Aspergillus are members of this group.)<br>Pyrenomycetes. Ascocarp usually a perithecium bearing oblong asci from one layer. | Coenocytic hyphae with simple perforated septa. Usually have an ascocarp. Always have ascus and ascospore. |

Ascus          Cleistothecium          Perithecium

— Ascus
— Ascospore

Discomycetes. Oblong ascus with or without
operculum in an (open) apothecium

## TABLE 1.   Overview of the Fungi *(Continued)*

| OLD | NEW | CHARACTERISTICS |
|---|---|---|

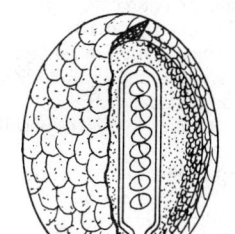

|  | 2. Loculoascomycetes (Class) | |

2. Loculoascomycetes (Class)
   Bitunicate (two-layered) ascus in a hollowed-out stroma. May resemble perithecium or black tar spots. Piedraia hortae on man.
3. Laboulbeniomycetes. Minute, on arthropod exoskeletons.

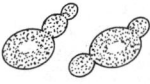

**Fungi Imperfecti**
(Most fungi growing on laboratory Petri plate cultures are Deuteromycotina or Zygomycetes).

**Deuteromycotina (Subdivision)**
(asexual fungi)
Blastomycetes (Class) yeasts
Hyphomycetes. Spores borne in open on hyphae
Coelomycetes. Spores borne in (enclosed) pycnidium or on acervulus cushion breaking plant tissue epidermis

Yeast or hyphal fungi without a sexual phase. If a sexual phase is found, both names can be used. Many are now known to be ascomycetes or to have ascomycetous affinities. Hyphae are coenocytic with perforated septa. Candida, Cryptococcus, Torulopsis, Pityrosporum.

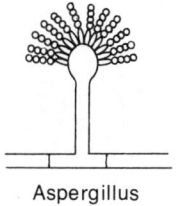 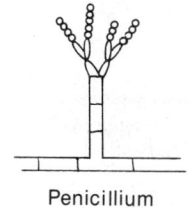 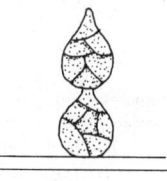 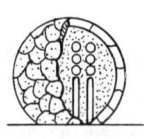 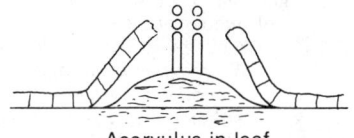

| Aspergillus | Penicillium | Alternaria | Phoma | Acervulus in leaf |

**Basidiomycetes**

**Basidiomycotina (Subdivision)**
Coenocytic hyphae with complex perforated septa and often with two nuclei per compartment.
Basidium and basidiospore, and often clamp connection characterize the Subdivision. The human pathogen *Cryptococcus neoformans* recently found to be asexual phase of the basidiomycete *Filobasidiella neoformans.*
   Teliomycetes (Class) Rusts and smuts.
      No basidiocarp.
   Hymenomycetes. Spores shot off. Mushrooms.
   Gasteromycetes. Spores not shot off; in an enclosed basidiocarp.

Basidium with spores

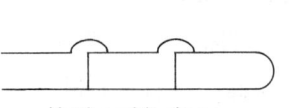 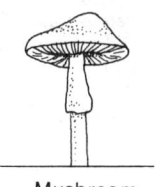 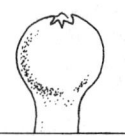

| Hypha with clamp connection | Mushroom | Puffball |

## TABLE 2.  Fungal Taxa That Cause Diseases of Man

Eumycota
  Mastigomycotina
    Chytridiomycete (?)
      *Rhinosporidium seeberi*
      *Emmonsia parva* and *Emmonsia crescens* ?
  Zygomycotina
  *Coccidioides immitis?* coccidioidomycosis. Taxonomic location uncertain
  Zygomycetes
    Mucorales
      *Absidia corymbifera*
      *Absidia ramosa*
      *Hyphomyces destruens* ?
      *Mortierella* sp. (questionable)
      *Mucor circinelloides*
      *Mucor pusillus*
      *Mucor ramosissimus*
      *Rhizopus arrhizus*
      *Rhizopus oryzae*
    Entomophthorales (usually grow on insects or in ground litter)
    *Basidiobolus haptosporus* (tropical)
    *Entomophthora coronata*
  Ascomycotina
  Euascomycete (unitunicate ascus; ascocarp wall built around developing asci)
    Hemiascomycete (yeast or yeast-like)
      Endomycetales
        *Endomyces geotrichum,* ascomycetous state of *Geotrichum candidum*
        *Pichia guilliermondii* (yeast). Sexual state of *Candida guilliermondii*
    Plectomycete (globose asci borne at different levels in ascocarp; asci dissolving)
      Eurotiales (cleistothecium)
        Gymnoascaceae
          *Ajellomyces dermatitidis*—ascomycetous state of *Blastomyces dermatitidis.* Blastomycosis
          *Arthroderma benhamiae*—ascomycetous state of the dermatophyte *Trichophyton mentagrophytes*
          *Arthroderma gertleri*—ascomycetous state of dermatophyte *Trichophyton vanbreuseghemii*
          *Arthroderma simii*—ascomycetous state of dermatophyte (?) *Trichophyton simii*
          *Allescheria boydii* (location ?)—ascomycetous state of *Monosporium apiospermum,* mycetoma
          *Emmonsiella capsulata*—ascomycetous state of *Histoplasma capsulatum,* histoplasmosis
          *Nannizzia cajetani*—ascomycetous state of dermatophyte (?) *Microsporum cookei*
          *Nannizzia fulva*—ascomycetous state of dermatophyte *Microsporum fulvum*
          *Nannizzia grubyia*—ascomycetous state of dermatophyte *Microsporum vanbreuseghemii*
          *Nannizzia gypsea*—ascomycetous state of dermatophyte *Microsporum gypseum*
          *Nannizzia incurvata*—ascomycetous state of dermatophyte *Microsporum gypseum* (same asexual state as above).
          *Nannizzia obtusa*—ascomycetous state of dermatophyte *Microsporum nanum*
          *Nannizzia persicolor*—ascomycetous state of dermatophyte *Microsporum persicolor*
        Eurotiaceae (Trichocomataceae?)
          *Sartorya fumigata* — ascomycetous state of *Aspergillus fumigatus,* aspergillosis
      Microascales (perithecium; asci at various levels, usually spheric, asci dissolving)
        Microascaceae
          *Microascus cinereus* — ascomycetous state of *Scopulariopsis cinerea.* Dermal. This genus placed by von Arx in
            Sphaeriales (see Muller & von Arx 1973).
          *Microascus manganii* — ascomycetous state of *Scopulariopsis albo-flavescens.* Dermal.
          *Microascus trigonosporus*—ascomycetous state of a *Scopulariopsis*
  Loculoascomycete (asci borne in locules of hollowed-out ascostroma; bitunicate ascus)
    *Leptosphaeria senegalenis.* Mycetoma
    *Neotestudina rosatii.* Mycetoma
    *Piedraia hortae.* Black piedra (tropical) nodules as ascostroma on hair
Deuteromycotina (asexual state, often, of ascomycetes; if sexual and asexual states are known, fungus will have two names with
  sexual name taking preference)
  Blastomycetes (asexual yeasts)
    Cryptococcaceae
      *Cryptococcus neoformans.* Cryptococcus. Asexual state of Basidiomycete *Filobasidiella neoformans.*
      *Pityrosporum* sp. (*Malassezia furfur*). In the stratum corneum; pityriasis versicolor
      *Candida albicans.* Candidiasis
      *Candida guilliermondii*
      *Candida parapsilosis*
      *Candida stellatoidea*
      *Candida tropicalis*
      *Trichosporon beigelii.* White piedra
      *Trichosporon cutaneum*

**TABLE 2.   Fungal Taxa That Cause Diseases of Man** (*Continued*)

*Geotrichum candidum* (white, moist colony but not a yeast—no buds). See below.
*Torulopsis glabrata.* Secondary invader
Hyphomycetes (filamentous, spores borne in open)
Moniliales
Moniliaceae (hyaline or light colored except for Aspergillus niger)
  Trichophyton (see also Arthroderma in Ascomycetes) dermatophyte
    *T. schoenleinii; T. rubrum; T. mentagrophytes; T. concentricum; T. verrucosum; T. violaceum; T. tonsurans; T. equinum; T. simii* (monkeys); *T. ajelloi* (?), *T. megninii*
  Microsporum (see also Nannizzia in Ascomycetes) dermatophyte
    *M. canis; M. gypseum; M. audouini; M. ferrugineum; M. fulvum; M. nanum; M. obtusa; M. vanbreuseghemii; M. persicolor; M. gallinae; M. distortum* (?); *M. cookei* (?)
  *Epidermophyton floccosum.* Dermatophyte
  *Geotrichum candidum* (wet, white growth with yeast-like arthrospores formed by fragmentation of hyphae
  *Cepahalosporium* (now *Acremonium*) mycetoma
  *Sporothrix schenkii* (white at first, becoming black with age) sporotrichosis (a yeast when growing in the body; hyphal otherwise)
  *Coccidioides immitis* (Phycomycete?) coccidioidomycosis. (Spherule in the body, hyphal otherwise)
  *Histoplasma capsulatum* (see Ascomycetes) (Yeast in the body; otherwise hyphal)
  *Blastomyces dermatitidis* (see Ascomycetes) (Yeast in the body; otherwise hyphal)
  *Paracoccidioides brasiliensis* (Chrysosporium?) (Yeast in the body; otherwise hyphal)
  *Penicillium commune.* Pulmonary
  *Aspergillus fumigatus* (see Ascomycetes) pulmonary, aspergillosis
  *Aspergillus niger.* Otomycosis, fungus balls
  *Scopulariopsis brevicaulis* (see Ascomycetes) in nails
  *Fusarium solani, F. oxysporum, F. nivale.* Keratitis
  *Madurella mycetomi, M. grisea.* Mycetoma
  *Monosporium apiospermum* (see Ascomycetes) mycetoma
Dematiaceae (hyphae black or black-green)
  *Cercospora apii* (also pathogen of celery and other crops) subcutaneous
  *Torula bantiana.* Banti's mycosis
  *Cladosporium carrionii*
  *Cladosporium trichoides.* Cladosporiosis
  *Cladosporium werneckii.* On hands
  *Curvularia lunata* and *C. geniculata.* Mycetoma
  Phialophora (at least one species pathogenic to both man and certain trees)
    *P. compacta* chromomycosis
    *P. dermatitidis* chromomycosis
    *P. gougerotii* phaeosporotrichosis
    *P. jeanselmei* mycetoma
    *P. parasitica.* subcutaneous
    *P. pedrosoi.* chromomycosis
    *P. repens.* mycetoma
    *P. richardsiae.* phaeosporotrichosis
    *P. spinifera.* granulomatous lesion
    *P. verrucosa.* chromomycosis
Coelomycetes (asexual spores in an enclosed pycnidium or on an acervulus)
Sphaeropsidales
  *Macrophoma* sp. keratitis
  *Pyrenochaeta romeroi.* Mycetoma
Loboa loboi (never cultured) Lobo's disease
*Prototheca zopfii.* Probably a fungus but may be an algal mutant

spheric asci are produced scattered throughout the ascocarp. Muller and von Arx (1973) place Microascus in the Sphaeriales to be considered below.

***Pyrenomycetes.*** This class houses those ascomycetes that produce oblong unitunicate asci in a perithecium that is an ascocarp containing an ostiole, or opening, at the top. Asci originate from one layer of cells rather than being distributed throughout the ascocarp as with Plectomycetes.

The spores are usually one celled. Some cleistothecial "analogs" or perithecial forms do exist, however. The ascospores of most pyrenomycetes are shot out of the ascus, but in a very few genera, such as Chaetomium and Melanospora, the asci dissolve and spores ooze out. Virtually all live on plant tissue or in the soil and probably none is a human pathogen if Microascus is considered to be a Plectomycete.

***Discomycetes.*** Cylindric unitunicate asci are

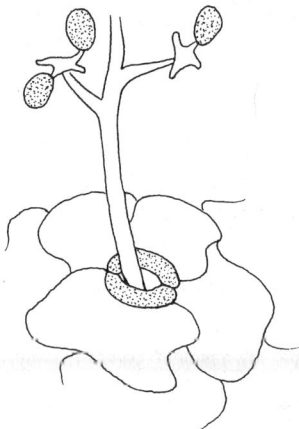

**FIGURE 4.** *Sporophore of a downy mildew protruding out of a stoma of an infected leaf.*

produced on, or supported on, an open saucer-like ascocarp, the apothecium (Table 1). None is known to be a human pathogen.

### Loculoascomycetes

Ascomycetes possessing bitunicate asci in the locule or cavity of a "hollowed-out" ascostroma are placed in this class (Luttrell, 1973). The asci are usually thick walled with an apical dimple and a distinct shoulder (Fig. 5). Ascopores are usually multiseptate and dark colored. *Testudina rosatti* causes mycetoma (Table 2) and *Piedraia hortae*, which grows as ascostroma on hair, causes black piedra.

### Laboulbeniomycetes

These are minute, nonmycelial ascomycetes that grow on the exoskeletons of insects. Benjamin (1973) reviews this unique group of fungi that may or may not be pathogens of insects and certain mites.

### *Basidiomycotina*

Basidiomycetes are those fungi that produce sexual spores, basidiospores, on a basidium (Table 1, Fig. 1). As with the ascus, nuclear fusion and meiosis takes place in this cell. Mating types occurring at one or two loci exist. These segregate as a result of meiosis, and the four basidiospores that are the direct product of meiosis contain the two or four different mating types. Germinated basidiospores are haploid and contain as a rule one nucleus per compartment. There are no sexual organs in the basidiomycetes (except rusts) and the nuclei differing in mating type are brought together as a result of fusion of hyphae derived from basidiospores of different mating types. These secondary hyphae usually contain two nuclei per compartment. The perforated septa dividing the coenocytic mycelium into compartments often possess ornamentations that distinguish them from the simple septa of the ascomycetes.

### Teliomycetes

This class unites basidiomycetes not having basidiocarps. The plant pathogens, rusts and smuts, and the sexual stage of *Cryptococcus neoformans* and *Filobasidiella neoformans* are members of this class.

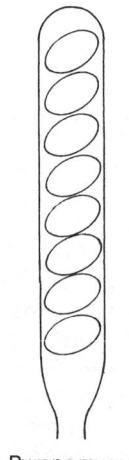
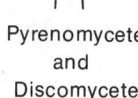
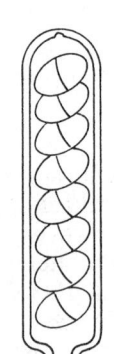

**FIGURE 5.** *Asci and ascospores.*

Plectomycete       Pyrenomycete        Loculoascomycete
                      and
                   Discomycete

## Hymenomycetes

Mushrooms (Fig. 1; Table 1) and other fleshy basidiomycetes bearing basidia on gills, pores, smooth surfaces, or spines are allocated to this class. In all cases, spores are shot off of the basidium.

## Gasteromycetes

Basidiomycetes producing spores that are not shot off are placed in this class. Basidia are contained within an enclosed basidiocarp, such as that of the puffball (Table 1).

### *Deuteromycotina*

The Class Deuteromycotina (Fungi Imperfecti) unites those fungi producing asexual spores or no spores at all. As indicated earlier, many are now known to produce sexual spores under conditions such as certain environmental conditions or presence of two mating types, and such fungi are assigned two names. Most fungi observed growing on Petri plate cultures will be Deuteromycotina or Zygomycotina. Probably the vast majority of Fungi Imperfecti are ascomycetes or were derived from ascomycetes. The pathogenic yeast *Cryptococcus neoformans* and the yeast *Candida scottii* along with a few others are asexual yeasts of basidiomycetes, however.

## Blastomycetes

Asexual yeasts are placed in this class. There are approximately 17 genera of asexual yeasts, 17 genera of ascomycete yeasts, and five genera of basidiomycete yeasts (Kreger-van Rij, 1973). This publication provides keys to genera of all yeasts. Identification keys are also given in the following publications (Lodder, 1970; Barnett and Pankhurst 1974; and DeHoog, 1977).

## Hyphomycetes

Most Fungi Imperfecti observed in the laboratory are members of this class, which embraces those asexual fungi producing spores on hyphae not contained within sporocarps (Table 1). Approximately 595 genera are recognized in the latest treatment (Kendrick and Carmichael, 1973). They do not assign genera to families and they base their classification of genera on four properties: 1) Saccardoan spore group, which indicates shape and number of compartments of the spore, 2) arrangement of conidia, 3) color of conidia, and 4) type of conidiogenous cell.

The Hyphomycetes can be divided into five form families: Moniliaceae — mycelia and spores colorless or bright colored (except for the black *Asper-*

*gillus niger,* which otherwise conforms to the characteristics of the moniliaceous Aspergillus); Dematiaceae — mycelia and spores black, dark green or dark brown; Stilbaceae — conidiophores united into vertical fascicles called synnemata or coremia; Tuberculariaceae — sporophores borne on an acervulus-like cushion of hyphae infecting a plant; Mycelia Sterilia — spores not produced.

*Aspergillus flavus* and *Aspergillus fumigatus* cause pulmonary diseases and are unique in being the only non-Zygomycete fungi that grow deep in tissue in mycelial rather than yeast form. The asexual forms of the dermatophytes are also placed in the Moniliaceae or Hyphomycetes. Dark-spored Phialophora and Cladosporium are dematiaceous fungi.

## Coelomycetes

Those fungi producing asexual spores in an enclosed sporocarp, the pycnidium, or in the cushion-like structure, the acervulus, are placed in this class (Table 1). There are approximately 500 genera (Sutton, 1973). *Macrophoma* sp. and *Pyrenochaeta romeroi* cause diseases in man.

## *HABITAT OF HUMAN PATHOGENIC FUNGI*

Fungal diseases can be divided into systemic mycoses, subcutaneous mycoses, and superficial mycoses. Of those causing systemic mycoses and subcutaneous mycoses (histoplasmosis, coccidioidomycosis, sporotrichosis, blastomycosis, aspergillosis, and candidiasis), only *Candida albicans*, the causal agent of candidiasis, normally lives in man. The rest live in soil or on plant products. Some of the dermatophytes live in soil and it is now believed (Emmons et al., 1977) that some of the dermatophytes have become so well adapted to man that they now normally live on him. This conclusion is based on the observation that some of the human dermatophytes have not been isolated from soil. Ainsworth (1968a) discusses the fungi parasitizing vertebrates.

### References

Ainsworth, G.C.: Fungal parasites of vertebrates. In Ainsworth, G.C., and Sussman, A.S. (eds): The Fungi. Volume III. New York, Academic Press, 1968a, p. 211.

Ainsworth, G.C.: The number of fungi. In Ainsworth, G.C., and Sussman, A.S. (eds): The Fungi. Volume III. New York, Academic Press, 1968b, p. 505.

Ainsworth, G.C.: The Dictionary of Fungi. 7th ed. Kew, Surrey, England, Commonwealth Mycological Institute, 1971.

Barnett, J.A., and Pankhurst, R.J.: A new key to the yeasts. A key for identifying yeasts based on physiological tests only. Amsterdam, North Holland Publishers, 1974.

Benjamin, R.K.: Laboulbeniomycetes. In Ainsworth, G.C., Sparrow, F.K., and Sussman, A.S. (eds): The Fungi. Volume IVA. New York, Academic Press, 1973, p. 223.

DeHoog, G.S., and Hermanides-Nijhof, E.J.: The black yeasts and allied genera. Baarn, Holland, Centraalbureau voor Schimmelcultures, 1977.

Emmons, C.W., Binford, C.H., Utz, J.P., and Kwon-Chung, K.J.: Medical Mycology. 3rd ed. Philadelphia, Lea & Febiger, 1977.

Hesseltine, C.W., and Ellis, J.J.: Mucorales. In Ainsworth, G.C., Sparrow, F.K., and Sussman, A.S. (eds): The Fungi. Volume IVB. New York, Academic Press, 1973, p. 187.

Kendrick, W.B., and Carmichael, J.W.: Hyphomycetes. In Ainsworth, G.C. Sparrow, F.K., and Sussman, A.S. (eds): The Fungi. Volume IVA. New York, Academic Press, 1973, p. 323.

Kreger-van Rij, N.J.W.: Endomycetales, basidiomycetous yeasts and related fungi. In Ainsworth, G.C., Sparrow, F.K., and Sussman, A.S. (eds): The Fungi. Volume IVA. New York, Academic Press, 1973, p. 11.

Lodder, J. (ed): The yeasts, a taxonomic study. Amsterdam, North Holland press, 1970.

Luttrell, E.S.: Loculoascomycetes. In Ainsworth, G.C., Sparrow, F.K., and Sussman, A.S. (eds): The Fungi. Volume IVA. New York, Academic Press, 1973, p. 135.

Martin, G.W., and Alexopoulos, C.J.: The Myxomycetes. Iowa City, The University of Iowa Press, 1969.

Muller, E., and von Arx, J.A.: Pyrenomycetes. In Ainsworth, G.C., Sparrow, F.K., and Sussman, A.S. (eds): The Fungi. Volume IVA. New York, Academic Press, 1973.

Sutton, B.C.: Coelomycetes. In Ainsworth, G.C., Sparrow, F.K., and Sussman, A.S. (eds): The Fungi. Volume IVA. New York, Academic Press, 1973, p. 513.

Taber, W.A., and Taber, R.A.: The Impact of Fungi on Man. Boulder, Col., Educational Programs Improvement Corporation, 1967.

Taber, W.A., and Taber, R.A.: Ascomycetes. In Lechevalier, H.A., and Laskin, A.I. (eds): Handbook of Microbiology. 2nd ed. West Palm Beach, Fl., CRC Press, 1978, p. 97.

# 15　FUNGAL TOXINS

## Makoto Enomoto, M.D.

*Mycotoxicosis* is a disease caused by fungal toxins (mycotoxins), and should be distinguished from *mycosis* caused by opportunistic infections of fungi. Fungi include mushrooms, molds, mildews, blights, rusts, and yeasts. Generally, fungi are valued for the organic fermentation they produce and as a source of many antibiotics. In addition, edible mushroms are used as human food. Toxin-producing fungi were occasionally encountered during exploration for antibiotics, but were given little attention. Except for griseofulvin, cancer production was usually found in animals only after parenteral administration of antibiotics, including mitomycin C, streptozotocin, penicillin G, azaserine, daunomycin, elaiomycin, and actinomycin D, L, and S. The hepatocarcinogenicity of griseofulvin was proved in mice by the oral administration of a daily dosage of 5000 to 10,000 ppm. In the bone marrow and small intestine there was no tumor, but cytotoxicity was observed in rats given a high dose of griseofulvin.

### MUSHROOM POISONS

Mycotoxicoses known to be related to human disease are shown in Table 1. Among them are ergotism and mushroom poisoning *(mycetismus)*, which are known in many countries. The poisonous principles of mushrooms of the genus Amanita are cell-destroying cyclic peptides, such as hepatotoxic "phalloidin" and "amanitin," each representing two groups of lethal sulfur-containing cyclopeptides, the phallotoxins and amatoxins. The phallotoxins act on the endoplasmic reticulum of liver cells, whereas the amatoxins act on the nucleus. After the isolation from *Amanita muscaria* of muscarine, which excites the parasympathetic nervous system, centrally active substances of isoxazole type, like "muscimol," "ibotenic acid," and "tricholomic acid," have been discovered in it and in other mushrooms (Wieland, 1968).

### ERGOT

Widespread epidemics of ergotism, popularly known as St. Anthony's fire, were caused by a fungus, *Claviceps purpura,* infecting rye and other cereal grains during the Middle Ages. When ingested, the ergotized grain produced either cardiovascular effects, such as vasoconstriction and gangrenous symptoms, or neurologic changes, including convulsions and confusion. It is an interesting fact that the ravages of ergotism during the Middle Ages in Europe were largely alleviated by the introduction of new dietary staples such as potatoes and maize.

The first chemically pure alkaloid exhibiting the typical biologic properties of ergot was named ergotamine by Stoll and Hofmann (1970). Ergot alkaloid is a highly variable mixture. The ergot alkaloids have been used as therapeutic agents because of their ability to cause vasoconstriction and contraction of the uterus, and to affect the central nervous system. One of the alkaloids, lysergic acid diethylamide (LSD), is a well-known prototype of hallucinogens.

## TABLE 1. Mycotoxicosis in Man

| DISEASE (Date of outbreaks) | LOCATION (Reported) | FUNGAL TOXINS | SPECIES OF FUNGUS | SYMPTOMS |
|---|---|---|---|---|
| Mushroom poisoning (sporadic) | Distributed | Phallotoxin, Amatoxin | Amanita (A. phalloides, verna, bisporigera, tenuifolia, A. muscaria) | Vomiting, diarrhea, jaundice |
| | | Muscarin | | Hallucination, excites parasympathic nervous system |
| Ergotism, "St. Anthony's fire" (Middle Ages) | Central Europe, U.S.A., India | Ergot alkaloids (ergotamine, ergostine, lysergic acid derivative) | Claviceps purpurea, pasali | Lassitude, muscular pain, gangrenous symptoms, convulsion, confusion |
| Alimentary toxic aleukia or specific angina (1913, 1942–1955) | USSR, Japan | Trichothecenes | Fusaria (F. poae, sporotrichoides, tricinctum, graminearum, etc.) Cephalosporium, Trichothecium, Stachybotrys, Myrothecium, Trichoderma | Vomiting, diarrhea, fever, hemorrhagic rash, necrotic angina, leukopenia, sepsis, etc. |
| Onyalai (1904–1975) | Africa | Not determined | Phoma sorghina | Hemorrhagic bullae in the mouth, thrombocytopenia |
| Aflatoxicosis | Africa, India, Thailand | Aflatoxins | Aspergillus flavus, parasiticus | Edema, anorexia, abdominal pain and distention (ascites), jaundice, Reye's syndrome (Thai children) |
| Luteoskyrin poisoning | Japan* | Luteoskyrin | Penicillium islandicum, Mycelia Sterilia | Anorexia, edema, jaundice |

*Accidental case

## CARCINOGENIC MYCOTOXINS

Mycotoxicosis received attention in recent years upon discovery of a number of carcinogenic mycotoxins contaminating human and animal foods. The infrequent reports of human intoxication attributable to fungal toxins in foods may be explained by the absence of dramatic acute effects. Acute mycotoxicosis is common in livestock, fish, birds, and experimental animals that eat moldy feed polluted by mycotoxins. A series of outbreaks of unexplained hemorrhage and/or hepatic injury in domestic animals and "spontaneous" hepatic tumors in hatchery-raised fish and laboratory animals resulted from mycotoxin contamination of feed. Of major importance in this regard is a group of hepatocarcinogenic aflatoxins produced by *Aspergillus flavus* (Detroy et al., 1971; Butler, 1974). Luteoskyrin and cyclochloritine isolated from culture of *Penicillium islandicum* were also shown to be responsible for acute hepatic damage, cirrhosis, and tumors of the liver in mice and rats. The type of injury depended on the amount of mold metabolites produced (Uraguchi, 1971; Enomoto and Ueno, 1974). Table 2 shows the animals susceptible to both the carcinogenic and the toxic actions of several important mycotoxins.

The *aflatoxins* are a group of secondary metabolites produced by *Aspergillus flavus* and *A. parasiticus*. They are a mixture of chemically related compounds, derivatives of difuranocoumarin. Aflatoxins $B_2$ and $G_2$ are dihydro derivatives of the parent aflatoxins $B_1$ and $G_1$. Aflatoxins $P_1$, $M_1$, and $Q_1$ are hydroxylated derivatives of aflatoxin $B_1$. Aflatoxin $M_1$ has been recovered from milk, feces, and urine of various mammals, including humans who ingested aflatoxin $B_1$. In monkeys and chickens, conjugates of aflatoxin $P_1$ have been detected in the urine in addition to $M_1$. Aflatoxin $B_1$ is the most potent carcinogen, followed by $G_1$, $B_2$, and $M_1$ in order of decreasing carcinogenic potency.

Aflatoxin $B_1$ suppresses synthesis of DNA, RNA, and protein and inhibits the polymerase in rat liver cells. These changes are reflected in the segregation of nucleolar granules and fibrils, capping of the nucleolus, and disruption of the cytoplasmic rough endoplasmic reticulum in liver cells. Aflatoxin $B_1$ also causes increased activity of DNase and other lysosomal enzymes in the liver or pancreas of rats. The active metabolite is thought to be an epoxide such as $B_1$-2,3-epoxide.

*Sterigmatocystin* was first isolated from a culture of *Aspergillus versicolor* and was also found to be a metabolite of *A. nidulans* and Bipolaris species. Sterigmatocystin is a derivative of difurano-xanthone and has a difuranmethoxy-benzene ring in its structure, just as aflatoxins have. Consequently, these two mycotoxins can be derived from a common intermediary in their biosynthesis (Van der Watt, 1974). Sterigmatocystin is carcinogenic to the rat and newborn mouse. A high incidence of liver cell carcinoma was observed in rats surviving a dose of 0.75, or 1.5 to 2.25 mg/rat/day (Van der Watt, 1974; Fujii et al., 1976). The relatively high carcinogenic potency of sterigmatocystin and the wider distribution of this mycotoxin in Japan and South Africa suggest that it may present a more formidable danger than aflatoxins. The metabolic fate of sterigmatocystin in mammals is unknown. The biologic activity of derivatives of sterigmatocystin has not been extensively studied, but O-acetylsterigmatocystin is more toxic and carcinogenic than sterigmatocystin (Terao, 1977). Various derivatives of sterigmatocystin are mutagenic for bacteria, including sterigmatocystin itself, demethylsterigmatocystin, stergmatin, O-acetylsterigmatocystin, 6, 8-dimethylversicolin A and B, 5-methoxysterigmatocystin, and versicolin A.

*Luteoskyrin* and *rugulosin* are anthraquinone pigments. Both induce acute hepatic centrilobular toxic lesions in mice and rats and liver cell adenoma or carcinoma in mice. Rugulosin has less carcinogenic activity than luteoskyrin, but rugulosin is produced by a number of common contaminants of foodstuffs, such as *Penicillium rugulosum, P. brunneum,* and *P. tardum* (Enomoto and Ueno, 1974).

## MYCOTOXINS AND HUMAN LIVER CANCER

Data from Thailand, Kenya, Mozambique, and Swaziland provide strong circumstantial evidence of a causal relationship between aflatoxin ingestion and liver cancer incidence in man (Wogan, 1976). The evidence for human aflatoxicosis has also been increasing. Outbreaks of hepatitis in both man and dogs in West India were traced to consumption of spoiled maize heavily contaminated with *Aspergillus flavus*. Aflatoxins were detected in these contaminated samples and in serum samples of a few patients (Krishnamachari et al., 1975). The symptoms of high fever and rapidly progressive jaundice and ascites and the morphologic changes in the liver suggested toxic hepatitis. There was centrilobular scarring with varying degrees of occlusion of the hepatic veins, severe cholangiolar proliferation with cholestasis, and syncytial giant cells of liver-cell origin (Tandon et al., 1977). In Thai children afla-

TABLE 2.   Mycotoxins Known to Produce Cancer in
Animals by Oral Administration

| CARCINOGENIC MYCOTOXIN | ANIMAL SPECIES SUSCEPTIBLE TO BOTH THE CARCINOGENIC AND TOXIC EFFECTS (target organs) | REGULAR* DOSAGE (ppm in diet) | ANIMAL SPECIES SENSITIVE ONLY TO THE TOXIC EFFECTS |
|---|---|---|---|
| Aflatoxin $B_1$ | Rat (liver, kidney, colon); trout, duck, guppy, ferret, newborn mouse, salmon, monkey, marmoset (liver); sheep (liver, nose) | 0.5–1.5 (rat) | Turkey, mink, cattle, guinea-pig, swine, dog, hamster, rabbit, pheasant, quail, chicken, cat, frog |
| Aflatoxin $G_1$ | Rat (liver, kidney); duck (liver) | 1–3 (rat) | |
| Aflatoxin $B_2$ | Rat, duck (liver) | | |
| Aflatoxin $M_1$ | Rat, trout (liver) | | Duckling |
| Sterigmatocystin† | Rat, velvet monkey, newborn mouse (liver) | 10–50 (rat) | Guinea pig |
| Luteoskyrin | Mouse, rat (liver) | 30–100 (mouse) | Rabbit, chicken, monkey |
| Rugulosin | Mouse (liver) | 200 (mouse) | Rat |
| Griseofulvin | Mouse (liver) | 5000–10,000 (mouse) | Rat |

*Oral carcinogenic dosage per day in the representative animal shown in parentheses.
†O-Acetylsterigmatocystin is more carcinogenic than sterigmatocystin in rats. Hepatocellular carcinomas were produced in 53 per cent of rats fed 10 ppm O-acetylsterigmatocystin for 52 weeks.
(From Enomoto, M.: Carcinogenicity of mycotoxin. In Uraguchi, K., and Yamayaki, M. (eds): Toxicology, Biochemistry and Pathology of Mycotoxins. Tokyo, Kodansha International, Ltd., 1977.)

toxin presents the picture of Reye's syndrome, i.e., fatty liver and encephalopathy (Shank et al., 1971). The chronic and carcinogenic effect of aflatoxins in man is potentially more important than acute toxicosis but is difficult to prove. Aflatoxin has been detected in human urine, milk, biopsy specimens of liver, and autopsied liver or other tissues by improved chemical methods of aflatoxin analysis (Pong et al., 1974) or immunoassay with antibody against aflatoxin $B_1$. Yet its role in neoplastic transformation of the liver is not proved by its presence in liver tissue any more than that of viruses that are frequently found in human livers with carcinomas.

In evaluating the danger from fungal toxins after long-term exposure, one must take into account the fact that experimental evidence linking cirrhosis and liver cancer has not been convincing, especially with respect to aflatoxins or sterigmatocystin. Liver cirrhosis and cancer were consistently associated with high incidence rates only in rats and mice fed moldy rice infested with *Penicillium islandicum*. The metabolites of this fungus contain both hepatocarcinogenic luteos-

kyrin and cirrhogenic cyclochlorotine (Miyake et al., 1960; Enomoto and Ueno, 1974). These facts suggest that in man liver cirrhosis itself is attributable to the combined effects of other factors, such as hepatitis virus, cirrhogenic mycotoxin, or nutritional agents. Further studies are needed to give definitive evidence of the relationship between liver cell cancer and carcinogenic mycotoxins other than aflatoxins. If prevention of mycotoxin contamination in human foodstuffs results in a decrease in human liver cancer it would be convincing evidence for the positive role of carcinogenic mycotoxins in human carcinogenesis (Fig. 1).

## ALIMENTARY TOXIC ALEUKIA (ATA)

Alimentary toxic aleukia has been endemic in Siberia and the Amur region of the U.S.S.R. since 1913. The causal agents are the Fusarium species, which grow on overwintered moldy cereals and other crops and produce burning sensations of the mouth, anorexia, vomiting, and diarrhea

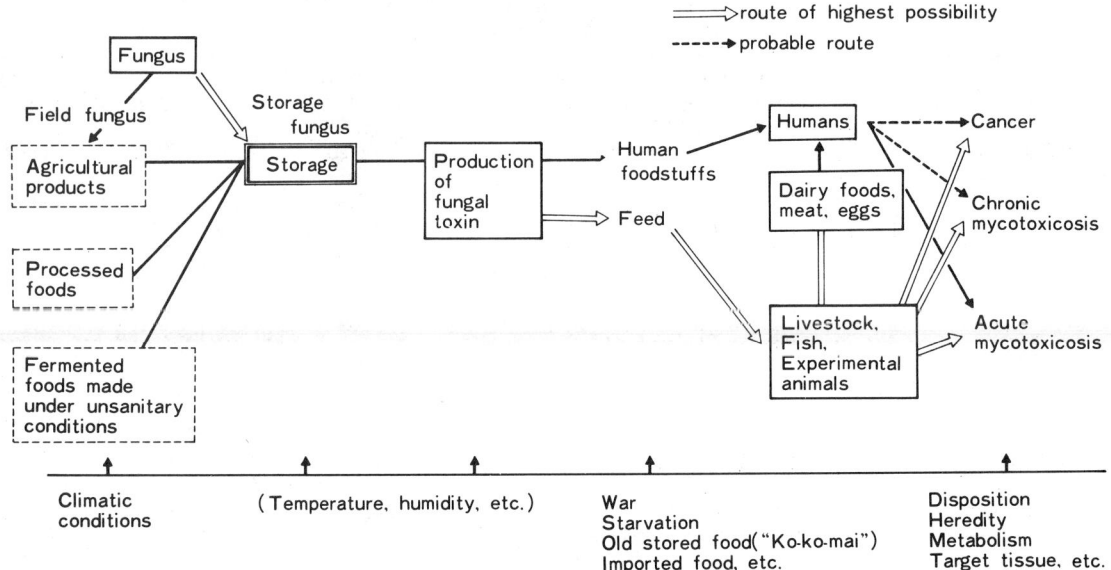

**FIGURE 1.** *Mycotoxin-induced diseases of man and animals: related conditions and causal relationships. (After Enomoto, M.: In Yamamura, Y., and Sugimura, T., (eds.): Cancer. Vol. 15. Tokyo, Iwanami Shoten, 1976. [Japanese].)*

(Stage I), followed by depression of all bone marrow and thrombopoiesis (Stage II). Fever, hemorrhagic rash, bleeding from gums and nose, necrotic angina, extreme leukopenia, and agranulocytosis with general sepsis occur in the final stage (Stage III) (Joffe, 1971). Death occurs six to eight weeks after ingestion of large amounts of toxin. Skin testing is reliable for toxic assay of overwintered grains. The only prophylactic measure against ATA is the elimination of polluted grain from food.

After the isolation of diacetoxyscirpenol from *Fusarium scirpi*, a number of trichothecene compounds, including T2-toxin, trichothecolon, nivalenol, fusarenon-X, verrucarin A, roridin A, and neosolaniol, have been isolated from imperfect fungi, including Cephalosporium, Fusarium, Trichoderma, Myrothecium, and Stachybotrys species (Bamburg and Strong, 1971; Smalley and Strong, 1974). At present these trichothecenes are considered to be responsible for human ATA because of their characteristic biologic activities in animals. Mice exhibit decreased activity shortly after administration of these trichothecene samples, followed by diarrhea, loss of reaction against skin stimulation, lowered body temperature, and lethargy. The animals usually die from 12 to 72 hours after administration of toxins. Histologic examination revealed marked cytotoxic changes in tissues with actively dividing cells, such as the mucosa of the gastrointestinal tract,

lymph follicles, thymus, and bone marrow (Saito et al., 1969, 1974).

## ONYALAI

Onyalai is an acute purpuric disease endemic in Africa since 1904. It is attributed to the mycotoxin of *Phoma sorghina* isolated from millet and grain sorghum (Rabie et al., 1975).

## CARDIAC BERIBERI

Acute cardiac beriberi was an enigmatic toxic disease prevalent in Japan until 1950. Many patients still suffer from this disease in Southeast Asia. Although the disease is considered a vitamin B$_1$ deficiency, Japanese investigators attribute it to a fungal toxin of rice and other staple foods. Citroviridin isolated from *Penicillium citroviride* Biourge causes an acute poisoning in the cat and monkey, characterized primarily by an ascending paralysis like that in human beriberi (Uraguchi, 1971; Ueno, 1974). Cardiac damage occurs in mice given xanthoascin (Takahashi et al., 1976) from *Aspergillus candidus*, a frequent contaminant of human foodstuffs in Southeast Asia. Cardiac muscle undergoes vacuolar degeneration and necrosis followed by cardiac dilatation (Ohtsubo et al., 1976).

# References

Bamburg, J. R., and Strong, F. M.: 12,13-Epoxytrichothecenes. In Kadis, S., Ciegler, A., and Ajl, S. J. (eds.): Microbial Toxins. Vol. 7. New York, Academic Press, 1971, p. 207.

Butler, W. H.: Aflatoxin. In Purchase, I. F. H. (ed.): Mycotoxins. Amsterdam, Elsevier Scientific Publishing Company, 1974, p. 1.

Detroy, R. W., Lillehoj, E. B., and Ciegler, A.: Aflatoxin and related compounds. In Ciegler, A., Kadis, S., and Ajl, S. J. (eds.): Microbial Toxins. Vol. 6. New York, Academic Press, 1971, p. 4.

Enomoto, M.: Carcinogenicity of mycotoxin. In Uraguchi, K., and Yamazaki, M. (eds.): Toxicology, Biochemistry and Pathology of Mycotoxins. Tokyo, Kodansha International, Ltd., 1977, p. 239.

Enomoto, M., Mabuchi, M., Miyata, K., Naoe, S., Takada, N., and Yamazaki, M.: Development of liver cell carcinoma in rats fed toxic rice culture *(Aspergillus versicolor)* containing 1 ppm of sterigmatocystin. St Marianna Med J 5:101, 1977.

Enomoto, M., and Ueno, I.: *Penicillium islandicum* (toxic yellowed rice) — luteoskyrin-islanditoxin-cyclochlorotine. In Purchase, I. F. H. (ed.): Mycotoxins. Amsterdam, Elsevier Scientific Publishing Company, 1974, p. 303.

Fujii, K., Kurata, H., Odashima, N., and Hatsuda, Y.: Tumor induction by a single subcutaneous injection of sterigmatocystin in newborn mice. Cancer Res 36:1615, 1976.

Joffe, A. Z.: Alimentary toxic aleukia. In Kadis, S., Ciegler, A., and Ajl, S. J. (eds.): Microbial Toxins. Vol. 7. New York, Academic Press, 1971, p. 139.

Krishnamachari, K. A. V., Baht, R. T., Nagarajan, V., and Tilak, T. B. G.: Hepatitis due to aflatoxicosis. Lancet 1:1061, 1975.

Miyake, M., Saito, M., Enomoto, M., Shikata, T., Ishiko, T., Uraguchi K., Sakai, F., Tatsuno, T., Tsukioka, M., and Sakai, F.: Toxic liver injuries and liver cirrhosis induced in mice and rats through long term feeding with *Penicillium islandicum* Sopp-growing rice. Acta Path Jap 10:75, 1960.

Ohtsubo, K., Horiuchi, T., Hatanaka, Y., and Saito, M.: Hepato- and cardiotoxicity of xanthoascin, a new metabolite of *A. candidus* Link, to mice. Japan J Exp Med 46:277, 1976.

Pong, R. T. L., Husaini, and Karyadi, D.: Aflatoxin and primary hepatic cancer in Indonesia. Presented at the V World Congress of Gastroenterology, 1974.

Rabie, C. G., Van Rensburg, S. J., Van der Watt, J. J., and Lübben, A.: Onyalai — the possible involvement of a mycotoxin produced by *Phoma sorghina* in the aetiology. S A Med J 49:1647, 1975.

Richer, C., Paccalin, J., Larcebeau, S., Faugeres, J., Morard, J-L, and Lamant, M.: Présence d'aflatoxine B₁ dans le foie humain. Biologie Générale 223, 1975.

Saito, M., Enomoto, M., and Tatsuno, T.: Radiomimetic biologic properties of the new scirpenol metabolites of *Fusarium nivale*. Gan 60:599, 1969.

Saito, M., and Ohtsubo, K.: Trichothecene toxins of *Fusarium* species. In Purchase, I. F. H. (ed.): Mycotoxins. Amsterdam, Elsevier Scientific Publishing Company, 1974, p. 263.

Shank, R. C., Bourgeois, C. H., Keshamra, N., and Cahndavimol, P.: Aflatoxins in autopsy specimens from Thai children with an acute disease of unknown aetiology. Food Cosmet Toxicol 9:501, 1971.

Smalley, E. B., and Strong, F. M.: Toxic trichothecenes. In Purchase, I. F. H. (ed): Mycotoxins. Amsterdam, Elsevier Scientific Publishing Company, 1974, p. 199.

Stoll, A., and Hofmann, A.: The chemistry of ergot alkaloids. In Pelletier, S. W. (ed.): Chemistry of the Alkaloids. New York, Van Nostrand Reinhold, 1970, p. 267.

Takahashi, C., Yoshihira, K., Natori, S., and Umeda, M.: Xanthoascin, a new metabolite isolated from *Aspergillus candidus*. Chem Pharm Bull 24:613, 1976.

Tandon, B. N., Krishnamurthy, L., Koshy, A., Tandon, H. D., Ramalingaswami, V., Mathur, M. M., and Mathur, P. D: Study of an epidemic of jaundice, presumably due to toxic hepatitis, in Northwest India. Gastroenterology 72:488, 1977.

Terao, K., and Ueno, Y.: Morphological and functional damage to cells and tissues. In Uraguchi, K., and Yamazaki, M. (eds.): Toxicology, Biochemistry and Pathology of Mycotoxins. Tokyo, Kodansha International, Ltd., 1977, p. 189.

Ueno, Y.: Citrioviridin from *Penicillium citreo-viride* Biourage. In Purchase, I. F. H. (ed.): Mycotoxins. Amsterdam, Elsevier Scientific Publishing Company, 1974, p. 283.

Uraguchi, K.: Pharmacology of mycotoxins. In Raskova, H. (ed.): International Encyclopedia of Pharmacology and Therapeutics. Section 71. Oxford, Permagon, 1971, p. 143.

Van der Watt, J. J.: Sterigmatocystin. In Purchase, I. F. H. (ed.): Mycotoxins. Amsterdam, Elsevier Scientific Publishing Company, 1974, p. 369.

Wieland, T.: Poisonous principles of mushrooms of the genus Amanita. Science 159:946, 1968.

Wogan, G. N.: The induction of liver cell cancer by chemicals. In Cameron, H. M., Linsell, D. A., and Warwick, G. P. (eds.): Liver Cell Cancer. Amsterdam, Elsevier Scientific Publishing Company, 1976, p. 121.

# Parasitology

# **16** *CLASSIFICATION AND ANATOMY OF PARASITES*

## *D. L. Lee, B.Sc., Ph.D.*

The parasites that will be mentioned in this chapter belong to the Protozoa, Platyhelminthes, Nematoda, and Acanthocephala.

# PHYLUM PROTOZOA

The Protozoa are regarded as a phylum within the animal kingdom but consist of a single cell, unlike the rest of the animal kingdom, in which the cells are grouped to form tissues and organs. The taxonomic position of the Protozoa is controversial, but the most commonly accepted scheme is that proposed by the Society of Protozoologists, as modified by Baker in 1973. Those groups that contain parasites of man are given below.

## *SUBPHYLUM I. SARCOMASTIGOPHORA*

Locomotor organs are flagella, pseudopodia, or both.

## Superclass 1.  Mastigophora (The Flagellates)

One or more flagella present on trophozoite; asexual reproduction by binary fission; sexual reproduction unknown in many groups. Free-living and parasitic classes.

### *Class Zoomastigophorea*

***Order Kinetoplastida.*** One to four flagella; kinetoplast.

SUBORDER TRYPANOSOMATINA.  One flagellum, free or attached to body by undulating membrane (Fig. 1); all species parasitic (*Trypanosoma, Leishmania*).

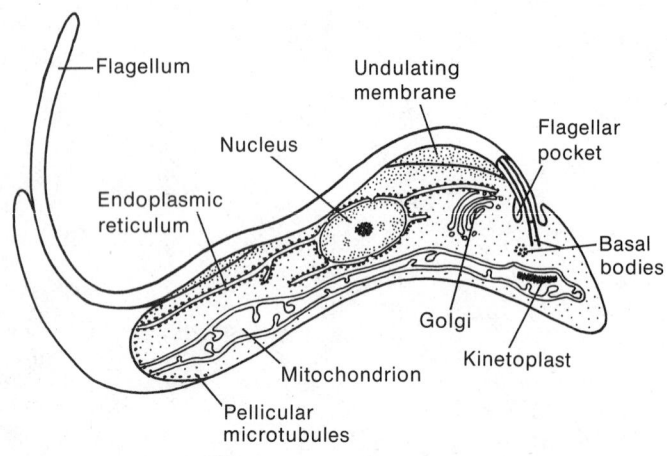

**FIGURE 1.** *Diagram to show the internal structure of a* Trypanosoma *species, as revealed by electron microscopy. Note the elongate mitochondrion with tubular cristae, the undulating membrane and the kinetoplast.*

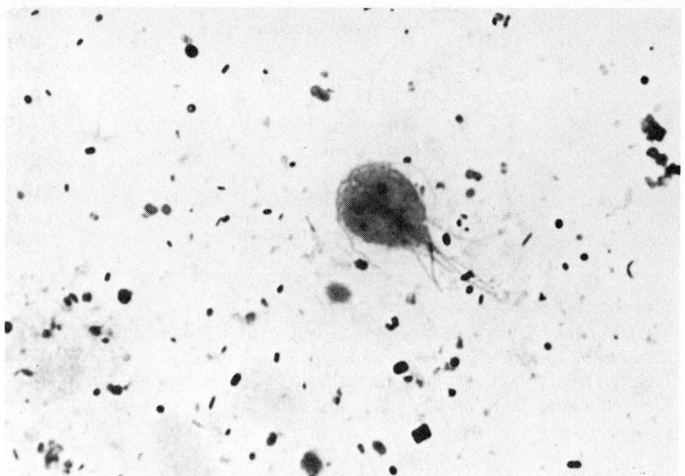

**FIGURE 2.** *Photomicrograph of* Giardia. *Note the two nuclei and four pairs of flagella.*

***Order Retortamonadida.*** One to four flagella, one runs posteriorly and is associated with a cytostome; harmless parasites of man (*Retortamonas, Chilomastix*).

***Order Diplomonadida.*** Four pairs of flagella; body bilaterally symmetric; two similar nuclei (*Giardia*) (Fig. 2).

***Order Trichomonadida.*** Four to six flagella, one trailing and associated with undulating membrane if present; axostyle and parabasal body; no cystic stage (*Trichomonas, Pentatrichomonas*) (Fig. 3).

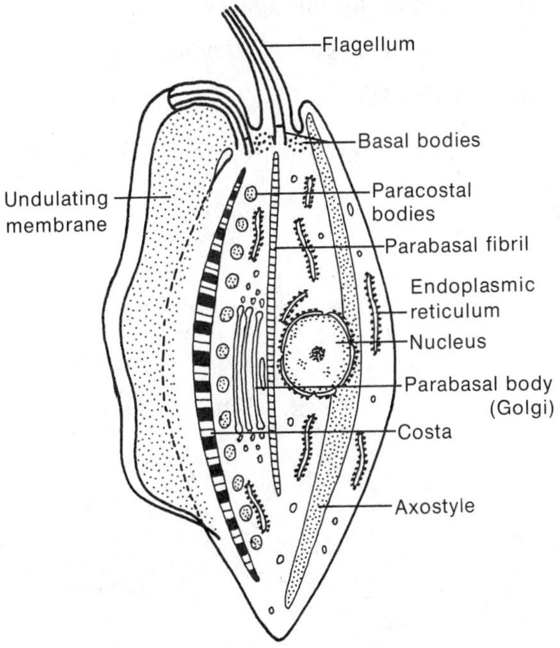

## Superclass 2.  Opalinata

Parasites of amphibia, fish, and snakes; numerous cilia in rows over body; two to many nuclei of one type.

## Superclass 3.  Sarcodina

The amebae; locomotion by means of pseudopodia.

### Class Rhizopodea

#### Subclass Lobosia

Pseudopodia broad and blunt (lobopods), rarely long and thin (filiform).

***Order Amoebida.*** Naked; single nucleus; multiply by binary fission; many produce resistant cysts (*Entamoeba, Hartmanella, Naegleria*) (Fig. 4).

## SUBPHYLUM II.  SPOROZOA

Produce simple spores containing one to many sporozoites (Fig. 5); cilia and flagella absent except on microgametes of some; single nucleus.

### Class 1.  Telosporea

Reproduction sexual and asexual; spores and sporozoites usually present; move by gliding or flexing body.

Flagellum

Basal bodies

Paracostal bodies

Parabasal fibril

Endoplasmic reticulum

Nucleus

Parabasal body (Golgi)

Costa

Axostyle

Undulating membrane

**FIGURE 3.** *Diagram to show the internal structure of a Trichomonas species as revealed by electron microscopy. Note the various rodlike structures (costa, parabasal fibril, axostyle), the anterior flagella (4 in* Trichomonas vaginalis*), the recurrent flagellum, which is associated with the undulating membrane, and the lack of mitochondria.*

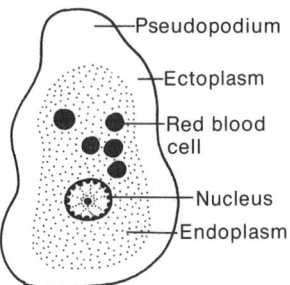

**FIGURE 4.** *Diagram to show the structure of a trophozoite of Entamoeba histolytica as revealed by light microscopy. Note the ingested red blood cells, the characteristic appearance of the nucleus, the ectoplasm, and the endoplasm.*

## Subclass Coccidia

Mature trophozoites are intracellular parasites.

*Order Eucoccidia.* Schizogony (a type of asexual reproduction) present; asexual and sexual phases in life cycle; parasitic in epithelial and blood cells of vertebrates and invertebrates.

SUBORDER EIMERIINA. Micro- and macrogam-

etes develop independently (no syzygy); zygote nonmotile; oocyst present; sporozoites (Fig. 5) enclosed in sporocyst. (*Eimeria, Isospora, Toxoplasma.*)

SUBORDER HAEMOSPORINA. Micro- and macrogamete develop independently (no syzygy); zygote motile; oocyst present; sporozoites naked; schizogony in vertebrate host and sporogony in invertebrate host (*Plasmodium, Haemoproteus, Hepatocystis*) (Fig. 6).

### Class 2.  Piroplasmea

No spores; small, nonpigmented parasites of erythrocytes of vertebrates, occasionally in other cells; transmitted by an invertebrate host, usually a tick.

*Order Piroplasmida.* (*Babesia, Theileria.*)

## SUBPHYLUM III.  CNIDOSPORA

Spores possess one or more polar filaments; parasites of fish and invertebrates, including the protozoa.

## SUBPHYLUM IV.  CILIOPHORA

Cilia are present in at least one stage of life cycle; two different types of nucleus (Fig. 7); sexual reproduction by conjugation.

### Class 1.  Ciliatea

#### Subclass Holotrichia

Cilia simple, uniform over body; buccal cilia usually absent.

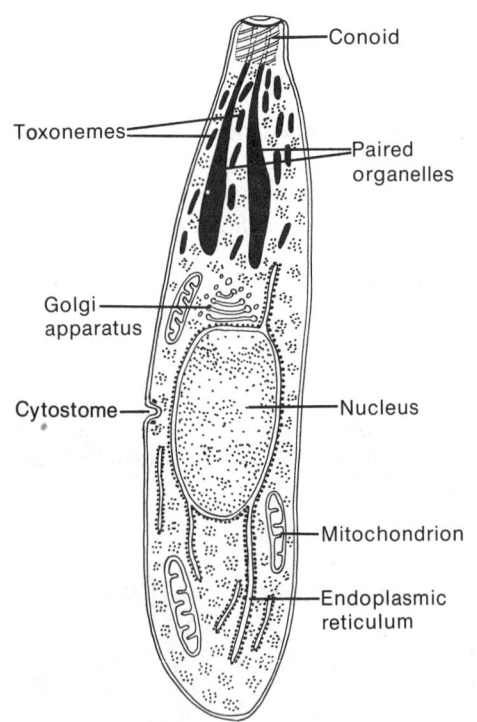

**FIGURE 5.** *Diagram to show the internal structure of a sporozoite, as revealed by electron microscopy. Note the paired organelles and associated taxonemes or dense bodies (the function of these is unknown but they may be concerned with penetration of the host cell, the conoid with its reinforcing rings, the mitochondria, and the cytostome.*

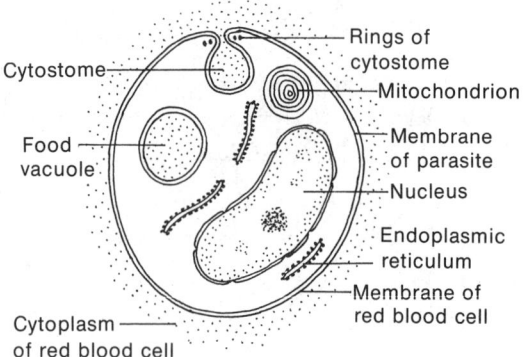

**FIGURE 6.** *Digram to show the internal structure of a trophozoite of Plasmodium as revealed by electron microscopy. Note the membrane of the red blood cell around the parasite, the cytostome, the food vacuole containing cytoplasm from the red blood cell, and the so-called "mitochondrion," which lacks cristae but sometimes contains whorls of membranes.*

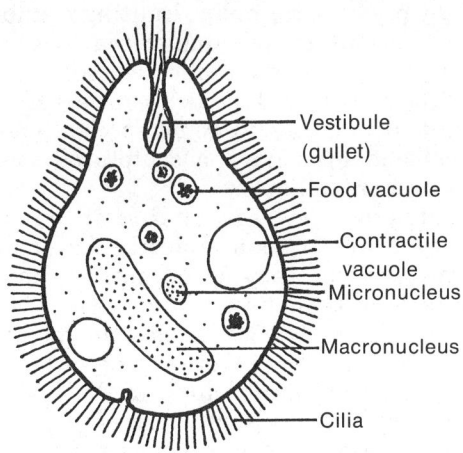

**FIGURE 7.**   *Diagram to show the structure of Balantidium coli as revealed by light microscopy. Note the uniform cilia over the surface, the micro- and the macronuclei, the two contractile vacuoles, the vestibule or gullet at the base of which lies a cytostome, and the food vacuoles.*

*Order Trichostomatida.*   Cytostome at base of a vestibule; cilia normally uniform but asymmetric in some (*Balantidium*) (Fig. 7).

*Order Hymenostomatida.*   Cilia of buccal cavity fused to form membranelles; cilia uniform over body (*Tetrahymena*). (Most species free living but much used in study of protozoan physiology.)

For general references to the classification of protozoa see Honigberg et al., 1964; Corliss, 1961; Kudo, 1966; Levine, 1961; Garnham, 1966; and Baker, 1973.

## ANATOMY OF PROTOZOA

The protozoan cell resembles cells of higher animals in that it may contain some, or all, of the structures (organelles) found in the metazoan cell. The protozoon consists of a mass of cytoplasm enclosed by a limiting membrane (plasmalemma or pellicle) and contains one or more nuclei, mitochondria, endoplasmic reticulum, ribosomes, Golgi apparatus (dictyosome, parabasal body), centrioles, flagella, cilia, microtubules, and fibrils. Some protozoa, and specific stages in the life cycle of others, lack certain of these organelles. In some groups — for example, the Sarcodina — the cytoplasm is divided into an outer, clearer ectoplasm and an inner, denser endoplasm that contains most of the organelles (Fig. 4). Some protozoa contain contractile vacuoles (Fig. 7) and some contain skeletal rods (Fig. 3), which do not occur in metazoan cells.

The nucleus is similar to that of the metazoan cell. The ciliates have two different types of nucleus; one is the sexual nucleus (micronucleus), and the other is the asexual nucleus (macronucleus) (Fig. 7). In *Entamoeba* the nucleoprotein is arranged around the periphery of the nuclear membrane in a characteristic pattern (Fig. 4).

The mitochondria are similar to those found in the cells of higher organisms, but the cristae (infoldings of the inner membrane) are usually tubular rather than plate-like (Figs. 1, 8). Certain species are apparently anaerobic and lack mitochondria (*Trichomonas* (Fig. 3), *Entamoeba*). Some species of malaria parasites lack true mi-

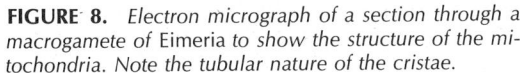

**FIGURE 8.**   *Electron micrograph of a section through a macrogamete of Eimeria to show the structure of the mitochondria. Note the tubular nature of the cristae.*

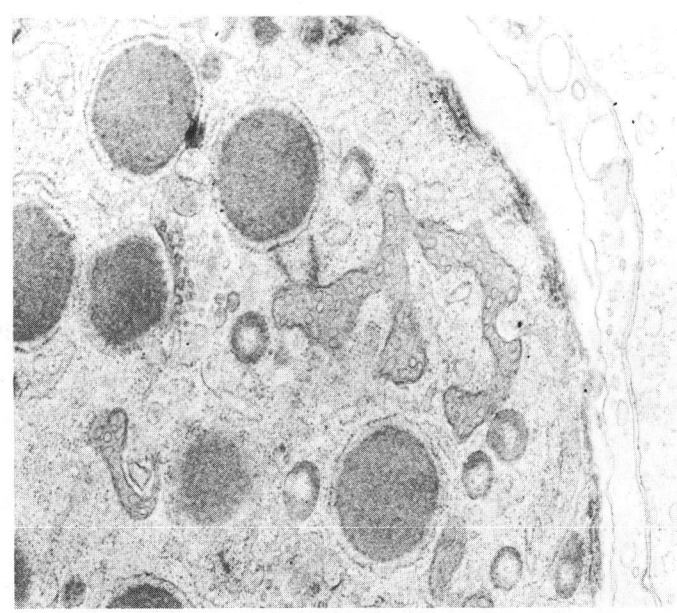

tochondria in their asexual stages but contain membranous organelles that may perform a similar function (Fig. 6). Members of the Trypanosomatina possess a spherical or rod-shaped structure called the kinetoplast; this contains DNA and lies within a single, large mitochondrion (Fig. 1).

Rough and smooth endoplasmic reticulum, ribosomes, and Golgi apparatus (dictyosome) are similar to those found in metazoan cells. The parabasal body found in the Mastigophora is apparently a type of Golgi apparatus (Figs. 1, 3).

Many protozoa possess contractile flagella or cilia on their body surface (Figs. 3, 7). These perform a locomotory, and sometimes an attachment, function. Cilia are usually shorter and more numerous than flagella, but they have a similar internal structure consisting of nine pairs of microtubules arranged around the periphery of the flagellum and two single fibrils in the center (Fig. 9); this is called the axoneme. The whole flagellum is enclosed by an extension of the limiting membrane of the protozoon. Cilia and flagella arise from a basal body or kinetosome within the cell (Figs. 1, 3). This basal body is a hollow cylinder, about 1.5 μm in diameter and is composed of nine outer double or triple microtubules that connect with the outer microtubules of the flagellum; the two central microtubules of the flagellum are not present in the basal body. A basal plate marks the junction of the basal body with the axoneme of the flagellum. In certain species (*Trypanosoma, Trichomonas*) an undulating membrane is associated with the flagellum and is an extension of the plasmalemma of the body surface (Figs. 1, 3).

In many protozoa the outer, limiting membrane is a typical membrane (plasmalemma), but in certain groups it is a more complicated structure and is called the pellicle. The pellicle consists of two or more unit membranes in some species (malaria parasites) and may have a sculptured appearance, as in many ciliates.

Cysts are produced by many parasitic protozoa, and the cyst wall forms a protective covering for the parasites when they spend part of their life cycle outside of their host (*Entamoeba, Eimeria, Isospora*). Granules arise inside the protozoan and are secreted to the exterior, where their contents coalesce and harden to form the cyst wall. Cysts are produced by some species of parasitic protozoa that use a vector as a means of transmission to another host (oocysts of malaria parasites) and by other species as a means of protecting the parasite from the defenses of the host (tissue cysts of *Toxoplasma*). These cysts usually have a softer and more flexible wall.

Skeletal structures, fibers, and microtubules are found in several groups of parasitic protozoa. Fibrils are present in the cytoplasm of many protozoa and may have a skeletal or contractile function. Microtubules are often found beneath the limiting membrane (Fig. 1) as well as in the flagellum (Figs. 1, 3, 9) and may have a skeletal or locomotory function. Some may also play a role in the transport of materials within the cell. Larger skeletal structures, such as the costa and the axostyle of *Trichomonas* (Fig. 3), are also found in certain groups of protozoa.

Contractile vacuoles are unusual in parasitic protozoa but they do occur in parasitic ciliates (*Balantidium*) (Fig. 7) and in the amebae *Naeg-*

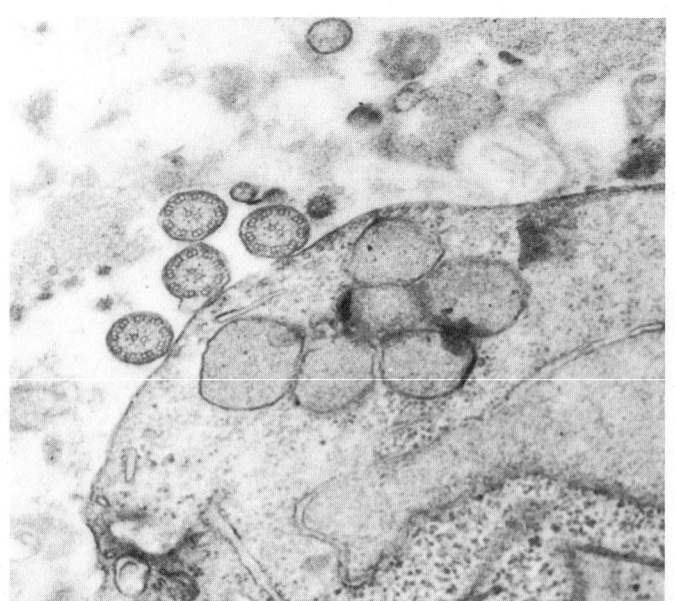

**FIGURE 9.** *Electron micrograph of a section through the flagella of* Trichomonas *to show the internal structure of the flagellum.*

*leria* and *Hartmanella*, which occasionally infect man. The contractile vacuole is a vesicle or vacuole that pulsates in a rhythmic manner and opens to the outside through a small pore in the limiting membrane.

Many parasitic protozoa possess a mouth, or cytostome, through which food particles are ingested. This cytostome may be a small depression on the surface of the body (Sporozoa) (Figs. 5, 6) or may lie at the base of a groove or cytopharynx, where it is usually associated with one or more flagella (Fig. 7).

Further reading on the structure of protozoa: (Baker, 1973; Dogiel, 1965; Mackinnon and Hawes, 1961; Adam *et al.*, 1971; Sleigh, 1973; Vickerman and Cox, 1967).

# PHYLUM  PLATYHELMINTHES

The platyhelminthes are worms that are usually flattened dorsoventrally, bilaterally symmetric, and without true segmentation. The digestive tract is incomplete or absent. The excretory system is the flame cell type and there is no body cavity, circulatory system, or respiratory system. The nervous system consists of a pair of anterior ganglia from which extend longitudinal nerves connected by transverse commissures. Individuals are hermaphroditic, with a few exceptions. The body is covered by a cytoplasmic epidermis or tegument (formerly thought to be a secreted cuticle in the Trematoda and Cestoidea).

The classification given here is incomplete because particular attention was given to parasites that attack man. For details of the complete classification see the references at the end of each section.

## Class Trematoda (Flukes)

### Subclass Digenea

Adult worms are typically leaf-shaped, but cylindric forms exist. A cup-shaped sucker surrounds the mouth (oral sucker) and a second sucker (acetabulum) is situated on the ventral surface. Almost all species are endoparasitic as adults and live in the alimentary tract, bile duct, blood vessels, lungs, bladder, or other organs of the vertebrate host.

The classification of the Digenea is controversial. The system described here is based on the system proposed by La Rue (1957) and used by Erasmus (1972) and by Noble and Noble (1976), but reference should be made to Yamaguti (1958) and to Dawes (1956).

### Superorder Anepitheliocystidia

Cercaria with thin excretory bladder; tails simple or forked; stylet absent.

*Order Strigeatoiida.* Miracidia with one or two pairs of flame cells; cercaria with forked tail.

#### SUBORDER STRIGEATA

*Superfamily Schistosomatoidea (=Bilharziidae).* Sexes separate; adults live in blood vessels of mammals and birds. (*Schistosoma.*)

### Order Echinostomida

#### SUBORDER ECHINOSTOMATA

*Superfamily Echinostomatoidea. (Fasciola hepatica, Fasciolopsis buski, Echinostoma ilocanum.)*

#### SUBORDER PARAMPHISTOMATA

*Superfamily Paramphistomatoidea. (Gastrodiscoides = Gastrodiscus hominis.)*

### Superorder Epitheliocystida

Cercaria with thick walled excretory bladder; tail of cercaria single, reduced in size, or absent; miracidium with a single pair of flame cells.

### Order Plagiorchiidae

#### SUBORDER PLAGIORCHIATA

*Superfamily Plagiorchioidea. (Dicrocoelium dendriticum; Paragonimus westermani.)*

### Order Opisthorchiida

#### SUBORDER OPISTHORCHIATA

*Superfamily Opisthorchioidea. (Opisthorchis = Clonorchis sinensis; Heterophyes heterophyes; Metagonimus yokogawai.)*

### ANATOMY OF THE DIGENEA

The life cycle of the digeneans consists of some or all of the following stages: egg, miracidium, mother sporocyst, daughter sporocyst, redia, cercaria, metacercaria, and adult.

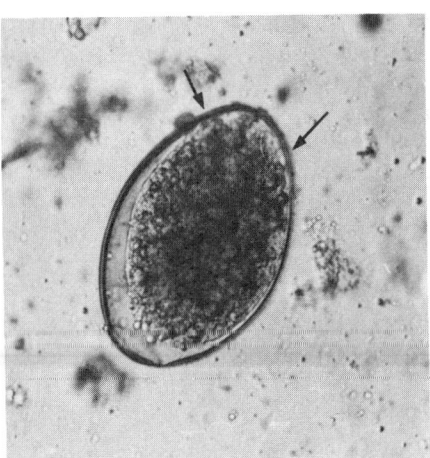

**FIGURE 10.** *Photomicrograph of the egg of* Fasciola hepatica. *Note the operculum at one end of the egg shell (arrows).*

The egg shell should correctly be referred to as an egg capsule. It is usually oval, light to dark brown, and operculated at one end (Fig. 10). The egg capsule of the human blood flukes (*Schistosoma*) is nonoperculate and bears a terminal spine (*S. haematobium*), a lateral spine (*S. mansoni*) (Fig. 11), or a lateral knob (*S. japonicum*).

The miracidium is a ciliated, bullet-shaped, free-swimming larva in most species (Figs. 12, 13). Ciliated epidermal plates on the outer surface are separated from each other by extensions of the subepidermal layer that lie beneath the plates (Fig. 13). The anterior end of the miracidium bears an apical papilla that lacks cilia but carries the openings of the apical and penetration glands. Most miracidia possess a pair of eyespots,

each of which is a pigmented cup containing a lens. The cerebral mass, which lies behind the eyespots, is connected by nerves to the eyespots, the sense organs, the apical papilla, and the posterior end of the larva. Sense organs occur on the apical papilla and also laterally on the body of the miracidium. The posterior part of the miracidium contains the germinal cells that may form clusters of cells called germ balls. The miracidium possesses one or more pairs of flame cells (Figs. 13, 21).

In most species the miracidium develops into a sporocyst (Fig. 14) after penetration of a suitable snail host. It loses its ciliated epidermal plates, the subepidermal layer develops into the new outer layer or tegument, and the larva becomes an elongated sac containing germinal cells. These germinal cells subsequently give rise to daughter sporocysts (as in the schistosomes) or to rediae that escape through a birthpore.

The redia is not present in all species. It is an elongate developmental stage that possesses a mouth, muscular pharynx, and a simple sac-like gut (Fig. 15). It usually bears a ridge-like collar around its anterior end and a pair of lobe-like lappets near the posterior end. The outer covering is a thin tegument (Fig. 16) that covers circular and longitudinal muscles and a cellular layer. The body cavity contains germinal cells, germinal masses, and developing daughter rediae or cercariae (Fig. 15). The excretory system consists of flame cells that open into two lateral excretory canals.

The cercaria arises from germinal masses within the daughter sporocysts (as in the schistosomes) or within the rediae. They vary in appear-

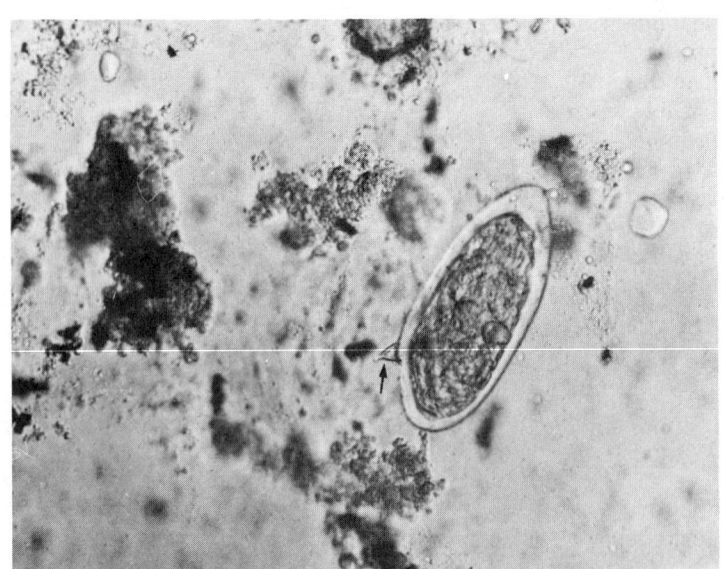

**FIGURE 11.** *Photomicrograph of the egg of* Schistosoma mansoni. *Note the lack of an operculum and the characteristic spine on the egg shell (arrow).*

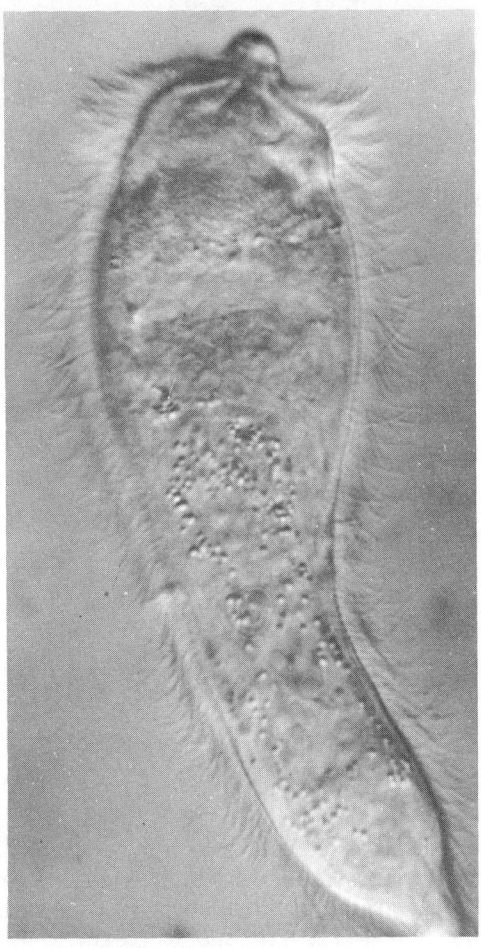

FIGURE 12. *Photomicrograph of the miracidium of* Schistosoma mansoni *(Nomarski interference microscopy). Note the ciliated epidermis and apical papilla.*

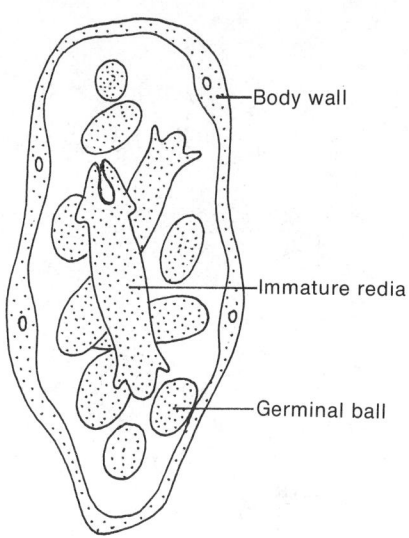

FIGURE 14. *Diagram of a sporocyst. Note the sac-like appearance and the germinal balls, which develop into rediae (or into daughter sporocysts or cercariae in those species that lack a redia stage).*

ance according to the species (Figs. 17 *A, B*) but have a cylindric or globular body and a muscular tail that is used in locomotion. The tail may be simple or forked (Figs. 17 *A, B*); both the body and the tail are covered by a cytoplasmic tegument. An oral sucker surrounds the mouth, and most species also have a ventral sucker. The rudimentary digestive system consists of a mouth, muscular pharynx, esophagus, and a pair of blind-ended ceca. A cerebral ganglion lies just behind the oral sucker and supplies nerves to various parts of the

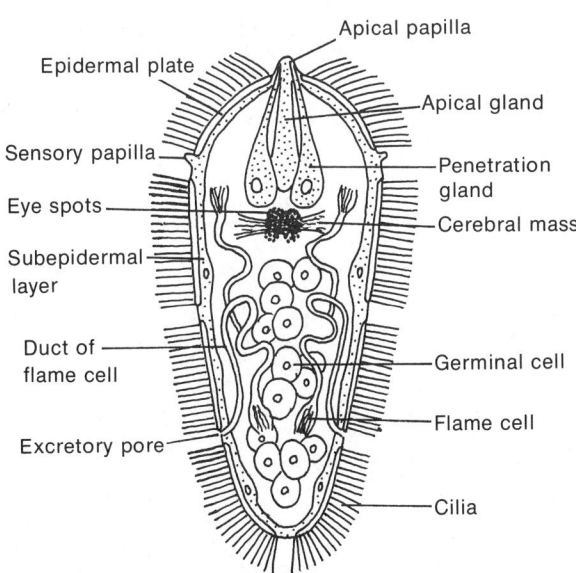

FIGURE 13. *Diagram of a miracidium. Not the ciliated epidermal plates, the subepidermal layer, which becomes the body wall of the sporocyst, the apical papilla with its associated glands, the flame cells with their collecting ducts, and the germinal balls.*

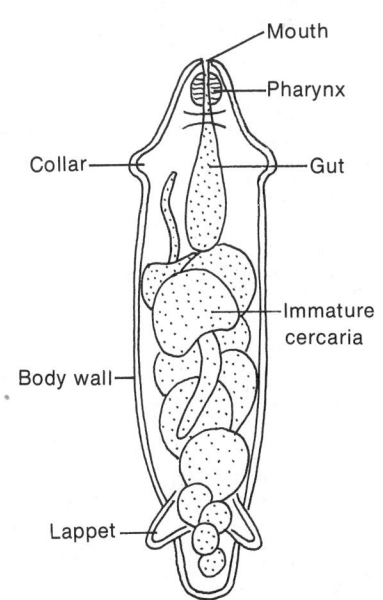

FIGURE 15. *Diagram of a redia. Note the presence of a simple gut, the collar, lappets (2), and germinal balls, which develop into cercariae.*

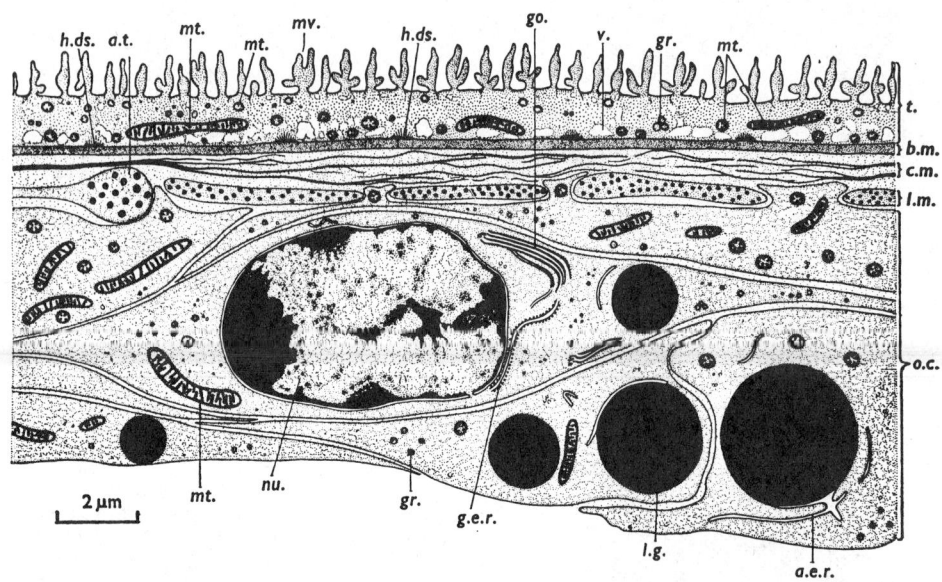

**FIGURE 16.** *Diagram of the ultrastructure of the body wall of a redia. Note the extension of the surface into branched microvilli. a.e.r., agranular endoplasmic reticulum; a.t., axon terminal; b.m., basement membrane; c.m., circular muscle; g.e.r., granular endoplasmic reticulum; go., Golgi complex; gr., granule; h.ds., half-desmosome; l.g., lipid globule; l.m., longitudinal muscle; mt., mitochondrion; mv., microvillus; nu., nucleus; o.c., overlapping cell; t., tegument; v., vacuole. (Reproduced with permission from G. Rees:* Parasitology *56, 1966.)*

cercaria. Some species possess pigmented eye-spots. The cercaria also possesses a well-developed excretory system of flame cells and collecting ducts.

Gland cells secrete the metacercarial cyst in those species that encyst, or secrete materials such as an adhesive substance or enzymes if the cercaria penetrates a second intermediate host or the final host. Penetration glands (Fig. 17 A) are a characteristic feature of the cercariae of schisto-

somes and they secrete several substances. Cystogenous gland cells, which are usually more widely scattered around the body of the cercaria, give rise to the wall of the metacercarial cyst (Fig. 17 B) in those species that form a cyst (*Fasciola hepatica*). The tail of the cercaria, which is well-supplied with muscles and mitochondria, is shed when the cercaria penetrates another host or encysts.

The cercaria of many species (*Fasciola hepati-*

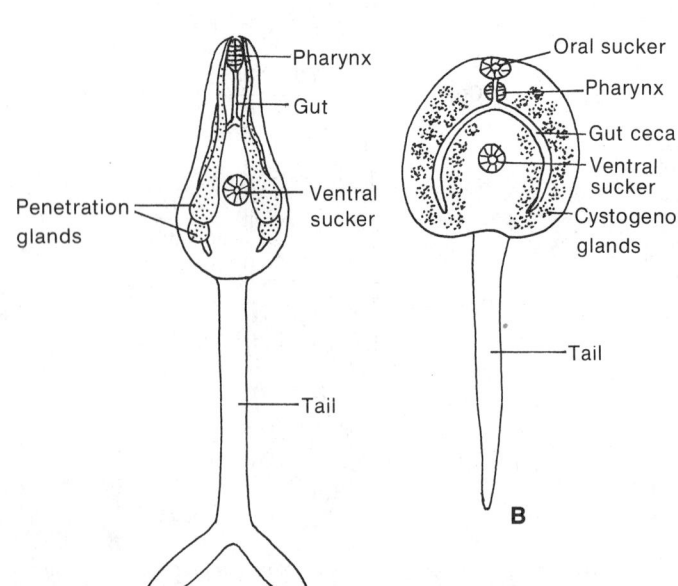

**FIGURE 17.** A, *Diagram of a schistosome-type cercaria. Note the bifurcate tail, the penetration glands, and the sucker. B, Diagram of a Fasciola-type cercaria. Note the unbranched tail, the lack of penetration glands, the cystogenous glands, which produce the wall of the metacercaria, and the suckers.*

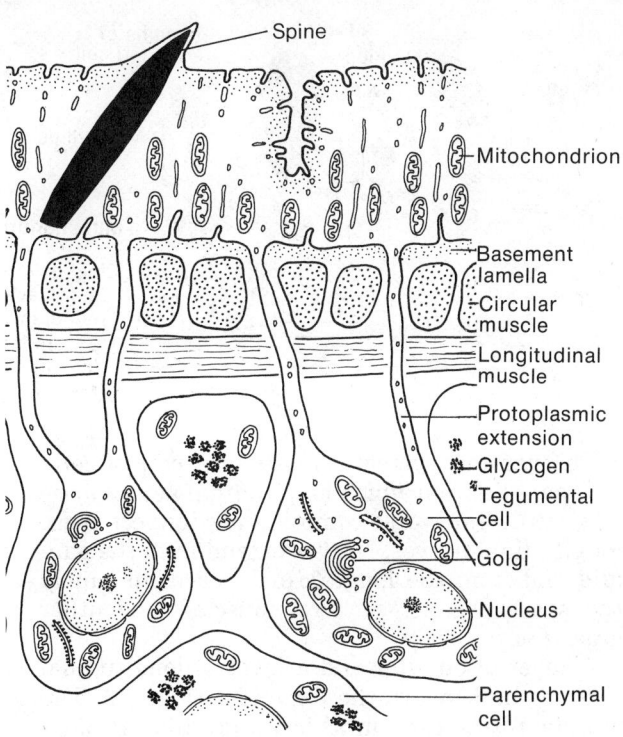

**FIGURE 18.** *Diagram to show the ultrastructure of the body wall of Fasciola hepatica. Note the syncytial cytoplasmic nature of the tegument, the tegumental cells, which lie below the tegument but connect with it by processes, the muscle layers, and the spine. The nuclei of the tegument lie in the tegumental cells and not in the tegument itself. (Based on Threadgold; Quart J Microscopical Sci. 104, 1963.)*

*ca*) encyst upon vegetation, whereas others penetrate a second intermediate host (*Opisthorchis sinensis*) and encyst inside the tissue; these stages are called the metacercaria. The cercaria of schistosomes penetrates the skin of the final host and becomes an active schistosomule; the schistosomule lacks the tail of the cercaria and has discharged its penetration glands.

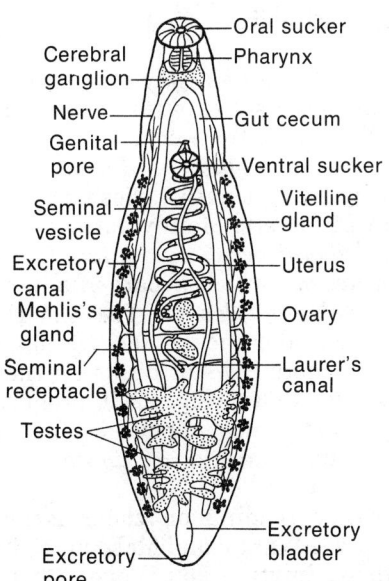

**FIGURE 19.** *Diagram to show the morphology of a digenetic trematode (Opisthorchis-Clonorchis sinensis).*

The adult digenean is covered with a syncytial cytoplasmic epidermis called the tegument, the nucleated portions of which lie below the main outer layer (Fig. 18). The tegument contains mitochondria, dense rod-shaped bodies of unknown function, endoplasmic reticulum, vacuoles, and, in some species, spines that extend from the surface of the tegument (Fig. 18). Nuclei and lateral cell walls are not present in the outer covering. Nucleated cells make contact with the main tegument by means of cytoplasmic tubes (Fig. 18). These cells contain endoplasmic reticulum, mitochondria, Golgi apparatus, and ribosomes. The tegument of adult schistosomes is covered by a series of membranes that may be important in evasion of the immune response of the host.

The terminal mouth of the adult leads to a muscular pharynx, esophagus, and a pair of blind-ending intestinal ceca in most species (Fig. 19). The wall of the ceca consists of a single layer of epithelial cells lying upon a basement lamella; a thin layer of muscle surrounds the cecal wall. The surface of the cells that line the cecal lumen is covered with long microvilli (Fig. 20). These intestinal cells are capable of secretion and absorption.

The excretory system consists of flame cells (Fig. 21) and collecting ducts, which open either directly to the outside from two large lateral excretory tubules or into a bladder that opens to the exterior (Fig. 19). A system of lymph channels occurs in some species but little is known about them.

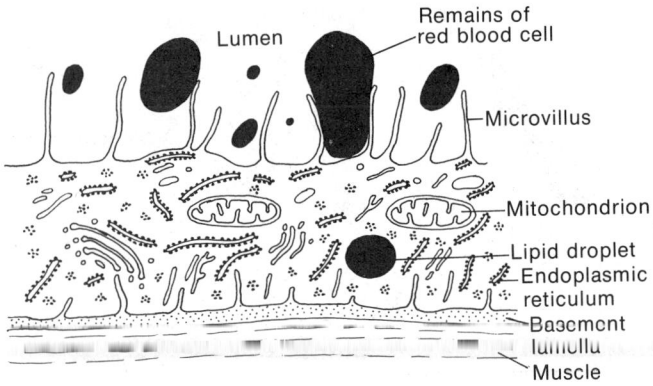

**FIGURE 20.** *Diagram to show the ultrastructure of part of the gut ceca of* Schistosoma mansoni. *Note the long, widely spaced microvilli and the partly broken-down red blood cells. (Drawn from an electron micrograph in Morris, A. P. Experientia,* 24, 1968).

The nervous system consists of a pair of cerebral ganglia from which longitudinal nerves arise (Fig. 19). Transverse commissures connect these longitudinal nerves. Nerves extend from the ganglia and from the longitudinal nerves to supply the sense organs, suckers, muscles, and other organs of the body.

A layer of circular and a layer of longitudinal muscles lie beneath the tegument (Fig. 18). The muscle fibers contain thick and thin myofilaments, and an extension of the sarcoplasm contains the nucleus, mitochondria, and endoplasmic reticulum of the muscle cell. The muscle fibers appear nonstriated in the adult worm, but the muscles in the tail of the cercaria are striated.

The parenchyma consists of large cells that lie in contact with the various tissues and organs of the body; there is no body cavity in the adult worm.

Most digeneans are hermaphroditic but the sexes are separate in the schistosomes. Figure 19 shows a diagram of the reproductive system of a typical digenean. There is usually a single ovary and one or more testes, which may be either compact or branched organs. Yolk for the eggs is produced by paired vitelline glands that may be branched or compact. A characteristic chamber called the ootype lies between the oviduct and the uterus. A series of small cells that form the Mehlis' gland are associated with the ootype. This combined structure is important in the formation of the egg capsule. The uterus, which is usually long and full of eggs, opens to the exterior at the genital atrium. Spermatozoa pass from the testes along the vas deferens to a seminal vesicle and an eversible cirrus.

For further reading on the structure and anatomy of trematodes see Hyman, 1951a; Erasmus, 1972; Smyth, 1966; Dawes, 1956; and Yamaguti, 1958.

### Class Cestoidea

The class Cestoidea consists of hermaphroditic worms, which, as adults, are parasitic in the alimentary tract of vertebrates. They are commonly called cestodes or tapeworms.

#### Subclass Eucestoda (= Cestoda)

The long, ribbon-like body consists of 4 to 4000 proglottids and a scolex with adhesive organs at the anterior end of the worm.

*Order Pseudophyllidea.* Scolex with two bothria (Fig. 22B); length varies from a few millimeters to 25 meters. Mainly parasites of fish except for *Dibothriocephalus latus* (= *Diphyllobothrium latum*), which is parasitic in man.

*Order Cyclophyllidea (= Taenoidea).* Scolex with four muscular suckers (acetabula) and often with one or more rows of hooks on the tip (rostellum) of the scolex (Fig. 22C); proglottids well defined. Includes most tapeworms of higher animals and man (*Taenia, Echinococcus, Hymenolepis*).

For further reading on the classification of tapeworms see Wardle and McLeod, 1952; Wardle et al., 1974; Smyth, 1969; Voge, 1969; Hyman, 1951; Joyeux and Baer, 1961; and Yamaguti, 1959.

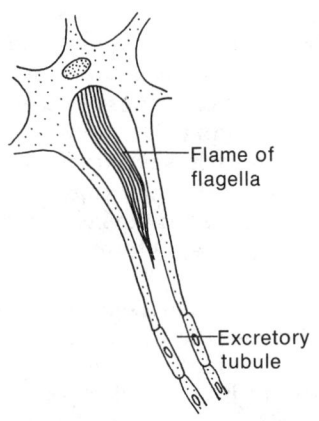

**FIGURE 21.** *Diagram of a flame cell (highly magnified).*

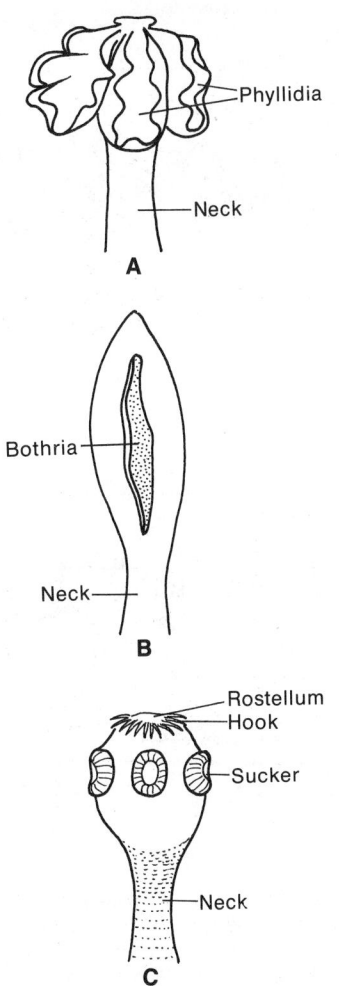

**FIGURE 22.** *Diagrams of scoleces of some cestodes. A, Tetraphyllidea-type, note the trumpet-like attachment organs (phyllidia); B, Pseudophyllidea-type (Dibothriocephalus latus), note the slit-like bothria, one of two; C, Cyclophyllidea-type (Taenia solium), note the rostellum bearing hooks (these are absent in some species) and the muscular suckers (acetabula).*

### ANATOMY OF CESTOIDEA

All tapeworms that parasitize man belong to the Eucestoda. They are mostly slender, elongate, white or cream-colored worms with a body consisting of few to many segments (proglottids). Each proglottid contains a complete set of male and female reproductive organs at some stage in development. There are no circulatory, respiratory, or skeletal organs and there is no alimentary system. Larval stages develop in one or more intermediate hosts.

The head is an attachment organ (scolex) that is armed with suckers of various sorts (bothria are slit-like grooves, Fig. 22B; phyllidia are trumpet-like or leaf-like structures, Fig. 22A; acetabula are muscular suction cups, Fig. 22C,

24) and may or may not also possess hooks. The anterior end of the scolex may be formed into a rostellum (Figs. 22C, 24). The neck lies behind the scolex and is a zone of proliferation from which immature proglottids are formed. These proglottids pass through a phase when they increase in size, develop gonads (mature proglottids), and fill the uterus with eggs (gravid proglottids) (Fig. 24). These proglottids form the thin, tape-like body of the worm and are constantly renewed from the neck region. Gravid proglottids drop off the end of the tape and are excreted in the feces of the host.

The adult tapeworm is covered by a cytoplasmic epidermis called a tegument (Figs. 23, 26) and not by a cuticle. The outer surface of the tegument is covered with numerous microvillus-like extensions (microtriches) that vary in length from species to species; each microthrix is tipped with an electron-dense, spine-like structure. The microtriches are covered with a membrane that is continuous with the limiting membrane of the tegument. The cytoplasm of the tegument contains mitochondria, small electron-dense bodies of unknown function, and vesicles, but no lateral cell walls or nuclei. Nucleated tegumental cells lie in the parenchyma beneath the tegument and con-

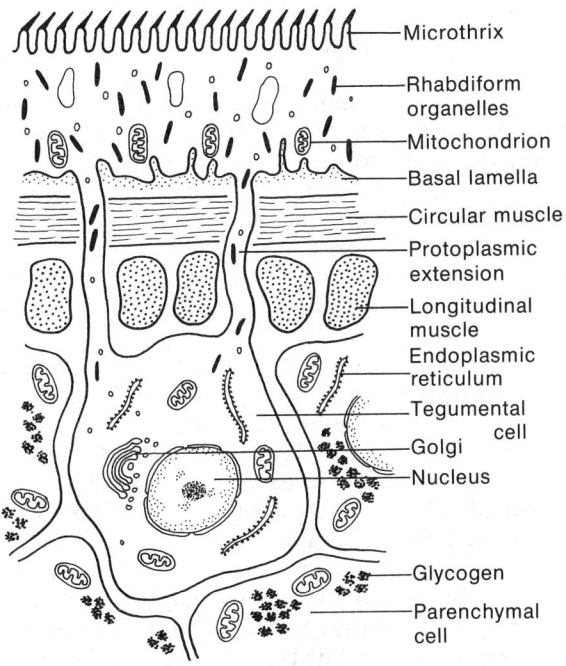

**FIGURE 23.** *Diagram to show the ultrastructure of the tegument of a typical cestode. Note the syncytial cytoplasmic outer layer which bears microvilli called microtriches (plural) or microtrix (singular), with spine-like tips; the nucleated tegumental cells, which are sunk in the parenchyma; and the muscles of the body wall.*

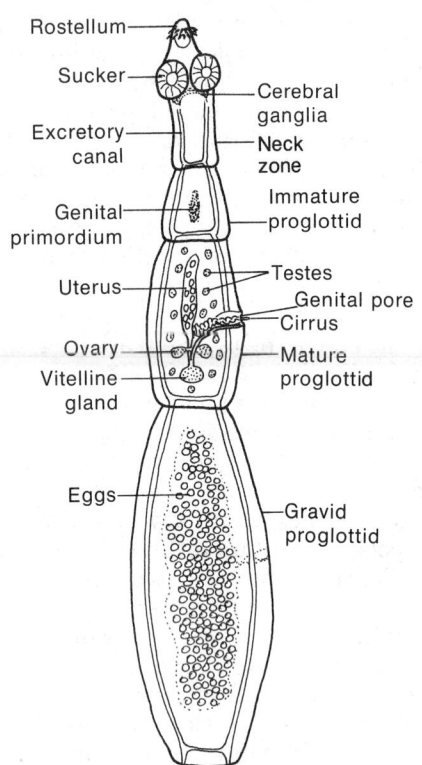

**FIGURE 24.** *Diagram of adult* Echinococcus granulosus *to show various anatomic features of a cyclophyllidean cestode.*

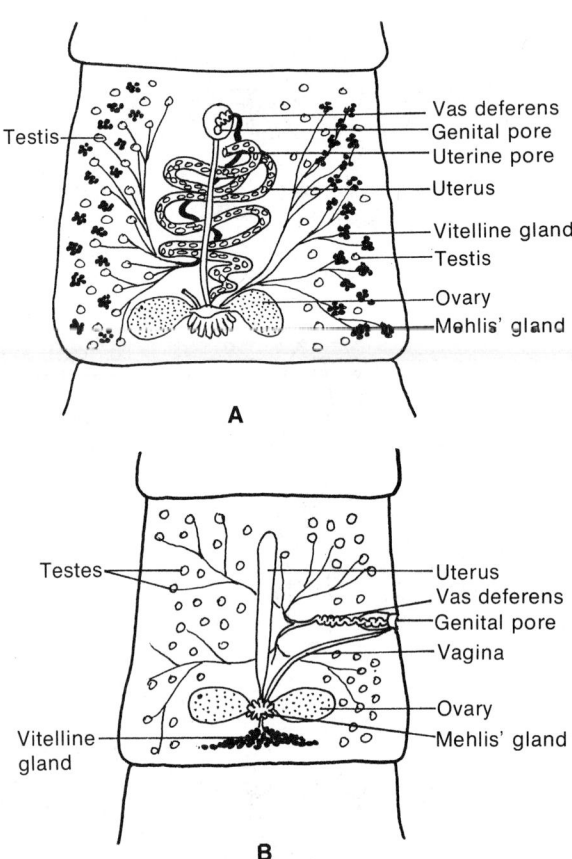

**FIGURE 25.** A, *Diagram of a mature proglottid of Dibothrio-cephalus latus to show the reproductive system. Note the scattered nature of the vitelline glands. Excretory canals and nerves omitted from the diagram. B, Diagram of a mature proglottid of* Taenia saginata *to show the reproductive system. Note the compact vitelline gland. Excretory canals and nerves omitted from the diagram.*

nect with it by means of cytoplasmic extensions (Fig. 23).

A layer of circular and a layer of longitudinal muscle lie beneath the tegument (Fig. 23), and transverse, diagonal, and dorsoventral muscles traverse the proglottid. The scolex is often very muscular. The nervous system consists of paired cerebral ganglia in the scolex and longitudinal nerves that run along the lateral margins of the worm. Sensory receptors are present on the scolex and on the proglottids. The excretory system consists of flame cells (Fig. 21), collecting vessels, and longitudinal excretory canals (dorsal and ventral) located along the lateral margins of the worm (Figs. 24, 26). Transverse canals link the longitudinal canals in each proglottid (Fig. 24).

All of the organs and tissues of the body are embedded in a cellular parenchyma (Fig. 26); there is no body cavity.

The worms are usually hermaphrodites (Figs. 25, 26), but in many species the male organs ripen before the female. The reproductive organs can be divided into two groups: the first group (Fig. 25A) has the vitellaria scattered throughout the proglottid or in laterally situated masses (Pseudophyllidea); the second group has compact vitelline glands usually situated toward the center of the proglottid (Cyclophyllidea) (Fig. 25B).

The egg of cestodes varies in different groups, but essentially it has four layers, or envelopes, enclosing the embryo. These layers are the capsule, outer envelope, inner envelope (which may be subdivided to form the embryophore), and oncospheral membrane (Fig. 27). The pseudophyllidean egg (Fig. 27) has an operculum, and a thick capsule composed of tanned protein. It usually

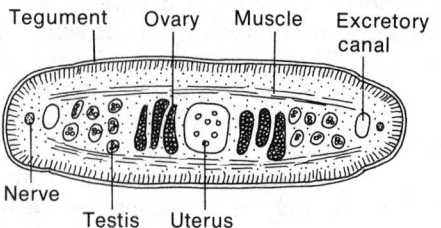

**FIGURE 26.** *Diagram of a transverse section through a mature proglottid of* Taenia solium *to show the arrangement of the excretory canals, nerve cords, and reproductive organs within the section.*

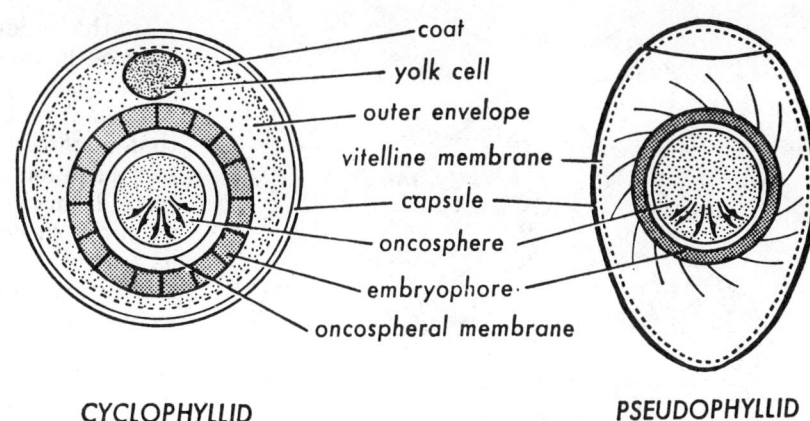

**FIGURE 27.** *Diagrams of a cyclophyllid-ean egg* (Taenia) *and a pseudophyllidean egg* (Dibothriocephalus). *Note the thick, toughened egg capsule with its operculum, and the ciliated embryophore (coracidium larva) in the pseudophyllidean egg, and the lack of a thick egg capsule in the egg of the cyclophyllidean but the presence of a thick, striated embryophore. (Reproduced, with permission, from Smyth: The Physiology of Cestodes, Oliver & Boyd 1969.)*

hatches in water to release a ciliated, free-swimming larva (coracidium). Embryonation of the egg occurs in water. The eggs of other tapeworms are usually embryonated when laid and do not have a free-living aquatic stage in the life cycle. They fall into three types: type 1 has a thin capsule and a thin embryophore *(Hymenolepis);* type 2 has an outer tanned protein capsule and a thick, striated embryophore (Fig. 27) *(Taenia, Echinococcus);* and type 3 has a shell formed by the egg and not by the vitellaria *(Stilesia).*

In the Pseudophyllidea, of which *Dibothriocephalus latus* is the most important species to man,

the egg hatches in water to release a ciliated larva (coracidium). This coracidium contains an oncosphere or hexacanth embryo (Fig. 27) that carries three pairs of hooks. The cilia are shed when the coracidium is eaten by a copepod and the oncosphere migrates to the body cavity, where it develops into a proceroid larva. This larval stage is a small worm-like creature that possesses a tail-like appendage containing the oncospheral hooks. When the infected copepod is eaten by a suitable fish, the larva migrates to the muscles of the fish and develops into a plerocercoid larva. The plerocercoid of *Dibothriocephalus latus* is an undifferentiated worm with a poorly developed

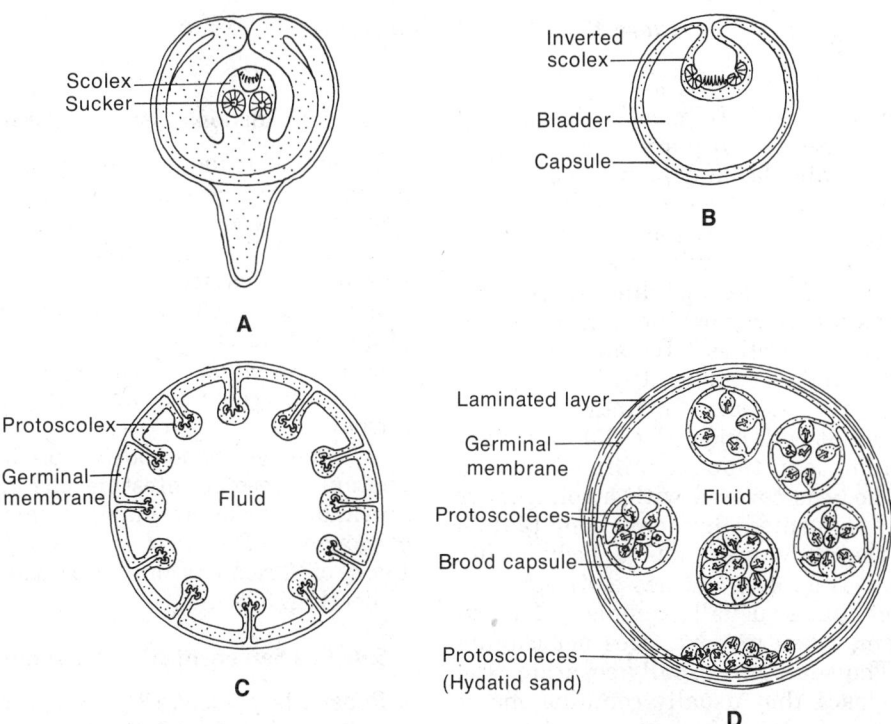

**FIGURE 28.** *Diagrams of A, cysticercoid larva; B, cysticercus larva; C, coenurus larva; and D, hydatid cyst.*

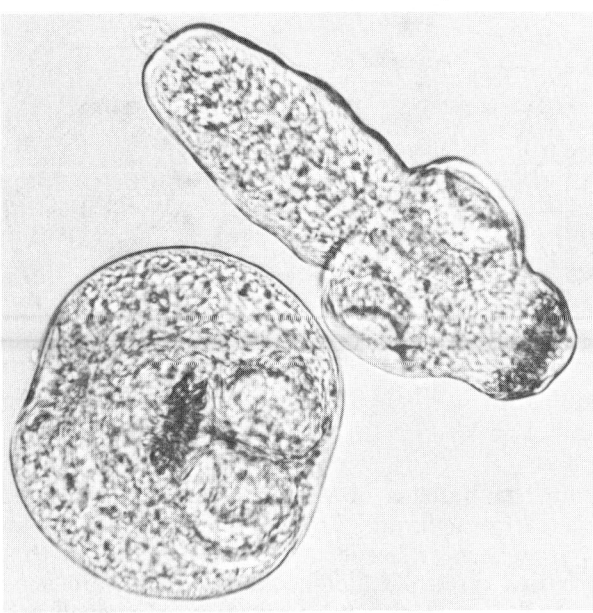

**FIGURE 29.** *Photomicrograph of protoscoleces of* Echinococcus granulosus, *one is evaginated and the other invaginated.*

scolex at the anterior end. When ingested by the final host, this larva differentiates into the adult worm.

In the order Cyclophyllidea, which includes most of the tapeworms parasitic in man, there are three types of larvae. The oncosphere (Fig. 27) hatches from the egg and is a six-hooked embryo that penetrates the tissues of the intermediate host. The oncosphere then develops into a cysticercoid larva or into a cysticercus, depending upon the species. The cysticercoid larva develops as a small cyst or bladder in which the scolex of the future adult is retracted (Fig. 28A) as in *Hymenolepis nana.* The cysticercus (often called the bladderworm) consists of a rounded, fluid-filled cyst or bladder within which the scolex of the future adult is invaginated (Fig. 28B) as in *Taenia solium.* A coenurus larva is a larger cysticercus in which several inverted scoleces (protoscoleces) develop from the inner (germinal) layer of the bladder wall (Fig. 28C) as in *Multiceps.* A hydatid cyst is a form of coenurus and is a large bladder that buds off numerous daughter cysts (brood capsules) from the germinal layer of the bladder wall. Each of these brood capsules contains several inverted scoleces (protoscoleces) (Figs. 28, 29).

For further reading on the structure and anatomy of cestodes see Wardle and McLeod, 1952; Wardle et al., 1974; Smyth, 1969; Voge, 1969; Hyman, 1951a; Joyeux and Baer, 1961; Yamaguti, 1959; Noble and Noble 1976.

# PHYLUM ASCHELMINTHES

## Class Nematoda (Roundworms)

Nematodes are found in most habitats and there are many species. They are important parasites of man, animals, and plants, but many species are free living. This classification will concentrate on those groups that are important in human disease. Some authorities regard the nematodes as a separate phylum (Maggenti, 1976), whereas others regard them as a class in the phylum Aschelminthes (Hyman, 1951b; De Coninck, 1965; Anderson et al., 1974).

Nematodes are slender, cylindric worms, usually tapered at both ends (Fig. 30), that vary in length from less than a millimeter to 9 meters. The body is covered with a collagenous cuticle, is unsegmented, has only longitudinal muscles in the body wall, has a body cavity (pseudocoelom) (Fig. 31), and has a straight alimentary tract that is usually complete. The excretory system, when present, does not contain flame cells. The sexes are usually separate. The male has a cloaca that usually contains one or two copulatory spicules.

### Subclass Adenophorea (= Aphasmidia)

Phasmids (caudal sensory organs) (Fig. 30) absent; excretory system without lateral canals; esophagus (should more correctly be called a pharynx) cylindric, esophageal glands may be free in body cavity and form a stichosome or a trophosome; eggs of some species have polar plugs (Fig. 32A).

***Order Enoplida.*** Esophagus cylindric, usually with anterior muscular and posterior glandular parts.

*Superfamily Trichuroidea.* Stichosome or trophosome present; intestine and rectum present; no caudal sucker in male; females with one set of gonads. *(Trichuris, Trichinella, Capillaria).* Eggs of *Trichuris* and *Capillaria* with polar plugs (Fig. 32A).

### Subclass Sercenentea (= Phasmidia)

Phasmids present (Fig. 30); excretory system usually with paired lateral canals (Fig. 34); sti-

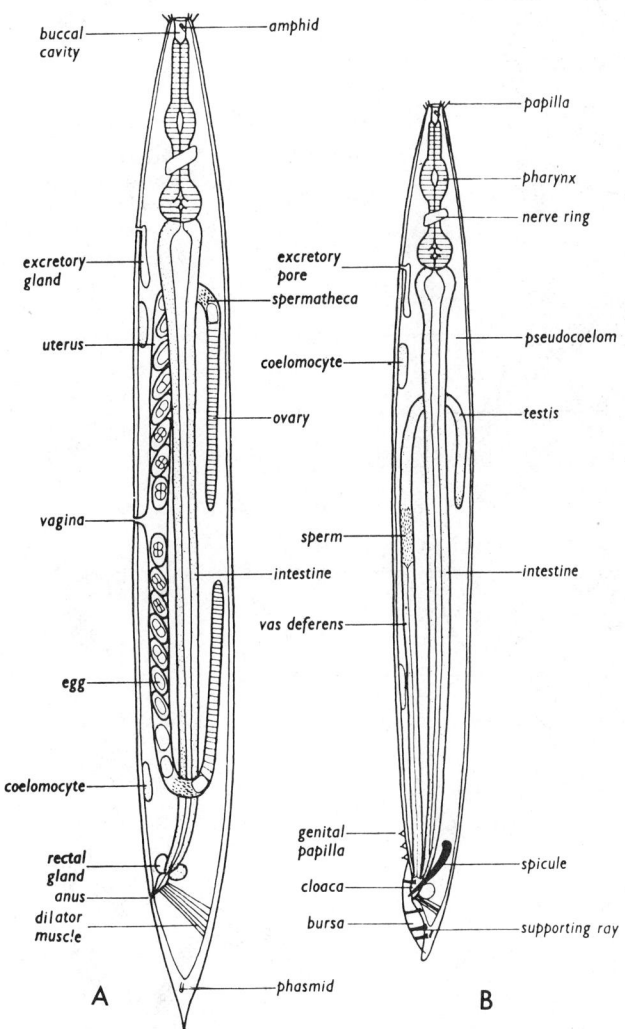

**FIGURE 30.**   *Diagram of a generalized female (A) and male (B) nematode to show their anatomy. (Reproduced, with permission, from Lee & Atkinson: Physiology of Nematodes, 2nd ed. Macmillan 1976.)*

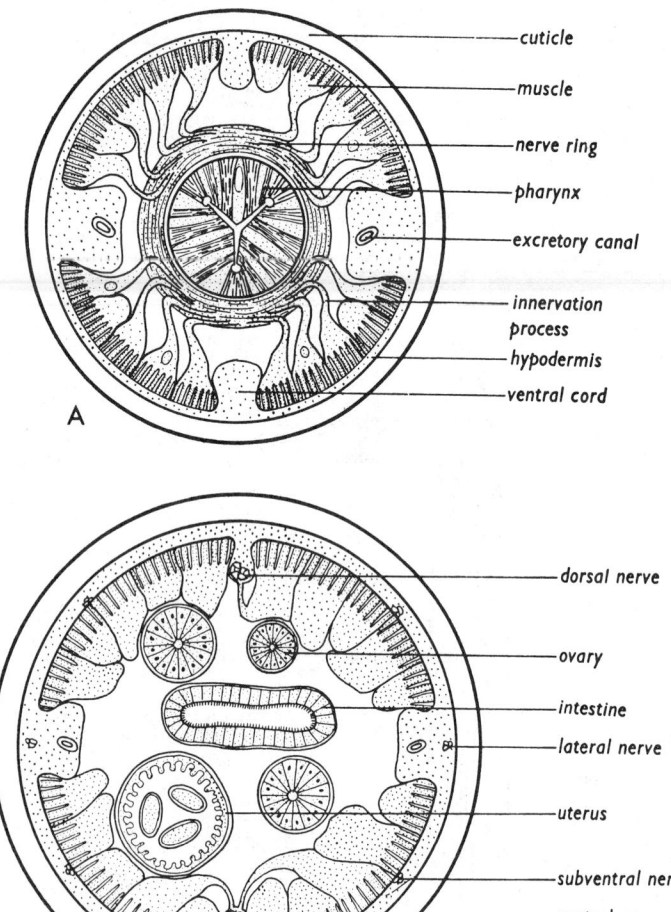

**FIGURE 31.** *Diagram of transverse sections through the esophageal (A) (should more correctly be called pharynx) and middle (B) regions of a female nematode to show the arrangement of the tissues and organs. (Reproduced with permission from Lee & Atkinson: Physiology of Nematodes, 2nd ed. Macmillan 1976.)*

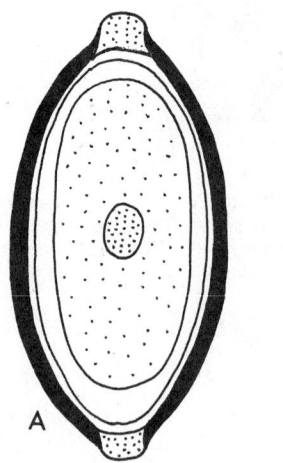
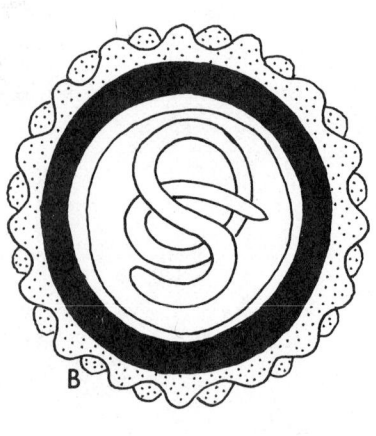

**FIGURE 32.** *Diagram of an egg of Trichuris (A) (note the polar plugs at each end), and Ascaris (B).*

chosome or trophosome absent; eggs without polar plug.

**Order Rhabditida.** Parasitic generation (females only) alternating with free-living generations (males and females); parasitic in lungs of amphibia or small intestine of vertebrates. (*Strongyloides stercoralis*).

**Order Tylenchida.** Stylet present in buccal cavity. Feed on plants or fungi; same species parasitic in body cavity of insects.

**Order Strongylida.** Male has copulatory bursa with supporting rays (Fig. 33); usually two spicules; ovejector of female with well-developed sphincter muscles. Mouth and buccal cavity variable in size and shape. Excretory system H-shaped and with two large glands (Fig. 34*A*, *B*). Parasitic in vertebrates.

*Superfamily Diaphanacephalodea.* Intestinal parasites of snakes and lizards.

*Superfamily Ancylostomatoidea.* Buccal capsule large, strongly cuticularized; lips absent; mouth with teeth and cutting plates (Fig. 35) or unarmed. Parasitic in intestine of mammals. (*Necator americanus, Ancylostoma duodenale.*)

*Superfamily Strongyloidea.* Buccal cavity variable, sometimes surrounded by ring of projections (corona radiata); no teeth or cutting plates. Parasites of intestine, respiratory tract, or urinary tract of mammals and birds. (*Strongylus, Oesophagostomum.*)

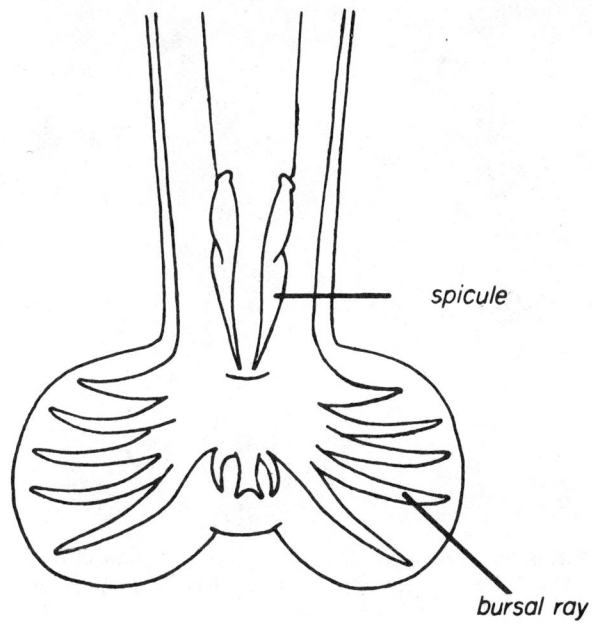

**FIGURE 33.** *Diagram of tail of a male trichostrongyle to show the copulatory bursa and spicules. (Reproduced with permission from Lee & Atkinson: Physiology of Nematodes, 2nd ed. Macmillan 1976.)*

*Superfamily Trichostrongyloidea.* Buccal cavity small (Fig. 36); cuticle around head often inflated; longitudinal cuticular ridges often present.

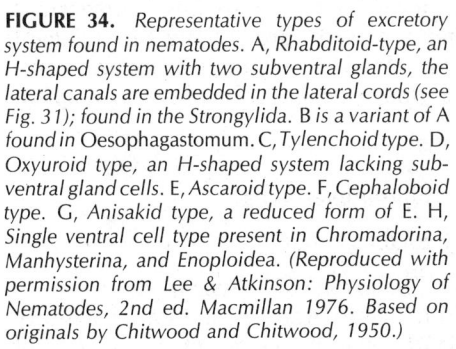

**FIGURE 34.** *Representative types of excretory system found in nematodes. A, Rhabditoid-type, an H-shaped system with two subventral glands, the lateral canals are embedded in the lateral cords (see Fig. 31); found in the Strongylida. B is a variant of A found in* Oesophagastomum. C, *Tylenchoid type.* D, *Oxyuroid type, an H-shaped system lacking subventral gland cells.* E, *Ascaroid type.* F, *Cephaloboid type.* G, *Anisakid type, a reduced form of E.* H, *Single ventral cell type present in Chromadorina, Manhysterina, and Enoploidea. (Reproduced with permission from Lee & Atkinson: Physiology of Nematodes, 2nd ed. Macmillan 1976. Based on originals by Chitwood and Chitwood, 1950.)*

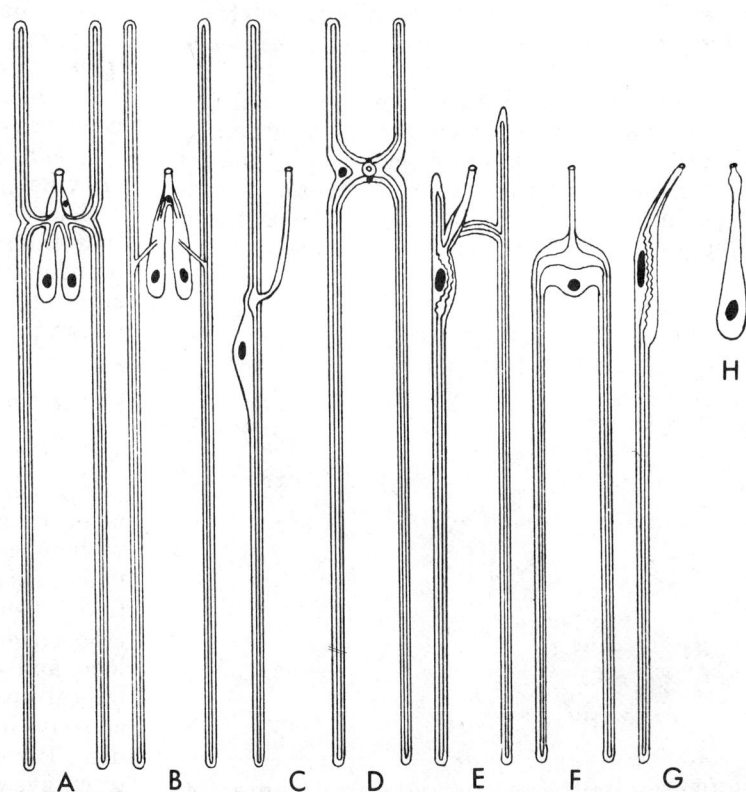

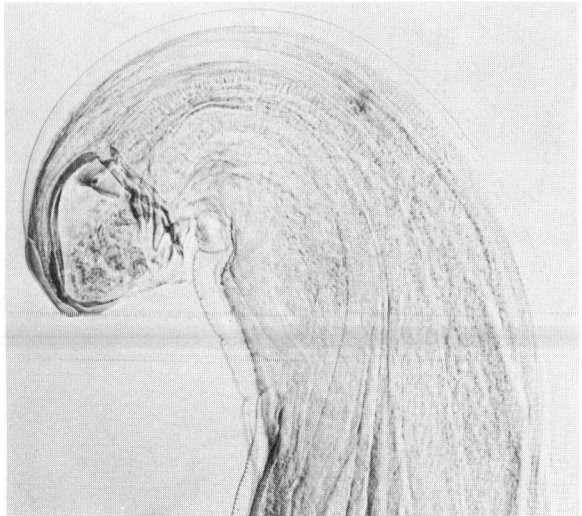

**FIGURE 35.** *Photomicrograph of the head end of Ancylostoma duodenale. Note the cutting plates at the opening of the mouth and the teeth at the base of the buccal cavity.*

Parasites of alimentary tract or respiratory tract of mammals. (*Trichostrongylus colubriformis.*)

*Superfamily Metastrongyloidea.* Buccal cavity small; copulatory bursa often reduced; vulva near anus; longitudinal cuticular ridges absent. Mainly parasites of respiratory tract of mammals. Intermediate host usually a gastropod, oligochaete, crustacean, or occasionally a vertebrate. (*Metastrongylus* spp., *Angiostrongylus cantonensis.*)

***Order Oxyurida.*** Male without copulatory bursa, one or two spicules; excretory system H-shaped (Fig. 34*D*); esophageal bulb present; body usually short and stout. Parasitic in lower intestine, colon, or rectum of vertebrates or hindgut of insects. (*Enterobius vermicularis.*)

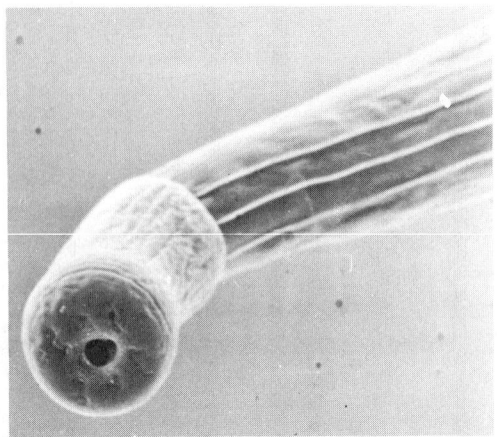

**FIGURE 36.** *Scanning electron micrograph of the head end of a trichostrongyle nematode. Note the small mouth.*

***Order Ascaridida.*** Usually three or six lips; esophagus variable in form but not divided into short muscular and long glandular parts; excretory system a modified "H" system (Fig. 34*E*). Usually parasitic in intestine of vertebrates.

*Superfamily Cosmocercoidea*

*Superfamily Seuratoidea*

*Superfamily Heterakoidea*

*Superfamily Ascaridoidea.* Mouth surrounded by three lips (Fig. 37); buccal cavity and esophagus simple. Tail of male usually curved or coiled. (*Ascaris lumbricoides, Toxocara canis.*)

*Superfamily Heterocheiloidea (= Anisakoidea).* Esophageal ventriculus (glandular modification of esophagus, which extends posteriorly beside the intestine) present; intestinal cecum often present. Parasitic in stomach of mammals (*Anisakis*).

***Order Spirurida.*** Usually two lateral lips surround mouth; esophagus with anterior muscular and posterior glandular part; most males have two unequal spicules.

SUBORDER CAMALLANINA. Larvae without cephalic hooks; esophageal glands usually uninucleate.

*Superfamily Camallinoidea.* Buccal cavity well developed. Parasites of gut.

*Superfamily Dracunculoidea.* Buccal cavity weakly developed; six conspicuous labial papillae present. Usually parasitic in tissues of host. (*Dracunculus medinensis.*)

SUBORDER SPIRURINA. Larvae with cephalic hooks; esophageal glands multinucleate.

*Superfamily Gnathostomatoidea.* Cuticular outgrowths (pseudolabia) overlie and replace lips; cuticle on inner face folded to form projections that interdigitate with projections on adjacent pseudolabium. Head sometimes bulbous. Parasites of gut and tissues. (*Gnathostoma spinigerum.*)

*Superfamily Physalopteroidea*

*Superfamily Rictularioidea*

*Superfamily Thelazioidea.* Buccal cavity variable, sometimes long and thin; mouth usually without definite lips. Parasites of eye cavity of mammals and birds, lungs of mammals, or intestine of fishes. (*Thelazia.*)

*Superfamily Spiruroidea.* Buccal cavity never long and cylindric, but well cuticularized; two lateral lips surround mouth. Vulva near middle of body; males usually have two unequal spicules. Parasites of alimentary tract, respiratory tract, eye cavity, nasal cavity, or sinuses of vertebrates. (*Gongylonema pulchrum.*)

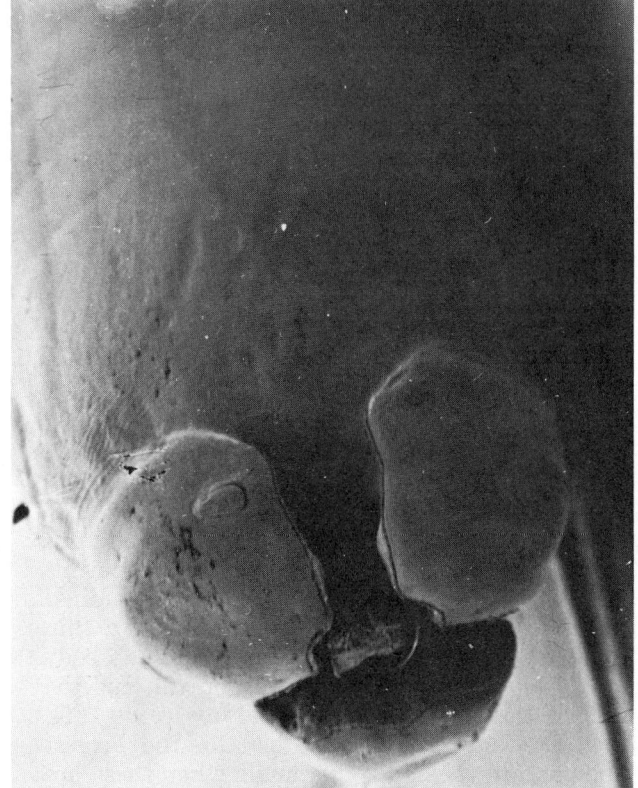

**FIGURE 37.** *Scanning electron micrograph of the head end of* Ascaris. *Note the three lips.*

*Superfamily Habronematoidea*

*Superfamily Acuarioidea*

*Superfamily Filarioidea.* **Lips absent; ovoviviparous; first larva a microfilaria. Parasites of tissues and tissue spaces of vertebrates; transmitted by arthropod vectors. (*Wuchereria bancrofti, Onchocerca volvulus, Loa loa*.)

*Superfamily Aproctoidea*

*Superfamily Diplotriaenoidea*

For further information on the classification of nematodes see Hyman, 1951b; de Coninck, 1965; Chitwood, 1969; Maggenti, 1976; Anderson, Chabaud, and Willmott, 1974; Yamaguti, 1961.

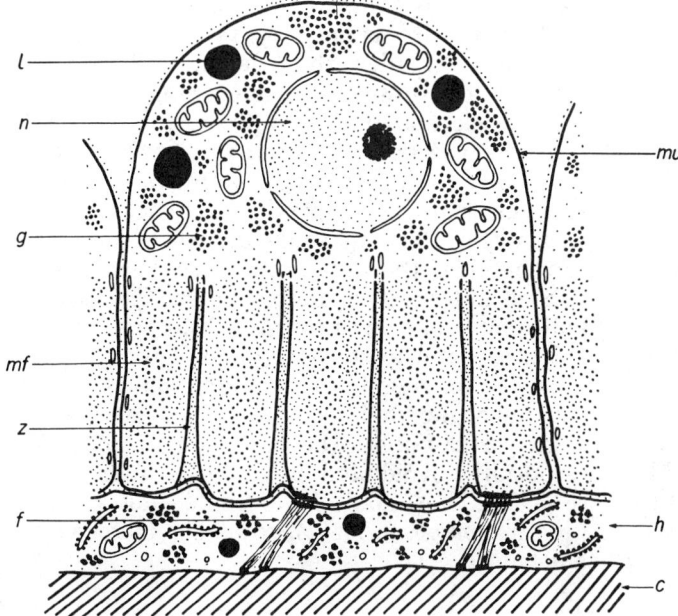

**FIGURE 38.** *Diagram of a section through a longitudinal muscle of the body wall of a nematode to show the internal structure of the muscle and the association with the hypodermis and the cuticle. c, cuticle;  f, fibres connecting muscle to cuticle; g, glycogen; h, hypodermis; l, lipid; mf, myofilaments; mu, muscle; n, nucleus; z, z-band region of muscle. (Reproduced with permission from Lee & Atkinson: Physiology of Nematodes. 2nd ed. Macmillan 1976.)*

## ANATOMY OF NEMATODA

The typical nematode is a spindle-shaped, unsegmented, and bilaterally symmetric worm (Fig. 30) that is round in cross-section (Fig. 31). The internal organs of the male and of the female are shown in Figures 30 and 31.

The body wall has an outer collagenous cuticle, a cellular or syncytial hypodermis, and a layer of longitudinal muscle (Fig. 31). The cuticle lines the buccal cavity, esophagus (more correctly called the pharynx), excretory pore, rectum, cloaca, and vulva. Teeth, cutting plates, stylets, and spicules are formed from toughened and hardened cuticle. The cuticle is basically three layered, but further subdivisions often occur. The outer surface of the cuticle is superficially annulated and may also be formed into fin-like structures (alae) or ridges that run along the length of the body. The hypodermis lies between the cuticle and the longitudinal muscles of the body wall. It is normally a thin layer of cytoplasm but it projects into the body cavity along the middorsal, midventral, and the lateral lines to form four ridges or cords (Fig. 31). The lateral cords are usually the largest and contain the excretory canals when these are present (Fig. 31).

The muscles of the body wall are spindle shaped, longitudinal cells that have a contractile and a noncontractile portion (Fig. 38). There are no circular muscles in the body wall. The muscles are innervated by arms that extend from the muscle to the nerves (Fig. 31).

The nervous system consists of a ganglionated circumesophageal ring with a large ventral, a smaller dorsal, and two or more lateral nerves running from it along the length of the hypodermal cords (Figs. 30, 31). Nerves extend forward from the nerve ring to innervate the sense organs around the mouth (Fig. 39). Sense organs occur elsewhere on the body, particularly around the tail of the male.

The body cavity is not a true coelom and is called a pseudocoelom. It is filled with fluid under pressure and forms the hydrostatic skeleton of the nematode.

The alimentary system is usually complete. There is a mouth surrounded by lips (Fig. 39) (these may be reduced in number from the normal six, or may be absent), a buccal cavity of varying shape and size, a muscular and glandular esophagus (pharynx), which usually has a triradiate lumen, a straight intestine, a rectum (cloaca in the male), and anus (Figs. 30, 31). The intestine consists of a single layer of epithelial cells that carry microvilli on the lumen side (Fig. 31B).

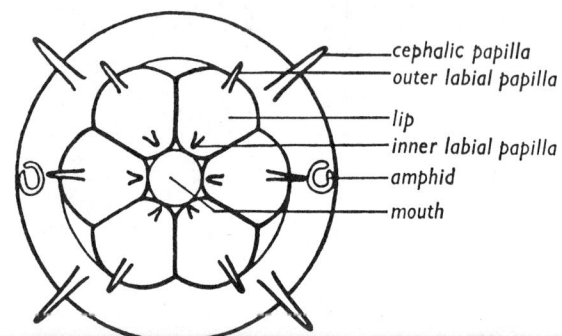

**FIGURE 39.** En face *view of a nematode head showing the position of the mouth, lips, amphids, labial sensillae, and cephalic sensilla (usually called papilla). (Redrawn from Jones:* Plant Nematology. *H.M.S.O. 1959.)*

The excretory system varies in structure from group to group and is absent in some species. There are two basic types — a glandular system and a tubular system (Fig. 34). The glandular system is found in many free-living nematodes and consists of a ventral gland cell situated in the body cavity near the base of the esophagus. It usually has a terminal ampulla that opens to the exterior on the ventral surface. The tubular system varies in structure but is basically an H-shaped system with a lateral canal in each lateral cord. It is united by a transverse canal in the anterior end of the nematode (Fig. 34D, E). This opens to the exterior through a common excretory duct and pore on the ventral surface. The Strongylida also contain a pair of glands in the pseudocoelom and these open into the transverse excretory canal just behind the excretory pore (Fig. 34A, B); although these are called excretory glands they appear to have a secretory rather than an excretory function. The excretory system contains no flagella or cilia.

The sexes are usually separate, and males are frequently smaller than females. The males have one or two testes, each opening into a seminal vesicle and then into a common vas deferens. The vas deferens open into a cloaca (Fig. 30). Many males possess one or two copulatory spicules that lie in pouches connected to the cloaca (Fig. 33). In some groups of nematode (Strongylida) the area around the cloaca is expanded to form a copulatory bursa (Fig. 33). Females have one or two ovaries that open into an oviduct(s) and a uterus or uteri (Fig. 30). The uterus often ends in an ovejector that is usually very muscular and opens to the exterior via the vagina and vulva. The eggs of nematodes are essentially ovoid and have three main layers (Fig. 32), the middle layer containing a chitin-protein complex. The sperm of nematodes are ameboid.

Nematodes have no circulatory or respiratory organs and lack true flagella.

The larval stages are really juveniles, since they are usually miniature adults with similar structure but without sex organs. All nematodes moult four times, and any structural changes that occur during the life cycle, such as modifications to the buccal cavity or to the cuticle, occur during the moult.

For further reading on the structure and anatomy of nematodes see Bird, 1971; Chitwood and Chitwood, 1950; Hyman, 1951b; Croll, 1976; and Lee and Atkinson, 1976.

# PHYLUM ACANTHOCEPHALA

These worm-like parasites live as adults in the intestine of vertebrates and as larvae in arthropods. They are distinguished by their spined anterior proboscis, which may be retracted into the main body of the worm. A digestive system is completely absent and there are no circulatory or respiratory structures. The sexes are separate; the males possess a posterior bell-like bursa.

*Order Archiacanthocephala.* Proboscis spines are concentric; contain protonephridia, eight cement glands in male. Parasitic in terrestrial hosts (*Moniliformis, Macracanthorhynchus*).

*Order Palaeacanthocephala.* Proboscis spine in alternate radial rows; no protonephridia; usually six cement glands in males. Parasitic mainly in aquatic hosts.

*Order Eoacanthocephala.* Proboscis spines arranged radially; no protonephridia; cement gland syncytial. Parasitic in aquatic hosts.

## ANATOMY OF ACANTHOCEPHALA

Adult acanthocephala are unsegmented worms in which the sexes are separate (Figs. 40A, B). Most species are 1 to 2 cm long, but a few, notably *Macracanthorhynchus hirudinaceus* from pigs, are longer and can reach 45 cm. The body is divided into an anterior praesoma that contains the retractable spiny proboscis together with its associated structures, and a larger posterior portion called the metasoma that includes the other organs and tissues of the body. The body wall consists of about five layers. There is a thin outer epicuticle, a tough cuticle penetrated by numerous pores that lead into canals of the striped layer. This striped layer merges into the fibrous felt layer. The innermost layer of the body wall is the thickest layer and is called the radial layer. It contains nuclei, mitochondria, ribosomes, and other cellular constituents, but has no lateral cell walls. The radial layer is separated from the circular and longitudinal muscles of the body wall by a basement lamella. There is a body cavity but it is not a true coelom. There is no alimentary tract in this group of worms. Food is taken up across the body wall. There are no circulatory or respiratory structures; nephridia are present in some groups but not in others. A nerve ganglion associated with the proboscis sheath sends nerves to various regions of the body. The male reproduction system consists of a copulatory bursa, a number of cement glands (usually six to eight), a pair of testes, and a sperm duct that leads to the genital pore. The female system has no persistent ovary; ova develop on a ligament in the body cavity and are set free in the body cavity, where they are fertilized. The eggs are sorted in a uterine bell and pass through a uterus to the genital pore.

For further reading on the Acanthocephala see Hyman, 1951b, and Crompton, 1970.

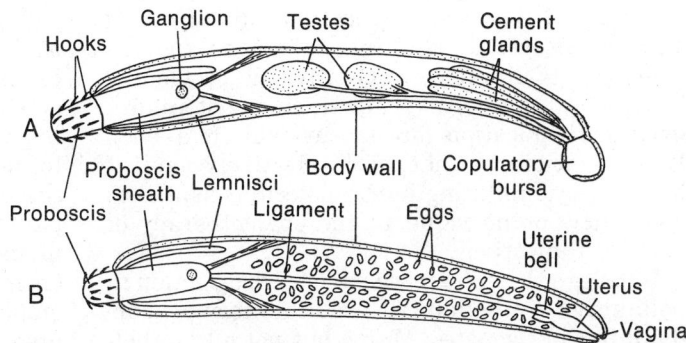

**FIGURE 40.** *Diagram of a male (A) and female (B) acanthocephalan to show their internal anatomy. Note the spiny proboscis and the lack of an alimentary system.*

## References

Adam, K. M. G., Paul, J., and Zaman, V.: Medical and Veterinary Protozoology. Edinburgh, Churchill Livingstone, 1971.

Anderson, R. C., Chabaud, A. G., and Willmott, S: CIH keys to the nematode parasites of vertebrates. No. 1. Commonwealth Agricultural Bureaux, Farnham Royal, Slough, U. K., 1974.

Baker, J. R.: Parasitic Protozoa. London, Hutchinson, 1973.

Bird, A. F.: The Structure of Nematodes. New York, Academic Press, 1971.

Chitwood, B. G., and Chitwood, M. B.: An Introduction to Nematology. Baltimore, Maryland, Monumental Printing Co., 1950.

Corliss, J. O.: The Ciliated Protozoa. Oxford, Pergamon Press, 1961.

Croll, N. A.: The Organization of Nematodes. New York, Academic Press, 1976.

Crompton, D. W. T.: An Ecological Approach to Acanthocephalan Physiology. Cambridge, Cambridge University Press, 1970.

Dawes, B.: The Trematoda. Cambridge, Cambridge University Press, 1956.

de Coninck, L.: Classe des nématodes. In Grassé, P-P (ed.): Traité de Zoologie. IV Némathelminthes (Nématodes). Paris, Masson et Cie, 1965.

Dogiel, V. A.: General Protozoology. Oxford, Clarendon Press, 1965.

Erasmus, D. A.: The Biology of Trematodes. London, Edward Arnold, 1972.

Garnham, P. C. C.: Malaria Parasites and Other Haemosporidea. Oxford, Blackwell Scientific Publications, 1966.

Honigberg, B. M., Balamuth, W., Bovee, E. C., Corliss, J. O., Gojdics, M., Hall, R. P., Kudo, R. R., Levine, N. D., Loeblich, A. R., Weiser, J., and Wenrich, D. H.: A revised classification of the Phylum Protozoa. Protozool, 11:7, 1964.

Hyman, L. H.: The Invertebrates. Vol. II. New York, McGraw-Hill, 1951a.

Hyman, L. H.: The Invertebrates. Vol. III. New York, McGraw-Hill, 1951b.

Joyeux, C., and Baer, J. G.: Classe des Cestodaires. In Grassé, P-P. (ed.): Traité de Zoologie, IV. Paris, Masson et Cie, 1961.

Kudo, R. R.: Protozoology. Springfield, Illinois, Charles C Thomas, 1966.

La Rue, G. A.: The classification of digenetic trematodes: a review and a new system. Exp. Parasitol 6:306, 1957.

Lee, D. L., and Atkinson, H. T.: Physiology of Nematodes. London, Macmillan Press, 1976.

Levine, N. D.: Protozoan Parasites of Domestic Animals and of Man. Minneapolis, Burgess Publishing Co., 1961.

Llwellyn, J.: The evolution of parasitic platyhelminths. Symposia of the British Society for Parasitology 3:47, 1965.

Mackinnon, D. L., and Hawes, R. S. J.: An Introduction to the Study of Protozoa. Oxford, Clarendon Press, 1961.

Maggenti, A. R.: Taxonomic position of Nematoda among the Pseudocoelomate Bilateria. In Croll, N. A. (ed.): The Organization of Nematodes. New York, Academic Press, 1976.

Noble, E. R., and Noble, G. A.. Parasitology. The Biology of Animal Parasites. Philadelphia, Lea and Febiger, 1976.

Sleigh, M.: The Biology of Protozoa. London, Edward Arnold, 1973.

Smyth, J. D.: The Physiology of Trematodes. Edinburgh, Oliver & Boyd, 1966.

Smyth, J. D.: The Physiology of Cestodes. Edinburgh, Oliver & Boyd, 1969.

Vickerman, K., and Cox, F. E. G.: The Protozoa. London, John Murray, 1967.

Voge, M.: Systematics of cestodes — present and future. In Schmidt, G. D. (ed.): Problems in Systematics of Parasites. Baltimore, University Park Press, 1969.

Wardle, R. A., and McLeod, J. A.: The Zoology of Tapeworms. Minneapolis, University of Minnesota Press, 1952.

Wardle, R. A., McLeod, J. A., and Radinovsky, S.: Advances in the Zoology of Tapeworms 1950–1970. Minneapolis, University of Minnesota Press, 1974.

Yamaguti, S.: Systema Helminthum. I. The Digenetic Trematodes of Vertebrates. New York, Interscience Publishers Inc., 1958.

Yamaguti, S.: Systema Helminthum II. Cestodes of Vertebrates. New York, Interscience Publishers Inc., 1959.

Yamaguti, S.: Systema Helminthum III. The Nematodes of Vertebrates. New York, Interscience Publishers Inc., 1961.

# 17 BIOCHEMISTRY OF PARASITES: HELMINTHS

*Howard J. Saz, Ph.D.*

In order to understand the mode of action of anthelmintic agents, it must be realized that the metazoan parasites differ from other disease-causing organisms in several important pharmacologic as well as biochemical respects. Pathogenesis of bacterial, viral, protozoan, and mycotic diseases depends on the replication or multiplication of the invading pathogens. Therefore, agents that inhibit pathogen replication will arrest or cure the disease. In helminth infections, the picture is quite different. Generally, the problem is to remove the adult worm, which is not reliant upon multiplication for its survival in a host. Hence, antibiotics that work effectively against bacteria by inhibiting macromolecular synthesis have little or no value in the chemotherapy of helminth infections.

What are the vulnerable sites for drug action in helminths? Anthelmintics are inhibitory primarily at one of two sites. Many, but not all, anthelmintics inhibit either muscle contraction or energy-generating processes within the parasites. Table 1 lists some anthelmintic compounds and their reported sites of inhibition. Although the inhibitions noted may account for the chemotherapeutic effect of each of these compounds, it is not established that these inhibitions represent their primary modes of chemotherapeutic action. At any rate, the importance of studying the biochemistry of the metazoan parasites now becomes more obvious. A better understanding of parasite biochemistry would help to explain the modes of action of anthelmintics. It would also aid in pointing out possible sites of inhibition that are unique to the parasite metabolism and therefore suggest the design of drugs that are more toxic for the parasite than they are for the host. In the remainder of this chapter we will discuss the biochemistry of the metazoan parasites with major emphasis on their energy metabolisms, since this area is quite susceptible to drug action.

Before 1950, most biochemists were concerned

**TABLE 1.   Reactions Inhibited by
Anthelmintic Compounds**

| ANTHELMINTIC AGENT | SITE OF INHIBITION |
|---|---|
| Trivalent antimonials | Phosphofructokinase |
| p-Rosaniline | Glycogen accumulation<br>Acetylcholine esterase |
| Cyanine dyes (Dithiazanine) | Respiration<br>Glucose uptake |
| Chlorsalicylamide (Yomesan)<br>Dichlorophen<br>Desaspidin<br>2,4-Dihexanoyl-6-methyl<br>  phloroglucinol | Electron transport phosphory-<br>  lation |
| Tetramisole | Neurotransmission<br>Fumarate reductase |
| Thiabendazole<br>Cambendazole | Fumarate reductase |
| Mebendazole | Glucose and amino acid<br>  uptake |
| Dibenzylamines | Glucose transport |

primarily with elucidating the concept of unity in biochemistry. They were struck by the biochemical similarities of all living tissues. However, small groups of scientists, particularly the pharmacologists and the immunologists, began to stress the fact that tissues even from related species were biochemically distinct in some respects. These considerations gave rise to studies of comparative biochemistry. It is now readily accepted that differences exist both at the subtle level of protein or enzyme structure and kinetics as well as at the more obvious metabolic level.

Krebs and Najjar (1948) were the first to report that enzymes carrying out the same reaction in different animal species could be antigenically different. Antisera to purified yeast glyceraldehyde-3-phosphate dehydrogenase inhibited the yeast enzyme, but not the corresponding enzyme isolated from rabbit muscle. Similarly, certain enzymes of *Schistosoma mansoni* were found to be immunologically distinct from the corresponding enzymes of rabbit muscle. It may be concluded, therefore, that the protein structure of the host and parasite enzymes is different.

Such structural differences between corresponding host and parasite enzymes may account for the specificity of some anthelmintics. For example, the trivalent organic antimonials, such as stibophen and potassium antimony tartrate, have been used to treat both schistosomiasis and filariasis. As with numerous other anthelmintics, the antimonials destroy the parasites by inhibiting energy metabolism; in this case by inhibiting

glycolysis. Specifically, in schistosomes, filariids, *Ascaris,* and the rat tapeworm *Hymenolepis diminuta,* the antimonials are known to be potent inhibitors of the glycolytic enzyme phosphofructokinase. Most important, and presumably because of differing protein structures, the mammalian phosphofructokinase is not affected by therapeutic concentrations of antimonials. Only slight inhibition of the mammalian enzyme occurs even at levels of drug 80- to 100-fold higher than those that inhibit the parasite enzyme almost completely (Mansour and Bueding, 1953; Saz and Dunbar, 1975).

In addition to the differences in protein structure, striking differences also exist between the metabolic pathways of the parasites and their hosts. This first became obvious at the level of overall metabolism. Although all helminths examined can consume oxygen, none can catalyze the complete oxidation of substrates to carbon dioxide and water. All helminths examined accumulate end products of metabolism other than, or in addition to, carbon dioxide and water. The same is true of the parasitic protozoans. Thus, in contrast to their mammalian hosts, terminal aerobic respiration in parasites is either absent or rate limiting. Similarly, it appears that many helminths surprisingly have lost their ability to synthesize long chain fatty acids de novo and must rely on their host to supply these important nutritional components (Meyer et al., 1966). Such an abbreviated lipid metabolism occurs in the cestodes *Spirometra mansonoides* and *Hymenolepis diminuta;* the nematode *Ascaris lumbricoides;* and the trematode *Schistosoma mansoni.*

Although the oxidative capacity of all helminths is limited, some are obligate aerobes and are destroyed rapidly by anaerobiosis. In contrast, others require no oxygen for energy metabolisms and survive equally well in the presence or absence of oxygen. Relatively few parasites have been cultured through their life cycles in vitro, making it difficult to assess their oxygen requirements for growth. Investigators have determined oxygen requirements mainly from survival time in air of a given stage of the parasite. Among worms that have been completely or partially cultured, a gradation of oxygen requirements exists ranging from highly aerobic to anaerobic. It has been suggested that oxygen may even inhibit the normal development of some parasites. In all helminths and in all stages of their development, however, oxygen can be consumed even though it may be deleterious to survival. In many instances, when the energy metabolism appears to be anaerobic, neither the physiologic significance nor the mechanism of this oxygen consumption is understood. It must be borne in mind that we are dealing with complex developmental stages in the life cycles of the helminths. In a given parasite, some of these stages may be aerobic while others are not. Shifts or changes in the metabolism of the parasites occur upon development from one stage to another. Almost nothing is known of the mechanisms by which these "switches" in metabolism occur. Examples of this "switching" phenomenon will be discussed below.

In many respects, the helminths resemble the facultative and obligate anaerobic bacteria. A wide range of fermentation products is formed, indicating the utilization of terminal electron acceptors other than oxygen. More simply stated, rather than oxygen being reduced to $H_2O$, other organic compounds take the place of oxygen and accept electrons, resulting in an accumulation of fermentation products. Some of the helminths are homolactate fermenters, accumulating lactate as the sole fermentation product. This also occurs in certain bacteria, rapidly contracting muscle, mammalian red blood cells, and numerous other organisms. Most helminths accumulate an array of fermentation products that might include volatile fatty acids, succinate, lactate, and neutral volatile compounds such as ethanol and acetylmethylcarbinol (acetoin). In general, all of these products arise from either pyruvate or succinate, or from both of these acids. Therefore, the carbohydrate metabolisms of most helminths studied might be divided into two categories. The first group would comprise those parasites, such as the schistosomes and filarial worms, that rely entirely on glycolysis and a few adjunct reactions for their energy metabolisms. Products of these fermentations would include lactate or ethanol and possibly acetate and acetylmethylcarbinol (acetoin). The second group of parasites, as exemplified by *Ascaris* and *Hymenolepis diminuta,* rely on a similar series of reactions, but can also fix carbon dioxide into phosphoenolpyruvate leading to the formation of a $C_4$ dicarboxylic acid, which in turn could give rise to succinate, propionate, and other volatile fatty acids. A representative sampling of a few parasites and their type of metabolism are listed in Table 2 together with the products formed by each worm. In the remainder of this chapter, examples of the "primarily glycolytic helminths" and the "$CO_2$-fixing helminths" will be discussed. A limited number of examples of each type of parasite will be examined.

## *PRIMARILY GLYCOLYTIC HELMINTHS*

### Schistosomes

The schistosomes constitute one of the most prevalent of the parasitic helminths that infect man. It is not surprising, therefore, that *Schisto-*

**TABLE 2.   Glycolytic and $CO_2$ Fixing Helminths and Products Formed**

| PARASITE | FERMENTATION PRODUCTS |
|---|---|
| **Glycolytic** | |
| *Schistosoma mansoni* | Lactate |
| *Schistosoma haematobium* | Lactate |
| *Schistosoma japonicum* | Lactate |
| *Brugia pahangi* | Lactate |
| *Dipetalonema viteae* | Lactate |
| *Litomosoides carinii* | Lactate, Acetate, $CO_2$ |
| *Dirofilaria uniformis* | Lactate |
| *Dracunculus insignis* | Lactate |
| *Angiostrongylus cantonensis* | Lactate |
| | |
| **$CO_2$ Fixing** | |
| *Ascaris lumbricoides* | Succinate, volatile fatty acids |
| *Heterakis gallinae* | Succinate, propionate |
| *Trichuris vulpis* | Succinate, volatile fatty acids |
| *Trichinella spiralis* (larvae) | Acetate, propionate, volatile fatty acids |
| *Hymenolepis diminuta* | Succinate, acetate, lactate |
| *Moniezia expansa* | Succinate, lactate |
| *Echinococcus granulosus* (cysts) | Succinate, lactate, acetate, ethanol |
| *Taenia taeniaformis* (adults and larvae) | Succinate, lactate, pyruvate, acetate, ethanol, glycerol |
| *Spirometra mansonoides* (spargana and adults) | Propionate, acetate, succinate, lactate |
| *Echinostoma liei* | n-Valerate, propionate, acetate, n-hexanoate |
| *Fasciola hepatica* | Acetate, propionate, lactate |
| *Paragonimus westermani* | Acetate, formate, propionate, n-valerate, 2-methylbutyrate, n-caproate |
| *Moniliformis dubius* | Succinate, lactate, acetate, ethanol |

*soma mansoni* was one of the first helminths whose pathway of carbohydrate metabolism was elucidated (Bueding, 1950). This blood fluke was found to utilize glucose very rapidly. In one hour an amount of glucose equivalent to approximately one fifth of its dry weight was dissimilated by a schistosome. Essentially all of the glucose carbon that disappeared from the medium was recoverable as lactate carbon, indicating that these organisms were homolactate fermenters, almost quantitatively converting the glucose utilized to lactate by the reactions of glycolysis (Fig. 1).

It is of particular interest that these blood flukes, living free in the aerobic environment of the bloodstream, should still employ the anaerobic reactions of glycolysis as their sole source of carbohydrate energy metabolism. Presumably, glucose concentrations in the blood are always sufficiently high to allow the parasite the extravagance of such a wasteful metabolism. Further evidence in support of the anaerobic nature of this energy metabolism comes from several sources. First, the rates of glucose utilization, as well as the rates of lactate formation, by the schistosomes are the same under either aerobic or anaerobic conditions of incubation. Second, a group of compounds referred to as the cyanine dyes (of which the anthelmintics dithiazanine and pyrivinium chloride are members) inhibits oxygen uptake almost completely in the schistosomes, but has no effect upon their rate of glycolysis or their surviv-

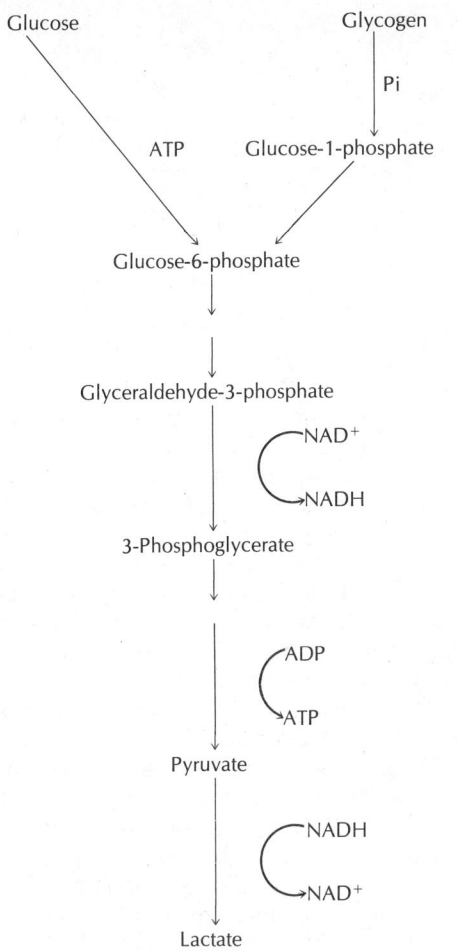

**FIGURE 1.** *The homolactate fermentation pathway in Schistosomes.*

al. Third, during in vitro incubation of adult schistosomes for 12 days, their gross morphology, motor activity, frequency of sex pairings, rates of glucose utilization, and lactate formation were the same in the presence or absence of oxygen. However, egg production was essentially stopped when oxygen was omitted. It is not known if oxidative metabolism is required for energy to produce eggs, or whether another non-energy-yielding reaction is essential for the developmental processes within the egg. Preliminary reports indicate that one non–energy-yielding reaction, tanning of the egg shell, is needed for maturation. Tanning requires the oxidation of some phenolic compounds with oxygen. There is little question, however, that for survival the adult parasite requires little or no oxygen.

The importance of carbohydrate metabolism to the schistosomes is indicated by more evidence than their rapid utilization of exogenous glucose and endogenous glycogen. As mentioned, the trivalent antimonials impair carbohydrate utiliza-

tion by inhibiting phosphofructokinase, which, in turn, destroys the parasite. Glycolysis, therefore, is vital for schistosomes. Another example concerns the antischistosomal drug niridazole. Its first detectable effect is to lower glycogen levels of the male *S. mansoni*. Glycogen is depleted through accelerated utilization. Glycogen phosphorylase catalyzes this degradation of glycogen in tissues, including those of the schistosomes. This enzyme has two rapidly interconvertible forms, the "inactive" b form and the "active" a form (Fig. 2). Phosphorylase a is formed by the phosphorylation of phosphorylase b. Normally, when glycogen utilization is no longer necessary, glycogen phosphorylase a is converted back to the "inactive" phosphorylase b by the removal of phosphate as catalyzed by phosphorylase phosphatase. Niridazole inhibits phosphorylase phosphatase, thereby preventing the removal of the "active" glycogen phosphorylase a. As a consequence, in the presence of niridazole the phosphorylase continues to break down glycogen, depletes the parasite of stored glycogen, and kills it. Unfortunately, niridazole also lowers muscle glycogen in patients and causes muscular weakness. These findings further indicate the importance of carbohydrate metabolism to schistosomes.

Relatively little is known of the metabolism of other developmental stages of the schistosomes. The cercariae appear to differ from the schistosomules and adults. Cercariae oxidize all three carbons of pyruvate to $CO_2$, indicating (but not proving) the operation of a tricarboxylic acid cycle. In support of this possibility, some of the intermediates of the tricarboxylic acid cycle also are utilized by cercariae. Schistosomules, on the other hand, show a much reduced pyruvate catabolism and appear to more closely resemble the adults. The factors that regulate this shift from an apparent aerobic metabolism of the cercariae to the more nearly anaerobic metabolism of the adults (and presumably the schistosomules) are obscure.

## Filarial Worms

Most filarial parasites that infect man are not amenable to biochemical studies, since they have not been reared in sufficient quantities in laboratory animals. This difficulty has been overcome partially by utilizing other filarial systems as models. Of these models, the three that have received most attention from the biochemical point of view are these: *Litomosoides carinii*, the adult form of which invades the pleural cavity of cotton rats or jirds; *Dipetalonema viteae*, which matures in the subcutaneous tissues of jirds or hamsters; and *Brugia pahangi*, which normally invades lymphatics but for experimental purposes is

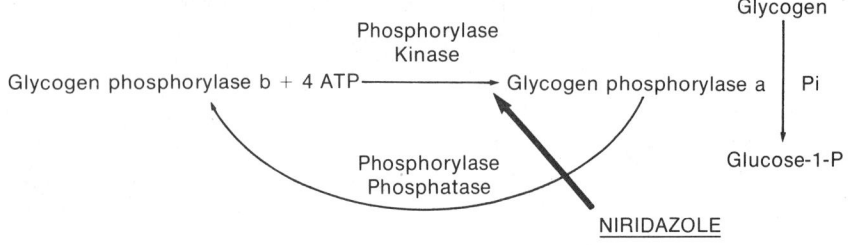

FIGURE 2. *The mechanism of the stimulation of glycogen breakdown by niridazole.*

much more readily recovered from the peritoneal cavity of jirds when they are infected intraperitoneally. Of these three species, only *B. pahangi* can infect man.

*L. carinii* was the first of this group of parasites to be reared in small animals, studied biochemically, and employed routinely for the screening of antifilarial compounds. Diethylcarbamazine (Hetrazan) was discovered by using this screen. Subsequently, another series of compounds, the cyanine dyes (for example, dithiazanine) was found to eliminate *L. carinii* infections in cotton rats. Cyanines strongly inhibit oxygen uptake of the parasite, which requires this gas for survival. Unfortunately, dithiazanine was without effect on those filariids that infect man. This disparity between the effectiveness of the cyanine dyes on these closely related species was disappointing and raised the question of the ways *L. carinii* differed from the other filariids.

A probable answer to this question has been arrived at by comparing the energy metabolisms of *L. carinii, B. pahangi,* and *D. viteae*. The motility of *L. carinii* adults ceases almost completely within one hour of anaerobic incubation, whereas aerobically, the parasites maintain good motility for several days. Therefore, *L. carinii* is an obligate aerobe. In contrast to this, both the motility and survival of *B. pahangi* and *D. viteae* is the same aerobically or anaerobically. Thus, oxygen does not appear to be required for motility or maintenence in either of these two parasites.

In accord with the apparent lack of an oxygen requirement for the motility of *B. pahangi* and *D. viteae,* subsequent studies have demonstrated that, in vitro, both of these parasites are homolactate fermenters, as was found with the schistosomes. All of the glucose carbons utilized could be accounted for as lactate. No other products were detected. If the filarial worms that infect man are similar in their energy metabolism to *B. pahangi* and *D. viteae* then they too would have no need for oxygen for survival, and depression of oxygen consumption by the cyanine dyes would be expected to have little or no effect upon them. On the other hand, the trivalent antimonials that inhibit the anaerobic reactions of glycolysis at the level of phosphofructokinase were once used for

treating filarial infections but later abandoned because of their high toxicity.

In contrast with *B. pahangi* and *D. viteae,* adult *L. carinii* are obligate aerobes. This pleural cavity-invading parasite is a heterolactate fermenter. That is, it accumulates other fermentation products in addition to lactate. Approximately 50 per cent of the glucose carbon it dissimilates aerobically is recovered as lactate. Acetate, $CO_2$ acetylmethylcarbinol (acetoin), and one or more unidentified products also accumulate. Presumably energy is derived from this further metabolism, since under anaerobic incubation the fermentation shifts toward a homolactate fermentation but the parasite dies. Studies employing various species of $^{14}C$-glucose as substrates indicate that essentially all of the respiratory $CO_2$ formed arises from the 3 and 4 carbons of glucose with very little arising from the other carbon atoms of glucose (Wang and Saz, 1974). According to the glycolytic sequence of reactions, the 3 and 4 carbons of glucose give rise to the carboxyl carbons of pyruvate, which, in turn, would be lost as $CO_2$ in the oxidative decarboxylation to acetate. Since almost no $CO_2$ arises from the 1,2 or 5,6 carbons of glucose, presumably acetate is not further oxidized and the tricarboxylic acid cycle is not a quantitatively significant energy-yielding pathway in *L. carinii*. The findings suggest that the aerobic requirement of *L. carinii* may reside completely in one system, the oxidative decarboxylation of pyruvate to acetate and $CO_2$. A summary of the metabolic energy pathways of the three filariids is outlined in Figure 3.

As might be expected, the metabolisms of the adult and microfilarial stages differ from each other. The microfilariae lose their motility in the absence of oxygen, but even after seven days of anaerobic incubation the reintroduction of air results in full restoration of motility. Therefore, although oxygen is required for motility, it does not appear to be required for survival of the microfilariids.

Under aerobic conditions, *B. pahangi* microfilariae switch to a heterolactate fermentation that resembles the process described for the adult *L. carinii,* forming lactate, acetate, and $CO_2$. Most of the pyruvate decarboxylated accumulates as the one step oxidation product, acetate. However, a small quantity of the acetate may be oxidized completely to $CO_2$, presumably via a tricarboxylic acid cycle mechanism. When the microfilariae are incubated anaerobically they become nonmotile and concurrently shift their metabolism toward total lactate accumulation (Rew and Saz, 1977).

A further indication of the coupling of motility with the aerobic metabolism of *B. pahangi* microfilariae is obtained when they are incubated with the anthelmintic levamisole. Levamisole inhibits neuromuscular transmission (possibly by ganglionic blockade) so that the parasites are paralyzed. Aerobic incubation in vitro in the presence of low concentrations of levamisole results in a rapid loss of motility. After this loss of motility, the energy metabolism shifts toward lactate production, mirroring an anaerobic metabolism. The effects of levamisole on the metabolism of the microfilariid appear to be secondary to the paralysis because loss of motility from tetramisole blockade reduces the energy requirement. The lowered energy requirement may cause a secondary shift toward an anaerobic lactate-forming metabolism. These findings indicate a tight coupling between motility and aerobiosis in these microfilariae.

## CO₂-FIXING HELMINTHS

### Ascaris lumbricoides

Although all helminths examined dissimilate carbohydrates to triose via the glycolytic pathway, many of them have evolved another sequence of reactions leading to the accumulation of succinate or products derived from succinate. This succinate-forming pathway requires the fix-

ation of carbon dioxide and has the potential of yielding additional energy (ATP) for the worm. *A. lumbricoides,* the parasitic intestinal roundworm, has served as the model system in elucidating this pathway. Increasing numbers of species of organisms that accumulate succinate under reduced oxygen tension and appear to obtain energy for survival by employing this "*Ascaris* pathway" are being reported. In addition to many of the parasitic helminths and protozoans, numerous free-living metazoans, such as the intertidal molluscs, which spend part of their life cycle under anoxic conditions burrowing in the sand, diving mammals such as seals and porpoises, and ischemic or anoxic rat hearts are all reported to use this pathway of succinate formation. Therefore, the pathway reported initially for *Ascaris* represents an important sequence in many organisms, including some mammals, in which it is a means of obtaining additional energy during oxygen deprivation to the tissues.

It has long been known that *Ascaris* survives equally well under aerobic or anaerobic conditions. The presence of $CO_2$ in the environment enhances survival. Adult *Ascaris,* therefore, can obtain energy for survival via anaerobic pathways. Accordingly, the organism is not sensitive to cyanide and levels of cytochrome c oxidase are so low as to be of doubtful physiologic significance. Accumulation of hydrogen peroxide in the presence of air indicates the existence of a flavin terminal oxidase rather than the usual cytochrome system, although it has been postulated that cytochrome o, which can react directly with oxygen to give hydrogen peroxide, may be involved in terminal respiration. Due to a deficiency of catalase, hydrogen peroxide accumulates and is toxic to the tissues of the worm.

Succinate and a mixture of volatile fatty acids

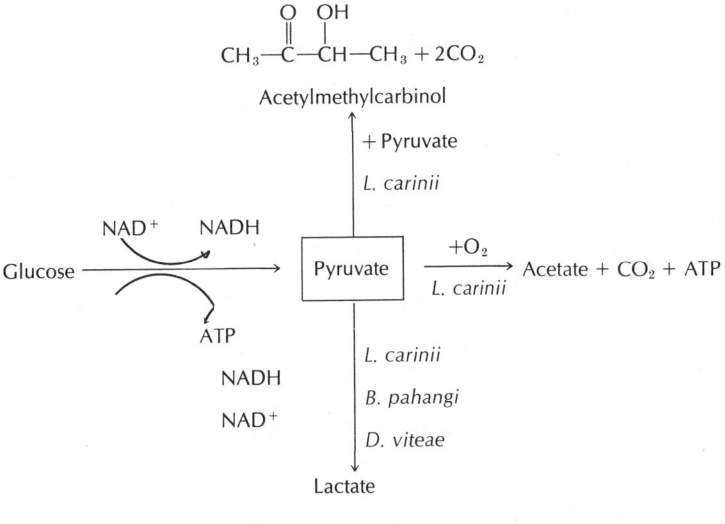

**FIGURE 3.** *Pathways of glucose dissimilation in L. carinii, B. pahangi, and D. viteae.*

comprise the major fermentation products of *Ascaris* metabolism. Volatile acids formed include acetate, propionate, traces of butyrate, pentanoate (valerate), tiglate (2-methylcrotonate), 2-methylbutyrate, and 2-methylvalerate. Lactate is not a fermentation product of intact *Ascaris* adults. The current concept of the carbohydrate fermentation pathway in *Ascaris* muscle is illustrated in Figure 4 (Saz, 1971). According to this pathway, the glycolytic enzymes of *Ascaris* muscle, which are present in the cytosol portion of the cell, function similarly to those of the host tissues up to the point of phosphoenolpyruvate (PEP) accumulation. At this point the metabolism of the parasite diverges from that of the host. In *Ascaris,* cytoplasmic pyruvate is not formed from PEP, since pyruvate kinase activity is barely detectable and of doubtful physiologic significance. Instead, the cytoplasmic PEP carboxykinase catalyzes the fixation of carbon dioxide into PEP to form oxalacetate according to the following reaction:

$$PEP + CO_2 + IDP(GDP) \rightleftharpoons$$
$$Oxalacetate + ITP(GTP)$$

In this reaction a substrate level phosphorylation of inosine diphosphate or of guanosine diphosphate takes place to form the corresponding energy-rich triphosphate. This conserves the energy of the phosphate bond of PEP as is accomplished by the pyruvate kinase reaction of the host tissues. Therefore, up to this point, identical amounts of energy are recovered from both pathways.

In order for glycolysis to continue, the NADH formed at the glyceraldehyde dehydrogenase level of glycolysis must be reoxidized back to $NAD^+$ so that another molecule of glyceraldehyde may be oxidized. In mammalian tissues this would be accomplished by the lactate dehydrogenase reaction, wherein pyruvate is reduced to lactate with NADH as the electron donor, thus reforming $NAD^+$. In *Ascaris*, however, cytoplasmic pyruvate is not formed and lactate is not an end product. Instead of employing lactate dehydrogenase, the parasite uses its cytoplasmic malate dehydrogenase for this function. Oxalacetate formed from the PEP carboxykinase reaction as illustrated above is reduced with NADH to form malate and regenerate $NAD^+$ as follows:

$$HOOC—CH_2—CO—COOH + NADH + H^+ \rightleftharpoons$$
$$(Oxalacetate)$$

$$HOOC—CH_2—CHOH—COOH + NAD^+$$
$$(Malate)$$

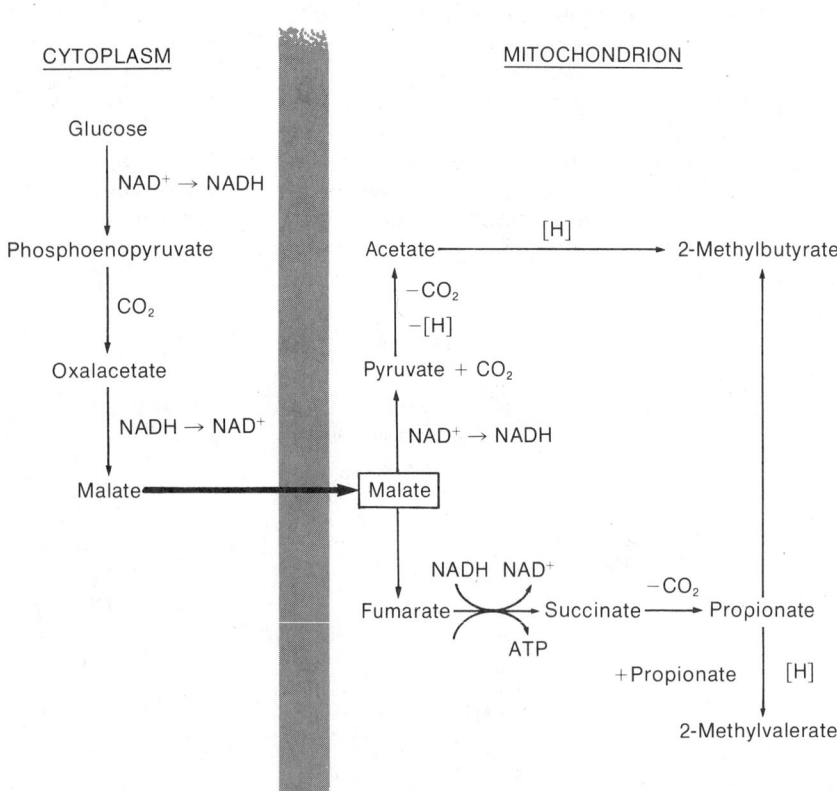

**FIGURE 4.** *Pathway for the dissimilation of glucose and the formation of succinate and volatile acids in* Ascaris lumbricoides *muscle.*

Malate then permeates through the mitochondrial membrane and serves as the substrate for the mitochondrion of the nematode. In contrast with mammalian mitochondria, evidence indicates that a functional tricarboxylic acid cycle is absent from the *Ascaris* organelles. The roundworm mitochondria function and generate energy anaerobically. Under these conditions, the malate that enters the mitochondrion cannot be oxidized directly, but rather must undergo a dismutation reaction. That is, for each mole of malate oxidized, a corresponding amount must be reduced simultaneously.

As illustrated in Figure 4, the oxidative leg of this dismutation is provided by the $NAD^+$-linked oxidation of malate to pyruvate and $CO_2$ catalyzed by the mitochondrial "malic" enzyme (malate dehydrogenase decarboxylating). This reaction proceeds as follows:

$$1\text{-Malate} + NAD^+ \rightleftharpoons Pyruvate + CO_2 + NADH + H^+$$

The "malic" enzyme reaction then serves to generate intramitochondrial reducing power in the form of NADH. This NADH will be subsequently employed in the ATP-generating reductive leg of the dismutation reaction.

An equivalent quantity of malate must now be reduced through fumarate to succinate as catalyzed by reactions (1) and (2):

(1) Fumarase:

$$HOOC-CH_2-CHOH-COOH \rightleftharpoons$$
$$\text{Malate}$$

$$HOOC-CH=CH-COOH + H_2O$$
$$\text{Fumarate}$$

(2) Fumarate Reductase:

$$HOOC-CH=CH-COOH + NADH + H^+ \xrightarrow{\text{ADP   ATP}}$$
$$\text{Fumarate}$$
$$HOOC-CH_2-CH_2-COOH + NAD^+$$
$$\text{Succinate}$$

NADH formed from the "malic" enzyme reaction donates electrons to fumarate, thereby accumulating succinate. The fumarate reductase reaction differs dramatically from the corresponding mammalian enzyme, succinate dehydrogenase. It does not catalyze a simple reversal of the succinate dehydrogenase system found in host tissues. The mammalian succinate dehydrogenase passes electrons directly to flavins, bypassing $NAD^+$. In contrast, the fumarate reductase of *Ascaris* couples with NADH, which, in turn, passes the electrons to a presumed flavin. This transfer of electrons from NADH to flavin would be analogous to

a site I phosphorylation of mammalian electron transport and, as would be expected, electron-transport–associated ATP is generated by the *Ascaris* fumarate reductase reaction. Therefore, this reaction provides energy for the cell in excess of that which would be obtained by the homolactate fermentation, providing an advantage to the succinate-forming organisms. For each glucose molecule fermented, two malates would enter the mitochondrion, but one half of the malate would be oxidized and one half would be reduced to succinate. Thus, 1 mole of ATP would be formed in the fumarate-reductase reaction for each mole of glucose dissimilated over this pathway.

The fumarate reductase and its associated reactions of electron transport are of great importance for chemotherapeutic and other reasons. A number of anthelmintic agents such as thiabendazole, cambendazole, and tetramisole inhibit the reduction of fumarate, although it is not clear whether this inhibition would constitute the primary site of action. A number of other anthelmintics uncouple the phosphorylation system associated with this reaction. Chlorsalicylamide (Yomesan), desaspidin, dichlorophen, and phloroglucinol derivatives constitute some examples. The fumarate reductase pathway of metabolism is by no means limited to *Ascaris*, but appears to be a means of anaerobic energy generation in numerous other parasitic and free living forms (Table 2).

Many helminths, including *Ascaris* adults, accumulate additional products that arise from succinate; that is, succinate serves as the precursor for these products. The most common is the three-carbon volatile acid propionate, which is formed by an overall decarboxylation of succinate (Fig. 4). The reaction occurs in two steps as it does in mammalian tissues and requires the coenzyme A derivatives as illustrated by reactions (A) and (B) below:

$$\text{(A) Succinyl-CoA} \underset{\text{Vitamin B}_{12}}{\overset{\text{Mutase}}{\rightleftarrows}} \text{Methylmalonyl-CoA}$$

$$\text{(B) Methylmalonyl-CoA} \underset{\text{Propionyl-CoA} + CO_2}{\overset{\begin{array}{c}\text{Propionyl-CoA}\\\text{Carboxylase}\end{array}}{\rightleftarrows}}$$

Mammalian tissues generally employ these reactions in a direction opposite to that shown. Propionate is utilized by means of $CO_2$ fixation to form succinate. As a consequence, propionate is a glycogenic fatty acid in mammals. That is, it can give rise to succinate that, in turn, can go on to form glycogen. In *Ascaris,* however, the reaction operates primarily in the reverse direction, toward propionate accumulation. What controls the direction of this sequence in *Ascaris* is not understood completely. However, the fact that propionyl-CoA is further metabolized by the nematode, as will be discussed below, may pull the reaction in the indicated direction. Since the methylmalonyl-CoA mutase requires vitamin $B_{12}$, those parasites that form propionate contain high levels of this vitamin (Tkachuck et al., 1977). In contrast, those helminths that form primarily succinate, lactate, or products unrelated to propionate do not contain appreciable amounts of vitamin $B_{12}$.

Pyruvate, formed as a product of the "malic" enzyme reaction (Fig. 4), is a precursor of acetate that arises within the mitochondrion. In mammalian tissues the oxidative decarboxylation of pyruvate to acetate and $CO_2$ results in the generation of ATP, since the reaction is linked to the electron transport system with oxygen acting as the terminal electron acceptor. Pyruvate utilization by *Ascaris* is particularly interesting in that acetate is formed anaerobically. What substitutes for oxygen as the electron acceptor is still not known, but it is possible that the oxidation of pyruvate may be coupled to the formation of the volatile fatty acids, 2-methylbutyrate and 2-methylvalerate. Whether or not ATP is generated

in the nematode by this anaerobic oxidative decarboxylation is unknown.

The mechanism by which *Ascaris* muscle forms its major fermentation products, 2-methylbutyrate and 2-methylvalerate, is not completely understood. However, acetate and propionate, presumably as the coenzyme A derivatives, are precursors to these volatile fatty acids. Incubating various radioactive substrates with *Ascaris* muscle preparations, then isolating the fermentation products formed and chemically degrading these products to determine the distribution of isotope in the carbon atoms of each have led to a postulation of the pathways for the formation of the two branched chain volatile acids (Fig. 5). Observations are consistent with the hypothesis that 2-methylbutyrate is formed after a condensation of the carboxyl carbon of acetyl-CoA with the number-two carbon of propionyl-CoA. The condensation product would be the coenzyme A derivative of methylacetoacetate, which possesses the appropriate carbon skeleton and could be reduced to 2-methylbutyrate. A similar series of reactions appears to account for the formation of the six carbon branched chain volatile acid, 2-methylvalerate. In this case, two molecules of propionyl-CoA condense to form the corresponding $C_6$ keto acid, which would then be reduced to 2-methylvalerate. Although it was thought that these reactions were unique to *Ascaris,* it was

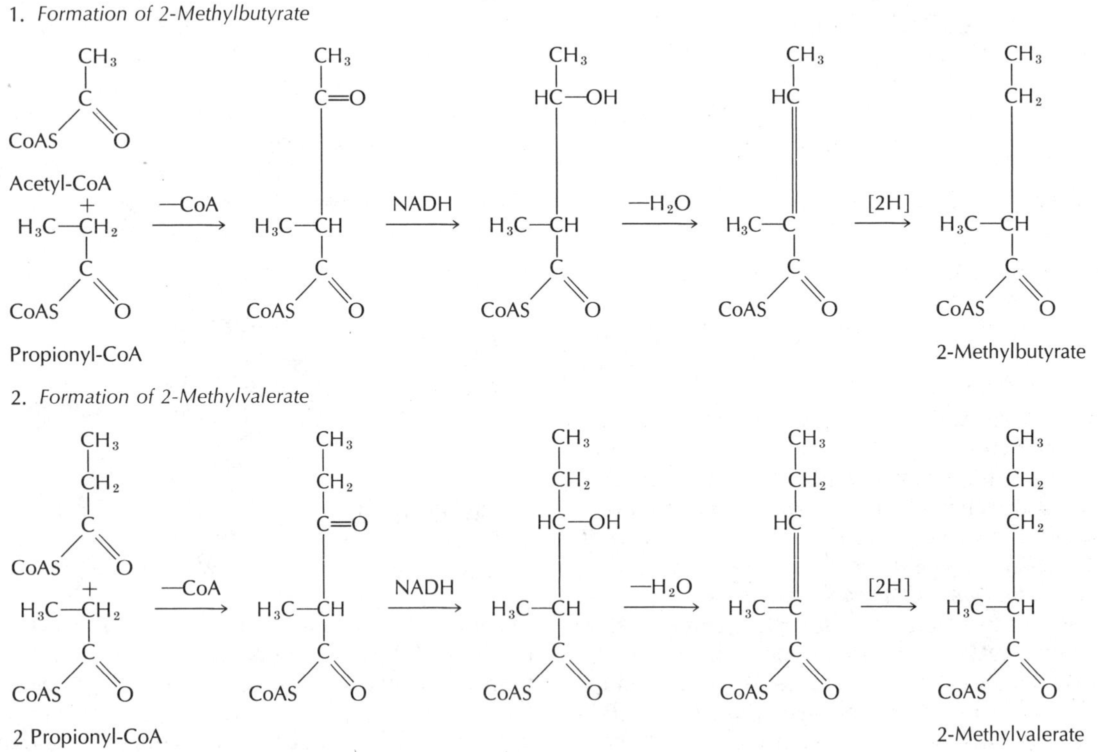

**FIGURE 5.** *Proposed pathways for the formation of 2-methylbutyrate and 2-methylvalerate by* Ascaris lumbricoides *muscle.*

reported recently that the clinically important lung fluke *Paragonimus westermani* also accumulates 2-methylbutyrate as a fermentation product.

Although many of the reactions in the energy pathways of *Ascaris* and its host are similar or almost identical, others are distinct and therefore vulnerable to chemotherapeutic attack. The fumarate reductase system is vital to the adult ascarids, but of minor, if any, physiologic importance to the mammalian host. Thus, interference with the fumarate reductase reaction should be detrimental to the parasite, but not to the host. As stated above, many anthelmintics inhibit some component of the fumarate reductase electron transport system. Accordingly, succinate formation and the fumarate reductase pathway are common among other parasites and invertebrates (Table 2). On the other hand, the formation of the branched-chain volatile acids seems to be of great importance in the overall economy of *Ascaris* and *Paragonimus,* but may be unique to these two helminths. Therefore, each parasite may have unique as well as common features in its biochemical arsenal of reactions. Each parasite is in some ways similar to and in some ways different from other parasites and from the host tissues, indicating that each worm should be examined independently.

In contrast to the adult *Ascaris,* fertilized eggs laid by the female in the intestines cannot develop past the single cell stage until they are passed out and gain access to oxygen. The eggs require oxygen to initiate and maintain development. At any stage, growth and differentiation may be arrested by removing oxygen. Yet, the potential for continued development remains even after extended periods of anaerobiosis, and normal maturation may be resumed merely by the introduction of air. Unlike adults, respiration of the eggs is highly sensitive to the cytochrome oxidase inhibitors, cyanide, azide, and carbon monoxide in the dark. Cytochrome oxidase activity is not detectable in unembryonated eggs. After exposure to air, however, the cytochrome oxidase activity increases continuously throughout development and high levels of activity are attained. Metabolic pathways in the egg are switched from those of the adult to one more closely resembling the aerobic metabolism of the host. The eggs are cleidoic; that is, only gases and water can permeate the vitelline membrane. As a consequence, all of the substrates for development are contained and utilized within the egg. Interestingly, *Ascaris* eggs were the first cells unequivocally shown to catalyze the net conversion of lipid into carbohydrate (Passey and Fairbairn, 1957). Most tissues cannot accomplish this transformation, since acetate formed from long chain fatty acids is oxidized by the mechanism of the tricarboxylic acid cycle, which results in the complete oxidation of the equivalent of both carbons of acetate to $CO_2$, leaving no carbons for a net synthesis of glycogen. Hence, no *net* synthesis of carbohydrate can take place from lipid. However, the glyoxylate cycle pathway in certain bacteria, plant cells, and in *Ascaris* eggs allows for this conversion of lipid into carbohydrate (Fig. 6), thereby allowing the egg to utilize its stored lipids to replenish depleted carbohydrate stores for subsequent use.

The first molt in the *Ascaris* life cycle occurs within the eggs, resulting in formation of the second stage larvae that are released from the eggs on hatching in the upper intestine. The second molt occurs in the lungs of the host and the third stage larvae make their way up the bronchial tree to the esophagus to be swallowed back down to the intestine. Before or shortly after entering the intestine the third molt to the fourth stage occurs. Cytochrome c oxidase activity is present in each stage from the developing egg through the third (lung stage) larvae. When the larvae molt to the fourth stage, the cytochrome c oxidase activity is lost, indicating a shift from aerobic to an anaerobic metabolism. Factors that control the "switchovers" from anaerobic to aerobic metabolism in the developing egg and from aerobic to anaerobic in going from the third to the fourth larval stages are unknown.

### Hymenolepis diminuta

The large intestinal tapeworm of the rat, *Hymenolepis diminuta,* also has served as a biochemical model for studying parasitic helminths. There is little doubt that this cestode is an anaerobe, since it has been cultivated from larva through adult in a $CO_2$-containing anaerobic environment. Oxygen may be detrimental to normal development. Another cestode, *Hymenolepis nana,* which infects humans, has also been cultivated. This cultivation also requires a $CO_2$-containing anaerobic gas phase. It is noteworthy that both the adult and larval stages were cultivated anaerobically. This is different from the larval stages of *Ascaris,* most of which require oxygen.

*Hymenolepis diminuta* adults accumulate succinate as the major fermentation product. Smaller quantities of acetate and lactate also are produced. Succinate is formed by a pathway involving $CO_2$ fixation, a "malic" enzyme, and fumarate reductase, as was described in *Ascaris.* The tapeworm also is similar to *Ascaris* in other respects. The tricarboxylic-acid cycle does not appear to be of physiologic significance as an energy

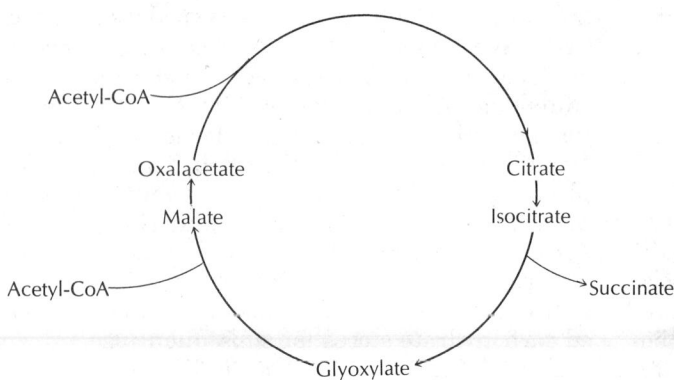

(a) $\text{ATP} + \text{CoA} + \text{Acetate} \longrightarrow \text{Acetyl CoA} + \text{AMP} + \text{P-P}$

(b) $\text{Isocitrate} \longrightarrow \text{Glyoxylate} + \text{Succinate}$

(c) $\text{Glyoxylate} + \text{Acetyl CoA} \longrightarrow \text{Malate} + \text{CoA}$

**FIGURE 6.** *The glyoxylate cycle for the net synthesis of carbohydrates from lipids in Ascaris eggs.*

(d) $= (a) + (b) + (c)$

$\text{ATP} + \text{Isocitrate} + \text{Acetate} \longrightarrow \text{Malate} + \text{Succinate} + \text{AMP} + \text{P-P}$

(e) From TCA cycle reactions:

$\text{ATP} + \text{Malate} + \text{Acetate} \longrightarrow \text{Isocitrate} + 2\,(\text{H}) + \text{AMP} + \text{P-P}$

(f) $= (d) + (e)$

$2\,\text{ATP} + 2\,\text{Acetate} \longrightarrow \text{Succinate} + 2\,(\text{H}) + 2\,\text{AMP} + 2\,\text{P-P}$

yielding pathway in *H. diminuta*. Mitochondrial ATP generation from the fumarate reductase reaction is inhibited by chlorosalicylamide (Yomesan), desaspidin, dichlorophen, and some of the phloroglucinol derivatives, and the cestode has lost its ability to synthesize long-chain fatty acids de novo.

Unlike *Ascaris* metabolism, succinate is a terminal fermentation product in *H. diminuta* in that it is not further utilized. The adult cestode does not form propionate from succinate, and in accordance with this does not contain appreciable levels of vitamin $B_{12}$. Another interesting difference between *Ascaris* and *H. diminuta* was uncovered upon comparing their respective "malic" enzymes. In the case of the former, the oxidative decarboxylation of malate is coupled with $NAD^+$ (see text above for reaction). In the cestode, the reaction is coupled specifically with $NADP^+$. This is important because the reducing power generated by these mitochondrial reactions must be further employed in the specific NADH-requiring fumarate reductase reaction, which presumably will not accept directly from NADPH. To overcome this discrepancy, *H. diminuta* adults con-

tain an active $NADP^+:NAD^+$ transhydrogenase as a constituent of their inner mitochondrial membranes. This activity is not detectable in *Ascaris*. The $NADP^+:NAD^+$ transhydrogenase provides the *H. diminuta* fumarate reductase with NADH by reaction with the NADPH formed in the "malic" enzyme reaction as follows:

1. $\text{1-Malate} + NADP^+ \rightleftharpoons$
$\text{Pyruvate} + CO_2 + NADPH + H^+$

2. $NADPH + NAD^+ \xrightleftharpoons{\text{Transhydrogenase}} NADH + NADP^+$

3. $\text{Fumarate} + NADH + H^+ \xrightarrow[\text{Succinate} + NAD^+]{\text{ADP} \quad \text{ATP}}$

**Fasciola hepatica**

Although it seems clear that some of the helminths possess primarily, if not solely, an anaerobic energy metabolism as in the cases of the homolactate fermenters and the cestodes that have been cultured anaerobically, it is difficult to assess the physiologic significance of oxygen in the energy metabolisms of many other worms. One of the indications that oxygen plays a role in the metabolism of an organism is when the presence of oxygen alters the rate or type of metabolic products formed (for example, Pasteur effect). It has been known for many years that the liver fluke *Fasciola hepatica* exhibits such an effect of oxygen, but it has only recently been indicated that oxygen may serve as a terminal electron acceptor in the energy metabolism of the parasite.

During the adult phase of its life cycle, *F. hepatica* resides in a habitat of low oxygen tension. Therefore, the major part of the trematode's energy metabolism may be expected to be anaerobic. The major end products of either aerobic or anaerobic incubation are acetate and propionate, with considerably smaller quantities of lactate. Incubation of the fluke in air, however, decreases the amount of propionate formed but does not alter acetate formation. Therefore, oxygen may play a role in the energy metabolism of this parasite even though it appears to be predominantly anaerobic in this respect. Recent evidence indicates that either fumarate or oxygen may serve as the terminal respiratory acceptor of electrons. In both cases, phosphorylation of ADP to ATP is associated with the transport of electrons. If oxygen competes with fumarate as terminal acceptor, then aerobically less fumarate and hence less propionate would accumulate. Therefore, although the liver fluke is similar to *Ascaris* in most of its energy-forming pathway, aerobic oxidations may be of considerably greater physiologic significance to this trematode than they are to the nematode.

### SUMMARY

Chemotherapy of most helminth infections of man is still inadequate. Agents employed in the therapy of other infectious diseases are almost universally without effect on helminth infestations. Therefore, the therapy of the metazoan diseases has lagged far behind other therapies and must rely upon its own unique arsenal of drugs. Of those anthelmintics whose mode of action has been examined, most appear to act by inhibiting either neurotransmission or interrupting the energy-yielding reactions of the parasites. These inhibitions are possible because many of the components of the parasite tissues differ from those of the host. It is of both academic and practical importance to understand the biochemistry of the parasitic helminths.

It should be clear that no two helminths will have completely identical biochemical reactions. Differences exist not only between parasite and host, but also between any two parasites. These differences may be at the subtle level of enzyme or protein structure and kinetics or at a more obvious level of pathways, reactions, and products. The key, in examining the energy metabolism of the parasites, is that each organism is different and is a separate biochemical entity. Some helminths, such as *Hymenolepis diminuta* and *Hymenolepis nana,* appear to be anaerobic in all stages of development. Others are capable of a complete or major anaerobic energy metabolism in one or more developmental stages, but require aerobiosis during other parts of the life cycle. Still other parasites are obligate aerobes in one or more of their developmental forms.

Most parasitic worms possess one of two types of energy metabolism; either they are primarily glycolytic, or they are glycolytic but also depend, for part of their energy supply, on the fixation of $CO_2$ and the formation of succinate or products arising from succinate. Many worms employ both pathways and accumulate lactate as well as succinate. Generally, where this is found, the succinate pathway is dominant. Schistosomes and the filarial worms *Brugia pahangi* and *Dipetalonema viteae* are the best examples of glycolyzing helminths, since in vitro they are all homolactate fermenters and do not appear to require oxygen for energy generation. *Litomosoides carinii,* another filarial worm, is an example of a primarily glycolyzing parasite that forms mostly lactate but also requires oxygen for survival, presumably for the single-step energy-yielding oxidative decarboxylation of pyruvate to acetate and $CO_2$. Many other parasites accumulate acetate; some require air for this reaction, others accomplish this oxidative decarboxylation anaerobically. Little is known about the mechanism or energetics of the anaerobic oxidative decarboxylation of pyruvate to acetate in the helminths.

*Ascaris* and to some extent *Hymenolepis diminuta* have served as models for parasites that require $CO_2$ fixation and succinate formation for their energy needs. Many anthelmintics act by inhibiting either the fumarate reductase reaction or the ATP-generating electron transport system associated with it. The role of oxygen in the parasites that form succinate is still not clear. In some — for example, *F. hepatica* — oxygen appears capable of partially competing with fumarate as the terminal electron acceptor. Other parasites, such as *Ascaris* and *Hymenolepis,* will take up oxygen, but the parasites survive equally well without air.

Progress has been slow in the field of parasite biochemistry for many reasons, but some of the biochemical relationships that exist between the host and parasite systems are emerging. Pathways and reactions of greater physiologic significance to the parasite than to the host are being recognized, thereby designating areas that may be amenable to chemotherapeutic attack. However, the giant void between recognizing vulnerable pathways and designing specific inhibitors of these pathways must still be bridged.

### References

Bueding, E.: Carbohydrate metabolism of *Schistosoma mansoni*. J Gen Physiol 33:475, 1950.

Krebs, E. G., and Najjar, V. A.: The inhibition of d-glyceraldehyde 3-phosphate dehydrogenase by specific antiserum. J Exp Med 88:569, 1948.

Mansour, T. E. and Bueding, E.: The actions of antimonials on glycolytic enzymes of *Schistosoma mansoni*. Br J Pharmacol 9:459, 1954.

Meyer, F., Kimura, S., and Mueller, J. F.: Lipid metabolism in the larval and adult forms of the tapeworm *Spirometra mansonoides*. J Biol Chem 241:4224, 1966.

Passey, R. F., and Fairbairn, D.: The conversion of fat to carbohydrate during embryonation of *Ascaris* eggs. Can J Biochem Physiol 35:511, 1957.

Rew, R. S., and Saz, H. J.: The carbohydrate metabolism of *Brugia pahangi* microfilariae. J Parasitol 63:123, 1977.

Saz, H. J.: Facultative anaerobiosis in the invertebrates: Pathways and control systems. Am Zoologist 11:125, 1971.

Saz, H. J. and Dunbar, G. A.: The effects of stibophen on phosphofructokinases and aldolases of adult filariids. J Parasitol 61:794, 1975.

Tkachuck, R. D., Saz, H. J., Weinstein, P. P., Finnegan, K., and Muller, J. F.: The presence and possible function of methylmalonyl CoA mutase and propionyl CoA carboxylase in *Spirometra mansonoides*. J Parasitol 63:769, 1977.

Wang, E. J., and Saz, H. J.: Comparative biochemical studies of *Litomosoides carinii, Dipetalonema viteae,* and *Brugia pahangi* microfilariae. J Parasitol 60:361, 1974.

# 18 *ARTHROPODS OF MEDICAL IMPORTANCE*

### A. L. Dohany, Ph.D.
### John J. S. Burton, Ph.D.

The animals within the phylum Arthropoda are characterized by bilateral symmetry, a chitinous exoskeleton, and paired jointed appendages (Borror et al., 1976). This phylum, the largest of all animal phyla, contains species that transmit some of the most important diseases known to man, including malaria, yellow fever, plague, dengue, typhus, and the encephalitides. The majority of the arthropods of medical importance are contained within two large classes: Insecta (insects) and Arachnida (mites, ticks, spiders, and scorpions) (Furman and Catts, 1970).

The purpose of this chapter is to provide an overview of the arthropods of medical importance. Specific relationships between the arthropods and their animal hosts will be covered in chapters pertaining to the diseases they cause or transmit.

## CLASS: INSECTA

### Order: Diptera

### Flies and Mosquitoes

Adult Diptera or true flies have only a single pair of wings. The hind wings are modified into a pair of small stalked knobs called halteres (balancing organs). The mouth parts of adult biting Diptera are broadly classed as piercing-sucking, and those of filth flies as sponging-lapping.

The Diptera are the most important arthropods medically, and Culicidae (mosquitoes) is the most important family within the group. The activities of Diptera in relation to man can be placed in three categories. (1) As *disease vectors*, they are capable of rapid dissemination of infection either by biologic transmission (e.g., malaria, filariasis) or by mechanical transmission (e.g., typhoid, anthrax) (Chamberlain and Sudia, 1961). (2) As *pests*, the persistence of flies can interrupt and interfere with human activity over broad geographic areas. (3) As *allergens*, biting Diptera sometimes produce rather severe reactions in man, depending on the immune system of the individual (Feingold, 1973). Scratching the site of the reaction can lead to secondary infection.

### *Family: Culicidae*

### *Mosquitoes*

Mosquitoes can be recognized by their relatively long and slender wings, with scales along the wing veins and posterior margin, and by their long, forward-projecting sucking proboscis. Only the females suck blood. The males can be distinguished by the much greater plumosity of the antennae.

There are a number of medically important genera. Living specimens of *Anopheles* (subfamily Anophelinae) are readily distinguishable by their resting and biting posture (Fig. 1). Their body plane is generally at a considerable angle to the substrate, giving the impression that they are standing on their heads. The palpi of both sexes are long like the proboscis. The eggs float singly on the water surface, and the larvae lie parallel to and just below the surface. Certain species in this genus are exclusively responsible for the biologic transmission of the four species of human malaria (*Plasmodium*) as well as simian malaria. They are also known to transmit filariasis (both *Wuchereria* and *Brugia*), as well as some viruses of man, notably that producing O'nyong-nyong fever in Africa.

The genera *Aedes* and *Culex* (subfamily Culicinae) hold their thoracic-abdominal plane essentially parallel to the substrate during resting and biting (Figs. 2 and 3). Palpi of the male are long like the proboscis; those of the female are short. The eggs of *Aedes* are laid singly, most commonly on moist substrate above the water line; those of *Culex* are laid in groups (rafts) on the water. The larvae of this subfamily hang head down into the water and contact the surface film only with an elongated respiratory siphon. *Aedes* mosquitoes are best known for transmitting viral diseases, and *A. aegypti* is clearly the most important disease vector in this genus. Yellow fever and dengue are the major viral diseases transmitted by *Aedes*, but they are also known to transmit chikungunya and encephalitis viruses. Several species also transmit filariasis. *Culex* mosquitoes may be most important as vectors of filariasis (*Wuchereria*), but they also have significant roles in the transmission of viral encephalitis, including Japanese encephalitis, western and eastern equine encephalitides, and St. Louis encephalitis.

Some other genera are important vectors of *specif*ic diseases; e.g., *Mansonia* mosquitoes are the principal vectors of *Brugia*. Larvae of this genus obtain oxygen peculiarly by attaching to the submerged parts of aquatic plants rather than at the water surface, a characteristic that complicates control measures.

*Toxorhynchites* mosquitoes (subfamily Toxorhynchitinae) are beneficial. The adults do not suck blood; instead they live on plant juices. The larvae are predaceous and may partially control the larvae of other mosquito genera locally.

### Family: Simuliidae

### Black Flies

Black flies are small (1 to 5 mm) and have stout bodies that are usually dark in color (Fig. 4).

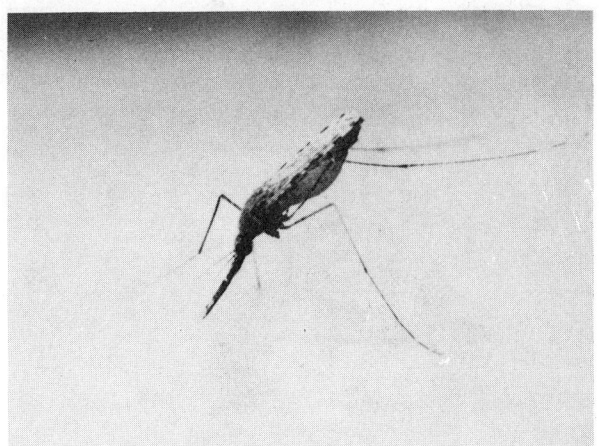

**FIGURE 1**

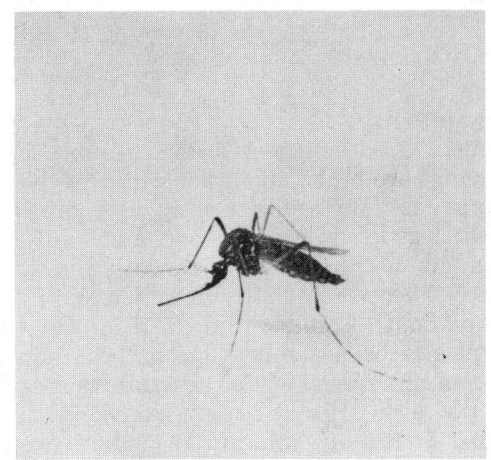

**FIGURE 2**

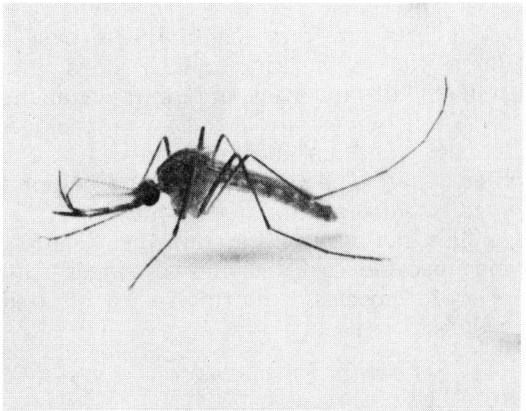

**FIGURE 3**

**FIGURES 1–3.**  Anopheles, Aedes and Culex *mosquitoes in typical resting positions.*

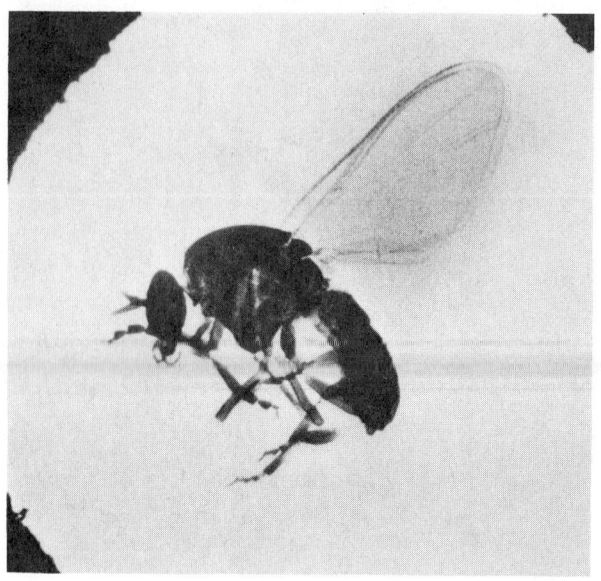

**FIGURE 4.** *A slide-mounted specimen of the family Simuliidae, black flies.*

Their antennae contain 9 to 12 segments (usually 11) and are without arista (long sensory hairs). The wings are broad and are folded over the body when at rest. The anterior wing veins are strong and the legs are relatively short and stout.

The genus *Simulium* transmits the filarial worm *Onchocerca volvulus* in Africa and in Central and South America (Smith, 1973). *Onchocerca* typically causes subcutaneous swellings and may cause blindness when the organism migrates into the eyes. Black fly attacks may also be serious. Irritation, allergic reactions, toxemia, and secondary infections may complicate the bites of simulia (Smith, 1973).

### Family: Ceratopogonidae

### Biting Midges

Biting midges are very small (0.6 to over 4 mm), have piercing-sucking mouth parts, and usually have 14 apparent antennal segments (Fig. 5). Their wings are sometimes speckled, have reduced venation, and are folded over the body when at rest. The most important genera are *Culicoides, Lasiohelea,* and *Leptoconops*.

These flies can be a major nuisance to man. Bites may become irritated and secondarily infected. Several species of filaria are transmitted by *Culicoides*.

### Family: Psychodidae

### Sand Flies and Moth Flies

The Psychodidae are small flies (1.5 to 4 mm) with hairy bodies (Fig. 6). They usually have

rounded wings that are pointed at the tip. The wings have numerous longitudinal veins but few if any basal cross veins.

Moth flies are important only for their nuisance effects. They are often found around sewage treatment plants or in kitchen or bathroom drains. They hold their wings rooflike over the body when at rest.

Phlebotomine sand flies, of which *Phlebotomus* is the important genus, are best known as vectors of visceral and dermal leishmaniasis throughout Central and South America, Africa, southern Europe, and eastward through India and China. Bartonellosis *(Bartonella)* is transmitted by sand flies in South America. Sand fly fever, a nonfatal viral disease, occurs from the Mediterranean area eastward to Sri Lanka and China.

### Family: Tabanidae

### Horse Flies and Deer Flies

The Tabanidae have medium to stout bodies and large convex heads. The overall length of Tabanidae varies from 5 to 30 mm. Their piercing-sucking mouth parts have broad, blade-like stylets. Their wing venation is very characteristic (Figs. 7 and 8).

Horse flies and deer flies are vicious biters of

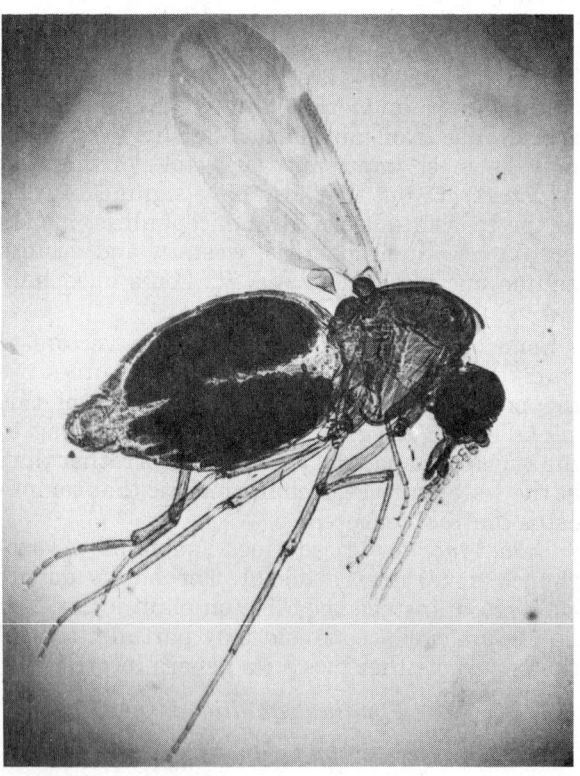

**FIGURE 5.** *A slide-mounted specimen of a biting midge, Culicoides.*

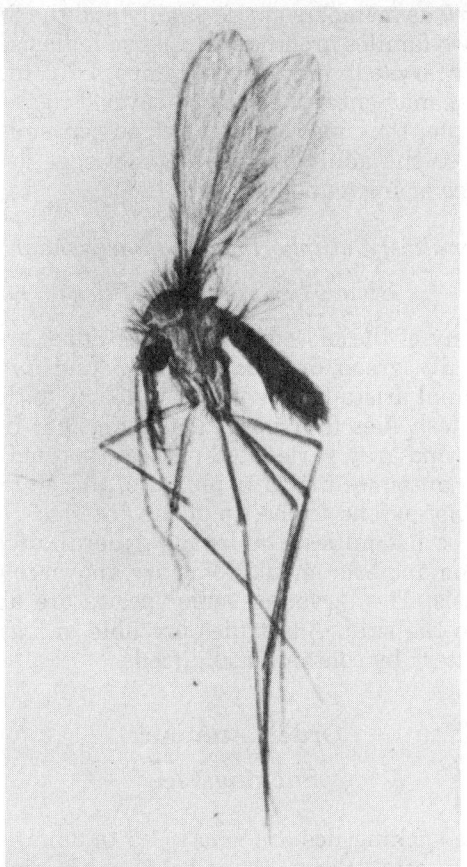

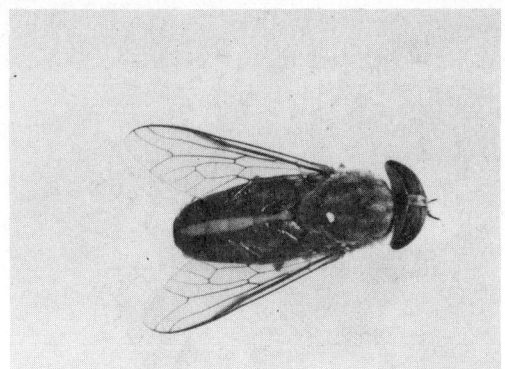

**FIGURE 7**

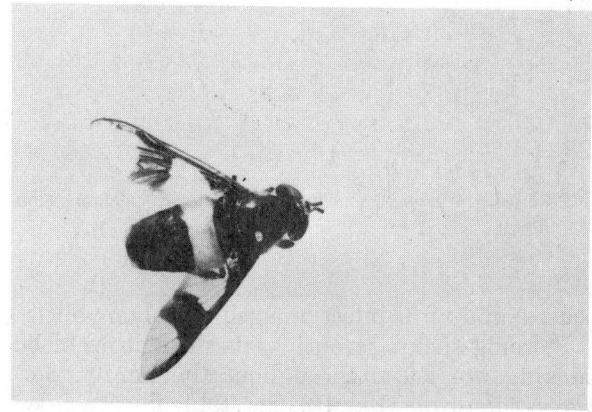

**FIGURE 8**

**FIGURE 6.** *A slide-mounted specimen of a phlebotomine sand fly.*

**FIGURES 7–8.** *Pinned specimens of a horse fly,* Tabanus, *and of a deer fly,* Chrysops, *showing their stout bodies and large convex heads.*

man and animals, producing a large wound that can become secondarily infected. They can be efficient mechanical vectors of disease when their mouth parts have been recently contaminated with pathogenic organisms. Anthrax (*Bacillus anthracis*) and tularemia (*Pasteurella tularensis*) are diseases known to be transmitted in that manner (Krinsky, 1976). In Africa, several species of deer flies (*Chrysops*) are responsible for the biologic transmission of loiasis caused by the filaria *Loa loa*.

### Family: Muscidae

### House Flies, Tsetse Flies, and Relatives

The Muscidae are usually dull-colored and medium to small in size. Their mouth parts vary considerably.

Most species of the genus *Musca*, including *M. domestica*, the common house fly (Fig. 9), have sponging-lapping mouth parts. The larvae breed in filth and the adults frequent feces and garbage. Their sponging-lapping mouth parts and regurgitation of food make them efficient transmitters of

various diseases by food contamination. The diseases that house flies are known to transmit include: many bacterial diseases such as dysenteries, typhoid, and paratyphoid; protozoan diseases including amebic dysentery; helminthic dis-

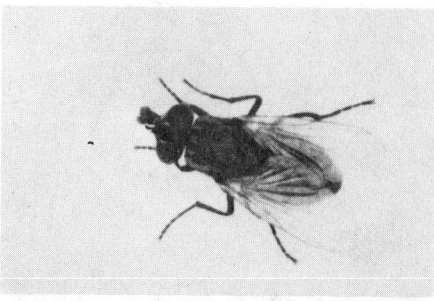

**FIGURE 9.** *A specimen of the common house fly,* Musca domestica.

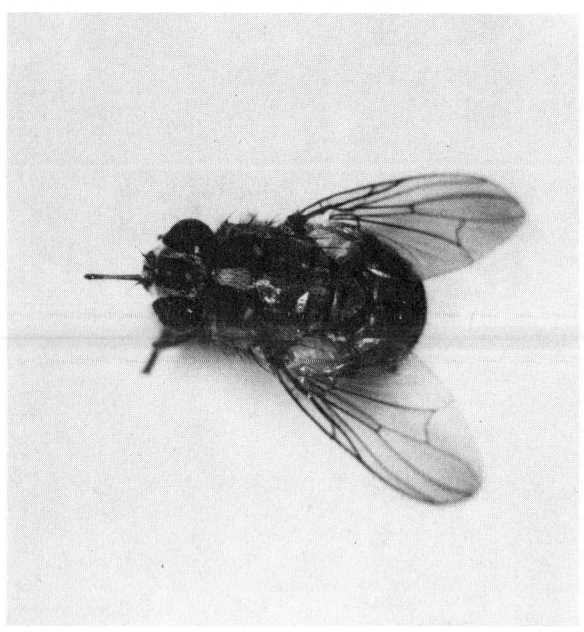

**FIGURE 10.** *A pinned specimen of* Stomoxys calcitrans, *the stable fly.*

Various members of this family and the following two familes are known to cause myiasis, with the fly larvae living, at least temporarily, in man. Larvae may enter the body by several routes. For example, they may be ingested in contaminated food, or the adult fly may deposit eggs at body orifices or in wounds.

### *Families: Calliphoridae and Sarcophagidae*

### *Blow Flies and Flesh Flies*

Many of the blow flies (Calliphoridae) are metallically green or blue (Fig. 12) and have an antennal arista that is plumose nearly to the tip. The flesh flies (Sarcophagidae) (Fig. 13) have a black and gray variegated pattern (not metallic). If the antennal arista is plumose, the plumosity does not extend to the tip of the antenna.

In both families, the larvae generally feed on carrion and excrement. Some are known to cause myiasis. The larvae of some species are able to pierce the skin. Adult flies are able to transmit dysentery by contaminating food.

eases; and viral infection such as poliomyelitis.

Piercing-sucking mouth parts suitable for blood sucking are found throughout the family. *Stomoxys calcitrans* (Fig. 10), the stable fly, is a blood sucker that may transmit pathogens to man. Members of the genus *Glossina* (Fig. 11), the tsetse flies, are well known for their ability to transmit African sleeping sickness (*Trypanosoma rhodesiense* and *T. gambiense*).

### Order: Anoplura

### Sucking Lice

The sucking lice are small (1.5 to 3mm) wingless insects (Figs. 14 and 15) with piercing-sucking mouth parts. The tarsi of the legs are usually reduced. The single tarsal claw is opposed by a toothed projection on the tibia. These two structures provide an excellent means of grasping hairs of their hosts.

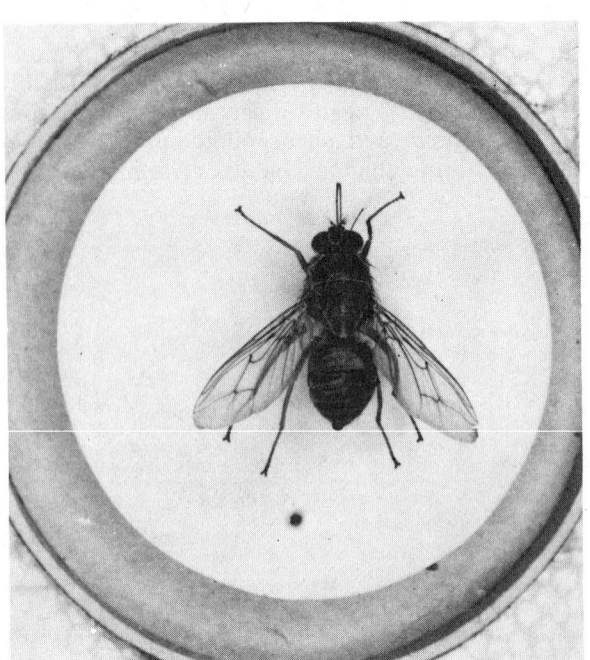

**FIGURE 11.** *A pinned specimen of* Glossina, a tsetse fly, showing a distinct hatchet-shaped wing cell.

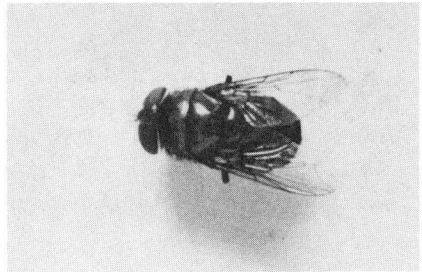

**FIGURE 12.** *A pinned specimen of a blow fly, Calliphoridae.*

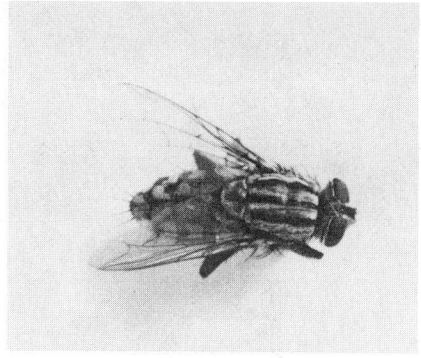

**FIGURE 13.** *A pinned specimen of a flesh fly, Sarcophagidae, showing a non-metallic black and gray color-pattern.*

Two varieties of the species, *Pediculus humanus*, the head and the body louse, and *Pthirus pubis*, the crab louse, are important to man.

Louse infestation, pediculosis, may cause extreme irritation and discomfort. Red papules, swelling, and sensitization may result from the feeding of sucking lice. Often the egg or nit may be easily found (Fig. 16).

Epidemic relapsing fever (*Borrelia recurrentis*) is transmitted by crushing an infected body louse on the skin. Epidemic typhus or louse-borne typhus (*Rickettsia prowazekii*) and trench fever (*R. quintana*) may be transmitted to humans either by the feces of the louse or by crushing of the body of the louse (Hunter et al., 1976). Transmission from the salivary glands of the louse is not involved in any of these diseases.

### Order: Siphonaptera

### Fleas

Fleas, which are well known for their jumping ability, are wingless insects (Fig. 17) with lateral-

ly compressed bodies. The usual size varies from 1.5 to 4 mm. Their mouth parts are adapted for piercing-sucking. Only adult fleas feed on mammals. The larvae and pupae are normally found in soil or bedding.

Fleas are the vector of the bacterium *Yersinia pestis*, which causes plague. Plague, an infection of rodents, is transmitted to humans when conditions become favorable. Fleas that have fed on an infected animal often develop a blocked proventriculus. Then, when they try to feed on another host, the plague bacilli are forced into the uninfected host. Plague bacilli have also been shown to be transmitted by the flea's feces. The major flea involved in urban plague is *Xenopsylla cheopis*; a large number of other species have been incriminated, however, especially in sylvatic or campestral plague (Hunter et al., 1976).

*Xenopsylla cheopis* is the main vector of murine typhus (*Rickettsia typhi*), although *Nosopsyllus*

**FIGURE 14.** *A slide-mounted specimen of the human body louse, Pediculus humanus.*

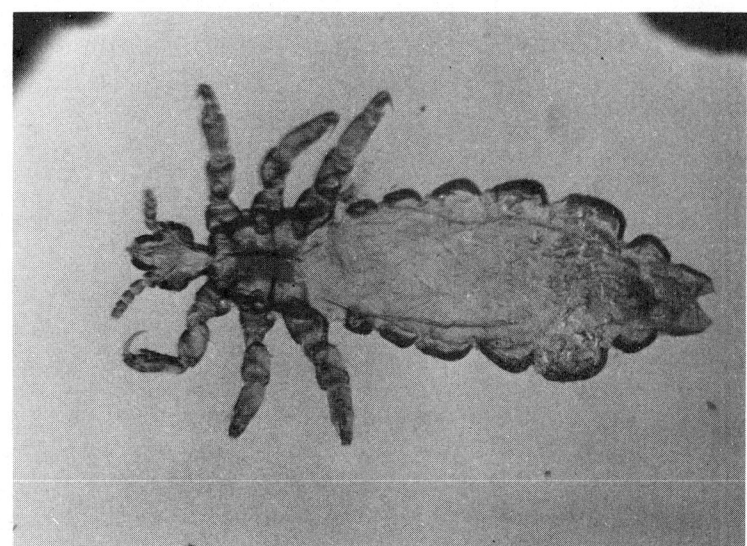

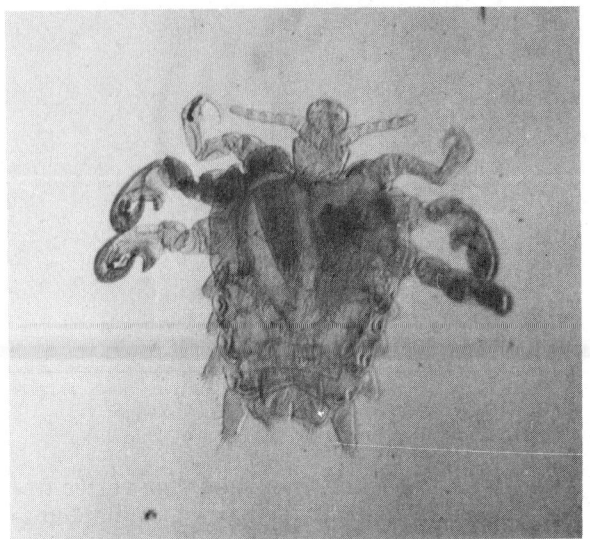

**FIGURE 15.** *A slide-mounted specimen of the pubic louse,* Pthirus pubis, *showing the distinctive tarsal claws used for grasping hairs.*

*fasciatus* and *Leptopsylla segnis* are also known to be vectors (James and Harwood, 1969). The mode of infection is scratching of the vector's feces into the skin.

## Order: Orthoptera

### Cockroaches

Cockroaches are normally flattened dorsoventrally and have a smooth but tough integument (Fig. 18). Adults are characterized by leathery outer wings and membranous inner wings. Their color varies from green to orange in tropical species to dark brown to black in the more common household species. The size of adults varies from 12 to 40 mm. Most species remain in dark locations during the day and can be seen feeding only during the night, usually in kitchens and food storage areas when lights are suddenly turned one.

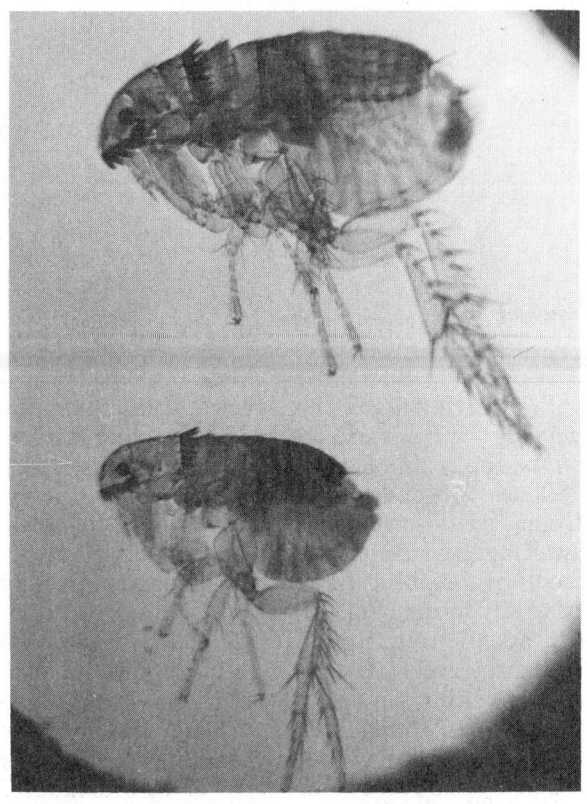

**FIGURE 17.** *Male (top) and female (bottom) adult Siphonoptera, showing their lack of wings and their strong hind legs.*

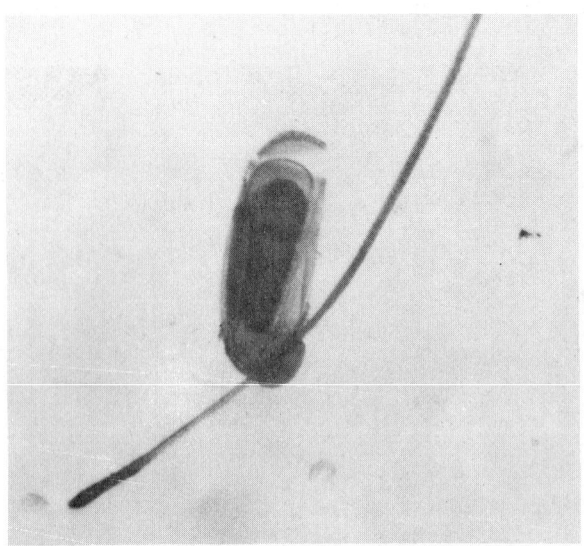

**FIGURE 16.** *Egg of a sucking louse cemented to a hair.*

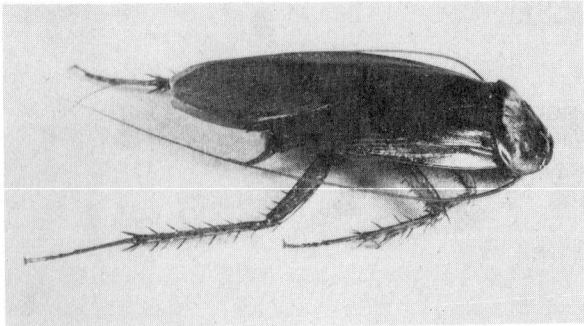

**FIGURE 18.** *Specimen of the cockroach,* Periplaneta americana.

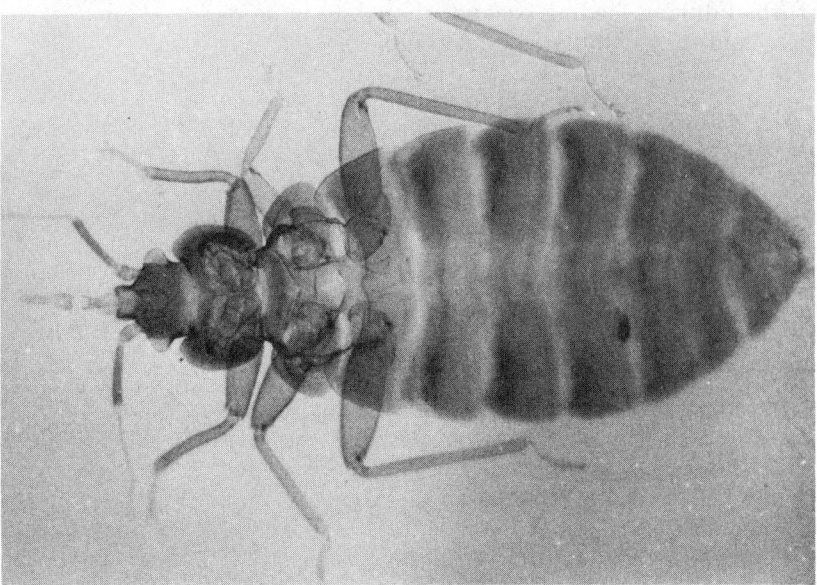

**FIGURE 19.** *A slide-mounted specimen of* Cimex, *showing rudimentary wings.*

Circumstantial and experimental evidence indicates that cockroaches could be involved in the mechanical transmission of several organisms. They are omnivorous feeders and have the habit of disgorging partially digested food and feces as they feed. Thus, the medical importance of cockroaches lies in their ability to contaminate food and foodstuffs.

Numerous viruses, pathogenic bacteria, pathogenic fungi, and protozoa have been isolated from cockroaches. Additionally, the list of different organisms that cockroaches may harbor experimentally is quite long (James and Harwood, 1969). Cockroaches are also known to be intermediate hosts for several rat nematodes.

## Order: Hemiptera

### True Bugs

The fore wing of the adult Hemiptera is usually divided into a leathery basal portion and a membranous apical portion. The hind wing is totally membranous. The bed bug, which has only rudimentary wings, is an exception to this general rule. The mouth parts of the order are adapted for piercing and sucking.

Bed bugs, family Cimicidae (4 to 5 mm) (Fig. 19), are not known to be vectors of human pathogens, but their bite does cause extreme irritation and swelling in individuals who are allergic to the saliva that is introduced at the time of feeding. Bed bugs are nocturnal. They spend the daylight hours hidden in cracks, crevices, or bedding. *Cimex lectularius* is normally found in the temperate regions, whereas *C. hemipterus* is usually

restricted to the tropics. A third species, *Leptocimex boueti*, is limited to Africa (James and Harwood, 1969).

The bite of the assassin bugs (Fig. 20), family Reduviidae, can cause extreme local irritation and swelling. Systemic reactions may also occur as a result of the injection of foreign protein.

Chagas' disease (*Trypanosoma cruzi*), normally found in South and Central America, is transmitted by several genera of reduviids. This disease is transmitted when the reduviid defecates while feeding (Faust et al., 1968). The feces are then transported by the fingers to the conjunctiva of the eye or the mucosa of the mouth or nose. Although these bugs are large (up to 25 mm) and formidable in appearance, they are seldom dis-

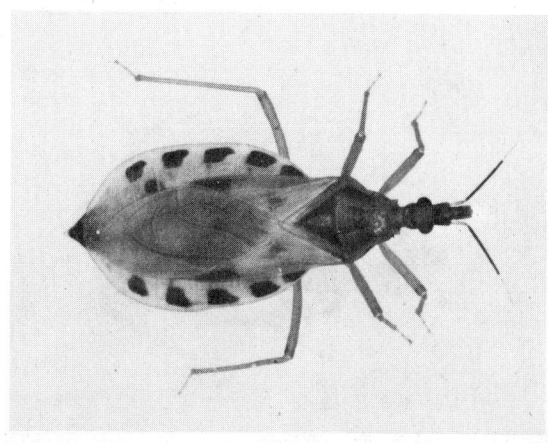

**FIGURE 20.** *A specimen of a reduviid,* Triatoma.

turbed during feeding because their bite is painless and they usually feed at night.

## Order: Coleoptera

### Beetles

The adults of the order Coleoptera have two pairs of wings. The outer pair is thickened to form wing covers called elytra, while the inner pair is membranous (Fig. 21). The mouth parts are formed for chewing.

Some families of beetles are known for their ability to produce blisters by discharging their body fluids onto the skin. The "Spanish fly" (*Lytta vesicatoria*) (10 to 15 mm) is perhaps the best known vesicating beetle. Blisters are formed when this beetle is crushed on the skin.

## Order: Lepidoptera

### Butterflies and Moths (Caterpillars)

The adults of the Lepidoptera (butterflies and moths) may be separated from other insects by their two pairs of membranous wings that are covered with overlapping scales. Their mouth parts are adapted for siphoning. Larvae and caterpillars are usually cylindrical in shape and have three pairs of thoracic legs and two to five pairs of abdominal legs or prolegs (Fig. 22).

Contact with poison hairs on the external surface of caterpillars causes a stinging dermatitis. The urticating fluid is released when the tips of the hairs are broken upon contact.

## Order: Hymenoptera

### Bees, Wasps, Hornets, and Ants

The Hymenoptera usually have two pairs of membranous wings with hind wings that are

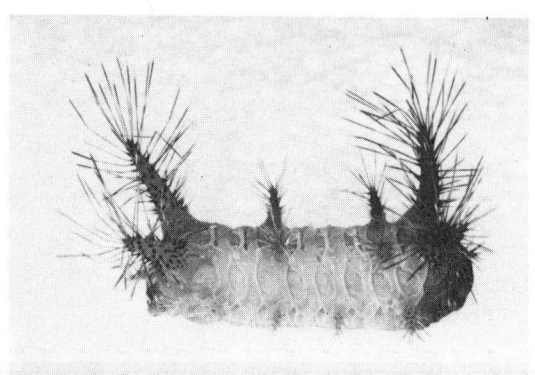

**FIGURE 22.** *A specimen of a lepidopterous larva, showing its urticating hairs.*

smaller than the fore wings (Fig. 23), but some members of the order, notably the ants, are wingless. The abdomens of the females are usually provided with a stinging apparatus.

The effects of a Hymenoptera sting may range from moderate, temporary pain and slight local swelling to shock and death.

## CLASS: ARACHNIDA

### Subclass: Acari

### Mites and Ticks

The subclass Acari is composed of the arthropods that are commonly referred to as ticks and mites. These arthropods are distinctive in that they have two body regions, an idiosoma (fused abdomen and cephalothorax) and a gnathosoma (mouth parts) (Krantz, 1978). Adult Acari usually have four pairs of legs, but larvae have only three.

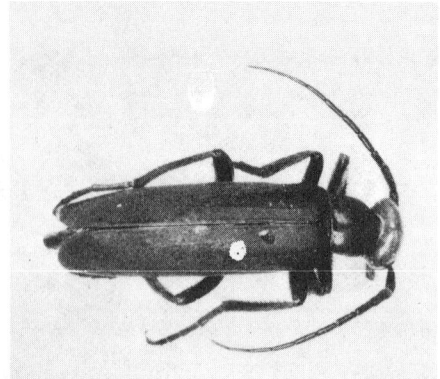

**FIGURE 21.** *A pinned specimen of a blister beetle, showing its thick wing covers or elytra.*

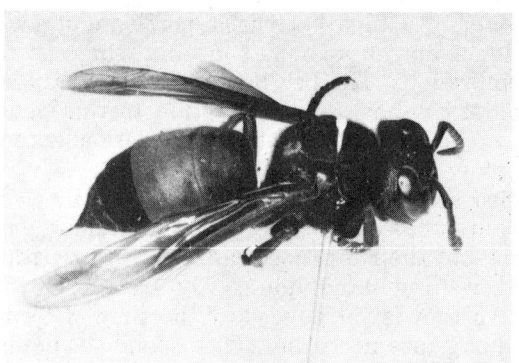

**FIGURE 23.** *A pinned specimen of an adult hymenopteran, showing a stinger on the terminal abdominal segment.*

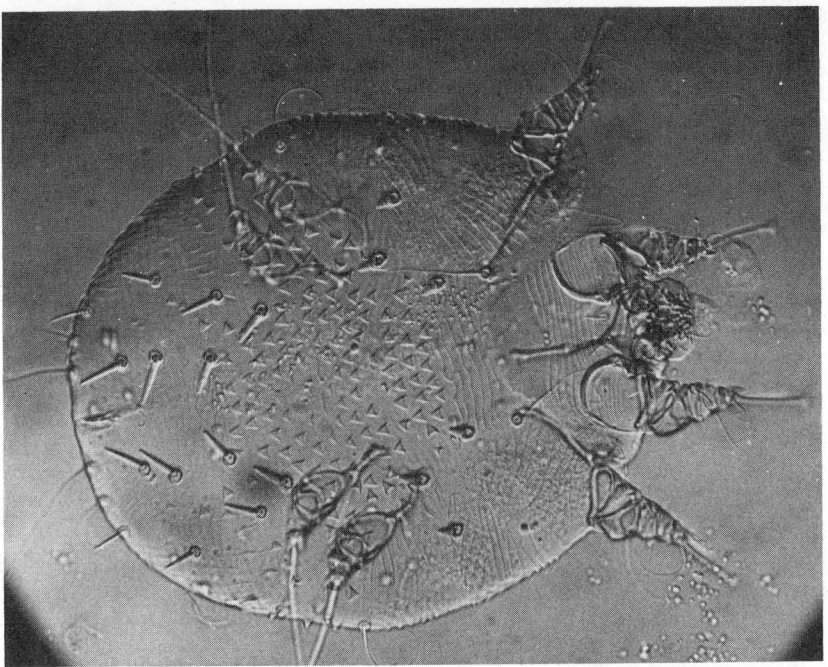

**FIGURE 24.** *A slide-mounted specimen of* Sarcoptes scabiei.

Only two species of mites are parasites of man: the skin mite, *Sarcoptes scabiei* (0.3 to 0.5 mm) (Fig. 24), and the follicle mite, *Demodex folliculorum* (0.4 mm) (Fig. 25). *Demodex folliculorum* may not cause any disease in man; it may only be a commensal. However, *Sarcoptes scabiei* can cause extreme itching and keratotic crusts covering large numbers of mites. *Demodex* and *Sarcoptes* cause the condition commonly known as mange in animals.

A large number of mites and ticks can parasitize man if their normal host is not available. Additionally, another large group of mites may affect many by biting and causing dermatitis (Krantz, 1978). This group includes many mites that feed on plants and organic matter and that come into contact with man only accidentally.

Scrub typhus or chigger-borne rickettsiosis (*Rickettsia tsutsugamushi*) is transmitted by the larvae of the trombiculid mite or chigger (Fig.

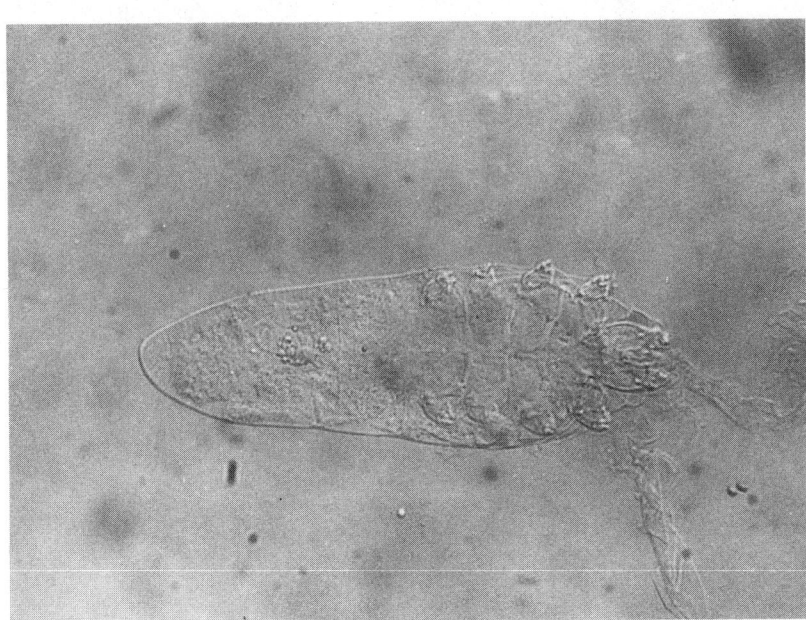

**FIGURE 25.** *A slide-mounted specimen of* Demodex folliculorum.

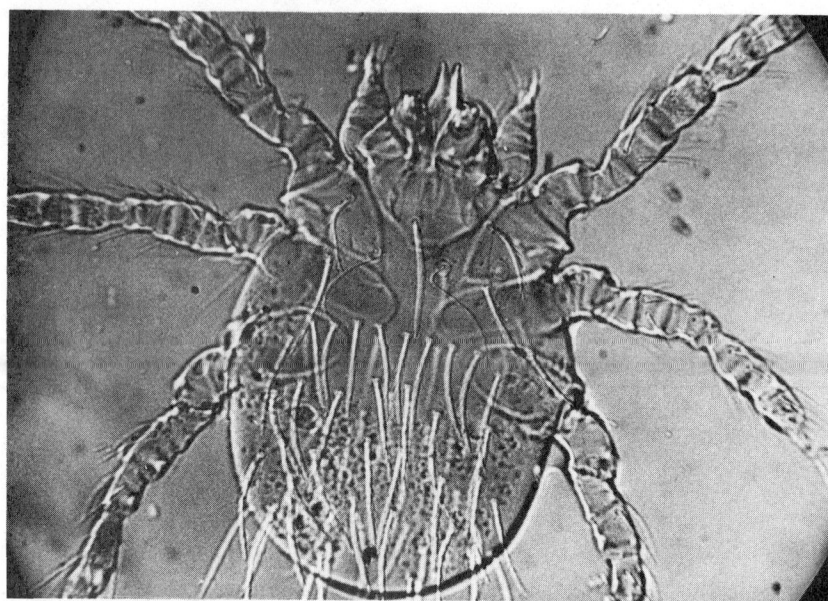

**FIGURE 26.** *A slide-mounted specimen of a* Leptotrombidium *chigger.*

26). The disease occurs throughout Asia in a triangle roughly bound by India, northern Australia, and northern Japan. All known vectors are in the genus and subgenus *Leptotrombidium* (Traub and Wisseman, 1974). The small (0.2 to 0.4 mm), six-legged larvae normally feed on small rodents but will attack man if he is in the chiggers' habitat. Feeding by these mites is often inapparent until the onset of the disease.

Rickettsialpox (*Rickettsia acari*) reported from the United States and Russia is transmitted by nymphs and adults of the house mouse mite, *Liponyssoides sanguineus*. Although this disease is apparently uncommon, it may be more widely spread than has been reported, since a similar disease has been described from Africa and the causative organism has been isolated from wild rodents in Korea.

A number of mites commonly referred to as house dust mites have been associated with the

**FIGURE 27.** *A slide-mounted specimen showing the hypostome (arrow) of a tick.*

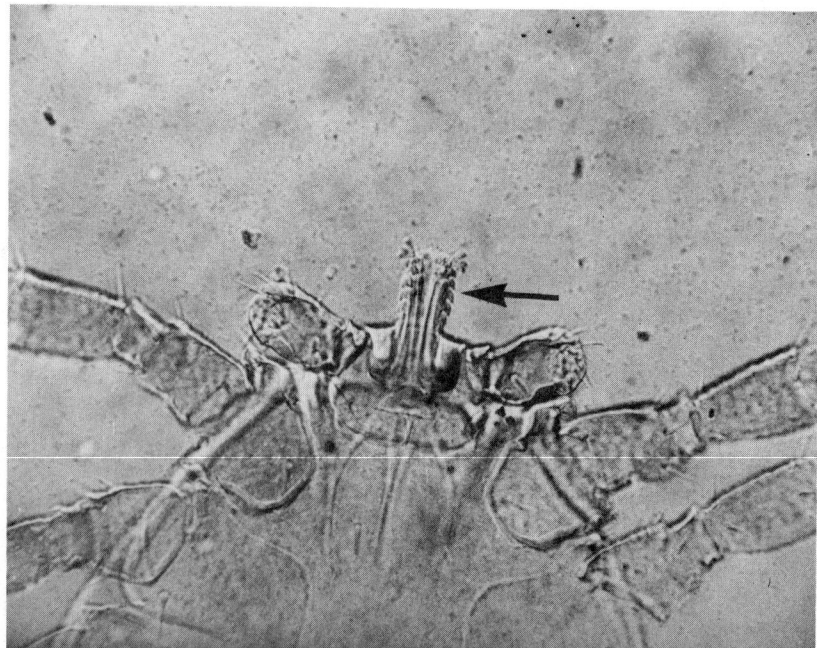

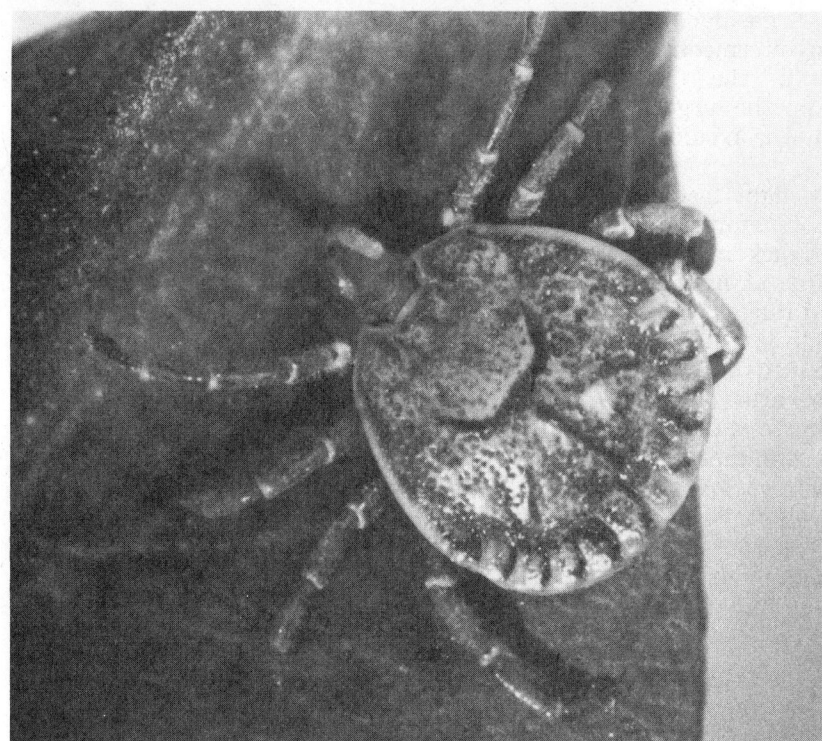

**FIGURE 28.** *A specimen of an adult tick, Ixodidae.*

production of allergens that cause bronchial asthma and rhinitis (Wharton, 1976). Although a large number of different genera may occur in dust samples, species of the genus *Dermatophagoides* (0.2 to 0.4 mm) have proved to be the most important in relation to allergies. Dust mites are normally found in beds and furniture and under beds, feeding on human dander.

Ticks (superfamily Ixodoidea) can be differentiated from the other acari by the presence of a sensory structure known as Haller's organ on the first pair of tarsi. Also, many species have a toothed hypostome (Fig. 27). Generally, adult ticks are relatively large (0.3 to 5 mm) in comparison to other acari and have a leathery appearance (Fig. 28). Ixodoidea is composed of three

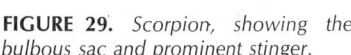

**FIGURE 29.** *Scorpion, showing the bulbous sac and prominent stinger.*

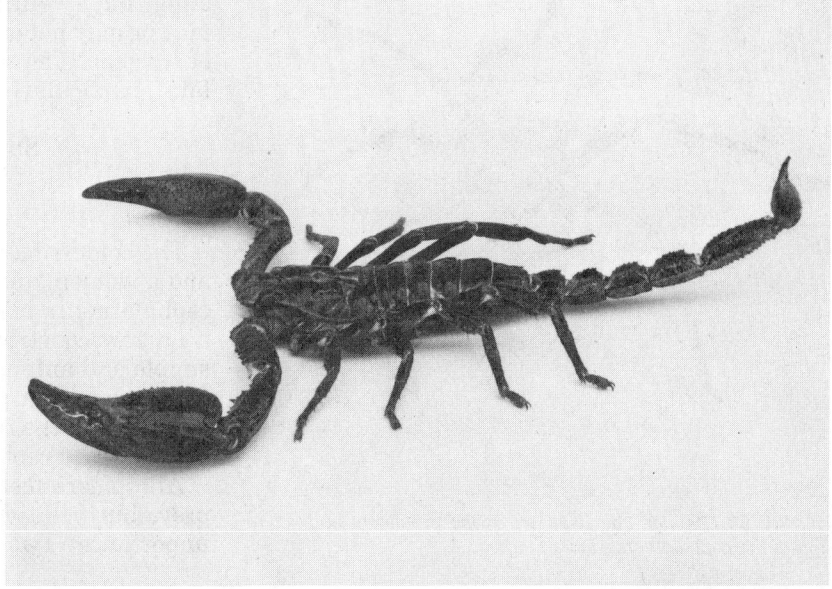

families: Ixodidae, or hard ticks; Argasidae, or soft ticks; and Nuttalliellidae, an intermediate represented by a single species. Of the vast number of tick-borne diseases, by far the largest number are transmitted to man by the Ixodidae (Balashov, 1972).

James and Harwood (1969) list eight factors that make ticks such good vectors of mammalian diseases. Ticks are persistent bloodsuckers, slow feeders, highly sclerotized, and free of natural enemies. They also have a wide host range, a long life span, ability to transmit the disease agents transovarially, and a great reproductive potential. Ticks are known to transmit arboviruses, rickettsiae, bacteria, and piroplasms to man. Additionally, ticks may cause paralysis in man.

By far the largest number of diseases transmitted to man by ticks are caused by arboviruses. The majority fall into the category known as the Russian spring-summer complex (flavivirus or antigenic group B).

### Subclass: Scorpiones

### Scorpions

Scorpions are easily recognizable by their long, five-segmented, tail-like post-abdomen that terminates in a bulbous sac with a prominent stinger. Anteriorly, the pedipalps are enlarged and resemble an additional pair of legs, and the

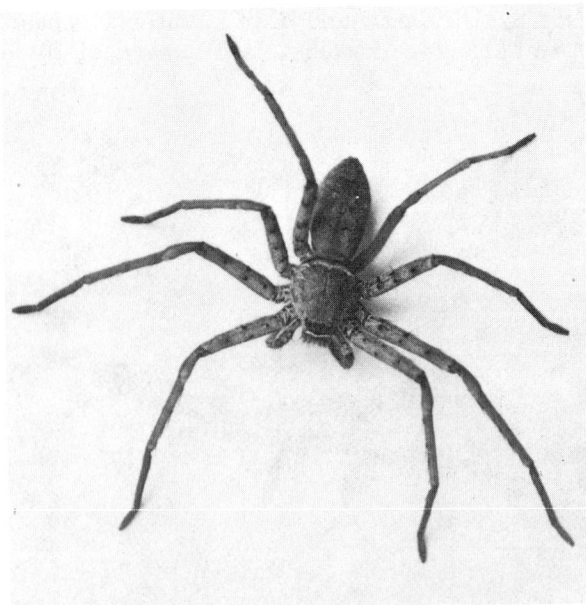

**FIGURE 30.** *Spider, characterized by the prominent body division of the cephalothorax and abdomen.*

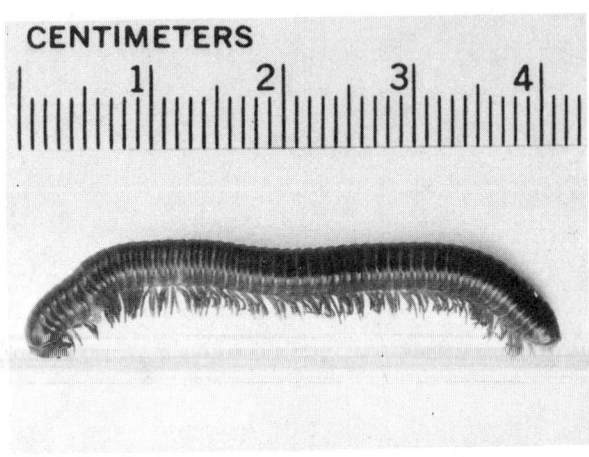

**FIGURE 31.** *Millipede, bearing 2 pairs of legs per body segment.*

last two segments are modified to form pincers (Fig. 29).

Scorpions are nocturnal by nature, remaining hidden in the daytime under stones, litter, and lumber. The sting usually results from accidental contact with a scorpion, such as accidentally stepping on it, placing one's foot in its hiding place (e.g., a boot), or disturbing its habitat. The sting of the scorpion can be very dangerous, depending upon the species. Areas such as Mexico, southwestern United States, parts of South America, and North Africa west of Egypt are known to have particularly dangerous species. The severity of the sting is not necessarily related to the size of the scorpion; the smaller species are often more dangerous. Children are more seriously affected. Pain is usually associated with the sting, but swelling and discoloration at the site may or may not occur, depending upon the species of scorpion. The sting of dangerous species can be fatal, particularly to children.

### Subclass: Araneae

### Spiders

The spiders have two body parts, cephalothorax and abdomen, and four pairs of legs (Fig. 30). The cephalothorax is separated from the abdomen by a narrow constriction, the pedicel. The eyes are simple and antennae are absent. All spiders have silk glands that produce silk through spinnerets located near the rear of the abdomen. The legs are borne on the cephalothorax.

All spiders feed by injecting venom into their prey, but relatively few species are of medical importance. Two types of effects are commonly noted from spider bites: the formation of a necrotizing ulcer and systemic symptoms. The bite of *Loxosceles* spp., brown recluse or fiddle-back spiders, causes necrotic ulcers on the skin, a condition termed loxoscelism. In mild cases the necrotic ulcer may be slow to heal, leaving a disfiguring scar. In severe cases erosion of all mucous membranes, hemorrhage, and death may occur (Southcott, 1976). Systemic reactions from spider bites are particularly well known from the hairy spiders known as tarantula, Theraphosidae, and the "black widows," *Latrodectus* spp. Swelling and pain may occur at the site of the bite, followed by burning and aching in the general area of the bite. Circulating venoms may induce abdominal cramps. Untreated bites may cause convulsions, shock, and death.

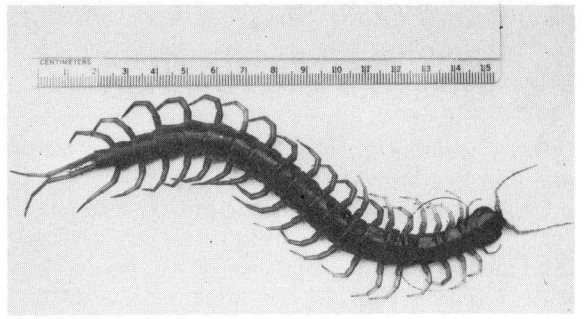

**FIGURE 32.**   *Centipede, bearing a single pair of legs per segment.*

Erythema and edema may occur and persist for several weeks.

## CLASS: *DIPLOPODA*
### *MILLIPEDES*

Members of the class Diplopoda are multi-segmented and multi-legged arthropods. Each body segment bears two pairs of legs (Fig. 31). Most species of millipedes feed on decaying organic matter and many species are equipped with offensive stink glands.

The stink glands of the millipede may have the capability of forcefully ejecting secretions. This liquid may cause severe pain and staining of the skin at the site of contact. The lining epithelium of the eye and mouth are particularly susceptible.

## CLASS: *CHILOPODA*
### *CENTIPEDES*

The Chilopoda have a single pair of antennae and a multi-segmented trunk. Each segment bears a single pair of legs (Fig. 32). Paired poison claws arise from the first trunk segment.

The venom of the poison claws of centipedes is used to kill prey, usually insects, but occasionally small reptiles, mammals, and birds. Some species of centipedes are able to pierce human skin and cause severe pain and localized swelling. The severity of a centipede bite is often compared with that of a bee or wasp sting.

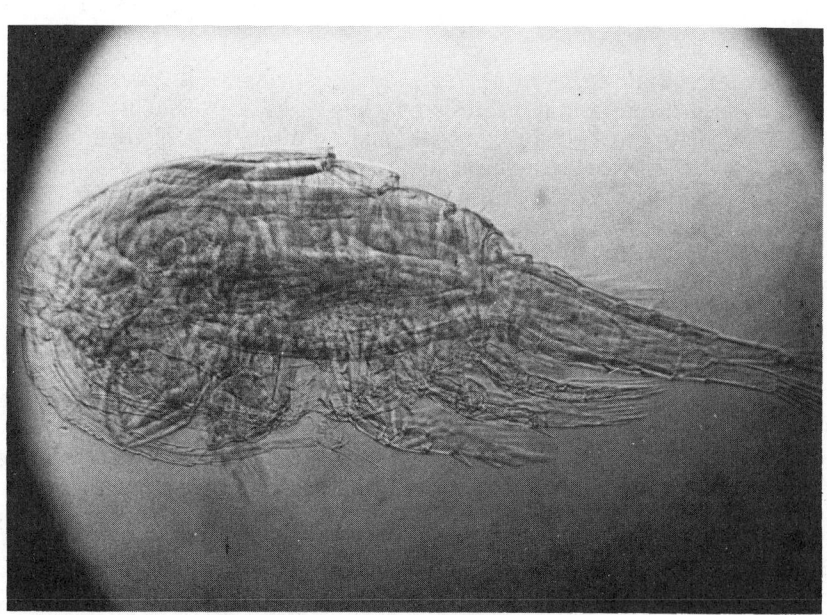

**FIGURE 33.**   *A slide-mounted specimen of a copepod,* Cyclops.

## CLASS: CRUSTACEA

### CRAYFISH, SHRIMP, CRABS, LOBSTERS, AND COPEPODS

Crustaceans typically have two pairs of antennae and five or more pairs of legs.

Crustaceans play an important part in the life cycle of a number of helminths by acting as intermediate hosts. Species of copepods, especially *Cyclops* (Fig. 33), are intermediate hosts for the broad tapeworm *Diphyllobothrium latum* and for the guinea worm of Africa, *Dracunculus medinensis*.

### References

Balashov, Y.S.: Bloodsucking ticks (Ixodoidea) — vector of diseases of man and animals (1968). Misc Pub Entomol Soc Am 8:161, 1972.

Borror, D.J., DeLong, D.M., and Triplehorn, C.A.: An Introduction to the Study of Insects. 4th ed. New York, Holt, Rinehart & Winston, 1976.

Chamberlain, R.W., and Sudia, W.D.: Mechanism of transmission of viruses by mosquitoes. Ann Rev Entomol 6:371, 1961.

Faust, E.C., Beaver, P.C., and Jung, R.C.: Animal Agents ;and Vectors of Human Disease. 3rd ed. Philadelphia, Lea & Febiger, 1968.

Feingold, B.F.: Introduction to Clinical Allergy. Springfield, Ill., Charles C Thomas, 1973.

Furman, D.P., and Catts, E.P.: Manual of Medical Entomology. 3rd ed. Palo Alto, Calif., National Press Books, 1970.

Hunter, G.W., III, Swartzwelder, J.C., and Clyde, D.F.: Tropical Medicine. 5th ed. Philadelphia, W.B. Saunders Co., 1976.

James, M.T., and Harwood, R.F.: Herms's Medical Entomology. 6th ed. New York, Macmillan, 1969.

Krantz, G.W.: A Manual of Acarology. 2nd ed. Corvallis, Ore., State University Book Stores, Inc., 1978.

Krinsky, W.L.: Animal disease agents transmitted by horse flies and deer flies (Diptera: Tabanidae). J Med Entomol 13:225, 1976.

Smith, K.G.V. (Ed.): Insects and Other Arthropods of Medical Importance. London, Trustees of the British Museum (Natural History), 1973.

Southcott, R.V.: Arachnidism and allied syndromes in the Australian Region. Records Adelaide Children's Hosp 1:97, 1976.

Traub, R., and Wisseman, C.L., Jr.: The ecology of chigger-borne rickettsiosis (scrub typhus). J Med Entomol 11:237, 1974.

Wharton, G.W.: House dust mites. J Med Entomol 12:577, 1976.

# Principles of Antimicrobial Chemotherapy of Infections

# 19 DESCRIPTION OF ANTIMICROBIAL DRUGS

Abraham I. Braude, M.D., Ph.D.

# CLASSIFICATION

Antimicrobial drugs may no longer be classified according to the organisms they inhibit because their spectra can be broadened by minor adjustments in structure or dosage. Classification of antibiotics and synthetic antimicrobial drugs is based instead on chemical structure or biochemical effects. Since the biochemical effects are considered in the next chapter, "Mechanisms of Action of Antimicrobial Drugs," a chemical classification will be presented here. All antimicrobial drugs are ring compounds; otherwise, the various groups have little structural similarity.

## THE PEPTIDES

The penicillins, cephalosporins, bacitracin, and polymyxins are the most important peptide antibiotics. Their molecular weight seldom exceeds 3000. For this reason they are too small to be antigenic and stimulate neutralizing antibodies that would cause them to lose activity with continued administration. Small nonantigenic peptide antibiotics are a lucky evolutionary by-product in the molds and bacteria that produce these antimicrobial agents. They are small because they are synthesized by a pathway that does not depend on the elaborate system for coding amino acids and their sequences required for protein synthesis. It is likely that microbial peptides, including peptide antibiotics, evolved before the process of protein synthesis via nucleic-acid coding on ribosomes. Since the functions performed by peptides were later taken over by microbial proteins, the peptides can be regarded as "fossils."[1] The fact that the majority of these antibiotics have a cyclic structure is also consistent with the idea that they once performed a functional role in microbial metabolism because cyclic structures are found in enzymes and other functional proteins.

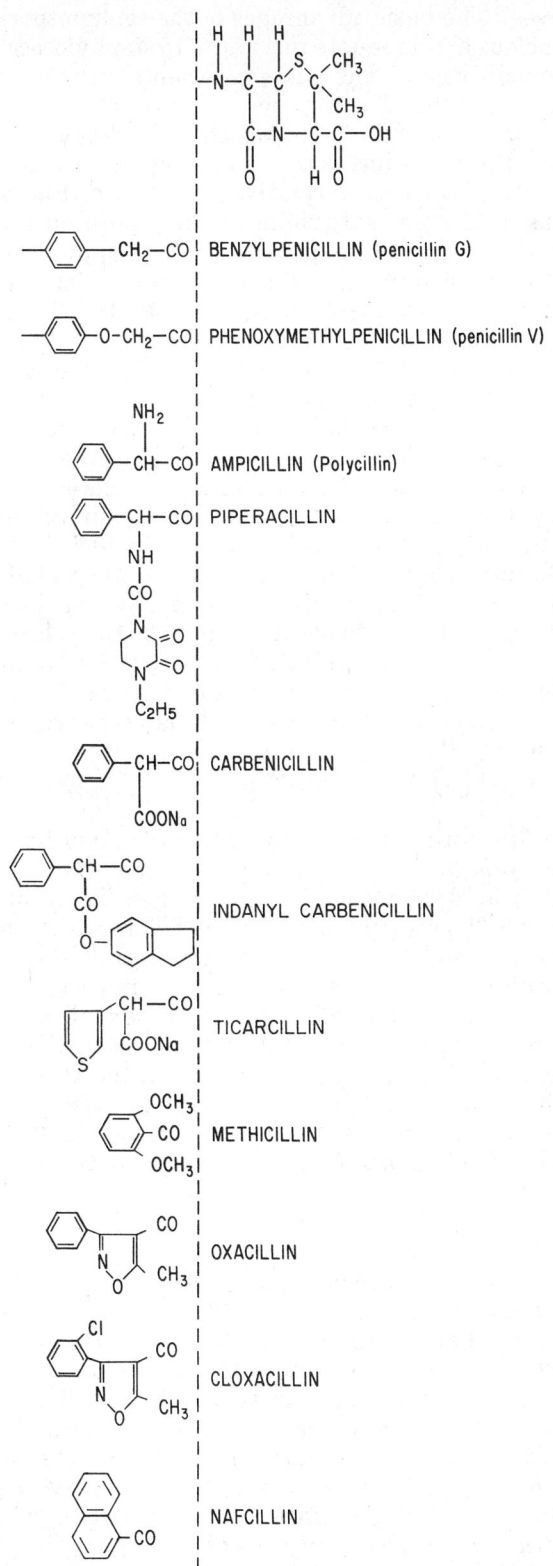

**FIGURE 1.**  *The side chains responsible for the biologic differences in each of the penicillins are shown to the left of the dotted line, and 6-aminopenicillanic acid is on the right. The last four side chains protect the β-lactam ring from the action of penicillinase.*

## The Penicillins

The common nucleus of the penicillins is 6-aminopenicillanic acid, a cyclic dipeptide of L-cysteine and D-valine (Fig. 1). These are arranged in a basic structure consisting of a thiazolidine ring joined to a β-lactam ring. Individual penicillins differ with respect to the side chains attached to the common nucleus. The most important of the naturally occurring penicillins is penicillin G, containing a benzyl side chain (Fig. 1). Penicillin V is obtained when phenoxyacetic acid is added as a precursor to the fermentation medium so that a phenoxymethyl side chain becomes attached to the penicillin nucleus. This compound is well suited for oral use because of its resistance to gastric acid. Other penicillins are prepared by the synthetic addition of various groups as side chains to 6-aminopenicillanic acid after it has been isolated from *Penicillium* fermentation media. Depending on their chemical structure, these side chains can broaden the antimicrobial spectrum, protect the penicillin nucleus from acid hydrolysis, or protect it against penicillinase. In ampicillin, for example, the presence of an amino group in the phenyl radical of benzylpenicillin produces a compound both resistant to acid and more active against gram-negative bacteria than penicillin G. If a carboxyl group is introduced instead, as in carbenicillin, the spectrum is altered so that the compound becomes the only penicillin derivative with activity against *Pseudomonas aeruginosa*. None of these modifications, however, confers resistance to staphylococcal penicillinase. This was first accomplished in the synthesis of methicillin by the introduction of methoxy groups at positions 2 and 6 on the benzyl ring so that affinity of the substrate site for penicillinase is reduced 10,000 times.[13] This modification did not achieve acid resistance, but the synthesis of isoxazolyl penicillin introduced a series of products with combined resistance to penicillinase and gastric acid. Oxacillin and dicloxacillin are the most widely used of these doubly resistant penicillins.

These and other penicillin derivatives have been modified further to improve their blood levels, broaden their antimicrobial spectrum and reduce side effects. The conversion of ampicillin to amoxicillin, by the introduction of a hydroxyl radical at the para position in the benzyl side chain, improves absorption. Absorption is also improved by conversion of amoxicillin to pivampicillin, the pivaloyloxymethyl ester of ampicillin. After absorption, pivampicillin is hydrolyzed first to pivalic acid and the hydroxymethyl ester of ampicillin; these are then hydrolyzed within 15 minutes to ampicillin and formaldehyde. Either

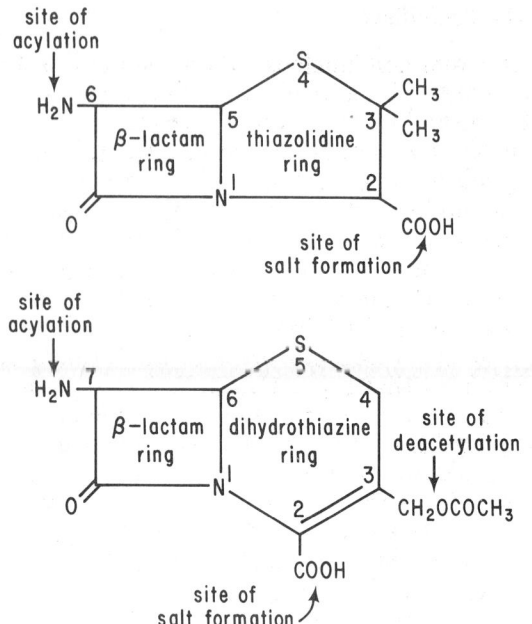

**FIGURE 2.** *Comparison of penicillin nucleus, 6-aminopenicillanic acid (upper figure), with cephalosporin nucleus, 7-aminocephalosporanic acid (lower diagram). The main difference in the two compounds is the thiazolidine ring in penicillin and the dihydrothiazine ring in the cephalosporins. Most penicillin derivatives are produced by addition of side chains at the acylation site. Cephalosporin derivatives vary in the chemical groups at the acylation site, and at the deacetylation site as well.*

modification provides blood levels after oral administration that are approximately twice that obtained with ampicillin.[12]

The acid lability of carbenicillin in the stomach has been overcome by converting it to the 5-indanyl ester, as indanyl-carbenicillin. In this compound the α-carboxylic acid moiety of carbenicillin is bound through ester linkage to 5-indanol and hydrolyzed after ingestion to active carbenicillin. The carbenicillin is then well absorbed. If the benzyl group in carbenicillin is replaced with the 5-carbon thienyl ring, the resulting compound, ticarcillin, is two to four times more active against *Pseudomonas aeruginosa,* but remains acid labile and must be given parenterally. Even greater activity against *P. aeruginosa* is obtained with piperacillin. In this antibiotic, ampicillin is bound through its amino group to a derivative of piperazine.

The structural modifications of semisynthetic penicillins are illustrated in Figure 1.

### The Cephalosporins

The common nucleus of the cephalosporins resembles 6-aminopenicillanic acid but differs by having a dihydrothiazine ring, instead of a thiazolidine ring, attached to the β-lactam ring (Fig. 2). The active nucleus, known as 7-aminocephalosporanic acid, can also be manipulated chemically to yield more active and useful deriva-

tives.[6] The basic advantages of the cephalosporin nucleus are its innate resistance to staphylococcal penicillinase and its safety in patients with allergy to penicillin. These properties are retained in cephalothin (Fig. 3), in which the side chain at the 7-position increases its potency and range of activity. Another derivative, cephalexin (Fig. 3), has a different side chain at the 7-position that confers resistance to gastric acid and allows good absorption from the alimentary tract. Cefazolin (Fig. 3), with substitutions at both the 7- and 3-positions, can be injected intramuscularly without pain and possesses greater activity than cephalothin against certain bacteria.

Two newer cephalosporins, cefamandole and cefoxitin, are more resistant to the β-lactamase of *Bacteroides fragilis* and more active against that organism than cephalothin and cefalexin. Cefoxitin is derived from cephamycin C, which has a methoxy group at position 7 in 7-aminocephalosporanic acid. The methoxy group may be responsible for the resistance of this drug to the β-lactamase of *B. fragilis* and other gram-negative bacilli. Cefoxitin also appears to be able to reach higher levels in the cerebrospinal fluid than other cephalosporins.[11]

### Bacitracin

This antibiotic is produced by a strain of *Bacillus subtilis,* which was isolated from the dirty compound fracture of a girl named Tracy and called "bacitracin" out of joint deference to the bacillus and patient.[8] The antibiotic consists of a mixture of polypeptides, the most important of which is bacitracin A. Like the penicillins, it contains a thiazolidine ring but does not have their β-lactam ring. In bacitracin A the thiazolidine ring is a condensation product of isoleucine and a cysteine residue and is attached through L-leucine to a peptide composed of D- and L-amino acids (Fig. 4).

### The Polymyxins

These cyclic polypeptides are also produced by a spore-forming aerobic bacillus, *Bacillus polymyxa.* Their detergent activity on bacteria can be attributed to two unique components: an amino acid, α,γ-diaminobutyric acid (DAB), and a C9 fatty acid, 6-methyloctanoic acid (Fig. 5). The cationic α-amino groups of DAB and the hydrophobic side chain of the fatty acid give the polymyxins the surface-active properties of a cationic detergent. Only two of the polymyxins, B and E, are used in clinical medicine. Polymyxin E is generally known as colistin.

### THE AMINOGLYCOSIDES

The aminoglycosides are derived from different species of *Streptomyces* and are composed of

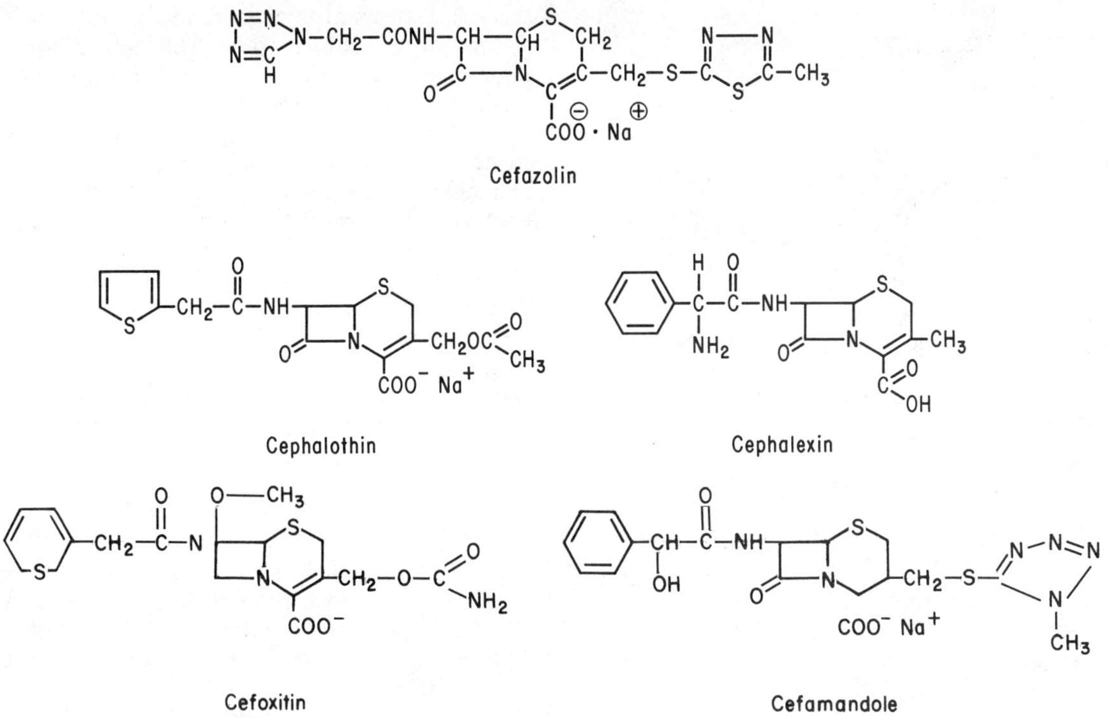

Cefazolin

Cephalothin

Cephalexin

Cefoxitin

Cefamandole

**FIGURE 3.** *Structural formulas of five important cephalosporin derivatives illustrate differences in side chains at acylation and deacetylation sites.*

amino sugars. In contrast to penicillin, they are organic bases rather than acids. Streptomycin, neomycin, kanamycin, and paromomycin — listed in order of discovery — are all members of this group. They resemble each other because of the inositol residue and the prominent basic groups, ranging from three in streptomycin to six in neomycin. They differ in the sugars attached to inositol and in the guanidine groups of streptomycin (Fig. 6). This similarity in structure accounts for common toxic effects on patients and bacteria.

Gentamicin is structurally similar to these aminoglycosides but is produced by a species of *Micromonospora* rather than *Streptomyces*. It has an inositol residue with two amino sugars and is a

complex of three antibiotics (designated $C_1$, $C_2$, and $C_{1A}$) which differ in structure only by one or two methyl groups.

## THE TETRACYCLINES

The tetracyclines are so named because their common hydronaphthacene nucleus contains four

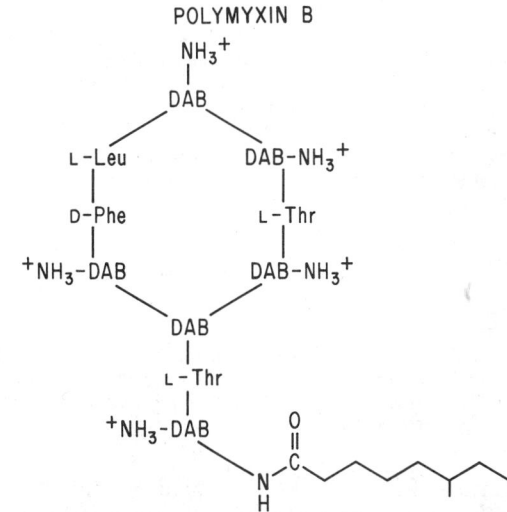

POLYMYXIN B

**FIGURE 5.** *Diaminobutyric acid (DAB) is present in all polymyxins, including colistin (polymyxin E). The terminal residue of DAB is acetylated by 6-methyloctanoic acid, the C9 fatty acid at the bottom of the structural formula. The cationic α-amino group of DAB and the hydrophobic fatty acid are responsible for the surface-active properties of the cationic detergent.*

BACITRACIN A

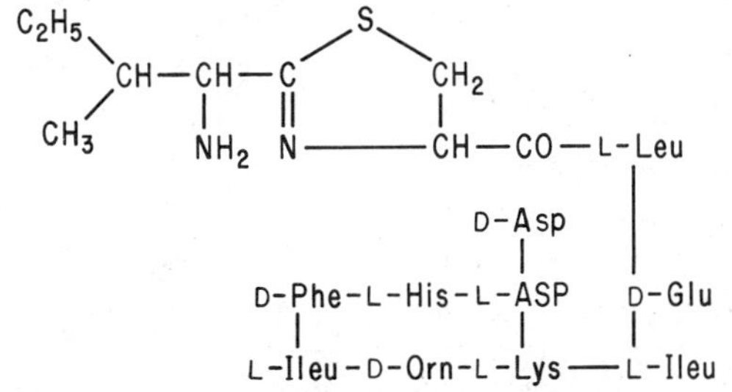

**FIGURE 4.** *Like penicillin, bacitracin A contains a thiazolidine ring. It is a condensation product of isoleucine and cysteine, in contrast to that of penicillin which contains D-valine and L-cysteine. Bacitracin lacks the β-lactam ring of penicillin.*

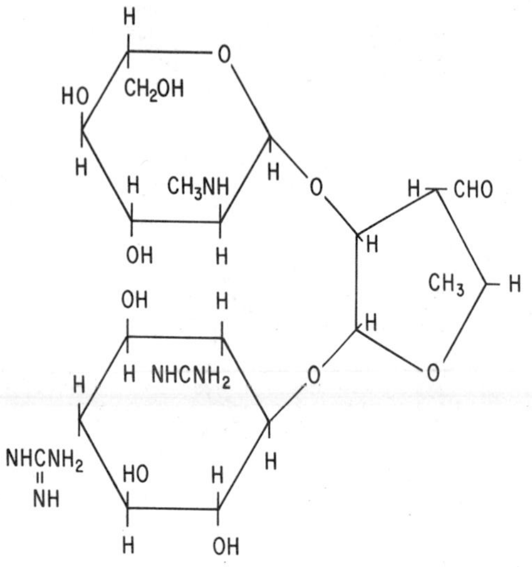

STREPTOMYCIN

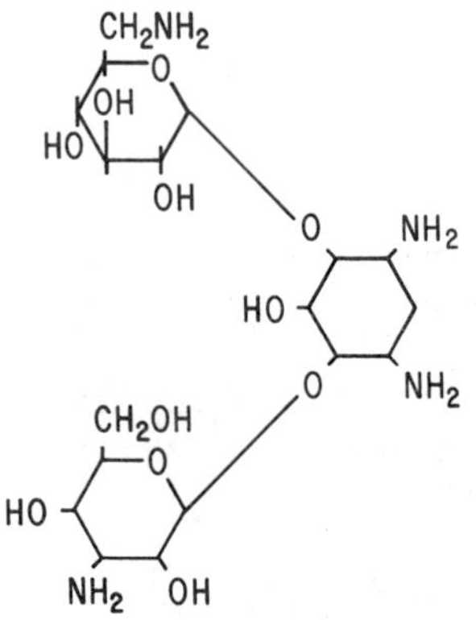

KANAMYCIN

**FIGURE 6.** *The basic structure of the aminoglycosides, illustrated by kanamycin and streptomycin, is that of a polycationic compound composed of amino sugars and connected by glycosidic linkages. In streptomycin, the inositol residue common to both compounds is in the form of streptidine (the bottom sugar with two guanido groups), and in kanamycin it is deoxystreptamine (the central sugar with two amino groups). Amikacin and tobramycin are related structurally to kanamycin. In amikacin the lower amino group in the diagram of the deoxystreptamine nucleus (position 1) is replaced with a side chain consisting of:*

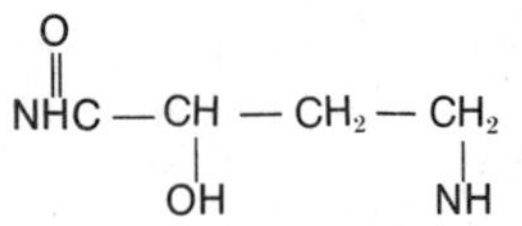

*in order to increase its resistance to bacterial inactivating enzymes. In tobramycin the main differences from kanamycin are the absence of the first two hydroxyl groups in the upper ring and the presence of an amino group at position 1.*

fused rings (Fig. 7). Chlortetracycline (Aureomycin) was the first tetracycline compound described, and oxytetracycline (Terramycin) was discovered 2 years later, in 1950. Both compounds were produced by strains of *Streptomyces*. Al-

though tetracycline was made by the catalytic reduction of chlortetracycline, all other compounds in this group are named in relation to the basic structure of tetracycline. In chlortetracycline a hydrogen is replaced by chlorine, and in oxytetracycline it is replaced by a hydroxyl ion. Demeclocycline (Declomycin) is chlortetracycline without the 6-methyl group, and doxycycline is oxytetracycline without the 6-hydroxyl group. These minor structural differences have less effect on their antimicrobial spectra than on stability in solution and pharmacologic properties. Chlortetracycline not only is less stable than the other tetracyclines but is the least stable of any important antibiotic.

## CHLORAMPHENICOL

Chloramphenicol is the only naturally occurring antibiotic with nitrobenzene in its structure (Fig. 8). This chemical grouping probably accounts for its toxicity to both bacteria and patients. Its tendency to cause aplastic anemia is explained by its benzene ring, a component of most organic substances involved in that disorder. Its ability to compete with messenger RNA for ribosomal binding is explained by its spatial similarity to uridine-5-phosphate.

## THE MACROLIDES

Erythromycin, isolated from *Streptomyces erythreus,* is the only important member of the

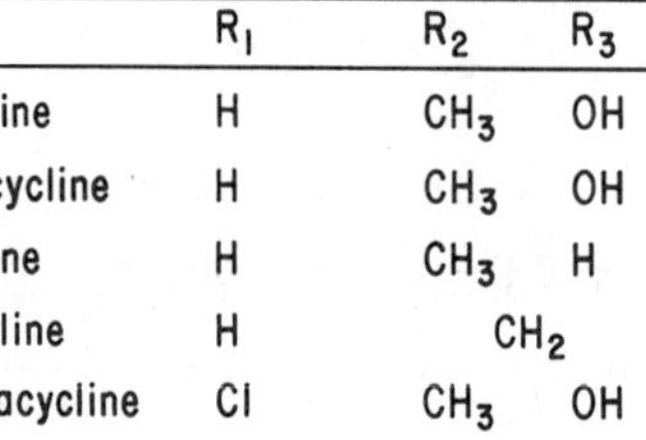

| | $R_1$ | $R_2$ | $R_3$ | $R_4$ |
|---|---|---|---|---|
| Tetracycline | H | $CH_3$ | OH | H |
| Oxytetracycline | H | $CH_3$ | OH | OH |
| Doxycycline | H | $CH_3$ | H | OH |
| Methacycline | H | $CH_2$ | | OH |
| Chlortetracycline | Cl | $CH_3$ | OH | H |
| Demethylchlor-tetracycline | Cl | H | OH | H |
| Minocycline | $N(CH_3)_2$ | H | H | H |

**FIGURE 7.** *The compounds of this group are named in relation to the basic structure of tetracycline and on the basis of substituted chemical groups at one or more of the four R positions.*

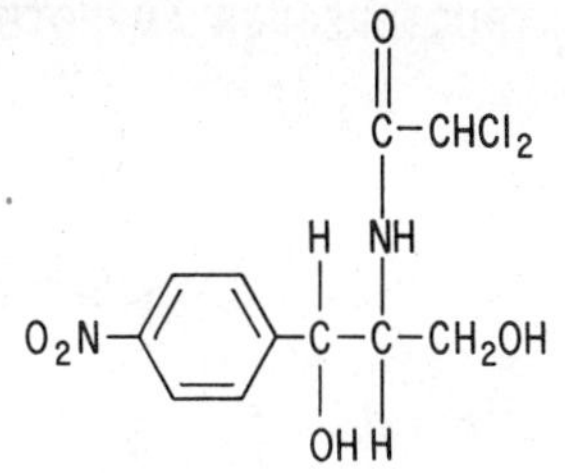

CHLORAMPHENICOL

**FIGURE 8.** *Chloramphenicol is the only naturally occurring antibiotic with nitrobenzene in its structure, a property that may account for its tendency to cause aplastic anemia.*

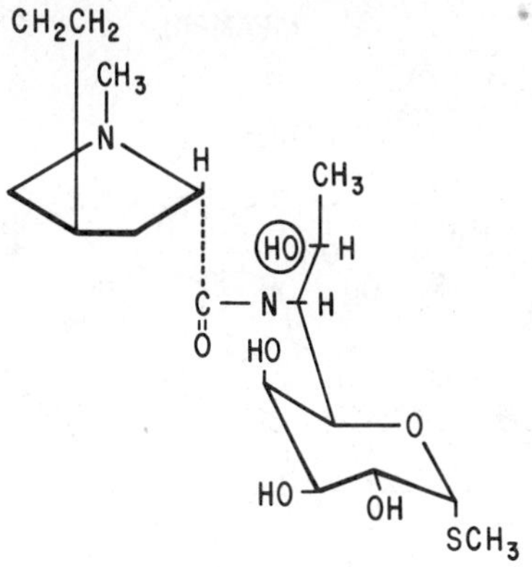

LINCOMYCIN

**FIGURE 10.** *The sulfur-containing amino acid, methyl-α-thiol lincosamide, is named for the parent compound which was obtained from a mold growing in Lincoln, Nebraska. Note total dissimilarity of lincomycin from macrolides (Fig. 9). The circle indicates the 7-hydroxyl group where a chloro group is substituted in clindamycin.*

macrolides. The basic structure is a large lactone ring to which unusual sugars are attached (Fig. 9). The term "macrolide" refers to the large ring, formed from a chain of 14 to 20 carbon atoms by lactone condensation of a carboxyl and hydroxyl group. The other 37 macrolides, such as oleandomycin, spiramycin, kitasamycin, and carbomycin, differ from erythromycin both in the structure of the lactone ring and in the attached sugars. Since the other macrolides have the same spectrum but are less potent than erythromycin, they are not widely used.

## LINCOMYCIN

Despite striking similarity in the biologic effects of lincomycin and erythromycin, their chemical structures are totally dissimilar. In contrast to the macrolides, lincomycin consists of an amino acid joined to a sulfur-containing amino sugar. The amino acid is trans-L-4-*n*-propyl hygric acid,

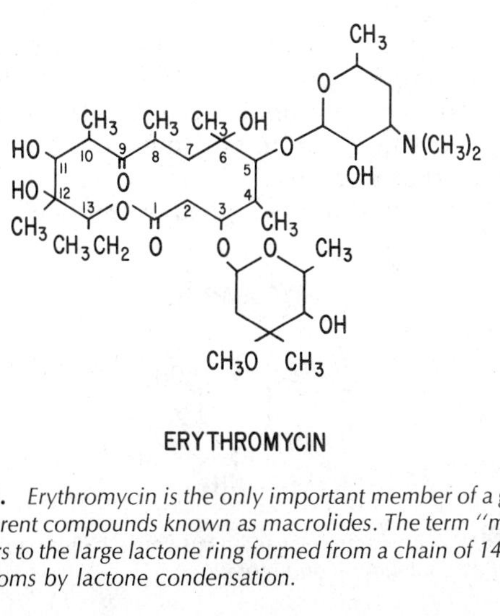

and the amino sugar is methyl-α-thiol lincosaminide (Fig. 10).

Clindamycin is a synthetic modification of lincomycin. As indicated by its chemical name, 7-chloro-7-deoxylincomycin, clindamycin is produced by a 7-chloro substitution of the 7(R)-hydroxyl group of the parent compound, lincomycin. These modifications in structure appear to increase absorption, blood levels, and antibacterial activity.

## THE RIFAMYCINS

The rifamycin antibiotics are fermentation products of *Streptomyces mediterranei*. Their basic structure is an aromatic ring compound spanned by an aliphatic bridge. The most active of the original compounds, rifamycin B, was not well absorbed after ingestion. After the chemical structure of various rifamycins was determined in 1963, it was possible to synthesize a great many semisynthetic derivatives.[16] At the time of this writing, rifampin is the most important of these because it is orally effective in tuberculosis and leprosy, and in infections by various gram-negative and gram-positive bacteria. The special features of rifampin, shown in Figure 11, are the double ring compound, the long aliphatic bridge, and the side chain: $CH = N - N \subset\supset N - CH_3$. The ring is a naphthohydroquinone and is the chemical grouping responsible for the red color of the antibiotic. The importance of the rifamycins lies not only in their currently important derivative, rifampin, but also in the great potential for new derivatives with activity against many different microorganisms, including viruses and fungi.

ERYTHROMYCIN

**FIGURE 9.** *Erythromycin is the only important member of a group of 37 different compounds known as macrolides. The term "macrolide" refers to the large lactone ring formed from a chain of 14 to 20 carbon atoms by lactone condensation.*

RIFAMPIN

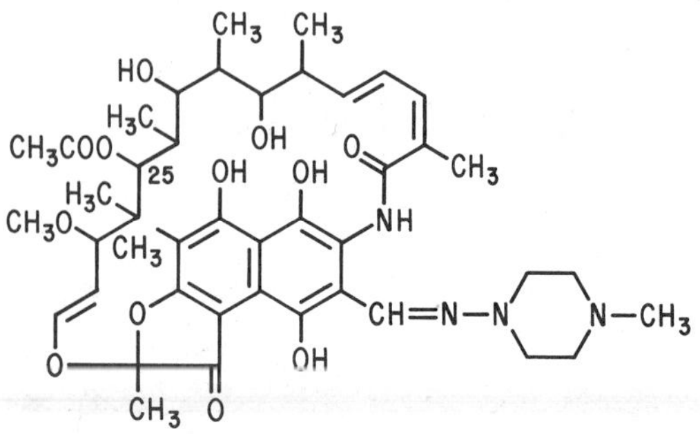

**FIGURE 11.** *The basic structure of rifampin is the double ring compound spanned by a long aliphatic bridge, and the side chain.*

## VANCOMYCIN

Vancomycin is a bactericidal antibiotic produced by *Streptomyces orientalis*. The structure of vancomycin has recently been determined by x-ray analysis.[15] The principal units in the structure are a disaccharide linked to three aromatic rings: N-methylleucine, aspartic acid, and a biphenyl system. These units are connected by secondary amide bonds to form a tricyclic molecule containing N-terminal N-methylleucine and two free carboxyl groups.

## GRISEOFULVIN

Although derived from *Penicillium* molds, griseofulvin is active against fungi rather than bacteria. Discovered in 1939 in London, griseofulvin was used against plant fungi before its value against human dermatophytes was demonstrated.[14] It has a spirocyclic structure formed from acetate units (Fig. 12).

## THE POLYENES

Amphotericin B, nystatin, and pimaricin are polyenes. These antifungal antibiotics are clas-

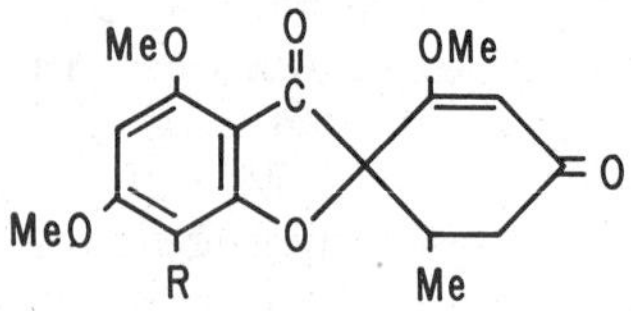

GRISEOFULVIN

**FIGURE 12.** *Griseofulvin is a spirocyclic compound formed from acetate units.*

PARTIAL STRUCTURE FOR AMPHOTERICIN B

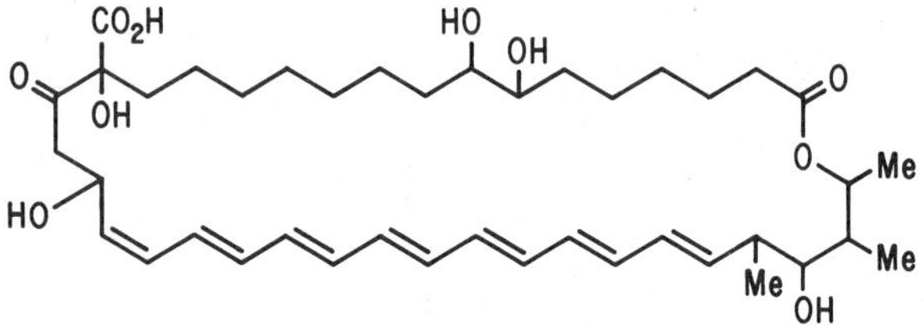

**FIGURE 13.** *Amphotericin B is called a polyene because it contains a series of carbon atoms with multiple conjugated double bonds.*

sified as polyenes because the molecules contain a series of carbon atoms with four or five conjugated double bonds. Nystatin and amphotericin also possess the aminodeoxyhexose, mycosamine (Fig. 13), which is not present in many of the polyenes that are unsuitable for medical use.[3] Their extensive unsaturation makes them unstable compounds, especially in acid or alkaline solutions. They are also unstable in light and air. Although the exact formula has not been worked out for either one, amphotericin B is known to be a conjugated heptaene lactone linked with mycosamine and has the tentative formula $C_{46}H_{73}O_{20}N$ (Fig. 14).

## SYNTHETIC ANTIMICROBIAL DRUGS

### The Sulfonamides

The term "sulfonamide" refers to derivatives of sulfanilamide, or $\pi$-aminobenzenesulfonamide (Fig. 15), the first antimicrobial shown to be effective systemically for the treatment of human bacterial infection.[10] Thousands of sulfonamides have been synthesized, but only a dozen are of value for patients.

Most derivatives are made by substitutions on the sulfonamide group ($SO_2NH_2$), since these increase the antimicrobial activity. The para-$NH_2$ group, on the other hand, must remain free, or become free, after hydrolysis. Succinylsulfathiazole (Sulfasuxidine) is a good example of how the

MYCOSAMINE

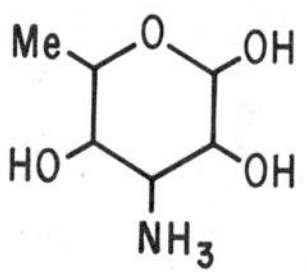

**FIGURE 14.** *This amino sugar, mycosamine, is linked to a polyene in both amphotericin B and nystatin.*

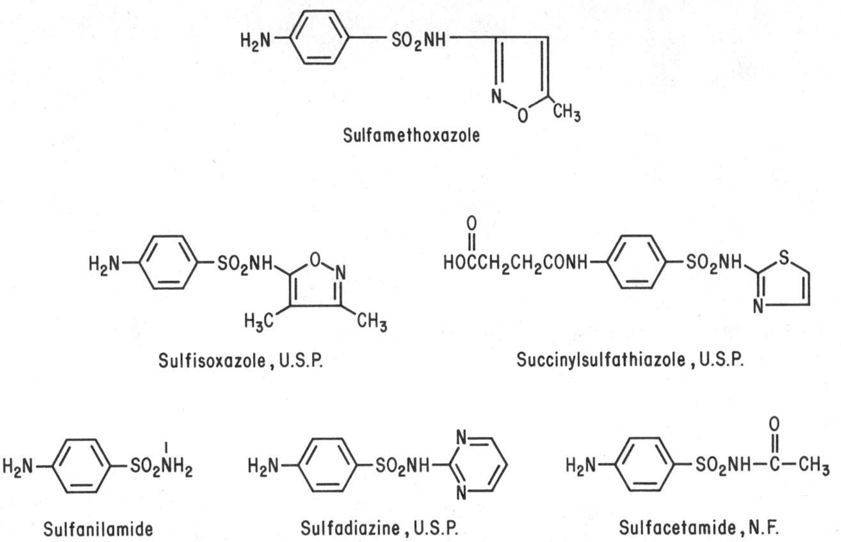

Sulfamethoxazole

**FIGURE 15.** *These and other sulfonamide derivatives are made by substitutions on the $SO_2NH_2$ group of the parent compound sulfanilamide. The para-$NH_2$ group must remain free.*

Sulfisoxazole, U.S.P.

Succinylsulfathiazole, U.S.P.

Sulfanilamide

Sulfadiazine, U.S.P.

Sulfacetamide, N.F.

para-$NH_2$ group becomes free after slow hydrolysis from its inactive form to the active sulfathiazole. The substitutions on the $SO_2NH_2$ group of other sulfonamides are shown in Fig. 15.

### The Sulfones

As is evident from the structural formula of dapsone in Figure 16, sulfones are related to sulfonamides but lack the sulfonamide group and its broad antibacterial spectrum. Instead, the sulfones are limited in antibacterial activity to the leprosy bacillus.

### Isoniazid and Ethionamide

Isoniazid was the first modern chemotherapeutic agent synthesized (1912), but its value in tuberculosis was not appreciated until 1952.[4] It is the hydrazide of isonicotinic acid (Fig. 17). Ethionamide is also a derivative of isonicotinic acid.

### The Diaminopyrimidines

The diaminopyrimidine compounds were first synthesized as analogs of the nitrogenous bases found in DNA. Pyrimethamine, for example, was prepared as a thymine analog. This drug and trimethoprim are the only two members of this group that are of practical medical importance. Their formulas are given in Figure 18. Both are

useful in protozoal infections, and trimethoprim in bacterial infections.[7]

### The Fluorinated Pyrimidines

The substitution of fluorine for hydrogen in the 5-position on pyrimidines was first made in order to produce the pyrimidine analog 5-fluorouracil, a potent antimetabolite for mammalian cells and useful in cancer chemotherapy. Another fluorinated pyrimidine, 5-fluorocytosine (5FC), does not seem to be metabolized in mammalian cells and has no activity against cancer cells. The activity of 5FC against microorganisms seems to be related to its conversion to 5-fluorouracil by deamination[9] (Fig. 19).

### The Nitrofurans

The nitrofurans are derivatives of the 5-membered ring sugars known as furans and possess a nitro group in the 5-position. The chief nitrofuran available for clinical application is shown in Figure 20 and is the only sugar derivative with clinically important antibacterial properties.

### The Aminoquinolines

The most important member of the aminoquinolines is chloroquine, a 4-aminoquinoline with

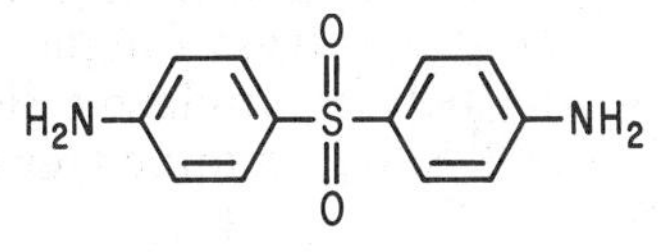

Dapsone, U.S.P.

**FIGURE 16.** *Note structural relationship of dapsone to sulfonamides.*

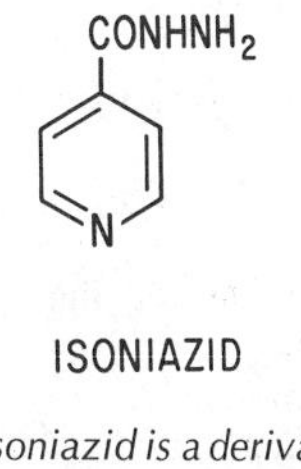

ISONIAZID

**FIGURE 17.** *The drug isoniazid is a derivative of isonicotinic acid.*

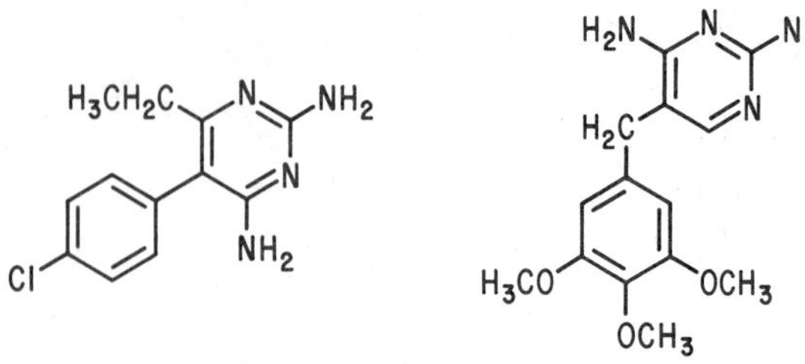

Pyrimethamine Trimethoprim

**FIGURE 18.** *These diaminopyrimidines were first synthesized as analogs of the nitrogenous bases found in DNA.*

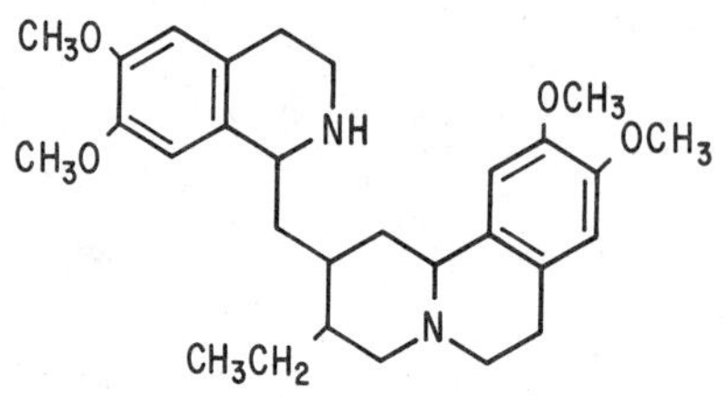

EMETINE

**FIGURE 22.** *Emetine. This is the structure of the active principle of ipecac.*

DEAMINATION OF
5-FLUOROCYTOSINE TO 5-FLUOROURACIL

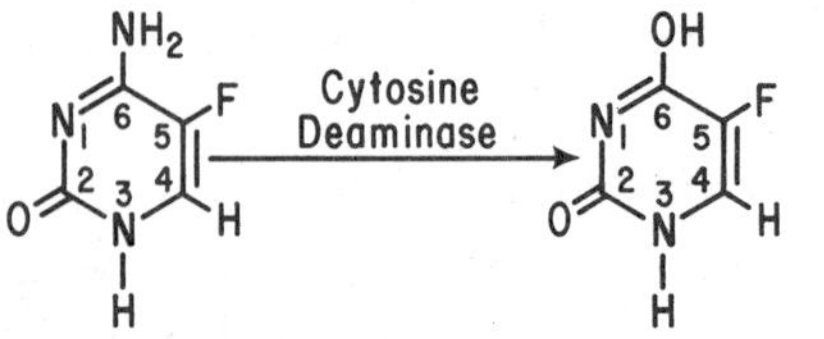


5-Fluorocytosine 5-Fluorouracil

**FIGURE 19.** *The activity of 5-fluorocytosine against microorganisms seems to be related to its conversion to 5-fluorouracil.*

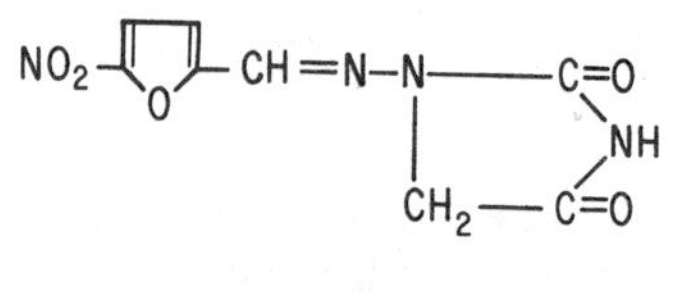

FURADANTIN

**FIGURE 20.** *The nitrofurans are the only synthetic sugar derivatives with clinically useful antibacterial properties.*

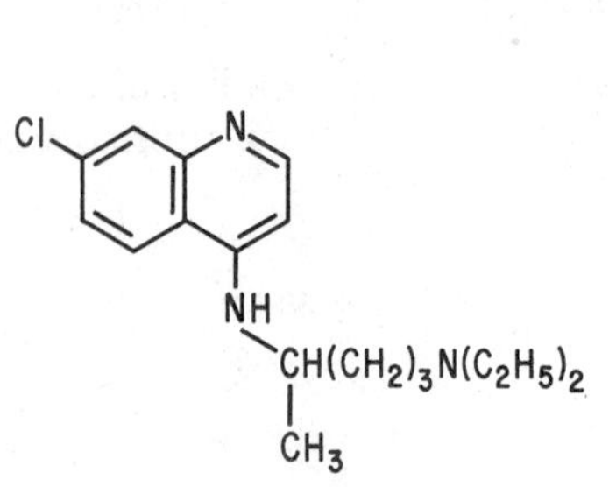

Chloroquine

**FIGURE 21.** *The Cl atom in position 7 is necessary for maximum antimalarial activity of chloroquine.*

the structure shown in Figure 21. The main parts of the molecule are the quinoline nucleus composed of a double ring and the alkyl side chain. The chlorine atom in position 7 of the quinoline nucleus appears necessary for maximum antimalarial activity.

Although first used as an antimalarial, chloroquine was later found to be valuable in the treatment of amebic liver abscess and giardiasis.

### Emetine

Emetine is the oldest amebicidal drug and the active principle chiefly responsible for the clinical efficacy of ipecac in amebic infections. Emetine hydrochloride is obtained from ipecac as a hydrated hydrochloride[5] (Fig. 22).

### Nitroimidazoles

Metronidazole (Fig. 23) is the newest amebicidal drug in clinical use. It is a nitroimidazole derivative active against two groups of anaerobic organisms, the anaerobic bacteria and the pathogenic protozoa, including amebae, *Trichomonas, Giardia,* and *Balantidium.* Trinidazole, another promising nitroimidazole drug, has been effective in amebic dysentery and trichomonas infections.

### Imidazoles

Three antifungal drugs, clotrimazole, miconazole, and ketoconazole, are imidazoles that are related to the nitroimidazoles used for anaerobic bacteria and protozoa (Fig. 23). The benzimidazoles (see Fig. 27) are potent anthelmintics. Clotrimazole is limited to topical use for ringworm and moniliasis of the skin, but miconazole can be given intravenously for generalized fungus infections. Ketoconazole, the newest imidazole, is well absorbed orally and is being examined for its clinical effectiveness.

### The Anthelmintics[2]

The simplest structure of the anthelmintics, a group of nitro ring compounds, is that of pipera-

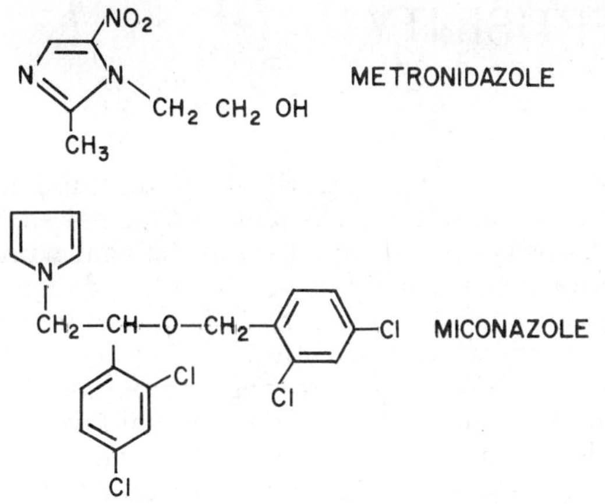

**FIGURE 23.** *Comparison of the nitroimidazole, metronidazole, with the imidazole, miconazole. Metronidazole attacks anaerobic organisms only (bacteria and protozoa) after the nitro group is reduced, whereas miconazole acts against fungi, which are strictly aerobic. Compare also the benzimidazoles (Fig. 27), which are also active against anaerobes—the intestinal worms.*

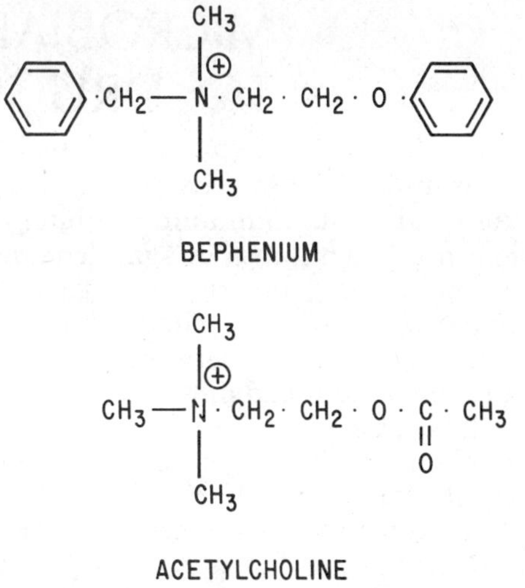

**FIGURE 25.** *The anthelmintic bephenium resembles acetylcholine in structure and action. Bephenium paralyzes nematodes by causing membrane depolarization of muscle in the worms.*

zine, a drug used unsuccessfully at first for the treatment of gout but later found to be highly effective against *Ascaris* and *Enterobius* worms. Modification of piperazine (Fig. 24) by substituting a diethylcarbamyl group at the 1-position and a methyl group at the 4-position created diethylcarbamazine, a drug that can kill adult filaria and microfilaria. Bephenium is a quaternary amine and resembles acetylcholine in both structure and function (Fig. 25). The anticestodal drug, niclosamide (chlorsalicylamide), resembles closely the structure of desaspidin, the active principle of oleoresin of aspidium, the oldest remedy for tapeworms (Fig. 26). Another important group of anthelmintics are the substituted benzimidazole compounds. One of these, thiabendazole, is effective against various round worms, while mebendazole is the only anthelmintic effective against both tapeworms and round worms. The formula of thiabendazole is shown in Figure 27. The only compound with a close structural resemblance to antibacterial drugs is niridazole, which is derived from a nitrothiazole nucleus (Fig. 28). Its structure is related to that of nitrofurantoin and metronidazole, two agents with antibacterial activity.

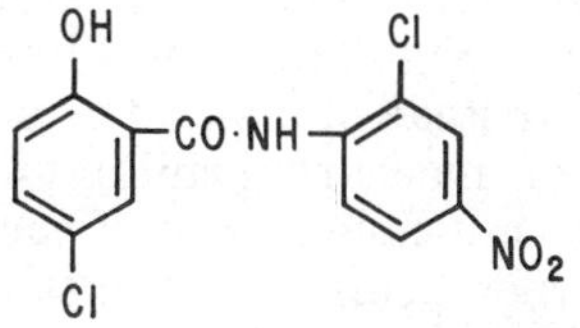

**FIGURE 26.** *Niclosamide resembles in structure desaspidin, the active principle of oleoresin of aspidium, an old remedy for tapeworms.*

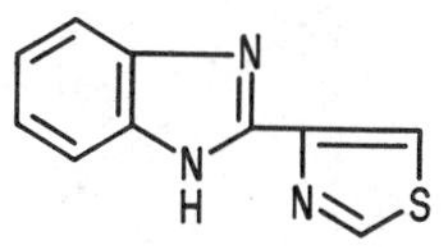

Thiabendazole

**FIGURE 27.** *Thiabendazole is the best anthelmintic among several hundred substituted benzimidazole compounds.*

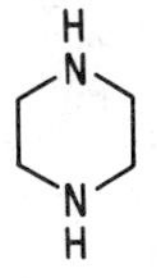

PIPERAZINE

**FIGURE 24.** *Piperazine has the simplest structure of the anthelmintics.*

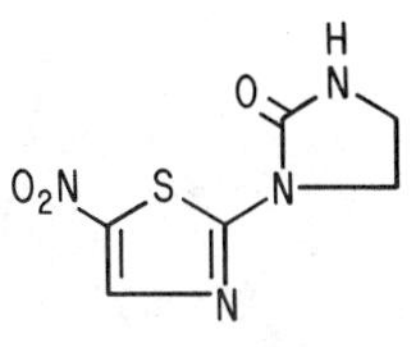

NIRIDAZOLE

**FIGURE 28.** *Niridazole. Note structural similarity of this anthelmintic to the antibacterial drug nitrofurantoin.*

# MICROBIAL SUSCEPTIBILITY TO DRUGS

The antimicrobial activity of a drug is generally expressed as its minimum inhibitory concentration in nutrient broth or agar. The test conditions would seem far removed from those in infected tissues or body fluids, but there is a remarkable correlation between successful treatment of the patient and inhibitory concentrations in the laboratory.

Microbial inhibition is measured either by serial dilution or by diffusion of antibiotics.[41] In the dilution tests the antibiotic is diluted serially in broth or agar, and results are expressed as the lowest concentration that inhibits growth of a standard bacterial inoculum at 37° C. Three diffusion tests are used: the disk test, the filter strip, and the gradient plate. In the disk test, antibiotics are incorporated into filter paper disks, and the minimum inhibitory concentration is calculated indirectly from the diameter of the inhibitory zone.[5, 17] (Fig. 29). Long filter paper strips can be used instead of disks. The strips have the advantage of measuring inhibitory concentrations against multiple strains of bacteria that are streaked perpendicularly to the strip.

The gradient plate is prepared by pouring agar with a given concentration of antibiotic in square Petri dishes that are tilted so that the agar solidifies on a slant. The plate is then placed on a flat surface and an equal volume of agar without antibiotic is poured over the slanted agar to provide a horizontal layer, as shown in Figure 30. The antibiotic diffuses into the upper layer to give a perfect linear gradient ranging from zero to the concentration present in the original layer. Multiple strains can be streaked on the agar surface along the gradient. The minimum inhibitory concentration is directly related to the distance bacterial growth extends from the zero end of the gradient.

The gradient plate method is the best method for laboratories that need to perform sensitivity on many strains because multiple organisms can be examined on one plate and there is little room for error.[7] The disk test is the most widely used (despite a number of disadvantages) because it lends itself to commercial distribution and has been publicized. The most serious problem encountered with the disk method is the occasional failure to detect strains of staphylococci that are resistant to penicillin. These resistant staphylococci are easily recognized by tests for penicillinase. The simplest is a rapid capillary tube assay

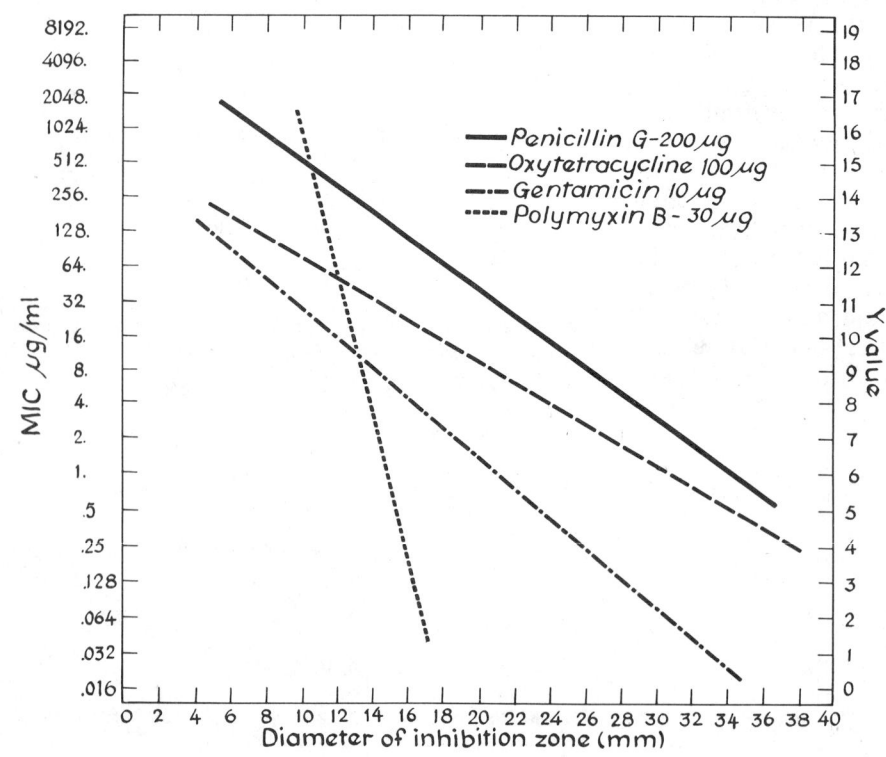

FIGURE 29. *Determination of antibiotic sensitivity by disk method is based on correlation between zone diameter and minimum inhibitory concentration. Regression lines for minimum inhibitory concentrations and inhibitory zone diameter are shown for penicillin G (200 µg), oxytetracycline (100 µg), gentamicin (10 µg), and polymyxin B sulfate (30 µg). (From Stamey, T. A.: Urinary Infections. © 1972, The Williams and Wilkins Co., Baltimore, p. 45.)*

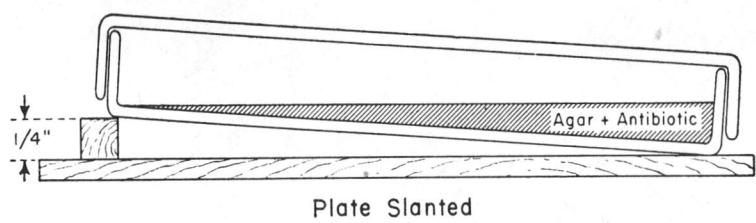

Plate Slanted

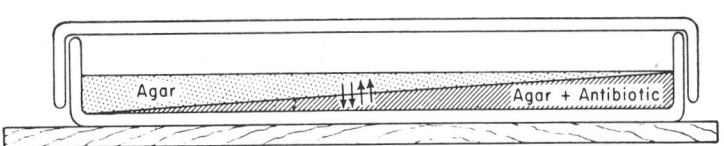

Plate Level

**FIGURE 30.** *Diagram of procedures used for preparing gradient plates. The extreme right end of the completed plate (bottom) is where the gradient begins; there is initially no dilution of antibiotic at this point. Halfway across the plate (arrows) there is a twofold dilution of antibiotic. At the extreme left there is virtually no antibiotic and its concentration is zero. Thus a uniform linear gradient is formed by the vertical diffusion of antibiotic. (From Braude, A. I., Banister, J., and Wright, N.: Use of the gradient plate for routine clinical determinations of bacterial sensitivities to antibiotics. Antibiot Annu p. 1134, 1954–1955.)*

that should be carried out routinely in all laboratories.[44] It is based on the change in pH that occurs when staphylococcal penicillinase hydrolyzes penicillin to penicilloic acid.

The values given below for antibiotic sensitivity are derived from either dilution methods or the gradient plate and are a composite of results from our laboratory and several other representative laboratories.

### THE COCCI

With the exception of certain staphylococci, gonococci,[11, 42] and enterococci, cocci remain exquisitely sensitive to penicillin G (benzylpenicillin). Pneumococci, hemolytic streptococci, meningococci, anaerobic streptococci, and *Streptococcus viridans* are usually inhibited by less than 0.1 microgram ($\mu$g) per ml and frequently by as little as 0.01 $\mu$g/ml[18, 34, 46] (Table 1). Gonococci and staphylococci are no longer uniformly sensitive to penicillin. Staphylococci that produce penicillinase cannot be treated with benzylpenicillin at any dosage. The number of staphylococci that produce penicillinase varies among hospitals. At the University Hospital in San Diego 90 per cent do so. Before 1960, 95 per cent of gonococci were sensitive to 0.1 $\mu$g/ml benzylpenicillin, but now less than half are inhibited by this concentration, and 1.0 $\mu$g/ml is necessary to inhibit 95 per cent of gonococcal strains in many communities.[32]

In contrast to those gonococci and staphylococci which have lost initial sensitivity, enterococci have always been relatively resistant to penicillin G. Enterococci generally grow readily in 1.0 $\mu$g/ml and usually require 3 to 6 $\mu$g/ml for inhibition.[18]

Modification of penicillin G to acid-resistant or

penicillinase-resistant compounds causes loss in antibacterial power. In penicillin V and ampicillin the loss of activity against most cocci is usually slight; in fact, ampicillin is more active than penicillin G against the enterococci. *Neisseria* show the biggest differences in sensitivity between penicillin V and G, with the meningococcus and penicillin-sensitive gonococci requiring concentrations of penicillin V four times greater than those of penicillin G for inhibition.

The penicillinase-resistant penicillins show greater loss of activity against penicillin-sensitive cocci. Methicillin is 35 to 40 times less active than penicillin G against streptococci and penicillinase-negative staphylococci. Cloxacillin, oxacillin, and dicloxacillin are approximately 8 to 12 times less active than penicillin G against pneumococci, various streptococci, and penicillinase-negative staphylococci.[22, 58] The same, except for a little more activity against the pneumococcus, is true for nafcillin. All four inhibit penicillinase-producing staphylococci in a range of 0.15 to 1 $\mu$g/ml.

The related group of penicillinase-resistant antibiotics, the cephalosporins, are also less active than penicillin against all cocci (Table 2). Cephaloridine approaches benzylpenicillin in potency in vitro against the pneumococcus and group A streptococcus but otherwise the cephalosporins are considerably less active against cocci than is benzylpenicillin.[25] The cephalosporins are so inactive against the enterococcus and meningococcus that they are virtually useless in infections with those organisms.[6, 47]

Tetracyclines are losing some of their potency against cocci.[18, 34] In all species of cocci, strains have appeared that are too resistant for treatment with this group of antibiotics. Resistance to tetracyclines has been most marked among the

TABLE 1. Usual Minimum Inhibitory Concentrations (μg/ml) of Penicillin Derivatives Against Cocci

| | BENZYL-PENICILLIN | PHENOXYMETHYL-PENICILLIN | AMPICILLIN* | METHICILLIN | OXACILLIN | DICLOXACILLIN | NAFCILLIN |
|---|---|---|---|---|---|---|---|
| Pneumococcus | 0.01 | 0.03 | 0.02 | 0.1 | 0.5 | 0.15 | 0.04 |
| Group A streptococcus | 0.005 | 0.015 | 0.02 | 0.2 | 0.02 | 0.05 | 0.02 |
| Staphylococcus aureus (penicillinase-negative) | 0.03 | 0.03 | 0.05 | 1.0 | 0.30 | 0.15 | 0.40 |
| S. aureus (penicillinase producer) | R | R | R | 1.0 | 0.40 | 0.10 | 0.50 |
| Streptococcus faecalis | 3.6 | 3.2 | 1.6 | >25.0 | >25.0 | — | 25.0 |
| Streptococcus viridans | 0.01 | 0.01 | 0.1 | 0.1 | — | — | 0.06 |
| Gonococcus | 0.01–3.0 | 0.03–>3.0 | 0.3 | 12.0 | 12.0 | 0.06–4.0 | — |
| Meningococcus | 0.03 | 0.25 | 0.05 | 6.0 | — | 6.0 | 6.0 |
| Peptostreptococcus | 0.2 | 0.5 | 0.2 | 2.0 | 0.6 | 2.0 | <25.0 |

*The activity of amoxicillin is very similar to that of ampicillin, except for *Streptococcus faecalis*. Amoxicillin inhibits most strains of *S. faecalis* at 0.6 μg/ml.
R = Resistant at all concentrations.
— = Inadequate data.

**TABLE 2.  Usual Minimum Inhibitory Concentrations ($\mu$g/ml) of Cephalosporin Antibiotics Against Cocci[29, 47]**

|  | CEPHALOTHIN | CEPHALEXIN | CEFACLOR | CEFAZOLIN | CEFOXITIN |
|---|---|---|---|---|---|
| Pneumococcus | 0.4 | 3.1 | 1.0 | 0.1 | 2.0 |
| Group A streptococcus | 0.1 | 1.0 | 0.8 | 0.2 | 0.8 |
| *Staphylococcus aureus* | 0.6 | 6.0 | 4.0 | 0.6 | 2.5 |
| *Staphylococcus epidermidis* | 0.6 | 12.0 |  | 1.0 | 3.0 |
| *Streptococcus faecalis* | 50.0 | 50.0 | 60.0 | 50.0 | >50.0 |
| *Streptococcus viridans* | 2.0 | 6.25 |  | 0.3 | 12.0 |
| Gonococcus | 4.0 | 6.0 | 0.02–2.0 | 4.0 | 0.5–1.0 |
| Meningococcus | 1.6 | 100.0 |  | — | 0.5–1.5 |

− = Inadequate data.

enterococci, but many staphylococci have also developed resistance beyond the limits of clinical efficacy. In certain hospitals as many as 50 per cent of staphylococci show such resistance while staphylococci from patients in outpatient clinics remain sensitive. So much resistance has developed among strains of pneumococci (5 to 23 per cent) and group A streptococci (20 to 40 per cent)[34] that tetracyclines cannot be relied on for the treatment of pneumonia or sore throat unless sensitivity tests establish their susceptibility. Among anaerobic gram-positive cocci, tetracycline resistance is a lesser problem. In contrast to the aerobic gram-positive cocci, over 90 per cent of *Neisseria* remain sensitive to the tetracyclines, which can cure most cases of gonorrhea. One tetracycline, minocycline, has also been somewhat effective in treating pharyngeal carriers of meningococci.[21] The in vitro susceptibility of sensitive strains of cocci to the tetracyclines is shown in Table 3.

Certain tetracycline analogues seem to be more active in vitro against cocci that are resistant to other tetracyclines.[57] Minocycline is the best example of this phenomenon since it inhibits in low concentrations staphylococci, group A streptococci, and enterococci that are resistant to tetracycline.

Lincomycin and clindamycin inhibit most of the gram-positive cocci, but not the *Neisseria*. Clindamycin is 4 to 16 times more active than lincomycin against staphylococci, and the minimum inhibitory concentration (MIC) against hemolytic streptococci (groups A, B, and C), pneumococci, and *Streptococcus viridans* is less than 0.05 $\mu$g/ml.[12] Among gram-positive cocci, only enterococci are resistant. Anaerobic cocci are almost all sensitive to 1.0 $\mu$g/ml or less of clindamycin.

The spectrum of erythromycin resembles that of lincomycin and clindamycin except for the *Neisseria*.[12, 20] Most strains of gonococci and meningococci are inhibited by 1.0 $\mu$g/ml of erythromycin.[46] The pyogenic streptococci and pneumococci are inhibited by 0.04 $\mu$g/ml, and sensitive staphylococci by 0.4 $\mu$g/ml. Staphylococci sometimes become resistant to erythromycin, especially in the hospital, and may show cross resistance to lincomycin. Strains of group A streptococci[48] and pneumococci are rarely resistant, but in some large hospitals over half the strains of enterococci are resistant to erythromycin.[60] Other enterococci range in sensitivity from 0.1 to 1.5 $\mu$g/ml erythromycin. Most anaerobic streptococci also fall in this range of sensitivity.[33]

The cocci do not show the exquisite sensitivity to chloramphenicol often found with other antibiotics, but most cocci are inhibited by 1 to 4 $\mu$g/ml and acquired resistance is unusual. The average pneumococcus or group A streptococcus, for example, is inhibited by 3.0 $\mu$g/ml of chloramphenicol. Meningococci tend to be more sensitive, with the average strain inhibited by 1.0 $\mu$g/ml. Staphylococci, anaerobic cocci, enterococci, gonococci, and *Streptococcus viridans* are generally sensitive to 4 $\mu$g/ml or less.[18, 46]

The aminoglycosides are less active against cocci than other antibiotics that interfere with protein synthesis. Streptococci and pneumococci are naturally resistant, and the *Neisseria* generally show only marginal sensitivity. The staphylococci are an exception, because kanamycin and gentamicin are both highly active against them, and some strains are sensitive to streptomycin.[52]

**TABLE 3.  Usual Minimum Inhibitory Concentrations ($\mu$g/ml) of Tetracyclines Against Sensitive Strains of Cocci**

|  | TETRA-CYCLINE | DOXY-CYCLINE | MINO-CYCLINE |
|---|---|---|---|
| *Staphylococcus aureus* | 0.3 | 0.8 | 0.8 |
| Group A streptococcus | 0.3 | 0.2 | 0.2 |
| Pneumococcus | 0.3 | 0.1 | 0.1 |
| *Peptostreptococcus* | 1.6 | 0.8 | 0.8 |
| Gonococcus | 0.8 | 0.8 | 0.8 |
| Meningococcus | 0.8 | 0.8 | 0.8 |

**TABLE 4.  Usual Minimum Inhibitory Concentrations ($\mu$g/ml) of Benzylpenicillin Against Sensitive Bacilli**

| | |
|---|---|
| Gram-positive rods | |
| Listeria monocytogenes | 0.2 |
| Actinomyces israelii | 0.06 |
| Clostridium perfringens | 0.16 |
| Bacillus anthracis | 0.02 |
| Corynebacterium diphtheriae | 0.08 |
| Erysipelothrix rhusiopathiae | 0.03 |
| Bordetella pertussis | 0.5 |
| | |
| Gram-negative rods | |
| Hemophilus influenzae | 0.8 |
| Hemophilus ducreyi | 1.0 |
| Pasteurella multocida | 0.4 |
| Streptobacillus moniliformis | 0.01 |
| Bacteroides oralis | 1.6 |
| Bacteroides melaninogenicus | 1.0 |
| Fusobacterium nucleatum | 0.8 |

Staphylococci range in sensitivity to gentamicin from 0.1 to 1.0 $\mu$g/ml, and to kanamycin from 0.4 to 4.0 $\mu$g/ml. Spectinomycin is the only aminoglycoside with enough activity against the gonococcus to warrant its use for the routine treatment of gonorrhea. Gonococci range in sensitivity from 6.2 to 25 $\mu$g/ml.[24]

One of the most active antibiotics against cocci is rifampin. The MIC for group A streptococci, staphylococci, and pneumococci is 0.02 $\mu$g/ml or less, while meningococci are inhibited by 0.2 $\mu$g/ml, gonococci by 0.5 $\mu$g/ml, and anaerobic streptococci by 1.6 $\mu$g/ml.[28, 49] Only enterococci have too much innate resistance for clinical effectiveness of the drug. Acquired resistance to rifampin among staphylococci and other cocci occurs readily and limits its usefulness.

Only one other antibiotic, vancomycin, deserves brief mention for its use against cocci. Its main value is for enterococcal endocarditis in patients with severe penicillin allergy.[19] The MIC for vancomycin against enterococci is 0.3 to 3.0 $\mu$g/ml.

Most other antimicrobials have little place in the treatment of coccal infections. The polymyxins are inactive against cocci, and antimicrobials other than antibiotics are of such limited value that they need not be discussed here. An exception is trimethoprim, whose antimicrobial spectrum is described later.

## THE BACILLI

Penicillin G is highly effective against all gram-positive bacilli and many gram-negative bacilli. Most enteric bacilli are relatively resistant but the penicillin derivatives, ampicillin, carbenicillin, and pipericillin usually inhibit these gram-negative rods in concentrations that can be reached in infected body fluids. The gram-positive rods, *Listeria monocytogenes, Actinomyces israelii,* the clostridia, *Erysipelothrix rhusiopathiae, Bacillus anthracis,* and *Corynebacterium diphtheriae,* are all very sensitive to penicillin, and most are inhibited by less than 0.1 $\mu$g/ml. Certain important gram-negative rods such as *Hemophilus influenzae, Pasteurella multocida, Streptobacillus moniliformis,* and most *Bacteroides* other than *Bacteroides fragilis* are also sensitive to penicillin in a range of 0.5 to 2.0 $\mu$g/ml (Table 4). Despite impressions to the contrary, ampicillin is not superior to penicillin G against *H. influenzae.* Most careful studies in the United States have shown that the MIC of both antibiotics against *H. influenzae* ranges from 0.2 to 1.6 $\mu$g/ml, with a median near 0.8 $\mu$g/ml.[35, 46] A few strains have developed resistance, but since this is mediated by a $\beta$-lactamase, both drugs are ineffective against them.

**TABLE 5.  Comparison of Usual Minimum Inhibitory Concentrations ($\mu$g/ml) of Penicillin G, Ampicillin, and Carbenicillin for Enteric Gram-Negative Rods**

| | BENZYLPENICILLIN | AMPICILLIN* | CARBENICILLIN | PIPERICILLIN |
|---|---|---|---|---|
| E. coli | 100.0 | 1.6–500 | 12.0 | 3.1–500 |
| P. mirabilis | 50.0 | 1.0–32.0 | 1.6 | 0.8 |
| K. pneumoniae | >100.0 | 25.0–400.0 | >200.0 | >200.0 |
| Enterobacter species | >500.0 | 20.0–250.0 | 6.0 | 50.0 |
| S. marcescens | >500.0 | 40.0–100.0 | 12.0–400.0 | 3.1–500 |
| P. aeruginosa | >500.0 | >200.0 | 50.0–100.0 | 12.0 |
| Proteus vulgaris | >100.0 | 3.0–100.0 | 2.0–25.0 | — |
| Other indole + Proteus | >100.0 | 3.0–50.0 | 1.0–12.0 | 1.6–500 |
| Salmonella species | 12.0 | 6.0 | 12.0 | 1.6–500 |
| Pseudomonas pseudomallei | 25.0 | 10.0 | >100.0 | — |

*Amoxicillin activity against gram-negative rods is very similar to that of ampicillin except that amoxicillin is approximately four times as active against *Salmonella* strains.[38]
— = Inadequate data.

**TABLE 6.**  Usual Minimum Inhibitory Concentrations (μg/ml)
of Cephalosporins for Pathogenic Bacilli

|  | CEFAZOLIN | CEPHALOTHIN | CEFACLOR | CEPHALEXIN | CEFOXITIN |
|---|---|---|---|---|---|
| **Gram-positive rods** | | | | | |
| *Listeria monocytogenes* | — | 2.0 | — | 64.0 | — |
| *Actinomyces israelii* | — | 2.0->100 | — | — | 0.5–32.0 |
| *Clostridium perfringens* | — | 0.6 | 12.0 | 1.2 | 1.2 |
| *Bacillus anthracis* | — | 0.6 | — | 2.0 | — |
| **Gram-negative rods** | | | | | |
| *Hemophilus influenzae* | 25.0 | 6.0–10.0 | 1.0 | 6.0–20.0 | 7.0 |
| *Pasteurella multocida* | — | 0.6 | — | 2.0 | — |
| *Bacteroides fragilis* | >200.0 | 25.0 | >100 | 25.0 | 10.0 |
| *Bacteroides oralis* | — | 0.1 | — | — | — |
| *Bacteroides melaninogenicus* | — | 0.2–6.0 | — | — | 1.0 |
| *Fusobacterium nucleatum* | 2.0 | 1.0 | — | — | 2.5 |
| *E. coli* | 0.8 | 6.0 | 3 | 12.0 | 2.0 |
| *P. mirabilis* | 3.0 | 6.0 | 6 | 20.0 | 2.0 |
| *K. pneumoniae* | 3.0 | 6.0 | 12 | 20.0 | 2.5 |
| *E. aerogenes* | 6.0–400.0 | 50.0->400.0 | >100 | >100.0 | >75.0 |
| *S. marcescens* | >400.0 | >100.0 | — | >100.0 | >40.0 |
| *P. aeruginosa* | >400.0 | >400.0 | — | >100.0 | >100.0 |
| Indole + *Proteus* | 200.0 | 100.0–400.0 | >100 | >100.0 | 5.0 |
| *Salmonella* spp. | 1.0 | 2.0 | 0.8 | 4.0 | 3.0 |
| *Shigella* spp. | 1.0 | 8.0 | 0.8 | 12.0 | — |
| *Pseudomonas pseudomallei* | — | >1000.0 | — | — | — |

— = Inadequate data. The antibacterial activity of cephradine is nearly identical to that of cephalexin.

Enteric bacilli are considerably less sensitive to penicillin G than the rods listed in Table 4.[18, 47, 56] Table 5 shows the greater susceptibility of these organisms to ampicillin and carbenicillin. Ampicillin inhibits sensitive strains of *Proteus mirabilis* and *E. coli* at a concentration of 3.0 μg/ml or less, and salmonellae at 6μg/ml. Carbenicillin is active in a range achieved clinically against all gram-negative bacilli listed except for certain strains of *Serratia*.[10, 53]

The cephalosporins differ from the penicillins in the poor activity of the former against *H. influenzae* (Table 6). Another notable difference is the greater activity of cephalothin, cefoxitin, cefa-

mandole, and cefazolin against *Klebsiella pneumoniae* than that shown by ampicillin and penicillin G. *Enterobacter aerogenes, Serratia*, indole + *Proteus,* and *Pseudomonas* are resistant to the older cephalosporins,[15] but indole + *Proteus* is inhibited by 5 μg/ml of cefamandole or cefoxitin, and many strains of *Enterobacter* are inhibited by 2.5 μg/ml cefamandole.

Erythromycin, lincomycin, and clindamycin are effective in vitro against *Bacteroides*[33] and the gram-positive rods, but not against enteric gram-negative bacilli. Erythromycin also shows activity against *H. influenzae* and *B. pertussis,* but lincomycin does not. Table 7 compares the activi-

**TABLE 7.**  Usual Minimum Inhibitory Concentrations (μg/ml)
of Erythromycin, Lincomycin, and Clindamycin Against
Susceptible Bacilli

|  | ERYTHROMYCIN | LINCOMYCIN | CLINDAMYCIN |
|---|---|---|---|
| *A. israelii* | 0.12 | 0.25 | — |
| *L. monocytogenes* | 2.0 | — | — |
| *C. diphtheriae* | 1.6 | — | — |
| *C. perfringens* | 1.5 | 2.0 | 0.8 |
| *B. anthracis* | 0.6 | 6.0 | — |
| *H. influenzae* | 3.0 | 20.0 | 6.0 |
| *P. multocida* | 3.1 | — | — |
| *B. fragilis* | 2.0 | 2.0 | 0.2 |
| *B. oralis* | 0.1 | 0.1 | 0.1 |
| *B. melaninogenicus* | 0.4 | 0.1 | 0.01 |
| *F. nucleatum* | 1.6 | 3.1 | 0.4 |
| *C. fetus (jejuni)* | 3.1 | 12.5 | 0.8 |

— = Inadequate data.

**TABLE 8.** Usual Minimum Inhibitory Concentrations ($\mu$g/ml) of Chloramphenicol and Tetracycline Against Gram-Positive and Gram-Negative Rods

| | CHLORAMPHENICOL | TETRACYCLINE |
|---|---|---|
| A. israelii | 3.0 | 3.0 |
| L. monocytogenes | 5.0 | 1.0 |
| C. diphtheriae | 0.5 | 0.3–1.0 |
| C. perfringens | 3.0 | 3.0 |
| B. anthracis | 1.5 | 4.0 |
| H. influenzae | 2.0 | 2.0 |
| H. ducreyi | <1.0 | <1.0 |
| B. pertussis | 2.0 | 2.0 |
| P. multocida | 1.5 | 3.0 |
| B. fragilis | 6.0 | 1.0–25.0 |
| B. oralis | 1.5 | 0.5 |
| B. melaninogenicus | 1.5 | 1.0 |
| F. nucleatum | 3.1 | 6.2 |
| E. coli | 6.0–12.0 | 6.0–50.0 |
| E. aerogenes | 20.0 | 50.0–>100.0 |
| K. pneumoniae | 10.0 | 50.0–>100.0 |
| S. marcescens | 25.0 | 100.0 |
| P. mirabilis | 6.0–12.0 | 50.0–100.0 |
| Indole + Proteus | 50.0 | 25.0 |
| P. aeruginosa | >100.0 | >100.0 |
| Y. enterocolitica[64] | 3.0 | 6.0 |
| B. abortus[63] | 3.0 | 1.0 |
| P. pseudomallei[16] | 6.4 | 1.6 |
| Salmonella spp. | 2.0 | 1.0 |
| Shigella spp. | 2.0 | 8.0 |
| Vibrio cholerae[30] | 1.25 | 1.05 |
| Vibrio parahemolyticus | 3.1 | 3.1 |

ties of these three antibiotics against bacilli. The activity of clindamycin against *Campylobacter fetus* subsp. *jejuni* is noteworthy.

All the rods, both gram-positive and gram-negative, were initially sensitive to the tetracyclines and chloramphenicol, but some resistance has developed among the enteric bacilli. Table 8 shows that *Pseudomonas aeruginosa, Yersinia enterocolitica,* indole + *Proteus,* and most *Serratia* are beyond the reach clinically of chloramphenicol and tetracycline.

The aminoglycosides differ from other antibiotics in the weakness of their inhibitory action against anaerobes[33] but show potent in vitro activity against nearly all other bacilli. The usual MIC of streptomycin, kanamycin, and gentamicin against aerobic gram-negative bacilli is given in Table 9. Two MIC values are given for a number of enteric bacteria because of differences in susceptibility between "street" and "hospital" strains and because of variations from one community or hospital to another. The in vitro sensitivities of *Salmonella* and *Brucella* are misleading because streptomycin and kanamycin are not effective in treating brucellosis or *Salmonella* infections.

The polymyxins — polymyxin B and colistin methane sulfonate — are also impotent against the anaerobes, as well as the gram-negative bacilli, *Proteus, Serratia, Brucella,* and *P. pseudomallei.* Most strains of *E. coli, K. pneumoniae,* and *P. aeruginosa* are inhibited by 2.5 $\mu$g/ml or less of either drug. *Salmonella, Shigella,* and *H. influenzae* are even more sensitive (0.2 to 0.4 $\mu$g/ml), but the polymyxins are seldom used to treat infections by these three groups of organisms.

Rifampin is effective to some degree against all the enteric rods, *H. influenzae,*[2, 26, 49] and *H. ducreyi* (Table 10).

Among the sulfonamides, sulfadiazine and sulfisoxazole will inhibit most enteric bacilli in con-

**TABLE 9.** Sensitivity in vitro of Gram-Negative Bacilli to Aminoglycosides

| | USUAL MINIMUM INHIBITORY CONCENTRATIONS ($\mu$g/ml) | | | |
|---|---|---|---|---|
| | Streptomycin | Kanamycin | Gentamicin* | Amikacin |
| H. influenzae | 8.0 | 4.0 | 2.0 | – |
| B. pertussis | 4.0 | 2.0 | 1.0 | – |
| P. multocida | 25.0 | – | – | – |
| E. coli | 4.0–25.0 | 3.0 | 2.0 | 2.0–4.0 |
| E. aerogenes | 4.0–25.0 | 2.0–10.0 | 0.5–2.0 | 1.4–2.0 |
| K. pneumoniae | 6.0–100.0 | 2.0–10.0 | 1.0–4.0 | 1.8 |
| S. marcescens | >100.0 | 10.0 | 4.0 | 3.2 |
| P. mirabilis | 6.0–>100.0 | 2.0–>100.0 | 0.3–5.0 | 1.2–2.0 |
| Indole + Proteus | 6.0–>100.0 | 2.0–>100.0 | 2.0 | – |
| P. aeruginosa | 50.0 | >100.0 | 1.0–4.0 | 3.0–6.0 |
| P. pseudomallei | >200.0 | 25.6 | 50.0 | – |
| Y. enterocolitica[64] | 6.0–>100.0 | 6.0 | – | – |
| B. abortus[63] | 2.0 | 1.5 | 0.3 | – |
| Salmonella spp. | 4.0–16.0 | 3.0 | 0.8 | – |
| Shigella spp. | 3.0–10.0 | 5.0 | 2.0 | – |
| Francisella tularensis[3] | 0.4 | – | – | – |
| Vibrio cholerae | 20.0 | – | – | – |

*Tobramycin activity against gram-negative bacilli is similar to that of gentamicin except that tobramycin is twice as active against *P. aeruginosa* and less active against some *Serratia.*
— = Inadequate data.

**TABLE 10.   Sensitivity of Gram-Negative Bacilli to Rifampin**

| ORGANISM | USUAL MINIMUM INHIBITORY CONCENTRATIONS ($\mu$g/ml) |
|---|---|
| E. coli | 2.5–10.0 |
| P. mirabilis | 1.0 |
| Indole + Proteus | 3.0 |
| P. aeruginosa | 10.0 |
| Salmonella spp. | 7.5 |
| Shigella spp. | 2.5 |
| K. pneumoniae | 10.0 |
| P. pseudomallei | 50.0 |
| H. influenzae | 0.2–0.8 |
| H. ducreyi | 0.02 |

centrations of 8 to 64 $\mu$g/ml in the absence of acquired resistance. Of the gram-negative rods, P. aeruginosa is most likely to be innately resistant to these concentrations. Acquired resistance to sulfonamides is so common among all bacteria, however, that sensitivity tests are usually needed to predict results.

Many gram-negative bacilli are also susceptible to nalidixic acid in concentrations of 20 to 50 $\mu$g/ml. Klebsiella, E. coli, P. mirabilis, and indole + Proteus organisms are often sensitive, while P. aeruginosa is uniformly resistant. Resistance tends to develop so rapidly, however, that it can appear overnight during treatment with nalidixic acid.[43, 54]

Metronidazole, a drug with interesting potential activity in anaerobic infections, can inhibit B. fragilis and other species of the family Bacteroidaceae. Concentrations of 3.1 $\mu$g/ml inhibit most B. fragilis.[59]

## OTHER PATHOGENIC MICROORGANISMS

### Mycobacteria and Nocardia

Mycobacteria show a different pattern of drug susceptibility than that of most bacteria (Table 11). Among antibiotics in general use in various bacterial infections, only the aminoglycosides and rifampin are active enough to warrant extensive use in tuberculosis and other mycobacterial infections.[28, 40] In fact, the most important antituberculosis drug, isoniazid, has no significant inhibitory effect on any other group of bacteria. The same is true of ethambutol and pyrazinamide. Despite its spectacular activity against human and bovine tubercle bacilli, isoniazid is inactive against most mycobacteria. Some other mycobacteria, especially Mycobacterium kansasii, are very sensitive to rifampin (but not rifamycin) and

are moderately sensitive to streptomycin.[31] This organism is also sensitive in vitro to erythromycin. The major difference in susceptibility between the human and bovine tubercle bacillus is that M. tuberculosis var. bovis is resistant to pyrazinamide while M. tuberculosis var. hominis is sensitive. The slight sensitivity of the human tubercle bacillus to tetracycline has had some practical implications in combined drug therapy for preventing resistance to another antituberculous drug, but not for primary treatment.

Nocardia asteroides, the only important acid-fast bacillus other than the mycobacteria, is resistant to most antimycobacterial drugs. In general, strains of Nocardia show considerable variation in susceptibility to a given drug but are usually sensitive in vitro to the sulfonamides, tetracyclines, and cycloserine. The most consistently active antibiotic in vitro is minocycline, which inhibits 90 per cent of nocardial strains at a concentration of 3.1 $\mu$g/ml.[4] Erythromycin inhibits 40 per cent of strains at 0.8 $\mu$g/ml, but the others are resistant to >100 $\mu$g/ml. These in vitro results, based on standard testing methods, are probably not applicable to clinical therapy because the sulfonamides have been the most consistently successful drug for treating human nocardiosis even though Nocardia strains are highly resistant (>1600 $\mu$g/ml) to sulfonamides in vitro unless tiny inocula (<100 organisms) are used. Likewise, a number of patients have not responded to antibiotics that inhibited the infecting strain of Nocardia in low concentrations in vitro.

### Mycoplasma

Mycoplasma pneumoniae, the cause of primary atypical pneumonia, is the only mycoplasma which has been proved to cause human infection, although Ureaplasma has been implicated in nongonococcal urethritis. Both organisms are resistant to drugs that affect the mucopeptide of bacteria because this structure is not present in mycoplasma. Their in vitro sensitivities are given in Table 12.[8, 39] Erythromycin and tetracycline are active against them, while lincomycin and clindamycin are ineffective.

### Yeasts and Fungi

Amphotericin B, 5-fluorocytosine, nystatin, miconazole, and griseofulvin are the major drugs given for treating fungus infections. Amphotericin B, 5-fluorocytosine, and miconazole are active against the fungi causing deep mycoses, and griseofulvin against dermatophytes. Nystatin is used only topically. The sulfonamides, clotrimazole, and hydroxystilbamidine have some antifungal properties, but toxicity (clotrimazole,

#### TABLE 11.  Drug Sensitivity of Mycobacteria

| | USUAL MINIMUM INHIBITORY CONCENTRATIONS ($\mu$g/ml) | | | | |
|---|---|---|---|---|---|
| | M. tuberculosis var. hominis | M. kansasii | M. marinum | M. intracellulare | M. fortuitum |
| Isoniazid | 0.2 | >25.0 | >25.0 | >25.0 | >25.0 |
| Rifampin | 0.1 | 0.1–0.5 | 0.6 | 10.0 | >20.0 |
| Ethambutol | 1.0 | 5.0 | — | — | >20.0 |
| Streptomycin | 0.3–6.0 | 12.0–25.0 | 2.0–10.0 | 12.0–25.0 | >100.0 |
| Kanamycin | 8.0 | >5.0 | 5.0 | — | — |
| Erythromycin | >32.0 | 1.0–2.0 | — | 32.0 | >32.0 |
| Tetracycline | 10.0 | — | — | — | — |
| PAS | 1.0 | >10.0 | >2.0 | — | >10.0 |
| Pyrazinamide | 18.0–20.0 | >100.0 | 50.0 | >100.0 | — |
| Cycloserine | 5.0–20.0 | >50.0 | 50.0 | — | >100.0 |
| Gentamicin | 3.0–6.0 | 3.0 | — | 3.0 | 25.0 |

— = Inadequate data.

#### TABLE 12.  In Vitro Sensitivity of Mycoplasmas to Antibiotics

| | USUAL MINIMUM INHIBITORY CONCENTRATIONS ($\mu$g/ml) | |
|---|---|---|
| | M. pneumoniae | Ureaplasma |
| Tetracycline | 1.6 | 0.4 |
| Erythromycin | 0.025 | 1.6 |
| Lincomycin | 20.0 | 200.0 |
| Chloramphenicol | 12.0 | 1.6 |
| Streptomycin | 1.0 | 1.6 |
| Polymyxin | — | 500.0 |
| Kanamycin | — | 3.1 |
| Gentamicin | — | 6.2 |
| Clindamycin | — | 6.2–50.0 |

— = Inadequate data.

hydroxystilbamidine) or narrow spectrum (sulfonamides) greatly limit their use. Their activity against sensitive strains in vitro[1, 13, 14, 23, 27, 50, 51, 55, 61] is summarized in Table 13.

Griseofulvin inhibits virtually all dermatophytes at a concentration of less than 0.5 $\mu$g/ml. *Microsporum canis, M. gypseum, M. audouinii, Epidermophyton floccosum, Trichophyton mentagrophytes, T. rubrum, T. tonsurans, T. versicolor,* and all other clinically significant dermatophytes are susceptible in tube dilution tests to this concentration, or less, of griseofulvin.[45] Miconazole is less active against dermatophytes than griseofulvin, inhibiting most of these skin fungi at 32 $\mu$g/ml or less; it is especially active against *E. floccosum* (<0.125 $\mu$g/ml). Miconazole is useful when applied topically in ringworm.

### SYNERGISM

A few important drugs are more active in the presence of another. The second drug can potentiate by increasing permeability. Thus, the aminoglycosides are more active with penicillin, while rifampicin, 5-fluorocytosine, and tetracycline are potentiated against fungi by amphotericin B. By injuring the mucopeptide of the cell wall, penicillin facilitates entry so that more of the aminoglycoside can reach the ribosomes.[37, 65] Amphotericin B alters permeability by binding with sterols so that more 5-fluorocytosine can enter the cells and inhibit nucleic acid synthesis through its action on pyrimidine biosynthesis.[36] This idea is the basis for the combined treatment of cryptococcosis with amphotericin B plus 5-fluorocytosine, and of enterococcal endocarditis with streptomycin and penicillin. More than 50 $\mu$g/ml streptomycin and more than 100 $\mu$g/ml

#### TABLE 13.  Usual Minimum Inhibitory Concentrations ($\mu$g/ml)

| | AMPHOTERICIN | 5-FLUOROCYTOSINE | CLOTRIMAZOLE | NYSTATIN | MICONAZOLE |
|---|---|---|---|---|---|
| *Cryptococcus neoformans* | 0.4–3.0 | 0.5–4.0 | 1.6 | 1.5 | 0.5 |
| *Coccidioides immitis* | 0.5 | >100.0 | 0.4 | 1.5 | 3.0 |
| *Aspergillus fumigatus* | >40.0 | 50.0->100.0 | 1.6 | 3.0 | 8.0–16.0 |
| *Blastomyces dermatitidis* | 0.4–0.8 | 25.0 | 0.2 | 0.8 | 1.0 |
| *Candida albicans* | 2.0–4.0 | 0.5–500.0 | 4.0–16.0 | 3.0 | 30.0 |
| *Torulopsis glabrata* | 0.5–2.0 | 0.5–5.0 | 2.0–8.0 | — | 16.0–64.0 |
| *Histoplasma capsulatum* | 0.1–0.8 | >100.0 | 3.0 | 1.5 | 0.5 |
| *Sporothrix schenckii* | 0.1–0.6 | >100.0 | — | 12.0 | 2.0 |
| *Mucoraceae* | 0.03->2.5 | >100.0 | 0.8 | 12.0 | 1000.0 |

— = Inadequate data.

**TABLE 14.   Synergism between Trimethoprim and Sulfamethoxazole[9]**

| | USUAL MINIMUM INHIBITORY CONCENTRATIONS (μg/ml)* | | | |
| --- | --- | --- | --- | --- |
| | Sulfamethoxazole Alone | Trimethoprim Alone | Sulfamethoxazole in Combination | Trimethoprim in Combination |
| *Streptococcus pyogenes* | 100.0 | 1.0 | 1.0 | 0.05 |
| Pneumococcus | 30.0 | 2.0 | 2.0 | 0.1 |
| *S. aureus* | 3.0 | 1.0 | 0.3 | 0.015 |
| *H. influenzae* | 10.0 | 1.0 | 0.3 | 0.015 |
| *K. pneumoniae* | 100.0 | 3.0 | 4.0 | 0.2 |
| *E. coli* | 3.0 | 0.3 | 1.0 | 0.05 |
| *Salmonella typhimurium* | 10.0 | 1.0 | 0.3 | 0.05 |
| *Shigella sonnei* | >10.0 | 1.0 | 0.3 | 0.05 |
| *N. gonorrhoeae* | 5.0 | 18.3 | 4.0 | 2.3 |
| *B. fragilis* | 6.0 | 25.0 | 4.0 | 0.2 |
| *Fusobacterium* spp. | 40.0 | 100.0 | 15.0 | 1.0 |
| *Peptostreptococcus* spp. | >100.0 | >100.0 | 30.0 | 2.0 |

*The levels of sulfamethoxazole usually reached in serum are 16 to 32 μg/ml and those of trimethoprim are 0.8 to 1.6 μg/ml.

penicillin are required to kill most enterococci, but many of these are killed by 6.25 μg of streptomycin in the presence of 6.25 μg penicillin or less.[62] In other words, one-fourth or less of the minimum bactericidal concentration of each drug alone killed enterococci in combination. Similar synergism against enterococci occurs with penicillin plus kanamycin and with penicillin plus gentamicin.

A second drug can also potentiate by reinforcing the metabolic disturbance of the first. This approach is used for synergism between trimethoprim and sulfonamides, two drugs that block two sequential steps in folinic acid synthesis.[9] Maximum potentiation occurs when the two drugs are present in proportions corresponding to their respective MIC when acting singly. Trimethoprim is usually about 20 times more active than sulfamethoxazole, the sulfonamide with which it is usually combined. When the two drugs are mixed according to this ratio (20 sulf:1 trimethoprim), they potentiate each other against many organisms, including streptococci, pneumococci, *S. aureus, H. influenzae, B. pertussis, K. pneumoniae, E. coli, Salmonella, Shigella, Proteus,* and gonococci. Examples are given in Table 14 and Figure 31, which give the minimum inhibitory concentrations of each drug when they are combined in a ratio of 1 part trimethoprim and 20 parts sulfamethoxazole.[9] The results show a po-

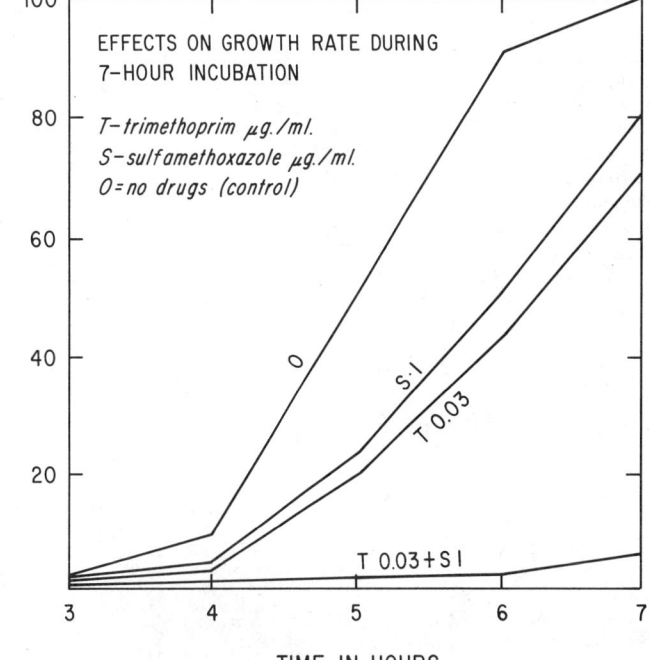

**FIGURE 31.** *Synergism between trimethoprim and sulfamethoxazole on growth inhibition of E. coli. (Modified from Bushby, S. R. M.: Combined antibacterial action in vitro of trimethoprim and sulphonamides. Postgrad Med J 45:17, Nov. 1969.)*

**TABLE 15.  Average Serum Concentrations After Single Oral Doses in Fasting Subjects**

| | DOSE (mg) | AVERAGE PEAK SERUM LEVEL (µg/ml) | AVERAGE SERUM HALF-LIFE (hours) | AVERAGE PERCENTAGE EXCRETED IN URINE IN 6 HOURS |
|---|---|---|---|---|
| Benzylpenicillin (penicillin G) | 500 | 0.5 | 4.0 | 10.0 |
| Phenoxymethyl penicillin (penicillin V) | 500 | 2.9 | 2.0 | 35.0 |
| Ampicillin | 500 | 3.0 | 5.0 | 30.0 |
| Amoxicillin | 500 | 7.5 | 1.0 | 60.0 |
| Oxacillin | 500 | 2.6 | 1.5 | 20.0 |
| Dicloxacillin | 500 | 11.5 | 3.0 | 40.0 |
| Cloxacillin | 500 | 8.0 | 2.0 | 20.0 |
| Indanyl carbenicillin | 500 | 12.0 | 3.5 | 22.0 |
| Cephalexin | 500 | 17.0 | 2.0 | 95.0 |
| Erythromycin base | 500 | 1.0 | 3.0 | 0.5 |
| Erythromycin base | 250 | 0.35 | 5.5 | 0.5 |
| Erythromycin stearate | 500 | 1.1 | 5.0 | 0.5 |
| Erythromycin stearate | 250 | 0.4 | 6.0 | 0.5 |
| Erythromycin estolate | 500 | 2.5 | 3.5 | 0.9 |
| Lincomycin | 500 | 3.5 | 5.0 | 5.0 |
| Clindamycin | 450 | 4.5 | 3.5 | 5.0 |
| Tetracycline | 500 | 3.0 | 8.5 | 17.0 |
| Tetracycline | 250 | 2.2 | 8.0 | 25.0 |
| Oxytetracycline | 500 | 2.2 | 5.6 | — |
| Chlortetracycline | 500 | 1.4 | 8.0 | — |
| Minocycline | 300 | 4.0 | 15.0 | 2.0 |
| Doxycycline | 100 | 1.6 | 18.0 | 10.0 |
| Doxycycline | 200 | 2.8 | 20.0 | 10.0 |
| Chloramphenicol | 500 | 11.0 | 3.5 | <5.0 (as active drug) |
| Rifampin | 600 | 7.0 | 3.3 | <5.0 (as active drug) |
| Sulfadiazine | — | — | — | 7.0 (as active drug) |
| Sulfamethoxazole | 800 | 53.8 | 12.0 | 10.0 |
| Trimethoprim | 160 | 1.58 | 12.0 | 16.0 |
| Chloroquine | 500 | 0.2 | 72.0 | — |
| Isoniazid | 600 | 8.5 | 2.6 | 30.0 (as active drug in 24 hr) |
| 5-Fluorocytosine | 2000 | 25.0 | 6.0 | 70.0 (24 hr) |
| Griseofulvin | 500 | 1.25 | — | <0.5 |
| Neomycin | 2000 | 0.95 | 8.0 | 0.85 (48 hr) |
| Ethambutol | 1750 | 3.5 | — | 50.00 (24 hr) |

— = Inadequate data.
See references 11, 21, 26, 35–38, 57, 60.

**TABLE 16.   Average Serum Concentrations After Single Intramuscular Dose**

| | DOSE (gm) | AVERAGE PEAK SERUM LEVEL (µg/ml) | AVERAGE SERUM HALF-LIFE (hours) | AVERAGE PERCENTAGE EXCRETED IN URINE IN 6 HOURS |
|---|---|---|---|---|
| Benzylpenicillin | 0.6 | 12.0 | 0.5 | 70.0 |
| Procaine penicillin G | 0.2 | 1.0 | 18.0 | 70.0 |
| Benzathine penicillin G | 0.75 | 0.01 | — | — |
| Ampicillin trihydrate | 0.5 | 4.3 | 4.0 | — |
| Sodium methicillin | 1.0 | 16.0 | 1.5 | 66.0 |
| Sodium oxacillin | 0.5 | 10.9 | — | — |
| Sodium nafcillin | 0.5 | — | — | 10.0 |
| Carbenicillin disodium | 1.0 | 19.0 | 3.5 | 65.0 |
| Sodium cephalothin | 0.5 | 10.0 | 2.0 | — |
| Sodium cefazolin | 0.5 | 42.2 | 1.8 | 60.0 |
| Cephaloridine | 0.5 | 18.0 | 1.1 | 85.0 (24 hr) |
| Erythromycin ethylsuccinate | 0.1 | 0.6 | 2.5 | — |
| Clindamycin | 0.6 | 5.1 | 8.0 | 15.0 (24 hr) |
| Lincomycin hydrochloride | 0.6 | 9.5 | 8.0 | 30.0 (24 hr) |
| Streptomycin | 0.5 | 18.0 | 5.0 | 60.0 (12 hr) |
| Kanamycin sulfate* | 0.5 | 21.0 | 4.0 | 60.0 |
| Gentamicin* | 0.06 | 4.7 | 4.0 | 60.0 (24 hr) |
| Chloramphenicol sodium succinate | 1.0 | 5.0 | 6.0 | 1.0 (as active drug) |
| Polymyxin B sulfate | 0.05 | 3.0 | 7.0 | — |
| Sodium colistimethate | 0.15 | 3.0 | 3.0 | — |
| Spectinomycin | 2.0 | 100.0 | 5.0 | — |
| Pentamidine isethionate | 0.280 | 0.5 | >24.0 | 15.0 (24 hr) |

— = Inadequate data.
*The peak level, half-life, and urinary excretion of tobramycin are approximately the same as those of gentamicin, whereas these properties of amikacin are similar to those of kanamycin.
See references, 8, 10, 16, 21, 28, 32, 37, 44, 46, 48–50.

**TABLE 17.  Average Serum Concentrations After Single Intravenous Dose**

| | DOSE (gm) | AVERAGE PEAK SERUM LEVEL ($\mu$g ml) | AVERAGE SERUM HALF-LIFE (hours) | PERCENTAGE OF ACTIVE DRUG EXCRETED IN URINE IN 6 HOURS |
|---|---|---|---|---|
| Benzylpenicillin | 0.5 | 5.5 | 0.15 | 90.0 |
| Ampicillin | 0.5 | 9.0 | 1.5 | 70.0 |
| Sodium methicillin | 0.5 | 16.2 | 0.7 | 80.0 |
| Sodium oxacillin | 0.5 | 60.0 | 0.4 | 45.0 |
| Sodium nafcillin | 0.5 | 40.0 | 0.5 | 35.0 |
| Carbenicillin disodium | 1.0 | 125.0 | 1.0 | 70.0 |
| Sodium cephalothin | 1.0 | 70.0 | 0.5 | 52.0 (24 hr) |
| Sodium cefazolin | 0.5 | 118.0 | 1.8 | 95.0 (24 hr) |
| Sodium cephapirin | 1.0 | 36.7 | 0.6 | — |
| Erythromycin lactobionate | 0.2 | 3.5 | 1.0 | 8.0 |
| Clindamycin | 0.6 | 8.5 | 3.0 | 20.0 |
| Streptomycin | 0.6 | 32.8 | 3.0 | 60.0 (12 hr) |
| Gentamicin sulfate | 0.08 | 11.0 | 2.0 | — |
| Amikacin | 1.0 | 20.0 | 2.5 | 60.0 |
| Sodium colistimethate | 0.15 | 20.0 | 2.5 | 75.0 |
| Doxycycline hyclate | 0.2 | 4.0 | 18.0 | 71.4 (48 hr) |
| Tetracycline hydrochloride | 0.5 | 8.5 | 8.5 | 45.0 (24 hr) |
| Oxytetracycline hydrochloride | 0.5 | 7.0 | 9.2 | 60.0 (24 hr) |
| Chlortetracycline hydrochloride | 0.5 | 9.0 | 5.6 | 15.0 (24 hr) |
| Amphotericin B | 0.7 | 5.0 | 24.0 | — |
| Chloramphenicol sodium succinate | 1.0 | 11.0 | 3.5 | 5.0 |
| Rifampin | 0.6 | 7.0 | 3.3 | 5.0 (as active drug) |
| Vancomycin | 0.5 | 33.0 | 6.0 | 80.0 (24 hr) |
| Sulfadiazine | — | — | — | 7.0 (as active drug) |
| Sulfamethoxazole | 0.8 | 53.8 | 10.0 | 10.0 |
| Trimethoprim | 0.16 | 1.58 | 10.0 | 16.0 |
| Chloroquine | 0.5 | 0.2 | 72.0 | — |
| Isoniazid | 0.6 | 8.5 | 6.0 | 30.0 (as active drug in 24 hr) |
| 5-Fluorocytosine | 2.0 | 25.0 | 6.0 | 70.0 (24 hr) |
| Griseofulvin | 0.5 | 1.25 | — | 0.5 |
| Miconazole | 1.0 | 1.5 | 1.0 | 2.0 |

— = Inadequate data.
See references 21, 28, 30, 31, 44, 48, 50, 62.

tentiation of at least 20-fold for each drug against most organisms when used in combination.

## SERUM CONCENTRATIONS OF ANTIMICROBIAL DRUGS

The aim of chemotherapy is to get enough drug into the infected tissues to inhibit or kill the pathogenic organism. In other words, the drug level must exceed the minimum inhibitory concentration. The levels of drug that can be anticipated in serum after different routes of administration are listed in Tables 15, 16, and 17. By comparing these levels to the minimum inhibitory concentrations given in the preceding tables, an estimate can then be made of appropriate drugs and dosage for a given infection. These estimates will be modified, in turn, by the pharmacologic considerations discussed in the next chapter. Renal failure, diffusion barriers, and the type of inflammatory reaction, if any, must be taken into account in selecting a drug and deter-

mining its dose. The interval between doses is a function of half-life, and the effect of renal failure can be predicted by the percentage of drug excreted in the urine.

## References

*Classification*

1. Bodanszky, M., and Perlman, D.: Peptide antibiotics. Science 163:352, 1969.
2. Bueding, E.: Some biochemical effects of anthelmintic drugs. Biochem Pharmacol 18:1541, 1969.
3. Dutcher, J. D., Young, M. B., Sherman, J. H., et al.: Chemical studies on amphotericin B. I. Preparation of the hydrogenation product and isolation of mycosamine, an acetolysis product. Antibiot Annu 866, 1956–1957.
4. Fox, H.: The chemical attack on tuberculosis. Trans. NY Acad Sci 15:234, 1953.
5. Grollman, P.: Structural basis for inhibition of protein synthesis by emetine and cycloheximide based on an analogy between ipecac alkaloids and glutarimide antibiotics. Proc Nat Acad Sci USA 56:1867, 1966.
6. Hewitt, L.: The cephalosporins — 1973. J Infect Dis 128: Suppl:S312, 1973.
7. Hitchings, H.: Species differences among dihydrofolate reductases as a basis for chemotherapy. Postgrad Med J 45(Suppl):7, 1969.
8. Johnson, A., Anker, H., and Meleney, L.: Bacitracin; new antibi-

otic produced by member of *B. subtilis* group. Science 102:376, 1945.

9. Lacroute, F.: Regulation of pyrimidine biosynthesis in Saccharomyces cerevisiae. J. Bacteriol 95:824, 1968.

10. Long, H., and Bliss, A.: Para-amino-benzene-sulfonamide and its derivatives; experimental and clinical observations on their use in treatment of beta-hemolytic streptococcic infection: preliminary report. JAMA 108:32, 1937.

11. Nair, S., and Cherubin, C.: Use of cefoxitin, new cephalosporin-like antibiotic, in the treatment of aerobic and anaerobic infections. Antimicrob Agents Chemother 14:866, 1978.

12. Neu, H. D.: Antimicrobial activity and human pharmacology of amoxicillin. J Infect Dis 129 (Suppl):123, 1974.

13. Novick, P.: Staphylococcal penicillinase and the new penicillins. Biochem J 83:229, 1962.

14. Oxford, E., Raistrick, H., and Simonart, P.: XXIX. Studies in the biochemistry of microorganisms: LX: Griseofulvin, $C_{17}H_{17}O_6Cl$, a metabolic product of *Penicillium griseofulvum* Dierckx. Biochem J 33:240, 1939.

15. Sheldrick, G., Jones, P., Kennard, O., Williams, D., and Smith, G.: Structure of vancomycin and its complex with acetyl-D-alanyl-D-alanine. Nature 271:223, 1978.

16. Wehrli, W., and Staehelin, M.: Actions of the rifamycins. Bacteriol Rev 35:290, 1971.

*Microbial Susceptibility to Drugs*

1. Artis, D.,and Baum, G. L.: In vitro susceptibility of 24 strains of *Histoplasma capsulatum* to amphotericin B. Antibiot Chemother 11:373, 1961.

2. Atlas, E. and Turck, M.: Laboratory and clinical evaluation of rifampicin. Am J Med Sci 256:47, 1968.

3. Avery, F. W., and Barnett, T. B.: Pulmonary tularemia. A report of five cases and consideration of pathogenesis and terminology. Am Rev Resp Dis 95:584, 1967.

4. Bach, M.C., Sabath, L. D., and Finland, M.: Susceptibility of *Nocardia asteroides* to 45 antimicrobial agents in vitro. Antimicrob Agents Chemother 3:1, 1973.

5. Bauer, A. W., Kirby, W. M., Sherris, J. C., et al.: Antibiotic susceptibility testing by a standardized single disk method. Am J Clin Pathol 45:493, 1966.

6. Benner, E. J.: The cephalosporin antibiotics. Pediatr Clin North Am 15:31, 1968.

7. Braude, A. I., Banister, J., and Wright, N.: Use of the gradient plate for routine clinical determinations of bacterial sensitivites to antibiotics. Antibiot Annu 1133, 1954–1955.

8. Braun, P., Klein, J. O., and Kass, E. H.: Susceptibility of genital mycoplasmas to antimicrobial agents. Appl Microbiol 19:62, 1970.

9. Bushby, R. S.: Combined antibacterial action in vitro of trimethoprim and sulphonamides. The in vitro nature of synergy. Postgrad Med J 45 (Suppl):10, 1969.

10. Butler, K., English, A. R., Ray, V. A., et al.: Carbenicillin: chemistry and mode of action. J Infect Dis 122:(Suppl):51, 1970.

11. Cave, V. G., Hurdle, E. S., and Catelli, A. R.: Sensitivity of *Neisseria gonorrhoeae* to penicillin and other drugs. NY State J Med 70:844, 1970.

12. Chadwick, P.: Bacteriological assessment of clindamycin, a new lincomycin derivative. J Med Microbiol 4:529, 1971.

12a. Dixon, D., Shadomy, S., Shadomy, H., Espinel-Ingroff, A., and Kerkering, T.: Comparison of the *in vitro* antifungal activities of miconazole and a new imidazole, R 41,400. J Infect Dis 138:245, 1978.

13. Drouhet, E.: Basic mechanisms of antifungal chemotherapy. Mod Treat 7:539, 1970.

14. Drutz, D. J., Spickard, A., Rogers, D. E., et al.: Treatment of disseminated mycotic infections. A new approach to amphotericin B therapy. Am J Med 45:405, 1968.

15. Edmondson, E. B., and Sanford, J. P.: The Klebsiella-Enterobacter (Aerobacter)-Serratia group. A clinical and bacteriological evaluation. Medicine (Balt) 46:323, 1967.

16. Eickhoff, T. C., Bennett, J. V., Hayes, P. S., et al.: *Pseudomonas pseudomallei*: susceptibility to chemotherapeutic agents. J Infect Dis 121:95, 1970.

17. Ericsson, H., Hogman, C., and Wickman, K.: Paper disc method for determination of bacterial sensitivity to chemotherapeutic and antibiotic agents. Scand J Clin Lab Invest 6 (Suppl):21, 1954.

18. Finland, M.: Changing patterns of susceptibility of common bacterial pathogens to antimicrobial agents. Ann Intern Med 76:1009, 1972.

19. Friedberg, C. K., Rosen, K. M., and Bienstock, P. A.: Vancomycin therapy for enterococcal and *Streptococcus viridans* endocarditis. Successful treatment of six patients. Arch Intern Med (Chicago) 122:134, 1968.

20. Griffith, R. S., and Black, H. R.: Erythromycin. Med Clin North Am 54:1199, 1970.

21. Guttler, R. B., Counts, G. W., Avent, C. K., et al.: Effect of rifampin and minocycline on meningococcal carrier rates. J Infect Dis 24:199, 1971.

22. Hammerstrom, C. F., Cox, F., McHenry, M. C., et al.: Clinical laboratory, and pharmacological studies of dicloxacillin. Antimicrob Agents Chemother 69, 1966.

23. Hildick-Smith, G.: Antifungal antibiotics. Pediatr Clin North Am 15:107, 1968.

24. Judson, F. N., Allaman, J., and Dans, P. E.: Treatment of gonorrhea — Comparison of penicillin G procaine, doxycycline, spectinomycin, and ampicillin. JAMA 230:705, 1974.

25. Kayser, F. H.: In vitro activity of cephalosporin antibiotics against gram-positive bacteria. Postgrad Med J 47 (Suppl):14, 1971.

26. Kunin, C. M., Brandt, D., and Wood, H.: Bacteriologic studies of rifampin, a new semisynthetic antibiotic. J Infect Dis 119:132, 1969.

27. Larsh, H. W., Hinton, A., and Silberg, S. L.: The use of the tissue culture method in evaluating antifungal agents against systemic fungi. Antibiot Annu 988, 1957–1958.

28. Lester, W.: Rifampin: a semisynthetic derivative of rifamycin — a prototype for the future. Am Rev Microbiol 26:85, 1972.

29. Levison, M.E., Johnson, W. D., Thornhill, T. S., et al.: Clinical and in vitro evaluation of cephalexin. A new orally administered cephalosporin antibiotic. JAMA 209:1331, 1969.

30. Lindenbaum, J., Greenough, W. B., and Islam, M. R.: Antibiotic therapy of cholera. Bull WHO 36:871, 1967.

31. Lorian, V., and Finland, M.: In vitro effect of rifampin on mycobacteria. Appl Microbiol 17:202, 1969.

32. Martin, J. E., Jr., Lester, A., Kellogg, D. S., Jr., et al.: In vitro susceptibility of *Neisseria gonorrhoeae* to nine antimicrobial agents. Appl Microbiol 18:21, 1969.

33. Martin, W. J., Gardner, M., and Washington, J. A. II: In vitro antimicrobial susceptibility of anaerobic bacteria isolated from clinical specimens. Antimicrob Agents Chemother 1:148, 1972.

34. Matsen, J. M., Blazevic, D. J., and Chapman, S. S.: In vitro susceptibility patterns of beta-hemolytic streptococci. Antimicrob Agents Chemother 485, 1969.

35. McLinn, S. E., Nelson, J. D., and Haltalin, K. C.: Antimicrobial susceptibility of *Hemophilus influenzae*. Pediatrics 45:827, 1970.

36. Medoff, G., Comfort, M., and Kobayashi, G. S.: Synergistic action of amphotericin B and 5-fluorocytosine against yeast-like organisms. Proc Soc Exp Biol Med 138:571, 1971.

37. Moellering, R. C., Jr., Wennersten, C., and Weinberg, A. N.: Studies on antibiotic synergism against enterococci. I. Bacteriologic studies. J Lab Clin Med 77:821, 1971.

38. Neu, H.: Antimicrobial activity and human pharmacology of amoxicillin. J Infect Dis 129 (Suppl):S123, 1974.

39. Niitu, Y., Hasegawa, S., Suetake, T., et al.: Resistance of *Mycoplasma pneumoniae* to erythromycin and other antibiotics. J Pediatr 76:438, 1970.

40. Raleigh, J. W.: Rifampin in treatment of advanced pulmonary tuberculosis. Report of a VA cooperative pilot study. Am Rev Respir Dis 105:397, 1972.

41. Ribble, J. C.: Laboratory assistance in the treatment of bacterial infections. Pediatr Clin North Am 18:115, 1971.

42. Ronald, A. R., Eby, J., and Sherris, J. C.: Susceptibility of *Neisseria gonorrhoeae* to penicillin and tetracycline. Antimicrob Agents Chemother 431, 1968.

43. Ronald, A. R., Turck, M., and Petersdorf, R. G.: A critical evaluation of nalidixic acid in urinary-tract infections. N Engl J Med 275:1081, 1966.

44. Rosen, I. G., Jacobsen, J., and Rudderman, R.: Rapid capillary tube method for detecting penicillin resistance in *Staphylococcus aureus*. Appl Microbiol 23:649, 1972.

45. Roth, F. J., Sallman, B., and Blank, H.: In vitro studies of the antifungal antibiotic griseofulvin. J Invest Dermatol 33:403, 1959.

46. Sabath, L. D., Stumpf, L. L., Wallace, S. J., et al.: Susceptibility

of *Diplococcus pneumoniae, Hemophilus influenzae,* and *Neisseria meningitidis* to 23 antibiotics. Antimicrob Agents Chemother 53, 1970.

47. Sabath, L. D., Wilcox, C., Garner, C., et al.: In vitro activity of cefazolin against recent clinical bacterial isolates. J Infect Dis 128 (Suppl):S320, 1973.

48. Sanders, E., Foster, M. T., and Scott, D.: Group A beta-hemolytic streptococci resistant to erythromycin and lincomycin. N Engl J Med 278:538, 1968.

49. Sensi, P., Maggi, N., Füresz, S., et al.: Chemical modifications and biological properties of rifamycins. Antimicrob Agents Chemother 699, 1966.

50. Shadomy, S.: Further in vitro studies with 5-fluorocytosine. Infect Immun 2:484, 1970.

51. Shadomy, S., Kirchoff, C. B., and Ingroff, A. E.: In vitro activity of 5-fluorocytosine against *Candida* and *Torulopsis* species. Antimicrob Agents Chemother 3:9, 1973.

52. Simon, H. J.: Streptomycin, kanamycin, neomycin, and paromomycin. Pediatr Clin North Am 15:73, 1968.

53. Smith, C. B., Wilfert, J. N., Dans, P. E., et al.: In-vitro activity of carbenicillin and results of treatment of infections due to *Pseudomonas* with carbenicillin singly and in combination with gentamicin. J Infect Dis 122 (suppl):S14, 1970.

54. Stamey, T. A., Nemoy, N. J., and Higgins, M.: The clinical use of nalidixic acid. A review and some observations. Invest Urol 6:582, 1969.

55. Sterr, P. L., Marks, M. I., Klite, P. D., et al.: 5-Fluorocytosine: an oral antifungal compound. A report on clinical and laboratory experience. Ann Intern Med 76:15, 1972.

56. Steigbigel, N. H., McCall, C. E., Reed, C. W., et al.: Antibacterial action of "broad spectrum" penicillins, cephalosporins and other antibiotics against gram-negative bacilli isolated from bacteremic patients. Ann NY Acad Sci 145:224, 1967.

57. Steigbigel, N. H., Reed, C. W., and Finland, M.: Susceptibility of cillin, a new isoxazolyl penicillin, compared with oxacillin, in vitro. Am J Med Sci 255:179, 1968.

58. Sutherland, R., Croydon, E. A., and Rolinson, G. N.: Flucloxacilin, a new isoxazolyl penicillin, compared with oxacillin, cloxacillin, and dicloxacillin. Br Med J 4:455, 1970.

59. Tally, F. P., Sutter, V. L., and Finegold, S. M.: Metronidazole versus anaerobes. In vitro data and initial clinical observations. Calif Med 117:22, 1972.

60. Toala, P., McDonald, A., Wilcox, C., et al.: Comparison of antibiotic susceptibility of group D streptococcus strains isolated at Boston City Hospital in 1953–54 and 1968–69. Antimicrob Agents Chemother 479, 1969.

61. Watson, D. C., and Neame, P. B.: In vitro activity of amphotericin B on strains of *Mucoraceae* pathogenic to man. J Lab Clin Med 56:251, 1960.

62. Wilkowske, C. J., Facklam, R. R., Washington, J. A., II., and Geraci, J.: Antibiotic synergism: enhanced susceptibility of group D streptococci to certain antibiotic combinations. Antimicrob Agents Chemother 195, 1970.

63. Yow, E. M., and Spink, W. W.: Symposium on antibiotics; experimental studies on the action of streptomycin, aureomycin, and chloromycetin on brucella. J Clin Invest 28:871, 1949.

64. Zen-Yoji, H., and Maruyama, T.: The first successful isolations and identification of *Yersinia enterocolitica* from human cases in Japan. Jap J Microbiol 16:493, 1972.

65. Zimmermann, R. A., Moellering, R. C., Jr., and Weinberg, A. N.: Mechanism of resistance to antibiotic synergism in enterocci. J Bacteriol 105:873, 1971.

# 20 MECHANISMS OF ACTION OF ANTIMICROBIAL DRUGS

## *Abraham I. Braude, M.D., Ph.D.*

The key to antibiotic action is a selective toxicity for the infecting organism but not for the patient. Antibiotics can hit at least four targets in bacteria and other organisms that are either missing or less vulnerable in human cells: the cell wall, the cytoplasmic membrane, the ribosomes, and the molecules involved in transcription of genetic information.

### CELL WALL

The cell wall is where the penicillins and cephalosporins do their damage. It is the most important target for antibiotics because it is absent in human cells. The cell wall of bacteria is a thick rigid envelope that surrounds the cell membrane, maintaining the shape of the bacteria and keeping them from osmotic damage in water and body fluids. The internal pressures of pathogenic bacteria are somewhat higher than serum and other extracellular fluids so that the organisms would imbibe water, swell, and burst if the cell wall became defective. The rigid portion of the cell wall, known as the sacculus, is reminiscent of grape hulls in cocci and balloons in bacilli. The rigid material in the sacculus is a material composed of sugar and peptides and called mucopeptide or murein. The mucopeptide is at least four times thicker in gram-positive cells than in gram-negative cells. In *E. coli* the layer of mucopeptide is made up of polysaccharide chains linked together by peptides. The polysaccharide chains are composed of repeating units of two sugars, muramic acid and *N*-acetylglucosamine, as indicated in Figure 1. The cross-linking peptide strands are attached to the polysaccharide chains by a peptide bond between the carboxyl group in each muramic acid unit and the amino group of L-alanine. Another peptide bond connects L-alanine to D-glutamic acid, followed in turn by $\alpha$, $\epsilon$-diaminopimelic acid, and finally D-alanine to form a tetrapeptide. The free carboxyl groups on the D-alanine residues are also attached to the $NH_2$ group of the $\alpha$, $\epsilon$-diaminopimelic acid in adjacent tetrapeptides to produce a cross-linked

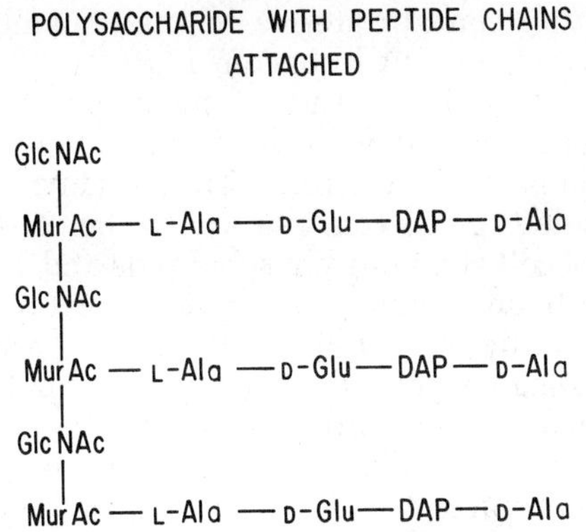

POLYSACCHARIDE WITH PEPTIDE CHAINS
ATTACHED

GlcNAc
|
MurAc — L-Ala — D-Glu — DAP — D-Ala
|
GlcNAc
|
MurAc — L-Ala — D-Glu — DAP — D-Ala
|
GlcNAc
|
MurAc — L-Ala — D-Glu — DAP — D-Ala

**FIGURE 1.** *The rigid structure in bacterial cell walls is a sugar peptide called mucopeptide or murein. The sugar is a polysaccharide of muramic acid (MurAc) and glucosamine (GlcNAc). The peptides are composed of four amino acids: L-alanine (L-Ala), D-glutamic acid (D-Glu), α, ε-diaminopimelic acid (DAP), and D-alanine.*

structure (Fig. 2). In staphylococci a second chain composed of five glycine molecules is used to connect neighboring peptides so that the structure is more like that in Figure 3. The peptide group in staphylococci is also different from that in *E. coli*, as shown in Figure 4. The staphylococcal peptide lacks diaminopimelic acid and, instead, has L-lysine as the third amino acid. This is followed by D-alanyl-D-alanine at the end of the chain. The murein network in the *Staphylococcus* is completed when D-alanine is split from D-alanyl-D-alanine so that a peptide bond can form between the carboxyl group of the residual D-alanine and the terminal amino group of the pentaglycine chain (Fig. 4).

Penicillin is thought to prevent the final peptide bond between D-alanine and glycine.[30] It has been suggested that penicillin combines with the enzyme responsible for this final cross linkage (the cross-linking enzyme). Since the stearic configuration of penicillin is like that of D-alanyl-D-alanine, penicillin might react with the cross-linking enzyme and inactivate it so that it could not complete the transpeptidation reaction (Fig. 5). By preventing this final step in murein synthesis, penicillin seems to have at least two del-

eterious effects on bacteria: (1) it inhibits multiplication; and (2) it creates weak points in the cell wall through which the growing cytoplasm can bulge. There is also evidence that penicillin binds to proteins that suppress murein hydrolases. It has been suggested that binding of penicillin by the proteins releases hydrolases from suppression, allows them to destroy the mucopeptide, and thus kills the bacterium by autolysis.[29]

An important feature of penicillin action is its ability to kill growing bacterial cells, but not stationary organisms. During growth of certain bacteria hydrolases seem to produce gaps in the mucopeptide that are filled with new structural units. These units are tied into the mucopeptide by the transpeptidation (cross-linking) reaction and can therefore be blocked by penicillin so that open gaps remain in the mucopeptide. The cell membrane extends through these gaps and ruptures under osmotic stress, and the cell dies (Fig. 6). Cells that are not undergoing multiplication, or cells that have no murein hydrolases ("penicillin-tolerant"), can survive in the presence of penicillin because their mucopeptide is unbroken and there is no reparative cross-linking activity for the penicillin to block. These cells are known as "persisters" and may be responsible for recurrence of infection after penicillin treatment has been stopped.[12] Penicillin and cephalosporin derivatives attack bacteria by similar mechanisms.

While penicillins block the terminal cross-linking reaction of mucopeptide formation, it is also theoretically possible for antibiotics to prevent the synthesis or transfer of mucopeptide precursors. Such action against precursors by certain antibiotics does, in fact, take place but these are of minor clinical importance. Cycloserine is a structural analog of D-alanine and competitively inhibits the enzyme responsible for synthesis of D-alanyl-D-alanine, an essential component of the pentapeptide.[22] Bacitracin[28] and vancomycin[1] both block the stages of cell wall construction which involve the transfer of the sugar pentapeptide from the site of synthesis in

**FIGURE 2.** *Cross linking of peptide chains in gram-negative bacilli by bonds between the free carboxyl groups of D-alanine and the NH₂ groups of α,ε-diaminopimelic acid. (Modified from Rogers, H. J.: The mode of action of antibiotics. In Bittar, E. E. (ed.): The Biological Basis of Medicine. Vol. 2. New York, Academic Press, 1968, p. 427.)*

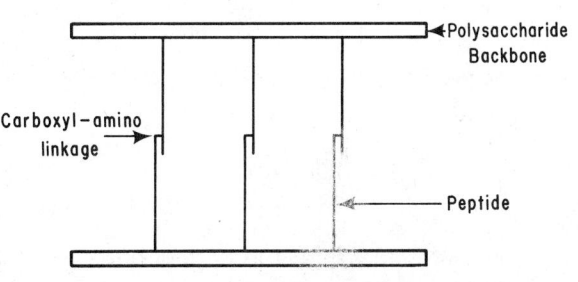

BASIS OF GRAM-NEGATIVE
MUCOPEPTIDE

STAPHYLOCOCCAL MUCOPEPTIDE

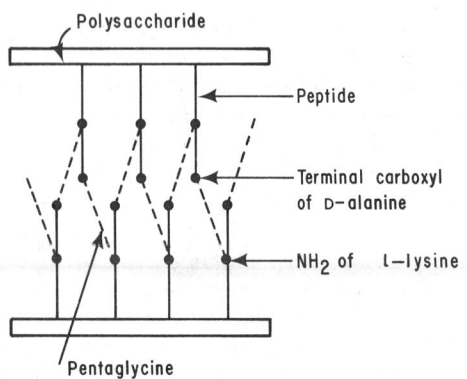

**FIGURE 3.** *In staphylococci a second chain composed of 5-glycine (pentaglycine) molecules connects the neighboring peptides. (Modified from Rogers, H. J.: The mode of action of antibiotics. In Bittar, E. E. (ed.): The Biological Basis of Medicine. Vol. 2. New York, Academic Press, 1968, p. 428.)*

the cytoplasm to its attachment to a lipid in the cell membrane.

## CYTOPLASMIC MEMBRANE

Beneath the rigid cell wall is a membrane that totally encloses the cytoplasm (Fig. 7A). This cytoplasmic membrane resembles that of human cells in possessing lipid and protein structural elements. Bacterial lipids are mainly phospholi-

pids. Fungi contain sterols in their membranes that are not present in bacteria.

The lipoproteins in the cytoplasmic membrane of all cells account for selective permeability to water, ions, and nutrients. The polymyxins are cationic detergents that react with the phosphate groups of cell envelope phospholipids and disorganize the lipoproteins in the bacterial cytoplasmic membrane by inserting the lipophilic portion of their molecule into the membrane lipid. This causes leakage of amino acids, purines, pyrimidines, and other small molecules from inside the cell so that nucleic acids and proteins break down and the cell dies.[11, 23]

Amphotericin and other polyene antibiotics also alter the permeability of sensitive cells, but only in organisms whose membranes contain sterols. For this reason they do not affect bacteria and are limited in their action against pathogenic organisms to yeasts, fungi (Fig. 7B), and certain amebae. After reacting with polyenes, sterols probably become reoriented within the membranes so that permeability is altered.[18] If sterol synthesis is blocked in fungi, the polyenes lose their target and are no longer effective. This occurs in fungi exposed to miconazole, which inhibits ergosterol synthesis and thus interferes with the antifungal action of amphotericin B. For this reason amphotericin is of no value in patients under treatment with miconazole.[32] By itself, however, miconazole and other imidazoles impair membrane structure and function of fungal membranes by depriving them of ergosterol. Electron microscopy in vitro and in vivo discloses that the first effect of imidazole on fungi is a disturbance in the cell membrane structure.[33]

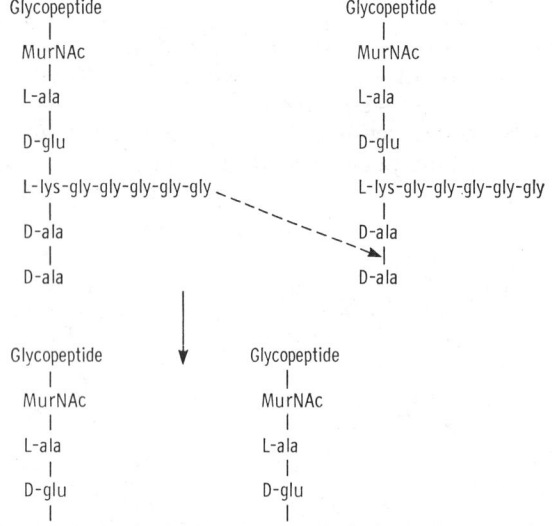

**FIGURE 4.** *Mucopeptide from staphylococci. The peptide chain differs from that in E. coli (Fig. 1) in that staphylococcal peptide lacks diaminopimelic acid and instead has L-lysine as the third amino acid. The murein network is completed when D-alanine is split from D-alanyl-D-alanine so that a peptide bond can form between the carboxyl group of the residual D-alanine and the terminal group of the pentaglycine chain. Penicillin is thought to act by inhibiting the enzyme (transpeptidase) responsible for this cross linkage. (From Strominger, J. L.: Enzymatic reactions in bacterial cell wall synthesis sensitive to penicillins and other antibacterial substances. In Guze, L. B. (ed.): Microbial Protoplasts, Spheroplasts and L-Forms. © 1968, The Williams & Wilkins Co., Baltimore, p. 57.)*

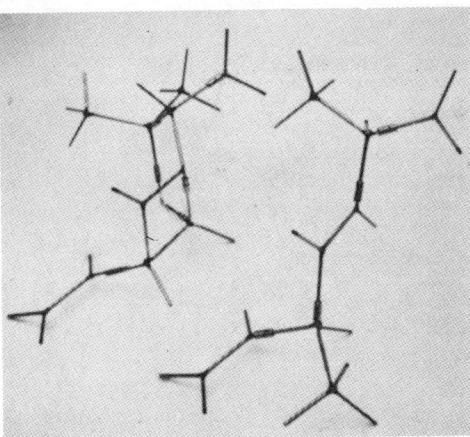

## RIBOSOMES

Ribosomes act as an assembly line where amino acids are strung together in peptide chains and proteins. The process is directed by messenger RNA (mRNA), which carries the code for protein synthesis from nuclear DNA. The message in the code is *transcribed* from DNA to RNA (Fig. 8A) and translated into the appropriate amino acid sequence by the four types of ribonucleotides in mRNA. These four ribonucleotides are prearranged in $4^3$ (or 64) different triplet combinations that are able to specify different amino acids. Since there are 64 triplets and only 20 amino acids used in protein synthesis, many amino acids are selected by more than one triplet (or codon). Three of the codons (UAA, UAG, and UGA) code for chain termination only and do not select amino acids. Each amino acid specified by the triplet is carried to the ribosome for incorporation into the growing peptide chain by a second type of RNA, transfer RNA (tRNA). The triplet AUG (adenylyl-uridylyl-guanylyl) or GUG initiates peptide chain formation by directing tRNA carrying methionine (as N-formylmethionine) to attach to the ribosome.

The bacterial ribosomes are spherical particles with a molecular weight of nearly 3 million. They sediment in the Svedberg ultracentrifuge at a rate expressed as 70S (Svedberg units). Before protein synthesis is started, the ribosome dissociates into a 30S subunit and a 50S subunit (Fig. 8B). Protein synthesis starts when mRNA attaches to the 30S subunit and tRNA carrying methionine is bound (Fig. 8C). This is followed by recombination with the 50S subunit to form the functioning 70S ribosome (Fig. 8D). The complete 70S ribosome has another binding site for tRNA, so that a second tRNA molecule carrying another

**FIGURE 5.** *Stereomodels of penicillin (left) and the end of the peptide D-alanyl-D-alanine have suggested that penicillin is a structural analog of the D-alanyl-D-alanine end of the peptide and thereby can react with the transpeptidase to prevent the transpeptidation reaction required for closure of the glycine bridges between peptide chains. (From Strominger, J. L.: Enzymatic reactions in bacterial cell wall synthesis sensitive to penicillins and other antibacterial substances. In Guze, L. B. (ed.): Microbial Protoplasts, Spheroplasts and L-Forms. ©1968, The Williams & Wilkins Co., Baltimore, p. 58.)*

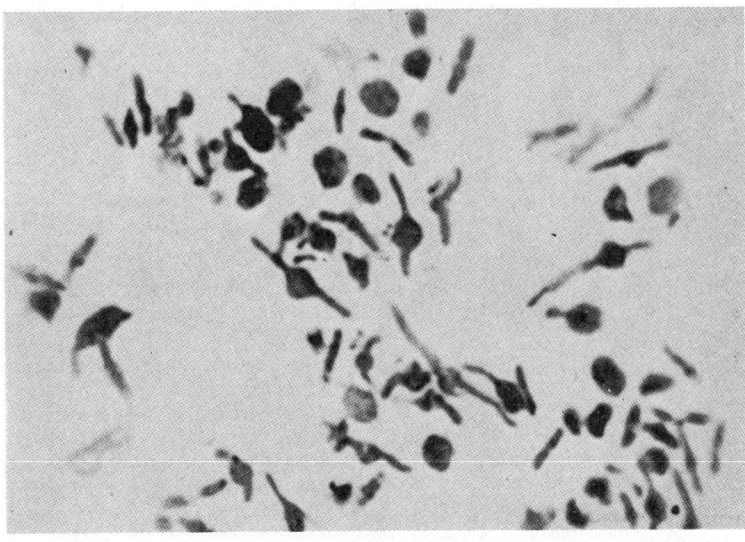

**FIGURE 6.** *Effect of penicillin on cell wall of Klebsiella pneumoniae. Defective portions of the mucopeptide allow the high internal osmotic pressure to cause swellings in both the central and terminal portions of the rods. (From Braude, A. I., Siemienski, J., and Jacobs, I.: Protoplast formation in human urine. Trans Assoc Am Physicians 74:238, 1961.)*

GRAM-NEGATIVE BACILLUS

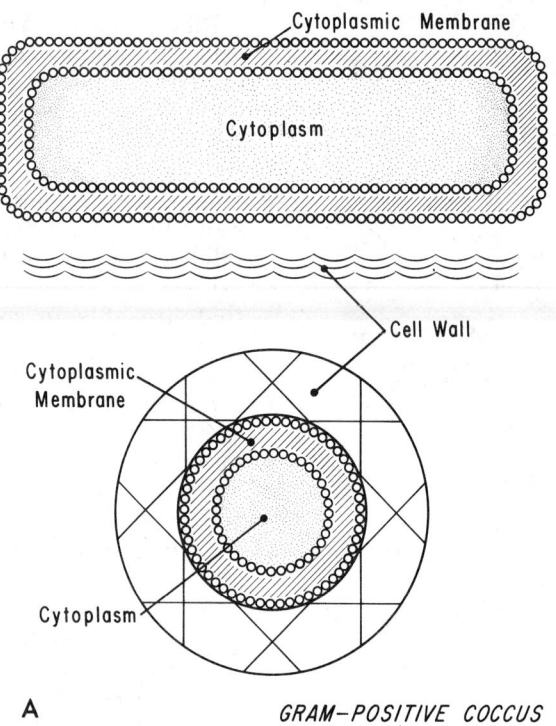

A

GRAM-POSITIVE COCCUS

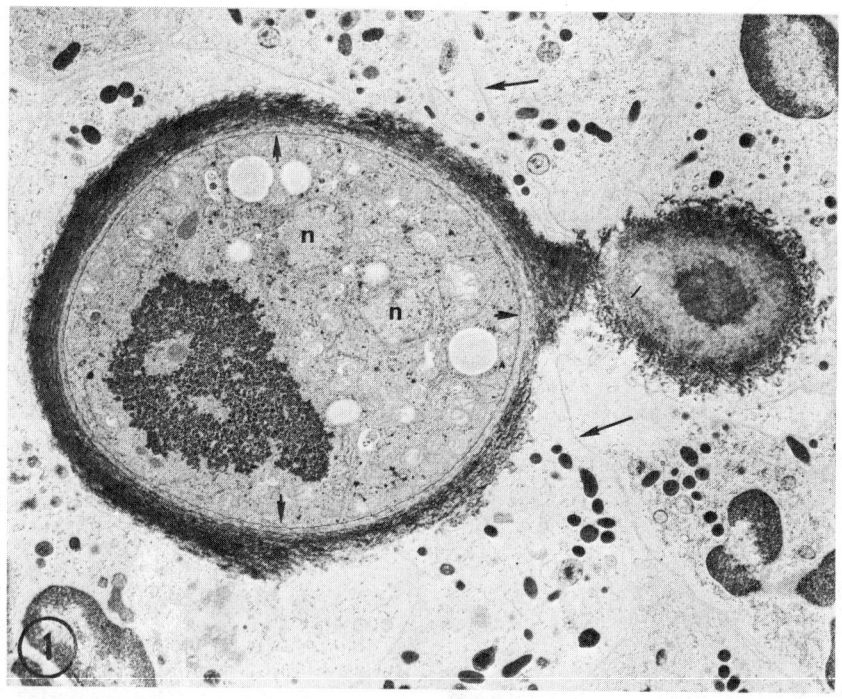

**FIGURE 7.** A, *Bacterial cell wall and underlying cytoplasmic membrane. The circles indicate the protein, and the adjacent diagonal lines represent the lipid in the lipoprotein cytoplasmic membrane. The cytoplasmic membrane is drawn out of proportion to its true relationship to the rest of the cell for purposes of illustration. In gram-negative bacilli the cytoplasmic membrane is the site of action of the polymyxins, but in gram-positive cocci it is not damaged by those drugs in usual doses. Differences in accessibility to the membrane, related to differences in cell wall, may account for these differences in susceptibility between gram-positive and gram-negative organisms.*

*B, Effect of amphotericin B on cytoplasmic membrane of fungi. 1, 2, 3, and 4 show in vivo effect of amphotericin during treatment of human North American blastomycosis. (Courtesy Dr. Henry C. Powell.)*

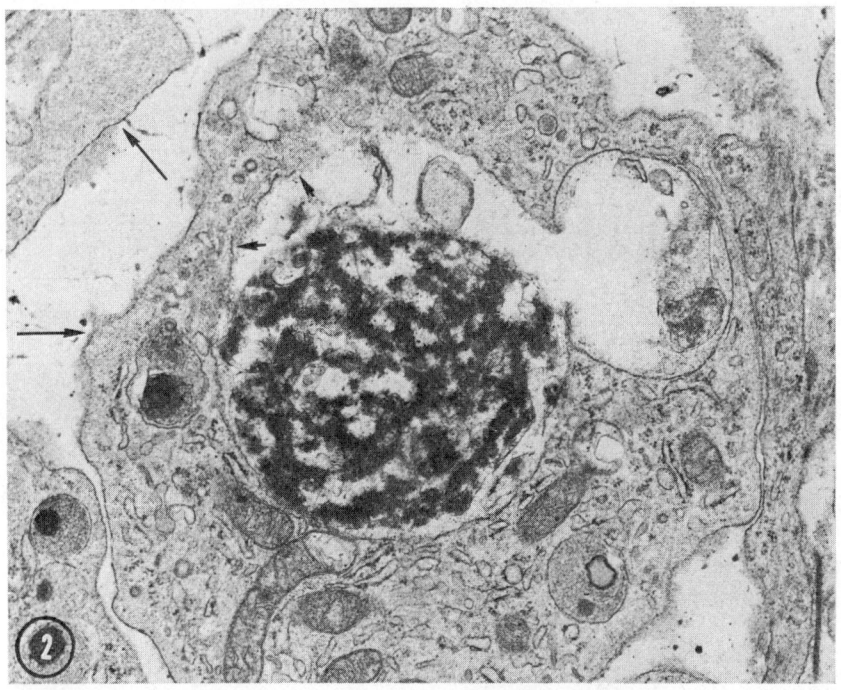

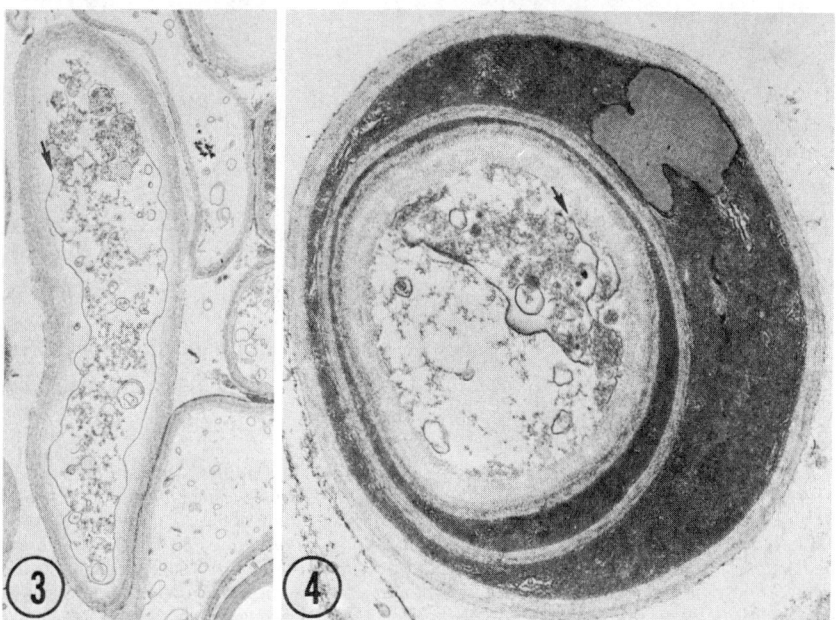

**FIGURE 7** continued.

*1. Skin biopsy, North American blastomycosis. Budding organism: the parent cell shows two nuclei (n), numerous mitochondria, and aggregates of electron-dense material (probably glycogen) enclosed by cell membrane (arrowheads) and the rough outer coat. The surfaces of surrounding macrophages are closely apposed (arrows). ×20,000. 2. Skin biopsy, North American blastomycosis, after amphotericin treatment. Rupture of the cell membrane (arrowhead) and cytolysis. ×20,000. 3. North American blastomycosis. Fungal cells in vitro after incubation with amphotericin and 5-fluorocytosine. Note lysis of the cell membranes (arrow) and cytoplasmic degeneration. ×7000. 4. Degenerating fungal cell with electron-dense deposits in the cell wall. ×20,000.*

DNA

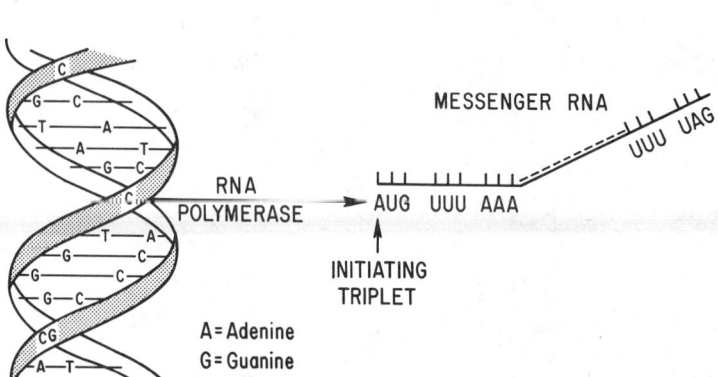

A=Adenine
G=Guanine
T=Thymine
C=Cytosine
U=Uracil

A. Transcription

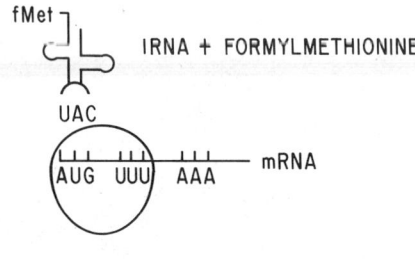

C. Formation of initiation complex
between mRNA, fMet and tRNA

C

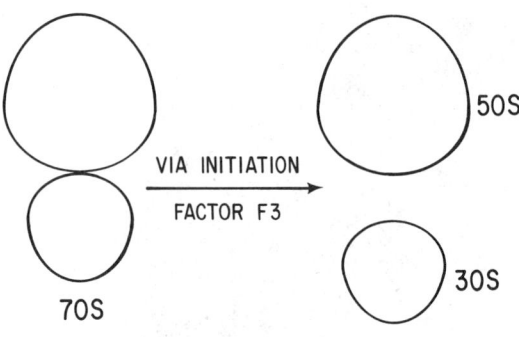

B. Dissociation of 70S ribosome

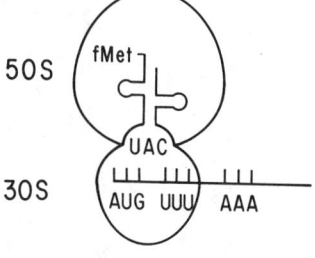

D. Reassociation of 50S and 30S
subunits to form functional 70S
ribosome

**FIGURE 8.** A, *Messenger RNA receives the code for amino acid sequence (and thus protein synthesis) from DNA in a process known as transcription. The message is carried to the ribosomes in the form of nucleotide triplets. Since there are four nucleotides in mRNA, they can be arranged in 4³, or 64, different triplet combinations, and each can specify one of the 20 amino acids. As each triplet reaches the ribosome it directs the attachment of a specific amino acid. Rifampin, chloroquine, 5-iodo-2'-deoxyuridine, 5-fluorocytosine, sulfonamides, pyrimethamine, and trimethoprim all interfere with transcription by one or more mechanisms as described in the text. B, Dissociation of the 70S ribosome is the first step in protein synthesis on ribosomes. C, Protein synthesis starts when mRNA attaches to the 30S subunit and then tRNA + formylmethionine are bound. The 50S subunit then reassociates and the initiation complex is completed. Streptomycin binds the 30S subunit and inactivates the initiation complex so that it cannot form peptide bonds. The tetracyclines also bind to the 30S subunit and prevent binding of tRNA. D, Reassociation of 50S and 30S subunits to form functional 70S ribosome.*

# ELONGATION (GROWTH) OF PEPTIDE

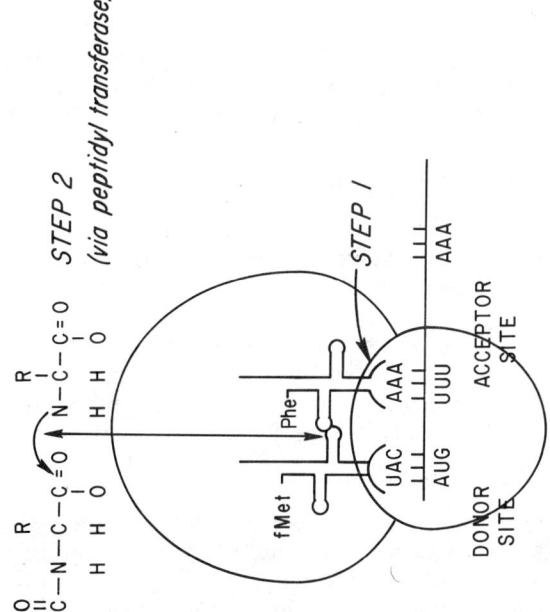

*STEP 1:* Binding of tRNA + 2nd amino acid (e.g. phenylalanine) to acceptor site of 70S ribosome, as directed by 2nd triplet on mRNA (e.g. UUU).

*STEP 2:* Formation of peptide bond by reaction of amino group of newly bound amino acid (e.g. phenylalanine) with carboxyl group of methionine. The enzyme peptidyl transferase in the 50S subunit catalyzes this reaction.

E

# ELONGATION OF PEPTIDE

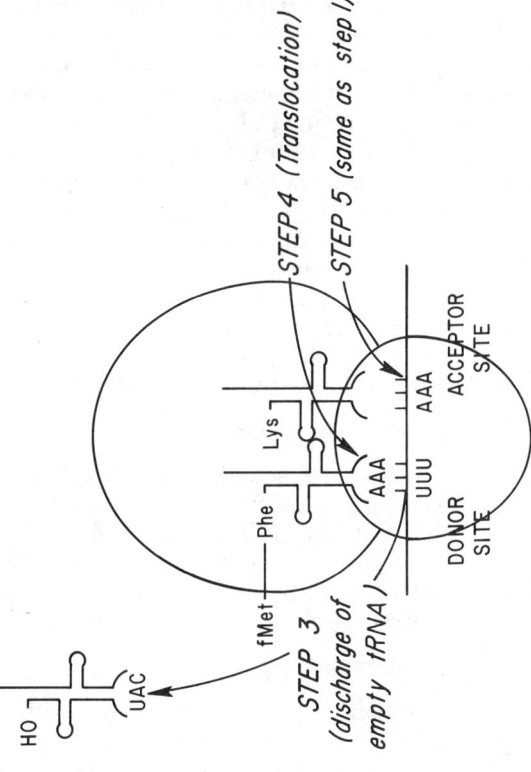

*STEP 3:* Discharge of empty tRNA (formerly carrying formylmethionine) from donor site on 70S ribosome.

*STEP 4:* Translocation of mRNA and tRNA with new peptide bond (between methionine and e.g. phenylalanine) to donor site on 70S ribosome.

E

**FIGURE 8** Continued.  E, Step 1: The second amino acid is brought in by tRNA after the initiation complex is completed. Step 2: This binds the two amino acids by a peptide bond and is blocked by chloramphenicol and lincomycin. Steps 3 and 4: The first tRNA is ejected from the ribosome and the second tRNA with its dipeptide is translocated to the site vacated by the first tRNA. The ribosome then moves along the chain of mRNA to the next triplet codon for instruction on the identity of the third amino acid to be introduced into the growing peptide chain. Erythromycin blocks the translocation step.

amino acid becomes attached (Fig. 8E, step 1). The first amino acid (methionine) is linked to the second amino acid by the enzyme peptidyltransferase, the two being joined by a peptide bond between the carboxyl group of formylmethionine and the amino group of the second amino acid (Fig. 8E, step 2). This beginning chain with its tRNA is translocated to the first site (donor site) after it has been vacated by the release of tRNA that had formerly carried formylmethionine (Fig. 8E, steps 3 and 4). The ribosome then moves along the chain of mRNA to the next triplet codon for further instruction. Here directions are given for the attachment of the unoccupied acceptor site of a third tRNA with its amino acid. The dipeptide on the donor site is transferred to the third amino acid, and the process of chain elongation is continued until a termination code triplet in mRNA announces that the protein chain is complete.

Since the mRNA strand is "read" by several ribosomes simultaneously, multiple proteins are synthesized simultaneously. A connecting mRNA fiber between adjacent ribosomes, which forms an assembly of as many as 100 ribosomes on a single mRNA strand, can be seen in the electron microscope. This arrangement of multiple ribosomes, each producing its own protein, is called a polyribosome.

Antibiotics that bind to ribosomes cure infections by interfering at certain points with peptide chain formation in bacteria. Thus, they may interfere with initiation of the peptide chain, the attachment of tRNA after initiation, peptide-bond formation, translocation, and the movement of ribosomes along mRNA. Among antimicrobials important in clinical medicine, the mechanism of such interference has been worked out best for five groups: the aminoglycosides, the tetracyclines, chloramphenicol, erythromycin, and emetine.

### The Aminoglycosides

The mode of action of streptomycin has been examined far more than that of other aminoglycosides. Streptomycin binds to the 30S subunit of the ribosome by irreversibly combining with a specific ribosomal protein, designated P10. At this site it has three effects on protein synthesis: (1) It permits formation of the initiation complex but blocks its normal activity. When streptomycin attaches to ribosomes, they fall off the "assembly line"; i.e., they leave mRNA prematurely. These ribosomes dissociate into 30S and 50S subunits which subsequently reassociate at the normal initiation sites on mRNA, but they remain irreversibly inactivated initiation complexes that cannot form peptide bonds. (2) It

interferes with the attachment of tRNA. (3) It distorts the triplet codons of mRNA so that the message is misread, the wrong amino acids are inserted into the peptide chain, and faulty proteins are produced. Of these three effects, the first is the most important cause of bacterial killing by streptomycin. Cells are killed by the accumulation of aberrant inactive initiation complexes.[19, 24] The third occurs only at borderline inhibitory concentrations of streptomycin.[6]

Other aminoglycosides such as kanamycin, neomycin, and gentamicin probably act similarly, but more research is necessary to establish their mode of action. There is some evidence that amikacin, neomycin, and gentamicin have binding sites on both 30S and 50S ribosomes.

### The Tetracyclines

These drugs also bind to the 30S subunit of bacterial ribosomes and block the binding of tRNA to the mRNA 30S ribosomal subunit.[5] In other words, tetracyclines prevent the introduction of new amino acids into the peptide chain so that protein synthesis cannot proceed.

### Chloramphenicol

In contrast to the aminoglycosides and tetracyclines, chloramphenicol attaches exclusively to the larger (50S) moiety of the ribosome. The drug prevents peptide-bond formation by inhibiting the enzyme peptidyltransferase. This enzyme is located in the 50S subunit, so that it is blocked when chloramphenicol binds to that portion of the ribosome.[25]

### Erythromycin

Like chloramphenicol, erythromycin binds to 50S ribosomal subunits and can compete with chloramphenicol for binding sites on 50S ribosomes. Like chloramphenicol, it interferes with peptidyltransferase activity.[20]

### Lincomycin

This antibiotic resembles erythromycin in its antibacterial spectrum and also acts like chloramphenicol in inhibiting protein synthesis. Thus, lincomycin binds to 50S ribosomes (but not ribosomes of *E. coli,* organisms whose growth is not inhibited by lincomycin) and also appears to block the peptidyltransferase reaction necessary for peptide-bond formation.

### Emetine

This ancient amebicidal drug has only recently been found to be an inhibitor of protein synthesis. It inhibits the transfer of amino acids from tRNA to the polypeptide on the ribosome and prevents elongation, rather than initiation, of peptide chains. Emetine also inhibits protein synthesis in bacteria and mammalian cells. This lack of selectivity may explain the toxicity of emetine for patients during treatment of amebic dysentery or liver abscess.[13]

### The Thiosemicarbazones (Methisazone)

If polyribosomes are disrupted, protein synthesis stops. At least one group of antimicrobials, the thiosemicarbazones, seem to interfere with protein synthesis of smallpox virus by breaking up the mRNA into smaller fragments and disrupting the ribosomes.[2]

## TRANSCRIPTION MECHANISMS

The information that determines the sequence of amino acids in a given protein is coded in the DNA and *transcribed* into messenger RNA (see Fig. 8A). Messenger RNA then becomes attached to ribosomes, where the code is translated into protein synthesis. Antibiotics interfering with translation act on the ribosomes, as described in the preceding section. Drugs acting on transcription may interfere either with separation of DNA strands or with the synthesis of RNA. DNA consists of two polynucleotide chains twisted about each other in the form of a double helix. During transcription these strands of the double helix separate, and one of them serves as a specific surface or *template* upon which a complementary strand of RNA is synthesized through the action of RNA polymerase. The complementary RNA strand and its template DNA differ in only two respects: the presence of deoxyribose in DNA in place of ribose, and of thymine, in place of uracil, as one of the four major bases.

A drug can interfere with the transcription process by preventing strand separation of DNA, by breaking a strand, by introducing an improper component into the replicating RNA strand, or by blocking access of RNA polymerase to the template strand. Only one clinically valuable antibiotic, rifampicin, interferes with transcription. Other antimicrobial drugs, however, active against protozoa, fungi, and viruses act by interfering with transcription.

### Rifampicin

This antibiotic is the most potent inhibitor of DNA-dependent RNA polymerase in bacteria. Human DNA-dependent RNA polymerase, on the other hand, is resistant to rifampicin, so that the drug is selectively toxic for bacterial but not human cells. By binding to RNA polymerase, rifampicin inhibits the formation of all forms of RNA in bacteria.[34]

### Chloroquine

This important antiprotozoal drug inhibits nucleic acid synthesis by interfering with the ability of DNA to act as a template.[15] Chloroquine is inserted (intercalated) between the stacked base pairs of the double helix. This drug inhibits nucleic acid synthesis in mammalian cells as well, but protozoa concentrate chloroquine so that their intracellular level is much higher than that in the body fluids of the patient.

### Nitroimidazoles

The selective toxicity of metronidazole and other 5-nitroimidazoles against anaerobic bacteria and protozoa probably involves reduction of the nitro group to a nitrosohydroxyl amino group. This is carried out by a reduced electron transport protein similar to ferredoxin, which is important in the terminal energy metabolism of susceptible organisms. The intracellular concentration of the unreduced nitroimidazole is kept low by its metabolism so that the drug is taken up by simple diffusion to reach intracellular concentrations 50 to 100 times that in the environment.[14] The reduced drug is lethal to anaerobic organisms because it causes strand breaks in DNA.[9] Mammalian cells are unharmed because they lack the enzymes required for reduction of the nitro group.

### 5-Iodo-2′ deoxyuridine (IUDR)

This nucleoside analog is widely used in the treatment of herpes simplex infections of the cornea. The drug is incorporated into *viral* DNA instead of thymidine.[17] Normally, deoxuridilic acid is converted to thymidilic acid by the enzyme thymidilic acid synthetase. IUDR inhibits this enzyme so that insufficient thymidine phosphate is available for DNA synthesis. Strands of DNA containing IUDR in place of thymidine are more easily broken. In addition, the presence of IUDR in DNA could lead to abnormal base pairing and the consequent production of nonfunctional proteins that are not assembled into virus particles.[2]

### 5-Fluorocytosine

Like IUDR, this halogenated (fluorinated) pyrimidine probably acts by eventually inhibiting the action of the enzyme thymidilic acid synthetase. Cytosine is first deaminated to uracil by cytosine deaminase. 5-Fluorouracil is then converted to 5-fluorodeoxyuridylate. This fluorinated compound causes a lethal thymine deficiency by blocking the conversion of the normal deoxyribonucleotides to deoxythymidylate by thymidylate synthetase. 5-Fluorouracil is also incorporated into mRNA so that errors are produced in translation of information from DNA into protein.[7]

### The Sulfonamides

This group of drugs is placed here among transcription inhibitors because sulfonamides block the synthesis of thymidine and all purines. Thymidine is necessary for DNA synthesis, and the purines for nucleic acid synthesis. This action of sulfonamides is accomplished by preventing the synthesis of folic acid (pteroylglutamic acid) by microbial cells. Sulfonamides are structural analogs of para-aminobenzoic acid (PABA), an essential ingredient of folic acid (Fig. 9). Competitive inhibition of PABA utilization by sulfonamides interferes with folic acid synthesis. Since folic acid functions as a coenzyme for transporting 1-carbon units from one molecule to another, the sulfonamides block these reactions which are necessary for the synthesis of thymidine, purines, methionine, and serine. Folic acid metabolism in patients is not affected by sulfonamides because human cells cannot synthesize folic acid. Instead, patients must obtain folic acid in their diets. Since bacteria cannot transport exogenous folic acid into their cells, dietary folate does not interfere with the action of sulfonamide drugs. In pus, however, the breakdown of cells may cause a considerable accumulation of thymidine, purines, methionine, and serine which reverse the inhibitory effect of sulfonamides on bacteria by replenishing the end products of folic acid metabolism. In this way, the sulfonamides may lose therapeutic effectiveness.[10]

In addition to the sulfonamides, para-aminosalicylic acid (PAS) and the sulfones (both active against certain mycobacteria) are PABA analogs and block folic acid synthesis by competitive inhibition.

### The Diaminopyrimidines

Both pyrimethamine and trimethoprim, the two important members of this group, are folic

Structural relationship between
p-aminobenzoic acid (left) and
sulfanilamide (right)

**FIGURE 9.** *The close structural relationship of sulfonamides to para-aminobenzoic acid (PABA) is used to explain their antibacterial effect. The competitive inhibition of PABA utilization by sulfonamides interferes with folic acid synthesis in bacteria but not in man.*

acid antagonists ("antifols"). Their site of action is different from that of the sulfonamides, however. The diaminopyrimidines are structurally similar to the pteridine portion of dihydrofolate; therefore, instead of blocking PABA utilization, they prevent the conversion of folic acid to tetrahydrofolic acid by depression of the enzyme dihydrofolic reductase, as indicated in the following reactions:

$$PABA \rightarrow folic\ acid \xrightarrow[reductase]{folic} dihydrofolic\ acid$$

$$dihydrofolic \xrightarrow[reductase]{} tetrahydrofolic\ acid\ (H_4FA)$$

$$Precursors \xrightarrow{H_4FA} components\ of\ nucleic\ acids$$

The dihydrofolic acid reductase of protozoa and certain other pathogenic organisms is far more sensitive to trimethoprim than that of man, so that folic acid deficiency in patients given trimethoprim is not a serious problem.[16]

In order to take advantage of the two vulnerable metabolic sites in protozoa and other pathogens, the diaminopyrimidines are usually given in conjunction with sulfonamides. This combination has a much greater antifol action than a simple summation of the two, and, since the two sequential depression steps are present only in the parasite, the combination has markedly increased activity against infection without an increased toxicity for patients.

## MECHANISM OF ACTION OF ANTHELMINTIC DRUGS

Chemotherapy for worms is based on physiologic damage rather than protein inhibition. This is because pathogenic worms are fully grown when treatment is needed. Drugs that interfere with growth through inhibition of protein synthesis can stop egg production, but egg production is not needed for worm survival.

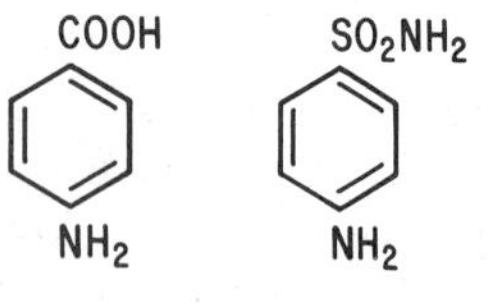

Anthelmintics kill worms by blocking energy metabolism or by paralysis.[3] Pyrvinium and mebendazole, for example, interfere with energy metabolism by blocking uptake of glucose, while thiabendazole inhibits fumaric reductase, a key enzyme in fermentation of glucose.[31] Like other intestinal microflora, worms are anaerobic and do not have the enzymes that mammalian cells use for terminal oxidation of glucose.[26] In the generation of energy-rich phosphate during glucose metabolism in worms, electron transfer is characterized by the reduction of fumarate to succinate through the action of fumarate reductase, which serves as an electron carrier from flavoproteins to fumarate. In other words, fumarate, instead of $O_2$, becomes the ultimate electron acceptor in worms as in the following schema of electron transfer in worms and man:

Worms: Flavoprotein → fumaric reductase → fumarate
Man:     Flavoprotein → cytochrome oxidase → $O_2$

This selective inhibition of fumaric reductase explains the toxicity of thiabendazole for worms, but not man.

Niclosamide, another important anthelmintic, interferes with energy metabolism by blocking the phosphorylation of adenosine diphosphate (ADP) and thus the formation of adenosine triphosphate (ATP) during electron transport. In other words, the high-energy phosphate required for energy by the worm is not generated in the presence of niclosamide. Niclosamide would, no doubt, show the same effect on human ATP formation, but fortunately the drug is not absorbed from the intestine. Niridazole, a powerful new remedy for schistosomiasis, affects energy metabolism by depleting glycogen reserves. It blocks the inhibitor of glycogen phosphorylase so that glycogenolysis becomes excessive.[4]

Two important paralyzing anthelmintics are piperazine and bephenium hydroxynaphthoate.[27] Piperazine produces flaccid paralysis of *Ascaris* so that the worm can be expelled from the patient by intestinal peristalsis.[8, 21] It stabilizes the membrane potential of *Ascaris* muscle by hyperpolarization, but has no effect on human muscle. Hence its toxicity is fully selective for the parasite. Bephenium, which resembles acetylcholine in

## TABLE 1.   Mechanisms of Action of Antimicrobial Drugs

| NATURE OF INJURY | ANTIMICROBIAL DRUG | MODE OF ACTION |
|---|---|---|
| Defective cell wall mucopeptide | Penicillins and cephalosporins | Prevent final peptide bond between D-alanine and glycine |
| | Cycloserine | As structural analogue of D-alanine, it inhibits enzymes responsible for synthesis of D-alanyl-D-alanine, an essential component of mucopeptide |
| | Bacitracin and vancomycin | Block transfer to cell membrane of sugar pentapeptide from site of synthesis in cytoplasm |
| Damaged cytoplasmic membrane | Polymyxins | Disorganize lipoproteins by inserting lipophobic moiety into membrane lipid |
| | Polyenes | React with steroids in fungal membranes so that permeability is altered |
| Impaired function of ribosomes | Aminoglycosides | Bind to 30S ribosomal unit, causing ribosomes to leave mRNA prematurely; also interfere with attachment of tRNA and distort triplet codons so that message is misread |
| | Tetracyclines | Bind to 30S unit and block binding of tRNA so that new amino acids cannot be introduced into peptide chain |
| | Chloramphenicol | Attaches to 50S subunit of ribosomes and prevents peptide-bond formation by inhibiting enzyme peptidyltransferase |
| | Erythromycin and lincomycin | Same as chloramphenicol |
| | Emetine | Prevents elongation of peptide chain by inhibiting transfer of amino acids from tRNA to polypeptide on ribosome |
| | Thiosemicarbazones | Disrupt polyribosomes |
| Impaired nucleic acid function | Rifampicin | Blocks bacterial RNA formation by inhibiting DNA-dependent RNA polymerase |
| | Chloroquine | Inserted between stacked base pairs in double helix and thus interferes with ability of DNA to act as a template for nucleic acid synthesis |
| | 5-Iodo-2'deoxyuridine | Incorporated into viral DNA instead of thymidine so that nonfunctional proteins are synthesized |
| | 5-Fluorocytosine | Converted to 5-fluorouracil which blocks thymidylate synthetase so that lethal thymine deficiency results |
| | Sulfonamides and diaminopyrimidines | By preventing synthesis of folic acid, they block formation of thymidine and purines needed for nucleic acid synthesis |
| | Metronidazole | After partial reduction of the nitro group, the activated drug causes strand breaks in DNA |
| Impaired energy metabolism | Pyrvinium and mebendazole | Block glucose uptake |
| | Thiabendazole | Inhibits fumaric reductase so that glucose fermentation is impaired |
| | Niclosamide | Blocks phosphorylation of ATP |
| | Niridazole | Depletes glycogen reserves |
| Paralysis | Piperazine | Stabilizes membrane potential of *Ascaris* muscle by hyperpolarization |
| | Bephenium | Depolarizes membranes (i.e., reverse of piperazine) |

structure and function, has the reverse effect on nematodes. Instead of hyperpolarization and flaccid paralysis, it causes depolarization and contraction. Since the cuticle of many worms is impervious to bephenium, the drug is effective against only a few nematodes of clinical importance, including *Necator americanus, Ancylostoma duodenale,* and *Ascaris lumbricoides.* The mucosa of the human gastrointestinal tract is also impervious to bephenium, as it is to acetylcholine, presumably because these two compounds possess a quarternary nitrogen, i.e., a central nitrogen attached to four methyl groups. The poor absorption explains the low toxicity of this anthelmintic.

## References

1. Anderson, J. S., Meadows, P. M., Haskin, M. A., et al.: Biosynthesis of the peptidoglycan of bacterial cell walls. I. Utilization of uridine diphosphate acetylmuramyl pentapeptide and uridine diphosphate acetylglucosamine for peptidoglycan synthesis by particulate enzymes from *Staphylococcus aureus* and *Micrococcus lysodeikticus.* Arch Biochem 116:487, 1966.
2. Appleyard, G.: Chemotherapy of viral infections. Br Med Bull 23:114, 1967.
3. Bueding, E.: Some biochemical effects of anthelmintic drugs. Biochem Pharmacol 18:1541, 1969.
4. Bueding, E., and Fisher, J.: Biochemical effects of niridazole on *Schistosoma mansoni.* Molec Pharmacol 6:532, 1970.
5. Craven, G. R., Gavin, R., and Fanning, T.: The transfer RNA binding site of the 30 S ribosome and the site of tetracycline inhibition. Sympos Quant Biol 34:129, 1969.
6. Davis, B. D.: Streptomycin resistance and the study of ribosomal structure and function. N Engl J Med 83:1405, 1970.
7. De Kloet, S. R.: Effects of 5-fluorouracil and 6-azauracil on the synthesis of ribonucleic acid and protein in *Saccharomyces carlsbergensis.* Biochem J 106:167, 1968.
8. Del Castillo, J., De Mello, W. C., and Morales, T.: Mechanism of the paralysing action of piperazine on ascaris muscle. Br J Pharmacol 22:463, 1964.
9. Edwards, D. I.: The action of metronidazole on DNA. J Antimicrob Therap 30:43, 1977.
10. Feingold, D. D.: Antimicrobial chemotherapeutic agents: the nature of their action and selective toxicity. N Engl J Med 269:957, 1963.
11. Few, A. V.: Interaction of polymyxin E with bacterial and other lipids. Biochim Biophys Acta 16:137, 1955.
12. Greenwood, D.: Mucopeptide hydrolases and bacterial "persisters." Lancet 2:465, 1972.
13. Grollman, A. P.: Structural basis for inhibition of protein synthesis by emetine and cycloheximide based on an analogy between ipecac alkaloids and glutarimide antibiotics. Proc Nat Acad Sci USA 56:1867, 1966.
14. Gutteridge, W., and Coombs, G.: Biochemistry of Parasitic Protozoa. Baltimore, University Park Press, 1977.
15. Hahn, F. E., O'Brien, R. L., Ciak, J., et al.: Studies on modes of action of chloroquine, quinacrine, and quinine and on chloroquine resistance. Milit Med 131(Suppl):1071, 1966.
16. Hitchings, G. H.: Species differences among dihydrofolate reductases as a basis for chemotherapy. Postgrad Med J 45(Suppl):7, 1969.
17. Kaplan, A. S., and Ben-Porat, T.: Differential incorporation of iododeoxyuridine into the DNA of pseudorabies virus-infected and noninfected cells. Virology 31:734, 1967.
18. Kinsky, S. C.: Nystatin binding by protoplasts and a particulate fraction of *Neurospora crassa,* and a basis for the selective toxicity of polyene antifungal antibiotics. Proc Nat Acad Sci USA 48:1049, 1962.
19. Luzzato, L., Apirion, D., and Schlessinger, D.: Mechanism of action of streptomycin in *E. coli*: interruption of the ribosome cycle at the initiation of protein synthesis. Proc Nat Acad Sci USA 60:873, 1968.
20. Mao, J. C., and Robishaw, E. E.: Erythromycin, a peptidyltransferase effector. Biochemistry 11:4864, 1972.
21. Mansour, T. E.: Chemotherapy of parasitic worms: New Biochemical Strategies 205:462, 1979.
22. Neuhaus, F. C., and Lynch, J. L.: The enzymatic synthesis of D-alanyl-D-alanine. 3. On the inhibition of D-alanyl-D-alanine synthetase by the antibiotic D-cycloserine. Biochemistry (Wash) 3:471, 1964.
23. Newton, B. A.: The properties and mode of action of the polymyxins. Bacteriol Rev 20:14, 1956.
24. Ozaki, M., Mizushima, S., and Nomura, M.: Identification and functional characterization of the protein controlled by the streptomycin-resistant locus in *E. coli*. Nature (London) 222:333, 1969.
25. Pongs, O., Bald, R., and Erdmann, V. A.: Identification of chloramphenicol-binding protein in *Escherichia coli* ribosomes by affinity labeling. Proc Nat Acad Sci USA 70:2229, 1973.
26. Saz, H. J.: Comparative energy metabolisms of some parasitic helminths. J Parasitol 56:634, 1970.
27. Saz, H. J., and Bueding, E.: Relationships between anthelmintic effects and biochemical and physiological mechanisms. Pharmacol Rev 18:871, 1966.
28. Siewert, G., and Strominger, J. L.: Bacitracin: an inhibitor of the dephosphorylation of lipid pyrophosphate, an intermediate in biosynthesis of the peptidoglycan of bacterial cell walls. Proc Nat Acad Sci USA 57:767, 1967.
29. Thomasz, A.: The mechanism of the irreversible antimicrobial effects of penicillins. How the beta-lactam antibiotics kill and lyse bacteria. Ann Rev Microbiol 33:113, 1979.
30. Tipper, D. J., and Strominger, J. L.: Mechanism of action of penicillins: a proposal based on their structural similarity to acyl-D-alanyl-D-alanine. Proc Nat Acad Sci USA 54:1133, 1965.
31. Van den Bossche, H.: Biochemical effects of the anthelmintic drug mebendazole. In Van den Bossche, H. (ed.): Comparative Biochemistry of Parasites. New York, Academic Press, 1972, pp. 139–157.
32. Van den Bossche, H., Willemsens, G., Couls, W., Lauwers, W., and Le June, L.: Inhibition of ergosterol biosynthesis in *Candida albicans* by miconazole. Curr Chemother 3:228, 1978.
33. Voigt, W.: On the mode of action of antimycotics, especially of clotrimazole (canesten) on the ultrastructural level of human pathogenic fungi. Scand J Infect Dis Suppl 16:51, 1978.
34. Wehrli, W., and Staehelin, M.: Actions of the rifamycins. Bacteriol Rev 35:290, 1971.

# RESISTANCE TO **21**
## ANTIMICROBIAL DRUGS

Microbial resistance is acquired after a change in DNA. This change may occur by alteration in the structure of chromosomal DNA or by acquisition of extrachromosomal DNA. The alteration of chromosomal DNA is called mutation, and the acquisition of extrachromosomal DNA is the result of genetic exchange. These changes lead to the formation of enzymes or other proteins that inactivate drugs or hinder access to their site of action.

## GENETIC EXCHANGE: R FACTORS

### Susumu Mitsuhashi

### *GENERAL PROPERTIES OF R FACTORS*

Genetic exchange is the more important cause of clinical drug resistance because it produces epidemic resistance to multiple drugs. The extrachromosomal DNA that is responsible for such resistance can reproduce itself within the bacterial cell and then spread to other bacteria by transduction or mating (conjugation) (Mitsuhashi et al., 1965; Novick, 1969). Transduction is a type of gene transfer in which DNA from one bacterial cell is introduced into another bacterial cell by bacteriophage infection. The transmission of resistance from one bacterial cell to another is known as "infectious" drug resistance, because sensitive bacteria become "infected" with resistance determinants. By this process, resistance to one or multiple antibiotics may spread from one bacterium to another during mating, even in the absence of antibiotics. In other words, bacteria may become resistant to multiple drugs without ever having been exposed to them.

The genetic elements that control infectious drug resistance are a form of DNA known as plasmids. Plasmids are not part of the large circular bacterial chromosome but exist as small cyclic DNA molecules that are capable of reproducing themselves independently. The extrachromosomal resistance factors in gram-negative bacteria are called R factors (Mitsuhashi, 1977B). R factors are composed of two kinds of genes: those that carry determinants for antibiotic resistance and those that promote transfer from one cell to another. The first are called resistance determinants (RD) and the second are called resistance transfer factors (RTF). The transfer of the R factor during mating depends on external hair-like appendages — the sex pili. They facilitate plasmid transfer from male bacteria (donors) to female bacteria (recipients), which have no pili (Fig. 1). The number of RD attached to the RTF determines the number of drugs to which the bacteria become resistant. One R factor may have many genes, each of which is responsible for resistance to a different antibiotic (Fig. 2).

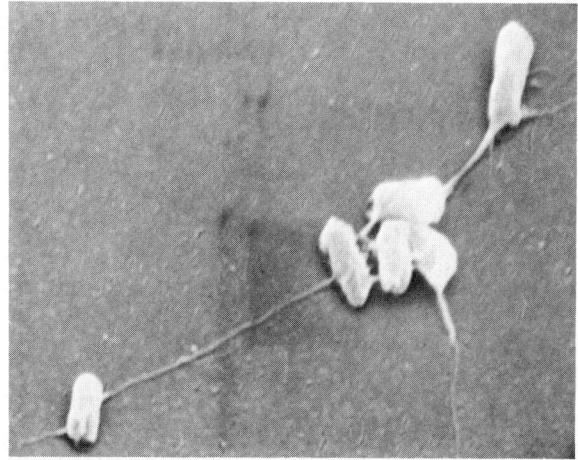

**FIGURE 1.** *Sex pili in* E. coli *06. The sex pili are the long, hairlike appendages that extend from one bacillus to another. The sex pilus is about 90 Å across, and of variable length (mean 1 to 2 μm). The first step in conjugation is the formation of a mating pair by interaction between the tip of one pilus and a receptor site on the surface of the recipient cell. According to one concept, the pilus then serves as the bridge along which R-factor DNA passes. In an alternative postulate for DNA transfer, the pilus may retract by sequential depolymerization of its subunits into the donor cell membrane. This draws the surfaces of the 2 bacterial cells together and allows formation of a conjugation bridge not involving the pilus (× 8000 scanning electron micrograph made by Dr. R. Weller, Univ. Calif., San Diego).*

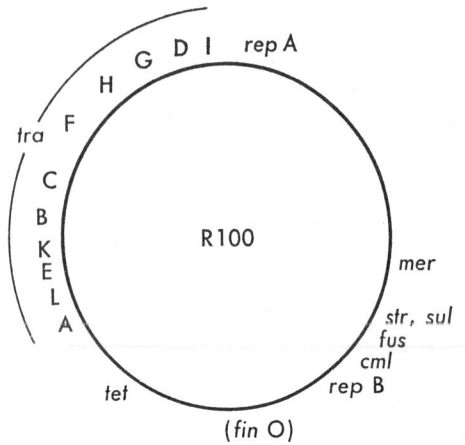

**FIGURE 2.** *Circular map of an R factor (R100 factor, a conjugative plasmid in E. coli K12). Distance between each marker is drawn arbitrarily. The following genetic determinants are represented: tet = tetracycline resistance; str = streptomycin resistance; sul = sulfonamide resistance; mer = mercury resistance; cml = chloramphenicol resistance; fus = fusidic acid resistance; tra (A→L inclusive are each required for the different steps in this complex process. Thus 9 of the 12 cistrons are required for synthesis of the sex pilus and others for penetration of plasmid DNA during conjugation; rep determines the ability to replicate in the host cell; fin = fertility inhibition by repressing piliation.*

When a bacterium becomes infected with an R factor, the cell develops sex pili and becomes a donor cell. Donor competence, or the capacity to transfer resistance by conjugation, is greatest in bacteria that have recently acquired an R factor. The number of cells that are competent donors declines after a few generations as the capacity to produce sex pili is repressed.

## DISCOVERY OF R PLASMID

The appearance and rapid increase in number of multiply resistant *Shigella* strains in Japan attracted the attention of microbiologists — from the standpoint of epidemiology especially, and later from the standpoint of genetics (Mitsuhashi, 1977B).

Evidence for the existence of drug resistance genes in the cytoplasm of resistant bacteria was first obtained in Japan (Mitsuhashi, 1977B) by demonstrating the properties of resistant bacteria that would be indicative of conjugative plasmids: 1) transmission of drug resistance by mixed cultivation of resistant and sensitive strains; 2) interruption of the transmission with a fritted glass disk to separate the two parental cultures; and 3) spontaneous and induced loss of drug resistance from drug-resistant cells. The artificial elimination of R plasmids is carried out with drugs (ethylenediaminetetraacetate [EDTA], do-

decyl sodium sulfate) that kill bacteria carrying such plasmids, or with DNA intercalating agents (acriflavine) that inhibit DNA synthesis. Drug resistance was transmitted by mixed cultivation from drug-resistant *Escherichia coli* K12 F⁻ or Hfr to drug-sensitive *Shigella,* regardless of the polarity of the F agent. Between substrains of *E. coli* K12, drug resistance was found to be transmitted similarly by mixed cultivation without regard to the polarity of the F agent. These facts indicated that transferable drug resistance is transmitted independently of the chromosomal transmission of the donor strain and that this agent is different from the F factor. Direct proof of the cytoplasmic existence of drug resistance genes was obtained by physical isolation of plasmid DNA. The R plasmids were isolated as a satellite DNA different from the chromosomal DNA by centrifugation, and were demonstrated by electron microscopy as covalently closed circular or open circular DNA (Falkow, 1975). A mixed incubation of a small number of bacterial cells carrying transmissible drug resistance results in the rapid acquisition of multiple drug resistance by a majority of the recipient cells. R factors are transferable among all species of the family Enterobacteriaceae, as well as among *Neissaria gonorrhoeae, Hemophilus influenzae,* the *Vibrio* group, *Pasteurella pestis, Bordetella bronchiseptica,* and the *Pseudomonas* group (Iyobe et al., 1974). They can also be transferred from *Bacteroides* to *E. coli* (Guiney and Davis, 1978). These properties of the R factor (i.e., autonomous replication and a wide range of transmission among various species of bacteria) are of great importance in public health and animal husbandry.

From these studies, and others, it can be concluded that R factors are self-replicating genetic elements that 1) confer drug resistance on the host; 2) possess plasmid characteristics, including autonomous replication, self-regulation, conjugal transferability, and stable residence within the host; and 3) interfere with other genetic elements, such as the F, R, and Col factors, and bacteriophages.

## RESISTANCE MARKERS

Transfer between gram-negative enteric bacteria of multiple drug resistance — i.e., resistance to tetracycline (TC), chloramphenicol (CM), streptomycin (SM), and sulfanilamide (SA) — was first described in 1959. An R factor carrying kanamycin (KM) resistance was isolated in 1963 and later was found also to confer resistance to both neomycin (NM) and paromomycin (PM). In 1965, ampicillin (APC) resistance conferred by an R factor was reported, APC inactivation resulting from the production of a $\beta$-lactamase. R factors have been found that are capable of conferring resistance to aminoglycosidic antibiotics, such as the gentamicin C (GM) complex. In addition to conferring resistance to antibacterial agents, R factors are capable of causing resistance to heavy metal ions, such as $Ni^{2+}$, $Hg^{2+}$, and $Co^{2+}$.

## R FACTOR PROPERTIES OTHER THAN DRUG RESISTANCE

R factors can control many genetic properties other than those responsible for drug resistance, e.g., conjugal transferability, autonomous replication, stable maintenance in the host, maleness of the host (R mating), and interference with other plasmids and bacteriophages. It has been demonstrated that R factors, like the F factor, carry structural genes for pili formation, which govern conjugation, R factor transfer, and R mating. However, R factors, unlike the F factor, have a regulator gene that can repress piliation due to R and F factors; thus, when R factors and F factor coexist within the same cell, F mating is inhibited. At the present time, the locus that governs R mating (the ability of R factors to promote the transfer of the host chromosome) has not been separated genetically from the locus *tra,* which is responsible for the transfer of R factors.

One R factor interferes with superinfection with another R factor by the phenomena of entry exclusion and incompatibility. Superinfection inhibition occurs when the frequency of R factor transfer is decreased by the presence of an R factor within the cell, i.e., in an $R^+$ recipient. Mutual exclusion occurs in cells that contain two incompatible R factors. The factors become labile, and either one or both are easily lost during subsequent growth of the bacteria. R factors can also suppress plaque formation by bacteriophages. This trait is designated as *spp.* The suppression is not caused by an inhibition of phage adsorption, but is the result of degradation of the injected phage DNA.

The genetic properties of R factors are summarized in Table 1, and the genetic structure of an R factor is shown in Figure 2.

## BIOCHEMICAL MECHANISMS OF R-MEDIATED RESISTANCE

Drug resistance that is conferred by R factors is achieved in some instances by the production of inactivating enzymes, as has been demonstrated in *E. coli* strains that are resistant to CM, KM, and SM. Chloramphenicol is inactivated by an *o*-acetyltransferase that in the presence of acetyl CoA and CM forms 3-0-acetyl CM and 1-3-0-0-diacetyl CM (Fig. 3A). Streptomycin can be inac-

**TABLE 1.   Genetic Properties of R Factors**

| GENETIC PROPERTY | | MECHANISM |
|---|---|---|
| Drug resistance | Tetracycline | Impermeability |
| | Chloramphenicol | Acetylation |
| | | Impermeability |
| | Aminoglycoside antibiotics | Phosphorylation |
| | | Adenylylation |
| | | Acetylation |
| | | Impermeability |
| | Sulfonamides | Impermeability, production of sulfonamide-resistant dihydropteroate synthetase |
| | Ampicillin | $\beta$-Lactamase |
| Resistance to metal ions | $Hg^{2+}$ | Mercury vaporization |
| | $Co^{2+}$ | |
| | $Ni^{2+}$ | |
| Conjugal transfer(*tra*) | R transfer | Pili formation |
| | Chromosome transfer | |
| | Repression | Repressor of pili formation |
| Replication | | |
| Stable inheritance | | |
| Superinfection inhibition | Entry exclusion | |
| | Incompatibility | |
| Phage interference | | Restriction enzyme |

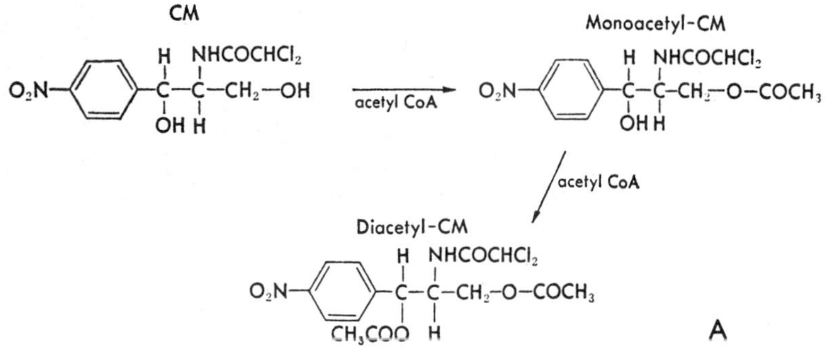

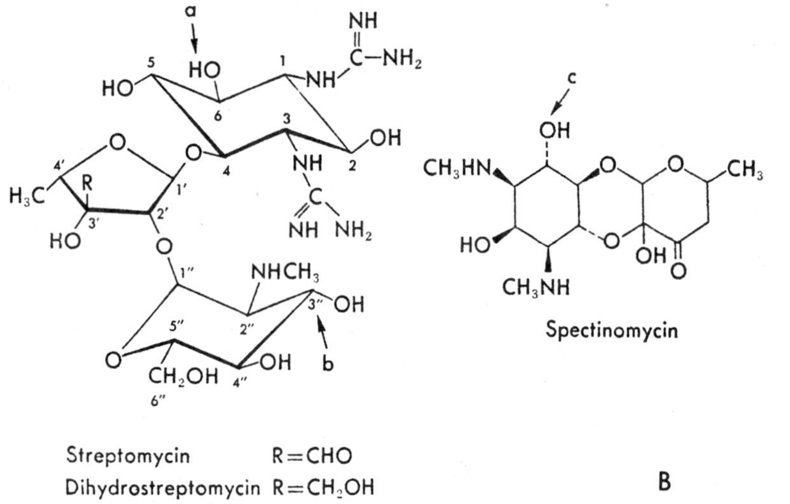

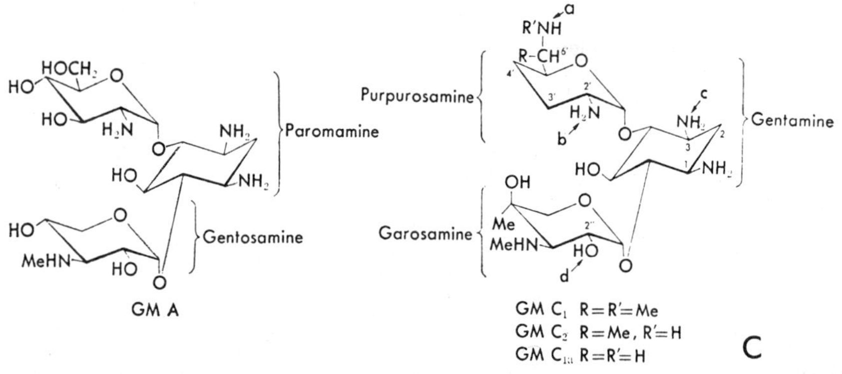

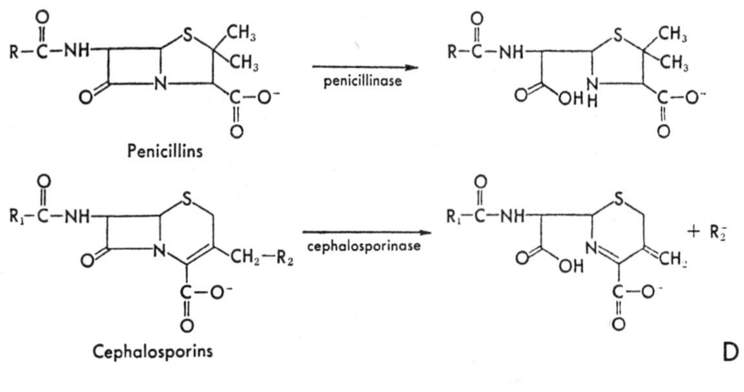

**FIGURE 3.** *Mechanisms responsible for resistance in bacteria carrying R factors. A, Inactivation of chloramphenicol (CM) by CM acetyltransferase. B, Arrows indicate site of inactivation of streptomycins and spectinomycin by adenylylation (a,b,c), and phosphorylation (a,b). C, Chemical structures of gentamicins; arrows indicate the site of inactivation, acetylation (a,b,c), and adenylylation (d). D, Inactivation of penicillins and cephalosporins by the beta-lactamases.*

tivated by adenylylating or phosphorylating enzymes in the presence of adenosinetriphosphate (ATP), resulting in the formation of adenylyl-streptomycin (Fig. 3B) or phosphorylstreptomycin. Kanamycin can also be inactivated either by acetylation in the presence of acetyl CoA, which produces 6'-N-acetylkanamycin, or by phosphorylation in the presence of ATP, which produces 3'-phosphorylkanamycin.

The newly introduced aminoglycoside gentamicin C lacks a 3-hydroxyl group in its amino sugars and consequently is not inactivated by the KM or SM phosphorylating enzyme previously isolated from resistant R factor–carrying strains. Enzymes isolated from bacterial cells harboring new types of R factors can inactivate gentamicin C components either by acetylation or by adenylylation (Fig. 3C).

Hydrolytic enzymes can also mediate R factor resistance. Penicillin, ampicillin, and cephalosporin resistance, for example, are produced by enzymes that hydrolyze the C-N bond of the $\beta$-lactam ring (Fig. 3D). There are two general types of $\beta$-lactamases that differ in antigenic and substrate specificity but have similar molecular weights in the range of 20,000 to 25,000 (Table 2). Type I is more active against cephaloridine than is type II, and type II is more active against ampicillin, cloxacillin, methicillin, and oxacillin than is type I. These penicillinases elaborated by R factors thus differ from staphylococcal penicillinase, which is relatively inactive against the cephalosporins, oxacillin, cloxacillin, and methicillin. In fact, the clinical success of the cephalosporins and these three semisynthetic penicillins is primarily related to their continued effectiveness against serious infections by $\beta$-lactamase-producing staphylococci. In addition to the gram-negative enteric bacteria, the R plasmids mediating type I penicillinase have been demonstrated in *Pseudomonas aeruginosa*, gonococci, and *H. influenzae*. These R factor penicillinases are found between the cell wall and the cell membrane. They are all constitutive.

Drug resistance due to a decrease in permeation of the drug into the bacterial cell has also

**TABLE 2.  Summary of Comparison between Types I and II Penicillinases Mediated by R Plasmids**

| PROPERTIES | PENICILLINASE | | |
|---|---|---|---|
| | Type Ia Penicillinase ($R_{GN14}$, Renamed $R_{ms212}$) | Type Ib Penicillinase ($R_{GN823}$) | Type II Penicillinase ($R_{GN238}$, Renamed $R_{ms213}$) |
| Penicillinase activity* per mg of dry weight of bacteria | 0.6 | 16.7 | 0.025 |
| Specific penicillinase activity per mg of enzyme protein | 1330 | 1670 | 20 |
| pH optimum | 6.5–7.0 | 6.5–7.0 | 7.6 |
| Temperature optimum (°C) | 45 | 40–45 | 30 |
| Inhibition of activity by chloride ion | No | No | Yes |
| Inhibition of activity by anti-serum (Type Ia penicillinase) | Yes | Yes | No |
| Molecular weight† | 20,600 | 24,000 | 25,400 |
| Isoelectric point‡ | 5.1 | 6.9 | 8.3 |
| | (5.4) | (5.6) | (7.4) |
| $s_{20,w}$ | — | 2.45 | 2.66 |
| Secondary structure§ | $\alpha 25\%$ | $\alpha 25\%$ | $\alpha + \beta$ |
| Substrate specificity ▶ and *Km* | | | |
| Substrate | | | |
| Benzylpenicillin | 100 ( 27 $\mu$M) | 100 ( 24 $\mu$M) | 100 ( 5 $\mu$M) |
| Phenethicillin | 33 ( 32 $\mu$M) | 27 ( 14 $\mu$M) | 155 ( 6 $\mu$M) |
| Ampicillin | 115 ( 30 $\mu$M) | 112 ( 32 $\mu$M) | 450 ( 16 $\mu$M) |
| Cloxacillin | 2 | 1 | 292 ( 13 $\mu$M) |
| 6-Aminopenicillanic acid | 87 (222 $\mu$M) | 89 (200 $\mu$M) | 363 ( 26 $\mu$M) |
| Cephaloridine | 130 (400 $\mu$M) | 111 (500 $\mu$M) | 36 (111 $\mu$M) |

*Penicillinase activity is expressed in units; one unit of the enzyme activity is defined as the activity which hydrolyzes 1 $\mu$mole of benzylpenicillin per min at 30 °C.

†The molecular weight was estimated by the gel filtration method.

‡Isoelectric points were determined by the use of agar-gel electrophoresis. The values in parenthesis were taken from the data of Matthew, which were determined by the use of analytical isoelectric focusing.

§$\alpha$-Helix content was determined by ORD spectrum.

▶Substrate specificity is expressed as the percentage of hydrolysis of benzylpenicillin.

been reported. Tetracycline and its derivatives have been shown to inhibit, to the same degree, protein synthesis in cell-free systems prepared from TC-sensitive and R factor–carrying TC-resistant strains. Strains resistant to TC by virtue of an R factor also have been shown to be incapable of inactivating tetracycline. This suggests that the mechanism of TC resistance involves a decrease in the permeability of the drug. R factors causing CM resistance by decreasing CM penetration into the cell have also been found. Similarly, the mechanism of sulfonamide (SA) resistance in strains of *E. coli* containing an R factor has been explained by a decrease in the permeability of the cell membrane to sulfanilamide. Plasmid-mediated SA resistance is also achieved by the formation of SA-resistant dihydropteroate synthetase. Resistance to $Hg^{2+}$ in R-carrying strains has been attributed to mercury vaporizing activity (Mitsuhashi et al., 1977).

## CLASSIFICATION OF R PLASMIDS

The R factors of the *Enterobacteriaceae* are diverse and distributed all over the world — in hospitals, livestock farms, and fish ponds. Classification of R plasmids is useful in epidemiologic studies (Mitsuhashi, 1977A). Resistance patterns of R plasmids and their biochemical mechanisms of resistance can be used for their classification. Another classification of these plasmids is based on their compatibility properties. The closely related plasmids are incompatible; i.e., they cannot coexist in their bacterial host. The unknown R factor to be tested is transferred from its wild host to an auxotrophic strain of *E. coli* K12. The $R^+$ strain is used as the donor in matings with a set of K12 cultures, each of which carries a plasmid of known compatibility group (Datta, 1977).

Most R plasmids from *P. aeruginosa* strains are nontransferable to *E. coli* strains and are conjugally transferred only between *P. aeruginosa* strains. Therefore, the R factors of *P. aeruginosa* strains can be classified by an intraspecies conjugation system (Sagai et al., 1976).

## NONCONJUGATIVE RESISTANCE (r) PLASMIDS

Nonconjugative resistance (r) plasmids were discovered after R plasmids in multiply resistant *Staphylococcus aureus* strains by the irreversible loss of resistance (Mitsuhashi, et al., 1963) and by genetic analysis of staphylococcal resistance (Novick, 1963). The r plasmids are self-replicating genetic elements that confer drug resistance to

the host and possess plasmid characteristics, including autonomous replication and stable residence within the host. A big difference from the conjugative R plasmids is a lack of conjugal transferability with r plasmids because staphylococci do not mate. The r plasmids are usually smaller than R plasmids, because a *tra* (transferability) region is absent from the r molecule (Fig. 4). The transmission of r plasmids in staphylococci is mediated by transduction with bacteriophages, by which staphylococci are lysogenized (Mitsuhashi et al., 1965). It has been found that the drug resistance of *Streptococcus pyogenes* is mostly due to the presence of a nonconjugative plasmid (Mitsuhashi, 1979).* Further studies have disclosed that nonconjugative resistance (r) plasmids are widely distributed even in gram-negative bacteria, and drug resistance of naturally occurring resistant strains is mostly caused by the presence of conjugative (R) or nonconjugative (r) plasmids, or both. Nonconjugative plasmids confer single resistance on *S. aureus* and other host bacteria, and those carrying multiple resistance are very exceptional in contrast to R plasmids, which confer multiple resistance.

In staphylococci with r factors, penicillin resistance is caused by an inducible $\beta$-lactamase. The $\beta$-lactamases of enteric bacteria are not inducible. The enzyme responsible for chloramphenicol resistance in r-bearing staphylococci is also inducible. Chloramphenicol resistance in these staphylococci is produced by an acetyltransferase like that in enteric bacteria, but the chloramphenicol-acetylating enzyme of enteric bacteria is constitutive (noninducible).

## MOLECULAR NATURE OF R FACTOR DNA

The relatively small size of plasmids permits their isolation as intact DNA molecules in both the resting and replicating states, and allows a definitive analysis of their molecular structure. Fragmentation during this manipulation is much less of a problem than in the case of bacterial chromosomes whose large size makes them vulnerable to shearing. The DNA of R plasmids has a molecular weight in the range of $60 \times 10^6$ and a buoyant density of 1.710 to 1.712 g/ml (Rownd and Womble, 1977). This is similar to the density of chromosomal DNA in *E. coli* and *Shigella,* so that the plasmid DNA cannot be distinguished by a satellite band in CsCl gradients. The molecular weight of nontransmissible r plasmids is only 5 to $10 \times 10^6$ because they have only one or two

---

*In group D streptococci (enterococci) conjugative plasmids confer resistance to erythromycin, kanamycin, tetracycline, and streptomycin.

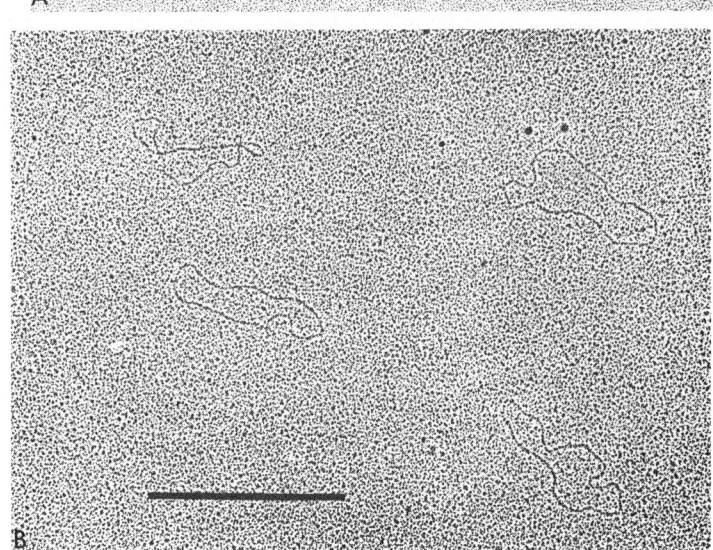

**FIGURE 4.** *Electron micrograph of the open circular molecules of plasmid DNA from a conjugative (A) and nonconjugative (B) plasmid to illustrate that conjugative plasmids are larger because they have more resistance genes and transfer genes. Bar represents 1 μm. (A) a conjugative RMS201 plasmid DNA (about 31 μ) encoding resistance to TC, CM, SM, SA and APC; (B) a nonconjugative rMS31 plasmid DNA (about 2 μ) encoding resistance to SA.*

resistance determinants and no transfer factor (Fig. 5).

Like the bacterial chromosome, R factors are circular molecules of DNA. The circular R factors are twisted (super coiled) double strands closed by covalent bonding. Through various physicochemical manipulations (e.g., pH 12.5) the covalently bonded R factor becomes more compact and can be separated in density gradients from the separated chromosomal strands by its faster sedimentation. Such maneuvers overcome the problem of separating the R factor from the chromosome that results from their uniform buoyant density under normal conditions.

# CHROMOSOMAL DRUG RESISTANCE

### Abraham I. Braude

In contrast to infectious drug resistance, resistance after mutation involves chromosomal genes. Spontaneous mutation to drug resistance is infrequent, generally occurring in only 1 of 10 million to 1 trillion bacterial cells. The resistant mutants are difficult to detect unless the drug is present as a selective agent to suppress the overwhelming number of nonmutated cells and to allow the multiplication of resistant ones. The multiplication of resistant organisms during antibiotic therapy usually occurs on mucous membranes, in urine, or in lung cavities, where no immune mechanisms can check the growth of the organisms. Streptomycin has been the most important antibiotic responsible for selecting resistant mutants during treatment. Resistance develops in *E. coli* mutants because of a change in the gene that specifies the P10 protein in 30 S ribosomes (Ozaki et al., 1969).

The P10 protein of sensitive strains allows the attachment of streptomycin to the 30 S ribosome, but in resistant strains the attachment sites for streptomycin are masked so that streptomycin is not bound to the ribosome. The loss of binding to the ribosome produces more or less total resistance to streptomycin and occurs in a single mutational step. Hence, there can be an abrupt appearance of resistant organisms during treatment with streptomycin after the original sensitive organisms have been rapidly eliminated. In urinary tract infections, for example, massive resistance to streptomycin can develop after five days of treatment. High-level resistance also occurs after exposure to erythromycin, apparently due to the modification of 23 S ribosomal RNA by mutation so that binding of the drug is reduced (Lai et al., 1973). High-level resistance is not confined to drugs acting on ribosomes, since it develops to antituberculous drugs such as isoniazid and rifampin (Guttler et al., 1971) that do not interfere directly with ribosomal function.

Mutation appears to be responsible for one type of gonococcal resistance to penicillin, but the level of such resistance is much lower than that seen in gonococci possessing R factors. The reason for this is that chromosomal resistance in gonococci to penicillin increases slowly by succeeding mutational steps. Similar low-level resistance to tetracycline has occurred in gonococci, in occasional strains of pneumococci, and in group A streptococci. A higher level of resistance of pneumococci to penicillin has recently been reported in South Africa (see later discussion).

Drug resistance can also occur in fungi and protozoa. Among fungi, resistance to 5-fluorocytosine in *Cryptococcus neoformans, Candida albicans,* and other species of *Candida* has limited the usefulness of this important new drug. High-level resistance of cryptococci and *Candida* to 5-fluorocytosine can develop by single-step mutation, so that a strain that was sensitive to 3.0 $\mu$g/ml is no longer inhibited by 1000 $\mu$g/ml after short periods of treatment (Weese, 1972).

The most important example of drug resistance in protozoa is that of *Plasmodium falciparum* (the cause of malignant subtertian malaria) to chloroquine (Peters, 1970). The major difference between chloroquine-sensitive and chloroquine-resistant malarial parasites is the loss of high-affinity binding of chloroquine by red cells infected with chloroquine-resistant parasites. Chloroquine resistance is thus attributed to a decrease in the number, affinity, or accessibility of chloroquine receptors at the site of action within the malaria parasite. The nature and subcellular location of substances that bind chloroquine are still under study.

The mechanism of acquired resistance of cryptococci or *Candida* to 5-fluorocytosine can be inferred from studies of the nonpathogenic yeast, *Saccharomyces cerevisiae* (Jund and Lacroute 1970). By such an analogy it has been suggested that resistance could occur through one of three processes: 1) failure of the deamination of cytosine to 5-fluorouracil — the product responsible for blocking nucleic acid synthesis; 2) loss of the permeases required for permeation of the drug into the yeast cell; or 3) the absence of uracil-binding sites. The first of these mechanisms, loss of cytosine deaminase activity, was responsible for acquired resistance to 5-fluorocytosine in a strain of *Candida parapsilosis,* causing fatal endocarditis (Hoeprich et al., 1974).

## PRACTICAL IMPLICATIONS OF DRUG RESISTANCE

Gram-negative bacteria carrying R factors are the most serious problem among antibiotic-resistant organisms because their resistance to multiple drugs can be spread in epidemic proportion throughout hospitals and whole communities. In Japan the situation became so bad that in 1966 to 1967, 79 per cent of *Shigella* strains were resistant to one or more drugs, and at least half of these strains carried R factors (Mitsuhashi, 1969). Similar outbreaks have occurred in other parts of the world and with other enteric pathogens (Jonsson, 1972; Lowbury et al., 1972; Anderson and Smith, 1972). In Mexico, for example, multiresistant *Salmonella typhi* recently produced the worst epidemic of typhoid fever in modern history (Gangarosa et al., 1972).

*Shigella* and *Salmonella* resistance is primarily an epidemiologic problem outside the hospital. In hospitals, as many as 60 to 70 per cent of all enteric bacteria (other than *Salmonella-Shigella*) carry R factors for multiple antibiotics. The high prevalence of infectious drug resistance can be traced directly to the increased use of antibiotics both in and out of the hospital. The importance of selective pressure by antibiotics in promoting infectious drug resistance in hospitals can be shown by the parallel rise in resistance with drug use and by the disappearance of gram-negative bacilli transferring drug resistance when antibiotic therapy is sharply restricted (Lowbury et al., 1972). Outside the hospital, when antibiotics are used in animal feed and sold without restriction, selective antibiotic pressure encourages the spread of R factors. Feed containing a penicillin or tetracycline for growth stimulation of livestock has led to the widespread distribution of enteric bacteria containing R factors. In Great Britain, the extensive use of antibiotics for preventing *Salmonella* infections in cattle was followed by a human epidemic of antibiotic-resistant *Salmonella typhimurium* infection (Anderson, 1968). In Mexico, the recent epidemic of chloramphenicol-resistant typhoid fever can be related to the unrestricted sale of chloramphenicol in pharmacies to patients without prescriptions.

Although antibiotics have generated the problem, they did not create the R factor. Davis and Anandan (1970) have shown that R factors existed in communities that had never been exposed to commercial antibiotics (Fig. 5). Their evolutionary development can be explained as a survival mechanism in the presence of antibiotics produced by other organisms in the bowel or soil. After the introduction of commercial antibiotics, these bacteria with R factors possessed a selective advantage and became predominant. They can transfer multiple resistance in the bowel to pathogenic enteric bacteria. Multiple resistance in one organism may involve as many as seven antibiotics. Determinants for resistance to kanamycin, for example, tend to occur on R factors in conjunction with determinants for resistance to sulfonamides, streptomycin, tetracycline, and chloram-

phenicol. The use of kanamycin, therefore, could promote the simultaneous spread of resistance to itself and to four other antibiotics (Cohen, 1969).

Penicillinase plasmids in staphylococci have created a less serious clinical problem than the R factors in gram-negative bacteria, because multiple resistance is not usually transmitted by penicillinase plasmids. Antibiotics that are resistant to penicillinase can therefore successfully treat infections caused by penicillinase-producing staphylococci. An exception to this is the resistance to methicillin in 10 to 17 per cent of staphylococcal infections in England, France, and Switzerland occurring in hospitalized patients with chronic debilitating diseases (Benner and Kayser, 1968). This resistance may cross over to other penicillinase-resistant penicillins and is not caused by inactivation of the drug. Because methicillin-resistant staphylococci are confined to extremely debilitated patients, they have probably lost virulence, even though they cause serious and even fatal infections. They are becoming a problem in the United States, where such strains have been isolated recently in growing numbers.

Chromosomal drug resistance is a major clinical problem in the treatment of tuberculosis, cryptococcosis, candidiasis, and gram-negative urinary infections. In cavitary pulmonary or genitourinary infections, any of the antituberculous drugs can select resistant mutants, which then produce relapses during treatment. In contrast to

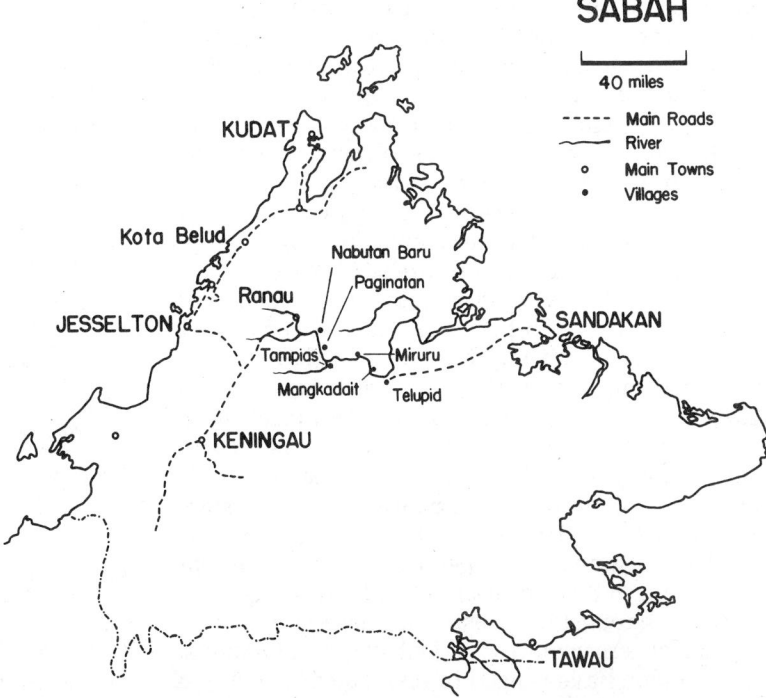

**FIGURE 5.** *A remote locale in Borneo was used for exploring the existence of R factor before the introduction of commercial antibiotics. Davis found that R factors existed in Miruru, a community that had never been exposed to commercial antibiotics. From his discovery, it is reasonable to infer that the evolutionary development of R factor can be explained as a survival mechanism in the presence of antibiotics produced by other organisms in the bowel or soil. (From Davis, C. E., Anandan, J.: The evolution of R factor. A study of a preantibiotic community in Borneo. N Engl J Med 282:118, 1970.)*

plasmids, which produce multiple drug resistance, chromosomal mutations affect susceptibility to only one drug. Clinical resistance can, therefore, be prevented by combination treatment with two drugs. Since the mutation rate of the tubercle bacillus to streptomycin resistance is approximately $10^{-10}$, and $10^{-6}$ to isoniazid, the chance of developing resistance to both is only one in $10^{16}$ cell divisions. This probability is so small that the combined use of streptomycin and isoniazid in treating cavitary pulmonary tuberculosis is almost never followed by the development of resistance to either drug. This principle is also used in cryptococcosis by giving amphotericin with 5-fluorocytosine to prevent resistance to 5-fluorocytosine; in protozoal infections by giving sulfonamides with trimethoprim to prevent resistance to trimethoprim; and in *E. coli* urinary infections by giving small doses of tetracycline with streptomycin to prevent resistance to streptomycin.

Except for the foregoing examples, chromosomal drug resistance has not been a serious clinical problem. Clinical resistance to penicillin, the most important antimicrobial, probably never occurs during the course of treating a specific infection with penicillin. Despite the high frequency of infection by penicillinase-producing staphylococci in hospitals, these organisms do not arise from penicillin-sensitive staphylococci in patients undergoing treatment with penicillin. Their exact origin is unknown, but it is more likely that penicillinase-producing staphylococci are selected out in the nasopharynx of staphylococcal carriers among hospital personnel who are exposed to low concentrations of penicillin in aerosols that develop from open vials or syringes. Penicillin resistance rarely occurs among pyogenic streptococci, but it is becoming a serious problem among pneumococci in certain parts of the world. The resistance was first observed in a type 23 pneumococcus isolated in 1967 from Australian patients with hypogammaglobulinemia and in type 4 pneumococci recovered from 15 asymptomatic carriers in remote areas of New Guinea where penicillin was in frequent use (Hansman et al., 1971). Although these strains apparently lost the extreme sensitivity to penicillin that characterizes pneumococci, they were still sensitive to 0.5 $\mu$g/ml — a level easily reached in treatment. More recently, high-level resistance to penicillin led to fatal infection from pneumococcal bacteremia in Johannesburg, South Africa. Carriers of types 6A and 19A penicillin-resistant pneumococci were found in 29 per cent of pediatric patients and in 2 per cent of hospital staff members in the Johannesburg Hospital. These pneumococci and others isolated in Durban, Minneapolis, and London have ranged in resistance from 2.5 to 4 $\mu$g/ml. However, the new South African strains were multiply resistant to other $\beta$-lactam antibiotics as well as erythromycin, clindamycin, tetracycline, and chloramphenicol. The Durban strains of resistant pneumococci caused 14 deaths among 29 patients with systemic infections. These episodes emphasize the importance of testing the sensitivity of pneumococci in certain parts of the world. The mechanism of this resistance is unknown, but it is probably chromosomal because the resistant pneumococci do not produce penicillinase.

## References

Anderson, E. S.: The ecology of transferable drug resistance in the enterobacteria. Annu Rev Microbiol 22:131, 1968.

Anderson, E. S., and Smith, H. R.: Chloramphenicol resistance in the typhoid bacillus. Br Med J 3:329, 1972.

Benner, E. J., and Kayser, F. H.: Growing clinical significance of methicillin-resistant *Staphylococcus aureus*. Lancet 2:741, 1968.

Cohen, S.: A decade of R factors. J Infect Dis 119:104, 1969.

Datta, N.: R factors in Enterobacteriaceae. In Mitsuhashi, S. (ed.): Transferable Drug Resistance Plasmid—R Factor. Tokyo, University of Tokyo Press; Baltimore, University Park Press, 1977, p. 109.

Datta, N., and Richmond, M. H.: The purification and properties of a penicillinase whose synthesis is mediated by an R-factor in *Escherichia coli*. Biochem J 98:204, 1966.

Davis, C. E., and Anandan, J.: The evolution of R factor. A study of a "preantibiotic" community in Borneo. N. Engl J Med 282:117, 1970.

Falkow, S.: Infectious Multiple Drug Resistance, London, Pion Limited Publishing Company, 1975.

Gangarosa, E. J., Bennett, J. V., Wyatt, C., et al.: An epidemic-associated episome? J Infect Dis 126:215, 1972.

Guiney, D., and Davis, C.: Identification of a conjugative R plasmid in *Bacteroides ochraceus* capable of transfer to *Escherichia coli*. Nature 274:181, 1978.

Guttler, R. B., Counts, G. W., Avent, C. K., et al.: Effect of rifampin and minocycline on meningococcal carrier rates. J Infect Dis 24:199, 1971.

Hansman, D., Glasgow, H., Sturt, J., et al.: Increased resistance to penicillin of pneumococci isolated from man. N Engl J Med 284:175, 1971.

Hoeprich, P. D., Ingraham, J. L., Kleker, E., et al.: Development of resistance to 5-fluorocytosine in *Candida parapsilosis* during therapy. J Infect Dis 130:112, 1974.

Iyobe, S., Hasuda, K., Fuse, I., and Mitsuhashi, S.: Demonstration of R factors from *Pseudomonas aeruginosa*. Antimicrob Ag Chemother 5:547, 1974.

Jonsson, M.: Antibiotic resistance and R factors in gram-negative bacteria. A study from Sweden. Scand J Infect Dis 5(Suppl):1, 1972.

Jund, R., and Lacroute, F.: Genetic and physiological aspects of resistance to 5-fluoropyrimidines in *Saccharomyces cerevisiae*. J Bacteriol 102:607, 1970.

Lai, C. J., Weisblum, B., Fahnestock, S. R., et al.: Alteration of 23 S ribosomal RNA and erythromycin-induced resistance to lincomycin and spiramycin in *Staphylococcus aureus*. J Mol Biol 74:67, 1973.

Lowbury, E. J., Babb, J. R., and Roe, E.: Clearance from a hospital of gram-negative bacilli that transfer carbenicillin-resistance to *Pseudomonas aeruginosa*. Lancet 2:941, 1972.

Mitsuhashi, S.: The R factors. J Infect Dis 119:89, 1969.

Mitsuhashi, S.: Epidemiology of bacterial drug resistance. In Mitsuhashi, S. (ed.): Transferable Drug Resistance Plasmid — R Factor. Tokyo, University of Tokyo Press; Baltimore, University Park Press, 1977A, P. 3.

Mitsuhashi, S.: Discovery of R factors. In Mitsuhashi, S. (ed.): Transferable Drug Resistance Plasmid — R Factor. Tokyo, University of Tokyo Press; Baltimore, University Park Press, 1977B, p. 18.

Mitsuhashi, S.: Drug Resistance Plasmids. Mol Cell Biochem 26:135, 1979.

Mitsuhashi, S., Morimura, M., Kono, M., and Oshima, H.: Elimination of drug resistance of *Staphylococcus aureus* by treatment with acriflavine. J Bacteriol 86:162, 1963.

Mitsuhashi, S., Oshima, H., Kawarada, U., and Hashimoto, H.: Drug resistance of staphylococci. I. Transduction of tetracycline resistance with phage lysates obtained from multiply resistant staphylococci. J Bacteriol 89:988, 1965.

Mitsuhashi, S., Yamagishi, S., Sawai, S., and Kawabe, H.: Biochemical mechanisms of plasmid-mediated resistance. In Mitsuhashi, S. (ed.): Transferable Drug Resistance Plasmid — R Factor. Tokyo, University of Tokyo Press; Baltimore, University Park Press, 1977, p. 195.

Novick, R. P.: Analysis by transduction of mutation affecting penicillinase formation in *Staphylococcus aureus*. J Gen Microbiol 33:121, 1963.

Novick, R. P.: Extrachromosomal inheritance in bacteria. Bacteriol Rev 33:210, 1969.

Ozaki, M., Mizushima, S., and Nomura, M.: Identification and functional characterization of the protein controlled by the streptomycin-resistant locus in *E. coli*. Nature 222:333, 1969.

Peters, W.: Chemotherapy and Drug Resistance in Malaria. New York and London, Academic Press, 1970.

Rownd, R. H., and Womble, D. D.: Molecular nature and replication of R factors. In Mitsuhashi, S. (ed.): Transferable Drug Resistance Plasmid — R Factor. Tokyo, University of Tokyo Press; Baltimore, University Park Press, 1977, p. 161.

Sagai, H., Hasuda, K., Iyobe, S., et al.: Classification of R plasmids by incompatibility in *Pseudomonas aeruginosa*. Antimicrob Ag Chemother 10:573, 1976.

Watanabe, T.: The origin of R factors. Ann NY Acad Sci 182:126, 1971.

Weese, W. C.: 5-Fluorocytosine therapy. Ann Intern Med 77:1003, 1972.

# THE PHARMACOLOGY AND TOXICOLOGY OF ANTIMICROBIAL AGENTS

# 22

*Harold C. Neu, M.D.*

There has been great progress in understanding the pharmacology of antibiotics. Unfortunately, it is not always possible to apply data about the biologic half-life, plasma and renal clearance, and bioavailability to clinical practice in a way that improves on the results of empirical antimicrobial therapy. Unlike the situation with anesthetics and anticonvulsants, in which serum concentrations of an agent correlate well with therapeutic effect, there has been little substantiation that serum or tissue concentrations of antibiotics correlate well with successful therapy. The reason for this is that response to therapy with antimicrobials is the result of many disparate factors in addition to the antimicrobial effect of the drugs, including the infectious and pathogenic abilities of the particular microorganism and the resistance of the patient.

Knowledge of the pharmacology of antimicrobials can, however, be used to minimize drug toxicity. Close attention to certain pharmacokinetic properties of antibiotics results in fewer adverse side effects, since many of the toxic reactions of antimicrobials are due to the accumulation of drugs in patients who have renal or hepatic dysfunction, which can be avoided by adjustments in dosage programs.

## GENERAL CONSIDERATIONS

Antibiotics can be administered by oral, intramuscular, intravenous, or topical routes. After absorption, they dissolve in the plasma water.

They are bound to plasma proteins and occasionally are absorbed into erythrocytes. In the plasma, they are distributed to various extravascular tissues and fluids in which they may be free or bound. As the antibiotic is distributed into extravascular compartments, there is an initial rapid fall in plasma concentration. This initial fall in the plasma level occurs at the end of an I.V. infusion. After intramuscular injection and after oral ingestion, the initial distribution phase is obscured by the combination of slow absorption and simultaneous excretion. The continued decrease in serum levels of antibiotics is related to renal and biliary excretion as well as to biotransformation in the case of some drugs. The amount of drug that reaches extravascular tissue depends not only upon the concentration gradient from serum to tissue fluid, but also on the degree of protein binding in serum and in tissues, as well as on the diffusibility of the agent. Diffusibility of a drug is a function of its molecular size, dissociation constant, and lipid solubility.

Although blood and tissue levels both decline after each dose, the decline in the two compartments is not usually parallel. Some tissues may even avidly bind the drug, although the amount of drug bound in relation to the total dose is usually small, and the rate of decline of drug concentration is not usually affected. Locally bound drug may be extremely important from a toxicologic viewpoint, however.

The pharmacokinetics of most antibiotics are first or second order. Thus, a plot of antibiotic concentration in serum on a logarithmic scale versus time on a linear scale yields a straight line after the initial phase of absorption and distribution. The slope of the linear phase is a measure of biologic life of the antibiotic. The most commonly used measure is the time required for a 50 per cent decrease from the peak value; this is the half-life of the antibiotic. For most antibiotics, the half-life is independent of the dose, initial concentration, or route of administration.

## ABSORPTION

### Penicillins

There has not been any demonstration of an active transport of penicillins across the lipid protein barrier of the intestinal mucosal cell. Penicillin G is not stable in the presence of gastric acid at pH 1-2, and 50 per cent of the drug is destroyed in 20 minutes. In contrast, at pH 4-5, penicillin G is stable for four hours. Other forms of penicillin are more acid-stable, such as penicillin V, and they are well absorbed by mouth (McCarthy and Finland, 1960). Oral absorption of the semi-synthetic penicillinase-resistant penicillins (cloxacillin, dicloxacillin, and flucloxacillin) is excellent. Oral absorption of nafcillin is erratic, and the oral absorption of oxacillin is so much less than the other penicillins that it probably should not be used orally. Methicillin is not orally absorbed owing to its acid liability. Wide variations in oral absorption exist among the aminopenicillins. Amoxicillin is well absorbed, approximately twice as well as ampicillin. The acetone derivative of ampicillin, hetacillin, is no better absorbed orally than is the parent compound. Pivampicillin, talampicillin, and bacampicillin are esters of ampicillin that are covered in the intestinal mucosa and in serum to ampicillin. These compounds produce blood levels twice those achievable with ampicillin. Cyclacillin, azidocillin, and epicillin are adequately absorbed after oral ingestion. Pivmecillinam, a pivolyl ester of mecillinam, is absorbed and converted immediately to the parent compound. None of the extended spectrum or anti-*Pseudomonas* penicillins (carbenicillin, ticarcillin, azlocillin, mezlocillin, and piperacillin) are absorbed orally. An indanyl ester of carbenicillin, indanylcarbenicillin, is well absorbed (Butler et al., 1972), but the serum and tissue levels are too low to treat systemic *Pseudomonas* infections. It does achieve adequate urinary levels. Ingestion of food at the same time as the pencillin decreases the absorption of ampicillin but not of amoxicillin, pivampicillin, or pivmecillinam; and it may increase the absorption of indanylcarbenicillin.

### Cephalosporins

The orally absorbed cephalosporins are cephalexin, cephradine, cephaloglycin, cefaclor, cefatrizine, and cefadroxil. Cephalexin is extremely well absorbed even in the presence of food (Kirby and Regamy, 1973). Cephaloglycin is poorly absorbed, which results in inadequate serum levels, although urinary concentrations are adequate for the treatment of infections with susceptible bacteria. Cephradine appears to behave almost identically to cephalexin. None of the other cephalosporins are absorbed after oral ingestion.

### Tetracyclines

With the exception of chlortetracycline, the tetracyclines are well absorbed when taken by mouth (Fabre et al., 1973). Food, divalent cations (such as those found in antacids and milk), and iron interfere with absorption of the tetracyclines. If a patient ingests a tetracycline on an empty stomach, about 75 per cent of tetracycline hydrochloride, 55 per cent of oxytetracycline, 30 per cent of chlortetracycline, 65 per cent of demeclocycline, and 95 per cent of minocycline and doxycycline are absorbed. The absorption of both of the latter compounds is less affected by food, but iron and calcium decrease their absorption.

### Macrolides and Lincinoids

Because erythromycin base is destroyed by acid it must be coated with an acid-resistant coating if it is taken by mouth. Since absorption of the coated antibiotic occurs in the duodenum and ileum, peak levels occur later than with erythromycin estolate or stearate, which are absorbed by the stomach. Food does not appreciably alter the absorption of erythromycin estolate, but absorption of erythromycin stearate is decreased if it is given with food. Spiramycin, oleandomycin, and triacetyloleandomycin (all macrolides) are all absorbed orally, as are rosamicin and kitasamycin. Lincomycin is absorbed after oral ingestion but not as well as clindamycin, which produces blood levels five-fold greater. Furthermore, although the presence of food markedly impairs lincomycin absorption, food does not decrease clindamycin absorption.

### Other Agents

Chloramphenicol is well absorbed orally, yielding levels equal to those after intravenous injection (Dupont et al., 1970). However, in the form of palmitate ester, unless particle size is well controlled, absorption may be erratic.

Fusidic acid is usually administered by the oral route. There is considerable variation in the amount of absorption of fusidic acid from one individual to another.

None of the aminocyclitol-aminoglycoside antibiotics yield levels adequate for therapeutic purposes after oral ingestion, although ototoxic serum levels of neomycin can be reached after chronic oral ingestion or after rectal dosing. Some aminoglycosides are, in fact, now used primarily to suppress microflora, e.g., neomycin and paromomycin. The same is true of vancomycin, which is not an aminoglycoside.

All the sulfonamides (except sulfaguanidine, succinylsulfathiazole, and phthalylsulfathiazole) are well absorbed after oral administration. Trimethoprim and pyrimethamine are also well absorbed orally. All of the urinary "antiseptics" (such as methenamine, furadantoin, nalidixic acid, oxolinic acid, and cinoxacin) are absorbed when taken orally but yield inadequate serum levels to treat infections outside the urinary tract. Urinary levels are, however, adequate to treat urinary tract infections.

Among the antituberculosis drugs (isoniazid, para-amino salicylic acid, ethambutol, pyrazinamide, ethionamide, thiacetazone, and rifampin), all are absorbed orally.

Antifungal agents that can be given orally are 5-fluorocytosine, clotrimazole, and griseofulvin. However, the orally absorbed clotrimazole is rapidly converted to an inactive form. There are two antiviral agents that are taken orally: amantadine and methisazone.

### Parenterally Administered Agents

In general, intramuscular (I.M.) administration of antibiotics is safe and effective. However, a number of the antibiotics cannot be given frequently by intramuscular administration because of pain on injection, and others probably should not be used this way since oral administration yields levels greater than those achieved by I.M. injection. Intramuscular routes should not be relied on in individuals in shock nor in obese individuals or in diabetics because there may be altered absorption due to poor perfusion from the injection sites.

Among the penicillins, crystalline penicillin G, given I.M., is so rapidly cleared from the body that it yields inadequate serum levels unless given frequently. Indeed, when used in prophylaxis for dental procedures to prevent endocarditis in individuals with valvular heart disease, it should be given no more than 30 minutes before dental work is begun. Penicillin combined with procaine produces low levels for 12 hours and is satisfactory to treat hemolytic streptococcal or pneumococcal infections. Doubling the dose of procaine penicillin does not double the serum level unless the dose is given at two sites. Benzathine penicillin G is a repository salt of penicillin that provides tissue and serum levels for 15 to 30 days (depending upon the size of the dose used) that will treat syphilis or streptococcal pharyngitis and will prevent recurrences of rheumatic fever. In general, in adults the levels of penicillinase-resistant penicillins produced by I.M. injection are below those needed for serious systemic staphylococcal illness. Ampicillin, carbenicillin, ticarcillin, and the newer broad spectrum penicillins yield serum levels after I.M. injection that are adequate to treat gram-positive infections or urinary infections but not to treat systemic infections with gram-negative bacteria such as *E. coli, Pseudomonas, Klebsiella,* and *Enterobacter.* Indeed, relatively high serum levels are needed to treat most gram-negative infections with agents such as carbenicillin, so they should be administered every four hours by intravenous infusion.

Cephalothin, cephapirin, cephacetrile, and cefoxitin are too painful to be given by the I.M. route. Cefamandole can be given by I.M. injection, but cephaloridine and cefuroxime yield slightly higher serum levels. Cefazolin yields the highest serum levels of all the cephalosporins after either intravenous or intramuscular administration (Kirby and Regamey, 1973). Cefotaxime, ceftizoxime, and moxalactam all can be given by the I.M. route but it is preferable to administer cefoperazone intravenously.

Most of the tetracyclines can be given by either intramuscular or intravenous routes, although the acid pH of tetracycline solutions causes phlebitis. Chloramphenicol as an ester with succinate can be used intravenously, but, given intramuscularly, the ester is not hydrolyzed, and blood levels are inadequate. Lincomycin and clindamycin can be given by either the I.M. or the I.V. route, but rapid infusions should be avoided. Erythromycin is usually too painful to use by the I.M. route, but, as lactobionate or gluceptate, it can be given intravenously. Vancomycin can be given only intravenously since I.M. injection produces sterile abscesses.

All of the aminoglycosides (amikacin, dibekacin, gentamicin, kanamycin, netilmicin, sisomicin, and tobramycin) yield effective serum levels after I.M. injection or I.V. infusion. Streptomycin and spectinomycin are given only by the I.M. route. Rifamide is administered by I.M. injection. It is also possible to give isoniazid by I.M. injection. Amphotericin is given only by I.V. infusion. Pentamidine isoethenate is given I.M. since there is an increased risk of hypotension when it is given intravenously. Adenosine arabinoside is given by intravenous infusion.

Nearly all antibiotics that can be administered I.M. can be given intravenously (some exceptions are mentioned above). In general, higher peak blood levels are produced by equal doses of intravenously administered antibiotics. If a drug can be safely administered by either route, intravenous administration is preferred when: (1) absorption from I.M. sites cannot be relied upon; (2) the volume of the required dose precludes I.M. injection; or (3) there is a risk of hemorrhage from the trauma of the infection.

### Topical Absorption of Antibiotics

Antibiotics can exert their antibacterial effect when used as topical agents. The degree of absorption of antibiotics from the skin varies widely, but in the presence of denuded or burned skin, even poorly absorbed agents may be absorbed sufficiently to accumulate and produce toxic reactions. Topical administration of penicillins and cephalosporins is probably unwise, since not only does it promote the selection of resistant bacterial species, but it is also a means of sensitization of the patient by coupling the beta-lactam to body proteins. Aminoglycosides can be absorbed through burned skin to a degree sufficient to produce renal toxicity and ototoxicity if combined with parenteral use of the agents. In contrast, topical use of silver sulfadiazine, mafenide, and silver nitrate has been effective and safe as a therapeutic maneuver in reducing bacterial colonization of the wound eschar and thereby preventing wound sepsis. Compounds such as bacitracin, vancomycin, and aminoglycosides, which can be incorporated into fibrin material but are not bound to the protein, are able to inhibit entrapped bacteria. In general, however, the topical use of antibiotics should be avoided.

## ELIMINATION OF ANTIBIOTICS

Antibiotics may be removed from the body by renal mechanisms (glomerular filtration, tubular secretion, or both), by secretion into the bile, or by enzymatic inactivation in the liver.

### Renal Excretion

Most antimicrobials are excreted by the kidney as active compounds (Table 1). The renal clearance of compounds within the same class of drug may vary widely. All penicillins, which are weak anions, are cleared from the body by proximal tubular secretion, but the rate of clearance of the penicillins varies somewhat. Thus the half-lives of the penicillins vary from a half-life for penicillin G of 40 minutes to that of carbenicillin, 66 minutes. Renal clearance of oxacillin is half that of dicloxacillin, accounting to some extent for differences in serum levels. Amoxicillin and ampicillin are cleared equally by the kidney, and the clearances of carbenicillin, ticarcillin, azlocillin, mezlocillin, and piperacillin are similar. Some of the difference in the half-lives of penicillin is due

not only to differences in renal clearance but to differences in metabolism. For example, only 5 per cent of carbenicillin is metabolized to penicilloic acid versus 17 per cent of penicillin G.

The renal clearance of cephalosporins is accomplished by tubular secretion for the most part, although some are also metabolized. Cefazolin is cleared most slowly, followed by cephaloridine and cefuroxime. Cephaloridine differs from the other cephalosporins because it is both excreted by glomerular filtration and actively transported into the proximal tubule cell, where it can accumulate to toxic levels. The newer cephalosporins (cefamandole, cefuroxime, cefoxitin, cefotaxime, and ceftizoxime) all are rapidly secreted by renal tubular cells. Moxalactam and cefoperazone are excreted more slowly with $T^{1/2}$ of about 2h compared with 1h or less for the previous agents.

The excretion of beta-lactam compounds, both penicillins and cephalosporins, can be blocked by probenecid, which seems to bind to the transport protein in the renal tubule and thereby competitively interferes with the tubular transport of the antibiotics.

All the aminoglycosides are excreted by glomerular filtration. There may be a minor role for tubular secretion. In the presence of decreased renal function, the aminoglycosides accumulate. Even in normal individuals, not all of a dose is excreted, and variable amounts, depending on the particular aminoglycoside, bind to renal cortical tissue. Vancomycin is also excreted by the kidney via glomerular filtration. Polymyxins, polymyxin B and colistimethate, are excreted by the kidney, but the precise mechanism is unclear. Polymyxins also bind to renal tissue.

That amount of tetracycline not eliminated in the feces is excreted by the kidney with the exception of chlortetracycline, which is metabolized, and doxycycline, which is excreted into the intestine.

Renal excretion accounts for only a small fraction of the elimination of erythromycin, other macrolides, chloramphenicol, lincomycin, and clindamycin.

Sulfonamides are partly filtered and partly reabsorbed and secreted, depending on the nature of the individual drug. The solubility of sulfonamides in the urine depends on the drug concentration, which is a function of the plasma concentration and state of hydration, the urinary pH, and the temperature and inherent solubility of the drugs and their acetylated derivatives. Trimethoprim appears to be handled by both glomerular filtration and tubular secretion, and renal clearance increases with acidity.

If the hepatic clearance of rifampin is exceeded, the excess drug, as well as the desacetyl derivative, is cleared by the kidney. Isoniazid, both the free form and the acetylated derivative, is cleared by the kidney.

### Hepatic Elimination

Although the liver can secrete weak anions such as the beta-lactam compounds, hepatic clearance of penicillins (except for nafcillin and dicloxacillin) is not significant. In the presence of combined hepatic and renal insufficiency, however, carbenicillin and ticarcillin do accumulate.

Many antibiotics are converted in the liver to compounds that are either less active or inactive. Cephalothin, cephapirin, and cephacetrile are all converted by hepatic esterases to desacetyl derivatives, which are much less active than the parent compounds. Isoniazid is also modified in the liver by acetylation, as are sulfonamides (Hughes, 1953). Chloramphenicol is converted by glucuronyltransferase to the inactive glucuronide, which is then excreted by renal tubular secretion. Although rifampin is converted in the liver to a desacetyl derivative, this metabolite retains significant activity against bacteria and mycobacteria. The desacetyl rifampin is excreted in bile but is reabsorbed in the intestine to reenter the enterohepatic circulation and thereby maintain prolonged serum levels (Cohn, 1969). Rifampin induces the microsomal liver enzymes responsible for its excretion, thereby resulting in a shorter half-life and lower peak blood levels after chronic therapy. Cefotaxime is converted to a desacetyl derivative that is as active as the parent compound except against *Morganella* and *Pseudomonas*. Cefoporazone is excreted to a major degree by the liver.

Although erythromycin, lincomycin, clindamycin, fusidic acid, and doxycycline are excreted in bile, this route does not account for all of the drug excreted, and it seems probable that there are other mechanisms of inactivation.

Some drugs may be bound to tissues, as appears to be the case with amphotericin, aminoglycosides, and certain quinolines that disappear from serum but can be detected in urine for months after the last dose has been administered.

The metabolism of antibiotics can be altered by other drugs that diminish the microsomal degradation system of the liver or by intrinsic liver disease. Thus, toxic concentrations of free drug may develop in patients with liver failure. There is no way to predict the blood level of hepatically excreted or metabolized antibiotics in patients with liver disease.

## *DISTRIBUTION*

The tissue distribution of antibiotics can be considered as consisting of three major areas: (1) highly perfused lean tissues, such as the heart, lung, and hepatoportal system; (2) less well perfused tissues, such as muscle and skin, representing lean tissue mass; and (3) adipose tissues of negligible perfusion, such as ligaments, cartilage, and some areas of bone. Concentrations of antibiotics in the heart, lung, and liver are equivalent to the levels in serum. However, the level of antibiotic found in normal tissues may not be representative of the amount in an area of infection since the inflammation alters blood flow. Certain "barriers" in the body markedly alter the concentration of antibiotic in a compartment such as the brain and CSF (blood-brain and blood-cerebrospinal fluid barriers) and the aqueous and vitreous barriers in the eye between the ocular fluid and plasma water). Some agents, because of ionization, cannot cross tissue barriers such as the prostatic acini.

Many of the commonly used antibiotics are bound to serum proteins, principally to albumin. The amount of an antibiotic bound to protein usually represents only a small fraction of the antibiotic in the body. If a drug is 50 per cent bound to albumin, only 10 per cent of the total drug is bound. The precise effect that protein binding of antibiotics has on biologic activities is poorly understood. Only the free antibiotic has antibacterial action. Most antibiotic receptor sites lie below the outer membrane of the bacterial cell wall and, if an antibiotic is bound to a protein the size of albumin, it cannot reach its receptor, e.g., penicillin receptors of the inner wall or aminoglycoside receptors on ribosomes in the cytoplasm of the bacterium. On the other hand, protein binding of some antibiotics acts as a temporary store of the agents and thereby prevents large fluctuations in the concentrations of free drug in the body fluids. Indeed, some penicillins have never been used clinically since, as a result of low protein binding, there is rapid tubular secretion, and they are cleared from the body too rapidly to be effective.

Antibiotics differ greatly in protein binding from one class to another and markedly within a class, as illustrated in Table 1. For example, aminoglycosides are not protein-bound, while penicillins range in protein binding from 17 per cent for ampicillin and amoxicillin to 97 per cent for dicloxacillin. The values given in the literature for the protein binding of antibiotics show a marked variation from one study to another, depending upon the technique used to measure protein binding. Protein concentration, pH, and presence of other substances alter the binding and probably do so in vivo since the serum binding of antibiotics in uremic patients is markedly less for certain agents, and uremic patients have higher levels of free drug. If other competing

**TABLE 1.  Pharmacokinetic Properties of Antibiotics**

| ANTIBIOTIC | ORAL ABSORPTION | MAJOR EXCRETION ROUTE | PROTEIN BINDING (%) | SERUM HALF-LIFE Normal (h) | SERUM HALF-LIFE $C_{cr} < 10$* (h) | HEPATIC METABOLISM-EXCRETION | DOSE ADJUSTMENT IN RENAL FAILURE | SERUM LEVEL AFFECTED BY Hemodialysis | SERUM LEVEL AFFECTED BY Peritoneal Dialysis |
|---|---|---|---|---|---|---|---|---|---|
| Amikacin | No | R–G | 0 | 2 | 35–50 | No | Major | Yes | Yes |
| Amoxicillin | Yes | R–T | 17 | 1 | 6–18 | No | Yes | Yes | Yes |
| Amphotericin | No | Nonrenal | 90 | 24 | 24 | No | Minor | No | No |
| Ampicillin | Yes | R–T | 17 | 1 | 6–18 | No | Yes | Yes | Yes |
| Azlocillin | No | R–T | 50 | 1 | 10–15 | Yes | Major | Yes | Yes |
| Carbenicillin | No | R–T | 50 | 1 | 10–15 | Yes | Major | Yes | Yes |
| Cefaclor | Yes | R–T | 15 | 1 | 20 | No | Yes | Yes | Yes |
| Cefamandole | No | R–T | 70 | 0.5 | 9 | No | Yes | Yes | Yes |
| Cefazolin | No | R–T | 85 | 1.9 | 30–50 | No | Major | Yes | Yes |
| Cefoperazone | No | R, L | 90 | 2 | 3–6 | Yes | Minor | Yes | |
| Cefotaxime | No | R–T | 50 | | 2–4 | Yes | Minor | Yes | Yes |
| Cefoxitin | No | R–T | 70 | 0.5 | 9 | No | Yes | Yes | Yes |
| Ceftizoxime | No | R–T | 50 | 1.5 | | No | Minor | Yes | |
| Cefuroxime | No | R–T | 50 | 1 | | No | Yes | Yes | Yes |
| Cephacetrile | No | R–T | 70 | 0.5 | 3–8 | Yes | Yes | Yes | Yes |
| Cephalexin | Yes | R–T | 15 | 1 | 8–20 | No | Yes | Yes | Yes |
| Cephaloridine | No | R–G, T | 50 | 1.5 | 25 | No | Avoid | Yes | Yes |
| Cephalothin | No | R–T | 70 | 0.5 | 3–8 | Yes | Yes | Yes | Yes |
| Cephapirin | No | R–T | 70 | 0.5 | 3–8 | Yes | Yes | Yes | Yes |
| Cephradine | Yes | R–T | 15 | 1 | 8–20 | No | Yes | Yes | Yes |
| Chloramphenicol | Yes | L | 25 | 1–2 | 3–5 | Yes | Minor | Yes | Yes |
| Chlortetracycline | Yes | L | 55 | 6 | 7–11 | Yes | Avoid | No | No |
| Clindamycin | Yes | L | 94 | 2–2.5 | 6–10 | Yes | Minor | No | No |
| Cloxacillin | Yes | R–T | 94 | 0.5 | 1–2 | Yes | Minor | No | No |
| Colistimethate | No | R | <10 | 5 | 50–70 | No | Avoid | Yes | Yes |
| Demethylchlortetracycline | Yes | R | 50 | 10 | 50 | Yes | Avoid | No | No |
| Dicloxacillin | Yes | R–T | 97 | 0.5 | 1–2 | Yes | Minor | No | No |
| Doxycycline | Yes | L | 90 | 15–20 | 15–20 | Yes | No | No | No |
| Erythromycin | Yes | L | 18 | 1.5 | 4–6 | Yes | No | No | No |
| Ethambutol | Yes | R–G | <10 | 4 | 7–10 | No | Major | Yes | Yes |
| Flucloxacillin | Yes | R–T | 96 | 0.5 | 1–2 | Yes | No | No | No |
| 5-Fluorocytosine | Yes | R–G | <10 | 3–6 | 70 | No | Yes | Yes | Yes |
| Gentamicin | No | R–G | 0 | 2 | 35–50 | No | Major | Yes | Yes |
| Isoniazid | Yes | L, R | <10 | 1–4 | 1–4 | Yes | Minor | Yes | Yes |

| Drug | | Route | | | | | | | | |
|------|------|-------|----|------|------|-----|-------|------|------|
| Kanamycin | No | R-G | 0 | 2 | 35–50 | No | Major | Yes | Yes |
| Lincomycin | Yes | L | 70 | 4 | 10–15 | Yes | No | No | No |
| Methenamine | Yes | R | 35 | 4 | | No | Avoid | No | – |
| Methicillin | No | R-T | 20 | 0.5 | 4 | No | Minor | Yes | No |
| Metronidazole | Yes | R, L | 50 | 6–14 | | No | Major | Yes | Yes |
| Mezlocillin | No | R-T | 90 | 1 | 10–15 | Yes | Major | No | No |
| Minocycline | No | R, L | 60 | 15 | 35 | No | Major | Yes | |
| Moxalactam | No | R-T | 90 | 2 | 19 | Yes | Major | Yes | |
| Nafcillin | Yes | R-T | 93 | 0.5 | 1–2 | No | Minor | No | No |
| Nalidixic acid | Yes | R | | 1–2 | 6 | No | Avoid | | |
| Neomycin | No | R-G | 0 | 2 | 50 | No | Avoid | Yes | Yes |
| Netilmicin | No | R-G | 0 | 2 | 35–50 | No | Major | Yes | Yes |
| Nitrofurantoin | Yes | R | | 0.3 | 1 | No | Avoid | Yes | No |
| Oxacillin | Yes | R-T | 94 | 0.5 | 1–2 | No | Minor | Yes | No |
| Oxytetracycline | Yes | R | 35 | 10 | 50 | Yes | Avoid | No | No |
| Para-aminosalicylic acid | Yes | R | 70 | 1 | 25 | Yes | Avoid | No | No |
| Paromomycin | No | R-G | 0 | 2 | 50 | No | Avoid | Yes | Yes |
| Penicillin G | Yes | R-T | 60 | 0.5 | 2–6 | No | Minor | Yes | No |
| Penicillin V | Yes | R-T | 80 | 1 | 1–2 | No | Minor | No | |
| Pentamidine | No | R | | – | – | No | – | Yes | Yes |
| Piperacillin | No | R-T | 50 | 1 | 10–15 | Yes | Major | Yes | No |
| Polymyxin B | No | R | <10 | 5 | 40–70 | No | Avoid | No | |
| Pyrimethamine | Yes | Nonrenal | | 2–5 | 20 | No | Major | Yes | No |
| Quinine | Yes | Nonrenal | 70 | 4 | | Yes | Major | No | No |
| Rifampin | Yes | L | 70 | 1.5–5 | 1.5–5 | Yes | Minor | Yes | Yes |
| Sisomicin | No | R-G | 0 | 2 | 35–50 | No | Major | Yes | – |
| Spectinomycin | No | R-G | 0 | 2 | | No | Avoid | Yes | Yes |
| Streptomycin | No | R-G | 0 | 2 | 25 | No | Major | Yes | Yes |
| Sulfadiazine | Yes | R | 50 | 2–5 | 12–25 | Yes | Major | Yes | Yes |
| Sulfamethoxazole | Yes | R | 50 | 5–7 | 12 | Yes | Major | Yes | No |
| Sulfisoxazole | Yes | R | 50 | 5–7 | 12 | Yes | Major | Yes | No |
| Tetracycline-HCl | Yes | R | 55 | 6–8 | 50 | Yes | Avoid | No | Yes |
| Thiamphenicol | Yes | L | 25 | 1–2 | 3–5 | Yes | Minor | Yes | Yes |
| Ticarcillin | No | R-T | 50 | 1 | 12–17 | Yes | Major | Yes | Yes |
| Trimethoprim | Yes | R | 60 | 10 | 25 | No | Major | Yes | Yes |
| Tobramycin | No | R-G | 0 | 2 | 35–50 | No | Major | Yes | Yes |
| Vancomycin | No | R | <10 | 6 | 240 | No | Major | No | No |

*Creatinine clearance less than 10.
R = renal, T = tubular, G = glomerular
L = liver

compounds are present in the serum, the amount of each substance bound to protein depends on the relative affinity of each agent for the particular protein receptor site.

Florey and associates studied the distribution of penicillin into tissues in 1946 and showed that there was penicillin in wound exudates eight hours after an intramuscular injection of penicillin. This observation has been confirmed and extended by recent studies utilizing a variety of model systems that have shown that antibiotics that are not highly protein-bound reach peak levels in tissue one to two hours after administration, but highly protein-bound antibiotics reach peak levels later and remain in the tissue for longer periods. Using a fibrin clot model, Barza and colleagues (1974) found that there was an inverse correlation between penetration of beta-lactam antibiotics into the clot and the degree of protein binding. With a chamber implanted in an animal, it has been shown that highly protein-bound agents penetrate the chambers best and remain for the longest period.

Although protein-bound drug is also carried to tissue sites, the amount of free drug in serum governs the level of free drug in tissues. This is important since it might be thought that leakage of serum into an area of inflammation would provide a higher concentration of drug than one could achieve on the basis of diffusion of unbound drug. However, it is unlikely that inhibitory levels of an antibiotic will be achieved at sites of infection if the concentration of free drug in serum never reaches inhibitory levels.

Highly protein-bound agents tend to be excluded from areas of the body in which a complex carrier system across a lipid-protein barrier is needed to transport antibiotics. Protein binding also delays the removal of drugs handled by glomerular filtration, but, in the case of tubular secretion, even a highly protein-bound antibiotic can be eliminated rapidly without eliminating a volume of plasma fluid that contains the drug.

## TISSUE BINDING

Many body tissues can inactivate antibiotics by binding them and releasing such small amounts so slowly that the agent is rendered ineffective. This is particularly true of the polymyxin class and the antifungal polyene antibiotics. Polymyxin B and E bind to acid phospholipids present in mammalian tissues. Polyene antibiotics are taken up in the reticuloendothelial system. Recently it has been shown that intracellular ligands in liver tissue bind penicillins, cephalosporins, tetracyclines, and chloramphenicol. Nucleic acid debris, acid proteins, and high con-

centrations of divalent cations, such as calcium and magnesium, decrease the activity of aminoglycosides. Inert materials, such as fecal material, can inactivate aminoglycosides; and calcium, iron, or magnesium salts in the intestine chelate tetracyclines, rendering them inert.

## DISTRIBUTION OF ANTIBIOTICS TO SPECIFIC BODY AREAS

### Pulmonary

Concentrations of most antibiotics within the lung are satisfactory, provided there is some blood flow. There is a wide variation in the concentrations of penicillins and tetracyclines in sputum. Peak sputum levels occur about two hours after the drugs are administered and are dose-dependent, although disproportionately higher sputum concentrations are achieved at higher doses. Levels of carbenicillin and ticarcillin are only 5 per cent of simultaneous serum levels. Appreciable levels of the newer cephalosporin antibiotics, cefoxitin and cefuroxime, are reached in bronchial secretions within one hour after an intravenous dose. Cephalothin concentrations in sputum are approximately 25 per cent of the serum level. Tetracycline concentrations in sputum are generally low and do not seem to vary with the degree of purulence. Although sputum concentrations of tetracyclines are low, levels in bronchial epithelium and lung are close to serum levels. Aminoglycoside levels in bronchial secretions are appreciable, but, because of charge properties, they may be less effective in sputum than other agents. Chloramphenicol, because of its lipid solubility and small size, achieves high concentrations in sputum and bronchial secretions. Trimethoprim also has chemical properties that cause it to achieve effective levels in sputum and bronchial secretions. All of the antituberculosis agents (isoniazid, ethambutol, rifampin, and others) achieve appreciable levels in pulmonary tissue.

It has not been established that either sputum or bronchial concentrations of antibiotics influence therapy of pneumonia.

### Pleural, Pericardial, and Ascitic Fluid

Most of the penicillins, cephalosporins, sulfonamides, macrolides, clindamycin, chloramphenicol, fusidic acid, and antituberculosis drugs diffuse into serous cavities. Aminoglycosis, such as tobramycin and gentamicin, diffuse slowly into the peritoneal cavity, but, once equlibrium with extracellular fluid is achieved, the serum levels are lower than predicted because of the increased volume of distribution. Peritonitis increases the rate at which aminoglycosides enter ascites. In most cases, it is unnecessary to inject antibiotics into the peritoneum, but penicillins, cephalosporins, and aminoglycosides can be added safely to peritoneal dialysis fluids.

### Bone

Penicillins, tetracyclines, cephalosporins, and the lincomycin-clindamycin antibiotics penetrate bone and bone marrow. Levels of these antibiotics in infected bone are greater than in normal bone. Administration of semisynthetic penicillinase-resistant penicillins or cephalosporins at the time of surgery yields bone hematoma levels adequate to inhibit most staphylococci. Further injection over the next 24 to 48 hours causes continued incorporation of antibiotic into the wound site hematoma, which, during this period, continues to develop. Tetracycline binds to bone in areas in which bone is being laid down. Tetracyclines temporarily depress normal skeletal growth, but permanent effects on the skeleton have not been seen. It is not established whether the high calcium environment of bone depresses aminoglycoside activity, but these drugs have been used successfully to treat osteomyelitis due to *Pseudomonas* and *Serratia*. Antituberculosis drugs (isoniazid, rifampin, and ethambutol) all achieve therapeutic concentrations in bone.

### Synovial Fluid

Most antibiotics used in the treatment of joint infections enter inflamed joints adequately so that intra-articular instillation of antibiotic is unnecessary (Parker and Schmid, 1971). The penicillins, cephalosporins, chloramphenicol, tetracycline, lincomycin, and clindamycin reach peak levels in joint fluid about one to two hours after administration and are present in the synovial fluid at levels equal to or in excess of those in serum for the next four to six hours. Aminoglycosides (kanamycin, gentamicin, tobramycin, and amikacin) all reach therapeutic levels in synovial fluid in the presence of inflammation. Measurement of antibiotic activity in joint fluid should be done and the drugs instilled only if patients do not respond to treatment. Polymyxins are not transported into synovial fluid in adequate concentrations and must be injected into the joint.

### Ear, Sinuses, and Tears

Most of the penicillins, including penicillin G, penicillin V, ampicillin, and amoxicillin, reach levels in middle ear fluid in acute otitis adequate to eradicate the major organisms involved in this infection. Amoxicillin and bacampicillin yield higher middle ear fluid levels than ampicillin. Cephalosporins reach the middle ear but, with the exception of cefaclor, their concentrations are too low to inhibit most strains of *Haemophilus influenzae*. Erythromycin, sulfonamides, and trimethoprim achieve adequate middle ear fluid levels. In chronic otitis in which there is a great deal of scarring, middle ear fluid levels of penicillins are often inadequate, and perhaps in these situations large doses of the drugs are needed. In such situations benzathine penicillin does not yield adequate levels.

Concentrations of antibiotics in sinuses have been shown to be adequate for ampicillin, amoxillin (and the other aminopenicillin esters), tetracyclines, erythromycin, sulfonamides, and trimethoprim. High concentrations of sulfonamides, minocycline, and rifampin are present in the lacrimal secretions, which bathe the posterior pharynx where meningococci are harbored, explaining the value of these agents for the prophylaxis of meningococcal disease.

### Eye

Very few antibiotics penetrate the eye well. Measurements in patients undergoing cataract extraction or rabbit models to determine tissue levels in the eye have been disparate. In general, the levels of penicillins and cephalosporins in the aqueous are less than 10 per cent of the peak serum level and so inhibit only highly sensitive bacteria such as pneumococci or streptococci (Records, 1968). The penicillinase-resistant penicillins (methicillin, oxacillin, and others) do not penetrate the aqueous of noninflamed eyes, but, in the presence of infection, achieve levels adequate to inhibit staphylococci, provided large doses are given intravenously. Cefamandole can reach levels in the aqueous high enough to inhibit streptococci and staphylococci. Aminoglycosides do not achieve adequate aqueous levels when given by I.M. or I.V. injection. Chloramphenicol given orally or I.V. yields measurable levels in the aqueous, but not if injected subconjunctivally as the succinate salt (McPherson et al., 1968). Amphotericin concentrations are not measurable when the drug is administered parenterally.

Subconjunctival instillation of aminoglycosides, gentamicin, or tobramycin has produced levels adequate to treat experimental *Pseudomonas* infection in the rabbit eye. Amphotericin has also been administered by this technique. No significant penetration of any antibiotic into the vitreous has been demonstrated, and intracameral injection of aminoglycosides has been used on rare occasions.

### Skin

Highly protein-bound penicillins and cephalosporins have not achieved high concentrations in skin windows. Tetracyclines and clindamycin concentrate in skin tissue, accounting for their effectiveness in the treatment of acne. Minocycline, because of its high lipid solubility, has the greatest concentration in skin among the tetracyclines. Chloramphenicol also achieves excellent levels in skin tissues but obviously should not be used for skin infections unless other agents are not available. In second and third degree burns, antibiotics do not penetrate the subeschar level, and even sensitive bacteria can proliferate in this area although serum levels are very high.

### Kidney

Renal parenchymal concentrations of antibiotics differ in relation not only to renal blood flow but also to the state of hydration and the presence of other drugs within the kidney that compete for transport mechanisms. In general, it has been stated that cure of urinary tract infection is related to urinary levels rather than to serum levels (Whelton et al., 1972). This is well substantiated by compounds such as nalidixic acid or the nitrofurantoins that are effective in the treatment of urinary tract infections in spite of inadequate serum levels. In the treatment of pyelonephritis, high concentrations within medullary, cortical, and papillary interstitial fluid may be important. Penicillin G and ampicillin levels are two to eight times the serum level. Similar findings have been made for cephalosporins. Aminoglycosides concentrate in the renal cortical tissue, which undoubtedly contributes to the development of proximal tubular cell damage. Bound gentamicin may also function as an antibiotic, however. The renal cortical concentrations of tobramycin and netilmicin are considerably less than those of gentamicin.

In the presence of markedly decreased renal function, oral ampicillin, cephalexin, and trimethoprim-sulfamethoxazole still give urinary concentrations adequate to treat infections by most urinary bacteria. In contrast, nitrofurantoins (Sachs et al., 1968), methenamine, and nalidixic acid do not yield urine levels in renal failure necessary to treat urinary infection unless toxic serum levels are achieved. The parenterally administered penicillins (carbenicillin and ticarcillin) and parenteral cephalosporins (such as cephalothin, cefazolin, cefamandole, and cefoxitin) yield adequate intrarenal and urinary concentrations even in the presence of markedly decreased renal function.

### Prostate

The high degree of ionization and protein binding of most antibiotics excludes most antibiotics from the prostate (Stamey, 1972). In acute inflammatory prostatic infections, this is not a consideration since the acute inflammatory process allows the antibiotics to enter the infected gland. Although some sulfonamides, erythromycin, and rifampin enter the normal gland, these agents are usually not effective against the microorganisms that cause chronic prostatitis. Trimethoprim achieves prostatic fluid levels eightfold greater than serum levels, and doxycycline (Garnes, 1973) and minocycline also achieve high prostate levels.

### Placenta

Penicillin G, ampicillin, amoxicillin, tetracyclines, clindamycin, lincomycin, erythromycin, cephalothin, and cephaloridine reach effective levels in fetal blood within a short time after administration to the mother. Penicillins cross the placental barrier poorly if they are very highly bound to proteins. Aminoglycosides, trimethoprim, and metronidazole cross the placenta, as do the antimalarial quinolines. Penicillin G, ampicillin, erythromycin, and clindamycin reach therapeutic concentrations in amniotic fluid readily, but only negligible amounts of streptomycin, tetracycline, and chloramphenicol are found there (Duignan et al., 1973).

### Central Nervous System

Only lipid-soluble compounds reach the brain readily because of the blood-brain barrier created by tight intracellular junctions and specialized cells surrounding the brain capillaries (Rall, 1971). Chloramphenicol achieves high brain tissue levels. In the presence of inflammation, such as a brain abscess, penicillin G, ampicillin, methicillin, oxacillin, and nafcillin achieve levels of antibiotic high enough to be measured. Lincomycin and clindamycin do not produce adequate brain tissue levels nor do the aminoglycosides. Vancomycin does achieve levels in the brain in the presence of inflammation. Trimethoprim and many of the sulfonamides achieve adequate levels in brain tissue. Unfortunately, with most of the antibiotics, the kinetics of entry into the brain and the rate of decline of brain levels are unknown.

The level of antibiotics in the cerebrospinal fluid (CSF) is a function of lipid permeability, protein binding, and the secretion and removal of weak anions by the transport systems of the choroid plexus and other sites in which CSF is formed. CSF levels of most agents except chloramphenicol, trimethoprim, some sulfonamides, isoniazid, and 5-fluorocytosine are low in the absence of inflammation. Penicillins not only have difficulty passing through the blood-brain barrier into the CSF but are removed from the CSF by active transport. Penicillin G and ampicillin can achieve adequate CSF levels in the presence of inflammation (Barrett et al., 1966). Oxacillin, nafcillin, and methicillin administered at high doses (12 g/day) yield CSF levels adequate for the treatment of staphylococcal meningitis. Vancomycin also achieves adequate CSF levels, but most cephalosporins do not. Relapses of meningitis due to pneumococcus and meningococcus have occurred in patients being treated with cephalothin. Recent studies suggest that cefamandole and cefuroxime may yield CSF levels adequate to treat selected organisms, but the data are not firm enough to advocate their use. The tetracyclines enter CSF but to a lesser extent than does chloramphenicol. The concentration of a tetracycline is about 10 per cent of the serum level. Minocycline penetrates normal CSF more readily than the other tetracyclines. Erythromycin does not enter the CSF in the absence of inflammation. Although chloramphenicol produces CSF levels adequate to treat pneumococci, meningococci, and *Haemophilus*, the levels needed to eradicate some gram-negative bacteria may be higher than those that are usually achieved. Aminoglycosides do not penetrate the CSF adequately, and administration via the intrathecal route or intraventricular injection via an Omaya reservoir is necessary to treat *Pseudomonas* or multi-resistant Enterobacteriaceae. Polymyxins do not enter the CSF and must be given intrathecally if they are to be used in the treatment of central nervous system infections. Cefotaxime, moxalactam, ceftizoxime and cefoperazone enter the CSF in the presence of inflammation in concentrations adequate to inhibit *S. pneumoniae, H. influenzae, N. meningitidis,* and even many *E. coli* and *K. pneumoniae.*

Amphotericin achieves concentrations in CSF that are sufficient to treat cryptococcal meningitis but not meningitis due to *Coccidioides immitis* or amebas. Rifampin and ethambutol enter the CSF with inflammation of levels adequate to treat most mycobacteria. Quinine and pyrimethamine enter CSF and brain tissue in concentrations that inhibit Plasmodia. Adenosine arabinoside enters both brain tissue and CSF in concentrations adequate to inhibit growth of herpes simplex virus.

### Intracellular

Many antibiotics do not enter phagocytic cells, such as polymorphonuclear cells and macrophages. Chloramphenicol, tetracycline, trimethoprim, rifampin, and isoniazid all enter these cells, and this property may be important in the eradication of intracellular bacteria. The uptake of amphotericin by the reticuloendothelial system may contribute to its destruction of fungi within these cells.

## MODIFICATION OF ANTIBIOTIC PROGRAMS IN THE PRESENCE OF RENAL FAILURE

For some antibiotics, little or no dosage adjustment is required in the presence of renal failure, either because they are eliminated by extrarenal mechanisms or because the margin of safety is so great that accumulation does not result in toxicity. With the aminoglycosides, vancomycin, anti-*Pseudomonas* penicillins, sulfonamides, and trimethoprim, major adjustments in dosage are necessary. There are a number of methods available to adjust dosage in the presence of renal failure. These are based on the assumption that the drugs are eliminated in an exponential fashion and that the rate of elimination is proportional to the glomerular filtration rate. In order to reach a therapeutic level in critically ill patients with a decreased renal function, it may be necessary to administer a loading dose of antibiotics. Dosage adjustments may be made by giving an initial dose and then subsequent doses at prolonged intervals, which are calculated from the serum creatinine or creatinine clearance. The alternative method is to give the loading dose and then a fraction of the usual dose at the usual interval for the drug. This method avoids the high peak and low trough concentrations that result from the former, but, in some animal studies, aminoglycosides administered this way are more nephrotoxic.

Aminoglycosides require dose adjustment most commonly even when there is only moderate renal insufficiency because their toxic to therapeutic ratio is so narrow. Since, in hospitalized patients, medications are conveniently administered at certain regular intervals, Table 2 shows a method for estimating the dose to be given at fixed intervals to provide effective but safe peak blood levels for all degrees of renal insufficiency. The creatinine clearance can be estimated from the serum creatinine as follows:

$$C_{cr} = \frac{(140 - \text{Age})\, Wt^*}{72\, Cr}$$

This method provides only an estimate of the serum levels that will be obtained, and these levels should be measured. If this method is followed, the blood levels may fall below the minimal inhibitory concentration toward the end of the interval between doses, but there is no evidence that sustained levels above the MIC are necessary.

All techniques for dosage adjustment are guides to therapy and should be confirmed by

---

*Weight in kilograms.

**TABLE 2.  Aminoglycoside Dosing Chart**

1. Select loading dose in mg/kg [ideal weight] to provide peak serum levels in range listed below for desired aminoglycoside.

| AMINOGLYCOSIDE | USUAL LOADING DOSES | EXPECTED PEAK SERUM LEVELS |
|---|---|---|
| Tobramycin Gentamicin | 1.5 to 2.0 mg/kg | 4 to 10 μg/ml |
| Amikacin Kanamycin | 5.0 to 7.5 mg/kg | 15 to 30 μg/ml |

2. Select maintenance dose (as percentage of chosen loading dose) to continue peak serum levels indicated above according to desired dosing interval and the patient's corrected creatinine clearance.

**PERCENTAGE OF LOADING DOSE REQUIRED FOR DOSAGE INTERVAL SELECTED**

| C(c)cr (ml/min) | Half Life† (hr) | 8 hr | 12 hr | 24 hr |
|---|---|---|---|---|
| 90 | 3.1 | 84% | — | — |
| 80 | 3.4 | 80 | 91% | — |
| 70 | 3.9 | 76 | 88 | — |
| 60 | 4.5 | 71 | 84 | — |
| 50 | 5.3 | 65 | 79 | — |
| 40 | 6.5 | 57 | 72 | 92% |
| 30 | 8.4 | 48 | 63 | 86 |
| 25 | 9.9 | 43 | 57 | 81 |
| 20 | 11.9 | 37 | 50 | 75 |
| 17 | 13.6 | 33 | 46 | 70 |
| 15 | 15.1 | 31 | 42 | 67 |
| 12 | 17.9 | 27 | 37 | 61 |
| 10 | 20.4 | 24 | 34 | 56 |
| 7 | 25.9 | 19 | 28 | 47 |
| 5 | 31.5 | 16 | 23 | 41 |
| 2 | 46.8 | 11 | 16 | 30 |
| 0 | 69.3 | 8 | 11 | 21 |

†Alternatively, one half of the chosen loading dose may be given at an interval approximately equal to the estimated half life.
Modified from Sarubii, F.A., and Hull, J.H.: Amikacin serum concentrations: prediction of levels and dosage guidelines. Ann Intern Med 89:612, 1978.

measuring serum levels. Checking the serum level at the time of anticipated peak concentrations (just after an I.V. dose or 30 to 60 minutes after an I.M. dose) and just before the next dose establishes both whether the levels are adequate and if the agents are accumulating unduly.

### Effects of Peritoneal Dialysis and Hemodialysis

Because patients who are treated by dialysis have minimal or no renal function, no antibiotic is eliminated in the urine. However, many antibiotics are removed by dialysis, and during that procedure they are eliminated at a constant rate. The exact rate of elimination depends both on the characteristics of the drug (i.e., protein binding, charge, and molecular weight) and on the conditions of dialysis (such as the machine that is used,

the flow-pressure relationships, and the duration of dialysis). Table 1 provides data on which antibiotics can be removed by dialysis. If a drug is removed, it is necessary to administer an additional dose after dialysis. It is possible to add the antibiotic to the peritoneal dialysate at the same concentration that is desired in the blood. If that is done, it is not necessary to administer additional doses of the antibiotic. If the toxic to therapeutic ratio is narrow, it should be measured just before and just after dialysis to determine whether safe but effective concentrations have been attained. If that is not possible, then drugs with a wider margin of safety should be used.

## TOXICOLOGY OF ANTIMICROBIAL AGENTS

Antimicrobial agents cause direct toxicity, can interact with other drugs to influence the toxicity of the other agent, or can by alteration of microbial flora result in infection with organisms that are normally saprophytic (Table 3).

### Hypersensitivity Reactions

Almost any antimicrobial agent has the potential of being an antigenic stimulus and provoking an immunologic reaction due either to immuno-

**TABLE 3.  Major Toxicities of Selected Antimicrobial Agents**

| AGENT | MECHANISM | SIGNS |
|---|---|---|
| *Hematologic* | | |
| Chloramphenicol | Inhibits protein synthesis | Reversible anemia, leukopenia |
| Chloramphenicol | Damages stem cell | Aplastic anemia |
| Sulfonamides | G-6-PD deficiency | Hemolytic anemia |
| Carbenicillin and ticarcillin | Platelet aggregation inhibited | Bleeding |
| *Nervous System* | | |
| Aminoglycosides | Binds hair cells of organ of Corti | Deafness |
| Aminoglycosides | Binds vestibular cells | Vertigo |
| Aminoglycosides | Competitive neuromuscular blockade | Respiratory paralysis |
| Polymyxins | Noncompetitive neuromuscular blockade | Respiratory paralysis |
| Penicillins and cephalosporins | Cortical stimulation | Myoclonic seizures |
| *Gastrointestinal* | | |
| Rifampin, isoniazid and tetracyclines | Liver cell damage | Hepatitis |
| Neomycin | Villous damage | Malabsorption |
| Clindamycin, lincomycin | Clostridium difficile | Diarrhea |
| All agents | Altered bowel flora | Diarrhea |

globulins or to sensitized lymphocytes, but in fact the most common agent to do this has been penicillin G or one of the other penicillins. Penicillins are widely dispersed in nature and contaminate milk products and other foods so that individuals who have never received penicillin for medical reasons have been otherwise exposed to them. Penicillin G and its derivatives act as haptens that can combine either with proteins contaminating the penicillin solution or with human proteins. The most important antigenic component of penicillin is the penicilloyl determinant. This hapten develops after the beta-lactam ring opens and allows formation of an amide linkage with cellular and serum proteins. Penicillenic acid is produced by normal breakdown in solution of penicillin G, ampicillin, and carbenicillin, and this material also makes amide linkages with serum proteins. Both compounds are the major determinants of penicillin allergy. Minor determinants of allergy are benzylpenicillin itself and benzylpenicilloate (Levine et al., 1966). Both major and minor determinants may be involved in anaphylactic reactions and urticaria. These reactions are due to IgE antibodies. Immediate anaphylactic reactions are uncommon, occurring in 0.04 to 0.004 per cent of patients treated with penicillin.

Positive skin tests with benzylpenicilloyl polylysine and with penicillin G, benzylpenicilloic acid, and benzylpenicilloate predict who will have immediate reactions to penicillins (Voss et al., 1966). An immediate wheal and flare reaction to the major and minor determinants after skin pricks or intradermal injection indicates a high probability of immediate (2 to 30 minutes) anaphylactic or accelerated (1 to 72 hours) urticarial reactions (with wheezing, pharyngeal edema, or local inflammation) to penicillins. Negative skin tests virtually rule out an anaphylactic reaction, although they do not exclude late cutaneous reactions. These later skin reactions probably are mediated by IgM antibodies. Indeed, continued administration of penicillin during the development of the skin eruption may elicit production of blocking IgG antibodies that prevent allergic reactions. Serum sickness from immune complexes containing IgG antibodies can develop, but it appears to be rare now that purer preparations of penicillin, made with improved production methods, are being used.

Ampicillin produces rashes twice as frequently as do other penicillins (7 per cent versus 3 per cent). The mechanism of this reaction is not understood. The rash occurs in almost all individuals with Ebstein-Barr virus infection (infectious mononucleosis) and cytomegalovirus infections. Rechallenge of these individuals with penicillin does not elicit a reaction. Allergic cross-reactions with cephalosporins in patients allergic to penicillins are uncommon.

Anaphylaxis and serum sickness have been associated with most of the other antimicrobial agents but are uncommon for erythromycin, clindamycin, and chloramphenicol. Serum sickness due to antigen-antibody complexes has complicated treatment with sulfadiazine and sulfathiazole.

Drug fever mediated via sensitized lymphocytes has been associated with all antimicrobials. Indeed, allergy to cephalosporins is manifest more often as fever than as a rash. Isoniazid can produce a syndrome indistinguishable from systemic lupus erythematosus that is presumably on an allergic basis. Both penicillins and sulfonamides have produced a nonspecific vasculitis similar to Henoch-Schönlein purpura.

### Skin Reactions

Cutaneous reactions ranging from urticaria, fixed drug eruptions, and photodermatitis to exfoliative dermatitis, toxic epidermal necrolysis, and erythema nodosum have been reported with antimicrobial agents of every class. Sulfonamides and penicillins are the most common offenders. Tetracyclines and antituberculosis medications (such as isoniazid, ethambutol, rifampin, and particularly para-aminosalicylic acid) have produced dermatologic reactions. Antimalarials have produced alopecia. Nalidixic acid, griseofulvin, chlortetracycline, and demethylchloretetracycline (Saslaw, 1961) cause photosensitivity. This reaction is probably phototoxic rather than photoallergic and apparently results from conversion of the drug by light to a noxious agent. It can range from intense sunburn and loosening of the nails with tetracyclines to bullous skin eruptions with nalidixic acid. For unknown reasons, chlorination makes the tetracyclines phototoxic.

### Hematologic Reactions

Pancytopenia and aplastic anemia have been produced by chloramphenicol. The incidence of aplastic anemia is estimated at one in 60,000. There are two types of marrow reaction to chloramphenicol. In one type, which occurs in nearly everyone after prolonged serum levels over 25 $\mu$g/ml, there is gradual development of anemia and mild thrombocytopenia. Serum iron increases, and the reticulocyte count falls. Bone marrow cells show maturation arrest with vacuolization of the cytoplasm of erythroid cells. These changes reverse if chloramphenicol is discontinued. The second type of marrow depression is not reversible or dose-related. It has occurred in individuals who have had multiple exposures to the drug and is characterized by fatal aplastic anemia. Its occurrence in identical twins raises the question of genetic predisposition (Nagao and Mauer, 1969).

Hemolytic anemia occurs in individuals with glucose-6-phosphate dehydrogenase deficiency who take eight aminoquinolines, such as quinacrine, sulfonamides, nitrofurans, sulfones, nalidixic acid, and chloramphenicol. Immune hemolysis has developed during treatment with PAS, penicillins, and cephalosporins. With cephalosporins, most positive Coombs' tests are false-positives, and hemolysis is very rare. Hemolysis due to membrane damage occurs with amphotericin, but most of the anemia seen with amphotericin results instead from marrow suppression (Brandiss et al., 1964).

Leukopenia and agranulocytosis have followed use of chloramphenicol, penicillins, cephalosporins, sulfonamides, dapsone, trimethoprim, and 5-fluorocytosine. In most instances, the reaction is reversible. In some cases leukopenia due to penicillins and cephalosporins is dose-related, and reduction in dose causes the white count to become normal. Sulfisoxazole has produced a pseudo Pelger-Huët anomaly of white cells.

Thrombocytopenia can result from an immunologic reaction with penicillins, sulfonamides, cephalosporins, and rifampin. Direct damage to platelets has occurred with other antibiotics. Trimethoprim produces thrombocytopenia, leukopenia, and megaloblastic anemia by interference with the dihydrofolate reductase enzyme (Kahn et al., 1968). A serious platelet injury is caused by carbenicillin and other penicillins through unknown mechanisms. When carbenicillin is given in therapeutic doses, all recipients develop defective platelet function within 12 to 24 hours. The drug or a metabolite appears to impair the function of platelets by decreasing their sensitivity to aggregation by adenosine diphosphate (ADP). Since ADP is the physiologic agent responsible for aggregation of platelets into plugs that repair blood vessels, it is not surprising that carbenicillin frequently causes prolonged bleeding and that it is responsible for bleeding problems after surgery (Brown et al., 1974).

### Cardiovascular Toxicity

Most cardiovascular toxicity occurs with antiparasitic drugs. Emetine and pentamidine can cause hypotension and electrocardiographic changes. Quinine depresses conduction velocity. Rapid injection of large doses of a potassium salt of penicillin can produce cardiac arrest. Miconazole has produced hypotension and arrhythmias.

### Gastrointestinal Toxicity

Many antibiotics produce gastrointestinal complaints that vary from hairy tongue to enterocolitis. Severe diarrhea progressing to pseudomembranous enterocolitis has occurred with ampicillin, indanylcarbenicillin, tetracyclines, and chloramphenicol, but more frequently with lincomycin and clindamycin. The mechanism for this toxicity appears to be alteration of intestinal flora. Proliferation of Clostridium difficile and accumulation of toxin within the colon has been established as one cause of this syndrome (Bartlett et al., 1978). Nonabsorbable aminoglycosides, such as neomycin, produce malabsorption of fat, protein, and carbohydrates. Oral neomycin causes striking villous shortening, round cell infiltration of the upper small bowel, and crypt-cell damage. This mucosal injury, plus an interaction of neomycin with bile salts, are responsible for malabsorption.

## HEPATIC TOXICITY

Cholestatic jaundice has followed use of tetracyclines, erythromycin estolate, oxacillin, nitrofurans, and sulfonamides. Tetracyclines, taken in doses above 2 g/day during the third trimester of pregnancy or postpartum, have produced hepatic damage with extensive fatty changes in the liver and a fatality rate of 80 per cent (Schultz et al., 1963).

Antituberculosis agents are the antimicrobials most often associated with hepatocellular toxicity. Isoniazid produces hepatitis, but the incidence of this side effect varies with the age of the patient (Brummer et al., 1971). The risk of individuals below 20 years of age developing hepatitis due to isoniazid is 0.03 per cent, while those above 35 years, the risk is over 1 per cent. Approximately 10 per cent of children receiving isoniazid develop abnormal liver chemistry values, but clinical signs of hepatitis are extremely rare in children. Toxicity due to isoniazid is not related to previous hepatic disease but is more common in rapid acetylators of isoniazid, suggesting that the toxic component is the acetyl derivative. Para-aminosalicylic acid, ethionamide, and pyrazinamide have produced fulminant hepatic necrosis. Rifampin is infrequently associated with liver toxicity but seems to increase the likelihood of isoniazid toxicity.

Sulfonamides may produce both hepatocellular and cholestatic liver damage. Penicillins (penicillin G, ampicillin, oxacillin, and carbenicillin) rarely produce a hepatitis and usually in association with a general allergic reaction. Erythromycin, many of the penicillins, and cephalosporins produce elevations in serum glutamic-oxaloacetic transaminase by mechanisms that are unexplained.

### Respiratory Toxicity

Nitrofurantoin produces two forms of pulmonary reaction (Hailey et al., 1969). In the acute form, chills, fever, cough, and dyspnea begin 2 to 10 days after the antibiotic is started. X-rays reveal diffuse alveolar infiltrates, and there usually is an eosinophilia. This reaction resolves when the drug is stopped. The second reaction to nitrofurans is a chronic one that occurs after the patient has taken the drug for a prolonged period, usually months. Dyspnea, cough, and cyanosis develop gradually. The x-ray shows diffuse basilar interstitial infiltrates, and pulmonary function studies show restrictive lung disease. Partial recovery occurs if the drug is stopped.

### Metabolic Toxicity

Hypoglycemia can follow pentamidine administration. Use of large doses of penicillins, particularly the anti-*Pseudomonas* agents like carbenicillin, present such a large load of nonreabsorbable anion to the distal tubule that hypokalemia results. Carbenicillin also can produce sodium overload since it contains 4.7 mEq/g and is given in doses of 24 to 40 g/day. Demethylchlortetracycline produces nephrogenic diabetes insipidus (Singer and Rotenberg, 1973). Amphotericin B and stale (outdated) tetracyclines produce renal tubular acidosis and hypokalemia.

### Renal Toxicity

Many factors intrinsic to the kidney make it particularly vulnerable to nephrotoxic reactions to antimicrobial agents (Fig. 1). The most common form of renal damage due to penicillins is an acute interstitial nephritis that has been associated with methicillin therapy but can occur with any penicillin. Fever, eosinophilia, and rash commonly antedate or accompany the renal lesion. Urinalysis may reveal white cells, casts, and proteinuria, but microscopic hematuria is most common. Urinary output is normal at first, although the serum creatinine and urea nitrogen increase. With discontinuation of the drug, the renal function of most patients returns to normal. Renal biopsy shows patchy tubular damage with interstitial edema, accumulation of lymphocytes, monocytes, eosinophils, and plasma cells. Glomeruli are normal. Most of the evidence suggests that this is a hypersensitivity reaction. Antitubular basement membrane antigens have been demonstrated in the serum in methicillin nephritis; and IgG, $C_3$, and a methicillin antigen were present in a linear pattern along the tubular basement membrane (Border et al., 1974).

Nephrotoxicity due to cephaloridine is dose-related (Silverblatt et al., 1973). There is proximal tubular damage due to accumulation of high

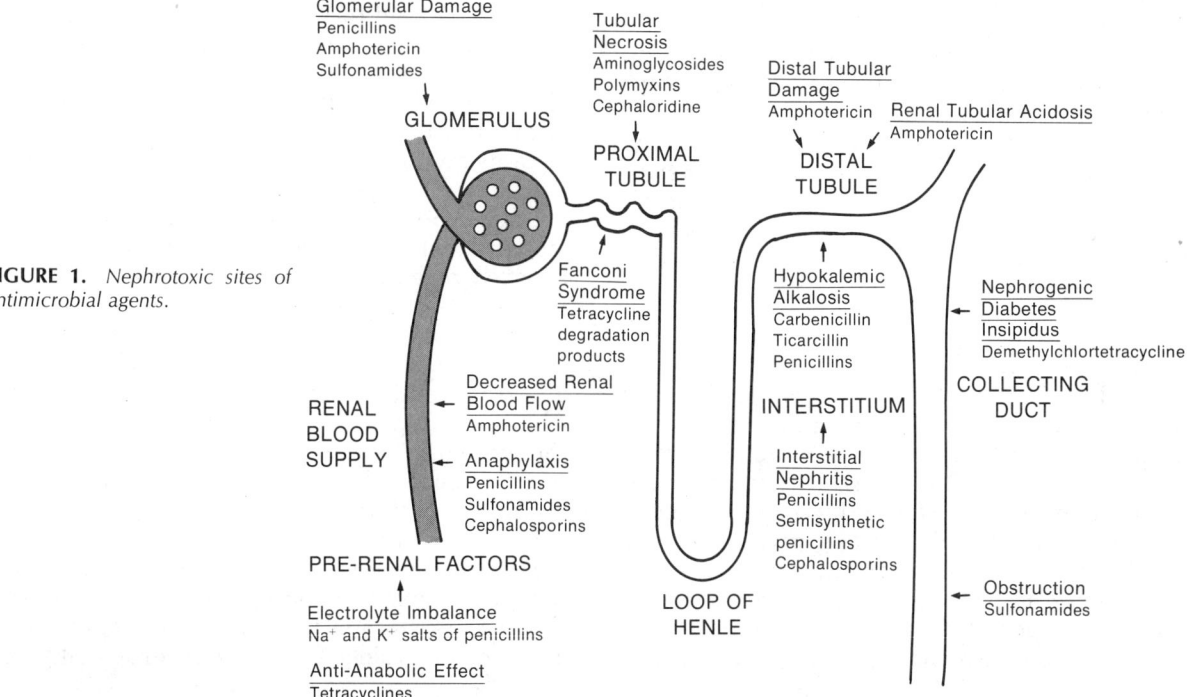

**FIGURE 1.** *Nephrotoxic sites of antimicrobial agents.*

intracellular concentrations of the drug in cortical tubular cells. The other cephalosporins have not been convincingly shown to be nephrotoxic.

Polymyxins bind to proximal tubular cells and damage cellular membranes. The aminoglycosides vary in their nephrotoxic potential ranging from neomycin, the most toxic agent, to streptomycin, the least toxic. Gentamicin and amikacin appear to be more nephrotoxic in animals than tobramycin, but clinical differences among the agents are difficult to establish. Gentamicin damages proximal tubules with loss of renal tubular enzymes, concentrating ability, and the development of intracytoplasmic bodies that seem to be injured cellular organelles. Aminoglycoside nephrotoxicity is dose-related and seems to be increased by simultaneous administration of cephalosporins. The overall incidence of nephrotoxicity due to aminoglycosides is about 5 to 10 per cent.

Crystallization-producing obstructive nephropathy, allergic and hypersensitivity reactions, precipitation of hemoglobin casts secondary to drug-induced hemolysis, and an intrinsic toxic effect have all been reported as secondary to sulfonamide therapy. Whether trimethoprim produces nephrotoxicity is unclear, but it does seem to alter handling of creatinine by the kidney.

Amphotericin can cause renal vasoconstriction and damage to proximal and distal tubular cells with intratubular calcium deposits. Renal abnormalities occur in about 25 per cent of patients who receive the drug. Most of the toxicity due to amphotericin is reversible, provided less than 5 g have been given. The primary disturbance is distal tubular acidosis (Burgess and Birchall, 1972). The drug seems to produce a permeability defect that allows the tubular cells to leak potassium and become permeable to hydrogen ions. Hydrogen ions then pass from tubular urine into the cells. The overall picture of amphotericin toxicity to the kidney is one of azotemia, acidosis, hypokalemia, and polyuria. Daily supplements of 100 mg of potassium are often needed after even small doses of amphotericin.

### Neurologic Toxicity

Peripheral neuropathy has been produced by isoniazid most often in patients who acetylate the drug slowly. It is dose-related and can be reversed by pyridoxine (La Du, 1972). Ethionamide also produces peripheral neuropathy. High concentrations in the blood of nitrofurans, polymyxins, and emetine cause peripheral neuropathy in patients with decreased renal function. Polymyxins and aminoglycosides produce a reversible neuromuscular blockade resembling myasthenia gravis

(Warner and Sanders, 1971). This toxicity is dose-related and has followed use of the agents as a peritoneal lavage. The drug produces a competitive blockade at the myoneural end-plate. Aminoglycosides probably compete with acetylcholine for receptor sites so that the end-plate is not depolarized. Neostigmine reverses this paralysis (Ream, 1963). Polymyxins also produce a noncompetitive prolonged depolarization due to calcium depletion, which can be reversed by calcium (Zauder et al., 1966).

Central nervous system excitation and seizures can be induced by isoniazid, amantadine, and penicillin. Penicillin-induced seizures are a myoclonic type and are more frequent in elderly patients and following cardiopulmonary by-pass (Seamans et al., 1968). Direct instillation of methicillin, oxacillin, or cephalosporins into the ventricles when CSF shunts are installed usually does not produce seizures. Cycloserine also causes seizures.

### Ototoxicity

Aminoglycosides vary in their potential to produce deafness. Neomycin is the most ototoxic, followed by kanamycin, gentamicin, and amikacin. Tobramycin and netilmicin are less ototoxic. Deafness is the result of damage to the hair cells of the organ of Corti (Friedman et al., 1966). The mechanism for this reaction is unknown. Sensory cells of the vestibular system are also damaged by aminoglycosides, and, although it was originally thought that certain aminoglycosides produced only vestibular damage and other agents produced only auditory damage, it is clear that individual drugs can injure both vestibular and auditory function. Streptomycin and gentamicin also seem to have a greater propensity to produce vestibular toxicity than auditory toxicity, but kanamycin, neomycin, tobramycin, and any of the agents can produce either or both forms of toxicity. Both forms of ototoxicity seem to occur most frequently in older people, those who have received repeated doses of aminoglycosides, and individuals with decreased renal function in whom the drugs accumulate. The exact incidence of ototoxicity is not known, since hearing loss first affects perception of sounds above 2000 cycles/sec, which is outside the conversational range and therefore overlooked by patients and physicians, and the body adjusts for minor damage to the vestibular system, making its recognition difficult.

The other antibiotic that causes vestibular dysfunction is minocycline (Williams et al., 1974). This occurs more often in females. This toxicity can often be avoided by giving the drug in divided

## TABLE 4. Drug Interactions of Antimicrobial Agents With Other Compounds

| INTERACTING DRUGS | ADVERSE EFFECT |
| --- | --- |
| *Aminoglycoside antibiotics with:* | |
| Cephaloridine | Nephrotoxicity |
| Cephalothin and other cephalosporins | Nephrotoxicity |
| Curariform drugs | Neuromuscular blockade |
| Digoxin | Possible decreased digoxin effect |
| Ethacrynic acid | Ototoxicity |
| Furosemide | Ototoxicity |
| Methoxyflurane | Nephrotoxicity |
| Polymyxins | Nephrotoxicity |
| *Aminosalicyclic acid (PAS) with:* | |
| Probenecid | Aminosalicylic acid toxicity |
| *Amphotericin B with:* | |
| Curariform drugs | Curare effect |
| Digitalis | Digitalis toxicity |
| *Cephaloridine with:* | |
| Aminoglycoside antibiotics | Nephrotoxicity |
| Ethacrynic acid | Nephrotoxicity |
| Furosemide | Nephrotoxicity |
| *Cephalosporins with:* | |
| Aminoglycoside antibiotics | Nephrotoxicity |
| *Chloramphenicol with:* | |
| Dicoumarol | Excessive anticoagulation |
| Phenytoin | Phenytoin toxicity |
| Hypoglycemics, oral | Hypoglycemia |
| *Griseofulvin with:* | |
| Anticoagulants, oral | Decreased anticoagulant effect |
| *Isoniazid with:* | |
| Aluminum antacids | Decreased isoniazid effect |
| Disulfiram | Psychotic episodes, ataxia |
| Phenytoin | Phenytoin toxicity |
| *Lincomycin with:* | |
| Kaolin-pectin | Decreased lincomycin effect |
| *Metronidazole with:* | |
| Alcohol | Antabuse-like reaction |
| Disulfiram | Psychosis |
| *Nalidixic acid with:* | |
| Dicoumarol | Prolonged prothrombin time |
| *Polymyxins with:* | |
| Aminoglycoside antibiotics | Nephrotoxicity |
| Curariform drugs | Neuromuscular blockade |
| *Rifampin with:* | |
| Anticoagulants, oral | Decreased anticoagulant effect |
| Contraceptives, oral | Decreased contraceptive effect |
| Corticosteroids | Decreased corticosteroid effect |
| Hypoglycemics, oral | Possible decreased effect |
| Methadone | Methadone withdrawal symptoms |
| *Sulfonamides with:* | |
| Anticoagulants, oral | Anticoagulant effect |
| Hypoglycemics | Sulfonylurea hypoglycemia |
| *Tetracyclines with:* | |
| Antacids, oral | Decreased effect of tetracyclines |
| Barbiturates | Decreased doxycycline effect |
| Carbamazepine | Decreased tetracycline effect |
| Iron, oral | Decreased effect of tetracyclines |
| Methoxyflurane | Nephrotoxicity |

## ALTERATION OF MICROBIAL FLORA

Alteration of intestinal flora by use of antibiotics allows overgrowth of *Candida*, which often results in thrush (Solomon, 1961) or vaginitis and may cause disseminated candidiasis in patients with depressed resistance. Prolonged use of oral penicillins as prophylaxis against recurrent rheumatic fever has been complicated by colonization of the oropharynx with streptococci that are relatively resistant to penicillin. Administration of antibiotics in *Salmonella* gastroenteritis results in prolongation of the carrier state and occasionally increases the risk of bacteremia (Aserkoff and Bennett, 1969). Pseudomembranous colitis due to overgrowth of *C. difficile* has been discussed.

## DRUG INTERACTIONS

Penicillins can inactivate aminoglycosides when the two are mixed in the same solution. Drug interactions within the patient are numerous and may result in increased toxicity of an agent or a decreased effect of a drug (Table 4). These antibiotic reactions with other agents in vivo involve a change in the metabolism of a compound. Microsomal enzymes that destroy more drug may be induced or there may be competition for enzymes involved in inactivation of both drugs. Binding to receptor sites on proteins or tissues, so that the second drug is blocked, may make more drug available. Competition for excretory pathways in the kidney or liver may result in accumulation of a drug.

### References

Aserkoff, B., and Bennett, J. V.: Effect of antibiotic therapy in acute salmonellosis on the fecal excretion of salmonellae. N Engl J Med 281:636, 1969.

Barrett, F. F., Eardley, W. A., Yow, M. D., et al.: Ampicillin in the treatment of acute suppurative meningitis. J Pediatr 69:343, 1966.

Bartlett, S., Chang, T., Gururth, M., Gorback, S. L., and Guderdonk, S.: Antibiotic-associated pseudomembranous colitis due to toxin-producing clostridia. N Eng J Med 298:531, 1978.

Barza, M., Brusch, J., Bergeron, M., et al.: Penetration of antibiotics into fibrin loci in vivo. III. Intermittent vs. continuous infusion and the effect of probenecid. J Infect Dis 129:73, 1974.

Border, W. A., Lehman, D. H., Egan, J. D., et al.: Antitubular basement-membrane antibodies in methicillin-associated interstitial nephritis. N Engl J Med 291:381, 1974.

Brandiss, M. U., Wolff, S. M., Moores, R., et al.: Anemia induced by amphotericin B. JAMA 189:663, 1964.

Brown, C. H., Natelson, E. A., Bradshaw, W., et al.: The hemostatic defect produced by carbenicillin. N Engl J Med 291:265, 1974.

Brummer, D. L., et al.: Summary of the report of the Ad Hoc Advisory Committee on isoniazid and liver disease. Morbidity and Mortality Weekly Report, 20:231, 1971.

Burgess, J. L., and Birchall, R.: Nephrotoxicity of amphotericin B, with emphasis on changes in tubular function. Am J Med 53:77, 1972.

Butler, K., English, A., Knirsch, A., and Korst, J.: Metabolism and laboratory studies with indanylcarbenicillin. In Holloway, W. J.

doses rather than at a single time. Vancomycin can also produce deafness, and erythromycins at very high concentrations can cause temporary decrease of hearing.

(ed.): Infectious Disease Reviews. Wilmington, Futura Publishing Company, 1972, pp. 157–166.

Cohn, H. D.: Clinical studies with a new rifamycin derivative. J Clin Pharmacol 9:118, 1969.

Duignan, N. M., Andrews, J., and Williams, J. D.: Pharmacological studies with lincomycin in late pregnancy. Br Med J 3:75, 1973.

DuPont, H. L., Hornick, R. B., Weiss, C. F., et al.: Evaluation of chloramphenicol acid succinate therapy of induced typhoid fever and Rocky Mountain spotted fever. N Engl J Med 282:53, 1970.

Fabre, J., Milek, E., Kalfopoulos, P., et al.: The kinetics of tetracyclines in man. I. Digestive absorption and serum concentrations. In Doxycycline, A Compendium of Clinical Evaluations. New York, Pfizer Laboratories Division, Pfizer Inc., 1973, pp. 13–18.

Florey, T. E., Turton, E. C., and Duthe, E. S.: Penicillin in wound exudates. Lancet 2:405, 1946.

Friedmann, I., Dadswell, J. V., and Bird, E. S.: Electronmicroscope studies of the neuroepithelium of the inner ear in guinea-pigs treated with neomycin. J Pathol Bacteriol 92:415, 1966.

Garnes, H. A.: Doxycycline levels in serum and prostatic tissue in man. Urology 1:205, 1973.

Hailey, F. J., Glascock, H. W., Jr., and Hewitt, W. F.: Pleuropneumonic reactions to nitrofurantoin. N Engl J Med 281:1087, 1969.

Hughes, H. B.: On the metabolic fate of isoniazid. J Pharmacol Exp Ther 109:444, 1953.

Kahn, S. B., Fein, S. A., and Brodsky, I.: Effects of trimethoprim on folate metabolism in man. Clin Pharmacol Ther 9:550, 1968.

Kirby, W. M., and Regamey, C.: Pharmacokinetics of cefazolin compared with four other cephalosporins. J Infect Dis 128: Suppl. S341–346, 1973.

La Du, B. N.: Pharmacogenetics: Defective enzymes in relation to reactions to drugs. Annu Rev Med 23:453, 1972.

Levine, B. B., Redmond, A. P., Fellner, M. J., et al.: Penicillin allergy and the heterogeneous immune responses of man to benzylpenicillin. J Clin Invest 45:1895, 1966.

McCarthy, C. G., and Finland, M.: Absorption and excretion of four penicillins: penicillin G, penicillin V, phenethicillin, and phenylmercaptomethyl penicillin. N Engl J Med 263:315, 1960.

McPherson, S. D. Jr., Presley, G. D., and Crawford, J. R.: Aqueous humor assays of subconjunctival antibiotics. Am J Ophthalmol 66:430, 1968.

Nagao, T., and Mauer, A. M.: Concordance of drug-induced aplastic anemia in identical twins. N Engl J Med 281:7, 1969.

Parker, R. H., and Schmid, F. R.: Antibacterial activity of synovial fluid during therapy of septic arthritis. Arthr Rheum 14:96, 1971.

Rall, D. P.: Drug entry into brain and cerebro-spinal fluid. In Brodie, B. B., and Gillette, J. R. (eds.): Handbook of Experimental Pharmacology: Concepts in Biochemical Pharmacology, Part. 1. New York, Springer-Verlag, 1971, pp. 240–248.

Ream, C. R.: Respiratory and cardiac arrest after intravenous administration of kanamycin with reversal of toxic effects by neostigmine. Ann Intern Med 59:384, 1963.

Records, R. E.: Intraocular penetration of cephalothin. Am J Ophthalmol 66:436, 1968.

Sachs, J., Geer T., Noell, P., et al.: Effect of renal function on urinary recovery of orally administered nitrofurantoin. N Engl J Med 278:1032, 1968.

Saslaw, S.: Demethylchlortetracycline phototoxicity. N Engl J Med 264:1301, 1961.

Schultz, J. C., Adamson, J. S., Jr., Workman, W. W., et al.: Fatal liver disease after intravenous administration of tetracycline in high dosage. N Engl J Med 269:999, 1963.

Seamans, K. B., Gloor, P., Dobell, R. A. R., et al.: Penicillin-induced seizures during cardiopulmonary bypass. A clinical and electroencephalographic study. N Engl J Med 278:861, 1968.

Silverblatt, F., Harrison, W. O., and Turck, M.: Nephrotoxicity of cephalosporin antibiotics in experimental animals. J Infect Dis 128: Suppl. S367–377, 1973.

Singer, I., and Rotenberg, D.: Demeclocycline-induced nephrogenic diabetes insipidus. In vivo and in vitro studies. Ann Intern Med 79:679, 1973.

Solomon, P.: Oral moniliasis complicating combined broad-spectrum antibiotic and antifungal therapy. N Engl J Med 265:847, 1961.

Stamey, T.: Urinary infections. Baltimore, The Williams & Wilkins Company, 1972, pp. 161–200.

Voss, H. E., Redmond, A. P., and Levine, B. B.: Clinical detection of the potential allergic reactor to penicillin by immunologic tests. JAMA: 196:679, 1966.

Warner, W. A., and Sanders, E.: Neuromuscular blockade associated with gentamicin therapy. JAMA 215:1153, 1971.

Whelton, A., Sapir, D. G., Carter, G. G., et al.: Intrarenal distribution of ampicillin in the normal and diseased human kidney. J Infect Dis 125:466, 1972.

Williams, D. N., Laughlin, L. W., and Lee, Y.: Minocycline: Possible vestibular side-effects. Lancet 2:744, 1974.

Zauder, H. L., Barton, N., Bennett, E. J., et al.: Colistimethate as a cause of postoperative apnoea. Canad Anaesthiol Soc J 13:607, 1966.

# B. SPECIFIC MICROBIAL AGENTS OF DISEASE

# 1 AEROBIC BACTERIA OR FACULTATIVELY ANAEROBIC BACTERIA

## Gram-Positive Cocci

## STAPHYLOCOCCI    23

### Stephen I. Morse, M.D. *

The staphylococci make up the medically most important genus in the family *Micrococcaceae*. There are three species: *Staphylococcus aureus* is responsible for most cases of staphylococcal disease in man; *S. epidermidis* usually causes minor skin lesions; and the newly recognized species *S. saprophyticus* may produce bladder infection.

### MORPHOLOGY

Staphylococci are nonmotile, nonspore forming, gram-positive cocci; in old cultures, or after ingestion by phagocytes, they may appear gram negative. Individual cells have a diameter of 0.7 to 1.2 $\mu$m and are characteristically grouped in irregular aggregates that resemble clusters of grapes, hence the name *staphylo* from the Greek *staphylē* — bunch of grapes (Fig. 1). Cell division takes place in successive perpendicular planes, but there is incomplete separation of the daughter cells and, instead of residual attachment along the division plane, the attachment point is usually eccentric to the division plane, resulting in irregular aggregates (Tzagaloff and Novick, 1977). Moreover, daughter cells may shift from their original site of attachment. Although clusters are usually seen in pathologic material and in growth on solid media, staphylococci often form short chains in liquid culture.

Some *S. aureus* strains possess distinct capsules, as demonstrated by the India ink method,

electron microscopic techniques, or the Quellung reaction with specific capsular antiserum (Morse, 1978). Encapsulation may be more frequent in vivo than after cultivation in vitro.

The peptidoglycan of staphylococcal cell walls is characterized by unique pentaglycine bridges that link the tetrapeptides attached to the muramic acid residues (see Chapter 20). The pentaglycine bridges are specifically susceptible to the action of the enzyme lysostaphin, thereby providing a useful means of identifying the genus.

Osmotically unstable L forms, deficient in cell wall material, can be induced by agents that affect cell wall synthesis or structure — for example, penicillin or lysostaphin — and can be propagated in vitro in hypertonic medium. Small colony variants of *S. aureus* (G forms) occur when microbial growth is inhibited by a variety of agents, including antimicrobials, but also may appear spontaneously. Both L and G forms are resistant to many drugs, especially those affecting the cell wall, and it has been postulated that recrudescent *S. aureus* disease is sometimes due to reversion of persisting dormant L or G forms to invasive parental organisms.

On solid media, most strains of *S. aureus* produce a characteristic golden-yellow (*aureus*) carotenoid pigment; however, colonial coloration may vary from white to orange. *S. epidermidis* colonies usually are white and those of *S. saprophyticus* are white to greyish-white. Colonies of staphylococci are sharply defined, round, con-

---

*Deceased.

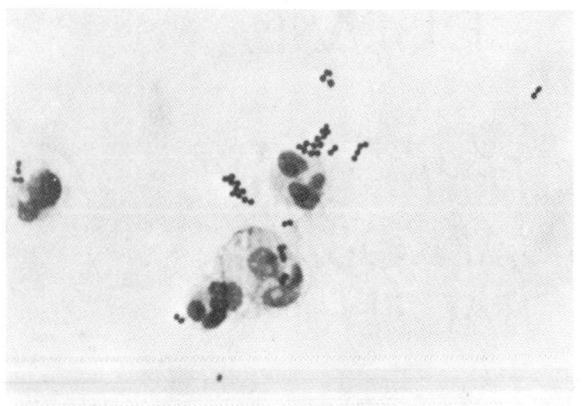

**FIGURE 1.** *Gram stain of exudate containing intracellular and extracellular staphylococci × 650. (From White, A., and Brooks, G. F.: Furunculosis, pyoderma, and impetigo. In Hoeprich, P. D. (ed.): Infectious Diseases. 2nd ed. Hagerstown. Harper and Row, 1977, p. 786.)*

vex, and measure 4 mm in diameter. On blood agar, *S. aureus* is usually surrounded by a zone of clear (β) hemolysis. Strains of *S. aureus* may produce one or more of four distinct hemolysins with different hemolytic specificities; therefore, the occurrence and extent of hemolysis depends upon both the strain and the source of blood. Some *S. epidermidis* strains are also hemolytic, whereas *S. saprophyticus* is nonhemolytic.

## *ANTIGENIC COMPOSITION*

### Species Antigens

The species-specific antigens of staphylococci are cell wall teichoic acids. In *S. aureus*, the antigen is a ribitol teichoic acid composed of a linear backbone of ribitol linked by phosphodiester bridges. *N*-acetylglucosamine is attached to the C4 position of the ribitol residues, and ester-linked *D*-alanine is attached to approximately 50 per cent of the C2 residues. The antigenic determinant is the glucosamine moiety, which may be in either α or β glycosidic linkage to ribitol. In most strains both types of glycosidic linkage are found, but in some only one is present. Therefore, antisera that will react with both anomers must be used for immunochemical determination of the species. Similarly, teichoic acids with both specificities must be used when testing for the presence of serum antibodies.

The *S. epidermidis* species-antigen is a glycerol teichoic acid in which glucose residues, in either α or β glycosidic linkage, are attached to a glycerol phosphate backbone and constitute the antigenic determinant. Cell walls of *S. saprophyticus* contain ribitol teichoic acid of two types. One has *N*-acetylglucosamine residues, whereas the other has glucose residues. Both may be present in the same strain.

### Cellular Antigens of S. Aureus

***Capsules.*** The few strains of *S. aureus* that are encapsulated in vitro tend to be more virulent in animals, and anticapsular antibodies protect against experimental disease. The capsule of one group of strains is a polymer of glucosaminuronic acid; that of another contains mannosaminuronic acid; and components characteristic of the peptidoglycan, e.g., glycine, alanine, and glucosamine, are found in the capsules of other strains.

***Protein.*** Protein A (agglutinogen A) is a surface component of most strains of *S. aureus*. Depending upon the method of isolation, the molecular weight of protein A ranges between 13,000 and 42,000. Although the bulk of protein A is covalently linked to the peptidoglycan, approximately one third is released extracellularly. The most striking property of protein A is its nonspecific interaction with the Fc portion of the IgG of a wide range of mammalian species. The result of the interaction may be either precipitation or the formation of soluble complexes. In the case of human IgG, protein A reacts with subclasses $IgG_1$, $IgG_2$, and $IgG_4$, but not $IgG_3$. Protein A also binds to some samples of human IgM and $IgA_2$. The interaction with the Fc portion of IgG produces a variety of biologic effects, including: activation of complement by both the classical and the alternative pathways; local wheal and flare reaction; the Arthus phenomenon; local and systemic anaphylaxis; inhibition of phagocytosis of opsonized particles through competition with the Fc receptors of phagocytes for the Fc portion of opsonic antibody (Peterson et al., 1977); and in vitro induction of proliferation of both human T lymphocytes and B lymphocytes (Sakane and Green, 1978). Protein A is also a true antigen and reacts with the Fab portion of specific antibody.

***Clumping Factor (Bound Coagulase).*** Unencapsulated strains of *S. aureus* clump when suspended in fibrinogen-containing solutions. There are apparently specific receptors on the bacterial surface for fibrinogen and the clumping is due to cross-linkage of the cells by fibrinogen. The receptors have not been characterized.

### Extracellular Antigens and Products of S. aureus

***Coagulase.*** *S. aureus* has the unique ability to clot a variety of mammalian plasmas. Clotting is caused by an extracellular product, coagulase (or free coagulase), which exists in several antigenically different forms, all having the same mechanisms of action. Virtually all naturally occurring strains of *S. aureus* produce coagulase, and since tests for coagulase are simple to perform, the *aureus* species is usually identified by coagulase production rather than by seriologic, physiologic, or biochemical tests. Coagulase-positive staphylococci are by definition *S. aureus*.

Coagulase does not clot fibrinogen directly but first reacts with a plasma constituent, coagulase-reacting factor (CRF), which is most probably prothrombin, to form a thrombin-like substance. The fibrinopeptides formed during clotting are identical to those produced by the action of thrombin on fibrinogen and, as in the case of thrombin-mediated clotting, diisopropylfluorophosphate (DFP) blocks the reaction.

**Hemolysins.** Four distinct hemolysins are produced by *S. aureus* and many strains manufacture more than one type (Wiseman, 1975). All cause β (clear) hemolysis. They have different lytic spectra with respect to the susceptibility of various erythrocyte species and are also cytotoxic for cells other than erythrocytes. The hemolysins are antigenic proteins; activity is neutralized by specific antiserum.

α-Hemolysin (α-toxin) is the most commonly encountered hemolysin in clinical isolates of *S. aureus*. Rabbit erythrocytes are highly susceptible, whereas human erythrocytes are unaffected. In experimental animals, α-hemolysin causes dermonecrosis at the site of local injection and is lethal when injected intravenously. The mode and site of action of α-hemolysin are unknown.

β-Hemolysin is found in many strains of animal origin but is produced by less than 20 per cent of human strains. It is a "hot-cold" hemolysin; lysis is maximal only after blood agar plates or toxin-erythrocyte mixtures are held at low temperatures after incubation at 37°C. β-hemolysin is a sphingomyelinase, which, in the presence of magnesium ions, catalyzes the breakdown of sphingomyelin to *N*-acylsphingosine and phosphorylcholine. Erythrocyte susceptibility is directly correlated with sphingomyelin content. Sheep, human, and guinea pig erythrocytes contain decreasing amounts of sphingomyelin and are decreasingly susceptible to β-hemolysin. β-Hemolysin is toxic for experimental animals only in high doses.

γ-Hemolysin consists of two components that act in concert to induce hemolysis. γ-Hemolysin is inhibited by sulfonated polymers, including agar, and hence its activity is not readily seen on blood agar plates. Rabbit, human, and sheep erythrocytes are susceptible to lysis.

δ-Hemolysin consists of aggregates of low molecular weight subunits and has a broad range of lytic and cytotoxic activity probably due to a nonspecific detergent-like action. Since serum phospholipids inhibit δ-hemolysin, it is not clear whether it functions in vivo.

**Leucocidin.** In addition to the leukocytoxic effects of some of the hemolysins, *S. aureus* also produces a distinct nonhemolytic leukocytotoxic substance, Panton-Valentine (P-V) leucocidin. P-V leucocidin contains two components, F (electrophoretically fast moving) and S (slow moving). Both are required for activity, and antibody to either component neutralizes toxicity. Human and rabbit polymorphonuclear leukocytes and macrophages are the only susceptible cells.

**Enterotoxins.** Five chemically and immunologically related enterotoxins (designated a-e) are produced by *S. aureus*. These proteins have a molecular weight of $3.5 \times 10^4$, are relatively heat stable, and only moderately susceptible to trypsin digestion (Bergdoll et at., 1974). They are responsible for many cases of food poisoning, but the mechanism of action has not been completely elucidated. It appears that both the bowel itself and neural innervation are affected.

**Exfoliatin.** Exfoliatin is an extracellular product that cleaves the stratum granulosum layer of the epidermis and causes several clinical syndromes. It is produced by many *S. aureus* strains in phage group II, and it is probable that more than one antigenic type exists.

A number of other extracellular substances with biologic activity are also produced by *S. aureus*. These include staphylokinase (fibrinolysin). hyaluronidase, and phospholipase.

The wide variety of antigenic components and extracellular products found in *S. aureus* is not seen in either *S. epidermidis* or *S. saprophyticus*. Some strains of *S. epidermidis* cause β-hemolysis owing to a hemolysin termed ε-hemolysin, which is similar to the *S. aureus* δ-hemolysin. *S. saprophyticus* is not hemolytic.

## METABOLISM

*S. aureus* and *S. epidermidis* are facultative anaerobes that ferment sugars with the formation of large amounts of lactic acid, as occurs in lactic acid bacteria (Baird-Parker, 1974). They also resemble the spherical lactic acid bacteria in the low G + C content (30 to 35 moles per cent) of their DNA, but staphylococci possess heme-containing enzymes that allow normal respiratory metabolism, which is absent in lactic acid bacteria. The most important of these respiratory enzymes in staphylococci are cytochromes a, b, and o, which contain firmly bound prosthetic groups capable of donating or accepting electrons as they undergo oxidation or reduction. They are bound to the cell membrane of the staphylococcus and, with a group of quinones (menaquinones), form the membrane-bound electron transport system. The quinones are nonprotein carriers of relatively low molecular weight. Catalase, another heme enzyme possessed by staphylococci, is important for splitting hydrogen peroxide and preventing accumulation of this highly toxic compound. In the diagnostic laboratory, catalase activity helps distinguish staphylococci from streptococci, which are catalase deficient. Of particular usefulness in species differentiation is the capacity of S. aureus to ferment mannitol and to grow in concentrations of sodium chloride that are inhibitory for other microorganisms — for example 7.5 per cent NaCl. S. aureus also produces a heat-stable nuclease, not found in the other species. In contrast to S. aureus and S. epidermidis, S. saprophyticus grows very poorly under anaerobic conditions.

Although capable of anaerobic growth, S. aureus and S. epidermidis grow better aerobically. Moreover, they exhibit different metabolic activities under aerobic and anaerobic conditions. For example, oxygen is necessary for pigment production, and nonpigmented colonies of S. aureus grown anaerobically will develop their characteristic yellow color upon exposure to air (aerochromogens; compare with photochromogens among mycobacteria, Chapter 40). Glucose, lactose, maltose, and mannitol are energy sources for staphylococci anaerobically. These sugars are also metabolized in air, and so are other hexoses, pentoses, disaccharides, and sugar alcohols. The products of glucose metabolism change from lactic acid during fermentation to acetate and $CO_2$ in air. S. epidermidis produces nitrite from nitrate when grown in air but may not do so under anaerobic conditions because nitrate reductase does not function in the absence of air. For reduction of nitrate, oxygen is required not as a terminal electron acceptor but for the biosynthesis of a cytochrome, which mediates in electron transfer to nitrate.

## GENETICS

Many of the properties and products of S. aureus are genetically controlled by plasmids. Plasmid regulation of antibiotic resistance, especially through the production of penicillinase ($\beta$-lactamase), is of profound clinical importance (Lacey, 1975).

In contrast to R-factors in gram-negative bacteria, penicillinase plasmids do not tend to carry other antibiotic resistance markers, with the exception of erythromycin. Hence, multiple drug resistance mediated by plasmids is unusual in S. aureus. There appear to be two molecular classes of staphylococcal resistance plasmids. The larger of these has a molecular weight of $20 \times 10^6$, may be isolated as a covalently closed ring molecule, and its replication appears to depend on cell division so that only one (or at most a few) copy occurs in each cell. The other type is much smaller and has a molecular weight in the range of $3 \times 10^6$. The smaller type may carry resistance determinants for tetracycline or chloramphenicol and multiply independently of cell division so that multiple copies are produced in each cell. As with gram-negative bacteria, chloramphenicol resistance is mediated by staphylococcal plasmids through the enzyme chloramphenicol acetyltransferase. In contrast, however, to the constituent enzymes of gram-negative R-factors, the penicillinase and acetyltransferase of resistant staphylococci are inducible (see Chapter 4). Transfer of genetic material between strains of S. aureus occurs by transduction. Most strains of S. aureus are lysogenic, and lysogenic bacteriophages belonging to serologic group B are capable of generalized transduction, in which bacterial DNA (rather than phage DNA) is incorporated with the phage particle. Spontaneous prophage induction and subsequent transduction occurs in mixed cultures in vitro and more importantly transduction occurs in vivo in animals and humans carrying an appropriate lysogenic donor and a suitable recipient strain of S. aureus (Novick and Morse, 1968). In addition to transduction, bacteriophages also exert genetic control by the process of phage conversion as in the production of staphylokinase and $\beta$-hemolysin. Under highly specialized circumstances, transformation reactions can occur, but conjugation as a means of genetic transfer in staphylococci is not seen.

## PATHOGENIC PROPERTIES

Two types of disease are produced by S. aureus, invasive and toxinogenic. The hallmark of invasive disease is abscess formation. Most often the abscesses are superficial (furuncle), but in some cases the furuncles develop into burrowing lesions consisting of a number of interconnecting abscesses (carbuncle). Serious deep-seated disease usually is not seen in healthy people, but may occur in those debilitated by disease, malnutrition, extensive surgical procedures, and immunosuppression. In these instances, abscesses may occur in almost any organ; bacteremia is frequent with metastatic lesions appearing most commonly in the lung, bones, and kidney. Approximately two-thirds of patients with bacteremia may develop endocarditis due to *S. aureus* and the course is often fulminating. Inhalational staphylococcal pneumonia generally is a complication of viral pneumonia, particularly influenza.

No single component or product of *S. aureus* has been shown to be the primary determinant of either the initiation or the progression of invasive lesions. It appears, therefore that a number of factors may be involved. These include the intraphagocytic survival of a few cells; inhibition of phagocytosis by capsules and protein A (Peterson et al., 1977); and the toxic effects on cells and tissues of the hemolysins, leucocidin, and enzymatic products. Some strains of *S. aureus* appear to be more virulent for man than others, but the reasons for this difference are unknown.

There are two clinical syndromes produced by *S. aureus* that are not the consequence of invasion of host tissues. *S. aureus* is a major cause of food poisoning due to ingestion of preformed enterotoxin. Typically, staphylococcal food poisoning follows consumption of food such as custards, meats, pastries, or salad dressings that have been contaminated by enterotoxin-producing organisms from a food handler. If the food is kept at a temperature that permits bacterial multiplication, enterotoxin production occurs. If the foods are then heated, the organisms may be killed but the heat-stable enterotoxin persists. Alternatively, contamination occurs after cooking, in which case live organisms may also be ingested. Nausea, vomiting, and sometimes diarrhea appear one to six hours after ingestion of enterotoxin. Prompt recovery without therapy is the rule except in the case of infants and the elderly, where replacement of fluid and electrolytes may be required.

In patients with syndromes caused by exfoliation, viable phage group II organisms are present, with or without overt lesions. There are three basic syndromes that together are termed the staphylococcal scalded skin syndrome (Melish and Glasgow, 1970). The term derives from the most serious manifestation that occurs in infants and young children. Wide areas of skin are denuded and generalized bullous formation occurs (toxic epidermal necrolysis or Ritter's disease) (Fig. 2). In older children or adults the disorder is characterized by the formation of local bullae (Lyell's disease) or by a scarlatina-like rash that mimics streptococcal scarlet fever except that the tongue and palate are spared. The different clinical manifestations may be related to the individual's state of immunity to exfoliatin. Fatalities are unusual, since the lesions are at the stratum granulosum and severe exudation and transudation do not occur.

*S. epidermidis* is often responsible for minor skin abscesses, but in the compromised host and after major surgery, particularly involving the insertion of an intravascular prosthetic device, bacteremic disease may occur. *S. saprophyticus* may cause infection of the urinary bladder in man.

## IMMUNITY

The roles of humoral antibodies and cell-mediated immunity in invasive *S. aureus* disease are controversial. In experimental animals, except for the uncommon encapsulated organisms, there is little evidence for protection against invasive disease by humoral anticellu-

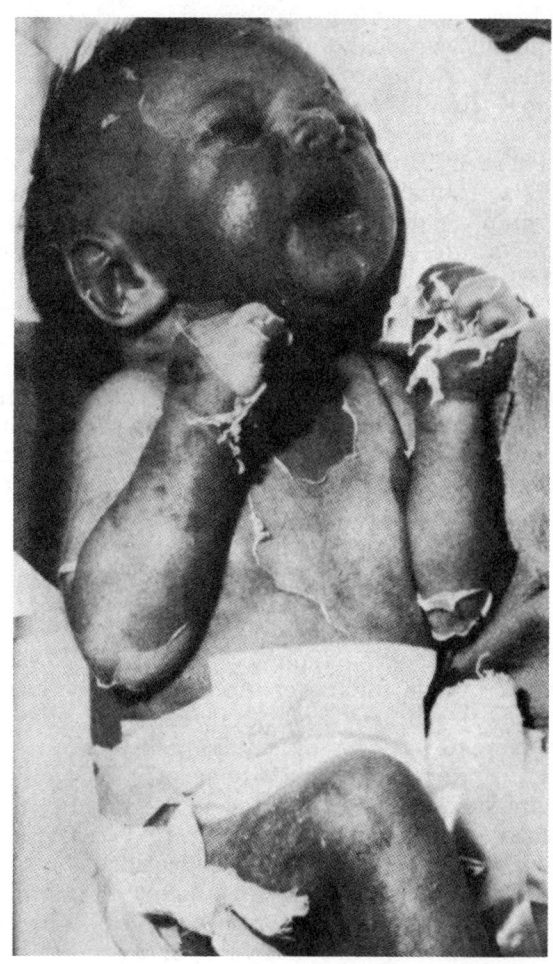

**FIGURE 2.** *Staphylococcal scalded skin syndrome in an infant. (From Melish, M. E., and Glasgow, L. A.: N Engl J Med 282:1114, 1970. Reprinted by permission from the N Engl J Med.)*

lar antibodies. Although toxic effects such as those produced by $\alpha$ toxin are diminished in experimental animals by antitoxin, toxic effects in man are usually not primary, and antitoxins do not appear to protect. Moreover, antibodies to a variety of components and products of S. aureus are found in normal humans, but there is no correlation between the presence of these antibodies and the occurrence and progression of disease.

In experimental animals, cell-mediated immunity may restrict the spread of organisms from the inoculation site but, as in the case of tuberculosis, local reactions are often more severe. Thus, the characteristic morphology and confinement of the staphylococcal abscess may be related to the effects of cell-mediated immunity.

Man has a high innate resistance to S. aureus disease, but resistance can be readily decreased by local factors. For example, intradermal injection of as many as $10^8$ to $10^9$ organisms usually causes no abscess, but if a suture containing as few as $10^2$ organisms is passed through the skin and tied, marked abscess formation occurs, often requiring surgical and antimicrobial therapy. Other local factors, particularly those that impeded circulation, enhance susceptibility to staphylococcal disease.

There is considerable evidence that colonization of normal human skin or mucosa with one strain of S. aureus inhibits colonization with another strain, a phenomenon known as bacterial interference. This has been used therapeutically in the case of epidemics in newborn nurseries. The neonate is purposefully colonized in the nares with an avirulent strain of S. aureus, and suprainfection with an epidemic virulent strain is thereby prevented. The nature of the inhibition is unknown but may be based upon competition for nutrients, or, more likely, the production of bactericidins.

## LABORATORY DIAGNOSIS

The diagnosis of staphylococcal disease is suggested by the finding of gram-positive cocci in clumps in pathologic material, but final diagnosis is achieved only by culture and appropriate tests. The characteristic $\beta$-hemolysis and yellow pigmentation strongly point to S. aureus, and selective media are useful. But, a positive coagulase test is required for identification. The test is performed by adding an aliquot of a broth culture or an inoculum from agar to 0.5 ml of rabbit plasma (either undiluted or diluted 1:10). Most strains produce clotting within three hours of incubation at 37°C, but cultures should be

held overnight before a negative result is reported.

Identification of individual strains of S. aureus is often epidemiologically useful. Serologic tests are complex and typing sera are not readily available for routine use. Determining the spectrum of antibiotic resistance (resistogram) is simple but imprecise. Phage typing is the most useful technique and is based upon the susceptibility of S. aureus to lytic phages. The phages used for typing are divided into groups that have similar, but not identical, host range. An agar plate, subdivided into sections, is heavily swabbed with a suspension of the test strain and a standard drop of typing phage is placed onto each section. After overnight incubation, the areas of lysis are noted and the strain is designated by the identification number of the typing phages to which it is susceptible and by the phage group of the lytic phages. On the basis of phage susceptibility S. aureus strains are divided into four groups. Phage group II is distinctive in that production of bacteriocins and exfoliatin are limited to this group.

Typing phages for S. epidermidis strains are at present not available for general use and strains are usually distinguished by their patterns of resistance to antimicrobials, or their metabolic and biochemical properties (biotypes).

Strains of coalgulase-negative staphylococci, isolated from urine, can be identified as S. saprophyticus by their poor growth anaerobically and their resistance to novobiocin (M.I.C. > 2.0 $\mu$g/ml, Baird-Parker, 1974).

## DRUG SUSCEPTIBILITY

When penicillin was first introduced, the vast majority of strains of S. aureus were susceptible. Depending upon the geographic area, as many as 50 per cent or more of strains occurring in the population-at-large are now penicillin-resistant, and 80 per cent of strains responsible for hospital-acquired disease may be resistant. Resistance is due to the plasmid-mediated enzyme penicillinase, which is a $\beta$ lactamase that splits that $\beta$ lactam ring of the penicillin nucleus (Lacey, 1975). In severe staphylococcal disease, unless the strain is sensitive to penicillin, penicillinase-resistant penicillins such as oxacillin and methicillin are the drugs of choice. In patients allergic to penicillin, cephalosporin derivatives may be used. Combined therapy with an aminoglycoside such as gentamycin is often employed, but there is no clear evidence that such combinations are more effective than the use of the bactericidal penicillins or cephalosporins alone. Vancomycin is used in patients who are allergic to the penicillins and cephalosporins.

Infections due to *S. epidermidis* are often caused by strains resistant to a variety of antimicrobial agents, and therapy of deep-seated disease may be very difficult. Strains of *S. saprophyticus* are generally sensitive to penicillin.

Superficial staphylococcal abscesses generally do not require antimicrobial therapy. Local application of moist heat, immobilization, and incision and drainage usually suffice. In both serious and minor staphylococcal disease, infected foci such as foreign bodies or necrotic bone or tissue must be removed.

## EPIDEMIOLOGY

*S. aureus* is ubiquitous. Approximately 30 to 40 per cent of adults are asymptomatic carriers. Colonization begins in the neonatal period and approximately 90 per cent of infants discharged from hospital nurseries are carriers. The carrier rate in infants delivered at home is less but still substantial. The prevalence drops in the ensuing several years and then rises again to the adult level. The nares are the usual carrier site, but organisms can be found on skin and mucous membranes, and occasionally in the gut. *S. aureus* is extremely hardy and survives in the air and on inanimate objects and surfaces for long periods of time, but it is likely that person-to-person transmission is more important than environmental contamination.

Because of the widespread occurrence of *S. aureus,* it is inappropriate to consider methods to prevent acquisition of strains in a normal population. However, in "at risk" patients, such as newborns and patients in hospitals with serious underlying disorders, it is imperative that individuals with open lesions be isolated from the patient. In the face of hospital epidemics, which appear to be much less frequent than a decade ago, personnel who are carriers of the epidemic strain also should be removed from contact with such patients.

### References

Baird-Parker, A.C.: *Micrococcaceae.* In Buchanan, R.E. and Gibbons, N.W. (eds.): Bergey's Manual of Determinative Bacteriology. 8th ed. Baltimore, Williams and Wilkins, 1974, p. 483.

Bergdoll, M.S., Huang, I.Y., and Schantz, E.J.: Chemistry of the staphylococcal enterotoxins. J Agr Food Chem 22:9, 1974.

Bernheimer, A.W.: Interactions between membranes and cytolytic bacterial toxins. Biochim et Biophysica Acta 344:27, 1974.

Cohen, J.O.: The Staphylococci. New York, John Wiley and Sons Incorporated, 1972.

Forsgren, A.: Immunological aspects of protein A. In Schlessinger, D., (ed.): Microbiology-1977. Washington, D.C., American Society for Microbiology, 1977, p.353.

Jeljaszewiez, J. (ed.): Staphylococci and Staphylococcal Diseases. New York, Gustav Fischer Verlag, 1976.

Lacey, R.W.: Antibiotic resistance plasmids of *Staphylococcus aureus* and their clinical importance. Bacteriol Rev 39:1, 1975.

Melish, M.E., and Glasgow, L.A.: The staphylococcal scalded-skin syndrome: development of an experimental model. N Engl J Med 282:1114, 1970.

Morse, S.I.: Staphylococci. In Davis, B.D., Dulbecco, R., Eisen, H.N., and Ginsberg, H.S. (eds.): Microbiology. 3rd ed. Hagerstown, Harper and Row, 1978.

Novick, R.P., and Morse, S.I.: In vivo transmission of drug resistance factors between strains of *Staphlococcus aureus*. J Exp Med 125:45, 1968.

Peterson, P.K., Verholf, J., Sabbath, L.D., and Quie, P.G.: Effect of protein A on staphylococcal opsonization. Infect Immun 15:760, 1977.

Sakane, T., and Green, I.: Protein A from *Staphylococcus aureus* — a mitogen for human T lymphocytes and B lymphocytes but not L lymphocytes. J Immun 120:302, 1978.

Tzagaloff, H., and Novick, R.P.: Geometry of cell division in *Straphylococcus aureus*. J Bact 129:343, 1977.

Wiseman, G.M.: The hemolysins of *Staphylococcus aureus*. Bacteriol Rev 39:317, 1975.

# STREPTOCOCCUS **24**

## Isaac Ginsburg, M. Sc., Ph.D.

Since the discovery of the streptococcus by Billroth and Ehrlich in 1877, it has received special attention because it is involved in numerous diseases of humans and lower animals. Few other microorganisms of medical importance can elaborate as many exotoxins and enzymes and also produce serious infections in virtually any tissue. Certain streptococci are notorious for inducing nonsuppurative sequelae that affect the heart, kidney, joints, and brain, and take the form of rheumatic fever, acute glomerulonephritis (AGN), and chorea.

Although certain streptococci are human pathogens, others are integral parts of the normal flora of the mouth and intestinal tracts. The normal streptococcal flora may, however, on occasion invade the bloodstream and cause septicemia, usually associated with endocarditis. Certain streptococci that inhabit the mouth are involved in the pathogenesis of dental caries.

The genus *Streptococcus* belongs to the family Streptococcaceae. The most important species of streptococci with pathogenic properties for man are *Streptococcus pyogenes* (group A streptococci),

*Streptococcus pneumoniae, Streptococcus agalactiae* (group B), *Streptococcus faecalis* (enterococci — group D) and *Streptococcus viridans* (a heterogenous group of different species). The guanine + cystosine content of streptococcal DNA ranges from 33 to 44 moles per cent. Analysis of DNA-RNA homology among streptococci (including pneumococci) discloses a close relationship except for *S. faecalis* (Weissman et al., 1966).

# GROUP A STREPTOCOCCI

## *MORPHOLOGY*

Streptococci are gram-positive, usually nonmotile cocci that are arranged in chains. Growth occurs by elongation on the axis parallel to the chain and division is at right angles in the equatorial plane. Whereas certain streptococci — that is, pneumococci and the oral streptococci — grow in pairs or relatively short chains in liquid medium, the hemolytic streptococci grow in longer chains. These do not elongate indefinitely, since in some cases the streptococci produce a "dechaining factor."

The most typical colonies of *S. pyogenes* are disk-like, matt (dull), and 0.5 to 2.0 mm in diameter. The matt colonies are derived from younger mucoid colonies whose hyaluronic acid capsules become dehydrated. If plate cultures are sealed to prevent dehydration, the colonies of group A streptococci remain mucoid. With loss of virulence the matt form reverts to small, smooth colonies with a dry, glistening surface or a typical rough colony.

When grown on blood agar, various streptococcal groups can modify hemoglobin. Thus, most *S. faecalis* species do not modify hemoglobin and no discrete zones are formed around colonies on blood agar. Most oral streptococci and pneumococci modify hemoglobin to green pigments (biliverdin and other heme compounds) and are designated $\alpha$-hemolytic, whereas most Lancefield groups A, B, C, and G streptococci (see below) produce a discrete clear zone of true hemolysis around the colonies; this is known as $\beta$-hemolysis. These characteristics greatly aid in a rapid preliminary screening of different streptococcal groups, but final classification depends on detailed biochemical, serologic, and genetic analysis of streptococci.

### L-forms

Protoplasts may be induced by penicillin or by the group C streptococcus phage-associated lysin and may be propagated on hypertonic media to produce L-forms (see Chapter 54). Removal of penicillin usually allows reversion to the parent strain. However, there are many stable L-form strains that are no longer capable of reversion. Certain L-forms can also be propagated in isotonic media. The role played by L-forms in disease or in the persistence of streptococci in tissues is not known (Ginsburg, 1972).

## *METABOLISM*

Streptococci are facultatively anaerobic, acidogenic, and acidophilic. Growth in media that lack body fluids is usually poor but it may be greatly enhanced by the addition of serum proteins and reducing agents in the form of sulfhydryl compounds. Most streptococci virulent for humans show an absolute demand for at least 12 amino acids, 3 purines and pyrimidines, 4 vitamins, certain divalent metals, and an energy source like glucose. Growth is sometimes enhanced by certain peptides (strepogenin).

Luxurious growth in fluid media always forms aggregates (floccules) that fall to the bottom, leaving a relatively clear supernatant fluid. Growth of bacteria in the submerged floccules is inhibited by lactic acid, which is formed from glucose by glycolysis. Excellent growth is usually obtained on brain heart infusion media or trypticase-soy broth. Growth is also facilitated by constant neutralization of the lactic acid and rich growth is achieved in a chemostat (steady-state culture) in a complete synthetic medium.

All streptococci ferment glucose, maltose, and most of them ferment lactose and sucrose. They all give a negative catalase reaction, since they all lack cytochrome systems. The major end product of fermentation is lactic acid. A most important characteristic of certain viridan streptococci (normal flora of the oral cavity) is the synthesis of polysaccharides from sucrose (dextrans) and fructose (levans). The mucoid appearance of streptococcal colonies grown on 5 per cent sucrose is used to classify these streptococci (Table 1). Certain streptococci liquify gelatin and about half of the *S. pyogenes* strains hydrolyze casein. Production of ammonia from arginine and hydrolysis of hippuric acid and esculin characterize certain streptococci that grow in the colon. Strong reducing activity (for example, early reduction of litmus

**TABLE 1.  Distinguishing Feature Among Members of
Viridans Group of Streptococci**

| SPECIES | LANCEFIELD GROUP ANTIGENS | LEVAN (L) OR DEXTRAN (D) FROM SUCROSE | Inulin | Raffinose | Salicin | Lactose | Trehalose |
|---------|---------------------------|---------------------------------------|--------|-----------|---------|---------|-----------|
| | | | | FERMENTATION OF | | | |
| *S. sanguis* | H | + (D) | ± | 0 | + | + | + |
| *S. salivarius* | K(?) | + (L) | + | + | + | ± | ± |
| *S. mitis* | O(?),N(?) | ∓ | 0 | ∓ | ± | ± | ∓ |
| *S. milleri* | A,C,F,G | 0 | ? | 0 | + | + | + |
| *S. anginosus* | F,G,L | 0 | ? | ± | + | + | + |
| *S. mutans* | none | + (D) | ? | ± | + | + | + |

± = usually +
∓ = rarely +
0  = never
?  = questionable

milk), black colonies on tetrazolium agar, and growth in media with high NaCl content and at high pH help identify *S. faecalis* species.

### Cell Wall Structure

The rigid cell of streptococci has several layers of a linear polymer that is composed of *N*-acetylglucosamine-*N*-acetylmuramic acid (the peptidoglycan, PPG) held together by peptide bridges (Wannamaker and Matsen, 1972) and forming a three-dimensional lattice. The PPG accounts for about 40 to 80 per cent of the wall. In most β-hemolytic strains the PPG is attached covalently to a surface polysaccharide, the C carbohydrate.

Many strains of hemolytic streptococci produce a prominent capsule in young cultures and is composed of hyaluronic acid in Group A streptococci. It is not immunogenic and is susceptible to streptococcal hyaluronidase.

Streptococci also possess characteristic surface polymers known as teichoic (TA) and teichuronic acids. These acids contain polyglycerol phosphate and alanine and are covalently linked to the PPG. Certain strains belonging to Lancefield's groups A, B, C, D, and G possess an immunoglobulin (Ig) receptor responsible for the interaction with the Fc fragment and possibly with the CH2 domain. This Ig receptor is heat labile and trypsin sensitive, and is probably responsible for the agglutination of streptococci by sera devoid of specific antistreptococcal antibodies. The IgG receptor is different from many known surface components of streptococci and its role in the biology of the streptococcus is unknown.

The cellular membrane, which is triple layered (75 to 90 Å), is composed of lipoprotein that differs in structure and content from that of L-forms. The cell membrane is attached by hydrophobic interaction with the glycolipid moiety of lipoteichoic acid (LTA). LTA consists of chains of polyglycerol phosphate units that may contain sugar or amino sugar substituents covalently linked to a glycolipid. The LTA extends through the width of the wall and appears on its surface. The LTA is haptenic when extracted from the streptococci by phenol, but is highly immunogenic when bound to the streptococcal cells. Although only a fraction of the LTA is spontaneously released into the medium during growth, the bulk of LTA may be released by phenol, lysozyme, extracts of human leukocytes, and a variety of cationic polyelectrolytes. Although LTA's function is not fully known, it is possible that, like M-protein, it is involved in the attachment of the streptococci to cell surfaces. LTA of all streptococci cross-react immunologically among themselves and with LTA of other gram-positive bacteria.

The cytoplasm of streptococci contains proteins (including enzymes) and nucleic acids. At least 11 distinct components have been detected in the cytoplasm. A high degree of antigenic heterogeneity is a particular characteristic of the nucleoprotein fraction.

### *ANTIGENIC COMPOSITION*

#### Group-Specific Carbohydrate

The work of Rebecca Lancefield laid the ground for the serologic classification of streptococci into at least 18 groups (A–R) on the basis of the group-specific carbohydrate, the "C carbohydrate." Groups A, B, and C "C carbohydrates" are composed of branched polymers. The carbohydrate is covalently linked to the PPG. They can be extracted with either hot formamide, hot TCA autoclaving, or enzymatic digestion with lysozyme and *Streptomyces albus* enzymes. The carbohydrate probably protects the peptidoglycan against lysozyme. It accounts for approximately 30 to 50 per cent of the dry weight of the cell wall and about 10 per cent of the intact cell, and may be found on both sides of the PPG. The polysaccharide of group A streptococci, which is composed of a terminal *N*-acetyl glucosamine (NAGA) and rhamnose, may be cleaved by *N*-acetylglucosaminidase of human macrophages. Upon cleavage of the terminal NAGA a structure known as the A-variant antigen is left; rhamnose is the antigenic determinant.

The group-specific antigen of Group D streptococci is a teichoic acid, not a carbohydrate, and it is a component of the cytoplasmic membrane, not of the cell wall.

### Type-Specific M-Proteins

These proteins are almost exclusively found in group A streptococci. M-proteins are surface antigens (Fox, 1974). They are responsible for the virulence of group A streptococci by virtue of their unique antiphagocytic characteristic and are lost when virulence is lost. The large M-protein complex contains hair-like structures (fimbria or pili) on the cell wall that are probably attached to it by covalent bonds. They are attachment structures for colonization of the susceptible patient. As protein antigens, they confer type specificity upon Group A streptococci; about 80 types are known. M-protein has been released from the streptococci by extraction with HCl, sonic oscillation, pepsin digestion; phage lysis, extraction with guanidine, and by nonionic detergents. The M-protein molecule has been purified. It is a heat- and acid-stable protein, soluble in alcohol, has a molecular weight of 40,000, and an isoelectric point of 5.3. It possesses multiple subunits, all having identical serologic activity. M-protein is susceptible to proteases, including streptococcal proteinase, which can prevent typing by digesting this antigen.

Until recently, all preparations of M-protein were contaminated with non–type-specific polypeptides. These strongly associated proteins give rise to non–type-specific antibodies and also elicit local and systemic hypersensitivity reactions. Beachey and his colleagues have separated M-protein from these contaminants and their preparation is both immunogenic and nontoxic.

### T Antigen

In addition to the type-specific M-protein, streptococci possess another set of protein antigens known as the T-system. The T-protein can be isolated by peptic, tryptic, or pancreatic digestion of heat-killed streptococci. It is protease-resistant, insoluble in alcohol, antigenic in the cell, and antigenic when cell free. It is not related to virulence, and antibodies against it are not protective. Some T-antigens are restricted to a single M-type whereas others may be shared by several M-types. The T-system is employed for typing those group A strains that either fail to synthesize M-

protein or to which no anti-M-type serum is available (see *Laboratory Diagnosis*).

### R Antigen

Certain types of group A streptococci possess R antigens that can also be found among groups B, C, G, and L streptococci. The antigen is a nonprotective protein that cross-reacts with grouping and typing antisera that contain antibodies to the R protein. This antigen is not commonly employed for classification and its biologic significance is still not known.

## PATHOGENETIC PROPERTIES

The most prominent pathogen for humans is *Streptococcus pyogenes* belonging to Lancefield's groups A and C (See also *Infections by Other Streptococci*). Pyogenic streptococci (Groups A and C) produce large amounts of extracellular products during growth in vitro in defined media or in human tissues. At least 25 different antigens are detected in concentrated culture supernatants by immunoelectrophoresis with pooled human γ-globin or rabbit sera hyperimmune to streptococcal extracellular products (Ginsburg, 1972). Only a few of these products have been identified, and a small number purified. Of the numerous factors elaborated by the Group A streptococcus, few have been implicated in the pathogenesis of tissue damage in animal models.

The major virulence factor of group A streptococci is the type-specific M-protein that deters phagocytosis. Whether the hyaluronic acid capsule also has significant antiphagocytic activity in natural infections is less certain.

Purified M-protein precipitates fibrinogen and interacts with fibrin lysates and fibrinomonomer complexes. It clumps platelets and leukocytes, it lyses PMN, and inhibits the migration of leukocytes in capillary tubes. The cytotoxic effect of M-protein requires both heat-stable and heat-labile serum factors, probably related to complement. It is highly immunogenic, and complexes of M-protein and antibodies can localize in the glomeruli and may be associated with glomerulonephritis (see below). M-positive strains can adhere to mucosal epithelial cells in vitro, whereas M-negative streptococci do not. The adherence of virulent streptococci to mucosal surfaces can be inhibited with type-specific antibody (including secretory IgA).

### Extracellular Toxins

Streptococcal infection is probably facilitated by extracellular products, some of which possess cytopathic properties (Ginsburg, 1972).

***Streptolysins.*** The majority of group A, C, and G streptococci elaborate two distinct hemolysins called Streptolysins O and S. The hemolytic zones around streptococcal colonies on blood agar, under aerobic conditions, are primarily due to streptolysin S (SLS). Both hemolysins are cytopathic for mammalian cells and block phagocytosis, presumably by impairing chemotaxis and ingestion by leukocytes and disrupting their lysosomes.

***Streptolysin O (SLO).*** This oxygen-labile protein antigen has a molecular weight of approximately 70,000. It is synthesized only by growing streptococci. It possesses a labile SH-group and is hemolytic or cytolytic only under reducing conditions. Its activity is strongly inhibited by cholesterol and other sterols. SLO is also cardiotoxic. It may cause interstitial myocarditis in experimental animals and systolic arrest of perfused mammalian hearts. Its cardiotoxicity is probably caused by inducing the release from atria of acetylcholine, which poisons the ventricles.

***Streptolysin S (SLS).*** This is an oxygen-stable nonantigenic peptide with a molecular weight of approximately 2800. It is synthesized by both growing and resting cells and is found on the surface of washed streptococcal cells as a cell-bound hemolysin. This loosely bound peptide can, however, be released into the surrounding medium by a variety of carrier molecules (for example, serum albumin, $\alpha$-lipoproteins, yeast RNA, and nonionic detergents like tweens and tritons). Upon release by the carriers, the hemolysin becomes recognized as SLS. Extracellular SLS is thus a complex between a nonspecific carrier molecule and the specific hemolytic peptide. The peptide can be transferred among the various carriers and finally to the surface of mammalian cells. After the interaction with membrane phospholipids the hemolytic peptide is inactivated. SLS activity is strongly inhibited by lecithin and $\beta$-lipoproteins but not by cholesterol. RBC treated with SLO show distinct "lesions" similar to those caused by complement; no such lesions have been shown to be induced by SLS. Upon intravenous injection, SLS causes necrosis of liver and kidney tubuli and massive intravascular hemolysis. It can induce a chronic arthritis when injected intraarticularly. Group A streptococci also possess an intracellular hemolysin with properties similar to SLS. This hemolysin can be released only after prolonged bacterial sonication (Ginsburg, 1972).

***Erythrogenic Toxin (ET).*** Most group A streptococci produce one (or more) of three immunologically distinct erythrogenic toxins (ET) known today as Streptococcal Pyrogenic Toxin (SPT), which were first described by the Dicks. In addition to causing fever and rash, SPT enhances susceptibility to lethal endotoxin shock, injures macrophages, alters antibody response to red blood cells, and is mitogenic for lymphocytes. SPT has been purified and crystallized from culture supernatant fluid of certain streptococcal strains. It has $1 \times 10^7$ rabbit skin doses per 20/mg N and a molecular weight of approximately 29,000. It contains 80 per cent protein and hyaluronic acid; the latter probably acts as a carrier and is not associated with toxicity. The symptoms of scarlet fever are believed due to both the primary toxicity of SPT and the secondary effects of hypersensitivity; the typical scarlatinal rash is due to the latter. The role, if any, played by SPT in the pathogenesis of streptococcal infections and their sequelae is not established. SPT is probably produced under the direction of a temperate phage (Wannamaker and Matsen, 1972).

***Proteinase.*** Most group A streptococci elaborate an SH-dependent proteinase precursor (M.W. = 44,000), which can be converted to an active proteinase by reducing agents and by proteases. Proteinase paradoxically destroys M-protein. This protease acts on several naturally-occurring proteins as well as on some synthetic substrates. The intravenous injection of reduced proteinase causes massive myocardial and skeletal muscle necrosis in rabbits. It is immunogenic and the specific antibodies that develop neutralize the proteolytic activity of this enzyme. Its role in the pathogenesis of streptococcal infections is not known.

***Streptokinase (SK).*** Most group A and C strains produce SK, an activator of the fibrinolytic system of human blood. SK is a protein with a molecular weight of approximately 47,000. It converts a proactivator present in plasma to an activator, which converts plasminogen to the proteolytic enzyme, plasmin. Plasmin splits fibrinogen, fibrin, and other proteins. A small amount of plasmin activates more plasminogen. SK may be a virulence factor of streptococci by lysing blood clots and fibrin precipitates. Together with hyaluronidase and the nucleases it may function as a "spreading factor" (see below). Preparations of SK have been widely employed for debriding surface infections, for enhancement of wound healing, for treatment of fibrinous exudates, and for the lysis of intravascular thrombi.

***The Spreading Factors.*** Several extracellular products of streptococci are regarded as "spreading factors" because they promote spread of streptococci in tissues by liquifying and reducing the viscosity of inflammatory exudates. Group A strains elaborate hyaluronidase, four serologic varieties of deoxyribonucleases (A, B, C, and D), and a ribonuclease. All these enzymes are immunogenic.

***Nicotinamide adenine dinucleotide glycohydrolase (NADG).*** Some strains belonging to groups A, C, and G elaborate NADG. At one time this enzyme was thought to be associated with leukotoxicity of streptococci, presumably because of its ability to affect leukocyte metabolism. Now it is believed that leukotoxicity is due to cell-bound SLS. The role of NADG in pathogenicity of streptococci is not known. Production of NADG by streptococci is sometimes used in serologic differentiation of certain strains (see below).

*Cardiohepatic Toxin (CHT).* Injection of viable group A streptococci into tonsils is followed within 24 hours by interstitial myocarditis of rabbits with granulomatous lesions in the myocardium of some animals that resemble Aschoff bodies.

An active principle isolated from supernatant culture fluids of group A streptococci, called "cardiohepatic toxin," causes myocardial and diaphragmatic lesions in rabbits similar to those induced by tonsilar infection. It also produces giant cell granulomas in the liver. Animals injected with CHT develop hyperlipemia and high blood levels of glutamicoxaloacetic transaminase, sorbitol-dehydrogenase, and creatine phosphokinase. The chemical nature of CHT is not known.

### Cell-Associated Toxins

*Peptidoglycan-Polysaccharide Complexes (PPGPS).* Although streptococci are killed after phagocytosis by PMN and macrophages, intracellular digestion (degradation) of their cell walls is extremely slow. It is claimed that mammalian cells lack specific enzymes capable of degrading streptococcal wall components. The extreme resistance to degradation is due either to the C-polysaccharide or to the presence on the cell surface of teichoic acid, which hinders the interaction of lysozyme with the PPG.

Cell-wall components of group A streptococci persist for many months within macrophages in granulomatous lesions in the heart, synovium, and liver of laboratory animals. Since the persistence of cell wall components within macrophages leads to secretion of lysosomal enzymes, it was postulated that enzyme secretion initiated these chronic lesions (Davies et al., 1974; Ginsburg and Sela, 1976).

Undegraded streptococcal cell-wall components have also been shown to localize selectively in tissue sites remote from the original focus of infection after transport within phagocytic cells. Several investigators suggest that the pathogenesis of rheumatic fever may be associated with the localization and persistence of undegraded PPGPS in the cardiac muscle (Ginsburg and Sela, 1976). Wall components of streptococci may also activate complement.

BIOLOGIC PROPERTIES OF PEPTIDOGLYCANS (PPG). Isolated and partially purified PPG can cause the following: fever, the localized Shwartz-

man reaction, nonspecific resistance to infections, enhancement of lesions induced by pyogenic bacteria, enhanced immunologic response to other antigens (adjuvant effect), inhibition of macrophage migration, tumor inhibition, impaired phagocytosis by PMN, activation of complement, and lysis of platelets. Undegraded complexes of PPG and other polysaccharide moieties have induced granulomatous inflammation in the skin, heart, joints, and liver of laboratory animals. It appears that the size of the PPG molecule and its association with the naturally occurring polysaccharide moiety of the cell wall is of utmost importance for the expression of toxicity, immunogenicity, and persistence in tissues. The probability that different individuals may degrade streptococcal cell walls to different entities may explain the enigma that poststreptococcal sequelae affect only certain patients (see below).

*Lipoteichoic Acid (LTA).* This membrane-associated haptene can sensitize mammalian cells to lysis in the presence of antistreptococcal IgM antibodies and complement. LTA can cause chronic arthritis after intraarticular injection into animals preimmunized with group A streptococci. It can cause resorption of bone (via cyclic AMP and prostaglandins) in culture and nephrocalcinosis in laboratory animals. LTA is the adherence factor that accounts for the affinity of streptococci for mucous membranes. Both LTA and M-protein, which had been thought to be the adherence factor, are components of the hairy fibrils on the surface of the streptococcus. The nature of the epithelial cell receptor is unknown except that it is trypsin sensitive.

## SEQUELAE OF ACUTE STREPTOCOCCAL INFECTIONS

A unique characteristic of group A streptococci is their ability to induce nonsuppurative sequelae in susceptible individuals. These are rheumatic fever (RF), chorea, and acute glomerulonephritis (AGN) and they may follow overt or inapparent infections. The onset of these complications may start two to three weeks after infection. The common denominator among these diverse late complications of Group A streptococcal infections is the failure to isolate living streptococci from the affected tissue. The failure to duplicate these sequelae in lower animals has hampered research into the pathogenesis of these syndromes. Our present concepts are based on circumstantial evidence and no mechanism can be considered proved or accepted by most investigators in this field.

There are several absolute requirements for the development of rheumatic carditis and arthritis.

First, group A streptococci must have been present; second, the infection must be localized in the upper respiratory tract; third, the bacteria must persist for complication to occur; and fourth, a streptococcal antibody response indicative of a recent infection must be known.

The importance of the site of infection for the development of RF has been stressed; many observations suggest that RF does not develop after streptococcal infection of the skin. The factors that localize streptococci to the throat are not fully understood, but M-protein and LTA are both implicated in anchoring streptococci to the surface of epithelial cells.

### Current Theories of Pathogenesis

The numerous theories proposed to explain how group A streptococci initiate sequelae fall under several headings: (Wannamaker and Matsen, 1972; Ginsburg, 1972; Stollerman, 1975; Glynn, 1975) (a) The "rheumatic" toxin; (b) autoimmunity and immunopathology; (c) genetic and anatomic abberations; (d) a combination of these theories.

*Is There a "Rheumatic Toxin"?* Several extracellular substances elaborated by group A streptococci can induce myocardial, endocardial, hepatic, articular, and renal lesions in laboratory animals (see above). As a rule, none of the lesions fully resemble the human lesions of RF, and no clinical manifestations similar to those seen in humans have been duplicated in the animals. Undegraded peptidoglycan-polysaccharide complexes (PPGPS) of the cell wall have produced rheumatic-like granulomatous lesions in mice and rabbits. Another approach suggests that in early streptococcal pharyngitis certain susceptible patients develop acute myocardial and articular injuries explainable by diffusible "toxins." None of the "toxic" theories have been based on firm ground and all data have been obtained from experimental models (Wannamaker and Matsen, 1972; Ginsburg, 1972; Glynn, 1975; Ginsburg and Sela, 1976).

*Immunopathology and Autoimmunity.* Several investigations have proposed that complexes formed between streptococcal products and autologous antibodies (for example, SLO–anti-SLO complexes) may localize in tissues and damage them by activating complement (serum sickness type), or through cell-mediated immunity (CMI). Sensitized T lymphocytes may then interact with streptococcal antigens to cause the release of lymphokines. Cell-sensitizing agents (lipoteichoic acids) have also been implicated in tissue damage. These agents can sensitize mammalian cells to passive lysis in the presence of antistreptococcal antibodies and complement. This theory suffers from lack of evidence for the localization of streptococcal antigens in the heart or in joint lesions.

The theory of autoimmunity gained favor because substances in mammalian cardiac tissue can act as autoantigens and because certain streptococcal toxins can release such antigens. However, the theories implicating autoimmunity in RF have been stated only in general terms, with no focus on precise mechanisms, and have been overshadowed by theories implicating immunologic cross-reaction between streptococcal antigens and components of mammalian tissues.

The phenomenon of crossed immunity between mammalian and bacterial constituents (the concept of molecular mimicry) is well established (Kaplan, 1976; Zabriskie, 1976). Several antigens in group A streptococcal cell walls and protoplast membrane have been isolated. These cross-react with glycoproteins of the heart valves, sarcolemma of cardiac and skeletal muscle, bundle of His, glycoprotein of glomerular basement membrane, human fibroblasts, endothelial cells, astrocytes, cytoplasm of subthalamic and caudate nuclei, and histocompatibility antigens (Kaplan 1976; Zabriskie, 1976). Despite the presence in human sera of cross-reactive antibodies and their elution from myocardium of patients with RF there is no evidence that such antibodies have any relationship to the lesions of rheumatic fever. It is interesting that no bound cross-reactive globulin is found in Aschoff bodies. There is no evidence that the cross-reactive antibodies are cytotoxic to mammalian cells.

*Genetic and Anatomic Abberations.* Certain investigators claim that the "rheumatic patient" may possess direct anatomic routes (probably lymphatic channels) that connect the tonsils with the heart. It is proposed that through such channels streptococci, streptococcal L-forms, and their diffusible extracellular products (toxins) and undegraded cell-wall components may freely migrate and localize in the heart to cause tissue damage (Wannamaker, 1973). Others favor the theory that the rheumatic patient is predetermined genetically to develop abnormal cellular and humoral responses to streptococcal antigens (Zabriskie, 1976).

### Arthritis

Migratory arthritis is part of the rheumatic syndrome. The similarity of the tissue alterations in the joints of rheumatic patients to those induced experimentally by anaphylactic and delayed hypersensitivity reactions suggest that the human joint disease may be caused by such mechanisms. As a rule, neither viable streptococci nor their extracellular or cellular constituents are found within the inflamed joints. A decrease in both early and late components of complement within the synovial fluid of RF patients suggest local activation by immune complexes. Although the streptococcus antigen that could be present in these complexes has not been identified, this phenomenon may point to the mechanism of arthritis in rheumatic fever. Arthritic lesions can be induced in laboratory animals by the intra-articular injection of Streptolysin S, by a pool of extracellular products, by soluble cell wall components, by L-forms, and by lipoteichoic acid (LTA) (Ginsburg et al., 1977).

## Acute Glomerulonephritis (AGN)

One of the most common complications of upper respiratory and skin infections with group A streptococci is AGN. It is an old observation that acute RF and AGN rarely, if ever, occur in the same person at the same time (Stollerman, 1975). AGN is probably caused by special nephritogenic strains. The pharyngeal M-types 12, 14, and 49 and a family of "impetigo" streptococcal strains belonging to the following serologic complexes: T-3/13/B3264/12 (related to the M serotypes (22, 33, 39, 41, 43, 52, 56); T8/25/Dmp19(M-types 2, 8, 25, 55, 57, 58); and T5/11/12/27/44 (M-types 11, 59, 61) are all associated with AGN. The latter pyodermia strains were previously unrecognized owing to lack of specific antisera for typing them. The factors elaborated by these skin strains, which endow them with nephritogenicity, is not understood. Furthermore, in spite of the detailed serologic, epidemiologic, and renal morphologic studies, the pathogenesis of nephritis remains unknown. The theories regarding pathogenesis of AGN can be summarized under four main headings and are based primarily on experimental models (Ginsburg, 1972).

*The Nephrotoxin.* Streptococcal agents like Streptolysin S, M-protein, autolysates of nephritogenic streptococci, extracts of streptococcal cell walls, solubilized protoplast membranes, and undefined diffusible agents released by certain nephritogenic streptococci (nephrotoxin) can cause renal disease in laboratory animals but not the full spectrum of clinical and pathologic changes seen in humans.

*Immunologic Cross-Reactivity.* Cross-reactive antigens between soluble components of glomerular basement membranes are chemically and immunologically similar to antigens of protoplast membranes of nephritogenic streptococci. Antibodies to protoplast membranes can cause glomerular lesions.

*Autoantibody.* Extracts of kidneys that had been mixed with streptococci were claimed to give rise to nephrotoxic antibodies. Although this theory was favored by several investigators, the results were controversial and could not be duplicated in several other laboratories.

*Immune Complex Disease.* Immunofluorescent and electron microscopic analysis of kidneys obtained from patients with AGN showed localized immune complexes and complement in the glomeruli. The nature of the antigenic substance in these complexes and its possible relationship to streptococci is still controversial. It has also been suggested that immune complexes can be obtained when streptococcal enzymes modify the chemical composition of IgG; the altered IgG then interacts with autoantibodies that recognize both native and altered globulin. Such complexes can cause glomerular lesions.

Despite the numerous models established, none are satisfactory analogs to the human disease (Wannamaker and Matsen, 1972).

*Immunity.* Infections with group A streptococci that possess M-antigen are usually followed by a type-specific humoral immunity. If the anti-M antibodies disappear, they can be recalled by small booster doses of homologous M antigen. The anti-M antibodies are mainly IgG. They appear slowly (over 30 to 60 days) and are opsonins (Stollerman, 1975). None of the antibodies that are regularly produced against C-polysaccharide, T antigen, teichoic acid, or the numerous extracellular enzymes and other factors can prevent infection. Type-specific antibody can be detected by opsonization, mouse protection, or chain elongation in vitro. These tests are difficult to perform in a routine bacteriologic laboratory.

### Streptococcal Vaccine

Since the immunity to Group A streptococci is type-specific, and since about 80 types are known to be present in different populations, the rationale for preparing an adequate vaccine depends on the distribution of the major M-types in a particular population. Immunization, if available, should aim to prevent both suppurative and nonsuppurative complications. The preparation of a vaccine should also take into consideration the risk of inducing delayed hypersensitivity reactions, the elimination from the M-protein of antigens cross-reactive with heart, and the elimination from M-protein of covalently bound lipoteichoic acid (LTA). Preliminary field trials have used M-protein in alum given either subcutaneously (Sc) or intrapharyngeally. The patients were then challenged by smearing the homologous M-types on their tonsils. Seventy-five per cent of the subjects immunized revealed a primary opsonic response to the vaccine with no reactions. Although the parenteral immunization did not prevent colonization of the throat, it protected against clinical illness. The main questions to be answered are these: how many serologic types warrant inclusion in the vaccine; how often do prevalent M-types change under natural circumstances; and how much variation in prevalence of specific M-types is there in different parts of the world.

Recent experiments have been conducted on a vaccine against dental caries by employing strains of *S. mutans*. Monkeys injected with this streptococcus developed antibodies that could be detected in gingival fluid. Such antibodies (mostly IgG) may be responsible for the substantial decrease in the incidence of cervical caries but had no effect on the incidence of carious lesions on smooth surfaces (Lehner et al., 1976).

### Pneumococcal Vaccine

See section of *S. pneumoniae*.

## *LABORATORY DIAGNOSIS*

### Tests for Streptococcal Antibodies

Antibodies against streptolysin O, streptokinase, hyaluronidase DNase-B, NADase, and proteinase are routinely measured to diagnose recent streptococcal infections. Proof of a streptococcal infection is based, in part, upon an increase in one or more of these antibodies. Although antistreptolysin O (ASO) titration in patients' sera is the most common test, it is often advantageous to measure other antistreptococcal antibodies. The streptozyme test is a two-minute slide hemagglutination procedure that quantitatively measures multiple antibody (A-STZ) to streptococcal extracellular products. The reagents are sheep RBC sensitized simultaneously with streptolysin-O, deoxyribonuclease-B, hyaluronidase, streptokinase, and nicotinamide adenine dinucleotide glycohydrolase. A-STZ correlates well with ASO in the sera of rheumatic fever patients. Moreover, it has been found that the A-STZ test detects a higher incidence of elevated antistreptococcal antibodies than does one ASO test. The specificity of the test (no antibodies to cellular elements of streptococci are detected with this reagent), its high reproducibility, the ease of performance, and the minimal quantities of patient serum required indicate that the test is helpful in estimating antibody response to streptococcal infection whenever the performance of a battery of tests for individual antibodies is impractical and expensive.

### Culture of Group A Streptococci

For the diagnosis of a group A streptococcal infection, the Streptococcus must be isolated and identified. Specimens must be transported to the laboratory without delay, because cotton swabs may contain substances that inhibit group A streptococci. Viability is well maintained in swabs transported in a silica-gel. Use of enrich-ment media (for example, Pike's broth) increases the isolation rate of Group A streptococci compared with direct plating on blood agar. The growth on blood agar is screened for complete ($\beta$) hemolysis. Sheep blood is preferred because it inhibits the growth of *Hemophilus hemolyticus,* a $\beta$-hemolytic saprophyte commonly found in the throat. Overgrowth of other microorganisms can be prevented by various selective agents in the media. Group A streptococci can be tentatively identified, rapidly and easily, with bacitracin disks. About 90 per cent of Group A streptococci are inhibited by disks containing 0.04 unit of bacitracin, whereas most Group B, C, and G streptococci are resistant. Definitive identification is made by demonstrating the C carbohydrate of Group A by immunofluorescence with group-specific antiserum, or by precipitin tests with C carbohydrate extracted from the bacteria.

## *DRUG SUSCEPTIBILITY*

Unlike staphylococci, no group A streptococcus strain has been resistant to penicillin. This makes penicillin the drug of choice in the treatment of streptococcal infections and in prevention of rheumatic fever. The MIC for penicillin G is usually 0.001 $\mu$g/ml. About 40 per cent of strains are resistant to tetracycline and sulfadiazine. Resistance to erythromycin is uncommon and is mediated by a plasmid. Streptococci are resistant to polymyxins, kanamycin, and streptomycin.

## *EPIDEMIOLOGY*

### Upper Respiratory Infections

Understanding of the pathogenesis of streptococcal infections, its nonsuppurative sequelae, and its epidemiology depends on the distinction between a "carrier" state and acute streptococcal upper respiratory infection. Group A streptococci cultured from acute sore throats contain large amounts of M-protein. Pharyngitis and tonsillitis occur most frequently in children from 5 to 15 years of age. It is unlikely for a child to reach the age of ten without having encountered the Group A streptococcus.

Transmission occurs via droplets from respiratory secretion of patients or from healthy carriers. Both food and milk may be sources for occasional outbreaks. Organisms recovered from clothing, bed, or house dust are usually noninfective. Control of hemolytic streptococcal disease is difficult because many infections are either exceedingly mild or inapparent, and persons with subclinical infections can disseminate streptococci. Overcrowding allows the explosive spread of single serotypes, especially among civilians.

Peak incidence occurs between December and May in temperate zones.

## Pyoderma

Occurrence is usually confined to the summer and early fall in hot and tropical climates. It mostly affects preschool children and infants. Transmission may be aided by insects. Poverty, filth, and overcrowding are major predisposing factors. The same streptococcus type is often found in throats and in pyoderma lesions.

## PREVENTION

Infections with Group A streptococci may be prevented by therapeutic intervention during epidemics or by prophylactic drugs given to those at high risk, such as in boarding schools, orphanages, and military camps in which infections are endemic. Immunization with M-protein has been tested on a relatively small scale and was found to be effective, but the use of vaccine in general or in selected population needs to be explored (see above). Impetigo may be prevented by improved skin hygiene. Epidemics are best halted by antibiotic treatment of all cases.

# OTHER β-HEMOLYTIC STREPTOCOCCI PATHOGENIC FOR HUMANS

## ANTIGENIC STRUCTURE

### Group B Streptococci (Streptococcus agalactiae)

Group B streptococci contain as a major constituent of the cell wall, a group-specific carbohydrate (C-substance) composed of rhamnose, N-acetylglucosamine, and galactose. L-rhamnose is the significant component of the antigenic determinant. The capsule antigen (S-substance) can serve to classify further the group into four serologic separate and distinct types, Ia, Ib, II, and III. A fifth type, Ic, contains the Ia carbohydrate antigen plus a protein antigen. Both human and bovine strains are found in all these types but with different frequencies.

### Groups C and G streptococci (S. equisimilis, S. zooepidemicus, S. equi, S. dysgalactiae)

These differ from group A by causing neither glomerulonephritis nor rheumatic fever and by possessing a group-specific carbohydrate polymer of L-rhamnose and NAGA (in group C) and galactose, galactosamine, and rhamnose (group G). Neither group contains type-specific protein antigens like the M-protein of group A.

### Group D streptococci (S. faecalis-enterococci, S. faecium, S. durans, S. bovis, S. equinus)

The Group D antigen is unique among the streptococci in that it is a glycerol teichoic acid containing D-alanine and glucose, is probably located in the region of the wall, and may not be linked through a primary bond with the wall components. The type-specific antigen is a cell-wall carbohydrate that is composed of D-glucose and NAGA and that also contains rhamnose. In order to preserve the type-specific antigens of Group D streptococci, they must be released from the cells not by the routine hot HCl method but by lysozyme or by lytic or autolytic enzymes.

## METABOLISM

Carbohydrate metabolism is chiefly homofermentative in all these groups. Glucose is fermented to lactic acid. An oxidative pathway also can be utilized by S. agalactiae, which yields lactic acid, acetic acid, acetylmethylcarbenol, and carbon dioxide. A noncytochrome iron-containing chromophore appears to be utilized, and oxygen is the terminal electron receptor in this reaction.

## PATHOGENIC PROPERTIES

S. agalactiae (Group B) has long been recognized as an important bovine pathogen. Recently it has been recognized as a frequent cause of meningitis and pneumonia in neonates (Patterson and Hafeez, 1976). Meningitis is caused almost exclusively by type III, and pneumonia by type Ia. Sporadic infections in adults show no type predilection. The explanation for the organotropism in infants of these two serotypes is obscure. Nevertheless, the type-specific antigens are the most important virulence factors known. *S. agalactiae* produces a hemolysin distinct from streptolysins O and S and a hyaluronidase, but their pathogenic significance is unknown. Group C streptococci have a hyaluronic acid capsule that deters phagocytosis. Many Group C and G strains produce streptolysin O, but its pathogenic significance is as uncertain for these groups as it is for Group A streptococci.

## IMMUNITY

It has been shown in mice that antibody to the type-specific antigens of *S. agalactiae* is protective. Furthermore, transplacental passage of antibody to capsular type III protects newborns from Group B streptococcal meningitis. Both type-specific antibody and a heat labile component (presumably complement) are opsonic for type Ia strains. Most maternal sera and cord sera lack opsonins for that strain. Leukocytes from neonates have diminished bactericidal activity for Group B streptococci but this defect is probably not specific for these bacteria.

## LABORATORY IDENTIFICATION

Non–Group A hemolytic streptococci are usually distinguished from Group A by their resistance to an 0.04 unit bacitracin disk. However, because up to 5 per cent of Group A streptococci are also resistant and a like percentage of other Groups are sensitive, this is not a definitive test. β-Hemolytic streptococci are identified with specific antibody against the C carbohydrate. It is often difficult to identify the Group D strains by this reaction and they are identified by their hydrolysis of esculin in the presence of 40 per cent bile (Table 2). Group D streptococci are divided into enterococci (including *S. faecalis, S. faecium, S. zymogenes*) and nonenterococcal species (*S. bovis, S. equinis*).

This distinction, which is based on their ability to grow in hypertonic salt media, has therapeutic implications. Group B strains hydrolyze hippurate and produce a soluble hemolysin that acts synergistically with the β-hemolysis of *Staphylococcus aureus* (CAMP phenomenon).

## DRUG SUSCEPTIBILITY

β-Hemolytic streptococci, other than Group D, are uniformly susceptible to less than 1.0 unit/ml of penicillin G. Ninety per cent are also susceptible to erythromycin and clindamycin, but up to 50 per cent of recently isolated strains of Group B are resistant to tetracycline. Nonenterococcal Group D streptococci are also susceptible to penicillin, but enterococci are much less so. Enterococci are somewhat more susceptible to ampicillin than to penicillin G and show variable susceptibilities to chloramphenicol, tetracycline, and erythromycin. They are susceptible to vancomycin. Synergism between penicillin and aminoglycoside antibiotics is important in the treatment of enterococcal endocarditis. The combination is bactericidal in concentrations of each drug that are only one tenth that required to kill the enterococcus when either acts alone.

## EPIDEMIOLOGY

Group B, C, and G streptococci are often isolated from the nasopharynx. Group D predominates in the gastrointestinal tract, but as many as 30 per cent of normal people have Group B streptococci in their feces. Group B streptococci can also be isolated from the genital tract of 30 per cent of normal women. Neonatal colonization with Group B streptococci is common, but the risk of disease is probably less than 5 per cent. Serotype III Group B streptococci are often acquired by infants in the nursery as well as in utero or at delivery. These bacteria may spread from infant to infant or from nurses to infants, because many nurses may be colonized.

**TABLE 2.   Reactions That are Useful for the Differentiation of Several Groups of Streptococci**

| GROUP | HEMOLYSIS | BACITRACIN SENSITIVITY | HIPPURATE | ESCULIN | 6.5% NaCl | CAMP |
|---|---|---|---|---|---|---|
| A | β | + | − | − | − | − |
| B | β | − | + | − | + | + |
| D enterococci | α, β | − | − | + | + | − |
| D nonenterococci | − | − | − | + | − | − |

# THE VIRIDANS GROUP

This is a heterogenous group of very poorly defined α-hemolytic organisms that are commonly found in the mouth and pharynx. About 50 per cent of bacterial endocarditis is caused by these bacteria. Since they do not have a defined group carbohydrate antigen, no correlation exists between serologic and physiologic characteristics of these strains.

## MORPHOLOGY

Viridans streptococci usually form a narrow zone of α-hemolysis around their pinhead colonies. No exotoxins or hydrolytic enzymes similar to those produced by pyogenic streptococci are found in culture supernatants. Several of the streptococci elaborate a constitutive extracellular glycosyltransferase and fructosyltransferase responsible for the synthesis from sucrose of large capsules of dextran and levan respectively. Certain of the streptococci also accumulate intracellular polysaccharides of the amylopectin type.

Their cell wall structure is essentially that of the pyogenic streptococci. They possess peptidoglycan, wall teichoic acid, and membrane-associated lipoteichoic acid.

## METABOLISM

Viridans streptococci resemble pneumococci both culturally and in Gram stains, but unlike pneumococci they do not possess well-developed autolytic systems and are not lysed by bile salts. The viridans streptococci are fastidious and grow luxuriantly only in heart infusion broth or in media rich in protein. They are microaerophilic and acidophilic, and the major product of fermentation is lactic acid. This heterogenous group can, however, be classified by its ability to ferment inulin, raffinose, salicin, lactose, and trehalose, and to release ammonia from arginine. The most common species recognized are *S. salivarius, S. milleri, S. M. G. (anginosus), S. mitis, S. sanguis,* and *S. mutans* (Table 1).

## PATHOGENIC PROPERTIES

### Dental Caries

Four recognized species, *S. sanguis, S. mitis, S. salivarius,* and *S. mutans,* are associated with dental caries in humans, rats, and in monkeys. *S. mutans* appears to be the most virulent and is the only species recognized that consistently initiates decay affecting smooth enamel surfaces. This pathogenic potential is probably related to its ability to adhere and accumulate on the surface of the teeth and to form large bacterial plaque deposits. It can synthesize high molecular weight dextrans and other glucans from sucrose but not from other sugars. The extracellular polysaccharides enable them to adhere to surfaces. It has the unique property of aggregating in the presence of very small amounts of high molecular weight dextran, indicating the presence on its surface of specific receptors. Small fragments of dextran prevent plaque formation and tooth decay in laboratory animals presumably by functioning as glucosyl acceptors for dextransucrase, thereby inhibiting synthesis of high molecular weight polymers.

Dental caries may be looked upon as an infectious disease and studies with monoinfected gnotobiotic animals show that *S. mutans* can spread among members of hamster or rat colonies, colonize the mouth, and induce carious lesions in animals fed high sucrose diets. Thus, the unique combination of streptococci, sucrose, and tooth surface are prerequisite for the initiation of caries.

### Bacterial Endocarditis

Most strains of viridans streptococci can adhere to human heart valves. The chemical nature of the receptors has not been identified.

# STREPTOCOCCUS PNEUMONIAE (PNEUMOCOCCUS)

The pneumococcus is a *Streptococcus* that forms α-hemolytic zones on blood agar and readily undergoes spontaneous autolysis. It causes pneumococcal pneumonia, septicemia, and meningitis.

## MORPHOLOGY

The cell is characteristically ovoid or lanceolate and is usually arranged in pairs, but chains are also present in infected secretions and in cultures.

Pneumococci grow well on meat infusions supplemented with serum or blood under reducing conditions. Pneumococcal colonies are 1 mm in diameter, raised, smooth, and circular. Type 3 strains grow as larger mucoid colonies. When autolysis occurs, the center of the pneumococcal colony becomes depressed. Growth in the presence of antiserum may yield chains of unencapsulated variants that produce small, granular, rough colonies.

## ANTIGENIC STRUCTURE

About 82 pneumococcal types are recognized. Typing is based on variation of the chemical composition of the capsular polysaccharide. Eighty per cent of strains isolated from cases of lobar pneumonia in adults fall into types 1 to 8.

The different types of capsular polysaccharides differ serologically and chemically. Thus, the polysaccharide antigen of Type 1 pneumococci contains galacturonic acid, galactose, fucose, and glucosamine; that of type 2 contains rhamnose, glucose, and glucuronic acid; type 3 is a polymer of cellobiuronic acid that consists of alternate residues of glucose and glucuronic acid. The isolated capsular polysaccharides are immunogenic in man and mice, but not in horses or in rabbits unless they are injected with a protein carrier. Human beings injected with 30 to 60 $\mu$g of pneumococcal polysaccharide produce antibodies that protect them against pneumonia.

Some capsular surface polysaccharides cross-react immunologically with other α-hemolytic streptococci, with capsular polysaccharides of *Klebsiella* or *Salmonella,* and with blood group substances. The capsule swells when reacting with specific antibodies (the Quellung reaction). The cell wall of pneumococci is composed of a peptidoglycan similar in structure to the group A streptococci. In addition, a carbohydrate C-substance is present that reacts with C-reactive protein, a protein that appears in the blood during acute inflammatory conditions. The pneumococcal cell wall also contains choline, which forms part of the wall teichoic acid. The key role of choline in susceptibility to lysis by bile salts and penicillin is evident when pneumococci are grown in the presence of ethanolamine instead of choline. With ethanolamine they form chains and are no longer solubilized by bile salts nor lysed by penicillin. The choline-containing lipoteichoic acid is a powerful inhibitor of the homologous autolytic enzyme N-acetylmuramyl-L-alinine amidase and is lost from the cell in the presence of penicillin so that autolysis is no longer inhibited. The C-substance may be identical with the wall teichoic acid. Pneumococci also possess protein antigens similar to the streptococcal M-proteins, but unlike the streptococcus this pneumococcal protein antigen is not associated with virulence.

## LABORATORY DIAGNOSIS

*Streptococcus pneumoniae* is bile soluble and inhibited by optochin (ethylhydrocuprine). The nutritional requirements are complex, but they can be grown readily on infusion agars supplemented with 5 per cent blood. The white mouse is exquisitely sensitive to many pneumococcal types (type 14 is a notable exception) and pneumococci are isolated from sputum by injecting it intraperitoneally into a mouse. The mouse will eliminate other bacteria but die from pneumococcal septicemia and its heart blood will contain only pneumococci. This is the most sensitive way of isolating the pneumococcus from sputums, but it is rarely necessary if blood agar is inoculated and the growth examined with a dissecting microscope. Acid is formed from lactose, sucrose, trehalose, and raffinose and the fermentation of inulin is considered a diagnostic characteristic.

Pure cultures are identified as *S. pneumoniae* by capsular swelling. A diagnostic reagent,

"Omni-serum," which contains antibodies to all 82 capsular polysaccharides, has been employed for rapid identification (obtained from Statens Serum Institut, Copenhagen, Denmark). This serum can also be used to identify by counterimmunoelectrophoresis (CIE) capsular polysaccharide in the blood and urine of patients with pneumonia and the cerebrospinal fluid (CSF) of patients with meningitis. The CIE technique gives rapid diagnosis and identifies pneumococcal infection in patients whose CSF has been sterilized by antibiotics.

## PATHOGENICITY

The capsular polysaccharide makes the pneumococcus virulent. Like the M-protein of group A streptococci, this surface polysaccharide deters phagocytosis by both polymorphonuclear leukocytes and macrophages. On the other hand, decapsulated pneumococci or encapsulated organisms opsonized with specific antibodies are readily taken up by phagocytes. Complement may also be opsonic for some types, even in the absence of specific antibody. Solubilized polysaccharide may overcome host resistance by binding with circulating antibodies. The polysaccharide, being resistant to degradation by host enzymes, may also contribute to immune paralysis by overwhelming the mononuclear phagocytic system. The polysaccharide may thus remain within phagocytic cells for the life of the animal without inciting an inflammatory response. "Surface phagocytosis" is a phenomenon in which encapsulated pneumococci can be phagocytosed when trapped by phagocytes in vitro on rough surfaces. Its role, if any, in the phagocytosis of encapsulated pneumococci in the alveoli has not been established.

No pneumococcal toxin is known to be definitely related to pathogenicity. Upon washing and autolysis, pneumococci release a cell-bound lysin that is antigenically related to streptolysin O. A neuraminidase, which cleaves terminal N-acetyl-neuraminic acid from glycoprotein substrates on cell membranes, may be involved in the neurotoxicity of meningeal infections. In the presence of immunoglobulin, platelets are aggregated by heat-killed bacteria; this may play a role in the pathogenesis of disseminated intravascular coagulation seen in severe infections. It is believed that lethality depends entirely on the ability of the organism to grow extracellularly and that toxins are not significant lethal factors.

## DRUG SUSCEPTIBILITY

Although most pneumococci are susceptible to less than 0.03 $\mu$g/ml penicillin G, acquired resistance to this antibiotic has been described in South Africa, New Guinea, and elsewhere. Tetracycline, erythromycin, and vancomycin resistance have also been reported. Multiple drug resistance, not associated with $\beta$-lactamase production, has also been described (see Chapter 21).

## EPIDEMIOLOGY

Infection with pneumococci occurs through droplets released from infected patients. Whether or not soiled clothing and blankets can serve as infective material has not been established. There is no animal reservoir. Intrafamily spread and asymptomatic infection occurs frequently, especially in association with viral upper respiratory infections.

### References

Davies, P., Page, R. C., and Allison, A. C.: Changes in cellular enzyme levels and extracellular release of lysosomal acid hydrolases in macrophages exposed to group A streptococcal cell wall substance. J Exp Med 139:1962, 1974.

Fox, E. N.: M Proteins of group A streptococci. Bact Rev 38:57, 1974.

Ginsburg, I.: Mechanism of cell and tissue injury induced by group A Streptococci: Relation to poststreptococcal sequelae. J Infect Dis 126:294, 1972.

Ginsburg, I., and Sela, M. N.: The role of leukocytes and their hydrolases in the persistence, degradation and transport of bacterial constituents in tissues: Relation to chronic inflammatory processes in staphylococcal, streptococcal and mycobacterial infections and in chronic periodontal disease. Critical Reviews in Microbiology, 4:249, 1976.

Ginsburg, I., Zor, U., and Floman, Y.: Experimental Models of Streptococcal arthritis: Pathogenetic role of streptococcal products and prostaglandins and their modification by anti-inflammatory agents. In Glynn, L. E., and Schlumberger, H. D. (eds.): Experimental Models in Chronic Inflammatory Diseases. Berlin, Springer Verlag, 1977, 256.

Glynn, L. E.: Rheumatic Fever. In Gell, P. G. H., Combs, R. R. A., and Lachmann, P. J. (eds.): Clinical Aspects of Immunology. 3rd ed. Oxford, London, Blackwell Scientific Publications, 1975, p. 1079.

Kaplan, M. H.: Antoimmunity in Rheumatic Fever: Relationship to Streptococcal antigens cross-reactive with valve fibroblasts, myofibers and smooth muscle. In Dumonde, D. C. (ed): Infection and Immunity in the Rheumatic Disease. Oxford, Blackwell, Scientific Publication, 1976, p. 113.

Lehner, T., Challacombe, S. J., and Caldwell, J.: Immunologic basis for vaccination against dental caries in rhesus monkeys. J Dent Res 55:c166, 1976.

Patterson, M. J., and Hafeez, A. El.B. Group B streptococci in human disease. Bact Rev 774:40, 1976.

Stollerman, G. H.: Rheumatic fever and streptococcal infection. New York, Grune and Stratton, 1975.

Wannamaker, L. W., and Matsen, J. M.: Streptococci and Streptococcal Diseases. Recognition, Understanding and Management. New York, Academic Press, 1972.

Wannamaker, L. W.: The chain that links the heart and the throat. Circulation 48:9, 1973.

Weissman, S. M., Reich, P. R., Somerson, N., and Cole, R.: Genetic differentiation by nucleic acid homology. IV. Relationships among Lancefield groups and serotypes of Streptococci. J Bacteriol 92:1372, 1966.

Wilson, G. S., and Miles, A. A. (eds.): The Streptococci. In Topley and

Wilson's Principles of Bacteriology, Virology and Immunity. 6th ed. London, Edward Arnold, 1975, p. 712.

Zabriskie, J. B.: Rheumatic Fever: A streptococcal-induced autoimmune disease? In Dumonde, D. C. (ed.): Infection and Immunology in the Rheumatic Diseases. Oxford, Blackwell Scientific Publications, 1976, p. 97.

# Gram-Positive Rods

## *DIPHTHERIA BACILLI* 25
## *AND OTHER*
## *CORYNEBACTERIA*

### Lane Barksdale, Ph.D.

Diphtheria is a contagious disease of man in which *Corynebacterium diphtheriae* colonizes the mucous membranes of the fauces and pharynx (sometimes extending to the larynx and the trachea). This is *faucial (laryngeal,* etc.) *diphtheria.* When colonization occurs on the subcutaneous tissue (of the skin) *cutaneous diphtheria* may result.

### THE DISCOVERY OF DIPHTHERIA, CORYNEBACTERIUM DIPHTHERIAE, DIPHTHERIAL TOXIN, AND ANTITOXIN

Just one century ago, in most countries of the world, diphtheria was a dreaded disease with a case fatality rate of about 8 per cent (see Table 1).

**TABLE 1.** Decline in the Case Fatality Rate for Diphtheria in England According to Returns from the Hospitals of the Metropolitan Asylums Board*

| YEAR | CASE MORTALITY PER CENT | YEAR | CASE MORTALITY PER CENT |
|---|---|---|---|
| 1889 | 40.7 | 1909 | 9.4 |
| 1890 | 33.5 | 1910 | 7.8 |
| 1891 | 30.6 | 1911 | 8.4 |
| 1892 | 29.3 | 1912 | 6.2 |
| 1893 | 30.4 | 1913 | 6.2 |
| 1894 | 29.3 | 1914 | 7.9 |
| 1895 | 22.8 | 1915 | 8.4 |
| 1896 | 21.2 | 1916 | 6.8 |
| 1897 | 17.7 | 1917 | 6.7 |
| 1898 | 15.4 | 1918 | 7.7 |
| 1899 | 13.9 | 1919 | 9.3 |
| 1900 | 12.3 | 1920 | 8.6 |
| 1901 | 11.1 | 1921 | 8.8 |
| 1902 | 11.0 | 1922 | 8.7 |
| 1903 | 9.7 | 1923 | 6.8 |
| 1904 | 10.0 | 1924 | 7.0 |
| 1905 | 8.3 | 1925 | 5.0 |
| 1906 | 8.8 | 1926 | 4.9 |
| 1907 | 9.6 | 1927 | 4.0 |
| 1908 | 9.7 | | |

*Antitoxin came into general use in the treatment of diphtheria in 1895. During the same period the diagnosis of diphtheria began to pick up mild cases that previously may have fallen into some other clinical category. There was probably a slow but general improvement in living standards including personal hygiene. Mandatory immunization with toxoid was not begun until more than 20 years after the gathering of the data in this table. (Data from Wilson, G. S., and Miles, A. A.: Topley and Wilson's Principles of Bacteriology and Immunity. 4th ed. Baltimore, The Williams and Wilkins Company, 1955.)

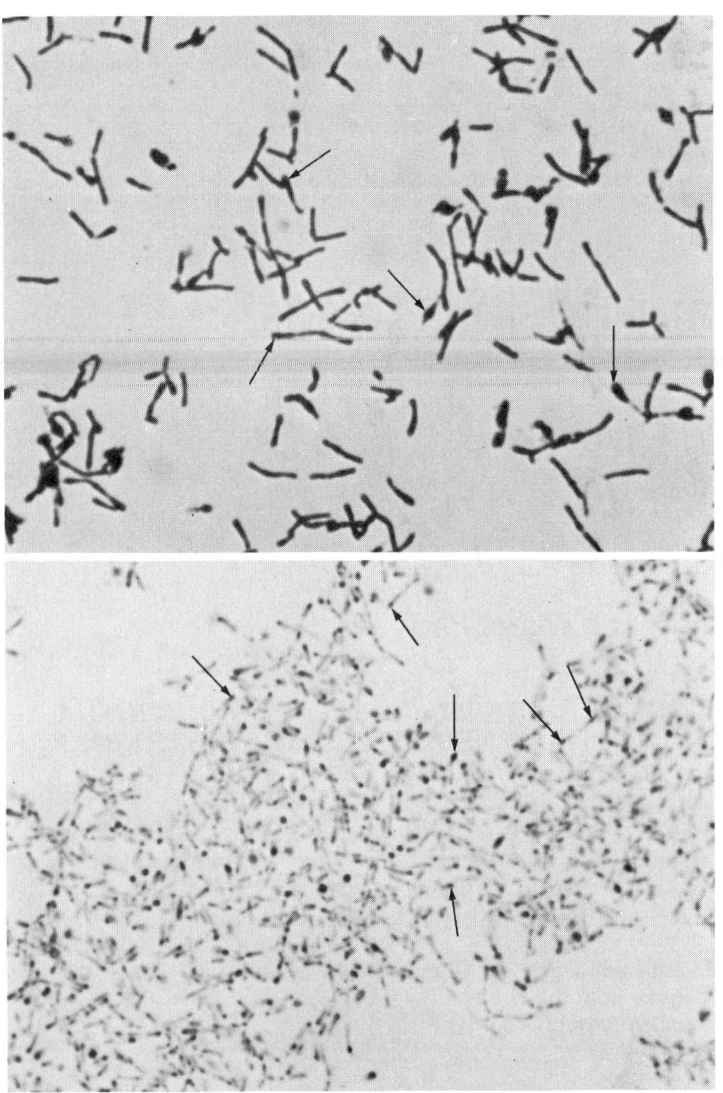

**FIGURE 1.** *Corynebacterium diphtheriae, strain* $C7_S(-)^{tox-}$ *grown on Loeffler's Medium with added phosphate. Upper, Cells stained by the method of Gram. Arrows indicate swollen areas, "club shapes." See text. Lower, Cells stained with alkaline methylene blue. Arrows indicate metachromatic granules. Compare these shapes with those found in tissue culture (Fig. 2) and those found under conditions ideal for maximal growth (Fig. 3, upper).* ×2000. *Courtesy K.-S. Kim.*

The history of our coming to understand diphtheria and to devise a means of combating *diphtheritic death* stands as a model investigation of the etiology of an infectious disease and as a lasting tribute to the clinicians and microbiologists concerned (Andrewes et al., 1923). It was the astute French physician Pierre Fidèle Bretonneau who (from 1821 to 1826) conceived the clinical entity diphtheria to be characterized by the formation of a tightly adhering membranous growth (the pseudomembrane) on the mucous membranes of the throat, sometimes extending into the trachea. At that time, before bacterial agents of disease were known, Bretonneau's clear delineation of the specific clinical condition of diphtheria was the beginning of separation of one throat infection from another, for example, diphtheria from streptococcal pharyngitis. The question "can diphtheria be transmitted from one human subject to another?" was asked by Bretonneau and answered by Tren-

delenburg (1879), who showed that injection of pseudomembranous material from human cases of diphtheria into pigeons and rabbits gave rise to pseudomembranes. Thus the pseudomembrane of diphtheria was transmissible. With these important facts to go on, Friedrich Loeffler began a painstaking investigation into the cause(s) of diphtheria. Being a student in the laboratory of Robert Koch (see *Mycobacterium tuberculosis*), he was disposed to think that diphtheria might have a bacterial etiology. He also accepted the idea of Bretonneau that diphtheria was a singular disease, in the sense that physicians of Bretonneau's day considered smallpox to be singular.

Loeffler's approach to the microscopic examination of material from diphtheritic lesions was essentially that employed today. The staining of smears from some pseudomembranes with alkaline methylene blue revealed to him club-shaped bacilli containing reddish, spheroidal inclusions (metachromatic granules), as shown in Figure 1. Loeffler also knew that diphtheria bacilli growing in vitro often assumed a unique shape (Fig. 2). In smears from 22 cases of clinical diphtheria *he was able to demonstrate bacilli in only 13.* From 6 of these he isolated diphtheria bacilli in culture (on inspissated serum slants). Thus, it was not possible for Loeffler to isolate the causal agent in every case of diphtheria. To the present day, such has been a common experience of bacteriologists. He also isolated diphtheria bacilli from one normal child. Thus, he realized that *the isolation of diphtheria bacilli from the human throat does not necessarily mean that that throat is a diphtheritic one.* He observed that diphtheria and streptococcal pharyngitis *could occur together.* To this day *streptococcal infections sometimes occur simultaneously with diphtheria.* Thus, a diagnosis of diphtheria may require sophisticated clinical judgment backed up with careful bacteriology.

Loeffler's experimental infections in animals led to the discovery that diphtheria bacilli tended to remain at the site where they had been injected, although autopsy of those animals revealed damage to organs far from that site. The *connection* between diphtheria bacilli at a superficial location (in experimentally infected animals) and damage to distant organs with subsequent death was shown by Roux and Yersin (1888) to be the filterable poison diphtherial toxin. It remained for Behring and Kitasato (1890) to discover that antibodies prepared against diphtherial toxin could neutralize its toxicity, thus providing a means of

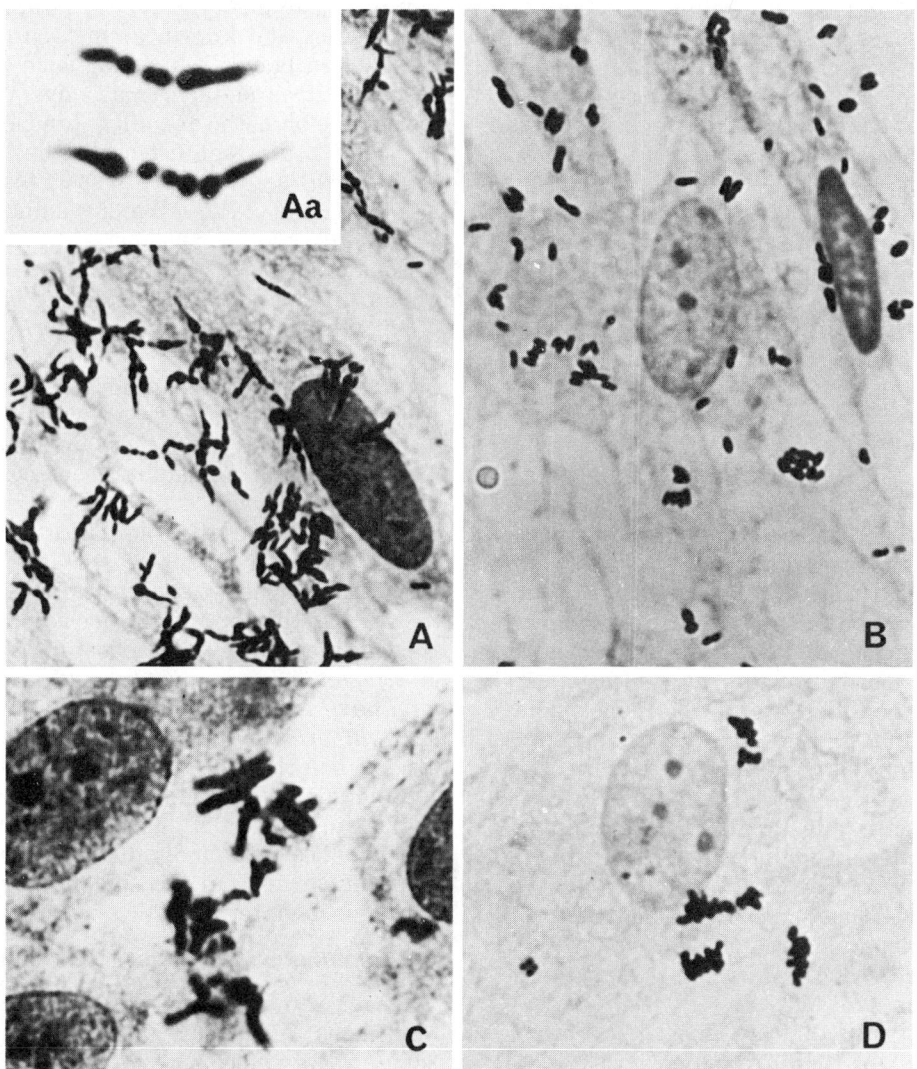

**FIGURE 2.** Corynebacterium diphtheriae *strain C7*$_s$*(−)*$^{tox-}$ *growing in tissue culture,* A *and* Aa. B *and* C, diphtheriae gravis *growing as in* A. C, Bacterium sp. *strain 22M growing as in* A. D *and* C, xerosis *growing as in* A. ×*3,000. Courtesy K.-S. Kim.*

rescuing patients from diphtheritic death by *passively* immunizing them against diphtherial toxin.

## CHEMICAL BASIS OF TAXONOMY OF THE GENUS CORYNEBACTERIUM AND C. DIPHTHERIAE

*Corynebacterium* is the Latin name applied to a variety of tapered, gram-positive, nonmotile, nonspore-forming, rod-shaped bacteria. Their closest relatives are in the genus *Nocardia* and the genus *Mycobacterium,* collectively known as the CMN group (Barksdale, 1970). This group of organisms share a basic cell wall peptidoglycan of cross-linked subunits containing *meso*diaminopimelic acid, L-alanine, and D-alanine to which are covalently bonded polysaccharides consisting of arabinose and galactose (arabinogalactan) and some mannose as arabinomannan. In addition, the cell walls of organisms of each of the three genera contain ester-linked, $\beta$-hydroxylated, $\alpha$-branched, long-chain fatty acids of characteristic carbon lengths ranging from about $C_{28}$ to $C_{90}$ (corynomycolic, $C_{28}$ to $C_{40}$, nocardomycolic, $C_{40}$ to $C_{56}$ and mycolic (mycobacterial), $C_{60}$ to $C_{90}$, acids). These mycolic acids are important constituents of the outer cell walls and such cell-surface-associated conjugates as trehalose dimycolates (cord factors) (Fig. 3). Members of the CMN group can be used as adjuvants in experimenal immunization.

## MORPHOLOGY

Diphtheria bacilli may be separated primarily into different kinds on the basis of the size, shape, and texture of the colonies they form (colonial types). They can be further characterized according to the various biochemical properties discussed under The Laboratory Identification of *C. diphtheriae*. The difference in colony morphology reflects certain essential differences in the ·cell surfaces of individual diphtheria bacilli. These surface peculiarities affect the manner in which individual bacilli pile up to form a colony. To identify diphtheria bacilli, knowledge of the colonial type is useful. The three most common types of colony are (1) smooth, (2) dwarf-smooth, and (3) semirough. (Rough strains of *C. diphtheriae* lack characteristic surface antigens present in semirough organisms.)

When the strains that are smooth also produce diphtherial toxin, they are called *mitis* (Fig. 4) (McLeod, 1943; Robinson, 1934). Similarly, toxin-producing strains of the dwarf-smooth variety

have been termed *intermedius* and certain starch-fermenting, toxin-producing rough strains have been designated *gravis* (Fig. 4). Each of these colonial categories can be further subdivided on the basis of phage types (specific patterns of sensitivity to selected corynebacteriophages) and antigenic types identifiable with specific antisera (serotypes). Some public health laboratories have also typed strains according to their sensitivity to bacteriocins (see Chapter 4). Individuals cells of semirough strains of *C. diphtheriae* tend to be short and stubby. Cells of smooth strains are much longer, whereas the cells of dwarf-smooth strains are intermediate in length.

Common to cells of diphtheria bacilli and most other corynebacteria are certain properties which can be observed with the light microscope: (1) When growing in tissue their cell walls have in them thin spots that are leaky to the Gram stain; they are gram-variable. (2) Old cells store phosphate as polymetaphosphate, localized as phosphate glass and known as metachromatic granules. When bacilli containing such granules are stained with a metachromatic dye, e.g., alkaline methylene blue, the granules stand out as reddish refractile bodies against a blue background (see Fig. 1). (3) Bacilli with thin spots tend to balloon out at one end of the cell and assume a shape like a club (coryne-, coryneform, corynebacterium). Misshapenness of this sort is called pleomorphism. In smears from tissue, the pleomorphism of smooth strains is more exaggerated than that of dwarf-smooth and rough strains. Thus, the bizarre morphology of diphtheria bacilli from a pseudomembrane associated with infection by a *mitis* strain could be more readily recognized than that from a membrane associated with a *gravis* infection.

Since in each of the colonial categories (*gravis, mitis,* and *intermedius*) there are a number of serologic and phage types, the species *C. diphtheriae* has the potentiality for accommodating to the defenses of the human host much as do Group A *streptococci* and *pneumococci*. Thus, persons who have experienced infection with one type of *C. diphtheriae* may later be infected with another type. When this happens in young adults or older individuals having adequate levels of circulating antitoxin, the second infection is apt to be of little consequence to the individual though it may be of some importance in the epidemiology of the disease (see Chapter 90).

### C. diphtheriae and Salts of Tellurium

Most corynebacteria share with certain other organisms, including some staphylococci and some yeasts, the capacity to grow in the presence of 100 $\mu$g/ml potassium tellurite, to reduce the tellurite to tellurium and to concentrate the tel-

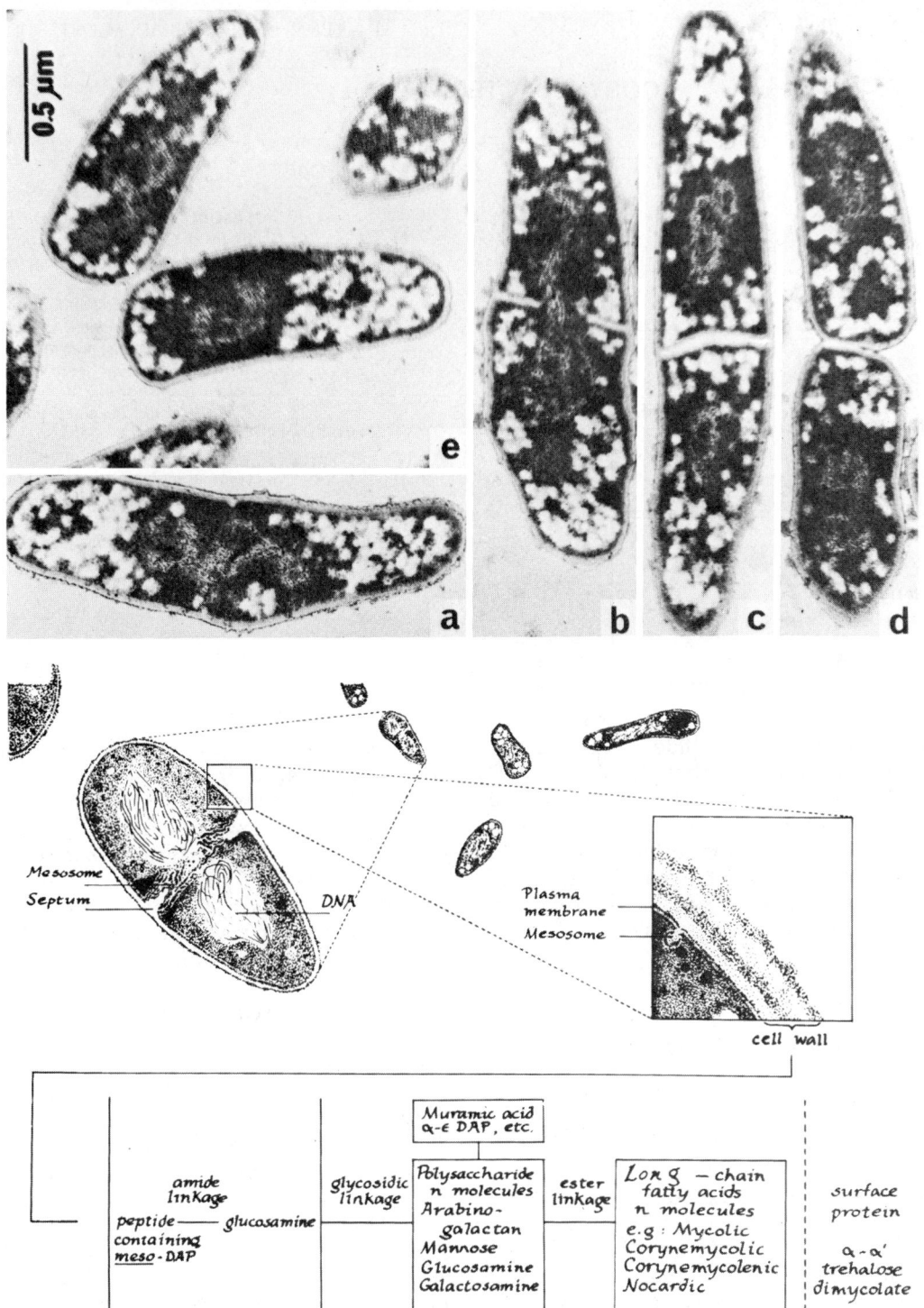

**FIGURE 3.** Upper, *An electron micrographic record of cell division as it occurs in logarithmically growing* C. diphtheriae, *C7*$_S$*(−)*$^{tox-}$*. Division time = 60 minutes. A, Initiation of septum formation by ingrowth of membrane. B, Well-developed septal initials showing "layers" of the components of the cell envelope. C, Two cells still connected showing that the septum consists of two full complements of membrane and envelope components. D, Beginning of separation of cell doublets. E, The "snapping" involved in the pulling apart of two corynebacterial cells, showing the characteristic taper from septal to distal end. Electronopaque areas, peculiar to actively growing cells, seem not to be glycogen but may represent lipid associated with loci of intense biosynthetic activity. ×51,000. Bar = 0.5 μm. From data of Sheila Heitner.*

Lower, *Diagrammatic sketch of an actively growing bacterial cell representing a composite of the CMN group. A "resting" cell with metachromatic granule is shown. A portion of the envelope of an actively growing cell has been expanded to show the relation of the complex envelope to the cytoplasmic membrane. A portion of the wall is shown to consist of murein, arabinogalactan-mannan linked to species of long-chain, α-branched, β-hydroxylated fatty acids, the mycolic acids, and to dimycolates of trehalose and to a surface protein antigen. The mureins and arabinogalactans are distinctive from genus to genus as are the mycolic acids — for example, mycolic (Mycobacterium), corynemycolic and corynemycolenic (Corynebacterium), and nocardomycolic (Norcardia). In general terms, the murein-arabinogalactan is a heat-stable O antigen; the heat-labile surface protein antigen is the K antigen. Drawing by James E. Ziegler. Rearrangement by Kwang-Shin Kim. Reproduced with permission of Bacteriological Reviews.*

## CORYNEBACTERIA

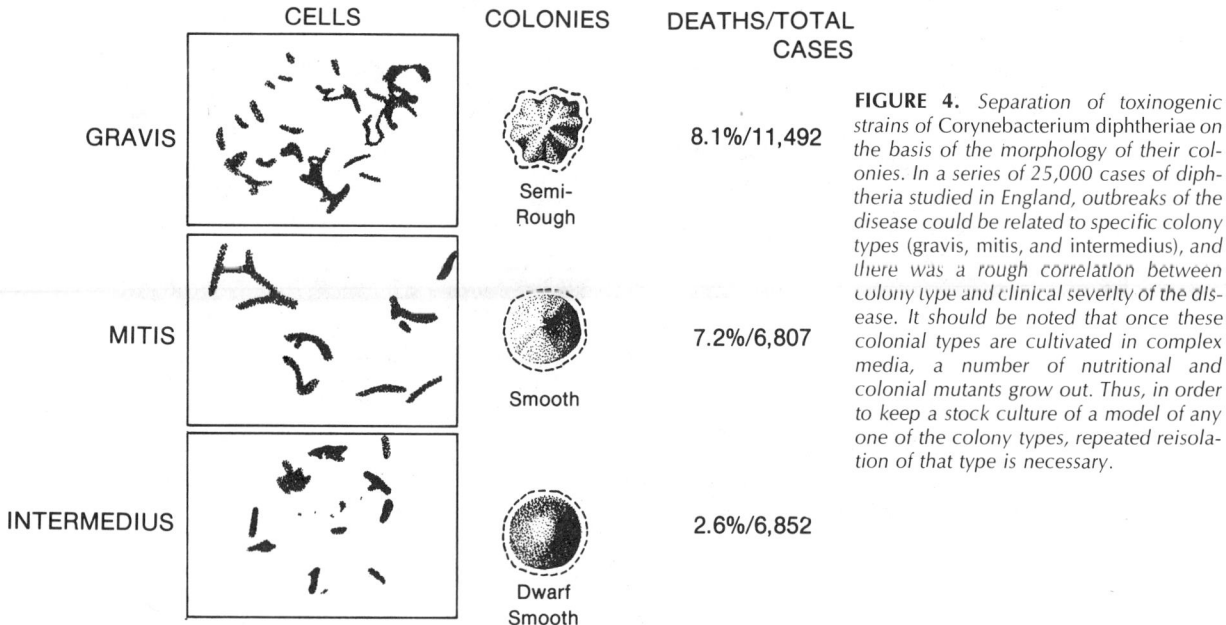

**FIGURE 4.** *Separation of toxinogenic strains of* Corynebacterium diphtheriae *on the basis of the morphology of their colonies. In a series of 25,000 cases of diphtheria studied in England, outbreaks of the disease could be related to specific colony types (gravis, mitis, and intermedius), and there was a rough correlation between colony type and clinical severity of the disease. It should be noted that once these colonial types are cultivated in complex media, a number of nutritional and colonial mutants grow out. Thus, in order to keep a stock culture of a model of any one of the colony types, repeated reisolation of that type is necessary.*

lurium (as the metal or its sulfide) in the cells, so that the bacterial colonies that develop on tellurite agar appear grayish black to jet black. The growth of most streptococci, some staphylococci, and other members of the throat flora is inhibited on tellurite agar. For over 60 years a variety of tellurite media have been used for the selective cultivation of *C. diphtheriae* (see The Laboratory Identification of *C. diphtheriae*).

## *PATHOGENIC PROPERTIES*

### Diphtherial Toxin

Diphtherial toxin is a simple protein with a molecular weight of about 62,000 daltons. It is lethal for man in amounts of 130 ng/kg of body weight. Toxin is liberated into the extracellular milieu by growing cells of *C. diphtheriae* and is therefore called an exotoxin. It consists of a single polypeptide chain cross-connected by two disulfide bridges, as shown in Figure 5. Mild treatment of toxin with trypsin (termed "nicking"), followed by reduction of its disulfide bridges with dithiothreitol, yields two fragments: an N-terminal fragment A (m.w. 21,000) and a C-terminal fragment B (m.w. 39,000); see Pappenheimer (1977).

Although the only biologic activity directly associated with the intact toxin molecule is the ability to inactivate a variety of animal cells, fragment A behaves as a diphosphopyridine nucleotidase (NADase) as well as an adenosine diphosphoribosyl transferase. This latter function

of fragment A stops protein synthesis in the test tube by covalently linking the adenosine diphosphoribose moiety of nicotinamide adenine dinucleotide to eukaryotic elongation factor 2 (EF2) (Collier, 1975). This *enzymatic activity of fragment A* (liberated from diphtherial toxin) operationally places toxin in the category of a proenzyme. There is good evidence to suggest that toxin fixes to the sensitive animal cells by its carboxy terminal end (Fig. 5) and that proteolytic and reductive steps occurring near the cell surface (or infolds related to the process of endocytosis) liberate fragment A, which, once inside the cell, inactivates EF2. Enough such inactivation would stop protein synthesis, leading to cell death.

*The Genetic Control of Toxin Production.* The genetic information required for the synthesis of diphtherial toxin is carried in the genomes of certain temperate corynebacteriophages as the gene *tox*. This information gains expression in strains of *C. diphtheriae* undergoing lysis by the phage as well as in lysogenic strains that carry *tox*[+] in the prophage state (Fig. 6). Integration of *tox*-containing prophages into the corynebacterial nucleoid assures perpetuation of the toxinogenic character from one generation of toxinogenic corynebacteria to the next.

### Toxoid

The early efforts at immunizing against diphtherial toxin with graded doses of toxin and, later, with mixtures of toxin and antitoxin (horse) sometimes led to unfortunate accidents. A satisfactory nontoxic antigen was obtained by Ramon

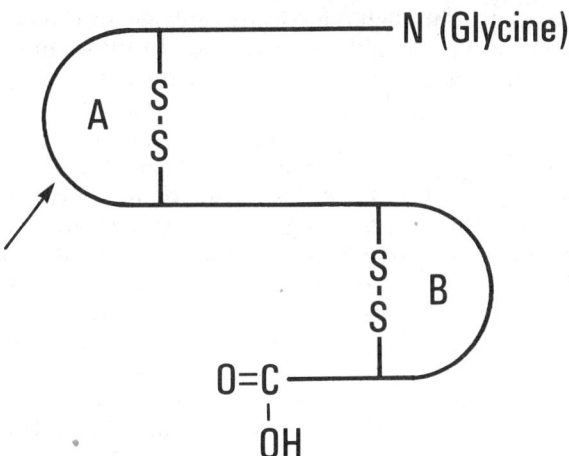

**FIGURE 5.** *A molecule of diphtherial toxin schematically represented as a single polypeptide chain. At one terminus is the amino group of glycine; the amino acid functioning as the*

$$\overset{O}{\underset{\|}{carboxy\ (-C-OH)}}\ terminal\ is\ not\ known.$$

*carboxy (—C—OH) terminal is not known. The molecule is interconnected by disulfide bridges between cystine residues. At the bend shown by the arrow is a sequence of three arginines. Trypsin acts to nick toxin at the arrow point. When such nicking action is followed by exposure of the molecule to dithiothreitol, the disulfide bridges are broken and two fragments of toxin result. The smaller piece (from the arrow point back to the terminal glycine residue) has been designated fragment A. The larger piece (from the arrow point to the carboxy terminus) has been designated fragment B. Fragment A is the enzymically active fragment responsible for the following group transfer reactions:*

*1. $NAD^+ + EF2 \leftrightarrows ADP\text{-}ribosyl\ EF2 + nicotinamide + H^+$*
*2. $NAD^+ + HOH \leftrightarrows ADP\text{-}ribose + nicotinamide + H^+$*
*3. $NAD^+ + toxin \leftrightarrows ADP\text{-}ribosyl\text{-}toxin + nicotinamide + H^+$*
*$EF\text{-}2$ = elongation factor 2. See text. Fragment B is thought to be important for the fixing of diphtherial toxin to receptors on toxin-sensitive cells.*

and Glenny, who found that prolonged incubation of diphtherial toxin with formalin under alkaline conditions converted it into a nontoxic antigen which, when injected into laboratory animals, stimulated the production of antitoxin. Formalin interacts with the tyrosine residues of toxin, effecting their cross-linkage with the ε-amino groups of constituent molecules of lysine. Toxoid is unable to fix to animal cells and it cannot be split into A and B fragments. It lacks, therefore, all of the properties of toxin except antigenicity and the capacity to interact with antitoxic antibody. This remarkably stable antigen has served for more than 50 years as satisfactory prophylactic agent against death from diphtheritic intoxication (see also Schick Test).

In the early days of production of toxoid for immunization, it was necessary to find an exceptional strain of *C. diphtheriae* that produced large amounts of toxin. Park and Williams discovered an *avirulent* diphtheria bacillus, the Park-Williams number 8 strain (PW8), which is used throughout the world in the "manufacture" of diphtherial toxoid. In suitable media the PW8 strain can produce 300 μg toxin protein/$10^9$ bacilli/ml, or around 300 mg per liter.

### Invasiveness of Virulence of C. diphtheriae

In Figure 6 are listed the properties of a smooth strain of *C. diphtheriae*, $C7_S(-)^{tox}$, carrying no $tox^+$ prophage and the properties of $C7_S(\beta)^{tox+}$, a lysogenic strain carrying prophage $\beta^{tox+}$. Antigenically, these two strains are identical except

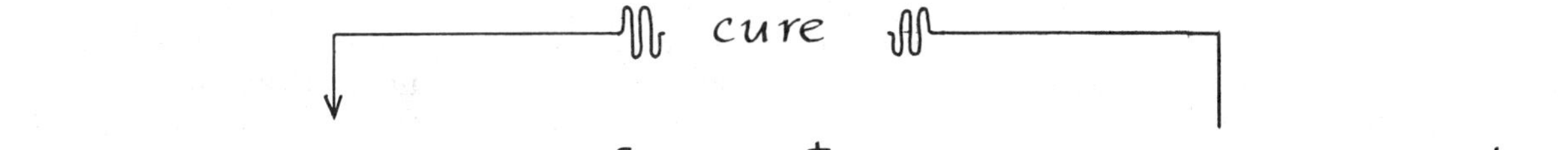

$$C.\ diphtheriae\ C7_S(-)^{tox^-} + \phi^{tox+} \longrightarrow C.\ diphtheriae\ C7_S(\phi)^{tox+}$$

*cure*

Invasive
Nontoxinogenic
Sensitive to phage φ

May cause nontoxaemic diphtheria

Invasive
Toxinogenic
Immune to phage φ
Lysogenic for phage φ

May cause toxaemic diphtheria

**FIGURE 6.** *Changes brought to Corynebacterium diphtheriae, strain $C7_S(-)^{tox-}$, following integration (into its genome) of a probacteriophage that carries the tox gene. Presumably, the indicator strain $C7_S$ is nonlysogenic, hence the designation $(-)$, and is nontoxinogenic, $tox.^-$ When nontoxinogenic, nonlysogenic C7 is lysed by a phage carrying the $tox^+$ marker, such as $\phi^{tox-}$ or $\beta^{tox-}$, toxin is produced during the course of phage multiplication and lysis of the cell. When lysogenized by such phages, the genome of $C7_S(\phi)^{tox+}$ includes phage genes that endow it with immunity to homologous phage (lysogenic immunity = synthesis of specific repressor) and the ability to synthesize diphtherial toxin. The subscript s refers to the smooth (surface) antigen of the strain. See text for those corynebacterial products that play a role in invasiveness. From Barksdale, L.:* Corynebacterium diphtheriae *and its relatives.* Bacteriological Reviews *34:378, 1970. Reproduced with permission of the publisher.*

for the synthesis of diphtherial toxin by the toxinogenic strain. Each of the strains can colonize the pharyngeal mucous membranes of susceptible people and produce a pseudomembrane. Invasiveness in *C. diphtheriae* is associated with production of a dimycolate of trehalose, a so-called cord factor (see Chapter 40), which can inactivate the mitochondria of mammalian cells. *C. diphtheriae* can survive in pharyngeal mucus by producing a neuraminidase (sialidase) capable of cleaving residues of *N*-acetylneuraminic acid, NANA (sialic acid), from parent molecules such as mucins, the glycoproteins of cell surfaces, and gangliosides. In addition, these corynebacteria liberate an *N*-acetylneuraminic acid lyase which can split NANA into its constituents, *N*-acetyl mannosamine and pyruvate. Pyruvate markedly stimulates growth of corynebacteria and other members of the CMN group.

## THE LABORATORY IDENTIFICATION OF *C. DIPHTHERIAE*

At present, *C. diphtheriae* is not sought in the average diagnostic laboratory *unless* a death from diphtheria has occurred. In many countries there are few if any laboratory technicians who have had first-hand experience with *C. diphtheriae*. Yet diphtheria occurs in at least one major city of the world each year. The problem of diagnostic inadequacy of laboratories is compounded by deficiencies in contemporary textbooks regarding the characterization of diphtheria bacilli. The deficiencies include (1) inadequate definitions of "pleomorphism" in general and with regard to *C. diphtheriae* in particular; (2) absence of a clear statement of the relationship existing between nontoxinogenic and toxinogenic *C. diphtheriae* (see Fig. 6); and (3) erroneous fermentation patterns (repeated from earlier textbooks) by which various corynebacteria are identified.

### Procedures

Smears are prepared from diphtheritic membrane, and media are inoculated for enrichment of numbers of diphtheria bacilli and for primary isolation. *Note*: Corynebacteria thrive in a $CO_2$-rich environment, e.g., 10 per cent in air. A candle jar provides satisfactory levels of $CO_2$.

The diphtheritic membrane (pseudomembrane, see Figs. 1 and 2 in Chapter 90) is usually so tenacious that rubbing it with a cotton swab will remove only some of its outermost material. More of the fibrinous exudate may be obtained by using a bacteriologic loop (steel) that has been opened into a hook. Pulling away bits of pseudomembrane with such a device often results in slight

bleeding. This behavior is in contrast to that of the easily removable exudate found in uncomplicated streptococcal pharyngitis. Some of the pseudomembrane so obtained is used for inoculating (1) a slant of Loeffler's medium supplemented with 2.5 gm $K_2HPO_4$/liter, (2) a blood agar plate, and (3) a Mueller-Miller tellurite or Tinsdale tellurite agar plate. From the remainder, smears should be prepared for future reference and for (1) the Gram stain and (2) staining with alkaline methylene blue. The former should provide an assessment of the different kinds of bacteria present in the exudate; the latter indicates whether or not any of the tapered, pleomorphic rods present contain polyphosphate (metachromatic) granules. Corynebacteria growing in a low phosphate environment produce very few metachromatic granules. This probably explains the limited numbers of granules found in *C. diphtheriae* in smears from tissues. The tapered ends of *C. diphtheriae* (see Figs. 1 and 2) will appear more exaggerated with the methylene blue stain than with the Gram stain. The exaggeration of the taper is most striking with *mitis* strains and less so with *intermedius* and *gravis* strains. Tapering of these rods is stressed here because it represents a particular kind of misshapenness or pleomorphism. Pleomorphism per se is not uncommon among gram-positive bacteria such as α-hemolytic streptococci, certain group G streptococci, propionibacteria, lactobacilli, and corynebacteria. In addition, fusobacteria, ordinarily gram-negative, in mixed cultures sometimes do not decolorize properly and may be mistaken for pleomorphic gram-positive rods. Any one of these bacteria might grow well in and about a streptococcal sore throat or a diphtheritic membrane. Since the normal pharyngeal flora varies as to numbers and kinds of bacteria from one individual to another, the secondary organisms in a pseudomembrane vary greatly as to both kind and absolute numbers. Their numbers more often than not obscure the presence of *C. diphtheriae*. However, *C. diphtheriae*, particularly *mitis* strains, when present may be presumptively singled out on the basis of the taper of the cells and the presence of metachromatic granules in a few cells.

A presumptively positive set of smears should correlate with the growth of similar bacteria on the inoculated Loeffler's slant, in use all of these years because it favors the outgrowth of *C. diphtheriae*, and the morphologic characteristics of the organisms growing on it are closer to those seen in vivo (e.g., in smears from diphtheritic exudates). Compare cells in Figure 3 with those in Figures 1 and 2. From rich inocula *C. diphtheriae* may show considerable increase in numbers as early as 7 hours after incubation.

## Final Identification

Colonies of suspected corynebacteria are picked, suspended in sterile broth, and restreaked onto sterile plates. Once isolated colonies have grown up, one (or more) is selected for the preparation of stock cultures for further propagation and identification. Identification is made possible by determining, for the strain under study, the reactions given in Table 2. The way in which the reactions obtained identify the organism under study is shown in Table 3.

## Methods for Detecting Diphtherial Toxin and Antitoxin

*Agar Gel Diffusion (The Ouchterlony-Elek Plate).* Elek and Ouchterlony independently found that precipitates of diphtherial toxin and antitoxin, formed in agar gels, could be used as a means for the in vitro detection of toxinogenic

**TABLE 2.   Ten Properties Useful for Separating Members of the Genus *Corynebacterium*\***

1. Fermentation of lactose
2. Production of catalase†
3. Formation of iodinophilic polymer from glucose-1-phosphate
4. Production of disulfide reductase
5. Fermentation of dextrose
6. Fermentation of maltose
7. Fermentation of starch
8. Production of urease
9. Production of pyrazinamidase
10. Hydrolysis of gelatin

*The author is much indebted to M. C. Pollice and Ioan T. Sulea for data supporting this Table.
†In the absence of exogenous hemin.

strains of *C. diphtheriae*. A horse serum agar plate (Petri dish) is poured and, before the agar has hardened, a strip of filter paper (1.6 × 8 cm),

**TABLE 3.   Formulation of Species of *Corynebacterium* According to the 10 Properties Listed in Table 2\***

*C. diphtheriae mitis:* $\dfrac{2\quad 3\quad 4\quad 5\quad 6}{1\qquad\qquad\qquad 7\quad 8\quad 9\quad 10}$

*C. diphtheriae gravis:* $\dfrac{2\quad 3\quad 4\quad 5\quad 6\quad 7}{1\qquad\qquad\qquad\qquad 8\quad 9\quad 10}$

*C. diphtheriae intermedius:* $\dfrac{2\quad 3\quad 4\quad 5\quad 6}{1\qquad\qquad\qquad 7\quad 8\quad 9\quad 10}$

*C. diphtheriae* variety *ulcerans:* $\dfrac{2\quad 3\quad 4\quad 5\quad 6\quad 7\quad 8\qquad 10}{1\qquad\qquad\qquad\qquad\qquad 9}$

*C. kutscheri:* $\dfrac{2\quad 3\quad 4\quad 5\quad 6\qquad 8\quad 9}{1\qquad\qquad\qquad 7\qquad 10}$

*C. minutissimum:* $\dfrac{2\quad 3\quad 4\quad 5\quad 6\qquad 9}{1\qquad\qquad\qquad 7\quad 8\qquad 10}$

*C. pseudotuberculosis (ovis):* $\dfrac{2\quad 3\quad 4\quad 5\quad 6\qquad 8}{1\qquad\qquad\qquad 7\qquad 9\quad 10}$

*C. pseudodiphtheriticum: (hofmanni)* $\dfrac{2\quad 3\quad 4\qquad\qquad 8\quad 9}{1\qquad\qquad 5\quad 6\quad 7\qquad 10}$

*C. renale:* $\dfrac{2\quad 3\quad 4\quad 5\qquad\qquad ⑨}{1\qquad\qquad 6\quad 7\quad 8\qquad 10}$

*C. xerosis:* $\dfrac{2\quad 3\quad 4\quad 5\qquad 9}{1\qquad\qquad ⑥\quad 7\quad 8\qquad 10}$

*Numbers above the line indicate positive traits. Numbers below the line indicate negative traits. Circled numbers below the line indicate that a very occasional strain may be positive; circled numbers above the line indicate that a very occasional strain may be negative. Sucrose has not been included. Most *C. xerosis* are sucrose positive; some *C. diphtheriae mitis* are sucrose positive, as are some strains of *C. minutissimum* and *C. kutscheri*. Note that the

pattern $\dfrac{2\quad 3\quad 4}{1}$ is common to each of the 10 species. The three types of *C. diphtheriae* differ only with regard to starch fermentation. However, when

this pattern is supplemented with colonial morphology on tellurite agar and cellular morphology (under the microscope), as shown in Figure 4, precise identification can readily be accomplished. Those laboratories using sheep's blood agar plates with a concentration of erythrocytes low enough to reveal feeble hemolysis will be able to separate hemolytic *mitis* strains from nonhemolytic *gravis* and *intermedius* strains. Note: To obtain the most prompt and reliable test reactions, actively growing corynebacteria should be washed with saline, resuspended as a thick slurry and inoculated into test media so that each tube receives 100 million or more bacteria.

The author is much indebted to M. C. Pollice and Ioan T. Sulea for data supporting this table.

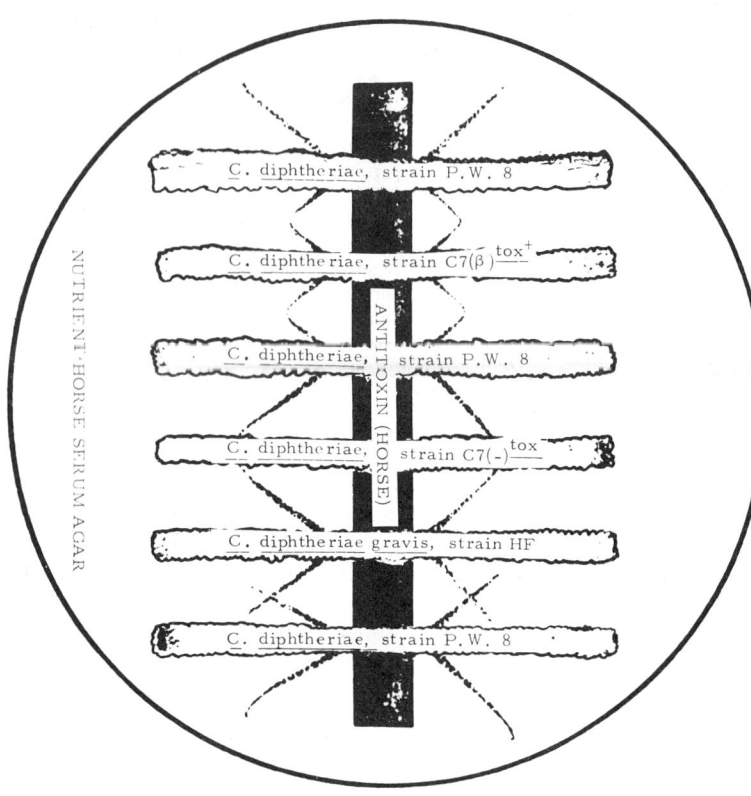

**FIGURE 7.** *Diagram of an Elek/Ouchterlony plate (see text for details) for the in vitro detection of diphtherial toxin. Cultures of strains of C. diphtheriae have been streaked at right angles to the central strip of filter paper soaked in antitoxin. See text for information concerning each of the different strains of diphtheria bacilli and the antigen-antibody precipitates formed in their vicinities.*

previously dipped into horse antitoxin (500 au/ml) and drained of excess liquid, is placed across the center of the agar surface. The Petri dish, its lid ajar, is kept in a 37° C incubator until dry. Onto the dry surface of the plate in well separated parallel lines (Fig. 7) are streaked known toxinogenic and nontoxinogenic strains of *C. diphtheriae* and the unknown organisms being tested. Cotton swabs, soaked in heavy bacterial cultures and then freed of excess liquid by expression against the sides of the culture tubes, are useful for introducing each of the bacterial cultures onto the plate. A satisfactory positive control is the toxinogenic avirulent PW8 strain, and a suitable negative control is the nontoxinogenic mutant of *C. diphtheriae gravis,* HF. Consider as unknown organisms to be tested strains $C7_s(-)^{tox-}$ and $C7_s(\beta)^{tox+}$. Each is streaked so that it is growing next to the known toxinogenic strain, PW8. If, during growth on the antitoxin-containing agar plate, toxin is produced, then a line of toxin-antitoxin precipitate will become visible in the agar, as can be seen to the left of the PW8 strain. When gradients of identical precipitates of antigen-antibody are formed from different loci in agar gels, they will fuse, producing an arc of identity. Thus, between C7 ($\beta$) and PW8 the diffusing toxins interacting with antitoxin in the agar have produced arcs between toxin (C7 ($\beta$))· antitoxin from one side to toxin (PW8)· anti-

toxin from the other. Diphtheria bacilli produce various proteins other than toxin. In most preparations of antitoxin there are antibodies to some of these proteins. In the case of $C7(-)^{tox-}$ (Fig. 7) an anomalous protein has formed a precipitate with its antibody. Between strain PW8 and strain HF anomalous antigen-antibody precipitates have formed showing no arc of identity.

### Intradermal Skin Tests

Necrosis by diphtherial toxin can readily be seen following the introduction of minute amounts of toxin into the skin of shaved rabbits or guinea pigs. Neutralization of toxicity by antitoxin specifically identifies the toxin. Bacterial cultures may similarly be tested intradermally for their capacity to produce toxin. For example, at numbered multiple sites on the back of a rabbit, *known* and *test cultures* are injected at time zero, antitoxin is given intravenously at time $t$ (usually 3½ hours later), and at time $t + 30$ minutes *the same cultures* are injected at new (prime) sites. The reactions are read daily up to 96 hours. When diphtherial toxin is present, necrosis will occur at the sites inoculated at time $t$ but not at the sites inoculated 30 minutes after the administration of antitoxin. Necrosis at both sites indicates the production of a toxin not neutralized by diphtherial antitoxin, i.e., a toxin immunologically distinct from diphtherial toxin.

## IMMUNITY: THE SCHICK TEST

In 1913 Bela Schick described a skin test for the detection of circulating antitoxin in human subjects. Once in use, it became clear that a modified Schick test would also detect delayed hypersensitivity to other products of *C. diphtheriae*. In the modified Schick test used at New York University Medical School for over 30 years, minute amounts of toxin are injected at one site (on the forearm) and toxoid at a second site. There are five pairs of reactions possible. (1) If at 48 to 96 hours there is no reaction at either site, the subject has sufficient circulating antitoxin to neutralize the dose of toxin and shows no allergy to corynebacterial products. This rather positive capacity has been designated as *the Schick-negative reaction*. (2) If there is *necrosis* at the toxin site and no reaction at the toxoid site, the subject has insufficient circulating antitoxin to neutralize the toxin. This relatively negative condition is designated as *the Schick-positive reaction*. (3) An *immediate wheal* and *erythematous reaction* at both sites at about 35 minutes post injection indicates circulating IgE specific for the injected products. (4) An *erythematous reaction* at *48 to 96 hours* at both sites indicates that there has been enough circulating antitoxin to neutralize the toxin administered and that in addition the subject shows delayed allergy to corynebacterial products. This has been called *the pseudoreaction*. (5) *Necrosis* at the test site and *delayed allergy* at both sites indicate insufficient circulating antitoxin to neutralize the toxin and an allergy to corynebacterial products. This has been called *the combined reaction*.

Over the years the examination of human populations with the Schick test has given various insights into immunobiology (Barksdale, 1980). It has revealed that carriers of *C. diphtheriae* do not necessarily have detectable levels of circulating antitoxin. It has revealed that circulating antitoxin per se does not prevent the onset of a diphtheritic infection. And, most recently, it has led to the discovery that about 1.5 to 2 per cent of the human population cannot respond to immunizing doses of toxoid with the production of detectable levels of circulating antitoxin. As long as these people are around and as long as diphtheria bacilli continue to be carried in populations, there will probably be occasional deaths from diphtheria.

## SENSITIVITY OF DIPHTHERIA BACILLI TO COMMONLY AVAILABLE ANTIBIOTICS

Although *C. diphtheriae* is sensitive to a variety of antibiotics active on gram-positive organisms, including chloramphenicol, erythromycin, kanamycin, methicillin, penicillin G, rifampin, streptomycin, and tetracycline, the antibiotics that have been most thoroughly examined in relation to cases of diphtheria and carriers of diphtheria bacilli are penicillin G and erythromycin. In a recent study of the antibiotic sensitivity of 337 strains of *C. diphtheriae* isolated from cases of diphtheria, 90 per cent were sensitive to the aforementioned antibiotics, and 100 per cent of the strains were sensitive to gentamicin. The minimal inhibitory concentrations of antibiotics for *C. diphtheriae* are as follows ($\mu$g/ml): penicillin G, 0.08; erythromycin, 1.6; chloramphenicol, 0.5; and tetracycline, 1.0.

## OTHER CORYNEBACTERIA

Listed in Table 3 are most of the species of *Corynebacterium* encountered in material from human and animal sources. Those that are of significance in diphtheritic infections are *C. diphtheriae* and sometimes *C. ulcerans*. Rare infections with *C. pseudotuberculosis (ovis)* have been reported in human subjects whose occupation put them into intimate contact with animals. *C. pseudotuberculosis (ovis)* causes infections in sheep and horses. *C. xerosis*, originally isolated from the conjunctiva, is one of those "background" corynebacteria from which *C. diphtheriae* must be differentiated. Aside from its distinguishing properties given in Table 3, *C. xerosis* tenaciously retains crystal violet, in contrast to the leaky, gram-variable reaction given by *C. diphtheriae* to the Gram stain. *C. pseudodiphtheriticum (C. hofmanni)* (Table 3) is another species of *Corynebacterium* that was originally isolated from normal throats and sometimes is encountered in routine bacteriologic study of the throat and upper respiratory tract. Among corynebacteria associated with genitourinary infections is a group recently designated *C. genitalium*. *C. kutscheri* is found in overt and latent infections of mice. *C. renale* is the cause of pyelonephritis in cattle.

Organisms that have been wrongly listed as belonging in the genus *Corynebacterium* include the group G streptococcus originally designated *C. pyogenes*, and the propionibacterium called *C. acnes*. The group G streptococcus (*C. pyogenes*), which under natural conditions produces suppurative lesions in cattle, sheep, pigs, and goats, has been associated with pharyngitis and skin ulcers occurring in humans. In these latter cases, the bacillary shape assumed by this streptococcus has led to its confusion with *Corynebacterium*. However, the absence of an obvious taper to its cells and the absence of metachromatic granules in them readily suggests that these *lactose-fermenting* streptococci are not corynebacteria.

## References

Andrewes, F. W., Bulloch, W., Douglas, S. R., Dreyer, G., Gardner, A. D., Fildes, P., Ledingham, J. C. G., and Wolf, C. G. L.: Diphtheria, Its Bacteriology, Pathology and Immunology. London, Medical Research Council, His Majesty's Stationery Office, 1923.
Barksdale, L.: *Corynebacterium diphtheriae* and its relatives. Bacteriol Rev 34:378, 1970.

Barksdale, L.: The immunobiology of diphtheria. In Nahmias, A. J., and O'Reilly, R. J. (eds.): Immunology of Human Infection. Part I in Comprehensive Immunology, Vol. 8. R. A. Good and S. B. Day (eds.) New York, Plenum Medical Book Company, 1980.
Collier, R. J.: Diphtheria toxin: mode of action and structure. Bacteriol Rev 39:54, 1975.
McLeod, J. W.: The types mitis, intermedius and gravis of *Corynebacterium diphtheriae*, a review of observations during the past ten years. Bacteriol Rev 7:1, 1943.
Pappenheimer, A. M., Jr.: Diphtheria toxin. Ann Rev Biochem 46:69, 1977.
Robinson, D. T.: Further investigations on the *gravis, mitis* and "intermediate" types of *C. diphtheriae*: type stability. J Path Bact 39:551, 1934.

# 26 *LISTERIA MONOCYTOGENES*

## H. P. R. Seeliger, M.D.

### MORPHOLOGY

*Listeria monocytogenes* (Murray, et al., 1926) represents a bacterial species consisting of gram-positive to gram-variable asporogenous, acapsular, aerobic to microaerophilic rods. At temperatures of around 20° C the cells show peritrichous flagellation. At 37° C usually only one polar flagellum is apparent. Motility is best at around 20° C. The growth range is between +4° C and 42° C with most rapid growth of delicate colonies at around 36° C on ordinary media at slightly alkaline pH preferably in the presence of 5 per cent sheep or rabbit blood. Dissociation of colonies occurs with formation of S− and R− and several intermediary forms. Culturally, *L. monocytogenes* may be confused with streptococci, notably motile enterococci.

### ANTIGENIC COMPOSITION

By means of antigenic analysis, various somatic and flagellar antigens allow the differentiation of several serogroups with one to several serovarieties in each of these groups. This forms the basis for serologic identification (Table 1). It should be noted that the former serovariants 4f and 4g with numerous subvarieties do not belong to *L. monocytogenes* proper, but rather to a related apathogenic species of *Listeria* that has been named *L. innocua* (Seeliger and Schoofs, 1978).

### METABOLISM

Glucose and other carbohydrates are attacked by production of acid, but not of gas. Contrary to the biovarieties of *Murraya grayi*, mannitol is not acidified (see Table 2). $NO_3$ is not reduced to $NO_2$. All strains that have been isolated from pathologic specimens of human and animal origin produce a β-hemolysin. β-hemolysis is most pronounced with strains representing serovar 5. Nonhemolyzing strains usually belonging to *L. innocua* and related subvarieties (cf., Table 2) are otherwise biochemically identical with *L. monocytogenes*, but, because of complete lack of virulence, absent β-hemolysis, and failure to produce an experimental monocytosis in rabbits, do belong to a different species. *L. monocytogenes*, including this closely related group of organisms, is differentiated from similar gram-positive rods classified with the genus *Murraya* by a set of biochemical tests as outlined in Table 2, although their G + C ratio of 38 to 40 moles per cent is identical.

### PATHOGENIC PROPERTIES

Strains of human and animal origin do not show any differences in pathogenic properties. Smooth virulent cultures can stimulate in rodents an experimental monocytosis through the action of extractable lipids. Instillation of *L. monocytogenes* into the conjunctiva of rabbits provokes a characteristic keratoconjunctivitis. In warm-blooded animals, parenteral inoculation causes a septic disease with varying clinical and organic manifestations. Liver, spleen, central nervous system, and the reproductive organs are most commonly attacked. Infections via the oral route usually are successful only in young or pregnant animals. Typical focal granulomas (listerioma) are prominent; suppuration and abscess formation occur less frequently.

**TABLE 1.   Serovars of Listeria monocytogenes, Murraya grayi, and Related Species**

| DESIGNATION Paterson | Seeliger-Donker-Voet | O-ANTIGENS | | | | | | | H-ANTIGENS |
|---|---|---|---|---|---|---|---|---|---|
| 1 | 1/2 a | I II (III) | | | | | | | A B |
| | 1/2 b | I II (III) | | | | | | | A B C |
| 2 | 1/2 c | I II (III) | | | | | | | B  D |
| 3 | 3 a | II (III) IV | | | | | | | A B |
| | 3 b | II (III) IV | | | | | | | A B C |
| | 3 c | II (III) IV | | | | | | | B  D |
| 4 | 4 a | (III) | (V) | VII | | IX | | | A B C |
| | 4 ab | (III) | V VI VII | | | IX | | | A B C |
| | 4 b | (III) | V VI | | | | | | A B C |
| | 4 c | (III) | V | VII | | | | | A B C |
| | 4 d | (III) | (V) VI | | VIII | | | | A B C |
| | 4 e | (III) | V VI | | (VIII)(IX) | | | | A B C |
| | 5 | (III) | (V) VI | | VIII | X | | | A B C |
| | 7? | (III) | | | | | XII XIII | | A B C |
| Listeria innocua* | 6a (4f) | (III) | V VI VII | | | IX | | XV | A B C |
| | 6b (4g) | (III) | V VI VII | | | IX X XI | | | A B C |
| M grayi (ssp. grayi) | | (III) | | | | | XII | XIV | E |
| (spp. murrayi) | | (III) | | | | | XII | XIV | E |

*nonhemolytic strains, additional antigen combinations are known but not listed.
†nonhemolytic serovar, strongly related to serovars 4 f and 4 g.

**TABLE 2.   Nitrate Reduction and Acid Production from Carbohydrates by Species of Genus Listeria* and Murraya**

| | L. MONO-CYTOGENES† | MURRAYA subspec. *grayi* | subpec. *murrayi* |
|---|---|---|---|
| NO₃ → NO₂ | − | − | + |
| L-arabinose | − | − | − |
| D-galactose | d | + | (+) |
| glycogen | − | − | − |
| lactose | (d) | + | + |
| mannitol | − | + | + |
| melezitose | d | − | − |
| melibiose | − | − | − |
| rhamnose | d | − | d |
| sucrose | (d) | − | − |
| xylose | d | − | − |

Key:  + = acid produced 24-48 hrs (90% or more strains)
    − = no acid produced 21 days (90% or more strains)
    d = some strains positive, some negative
    (+) = acid produced slowly (3-7 days)
    (d) = some strains produce acid slowly (3-7 days), other strains negative.
*All species produce acid but no gas in 24-48 hours from amygdalin, esculin, cellobiose, dextrin, fructose, glucose, maltose, mannose, salicin, starch and trehalose. No acid in 21 days from adonitol, dulcitol, erythritol, inositol, inulin or raffinose.
†Including nonhemolyzing, serologically identifiable strains that represent a different nonpathogenic species named *L. innocua.*

*L. monocytogenes* is the cause of sporadic enzootic and epizootic disease of numerous small and large animals. It is globally spread. The infection may follow the course of a septicemia or may localize in certain organs, especially the central nervous system.

Septicemia occurs mainly in rodents, poultry, and young animals. The central nervous system is involved predominantly in large adult animals. Atypical and silent forms of the disease are not rare. The maturity grade, the resistance of the animals, and the portal of entry probably play a decisive role in the course of the disease. In general, young animals are known to have an increased susceptibility to listeriosis. In older animals, *L. monocytogenes* often is a secondary invader after primary damage from another disease. Only sheep seem to be an exception, since the disease in them often runs a fulminating course with a high mortality.

*L. monocytogenes* sometimes invades the reproductive organs of wild and domestic animals. Infection of the pregnant animal may result in damage and death of the fetus or abortion. The extent of listeriosis as a cause of infectious abortion in cattle, sheep, and other animals needs more study. Permanent damage to the reproductive organs has been noted only infrequently. Under natural conditions infections occur sporadically and in epizootics; however, they seem to be more frequent than is generally appreciated.

Mortality is high in clinically manifest cases. Epizootics in breeding stocks and live stocks may cause severe economic losses.

In human listeriosis there are many symptoms that may easily lead to confusion with diseases of different etiology. The symptomatology comprises "grippe-like" infections, sore throat with glandular swelling and monocytosis, severe septicemia with predominant involvement of the liver, disease of the central nervous system, and localized purulent inflammations of the mucous membranes. The infected tissues develop granulomatous reactions.

All age groups are affected, but predominantly the newborn and infants, and to a lesser degree the aged. Inapparent infections during pregnancy are transmitted transplacentally to the fetus and may result in abortion or stillbirth owing to infection of the fetus. In other cases, sick infants die shortly after birth. The newborn may also be infected during delivery either by infected vaginal secretions or by swallowing infected amniotic fluid. The immaturity of the neonatal tissues, especially of the intestinal tract, facilitates the penetration of the causative organisms into the body of the newborn. A purulent acute meningitis frequently kills the baby. Apparently, listeriosis is a more frequent cause of fetal damage, abortions, and neonatal death than is generally recognized. In adults, meningitis and meningoencephalitis compose the main clinical syndrome. The disease has also been observed as a secondary infection during corticosteroid therapy or repeated hemodialysis.

In newborns and the aged listeriosis has a fatality rate of 70 per cent and higher. Other forms of the disease are somewhat more benign; asymptomatic infections and a carrier state (fecal, genital, and oropharyngeal) have been observed.

## IMMUNITY

Little is known about immunity to listeriosis. Passive protection has not been achieved experimentally by treatment of animals with homologous antiserum. Vaccination with killed suspensions of L. monocytogenes has not afforded protection. However, experiments with living vaccines have given more promising results.

Present research indicates that protection may depend on cell-mediated immunity. Although in rare cases circumstantial evidence points to repeated attacks of Listeria infection in subsequent pregnancies endangering the fetus, no second clinical Listeria infection has been observed in individuals or animals who had been cured of proven listeriosis.

## LABORATORY DIAGNOSIS

The diagnosis of listeriosis is made primarily by culture. With certain restrictions, serologic procedures are applicable for case finding and retrospective diagnosis. Blood, sternal bone-marrow, spinal fluid, amniotic fluid, meconium, placenta, throat swabs, and all kinds of discharge should be examined by smear and culture. L. monocytogenes may also be found postmortem in the liver, spleen, lymph nodes, cerebrum, cerebellum, and medulla.

Primary culture of Listeria is occasionally difficult. Most of the difficulties may be overcome by cultivating the specimens in tryptose or sodium thioglycollate broth, and by use of Gray's enrichment technique — that is, by several weeks' storage at $+4°$ C with repeated subcultures on blood agar or tryptose agar. Media containing nalidixic acid and trypaflavine are helpful in the isolation of Listeria from contaminated samples. The recognition of suspicious colonies is facilitated by use of Henry's illumination technique. Owing to morphologic, cultural, biochemical, and serologic similarities with other bacterial species, accurate identification of the organism is required in every suspected case. There are many sources of error and often Listeria is overlooked or wrongly classified. Similar organisms may be mistaken for L. monocytogenes. This applies particularly to nonhemolytic L. innocua and to certain strains of enterococci and corynebacteria. Hemolysis, characteristic tumbling (end over end) motility, and ability to produce keratoconjunctivitis in rabbits are among the most useful diagnostic features.

During and after Listeria infections serum antibodies are found in animals and human patients by agglutination reactions with somatic and flagellar antigens. However, Listeria agglutinins are frequently found in sera of healthy animals and man without a history of listeriosis. Whether those agglutinins are "specific" is still an unsolved problem. Newborn and infants up to the sixth month may lack serum antibodies against L. monocytogenes, even in proven infections. The distribution of agglutinin titers varies with age and reaches its maximum between the third and fifteenth year of life. Whether this is due to subclinical infections is a matter of conjecture.

Cross-reactions with enterococcal and especially with staphylococcal antigen create a serious handicap. Therefore, the interpretation of agglutination reactions requires great caution and a critical approach. Only titers of 1:200 and above, or rises in titer by at least two dilutions are considered of some diagnostic significance. Recently the serodiagnosis of *Listeria* infections has been improved by a complement-fixation test. Positive findings with this test must, however, in many instances be checked for specificity by absorption of the serum samples with staphylococcal antigens. About two thirds of patients above the age of six months show rises in antibody titers during the disease and in convalescence. Serologic tests are inferior to the bacteriologic methods for establishing diagnosis. Skin tests have been tried repeatedly. A "polypeptide" skin test antigen has been developed that has given specific results in some suspected human cases.

## *DRUG SUSCEPTIBILITY*

Chemotherapy with sulfonamides, and recently with certain antibiotics, may be successful. Ampicillin, tetracyclin, chloromycetin, and erythro-

mycin have reduced the case fatality rate of the severe forms of human listeriosis. But treatment is usually successful only if it is instituted early in the disease. Occasional relapses require a second course of antibiotic therapy.

Although the sensitivity pattern of *L. monocytogenes* as found with several thousand isolates from human and animal sources is rather uniform, in vitro sensitivities should be determined for all strains isolated from clinical material. *L. monocytogenes* is usually inhibited by the following concentrations of antibiotics ($\mu$g/ml): benzylpenicillin 0.2, cephalothin 2.0, erythromycin 2.0, chloramphenicol 5.0, tetracycline 1.0.

## *EPIDEMIOLOGY*

The epizootology remains largely unknown. Direct contact, aerogenous transmission, mating infection, and rhinogenous as well as otogenous infections have been considered as essential modes of infection. Susceptibility is definitely influenced by the state of general resistance and by many environmental and climatic factors. Inade-

FIGURE 1.

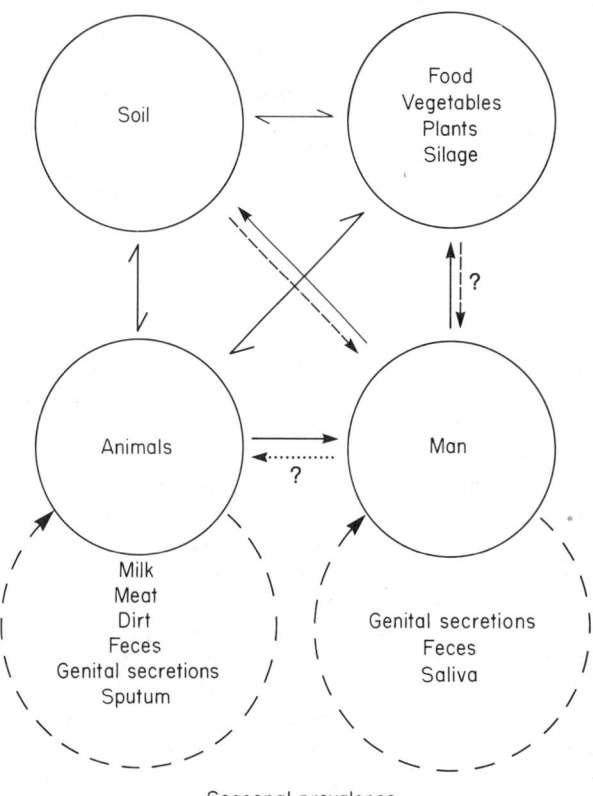

| Seasonal prevalence | |
|---|---|
| Animal | Man |
| Autumn–Winter | Spring–Summer |

quate food seems to be essential in lowering resistance. In sheep and cows the consumption of poorly fermented silage has been shown to be the main source of infection during the stabling period. Most cases among domestic animals occur in late autumn and winter.

A risk exists for anyone dealing with animals or animal products, meat, game, and nonpasteurized milk and milk products in particular. Like other zoonoses listeriosis is transmissible from animals to humans. The chains of infection usually end "blind"; that is, in most cases the organisms are not known to be transmitted from a human host to others, with the exception of neonatal listeriosis, which is transmitted from mother to fetus. Transmission has taken place by direct contact with diseased animals or their excretions, possibly by consumption of contaminated food and by inhalation of infected dust. In most cases, however, the origin of the infection and the mode of transmission are unknown.

In view of the increased isolation of *L. monocytogenes* from environmental sources and its psychrophile nature, soil, plants, and certain vegetables would seem to be an important reservoir. The present view on the epizootic and epidemiologic pattern of listeriosis is outlined in Figure 1. In humans, listeriosis occurs more frequently in spring and summer than in the other seasons.

Prophylactic measures comprise a general improvement in sanitation with particular reference to an enforced control of raw material products destined for human use and consumption. Warnings and instruction are necessary for exposed individuals, particularly the pregnant, the obstetrician and his staff, including midwives and nurses, the veterinary profession, and all animal keepers and animal breeders. If listeriosis is suspected during pregnancy, prophylactic short-term antibiotic treatment is advised.

### References

Gray, M. L., and Killinger, M. H.: Listeria monocytogenes and listeric infections. Bacteriol Rev 30:309, 1966.
Murray, E. G. D., Webb, R. A., and Swann, M. B. R.: A disease of rabbits characterized by a large mononuclear leukocytosis caused by a hitherto undescribed bacillus: Bacterium monocytogenes (n.sp.). J Path Bact 29:407, 1926.
Paterson, J. St.: The antigenic structure of organisms of the genus Listerella. J Path Bact 48:25, 1940.
Seeliger, H. P. R., and Finger, H.: Analytical serology of Listeria. In Kwapinski, J. B. G. (Ed.): Analytical serology of microorganisms. J. S. Wiley and Sons, Inc., vol. 2, 1969.
Seeliger, H. P. R., and Höhne, K.: Determination of serovars of Listeria. In Bergan, T. (ed.): Methods in microbiology. vol. 10 (in press).

# 27 ERYSIPELOTHRIX RHUSIOPATHIAE

## Charles E. Davis, M.D.

*Erysipelothrix rhusiopathiae* is a facultatively anaerobic, gram-positive bacillus that shares many characteristics with *Listeria monocytogenes* (Chapter 26), corynebacteria, lactobacilli, and certain streptococci. The technique of numerical taxonomy, and the guanine plus cytosine content of its DNA indicate a closer relationship to *Listeria*, lactobacilli, and some streptococci than to coryneform bacteria but no definite relationship to any family of bacteria. In the eighth edition of Bergey's Manual of Determinative Bacteriology (1974), *Erysipelothrix* and *Listeria* have been removed from the chapter on coryneform bacteria and placed in the *Lactobacillus* chapter as genera of uncertain affiliation.

*Erysipelothrix* was first recovered from mice in 1880 by Koch. In 1882, Löffler and Pasteur and Thuillier independently isolated *Erysipelothrix* from pigs with erysipelas. Only two years later, Rosenbach isolated the same organism from an erysipeloid lesion of a patient and established it as the cause of erysipeloid by inoculating himself with the isolate. Although *Erysipelothrix* is still isolated from zoonotic skin infections of patients and from rare cases of septicemia and endocarditis, its major importance is the economic loss associated with outbreaks of swine erysipelas.

### MORPHOLOGY

*Erysipelothrix rhusiopathiae* is a gram-positive, nonmotile, nonsporulating bacillus that may form either smooth or rough colonies on primary isolation. Smooth colonies are entire, convex, transparent, and about 1.0 mm in diameter. There may be a blue sheen by reflected light. Broth cultures are uniformly turbid. Rough colonies are larger and granular with a matt appearance on agar and flocculent with hair-like projections in broth. Cells from smooth colonies are small, slender, straight or slightly curved bacilli that measure from 0.2 to 0.4 $\mu$m in width by 0.5 to 2.5 $\mu$m in length. Cells from rough colonies vary from short forms to long chains of bacilli. Some are filamentous and beaded like the actinomycetes. Others may have large, fundus-like swellings.

Fully developed colonies on blood agar are surrounded by a zone of greening that may clear on further incubation. Colonies on tellurite agar are pinpoint and gray at 24 hours, but they become larger and jet black by 48 to 72 hours.

## ANTIGENIC COMPOSITION

*Erysipelothrix* has been divided into at least 20 serotypes according to cross-agglutination studies against heat-resistant, acid-soluble antigens (Dedie, 1949; Kucsera, 1973; Wood et al., 1978). These antigens have not been further characterized but are thought to be peptidoglycans of the cell wall.

Although Pasteur and Thuillier successfully immunized swine against *Erysipelothrix* in 1883 with live organisms attenuated by passage through rabbits, little was known about the protective antigen until recently. Traub (1947) and Gledhill (1952) showed that at least part of the protective activity of the vaccine was a result of antibody directed at a soluble antigen found in the supernatants of cultures. White and Verway (1970 and 1970a) extended these observations and found that the soluble protective antigens contained a glycolipoprotein that was probably derived from the cell wall, since 75 per cent of the protective activity was destroyed by pretreatment of the antigen with muramidase. Trypsin and heat also destroyed part of the protective activity of this antigen, which was soluble in butanol but unaffected by lipase or ribonuclease.

Animals immunized with either the vaccine of Pasteur and Thuillier or cell-free culture supernatants develop agglutinins to whole bacteria.

## METABOLISM

*Erysipelothrix rhusiopathiae* is microaerophilic. It will grow when exposed to atmospheric concentrations of oxygen but grows best in reduced oxygen tension with 5 to 10 per cent carbon dioxide. *E. rhusiopathiae* multiplies at temperatures of 16 to 41° C. Optimum growth occurs at 33 to 37° C. It obtains the energy for growth by glycolysis and does not produce catalase, even when grown aerobically. All strains produce acid but no gas from glucose, galactose, fructose, and lactose.

Riboflavin and oleic acid are required for growth. Acid production from carbohydrates is poor in 1 per cent peptone water. Five per cent rabbit serum or yeast autolysate should be added to the sugar in 1 per cent peptone water.

One of the unique metabolic properties of *Erysipelothrix* is the production of hydrogen sulfide. Among gram-positive organisms, only a few species of streptococci and *Bacillus* show this characteristic. *Erysipelothrix* acidifies the butt of Kligler's iron agar by producing organic acids from glucose by the process of anaerobic respiration with thiosulfate as the electron acceptor. In this acid environment, thiosulfate is broken down to sulfite and $H_2S$ gas by the enzyme thiosulfate reductase, which is produced in most bacteria that generate $H_2S$.

## PATHOGENIC PROPERTIES

*Erysipelothrix* is a natural pathogen primarily of mice, fish, swine, and man. Sheep and turkeys are also susceptible to natural infections. In swine, *Erysipelothrix* produces three clinical types of disease: acute fatal septicemia, red rhomboid-shaped skin lesions ("diamond skin disease"), and chronic disease with endocarditis of the mitral valves. Arthritis is a frequent complication of all forms of swine erysipelas and may also occur independently of the other manifestations. Laboratory mice die of overwhelming septicemia after intraperitoneal inoculation.

*Erysipelothrix* causes skin infections in man that are called erysipeloid because they resemble streptococcal erysipelas. These lesions usually occur on the hand after contact with infected animals or animal products. Arthritis of nearby joints is common (see Chapter 245).

The virulence of different strains of *Erysipelothrix* for mice varies, but most strains kill mice. Variations in virulence are independent of serotype, biochemical properties, and protein composition as determined by patterns on electrophoresis and electrofocusing (White and Mirikitani, 1976). The virulence factors have not been determined, but virulence is related to rapid growth and the production of neuraminidase (Krasemann and Muller, 1975). Inoculation of a partially purified glycoprotein from culture filtrates into the skin of rabbits causes necrosis. Intravenous inoculation of this product also causes high fevers in rabbits (Leimbeck et al., 1975).

The pathogenesis of *Erysipelothrix* arthritis has been extensively studied because it is a prominent feature of swine erysipelas and erysipeloid in man (Chapter 245). It has been used as a laboratory model of relapsing, erosive arthritis because its histopathology and course are similar

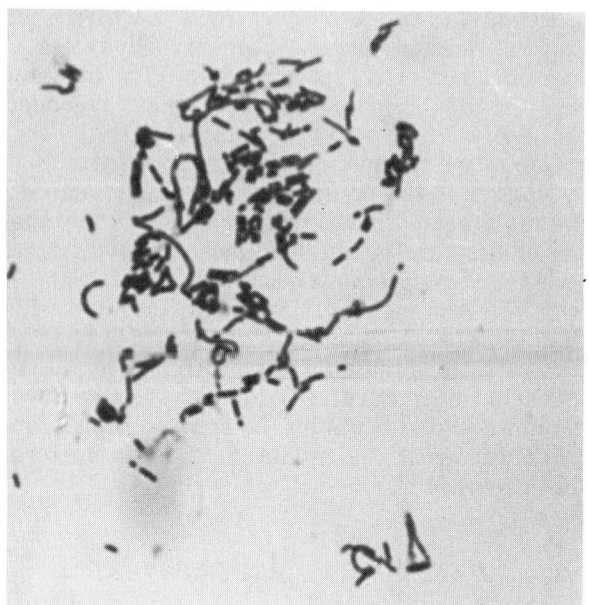

**FIGURE 1.** *Gram stain appearance of rough colony of* E. rhusiopathiae. *Note predominance of filamentous beaded bacilli.*

to rheumatoid arthritis (Hadler, 1976). Intravenous inoculations of whole live organisms causes
polyarthritis in swine, dogs, and rabbits. Rabbits
develop heterologous rheumatoid factor (Astorga,
1969) and polyarthritis after injection of dead
organisms and cell-free culture extracts (White et
al., 1971). This cell-free extract contains murein
and many proteins. Some of these products bind
rapidly to the synovium, persist for as long as six
months, and cause cytopathic changes in synovial
cell cultures after a single brief exposure (White
et al., 1976). The exact antigen or antigens responsible for this effect have not been isolated,
but it is clear that the pathogenic factors do not
require the continuing presence of the organism.

## IMMUNITY

Active immunization with the live attenuated
vaccine of Pasteur and Thuillier protects against
swine erysipelas. This protection is probably mediated by antibody because passive protection
with antiserum provides effective prophylaxis for
at least two weeks. The protective antigen in this
preparation is a glycolipoprotein that is destroyed
by lysozyme (White and Verway, 1970 and
1970a). The immune response after vaccination
with either whole cells or cell-free culture extracts may be monitored by the titer of agglutinins to *Erysipelothrix*. Immunization is effective
after a single inoculation. Swine do not develop
clinical arthritis after immunization. Polyarthri-

tis from culture extracts develops only after multiple intravenous inoculations. This arthritis does
not seem to be primarily an antibody-mediated
autoimmune phenomenon, since persistence of
bacterial antigens in the synovium has been
demonstrated (White et al., 1976).

Natural human infection with *E. rhusiopathiae*
also stimulates the production of agglutinins, but
patients undergo relapses and reinfections. Immunization of swine probably does not prevent
colonization of the tonsils and gastrointestinal
tract. It is possible that swine are more effectively
immunized by vaccination than man is by natural
infection because swine are reimmunized by colonization with *Erysipelothrix* (see Epidemiology,
below).

Crude culture extracts are cytopathic for synovial cells and probably mitogenic for lymphocytes (White and Mirikitani, 1976), but the role of
cellular immunity against this bacterium has not
been determined.

## LABORATORY DIAGNOSIS

Gram stains of aspirates or biopsies from erysi-
eloid or blood cultures from patients with septicemia and endocarditis may reveal coccobacillary, coryneform, or filamentous gram-positive
bacilli. Forms that are almost indistinguishable
from streptococci are not uncommon either from
infected material or from primary isolation plates
(Seeliger, 1961). Growth is enhanced by carbon
dioxide, reduced oxygen tension, and 5 per cent
serum. Both smooth and rough colonies (see Morphology, above) usually produce a zone of greening on blood agar. This zone may clear on further
incubation. Gram stains of smooth colonies usually reveal coccobacillary or coryneform bacilli,
while smears of the larger rough colonies often
show a predominance of filamentous, beaded bacilli that may resemble actinomycetes or lactobacilli (Fig. 1).

Two unique cultural features of *Erysipelothrix*
should prevent confusion with any other gram-
positive rod. Except for a few species of *Bacillus*
and a few streptococci, *E. rhusiopathiae* is the
only gram-positive bacterium that will produce
$H_2S$ in Kligler's iron agar incubated in air (Fig.
2). It also produces a unique appearance in gelatin stab cultures if the tube is incubated at
temperatures low enough to keep the gelatin in a
solid state. Bead-like colonies with lateral filamentous growth develop and resemble a test-tube
brush (Fig. 3).

*Erysipelothrix* is nonmotile, and is negative for
catalase, oxidase, and indole production; it does not
reduce nitrate to nitrite. It makes acid but not gas

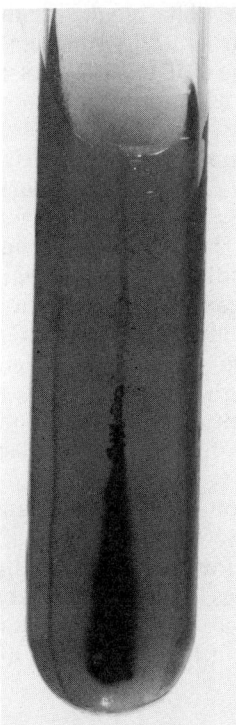

**FIGURE 2.**  *Twenty-four-hour culture of* E. rhusiopathiae *in Kligler's iron agar. Note $H_2S$ production along stab line.*

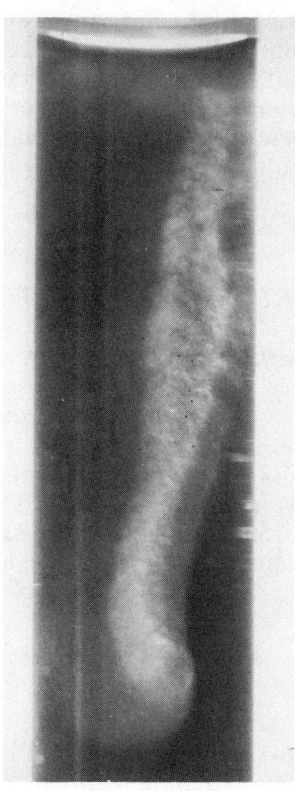

**FIGURE 3.**  *Forty-eight-hour gelatin stab culture of* E. rhusiopathiae *with lateral filamentous growth that resembles a test tube brush.*

from glucose, lactose, galactose, and fructose. Some strains make acid from mannose (10/14) and xylose (4/14) (White and Mirikitani, 1976). It makes an acid slant and butt in Kligler's iron agar and triple sugar iron agar with enough $H_2S$ formation to blacken the butt. Key biochemical reactions are shown in Table 1.

*Erysipelothrix* can be easily differentiated from *Listeria* (Chapter 26) because *Listeria* is motile

and beta-hemolytic and does not produce $H_2S$ (Table 1). *Erysipelothrix* is resistant to neomycin and kanamycin, but *Listeria* is not. Intraperitoneal inoculation of mice with a 24- to 48-hour culture of *Erysipelothrix* kills mice within two to three days but will not cause keratoconjunctivitis when dropped into the eye of a rabbit. *Listeria* is

**TABLE 1.**   Characteristics of *Erysipelothrix rhusiopathiae*

| TEST OR COMPOUND | REACTION | COMMENT |
|---|---|---|
| Alpha-hemolysis | + | |
| Beta-hemolysis | − | *Listeria, C. pyogenes,* and *C. haemolyticum* are + |
| Motility | − | *Listeria* is + |
| $H_2S$ in KIA or TSI | + | *Listeria,* corynebacteria and lactobacilli are − |
| Nitrate reduction | − | *Listeria* is + |
| Catalase | − | *Listeria* and most corynebacteria are + |
| Esculin hydrolysis | − | *Listeria* is + |
| Glucose | A[a] | *Erysipelothrix* produces acid without gas from carbohydrates |
| Lactose | A | |
| Fructose | A | |
| Galactose | A | |
| Mannose | A(10/14) | (White and Mirikitani, 1976) |
| Xylose | −(10/14) | (White and Mirikitani, 1976) |
| Resistance to neomycin and kanamycin | + | *Listeria* is sensitive |
| Pathogenic for mice | + | *Listeria* is − |
| Keratoconjunctivitis in rabbits | − | *Listeria* is + |
| Per cent G + C | 36.5% | *Listeria* is 38% |

[a]A few drops of rabbit serum or yeast autolysate should be added to carbohydrate tests if the base is 1 per cent peptone water.

not pathogenic for mice but causes keratoconjunctivitis in rabbits. *Erysipelothrix* can be differentiated from all lactobacilli and corynebacteria by the production of $H_2S$ in KIA or TSI slants. Corynebacteria also produce catalase except for *C. pyogenes* and *C. haemolyticum*, which are beta-hemolytic.

## DRUG SUSCEPTIBILITY

*E. rhusiopathiae* is exquisitely sensitive to penicillin (0.0025 to 0.02 $\mu$g/ml), ampicillin, the semisynthetic penicillins, the cephalosporins, erythromycin, and clindamycin. It is also susceptible to readily achievable levels of tetracycline. Some strains are only moderately sensitive to chloramphenicol. It is resistant to the aminoglycosides, vancomycin, sulfonamides, and polymyxin.

## EPIDEMIOLOGY

*Erysipelothrix* lives on dead and dying organic matter in the environment. It can be isolated in large numbers from the slime covering the bodies of fish and has been isolated from the soil of pig pens as long as five years after an outbreak of swine erysipelas. The organism tolerates high salt concentrations and develops as well in sea water as it does in fresh water.

*Erysipelothrix* also colonizes many animals including fish, crustaceans, wild and domestic birds, and rodents, especially mice and rats. Its primary economic importance is in agriculture, in which significant losses of poultry and swine are common. *Erysipelothrix* colonizes a high percentage of apparently normal swine. In one recent study (Stephenson and Berman, 1978), the tonsils of 62 out of 63 normal pigs were colonized by *Erysipelothrix* at slaughter. The organism is widely distributed throughout Europe and the United States. Tissue (primarily spleens) of hogs from 2633 herds in 46 states of the United States were contaminated with *E. rhusiopathiae* in another recent study (Harrington and Ellis, 1975). In this study, the swine came from herds in which hog cholera was suspected, and 21.1 per cent were infected with *Erysipelothrix*.

Hogs and other wild and domestic animals can probably be infected either through the skin or through the alimentary canal. The tonsils may be one of the major foci of infection in hogs. Hogs and poultry probably acquire Erysipelothrix primarily from the soil of their pens, but uncooked garbage and rodents may also be a major source of swine infection. The peak incidence of swine erysipelas occurs in the summer. The peak incidence of human disease occurs in the fall and winter shortly after outbreaks of swine erysipelas.

*E. rhusiopathiae* infection is primarily an occupational disease in humans. Farmers, abbatoir workers, poultry workers, fishermen, and housewives acquire the infection through skin abrasions while handling infected meat. Occasionally, cases of septicemia and endocarditis have no apparent preceding skin infection. Some investigators believe that these infections may be acquired through the gastrointestinal tract after ingestion of improperly prepared infected meat or fish. Human-to-human transmission has never been proved.

Disease in domestic animals and humans can be prevented by immunization of animals with the vaccine of Pasteur and Thuillier and by improved practices of animal husbandry. Housewives and those at occupational risk should handle meat and fish cautiously and wear gloves when possible.

## References

Astorga, G.P.: Immunologic studies of an experimental chronic arthritis resembling rheumatoid arthritis. Arthritis Rheum. 12:589–596, 1969.

Dedie, K.: Die Säurelöslichen Antigene von *Erysipelothrix rhusiopathiae* Mh. Vet. Med. 4:7, 1949.

Gledhill, A. W.: The immunizing antigen of *Erysipelothrix*-the role of the L-antigen. J. Gen. Microbiol. 7:179–191, 1952.

Hadler, Nortin H.: A pathogenetic model for erosive synovitis. Lessons from animal arthritidies. Arthritis and Rheumatism 19:256–266, 1976.

Harrington, R., and Ellis, E. M.: Salmonella and Erysipelothrix infection in swine: A laboratory survey. Am. J. Vet. Res. 36:1379–80, 1975.

Jones, D.: The taxonomic position of *Listeria*. *In* M. Woodbine (ed.): *Problems of Listeriosis*. Leicester University Press, Leicester, 1975, pp. 4–17.

Krasemann, C., and H.E. Muller: The virulence of *Erysipelothrix rhusiopathiae* strains and their virulence production. Zentrabl. Bakteriol. [ORIG A] 231 (1-3), 206–213, 1975.

Kucsera, G.: Proposal for standardization of the designations used for serotypes of *Erysipelothrix rhusiopathiae* (Migula) Buchanan. Int. J. Syst. Bacteriol. 23:184–188, 1973.

Leimbeck, R., K.H. Bohm, H. Ehard, and L.-Cl Schulz: Studies of the toxic components of *Erysipelothrix rhusiopathiae*: Detailed characterization of an extracted endotoxin. Zentrabl. Bakteriol. [ORIG A] 232 (2–3), 266–286, 1975.

Seeliger, H.P.R.: *Listeriosis*. Karger Co., Basle, Switzerland, 1961.

Stephenson, E. H., and D.T. Berman: Isolation of *Erysipelothrix rhusiopathiae* from tonsils of apparently normal swine by 2 methods. Am. J. Vet. Res. 39:187–188, 1978.

Traub, E.: Immunisierung gegen Schweinerotlauf mit konzentrientem Adsorbatimpstoffen. Monatsh. Veterinaermed. 10:165–173, 1947.

White, R.R., and W.F. Verway: Isolation and characterization of a protective antigen-containing particle from culture supernatant fluids of *Erysipelothrix rhusiopathiae*. Infect. Immun. 1:380–386, 1970.

White, R.R., and W.F. Verway: Solubilization and characterization of a protective antigen of *Erysipelothrix rhusiopathiae*. Infect. Immun. 1:387–393, 1970(a).

White, T.G., J.L. Puls, and F.K. Mirikitani: Rabbit arthritis induced by cell-free extracts of *Erysipelothrix*. Infect. Immun. 3:715–722, 1971.

White, T.G., F.K. Mirikitani, and Patricia Hargrove: The effect of bacterial extracts on synovial cells in tissue culture. *In Vitro* 12:702–707, 1976.

White, T.G., and F.R. Mirikitani: Some biological and physical-chemical properties of *Erysipelothrix rhusiopathiae*. Cornell Vet. 66:152–163, 1976.

Wood, R.L., and R.A. Packer: Isolation of *Erysipelothrix rhusiopathiae* from soil and manure of swine-raising premises. Am. J. Vet. Res. 33:1610–1620, 1972.

Wood, R.L., D.R. Haubrich, and R. Harrington: Isolation of previously unreported serotypes of *Erysipelothrix rhusiopathiae* from swine. Am. J. Vet. Res. 39:1958–1961, 1978.

# *BACILLUS ANTHRACIS* **28** *AND OTHER AEROBIC SPORE-FORMING BACILLI*

*Robert P. Williams, Ph.D.*

## *MORPHOLOGY*

The genus *Bacillus* is a member of the family Bacillaceae. The bacteria are rod-shaped, and the majority are motile by means of lateral flagella. An important exception is *Bacillus anthracis,* which lacks flagella and is not motile. Formation of a single endospore in the vegetative bacterium is a dominant feature of the genus. Spores may be oval or spherical, and may be located centrally, subterminally, or terminally. The presence of spores causes the vegetative cell to swell in some species. Capsules are present in a few species, particularly *Bacillus anthracis,* whose virulent strains synthesize a polypeptide capsular material composed of repeating units of D-glutamic acid.

The bacteria can be divided into two groups depending on the size of the vegetative cell (Table 1). In small cell species, the bacterium has a width of 0.6 to 0.8 $\mu$m and a length of 1.5 to 3 $\mu$m; in large cell species, the width is 1.0 to 1.5 $\mu$m and the length 2 to 5 $\mu$m. Although the Gram reaction is usually positive, some species show a variable reaction, particularly if the stain is made from samples taken in the later stages of growth. Sometimes globules of a reserve metabolic material, poly-beta-hydroxybutyrate, are seen in vegetative bacteria of *B. anthracis, B. cereus,* and related species.

The structure of the endospore and its location within the vegetative cell are characteristics useful for taxonomy (Table 1). In group I, which includes *B. anthracis, B. cereus,* and *B. subtilis,* the spore is oval, has a central location, and does not distend the vegetative cell. Vegetative cells of *B. subtilis* do not contain globules of poly-beta-hydroxybutyrate. Spores of group II, including *B. macerans* and *B. polymyxa,* cause the vegetative cell to swell. These spores usually are located centrally but also may be found subterminally or terminally. When thin sections of these spores are examined with the electron microscope, they show a thick spore coat with several prominent longitudinal, parallel ridges on the surface. The ridges are not seen on spores of other species. *B. sphaericus* is included in Group III, in which the spores are round, are located terminally, and cause the vegetative cell to swell. The endospores of *B. cereus, B. anthracis,* and *B. thuringiensis* are enclosed within a loose outer coat, the exosporium.

The different species have an enormous range of colonial morphology that can vary according to the composition of the medium. Isolated colonies may be quite rough and may spread over the surface, particularly if the agar is moist. Pigments sometimes color colonies yellow, pink, red, or even black.

*B. anthracis* grows in vitro in long chains that look like a jointed bamboo rod. In vivo, the chains are shorter, and single bacilli or pairs of rods may be seen (Fig. 1). When grown in culture, no capsule can be seen around anthrax bacteria unless they are grown under an increased tension of carbon dioxide. Capsules are readily apparent around the bacteria when smears from infected animals are examined, particularly if a polychrome stain is used (Fig. 1). When grown on conventional media in air, encapsulated anthrax bacteria, the virulent form, grow as rough colonies. But when the same bacteria are incubated on media containing bicarbonate in an atmosphere of increased carbon dioxide, the colonies are mucoid and smooth (Fig. 2), and capsules are readily seen around the rods (Fig. 3). No other species of *Bacillus* grows in this fashion under these conditions. *B. anthracis* forms spores only under aerobic conditions; thus, spores are not seen in the circulating blood of infected animals.

**TABLE 1.  Characteristics Useful to Differentiate Between Some Species of *Bacillus* [a]**

| CHARACTERISTIC | anthracis | alvei | brevis | cereus | circulans | coagulans | firmus | laterosporus | licheniformis | macerans | megaterium | polymyxa | pumilus | sphaericus | subtilis |
|---|---|---|---|---|---|---|---|---|---|---|---|---|---|---|---|
| *Morphologic* | | | | | | | | | | | | | | | |
| Gram stain | + | v | v | + | v | + | + | v | + | v | + | v | + | v | + |
| Size[c] | l | s | s | l | s | s | s | s | s | s | l | s | s | s | s |
| Motility | − | + | + | v | v | + | v | + | + | + | v | + | + | + | + |
| Spore shape[d] | o | o | o | o | o | o | o | o | o | o | o | o | o | r | o |
| Spore location[e] | c | cts | cts | c | cts | cts | c | c | c | t | c | cts | c | t | c |
| Swelling of vegetative cell | − | + | + | − | + | v | − | + | − | + | − | + | − | + | − |
| Capsule | + | − | − | − | − | − | − | − | + | − | v | + | − | − | − |
| | | | | | | | | | | | | | | | |
| *Biochemical* | | | | | | | | | | | | | | | |
| Catalase | + | + | + | + | + | + | + | + | + | + | + | + | + | + | + |
| Fermentations (acid)[f] | | | | | | | | | | | | | | | |
|   Arabinose | − | − | − | − | + | v | v | − | + | + | v | + | + | − | + |
|   Glucose | + | + | + | + | + | + | d | + | +[g] | +[g] | + | +[g] | + | − | + |
|   Mannitol | − | − | v | − | + | v | + | + | + | + | v | + | + | − | + |
|   Xylose | − | − | − | − | + | v | v | − | + | + | v | + | + | − | + |
| Citrate utilization | v | − | v | v | v | v | − | − | + | v | + | − | + | v | + |
| Nitrate reduction | + | − | v | + | v | v | v | + | + | + | v | + | − | − | + |
| Gelatin liquefaction | + | + | + | + | + | − | + | + | + | + | + | + | + | v | + |
| Hemolysis on sheep blood agar[h] | − | n | n | + | n | n | n | n | n | n | n | n | n | n | ± |
| Lecithinase activity | + | − | − | + | − | − | − | + | − | − | − | − | − | v | − |
| Starch hydrolysis | + | + | − | + | + | + | + | − | + | + | + | + | − | − | + |
| Voges-Proskauer reaction | + | + | − | + | − | v | − | − | + | − | − | + | + | − | + |
| Anaerobic growth[i] | + | + | − | + | v | + | − | + | + | + | − | + | − | − | + |
| Growth at pH <6 | + | − | v | + | v | + | − | − | + | + | + | + | + | v | + |
| Growth in 7% NaCl | + | − | − | v | v | − | + | − | + | − | + | − | + | v | + |
| Growth at 50° C | − | − | + | − | + | + | − | v | + | v | − | − | + | − | + |

[a]Data obtained principally from Bergey's Manual of Determinative Bacteriology, 8th ed., and Cowan and Steel, Manual for the Identification of Medical Bacteria, 2nd ed.
[b]Variable reactions indicated by v; d indicates delayed reaction; n indicates reaction not reported in manuals.
[c]l represents large (width 1.0 to 1.5 $\mu$m and length 2 to 5 $\mu$m); s represents small (width 0.6 to 0.8 $\mu$m and length 1.5 to 3 $\mu$m).
[d]o represents oval; r, round.
[e]c represents central; t, terminal; and s, subterminal.
[f]In media containing $(NH_4)_2HPO_4$ and the appropriate sugar.
[g]Gas is also produced.
[h]Presence of hemolysis eliminates possibility of *B. anthracis,* but lack of hemolysis may be characteristic of other species also.
[i]In broth containing glucose.

## ANTIGENIC COMPOSITION

The genus *Bacillus* forms an antigenically heterogeneous group. However, data about the definitive antigenic composition of the various species are scant. Vegetative cells and spores contain different antigens. Since the bacteria usually are motile, flagellar or H antigens are also present. Unfortunately, except for *B. cereus* and *B. thuringiensis,* in which serotyping schemes have been developed based upon agglutinins formed against the H antigens, the antigenic composition of the genus has been of little help in distinguishing species or strains from one another.

Spores and vegetative cells are antigenically distinct, although some investigators claim that vegetative antigens can be found in spores. Spore antigens can distinguish among the small cell species of the genus, but differentiation among large cell species is less successful. Injection of autoclaved spores into animals produces agglutinins and precipitins. If live spores are injected, antibodies against both the spore and the vegetative cell develop. The precipitinogens seem to be mainly species-specific, while the agglutinogens show subspecies distribution.

Vegetative cell, spore, and flagellar antigens show different levels of specificity. Considerable cross-reaction occurs among species with respect to vegetative cell antigen. Spore antigens seem to provide the highest species specificity, whereas flagellar antigens show the greatest strain specificity within species.

A serotyping scheme has been developed based

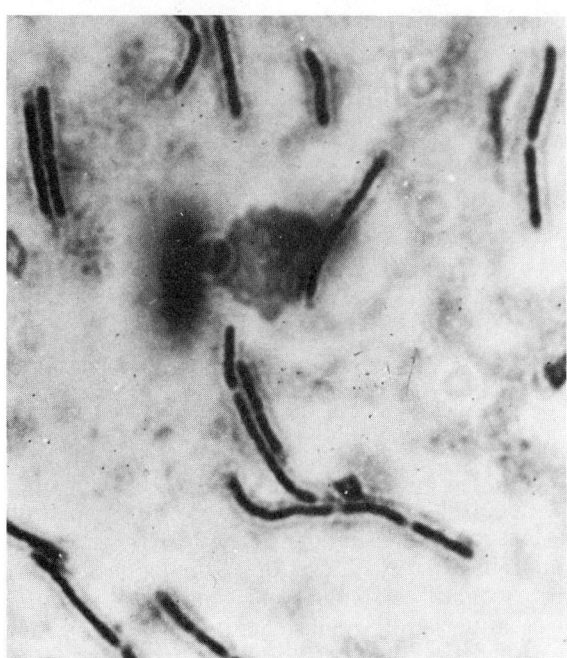

**FIGURE 1.**  *Blood smear from a moribund guinea pig infected with* B. anthracis. *Smear was stained with polychrome methylene blue.*

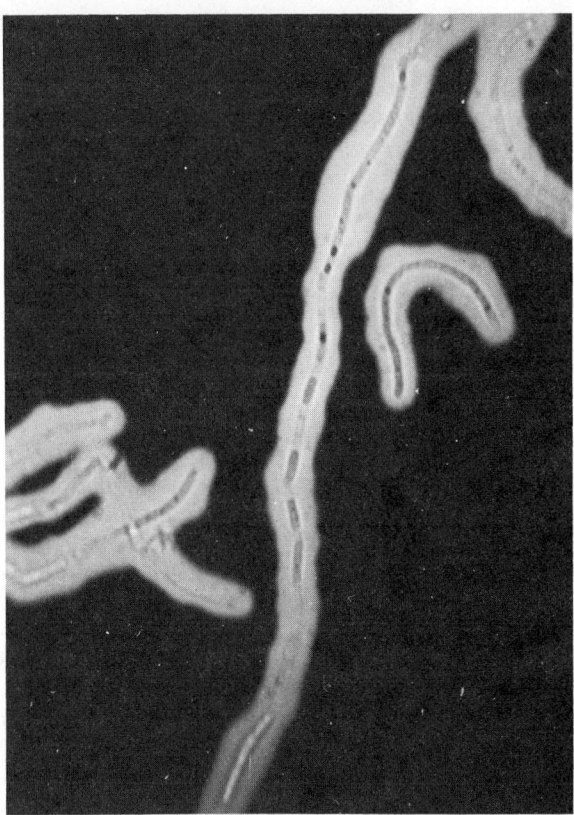

**FIGURE 3.**  *Smear of bacteria stained with India ink from colonies of* B. anthracis *grown in a candle jar on bicarbonate medium. Note the abundant capsule around the bacteria.*

on agglutination with the H antigen of *B. cereus* and has been used in epidemiologic studies of outbreaks of food poisoning caused by the bacteria. Strains of *B. cereus* were classified into 23 serotypes, but about half of the strains isolated

could not be typed. Strains isolated from infections other than food poisoning often were not typable.

The capsular polypeptide of *B. anthracis* is antigenic, although antibodies against it are not protective against infection. Only one capsular type of *B. anthracis* is known. An antigenic polysaccharide is a component of the cell wall of *B. anthracis*. Antibodies to the polysaccharide cross-react with sera prepared from vegetative cells of *B. cereus*. Whereas *B. anthracis* seems to possess only one type of cell-wall antigen, several types are present in *B. cereus* and *B. megaterium*. However, little success has been achieved in the serologic identification of strains of *B. cereus* on the basis of cell-wall antigens. The complex protein toxin produced by *B. anthracis* also is antigenic (Table 2).

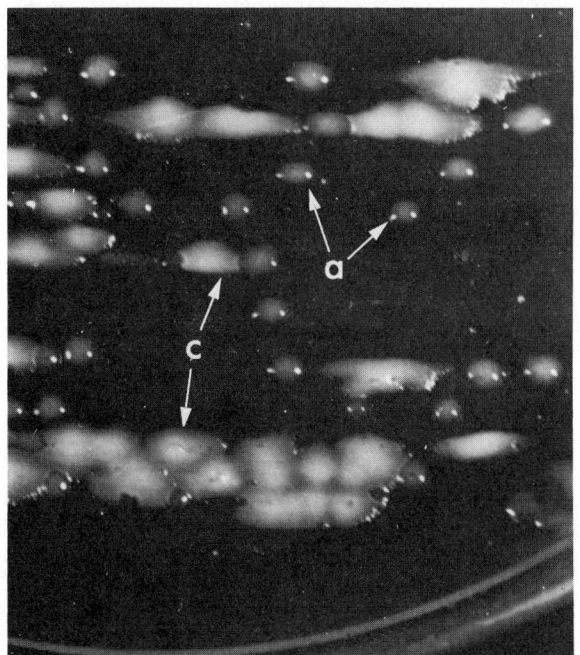

**FIGURE 2.**  *Colonial morphology of virulent* B. anthracis *(smooth colonies, a) and* B. cereus *(rough colonies, c) when grown on nutrient agar containing 0.7 per cent of sodium bicarbonate and incubated at 35° C in a candle jar.*

## METABOLISM

The great diversity among species of *Bacillus* is exemplified by their metabolism. The bacteria are classified as aerobes, but most species are facultative anaerobes, although growth occurs best aero-

**TABLE 2.  Anthrax Toxin: Composition and Biological Effects**

| FACTOR[a] | CHEMICAL NATURE | TOXIC EFFECT[b] | | ANTIGENIC ACTIVITY | IMMUNOGENIC ACTIVITY |
|---|---|---|---|---|---|
| | | Edema | Lethal | | |
| Edema factor (EF); I | Protein, carbohydrate | − | − | + | − |
| Protective antigen (PA); II | Protein | − | − | + | + |
| Lethal factor (LF); III | Protein | − | − | + | − |
| EF + PA | | + | + | + | + |
| EF + LF | | − | − | + | + |
| PA + LF | | − | + | + | + |
| EF + PA + LF[c] | | + | + | + | + |

[a]The descriptive terms and acronyms are the American terminology. The Roman numerals are the British terms.
[b]Edema tested in guinea pig skin; lethal effect in mice.
[c]Complete toxin that would simulate the substances present in infected animals.

bically. All are chemoheterotrophs and can dissimilate a variety of organic substrates such as amino acids, organic acids, and sugars to obtain carbon and energy by aerobic respiration, anaerobic respiration, or fermentation. Adenosine triphosphate (ATP) usually is generated from an aerobic electron transport chain.

Growth requirements range from simple to complex. Most species grow readily on nutrient agar or peptone media. *B. subtilis* grows on a minimal medium containing glucose, citrate, ammonium phosphate, and the usual mineral salts. *B. cereus* requires the addition of certain amino acids, whereas *B. anthracis* needs in addition thiamine, and its growth is stimulated by adenine, guanine, and uracil. Some of the insect pathogens have a more fastidious nutrition and require factors for growth that have not been identified.

Most species grow optimally at pH 7, but some species can grow under alkaline conditions at pH 9, while a few tolerate acidic conditions as low as pH 2. The optimal temperature for growth of the majority of species is 30 to 45° C. *B. stearothermophilus* is thermophilic and grows vigorously at 65° C. Other extreme thermophiles occur in the genus, but these species have not been well characterized. They grow in hot, moist environments such as hay stacks, where they decompose plant material. A few species are psychrophiles and grow at temperatures below 25° C.

Fermentation of glucose can yield a mixture of end products depending upon the species. Initial dissimilation of the sugar is through the Embden-Meyerhof pathway. *B. cereus* and other large cell species of group I convert 2-glyceraldehyde-3-phosphate (triose phosphate) into pyruvate that then is metabolized through acetoin to 2,3-butanediol and carbon dioxide. The reduced nicotinamide adenine dinucleotide (NADH) remaining from the latter reaction is used to reduce another molecule of triose phosphate to glycerol. In addition to 2,3-butanediol, glycerol, and carbon

dioxide, these species also produce small amounts of lactate and ethanol. *B. anthracis* can grow anaerobically on sugars, but *B. megaterium* cannot. A small cell variety of group I, *B. subtilis*, also cannot grow anaerobically on glucose, perhaps because the enzyme for reduction of triose phosphate to glycerol is missing, but in air this bacterium does produce large quantities of 2,3-butanediol. *B. licheniformis* is unique in the genus because it can carry out denitrification. Under anaerobic conditions, this bacterium can grow on nonfermentable organic substrates if furnished with nitrate. Another unique member of group I, *B. fastidiosus*, a species of no medical importance, utilizes uric acid as the only source of energy, carbon, and nitrogen, producing ammonia, carbon dioxide, and cell material.

Good growth of species in group II occurs only on utilizable carbohydrates. Although *B. polymyxa* produces 2,3-butanediol from glucose, the fermentation is different from that carried out by bacilli in group I because no glycerol is formed. *B. macerans* ferments glucose with the formation of ethanol, acetone, acetate, formate, carbon dioxide, and $H_2$. Both species can dissimilate starch and pectins, and they participate in the retting of flax. When grown anaerobically, both species can fix atmospheric nitrogen.

Species of group III such as *B. sphaericus* do not use carbohydrates effectively as sources of energy because they lack fermentative ability. They utilize amino and organic acids as oxidizable substrates. Many strains produce urease, which hydrolyzes urea to form ammonia, and during growth of these bacteria the pH of the medium rapidly becomes alkaline. Growth of these strains usually does not occur unless the medium is initially alkaline and contains urea or ammonium salts. Actively growing cultures of these bacteria can decompose three g of urea per liter of medium per hour.

The different species produce an abundance of

extracellular products including antimicrobial substances, enzymes, pigments, and in some cases toxins. With few exceptions, primarily among the insect pathogens and thermophiles, catalase is formed. Amylase, collagenase, hemolysin, lecithinase, phospholipase, protease, and urease are some of the other enzymes that can be found in cultures. The hemolysin of *B. cereus* can be separated into two components: one, termed cereolysin, has a molecular weight of 52,000; the other has a molecular weight of 31,000. These hemolysins appear similar to those produced by *B. thuringiensis*. *B. anthracis* does not synthesize hemolysin, and this deficiency is used to separate this pathogen from other members of the genus. The enzyme activities, fermentation reactions, and other characteristics of metabolism form the basis for the differentiation of the several species of *Bacillus* (Table 1, Fig. 4).

Several species produce pigments, two of which have been identified. Pulcherrimin, the ferric salt of the pyrazine compound pulcherriminic acid, is synthesized by strains of *B. cereus, B. licheniformis,* and *B. subtilis.* An aromatic compound, protocatechuic acid, is formed by *B. anthracis,* proba-

bly as a derivative of shikimic acid. When complexed with iron in various proportions, protocatechuic acid causes liquid cultures to vary in color from brown to pink to red. Virulent strains of *B. anthracis* reportedly produce more protocatechuic acid than avirulent strains. Unidentified pigments formed by some species are black, tan, or yellow.

*B. cereus* and *B. anthracis* synthesize toxins that cause disease in humans (Tables 2 and 3). Cultural conditions, particularly the tension of carbon dioxide, are critical for synthesis of anthrax toxin. If cultures of *B. cereus* are rapidly transferred in broth, they produce an uncharacterized toxin that is extremely lethal for guinea pigs and mice. Toxins from *B. lentimorbus, B. popilliae,* and *B. thuringiensis* are lethal for insects.

Production of antimicrobial substances prior to the onset of sporulation is characteristic of the genus. These compounds are linear or cyclic polypeptides with a molecular weight of about 1400. Many of the amino acids in the peptides are of the D configuration. Biosynthesis of the peptides does not involve transfer ribonucleic acid (tRNA) and

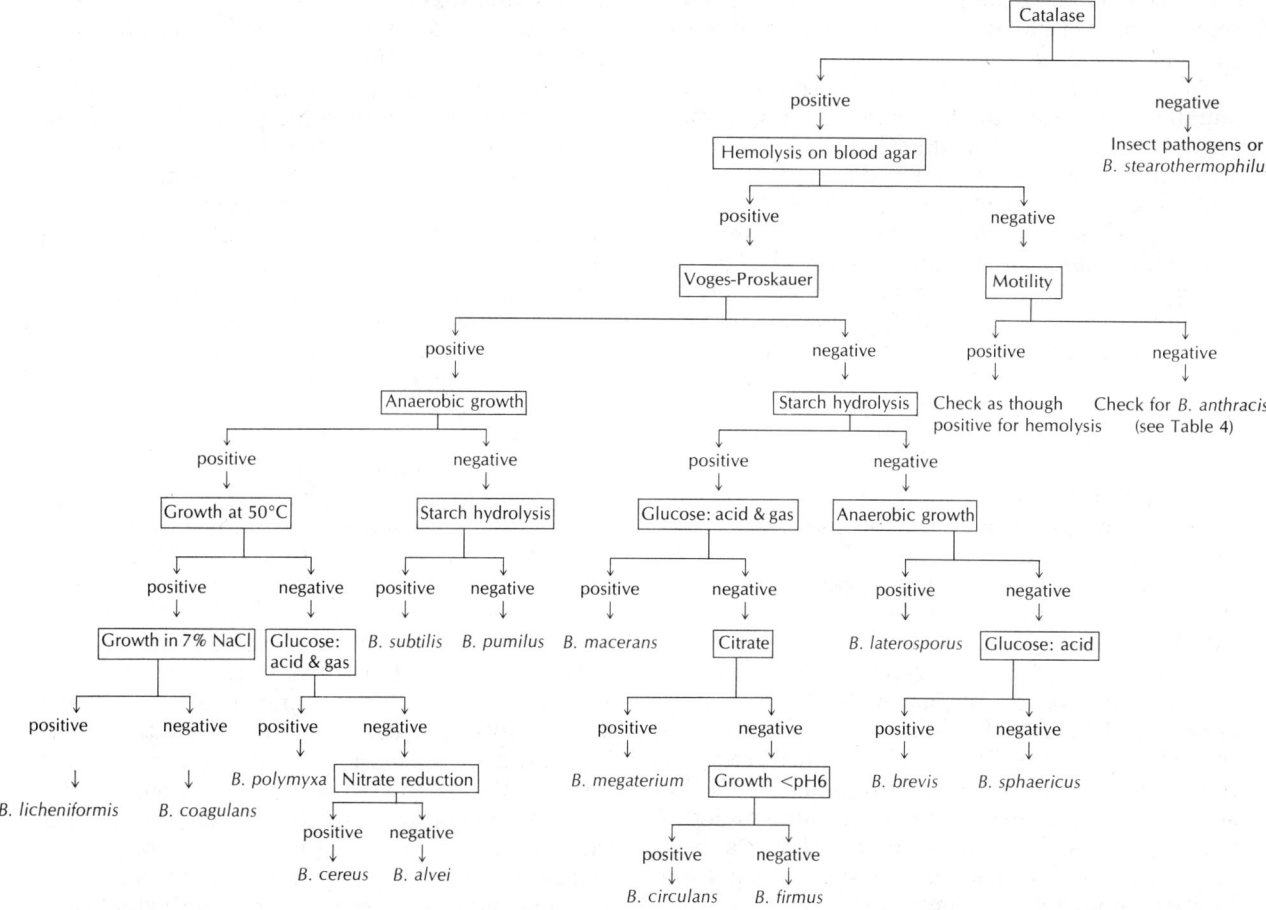

**FIGURE 4.**  *Schema for identification of some species of* Bacillus. *Modified from Dr. D. H. M. Gröschel.*

**TABLE 3.** Comparison of Two Enterotoxins Produced by *Bacillus cereus* [a]

| CHARACTERISTIC | TYPE OF ENTEROTOXIN | |
| --- | --- | --- |
| | Diarrheal | Emetic |
| *Clinical syndrome* | | |
| Incubation period | 8 to 16 hr | 1 to 5 hr |
| Diarrhea | Very common | Fairly common |
| Vomiting | Occasional | Very common |
| Duration of illness | 12 to 24 hr | 6 to 24 hr |
| Foods implicated | Meat products, soups, vegetables, puddings, sauces | Fried or boiled rice |
| Serotypes of *B. cereus* involved | 1, 2, 6, 8, 9, 10, 12, 19 | 1 (majority) 3, 4, 5, 8, 12, 19 |
| *Enterotoxin* [b] | | |
| Molecular weight | *ca.* 50,000 | <5,000 |
| Stability to heat | − | + |
| Fluid accumulation in ligated rabbit ileal segment | + | − |
| Increased vascular permeability in guinea pig or rabbit skin | + | − |
| Lethal for mice after intravenous injection | + | − |
| Stimulation of adenylate cyclase-cAMP system in intestinal epithelial cells | + | − |
| Response when fed to rhesus monkeys | Diarrhea | Vomiting |

[a] From Terranova and Blake, 1978; Gilbert, 1979.
[b] Except for molecular weight, data obtained from cell-free culture filtrates.

ribosomes; their assembly instead is directed by a protein enzyme. Examples of these antimicrobial compounds are bacitracin, gramicidin, polymyxin, and tyrocidine.

The peptidoglycan of the vegetative cell wall usually is similar to the type found in gram-negative bacteria. The diamino acid, *meso*-diaminopimelic acid, is present and is cross-linked to D-alanine to form the interpeptide bridge. In some species, L-lysine replaces diaminopimelic acid, and additional amino acids are present in the interpeptide bridge. The cortex of spores contains a unique peptidoglycan that contains three repeating subunits: a muramic acid unit without attached amino acids; a muramic acid unit attached to an alanine residue; and a muramic acid unit attached to L-alanine, D-glutamic acid, *meso*-diaminopimelic acid, and D-alanine.

The guanine plus cytosine content of the DNA of species ranges from 32 to 53 moles per cent. The DNA base composition of *B. cereus* and *B. anthracis* is similar but not the same, indicating that these two species are related but not identical. Relationships between some species have been studied by use of genetic recombination mediated by transformation or by transduction, or by use of DNA-to-DNA hybridization. Because the DNA of *B. subtilis* is readily transferred, and the bacteria grow well on a minimal medium, this species has been used extensively for studies of bacterial physiology and genetics. Mutants, both natural and induced, of various species can differ in nutritional requirements, sensitivity to drugs and bacteriophage, heat resistance, and, in the

case of *B. anthracis,* virulence and production of capsule and toxin.

Formation of endospores is one of the most salient characteristics of *Bacillus*. The process is complex. Essentially, the phenomenon involves cell differentiation in which morphologic, biochemical, genetic, and physical changes occur in the bacteria. Endospores are a normal stage in the life history of *Bacillus,* but their biologic function is unknown. Their high resistance to inimical environments has survival value, and the mode of life of these bacteria depends upon the accumulation of spores in nature. Asporogenous mutants have little capacity to survive.

The initiation of endospore formation begins as the exponential growth of vegetative cells ends and the cultures approach the stationary phase as a result of limitation of nutrients, particularly sources of nitrogen and carbon. Synthesis of polypeptide antimicrobial substances commences, and cytologic changes begin in the vegetative cell. The two nuclear bodies in a vegetative cell condense to form a single filament. Near the terminal end of the bacterium, a transverse septum forms from the cytoplasmic membrane, probably in conjunction with development of a mesosome. This septum divides the nuclear material and cytoplasm to form a smaller cell, which will become the spore, from a larger cell that is destined eventually to lyse. The cytoplasmic membrane and the cytoplasm of the larger cell engulf the smaller cell and its membrane so that the forespore is surrounded by two cytoplasmic membranes, one from the larger cell and the other from growth of the septum that originally developed to separate the smaller cell. The process is irreversible at this stage, and the vegetative cell is committed to sporulation.

Synthesis and deposition of new structures distinctive to the spore then ensue. A cortex composed of a unique peptidoglycan develops from the two membranes. Exterior to the cortex, a spore coat is synthesized. The coat is a protein like keratin that is resistant to the usual procedures for solubilization of protein. It represents about 80 per cent of the spore protein. In some species, such as *B. cereus,* the exosporium, a loose, thin layer composed of lipoprotein and carbohydrate, surrounds the spore coat. As the spore coat forms, the spores become more refractile. Heat resistance then develops and is associated with an uptake of calcium ions by the spores and synthesis of dipicolinic acid, 2,6-dicarboxylpyridine, which is synthesized by spores from aspartic acid as an offshoot of the lysine pathway. The calcium salt of dipicolinic acid accounts for 10 to 15 per cent of the dry weight of spores and probably is a major factor in heat resistance. After development through the above stages, the mature spore is liberated from the parent cell by autolysis.

Morphologically, the mature endospore consists of a core, the spore protoplast, which contains the nucleus and the enzymes needed for subsequent germination. A complex envelope surrounds and protects the core. The innermost layer is the spore membrane, the original cytoplasmic membrane of the forespore, which contains normal peptidoglycan. External to this membrane is the cortex, the thickest layer of the envelope. The relatively impermeable spore coat is the most superficial layer of most spores, although it may be enclosed by an exosporium in some species.

Mature endospores are less easily stained than vegetative cells and are highly refractile. They have no detectable metabolism, are highly dehydrated, and can survive for decades in a state of dormancy. Spores are highly resistant to deleterious treatment by chemical agents, enzymes, heat, ionizing radiation, and ultraviolet light. Boiling for 10 minutes, dry heat at 140° C for three hours, or autoclaving for 20 to 30 minutes at 15 pounds of steam pressure kills most spores. Alcohols, phenols, heavy metal ions, and detergents are poor agents for killing spores.

When an endospore is placed in an environment with favorable nutritional conditions, it germinates to produce a single vegetative cell. Germination takes place in three stages. First, the spores must be activated by chemical or mechanical agents that damage the spore coat. Abrasion with glass beads, a low pH, or contact with compounds that contain free sulfhydryl groups activates spores. A common laboratory

procedure for activation is called "heat shock," in which a suspension of spores is heated to 65° C for a few minutes to activate them. After the dormancy of spores is broken by activation, initiation of germination commences if environmental conditions are favorable. Water and an effector compound that activates spore enzymes are required. The effector agent varies with different species. L-alanine or adenosine or other amino acids or compounds can serve. Enzymes in the spore are activated to degrade spore constituents, in particular the peptidoglycan of the cortex. Water is taken up by the spores, and calcium dipicolinate is released. Respiration commences, and the spores lose their refractility and heat resistance. If the nutrients required for growth of vegetative cells are present, outgrowth of the spore occurs. Cell wall is synthesized from the spore membrane, and other biosyntheses rapidly develop, culminating in cell division.

During sporulation, the genes for spore formation are activated, while the genes for vegetative cell growth are repressed. The pattern of gene transcription is shifted, and the specificity of RNA polymerase is altered so that different regions of DNA are selected for transcription into messenger RNA. The new gene products direct the formation and composition of the spore. Linkage maps constructed for *B. subtilis* show that the genes for sporulation are clustered in about five widely dispersed regions of the chromosome. A variety of asporogenous mutants exist that are blocked at different stages in the development of endospores. Study of these mutants has contributed enormously to knowledge about sporulation. At least 20 genes are known to be involved in sporulation, and the total number may be several times that. Sporulation provides a relatively simple model in which cell differentiation and morphogenesis can be studied.

## PATHOGENIC PROPERTIES

Susceptible animals injected with *B. anthracis* develop a massive septicemia. Even in the natural infection, the number of bacilli in the blood is so great that they can be seen in stained smears. These observations led to the early conjecture that death from anthrax was caused by blockade of capillaries that prevented oxygenation of tissues. In 1955, British investigators demonstrated that sterile plasma obtained from guinea pigs dying of anthrax was lethal when injected into guinea pigs or mice. The presence of masses of bacteria in the blood was not required, because termination of bacteremia by administration of streptomycin did not prevent death of guinea pigs once the critical number of *B. anthracis* was

322

I — SPECIFIC MICROBIAL AGENTS OF DISEASE

reached. This number was about 1/300 of the number of bacteria present at death in untreated animals.

Anthrax toxin is a complex substance that contains three factors (Table 2): edema factor (EF), protective antigen (PA), and lethal factor (LF), or factors I, II, and III respectively. Various combinations cause edema or are lethal. The most lethal is a combination of the three. Problems arise in precise interpretations of the effects of mixtures because of the difficulty of recombining three relatively unstable proteins 'in the appropriate proportions. Purified protective antigen is immunogenic and has been used as a vaccine for humans. The toxin complex is produced by virulent, encapsulated and avirulent, nonencapsulated *B. anthracis.* For production of protective antigen, cultures of avirulent, nonencapsulated *B. anthracis* are used.

The purified toxin complex interferes with phagocytosis and the bacteriocidal activity of serum. The toxin also increases vascular permeability. The decrease in circulating blood volume plus capillary thrombosis produced by the toxin may account for death from anthrax. The virulence of *B. anthracis* apparently depends upon both the ability to produce the toxin complex and the possession of a capsule. The presence of bicarbonate or serum is required in the medium for production of both the capsule and the toxin. Although the capsule is antigenic, it is not immunogenic. However, the capsule does interfere with phagocytosis and probably plays a role in the pathogenicity of anthrax.

The complex nature of anthrax toxin has left unresolved the ·precise nature of its pathogenic effects. Paradoxically, some animals such as mice are very susceptible when challenged with spores but relatively resistant when toxin is given intravenously. In contrast, dogs and rats are resistant when injected parenterally with spores but succumb to small doses of toxin. In addition, various animal species show different pathophysiologic responses to injection of the substance. Other factors with pharmacologic activity are produced by *B. anthracis,* such as a material with epinephrine-like activity and a cardioactive substance. The bacteria also produce protocatechuic acid that combines with iron to form pigment in liquid cultures of *B. anthracis.* The role, if any, of these substances in the pathophysiology of anthrax is unknown. Other species of *Bacillus* produce a variety of extracellular metabolites with antibiotic, hemolytic, lethal, lipolytic, or proteolytic activity, but their association with the occasional pathogenicity of the bacteria is unknown.

Two enterotoxins are produced by *B. cereus* during exponential growth (Table 3), one that causes diarrhea and the other vomiting. The diarrheal toxin is produced readily on media such as brain-heart infusion broth containing added glucose. Detection of emetic toxin was difficult at first because ordinary media did not support its production, but growth on a medium prepared from rice permitted its isolation. The diarrheal toxin causes fluid accumulation in rabbit ileal loops, promotes vascular permeability in rabbits, and is lethal for mice when injected intravenously. Purulent, pyrogenic, lethal, and necrotic activities are associated with strains of *B. cereus* isolated from patients with severe infections not associated with the gastrointestinal tract. These various activities and the diarrheal toxin may be manifestations of a single substance. Hemolytic and phospholipolytic activities are not associated with pathogenicity of *B. cereus* or with the enterotoxins. Strains of *B. cereus* produce amounts of the diarrheal toxin that vary from undetectable to considerable. Loss of the capacity to produce toxin after transfer in the laboratory led to the speculation that elaboration of the toxin might be under the control of plasmids or bacteriophages. This speculation has not been confirmed.

Some species of *Bacillus* are pathogenic for insects but not for vertebrates. *B. lentimorbus* and *B. popilliae,* which grow readily and produce large numbers of spores in the hemolymph of Japanese beetles, cause milky disease that is lethal for the insects. During sporulation, *B. thuringiensis* forms a crystalline protein that lies adjacent to the spore. After ingestion by larvae of *Lepidoptera,* this parasporal protein dissolves in the gut and effects paralysis of the caterpillar. A specific strain of *B. thuringiensis* also is lethal for larvae of *Diptera,* and its use as a bacterial pesticide may provide means to control mosquitoes and flies.

## IMMUNITY

Louis Pasteur in 1881 dramatically established that herbivorous animals developed immunity to anthrax. He immunized a group of sheep with a vaccine made from an attenuated strain of *B. anthracis.* When later challenged with virulent *B. anthracis,* all 25 vaccinated animals survived, while an equal number of unvaccinated controls did not. Because the attenuated Pasteur vaccine sometimes caused severe disease in vaccinated animals, its use has been supplanted by a suspension of viable spores prepared from a nonencapsulated, avirulent strain of *B. anthracis.* This vaccine is not approved for human use, and occasional cases of disease still occur in vaccinated animals. Both of these vaccines probably produce immunity by release of toxin by growing bacteria.

Second attacks of anthrax in man are rare, and humans probably are relatively resistant to the disease. Manufacturing plants that process wool have large numbers of spores in the air and dust that is inhaled by workers, yet few cases of inhalation anthrax occur in spite of the fact that some of the particles in the dust are of a size that could reach the alveoli. Nor is cutaneous anthrax common in such plants. Antibodies to protective antigen were found in workers who were not immunized and who had no history of anthrax. This serologic evidence suggests that inapparent or mild forms of anthrax occur in humans to provide an antibody response and immunity.

Vaccines of killed bacilli evoke no significant immunity probably because they cannot grow and produce anthrax toxin. Antibody against the polypeptide capsule is not protective except in mice. The complex, purified anthrax toxin is both antigenic and immunogenic, but isolated edema and lethal factors are only antigenic (Table 2). Protective antigen is immunogenic. A vaccine prepared by precipitation and concentration of protective antigen by addition of aluminum potassium sulfate to sterile culture filtrates was calculated to be 92 per cent effective in an exposed, susceptible population of humans. Antibody can be measured by complement fixation, agar gel precipitation, or indirect microhemagglutination tests. The latter procedure is the most sensitive.

Acquired immunity to anthrax apparently involves primarily antibody to the toxin, although the antiphagocytic nature of the capsule suggests that it also may be important. Some animals have a high natural immunity to anthrax. Rats and dogs are only slightly susceptible to infection, but the nature of their immunity is unknown. Guinea pigs, mice, and rabbits are very susceptible, and reportedly one virulent *B. anthracis* organism is lethal after injection into a mouse. The natural disease occurs primarily in herbivorous animals such as cattle, sheep, and horses, who possess little immunity.

Whether other species of *Bacillus* evoke an immune response is unknown. Except for food poisoning, primarily by *B. cereus,* other species cause no well-defined infection. Apparently there is little or no immunity to the enterotoxin produced by *B. cereus* (Table 3).

## LABORATORY DIAGNOSIS

An isolated, hemolytic colony of an aerobic, spore-forming, gram-positive, motile bacillus often is dismissed by the microbiology laboratory as an unimportant contaminant. But the increasing frequency with which severe infections caused by *Bacillus* is being reported mandates that the laboratory consult with the clinician before discarding such cultures. If the specimen originated from a seriously ill patient or from an unusual source or was isolated in large numbers in repeated specimens, the physician should be notified so that the results can be interpreted in terms of the clinical findings.

Identification of the species of *Bacillus* usually can be made by evaluation of several morphologic and biochemical characteristics (Table 1, Fig. 4), although speciation may not be made quickly because of the number of species and the fact that variant strains are common. The bacteria most often encountered in humans grow readily on common nutrient media. Specimens should be obtained from patients prior to administration of antimicrobial therapy and inoculated onto 5 per cent horse or sheep blood agar. The cultures are incubated at 35 to 37° C in air for 24 to 48 hours. Hemolytic, catalase-positive colonies of gram-positive bacilli that contain spores can then be identified by a series of commonly used biochemical tests that include the Voges-Proskauer reaction, starch hydrolysis, glucose fermentation, and anaerobic growth (Table 1, Fig. 4). Experienced technicians may make a preliminary identification from the morphologic appearance of the colonies.

When *B. cereus* is suspected as a cause of food poisoning, the food can be cultured to isolate the bacteria, or isolation of *B. cereus* from the stool of patients can be attempted. If more than $10^5$ bacteria per gram of food are identified as *B. cereus,* the diagnosis is confirmed. Serologic typing of isolated strains can be done for epidemiologic purposes, but the antisera developed by the Food Hygiene Laboratory in London are available only in a few centers. *B. licheniformis* and *B. subtilis* also may be isolated from foods and incriminated as causes of food poisoning.

Although *B. anthracis* is seldom encountered in an average hospital or public health laboratory, it can be confused with the more common *B. cereus* or encapsulated *B. megaterium*. The three species can be differentiated easily (Table 4). The "string of pearls" phenomenon is observed when *B. anthracis* is inoculated onto agar containing penicillin (0.05 to 0.5 units per ml). After incubation for about three to six hours, the areas where growth might occur are examined microscopically for the presence of large spherical bacilli in chains, the "string of pearls." Animals injected subcutaneously with *B. anthracis* develop an overwhelming infection within 36 to 48 hours, and smears from the blood or spleen show numerous encapsulated bacteria. Suspensions should be diluted and made in saline to avoid nonspecific deaths.

**TABLE 4.  Characteristics Useful for Distinguishing *B. anthracis*, *B. cereus*, and *B. megaterium***

| CHARACTERISTIC | *B. anthracis* | *B. cereus* | *B. megaterium* |
|---|---|---|---|
| Hemolysis on sheep's blood agar | − | + | − |
| Peptonization of litmus milk | − | + | ± |
| Fermentation of salicin | − | ± | − |
| Specific fluorescent antibody stain | + | − | − |
| Appearance of colonies grown on bicarbonate (0.7%) nutrient agar[a] | | | |
|    In air | (Rough)[b] | Rough | No growth |
|    In 5% $CO_2$ or candle jar | Smooth | Rough | Rough |
| Growth in penicillin (10 $\mu$/ml) agar | − | + | − |
|    String of pearls reaction | + | − | − |
| Pathogenicity for mice | + | − | − |
|    Positive capsular stain for bacteria from spleen[c] | + | − | − |
| Susceptibility to specific gamma bacteriophage | + | − | − |

All cultures incubated at 35 to 37° C.
[a]Bicarbonate must be sterilized separately by filtration and added to agar.
[b]*B. anthracis* may not grow under these conditions.
[c]Stained by Loeffler's methylene blue stain (polychrome methylene blue stain).

Samples from cutaneous anthrax lesions should be obtained carefully. Fluid can be taken from the vesicles with a Pasteur pipette, or less preferably, with a syringe and needle or swab, and used for smear and culture. Tentative identification can be made if a smear shows short chains of large gram-positive rods, perhaps with a few spores. Pulmonary anthrax cannot be diagnosed by culture because the sputum rarely contains bacteria; a blood culture usually is positive. Blood cultures also should be obtained to diagnose intestinal anthrax. Specimens for diagnosis in animals are best taken from the jugular vein.

The fluorescent antibody stain for *B. anthracis* is presumptive because *B. megaterium* and *B. cereus* also fluoresce with the antiserum. Cultures for fluorescent staining must be grown in carbon dioxide to permit capsule production. This test and the test for susceptibility to gamma bacteriophage are obtainable only in certain laboratories such as the Center for Disease Control in the United States. Serologic diagnosis for anthrax is not valuable because the disease is of short duration, although procedures such as an agar gel precipitation test, complement fixation, and indirect microhemagglutination have been used to detect antibody. Selective media for isolation have been unsatisfactory because they inhibit growth of *B. anthracis*.

*B. anthracis* can be isolated from contaminated wool and hair. The material should be soaked in detergent or dilute potassium hydroxide. After thorough soaking, the sample is teased, heated to 65° C for five minutes, and centrifuged. The sediment is cultured, and suspicious colonies are identified.

Any competent microbiology laboratory can handle *B. anthracis* safely. Aerosols should be avoided, and use of a biological safety hood is advisable, particularly if contaminated materials are examined. Animals should be inoculated only when adequate facilities are available for isolation, but reasonable identification of *B. anthracis* can be made without use of animals. Benches should be washed with 5 per cent carbolic acid (phenol) or 5 per cent hypochlorite, and instruments should be autoclaved to reduce the possibility of contamination.

## DRUG SUSCEPTIBILITY

With one exception, broad spectrum antimicrobial agents are usually effective against species of *Bacillus*. The exception is penicillin. *B. cereus* in particular produces a beta-lactamase that renders penicillin ineffective for treatment. Chloramphenicol, erythromycin, penicillin, tetracyclines, and sulfonamides have been used to treat anthrax. About 24 to 48 hours after treatment with penicillin, *B. anthracis* disappears from cutaneous lesions. The bacteria are reported to persist longer after treatment with chloramphenicol or tetracycline. However, some patients with cutaneous anthrax recover without treatment, another indication that humans are relatively resistant to the disease. *B. anthracis* is resistant to neomycin and polymyxin. Other species of *Bacillus* are sensitive to chloramphenicol, gentamicin, kanamycin, and tetracyclines. Treatment of infections caused by these organisms usually involves initial treatment with a broad spectrum antibiotic, followed by laboratory tests on the isolated organism to determine sensitivities. *B. subtilis* is susceptible, *B. pumilus* less so, to ampicillin, cephalothin, methicillin, and penicillin G. *B. cereus* is resistant to these drugs as well as to sulfonamides and trimethoprim.

## *EPIDEMIOLOGY*

Gram-positive, aerobic, spore-forming bacilli are ubiquitous in the environment. They are found in decaying organic matter, dust, soil, vegetables, and water, and some species are part of the normal flora. From these sources, the bacteria can readily cause infections in debilitated, immunosuppressed, or traumatized patients. However, except for *B. anthracis,* members of the genus usually are not considered pathogenic. But the opportunity for infection with other species is increasing with the prolonged survival of patients with severe illnesses. When the bacteria are isolated from blood, body fluids, or infections of closed spaces, they should not be dismissed as contaminants, particularly if patients are receiving immunosuppressive or myelosuppressive drugs, are undergoing hemodialysis, or are drug addicts. Although the true prevalence is unknown, infection caused by the bacteria occurs more frequently than is appreciated. They have been documented as causes of bronchopneumonia, meningitis, ocular infections, septicemia, osteomyelitis, endocarditis, abscesses, and several other types of infections.

The diarrheal type of gastroenteritis caused by *B. cereus* is associated with a wide range of foods, whereas boiled and fried rice is primarily implicated in the emetic disease (Table 3). Several serotypes are found in outbreaks of diarrhea, but Serotype 1 predominates in cases of vomiting, perhaps because the spores of this type are more resistant to heat, and they survive in cooked rice. Outbreaks of food poisoning caused by *B. cereus* have been reported from Asia, Australia, Europe, and North America. The diseases may be more common than reported because they are easily confused with the more frequent outbreaks of food poisoning caused by staphylococci and *C. perfringens.* Thorough cooking and refrigeration of foods help control gastroenteritis effected by *B. cereus.*

*B. anthracis* is a saprophytic bacterium that can become a facultative parasite. The bacteria probably survive in soil in a dynamic state in which they undergo cycles of germination and sporulation depending upon conditions in the microenvironment. Contamination of the soil originally occurs when infected animals soil the ground with blood and excreta that contain vegetative bacteria. Sporulation ensues in the aerobic environment outside of the body. In an alkaline, calcareous soil that is poorly drained, the spores germinate in decayed vegetation. When the weather becomes dry, spores form, and, if grazing animals inadvertently ingest them, an outbreak of anthrax can occur. Such focal areas may remain contaminated indefinitely, with *B. anthra-*cis undergoing cycles of germination and sporulation. The dependency of the cycle upon the environment may account for the seasonal occurrence of anthrax in the late summer and early fall subsequent to previous rain, as well as for the sporadic outbreaks of the disease.

Anthrax primarily afflicts herbivorous animals. It is one of the major livestock diseases in the world and affects thousands of cattle, goats, horses, and sheep annually. Carnivorous animals can be infected secondarily if they feed on infected carcasses, but the disease is not spread from animal to animal. About a third of the cases in animals occur in Europe, with the major portion of infections occurring in Asia and Africa. The disease is enzootic in Asia Minor, Central and South America, Africa, and Southeast Asia, from whence epizootics periodically are reported in wild and domestic animals. In the United States, sporadic cases occur in the Gulf coast and midwest states and in California. The disease may be more prevalent than reported because many sudden deaths in animals, the typical outcome of an infection, may not be recognized as anthrax.

As many as 20,000 to 100,000 cases of anthrax in humans are estimated to occur worldwide per year, but such figures are unreliable because many countries do not report the disease. Anthrax was a formidable scourge in England in the mid-19th century, when fatal outbreaks of "woolsorter's disease" (inhalation anthrax) among textile workers led to legislation to control the disease. Today in industrial countries anthrax still is predominantly an occupational disease in the textile and tanning industries. Wool, hair, hides, and bone meal imported from countries where the disease is prevalent in animals contain large numbers of spores. Workers are exposed to the spores in the air and dust of plants and while handling the contaminated materials. However, although the bacteria are widespread, the number of cases of disease is few. Cutaneous infections are most common when spores invade the skin of the head, neck, or arms through cuts or abrasions, but if properly treated, the mortality is nil. Inhalation anthrax is rare but almost uniformly fatal. Although industrial anthrax is the most commonly reported form of the disease, agricultural anthrax may be widespread among farmers in countries where the disease is epizootic. Intestinal anthrax that has a high mortality occurs when meat from diseased animals is eaten. Veterinarians occasionally develop anthrax from contact with infected animals or carcasses. Cases of disease now occur in amateur craftsmen who use raw wool contaminated with anthrax spores. There are no age or sex differences in cases. Industrial anthrax has no seasonal incidence, but agricultural cases are most common in the late summer and early fall. No human anthrax was reported in the United States in 1979.

Control of anthrax requires elimination or reduction of contact with infected animals. Carcasses of animals that died from anthrax must be incinerated or buried with lime deep in the soil. Autopsies should not be done if anthrax is suspected to avoid recontamination of the soil. Potential focal areas for growth of *B. anthracis* can be eliminated by proper drainage or tillage. If anthrax does occur, infected animals must be treated, and the exposed herd quarantined and vaccinated with the viable spore vaccine. This vaccine protects for about one year. Immunization and improved working conditions in industry seem to be responsible for the progressive decline of human cases of anthrax, so that the disease now is rare in the United States and Europe. Vaccine prepared from protective antigen can be used to immunize exposed individuals who handle materials contaminated with anthrax spores. Antibody titer declines rapidly; booster doses of the vaccine are suggested at six months or one year to maintain immunity.

### References

Gilbert, R. J.: *Bacillus cereus* gastroenteritis. In Riemann, H., and Bryan, F. L. (eds.): Foodborne Infections and Intoxications. 2nd ed. New York, Academic Press, 1979.

Gilbert, R. J., Turnbull, P. C. D., Parry, J. M., and Kramer, J. M.: Food poisoning and other clinical infections associated with *Bacillus* species with particular reference to *B. cereus*. In Berkeley, R., and Goodfellow, M. (eds.): The Aerobic Endospore-Forming Bacteria: Classification and Identification. Soc Gen Microbiol Special Publications Series. New York, Academic Press, 1980.

Nungester, W. J.: Proceedings of the conference on progress in the understanding of anthrax. Fed Proc 26:1485, 1967.

Terranova, W., and Blake, P. A.: *Bacillus cereus* food poisoning. N Engl J Med 298:143, 1978.

Tuazon, C. U., Murray, H. W., Levy, C., Solny, M. W., Curtin, J. A., and Sheagreen, J. N.: Serious infection from *Bacillus* species. JAMA 241:1137, 1979.

Turnbull, P. C. B., Jorgensen, K., Kramer, J. M., Gilbert, R. J., and Parry, J. M.: Severe clinical conditions associated with *Bacillus cereus* and the apparent involvement of exotoxins. J Clin Pathol 32:289, 1979.

Van Ness, G. B.: Ecology of anthrax: Anthrax undergoes a propagation phase in soil before it infects livestock. Science 172:1303, 1971.

Wright, G. G.: Anthrax toxin. In Schlessinger, D. (ed.): Microbiology — 1975. Washington, D. C., American Society for Microbiology, 1975, p. 272.

# Gram-negative Cocci and Coccobacilli

# 29 NEISSERIA

*Stephen A. Morse, Ph.D.*

## NEISSERIA

The genus *Neisseria* is one of four genera included in the family *Neisseriaceae*. The other genera in the family are *Branhamella, Moraxella,* and *Acinetobacter* (see Table 1). Members of the genus *Neisseria* inhabit the mucosal surfaces of warm-blooded animals. The genus includes two species that are pathogenic for man: *Neisseria gonorrhoeae* (the gonococcus) and *Neisseria meningitidis* (the meningococcus). It also includes several nonpathogenic species (*N. flavescens, N. mucosa, N. perflava, N. sicca,* and *N. lactamica*) that may be part of the normal flora and therefore can be confused with gonococci and meningococci.

Descriptions of a condition resembling gonococcal urethritis can be found in the earliest recorded histories of man. The disease, gonorrhea, was named by Galen in about A.D. 130 (*gonos*, seed; *rhoia*, flow). Galen had the mistaken impression that the disease was due to a morbid loss of semen. Gonorrhea was known to be of venereal origin in the 13th century, but was thought to be an early symptom of syphilis. It was not until the middle of the 19th century that gonorrhea and syphilis were clearly differentiated. *N. gonorrhoeae*, the causative agent of gonorrhea, was first described by Neisser in 1879 in smears of purulent exudates from patients with acute gonorrhea and from newborn infants with conjunctivitis. The gonococcus was first cultivated by Leistikow and Loeffler in 1882. Bumm showed that the gonococcus fulfilled Koch's postulates in 1885.

*N. meningitidis* is the causative agent of men-

## TABLE 1. Taxonomy and Nomenclature of the Neisseriaceae

Genus I.  Neisseria
Species:  *N. gonorrhoeae*
          *N. meningitidis*
          *N. lactamica*
          *N. sicca*
          *N. flavescens*
          *N. subflava* (includes *N. flava, N. perflava*)
          *N. mucosa*

Genus II.  Branhamella
Species:  *B. catarrhalis* (formerly *N. catarrhalis*)
          *B. ovis* (formerly *N. ovis*)
          *B. caviae* (formerly *N. caviae*)

Genus III.  Moraxella
Species:  *M. lacunata*
          *M. nonliquifaciens*
          *M. bovis*
          *M. osloensis*
          *M. phenylpyruvica*
          *M. kingii*
          *M. urethralis*\* (formerly *Mima polymorpha* var *oxidans*)

Genus IV.  Acinetobacter
Species:  *A. calcoaceticus* (formerly *Bacillus anithratum, Herrelea vaginicola,* or *M. lwoffi*)

*Tentatively placed in this genus.

Thin sections of gonococci or meningococci grown in vitro exhibit cell structures in electron micrographs similar to those of other gram-negative bacteria (Fig. 1). An undulating outer membrane, approximately 7.5 to 8.5 nm in thickness, appears as a bilayered structure. The periplasmic space, between the cytoplasmic membrane and the outer membrane, contains a thin, electron-dense layer, approximately 6.0 nm in diameter, which corresponds to the peptidoglycan layer of the bacterial cell envelope. The chemical composition of the purified peptidoglycan from *N. gonorrhoeae* consists of muramic acid, glutamic acid, alanine, *meso*-diaminopimelic acid, and glucosamine in approximate molar ratios of 1:1:2:1:1 respectively (Morse, 1978; Roberts, 1977). The peptidoglycan layer and the outer membrane adhere to each other at regular intervals around the periphery of the cell.

Cell wall blebs produced by budding of the outer membrane have been seen both in lag phase broth- or agar-grown cultures of *N. meningitidis* and *N. gonorrhoeae*. The blebs consist of outer membrane components, including lipopolysaccharide. The production of these blebs occurs on rapidly growing cells since no blebs are seen on stationary phase cells.

ingococcal meningitis (formerly called epidemic cerebrospinal meningitis). The disease has the potential for occurring in epidemic form. It was first recognized as a contagious disease early in the 19th century. Outbreaks were eventually described on all continents, and the prevalence of the disease, particularly among military personnel, became apparent. The causative organism was first described by Marchiafava and Celli (1884) in meningeal exudate. In 1887, Weichselbaum isolated the organism in pure culture and described it in detail as the characteristic bacterium found in six cases of acute cerebrospinal meningitis.

### Morphology

*Neisseria* are gram-negative cocci, 0.6 to 1.0 μm in diameter. The organisms are usually seen in pairs with their adjacent sides flattened. Tetrads or clusters are occasionally seen. Negatively stained cells display a rugose outer cell surface that is characteristic of many gram-negative bacteria. Fresh isolates of most *N. meningitidis* serogroups are encapsulated. Gonococci also possess a capsule; however, the capsule is most evident on recent isolates (Hendley et al., 1977; Richardson and Sadoff, 1977). *Neisseria* do not possess flagella; however, twitching motility may sometimes be observed with piliated organisms.

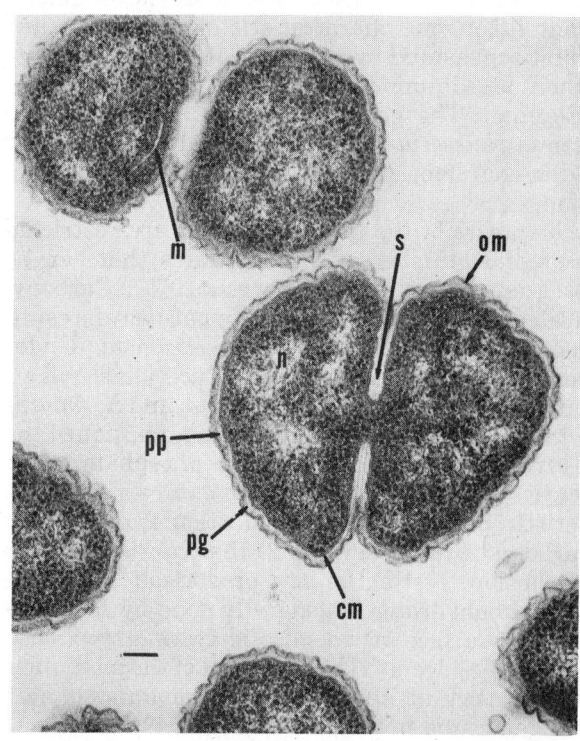

**FIGURE 1.** *Electron micrograph of a thin section of* N. gonorrhoeae *stained with uranyl acetate and lead citrate. Symbols: om, outer membrane; pg, peptidoglycan; pp, periplasmic space; cm, cytoplasmic membrane; s, septum; n, nucleoid zone; m, mesosome. Bar + 0.1 μm. (Used with permission of the American Society for Microbiology.)*

**TABLE 2.  Differential Characteristics of the Genus Neisseria***

| | N. gonorrhoeae | N. meningitidis | N. lactamica | N. sicca | N. subflava† | N. flavescens | N. mucosa |
|---|---|---|---|---|---|---|---|
| Acid from: | | | | | | | |
| Glucose | + | + | + | + | + | − | + |
| Maltose | − | + | + | + | + | − | + |
| Lactose | − | − | + | − | − | − | + |
| Fructose | − | − | − | + | v | − | + |
| Sucrose | − | − | − | + | v | − | + |
| Starch | − | − | − | v | v | − | + |
| Glycogen synthesis from 5% sucrose | Ø | Ø | ? | +‡ | d | + | + |
| Growth at 22° C | − | − | − | d | d | + | + |
| Presence of capsule | v | d | ? | v | + | − | + |
| Production of $H_2S$ | − | − | − | + | + | + | + |
| Pigment | − | − | − | d | + | + | − |
| Reduction of nitrate | − | − | − | − | − | − | + |
| Reduction of nitrite | = | d | ? | + | + | + | + |

*+, most strains positive (≧ 90%); −, most strains negative (≧ 90%); d, some strains positive, some negative; v, character inconstant within single strain; Ø, no growth on medium with 5% sucrose.

†New species consisting of N. subflava, N. flava, and N. perflava.

‡N. sicca forms an iodine-positive product when grown on trypticase soy agar without 5% sucrose. This reaction, which does not occur with N. subflava, may be used as a differentiating characteristic.

## Metabolism

*Neisseria* are aerobic and contain high levels of cytochrome *c* oxidase activity (Morse, 1978; Roberts, 1977). Cytochrome *c* oxidase is an important taxonomic characteristic of this genus and can be measured by reduction of *N,N*-dimethyl-*p*-phenylenediamine (or tetramethyl-*p*-phenylenediamine). The principal species included in the genus *Neisseria* are listed in Table 2, together with characteristics used in species differentiation.

Members of the genus *Neisseria* are restricted as to the number of carbohydrates that can be utilized (Morse, 1978; Roberts, 1977). Carbohydrates are utilized by oxidative pathways, resulting in the accumulation of acetic acid. Under some conditions, lactic acid and acetylmethylcarbinol are produced. *N. gonorrhoeae* and *N. meningitidis* dissimilate glucose by a combination of the Entner-Doudoroff and pentose phosphate pathways. Each species of *Neisseria* exhibits a characteristic pattern of acid production from specific carbohydrates (see Table 2) that can be used for speciation. Testing for acid production from various carbohydrates is generally done by inoculating the surface of a semisolid cystine trypticase agar (CTA) deeply. The initial pH of the medium is very important, since only small amounts of acid are generated in positive reactions.

Both the gonococcus and meningococcus have a functional tricarboxylic acid cycle (Morse, 1978; Roberts, 1977). However, the utilization of this pathway is markedly influenced by growth conditions.

*N. gonorrhoeae* and *N. meningitidis* are fastidious organisms (the gonococcus more so than the meningococcus) with complex nutritional growth requirements. Both organisms are sensitive to growth inhibition by free fatty acids present in various peptones or in agar. The toxic effect of the free fatty acids can be eliminated by adding a binding agent, such as soluble starch, serum, or charcoal, to the medium. Gonococci and meningococci are unique among gram-negative bacteria because they are inhibited by low concentrations of gonadal steroids (Morse, 1978; Roberts, 1977).

Many strains of *N. gonorrhoeae* require increased atmospheric carbon dioxide concentrations (ca 4 to 8 per cent) for initial isolation. This requirement is often lost after repeated subculture. An exogenous source of carbon dioxide is required during the lag phase. This requirement may be met by either the addition of bicarbonate ions or gaseous carbon dioxide. During exponential growth, the exogenous source is replaced by metabolically generated carbon dioxide. Meningococci are less stringent in their requirement for carbon dioxide.

Gonococci and meningococci typically undergo autolysis in older cultures or when suspended in appropriate buffers. In *N. gonorrhoeae*, autolysis results from a combination of peptidoglycan hydrolysis and destabilization of the cell membranes (Morse, 1978; Roberts, 1977). The presence of divalent cations ($Mg^{2+}$ or $Ca^{2+}$) will prevent cellular lysis but will not inhibit peptidoglycan hydrolysis.

The pathogenic *Neisseria* have an optimum growth temperature that ranges from 36 to 39°C.

The maximum growth temperature is ca 41°C and the minimum growth temperature is ca 24°C. The inability of *N. gonorrhoeae* and *N. meningitidis* to grow at 22°C distinguishes these species from most of the nonpathogenic species of *Neisseria*. The pH range for growth varies from strain to strain. Many strains will grow in media buffered over a pH range of 6.0 to 8.0.

## NEISSERIA GONORRHOEAE

### Colonial Types

As early as 1904 differences were noted in the colonial appearance of *N. gonorrhoeae*. More recently, an association was observed between virulence and colonial morphology. Four morphologically distinct colonial types were initially described and designated 1, 2, 3, and 4 (T1, T2, T3, T4). Later, other colonial types, such as T5, were reported. The properties of these colonial variants are summarized in Table 3.

Freshly isolated strains consist of type 1 and type 2 colonies. The type 1 and type 2 colonial morphology can be maintained by selective subculture at daily intervals. Organisms from type 1 and type 2 colonies are piliated and retain virulence when they are inoculated experimentally into the urethra of the human or chimpanzee male, or intravenously into chicken embryos. During nonselective transfer, the predominant colonial types (T1 or T2) may be rapidly replaced by the less virulent colonial types T3, T4, and T5. Organisms from these colonial forms lack pili.

### Antigenic Composition

Strains of *N. gonorrhoeae* differ not only when freshly isolated, but also change antigenically on continued subculture. Recent evidence suggests that some antigens may be expressed only in vivo or in response to specific environmental factors. The gonococcus also shares antigens with the meningococcus and other gram-negative bacteria. Most current knowledge concerns antigens associated with the cell envelope.

*Capsules.* Encapsulation of gonococci is suggested by the finding that meningococci have a polysaccharide capsule that provides a basis for grouping. It has been demonstrated by negative staining and by electronmicroscopy of cells exposed to hyperimmune serum that freshly isolated strains of *N. gonorrhoeae* possessed a capsule (Hendley, 1977; Richardson and Sadoff, 1977). Environmental and nutritional factors are important in capsule synthesis. The capsule is loosely associated with the cell surface and can be easily removed by mild shearing. Although the capsule is most evident on recent isolates or on organisms recently grown in vivo, it is also present on the surface of laboratory strains. Cells from all colony types produce capsules. The capsules are antiphagocytic; however, anticapsular antibodies promote phagocytosis. The chemical nature of the capsule and homo- or heterogeneity of capsular types are still unknown (Richardson and Sadoff, 1977).

*Pili.* Metal-shadowed electronmicrographs of *N. gonorrhoeae* reveal hairlike filaments, known as pili, extending from the surface. Pili have a

**TABLE 3.  Morphology and Other Properties of Colonial Types of N. gonorrhoeae**

| | COLONIAL TYPE | | | | |
|---|---|---|---|---|---|
| | 1 | 2 | 3 | 4 | 5 |
| Average diameter (mm) | 0.5–0.7 | 0.5–0.7 | 1.0–1.4 | 1.0–1.4 | 1.4 |
| Elevation (convexity) | ++ | ++ | + | + | + |
| Reflection of light | + | ++ | − | − | + |
| Surface granularity | − | + | + | − | ++ |
| Edge | Entire | Entire | Entire | Entire | Slightly crenated |
| Opacity | Translucent | Translucent | Translucent | Translucent | Opaque |
| Color* | Gray-Gold | Dark Gold | Light Brown | Colorless | Brown |
| Structure | Amorphous | Amorphous | Granular | Amorphous | Granular |
| Consistency | Viscid | Friable | Viscid | Viscid | ? |
| Autoagglutinability in saline | + | + | − | − | ++ |
| Hemadsorption with rabbit erythrocytes | + | + | − | − | − |
| Hemagglutination | + | + | − | − | +/+ |
| Clumping during growth in liquid medium | Slight or moderate | Marked | Moderate | None | ? |
| Presence of visible pili | + | + | − | − | − |
| Presence of rhamnose in LPS | − | − | + | + | + |
| Competent for transformation | + | + | − | − | ? |
| Cryptic $2.6 \times 10^6$ dalton plasmid | + | + | + | + | ? |
| Self-transmissible $24.5 \times 10^6$ dalton plasmid | + | + | + | + | − |
| Approximate $LD_{50}$ for chick embryos inoculated intravenously (colony-forming units) | $<10^4$ | $<10^2$ | $<10^7$ | $<10^7$ | $<10^7$ |

*Light variants of colonial types 1 and 2 have been reported.

diameter of ca 7 nm and are found on the surface of gonococci from colony types 1 and 2; gonococci from colony types 3 and 4 are devoid of visible pili. The presence of pili on *N. gonorrhoeae* is not unique. Nonpathogenic *Neisseria* spp and *N. meningitidis* also possess pili. Short pili (175 to 210 nm in length) are seen only on nonpathogenic species, whereas long pili (up to 4300 nm) are seen on organisms of both nonpathogenic and pathogenic species. There is no consistent relationship between colonial morphology and pili among the nonpathogenic *Neisseria* spp and *N. meningitidis*.

Gonococcal pili have been purified and are primarily protein in nature. Neutral sugar and phosphate residues have also been reported in them. Pilar subunit molecular weights vary among strains and range between 18,000 and 20,000. Pili also exhibit antigenic heterogeneity. The amino-terminal amino acid sequence is identical for the first 24 residues in pili purified from three strains of *N. gonorrhoeae* and one strain of *N. meningitidis*. This finding was unexpected in that the three sources of gonococcal pili exhibited less than 1 per cent shared antigenicity.

A potential antiphagocytic role for pili has been proposed to explain the decreased association of piliated gonococci with human polymorphonuclear leukocytes as compared with nonpiliated gonococci. This role has been challenged, and the association of the gonococcus with polymorphonuclear leukocytes has been ascribed to another protein surface factor (leukocyte association (LA) factor). On the other hand there is considerable evidence that gonococcal pili play an important role in the attachment of the gonococcus to host cells. Pili appear to recognize specific binding sites on host cell surfaces. It is noteworthy that the greatest attachment of purified pili is to cells that are histologically the most similar to the actual sites of gonococcal infection. It has been postulated that pili overcome the long-range electrostatic repulsion between the negatively charged gonococcal and host cell surfaces.

***Outer Membrane Proteins.*** The outer membrane of *N. gonorrhoeae* contains relatively few proteins, with one protein accounting for as much as 66 per cent of the total outer membrane protein. This protein varies antigenically among strains and can be used to divide the gonococcus into serotypes. At least 16 serotypes have been isolated. Antibodies against the principal outer membrane protein are bactericidal in a complement-dependent assay.

***Lipopolysaccharides.*** The lipopolysaccharide (LPS) from *N. gonorrhoeae* has been isolated and characterized by several groups of investigators. There is some controversy as to whether the gonococcus possesses a smooth-type or rough-type LPS. A smooth-type LPS has been reported in organisms from type 1 and type 2 colonies. However, growth conditions may alter the type of LPS synthesized. The LPS from types 3 and 4 organisms contains rhamnose. The gonococcus also produces an enzyme that degrades the polysaccharide portion of its LPS. The core region of the LPS is antigenic and antibodies are bactericidal.

### Genetics

The chromosome of the gonococcus has approximately $1.5 \times 10^6$ nucleotide pairs and a molecular weight of $9.8 \times 10^8$. Most strains of *N. gonorrhoeae* contain a $2.4 \times 10^6$ dalton plasmid. There has been no function ascribed to the presence of this plasmid and it remains phenotypically cryptic. A smaller percentage of gonococcal strains contains a $24.5 \times 10^6$ dalton plasmid. It has been recently shown that this plasmid is a sex factor capable of promoting the transfer of chromosomal genes and R-plasmids via conjugation.

Genetic transformation readily occurs with *N. gonorrhoeae*. Unlike most bacteria, the gonococcus is competent for transformation throughout the growth cycle. All strains of *N. gonorrhoeae* examined have been found competent for genetic transformation. Transformation frequencies are significantly higher ($>10^3$-fold higher) with piliated cells from type 1 or type 2 colonies than with nonpiliated cells from type 3 or type 4 colonies.

Conjugation has recently been described in *N. gonorrhoeae*. Only strains harboring the $24.5 \times 10^6$ dalton plasmid serve as donors. There is no relationship between colony type (and presumably the presence of pili) and the ability to serve as donor.

No bacteriophage has been described for *N. gonorrhoeae*, and transduction has not been reported in the gonococcus.

### Epidemiology

The only natural host for *N. gonorrhoeae* is the human. An estimated 3 million cases of gonorrhea were treated in the United States during 1977. The annual incidence of reported gonorrhea in the United States tripled between 1963 and 1975. This increase in incidence has apparently leveled off in the last few years. Gonorrhea is a worldwide problem. Significant increases in incidence have been reported from Argentina, Austria, Bolivia, Canada, Chad, Colombia, Costa Rica, Denmark, El Salvador, Ecuador, Finland, Gabon, Germany, Hong Kong, Israel, Iran, Iraq, Jamaica, Mali, Norway, Panama, the Philippines, Poland, Rwanda, Swaziland, Trinidad and Tabago, the United Kingdom, and Venezuela.

The incidence has leveled off in the United Kingdom and is apparently falling in the Scandinavian countries.

The gonococcus is susceptible to drying and will die within one to two hours. Because it cannot survive for long away from its host, and because it can produce primary infection only on certain specific epithelial surfaces, the gonococcus is almost always venereally transmitted.

The highest attack rate for gonorrhea in both men and women occurs in the 20 to 24 year old age group. The second highest attack rate is in the 15 to 19 year old age group. Because of numerous biases in case detection and reporting, the true male-female ratio for new cases of gonorrhea is unknown but is probably close to 1:1 in large populations.

There are several factors that contribute to the incidence of uncomplicated gonorrhea. Some host-related factors are as follows: the number of sexual partners; patterns of contraceptive use; population mobility; homosexuality; recidivism; and individuals with blood group B. An increase in the resistance of the gonococcus to therapeutic antibiotics may also be an important factor.

Behavioral factors predisposing to gonococcal infection also increase the risk of acquiring other sexually transmitted diseases. Such diseases are prevalent in groups with a high incidence of gonorrhea, and populations or individuals with any sexually transmitted disease should be screened for gonorrhea.

## Pathogenic Properties

Not everyone exposed to gonorrhea acquires the disease. It is uncertain whether this is due to variations in virulence or in the size of the inoculum, to nonspecific resistance, or to specific immunity. Several potential virulence factors (pili, capsule, lipopolysaccharide) have been discussed in a preceding section. The gonococcus elaborates a cytotoxic factor that damages ciliated epithelial cells in fallopian tube cultures. In addition, gonococci and meningococci produce an extracellular protease that cleaves a pro-thr bond on the heavy chain of the $IgA_1$ subclass of IgA. Cleavage of this bond results in a loss of antimicrobial activity. Because IgA is the antibody subclass that predominates in secretions, this enzyme may be important in pathogenesis of infection.

There is considerable controversy as to the intracellular survival and multiplication of the gonococcus. Gonococci are present both on and within PMN leukocytes soon after phagocytosis. Although most of the ingested gonococci are killed, gonococci may survive and multiply within phagocytes. Acquired IgA and IgG serum antibody enhances the association of gonococci with PMN leukocytes in vitro. However, piliated cells tend to remain extracellular, whereas nonpiliated cells are readily ingested and killed.

## Drug Susceptibility

Sulfonamides were used extensively to treat gonorrhea until the end of World War II, when sulfonamide resistance of gonococci became extensive. Fortunately, penicillin was introduced at about the same time as the sulfa drugs were losing effectiveness. Initially, gonococci were extremely sensitive to penicillin with minimum inhibitory concentrations (MIC) ranging from 0.003 to ca 0.03 units/ml. Treatment with a single injection of 150,000 units of penicillin produced cure rates of 90 per cent or more.

By the mid-1950s, gonococci with reduced sensitivity to penicillin were isolated from various parts of the world. This low-level resistance was not due to a β-lactamase but necessitated higher doses of penicillin. At the same time, gonococci developed low-level resistance to several other antibiotics, including tetracycline, chloramphenicol, and erythromycin. The use of streptomycin for therapy has resulted in resistance to levels of streptomycin far in excess of achievable serum levels of this drug.

β-Lactamase-producing strains of *N. gonorrhoeae* were first reported in 1976. The β-lactamase was active against penicillin G, ampicillin, and cephalosporins. The β-lactamase-producing strains possess either a $3.2 \times 10^6$ or $4.4 \times 10^6$ dalton plasmid. Loss of this plasmid results in loss of β-lactamase production. Some strains which possess the $4.4 \times 10^6$ dalton plasmid also possess a $24.5 \times 10^6$ dalton sex factor capable of mediating the conjugal transfer of the resistance factor. It is generally believed that the $4.4 \times 10^6$ and $3.2 \times 10^6$ dalton plasmid are genetically related and originated in an enteric bacterium. Penicillin-resistant strains of *N. gonorrhoeae* may be successfully treated with other drugs, including spectinomycin. However, spectinomycin resistance has also been reported.

## Immunity

The natural route of infection by *N. gonorrhoeae* brings the organism into direct contact with mucosal surfaces. However, it is still not clear to what extent gonococcal infection stimulates local immunity and whether any subsequent secretory immune response will protect against subsequent infection (Griffiss, 1976).

Repeated infections with *N. gonorrhoeae* are common. The development of serologic and biochemical typing schemes will allow differentiation between reinfection and infection with a new strain. It is also not clear whether disseminated infection elicits protective antibody. There is no vaccine against gonorrhea.

Gonococci in urethral exudates are resistant to the bactericidal activity of the patients' serum, but lose this resistance upon subculture on laboratory medium. Serum resistance can be maintained by subculture on a medium resembling the chemical environment of the host. Virulent colonial types are generally more resistant to killing by serum than the avirulent colonial types. After exposure to killing by serum, virulent colonial types can acquire complete resistance to serum. This acquired resistance is rapidly lost upon subculture on serum-free medium. The loss and gain of serum resistance is due to phenotypic variation.

### Laboratory Diagnosis

*Men.* Gram-stained smears of urethral exudate will often reveal gram-negative intracellular diplococci. This finding is sufficient for a diagnosis of gonorrhea. Culture specimens should be obtained from the anterior urethra and inoculated onto a selective medium (modified Thayer-Martin). Plates should be incubated in a candle jar or $CO_2$ incubator. Oxidase-positive colonies composed of gram-negative diplococci are presumed to be *N. gonorrhoeae*. Fluorescent antibody staining or the production of acid from glucose, but not from maltose, sucrose, or fructose, may be used for confirmation. In homosexuals, an additional specimen should be obtained from the anal canal and pharynx and processed as above.

*Women.* Gram-stained smears of exudate are not recommended for diagnosis of gonorrhea in women. Culture specimens should be obtained from the cervix and anal canal and inoculated on modified Thayer-Martin plates. The criteria for presumptive and confirmatory identification are as above. Serologic tests for gonorrhea have not proved satisfactory for either women or men.

## *NEISSERIA MENINGITIDIS*

### Antigenic Composition

*Capsule.* The capsular polysaccharides of *N. meningitidis* provide the basis for grouping these organisms (Bhattacharjee and Jennings, 1974; Bhattacharjee et al., 1976; Gotschlich et al., 1969). The serogroups and the chemical composition of their capsular polysaccharide, where known, are listed in Table 4. Meningococcal capsular polysaccharides are immunogenic when the intact bacterium is presented either to man or to

**TABLE 4. Chemical Composition of the Capsular Polysaccharides of N. meningitidis**

| SEROGROUP | COMPOSITION |
|---|---|
| A | Partially 0-acetylated comopolymer of 2-acetamido-2-deoxy-D-mannose-6-phosphate |
| B | N-acetyl neuraminic acid ($2 \rightarrow 8$-$\alpha$-linked) |
| C | 0-acetylated N-acetylneuraminic acid ($2 \rightarrow 9$-$\alpha$-linked) |
| X | 2-acetamido-2-deoxy-D-glucose-4-phosphate |
| Y | Partially 0-acetylated alternating sequence of D-glucose and N-acetylneuraminic acid |
| Z | Not determined |
| 29E | Equimolar amounts of 3-deoxy-D-*manno*-octulosonic acid and 2-acetamido-2-deoxy-galactosamine |
| W-135 | Alternating sequence of D-galactose and N-acetylneuraminic acid |

rabbits. Highly specific anticapsular antibodies produced by rabbits are used in an agglutination test to group meningococci.

*Outer Membrane Proteins.* Serogroups B and C meningococci have been subdivided into serotypes based upon the presence of outer membrane proteins. The majority of both group B and group C disease is caused by one serotype, type 2. The type 2 antigens from groups B and C meningococci are chemically and serologically identical. Antibodies against the serotype antigens are bactericidal in the presence of complement.

*Lipopolysaccharide.* Purified meningococcal LPS is highly toxic, and is as lethal for mice as is the LPS from *Escherichia coli* or *Salmonella typhimurium*. However, meningococcal LPS is five- to tenfold more effective than enteric LPS in eliciting a dermal Schwartzman reaction in rabbits (Davis and Arnold, 1974). Humans develop antibodies against meningococcal LPS during systemic disease. However, a role for these antibodies in immunity to meningococcal infection has yet to be demonstrated.

### Pathogenic Properties

Untreated meningococcal meningitis has a mortality rate of approximately 85 per cent. The virulence of *N. meningitidis* depends in part upon the antiphagocytic properties of its capsule. Antibodies directed against the capsular polysaccharide are bactericidal. In the animal, meningococci behave as extracellular parasites. Although they are often visible within PMN leukocytes, there is no evidence that they can multiply intracellularly. The toxic properties of the meningococcus reside in its LPS (Davis and Arnold, 1974).

## Epidemiology

The meningococcus usually inhabits the human nasopharyngeal area without causing disease (Griffiss, 1976). This carrier state may last for days or months and is important because it provides a reservoir for meningococcal infections and enhances the immunity of the host. From 3 to 30 per cent of normal individuals are carriers at any given time, yet few develop meningococcal disease. Even during epidemics of meningococcal meningitis in military recruits, when the carrier rate may reach 95 per cent, the incidence of systemic disease is less than 1 per cent (Goldschneider et al., 1969, 1969a). Carriers of meningococci are usually over 21 years of age, but the attack rates of disease are highest in children: with group B, under 5 years of age; with group C, 4 to 14 years of age. The low incidence of disseminated disease after colonization suggests that host rather than bacterial factors play an important determining role.

Meningococcal meningitis occurs sporadically and in epidemics, with highest incidence during the late winter and early spring. The disease appears to be declining in frequency in the United States and in Great Britain, whereas there has been an increased frequency in Finland and in Brazil. Most epidemics are caused by group A strains, but small outbreaks have occurred with both group B and group C strains. Sporadic cases are generally caused by group B, group C, and group Y strains, with groups B and C alternating in predominance. Whenever group A strains become prevalent, the incidence of meningitis increases markedly.

## Drug Susceptibility

The usual minimal inhibitory concentrations of antibiotics against the meningococcus are as follows ($\mu$g/ml): benzylpenicillin 0.03, ampicillin 0.05, methicillin 6.0, dicloxacillin 6.0, cephalothin 1.6, cephalexin 10.0, tetracycline 0.8, minocycline 0.8, rifampin 0.2, chloramphenicol 1.0, and erythromycin 1.0. Penicillin is the most potent and is the drug of choice in treatment, although useless in prophylaxis (see Chapter 180). Chloramphenicol has less in vitro activity than penicillin but penetrates the cerebrospinal fluid so well that it is an acceptable alternative in meningococcal meningitis for patients who cannot take penicillin. Rifampin, minocycline, and sulfonamides are sometimes used for eliminating meningococci from pharyngeal carriers. During World War II sulfonamides were remarkably effective in eliminating the carrier state but many strains of meningococci are now resistant to that drug.

## Immunity

Group A and group C capsular polysaccharide vaccines are available (Gotschlich et al., 1969, 1969a). These vaccines are highly protective against strains of these serogroups. Protection is provided through complement-mediated bactericidal antibodies that persist for at least five years after a single parenteral injection of vaccine. The capsular polysaccharide from serogroup B organisms is not immunogenic for humans.

## Laboratory Diagnosis

Specimens of blood, spinal fluid, and nasopharyngeal secretions should be examined for the presence of N. meningitidis in cases of suspected meningococcal disease. Specimens should be collected before treatment with antimicrobial agents because they reduce cultural isolation. However, smears may still show gram-negative diplococci, and counter-immunoelectrophoresis will detect meningococcal capsular polysaccharide. The CSF should be cultured on chocolate or blood agar in either a candle jar or a $CO_2$ incubator. The presence of oxidase-positive colonies consisting of gram-negative diplococci provides a presumptive identification of N. meningitidis. Production of acid from glucose and maltose, but not from sucrose, lactose, or fructose, may be used for confirmation. The serologic group may be determined by a slide agglutination test, using first polyvalent then monovalent antisera.

Nasopharyngeal specimens must be obtained from the posterior nasopharyngeal wall behind the soft palate. Specimens should be inoculated onto selective medium (modified Thayer-Martin) and processed as above.

Gram-stained smears of CSF may be diagnostic. However, organisms in CSF smears are often more difficult to find than in pneumococcal meningitis. Quellung tests may be of value.

## References

Bhattacharjee, A.K., and Jennings, H.J.: Characterization of 3-deoxy-D-*manno*-octulosonic acid as a component of the capsular polysaccharide antigen from *Neisseria meningitidis* serogroup 29-e. Biochem Biophys Res Commun 61:489, 1974.
Bhattacharjee, A.K., Jennings, H.J., Kenny, C.P., Martin, A., and Smith, I.C.P.: Structural determination of the polysaccharide antigens of *Neisseria meningitidis* serogroups Y, W-135, and BO. Canad J Biochem 54:1, 1976.
Davis, C. E., and Arnold, K.: Role of meningococcal endotoxin in meningococcal purpura. J Exp Med 140:159, 1974.
Goldschneider, I., Gotschlich, E.C., and Artenstein, M.S.: Human immunity to the meningococcus. I. The role of humoral antibodies. J Exp Med 129:1307, 1969.
Goldschneider, I., Gotschlich, E.C., and Artenstein, M.S.: Human immunity to the meningococcus. II. Development of natural immunity. J Exp Med 129:1327, 1969a.
Gotschlich, E.C., Goldschneider, I., and Artenstein, M.S.: Human im

munity to the meningococcus. IV. Immunogenicity of group A and group C meningococcal polysaccharides in human volunteers. J Exp Med 129:1367, 1969.

Gotschlich, E.C., Goldschneider, I., and Artenstein, M.S.: Human immunity to the meningococcus. V. The effect of immunization with meningococcal group C polysaccharide on the carrier state. J Exp Med 129:1385, 1969a.

Gotschlich, E.C., Liu, T.Y., and Artenstein, M.S.: Human immunity to the meningococcus. III. Preparation and immunochemical properties of the group A, group B, and group C meningococcal polysaccharides. J Exp Med 129:1349, 1969.

Griffiss, J.M., and Artenstein, M.S.: The ecology of the genus Neisseria. Mt Sinai J Med 43:746, 1976.

Hendley, J.O., Powell, K.R., Rodewald, R., Holzgrefe, H.H., and Lyles, R.: Demonstration of a capsule on Neisseria gonorrhoeae. N Engl J Med 296:608, 1977.

Morse, S.A.: The biology of the gonococcus. Crit Rev Microbiol 7:000, 1978.

Richardson, W.P., and Sadoff, J.C.: Production of a capsule of Neisseria gonorrhoeae. Infec Immun 15:663, 1977.

Roberts, R. B. (ed.): The Gonococcus. New York, John Wiley and Sons, 1977.

# 30 *MORAXELLA AND ACINETOBACTER*

## *Herman Baer, M.D.*

Organisms of *Moraxella* and *Acinetobacter* are gram-negative, strictly aerobic, coccobacillary rods that do not produce flagella or spores. Their classification has changed repeatedly and there are numerous synonyms for some of the species. The most recent reclassification in the eighth edition of *Bergey's Manual*, 1974, lists five species of *Moraxella: M. lacunata* (the diplobacillus of Morax and Axenfeld), *M. bovis, M. nonliquefaciens, M. phenylpyruvica,* and *M. osloensis.* The validity of these species, which are very similar phenotypically, has been confirmed genetically by transformation studies. *M. kingii* and *M. urethralis* (formerly *Mima polymorpha*, variety oxidans) have been tentatively grouped with the five valid species of *Moraxella. Acinetobacter* is considered in *Bergey's Manual* to consist of one species, *A. calcoaceticus.* This species includes both saccharolytic (formerly *Herellea vaginicola)* and nonsaccharolytic strains (formerly *Mima polymorpha,* variety nonoxidans).

Both genera are currently included in the family Neisseriaceae (see Chapter 29, Table 1). *Moraxella* is genetically and phenotypically related to the other members of this family, especially *Branhamella,* but *Acinetobacter* is a hardier, nutritionally versatile organism that shows no significant genetic homology with the other Neisseriaceae. Although the G + C content of both *Moraxella* and *Acinetobacter* is in the range of 40 to 47 per cent, DNA hybridization studies show very limited homology (Henriksen, 1976).

# MORAXELLA

## *MORPHOLOGY*

The chief reason for considering *Moraxella* and *Acinetobacter* as closely related bacteria is their microscopic morphology. In stained smears of wild organisms obtained directly from patients or the environment, *Moraxella* and *Acinetobacter* are short, plump bacteria that tend to occur in pairs and to be so coccoid that they may be confused with *Neisseria.* Careful examination almost always reveals some bacillary forms that increase in number with repeated passages in culture. *Moraxella* are usually fastidious and produce small colonies. Colonies from freshly isolated strains of *M. nonliquefaciens, M. bovis,* and *M. kingii* spread and corrode agar surfaces after incubation for several days in a humid environment. This type of growth is associated with polar fimbriae of about 5 nm diameter. Fimbriated cells show twitching motility that appears to cause the spreading phenomenon. Nonfimbriated bacteria neither corrode agar surfaces nor exhibit twitching motility (Henriksen, 1976). Because the twitching motility and corrosion are difficult to demonstrate by routine procedures, *Moraxella* are still considered nonmotile for purposes of differentiation from flagellated bacteria in the diagnostic laboratory. The polar fimbriae appear to determine competence in transformation.

Capsules may or may not be present. The cell walls of *Moraxella* have not been extensively studied.

## ANTIGENIC COMPOSITION

Because *Moraxella* are not important pathogens, few studies of antigenic composition have been undertaken. Instead, the purpose of serologic studies has been to confirm taxonomic relationships. Studies of a collection of *Moraxella* species and a few Acinetobacter strains showed serologic relationships between *M. lacunata, M. bovis,* and *M. nonliquefaciens.* There was no cross-reactivity with the other *Moraxella* species or *Acinetobacter.*

## METABOLISM

All *Moraxella* are relatively fastidious and grow best on rich media such as blood agar. In the case of *M. lacunata,* this fastidiousness is due in part to inhibition by fatty acids and other media components that can be neutralized by the addition of binding agents such as starch, charcoal, or serum. *Moraxella* are mesophilic and obligately aerobic. They grow poorly at room temperature and not at all at 5° C. They do not attack sugars. All *Moraxella* are oxidase positive when tested by *N,N*-dimethyl-*p*-phenylenediamine, a characteristic demonstrated by Baumann et al. (1968) to be associated with the presence of cytochrome C in the electron transport system. *Moraxella* species are chemoorganotrophs that utilize only a limited number of organic acids, alcohols, and amino acids as carbon and energy sources. Little is known about specific growth requirements. *M. osloensis,* but not the other species, will grow in mineral medium with acetate and ammonium salts. Only *M. bovis* produces a β-hemolysin. It is also the only species that does not produce detectable catalase activity.

Nitrogen can be obtained from reduction of nitrate by *M. lacunata, M. nonliquefaciens,* most strains of *M. phenylpyruvica,* and occasional strains of *M. osloensis. M. bovis* and *M. lacunata* are proteolytic and digest blood serum in Loeffler's medium. The other species are nonproteolytic. Only *M. phenylpyruvica* degrades urea. *M. osloensis* can utilize ammonium as the sole nitrogen source.

## PATHOGENIC PROPERTIES

*Moraxella* are obligate parasites of the mucous membranes of animals. They rarely cause systemic disease even when defense mechanisms are impaired. In the last century, *M. lacunata* was described by Morax and Axenfeld as a cause of keratoconjunctivitis in man, but this infection has essentially disappeared. *M. bovis* causes epizootic keratoconjunctivitis in cattle. *M. caprae* and *M. equi,* which are indistinguishable bacteriologically from *M. lacunata,* are isolated from keratoconjunctivitis of goats and horses, respectively. *M. phenylpyruvica, M. osloensis,* and *M. nonliquefaciens* are part of the indigenous flora of mammals and are virtually nonpathogenic. *M. urethralis,* which includes some of the strains formerly called *Mima polymorpha* var. *oxidans,* is a rare cause of local and systemic infection in compromised patients.

Because *Moraxella* rarely cause disease, there have been few studies of possible pathogenic properties. Possession of fimbriae is a prerequisite for the ability of *M. bovis* to colonize mucous membranes and cause bovine disease. Fimbriae are probably also responsible for the adhesiveness of *M. nonliquefaciens* and *M. kingii,* but the nonfimbriated *M. osloensis* and *M. lacunata* also adhere readily to mucosal surfaces. Because *Moraxella* possess a typical gram-negative wall, they presumably contain LPS but its toxicity has not been studied.

## IMMUNITY

Immune mechanisms do not prevent colonization of mucous membranes by *Moraxella.* If the limited pathogenicity of these bacteria were related to immunity against invasion stimulated by colonization, *Moraxella* should be a more common cause of infection in the immunocompromised patient. It seems likely, therefore, that *Moraxella* rarely cause infection because they lack pathogenic properties, not because they are limited to the mucous membranes by acquired immunity.

## LABORATORY DIAGNOSIS

*Moraxella* should be suspected when the Gram stain reveals deep-staining, gram-negative diplococci accompanied by definite bacillary forms. Colonies are small and delicate, and some strains may grow only on agar enriched with blood or serum *(M. lacunata* and *M. bovis).* All species are oxidase positive, nonmotile by standard tests, indole negative, nonsaccharolytic, and penicillin sensitive. They are differentiated from *Acinetobacter* with 100 per cent accuracy by their oxidase positivity and penicillin sensitivity. They are more difficult to differentiate from several unnamed bacteria that resemble *Moraxella* phen-

TABLE 1. Diagnostic Characteristics of Moraxella and Acinetobacter

| TEST OR SUBSTRATE | MORAXELLA | | | | | ACINETOBACTER | |
|---|---|---|---|---|---|---|---|
| | lacunata | bovis | nonlique-faciens | osloensis | phenyl-pyruvica | var. anitratus (Herellea) | var. lwoffi (Mima) |
| Enrichment[1] | [required] | ± | 0 | 0 | 0 | 0 | 0 |
| β-Hemolysis | 0 | [+] | 0 | 0 | 0 | partial[2] | partial[2] |
| Oxidase | + (w) | + | + | + | + | [0] | [0] |
| Catalase | + | 0 | + (w) | + (w) | + (w) | + | + |
| $CO_2$ enhancement | + | 0 | | | | 0 | 0 |
| MacConkey agar | NG | NG | NG | + (w) or NG | + (w) or NG | [+] | [+] |
| $H_2S$ (Pb ac paper) | 0 or + (w) | + (w) | + (w) or − | + (w) or − | − or + (w) | 0 | 0 |
| Citrate | 0 | 0 | 0 | 0 | 0 | + (90%) | + (50%) or − |
| Nitrate reduction | + | 0 | + | − or + (28%) | + (64%) or − | [0] | 0 |
| Phenylalanine deaminase | 0 | 0 | 0 | 0 | [+] | 0 | 0 |
| Urease (Christensen's) | 0 | 0 | 0 | 0 | [+ (95%)] | − or + (40–50%) | − or + (15%) |
| Acid from glucose | 0 | 0 | 0 | 0 | 0 | [+[3]] | 0 |
| xylose | 0 | 0 | 0 | 0 | 0 | [+] | 0 |
| lactose | 0 | 0 | 0 | 0 | 0 | [+] | 0 |
| OF media | − | − | − | − | − | [oxid.] | − |
| Penicillin sensitivity | S | S | S | S | S | [R] | [R] |

[1] with blood or 3% rabbit serum

[2] Most strains of Acinetobacter cause indeterminate, partial hemolysis. About 12.5% of each variety produce complete hemolysis. These strains differ from other Acinetobacter in that they grow on SS agar, liquefy gelatin, and peptonize peptone milk.

[3] Reactions clearer in OF media than in liquid peptone media; (w) = weak; NG = no growth; 0 = negative; K = alkaline; N = no change; R = resistant; TSI = triple sugar iron agar. [ ] = reaction of major importance in identification.

otypically (M-3, M-4, M-4f, M-5, and M-6). Careful attention to yellow pigment production (M-4f, M-5, and M-6), and alkalinization of citrate media (M-4) will usually separate these unusual isolates. *Moraxella* are differentiated from one another and from *Acinetobacter* by the diagnostic characteristics shown in Table 1. *M. lacunata* is recognized by its requirement for enrichment with blood or serum and enhancement of growth by $CO_2$; *M. bovis* by its $\beta$-hemolysis and catalase negativity; and *M. phenylpyruvica* by production of urease and phenylalanine deaminase. *M. nonliquefaciens* can usually be separated from *M. osloensis* by failure to grow on MacConkey agar and by production of nitrate reductase. *M. osloensis* is a hardier organism than the other *Moraxella* and produces colonies that approach those of *Acinetobacter* in size and character. *M. phenylpyruvica* is a very fastidious organism that grows poorly even in complex media.

Both the species tentatively grouped with the *Moraxella* are easy to separate from the valid members of this genus. Except for oxidase positivity, the biochemical reactions of *M. urethralis* are identical to those of *A. lwoffi* (Mima). *M. kingii* is catalase negative and $\beta$-hemolytic, grows without enrichments, and makes acid from glucose and maltose on ascites agar medium.

## DRUG SUSCEPTIBILITY

*Moraxella* species are uniformly sensitive to penicillin and most other antibiotics.

## EPIDEMIOLOGY

*Moraxella* species are part of the indigenous flora of the mucosal surfaces of man and other warm-blooded animals. Colonization probably occurs after transmission by droplets or direct contact. Fimbriae are a prerequisite for colonization of mucous membranes by *M. bovis* and are probably important colonization factors for *M. nonliquefaciens* and *M. kingii*. The other *Moraxella* colonize successfully without fimbriae, however. *M nonliquefaciens* and *M. osloensis* colonize the upper respiratory tract, and *M. urethralis* the urogenital tract. These and the other species also inhabit other mammalian mucosal surfaces including the conjunctivae.

# ACINETOBACTER

*Acinetobacter calcoaceticus* is the only species recognized in *Bergey's Manual*, but it is customary to divide the species into strains that oxidize carbohydrates and strains that fail to attack carbohydrates. The oxidative strains have been known under a variety of names, including *Herellea vaginicola, Moraxella glucidolytica, Bacterium anitratum,* and *Acinetobacter anitratus.* Synonyms for the nonoxidizing strains include *Moraxella lwoffi, Mima polymorpha* var. nonoxidans, *B5W*-organism, and *Acinetobacter lwoffi.*

## MORPHOLOGY

The microscopic morphology of *Acinetobacter* strains is indistinguishable from that of *Moraxella*. The nonsaccharolytic members of *A. calcoaceticus* were presumably named *Mima* because they mimicked *Neisseria*. Larger cells, typical bacilli, and filamentous forms can be found in most cultures. *Acinetobacter* strains generally grow more vigorously than *Moraxella* and produce butyrous colonies resembling those of the Enterobacteriaceae.

Electron microscopy of thin sections of Acinetobacter has revealed a multilayer cell envelope typical of gram-negative bacilli. Chemical studies of the LPS and peptidoglycan confirm their similarity to the equivalent cell wall structures of Enterobacteriaceae. Capsules have been seen in electron micrographs and have been characterized chemically and serologically. Some strains of *Acinetobacter* display twitching motility that is dependent on the production of polar fimbriae. The relationship of genetic competence to fimbriae has not been studied.

## ANTIGENIC COMPOSITION

Fluorescein-labeled antisera to capsular antigens have identified 28 serotypes of saccharolytic acinetobacters and suggested that there are different serotypes of nonsaccharolytic acinetobacters (Marcus et al., 1969). Juni (1978) has studied the capsules of two strains of *Acinetobacter* and shown that one was composed of L-rhamnose and D-glucose and the other of glucose and galactose. The capsule that was composed of rhamnose and glucose cross-reacted in precipitin studies with antisera to groups B and G streptococci and type XIII pneumococci.

The peptidoglycan of saccharolytic and nonsaccharolytic strains is similar and contains muramic acid, glucosamine, alanine, D-glutamic acid, and $m_i$-diaminopimelic acid, a composition characteristic of peptidoglycans of chemotype I (Horisberger, 1977). Neither the LPS nor the polar fimbriae of *Acinetobacter* have been characterized antigenically.

## METABOLISM

Acinetobacters are strictly aerobic chemoorganotrophs that are versatile in the utilization of organic compounds for carbon and energy sources. None has specific growth requirements and most can grow in a mineral medium containing a single organic carbon and energy source. Nitrate is not reduced to nitrite or other reduced compounds but ammonium and nitrate salts can be used as nitrogen sources. Urease-producing strains can substitute urea for these compounds.

Acinetobacters capable of using glucose as a source of carbon and energy degrade this compound exclusively via the Entner-Doudoroff pathway. Acinetobacters lack enzymes for the direct phosphorylation of hexoses, and the first step for entry into the Entner-Doudoroff pathway is the oxidation of glucose to gluconic acid (Juni, 1978).

Acinetobacters that produce acid from glucose, lactose, mannose, arabinose, and xylose produce a glucose dehydrogenase that oxidizes D-glucose to D-gluconolactone. Oxygen is the ultimate electron acceptor for the particulate form of this enzyme which is tightly complexed to cytochrome b (Hauge, 1960). Nonsaccharolytic acinetobacters lack glucose dehydrogenase (Juni, 1978).

All the enzymes of the tricarboxylic and glyoxylate cycles have been demonstrated in either cell-free extracts or ethanol-grown cells of *Acinetobacter*. Acinetobacters contain functional electron transport pathways consisting of cytochrome $a_1$, $a_2$, and b as well as flavin. All can be reduced with NADH or succinate and re-oxidized by oxygen. As expected for an oxidase negative organism, *Acinetobacter* does not contain cytochrome C.

Pathways used by this versatile organism for biosynthesis and for the degradation of aromatic and alicyclic compounds, hydrocarbons, and 2,3-butanediol are similar to those of the pseudomonads and have recently been extensively reviewed by Juni (1978).

Most strains grow well at mesophilic temperature ranges of 35 to 37° C but have an optimal temperature range of 30 to 32° C. Some strains grow well at 5° C. The optimal pH for growth is about 7.

## PATHOGENIC PROPERTIES

*Acinetobacter* is common in the environment and has been isolated from a nearly unlimited variety of clinical specimens. In most cases *Acinetobacter* can be dismissed as a contaminating or colonizing strain, but it is occasionally isolated from patients in whom its pathogenic role is indisputable. When *Acinetobacter* is isolated in mixed culture, the clinical situation and the culture results must be carefully evaluated before the diagnosis of *Acinetobacter* infection is accepted.

*Acinetobacter* behaves essentially like any other gram-negative, aerobic, opportunistic pathogen. Because of its low pathogenicity, the organism rarely, if ever, causes infection in otherwise healthy individuals. The number of nosocomial infections by *Acinetobacter* has increased in recent years. Several outbreaks of nosocomial *Acinetobacter* septicemia have been reported, and indwelling intravenous catheters were suspected as the portal of entry of the organisms. Nosocomial *Acinetobacter* pneumonia most often affects patients who are severely debilitated and have undergone major surgery or trauma. The pneumonia may be necrotizing. Abscesses, pleural effusions, and septicemia are occasional complications. *Acinetobacter* urinary tract infection is usually associated with the presence of an indwelling bladder catheter. When postoperative infections of the surgical area have been observed, they usually involve complicated procedures in severely ill patients or orthopedic procedures with implantation of a prosthetic device (Glew et al., 1977).

Some strains of *Acinetobacter* produce fimbriae. The role of these structures in the usual habitat of this free-living bacterium is unknown. It is not clear whether fimbriae promote nosocomial colonization of severely ill, hospitalized patients who are colonized more frequently than healthy people.

Since *Acinetobacter* causes disease uncommonly, there have been few studies of possible pathogenic properties. The heteropolysaccharide capsules may prevent phagocytosis by the severely ill patient who may be deficient in opsonins or phagocytes.

*Acinetobacter* contains a typical trilaminar, gram-negative cell wall, and LPS has been isolated and partly characterized chemically. Biologic studies of the endotoxic potency of this LPS have not been reported.

## IMMUNITY

Healthy people resist colonization and infection by *Acinetobacter*. Since severely ill, immunocompromised patients are frequently colonized and occasionally infected, it is likely that normal resistance mechanisms play a role in preventing *Acinetobacter* infection. The relative importance of natural versus acquired immunity is unknown. The heteropolysaccharide capsule is antigenic in animals and it is likely that both the *Acinetobacter* capsule and LPS stimulate antibody production in human beings. It is possible that natural resistance to infection is partly related to the known cross-reactions between *Acinetobacter* capsules and those of Streptococcus B and G and *S. pneumoniae* type XIII.

## LABORATORY DIAGNOSIS

Although the microscopic morphology of *Acinetobacter* is indistinguishable from that of *Moraxella*, the colonial morphology is usually quite different. Acinetobacters produce larger, butyrous colonies on most standard laboratory media; *Moraxella* produce smaller, more fragile colonies that may require media enriched with blood or serum. Unlike *Moraxella*, acinetobacters are strongly catalase positive, oxidase negative, and resistant to penicillin. They are easily differentiated from *Pseudomonas* by the oxidase reaction and from Enterobacteriaceae by their failure to reduce nitrate and their lack of reactivity in triple sugar iron agar or Kligler's iron agar. Acinetobacters also give uniformly negative results in the following tests: indole, $H_2S$, decarboxylation of lysine, ornithine, and arginine, and deamination of phenylalanine. The remainder of the laboratory characteristics of the saccharolytic (var. anitratus) and the nonsaccharolytic (var. lwoffi) strains are given in Table 1.

## ANTIBIOTIC SUSCEPTIBILITY

*Acinetobacter* is resistant to penicillin, ampicillin, the cephalosporins, and chloramphenicol. The susceptibility to tetracycline varies. Most strains are sensitive to the aminoglycosides, colistin, and carbenicillin. However, R-factor-mediated resistance to carbenicillin, kanamycin, and gentamicin is becoming increasingly prevalent.

## EPIDEMIOLOGY

*Acinetobacter* is not part of the indigenous flora of man or animals, but it is commonly found in soil and water. The organism is occasionally recovered in specimens obtained from nonhospitalized patients, but it is much more prevalent in hospitalized patients. *Acinetobacter*, like many other aerobic gram-negative organisms, is a frequent contaminant of moist environments in the hospital, e.g., respirators, humidifiers, and sinks (Smith and Massanari, 1977). Patients acquire the organism either by direct contact with an environmental reservoir of the organism, or indirectly from members of the hospital staff who carry the organism on their hands. Nosocomial colonization by *Acinetobacter* may involve the respiratory tract, intestinal tract, urogenital tract, and the moist intertriginous areas of the skin. The severity of illness seems to be the most important risk factor for nosocomial colonization.

Fluorescein-labeled antisera to capsular antigens can be used as an epidemiologic marker for tracing the source of nosocomial infections.

### References

Baumann, P., Doudoroff, M., and Stanier, R. Y.: Study of the Moraxella group. I. Genus Moraxella and the Neisseria catarrhalis group. J Bacteriol 95:58, 1968.

Buchanan, R. E., and Gibbons, N. E. (eds.): Bergey's Manual of Determinative Bacteriology. 8th ed. Baltimore, The Williams and Wilkins Company, 1974, pp. 426–438.

Glew, R. H., Moellering, R. C., and Kim, L. J.: Infections with Acinetobacter calcoaceticus (Herellea vaginicola): Clinical and laboratory studies. Medicine 56:79, 1977.

Hauge, J. G.: Purification and properties of glucose dehydrogenase and cytochrome b from Bacterium anitratum. Biochim Biophys Acta 45:250, 1960.

Henriksen, S. D.: Moraxella, Neisseria, Branhamella, and Acinetobacter. Annu Rev Microbiol 30:63, 1976.

Horisberger, M.: Structure of the peptidoglycans of Moraxella glucidolytica and Moraxella lwoffi grown on hydrocarbons. Arch Microbiol 112:297, 1977.

Juni, E.: Genetics and physiology of Acinetobacter. Annu Rev Microbiol 32:349, 1978.

Marcus, B. B., Samuels, S. B., Pittman, B., and Cherry, W. B.: A serologic study of Herellea vaginicola and its identification by immunofluorescent staining. Am J Clin Pathol 52:309, 1969.

Smith, P. W., and Massanari, M.: Room humidifiers as the source of Acinetobacter infections. JAMA 237:795, 1977.

# Gram-Negative Rods

# 31 *ENTEROBACTERIACEAE*

## *Frits Ørskov, M.D., and Ida Ørskov, M.D.*

Enterobacteriaceae are a family of five tribes (Table 1) of closely related, nonspore-forming gram-negative bacilli that ferment glucose and, except for some strains of *Erwinia*, reduce nitrates to nitrites. Many genera are important normal inhabitants of the intestinal flora of mammals. Others, like the typhoid bacillus, the Shiga bacillus, and the plague bacillus, are historically and medically among the most important bacterial pathogens encountered by man. The plague bacillus, *Yersinia pestis,* and the other *Yersinia* species are discussed more extensively in Chapter 37 for historical reasons and because they cause clinical syndromes similar to those caused by *Francisella* and *Pasteurella.*

## *MORPHOLOGY*

Enterobacteriaceae are relatively short, 2 to 3 $\mu$ by 0.4 to 0.6 $\mu$, rod-shaped, gram-negative bacteria. Most genera are so similar microscopically and colonially that they cannot be differentiated from one another reliably without the use of differential media or a battery of biochemical tests. Most Enterobacteriaceae are motile, and motility is always dependent upon the production of peritrichous flagella. Many strains produce common pili or fimbriae. Strains that can serve as donors of plasmid DNA during conjugation also produce sex pili. Several members of the family produce capsules or microcapsules that are composed of repeating units of acidic polysaccharides. The capsules of *Klebsiella* and the microcapsules that are more typical of *Escherichia coli* and some other Enterobacteriaceae can be recognized by electron-microscapsules of Enterobacteriaceae are referred glutination or capsular swelling. The capsules and microcapsules of Enterbacteriaceae are referred to as K antigens except for the microcapsule of *Salmonella typhosa,* which is called the Vi (virulence) antigen.

Enterobacteriaceae contain the typical, lipid-rich multilayered cell wall of gram-negative bacteria. The outer layer contains the lipopolysaccharide (LPS) that is responsible for many of the toxic and biologic properties of these organisms. LPS also contains complex oligosaccharide side chains that determine O antigen specificity. The peptidoglycan forms a distinct layer of the cell wall between the LPS and the cytoplasmic membrane but is neither as thick nor as complex as that of gram-positive bacteria. Enterobacteriaceae contain 5 to 10 per cent lipoprotein in the cell wall. This substance is intermixed with the LPS and covalently linked to the peptidoglycan. It does not form a distinct layer. Unlike gram-positive bacteria, Enterobacteriaceae do not produce teichoic acid.

Enterobacteriaceae grow on most common media and on media with concentrations of bile salts and aniline dyes that inhibit most gram-positive bacteria. Colonies are circular, convex, entire, and more or less glistening and mucoid, depending partly on the production of polysaccharide surface structures. Unencapsulated forms, which have also lost the hexose epimerases necessary for synthesis of the O antigenic polysaccharide side chains of the LPS, produce flat, granular, irregular colonies that are referred to as "rough." The highly motile *Proteus* spp. may move away from the original point of inoculum on solid media and produce the unique, poorly understood swarming phenomenon. Only *E. coli* frequently produce hemolysins on blood agar. Some strains of *Serratia* produce a nondiffusible red pigment called prodigiosin. *Enterobacter agglomerans* (classified by some taxonomists as the Herbicola group of *Erwinia*) produces yellow colonies. Other *Erwinia* strains that are infrequently isolated from man produce blue or pink pigments. The rest of the Enterobacteriaceae are unpigmented.

**TABLE 1.    Family Enterobacteriaceae**

| TRIBES | GENERA |
|---|---|
| I   Escherichieae | Escherichia<br>Edwardsiella<br>Citrobacter<br>Salmonella<br>Shigella |
| II   Klebsielleae | Klebsiella<br>Enterobacter<br>Hafnia<br>Serratia |
| III   Proteeae | Proteus<br>Providence (*Proteus inconstans*) |
| IV   Yersinieae[a] | Yersinia |
| V   Erwinieae | Erwinia |

[a]This tribe is discussed in depth in Chapter 37.

## *ANTIGENIC COMPOSITION*

### General

Most genera of Enterobacteriaceae can be subdivided into serotypes by antibody raised against their antigenic surface components. The O, K, and H antigens are the fundamental serotyping antigens because of the great variety of their chemical composition and their antigenic stability. The properties of these antigens are relatively stable because they are chromosomally determined. Serotyping is used to establish the precise identification of strains isolated during outbreaks and epidemics. As certain serotypes have special pathogenic properties, antigenic analysis may also be important diagnostically.

### O Antigens

The O antigens that are the polysaccharide side chains of the LPS are the backbone of analytic antigenic systems. LPS is a highly complex molecule (see Chapter 6), which consists of three regions (Luderitz et al., 1971): (1) Lipid A, which is buried in the outer membrane of the cell wall, is responsible for many of the biologic properties of LPS. (2) The LPS core, which is linked to lipid A and expresses R (rough) specificity, is partly hidden in S (smooth) forms by the attachment to the core of O antigens. (3) The O-specific polysaccharides of the bacterial S forms are the chemical basis for the serologic classification of Enterobacteriaceae into hundreds of complex O antigen groups, e.g., *Salmonella* into 60 and *E. coli* into more than 160 such groups (Ørskov et al., 1977).

O antigenic analysis is carried out by bacterial agglutination.

### K Antigens

K antigens are polysaccharides that usually contain acidic groups. When well developed, they form microscopically distinct capsules. K antigens are determined by the capsular swelling technique, in which the capsule is made visible by the addition of specific antiserum or by the development of precipitin lines when tested against specific antisera by countercurrent immunoelectrophoresis (CIE). Bacterial agglutination can also be used, but the results may be difficult to interpret because of the many other surface antigens (Ørskov and Ørskov, 1978). Capsules interfere with phagocytosis and serum bactericidal activity.

### H Antigens

Flagella are protein organelles that determine the H antigen specificity of motile members of the family. Many *Salmonella* strains show phase variation, i.e., the H antigens of a single strain may occur in either one or both of two serologically different phases called Phase 1 and Phase 2. Serologic determination is performed by agglutination techniques.

### Fimbrial or Pili Antigens

Most Enterobacteriaceae may develop fimbriae (or pili). These will usually be the so-called type 1 fimbriae. General serologic analysis of fimbrial antigens is not yet available.

The K88 and K99 antigens of *E. coli* are fimbrial, proteinaceous antigens that are important colonization factors of strains associated with diarrhea in young pigs and calves. They received the K label at a time when their true nature was not recognized and may, therefore, soon receive a new designation that will also be an appropriate term for other fimbrial antigens.

### Serotypes

Serotyping schemes, such as the Kauffmann-White scheme (Kauffmann, 1966), are based on the systematic examination of the antigenic specificities and cross-reactions between the surface antigens. Complete analysis may require numerous cross-absorption and cross-reaction tests.

The table below shows the basic agglutination-absorption experiment used in Enterobacteriaceae serology. Two strains, A and B, react mutually in antisera A and B. By reciprocal absorption followed by agglutination, it is shown that both strains contain a common and a specific antigenic factor. The two absorbed sera are called factor sera. Strain A might be given the antigenic designation of 1,2 and Strain B the designation of 1,3, where 1 represents the common factor and 2 and 3 the specific factors.

| | ANTISERUM A | | ANTISERUM B | |
|---|---|---|---|---|
| | Unabsorbed | Absorbed by B | Unabsorbed | Absorbed by A |
| Antigen A | + | + | + | 0 |
| Antigen B | + | 0 | + | + |

Some typical examples of serotypes are:

*Salmonella* 1,4,5,12:b:1,2 (*S. paratyphi* B), where 1,4,5,12 represents the O antigen and b:1,2 the two phases of the H antigen.

*Klebsiella* O1:K1, or just K1, because the O antigens of *Klebsiella* are not usually determined.

*Escherichia coli* O1:K1:H5 or 1:1:5.

*Shigella* II:1,3,4 (*Shigella flexneri* 2a), where both II and 1,3,4 stand for O antigen determinants, II for the so called type-specific O factor and 1,3,4 for the group factors.

Simplified serologic labels can be found in the literature, e.g., when *E. coli* O111 and O75 are described as serotypes, even though they are O groups. The serotype of strains belonging to these O groups could be O111:H2 or O75:K100:H5.

## Special

### Escherichia Coli

A recent list of all the antigenic test strains that have been published contains 164 O antigens, 103 K antigens, and 75 H antigens. Most of the K antigens are polysaccharides, but a few proteinaceous, fimbrial antigens, which confer adhesiveness on enterotoxigenic E. coli, are presently listed as K antigens. They may be established as a special group of antigens (F antigens). Since many O, K, and H antigens can be combined in different ways, the number of possible serotypes is very high. Fortunately, some are more common than others, both among the special serotypes associated with disease and among the flora of the normal colon. Consequently, most routine laboratories use only a limited number of antisera that correspond to certain "pathogenic" serotypes. More detailed serologic analysis should be carried out in specialized national or international centers.

### Salmonella

Salmonella strains are serotyped by the Kauffmann-White scheme, which has divided this genus into more than 1500 serotypes (Kauffmann, 1966). The O and H antigens in this highly complex scheme were defined only after extensive cross-absorption and cross-agglutination tests. More than 65 O-antigenic groups have been described. Several strains contain more than one O antigen factor. This means that more than one determinant has been found on the O-specific side chain of the LPS molecule, e.g., O factors 1,2,12 in Salmonella paratyphi A. Lysogenization by converting bacteriophages can bring about modification of certain O antigens.

Only one K antigen, the Vi antigen, is important for Salmonella serotyping, and it is usually associated only with S. typhi.

H antigens, the flagellar antigens, can be found in two alternative phases in many Salmonella cultures. One is called "specific phase," or Phase 1, and the other "non-specific phase," or Phase 2. During subculture of the two types, the population of each gives rise to cells of the alternative phase. The Kauffmann-White scheme first divides Salmonella into O groups. Strains of the same O group are then subdivided according to their H antigen.

Fimbriae can interfere with serotyping by blocking antigenic sites of the other surface antigens.

### Shigella

Shigella is closely related to E. coli phenotypically and genetically. When these groups were given taxonomic status, Shigella strains had been isolated primarily from patients with severe dysentery, while E. coli was considered to be a harmless, normal inhabitant of the mammalian intestinal tract. The fact that otherwise typical Escherichia strains may cause dysentery has underscored the similarities between the two groups. By agglutination with O antiserum and minor biochemical differences Shigella is subdivided into four subgroups: S. dysenteriae, S. flexneri, S. boydii, and S. sonnei. The first three of these can be subdivided into several serotypes based on further analysis of O antigens. Capsular polysaccharide antigens have not been demonstrated in Shigella. Fimbrial antigens have been described but are not used for serotyping.

Edwardsiella and Citrobacter, the other two genera of Tribe I, are usually not serotyped.

### Klebsiella

This genus is characterized by a rich variety of K antigens but a small number of different O antigens. Thus, antigenic analysis of Klebsiella strains is based on testing the organism against about 80 antisera to different K types.

Enterobacter, Hafnia, Serratia, and Proteus are usually not serotyped.

### Yersinia

Yersinia enterocolitica has attracted much interest in recent years because of its possible relationship to certain enteric diseases and to rheumatic conditions. Serotyping is based on O and H antigens.

## METABOLISM

Enterobacteriaceae organisms are facultative anaerobes. They possess a respiratory electron transport system that enables them to grow aerobically at the expense of a rich variety of oxidizable organic compounds. Organic acids, amino acids, and carbohydrates are utilized by all members of the family, and some can use aromatic compounds. They are oxidase negative because their electron transport system does not include cytochrome C. All except one species of Shigella produce catalase. Under anaerobic conditions, growth becomes strictly dependent upon carbohydrate fermentation. Many monosaccharides, disaccharides, and polyalcohols can be fermented by members of this group. Polysaccharides are utilized less commonly, but some plant pathogens (*Erwinia*) do attack pectin. All, except some species of *Erwinia*, reduce nitrates to nitrites.

Enterobacteriaceae ferment sugars by the Embden-Meyerhof pathway (Chapter 3). The pyruvic acid produced by this fermentation can be catabolized through several different pathways. All Enterobacteriaceae cleave pyruvate to formic acid. This unique cleavage is not encountered in any other bacterial fermentation. Formic acid does not always accumulate because many Enterobacteriaceae synthesize formic hydrogenylase, which converts formic acid to hydrogen and carbon dioxide. The remainder of the pyruvic acid is broken down either by mixed-acid fermentation or by butylene glycol (butanediol) fermentation. Enterobacteriaceae that metabolize glucose by the mixed-acid fermentation produce succinic acid by one pathway, lactic acid by another, and acetic acid and ethanol by the third. Enterobacteriaceae that use the butylene glycol fermentation convert a major portion of the pyruvate to a different end product, 2,3-butanediol, which is formed by an additional independent pathway. Although bacteria that use the butylene glycol pathway also produce succinic, lactic, and acetic acids, the neutral end products (butanediol and ethanol) predominate, and the total amount of acid formed per mole of glucose is much less than in the mixed-acid fermentation. Two simple tests on cultures in glucose-peptone broth divide the Enterobacteriaceae into two groups according to which fermentation pathway they use. The methyl red test detects those that use the mixed-acid fermentation because they produce enough acid from glucose to convert this indicator to its red, acidic form. The Voges-Proskauer test detects the butylene-glycol fermentation because acetoin, an intermediate in this pathway, is oxidized to a diacetyl form at an alkaline pH and complexes with creatine in the media to form a pink compound. The mixed-acid pattern is typical of the Escherichieae and Yersinieae tribes, and the butylene glycol pattern is typical of the Klebsielleae tribe.

All Enterobacteriaceae produce formic acid, but only those that synthesize formic hydrogenylase produce gas. The production of butanediol also results in a net production of $CO_2$, but the $CO_2$ is very soluble in water and does not cause observable gas in the medium. Gas formation is a property of differential value in identification of Enterobacteriaceae, since it differentiates the gas formers of the genus *Escherichia* from *Salmonella typhosa* and *Shigella* spp. and the gas forming *Enterobacter* from *Serratia*.

The ability to ferment lactose, a disaccharide, depends on the possession of $\beta$-galactosidase and is a characteristic of considerable diagnostic importance in this family. Utilization of lactose also depends upon a specific galactoside permease, which facilitates the entry of lactose into the cell. Lactose fermentation is characteristic of *E. coli* and *Enterobacter* and is absent from *Shigella*, *Salmonella*, and *Proteus*. Some *Shigella* species produce $\beta$-galactosidase but cannot ferment lactose because they lack a permease.

## PATHOGENIC PROPERTIES

### General

The natural habitat of many Enterobacteriaceae is the mammalian intestine. Some, like *E. coli*, are found in the normal healthy intestine; others, like *Salmonella*, *Shigella*, and enteropathogenic *E. coli*, can be considered to be pathogenic.

Although many Enterobacteriaceae are part of the normal intestinal flora, they are also "opportunistic" pathogens that may cause fatal infections when the normal host defenses are insufficient, e.g., in newborns, in patients in terminal stages of disease or in patients receiving immunosuppressive therapy. Enterobacteriaceae are the most common causes of infection of the obstructed biliary and urinary tracts and, along with the intestinal anaerobes, the major cause of infection of the soiled peritoneum. Enterobacteriaceae, especially *E. coli* and *Klebsiella*, are now the most common cause of septicemia in hospitalized patients.

### Endotoxin

All Enterobacteriaceae synthesize endotoxin. Lipid A seems to be responsible for most of the potent biologic activities of endotoxin. Endotoxin is extensively discussed in Chapter 6, but it is important to point out in this chapter that many of the symptoms of invasive disease caused by Enterobacteriaceae can be ascribed to endotoxin.

Among these effects are: (1) pyrogenicity: microgram doses of LPS given intravenously cause a diphasic rise of the temperature of humans and many experimental animals; (2) consumption of complement: the survival rate of patients with enterobacterial septicemia is inversely related to the complement level; (3) consumption of coagulation factors: hemorrhage and fibrin deposition occur in patients and are equivalent to the Shwartzman phenomenon in experimental animals; and (4) shock: injection of larger doses of LPS causes hypotension, irreversible shock, and death. Similar symptoms can be caused by the presence of large numbers of Enterobacteriaceae in the blood.

## Enterotoxins

Enterotoxin-producing *E. coli* strains have been the subject of intensive investigation in recent years (Sack, 1975). These protein exotoxins, which are genetically determined by transferable plasmids, play a prominent role in the pathogenesis of diarrhea in animals and man. Enterotoxin-positive strains colonize but do not invade the small intestine. Toxin-producing strains of other members of the family Enterobacteriaceae have been reported recently. There at least two types of enterotoxins; one is called ST (thermostable toxin) and the other LT (thermolabile toxin). Diarrhea occurs as a result of water and electrolyte loss caused by enterotoxin-induced adenyl cyclase activity of the epithelial cells. LT (the thermolabile toxin) is immunogenic but ST is not. Enterotoxigenic *E. coli* also affects infant pigs and calves, causing great economic loss to farmers.

## Colonization Factors

Many enterotoxigenic strains produce special, plasmid-determined fimbriae (or pili) that play an important pathogenic role as adhesive structures. Experimental evidence suggests that these structures make it possible for enterotoxin-producing *E. coli* to deliver their toxin close to the intestinal epithelial cells.

The best known colonization factor is the K88 antigen of the *E. coli* strains that cause diarrhea in piglets. Enterotoxin-producing strains are not virulent for piglets if they have lost the K88 antigen or if the pigs have been immunized with K88. Studies of the K99 antigen suggest that it plays a similar role in diarrhea of calves. Similar colonization factors have been identified in human enterotoxigenic strains. K88 and K99 are both mediated by transferable plasmids.

## K Antigens

K antigens are acidic polysaccharides that probably promote pathogenicity primarily by interfering with phagocytosis.

*E. coli* K1 strains cause a very high percentage of neonatal meningitis without an equivalent increase in either gastrointestinal colonization or septicemia. The sialic acid-containing K1 capsule cross-reacts immunologically with the capsule of serogroup B meningococci (Robbins et al., 1975). The reasons for this unique predilection for the meninges are not known. K1, K2, K3 K5, K12, and K13 are the most common K types associated with infections of the urinary tract. Certain O types — O1, O2, O4, O6, O7, O8, O9, O11, O18, O22, O25, and O75 — are also more commonly associated with urinary tract and other extraintestinal infections. These O and K groups are commonly found in the intestine, and it is uncertain whether they are especially virulent or are just more prevalent.

## Special

*E. Coli Diarrhea.* Three groups of special-*Escherichia* strains are associated with three types of intestinal disease (Table 2). The enterotoxigenic *E. coli* species (ETEC), which were discussed above, cause diarrhea in piglets and calves, traveler's diarrhea in man, and a cholera-like disease in the people living in the warm climates of developing countries.

Another group of special *Escherichia* serotypes (EIEC), which are related to certain serotypes of *Shigella*, is invasive into the epithelial cells of the human colon and can cause dysentery-like disease. These serotypes have also been associated with food poisoning.

A third group of special serotypes is associated with diarrhea in institutionalized infants in developed countries. These special serotypes, which are not commonly found in the normal intestine, have been called the enteropathogenic *E. coli* (EPEC). Because they do not invade the epithelial cells of the small intestine and do not produce readily detectable enterotoxins, there has been doubt about their pathogenic role. However, the close association of these highly specialized serotypes with severe outbreaks of diarrhea cannot be disputed. Only future research will reveal their actual role in the pathogenesis of infantile diarrhea.

## Salmonella

More than 1500 different serotypes have been

TABLE 2. *Escherichia Coli* and Acute Diarrhea

|  | ENTEROPATHOGENIC EPEC | ENTEROTOXIGENIC ETEC | ENTEROINVASIVE EIEC |
|---|---|---|---|
| Pathogenic mechanism | Unknown | Enterotoxin (LT, ST) | Epithelial cell invasion |
| Age groups affected | Infants | Infants and adults | Adults and infants |
| Epidemiology | Sporadic cases and outbreaks | Sporadic cases and outbreaks | Sporadic cases and outbreaks |
| O groups associated | 26, 55, 86, 111, 114, 119, 125, 126, 127, 128, 142 | 6, 8, 15, 25, 27, 78, 148, 159 | 28ac, 112ac, 124, 136, 143, 144, 152, 164 |

From Rowe, B.: *Escherichia coli* in acute diarrhoea. Lab-Lore 7:449, 1977.

described, all of which should be considered as potentially pathogenic to man. Several cause generalized infection in specific animals, such as *S. typhimurium* in mice and *S. typhi* in man. Most serotypes can cause enteritis in many different animals when large numbers of organisms are ingested.

*Enteric Fever.* In humans, enteric fever is caused by *S. typhi* or *S. paratyphi* A, B, and C, depending on the geographic location. Other *Salmonella* serotypes are occasionally isolated from cases of enteric fever. A relatively small oral inoculum of the strains of *Salmonella* that cause enteric fever can initiate disease. The organisms invade the mucosa and the mucosal macrophages of the small intestine, multiply in local lymph nodes, spread through the lymphatics to the bloodstream, and disseminate to many organs. *S. typhi* and *S. paratyphi* C (*S. hirschfeldii*) frequently produce the Vi antigen, which is composed of a simple polymer of *N*-acetyl galactosaminuronic acid. This substance is elaborated as a thin, outermost layer and is equivalent to K antigen.

*Salmonella* septicemia may be caused by some other serotypes, notably *S. choleraesuis*. This infection is characterized by high remittent fever and bacteremia usually without involvement of the intestinal tract. Focal suppuration, meningitis, osteomyelitis, pneumonia, and endocarditis may occur.

*Enteritis (Food Poisoning).* Most other *Salmonella* serotypes can cause enteritis in man when ingested in large numbers. Typically, these strains cause disease after ingestion of food in which the *Salmonella* strain has had the opportunity to multiply. The disease is often labeled food poisoning, but invasion and multiplication are probably a necessary part of the pathogenesis. The incubation period ranges from 8 hours to 3 days. The disease is usually limited to the local intestinal lymph nodes. Some serotypes, e.g., *S. typhimurium, S. enteritidis, S. heidelberg,* and *S. adelaide,* are more frequently associated with this disease, but almost all strains have caused enteritis.

### Shigella

*Shigella* causes bacillary dysentery in man and higher apes. This enteritis is localized to the mucosa of the terminal ileum and colon. The bacteria invade the colonic epithelial cells, where they multiply and cause mucosal ulcerations. One of the serotypes, *Shigella dysenteriae* Type 1 (the Shiga bacillus), also produces a special exotoxin that was earlier described as a neurotoxin.

### Yersinia

*Yersinia pestis,* the cause of plague, is discussed in Chapter 37. *Y. pseudotuberculosis* and *Y. en-*terocolitica* may cause dysentery, mesenteric adenitis and an interesting syndrome consisting of dysentery and inflammatory noninfectious arthritis. The pathogenesis of this disease is not known, but it appears to be more frequent in certain geographic areas, and perhaps in certain HLA types (Chapter 129).

### Other Enterobacteriaceae

The other members of the family are primarily causes of opportunistic infections. Several reports have suggested an association of the *Klebsiella* group with enterotoxic diarrhea, but there is no current evidence to suggest that there is a regular association of the enterotoxin plasmid with any serotype of *Klebsiella.*

*Proteus* species are found regularly in the mammalian intestine. These urease-producing bacteria, which break down urea to ammonium, are so frequently associated with stones of the urinary tract that the isolation of *Proteus* from the urine alerts clinicians to this possibility.

## IMMUNITY

The intestinal tract of the newborn mammal is colonized shortly after birth by several different groups of bacteria including the Enterobacteriaceae. Of the many bioserotypes or clones of *E. coli,* only a limited number are highly prevalent. Immune reactions take place, and low titers of anti-Escherichia antibodies develop against the more common serogroups. The *E. coli* flora undergoes changes with time, age, and diet and is also dependent on the bacteria that are continuously taken in by mouth. Thus, some of the so-called natural antibodies are determined by immune reactions to the gram-negative intestinal bacteria. Antigenic cross-reactions that occur between different species of Enterobacteriaceae may be of importance for protection against intestinal diseases, and similar cross-reactions also exist between Enterobacteriaceae and pathogenic organisms from quite different bacterial groups. Thus, immune reactions to normal intestinal *E. coli* may protect against the invasion of many different bacteria; for example, *Haemophilus influenzae* Type b, which has a capsule that is serologically similar to the capsular antigen K100 of *E. coli* (Robbins et al., 1975).

### Escherichia Coli

People living in an area in which enterotoxigenic *E. coli* strains are widely distributed are more resistant to disease from this type of organism than visitors coming from areas with few enterotoxigenic strains. Experimental evidence suggests that this immunity may be mediated by antibody production either to the heat-labile toxin or to colonization factors such as pili or K antigens. Experimental vaccines against enterotoxigenic *E. coli* are being tried in animals and may eventually be available for human beings.

### Salmonella

Enteric fever provides some protection against the infecting serotype. Vaccination with TAB vaccine against *S. typhi* and *S. paratyphi* A and B has been given for more than 50 years to travelers going to parts of the world in which these diseases are endemic. The vaccine provides some protection against exposure to smaller doses of *S. typhi*.

### Shigella

People living in geographic areas in which *Shigella* species are endemic acquire some immunity to the disease. There are no effective vaccines, probably because most *Shigella* vaccines have not been able to increase the local intestinal defenses.

## *LABORATORY DIAGNOSIS*

Enterobacteriaceae are easy to cultivate either directly from feces, urine, or blood or from swabs of feces held in Stuart's medium. In addition to blood agar or nutrient agar, specimens that may contain Enterobacteriaceae are plated onto media that are both selective and differential. These media incorporate bile salts (MacConkey's agar, deoxycholate agar) or dyes (eosin-methylene blue or bromthymol blue) to inhibit gram-positive bacteria, lactose as the sole fermentable substrate, and a pH indicator (e.g., methylene blue), so that colonies that make acid from lactose are colored. Strains that do not ferment lactose are able to grow on the

peptone provided in the media but are colorless because they do not produce acid.

*Salmonella* and *Shigella* are very resistant to bile salts and certain dyes and can be selected by plating directly on media (e.g., Salmonella-Shigella agar, Hektoen agar) that partly inhibit *E. coli* and the other Enterobacteriaceae. Further selection is accomplished by culturing feces into selenite or tetrathionate broth for 18 to 24 hours before subculturing onto the selective solid media.

Final identification of Enterobacteriaceae is established by a battery of biochemical tests, agglutination with appropriate O, K (Vi), and H antisera, and occasionally by phage typing. A limited number of biochemical tests (Table 3) separates the five tribes. In practice, identification to the species level is usually accomplished easily in one step by selecting certain differential tests from the major biochemical characteristics of Enterobacteriaceae listed in Table 4. A typical battery of these tests, which will differentiate between the major species of the *Escherichia* and *Klebsiella* groups, is given in Table 5. Tables 6 and 7 highlight the limited number of tests necessary to separate the species of *Klebsiella* and *Enterobacter*, respectively. Most *Klebsiella* isolates are typical strains of *K. pneumoniae; K. ozaenae* and *K. rhinoscleromatis* are unusual isolates. *Enterobacter aerogenes* is the most commonly isolated *Enterobacter* species, but *E. cloacae* and *E. agglomerans* are isolated fairly frequently. *E. agglomerans* (*Erwinia herbicola*) is still classified with the *Erwinia* in the 8th edition of Bergey's Manual (1974), but many medical diagnostic laboratories have followed the suggestion of Ewing and Fife (1972) and classified it with *Enterobacter*.

There are three species or biotypes of *Citrobacter* (*Escherichia* tribe) that can be separated from one another by a limited number of biochemical tests (Table 8). *Citrobacter freundii* is by far

**TABLE 3.  Distinguishing Characteristics of the Five Primary Groups (Tribes)**

|  | TRIBE I ESCHERICHIEAE | TRIBE II KLEBSIELLEAE | TRIBE III PROTEEAE | TRIBE IV YERSINIEAE | TRIBE V ERWINIEAE |
|---|---|---|---|---|---|
| Fermentation pattern | Mixed acid | 2,3-Butanediol |  | Mixed acid | Mixed acid and 2,3-butanediol |
| M.R. | + | D | + | + |  |
| V.P. | − | D | D | − | D |
| Phenylalanine deamination | − | − | + | − | D |
| Nitrate reduction | + | + | + | + | D |
| Urease | − | D | D | D | − |
| KCN, growth in | D | + | + | − | D |
| Optimal temp. for growth | 37 C | 37 C | 37 C | 30–37 C | 27–30 C |
| G + C, % | 50–53 | 52–59 | 39–42 | 45–47 | 50–58 |

From Buchanan, C. E., and Gibbons, N. E. (eds.): Bergey's Manual of Determinative Bacteriology, 8th ed. Baltimore, The Williams & Wilkins Company, 1974.
G + C = Guanine + cytosine
D = different reactions from different genera or species

## TABLE 4.   Main Biochemical Characters of Primary Groups I to IV

| | GROUP I | | | | | GROUP II | | | | GROUP III PROTEUS | GROUP IV YERSINIA |
|---|---|---|---|---|---|---|---|---|---|---|---|
| | Escherichia | Edwardsiella | Citrobacter | Salmonella | Shigella | Klebsiella | Enterobacter | Hafnia | Serratia | | |
| Catalase | + | + | + | + | Dᵃ | + | + | + | + | + | + |
| Oxidase | − | − | − | − | − | − | − | − | − | − | − |
| β-Galactosidase | + | − | + | − | d | + | + | + | + | − | + |
| Gas from glucose at 37 C | + | + | + | D | − | d | + | + | d | D | − |
| KCN (growth on) | − | − | + | + | − | + | + | + | + | + | − |
| Mucate (acid) | + | − | + | D | − | d | d | − | − | − | |
| Nitrate reduced | + | + | + | + | + | + | + | + | + | + | + |
| G + C, moles % | 50–51 | | | 50–53 | | 52–56 | 52–59 | 52–57 | 53–59 | 39–42 (one species = 50) | 45–47 |
| **Carbohydrates (acid from)** | | | | | | | | | | | |
| Adonitol | − | − | − | − | − | d | + | − | d | − | D |
| Arabinose | + | − | + | + | d | + | + | + | − | D | + |
| Dulcitol | d | − | d | D | − | + | − | − | − | − | − |
| Esculin | d | − | d | − | − | d | D | − | d | d | D |
| Inositol | − | − | − | d | − | + | D | − | − | D | − |
| Lactose | + or × | − | + or × | − | D | D | + | − | + | − | − |
| Maltose | + | + | + | D | D | + | + | + | + | D | + |
| Mannitol | + | − | + | + | − | + | + | + | + | D | + |
| Salicin | d | − | d | − | − | + | + | − or × | + | d | D |
| Sorbitol | + | − | + | + | D | + | + | − | + | − | D |
| Sucrose | d | − | d | − | − | + | + | + | d | D | D |
| Trehalose | + | − | + | + | D | + | + | + | + | d | + |
| Xylose | d | − | + | + | D | + | + | + | + | D | D |
| **Related C sources** | | | | | | | | | | | |
| Citrate | − | − | + | + | − | d | + | + | + | D | − |
| Gluconate | − | − | d | − | − | + | + | + | + | − | d |
| Malonate | − | − | d | D | − | D | + | − | − | d | + |
| d-Tartrate | d | − | + | D | − | d | − | − | − | D | − |
| M.R. | + | + | + | + | + | D | − | − | D | − | + |
| V.P. | − | − | − | − | − | D | + | + | + | d | − |
| **Protein reactions** | | | | | | | | | | | |
| Arginine | d | − | d | + | − | (d) | D | − | − | − | − |
| Gelatin hydrolysis | − | − | − | − | − | − | (+) | − | + | D | − |
| H₂S from TSI | − | + | D | D | − | d | − | − | − | D | D |
| Indole | + | + | D | + | D | d | − | − | − | D | D |
| Lysine decarboxylated | + | + | − | + | − | + | D | + | + | d | − |
| Ornithine | d | + | d | + | d | − | + | + | + | D | D |
| Urea hydrolyzed | − | − | (+) | − | − | d | (d) | − | − | + | D |
| Glutamic acid | − | − | − | − | − | − | − | − | − | + | D |
| Phenylalanine | − | − | − | − | − | − | − | − | − | + | − |

ᵃD = different reactions given by different species of a genus; d = different reactions given by different strains of a species or serotype; × = late and irregularly positive (mutative).

From Buchanan, C. E., and Gibbons, N. E. (eds.): Bergey's Manual of Determinative Bacteriology, 8th ed. Baltimore, The Williams & Wilkins Company, 1974.

**TABLE 5.  Differentiation of Major Genera of Escherichieae and Klebsielleae**

| | E. COLI | EDWARD-SIELLA | SHIGELLA | SAL-MONELLA | CITRO-BACTER | KLEBSIELLA PNEU-MONIAE | ENTERO-BACTER AEROGENES | HAFNIA | SERRATIA MAR-CESCENS |
|---|---|---|---|---|---|---|---|---|---|
| KIA | A/AG | K/AG | K/A | K/AG | K or A/AG | A/AG | A/AG | K/AG | K/A or AG |
| H₂S (KIA) | − | + | − | + | + or − | − | − | − | − |
| Indole | + | + | − or + | − | − | − or + | − | − | − |
| Methyl red | + | + | + | + | + | − | − | + or − | − or + |
| Voges-Proskauer | − | − | − | − | − | + | + | + or − | + |
| Citrate (Simmons) | − | − | − | d | + | + | + | (+) or − | + |
| Motility | + | + | − | + | + | − | + | + | + |
| Urease | − | − | − | − | − | + | − | − | − |
| KCN | − | − | − | − | + or − | + | + | + | + |
| Lysine decarboxylase | d | + | − | + | − | + | + | + | + |
| Ornithine decarboxylase | d | + | d | + | d | − | + | + | + |
| Gas from glucose | + | + | − | + | + | + | + | + | − or + |
| Lactose | + | − | − | − | d | + | + | − or (+) | − or (+) |
| Salicin | d | − | − | − | d | + | + | d | + |
| Sorbitol | + | − | d | + | + | + | + | − | + |
| Raffinose | d | − | d | − | d | + | + | − | − |
| Rhamnose | d | − | d | + | + | + | + | + | − |
| Gelatin liquefaction (22°C) | − | − | − | − | − | − | − or (+) | − | + |

+ = 90% or more positive in 1 to 2 days; − = 90% or more negative; d = different biochemical types; (+) delayed positive; − or + = majority of cultures negative; + or − = majority positive; KIA = Kligler's iron agar; K = alkaline or no change; A = acid; G = gas.

Modified from Edwards, P. R., and Ewing, W. H.: Identification of Enterobacteriaceae, 3rd ed. Minneapolis, Burgess Publishing Co., 1972.

the most common isolate. Most laboratories do not recognize *Citrobacter intermedius* (not listed in Table 8 — see 8th ed. Bergey's Manual of Determinative Bacteriology) and regard strains that are either H₂S negative, indole positive, or ornithine-positive as variants of *C. freundii*. *C. diversus* is the biotype of Citrobacter that combines these 3 divergent characteristics with the inability to grow in KCN and inability to decarboxylate lysine.

The biochemical reactions used to differentiate between *Salmonella* and *Shigella* species are listed in Tables 9 and 10. *Shigella* can be differentiated to the species level by a combination of the indicated biochemical tests and simple agglutination tests with four O antisera. Speciation of *Salmonella* is an entirely different matter. The Salmonella species *S. typhi*, *S. paratyphi* A, *S. arizona* (formerly Arizona), and *S. choleraesuis* can be identified biochemically but have distinct serotypes. More than 1500 other bioserotypes are now grouped together as *S. enteritidis* and differentiated mainly by serologic methods (see below).

Biochemical differentiation of the *Proteus* tribe is usually easily accomplished by the tests listed in Table 11. The Providencia species have been renamed *Proteus inconstans*, which appropriately points out their close relationship to the other *Proteus* spp.

Table 12 lists the major differential charac-

**TABLE 6.  Differentiation of Klebsiella Species**

| | K. PNEU-MONIAE | K. OZAENAE | K. RHINO-SCLEROMATIS |
|---|---|---|---|
| Urease | + | − or + | − |
| Methyl red | − or + | + | + |
| Voges-Proskauer | + | − | − |
| Citrate (Simmons) | + | − or + | − |
| Malonate | + | − | + or − |
| Lysine decarboxylase | + | − or + | − |
| Gas from glucose | + | + or − | + |
| Lactose | + | (+) or − | (+) or − |

+ = 90% or more positive in 1 to 2 days; − = 90% or more negative; − or + = majority of cultures negative; + or − = majority positive; (+) = delayed positive.

Modified from 8th ed., Bergey's Manual of Determinative Bacteriology, 1974; and Lannette et al., Manual of Clinical Microbiology, 2nd ed., Am Soc Microbiol, Wash., D.C., 1974. Some bacteriologists recognize the oxytoca variant of *K. pneumoniae* as a separate species. These strains differ from other Klebsiella because they produce indole, liquefy gelatin, and produce a brown pigment when grown on defined medium containing gluconate and ferric citrate (Korth et al., 1969).

**TABLE 7.  Differentiation of Enterobacter Species**

| | E. AEROGENES | E. CLOACAE | E. AGGLO-MERANS |
|---|---|---|---|
| Urease | − | + or − | − or + |
| Lysine decarboxylase | + | − | − |
| Ornithine decarboxylase | + | + | − |
| Adonitol | + | − or + | − |
| Inositol (acid) | + | − or + | − or + |
| Inositol (gas) | + | − | |
| Esculin | + | − or + | d |
| Yellow pigment | − | − | + or − |

+ = 90% or more positive in 1 to 2 days; − = 90% or more negative; − or + = majority of cultures negative; + or − = majority positive; d = different biochemical types.

Modified from Edwards, P. R., and Ewing, W. H.: Identification of Enterobacteriaceae. 3rd ed., Minneapolis, Burgess Publishing Co.; and Ewing, W. H., and Fife, M. A.: *Enterobacter agglomerans* (Baijerinck) Comb. Nov. (The Herbicola-hathyri Bacteria.) Int J Syst Bacteriol 22(1):4–11, 1972.

**TABLE 8. Differentiation of Citrobacter Species**

|  | C. FREUNDII | C. DIVERSUS |
|---|---|---|
| Citrate (Simmon's) | + | + |
| Indole | − | + |
| H₂S (KIA) | + | − |
| Ornithine decarboxylase | − or + | + |
| Lysine decarboxylase | − | − |
| KCN | + | − |

+ = 90% or more positive in 1 to 2 days; − = 90% or more negative; d = different biochemical types; − or + = majority negative; KIA = Kligler's iron agar.
Modified from 8th ed. Bergey's Manual of Determinative Bacteriology, 1974; and Ewing, W. H.: Differentiation of Enterobacteriaceae by Biochemical Reactions, Revised. DHEW Publication No. (CDC) 74-8270, May, 1974.

teristics of the *Yersinia* species, which are discussed more extensively in Chapter 37. Although *Yersinia* has recently been reclassified in the family Enterobacteriaceae, it is discussed separately for historic reasons and because it causes clinical syndromes similar to those of *Francisella* and *Pasteurella*.

*Erwinia*, another recent addition to the family of Enterobacteriaceae, also cause classification problems. These organisms are plant pathogens or commensals and are isolated infrequently from human sources except for the Herbicola group (*Enterobacter agglomerans*). *Erwinia* are usually divided into three groups: the Amylovora group (sometimes referred to as "true *Erwinia*"), the Herbicola group (*E. agglomerans*), and the Carotovora group (pectobacteria). The Amylovora group is frequently nitrate-negative, attacks glucose primarily oxidatively, fails to grow at 37°C, and is isolated very infrequently from humans. Since this group fits the definition of Enterobacteriaceae poorly and is rarely isolated from humans, we will not deal with it further in this chapter. *E. agglomerans* (Herbicola group) is characterized in Table 7. The Carotovora group (pectobacteria) is occasionally isolated from man and is biochemically similar to the *Klebsiella* tribe but also grows better at room temperature than at 37° C; reactions are given at both temperatures.

As indicated in the tables, most Enterobacteriaceae can be differentiated to the species level by biochemical tests. Serologic methods are used most frequently for the identification of *Shigella*, *Salmonella*, and certain serotypes of *E. coli*. Although *Shigella* can frequently be speciated by the tests shown in Table 10, the identification is always confirmed by agglutination with O antisera. Shigellae have no special capsular antigens and no H antigens since they are nonmotile. Salmonellae are speciated by the Kaufmann and White scheme described previously under Antigenic Composition. Most laboratories use only O

and Vi antisera for preliminary identification of salmonellae and send their isolates to reference laboratories for final identification. If *S. typhi* is suspected in the clinical laboratory, it is important to attempt agglutination with Vi antisera, because the Vi antigen may block access to the O antigenic sites by O antisera. Blocking of O agglutination by either Vi or H antigens may be removed by boiling. *S. typhi* should be suspected when a *Salmonella*-like organism (Table 10) fails to utilize citrate as the sole carbon source, produces no gas from glucose, produces little or no H₂S, and fails to decarboxylate ornithine. A *Salmonella* with these biochemical reactions that agglutinates with Vi antisera before boiling and with O antisera after boiling should be identified as *S. typhi*. A *Salmonella* that agglutinates with C₁ antisera and has typical *Salmonella* reactions, except for failure to produce H₂S, is identified as *S. choleraesuis*. All other salmonellae are customarily identified as *S. enteritidis*, Group — according to the group of O antisera with which they agglutinate, and are sent to reference laboratories for final identification.

### Enteropathogenic E. Coli

The *E. coli* bioserotypes associated with diarrhea constitute a special problem because they cannot be differentiated from other *E. coli* on existing media.

Enterotoxigenic *E. coli* isolated from diseases of pigs are usually hemolytic, so that only hemolytic colonies are tested with agglutinating antisera against the serotypes that cause piglet diarrhea. No similar characteristic trait is known for strains that are enteropathogenic to human beings. Recent studies suggest that some serotypes harbor enterotoxin plasmids more frequently than others. This finding may simplify the screening for enterotoxigenic strains, but it will not represent a definitive test.

The laboratory identification of enterotoxigenic strains is very time-consuming and is ordinarily a research procedure. Single colonies of each specimen are tested for LT (heat-labile) enterotoxin by determining their influence on the morphology of adrenal (Y1) or Chinese hamster ovary cells (CHO) in tissue culture. ST (heat-stable) enterotoxin is detected in infant mice by peroral or intragastric injections of suspected colonies followed by measurement of fluid accumulation (weight gain) of the total intestinal tract. Both toxins can be detected by fluid accumulation in the "rabbit ileal loop," which is even more forbidding as a routine test. The recent isolation in several laboratories of pure LT has brought simple serologic tests for LT within reach. A similar approach for ST will not be possible because it is nonimmunogenic.

**TABLE 9.   Differentiation of Major Species of Salmonella**

|  | S. TYPHI | S. CHOLERAESUIS[a] | S. ENTERITIDIS | S. PARATYPHI A | S. ARIZONAE |
|---|---|---|---|---|---|
| H₂S (KIA or TSI) | +[w] | d | + | − or + | + |
| Citrate (Simmons) | − | (+) | + | − or (+) | + |
| Lysine decarboxylase | + | + | + | + | + |
| Ornithine decarboxylase | − | + | + | + | + |
| Gas from glucose | − | + | + | + | + |
| Dulcitol | − or(+) | − or + | + | + | − |
| Trehalose | + | − | + | + |  |
| Arabinose | − | − | + | + | + |
| Rhamnose | − | + | + |  | + |
| Malonate | − | − | − | − | + |
| O group | D | C₁ | All groups | A | Arizona[b] |

[a]H₂S positive strains are referred to as *S. choleraesuis* var. *Kunzendorf.*

Salmonella are now named either *S. typhi, S. choleraesuis,* or *S. enteritidis,* serogroup−. *S. paratyphi* A and *S. arizonae* are included in this table because they can be identified biochemically and because *S. arizonae* was considered a separate species until recently.

Precise identification is made in reference centers by extensive cross agglutination tests and occasionally by phage typing.

+ = 90% or more positive in 1 to 2 days; − = 90% or more negative; d = different biochemical types; (+) = delayed positive; − or + = majority of cultures negative; + or − = majority positive; A = acid, KIA = Kligler's iron agar; TSI = triple sugar iron agar.

[b]*S. arizona* is agglutinated by commercial Arizona antisera and by some specific salmonella antisera.

Modified from 8th ed. Bergey's Manual of Determinative Bacteriology, 1974; and Edwards, P. R., and Ewing, W. H.: Identification of Enterobacteriaceae, 3rd ed., Minneapolis, Burgess Publishing Co., 1972.

Invasive *E. coli* can be detected by the capacity of a few drops of an overnight culture to cause keratoconjunctivitis in guinea pigs or rabbits. The so-called enteropathogenic serotypes (EPEC) from infantile diarrhea can be detected by screening colonies with appropriate antisera.

## DRUG SENSITIVITY

Except for benzyl penicillin, Enterobacteriaceae are intrinsically sensitive to achievable serum and tissue concentrations of most antimicrobials when they are first introduced. Resistant strains are selected quickly, however, because the Enterobacteriaceae in the normal intestinal tract are frequently exposed to antibiotics directed at other, more invasive bacteria. Furthermore, some genera of Enterobacteriaceae are in-

trinsically resistant to certain antimicrobials. Some examples of this property include the resistance of *Proteus* spp. and *Serratia* to polymyxins, the resistance of *Proteus* spp. to tetracycline, and the resistance of *Enterobacter* to cephalothin. *Klebsiella* is usually resistant to aminobenzylpenicillin (ampicillin) but sensitive to the cephalosporins. *Proteus mirabilis* is unique among the Enterobacteriaceae species for its sensitivity to benzylpenicillin. Rapid selection of resistant mutants may occur when Enterobacteriaceae are exposed to nalidixic acid, rifampin, or the aminoglycosides as single antimicrobial therapy. All Enterobacteriaceae are intrinsically resistant to achievable levels of erythromycin and the other macrolides.

Most of the genetic determinants of resistance, however, are carried on transferable plasmids that have been responsible for the appearance of

**TABLE 10.   Differentiation of Shigella Species**

|  | S. DYSENTERIAE | S. FLEXNERI | S. BOYDII | S. SONNEI |
|---|---|---|---|---|
| Indole | d | d | d | − |
| Lactose (acid) | − | − | − | (+) |
| Mannitol | − | d | + | + |
| Sucrose | − | − | − | (+) |
| Dulcitol | d | d | d | − |
| Xylose | d | d | d | − |
| Ornithine decarboxylase | − | − | − | + |
| Rhamnose | d | d | d | + |
| Raffinose | − | d | − | d |
| O groups | A | B | C | D |

+ = 90% or more positive in 1 to 2 days; − = 90% or more negative; d = different biochemical types; (+) = delayed positive.

Modified from 8th ed. Bergey's Manual of Determinative Bacteriology, 1974; and Edwards, P. R., and Ewing, W. H.: Identification of Enterobacteriaceae, 3rd ed., Minneapolis, Burgess Publishing Co., 1972.

**TABLE 11.   Differentiation of Proteus Species[a]**

| | P. VULGARIS | P. MIRABILIS | P. MORGANII | P. RETTGERI | P. INCONSTANS[a] A | P. INCONSTANS[a] B |
|---|---|---|---|---|---|---|
| Phenylalanine deaminase | + | + | + | + | + | + |
| Urease | + | + or (+) | + | + | − | − |
| Indole | + | − | + | + | + | + |
| H$_2$S (KIA or TSI) | + | + | − | − | − | − |
| Lysine decarboxylase | − | − | − | − | − | − |
| Ornithine decarboxylase | − | + | + | − | − | − |
| Moles % G + C | 39 | 39 | 50 | 39 | 41 | 41 |
| Gas from glucose | + | + | + or − | − or + | + or − | − |
| Esculin | d | − | − | + | − | − |
| Inositol | − | − | − | + | − | + |
| Maltose | + | − | − | − | − | − |
| Mannitol | − | − | − | + or − | − | − or + |
| Mannose | − | − | + | + | + | + |
| Rhamnose | − | − | − | + or − | − | − |
| Adonitol | − | − | − | + or − | + | − |
| Spontaneous swarming | + | + | − | − | − | − |
| Penicillin sensitivity | − | + | − | − | − | − |

[a]*P. inconstans* subgroups A and B (8th ed., Bergey's Manual of Determinative Bacteriology) were formerly known as *Providencia alcalifaciens* and *Providencia stuartii*.

+ = 90% or more positive in 1 to 2 days; − = 90% or more negative; d = different biochemical types; (+) = delayed positive; − or + = majority of cultures negative; + or − = majority positive.

Modified from Edwards, P. R., and Ewing, W. H.: Identification of Enterobacteriaceae. 3rd ed. Minneapolis, Burgess Publishing Company, 1972, and 8th ed., Bergey's Manual of Determinative Bacteriology, 1974.

an increasing number of multiresistant Enterobacteriaceae. The use of antibiotics for treatment of disease and as food additives in animal breeding has exerted a powerful selection pressure for antibiotic-resistant strains. When the use of antibiotics is restricted, the number of resistant strains in that area decreases (Falkow, 1975).

Thus, the antimicrobial sensitivities of individual species of this important family of bacteria are unpredictable. They vary from broad sensitivity to complete resistance to the tetracyclines, aminoglycosides, the sulfonamides, cephalosporins, polymyxins, chloramphenicol, ampicillin, and carbenicillin. For this reason, antimicrobial sensitivity tests must be conducted quickly and accurately to ensure effective therapy against enterobacterial infections.

## EPIDEMIOLOGY

### Escherichia Coli

The source of infection with the three types of *E. coli* diarrhea described above is human. Few cases exist that point to direct transfer of pathogenic strains from domestic animals to human beings. The enteropathogenic types (EPEC), are transferred nosocomially in nurseries and wards directly or indirectly from one child to another. The ultimate source of human enterotoxigenic strains (ETEC) is probably the infected patient, but transmission is indirect, possibly through

contaminated food. The finding of the same highly defined serofermentative types among enterotoxigenic strains isolated all over the world indicates that the same clones of bacteria have spread around the world. Enterotoxigenic piglet diarrhea strains spread from country to country within a short period of time and demonstrated how easily special pathogenic strains can be globally disseminated.

The epidemiologic characteristics of *E. coli* strains from dysentery-like disease (EIEC) are the same as those of *Shigella* (see below).

**TABLE 12.   Differentiation of Yersinia Species**

| | Y. PESTIS | Y. PSEUDO-TUBERCULOSIS | Y. ENTEROCOLITICA |
|---|---|---|---|
| Motility | | | |
| 22 °C | − | + | + |
| 37 °C | − | − | − |
| Urease | − | + | + |
| Esculin | + | + | − or + |
| Rhamnose | − or + | + | − |
| Salicin | + or − | + | − |
| Sucrose | − | − | + |
| Ornithine decarboxylase | − | − | + |
| Indole | − | − | + or − |

+ = 90% or more positive in 1 to 2 days; − = 90% or more negative; − or + = majority negative; + or − = majority positive.

Modified from 8th ed., Bergey's Manual of Determinative Bacteriology; and Lennette et al., Manual of Clinical Microbiology, 2nd ed., Am Soc Microbiol, Wash., D.C., 1974.

## Salmonella

Typhoid and paratyphoid bacteria are primarily human parasites, and the corresponding diseases originate from human sources, i.e., either sick patients or carriers. Some geographic differences occur, e.g., *S. paratyphi* C is found primarily in Eastern Europe and Asia, while *S. paratyphi* A is found in the Americas and India.

Typhoid fever in developing countries is often waterborne in contrast to paratyphoid fevers. Shellfish, especially oysters, are an important source of typhoid fever but are rarely the source of paratyphoid fever. Milk and other diary products are often vehicles for typhoid and paratyphoid infections. A small percentage of clinical cases of typhoid fever become chronic carriers and excrete the organism indefinitely. In developed countries, it is often possible to trace nonimported cases of typhoid fever to such carriers.

*Salmonella* enteritis, associated with many different serotypes, such as *S. typhimurium, S. newport, S. adelaide,* and others, is often described under the heading of food poisoning. It is true that large infectious doses are generally necessary to cause disease, but the pathogenesis includes inflammation of the mucosal tissues and often involves the local lymph nodes. Human *Salmonella* enteritis is associated with consumption of food contaminated either directly or indirectly by an infected animal, e.g., pig, fowl (eggs), cattle, and others. *S. typhimurium* is the most widespread of the serotypes causing enteritis, but the predominant *Salmonella* serotype varies in different geographic areas. Patterns of prevalence change with time as new serotypes are introduced and spread within certain geographic locations. The present close contact between countries and the extensive exchange of travelers and food products have also increased the exchange of pathogenic *Salmonella* serotypes. The same applies, of course, to other pathogenic (and nonpathogenic) Enterobacteriaceae.

## Shigella

Human cases are always the source of infection, so the prevalence of bacterial dysentery is highly dependent on sanitary conditions. Bacillary dysentery is endemic in many developing countries. In countries with better conditions of public health, this disease is often confined to institutions or to outbreaks caused by contamination of dairy products. In the highest developed countries, shigellosis is rare and often imported. Chronic carriers are uncommon. *Shigella dysenteriae* Type 1 (the Shiga bacillus) causes the most severe disease.

## PREVENTIVE MEASURES

Sanitary measures are all important to control enteric diseases caused by *Salmonella, Shigella,* pathogenic *E. coli,* and other Enterobacteriaceae, e.g., control of water, food, milk, and sewage disposal. Carriers (of *Salmonella*) must not be allowed to work as food handlers.

## References

Buchanan, C. E., and Gibbons, N. E. (ed.): Bergey's Manual of Determinative Bacteriology. 8th ed. Baltimore, The Williams & Wilkins Company, 1974, pp. 290–340.

Edwards, P. R., and Ewing, W. H.: Identification of *Enterobacteriaceae.* 3rd ed. Minneapolis, Burgess Publishing Company, 1972.

Ewing, W. H.: Differentiation of Enterobacteriaceae by Biochemical Reactions, Revised. DHEW Publication No. (CDC) 74-8270, May, 1974.

Ewing, W. H., and Fife, M. A.: Enterobacter agglomerans (Beijernick) Comb. Nov. (the Herbicola-Lathyri bacteria). Int J. System Bacteriol 22(1):4, 1972.

Falkow, S.: Infectious Multiple Drug Resistance. London, Pion Limited, 1975.

Kauffmann, F.: The Bacteriology of *Enterobacteriaceae.* Copenhagen, E. Munksgaard, 1966.

Korth, H., Ørskov, I., and Pulverer, G.: Farbstoffbildende *Klebsiella*-Stamme. Zentrabl. Bacteriol Parasitenk Infectionskr Abt Orig I 211 (1):105–107, 1969.

Lennette, E. H., Spaulding, E. H., and Truant, J. P.: Manual of Clinical Microbiology, 2nd ed. American Society of Microbiology. Washington, D.C. 1974.

Lüderitz, O., Westphal, O., Staub, A. M., and Nikaido, H.: Isolation and chemical and immunological characterization of bacterial lipopolysaccharides. In Weinbaum, G., Kadis, S., and Ajl, S. J. (eds.): Microbial Toxins. Vol. 4. New York and London, Academic Press, 1971, pp. 145–233.

Ørskov, F., and Ørskov, I.: Serotyping of *Enterobacteriaceae* with special emphasis on K determination. In Norris, J. R., and Bergan, T. (eds.): Methods in Microbiology. Vol. 11. London and New York, Academic Press, 1978.

Ørskov, I., Ørskov, F., Jann, B., and Jann, K.: Serology, genetics and chemistry of O and K antigens of *Escherichia coli.* Bacterial Rev 41:667, 1977.

Robbins, J. B., Schneerson, R., Liu, T., Schiffer, M. S., Schiffman, G., Myerowitz, R. L., McCracken, G. H., Jr., Ørskov, I., and Ørskov, F.: Cross reacting bacterial antigens and immunity to disease caused by encapsulated bacteria. In Neter, E., and Milgrom, F. (eds.): The Immune System and Infectious Disease. Buffalo, Fourth International Convocation on Immunology, 1975, pp. 218–241.

Rowe, B.: *Escherichia coli* in acute diarrhoea. Lab-Lore 7:499, 1977.

Sack, R. B.: Human diarrhea disease caused by enterotoxigenic *Escherichia coli.* Ann Rev Microbiol 29:333, 1975.

# VIBRIOS 32

## Barun Deb Chatterjee, M.B.B.S., Ph.D., Dip. Bact.

Curved bacteria with polar flagellation are called *vibrios*. These chem-organotrophic bacteria are grouped as follows: I. Family Vibrionaceae (respiratory and fermentative metabolism) — (a) *Vibrio cholerae*, (b) Noncholera vibrios (NCV) or Nonagglutinating (NAG) vibrios, (c) *Aeromonas hydrophila*, (d) *Plesiomonas shigelloides;* and II. Family Spirillaceae (respiratory metabolism) — *Campylobacter fetus.* The earliest designation, *Vibrio gindha*, Pfeiffer 1896 (Chalmers and Waterfield, 1916),. is preferred to NCV or NAG vibrios, since these organisms produce cholera-like disease and agglutinate in homologous antisera (although not in anticholera serum). The taxonomic position of *Vibrio parahaemolyticus* is unsettled: being peritrichous, it is not a vibrio. Although related to different genera, as shown in Table 1, *V. parahaemolyticus* and *C. fetus* are provisionally described here until their taxonomy is clarified.

In the tropics, cholera vibrios are the principal but not the sole agents of acute dehydrating rice water diarrhea. Cholera syndrome may be related to a range of pathogens of widely different taxons — for example, NCV, *V. parahaemolyticus, A. hydrophila, Pl. shigelloides,* and enterotoxigenic *E. coli* (Chatterjee and Neogy, 1972).

**TABLE 1. Alliance of *V. parahaemolyticus* to different Fermentative, Gram-Negative Bacteria**

| Characters | V.parahaemo-lyticus | Pasteurella | Yersinia | Lucibac-terium | Aeromonas | Vibrio ‡ |
|---|---|---|---|---|---|---|
| Cells : coccoid | + | + | + | − | −* | − |
| Capsule | + | + | − | − | + | − |
| Flagella : polar and peritrichous | + | − | − | + | − | − |
| Swarming | + | − | + | + | − | − |
| Growth in 0% NaCl conc. | − | + | + | − | + | + |
| Oxidase | + | + | − | + | + | + |
| β-galactosidase | − | − | + | ? | + | + |
| Lysine decarboxylase | + | d | − | + | − | + |
| Zoonosis | + | + | + | − | + | − |
| Tissue invasion | + | + | + | ? | + | − |
| Luminescence | − | − | − | + | − | − |
| GC ratio : 46 | + | +† | + | + | − | − |

+ = more than 90% strains positive
− = more than 90% strains negative
*occasionally positive
† top range
‡ type species
d = 11-89% strains positive

# VIBRIO CHOLERAE
(*vibrio,* which vibrates; *cholerae,* an intestinal disease)

### MORPHOLOGY

Cells are slightly curved, gram negative, 0.5 by 1.5 to 3.0 $\mu$m, and occur singly (Fig. 1). Bacilli rarely appear straight, spherical, and, if joined, S- or C-shaped and as spirilla. The cholera vibrios are fimbriated and show fast linear motility by a long wavy polar flagellum (Fig. 2). They are essentially noncapsulated, but occasionally a cell may look encapsulated. In smears from mucus flakes of rice water stool, bacilli lie parallel to each other like "fish in a stream," presumably

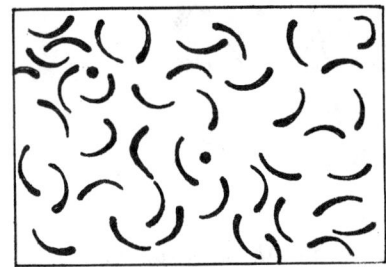

**FIGURE 1.** *Cell morphology of cholera vibrios.*

because of the degenerating spirilla forms. Cells are vividly stained by dilute carbol fuchsin.

On nutrient agar, the organism produces semi-transparent, low convex, 2 to 3 mm round colonies that suspend uniformly in saline. In one week, the growth is overlaid by minute secondary colonies and develops needle-shaped crystals underneath. Colonies may undergo variations to (1) dwarf, (2) entirely opaque, (3) centrally opaque with smooth periphery, and (4) reversible rugose colonies.

After primary isolation in bile salt agar (BSA) and lactose teepol agar (LTA), the conspicuously transparent, flat colonies of cholera vibrios are readily differentiated from the opaque raised ones of coliforms. Under stereo-plate microscopy, the cholera vibrios on BSA exhibit greenish to red-bronze iridescence with fine granular transparency.

Colonies appear opaque-yellow on thiosulfate citrate bile salts-sucrose (TCBS) agar, translucent-yellow on sucrose teepol tellurite (STT) agar (Chatterjee et al., 1977), translucent bluish gray on thiosulfate citrate bile salts-sucrose lauryl sulfate agar (Vibrio agar), grayish translucent on lauryl sulfate tellurite agar (Cholera medium), and gelatin taurocholate tellurite (GTT) agar. While BSA and LTA inhibit gram-positive bacilli, others suppress coliforms as well, thus permitting vibrios to grow in pure form. The slide agglutination with antisera can be done from isolates of all media except TCBS and vibrio agar, for which, because of the stickiness, subculture on nutrient agar is necessary.

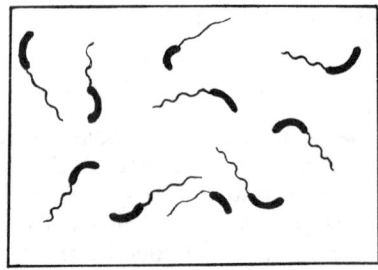

**FIGURE 2.** *Long, wavy polar flagella of cholera vibrios.*

## ANTIGENIC COMPOSITION

Cholera vibrios possess heat labile flagellar (H) and heat stable somatic (O) antigens. The former is a protein, the latter a lipopolysaccharide. Three fractions of the O antigen: A, B, and C determine Ogawa (AB), Inaba (AC), Hikojima (ABC), and one unusual (A) serotypes. In vivo conversion from Ogawa to Inaba and the reverse is a rare possibility. The isolates from chronic carriers even if appearing smooth may lack O antigen because of S-R variation. Detection of such a variant is facilitated by the "rough" antiserum, made against O antigen-deficient strain. Minor proportions of cholera H antigen are present in certain strains of NCV and *S. enteritidis*. A common O antigenic factor being shared by cholera vibrios, brucella species, *Y. enterocolitica* serotype IX, and *C. terrigena* may confuse serologic diagnosis.

## METABOLISM

Cholera vibrios are facultative anaerobes and can multiply at 16 to 42°C and pH 6.4 to 9.6. Optimum growth occurs aerobically, at 37°C, pH 8.0 to 8.2, in ordinary media and even on minimal synthetic medium containing sources of carbon, nitrogen, and salts. Higher pH (8.5 to 9.5) is beneficial but a lower one (pH 4.0) is lethal, so that strains grown in media containing glucose do not survive. In Table 2, the various distinctive characters of *V. cholerae* are presented. The positive oxidase, catalase, and nitrate reduction tests should be noted.

*V. cholerae* differs from *V. cholerae* biotype El Tor (El Tor vibrio, named for its discovery in El Tor lazeret of Sinai Peninsula). The *V. cholerae* (classic vibrio) is sensitive to 50 IU polymyxin B disk (or 15 μg/ml in nutrient agar) and 1 RTD group IV cholera phage, whereas the El Tor is resistant to these. Only El Tor produces acetoin and agglutinates with chicken, sheep, and human erythrocytes. Further, El Tor causes distinct opacity and a pellicle in nutrient broth, whereas the *V. cholerae* creates minimum turbidity and no pellicle. Until 1962, El Tor strains were hemolytic, but subsequent isolates have not been.

With four lytic phages and standard laboratory strains, classic vibrios exhibit five lytic patterns and El Tor is distributed into six types by five phages. However, phage typing provides limited information in tracing the source of infection, because in actual practice, wild strains of the classic and El Tor strains comprise only two phage types, and the El Tor phages are unstable. Strains of El Tor vibrio isolated from clinical cases from the year 1961 onward, almost invariably show ly-

**TABLE 2.  Distinguishing Features of Vibrio and Allied Pathogens
(All single polar flagellated, rapidly motile, positive to catalase, oxidase
and nitrate reduction tests)**

| Characters | V.cholerae | NCV | A.hydrophila | Pl.shigell-oides | V.para-haemolyticus | C.fetus |
|---|---|---|---|---|---|---|
| Cells: | | | | | | |
| curved | + | + | − | − | − | + |
| coccoid | − | −* | −* | − | + | − |
| Flagella | | | | | | |
| lophotrichous | − | − | + | + | + | − |
| peritrichous | − | − | − | − | + | − |
| Capsule | − | + | + | + | + | − |
| Motility: corkscrew-like | − | − | − | − | − | + |
| | | | | | | |
| Facultative anaerobic | + | + | + | + | + | − |
| Microaerophilic | − | − | − | − | − | + |
| | | | | | | |
| Growth: | | | | | | |
| TCBS agar | + | + | − | − | + | NT |
| SS agar | − | − | + | + | − | − |
| 0% NaCl in gelatin agar | + | + | + | + | − | NT |
| 7% NaCl in gelatin agar | − | − | − | − | + | NT |
| KCN broth | d | d | + | − | − | NT |
| | | | | | | |
| O-F test: fermentative | + | + | + | + | + | − |
| Gas from: glucose | − | − | d | − | − | − |
| Acid from | | | | | | |
| glucose | + | + | + | + | + | − |
| mannitol | + | + | + | − | + | − |
| inositol | − | − | − | + | − | − |
| Current Heiberg groups | I | (I II V) | (I III IV V) | VI | VII | − |
| Acid from | | | | | | |
| mannose | + | + | − | + ++ − + | − | + |
| sucrose | + | + | + | − ++ + − | − | − |
| arabinose | − | − | − | − −+ + − | − | + |
| | | | | | | |
| β-galactosidase | + | + | + | + | − | NT |
| | | | | | | |
| Arginine dihydrolase | − | − | + | + | − | − |
| Lysine decarboxylase | + | + | − | + | + | − |
| Ornithine decarboxylase | + | + | − | + | + | − |
| | | | | | | |
| Methyl red | d | d | + | + | − | − |
| Voges-Proskauer | − | d | d | − | − | − |
| Indole | + | + | + | + | d(weak) | − |
| Citrate utilization | d | + | d | − | − | − |
| | | | | | | |
| Hydrolysis | | | | | | |
| gelatin | + | + | + | − | + | − |
| casein | + | + | + | − | + | − |
| Tween 80 | + | + | ? | − | + | − |
| starch | + | + | + | − | + | − |
| esculin | − | − | d | − | + | − |
| | | | | | | |
| Hemolysis | | | | | | |
| sheep cell suspension | − | d | d | − | − | − |
| | | | | | | |
| 0/129 sensitivity | + | + | − | + | + | − |
| | | | | | | |
| Moles per cent GC | 47 | 46–48 | 57–63 | 51 | 46 | 32–35 |
| | | | | | | |
| Mice: s.c. injection bacteremia | − | + | + | + | + | NT |
| | | | | | | |
| Saprophytic existence | − | + | + | − | + | − |

+ = more than 90% strains positive
d = 11–89% strains positive
− = more than 90% strains negative
NT = not tested
*occasionally positive
S.C. = subcutaneous

sogenization by a specific temperate phage called the "kappa" phage. Such strains are identified by their capacity to elicit turbid plaques on *V. cholerae* H 218. By detecting "kappa" phage lytic mutants in their feces, bacteriologically negative cases of El Tor cholera and their contacts can be identified. The *V. cholerae* is resistant to "kappa" phage; El Tor acquires susceptibility after eliminating the temperate phage.

## PATHOGENIC PROPERTIES

Evidence suggests that low gastric acid predisposes to attacks of cholera, a finding in keeping with the susceptibility in vitro of *V. cholerae* to low pH. The infective dose in natural infections is probably less than that causing disease in volunteers ($10^6$), since the organism is short-lived in soil, impure water, saprophytic contaminants, and chlorinated water, and perishes when desiccated, gently heated, or exposed to sunlight.

After bypassing the acid gastric barrier, the organisms reach the favorable alkaline medium in the small bowel, where they anchor to the gut mucosa and colonize, and liberate enterotoxin to cause acute rice water diarrhea. The toxin, irreversibly fixed to the intestinal mucosa, stimulates adenyl cyclase, which in its turn builds up cAMP to trigger outpouring of isotonic fluid. Cholera toxin is a protein of molecular weight 84,000 and comprises synergistically acting toxin and toxoid moieties. Experimentally, the toxin produces diarrhea in nine day old rabbits and mongrel dogs. It causes dilatation and fluid accumulation in the ligated loops of adult rabbits, induces rounding of cells and steroidogenesis in clonal cell lines of Y-1 and OS-3 adrenal tumor cells in tissue culture, and elongation of Chinese hamster ovarian (CHO) cell line.

The toxin moiety consists of six light subunits (L) and one heavy subunit (H). While the former helps adherence to the receptor (ganglioside) of the cell membrane, the latter performs the toxic activity.

However, other metabolites of cholera vibrios, like vascular permeability factor, cytolysin, hemolysin, and mucinase do not appear to be related to the pathogenesis of cholera.

## IMMUNITY

An attack of cholera confers short-lived immunity to reinfection. Within a few weeks after onset of the disease, there is rise of both serum antibodies (agglutinins [IgM], vibriocidal antibody [IgM], antitoxin [IgG]) and coproantibody (IgA), which persists for three months, but shortly afterward falls to low titer. It is well known that the IgM and IgG lose their normal functions within the gut lumen because of enzymatic inactivation, and because complement-mediated bactericidal activity as well as complement-dependent phagocytosis are not operative in the anticomplementary intestinal contents. However, it is believed that the antibacterial antibody prevents attachment of the organism to the gut mucosa, whereas the antitoxic immunity inhibits fixation of the toxin.

Likewise, the cholera vaccines, killed parenteral (with or without adjuvant) and live or killed oral varieties, without exception impart short-term (three to nine months) protection. The efficacy of vaccines is further limited by their failure to prevent epidemics, death, and inapparent cases and carriers.

## LABORATORY DIAGNOSIS

### Collection

Fecal samples are collected aseptically in sterile containers with soft rubber catheters (No. 22 or 24), previously lubricated in sterile liquid paraffin. Rectal swabs are not recommended because they often become dry if sampling is inadequate or if the interval between collection and inoculation is too long. If cotton swabs are used they should be soaked in Sorensen's buffer, pH 7.4, before autoclaving. A sample that cannot be inoculated soon after collection should be kept in Cary-Blair's transport medium, which is ideal for vibrios, shigella, salmonella, and *E. coli*.

### Culture

Since a range of pathogens are expected in a rice water stool, a semiquantitative approach sheds light on the role of organisms, especially in mixed infections (Chatterjee and Neogy, 1972). Usually one of these agents is found in high numbers ($10^6$ to $10^9$/ml), whereas others constitute a minor proportion ($10^1$ to $10^4$/ml). A calibrated loop (0.01 ml; 4 mm internal diameter) is filled with neat, 1/10 and 1/100 dilutions of feces in sterile saline containing 0.1 per cent peptone, and streaked on selective media as for a urine culture.

Six hours of enrichment in alkaline peptone water (with 3 per cent NaCl), pH 9.2 enhances isolation of cholera vibrios, NCV, and *V. parahaemolyticus*. For the salmonella, aeromonas, and plesiomonas species, 18 hour enrichment in selenite F broth is recommended. Subculture on selective media after preliminary enrichment allows identification of pathogens.

## Media

Colony counts of cholera vibrios, NCV, and *V. parahaemolyticus* are done from TCBS or STT agar. The SS agar provides similar information on salmonella, aeromonas, plesiomonas, and pseudomonas; the desoxycholate citrate agar (DCA) is primarily used for salmonella and shigella species, and the MacConkey agar is used for *E. coli.*

## Identification

Oxidase-positive isolates on TCBS or STT agar that ferment sucrose are tested in cholera polyvalent and (if necessary) "rough" antisera. Cholera vibrios showing agglutination are divided into Inaba, Ogawa, or (rarely) Hikojima serotypes by specific sera and classic or El Tor biotypes after noting sensitivity to phage IV and polymyxin B (and/or hemagglutination in sheep cells). Contrarily, the sucrose fermenters not reacting with cholera sera are identified as NCV on the basis of decarboxylase-dihydrolase tests. Of the sucrose nonfermenting colonies, the Heiberg group VII strains, showing growth at 7 per cent but not in 0 per cent NaCl concentrations and a negative $\beta$-galactosidase reaction are identified as *V. parahaemolyticus* biotype 1; whereas those of Heiberg group V, lacking the halophilic property with a positive $\beta$-galactosidase test are regarded as NCV (Table 2). *V. parahaemolyticus* is subjected to serotyping and the Kanagawa test (see below). The oxidase-positive colonies of MacConkey agar and DCA are treated in a similar manner.

The nonlactose-fermenting, oxidase-positive colonies from SS agar are tested for their oxidation-fermentation (O-F) reaction: *C. terrigena* is negative, whereas *P. aeruginosa* is oxidative. The fermentative breakdown of glucose suggests aeromonas and plesiomonas species. They are identified from the results of mannitol and inositol fermentation and decarboxylase tests (Table 2, Fig. 3).

## DRUG SUSCEPTIBILITY

The mean inhibitory concentrations (MIC) in $\mu$g/ml for cholera vibrios are as follows: tetracycline 2.5, chloramphenicol 1.5, streptomycin 25, paromomycin 25, viomycin 200, and neomycin 20 to 30. The cholera vibrios are also sensitive to disks of ampicillin (2 $\mu$g), sulfisoxazole (4 $\mu$g), and polymyxin B (100 IU). Only 2.5 per cent of the global strains are not susceptible to one of these agents. The resistance is chromosomal in origin and seldom, if ever, mediated by plasmids.

## EPIDEMIOLOGY

From remote times, *V. cholerae,* the pathogen of Asiatic cholera had been endemic in the vicinity of the Ganges and Brahmaputra rivers in Eastern India and Bangladesh. Over the 19th and early part of the present century, a series of six pandemics originated from the endemic focus in which areas of Asia, Europe, Africa, and America were devastated. During 1923 to 1960, it produced seasonal epidemics within India and Bangladesh with occasional extensions to the neighboring countries.

In 1961, the biotype El Tor was implicated in the seventh pandemic, which, since 1937 had been causing bouts of mild cholera in the Sulawesi island of Indonesia. It spread to all states of Southeast Asia in 1961 to 1962, states of mainland Asia within 1963 to 1969, and, almost replaced classic vibrio. Lately, it also invaded Africa, Europe, and South USSR, and, to a minor extent, Canada and Australia. There have been cases of imported cholera in nonendemic areas owing to rapid air travel.

Under natural conditions, cholera vibrios produce attacks of diarrhea, inapparent cases, and carrier states in no other animals than man. Incubation period ranges from one to five days, and, the infectivity 5 to 14 days. The bacterium is transmitted from man to man by the fecal oral route through food and drink. It is particularly prevalent in overcrowded and unsanitary conditions with sharing of common water sources and latrines.

In endemic areas, such as India, Philippines, and Bangladesh, the outbreak occurs before, during, and after the monsoon. In the interepidemic periods, the endemicity continues through a sort of "silent epidemic," moving from the carriers to inapparent cases or vice versa.

In comparison to the classic biotype, El Tor proliferates faster, is more resistant to environmental conditions, and produces many more cases, carriers, and newer foci of infections. An El Tor epidemic runs a protracted course rather than the explosive pattern of the Asiatic cholera. The Inaba and Ogawa serotypes, respectively, predominate among the isolates of *V. cholerae* and *V. cholerae* biotype El Tor. Quite recently, the latter has revealed more strains of Inaba type.

Cost benefit analyses point to the superiority of hygiene and improved sanitation over cholera vaccines. Vaccination is economically justified only when the case incidence exceeds 8 per 1000 population, which is hardly seen in practice. Although the immunity is serotype specific, one biotype induces nearly equal protection against the other. However, vaccination is indicated in persons moving from a cholera-free area to the endemic zone.

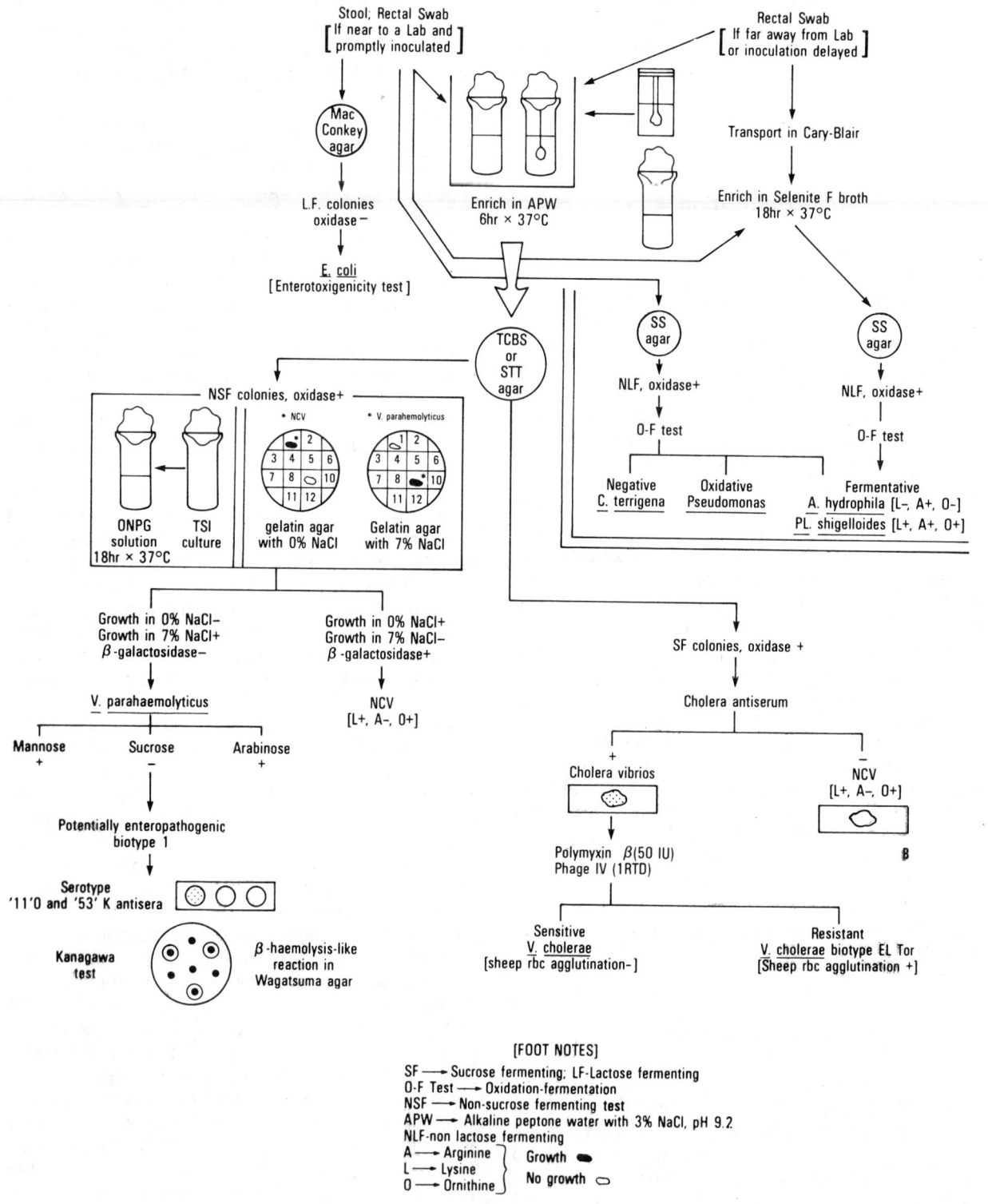

**FIGURE 3.** *Laboratory diagnosis of cholera syndrome.*

# NONCHOLERA VIBRIOS (NCV)

## *MORPHOLOGY*

The features are identical with *V. cholerae*, except that all NCV are thinly capsulated and a few are coccobacillary. Fimbriated forms of NCV are not known. Colonies on BSA and nutrient agar may mimic those of cholera vibrios.

In TCBS and STT agar, the colonies are slightly mucoid and yellow or bluish green. Rough colonies have not been recognized.

## *ANTIGENIC COMPOSITION*

On the basis of heat stable somatic antigens, the strains of human diarrhea fall under 40 O-groups. The flagellar (H) and capsular (K) antigens are heat labile and heterogenous. Smith (1974) disclosed major differences between the H antigens of cholera vibrios and NCV, although previously they were thought to be identical.

## *METABOLISM*

Characteristics do not differ from *V. cholerae* (Table 2), but NCV in order of prevalence belong to Heiberg groups I, II and V.

## *PATHOGENIC PROPERTIES*

The NCV cause mild gastroenteritis or illness simulating cholera and dysentery. Some strains elaborate enterotoxin that produce fluid accumulation and dilatation in the ligated loops of adult rabbits and diarrhea in 9 day old rabbits.

## *DRUG SUSCEPTIBILITY*

The MIC in $\mu$g/ml: tetracycline 1.5, chloramphenicol 1.5, streptomycin 75, paromomycin 50, viomycin 500, and neomycin 30. It is also sensitive to disks of polymyxin B (100 IU) and ampicillin (25 $\mu$g). Sometimes drug resistance is found.

## *EPIDEMIOLOGY*

NCV can be isolated usually from natural waters, sewage, flies, and the feces of cold-blooded and hot-blooded animals, but not from normal human stool. These organisms produce sporadic human diarrhea in different regions of the world. The incidence commonly rises before and after the cholera outbreak in eastern India. NCV do not produce epidemics.

# AEROMONAS HYDROPHILA
(*aer,* gas; *monad,* unit; *aeromonas,* gas-producing one; *hydrophila,* water loving)

## *MORPHOLOGY*

Cells are gram-negative, thinly capsulated, straight rods, or coccobacilli, 1.0 to 4.4 $\mu$m, arranged singly, in pairs and short chains, and rapidly motile by one or more terminal flagella.

On nutrient agar, the colonies are 2 to 3 mm, translucent, smooth, round, and convex after 18 hrs at 30° to 37° C. Broth culture shows diffuse turbidity with or without pellicle.

## *METABOLISM*

*A. hydrophila* is a facultative anaerobe and is nonfastidious. Its generation time is short. Growth occurs at 21° to 40° C, pH 5.5 to 9.0, but some biochemical characters (Table 2) are better elicited at 22°C than 37°C — for example, gas from carbohydrates, production of acetoin, and utilization of citrate. Whereas the aerogenic biotype produces acetoin and $H_2S$ from cysteine, the anaerogenic one is negative to these tests.

## PATHOGENIC PROPERTIES

*A. hydrophila* causes mild gastroenteritis, choleraic diarrhea, and dysentery in man. Its enterotoxin is heat labile, neutralized by the cholera antitoxin and gives positive reaction in rabbit loops and adrenal tumor cells (Wadström et al., 1976). The enteropathogenic serotypes remain uncharacterized.

The organism may also be associated with bacteremia, osteomyelitis, cutaneous ulcers, and urinary tract infection. It is pathogenic to amphibians and reptiles.

## DRUG SUSCEPTIBILITY

*A. hydrophila* is sensitive to disks of streptomycin (10 μg), tetracycline (30 μg), chloramphenicol (30 μg), erythromycin (15 μg), nalidixic acid (100 μg), furadantin (100 μg), kanamycin (5μg), and polymyxin B (100 IU), but resistant to ampicillin (25 μg). Resistance is rarely noted to streptomycin and tetracycline. The organism may possess drug-resistant plasmids.

# PLESIOMONAS SHIGELLOIDES
*(Plesios,* nearer to *(aeromonas); shigelloides,* like
*shigella)*

## MORPHOLOGY

Cells are rod shaped with rounded ends, 0.8 to 1.0 by 3.0 μm, thinly capsulated, arranged singly, in pairs, short chains, and are rapidly motile with single polar or lophotrichous (tufted) flagella. Colonies appear small, 1 to 1.5 mm, almost transparent, convex, and glossy.

## ANTIGENIC COMPOSITION

Strains are classified into 16 O-groups, of which one reveals major sharing with *Sh.sonnei.* The H antigen is divided into four types.

## METABOLISM

*Pl. shigelloides* is a facultative anaerobe and grows on ordinary media at 18 to 37°C. Unlike the vibrios and aeromonas, it lacks diastase, lipase, DNase, proteinase, hemolysin (Table 2), and has no biotypes.

## PATHOGENIC PROPERTIES

The organism is suspected as an enteropathogenic agent in Japan, India, and Africa, but enteric effects have yet to be reproduced in laboratory models. It may be isolated from blood, cerebrospinal fluid, and feces of animals. Its significance for man is not known.

## DRUG SUSCEPTIBILITY

It is usually sensitive to disks of streptomycin (10 μg), tetracycline (10 μg), chloramphenicol (25 μg), kanamycin (30 μg), gentamycin (10 μg), paromomycin (30 μg), furazolidone (100 μg), but resistant to ampicillin (25 μg).

# VIBRIO PARAHAEMOLYTICUS
*(para,* like; *haema,* blood; *parahaemolyticus,* like
*haemolytica)*

## MORPHOLOGY

Cells are ellipsoidal, gram-negative, capsulated rods, 0.5 to 1.4 μm by 0.4 to 0.6 μm, slightly pleomorphic, arranged singly, in pairs, short chains and small clusters; filaments are rare but consistent (Fig. 4). Adverse conditions or aging produces marked pleomorphism. Strains grown on nutrient agar containing 3 per cent NaCl after two or three days show involution forms — for example, bipolar staining, spheroplasts, slender rods with tapering ends, and clubs. Broth culture at 37° C reveals polar flagellated cells with rapid linear motility. Contrarily, 18-hr growth at 22 to

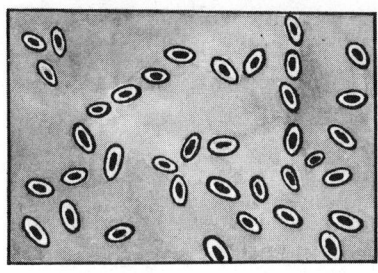

**FIGURE 4.** *Well formed capsule of* V. parahaemolyticus.

28°C on semisolid agar and 5-hr nutrient agar culture at 37°C disclose feebly motile peritrichous and polar flagellated cells (Fig. 5). The polar flagella are thick and wavy but the lateral ones are thin, fragile, and curly (Chatterjee, 1974).

The organism produces dome-shaped, off-white, sticky colonies in meat extract agar that measure 2 to 3 mm in diameter. With time, the culture is slowly covered by minute daughter colonies. Colonies of the enteropathogenic variety are bluish green on TCBS and STT agar but others are yellow. Sometimes a smooth colony exhibits wrinkled opaque transformation at the center with unaltered periphery; this is reversed on subculture at 22°C. An old culture in agar slant may show brown coloration of the medium and a bunch of needle shaped crystals underneath. Growth on semisolid agar at 22°C may show swarming.

## ANTIGENIC COMPOSITION

*V. parahaemolyticus* possess flagellar (H) capsular (K) and somatic (O) antigens, each having 2, 53, and 11 types respectively. Flagellar antigenicity and agglutinability are better developed at 22 to 28°C than 37°C. Since these H antigens are shared by all strains, they do not help in classification. Serotyping is based on O and K antigens. The enteropathogenic serotypes are: 01:K38, 01:K56, 02:K3, 03:K4, 03:K33, 04:K8, 04:K9, 04:K11, 04:K12, 04:K13, 04:K55, 05:K12, 05:K15, 05:K17, 05:K30, 05:Cal/Ka, 05:K47, 08:K20, 08:K21, 08:K22, 09:K23, 010:K19, and

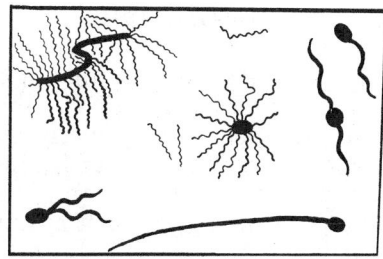

**FIGURE 5.** *Polar and peritrichous flagella of* V. parahaemolyticus.

010:K24; they are rarely distributed in the fish and water.

## METABOLISM

*V. parahaemolyticus* differs sharply from the other members in that it gives a negative test for β-galactosidase and fails to grow in NaCl-deficient media. In order to cultivate the organism in gelatin agar, at least 0.1 per cent NaCl is needed. Table 2 shows characteristics of enteropathogenic strains grouped under the biotype 1. It differs from the biotype 2 (*V. parahaemolyticus* biotype *alginolyticus),* which ferments sucrose, produces acetoin, and grows in 10 per cent NaCl. There are intermediate forms between the biotypes 1 and 2. *V. parahaemolyticus* is proteolytic, saccharolytic but essentially nonhemolytic for suspended red cells of different species. Yet, most (> 90 per cent of strains from human cases of diarrhea and their contacts show the Kanagawa phenomenon — that is, a reaction resembling β-hemolysis in Wagatsuma agar during overnight incubation at 37°C. On the other hand, the isolates of fish, food, and water are Kanagawa-negative after overnight incubation and positive only after 48 hours. Growth on Wagatsuma agar, with its high pH, excess NaCl, and fermentable carbohydrate-like mannitol is a test for hemodigestion rather than true hemolysis.

The media for methyl red (MR), V–P, and decarboxylase-dihydrolase tests being salt free are supplemented with 0.5 per cent NaCl. Results of the MR test, KCN tolerance, and citrate utilization are negative in media having 0.5 per cent NaCl (Table 2), but can be reversed if the same media are modified with 3 per cent NaCl (Chatterjee, 1974).

## PATHOGENIC PROPERTIES

*V. parahaemolyticus* causes attacks of food poisoning, sporadic rice water diarrhea, and dysentery. It may also cause fulminating septicemia that is manifested by hemolytic anemia, hypotension, thrombophlebitis, erythema multiforme, and vasculitis leading to gangrene. Live cultures fed orally to infant rabbits cause bacteremia. Factors determining pathogenicity are not known.

An "aberrant biotype" of *V. parahaemolyticus* ("group F vibrio") ferments sucrose but reacts negatively to lysine and ornithine decarboxylase reactions and V-P test. Like *A. hydrophila,* it reveals arginine dihydrolase activity. This organism can be isolated from cold blooded animals and water. (Chatterjee, 1974; Furniss *et al,* 1977). It caused sporadic and epidemic forms of gastroenteritis in Bangladesh.

## LABORATORY DIAGNOSIS

The steps of investigating *V. parahaemolyticus* food poisoning are shown below in addition to those already indicated in connection with the cholera syndrome.

### Food Bacteriology

Demonstration of numerous organisms in the food strongly supports the diagnosis. Accordingly, 50 g of food are homogenized and diluted 1/10 and 1/100 in sterile saline with 0.1 per cent peptone. The neat and diluted samples are streaked on TCBS or STT agar with a calibrated loop for quantitation. A similar quantity of homogenized food is also put up for enrichment in alkaline peptone water (pH 9.2) containing 3 per cent NaCl.

Isolation and identification of *V. parahaemolyticus* from feces are already discussed under *V. cholerae*. The isolates of food and feces are compared by serotyping and the Kanagawa test; they may reveal multiple serotypes, of which one remains the dominant type.

## DRUG SUSCEPTIBILITY

MIC in $\mu$g/ml are as follows: streptomycin 15 to 25, tetracycline 2.5 to 6, and chloramphenicol 0.5 to 2.5. It is also sensitive to disks of kanamycin (5 $\mu$g), polymyxin B (50 IU), colistin (10 $\mu$g), cepha-lothin (30 $\mu$g), furazolidone (100 mg), but resistant to ampicillin (25 $\mu$g). The organism produces $\beta$-lactamase.

## EPIDEMIOLOGY

*V. parahaemolyticus* is a free-living bacterium. It is distributed all over the world in offshore sea water and marine animals. In eastern India where the inland water is slightly brackish it is found in pond water and its fish; it is also recovered from flies and sewage.

The organism produces sporadic diarrhea and food poisoning in Japan, Southeast Asia, Australia, and the United States. The food poisoning may break out suddenly in a community after sharing common meals. It is occasionally lethal in Japan. It may also be confined within a family.

Fish are most often responsible for infection. In Japan more than 70 per cent of summer food poisoning cases are produced by *V. parahaemolyticus* after eating uncooked or undercooked fish. Since adequate cooking reduces the risk of infection, the incidence of food poisoning is much lower in other countries. However, the food may be recontaminated by the pathogen after cooking by exposure to kitchen utensils or food handlers. Its short generation time (ten minutes) allows it to attain infective numbers ($10^5$ to $10^7$ viable cells in human volunteers) rapidly at ambient temperatures.

# CAMPYLOBACTERS
(*campylo*, curved; *bacter*, rod)

## MORPHOLOGY

Cells are curved, S- or gull-shaped, gram-negative, slender rods, 1.5 to 5 $\mu$m by 0.2 to 0.5 $\mu$m and occur in chains with three to five spirals. The organism bears a polar flagellum at one or both ends and displays rapid linear or corkscrew-like motility (Smibert, 1978). It is not encapsulated.

On primary isolation, the colonies are small (0.5 to 1 mm) and vary in appearance from smooth to rough forms and in color from white to cream. Upon further incubation, the smooth colonies become mucoid. Subculture may produce "cut glass" colonies with reflecting facets. Broth culture shows uniform turbidity with a powdery deposit.

## ANTIGENIC COMPOSITION

On the basis of heat-stable somatic antigens, *C. fetus* and *C. fetus* biotype *intestinalis* have two serotypes each, whereas *C. fetus* biotype *jejuni* shows one serotype. *C. fetus* may cross-react among its biotypes and with *Brucella abortus*.

## METABOLISM

The organism needs a microaerophilic condition for growth in solid medium at 37° C, which is provided by an atmosphere of 5 per cent $O_2$, 10 per cent $CO_2$, and 85 per cent $N_2$. Aerobic incubation in 10 per cent $CO_2$ yields growth on semisolid media (0.16 per cent agar), such as thiol agar, yeast extract agar, *Brucella* agar, and also in a liquid medium like *Brucella* broth. It is not very active biochemically (Table 2).

Lately, the organism is grown in 10 per cent $CO_2$ and 90 per cent $H_2$ or air. The tests for characterizing the species and the biotypes of campylobacters are shown in Table 3.

## PATHOGENIC PROPERTIES

*C. fetus* biotype *jejuni* causes acute diarrhea in children (5.8 per cent) and in adults (2.3 per cent). In children below 8 months, it can account for 30 per cent of the cases of acute diarrhea in developing countries. It is sometimes related to bacteremia. Debilitated patients are prone to infections with *C. fetus* biotype *intestinalis,* which produces septicemia (without splenomegaly), meningitis, meningoencephalitis, abortion, enteritis, thrombophlebitis, septic arthritis, and jaundice with hepatomegaly. Other species and biotypes are not pathogenic to man (Table 3). *C. fetus* biotype *jejuni* and *C. sputorum* may be rarely isolated respectively from the feces and mouth of normal persons.

## IMMUNITY

In older children (above 8 months) and adults, *C. fetus* biotype *jejuni* appears to impart immunity localized to the gut. Information from animal diseases may help us to understand the mechanism of protection of man. It is well known that *C. fetus* infection remains confined to the reproductive organs of cattle. On the other hand, *C. fetus* biotype *intestinalis* in sheep produces bacteremia before localization in the placenta. The cattle develop a local immune response (usually IgA antibody against 0 antigen), whereas the infection of sheep produces a generalized immune response. Live or heat-killed vaccine prevents bovine infection, but the ovine disease is averted by the purified, heat-labile surface protein or the live bivalent-type vaccine.

## LABORATORY DIAGNOSIS

A spiral organism in blood culture should arouse suspicion of *Campylobacter,* since *Spirillum minus,* the pathogen of relapsing fever fails to grow

#### TABLE 3.   Differential Features of Campylobacters

| SPECIES CHARACTERIZED BY TESTS | BIOTYPES KNOWN TO GROW ON | | | | RESERVOIR HOSTS | PATHOGENICITY |
|---|---|---|---|---|---|---|
| | Glycine 1% | NaCl 3.5% | Bile 1% | 25° C | | |
| Catalase + $H_2S$ nitrate reduction<br>C. fetus | − | − | + | + | Bulls: genital tract. | Cattle: abortion, infertility, venereally transmitted. |
| C. fetus biotype *intestinalis* | + | − | + | + | ? | Man: infections (see text) orally transmitted; cattle, sheep: abortion. |
| C. fetus biotype *jejuni* | + | − | + | − | Man, cattle, sheep, goats, pigs, birds: gut lumen. | Man: infections (see text) orally transmitted;<br>sheep: abortion;<br>turkeys: bluecomb disease, enteritis;<br>pigs: dysentery. |
| Catalase $H_2S$ + nitrate reduction + : C. sputorum | + | − | + | + | Man: oral cavity. | ? |
| C. sputorum biotype *bubulus* | + | + | − | + | Cattle, sheep: genital tract. | ? |
| C. sputorum biotype *mucosalis* | − | − | − | ? | Pigs: oral cavity. | Pigs: intestinal adenomatosis, necrotic enteritis, regional ileitis, proliferative enteropathy. |
| Catalase + $H_2S$ + nitrate reduction<br>C. fecalis | + | V | V | − | Sheep: genital tract, gut. | ? |

v, variable; ? unknown.

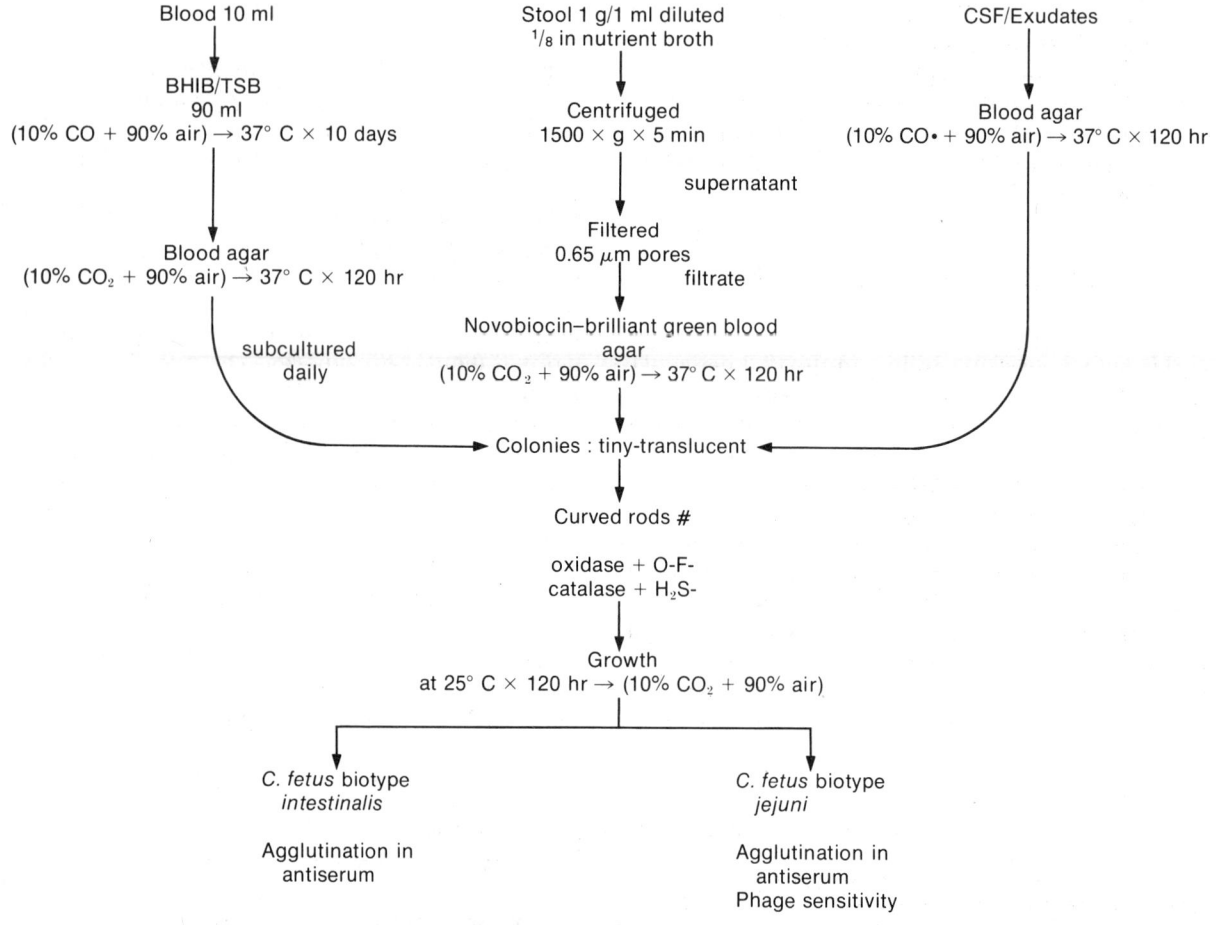

BHIB, brain heart infusion broth; TSB, trypticase soy broth; O-F, oxidation-fermentation. Five to 7 days' old culture show coccoid cells.

**FIGURE 6.** *Laboratory diagnosis of human campylobacteriosis.*

on artificial medium. *Campylobacter* can be easily isolated from blood or body fluids under microaerophilic conditions. In case of stools, the normal fecal flora are first partially removed by millipore filtration (0.65 $\mu$m pores) and then suppressed on selective-inhibitory media for *Campylobacter* (Fig. 6). Rising titers of complement-fixation and indirect hemagglutination tests suggest infection.

## DRUG SUSCEPTIBILITY

The MIC in $\mu$g/ml for *C. fetus* biotypes *intestinalis* and *jejuni* are: clindamycin, 0.4 to 1.6; tetracycline, 0.8; streptomycin, 2 to 4; neomycin, 8; kanamycin, 0.01 to 3.12; gentamicin, 0.19 to 1.56; ampicillin, 1.56 to 25; erythromycin, 2 to 8; chloramphenicol, 4; cephalothin, 50; and carbenicillin, 200. They are resistant to penicillin (5 units), polymyxin B (1024 units), and bacitracin (120 units). Tetracycline and trimethoprim resistance is sometimes encountered.

## EPIDEMIOLOGY

Human campylobacteriosis until lately was reported from the United States, Europe, and Africa. Awareness of the disease has resulted in increasing recognition from many other places in the world. It is suspected that the organism is transmitted from animals to man, but the exact mode of acquisition is obscure.

## References

Chalmers, A. J., and Waterfield, N. E.: Paracholera caused by *Vibrio gindha*. Pfeiffer 1896. J Trop Med Hyg 19:165, 1916.
Chatterjee, B. D.: Epidemiologic and taxonomic status of *Vibrio parahaemolyticus*. In Fujino, T., Sakaguchi, G., Sakazaki, R., and Takeda, Y. (eds.): International Symposium on *Vibrio parahaemolyticus*. Tokyo, Saikon Publ. Co., 1974, p. 177.
Chatterjee, B. D., and Neogy, K. N.: On the etiology of choleraic diarrhoea. Indian J Med Res 60:531, 1972.
Chatterjee, B. D., De, P. K., and Sen, T.: Sucrose teepol tellurite agar: A new selective indicator medium for isolation of *Vibrio* species. J Infect Dis 135:654, 136:716.
Furniss, A. L., Lee, J. V., and Donovan, T. J.: Group F, a new vibrio? Lancet ii:565, 1977.

Smith, H. L., Jr.: Antibody responses in rabbits to injections of whole cell, flagella and flagellin preparations of cholera and non-cholera vibrios. J Appl Microbiol 27:375, 1974.

Wadström, T., Ljungh, A., and Wretlind, B.: Enterotoxin, haemolysin and cytotoxic protein in *Aeromonas hydrophila* from human infections. Acta Path Microbiol Scand Sec B 84:112, 1976.

# GENUS **33**
# *PSEUDOMONAS* *

## M. J. Pickett

## DEFINITION

Pseudomonads are nonsporulating, gram-negative rods. Most species are polarly flagellated, and a few also have lateral flagella. The cells of some species may contain granules of poly-$\beta$-hydroxybutyrate (PHB). These PHB granules may be evident in Gram-stained preparations and, by special staining procedures, can be used as an aid in identification. Most pseudomonads are oxidase-positive and noncapsulated. Excluding *P. vesicularis,* which may be negative, all are catalase-positive. With few exceptions, they grow readily on nutrient and blood agar media at both room ($22\pm2^{\circ}$ C) and incubator (35 to 37 $^{\circ}$ C) temperatures. They are obligatively aerobic and non-fermentative. Most species oxidatively acidify carbohydrates. All are anaerogenic. One species, *P. putrefaciens,* produces hydrogen sulfide in Kligler iron agar (KIA) and triple sugar iron agar (TSIA) media. None forms indole or gives a positive Voges-Proskauer test for acetoin. With few exceptions, they are resistant to penicillin. The moles percentage of guanine plus cytosine (percentage GC) in their chromosomal DNA ranges from 48 to 70.

## Habitat, Resistance

Many of the species, including those associated with human disease, are commonly present in soil and in the hospital environment and may be a part of the normal flora of the body. Plants and both wild and domestic animals may harbor pseudomonads, but rarely play a significant role as reservoirs and vectors for transmission to humans. One species, *P. fluorescens,* can grow at 4° C and has been associated with endotoxemia following administration of contaminated intravenous fluids. Others, such as *P. cepacia,* can grow in commercial distilled water. Several have been recovered from cosmetics and other toiletries. Most are relatively resistant to several common germicides, particularly quaternary ammonium compounds such as Zephiran. They display both species and strain variation in respect to susceptibility to antimicrobials.

More than 25 different species of pseudomonads are associated with man and his immediate environment, but only two of these, *P. aeruginosa* and *P. maltophilia,* account for more than 75 per cent of those recovered from clinical specimens (Tables 1 and 2).

## PATHOGENICITY

Only two species of pseudomonads are uniquely associated with specific diseases of man; *P. mallei* is the etiologic agent of glanders and *P. pseudomallei* of melioidosis. However, many of the species, notably *P. aeruginosa,* are opportunistic pathogens. They may be etiologically significant, usually in previously compromised patients, in wounds and postburn sepsis, postsurgical infections, septicemia, and respiratory and urinary tract infections, among others.

**TABLE 1.   Distribution of Aerobic Gram-Negative Bacilli in Clinical Specimens**[a]

| GROUP | % (APPROX.) |
|---|---|
| Enterobacteriaceae | 73 |
| *Haemophilus* | 12 |
| Nonfermentative bacilli | 14 |
| Other[b] | 1 |

[a]Unpublished data from Pickett and Martin, 1032 strains, June, 1976, UCLA Hospital and Clinics, Los Angeles, California, and Blachman, 768 strains, March-April, 1976, Olive View Medical Center, Sylmar, California.

[b]E.g., *Aeromonas, Cardiobacterium, Eikenella.*

---

*This chapter is not documented with an exhaustive list of references. Readers wishing such documentation should consult the references given in the manual of Lennette et al. (1974), the textbook of Wilson and Miles (1975), and the monograph of Gilardi (1978a).

**TABLE 2.** Distribution of Nonfermentative Bacilli in Clinical Specimens[a]

| | % (APPROX.) | | % (APPROX.) |
|---|---|---|---|
| Pseudomonas aeruginosa | 73 | P. alcaligenes | <1 |
| (pyocyanin-positive) | (64) | P. denitrificans | <1 |
| (pyocyanin-negative) | (9) | P. diminuta | <1 |
| Acinetobacter | 9 | P. pseudoalcaligenes | <1 |
| P. maltophilia | 6 | P. putrefaciens | <1 |
| Flavobacterium | 3 | P. vesicularis | <1 |
| P. cepacia | 1 | Pseudomonas, IIk group | <1 |
| P. fluorescens | 1 | Pseudomonas, Ve group | <1 |
| P. pickettii | 1 | Achromobacter | <1 |
| P. putida | 1 | Alcaligenes | <1 |
| P. stutzeri | 1 | Bordetella | <1 |
| Moraxella | 1 | Kingella | <1 |
| P. acidovorans | <1 | | |

[a]Unpublished data from Pickett and Pedersen, 486 strains, 1968, and Greenwood and associates, 525 strains, 1978, UCLA Hospital and Clinics, Los Angeles, California.

**TABLE 3.** Differential Features for Fluorescent Pseudomonads[a,b]

| | P. AERUGINOSA | P. FLUORESCENS | P. PUTIDA |
|---|---|---|---|
| Moles % GC | 67 | 59–64 | 60–63 |
| Flagella | 1 | >1 | >1 |
| Growth at 42°C*[c] | +[d] | 0 | 0 |
| Pyocyanin | (+) | 0 | 0 |
| Acidification of | | | |
| Lactose | 0 | (+) | (−) |
| Sorbitol | 0 | (+) | 0 |
| Sucrose | 0 | (+) | − |
| Alkalinization of | | | |
| Acetamide* | + | 0 | − |
| Tartrate | 0 | 0 | (+) |
| Nitrate → gas | (+) | (−) | 0 |
| Gelatin* | (+) | + | 0 |
| Hippurate | 0 | 0 | (+) |

[a]P. aeruginosa occasionally fails to show fluorescence at 20 to 25°C; P. fluorescens and P. putida frequently fail to show fluorescence at 35 to 37°C.

[b]All three species are oxidase-positive and glucose-positive, grow on MacConkey agar medium, and are susceptible to polymyxin; none contains PHB granules.

[c]Asterisk indicates features that are most useful for identification.

[d]+, 90 per cent (or more) of strains are positive; (+), usually positive; (−), usually negative; −, 10 per cent (or less) of strains are positive; 0, never positive.

## DETECTION AND IDENTIFICATION

Initial detection is similar to that for Enterobacteriaceae, namely, in broth medium for blood specimens or on a blood agar plate for other specimens. Since they are obligatively aerobic, most strains fail to grow when these media are incubated anaerobically. Most species, including the two most commonly encountered, grow rapidly and present 0.5 to 2 mm colonies on 24-hour blood agar plates. Confirmation that a clinical isolate is an obligatively aerobic, nonfermentative bacillus (NFB) is commonly effected by demonstrating its failure to grow in a tube of oxidation-fermentation (OF) medium overlayed with petrolatum. Alternatively, its identity as an NFB may be confirmed by demonstrating growth on the slant but neither growth nor acidification in the butt of KIA or TSIA medium.

Many of the features used for identification of enteric bacteria are equally applicable to the pseudomonads, but since the latter not only are obligate aerobes but also usually alkalinize media containing peptone, special methods are usually used for biochemical tests (Tatum et al., 1974; Gilardi, 1978b). Features for identification of the more commonly encountered pseudomonads include (1) colonial and microscopic morphology including pigmentation, if any; (2) production of fluorescein; (3) production of gas from nitrate; (4) growth at 42° C; (5) acidification of carbohydrates, particularly glucose, lactose, mannitol, and sucrose; (6) decarboxylation of lysine (the LDC test); and (7) alkalinization of acetamide and urea. Tables 3 through 5 present the principal differential features of these bacilli. "Antibiograms" are also useful guides for identification (Table 6).

# PSEUDOMONAS AERUGINOSA

P. aeruginosa (Pseudomonas pyocyanea) is more frequently encountered and more important as an agent of human disease than all the other nonfermentative bacilli. Understandably, many of its features have been studied in considerable detail.

## MORPHOLOGY

Microscopically, P. aeruginosa is a slender, nonsporulating, usually noncapsulated rod bearing a single polar flagellum. The cells do not contain PHB inclusions. This bacterium presents three types of colonies. The most common, on a 24-hour blood agar plate, is low convex to flat and 1 to 5 mm in diameter with a rough or frosted glass surface and an undulate or erose periphery. It may be β-hemolytic on a 24-hour plate and usually shows diffuse β-hemolysis on a 48-hour plate. Most strains form a water- and chloroform-soluble phenazine pigment, pyocyanin (from the Greek, blue pus), which usually imparts a green or blue-green color to the medium surrounding

TABLE 4.  Differential Features for Nonfluorescent, Glucose-Positive Pseudomonads

| | P. CEPACIA | P. MALTOPHILIA | P. PAUCIMOBILIS (BIOGROUP IIk-1) | P. PICKETTII (BIOTYPE Va-1) | P. PICKETTII (BIOTYPE Va-2) | P. PSEUDOMALLEI | P. PUTREFACIENS | P. STUTZERI | P. VESICULARIS | PSEUDOMONAS (BIOGROUP Ve-1) | PSEUDOMONAS (BIOGROUP Ve-2) |
|---|---|---|---|---|---|---|---|---|---|---|---|
| Moles % GC | 68 | 67 | 65 | 63 | 64 | 70 | 48–59 | 65 | 66 | 57 | 67 |
| Flagella | >1 | >1 | 1 | 1 | 1 | >1 | 1–2 | 1–2 | 1 | >1 | 1 |
| PHB granules | + | − | + | + | + | + | ND[d] | − | + | ND | ND |
| Pigmented growth[a] | (−) | (−) | + | 0 | 0 | (−) | (−) | (−) | (−) | + | + |
| Oxidase*[b] | + | − | + | + | + | + | + | + | + | − | − |
| MacConkey, growth | (+) | + | (+) | + | + | + | + | + | (+) | + | + |
| Growth at 42°C | (+) | (+) | − | (−) | (+) | + | (+) | + | − | (+) | (−) |
| Polymyxin susceptible[c] | − | + | (+) | − | − | − | + | + | + | + | + |
| Acidification of | | | | | | | | | | | |
| Arabinose* | + | − | + | + | + | + | (+) | + | + | + | + |
| Cellobiose | + | + | + | + | 0 | + | (−) | 0 | + | 0 | (−) |
| Ethanol | (+) | − | + | 0 | 0 | (+) | − | + | + | + | + |
| Lactose* | + | + | + | + | 0 | + | (−) | 0 | 0 | − | − |
| Maltose* | + | + | + | + | 0 | + | (−) | + | + | + | + |
| Mannitol* | (+) | 0 | 0 | 0 | 0 | + | 0 | (+) | 0 | + | + |
| Sorbitol | + | 0 | 0 | 0 | 0 | + | − | 0 | 0 | − | (+) |
| Sucrose* | (+) | + | + | 0 | 0 | (+) | (−) | 0 | 0 | − | (−) |
| Amylase | 0 | 0 | (+) | 0 | 0 | (+) | 0 | + | − | (−) | (+) |
| Citrate (Simmons) | + | (−) | (−) | + | + | + | (−) | + | − | + | (+) |
| Esculin | (+) | + | + | 0 | 0 | (+) | (−) | 0 | + | + | − |
| H₂S (in KIA or TSIA)* | 0 | 0 | 0 | 0 | 0 | 0 | + | 0 | 0 | 0 | 0 |
| Lysine (LDC)* | + | + | 0 | 0 | 0 | 0 | 0 | 0 | 0 | 0 | 0 |
| Nitrate → gas* | 0 | 0 | 0 | + | + | + | 0 | + | 0 | 0 | 0 |
| Nitrate → nitrite | (−) | (−) | − | + | + | (+) | (+) | (+) | − | (+) | (−) |
| Urea (Christensen)* | (−) | − | − | + | + | (−) | − | (−) | − | (+) | (+) |

[a]Growth tan, yellow, or orange on a 24- to 48-hr blood agar plate. Other notations as for Table 3.
[b]Asterisk indicates features that are most useful for identification.
[c]300 unit disk.
[d]ND, no data.


TABLE 5.  Differential Features for Glucose-Negative Pseudomonads[a]

| | P. ACIDOVORANS | P. ALCALIGENES | P. DIMINUTA | P. PSEUDO-ALCALIGENES | P. TESTOSTERONI |
|---|---|---|---|---|---|
| Moles % GC | 67 | 66 | 67 | 63 | 62 |
| Flagella | >1 | 1 | 1 | 1 | >1 |
| PHB granules | + | − | + | (+) | + |
| Growth at 42°C | 0 | + | (+) | + | 0 |
| Polymyxin susceptible | (+) | + | (−) | + | (+) |
| Acidification of | | | | | |
| Arabinose | 0 | 0 | (−) | (−) | 0 |
| Ethanol*[b] | + | − | (+) | + | (−) |
| Fructose* | + | 0 | 0 | + | 0 |
| Mannitol | (+) | 0 | 0 | 0 | 0 |
| Alkalinization of | | | | | |
| Acetamide* | + | 0 | 0 | 0 | 0 |
| Allantoin | + | 0 | 0 | 0 | (+) |
| Formate* | + | (+) | 0 | + | + |
| Nicotinamide | + | 0 | 0 | 0 | 0 |
| Tartrate | + | (−) | 0 | 0 | − |
| Citrate (Simmons)* | + | (+) | − | (+) | (+) |
| Nitrate → nitrite | + | + | (−) | + | (+) |

[a]All are oxidase-positive and grow on MacConkey agar medium; none is pigmented, fluorescent, or forms gas from nitrate. Other notations as for Table 3.
[b]Asterisk indicates features most useful for identification.

TABLE 6.  In vitro Antimicrobial Susceptibility of Pseudomonads[a]

| SPECIES/GROUP | NUMBER OF STRAINS | CARBENI-CILLIN | GENTAMICIN | NOVO-BIOCIN | POLYMYXIN | STREPTO-MYCIN | TRIMETHO-PRIM/SULFA-METHOX-AZOLE |
|---|---|---|---|---|---|---|---|
| P. acidovorans[b] | 81 | 37[e] | 7 | 39 | 70 | 4 | 99 |
| P. aeruginosa[c] | 72 | 63 | 93 | 0 | 97 | 36 | 76 |
| P. alcaligenes[d] | 71 | 75 | 73 | 10 | 94 | 37 | 62 |
| P. cepacia | 132 | 10 | 13 | 48 | 0 | 2 | 100 |
| P. diminuta | 33 | 97 | 100 | 100 | 49 | 15 | 94 |
| P. fluorescens | 137 | 4 | 96 | 0 | 96 | 53 | 47 |
| P. maltophilia | 390 | 38 | 43 | 1 | 95 | 20 | 95 |
| P. paucimobilis | 61 | 90 | 80 | 77 | 70 | 13 | 95 |
| P. pickettii |  |  |  |  |  |  |  |
|   biotype Va-1 | 15 | 20 | 53 | 0 | 0 | 20 | 100 |
|   biotype Va-2 | 22 | 36 | 0 | 0 | 0 | 0 | 100 |
| P. pseudomallei | 7 | 0 | 0 | 86 | 0 | 0 | 0 |
| P. putida | 180 | 13 | 96 | 1 | 99 | 58 | 9 |
| P. putrefaciens | 44 | 80 | 100 | 0 | 100 | 89 | 100 |
| P. stutzeri | 116 | 89 | 100 | 0 | 100 | 90 | 70 |
| P. vesicularis | 19 | 95 | 100 | 100 | 90 | 90 | 90 |
| Biogroup Ve-1 | 16 | 100 | 100 | 0 | 100 | 100 | 60 |
| Biogroup Ve-2 | 39 | 100 | 100 | 0 | 100 | 54 | 39 |

[a]Data adapted from Gilardi (1979, personal communication).
[b]Includes closely related P. testosteroni.
[c]Apyocyanogenic strains.
[d]Includes closely related P. pseudoalcaligenes.
[e]Per cent of strains susceptible.

the colony. Other brown to black, phenazine pigments are also occasionally formed. Fluorescein (pyoverdin), a water-soluble, pale yellow-green pigment, is formed by nearly all strains of *P. aeruginosa* and is an important feature for identification of this species. Fluorescein is not apparent on blood agar medium; a special medium enriched with magnesium and phosphate should be used, and detection is by fluorescence under ultraviolet light.

A second type of colony, commonly displayed by strains recovered from the sputum of patients suffering from cystic fibrosis, is relatively large and markedly mucoid, particularly on MacConkey agar medium. Such strains, when repeatedly subcultured, may yield a third small and smooth type colony. This third phenotype, in turn, may yield the familiar large rough colony upon repeated subculture. Qualitatively identical biochemical features obtain for the three colonial varieties of *P. aeruginosa*, although the reactions (e.g., acidification of sugars and alkalinization of acetamide) are frequently weak and delayed with mucoid strains.

The characteristic rough or mucoid colony, β-hemolysis, blue-green pigmentation, and fruity odor represent tentative identification of this species in the clinical laboratory. Approximately 12 per cent of strains are nonpigmented, but these, too, can easily be identified by their fluorescence and alkalinization of acetamide (Table 3).

## NUTRITION AND GROWTH

*P. aeruginosa*, like most pseudomonads, is not nutritionally fastidious. It grows in an inorganic basal medium supplemented with a single organic compound such as acetate or glucose (Stanier et al., 1966). As noted above, it is nonfermentative. Electron acceptors other than oxygen (e.g., nitrate) permit growth in an otherwise anaerobic environment. It grows readily at 20 to 42° C; in contrast, another fluorescent species, *P. fluorescens*, grows at 4° C but not at 41 to 42° C (Table 3). All strains of *P. aeruginosa* grow readily on MacConkey agar medium. Most strains also grow on a selective medium containing hexadecyltrimethylammonium bromide ("cetrimide agar").

## PHYSIOLOGY

All of the three fluorescent pseudomonads (*P. aeruginosa*, *P. fluorescens*, and *P. putida*) are oxidase-positive. All are relatively versatile in their oxidative attack of amides, amino acids, carbohydrates, and organic salts (Stanier et al., 1966; Gilardi, 1978b). They rarely hydrolyze starch and esculin; never decarboxylate lysine and ornithine; and never produce acetoin, indole, and $H_2S$ (in KIA or TSIA medium). Most strains of the fluorescent group, but not other pseudomonads, oxidize gluconate to 2-ketogluconate. All alkalinize Simmons citrate medium. Most strains of *P. aeruginosa,* but not of the other two species, produce gas from nitrate and rapidly digest gelatin, casein (skim milk medium), and serum (Loeffler's slant). *P. aeruginosa* acidifies glucose, arabinose, and xylose but not lactose, maltose, and sucrose.

## PATHOGENICITY

*P. aeruginosa* is etiologically significant in many diseases and is particularly associated with postburn sepsis and other nosocomial infections, cystic fibrosis, and septicemia in patients with immunodeficiencies, including those common to neoplastic disease. Neonates are particularly prone to *P. aeruginosa* infection, although this may be referable more to the high humidity and contaminated equipment of the nursery than to high susceptibility. Infection of neonates commonly occurs as otitis media, meningitis, septicemia, and infection of the umbilicus.

*P. aeruginosa* may be a primary infectious agent but may also emerge following eradication of other bacteria by antibiotics. The normal eye is usually resistant, but following physical trauma may become infected with this bacterium, frequently with resultant blindness. Infection of the eye may also arise from contact lenses that have been stored in contaminated solutions. Normal skin, too, is relatively resistant, but a soggy dermatitis may occur on chronically moist surfaces of the body. Mucoid strains are particularly associated with patients suffering from cystic fibrosis and bronchiectasis. Such strains are only rarely recovered from other patients; indeed, there is suggestive evidence that the in vivo environment of these patients favors the mucoid phenotype of *P. aeruginosa.*

## ANTIGENS, TOXINS, AND PATHOGENESIS

A broth culture of *P. aeruginosa* contains not only bacteria but also extracellular factors proliferated by this bacterium. Peripheral to the bacterial cell envelope, at least with some strains, are a capsule-like slime layer, pili, and a flagellum. In vivo, flagella elicit antibodies, and these may be useful for serotyping this species, but there is no evidence that flagella are significant in host-parasite interactions. Though pili (fimbriae) are frequently present on strains recently recovered from clinical specimens, there is no evidence that these are significant for attachment to mammalian cells or for phage-mediated genetic transfer,

thus differing from observations on *Escherichia coli.* The extracellular slime surrounding the bacterial cell contains polysaccharide that is both toxic and antigenic (see Sadoff in Artenstein and Sanford, 1974). In experimental animals, both active and passive immunization against slime protect against lethal challenge with live bacteria.

The cell envelope, consisting of cytoplasmic membrane, the intermediate peptidoglycan layer, and the outer cell wall, is typical of that associated with other gram-negative bacteria. Endotoxicity, O-antigen, and lipopolysaccharide (LPS) are resident in the outer cell wall. As with Enterobacteriaceae, advantage is taken of the O-antigens in serotyping. At present there are several nomenclatures for these O-antigens, and a universal system has been proposed (Serotyping Committee, 1979). It is not clear whether O-specificity resides in the polysaccharide or in the lipid moiety of LPS. Opsonizing antibody directed against LPS appears to play an important role in immunologic defense against *P. aeruginosa,* but high titer antibody in patients with cystic fibrosis usually does not lead to its eradication from the respiratory tract (see Neter in Artenstein and Sanford, 1974). The LPS is similar to that of the Enterobacteriaceae, but there are differences in the hydroxy acids of its lipid A moiety (see Eagon in Artenstein and Sanford, 1974).

Among the several extracellular substances associated with *P. aeruginosa* are proteases, phospholipase, hemolysin, and exotoxin A (see Liu in Artenstein and Sanford, 1974). According to Liu, the "collagenase" of *P. aeruginosa* appears to be a nonspecific activity of proteases. In vitro, purified proteases cause clumping and vacuolization of rabbit alveolar macrophages (Leake et al., 1978). Injected intratracheally into rabbits, they elicit hemorrhage histopathologically resembling that occurring in *P. aeruginosa* pneumonia of man. Exotoxin A is a protein of more than 10,000 daltons. Injected intravenously, the $LD_{50}$ for mice is approximately 7 $\mu$g (see Pavlovskis et al. in Artenstein and Sanford, 1974). Injected intradermally, it causes edema and necrosis. Injected intraperitoneally, 5 to 10 $LD_{50}$ causes leukopenia and death; autopsy discloses necrosis of the liver, edema and hemorrhage of the lungs, and necrosis and hemorrhage in the kidneys. Its mode of action appears to be similar to that of diphtheria toxin (Chung and Collier, 1977; Leppla et al., 1978).

To summarize, all of the following are associated with *P. aeruginosa,* and all may be significant in the pathogenesis of disease referable to this bacterium: lipopolysaccharide, a slime layer consisting of polysaccharide and protein, proteases, phospholipase, and exotoxin A.

## THERAPY AND CONTROL

Most strains of *P. aeruginosa* are susceptible to one or more of the aminoglycosides, amikacin, gentamicin, kanamycin, netilmicin, sisomycin, and tobramycin (Artenstein and Sanford, 1974; Neu, 1978). Resistance to one aminoglycoside is not necessarily accompanied by resistance to others. Resistance, when present, may be attributed either to failure of the agent to enter the bacterium or to enzymatic inactivation. Both chromosomal and plasmid DNA are involved in the mediation of resistance.

The uniform resistance to penicillin appears referable to both exclusion by the cell membrane and chromosomally mediated $\beta$-lactamase. Penicillin derivatives such as carbenicillin and ticarcillin presently are effective therapeutic agents since they do cross the membrane and are relatively resistant to the $\beta$-lactamases. Mucoid strains are exceptional in that they frequently are resistant to both carbenicillin and tobramycin but are susceptible to tetracycline (Govan and Fyfe, 1978). Most strains of *P. aeruginosa* are susceptible to polymyxin B and E (colistemethate) but are resistant to other antimicrobials.

Attempts to control *P. aeruginosa* infections call to mind similar problems with another ubiquitous bacterium, *Staphylococcus aureus,* and have been met with limited success. Routine monitoring and rigorous control of the entire hospital environment suppress but seldom eradicate nosocomial infections. Particular attention to epidemic strains should be a significant factor in controlling *P. aeruginosa* but has not been extensively practiced. Phage-, pyocin-, and serotyping do permit delineation of strains within this species (Zierdt, 1978). Nevertheless, none of these methods has disclosed types with unique antibiograms, epidemic propensities, or anatomic specificities. Additionally, and although there has been one recent favorable report (Shivananda et al., 1978), there is little evidence that either prophylactic antimicrobials or vaccines significantly control nosocomial infections.

## DIAGNOSTIC PROCEDURES

As in the search for other pathogenic bacteria, body fluids such as blood and aspirates are transferred to a fluid medium. *P. aeruginosa* requires an aerobic environment for optimal growth, and hence commercial blood-broth bottles containing an inert gas are "vented" to admit air if this bacterium is anticipated. Secondary culture of such specimens and primary culture of swabs, exudates, and urine are made on blood agar plates, and frequently also on a differential medium such as MacConkey agar. A selective medium such as a cetrimide agar plate is also used in environmental and epidemiologic surveys when only this species is being sought.

In the routine clinical laboratory most isolates of *P. aeruginosa* are, as noted above, pyocyanin-positive; this feature, along with characteristic colonial morphology (large, flat, frosty) and odor permit tentative identification. When the pigment is not obvious and the colony is mucoid or smooth, thus mimicking enteric bacilli, a colony should be transferred to KIA or TSIA medium. Failure to grow in, or acidify, the butt of this medium and good growth on the slant is confirmatory of a nonfermentative bacterium. The following tests, along with appropriate microscopic morphology as seen in Gram stain, confirm its identification as *P. aeruginosa:* fluorescence +, acetamide +, and growth at 41 to 42° C (Table 3). Identification to the subspecies level may be desirable for epidemiologic purposes; this can be effected by sero-, phage-, or pyocin-typing (Zierdt, 1978).

## SUMMARY

*P. aeruginosa* is widely distributed in nature and the hospital environment. This obligatively aerobic, gram-negative, oxidase-positive, nonsporulating motile rod is more common than all other nonfermentative bacilli in clinical specimens, and is etiologically significant as both a primary and a secondary opportunistic pathogen. Although *P. aeruginosa* is resistant to many antimicrobials, it is usually susceptible to one or more of the aminoglycosides. Easily grown and identified, its salient features are blue-green pigmentation, colonial morphology, odor, fluorescence, growth at 42° C, and alkalinization of acetamide.

# PSEUDOMONAS
# MALTOPHILIA

Approximately 7 per cent of the pseudomonads recovered from hospital specimens are *P. maltophilia (Alcaligenes bookeri)*. This species is strongly proteolytic and only weakly saccharolytic and hence is frequently misidentified as *Alcaligenes faecalis*. As the "maltose-loving" name suggests, it readily acidifies this sugar.

## MORPHOLOGY

Microscopically, *P. maltophilia* is a slender, gram-negative rod bearing a tuft of polar flagella. Colonies on a 24-hour blood agar plate are small (0.2 to 0.5 mm), convex, smooth, colorless, and entire. On a 48-hour plate, the colonies are 1 to 2 mm in diameter, slightly brown, and surrounded by a zone of diffuse $\beta$-hemolysis.

## NUTRITION AND GROWTH

Like *P. aeruginosa*, *P. maltophilia* grows luxuriantly on nonselective media routinely used in the clinical laboratory. Though most strains require methionine for growth, this amino acid is already present in such media. Growth occurs on MacConkey agar but is frequently less luxuriant than on nonselective media. *P. maltophilia* does not grow on salmonella-shigella and cetrimide agar and, like the fluorescent pseudomonads, rarely grows on media containing 6.5 per cent sodium chloride. Good growth and motility are obtained in OF basal medium, and such cultures remain viable for months at 4° C.

## PHYSIOLOGY

*P. maltophilia* is usually oxidase-negative, but nearly 5 per cent of strains are weakly to moderately oxidase-positive. Though it is a saccharolytic pseudomonad, acidification of carbohydrates is masked in media containing 0.5 per cent or more of organic nitrogen. However, in suitable basal medium containing 0.2 per cent or less of peptone, not only maltose but usually also glucose, lactose, and sucrose are acidified (Otto and Pickett, 1976; Gilardi, 1978b). It hydrolyzes esculin and deoxyribonucleic acid but not starch and urea. It is one of only two pseudomonads that are LDC-positive.

These two, *P. cepacia* and *P. maltophilia,* are easily distinguished by other features, particularly their differential acidification of mannitol and arabinose (Table 4).

## HABITAT

*P. maltophilia* has been recovered from an impressive variety of sites both within and outside the hospital environment (Hugh and Gilardi, 1974), and therefore it appears to be readily available to colonize compromised hosts. Among these sites are deionized water, eggs, feces, fish, milk, normal nasopharynges, sewage, soil, and therapeutic baths.

## PATHOGENICITY AND THERAPY

This species has been etiologically associated, in both mixed and pure cultures, with lymphadenopathy, infected wounds, pulmonary disease, septicemia, superficial ulcers, and urinary tract infections. Most strains are susceptible in vitro to chloramphenicol, colistin, nalidixic acid, polymyxin B, and trimethoprim/sulfamethoxazole but are resistant to ampicillin, cephalothin, erythromycin, nitrofurantoin, and novobiocin. The trimethoprim-sulfamethoxazole combination has been favorably reported as a therapeutic agent (Moody and Young, 1975; von Graevenitz, 1978).

## SUMMARY

*P. maltophilia* is widely distributed in nature. This obligatively aerobic, gram-negative, usually oxidase-negative, nonsporulating, noncapsulated rod grows well on blood, infusion, and Kligler iron agar media. The small, smooth, weakly pigmented colonies are strongly proteolytic but weakly saccharolytic and LDC-positive. Maltose is acidified, but arabinose and mannitol are not. Among the pseudomonads, *P. maltophilia* is second only to *P. aeruginosa* as an opportunistic pathogen. Although it is resistant to many antimicrobials, it is usually susceptible to chloramphenicol and trimethoprim/sulfamethoxazole.

# OTHER PSEUDOMONADS

*Pseudomonas (Bacillus, Actinobacillus, Loefflerella, Malleomyces, Pfeifferella) mallei* is almost never encountered today in the Western world. It is the etiologic agent of glanders in ungulates, particularly equines, and only rarely in other animals, but this disease is largely controlled today in most areas of the world. Human infections, frequently fatal, were acquired from the nasal discharge of diseased animals, commonly horses and donkeys (Wilson and Miles, 1975). In man, glanders is usually an acute, though sometimes chronic respiratory disease. In the acute form there is usually fever, prostration, a mucopurulent discharge, and death within 2 weeks of onset. The chronic form may persist for months or years, usually with lymphadenopathy.

*P. mallei* differs from other pseudomonads in its parasitic habitat, slow growth in both defined and complex media, and absence of flagella, but many of its features, including oxidase positivity, aerobic metabolism, and moles per cent GC (69) in its chromosomal DNA are those of the genus *Pseudomonas* (Redfearn et al., 1966; Mandel, 1966). It resembles *P. pseudomallei* in its production of gas from nitrates, moles per cent GC, antigenic composition, oxidative assimilation of organic substrates, and sensitivity to temperate *P. pseudomallei* phages. Features that serve to distinguish these two species are shown in Table 7.

*Pseudomonas (Loefflerella, Malleomyces, Pfeifferella) pseudomallei,* formerly called Whitmore's bacillus, is the etiologic agent of melioidosis. Its normal habitat appears to be tropical soils throughout the world, but subclinical colonization of man may occur months prior to overt disease. Hence cases of melioidosis, often fatal, have been reported from temperate and subtropical as well as tropical areas of the world. There is suggestive evidence that both overt and covert infections exist in rodents and domestic animals in the tropics, but there is little evidence that these serve as a source of human infections. In man, pulmonary infection is the more common form of melioidosis, and the x-ray picture may mimic that of tuberculosis or mycotic disease. It may occur as a rapidly progressive and fatal septicemia, despite antimicrobial therapy. Chloramphenicol, tetracycline, and trimethoprim/sulfamethoxazole have been reported as effective therapeutic agents (Howe et al., 1971; John, 1976; Girard et al., 1976). It is usually not susceptible to penicillin, its derivatives, and the aminoglycosides.

*P. pseudomallei* is a slender, relatively short, noncapsulated, gram-negative rod bearing two or more polar flagella. When grown on a suitable medium, the rods contain PHB granules, visible by Sudan black staining or phase microscopy. On a 24-hour blood agar plate, colonies are 0.2 to 0.6 mm in diameter, translucent, convex, entire, nonpigmented, and oxidase-positive. At 48 to 72 hours the colonies are usually 3 to 4 mm in diameter, opaque, and yellow-brown with a uniquely corrugated appearance. Note that this unique, rugose, "textbook" description refers to aged, not 24-hour, colonies. Strains may vary from rough to mucoid and in color from cream to orange; this heterogeneity in colonial morphology is in contrast to the homogeneity of other features (Redfearn et al., 1966). Useful features for identification of this species, in addition to unique colonial morphology when present, are gas from nitrate; growth at 42° C, acidification of mannitol, sorbitol, and sucrose; and hydrolysis of gelatin, casein (milk), and serum proteins (Loeffler's slant). Denitrification may not occur in peptone-rich media and with stock cultures, and such cultures may also fail to acidify sucrose (Table 4).

*Pseudomonas cepacia (P. multivorans,* biogroup EO-1) was first associated with skin rot of the onion, *Allium cepa.* Later EO-1, associated with humans, and *P. multivorans,* recovered from soil, were shown to be synonymous with *P. cepacia.* Though strains of both plant and clinical origin are now given a common species designation, they do have distinguishing features, particularly their sensitivity to bacteriocins (Gonzalez and Vidaver, 1979). This species is particularly important as an opportunistic pathogen in that it can cause fulminating septicemia. It has also been implicated in endocarditis, necrotizing vas-

**TABLE 7.    Differential Features for Pseudomonas mallei and P. pseudomallei[a]**

|  | P. MALLEI | P. PSEUDO-MALLEI |
|---|---|---|
| Flagella | 0 | >1 |
| Colonies, rugose | — | V[b] |
| Growth, MacConkey agar | — | + |
| Amylase | V | + |
| Assimilation of |  |  |
| L-Arabinose | V | 0 |
| Erythritol | 0 | + |
| D-Ribose | 0 | + |
| D-Xylose | + | 0 |

[a]Adapted from Redfearn et al., 1966, and Wilson and Miles, 1975.
[b]V, variable.

culitis, pneumonitis, and urinary tract and wound infections. Differing from *P. aeruginosa,* it is usually highly resistant to the aminoglycosides. Trimethoprim/sulfamethoxazole, trimethoprim/sulfisoxazole, and chloramphenicol have been effective therapeutic agents.

This species appears to be widely distributed in nature. It has been recovered from cannulas, catheters, distilled water, the eye, feces, nose, plants, soil, solutions of disinfectants (chlorhexidine, Zephiran), throat, and the urinary tract. The two synonyms for *P. cepacia* reflect its features. It grows luxuriantly (eugonically) on routine laboratory media and oxidatively acidifies carbohydrates; "multivorans" indicates its utilization of many substrates, particularly sugars. It is a slender, gram-negative, noncapsulated rod bearing two or more polar flagella and, like *P. pseudomallei,* forms PHB inclusions. Many strains are yellow to orange on iron-rich media such as KIA, but pigmentation is rare on blood agar plates. On such plates, 24-hour colonies are 0.2 to 0.8 mm in diameter, translucent, convex, smooth, entire, and oxidase-positive (frequently weak). At 48 hours, the colonies are 1 to 2 mm in diameter, opaque, and occasionally pigmented. Though sharing many features with *P. pseudomallei,* it differs in acidifying adonitol, never producing gas from nitrate, never attacking arginine (ADH-negative), and always decarboxylating lysine (Table 4).

*Pseudomonas vesicularis (Corynebacterium vesiculare),* initially recovered from a medicinal snail, has recently been implicated in genitourinary tract infections, particularly cervicitis (Otto et al., 1978). Its normal habitat is not known. Like *P. diminuta,* it differs from other pseudomonads in having specific nutritional requirements (biotin, cyanocobalamin, and pantothenate) and bearing a polar flagellum of exceptionally short wavelength (Ballard et al., 1968; Gilardi, 1978b). It has been recovered from cervical and urethral swabs inoculated onto Thayer-Martin medium and grows poorly on initial isolation. Salient features for identification of this species are orange pigmentation; acidification of glucose and maltose but not fructose, lactose, mannitol, or sucrose; and hydrolysis of esculin (Table 4).

the hospital environment but, excepting an occasional genitourinary tract infection is rarely implicated in human disease. Like *P. putida, P. pickettii* appears to be present in the hospital environment but only rarely is etiologically significant. Among its salient features (Table 4) are hydrolysis of urea and production of gas from nitrate (at 20 to 30° C but usually not at 35 to 37° C). *P. putrefaciens,* a frequent cause of spoilage in marine foods, is occasionally recovered from clinical specimens and may have etiologic significance (Vandepitte and Debois, 1978). Presently it is a heterogeneous species but nevertheless is easily identified, since it is the only H₂S-positive pseudomonad and also decarboxylates ornithine (ODC-positive), a feature shared with only one other species, *P. cepacia. P. stutzeri,* an occasional opportunistic pathogen in compromised patients, particularly drug addicts, is well known as a resident in the soil and on plants. Though commonly described as presenting a unique colonial morphology and producing gas from nitrate, neither of these features may be evident with clinical isolates. Other features permit identification of this species (Table 4); among these are hydrolysis of starch and acidification of glucose, maltose, and mannitol but not lactose and sucrose.

Pseudomonads presenting lemon-yellow colonies are occasionally recovered from clinical specimens. These are usually biogroups IIk and Ve. Some investigators have equated IIk with genus *Xanthomonas,* a phylogenetic group of plant pathogens, but this synonymy remains controversial (Gilardi, 1978b). Two biotypes of the IIk group are recognized. IIk-1 has the features of a pseudomonad (65 moles per cent GC, oxidative metabolism, one polar flagellum) and has recently been named *P. paucimobilis* (Holmes et al., 1977). IIk-2 differs in having 40 moles per cent GC; this appears to exclude it from genus *Pseudomonas* (48 to 70 moles per cent GC). IIk-2 also differs from IIk-1 in not being strongly pigmented and in several biochemical features. The Ve group (*"Chromobacterium" typhiflavum*) similarly contains two biotypes that can easily be distinguished (Table 4). Both appear to be pseudomonads (Gilardi et al., 1975), but neither has been assigned a species epithet.

## OTHER SACCHAROLYTIC PSEUDOMONADS

*P. fluorescens* and *P. putida,* like *P. aeruginosa,* are fluorescent pseudomonads (Table 3). As noted above, *P. fluorescens* has been implicated in endotoxemia following intravenous administration of contaminated solutions. *P. putida* is present in

## GLUCOSE-NEGATIVE PSEUDOMONADS

These organisms (Table 5) are infrequently encountered in clinical specimens, are rarely etiologically significant, and are commonly misidentified as *Alcaligenes faecalis;* indeed, the latter species is almost never present in such specimens.

Although they almost never acidify glucose, other features permit their identification. *P. acidovorans* acidifies fructose and usually mannitol; some strains weakly acidify glucose. *P. pseudoalcaligenes* acidifies fructose and, rarely and weakly, arabinose, glucose, and xylose. Additionally, growth at 42° C and alkalinization of acetamide are useful features for identification of these species. These two species and *P. alcaligenes* are the more commonly encountered glucose-negative pseudomonads; *P. denitrificans* (gas from nitrate), *P. diminuta,* and *P. testosteroni* are far less commonly encountered.

## References

Artenstein, M. S., and Sanford, J. P. (eds.): Symposium on *Pseudomonas aeruginosa.* J Inf Dis 130(Supplement):51, 1974.

Ballard, R. W., Doudoroff, M., Stanier, R. Y., and Mandel, M.: Taxonomy of the aerobic pseudomonads: *Pseudomonas diminuta* and *P. vesiculare.* J Gen Microbiol 53:349, 1968.

Chung, D. W., and Collier, R. J.: Enzymatically active peptide from the adenosine diphosphate-ribosylating toxin of *Pseudomonas aeruginosa.* Infect Immun 16:832, 1977.

Gilardi, G. L. (ed.): Glucose Nonfermenting Gram-Negative Bacteria in Clinical Microbiology. West Palm Beach, CRC Press, Inc., 1978a.

Gilardi, G. L: Identification of *Pseudomonas* and related bacteria. In Gilardi, G. L. (ed.): Glucose Nonfermenting Gram-Negative Bacteria in Clinical Microbiology. West Palm Beach, CRC Press, 1978b.

Gilardi, G. L., Hirschl, S., and Mandel, M.: Characteristics of yellow-pigmented nonfermentative bacilli (groups VE-1 and VE-2) encountered in clinical bacteriology. J Clin Microbiol 1:384, 1975.

Girard, D. E., Nardone, D. A., and Jones, S. R.: Pleural melioidosis. Am Rev Resp Dis 114:1175, 1976.

Gonzalez, C. F., and Vidaver, A. K.: Bacteriocin, plasmid and pectolytic diversity in *Pseudomonas cepacia* of clinical and plant origin. J Gen Microbiol 110:161, 1979.

Govan, J. R. W., and Fyfe, J. A. M.: Mucoid *Pseudomonas aeruginosa* and cystic fibrosis: Resistance of the mucoid form to carbenicillin, flucloxacillin and tobramycin and the isolation of mucoid variants *in vitro.* J Antimicrob Chemother 4:233, 1978.

Holmes, B., Owen, R. J., Malnick, A. E. H., and Willcox, W. R.: *Pseudomonas paucimobilis,* a new species isolated from human clinical specimens, the hospital environment, and other sources. Int J System Bacteriol 27:133, 1977.

Howe, C., Sampath, A., and Spotnitz, M.: The pseudomallei group: A review. J Inf Dis 124:598, 1971.

Hugh, R., and Gilardi, G. L.: *Pseudomonas.* In Lennette, E. H., Spaulding, E. H., and Truant, J. P. (eds.): Manual of Clinical Microbiolo-

gy. 2nd ed. Washington, D.C., American Society for Microbiology, 1974.

John, J. F., Jr.: Trimethoprim-sulfamethoxazole therapy of pulmonary melioidosis. Am Rev Resp Dis 114:1021, 1976.

Leake, E. S., Wright, M. J., and Kreger, A. S.: *In vitro* effect of purified proteases of *Pseudomonas aeruginosa* on rabbit lung macrophages. Exp Mol Pathol 29:241, 1978.

Lennette, E. H., Spaulding, E. H., and Truant, J. P. (eds.): Manual of Clinical Microbiology. 2nd ed. Washington, D.C., American Society for Microbiology, 1974.

Leppla, S. H., Martin, O. C., and Muehl, L. A.: The exotoxin of *P. aeruginosa:* A proenzyme having an unusual mode of activation. Biochem Biophys Res Commun 81:532, 1978.

Mandel, M.: Deoxyribonucleic acid base composition in the genus *Pseudomonas.* J Gen Microbiol 43:273, 1966.

Moody, M. R., and Young, V. M.: In vitro susceptibility of *Pseudomonas cepacia* and *Pseudomonas maltophilia* to trimethoprim and trimethoprim-sulfamethoxazole. Antimicrob Agents Chemother 7:836, 1975.

Neu, H. C.: Clinical role of *Pseudomonas aeruginosa.* In Gilardi, G. L. (ed.): Glucose Nonfermenting Gram-Negative Bacteria in Clinical Microbiology. West Palm Beach, CRC Press, Inc., 1978.

Otto, L. A., Deboo, B. S., Capers, E. L., and Pickett, M. J.: *Pseudomonas vesicularis* from cervical specimens. J Clin Microbiol 7:341, 1978.

Otto, L. A., and Pickett, M. J.: Rapid method for identification of gram-negative, nonfermentative bacilli. J Clin Microbiol 3:566, 1976.

Redfearn, M. S., Palleroni, N. J., and Stanier, R. Y.: A comparative study of *Pseudomonas pseudomallei* and *Bacillus mallei.* J Gen Microbiol 43:293, 1966.

Serotyping Committee, Japan *Pseudomonas aeruginosa* Society: Proposal of an International Standard for the infra-specific serologic classification of *Pseudomonas aeruginosa.* Jpn J Exp Med 49:89, 1979.

Shivanananda, P. G., Nayak, M. N., Mohan, M., Rao, K. N. A., and Singh, Y. I.: Therapeutic trial of pseudomonas vaccine — a preliminary report. Indian J Med Res 68:580, 1978.

Stanier, R. Y., Palleroni, N. J., and Doudoroff, M.: The aerobic pseudomonads: A taxonomic study. J Gen Microbiol 43:159, 1966.

Tatum, H. W., Ewing, W. H., and Weaver, R. E.: Miscellaneous gram-negative bacteria. In Lennette, E. H., Spaulding, E. H., and Truant, J. P. (eds.): Manual of Clinical Microbiology. 2nd ed. Washington, D.C., American Society for Microbiology, 1974.

Vandepitte, J., and Debois, J.: *Pseudomonas putrefaciens* as a cause of bacteremia in humans. J Clin Microbiol 7:70, 1978.

Von Graevenitz, A.: Clinical role of infrequently encountered nonfermenters. In Gilardi, G. L. (ed.): Glucose Nonfermenting Gram-Negative Bacteria in Clinical Microbiology. West Palm Beach, CRC Press, Inc., 1978.

Wilson, G. S., and Miles, A.: Topley and Wilson's Principles of Bacteriology, Virology and Immunity. 6th ed. Baltimore, The Williams & Wilkins Company, 1975.

Zierdt, C. H.: Systems for typing *Pseudomonas aeruginosa.* In Gilardi, G. L. (ed.): Glucose Nonfermenting Gram-Negative Bacteria in Clinical Microbiology. West Palm Beach, CRC Press, Inc., 1978.

# 34 *BRUCELLA*

## *Wesley W. Spink, A.B., M.D.*

### *MORPHOLOGY*

Members of the genus *Brucella* occur as small, nonmotile, noncapsular, gram-negative bacilli or coccobacilli that do not form spores and are not acid-fast. They vary from 0.4 to 1.5 $\mu$m in length and 0.4 to 0.8 $\mu$m in width. Young colonies are pinpoint in size, moist, translucent, and glistening. Six species of *Brucella* are recognized, some with several biotypes. The most significant species in human disease are *Brucella melitensis,* *Brucella abortus,* and *Brucella suis,* which cause contagious abortion in goats (melitensis), cattle (abortus), and swine (suis), and are shed in their milk. *Brucella neotomae* has been identified in the desert wood rat *(Neotoma lepida)* in the western United States. *Brucella ovis* is an important pathogen in sheep, causing chiefly ram epididymitis. *Brucella canis* is found in dogs, especially in the beagle family, and causes epidemic abortions in kennels. Neither *B. neotomae* nor *B. ovis* has been known to cause human illness, and *B. canis* has resulted in only a few recognized human cases. *Brucella neotomae* grows as smooth colonies on solid media and is probably a derivative of *B. abortus*. *Brucella ovis* and *B. canis* reproduce as rough colonies, and both are probably variants of *B. suis*. Further discussion centers on the three classic species: *melitensis, abortus,* and *suis,* and some of their biotypes. These and other members of the genus are closely related as determined by DNA hybridization. The G & C content of their DNA ranges from 56 to 58 moles per cent (Brinley-Morgan and McCullough, 1974).

*Brucella* cells contain nucleoprotein, protein, lipopolysaccharide, and polysaccharide antigens. A soluble polysaccharide fraction elicits an immediate localized reaction when injected intradermally into an infected subject, whereas the nucleoprotein material produces a delayed response.

## METABOLISM

Although *Brucella* may sometimes be cultivated on chemically defined media containing amino acids, glucose, and B vitamins (nicotinic acid, thiamine, and biotin), the fastidious nutritional requirements of *Brucella* are ordinarily met by tryptose or trypticase broth and agar. Aerobic growth at 37° C requires several days, and for some strains (*abortus*) added carbon dioxide is essential. Neither acid nor gas is produced from carbohydrates in peptone media, catalase activity is variable, and urease is present in *B. suis* and *B. melitensis*. Hydrogen sulfide is produced by all three species, but in variable amounts. All species except *B. neotomae* and *B. ovis* are usually oxidase-positive (Brinley-Morgan and McCullough, 1974). The differential metabolic requirements of the three species and their subtypes are discussed later under Laboratory Diagnosis.

*Brucella* organisms are killed in 3 minutes at 143° to 145° F, that is, at temperatures used for pasteurization. They are also killed by gastric juice so that persons who ingest the organism are infected by *Brucella* less easily than those who are exposed through skin abrasions (Garrod, 1939; Morales-Otero, 1929).

## PATHOGENIC PROPERTIES

The three classic species of *Brucella* are highly invasive, gaining entrance into the body through the oral or ocular mucosae or through abrasions of the skin. Controversy exists as to whether the organisms invade the respiratory tract. A state of

bacterial hypersensitivity much like that in tuberculosis is induced. Strains having attenuated virulence such as those used in immunization programs in cattle (*B. abortus* strain 19) can cause human illness when accidentally injected through the skin during the procedure of vaccination. When this occurs in veterinarians having a previous history of brucellosis, an immediate localized reaction takes place at the site of entry of the organisms, which is accompanied by a systemic response with chills and fever. This is due to the acquired *Brucella* hypersensitivity caused by the previous infection (Spink, 1956).

## ANTIGENIC COMPOSITION

The basic antigenic components of *Brucella* as defined by Wilson and Miles (1932) with quantitative agglutinin-absorption tests distinguish *B. melitensis* from *B. abortus* and *B. suis*. These species all possess A and M antigen in different proportions; in *B. melitensis* the ratio of A and M is 1:20 and in *B. abortus* it is 20:1. This permits the production of specific monovalent sera for agglutination tests with *melitensis* or *abortus*. From a practical point of view a standardized *Brucella* antigen for diagnostic agglutination tests can be prepared from cultures of any one of the three species.

*Brucella* organisms produce no exotoxins but, as in all gram-negative bacteria, the lipopolysaccharide (LPS) in their cell wall is an endotoxin. *Brucella* endotoxins have the same chemical and biologic properties as the endotoxins of enteric bacilli (see Chapter 6). The O-specific side chains of *Brucella* LPS are lost when smooth (S) strains undergo dissociation to rough (R) strains. This S→R transformation occurs more readily than in enteric bacteria and is accompanied by loss in virulence and serologic specificity. The loss in virulence implies that the complete LPS is a virulence factor. This implication is supported by the fact that patients with brucellosis uniformly develop hypersensitivity to *Brucella* LPS, and that certain important clinical manifestations can be reproduced in these patients with LPS (Spink, 1956).

A prominent feature of *Brucella* infection is intracellular parasitism of the macrophages and histiocytes of the reticuloendothelial system. Focal aggregates of the parasitized cells produce granulomas of the liver, spleen, and bone marrow. In experimental animals the pathologic response varies with the species (Braude, 1951). In infections of guinea pigs caused by *B. abortus,* there is marked splenomegaly, little if any suppuration, and no discernibly ill health. Guinea pigs infected with *B. suis*, on the other hand, develop extensive suppurating granulomas of the liver, bones, and testicles. *B. melitensis* infections are intermediate in their tissue damage, but more disabling than the other two.

## IMMUNITY

Recovery from brucellosis is accompanied by an effective, but not total, acquired immunity to subsequent attacks of the disease. The humoral immune response can be evaluated by measuring bacteriolysins, precipitins, and agglutinins in the serum. Cellular immunity is associated with acquired hypersensitivity, as it is in tuberculosis, and can be detected with the use of *Brucella* antigens for skin tests.

Evidence for immunity against brucellosis has been demonstrated by the remarkable protection afforded cattle, sheep, and goats through the use of vaccines containing living organisms with attenuated virulence.

## LABORATORY DIAGNOSIS

### Bacteriologic

A definitive diagnosis of brucellosis is made through the isolation of *Brucella* from body fluids or tissues (Alton et al., 1975). For this purpose the culture media of tryptose or trypticase broth and agar is recommended. Liquid media are employed for primary isolation and subcultures on agar slants and plates are used for identification. For the majority of specimens such as blood, cerebrospinal fluid, urine, and minced tissue suspensions, the double medium of Castaneda is recommended. The medium is prepared under sterile conditions and stored in 4 oz rubber-stoppered glass bottles until ready for use. Twenty ml of broth are added to each bottle and then 10 ml of melted agar are layered on one of the narrow edges. Ten per cent of the bottled air should be displaced with $CO_2$. After the bottle is inoculated with suspected material, it is incubated at 37° C for a minimum of 2 to 3 weeks. After 48 to 72 hours minute colonies of *Brucella* may be detected on the agar surface. Subcultures should be made on agar plates by withdrawing material through the rubber stopper with a needle and syringe every 4th, 7th, 15th, and 21st day. The agar plates should be placed in a jar containing 10 per cent $CO_2$. Usually organisms can be detected for identification within a week after the primary culture is made.

The isolation of *Brucella* from heavily contaminated substances is possible by the intraperitoneal injection of the material into guinea pigs.

Colonies appearing on the agar surface should be transferred to agar plates and to broth suspensions. A suspected culture of *Brucella* reveals small gram-negative bacilli or coccobacilli. Discrete colonies appearing within 48 to 72 hours should be examined by indirect light. Freshly isolated smooth colonies are gray, translucent, sharply edged, and about 0.5 mm in size. *Brucella* organisms tend to dissociate, especially in broth cultures, from smooth to rough forms, revealing morphologic changes and a decrease in virulence. Rough colonies are flat, dull, opaque, and granular. Mucoid colonies are slimy in consistency.

The observations made by direct examination of the colonial morphology can be supplemented quickly by exposing the organisms to acriflavine and to crystal violet. After a drop of fresh acriflavine solution in a concentration of 1:1000 is added to a loopful of suspended smooth colonies on a slide, examination under low-power magnification shows that the colonies remain in suspension, but rough colonies are immediately agglutinated, and mucoid variants form threads. When a fresh culture of *Brucella* on a plate is flooded with a fresh 1:40 dilution of crystal violet, the smooth colonies are not stained, whereas dissociated rough forms appear red and purple with radial cracks on the surface. Only smooth forms should be used for identification with *Brucella* antiserum because rough variants not only lose their antigenic specificity but also become autoagglutinable owing to loss of their O side chains.

A presumptive identification of *Brucella* can be readily made by mixing a drop of high titer human or rabbit anti-*Brucella* serum with a suspended drop of smooth organisms on a slide when agglutination of *Brucella* occurs. Further substantiation is obtained with the tube-agglutination test and by using appropriate controls of a known *Brucella* culture, anti-*Brucella* serum, and a serum without *Brucella* antibody.

Having identified a culture as belonging to the genus *Brucella*, it is necessary to determine the species of *Brucella*. For practical purposes the aim is to distinguish between the three principal species: *melitensis*, *abortus*, and *suis*. Methods that are used are indicated in Table 1.

**TABLE 1.   Tests for Distinguishing Among the Species of Brucella**

1. Requirement of added $CO_2$ for growth
2. Inhibitory action of basic fuchsin and thionin on growth
3. Production of $H_2S$
4. Urease activity
5. Inhibitory action of bacteriophage on growth
6. Agglutination with monospecific serum
7. Oxidative-metabolic tests

**TABLE 2.   Inhibiting Action of Fuchsin and Thionin on Brucella**

| | |
|---|---|
| B. melitensis | Growth on all six plates |
| B. abortus | Growth only in $CO_2$ and with fuchsin |
| B. suis | Growth with and without $CO_2$ but only with thionin |

***$CO_2$ Requirement.***   The vast majority of the initial isolates of *B. abortus* strains require the addition of 10 per cent $CO_2$ for optimal growth. After many subsequent subcultures, particularly in broth, this requirement is reduced or lost. Strain 19 *B. abortus,* used widely in the United States for vaccinating cattle, does not require added $CO_2$.

***Inhibitory Action of Fuchsin and Thionin.***   Freshly prepared agar plates with either of these dyes from a stocked solution should be used. The test is performed by dividing a plate into four segments and streaking suspensions of each of the known three species on three segments, and the unknown on the fourth. One set of two plates, one with fuchsin and one with thionin, is placed in a jar with 10 per cent $CO_2$ added and incubated at 37° C. A second set of plates is incubated without added $CO_2$. Growth is checked at 48 and 72 hours. The following results in Table 2 distinguish among the three species.

***$H_2S$ Production.***   The three species can be differentiated by the amount of S liberated from agar slants by reproducing organisms. This is determined by suspending in tubes dried filter strips that have been soaked in a 10 per cent solution of lead acetate and then noting the intensity of the black precipitated sulfide on the paper. Each of three tubes contain one of the known species of *Brucella* and the fourth has the unknown culture. The tubes are incubated at 37° C for 4 days with 10 per cent $CO_2$ added to each tube. Every 24 hours the strips are examined and replaced by fresh ones. The degree of blackening is measured from 0 to 4+. A typical series of observations is as follows:

| DAY | ABORTUS | MELITENSIS | SUIS | UNKNOWN |
|---|---|---|---|---|
| 1 | + | 0 | ++ | + |
| 2 | ++ | 0 | +++ | + |
| 3 | ± | 0 | ++++ | ± |
| 4 | 0 | 0 | +++ | 0 |

The "unknown" is *B. abortus.* $H_2S$ production is most intense with *B. suis* and is not observed with *B. melitensis.*

***Urease Activity.***   Most *Brucella* strains split urea to form ammonia. This activity can be measured by adding urea to the media along with phenol red as an indicator. A loopful of known

*Brucella* organisms and an unknown culture is added to the surface of an agar slant and observed at room temperature. *Brucella suis* produces a pink color of the medium almost immediately, reaching a maximum intensity within 15 to 30 minutes, whereas the color change with *B. abortus* takes several hours. The color change with *B. melitensis* occurs more slowly than with *B. abortus* and the overall results are variable.

Thus, the $H_2S$ and urease tests are most specific in identifying strains of *B. suis.*

***Inhibitory Action of Brucella Bacteriophage.***   Tb (Tbsili) phage, originally isolated in the U.S.S.R., is specific for most *abortus* strains. This test is rarely necessary in a routine diagnostic laboratory. If it is necessary, assistance should be sought from one of the FAO/WHO Research Centers for Brucellosis.

***Agglutination with Monospecific Serum.***   For practical purposes the foregoing procedures for the differentiation of *Brucella* species can be adapted to a diagnostic laboratory. Thus, *B. suis* can be readily distinguished from *abortus* and *melitensis* cultures. The vast majority of fresh isolates of *B. abortus* can be differentiated from *melitensis* and *suis* cultures because of the requirement of added $CO_2$ for optimal growth of *abortus.* However, on rare occasions some difficulty may be encountered in differentiating *abortus* cultures from those of *melitensis,* especially if the $CO_2$ requirement for the former is not definite. For this reason the use of monospecific absorbed agglutinating serum can be helpful. An example from our laboratory using monospecific anti-*abortus* and anti-*melitensis* sera is shown in Table 3.

The "unknown" in Table 3 is not *B. melitensis,* but it still could be *B. suis* on the basis of this single procedure. The $H_2S$ and urease tests will make the final distinction.

Although many *Brucella* isolates have been studied intensively on a world-wide basis, the taxonomy of the *Brucella* species is focused on three basic species. Nevertheless, on the basis of biologic and metabolic studies, some strains cannot be strictly assigned to *abortus, suis,* or *melitensis.* These strains have not been classified as new species but rather as biotypes of one of the three. Three biotypes of *B. melitensis* are recognized, two of which have antigenic properties of *abortus* strains as determined with monospecific agglutination sera. Some isolates of *abortus* strains do not require additional $CO_2$ for growth; in others agglutinins for *melitensis* predominate. Nine types of *abortus* are known. There are four biotypes of *suis.* Although the classic strain forms $H_2S$ readily, three do not, including type 4, which is found in reindeer, and type 2, found in the Danish hare and swine.

**Table 3.** Differentiation of Abortus and Melitensis Cultures Using Monospecific Serum

| | MONOSPECIFIC ANTI-ABORTUS SERUM | | | | MONOSPECIFIC ANTI-MELITENSIS SERUM | | | |
|---|---|---|---|---|---|---|---|---|
| | 1:20 | 1:40 | 1:80 | 1:160 | 1:20 | 1:40 | 1:80 | 1:160 |
| B. abortus | +++[a] | +++ | +++ | +++ | 0 | 0 | 0 | 0 |
| B. melitensis | 0 | 0 | 0 | 0 | ++++ | +++ | +++ | +++ |
| Unknown | +++ | +++ | +++ | +++ | 0 | 0 | 0 | 0 |

[a]Degree of agglutination ranges from 0 to ++++.

Additional information useful for differentiating the strains has been derived from oxidative-metabolic studies. These studies involve a measurement of the utilization of oxygen with individual sugars or amino acids used as substrates (Meyer, 1974). This procedure is performed in brucellosis research centers such as the U.S. Department of Agriculture, Veterinary Services Laboratories, Box 70, Ames, Iowa 50010, U.S.A.; FAO/WHO Collaborative Centre for Brucellosis, Central Veterinary Laboratory, Weybridge, England; and the Pan American Zoonoses Center, Casella 23, Ramos Mejía, Buenos Aires, Argentina.

### Serologic

If Brucella organisms are not isolated, the diagnosis can sometimes be made by testing the serum of patients for antibody. The most reliable serologic test is the tube-dilution, saline-agglutination test using a standardized B. abortus antigen. The test has minor limitations as far as specificity is concerned. Cross-agglutination with Vibrio cholera and Pasteurella tularensis occurs in the sera of patients who have either had these diseases or have been vaccinated for them. The antigen-serum mixtures should be incubated for 48 hours at 37° C and then examined. Titers of 1:100 and above are significant, though on occasion healthy individuals who have had the disease months and years previously may have titers of 1:100 or below, rarely higher. "Blocking antibodies" may interfere with a clear-cut reading so that the lower dilutions reveal little or no agglutination, and the higher dilutions show incomplete agglutination. When such blocking is present, centrifuging the mixtures at 3000 rpm may reveal further clumping. The presence of blocking antibody can also be detected by incubating the suspect serum with a known serum of high antibody content. The known serum is then diluted with antigen and incubated, and if blocking is occurring the titer will be lower than in the untreated serum.

Although agglutinins are rarely absent in patients with active disease, especially in those with blood cultures that reveal Brucella organisms,

the interpretation of agglutinin titers of 1:100 or less is often difficult when the cultures remain sterile. The Brucella agglutinin in active disease is IgG antibody, whereas in those who have recovered from the disease it is IgM. The type of antibody present in the serum may be differentiated by adding 2-mercaptoethanol to the antigen-antibody mixtures. Under these circumstances IgM dissociates and no agglutination occurs.

Other serologic tests carried out in some laboratories include the complement-fixation, the Coombs'-antiglobulin, and the fluorescent antibody tests.

### Drug Susceptibility

It is not necessary to carry out routinely in vitro drug sensitivity tests on isolated strains of Brucella for the purposes of human therapy. Extensive clinical experience in several areas of the world has shown that tetracycline is the drug of choice for the treatment of brucellosis. In severe illness tetracycline can be supplemented with streptomycin. An alternate drug for tetracycline is chloramphenicol.

Tests in vitro also show that the tetracycline antibiotics are the most effective. Tetracycline, for example, inhibits 95 per cent of strains in a concentration of 0.02 $\mu$g/ml, and is more bactericidal for Brucella than is generally appreciated (Hall and Manion, 1970). Chloramphenicol is approximately 100 times less active against Brucella than tetracycline. Streptomycin is as active in vitro as chloramphenicol but the aminoglycoside is not effective in clinical therapy, presumably because it does not effectively enter the cells in which Brucella organisms are living.

### EPIDEMIOLOGY

Brucellosis is one of the zoonoses — that is, a disease transmitted directly or indirectly from animals to man. The disease is very rarely transmitted from one person to another. The most common animal reservoirs are sheep, goats, cattle, hogs, and caribou, although other domestic animals can harbor the organisms. The prevalence of human disease will depend on the concentration of the animal populations just mentioned, the incidence of animal disease, and the efficiency of disease eradication programs in animals.

Where disease is prevalent in sheep and goats (*B. melitensis*) there will be a high incidence of human infection transmitted through the milk and cheese of these animals. Likewise, brucellosis in cattle (*B. abortus*) results in human disease by ingestion of unpasteurized dairy products. Hogs and caribou infected with *Brucella (B. suis)* transmit disease to veterinarians, farmers, and packing-house workers who handle infected tissues and vaginal discharges of aborting animals. The frequent association of *B. abortus* with fistulous withers in horses provides another source of potential infection. *Brucellae* will survive in dry soil for 40 to 60 days after it is soiled by animal discharges or tissues, and in milk for 10 days at 10° C. Unpasteurized cheese preserves the vitality of these organisms for up to 2 months, but they do not survive in ripened, aged cheeses.

Eradication programs in domestic animals include testing and slaughtering infected animals. Vaccination has been successful in sheep and goats, and in cattle. Prophylactic vaccines in humans are not feasible. The successful eradication program of bovine brucellosis in the United States has markedly reduced the incidence of human brucellosis from 3500 cases reported in 1950 to several hundred in 1970. In other parts of the world, however, animal and human brucellosis is still widespread. The disease is still prevalent in Mexico, Central and South America, much of Africa, France, Italy, Spain, the Middle East, India, Australia, Polynesia, and New Zealand.

### References

Alton, G. G., Jones, L. M., and Pietz, D. E.: Laboratory Techniques in Brucellosis. 2nd ed. Geneva, World Health Organization, 1975.

Braude, A. I.: Studies on the pathology and pathogenesis of experimental brucellosis. I. A comparison of the pathogenicity of *Brucella abortus, Brucella melitensis,* and *Brucella suis* for guinea pigs. J Inf Dis 89:76, 1951.

Brinley-Morgan, W. J., and McCullough, N. B.: *Brucella. In* Bergey's Manual of Determinative Bacteriology. 8th ed. Baltimore, The Williams & Wilkins Company, 1974, p. 278.

Garrod, L. P.: A study of the bactericidal power of hydrochloric acid and of gastric juice. St. Barth Hosp Rep 72:145, 1939.

Hall, W., and Manion, R.: In vitro susceptibility of *Brucella* to various antibiotics. Appl Microbiol 20:600, 1970.

Meyer, M. E.: Advances in research on brucellosis, 1957–1972. In Bradley, C. A., and Cornelius, C. E. (eds.): Advances in Veterinary Science and Comparative Medicine. Vol. 18. New York, Academic Press, 1974, p. 231.

Morales-Otero, P.: Experimental infection of *Brucella abortus* in man: Preliminary report. Puerto Rico J Public Health and Trop Med 5:144, 1929.

Spink, W. W.: The Nature of Brucellosis. Minneapolis, University of Minnesota Press, 1956.

Wilson, G., and Miles, A. A.: The serologic differentiation of smooth strains of the *Brucella* group. Br J Exp Pathol 13:1, 1932.

# *BORDETELLA* 35

### Jean M. Dolby, Ph.D.

*Bordetella pertussis* is virulent for man and is the cause of whooping cough. *B. parapertussis* also causes whooping cough in children, and *B. bronchiseptica* is an animal pathogen of the upper respiratory tract rarely transmissible to man.

## MORPHOLOGY

All three species are minute, gram-negative, nonacidfast coccobacilli 1 × 0.3 to 0.5 μm; *B. pertussis* is shown in Figure 1. *B. bronchiseptica* is the only motile species, and *B. pertussis* is the only one that is capsulated. Pili have been demonstrated on *B. pertussis* (Morse and Morse, 1976).

## ANTIGENIC COMPOSITION

The three members of the species are more closely related antigenically to each other than to *Haemophilus* and *Brucella*, with which one or the other has been classified. Some of the antigens are common to the genus *Bordetella*, some are shared by only two of the three species, and some are species- or even strain-specific. Most antigens are protein or lipopolysaccharide components of the bacterial cell wall.

When freshly isolated, *B. pertussis* organisms are nutritionally exacting; they can be slowly adapted to grow on less complex media. The derivative strains, growing on nutrient agar or in nutrient broth, are called Phase IV; they have lost most of the Phase I antigens (Leslie and Gardner, 1931; Standfast, 1951). Phase IV organisms can still be identified, however, because the lipopolysaccharide or their cell walls retains the ability to elicit "bactericidal antigen" as do Phase I cells (Dolby and Ackers, 1975).

More rapid loss of Phase I properties occurs in cells grown in a medium containing (a) magnesium sulfate, to give C-model cells (Lacey, 1960) or

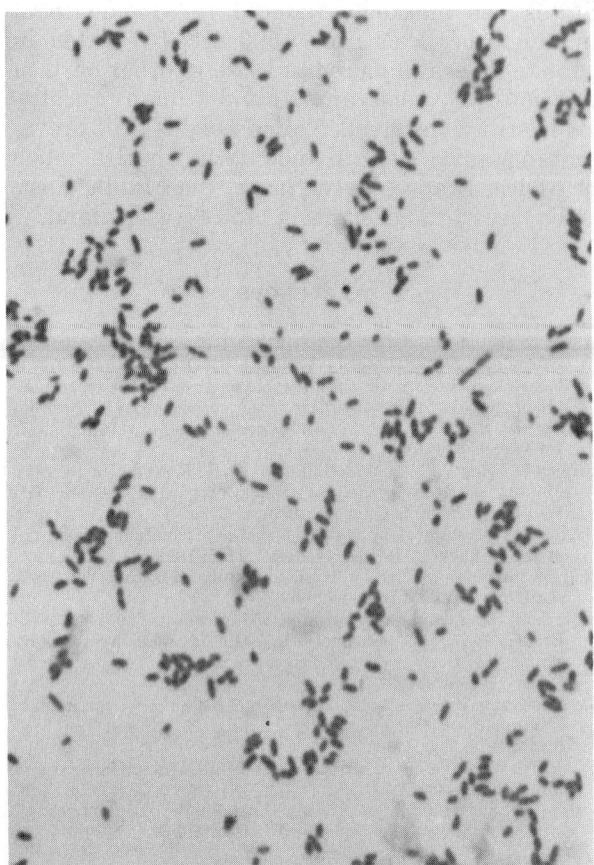

**FIGURE 1.** B. pertussis, *phase I, grown 18 hours on Bordet-Gengou agar medium at 36° C and stained with carbol-fucshin (× 3000).*

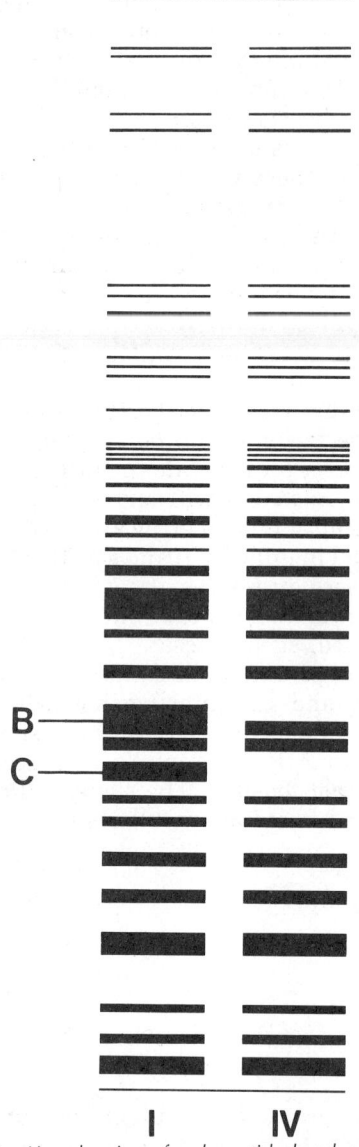

**FIGURE 2.** *Line drawing of polypeptide band patterns of SDS-polyacrylamide gel electrophoresis preparations of the cell envelopes of phase I and phase IV B. pertussis. (From Parton, R., and Wardlaw, A. C.: J Med Microbiol 8:47, 1975.)*

(b) 500 μg/ml nicotinic acid (Pusztai and Joo, 1967). Phase IV cells and C-mode cells may be similar; Phase IV cells and cells grown in high concentrations of nicotinic acid are not (Table 1). Initially at least, the loss of antigens is reversible, and cultivation on complex media causes reversion to typical Phase I cells.

By simple immunodiffusion techniques, about 20 precipitin lines denoting antigen-antibody systems of Phase I antigens can be demonstrated. By chemical methods, 35 proteins can be demonstrated in the cell walls of Phase I *B. pertussis;* Phase IV cells have only two less protein bands (Fig. 2),

which cannot account for all the antigens lost (Wardlaw et al., 1975). Electronmicroscope photographs show more differences between Phases I

**TABLE 1.  Antigenic Relationship of *B. pertussis* and Derivatives**

| ANTIGEN | PHASE I | PHASE IV | NICOTINIC-ACID-GROWN | C-MODE |
|---|---|---|---|---|
| K agglutinogens 1–6 | + | − | − | − |
| HSF, LPF[a] | + | −? | − | |
| "Bactericidal antigen" | + or ± | as ph I | as ph I | |
| "Protective antigen" | + | − | − | − |
| "Adhesion antigen" | + | − | + | |
| Antigen-stimulating opsonin | + | + | − | |
| Hemagglutinin (pili) | + | − | − | |

[a]HSF = histamine-sensitizing factor; LPF = lymphocytosis-promoting factor.

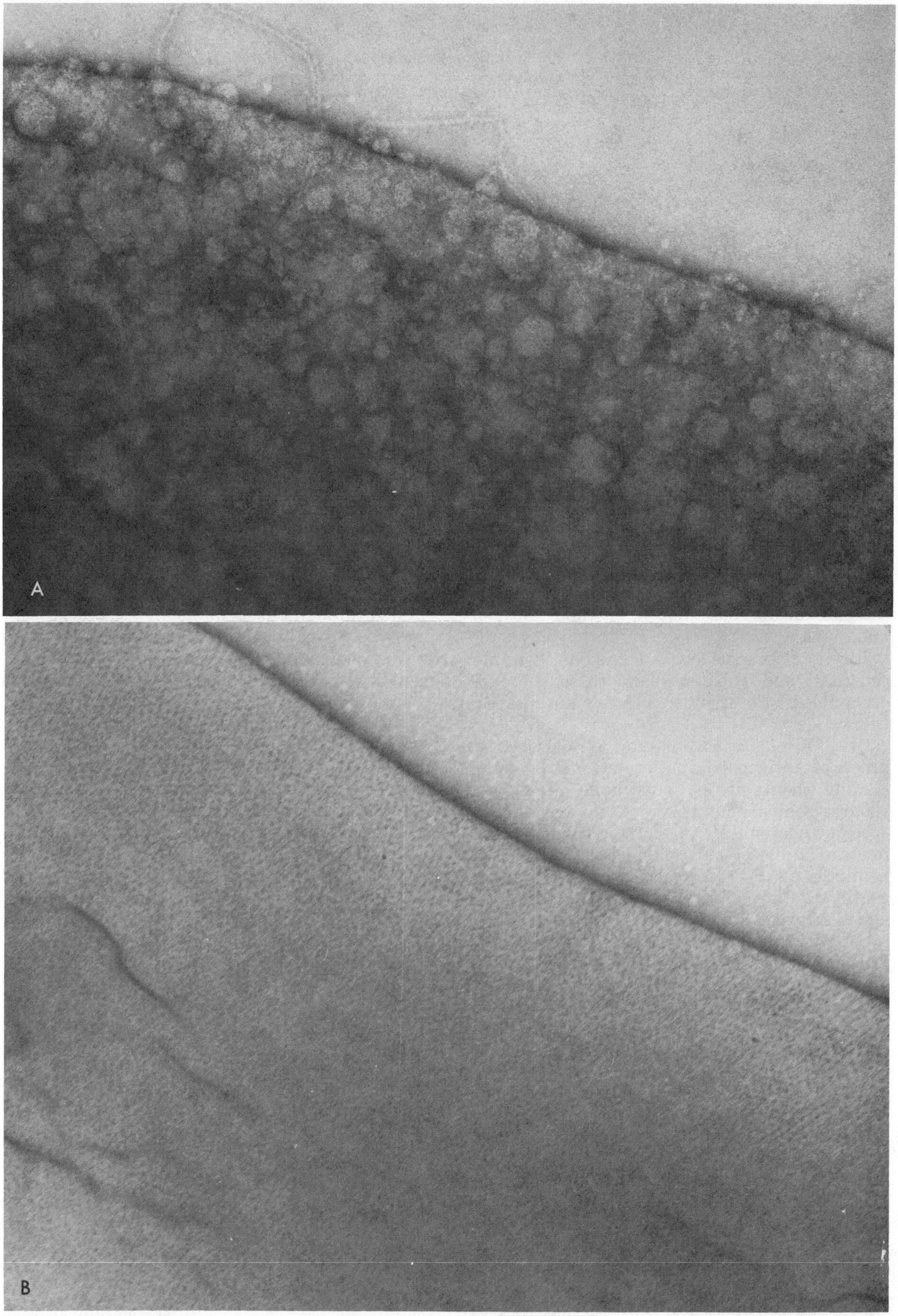

**FIGURE 3.** *Electron micrographs of B. pertussis. A,* Phase I, *and B,* Phase IV *fixed in formalin and negatively stained in uranyl acetate (× 189,900). (By permission of Dr. Alan Lawn, Poultry Research Station, Houghton, Cambridgeshire—from the Lister Institute collection.)*

**TABLE 2.  Antigenic Relationships in the Genus *Bordetella***

| | ANTIGEN | B. PERTUSSIS | B. PARAPERTUSSIS | B. BRONCHISEPTICA |
|---|---|---|---|---|
| | K agglutinogens 7–14 | 7, 13 | 7–11, 14 | 7–11, 12, 13 |
| | Toxin | + | + | + |
| | Antigen-stimulating opsonin | + | + | + |
| | Pertussis "bactericidal antigen" | + or ± | – | – |
| **Precipitinogen** | Pertussis LPS[a] | + | – | variable |
| | Parapertussis LPS | – | + | variable |
| | Bronchiseptica LPS | variable | variable | + |
| **Protection by Vaccine** | Pertussis | + | – | variable |
| | Parapertussis           against | – | + | variable |
| | Bronchiseptica | variable | variable | + |

[a]LPS = lipopolysaccharide.

and IV than are apparent from protein analysis (Fig. 3).

*B. parapertussis* and *B. bronchiseptica* grow on simple media upon isolation, and cultivation on complex media does not alter their antigenic make-up.

Table 1 lists some of the defined antigens of *B. pertussis*, and Table 2 shows those shared by other *Bordetella* organisms. A few are discussed below.

(1) The agglutinogens are a heterogeneous group of antigens that stimulate antibodies including the relatively heat-labile K antigens, protein components of the wall, and the less specific heat-stable lipopolysaccharide components. The K antigens are demonstrable in cells heated at 56° C and in vaccine but are destroyed at 100° C; they are numbered 1 through 14, of which 1 through 7 and 13 are found in *B. pertussis*, 1 through 6 being specific (Andersen, 1953; Eldering et al., 1957). Agglutinogen 1 is found in all *B. pertussis* organisms together with one or more of all of the others, usually in the combinations 3 and 6, 2 and 4. Serotypes are distinguished on the basis of agglutinogens (K antigens), which are stable characteristics with the exception of variable strains of serotypes 1,2,3 (Bronne-Shanbury and Dolby, 1976).

(2) The histamine-sensitizing factor (HSF) and lymphocyte-promoting-factor (LPF) appear to be one antigenic moiety, distinct from the hemagglutinating pili and responsible for several different biologic effects. The responsible moiety appears to be a protein in the cell wall and is composed of four subunits. When injected into mice, it produces leukocytosis and lymphocytosis (LPF) and sensitizes the mice so that they are

more susceptible to killing by histamine (HSF). This moiety also prevents the hyperglycemia that follows epinephrine injection and causes fasting hypoglycemia. The four phenomena may be mediated through effects on adenylate cyclase. This protein may also promote the formation of IgE (reaginic antibody) by eliminating the suppressor activity of T-lymphocytes (Munoz and Bergman, 1968; Morse, 1976).

(3) Hemagglutinin has been isolated as pili (Morse and Morse, 1976) and separated from the LPF with which it was thought to be associated (Sato et al., 1974). Others, however, report two hemagglutinins, one associated with LPF and one with fimbriae (Arai and Sato, 1976; Irons and MacLennan, 1978).

(4) Protective antigen (PA) is part of the cell wall and is so called because it induces immunity to infection. It was reported to be a protein 22S antigen (Sato and Nagase, 1967), but this has not been confirmed. This is the most important antigen from the standpoint of conferring immunity to whooping cough.

By the standard assay for PA in mice (see below) it has been shown not to be agglutinogen 1 (Ross and Munoz, 1971), agglutinogens 2 through 6 (Dolby and Bronne-Shanbury, 1975), HSF (Dolby, 1958), LPF (Morse, 1976), hemagglutinin (Pillemer, 1950; Masry, 1952), or the cell wall lipopolysaccharide (Ackers and Dolby, 1972). Evidence that agglutinogens may be involved in protection has been taken from experiments using other assays (Preston and Evans, 1963; Stanbridge and Preston, 1974). Recent work has suggested that a protective property is associated with the fimbrial hemagglutinin.

The antigens of *B. parapertussis* and *B. bron-*

*chiseptica* that are shared with *B. pertussis* and the species-specific ones are shown in Table 2. *B. bronchiseptica* is antigenically heterogeneous.

## METABOLISM

Phase I *B. pertussis* requires a complex medium; the original solid one of Bordet and Gengou (1906) and still used in a modified form contains starch, peptone glycerol, and 33 per cent blood. Increasingly defined liquid ones have been suggested (Cohen and Wheeler, 1946; Lacey, 1954; Stainer and Scholte, 1970) on which *B. pertussis* may be grown for a vaccine. *B. parapertussis* and *B. bronchiseptica* present no problems and can be grown on nutrient agar, broth, and citrate agar. None of them ferment carbohydrates or reduce nitrates to nitrites. *B. pertussis* does not possess a urease, but the other two do.

All three species derive energy from oxidative deamination so that suitable buffering is necessary to retain the optimum pH at about 7.6. Amino acids essential to the metabolism of *B. pertussis* are cysteine and glutamic acid or proline, without which the others cannot be utilized. Growth factors nicotinic acid, glutathione, and ferrous salt are necessary (Rowatt, 1955).

The blood in the agar medium absorbs inhibiting substances and allows growth from small inocula of *B. pertussis*. Albumin or charcoal can be used instead.

The subject has been reviewed by Rowatt (1957) and Parker (1976).

## PATHOGENIC PROPERTIES

*B. pertussis* is virulent for humans (Bordet and Gengou, 1906) and so is *B. parapertussis* (Bradford and Slavin, 1937; Eldering and Kendrick, 1938). The organisms are not invasive but attach themselves to the ciliated epithelium of the upper respiratory tract (Rich, 1932) causing catarrh, lasting about 2 weeks, and then paroxysmal coughing and "whooping," which may last 4 to 6 weeks. *B. bronchiseptica,* mainly a disease of animals, attaches to ciliated epithelium in the same way (Bemis et al., 1977). In exposed humans, it causes chronic catarrh and spasmodic cough (McGowan, 1911; Brown, 1926). In experimental situations, ciliated epithelium elsewhere can become the target of *B. pertussis,* as shown in Figure 4. The surface component of the bacterial cell upon which this attachment depends is obviously of great importance in pathogenicity. It may be the adherence antigen (Holt, 1972), hemagglutinin, or some other antigen. Toxin, common to all three species, that paralyzes the cilia

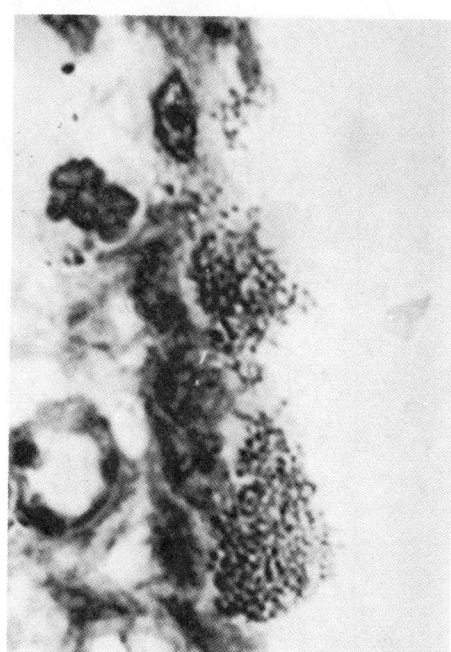

**FIGURE 4.**  B. pertussis *on the ependymal cells of mouse brain 24 hours after infection, Giemsa stain (× 1500). (From Iida, T., et al.: Jap J Exp Med 32:490, 1962.)*

may be only a minor factor in aiding lodgment (Standfast, 1958a).

Toxin may be responsible for the cough and lung tissue damage either directly or indirectly and perhaps also brain damage (Munoz, 1971; Lehrer et al., 1977).

## IMMUNITY

Successful immunization has been achieved with parenteral vaccination of children with a whole cell *B. pertussis* vaccine (Medical Research Council, 1951; 1956), and the incidence of whooping cough has been reduced to a very low level in communities with a high acceptance of vaccine (Kendrick, 1975). A cell-free but not purified absorbed bacterial extract (Pillemer, 1950) has also been effective (Medical Research Council, 1959). The effect of vaccination on pertussis in the United Kingdom is shown in Figure 5. *B. parapertussis* vaccine is similarly used with success in areas in which parapertussis is prevalent. An experimental study on vaccination in dogs with *B. bronchiseptica* has been reported (Bemis et al., 1977).

The ability of vaccine to protect mice against an intracerebral but not an intranasal challenge was correlated with the success of the vaccine in children (Standfast, 1958b), as shown in Figure 6. This correlation is the basis of the international assay of vaccine in mice (World Health Organization, 1964).

**384**

Annual live births and average whooping-cough notifications.

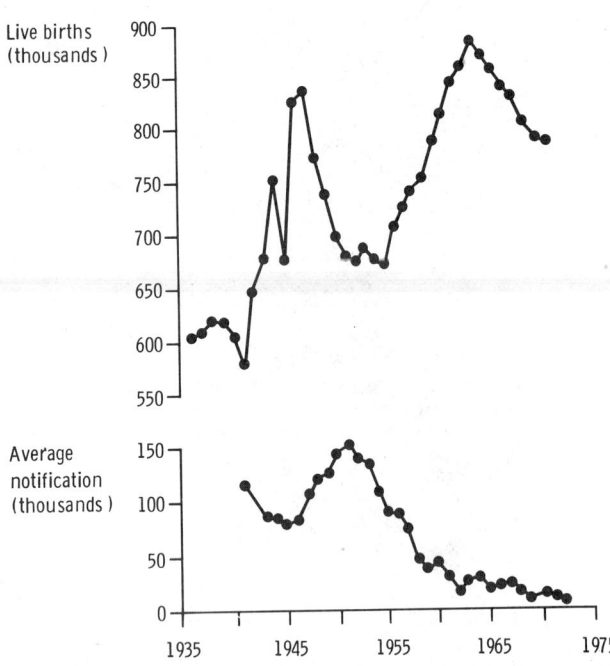

FIGURE 5. *Annual live births and average whooping cough notifications in the United Kingdom from 1940 to 1975. Wide-spread vaccination was introduced in 1957 at the time that the number of births increased — whooping cough notifications continued to decrease. (From Miller, C. L., et al.: Lancet 2:510, 1974.)*

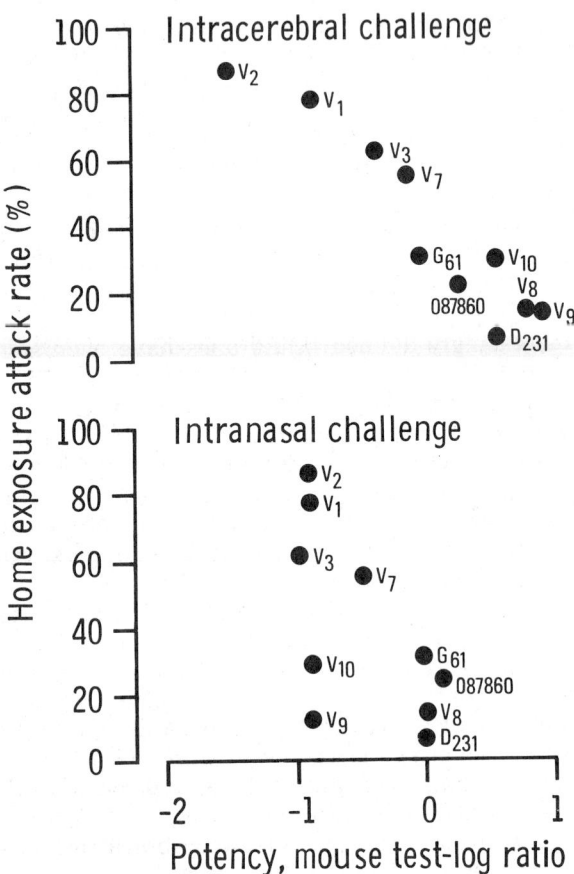

FIGURE 6. *The relationship between mouse protection tests and home exposure attack rate for ten pertussis vaccines: (top), close relationship by intracerebral mouse challenge (bottom), no relationship by intranasal mouse challenge. (From Standfast, A. F. B.: Immunology 1:135, 1958.)*

The vaccine is a suspension of inactivated cells of *B. pertussis* in Phase I, which is free from unacceptable amounts of endotoxin, heat-labile toxin, and LPF. A course consisting of a minimum of 12 units in three doses is recommended. The addition of alum, which increases antibody response and potency, is not recommended in areas in which poliomyelitis is prevalent.

Protection of the mouse against an intranasal challenge follows vaccination by all *B. pertussis* organisms, including Phase IV (Logan et al., 1959) and is due to antibody against lipopolysaccharide. Protection against an intracerebral challenge, which is correlated with child protection, can be achieved only with Phase I vaccine (Fig. 6). Both 7S and 11S immunoglobulins protect mice against intracerebral infection. Antibody in the 19S fraction is not effective unless injected intracerebrally along with the bacteria. Passive transfer of lymph node cells from immune animals is also protective, but the responsible cell type is unknown (Adams and Hopewell, 1970; Dolby et al., 1975). These antibodies may function as opsonins (Holt, 1972), but not all opsonic antibodies give protection. Mice can be immunized by repeated oral vaccine. This route may offer a new approach to human immunization (Hof et al., 1976). Host-parasite relationships in

pathogenesis and immunity to the disease have been reviewed by Pittman (1970).

## LABORATORY DIAGNOSIS

Organisms can be cultured in the 1st or 2nd week of the disease from the posterior nasopharynx by using swabs made from 16-cm lengths of thin wire wrapped with cotton wool. Unless plated immediately, the swabs should be held in a tube containing 0.2 ml of 1 per cent casamino acids and plated within 4 to 6 hours onto solid media (Bordet-Gengou or blood-charcoal medium) containing 0.25 to 0.3 unit of benzyl penicillin per ml and, if possible, 2 μg/ml of M&B 938 (4:4 diamidino phenylamine dihydrochloride) (Lacey, 1954). The identity of the isolated *Bordetella* can be checked by agglutination and growth characteristics: *B. parapertussis* grows on nutrient agar with brown pigment formation; *B. bronchiseptica* grows on nutrient agar without forming pigment.

Fluorescent-labeled antipertussis serum to a strain of 1,2,3,4 serotype has given good diagnostic results on smears from nasopharyngeal swabs (Kendrick et al., 1961). A greater success rate has been obtained by using a combination of culture and labeled antibody than by either method alone (Chalvardjian, 1966).

## DRUG SUSCEPTIBILITY

*B. pertussis* is sensitive in vitro to several antibiotics; erythromycin is best, but chloramphenicol, kanamycin, and oxytetracycline are moderately effective (Bass et al., 1969a). None of these has any effect on the course of the disease, but they reduce the infectivity of the patients (Bass et al., 1969b).

## EPIDEMIOLOGY

Pertussis and parapertussis are spread by droplet infection, particularly during the catarrhal stage. *B. parapertussis* may account for 0.5 to 5 per cent of all whooping cough (Linneman, 1977). *B. bronchiseptica* is very rare in man.

*B. pertussis* infection occurs sporadically the world over (Raska, 1970), mainly in children up to 8 to 10 years old, and an attack probably confers immunity of 15 to 20 years, or the same duration as vaccination. The disease incidence undulates (Fig. 7). Newborns are particularly susceptible, but it is still not known whether transfer of immunity from the mother to her baby is impossible, or whether transmissible immunity at child-bearing age is low (Kendrick et al., 1945).

Adult vaccination is not recommended, even though the adult population may be susceptible in countries with successful vaccination campaigns (Linneman et al., 1975). Partial immunity decreases the severity of the disease (Miller and Fletcher, 1976), which may pass undiagnosed and may be a source of subsequent infection (Kurt et al., 1972). There is probably no completely asymptomatic carrier state.

A high vaccination rate (greater than 80 per cent) can protect a community. At the beginning of a vaccination campaign, babies should be inoculated at 1, 2, and 3 months of age, but, as these grow up to be immune siblings, the vaccination of the newborn can be postponed to begin at 3 months. Later vaccination produces less general reaction to the vaccine and enables pertussis to be combined with diphtheria and tetanus toxoids (Dudgeon, 1976).

There has been concern in Northern Europe about the rare (1:100,000) brain damage to vaccinated children (Strom, 1967; Kulenkamphff et al., 1974). Such reactions are idiosyncratic and can occur after vaccine or infection (Byers and Moll, 1948). Less rare reactions from which the child recovers are shock and screaming. Decline in the acceptance of vaccine because of the ensuing reactions is an obstacle to any vaccination program. The balance of benefits and hazards in the United Kingdom has been reviewed (Department of Health and Social Security, 1977).

Over the last 30 years, there has been a change in the infecting serotype of *B. pertussis* in some countries, from predominantly 1,2,4 to 1,3,6 (Blaskett et al., 1971; Bronne-Shanbury et al., 1976). It has been suggested that this may be influenced by vaccination (Preston, 1976), particularly

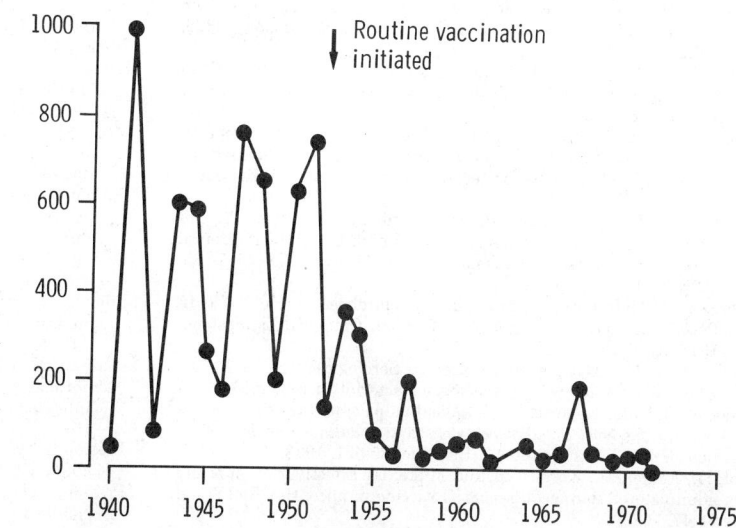

City of Oxford annual notifications of whooping cough (1940-1972)

**FIGURE 7.** *The seasonal fluctuation of* B. pertussis *in Oxfordshire, England. (From Warin, J. F.: Proc Roy Soc Med 67:374, 1974.)*

by vaccine from which one serotype is missing. Vaccine containing the main serotypes is now made, and the consequences are awaited with interest.

# References

Ackers, J. P., and Dolby, J. M.: The antigen of *Bordetella pertussis* that induces bactericidal antibody and its relationship to protection in mice. J Gen Microbiol 70:371, 1972.

Adams, G. J., and Hopewell, J. W.: Enhancement of intracerebral infection of mice with *Bordetella pertussis*. J Med Microbiol 3:15, 1970.

Andersen, E. K.: Serological studies on *H. pertussis, H. parapertussis* and *H. bronchisepticus*. Acta Pathol Microbiol Scand 33:202, 1953.

Arai, H., and Sato, Y.: Separation and characterization of two distinct haemagglutinins contained in purified leukocytosis-promoting factor from *Bordetella pertussis*. Biochem Biophys Acta 444:765, 1976.

Bass, J. W., Crast, F. W., Kotheimer, J. B., and Mitchell, I. A.: Susceptibility of *Bordetella pertussis* to 9 antimicrobial agents. Am J Dis Child *117*:276, 1969a.

Bass, J. W., Klenk, E. L., Kotheimer, J. B., Linneman, C. C., Smith, M. H. D.: Antimicrobial treatment of pertussis. J Pediatr 75:768, 1969b.

Bemis, D. A., Greisen, H. A., and Appel, M. J. G.: Pathogenesis of canine Bordetellosis. J Infect Dis 135:753, 1977.

Blaskett, A. C., Gulasekharam, L. M. S., and Fulton, L. C.: The occurrence of *Bordetella pertussis* serotypes in Australia, 1950–70. Med J Aust 1:781, 1971.

Bordet, J., and Gengou, O.: Le microbe de la coquelucheuse. Ann Inst Pasteur 23:415, 1906.

Bradford, W. C., and Slavin, B.: An organism resembling *Hemophilus pertussis*. Am J Public Health 27:1277, 1937.

Bronne-Shanbury, C. J., and Dolby, J. M.: The stability of serotypes of *Bordetella pertussis* with particular reference to serotypes 1,2,3,4. J Hyg (Camb) 76:277, 1976.

Bronne-Shanbury, C. J., Miller, D., and Standfast, A. F. B.: The serotypes of *Bordetella pertussis* isolated in Great Britain between 1941 and 1968 and a comparison with serotypes observed in other countries over this period. J Hyg (Camb) 76:265, 1976.

Brown, J. H.: *Bacillus bronchisepticus* infections in a child with symptoms of pertussis. Bull Johns Hopkins Hosp 38:147, 1926.

Byers, R. K., and Moll, F. C.: Encephalopathies following prophylactic pertussis vaccine. Pediatrics 1:437, 1948.

Chalvardjian, N.: The laboratory diagnosis of whooping-cough by fluorescent antibody and by culture methods. Can Med Assoc J 95:263, 1966.

Cohen, S. M., and Wheeler, M. W.: Pertussis vaccine prepared with Phase-I cultures grown in fluid medium. Am J Public Health 36:371, 1946.

Department of Health and Social Security: Whooping Cough Vaccination. London, Her Majesty's Stationery Office, 1977.

Dolby, J. M.: The separation of the histamine-sensitising factor from the protective antigens of *Bordetella pertussis*. Immunology 1:328, 1958.

Dolby, J. M., and Ackers, J. P.: Taxonomic distribution of the antigen eliciting bactericidal antibody for *Bordetella pertussis*. J Gen Microbiol 87:239, 1975.

Dolby, J. M., and Bronne-Shanbury, C. J.: The use of spheroplast-derived strains to differentiate between *Bordetella pertussis* heat-labile agglutinogens and protective antigen for mice. J Biol Stand 3:89, 1975.

Dolby, J. M., Dolby, D. E., and Bronne-Shanbury, C. J.: The effects of humoral, cellular and non-specific immunity on intracerebral *Bordetella pertussis* infections in mice. J Hyg (Camb) 74:85, 1975.

Dudgeon, J. A.: Immunising procedures in childhood. In Hull, D. (ed): Recent Advances in Paediatrics. London, Churchill-Livingstone, 1976, p. 169.

Eldering, G., Hornbeck, C., and Baker, J.: Serological study of *Bordetella pertussis* and related species. J Bacteriol 74:133, 1957.

Eldering, G., and Kendrick, P. L.: Bacillus para-pertussis: A species resembling both *Bacillus pertussis* and *Bacillus bronchisepticus* but identical with neither. J. Bacteriol 35:561, 1938.

Hof, H., Finger, H., Korner, L., and Milke, L.: Effectiveness of orally administered *Bordetella pertussis* vaccine in mice. Dev Biol Stand 33:47, 1976.

Holt, L. B.: The pathology and immunology of *B. pertussis* infections. J Med Microbiol 5:407, 1972.

Iida, T., Kusano, N., Yamamoto, A., and Shiga, H.: Studies on experimental infection with *Bordetella pertussis*. Bacteriological and pathological studies on the mode of infection in the mouse brain. Jpn J Exp Med 32:471, 1962.

Kendrick, P. L.: Can whooping cough be eradicated? J Infect Dis 132:707, 1975.

Kendrick, P. L., Eldering, G., and Eveland, W. C.: Fluorescent antibody techniques. Am J Dis Child 101:149, 1961.

Kendrick, P. L., Thompson, M., and Eldering, G.: Immunity response of mothers and babies to injections of pertussis vaccine during pregnancy. Am J Dis Child 70:25, 1945.

Kulenkampff, M., Schwartzmann, J. S., and Wilson, J.: Neurological complications of pertussis inoculation. Arch Dis Child 49:46, 1974.

Kurt, T. L., Yeager, A. S., Guenette, S., and Dunlop, S.: Spread of pertussis by hospital staff. J Am Med Assoc 221:264, 1972.

Lacey, B. W.: A new selective medium for *Haemophilus pertussis* containing a diamidine, sodium fluoride and penicillin J. Hyg (Camb) 52:273, 1954.

Lacey, B. W.: Antigenic modulation of *Bordetella pertussis*. J Hyg (Camb) 58:57, 1960.

Lehrer, S. B., Nakamura, R. M., and Tan, E. M.: Histopathological changes in mice treated with extracts of histamine sensitising factor of *Bordetella pertussis*. Int Arch Allergy Appl Immunol 54:129, 1977.

Leslie, P. H., and Gardner, A. D.: The phases of *Haemophilus pertussis*. J Hyg (Camb) 31:423, 1931.

Linneman, C. C.: *Bordetella parapertussis*. Recent experience and review of literature. Am J Dis Child 131:560, 1977.

Linneman, C. C., Ramundo, N., Perlstein, P. H., Minton, S. D., Englender, G. S., McCormick, J. B., and Hayes, P. S.: Use of pertussis vaccine in an epidemic involving hospital staff. Lancet 2:540, 1975.

Logan, J. E., Griffiths, B. W., and Mason, M. A.: Specificity of the clearance phenomenon in the lungs of pertussis-immunised mice following intratracheal administration of radio-iodinated pertussis vaccine. Can J Microbiol 5:405, 1959.

McGowan, J. P.: Some observations on a laboratory epidemic principally among dogs and cats in which animals affected presented the symptoms of the disease called 'distemper.' J Pathol Bact 15:372, 1911.

Masry, F. L. G.: Production, extraction and purification of the haemagglutinin of *Haemophilus pertussis*. J Gen Microbiol 7:201, 1952.

Medical Research Council: Vaccination against whooping cough. Investigation. Br Med J 1:1464, 1951; Relation between protection of children and laboratory tests. Ibid 2:454, 1956; Final report. Ibid 1:994, 1959.

Miller, C. L., and Fletcher, W. B.: Severity of notified whooping cough. Br Med J 1:117, 1976.

Miller, C. L., Pollock, T. M., and Clewer, A. D. E.: Whooping cough vaccine, an assessment. Lancet 2:510, 1974.

Morse, S. I.: Biologically active components and properties of *Bordetella pertussis*. Adv Appl Microbiol 20:9, 1976.

Morse, S. I., and Morse, J. H.: Isolation and properties of the leukocytosis- and lymphocytosis-promoting factor of *Bordetella pertussis*. J Exp Med *143*:1483, 1976.

Munoz, J. J.: Protein toxins from *Bordetella pertussis*. In Kadis, S., Montie, T. C., and Ajl, S. J. (eds.): Microbial Toxins. Vol. IIA. New York, Academic Press, 1971, p. 271.

Munoz, J. J., and Bergman, R. K.: Histamine-sensitising factors from microbial agents, with special reference to *Bordetella pertussis*. Bacteriol Rev 32:103, 1968.

Parker, C.: Role of the genetics and physiology of *Bordetella pertussis* in the production of vaccine and the study of host-parasite relationships in pertussis. Adv Appl Microbiol 20:27, 1976.

Parton, R., and Wardlaw, A. C.: Cell envelope proteins of *Bordetella pertussis*. J Med Microbiol 8:47, 1975.

Pillemer, L.: Adsorption of protective antigen of *Hemophilus pertussis* on human red cell stromata. Proc Soc Exp Biol Med 75:704, 1950.

Pittman, M.: *Bordetella pertussis* — bacterial, and host factors in the pathogenesis and prevention of whooping cough. In Mudd, S. (ed.): Infectious agents and host reactions. W. B. Saunders Co., p. 239, 1970.

Preston, N. W.: Prevalent serotypes of *Bordetella pertussis* in nonvaccinated communities. J Hyg (Camb) 77:85, 1976.

Preston, N W., and Evans, P.: Type specific immunity against intracerebral pertussis infection in mice. Nature 197:508, 1963.

Pusztai, S., and Joo, I.: Influence of nicotinic acid on the antigenic structure of *Bordetella pertussis*. Ann Immunol Hung 10:63, 1967.

Raska, K.: Whooping cough: Epidemiological situation in the world. Symposia Series in Immunobiological Standardisation 13:4, 1970.

Rich, A. R.: On the aetiology and pathogenesis of whooping cough. Bull Johns Hopkins Hosp 51:346, 1932.

Ross, R. F., and Munoz, J. J.: Antigens of *Bordetella pertussis*. V. Separation of agglutinogen 1 and mouse-protective activity. Infect Immun 3:243, 1971.

Rowatt, E.: Amino-acid metabolism in the genus *Bordetella*. J Gen Microbiol 13:552, 1955.

Rowatt, E.: Growth requirements of *Bordetella pertussis:* A review. J Gen Microbiol 17:279, 1957.

Sato, Y., Arai, H., and Suzuki, K.: Leucocytosis-promoting factor of *Bordetella pertussis*. III. Its identity with protective antigen. Infect Immun 9:801, 1974.

Sato, Y., and Nagase, K.: Isolation of protective antigen from *Bordetella pertussis*. Biochem Biophys Res Commun 27:195, 1967.

Stainer, D. W., and Scholte, M. J.: A simple, chemically defined medium for the production of phase I *Bordetella pertussis*. J Gen Microbiol 63:211, 1970.

Stanbridge, T. N., and Preston, N. W.: Experimental pertussis infection in the marmoset: Type specificity of active immunity. J. Hyg (Camb) 72:213, 1974.

Standfast, A. F. B.: The phase I of *Haemophilus pertussis*. J Gen Microbiol 5:531, 1951.

Standfast, A. F. B.: Some factors influencing the virulence in mice of *Bordetella pertussis* by the intracerebral route. Immunology 1:123, 1958a.

Standfast, A. F .B.: Comparison between field trials and mouse protection tests against intranasal and intracerebral challenges with *Bordetella pertussis*. Immunology 1:135, 1958b.

Strom, J.: Further experience of reactions, especially of a cerebral nature in conjunction with triple vaccination. Br Med J 4:320, 1967.

Wardlaw, A. C., Parton, R., and Hooker, M. J.: Loss of protective antigen, histamine sensitising factor and envelope polypeptides in cultural variants of *Bordetella pertussis*. J Med Microbiol 9:89, 1975.

Warin, J. F.: Immunisation: Balancing the risks. Proc R Soc Med 67:374, 1974.

World Health Organisation: Requirements for pertussis vaccine. Technical Reports Series No. 274, 25–40, 1964.

# HAEMOPHILUS 36

## Mogens Kilian, D.D.S., Ph.D.

The organisms of the genus *Haemophilus* are small, gram-negative, nonmotile, and nonspore-forming, facultatively anaerobic rods, which require accessory factors for in vitro growth. The name of the genus refers to the fact that these growth factors are contained in blood cells and may be supplied to ordinary growth media by the addition of blood or its derivatives.

### HISTORY

The German bacteriologist Robert Koch was the first to observe bacteria of the genus *Haemophilus* during his examinations of conjunctivitis exudates in Egypt (Koch, 1883). However, the isolation and description of another Haemophilus organism in 1892 by Koch's colleague Richard Pfeiffer caused more sensation (Pfeiffer, 1892). Pfeiffer's bacillus was isolated from purulent sputum and postmortem lung cultures of patients succumbing to influenza during the pandemic of 1889 through 1892. The discovery was published as "the exciting cause of influenza," and the organism was accordingly designated *Haemophilus influenzae* by a committee of the American Society of Bacteriologists. Following the discovery in 1933 of the influenza virus, the actual etiologic agent of epidemic influenza, interest in *H. influenzae* vanished for several years.

The precise role played by *H. influenzae* in the pandemic of 1890 and again in that of 1918 through 1919 is still not clear. The view was held by a number of investigators of the 1918 pandemic that the unprecedented severity of the disease reflected the concurrent interplay of a virus and Pfeiffer's bacillus. This thesis was strengthened by the subsequent demonstration by Shope (1931) that the synergistic effect of a Haemophilus organism (*H. suis*) and swine influenza virus is essential for both natural and experimental swine influenza. Because *H. influenzae* has clearly not played a similar part in more recent pandemics, the importance of viral and bacterial synergism in the pathogenesis of the human disease needs further study (Michaels et al., 1977).

### MORPHOLOGY

Bacteria of the genus *Haemophilus* tend to be pleomorphic (Fig. 1). In samples of pathologic material such as cerebrospinal fluid, the bacteria are predominantly coccobacillary, sometimes simulating diplococci and erroneously suspected of being meningococci or pneumococci. In older cultures, or when grown under unfavorable conditions, the rods become elongated and frequently appear filamentous. The pleomorphic appearance is most prominent among the X-factor independent species.

Strains of *H. influenzae* may have capsules that are readily demonstrable only in young cultures. After 24 hours of incubation, the capsules often

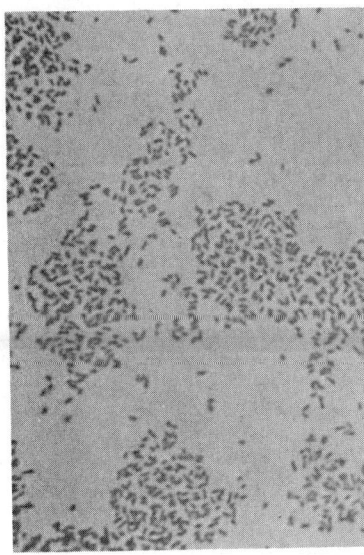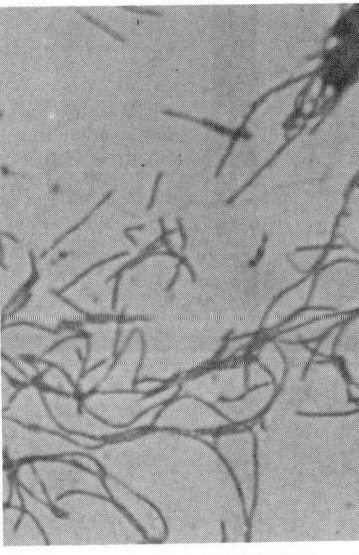

**FIGURE 1.** *Variations in microscopic appearance of Hemophilus organisms (Gram-stained smears × 800).*

disappear. Capsular material is shed into liquid culture media during growth.

Colonies formed on solid media are 1 to 3 mm long after incubation for 24 hours. Young cultures (8 to 18 hours) of encapsulated strains on translucent solid media are characteristically iridescent (produce a rainbow effect) when examined in obliquely transmitted light. Strains of some species are β-hemolytic (Table 1).

## ANTIGENIC COMPOSITION

Virtually all strains of *H. influenzae* isolated from invasive infections possess capsules. The capsular material evokes antibodies that protect against infection. Six distinct antigenic types, designated a through f, have been described by Pittman (1931). The capsular material of all six types are polysaccharides, and all except those of Types d and e contain phosphorus. Strains causing meningitis and other acute illnesses virtually all belong to serotype b. The capsule of this serotype is a polymer of ribose- and ribitolphosphate. It is structurally and serologically closely related to the cell-wall teichoic acid of grampositive bacteria and the capsular polysaccharides of certain serotypes of pneumococci and certain enterobacteria (Table 2) (Alexander, 1958; Argaman et al., 1974; Bradshaw et al., 1971).

Very little is known about the somatic antigens of *H. influenzae*. A protein common to all types has been described, as well as an endotoxin that resembles those from other gram-negative bacteria.

## METABOLISM

Haemophilus organisms grow very poorly on ordinary laboratory media. The hemophilic nature of these bacteria is due to their inability to carry out the biosynthesis of either one or two substances present in blood cells (as well as in most other cells). The two growth factors were first recognized as a heat-stable substance referred to as the *X-factor* and a heat-labile substance referred to as the *V-factor*. The requirement for these factors has been used for the definition of the genus as well as for its internal subdivision into species. *H. influenzae* thus requires both X- and V-factors for growth, whereas most other species require only one (Table 1).

Both X- and V-factors are of vital importance in the metabolism and growth of living cells. The X-factor is used in the biosynthesis of respiratory cytochromes and has been identified as hematin or certain precursors. The V-factor, which is involved in oxidation-reduction processes, can be replaced by one of the two co-dehydrogenases, NAD or NADP (Lwoff and Lwoff, 1937a, b).

Optimal growth occurs in rich media to which the two growth factors have been added. The growth on ordinary blood agar is very poor, since only the X-factor is directly available to the bacteria in satisfactory quantities. Both growth factors may be liberated into the medium either by peptic digestion of the blood (Fildes medium) or by briefly heating the medium (chocolate agar and Levinthal's medium).

Various microorganisms (e.g., staphylococci) excrete the V-factor and may support the growth of haemophili on media deficient in this growth

**TABLE 1.  Principal Differential Characteristics and Primary Habitat
of the Common Species of the Genus *Haemophilus***

|  | X-FACTOR REQUIRED[a] | V-FACTOR REQUIRED | HEMOLYSIS | INDOLE | GLUCOSE, ACID | SUCROSE, ACID | LACTOSE, ACID | XYLOSE, ACID | NITRATE REDUCTION | PRIMARY HABITAT |
|---|---|---|---|---|---|---|---|---|---|---|
| *H. influenzae* | + | + | − | d[b] | + | − | − | + | + | pharynx |
| *H. haemolyticus* | + | + | + | d | + | − | − | + | + | pharynx |
| *H. ducreyi* | + | − | − | − | − | − | − | − | + | (genital organs) |
| *H. parainfluenzae* | − | + | d | − | + | + | − | − | + | oral cavity and pharynx |
| *H. aphrophilus* | − | − | − | − | + | + | + | − | + | oral cavity |
| *H. paraphrophilus* | − | + | − | − | + | + | + | − | + | oral cavity |

[a]X-factor requirement as determined by the porphyrin test (Kilian, 1974). Ref.: Kilian, 1976.
[b]d = differences observed

factor. This satellite phenomenon, which is illustrated in Figure 2, is widely used for the demonstration of this growth requirement.

All *Haemophilus* species reduce nitrate, and all, except for *H. ducreyi*, are heterofermentative. In addition to the requirement for growth factors, fermentation reactions and other biochemical characteristics are useful for the identification of the *Haemophilus* species (Table 1). Virtually all strains of *H. influenzae* isolated from meningitis produce indole and ornithine decarboxylase, characters that are rarely encountered concurrently among nasopharyngeal commensals of the same species (Kilian, 1976).

## PATHOGENIC PROPERTIES

### H. Influenzae

The infections in which *H. influenzae* is a primary etiologic agent are almost invariably due to encapsulated strains of serotype b, and they are diseases usually associated with bacteremia. The most important of these are meningitis and epiglottitis.

*H. influenzae* (serotype b) is among the three leading causes of bacterial meningitis, the two others being meningococci and the pneumococci. *Haemophilus* meningitis is, however, more strictly a disease of early childhood than are the two other forms. About 80 per cent of all cases occur between the age of 2 months and the end of the 3rd year, and most of the rest occur during the next few years (Fig. 3). Adults are rarely affected.

Epiglottitis is another serious disease caused by *H. influenzae* serotype b, although less common. As with meningitis, the patients are children but usually somewhat older.

Invasion of the bloodstream by *H. influenzae* (usually serotype b) frequently results in suppurative arthritis, osteomyelitis, and pericarditis. Primary *H. influenzae* pneumonia occurs in children as well as in adults but is an uncommon condition.

*H. influenzae* is a common and important cause of surface infection of mucous membranes of the respiratory tract and attached sinuses. Such in-

**TABLE 2.  Bacterial Species Possessing Antigens
Cross-Reactive with the Capsular Material of
*H. influenzae* Type b**

*Bacillus alvei*
*Bacillus pumilus*
*Escherichia coli* K 100
*Lactobacillus plantarum*
*Staphylococcus aureus*
*Staphylococcus epidermidis*
*Streptococcus faecalis*
*Streptococcus pneumoniae* types 6, 15a, 29, 35a
*Streptococcus pyogenes* (group A)

Refs.: Alexander, 1965; Argaman *et al.,* 1974; Bradshaw *et al.,* 1971.

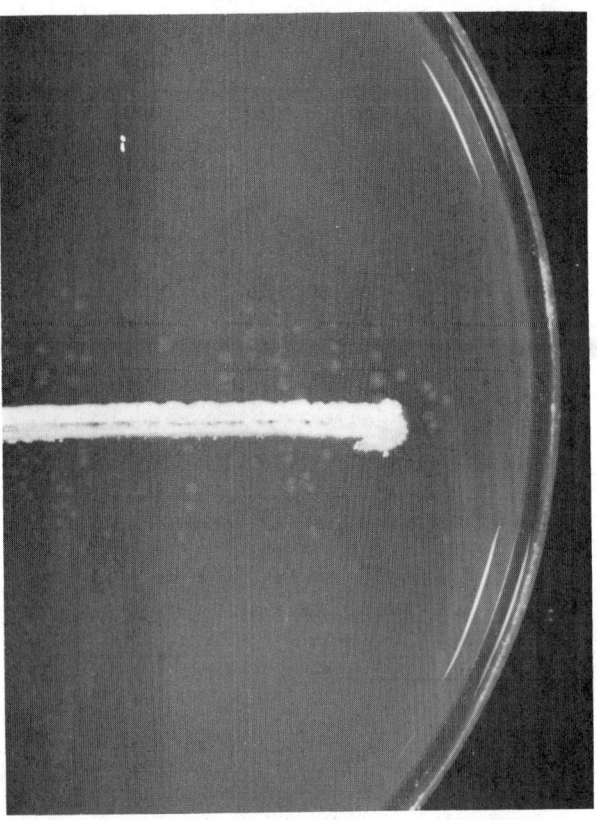

**FIGURE 2.** *Satellite phenomenon: Colonies of H. influenzae growing on an agar plate cross-inoculated with a staphylococcus. The agar medium is autoclaved blood agar that lacks the V-factor.*

fections are secondary to the breakdown of local resistance, as in bronchitis, bronchiectasis, cystic fibrosis, otitis media, and chronic sinusitis. The responsible organisms are usually noncapsulated nasopharyngeal commensals, which enter the normally sterile locations after viruses, allergic reactions, or dysfunctions have initiated the inflammatory processes. The conditions, which appear as acute exacerbations of chronic inflammation, usually respond to chemotherapy. Infection often recurs owing to recolonization with the same or other commensals.

Likewise, lowered resistance of the conjunctival mucosae due to trachomatous or viral infection or obstruction of the lacrimal duct may lead to colonization with noncapsulated *H. influenzae* organisms from the respiratory tract. A hemagglutinating variety of *H. influenzae,* the Koch-Weeks bacillus ("*H. aegyptius*") is associated with a more acute, purulent, and contagious form of conjunctivitis. This disease occurs as seasonal endemics, especially in hot climates.

Capsulation has a bearing upon pathogenicity in the invasive diseases caused by *H. influenzae.* As with pneumococci and meningococci, the polysaccharide capsule protects the organism against phagocytosis. However, the properties that determine the ability of *H. influenzae* serotype b strains to colonize and invade the mucosa of the respiratory tract are largely unknown. There is no evidence that haemophili produce an exotoxin.

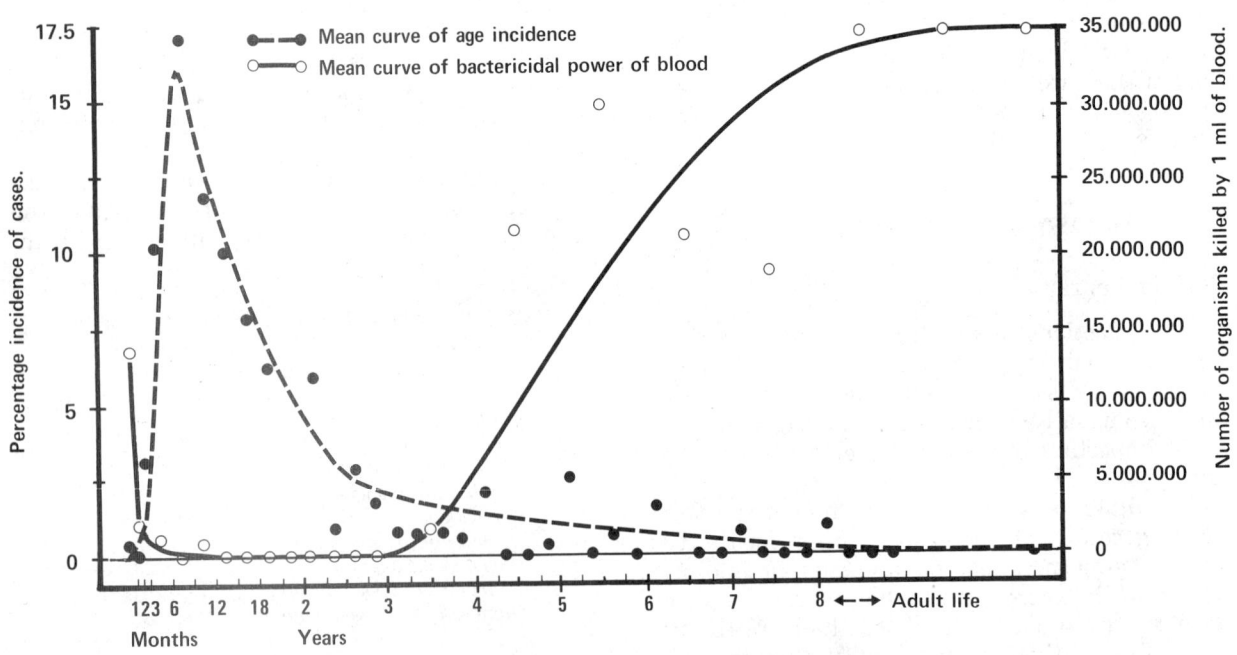

**FIGURE 3.** *Relation of the age incidence of* H. influenzae *meningitis to bactericidal activity in the blood. (From Fothergill, L. D., and Wright, J.: J Immunol 24:281, 1933. © (1933) The Williams & Wilkins Co., Baltimore.)*

The endotoxin of some strains may cause lethal toxic injury in animals when it is injected in large doses, but there is no conclusive evidence that it plays a significant role in the pathogenicity for humans.

It has recently been discovered that strains of *H. influenzae,* meningococci, and pneumococci produce an enzyme that specifically cleaves immunoglobulin A (subclass 1). This property, which is lacking in nonpathogenic species of the same genera, may prove to be an important virulence factor.

### H. ducreyi

This organism was first described by Ducrey (1889) in purulent discharge from the venereal disease "soft chancre" or "chancroid." The organism is recognized as the etiologic agent of the disease. However, it is often isolated together with poorly staining, gram-positive rods, which have been misidentified as *H. ducreyi.* In purulent material collected from ulcerative lesions or bubonic lymph nodes, the organism appears as chains of small gram-negative coccobacilli often located intracellularly.

### Other Haemophilus Species

The species found indigenously in the oral cavity, *H. parainfluenzae, H. aphrophilus,* and *H. paraphrophilus,* like other oral bacteria, occasionally cause subacute endocarditis and brain abscesses in predisposed patients. *H. haemolyticus* occurs in the healthy upper respiratory tract and is nonpathogenic. Its β-hemolytic colonies may be mistaken for those of hemolytic streptococci on blood agar.

## *IMMUNITY*

Both *H. influenzae* meningitis and epiglottitis are caused by strains possessing a capsule of serotype b, and anticapsular antibodies, which promote phagocytosis, are protective against disease. Apart from showing distinctive clinical and epidemiologic features, patients who develop meningitis and epiglottiditis also show different serum antibody responses (Whisnant et al., 1976). Children with *H. influenzae* meningitis develop surprisingly low levels of antibodies against the capsular material (Norden et al., 1976). The convalescent-phase levels of antibody after meningitis are even lower than levels found in healthy, age-matched siblings. In patients less than 2 years of age, an antibody response is even undetectable (Anderson et al., 1972; Sell and Karzon, 1973). However, this apparent failure of some children to respond to the invasion of this organism is not due to a general deficiency in immunoglobulin production and may, therefore, suggest some limited and genetically determined specific deficiency in immune response to this particular antigen.

The characteristic age distribution of *H. influenzae* meningitis has been shown by Fothergill and Wright (1933) to be inversely related to that of a serum factor bactericidal to the causative organism (Fig. 3). This finding was used to support the hypothesis that immunity in the newborn is passively acquired from the mother transplacentally, is lost within the first months of life, and then is gradually restored by natural immunization during childhood. However, the serum bactericidal activity detected by these authors does not seem to be caused only by anticapsular antibodies but also by antibodies directed against somatic antigens (Mpairwe, 1971). Although the evaluation of the importance of these latter antibodies is still indirect, resistance to *H. influenzae* Type b meningitis is probably determined by a combined action of anticapsular antibodies, which promote phagocytosis, and complement-dependent bacteriolytic antibodies directed against one or more somatic antigens.

In contrast to meningitis patients, children with epiglottiditis react with high levels of antibody to the capsular antigen of *H. influenzae* Type b. The magnitude of the antibody response correlates with increasing age of the patients. Although the pathogenesis of the disease is largely unknown, the dramatic changes taking place in the epiglottis are likely to be a result of a local allergic reaction.

Acute sinusitis, otitis media, or bronchial infection due to noncapsulated *H. influenzae* strains results in significantly raised serum levels of complement-fixing antibodies against somatic antigens. Detection of this antibody response may be used as a diagnostic tool (Turk and May, 1967).

The contribution of secretory antibodies of the IgA type to resistance against *H. influenzae* infection is still unknown.

Because of the relative rarity of *H. influenzae* Type b in the normal population, the wide prevalence of anticapsular antibodies in normal adults has been difficult to explain. However, there is growing evidence that "natural" antibodies, and hence protective immunity to this organism, is due in part to antigenic stimulation by cross-immunogenic substances in the normal bacterial flora of the body (Table 2).

## *LABORATORY DIAGNOSIS*

Haemophili do not survive well in clinical specimens. Whenever possible a suitable transport medium should be used for transportation of swabs for throat or nose cultures or scrapings from the conjunctivae or chancroid lesions.

If gram-negative rods resembling *H. influenzae* are found in normally sterile material, such as cerebrospinal fluid or pleural fluid, an immediate diagnosis can be made by exposing the organisms in the fluid to a specific anticapsular antiserum. The diagnosis is established if capsular swelling (positive quellung-reaction) is observed. Even in the absence of visible bacteria, a precipitin test (counter immunoolectrophoresis) for free capsular material may give the diagnosis. Blood culture is important in establishing the diagnosis in the invasive diseases caused by *H. influenzae*, especially in epiglottiditis, since recovery of *H. influenzae* by swabbing the epiglottis is unreliable.

Likewise, smears of scrapings from conjunctivae or chancroid lesions, although not diagnostic, are clinically useful, since recovery of the infectious agent of these diseases is often unsuccessful.

Cultivation of clinical samples for *H. influenzae* is performed on chocolate (heated blood) agar, (Fildes enrichment agar), or ordinary blood agar cross-inoculated with a staphylococcus (Fig. 2). For primary isolation from sources such as the respiratory tract, advantage may be taken of the selective action of bacitracin (300 mg/l). *H. ducreyi* may be cultivated on an agar medium containing 30 per cent freshly drawn rabbit blood or chocolate agar supplemented with 10 per cent Iso-Vitalex plus vancomycin 5 $\mu$g/ml (Hammond et al., 1978). Incubation of agar plates is performed in a mixture of air plus 5 to 10 per cent extra carbon dioxide (candle jar).

Identification of isolated strains is done by determining the growth factor requirements and by performing selected biochemical tests (Table 1). The V-factor requirement can be demonstrated by observing the satellite phenomenon, preferably on autoclaved blood agar. The X-factor requirement is difficult to determine on agar media, since most media contain small quantities of hematin. It is most clearly established by a biochemical detection of the in vitro ability of strains to carry out some of the steps involved in the biosynthesis of hematin (porphyrin test) (Kilian, 1974).

## DRUG SUSCEPTIBILITY

Most Haemophilus strains are susceptible to penicillin and its derivatives, chloramphenicol, sulfonamides, trimethoprim, and the tetracycline group. These antibiotics have been extensively used to treat infections caused by these organisms. For the treatment of *Haemophilus* meningitis, chloramphenicol and ampicillin are particularly effective. However, since 1974 an increasing number of *Haemophilus* isolates have been found to be resistant to ampicillin due to plasmid-mediated $\beta$-lactamase production (Katz, 1975; Sykes et al., 1975). In areas of the world with extensive use of antibacterial drugs, the prevalence of ampicillin resistance among *Haemophilus* strains is approaching 10 per cent. More recently, plasmid-mediated resistance against chloramphenicol and tetracycline have likewise been recorded. The choice of initial therapy in acute *Haemophilus* infections should, at present, depend on the prevalence of resistance to ampicillin and chloramphenicol in the particular area. Subsequent revision of the chemotherapy is done according to the results of the bacteriologic examination.

## EPIDEMIOLOGY

Haemophili form part of the normal flora of the upper respiratory tract and oral cavity soon after birth. The predominant species in the pharynx is *H. influenzae*, which is virtually absent from the oral cavity (Table 1). The majority of *H. influenzae* strains found in the indigenous flora are noncapsulated and differ biochemically from strains producing invasive diseases. The carriage rate of capsulated strains of *H. influenzae* seldom exceeds 5 per cent, although it may be considerably higher in closed communities of children (Kilian, 1976).

Over a recent 25-year period, *H. influenzae* Type b infection has shown both relative and absolute increases in incidence (Sell and Karzan, 1973). Statistics from the United States indicate that, before the age of 5 years, one in 400 to 500 children will contract *Haemophilus* meningitis. The attack rate in blacks appears to be higher.

*Haemophilus* meningitis occurs almost always sporadically. The infectious organism spreads from healthy carriers, but case-to-case spread of *Haemophilus* meningitis is very rare. Asymptomatic nasopharyngeal carriage of *H. influenzae* Type b is common in homes in which *Haemophilus* meningitis occurs. It seems that the organism must pass through one or two partially immune contacts before it can cross the meningeal barrier.

The unpredictability of *Haemophilus* meningitis deprives us of any practicable means of preventing it. Prophylactic chemotherapy is indicated only in special situations in which younger children are at high risk. The effect of an experimental vaccine prepared from purified polyribophosphate from the capsule of *H. influenzae* Type b has been studied. Immunization is well tolerated, but a significant antibody response is only achieved in adults and children older than 2 years (Anderson et al., 1972).

## References

Alexander, H. E.: The Hemophilus group. In Dubos, R. J. (ed.): Bacterial and Mycotic Infections in Man. 3rd ed. Philadelphia, J.B. Lippincott Company, 1958, p. 470.

Anderson, P., Peter, G., Johnston, R., Jr., Wetterlow, L. H., and Smith, D. H.: Immunization of humans with polyribophosphate, the capsular antigen of *Hemophilus influenzae*, type b. J Clin Invest 51:39, 1972.

Argaman, M., Liu, T-Y., and Robbins, J. B.: Polyribitolphosphate: An antigen of four gram-positive bacteria cross-reactive with the capsular polysaccharide of *Haemophilus influenzae* type b. J Immunol 112:649, 1974.

Bradshaw, M. W., Schneerson, R., Parke, F. C., and Robbins, F. B.: Bacterial antigens cross-reactive with the capsular polysaccharide of *Haemophilus influenzae* type b. Lancet 1:1095, 1971.

Fothergill, L. D., and Wright, J.: Influenzal meningitis: The relation of age-incidence to the bactericidal power of blood against the causal organism. J. Immunol 24:273, 1933.

Hammond, G. W., Lean, C. J., Wilt, S. C., and Ronald, A. R.: Comparison of specimen collection and laboratory techniques for the isolation of *Haemophilus ducreyi*. J Clin Microbiol 7:39, 1978.

Katz, S. L.: Ampicillin-resistant *Haemophilus influenzae* type b: A status report. Pediatrics 55:6, 1975.

Kilian, M.: A rapid method for the differentiation of *Haemophilus* strains. The porphyrin test. Acta Pathol Microbiol Scand [8] 82:835, 1974.

Kilian, M.: A taxonomic study of the genus *Haemophilus*, with the proposal of new species. J Gen Microbiol 93:9, 1976.

Koch, R.: Bericht über die Thätigkeit der deutschen Cholerakommision in Aegypten und Ostindien. Wien Med Wochenschr 33:1548, 1883.

Lwoff, A., and Lwoff, M.: Role physiologique de l'hémine pour *Haemophilus influenzae*. Pfeiffer. Ann Inst Pasteur 59:129, 1937a.

Lwoff, A., and Lwoff, M.: Studies on codehydrogenases. I. Nature of growth factor "V". Proc Royal Soc B 122:352, 1937b.

Michaels, R. H., Myerowitz, R. L., and Klaw, R.: Potentiation of experimental meningitis due to *Haemophilus influenzae* by influenza A virus. J Infect Dis 135:641, 1977.

Mpairwe, Y.: Immunity to *Haemophilus influenzae* type b: The nature of the bactericidal antibody in human blood. J Med Microbiol 4:43, 1971.

Norden, C. W., Michaels, R. H., and Melish, M.: Serologic responses of children with meningitis due to *Haemophilus influenzae* type b. J Infect Dis 134:495, 1976.

Pfeiffer, R.: The influenza bacillus. I. Preliminary communication on the exciting causes of influenza. Br Med J:i:128, 1892.

Pittman, M.: Variation and type specificity in the bacterial species *Haemophilus influenzae*. J Exp Med 53:471, 1931.

Sell, S. H. W., and Karzon, D. T. (eds.): *Hemophilus influenzae*. Nashville, Vanderbilt University Press, 1973.

Shope, R. E.: Swine influenza: Experimental transmission and pathology. J Exp Med 54:349, 1931.

Sykes, R. B., Matthew, M., and O'Callaghan, C. H.: R-factor mediated β-lactamase production by *Haemophilus influenzae*. J Med Microbiol 8:437, 1975.

Turk, D. C., and May, J. R.: *Hemophilus influenzae*. Its clinical importance. London, The English Universities Press Ltd., 1967.

Whisnant, J. K., Rogentine, G. N., Gralnick, M. A., Schlesselman, J. J., and Robbins, J. B.: Host factors and antibody response in *Haemophilus influenzae* type b meningitis and epiglottitis. J Infect Dis 133:448, 1976.

# *YERSINIA, PASTEURELLA, AND FRANCISELLA* **37**

## T. H. Chen, M.D., and
## Sanford S. Elberg, Ph.D.

The new genus *Yersinia*, of the family Enterobacteriaceae, comprises the species *Y. pestis*, *Y. pseudotuberculosis*, and *Y. enterocolitica* (Bergey's Manual of Determinative Bacteriology, 1974). *Pasteurella* is now restricted to the type species *P. multocida* and a number of other closely related animal pathogens. *Francisella tularensis* is a species of another new genus, *Francisella*. These microorganisms are the causes of plague (*Y. pestis*), yersiniosis (*Y. pseudotuberculosis* and *Y. enterocolitica*), pasteurellosis (*P. multocida* et al.), and tularemia (*F. tularensis*). Although they are primarily rodent, other mammalian, and fowl parasites, they are also responsible for severe human infections.

# YERSINIA PESTIS AND PLAGUE

### *MORPHOLOGY*

*Yersinia pestis*, the causative agent of plague, was independently discovered by Kitasato and Yersin during the great epidemic in Hong Kong in 1894 (Bibel and Chen, 1976). The bacilli (small, oval, pleomorphic rods with rounded ends) are nonmotile and form no spores. They vary considerably in size (average $1.5 \times 0.7$ $\mu$m), stain readily with the basic aniline dyes, and are gram-

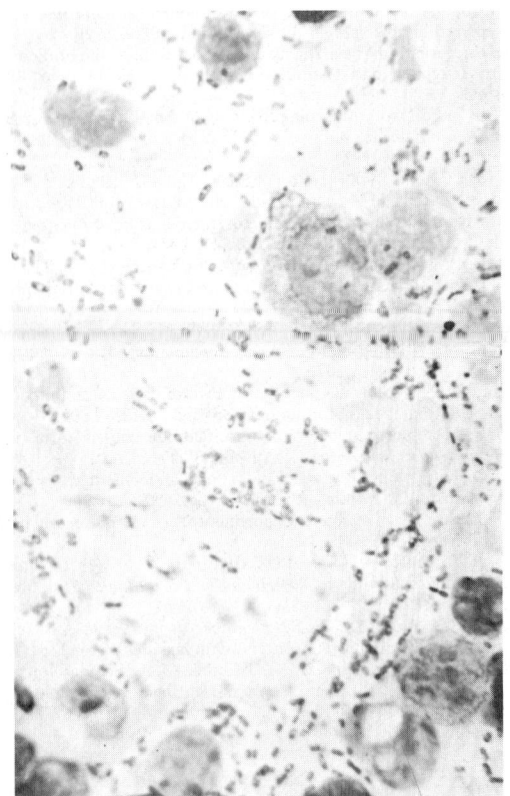

**FIGURE 1.** Y. pestis *from impression smear of spleen of experimental guinea pig. Wayson's stain.* × 1050.

negative. With the use of such stains as Wayson's, Giemsa, and Gram's, the central part of the bacillus is often left colorless, yielding the so-called bipolar staining. Thus, the overall morphology of plague bacilli in a smear resembles a scattering of various sized "safety pins" (Fig. 1). In cultures grown at 37° C, envelopes can be demonstrated by negative staining with India ink (Fig. 2). When the organisms are cultivated under suboptimal conditions (with media containing 2 to 4 per cent sodium chloride, i.e., "salt agar"), these involuted forms become very large and take on a striking diversity of shapes, becoming large globular, oval, or pyriform yeastlike bodies (Fig. 3).

On blood agar plates Y. pestis grows well but slowly. The pinpoint, transparent colonies become gray and grossly visible after 48 hours and, following 72 hours of incubation, enlarge up to 3 to 4 mm in diameter. If growth is prolonged, particularly at lower temperatures, the colonies have a "fried egg" appearance. Those grown at 37° C for 72 hours, because of the gelatinous surface antigen (envelope) of this organism, are more abundant and have a stringy consistency when tested with a wire loop. In broth Y. pestis

causes little turbidity, appears slightly granular, and collects at the bottom and sides of the container, illustrating its stalactiform growth property. A feathery vortex can be seen when the culture is gently shaken. In smears from young broth cultures, the bacilli generally emerge in chains, sometimes of considerable length, exhibiting a streptobacillary configuration (Fig. 4).

## METABOLISM

Although biochemical tests are not used extensively to identify this microorganism, they may help to distinguish it from other species of *Yersinia* (Buchanan and Gibbons, 1974) (Table 1). The two most important distinctive characteristics of *Y. pestis* are (1) slower alkali production from nitrogenous constituents than other species of *Yersinia* and (2) no hydrolysis of urea. Thus this strain, cultivated on deoxycholate citrate agar plates for 48 hours at 37° C, grows rather scantily in reddish, pinpoint colonies while the medium retains its original pink hue. *Yersinia pseudotuberculosis* bacilli, in contrast, grow plentifully within this period of time in large opaque colonies that (like the medium in general) become yellow. *Yersinia pestis* growth occurs in urea medium without hydrolyzing it. The urease of *Y. pseudotuberculosis* strains reddens the urea medium within 24 hours (Thal and Chen, 1955).

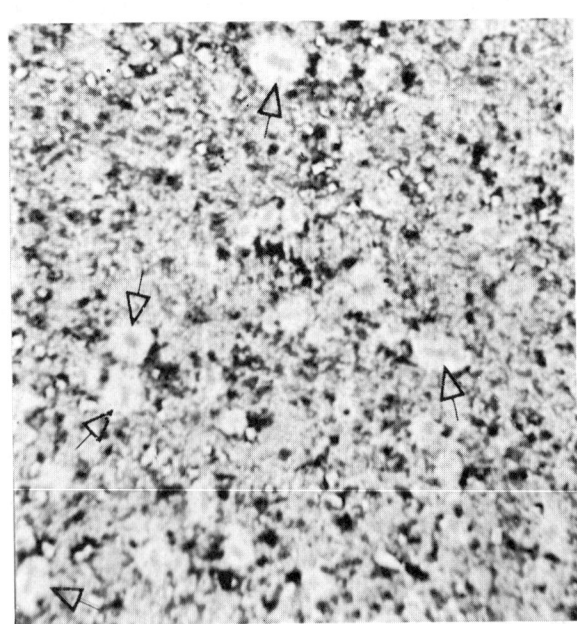

**FIGURE 2.** Y. pestis *grown on blood agar at 37° C for 72 hours. India ink preparation. Note the envelope antigen around the organisms (arrows).* × 1050.

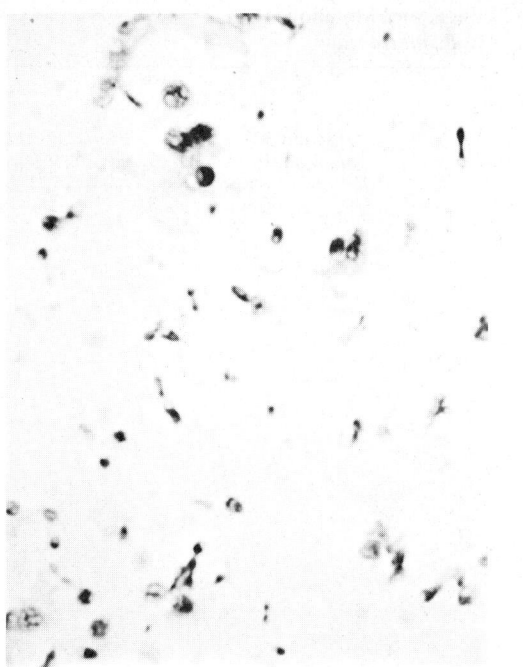

**FIGURE 3.**  Y. pestis *grown on 3 per cent salt agar. Wayson's stain.* × 1050. *Note the involution forms.*

## ANTIGENIC COMPOSITION

*Yersinia pestis* contains at least 19 different antigenic components recognizable by gel diffusion and/or biochemical methods (Albizo and Surgalla, 1970; Chen, 1965; Chen, 1972), 15 of which are shared by the closely related *Y. pseudotuberculosis.* Some of these 19 antigenic constituents of *Y. pestis* have been isolated in pure form, and five components (Fraction 1, the V and W antigens, exotoxin, and endotoxin) correlate well or at least somewhat with immunogenic activity and virulence (see Pathogenic Properties later in this chapter), whereas the remainder bear little or no relationship to plague immunity and infection.

### Fraction 1

Fraction 1 or "envelope antigen," which was first isolated in a highly purified state by Baker et al. (Baker et al., 1974), is a principal antigen involved with both virulence and immunity. Envelope antigen consists of two serologically identical components, 1A and 1B, which appear to differ chemically only in respect to the presence of a carbohydrate moiety in the former and its absence in the latter (Bennett and Tornabene, 1974). Bennett and Tornabene reported that the soluble Fraction 1 antigen of *Y. pestis* exists in the form of aggregates more than 300,000 in molecular weight, and that each aggregate can be further separated into a single antigenic subunit

of 15,000 to 17,000 MW by dissociation treatment with 0.1 per cent mercaptoethanol in 0.25 per cent sodium dodecyl sulfate (SDS) at 95° C for 5 minutes. These subunits reaggregate into a variety of large molecular weight structures upon removal of the SDS (Bennett and Tornabene, 1974). Chen and Elberg have confirmed these physicochemical observations by scanning electronmicroscopy (Chen and Elberg, 1977).

### V and W

In 1956, Burrows and Bacon demonstrated that the virulent *Y. pestis* strain contains two additional antigens, designated V and W, which are not produced by most avirulent strains of *Y. pestis* (Burrows and Bacon, 1956). It was their belief that these components were responsible for the virulence of a strain. V antigen is a protein with a molecular weight of 90,000, and the W antigen is a lipoprotein of 145,000 MW. The titers of both antigens fall upon prolonged storage at 5° C or after lyophilization, but not upon storage at −20° C. Thus, V and W are unstable antigens.

## PATHOGENIC PROPERTIES

In experimental plague, the term "virulence" is used to define the comparative lethality of different strains as measured in $LD_{50}$. Virulent strains have lower $LD_{50}$ levels than avirulent strains. Low virulence resulting from repeated cultivation in artificial media will be restored to full virulence by passage through susceptible animals (guinea pigs), in which selection occurs and the nonvirulent organisms are killed by phagocytes.

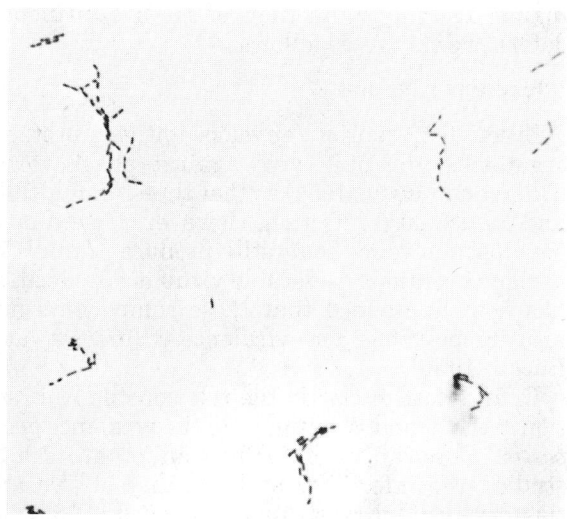

**FIGURE 4.**  Y. pestis *grown in broth for 24 hours at 37° C. Wayson's stain.* × 1050.

**TABLE 1.** Comparison of the Physical and Metabolic
Characteristics of *Yersinia* and *P. multocida*[a]

| | YERSINIA | | | PASTEURELLA MULTOCIDA |
| | pestis | enterocolitica | pseudo-tuberculosis | |
|---|---|---|---|---|
| Growth in MacConkey's | + | + | + | − |
| Growth at 5 °C | − | ⊕ | − | − |
| Motile | ⊖ | + (22°) | + (22°) | − |
| Nitrate | + | + | + | + |
| Citrate | − | − | − | − |
| Oxidase | − | − | − | v |
| Indole | − | d | − | + |
| Urease | − | ⊕ | ⊕ | − |
| β-Galactosidase | + | + | + | − |
| Ornithine decarboxylase | − | ⊕ | − | + |
| Phenylalanine deaminase | · | − | − | · |
| Fermentations | | | | |
|   lactose | − | − | − | − |
|   glucose | · | · | · | + |
|   galactose | (+) | + | + | + |
|   sucrose | − | ⊕ | − | + |
|   rhamnose | v | − | + | − |
|   salicin | v | − | + | − |
|   inositol | · | · | · | − |
|   sorbose | − | − | + | − |
|   adenitol | − | − | + | − |
|   esculin | + | ⊖ | + | − |

[a]v, variable reaction; >50% of stains are +; circled reactions are most helpful in differentiating between species.

The virulence determinants of a strain are complex and are associated with its specific antigens (see Antigenic Composition) and nutritional factors. In *Y. pestis*, the five generally established determinants of virulence consist of the capacity to (1) develop an elaborate envelope of Fraction 1 antigen, (2) produce V and W antigens, (3) synthesize a surface structure that permits absorption of hemin from the medium and pigments, (4) synthesize purines, and (5) generate toxins. The major functions of the five virulence determinants are as follows:

### Fraction 1, V, and W

Fraction 1, a surface envelope antigen, protects organisms grown in vivo against phagocytosis (Chen and Meyer, 1954) so that they can multiply and induce fatal infection. However, certain nonenveloped strains that still produce V and W antigens retain considerable virulence. Indeed, it has been contended that these components are also responsible for virulence (Burrows and Bacon, 1956).

In an effort to clarify the relationship of Fraction 1 and V and W antigens to the virulence of *Y. pestis*, Donovan et al. (Donovan et al., 1961) studied the infectivity and lethality of two antigenically different strains, enveloped MP6 (wild strain, F+, V and W+), and nonenveloped M23 (mutant strain, F−, V and W+). They found that a single bacterium of the enveloped strain, intradermally injected, could cause fatal infection in the guinea pig. Nonenveloped strains possessing the ability to produce V and W antigens lose their lethality but maintain the capacity to establish infection (skin lesions, buboes, and fever); death does not ensue if the organism is injected in nontoxic dosages. Thus the strain possessing the envelope antigen would appear to be more virulent.

Further studies of the Fraction 1 and V and W antigens by Cavanaugh and Randall (1959) have elucidated the process of plague infection. Following the injection of bacilli in the phagocytosis-sensitive state from the blocked flea into a host (plague-blocked fleas contain nonenveloped [F−, V and W+] virulent *Y. pestis* because the organisms are grown at a temperature lower than 37° C), the majority of organisms were ingested by polymorphonuclear leukocytes (PMN) and destroyed, while the minority, engulfed by monocytes, survived and multiplied. Later the pathogens were released in a well-enveloped form (F+, V and W+) that was resistant to phagocytosis by both PMN and monocytes. These phagocytosis-resistant, enveloped organisms account for the establishment of fatal infection.

Janssen et al. (1963) found no strict correlation between virulence and the envelope antigen's ability to resist phagocytosis. The well-enveloped avirulent strains (F+, V and W−) were more resistant to ingestion by nonsessile phagocytes than nonenveloped strains that produced V and W antigens. Hence these authors concluded that the primary factors in determining the virulence of *Y. pestis* were, rather, the V and W antigens, which permit survival and multiplication of the organisms within the phagocytic cells (monocytes). Apparently the factors determining virulence are Fraction 1, associated with resistance to phagocytosis, and the V and W antigens, associated with the capacity for intracellular multiplication. In contrast, an avirulent (F+, V and W−) strain of *Y. pestis* cannot multiply extensively and is destroyed by phagocytic activity.

### Pigmentation

Virulent strains grown on a defined medium ("pigmentation medium" containing hemin) (Jackson and Burrows, 1956) form dark brown (P+) colonies; others produce whitish or straw-colored (P−) colonies in the same medium. To demonstrate high virulence, both for guinea pigs and mice, it is insufficient for a strain to produce only Fraction 1 and V and W antigens (F+, V and W+); it must also be capable of absorbing hemin (P+) from the medium. Nonpigmented colonies consist of avirulent organisms. Loss of pigmentation will result in the loss of virulence. For example, the avirulent, living vaccine strain EV76 is F+, V and W+ but P−.

## PURINE

Many nutritional factors can differentiate virulent from avirulent *Y. pestis*. As noted above, fully virulent strains possessing the properties of F+, V and W+, and P+ must also synthesize purine (Pu+) to grow in the host. If a mutant strain derived from a fully virulent one loses the ability to synthesize purine (Pu−), a considerable loss of virulence and failure to produce disease result. However, if purine is injected into mice simultaneously with the bacilli, disease develops (Burrows, 1955).

## TOXINS

All of the fully virulent strains have produced toxins (Ts+), which are doubtless responsible for death from plague, suggesting that toxigenicity is a significant virulence determinant.

Two classes of toxins have been isolated and characterized from the plague bacillus. One, a soluble, heat-labile, formalin-sensitive exotoxin, is composed of two active proteins of toxin A (associated with the cytoplasmic membrane) and toxin B (within the cytoplasm) with molecular weights of 240,000 and 120,000, respectively (Montie et al., 1966). These two proteins are highly toxic for rats and mice: the $LD_{50}$ is less than 1 $\mu g$ in the mouse, as determined via the intravenous route (Ajl et al., 1958). The other, an insoluble, heat-stable lipopolysaccharide endotoxin contained in the cell wall (Albizo and Surgalla, 1970), has an intraperitoneal $LD_{50}$ of about 500 $\mu g$ in guinea pigs and mice and an intravenous $LD_{50}$ of 32 $\mu g$ in rabbits. Both the exotoxin and the endotoxin contribute to or account for death in plague, acting respectively on the peripheral vascular system to produce hemoconcentration and shock and on the liver to produce gross pathologic changes and endotoxic shock.

Yet many avirulent strains produce about the same amount or more toxin than the virulent strains (Englesberg et al., 1954); none are fatal, however, if the number of injected bacilli is below the toxic death level. Toxicity alone, then, is inadequate to render an organism virulent.

In summary, the pathogenic properties of *Y. pestis* are complex. To cause fatal infection, a strain should possess all virulent features, i.e., F+, V and W+, P+, Ts+ and Pu+. Absense of one or more factors will cause loss of virulence. Still, there are some strains with all of the known determinants of virulence that, surprisingly, remain not fully virulent. Perhaps the final determinant of virulence is the *quantity* in which these substances are present.

## IMMUNITY

Those who recover from plague appear to be protected from a second attack or at least incur a milder form on reinfection. Antibodies to three of nineteen recognized antigens correlate well with immunity, and the remainder have no bearing on plague immunity. The three most important immunogens are Fraction 1, exotoxin, and endotoxin.

A variety of antibodies present in immunized animals cannot eradicate *Y. pestis* in the absence of phagocytic cells. In the blood of immune hosts, plague bacilli are more readily phagocytized than in the blood of the nonimmune host. This is because Fraction 1 antibodies react to the surface envelope of the organisms and act as opsonins. Antibody to Fraction 1 is the principal protective factor against plague in animals as well as in man, as concluded from the positive correlation found between Fraction 1 antibody (CF and PHA titers), the opsonocytophagic index, and resistance to virulent infection following immunization by Fraction 1. Phagocytosis by neutrophils and macrophages of virulent *Y. pestis* directly parallels the development of Fraction 1 antibodies. Immunity to *Y. pestis* infection ultimately depends upon the ability of the macrophage to inactivate and to resist cytotoxic effects of the intracellular organism. Factors other than antibody that are produced by a subpopulation of lymphocytes from spleens of specifically immunized animals are essential for this macrophage function (Wong and Elberg, 1977).

Albizo and Surgalla (1970) isolated and purified the endotoxin and showed that endotoxin can contribute significantly to death in plague. Rabbits can be immunized and develop monospecific antibody that reacts with *Y. pestis* endotoxin. Although we do not understand the neutralizing effect of this antitoxin, it has a curative value, despite the fact that the antitoxic antibodies of exotoxin and endotoxin are not considered essential for serotherapy. Only in near-terminal cases, or when excessive antibiotic therapy may have caused the lysis of numerous bacilli, is antitoxin needed to neutralize the toxin.

Prevention of plague by vaccination has been practiced since the advent of the Haffkine vaccine in 1897. Thereafter, many investigators developed various vaccines, which were prepared as (1) killed broth cultures of *Y. pestis*, (2) chemically inactivated, agar-grown cultures of *Y. pestis*, (3) certain antigenic fractions of *Y. pestis*, or (4) live, attenuated plague strains. At present, the recommended regimen of immunization consists of administering two intramuscular injections, one month apart, of $1 \times 10^9$ formalin-killed plague bacilli preserved with phenol in physiologic saline (0.5 ml), followed by a booster dose of $4 \times 10^8$ bacilli (0.2 ml) 4 to 12 weeks after the second dose. Measurable levels of antibody can be maintained by booster inoculations given at intervals of not less than six months apart. When administered parenterally, attenuated live *Y. pestis* in repeated revaccinations has been effective during interepidemic periods (Payne et al., 1956). Severe local and systemic reactions have occurred, however, and there is no proof of the efficacy of this vaccine in preventing pneumonic plague. Oral administration of live attenuated EV76 (Paris) F vaccine is efficacious against both bubonic and pneumonic plague in the very susceptible vervet (*Cercopithecus aethiops*) (Chen et al., 1976, 1977). Thus the prospect that an oral, live, avirulent vaccine will be effective for human immunization is promising.

### LABORATORY DIAGNOSIS

The clinical diagnosis of plague must be confirmed by conventional bacteriologic procedures.

Smears from bubo aspirates, sputum, and blood should be stained with Gram's stain and also with Wayson's reagent. The direct smear should show gram-negative bipolar staining bacilli. A pure culture may be obtained after 48 to 72 hours from such material, with the use of the blood agar plate and infusion broth tube. *Yersinia pestis* grows slowly on blood agar, requiring 48 hours for macroscopic visibility, especially at 37° C. Touched with a wire loop, the 72-hour-growth colonies exhibit some stickiness. *Yersinia pestis* is nonmotile and never displays turbidity in standing broth culture tubes. A feathery vortex can be seen when the tube is gently shaken. Confirmation can also be achieved by specific bacteriophage lysis at 20° C. At a temperature of 37° C, but not 20° C, this phage can also lyse *Y. pseudotuberculosis*. Passive hemagglutination is the most specific and sensitive serologic procedure (Chen and Meyer, 1954, 1966). Positive results can usually be obtained after about five to seven days of illness.

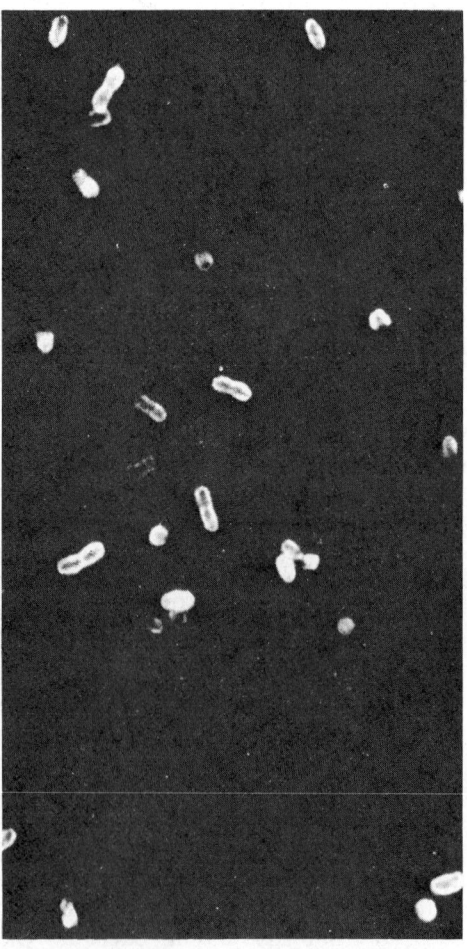

**FIGURE 5.** *Smear of* Y. pestis *strain 195/P stained with fluorescent Fraction I specific antibody.* × 1000. (From Quan, S. F., et al., Am J Trop Med Hyg 14:424, 1965.)

Inoculation of the plague specimens into mice and guinea pigs produces bacteremia and death within two to seven days. The appearance of the bacilli in these animals, combined with the pathologic changes induced by the infection, helps identify *Y. pestis*. Direct fluorescent antibody techniques allow screening of the cultures and detection of the organisms in infected material (Moody and Winter, 1959) (Fig. 5).

## DRUG SUSCEPTIBILITY

*Yersinia pestis* is susceptible to sulfonamides and antibiotics, including streptomycin, tetracycline, kanamycin (Cantey, 1974), and chloramphenicol. The in vitro and in vivo effects of trimethoprim-sulfamethoxazole on *Y. pestis* are at least equal to those of streptomycin and chloramphenicol (Nguyen Van Ai et al., 1972a, b).

## EPIDEMIOLOGY

Plague, primarily a naturally occurring disease of rodents and mammals, infects over 200 species of wild rodents, which are frequently incriminated hosts for *Y. pestis* (Pollitzer and Meyer, 1961). Humans may become victim to the disease through an aberrant interruption of the rodent-flea-rodent sequence or through the handling of infected animals. Usually bubonic plague in humans is transmitted by a bite from fleas (*Xenopsylla cheopis*, rat flea; *Pulex irritans*, human flea) that have previously sucked blood from a plague-infected animal or human. Plague bacilli (as many as $10^7$/ml) are present in rat blood during the acute stage, and the flea becomes infected by feeding on the diseased rat (Douglas and Wheeler, 1943). As ingested bacilli multiply in the midgut of the flea, massive infection eventually blocks the proventriculus to the extent that little or no blood can pass. During feeding, some bacilli mix with the blood of the new host and are regurgitated into the wound of the bite, transmitting about 25,000 to 100,000 bacilli. Thus, under natural conditions, transmission from rodent to rodent or human is always mediated by infected fleas. Generally the bubonic form proceeds to the secondary pneumonic form and may lead to person-to-person "droplet" transmission of primary pneumonic plague without the insect vector.

The most prevalent vector species for transmitting plague is *Xenopsylla cheopis*, the rat flea, because of its longevity as a reservoir of plague bacilli and the more frequent impediment of its proventriculus than in other types of fleas. Infected fleas can sometimes survive for 396 days (Pollitzer and Meyer, 1961), suggesting that possibly fleas carry infection from one epizootic season to another, even in the absence of definitive hosts. The human flea, *Pulex irritans*, is a relatively ineffective vector but can transmit plague from person to person under certain circumstances. *Diamanus montanus*, the common squirrel flea, is also an important vector and is a far more serious threat in introducing plague into rat populations in rural and perhaps urban areas (Meyer and Holdenride, 1949). The danger of human plague in an area can be measured by the "flea index" (the average number of fleas per rat). An *X. cheopis* index of at least 3 appears to prevail during epidemics.

Plague now occurs in Central and South Africa, South America, and Asia. In the United States, rural plague has been discovered in ground squirrels, prairie dogs, jack rabbits, voles, pack rats, and other animals in 15 states. A minimum of 50 rodent species is involved in enzootic and epizootic plague (Meyer, 1965). Under natural conditions, camels, sheep, coyotes, deer, dogs, and cats can contract plague infection, either by feeding on infected carcasses or, as in the case of dogs and cats, by acting as mechanical conveyances transporting the infected fleas to their owners. Seventy-eight cases were recognized in the United States from 1966 to 1976, all acquired from areas of wilderness in the enzootic western states (Center for Disease Control, 1975, 1977).

The incidence of plague continues to decline only because the epidemics are under control, rather than because the disease has been eradicated. It is now, in fact, firmly established in endemic foci. Plague is still a potential danger, due to the vast areas of wilderness in which infection persists and the increasing use of wilderness areas for recreational purposes.

# YERSINIA PSEUDOTUBERCULOSIS AND YERSINIOSIS

## MORPHOLOGY

*Yersinia pseudotuberculosis*, a pleomorphic, coccoid-appearing, oval or rod shaped microorganism, is gram-negative and measures 0.8 to 6.0 ⋈ 0.8 μm. Some strains disclose bipolar staining with Wayson's stain. Neither spores nor definite capsules are detectable, but at 22° C a viscous layer may be visible in India ink preparations. When cultured between 20 and 30° C, the organism is motile, and examination by scanning electronmicroscopy reveals peritrichous flagella (Fig. 6) (Chen and Elberg, 1977).

## METABOLISM

A facultative anaerobe, *Yersinia pseudotuberculosis* ferments rhamnose, esculin, salinigrin, adonitol, arabinose, arbutin, dextrin, galactose,

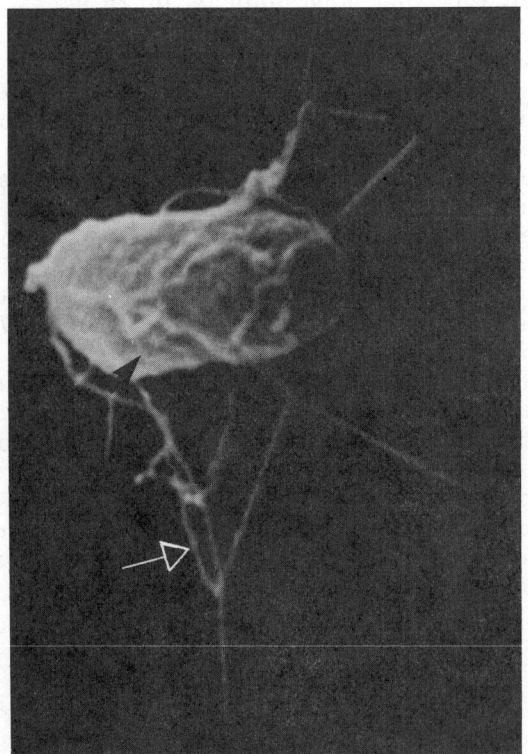

**FIGURE 6.** Y. pseudotuberculosis *Type I bacillus cultured at 22° C for 48 hours. Note the prominent flagella (arrows). Scanning Electron Micrograph. × 43,000. (From Chen, T. H., and Elberg, Sanford S.: Infect Immun 15:972, 1977.)*

and melibiose, producing acid (but no gas). It has both a urease and a β-galactosidase. It can be distinguished from *Y. enterocolitica* and *Y. pestis* by its fermentation of adonitol (Table 1).

## ANTIGENIC COMPOSITION

The multiplicity of antigens in *Y. pseudotuberculosis* is exemplified by the variety of somatic (O) antigens present in different strains. Fifteen somatic and five flagellar (H) antigens have been defined by Thal and Knapp (1969), and a diagnostic antigenic scheme of ten serotypes has been proposed. In diagnostic work it is sufficient to identify the O group.

Many of the antigenic components of *Y. pseudotuberculosis* are shared with those of *Y. pestis*. Indeed, extensive investigation of the antigenic structure of both *Yersinia* species has revealed 17 antigenic components, 15 of which are common to both (Burrows and Bacon, 1956, 1960; Lawton et al., 1960; Larrabee et al., 1965). A protein-lipopolysaccharide complex, protective factor (PF), has been isolated from avirulent *Y. pseudotuberculosis* type IV and *Y. pestis* strains (Lawton and Surgalla, 1963). Burrows and Bacon (1960) demonstrated that only newly isolated *Y. pseudotuberculosis* strains also produce V and W antigens identical to those of *Y. pestis*. (The importance of these two antigens is discussed in the preceding section on the antigenic composition of *Y. pestis*.)

Exotoxins have been isolated mainly in group III strains of *Y. pseudotuberculosis*, although they may also be found in some other groups. Despite the fact that each of these exotoxins is unique, they are nevertheless immunologically identical (Thal, 1954, 1966).

Certain O antigens of *Y. pseudotuberculosis* are related to *Salmonella* antigens, and group II and IV strains can be agglutinated by sera from patients infected with *Salmonella*.

## PATHOGENIC PROPERTIES

In humans, yersiniosis, which is characterized by diarrhea and lymphadenopathy with necrosis and septicemia, may be severe and even fatal. Generally, however, the human disease is localized to the mesenteric lymph nodes and commonly has a benign course. The capacity of *Y. pseudotuberculosis* for intracellular survival and reproduction represents a significant factor in the virulence of the organism (Besednova et al., 1975).

## IMMUNITY

Immunization against yersiniosis caused by *Y. pseudotuberculosis* has been of wide interest because this pathogen is intimately related antigenically to *Y. pestis* (see Antigenic Composition). Guinea pigs recovered from yersiniosis become immune to reinfection, and active immunity in these animals can be induced by inoculation with suspensions of avirulent, live Type IV strain 32 *Y. pseudotuberculosis* (Thal, 1962). Such immunization will also protect them from infection with *Y. pestis*. Yet guinea pigs so immunized or recovered from *Y. pestis* remain susceptible to yersiniosis. The relationship of the PF antigen to plague and yersiniosis immunity is still unclear. Injection of PF antigen protects guinea pigs as early as the first day by increasing nonspecific resistance to infection. Anti-*Y. pestis* serum usually agglutinates a variety of strains of *Y. pseudotuberculosis*, and anti-*Y. pseudotuberculosis* R serum also reacts with nonenveloped *Y. pestis* strains.

## LABORATORY DIAGNOSIS

The diagnosis of yersiniosis is confirmed by isolating *Y. pseudotuberculosis* from the affected blood, liver, spleen, lymph nodes, or feces, or by demonstrating the presence of specific antibodies in the serum. *Y. pseudotuberculosis* is easily cultured in ordinary media. The smooth phase produces a uniform turbidity in broth and a sediment after 24 hours. The rough phase strains grow without generating turbidity. On solid media, transparent colonies reach diameters of 0.5 to 1.0 mm in 24 hours. The pathogen grows abundantly in large opaque colonies on deoxycholate citrate agar, whereas *Y. pestis* grows scantily in reddish pinpoint colonies (Thal and Chen, 1955).

Biochemical and growth characteristics (discussed under Metabolism) also should be assayed (Table 1). The commercial specific typing sera containing agglutinins for types of *Y. pseudotuberculosis* will not agglutinate *Y. pestis*. Likewise, *Y. pseudotuberculosis* bacteriophage will lyse all strains of this organism but will not lyse *Y. pestis*. Further, *Y. pestis* phage will lyse *Y. pseudotuberculosis* at 37° C but not at 22° C. For these reasons, two sets of cultures should be prepared for incubation at two different temperatures (Gunnison et al., 1951). The two simple media that are used to differentiate plague and *Y. pseudotuberculosis* bacilli, namely urea and deoxycholate citrate agar, are extremely useful (Thal and Chen, 1955). *Yersinia pseudotuberculosis* grown below 30° C, but not at 37° C, is motile.

## DRUG SUSCEPTIBILITY

*Yersinia pseudotuberculosis* is sensitive to chloramphenicol, kanamycin, tetracycline, and streptomycin, and some strains are sensitive to penicillin or ampicillin.

## EPIDEMIOLOGY

Rodents and birds constitute the primary reservoirs of yersiniosis. Mice and rats, although apparently resistant to natural infection, shed the organisms for weeks in their urine and feces. Thus the resistant rodents may be the carriers and would seem to play an important epidemiologic role in spreading the disease (Mair, 1973).

*Yersinia pseudotuberculosis* inhabits a diversity of mammals, which are probably the main sources of most human infections. Evidence indicates that the strains isolated from man and animals possess the same cultural, biochemical, and pathologic characteristics. The majority of human cases can be attributed to contact with or ingestion of contaminated food and drinking water, and the consistent involvement of the abdominal organs in this disease also suggests that the mode of transmission may be via the oral route.

# YERSINIA ENTEROCOLITICA AND YERSINIOSIS

## MORPHOLOGY, METABOLISM, AND ANTIGENIC COMPOSITION

*Yersinia enterocolitica* was originally isolated by Hässing et al. in 1949 from abscesses at autopsy in two cases of human septicemia. The microorganism is a facultative anaerobe, grows well in air, is gram-negative and oval or coccoid-shaped, and has dimensions of 0.5 to 1.0 × 1.0 to 3.0 $\mu$m. It is easily grown on both blood agar and selective media and demonstrates motility by peritrichous flagella when cultivated at less than 30° C. The optimal temperature for the growth of *Y. enterocolitica* is 30 to 37° C, and it has a somewhat slower growth rate at this temperature than other enteric pathogens. The outstanding multiplication feature of the organism is its ability to increase at lower temperatures ($\pm5°$ C) (other kindred organisms do not). Refrigeration in 2 per cent peptone water of the specimen (from feces, lymph nodes, etc.) therefore results in selective enrichment. Upon primary isolation this bacterium produces smooth colonies, 0.5 to 2.0 mm in diameter, that often exhibit R forms in subculture. When cultivated in broth, either turbidity or a pellicle with clear supernatant and sediment is visible. Arbutin, cellobiose, galactose, sorbitol, and sorbose are fermented, forming acid but no gas. Urease, $\beta$-galactosidase, and ornithine decarboxylase are all produced by this organism. *Yersinia enterocolitica* can be distinguished from *Y. pestis* and *Y. pseudotuberculosis* by its fermentation of sucrose, cellobiose, and sorbose as well as by its production of ornithine decarboxylase, which the other organisms do not produce; *Y. enterocolitica* in some instances also forms indole.

On the basis of experimental evidence of heat-stable O-antigen types, a total of 34 different O antigens has lately been established in *Y. enterocolitica* (Wauters et al., 1972). In 1973 Knapp and Thal proposed a revision of the serologic scheme of *Y. enterocolitica* on the basis of six O-antigen groups. Serotype O9 (now known as O-group V) cross-reacts with *Brucella abortus*. The cross-reacting antigens were isolated by hot phenol water extraction of the respective bacteria and identified as lipopolysaccharides.

## PATHOGENIC PROPERTIES AND IMMUNITY

O-antigen Types 3 and 9 of *Y. enterocolitica* are pathogenic for humans and are the most common types isolated from humans and swine in Europe. In the United States, Serotype 8 has been isolated from patients, and Canadian strains contain Type 3. Clinical infections with this organism take the form of either acute mesenteric lymphadenitis or enterocolitis. Usually enterocolitis provokes nonbloody diarrhea and abdominal pain due to enlargement of the lymph nodes, while mesenteric lymphadenitis or acute, terminal ileitis elicits appendicitis-like symptoms. Maximal antibody titers are demonstrable in patients by the agglutination test within one or two weeks, declining within one or two months.

## LABORATORY DIAGNOSIS AND DRUG SUSCEPTIBILITY

*Yersinia enterocolitica* has been confirmed as the causative infection by isolation of the organisms from the affected blood, urine, feces, lymph nodes, wounds, or abscesses, or by demonstrating the presence of specific antibodies in the serum. The *Yersinia* species, *enterocolitica* and *pseudotuberculosis*, can be differentiated by their biochemical reactivity, bacteriophage susceptibility, and pathogenicity for laboratory animals. Whereas *Y. enterocolitica* is nonpathogenic for mice, guinea pigs, and rabbits by subcutaneous, intraperitoneal, or intravenous injection (Knapp and Thal, 1963), *Y. pseudotuberculosis* is pathogenic for all these animals. Both species are motile at 22° C, but not at 37° C.

Generally *Y. enterocolitica* and *Brucella abortus* infections result in cross-reacting antibodies, so that yersiniosis and brucellosis are indistinguishable by the agglutination and complement fixation tests, a situation that has caused great confusion in brucellosis eradication work in cattle. However, the two diseases can now be differentiated by electroimmunoassay (Hurwell, 1975).

## DRUG SUSCEPTIBILITY

Most strains of *Y. enterocolitica* are sensitive to polymyxin, gentamicin, kanamycin, chloramphenicol, and streptomycin.

## EPIDEMIOLOGY

Apparently *Y. enterocolitica* is worldwide in distribution. Extensive animal reservoirs of this organism exist, and it has been isolated from both sick and healthy animals throughout Europe and the United States. Such animals include horses, swine, sheep, goats, cows, dogs, deer, monkeys, and chinchilla. A common source of human infec-tion is food, especially fluids (milk, ice cream, water), contaminated by feces and urine from infected animals. Yersiniosis in both animals and humans is more prevalent in the colder months, possibly because it grows at lower temperature.

# PASTEURELLA MULTOCIDA AND PASTEURELLOSIS

## *MORPHOLOGY*

*Pasteurella multocida* appears as an ellipsoid gram-negative rod or a coccobacillus, ranging from 1.0 to 1.8 × 0.3 to 0.5 $\mu$m in size with bipolar-staining capsules (when present), which are best demonstrated by negative staining, as with India ink or Giesma stain. *Pasteurella multocida* is nonsporogenous and nonmotile at both 22 and 37° C. Its optimal growth temperature is 37° C. Small, nonhemolytic, gray colonies form on blood agar, but most nonhemolytic strains create a brownish discoloration in the blood medium. Broth cultures of smooth or mucoid strains are evenly turbid, while the rough strain produces floccular or granular deposits.

## *METABOLISM*

*Pasteurella multocida* is an aerobe (or facultative anaerobe) that will not grow in MacConkey's agar. It produces acid from galactose, mannose, and sucrose, and most strains ferment mannitol, sorbitol, and xylose (lactose is not fermented). Indole and $H_2S$ are also usually produced, as well as ornithine decarboxylase. The organism is urease-negative and catalase-positive.

## *ANTIGENIC COMPOSITION*

*Pasteurella multocida* has both capsule polysaccharide and somatic lipopolysaccharide antigens, which can be used to serotype the pathogen. The antigenic structure correlates with strain virulence and host susceptibility (Collins, 1977). Bain (1955) and Dhanda (1960) both isolated a mouse-protective protein antigen from some of their strains of *P. multocida*. On the basis of the capsular antigen, Carter (Carter and Annau, 1953; Carter, 1972a), using the indirect hemagglutination (IHA) test, separated *P. multocida* into four serotypes (A to D). Later, a new type (E) was added (Carter, 1961, 1963) and type C was discarded, narrowing the serotypes to A, B, D, and E.

*P. multocida* also contains a number of smooth, somatic, lipopolysaccharide antigens. The rapid agglutination test (Carter, 1972b) has been used for subtyping strains classified in the same capsular serotype category. The arabic numeral is utilized for the specific somatic antigen, followed by a capital letter designating the capsular antigen. So far, 11 specific O antigens have been identified, e.g., 1:A, 3:A, 11:B (Namioka and Bruner, 1963).

Endotoxins and their component lipopolysaccharides have been isolated from whole cells and cell walls. They are toxic for mice and pyrogenic in rabbits (Bain and Knox, 1961). Type E lipopolysaccharide is antigenic for rabbits, and mice can be passively immunized with this antiserum (Perreau and Petit, 1963).

## *PATHOGENIC PROPERTIES AND IMMUNITY*

*P. multocida* represents an animal parasite of considerable economic and veterinary importance, especially to cattlemen and fowl ranchers (Collins, 1977). This microorganism is so highly pathogenic for mice and rabbits that only one to ten cells of a smooth or mucoid variant are usually fatal in the mouse. Infrequently, it may be found in the throats of healthy humans (Smith, 1959), and under conditions of stress or debilitation of the host, the parasite, previously benign, may penetrate beneath the mucous membrane and result in frank disease. Most infections take one of three clinical patterns: local infection by cat scratch or animal bite, respiratory tract infection, or systemic infections such as meningitis and bacteremia.

Agglutinins in the sera of patients with generalized infection can be detected by the hemagglutination test. (Normally, no antibodies are present in the patient with a localized wound infection.) It is not known if these antibodies are bactericidal or antitoxic, although evidence indicates that the immunity is humorally mediated (Collins, 1973). The immunization of domestic animals (cattle) and birds (poultry) with a killed vaccine conveying protection against pasteurellosis is often practiced. Viable, attenuated, oral vaccines have also proved effective in turkeys and chickens. No vaccine exists for man.

## LABORATORY DIAGNOSIS

Specimens from infected wounds, sinuses, sputum, pleural or spinal fluid, blood and postmortem tissues should be placed on 5 per cent blood agar. Pure cultures can be further identified as *P. multocida* by their inability to grow in MacConkey's agar, biochemical reactions, lack of motility at both 22 and 37° C, sensitivity to penicillin, and high pathogenicity for mice. Bacteriophage can also be used for identification of *P. multocida* (Gadberry and Miller, 1977).

## DRUG SUSCEPTIBILITY

*P. multocida* is inhibited by drugs at the following average concentrations (mg/ml): chloramphenicol (1.5), tetracycline (3.0), penicillin (0.4), and erythromycin (3.1). Chang and Carter (1976), studying the multiple drug resistance of *P. multocida* and *P. hemolytica,* observed that penicillin and tetracycline may not always be effective. Chloramphenicol proved most efficacious; only 4 of 403 isolates were resistant to this agent.

## EPIDEMIOLOGY

*P. multocida* can survive for only a short time outside the host; thus, the reservoir of infection is probably a healthy carrier. Mammals, birds, and people have been found to be reservoirs for *P. multocida*. In general, human infections are acquired from animal bites, and 15 per cent of cat bites and dog bites treated in United States and Russian hospitals have yielded positive cultures of *P. multocida* (Francis et al., 1975). Most human respiratory and septicemic infections occur in farmers. Most human isolates are Serotype A or D (Carter, 1962). On occasion, the organism is discovered in the throats of healthy individuals exposed to infected animals (Smith, 1959), so the possibility of interhuman spreading by nasopharyngeal excretions, urine, and feces must be considered (Hubbert and Rosen, 1970). *P. multocida* may remain in the host for a long time, later asserting its pathogenic properties when resistance to the infection diminishes. In animals, pasteurellosis has been characterized as a disease of debility. In fact, stress in livestock during transportation is responsible for the illness known as "shipping fever."

# FRANCISELLA TULARENSIS AND TULAREMIA

In 1911, McCoy, exploring plague in California ground squirrels, discovered a disease characterized by lesions similar to those of plague. The following year, he and Chapin isolated the causative organism of this plaguelike disease by means of coagulated egg yolk medium and named it *Bacterium tularense,* after Tulare County, California. After previous assignment to several genera, this organism is now known by its own genus name, *Francisella,* in honor of Francis, a pioneer investigator of the disease in humans (Francis, 1921a, b), who infelicitously termed it "tularemia" to indicate its ability to cause septicemia.

## MORPHOLOGY

*Francisella tularensis* is small and aerobic, measuring 0.2 × 0.2 to 0.7 μm. A gram-negative, nonmotile, noncapsular, nonspore-forming bacillus, it is highly pleomorphic, often appearing as a rod or coccus and always singly. The bacterium forms minute, transparent droplike colonies on blood-glucose-cystine agar. Colonies may reach a diameter of 4 mm after two to five days of incubation and are readily emulsified. They require more cystine than is present in the ordinary nutrient medium.

## METABOLISM

The optimal growth temperature of *F. tularensis* is 37° C. Most strains ferment glucose, maltose, mannose, fructose, and dextrose, creating acid without gas. The organism is grown in medium containing cystine or cysteine and produces $H_2S$ (Table 1). Enriched media with incorporated antibiotics (penicillin, polymyxin B, and cycloheximide) may be of value when clinical specimens harboring normal flora are cultured for *F. tularensis.*

## ANTIGENIC COMPOSITION

Several strains of *F. tularensis* have been studied by serologic methods, but no immunologic types have emerged. Agglutinins appear during the 2nd and 3rd weeks of illness and reach a peak two or three months after infection. Cross-reactions with *Brucella melitensis* and *B. abortus* do occur, but rising titers for *F. tularensis* in the convalescent phase will confirm this infection.

Jellison (1970) and Russian scientists have observed and discussed the fact that two basic types of *F. tularensis* occur in nature; they are distinguishable by differences in virulence and biochemical reactions but cannot be antigenically differentiated. The highly virulent strains, mainly isolated in North America, can cause fatality in mice, guinea pigs, and rabbits (Bell et al., 1955). They are usually isolated from tick-borne tularemia in rabbits. They utilize glycerol and produce citrulline ureidase. In doses of 1 to 100 organisms, these highly virulent strains result in necrotic nodules of the lung, spleen, and liver. The low-virulent strains are lethal for rabbits only when the dose is at least $5 \times 10^9$ organisms; these strains do not utilize glycerol or generate citrulline ureidase. This type is primarily associated with rodents; it may also be transmitted by ticks but is frequently associated with water and occurs in both the western and eastern hemispheres.

Treatment of aqueous suspensions of *F. tularensis* with ethyl ether yields an ether-soluble, immunogenic antigen that protects mice from death following challenge with more virulent strains of *F. tularensis* (Larson, 1945; Bell et al., 1952). This ether-soluble antigen has been further purified by salt precipitation, differential centrifugation, and dialysis, resulting in a uniform immunogenic activity. The immunizing antigens appear to be composed of pure cell wall material (Ormsbee and Larson, 1955). Ether-water extracts of strain SCHU S4 from stationary-phase, liquid-grown, saline suspensions have been demonstrated to stimulate better antibody formation in rabbits than do antigens obtained by other chemical procedures. Thus they provide a good crude antigenic mixture for further purification and the production of related monospecific antisera (Nutter, 1971). It has been reported that *F. tularensis* yields both a toxic filtrate and an endotoxin (Meyer, 1965).

## PATHOGENIC PROPERTIES

*F. tularensis* is a facultative, intracellular parasite that may persist for many years in the organs (Carr and Kadull, 1957). Direct human contact with infected vertebrates and the discharges or bites of arthropods (deerflies and ticks) generally evoke tularemia. The persistent immune response and the occasional tendency of the disease toward relapse and chronicity are probably attributable to the prolonged intracellular survival of the microorganisms.

## IMMUNITY

An attack of tularemia confers solid lifelong immunity. Agglutinins appear during the 2nd or 3rd week of illness and persist for years. The tendency of the disease to progress (and sometimes relapse) despite high antibody titers is probably due to the ability of the organism to survive and multiply intracellularly. Although the inactivated vaccines do not offer complete resistance, they modify the course of the infection favorably. A live, attenuated strain of *F. tularensis* has been used to immunize both animals and people and has afforded significant protection against the pathogen (Eigelsbach and Downs, 1961). In the United States, live vaccine in volunteers protected 10 of 14, whereas the cell wall antigen and the killed vaccine protected few or none against intracutaneous or respiratory-route challenge infection (McCrumb, 1961; Saslaw et al., 1961a, b). Burke (1977), in an effort to determine the incidence of tularemia in laboratory workers, compared the number of individuals vaccinated with the phenol-killed Foshay vaccine and those given the live, avirulent vaccine and demonstrated that the live vaccine was more protective; the incidence of typhoidal tularemia fell from 5.70 to 0.27 cases per 1000, whereas the incidence of ulceroglandular tularemia remained constant, although the clinical signs and symptoms were much milder than in those vaccinated with the killed vaccine. At present, vaccination with the live, attenuated vaccine is indicated only for persons at high risk, such as laboratory workers.

## LABORATORY DIAGNOSIS

A definitive diagnosis of tularemia is usually achieved by a combination of bacteriologic, serologic, and animal inoculation methods. *F. tularensis* cannot be grown in ordinary media but thrives on coagulated egg yolk, enriched blood glucose-cystine agar, and thioglycollate broth. It can be isolated from sputum, pharyngeal exudate, scrapings, and biopsy material from local lesions or gastric washings when it is cultured on specific media, such as blood-glucose-cystine agar, or when guinea pigs are inoculated. Colonies may appear in two to four days and should be identified by the rapid slide agglutination test with specific antiserum. For fast screening of cultures and detection of the organism in infected material, it is possible to use fluorescent antibody techniques (Yager et al., 1960). Cultures should be incubated for two weeks before being discarded as negative, and culture plates should be enclosed in polyethylene bags to reduce desiccation during the prolonged incubation period. It is also of value to determine the dependence of the organism upon special media (the possible requirement for extra cystine or sulfhydryl compound) for growth.

Guinea pigs, mice, and hamsters are susceptible to F. tularensis and die with characteristic lesions two to seven days after subcutaneous or intraperitoneal inoculation. Animal inoculation is particularly valuable when the specimen is contaminated with other organisms that tend to overgrow F. tularensis in culture. At autopsy there is hemorrhagic edema at the site of inoculation and whitish necrotic lesions of the liver, spleen, lung, and bone marrow, each capable of yielding positive culture.

Berdal and Søderlund (1977) observed that specimens grown on selective chocolate agar (containing 7.7 µg/ml colistin, 12.5 µg/ml nystatin, 0.5 µg/ml lincomycin, and 5 µg/ml trimethoprim lactate) at 37° C in an atmosphere of 5 per cent $CO_2$ for two to three days disclosed smooth colonies of F. tularensis, 0.1 to 1.0 mm in diameter, cultures that were either pure or only slightly contaminated. Thus, the selective chocolate agar medium might be a practical supplement to nonselective media.

Serologic tests are also of value in diagnosis. Agglutinins appear during the 2nd or 3rd week of illness and reach peak titer at two to three months. Only rising titers are indicative of recent infection, since previous infections with the same or other organisms can cause detectable antibody titers which may persist for years. Cross-reactions with Brucella immune sera may occur, but they can be distinguished by comparative agglutination tests performed with antigens of both species, since the homologous titers are much higher than the heterologous ones.

Delayed hypersensitivity reactions to the tularemia skin test may be an early diagnostic aid because the positive reaction may be obtained during the first week of illness (Buchanan et al., 1971).

## DRUG SUSCEPTIBILITY

F. tularensis is susceptible to streptomycin, kanamycin, tetracycline, and chloramphenicol.

## EPIDEMIOLOGY

Tularemia is a sporadic disease, largely limited to lagomorphs (rabbits, hares) and rodents in certain areas of enzootic infection. Humans are an accidental end host. Human infections have been traced to a broad variety of sources, including ectoparasites, vertebrates, aerosols and contaminated water. F. tularensis, originally isolated from California ground squirrels in 1912, has since been found in innumerable species of wild animals (muskrats, beavers, woodchucks, water rats, voles, skunks, deer, dogs, cats, and rabbits) throughout North America and primarily in Europe, Russia, Turkey, and Japan. The insects that are most significant in the transmission of tularemia and that keep the infection active in vertebrates are lice, mites, and ticks (Meyer, 1965).* The propagation of F. tularensis in nature depends upon the wood tick and dog tick, feeding on cottontail and jack rabbits and many other rodents. Animals naturally infected with F. tularensis can therefore serve as reservoirs. The tick efficiently maintains the chain of infection by transmitting the organisms via the ovary to the eggs, through the larva and nymph, and finally to the adult, which is then capable of infecting rodents.

In the United States, there are two distinct types of tularemia, the highly virulent and the low-virulent forms. The former is tick-borne from the rabbit; the low-virulent, rodent form is contracted from water contaminated by water rats. Low-virulent strains growing in water and mud can infect muskrats and then trappers. Tularemia in humans, however, is largely transmitted by direct contact with the blood or other tissue fluids of infected rodents. Vector-borne tularemia in the United States, mainly conveyed by ticks and deerflies (Boyce, 1975), has a mortality rate of 7.5 per cent in untreated cases.

## References

*Yersinia pestis*

Ajl, J., Jr., Rust, J., Jr., Hunter, D., Woebke, J., and Bent, D. F.: Preparation of serologically homogeneous plague murine toxin and its reactions with physical, chemical and enzymatic agents. J Immun 80:435, 1958.
Albizo, J. M., and Surgalla, M. J.: Isolation and biological characterization of *Pasteurella pestis* endotoxin. Infect Immun 2:229, 1970.
Baker, E. E., Somer, H., Foster, L. E., Meyer, E., and Meyer, K. F.: Antigenic structure of *Pasteurella pestis* and the isolation of a crystalline antigen. Proc Soc Exp Biol Med 64:139, 1947.
Bennett, L. G., and Tornabene, T. G.: Characterization of the antigenic subunits of the envelope protein of *Yersinia pestis*. J Bacteriol 117:48, 1974.

*Haemaphysalis leporispalustris,* rabbit tick; *Amblyomma americanum,* Lone Star tick; *Dermacentor andersoni,* common wood tick; *D. variabilis,* dog tick; *Chrysops discalis,* bloodsucking deerfly.

Bibel, D. J., and Chen, T. H.: Diagnosis of plague: An analysis of the Yersin-Kitasato controversy. Bacteriol Rev 40:633, 1976.

Buchanan, R. E., and Gibbons, N. E. (eds.): Bergey's Manual of Determinative Bacteriology. 8th ed. Baltimore, The Williams & Wilkins Company, 1974.

Burrows, T. W.: The basis of virulence for mice of *Pasteurella pestis. In* Mechanisms of Microbial Pathogenicity. Fifth Symposium of the Society for General Microbiology. Cambridge, Cambridge University Press, 1955, p. 152.

Burrows, T. W., and Bacon, G. A.: The basis of virulence in *Pasteurella pestis.* An antigen determining virulence. Br J Exp Pathol 37:481, 1956.

Burrows, T. W., and Bacon, G. A.: V and W antigen in strains of *Pasteurella pseudotuberculosis.* Br J Exp Pathol 41:38, 1960.

Cantey, J. R.: Plague in Vietnam. Clinical observation and treatment with kanamycin. Arch Intern Med 133:280, 1974.

Cavanaugh, D. C., and Randall, R.: The role of multiplication of *Pasteurella pestis* in mononuclear phagocytes in the pathogenesis of fleaborne plague. J Immunol 83:348, 1959.

Center for Disease Control: Annual Supplement Summary 1975. Morbid Mortal Weekly Rep 24(54):1, 1975.

Center for Disease Control: Morbid Mortal Weekly Rep 26:159, 1977.

Chen, T. H.: The antigenic structure of *Pasteurella pestis* and its relationship to virulence and immunity. Acta Trop (Basel) 22:97, 1965.

Chen, T. H.: The immunoserology of plague. In Kwapinski, J. B. (eds.): Research in Immunochemistry and Immunobiology. Vol. 1. Baltimore, University Park Press, 1972, p. 223.

Chen, T. H., and Elberg, S. S.: Scanning electron microscopic study of virulent *Yersinia pestis* and *Yersinia pseudotuberculosis* Type I. Infect Immun 15:972, 1977.

Chen, T. H., Elberg, S. S., and Eisler, D. M.: Immunity in plague: Protection induced in *Cercopithecus aethiops* by oral administration of live, attenuated *Yersinia pestis.* J Infect Dis 133:302, 1976.

Chen, T. H., Elberg, S. S., and Eisler, D. M.: Immunity in plague: Protection of the vervet *(Cercopithecus aethiops)* against pneumonic plague by the oral administration of live attenuated *Yersinia pestis.* J Infect Dis 135:289, 1977.

Chen, T. H., and Meyer, K. F.: Studies on immunization against plague. VII. A hemagglutinin test with the protein fraction of *Pasteurella pestis:* A serologic comparison of virulent and avirulent strains with observations on the structure of the bacterial cells and its relationship to infection and immunity. J Immunol 72:282, 1954.

Chen, T. H., and Meyer, K. F.: An evaluation of *Pasteurella pestis* Fraction-I-specific antibody for the confirmation of plague infections. Bull WHO 34:911, 1966.

Donovan, J. E., Han, D., Fukui, G. M., and Surgalla, M. J.: Role of the capsule of *Pasteurella pestis* in bubonic plague in the guinea pig. J Infect Dis 169:154, 1961.

Douglas, J. R., and Wheeler, C. M.: Sylvatic plague studies. II. The fate of *Pasteurella pestis* in the flea. J Infect Dis 72:18, 1943.

Englesberg, E., Chen, T. H., Levy, J. B., Foster, L. E., and Meyer, K. F.: Virulence in *Pasteurella pestis.* Science 119:413, 1954.

Jackson, S., and Burrows, T. W.: The pigmentation of *Pasteurella pestis* on a defined medium containing hemin. Br J Exp Pathol 37:570, 1956.

Janssen, W. A., Lawton, W. D., Fukui, G. M., and Surgalla, M. J.: The pathogenesis of plague: A study of the correlation between virulence and relative phagocytosis resistance of some strains of *Pasteurella pestis.* J Infect Dis 113:139, 1963.

Meyer, K. F.: *Pasteurella* and *Francisella.* In Dubos, R. J., and Hirsch, J. G. (eds.): Bacterial and Mycotic Infections. 4th ed. Philadelphia, J. B. Lippincott Company, 1965, p. 659.

Meyer, K. F., and Holdenride, R.: Rodents and fleas in a plague epizootic in a rural area of California. Puerto Rico J Public Health Trop Med 24:201, 1949.

Montie, T. C., Montie, D. B., and Ajl, S. J.: A comparison of the characteristics of two murine-toxic proteins from *Pasteurella pestis.* Biochim Biophys Acta 130:406, 1966.

Moody, M. D., and Winter, C. C.: Rapid identification of *Pasteurella pestis* with fluorescent antibody. III. Staining *Pasteurella pestis* in tissue impression smears. J Infect Dis 104:288, 1959.

Nguyen Van Ai, Nguyen Duc Hanh, Pham Van Dien, and Nguyen Van Le: Action *in vitro* and *in vivo* of trimethoprim-sulfamethoxazole on *Yersinia pestis.* Bull Soc Pathol Exot 65:759, 1972a.

Nguyen Van Ai, Nguyen Duc Hanh, Pham Van Dien, and Nguyen-Van Le: Successful treatment of bubonic and septicaemic plague by trimethoprim-sulfamethoxazole. Preliminary note. Bull Soc Pathol Exot 65:770, 1972b.

Payne, F. E., Smadel, J. E., and Courdurier, J.: Immunologic studies on persons residing in a plague epidemic area. J Immunol 77:24, 1956.

Pollitzer, R., and Meyer, K. F.: The ecology of plague. In May, J. M. (ed.): Studies in Disease Ecology. New York, Hafner Publishing Company, 1961, p. 433.

Thal, E., and Chen, T. H.: Two simple tests for the differentiation of plague and pseudotuberculosis bacilli. J Bacteriol 69:103, 1955.

Wong, J. F., and Elberg, S. S.: Cellular immune response to *Yersinia pestis* modulated by product(s) from thymus-derived lymphocytes. J Infect Dis 135:67, 1977.

## *Yersinia pseudotuberculosis*

Besednova, N. N., Timchenko, N. F., Gorshknova, R. P., and Somov, G. P.: An interaction of the causative agent of pseudotuberculosis with the peritoneal macrophages of the immune and nonimmune organism. Zh Mikrobiol Epidemiol i Immunobiol (10):39, 1975.

Burrows, T. W., and Bacon, G. A.: The basis of virulence in *Pasteurella pestis.* An antigen determining virulence. Br J Exp Pathol 37:481, 1956.

Burrows, T. W., and Bacon, G. A.: V and W antigens in strains of *Pasteurella pseudotuberculosis.* Br J Exp Pathol 41:38, 1960.

Chen, T. H., and Elberg, S. S.: Scanning electron microscopic study of virulent *Yersinia pestis* and *Yersinia pseudotuberculosis* Type I. Infect Immun 15:972, 1977.

Gunnison, J. B., Larson, A., and Lazarus, A. S.: Rapid differentiation between *Pasteurella pestis* and *Pasteurella pseudotuberculosis* by action of bacteriophage. J Infect Dis 88:254, 1951.

Larrabee, A. R., Marshall, J. D., and Crozier, D.: Isolation of antigens of *Pasteurella pestis.* I. Lipopolysaccharide-protein complex and R and S antigens. J Bacteriol 90:116, 1965.

Lawton, W. D., Fukui, G. W., and Surgalla, M. J.: Studies on the antigens of *Pasteurella pestis* and *Pasteurella pseudotuberculosis.* J Immunol 84:476, 1960.

Lawton, W. D., and Surgalla, M. J.: Immunization against plague by a specific fraction of *Pasteurella pseudotuberculosis.* J Infect Dis 113:39, 1963.

Mair, N. S.: Yersiniosis in wildlife and its public health implications. J Wildlife Dis 9:64, 1973.

Thal, E.: Untersuchungen über *Pasteurella pseudotuberculosis* und besonderer Berücksichtigung ihres immunologischen Verhaltens. Nord Vet Med 6:829, 1954.

Thal, E.: Oral immunization of guinea pigs with avirulent "*Pasteurella pseudotuberculosis.*" Nature 194:490, 1962.

Thal, E.: Immunobiologische Studien an *Yersinia pseudotuberculosis* (Syn. *Pasteurella pseudotuberculosis*). Schweiz Arch Tierheilkd 108:372, 1966.

Thal, E., and Chen, T. H.: Two simple tests for the differentiation of plague and pseudotuberculosis bacilli. J Bacteriol 69:103, 1955.

Thal, E., and Knapp, W.: The revised antigenic scheme of *Yersinia pseudotuberculosis.* Symposia Series in Immunobiological Standardization, Bern 15:219, 1969.

## *Yersinia enterocolitica*

Hässig, A., Karrer, J., and Pusterla, F.: Über Pseudotuberkulose beim Menschen. Schweiz Med Wochenschr 79:971, 1949.

Hurwell, B.: Differentiation of cross-reacting antibodies against *Brucella abortus* and *Yersinia enterocolitica* by electroimmunoassay. Acta Vet Scan 16:318, 1975.

Knapp, W., and Thal, E.: Untersuchungen über die kulturell-biochemischen, serologischen, tierexperimentellen und immunologischen Eigenschaften einervorläufig "*Pasteurella* X" benannten Bakterienart. Zbl Bakt (Abt I, orig.) 190:472, 1963.

Knapp, W., and Thal, E.: Die biochemische Charakterisierung von *Yersinia enterocolitica* (Syn. "*Pasteurella* X") als Grundlage eines vereinfachten O-Antigenschemas. Zbl Bakt (Abt I, orig.) 223:88, 1973.

Wauter, G., Le Minor, L., Chalon, A. M., and Lassen, J.: Supplément au schéma antigénique de "*Yersinia enterocolitica.*" Ann Inst Pasteur Lille 122:951, 1972.

## *Pasteurella multocida*

Bain, R. V. S.: Studies on hemorrhagic septicemia of cattle. IV. A preliminary examination of antigens of *Pasteurella multocida* Type I. Br Vet J 111:492, 1955.

Bain, R. V. S., and Knox, K. W.: The antigens of *Pasteurella multocida* Type I. II. Lipopolysaccharides. Immunology 4:122, 1961.

Carter, G. R.: A new serological type of *Pasteurella multocida* from central Africa. Vet Rec 73:1052, 1961.

Carter, G. R.: Animal serotypes of *Pasteurella multocida* from human infections. Can J Public Health 53:158, 1962.

Carter, G. R.: Immunological differentiation of Type B and E strains of *Pasteurella multocida*. Can Vet J 4:61, 1963.

Carter, G. R.: Improved hemagglutination test for identifying Type A strains of *Pasteurella multocida*. Appl Microbiol 24:162, 1972a.

Carter, G. R.: Agglutinability of *Pasteurella multocida* after treatment with hyaluronidase. Vet Rec 91:150, 1972b.

Carter, G. R., and Annau, E.: Isolation of capsular polysaccharides from colonial variants of *Pasteurella multocida*. Am J Vet Res 14:474, 1953.

Chang, W. H., and Carter, G. R.: Multiple drug resistance in *Pasteurella multocida* and *Pasteurella hemolytica* from cattle and swine. J Am Vet Med Assoc 169:710, 1976.

Collins, F. M.: Growth of *Pasteurella multocida* in vaccinated and normal mice. Infect Immun 8:868, 1973.

Collins, F. M.: Mechanisms of acquired resistance to *Pasteurella multocida* infections: A review. Cornell Vet 67:103, 1977.

Dhanda, M. R.: Purification and properties of the soluble antigen of *Pasteurella septica*, Type I. Indian J Pathol Bacteriol 2:59, 1960.

Francis, D. P., Holmes, M. A., and Brandon, G.: *Pasteurella multocida*. Infections after domestic animal bites and scratches. JAMA 233:42, 1975.

Gadberry, J. L., and Miller, N. G.: Use of bacteriophages as an adjunct in the identification of *Pasteurella multocida*. Am J Vet Res 38:129, 1977.

Hubbert, W. T., and Rosen, M. N.: II. *Pasteurella multocida* infection in man unrelated to animal bite. Am J Public Health 60:1109, 1970.

Namioka, S., and Bruner, D. W.: Serological studies on *Pasteurella multocida*. IV. Type distribution of organisms on the basis of their capsular and O groups. Cornell Vet 53:41, 1963.

Perreau, P., and Petit, J. P.: Lipopolysaccharide antigens of *Pasteurella* Type E. Rev Élèvage Med Vet Pays Trop 16:5, 1963.

Smith, J. E.: Studies on Pasteurella septica. III. Strains from human beings. J Comp Pathol 69:231, 1959.

*Francisella tularensis*

Bell, J. F., Larson, C. L., Wight, W. C., and Ritter, S. S.: Studies on the immunization of white mice against infections of *Bacterium tularense*. J Immunol 69:515, 1952.

Bell, J. F., Owen, C. R., and Larson, C. L.: Virulence of *Bacterium tularense*. I. A study of the virulence of *Bacterium tularense* in mice, guinea pigs, and rabbits, J Infect Dis 97:162, 1955.

Berdal, B. P., and Søderlund, E.: Cultivation and isolation of *Francisella tularensis* on selective chocolate agar as used routinely for

the isolation of gonococci. Acta Pathol Microbiol Scand (B) 85:108, 1977.

Boyce, J. M.: Recent trends in the epidemiology of tularemia in the United States. J Infect Dis 131:197, 1975.

Buchanan, T. M., Brooks, G. F., and Branchman, P. S.: The tularemia skin test. 325 skin tests in 210 persons: Serologic correlation and review of the literature. Ann Intern Med 74:336, 1971.

Burke, D. S.: Immunization against tularemia: Analysis of the effectiveness of live *Francisella tularensis* vaccine in prevention of laboratory acquired tularemia. J Infect Dis 135:55, 1977.

Carr, E. A., Jr., and Kadull, P. J.: Persistence of *Bacterium tularense* in man in the absence of serious clinical illness. Arch Pathol 64:382, 1957.

Eigelsbach, H. T., and Downs, C. M.: Prophylactic effectiveness of live and killed tularemia vaccines. I. Production of vaccine and evaluation in the white mouse and guinea pigs. J Immunol 87:415, 1961.

Francis, E.: Tularemia Francis 1921. I. The occurrence of tularemia in nature as a disease of man. Public Health Rep 36:1731, 1921a.

Francis, E.: Tularemia Francis 1921. A new disease of man. JAMA 78:1015, 1921b.

Jellison, W. L.: Tularemia in Montana. *In* Montana Wildlife, Series 2 of Montana Animals, Montana Fish and Game Commission. Butte, McKee Printing Company, 1970.

Larson, C. L.: Immunization of white rats against infections with *Pasteurella tularensis*. Public Health Rep 60:725, 1945.

McCoy, G. W.: A plague-like disease of rodents. Public Health Bull 43:53, 1911.

McCoy, G. W., and Chapin, G. W.: Further observations on a plague-like disease of rodents with a preliminary note on the causative agent, *Bacterium tularense*. J Infect Dis 10:61, 1912.

McCrumb, F. R.: Aerosol infection of man with *Pasteurella tularensis*. Bacteriol Rev 25:262, 1961.

Meyer, K. F.; *Pasteurella* and *Francisella*. In Dubos, R. J., and Hirsch, J. G. (eds.): Bacterial and Mycotic Infections of Man. Philadelphia, J. B. Lippincott Company, 1965, p. 659.

Nutter, J. E.: Antigens of *Pasteurella tularensis:* Preparative procedures. Appl Microbiol 22:44, 1971.

Ormsbee, R. A., and Larson, C. L.: Studies on *Bacterium tularense*. II. Chemical and physical characteristics of protective antigen preparations. J Immunol 74:359, 1955.

Saslaw, S., Eigelsbach, H. T., Wilson, H. E., Prior, J. A., and Carhart, S.: Tularemia vaccine study. I. Intracutaneous challenge. Arch Intern Med 107:689, 1961a.

Saslaw, S., Eigelsbach, H. T., Prior, J. A., Wilson, H. E., and Carhart, S.: Tularemia vaccine study. II. Respiratory challenge. Arch Intern Med 107:702, 1961b.

Yager, R. H., Spertzel, O. R., Yaeger, R. F., and Tigertt, W. D.: Domestic fowl: Source of high titer *P. tularensis* serum for the fluorescent antibody technique. Proc Soc Exp Biol Med 105:651, 1960.

# **38** *STREPTOBACILLUS MONILIFORMIS*

## *Joshua Fierer, M.D.*

*Streptobacillus (Actinobacillus) moniliformis* is a pleomorphic bacterium. It is nonmotile, unencapsulated, and nonacid-fast. Gram-stained smears of exudate show small rods or short filaments. When grown in serum-enriched broth, they are branching filaments that form interwoven masses. There usually is marked pleomorphism. Many filaments contain cells with rounded or fusiform swellings. After prolonged culture, tiny curved and ring forms appear.

Much of the pleomorphism of this bacterium is due to the spontaneous appearance of variants with defective cell walls, called L-phase variants (after the Lister Institute where this observation was first made). These are stable variant bacteria that lack a rigid cell wall. As a consequence, in broth they grow as small round cells, and on agar the colonies are flat and grow into the agar like *Mycoplasma* colonies. For many years this similarity in colonial morphology and in osmotic fragility between L-forms and mycoplasmatales obscured the large and fundamental differences between these disparate microorganisms (see Chapters 53 and 54. Stable L-forms lack the mucopeptide that confers on the parent bacteria their rigidity and rod-like shape. The L-forms divide and propagate by binary fission as cell-deficient forms. Unstable L-forms revert back to parental bacteria. Protoplasts, in contrast to L-forms, are cell wall-deficient forms that are created artificially by exposing gram-positive bacteria to enzymes (e.g., lysozyme) or antibiotics such as penicillin that directly interfere with cell wall synthesis. Sometimes a stable protoplast is produced by these manipulations that can multiply without synthesizing a cell wall in the absence of the inducing agent.

## ANTIGENIC COMPOSITION

The L-phase variant and the bacillus share a common antigen, but the L-phase lacks antigens present in the latter. There appears to be only one serotype of the bacillus, but the chemical nature of the antigen has not been established.

## METABOLISM

Growth can occur aerobically but is equally good or better under anaerobic conditions (Wittler, 1974). A 10 per cent $CO_2$ atmosphere probably enhances growth. Optimum temperature for growth is 37° C. The metabolic characteristics of the organism have not been studied in detail. It is both catalase and oxidase negative and does not reduce nitrate to nitrite, nor produce idole. Urea is not hydrolyzed nor is phenylalanine deaminated. Acid but not gas is produced from dextrin, fructose, galactose, glucose, maltose, mannose, starch, and glycogen. No acid is produced from glycerol, inositol, inulin, sorbitol, rhamnose, or mannitol. Tetrazolium salt and tellurite are reduced aerobically and anaerobically though the tellurite reduction test may be only weakly positive.

## IMMUNITY

The pathogenic properties of this organism have not been studied in detail. The stable L-forms do not produce disease in mice whereas bacilli do. If injected into mice, unstable L-forms revert to the bacterial form and cause disease. Vaccination with the L-form does not protect mice against challenge with the bacterial form, but a killed bacterial vaccine is protective.

## LABORATORY DIAGNOSIS

Diagnosis of infection is made by isolating the bacteria from a lymph node, pus, joint fluid, or blood. Bacteria grow in ordinary blood culture media (Rogosa, 1974). This organism does not grow on nutrient agar, but on sheep blood agar it produces very small, gray, translucent, nonhemolytic colonies with entire edges after 48 to 72 hours of incubation. In serum or ascitic fluid broth, it grows as white granules or flocculent balls that sediment rapidly or stick to the side of the glass tube. Nutrient broth supplemented with 20 per cent horse serum is useful for primary isolation. Injection of pus into mice can also be used to isolate the bacterium, but care must be taken not to use naturally infected animals for such isolation.

The tube-agglutination test with whole bacterial antigen can be used for serologic diagnosis. Demonstration of a rising titer is significant. A negative test does not exclude the diagnosis.

## DRUG SUSCEPTIBILITY

The organism is susceptible to penicillin (0.05 unit/ml), streptomycin, and tetracycline. The L-phase variant is resistant to penicillin, and persistent symptoms and signs may be associated with the presence of L-phase organisms in the blood during penicillin therapy. Tetracycline or streptomycin can be used in that circumstance.

## EPIDEMIOLOGY

The distribution of this organism is worldwide, although human infections are rare in Europe and North America. The reservoir is infected rats or, rarely, other rodents. It may cause an epizootic disease in mice characterized by arthritis and lymphadenitis. Most human infections are acquired as the result of a rat bite (Cole et al., 1979). Consequently, it is an occupational hazard of research laboratory workers. After a bite, the incubation period is 3 to 10 days. Infection can occur as a consequence of ingesting contaminated milk (Haverhill fever or erythema arthriticum epidemicum). Some patients who live in rat-infested environments have had no history of a bite, and infection may have been food-borne.

## References

Cole, J. S., Stoll, R. W., and Bulger, R. J.: Rat bite fever, report of three cases. Ann Intern Med 71:979, 1969.

Rogosa, M.: Streptobacillus moniliformis and Spirillum minus. In Manual of Clinical Microbiology, 2nd ed. American Society for Microbiology, Washington, 1974.

Wittler, R. G.: In Bergey's Manual of Determinative Bacteriology, 8th ed. Baltimore, The Williams & Williams Company, 1974.

# 39 ACTINOBACILLUS AND CARDIOBACTERIUM

*Irving J. Slotnick, Ph.D.*

# ACTINOBACILLUS

Only one species in the genus *Actinobacillus*, *Actinobacillus actinomycetemcomitans*, has been consistently associated with human infection. The other species are pathogenic in cattle, horses, and pigs, but only rarely in man.

## MORPHOLOGY

Members of the genus *Actinobacillus* are gram-negative rods, coccoid to coccobacillary in shape, 0.3 to 0.5 µm wide and 0.5 to 1.5 µm long, nonspore-forming and nonacid-fast. They often present pleomorphic coccal and long bacillary and filamentous forms. They are not distinguishable morphologically from organisms in the genera *Brucella*, *Haemophilus*, and *Pasteurella* (Figs. 1 and 2).

In infections of animals, grayish white granules may appear in pus that are similar to but smaller (0.4 mm diameter) than the "sulfur" granules of actinomycosis. The granules contain

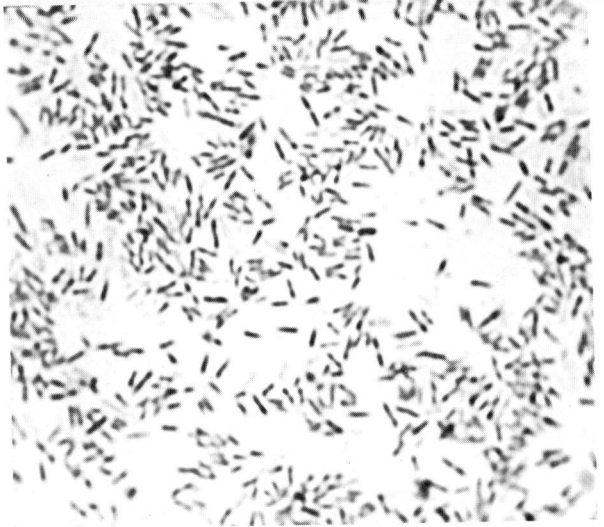

**FIGURE 2.** Actinobacillus actinomycetemcomitans #CS-G. Gram stain. Blood agar. 48-hours growth. 1800×.

clublike bodies emanating radially from the center, which is made up of the gram-negative bacilli and cell deposits. Care must be taken to differentiate these from granules caused by *Actinomyces* spp, *Nocardia* spp, staphylococci, *Monosporium* spp, fragments of caseous material, and clumps of pus cells and fibrin. A Ziehl-Neelsen stain colors the granule interior blue whereas the clubs are weakly acid-fast.

Growth is improved in the presence of increased carbon dioxide and by adding blood (5 per cent) or serum (10 per cent) to any of the common agar media. No growth occurs on *Salmonella-Shigella* (SS) or eosin-methylene blue (EMB) agar. *A. lignieresii* and *A. equuli* grow on MacConkey agar, whereas *A. actinomycetemcomitans* grows only slightly at best. Both rough and smooth types of colonies occur in primary cultures. Rough colonies are tiny at 24 hours, ranging up to 1.0 mm in diameter, they are raised, grayish, opaque, convex, tenacious, and firmly adherent to the medium. The surface appears dry and dull. In 72 hours the colony increases to 3.4 mm in diameter.

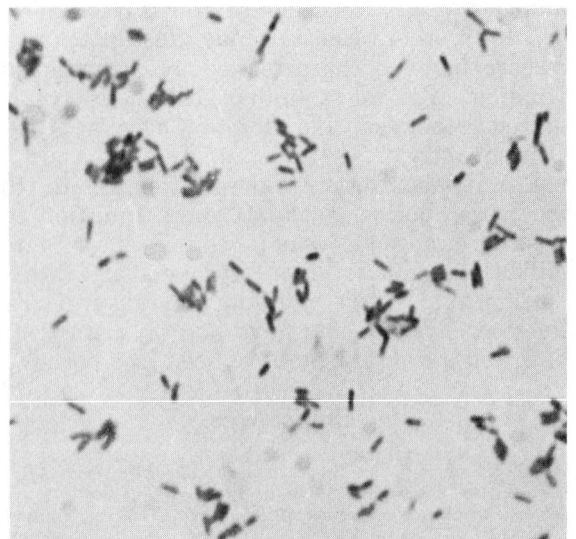

**FIGURE 1.** Actinobacillus lignieresi. ATCC #10811. Gram stain. Blood agar. 48-hours growth. 1800×.

Smooth colonies are the same size as rough forms. They are small, discrete, convex, and semi-opaque, with entire edges and glistening surfaces. The colonies appear gray but may have a blue to yellowish hue when viewed by transmitted light. After four to five days of incubation, the colony has a domed appearance when examined microscopically. The formation of smooth colony variants is favored on continued subculture (Alexander, 1974).

The central area of the colonies may, after three to five days of incubation, appear to contain a four- to six-pointed star formation. This portion of the colony grows into the agar, and when the colony is scraped away, the star formation remains. This is more readily observed on clear media than on blood agar.

The consistency of bacterial growth on agar is strain-dependent. On blood agar growth may be butyrous and can be scraped up easily, or it may be adherent and difficult to remove with a loop.

Serum enriched thioglycollate, soy broths, cooked meat, and other infusion media show growth at the end of 24 hours in air. Granular growth may follow uniform turbidity. The granules tend to adhere to the walls of the tubes, leaving the broth fairly clear. A surface film and a heavy tenacious sediment also occur in old broth cultures.

## ANTIGENIC COMPOSITION

Heat-stable polysaccharide agglutinating antigens associated with extracellular slime and several agglutinogens are formed by the actinobacilli. Antigenic relationships exist between *A. lignieresii* and *A. equuli*. Cross-reactions between *Pseudomonas mallei*, *Pseudomonas pseudomallei*, and *A. equuli* are well known. Phillips (1967) defined six types (1 through 6) and two subtypes (1a and 4c) of *A. lignieresii* on the basis of heat-stable somatic antigens. Some host specificity in the distribution of serotypes seems to be involved, because most cattle strains belong to Type 1 and most sheep strains belong to Types 2, 3, and 4. Heat-labile antigens common to different antigenic types also occur.

Pulverer and Ko (1972) examined 100 strains of *A. actinomycetemcomitans* by a variety of serologic procedures and delineated 6 heat-stable agglutinating antigens and 24 agglutinating patterns. Ouchterlony agar-gel diffusion tests proved to be inferior to the agglutination procedures for typing purposes.

## METABOLISM

The actinobacilli are representative chemoorganotrophs, using only organic compounds as their source of energy. Growth is aerobic and facultatively anaerobic. Carbohydrates are fermented with production of acid and usually no gas. Fermentation reactions are weak, variable, and often delayed. Glucose, maltose, mannitol, sucrose, xylose, galactose, trehalose, and dextrin can be used as substrates. Lactose fermentation is variable. Dulcitol, rhamnose, and inositol are not attacked. The OF medium of Hugh and Leifson is not recommended for fermentation reactions because it does not support the growth of most strains of actinobacilli. Carbohydrate broths used to test reactions should be supplemented with 5 to 10 per cent sterile horse serum and not incubated more than 14 days to minimize nonspecific reactions.

Pulverer and Ko (1970) classified eight fermentative biotypes of *A. actinomycetemcomitans* on the basis of galactose, mannitol, and xylose reaction patterns. Biotypes I through IV make up the majority of strains isolated from cases in the United States reported to the Center for Disease Control.

Optimal temperature for growth is 37° C, with a range of 20 to 42° C. Optimal pH is 7.6, and no growth occurs at pH below 6.5. The guanine plus cytosine (G+C) content of the DNA ranges from 40.6 to 42.0 moles per cent. Capsules are not produced, but some strains produce extracellular slime. Flagella are not synthesized, and the bacilli are nonmotile.

## PATHOGENIC PROPERTIES

Localized purulent granulomatous lesions, abscess formation in soft tissues, septicemia, endocarditis, and occasionally meningitis characterize the disease spectrum of the actinobacilli. No exotoxins have been demonstrated. Subcutaneous inoculation of a pure culture of *A. lignieresii* or *A. equuli* into cattle leads to the formation of an abscess similar to that occurring in the natural disease, but not all strains are virulent. Experimental studies have been limited due to absence of another animal model and lack of pathogenicity for rabbits, mice, or guinea pigs.

## IMMUNITY

Definitive data concerning the immune state following an overt case of actinobacillosis are meager. Repeated attacks have been singularly rare, although chronic cases can occur. Serum antibodies are formed in animals and humans, but it is not known if they are protective. Horse antiserum has been employed in the treatment of animals without conspicuous success.

Nonspecific agglutination reactions with sera from normal hosts and seronegative reactions in proven cases make serodiagnostic testing unsatisfactory (Phillips, 1967). Agglutination tests with known organisms or known antisera can be used to identify antibody or species, but commercial sources for either are not available. However, it is possible to follow antibody development in individuals from whom an isolate has been obtained (Pathak and Ristic, 1962). The serum of animals suffering from actinobacillosis frequently agglutinates the causative organism agent to a titer of 1:160 or higher. We observed a transitory rise to a titer of 1:320 in a human case of *A. actinomycetemcomitans* endocarditis and found no rise in a second case.

## LABORATORY DIAGNOSIS

Identification of culture isolates is based on biochemical reactions in Table 1.

## DRUG SUSCEPTIBILITY

Streptomycin, tetracycline, and chloramphenicol inhibit all strains tested in reasonably low concentrations (Page and King, 1966). Less than 50 per cent of *A. actinomycetemcomitans* organisms are inhibited by 12.5 $\mu$g/ml of penicillin, only 35 per cent are inhibited by 3.12 $\mu$g/ml of ampicillin, and all are resistant to methicillin.

Potassium iodide is very effective and is the drug of choice in the treatment of spontaneous actinobacillosis. The response is dramatic and permanent. It has been used with some success in the more chronic cases of disease in humans. The iodides have little bactericidal effect against *A. lignieresii*. The sulfonamides, penicillin, streptomycin, and broad-spectrum antibiotics are used to treat *A. lignieresii* and *A. equuli* infection.

## EPIDEMIOLOGY

Even though actinobacilli are recognized obligate parasites of animals and humans, their eco-

**TABLE 1. Identification Characteristics of Suspected Actinobacilli and Cardiobacterium Strains**

|  | ACTINOBACILLUS ACTINOMYCETEM-COMITANS | ACTINOBACILLUS LIGNIERESII | ACTINOBACILLUS EQUULI | CARDIOBACTERIUM HOMINIS |
|---|---|---|---|---|
| Oxidase activity | −/weak | + | + | + |
| Growth on MacConkey's agar | −/slight | + | + | − |
| Acetyl-methylcarbinol (VP test) | − | v | − | − |
| Catalase activity | + | −/weak | −/weak | − |
| Indole production | − | − | − | +/weak |
| Citrate utilization | − | − | − | − |
| Nitrate reductase | + | + | + | − |
| H₂S production (TSI)[a] | − | − | − | − |
| H₂S: lead acetate paper | +/weak | +/weak | +/weak | +/weak |
| β-galactosidase (ONPG)[a] | − | + | + | − |
| Urease activity | − | + | + | − |
| LDC/ODC[a] | − | − | − | − |
| TSI, acid butt | + | + | + | + or NG[a] |
| Gelatin hydrolysis | − | − | + | − |
| Hippurate hydrolysis | − | − | + | − |
| *Carbohydrates* attacked |  |  |  |  |
| arabinose | − | d | − | − |
| lactose | − | + | + | − |
| maltose | + | + | + | + |
| mannitol | d[a] | + | + | d |
| raffinose | − | − | + | · |
| salicin | − | − | − | − |
| sorbitol | − | d | − | + |
| sucrose | − | + | + | + |
| trehalose | − | − | + | − |
| xylose | d | + | + | − |
| galactose | d |  |  | − |
| glucose | + | + | + | + |

Data adapted from Weaver et al. (1972) and Cowan and Steele (1974). Both references cite excellent sets of key reactions to differentiate other fastidious gram-negative fermentative bacteria.
[a]TSI, triple sugar iron agar; LCD, lysine decarboxylase; ODC, ornithine decarboxylase; ONPG, O-nitrophenyl−$\beta$−D-galactopyranoside (test for $\beta$-galacto-sidase); NG, no growth; d, some strains positive but may be delayed.

logic habits are not fully known. They are recovered with ease from the normal mouth, tonsillar area, and intestinal tract of all hosts. The genital tract may also be colonized. The oral cavity and upper respiratory tract are primary portals of entry and serve as a focal endogenous habitat.

Human infection caused by *A. actinomycetemcomitans* develops as endocarditis in rheumatic or congential heart disease or as opportunistic invaders in malignant lymphoma and acute leukemia. Infections have followed dental manipulations, but soft tissue *A. actinomycetemcomitans* abscesses have also been seen without evidence of

trauma to the area of infection (Burgher et al., 1973). A human urinary tract infection has been reported (Townsend and Gillenwater, 1969).

*A. lignieresii* and *A. equuli* are chiefly the cause of actinobacillosis in animals and can cause epidemics. The disease can spread rapidly in a herd, attacking up to 50 per cent of the animals in a matter of weeks. When human infections have been caused by *A. lignieresii* or *A. equuli*, they occurred in persons whose occupations required heavy contact with animals, such as farmers, animal husbandmen, veterinarians, and abbatoir personnel (Custus et al., 1944).

# CARDIOBACTERIUM

### *MORPHOLOGY*

The only species in this genus is *Cardiobacterium hominis*. It is a gram-negative rod, 0.5 $\mu$m wide and 1.0 to 2.2 $\mu$m long, arranged singly, in pairs, short chains, or clusters. The rods may be uniform or pleomorphic. The pleomorphic forms have one or both ends enlarged, tear-drop forms, or rosette clusters (Figs. 3, 4, and 5). There is evidence that pleomorphism is related to the yeast extract content of the medium. Organisms appear homogeneously stained and of *uniform dimensions* on blood agar containing yeast extract. The organism is nonspore-forming and nonacid-fast. Sudanophilic bodies and metachromatic inclusions are demonstrable.

Thin sections of *C. hominis* show a cell wall of gram-negative type with a cytoplasm containing

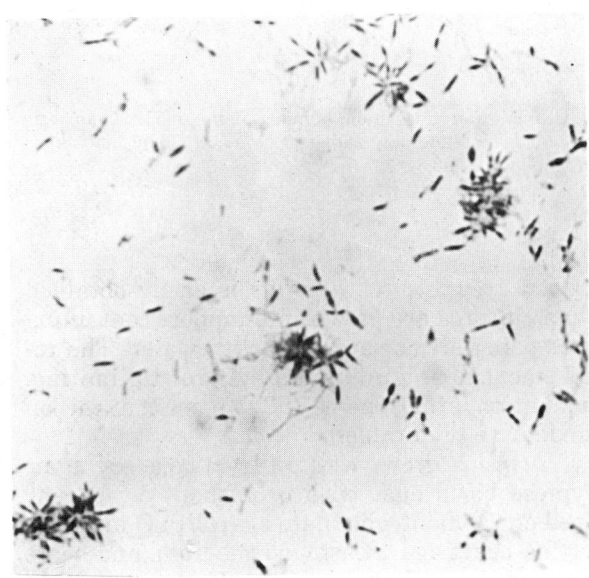

FIGURE 4.  Cardiobacterium hominis.  Strain #6573. Rosette-clusters in a Gram stain preparation of a blood agar culture. 1800 ×.

numerous intrusive membranes disposed around the periphery of the cells, especially at the poles (Reyn et al., 1971). The cell wall consists of a unit membrane sandwiched between dense outer and inner layers. Polar caps are seen on the ends of cells. The substructure of the surface layer is unusual for a gram-negative bacterium.

*C. hominis* colonies on blood agar are punctiform after 24 hours, and attain a maximum size of one to two mm in 48 to 72 hours. Colonies are circular, convex, smooth, entire, glistening, opaque, and butyrous. In older cultures, the center of the colony appears more opaque and grayish white in contrast to the edges. A slight greening of blood agar, which develops around dense areas of growth in two to three days, becomes brownish with further incubation. Clear hemolytic zones are not observed.

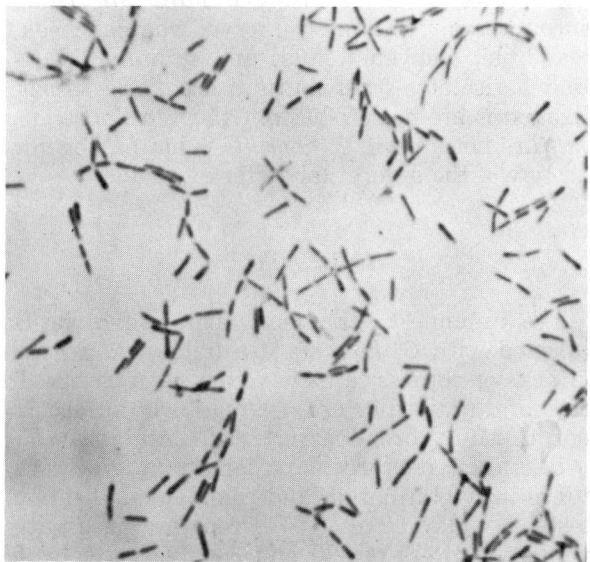

FIGURE 3.  Cardiobacterium hominis. Strain #6518. Blood agar culture illustrative of a culture with singular lack of pleomorphic cell-types. Rod shape cells predominate. 1800 ×.

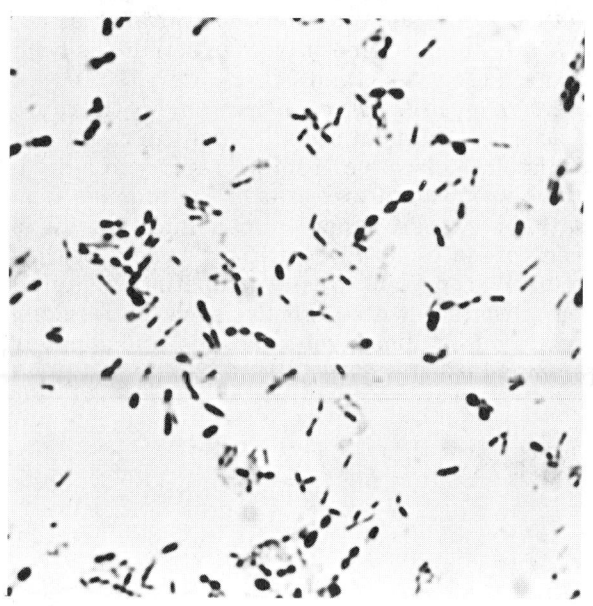

**FIGURE 5.** Cardiobacterium hominis. *Strain #6573. Gram stain of blood agar culture illustrating tear-drop morphology and chaining tendency. 1800×.*

## METABOLISM

*C. hominis*, like the actinobacilli, is an aerobic, facultative anaerobic, chemoorganotroph with a fermentative, albeit weak, type of metabolism.

*C. hominis* ferments carbohydrates without gas production. Fermentable substrates include glucose, sucrose, levulose, mannose, and sorbitol. Maltose and mannitol breakdown varies with individual strains. Fermentation is late and irregular in raffinose, dextrin, glycogen, and starch. Xylose, lactose, glycerol, salicin, inulin, arabinose, adonitol, dulcitol, galactose, rhamnose, trehalose, inositol, cellobiose, erythritol, melibiose, and melezitose are not attacked. Glucose is converted primarily to lactate and smaller amounts of pyruvate, formate, and propionate.

Optimal temperature for growth is 37° C. No growth occurs at 42° C or above, and only sporadic light growth occurs at 25° C. Optimal pH range 7.0 to 7.2. The G+C content of the DNA is 61.7 moles per cent (Hill and LaPage, 1969). Neither capsules nor flagella are produced.

Good growth of *C. hominis* is easily obtained when cultures are grown in humidors containing filter paper strips saturated with water. The requirement for high humidity is growth-limiting. In addition, atmospheres of 3 to 5 per cent carbon dioxide are preferable.

*C. hominis* grows well on trypticase soy agar, tryptose blood agar with or without 5 per cent blood enrichment, chocolate agar, PPLO medium, cystine-heart agar, Casman's medium, and heart infusion agar. Moderate growth occurs on nutrient agar and Lowenstein-Jensen's medium. The organism does not grow on MacConkey's agar, Simmon's citrate, SS agar, tellurite medium, potato medium, Sabouraud's dextrose agar, phenylethylalcohol medium, EMB medium, or endo agar medium.

## PATHOGENIC PROPERTIES

Infections with *C. hominis* have been primarily associated with human endocarditis (Tucker et al., 1969; Midgley et al., 1970; Snyder and Ellner, 1969; Weiner and Werthamer, 1975; Savage et al., 1977; Perdue et al., 1974). Their low intrinsic virulence is in keeping with the subacute course of the endocarditis. Infection occurs most frequently in patients with pre-existing cardiovascular defects or disease. However, an ever increasing number of diseased sites are being encountered, including the cervix, vagina, cheek, mandible, empyema fluid, and spinal fluid, as well as isolates from sputum, nose, and throat. Exotoxins are not produced. Other virulence factors are not known. *C. hominis* is not pathogenic for any of the several laboratory animals.

## ANTIGENIC COMPOSITION

Antigenically, *C. hominis* is relatively homogeneous. The organisms cross-agglutinate to high titer in unabsorbed immune antisera. Antiserum absorption with heterologous strains gives residual titers indicative of varied as well as common antigenic groupings. Fluorescent-isothiocyanate-labeled antibody detects the same antigenic relationships (Slotnick and Dougherty, 1964).

## IMMUNITY

The immune mechanisms operative in hosts infected with *C. hominis* are unknown. Second attacks or chronic cases have not been observed. Humoral antibodies are not regularly formed in normal adult throat carriers of *C. hominis*.

Serum of endocarditis patients may give high titers in agglutination and complement fixation tests. Midgley et al. (1970) report a case with admission titers of 320 and 640 respectively in agglutination and complement fixation tests. Serum obtained nine months later gave an agglutination titer of 160, showing little change, whereas the complement fixation titer had fallen considerably to 20. Neither of these sera produced agglutination with a variety of other organisms isolated in the authors' laboratory, and conversely, numerous sera from other patients failed to agglutinate *C. hominis* in slide agglutination tests.

## LABORATORY DIAGNOSIS

Conventional blood culture media containing 10 per cent carbon dioxide are suitable for recovering *C. hominis*. The biochemical identification of this organism is based on reactions given in Table 1 and is confirmed serologically with specific agglutinating or immunofluorescent antisera.

## DRUG SUSCEPTIBILITY

*C. hominis* is susceptible to a wide range of antibiotics. Penicillin and streptomycin, either singly or in combination, should be considered the drugs of choice. Drug resistance in treatment has not been a problem.

## EPIDEMIOLOGY

*C. hominis* is part of the indigenous commensal human respiratory flora. A large proportion of normal individuals of all ages and both sexes harbor these organisms. Their presence in the stool is easily detectable with direct fluorescent antibody staining. An extremely low incidence in cervical and vaginal cultures coupled with complete absence in urine supports the conclusion that they are only transient contaminants of the genitourinary tract.

In contrast to actinobacillosis, *C. hominis* infection does not occur in epidemics. It is primarily an infection of compromised persons.

No animal host or reservoir is known, and extensive sampling of several soil and hospital environments has failed to detect these organisms.

## References

Alexander, A. D.: Actinobacillus. In Lennette, E. H., Spaulding, E. H., and Truant, J. P. (eds.): Manual of Clinical Microbiology. 2nd ed. Washington, D.C., American Society for Microbiology, 1974, p. 320.

Burgher, L. W., Loomis, G. W., and Ware, F.: Systemic infection due to *Actinobacillus actinomycetemcomitans*. Am J Clin Pathol 60:412, 1973.

Custus, D. L., Halley, H., and Bacon, C. M.: *Actinobacillus lignieresii* endocarditis. Arch Pathol 38:332, 1944.

Hill, L. R., and LaPage, S. P.: The DNA base compositions and taxonomy of *Bacteroides corrodens* and *Cardiobacterium hominis*. Brno Conference on the Taxonomy of Bacteria, 24–27 September, 1969.

Midgley, J., LaPage, S. P., Jenkins, B. A. G., Barrow, G. I., Roberts, M. E., and Buck, A. G.: *Cardiobacterium hominis* endocarditis. J Med Microbiol 3:91, 1970.

Page, M. I., and King, E. O.: Infection due to *Actinobacillus actinomycetemcomitans* and *Haemophilus aphrophilus*. N Engl J Med 275:181, 1966.

Pathak, R. C., and Ristic, M.: Detection of an antibody to *Actinobacillus lignieresii* in infected human beings and the antigenic characterization of isolates of human and bovine origin. Am J Vet Res 23:310, 1962.

Perdue, C. D., Dorney, E. R., and Ferrier, F.: Embolomycotic aneurysm associated with bacterial endocarditis due to *Cardiobacterium hominis*. Am Surg 34:901, 1974.

Phillips, J. E.: The incidence of agglutinating antibodies to *Actinobacillus lignieresii* in the sera of normal and infected cattle. J Pathol Bacteriol 90:557, 1965.

Phillips, J. E.: Antigenic structure and serological typing of *Actinobacillus lignieresii*. J Pathol Bact 93:463, 1967.

Pulverer, G., and Ko, H. L.: *Actinobacillus actinomycetemcomitans*: Fermentative capabilities of 140 strains. Appl Microbiol 20:693, 1970.

Pulverer, G., and Ko, H. L.: Serological studies on *Actinobacillus actinomycetemcomitans*. Appl Microbiol 23:207, 1972.

Reyn, A., Birch-Anderson, A., and Murray, R. G. E.: The fine structure of *Cardiobacterium hominis*. Acta Pathol Microbiol Scand [B]72:51, 1971.

Savage, D. D., Kagan, R. L., Young, A. N., and Horvath, A. E.: *Cardiobacterium hominis* endocarditis: Description of two patients and characterization of the organism. J Clin Microbiol 5:75, 1977.

Slotnick, I. J., and Dougherty, M.: Further characterization of an unclassified group of bacteria causing endocarditis in man: *Cardiobacterium hominis* gen. et sp.n. Antonie van Leeuwenhoek 30:261, 1964.

Snyder, A. I., and Ellner, P. D.: *Cardiobacterium hominis* endocarditis. NY State J Med 69:704, 1969.

Townsend, T. R., and Gillenwater, J. Y.: Urinary tract infection due to *Actinobacillus actinomycetemcomitans*. JAMA 210:558, 1969.

Tucker, D. N., Slotnick, I. J., King, E. O., Tynes, B., Nicholson, J., and Crevasse, L.: Endocarditis caused by *Pasteurella*-like organism: Report of four cases. N Engl J Med 267:913, 1962.

Weiner, M., and Werthamer, S.: *Cardiobacterium hominis* endocarditis: Characterization of the unusual organisms and review of the literature. Am J Clin Pathol 63:131, 1975.

# Acid-Fast Rods

# 40 MYCOBACTERIA
### Donald W. Smith, Ph.D.

The genus *Mycobacterium* includes the causative agents of tuberculosis and leprosy, two diseases that, according to the World Health Organization, are among the main public health priorities of many of the developing countries of the world. For example, the global tuberculosis problem is estimated to be the following: 1500 million persons infected with tubercle bacilli; 20 million sputum-positive persons capable of disseminating the disease; 3 to 5 million new cases each year; and 600,000 deaths per year.

The principal species of mycobacteria that cause disease in man and other animals are listed in Table 1, along with the most common saprophytic (free-living) mycobacteria.

## TABLE 1. Pathogenic and Saprophytic Mycobacteria

### PATHOGENIC MYCOBACTERIA

| Microorganism | Disease Produced |
|---|---|
| M. tuberculosis | Tuberculosis in man and subhuman primates |
| M. bovis | Tuberculosis in cattle, man and subhuman primates |
| M. avium intracellulare* | Tuberculosis in birds and swine; tuberculosis-like disease in man |
| M. kansasii* | Tuberculosis-like disease in man |
| M. fortuitum complex* (including M. chelonei) | Wound infection in man |
| M. marinum* | Tuberculosis in fish and cutaneous disease in man |
| M. ulcerans* | Ulcerative lesions in man |
| M. leprae | Leprosy in man |

### SAPROPHYTIC MYCOBACTERIA

| Microorganism | Source in Nature |
|---|---|
| M. gordonae | Soil, water Not responsible for human disease but may be isolated from sputum, gastric washings, etc. |
| M. terrae complex (includes M. terrae, M. triviale, M. novum, and M. nonchromogenicum) | Soil, water |
| M. flavescens | Soil, water |
| M. gastri | Soil, water |

*Atypical mycobacteria.

## MYCOBACTERIUM TUBERCULOSIS AND ATYPICAL MYCOBACTERIA

### Morphology

Mycobacteria are slender, rod-shaped organisms that cannot be distinguished from each other on the basis of morphology. Tubercle bacilli in tissue and in sputum smears frequently have an irregularly staining, beaded appearance. The unstained regions of the cell are presumably areas containing inclusion bodies such as glycogen and polymetaphosphate. Electron microscopic examination of mycobacteria shows a thick cell wall, the presence of mesosomes, and inclusions of lipid (Fig. 1). Mycobacteria do not form spores. They have an unusually high lipid content, greater than 25 per cent in contrast to 0.5 per cent lipid in gram-positive and 3 per cent lipid in gram-negative bacteria. The high lipid content is presumed to be responsible for their characteristic resistance to drying, alcohol, acids, alkali, and certain germicides. The high lipid content also renders the Gram stain invalid for mycobacteria. On the other hand, mycobacteria are acid-fast; this property is shared with certain species of only one other genus of bacteria, *Nocardia*. Once stained with basic fuchsin dyes, acid-fast organisms resist decolorization even with alcohol containing 3 per cent mineral acid. Acid-fastness is an important characteristic useful in the laboratory diagnosis of all mycobacterial diseases. Although the lipids extracted from mycobacteria are weakly acid-fast and the lipid-free cell residue is not acid-fast, tubercle bacilli also become non-acid-fast after such damage as crushing the cells between glass slides or exposure to ultrasound. According to Barksdale and Kim (1977), the acid-fastness of intact mycobacterial cells depends on trapping of intracellular fuchsin. A barrier results from mycolate-fuchsin complexes that form in the cell wall.

### Growth

Most pathogenic mycobacteria grow unusually slowly. The doubling time for *M. tuberculosis* is

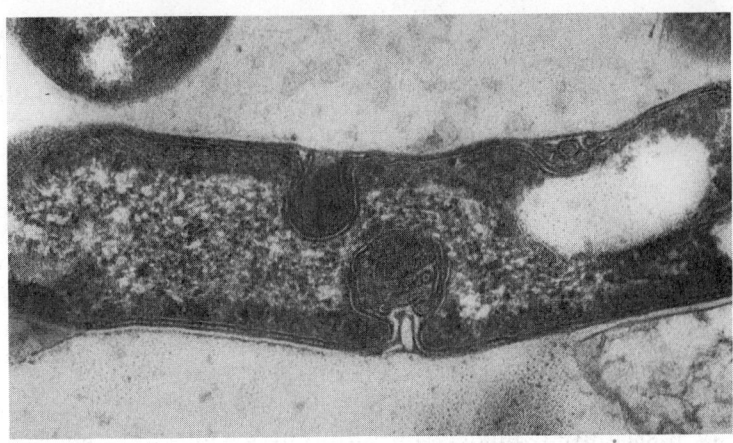

**FIGURE 1.** *Section of actively growing cell of M.* tuberculosis *strain H37Rv. Note the presence of mesosomes at the initiation of cross-wall formation and the presence of vacuole-like fatty inclusion bodies. ×78,000. (From Barksdale, L., and Kim, K. S.: Mycobacterium. Bacteriol. Rev. 41:217, 1977.)*

12 to 18 hours, in contrast to 15 minutes for the Enterobacteriaceae. Although tubercle bacilli can grow on simple synthetic media, their isolation from clinical specimens requires complex media. The organism is a strict aerobe, an attribute that appears to play an important role in the pathogenesis of tuberculosis.

Virulent (but not avirulent) strains of *M. tuberculosis* grown on the surface of liquid or solid media characteristically form strands or cords, and this is reflected in a difference in the appearance of the colonies on solid media (Fig. 2).

### Drug Susceptibility

Tubercle bacilli are inhibited in vitro and in vivo by isonicotinic acid hydrazide (INH), streptomycin (ST), para-aminosalicylic acid (PAS), thiacetazone (TH), ethambutol (EMB), and rifampin (RIF), as well as by several other more toxic drugs (e.g., ethionamide, kanamycin, cycloserine) that are used primarily in patients whose organisms are resistant to the first-line drugs (INH, ST, PAS, TH, EMB, RIF). RIF inhibits DNA-dependent RNA polymerase in prokaryotic cells; ST inhibits func-

tion of the 30 S ribosomal subunit. The mode of action of INH is unclear but may involve suppression of mycolic acid synthesis. Although antituberculosis drugs administered singly to experimentally infected animals bring about bacteriostasis, the combination of RIF and INH has been demonstrated to have bactericidal activity in vivo. Tubercle bacilli isolated from the sputum of inadequately treated patients may be resistant to one or more of the drugs used. This resistance is not associated with plasmids (no R-factor) and is due to the selection and the eventual predominance of naturally occurring resistant mutants present in small numbers among the high populations of bacilli that develop in cavitary tuberculosis.

### Lipids

Mycobacteria contain a number of unusual high molecular weight complex lipids, for example, mycolic acid, mycosides, waxes D, trehalose-6,6'-dimycolate, and sulfolipid. A number of the complex lipids of mycobacteria contain mycolic acid, which has the general formula

**FIGURE 2.** *Colonies of virulent (H37Rv) and attenuated (H37Ra) M.* tuberculosis *grown on the surface of agar medium. A, H37Ra: 12-day-old culture illustrating the nonoriented heaped-up structure of the colony. B, H37Rv: the colonies are flat with a serpentine structure. Cording is visible at the edge of the colony as thin strands and loops. (From Middlebrook, G., Dubos, R. J., and Pierce, C.: Virulence and morphological characteristics of mammalian tubercle bacilli. J. Exp. Med. 86:175, 1947.)*

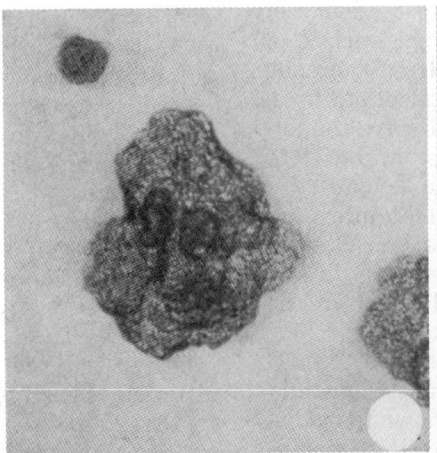
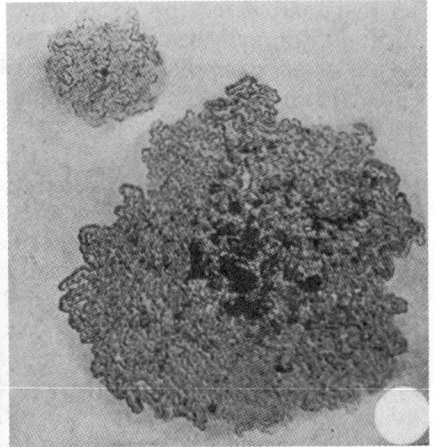

$C_{88}H_{176}O_4 \pm 5CH_2$. The general structure of mycolic acid from *M. tuberculosis* is:

$$\underset{\underset{C_{24}H_{49}}{|}}{R-CH-\overset{\overset{OH}{|}}{CH}-COOH}$$

The R group in the formula contains about 60 carbon atoms and an undetermined oxygen function and occurs in the molecule in three chains.

The mycosides, a series of mycolic acid–containing glycolipids or glycolipid peptides, are uniquely distributed among the different species of mycobacteria, a chemically distinct mycoside associated with each species (Randall and Smith, 1964). Some of the mycosides have been shown to occur on the outer surface of the cell and to act as mycobacteriophage receptors. Although determination of the specific mycoside present in an isolate could contribute to its identification, the steps involved are too complex for routine application.

Waxes D are a family of closely related substances composed of mycolic acid, peptides, and polysaccharides. When extracted from *M. tuberculosis*, these substances have unique adjuvant properties in that they not only enhance antibody production against a protein antigen incorporated in a wax D oil emulsion, but also induce a cell-mediated immune (CMI) response against the protein (White et al., 1958). Because of this attribute, waxes D may contribute to the pathogenesis of tuberculosis through enhancement of the CMI response (specifically, delayed-type hypersensitivity) against mycobacterial proteins. Recent work from several laboratories indicates that the adjuvant-active component of waxes D (and the mycobacterial cell wall) is an N-acetylmuramyl dipeptide (see Barksdale and Kim, 1977).

Cord factor, so named because it was thought to be responsible for the cord-forming tendency of virulent tubercle bacilli grown on the surface of liquid or solid media, can be extracted from the cells with hexane. The purified material has been reported by various investigators to have the following properties: lethality for mice; inhibition of migration of polymorphonuclear leukocytes; induction of protection against virulent infection; and induction of granuloma formation. Despite this impressive array of potential contributors to virulence, the role played by cord factor in the pathogenesis of tuberculosis is unknown.

Binding of the dye neutral red, another property reported to distinguish between virulent and avirulent mycobacteria, has been shown to be due to the presence of a sulfonated glycolipid characterized as a tetraester of trehalose; again, the role of this substance in the disease process has not been elucidated.

### Antigenic Structure

As is true of all other microbes, mycobacteria contain many antigens and antigenic determinants. Antibody-mediated immunity (AMI) and cell-mediated immunity (CMI) develop against many of these determinants during the course of infection; however, no association between a particular antigenic structure and virulence has been established. Various species of mycobacteria share antigenic determinants, and this is responsible for the cross-reactions observed in tuberculin skin test responses.

### Pathogenic Properties

Tuberculosis epitomizes the pathogenesis of chronic infectious diseases. Virulent mycobacteria produce no potent toxins or tissue-destructive enzymes. The principal basis for their virulence lies in the fact that, though readily phagocytosed, the organisms resist the destructive properties of normal macrophages and are capable of multiplying intracellularly. This process damages tissue once CMI is activated.

The principal features in the initiation of tuberculous infection and its evolution to tuberculous disease, as revealed by studies of the disease in man and in an experimental model of tuberculosis in guinea pigs, can be summarized as follows. The organism (usually one to three), airborne as droplet nuclei coming from an individual with cavitary tuberculosis (or in the case of the guinea pig model, from an aerosol-generating device) is inhaled by a susceptible individual. Droplet nuclei less than 5 $\mu$m in diameter escape the defense mechanisms of the upper respiratory tract, and usually one such particle is carried into a terminal alveolar space in the well-ventilated mid to lower lung. The small number of organisms present in the particle is readily ingested by an alveolar macrophage.

After a lag period of about three days, the organism begins to multiply slowly, with one generation occurring each 12 to 18 hours. The bacilli, accumulating intracellularly, kill the initial alveolar phagocyte, and the organisms released are readily ingested by macrophages (transformed from blood monocytes) carried to the site and replicating in response to the developing inflammatory process. This slowly evolving local lesion continues to enlarge, and about two weeks after initiation of the infection, bacilli are transported via the lymphatics to the lymph node draining that region of the lung. The fixed macrophages in the lymph node ingest the organisms, but again they continue to multiply intracellularly.

A few days later, organisms leave the lymph node and are carried via the efferent lymphatics and thoracic duct to the bloodstream. This bacillemic phase of the infection leads to the dissemination of organisms throughout the body, where they are again trapped by macrophages already present, or they are ingested by macrophages carried to the sites of deposition. Again, evidence suggests that the bacilli likely multiply inside cells at each of these sites.

About three to four weeks after infection, the CMI response has been initiated, and immune (sensitized) lymphocytes coming from lymph nodes and spleen are carried by the bloodstream to the sites of the developing microscopic lesions. The interaction between lymphocytes sensitive to mycobacterial antigens and the corresponding specific antigen presumably leads to the release of mediators (lymphokines) and in turn to the activation of macrophages and to the initiation of caseation necrosis. The joint action of the activated macrophages and the unfavorable oxygen tension at most of the sites of hematogenous dissemination are presumably responsible for the death of the mycobacteria. In contrast, the organisms that by chance lodge in the apex or the subapical area of the lungs, the kidney, or the growing ends of long bones (in children) are favored by the high $pO_2$ in these sites (the high $pO_2$ in the apical and subapical areas of the lungs results from a high ventilation-perfusion ratio). The tubercle bacillus, a strict aerobe, may survive in small numbers in these sites of high $pO_2$ in a slowly metabolizing, relatively dormant state.

These events can all occur without the development of symptoms; that is to say, this is tuberculous infection, but not tuberculous disease. The host-parasite interaction terminates at this stage in about 90 per cent of infected persons. The only evidence that infection has taken place is conversion of the tuberculin reaction from negative to positive (tuberculin conversion) and perhaps the later development of a calcified focus at the site of the primary respiratory implantation and perhaps at the site of the draining lymph node in the hilus of the lung. These calcified sites are called the primary complex or Ghon complex. There may also be radiologic abnormalities and even calcification in the apical and subapical areas of the lung. These are sometimes referred to as Simon's foci.

Paradoxically, if tuberculous infection is to progress to tuberculous disease, the subsequent critical events usually take place at the apical or subapical site seeded during the bacillemia (Fig. 3), rather than at the site of the primary respiratory implantation (primary complex). This pro-

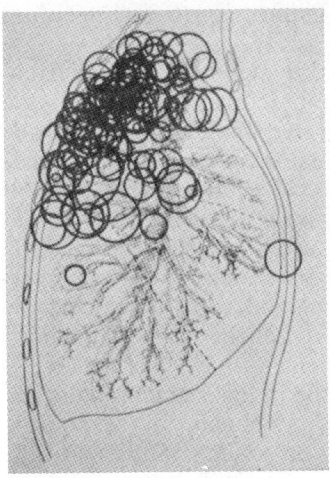

**FIGURE 3.** *Location of 268 cavities in the lungs of 204 tuberculosis patients as revealed by stereoscopic radiographs. Note the tendency for cavities to occur in the apical and subapical areas of the lungs. (From Sweaney, H. C., Cook, C. E., and Kegerreis, R.: A study of the position of primary cavities in pulmonary tuberculosis. Am. Rev. Tuberc. 24:558, 1931.)*

gression occurs during the first two years of infection in about 5 per cent (recent experience in India suggests a lower percentage) of those infected and much later in life in another 5 per cent. One can postulate the following events.

There is an antecedent temporary suppression of the CMI response, perhaps due to another infection or therapy for another disease. Activated macrophages are no longer produced, and the organisms that had been dormant in the apical focus begin to multiply and within several weeks are present in relatively high numbers. Later, when the CMI response is restored, sensitive lymphocytes reappear at the site of the developing lesion, lymphokines are released, and macrophages are activated. However, because of the high level of bacillary antigen, the entire process is exaggerated, and although the population of bacilli is temporarily reduced, caseation necrosis is extensive. Some change in the lesion, which is not yet fully understood, causes the caseous mass to undergo liquefaction. This creates a favorable environment for the bacillus, and massive growth ensues, more lymphocytes infiltrate, more lymphokines are released, and the lesion enlarges. As the developing lesion erodes through a bronchus, the liquid caseum is released into the bronchial tree, coughed up, and expectorated or swallowed. This leaves a cavity in the lung, and bacilli continue to multiply in the lining of the cavity. This process is usually accompanied by low-grade fever, cough, and malaise — that is, the symptoms of tuberculous disease.

## Immunity to Tuberculosis

Substantial evidence from work with animal models of tuberculosis, as well as work with other diseases caused by facultative intracellular pathogens, indicates that immunity to these microbial agents is most likely due to the CMI response. Macrophages, activated as a result of the lymphokines released from the interaction of immune lymphocytes and specific mycobacterial antigen, are apparently altered so that they become competent to control the intracellular organism. The process of macrophage activation results in increases in the following: metabolic activity; membrane activity; phagocytic activity; and granule (lysosomal) enzymes (Dannenberg, 1968). It has not been established, however, which if any of these changes is responsible for the ability of the activated macrophage to limit the intracellular multiplication of tubercle bacilli. The role of CMI in the tissue-destructive aspects of the disease and in acquired resistance to tuberculosis is a clear example of the immune response as a "double-edged sword."

Human field trials have revealed that injection of bacille Calmette-Guérin (BCG) vaccine, a viable attenuated strain of *M. bovis*, leads to as much as 70 to 80 per cent reduction in the incidence of tuberculosis in vaccinated subjects (Hart, Sutherland, and Thomas, 1967). It is theorized that the protective effect of BCG stems from an interference with the bacillemic phase of the infection in vaccinated persons. This hypothesis is directly supported by studies in a guinea pig model of tuberculosis constructed so as to mimic the conditions under which tuberculosis is initiated in humans (Fok et al., 1976). Many reports indicate that killed mycobacterial vaccines or bacillary fractions induced protective immunity in experimental animals (Smith, Wiegeshaus, and Grover, 1968); however, none of these substances has been shown yet to have application for the prevention of human disease.

## Epidemiology of Tuberculosis (Prevalence, Mode of Spread, Prevention)

The *prevalence* of tuberculous infection is estimated by tuberculin test surveys of sample populations. The *incidence* of tuberculous disease is obtained from data giving the number of new cases of tuberculosis, as revealed by laboratory studies and clinical findings, or from the frequency of individuals shown to have tubercle bacilli in their sputum. The incidence of tuberculosis varies greatly from one country to another. In several of the developing countries, tuberculous infection rates are as high as 85 to 90 per cent of the

general population. In these same areas the prevalence of tuberculous disease may be as frequent as one to two per hundred. In contrast, in some of the developed countries, rates of tuberculous infection have fallen to as low as 10 to 15 per cent, and of tuberculous disease as low as 10 to 15 per 100,000.

As was indicated earlier, transmission of tuberculosis occurs when an individual with tubercle bacilli present in his or her sputum (sputum-positive tuberculosis) coughs, sings, or otherwise creates an aerosol and a few organisms are inhaled by a nearby susceptible individual. This situation, referred to as a primary aerosol, is one in which droplet nuclei containing bacilli are transmitted via the air directly from the diseased person to a susceptible person. It is this primary aerosol that is most likely to be associated with transmission of the infection. In contrast, droplets of sputum that fall to the floor, bedding, or furniture are less likely to result in transmission even if they become airborne once again. This situation is referred to as a secondary aerosol, and successful transmission is less likely for several reasons. The most important is that the bacilli in the secondary aerosol are almost always associated (by electrostatic forces) with particles of dust or lint, and the particle size is thereby increased. Because the defense mechanisms of the upper respiratory tract are very effective in trapping and eliminating particles greater than 5 $\mu$m in diameter, the organisms in the secondary aerosol are removed before they reach susceptible tissues deep in the lung. Moreover, bacilli in the secondary aerosol usually have had longer exposure to the inactivating influence of ultraviolet light. It has been shown experimentally that tubercle bacilli in an aerosol are rapidly killed upon exposure to ultraviolet light. The importance of the contrast between primary and secondary aerosol is that it focuses attention on the most important source of transmission, namely, the infectious person. It is possible to reduce transmission of tuberculosis to direct contacts of patients with positive sputum by lowering the concentration of infectious particles in the air. This can be done by means of an adequate number of air changes and by ultraviolet irradiation of the upper air in the patient's room. The concept of primary aerosol indicates that less attention need be given to the handling of bedding and objects used by the patient.

The most effective means of preventing tuberculosis is to block the transmission of the organism. This is best accomplished by early detection and treatment of patients with tubercle bacilli in their sputum. Treatment for only several weeks with isoniazid alone (despite the need for two or more drugs to prevent drug resistance) will greatly reduce the number of secondary cases among close contacts of a patient under treatment, even though organisms may still be recovered from his sputum.

A second means of reducing the tuberculosis problem in a given area is vaccination with BCG. As was indicated earlier, field trials have shown that use of an effective BCG vaccine is accompanied by a 70 to 80 per cent reduction in the incidence of tuberculous disease.

## Laboratory Diagnosis

### Direct Microscopy

Sputum collected from the diseased person should be examined after the preparation of an acid-fast stain. A loopful of material from the sediment in the sputum container (the maximal chance of finding bacilli is realized from a study of the solid particles) is smeared on a glass slide, air-dried, and heat-fixed. Some modification of the Ziehl-Neelsen acid-fast stain is usually employed. The smear is flooded with carbol-fuchsin and then heat is applied to cause the stain to steam. After five minutes of steaming, the carbol-fuchsin is washed off with water and the smear is decolorized for up to two minutes with a reagent consisting of 3 ml of hydrochloric acid in 97 ml of 95 per cent ethanol or with 25 per cent sulfuric acid. The preparation is then washed with water and counterstained for one minute with methylene blue. After a final water wash, the slide is air-dried and examined under the oil-immersion lens of a microscope. Tubercle bacilli appear as deep-red–staining, thin-beaded, often curved rods in a blue background. The number of tubercle bacilli in a positive sputum smear could vary from a few in 20 to 30 oil-immersion fields to many in each oil-immersion field. *Fluorochrome staining* may be superior to Ziehl-Neelsen staining for the detection of tubercle bacilli in sputum. The staining reagent is tetramethyldiaminodiphenyl ketoimine (auramine O), and although most laboratories examine auramine-stained smears under ultraviolet light with a special microscope, techniques have been developed that permit use of a standard microscope and an illuminator with a special filter (Runyon et al., 1974). The fluorochrome staining procedure has the advantage of permitting the survey of a sputum smear at a lower magnification, and this speeds up the examination and increases the sensitivity of the detection of acid-fast organisms.

### Digestion and Concentration

If the laboratory has resources for culture of the specimen, acid-fast stains would be made after the specimen has been subjected to digestion and concentration. The primary objectives of the digestion-concentration step are to break up tissue debris, to kill nonmycobacterial organisms present as contaminants, and to concentrate tubercle bacilli in a smaller volume of specimen. Digestion can be accomplished by vigorous shaking of a mixture of equal parts of specimen and 3 per cent sodium hydroxide for 30 minutes. The process can be accelerated by incorporating 0.5 per cent acetyl cysteine in 2 to 4 per cent sodium hydroxide, mixing, and allowing the suspension to stand for 15 minutes. The shorter contact time increases the number of surviving mycobacteria and thus increases the sensitivity of the technique for detection of a positive specimen. After digestion, the specimen is centrifuged, the supernatant fluid is decanted, and the sediment is used for smears and stains and for culture.

### Culture

Recovery of mycobacteria from clinical specimens requires an enriched medium. Ordinarily this is some modification of Löwenstein-Jensen's (L-J) medium containing egg, potato extract, glycerine, and an inhibitory dye (often malachite green) added to retard the growth of contaminants that have survived the decontamination step. Slants of L-J medium are inoculated with the concentrated sediment. The cultures are incubated at 37° C for as long as eight weeks and are examined weekly for the appearance of colonies. If viable *M. tuberculosis* organisms were present in the specimen, small buff-colored, rough colonies could appear in about three weeks but may take as long as six to eight weeks to appear. Acid-fast stains made from these colonies will reveal a morphology like that described above. If growth appears within one week, the organism could be *M. fortuitum* or one of the saprophytic mycobacteria. Although a slow-growing, nonpigmented, acid-fast organism may be *M. tuberculosis*, it could also be one of the atypical mycobacteria.

### Atypical Mycobacteria

Depending on the region of the world, mycobacteria other than *M. tuberculosis* are recovered from less than 0.1 per cent to as many as 50 per cent of individuals with tuberculosis-like diseases.* These organisms, collectively called "atypical mycobacteria," are indicated by an asterisk

---

*The high levels are based on recent reports from the low-prevalence areas of developed countries. In contrast, in a recent report from Madras, only one case of disease due to atypical mycobacteria was found among many thousands of cases of tuberculosis.

in the list of mycobacteria given in Table 1. Recent reports suggest that atypical mycobacteria more frequently cause disease in patients whose lung or immune response is already damaged by another disease. Atypical mycobacteria and the disease they produce differ in several important respects from classic tuberculosis. Of primary significance is that examination of close contacts of patients with disease due to an atypical mycobacterium reveals *no evidence of human to human transmission* (atypical mycobacteria have been recovered from the soil and from water). Atypical mycobacteria are more likely to be *resistant to the first-line antituberculous drugs* than is *M. tuberculosis*. Patients infected with atypical mycobacteria usually give a *negative tuberculin test* to the 5-TU test dose of tuberculin prepared from *M. tuberculosis*. Finally, atypical mycobacteria can be distinguished from *M. tuberculosis* by a series of laboratory tests, primarily biochemical tests.

### Identification of the Species of Mycobacteria (Speciation)

When laboratory resources are available, the identification of the species of mycobacteria causing disease in a given patient is important because of the implications for the treatment regimen employed and for the need to search for other diseased persons among the contacts of the patient. Speciation is accomplished by examining the results of a series of differential tests. Although complete speciation requires a comprehensive series of tests, the 12 characteristic tests shown in Table 2 permit a satisfactory identification of most species. (Note, for example, that *M. avium* and *M. intracellulare* differ primarily in the proportion of strains showing photo-inducible pigmentation and the proportion that grow on Mac-Conkey agar. This is the reason why these species were listed in Table 1 as the *M. avium intracellulare* complex.)

### Drug Susceptibility Tests

As many as 5 to 10 per cent or even more of cultures isolated from human specimens may contain bacilli resistant to one or more of the first-line antituberculosis drugs. Therefore, pathogenic mycobacteria recovered from clinical material should be examined for susceptibility to the first-line antituberculosis drugs. If acid-fast organisms are still grown from the sputum six months after the initiation of therapy, susceptibility tests should be repeated to look for drug-resistance. The drugs to be tested are added to slants of L-J medium, and the drug-containing media and suitable control media are then inoculated with standardized suspensions of organisms prepared

from the primary L-J culture. The appearance of colonies on drug-containing media is indicative of the presence of drug-resistant mycobacteria. In this event, it may be necessary to determine the susceptibility of the organism to the second-line (more toxic, less effective, and often more expensive) antituberculosis drugs.

## MYCOBACTERIUM LEPRAE

*Mycobacterium leprae*, the causative agent of leprosy, was discovered by Hansen in 1874. In honor of his discovery and in part to circumvent the stigma associated with leprosy, the affliction is sometimes referred to as Hansen's disease and the organism as Hansen's bacillus.

### Morphology

*M. leprae* is morphologically indistinguishable from the other mycobacteria; they are rod-shaped organisms approximately 0.3 to 0.5 $\mu$m wide and 2 to 5 $\mu$m in length. *M. leprae* is acid-fast and can be stained by the Ziehl-Neelsen method.

### Metabolism and Drug Susceptibility

Of paramount importance is that *M. leprae* is an obligate intracellular parasite. The microbe has not been cultured in the absence of living tissues and is therefore referred to as a noncultivable mycobacterium. *M. leprae* appears to require something in the parasitized host cell in order to replicate. Even when multiplying intracellularly, the generation time of the organism is exceptionally long. Estimates based on experimental infection of mouse foot pads (Shepard, 1971) indicate a generation time of 13 days. *M. leprae* is susceptible to diaminodiphenylsulfone (dapsone) and to rifampin. Inoculation tests in the mouse food pad indicate that *M. leprae* present in the circulation of lepromatous patients is killed faster after rifampin therapy than dapsone therapy.

### Antigenic Composition

*M. leprae* contains no unusual antigens. Patients infected with *M. leprae* may undergo both an antibody-mediated immune (AMI) response and a cell-mediated immune (CMI) response. Because the organism is noncultivable, the skin test reagent, called lepromin, is prepared from organisms concentrated from diseased tissue.

### Pathogenic Properties

Like the tubercle bacillus, *M. leprae* produces no potent toxins or extracellular factors contrib-

## TABLE 2. Characterization of Clinically Significant Mycobacteria According to Twelve Key Properties*

**TWELVE PROPERTIES**[a]

(1) Rate of growth (S = slow; F = fast)
(2) Secretion of niacin
(3) Reduction of nitrate ($NaNO_3$)
(4) Semiquantitative test for hyperproduction of catalase (column of gas bubbles, >45 mm)
(5) Stability of catalase to 68°C, 20 min
(6) Carotenogenesis constitutive (scotochromogenic)
(7) Carotenogenesis photoinducible (photochromogenic)

(8) Hydrolysis of Tween 80 after 10 days
(9) Reduction of tellurite ($KTeO_2$), 3 days
(10) Growth on media containing 5% (wt/vol) NaCl
(11) Hydrolysis of tripotassium phenolphthalein disulfate by arylsulfatase, 3 days
(12) Growth on MacConkey agar

### FORMULAE FOR 17 MYCOBACTERIAL TAXA AND 1 SPECIES COMPLEX[a]

*From Barksdale, L., and Kim, K. S.: Mycobacterium. Bacteriol Rev *41*:217, 1977.

[a]Key for reading formulae. When number N is unboxed, N (number above the line) = 100% strains tested was positive (e.g., *11* in *M. chelonei*); Ⓝ = 70 to 99% strains tested, positive (e.g., ⑤ in *M. avium*); [N] = 15 to 60% strains tested, positive (e.g., |7| in *M. avium*); N (number below the line) = 0.4 to 14% strains tested, positive (e.g., 3 in *M. avium*). Absence if N = 100% strains tested, negative (e.g., 11 absent in *M. avium*).

[b]*M. chelonei* subsp. chelonei fails to grow in 5% NaCl.

[c]*M. fortuitum* includes strains designated as *M. peregrinum*.

[d]*M. terrae* complex includes *M. terrae, M. nonchromogenicum* and *M. novum.*

uting to the disease process. The pathogenesis of leprosy appears to derive from the ability of the microbe to survive and replicate in macrophages and other host cells, especially nerve cells, and the consequent immune response to the invader. In one polar form of leprosy, lepromatous leprosy, the CMI response appears to be suppressed, and consequently the organisms accumulate in the tissues in large numbers. On the other hand, the AMI response in the lepromatous patient is not suppressed (and perhaps not even controlled), and excessive quantities of antibody are produced. The sera of lepromatous patients often contain circulating immune complexes composed of an-

tibacillary antibody and anti-immunoglobulin. These immune complexes, which precipitate in the cold (+4° C) and therefore are called cryoglobulins, contribute to the pathogenesis of the disease. In patients with the other polar form of leprosy, tuberculoid leprosy, the CMI response appears to be intact and the bacillary population in the tissues is very low or even nondemonstrable.

Experimental infections have been produced in the foot pads of mice and in the nine-banded armadillo. Mice that have been thymectomized and x-irradiated develop a more rapidly progressing infection upon inoculation with *M. leprae*. A recent report suggests that a naturally occurring infection in armadillos in the United States is caused by an organism indistinguishable from *M. leprae* (Walsh et al., 1975).

## Immunity to Leprosy

The patient with tuberculoid leprosy appears to be making an effective immune response against *M. leprae*, and bacillary populations are reduced to a very low level. On the other hand, the patient with lepromatous leprosy appears to have either a specific or a general defect in CMI responsiveness, and bacillary populations in the tissues reach very high levels. The increased frequency of leprosy in certain families in endemic areas and the studies of Jamison and Vollum (1968) suggest that the CMI defect in lepromatous leprosy has a genetically determined component. They compared tuberculin-negative children with a family history of leprosy and tuberculin-negative children with no family history of leprosy for their response to a vole bacillus vaccine (a live attenuated antituberculosis vaccine about equal in potency to BCG). Whereas 90 per cent of the children with no family history of leprosy responded to the vaccine by converting to a positive tuberculin test, tuberculin conversion was observed in less than 20 per cent of children with a family history of leprosy.

Considering all lines of evidence, it appears that the protective host response in leprosy is the CMI response. No vaccine has been developed from *M. leprae*. Field trials with BCG vaccine have yielded discouraging results in reducing the extent of leprosy (only 20 per cent over a nine year follow-up — Bechelli et al., 1974).

## Laboratory Diagnosis of Leprosy

The bacteriological diagnosis of leprosy is based on finding acid-fast organisms in scrapings from nasal mucosa and skin lesions or in biopsy specimens. Leprosy is differentiated from other mycobacterial diseases by demonstrating the lack of cultivability and by showing nerve involvement in histologic examination of tissue biopsies.

## Epidemiology of Leprosy

Leprosy appears to be transmitted by direct contact. The disease is not highly contagious, and prolonged contact with infected persons may be required before transmission occurs. It is estimated that approximately 35 million persons have leprosy, most of them living in states in central Africa and certain regions in Asia. Prevention of leprosy in endemic areas is based on diagnosis, isolation, and treatment of infected persons.

## References

Barksdale, L., and Kim, K.S.: Mycobacterium. Bacteriol Rev 41:217, 1977.

Bechelli, L.M., Lwin, K., Garbajosa, P.G., Gyi, M.M., Uemura, K., Sundaresan, T., Tamondong, C., Matejka, M., Sansarricq, H., and Walter, J.: BCG vaccination of children against leprosy: Nine-year findings of the controlled WHO trial in Burma. Bull WHO 51:93, 1974.

Dannenberg, A. M., Jr.: Cellular hypersensitivity and cellular immunity in the pathogenesis of tuberculosis: Specificity, systemic and local nature, and associated macrophage enzymes. Bacteriol Rev 32:85, 1968.

Fok, J.S., Ho, R.S., Arora, P.K., Harding, G.E., and Smith, D.W.: Host-parasite relationships in experimental airborne tuberculosis. V. Lack of hematogenous dissemination of *Mycobacterium tuberculosis* to the lungs in animals vaccinated with bacille Calmette-Guerin. J. Infect Dis 133:137, 1976.

Hart, P.D., Sutherland, I., and Thomas, J.: The immunity conferred by effective BCG and vole bacillus vaccines, in relation to individual variations in induced tuberculin sensitivity and to technical variations in the vaccines. J Brit Tuberc Assoc 48:201, 1967.

Jamison, D.G., and Vollum, R.L.: Tuberculin conversion in leprous families in northern Nigeria. Lancet 11 (no.7581):1271, 1968.

Middlebrook, G., Dubos, R.J., and Pierce, C.: Virulence and morphological characteristics of mammalian tubercle bacilli. J Exp Med 86:175, 1947.

Randall, H.M., and Smith, D.W.: Characterization of mycobacteria by infrared spectroscopic examination of their lipid fractions. Zentralbl Bakteriol 194:686, 1964.

Runyon, E.H., Karlson, A.G., Kubica, G.P., and Wayne, L.G.: Mycobacterium. In Lennette, E.H., Spaulding, E.H., and Truant, J.P. (eds.): Manual of Clinical Microbiology, 2nd ed. Washington, D.C., American Society for Microbiology, 1974, pp. 148–174 (pertinent section, p. 155).

Shepard, C.C.: The first decade in experimental leprosy. Bull WHO 44:821, 1971.

Smith, D.W., Grover, A.A., and Wiegeshaus, E.: Nonliving immunogenic substances of mycobacteria. Adv Tuberc Res 16:191, 1968.

Sweany, H.C., Cook, C.E., and Kegerreis, R.: A study of the position of primary cavities in pulmonary tuberculosis. Am Rev Tuberc 24:558, 1931.

Walsh, G.P., Storrs, E.E., Burchfield, H.P., Cottrell, E.H., Vidrine, M.F., and Binford, C.H.: Leprosy-like disease occurring naturally in armadillos. J Reticuloendothel Soc 18:347, 1975.

White, R.G., Bernstock, L., Johns, R.G.S., and Lederer, E.: The influence of components of *M. tuberculosis* and other mycobacteria upon antibody production to ovalbumin. Immunology 1:54, 1958.

# NOCARDIA AND  **41**
# STREPTOMYCES

## Saroj K. Mishra
## and Ruth E. Gordon

*Nocardia* and *Streptomyces* are important aerobic actinomycetes known mainly for the causation of serious diseases of man and animals, for the production of potent antibiotics as well as toxic metabolites, and for their decomposition of organic matter in the soil (Waksman, 1959). The infections caused by members of the two genera are broadly classified into two categories: 1) Nocardiosis, a generalized or systemic disease due to members of the genus *Nocardia*, principally *N. asteroides,* and occasionally to *N. caviae* (Causey, 1974) and *N. brasiliensis* (Berd, 1973, see Chapter 112). The disease is usually characterized by primary pulmonary involvement that may be pneumonic or subclinical, chronic or transitory (Emmons et al., 1977). A hematogenous dissemination may occur from the lungs or other parts of the body, especially the brain, for which the pathogen seems to have a predilection. 2) Actinomycetoma, a localized swollen lesion, usually on the foot, hand, or back, and involving the skin, subcutaneous tissues, fascia, and bone (Mariat et al., 1977, see Chapter 238). The pus draining through the sinuses contains granules (compact colonies of the causative microorganism surrounded by reactive cells), the size, shape, and color of which may suggest specific etiology. The chief etiologic agents are strains of *N. madurae,** N. pelletieri, N. brasiliensis, N. caviae, N. asteroides,* and *Streptomyces somaliensis.* In addition, strains belonging to other species (Table 1), namely *N. dassonvillei, N. autotrophica, S. griseus, S. albus,* etc., are isolated from clinical specimens. But their actual role in the causation of disease is uncertain owing to the lack of supporting clinical, experimental, and histologic evidence. With increasing use of immunosuppressants in modern medicine, their role as "possible opportunistic invaders" should be judiciously considered.

## *MORPHOLOGY*

Cultures of nocardiae and streptomycetes are composed of branching filaments (hyphae) ap-

---

*The authors prefer the retention of *N. madurae, N. pelletieri,* and *N. dassonvillei* in the genus *Nocardia* to their assignment to *Actinomadura.*

proximately 1 $\mu$ in width. In stained smears the growth appears as gram-positive filaments (Fig. 1) or as fragmented forms (rods and/or coccoid bodies). Motile forms have not been reported.

In infections caused by some species of *Nocardia* (mainly *N. asteroides, N. caviae,* and *N. brasiliensis*), the microorganisms observed in clinical specimens are generally acidfast. Acidfastness (See *Appendix* in this chapter) of cultures of the same species grown in vitro is, however, a variable characteristic. In some cultures of these few species of *Nocardia,* usually those recently isolated, a high percentage (85 to 100 per cent) of the filaments and fragments retain the carbol fuchsin. Smears of other cultures reveal a decreasing range of acidfastness with only portions of the filaments resisting decolorization (Fig. 1), and many nonacidfast cultures have been observed.

Routinely, the best observation of morphologic characteristics of the nocardiae and streptomycetes is by microscopic examination (100, 200, and 400 ×) of individual, mechanically undisturbed colonies. After three to five days of incubation at 28° C, individual colonies of cultures streaked on plates of tap water agar (see *Appendix*) display a network of branching filaments (vegetative or substrate hyphae) that spread over the surface of the agar. (Caution: The microorganisms must be killed by formalin fumigation before opening the plate.) The vegetative hyphae normally give rise to aerial hyphae that project into the air and, therefore, appear wider and darker than the substrate hyphae (Fig. 2). Junctures of a substrate hypha and an aerial hypha can usually be clearly seen at the periphery of the colony. At the center of the colony, longer and more abundant aerial hyphae hide the substrate hyphae. After longer incubation (7 to 14 days), the aerial hyphae generally are more extensive and branching. Some are straight; some flexuous; and some form loose spirals or a variety of other forms. Under these conditions of growth, the aerial hyphae of cultures of nocardiae and streptomycetes may or may not segment into bead-like conidia (spores).

In the routine diagnostic laboratory, the microscopic appearance of the individual colonies of nocardiae and streptomycetes offers the best

**TABLE 1.  Some Properties of Typical Strains of Species of Nocardia and Streptomyces of Medical Importance**

| PROPERTY | N. asteroides | N. carnea | N. caviae | N. brasiliensis | N. transvalensis | N. autotrophica | N. orientalis | N. aerocolonigenes | N. dassonvillei | N. madurae | N. pelletieri | S. somaliensis | S. lavendulae | S. albus | S. rimosus | S. griseus |
|---|---|---|---|---|---|---|---|---|---|---|---|---|---|---|---|---|
| Acidfastness | v* | v | v | v | v | − | − | − | − | − | − | − | − | − | − | − |
| **Decomposition of** | | | | | | | | | | | | | | | | |
| Adenine | − | − | − | − | v | + | − | | + | | | | | | + | + |
| Casein | − | − | − | + | − | − | + | + | + | + | + | + | − | − | + | + |
| Hypoxanthine | − | − | + | + | + | + | + | + | + | + | v | + | − | + | + | + |
| Tyrosine | − | − | − | + | + | + | + | + | + | + | + | + | + | + | + | + |
| Urea | + | − | + | + | + | + | + | + | v | − | | | v | + | v | + |
| Xanthine | − | − | + | − | v | v | v | − | + | | | | v | v | + | + |
| **Resistance to** | | | | | | | | | | | | | | | | |
| Lysozyme | + | + | + | + | + | − | − | + | | − | | | | + | v | + | − |
| Rifampin | + | + | + | + | + | − | v | − | − | v | v | − | | + | + | − |
| **Hydrolysis of** | | | | | | | | | | | | | | | | |
| Hippurate | v | − | v | − | − | v | v | v | + | − | − | − | − | v | v | v |
| Starch | v | v | v | v | + | + | + | + | + | + | | v | + | − | + | + |
| Nitrite from nitrate | + | + | + | + | + | v | v | v | + | + | + | − | v | v | v | v |
| Survival at 50°C, 8 hr | + | + | + | − | + | v | v | v | + | + | + | v | − | + | + | + |
| **Acid from** | | | | | | | | | | | | | | | | |
| Adonitol | − | − | − | | + | + | + | v | − | + | | | | − | + | + |
| 1(+)Arabinose | − | − | v | | | v | + | + | v | + | − | | v | − | v | v |
| Cellobiose | − | − | − | | v | + | + | + | + | − | | v | v | v |
| 1-Erythritol | − | − | − | + | + | + | − | | − | − | | | v | + | + | + |
| Glucose | + | + | + | + | + | + | + | + | + | + | | | + | + | + | + |
| Glycerol | + | + | + | + | + | + | + | + | + | + | + | v | + | + | + | + |
| i-Inositol | − | v | + | + | v | v | + | + | + | − | − | | + | + | + | + |
| d(+)Lactose | − | − | − | − | − | − | + | + | v | − | | | v | v | + | v |
| d(+)Maltose | − | − | − | − | − | + | v | + | + | v | − | | v | + | + | + |
| d(−)Mannitol | − | + | v | + | v | + | + | + | + | + | − | | v | + | + | + |
| d(+)Melezitose | − | − | − | − | + | v | − | − | − | − | − | | − | + | − | + |
| α-Methyl-D-glucoside | − | − | − | | v | + | − | v | | | | | − | v | − | + |
| d(+)Raffinose | − | − | − | − | v | v | − | v | − | | | | − | + | − | v |
| 1(+)Rhamnose | v | − | − | − | − | v | v | v | + | | | | − | − | + | v |
| d-Sorbitol | − | + | − | | v | + | v | − | − | − | | | − | − | − | v |
| d(+)Trehalose | v | + | v | + | v | + | + | + | v | + | + | − | v | + | + | v |
| d(+)Xylose | − | − | − | − | − | + | + | + | v | + | − | | v | + | v | + |

*v, variable property; +, positive property; −, negative property of typical strains.

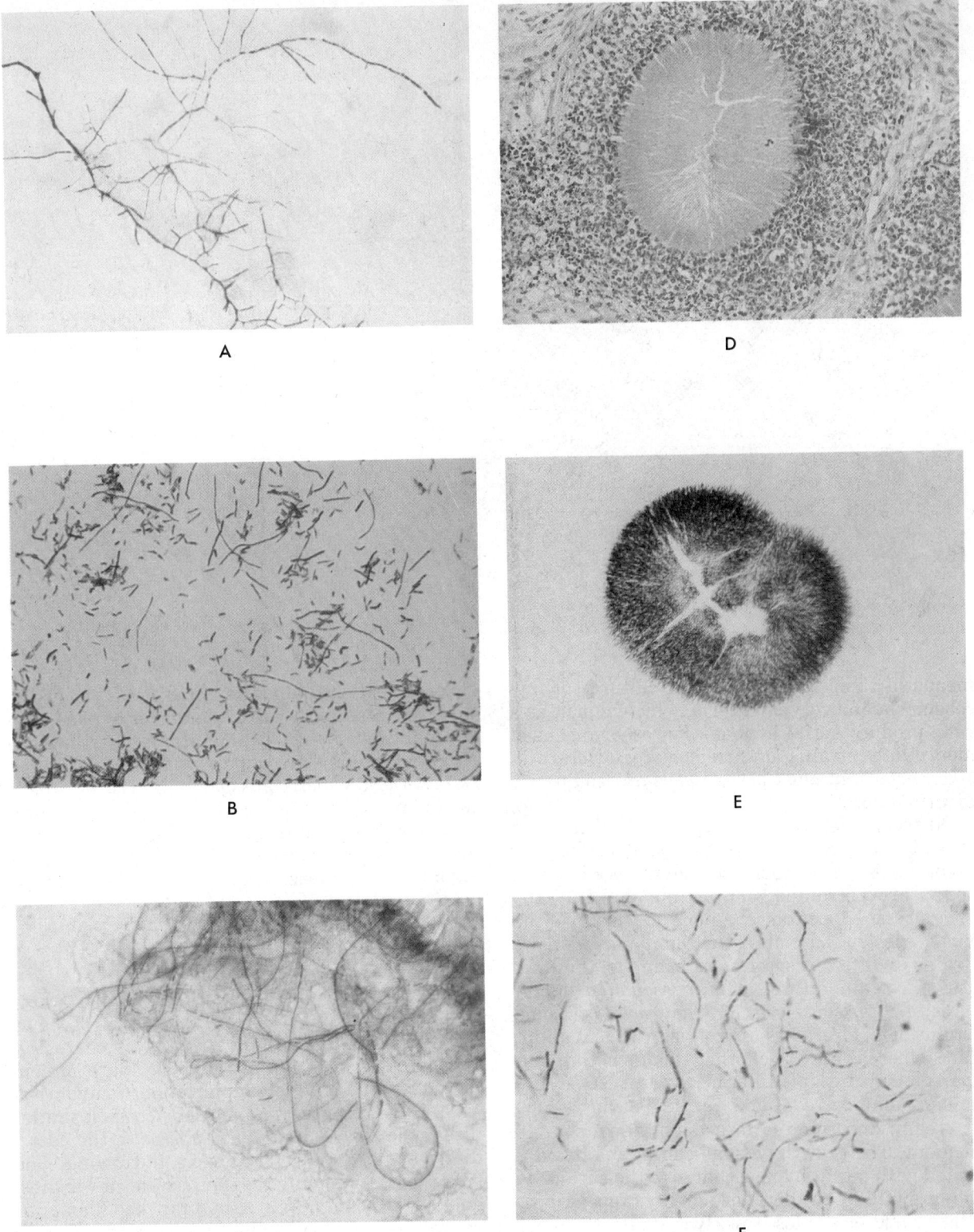

**FIGURE 1.** *Microscopic morphology of some Nocardiae in culture (A–C) and in tissue (D–F).*

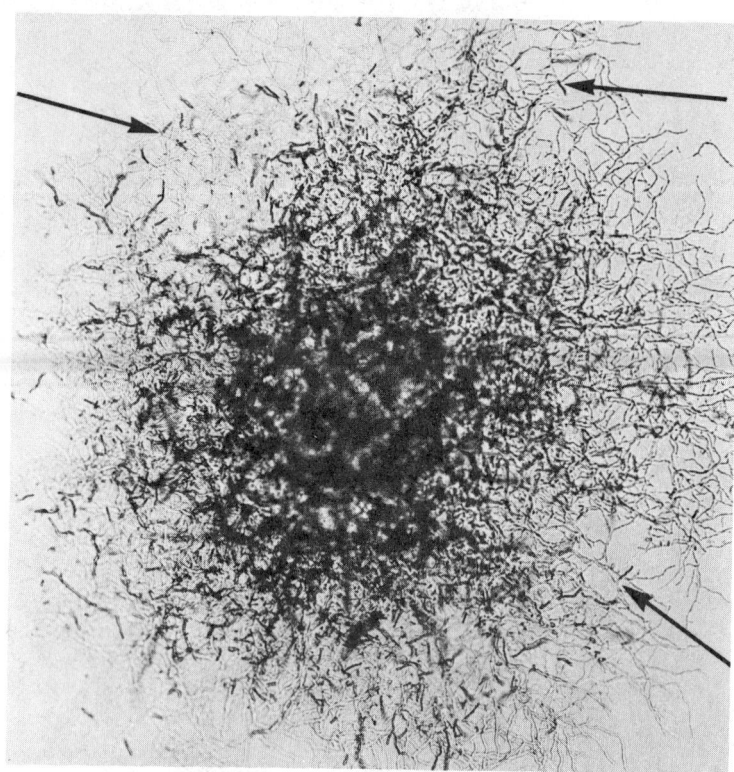

**FIGURE 2.** *Colony grown on tap water agar for 4 days at 28° C, showing vegetative and aerial hyphae. Arrows point to juncture of a vegetative and an aerial hypha. ×700.*

means of their separation from cultures of mycobacteria and corynebacteria, which do not, as a rule, produce aerial hyphae. (For other means of identifying strains of *Streptomyces, Nocardia, Mycobacterium,* and *Corynebacterium* see Species Identification.)

On the whole, the gross appearance of cultures of strains of *Nocardia* and *Streptomyces* belonging to the same species varies considerably. Figures 3 and 4 are presented to illustrate not only the diversity in appearance among cultures of the same species but also the similarity among strains of different species, for example, the likeness of certain cultures of *N. dassonvillei* to cultures of *S. griseus* (Fig. 3). The growth of some strains of *N. asteroides* (Fig. 4) is thick and abundant, whereas growth of other strains is thin and sparse. Cultures of different strains of *N. asteroides* may be red, pink, purple, peach, yellow, or cream, and some form a dark brown soluble pigment. The growth of some cultures is heavily coated with aerial hyphae that give the surface of the growth a powdery or chalky appearance. Other cultures are less thickly coated with aerial hyphae and varying amounts of the substrate growth can be seen. The aerial hyphae of other strains cannot be seen without the aid of a microscope.

Despite this quantitative variation, the formation of aerial hyphae, with few exceptions, is a taxonomically reliable characteristic of the nocardiae and streptomycetes; the aerial hyphae may be sparse and even rudimentary, but they are there. Exceptions are some strains of *N. madurae, N. pelletieri, N. aerocolonigenes,* and *S. somaliensis.* Strains that do not produce aerial hyphae are, however, identifiable by a distinctive pattern of physiologic, chemotaxonomic, and other morphologic properties (see section on *Laboratory Diagnosis*).

## PATHOGENIC PROPERTIES

Nocardiosis due to *N. asteroides* is characterized by the formation of multiple and confluent abscesses and intense suppuration (Emmons et al., 1977). In contrast to actinomycosis, a similar disease caused by *Actinomyces israelii,* the nocardial lesions show less fibrosis, burrowing, and sinus formation; sulfur granules are never present. The lesions contain thin, branched filaments, as well as bacillary bodies, which can be demonstrated only when the sections are properly stained. Loose conglomeratory growth may sometimes be observed in the tissues, but granules and the giant cell granulomatous tissue reaction, as seen in actinomycetoma or in organs of mice experimentally infected with nocardiae (Fig. 1), are

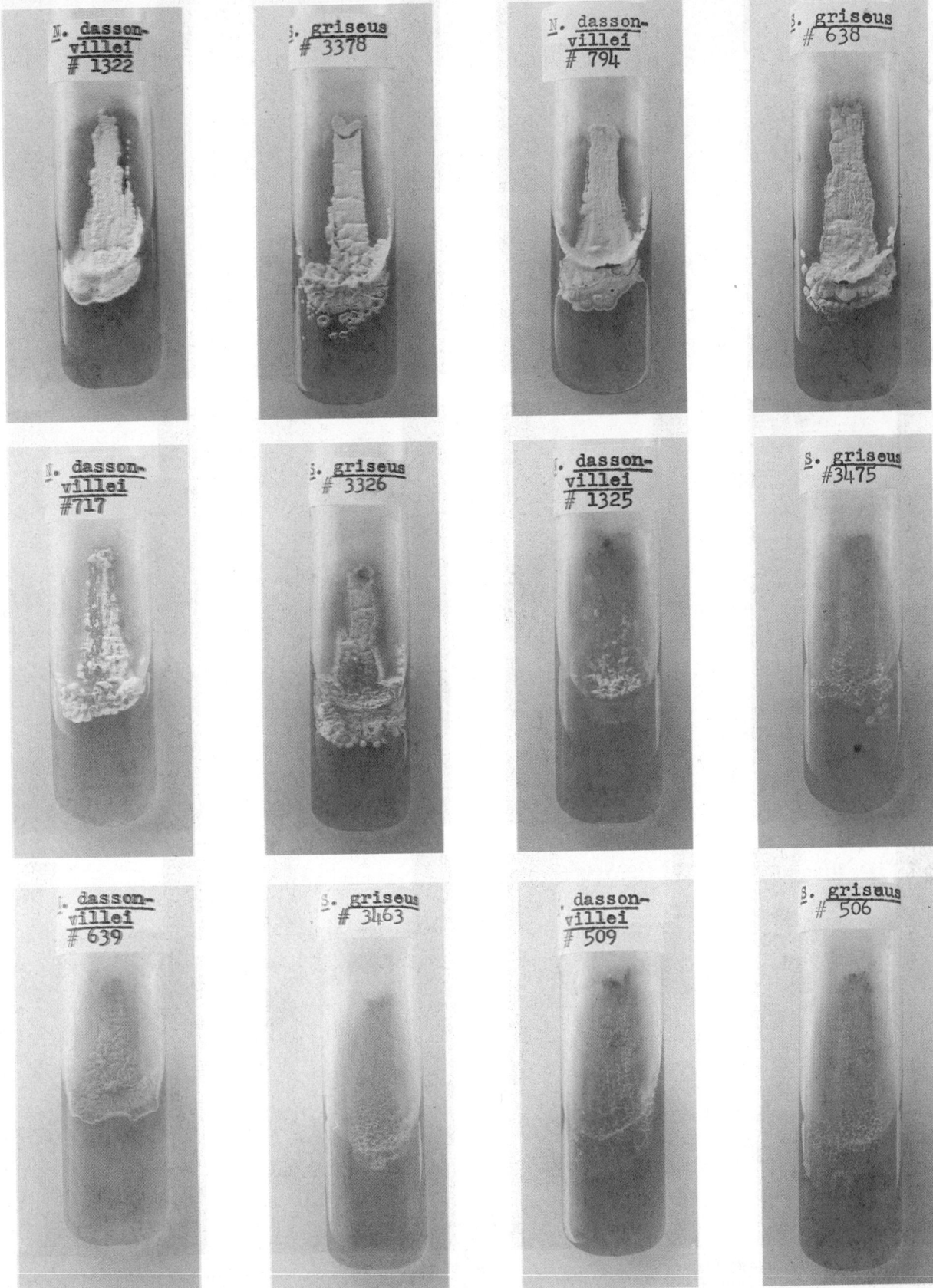

**FIGURE 3.** *Gross appearance of cultures of* Nocardia dassonvillei *and of* Streptomyces griseus. *Cultures of* N. dassonvillei *and* S. griseus *grown on yeast dextrose agar for 2 weeks at 28° C and forming varying amounts of aerial hyphae. (Reproduced from J Gen Microbiol 50:235–240, 1968, with the kind permission of the editors).*

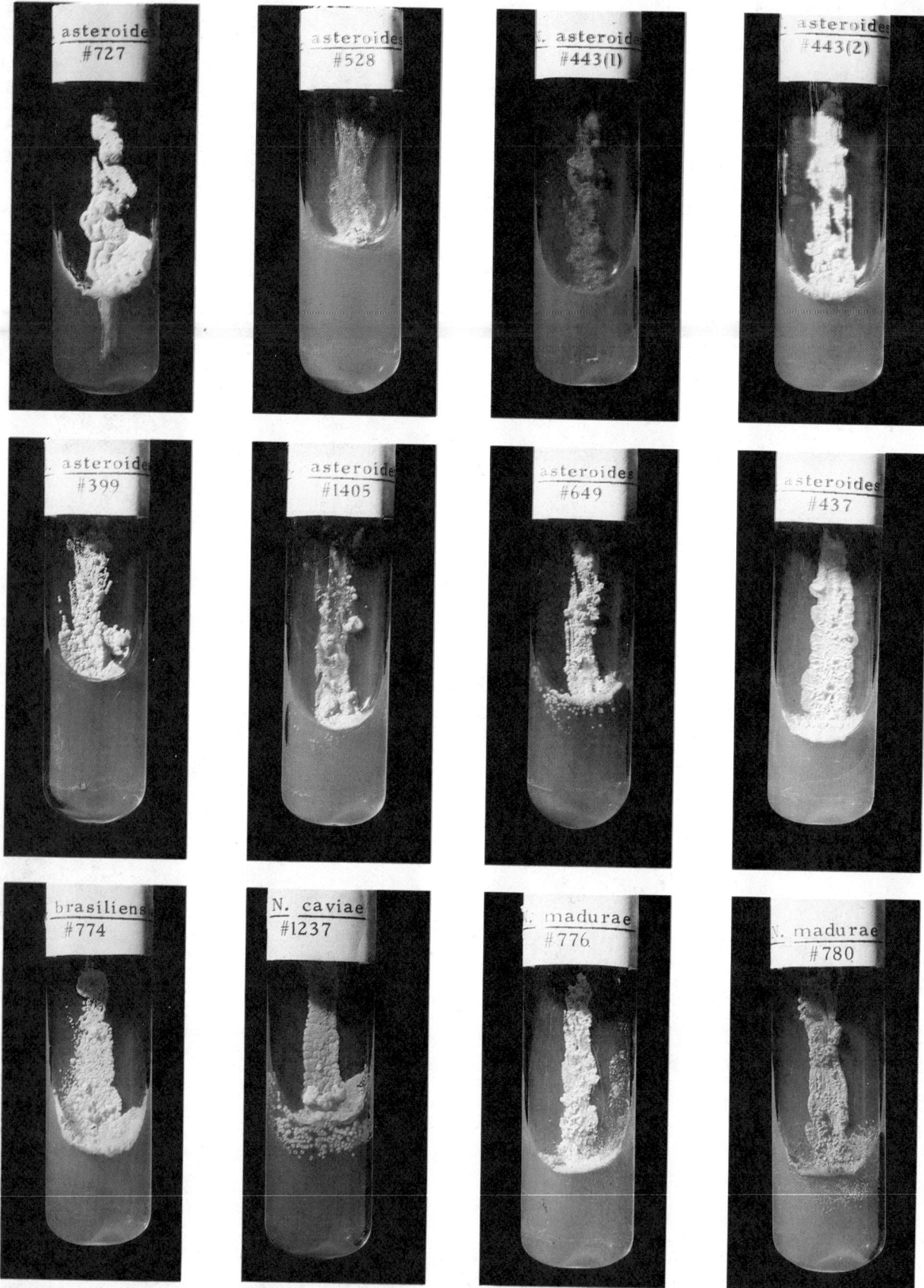

**FIGURE 4.** *Gross appearance of some cultures of* Nocardia asteroides, Nocardia brasiliensis, Nocardia caviae, *and* Nocardia madurae. *Cultures grown on yeast dextrose agar for 1 week at 28° C. N. asteroides: no. 727, heavy growth thickly covered with aerial hyphae; no. 528, thin growth covered with aerial hyphae; no. 443(1), red-pigmented growth without macroscopically visible aerial hyphae; no. 443(2), variant of red strain with abundant aerial hyphae; nos. 399, 1405, 649, and 437, cultures forming decreasing amounts of aerial hyphae; nos. 399 and 649, cultures producing dark brown soluble pigment. N. brasiliensis: no. 774. N. caviae: no. 1237. N. madurae: nos. 776 and 780, cultures with different pigments.*

seldom present in generalized or systemic nocardiosis in man.

For demonstrating nocardiae in the tissue, best results are obtained when the sections are stained by the method of Brown and Brenn or McCallum-Goodpasture-Gram. They can also be demonstrated by Gomori's methenamine-silver stain by extending the staining time. Periodic acid-Schiff or Gridley stains are not satisfactory, and the microorganisms cannot be detected by hematoxylin and eosin stain. Although most strains of *N. asteroides*, *N. caviae*, and *N. brasiliensis* possess a certain degree of acidfastness, this property is hard to demonstrate in sections of formalin-fixed tissue.

Generalized nocardiosis can be successfully produced in laboratory animals, although suitability of animal species varies and the degree of virulence may differ from microbial strain to strain. In our experience, albino mice are the most suitable for testing pathogenicity of nocardiae. Usually a heavy inoculum prepared in 5 per cent, sterile, gastrin mucin and injected intraperitoneally can cause multiple abscess formation involving most of the peritoneal organs. Dissemination to the lungs and brain may occur and the majority of animals die within one to two weeks. Alternatively, the infection may heal spontaneously with indefinite survival of most of the animals. The age of the culture (three to five days), amount of inoculum, and use of adjuvant are important factors. *N. brasiliensis* is reportedly more virulent than *N. asteroides* when injected intraperitoneally (Kurup et al., 1970A) or in the footpads of the mice (Gonzalez Ochoa, 1973). When injected intravenously, however, *N. asteroides* and *N. caviae* cause much higher mortality and morbidity than *N. brasiliensis* (Mishra et al., 1973B). Mishra and coworkers also demonstrated that cortisone administration can significantly lower the host resistance to the infection by the three species. The histopathologic picture in experimental nocardiosis is similar to that observed in generalized nocardiosis in man and animals. Attempts to infect mice or other laboratory animals with *N. madurae*, *N. pelletieri*, *N. dassonvillei*, and *S. somaliensis* have been, so far, unsuccessful.

## *LABORATORY DIAGNOSIS*

Due to the lack of a characteristic clinical syndrome and specific immunologic tests, the laboratory diagnosis of nocardiosis demands greater attention and effort than most of the other common bacterial and fungal infections. The problem is also aggravated by the in vitro sensitivity of cultures of *Nocardia* and *Streptomyces* to most of the commonly used antibiotics that are incorporated into culture media to suppress the fast-growing saprophytic or commensal bacteria and fungi. On the other hand, filaments of *N. asteroides* may occasionally survive the concentration procedure commonly used for the isolation of *Mycobacterium tuberculosis* and grow on Lowenstein-Jensen medium. Because the filaments may be very fragile and may show strong acidfastness, nocardiae may easily be mistaken for *M. tuberculosis*.

### Collection of Clinical Specimens

Samples of sputum, bronchial aspirates, gastric lavage (in the case of young children who tend to swallow their sputum), surgically removed tissues (biopsies and resected lungs), cerebrospinal fluid, and midstream urine are collected under aseptic conditions. A fresh morning sample of sputum, collected in a wide mouthed, glass stoppered bottle, after the patient has thoroughly cleaned his teeth and mouth, is more productive than a 24-hour specimen. The specimen is promptly brought to the laboratory and processed immediately. Sputum is homogenized by vigorous shaking with sterile glass beads. The biopsied tissues may be homogenized with the help of glass tissue grinders. Samples of cerebrospinal fluid and urine must be concentrated by centrifugation.

### Direct Examination

Smears prepared from the homogenized or concentrated specimen are stained and examined microscopically. Several fields should be searched for the presence of filaments and coccobacillary bodies. The filaments are gram positive but often take the stain irregularly, look beaded, and may sometimes be 50 $\mu$ in length. Branching is usually at right angles and tends to be at long intervals. Acidfastness, if demonstrable, is particularly helpful in differentiating *N. asteroides*, *N. caviae*, and *N. brasiliensis* from *N. madurae*, *N. pelletieri*, and *S. somaliensis*.

### Direct Culture

After the initial processing, the specimens are streaked upon neutral Sabouraud's dextrose agar and yeast dextrose agar plates (see *Appendix*) and incubated at 37° C (anaerobic or microaerophilic conditions are not required for growth). These media are useful for isolating nocardiae and streptomycetes from relatively less contaminated clinical specimens such as biopsied tissues, washed grains from actinomycetoma, and cerebrospinal fluid. If the specimens are suspected of harboring a wide spectrum of contaminating microbial flora, for example, gastric lavage and sputa of patients with chronic pulmonary diseases, the chances of isolating some nocardiae are enhanced by the use of the paraffin bait technique (see *Appendix*) as described by Mishra and Randhawa (1969) and Mishra et al. (1973A). It depends on the ability of nocardiae to use as energy sources certain organic compounds, such as paraffin, which are not attacked by other aerobic bacteria.

*N. asteroides* and other pathogenic nocardiae and streptomycetes, although widespread in nature, are surprisingly seldom encountered as laboratory contaminants or as constituents of normal microbial flora of the human body. Isolation of *N. asteroides* from a clinical specimen, therefore, has a definite diagnostic value. An unequivocal diagnosis of systemic nocardiosis depends upon repeated demonstration of gram-positive and partially acidfast branching filaments in the direct smear and isolation of the pathogen in culture.

Laboratory diagnosis of actinomycetoma is relatively easier. Biopsied tissue or the pus collected from the draining sinuses should be examined carefully for the presence of granules. If present,

the granules should be separated from the pus and washed carefully in sterile physiologic saline. In the case of *N. brasiliensis, N. caviae,* and *N. asteroides,* the granules are soft, white to cream colored, and range from 0.5 to 1 mm in size. The grains produced by *N. pelletieri* in tissue are hard, red, pink, or occasionally yellowish in color and measure about 1 mm. The granules produced by *N. madurae* are soft, big in size, mostly white or cream, rarely pink. *S. somaliensis* produces yellowish to brown, hard granules, 0.5 to 2 mm in diameter. After gross examination, the granules are crushed, examined microscopically, and inoculated on Sabouraud's dextrose agar and yeast dextrose agar. (The paraffin bait technique is not suitable for the isolation of *N. madurae, N. pelletieri,* and *S. somaliensis* because they do not utilize paraffin as the sole source of carbon.) Although morphology of the granules and staining characteristics of the filaments present therein are fairly distinctive of some of the etiologic species, the organism must be grown in culture for its specific identification.

Single colonies, morphologically compatible with the cultures of *Nocardia* and *Streptomyces,* should be picked from the plates or tubes directly

A KEY TO THE TENTATIVE IDENTIFICATION OF NOCARDIAE AND
STREPTOMYCES OF MEDICAL IMPORTANCE

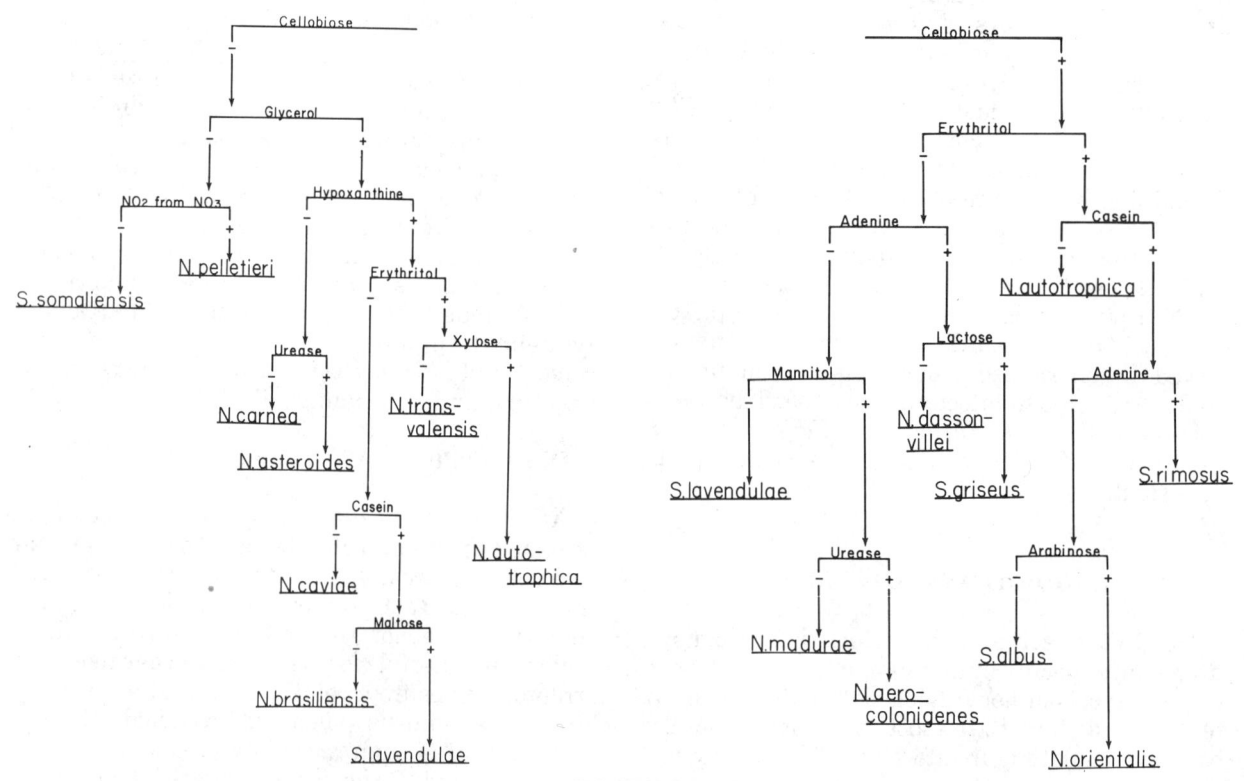

FIGURE 5.

inoculated with the clinical specimens or isolated from the growth on paraffin-coated rods. After purifying the culture by serial dilution or by repeated streaking on yeast dextrose agar plates, the growth, microscopic morphology, and physiologic characteristics are studied.

### Species Identification

In the absence of a reliable morphologic feature, or features, for the separation of the genera *Nocardia* and *Streptomyces*, the form of diaminopimelic acid (DAP) in the cell wall or in whole-cell hydrolysates is used to divide the genera (Lechevalier, 1977). Strains of *Nocardia* species have the *meso*-form of DAP and strains of *Streptomyces* species, the L-form.

Other properties — pigment formation, fragmentation of substrate hyphae, development of conidia, and production of an earthy odor — are possessed by some strains of nocardiae and by some strains of streptomycetes. Nor have we found any physiologic test that differentiates strains of the two genera. The key (Fig. 5) presented here for the tentative identification of strains of nocardiae and streptomycetes includes the species represented by the strains received here as isolations from patients. It is designed to permit the user, in whose laboratory chromatographic determination of DAP is not feasible, to arrive at species identifications of unknown isolations with the morphologic characteristics of nocardiae and streptomycetes as though the species belonged to one genus (Gordon, 1976). If the 13 tests employed in the key (see *Appendix*) are applied to an unknown isolate and the strain is found to be, for example, cellobiose negative, glycerol positive, hypoxanthine negative, and urease positive, the strain may be tentatively identified as one of *N. asteroides*. If the remaining properties of the strain are as follows: acid formation negative from arabinose, erythritol, lactose, maltose, mannitol, and xylose; inability to decompose adenine and casein; and positive reduction of nitrate to nitrite, the tentative identification of the strain as one of *N. asteroides* is partially confirmed.

Further confirmation may be obtained by studying additional physiologic characteristics listed in Table 1 and described in detail by Gordon et al. (1974, 1977, 1978).

If chemotaxonomic examinations are feasible in the laboratory, the presence of *meso*-DAP, arabinose, and galactose in the cell walls or in hydrolysates of whole cells will provide further evidence of the strain's identity as one of *N. asteroides*. The lipids (mycolic acids) of strains of mycobacteria and of some nocardiae offer another valuable chemotaxonomic property (Lechevalier,

1976). Species lacking mycolic acids are usually nonacidfast. Among the species described in Table I, cultures of *N. asteroides, N. carnea, N. caviae, N. brasiliensis,* and *N. transvalensis* contain LCN-A (lipid characteristic of *Nocardia* species-asteroides type) that distinguishes them from the other species in Table I and from strains of mycobacteria and corynebacteria. Mycolic acids apparently have no significant role in the pathogenicity of nocardiae and streptomycetes. Certain nonpathogenic species, e.g., *N. amarae,* are known to have LCN-A, whereas some of the well known pathogenic species, such as *N. madurae, N. pelletieri,* and *S. somaliensis,* do not have LCN-A or any other mycolic acids.

The importance of comparing unknown isolates with as many named strains of the various species as possible cannot be overstressed to anyone attempting to identify strains of nocardiae and streptomycetes for the first time. By applying the tests to known strains, the investigator soon learns whether each test as applied in his laboratory yields results comparable with those given here or elsewhere in the literature (Ajello et al., 1963; Goodfellow, 1971). If only a tentative identification of an isolate can be made or if the strain cannot be identified by the information provided, it should be sent to a reference laboratory (our Institute, the Waksman Institute of Microbiology, Piscataway, New Jersey; the Center for Disease Control, Atlanta, Georgia; or any other laboratory actively engaged in the identification of aerobic actinomycetes).

The name *N. farcinica,* the type species of the genus *Nocardia,* is not used here because its status is uncertain. Diversity of interpretations of Nocard's description (1888) of his strain isolated from a case of bovine farcy in Guadeloupe, the different species identity of strains purported to be Nocard's original isolation, and the assignment of causal agents of African cases of bovine farcy to the genus *Mycobacterium* (Asselineau et al., 1969) confuse present-day significance of the name.

### ANTIGENIC COMPOSITION, SEROLOGY AND IMMUNITY

The immunology of *Nocardia* and *Streptomyces* is still poorly understood. Cross-reaction with mycobacteria and members of related genera is frequently observed. Strains of *Nocardia, Mycobacterium,* and *Corynebacterium,* which have identical cell wall sugars, seem to have some common antigenic components. Crude and purified polysaccharides, protein derivatives, and polypeptide preparations are immunologically active but both homologous and heterologous reactions may occur. Pier and Fichtner (1971), using a gel diffusion precipitin test and soluble extracellular antigens, distinguished four serotypes in nocardiae. Type I, II, and III antigens were confined to *N. asteroides;* the type IV antigen occurred in strains of *N. caviae* and *N. brasiliensis* as well as in several strains of *N. asteroides.* By comparative reciprocal intradermal sensitin tests in guinea pigs, some success has been reported in delineating *Nocardia* at the species level but not at the generic level (Magnusson, 1976). Despite the promising value of immunologic methods in demonstrating homologous antigenicity in experimental models, the diagnostic worth of sensitin tests in demonstrating immediate or delayed hypersensitivity is limited. Skin test with purified protein derivatives (nocardin-PPD) derived from *N. brasiliensis,* is reported to elicit a positive reaction in patients with actinomycetoma caused by *N. brasiliensis* and to be negative in healthy individuals and patients with tuberculosis and various other diseases (Bojalil and Zamora, 1963). Similar convincing results, however, are lacking in cases of actinomycetoma caused by other species, and in cases of systemic or generalized nocardiosis.

The relationship of antibodies to immunity against infection by nocardiae and streptomycetes is not clear. Since members of the two genera are widely distributed in nature, it is logical to assume that more people are frequently exposed to these microorganisms than acquire clinical disease. The immunity may develop after a very mild or subclinical infection that diminishes spontaneously if host-defense mechanisms are not impaired.

## DRUG SUSCEPTIBILITY

Strains of *Nocardia* and *Streptomyces* are sensitive to a number of antibiotics in vitro, but there is considerable strain variation and lack of correlation between the in vitro and in vivo effects. Since the first successful use of sulphadiazine in the treatment of subcutaneous nocardiosis (Lyons et al., 1943) and the demonstration of its in vitro inhibitory effect on aerobic actinomycetes (Cutting and Gebhardt, 1941), sulphonamides have remained the drug of choice in the treatment of nocardial infections. *N. asteroides* is demonstrably more sensitive to chlortetracycline, oxytetracycline, and chloramphenicol than to sulphadiazine in vitro, but sulphadiazine is more effective in vivo (Strauss et al., 1951). Sensitivity to penicillin is poor, whereas ampicillin, streptomycin, erythromycin, neomycin, gentamycin, and many other antibiotics and chemotherapeutics

are quite active against nocardiae and streptomycetes (Bach et al., 1973; Pridham and Tresner, 1974). Some of these, alone or in combination with sulphonamides, have been used in the treatment of nocardiosis and actinomycetoma. A combination of trimethoprim and sulphamethoxazole has in vitro inhibitory effect on strains of *N. asteroides* and *N. brasiliensis* at a relatively low concentration and appears to be more useful in the treatment of actinomycetoma. Minocycline and fusidic acid have been recently reported to inhibit growth in vitro of all strains of *N. asteroides* tested at an impressively low concentration of 6.2 $\mu$g/ml and 3.1 $\mu$g/ml, respectively (Schaal and Heimerzheim, 1974; Wallace et al., 1977). There are not enough data, however, on the in vivo effect of these two drugs, as well as amikacin and tobramycin, which are also very active in vitro. Antifungal antibiotics, such as nystatin, cycloheximide, griseofulvin, and amphotericin B, are by and large not effective against *Nocardia* and *Streptomyces* infections, although occasional clinical success and in vitro inhibitory action have been reported.

## EPIDEMIOLOGY

*Nocardia* and *Streptomyces* are soil-inhabiting, ubiquitous microorganisms, commonly present in the human environment. After the first report on the isolation of *N. asteroides* from soil by Gordon and Hagan (1936), several investigators have demonstrated the occurrence of *N. asteroides, N. caviae, N. brasiliensis,* and other medically important aerobic actinomycetes in the soil in many different parts of the world (Cross et al., 1976). Since their filaments are delicate and highly fragile, they are easily airborne. Systemic or primary pulmonary infection is usually acquired by inhalation of the airborne mycelial fragments or spores. Occasionally, primary lesions may develop in the gastrointestinal tract through ingestion of food contaminated with dust or water harboring nocardiae. In the case of actinomycetoma or subcutaneous manifestations, traumatic implantation of the pathogen directly into the skin is the commonest mode of infection. These microorganisms have no special affinity for any particular race, sex, age, or geographic region. Cases of systemic nocardiosis are reported from all over the world (Kurup et al., 1970B) although more frequently from America and Europe than from Asia and Africa. The differences are mainly due to the greater availability of highly specialized laboratory diagnostic facilities and an increased awareness among the investigators in the more developed countries. Occupational relationship is not established, but farmers and laborers heavily exposed to the soil and dust are more likely to contract the infection, especially in the presence of debilitating metabolic diseases and poor nutritional and working conditions.

The etiologic agents of actinomycetoma also have a worldwide distribution, although the disease is more frequently observed in Sudan, Mexico, and certain other arid regions lying between the equator and the Tropic of Cancer. Incidentally, *N. pelletieri* and *S. somaliensis* are more commonly incriminated in the etiology of actinomycetoma in Sudan and other African countries, whereas *N. brasiliensis* and *N. madurae* are more frequently reported in Mexico. Strains of almost all the species have been isolated from cases in other countries but no etiologic or regional significance could be attached to any particular species.

## APPENDIX

### Acidfastness

Slides with air-dried smears of the cultures are immersed in carbolfuchsin (saturated ethanol solution of basic fuchsin, 10 ml; 5 per cent aqueous solution of phenol, 90 ml). Heat is applied and the fuchsin boiled for five minutes. The slides are washed in water, quickly dipped once in acid alcohol (concentrated HCl, 3 ml; 95 per cent ethanol, 97 ml), immediately washed again in water, and counterstained with methylene blue (saturated solution of methylene blue in 95 per cent ethanol, 30 ml; 0.01 per cent aqueous solution of KOH, 100 ml). Use of 0.5 per cent $H_2SO_4$ instead of acid alcohol was abandoned in this laboratory because filaments of some strains of *S. griseus* were not decolorized.

### Tap Water Agar

This medium contains only 1.5 g of agar in 100 ml of tap water.

### Neutral Sabouraud's Dextrose Agar

The ingredients of this agar are: glucose, 20 g; neopeptone, 10 g; agar, 20 g; distilled water, 1000 ml; pH 7.0.

### Yeast Dextrose Agar

This agar comprises 10 g of yeast extract, 10 g of glucose, 15 g of agar, 1000 ml tap water, and the pH is adjusted to 7.0.

### Paraffin Bait Technique

Mix 2 ml of the homogenized specimen with 5 ml of carbon-free broth ($NaNO_3$, 2 g; $K_2HPO_4$, 0.8 g; $MgSO_4 \cdot 7H_2O$, 0.5 g; $FeCl_3$, 10 mg; $MnCl_2 \cdot 4H_2O$, 8 mg; $ZnSO_4$, 2 mg; distilled water, 1000 ml; pH 7.0). Introduce into the tube a paraffin-coated glass rod (sterilized by storing overnight in 95 per cent alcohol), after the alcohol has drained off. Incubate the tubes at 37° C and observe regularly up to four weeks before discarding as negative. Cream to orange growth on the paraffin rod, just above the surface of the medium, is removed and streaked on Sabouraud's dextrose agar (pH 7.0). Single colonies morphologically compatible with those of nocardiae are picked and processed further for specific identification. Better results can be obtained if, after 1 week, the paraffin rod is carefully removed from the inoculated tube and transferred to another tube containing only 6 ml of carbon-free broth.

### Acid from Carbohydrates

The basal inorganic nitrogen medium contains $(NH_4)_2HPO_4$, 1 g; KCl, 0.2 g; $MgSO_4 \cdot 7H_2O$, 0.2 g; agar, 15 g; distilled water, 1000 ml. The pH value of the medium is adjusted to 7.0 before the addition of 15 ml of a 0.04 per cent solution (w/v) of bromcresol purple. After this agar is tubed and sterilized by autoclaving, 0.5 ml of a 10 per cent solution (w/v) of each carbohydrate (autoclaved separately) is added aseptically to the tubes. Cultures on slants of these carbohydrate agars are observed for acid color of the indicator after 7 and 28 days of incubation at 28° C. Tubes showing a negative reaction at 28 days are retained 4 more weeks and observed again.

### Decomposition of Adenine and Hypoxanthine

Adenine (0.5 g), suspended in 10 ml of distilled water, is autoclaved, mixed carefully with 100 ml of sterile nutrient agar (peptone, 5 g; beef extract, 3 g; agar, 15 g; distilled water, 1000 ml; adjusted to pH 7.0), cooled to 45° C, mixed again, and poured into sterile plates (60 mm diameter). Care must be taken to obtain an even distribution of the crystals of adenine throughout the solidified agar. Each culture is streaked once across a plate, incubated at 28° C, and observed at 14 and 21 days for the disappearance of the crystals underneath and around the growth. Plates of hypoxanthine are prepared, inoculated, incubated, and observed in the same way.

### Decomposition of Casein

A suspension of 5 g of skim milk powder in 50 ml of distilled water and a suspension of 1 g of agar in 50 ml of distilled water are autoclaved separately and cooled to 45° C. The two suspensions are then mixed and poured into plates. Each culture is streaked once across a plate and incubated at 28° C. At 7 and 14 days the plates are examined for clearing of the casein underneath and around the growth.

A heavy inoculum is necessary in testing for the decomposition of casein, adenine, and hypoxanthine. Some cultures grow well but do not dissolve the casein or the crystals of adenine and hypoxanthine except around the larger clumps of inoculum.

## Decomposition of Urea

A 10 ml amount of 15 per cent solution of urea (w/v), sterilized by filtration, is added to 75 ml of sterile urease broth ($KH_2PO_4$, 10 g; $Na_2HPO_4$, 9.5 g; yeast extract, 1 g; 0.04 per cent solution of phenol red (w/v), 20 ml; distilled water, 1000 ml; adjusted to pH 7.0). The mixture is pipetted aseptically in 2.5 ml amounts into sterile, capped tubes and inoculated with actively growing cultures. An alkaline reaction after 28 days of incubation at 28° C demonstrates the presence of urease.

## Reduction of Nitrate to Nitrite

Cultures in nitrate broth (peptone, 5 g; beef extract, 3 g; $KNO_3$, 1 g; distilled water, 1000 ml; pH 7.0) are tested for nitrite at 5, 10, and 14 days by mixing 1 ml of culture with three drops of each of the following solutions: 1) sulfanilic acid, 8 g; 5 N acetic acid (glacial acetic acid and water 1:2.5), 1000 ml; and 2) dimethyl-$\alpha$-naphthylamine, 6 ml; 5 N acetic acid, 1000 ml. (Caution: Dimethyl-$\alpha$-napthylamine is carcinogenic and should be used with care.) Development of red or yellow (high concentration of nitrite) is proof of the presence of nitrite. In the absence of a positive reaction for 14 days, 4 to 5 mg of zinc dust are added to the tube previously tested for nitrite. The presence of nitrate (absence of reduction) is demonstrated by the development of a red color.

We thank the Foundation for Microbiology for providing color Figures 1 and 4 and Dr. A. H. McIntosh and Mrs. R. Shamy for Figures 2 and 5. Permission of the *Journal of General Microbiology* to reproduce Figure 3 is gratefully acknowledged.

## References

Ajello, L., Georg, L. K., Kaplan, W., and Kaufman, L.: Laboratory Manual for Medical Mycology. Public Health Service Publication No. 994. Washington, U. S. Government Printing Office, 1963, p. G65.

Asselineau, J., Lanéele, M. A., and Chamoiseau, G.: De l'étiologie du farcin de zébus tchadiens: nocardiose ou mycobactériose? II. Composition lipidique. Rev. Élev Méd Vét Pays Trop 22:205, 1969.

Bach, M. C., Sabath, L. D., and Finland, M.: Susceptibility of *Nocardia asteroides* to 45 antimicrobial agents *in vitro*. Antimicrob Agents Chemother 3:1, 1973.

Berd, D.: *Nocardia brasiliensis* infection in the United States: A report of nine cases and a review of the literature. Am J Clin Path 60:254, 1973.

Bojalil, L. F., and Zamora, A.: Precipitin and skin tests in the diagnosis of mycetoma due to *Nocardia brasiliensis*. Proc Soc Exp Biol Med 113:40, 1963.

Causey, W. A.: *Nocardia caviae:* a report of 13 new isolations with clinical correlation. Appl Microbiol 28:193, 1974.

Cross, T., Rowbotham, T. J., Mishustin, E. N., Tepper, E. Z., Antoine-Portaels, F., Schaal, K. P., and Bickenbach, H.: The ecology of nocardioform actinomycetes. In Goodfellow, M., Brownell, G. H., and Serrano, J. A. (eds.): The Biology of the Nocardiae. London, Academic Press, 1976, p. 337.

Cutting, W. C., and Gebhardt, L. P.: Inhibitory effect of sulphonamides on cultures of *Actinomyces hominis*. Science 94:568, 1941.

Emmons, C. W., Binford, C. H., Utz, J. P., and Kwon-Chung, K. J.: Medical Mycology, 3rd ed. Philadelphia, Lea and Febiger, 1977.

Gonzalez Ochoa, A.: Virulence of nocardiae. Canad J Microbiol 19:901, 1973.

Goodfellow, M.: Numerical taxonomy of some nocardioform bacteria. J. Gen Microbiol 69:33, 1971.

Gordon, R. E.: A taxonomist's obligation. In Goodfellow, M., Brownell, G. H., and Serrano, J. A. (eds.): The Biology of Nocardiae. London, Academic Press, 1976, p. 66.

Gordon, R. E., and Barnett, D. A.: Resistance to rifampin and lysozyme of strains of some species of *Mycobacterium* and *Nocardia* as a taxonomic tool. Int J Syst Bacteriol 27:176, 1977.

Gordon, R. E., Barnett, D. A., Handerhan, J. E., and Pang, C. H-N.: *Nocardia coeliaca, Nocardia autotrophica*, and the nocardin strain. Int J Syst Bacteriol 24:54, 1974.

Gordon, R. E., and Hagan, W. A.: A study of some acid-fast actinomycetes from soil with special reference to pathogenicity for animals. J Infect Dis 59:200, 1936.

Gordon, R. E., Mishra, S. K., and Barnett, D. A.: Some bits and pieces of the genus *Nocardia: N. carnea, N. vaccinii, N. transvalensis, N. orientalis*, and *N. aerocolonigenes*. J. Gen Microbiol 109:69, 1978.

Kurup, P. V., Randhawa, H. S., Sandhu, R. S., and Abraham, S.: Pathogenicity of *Nocardia caviae, N. asteroides*, and *N. brasiliensis*. Mycopathologia 40:133, 1970A.

Kurup, P. V., Randhawa, H. S., and Gupta, N. P.: Nocardiosis: a review. Mycopathologia 40:193, 1970B.

Lechevalier, H. A.: The actinomycetales: Soil or oxidative actinomycetes. In Laskin, A. I., and Lechevalier, H. A. (eds.): Handbook of Microbiology, 2nd ed. Cleveland, CRC Press, 1977, p. 363.

Lechevalier, M. P.: The taxonomy of the genus *Nocardia:* Some light at the end of the tunnel? In Goodfellow, M., Brownell, G. H., and Serrano, J. A. (eds.): The Biology of the Nocardiae. London, Academic Press, 1976, p. 1.

Lyons, C., Owen, C. R., and Ayers, W. B.: Sulphonamide therapy in actinomycotic infections. Surgery 14:99, 1943.

Magnusson, M.: Sensitin tests as an aid in the taxonomy of *Nocardia* and its pathogenicity. In Goodfellow, M., Brownell, G. H., and Serrano, J. A. (eds.): The Biology of the Nocardiae. London, Academic Press, 1976, p. 236.

Mariat, F., Destombes, P., and Segretain, G.: The mycetomas: clinical features, pathology, etiology and epidemiology. Contr Microbiol Immunol 4:1, 1977.

Mishra, S. K., and Randhawa, H. S.: Application of paraffin bait technique to the isolation of *Nocardia asteroides* from clinical specimens. Appl Microbiol 18:686, 1969.

Mishra, S. K., Randhawa, H. S., and Sandhu, R. S.: Observations on paraffin baiting as a laboratory diagnostic procedure in nocardiosis. Mycopathologia 51:147, 1973A.

Mishra, S. K., Sandhu, R. S., Randhawa, H. S., Damodaran, V. N., and Abraham, S.: Effect of cortisone administration on experimental nocardiosis. Infect Immun 7:123, 1973B.

Nocard, E.: Note sur la maladie des boeufs de la Guadeloupe connue sous le nom de farcin. Ann Inst Pasteur 2:293, 1888.

Pier, A. C., and Fichtner, R. E.: Serologic typing of *Nocardia asteroides* by immunodiffusion. Am Rev Resp Dis 103:698, 1971.

Pridham, T. G., and Tresner, H. D.: Family VII. *Streptomycetaceae* Waksman and Henrici. In Buchanan, R. E., and Gibbons, N. E. (eds.): Bergey's Manual of Determinative Bacteriology. 8th ed. Baltimore, Williams and Wilkins Company, 1974, p. 747.

Schaal, K. P., und Heimerzheim, H.: Mikrobiologische Diagnose und Therapie der Lungennocardiose. Mykosen 17:313, 1974.

Strauss, R. E., Kligman, A. M., and Pillsbury, D. M.: Chemotherapy of actinomycosis and nocardiosis. Am Rev Tuberc 63:441, 1951.

Waksman, S. A.: The Actinomycetes. Vol. 1. Baltimore, Williams and Wilkins Company, 1959.

Wallace, R. J., Jr., Septimus, E. J., Musher, D. M., and Martin, R. R.: Disk diffusion susceptibility testing of *Nocardia* species. J Infect Dis 135:568, 1977.

# SPIROCHETES

## *LEPTOSPIRA* **42**

### A. D. Alexander, Ph.D.

## GENERAL CHARACTERISTICS AND MORPHOLOGY

The genus *Leptospira* consists of a large number of serologically heterogeneous strains that can be separated into two large complexes, the biflexa, or "saprophytic," leptospires and the parasitic leptospires. The biflexa leptospires are omnipresent in natural waters and wet soils, where apparently they are free-living. They are not known to produce infections in man or other mammalian hosts except for a few rare reports. The parasitic leptospires include the pathogenic strains known to infect man and other mammals. At present only one species, *Leptospira interrogans,* is recognized, although separate speciation has been proposed — *L. biflexa* for the saprophytic leptospires and *L. interrogans* for the parasitic types (International Committee on Systematic Bacteriology, 1974).

Biflexa strains are distinguishable from pathogenic strains in the following respects: inability to infect laboratory animals; relative resistance to growth-inhibitory effects of bivalent copper ions, 8-azaguanine and aniline dyes; less fastidious nutritional growth requirements; ability to grow at low temperatures; and serologic and genetic characteristics (Turner, 1976). Members of the two complexes share no nucleotide sequences as determined by DNA-DNA annealing tests. However, leptospires within each complex can be further separated into three groups that have partial DNA homology. A leptospire designated *illini* has been isolated which resembles the biflexa leptospires phenotypically but is genetically unrelated to any of the known genetic types (Brendle et al., 1974).

Morphologically the saprophytic and parasitic leptospires are indistinguishable. Leptospires are helicoidal, flexuous organisms with semicircular hooked ends (Fig. 1). Occasional strains are straight-ended or have only one hook. The organisms usually measure 6 to 20 $\mu$m in length (range 3 to 40 $\mu$m) and approximately 0.1 $\mu$m in diameter. The coils are tightly wound with an overall diameter of 0.2 to 0.3 $\mu$m and a wavelength of approximately 0.5 $\mu$m. When examined by electron microscopy the structure of leptospires consists of a helicoidal protoplasmic cylinder that is wound about two independent axial filaments (Fig. 2). The filaments are inserted subterminally at each end with their free ends positioned toward the middle, where they usually do not overlap. The axial filaments resemble bacterial flagella structurally, in chemical composition, and in method of attachment. The helicoidal body is delineated by a cytoplasmic membrane–cell wall complex similar to that of gram-negative bacteria. The flagella and protoplasmic cylinder are enclosed by a common outer envelope or sheath (Johnson, 1977).

In fluid media, leptopsires appear to rotate alternately along their longitudinal axis, moving forward or backward without polar differentiation. The movement is characteristic because of the spinning hooked ends. In semisolid media, serpentine, boring, and flexing movements are seen. Leptospires can be seen by dark-field or phase contrast but not by bright-field microscopy. They are not readily visualized when stained with aniline dyes but can be demonstrated by the

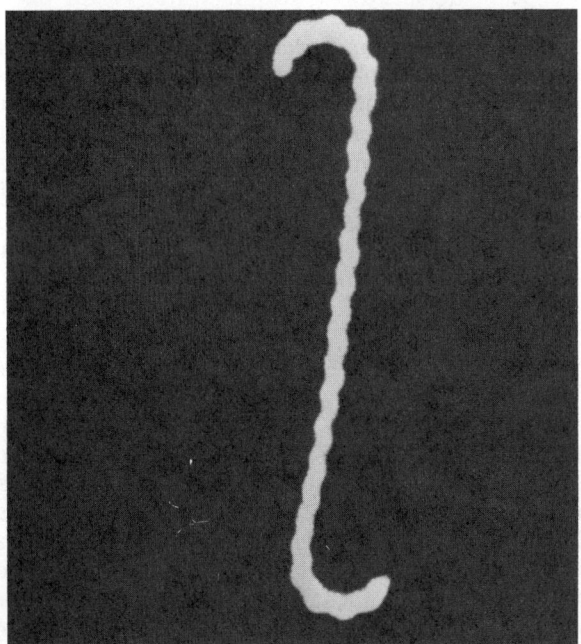

**FIGURE 1.** *Leptospira. Dark-ground illumination. (Courtesy C. D. Cox, University of Massachusetts, Amherst.)*

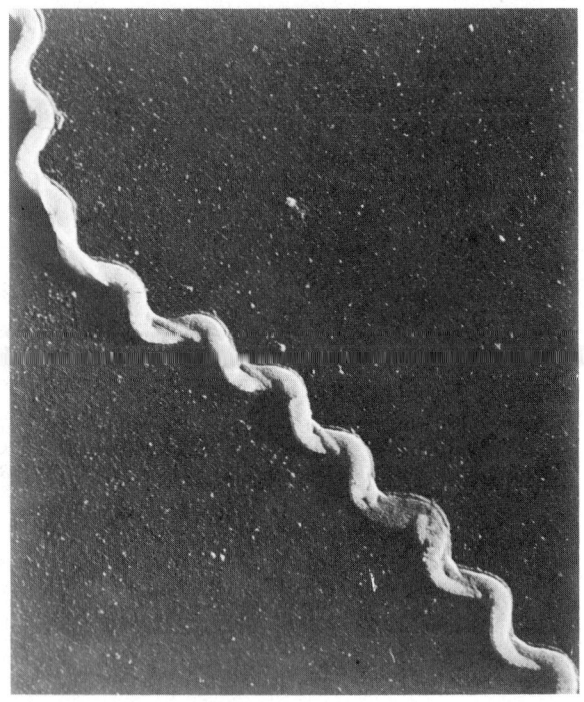

**FIGURE 2.** *Electron micrograph of a portion of a leptospire. (Courtesy Armed Forces Institute of Pathology, Washington, D.C.)*

use of silver deposition techniques. Leptospires are capable of penetrating bacterial retaining filters. These attributes coupled with the fact that they do not grow on conventional media have frequently led to the mistaken identification of leptospirosis as a viral disease.

## ANTIGENIC COMPOSITION

The pathogenic leptospires have distinct agglutinogenic properties that provide the basis for their differentiation. Otherwise they are indistinguishable by morphologic, cultural, and physiologic properties. The basic taxonomic group is the serovar (syn., serotype), which is included within a species. Currently, approximately 160 different serovars have been recognized on the basis of cross-agglutination and agglutinin-adsorption tests with serovar-specific rabbit antiserum (Turner, 1976). The serovars have been assembled into 18 serogroups on the basis of shared major agglutinogens. The serogroup has no taxonomic status but is used as an expedient for selection of antisera or antigens to identify isolates and to test sera. The agglutinogenic relationships do not necessarily correlate with genetic groupings. Each genetic group contains serologically diverse serovars. However, strains with major antigenic affinities appear to be genetically homologous (Brendle et al., 1974).

The agglutinogen, not surprisingly, has been associated with the enveloping sheath, which is composed of lipids, carbohydrates, and proteins (Johnson, 1977). Flagellar antigens have been isolated and shown to fall into eight antigenic groups by immunodiffusion techniques. They appeared to correlate best with genetic groupings (Chang et al., 1974). A variety of other antigenic substances have been extracted from leptospires by various chemical or physical treatments and have been shown to have specific or generic activity by the use of various serologic techniques. Their exact location and role in immunity and virulence needs additional study. An extract from biflexa serovars that is soluble in 50 per cent but insoluble in 95 per cent ethanol has proved to be particularly useful as a genus-specific, erythrocyte-sensitizing antigen in indirect hemagglutination and hemolytic tests (Cox et al., 1957; Sulzer et al., 1975).

## METABOLISM

The pathogenic leptospires are aerobic organisms that can be grown in media containing serum, or serum components and fatty acids, at pH 6.8 to 7.8 (optimally at pH 7.2 to 7.4). Long-chain fatty acids (not carbohydrates or amino acids) are used as a source of carbon and energy. They can utilize ammonium salts or urea but not amino acids for their nitrogen requirements. Exogenous purines but not pyrimidines can be incorporated. They require thiamin and vitamin $B_{12}$ in media. Cultures are usually incubated at 30° C. Incubation time for optimal growth ranges from a few days to 4 weeks or longer but is usually 6 to 14 days. At time of optimal growth the concentration of organism ranges from 1 to 4 $\times$ 10⁸/ml. Cytochrome enzymes, catalase, and enzymes of the citric acid cycle, glycolytic, and pentose pathways, and an acyl-coenzyme A dehydrogenase for $\beta$-oxidation of fatty acids have been demonstrated (Smibert, 1973).

## PATHOGENIC PROPERTIES

The clinical and histopathologic findings in leptospirosis are consistent with the action of a toxin. However, attempts to isolate and identify a toxic component or product of leptospires has been elusive. Endotoxic properties of leptospires have been reported but not confirmed, nor were findings of toxic substances in lysed cultures or culture filtrates consistent (Johnson, 1976). Toxic substances have been demonstrated in extracts of infected tissues of experimental animals (Arean et al., 1964; Hanson, 1976). The nature of these toxins has not been defined. A hot-cold heat-labile, oxygen-stable hemolysin with specific activity for ruminant red blood cells is produced by some pathogenic leptospires and may be a significant factor for the hemolytic manifestations in bovine and other ruminant species (Alexander, 1976b). Association of virulence with the outer envelope is suggested by findings that it is the site of the cidal action of antibody and complement and that virulent leptospires are more resistant to the antibody complement system than avirulent cells (Bey et al., 1974; Johnson and Harris, 1967). Pathogenicity has also been associated with production of catalase (Baseman and Cox, 1969). Pathogenic leptospires produce hyaluronidase (Yanagihara et al., 1973), which may contribute to the high invasiveness of these organisms.

## IMMUNITY

Immunity in leptospirosis is best correlated with specific agglutinogenic characteristics of serovars (Alexander, 1976b). Individuals who recover from infection with a specific serovar develop immunity against the same serovar but are susceptible to frank infection with antigenically different serovars. Where cross-protection was observed, it was related to common major agglutinogenic components. In accordance with this observation, the outer sheath has been found to be highly immunogenic and to have the same serologic specificity as agglutinogens (Auran et al., 1978). Intertype immunity against disease but not against infection has been demonstrated for certain serologically heterologous strains in experimental infections in hamsters and guinea pigs, and appeared to occur only between genetically homologous serovars (Alexander, 1976b).

The protection afforded by specific immunoglobulins reflects their agglutinating and opsonizing properties, which enhance destruction of the organisms by phagocytosis. Cell-mediated immunity does not appear to be important in combating acute disease but its role in the development or prevention of the renal carrier state and other persistent forms of infection cannot be ruled out (Adler and Faine, 1977). Immunologic factors may be important in some of the pathogenetic features of leptospirosis. Antigen-antibody complex reactions have been suggested to explain neurologic, renal, and ocular complications that occur after the first week of disease. Autoimmune reactions have been postulated to explain lesions in the kidney and eye. Various immediate and delayed-type hypersensitivity reactions have been elicited in experimental animals (Alexander, 1976b).

Vaccines are usually prepared from fixed cells. In man, vaccines have been extensively used in Japan, Italy, USSR, and other Eastern European countries. Vaccine prophylaxis for livestock and pets is carried out in the United States and in many other countries throughout the world. Vaccines are serovar specific and usually incorporate two or more serovars, depending on the types of prevailing leptospiral infections.

## LABORATORY DIAGNOSIS

Various microscopic, cultural, and serologic procedures are available for the laboratory diagnosis of leptospirosis. The selection and use of a suitable test depend on knowledge of the course of infection. After an incubation period, usually of 10 to 12 days, the disease appears abruptly, ushering in a septicemic stage persisting approximately 1 week. During this period the organisms may be found in the cerebrospinal fluid as well as in blood. The septicemic period usually ends with the appearance of detectable antibodies. Maximal antibody levels occur the third or fourth week of disease. Thereafter antibody levels gradually decline but may be detectable for years. Leptospires may be found in the urine after the first week of disease. Shedding is more pronounced during the first few weeks of convalescence; thereafter it may persist intermittently for two to three months in many cases and longer in some.

### Culture

Leptospires are best demonstrated during the acute stage by culture of blood on such media as Stuart's liquid or Fletcher's semisolid, which contain rabbit serum, or EMJH medium, which contains albumin and fatty acid in lieu of serum (Vera and Dumoff, 1974). Media are usually dispensed in test tubes in 5 ml amounts and inoculated with one or two drops of blood. At least four tubes of media, preferably from two different lots, should be used for each sample. Repeated blood cultures during the acute phase of disease are recommended. If culture medium is not immediately available at time of collection, blood may be defibrinated or mixed with anticoagulants, and subsequently cultured. Triturated clotted blood can also be used as inoculum. Spinal fluid, if available, may be cultured during the acute stage.

After the first week of disease, cultural recovery of leptospires from urine is possible in many cases. A midstream urine sample is carefully collected from cleansed genitalia and diluted 1:10 and 1:100 with media. Undiluted and diluted samples are cultured by using one to two drops of inoculum. In fatal cases leptospires may be isolated from suspensions of triturated liver and kidney. Minimal inocula of blood, urine, and tissue samples are recommended to dilute out growth-inhibitory substances. To inhibit the growth of contaminating organisms that may be present in urine or other samples, media may be supplemented with 5-fluorouracil, or with various antibiotics such as neomycin, furazolidone, cyclohexamide, or sulfathiazole, used singly or in combination (Alexander, 1974; Sulzer and Jones, 1976).

Cultures are incubated at 30° C or in the dark at room temperature, examined at five- to seven-day intervals, and discarded if negative after six weeks of incubation.

In semisolid media a linear disk of growth is usually seen 1 to 3 cm below the surface. Fluid media becomes slightly turbid. On plating media containing 1 per cent agar, many strains form subsurface colonies. Plating media are useful for purifying cultures but are less satisfactory than tubed media for primary isolation. To examine cultures, a drop is placed on a slide, covered with a coverslip, and examined by dark-ground microscopy at high dry magnification (450 times). Leptospires are recognized by their characteristic morphology and motility. Cultures can be stored in screw-capped or other airtight tubes. Transfers are made at two- or three-month intervals from semisolid media, and at three to six weeks if kept in fluid media. Cultures are typed by the use of microscopic agglutination techniques. Initially the isolate employed as antigen is tested against a battery of different serovar antisera to determine serogroup affinities. They are then tested with additional antisera to elucidate further relationships. For definitive identification, agglutinin-adsorption tests are carried out. Culture typing is usually carried out in state or national laboratories, or in special WHO Leptospirosis Reference Laboratories (Sulzer and Jones, 1976).

## Microscopic Examination

The concentration of leptospires in the blood of human patients is low and may not be demonstrated by dark-ground microscopic examination. In a small proportion of cases the chance of demonstrating leptospires may be increased by differential centrifugation of whole unclotted blood, first to remove cellular elements, and then to concentrate organisms in plasma (Wolff, 1954). Although the method may be valuable in establishing a rapid diagnosis, it is not recommended as a routine diagnostic procedure because artifacts such as cellular extrusions and fibrils are frequently mistaken for spirochetes. Direct microscopic methods are of value in examination of specimens in which a profuse number of leptospires may be present, such as blood and liver suspensions of hamsters or guinea pigs infected with clinical material or urine or kidney suspensions of natural animal hosts. Fluorescent-antibody staining techniques and silver deposition techniques have been used to demonstrate organisms in postmortem tissues and are especially useful if cultural and serologic tests are not possible (Alexander, 1974; Sulzer and Jones, 1976).

## Animal Inoculation

The use of laboratory animals offers no greater chance than direct culture for recovery of leptospires from blood or from other materials that can be obtained aseptically. Weanling hamsters and young guinea pigs are most commonly preferred because of their greater susceptibility to frank infection with a broad range of serovars (Wolff, 1954). The course of disease in laboratory animals varies with different serovars and also with different strains of the same serovar, and range from inapparent to lethal. Material is inoculated intraperitoneally. Heart blood for culture is taken on the fourth and sixth day after inoculation or whenever disease signs appear, and if necessary, at periodic intervals up to the twentieth day. On the twentieth day kidneys should also be cultured.

## Serologic Diagnosis

The microscopic agglutination test has been most widely used. It is highly sensitive for diagnosis of recent as well as past infections and can be applied to animal as well as human sera. However, it has high specificity. Consequently, to ensure detection of antibodies that may be provoked by any of the large number of different serovars, it is necessary to use multiple serovar antigens that would cross-react with most of the known serovars that may be present. The number of test serovars may range from a few to 15 or more, depending on the number of serovars and their relative occurrence in specific geographic regions (Alexander, 1976a). Young cultures of leptospires in fluid media are used as antigen. These may be used live or be treated with Formalin. Test sera are serially diluted two- to four-fold with physiologic salt solution to provide serum dilutions from 1:50 to 1:3200. Two-tenths-milliliter amounts of serum in each dilution are distributed in a series of agglutination tubes, to which is added an equal volume of antigen. The reaction mixtures are shaken, incubated at room temperature for two to three hours, shaken again, and examined for agglutination by dark-ground microscopic examination. The test has been adapted for use with microtitration techniques (Sulzer and Jones, 1976). Titers of 1:100 are considered to be significant, and may range as high as 1:25,600 or greater.

The laboriousness of the microscopic agglutination test limits its usefulness by the small laboratory. To circumvent this drawback, macroscopic-agglutination slide tests incorporating single or pooled antigens were developed and are commercially available (Alexander, 1976a). These tests are simple to perform and have good sensitivity for detecting recently or previously formed antibodies. "Genus-specific" tests have been proposed, which entail the use of specific biflexa strains known to cross-react frequently with leptospiral antibodies elicited by a large variety of pathogenic serovars (Alexander, 1976a; Turner, 1968). A hemolytic test with a "genus-specific" biflexa erythrocyte-sensitizing antigen has been used advantageously in areas of multiple leptospirosis (Cox et al., 1957; Tan, 1974). The test has been simplified by use of glutaraldehyde-fixed sensitized erythrocytes (Sulzer et al., 1975). Complement-fixation tests with biflexa antigens are in use in some European countries (Turner, 1968). Various fluorescent-antibody techniques have been reported for diagnosing leptospirosis but have not been widely adopted.

## DRUG SUSCEPTIBILITY

Penicillin, streptomycin, tetracycline, and macrolide antibiotics are all active against leptospires in experimental animals and in vitro. Leptospires are resistant to chloramphenicol, sulfa drugs, neomycin, actidione, and isoniazid (Stahlheim, 1973).

## EPIDEMIOLOGY

Leptospiroses are zoonoses that are globally distributed in a large variety of rodents and other feral and domestic mammals. Approximately 160 different mammalian species have been found to harbor leptospires (Leptospire Serotype Distributions Lists, 1966, 1975). Pathogenic leptospires have occasionally been isolated from birds, amphibians, reptiles, and ticks. The epidemiologic importance of nonmammalian hosts for leptospires has not been demonstrated. The distribution of the various serovars in mammalian hosts varies according to geographic region. The host range of selected serovars that are frequent causes of human disease in many parts of the world is shown in Table 1. Many serovars appear to be preferentially adapted to select mammalian hosts. For example, serovar *icterohaemorrhagiae* is primarily associated with the Norway rat, *canicola* with dogs, and *pomona* with swine and cattle. The occurrence of a specific serovar in a select host is not exclusive. The same mammalian species may be the primary reservoir for several serovars. In addition, this species may be infected and serve as a carrier of serovars that occur predominantly in other hosts. Infections in natural hosts are usually inapparent, but may be morbid. Naturally occurring disease in animals has been principally observed in dogs, swine, cattle, and other livestock. Cats appear to be relatively resistant to disease. In many countries leptospirosis is an important veterinary medical problem.

In natural hosts, leptospires nest in the lumen of convoluted tubules within the kidneys, whence they are shed in the urine. The degree and duration of leptospiruria vary with the host and infecting serovar. The Norway rat infected with *ic-*

**TABLE 1.   Host Range\* for Some Widely Distributed, Commonly Occuring Serovars Causing Human Leptospirosis†**

| SEROVAR | HOSTS | |
| --- | --- | --- |
| | **Domestic** | **Wild** |
| *Icterohaemorrhagiae* | dog, pig, horse, cattle | rats,‡ mice, mongoose, raccoon, muskrat, foxes, opossum, skunk, woodchuck, nutria, cavy, hedgehog, civet, apes |
| *canicola* | dog,‡ pig, cattle, cat, horse | skunk, raccoon, armadillo, mongoose, hedgehog, jackal, bandicoot, nutria, rats, vole |
| *pomona* | pig,‡ cattle,‡ goat, dog, cat, horse, sheep, water buffalo | skunk, opossum, foxes, raccoon, deer, hedgehog, mice, civet, cavy, woodchuck, vole, souslik, wolf, rabbit, sea lion |
| *grippotyphosa* | cattle, goat, sheep, swine, dog, cat | vole,‡ mice, rats, shrew, hedgehog, raccoon, skunk, fox, opossum, cavy, muskrat, weasel, mole, bobcat, leopard cat, bandicoot, rabbit, gerbil, squirrel, polecat |
| *batavlae* | dog,‡ cat, cattle | rats,‡ mice,‡ bandicoot, leopard cat, armadillo, vole, hedgehog, shrew |
| *autumnalis* | cattle, dog | mice,‡ rat, bandicoot, raccoon, opossum |
| *australis* | cattle, dog, horse | rats,‡ hedgehogs, mice, skunk, nutria, raccoon, vole, opossum, weasel, fox, bandicoot |

\*Based on cultural isolation.
†Source: Leptospiral Serotype Distribution Lists, 1966, 1975.
‡Known major maintenance host.

*terohaemorrhagiae* sheds profuse numbers of organisms, apparently for the remainder of its natural life. Strains of *canicola* are less efficient in colonizing rat kidneys. On the other hand, in the dog *canicola* is better able to establish leptospiruria than is *icterohaemorrhagiae* (Babudieri, 1958). Shedding in infected dogs, swine, cattle, and other domestic animals may be heavy for several months after infection but is usually sparse or absent after six months. The prevalence of infection in natural hosts can be remarkably high. Carrier rates of 50 per cent or greater in Norway rats and other feral mammals, and of 10 to 50 per cent in domestic animals, are common findings in many parts of the world.

Leptospires are transmitted through contact with urine of animal carriers, either directly or by contact with damp soil or natural waters soiled by carriers. Pathogenic leptospires can survive for three months or more in neutral or slightly alkaline waters. They do not persist in brackish or acid waters. Organisms enter hosts through abrasions of the skin or through mucosal surfaces of the mouth, nasopharynx, eye, or esophagus. Individuals of all ages and both sexes are susceptible. Infection in man is accidental and is related to occupational or avocational exposure, or to contact with infected pets. Man is usually a dead-end host. Sewer workers, butchers, fish and poultry processors, miners, ditch diggers, and other individuals who work or live in rat-infested areas are at risk. Cases in dairymen, swineherds, and in abattoir workers are usually epidemiologically related to infection in livestock. Sporadic cases or epidemics have occurred in various parts of the world in agricultural workers engaged in raising flax, rice, vegetables, or sugar cane, in rubber plantation workers, and in soldiers exposed to natural waters contaminated by carriers. Common-source epidemics have occurred repeatedly in children and young adults who bathe or swim in ponds or streams located in pasturelands.

## References

Adler, B., and Faine, S.: Host immunological mechanisms in the resistance of mice to leptospiral infections. Infect Immun 17:67, 1977.

Alexander, A. D.: *Leptospira*. In Lennette, E. H., Spaulding, E. H., and Truant, J. P. (eds.): Manual of Clinical Microbiology. 2nd ed. Washington, D. C., American Society for Microbiology, 1974, p. 347.

Alexander, A. D.: Serological diagnosis of leptospirosis. In Rose, N. R., and Friedman, H. (eds.): Manual of Clinical Immunology. Washington, D. C., American Society for Microbiology, 1976a, p. 352.

Alexander, A. D.: Immunity in leptospirosis. In Johnson, R. C. (ed.):

The Biology of Parasitic Spirochetes. New York, Academic Press, 1976b, p. 339.

Arean, V. M., Sarasin, G., and Green, J. H.: The pathogenesis of leptospirosis: Toxin production by *Leptospira icterohaemorrhagiae*. Am J Vet Res 25:836, 1964.

Auran, N. E., Johnson, R. C., and Alexander, A. D.: Chemical composition and serological activity of leptospiral outer envelope. In Proceedings of the National Symposium on Leptospirosis, *Leptospira*, and other *Spirochaeta*, 25-27 September, 1975. Cantacuzino Institute, Bucharest. Ilexum Editure Medicala, 1978, p. 277.

Babudieri, B.: Animal reservoirs of leptospires. Ann NY Acad Sci 70:393, 1958.

Baseman, J. B., and Cox, C. D.: Terminal electron transport in Leptospira. J Bacteriol 97:1001, 1969.

Bey, R. F., Auran, N. E., and Johnson, R. C.: Immunogenicity of whole cell and outer envelope leptospiral vaccines in hamsters. Infect Immun 10:1051, 1974.

Brendle, J. J., Rogul, M., and Alexander, A. D.: Deoxyribonucleic acid hybridization among selected leptospiral serotypes. Int J Systematic Bacteriol 24:205, 1974.

Chang, A., Faine, S., and Williams, W. T.: Cross-reactivity of the axial filament antigen as a criterion for classification of *Leptospira*. Aust J Exp Biol Med Sci 52:549, 1974.

Cox, C. D., Alexander, A. D., and Murphy, L. C.: Evaluation of the hemolytic test in the serodiagnosis of human leptospirosis. J Infect Dis 101:203, 1957.

Hanson, H. E.: Pathogenesis of leptospirosis. In Johnson, R. C. (ed.): The Biology of Parasitic Spriochetes. New York, Academic Press, 1976, p. 295.

van der Hoeden, J.: Epizootiology of leptospirosis. Adv. Vet Sci 4:277, 1958.

International Committee on Systematic Bacteriology. Subcommittee on the Taxonomy of *Leptospira*. Minutes of the meetings, 30 August-4 September 1973, Jerusalem, Israel. Int J. Systematic Bacteriol 24:381, 1974.

Johnson, R. C.: Comparative spirochete physiology and cellular composition. In Johnson, R. C. (ed.): The Biology of Parasitic Spirochetes. New York, Academic Press, 1976, p. 39.

Johnson, R. C.: The spirochetes. Annu Rev Microbiol 31:89, 1977.

Johnson, R. C., and Harris, V. G.: Antileptospiral activity of serum. II. Leptospiral virulence factor. J. Bacteriol 93:513, 1967.

Leptospiral Serotype Distribution Lists According to Host and Geographic Area. Atlanta, Georgia, U.S. Dept. Health, Education and Welfare, Center For Disease Control, 1966 (Supplement 1975).

Smibert, R. M.: *Spirochaetales*, a review. CRC Critical Reviews in Microbiol 2:491, 1973.

Stahlheim, O. H. V.: Chemical aspects of leptospirosis, CRC Critical Reviews in Microbiol 2:423, 1973.

Sulzer, C. R., Glosser, J. W., Roger, F., Jones, W. L., and Tiex, M.: Evaluation of an indirect hemagglutination test for the diagnosis of human leptospirosis. J Clin Microbiol 2:218, 1975.

Sulzer, C. R., and Jones, W. L.: Leptospirosis. Methods in Laboratory Diagnosis. Revised ed. U.S. Dept. Health, Education, and Welfare, Public Health Service, Center for Disease Control, HEW Publ. No. (CDC) 76-8275, 1976.

Tan, D. S. K., and Welch, Q. B.: Evaluation of *Leptospira biflexa* antigens for screening human sera by the microscopic agglutination (MA) test in comparison with the sensitized-erythrocyte-lysis (SEL) test. Southeast Asian J Trop Med Publ Hlth 5:12, 1974.

Turner, L. H.: Leptospirosis. II. Serology. Trans R Soc Trop Med Hyg 62:880, 1968.

Turner, L. H.: Classification of spirochaetes in general and of the Genus *Leptospira* in particular. In Johnson, R. C. (ed.): The Biology of Parasitic Spirochetes. New York, Academic Press, 1976, p. 95.

Vera, H. D., and Dumoff, M.: Culture media. In Lennette, E. H., Spaulding, E. H., and Truant, J. P. (eds.): Manual of Clinical Microbiology. 2nd ed. Washington, D. C., American Society for Microbiology, 1974, p. 881.

Wolff, J. W.: The Laboratory Diagnosis of Leptospirosis. Springfield, Ill., Charles C Thomas, 1954.

Yanagihara, Y., Taniyama, T., and Mifuchi, I.: Separation and purification of hyaluronidase of Leptospira (in Japanese). Medicine and Biology 86:83, 1973.

# 2. ANAEROBIC BACTERIA

## GRAM-POSITIVE COCCI: **43**
## PEPTOCOCCUS, PEPTOSTREPTOCOCCUS, STREPTOCOCCUS (ANAEROBIC), and SARCINA

*Howard Robert Attebery, D.D.S.*

The anaerobic gram-positive cocci are a controversial and difficult group of organisms in clinical microbiology. Their pathogenicity is doubted by some (Facklam and Smith, 1976) and respected by others (Finegold, 1977; Lambe et al., 1973; Pien et al., 1972). Their classification has been difficult.

Gram-positive cocci that upon isolation grow both in a mixture of 10 per cent carbon dioxide gas in air and in an anaerobic environment are microaerophilic cocci and are not classified with anaerobic cocci. However, some strains of anaerobic cocci can become tolerant of air upon subculturing and confuse classification efforts. Many other strains of anaerobic cocci, on the other hand, are fastidious in their anaerobic requirements, and good transport and anaerobic methods are needed for their recovery.

### MORPHOLOGY

It is not possible to classify anaerobic cocci to genera by using only cellular morphology. Though peptococci are usually clumped, they do occur singly or in pairs and are frequently found as short chains. Peptostreptococci and anaerobic streptococci cannot be differentiated by a Gram stain. Peptostreptococci may cluster as do peptococci with only short chains being evident. Chaining is best demonstrated in liquid cultures.

Many strains of anaerobic gram-positive cocci destain easily and have a gram-negative appearance. However, *Veillonella,* an anaerobic gram-negative coccus, is much smaller than the anaerobic gram-positive cocci, with the exception of *Peptostreptococcus micros.* Also, the anaerobic gram-positive cocci may be gram-variable during their life cycle. Anaerobic gram-positive cocci may elongate, so that they appear as short rods. This is common with *Peptostreptococcus productus* but may occur with other species. Cells may appear to be of unequal size in a culture. This size differential may be so great that it gives the appearance of budding.

The cellular morphology of *Sarcina ventriculi* is distinctive from that of the other anaerobic gram-positive cocci. The cells are usually about 2.0 mm in diameter and nearly spherical with their adjacent sides usually flattened. These cells occur in packets of eight or more.

*Peptococcus* (Pc.), *Peptostreptococcus* (Ps.) and the anaerobic members of the genus *Streptococcus* (S.) have no distinguishing colonial morphology. On blood agar plates, colonies of these anaerobic cocci are small (0.5 mm after 48 hours of incubation), convex, opaque, have an entire edge, and are either shiny or dull. Most colonies are gray to white in color. However, some strains of *Ps. micros* and *Ps. anaerobius* produce black colonies.

*S. constellatus* and *S. morbillorum* usually show alpha hemolysis. *S. intermedius* is usually not hemolytic; however, some strains are alpha-hemolytic. *Ps. productus* may be nonhemolytic or may give alpha or beta reactions. The other peptococci and peptostreptococci are not hemolytic except for some strains of *Ps. micros* and *Pc. prevotii* that may produce a beta hemolysin.

Surface colonies of *S. ventriculi* are 1 to 3 mm after 24 hours of incubation, colorless, circular, and opaque with an irregular edge. Most strains are not hemolytic; a few are alpha hemolytic. Subsurface colonies are frequently star-shaped or irregular in appearance.

## ANTIGENIC COMPOSITION

Few studies have been done on the antigens of the anaerobic gram-positive cocci. Agglutination and precipitation tests for the immunologic classification of anaerobic cocci were not successful (Stone, 1940). Another study showed no indication of a common *Peptococcus* or a *Peptostreptococcus* antigen but did show that antigens of *Pc. magnus* may be distinct from the other anaerobic gram-positive cocci. Identification of this species may therefore be practical by fluorescence technique (Porschen and Spaulding, 1974). A recent study of three strains of *Pc. magnus* and one strain of *Ps. anaerobius* using counterimmunoelectrophoresis also indicated that *Pc. magnus* isolates were immunologically distinct (Markowitz and Lerner, 1977).

## METABOLISM

The clinically important species of the anaerobic gram-positive cocci are listed in Table 1, together with their major end-products of amino acid and glucose metabolism.

Peptococci and peptostreptococci are heterofermentative, not producing lactic acid as the sole major end-product from glucose metabolism. They utilize amino acids as their main sources of nitrogen and energy. The anaerobic streptococci are homofermentative, producing only lactic acid as the major end product of carbohydrate fermentation.

Table 2 lists some of the metabolic activities of the anaerobic gram-positive cocci. Peptococci are not very active biochemically. *Pc. asaccharolyticus* is the only clinically important anaerobic gram-positive coccus that produces indole.

**TABLE 1.  Clinically Important Anaerobic Gram-Positive Cocci and Their Major Metabolic End-Products from Amino Acid and Glucose Metabolism**[a]

| NAME | MAJOR END PRODUCTS | | MINOR END PRODUCTS |
|---|---|---|---|
| Pc. asaccharolyticus | A | H | B(SLF) |
| Pc. magnus | A | H | (LSF) |
| Pc. prevotii | A | H | B(L) |
| Pc. saccharolyticus | FA2 | | |
| Ps. anaerobius | A | H | (2BL, et al.) |
| Ps. micros | A | | (LSF) |
| Ps. parvulus | LA | | (S) |
| Ps. productus | A | (H) | S(LP) |
| St. constellatus | L | | |
| St. intermedius | L | | |
| St. morbillorum | L | | |
| S. ventriculi | A2 | H,CO$_2$ | |

[a]Pc., *Peptococcus*; Ps., *Peptostreptococcus*; St., *Streptococcus*; S., *Sarcina*; A, acetic acid; B, butyric acid; F, formic acid; L, lactic acid; P, propionic acid; S, succinic acid; H, hydrogen gas; CO$_2$, carbon dioxide gas; ( ), variable; 2, ethyl alcohol.

*Sarcina ventriculi* has a fermentative metabolism; the principal products from glucose metabolism are carbon dioxide, hydrogen, ethyl alcohol, and acetic acid. This organism has available two pathways for conversion of pyruvate to ethyl alcohol. One is the same as that used by yeast and the other is similar to that of *Escherichia coli* (Canale-Parola, 1970).

## PATHOGENICITY

Evidence for the pathogenicity of anaerobic gram-positive cocci comes from clinical studies that show that only pure cultures of anaerobic gram-positive cocci are obtained from some infections. Pure cultures have been reported from

**TABLE 2.  Metabolic Reactions of Clinical Gram-Positive Anaerobic Cocci**[a]

| | FERMENTATION | | | | INDOLE | NITRATE REDUCTION | GELATIN HYDROLYSIS | ESCULIN HYDROLYSIS | CATALASE |
|---|---|---|---|---|---|---|---|---|---|
| | Glucose | Lactose | Maltose | Sucrose | | | | | |
| Pc. asaccharolyticus | − | − | − | − | + | − | − | − | − |
| Pc. magnus | −$^w$ | − | − | − | − | − | V | − | − |
| Pc. prevotii | −$^w$ | − | −$^\cdot$ | − | − | −$^+$ | − | − | −$^+$ |
| Pc. saccharolyticus | A$^w$ | − | − | − | − | +$^-$ | − | − | + |
| Ps. anaerobius | W$^{a-}$ | − | −$^w$ | − | − | −$^+$ | −$^w$ | − | −$^+$ |
| Ps. micros | −$^w$ | − | − | − | − | − | − | − | +$^-$ |
| Ps. parvulus | A | A | A | − | − | − | − | + | − |
| Ps. productus | A | A | A | A | − | − | − | + | − |
| St. constellatus | A | − | A | A | − | − | − | + | − |
| St. intermedius | A | A | A | A | − | − | − | + | − |
| St. morbillorum | A | − | A$^w$ | A | − | − | − | + | − |
| S. ventriculi | A | A | A$^w$ | A | − | +$^-$ | − | + | − |

[a]−, negative reaction; +, positive reaction; A, acid; W, weak acid; V, variable.
From Holdeman, L. V., Cato, E. P., and Moore, W. E.: Anaerobe Laboratory Manual. Blacksburg, Va., Virginia Polytechnic Institute and State University, 1977.

breast abscess, prostatitis, liver abscess, pleuro-pulmonary infections, epidermoid cysts, finger infections, osteomyelitis, and other infections. *Pc. magnus* was found in pure culture in four postoperative wound infections, a thigh abscess, and one case of septicemia (Lambe et al., 1973). Reports also show a high incidence of *Peptostreptococcus* isolated in pure cultures from brain abscess, meningitis, and extradural and subdural empyema. *Peptococcus* is not isolated as frequently in pure culture from clinically significant infections as are peptostreptococci.

The anaerobic gram-positive cocci are more commonly found in infections together with other anaerobes or with facultative bacteria. The pathogenic role of the anaerobic gram-positive cocci in such conditions is unproven. About one third of intraabdominal infections have a mixed flora in which anaerobic cocci are found together with either *Bacteroides fragilis* or clostridia or both. Anaerobic streptococci and clostridia are the most frequent anaerobes isolated from biliary tract infections. The pathogenic potential of the anaerobic cocci in these infections is unknown.

Certain bacteria act together in a synergistic manner to produce infections. For example, a synergistic gangrene is produced by a microaerophilic *Streptococcus* together with a hemolytic *Staphylococcus aureus*. If animals are monoinoculated with individual cultures no disease is produced, but if the organisms are combined and then inoculated, typical necrotic ulcers are formed (Meleney, 1949). The synergy involves hyaluronidase production by the *Staphylococcus* plus a growth factor that makes the microaerophilic *Streptococcus* invasive.

Little has been done to determine the mechanisms of pathogenicity in the anaerobic cocci. The hemolytic activity of the group has been mentioned. Most anaerobic cocci produce ammonia that causes inflammation.

*Sarcina ventriculi* is not considered a pathogen. It is a free-living form that enters the stomach frequently. Prolonged gastric retention allows *Sarcina* to grow rapidly and produces so much gas from fermentable substrates that abdominal discomfort results.

*S. ventriculi* is occasionally found in infections, especially of the gallbladder and bile duct, but never in pure culture. *S. ventriculi* is a minor member of the normal flora in humans.

## IMMUNITY

The role of immunologic mechanisms against specific anaerobic gram-positive cocci is unknown. Intact epithelium affords a high degree of resistance to the endogenous peptococci, pepto-streptococci, and anaerobic streptococci. Also, the essential exogenous *Sarcina ventriculi* is usually denied entrance to the body surface. Leukocytes can ingest and kill *Pc. magnus* and *Ps. anaerobius* in the absence of oxygen.

## LABORATORY DIAGNOSIS

Differentiation between the genera *Peptococcus* and *Peptostreptococcus* is difficult because the species are variable in morphologic, cultural, and metabolic properties and are relatively inert biochemically. Criteria established by the Anaerobe Laboratory of the Virginia Polytechnic Institute (Holdeman et al., 1977) are used by most laboratories for the identification of the anaerobic gram-positive cocci. Their method requires determination of the end-products of metabolism of glucose and amino acids in the base medium by gas-liquid chromatography.

Peptococci can be differentiated from peptostreptococci on the basis of the guanine plus cytosine content of their DNA. Peptostreptococci have 33.5 moles per cent, peptococci 35.7 to 36.7 moles per cent. However, anaerobic streptococci range from 33 to 44 moles per cent, making it necessary to use fermentation end-product analysis for the differentiation of anaerobic streptococci.

Anaerobic streptococci and peptostreptococci give negative catalase tests. Peptococci may give weak and variable catalase reactions. Therefore, a negative catalase test does not separate this group of organisms. A positive test does suggest the genus *Peptococcus*.

Members of the *Peptococcus* group usually do not form long chains. Peptostreptococci and anaerobic streptococci both have a strong chaining tendency. Absence of chaining, then, suggests peptococci. If long chains are present, end-product analysis of glucose fermentation is needed to differentiate peptostreptococci from anaerobic streptococci and to confirm members of the genus *Peptococcus*.

Two species common in clinical specimens may be identified by simple tests. *Pc. asaccharolyticus* is the only gram-positive anaerobic coccus found in clinical infections that produces indole. *Ps. anaerobius* is the only anaerobic gram-positive coccus that is susceptible to sodium polyanetholsulfonate (SPS), which can be used easily to differentiate it from the other anaerobic gram-positive cocci (Wideman et al., 1976).

*Sarcina ventriculi* can easily be distinguished by microscopic morphology. Large round cells with adjacent sides flattened and in packets of eight or more are characteristic of this species, the only anaerobic *Sarcina* found in man.

A key for the identification of the clinically

**TABLE 3.  Identification Key to The Clinically Important Anaerobic Gram-Positive Cocci**

| | |
|---|---|
| Lactic acid the sole major end-product | |
|   Esculin hydrolysis + | |
|     Lactose + | Streptococcus intermedius |
|     Lactose − | Streptococcus constellatus |
|   Esculin hydrolysis − | Streptococcus morbillorum |
| Lactis acid not the sole major end-product | |
|   Indole + | Peptococcus asaccharolyticus |
|   Indole − | |
|     Sensitive to SPS[a] | Peptococcus anaerobius |
|     Resistance to SPS | |
|       Lactose | |
|         Maltose + | Peptococcus productus |
|         Maltose − | Peptococcus parvulus |
|       Lactose − | |
|         Glucose + | Peptostreptococcus micros |
|         Glucose − | |
|           Butyric acid produced | Peptococcus prevotii |
|           Butyric acid not produced | Peptococcus magnus |

[a]Sodium polyanethol sulfonate.

important anaerobic gram-positive cocci is given in Table 3. This is one of several schemes that have been proposed for the identification of these bacteria.

Not all anaerobic gram-positive cocci isolates can be identified. On occasion, what are usually facultative gram-positive cocci grow only anaerobically upon isolation and initial subculture (Yatabe et al., 1977). Facultative cocci may also mutate to form obligate anaerobes that retain all their characteristics except anaerobiosis.

## DRUG SUSCEPTIBILITY

Tables 4 and 5 show the minimum inhibitory concentrations of ten antibiotics for the genus *Peptococcus* and *Peptostreptococcus*. Published information is lacking about the bactericidal activity of these drugs against the anaerobic gram-positive cocci.

The anaerobic gram-positive cocci are susceptible to the drugs listed except the aminoglycoside kanamycin and the structurally related antibiotic gentamicin. Many strains of anaerobic gram-positive cocci are resistant to tetracycline and erythromycin. Penicillin G is the drug of choice for most anaerobic gram-positive cocci infections. Clindamycin and cephalothin are alternate choices (Braude, 1976).

## EPIDEMIOLOGY

Peptococci, peptostreptococci, and anaerobic streptococci are part of the indigenous microbiota of the human oral cavity, gastrointestinal tract, genitourinary system, and skin. These opportunist bacteria are commonly found in infections that are closely associated with these organ systems.

*Sarcina ventriculi* is commonly found in soil and mud, and on grain, but only infrequently and in low numbers in the normal human fecal flora.

A 14-year study on the incidence of anaerobes in clinical specimens showed that 58.5 per cent yielded anaerobes (Holland et al., 1977). Anaerobic gram-positive bacteria were present in 66 per cent of these specimens and were second only to *Bacteroides,* which occurred in 70 per cent of the specimens. This is a major clinical concern, especially since 15 per cent of the specimens contained anaerobic cocci as the only anaerobe present.

*Pc. asaccharolyticus* is found in about 10 per cent of human infections. *Ps. anaerobius* occurs in about 9 per cent of the cases, and the third most numerous isolate, *S. intermedius,* in about 5 per cent of infections. *Pc. prevotti* and *Pc. magnus* are both found in about 4 per cent of infections.

In a study of 100 anaerobic pleuropulmonary infections, peptostreptococci were recovered 19

**TABLE 4.  In Vitro Susceptibility of 145 Clinical Isolates of Peptococcus to 10 Antibiotics[a]**

| | CUMULATIVE PERCENTAGE SUSCEPTIBLE AT INCREASING CONCENTRATION ($\mu$g/ml) | | | | | | | | | |
|---|---|---|---|---|---|---|---|---|---|---|
| | 0.1 | 0.2 | 0.4 | 0.8 | 1.6 | 3.1 | 6.2 | 12.5 | 25 | >25 |
| Penicillin G | 48 | 91 | 95 | 96 | 97 | 99 | | 100 | | |
| Erythromycin | 9 | 10 | 16 | 24 | 58 | 79 | 80 | 86 | 87 | 100 |
| Cephalothin | 22 | 38 | 56 | 78 | 88 | 89 | 97 | 98 | 99 | 100 |
| Tetracycline | 12 | 15 | 29 | 52 | 56 | 59 | 62 | 74 | 89 | 100 |
| Lincomycin | 29 | 45 | 69 | 92 | 95 | 96 | | | 97 | 100 |
| Clindamycin | 62 | 76 | 87 | 94 | 95 | 96 | 97 | | | 100 |
| Kanamycin | 1 | | | | 2 | | 4 | 13 | 44 | 100 |
| Chloramphenicol | 5 | 6 | 8 | 25 | 67 | 97 | 98 | | 99 | 100 |
| Gentamicin | 2 | 3 | | 5 | 7 | 11 | 30 | 62 | 95 | 100 |
| Rifampin | 47 | 50 | 62 | 76 | 96 | 98 | 99 | | | 100 |

[a]From Pien, F. D., Thompson, R. L., and Martin, W. J.: Mayo Clin Proc 47:251, 1972.

**TABLE 5.** In Vitro Susceptibility of 72 Clinical Isolates of Peptostreptococcus to 10 Antibiotics

| | CUMULATIVE PERCENTAGE SUSCEPTIBLE AT INCREASING CONCENTRATION ($\mu$g/ml) | | | | | | | | | |
|---|---|---|---|---|---|---|---|---|---|---|
| | 0.1 | 0.2 | 0.4 | 0.8 | 1.6 | 3.1 | 6.2 | 12.5 | 25 | >25 |
| Penicillin G | 58 | 91 | 97 | 98 | 100 | | | | | |
| Erythromycin | 37 | 39 | 46 | 56 | 73 | 88 | 92 | 99 | | 100 |
| Cephalothin | 40 | 57 | 70 | 78 | 96 | | 99 | | 100 | |
| Tetracycline | 18 | 26 | 44 | 55 | 65 | 73 | 77 | 83 | 96 | 100 |
| Lincomycin | 39 | 58 | 72 | 85 | 96 | 100 | | | | |
| Clindamycin | 81 | 85 | 90 | 98 | 100 | | | | | |
| Kanamycin | | | | 1 | 5 | 11 | 12 | 23 | 44 | 100 |
| Chloramphenicol | | 3 | 11 | 37 | 63 | 96 | 100 | | | |
| Gentamicin | 1 | 2 | 9 | 13 | 78 | 20 | 33 | 58 | 78 | 100 |
| Rifampin | 68 | | | 72 | | | 94 | | 96 | 100 |

[a]From Pien, F. D., Thompson, R. L., and Martin, W. J.: Mayo Clin Proc 47:251, 1972.

times, 3 times in pure culture. Peptococci were recovered 15 times, always in a mixed culture.

Anaerobic cocci are found in about 1 per cent of blood cultures. They make up approximately 7 per cent of the anaerobic isolates from blood cultures. The foci of infection in anaerobic gram-positive cocci bacteremias are usually infections of the soft tissue, gastrointestinal tract, liver, female genital tract, and oropharynx.

Anaerobes have been found in about 3 per cent of bacterial endocarditis. Anaerobic and microaerophilic streptococci make up over 90 per cent of these anaerobes.

Anaerobic cocci have been reported in about one third of all abdominal infections. The anaerobic gram-positive cocci are associated with *Bacteroides fragilis* and clostridia. Anaerobic cocci and clostridia are the dominant anaerobes in biliary tract infections, but overall they represent a minor cause of these infections.

The anaerobic gram-positive cocci are frequently found in liver abscesses and brain abscesses, and 40 per cent of abscesses of the female pelvis contain anaerobic streptococci. In septic abortions, *B. fragilis, B. melaninogenicus,* and anaerobic streptococci are isolated in greatest number. Bacteremias from septic abortions most frequently yield anaerobic streptococci and *Bacteroides*. These two anaerobic groups are also the most frequent isolates from postpartum endometritis.

One study of brain abscess reported recovery of anaerobes in 89 per cent of the cases, with peptostreptococci being the predominant organism (Heinemann and Braude, 1963). The most common isolates from chronic sinusitis are peptostreptococci.

The bacteria seen in synergistic necrotizing cellulitis are gram-negative bacilli, peptostreptococci, and *Bacteroides*. Peptostreptococci are the anaerobes most frequently found in necrotizing fasciitis.

## References

Braude, A. I.: Antimicrobial Drug Therapy. Philadelphia, W. B. Saunders Company, 1976.

Canale-Parola, E.: Biology of the sugar-fermenting sarcinae. Bacterial Rev 34:82, 1970.

Facklam, R. R., and Smith, P. B.: The gram positive cocci. Human Pathol. 7:187, 1976.

Finegold, S. M.: Anaerobic Bacteria in Human Disease. New York, Academic Press, 1977.

Heineman, H. S., and Braude, A. I.: Anaerobic infection of the brain: Observations on eighteen consecutive cases of brain abscess. Am J Med 35:682, 1963.

Holdeman, L. V., Cato, E. P., and Moore, W. E.: Anaerobe Laboratory Manual. Blacksburg, Va., Virginia Polytechnic Institute and State University, 1977.

Holland, J. W., Hill, E. O., and Altemeier, W. A.: Numbers and types of anaerobic bacteria isolated from clinical specimens since 1960. J Clin Microbiol 5:20, 1977.

Lambe, D. W., Vroon, D. H., and Rietz, C. W.: Infections due to anaerobic cocci. In Ballows, A., et al. (eds.): Anaerobic Bacteria: Role in Disease. Springfield, Ill., Charles C Thomas, 1973.

Markowitz, A., and Lerner, A. M.: Differentiation of several isolates of *Peptococcus magnus* by counterimmunoelectrophoresis. Infect Immun 16:152, 1977.

Meleney, F. L.: Clinical Aspects and Treatment of Surgical Infections. Philadelphia, W. B. Saunders Company, 1949.

Pien, F. D., Thompson, R. L., and Martin, W. J.: Clinical and bacteriologic studies of anaerobic gram-positive cocci. Mayo Clin Proc 47:251, 1972.

Porschen, R. K., and Spaulding, E. H.: Fluorescent antibody study of the gram-positive anaerobic cocci. Appl Microbiol 28:851, 1974.

Stone, M. L.: Studies on the anaerobic streptococcus. I. Certain biochemical and immunological properties of anaerobic streptococci. J Bacteriol 39:559, 1940.

Wideman, P. A., Vargo, V. L., et al.: Evaluation of the sodium polyanethol sulfonate disk test for the identification of *Peptostreptococcus anaerobius*. J Clin Microbiol 4:330, 1976.

Yatabe, J. H., Baldwin, K. L., and Martin, W. J.: Isolation of an obligately anaerobic *Streptococcus pneumoniae* from blood culture. J Clin Microbiol 6:181, 1977.

# 44 *ACTINOMYCES AND MICROAEROPHILIC ACTINOMYCETES*

## *Leo Pine, Ph.D.*

Perhaps the earliest description of the actinomycotic organism was made by von Graefe (1854), who described fungal masses he observed in granules taken from infections of the lacrimal canal. Cohn (1875) also observed a fine branching fungus in lacrimal concretions, which he named *Streptothrix foersteri*. In 1877, Bollinger published the first description of actinomycosis in cattle. This organism, resembling *Streptothrix*, was described in the tissues by Hartz (1879), who named it *Actinomyces bovis*. Israel described actinomycosis in man in 1878, and Ponfick (1880) compared human and bovine actinomycosis. Although Bujwid (1889) first isolated *Actinomyces* from human actinomycosis, it was the classic description of the morphology and physiology of this bacterium by Wolff and Israel (1891) that permitted subsequent workers to identify and establish this organism as the cause of actinomycosis in man.

Silberschmidt first cultured the anaerobic actinomycete from lacrimal concretions; he compared the organisms isolated from maxillary actinomycosis of a cow, from human lacrimal concretions, and from maxillary and thoracic infections in man (Silberschmidt, 1901). Because all strains appeared identical, Silberschmidt concluded that *Streptothrix* was the correct name on the basis of taxonomic priority. Thus *Streptothrix* and names such as *Leptothrix, Cladothrix,* and *Leptotrichia* were all commonly used in early ophthalmologic and dental literature to refer to long filamentous or branching organisms. These names were used so commonly that some investigators no longer associated the *Streptothrix* or *Leptothrix* of lacrimal canaliculitis or of dental plaque with the *Actinomyces* of thoracic infections. To add to the confusion, Bostroem (1891) had earlier isolated aerobic forms of filamentous bacteria not only from human and bovine cases of actinomycosis but also from plant materials and soil. Although years later these aerobic forms were given the name *Streptomyces*, the generic name *Actinomyces* is still used today in certain countries to describe the aerobic nonpathogenic streptomycetes.

The source of the infections became apparent when Naeslund (1925) identified the bacterium as part of the normal flora of the mouth; Emmons (1935) later found *Actinomyces* in granules in tonsillar crypts. Although Erikson (1940) believed that human and bovine strains were sufficiently different to warrant separation as *Actinomyces israelii* and *Actinomyces bovis*, respectively, these species were not accepted by other workers until after World War II (Thompson, 1950; Pine et al., 1960). *A. naeslundii*, originally isolated from the mouth by Thompson and Lovestedt (1951) and Howell et al. (1959), was later found to be pathogenic for animals and man (Colemen et al., 1969).

Of great importance for taxonomy and for laboratory diagnosis was the observation that the pathogenic *Actinomyces* had no catalase, whereas coryneforms were catalase positive (Suter, 1956). Analysis of fermentation products and cell wall composition helped delineate those actinomycetes that showed true branching or mycelial microcolonies (Cummins, 1962).

The 8th edition of *Bergey's Manual of Determinative Bacteriology* (Buchanan and Gibbons, 1974) describes five genera in the family. Five species of *Actinomyces* are accepted and an additional three species are described, although their present taxonomic status is uncertain (Table 1). All species of *Actinomyces* were originally isolated from patients with actinomycosis, actinomycosis-like disease, periodontal plaque, or dental caries. The exception is *Actinomyces humiferus*, which was isolated from the soil and is nonpathogenic. Similarly, *Bacterionema matruchotii*, a commensal in the mouth of animals, has not been associated with disease. The most definitive discussion of these organisms appears in *Actinomyces, Filamentous Bacteria: Biology and Pathogenicity* (Slack and Gerencser, 1975).

## *MORPHOLOGY*

The species of bacteria in the families Actinomycetaceae and Propionibacteriaceae have gram-positive, straight or curved, branching, pleomorphic rod-like cells that are nonacid-fast, nonmotile, and nonspore-forming (Figs. 1 and 2). The organisms are generally 0.2 to 0.3 $\mu m$ in

**TABLE 1.** Taxonomic Relationships of Fermentative Actinomycetes and Similar-Form Organisms Associated with Human or Animal Disease

| FAMILY[a] | GENUS (SPECIES) | SYNONYM | DISEASE | HABITAT | MORPHOLOGY IN DISEASE TISSUE | CELLULAR MORPHOLOGY[c] | PATHOGENICITY IN LABORATORY ANIMALS |
|---|---|---|---|---|---|---|---|
| Actinomycetaceae (microaerophilic, fermentative) | Actinomyces[b] bovis, A. israelii, A. naeslundii, A. suis, A. viscosus, A. odontolyticus | Streptothrix, Cladothrix, Leptothrix, Actinobacterium | Actinomycosis, lacrimal canaliculitis | Oral cavity, tonsillar crypts, dental plaque, calculus | Long branching mycelium or filamentous cells, sulfur granules, mycelial masses, streptococcal-like chains | Filaments, long rods, branching rods, clubs, small rods, diphtheroids | Pathogenic for mice and hamsters; forming limited or progressive abscesses in most animals when injected intraperitoneally |
| | Arachnia propionica | Actinomyces propionicus | Actinomycosis, lacrimal canaliculitis | Oral cavity, dental plaque, tonsillar crypts | Long threadlike filaments, sulfur granules; branching mycelial masses | Long branching rods, nonbranching filaments, coccoid bodies (spheroplasts) | Same as Actinomyces |
| | Bifidobacterium adolescentis[d] | Actinomyces eriksonii | Lung abscess, pleural fluid | Oral cavity, tonsils, intestinal tract | Small bifid rods; club-shapes; curved rods | Small singly branched rods, clubs, unbranched rods | Nonpathogenic; forms limited abscesses |
| | Bacterionema matruchotii | Leptotrichia dentium, L. buccalis | None | Dental plaque, calculus | None | Branching filaments, long filaments with terminal bacillary head | Nonpathogenic |
| | Rothia dentocariosa | Nocardia salivae | None | Dental plaque, calculus | Beaded filaments, short branching rods | Short or long branching rods, cocci, filaments | Nonpathogenic; forms limited abscesses |
| Propionibacteriaceae (microaerophilic, fermentative) | Propionibacterium acnes | Corynebacterium acnes | Skin abscess | Gingival plaque, skin abscesses, intestinal contents, lacrimal canal | "Diphtheroid" rods, curved rods, branched rods, irregular shapes | Diphtheroid rod-like cells | Forms limited abscesses when inoculated into mice subcutaneously or intraperitoneally |
| Nocardiaceae (aerobic, oxidative) | Nocardia asteroides, N. brasiliensis, Actinomadura madurae, Actinomadura pelletiera | Streptothrix, Proactinomyces, Actinomyces, Streptomyces, Nocardia | Maduromycosis | Soil | Long branching mycelial elements, granules | Nonsporulating fragmenting mycelium gives rise to rod-shaped and coccoidal elements | Pathogenic for laboratory animals depending on route of inoculation and species |
| Streptomycetaceae (aerobic, oxidative) | Streptomyces somaliensis, S. paraguayensis | Actinomyces | Maduromycosis | Soil | Long branching mycelial elements, granules | Nonfragmenting surface mycelium; may form chains of spores | May cause limited progressive abscesses with intraperitoneal inoculation |

[a]Based primarily on the data in Bergey's Manual of Determinative Bacteriology (Buchanan and Gibbons, 1974) and Slack and Gerencser (1975). Actinomyces humiferus, not listed above, is isolated from the soil and is not pathogenic.
[b]A. odontolyticus is nonpathogenic.
[c]Grown for 24 to 72 hours in semisolid thioglycolate or Trypticase Soy Broth.
[d]Mitsuoka et al. (1974).

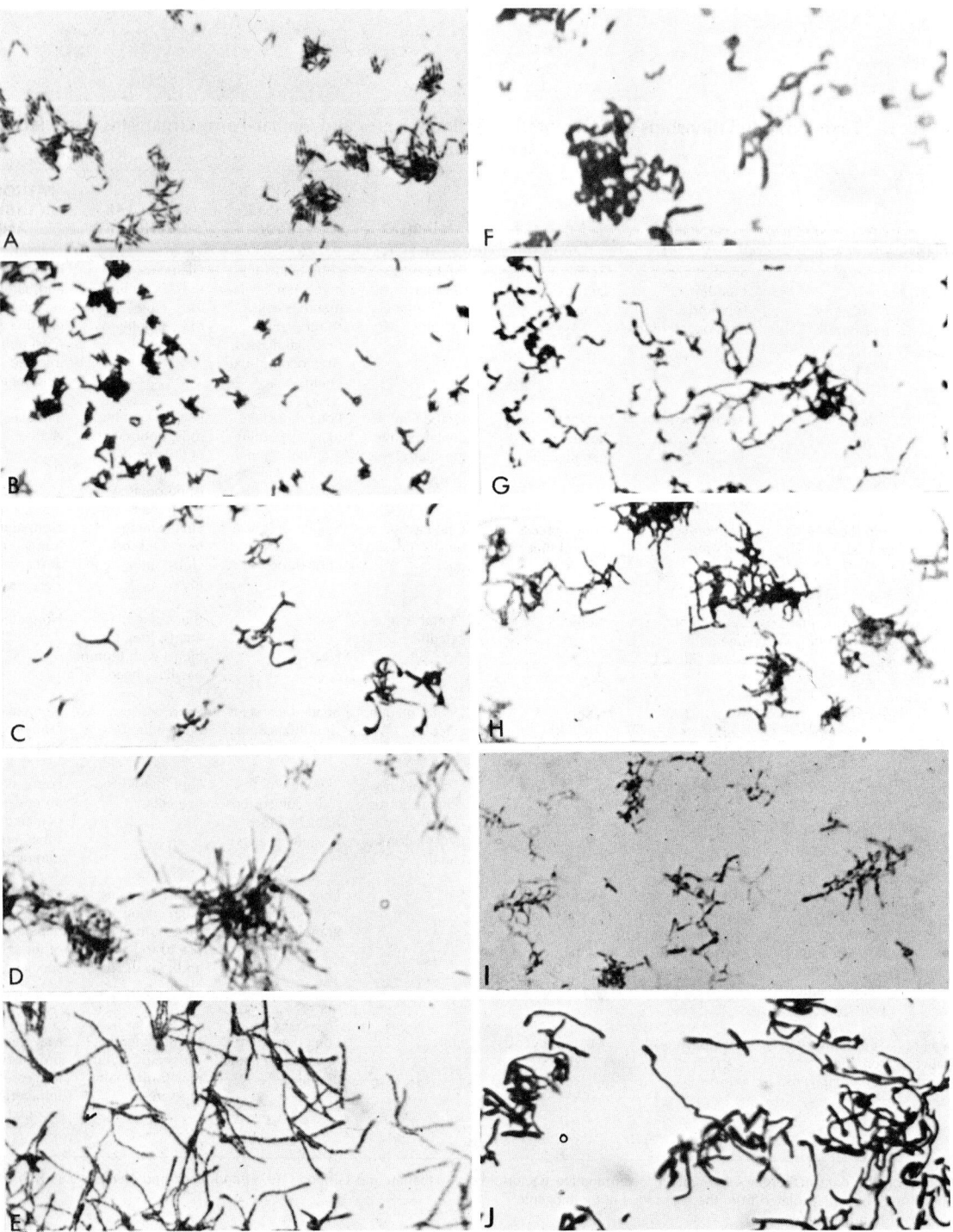

**FIGURE 1.** *Cellular morphology of* Actinomyces *species grown in thioglycollate broth, Gram stain, (1200 ×) (Mycology Division, Center for Disease Control, Atlanta, Georgia). (A)* Actinomyces bovis, *(B)* A. odontolyticus, *(C)* Bifidobacterium adolescentis (A. eriksonii), *(D)* A. naeslundii, *(E)* A. israelii, *(F)* A. israelli, *(G)* Arachnia propionica, *(H)* Propionibacterium acnes, *(I)* Rothia dentocariosa, *(J)* Bacterioma matruchotii. *Most species exhibit the range of cellular morphologies seen in Figure 2. However, the long filamentous form terminating in a bacillary head is characteristic only of* Bacterionema matruchotti *(J), whereas the bifid branching of* B. adolescentis *(C) is characteristic of the genus* Bifidobacterium. *Within the remaining species, short cells, often in pairs as V forms (A, F, and G) to long filamentous branching cells are often seen (E and F). The morphology of* P. acnes *cannot be distinguished from that of the* Actinomyces *species.*

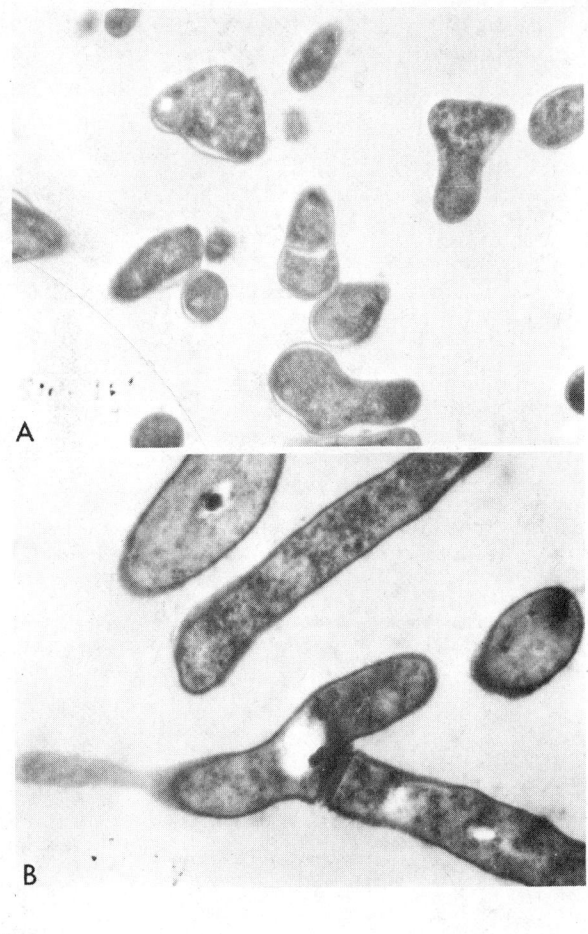

**FIGURE 2.** *Comparative cellular morphology of "diphtheroid" and filamentous forms (23,000 ×) (J. L.Overman).*
  *A.* Actinomyces bovis
  *B.* Arachnia propionica

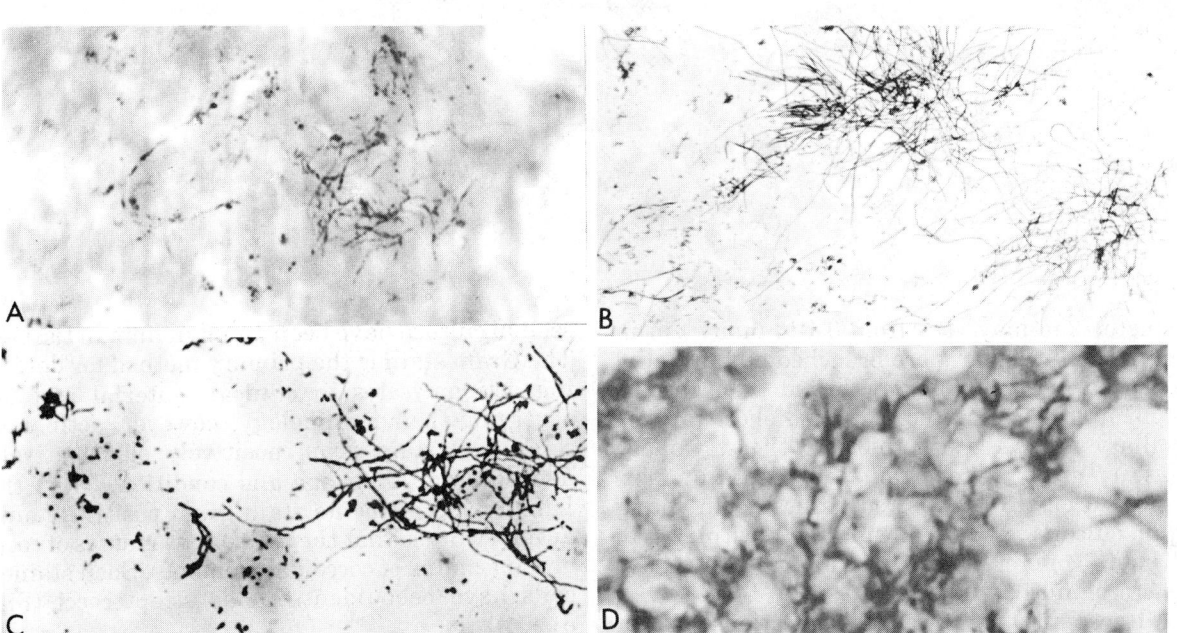

**FIGURE 3.** *Morphologic aspects of microaerophilic actinomycetes in tissues.*
  *A.* Actinomyces bovis *in pus from inoculated hamster. Gram stain (900 ×). Note streptococcal-like chains.*
  *B.* Arachnia propionica *in pus from inoculated hamster. Gram stain (900 ×). (Pine and Hardin, 1959.)*
  *C.* Actinomyces bovis *in pus from inoculated hamster. Gram stain (900 ×). (Pine et al., 1960.) Note coccal forms and filamentous forms without branching.*
  *D.* Actinomyces israelii *in lung, human infection. Brown and Brenn stain (1000 ×).*

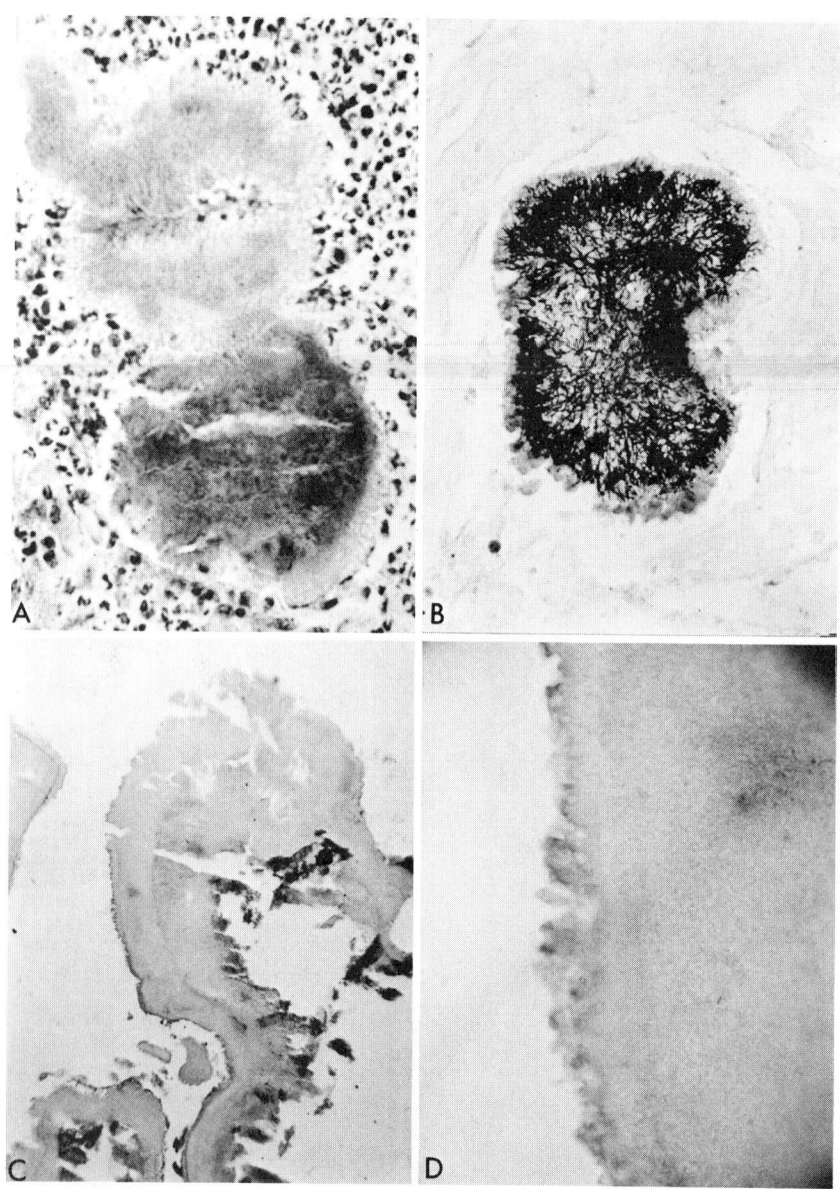

**FIGURE 4.** *Morphologic aspects of the sulfur granule.*

*A. Sulfur granule from human infection, H & E stain. (Mycology Division, Center for Disease Control, Atlanta, Ga.)*

*B. Sulfur granule from human infection. Brown and Brenn (Gram) stain (315 ×). (Mycology Division, Center for Disease Control, Atlanta, Ga.)*

*C. Sulfur granule from bovine lumpy jaw. Colloidal iron stain (100 ×)). (Pine and Overman, 1963.)*

*D. As C above (800 ×) showing peripheral arrangement of clubs.*

diameter and may vary from 0.4 to many μm in length. Cells appear more branched and mycelial in the early stages of growth and then become fragmented, forming coccoidal and short tapered bacillary forms (diphtheroids) in the stationary phase of growth. Important differences in morphology occur (1) in infected tissues (2) in young liquid cultures, and (3) on agar plate within 24 to 72 hours (microcolonies) and after 3 to 14 days (macrocolonies).

All species that cause deep infections (except *Bifidobacterium adolescentis*) are seen in pus or infected tissues as long, nonbranching filaments or as complexes of loosely or tightly interwoven branching mycelial elements (Fig. 3). Masses of *B. adolescentis* with a morphology similar to that

seen in culture have been found in human tissues. The Gram stain is the primary method for detecting actinomycetes in clinical material and for observing their morphology; however, actinomycetes may stain gram positively or negatively depending on their age and condition. Often the long hyphal elements stain gram positively only at intervals, so that they appear as masses of cocci or long chains of coccoidal elements. Such stained cells have been identified as streptococci (Fig. 3).

The various *Actinomyces* or *Arachnia* species form special structures, called drusen, sulfur granules, or mycelial granules within the tissues. Only trace amounts of sulfur are present in sulfur granules, so the term probably derived from their

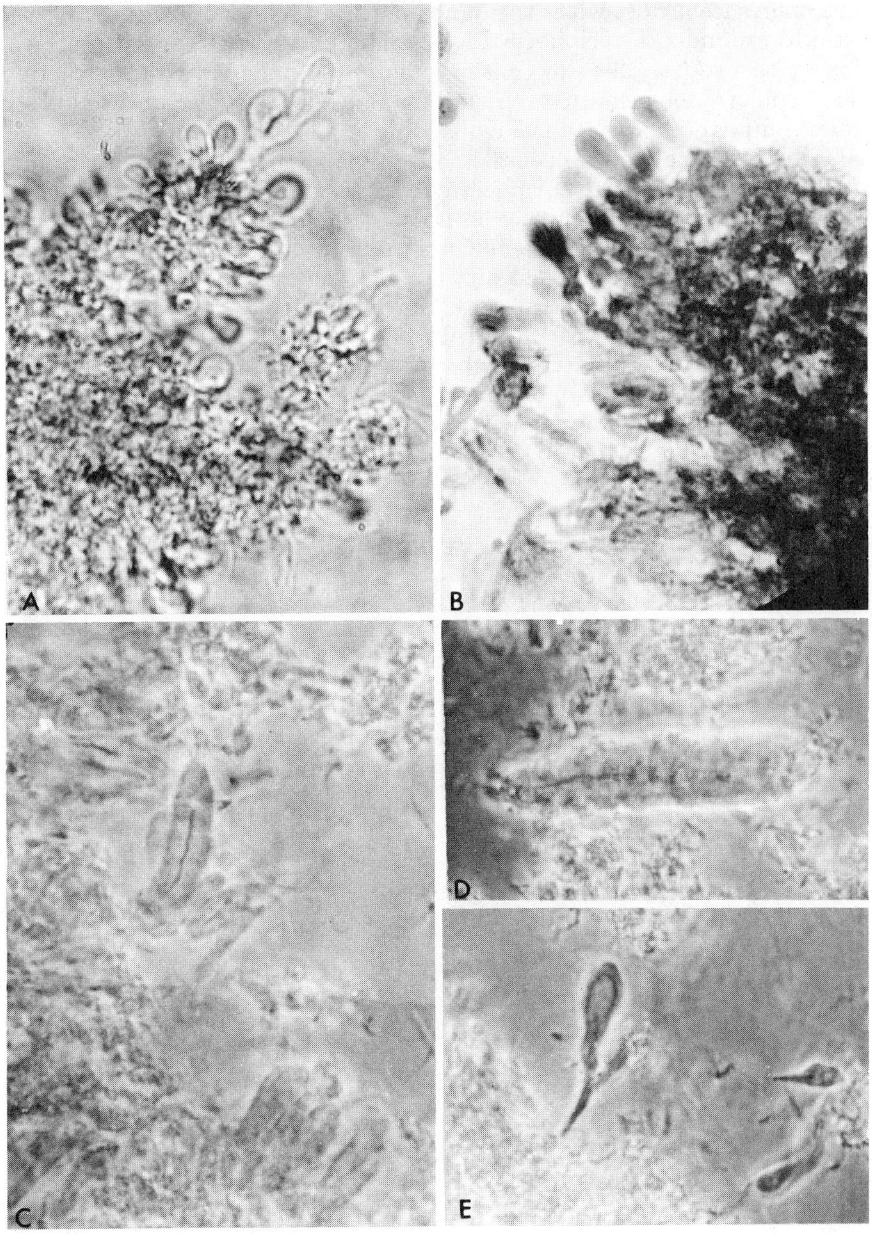

**FIGURE 5.** *Sulfur granule —structure of clubs.*

*A. Crushed granule mounted in 10 per cent KOH showing multibranched hyaline clubs (970 ×).*

*B. Periodic acid-Schiff stain of sectioned granule (970 ×). Note hyaline nature of clubs and absence of clearly defined mycelium.*

*C. Crushed granule, digested in 10 per cent KOH; phase contrast, (970 ×). Note presence of filaments within clubs. (Pine and Overman, 1966.)*

*D. Large intact club showing internal filament after successive treatments with trichloracetic acid and proteolytic enzymes (970 ×). (Pine and Overman, 1963.)*

*E. Crushed granule, lactophenol mount; phase contrast (970 ×). Note successive layers of capsular material.*

yellow color in pus. *A. odontolyticus* does not invade the tissues and does not make granules. *B. adolescentis* does not form granules, although it does form compact masses of bacterial cells in human infections (Georg et al., 1965). Characteristically, sulfur granules are seen in the pus or tissue as discrete yellow grains of relatively hard consistency (Fig. 4). They are 40 to 400 $\mu$m in diameter and can be seen by eye, trapped in the gauze of surgical dressings.

When placed in a water or 5 per cent postassium hydroxide mount and crushed between the coverslip and the glass slide, the mycelial and cellular elements can be seen directly with phase optics or with the use of Gram, methylene blue,

periodic acid-Schiff, or silver methenamine stains. The sulfur granules generally have peripheral clubs that with proper chemical treatment can be shown to contain an internal mycelial filament (Fig. 5). The sulfur granules of *A. bovis* have been analyzed by a combination of histochemical stains of thin sections, chemical analyses, and electron microscope studies (Pine and Overman, 1963, 1966). Whereas the overall chemical composition of the granules was similar to that of the organism grown on culture medium, they contained some 40 to 60 per cent $Ca_3(PO_4)_2$. Some of the $Ca_3(PO_4)_2$ was poorly crystallized apatite (Frazier and Fowler, 1967). The mycelial elements of the granule are cemented together by mucopolysaccharide with the clubs forming a rosette around the periphery (Fig. 4). The clubs may measure from 3 to 20 times the diameter of the hyphae embedded within them. The $Ca_3(PO_4)_2$ may completely saturate the embedding material, simply fill certain individual cells, or form a layer at their internal periphery. Coupled with Wright's (1905) demonstration of the production of typical sulfur granules in cultures containing serum, these findings suggest that $Ca_3(PO_4)_2$ deposition within the cells is caused by the biochemical activities of the bacterium itself. The normal hyphal elements within the center of a granule are readily see with Gram or silver methenamine stains (Fig. 5). However, heavily calcified granules or clubs do not stain intensely, and clear

observation of the cellular elements that are either within the club or embedded in the granule requires extraction of the granule with trichloracetic acid or treatment by other chemical means (Fig. 5).

Although the presence of sulfur granules strongly suggests *Actinomyces* infection, *Staphylococcus, Nocardia, Streptomyces,* and *Actinobacillus lignieresii* may also form "granules." The bacterium of the granule must therefore be identified by histopathologic and bacteriologic procedures.

Morphology of strains even within the same species may vary greatly (Fig. 6). In one medium a strain may be rod-shaped, and in another it may be a longer branched cell or even a coccus. Simi-

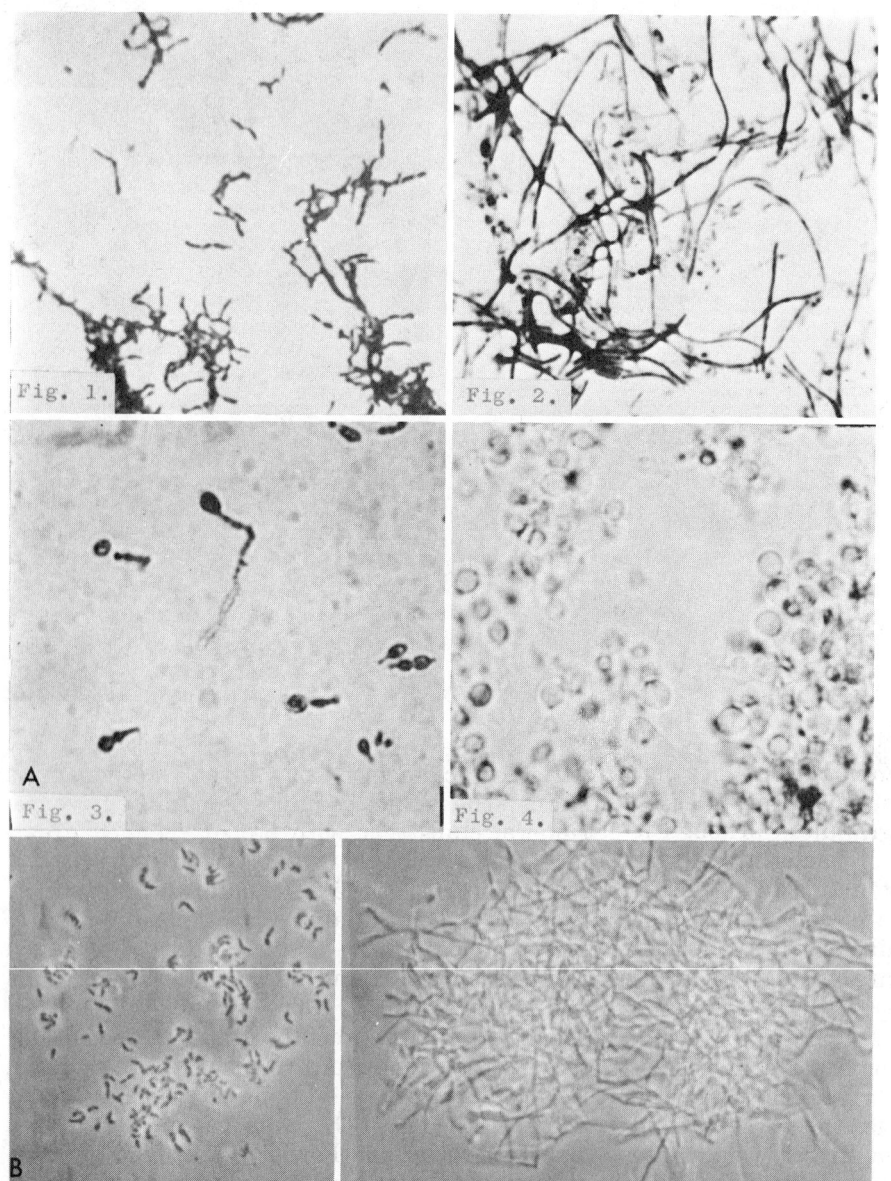

**FIGURE 6.** *Variation in cellular morphology during growth.*

*A. Variation of* Arachnia propionica *during growth in broth media. Changes from diphtheroidal morphology to filament and coccoidal forms, and formation of spheroplasts in glucose casitone broth (Figs. 1–3); formation of spheroplasts in rhamnose broth (Fig. 4), phase contrast (970 ×).*

*B.* Actinomyces bovis *diphtheroid and mycelial forms; phase contrast, (970 ×)). The mycelial form upon transfer may give rise to the diphtheroid morphology observed on the left.*

larly, morphology may change radically as the bacterium goes through its various phases of growth and the medium becomes depleted (Fig. 6).

The various strains of a given species may have cellular characteristics in common with all members of that species (Fig. 1; Table 2). Cellular morphology is best characterized in fluid (0.075 per cent agar) thioglycolate medium with 0.1 per cent sugar. Long incubation periods lead to fragmentation of branched hyphae, conversion to atypical forms, and loss of gram-positivity.

The two basic cell morphologies are: (1) diphtheroids, which are small branched or unbranched forms of comma-shaped cells or V- or

Y-forms with two or three cells connected, and (2) long rods, sometimes branching (Table 2). *A. bovis,* and *A. odontolyticus* are most often diphtheroids or short rods. *B. adolescentis* has the characteristic Y-branched form (Fig. 1). *A. israelii, A. naeslundii, A. viscosus,* and *A. suis* are V-forms, whereas *Arachnia propionica* and *Rothia dentocariosa* are mixed rods and long filaments with numerous coccoid forms. *Bacterionema matruchotii* has a long filament that gradually increases in diameter and terminates in a bacillary-shaped body (Fig. 1). *Propionibacterium acnes* and *Actinomyces* species are often found together in clinical materials and cannot be distinguished morphologically.

**TABLE 2.  Morphologic Aspects of the Microaerophilic Actinomycetes**

| | CELLULAR AND COLONY MORPHOLOGY IN CULTURE | | | | |
|---|---|---|---|---|---|
| | | | | Solid Medium[b] | |
| SPECIES | Morphology in Pus or Infected Tissue | Sulfur Granules | Liquid Medium[a] | *Microcolony* | *Macrocolony* |
| *Bifidobacterium adolescentis* | Short filaments | None | Short rods, branched V and Y shape | Smooth glistening entire edge, no mycelium | Large, shiny convex colonies; circular or irregular; surface smooth or granular |
| *Actinomyces odontolyticus* | None | None | Diphtheroid, very short, pleomorphic | Smooth circular granular colonies, no mycelium | Large, circular, glistening, white, opaque colonies; red colonies on blood |
| *A. bovis* | Long filaments, branching mycelium | Typical sulfur granules, clubs calcified | Short (rarely long) branching rods | Round streptococcal-like, smooth glistening colony, no mycelium or small compact mycelium | Colonies of a wide range of morphology (see Figs. 8 and 9); white to yellow; generally adherent to agar; roughly circular with smooth, granular, raspberry or molar tooth morphology |
| *A. suis* | Long filaments, branching mycelium | Typical sulfur granules, clubs | Short branching rods | Like *A. bovis* | As above |
| *A. israelii* | Long filaments, branching mycelium | Typical sulfur granules, clubs calcified | Long branching rods | Large mycelial colonies, spider colonies | As above |
| *A. naeslundii* | Long filaments, branching mycelium | Granules, no clubs reported | Short to long branching rods | Mycelial colonies with dense centers | As above |
| *A. viscosus* | Filamentous coccoidal | Granules, no clubs reported | Short branching rods | Like *A. bovis* | As above |
| *Arachnia propionica* | Long filaments, branching mycelium, short rods, coccoidal cells | Typical sulfur granules, clubs | Short branching rods, coccoidal cells, long unbranched filaments | Mycelial colonies, spider colonies | As above |
| *Rothia dentocariosa* | None | None | Short to long branched filaments, coccoidal forms | Diffuse mycelial colonies, branching filaments | As above |
| *Bacterionemia matruchotii* | None | None | Long filaments with bacillary or club-shaped terminal ends, short rods | Small diffuse clumps of branching filamentous cells | As above |
| *Propionibacterium acnes* | None | None | Short pleomorphic rods, resembles *Actinomyces* | Smooth on entire edges, glistening colony, streptococcal or micrococcal-like | Small, circular, white to pink colonies |

[a]Thioglycolate medium, 10 ml per tube.
[b]Brain Heart Infusion agar, incubated anaerobically or under microaerophilic conditions.

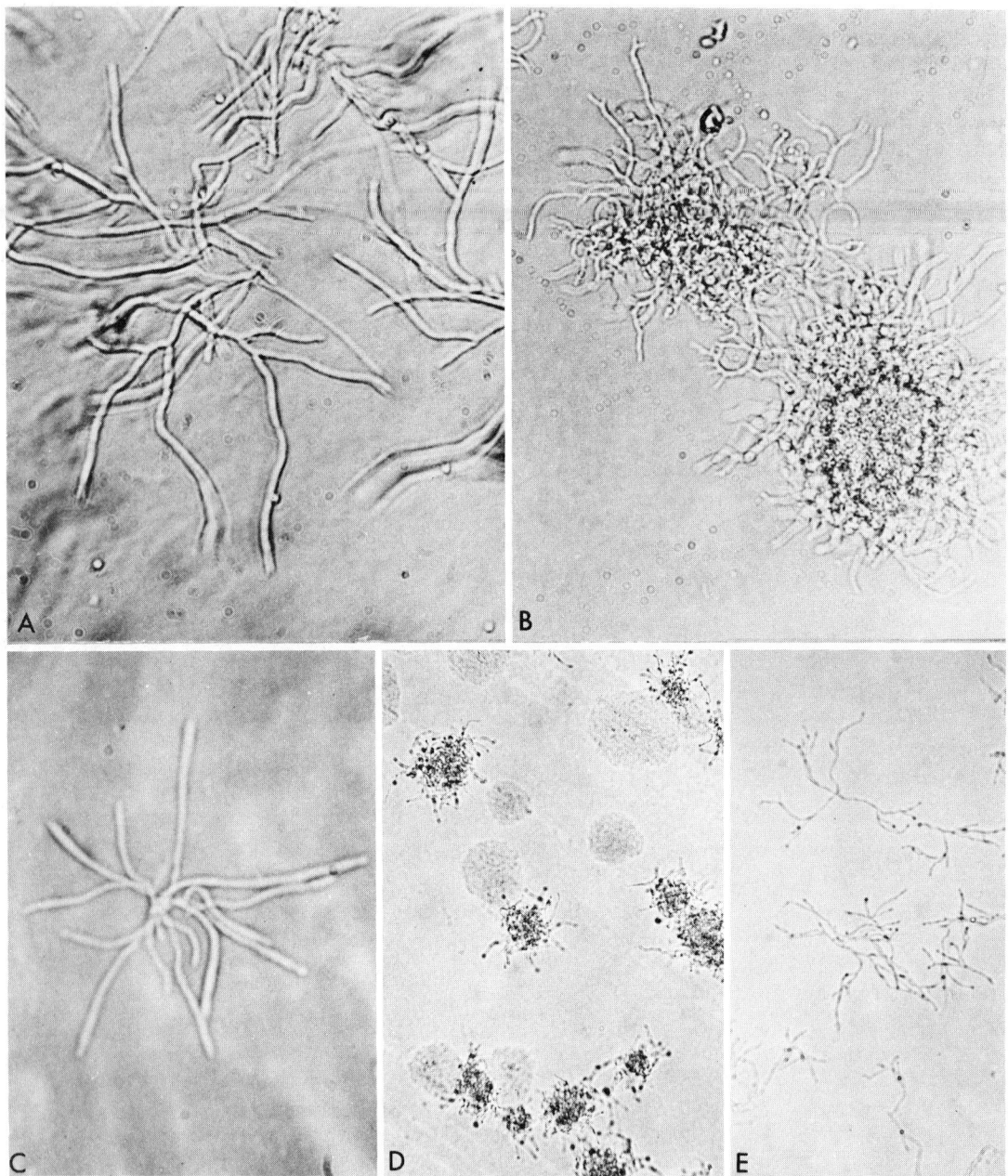

**FIGURE 7.** *Microcolonies of the microaerophilic actinomycetes.*

*A. Actinomyces israelii (Howell et al., 1959). The diffuse branching colony is characteristic of the species.*

*B. A. naeslundii (Howell et al., 1959). The tightly interwoven compact mycelium of the central portion of the colony is characteristic of this species.*

*C. A. viscosis (Howell, 1963).*

*D. A. bovis (Pine et al., 1960). Spider-like and smooth circular colonies isolated from the same case of bovine lumpy jaw. Transmitted light (290 ×).*

*E. Arachnia propionica (Buchanan and Pine, 1962). Web-like mycelial colonies (430 ×).*

Colonial morphology is best seen on agar plates at 24 to 48 hours by transmitted light. Young colonies have two basic forms (Fig. 7): (1) small mycelial colonies, and (2) smooth streptococcal-like colonies without true filaments. In general, microcolonies of *A. bovis* are small, circular, translucent or opaque, and have an entire edge with a smooth or granular surface. They cannot be distinguished from similar colonies of *Streptococcus pyogenes* (Fig. 7D). Although colonies of *A. odontolyticus* and *B. adolescentis* have characteristics very similar to those of *A. bovis* described above, some isolates of *A. bovis* are petite mycelial microcolonies (Fig. 7). No mycelial colonies have been reported for *A. odontolyticus* or *B. adolescentis*. Mycelial-like colonies may be formed by *Propionibacterium* species, although *P. acnes* forms only a smooth circular colony similar to that of *A. bovis*.

After incubation for three to seven days the microcolonies of the Actinomycetaceae develop into 1- to 3-mm diameter macrocolonies, which are often described as raspberry, molar tooth, or rough colonies. The forms vary considerably (Figs. 8 and 9) with no one morphologic pattern specific for a given species. Furthermore, the so-called smooth and matt strains of *Streptococcus pyogenes* may be confused with the macrocolonies formed by *Actinomyces* and *Arachnia* species (Fig. 8). In summary, various features of cellular or colonial morphology in tissues or in media that strongly suggest *Actinomyces* or *Arachnia* may instead indicate the genera *Streptococcus, Propionibacterium, Nocardia,* and *Streptomyces* (Table 2).

## *ANTIGENIC STRUCTURE*

*Actinomyces* antigens prepared from formalized whole cells, cell walls, soluble semipurified cell walls, or culture supernate precipitates have been used for taxonomy and serotyping (Bowden and Hardie, 1973). Also, formalized whole cells have been used to prepare hyperimmune fluorescein-tagged rabbit serum which very effectively demonstrates actinomyces in infected tissue, human saliva, and dental plaque. Because of cross-reactions with sera from cases of streptococcal infections, nocardiosis, and tuberculosis (Holm and Kwapinski, 1959; Georg et al., 1968), no satisfactory routine complement fixation, immunodiffusion, or hemagglutination test has been developed.

Species differentiation has relied principally on immunodiffusion, whole cell or cell wall agglutination, and fluorescent antibody staining of whole cells. Agar gel immunodiffusion has used soluble antigens either precipitated from the cul-

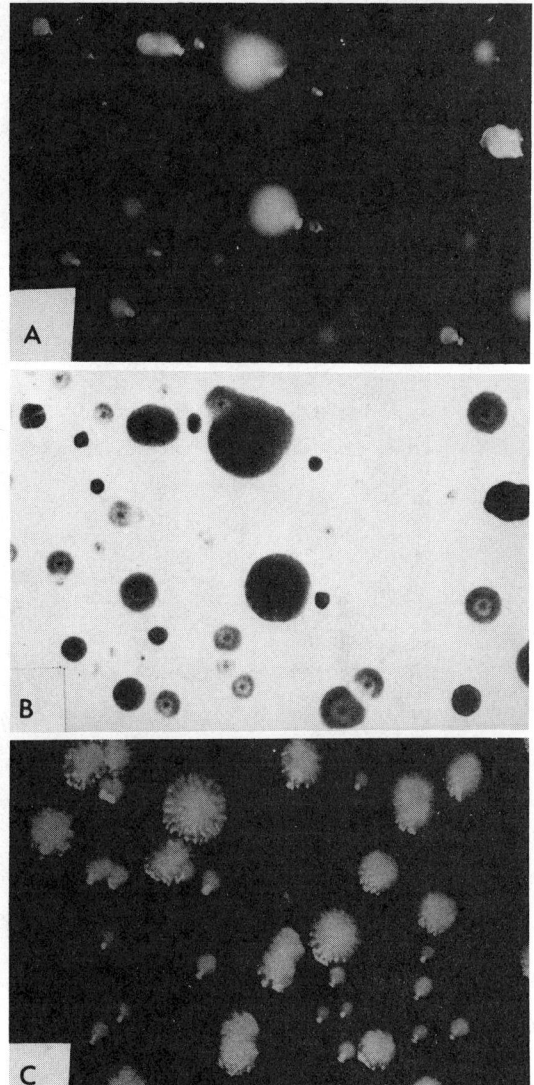

**FIGURE 8.**   *Macrocolony morphology of Actinomyces bovis (Pine et al., 1960).*

*A. Rough and smooth colonies; reflected light (13 ×).*

*B. Same field as A, viewed by transmitted light. Note "doughnut" aspect of smooth colonies of A. bovis.*

*C. A. bovis, strain P3, smooth and rough colonies; reflected light, (13 ×). Both colony forms are indistinguishable from the smooth and matt colonies of some strains of Streptococcus pyogenes.*

ture supernate by acetone or extracted from whole cells with formamide and trichloracetic acid. The protein associated with carbohydrate seems to be the serologically reactive component. Identification of species by agar gel immunodiffusion has not been entirely successful. Brock and Georg (1969) clearly separated *A. naeslundii* and *A. israelii* by agar gel diffusion, and Cummins (1968) distinguished the two serotypes of *A. israelii* using trichloracetic acid-acetone precipitated antigens from strains of *A. israelii*. These sero-

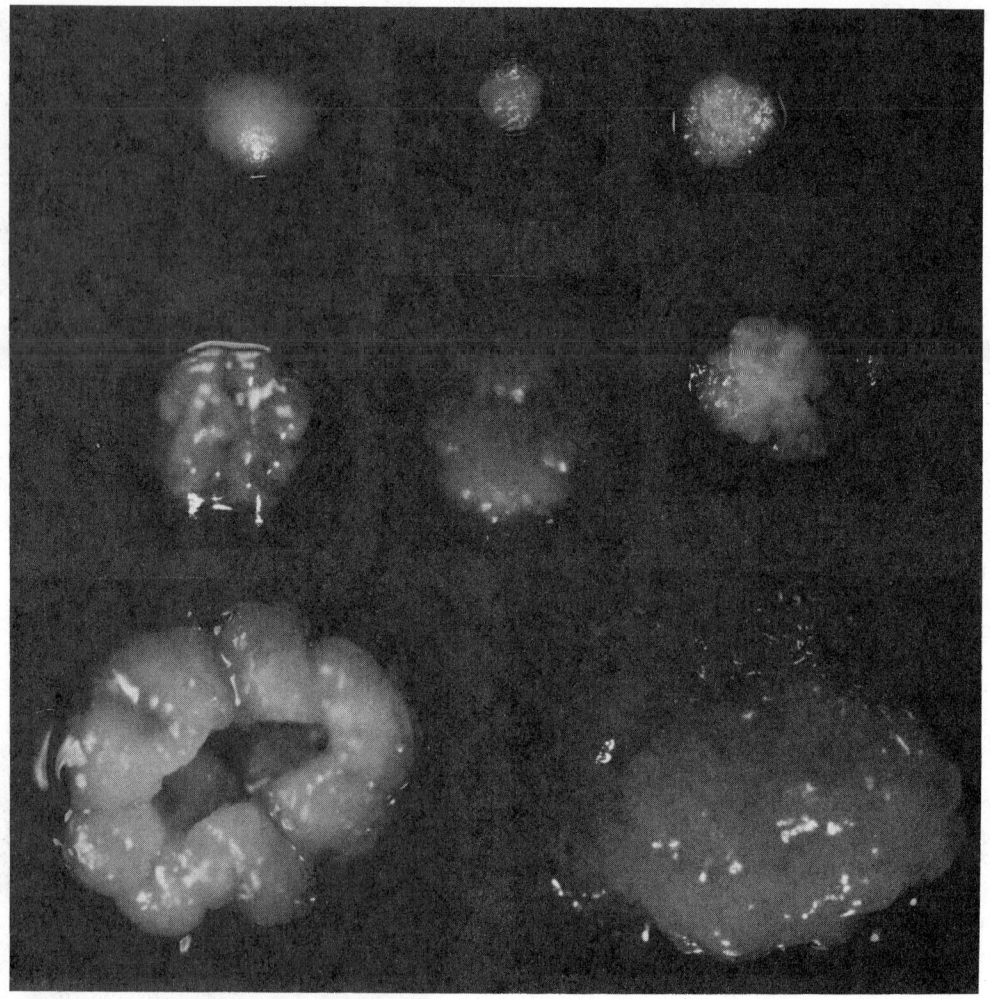

**FIGURE 9.** *Macrocolonies of Actinomyces israelii; reflected light (23 ×) (Howell et al., 1959). The diverse colony forms shown may be formed by strains of all the species of Actinomyces and Arachnia.*

types were confirmed with fluorescent antibody (Brock and Georg, 1969).

Chemical differentiation of purified cell walls (Cummins and Harris, 1958) combined with the use of whole cells for cell wall agglutination studies (Cummins, 1962) provided a definitive basis for species identification. What was once an extremely complex heterogeneous mixture of overlapping morphologic and physiologic groups was now organized primarily on the basis of a definitive chemical cell wall composition (Table 3). After delineation of these groups, their serologic relationships became clear.

The fluorescent antibody technique, which became the most fruitful and least complex serologic procedure for identifying species and serotypes, was first used by Slack and his colleagues (1966) to identify *A. israelii* from two patients with actinomycosis. The technique, tested with pure cultures and specific sera, has led to serologic separations and identification of species that correlate with species designations determined by other means. Nevertheless, cross-reactions occur, and sera specific for the species *A. israelii, A. naeslundii,* and *A. viscosus* interact in a complex manner (Slack and Gerencser, 1975). All *Actinomyces* species and *Ar. propionica* have had two serotypes described; the exceptions are *A. naeslundii,* which has one, and *R. dentocariosa,* which has four or more.

## METABOLISM

All members of the family Actinomycetaceae are fermentative, and their substrates are largely converted to volatile and nonvolatile acids in anaerobic, microaerophilic, or strongly aerobic conditions. Alcohols are not formed. The fermentative actinomycetes do not contain a sequence of

TABLE 3. Cell-Wall Composition of the Pathogenic *Actinomyces* and Related Species[a]

| | AMINO ACIDS[b] | | | | | | | | | | | | | |
|---|---|---|---|---|---|---|---|---|---|---|---|---|---|---|
| | Aspartic Acid | Lysine | Ornithine | Glycine | LL Diaminopimelic Acid | DL Diaminopimelic Acid | GALACTOSE | GLUCOSE | MANNOSE | RHAMNOSE | DEOXYHEXOSE | DEOXYTALOSE | FUCOSE | ARABINOSE |
| **Actinomyces** | | | | | | | | | | | | | | |
| A. bovis ATCC13683 | + | + | − | − | − | − | − | + | + | + | + | + | + | − |
| A. bovis P2R | − | + | − | − | − | − | − | + | + | + | + | + | + | − |
| A. humiferus | + | + | + | − | − | − | − | + | − | + | − | − | − | − |
| A. odontolyticus | − | + | + | − | − | − | + | + | − | + | − | − | − | − |
| A. suis | − | + | + | − | − | − | − | − | − | + | − | − | − | − |
| A. israelii/1 | − | + | + | − | − | − | + | − | − | − | − | − | − | − |
| A. israelii/2 | − | + | + | − | − | − | + | − | − | − | − | − | − | − |
| A. naeslundii | − | + | + | − | − | − | − | + | + | + | + | + | − | − |
| A. viscosus/1 | − | + | + | − | − | − | + | + | − | + | + | + | − | − |
| A. viscosus/2 | − | + | + | − | − | − | + | + | − | + | + | + | − | − |
| Bifidobacterium adolescentis | + | + | + | − | − | − | + | + | − | − | − | − | − | − |
| Rothia dentocariosa | − | + | − | − | − | − | + | + | − | − | − | − | − | − |
| Bacterionemia matruchotii | − | − | − | + | − | + | + | + | − | − | − | − | − | + |
| **Arachnia** | | | | | | | | | | | | | | |
| A. propionica/1 | − | − | − | + | + | − | − | + | − | − | − | − | − | − |
| A. propionica/2 | − | − | − | + | + | − | + | + | − | − | − | − | − | − |
| **Propionibacterium** | | | | | | | | | | | | | | |
| P. acnes/1 | − | − | − | + | + | − | + | + | ± | − | − | − | − | − |
| P. acnes/2 | − | − | − | + | + | − | − | + | ± | − | − | − | − | − |

[a]Based on data and references in Cummins (1968), Johnson and Cummins (1972), Schleifer and Kandler (1972), Pine (1973), and Cummins (personal communication).
[b]All strains have alanine and glutamic acid.

cytochromes to oxidize the substrate for utilizable energy. A carbohydrate energy source such as sugar, alcohol, pentose, hexose, di- or trisaccharide, or starch is required for growth, but amino acids or proteins are not used. In contrast with this family, which accumulates acids in the medium, strictly aerobic genera such as *Mycobacterium, Nocardia, Actinomadura,* and *Streptomyces* oxidize their substrates mainly to carbon dioxide and water; in addition, these genera may also use amino acids and proteins for growth once the carbohydrate is completely metabolized.

Within the family Actinomycetaceae, the fermentations of glucose are best described as homolactic, heterolactic, or propionic acid (Pine, 1970). All species of *Actinomyces* are homolactic acid organisms because, given the correct conditions of growth and medium, they will ferment glucose primarily to lactic acid. Therefore, they have fructose diphosphate aldolase and use primarily the Embden-Meyerhof glycolytic scheme for catabolizing sugar. However, under anaerobic conditions when carbon dioxide is present, all species form acetic, lactic, and succinic acids, and traces of formic acid (Table 4). Some species use large amounts of carbon dioxide to synthesize succinic acid and form aspartic acid internally. Since these carbon dioxide-fixing strains lack a permease for the uptake of aspartic acid (Buchanan

and Pine, 1965), carbon dioxide is a factor required for growth. But once growth is initiated, some members of the genus can grow aerobically, converting glucose primarily to acetic acid and carbon dioxide.

The genus *Bifidobacterium*, however, does not have fructose diphosphate aldolase or glucose-6-phosphate dehydrogenase, and glucose is degraded by the fructose-6-phosphate shunt to acetic and lactic acids (DeVries and Stouthamer, 1967). Since two moles of lactic acid cannot be formed from one mole of glucose, this fermentation is heterolactic. Acetate and lactate are formed in molar ratios approximating 3:2; only traces of other products such as formic or succinic acid are formed.

Although they contain fructose diphosphate aldolase, the species of the third group (*Ar. propionica* and *B. matruchotii*) ferment glucose to form propionic and acetic acids as the major products. Small amounts of lactic and succinic acids with considerable amounts of carbon dioxide are also formed in the single anaerobic fermentation within the family in which carbon dioxide is a major product. Although the fermentations resemble those of the propionobacteria, they can differ significantly in the relative quantities of the products formed.

There is an excellent correlation of the cell wall

**TABLE 4.** Fermentative Characteristics Differentiating Genera of *Actinomycetaceae* and *Propionibacterium*

| GENUS | OXYGEN RELATIONSHIP | CELL-WALL MUCOPEPTIDE[a] | FERMEN-TATION | MAJOR ACIDS FORMED FROM GLUCOSE | |
|---|---|---|---|---|---|
| | | | | Anaerobic | Aerobic |
| *Actinomyces* | Anaerobe, facultative anaerobe | Lysine, ornithine, glutamic acid (1:1:2) | Homolactic | (Formic), acetic, lactic, succinic | $CO_2$, acetic |
| *Rothia* | Aerobe | Lysine | Homolactic | Lactic | Acetic, lactic |
| *Bifidobacterium* | Anaerobe | Alanine, lysine (ornithine): glutamic acid (1:1) | Heterolactic | Acetic, lactic | No growth |
| *Arachnia* | Facultative anaerobe | Glycine, alanine, glutamic acid (2:1:1) plus LL diaminopimelic acid | Propionic | $CO_2$, acetic, propionic, lactic, succinic | $CO_2$, acetic |
| *Propionibacterium* | Anaerobe | Glycine, alanine, glutamic acid (1:2:1) plus LL diaminopimelic acid | Propionic | $CO_2$ acetic, propionic (lactic, succinic) | $CO_2$, acetic |
| *Bacterionema* | Aerobic, facultative anaerobe | Glycine, DL diaminopimelic acid | Propionic | $CO_2$, propionic, lactic | $CO_2$, acetic, propionic |

[a]Data based on Schleifer and Kandler (1972).

mucopeptide components to the fermentation. All *Actinomyces* species except *A. bovis* have lysine, ornithine, and glutamic acid in their cell walls in a ratio of 1:1:2, and all ferment glucose homolactically. However, in *B. adolescentis (A. eriksonii)* ornithine or lysine occurs in a ratio of 1:1 with glutamic acid, replacing one or the other within the peptide subunit (Schleifer and Kandler, 1972). The propionic acid-forming species, however, have diaminopimelic acid instead of lysine or ornithine as the dibasic component of the cell wall. These relationships of fermentation to cell wall composition are summarized in Table 4.

The general identifying physiologic characteristics of the various species of Actinomycetaceae are listed in Table 5. Basically, all organisms are anaerobic or facultatively anaerobic; the latter can grow in oxygen when growth is initiated with larger inocula. Carbon dioxide stimulates growth and increases the fermentation products of glucose from only lactic acid to volatile and nonvolatile acids that are more characteristic of the species. Under strongly aerobic conditions, certain species ferment glucose to acetate and carbon dioxide; the cell yields under these conditions are doubled, indicating that the use of oxygen is energy yielding and linked to growth. *Ar. propionica, B. matruchotii, A. viscosus,* and *R. dentocariosa* are aerobic or facultatively aerobic and may not require carbon dioxide to initiate growth. In general, the presence of carbon dioxide improves the primary isolation from small numbers of cells whether the incubation is anaerobic or aerobic.

Although numerous primary colonies of species defined as aerobic may grow on isolation plates, incubated anaerobically, they cannot be transferred under anaerobic conditions. Conversely, particularly when the inoculum is heavy, anaerobic species may sometimes grow under aerobic conditions. On occasion microcolonies of even the aerobic *Nocardia asteroides* may grow on primary isolation plates incubated anaerobically. Thus these results suggest that for primary isolation of an actinomycete, both aerobic and anaerobic isolations should be made in the presence of carbon dioxide.

The definition of a species as aerobic is strongly supported by the presence of catalase or of cytochromes, as shown by the benzidine test. *R. dentocariosa* is aerobic and catalase-positive. *P. acnes* and *A. viscosus* are anaerobic and facultatively anaerobic respectively, but both have catalase. This distinguishes them from all other facultative or anaerobic species within the family Actinomycetaceae.

The growth requirements of this family of organisms are complex and resemble those of lactobacilli and streptococci. A few strains of *A. israelii* require cysteine, glutamic acid, lysine, leucine, isoleucine, and tryptophan (Keir and Porteus, 1962).

Of the physiologic characteristics in Table 5, acid is formed by certain strains, listed as acid-negative, only with prolonged incubation of 14 days or more. The results given in Table 5 should be apparent within seven or eight days. Thus, hydrolysis of starch by *A. bovis* and *B. adolescen-*

**TABLE 5.** Physiologic Characteristics of Species of *Actinomycetaceae* and *Propionibacterium acnes* [a]

| ORGANISM | CATALASE | NITRATE REDUCTION | NITRATE REDUCED | CASEIN AND GELATIN HYDROLYSIS | STARCH HYDROLYSIS | GLUCOSE | STARCH | MANNITOL | XYLOSE | ARABINOSE | GLYCEROL | OXYGEN REQUIREMENTS | CO₂ REQUIRED | %G+C COMPOSITION OF DNA |
|---|---|---|---|---|---|---|---|---|---|---|---|---|---|---|
| *Actinomyces* | | | | | | | | | | | | | | |
| A. humiferus | − | − | − | + | + | A | A | A | A | A | A(−) | Ae | − | 73 − |
| A. bovis | − | − | nr | − | + | A | A | − | −(A) | − | − | An | + | 57–63 |
| A. suis | − | nr | nr | − | + | A | A | A(−) | nr | A(−) | −(A) | An | + | nr |
| A. odontolyticus | − | +(−) | − | − | − | A | − | − | A | −(A) | (A) | FacAn | + | 62 |
| A. israelii | − | +(−) | − | − | − | A | − | A | A | A− | − | An | + | 57–60 |
| A. naeslundii | − | + | − | − | − | A | − | − | − | − | A,− | FacAn | + | 63–64 |
| A. viscosus | + | + | +− | − | + | A | A− | − | − | A− | A,− | FacAn | + | 63–70 |
| Rothia dentocariosa | + | + | + | − | − | A | − | − | − | − | A,− | FacAn | + | 63–70 |
| Bifidobacterium adolescentis | − | − | − | − | + | A | A | A | A | A | − | An | − | 62 |
| Arachnia propionica | − | + | nr | − | − | A | − | A | − | − | −(A) | FacAn | − | 63–65 |
| Bacterionemia matruchotii | +− | + | + | − | +(−) | A | nr | − | A(−) | − | − | An | − | 50–56 |
| Propionibacterium acnes | + | + | nr | + | − | A | − | A(−) | − | − | A(−) | An | − | 57–60 |

[a] +, positive reaction; −, negative reaction; +−, positive and negative reactions among strains; A, acid formed but no gas; nr, not reported; Ae, aerobic; An, anaerobic; FacAn, facultative anaerobe; ( ), occurs in a few strains.

Data compiled from Pine (1973), and Slack and Gerencser (1975).

*tis* is rapidly apparent. Although a few strains of *Ar. propionica* may ferment glycerol or lactic acid after prolonged incubation, they do so less readily than *P. acnes* or other propionibacteria. Gelatin liquefaction or casein hydrolysis differentiates *P. acnes* and *A. humiferus* from all other species. Catalase production may require a short period of aerobic induction. A major source of confusion in identification of pathogenic species in actinomycosis is *P. acnes,* because it is often present as a contaminant or commensal. However, *P. acnes* can be differentiated from the other species by the catalase test and gelatin liquefaction.

## PATHOGENIC PROPERTIES

*A. humiferus,* which was isolated from the soil, is the only *Actinomyces* species that is not resident in the animal body. *A. bovis* has been isolated only from infected cows and *A. suis* has been described only in pigs, primarily as a cause of mammary actinomycosis. In the cases of bovine and swine actinomycosis, it would appear that both species inhabit the oral cavity of their host as do the other species in this genus. *A. israelii* is reported to be the major cause of actinomycosis in man; although actinomycosis has been reported in dogs, deer, and other animals, species identification has been minimal. *A. israelii* causes lacrimal canaliculitis, which is not a true actinomycosis because the deeper tissues are not penetrated. In this infection, large mycelial masses of the organism block the lacrimal canal and may erode the surface membrane without invading the underlying tissues. *Ar. propionica* also shares these characteristics with *A. israelii.* Typical actinomycosis, i.e., progressive chronic inflammatory disease, suppuration, and sinus and sulfur granule formation, is rarely caused by the other species of the family (Table 6).

Transmission of these diseases from man to man or animal to animal is unknown except in cases of human or animal bite; this mode of transmission is suspected in cases of swine actinomycosis. Bovine actinomycosis is attributed to injury of the tissues surrounding the mandible during the chewing of roughage by the cow. In lacrimal canaliculitis the assumption is that the organisms spread from the mouth or nasopharynx to the lacrimal duct by a stifled sneeze or by transfer of saliva to the eye from which it drains into the lacrimal canal. There is no evidence that *Actinomyces* normally inhabits the lacrimal canal. All other cases of actinomycosis are attributed to the direct introduction of the organism from its normal habitat in the mouth into the deeper tissues or bloodstream as a result of some physical injury. Thus, tooth extraction or dental surgery may be followed by actinomycosis of the jaw. Appendectomy, cholecystectomy, or other operations were the major factors preceding actinomycosis in most patients reported by Brown (1973). Disseminated infections are best explained by spread of the organism from the mouth or bowel into the bloodstream (Bowden and Hardie, 1973).

Of the species examined for pathogenicity

**TABLE 6.** Pathogenicity of Microaerophilic Actinomycetes in Man and Experimental Animals

| | NATURAL INFECTION | EXPERIMENTAL INFECTION | | |
|---|---|---|---|---|
| ORGANISM | Number of Cases and Characteristics in Man | Animal | Lesions | Abscesses Formed with Mycelium, Sulfur Granules[h] |
| *Actinomyces* | | | | |
| *A. bovis* | None | Hamster, mouse | Progressive | 6/10 |
| *A. israelii* | Numerous cases[a] (true actinomycosis) | Hamster, mouse | Progressive | 52/66 341/397 |
| *A. naeslundii* | Three cases[b] (atypical actinomycosis) | Mouse | Progressive | 111/129 |
| *A. odontolyticus* | One case[a] (atypical actinomycosis) | Mouse | Regressive | 6/68 |
| *A. viscosus* | One case[d] (atypical) | Mouse | Progressive | 23/24 |
| *Arachnia propionica* | Numerous cases[e] (true actinomycosis) | Mouse | Progressive | 28/28 |
| *Bifidobacterium adolescentis* | Several cases[f] (abscess formation) | Mouse | Regressive | 34/49 |
| *Rothia dentocariosa* | One case[g] | Mouse | Regressive | 0/32 |
| *Bacterionema matruchoti* | None | Hamster | Regressive | 0/6 |

[a]Brown, J. R. (1973); Bowden and Hardie (1973).
[b]Coleman et al. (1969).
[c]Morris and Kilbourn (1974).
[d]Adeniyi-Jones et al. (1973).
[e]Slack and Gerencser (1975).
[f]Georg et al. (1965).
[g]Sharfen, J.: Zentralbl Bakterial [Orig A] 233:80, 1975.
[h]Data taken in part from Slack and Gerencser (1975); Animals positive/animals inoculated.

Data partially compiled from Table 11–3 in Slack and Gerencser (1975).

(Table 6), *A. israelii, A. naeslundii, A. viscosus,* and *Ar. propionica* were equally effective in causing actinomycotic lesions in mice. These four species usually produced progressive lesions with mycelial filaments, mycelial clumps, and occasionally sulfur granules, unlike the abscesses formed by other species. From the table and the results of population studies in dental calculus it is evident that *A. israelii* and *Ar. propionica* are the most pathogenic species for man regardless of their relative population in the oral cavity or on calculus. In mice and other animals all four species appear to be equally infectious and pathogenic.

The mechanisms by which species of *Actinomyces* establish a progressive infection in humans are unknown. In humans the disease is degenerative and may be accompanied by destruction of tissue and dissolution of bone. In cattle, lumpy jaw may destroy bone, although it most often stimulates bone growth in the upper or lower jaw. No toxin has been implicated in the pathogenesis of actinomycosis, nor is there any evidence that sulfur granules protect the bacterium from the defensive mechanisms of the host. There are sufficient reports of successful vaccine therapy to support the contention that high levels of antibody may limit the progress of the disease (Buchs, 1963). It is often stated but not proved that other organisms contribute to the pathogenesis of *A. israelii* infections.

The oral actinomycetes are strongly associated with the formation of cavities and periodontal disease. *A. naeslundii* and *A. viscosus* are implicated in gingivitis in man and cause extensive periodontal disease in hamsters and germ-free rats (Jordan et al., 1972).

From studies with *Streptococcus mutans*, it is believed that dental plaque forms as a result of bacterial adherence to the tooth surface, where the bacteria colonize the salivary glycoproteins coating the enamel. The bacterium has both a soluble and a cell-associated glycosyltransferase that converts sucrose to insoluble glucans and oligosaccharides of low molecular weight. The insoluble polysaccharide precipitates on the tooth surface and, because of the affinity of the cell-bound enzyme with its substrate, the streptoccocus adheres to the polysaccharide. Other bacteria also adhere to the insoluble polysaccharides, which may be used for further bacterial growth and colonization. The final result is the formation of plaque.

Within the plaque the fermenting bacteria form their characteristic volatile and nonvolatile acids that cause localized areas of low pH and subsequent dissolution of enamel; this latter process initiates the formation of dental caries. When the plaque becomes calcified by mechanisms not fully understood, it is converted to calculus, and both are colonized by all the *Actinomyces* species, which become the predominant populations. At this point, intimate contact or abrasion of the periodontal tissue by the calculus exposes the tissue to both the organism and its products, without being invaded by them.

Baker et al. (1976) summarized the immunologic events leading to the pathogenesis of gingivitis or periodontosis of 11 common oral bacteria. They strongly implicated *A. israelii, A., naeslundii, A. viscosus, Ar. propionica, P. acnes,* and a gram-negative rod as the primary causes of lymphocyte transformation. The immunologic responses to the organisms or their products result in the production of sensitized lymphocytes that release cell products. These products enhance antibody production, attract phagocytic cells, and initiate processes that resorb bone and damaged tissue. Ivanyi and Lehner (1970) showed a direct correlation between the severity of periodontal disease and the degree of blastogenesis of the host's lymphocytes when the host is exposed to oral bacteria. Baker et al. (1976) showed that the lymphocytic transformations caused by the above species were the result of antigenic sensitivity and not of the bacterial walls acting as mitogens. Thus, in general, leukocyte transformation induced by *Actinomyces* requires the sensitized leukocyte of the diseased host or immune serum. Leukocytes of patients with periodontal disease respond to sonicated dental plaque, whole *Actinomyces* cells and cell walls, and soluble cytoplasmic components. These components contain protein and neutral sugars and act as specific antigens for the immune cellular response (Reed et al., 1976). These data strongly implicate the four species above as major causes of periodontal disease by mechanisms linked with bacterial hypersensitivity. This mechanism may also be involved in pathogenesis of actinomycosis when the living actinomycete is introduced into the tissues.

## IMMUNITY

In the early 1920s, opsonins and agglutinins were observed in actinomycosis; more recently agar gel precipitins, hemagglutinins, and complement-fixing antibodies have been described. In a few cases, the serum precipitin response corresponded with the course of the disease in patients with actinomycosis. Thus recovery after treatment was accompanied by a decline in precipitins.

There is also a suggestion that vaccine therapy can control the disease when used alone or in combination with surgical procedures or antibiotic therapy. Colebrook (1921) found that vaccine therapy was particularly successful in treating cervico-facial actinomycosis. There are no reports of immunity to reinfection.

## DRUG SUSCEPTIBILITY

The susceptibility of pathogenic *Actinomyces* and *Arachnia* species to drugs is shown in Table 7. The correlation of such results with treatment of actinomycosis is summarized by Lerner (1974). The effectivenss of penicillin is well-established in human actinomycosis (Brown, 1973; Weese and Smith, 1975). The antifungal agents amphotericin B, nystatin, and griseofulvin are not effective.

Clinical failures with penicillin and other drugs active in vitro against *A. israelii* are attributed to secondary infections with Gram-negative organisms. Weese and Smith (1975) reported that 65 per cent of 57 cases over a 36-year period had *Actinomyces* in association with other bacteria, the majority of which were Gram-positive. There have been no extensive reports of antibiotic resistance of *Actinomyces* developing during therapy. Garrod (1952) found eightfold and twentyfold increases respectively in the resistance of two strains during treatment.

## LABORATORY DIAGNOSIS

### Media

For primary isolation of *Actinomyces* and related organisms, Brain Heart infusion agar plates both without blood and with 5 per cent whole defibrinated animal blood should be used. Rabbit, sheep, or horse blood is recommended; human blood is not. However, *Actinomyces* broth (BBL Division of BioQuest, Becton, Dickinson and Company) with 1.5 per cent agar can be used for isolation plates or with 0.7 per cent agar for dilution tubes and for maintenance. The recom-

**TABLE 7.  In Vitro Sensitivity of Pathogenic Species in the Family Actinomycetaceae**

| | A. ISRAELII | A. NAESLUNDII | A. ODONTO-LYTICUS | A. VISCOSUS | A. BOVIS | A. ERIKSONII [a] | ARACHNIA PROPIONICA |
|---|---|---|---|---|---|---|---|
| No strains tested | 32 | 5 | 5 | 15 | 4 | 6 | 7 |
| | | | μg/ml for total inhibition of colony growth | | | | |
| Penicillin G | 0.5 | 1.0 | 0.15 | 0.5 | 1.0 | 0.5 | 0.5 |
| Ampicillin | 2.0 | 2.0 | 2.0 | 1.0 | 2.0 | 2.0 | 1.0 |
| Cephaloridine | 0.5 | 0.5 | 0.5 | 1.0 | 2.0 | 0.5 | 1.0 |
| Cephalothin | 2.0 | 2.0 | 0.25 | 0.5 | 1.0 | 2.0 | 1.0 |
| Cephalexin | 8.0 | 16.0 | 4.0 | 8.0 | 8.0 | 16.0 | 4.0 |
| Minocycline | 1.0 | 1.0 | 0.5 | 1.0 | 0.5 | 0.5 | 0.5 |
| Doxycycline | 2.0 | 4.0 | 0.5 | 2.0 | 1.0 | 4.0 | 4.0 |
| Tetracycline | 2.0 | 8.0 | 8.0 | 2.0 | 2.0 | 4.0 | 2.0 |
| Clindamycin | 0.5 | 8.0 | 0.5 | 2.0 | 0.5 | 0.25 | 4.0 |
| Lincomycin | 1.0 | 4.0 | 0.5 | 2.0 | 2.0 | 0.5 | 2.0 |
| Oxacillin | 8.0 | 4.0 | 4.0 | 4.0 | 16.0 | 8.0 | 8.0 |
| Dicloxacillin | 3.2 | 16.0 | 8.0 | 16.0 | 32.0 | 16.0 | 16.0 |
| Erythromycin | 0.25 | 0.12 | 0.06 | 0.12 | 0.06 | 0.06 | 0.12 |
| Chloramphenicol | 8.0 | 8.0 | 4.0 | 8.0 | 32.0 | 4.0 | 8.0 |
| Vancomycin | 20.0 | 10.0 | 10.0 | 20.0 | 10.0 | 20.0 | 10.0 |
| Rifampin | >0.5 | >0.5 | 0.03 | >0.5 | 0.6 | >0.5 | >0.5 |
| Fusidic acid | 20.0 | >20.0 | 5.0 | >20.0 | >20.0 | >20.0 | >20.0 |
| Novobiocin | 8.0 | >25.0 | 16.0 | >25.0 | 16.0 | >25.0 | 16.0 |

[a]*A. eriksonii = Bifidobacterium adolescentis.*

Data from Lerner (1974).

mended formula for the *Actinomyces* broth is: potassium dihydrogen phosphate, 15.0 g/L; ammonium sulfate, 1.0 g/L; magnesium sulfate, 0.2 g/L: calcium chloride (anhydrous), 0.01 g/L; heart infusion broth, 25.0 g/L; dextrose, 5.0 g/L; cysteine hydrochloride, 1.0 g/L; casitone, 4.0 g/L; yeast extract, 5.0 g/L; insoluble potato starch (preferred) or soluble starch, 1.0 g/L; final pH adjusted to 6.5 to 6.8 with potassium hydroxide.

Fluid thioglycolate broth may also be used for dilution tubes. However different commercial products vary in sugar concentrations and in the presence or absence of cystine or phosphate as buffer, and also in their basic complex protein extracts. Media with cystine and phosphate are preferred. For best results the commercial fluid thiglycolate medium should be fortified with 0.2 per cent sterile rabbit serum just before use.

Although the Brain Heart infusion media are excellent for isolation, they are not satisfactory for maintenance. For maintenance, deep cultures are made in *Actinomyces* broth with 0.7 per cent agar. Tubes of the medium are sealed with the standard pyrogallol-sodium carbonate seal described below. For the maintenance of the aerobic species *R. dentocariosa,* 1.5 per cent agar slants of Brain Heart Infusion agar or Trypticase Soy Agar (BBL, BioQuest) are used.

The medium used for fermentation tests is Thiglycolate Fermentation Medium without added dextrose (BBL, BioQuest) or indicator to

which 2.0 g of yeast extract (glucose free) and 2.0 ml of 1.0 per cent Brom cresol purple have been added (Slack and Gerencser, 1975). This medium is used for all species except *R. dentocariosa,* for which meat-extract peptone base is used. The formula for this medium is: meat extract, 3.0 g/L; bactopeptone, 10.0 g/L; sodium chloride, 5.0 g/L; Andrade's indicator, 10 ml/L, pH adjusted to 7.4.

All media may be prepared and stored; before use, however, they should be fresly melted or heated to eliminate absorbed oxygen. For isolation or stock cultures, the *Actinomyces* maintenance medium with 0.7 per cent agar can be tubed in 10 ml quantities and stored in anaerobic containers or with pyrogallol-sodium carbonate seals at 5°C for one year.

**Steps in Laboratory Diagnosis**

*1.  Examination of Clinical Materials.* All materials should be examined under wet mounts in dilute KOH, and by Gram and acid-fast stains of thinly prepared smears. Acid-fast cells should be regarded as potential *Nocardia* or *Mycobacteria.*

Pus is examined for mycelium or sulfur granules by adding a few drops of it to 5 ml of sterile distilled water and shaking the mixture well to make a fine suspension and to lyse tissue cells. The sediment is examined in KOH mounts and by Gram stains. Granules are washed several times by passage through 4 or 5 ml of sterile distilled water and then crushed in 0.5 ml of liquid. This suspension is used to streak plates or make dilution tubes. Sulfur granules or mycelial colonies are characteristic of *Actinomyces* and *Arachnia*.

**2. Preparation and Examination of Primary Isolation Cultures** Two plates each of Brain Heart Infusion agar with and without blood should be made; a series of dilution tubes in the 0.7 per cent agar-*Actinomyces* medium or in thioglycolate broth are also made. One plate each, with and without blood, should be incubated anaerobically with carbon dioxide, and one set should be incubated aerobically with carbon dioxide. A candle jar or Gaspak (BBL, BioQuest) is adequate for the anaerobic carbon dioxide systems. However, anaerobic chambers that can be evacuated and flushed with the nitrogen-5 per cent carbon dioxide are preferred. A desiccator to which a few pea-sized granules of dry ice are added can be used for aerobic incubation with carbon dioxide. Dilution tubes made with *Actinomyces* medium are extremely effective for primary isolation, particularly if the tubes are sealed with pyrogallol-sodium carbonate. Once the tubes are inoculated, the top half of the cotton plug is cut off, and the plug is pushed into the tube, care being taken to keep the plug several inches above the agar. A second snug fitting stopper of absorbent cotton is inserted; five drops of a saturated pyrogallol solution and five drops of a 10 per cent sodium carbonate solution are added in that sequence, and the tube is rapidly sealed with a tight rubber stopper. Dilution tubes made in fluid thioglycolate medium may be used without the anaerobic seals. All cultures are incubated at 37° C.

All plates should be examined after 24 to 48 hours by transmitted or reflected light to observe the spider-like microcolonies of *A. israelii*, or the round entire microcolonies characteristic of *A. bovis, A. odontolyticus,* and *B. adolescentis*. Beta hemolysis or strong alpha hemolysis is not produced by the actinomycetes. After four to five days the macrocolonies are examined by Gram stain and for catalase.

To test for catalase one drop of a cell suspension is added to one drop of 1.5 per cent hydrogen peroxide on a microscope slide and immediately covered with a coverslip. If catalase is present, bubbles will form beneath the coverslip within 30 seconds and stream continuously to the edges. Blood agar media must not be transferred with the colony, since the red cells themselves contain catalase. Also, metallic ions such as iron can catalyze the breakdown of peroxide. In a positive test gas formation continues for at least 20 to 30 seconds after bubbling begins. A positive catalase test suggests *A. viscosus, R. dentocariosa,* or contaminating bacteria.

Primary cultures should be restreaked before a stock culture is made. Cultures that appear pink and are catalase-positive may contain *P. acnes*. After moderate growth in *Actinomyces* agar deeps, the cultures may be stored at 5° C for 6 to 12 months.

**3. Differential Physiologic Characteristics.** The identification of species rests on the characteristics summarized in Tables 3, 4, and 5. The physiologic and fermentation tests of Table 5 are the minimum required for generic if not species identification. Identification of species may also be made by the fluorescent antibody test (Slack and Gerencser, 1975). Volatile and nonvolatile acids are identified by chromatography; cell wall sugars and amino acids are identified by paper chromatography after enzymatic digestion or sodium hydroxide extraction of cell walls followed by acid hydrolysis (Cummins, 1962; Boone and Pine, 1968).

## *EPIDEMIOLOGY*

There have been no recorded epidemics of *Actinomyces* infections. In humans the disease occurs throughout the world and shows no propensity for any given racial group. One clinic reported an average incidence of from one to three cases per year over a 36-year period, with one three-year period averaging five cases per year (Weese and Smith, 1975). Another reported about five cases per year over a ten-year period (Buchs, 1963). Distribution does not seem to be age-related, although approximately 80 per cent of the patients were over 20 years old. In a study of 181 cases, Brown (1973) observed that two thirds of the patients were between 30 and 60 years old. A greater number of cases are reported in males, with only 20 to 40 per cent reported in females.

The incidence of human infections ranges from 35 to 55 per cent in the tissues of the head and neck, 14 to 33 per cent in the thorax, and 23 to 28 per cent in the pelvic and abdominal region, of which 10 per cent may occur in the pelvic organs alone (Brown, 1973). In cattle, where 0.03 to 0.5 per cent of the herds may have actinomycosis, the disease manifests itself primarily as lumpy jaw or as infections of the softer tissues of the head.

Because the organisms are commensals prevalent in the mouth of the adult, it is assumed that the young are colonized by direct oral contact or through some other physical vector. Once the organism is established in the host, an infection is most often associated with some physical trauma by which the organism gains entrance to the deeper tissues. Supporting the data on the effect of physical trauma are the reports of Henderson (1973), Schiffer et al. (1975), and Gupta et al. (1976), relating the presence of *Actinomyces* and pelvic actinomycosis to the use of intrauterine devices by women. These reports represent only a few of those published recently in America, England, and Canada on this subject. In recent observations, the description of abscesses with pus containing sulfur granules, the typical aspect of the sulfur granule stained with hematoxylin and eosin, and the typical gram-positive mycelium in sections stained by the Brown and Brenn stain all support the conclusion that *Actinomyces* is associated with infections that occur during the use of intrauterine devices. Even more significant, Spence et al. (1977) have observed organisms consistent with actinomycetes in 350 pancervicovaginal (Fast) smears of patients who used intrauterine devices. In 35 of these, *A. israelii* was identified by specific fluorescent antibody. Similar stains for *A. naeslundii* were negative. These reports of IUD-associated infections have been supported by isolations of *A israelii* from three cases by Luff and Gupta (1977) and by one fatality associated with *A. israelii* (Serotype 1) infection (Hager and Majmudar, 1979). The overall results strongly implicate *A. israelii* as a causal organism in infections resulting from the use of intrauterine devices and show that women who use IUDs or pessaries have an increased risk of infection by *A. israelii* (Christ and Haja, 1978).

## REFERENCES

Baker, J. J., Chan, S. P., Socransky, S. S., Oppenheim, J. J., and Mergenhagen, S. E.: Importance of *Actinomyces* and certain gram-negative anaerobic organisms in the transformation of lymphocytes from patients with periodontal disease. Infect Immun 13:1363, 1976.

Bollinger, O.: Ueber eine ne Pilzkrankheit beim Rinde. Zentralbl Med Weiss. 15:481, 1877.

Boone, C. J., and Pine, L.: Rapid method for characterization of actinomycetes by cell wall composition. Appl Microbiol 16:279, 1968.

Bostroem, E.: Untersuchungen über die Aktinomykose des Menschen. Beitr Pathol 9:1, 1891.

Bowden, G. H., and Hardie, J. M.: Commensal and pathogenic *Actinomyces* species in man. In Sykes, G., and Skinner, F. A. (eds.): Actinomycetales: Characteristics and Practical Importance. New York, Academic Press, 1973, p. 277.

Brock, D. W., and Georg, L. K.: Determination and analysis of *Actinomyces israelii* serotypes by fluorescent-antibody procedures. J Bacteriol 97:581, 1969.

Brown, J. R.: Human actinomycosis. A study of 181 subjects. Hum Pathol 4:319, 1973.

Buchanan, B. B., and Pine, L.: Relationship of carbon dioxide to aspartic acid and glutamic acid in *Actinomyces naeslundii*. J Bacteriol 89:729, 1965.

Buchanan, R. E., and Gibbons, N. E.: Bergey's Manual of Determinative Bacteriology. 8th ed. Baltimore, The Williams & Wilkins Company, 1974.

Buchs, H.: Zur klinik und therapei der cervicofaciaten aktinomykose. Dtsch. Zahnaerztl Z 18:1069, 1963.

Bujwid, O.: Ueber die Reinkulter des *Actinomyces*. Zentralbl Bakteriol [Orig. B] 6:630, 1889.

Cohn, F.: Untersuchungen über Bacterien. Beitr. Biol Pflanzen 1:141, 1875.

Colebrook, L.: A report on 25 cases of actinomycosis with special reference to vaccine therapy. Lancet 1:893, 1921.

Coleman, R. M., George, L. K., and Rozzell, A. R.: *Actinomyces naeslundii* as an agent of human actinomycosis. Appl Microbiol 18:420, 1969.

Christ, M. L., and Haja, J.: Cytologic changes associated with vaginal pessary use with special reference to the presence of *Actinomyces*. Acta Cytol 22:146, 1978.

Cummins, C. S.: Chemical composition and antigenic structure of cell walls of *Corynebacterium, Mycobacterium, Nocardia, Actinomyces* and *Arthrobacter*. J Gen Microbiol 28:35, 1962.

Cummins, C. S.: *Actinomyces israelii* type 2. In Prouser, H. (ed.): The Actinomycetales. Jena, Gustav Fischer Verlag, 1968.

Cummins, C. S., and Harris, H.: Studies on the cell wall composition and taxonomy of Actinomycetales and related groups. J. Gen. Microbiol 18:173, 1958.

DeVries, W., and Stouthamer, A. H.: Pathway of glucose fermentation in relation to the taxonomy of bifidobacteria. J Bacteriol 93:574, 1967.

Emmons, C. W.: *Actinomyces* and actinomycosis. Puerto Rico J Public Health Trop Med 11:63, 1935.

Erikson, D.: Pathogenic anaerobic organisms of the *Actinomyces* group. Med Res Council Spec Rep Ser 240:1, 1940.

Frazier, P. D., and Fowler, B. O.: X-ray diffraction and infrared study of the "sulphur granules" of *Actinomyces bovis*. J Gen Microbiol 46:445, 1967.

Garrod, L. P.: The sensitivity of *Actinomyces israelii* to antibiotics. Br Med J 1:1263, 1952.

Georg, L, K., Coleman, R. M., and Brown, J. M.: Evaluation of an agar gel precipitin test for the serodiagnosis of actinomycosis. J Immunol 100:1288, 1968.

Georg, L. K., Robertstad, G. W., Brinkman, S. A., and Hicklin, M. D.: A new pathogenic anaerobic *Actinomyces* species. J Infect Dis 115:88, 1965.

von Graefe, A.: Koncretionen in unteren Thränenröhrchen durch Pilzbildung. Arch Ophthalmol 1:284, 1854.

Gupta, P. K., Hollander, D. H., and Frost, J. K.: Actinomycetes in cervicovaginal smears: An association with IUD usage. Acta Cytol 20:295, 1976.

Hager, W. D., and Majmudar, B.: Pelvic actinomycosis in women using intrauterine devices. Am J Obstet Gynecol 156:60, 1979.

Hartz, C. O.: *Actinomyces bovis:* ein neuer Schimmel in dem Geweben des Rindes. Dtsche Z Tier-Med 5:125 (Suppl.) 1879.

Henderson, S. R.: Pelvic actinomycosis associated with an intrauterine device. Obstet Gynecol 41:726, 1973.

Holm, P., and Kwapinski, J. B.: Studies on the detection of *Actinomyces* antibodies in human sera by use of pure antigenic fractions of *Actinomyces israelii*. Acta Pathol Microbiol Scand [B] 45:107, 1959.

Howell, A., Jr., Murphy, W. C., Paul, F., and Stephan, R. M.: Oral strains of *Actinomyces*. J Bacteriol 78:82, 1959.

Israel, J.: Neue Beobachtungen auf dem Gebiete der Mykosen des Menschen. Arch Pathol Anat 74:15, 1878.

Ivanyi, L., and Lehner, T.: Stimulation of lymphocyte transformation by bacterial antigens in patients with periodontal disease. Arch Oral Biol 15:1089, 1970.

Jordan, H. V., Keyes, P. H., and Bellack, S.: Periodontal lesions in hamsters and gnotobiotic rats infected with *Actinomyces* of human origin. J Periodont Res 7, 21, 1972.

Keir, H. A., and Porteus, J. W.: The amino acid requirements of a single strain of *Actinomyces israelii* growing in a chemically defined medium. J Gen Microbiol 28:581, 1962.

Lerner, P. I.: Susceptibility of pathogenic actinomycetes to antimicrobial compounds. Antimicrob Agents Chemother 5:302, 1974.

Luff, R. D., and Gupta, P. K.: Actinomycetes-like organisms in wearers of intrauterine contraceptive devices. Am J Obstet Gynecol 129:477, 1977.

Morris, J. F., and Kilbourn, P.: Systemic actinomycosis caused by *Actinomyces odontolyticus*. Ann Int Med 81:700, 1974.

Naeslund, C.: Studies of *Actinomyces* from the oral cavity. Acta Pathol Microbiol Scand 2:110, 1925.

Pine, L.: Classification and phylogenetic relationship of microaerophilic actinomycetes. Int J System Bacteriol 20:445, 1970.

Pine, L.: Parasitic or fermentative actinomycetes. In Laskin, A. I., and Lechevalier, H. A. (eds.): Handbook of Microbiology. Cleveland, CRC Press, 1973, p. 212.

Pine, L., Howell, A., Jr., Watson, S. J.: Studies of the morphological, physiological and biochemical characters of *Actinomyces bovis*. J Gen Microbiol 23:403, 1960.

Pine, L., and Overman, J. R.: Determination of the structure and composition of the "sulphur granules" of *Actinomyces bovis*. J Gen Microbiol 32:209, 1963.

Pine, L., and Overman, J. R.: Differentiation of capsules and hyphae in clubs of bovine sulphur granules. Sabouraudia 5:141, 1966.

Ponfick, E.: Ueber Actinomykose. Berl Klin Wchnehr 17:660, 1880.

Reed, M. J., Potters, M. R., Mashimo, P. A., Genco, R. J., and Levine, M. J.: Blastogenic response of human lymphocytes to oral bacterial antigens: Characterization of bacterial sonicates. Infect Immun 14:1202, 1976.

Schiffer, M. A., Elguezabal, A., Sultana, M., and Allen, A. C.: Actinomycosis infections associated with intrauterine contraceptive devices. Obstet Gynecol 45:67, 1975.

Schleifer, K. H., and Kandler, O.: Peptidoglycan types of bacterial cell walls and their taxonomic implications. Bacteriol Rev 36:407, 1972.

Silberschmidt, W.: Über Actinomykose. Z Hyg 37:345, 1901.

Slack, J. M., and Gerencser, M. A.: *Actinomyces,* Filamentous Bacteria: Biology and Pathogenicity. Minneapolis, Burgess Publishing Company, 1975.

Slack, J. M., Moore, D. W., and Gerencser, M. A.: Use of the fluorescent antibody technique in the diagnosis of actinomycosis. W Va Med J 62:228, 1966.

Spence, M. R., Gupta, P. K., Frost, J. K., and King, T. M.: Cytological detection and clinical significance of *Actinomyces israelii* in women employing intrauterine contraceptive devices. Am J Obstet Gynecol 131(3):295, 1978.

Suter, V. L.: Evaluation of criteria used in the identification of *Actinomyces bovis* with particular reference to the catalase reaction. Mycopathologica 6:220, 1956.

Thompson, L.: Isolation and comparison of *Actinomyces* from human and bovine infections. Proc Staff Meet Mayo Clin 25:81, 1950.

Thompson, L., and Lovestedt, S. A.: An *Actinomyces*-like organism obtained from the human mouth. Proc Staff Meet Mayo Clin 26:169, 1951.

Weese, W. C., and Smith, I. M.: A study of 57 cases of actinomycosis over a 36-year period. Arch Intern Med 135:1562, 1975.

Wolff, M., and Israel, J.: Ueber Reincultur des *Actinomyces* und seine Uebertragbarkeit auf Theire. Virchow's Arch [Path Anat] 126:11, 1891.

Wright, J. J.: The biology of the microorganism of actinomycosis. J Med Res 13:349, 1905.

# THE CLOSTRIDIA   **45**

*Betty C. Hobbs, Ph.D., D.Sc., F.R.C.Path., Dip. Bact.*

## GENERAL CHARACTERISTICS

The *Clostridium* species are gram-positive, spore-forming bacilli, motile except for *C. perfringens* and obligate anaerobes. They vary in their requirements for reduced oxygen, and some species tolerate concentrations of oxygen not far below those found in the atmosphere.

The clostridia are biochemically active and may be saccharolytic, fermenting carbohydrate, such as *C. perfringens, C. septicum, C. oedematiens,* and *C. fallax,* and proteolytic, decomposing protein, such as *C. sporogenes, C. histolyticum,* and *C. botulinum.*

Most species are saprophytic, others exist as commensals in the human and animal intestine, and many are pathogenic. The pathogenic clostridia cause serious diseases such as tetanus *(C. tetani),* gas gangrene *(C. perfringens, C. oedematiens,* and *C. septicum),* and botulism *(C. botulinum).* *C. perfringens* also causes gastroenteritis, usually mild but sometimes fatal in elderly and debilitated persons, and also enteritis necroticans, which is a more serious disease and often fatal. In veterinary medicine clostridia are important intestinal pathogens. They cause enterotoxemia in sheep, calves, lambs, goats, and piglets. Dysentery in lambs *(C. perfringens* Type B) and piglets *(C. perfringens* Type C) may necessitate extensive vaccination programs. Toxemias in adult animals may follow a change of diet. High carbohydrate levels may encourage the growth of clostridia and toxin formation, as in the production of epsilon toxin by *C. perfringens* Type D in pulpy kidney disease. Similarly, it is suggested by Lawrence and Walker (1976) that in Papua New Guinea the sudden intake of pork during feasting encourages the growth of *C. perfringens* Type C and the production of beta toxin, which cannot be destroyed because of the low level of digestive proteases in the intestine; the staple diet is sweet potato that possesses a heat-stable trypsin inhibitor. The use of a *C. perfringens* Type C toxoid has given encouraging results in children (Leader, 1977).

The artificial feeding of 12 hospital-born neonates was followed by necrotizing enteritis of varying severity within ten days to six weeks. Evidence of the presence of *C. butyricum* was found in the blood of nine to ten babies examined; this organism was thought to be the invader responsible (Howard et al., 1977). Rifkin et al. (1977) described *C. sordellii* infection in adults with antibiotic-induced colitis. Thus it seems that clostridia can grow and produce toxin under con-

**TABLE 1.   Industrial Uses of the Clostridium Group**

| | |
|---|---|
| *C. pasteurianum* | Nitrogen fixation in the soil |
| *C. beijerinckii* | Anaerobic digestion |
| *C. cellobiofavum* | Cellulose degradation |
| *C. butyricum* | Butyric acid production in butter and cheese |
| *C. tyrobutyricum* | Butyric acid production in cheese |
| *C. butylicum* | Acetic and butyric acid production from glucose; also ethyl, butyl and propyl alcohols and acetone |
| *C. iodophilum* | Acetic and butyric acid production from glucose; also ethyl and butyl alcohols and acetone |
| *C. toanum* | Butyric acid; also ethyl, butyl and isopropyl alcohols and acetone |
| *C. acetobutylicum* | Acetic and butyric acids; also ethyl and butyl alcohols and acetone. Anaerobic digestion |
| *C. amylosaccharo-butylpropylicum* | Butyl and propyl alcohols from starch and sugar |

ditions favorable to them and in the absence of the usual flora or mechanisms that control them (Leader, 1977). It is suggested also that clostridia may be involved in the breakdown of bile salts to steroids during digestion and thus indirectly produce conditions that predispose toward cancer.

Aside from the medical and veterinary significance of the clostridia, many species are used commercially in the production of acids and alcohols in fermentative or digestive processes; some have been and could be used in the chemical industry when fossil fuels expire. Many species break down nitrogen and cellulose (denitrifying and degrading cellulose in the soil) and many fix nitrogen in the soil. They are prominent in decomposition processes such as silage maturation.

Table 1 lists the names of some clostridia and their uses.

In food technology, the presence of mesophilic clostridia in canned nonacid foods indicates that heating has been insufficient to destroy spores of *C. botulinum,* which are the greatest hazard in sterilized or pasteurized canned food. In chilled or dried foods, an unusually large number of viable clostridia might indicate a hazard from *C. perfringens* or *C. botulinum,* either in the food as preserved or in its future use. Spores of the more heat-resistant clostridia are also used to test the sterility of medical equipment.

*C. perfringens* is one of the more important members of the group, and its characteristics are described in detail.

# CLOSTRIDIUM PERFRINGENS

## *MORPHOLOGY*

The organism is a strongly gram-positive, nonmotile rod with blunt or square ends; it is not a strict anaerobe. On some media the bacilli may be longer and more slender. Human Type C strains may be larger with filaments and swollen forms. Sometimes there are short, almost coccoid, forms. Spores are rarely seen in laboratory media or in cooked foods. Sporulation may be encouraged in special media described by Ellner (1956), Duncan and Strong (1968), and Clifford and Annellis (1971); sporulating mutants have been induced. The spores are large, oval, and central and distend the organism. Capsules are mostly seen in the animal body.

The colonies are low, convex, semiopaque, and shiny; they may be round and entire, or somewhat irregular with a vine leaf appearance. Hemolysis is variable according to the strain and the animal source of the blood. It may be clear beta or partially clear alpha, sometimes with a double zone.

## *ANTIGENIC COMPOSITION*

*C. perfringens* is divisible into five serologic types, A to E, according to the kinds and proportions of exotoxins (soluble antigens) produced. Antitoxic sera are used in the routine typing of strains. The $\alpha$-toxin or lecithinase is produced by all types; it is antigenically related to the lecithinase of *C. bifermentans* and *C. sordellii.* Although agglutination is of little value in subdividing the species because of its heterogeneity, Type A strains nevertheless are further divided

into a large number of serotypes by simple agglutination. This is of value for the epidemiologic study of food poisoning and gas gangrene.

## *METABOLISM*

Glucose, lactose, maltose, and sucrose are fermented, and gelatinase is produced. $H_2S$ is formed, but not indole. *C. perfringens* may be differentiated from most other species of *Clostridium* by lactose fermentation, nitrate reduction, tests for motility and sporulation, and lecithinase activity; the Nagler reaction is a simple in vitro test for this substance.

## *PATHOGENIC PROPERTIES*

Types A, C, and D are pathogenic for man, Type A is responsible for gas gangrene and food poisoning, and Type C for enteritis necroticans; Type A has also been incriminated in necrotizing colitis. Types B, C, D, E, and possibly A affect animals. More than 80 per cent of environmental isolates have been shown to be Type A. Infection of experimental animals and patients causes extensive blood-stained edema fluid, often with gas in the tissues, and invasion of the bloodstream. A number of exotoxins are involved.

## *TOXICOLOGY*

There are at least 12 different soluble antigens described for *C. perfringens.* Alpha, beta, epsilon, and iota are the major lethal toxins in mice.

**TABLE 2. The Soluble Antigens of Clostridium perfringens**[a]

| | | $\alpha$ | $\beta$ | $\gamma$ | $\delta$ | $\epsilon$ | $\theta$ | $\iota$ | $\kappa$ | $\lambda$ | $\mu$ | $\nu$ |
|---|---|---|---|---|---|---|---|---|---|---|---|---|
| A | Gas gangrene, puerperal infection, septicemia, food poisoning: | | | | | | | | | | | |
| | Classical | ++++ | − | − | − | − | ++− | − | ++ | − | − | + |
| | Atypical | +− | − | − | − | − | − | − | +− | − | − | − |
| B | Lamb dysentery, foal enterotoxemia, goats and sheep: hemorrhagic enteritis | + | +++ | + | ++ | ++ | + | − | − | +++ | + | + |
| C | Sheep toxemia, calves and lambs: hemorrhagic enteritis, | + | +++ | + | ++ | − | + | − | + | − | − | + |
| | Man: enteritis necroticans | + | + | + | − | − | − | − | − | − | − | + |
| D | Sheep, lambs, goats, cattle: enterotoxemia | +++ | − | − | ++ | +++ | ++ | − | ++ | ++ | ++− | ++− |
| E | Sheep, cattle (? pathogenic) | +++ | − | − | − | − | ++ | +++ | ++ | ++ | (+) | +− |

[a]+++, produced by all strains; +, ++, produced in increasing quantities; ++−, +−, present in some strains only; −, not produced. Adapted from Willis (1977).

$\alpha$-toxin is common to all types of *C. perfringens*, but it is produced in largest amount by strains of Type A. It is lethal for mice 6 to 12 hours after intravenous inoculation. It also causes necrosis after intradermal injection in guinea pigs. The lecithinase activity of alpha toxin splits lecithin to phosphorylcholine and a diglyceride and can be demonstrated by production of opalescent clostridia on egg yolk agar (Nagler reaction) and by lysis of sheep or mouse erythrocytes.

$\beta$-toxin is produced by Types B and C. It is necrotizing and lethal, but not hemolytic; it is heat-labile. It is identified by the intradermal inoculation of depilated albino guinea pigs, in which it produces a purplish necrotic area.

$\delta$-toxin is lethal and hemolytic. It lyses sheep erythrocytes but not those of the horse or rabbit. It is produced by Types B and C.

$\theta$-toxin is produced in greatest amount by Type C strains but can be found also in culture filtrates of Types A, B, D, and E. It is an oxygen-labile hemolysin, active against sheep and horse red cells but not very active against those of the mouse.

$\epsilon$-toxin is produced by Types B and D. $\iota$-toxin is produced by Type E strains. Both toxins are lethal and necrotizing. They are detected in culture filtrates by intradermal tests in guinea pigs. Trypsinization must be used to ensure activation of the prototoxins. They are both absorbed from the intestinal tract.

$\kappa$-toxin is produced by Types A, C, E, and some strains of Type D. It is a collagenase and gelatin-ase and is also lethal and necrotizing.

$\lambda$-toxin is produced by Types B and E and some strains of Type D. It is a proteolytic enzyme that attacks gelatin and azocoll (commercial hide powder coupled to a dye) and also casein and hemoglobin (unlike $\kappa$-toxin).

$\gamma$- and $\eta$-toxins are lethal toxins without other demonstrable activity.

$\mu$- and $\nu$-antigens are a hyaluronidase and deoxyribonuclease; they may be estimated by the ACRA (acid-congo red-alcohol) test using horse synovial fluid (hyaluronic acid) ($\mu$) and sodium deoxyribonuclease ($\nu$) as the substrates (Oakley and Warrack, 1951).

Other soluble substances found in filtrates have included neuraminidase and fibrinolysis. The toxin patterns in relation to pathogenicity in man and animals are shown in Table 2 (Oakley and Warrack, 1953).

### Enterotoxin

This component of the sporulating cells of Types A and C is responsible for food poisoning and is produced and released in the large intestine during sporulation (Skjelkvåle and Duncan, 1975). Sporulation in cooked food as in laboratory media is poor, so that the toxin is unlikely to be detected either in the laboratory or by clinical manifestations. By means of ligated loop experiments, the association between a large intake of *C. perfringens*, sporulation, and enterotoxin production in the intestine was confirmed (Duncan and Strong, 1971).

Hauschild (1973, 1975) described the purified toxin as a protein of approximately 36,000 MW and isoelectric point 4.3, containing 19 amino acids with a predominance of aspartic and glutamic acids, serine, and leucine. The toxicity for mice was 2000 MLD/mg N. The enterotoxin is heat-labile with a decimal reduction time of 4 minutes at 60° C. The toxin has lethal and emetic properties and causes cutaneous erythema in the guinea pig and rabbit.

Antienterotoxin antibodies have been found in the blood of a high proportion of persons who yet remain sensitive to the enterotoxin (Torres-Anjel and Riemann, 1975).

Biologic assays are carried out with suckling mice and the ileum loop technique; the fluorescent antibody technique may be used also. Torres-Anjel et al. (1975) described a fluorescent antibody technique for the detection of enterotoxin-producing cells of *C. perfringens* Type A. Enterotoxin appeared at the end of the cell after four hours of growth and gradually spread throughout the cell (Niilo, 1977). Enterotoxin was demonstrated in the stools of patients by reversed-passive hemagglutination (Dowell et al., 1975).

## LABORATORY DIAGNOSIS

Pathologic material may be inoculated directly onto plates of blood agar and egg yolk agar and incubated anaerobically. Neomycin sulfate may be incorporated into the medium to suppress aerobic organisms. Cooked meat broth cultures may be subcultured onto the same two agar media after eight to ten hours growth. As the organism does not form spores in the tissue or in cooked foodstuffs, heat treatment is not required. The organism produces spores readily in feces, and heat treatment of fecal suspensions is an advantage for isolation of heat-resistant strains. Direct inoculation from a fecal sample onto blood agar (with neomycin sulfate) and subculture from cooked meat broth without heat treatment should also be carried out (Sutton et al., 1971).

*C. perfringens* is a minor component of the fecal flora in most, if not all, persons. The median count of *C. perfringens* in fecal samples from 50 healthy adults was $7.5 \times 10^3$ per g. The ratio of the spore count to the count of unheated material was generally of the order of 1/10 to 1/100 (Sutton, 1969). In outbreaks of *C. perfringens* food poisoning, counts of the organism in feces from patients are higher, usually $10^6$ to $10^7$, and the heat-resistant spore/vegetative cell count was found to be 1/2000 to greater than 1/60,000 in one outbreak reported by Sutton (1966). Thus quantita-

tion is useful in the assessment of the significance of *C. perfringens* in the stool. The Miles and Misra (1938) technique may be used on blood agar spread with neomycin sulfate; an approximately 1/10 suspension of the fecal sample may be used as the first dilution (Sutton et al., 1971). Heavily contaminated foods responsible for outbreaks may be cultured onto blood agar with and without neomycin sulfate and incubated anaerobically. For the enumeration of small numbers of *C. perfringens* for specification purposes, black colonies in pour plates of sulfite cycloserine agar may be preferred. The isolation of small numbers of *C. perfringens* through cooked meat or liver enrichment media may be of value in epidemiologic studies and when typing is carried out, but care must be taken in the interpretation of the results.

The simplest means of identification is by the reaction described by Nagler in 1939 and developed as a diagnostic test by McClung and Toabe (1947). Cultures growing on media incorporating lecithin, egg yolk agar with or without mannitol, and an indicator show an opalescent precipitate around colonies. The opalescence is due to the interaction between the lecithin in the medium and lecithinase ($\alpha$-toxin) produced by the organism. It is inhibited by antiserum to the $\alpha$-toxin. The antitoxin is usually spread over half the plate (half antitoxin egg yolk agar), so that single streaks of cultures across the plate show the precipitate on one half only. Several strains can be tested on one plate. Lecithinase-negative strains occur from time to time. Stringer et al. (1978) described five outbreaks due to lecithinase-negative strains, and found that in four, the serotype of the strains isolated was identical.

Other tests for identification include motility, proteolysis, nitrate reduction, and biochemical reactions; the action on litmus milk (stormy clot) is not always typical. Laboratory reactions used in differentiating *C. perfringens* from other pathogenic clostridia are summarized in Table 3.

## EPIDEMIOLOGY

The organism is widely distributed in nature in soil, sewage, water, and the intestinal tract of man and animals. Wounds may be infected from spores or cells in the environment or from contaminants on the skin surrounding the lesion. Serologic studies have indicated that *C. perfringens* in postoperational gangrene frequently originates from the intestine of the patient (Parker, 1967; Ayliffe and Lowbury, 1969).

*C. perfringens* is an important agent of food

TABLE 3. Differential Laboratory Reactions of Clostridia Pathogenic for Man

| | NAGLER REACTION (LECITHINASE) | SPORES | MOTILITY | β-HEMOLYSIS | LACTOSE FERMENTATION | GLUCOSE FERMENTATION | H₂S | INDOLE | UREASE | NITRATE REDUCTION |
|---|---|---|---|---|---|---|---|---|---|---|
| C. perfringens | + | C | 0 | + | + | + | + | 0 | 0 | + |
| C. tetani | 0 | T | + | + | 0 | 0 | 0 | + | 0 | 0 |
| C. botulinum | | | | | | | | | | |
| Types A, B, E, F | 0 | ST | + | + | 0 | + | + | 0 | 0 | 0 |
| Types C, D | 0 | ST | + | + | 0 | + | + | 0 | 0 | 0 |
| Type G | 0 | ST | + | + | 0 | 0 | + | 0 | 0 | 0 |
| C. novyi | | | | | | | | | | |
| Type A | + | ST | + | + | 0 | + | + | 0 | 0 | + |
| Type B | + | ST | + | + | 0 | + | + | 0 | 0 | + |
| C. histolyticum | 0 | ST | + | + | 0 | 0 | + | 0 | 0 | 0 |
| C. septicum | 0 | ST | + | + | + | + | + | 0 | 0 | + |
| C. sporogenes | + | ST | + | 0 | 0 | + | + | 0 | 0 | + |
| C. sordelli | + | C | + | + | 0 | + | + | + | + | + |

[a]T, terminal; C, central; ST, subterminal.

poisoning in the United States and the United Kingdom and perhaps (unrecognized) in many other countries also. It was reported as a cause of intestinal disturbances in hospital patients as early as 1895 (Klein, 1895). Knox and MacDonald (1943), McClung (1945), Zeissler and Rassfeld-Sternberg (1949), Hobbs et al. (1953), and many subsequent workers described the role of C. perfringens Type A in food poisoning. C. perfringens Type C was described by German investigators in a more serious and often fatal food-borne disease known as enteritis necroticans. Murrell et al. (1966) described the same disease in Papua, New Guinea. The β-toxin was thought to be responsible for the more severe intestinal lesions. The enterotoxin, which is distinct from the other toxins of C. perfringens, was later proved to be rsponsible for the milder type of food poisoning due to the Type A strains.

In humans symptoms of food poisoning from Type A strains develop 8 to 24 hours after eating food heavily contaminated with the organism. Symptoms include abdominal pain, nausea, and acute diarrhea lasting 12 to 24 hours; fever is rare. Occasionally there are fatalities among elderly debilitated patients. Deaths of some malnourished children with diarrhea may be due to terminal septicemia with C. perfringens. There were approximately 6500 cases of C. perfringens food poisoning in England and Wales during the years 1973 to 1975 (Vernon, 1977), representing between 15 and 32 per cent of the annual numbers reported from all bacterial causes. The outbreaks occurred mostly in hospitals, schools, and institutions and tended to be larger (50 persons average) than outbreaks due to other organisms. Outbreaks resulting from faults in the cooling and storage of foods cooked in bulk occurred repeatedly in hospitals and schools. Means for rapid cooling and adequate cold storage of meat and poultry, and other foods cooked in bulk ahead of requirements, should be incorporated into the design of canteen kitchens and other establishments preparing food on a large scale. The importance of this measure needs emphasis in teaching.

Statistics for enteritis necroticans due to the Type C strains are not available. The disease has been reported from Germany and Papua, New Guinea ("Pigbel"), but it is rarely noted in other countries. The factors leading to illness are similar to those for the Type A strains: the survival of spores resistant to heat and the multiplication of vegetative cells in the slow cooking and cooling of masses of meat. In New Guinea the slow spit roasting of pig carcasses eaten at feasts and the "cairn" cooking of meat by the heat of the sun have encouraged the multiplication of the organism to large numbers. Laurence and Walker (1976) suggest that the low protein diet of the people of the Highland of Papua, New Guinea, and the presence of heat-stable trypsin-inhibitor from sweet potatoes results in low levels of digestive proteases in the intestinal lumen. Thus there is no proteolytic activity, and the β-toxin from C. perfringens Type C that is normally susceptible to proteolysis is not destroyed and causes necrosis.

The heat resistance of the spores of C. perfringens Type A varies from strain to strain and also within strains. Some spores can survive for an hour or more in boiled meats, in which they may be protected by the meat or fat; others live for a few minutes only. Cooking stimulates (heat shock) most spores of C. perfringens to germinate; the activation of germination is detected at about 75 to 80° C. The optimum temperatures for growth in cooked meat are 43 to 47° C (Collee et al., 1961).

The rate of division or generation time at optimum temperatures is 10 to 12 minutes (Mead, 1969) in food favorable for growth, principally a meat medium. Cooking drives off dissolved oxygen and leaves an anaerobic environment suitable for the growth of *C. perfringens*. The resistance to heat and activation by heat of the spores during cooking, and the fast multiplication of the vegetative cells during cooling result in the food becoming a medium for an almost pure culture of *C. perfringens*. When many (millions per g) vegetative cells in cooked foods are swallowed, they survive passage through the gastric acid and become established in the intestine. In the United Kingdom and United States, outbreaks of *C. perfringens* food poisoning occur throughout the year with no seasonal prevalence. The fault lies in the prolonged storage at 30 to 50° C between cooking and eating. Without proper cooling and adequate cold storage facilities, the preparation of food in large catering establishments often leads to this type of food poisoning. In addition to outbreaks associated with hospitals, schools, and factories, there are many that follow banquets and meals prepared for touring groups. Kitchens designed to prepare a few meals are often expected to cater for many travelers, despite inadequate space and facilities.

Vegetative cells and spores of *C. perfringens* are common on raw meat and on and within poultry and fish. Their origin is assumed to be feces from man and animals. Because the spores are resistant to dehydration, they can survive for long periods in soil and dust. The ubiquitous nature of the organism makes epidemiologic investigation difficult without finer methods of typing the strains isolated. The serologic differentiation of Type A strains was originally described by Henderson (1940) and Hobbs et al. (1953). It has now been expanded widely into an international typing scheme (Hughes et al., 1976; Stringer et al., 1975; Stringer et al., 1978). Approximately 56 per cent of strains may be typed by simple slide agglutination method using a battery of 50 or more sera made up into polyvalent groups, each containing about five sera of different types. The antigenic specificity is thought to originate from the capsular material.

Serotyping is useful also for tracing the origin of infection in gas gangrene cases (Parker, 1967; Ayliffe and Lowbury, 1969).

# CLOSTRIDIUM TETANI

## MORPHOLOGY

The characteristic bacilli are slender, grampositive, motile, and strictly anaerobic. The mature spores are terminal and spherical so that the bacillus has a "drumstick" appearance; immature spores are oval and terminal. Sporefree forms occur, and older cultures may be gram-negative. The organism grows as a fine rhizoidal film with a finely filamentous edge of growth; the extremely fine growth may be missed. Nonmotile variants form discrete colonies with no swarming. Antitoxin will prevent swarming. There is alpha-to-beta hemolysis on horse blood agar.

## ANTIGENIC COMPOSITION

There are at least ten types of flagellar antigens. Antigenically identical neurotoxin is formed by all types. Nontoxigenic variants may be isolated from wounds of patients.

## METABOLISM

No sugars are fermented except glucose rarely. *C. tetani* is nonproteolytic but produces gelatinase. $H_2S$ is not produced, but most strains produce indole. A rennin-like enzyme gives zones of opacity around colonies on milk agar. Some strains produce deoxyribonuclease. Metabolic products include acetic, propionic, and butyric acids and ethanol and butanol.

## PATHOGENIC PROPERTIES

The pathogenicity of *C. tetani* for man arises from its neurotoxic exotoxin. The neurotoxin first causes local peripheral nerve and muscle spasms. The toxin (tetanospasmin) then spreads to the anterior horn cells via the bloodstream and causes generalized convulsions. A hemolysin (tetanolysin) is also produced but is less important; it is not related to the neurotoxin and may be produced by nontoxigenic strains. Tetanospasmin and *C. botulinum* neurotoxin are the most potent poisons known. In culture, tetanospasmin is produced after the phase of active growth; it is heat-labile and is destroyed at 65° C in five minutes.

## IMMUNITY

The disease may be prevented by active immunization with tetanus toxoid or passive immunization with antitetanus hyperimmune human periumglobulus. Recovered patients must be immunized because the disease is produced by amounts of toxin that are too small for immunization. Toxoid given to pregnant women prevents tetanus of the newborn.

## LABORATORY DIAGNOSIS

Pathologic material should be placed directly onto culture media and incubated in cooked meat broth for two to four days under anaerobic conditions. Fresh or heated blood agar is used for subculture, and the inoculum is placed near the edge of the plate so that the spreading or swarming growth may leave the contaminants behind. For purity, subcultures may be made from the edge of the growth. Neomycin sulfate and cautious heat treatment may be used to inhibit contaminants in material containing nonmotile variants of *C. tetani*.

## DRUG SUSCEPTIBILITY

The organism is sensitive to penicillin and its derivatives and to tetracycline.

## EPIDEMIOLOGY

*C. tetani* is widely distributed in soil, especially cultivated soil, and in the intestinal tract of man and animals. Infection of wounds and umbilical stumps of the newborn occurs after contamination with soil and human and animal feces. Military wounds, trauma among farm workers, and injuries from auto accidents are especially subject to soil contamination and thus to tetanus intoxication.

# CLOSTRIDIUM BOTULINUM

## MORPHOLOGY

The bacillii are large stout rods, motile and gram-positive, especially in young cultures. Sporulation may be sparse; the spores are oval and central or subterminal.

The colonies are irregular or circular and translucent with a granular surface; they may be lobular with an indefinte spreading edge. Growth may spread over the plate. There is hemolysis on horse blood agar.

## ANTIGENIC COMPOSITION

There are seven known toxicologic types, A to G, which produce antigenically distinct neurotoxins. There are minor antigenic relationships between the neurotoxins of Types C and D and between Types E and F. Walker and Batty (1964) found that the toxicologic types fell into three distinct serologic groups. Types A, B, and F are serologically related and are distinct from Types C, D, and F. Types C and D are related and are distinguishable from Type E. Walker and Batty also noted limited cross-reactions between strains of *C. botulinum* and *C. sporogenes*.

## METABOLISM

Types A, B, E, and F ferment glucose, maltose, and sucrose; Types C and D ferment glucose and maltose; Type G is nonsaccharolytic. All types produce gelatinase and $H_2S$; indole is not produced.

## PATHOGENIC PROPERTIES

*C. botulinum* Types A, B, E, and F cause botulism in man. Types C and D and more rarely A and B are pathogenic for mammals and birds. Type G has not been reported from outbreaks in man or animals. The exotoxin is responsible for the disease; the organisms do not multiply easily in the body. *C. botulinum* in wounds can give rise to botulism in a few cases (Mersam and Dowell, 1973). Toxin elaborated by *C. botulinum* in the bowel of infants can cause sudden death (Midura and Arnon, 1976).

The potent neurotoxins, although antigenically distinct, are pharmacologically similar; they are absorbed from the alimentary tract through the gastric and upper intestinal mucosa. They can be demonstrated in the blood, and they reach the peripheral nervous system. The toxin acts at the tips of the motor nerve endings at the neuromuscular junction and interferes with the release of acetylcholine. To be effective, antitoxin should be administered before the toxin becomes fixed to the tissues. The incubation period is usually less than 24 hours. Vomiting, thirst, and pharyngeal and ocular paresis occur. Voluntary muscles weaken, and death may occur within 24 hours from paralysis of the respiratory muscles. In poultry and wildfowl the condition known as limberneck gives rise to paralysis of the neck and leg muscles.

A fatal dose of toxin for man has been estimated to be between 0.1 and 1.0 $\mu$g (Schantz and Sugyama, 1974). The toxicity of the neurotoxin is about $10^3$ that of *C. perfringens* $\alpha$-toxin, $10^5$ that of crotactin (rattlesnake venom), and $10^6$ that of strychnine (van Heyningen, 1968, 1970). The toxin is described as a simple protein consisting of 19 amino acids, molecular weight about 150,000, and isoelectric point 5.6. The toxin is rapidly destroyed by boiling. Toxigenic strains may lose their toxigenicity, while naturally occurring nontoxigenic strains can revert to a toxigenic state after infection with certain phages.

## IMMUNITY

Natural immunity is unlikely to occur because the lethal dose of toxin is less than that required to elicit an antibody response. Laboratory workers may be immunized with polyvalent antitoxin (A, B, and E).

## LABORATORY DIAGNOSIS

The toxin in supernatants of food can be detected in mice injected with the extracts and identified by protection with antitoxin. The clinical diagnosis can be confirmed by demonstrating the toxin in blood and stool specimens. Reverse passive hemagglutination, immunofluorescence and agar plates containing specific antitoxins are also used for identification. The organism may be isolated from cooked meat cultured on to blood agar plates incubated anaerobically. Shaking the cooked meat culture with a little alcohol or benzol before subculture inhibits contaminants. Neomycin sulfate in culture media helps to repress aerobic organisms. However, low concentrations of neomycin sulfate may be inhibitory to *C. botulinum* Type E. Likewise, heat treatment should be used with caution. The selection of colonies is aided by the use of egg yolk agar; with the exception of type G, *C. botulinum* produces opalescence and a pearly layer. Culture on lactose egg yolk milk agar distinguishes proteolytic and non-

proteolytic variants. Types C, D, and E produce nonlactose, nonproteolytic fermenting lipolytic colonies. Also there are nonproteolytic variants of Types B and F.

## EPIDEMIOLOGY

*C. botulinum* is unevenly but widely distributed throughout the world. The natural habitat is the soil. Types A and B are the most common around the world. Type D has been found in Japan, Alaska, Canada, Russia, and also near the Baltic Sea. Type G was first isolated by Gimenez and Cicarrelli (1966, 1970) from Argentinian soil. Type E occurs in fish and in mud and shore waters; toxin production may increase to levels that affect fish. Intensive growth of *C. botulinum* may occur in overstocked fishfarms in which the fish are overfed. The infection is more difficult to control when the floor of the pond is earth rather than concrete.

Drought appears to encourage proliferation of the organism in mud and wildlife, such as fish, ducks, and seagulls. In foods, the germination of spores and the growth of vegetative cells are necessary for toxin production. The spores survive cooking, smoking, and salting; nitrite is required in the curing of salt meats to prevent the outgrowth of spores. Home-preserved foods are most frequently responsible for botulism. Examples are home-canned or salted low-acid vegetables, smoked or pickled fish, and pork products cured with salt without the addition of nitrite. Cheese can become toxigenic when acid production is deficient. Processes for commercially canned foods are usually calculated to destroy the spores of *C. botulinum* that are particularly resistant to heat. Outbreaks of botulism attributable to commercially canned foods have involved both underprocessing and postprocessing contamination. Micro-leaks in cans are significant even when chlorinated water is used for cooling, because vegetative cells may be destroyed by chlorine, but spores are not. Thus, adequate methods of food preservation are important in the prevention of botulism in both commercial and home processing of foods. Nonacid foods may be particularly dangerous.

# CLOSTRIDIUM NOVYI
# (C. OEDEMATIENS)

Type D is sometimes called *C. hemolyticum.*

## *MORPHOLOGY*

The organism is a fairly large gram-positive bacillus that is motile and strictly anaerobic. It sporulates freely, and the spores are large and subterminal and expand the rod. In young culture it resembles *C. perfringens.* Colonies are irregular or circular and semitranslucent with a finely lobulated or crenelated edge. The surface is finely granular. Growth may spread.

## *ANTIGENIC COMPOSITION*

There are four types: A, B, C, and D. All strains of *C. novyi* Types A, B, and C share two somatic antigens in varying proportions. Fluorescent-labeled antiserum prepared against Type B organisms stains strains of all types.

## *METABOLISM*

Glucose and maltose are fermented by Types A and B, but only glucose is fermented by Types C and D. All types produce gelatinase but do not attack more complex proteins. Type D produces large amounts of indole, and $H_2S$ is produced by all strains and especially by Type D. Products of metabolism include propionic and butyric acids and small amounts of acetic and valeric acids.

## *PATHOGENIC PROPERTIES*

Types A and B cause gas gangrene in man and animals; Types B and D are responsible for other diseases in animals. Type A is the most common clinical pathogen.

## *TOXICOLOGY*

Eight different soluble toxic antigens have been demonstrated in culture filtrates. Types A and B produce necrotizing lethal $\alpha$-toxin, which increases capillary permeability and causes the characteristic gelatinous edema of muscle seen in *C. novyi* gas gangrene. Production of $\alpha$-toxin is apparently bacteriaphage-dependent. Types A and B also produce lecithinase C enzymes that are hemolytic, necrotizing, and lethal (Type B).

## *LABORATORY DIAGNOSIS*

Isolation is often difficult and slow, particularly for Type D. Media should be freshly poured or prereduced. The cysteine dithiothreitol medium of Moore (1968) is recommended for Types B, C, and D. Before culture, the material may be heated at 80° to 100° C for 10 to 15 minutes. Preliminary enrichment in cooked meat broth is of value. Reactions on half-antitoxin lactose egg yolk milk agar is species specific and type specific for Type A strains; there is a diffuse lecithinase C opalescence and a restricted pearly layer due to lipolysis. Strains of Types B and D produce opalescence only, while Type C strains are egg yolk-negative. Animal inoculation and protection tests may be used. Neomycin sulfate may be used in culture media to suppress aerobic organisms.

## *EPIDEMIOLOGY*

The organism is widely distributed in soil and (Types A and B) in the livers of healthy animals. Approximately 42 per cent of the cases of gas gangrene in World War II were due to *C. novyi.*

# CLOSTRIDIUM HISTOLYTICUM

## *MORPHOLOGY*

The bacillus is gram-positive, motile, and not an exacting anaerobe. Spores are formed readily except under aerobic conditions. They are large and oval, subterminal, and distend the organism.

The colonies are small, circular, opaque, shiny with an entire edge, and grayish white. There is a narrow zone of hemolysis on horse blood agar.

## *ANTIGENIC COMPOSITION AND TOXICOLOGY*

There is no division into types. Oakley and Warrack (1950) demonstrated three separated soluble antigens in culture filtrates as follows:

$\alpha$-toxin, lethal and necrotizing.

$\beta$-antigen, collagenase attacking azocoll and gelatin.

γ-antigen, proteinase, attacks azocoll, gelatin, and casein also.

δ-antigen, an elastase (Oakley and Banerjee, 1963).

## METABOLISM

The organism ferments no sugars. It is strongly proteolytic and attacks gelatin and more complex proteins. $H_2S$ is produced but not indole. Acetic acid is produced as the only volatile product.

## PATHOGENIC PROPERTIES

The organism is pathogenic for man and animals. In man it is associated, together with other anaerobes, with gas gangrene infections.

## LABORATORY DIAGNOSIS

The organism grows slowly under aerobic conditions when it is atypical and pleomorphic without spores; growth is improved under anaerobic conditions. Colonies are easily recognised on lactose egg yolk milk agar. There is partial clearing, lactose is not attacked, and there is no typical egg yolk reaction. Neomycin sulfate may be used to eliminate aerobic organisms, and differential heating may be used for the same purpose. In cooked meat broth, there is vigorous proteolysis of the meat particles.

## EPIDEMIOLOGY

The organism is widely but sparsely distributed in soil and probably also in the intestinal tract of man and animals.

# CLOSTRIDIUM SEPTICUM AND CLOSTRIDIUM CHAUVOEI

Because the characteristics of these two organisms are similar, they are described together. Sometimes they are considered as a single species, C. septicum Types A and B (C. chauvoei).

## MORPHOLOGY

They are gram-positive bacilli, particularly in young culture. Spores are oval and subterminal, and they distend the organism. They are strict anaerobes. Colonies of C. septicum are small with a coarse rhizoidal edge; they may spread. There is beta hemolysis on horse blood agar. C. chauvoei colonies are small, umbonate, irregular or circular, shiny, and semitranslucent.

## ANTIGENIC COMPOSITION

C. septicum is divisible into two groups on the basis of the O antigen; neither group cross-reacts with C. chauvoei, which possesses a common O antigen (Moussa, 1959). Batty and Walker (1963) found that both organisms could be differentiated by the use of fluorescent antibodies. The swarming growth of C. septicum may be prevented by treating plates with a polyvalent C. septicum O antiserum before inoculation.

## METABOLISM

Both organisms ferment glucose, maltose, and lactose; in addition, C. septicum ferments salicin and C. chauvoei ferments sucrose. Both produce $H_2S$ but not indole. Both produce gelatinase and deoxyribonuclease. Acetic, butyric, and formic acids are formed.

## PATHOGENIC PROPERTIES

C. septicum is pathogenic for man and animals and is associated with gas gangrene in man. C. chauvoei is pathogenic for animals only, especially ruminants.

## TOXICOLOGY

C. septicum produces three exotoxins. The α-toxin is lethal, necrotizing, and hemolytic; the β-toxin is deoxyribonuclease; and the γ-toxin is hyaluronidase. A neuraminidase and hemagglutinin are also produced.

C. chauvoei also produces α- β- and γ-toxins and an oxygen-labile hemolysin; all appear to be related to the corresponding antigens produced by C. septicum.

## IMMUNITY

*C. septicum* antitoxin provides homologous protection and also protection against *C. chauvoei*. *C. chauvoei* antitoxin does not protect against *C. septicum* toxemia, because *C. septicum* produces additional toxins, in particular, the α-toxin, which is unrelated to the α-toxin of *C. chauvoei*.

## LABORATORY DIAGNOSIS

Both organisms are easy to grow; *C. chauvoei* is encouraged by the presence of liver in the medium. Preliminary enrichment is helpful and neo-mycin sulfate may be used to discourage growth of aerobic contaminants; initial heating is also useful. The organisms are egg yolk–negative. In clinical medicine, it is important to distinguish *C. septicum* from *C. chauvoei*. Animal protection tests may be used. In cooked meat medium, both organisms produce small amounts of gas, and the meat particles may become pink.

## EPIDEMIOLOGY

Both organisms are found chiefly in soil and also in the intestinal tract of herbivorous animals.

# CLOSTRIDIUM SPOROGENES

## MORPHOLOGY

The bacillus is strongly gram-positive. Sporulation is profuse, and the spores are oval and subterminal, and they distend the cell. Free spores are common. The colonies are umbonate, opaque with a grayish white center. They are flat, irregular or circular with a rhizoidal edge, and they may spread. There is no hemolysis.

## ANTIGENIC COMPOSITION

Soluble antigens of clinical significance are not produced.

## METABOLISM

Glucose and mannitol are fermented but not lactose or sucrose. Gelatin and more complex proteins are broken down. $H_2S$ is formed but not indole. A wide range of acids and alcohols are produced, particularly acetic, propionic, isobutyric, isovaleric, and isocaproic acids.

## PATHOGENIC PROPERTIES

In mixed clostridial infections *C. sporogenes* increases the virulence of pathogenic species such as *C. perfringens* and *C. septicum*. There are local putrefactive changes in inoculated muscles, especially after damage has occurred; occasionally guinea pigs may die after inoculation.

## LABORATORY DIAGNOSIS

Heat treatment and neomycin sulfate may be used to suppress contaminating aerobic organisms. On lactose milk yolk agar, there is restricted opalescence, and a pearly layer develops owing to lipase activity. Growth is surrounded by wide zones of clearing due to proteolysis of the milk. In cooked meat, broth meat particles are attacked and partly digested. A scum of fatty acids may develop on the surface. Cultures have an odor of skatol.

## EPIDEMIOLOGY

*C. sporogenes* is widely distributed in nature, both in soil and in the intestinal tract of man and animals. It is not easily distinguishable from nontoxic sporulating strains of *C. botulinum*.

# CLOSTRIDIUM BIFERMENTANS AND C. SORDELLII

## MORPHOLOGY

The organisms are strongly gram-positive bacilli, motile, and not exacting in their requirements. They spore readily, and the spores are large and cylindrical, usually central and slightly distending the cell. Chains of sporulating organims are formed, and free spores are common.

The colonies of both organisms are low, convex with an entire but irregular edge, and grayish white; they may swarm. There is a narrow zone of hemolysis on horse blood agar.

## ANTIGENIC COMPOSITION

Walker (1963) differentiated the two species on the basis of spore agglutinogens but not spore precipitinogens. There was no cross-agglutination or precipitation between the spores of the *C. bifermentans-sordellii* group and those of *C. sporogenes, C. histolyticum, C. sphenoides,* and *C. perfringens* Types A to D.

## METABOLISM

Glucose and maltose are attacked but not lactose or sucrose. In addition, *C. bifermentans* ferments mannose, sorbitol, and salicin; and *C. sordellii* is urease positive. Gelatin and more complex proteins are broken down by both organisms, and $H_2S$ and indole are produced.

Large amounts of acetic, isobutyric, and isovaleric and small amounts of propionic and isocaproic acids are formed.

## PATHOGENIC PROPERTIES

Intramuscular inoculation of a pathogenic strain of *C. sordellii* kills guinea pigs in one to two days. Proteolysis of tissues may progress in the same way as that of *C. histolyticum* infections; there is hemorrhage and gas production. Rifkin et al. (1977) describe infection by *C. sordellii* in colitis induced by antibiotics.

## TOXICOLOGY

Pathogenic strains of *C. sordellii* produce a lethal toxin for which antitoxic sera are available. All strains of *C. sordellii* and *C. bifermen-* *tans* produce a lecithinase C that is antigenically related to, but not identical with, the lecithinase C ($\alpha$-toxin) of *C. perfringens*. There are indications that at least one other soluble antigen is produced by these organisms.

## LABORATORY DIAGNOSIS

Heat treatment and neomycin sulfate in or on solid media help to inhibit aerobic organisms. On lactose egg yolk milk agar there is extensive opalescence that is inhibited by *C. perfringens* Type A antitoxin, but the inhibition is seldom complete. There is no pearly layer; lactose is not fermented; zones of partial clearing indicate that milk is attacked. In cooked meat broth, the meat particles are partially digested, and a viscous mucoid deposit is produced that is peculiar to these organisms.

## DRUG SUSCEPTIBILITY

*C. sordellii* is apparently resistant to clindamycin and sensitive to vancomycin. Thus, clindamycin treatment of patients may induce overgrowth of the bowel with *C. sordellii* and consequent clostridial colitis. This in turn can be treated successfully with orally administered vancomycin.

## EPIDEMIOLOGY

Both organisms are widely distributed in the soil and in the large bowel of man and animals.

### Acknowledgements

All those whose work and research have enabled this information to be assembled are acknowledged with gratitude. The author and editors are particularly grateful to Dr. A. T. Willis for his clear exposition of the facts in his book *Anaerobic Bacteriology: Clinical and Laboratory Practice,* third edition, and for his willingness to allow some of his material to be abstracted. We are grateful also to Butterworth and Co. (Publishers) Ltd. for their permission.

### References

Ayliffe, G. A. J., and Lowbury, E. J. L.: Sources of gas gangrene in hospital. Br Med J 2:333, 1969.
Batty, I., and Walker, P. D.: Differentiation of *Clostridium septicum* and *Clostridium chauvoei* by the use of fluorescent labelled antibodies. J Pathol Bacteriol 85:517, 1963.

Clifford, W. J., and Annellis, A.: *Clostridium perfringens*. I. Sporulation in a biphasic glucose-ion-exchange resin medium. Appl Microbiol 22:856, 1971.

Collee, J. G., Knowlden, J. A., and Hobbs, B. C.: Studies on the growth, sporulation, and carriage of *Clostridium welchii* with special reference to food poisoning strains. J Appl Bacteriol 24:326, 1961.

Dowell, V. R., Jr., Torres-Anjel, M. J., Reimann, H. P., Merson, M., Whaley, D., and Darland, G.: A new criterion for implicating *Clostridium perfringens* as the cause of food poisoning. Rev Lat-Am Microbiol 17:137, 1975.

Duncan, C. E., and Strong, D. H.: Improved medium for the sporulation of *Clostridium perfringens*. Appl Microbiol 16:82, 1968.

Duncan, C. E., and Strong, D. H.: *Clostridium perfringens* type A food poisoning. Response of the rabbit ileum as an indication of enteropathogenicity of strains of *Clostridium perfringens* in monkeys. Infec Immun 3:167, 1971.

Ellner, P. D.: A medium promoting rapid sporulation in *Clostridium perfringens*. J Bacteriol 71:495, 1956.

Gimenez, D. F., and Ciccarelli, A. S.: A new type of *Clostridium botulinum*. In Ingram, M., and Roberts, T. A. (eds.): Botulism. Proceedings of the 5th International Symposium on Food Microbiology, July 1966. London. Chapman and Hall, 1966, p. 455.

Gimenez, D. F., and Ciccarelli, A. S.: Another type of *Clostridium botulinum*. Zentralbl Bakteriol Parasitol Infektionskrankh Hyg Abt I [Orig] 215:221, 1970.

Hauschild, A. H. W.: Criteria and procedures for implicating *Clostridium perfringens* in food-borne outbreaks. Can J Public Health 66:388, 1975.

Hauschild, A. H. W.: Food poisoning by *Clostridium perfringens*. Can Inst Food Sci Technol J 6:106, 1973.

Henderson, D. W.: The somatic antigens of the *Cl. welchii* group of organisms. J Hyg Camb 40:501, 1940.

Hobbs, B. C., Smith, M. E., Oakley, C. L., Warrack, G. H., and Cruickshank, J. C.: *Clostridium welchii* food poisoning. J Hyg Camb 51:75, 1953.

Howard, F. M., Bradley, J. M., Flynn, D. M., Noone, P., and Szawatkowski, M.: Outbreak of necrotizing enterocolitis caused by *Clostridium butyricum*. Lancet 11:1099, 1977.

Hughes, J. A., Turnbull, P. C. B., and Stringer, M. E.: A serotyping system for *Clostridium welchii (Clostridium perfringens)* type A, and studies on the type-specific antigens. J Med Microbiol 9:475, 1976.

Klein, E.: On a pathogenic anaerobic intestinal bacillus, *Bacillus enteritidis sporogenes*. Zantralbl Bakteriol 1 Abt 18:737, 1895.

Knox, R., and MacDonald, E. J.: Outbreaks of food poisoning in certain Leicester institutions. Med Off 69:21, 1943.

Lawrence, G., and Walker, P. D.: Pathogenesis of enteritis necroticans in Papua New Guinea. Lancet 1:125, 1976.

Leader.: Clostridia as intestinal pathogens. Lancet ii:1113, 1977.

McClung, L. S.: Human food poisoning due to growth of *Clostridium perfringens (Cl. welchii)* in freshly cooked chickens: Preliminary note. J. Bacteriol 50:229, 1945.

McClung, L. S., and Toabe, R.: Egg-yolk plate reaction for presumptive diagnosis of *Clostridium sporogenes* and certain species of gangrene and botulinum groups. J. Bacteriol 53:139, 1947.

Mead, C. C.: Growth and sporulation of *Clostridium welchii* in breast and leg muscle of poultry. J. Appl Bacteriol 32:86, 1969.

Mersom, M. H., and Dowell, V. R.: Epidemiologic clinical and laboratory aspects of wound botulism. N. Engl J Med 289:1005, 1973.

Midura, T. F., and Arnon, S. S.: Infant botulism. Identification of *Clostridium botolinum* and its toxins in feces. Lancet 11:934, 1976.

Miles, A. A., and Misra, S. S.: The estimation of the bactericidal power of blood. J Hyg Camb 38:732, 1938.

Moore, W. B.: Solidified media suitable for the cultivation of *Clostridium novyi* type B. J Gen Microbiol 53:415, 1968.

Moussa, R. S.: Antigenic formulae for *Clostridium septicum* and *Clostridium chauvoei*. J Pathol Bacteriol 77:341, 1959.

Murrell, T. G. C., Egerton, J. R., Rampling, A., Samuels, J., and Walker, P. D.: The ecology and epidemiology of the pig-bel syndrome in man in New Guinea. J Hyg Camb 64:375, 1966.

Nagler, F. P. O.: Observations on a reaction between the lethal toxin of *Cl. welchii* (Type A) and human serum. Br J Exp Pathol 20:473, 1939.

Niilo, L.: Enterotoxin formation by *Clostridium perfringens* type A studied by the use of fluorescent antibody. Can J Microbiol 23:908, 1977.

Oakley, C. L., and Banerjee, N. G.: Bacterial elastases. J Pathol Bacteriol 85:489, 1963.

Oakley, C. L., and Warrack, G. H.: The ACRA test as a means of estimating hyaluronidase deoxyribonuclease and their antibodies. J Path Bact 63:45, 1951.

Oakley, C. L., and Warrack, G. H.: Routine typing of *Clostridium welchii*. J Hyg Camb 51:102, 1953.

Parker, M. T.; Clostridial sepsis. Br Med J 2:698, 1967.

Rifkin, G. D., Fekety, F. R., Silva, J., and Sack, R. B.: Antibiotic-induced colitis: Implications of a toxin neutralized by *Clostridium sordellii* antitoxin. Lancet ii:1103, 1977.

Schantz, E. J., and Sugyama, H.: Toxic proteins produced by *Clostridium botulinum*. Agric Food Chem 22:26, 1974.

Skjelkvåle, R., and duncan, C. L.: Enterotoxin formation by different toxigenic types of *Clostridium perfringens*. Infect Immun 11:563, 1975.

Stringer, M. F., Shah, N., and Gilbert, R. J.: Serological typing of *Clostridium perfringens* and its epidemiological significance in the investigation of food poisoning outbreaks. Proceedings of IAMS meeting in Szczecin, Poland, 1978.

Sutton, R. G. A.: The pathogenesis and Epidemiology of *Clostridium welchii* Food Poisoning. Thesis (Ph.D), University of London, 1969.

Sutton, R. G. A., Ghosh, A. C., and Hobbs, B. C.: Isolation and enumeration of *Clostridium perfringens*. In Shapton, D. A., and Board, R. G. (eds.): Isolation of Anaerobes. Soc Appl Bact Tech Ser No. 5. London, Academic Press, 1971, p. 39.

Torres-Anjel, M. J., Reimann, H. P., and Tsai, Che C.: A Fluorescent-Antibody Technique for the Detection of Enterotoxin-Producing Cells of *Clostridium perfringens* Type A. Scientific Publication No. 305. New York, Pan American Health Organization (World Health Organization), 1975.

Torres-Anjel, M. J., and Reimann, H. P.: Enterotoxic *Clostridium perfringens* in selected humans. II. A cohort study. Rev Lat Am Microbiol 17:199, 1975.

van Heyningen, W. E.: The pathogenic actions of exotoxins. Zentralbl Bacteriol Parasitol Infect Hyg Abt I [Orig] 212:191, 1970.

van Heyningen, W. E.: Tetanus. Sci Am 218:69, 1968.

Vernon, E.: Food poisoning and salmonella infections in England and Wales 1973–1975. An analysis of reports to the Public Health Laboratory Service. Public Health 91:225, 1977.

Walker, P. D.: The spore antigens of *Clostridium sporogenes, Cl. bifermentans* and *Cl. sordellii*. J Pathol Bacteriol 85:41, 1963.

Walker, P. D., and Batty, I: Fluorescent studies in the genus *Clostridium*. II. A rapid method for differentiating *Clostridium botulinum* types A, B, and F, types C and D, and type E. J Appl Bacteriol 27:140, 1964.

Willis, A. T.: Anaerobic Bacteriology: Clinical and Laboratory Practice. Third edition. Butterworth & Co. (Publishers) Ltd. 1977.

Willis, A. T., and Williams, K.: Prevention of swarming of *Clostridium septicum*. J Med Microbiol 5:493, 1972.

Zeissler, J., and Rassfeld-Sternberg, L.: Enteritis necroticans due to *Clostridium welchii* type F. Br Med J 1:267, 1949.

# **46** *BACTEROIDES*

## *Tor Hofstad, M.D.*

The genus *Bacteroides* comprises a heterogeneous group of nonspore-forming, obligately anaerobic rods that often are very pleomorphic. Their habitat is the mucous membranes of man and animals. They can be differentiated from *Fusobacterium* by their inability to produce substantial amounts of butyric acid from glucose.

The 8th edition of *Bergey's Manual of Determinative Bacteriology* (1974) lists 22 species of *Bacteroides*. A few of these, namely *B. fragilis, B. melaninogenicus,* and *B. corrodens,* are pathogenic in man. Strains of *Bacteroides* species of uncertain pathogenicity have been isolated from clinical specimens together with other anaerobic or facultative bacteria. At present, *B. fragilis* is subdivided into the subspecies ss. *fragilis,* ss. *distasonis,* ss. *vulgatus,* ss. *thetaiotaomicron,* and ss. *ovatus.* The different subspecies are, however, phenotypically and genotypically distinct. *B. melaninogenicus* is a heterogene species containing saccharolytic and nonsaccharolytic strains. *Bacteroides* strains classified as *B. oralis* are nonpigmented, saccharolytic *B. melaninogenicus* strains.

## *MORPHOLOGY*

Cells of *B. fragilis* are nonmotile, pale-staining, gram-negative straight or slightly curved rods with rounded ends, 0.5 to 1.0 $\mu$m in diameter and 0.5 to 5.0 $\mu$m long, occurring singly and in pairs (Fig. 1). Irregular staining, which is often bipolar, is frequently seen. Cells grown in fluid media containing a fermentable carbohydrate tend to be more pleomorphic than cells grown in solid media. Short filaments and, in particular, vacuolated cells may be seen in such cultures. Ovoid forms are common in some strains. *B. melaninogenicus* is a nonmotile, even-staining, gram-negative coccobacillus, 0.3 to 0.4 $\mu$m wide and 0.6 to 2.0 $\mu$m long (Fig. 2). Fluid cultures of some strains show larger, pale, and highly vacuolated cells, with some densely stained areas. Cells of *B. corrodens* are nonmotile, pale-staining, gram-negative rods, 0.5 to 0.7 $\mu$m in width and 1.0 to 3.0 $\mu$m long, occurring singly or in pairs. Filaments are occasionally seen. Most other *Bacteroides* species are characterized by short to medium-sized pleomorphic rods.

The ultrastructure of *Bacteroides,* as seen in the electron microscope, is that of a gram-

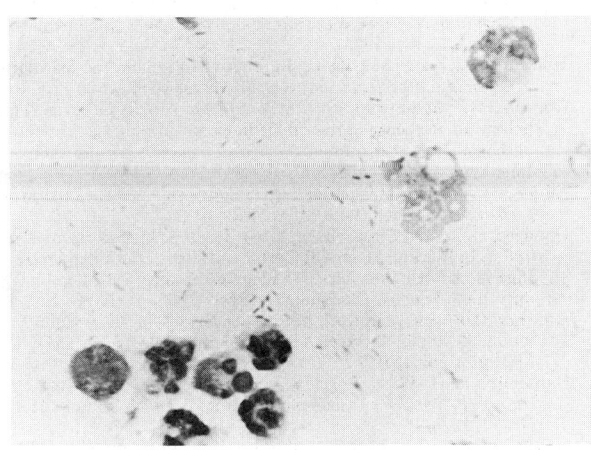

**FIGURE 1.** B. fragilis *in a smear from a liver abscess.*

negative bacterium. The cell wall has an electron-dense, solid layer containing the peptidoglycan and an outer, trilaminar membrane made up of protein, lipid, and polysaccharide.

## *ANTIGENIC COMPOSITION*

The best studied *Bacteroides* antigens are the cell wall lipopolysaccharides of *B. fragilis* and *B. melaninogenicus* (Hofstad, 1974). These are high molecular weight complexes composed of polysaccharide, lipid, and small amounts of protein. The lipopolysaccharides exhibit serologic specificity

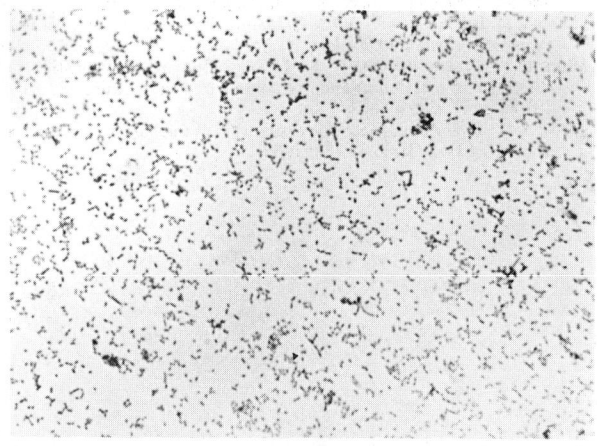

**FIGURE 2.** B. melaninogenicus *from blood agar.*

analogous to the O antigens of Enterobacteriaceae. Thus each *B. fragilis* strain shares several O-antigenic specificities with other *B. fragilis* strains and, occasionally, with other species of *Bacteroides*. All antigenic determinants are carried by the polysaccharide part of the lipopolysaccharide macromolecule. Beyond this, the chemical basis of the antigenic specificity is unknown. The lipopolysaccharides of *B. fragilis* and *B. melaninogenicus* seem to contain the same sugars, i.e., glucose, galactose, rhamnose, fucose, glucosamine, and galactosamine. Heptose and 2-keto-3-deoxyoctonate, which are essential constituents of most other bacterial lipopolysaccharides, are not present in these two or in any other species of *Bacteroides*. The O antigens are best examined by indirect hemagglutination and hemagglutination inhibition.

A group-specific capsular antigen from *B. fragilis* ss. *fragilis* has a molecular weight of 800,000 and is composed of hexose, hexosamine, methylpentose, and sialic acid (Kasper, 1976).

The outer membrane of *B. fragilis* contains a protein antigen that reacts with precipitation and is apparently group-specific. Several other precipitating antigens, the nature of which is unknown, have been observed in extracts of *B. fragilis* and *B. melaninogenicus* strains.

## GROWTH AND METABOLISM

The clinically important *Bacteroides* species grow well anaerobically on blood agar and in enriched media containing peptone and yeast extract. Surface colonies of *B. fragilis* on sheep or horse blood agar are after two days of incubation, 1 to 3 mm in diameter, circular, entire, convex, semiopaque, grayish to whitish, and nonhemolytic. Colonies of some strains may be soft and shiny. *B. melaninogenicus* organisms grow on blood agar with entire, circular, convex to pulvinate colonies, which after incubation for two days measure 0.5 to 2 mm in diameter. Old colonies are often surrounded by flattened margins. Colonies of some strains are shiny or slightly mucoid. Colonies are whitish or slightly gray in color when young, but after two or three days of incubation they take on a slightly tan to brownish pigment, and soon become jet black. The pigment is formed sooner on agar that contains laked blood rather than intact erythrocytes. The tan and light brown colonies fluoresce pink or orange, and the darker colonies show red under ultraviolet light (365 nm). Entirely black colonies do not fluoresce. The colonies of *B. melaninogenicus* are β-hemolytic or nonhemolytic. Surface colonies of *B. corrodens* range from barely visible to 0.5 mm in diameter after two days of incubation. Upon

continued incubation they grow to about 1 mm in diameter and are gray-white, convex or umbonate circular colonies with slightly undulating or entire margins that seem to disappear into the agar. Their ability to corrode, or pit, the agar may be lost after continued cultivation in fluid media. Colonies of most other *Bacteroides* species resemble those of *B. fragilis* but are usually smaller.

In fluid media growth of bacteroides causes turbidity and, frequently, a sediment that may be smooth, ropy or stringy. A small amount of gas is produced by most *B. fragilis* strains.

The bacteroides grow best at 37° C and at a pH of about 7.0. With some exceptions they are moderate anaerobes that grow maximally in oxygen tensions of up to 3 per cent. *B. fragilis* seems to be the most oxygen-tolerant species. *B. ochraceus,* a member of the normal oral microflora, grows in 5 to 10 per cent carbon dioxide in air.

The energy metabolism of *Bacteroides* is virtually unknown. There is evidence that *B. fragilis* has a primitive type of electron transport system with cytochrome B that is linked to the reduction of fumarate. The asaccharolytic *B. corrodens* seems to gain energy by the transfer of electrons from hydrogen or formate to fumarate.

*B. fragilis* has simple nutritional requirements. The organism has an obligate need of vitamin $B_{12}$, and the growth of most strains is stimulated by hemin and bile. Ammonium is the preferred nitrogen source rather than amino acids. A fermentable carbohydrate is essential for good growth. *B. melaninogenicus* and most other *Bacteroides* species are more fastidious anaerobes. *B. melaninogenicus* has an obligate requirement for hemin and for peptides, and many strains need vitamin K. The organism grows well in media based on tryptone and tryptose. Serum or L-asparagine often stimulates growth. Bile is growth-inhibitory. Fumaric acid has been found to stimulate growth of *B. corrodens*. This organism grows best in a liver digest medium with added yeast extract and blood. Strains of several *Bacteroides* species require carbon dioxide.

Most bacteroides metabolize carbohydrates. The fermentation products include combinations of acetic, lactic, succinic, propionic, isobutyric, isovaleric, and formic acids. Butyric acid is formed by a few species but not as a major product. *B. fragilis* is highly saccharolytic, giving a final pH in glucose broth of about 5.0 to 5.4. *B. corrodens* does not ferment carbohydrates. Asaccharolytic strains of *B. melaninogenicus* are highly proteolytic. The organism can hydrolyze casein, gelatin, plasma proteins, and collagen. Indole is produced by some *Bacteroides* species or subspecies. Catalase, lecithinase, and lipase are usually not produced. *B. fragilis* and most other bacteroides hydrolyze aesculin. Dehydrogenases specific for different amino acids and other organic acids are present in *Bacteroides* and have been used for differentiation between members of the species. β-Lactamase (Pinkus et al., 1968) and neuraminidase are produced by *B. fragilis*.

## PATHOGENIC PROPERTIES

The pathogenic *Bacteroides* species are part of the normal microflora of mucous membranes, particularly those of the gastrointestinal and upper respiratory tracts. They are harmless inhabitants unless the mucous membrane barrier is broken. The bacteroides, like other microorganisms on the mucosa, may then invade the adjacent tissue and cause localized infection or spread hematogenously to the liver, lung, or brain. Following aspiration they may be carried from the mouth into the lung. These endogenous infections are not communicable from one person to another.

A requisite for *Bacteroides* infection is lowering of the redox potential by tissue necrosis, impaired blood supply, and growth of facultative microorganisms in an infected area. The importance of underlying disease was illustrated in a study of 112 patients with bacteroidaceae bacteremia, caused mainly by *B. fragilis* (Chow and Guze, 1974). Forty-three per cent of the patients had either malignancy, arteriosclerosis, alcoholic liver disease, diabetes mellitus, or end-stage renal disease. Underlying disease was the overriding determinant of mortality. The most significant factors in nonfatal infections were old age and a history of trauma or surgery.

The most common serious anaerobic infections encountered are caused by members of the family Bacteroidaceae, especially *B. fragilis*. This organism may be implicated in suppurative lesions of almost every part of the human body, and is the anaerobic microorganism isolated most often from microbial infections. It is also the anaerobic gram-negative rod found most frequently in pure culture. Usually, however, *B. fragilis* and other bacteroides are accompanied by facultative or other anaerobic bacteria such as peptostreptococci. Other bacteria are almost universally present in infections with *B. melaninogenicus,* probably because they satisfy its need for vitamin K.

*B. fragilis* is now isolated from two thirds or more of intra-abdominal infections. Other *Bacteroides* species are isolated less often. *B. fragilis* and *B. melaninogenicus* are each found in 25 per cent of patients with anaerobic pleuropulmonary disease (empyema, lung abscess, pneumonitis), and in 25 per cent of those with infections of the female genital tract (Ledger et al., 1971). *Bacteroides* species are often isolated from abscesses of the liver and the brain. *B. fragilis* is the anaerobic organism isolated most often from soft tissue infections. In septicemic patients *B. fragilis* is isolated in 5 to 10 per cent of all positive blood cultures. The common portals of entry are the gastrointestinal and female genital tract. *Bacteroides* species may also be implicated in decubital ulcers (Rissing et al., 1974) and gangrene, in dental infections, and in chronic infections of the paranasal sinuses and the middle ear. Occasionally *Bacteroides* species are isolated from osteomyelitis, purulent arthritis, infective endocarditis, and urinary tract infections. *B. corrodens* has been found in oral and upper respiratory infections and in blood cultures.

Approximately 80 per cent of the *B. fragilis* strains isolated from anaerobic infections belong to subspecies ss. *fragilis*. The other four *B. fragilis* subspecies are less important as human pathogens. *B. fragilis* ss. *ovatus* does not seem to occur in systemic infections.

Pure cultures of *B. fragilis* or other *Bacteroides* species are noninfective or only slightly infective in experimental animals. Little is known, therefore, about the pathogenesis of *Bacteroides* infections. Synergistic mechanisms are thought to play a role in mixed infections. Two such mechanisms are known: production of a low oxidation-reduction potential by facultative organisms, and supply of an essential growth factor. A capsule in *B. fragilis,* particularly ss. *fragilis* and in some *B. melaninogenicus* strains may protect them from phagocytosis. The cell wall lipopolysaccharides of *B. fragilis* and *B. melaninogenicus* have low toxicity compared to endotoxins of the facultative enteric bacilli (Sveen et al., 1977). Certain enzymes, like neuraminidase, deoxyribonuclease, and heparinase may also contribute to pathogenicity. Heparinase may contribute to the septic thrombophlebitis observed in serious *B. fragilis* infections (Mitre and Rotheram, 1974). *B. melaninogenicus* is one of the few microorganisms that produce collagenase.

## IMMUNITY

Low titers of IgM antibodies against O antigens from *B. fragilis* and *B. melaninogenicus* are present in normal human serum, but their protective function is not known. Normal human serum kills *B. fragilis* isolated from stools, and polymorphonuclear leukocytes can phagocytose it with the help of heat-labile opsonins (Bjornson and Bjornson, 1978). A rise in IgM and IgG antibodies in patients has been observed after *B. fragilis* septicemia and local suppurative lesions. The significance of these humoral antibodies in recovery from infection is unknown.

## LABORATORY DIAGNOSIS

Pus tissue biopsies from normally sterile sites, transtracheal aspirates, pleural and ascitic fluids, aspirates from the nasal sinuses, carefully collected materials from the root canals and periapical tissues of teeth, cervical material collected by direct visualization, and specimens of blood should be cultured routinely for *Bacteroides* and other anaerobes. It is imperative to avoid contamination with normal flora. Whenever possible specimens should be taken by aspiration in large volumes. Purulent exudate is in itself a good transport medium.

### Processing of Specimens

A Gram-stained smear should always be examined for characteristic gram-negative rods that do not appear in aerobic culture. The specimen is streaked on a nonselective solid medium, preferably Brucella blood agar (tryptose agar with glucose added), and on laked blood agar containing 75 $\mu$g/ml of kanamycin and 7.5 $\mu$g/ml of vancomycin, which is selective for *Bacteroides*. The plates are incubated for two days in GasPak jars or in ordinary anaerobic jars in an atmosphere of nitrogen and hydrogen with 5 to 10 per cent carbon dioxide. An enriched liquid medium, for instance chopped-meat glucose, is also inoculated. If prereduced anaerobically sterilized (PRAS) media are not available, semifluid media can be used.

### Identification

A presumptive identification of *B. fragilis* and *B. melaninogenicus*, the *Bacteroides* species encountered most frequently, can be made on the basis of cellular morphology, colonial growth, antibiotic susceptibility patterns, and ability to grow in a medium containing 20 per cent ox bile. A scheme for the identification of *B. fragilis* subspecies and *B. melaninogenicus* is shown in Table 1. The scheme, which permits the distinction between the two *Bacteroides* species and the most common *Fusobacterium* species, can be used in any bacteriologic laboratory. Fermentation of carbohydrates and hydrolysis of esculin should be performed in media containing peptone and yeast extract. The indole reaction can be carried out as a spot test or in a medium containing tryptone or tryptose, which are peptones rich in tryptophan. Rapid fermentation of the *B. fragilis* subspecies can be tested by using large inocula in small volumes of carbohydrate-containing media. Also, micromethod multitest systems for identification of *Bacteroides* species and other anaerobic bacteria pathogenic in man are sold commercially. *B. corrodens* produces urease, reduces nitrate to nitrite, and pits the agar. The pitting may take days to develop or may not occur.

By means of indirect fluorescence, *B. fragilis* ss. *fragilis* may be identified with antiserum from rabbits immunized with capsular material from

**TABLE 1.** Distinguishing Characters of the Most Common *Bacteroides* and *Fusobacterium* Species

| SPECIES | MORPHOLOGY | | GROWTH INHIBITION | | BIOCHEMICAL TESTS | | | | | |
| | Cellular | Colony | Penicillin[a] (2 units/ml) | 20% Bile | Indole Production | Esculin Hydrolysis | Fermentation of | | | |
| | | | | | | | Glucose | Rhamnose | Mannitol | Trehalose |
|---|---|---|---|---|---|---|---|---|---|---|
| *B. fragilis* | Short rods with | Convex, white to gray, | | | | | | | | |
| ss. *fragilis* | rounded ends, | glistening. May be | − | − | − | + | + | − | − | − |
| ss. *vulgatus* | may be ovoid or | slightly hemolytic | − | − | − | + | + | + | − | − |
| ss. *thetaiotaomicron* | vacuolated, may | | − | − | + | + | + | V | − | + |
| ss. *distasonis* | show irregular | | − | − | − | + | + | V | − | + |
| ss. *ovatus* | staining | | − | − | + | + | + | V | + | V |
| *B. melaninogenicus* | Coccobacilli or short rods with rounded ends | Tan to black, or gray-white (*B. oralis*), hemolytic | + | + | V | − | V | − | − | − |
| *B. corrodens* | Slender rods with rounded ends | Pin-point, corroding, nonhemolytic | + | + | − | − | − | − | − | − |
| *F. nucleatum* | Slender, spindle-shaped bacilli with tapered ends (fusiform) | Convex, slightly irregular, grayish, glistening | + | + | + | − | − | − | − | − |
| *F. necrophorum* | Pleomorphic, often beaded, rods, with rounded to tapered ends | Convex, often raised opaque center and translucent entire edge. Hemolytic | + | + | + | − | − | − | − | − |

[a]Growth inhibition = zones <10 mm; +, positive; −, negative; V, variable.

Modified from Bartlett et al.: Anaerobic Bacteria and Disease. Kalamazoo, Mich., The Upjohn Company, 1975.

that organism. Most sera from rabbits immunized with whole bacterial cells appear to be species specific but do not discriminate among the subspecies. Double diffusion in agar and whole cell agglutination can differentiate only incompletely among the subspecies of *B. fragilis*.

## DRUG SUSCEPTIBILITY

All *B. fragilis* subspecies have a similar susceptibility pattern to antibacterial drugs. *B. fragilis* is the anaerobic microorganism most resistant to antimicrobial agents. Of particular importance is the fact that *B. fragilis* is resistant to the aminoglycoside antibiotics, and is resistant to penicillins and first generation cephalosporins. Clindamycin usually inhibits *B. fragilis* in a concentration of 0.2 $\mu$g/ml, and for the time being is the drug of choice for treatment of anaerobic infections with *B. fragilis*. The antibiotic is active also against most other anaerobes and has produced good results in the treatment of anaerobic infections. It is about ten times more active against *B. fragilis* than the parent compound lincomycin, but is not consistently bactericidal and does not penetrate well into the central nervous system. Serious colitis is seen sometimes in patients treated with clindamycin. Metronidazole, which inhibits *B. fragilis* at 3 $\mu$g/ml or less, is bactericidal in the same concentraction against anaerobic bacteria including *B. fragilis* (Finegold and Nastro, 1972) but inactive against aerobic bacteria. The drug has a low toxicity and crosses the blood-brain barrier, but prolonged administration in large doses has caused tumors in an animal model. It is also mutagenic in bacteria. *B. fragilis* is regularly inhibited by chloramphenicol at a level of 5 to 8 $\mu$g/ml and by erythromycin in concentrations of 2.0 $\mu$g/ml. The $\beta$-lactamase resistant cephalosporin, cefoxitin, is active against *B. fragilis* (Dailand and Birnbaum, 1977). A relatively small percentage of *B. fragilis* isolates, varying from one geographic area to another, is susceptible to tetracycline in a concentration of as low as 1.0 $\mu$g/ml.

The susceptibility pattern of other *Bacteroides* species is insufficiently known. Most isolates have been highly susceptible to the commonly used antibiotics, including penicillin. A few isolates of *B. melaninogenicus* and *Bacteroides* species other than *B. fragilis* have proved to be relatively or highly resistant to penicillin. Development of resistance to antimicrobial agents may occur among the *Bacteroides* and may be due to R-factors.

## EPIDEMIOLOGY AND ECOLOGY

In human subjects on a Western diet, *B. fragilis* is the predominant organism of the lower intestinal tract, amounting to $10^{11}$ or more organisms per gram dry weight of feces. The great majority is made up of ss. *vulgatus* and ss. *thetaiotaomicron*. Subspecies *fragilis* is present in a comparatively low number. *Bacteroides* is normally found in a small number in the terminal ileum. In patients with a continent ileostomy or with intestinal blind loops, there is a bacterial overgrowth, a substantial part of which is caused by *B. fragilis*. The overgrowth is regularly associated with vitamin $B_{12}$, malabsorption, and steatorrhea (stagnant loop syndrome) (Farrar et al., 1975). *B. fragilis* is present also in the normal urethral, vaginal, and cervical flora, and in the upper respiratory tract.

*B. melaninogenicus* constitutes 4 to 8 per cent of the cultivable microflora of the gingival crevices and is the predominating *Bacteroides* species of the mouth. It becomes established in the mouth upon eruption of the permanent teeth. The organism is a member of the normal flora of the upper respiratory tract, vagina, external male and female genitalia, and skin between the toes.

*B. corrodens* inhabits the mouth and the upper respiratory tract. The principal habitat of other *Bacteroides* species occasionally isolated from anaerobic infections seems to be the lower intestinal tract.

*Bacteroides* is frequently involved in hospital infections. Infection may be facilitated by radiation and surgery, and treatment with cytotoxic drugs. A substantial portion of *Bacteroides* infections is associated with surgery. The use of antibiotics that select resistant anaerobes such as *B. fragilis* is thought to predispose to infection.

A significant morbidity and mortality attend infections with *Bacteroides*. Prophylaxis would require avoidance of any condition that reduces the normal redox potential of the tissues and the introduction of the normal mucosal microflora into wounds, closed cavities, or other sites that are normally sterile. Prophylactic antimicrobial therapy may be of value in surgery involving the colon and the female genitalia.

## References

Bjornson, A., and Bjornson, H.: Participation of immunoglobulin and the alternative complement pathway in opsonization of *Bacteroides fragilis* and *Bacteroides thetaiotaomicron*. J Infect Dis 138:351, 1978.

Chow, A., and Guze, L.: Bacteroidaceae bacteremia: Clinical experiences with 112 patients. Medicine 53:93, 1974.

Dailand, G., and Birnbaum, J.: Cefoxitin resistance to beta-lactamase: A major factor for susceptibility of *Bacteroides fragilis* to the antibiotic. Antimicrob Agents Chemother 11:725, 1977.

Farrar, W., O'Dell, N., Achord, J., and Greer, H.: Intestinal microflora and absorption in patients with stagnation-inducing lesions of the small intestine. Am J Dig Dis 17:1065, 1975.

Finegold, S., and Nastro, L.: Bactericidal activity of five antimicrobial agents. J Infect Dis 126:104, 1972.

Hofstad, T.: Endotoxins of anaerobic gram-negative microorganisms. In Balows, A. (ed.): Anaerobic Bacteria. Springfield, Ill., Charles C Thomas, 1974, pp. 295–305.

Kasper, D. L.: The polysaccharide capsule of *Bacteroides fragilis* subspecies *fragilis:* Immunochemical and morphologic definition. J Infect Dis 133:79, 1976.

Ledger, W., Sweet, R., and Headington, J.: Bacteroides species as a cause of severe infections in obstetric and gynecologic patients. Surg Gynecol Obstet 133:837, 1971.

Mitre, R., and Rotheram, E.: Anaerobic septicemia from thrombophlebitis of the internal jugular vein. JAMA 230:1168, 1974.

Pinkus, G., Veto, G., and Braude, A. I.: Bacteroides penicillinase. J Bacteriol 96:1437, 1968.

Rissing, J., Crowder, J., Dunfee, T., and White, A.: Bacteroides bacteremia from decubitus ulcers. S Med J 67:1179, 1974.

Sveen, K., Hofstad, T., and Milner, K. C.: Lethality for mice and chick embryos, pyrogenicity in rabbits and ability to gelate lysate from amoebocytes of *Limulus polyphemus* by lipopolysaccharides from *Bacteroides, Fusobacterium* and *Veillonella.* Acta Pathol Microbiol Scand (B) 85:388, 1977.

# *FUSOBACTERIA* **47**

## *Howard Robert Attebery, D.D.S.*

Thirteen recognized species in the genus *Fusobacterium* have been found to be associated with human clinical infections (Moore and Holdeman, 1974). Four of these species, *F. mortiferum, F. necrophorum, F. nucleatum,* and *F. varium*, are of primary concern because they are the major isolates recovered from clinical infections. The other species are rarely or infrequently found and will not be discussed individually. For more information, refer to Moore and Holdeman, 1974; Holdeman, Cato, and Moore, 1977; and Finegold, 1977.

### *MORPHOLOGY*

Fusiform is the term used to describe thin, gram-negative anaerobic rods with pointed ends. Fusiforms are not all members of the genus *Fusobacterium*, and all fusobacteria are not fusiform shaped. *Fusobacterium nucleatum* organisms are fusiform, slender, and spindle shaped with tapered ends. *F. varium* organisms are coccobacillary to bacillary with rounded ends. The variability of size and shape may make one suspect a mixed culture. *F. necrophorum* and *F. mortiferum* are heavy bodied bacteria with rounded ends. Pleomorphic cells may be short or elongated. Terminal or central swellings are common. *F. mortiferum* is slightly larger than *F. necrophorum* and more pleomorphic.

The colonies and microscopic morphology of *F. nucleatum* offer a unique combination that assures recognition of this species. The colonies are circular, convex, and translucent with a "flecked" appearance. Mature colonies on blood agar produce a greenish discoloration of the surrounding agar when exposed to air for 15 minutes.

Colonies of *F. varium* are minute to 1 mm in diameter, circular with entire edges, flat to low convex, and translucent with gray-white centers and colorless edges. Colonies of *F. necrophorum* are 1 to 2 mm in diameter, circular with irregular to erose edges, convex to umbonate, frequently with an even surface. A mosaic interior can be seen with transmitted light.

Colonies of *F. mortiferum* are 1 to 2 mm in diameter, circular with entire to irregular edges, convex to umbonate, translucent, and smooth.

### *ANTIGENIC COMPOSITION*

There are few reports on the immunochemistry and the antigenic structure of *Fusobacterium*. Purified lipopolysaccharides with endotoxic activity exhibit a high degree of serologic specificity so that several serologic types can be distinguished (De Araujo et al., 1963). A carbohydrate, probably the O antigen, determines the serologic specificity (Kristoffersen et al., 1971). Protein containing antigens that may be associated with the outer membrane are responsible for broad cross-reactivity among strains of fusobacteria. The sera of a majority of normal people contain antibody to this antigen (Kristoffersen and Hofstad, 1970).

### *METABOLISM*

Fusobacteria obtain their energy for growth by metabolizing carbohydrates or peptones. Large amounts of butyric acids with small amounts of acetic and lactic acids are produced. Small amounts of propionic, succinic, and formic acids may be produced as well as short-chained alcohols. Pyruvate is converted predominantly to butyrate and acetate. Some strains convert threonine to propionate. All strains are strong ammonia producers. Some strains produce indole. Catalase is usually not produced. Nitrates are rarely reduced. The production of hydrogen sulfide gas, volatile amines, aldehydes, and large amounts of butyric acid give cultures a malodorous character and infections a putrid odor.

Fusobacteria are obligate anaerobes. Although they do not require an extremely low oxidation-reduction (redox) potential, some strains are very sensitive to peroxides and cannot survive exposure to air for even a few minutes. Carbon dioxide gas or bicarbonate stimulates growth. Some strains require purines, pantothenic acid, or tryptophan.

Some fusobacteria synthesize and store intracellular polysaccharides.

## PATHOGENIC PROPERTIES

Because fusobacteria are part of the normal mammalian flora, they are often isolated from mixed infections with facultative bacteria or other anaerobes such as *Bacteroides melaninogenicus, B. fragilis,* or anaerobic cocci. Although it is difficult to assess the pathogenic role of normal flora in mixed infections, it is clear that fusobacteria are capable of causing disease. Fusobacteria have been isolated many times in pure culture from the blood as well as from infections of the skin and mucous membranes. *F. nucleatum* was isolated from 18 per cent of anaerobic pleuropulmonary infections in one hospital series and was recovered four times in pure culture (Bartlett and Finegold, 1972). Fusobacteria are also one component of the fusospirochetal synergistic infection that has been demonstrated in experimental animals (Lewis and Barenberg, 1929; Smith, 1930), and *F. nucleatum* is one of the components of acute necrotizing ulcerative gingivitis (see Chapter 91, Vincent's infection). Another indicator of the pathogenicity of fusobacteria is the occurrence of metastatic lesions at sites distant from the primary lesion.

The only pathogenic factor of fusobacteria that has been studied is its lipopolysaccharide. Endotoxins have been isolated from several species of fusobacteria, and a recent study of the endotoxin of *F. necrophorum* has shown it to be very potent in all endotoxin assays (Garcia et al., 1975). The endotoxins of fusobacteria have been implicated in human periodontal disease and in fatal cases of septic shock in man and animals.

Hemolytic strains of *F. necrophorum* are isolated more frequently from serious infections than nonhemolytic strains and are more pathogenic in experimental infections of mice. It is not known whether hemolysin is directly responsible for the increased virulence.

The mechanism of symbiosis between fusobacteria and spirochetes in mixed infections is unknown, but these synergistic infections usually induce necrotic lesions. Purulent tissue reactions are more common when fusobacteria are isolated in pure culture or in association with other bacteria from infections such as periapical dental abscess, brain abscess, or mastoiditis.

## IMMUNITY

Little is known about specific immune responses to colonization or infection with fusobacteria. The sera of most people contain antibody to protein-containing antigens of fusobacteria (Kristoffersen and Hofstad, 1970), and the oligosaccharide side chains of fusobacterial endotoxins induce antibody production in experimental animals (De Araujo et al., 1963). The capacity of these antibodies to protect against invasion of the tissues by fusobacteria is unknown. Fusobacteria are probably sensitive to killing by serum complement and to ingestion and killing by phagocytes.

The most important defense against invasion of the tissues by all anaerobes is the redox potential of well-oxygenated tissue (about 150 microvolts). Obligate anaerobes like the fusobacteria cannot propagate at this redox potential. Consequently, death of tissue after trauma, surgery, arterial insufficiency, and infection by aerotolerant bacteria are important predisposing factors to fusobacterial infection.

The growth of facultative bacteria in the tissues may promote fusobacterial infection by lowering the redox potential, whereas other members of the normal flora may limit the growth of fusobacteria. The production of hydrogen peroxide and the superoxide ion during aerobic growth of competing microflora inhibits fusobacteria, since they have little or no catalase or superoxide dismutase.

## LABORATORY DIAGNOSIS

Fusobacteria are gram-negative obligate anaerobes that produce large amounts of butyric acid from fermentable carbohydrates or metabolized peptones (with little or no isobutyric or isovaleric acids). The differential reactions of the four major species are listed in Table 1.

*F. necrophorum* is the only *Fusobacterium* species that produces lipase. Not all *F. necrophorum* strains produce lipase, however. A lipase-

**TABLE 1.  Differential Culture Reactions of The Major Fusobacteria**[a]

| CULTURE REACTION | F. NECROPHORUM | F. NUCLEATUM | F. MORTIFERUM | F. VARIUM |
|---|---|---|---|---|
| Microscopic morphology | L-form like | spindle-shaped | L-form like | small, variable |
| Beta-hemolysis | + | − | − | − |
| Indole | + | + | − | $+^-$ |
| Esculin hydrolysis | − | − | + | − |
| Nitrate | − | − | − | − |
| Growth in 20% bile | $-^{2+}$ | $-^{2+}$ | 4+ | 4+ |
| Gas in glucose agar deeps | 4+ | $-^{2+}$ | 4+ | 4+ |
| Threonine → propionate | + | + | + | + |
| Lactate → propionate | + | − | − | − |
| Lipase | + | − | − | − |
| Fermentation | | | | |
|   glucose | $-^w$ | $-^w$ | $+^w$ | $w^+$ |
|   lactose | − | − | $w^+$ | − |
|   fructose | $-^w$ | $w^-$ | $W^+$ | w |
|   maltose | − | − | $w^-$ | − |

[a]Numbers refer to intensity of reaction. Superscripts refer to reactions of 10 to 40% of strains. +, 90% or more of strains positive; −, 90% or more of strains negative; w, weak reaction.

negative fusobacterium that is indole-positive and produces propionic acid from lactate is *F. necrophorum*. Most strains of *F. necrophorum* are hemolytic on horse and rabbit blood agar. Sheep red blood cells are less susceptible to this hemolysin.

*F. nucleatum* is the only *Fusobacterium* species with fusiform cells from colonies that show internal flecking. This species is indole-positive and does not produce propionic acid from lactate. Mannose is not fermented. Propionic acid is not produced from threonine.

*F. varium* is indole-variable. No propionic acid is produced from lactate. Mannose is fermented to a weak acid. Esculin is not hydrolyzed. Fructose is fermented. Propionic acid is produced from threonine.

*F. mortiferum* is indole-negative. Esculin is hydrolyzed. Acid is produced from lactose.

## DRUG SUSCEPTIBILITY

Penicillin G is the drug of choice in the treatment of fusobacterial infections (Table 2). However, an occasional strain of *F. varium* and *F. mortiferum* may be highly resistant to this drug. Occasional strains of *F. varium* are also highly resistant to clindamycin.

Erythromycin is relatively inactive against fusobacteria. At a level of 4 $\mu$g/ml only 30 to 50 per cent of the strains of fusobacteria tested were shown to be susceptible to erythromycin (Sutter and Finegold, 1976).

## EPIDEMIOLOGY

Fusobacteria live in the normal mucous membranes of the mouth, bowel, and urogenital tract, and often invade underlying tissue that has been damaged by biting, other accidental trauma, surgery, tumors, or another infection. They make up about 3 per cent of the anaerobes recovered from clinical infections (Finegold et al., 1977).

Fusobacteria in the mouth and throat frequently infect the teeth and throat. They may also infect any adjacent area such as the head, eyes, ears, mastoids, and sinuses. They may be aspirated into the terminal bronchioles, causing lung abscess, or spread by local or systemic circulation to cause brain abscess, meningitis, or pleuropulmonary disease. A recent literature survey showed that fusobacteria were the most common organisms isolated from brain abscesses (50 out of 142 cases), anaerobic meningitis (24 out of 104 cases), and from pleuropulmonary disease (Finegold, 1977).

Fusobacteria from the gastrointestinal tract, especially *F. necrophorum* and *F. varium*, may cause intra-abdominal and perineal infections and septicemia. They are the third most common isolate from these sites after *Bacteroides* and Peptostreptococci.

Fusobacteria are among the most common iso-

**TABLE 2.  Susceptibility of Fusobacteria to Antimicrobial Agents**[a]

|  | F. VARIUM | OTHER SPECIES |
|---|---|---|
| Penicillin G | $1^R$ | 1 |
| Lincomycin | 3 | 2 |
| Clindamycin | $3^R$ | 2 |
| Metronidazole | 3 | 2 |
| Chloramphenicol | 2 | 2 |
| Tetracycline | 3 | 2 |
| Erythromycin | 4 | 4 |
| Vancomycin | 4 | 4 |

[a]1, excellent activity, drug of choice; 2, good activity; 3, moderate activity; 4, poor activity; R, occasional strains may be resistant.

lates from the 70 per cent of normal postpartum uterine cavities that are culturally positive for anaerobes. They frequently colonize the genital tract of women and account for up to 20 per cent of serious pelvic infections (Gorbach and Barttlett, 1974).

Recent evidence suggests that the gastrointestinal tract is colonized with fusobacteria that are ingested in the diet. Japanese ingesting a Japanese diet have fusobacteria in their stools in concentrations of $10^8$ to $10^{10}$ (Ueno et al., 1974). *F. necrophorum* was present in ten out of ten studied, *F. varium* in two out of ten, and other fusobacteria in about five out of ten. Of 11 Americans (two black and nine Caucasian), only six had fusobacteria isolated from stool cultures. *F. varium* was present in three out of six and *F. nucleatum* in three out of six. None of the Americans had *F. necrophorum* in their stools. Two of the patients with *F. varium* ate rice regularly. Furthermore, the number of fusobacteria steadily declined in those Japanese who switched to American diets. Thus, diet determines whether fusobacteria appear in the stool and which species are present.

## References

Bartlett, J. G., and Finegold, S. M.: Anaerobic pleuropulmonary infections. Medicine 51:413, 1972.

De Araujo, W. C., Varan, E., and Mergenhagen, S. E.: Immunochemical analysis of human oral strains of *fusobacterium* and *leptotrichia*. J Bacteriol 86:837, 1963.
Finegold, S. M.: Anaerobic Bacteria in Human Disease. New York, Academic Press, 1977.
Finegold, S. M., Shepherd, W. E., and Spaulding, E. H.: Practical anaerobic bacteriology. Cumitech 5. American Society of Microbiology, April, 1977, p 14.
Garcia, M. M., Charlton, K. M., and McKay, K. A.: Characterization of endotoxin from *Fusobacterium necrophorum*. Infect Immun 11:371, 1975.
Gorbach, S. L., and Bartlett, J. G.: Anaerobic infections. N Engl J Med 290:1177, 1974.
Holdeman, L. V., Cato, E. P., and Moore, W. E.: Anaerobe Laboratory Manual. Blacksburg, Va., Virginia Polytechnic Institute and State University, 1977.
Kristoffersen, T., and Hofstad, T.: Antibodies in humans to an isolated antigen from oral fusobacteria. J Periodontol Res 5:110, 1970.
Kristoffersen, T., Maelund, J. A., and Hofstad, T.: Serologic properties of lipopolysaccharide endotoxins from oral fusobacteria. Scand J Dent Res 79:105, 1971.
Lewis, J. M., and Barenberg, L. H.: Pulmonary gangrene due to spirochetes and fusiform bacilli. Am J Dis Child 37:351, 1928.
Moore, W. E. C., and Holdeman, L. V.: Fusobacterium. In Buchanan, R. E., and Gibbons, N. E. (ed.): Bergey's Manual of Determinative Bacteriology, 8th ed. Baltimore, The Williams & Wilkins Co., 1974, p. 1268.
Smith, D. T.: Fuso-spirochetal disease of the lungs produced with cultures from Vincent's angina. J Infect Dis 46:303, 1930.
Sutter, V. L., and Finegold, S. M.: Susceptibility of anaerobic bacteria to 23 antimicrobial agents. Antimicrob Agents Chemother 10:736, 1976.
Ueno, K., Sugihara, P. T., Bricknell, K. S., Attebery H. R., Sutter, V. L., and Finegold, S. M.: Comparison of characteristics of gram-negative anaerobic bacilli isolated from feces of individuals in Japan and the United States. In Balows, A. (ed.): Anaerobic Bacteria, Role in Disease. Springfield, Ill., Charles C Thomas, Publisher, 1974.

# 48　*VEILLONELLA*

## *Howard Robert Attebery, D.D.S.*

Veillonella are gram-negative, obligately anaerobic cocci. They are universally present as part of the indigenous oral microbiota of man and are commonly found in the respiratory tract, intestine, and vagina of humans. By reason of their usual occurrence and high numbers as parasites on the mucous membranes of man, they can be found in infected sites when the indigenous flora are transported from the protective mucous membrane barrier into deeper tissues that can also support their growth.

Veillonella are not regarded as overt pathogens, although they do exhibit some pathogenic properties. They are not found in pure culture in any infections but are always mixed with facultative bacteria or other anaerobes or both. Veillonella are spoken of as "opportunists" because they share an infected site with more aggressive and more pathogenic microorganisms, and their role in the infectious process is considered minor.

Two species of *Veillonella* are commonly seen in the literature, *Veillonella parvula* and *Veillonella alcalescens*. These species have been found to be genetically homologous, and now only one species is recognized for the genus, *Veillonella parvula* (Holdeman et al., 1977).

### *MORPHOLOGY*

Veillonella are small cocci that measure 0.3 to 0.5 $\mu$m in diameter. They appear usually in masses or as diplococci and on occasion singly or as short chains.

On blood agar plates, colonies appear as small, convex, translucent, and glistening with an entire edge. Colony size is small unless pyruvate or lactate and carbon dioxide gas are added to the growth system.

## ANTIGENIC COMPOSITION

Rogosa found seven major serologic groups for the strains he tested (Rogosa, 1965). He could clearly distinguish 21 oral strains that were isolated from hamsters. These group I strains all possessed a distinctive antigen and were singularly homologous with each other. He placed 28 strains in group II, all oral isolates from hamsters, rats, and rabbits. Group III consisted of two oral strains isolated from rats. Group IV, *Veillonella alcalescens*, comprised 15 members, which included 3 from the rat, 1 from a rabbit, 4 from human bacteremias that followed dental operations, and 5 from the human mouth. Group V consisted of only two strains, one each from man and the rat. Group VI, *Veillonella parvula,* consisted of 28 strains. Most were oral strains from humans, but four were isolated from the intestinal tract of man. Group VII consisted of only three strains, two from the human mouth and one from the human respiratory tract.

A major antigenic component is associated with an endotoxin that induces pyrogenic and Shwartzman reactions and is structurally associated with an outer three-layered cell membrane (Bladen and Mergenhagen, 1964).

## METABOLISM

Veillonella has complex nutritional requirements. Carbohydrates are not fermented. D-ribose is, however, utilized biosynthetically and incorporated into nucleic acid (Kafkewitz and Delwiche, 1967).

For energy requirements, *Veillonella* utilizes pyruvate best but also lactate, oxaloacetate, malate, and fumarate. Veillonella also obtains energy by reducing nitrates to nitrites.

Lactate is metabolized to acetic and propionic acids and to carbon dioxide and hydrogen.

Hydrogen sulfide is produced from a number of sulfur-containing compounds such as thioglycolate, thiocyanate, thiosulfate, cysteine, cystine, and glutathione. Carbon dioxide is required for growth.

## PATHOGENICITY

Veillonella can produce disease in experimental animals. Its lipopolysaccharide is an endotoxin that produces fever and Shwartzman reactions in rabbits.

The role of *Veillonella* in human clinical infections is not clear. It appears that *Veillonella*, the parasite of mucous membranes, is an opportunist in human infection and does not play a major role in any infection. This view has evolved because of the relative infrequency of involvement of *Veillonella* in clinical infections and the fact that *Veillonella* is not present in pure culture in infections.

## LABORATORY DIAGNOSIS

Three genera of anaerobic, gram-negative cocci that belong to the family Veillonellocae may be found in infected material. These genera are easily differentiated. *Megasphaera* is fermentative and produces abundant acid from glucose, fructose, and maltose. *Veillonella* and *Acidaminococcus* are nonfermentative. In addition, *Megasphaera* produces butyric acid from carbohydrate growth media, while the others do not. *Megasphaera* has a large cell, between 1.7 and 2.5 $\mu$m, which also distinguishes this genus from *Veillonella* and *Acidaminococcus*. *Veillonella* reduces nitrates, whereas *Acidaminococcus* and *Megasphaera* do not.

The criteria separating *Veillonella* from the other anaerobes are as follows: small, gram-negative cocci, 0.3 to 0.5 $\mu$m, that reduce nitrate but do not ferment. Growth is stimulated by pyruvate and lactate, and carbon dioxide is required for growth.

One species is now recognized, *Veillonella parvula*. Commonly seen in the literature are two species that were separated by their catalase activity, *V. alcalescens*, which gives a positive catalase reaction, and *V. parvula*, which gives a negative reaction. Now both are classified as *V. parvula*.

## DRUG SUSCEPTIBILITY

*Veillonella* organisms are exquisitely sensitive to penicillin and clindamycin. Table 1 lists varying susceptibilities to ten antibiotics. Poor in vitro activity against *Veillonella* is seen with erythromycin, kanamycin, and gentamicin. In addition, *Veillonella* organisms are resistant to streptomycin, neomycin, and vancomycin.

## EPIDEMIOLOGY

*Veillonella* is part of the indigenous microbiota of the mouth, respiratory system, intestinal tract, and vagina of humans. The organisms are universally present in high numbers in the human mouth and might be expected in infections in which the oral flora is the primary infecting

**TABLE 1.    In Vitro Susceptibility of 13 Clinical Isolates of The Genus Veillonella to 10 Antibiotics\***

| ANTIBIOTIC | CUMULATIVE PER CENT SUSCEPTIBLE AT INCREASING CONCENTRATIONS ($\mu$g/m) | | | | | | | | | |
|---|---|---|---|---|---|---|---|---|---|---|
|  | 0.1 | 0.2 | 0.4 | 0.8 | 1.6 | 3.1 | 6.2 | 12.5 | 25 | >25 |
| Penicillin G | 23 | 77 | 100 | | | | | | | |
| Erythromycin | | 8 | 16 | | 23 | 31 | 38 | 69 | 77 | 100 |
| Cephalothin | 23 | 69 | | 84 | 100 | | | | | |
| Tetracycline | 23 | | 31 | 69 | 76 | 85 | | | 100 | |
| Lincomycin | 46 | 77 | | | 92 | | 100 | | | |
| Clindamycin | 100 | | | | | | | | | |
| Kanamycin | 8 | | | | | | 23 | 38 | 61 | 100 |
| Chloramphenicol | 15 | | 23 | 46 | 85 | 100 | | | | |
| Gentamicin | | | | | | 8 | | 31 | 46 | 85 | 100 |
| Rifampin | 23 | | | 31 | 100 | | | | | |

\*Adapted from Martin, W. J.: In Linnette, E. H., Spaulding,.. H., and Trauant, J. P. (eds.): Manual of Clinical Microbiology. Washington, D.C., American Society for Microbiology, 1974.

agent. *Veillonella* can on occasion be found in infections associated with the microbiota of the intestinal tract and vagina.

*Veillonella* can be found in transient bacteremias following dental extraction, in sinusitis, tonsillar and peritonsillar abscesses, otitis media, mastoiditis, and brain abscesses. The organisms are occasionally found in intra-abdominal infections and genitourinary infections. They are commonly found in the mixed infections in pneumonitis, necrotizing pneumonia, lung abscess, aspiration pneumonia, empyema, and pleuropulmonary infections. They can be seen in female genital tract infections, intrauterine infections, tubo-ovarian abscesses, and postoperative genitourinary infections.

*Veillonella* has been reported in bile. Some strains can dehydroxylate bile acids, and *Veillonella* organisms have the potential to be involved in the chain of microorganisms producing chemi-cal carcinogens from bile acids. Veillonella was found in 5 of 25 subjects with colonic polyps but not in 25 matched control subjects without polyps (Finegold et al., 1975).

### References

Bladen, H. A., and Mergenhagen, S. E.: Ultrastructure of *Veillonella* and morphological correlation of an outer membrane with particles associated with endotoxic activity. J Bacteriol. 88:1482, 1964.

Finegold, S. M., Flora, D. J., Attebery, H. R., and Sutter, V. L.: Fecal bacteriology of colonic polyp patients and control patients. Cancer Res 35:3407, 1975.

Holdeman, L. V., Cato, E. P., and Moore, W. E.: Anaerobe Laboratory Manual. Blacksburg, Va., Virginia Polytechnic Institute and State University, 1977.

Kafkewitz, D., and Delwiche, E. A.: Utilization of D-ribose by *Veillonella*. J Bacteriol 98:903, 1967.

Martin, W. J.: Anaerobic cocci. In Lennette, E. H., Spaulding, E. H., and Truant, J. P. (eds.): Manual of Clinical Microbiology. Washington, D.C., American Society for Microbiology, 1974, p. 970.

Rogosa, M.: The genus *Veillonella*. IV. Serological groupings, and genus and species emendations. J Bacteriol 90:704, 1965.

# 49 *SPIROCHETES: TREPONEMA AND BORRELIA*

*Daniel M. Musher, M. D.*

## DEFINITION

The order Spirochaetales includes the following five genera: *Treponema, Borrelia, Spirochaeta, Leptospira,* and *Cristispira*. This chapter will deal with the first two. The genus *Treponema,* which is pathogenic for man, includes *T. pallidum, T. pertenue,* and *T. carateum,* which cause syphilis, yaws, and pinta, respectively. These organisms have not been cultivated successfully in vitro, although recent studies have demonstrated that the viability and virulence of *T. pallidum* can be maintained for days to weeks in artificial media, and the organism may even have shown some degree of replication. Our inability to cultivate these bacteria in vitro is, to a great extent, responsible for our incomplete understanding of their properties. No differences between *T. pallidum, T. pertenue,* and *T. carateum* have been detected by microscopic, electronmicroscopic, or immunologic techniques, although the infections they produce in animals or humans are readily distinguishable (Turner and Hollander, 1957). *T. cuniculi* and *T. hyodysenteriae* cause dermal and systemic disease in rabbits and diarrheal disease in swine, respectively; *T. cuniculi* also produces experimental infection in primates. Neither of these organisms has been shown to infect people. *T. macrodentium* and *T. vincentii* may contribute to infections of the mouth and gums. Except for *T. cuniculi,* these other treponemes can all be cultivated in artificial media. This chapter will be confined to discussing the three treponemes that are pathogenic for man.

The genus *Borrelia* includes about 18 species or strains that are human pathogens. Some of these may be distinguished serologically, although formal classification is usually based on their arthropod vectors. Classification of these organisms is imprecise also, in part because in vitro cultivation of most strains has not been achieved.

## MORPHOLOGY

The pathogenic treponemes are so narrow ($\leq 0.15\ \mu$) that they are below the resolution of the light microscope; they are, therefore, considered gram-indeterminate. Electron microscopy shows them to be wavelike organisms with tapered ends (Fig. 1). They have tight, regular spirals with a wavelength of 1.1 $\mu$m and an amplitude of 0.2 to 0.3 $\mu$m; their length ranges from 6 to 15 $\mu$m, and is usually 10 to 13 $\mu$m. Examination of *T. pallidum* obtained from syphilitic rabbit testis reveals an amorphous outer layer. Recent electronmicroscopic studies of tissues have shown that *T. pallidum* in situ has an outermost layer that stains with ruthenium red and that may be the same as the amorphous external layer. The relation of these findings to a long-hypothesized slime layer that prevents phagocytosis and inhibits early antigen processing is not known. The virulent treponemes have three-sheathed flagella (also called axial fibrils) that emerge from electron-dense areas near each end of the organism; these flagella are contained between the three-layered outer membrane and an electron-dense layer (peptidoglycan) that is thought to be responsible for the wavelike configuration of treponemes. The cytoplasmic membrane is within and is adherent to the electron-dense layer. Although it might seem reasonable to assume that, by analogy to bacterial flagella, the axial fibrils are responsible for

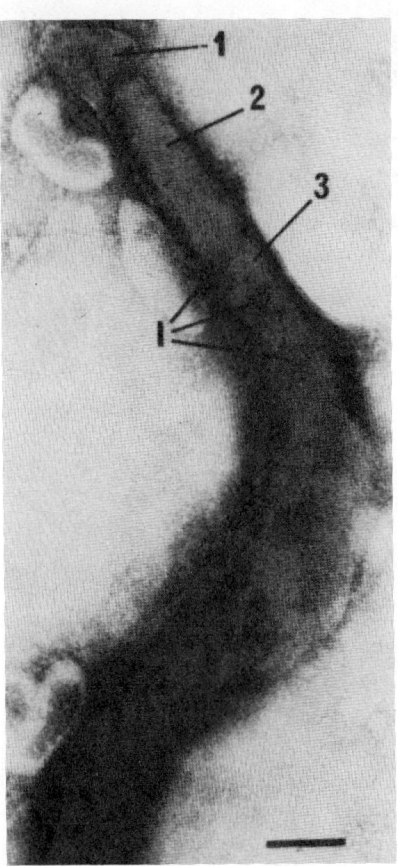

**FIGURE 1.** *Electron micrograph of Treponema pallidum (Nichols strain). Zone 1 is the outermost tip, which comes to a point. Zone 2 is the distal portion of the cytoplasm and tapers at its end beneath the outermost tip. Zone 3 is the region where flagella are inserted. Pathogenic treponemes have three flagella inserted in a row subterminally at each end. (From Hovind-Hougen, K.: Acta Pathol Microbiol (Scand) 255:1, 1976.)*

motility, their location within the outer membrane and the failure of antiflagellar antibody to immobilize certain spirochetes makes this assumption less certain. Intracytoplasmic tubules are present, but their function is unknown (Hovind-Hougen, 1976).

*Borreliae* are composed of pointed, helical organisms that usually are 10 to 20 $\mu$m in length. They have coarse irregular coils with variable amplitude. Because their width at the center is 0.4 to 0.5 $\mu$m, they are easily detectable in stained preparations as gram-negative, wavelike organisms. Wright's and Giemsa's stains also delineate them nicely, especially if prolonged staining is used. As is the case with *Treponema,* an outermost amorphous surface layer surrounds an outer membrane that has three distinct layers (Fig. 2). Between the outer and the cytoplasmic membrane may be found 15 to 20 flagella that lack sheaths; they are inserted at each end of the organism by means of basal knobs.

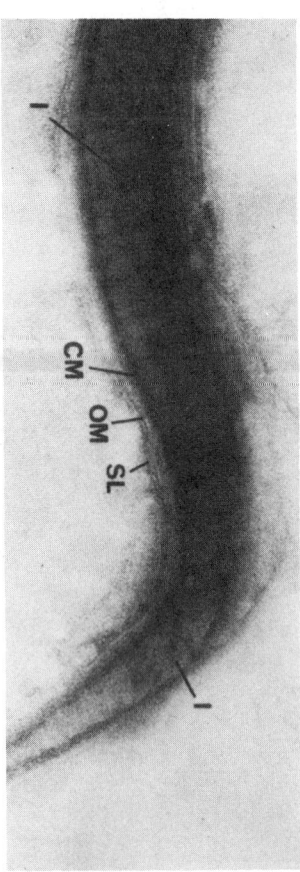

**FIGURE 2.** *Electron micrograph of Borrelia recurrentis. Note amorphous surface layer (SL), three-layered outer membrane (OM), and cytoplasmic membranes (CM). Flagella are inserted at I. The end is sharply pointed. (From Hovind-Hougen, K.: Acta Pathol Microbiol (Scand) 255:1, 1976.)*

## ANTIGENIC COMPOSITION

Little is known about the antigenic properties of the virulent treponemes because, as noted above, they must be obtained from infected tissue and because the problem of differentiating *Treponema* from mammalian antigens precludes precise analysis. It is not even known with certainty whether cardiolipin, the antigen that stimulates production of Wassermann (VDRL [Veneral Disease Research Laboratory]) antibody (see below), is a component of the treponeme or whether it is released from mammalian tissues during active treponemal infection. Favoring the former possibility is the observation that VDRL antibody follows clinically inapparent infection of primates with *T. cuniculi.* Favoring the latter is the association in experimental animals and humans between active lesions and the detection of this antibody, as well as its appearance in autoimmune disease states such as systemic lupus erythematosus. A recent study has shown that cardio-

lipin represents 13 per cent of the total lipid composition of *T. pallidum* (Matthews et al., 1979). However, since treponemes are unable to synthesize some fatty acids, their lipid composition may simply reflect that of the tissue in which they have grown. The outermost layer of *T. pallidum* has been shown to consist of mucopolysaccharides (Fitzgerald and Johnson, 1979) to which mammalian proteins readily adhere (Alderete and Baseman, 1979), further complicating studies of antigenicity of these organisms. Patients who have been infected with any of the pathogenic treponemes have antibodies against the others. Finally, because of cross-reactivity with nonpathogenic treponemes, it is necessary to absorb human serum with *T. phagedenis* (previously called *T. reiteri*) before performing tests to detect antibody to *T. pallidum.*

Antigenic properties of borreliae have not been studied thoroughly. Antiserum to one strain of *Borrelia* agglutinates other borreliae as well as *T. pallidum.* Typhus-immune serum may also contain complement-fixing antibodies that react with *Borrelia.* However, infection with one strain of *Borrelia* does not necessarily protect against others. Evidence related to "relapse strains" (see below) suggests that the antigens against which the host makes protective antibodies are unstable. Antibody to cardiolipin appears in a small percentage of cases of borreliosis. Both *Treponema* and *Borrelia* have ornithine and lack muramic and diaminopimelic acid in their cell walls, in contrast to *Leptospira.*

## METABOLISM

*T. pallidum* has traditionally been regarded as an obligate anaerobe because it best retains motility in vitro under anaerobic conditions. Recent studies, however, have shown that *T. pallidum* takes up oxygen and degrades glucose aerobically to carbon dioxide and acetate, as well as anaerobically to pyruvate and lactate, although of 22 carbon sources studied, only glucose and pyruvate were metabolized aerobically (Baseman et al., 1976). *T. pallidum* is better able to incorporate amino acids into proteins in the presence of 10 per cent oxygen than anaerobically. These studies are difficult to interpret because the organisms do not actively replicate in the in vitro systems utilized (Lysko and Cox, 1977).

The metabolic characteristics of most borreliae are unknown. *Borrelia duttoni* metabolizes glucose anaerobically via the Embden-Meyerhof pathway, with pyruvate acting as the terminal electron acceptor and reducing to lactate; aerobic respiration does not appear to play a role, and the borreliae are generally considered to be anaerobic or microaerophilic. Borreliae have been shown to metabolize lysolecithin (but not lecithin) to fatty acids and glycerol, and to incorporate cholesterol from culture medium in vitro.

## PATHOGENIC PROPERTIES

The means by which *Treponema* or *Borrelia* produces infection are unknown.

## IMMUNITY

By the time primary syphilis is diagnosed most patients have antibodies to *T. pallidum* that can be detected by immunofluorescent and hemagglutination techniques. Also present are antibodies that, together with complement, inhibit motility and eliminate infectivity of the organism (*T. pallidum* immobilizing [TPI] antibodies). Despite these antibodies, syphilis progresses and secondary lesions develop in virtually all patients unless specific therapy is given. Passive immunization with serum from rabbits that have recovered from experimental infection and are immune to rechallenge with *T. pallidum* delays and attenuates but does not prevent the development of syphilitic lesions (Bishop and Miller, 1976). An opsonizing effect of immune globulin has not been found, and phagocytosis of *T. pallidum* by polymorphonuclear leukocytes or macrophages has not been shown to contribute to resistance. Antibody to cardiolipin does not appear to contribute to immunity. Delayed hypersensitivity to treponemal antigens appears late in secondary syphilis and might, therefore, appear to be related to the onset of latency. Infection with *T. pallidum* stimulates cellular immune mechanisms, as demonstrated by enhanced ability of macrophages from syphilitic rabbits to suppress the growth of *Listeria monocytogenes;* this reaction is mediated by thymus-dependent lymphocytes (Schell et al., 1975). However, stimulation of acquired cellular resistance with unrelated organisms such as *Mycobacterium bovis* (BCG) or *Propionibacterium acnes* does not protect animals against challenge with *T. pallidum*. In addition, adoptive transfer of spleen cells from syphilis-immune rabbits fails to protect recipients against syphilitic infection. Several findings that suggest that thymus-dependent immune responses may be impaired early in syphilis might support the hypothesis that the failure of the host to control infection results from immune suppression: (1) in vitro blastogenic transformation of lymphocytes following stimulation with a variety of antigens is depressed, (2) paracortical (thymus-dependent) areas of lymph nodes are depleted, (3) delayed hypersensitivity to several antigens may be depressed, and (4) ability to be sensitized to sheep red blood cells with consequent production of IgG is markedly inhibited (Baughn and Musher, 1978). It is entirely possible that there is no complete immunity to *T. pallidum*. Active lesions may be brought under control and animals may be resistant to rechallenge with *T. pallidum,* but the host is unable to rid itself of the infecting organism, which continues to persist in lymph nodes. Human subjects have also been found to be resistant to rechallenge with *T. pallidum* during latency, although a number of observations indicate that they have not succeeded in eradicating the infecting organism (Magnuson, et al., 1956).

Humoral immunity is thought to be responsible for arresting borreliosis. Three to five days after the onset of symptoms, circulating antibodies appear that agglutinate, immobilize, and/or lyse borreliae; their appearance corresponds with clinical improvement and disappearance of these organisms from the bloodstream. Although these antibodies can be shown by some techniques to cross-react with other borreliae, immunity itself is species- and strain-specific. After the initial humoral response, and as a result of mechanisms that are not understood, the infecting organism undergoes a series of antigenic shifts, each one leading to the emergence of a new "relapse" serotype that is not immediately subject to humoral control. These serotypes cause a clinical relapse, which is then arrested within four days by a newly emerging set of specific antibodies. The shorter duration and the reduced intensity of the relapses suggest antigenic cross-reactivity with the original infecting strain. It is interesting that relapse strains appear to revert to parental forms on passage through insect vectors but not through mammalian hosts. Immunity to rechallenge with a particular strain of *Borrelia* may persist up to several years in experimental animals. In clinical reports that have described reinfection within a few months, the infecting strains have not been specifically identified. The physiologic role of phagocytosis in infection due to borreliae is thought to be minimal. Cell-mediated immunity has not been shown to play a role (Felsenfeld, 1965; Southern and Sanford, 1969).

## LABORATORY DIAGNOSIS

Three kinds of laboratory tests are important in diagnosing syphilis, yaws, or pinta: (1) Treponemes in exudates from suspicious lesions can be detected by darkfield microscopy. This method is sensitive if a good specimen has been obtained and is highly specific if care has been used to prevent contamination from oral or fecal sources. (2) Antibody to cardiolipin can be detected by a variety of flocculation tests. The most widely used is the VDRL reaction. The rapid plasma reagin (RPR) test or a modification thereof is particularly useful for screening large numbers of specimens. It is still considered best to verify and quantify positive RPR reactions by measuring VDRL antibodies. The VDRL test is reactive in about 80 per cent of patients at the time primary syphilis is diagnosed and in virtually all patients with secondary syphilis. Although VDRL reactivity is closely associated with active infection, this reaction may be negative in patients with cardiovascular or neurosyphilis. (3) Antibody to virulent treponemes can be detected by using an immunofluorescent technique (FTA-ABS, an acronym for *f*luorescent *t*reponemal *a*ntibody following *abs*orption with nonvirulent treponemes to remove nonspecific reactivity) or hemagglutination (TPHA, *T. pallidum h*emagglutination *a*ssay). Of these, the FTA-ABS technique is slightly more sensitive, being positive in more than 90 per cent of patients with primary syphilis. Both are positive in virtually all patients with secondary, latent, and late infections. The same antibodies are also detectable in yaws and pinta. These tests are highly specific for treponemal infection, although serum from patients with autoimmune diseases is rarely reactive. Despite the advantages of sensitivity and specificity, detection of antitreponemal antibody may not be useful in diagnosing active infection in an individual case because, once present, the antibody persists indefinitely; the FTA-ABS is most useful in excluding a treponemal cause for a chronic lesion (Rudolph, 1977).

Borreliosis is usually diagnosed by finding loosely coiled spirochetes during microscopic examination of Wright- or Giemsa-stained peripheral blood, or during darkfield microscopic examination of the whole fresh blood. This is highly specific but is relatively insensitive, being positive in one quarter to one half of patients who are found to have borreliosis. Injecting mice with blood from infected patients is helpful diagnostically because it produces an obvious spirochetemia, often within two to three days. Results in a recent outbreak suggested that agglutination of the *Proteus* Ox-K antigen is useful diagnostically because it was positive in at least two thirds of cases. Antibodies that agglutinate or kill *Borrelia* have been identified but have not been shown to be of practical clinical value. The VDRL test is negative in borreliosis.

## ANTIMICROBIAL SUSCEPTIBILITY

The virulent treponemes are highly susceptible to penicillins, cephalosporins, macrolides (erythromycin and clindamycin), tetracyclines, and chloramphenicol. They are resistant to sulfonamides and aminoglycosides. Borreliae are susceptible to penicillin, aminoglycosides, tetracycline, and chloramphenicol.

## EPIDEMIOLOGY

*T. pallidum, T. pertenue,* and *T. carateum* naturally infect only humans, although experimental infection has been produced in a variety of animals. *T. pallidum* infections have a world-wide distribution. Infection is spread primarily by venereal contact but may be acquired in utero. Yaws (*T. pertenue*) is limited to tropical areas and has largely been eradicated in recent years thanks to efforts of the World Health Organization. Infection appears to spread by direct contact, although flies may act as vectors. Pinta (*T. carateum*) is prevalent in areas of Central and South America and the Carribbean. It also appears to spread by contact from person to person. There is no known animal reservoir. Infection occurs sporadically in all age groups, although yaws generally begins in childhood.

In the United States borreliosis has almost always been acquired in areas above sea level where pine and fir trees predominate. The north rim of the Grand Canyon has become recognized as a highly endemic area with tick-infected log cabins playing the predominant role (Boyer et al., 1977). The reservoir of *B. recurrentis,* the classic cause of louse-borne relapsing fever, is unknown. Only human beings are clinically infected, and there is no transovarian transmission by the insect vector (*Pediculus humanus* var *humanus*). All the other borreliae infect rodents and small mammals; infection is transmitted to humans by *Ornithodorus* ticks. Elimination of rodent nests adjacent to human habitations and use of insecticide and insect repellents appear to control the spread of infection.

### References

Alderete, J. F., and Baseman, J. B.: Surface-associated host proteins on virulent *Treponema pallidum.* Infect Immun 26:1048, 1979.
Baseman, J. B., Nichols, J. C., and Hayes, N. S.: Virulent *Treponema pallidum:* Aerobe or anaerobe. Infect Immun 13:704, 1976.
Baughn, R. E., and Musher, D. M.: Altered immune responsiveness associated with experimental syphilis in the rabbit: elevated IgM and depressed IgG response to sheep erythrocytes. J Immunol 120:1691, 1978.
Bishop, N. H., and Miller, J. N.: Humoral immunity in experimental syphilis. I. The demonstration of resistance conferred by passive immunization. J Immunol 117:191, 1976.
Boyer, K. M., Munford, R. S., Maupin, G. O., Pattison, C. P., Fox, M. D., Barnes, A. M., Jones, W. L., and Maynard, J. E.: Tick-borne relapsing fever: an interstate outbreak originating at Grand Canyon National Park. Am J Epidemiol 105:469, 1977.
Canale-Parola, E.: Physiology and evolution of spirochetes. Bacteriol Rev 41:181, 1977.

Felsenfeld, O.: Borreliae, human relapsing fever, and parasite-vector-host relationships. Bacteriol Rev 29:46, 1965.

Fitzgerald, T. J., and Johnson, R. C.: Surface mucopolysaccharides of *Treponema pallidum*. Infect Immun 24:244, 1979.

Hovind Hougen, K.: Determination by means of electron microscopy of morphological criteria of value for classification of some spirochetes, in particular treponemes. Acta Pathol Microbiol (Scand) [B] Suppl 255:1, 1976.

Lysko, P. G., and Cox, C. D.: Terminal electron transport in *Treponema pallidum*. Infect Immun 16:885, 1977.

Magnuson, H. J., Thomas, E. W., Olansky, S., Kaplan, B. I., Demello, L., and Cutler, J. C.: Inoculation syphilis in human volunteers. Medicine 35:33, 1956.

Matthews, H. M., Yang, T.-K., and Jenkin, H. M.: Unique lipid com-

position of *Treponema pallidum* (Nichols virulent strain). Infect Immun 24:713, 1979.

Rudolph, A. H.: Laboratory diagnosis of syphilis. In Demis, D. J., Dobson, R. L., and McGuire, J. (eds.): Clinical Dermatology, vol. 3. Hagerstown, Md., Harper and Row, 1977, pp. 1–17.

Schell, R. F., Musher, D. M., Jacobson, K., and Schwethelm, P.: Induction of acquired cellular resistance following transfer of thymus-dependent lymphocytes from syphilitic rabbits. J Immunol 114:550, 1975.

Southern, P. M., Jr., and Sanford, J. P.: Relapsing fever: A clinical and microbiological review. Medicine 48:129, 1969.

Turner, T. B., and Hollander, D. H.: Biology of the Treponematoses. Geneva, World Health Organization, Monograph series No. 35, 1957.

# 3 UNIQUE INTRACELLULAR GRAM-NEGATIVE BACTERIA

## RICKETTSIA 50

### Garrison Rapmund, M.D.

## INTRODUCTION

Rickettsiae are small bacteria that are natural parasites of certain arthropods. Some of these arthropods can transmit rickettsiae to animals, including man. Most of our knowledge of rickettsiae come from studies of the few species that are pathogenic for man.

Rickettsiae are named after the American physician, H. T. Ricketts, who first recognized rickettsiae as the cause of typhus and spotted fever and who died of typhus in 1910 while investigating the disease in Mexico.

Rickettsiae are distinct from other bacteria because of their small size, their transmission by arthropods, and their obligate intracellular parasitism. Four groups of rickettsiae are pathogenic for man: the typhus group, of which the type species is *Rickettsia prowazekii;* the spotted fever group, of which the type species is *Rickettsia rickettsii;* the scrub typhus group, composed of one species complex, *Rickettsia tsutsugamushi*; and the Q fever group, *Coxiella burnetii*. The first three groups are similar in their growth and metabolism, fine structure, and pathogenic properties in man. They differ significantly, however, in size, intracellular location, extracellular behavior, and antigenic composition. These differences distinguish the species of rickettsiae and separate the organism that causes Q fever into a different genus, *Coxiella*. Several organisms that cause disease in man have been called rickettsiae in the past but have now been reclassified. *Rickettsia quintana*, the cause of louse-borne trench fever in man, is now placed in a separate genus, *Rochalimaea*, because of its ability to grow on artificial media. *Rickettsia sennetsu*, the cause of an infectious mononucleosis-like syndrome in

southern Japan and perhaps elsewhere, is now known to be related serologically to organisms of the genus *Ehrlichia*, which are pathogens of dogs and domestic ruminants. For reasons to be discussed later, *R. sennetsu* may require reclassification with the *Ehrlichia*.

## MORPHOLOGY

Rickettsiae are typically short rods 0.3 to 0.7 $\mu$m by 1.0 to 2.0 $\mu$m, a size just visible by light microscopy. Pleomorphism is common. Coccobacilli, diplobacilli, and individual rods are seen in infected tissue. A developmental cycle has never been identified in rickettsiae. Some investigators have postulated that morphologic variation represents a developmental cycle, but this view is not generally accepted. It is true that rickettsiae in the logarithmic growth phase are typically rod-shaped, while those in the stationary phase are often coccoid, filamentous, or swollen, but there is no evidence that this pleomorphism reflects a developmental cycle. *C. burnetii* is smaller than pathogenic rickettsiae and is filterable through certain pore filters that trap other bacteria.

Rickettsiae are gram-negative but stain poorly by the Gram technique. Rickettsiae stain red by the Macchiavello (Fig. 1) and Giminez techniques (Giminez, 1964) and purple by the Giemsa stain. Only specific immunofluorescent antisera can differentiate rickettsiae definitely from other microorganisms by means of a staining reaction.

The ultrastructure of rickettsiae is typical of gram-negative bacteria (Anacker et al., 1967). A five-layered cell wall-plasma membrane complex (Fig. 2) surrounds the cytoplasm, which contains a large array of ribosomes and fibrouslike strands

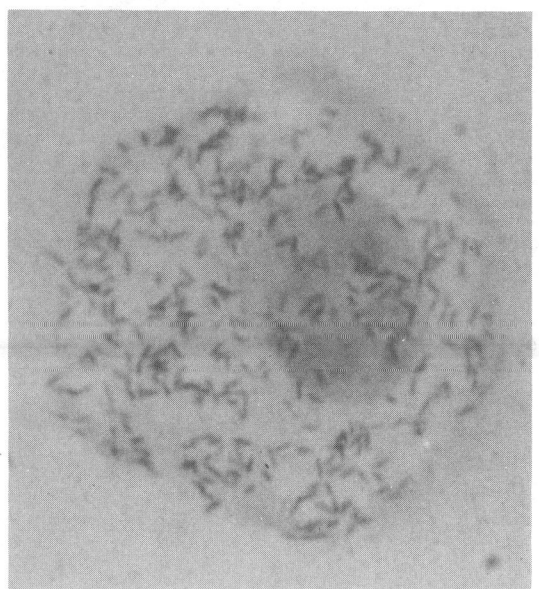

**FIGURE 1.** *Gimenez stain of R. conorii harvested 30 hours after infection of L929 cells in tissue culture.*

indicative of deoxyribonucleic acid. Intracytoplasmic vacuoles and invaginations of the plasma membrane are common (Figs. 2 and 3). Discrete, sharply defined nuclear structures have not been observed. *C. burnetii* contains a central fibrous body with radiating fibrils that are susceptible to treatment with ribonuclease. This suggests an organized DNA center that may be physically connected with RNA-containing ribosomes in the cytoplasm.

Several workers have demonstrated a zone on the outer surface of rickettsiae (Fig. 4). Silverman

and Wisseman (1978) called this a slime layer rather than a capsule because of its tendency to slough away. This extracellular layer corresponds to an electron-lucent zone surrounding *R. prowazekii* and *R. rickettsii* in infected host cells and appears to be a complex of three distinct zones: an inner layer at the cell surface of small projections with a periodicity of 13 nm radiating outward, an intermediate clear zone, and an outer fibrous slime layer that varies in width from 25 to 130 nm. The morphologic similarities to gram-negative bacteria are striking, but there seem to be significant functional differences. The presence of a capsule in other bacteria is associated with virulence, but the avirulent (Madrid E) strain of *R. prowazekii* contains the same extracellular structures as the fully virulent Breinl strain. Furthermore, the ultrastructure of rickettsiae in arthropod tissue is identical to that in mammalian tissue, and the ultrastructure of viable extracellular *R. prowazekii* in dried louse feces is identical to its intracellular morphology in the louse gut epithelium (Silverman et al., 1974). Thus, the ultrastructure of rickettsiae has not yet provided clues to the important functional

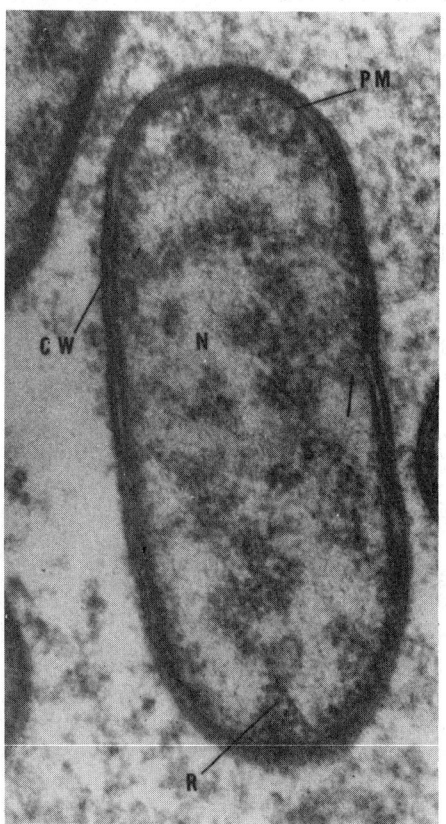

**FIGURE 3.** *Thin section through several R. quintana cells from the intestine of an infected louse. Cell wall (CW) and plasma membrane (PM) both appear trilaminar. Arrow indicates an invagination of the plasma membrane. R indicates granules that are presumed to represent ribosomes. The "nuclear" component (N) is composed of fine filaments between the granules. × 125,000. (From Ito, S., and Vinson, J. W.: J Bacteriol 89:481, 1965.)*

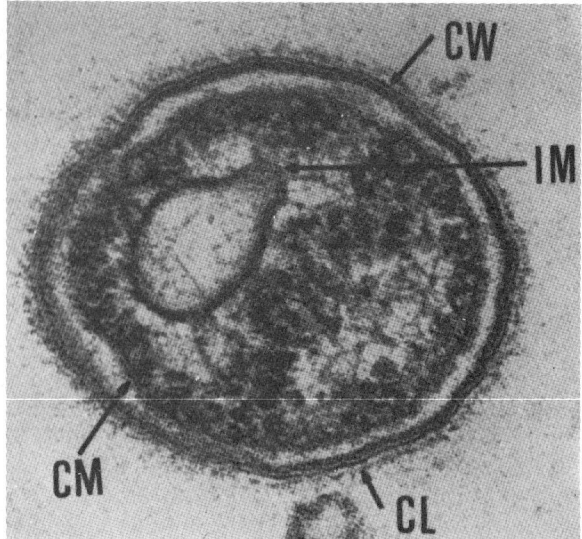

**FIGURE 2.** *Thin section of R. prowazekii. Note capsule-like layer (CL), five-layered cell wall (CW), and intracytoplasmic membrane (IM). × 185,000 (From Anacker, R. L., et al.: J Bacteriol 94:260, 1967.)*

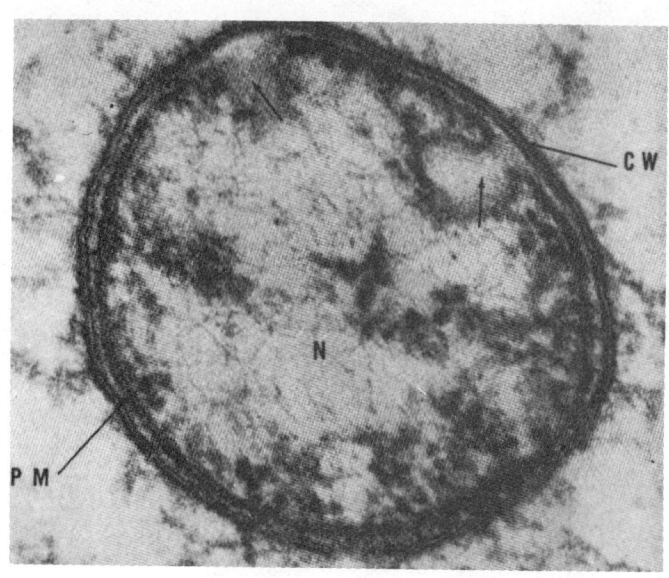

**FIGURE 4.** *Transverse section of R. quintana. Arrows designate multiple invaginations of the plasma membrane. Symbols are the same as those in Figure 3. × 190,000. (From Ito, S., and Vinson, J. W.: J Bacteriol 89:481, 1965.)*

properties of virulence and intracellular or extracellular survival.

The chemical composition of the rickettsial cell wall is similar to other gram-negative bacteria. It contains muramic acid, diaminopimelic acid, other amino acids, sugars, and amino sugars. Teichoic acid, a characteristic component of gram-positive bacteria, has not been found. Some years ago, Wood and Wisseman (1967) reported that *R. typhi* had endotoxic activity that suggested the possibility that it contained a lipopolysaccharide layer. More recently, Schramek and co-workers (1976) isolated lipopolysaccharide from the typhus group, the spotted fever group, and purified cells and soluble antigen preparations of the scrub typhus group. These workers have not yet reported a full chemical analysis of this rickettsial lipopolysaccharide, but they have analyzed similar preparations of lipopolysaccharide from purified phase 1 cells of *C. burnetii* (Schramek and Brezina, 1976). The lipopolysaccharide contains 17 fatty acids, including hydroxymyristic acid, which is a common constituent of most gram-negative bacterial lipopolysaccharides. The sugar moiety of *C. burnetii* lipopolysaccharide contains mannose, glucose, galactose, xylose, heptose, and 2-keto-3-deoxyoctonate (KDO). The presence of the amino sugars, glucosamine, galactosamine, and possibly fucosamine is further evidence of the similarity of this lipopolysaccharide to that of other gram-negative bacteria.

Rickettsiae contain both RNA and DNA. The RNA species include transfer RNA and ribosomal RNA. The size of the DNA genome is about one third that of *E. coli* and the same or slightly smaller than that of pathogenic *Neisseria*. Myers and Wisseman (1980) reported the genome to be about $1 \times 10^9$ daltons. Tyeryar et al. (1973) analyzed the base composition of rickettsial DNA and found a small but distinct difference in the molar percentage of guanine plus cytosine (G + C) between the typhus group (30 per cent) and the spotted fever group (32.5 per cent). Strains within each group show remarkable homogeneity of G + C content, even when isolated from widely separated geographic areas. *Rickettsia canada,* an organism that cross-reacts immunologically with members of both the typhus and the spotted fever groups, has a G + C content of 30 moles per cent, which suggests that it evolved from the typhus group. *C. burnetii* has a G + C content of 43 to 45 per cent (Schramek, 1968), distinctly different from other rickettsiae. *R. quintana's* G + C content of 38.6 moles per cent is also quite distinct. DNA-base composition can be identical in quite different organisms, however. The DNA-base ratio of typhus rickettsiae is identical to that of *Wolbachia persica,* a rickettsia-like symbiont of ticks, which has significant metabolic differences from typhus rickettsiae (Weiss, 1978).

## ANTIGENIC COMPOSITION

The typhus group of rickettsiae includes *R. prowazekii,* the cause of louse-borne epidemic typhus; *R. typhi,* also referred to as *R. mooseri,* the cause of flea-borne murine typhus; and *R. canada,* isolated from ticks in Canada. Members of this group possess common soluble antigens that are released into the aqueous phase during ether extraction of infected yolk sacs. These antigens cross-react in the complement fixation (CF) test. Members of the group can be distinguished from each other in the CF test by using washed whole rickettsial cells as the CF antigen.

The spotted fever group of rickettsiae includes representatives from all continents and Australia. Members of this group also possess common soluble antigens that are released into the aqueous phase by ether treatment of infected yolk sacs. The type species for the group, *R. rickettsii*, causes spotted fever in man in North America. Other members of this group that are pathogenic for man include Siberian tick typhus *(Dermacentroxenus sibericus)*, North Queensland tick typhus *(R. australis)*, fievre boutonneuse in the Mediterranean region *(R. conorii)*, and the cause of rickettsialpox *(R. akari)*. Washed rickettsial cells of each species are species-specific in the CF test. All spotted fever rickettsiae except *R. akari* cause acute toxic death of mice when inoculated live intravenously in high titer. In the so-called toxin neutralization test, rickettsiae and immune guinea pig sera are incubated together before inoculation. Neutralization of the toxic death is species-specific and distinguishes between members of the goup. A number of strains of spotted fever rickettsiae that are generally avirulent for guinea pigs have been isolated from different tick species in the West, Southwest, and Southeast regions of the United States. Some, like *R. parkeri* and *R. rhipicephalus,* have been given species designation (Burgdorfer et al., 1975). Other workers (Tarasevich et al., 1976; Urvolgyi and Brezina, 1978) have isolated from ticks spotted fever rickettsiae that are also distinguishable from the type species of their respective regions. A number of the tick and human strains of North American origin have been examined by Philip et al. (1978) by immunofluorescence with mouse antisera. They reported that all human isolates were identical to *R. rickettsii* and that the isolates from ticks can be sorted into one of eight other serotypes. None cross-reacted with *R. akari*. Rickettsiae of one serotype were not limited to one geographic locality. The serotypes may be grouped epidemiologically according to association with either one or more than one species of arthropod. Some serotypes were recovered from only one tick species and are apparently host-specific. They include *R. parkeri* from the Gulf Coast tick *Amblyomma maculatum;* an unclassified rickettsia from the rabbit tick, *Dermacentor parumapertus;* an unclassified rickettsia isolated many times from the Pacific Coast tick, *Ixodes pacificus;* and an unclassified rickettsia from another Pacific Coast tick, *Dermacentor occidentalis.* Rickettsiae of the five other serotypes were recovered from more than one species of ticks that were widely distributed in the United States. The tick species involved were *Haemaphysalis leporispalustris, Dermacentor andersoni, Dermacentor variabilis,* and *Rhipicephalus sanguineus.* The serotype to which all human isolates belonged was also recovered from the first three of the foregoing tick species. The stability of these antigenic characteristics is not known yet, but, if they prove to be genetically stable, they offer an interesting opportunity to search for antigenic markers of virulence for man among the spotted fever rickettsiae.

The scrub typhus group of rickettsiae is antigenically much more heterogeneous than the typhus and spotted fever groups. Yet, only one species, *R. tsutsugamushi,* is recognized. Soluble antigens extracted by ether treatment of infected yolk sacs are not group-reactive in the CF test. Therefore, members of the group are identified by a mouse vaccination-challenge procedure. A laboratory mouse that survives infection with one strain is immune to all other strains. Such broad heterologous immunity is unfortunately not seen in man, and an extraordinary amount of unsuccessful effort has been expended in attempts to overcome this vulnerability with a broadly protective vaccine. Three strains (Karp, Gilliam, and Kato), all isolated from human infections, have evolved into reference strains to which all other strains are compared. The full number of immunotypes of *R. tsutsugamushi* is still not known. Using the immunofluorescence procedure, Elisberg and co-workers (1968) identified six additional serotypes (as well as Karp, Gilliam, and Kato) from an array of human, larval mite, and wild small mammal isolates from Thailand. An immunofluorescence study of 74 isolates from Pakistan (Shirai and Wisseman, 1975) found almost all to be related to Karp. The remainder cross-reacted with Gilliam and/or Kato. Antigenic heterogeneity was also found by Russian workers in the Soviet Far East and in Tadjikistan and by Japanese workers throughout Japan. A single immunologic strain does not appear to be restricted to one species of mite vector. Implications of this strain diversity for the ecology of scrub typhus have been considered in a comprehensive review by Traub and Wisseman (1974).

## METABOLISM

Although rickettsiae produce some energy from independent metabolic activity, they are obligate intracellular parasites because their essential substrates must come from the host cell. Rickettsial respiration is stimulated most by glutamate, but less so by glutamine, which the rickettsia must deaminate to glutamate. Pyruvate and the dicarboxylic acid intermediates of the citric acid cycle support respiration to a much lesser extent. Glucose, glucose-6-phosphate, lactate, sucrose, and naturally occurring amino acids other than glutamate do not stimulate respiration. End products of glutamate metabolism include ammonia and carbon dioxide, but most of the amino group of glutamate is transaminated to form aspartate by glutamate-oxaloacetate transminase. Rickettsiae have a tricarboxylic acid cycle but not a complete glycolytic sequence and pentose shunt (Coolbaugh et al., 1976). In comparison with *Chlamydia*, *R. typhi* can generate appreciable amounts of energy. It has also been shown that typhus rickettsiae synthesize levels of monophosphate and diphosphate kinases comparable to those of *Salmonella typhimurium*. The fact that *C. burnetii* does catabolize glucose is further evidence of the great difference between this organism and other rickettsiae. All metabolic studies are hindered by the difficulties of harvesting viable undamaged whole cells or extracts free of host-cell material. The recent development of renografin density gradient centrifugation (Weiss et al., 1975) provides, for the first time, highly purified viable rickettsiae. Like other bacteria, rickettsiae have an electron-transport system, including nicotinamide adenine dinucleotide (NADPH) and NADPH-dependent enzymes. Oxidative energy can be converted into high energy phosphate bonds by formation of ATP. Rickettsiae can synthesize small amounts of protein as measured by incorporation of radiolabeled amino acids and the inhibition of this incorporation by chloramphenicol. The phosphorylation and stimulation of endogenous levels of adenine nucleotides by glutamate metabolism indicates that rickettsiae have the potential for sustained biosynthetic capabilities. However, the paucity of other nucleotides places severe restrictions on nucleic acid synthesis. Rickettsiae also synthesize lipids, but on a minute scale, similar to their synthesis of protein. These synthetic activities require the donation from outside the rickettsiae of complex energy-yielding substrates, including ATP.

One of the chief objectives of the studies of the metabolic pathways of rickettsiae is the definition and synthesis of an artificial medium that supports extracellular rickettsial growth. To date, this has not been achieved. Given the chemical composition and structural similarity between rickettsiae and other gram-negative bacteria, there is obviously some fundamental difference between the two that precludes extracellular growth of rickettsiae. Much attention has focused on the integrity and function of the rickettsial cell wall as a possible explanation for this difference. Moulder (1966) propounded the concept of "leakiness" of the cell wall. He suggested that rickettsial cell walls were nonspecifically porous and allowed passage of host-cell nutrients into intracellular rickettsiae, but allowed loss of essential nutrients from extracellular rickettsiae. Winkler (1976) disproved this thesis in a series of elegant experiments showing that rickettsial cell membranes are highly specialized and active rather than passive with respect to nutrient transport. He defined a carrier-mediated transport system that is very specific for ATP and ADP and the analog $\beta$, $\gamma$-methylene-ATP. The system is an obligatory exchange system in that a molecule can enter a cell only if another molecule can exit. The pool of ATP and ADP remains the same, but ATP can be acquired in exchange for ADP. Smith and Winkler (1977) defined a second system that actively transports lysine against a gradient. The system is highly specific only for L-lysine, D-lysine, and aminoethyl cysteine.

Rapid death of extracellular rickettsiae can be retarded by suspension in a medium composed of sucrose and glutamate in potassium phosphate buffered to pH 7.0 (SPG). This medium, devised years ago by Bovarnick et al. (1950), has been widely used to sustain rickettsiae during purification, metabolic studies, and titrations. Its performance was improved by the addition of serum albumin. Rickettsiae can be preserved for long periods frozen at minus 60° C, in whole yolk sac membranes or membranes triturated in SPG. In an effort to improve plaquing of rickettsiae, Wike et al. (1972) showed that extracellular infectivity and stability could be maintained more satisfactorily for short periods if rickettsiae were suspended in brain-heart infusion broth.

Rickettsiae multiply by transverse binary fission. Wisseman and Waddell (1975) have studied the kinetics of growth in irradiated chick embryo cells. As described by Weiss (1978), growth of *R. prowazekii* proceeded immediately if the inoculum was derived from rickettsiae harvested in the logarithmic phase of growth. There was a lag period of about 7.5 hours if rickettsiae were harvested in the stationary phase. The generation time of rickettsiae was slightly less than 9 hours at 34° C, and this rate continued for about 36 to 48 hours. After this period, heavily infected cells released their rickettsiae, and the cycle of growth became irregular.

Well-adapted strains of rickettsiae grow luxuriously in cell cytoplasm, often pushing the nucleus to one side, but they do not aggregate in the cytoplasm to form inclusion bodies like *Ehrlichia*. Spotted fever rickettsiae are distinguished by their ability to grow in the cell nucleus as well as the cytoplasm. *R. canada*, a member of the typhus group, also grows in the nucleus occasionally. Rickettsiae form plaques in monolayer cultures, and it is possible to clone strains. *R. rickettsii* forms plaques larger and faster than other rickettsiae. This is consistent with the independent observation that *R. rickettsii* is released from the cell and infects other cells at a much earlier stage of the growth cycle than either *R. prowazekii* or *R. tsutsugamushi*.

Rickettsiae require well-nourished host cells for growth, but the host cells do not need to multiply. It is possible, therefore, to stop host-cell metabolism with irradiation or colchicine and use these stationary cells as temporary microenvironments for the culture and study of rickettsiae. In such cells, rickettsiae may grow until the host cell bursts, but release of rickettsiae from actively metabolizing cells appears to occur also by extrusion. Schaechter et al. (1957) observed rickettsiae trapped in microfibrillar structures protruding from the edge of the cell. When the microfibrillae retracted, they either carried the rickettsiae back into the cytoplasm or released them to the outside. Stork and Wisseman (1976) have observed that *R. prowazekii* can infect and multiply in enucleated L and chicken embryo cells, but the rickettsiae do not achieve true exponential growth. This finding is consistent with the observations of Weiss (1973) that *R. typhi* continued to grow in cells that could not synthesize protein because of treatment with cycloheximide.

## PATHOGENIC PROPERTIES

Rickettsiae enter most mammalian cells by first attaching to the cell membrane and then being phagocytized. Attachment is not a casual process. Close contact is required; centrifugation of mixtures of entodermal cell cultures and rickettsiae increases penetration. Active participation of rickettsiae is also required. Ramm and Winkler (1973) have studied rickettsial red blood cell interactions as a possible model of cell penetrance. They showed that the lysis of sheep red blood cells required live rickettsiae. The erythrocyte was found to have a receptor for rickettsiae, a neutral lipid complex of cholesterol and palmitic acid. Energy poisons, such as potassium cyanide, inhibited both adsorption and lysis, and addition of ATP reactivated this rickettsial activity (Winkler, 1974). Scanning electronmicrographs revealed that rickettsiae adsorb end-on almost exclusively. Winkler and Ramm (1975) have also observed that rickettsiae harvested after lysing red blood cells can adsorb to other red blood cells. The mechanism of red blood cell lysis is unknown, but Winkler has observed in negative-stained preparations that lysed erythrocytes appear to be full of discrete holes. Hyperimmune rabbit serum inhibits adsorption but only by aggregation of rickettsiae. Hyperimmune serum enhances phagocytosis of rickettsiae by professional phagocytes, but it does not improve phagocytosis by such nonprofessional cells as endothelial cells and fibroblasts.

Once inside the cell, virulent rickettsiae can escape from the phagosome before it fuses with the lysosome and thus survive to multiply freely in the cell cytoplasm. By contrast, the avirulent Madrid E strain of *R. prowazekii* remains in the phagosome and is destroyed when the phagosome forms and the rickettsiae are exposed to lysosomal enzymes. Phagocytosed rickettsiae coated with immune serum are destroyed in professional phagocytes but survive in nonprofessional phagocytes. In contrast, *C. burnetii* remains in the phagosome and multiplies, protected by unknown means from the lysosomal hydrolases.

For experimental work, rickettsiae are usually cultivated in fertile hen eggs, tissue cultures, and small laboratory animals. The minimum infectious dose for eggs has been estimated to be one infectious rickettsia for the Madrid E strain of *R. prowazekii*. Ley et al. (1952) also estimated that only one *R. tsutsugamushi* organism could cause human disease. The optimum growth temperature for *R. rickettsii* is about 33.5° C and for other rickettsiae about 35° C. Large numbers of rickettsiae can be harvested from infected yolk sacs of chicken embryos (Cox, 1938), and this is usually the source of rickettsiae for a wide variety of investigations and for preparation of diagnostic antigens. Many host cell-parasite relationships have been worked out in explant and continuous-cell-line tissue cultures. Small laboratory animals are used chiefly for isolation of rickettsiae from patients. Guinea pigs are the animal of choice for typhus and the spotted fever group, and the laboratory mouse for scrub typhus (see *Laboratory Diagnosis*).

The basic lesion caused by rickettsiae is a vasculitis, localized to the endothelium and smooth muscle of the vessel wall. The lesion contains rickettsiae. There is endothelial swelling, thrombosis, and vascular and perivascular necrosis. Vascular permeability is increased. The infected host displays varying degrees of hemorrhage, tissue edema, and peripheral circulatory failure. Depending on the distribution of the vasculitis, the patient develops a petechial rash, frank hemorrhage into the skin, gangrene of appendages, interstitial inflammation of major viscera, lymph node hyperplasia, and meningoencephalitis. The circulatory failure of severe rickettsial disease has been studied by Harrell and Aikawa (1949). Plasma volume is decreased, and the extravascular fluid spaces are increased. The pathophysiology has been studied in experimental hosts including the guinea pig, rabbit, and monkey. Different species of rickettsiae have typical pathophysiologic manifestations, as shown by variations in the diseases they cause in man. Each pathogenic species causes some infections in man and experimental animals, however, that are entirely inapparent and others that are so severe as to be lethal. In some geographic regions, inapparent infection is the rule. As yet, there are no defined markers that distinguish virulent from avirulent rickettsiae in terms of host response to infection, nor is there clear evidence for any mechanism of rickettsiae-induced pathophysiology other than direct cell invasion and injury by live rickettsiae. De Brito et al. (1968) found gamma globulin and complement in late vascular lesions of guinea pigs infected with *R. rickettsii*, which suggests that immune complex vasculitis occurs in spotted fever. More recently, Walker and Henderson (1978) studied *R. rickettsii* infection in the immunosuppressed guinea pig. They found as severe a vasculitis in the immunosuppressed as in control animals and argued that rickettsiae damage cells without the participation of immune mechanisms.

Schramek, Brezina, and Tarasevich (1976) have reported isolation of lipopolysaccharide antigens from *R. prowazekii, R. typhi, R. canada, R. conorii,* and *R. tsutsugamushi.* From hypothermic reactions in intraperitoneally inoculated white rats and chemical analysis, they concluded that these antigens had endotoxic properties. Full characterization of a rickettsial endotoxin has not been reported. Nevertheless, the endotoxin hypothesis is attractive as an explanation of some aspects of rickettsial pathophysiology.

Yamada and co-workers (1978) reported activation of the kallikrein-kinin system in five patients with American spotted fever. Four had petechial rashes characteristic of vasculitis and then developed disseminated intravascular coagulation. They concluded that even if kinins do not initiate the early vascular changes, they may promote progression of the lesions.

Despite these studies of the basic pathology and pathogenic properties of rickettsiae, the virulence factors are still largely unknown. The attenuated Madrid E strain of *R. prowazekii* (Perez, 1963), in contrast to fully virulent strains, disappears quickly from the tissues of guinea pigs, so that serial passage is usually unsuccessful. It does not differ substantially from virulent strains, however, in a variety of other properties, including toxicity for mice, hemolytic activity, infectivity for body lice, antigenic characteristics, and quantity of slime layer. There is no difference in its

ability to infect and grow in chicken embryo cells and a variety of other cell lines. It does differ in one important respect: in human macrophages, the Madrid E strain cannot escape from the phagosome and is killed by lysosomal hydrolases. This may be the mechanism of its attenuation.

The stability of the E strain has been questioned by Russian (Balayeva and Nikolskaja, 1972) and Slovak (Kažar et al., 1973) workers who noted reversion to full virulence for guinea pigs after prolonged serial passage in the mouse lung and the guinea pig peritoneum. It is unclear whether this phenomenon represents selection of a virulent strain from a mixture that is predominantly avirulent or is a true back-mutation. Studies with cloned E strains have not been reported.

There have been many studies of the virulence of spotted fever rickettsiae. Long ago it was observed that inoculation of rickettsiae into guinea pigs from unfed adult ticks *(Dermacentor andersoni)* would produce immunity but no disease. If the ticks were given a blood meal before harvest and inoculation of rickettsiae, the guinea pigs became sick. Later, Spencer and Parker reexamined this phenomenon by inoculating a virulent strain of *R. rickettsii* into adult ticks and storing them for several months at refrigerator temperature. Inoculation at this point produced, as before, immunity but no disease in guinea pigs. If the ticks were warmed first or fed a blood meal, virulence for guinea pigs was restored. Close examination of this phenomenon showed that it was not caused by an increase in the number of rickettsiae (Gilford and Price, 1955). Addition of para-aminobenzoic acid (PABA), parahydroxybenzoic acid, or PABA plus coenzyme A to rickettsiae held for 60 hours at 25° C restored virulence to the stored rickettsiae. Virulence could also be restored by incubating the rickettsiae with recently fed and ground-up ticks.

Generally, the virulence of rickettsiae for laboratory animals does not parallel virulence for man. However, there does appear to be a consistent geographic difference in the virulence of scrub typhus rickettsiae for man. A strain from the Pescadores Islands, where disease is characteristically mild, was used as a live vaccine in Japan. Disease contracted during the winter months in Japan is said to be much milder than disease contracted in the warmer months. It is interesting that different mite vectors are involved in the Pescadores and during different seasons in Japan. Certainly, scrub typhus is commonly very mild in Southeast Asia, where the predominant vector mite is still another species. Because a good marker for virulence is lacking, it is not possible to examine the stability of rickettsial virulence during passage through different species of mites.

## IMMUNOLOGY

Natural host resistance to infection must be considered in assessments of rickettsial virulence. Groves and Osterman (1978) examined genetic resistance to lethal infections with *R. tsutsugamushi* in over 30 inbred strains of mice. They found some strains fully resistant, some fully susceptible, and a few selectively resistant to lethal infection with the Gilliam strain of scrub typhus rickettsiae. Resistance was genetically dominant and controlled by a single gene or a closely linked cluster of autosomal genes. Resistance was not due to an inability of host cells to support rickettsial growth. Susceptibility, on the other hand, was not due to inability to mount an immune response. Russian workers (Kokorin et al., 1976) analyzed the same phenomenon and noted a marked difference in the reaction of the macrophages of resistant and suceptible mice. Fatal infection was accompanied by death of macrophages and peritoneal necrosis. The resistant mice showed no clinical signs of infection but mounted an intensive macrophage reaction at the inoculation site. Most of the inoculated rickettsiae died at the inoculation site, and the macrophages remained viable. Some rickettsiae survive and persist in resistant mice for a long time without producing overt clinical disease. Recently, Anderson and Osterman (1980) have also observed a genetic basis for natural resistance to lethal infection with *R. akari* (rickettsialpox).

Rickettsiae stimulate both humoral and cellular immunity. The role of each in response to infection of man and animals is not completely understood. Humoral antibody appears in response to rickettsial infections between the seventh and fourteenth days of disease. Passive transfer of immune serum provides protection against clinical disease in animals challenged with the same strain. Persistence of rickettsiae in immune people and animals without recrudescence of disease may be the result of protection by humoral antibody, but humoral antibody is clearly not the sole factor in immunity to rickettsiae. Cellular immune processes also occur, as shown by the development of dermal hypersensitivity, lymphocyte transformation, and elaboration of migration-inhibiting factor.

Recent studies of *R. tsutsugamushi* and *C. burnetii* revealed some details of the immune process. Shirai and co-workers (1976) have shown that passive transfer of spleen cells from infected mice protects the recipient against challenge with homologous and heterologous strains of *R. tsut-*

*sugamushi*. The protective spleen cells were thymus-dependent lymphocytes. Subsequently, these investigators (Catanzaro et al., 1977) demonstrated that peritoneal exudate lymphocytes (PEL) were the mediators of this cellular protection. It was not possible to determine from their experiments whether PELs were the primary mediators, as they are in other bacterial infections. Subsequently, Nacy and Osterman (1979) determined that protective splenic lymphocytes elaborated lymphokines that activate the killer macrophages.

## LABORATORY DIAGNOSIS

Isolation of rickettsiae should ordinarily be attempted only in a research laboratory. Isolation is accomplished preferably by immediate (within one hour of collection) intraperitoneal inoculation of the specimen into a suitable experimental animal. The isolation host of choice for the typhus and spotted fever groups of rickettsiae is the guinea pig and for scrub typhus the laboratory mouse. The most appropriate isolation specimen for human diagnosis is blood clot prepared as a 10 per cent suspension in skim milk or brain-heart infusion broth. Other diluents adversely affect rickettsiae. Several passages of tissue from inoculated animals at approximately 14-day intervals may be necessary before symptomatic infection develops. In guinea pigs, the only indication may be an increase in rectal temperature, which must be recorded daily from the time of inoculation. On the first passage of typhus group rickettsiae, fever does not appear until the third week after inoculation. Either brain or spleen should be harvested from the febrile animal and inoculated intraperitoneally into other guinea pigs. If no fever or other evidence of infection occurs, animals in the second or third passage are bled on day 28 for antibody studies. Antibody may be the only evidence that rickettsiae have been isolated. The only gross evidence of *R. prowazekii* infection in the guinea pig is a fibrous exudate on the spleen surface. Examination of smears taken from scrapings of the spleen surface may show rickettsiae in serosal cells. If the inoculum of rickettsiae is large, the scrotum may enlarge, and the testes may adhere to the scrotal sac. This lesion is called the Neill-Mooser reaction after the investigators who discovered it. The lesion is much more often found in *R. typhi* infections and occurs at the time of fever. In other respects, *R. typhi* infections are like those of *R. prowazekii*, except that the incubation period of established infections is shorter (three to seven days), and the Neill-Mooser reaction is more severe. The isolated rickettsiae are identified by using the rickettsiae as antigen in the CF or other serologic test against various antisera and by cross-vaccination and challenge against known rickettsiae.

The response of guinea pigs to virulent spotted fever group rickettsiae is more severe. After several passages to establish the isolate, the incubation period is shortened to two to five days, the fever course is often prolonged, and the animals may die on the sixth to eighth day. A severe scrotal reaction usually begins on the third or fourth day of fever and first consists of edema and erythema. The scrotum becomes necrotic with eventual tissue sloughing. Gangrene of the ears and footpads may also occur. As in infections with the typhus group, necropsy findings consist chiefly of a fibrinous exudate on the spleen surface and the scrotal reaction.

Scrub typhus rickettsiae are isolated by intraperitoneal inoculation of the white laboratory mouse. Several passages of infected liver, spleen, or brain may be required to establish the agent. Gross signs of infection include ruffled fur and a swollen abdomen. Necropsy reveals an enlarged spleen and mucoid peritoneal fluid. Scrapings of the peritoneal lining yield mesothelial cells containing rickettsiae in the cytoplasm.

Rickettsiae can be isolated by inoculation either into the yolk sac of the hen eggs or into tissue cultures. Adaptation to these substrates is often slow, and small inocula may be lost. Laboratory acquired infection is a constant hazard, even in the most sophisticated laboratory (Oster et al., 1977), so isolation of rickettsiae should be attempted only by experienced personnel in well-equipped facilities. Identification of rickettsiae or rickettsial antigen in the first week of disease would greatly assist clinicians to diagnose atypical cases. DeShazo et al. (1976) diagnosed Rocky Mountain spotted fever by the fourth day of disease in rhesus monkeys upon identification of R. rickettsii by immunofluorescence in primary monocyte culture. Shirai et al. (1978) achieved similar results in R. tsutsugamushi infections of monkeys and dogs. Coolbaugh and colleagues (1978) have used this procedure for the early diagnosis of a human case of scrub typhus. For pathologic specimens, Walker and Cain (1978) have described a method allowing retrospective analysis of fixed, paraffin-embedded tissue by R. rickettsii-specific immunofluorescence. The diagnosis of R. rickettsii infection may also be suggested by examination of ticks taken from patients. Burgdorfer (1970) identified R. rickettsii by immunofluorescent examination of the hemolymph of live ticks. In desiccated ticks, rickettsial antigen may be detected by immunofluorescence for several weeks (Kurz and Burgdorfer, 1978).

Human rickettsial antibodies are detectable by many serologic procedures. Complement fixation has been the most widely used specific test because antigens for the typhus and spotted fever groups have been available commercially or from central reference laboratories. Group-specific soluble antigen is prepared by ether extraction of infected yolk sacs of embryonated hen eggs. The antigen is inactivated. Typhus group antigen is prepared from R. typhi, while spotted fever is usually prepared from R. akari. The CF test can be made species-specific by using washed rickettsial cell suspensions as antigen. For diagnosis of spotted fever infections in various parts of the world, it is best to use the prevalent rickettsial species as antigen since R. akari, while broadly group-reactive, does not detect CF antibody to all the spotted fevers. Scrub typhus-soluble CF antigens are principally strain-specific, and the CF test is unsuitable for group diagnosis.

The indirect microimmunofluorescence procedure (Bozeman and Elisberg, 1963) is increasingly employed for serologic diagnosis. Concentrated suspensions of rickettsiae from infected yolk sacs or cell culture are used as antigen. In the micro-technique, many antigen spots can be applied to one slide. After air drying and fixation in acetone, the slides may be stored at −70° C for later use. Philip and co-workers (1977) have compared this procedure with others for the diagnosis of both typhus and spotted fever group infections. In their hands, it was superior to the CF test for identifying disease.

Rickettsial agglutination has been used for many years for the diagnosis of a variety of rickettsial infections by French workers and has been widely used by others for the diagnosis of Q fever. A microagglutination procedure (Fiset et al., 1969) conserves antigen (washed rickettsial suspensions).

Chang et al. (1954) performed hemagglutination with an erythrocyte-sensitizing substance (ESS) from typhus and spotted fever group rickettsiae. This antigen, which depends for its activity on a carbohydrate moiety (Osterman and Eiseman, 1978), has not been isolated from R. tsutsugamushi. The hemagglutination and microagglutination procedures compare favorably with the microimmunofluorescence procedure for the diagnosis of North American spotted fever (Philip et al., 1977).

Because CF antibodies are not found until the third week of disease, much effort has been expended to develop procedures for early diagnosis. The indirect immunofluorescence procedure, the indirect hemagglutination test, and the ELISA (enzyme-linked immunosorbent assay) all detect antibodies as early as the sixth to seventh day of disease. Woodward et al. (1976) demonstrated R. rickettsii in skin biopsy specimens from two patients on days 4 and 8 of illness by direct immunofluorescence. While confirming this experience in some patients, other workers have failed to identify rickettsiae in skin biopsies from patients already treated with tetracycline or chloramphenicol. Years ago, Fleck et al. (1960) found murine typhus antigen in the urine by indirect hemagglutination, but this early diagnostic technique has not been evaluated by others.

Specific rickettsial antibody appears by the end of the first week of disease in human and animal infections and persists in some cases for years. Rickettsemia and circulating specific antibody are detectable in the same blood specimens during disease and convalescence. Humans respond early to primary typhus infection with IgM antibodies, but this class of antibody is not recalled in recrudescent typhus (Murray et al., 1965). Philip and co-workers (1976) found IgM antibodies by microimmunofluorescence early in American spotted fever patients but noted its absence in 15 per cent of them. IgM antibody usually disappears within three to four months. IgG antibody usually appears by the third week of disease and persists for one or more years.

The antibody response can be suppressed by antibiotics early in the disease. Patients with American spotted fever that were treated early, especially during the first two days of illness, were less likely to be seropositive and had lower titers of antibody by the CF test during convalescence (Philip et al., 1977). Smadel (1954) also observed delayed or diminished antibody production by patients who were treated for scrub typhus by the third day of disease but there was no effect when therapy was started on the sixth day or later. It is assumed that early treatment suppresses antibody production by reducing the antigenic mass.

Antigenic cross-reactions occur between the typhus and spotted fever groups. The degree of cross-reactivity reflects not only the extent of shared antigens but also the species of host involved. Ormsbee et al. (1978) found that most patients who were acutely ill with epidemic typhus produced IgG and IgM antibodies to purified antigens of *R. prowazekii, R. typhi,* and *R. canada.* They also produced IgG, but seldom IgM, antibodies to spotted fever rickettsiae. Similarly, patients acutely ill with spotted fever produced IgG and IgM antibodies to *R. rickettsii, R. conorii,* and *R. akari,* as well as both classes of antibody to the typhus group. By contrast, the mouse produces species-specific rickettsial antibody. Ormsbee et al. (1978) have speculated that the more specific rodent antibody response reflects the greater antiquity of this host-parasite relationship. Scrub typhus and Q fever rickettsiae do not share antigens with other rickettsiae. The degree of heterologous antibody response in spotted fever

and typhus infections is usually less than the homologous response, which helps clarify the serologic diagnosis of these infections. Prior immunization with epidemic typhus or spotted fever vaccine can cause confusion in the serologic findings because the anamnestic response of vaccine-induced antibody may exceed that stimulated by infection.

Rickettsiae share antigens with other bacteria. The antigens shared with *Proteus* organisms form the basis of the Weil-Felix agglutination test. For many years, this test was the only serologic test widely available for the diagnosis of rickettsial disease. The shared antigens have never been fully characterized, but years ago Castaneda (1934) described a carbohydrate antigen shared by *Proteus vulgaris* OX-19 and *R. prowazekii.* In human typhus, agglutinins occur chiefly against OX-19 and, to a much lesser extent, to the OX-2 strain. These agglutinins are rarely found in recrudescent typhus (Brill-Zinsser disease), although Ormsbee and co-workers (1977) found a brisk agglutinin response in two of five cases in Ethiopia. The cross-reactive antibody response stimulated by the spotted fever groups varies widely. Some patients produce chiefly OX-19 antibody, some chiefly OX-2, and some both. Therefore, the Weil-Felix agglutinins do not distinguish spotted fever from typhus group infections. Scrub typhus may stimulate production of agglutinins to *Proteus mirabilis* strain OXK. A titer of 1:200 or greater suggests infection. Because these antigens are commercially available, and the procedures are simple, physicians have relied on the Weil-Felix agglutination tests for rickettsial diagnosis. With the development of other procedures that use strain-specific antigens that are also noninfectious, the Weil-Felix test should be discarded. It is unreliable because agglutinins are often absent in proven rickettsial disease, especially scrub typhus. Furthermore, the presence of agglutinins may only indicate infection with *Proteus* or other bacteria (Hechemy et al., 1970). Infections with *R. akari* and *C. burnetii* do not produce Weil-Felix agglutinins.

## DRUG SUSCEPTIBILITY

The growth of rickettsiae is inhibited by chloramphenicol and the tetracyclines that are given for treatment of rickettsial diseases. Penicillin and streptomycin are of no clinical value but are slightly inhibitory to rickettsiae. Sulfonamides have no effect on rickettsiae. On the other hand, para-aminobenzoic acid, an antagonist of sulfonamides, inhibits most rickettsiae, but *R. tsutsugamushi* is affected only slightly and *C. burnetii* not at all. Ormsbee et al. (1955) studied the relative inhibitory effect of various antibiotics in infected chicken embryos and found that the inhibitory dose of oxytetracycline for typhus and spotted fever rickettsiae was about one-eighth that of chlortetracycline, which was one third as active as chloramphenicol. Erythromycin was highly inhibitory for *R. prowazekii,* less so for spotted fever rickettsiae, and almost not at all for *C. burnetii.* Chloramphenicol is also relatively inactive against *C. burnetii. R. tsutsugamushi* is as sensitive to chloramphenicol and the tetracyclines in laboratory culture as the spotted fever rickettsiae. Doxycycline, a long-acting tetracycline, is highly effective clinically against the typhus group and *R. tsutsugamushi.*

Growth-inhibiting antibiotics do not eliminate viable rickettsiae from infected people. *R. tsutsugamushi* can persist in lymph nodes for years after recovery from infection. Persistence of *R. prowazekii* in patients who had survived an attack of epidemic typhus in the preantibiotic era was dramatically illustrated by recrudescent disease long after they had emigrated from endemic areas of Europe to America. Recrudescent typhus is called Brill-Zinsser disease. In laboratory animals that survive a rickettsial infection, recrudescent disease can be provoked by administration of cortisone. It is assumed that cortisone in animals mimics stress in man, which seems to modify the steady-state host-parasite relationship and permit rickettsiae to proliferate. Clinical recrudescence of other rickettsial diseases long after recovery has not been observed, but persistence of viable rickettsiae after treatment indicates that these drugs are rickettsiostatic. Continous exposure of *R. tsutsugamushi* in cultured L-cells to high concentrations of chloramphenicol eventually sterilized the culture, but only after three weeks.

Antibiotic-resistant strains of rickettsiae have not been isolated from nature. Many serial passages of the Madrid E strain of *R. prowazekii* in the presence of increasing amounts of chloramphenicol did yield a substrain resistant to chloramphenicol (Weiss and Dressler, 1962). Resistance was not lost during 10 drugless egg passages. Weiss and Dressler (1960) isolated an erythromycin-resistant strain by the same procedure but could not induce resistance to tetracycline.

## HOST RANGE

The human pathogens among the rickettsiae are distributed widely in many arthropods and mammals. Among the typhus group, *R. prowazekii* parasitizes both the head and body varieties of the human louse, *Pediculus humanis.* The human body louse is the major vector of classic epidemic typhus. *R. prowazekii* infects only the gut epithelium of the louse, which acquires the rickettsiae by feeding on the blood of a rickettsemic human. After a few days, proliferating rickettsiae burst the epithelial cells of the gut and appear in the louse feces. The louse usually dies from the infection within 7 to 10 days. Its salivary glands are not infected. Man acquires the infection from the louse by scratching the skin that has become contaminated with rickettsiae-containing louse feces (autoinoculation). Until recently, it was believed that the only cycle of *R. prowazekii* in nature was man-louse-man. Man was thought to be the reservoir because the louse does not pass the rickettsiae from generation to generation transovarially like other rickettsiae of ticks and mites. Recently, Bozeman and co-workers (1975), in a remarkable series of studies, demonstrated the first nonhuman mammalian host of *R. prowazekii,* the American flying squirrel *(Glaucomys volans).* They found enzootic foci in flying squirrels from Florida, North Carolina, Virginia, and Maryland and also recovered rickettsiae from the squirrel lice and fleas. The squirrel flea is known to feed on man. The strains of rickettsiae isolated from flying squirrels have been identified as *R. prowazekii* (Dasch et al., 1978). McDade and co-workers (1980) have just reported that examination of sera from 7 of 1575 persons for rickettsial antibodies from 1976 through 1978 suggested recent infection with *R. prowazekii.* Two of the seven patients had had contact with flying squirrels. Reiss-Gutfreund (1966) reported infection with *R. prowazekii* in domestic animals and their ticks in Ethiopia that seemed to confirm earlier reports of epidemic typhus antibodies in domestic animals as well as man in the Upper Volta, Ruwanda-Burundi, and the Central African Republic. But other workers are skeptical (Burgdorfer et al., 1972).

*R. typhi* is found naturally in rats and mice. It is transmitted from rat to rat by the rat louse and the rat flea, *Xenopsylla cheopis,* which is usually the vector to man. Many other wild animals are also susceptible to *R. prowazekii.* The host range of *R. canada* is not well defined. It has been isolated in nature only from *Haemophysalis leporispalustris* ticks in Ontario, Canada (McKiel et al., 1967).

The host ranges of the spotted fever group and scrub typhus group are discussed in the chapters on each disease.

# Q FEVER RICKETTSIAE

*Coxiella burnetii* has been placed in a separate genus because it differs in many ways from other rickettsiae (Table 1). The differences have been summarized well by Ormsbee (1969). *C. burnetii* stains gram-positive when alcoholic iodine is used as mordant instead of aqueous iodine. Under these conditions, rickettsiae stain gram-negative. Rickettsiae release a soluble antigen when aqueous suspensions of cells are shaken in ether. *C. burnetii*, like other gram-negative bacteria, does not. Immunizing antigens of *C. burnetii* are very resistant to heat, whereas those of rickettsiae are heat-sensitive. The guanine plus cytosine molar per cent content of *C. burnetii* DNA is about 43 per cent, whereas rickettsiae have a G + C content in the range of 30 to 32.5 per cent. *C. burnetii* is remarkably resistant to physical and chemical agents. It survives in wool for seven to nine months at 20° C, at least two years in skim milk and tap water at 15 to 20° C, and for about six months in dried blood at room temperature. Disinfection of *C. burnetii* requires exposure to 5 per cent $H_2O_2$ or 2 per cent formaldehyde. Because of the extraordinary survival of *C. burnetii* in the extracellular environment, it probably infects man more often by the aerosol route than by tick transmission. Rickettsiae are generally transmitted to man by arthropods. The energy-producing metabolism of *C. burnetii* is quite different from that of rickettsiae. *C. burnetii* metabolizes pyruvate, synthesizes enzymes of the Embden-Meyerhof pathway, and contains many enzymes generally associated with the catabolism of glucose. Rickettsiae synthesize none of these enzymes.

The extraordinary extracellular resistance of *C. burnetii* may simply reflect its intracellular behavior, which is quite distinct from that of rickettsiae. *C. burnetii* enters the cell in phagosomes, remains there even as the phagosomes fuse with lysosomes, and can protect itself from the harsh action of lysosomal hydrolases. Rickett-

**TABLE 1.   Differences Between *Coxiella burnetii* and the Rickettsiae**

|  | C. burnetii | RICKETTSIAE |
|---|---|---|
| Gram stain (alcohol mordant) | Gram-positive | Gram-negative |
| Soluble antigen released with ether | No | Yes |
| Immunizing antigens | Heat-resistant | Heat-sensitive |
| Guanine plus cytosine molar per cent | 43 | 30 to 32.5 |
| Usual route of infection | Aerosol | Arthropods |
| Embden-Meyerhof pathway | Yes | No |
| Persistence in phagosomes | Yes | No |
| Susceptibility to chloramphenicol and erythromycin | ± | ++++ |
| Acute toxicity for mice | No | Yes |
| Phase variation | Yes | No |

siae quickly escape from the phagosome and exist free in the cell cytoplasm. Growth of *C. burnetii* in experimental yolk sac infections is only slightly affected by chloramphenicol and erythromycin, which are highly rickettsiostatic. *C. burnetii* is sensitive to the tetracyclines, however. Unlike certain rickettsiae, live *C. burnetii* do not cause acute toxic death of mice when inoculated intravenously in high titer. Finally, *C. burnetii* exhibits a unique phase variation, which is host-controlled. *C. burnetii* exists in nature only in Phase I. When cultivated in chick embryos, the organism shifts to Phase II but reverts to Phase I upon passage through laboratory animals. The significance of phase variation has been a topic of intense study since it was originally recognized by Stoker et al. (1955). Shift in phase is accompanied by changes in major antigenic components, pathogenicity, immunogenicity, buoyant density, agglutinability, staining properties, resistance to phagocytosis, and pyrogenicity. Phase variation appears to represent a phenotypic rather than a genotypic change. There is no discernible morphologic difference between phases of *C. burnetii*.

# ROCHALIMAEA QUINTANA

This organism causes trench fever in man. It was originally recognized as a natural inhabitant of the gut lumen of the human body louse in the course of studies undertaken to elucidate the etiology of louse-borne epidemic typhus during World War I. Although it was called a rickettsia for many years, this organism has been reclassified into its own genus because it is usually

located extracellularly and can be cultivated on cell-free media. The organism is named for the Brazilian scientist H. da Rocha-Lima, who was one of the early investigators of rickettsial diseases, and for the form of the disease, in which febrile episodes recur after every fifth (quintana) day without fever.

The organisms resemble rickettsiae in size and

cell structure. The cell wall is similar to that of rickettsiae in chemical composition (Osterman et al., 1974) and in structure by electron microscopy (Ito and Vinson, 1965). It multiplies by binary fission and, like rickettsiae, metabolizes glutamine and succinate but not glucose. It is gram-negative and stains like rickettsiae in the Giminez and Macchiavello stains. It is susceptible to inactivation by standard disinfectants, but it survives for months in dried louse feces, like *R. prowazekii.*

*R. quintana* is distinct from all other rickettsiae in its G + C content of 38.5 moles per cent. This characteristic contributed to the recent identification of Baker's vole agent as *R. quintana* (see Chapter 191). This was the first isolation of *R. quintana* in nature from a nonhuman mammalian source (Weiss et al., 1978).

The second major difference of *R. quintana* from rickettsiae is its capacity to grow on cell-free media. It was first cultivated by Vinson (1966) on a blood agar base enriched with 6 per cent horse serum inactivated at 56° C for 30 minutes and 4 per cent washed, hemolyzed horse erythrocytes incubated at 37° C in a moist atmosphere of 5 per cent $CO_2$ in air. After 12 to 14 days incubation, colonies are round, lenticular, translucent, mucoid, and 65 to 200 $\mu$ in diameter. Colonies develop only on the surface of the agar. Organisms do not multiply without added carbon dioxide nor under anaerobic conditions. Mason (1970) developed a liquid culture medium for study of the growth cycle of *R. quintana* and noted that fetal calf serum could be substituted for the erythrocyte lysate. The growth cycle was characterized by a lag phase of approximately 24 hours, an exponential growth phase of 72 hours, and a doubling time of approximately 4.5 hours. Myers and co-workers (1972) demonstrated a growth requirement for hematin and concluded that the hematin was required as a precursor in the synthesis of various heme-proteins. *R. quintana* would not grow on hematin substitutes that satisfied other hematin-requiring bacteria. Apparently, it absolutely requires hematin for the synthesis of heme-proteins. *R. quintana* does not appear to produce $H_2O_2$ and is catalase-negative (Myers et al., 1972).

The only experimental host for *R. quintana* is the rhesus monkey (Mooser and Weyer, 1953), but specific antibody can be produced in rabbits and guinea pigs immunized with soluble or whole cell antigens in Freund's adjuvant (Herrmann et al., 1977). A number of serologic procedures detect *R. quintana* antibody in man, including complement fixation, (Vinson and Campbell, 1968); passive hemagglutination (Cooper et al., 1976); enzyme immunoassay; and radioimmunoprecipitation tests (Herrmann et al., 1977). Hollingdale and co-workers (1978) examined sera by the enzyme immunoassay method from patients with various rickettsial infections. Nine of 15 sera from patients with typhus group infections, 2 of 7 sera from *R. rickettsii* infections, and 3 of 6 sera from scrub typhus infections produced antibody to *R. quintana* antigen. Cross-reactions also occurred in guinea pigs infected with scrub typhus. These findings suggest that *R. quintana* shares antigens with rickettsiae. Seroepidemiologic studies, which have not yet been undertaken on a broad scale, must take these cross-reactions into account.

# RICKETTSIA SENNETSU

In 1954, two Japanese groups (Fukuda, 1954; Misao and Kobayashi, 1954) reported the isolation of a rickettsia-like agent from patients with an infectious mononucleosis-like syndrome on the island of Kyushu. Subsequent studies established *R. sennetsu* to be immunologically distinct from *R. tsutsugamushi;* from *Neorickettsia helminthoeca,* the cause of salmon poisoning in dogs; and from Elokomin fluke fever agent, the cause of a similar lymphadenopathy in bears and raccoons in the Pacific Northwest of the United States (Kitao et al., 1973). Korb and co-workers (1966) in Czechoslovakia examined sera from 17 patients with clinical infectious mononucleosis. They, and other European workers, concluded that there was no good evidence to associate *R. sennetsu* with infectious mononucleosis in central Europe.

Electronmicrographs show that *R. sennetsu* resides within an intracytoplasmic vesicle (Fig. 5) in contrast to other rickettsiae, which lie free in the cytoplasm (Anderson et al., 1965). Huxsoll recognized that this property was similar to that of organisms of the genus *Ehrlichia,* which is taxonomically close to *Rickettsia* but pathogenic for animals. Recent studies by Huxsoll, Ristic, and colleagues (personal communication) suggest an immunologic relationship between *R. sennetsu* and *Ehrlichia canis,* a tick-borne disease agent of dogs found in many parts of the world. It is not yet known whether *R. sennetsu* is tick-transmitted to man, like *Ehrlichia,* or is transmitted by eating raw fish, like salmon poisoning in dogs. The discovery of this interesting disease agent and its possible relationship to *Ehrlichia*

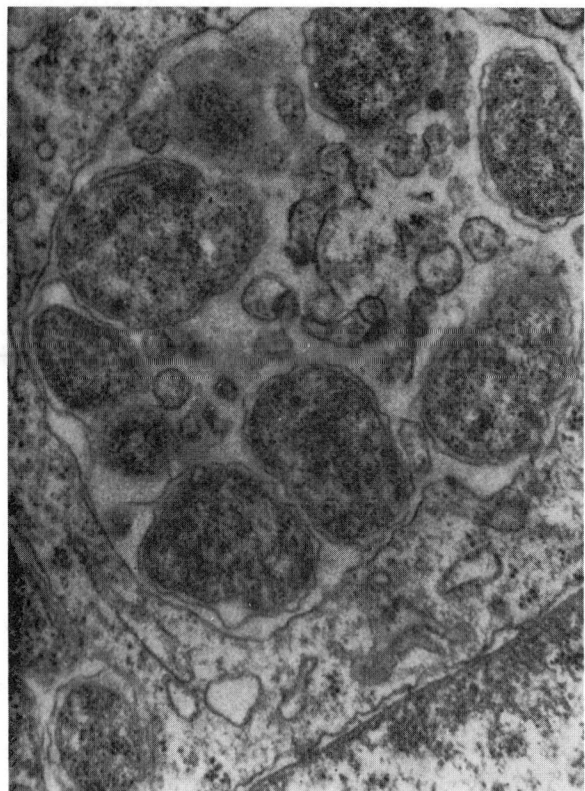

**FIGURE 5.** R. sennetsui *in a distended vacuole. Several organisms are enclosed in a membrane-lined vacuole. Note that each organism is enclosed by a cell wall and a plasma membrane. ×30,000. (From Anderson, D. R., et al.: J Bacteriol 90:1387, 1965.)*

underscores the importance of considering agents of animal disease when searching for the specific etiology of obscure human febrile diseases. These studies will not always be as rewarding as those on *R. sennetsu* mononucleosis. An example of one of these febrile diseases that still remains obscure is Kawasaki disease (or mucocutaneous lymph node syndrome of infants and children), first reported by Kawasaki on the basis of 50 cases in Tokyo (see Chapter 201). Hamashima et al. (1973) reported rickettsia-like bodies by electron microscopy of skin and lymph node biopsies, but others cannot confirm these results. The unresponsiveness of the disease to antibiotics suggests an alternate etiology.

## REFERENCES

Anacker, R. L., Pickens, E. G., and Lackman, D. B.: Details of the ultrastructure of *Rickettsia prowazekii* grown in the chick yolk sac. J Bacteriol 94:260, 1967.

Anderson, D. R., Hopps, H. E., Barile, M. F., and Bernheim, B. C.: Comparison of the ultrastructure of several rickettsiae, ornithosis virus, and mycoplasma in tissue culture. J Bacteriol 90:1387, 1965.

Anderson, G. W., and Osterman, J. V.: Host defenses in experimental rickettsialpox: Genetics of natural resistance to infection. Infect Immun 28:132, 1980.

Balayeva, N. M., and Nikolskaya, V. N.: Enhanced virulence of the vaccine strain E of *Rickettsia prowazekii* on passaging in white mice and guinea pigs. Acta Virol 16:80, 1972.

Bovarnick, M. R., Miller, J. C., and Snyder, J. C.: The influence of certain salts, amino acids, sugars, and proteins on the stability of rickettsiae. J Bacteriol 59:509, 1950.

Bozeman, F. M., and Elisberg, B. L.: Serological diagnosis of scrub typhus by indirect immunofluorescence. Proc Soc Exp Biol Med 112:568, 1963.

Bozeman, F. M., Masiello, S. A., Williams, M. S., and Elisberg, B. L.: Epidemic typhus rickettsiae isolated from flying squirrels. Nature 255:545, 1975.

Burgdorfer, W.: Hemolymph test. A technique for detection of rickettsiae in ticks. Am J Trop Med Hyg 19:1010, 1970.

Burgdorfer, W., Ormsbee, R. A., and Hoogstraal, H.: Ticks as vectors of *Rickettsia prowazekii* — a controversial issue. Am J Trop Med Hyg 21:989, 1972.

Burgdorfer, W., Sexton, D. J., Gerloff, R. K., Anacker, R. L., Philip, R. N., and Thomas, L. A.: *Rhipicephalus sanguineus*: Vector of a new spotted fever group rickettsia in the United States. Infect Immun 12:205, 1975.

Castaneda, M. R.: The antigenic relationship between proteus X-19 and typhus rickettsia. II. A study of the common antigenic factor. J Exp Med 60:119, 1934.

Catanzaro, P. J., Shirai, A., Agniel, L. D., and Osterman, J. V.: Host defenses in experimental scrub typhus: Role of spleen and peritoneal exudate lymphocytes in cellular immunity. Infect Immun 18:118, 1977.

Chang, R. S. M., Murray, E. S., and Synder, J. C.: Erythrocyte-sensitizing substances from rickettsiae of the Rocky Mountain spotted fever group. J Immunol 73:8, 1954.

Coolbaugh, J. C., Progar, J. J., and Weiss, E.: Enzymatic activities of cell-free extracts of *Rickettsia typhi*. Infect Immun 14:298, 1976.

Coolbaugh, J. C., Ho, C-M., and Fang, R. C. Y.: Diagnosis of scrub typhus by culture of blood monocytes. In Tan, D. S. K. (ed.): Proceedings of the 18th South East Asia Ministers of Education Organization Tropical Medicine Seminar. Bangkok, SEAMEO Regional Tropical Medicine Publishing Health Project, 1978.

Cooper, M. D., Hollingdale, M. R., Vinson, J. W., and Costa, J.: A passive hemagglutination test for diagnosis of trench fever due to *Rochalimaea quintana*. J Inf Dis 134:605, 1976.

Cox, H. R.: Use of yolk sac of developing chick embryo as medium for growing rickettsiae of Rocky Mountain spotted fever and typhus groups. Public Health Rep 53:2241, 1938.

Dasch, G. A., Samms, J. R., and Weiss, E.: Biochemical characteristics of typhus group rickettsiae with special attention to the *Rickettsia prowazekii* strains isolated from flying squirrels. Infect Immun 19:676, 1978.

deBrito, T., Tiriba, A., Godoy, C. V. F., Penna, D. O., and Jordao, F. M.: Glomerular response in human and experimental rickettsial disease (Rocky Mountain spotted fever group). A light and electron microscopy study. Pathol Microbiol (Basel) 31:365, 1968.

DeShazo, R. D., Boyce, J. R., Osterman, J. V., and Stephenson, E. M.: Early diagnosis of Rocky Mountain spotted fever. Use of primary monocyte culture technique. JAMA 235:1353, 1976.

Elisberg, B. L., Campbell, J. M., and Bozeman, F. M.: Antigenic diversity of *Rickettsia tsutsugamushi*: Epidemiologic and ecologic significance. J Hyg Epidemiol Microbiol Immunol 12:18, 1968.

Fiset, P., Ormsbee, R. A., Silberman, R., Peacock, M., and Spielman, S. H.: A microagglutination technique for detection and measurement of rickettsial antibodies. Acta Virol 13:60, 1969.

Fleck, L., Porat, S., Evenchik, Z., Klingberg, M. A.: The renal excretion of specific microbial substances during the course of infection with murine typhus rickettsiae. Am J Hyg 72:351, 1960.

Fukuda, T., Kitao, T., and Keida, Y.: Study on the causative agent of "Hyuga netsu" disease (infectious mononucleosis). Med Biol 32:200, 1954.

Gilford, J. H., and Price, W. H.: Virulent-avirulent conversions of *Rickettsia rickettsii* in vitro. Proc Nat Acad Sci 41:870, 1955.

Giminez, D. F.: Staining rickettsiae in yolk-sac cultures. Staining Technol 39:135, 1964.

Groves, M. G., and Osterman, J. V.: Host defenses in experimental scrub typhus: Genetics of natural resistance to infection. Infect Immun 19:583, 1978.

Hamashima, Y., Kishi, K., and Tasaka, K.: Rickettsia-like bodies in infantile acute febrile mucocutaneous lymph-node syndrome. Lancet 2:42, 1973.

Harrell, G., and Aikawa, J.: Pathogenesis of circulatory failure in Rocky Mountain spotted fever. Medicine 28:333, 1949.

Hechemy, K. E., Stevens, R. W., Sasowski, S., Michaelson, E. E.,

Casper, E. A., and Philip, R. N.: Discrepancies in Weil-Felix and microimmunofluorescence test results for Rocky Mountain spotted fever. J Clin Microbiol 9:292, 1979.

Herrmann, J. E., Hollingdale, M. R., Collins, M. F., and Vinson, J. W.: Enzyme immunoassay and radioimmunoprecipitation tests for the detection of antibodies to *Rochalimaea (Rickettsia) quintana*. Proc Soc Exp Biol Med 154:285, 1977.

Hollingdale, M. R., Herrmann, J. E., and Vinson, J. W.: Enzyme immunoassay of antibody to *Rochalimaea quintana*: Diagnosis of trench fever and serologic cross-reactions among other rickettsiae. J Inf Dis 137:578, 1978.

Ito, S., and Vinson, J. W.: Fine structure of *Rickettsia quintana* cultivated in vitro and in the louse. J Bacteriol 89:481, 1965.

Kazar, J., Brezina, R., and Urvolgyi, J.: Studies on the E strain of *Rickettsia prowazekii*. Bull WHO 49:257, 1973.

Kitao, T., Farrell, R. K., and Fukuda, T.: Differentiation of salmon poisoning disease and Elokomin fluke fever: Fluorescent antibody studies with *Rickettsia sennetsu*. Am J Vet Res 34:927, 1973.

Kokorin, I. N., Chyong, D. K., Kekcheeva, N. G., and Miskarova, E. D.: Cytological investigation on *Rickettsia tsutsugamushi* infection of mice with different allotypic susceptibility to the agent. Acta Virol 20:147, 1976.

Korb, J., Kouba, K., and Kulková, H.: *Rickettsia sennetsu* and the etiology of infectious mononucleosis. Čas lék Čes 105:975, 1966.

Kurz, J., and Burgdorfer, W.: Detection of the Rocky Mountain spotted fever agent, *Rickettsia rickettsii*, in dead ticks, *Dermacentor andersoni*. Infect Immun 20:584, 1978.

Ley, H. L., Smadel, J. E., Diercks, F. H., and Paterson, P. Y.: Immunization against scrub typhus. V. The infective dose of *Rickettsia tsutsugamushi* for men and mice. Am J Hyg 56:313, 1952.

Mason, R. A.: Propagation and growth cycle of *Rickettsia quintana* in a new liquid medium. J Bacteriol 103:184, 1970.

McDade, J. E., Shephard, C. C., Redus, M. A., Newhouse, V. F., and Smith, J. D.: Evidence of *Rickettsia prowazekii* infections in the United States. Am J Trop Med Hyg 29:277, 1980.

McKiel, J. A., Bell, E. J., and Lackman, D. B.: *Rickettsia canada*: A new member of the typhus group of rickettsiae isolated from *Haemophysalis leporispalustris* ticks in Canada. Can J Microbiol 13:503, 1967.

Misao, T., and Kobayashi, Y.: Studies on infectious mononucleosis: On the isolation of causative agents from blood, bone marrow fluid, and lymph gland with mice. Tokyo Med J 71:683, 1954.

Mooser, H., and Weyer, F.: Experimental infection of *Macacus rhesus* with *Rickettsia quintana*. Proc Soc Exp Biol Med 83:699, 1953.

Moulder, J. W.: The relation of the psittacosis group (chlamydiae) to bacteria and viruses. Ann Rev Microbiol 20:107, 1966.

Murray, E. S., Gaon, J. A., O'Connor, J. M., and Mulahasanovic, M.: Serologic studies of primary epidemic typhus and recrudescent typhus (Brill-Zinsser disease). 1. Differences in complement-fixing antibodies: High antigen requirement and heat lability. J Immunol 94:723, 1965.

Myers, W. F., and Wisseman, C. L., Jr.: Genetic relatedness among the typhus group of rickettsiae. Int J Syst Bacteriol 30:143, 1980.

Myers, W. F., Osterman, J. V., and Wisseman, C. L., Jr.: Nutritional studies of *Rickettsia quintana*: Nature of the hematin requirement. J Bacteriol 109:89, 1972.

Nacy, C. A., and Osterman, J. V.: Host defenses in experimental scrub typhus: Role of normal and activated macrophages. Infect Immun 26:744, 1979.

Ormsbee, R. A., Parker, H., and Pickens, E. G.: The comparative effectiveness of aureomycin, terramycin, chloramphenicol, erythromycin, and thiocymetin in suppressing experimental rickettsial infections in chick embryos. J Inf Dis 96:162, 1955.

Ormsbee, R. A.: Rickettsiae (as organisms). Ann Rev Microbiol 23:275, 1969.

Ormsbee, R., Peacock, M., Philip, R., Casper, E., Plorde, J., Gabre Kidan, T., and Wright, L.: Serologic diagnosis of epidemic typhus fever. Am J Epidemiol 105:261, 1977.

Ormsbee, R., Peacock, M., Philip, R., Casper, E., Plorde, J., Gabre Kidan, T., and Wright, L.: Antigenic relationships between the typhus and spotted fever groups of rickettsiae. Am J Epidemiol 108:53, 1978.

Oster, C. N., Burke, D. S., Kenyon, R. H., Ascher, M. S., Harber, P., and Pedersen, C. E., Jr.: Laboratory-acquired Rocky Mountain spotted fever. The hazard of aerosol transmission. N Engl J Med 297:859, 1977.

Osterman, J. V., Myers, W. F., and Wisseman, C. L., Jr.: Chemical composition of the cell envelope of *Rickettsia quintana*. Acta Virol 18:151, 1974.

Osterman, J. V., and Eisemann, C. S.: Rickettsial indirect hemagglu-

tination test: Isolation of erythrocyte-sensitizing substance. J Clin Microbiol 8:189, 1978.

Perez Gallardo, F.: Study of the E stain isolated in Madrid in 1941. Its antigenic properties, its avirulence. Bull Soc Pathol Exot 56:805, 1963.

Philip, R. N., Casper, E. A., Ormsbee, R. A., Peacock, M. G., and Burgdorfer, W.: Microimmunofluorescence test for the serological study of Rocky Mountain spotted fever and typhus. J Clin Microbiol 3:51, 1976.

Philip, R. N., Casper, E. A., MacCormack, J. N., Sexton, D. J., Thomas, L. A., Anacker, R. L., Burgdorfer, W., and Vick, S.: A comparison of serologic methods for diagnosis of Rocky Mountain spotted fever. Am J Epidemiol 105:56, 1977.

Philip, R. N., Casper, E. A., Burgdorfer, W., Gerloff, R. K., Hughes, L. E., and Bell, E. J.: Serologic typing of rickettsiae of the spotted fever group by microimmunofluorescence. J Immunol 121:1961, 1978.

Ramm, L. E., and Winkler, H. H.: Rickettsial hemolysis: Adsorption of rickettsiae to erythrocytes; effect of metabolic inhibitors upon hemolysis and adsorption. Infect Immun 7:93, 550, 1973.

Reiss-Gutfreund, R. J.: The isolation of *Rickettsia prowazekii* and *mooseri* from unusual sources. Am J Trop Med Hyg 15:943, 1966.

Schaechter, M., Bozeman, F. M., and Smadel, J. E.: Study on the growth of rickettsiae. II. Morphologic observations on living rickettsiae in tissue culture cells. Virology 3:160, 1957.

Schramek, S.: Isolation and characterization of deoxyribonucleic acid from *Coxiella burnetii*. Acta Virol 12:1822, 1968.

Schramek, S., and Brezina, R.: Characterization of an endotoxic lipopolysaccharide from *Coxiella burnetii*. Acta Virol 20:152, 1976.

Schramek, S., Brezina, R., and Tarasevich, I. V.: Isolation of a lipopolysaccharide antigen from *Rickettsia* species. Acta Virol 20:270, 1976.

Shirai, A. and Wisseman, C. L.: Serologic classification of scrub typhus isolates from Pakistan. Am J Trop Med Hyg 24:145, 1975.

Shirai, A., Catanzaro, P. J., Phillips, S. M., and Osterman, J. V.: Host defenses in experimental scrub typhus: Role of cellular immunity in heterologous protection. Infect Immun 14:39, 1976.

Shirai, A., Sankaran, V., Gan, E., and Huxsoll, D. L.: Early detection of *Rickettsia tsutsugamushi* in peripheral monocyte cultures derived from experimentally infected monkeys and dogs. Southeast Asian J Trop Med Public Health 9:11, 1978.

Silverman, D. J., Boese, J. L., Wisseman, C. L., Jr.: Ultrastructural studies of *Rickettsia prowazekii* from louse midgut cells to feces: Search for "dormant" forms. Infect Immun 10:257, 1974.

Silverman, D. J., and Wisseman, C. L., Jr.: Comparative ultrastructural study on the cell envelopes of *Rickettsia prowazekii*, *Rickettsia rickettsii*, and *Rickettsia tsutsugamushi*. Infect Immun 21:1020, 1978.

Smadel, J. E.: Influence of antibiotics on immunologic response in scrub typhus. Am J Med 17:246, 1954.

Smith, D. K., and Winkler, H. H.: Characterization of a lysine-specific active transport system in *Rickettsia prowazekii*. J Bacteriol 129:1349, 1977.

Stoker, M. G. P., and Fiset, P.: Phase variation of the Nine Mile and other strains of *Rickettsia burneti*. Can J Microbiol 2:310, 1956.

Stork, E., and Wisseman, C. L., Jr.: Growth of *Rickettsia prowazekii* in enucleated cells. Infect Immun 13:1743, 1976.

Tarasevich, I. V., Plotnikova, L. F., Fetisova, N. F., Makarova, V. A., Jablonskaja, V. A., Rehacek, J., Zupacico, M., Kovacova, E., Urvolgyi, J., Brezina, R., Zakarjan, A. V., and Kocinjan, M. E.: Rickettsioses studies. I. Natural foci of rickettsioses in the Armenian Soviet Socialist Republic. Bull WHO 53:25, 1976.

Traub, R., and Wisseman, C. L., Jr.: The ecology of chigger-borne rickettsioses (scrub typhus). J Med Entomol 11:237, 1974.

Tyeryar, F. J., Jr., Weiss, E., Millar, D. B., Bozeman, F. M., and Ormsbee, R. A.: DNA base composition of rickettsiae. Science 180:415, 1973.

Urvolgyi, J., and Brezina, R.: *Rickettsia slovaca*: A new member of the spotted fever group rickettsiae. In Kazar, J., Ormsbee, R. A., and Tarasevich, I. V. (eds.): Rickettsiae and Rickettsial Diseases. Bratislava, VEDA, 1978, pp. 299–306.

Vinson, J. W.: *In vitro* cultivation of the rickettsial agent of trench fever. Bull WHO 35:155, 1966.

Vinson, J. W., and Campbell, E. S.: Complement fixing antigens from *Rickettsia quintana*. Acta Virol 12:54, 1968.

Walker, D. H., and Cain, B. G.: A method for specific diagnosis of Rocky Mountain spotted fever on fixed paraffin-embedded tissue by immunofluorescence. J Inf Dis 137:206, 1978.

Walker, D. H., and Henderson, F. W.: Effect of immunosuppression on

*Rickettsia rickettsii* infection in guinea pigs. Infect Immun 20:221, 1978.

Weiss, E., and Dressler, H. R.: Selection of an erythromycin-resistant strain of *Rickettsia prowazekii*. Am J Hyg 71:292, 1960.

Weiss, E., and Dressler, H. R.: Increased resistance to chloramphenicol in *Rickettsia prowazekii* with a note on failure to demonstrate genetic interaction among strains. J Bacteriol 83:409, 1962.

Weiss, E.: Growth and physiology of rickettsiae. Bacteriol Rev 37:259, 1973.

Weiss, E., Coolbaugh, J. C., and Williams, J. C.: Separation of viable *Rickettsia typhi* from yolk sac and L cell host components by renografin density gradient centrifugation. Appl Microbiol 30:456, 1975.

Weiss, E.: In Kazar, J., Ormsbee, R. A., and Tarasevich, I. V. (eds.): Rickettsiae and Rickettsial Diseases. Bratislava, VEDA, Slovak Academy of Sciences, 1978.

Weiss, E., Dasch, G. A., Woodman, D. R., and Williams, J. C.: Vole agent identified as a strain of the trench fever rickettsia, *Rochalimaea quintana*. Infect Immun 19:1013, 1978.

Wike, D. A., Ormsbee, R. A., Tallent, G., and Peacock, M. G.: Effects of various suspending media on plaque formation by rickettsiae in tissue culture. Infect Immun 6:550, 1972.

Winkler, H. H.: Inhibitory and restorative effects of adenine nucleotides on rickettsial adsorption and hemolysis. Infect Immun 9:119, 1974.

Winkler, H. H., and Ramm, L. E.: Adsorption of typhus rickettsiae to ghosts of sheep erythrocytes. Infect Immun 11:1244, 1975.

Winkler, H. H.: Rickettsial permeability. An ADP-ATP transport system. J Biol Chem 251:389, 1976.

Wisseman, C. L., Jr., and Waddell, A. D.: In vitro studies on rickettsia-host cell interactions: Intracellular growth cycle of virulent and attenuated *Rickettsia prowazekii* in chicken embryo cells in slide chamber cultures. Infect Immun 11:1391, 1975.

Wood, W. H., Jr., and Wisseman, C. L., Jr.: Studies of *Rickettsia mooseri* cell walls. II. Immunologic properties. J Immunol 98:1224, 1967.

Woodward, T. E., Pedersen, C. E., Oster, C. N., Bagley, L. R., Romberger, J., and Synder, M. J.: Prompt confirmation of Rocky Mountain spotted fever: Identification of rickettsiae in skin tissues. J Inf Dis 134:297, 1976.

Yamada, T., Harber, P., Pettit, G. W., Wing, D. A., and Oster, C. N.: Activation of the kallikrein-kinin system in Rocky Mountain spotted fever. Ann Int Med 88:764, 1978.

# 51  *BARTONELLA BACILLIFORMIS*

## Manuel Cuadra, M.D.

### MORPHOLOGY

The morphology of *Bartonella bacilliformis* varies greatly with environmental conditions. In the red cells of blood smears from patients with Oroya fever, it appears as a pleomorphic organism (Fig. 1), varying from slender bacilli to coccoid forms. Although the bacillary forms usually have a smooth surface, there are also rosary-like forms that are considered to be produced by multisegmentation of the smooth forms; later the beaded forms disintegrate into coccoid forms. During the 1st week in typical cases of Oroya fever, when the rate of red cell parasitism increases geometrically, the bacillary (vegetative) forms predominate greatly over the coccoid forms (Fig. 1, top). In the 2nd week, both forms are found in approximately equal numbers. When the fever subsides in the 3rd week (usually by lysis), the coccoid forms greatly predominate over the bacillary forms. During convalescence (an afebrile stage with profound anemia), only coccoid forms are seen (Fig. 1, bottom). Electron microscopy shows that *B. bacilliformis* lies within the red cells (Fig. 2) and that its internal structure, showing a defined cell wall, resembles that of bacteria (Cuadra and Takano, 1969). Compact masses of organisms filling the cytoplasm of capillary endothelial cells have been found in the stage of Oroya fever (Strong, 1945; Aldana, 1929; Pinkerton and Weinman, 1937–38; Alzamora Castro, 1940; Urteaga, 1948).

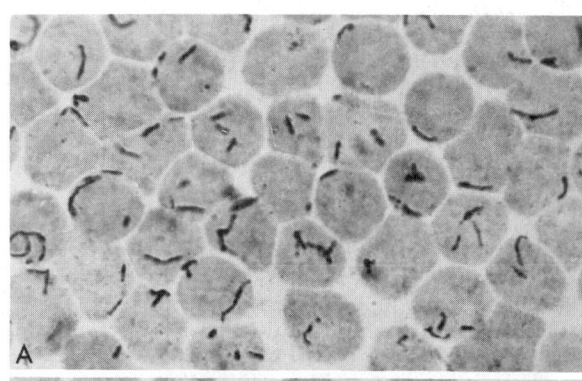
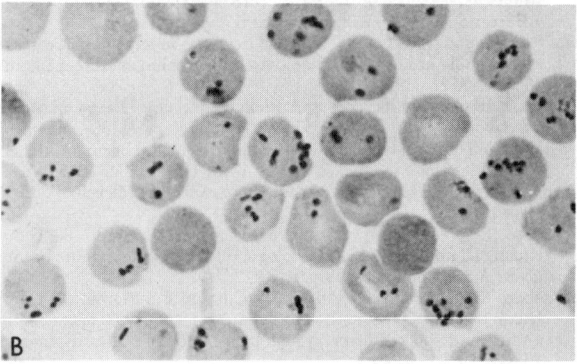

**FIGURE 1.** *Smears of peripheral blood from patients suffering from Oroya fever. A, Red cells parasitized by a bacillary (vegetative) type of* B. bacilliformis, *from a patient in acute febrile stage. B, Red cells parasitized by a coccoid (inactive) type of* B. bacilliformis, *from a patient in reconvalescence (nonfebrile) stage. Prior to performance of the smears the patients had received no antibiotics. Wright's stain.*

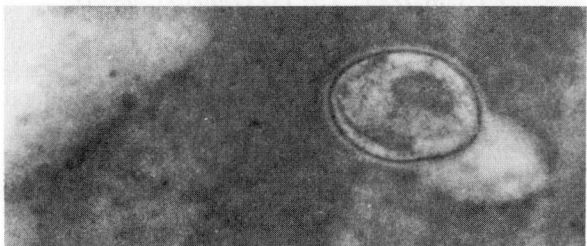

FIGURE 2. *Thin section of a red cell parasitized by B. bacilliformis. The organism lies within a cavity in the red cell and shows a dense cell wall. Lead hydroxide stain. ×50,000.*

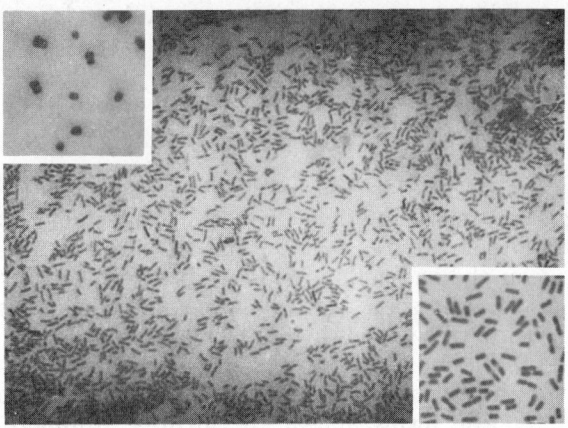

FIGURE 3. *Touch preparation from a blood agar culture of B. bacilliformis (4th day of incubation at 28° C) showing monomorphic rods. For comparison see insets: touch preparations of Staphylococcus epidermidis (top) and Escherichia coli (bottom). Giemsa stain. The three organisms are shown at the same magnification (×840).*

*B. bacilliformis* has been demonstrated within verruga nodules and experimental monkey nodules by light microscopy (Mackehenie and Weiss, 1926; Noguchi, 1926a, b; Noguchi, 1927a; Marquez da Cunha and Muniz, 1928; Weiss, 1932; Weinman and Pinkerton, 1937a; Alzamora Castro, 1945; Urteaga and Calderón, 1965) and electron microscopy (Recavarren and Lumbreras, 1972; Takano, 1970). Both extracellular (Recavarren and Lumbreras, 1972) and intracellular (Takano, 1970) organisms occur; they resemble those forms parasitizing red blood cells.

Inclusion-like bodies, consisting of aggregated organisms that are presumably in stages of intracellular digestion, have also been found in the cytoplasm of the verruga cells (angioblasts) (Mayer et al., 1913; Marquez da Cunha and Muniz, 1928; Weiss, 1932; Pinkerton and Weinman, 1937–38; Noguchi, 1927b; Kikuth, 1931). Both extracellular and intracellular bacterial forms and the inclusion-like bodies develop in cultured cells (Pinkerton and Weinman, 1937). The assumption that the inclusions are composed of a viral form of *B. bacilliformis* (Aldana, 1947) is speculative.

The morphology of *B. bacilliformis* in blood agar cultures is shown in Figure 3. During active growth (3rd to 6th day at 28° C), the organisms appear in Giemsa-stained touch preparations as small rods with parallel sides, straight or slightly curved axis, slightly rounded ends, moderate variation in length (monomorphism), and arranged as single elements or in palisades. Later, pleomorphism becomes marked and increases with time of incubation. Long and short bacilli, coccobacilli, coccoid forms, short chains, diplococcoid forms, diplobacilli, and bacilli with bipolar staining closely resembling *Pasteurella* are seen. In cultures more than seven days old, coccoid forms predominate over bacillary forms, and by the 9th day, ring-shaped organisms are predominant. The coccoid forms are derived either by segmentation of the rods or by dissolution of the midportion of bipolar rods, so that the poles become freestanding. Under electron microscopy,

many organisms show an envelope secondary to retraction of the cytoplasm (Fig. 4), and a defined cell wall is shown by thin sections (Cuadra and Takano, 1969) (Fig. 2). Most bacilli have single or multiple (up to 30 $\mu$m long and up to 10 in number) flagella (Fig. 4) at one pole (cephalotrica) (Peters and Wigand, 1951–1952; Perez Alva and Giustini, 1957). If transverse septation occurs centrally, two identical daughter cells result; if septation occurs eccentrically, the daughter cells are pleomorphic.

Growth of *B. bacilliformis* in liquid media produces no morphologic differences from the forms grown on solid media. Flagellated and nonflagel-

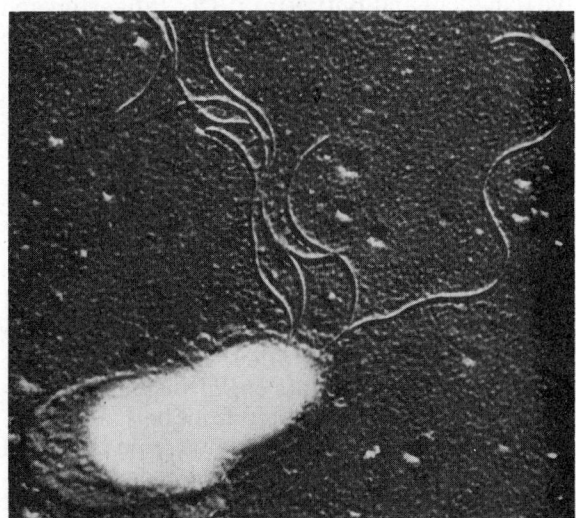

FIGURE 4. B. bacilliformis *as seen by electronmicroscope. The organism shows a pronounced retraction of the cytoplasm and flagella emerging from a pole. Coated with palladium. ×19,000. (From Peters, D., and Wigand, R.: Z. Tropenmed Parasitol 3:313, 1951.)*

lated forms appear in solid, semisolid, and liquid media.

## MOTILITY

Free forms in plasma (wet preparations) of patients suffering from Oroya fever have not been reported, but free forms lying in the spaces between the red cells of stained blood smears are occasionally seen. Most, however, lie in ghosts of erythrocytes (Cuadra, 1957). Old reports (Barton, 1909) that the organisms move inside the red cells have not been confirmed. Both motile and nonmotile forms appear in cultures. Nonmotile forms predominate markedly over motile ones, and paradoxically, flagellated forms predominate over nonflagellated ones. Hence, the flagellated organisms are not necessarily motile. This deduction is supported by the fact that *Bartonella* organisms growing in the semisolid medium of Noguchi may not be motile (Peters and Wigand, 1951–1952; Noguchi and Battistini, 1926) but are flagellated. Moreover, the yield of flagella increases with the time of incubation (Peters and Wigand, 1951–1952) as motility decreases.

Bartonellae can attach to red blood cells in cultures. The "parasitized" erythrocytes appear to rotate (dance) in a characteristic fashion (Cuadra, 1978). Dance is prevented, specifically, by antisera.

*B. bacilliformis* is gram-negative and readily takes the Romanowsky stains (Giemsa, Wright, Leishman) in smears from patients' blood or cultures and in histologic sections of organs and verruga nodules after fixation with Ragoud's fixative (Noguchi and Battistini, 1926; Pinkerton and Weinman, 1937–1938). Flagella stain by the method of Zettnow-Fontana (Noguchi and Battistini, 1926; Pinkerton and Weinman, 1937–1938).

## ANTIGENIC COMPOSITION

There have been no reports of flagellar or somatic antigens of *Bartonella*. Different clinical patterns in two different areas of Peru (Callejon de Huaylas and Rimac Valley) suggest that there are two antigenic variants of *Bartonella*. Morphologically, the strains isolated from both areas are indistinguishable. Strains isolated from the blood of Oroya fever patients cross-react in complement-fixation reaction with strains from verruga nodules (Noguchi, 1927c), and there is cross-immunity between Oroya fever and verruga (Noguchi, 1927d). No cross-reaction occurs with *Hemobartonella* or related organisms (Wigand, 1956, 1958).

## CULTURAL CHARACTERISTICS

*B. bacilliformis*, a nonsporing organism, grows slowly in different bacteriologic media. On blood-broth of Hercelles (1927), the first medium devised for cultivation of *B. bacilliformis*, the organism does not produce turbidity; the change in color of the medium from red to dark reddish violet is the only indicator of growth. Both single elements and clusters of them can be seen under the microscope from the 3rd to the 4th day of incubation. The organisms have a marked tendency to attach to red blood cells (Cuadra, 1978). Attachment is evidenced by) the "dance" of "parasitized erythrocytes" and by clumped red cells containing clusters of organisms arranged in a framework. We use both signs as indicators of growth. On blood agar, the colonies are too small for study by the naked eye. Under the stereoscopic microscope, the colonies appear from the 3rd to the 4th day of incubation to be variable in size, circular, transparent, and smooth. The colonies can also be studied microscopically on stained touch preparations (Fig. 3). A square piece of blood agar culture is removed from a Petri dish culture and placed, surface-to-surface, on a slide; when the piece is suddenly removed, a layer of organisms, arranged in colonies or singly, remains on the slide. On leptospirasemisolid medium of Noguchi (Noguchi and Battistini, 1926), which also contains blood factors essential for growth, *Bartonella* forms clusters; the organism, predominantly coccobacilli in form, are less motile than those on blood agar slants (Peters and Wigand, 1951-1952; Noguchi and Battistini, 1926). On liquid, semisolid, or solid media of Geiman (1941), which contain ascorbic acid and glutathione as key substances with animal serum, *Bartonella* grows well; in the liquid medium, it causes a fine dustlike deposit but neither turbidity nor clusters. The individual organisms are dispersed and are mainly nonmotile.

All media that support growth of *Bartonella* contain either whole blood or serum. Attempts to determine if the *Haemophilus influenzae* growth promoting V and X blood factors (Thjötta and Avery, 1921) are involved have given confusing results (Jimenes, 1940; Colichón and Bedón, 1973). In comparison with *H. influenzae* or any other current bacteria, *Bartonella* slowly reaches a moderate amount of growth.

### Metabolism

*B. bacilliformis* is an obligate aerobe (Noguchi and Battistini, 1926), but in blood broth the organism grows partly at the bottom on the mass of sedimented red cells and partly as a thin pellicle on the surface of the medium (Aldana,

1929, 1946). A difference in oxygen or carbon dioxide requirements therefore exists between the two populations. Growth occurs between about 20° and 37° C, but the optimal temperature is 28° C, and no growth occurs at 40° C. The pH range for growth is between 6.8 and 8.4, with an optimum level of 7.8 (Noguchi and Battistini, 1926). The organism ferments no carbohydrates (Noguchi and Battistini, 1926). No hemolysis occurs on blood agar, but in blood broth the erythrocytes attached to clusters of organisms become hemolyzed, and red cell ghosts can be seen by phase-contrast microscopy (Cuadra, 1978).

### Resistance and Viability

*B. bacilliformis*, a nonsporing organism, dies within seven minutes at 56° C. Formalin, phenol, mercurochrome, neosalvarsan, and neutroflavine inhibit growth in cultures. The inhibitory concentration varies. Thus, formalin is inhibitory at 1:100,000 and phenol at 1:100 concentrations (Aldana, 1929; Noguchi, 1928a).

Viability varies with the specimen, the cultural conditions, and the strain. Thus, in citrated blood from patients with Oroya fever, the organism remains viable for four months (Aldana, 1929), and in blood clots, for nine months (Herrer, 1948) at room temperature. In the excised verruga nodule from monkeys, *B. bacilliformis* survives for about 56 days at 4° C and 28 days at room temperature; on blood agar slants or leptospira semisolid medium, it remains viable for about 50 days at 37° C and four months at 4° C or room temperature (Noguchi, 1926c). On blood broth or blood agar slants, it survives for nine months at room temperature (Aldana, 1929). Protection of the cultures from drying by adequate stoppers, without impairing the oxygen supply (since *Bartonella* is an obligate aerobe), is essential to maintain viability. Under storage at −20° to −70° C, after freezing the cultures in the period of optimal growth (abundance of motile forms), *B. bacilliformis* remains viable for years and resists the process of lyophilization (Perez Alva et al., 1957).

## *PATHOGENIC PROPERTIES*

*B. bacilliformis* is pathogenic only for man and causes Oroya fever and verruga peruana, which represent two successive stages of the same disease (Carrión's disease).

Inoculations of *Bartonella* into human beings have given variable results. Carrión, a medical student, was inoculated intracutaneously with juice from a verruga nodule. After 21 days of incubation, he developed Oroya fever with severe anemia and died on the 16th day of disease (Rebagliati, 1940). Strong et al. (1945) inoculated a man intracutaneously with verruga material, and a local verruga nodule developed but no Oroya fever. Garcia Rosell, a physician, inoculated himself accidentally with the blood of an Oroya fever patient while giving a blood transfusion (Rebagliati, 1940). A febrile illness without anemia lasted for two weeks, and then a florid verruga eruption appeared. Another physician, Kuchinsky-Godard (Mackehenie, 1937), who inoculated himself voluntarily with a culture of bartonellae, developed verruga nodules locally and at distant sites but no Oroya fever. Urteaga (1950) could induce Oroya fever in splenectomized individuals, but not in normal ones, by inoculation of parasitized blood from Oroya fever patients.

Inoculations carried out in monkeys (*Macacus rhesus* is the animal of choice) have also given variable results (Jadassohn and Seiffert, 1910; Mayer et al., 1913; Arce et al., 1913; Noguchi and Battistini, 1926; Noguchi, 1926a, b; Marquez da Cunha and Muniz, 1928; Aldana, 1929; Weinman and Pinkerton, 1937a; Wigand and Weyer, 1952). In an effort to reproduce human bartonellosis with its two stages, infected blood from Oroya fever patients, juice from verruga nodules, infected wild sandflies, and cultures have been inoculated by all possible routes (intravenously, cutaneously by scarification, and intra- or subdermally). Local verruga nodules occur with relative ease after cutaneous inoculation of these materials. A mild Oroya fever characterized by fever, anemia, and parasitism of the red blood cells occurs in a limited number of cases after intravenous inoculation with cultures. With parasitized blood from Oroya fever patients as the inoculum, negative results are obtained as a rule. The high degree of parasitism that usually occurs in Oroya fever patients, involving nearly 100 per cent of red cells (Fig. 1) with associated severe anemia (one million erythrocytes/mm³), has never been obtained in monkeys (Weinman and Pinkerton, 1937a). The discrete Oroya fever induced in monkeys is very exceptionally followed by a generalized (endogenous) eruption (Noguchi, 1926a). However, it seems that anemia is produced more easily in splenectomized monkeys (Weinman and Pinkerton, 1937a).

According to old reports from Peruvian doctors, verruga peruana but not Oroya fever can be induced by inoculation of various animal species (Tamayo, 1899; Arce et al., 1913; Aldana, 1929). Noguchi confirmed the results in dogs and donkeys (Noguchi et al., 1929).

## IMMUNITY

Oroya fever is an acute disease. In most nonfatal cases, recovery occurs spontaneously within two to three weeks. It is followed first by an asymptomatic "intercalary period" of variable duration (one or more weeks) and then by the verruga peruana stage, which lasts about one to three months. Chronic Oroya fever with persistent anemia and *B. bacilliformis* in peripheral red blood cells has never been reported. After spontaneous remission of the verrucous eruption, a solid lifelong immunity is established. A second attack of Oroya fever has never been reported in patients who returned to endemic areas. However, two, three, or more episodes of verruga peruana, usually accompanied by rheumatoid manifestations (verrucous rheumatism) and mild fever may occur in some individuals (chronic verruga peruana). The fact that some subjects with or without a past history of Oroya fever or verruga peruana give positive blood cultures (Howe, 1943; Weinman and Pinkerton, 1937b; Herrer, 1959) supports the existence of a state of infection-immunity (i.e., immunity depending on existing but not prior infection).

## LABORATORY DIAGNOSIS

Blood smears stained with Giemsa, Wright, or Leishman stain reveal the organisms in the red cells of patients suffering from Oroya fever throughout the course of the fever and convalescent period (Fig. 1). The percentage of parasitized erythrocytes and the relative proportions of bacillary and coccoid forms should be estimated because bacillary forms, whatever the number of associated coccoid forms, are always related to the presence of fever. For this reason, the bacillary form is considered to be the active form. In contrast, in the convalescent period, when fever is absent, only coccoid forms, may be encountered, although they may be parasitizing 100 per cent of red cells (Fig. 1). Thus, the coccoid form, originating from the bacillary form, is considered to be an inactive (stationary) form. Parasitized erythrocytes disappear gradually during convalescence, which, in cases with a high rate of parasitism, may last up to three weeks. By this time, the residual red cells harboring coccoid forms are spherocyte-like microcytes. The finding of pure coccoid forms in febrile patients indicates that the fever is not caused by *Bartonella* but by an associated infection, usually caused by *Salmonella* (Cuadra, 1956).

In an atypical form of the disease characterized by little or no anemia, the organisms are found with difficulty. In these cases, the thick-blood technique is of great aid. Blood cultured in broth always produces growth of *B. bacilliformis* after a variable incubation period at 28° C. The incubation time is usually three to five days and depends on the degree of parasitism of red blood cells. Blood cultures are frequently positive for *Salmonella* after a shorter incubation time. *S. typhimurium* is encountered most frequently (Cuadra, 1956).

No bartonellae are found in blood films of patients suffering from verruga peruana, although the blood cultures, especially the cultures of excised verruga nodules, may be positive. The nodules have a characteristic histologic appearance (Rocha-Lima, 1913; Mackehenie, 1938).

The agglutination reaction was thoroughly studied by Howe (1942, 1943) in a group of 203 individuals. The titer of agglutinins appeared to be low but was of diagnostic significance. Practically all patients with Oroya fever had measurable agglutinins; in contrast, agglutinins were found in only 28 per cent (15 out of 54) of patients in the verruga stage. In both Oroya fever and verruga peruana, the titer showed a tendency to decline and to disappear within a relatively short time after remission of the symptoms. In many individuals, blood cultures were positive (with or without symptoms), and agglutination tests were negative; the reverse was uncommon. In a group of 21 apparently healthy residents of endemic areas, both blood cultures and agglutination tests were negative.

The complement fixation reaction (Strong et al., 1915; Noguchi, 1928b; Aldana, 1929; Reese et al., 1950) has not been evaluated by extensive clinical trials.

## DRUG SUSCEPTIBILITY

Penicillin, streptomycin, chloramphenicol, tetracycline, and erythromycin are highly effective against Oroya fever (Larrea, 1958). They produce defervescence within 24 hours, in parallel with morphologic changes of bartonellae and their disappearance from the peripheral blood cells. In vitro, *Bartonella* is highly susceptible to antibiotics and relatively resistant to sulphonamides (Wigand, 1952). Penicillin induces extraordinarily large coccoid forms in the cultures (Aldana and Tisnado Munoz, 1945; Wigand, 1952). Such forms correspond to L forms of *Bartonella* (Sharp, 1968). Resistance develops to streptomycin during treatment, whereupon the fever returns, the bacillary forms of bartonellae coincidentally reappear in the peripheral erythrocytes (Aldana et al., 1948; Cuadra, 1957).

The effectiveness of antibiotics on verruga peruana is doubtful. A comparative in vitro assay on drug susceptibility of strains isolated from Oroya fever patients with those isolated from verruga peruana patients is needed.

## EPIDEMIOLOGY

Bartonellosis occurs in certain Andean valleys of Colombia, Ecuador, and Peru between 2 degrees north and 13 degrees south latitude. In Peru, the most afflicted country, the endemic foci lie at altitudes of between 800 and 3500 meters above sea level. The most important foci lie in valleys watered by rivers that flow into the Pacific Ocean at about 30 km. distance from the sea Foci of minor importance are scattered in valleys with rivers that flow into the Amazon River (Rebagliati, 1940).

The inhabitants of the endemic areas constitute the reservoir. A high proportion of blood cultures of healthy individuals in those areas, with or without a past history of bartonellosis, is positive (Weinman and Pinkerton, 1937b; Howe, 1943; Herrer, 1959). Among animals, field mice have occasionally been found to harbor *Bartonella* in their blood (Hertig, 1948). The fact that some persons have contracted Oroya fever after spending the night in the forest supports the concept of the existence of an animal reservoir. Infection is transmitted by certain species of *Phlebotomus: Ph. verrucarum, Ph. pescei,* and *Ph. bicornutus* (Noguchi et al., 1929; Hertig, 1942; Herrer et al., 1959-1960). The bite of wild sandflies in the endemic areas can cause infection in monkeys (Battistini, 1931). However, the crucial experiment of transmission to man by *Phlebotomus* fed on Oroya fever patients failed. The cycle of bartonellae within *Phlebotomus* is unknown. In an epidemic area, Guaytara (Colombia), no *Phlebotomus* species were found, and only lice were present as a possible vector (Patino, Camargo, 1939). *Bartonella* can multiply within the celomic cavity of lice (Wigand and Weyer, 1952). Experimentally, the infection could be transmitted from infected to normal rhesus monkeys by the bite of the tick *Dermacentor andersoni* (Noguchi, 1926d).

## References

Aldana, L. D.: Bacteriologia de la enfermedad de Carrión. Cron Med Lima 46:237, 1929.

Aldana, L.: Estado actual del tratamiento de la enfermedad de Carrión por la penicilina. Rev Med Per Lima 19:617, 1946.

Aldana, L.: Estados biológicos de la Bartonella en la enfermedad de Carrión. Rev Sanid Polic Lima 7:391, 1947.

Aldana, L., and Tisnado Munoz, S.: Penicilina y enfermedad de Carrión. Rev Med Per Lima 18:343, 1945.

Aldana, L., Zubiate, P., and Contreras, F.: Un caso de verruga peruana

resistente a la estreptomicina. Arch Per Pat Clin Lima 2:553, 1948.

Alzamora Castro, V.: Contribución al estudio de la bartonellosis humana o enfermedad de Carrión. Grac Med Lima 2:78, 1945.

Alzamora Castro, V.: Enfermedad de Carrión: Ensayo de etiopatogenia. Anales Fac Cien Med 23:1, 1940.

Arce, J., Mackehenie, D., and Ribeyro, R.: Estudio experimental de la enfermedad de Carrión. I. Inoculabilidad de la verruga peruana a los animales. Cron Med Lima 30:394, 1913.

Barton, A.: Descripción de elementos endoglobulares en los enfermos de fiebre de verruga. Cron Med Lima 26:7, 1909.

Battistini, T.: La verrue péruviene. (Sa transmission par le phlébotome.) Rev Sud Amér Med Chirug 2:719, 1931.

Colichón, H., and Bedón, C.: Factores que la *Bartonella bacilliformis* requiere para su crecimiento. Rev Lat Am Microbiol 15:11, 1973.

Cuadra, M.: The ability of *Bartonella bacilliformis* growing in culture to attach to red blood cells. Abstracts of the Twelfth International Congress of Microbiology. Sept 3-8, 1978, München, p. 178.

Guadra, M.: Mecanismo de destrucción de los eritrocitos. La hemolisis intravascular. Anal Fac Med lima 40:872, 1957.

Cuadra, M.: Salmonellosis complication in human bartonellosis. Texas Rep Biol Med 14:97, 1956.

Cuadra, M.: Tratamiento con cloranfenicol de casos de bartonellosis aguda (enfermedad de Carrión) en periodo de inicio. Anal Fac Med Lima 40:147, 1957.

Cuadra, M., and Takano, J.: The relationship of *Bartonella bacilliformis* to the red blood cell as revealed by electron microscopy. Blood 33:708, 1969.

Geiman, Q. M.: New media for the growth of *Bartonella bacilliformis*. Proc Soc Exp Biol Med 47:329, 1941.

Hercelles, O.: El germen de la verruga peruana. Anal Fac Med Lima 10:231, 1927.

Herrer, A.: Estudios sobre la enfermedad de Carrión en el valle interandino del Mantaro. II. Incidencia de la infección bartonellósica en la población humana. Rev Med Exper Lima 23:47, 1959.

Herrer, A.: Supervivencia de la *Bartonella bacilliformis* en la sangre coagulada de los enfermos de verruga. Rev Med Exp Lima 7:70, 1948.

Herrer, A., Blancas, F., Cornejo Ubillús, J., Lung, J., Espejo, L., and Flores, M.: Estudios sobre la enfermedad de Carrión en el valle interandino del Mantaro. I. Observaciones entomológicas. Rev Med Exper Lima 13:27, 1959.

Hertig, M.: Phlebotomus and Carrión's disease. Am J Trop Med (suppl) 22:1942.

Hertig, M.: Sandflies of the genus *Phlebotomus*. A review of their habits, disease relationships, and control. Proceedings of the 4th International Congress of Tropical Medicine and Malaria, 1948; Washington, DC, USA, p. 1609.

Howe, C.: Carrión's disease. Immunologic studies. Arch Int Med 72:147, 1943.

Howe, C.: Demonstration of agglutinins for *Bartonella bacilliformis*. J Exp Med 75:65, 1942.

Jadassohn, W. E., and Seiffert, G.: Ein Fall von Verruga peruviana: Gelungene Übertragung auf Affen. Z Hyg Infec Krankh, 6:247, 1910.

Jimenes, J. F.: Carrión's disease. I. Some growth factors necessary for cultivation of *Bartonella bacilliformis*. Proc Soc Exp Biol Med 45:402, 1940.

Kikuth, W.: Experimentelle Untersuchungen über Oroyafieber und Verruga peruana. Z Immunforschg 73:1, 1931.

Larrea, P.: Los antibioticos en la bartonellemia humana. Arch Per Pat Clin 12:1, 1958.

Mackehenie, D.: Un caso de verruga humana por autoinoculación experimental. Ref Med Lima 23:741, 1937.

Mackehenie, D.: Estudio del noduloma verrucoso. Ref Med Lima 24:50, 1938.

Mackenhenie, D., and Weiss, P.: Contribución al estudio de la verruga peruana. Gac Med Per Lima 4:51, 1926.

Marquez de Cunha, A., and Muniz, J.: Pesquisas sobre la verruga peruana. Med Inst Oswaldo Cruz 21:161, 1928.

Mayer, M., Rocha-Lima, H., and Werner, H.: Untersuchungen über verruga peruviana. Münch Med Wochenschr 60:739, 1913.

Noguchi, H.: Comparative studies of different strains of *Bartonella bacilliformis* with special reference to the relation between the clinical types of Carrion's disease and the virulence of the infecting organism. J Exp Med 47:219, 1928b.

Noguchi, H.: Etiology of Oroya fever. II. Viability of *Bartonella bacilliformis* in cultures and in the preserved blood and an excised nodule of Macacus rhesus. J Exp Med 44:533, 1926c.

Noguchi, H.: Etiology of Oroya fever. III. The behavior of *Bartonella bacilliformis* in Macacus rhesus. J Exp Med 44:697, 1926a.

Noguchi, H.: Etiology of Oroya fever. IV. The effect of inoculation of anthropoid apes with *Bartonella bacilliformis*. J Exp Med 44:715, 1926b.

Noguchi, H.: Etiology of Oroya fever. VI. Pathological changes observed in animals experimentally infected with *Bartonella bacilliformis*. The distribution of the parasites in the tissues. J Exp Med 45:437, 1927a.

Noguchi, H.: Etiology of Oroya fever. VII. The response of the skin of Macacus rhesus and anthropoid apes to inoculation with *Bartonella bacilliformis*. J. Exp Med 45:455, 1927b.

Noguchi, H.: Etiology of Oroya fever. VIII. Experiments on cross-immunity between Oroya fever and verruga peruana. J Exp Med 45:781, 1927d.

Noguchi, H.: Etiology of Oroya fever. XIII. Chemotherapy in experimental *Bartonella bacilliformis* infection. J Exp Med 48:619, 1928a.

Noguchi, H.: The etiology of verruga peruana. J Exp Med 45:175, 1927c.

Noguchi, H.: The experimental transmission of *Bartonella bacilliformis* by ticks (*Dermacentor andersoni*). J Exp Med 44:729, 1926d.

Noguchi, H., Shannon, R. C., Tilden, E. B., and Tyler, J. R.: Etiology of Oroya fever. XIV. The insect vectors of Carrión's disease. J Exp Med 49:993, 1929.

Noguchi, H., Muller, H. R., Tilden, E. B., and Tyler, J. R.: Etiology of Oroya fever. XVI. Verruga in the dog and the donkey. J Exp Med 50:455, 1929.

Noguchi, H., and Battistini, T.: Etiology of Oroya fever. I. Cultivation of *Bartonella bacilliformis*. J Exp Med 43:851, 1926.

Patino Camargo, L.: Batonellosis del guaytara o fiebre verrucosa del guaytara. Ref Med Lima 24:649, 689, 1939.

Perez Alva, S., and Giustini, J.: La maladie de Carrión. Etude morphologique de *Bartonella bacilliformis* au microscope électronique. Bull Soc Path Exot 50:188, 1957.

Perez Alva, S., Roger, F., and Roger, A.: La maladie de Carrión. Resistance de *Bartonella bacilliformis* an processus de lyophilisation. Bull Soc Path Exot 50:243, 1957.

Peters, D., and Wigand, R.: Neue Untersuchungen über *Bartonella bacilliformis*. I. Morphologie der Kulturform. Z Tropenmed Parasitol 3:313, 1951.

Pinkerton, H., and Weinman, D.: Carrion's disease. I. Behavior of the etiological agent within cells growing or surviving in vitro. Proc Soc Exp Biol Med 37:587, 1937.

Pinkerton, H., and Weinman, D.: Carrión's disease. II. Comparative morphology of the etiological agent in Oroya fever and verruga peruana. Proc Soc, Exp Biol Med 37:591, 1937.

Rebagliati, R.: Verruga Peruana (Enfermedad de Carrión). Imprenta Lima, Torres Aguirre, 1940.

Recavarren, S., and Lumbreras, H.: Pathogenesis of the verruga of Carrión's disease. Am J Pathol 66:461, 1972.

Reese, J. D., Morrison, M. E., and Fowler, E. M.: Complement fixation and Weil-Felix reactions in rabbits inoculated with *Bartonella bacilliformis*. J Immunol 65:355, 1950.

Rocha-Lima, H.: Zur Histologie der Verruga peruviana. Verh Dtsch Path Ges 16:409, 1913.

Sharp, J. T.: Isolation of "L" forms of *Bartonella bacilliformis*. Proc Soc Exp Biol Med 128:1072, 1968.

Strong, R. P.: Verruga peruana and Oroya fever. In Stitt's Diagnosis, Prevention and Treatment of Tropical Disease, 7th ed. vol 2. Philadelphia, The Blakiston Company, 1945, pp. 997–1014b.

Strong, R. P., Tyzzer, E. E., and Sellards, A. W.: Differential diagnosis of verruga peruana. Fifth report. J Trop Med 18:122, 1915.

Takano, J.: Enfermedad de Carrión (bartonellosis humana). Estudio morfológico de la fase hemática y del período eruptivo con el microscopio electrónico. Doctoral thesis. Faculty of Medicine of the National University of San Marcos, 1970.

Tamayo, M. O.: Inoculabilidad de la verruga. Cron Med Lima 16:81, 1899.

Thjötta, T., and Avery, O. T.: Studies on bacterial nutrition. II. Growth accessory substances in the cultivation of hemophilic bacilli. J Exp Med 34:97, 1921.

Urteaga, O.: Histopatogenia de la anemia en la verruga peruana. Arch Per Pat Clin 2:355, 1948.

Urteaga, O.: Lecture at the Cathedra of Infectious, Parasitic and Tropical Diseases of the Faculty of Medicine, Lima, 1950.

Urteaga, O., and Calderón, J.: Ciclo biológico de reproducción de la *Bartonella bacilliformis* en los tejidos de pacientes de verruga peruana o enfermedad de Carrión. Arch Per Pat Clin Lima 19:1, 1965.

Weinman, D., and Pinkerton, H.: Carrion's disease. III. Experimental production in animals. Proc Soc Exp Biol Med 37:594, 1937a.

Weinman, D., and Pinkerton, H.: Carrion's disease. IV. Natural source of *Bartonella* in the endemic zone. Proc Soc Exp Biol Med 37:596, 1937b.

Weiss, P.: Contribución al estudio de la verruga peruana o enfermedad de Carrión. Rev Med Per Lima 4:5, 58, 1932.

Wigand, R.: Morphologische, biologische und serologische Eigenschaften der Bartonellen. Stuttgart. Georg Thieme Verlag, 1958.

Wigand, R.: Neue Untersuchungen über *Bartonella bacilliformis*. 2. Verhalten gegenüber Sulfonamide und Antibiotica in vitro. Z Tropenmed Parasitol 3:453, 1952.

Wigand, R.: Serologische Reaktionen an Haemobartonella muris und Eperythrozoon coccoides. Z Tropenmed 7:322, 1956.

Wigand, R., und Weyer, F.: Neue Untersuchungen über *Bartonella bacilliformis*. 3. Übertragungsversuche auf rhesus Affen und auf Kleiderläuse. Z Tropenmed Parasitol 4:243, 1952.

# 52 *THE CHLAMYDIAE*

## G. Philip Manire, Ph.D.

No other pathogenic microorganisms are better adapted for persistence and survival than the chlamydiae and no others are more widespread. Epidemiologic surveys suggest that some members of almost every species of birds and mammals may be infected with these organisms. Their ability to produce inapparent infections in these hosts is unexcelled, and individuals may be infected for extremely long periods of time without apparent harm. Estimates have been made that 10 to 20 per cent of the human population of the world is infected with chlamydiae. These organisms are ubiquitous, rarely kill their hosts, are generally highly infectious and easily trans-ferred to new hosts, and have a remarkable ability to escape normal host immune mechanisms.

### *CLASSIFICATION*

The genus *Chlamydia* is composed of two species, *C. trachomatis* and *C. psittaci* (Page, 1974). Although trachoma has been recognized as a specific disease for many centuries, and the first microscopic evidence of a specific causative agent was obtained early in the twentieth century, laboratory studies on these organisms began only in 1930 following the first successful isolation of

TABLE 1.  Differentiation of *C. trachomatis* and *C. psittaci*

| C. TRACHOMATIS | C. PSITTACI |
| --- | --- |
| Sensitive to sulfonamide | Resistant to sulfonamide |
| Rigid micro colonies | Diffuse micro colonies |
| Glycogen in inclusion | No glycogen in inclusion |
| Guanine + cytosine content of DNA ~ 44% | Guanine + cytosine content of DNA ~ 41% |

*C. psittaci* from infected humans and birds. Isolation of *C. trachomatis* was not achieved until 1957.

Since it was shown very quickly that chlamydiae are strict intracellular parasites, they were considered for many years to be the largest known viruses. As evidence regarding their growth and biochemical characteristics accumulated, it became obvious that these organisms are bacteria with unique characteristics. Like other bacteria they (1) contain both DNA and RNA, (2) possess a continuous cell envelope similar in most respects to that of gram-negative bacteria, (3) possess ribosomes similar to those of other bacteria and synthesize their own proteins and nucleic acids, (4) possess limited but definite numbers of metabolic systems, and (5) are susceptible to a wide range of antibiotics.

The characteristics separating the two species are shown in Table 1. This classification was further justified by the finding that there is a significant DNA homology within each species but very little homology between the two, suggesting a long-standing evolutionary separation.

## MORPHOLOGY

All members of the genus *Chlamydia* share a unique developmental cycle in which two distinct forms occur. These two forms are especially adapted for extracellular survival and transfer from cell to cell, and for intracellular growth. The extracellular form, generally referred to as an elementary body (EB), is a spherical bacterium 0.25 to 0.3 $\mu$m in diameter. It is surrounded by a rigid trilaminar cell envelope similar in composition to those of other gram-negative bacteria, except that the cell walls do not exhibit characteristic endotoxic properties. The inner side of the envelope is composed of a continuous layer of small subunit structures in a hexagonal array, and these subunits apparently serve to maintain envelope rigidity. The cytoplasm of the elementary body is surrounded by a typical plasma membrane. The DNA and ribosomes are condensed in the center of the organisms, and in electron micrographs of shadow-cast preparations these

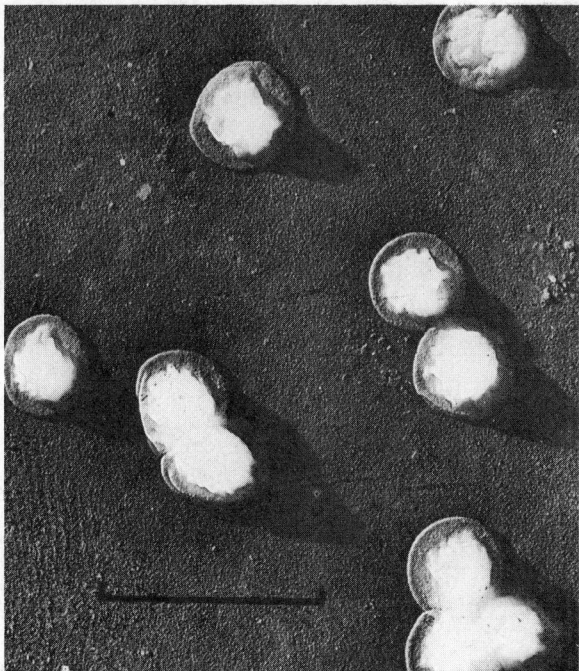

FIGURE 1.  *Shadowcast preparation of purified elementary bodies showing typical central condensation of cytoplasmic contents.*

assume a "derby hat" or "fried egg" appearance. Thin-section electron microscopy shows a similar central condensation.

The intracellular form of chlamydiae, referred to here as the reticulate body (RB), is much larger than the extracellular form and differs from it in many respects. It is surrounded by a trilaminar envelope that is very fragile and flexible so that pleomorphism results. The subunit layer found on the inside of the elementary body envelope is missing, and no sulfur-containing amino acids have been detected in the outer cell wall. Ribosomes and other cytoplasmic constituents are distributed homogeneously throughout the cytoplasm.

The genome of the organism has a molecular weight of $660 \times 10^6$ as estimated by electron-microscopic measurements. As in other bacteria, the chlamydiae contain numerous proteins, which comprise 60 per cent of dry weight of the organisms, and lipids, about 30 per cent of dry weight.

A summary of the differing characteristics of elementary bodies and reticulate bodies is shown in Table 2.

In a typical growth cycle, the elementary body attaches to a susceptible cell by a process that involves a heat-sensitive component on the surface of the organism and a trypsin-sensitive site on the host cell (Byrne, 1976). The organism enters the cell by phagocytosis, and the resulting

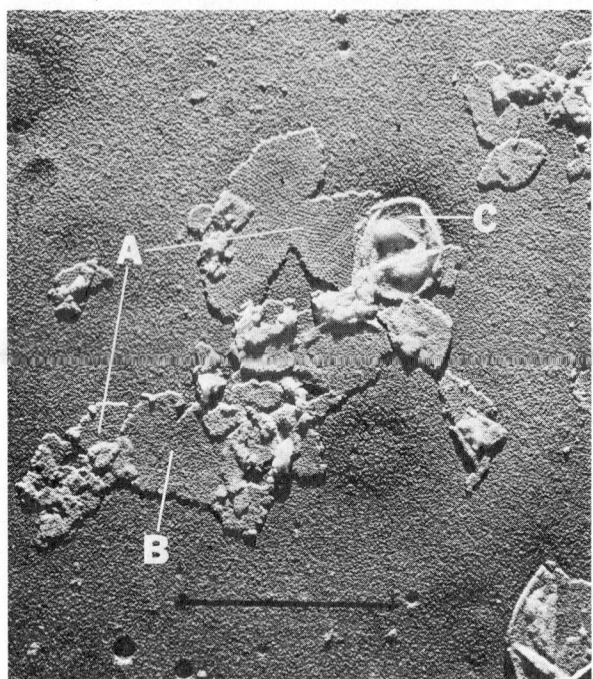

**FIGURE 2.** *Cell envelope fragments prepared from disrupted suspensions of C. psittaci. Fragment A illustrates the hexagonal array of subunit structure found on the inner side of the cell envelope. Fragment B illustrates the outer granular side of the envelope. The structure C is an intact envelope.*

phagosome membrane separates the developing colony of chlamydiae from the host cell cytoplasm throughout the active growth cycle. The developing phagosome membrane contains no protein synthesized by chlamydiae, but the membranes

continue to increase in size during colony development even when the host cell synthesis of protein is largely inhibited by cycloheximide. This suggests that chlamydiae play a role in control of phagosome membrane synthesis (Stokes, 1974).

By an unknown process the elementary bodies within the phagosome prevent lysosome activation and fusion of lysosomes and phagosomes, whereas when opsonized or heat-treated elementary bodies enter susceptible cells, there is rapid fusion of lysosomes and phagosomes, and the noninfectious chlamydiae are rapidly digested.

Within 6 to 8 hours after phagosome formation, the elementary bodies undergo a conversion to form reticulate bodies, and by 12 hours binary fission begins. In 20 to 24 hours some of the reticulate bodies have begun to show central condensation and conversion to elementary bodies, but most continue to undergo binary fission until about 40 hours, when large numbers of elementary bodies begin to appear. Following this the host cells begin to die and chlamydiae are released by lysis. It has been suggested that host cell lysosomes release into the cytoplasm hydrolytic enzymes that digest host cell constituents with consequent membrane lysis and release of chlamydiae (Todd and Storz, 1975).

## ANTIGENIC COMPOSITION

As with all bacteria, the chlamydiae have a complex antigenic structure. However, there are

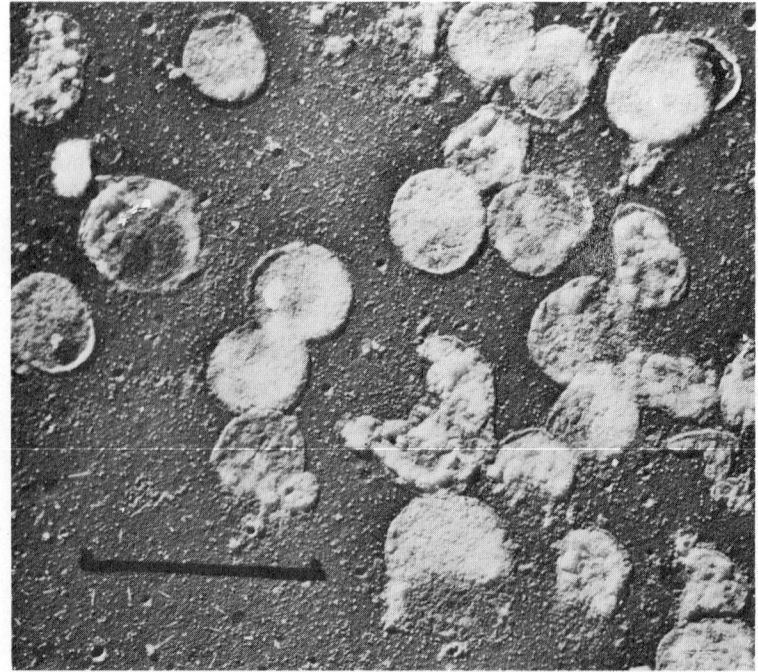

**FIGURE 3.** *Shadowcast preparation of purified reticulate bodies.*

**TABLE 2.  Characteristics of Elementary Bodies (EB) and Reticulate Bodies (RB)**

| CHARACTERISTICS | EB | RB |
| --- | --- | --- |
| Morphology | Small, dense centered | Large, homogeneous |
| RNA:DNA | 1:1 | 3:1 |
| Sonication | Resistant | Sensitive |
| Effect of trypsin | Resistant | Sensitive, lysis |
| Infectivity | + | − |
| Toxicity | + | − |
| Hemagglutinin | Present | Absent |
| Permeability | Slight | Marked |
| Envelope subunit | Present | Absent |
| Location | Extracellular | Intracellular |

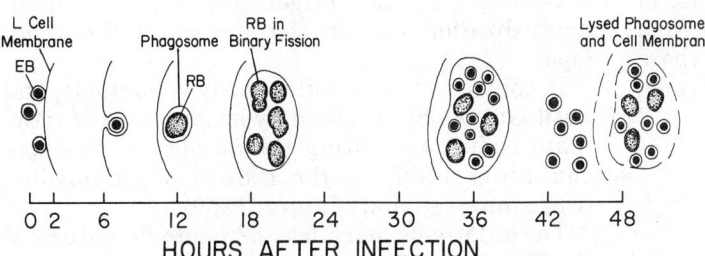

**FIGURE 4.** *Schematic representation of the reproductive cycle of C. psittaci in L cells. (EB = elementary body, RB = reticulate body).*

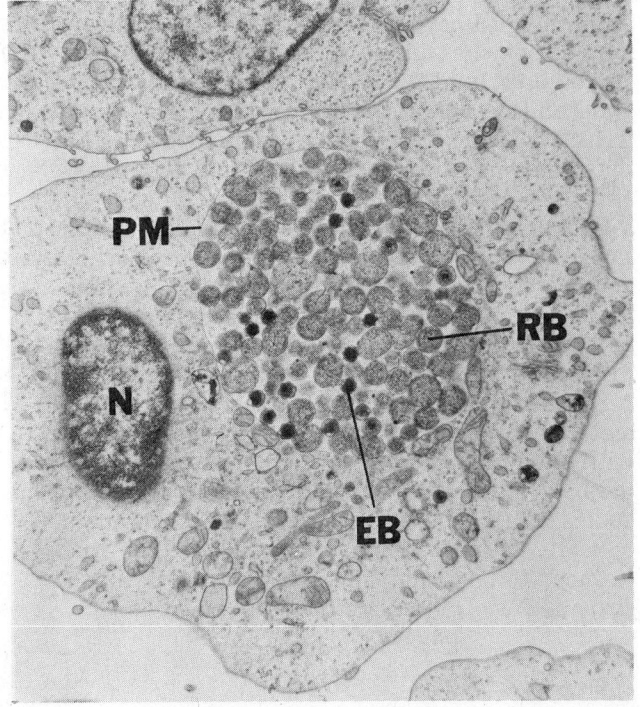

**FIGURE 5.** *Thin section of L cell 30 hours after infection with C. psittaci. Typical reticulate bodies (RB), newly formed elementary bodies (EB) and the continuous phagosome membrane (PM) are labeled.*

two general types of antigens, first recognized by Bedson in 1936. The first of these is the group antigen that is found in all chlamydiae and is usually demonstrated by complement fixation test. This antigen is a lipid-carbohydrate complex, stable when heated at 100° C for 30 minutes, and its antigenic determinant appears to be an acidic polysaccharide that is destroyed by periodic acid or acid hydrolysis.

There are a variety of specific antigens on or near the surface of the envelope of chlamydiae. In *C. psittaci* a large number of these have been demonstrated by toxin neutralization and plaque reduction tests. Among *C. trachomatis* strains, there are three serologically distinct types of lymphogranuloma venereum (LGV) agents, and 12 serotypes of the trachoma–inclusion conjunctivitis–urethritis group. The serotypes of *C. trachomatis* have been determined mostly by use of the microimmunofluorescence test (Wang and Grayston, 1970). Little is known about these antigens and none have been isolated for study, but they appear to be protein in nature.

## METABOLISM

The adaptation of chlamydiae for intracellular parasitism is well illustrated by their apparent total dependency on host cells for energy. They do synthesize their own macromolecules including DNA, RNA, and proteins, and they inhibit to varying degrees macromolecular synthesis in host cells, although the mechanism of this inhibition is not known. The chlamydiae contain numerous enzymes and can complete some metabolic processes, but they cannot complete the pentose cycle and do not utilize pyruvate by way of the tricarboxylic acid cycle. There is no evidence that they can generate high energy phosphate bonds, and they are completely dependent on the host cell for ATP. This dependence gives added significance to the microscopic evidence that mitochondria accumulate around the phagosome membrane of developing inclusions and are among the last cell organelles to distintegrate in the dying infected cell.

Essentially all of the in vitro studies done on metabolism of chlamydiae have been conducted with partially purified organisms prepared by methods that tend to destroy the reticulate bodies. Since the reticulate bodies are the metabolically active form of chlamydiae, further studies need to be done using purified and stabilized suspensions of reticulate forms.

## PATHOGENIC PROPERTIES

The chlamydiae do not possess demonstrable exotoxin and their cell envelopes, while similar in most characteristics of those of gram-negative bacteria, do not exhibit typical endotoxic properties. They do have several properties of significance in pathogenesis, one of which is toxicity of live elementary body preparations. Toxicity is usually measured by the intravenous injection of elementary body preparations into young mice. The component responsible for toxicity cannot be separated from the elementary body, and only live infectious elementary bodies exhibit this phenomenon. Toxicity can be neutralized by specific antisera, although the organisms may remain infectious. However, both live elementary bodies and their cell envelopes will absorb antitoxin, indicating that the antigen responsible for toxin neutralization lies on the surface of the envelope.

In contrast, the reticulate body is nontoxic, and antitoxin is not absorbed by suspensions of reticulate bodies, indicating the absence of this specific antigen during the growth of chlamydiae (Christoffersen and Manire, 1969).

The relatively harmless or nontoxic nature of the developing form may well contribute to another property of chlamydiae — the ease with which these organisms establish chronic inapparent carrier states in man and animals. This lack of specific antigenicity may allow reticulate bodies to reside intracellularly for long periods of time protected from host antibody.

Hypersensitivity may also play a role in *C. trachomatis* infection in that prior vaccination or infections often produce increasingly severe clinical symptoms.

In general, *C. trachomatis* tends to produce localized infections in mucous membranes with some extension in the case of genital infections. It may also produce pneumonitis in newborn infants. *C. psittaci*, in contrast, almost always produces generalized infections involving many organs in different animal hosts.

Little information is available to explain these differences or to answer other questions about the ability to chlamydiae to damage cells, establish latent or inapparent infections, or overcome immune mechanisms.

## IMMUNITY

Diseases produced by chlamydiae in animals and man tend to be chronic, and carrier states frequently develop following recovery from clinical disease. Neutralization of these organisms by specific antisera can be demonstrated in vitro, but the intracellular site of their growth and the absence of specific antigens on the surface of the dividing reticulate bodies apparently protect the organisms from specific antibody.

IgM, IgG, and IgA against chlamydiae are all detectable in infected animals and man, but the role of these antibodies and of cell-mediated immune mechanisms in recovery from infection is not known. Severe infection often occurs in healthy avian, and probably mammalian, carriers when they are subjected to stress, nutritional deprivation, and other traumatic events, indicating a delicate balance between host defense and chlamydial pathogenicity.

Since 1960 many trachoma vaccines produced by a variety of techniques have been tested in primates and humans. Short-term protection has been achieved in numerous instances, but subsequent susceptibility and development of hypersensitivity have been consistent long-term consequences.

## LABORATORY DIAGNOSIS

In *C. psittaci* infections, the complement fixation test using the heat-resistant group antigen has been the most commonly used serologic procedure. The organisms can be isolated without difficulty but with considerable hazard by injection of specimens into mice by various routes and into the chick embryo yolk sac, and many laboratory infections have occurred.

In *C. trachomatis* infections, recovery of the organisms by inoculation of specimens into ir-radiated or otherwise treated McCoy cells or by injection into chick embryo yolk sacs are well-established techniques. The examination of iodine- and/or Giemsa-stained smears has long been used to detect organisms in patients with trachoma. The more recently devised microimmunofluorescence test is rapidly replacing other serologic tests both for identification of specific antibody and for recognition of the organisms in cells removed from infected areas. A comparison of diagnostic methods currently available is shown in Table 3.

## DRUG SUSCEPTIBILITY

The first specific therapy for chlamydial infections followed the discovery that these organisms are sensitive to sulfonamides and penicillin. In general, *C. trachomatis* strains are sensitive to sulfonamides and these drugs have long been used in treatment of trachoma and LGV. *C. psittaci* strains are generally resistant to sulfonamides.

Penicillin has been used successfully in psittacosis infections, but its effect is to prevent conversion of reticulate forms to elementary bodies; it does not inhibit cell infection, conversion of elementary bodies to reticulate bodies, or growth of reticulate bodies.

Both of these drugs have been largely replaced by chloramphenicol, tetracycline, and rifamycin. The action of these drugs on chlamydiae is the same as with other bacteria.

A very useful observation in the studies on metabolism of chlamydiae is that cycloheximide will almost completely shut down host cell protein synthesis without effect on chlamydiae.

**TABLE 3.** Comparative Sensitivities of Diagnostic Laboratory Tests for *C. trachomatis* Infections

| | ANATOMIC SITE | | |
| --- | --- | --- | --- |
| **TEST** | **Conjunctiva (130)[a]** | **Male Urethra (200)[a]** | **Female Cervix (300)[a]** |
| Isolation | | | |
| Tissue culture | 95%[b] | 100 | 95 |
| Yolk sac | 38 | 26 | 40 |
| Stain of cell scrapings | | | |
| Giemsa | 45 | 15 | 41 |
| Fluorescent antibody | 85 | 60 | 66 |
| Serum antibody | | | |
| Complement fixation | 50 | 15 | 40 |
| Microimmunofluorescence | 100 | 90 | 99 |

[a]Number tested
[b]% positive
From Schachter, J.: N Engl J Med 298:545, 1978.

## EPIDEMIOLOGY

In 1967 Meyer presented a comprehensive review on the distribution of chlamydiae in humans and in wild and domestic mammals and birds. At that time more than 130 species of birds had been found to be infected, and it is probable that almost all bird species are carriers of *C. psittaci*. There is a wide range of mammals that are naturally infected. These include mice, cats, dogs, cattle, sheep, seals, and many other species. Various arthropods associated with infected animals also carry chlamydiae, but there is no evidence that arthropods play a role in disease transmission. The extent of infection in laboratory animals is illustrated by Meyer's finding that none of the colonies of mice and hamsters tested between 1940 and 1944 were free from chlamydiae.

Although clinical trachoma appears to have been diminishing since World War II, there are hundreds of millions of infected humans, primarily in Africa and Asia. Recent evidence that *C. trachomatis* is an important cause of nongonococcal urethritis and of cervicitis, and the finding of chlamydiae in 5 to 10 per cent of cervical specimens from asymptomatic women undergoing routine examinations, further confirm the extraordinarily widespread occurrence of these organisms and their role as a cause of infectious disease.

*C. psittaci* organisms spread from birds to man only sporadically, and outbreaks of human psittacosis occur mostly in persons processing carcasses of domestic turkeys, ducks, and other birds. There are several recorded instances of direct person-to-person transmission primarily involving hospital personnel.

Humans have been frequently infected following contact with apparently healthy birds. The organisms may be introduced from dust in bird cages and in other material contaminated with fecal materials from domestic or wild birds. Infection in humans most commonly results from inhalation of contaminated droplets or dust.

*C. trachomatis* is spread principally by three methods. The most common is direct contact by uninfected persons with eye secretions from infected carriers. In populations where hygiene is little practiced and where the carrier rate is very high, essentially every child is infected by contact with older carriers. The second method of transmission is sexual intercourse, resulting in acute, subacute, or inapparent infections of the genital tract of females and the genitourinary tract of males. The third method of transmission occurs during birth when the infant becomes infected during passage through the birth canal, with resulting conjunctivitis and/or pneumonitis.

### References

Bryne, G. I.: Requirements for ingestion of *C. psittaci* by mouse fibroblasts. Infect Immun 14:645, 1976.
Christoffersen, G., and Manire, G. P.: The toxicity of meningopneumonitis organism (*C. psittaci*) at different stages of development. J Immunol 103:1085, 1969.
Meyer, K. F.: The host spectrum of psittacosis-lymphogranuloma venereum agents. Am J Ophthalmol 63:1225, 1967.
Page, L. A.: Chlamydiales. In Buchanan, R. E., and Gibbons, N. E. (eds.): *Bergey's Manual of Determinative Bacteriology*, 8th ed. Baltimore, The Williams & Wilkins Company, 1974.
Schachter, J.: Chlamydial infections. N Engl J Med 298:428, 490, 540, 1978.
Stokes, G. V.: Cycloheximide-resistant glycosylation in L-cells infected with *C. psittaci*. Infect Immun 9:497, 1974.
Storz, J., and Spears, P.: Chlamydiales: Properties, cycle of development and effect on eukaryote host cells. Curr Topics Microbiol Immunol 76:167, 1977.
Todd, W., and Storz, J.: Ultrastructural cytochemical evidence for the activation of lysosomes in the cytocidal effect of *C. psittaci*. Infect Immun 12:638, 1975.
Wang, S. P., and Grayston, J. T.: Immunological relationship between genital TRIC, lymphogranuloma venereum and related organisms in a new microtiter indirect immunofluorescence test. Am J Ophthalmol 70:367, 1970.

# 4 MYCOPLASMAS AND L-FORMS

# 53 MYCOPLASMAS

Zell A. McGee, M.D.
David Taylor-Robinson, M.D.

Mycoplasmas, originally called pleuropneumonia-like organisms (PPLO), are the smallest of free-living organisms. In addition to their characteristic small size (smaller than some viruses), they all lack a cell wall and therefore are resistant to penicillin and other cell-wall active antimicrobials. The individual organisms are bounded by a pliable unit membrane that encloses the cyto-

**TABLE 1.** Characteristics of Mycoplasmas Compared to Those of Bacteria and Viruses

| CHARACTERISTIC | MYCOPLASMAS | BACTERIA | VIRUSES |
|---|---|---|---|
| Size (diameter) | 0.3 $\mu$m[a] | 1–2 $\mu$m | <0.5 $\mu$m |
| Lack a cell wall | Yes | No | Yes |
| Propagate on cell-free media | Yes | Yes | No |
| Usually require sterol and native protein for growth | Yes | No | No |
| Intrinsic energy metabolism | Yes | Yes | No |
| Usually narrow range of host specificity | Yes | No | Yes |
| Growth inhibited by specific antibody | Yes | No | Yes |
| Resistant to cell wall-active antibotics (e.g., penicillins) | Yes | No | Yes |
| Resistant to antibiotics that inhibit metabolism (e.g., tetracycline) | No | No | Yes |

[a]Smallest organism capable of propagation.

plasm, DNA, RNA, and other metabolic components necessary for propagation on cell-free media. Mycoplasmas have a number of other characteristics that distinguish them from bacteria and viruses (Table 1). They are not related to L-phase variants of bacteria (see Chapter 54) (Hayflick, 1969; McGee et al., 1967).

Despite the superficial similarities among mycoplasmas, they compose a heterogeneous assemblage of microorganisms that differ from one another in DNA composition, nutritional requirements, metabolic reactions, antigenic composition, and host species specificity. Taxonomically, the mycoplasmas are divided into two families: the Mycoplasmataceae, which require cholesterol for growth, and the Acholeplasmataceae, which do not. All the mycoplasmas commonly isolated from humans belong to the Mycoplasmataceae. This family comprises the genus *Mycoplasma*,

which contains organisms that do not hydrolyze urea, and the genus *Ureaplasma*, the organisms of which do hydrolyze urea. The latter were originally termed T strains or T mycoplasmas because of the tiny colonies they form.

Although the small size of their genome restricts the metabolic capabilities of mycoplasmas, certain species are important because they cause pneumonia, arthritis, keratoconjunctivitis, and mastitis among livestock and poultry in Africa, Australia, and other parts of the world. Eleven species constitute the normal flora or are pathogens of humans (Table 2). Many mycoplasma species are a laboratory nuisance as occult contaminants of tissue cultures. In addition, some mycoplasmas infect plants and insects (spiroplasmas), and others have been isolated from environments with a pH of less than 2 or with a temperature of 60° C (thermoplasmas).

**TABLE 2.** Mycoplasmas of Humans

| | SPECIES | FREQUENCY OF ISOLATION | USUAL SITE OF ISOLATION | NATURE OF DISEASE |
|---|---|---|---|---|
| Nonpathogenic | | | | |
| | M. orale | frequent | oropharynx | none |
| | M. salivarium | frequent | oropharynx | none |
| | M. buccale | rare | oropharynx | none |
| | M. faucium | rare | oropharynx | none |
| | M. lipophilum | rare | oropharynx | none |
| | A. laidlawii | very rare | oropharynx | none |
| | M. fermentans | infrequent | genitourinary tract | none[a] |
| | M. primatum | rare | genitourinary tract | none |
| Occasionally pathogenic | | | | |
| | M. hominis | frequent[b] | genitourinary tract | Septicemia, abscess, endometritis-salpingitis, reproductive disorders (sterility, abortion, prematurity)? |
| | U. urealyticum | frequent[b] | genitourinary tract | Nongonococcal urethritis, septicemia? endometritis-salpingitis? reproductive disorders |
| Frequently pathogenic | | | | |
| | M. pneumoniae | frequent[c] | oropharynx, respiratory tract | Tracheobronchitis, pneumonia, hemorrhagic bullous myringitis |

[a]Reports of isolation from joint fluids in rheumatoid arthritis remain unconfirmed.
[b]Colonization frequent, disease infrequent.
[c]During disease but otherwise infrequent.

## MORPHOLOGY

The morphology of individual organisms varies from one mycoplasma species to another, from time to time during the growth cycle, and from one environmental condition to another. Most mycoplasmas are spherical (0.3 to 0.8 μm in diameter) and divide by binary fission. Some mycoplasmas develop branching filaments 0.3 to 0.4 μm in diameter and up to 150 μm long. These divide to produce new spherical bodies.

The morphology of three species of mycoplasmas, *Mycoplasma pneumoniae*, *M. pulmonis* and *M. gallisepticum*, pathogens of the human, murine, and avian respiratory tracts respectively, is characterized by specialized structures at one or both ends of the organisms. *M. pneumoniae* has a tapered, filamentous tip that contains a dense, central rodlike core (Fig. 1). A specialized structure also has been observed in *M. pulmonis*. *M. gallisepticum* has a pear-shaped bleb at one or both ends of the organism. These structures may help attach the organism to the respiratory tract mucosa; they usually are the point of intimate contact of the mycoplasmas with the host cell membrane (Fig. 1). They also may be involved in motion, since these three mycoplasmas exhibit

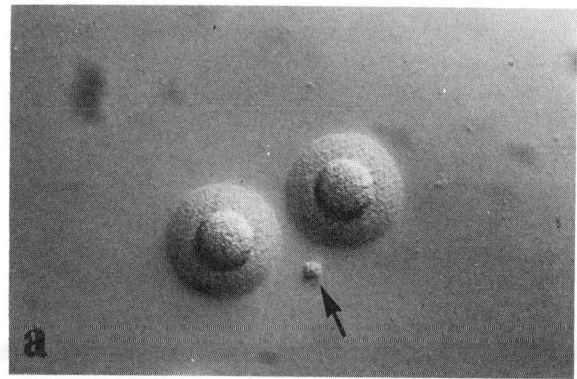

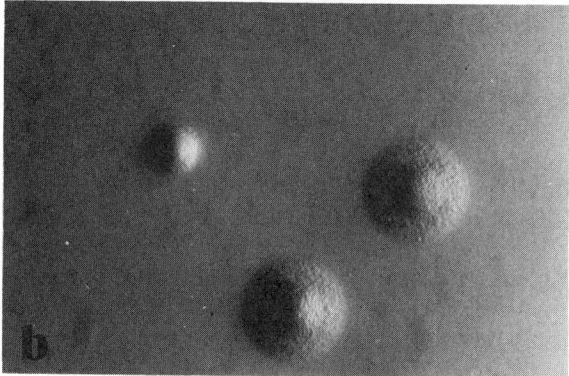

**FIGURE 2.** *Colonial morphology of mycoplasmas. (a) Two colonies (90 μm diameter) of* Mycoplasma hominis *and one colony (15 μm diameter) of* Ureaplasma urealyticum *or T-strain (tiny colony) mycoplasmas (arrow) from urethral exudate. (b) Three colonies of* Mycoplasma pneumoniae *from the sputum of a patient with pneumonia. Two colonies (80 μm diameter) have a poorly defined periphery and the third, more typical of* M. pneumoniae, *lacks a periphery.*

gliding motility in which the organisms move tip first.

Colonies of most mycoplasma species vary in size from 50 to 600 μm and are therefore most easily viewed through clear media with a dissecting microscope. The characteristic "fried egg" morphologic appearance of mycoplasma colonies on agar medium (Fig. 2a, large colonies) is caused by an opaque central zone of growth into the agar and a translucent peripheral zone on the surface. Such typical colonies do not always develop, since development depends on the species of mycoplasma, the constituents and degree of hydration of the medium, and atmospheric conditions. Ureaplasmas were originally called T-strains or T-mycoplasmas (T for tiny) because of the very small colonies they produce (15 to 30 μm in diameter—Fig. 2a, small colony); however, on medium buffered to pH 6, typical colonies up to 300 μm may develop. On primary isolation, *M. pneumoniae* usually produces mulberry-like colonies with no translucent peripheral zone, but larger colonies with a periphery sometimes develop (Fig. 2b).

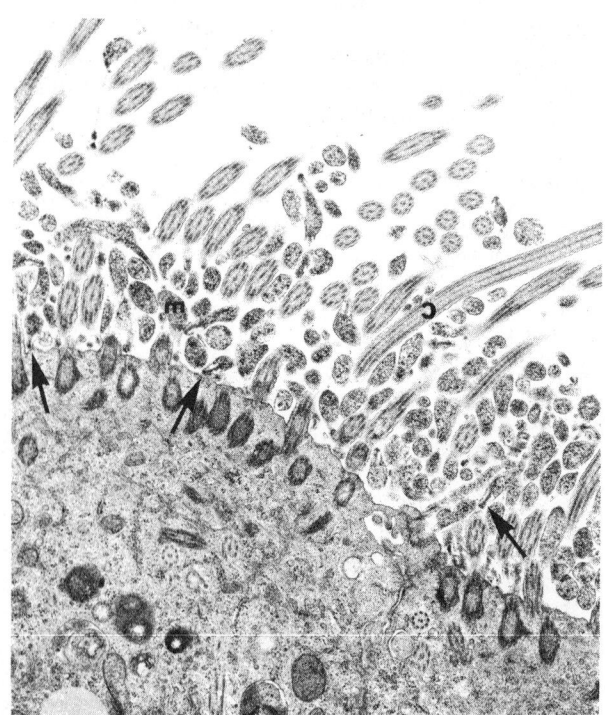

**FIGURE 1.** *Electron micrograph of ciliated epithelial cells in tracheal mucosa infected with* Mycoplasma pneumoniae. *Note cilia (c) and individual organisms of* M. pneumoniae (m) *with specialized terminal structure oriented toward the membrane of the host cell (arrows). (×13,000).*

## ANTIGENIC COMPOSITION

The major antigenic determinants of mycoplasmas are membrane proteins and glycolipids. The glucose- and galactose-containing glycolipids of *M. pneumoniae* are haptens, which are antigenic only when bound to membrane protein. They induce antibodies that react in tests of complement fixation, metabolism inhibition, and growth inhibition. Glycolipids of similar structure and activity are found in some other mycoplasmas, in most plants, and in human brains. The cross-reactivity of human brain tissue antigens with *M. pneumoniae* antibodies could account for the neurologic manifestations of *M. pneumoniae* infection. In contrast, a glycoprotein fraction of *M. pneumoniae*, rather than the glycolipid moiety, is involved in the development of a cell-mediated immune response to this mycoplasma species.

Several mycoplasma species, such as *M. mycoides* (bovine), *Acholeplasma laidlawii*, and *M. meleagridis* (avian), possess extracellular carbohydrates or capsule-like material. Although the function of these substances is not clear, the galactan of *M. mycoides,* which is similar to a substance found in bovine lung, may play an immunologic role in the production of pneumonia.

Antigenic relationships among mycoplasmas infecting humans have been defined by relatively specific serologic procedures (such as metabolism inhibition, growth inhibition, and immunofluorescence) that measure antibodies directed against mycoplasma membrane antigens. By means of these tests, mycoplasma "species" have been established. Species isolated from humans are distinct from each other and from those isolated from other animals. In contrast, tests employing mycoplasma cell extracts are less specific and show group relationships; thus, by immunodiffusion, common antigens are demonstrable among all the human mycoplasma species that have been tested except *M. pneumoniae*. Ureaplasmas of human origin comprise a single species, *U. urealyticum*, which has been subdivided into eight serotypes by such tests as metabolism and growth inhibition.

## NUTRITION AND METABOLISM

Mycoplasmas require lipids and lipid precursors for synthesis of the plasma membrane (Hayflick, 1969; Razin, 1978). Animal sera provide a complex of lipoprotein and cholesterol, the latter being incorporated into the lipid bilayer membrane of sterol-requiring mycoplasmas and functioning as a regulator of the bilayer fluidity. Acholeplasmas do not need exogenous cholesterol

**TABLE 3. Metabolic Properties of Common Human Mycoplasmas**

| | ARGININE HYDROLYZED | GLUCOSE FERMENTED TO ACID | UREA HYDROLYZED |
|---|---|---|---|
| M. orale | + | − | − |
| M. salivarium | + | − | − |
| M. hominis | + | − | − |
| M. pneumoniae | − | + | − |
| U. urealyticum | − | − | + |

because they synthesize saturated long-chain fatty acids and carotenoids that substitute for cholesterol in the membrane.

Mycoplasmas generally multiply at a slower rate than bacteria. The mean generation time for many mycoplasmas, including ureaplasmas, is one to three hours, and for some, six to nine hours. Most mycoplasmas are facultative anaerobes, but they will grow aerobically, some preferring this atmosphere. They utilize either glucose or arginine as a major source of energy. The carbohydrate-fermenting species catabolize glucose by glycolytic pathways, mainly to lactic acid. In most but not all mycoplasmas the respiratory pathways are flavin-terminated so that the heme compounds, cytochromes, and catalase are absent. Mycoplasmas that metabolize arginine use a three-enzyme system that converts it via ornithine to ammonia, and in so doing, supplies the organisms with ATP. A few species utilize both glucose and arginine, but ureaplasmas metabolize neither substrate. They convert urea to ammonia by means of a urease, although the need for urea as an energy source has not been established. Some metabolic properties of common human mycoplasmas are summarized in Table 3.

## PATHOPHYSIOLOGY

Although *M. hominis* and *U. urealyticum* have been associated with perinatal sepsis, endometritis-salpingitis, and other genitourinary infections, their pathogenic role in many cases is unclear, and little is known of their pathogenic mechanisms (McCormack et al., 1973; Bowie et al., 1976). The pathogenicity of *M. pneumoniae*, which has been studied in humans, hamsters, and tracheal organ cultures, seems to depend on attachment of the specific terminal structure to neuraminic acid receptor sites on the surface of mucosal cells in the trachea and bronchi (Fig. 1). Proteins on the membrane of *M. pneumoniae* play a role in the attachment (Hu et al., 1977). The organisms do not invade the mucosal cells but appear to damage them by a toxic factor. *M. neurolyticum,* a pathogen of mice, produces a soluble protein exotoxin, but the only toxic factor definitively identified in *M. pneumoniae* so far is hydrogen peroxide. Attachment is important in pathogenesis; disease is produced by strains of *M. pneumoniae* that produce peroxide and attach, but no disease is caused by strains that produce peroxide but do not attach. *M. pneumoniae* can also activate the classic and alternate pathways of complement and inhibit phagocytosis by alveolar macrophages.

Because fatal cases of *M. pneumoniae* pneumonia are rare, the histopathologic picture of this disease is derived mainly from experimental infection of hamsters and natural mycoplasmal disease in other animals. The pneumonic infiltrate is predominantly a peribronchiolar and per-

ivascular cuffing by lymphocytes (Fig. 3*a*). This tissue response is followed by a change of the exudate in the bronchioles from a predominance of lymphocytes to a predominance of polymorphonuclear leukocytes and macrophages. These latter cells may, in association with antibody, help clear mycoplasmas by immune phagocytosis. The rather slow development of these events in a primary infection contrasts with the markedly accelerated and often more intense response that occurs with reinfection. Some of the lymphocytes in the peribronchial infiltrate contain immunoglobulin, but most of these cells appear to be thymus-dependent. Ablation of the thymus in hamsters by various procedures prevents the development of peribronchial cuffing when these animals are challenged with *M. pneumoniae* (Fig. 3*b*). To at least some extent, therefore, the pneu-

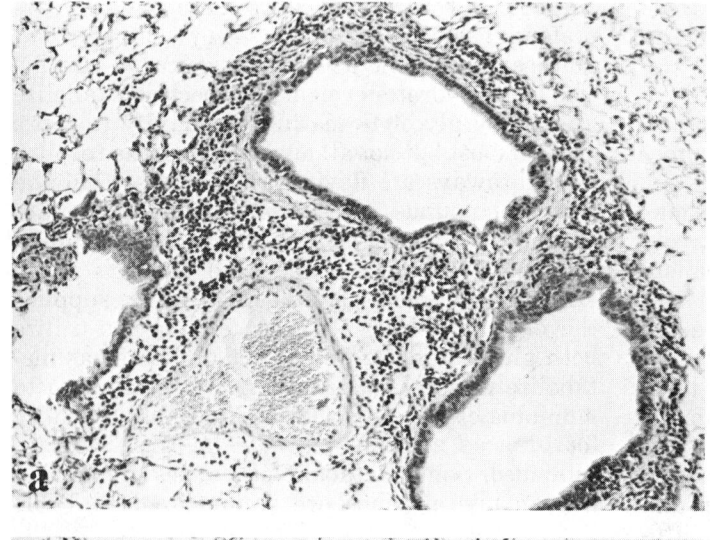

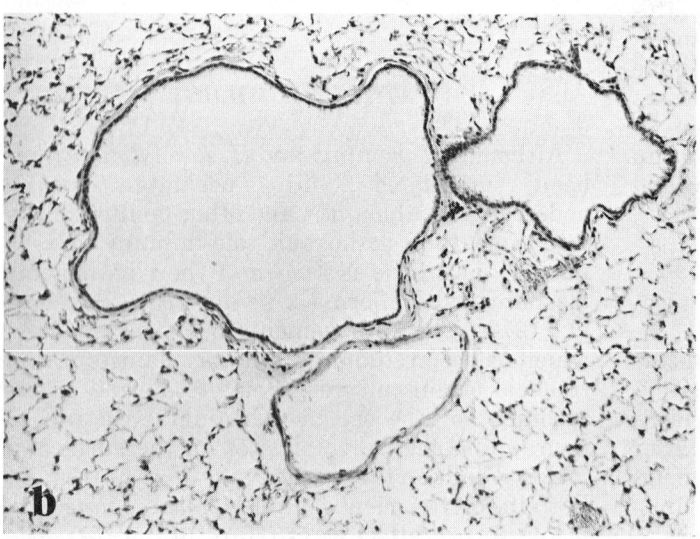

**FIGURE 3.** *Pathology of pneumonia caused by Mycoplasma pneumoniae. Pneumonia 2 weeks after intranasal inoculation with M. pneumoniae of (a) immunologically normal hamsters (note peribronchiolar and perivascular infiltrate of mononuclear cells, predominantly lymphocytes) and (b) hamsters previously depleted of T-lymphocytes (note virtual absence of infiltrate). (Hematoxylin and eosin, ×176).*

monia caused by *M. pneumoniae* is an immuno-pathologic process (Taylor and Taylor-Robinson, 1975). Since many young children possess *M. pneumoniae* antibody, it is possible that the pneumonia that occurs in older age groups is an immunologic overresponse to reinfection, the lung being infiltrated by previously sensitized lymphocytes.

The pathophysiology of the Stevens-Johnson syndrome (erythema multiforme), meningoencephalitis, and other conditions that sometimes complicate *M. pneumoniae* infections is not understood. No firm evidence supports a pathogenic role for the antiheart and antilung antibodies that are observed in some patients with *M. pneumoniae* pneumonia.

The localization of specific receptor sites, and thus the organisms of *M. pneumoniae*, in the trachea and bronchi with subsequent peribronchial infiltrates, contrasts with the localization of pneumococi in fluid-filled alveoli that are adjacent to the pleura. This may explain why pneumonia caused by *M. pneumoniae* is characterized by substernal burning and scanty production of sputum on coughing, whereas pneumococcal pneumonia is characterized by lateral pleuritic chest pain and generous production of sputum on coughing.

## IMMUNITY

Antibodies in serum may be detected during mycoplasma infections by a variety of techniques, the most sensitive of which are radioimmuno-precipitation, complement-dependent mycoplasmacidal and metabolism inhibition tests. Generally, the first antibodies produced are of the IgM class; later IgG predominates. Humoral antibodies, however, do not fully protect against infection or disease, since infection and development of pneumonia may occur despite high levels of, for example, mycoplasmacidal antibodies to *M. pneumoniae* in the serum. Furthermore, natural or experimental respiratory tract infection of animals may produce only low levels of serum antibodies, yet such local infection provides greater resistance to reinfection than does parenteral inoculation of organisms, which produces high levels of serum antibody. This suggests that local factors are crucial in resistance. Indeed, resistance of adult volunteers to *M. pneumoniae* has been related to the presence of specific IgA antibody in respiratory secretions. This antibody may function as the first line of defense by preventing the attachment of organisms to the respiratory epithelial cells. On the other hand, development of a cell-mediated immune response, which is detectable by lymphocyte transformation and macrophage migration inhibition, does not seem to be important in resistance.

In field trials, inactivated *M. pneumoniae* vaccines have prevented disease in only about half of those vaccinated. The inability of these and other killed mycoplasma vaccines to protect completely may be due to their failure to stimulate local antibody production. With this in mind, live but attenuated temperature-sensitive mutants of *M. pneumoniae* have been developed that multiply at the temperature of the upper respiratory tract but not at that of the lower tract. Some of the mutants have produced pulmonary infection both in the hamster and in human volunteers without causing disease and have induced resistance to challenge with virulent wild-type *M. pneumoniae*. Whether such mutants can be made sufficiently stable and attenuated for large-scale use as a human vaccine remains to be seen. However, permanent protection seems unlikely because naturally acquired *M. pneumoniae* infection does not provide lifelong immunity. Reinfection occurs with appreciable frequency, and second attacks of *M. pneumoniae* pneumonia also occur.

## LABORATORY DIAGNOSIS

Mycoplasmas grown in vitro are gram-negative. However, individual mycoplasma organisms are too small and do not take up the safranin counterstain well enough to be recognized on microscopic examination of gram-stained clinical specimens. The laboratory diagnosis depends, therefore, on cultural identification and on serologic tests. Details of these techniques have recently been outlined by Gump and Forsyth (1977).

The medium for primary isolation of *M. pneumoniae* consists of PPLO agar or broth, 20 per cent horse serum and 10 per cent vol/vol fresh yeast extract (25 per cent wt/vol). To enhance detection of *M. pneumoniae*, the medium is supplemented with thallium acetate and penicillin to inhibit bacteria and fungi, methylene blue to inhibit other human mycoplasmas, and glucose with phenol red as a pH indicator to detect acid produced by *M. pneumoniae*. A vial of diphasic medium (broth over agar) is inoculated with sputum or a pharyngeal swab and incubated at 37° C. A color change from purple to yellow-green, which usually occurs within 4 to 21 days, signals the fermentation of glucose with production of acid and the consequent change in color of the phenol red to yellow. This presumptive positive identification is confirmed by subculturing to agar medium and demonstrating inhibition of colony development with commercial disks impregnated with specific antiserum. Hemadsorption and rapid hemolysis of guinea pig red cells by colonies of *M. pneumoniae* on agar are also used to help in presumptive identification. The hemadsorption is attributed to neuraminic acid receptors on red cells.

A similar strategy, utilizing the metabolism of arginine or urea, has been employed to design media that select for and presumptively identify *M. hominis* and *U. urealyticum* in specimens from the genitourinary tract.

The most readily available specific serologic test for *M. pneumoniae* is the complement fixation test, for which reagents can be obtained commercially. It is positive in about 80 per cent of cases as indicated by a fourfold or greater rise in antibody titers between acute and convalescent specimens. The cold agglutinin test depends on nonspecific agglutination of O Rh-negative red blood cells at 4° C by antibodies to I antigen that arise in *M. pneumoniae* infection. The test is positive in only about 50 per cent of patients, usually those with more severe disease. Serologic tests that detect antibody to *M. hominis* and *U. urealyticum* are still research procedures.

## DRUG SUSCEPTIBILITY

Since the mycoplasmas lack a cell wall, they are resistant or indifferent to the penicillins, cephalosporins, and other antimicrobials that act on the cell wall. In contrast, mycoplasmas are generally sensitive to antimicrobials that inhibit protein synthesis. At clinically achievable concentrations, tetracycline is inhibitory for *M. pneumoniae*, *M. hominis*, and *U. urealyticum*. Whereas erythromycin has marked inhibitory and mycoplasmacidal activity against *M. pneumoniae*, it is only moderately active against *U. urealyticum* and is inactive against *M. hominis*. Both genital mycoplasmas, *U. urealyticum* and *M. hominis*, are sensitive to spectinomycin. Despite the sensitivity of *M. pneumoniae* to tetracycline and erythromycin and the good clinical responses to therapy that occur with these drugs, about 50 per cent of treated patients continue to harbor *M. pneumoniae* in the posterior pharynx for one to three months.

## EPIDEMIOLOGY

Infections with *M. pneumoniae* apparently occur world-wide and account for approximately 20 per cent of all cases of pneumonia in some cities. The disease is endemic with periodic epi-

demics. Spread of the organism, which occurs by aerosol transmission, is slow. Therefore, most infections occur in small groups of people who have frequent close contact such as families, military units, and college fraternities. The incubation period is two to three weeks. The disease is usually introduced into the family by a small child and moves from person to person over a period of months with an attack rate of greater than 50 per cent. Pneumonia is most frequent in persons aged 5 to 20. Thereafter, pneumonia occurs less frequently but is generally more severe as the patient's age increases.

Ureaplasmas are acquired by up to 30 per cent of infants at birth. Colonization of the genital tract is most common but is usually transient. The organisms are found again after puberty, and antibody is first detectable at this time. Thereafter, the frequency of occurrence is related to sexual activity; recovery rates of about 60 per cent and 80 per cent have been observed for men and women, respectively, attending venereal disease clinics (McCormack et al., 1973). The occurrence of ureaplasmas in apparently healthy persons has posed a problem in attributing a pathogenic role to them. However, the results of several studies, including the intraurethral inoculation of human volunteers with ureaplasmas, suggest that they cause some cases of nongonococcal urethritis (Bowie et al., 1976).

*M. hominis* is acquired at birth by about 6 per cent of infants. Most of these individuals lose these strains but become colonized later in life when sexual activity commences. *M. hominis* is unlikely to play a role in nongonococcal urethritis, but it has been associated with reproductive failure, low birth weight, recurrent abortions, and a variety of pelvic infections. It has been isolated from the blood in the absence of other microorganisms in 8 per cent of women with febrile abortions.

The frequent causation of arthritis and neurologic diseases by different mycoplasmas in various animal species has suggested that they might cause such diseases in humans. Although the search for mycoplasmas in rheumatoid arthritis and other diseases of unknown etiology continues, these studies have not yet yielded definitive evidence.

### References

Bowie, W. R., Floyd, J. F., Miller, Y., Alexander, E. R., Holmes, J., and Holmes, K. K.: Differential response of chlamydial and ureaplasma-associated urethritis to sulphafurazole (sulfisoxazole) and aminocyclitols. Lancet 2:1276, 1976.

Gump, D. W., and Forsyth, B. R.: Mycoplasma. In von Graevenitz, A. (ed.): Clinical Microbiology, vol. I. (CRC Handbook Series in Clinical Laboratory Science, Sec. E) Cleveland, CRC Press, 1977, p. 357.

Hayflick, L. (ed.): The Mycoplasmatales and the L-Phase of Bacteria. New York, Appleton-Century-Crofts, 1969.

Hu, P. C., Collier, A. M., and Baseman, J. B.: Surface parasitism by *Mycoplasma pneumoniae* of respiratory epithelium. J Exp Med 145:1328, 1977.

McCormack, W. M., Braun, P., Lee, Y. H., Klein, J. O., and Kass, E. H.: The genital mycoplasmas. N Engl J Med 288:78, 1973.

McGee, Z. A., Rogul, M., and Wittler, R. G.: Molecular genetic studies of relationships among mycoplasma, L-forms and bacteria. Ann N Y Acad Sci 143:21, 1967.

Razin, S.: The mycoplasmas. Microbiol Rev 42:414, 1978.

Taylor, G., and Taylor-Robinson, D.: The part played by cell-mediated immunity in mycoplasma respiratory infections. Develop Biol Stand 28:195, 1975.

# CELL WALL-DEFECTIVE 54 BACTERIA

## Zell A. McGee, M.D.

Susceptible bacteria that are exposed to penicillin or other substances that damage the bacterial cell wall are usually killed. Under certain conditions, however, bacteria can survive with damaged cell walls and multiply as organisms with markedly altered morphology, physiology, and cultural characteristics (Dienes and Weinberger, 1951; Gutman et al., 1967; Hayflick, 1969). These wall-defective bacteria are undetectable by routine cultural techniques, are not affected by penicillin and other cell wall-active antimicrobials, and may revert to the intact bacterium if the cell wall-active antibiotic is removed. These characteristics of elusiveness, indifference to the most frequently administered antimicrobials, and morphologic versatility have stimulated interest in the possibility that wall-defective bacteria may play a role in various chronic, recurrent, or culture-negative infections of humans (Clasener, 1972; Guze, 1967).

### MORPHOLOGY AND PHYSIOLOGY

The pliable bacterial cytoplasmic membrane is encased in a rigid peptidoglycan layer, which gives the bacterial cell its coccal or rod shape. In gram-negative bacteria, the intracellular osmotic pressure is 300 to 400 milliosmoles per kilogram water (mOsm/kg), and in gram-positive bacteria, it is 900 mOsm/kg or greater. When bacteria are suspended in serum or most bacteriologic media (270 to 300 mOsm/kg), the higher internal osmotic pressure of the bacteria favors the flow of water into their cytoplasm, but there cannot be a net gain of water because the peptidoglycan layer restricts any increase in volume. If the peptidoglycan layer is removed, water moves freely into the cytoplasm with increasing distention of the cytoplasmic membrane and dilution of the cytoplasm until the concentration of molecules

inside the membrane equals the concentration outside. Before this equalization occurs, however, the cytoplasmic membrane usually ruptures, and the organism is killed. This seems to be the way that bacteria die when their cell walls are damaged by penicillin.

If the concentration of molecules in the environment is increased so that it balances the concentration within the bacterium, removal of the peptidoglycan may result in a change of shape (e.g., from a rod to a spherical shape), but the organism will not rupture (see Fig. 1b). Bacteria with damaged or absent cell walls can survive in environments with osmolalities lower than their intracellular osmotic pressure, but their cytoplasmic membranes must be stabilized intrinsically by divalent cations or polyamines, or by an adaptive change to a higher ratio of saturated to unsaturated fatty acids in the membrane (Leon and Panos, 1976).

When bacteria are exposed to penicillin in a hypertonic medium (strictly, a medium with an osmolality greater than that of human serum [290 mOsm/kg] but conventionally, about 900 mOsm/kg), they may simply round up to become *spheroplasts* (which have partial loss of the cell wall) or *protoplasts* (which have complete loss of the cell wall) (Fig. 1a, b). Since bacteria in the spheroplast or protoplast phase cannot multiply and are lysed at physiologic osmolalities, they are unlikely to play a role in human infections. Bacteria may also undergo a more fundamental change, however, either directly or by further transition from spheroplasts or protoplasts to L-phase variants or L-forms (Fig. 1c,d) (L stands for the Lister Institute in London where they were first described in 1935). Some bacteria, such as *Neisseria gonorrhoeae* and *Bacteroides fragilis*, can undergo this transition to the L-phase spontaneously; others require the presence of penicillin, lysozyme, or other cell wall-active substances.

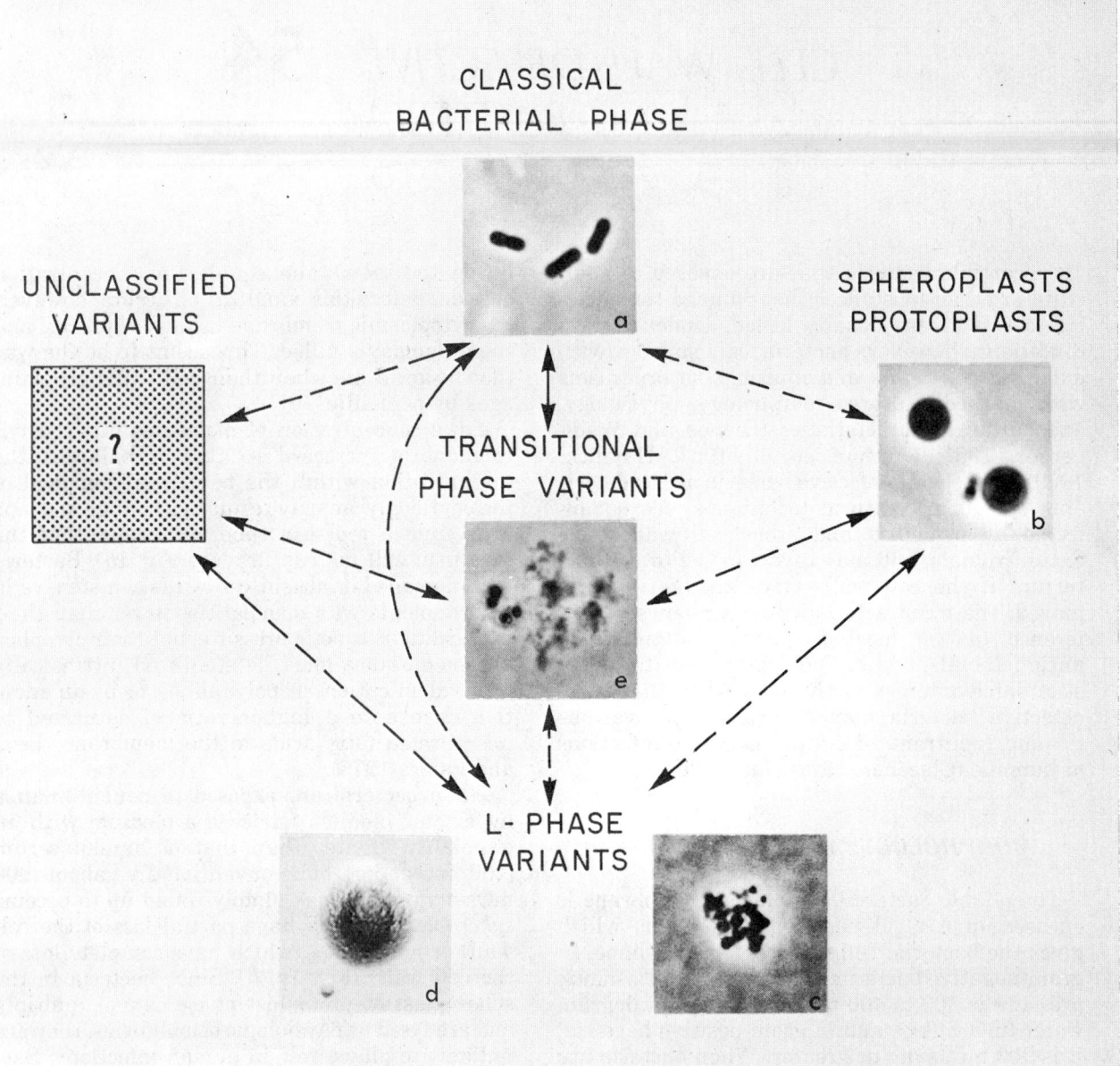

**FIGURE 1.** *Schematic representation of the transition of a bacterium to different variant phases. Photos a, b, and c demonstrate the contrasting morphology of the classic bacterial phase, spheroplast phase, and a clump of L-phase variants of* Proteus mirabilis *in identical media (900 mOsm/kg) and at the same magnification (phase contrast, × 3400). Photo d shows a "fried egg" colony of L-phase variants of* Proteus mirabilis *(× 150). Photo e shows a clump of transitional phase variants of* Staphylococcus albus *from the blood culture of a patient with an infected prosthetic heart valve (phase contrast, × 1600). (From McGee, Z.A., Wittler, R.G., Gooder, H., and Charache, P.: J Infect Dis 123:433, 1971.)*

Bacteria in the L-phase can replicate serially as nonrigid cells that are spherical or pleomorphic and vary in size from "large bodies," larger than some human cells, to elementary bodies, which may be as small as some viruses. On solid media, L-phase variants produce tiny colonies composed of a central core, which grows into the agar, and a superficial growth around the core, which gives them a "fried egg" appearance (Fig. 1d). L-phase variants that cannot revert to the classic bacterial phase are called "stable" L-phase variants. Bacteria that have reverted from the L-phase may be indistinguishable from the original bacteria, except that when exposed to the same or different inducing agents, they enter the L-phase more readily. L-phase variants resemble mycoplasmas in their individual and colonial morphology, but studies have failed to show any immunologic, biochemical or genetic relationship between these groups of microorganisms (Hayflick, 1969; McGee et al., 1971).

L-phase variants and bacteria undergoing transition to or from L-phase variants (*transitional phase variants*, Fig. 1e) are the types of wall-defective bacteria most likely to play a role in human disease.

## ANTIGENIC COMPOSITION

The antigenic composition of a bacterium in the L-phase is similar to that of its bacterial phase. Even L-phase variants that completely lack cell-wall antigens on their external surface may continue to elaborate them into the environment. Although L-phase variants sometimes show antigenic determinants that are different from those of the parental bacteria, these may not represent new antigens but merely greater accessibility of certain determinants to antibody-producing cells.

One type of antigen-antibody reaction that occurs with the L-phase but not with the classic bacterial phase is inhibition of growth by specific antibody (Braude and Siemienski, 1968). These growth-inhibiting antibodies, which may also be elicited by the bacterial phase, do not require complement and seem to be directed at antigens of the cytoplasmic membrane.

## METABOLISM

Transition to the L-phase is sometimes accompanied by loss of the ability to carry out certain metabolic reactions such as fermentation of a particular sugar or production of a hemolysin. The L-phase variants of a few bacterial species,

such as *Salmonella typhi,* require anaerobic conditions, whereas the parental bacterium can grow aerobically. Nevertheless, L-phase variants generally carry out metabolic reactions and generate products characteristic of the bacteria from which they were derived, although they may do so at a slower rate.

## HOST DEFENSES

A number of factors make the human body a potentially adverse environment for L-phase variants: (1) the osmolality of human serum and tissue fluid is approximately 290 mOsm/kg, well below the osmolality at which wall-defective variants of some bacteria undergo osmotic rupture; (2) normal human serum contains an antibody-complement system that rapidly disrupts the cytoplasmic membranes and kills L-phase variants of a variety of gram-positive and gram-negative pathogens; (3) growth-inhibiting antibodies may be elicited by L-phase variants or their parental bacteria; and (4) L-phase variants can be phagocytized by polymorphonuclear and mononuclear phagocytes.

## PATHOGENIC PROPERTIES

None of the defenses mentioned above precludes the survival and multiplication of L-phase variants in humans. L-phase variants of both gram-negative and gram-positive bacteria can survive at osmolalities comparable to those of serum or purulent exudates. The hypertonic milieu of the kidney provides osmotic protection and inactivates the antibody-complement system in serum that might otherwise be lethal to L-phase variants. These variants can be formed and can persist within certain host cells under experimental conditions in vitro and in vivo.

L-phase variants of toxigenic bacteria, such as *Clostridium tetani* or *Vibrio* species, also produce toxins and might thereby be pathogenic. The L-phase variants of some gram-negative bacteria elaborate endotoxin and can evoke the localized Shwartzman reaction. Infection of the urinary tract of experimental animals with L-phase variants of *Proteus mirabilis,* which produce urease, has been associated with formation of bladder stones (Braude and Siemienski, 1968). L-phase variants of group A beta-hemolytic streptococci have been shown to adapt to osmotic conditions like those in human tissues and to invade and kill human heart cells in tissue culture (Leon and Panos, 1976). However, L-phase variants have persisted for prolonged periods in the tissues of experimental animals with little evidence of damage. The greatest pathogenic potential of L-phase variants may reside in their ability to maintain a pathogenic organism in a host under conditions such as antibiotic therapy that might kill the bacterial phase. The L-phase variant may then revert to the pathogenic bacterial phase when conditions become favorable for its survival.

## ROLE IN INFECTIONS

Despite the varied methods of formation and survival of wall-defective variants in vivo under experimental conditions, it has been most difficult to prove that wall-defective variants play a role in human diseases. Koch's postulates have not been helpful in approaching this problem because they do not allow for a significant change in the nature of an organism during the course of an infection.

There are many reports of pyelonephritis, osteomyelitis, endocarditis, and other acute and chronic infections in which wall-defective variants were isolated on hypertonic but not on routine media. However, only a few of these studies provide evidence that L-phase variants were actually present in the patient and not merely induced on the media in the laboratory.

Microscopic examination of the urine from patients with pyelonephritis has revealed spheroplasts and other atypical bacteria during periods of antimicrobial therapy but only classic rod-shaped bacteria when therapy was not being administered. In one series of patients, the presence of viable cell-wall defective bacteria in the urine of 11 (16 per cent) of 57 patients with chronic pyelonephritis was documented by filtrating the specimens to remove bacteria and isolating L-phase variants from the filtrates on hypertonic but not on isotonic media. In three patients, who had only wall-defective variants in their urine and were not receiving antibiotics, the variants were apparently either induced by autolytic bacterial enzymes or by host factors.

One patient, a 10-year-old girl (described by Gutman et al., 1967), had recurrent bouts of urinary tract infection characterized by urgency, chills, fever, and more than $10^5$ P. mirabilis per ml. of urine. During ampicillin therapy, the patient's symptoms decreased and routine cultures became sterile, but L-phase variants of the Proteus were recovered from filtered urine cultured on hypertonic media. After therapy was discontinued, bacterial phase P. mirabilis returned, and cultures for L-phase variants became negative.

The bacterial phase was sensitive to ampicillin but resistant to erythromycin. The L-phase variant was resistant to ampicillin but sensitive to erythromycin. After ampicillin therapy was begun, routine cultures became negative, but cultures for L-phase variants became positive. When erythromycin was added to the regimen, cultures for L-phase variants became negative within three days. After completion of 12 days of combined therapy, all cultures remained negative and the patient was free of urinary tract infection for a follow-up period of 18 months.

Wittler and colleagues (1960) described the five-year course of a young girl with similar changes of symptoms and culture results during periods of penicillin therapy for Corynebacterium endocarditis. When penicillin was administered, she became asymptomatic and cultures on routine media became negative, but wall-defective variants were recovered on hypertonic media. The bacterial phase returned when penicillin was discontinued. This study was more convincing because the variants were visualized microscopically in peripheral blood cells when variants were recovered from hypertonic culture media and because penicillinase was used in the cultures to decrease the likelihood of producing variants in vitro.

These and a few other careful clinical studies as well as data from experimental animals strongly suggest that L-phase variants may be produced and persist in vivo. It is not clear whether such organisms are of clinical significance in more than rare cases.

## LABORATORY DIAGNOSIS

Cultures for wall-defective organisms can be performed by the laboratory on two different levels: (1) the laboratory may routinely include media that are appropriate for recovering wall-defective variants but will not determine whether organisms isolated were present in the patient as typical bacteria or as L-phase variants; or (2) the laboratory may perform on highly selected patients the specialized procedures necessary to isolate and identify wall-defective variants that do not revert on their first passage in vitro, determine their antimicrobial susceptibility, and establish whether the organism existed in a wall-defective form in the patient. The details of these procedures have recently been reviewed (McGee, 1977). Either or both approaches may be adopted, but the second requires experienced personnel, complex media, and a large commitment of time.

## DRUG SUSCEPTIBILITY

Bacteria undergoing transition to the L-phase always lose susceptibility to penicillins, cephalosporins, and other agents that act on the cell wall. Conversely, gram-negative bacilli, such as *Pseudomonas aeruginosa* become more susceptible to erythromycin, tetracycline, and other agents that act within the bacterial cytoplasm but are normally excluded by the gram-negative cell wall. These changes in susceptibility provide a rationale for the therapy of infections involving bacterial variants.

Therapy of infections with cell wall-defective variants has generally consisted of a combination of two drugs: (1) a cell wall-active agent such as penicillin that either kills residual bacteria or makes them wall-defective, and (2) an antimicrobial such as erythromycin or gentamicin that acts within the bacterial cell. Although this approach has been effective in controlled studies of infected experimental animals, reports of its success in human infections are anecdotal. Currently, the use of such therapy seems justified only in highly selected and closely monitored patients whose clinical specimens contain wall-defective variants (McGee, 1977).

## References

Braude, A. I., and Sieminski, J.: Production of bladder stones by L-forms. Trans Assn Amer Phys 81:323, 1968.

Clasener, H.: Pathogenicity of the L-phase of bacteria. Ann Rev Microbiol 26:55, 1972.

Dienes, L., and Weinberger, H. J.: The L-forms of bacteria. Bacteriol Rev 15:245, 1951.

Gutman, L. T., Schaller, J., and Wedgwood, R. J.: Bacterial L-forms in relapsing urinary-tract infection. Lancet 1:464, 1967.

Guze, L. B. (ed.): Microbial protoplasts, spheroplasts and L-forms. Baltimore, Williams and Wilkins, 1967.

Hayflick, L. (ed.): The mycoplasmatales and the L-phase of bacteria. New York, Appleton-Century-Crofts, 1969.

Leon, O., and Panos, C.: Adaptation of an osmotically fragile L-form of *Streptococcus pyogenes* to physiological osmotic conditions and its ability to destroy human heart cells in tissue culture. Infect Immun 13:252, 1976.

McGee, Z. A.: Cell-wall deficient bacteria. In von Graevenitz, Alexander (ed.): CRC Handbook Series in Clinical Laboratory Science, Section E: Clinical Microbiology, Vol. I. Cleveland, CRC Press, Inc., 1977, p. 367.

McGee, Z. A, Wittler, R. G., Gooder, H., and Charache, P.: Wall-defective microbial variants: terminology and experimental design. J Infect Dis 123:433, 1971.

Wittler, R. G., Malizia, W. F., Kramer, P. E., Tuckett, J. D., Pritchard, H. N., and Baker, H. J.: Isolation of a corynebacterium and its transitional forms from a case of subacute bacterial endocarditis treated with antibiotics. J Gen Microbiol 23:315, 1960.

# 5  VIRUSES

# DNA  Viruses

# ADENOVIRUS  55

*Lennart Philipson, M.D., Dr. Med. Sci.*

Adenoviruses constitute a family of viruses originally isolated from the respiratory tract of man and other animals. They were discovered in 1953. They are nonenveloped icosahedral viruses with DNA genomes of intermediate size ($20$ to $30 \times 10^6$ daltons). The adenovirus family has been subdivided in two genera, mastadenovirus and aviadenovirus, referring to viruses isolated from mammalian and avian hosts respectively (Norrby et al., 1976). There is no cross-reacting antigen between these two genera. The mastadenovirus comprises at least 80 different serotypes, of which 33 have been isolated from human sources. The aviadenovirus contains 14 distinct serotypes.

Precise biochemical tools to characterize adenovirus genomes have become available during recent years, including separated strands of the DNA, restriction enzyme fragments, and liquid hybridization methods to detect the viral transcription products. The structural and nonstructural proteins encoded by the adenovirus genome have also been extensively characterized with regard to both structure and function. The adenoviruses have therefore become a model virus to investigate the complex control mechanism involved in macromolecular synthesis in mammalian cells. Studies of the molecular biology of these viruses may help to elucidate mechanisms for transcription, processing of the transcripts to messenger RNA, and control mechanisms for protein synthesis in mammali-

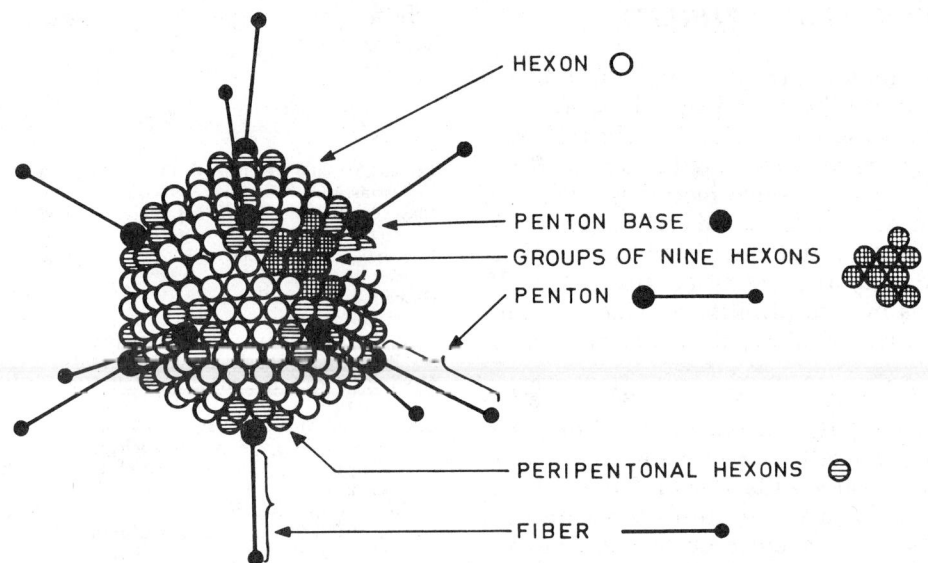

**FIGURE 1.** *Structure of the adenovirus capsid. Schematic drawing showing the icosahedral outline of the adeno-virus capsid and the location of various components. (Reprinted from Philipson et al., 1975.)*

an cells. The molecular biology of the adenoviruses has recently been reviewed (Philipson et al., 1975; Wold et al., 1978), but the role of these viruses in human infections has not been evaluated during recent years. Several reviews may provide a more detailed insight into the clinical aspects of adenovirus infections (Sohier et al., 1965; Potter, 1967; and Rose, 1969). This chapter will focus on some properties of adenoviruses and their role in infectious diseases in man.

## THE STRUCTURE OF THE VIRION

### Morphology

The adenoviruses are nonenveloped viruses with a diameter of 65 to 80 nm. The capsid has 252 capsomers arranged into an icosahedron with 20 triangular facets and 12 vertices, as schematically shown in Figure 1. Two hundred forty of the 252 capsomers have six neighbors, and they are called *hexons;* whereas the 12 capsomers at the vertices have five neighbors, and are therefore called *pentons.* Each penton unit consists of a penton base anchored in the capsid and a rod-like projection with a knob attached at the distal end. The rod-like portion is referred to as the *fiber.* Two types of hexons may be defined: (1) those 60 located in juxtaposition to the pentons, *peripentonal hexons* that have the penton base as one of their six neighbors, and (2) those 180 that form the triangular facets and the edges of the icosahedron. The lat-

ter may be released from the virions in aggregates of nine hexons, *ninemers,* which form a defined structure with threefold rotational symmetry. Inside the capsid there is a core with a diameter of 40 to 45 nm, which contains the DNA and additional proteins. It can be revealed by electron microscopy of thin sections of particles stained with uranyl acetate. A circular protein-DNA complex was recently observed after degradation of virions with guanidine, suggesting that the two termini of the DNA in the virion are linked to each other by proteins.

### Chemical Composition

The human adenovirus type 2 (ad2), which has been studied in detail, has an estimated particle weight of $175 \times 10^6$ daltons. It contains 13 per cent DNA corresponding to $23 \times 10^6$ daltons, and the additional components are all proteins. Unlike most other viruses the adenoviruses have capsid units that are soluble in nondenaturing solvent, which has facilitated the purification and characterization of the virus components. Methods have been developed for sequential disintegration of the virion. The pentons alone or together with peripentonal hexons can be selectively removed by dialysis at low pH. The release of pentons is accompanied by the release of additional antigens probably located in the peripentonal region. After treatment of the virus particle with sodium dodecyl sulfate (SDS), urea, or pyridine, the capsid is disrupted and the hexons from the triangular facets are released as ninemers. The polypeptide composition of adenoviruses has been studied by SDS-polyacrylamide electrophoresis. The virion of ad2, ad7, and ad12 contains a minimum of nine polypeptides that range in size from 7500 to 120,000 daltons. Eight of these are antigenically distinct and reside in different structures after sequential degradation of the virion. Five of the polypeptides are integral parts of the capsomers or the core. Thus, polypeptide II is the only polypeptide that is detected in purified hexons from infected cells. Polypeptide III resides in the penton base, IV, in the fiber, and polypeptide V and VII are associated with the core. The remaining polypeptides have been tentatively localized in the virion structure as indicated in Figure 2. The structural units observed in the virion as hexon, penton, and fiber are multimers of the integral polypeptide. Hexon contains three polypeptides, penton probably contains five, and fiber contains three polypeptides, and each unit must therefore be assembled independently.

The DNA of human adenoviruses has been extensively characterized. There is a difference in base composition between the different subgroups of the human adenoviruses (Table 1). In addition, there is considerable homology of the DNA sequence within each subgroup but only 10 to 20 per cent homology between DNA of members of different subgroups, regardless of whether filter hybridization or electron microscopic analysis of heteroduplexes was used to measure homology. The DNA for several types is infectious but the specific infectivity is at least $10^6$ times lower than for virions measured as number of infectious units/$\mu$g of DNA. The protein associated with the termini of the viral DNA appears to enhance the infectivity of viral DNA. Specific fragments of DNA representing around 7.5 per cent of the total genome can transform cells. The DNA has been cleaved by several restriction enzymes and fragment maps have been established (Fig. 3). The fragments have been used to map the position of tran-

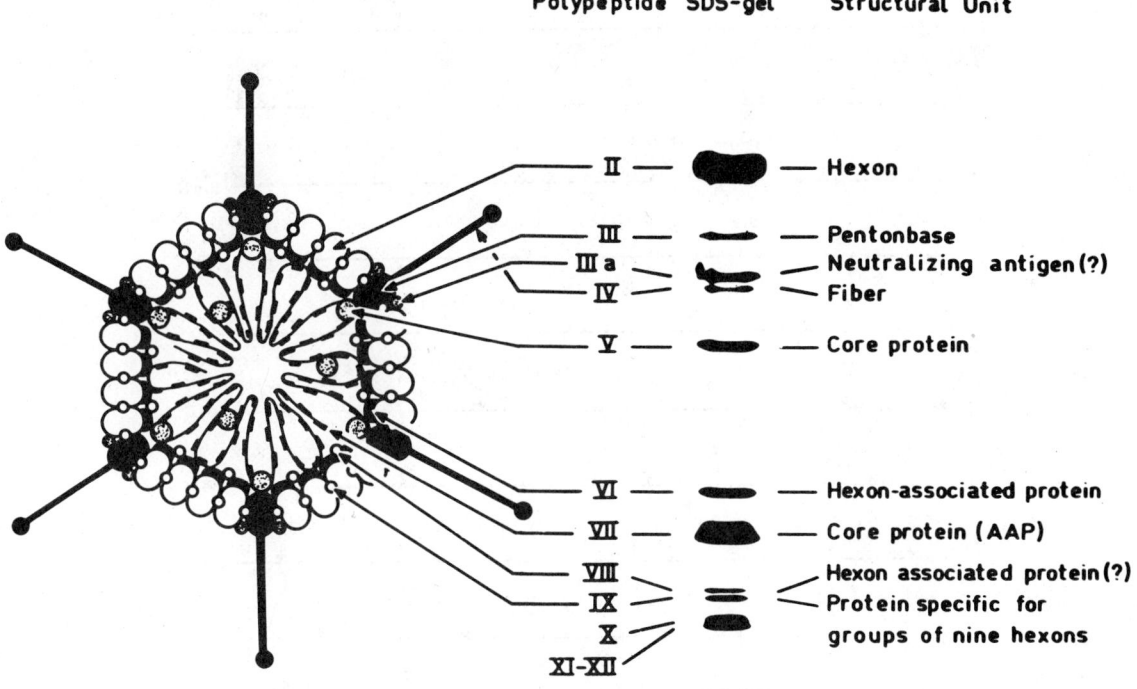

**FIGURE 2.** *A tentative model of the location of different proteins in the ad2 virion. The core protein V may be located inside at the vertices, since it is partially released with the peripentonal region. It has been estimated that core protein VII may neutralize about 50 per cent of all phosphate residues in the DNA. The molar ratio between polypeptide VI and the hexon polypeptide is about 2, and the native protein VI exists as a dimer. Protein VI is not iodinated in intact virions, which suggests that protein VI is located at the inner surface of the hexons. Peripentonal hexons also possess this protein. Protein IX appears to be the cementing substance between hexons from the facets, since it is associated with groups of nine hexons. Protein VIII is also associated with the hexons and may reside at the inner surface of the triangular facets, since it is not iodinated in intact virions. Polypeptide IIIa is probably located in the peripentonal region. The localization of protein X is unknown. The polypeptide composition of the virion proteins as identified in a stained exponential (10 to 16 per cent) SDS-polyacrylamide gel are also shown. (From Philipson et al., 1975.)*

**TABLE 1.   Classification of Human Adenoviruses***

| SUBGROUP | SEROTYPES | PER CENT GC IN DNA | PER CENT DNA HOMOLOGY BETWEEN TYPES | HEMAGGLUTI-NATION SUBGROUP | LENGTH OF FIBER (nm) | ONCOGENICITY† |
|---|---|---|---|---|---|---|
| A | 12,18,31 | 48–49 | 80–85 | IV | 28–31 | High |
| B | 3,7,11,14,16,21 | 50–52 | 70–95 | I | 9–11 | Weak |
| C | 1,2,4,5,6 | 57–59 | 85–95 | III | 23–31 | None but transform |
| D | 8,9,10,13,15,17,19, 20,22,23–28 | 57–61 | Not known | II | 12–13 | None but transform |

*Reprinted from Philipson et al., 1975, where the original references have been cited.
†Highly oncogenic types cause tumors within 2 months; weakly oncogenic types cause tumors in some animals in 4 to 18 months.

scripts and messenger RNA by nucleic acid hybridization. Isolated messenger RNAs have also been analyzed by in vitro translation in order to map the position of most of the gene products on the viral genome.

## CLASSIFICATION OF HUMAN ADENOVIRUSES

Human adenoviruses have been separated into four groups based on their ability to agglu-

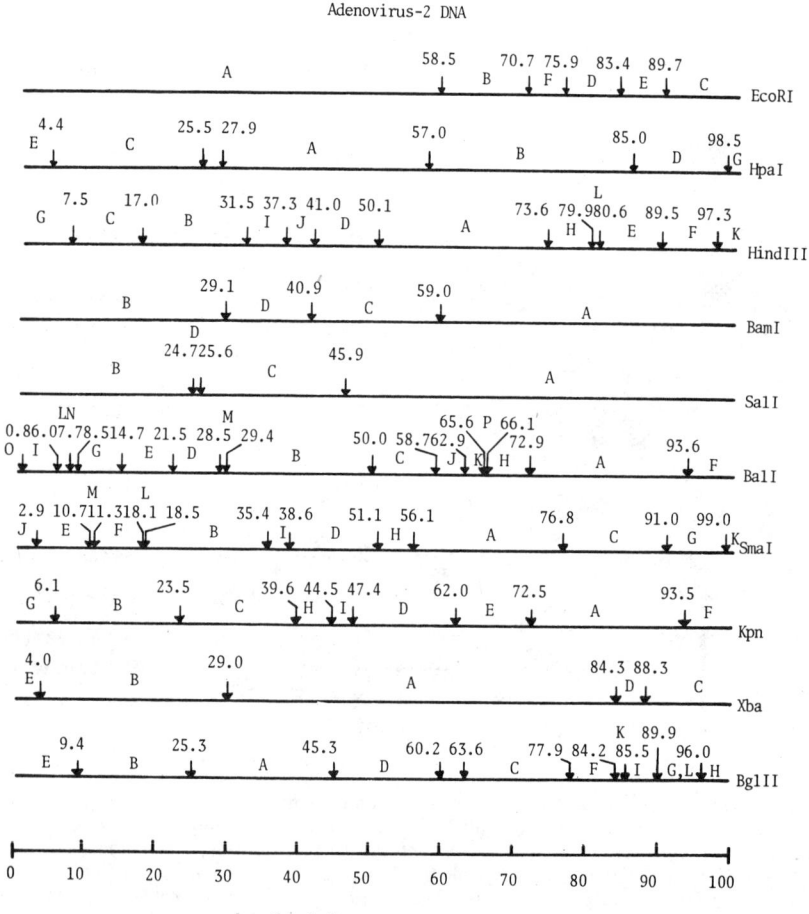

**FIGURE 3.**   *Restriction enzyme maps of adenovirus type 2 DNA. The restriction enzymes have been described by Roberts (1976) and the map positions of the different enzymes have been determined by several investigators at the Cold Spring Harbor Laboratory (Tooze, 1979). The presented maps were compiled by Dr. Marc Zabeau and distributed at the Cold Spring Harbor Tumor Virus Meeting, 1977.*

tinate monkey or rat erythrocytes. Group I viruses cause complete agglutination of monkey erythrocytes. group II complete agglutination of rat erythrocytes, group III incomplete agglutination of rat erythrocytes, and group IV viruses, which were originally reported to lack hemagglutinin, agglutinate rat erythrocytes with an incomplete pattern similar to group III viruses. Members of each subgroup have fibers of a characteristic length (Table 1). A classification based on oncogenicity into subgroups A to D has also been proposed, which also correlates well with the DNA homology. Not all types within each subgroup have been studied with regard to DNA homology or biologic parameters and the proposed classification in Table 1 remains tentative.

## ANTIGENIC COMPOSITION

Most of the antigens of adenoviruses reside in the outer capsid (Table 2). The hexons contain at least two different antigenic determinants, one is group specific ($\alpha$) and the other type specific ($\epsilon$). The penton base contains a dominant group-specific antigenic determinant ($\beta$). The fiber contains a type-specific determinant ($\gamma$) residing in the distal knob, which probably serves to anchor the virus to the cell at infection. An intrasubgroup determinant ($\delta$) is also present in the proximal part of the fiber of subgroups A, C, and D.

Hemagglutination by adenoviruses was first demonstrated in 1958. All human types display hemagglutinating capacity. The type-specific part of the fiber interacts with the red cell surface. Since the intact virion carries several vertex projections, they can establish a bridge between the erythrocytes and give a complete hemagglutination pattern. Multimers of pentons and fibers can in the same way give rise to hemagglutination. Monomers of penton and fiber can establish only a monovalent link with the cell and agglutination can be detected only when antibodies are used to bridge the fibers anchored with their type-specific moiety on the erythrocyte. Heterotypic antibodies must be used to link the group-specific determinants available on the surface of the cells. The short fibers of subgroup B viruses therefore cannot agglutinate, since they only contain type-specific determinants. This method to reveal adenovirus hemagglutination by heterotypic antisera has been called *hemagglutination enhancement*. Antibodies directed toward the fiber can be assayed by *hemagglutination inhibition*.

Adenoviruses carry a mosaic of antigenic specificities on their surface. Since, by definition, all types are distinct by neutralization, type-specific antigens should induce neutralizing antibodies. Both the fiber ($\gamma$) and the hexon ($\epsilon$) contain type-specific antigenic determinants and both have been claimed to induce neutralizing antibodies. The mechanism for adenovirus neutralization is still a matter of controversy. Antisera against crude hexon preparations induce neutralizing antibodies, and purified hexons from subgroup B and D viruses give rise to neutralizing antibodies, but hexons against subgroup C virions contain no or few exposed such determinants. Antisera against fibers from subgroup C viruses do not contain neutralizing activity when measured with the plaque assay. On the other hand, when neutralization is scored by the fluorescent focus assay, fiber anti-

TABLE 2. Antigens Associated with the Major Structural Proteins

| PROTEIN | CORRESPONDING POLYPEPTIDE (See Fig. 2) | DESIGNATION | ANTIGEN SPECIFICITY | REMARKS |
|---|---|---|---|---|
| Hexon | II | $\alpha$ | Group | Oriented toward the inside of the virion |
| | | — | Inter- and intrasubgroup | |
| | | $\epsilon$ | Type | Available at the surface of the virion from serotypes belonging to subgroups B and D |
| Penton base | III | $\beta$ | Group | Carries toxin activity |
| | | — | Inter- and intrasubgroup | |
| Fiber | IV | $\gamma$ | Type | Reacts with HI-antibody |
| | | — | Intersubgroup | Shared between members of subgroups C and D |
| | | $\delta$ | Intrasubgroup | At the proximal part of the fiber present only in subgroups A, C and D |

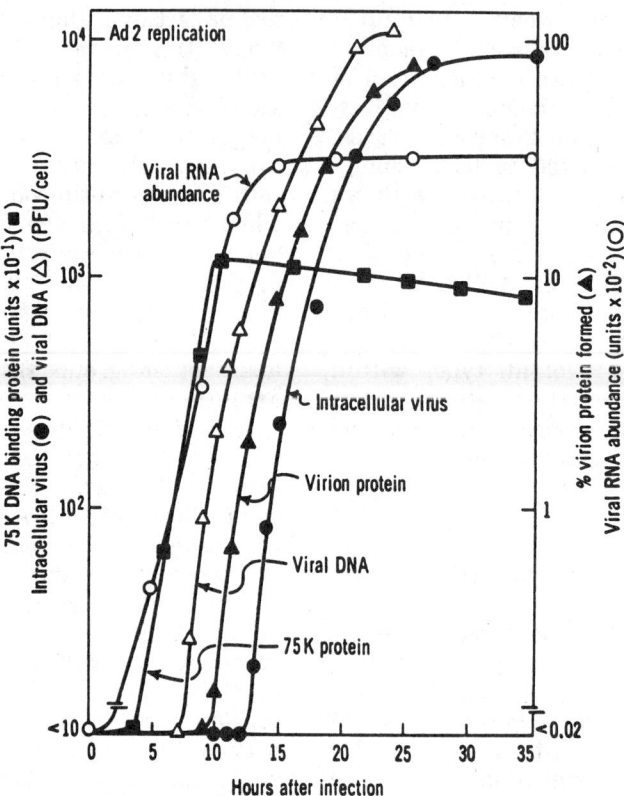

**FIGURE 4.** *The replication cycle of adenovirus type 2. Time course of synthesis of viral RNA, early viral 75K protein, viral DNA, virion protein, and intracellular virus. (From Wold, W.S.M., Green, M., and Büttner, W.: Adenoviruses. In Nayak, D.P. (ed.): The Molecular Biology of Animal Viruses. New York, Marcel Dekker, Inc., 1978. With permission.)*

sera contain high titers of neutralizing activity. In general antisera prepared against disrupted virions are more efficient in neutralization than antisera against purified capsid components. The neutralizing antigen of adenoviruses may therefore have escaped detection. It may be necessary to purify additional proteins in the peripentonal region to assess their capacity to induce neutralizing antibodies.

## SUSCEPTIBLE HOST CELLS

All adenoviruses of human origin produce cytopathic changes (CPE) when propagated in primary or continuous cell lines of human origin, such as diploid cells of human embryonic lung or kidney, HeLa, KB, or Hep-2 cells. Characteristic CPE manifests itself as rounding, enlargement, increased opacity, and aggregation of the cells into irregular clusters. The rapidity with which CPE occurs is a function of the dose of virus in the inoculum but the lower numbered types ad1 to ad7 produce CPE faster than do the other types. Monkey cells do support the early and most of the late expression of human adenovirus genomes but virions fail to assem-

ble. The block may be overcome by concurrent infection with SV 40 virus. Hamster cells are permissive for ad2 and ad5. Ad12, on the other hand, can express early products but fails to replicate its DNA and express late genes. Ad12, nevertheless, can induce CPE. Rat cells are semipermissive for ad2 in the sense that single cells may support replication but the majority of the cells fail to do so.

The lytic cycle of adenoviruses has been studied mostly in suspension cultures of KB or HeLa cells. The time course of the infection with ad2 is shown in Figure 4. When the cells are infected at high multiplicity (500 to 1000 PFU/cell), a synchronous response is observed with two functionally different phases of the infectious cycle. During the early phase that precedes viral DNA replication, about 40 per cent of the viral genome is expressed, exemplified with the 75K DNA-binding protein, which is one of the early proteins. In the late phase, beginning with the onset of viral DNA synthesis about six hours after infection, approximately, 90 per cent of the genome is expressed, and the amount of viral RNA increases about ten-fold. At about 14 hours postinfection the synthesis of host cell protein is, to a large extent, replaced by fabrication of viral products, mostly viral structural proteins. New virus particles begin to appear at 15 hours, and the infectious cycle for ad2 and ad5, both members of subgroup C, is completed within 20 to 25 hours. Similar time courses have been obtained with other serotypes although the growth cycle of group A viruses is longer than for ad2. The growth cycle in primary cells is prolonged at least for 12 to 15 hours even for group C viruses.

One system for subdivision of human adenovirus into subgroups A to D (Table 1) was originally based on the frequency with which newborn hamsters develop tumors after inoculation with virus. Several human adenoviruses as well as adenoviruses from other species can, in addition, transform cells in vitro, regardless of their oncogenic capacity in vivo. Cells that are nonpermissive for virus replication are more susceptible to transformation. The events leading to transformation may therefore occur also in permissive cells but it escapes detection because infected cells do not survive. The frequency of transformation is in all cases low for adenoviruses with only one transforming focus per $10^6$ cells or more. Only 4 to 8 per cent of the genome of ad5 is required for transformation, as revealed by transformation with DNA fragments. Accordingly, several cells transformed with ad2 and ad5 contain a limited amount of the viral DNA integrated into the host cell genome. With ad12, on the other hand, most of the viral genome appears to be integrated into the host genome of the transformed cell. Whether this difference could explain the varying oncogenic capacity of these viruses is unsettled.

## PATHOGENIC PROPERTIES

The human adenoviruses are almost exclusively pathogenic for man. A single type of adenovirus may cause different clinical syndromes and, conversely, more than one type may be responsible for the same clinical pattern. Four different syndromes of respiratory infection have been associated with adenoviruses.

1. *Acute febrile pharyngitis* is perhaps the most common clinical manifestation, especially in infants and children. It is difficult to distinguish the disease in individual cases from infections caused by influenza and parainfluenza viruses, respiratory syncytial virus, certain enteroviruses, and members of the rhinovirus group. It appears that subgroup C viruses are mainly responsible for infection in early life. The majority of children show serologic evidence of prior exposure to one or more of these antigenic types by the time they reach school age.

2. *Pharyngeal-conjunctival fever* is an infection usually observed in children and it may occur in epidemic form. It manifests itself as an acute febrile pharyngitis with concurrent conjunctivitis. Ad3 has been most frequently implicated as the etiologic agent, although ad7 and ad14 have also been involved. All belong to subgroup B. Subgroup C viruses may cause this syndrome in exceptional cases.

3. *Acute respiratory disease (ARD)* is prevalent in military recruits, although the same illness may be observed among other institutionalized young adults of similar age. Ad4 and ad7 are most frequently associated with this syndrome in recruit populations, but other types within subgroup B may periodically be involved as the responsible agent.

4. *Adenovirus pneumonia* is usually seen as a complications of ARD in patients infected with ad4 or ad7. The clinical course resembles that of pneumonia caused by *Mycoplasma pneumoniae* but the disease does not respond to treatment with antibiotics. Pneumonia may also be observed occasionally in infants and several adenovirus types have been isolated from fatal cases in infants.

Adenovirus may also cause acute follicular conjunctivitis. It is mainly seen in adults and principally is caused by ad3 and ad7, although other types have also been incriminated. Ad8 is the major cause of epidemic keratoconjunctivitis of the classic type with corneal infiltrates, but conjunctivitis may be caused by several adenovirus types. Adenoviruses may also be associated with gastroenteritis without respiratory disease and intussusception in infants and young children. Acute mesenteric lymphadenitis is thought to be caused by adenoviruses, although a causal relationship has not been established. Systemic infection with adenoviruses with involvement of several organs has mostly been observed in infants or young children.

## IMMUNITY

Susceptibility or resistance to most clinical infections by adenovirus appears to be correlated directly to the absence or the presence of circulating neutralizing antibodies. The adenoviruses are exceptionally good antigens for development of vaccines. One dose of vaccine apparently gives almost maximal antibody response. Several studies have demonstrated a reduction of 85 to 90 per cent in the attack rate of adenovirus infection in immunized groups. The low incidence of adenovirus infection in the civilian population, however, raises questions concerning the advisability of the indiscriminate use of adenovirus vaccines. It has been estimated from the incidence of adenovirus infections among civilians that a vaccine that completely prevented infection would lower by only 6 per cent the number of common respiratory illnesses experienced by an average child during the first 10 years of life. Since adenoviruses can transform cells and can be oncogenic to hamsters, adenovirus vaccines were abandoned. More recently, adenovirus vaccines that only contain purified protein components from infected cells have been reintroduced. Purified hexon or fiber preparations induce high levels of neutralizing antibodies in volunteers and a vaccine produced from these components was effective in a field trial. A vaccine of this type could be used for high risk military recruits. Successful vaccination has also been achieved by oral administration of live virus in capsules that decompose in the intestine.

## LABORATORY DIAGNOSIS

For virus isolation, throat and fecal samples are inoculated into primary cell cultures of human origin. Rapid diagnosis by immunofluorescence has more recently been introduced (Gardner and McQuillin, 1974). Aspirated cells from the nasopharynx are fixed and stained with group-specific immunofluorescent antibodies.

The complement fixation test is the most useful single procedure for serologic diagnosis of infection. One antigen detects antibodies to all human adenovirus strains and these antibodies increase significantly in titer (four-fold or greater) in the sera of adult patients within two weeks after onset of infection. The antigen may be prepared by propagating any virus type in cultures of human embryonic kidney, HeLa or KB cells, and purifying the hexon component. After primary isolation adenovirus is classified into groups by determining if the isolate will agglutinate monkey or rat red blood cells. Hemagglutination inhibition and virus neutralization tests with type-specific rabbit antisera can establish the virus type. To establish the type-specific serologic response in the patient, both hemagglutination inhibition and neutralization tests should be performed on acute phase and convalescent sera. In general, heterologous reactions occur more frequently in hemagglutination inhibition than in neutralization. The heterologous reactions observed with the neutralization test appear to be based on the presence of overlapping intertypic antigenic determinants more than on an anamnestic antibody response.

## EPIDEMIOLOGY

Adenoviruses exist in nearly all parts of the world. At least 33 antigenic types have been recovered from human sources, but not all are proven agents of disease. Serologic surveys indicate that most children become infected with one or more of the adenovirus types before the age of six years, but adenoviruses are probably responsible only for 2 or 3 per cent of acute febrile respiratory illness. The incidence may rise to 5 to 10 per cent of cases that require hospitalization. There is a general problem with estimating the incidence or significance of infections with adenoviruses, since infection leading to antibody response is not necessarily associated with clinical overt disease. Therefore, the recovery of the adenovirus from the respiratory tract or intestinal tract and a serologic response does not in itself permit the assumption that the virus is related to the observed disease. In general, adenoviruses do not cause more than 5 to 8 per cent of all cases of acute respiratory disease. Only sporadic cases have been observed in children and adults, but localized outbreaks may be encountered in boarding schools, summer camps, or colleges. Interestingly enough, the highest attack rates have been observed among military recruits where ad3, ad4, and ad7 have been responsible for major outbreaks. Ad14 and ad21 may also cause outbreaks among this population. The exceptional susceptibility of military recruits to these viruses is unexplained.

## References

Gardner, P. S., and McQuillin, J.: Rapid Virus Diagnosis. Application of Immunofluorescence. London, Butterworth and Co., Ltd., 1974, p. 181.
Norrby, E., Bartha, A., Boulanger, P., Dreizin, R. S., Ginsberg, H. S., Kalter, S. S., Kawamura, H., Rowe, W. P., Russell, W. C., Schlesinger, R. W., and Wigand, R.: Adenoviridae. Intervirology 7: 117, 1976.
Philipson, L., Pettersson, U., and Lindberg, U.: Molecular Biology of Adenoviruses. Virology Monographs, Vol. 14. Vienna and New York, Springer Verlag, 1975.
Potter, C. W.: Modern Trends in Medical Virology. Vol. 1., 1967, p. 162.
Roberts, R. J.: Restriction endonucleases. CRC Crit Rev Biochem 4:123, 1976.
Rose, H. M.: Adenoviruses. In Lennette, E. H., and Schmidt, N. J. (eds.): Diagnostic Procedures. 4th ed. American Public Health Association Inc., 1969, p. 205.
Sohier, R., Chardonnet, Y., and Prunieras, M.: Adenoviruses. Status of current knowledge. In Melnick, J. L. (ed.): Progress in Medical Virology, Vol. 7., New York, Karger Basel, 1965, p. 1.
Wold, W. S. M., Green, M., and Büttner, W.: Adenoviruses. In Nayak, D. P. (ed.): The Molecular Biology of Animal Viruses. Marcel Dekker, Inc., 1978, p. 673.

# THE HERPESVIRUSES 56

Joseph S. Pagano, M.D.
Stanley M. Lemon, M.D.

Few viruses have greater medical importance than the herpesviruses. These similar yet very different viruses are ubiquitous, infecting virtually everyone; they are all potentially pathogenic; and together they are responsible for a wide variety of diseases. Some of these viruses, especially the Epstein-Barr virus, have a special importance for developing nations. Once infection has taken place, these viruses or their genomes persist for life, usually silently. However, these latent infections are subject to reactivation, and they may cause serious illness, especially in immunosuppressed patients who receive modern therapies ranging from organ transplants to cancer chemotherapy.

Although over 70 viruses of the herpes group are known to infect many different animal species, there are only five distinct herpesviruses that commonly infect humans: herpes simplex virus (HSV) Types 1 and 2, varicella-zoster virus (VZV), cytomegalovirus (CMV), and Epstein-Barr virus (EBV). As a group these viruses are marked by both unity and diversity. All the herpesviruses resemble each other structurally and have biologic properties in common, particularly the hallmarks of latency and reactivation. However, pathogenetically and clinically they exhibit a spectrum of effects. On the molecular level the arrangement of genetic information is structured in herpesvirus genomes in a unique way.

All of these viruses may reactivate at any time during life upon natural or iatrogenic provocation. Curiously, the clinical manifestations of reactivated infection may be quite different from disease caused by primary infection. Finally, a most important property of these viruses is their oncogenic potential: Epstein-Barr virus is well known for its ability to "transform" or alter the growth potential of infected cells, and it is closely associated with two different human malignancies.

## VIRUS STRUCTURE

HSV, VZV, CMV, and EB virus particles are indistinguishable by electron microscopy. They are among the largest of viruses, with a diameter of approximately 150 to 200 nm. An inner core consisting of DNA intertwined with protein is surrounded by a protein capsid of symmetrical structure composed of 162 capsomeres. This nucleocapsid is covered by a loose amorphous envelope that is derived from the nuclear membrane of the host cell (Fig. 1). The nucleocapsid is assembled in the cell nucleus and is enveloped as it exits from the nucleus. Loss of this envelope greatly reduces virus infectivity. There are at least 33 polypeptides involved in the structure of the HSV virion including some that are included in the envelope. Other polypeptides are in the core of the virion intimately associated with the viral DNA and may affect regulation of viral gene expression. These viruses do not appear to contain polypeptides with enzymatic activities as part of their structure. They do code for several virus-specific enzymes, including DNA polymerases and thymidine kinases that are distinct from those found in mammalian cells.

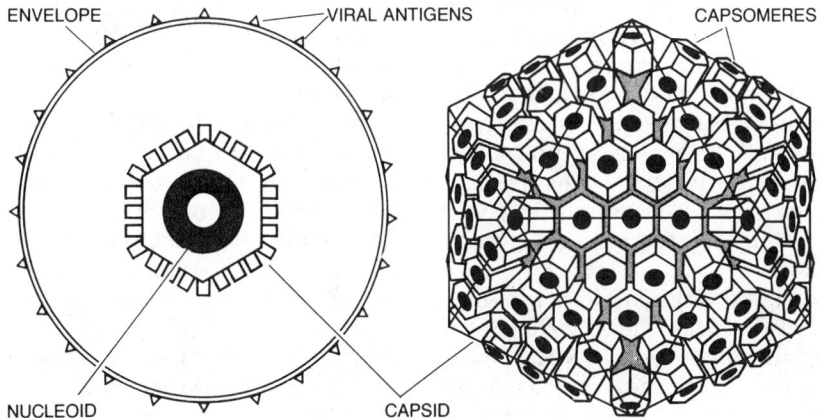

**FIGURE 1.** *Structure of herpes group viruses. The virion consists of a central core, or nucleoid, which contains the viral DNA; a capsid, which is icosahedral in shape and made of tubular protein subunits called capsomeres; and an envelope derived from cellular membranes. The envelope contains viral proteins or antigens. (From Henle, W., Henle, G., and Lennette, E. T.: The Epstein-Barr virus. Sci Am 24:48, 1979.)*

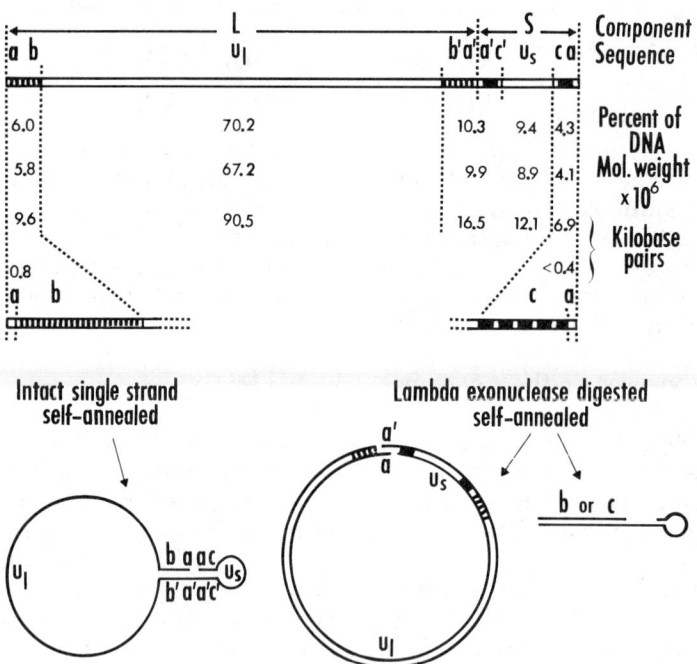

**FIGURE 2.** *Sequence arrangement in herpes simplex type 1 DNA. The HSV genome is divided into a long (L) and a short (S) segment. At the ends of the genome are nucleotide sequences that are also repeated within the genome at the junction of the L and S segments. The terminal sequences ab and ca of single strands anneal to their inverted repeats (b' a' and a' c') to produce the barbell structure on the lower left. The digestion of the DNA with a progressive exonuclease allows it to circularize. Most if not all members of the herpes group exhibit similar although not identical structural arrangements. (From Roizman, B.: The structure and isomerization of herpes simplex genomes. Cell 16:481, 1979.)*

Herpesvirus genomes consist of linear double-stranded DNA ranging from approximately 90 × 10⁶ daltons for certain EBV strains to 150 × 10⁶ daltons for CMV. Herpesvirus genomes possess terminal and internal stretches of repeated sequences. That is, in addition to the unique sequences, some of the nucleotide sequences found at the ends of the genome are also situated internally in the genome. The general structure of the herpesvirus genome is shown in Figure 2. A variety of such arrangements, ranging from simple to complex permuted structures, exist in the herpes group of viruses. Such sequence arrangements, the significance of which is unknown, appear to exist only in herpesvirus genomes and not in other genomes, viral or nonviral. These novel arrangements may relate to the generation of defective genomes.

Defective or incomplete virus particles are common among the herpesviruses. These virions possess less than the full complement of viral DNA. For example, in the case of cytomegalovirus many more virions contain only 100 × 10⁶ daltons of DNA than the full genome complement of 150 × 10⁶ daltons. Herpes simplex virions may possess a genome that is of normal unit length but is still defective in that many of the unique sequences are missing and are replaced by reiterations of a single segment of the genome. These defective forms may be important in some of the biologic effects of the herpesviruses such as persistent infection.

In addition to the linear form, the EBV genome can assume an entirely novel closed circular form within the cell. This supercoiled genome, called the EBV episome, is not encapsulated by virion structural protein (Fig. 3). It is found in the nuclei of latently infected cells within a nucleosomal structure similar to that of cellular chromatin. During latency the EBV episome is replicated as if it were a cellular constituent by host-cell DNA polymerase. This is the only episomal or plasmid DNA form known to exist in eucaryotic cells save for certain yeasts. Other herpesvirus genomes may be able to assume a similar episomal form, but thus far such closed circular genomes have been detected only in cells infected with an oncogenic herpesvirus of monkeys, *Herpesvirus samiri*. In the laboratory, however, linear HSV genomes can be circularized by exonuclease digestion of the ends of the DNA strands (Fig. 2). This digestion exposes homologous nucleotide sequences at either end of the genome, thereby permitting circularization. Some EBV DNA may also be directly integrated by covalent bonding into cellular DNA in latently infected cells.

With the exception of HSV Type 1 and HSV Type 2, the genomes of the human herpesviruses are completely or almost completely different as shown by cross-hybridization experiments. HSV Type 1 and HSV Type 2 share approximately 50 per cent of their genome content. A lesser degree of homology between, for example, the Epstein-Barr virus and cytomegalovirus — in the range of 5 per cent or less — has not yet been excluded. With the exception of certain simian EBV-like agents, the many herpes-group viruses of other animal species bear little if any genetic homologous relation to human herpes-group viruses. A few of the animal herpesviruses are capable of infecting man — herpes simiae and perhaps simian CMV — but do so rarely.

Sequence homology of DNA virus genomes can be analyzed by digestion with restriction endonucleases. These nucleases digest only at certain sites on different genomes, and thus generate specific DNA fragments which when examined by electrophoresis show characteristic patterns of sizes. Such patterns are a direct and precise reflection of virus strain differences that may be difficult to detect otherwise. Herpes simplex virus genomes and also CMV and EBV genomes isolated from various sources exhibit great diversity, especially in some regions of the genomes. Such analyses have demonstrated epidemiologic usefulness in tracing transmission of specific strains of virus.

## ANTIGENIC COMPOSITION

The relatively large herpesvirus genome contains sufficient genetic information to encode probably more than 50 different proteins, placing the herpesviruses among the more complex viruses of man. Many of these proteins, some of which are nonstructural (that is, not present in the intact virion), serve as efficient antigens. However, despite the identical morphologic appearance of the herpesviruses, there is little antigenic similarity among most members of this group.

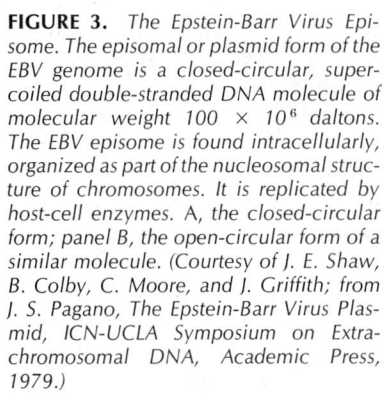

**FIGURE 3.** *The Epstein-Barr Virus Episome. The episomal or plasmid form of the EBV genome is a closed-circular, supercoiled double-stranded DNA molecule of molecular weight 100 × 10⁶ daltons. The EBV episome is found intracellularly, organized as part of the nucleosomal structure of chromosomes. It is replicated by host-cell enzymes. A, the closed-circular form; panel B, the open-circular form of a similar molecule. (Courtesy of J. E. Shaw, B. Colby, C. Moore, and J. Griffith; from J. S. Pagano, The Epstein-Barr Virus Plasmid, ICN-UCLA Symposium on Extrachromosomal DNA, Academic Press, 1979.)*

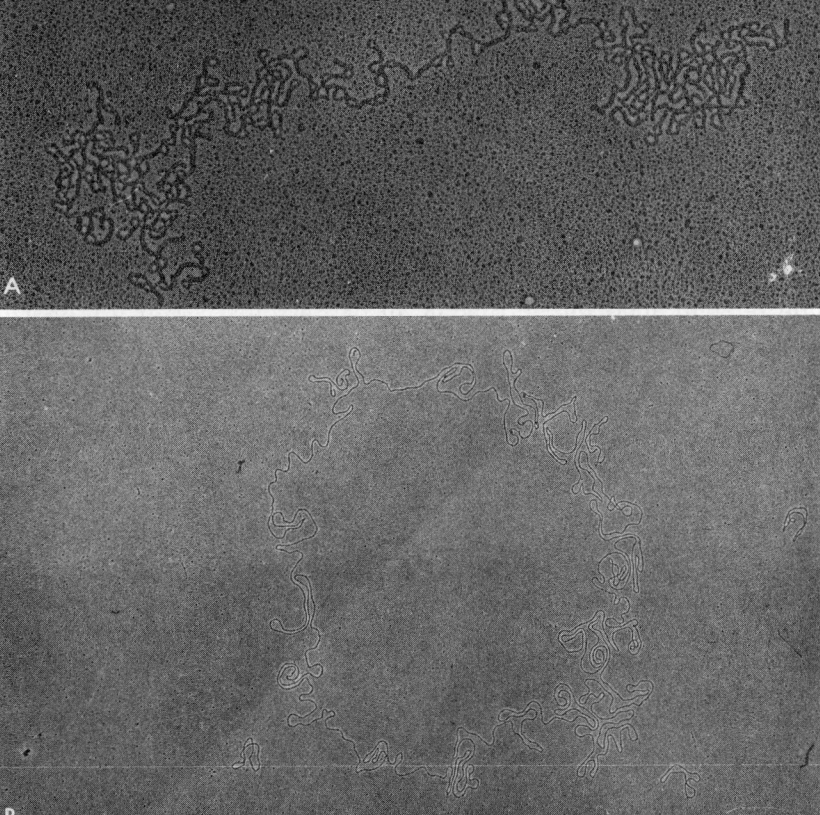

Among the human herpesviruses only HSV Type 1 and HSV Type 2 share a significant degree of antigenic relatedness. Although these two viruses are clearly separable by several different serologic techniques, antigenically related polypeptides common to both HSV Type 1 and HSV Type 2 have been identified by immunoprecipitation in gel-diffusion studies. This is not surprising in view of the high degree of nucleic acid homology (approximately 50 per cent) between these viruses. Heterologous neutralizing antisera are cross-reactive, which indicates that related antigenic sites exist on the envelope surface. Cross-reacting internal and nonstructural antigens have been identified as well. Antigenic diversity in HSV is not restricted to differences between Type 1 and Type 2 viruses; there is also considerable variation among strains of the same type. Such variation sometimes leads to the identification of an HSV strain as "intermediate" between Type 1 and Type 2.

Unlike strains of HSV, VZV isolates are relatively homogeneous in their antigenic make-up. There is no demonstrable cross-reactivity between VZV and HSV antigens despite the heterologous antibody rises that are occasionally observed following infection with one of the viruses.

Human cytomegalovirus strains are antigenically unrelated to other human herpesviruses, although they are related to CMV-like agents isolated from nonhuman primates. As with HSV, strains of CMV demonstrate considerable antigenic diversity when analyzed either by neutralization kinetics or complement fixation. However, no definitive grouping of strains on the basis of antigenic differences has yet emerged. Recent studies have identified "early" nonstructural CMV antigens that are distinct from "late" CMV antigens including virion components. Early and late refer to approximate time of appearance in the viral replicative cycle.

Several distinct antigens have been associated with EBV. None of these cross-reacts in any way with the other human herpesviruses, reflecting the general lack of nucleic acid homology among these agents. By fluorescent antibody technique, viral capsid antigen (VCA) activity has been recognized as part of the virion structure. However, additional antigenic activities have been identified that are nonstructural. EBV "early" antigen (EA) is found in cells that are abortively infected with virus and unable to produce mature infectious virions. "Membrane" antigen (MA) appears on the surface of some malignant cells grown in vitro from neoplasms associated with EBV. Such cells also contain EBV nuclear antigen (EBNA), the function of which is still unknown. Because of the superficial similarity between

EBNA and the T-antigens of the smaller DNA-containing tumor viruses, SV40 and adenovirus, there is a suspicion that EBNA may be involved in the transforming function of EBV. The appearance of antibodies to each of these distinct EBV antigens follows a characteristic temporal sequence after primary infection with the virus, and they are therefore of diagnostic significance.

## SUSCEPTIBLE HOST CELLS AND PATHOGENESIS

Many different types of cells become infected with herpesviruses. The type of cell susceptible to infection is to some extent dependent upon age, since infants seem to have a broader cellular susceptibility than adults. Primary infection, latency, and reactivation may involve different cell types even with the same virus. To add to the complexity, despite a common tendency to infect epithelial cells, each of the herpesviruses exhibits its own unique cellular interactions. Disease production may be linked directly to virus-caused cell death, or it may occur secondarily in relation to the immune response.

Both HSV Type 1 and Type 2 infect epithelial cells primarily. Type 1 virus is classically associated with oropharyngeal lesions, whereas Type 2 infects the genital mucosa and adjacent skin sites. Such territorial or organ-specific localization, while not absolute, is typical of herpes-group viruses. In severely affected infants and adults, HSV is found in the respiratory and gastrointestinal epithelium, the skin, and the parenchymal organs such as the liver. Such patients often have underlying immunocompromising conditions. HSV secondarily infects nervous tissue; Type 1 causes a latent infection in the trigeminal ganglion, and Type 2 infects the sacral ganglia. Reactivated infection occurs in mucosa and skin that the virus reaches from the ganglion by axonal spread. In addition to these silent ganglionic infections both viruses cause neurologic disease. In the United States, HSV Type 1 is the leading cause of sporadic and often fatal encephalitis. Whether the principal route of infection of the brain is directly from the trigeminal ganglion or through a cell-associated viremia is uncertain. However, it does seem likely that encephalitis can be produced not only by primary infection but also by reactivated infection. This view is supported by the occurrence of the condition at all ages. HSV Type 2 more commonly causes a benign aseptic meningitis. Herpes neonatorum is usually caused by Type 2 infections contracted during birth from active genital lesions in the mother. The majority of primary and secondary infections with HSV are probably asymptomatic.

Varicella-zoster virus primarily infects the respiratory epithelium, in which replication of the virus is for the most part asymptomatic. In adults who are infected for the first time with VZV, however, there is a high probability that a serious viral pneumonia will develop. The virus spreads to the skin by way of a cell-associated viremia. Virus may also spread to organs such as the liver in severe reactivated infection as well as in primary infection. Large amounts of infectious virus are replicated in the vesicles of chickenpox, but the virus seems to be transmitted primarily in respiratory aerosols. In the course of the infection peripheral sensory nerves in most parts of the body become infected asymptomatically. Here the virus persists for life, later to be reactivated in the form of herpes zoster, or "shingles." By all available criteria the viruses associated with varicella and with zoster are indistinguishable.

Cytomegalovirus replicates in the epithelial cells of the respiratory tract, salivary glands, and kidney; in the kidney the tubular cells shed virus for prolonged periods. In addition, CMV is frequently present in cervical secretions, especially late in pregnancy. Virus may also be found in the semen in CMV mononucleosis after its disappearance from other sites; the exact site of replication in the male genital tract is uncertain. As with other herpesviruses, spread via the bloodstream is accomplished by a cell-associated viremia, the virus being associated with both lymphocytes and polymorphonuclear leukocytes. Cell susceptibility to human CMV is strikingly affected by age. Infections in utero result in devastating destruction of the central nervous system, whereas encephalitis from postnatal CMV infection is exceedingly rare. CMV infection acquired later in life is usually asymptomatic, but occasionally it results in a mononucleosis-like syndrome with liver involvement. Cytomegalovirus infection exemplifies the different clinical forms infection may take upon reactivation. In patients who have received bone-marrow transplants CMV appears to cause an interstitial pneumonitis, whereas pneumonic involvement in primary CMV infection is virtually unknown. However, in recipients of renal allografts fever, leukopenia, and mild hepatitis may occur both in primary and in reactivated infection. Such infections appear to be more severe if they are primary.

Epstein-Barr virus probably replicates initially in the epithelial cells of the oropharynx and parotid gland. Subsequently, bone marrow-derived (B) lymphocytes are infected. Infected B lymphocytes do not appear to be a source of freely replicating virus in vivo, but they do harbor the episomal form of EBV DNA. Although symptoms of EBV infection arise from many organs, including the throat, lymphatic tissue, liver, and both the peripheral and central nervous systems, there is no direct evidence that the virus actually infects cells in parenchymal organs or the nervous system. Involvement of these organs may result from an intense immunologic response to the presence of EBV-bearing B lymphocytes and not from cellular invasion and destruction by virus itself.

In East and West Central Africa, EBV infection is closely associated with the development of Burkitt's lymphoma, a B-lymphocytic malignancy. Cells taken from African but not usually from the rarer North American Burkitt's lymphomas uniformly contain latent EBV DNA in its episomal form. In these areas of Africa, EBV infection takes place early in life. During the first year of life virtually 90 per cent of the children become infected, apparently asymptomatically, with EBV. This early exposure may be an important factor in the development of Burkitt's lymphoma. Persistently high EBV antibody titers early in life are predictive of the later development of Burkitt's lymphoma. Other factors, such as chronic infection with malaria, may be involved.

Several lines of evidence associate EBV with a second human malignancy, undifferentiated nasopharyngeal carcinoma. From a pathogenetic standpoint this association is especially interesting because this malignancy is epithelial in origin and points to the primary target cell of EBV replication. Although certain ethnic groups, especially Cantonese Chinese, are at high risk of developing this tumor, the association of the tumor with the virus is world-wide. EBV remains the prime candidate human tumor virus.

## LABORATORY DIAGNOSIS

HSV infection produces multinucleate giant cells and Cowdry type A intranuclear inclusion bodies. In cervical cytologic smears, such changes correlate well with isolation of virus. Similar cytologic changes occur with VZV infection (see Fig. 2 in Chap. 222), and the examination of Giemsa-stained smears of cells scraped from the floor of fresh vesicles is helpful in the diagnosis of vesicular disease due to these two herpesviruses. Intracytoplasmic as well as intranuclear inclusions occur with CMV infection. Cytologic examination of exfoliated cells in urine may lead to the diagnosis of cytomegaloviruria, but it is much less sensitive than virus isolation. Infection with other viruses, adenovirus and measles, for example, produce inclusion bodies and may cause confusion in the diagnosis.

HSV strains are easily isolated in a variety of cell cultures and can be recovered from the oropharynx, cervix, vesicular and ocular lesions, brain, and other tissues. Cytopathic effects caused by these virus strains develop rapidly and are usually obvious within 24 to 48 hours after inoculation of cell monolayers. VZV is less readily recovered but can be isolated from fresh vesicles (less than four days old) when fluid is inoculated into primary or diploid human cells. Cytopathic effects develop more slowly, and, unlike HSV, the virus remains tightly cell-associated. CMV can be recovered from urine, the cervix, semen, the oropharynx, and peripheral blood leukocytes. Replication of this virus in vitro is restricted to human diploid fibroblasts, despite the obvious presence of CMV within epithelial cells in vivo. Characteristic cytopathic effects may take several weeks to develop, and blind passage of infected cells may even be necessary. Final identification of these agents rests on fluorescent antibody tests or other immunologic procedures.

An in vitro cell system fully permissive for EBV replication has yet to be found. EBV biologic activity can, however, be detected by in vitro transformation assays with human cord-blood lymphocytes. Transforming EBV, found in oropharyngeal washings and parotid gland secretions, alters the growth potential of these lymphocytes so that they proliferate indefinitely in culture. Such transformed or "immortalized" lymphocytes contain EBNA. Transformation assays for EBV are complex and laborious, and are restricted to research laboratories. Clinical diagnosis depends on serologic techniques.

Antibodies to the herpesviruses can be detected by several methods. Serum neutralization tests have been developed for each virus and are both sensitive and specific. Following infection, neutralizing antibodies generally persist for the life of the individual. Neutralization tests are, however, time-consuming and expensive and are not suited for general clinical use. For detecting HSV antibodies the complement fixation technique is an excellent alternative because it is widely available, and complement-fixing antibodies to HSV are generally long-lasting. Significant antibody titer changes take place following severe recurrent infections as well as during primary infections. Because of the strong degree of antigenic relatedness between HSV Type 1 and HSV Type 2, however, neither of these techniques is able to distinguish type-specific antibodies unless special modifications are made.

Complement-fixing antibodies to VZV are short-lived, usually declining to undetectable levels within a year of infection. Antibodies to VZV antigen expressed on the membrane of infected cells may be detected by a fluorescent antibody technique. This assay is preferable for indicating immunity.

As with VZV, complement-fixing antibodies to CMV may disappear following primary infection only to reappear after reactivation or reinfection. Antibody detected by fluorescent antibody technique is more persistent and correlates better with neutralization test results. Detection of IgM antibody to CMV is important in the diagnosis of congenital infection.

Serodiagnosis of EBV infection depends on the detection of both virus-specific and heterophile antibodies. Paul-Bunnell-Davidsohn heterophile antibodies are predominantly IgM and are directed to surface antigens of erythrocytes from sheep and certain other animal species. These antigens do not cross-react with known EBV virion antigens; the reason for their occurrence in up to 90 per cent of cases of infectious mononucleosis due to EBV is unknown. In any case, such antibodies are highly suggestive of primary EBV infection. Indirect fluorescent antibody techniques may detect antibody to each of the several EBV-associated antigens. Antibodies to VCA and EA develop shortly after primary infection. VCA antibodies persist for life, whereas EA antibodies usually fall to low or undetectable levels within several months of infection. EBNA antibodies do not appear until one to three months after infection, but then they persist for life. This kind of antibody interplay is helpful in diagnosing and roughly dating EBV infection.

The promise of effective chemotherapy for some herpesvirus infections makes critical the need for rapid diagnostic procedures. The success of adenine arabinoside (Vidarabine) treatment of HSV encephalitis is highly dependent on how promptly therapy is begun. The most promising methods for rapid diagnosis of herpesvirus infections are based on the detection of virus antigen. A variety of techniques can be used to demonstrate virus antigens directly in fresh specimens. The techniques make use of virus-specific antibody labeled with fluorescein (direct and indirect IF tests), with radioisotopes (radioimmunoassays), or with enzymes (ELISA tests). Detection of HSV membrane antigens in the cerebrospinal fluid is an example of a new technique under evaluation. There appears to be a fairly good correlation with herpes encephalitis, although VZV infections sometimes give false-positive reactions for HSV antigens. A reliable test of this type would be welcome inasmuch as HSV is not shed into the cerebrospinal fluid. Fluorescent antibody techniques may demonstrate HSV antigens in brain-biopsy material and may shorten the time required to document cytomegaloviruria. Rapid diagnosis of congenital CMV infection also is possible with electronmicroscopy of urine specimens. However, the enzyme-linked (ELISA) tests appear to be potentially the most widely applicable.

A major problem in diagnosis is the tendency of herpesvirus to cause latent infection and the frequency with which reactivation of virus occurs. Many stimuli, including stress, fever, and immunosuppression, may lead to reactivation. For example, in patients with meningoencephalitis, the recovery of HSV from superficial mucosal sites does not correlate with its presence or absence in the brain. In severe or atypical herpesvirus infections the actual demonstration of virus in the affected organ is essential. Even then, the isolation of a herpesvirus must fit with the histopathologic findings and overall clinical pattern before an etiologic association can be made.

## IMMUNITY

Immunity to the herpesviruses is the result of a complex interplay between humoral and cell-mediated immune systems. Infection with the herpesviruses does not necessarily produce permanent immunity either to exogenous reinfection or to reactivation of endogenous virus. By and large the presence of circulating antibodies to EBV and VZV prevents full-fledged reinfection with these viruses, whereas the antibodies conferred by previous infection with CMV and HSV may modify disease but do not prevent reinfection, which may recur repeatedly. Reinfection from exogenous sources with HSV Type 1, HSV Type 2, and cytomegalovirus is common. Reinfection may in part be permitted by virus-strain differences inasmuch as some strains of herpes simplex virus and cytomegalovirus differ enough antigenically that there is suboptimal cross-protection. Probably more important, however, is the ability of these viruses to establish infection in local areas that are sheltered from immunologic response mechanisms because of their superficial location. There is some epidemiologic evidence to suggest that exogenous reinfection with VZV may occasionally occur as well, although it is clear that most cases of zoster are due to reactivation of latent virus. There is no evidence of reinfection with EBV.

Cell-mediated immune mechanisms are crucial for preventing or limiting reactivated infection and probably also limit primary infection once it is underway. Depressed or absent cellular immune responses to HSV and VZV correlate with the risk of reactivation of these viruses in recipients of organ transplants. Also, CMV reactivation occurs in transplant recipients with defective cellular immunity despite the presence of high complement-fixing or neutralizing antibody titers. Asymptomatic reactivation of EBV can also be detected in such patients. Thus, with each of the herpesviruses, intact humoral immunity is not by itself a deterrent to reactivation of endogenous virus. Although depressed cellular immunity certainly predisposes to reactivation, the common syndrome of reactivated oral or genital herpes is probably linked more to environmental effects that act as local triggers than to immunologic factors. Exposure to ultraviolet light, stress, fever, and local irritation are provocative factors. Pregnancy also seems to increase susceptibility to HSV and CMV infections.

Cellular immune mechanisms probably limit the extent of primary herpesvirus infections. For example, the proliferation of infected B lymphocytes that occurs during acute infectious mononucleosis appears to be held in check by a cytotoxic thymus-derived (T) lymphocytic response; this response is most intense shortly after primary infection. Cytotoxic cell-mediated response may be broadly reactive and may play a significant role in the production of disease. Thus, the atypical lymphocytosis that characterizes infectious mononucleosis is composed mainly of T lymphocytes responding to new antigens generated on the surface of B lymphocytes infected with EBV, although a nonspecific so-called "killer cell" (lymphocytic) response is also evoked.

## EPIDEMIOLOGY

Virtually everyone is infected with HSV Type 1, CMV, VZV, and EBV before middle life. There is a significant difference in the epidemiology of these viruses in developing and industrialized countries, however, in that infections occur considerably earlier in life in poorly developed areas. This difference in age-related incidence of infection is striking in the case of EBV in Kenya and Uganda, where virtually every inhabitant has acquired antibodies to EBV by the end of the first year of life. In contrast, only about 40 per cent of students entering college in the United States have antibodies to EBV, although lower socioeconomic groups living in crowded conditions are more likely to be infected with EBV at an earlier age. Infectious mononucleosis is a manifestation of EBV infection when acquired in the second or third decade of life, and it is therefore a disease that is virtually limited to the more highly developed nations.

Another epidemiologic difference is the striking incidence of Burkitt's lymphoma in endemic fashion in the so-called lymphoma belt of Africa. The pattern of occurrence of this tumor, including such features as its age-related incidence, geographic distribution according to elevation, and case-clustering in families and in districts, suggests a transmissible etiology. African Burkitt's lymphoma appears to be declining in incidence for unknown reasons. In the United States Burkitt's lymphoma is much rarer and is not invariably associated with EBV infection.

The very consistent association of EBV with nasopharyngeal carcinoma holds true both in populations with a genetic predisposition to this malignancy and in other groups without such a predisposition. There appears to be an association of nasopharyngeal carcinoma and an HLA-2 subtype in genetically susceptible groups.

Among the herpesviruses, only cytomegalovirus can infect in utero. It differs also in causing rather frequent perinatal infections. Thereafter the incidence of infection is related to age and socioeconomic status much like EBV infection. HSV Type 1 and VZV infections largely occur in childhood. HSV Type 2 and genital CMV infections occur mostly in late adolescence and early adulthood.

HSV Type 1 is spread primarily by exchange of oral secretions from person to person but also by direct contact with skin or mucous membranes infected with the virus. The disposition of HSV Type 1 to infect the mouth and lips and of HSV Type 2 to infect the genital region is by no means absolute. Both HSV Types 1 and 2 may be sexually transmitted. HSV is found not only in lesions of the external genitalia but also in cervical secretions where it may or may not be associated with cervicitis. The virus may be transmitted to infants during vaginal delivery and may cause disseminated neonatal infections. Obstetricians recommend cesarean section when there is active herpes genitalis.

Varicella is one of the most contagious of all human diseases. VZV infects children (or the rare adult who has escaped infection earlier in life) primarily by the respiratory route, although vesicular fluid is also infectious. Children incubating varicella are infectious for several days before the rash develops. Patients with herpes zoster are also a source of infection for susceptible children and adults.

Cytomegalovirus resembles HSV in that it is probably spread primarily from person to person by direct contact and exchange of secretions such as saliva. Venereal transmission is thought to occur because the virus is found in both semen and vaginal fluids, and because women with other venereal infections are much more likely to have CMV antibodies. Direct contact with virus results during the passage of an infant through an infected birth canal. Transplacental transfer of virus early in parturition is unfortunately all too common and frequently results in severe damage to the fetus. The presence of antibodies to CMV does not prevent reactivation of infection, nor do antibodies prevent reinfection with exogenous strains of CMV. Consequently, a mother who has given

birth to one infant with congenital CMV infection may, rarely, deliver a second child who has been infected in utero. Virus may be present in milk and be transmitted to the infant via breast feeding. Last, leukocyte-associated CMV can be transmitted by transfusion of fresh blood and result in mild hepatitis with or without a mononucleosis-like syndrome.

EBV infection is also thought to spread primarily by close contact with exchange of oral secretions containing infectious virus. The virus is shed from the throat intermittently for long periods — certainly for several months and possibly for as long as a year. The period of contagiousness is unknown; estimates of the incubation period are imprecise and range from two to four weeks.

## PREVENTION AND TREATMENT

There are as yet no accepted herpesvirus vaccines. The use of varicella hyperimmune globulin to ameliorate symptoms of VZV infection is well established, particularly in leukemic children who incur high mortality and morbidity. Experimental vaccines against cytomegalovirus and varicella-zoster virus, which are presumed to be attenuated by virtue of passage in vitro in tissue cultures, are now under study. These are live virus vaccines, and the virus is expected to persist in a latent form just as in natural infection. Inactivated vaccines, including so-called herpes simplex virus "subunit" vaccines, are also under investigation; these preparations consist of disrupted virus with the viral DNA removed. Preparations of this type require large amounts of virus, which are hard to obtain with the other herpes-group viruses, but they will not produce infection, either active or latent. Although herpesvirus vaccines present complicated and novel problems, their continued development is important, especially for the prevention of infections such as congenital CMV infection that elude early diagnosis and treatment.

Several specific HSV infections can be modified by available antiviral compounds. Iododeoxyuridine (IUdR) is of proven efficacy in herpes simplex keratitis. This is the only topical use for which IUdR and other such antiviral compounds is indicated. There is no consistent effect when such compounds by themselves are applied to lip or skin lesions, presumably because of failure of the drug to penetrate to the site of viral replication. Many nonspecific therapies have been proposed for the treatment of oral or genital herpes, but all have been unsuccessful when subjected to rigorous testings.

Although both IUdR and cytosine arabinoside

are either ineffective or even harmful in the treatment of HSV encephalitis, adenine arabinoside (Vidarabine) given intravenously early in the course of the illness appears to reduce mortality. The drug is now licensed for this use within the United States. Adenine arabinoside may also cause improvement in VZV infections in immunocompromised adults. Exogenous human interferon is of potential benefit in such cases of VZV infections because it tends to decrease the risk of dissemination. One striking feature of studies of these agents in VZV infection, however, is the surprisingly benign course of untreated disease in immunocompromised individuals. Interferon may also suppress CMV infection when administered prophylactically after renal transplantation.

New experimental drugs include phosphonoacetic acid and phosphonoformate, which are extremely effective in vitro against all herpesviruses and act by inhibiting the virus-induced DNA polymerases.

A new drug, acyclovir (9-(2-hydroxyethoxymethyl guanine), represents a novel class of antiviral agents. The mechanism of action of acyclovir in HSV infections requires that it first be phosphorylated in vivo to its mono-, di-, and triphosphorylated forms before it will act. The target of action of the drug appears to be confined to the infected cell where the drug is first phosphorylated and then interferes with virus-induced DNA polymerase activity and also may become inserted into DNA, acting as a terminator of DNA chain elongation. In laboratory tests the drug is highly specific for infected cells; it appears to derive this specificity from the requirement that the drug be phosphorylated by a virus-induced enzyme—in the case of herpes simplex virus infection, the virus-coded thymidine kinase. The second level of specificity may come in its selective inhibition of virus-induced DNA polymerase and lack of effect on normal host cellular DNA polymerases.

The drug is undergoing active clinical trials in herpes simplex encephalitis, disseminated herpes simplex infections, and disseminated varicella-zoster infections. In vitro the drug does not appear to be as effective against human cytomegalovirus; this relative insensitivity may be because CMV does not seem to induce the appearance of a new viral thymidine kinase in infected cells. In vitro the drug also has an effect against the freely replicating form of EBV but not against the latent episomal form of EBV. EBV DNA polymerase is especially sensitive to the phosphorylated drug in vitro. Preliminary studies in animals indicate that acyclovir is effective when applied topically or administered systemically against genital and oral herpetic lesions in animal models; the drug is soon to undergo tests in humans for these maladies.

## References

Epstein, M. A., and Achong, B. G.: Recent progress in Epstein-Barr virus research. Ann Rev Microbiol 31:421, 1977.

Henle, W., Henle, G. E., and Horwitz, C. A.: Epstein-Barr virus specific diagnostic tests in infectious mononucleosis. Human Pathol 5:551, 1974.

Huang, E. S., and Pagano, J. S.: Comparative diagnosis of cytomegaloviruses: New approach. In Kurstak, E. (ed.): Comparative Diagnosis of Viral Diseases. New York, Academic Press, 1977.

Kaplan, A. S. (ed.): The Herpesviruses. New York, Academic Press, 1973.

Nahamias, A. J., and Roizman, B.: Infection with herpes-simplex viruses 1 and 2. N Engl J Med 289:667, 719, 781, 1973.

Pagano, J. S.: Diseases and mechanisms of persistent DNA virus infection: Latency and cellular transformation. J Infect Dis 132:209, 1975.

Pagano, J. S., and Shaw, J. E.: Molecular probes and genome homology. In Epstein, M. A., and Achong, B. G. (eds.): The Epstein-Barr Virus. New York, Springer-Verlag, 1979.

Weller, T. H.: The cytomegaloviruses: Ubiquitous agents with protean clinical manifestations. N Engl J Med 285:203, 267, 1971.

Weller, T. H.: Varicella-herpes zoster virus. In Evans, A. S. (ed.): Viral Infections of Humans. New York, Plenum Medical Book Company, 1976, p. 457.

# POXVIRUSES  57

## Abraham I. Braude, M.D., Ph.D.

The poxviridae are a family of viruses composed of six genera. Five of the genera produce pox lesions or benign tumors of invertebrates and the sixth infects insects (Table 1). They have a similar morphology, a common nucleoprotein antigen, and the ability to recombine genetically. With the exception of ectromelia and myxoma viruses, the poxviruses are one of the most resistant groups of viruses. They are stable in storage under adverse conditions and remain infective in dried exudates and tissues for remarkably long periods.

### VIRAL STRUCTURE

The poxviruses have the greatest size and the most complicated structure of any animal virus. The double-stranded DNA virus has a molecular weight of approximately $150 \times 10^6$, the largest of any animal virus. It is enclosed in a dense, dumbbell-shaped core, which is covered by a closely adherent lipoprotein inner membrane. Two oval masses of obscure function known as lateral bodies fill the concavity of the dumbbell. A second outer membrane covers the entire struc-

**TABLE 1.  The Genera of Pox Viridae**

| GENUS | PRIMARY HOSTS | DISEASE |
|---|---|---|
| Orthopoxvirus | Man | Variola, vaccinia, alastrim |
| | Cows | Cowpox[a] |
| | Mice | Ectromelia |
| | Rabbits | Rabbitpox |
| | Monkeys | Monkeypox[a] |
| Capripoxvirus | Ungulates | Sheep-pox, goatpox |
| Leporipoxvirus | Rabbits and squirrels | Myxoma, fibroma |
| Parapoxvirus | Sheep | Orf[a] |
| | Cows | Papular stomatitis |
| | Cows | Milkers nodules[a] |
| Avipoxvirus | Birds | Fowlpox, canarypox |
| Entomopoxvirus | Arthropods | |

[a] Also produce human infections

ture. The resulting particle is oblong, and the surface is covered with ridges (see Chapter 7, Fig. 8). In contrast to other viral envelopes, the outer membrane of the virion is not derived from the cytoplasmic membrane of the infected cell but is synthesized by the virus. This difference in origin of the poxvirus envelopes accounts for a difference in sensitivity of the viruses to ether. Many poxviruses (ortho and poxviruses) are resistant to ether, whereas other enveloped viruses are inactivated by ether. Vaccinia virions measure 300 × 240 nm, whereas the parapoxvirus particles (Orf, papular stomatitis, and milkers nodes) are 260 × 160 nm.

In addition to DNA, poxviruses contain neutral lipid, phospholipid, protein, and carbohydrate. There are at least 75 proteins, but the function of most has not been identified. The core contains at least 17 structural proteins or polypeptides, and the inner membrane has two structural glycoproteins. Five other proteins are located at the surface of the viral particle. Seven enzymes have been identified in the core that are involved in RNA synthesis. One of these is a DNA-dependent RNA polymerase, the first to be demonstrated in any virion. All the phospholipid in the virion is located in the outer membrane. The predominant

phospholipid is lecithin. Poxvirus DNA ranges from 80 to 100 nm in length. Its guanine plus cytosine content of 35 to 40 per cent is the lowest of any vertebrate virus.

## ANTIGENIC COMPOSITION

In addition to the nucleoprotein antigen common to all members of the family, poxviruses contain a number of antigens derived from the structural components of the virion (structural antigens) and others known as soluble antigens (Table 2). The complex nucleoprotein antigen (NP), which is obtained by extraction with dilute alkali, constitutes over half the substance of the viral particle. NP contains 6 per cent DNA as well as certain core proteins. The structural antigens are demonstrated by chemical disruption of the virion or by neutralization of infectivity. At least 20 antigens are found in immunodiffusion tests after virion disruption, of which four have been localized to the core and one outside the core beneath the outer membrane. Two surface antigens have been identified by neutralization of infectivity. The antigens that produce neutralizing antibody are the basis for division of the poxvirus family into the genera listed in Table 1.

The soluble antigen known as LS is identified by complement fixation. It is found in virus-free extracts of tissue infected by vaccinia virus and appears to be a complex protein with a molecular weight of 240,000. The protein has both a heat-labile and a heat-stable antigen designated L and S, respectively. The L antigen is inactivated at 60 ° C and the S antigen is resistant to 100° C. The LS antigen seems to be derived from the viral surface because it stimulates neutralizing antibodies; it does not, however, immunize animals against vaccinia infection of the skin, and absorption with LS does not remove neutralizing antibody from protective sera obtained after vaccinia infection. Thus, it does not appear to be related to the protective structural surface antigens that delineate the orthopoxviruses. Another soluble antigen agglutinates chicken red cells. This hemagglutinin is a lipoprotein and is inactivated by

**TABLE 2.  Major Poxvirus Antigens**

| CATEGORY | ANTIGEN | COMPOSITION | SIZE | PROTECTIVE |
|---|---|---|---|---|
| Structural | NP | 6% DNA + core proteins | 50% of virion mass | 0 |
| | Surface antigens | Probably protein | ? | + |
| Soluble | LS | Protein | MW 240,000 | ± |
| | Hemagglutinin | Lipoprotein | 65 nm | 0 |

lecithinase. In contrast to hemagglutinin inhibition antibodies against influenza virus, antibodies that block hemagglutination of a poxvirus cannot neutralize infection by that virus. For this reason, the poxvirus hemagglutinin does not appear to be a structural unit of the viral surface.

## SUSCEPTIBLE HOST CELLS

Besides the primary hosts listed in Table 1, each poxvirus can infect other animals. The most extensive studies on the range of susceptibility of different animal tissues have been carried out with vaccinia virus. Calves, sheep, and rabbits can be infected with vaccinia virus and are used for the production of a smallpox vaccine composed of virus harvested from the skin lesions. Monkeys, rats, mice, guinea pigs, and hamsters are susceptible to vaccinia infection but less so than rabbits. Chick embryos are used to prepare smallpox vaccine by propagation of virus on the chorioallantoic membrane. Chick embryos can also be infected by inoculation of the amniotic cavity or yolk sac. Repeated propagation of vaccinia strains on the chorioallantoic membrane or in chick embryo tissue culture tends to lessen the virulence of vaccinia strains for man (Downie, 1965).

In contrast to their susceptibility to vaccinia virus, most animals other than primates are resistant to variola virus. It has not been possible to propagate variola virus serially in rabbits, guinea pigs, calves, sheep, and goats. Although smallpox virus can produce in rabbits a keratitis with the formation of Guarnieri bodies (intracytoplasmic spherical eosinophilic inclusions) and a local skin lesion, the virus cannot be propagated further in the rabbit skin. Variola virus is also less virulent than vaccinia virus upon intranasal inoculation of adult mice, but it kills suckling mice after intraperitoneal inoculation. On the cholioallantoic membrane, the pocks produced by variola virus are smaller and less heat-tolerant than those of vaccinia virus; variola pocks do not occur in embryos incubated at 39° C or above, whereas vaccinia pocks develop even at 41° C with some strains. Monkeypox virus shows the restricted host range of variola virus (Ho and Wenner, 1973), whereas the host range of cowpox virus resembles that of vaccinia virus.

Serial passage of poxviruses establishes an affinity for certain tissues, a phenomenon known as tropism. Passage of vaccinia virus, for example, in rabbit or calf skin creates dermotropic strains that have scant neurotropic properties. On the other hand, certain poxviruses are naturally neurotropic or become so after cerebral passage. Rabbitpox, cowpox, and vaccinia virus have all become neurotropic. The dermotropism of fowlpox

virus is evident from the extensive benign hyperplasia it produces in epithelial cells of the skin. Fibroma viruses have connective tissue tropism and produce benign connective tissue tumors in rabbits and squirrels.

Poxviruses multiply in cultured cells from many different tissues derived from rabbits, mouse, monkey, man, fowl, and cow. Variola virus, for example, can be propagated in HeLa, Hep 2, bovine kidney, bovine skin, human embryo skin, human embryo muscle, and L-cell cultures.

## PATHOGENIC PROPERTIES

In poxvirus infections, the cell dies after its ability to synthesize proteins is blocked during viral replication. From studies with vaccinia virus, it has been learned that the virion enters the cell by phagocytosis. The outer viral membrane and lateral basal bodies are degraded within the phagocytic vacuole so that the core is released into the cytoplasm. It is clear that this early step of removing the outer coat is carried out by constitutive enzymes of the cell because all of the phospholipid in the virion and half of the virion protein are released in a soluble form (Joklik, 1966). The inner viral core membrane, on the other hand, is degraded by viral enzymes. The DNA-dependent RNA polymerase within the core synthesizes mRNAs which are extruded into the cytoplasm by a mechanism that requires ATP (McAuslan, 1979). The mRNAs are translated on the ribosomes of the infected cell into proteins that direct the release of virus DNA from the core. One of these proteins is an uncoating enzyme that degrades the viral core membrane and allows the naked DNA to leave the core and enter the cytoplasm. The DNA-dependent RNA polymerase is heat-sensitive, so that poxviruses can be inactivated by heat. The heat-inactivated virus can be reactivated, however, by a viable poxvirus of any genus because all poxviruses appear to contain the RNA polymerase in their cores.

After the viral DNA leaves the core, viral growth begins with synthesis of viral DNA, virion enzymes, and structural proteins of the virion. This late phase of synthesis begins about 90 minutes after infection and lasts for about four hours. In contrast to other DNA viruses, the synthesis of poxvirus DNA takes place entirely in the cytoplasm in foci that are composed of dense granules and random fine threads and are independent of mitochondria or other cytoplasmic organelles. During this phase of viral growth, the virus blocks the ability of the host cell to transport RNA from its nucleus or to manufacture

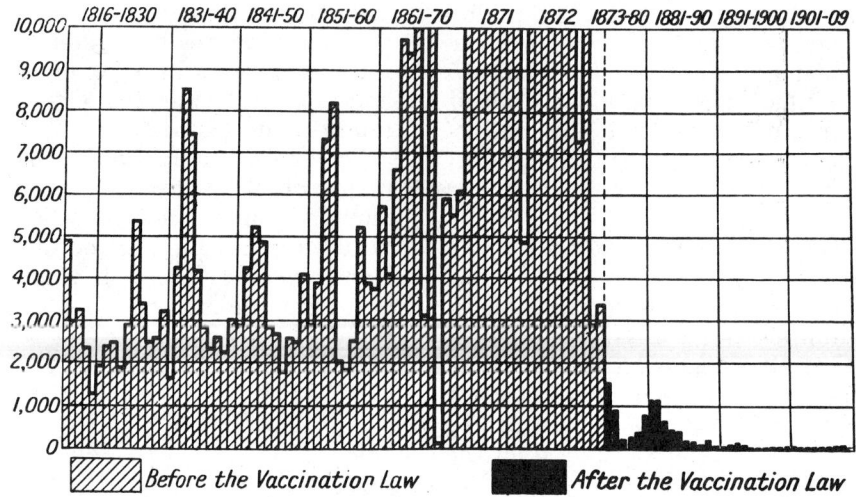

**FIGURE 1.** *The chart shows smallpox mortality during a period of a century in Germany. Vaccination was made compulsory in April, 1875, and in that year the total deaths from smallpox dropped to about 1500 compared with totals exceeding 10,000 in each of the years 1871 and 1872. Thereafter, the death totals fell nearly to zero. (After Jockmann: Pocken und Vaccinationlehre, Berlin, 1913.)*

protein. The synthesis of early virus proteins is also prevented.

Viral assembly begins after replication of viral DNA is completed and takes place on the cytoplasmic foci where viral DNA is synthesized. The virus synthesizes its own membrane, which encloses the viral DNA to form an "immature particle." These particles mature into the complex virion with its dumbbell-shaped core, lateral bodies, and outer membrane.

An interesting fluctuation in cell metabolism is seen in infections with rabbit fibroma virus. When cells are infected with this virus, cell DNA synthesis may be stopped for long periods, but the cells survive and DNA synthesis resumes after the virion matures (Tompkins et al., 1969).

From studies with other poxviruses, it has been proposed that in human infections variola virus first replicates at the portal of entry in the cells of the upper respiratory tract (Lancaster et al., 1966; Roberts, 1962). After spreading through the lymphatics, it multiplies in the regional lymphatic tissue and then enters the bloodstream. Virus is cleared from the blood by the reticuloendothelial system, where futher multiplication occurs. A second viremia occurs about 12 days after infection begins, marking the end of the incubation period. This viremia carries the infection to the skin and mucous membranes, where the virus first infects capillary endothelium and then epithelial cells. It has been suggested that the virus localizes in the skin because its lower temperature during fever is more conducive to viral replication than the temperature of visceral organs. Multiplication of virus in epithelial cells

causes cytolysis, intradermal fluid accumulation, release of lysosomal enzymes, hydrolysis of matrix proteins, and the development of vesicles. An inflammatory reaction to the infection and to cell necrosis delivers polymorphonuclear leukocytes into the lesions, converting the vesicles to sterile pustules.

## IMMUNITY

Observations on immunity were made in antiquity, when it was known that recovery from smallpox prevented another attack. Much later, a popular notion developed in Gloucestershire, England, that dairy maids who caught cowpox were afterwards immune to smallpox. The validity of this folklore was established by Jenner, who proved that vaccination of people with living cowpox virus produced solid immunity to smallpox (Fig. 1). Jenner had no idea of the mechanism of protection, let alone the nature of the material he was using, but he managed to discover the phenomenon of delayed hypersensitivity and its connection to smallpox immunity. This discovery was recorded in his description of the accelerated inflammatory reaction that occurred when smallpox material was injected into the skin of Mary Barge, who had once had cowpox. He wrote: 'It is remarkable that variolous matter, when the system is disposed to reject it, should excite inflammation more speedily than when it produces the smallpox. It seems as if a change which endures had been produced in the action, or disposition to action, in the vessels of the skin" (Jenner, 1798).

This observation that immunity to smallpox is related to a reaction that we now recognize as delayed hypersensitivity has been substantiated and elaborated by current research.

Contemporary observations on the response to smallpox vaccination have also given important insight into the mechanism of immunity in poxvirus infections. The relative importance of humoral and cellular immunity has been examined after vaccinating patients who have immune-deficiency diseases. Most patients with severe deficiencies in gamma globulin respond normally to smallpox vaccination and recover from it completely. On the other hand, vaccination of patients who have depressed cellular immunity but normal humoral antibody (autosomal recessive lymphopenia, or Nezelof's syndrome) usually causes disseminated vaccinia (Fulginiti et al., 1968). This finding in patients is supported by experiments that showed that administration of antithymocyte serum to mice markedly increased mortality from mousepox, even though humoral antibody levels were the same as those in controls (Blanden, 1970). Furthermore, immunity against mousepox was restored by transfer of immune T cells (Blanden, 1971).

These observations by themselves would imply that cellular immunity is more important than humoral immunity in vaccinia and mousepox. Other observations indicate that antibody may also contribute to protection against poxviruses. The most compelling of these is simply that passive immunity to pox infection can be transferred with virus-neutralizing antibody that develops after natural infection or after immunization with live virus. Neutralizing antibody can prevent skin lesions in animals and fatal encephalitis in mice.

## LABORATORY DIAGNOSIS

Now that smallpox has virtually disappeared and vaccination is no longer a standard practice, the laboratory diagnosis of smallpox or vaccinia should be confirmed in one of the few centers at which rapid reliable tests are available. Specimens from a suspected case of smallpox, vaccinia, and monkeypox should be examined by the electron microscope, inoculated into chick embryos and tissue cultures, and tested for pox antigens against specific antiserum by immunodiffusion in agar (Nakano and Bingham, 1974). Virus can be isolated earliest from heparinized blood during the pre-eruptive stage, and later from vesicular fluid and crusts. The vesicular fluid should be collected in capillary tubes and the crusts in screw-capped vials. Preparations of vesicle fluid or ground crusts are scanned in the electron

microscope at a magnification of 10,000 or 20,000, and the virion is examined in detail at 50,000 to 150,000. The brick-shaped smallpox virus is readily distinguishable from the enveloped icosahedrons of varicella virus. Variola virus must also be distinguished from nonviral particles and from herpes viruses, which can produce similar vesicles and crusts.

Examination of smears by light microscopy is less reliable. Smears are made by scraping material from the base of a vesicle or from papules with a scalpel blade and spreading it on a glass slide. After washing carefully with distilled water and ether, the smears are fixed with 95 per cent methyl alcohol and stained with a mixture of equal parts of 1 per cent gentian violet and 2 per cent sodium bicarbonate. The staining mixture is filtered onto the smeared slide and steamed for five minutes. The stained preparation is then examined for the characteristic elementary bodies of smallpox.

Isolation of the virus is carried out in fertile chicken eggs that have been incubated at 38 to 39° C for 11 to 13 days (World Health Organization, 1969). The chorioallantoic membrane (CAM) can be inoculated with plasma or buffy coat from blood samples or with vesicular fluid or scab material diluted in a buffered solution containing penicillin and streptomycin. The eggs are incubated at 35° C for 48 to 72 hours and the CAM examined for pocks. The pocks from vaccinia, variola, and monkeypox are differentiated from each other, and from those of herpesviruses by their appearance (Fig. 2).

Tissue cultures are also used for poxvirus isolation because the CAM method fails occasionally. Variola, vaccinia, and monkeypox viruses can all produce cytopathogenic effects in monkey kidney cells within 24 hours after inoculation.

Human poxvirus antigens in crusts or vesicle fluid can be detected in nearly 80 per cent of cases by agar gel precipitation. Antivaccinia antiserum is placed in the central well and the test specimens in outer wells. Upon incubation at 35° C, precipitin bands appear in a few hours between the wells containing antiserum and those containing pox antigen (Fig. 3). Antigens of smallpox, vaccinia, and human monkeypox viruses all react with vaccinia antiserum.

Serologic tests are of no practical value in smallpox because the antibody response is too slow for diagnostic help during the illness.

## EPIDEMIOLOGY

Man is the only host or reservoir of smallpox. He transmits the infection only when he has an outspoken illness in the active stage of the dis-

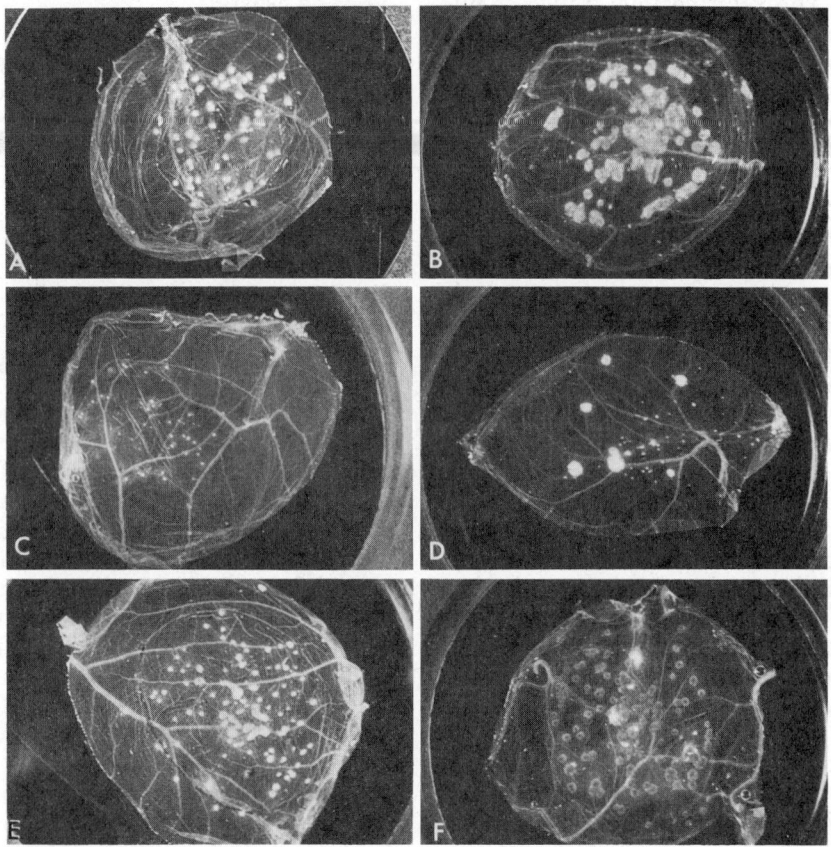

**FIGURE 2.** A, *Variola major lesions on chick chorioallantois (CAM) after three days at 35° C. Variola minor lesions are not distinguishable from those of variola major. B, Vaccinia lesions on CAM after three days at 35° C. Lesions are significantly larger than those of variola and are ulcerated. C, Variola major lesions on CAM after three days at 38.2° C. Inoculum was the same as that on CAM shown in Figure 1. Note that lesions are reduced in size and number.*

*D, Vaccinia lesions on CAM after three days at 35° C. Same virus as shown in Figure 3 but inoculated at a lower dose. Note the emergence of small secondary lesions. E, Herpes simplex lesions on CAM after three days at 35° C. Most strains of this virus give much smaller lesions, but strains isolated from genital lesions may have this appearance. The lesions in CAM resemble those of variola but are more irregular in size and some of them are ulcerated. After further incubation these lesions continue to increase in size, whereas those of variola do not (Barton, personal communication). F, Cowpox lesions on CAM after three days at 35° C. Most lesions are hemorrhagic, but a small portion of white variants are seen.*

*All chorioallantoic membranes shown were taken from eggs inoculated when the embryos were 12 days old. (From Dumbell, K. R.: Laboratory aids to the control of smallpox in countries where the disease is not endemic. Progr Med Virol 10:395, 1968.)*

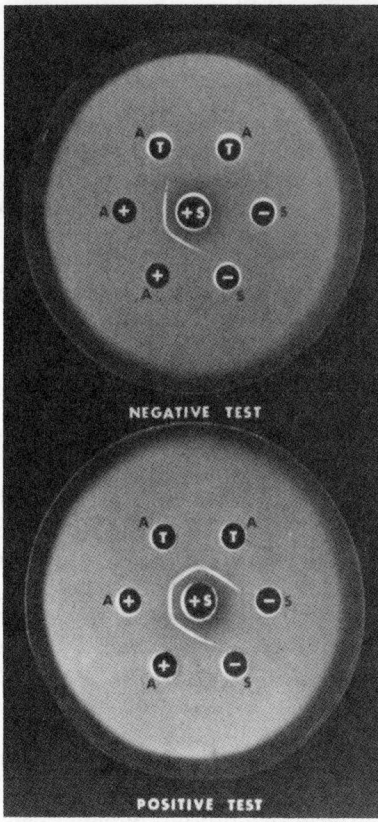

**FIGURE 3.** *+S (center wells): Positive rabbit antivaccinial serum; TA (top wells): test antigen made from material taken from the skin lesions of a case of smallpox; +A (left): positive antigen prepared from the crusts of a known case of smallpox; −S (right): Normal rabbit serum from an animal known to be devoid of antibodies to variola.*

*Above, A negative test. There is no precipitation between the test antigen (TA) and the positive serum (+S). The only lines of precipitation are between the positive serum and the positive control antigen (+A).*

*Below, A positive test. The lines of precipitation between the positive serum (+S) and the test antigen (TA) join the lines between the positive control antigen (+A) and the positive serum (+S). (From Swain, R., and Dodds, T.: Clinical Virology. Baltimore, The Williams & Wilkins Company, 1967, p. 106.)*

ease. Even in patients with partial immunity after vaccination, the attenuated infection still produces enough symptoms to identify the patient as a sick person so that direct contact with him is avoided. These features, plus the absence of asymptomatic carriers, have made smallpox easier to control than most other epidemic infections.

At first the eradication of smallpox was attempted through universal vaccination and revaccination. This approach was not entirely successful, however, because in many countries it was possible to vaccinate only three-fourths of the population. This might be enough with other

epidemic infections such as poliomyelitis, but not with smallpox because its relatively low infectivity does not generate herd immunity. Small pockets of smallpox can persist in villages and spread by close contact in families to susceptible individuals who have escaped natural immunization or vaccination. These characteristics make smallpox susceptible to control by surrounding each new case with a ring of immunized subjects (World Health Organization, 1968).

This change in approach from universal to selective (or strategic) vaccination came about in 1967 and involved two stages: First, the source of each outbreak was determined, and the chain of transmission was traced. Then the remaining susceptibles along the route of transmission were identified and vaccinated. This surveillance-containment program has been so successful that smallpox has been eradicated from all parts of the world.

## References

Blanden, R. V.: Mechanisms of recovery from a generalized viral infection: Mousepox. I. The effects of antithymocyte serum. J Exp Med 132:1035, 1970.

Blanden, R. V.: Mechanisms of recovery from a generalized viral infection: Mousepox. II. Passive transfer of recovery mechanisms with immune lymphoid cells. J Exp Med 133:1074, 1971.

Downie, A. W.: Poxvirus group. In Horsfall, G., and Tamm, I. (eds.): Viral and Rickettsial Diseases of Man. Philadelphia, J. B. Lippincott Company, 1965, p. 932.

Dumbell, K. R.: Laboratory aids to the control of smallpox in countries where the disease is not endemic. Progr Med Virol 10:388, 1968.

Fulginiti, V., Kempe, C., Hathaway, W., Pearlman, D., Seeber, O., Eller, J., Joyner, J., and Robinson, A.: Progressive vaccinia in immunologically deficient individuals. In Bergema, D. (ed.): Immunologic Deficiency Diseases in Man. Washington, D.C., The National Foundation, 1968, p. 128.

Ho, T., and Wenner, H. A.: Monkeypox virus. Bacterial Rev 37:1, 1973.

Jenner, E.: An inquiry into the causes and effects of the variolae vaccinae, a disease discovered in some of the western countries of England, particularly Gloucestershire, and known by the name of the cowpox. London, Sampson Low, 1798.

Jochmann, G.: Pocken und Vaccinationslehre, Vienna, Alfred Hölder, 1913.

Joklik, W. K.: The poxviruses. Bacteriol Rev 30:33, 1966.

Lancaster, M., Boulter, E., Westwood, J., and Randles, J.: Experimental respiratory infection with poxviruses. II. Pathological studies. Br J Exp Pathol 47:466, 1966.

McAuslin, B. R.: The biochemistry of poxvirus replication. In Levy, H. B. (ed.): Biochemistry of Viruses. New York, Dekker Publishing Company, p. 360, 1969.

Nakano, J., and Bingham, P.: Smallpox, vaccinia, and human infections with monkeypox viruses. In Lennette, E., Spaulding, E., and Truant, J. (eds.): Manual of Clinical Microbiology. Washington, D.C., American Society of Microbiology, 1974, p. 782.

Roberts, J. A.: Histopathogenesis of mousepox. I. Respiratory infection. Br J Exp Pathol 43:451, 1962.

Swain, R., and Dodds, T.: Clinical Virology. Baltimore, The Williams & Wilkins Company, 1967, p. 106.

Tompkins, G., Gelehter, T., Granner, D., Martin, D., Samuels, H., and Thompson, E.: Control of specific gene expression in higher organisms. Science 166:1474, 1969.

World Health Organization: Smallpox Eradication. Report of a WHO Scientific Report Group. Technical Report Series No. 393, Geneva, World Health Organization, 1968.

World Health Organization: Guide to the Laboratory Diagnosis of Smallpox for Smallpox Eradication Programmes. Geneva, World Health Organization, 1969.

# 58 *PAPOVAVIRUSES*

## *Michael N. Oxman, M.D.*

Papovaviruses are small DNA-containing viruses that characteristically produce latent and chronic infections in their natural hosts. When adequately tested, all papovaviruses appear to be capable of inducing neoplasms in at least some animal species. The name papovavirus is derived from the first two letters of the names of the viruses first placed in the group: *pa*pilloma virus, mouse *po*lyoma virus, and simian *va*cuolating virus (Melnick, 1962). Papovaviruses have been divided into two groups or genera, papillomaviruses and polyomaviruses (Table 1), primarily on the basis of the size of the viral genome (Melnick et al., 1974; Melnick, 1977).

The papillomavirus genus includes the human papilloma (wart) viruses, the Shope rabbit papilloma virus, and a number of other species-specific viruses that usually cause benign skin papillomas or warts in their natural hosts (Rowson and Mahy, 1967). Human warts were one of the first neoplasms shown to be caused by a transmissible agent with the properties of a virus (Rowson and Mahy, 1967; Ciuffo, 1907). Nevertheless, little is known about the multiplication of papillomaviruses or about their interactions with animal cells because there is no satisfactory tissue culture system for their propagation (Rowson and Mahy, 1967; Butel, 1972; zur Hausen, 1977.)

Simian vacuolating virus (simian virus 40, SV40) and mouse polyoma virus, members of the polyomavirus genus that can cause tumors and cell transformation, have been intensively studied as models of viral oncogenesis. As a consequence, we have an enormous amount of information about their structure, replication, genetics, and interactions with animal cells (Enders, 1965; Black, 1968; Benjamin, 1972; Sambrook, 1972; Levine, 1974; Eckhart, 1977; Salzman and Khoury, 1974; Kelly and Nathans, 1977; Fareed and Davoli, 1977; Fried and Griffin, 1977; Howley, 1980). In fact, the elucidation of the complete nucleotide sequence of SV40 DNA (Fiers et al., 1978; Reddy et al., 1978) is a major triumph of modern virology.

Interest in the potential role of papovaviruses in human disease was aroused in the early 1960s by the discovery that SV40 produced a latent infection of rhesus monkey kidneys and was a common but unrecognized contaminant of viral vaccines administered to millions of people in the 1950s (Sweet and Hilleman, 1960; Melnick and Stinebaugh, 1962; Shah and Nathanson, 1976). In 1965, particles resembling papovavirus virions were found within glial nuclei in the brains of patients with a rare demyelinating disease, progressive multifocal leukoencephalopathy (PML) (Zu Rhein and Chou, 1965; Silverman and Rubinstein, 1965; Howatson et al., 1965). In 1971, Padgett and his colleagues (Padgett et al., 1971) isolated a papovavirus, JCV, from the brain of a patient with PML, and Gardner and his associates (Gardner et al., 1971) isolated a papovavirus, BKV, from the urine of a renal allograft recipient. These two viruses, which are distinct from each other and from any previously recognized papovavirus (Padgett and Walker, 1976; Takemoto, 1978), commonly cause unrecognized infections in children. In 1972, Weiner et al. isolated papovaviruses SV40-PML$_1$ and SV40-PML$_2$ from the brains of two patients with PML. Surprisingly, these isolates were nearly indistinguishable from SV40 (Fareed and Davoli, 1977; Takemoto, 1978; Weiner et al., 1972). The almost exclusive relationship of JCV infection to PML and the prevalence of asymptomatic BKV infections in immunosuppressed patients are now established, and considerable progress has been made in characterizing these two human papovaviruses (Howley, 1980).

## *VIRAL STRUCTURE*

Papovaviruses are small, nonenveloped, icosahedral DNA viruses that replicate in the nuclei of susceptible vertebrate cells. Their virions

### TABLE 1. Papovaviruses

**PAPILLOMAVIRUS GENUS**
Human papilloma (wart) viruses
Shope rabbit papilloma virus
Rabbit oral papilloma virus
Bovine papilloma virus
Canine papilloma virus
Hamster papilloma virus
Papilloma viruses of horses, sheep, deer, and other species

**POLYOMAVIRUS GENUS**
Mouse polyoma virus
Simian vacuolating virus (SV40)[a]
Mouse K virus
Rabbit kidney vacuolating virus
Human BK virus
Human JC virus
Stumptailed macaque virus (STMV)
Papovavirus of chacma baboons (SA12)

[a]Includes two SV40-like viruses isolated from patients with progressive multifocal leukoencephalopathy (PML) that appear to be SV40 variants (Weiner et al., 1972).

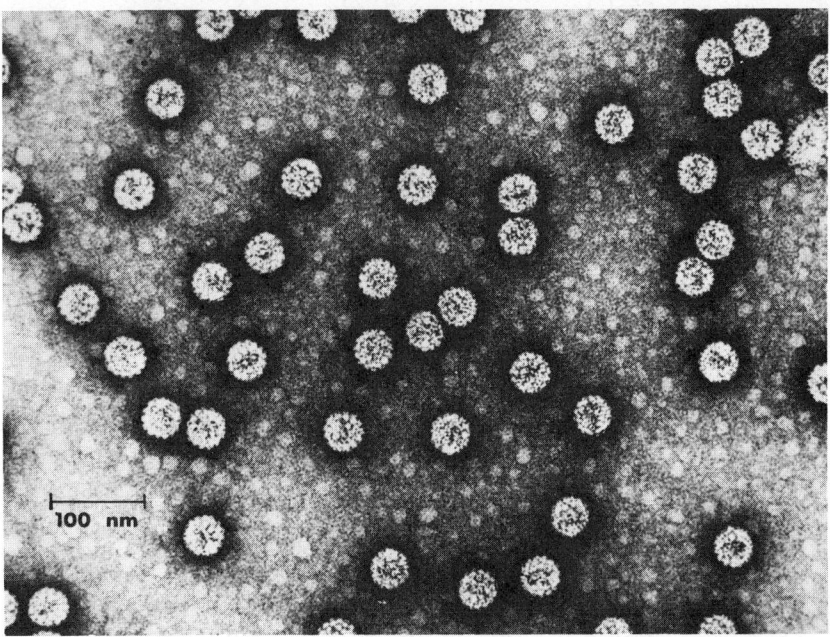

**FIGURE 1.** *Electron micrograph of purified SV40 virions (full particles: P = 1.34 g/cm³ in CsCl) negatively stained with sodium phosphotungstate (Bar = 100 nm).*

consist of a molecule of circular double-stranded DNA enclosed in a spherical protein coat or capsid composed of 72 morphologic subunits or capsomeres (Fig. 1). Many empty capsids are observed when unfractioned papovavirus preparations are examined electron-microscopically following negative staining with sodium phosphotungstate. The dense core of DNA is missing from these capsids, and they are thus penetrated by the stain. Filamentous or tubular forms may also be seen in the nuclei of infected cells and in preparations of extracellular virus (Finch and Klug, 1965; Mattern et al, 1967). The diameter of papillomaviruses is approximately 55 nm; they contain about $5 \times 10^6$ daltons of DNA. The polyomaviruses have diameters of 40 to 45 nm and contain approximately $3.3 \times 10^6$ daltons of DNA. The capsids of human papillomaviruses appear to be composed of one major protein that represents 60 to 80 per cent of the total viral protein and has an estimated molecular weight of between 54,000 and 63,000 (Gissman et al., 1977). The papillomavirus DNA within the capsid consists of a double-stranded, supercoiled, circular molecule closely associated with cellular histones.

In the case of the polyomaviruses, the major capsid protein VP-1 accounts for more than 75 per cent of the total virion protein and has an estimated molecular weight of 43,000 to 48,000. Two minor virus-coded proteins, VP-2 and VP-3, have estimated molecular weights of 32,000 to 39,000 and 23,000 to 31,000, respectively (Salzman and Khoury, 1974; Kelly and Nathans, 1977; Fareed and Davoli, 1977; Fried and Griffin, 1977). Within the polyomavirus virion the viral DNA is

a double-stranded, supercoiled, circular molecule closely associated with four cellular histones, H2A1, H2A2, H2B, and H3, in a structure resembling the chromatin of eukaryotic cells (Kelly and Nathans, 1977; Fareed and Davoli, 1977; Fried and Griffin, 1977; Howley, 1980).

## PHYSICAL AND CHEMICAL PROPERTIES

DNA accounts for 10 to 12 per cent of the weight of papovavirus virions, the remainder being protein. There is no essential lipid or carbohydrate. Complete virions have a buoyant density of 1.34 g/cm³ in CsCl; incomplete virions (empty capsids) have a buoyant density of 1.29 g/cm³. The infectivity of the polyomaviruses is resistant to lipid solvents (e.g., ether and chloroform) because they have no envelope; they are relatively resistant to irradiation, and are stable over a wide range of pH. These properties are exploited in extracting and purifying papovaviruses from tissues. Infectivity also resists heating at 50° C for one hour in distilled water but not at 50° C for one hour in 1M $MgCl_2$. Treatment with 0.1 per cent beta-propriolactone inactivates the infectivity of BK virus without destroying its hemagglutinating properties (Pitko et al., 1974), so that noninfectious BK virus hemagglutinin can be used in serologic tests.

When viral DNA is extracted from purified papovavirus virions or from infected cells, two species are generally found. Most of the viral DNA is in the form of a covalently closed circular

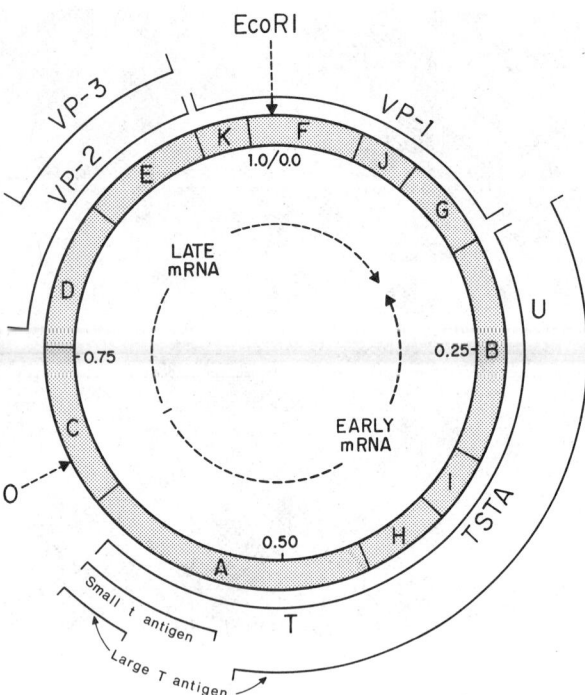

**FIGURE 2.** Hind II/III restriction endonuclease map of SV40 DNA. Map coordinates are oriented clockwise from the Eco RI restriction endonuclease cleavage site at 1.0/0.0. Letters refer to the Hind II/III fragments. Inner dashed lines indicate regions transcribed into early and late viral mRNA and the direction of transcription. Outer arcs indicate the approximate location of the genetic information for virus-coded proteins. The "O" indicates the approximate location of the origin of DNA replication in Hind II/III fragment C (prepared from information summarized in Fareed and Davoli, 1977; Fried and Griffin, 1977; Kelly and Nathans, 1977; Fiers et al., 1978; Reddy, et al., 1978; and Howley, 1980).

duplex molecule (DNA I) that, in SV40, consists of 5227 purine and pyrimidine bases and contains 26 negative superhelical turns. A small portion of the viral DNA is in the form of an open circular duplex molecule (DNA II), which is generated from DNA I by the rupture of one phosphodiester bond in either strand. Both forms of DNA are infectious. The degree of base sequence homology between various papovavirus isolates has been studied by nucleic acid hybridization. Bacterial restriction endonucleases, which recognize specific nucleotide sequences in duplex DNA and cleave both strands at these sites, have been used to construct physical maps of papovavirus genomes (Salzman and Khoury, 1974; Kelly and Nathans, 1977; Fareed and Davoli, 1977; Fried and Griffin, 1977; Padgett and Walker, 1976; Takemoto, 1978; Howley, 1980). With these techniques it is possible to compare the DNAs of different papovaviruses. An example of such a physical map of the SV40 genome is shown in Figure 2.

## VIRUS REPLICATION

In contrast to papillomaviruses, the replication of polyoma virus and SV40 has been extensively studied (Enders, 1965; Black, 1968; Benjamin, 1972; Sambrook, 1972; Levine, 1974; Eckhart, 1977; Salzman and Khoury, 1974; Kelly and Nathans, 1977; Fareed and Davoli, 1977; Fried and Griffin, 1977). When SV40 or polyoma virus infects the cells of its natural host (permissive cells), the usual result is a lytic (productive) infection characterized by extensive virus replication and cell lysis. These viruses can also infect cells of other species (termed nonpermissive cells) which do not support efficient virus replication. This results in an incomplete or abortive infection, in which only a part of the viral genome is expressed. Some abortively infected cells may be transformed to a malignant phenotype, a process that requires the persistence and expression of at least one viral gene.

Productive infection begins with the adsorption of virus to receptors on the cell surface. In the case of polyoma virus, and probably other hemagglutinating viruses such as BKV and JCV, adsorption can be prevented by treating cells with neuraminidase, which destroys sialic acid-containing cell receptors. After adsorption, the virus penetrates the cell membrane and is transported to the cell nucleus, where it is uncoated (Salzman and Khoury, 1974; Diacumakos and Gershey, 1977).

The replication cycle that follows can be divided into two phases: early and late. During the early phase, which precedes viral DNA replication (Fig. 3A), early viral mRNA is transcribed from approximately one half of one strand of the viral DNA, i.e., from the E strand of *Hind* fragments A, H, I, and B, counterclockwise from 0.65 to 0.17 on the map of the SV40 genome (Fig. 2). Transcription of early mRNA, which can be detected as early as six hours after infection, is followed by synthesis of virus-specific early proteins. Two of these, SV40 T antigen and SV40 U antigen, accumulate in the cell nucleus, where they can be detected by fluorescent antibody (FA) staining beginning about eight hours after infection (Fig. 4). A third early antigen, tumor specific transplantation antigen (TSTA), is transported to the cell membrane. The late phase begins with the onset of viral DNA replication 12 to 15 hours after infection (Fig. 3B). Late viral mRNA is transcribed from the remaining half of the genome (Fig. 2), its template being the opposite strand of the viral DNA from that involved in early mRNA synthesis (i.e., the L strand). Late structural viral proteins, VP-1, VP-2, and VP-3, are then synthesized and transported to the nu-

# PRODUCTIVE  PAPOVAVIRUS  INFECTION

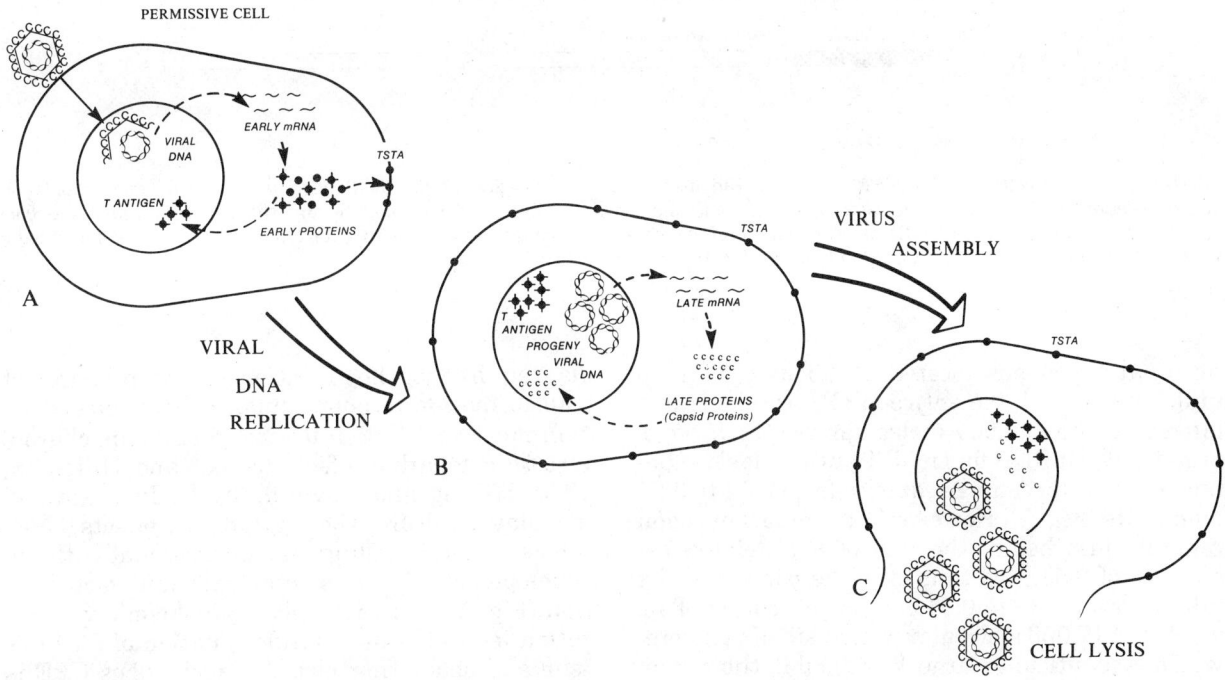

**FIGURE 3.** *Productive papovavirus infection as exemplified by SV40 infection of primary African green monkey kidney cells.*

cleus, where they can be detected by FA staining by about 15 hours after infection. Progeny virions assemble in the nucleus beginning about 18 hours after infection and accumulate for a prolonged period, usually for at least 40 hours, before cell lysis occurs.

It has recently been shown that there are actually two SV40 T antigens: large T antigen with a molecular weight of approximately 100,000 and small t antigen with a molecular weight of 17,000. The large T and small t proteins are immunologically related, and they have the same $NH_2$-terminal amino acids as well as several common methionine-tryptic peptides (Pauca et al., 1978; Simmons and Martin, 1978). The synthesis of each of these early proteins is directed by a distinct cytoplasmic 19S mRNA, but both mRNAs are derived from the same primary early RNA transcript by a process of splicing. The mRNAs for large T and small t both span almost the entire early region from approximately 0.65 counterclockwise to 0.15 on the map of the SV40 genome (Fig. 2), but they differ in the size and location of deleted intervening sequences (Berk and Sharp, 1978; Crawford et al., 1978). The mRNA coding for large T antigen lacks a 346-nucleotide intervening sequence from 0.59 to 0.535 map units (Fig. 5). Since

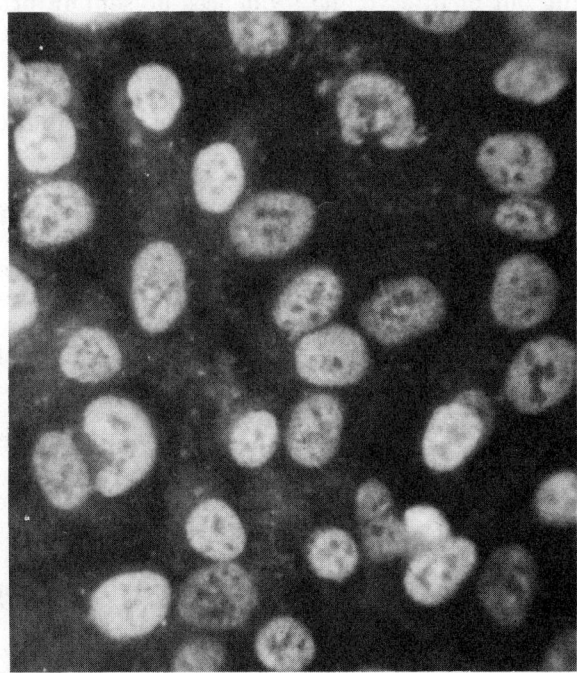

**FIGURE 4.** *SV40 T antigen demonstrated by fluorescent antibody staining of SV40 transformed cells. Note the finely granular staining confined to the nucleus and exhibiting characteristic nucleolar sparing (1000 ×).*

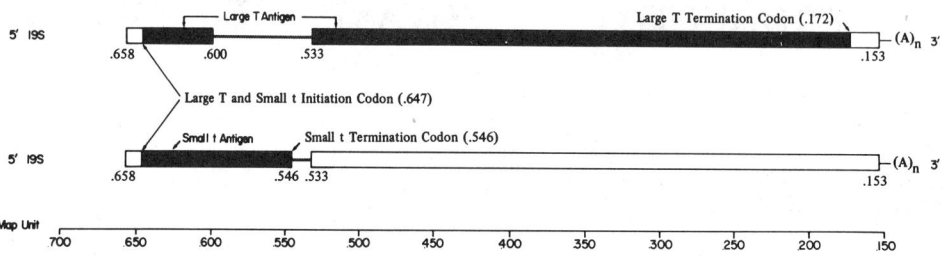

**FIGURE 5.** *The structure of SV40 early mRNAs. The map of the early region of the SV40 genome is shown counterclockwise below. The regions coding for the large T antigen and the small t antigen are indicated by the shaded areas within the bars that define the two early 19S mRNAs. The thin lines indicate regions of the SV40 genome that are spliced out of the mature poly-adenylated cytoplasmic mRNAs (from Howley, 1980).*

termination codons located at about 0.54 map units are deleted, the entire mRNA can be translated into the 100,000 molecular weight large T protein. The mRNA for small T antigen lacks a 65-nucleotide intervening sequence from 0.54 to 0.53 map units (Fig. 5). However, a termination codon remains just before the site of the deleted sequences of 0.54, and thus only the portion of the mRNA from 0.65 to 0.54 can be translated. This yields the 17,000 molecular weight small t protein, which is identical to large T antigen in the region encoded by sequences from 0.65 to 0.59 in the SV40 genome (Howley, 1980). The stable cytoplasmic late mRNAs, which direct the synthesis of VP-1, VP-2 and VP-3, are similarly formed by the splicing out of intervening sequences present in primary transcripts of the late region of the viral genome (Howley, 1980).

In contrast to many other viruses, papovavirus infection of permissive cells does not result in the early inhibition of host cell synthetic functions. Rather, there is an induction of host cell DNA, RNA, and protein synthesis during the early phase of infection. There are also changes in the surface properties of infected cells. These include increased uptake of sugars, enhanced agglutinability by plant lectins, and the appearance of new surface antigens, including TSTA. Most of these changes appear to be dependent upon the expression of the early portion of the papovavirus genome, and particularly upon the synthesis of large T antigen, a virus-coded early protein with a molecular weight of approximately 100,000. Large T antigen is required for productive infection. It is responsible for the initiation of viral DNA replication and late viral mRNA synthesis, as well as for the induction of host cell DNA replication (Howley, 1980). The large T protein contains an ATPase activity and binds specifically to SV40 DNA at the origin of replication. It also binds to host cell chromosomes. It may act by locally unwinding a portion of the duplex DNA, allowing polymerases to bind and initiate replication. Large T antigen is

also required for the initiation and maintenance of transformation in nonpermissive host cells.

Productive SV40 infection results in characteristic cytopathic effects (Sweet and Hilleman, 1960; Hsiung and Gaylord, 1961). In unstained monolayer cultures these cytopathic effects (CPE) consist of cell rounding and enlargement with the development of extensive cytoplasmic vacuolization (Fig. 6). This extensive cytoplasmic vacuolization led to the original designation of SV40 as "simian vacuolating virus." Papovavirus CPE is clearly visible when infected monolayer cultures are fixed and stained with hematoxylin and eosin. At about 24 hours after infection there is nuclear swelling, some clumping of chromatin, and the appearance of irregular patches of eosinophilic material within the nucleus. By about 48 hours after infection the nuclei show margination of chromatin and large basophilic Feulgen-positive intranuclear inclusions that, when examined by electron microscopy, are found to be composed of papovavirus virions. At about this time the extensive cytoplasmic vacuolization develops (Fig. 6). The fully developed intranuclear inclusions produced by papovaviruses of the polyomavirus genus may be basophilic, amphophilic, or eosinophilic, depending upon the virus strain, cell type, and method of fixation. Although productive infection results in cell lysis, progeny papovavirus virions are not always efficiently released. This is especially true of the hemagglutinating human papovaviruses, BKV and JCV, which remain associated with cells and cell debris. To achieve good yields of these viruses it is necessary to disrupt the infected cells mechanically and use receptor-destroying enzyme (RDE) to free the virions from cell debris.

Perhaps the most significant biologic property of the papovaviruses is their capacity to transform normal cells into tumor cells. Thus, while members of the polyomavirus genus are not associated with spontaneous tumors in their natural hosts, they regularly produce tumors experimentally. Moreover, they can transform normal cells in tissue culture into cells that closely resemble those derived from virus-induced tumors. Since transformation implies the survival and subsequent multiplication of the infected cell, it can occur only in the setting of abortive rather than lytic infection. Such abortive infections can result either from the infection of a nonpermissive cell or from the infection of a permissive cell with a defective viral genome (Black, 1968; Sambrook, 1972; Eckhart, 1977; Salzman and Khoury, 1974; Kelly and Nathans, 1977; Fareed and Davoli, 1977; Oxman, 1967). The common denominator appears to be the persistence and continued expression of early viral genetic information in the absence of virus replication.

When papovaviruses of the polyomavirus genus infect nonpermissive cells, e.g., when SV40 infects mouse 3T3 cells (Black, 1968; Sambrook, 1972; Eckhart, 1977; Salzman and Khoury, 1974; Kelly and Nathans, 1977; Fareed and Davoli, 1977; Oxman, 1967), the early phase of infection is similar to that described for infection of permissive cells. Virus adsorption, penetration, and un-

coating occur, and the early region of the viral genome is transcribed into early mRNA. The early viral proteins (T antigens, U antigen, and TSTA) are synthesized, the surface properties of the infected cell are altered, and cellular DNA, RNA, and protein synthesis are stimulated (Fig. 7A). However, the late phase of the replication cycle does not occur. There is little or no viral DNA replication, no synthesis of viral capsid proteins (V antigens), and no production of papovavirus virions. Such abortively infected cells are stimulated to divide and behave for a few generations like transformed cells, i.e., they become insensitive to the controls that regulate the multiplication of normal cells. This transient abnormal behavior, called "abortive transformation," is coincident with and dependent upon the expression of the early region of the viral genome, as evidenced by the synthesis of T antigens.

Gradually, and over several cell generations, most abortively transformed cells return to their original state because, in the absence of viral DNA replication, cell division and enzymatic destruction result in the loss of the early viral

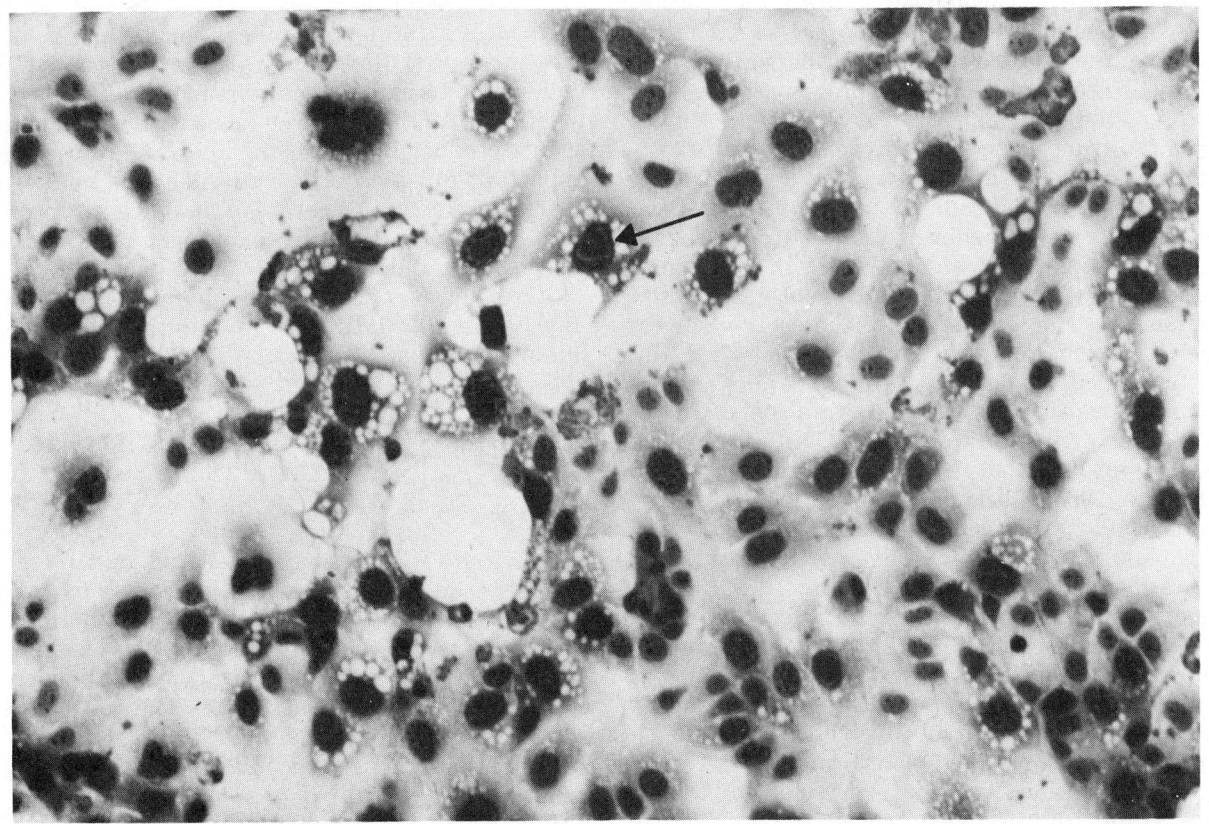

**FIGURE 6.** *SV40 infection of permissive (AGMK) cells. Monolayer cultures were fixed and stained with hematoxylin and eosin 3 days after infection with a multiplicity of approximately 5 plaque-forming units per cell. Note the extensive cytoplasmic vacuolization. The arrow indicates a cell with a typical basophilic intranuclear inclusion body (350 ×).*

# CELL TRANSFORMATION BY PAPOVAVIRUSES

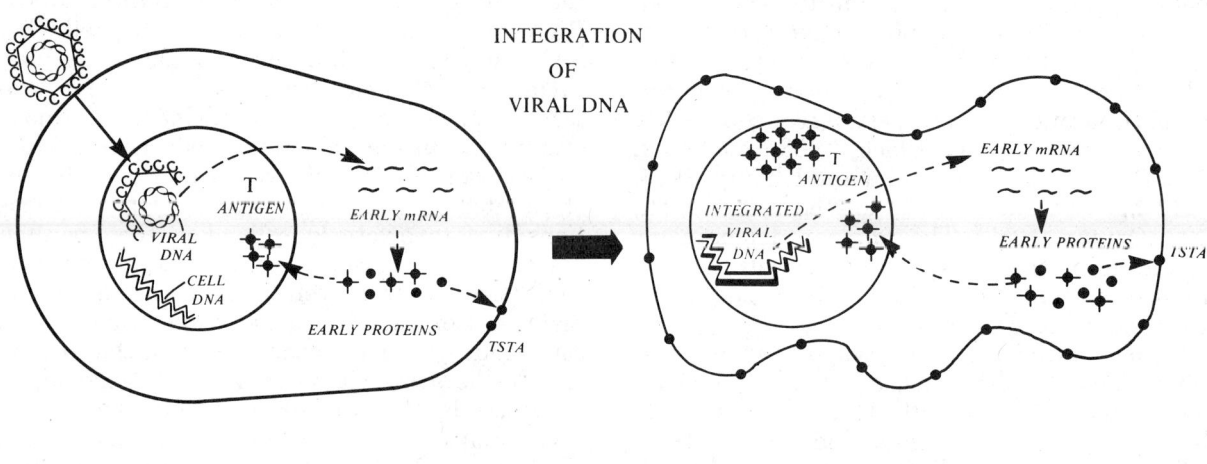

**FIGURE 7.** *Cell transformation by papovaviruses as exemplified by SV40 transformation of mouse 3T3 cells.*

gene(s) and gene product(s) responsible for the transformed phenotype (Sambrook, 1972; Oxman, 1967). However, abortive transformation is not the only possible outcome of abortive infection. Some of the infected cells are permanently transformed. These cells and their progeny continue to express the early papovavirus gene(s) and never lose the transformed phenotype. The critical difference between the permanently and the abortively transformed cells is the integration of the papovavirus genome (or at least the early region of the viral genome) into cell DNA in the permanently transformed cells. This event ensures the persistence and expression of the early viral genetic information that is responsible for the transformed phenotype (Fig. 7B). Thus, permanently transformed cells contain papovavirus DNA covalently linked to cell DNA, as well as early viral mRNA and early viral antigens (Enders, 1965; Black 1968; Benjamin, 1972; Sambrook, 1972; Levine, 1974; Eckhart, 1977; Salzman and Khoury, 1974; Kelly and Nathans, 1977; Fareed and Davoli, 1977; Oxman, 1967). Moreover, although they contain no infectious virus, transformed nonpermissive cells often contain one or more copies of the whole viral genome, and infectious virus can be rescued from them by cocultivation with permissive cells. It should be noted that papovavirus transformation (i.e., permanent transformation) is a very inefficient process; $10^4$ to $10^5$ infectious virions are required per transforming event (Sambrook, 1972).

Papovavirus transformation is of considerable importance to students of human disease. Be-

cause they contain early viral proteins, cells transformed by papovaviruses are extremely useful sources of antigens for serologic tests to detect antibodies to these viral gene products. Moreover, the capacity of the human papovaviruses, BKV and JCV, to induce malignancies in animals, together with the high frequency with which both agents produce infections in childhood, raises the important question of the possible role of these viruses in human cancers, especially those occurring in immunologically compromised individuals (Padgett and Walker, 1976; Takemoto, 1978). To date, however, there is no convincing evidence implicating SV40, BKV, or JCV in the etiology of human malignancies (Howley, 1980).

## VIRUS STRAINS AND ANTIGENIC PROPERTIES

### JC Virus

JC virus (JCV) was first isolated in 1971 by Padgett et al. from brain tissue of a case of PML that occurred in a 38-year-old man with Hodgkin's disease. Papovavirus virions were observed by electron microscopy in the nuclei of oligodendrocytes in the diseased tissue. The virus was isolated in primary human fetal glial (PHFG) cell cultures that had been inoculated with extracts of brain tissue.

JCV grows and produces CPE only in PHFG cell cultures that contain a high proportion of spongioblasts. Even in these cells the CPE is subtle, and the majority of the progeny virions remain cell-associated. In view of the restricted host range of JCV it is not surprising that earlier attempts to isolate virus from brain tissue of patients with PML failed in spite of the inoculation of multiple cell types and animals (Gardner et al., 1971; Weiner and Narayan, 1974). Recently, replication of JCV has been reported in primary human amnion and vascular endothelial cells in vitro (Howley, 1980). The amnion cells are readily available, and this should facilitate biologic and biochemical studies of JCV.

Since the original isolation of JCV, this virus has been identified in the brain tissue of more than 25 patients with PML (Padgett and Walker, 1976; Weiner and Narayan, 1974; Gardner, 1977; Takemoto, 1978; Padgett et al., 1977). JCV has also been isolated from patients without neurologic disease, including renal transplant recipients and a healthy 38-year-old pregnant woman (Gardner, 1977; Coleman et al., 1977; Hogan et al., 1980).

JCV agglutinates human, guinea pig, and chicken erythrocytes at 4° C, but not those of sheep, African green monkeys, rhesus monkeys, or hamsters (Padgett and Walker, 1976; Padgett et al., 1977). The hemagglutinin is associated with the virion, which has a buoyant density in CsCl of 1.34 g/cm³ (Osborne et al., 1977). The hemagglutination inhibition (HI) test detects antibody to JCV.

### BK Virus

BK virus (BKV) was first isolated in 1971 by Gardner et al. from the urine of a 39-year-old man receiving immunosuppressive therapy following a renal allograft. His urine contained abnormal epithelial cells with basophilic intranuclear inclusions. Electron-microscopic examination revealed papovavirus virions in the nuclei of these inclusion-bearing cells, as well as extracellular virions in the urine. Papovavirus virions were also detected in the nuclei of epithelial cells bordering the lumen of the donor ureter after its removal because of obstruction. BKV was isolated in the VERO monkey cell line, but primary human cells are considerably more susceptible to BKV than monkey cells, and thus human cells have been used to obtain many of the more recent isolates of BKV (Padgett and Walker, 1976; Gardner, 1977; Takemoto et al., 1974; Dougherty and Di Stefano, 1974; Takemoto and Mollarkey, 1973; Lecatsas et al., 1974). BKV grows very well in human embryonic kidney (HEK), human fetal fibroblast, and human fetal brain cultures, and produces a CPE like that produced by SV40 in AGMK cells (Fig. 6).

There is no serologic cross-reactivity between BKV and the human wart viruses or mouse polyoma virus, and only a very minor antigenic relationship between BKV and SV40. Since SV40 does not hemagglutinate and BKV agglutinates human O, chicken, and guinea pig cells to high titer, there is little likelihood of confusing BKV with SV40. Specific antibody to BKV inhibits hemagglutination, and thus the HI test provides a rapid and sensitive method for the detection and titration of antibody to BKV.

Since 1971 a number of investigators have isolated and identified BKV in the urine of renal allograft recipients, children and adults receiving chemotherapy for malignancies, and children with Wiskott-Aldrich syndrome, a congenital disorder involving defects in both cellular and humoral immunity (Padgett and Walker, 1976; Gardner, 1977; Takemoto, 1978; Hogan et al., 1980).

Although BKV is less oncogenic in vivo than JCV (see below), hamster and rat cells have been successfully transformed in vitro by BKV, as well as by BKV DNA (Padgett and Walker, 1976; Takemoto, 1978; Portolani et al., 1975; van der Noordaa, 1976; Takemoto and Martin, 1976; Howley and Martin, 1977). The transformed cells resemble cells transformed by SV40, and contain BKV T antigens and BKV DNA. In some cases, BKV can be rescued from them by fusion with permissive cells (Howley, 1980).

### Antigenic Relationships

*Virion Antigens.* Hyperimmune rabbit antisera to SV40, BKV, and JCV all show minor reciprocal cross-reactions at low dilutions. No cross-reactions have been observed between either BKV or JCV and other members of the polyomavirus genus (including other primate papovaviruses) or with human papilloma viruses. Neutralization and FA staining appear to be the most sensitive techniques for detecting these cross-reacting virion antigens. There is a genus-specific antigenic determinant on the major capsid protein, VP-1, which is shared by all members of the polyomavirus genus. It is not located on the surface of the virion, and antibodies to it are only produced after immunization with disrupted virions or purified VP-1.

*Nonvirion Antigens.* Like SV40, BKV and JCV induce T antigens that are detectable by FA staining in the nuclei of acutely infected and transformed cells; hamsters bearing tumors induced by these viruses develop anti-T antibodies (Padgett and Walker, 1976; Takemoto, 1978; Dougherty, 1976). The T antigens induced by all three viruses have been shown to be immunologically similar (Padgett and Walker, 1976; Takemoto, 1978; Dougherty, 1976). This is not unexpected, because they have some, but not all, of their methionine-tryptic peptides in common.

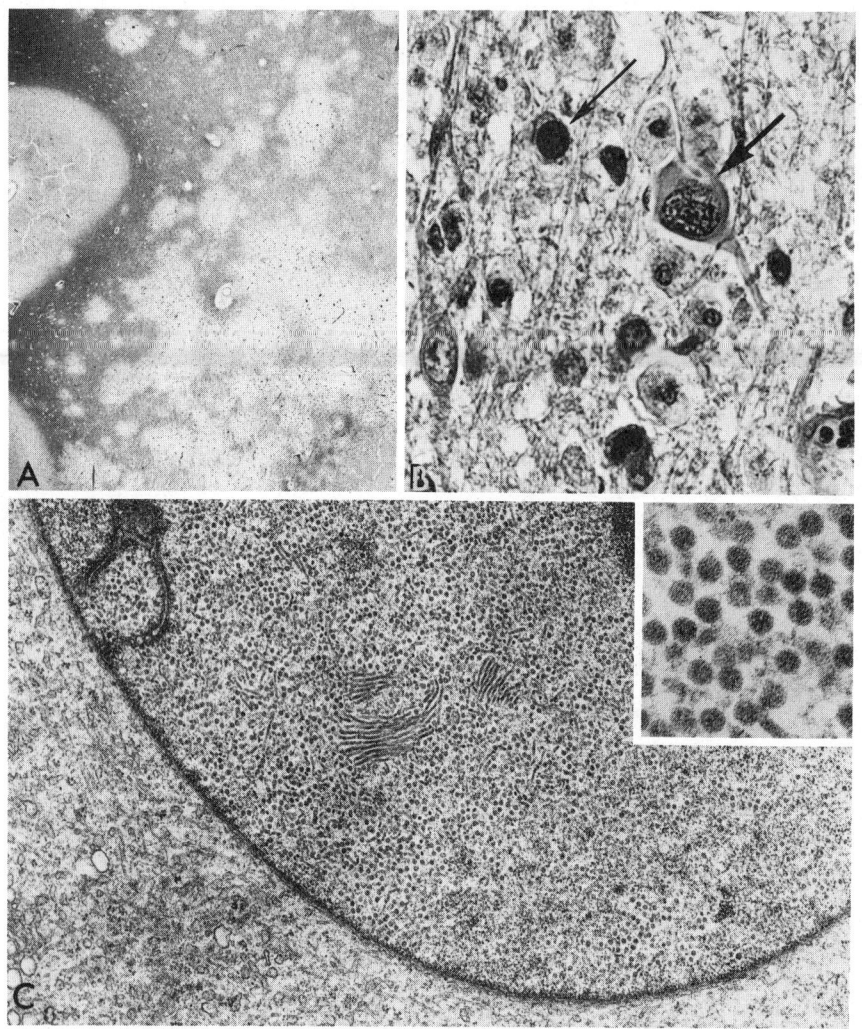

**FIGURE 8.** *The brain in a typical case of progressive multifocal leukoencephalopathy. A, Patchy demyelination unrelated to vessels merging into confluent lesions. Stained with Luxol fast blue (8 ×). B, The enlarged oligodendroglial nucleus showing margination of chromatin and effacement of nuclear structure by an intranuclear inclusion body (small arrow) and the hypertrophic astrocyte with a bizarre, giant nucleus (large arrow) are characteristic light microscopic findings. Stained with hematoxylin and eosin (350 ×). C, Oligodendrocyte with enlarged nucleus filled with spherical and filamentous virus particles (20,000 ×) that are enlarged in inset (80,000 ×). (Courtesy of Dr. Peter W. Lampert)*

## EPIDEMIOLOGY

### JC Virus

The consistent finding of JCV in the diseased brains of patients with progressive multifocal leukoencephalopathy (PML) and the localization of JCV virions in the abnormal oligodendrocytes that are the hallmark of the disease provide strong evidence that JCV is the cause of PML. PML is a rare disease that typically presents as a rapidly evolving neurologic illness in a patient with a long-standing systemic disease such as Hodgkin's disease, chronic lymphocytic leukemia, or lymphosarcoma that is associated with an impairment of immunity (Astrom et al., 1958; Richardson, 1961). The main clinical features are those of a diffuse but asymmetric disease of the cerebral hemispheres: mental aberrations, blindness and disturbances of ocular motility, abnormalities of speech, ataxia, hemiparesis, and other

focal neurologic deficits. The disease is relentlessly progressive in the absence of fever or abnormalities in the cerebrospinal fluid, and death usually occurs within three to six months of onset. Occasionally a patient may live for two years or longer.

The lesions in the central nervous system constitute the truly distinctive feature of PML (Zu Rhein and Chou, 1965; Silverman and Rubinstein, 1965; Howatson et al., 1965). These consist of multiple foci of demyelination of varying sizes and stages of evolution, which become confluent and may eventually involve the white matter of entire lobes (Fig. 8A). The lesions show no relationship to blood vessels and there is no inflammatory response. They do, however, show two characteristic cytopathologic abnormalities. The pathognomonic feature of PML is the presence of altered oligodendrocytes in and around the early foci of demyelination and at the periphery of the more advanced lesions. These oligodendrocytes are enlarged with markedly enlarged nuclei that are intensely basophilic and show effacement of their nuclear structure (Fig. 8B). These changes are followed by necrosis, and thus oligodendrocytes are generally absent from the central portions of more advanced lesions.

The other distinctive cytopathologic feature of PML is the presence, in the more advanced lesions, of giant astrocytes with bizarre hyperchromatic nuclei that resemble the malignant astrocytes of pleomorphic glioblastomas. These cells also resemble astrocytes that have been transformed in vitro by SV40. These changes, and especially the presence of inclusions in the nuclei of oligodendrocytes, led Cavanagh et al (Cavanagh et al., 1959) and Richardson (Richardson, 1961) to suggest that PML might represent an opportunistic viral infection involving oligodendrocytes in patients with impaired immunity. The demonstration in 1965 (Zu Rhein and Chou, 1965; Silverman and Rubinstein, 1965; Howatson et al., 1965) that nuclei of the affected oligodendrocytes in lesions of PML were packed with viral particles resembling papovavirus virions (Fig. 8C) lent strong support to this concept and set the stage for the subsequent isolation of JCV by Padgett et al. in 1971 (Padgett et al., 1971). It now seems likely that PML is due to an opportunistic infection by JCV of persons with impaired immunity, and that demyelination occurs because JCV produces a lytic infection of the oligodendrocytes.

Although PML is a rare disease, serologic studies indicate that JCV is widely disseminated in the human population (Padgett and Walker, 1976; Gardner, 1977; Padgett and Walker, 1973; Brown, Tsai, and Gajdusek, 1975). Infection is most frequently acquired in childhood, with HI antibody to JCV already present in 65 per cent of children aged 10 to 14 years (Padgett and Walker, 1973). Approximately 75 per cent of adults in the United States and England have antibody to JCV. There is no information about the route of transmission or the characteristics of the primary infection. However, excretion in the urine and infection via the oral or respiratory route seems likely in view of the isolation of JCV from urine and the epidemiology of other papovaviruses, such as polyoma virus in mice or SV40 in monkeys. Most members of the polyomavirus genus appear to be inhabitants of the urinary tract.

The highly restricted host range of JCV makes a nonhuman reservoir of infection very unlikely. Furthermore, Padgett et al. (Padgett et al., 1977) examined sera from a wide variety of animals for antibody to JCV and found that no species other than man had antibody to this virus. Thus, JCV appears to be a strictly human virus.

## BK Virus

BKV can be isolated from the urine of 15 to 40 per cent of renal allograft recipients, as well as from other immunosuppressed individuals, but there is no evidence of any significant disease resulting from BKV infection. There is no serologic evidence to suggest an association between BKV infection and malignancy. Furthermore, extensive studies have not confirmed early reports that BKV DNA could be detected by nucleic acid hybridization in certain human tumors (Howley, 1980).

Serologic surveys indicate that BKV infection is common throughout the world. Approximately 70 per cent of children have already acquired HI antibody to the virus by age 4 to 6 years. Thus, BKV is readily transmitted to children at an earlier age than JCV infection. As in the case of JCV, there is no information on the route of transmission or the characteristics of the primary infection. Furthermore, isolation of BKV has not yet been reported from normal children or adults. Like JCV, BKV is likely to be a strictly human virus.

## SV40

The isolation of papovaviruses indistinguishable from SV40 from brain tissue of two patients with PML (Weiner et al., 1972), the exposure of millions of individuals to SV40 in viral vaccines administered during the 1950s, the capacity of this virus to induce tumors in animals and transform human cells in vitro, and the presence of low titers of antibody to SV40 in a small proportion of human sera (Shah and Nathanson, 1976; Shah, 1972) have raised the question of the potential role of SV40 in human disease, especially cancer. However, no additional cases of PML have been associated with SV40-like viruses, and follow-up studies have not revealed any significant excess of malignancies in recipients of SV40-contaminated vaccines (Shah and Nathanson, 1976). Furthermore, it now appears that most or all of the antibody to SV40 that is not accounted for by exposure to SV40 in vaccines or contact with monkeys is due to cross-reacting antibody induced by the human papovavirus, BKV. Thus, there is no evidence that SV40 is a significant cause of disease in humans or that SV40 infects humans under natural conditions.

## Human Papillomaviruses

The human papillomaviruses cause a variety of hyperplastic lesions of the skin and mucous membranes. These papillomas or warts are generally benign and tend to spontaneously regress, but they may occasionally undergo malignant degeneration. Transmission of human papillomaviruses is by contact, either direct or indirect; and, since papillomaviruses appear to be highly species specific, humans are likely to be the only reservoir of infection. The peak incidence of warts occurs during the second decade of life, and most adults have been afflicted at least once. Cellular immunity is important in controlling papillomavirus infections, and patients treated with immunosuppressive drugs often have persistent and widely disseminated warts (Spencer and Anderson, 1970; Ingelfinger et al., 1977).

Although human papillomaviruses have not been propagated in cell culture, the ready availability of virus-containing papilloma tissue has permitted the extraction of sufficient quantities of virus to allow an analysis of human papillomavirus (HPV) DNA and capsid proteins. Restriction endonuclease analysis and nucleic acid hybridization of HPV DNA, together with immunologic and electrophoretic analysis of HPV proteins, has led to the identification of at least six distinct human papillomaviruses (Pass and Maizel, 1973; Favre et al., 1975; Gissmann et al., 1977; Orth et al., 1977; zur Hausen, 1977; Orth et al., 1978; Coggin and zur Hausen, 1979). Human papilloma virus type 1 (HPV-1) and HPV-4 are associated mainly, but not exclusively, with deep plantar warts. HPV-2 is associated with common hand warts and mosaic plantar warts. HPV-3 is associated with flat warts in normal individuals and in patients with epidermodysplasia verruciformis, a rare familial disease characterized by generalized warty lesions that persist and exhibit a tendency to become malignant. HPV-5 has been isolated from benign lesions in patients with epidermodysplasia verruciformis. HPV-6 is associated with condyloma acuminata (genital warts) and perhaps also with juvenile laryngeal papillomas. DNA hybridization under stringent conditions has revealed little if any nucleotide sequence homology between the DNAs of these different human papillomaviruses. This suggests that, in evolutionary terms, the different HPV types may have diverged as much from each other as they have from papillomaviruses of other species.

## LABORATORY DIAGNOSIS

### JC Virus

In view of our current lack of knowledge of the natural history of JCV infections, it would be desirable to attempt the isolation of virus from a variety of tissues and body fluids of patients with PML and of immunosuppressed patients without neurologic disease. Padgett and his associates

(Padgett and Walker, 1976; Padgett et al., 1977) have examined a wide variety of cells of human, nonhuman primate, and nonprimate origin, including primary human fetal cells derived from virtually every organ, but have been able to cultivate JCV only in cultures of primary human fetal glial (PHFG) cells. The isolation of JCV requires an enormous investment of time and energy, as well as the use of a cell culture that is not widely available. Thus the recent report that JCV can be propagated in primary human amnion cells is especially significant (Howley, 1980).

Fortunately, tissues and body fluids suspected of containing JCV can be examined directly by one or more of the following techniques. Tissue sections or cytologic preparations from urine, cerebrospinal fluid, or other body fluids may be stained with hematoxylin and eosin and examined by light microscopy for the presence of cells with typical intranuclear inclusion bodies (Rand et al., 1977; Coleman, 1975; Coleman et al., 1977). Tissue sections, cytologic preparations, and urine or other body fluids may also be examined by electron microscopy in search of papovavirus virions. When virions are observed in such specimens, they may be extracted and serotyped with monospecific rabbit sera by immune electron microscopy (Narayan et al., 1973). FA staining with specific antisera may be used to detect and identify virion antigens in tissue sections and cytologic preparations (Narayan et al., 1973). Finally, radiolabeled JCV DNA probes may be used to detect JCV DNA sequences in tissue specimens or cultured cells.

The HI test has been extensively used to detect and quantitate antibodies to JCV in human serum (Padgett and Walker, 1976; Padgett and Walker, 1973). Consideration should be given to the use of FA tests for the detection of antibody to JCV T antigens. However, the greatest need at present is to employ the HI test more widely in order to better define the natural history of JCV infections.

### BK Virus

As in the case of JCV, it would be desirable to attempt the isolation of BKV from a variety of tissues and body fluids of immunosuppressed patients. It would also be useful to screen children under 6 years of age for excretion of BKV in urine, feces, saliva, and respiratory secretions to determine the mode of transmission of BKV infection. Unfortunately, although the host range of BKV is not as restricted as that of JCV, this is still a formidable undertaking.

When VERO cells have been employed in the isolation of BKV from urine, the interval from inoculation to the development of CPE has generally ranged from one to five months, and the CPE has not been very distinctive (Gardner et al, 1971; Coleman et al, 1973; Takemoto and Mullarkey, 1973). Primary human cells, including primary HEK, fetal fibroblasts, and PHFG, are considerably more susceptible to BKV than VERO cells and exhibit a much more easily recognized CPE. However, CPE may not appear for five or more weeks following inoculation. Thus, it would be reasonable to employ a series of four blind passages, each of 21 days duration and initiated with sonicated RDE-treated cells from the preceding passage. Moreover, cultures in the final passage should be examined by electron microscopy, FA staining for BKV V antigens, and testing of supernatant fluids and sonicated RDE-treated cell extracts for hemagglutination before being discarded as negative. BKV may be assayed by CPE end-point dilution, plaque formation in HEK monolayers, or the formation of foci of infected cells detectable by FA staining with antibody to V antigen (Padgett and Walker, 1976; Gardner, 1977; Takemoto, 1978). Although the isolation of BKV is not as difficult as that of JCV, it is still a costly and time-consuming endeavor.

Fortunately, tissues and body fluids suspected of containing BKV can be examined directly. Tissue sections, or cytologic preparations from urine, cerebrospinal fluid, or other body fluids may be stained with hematoxylin and eosin and examined by light microscopy for the presence of cells with typical basophilic intranuclear inclusion bodies. Tissue sections, cytologic preparations, and urine or other body fluids may also be examined by electron microscopy in search of papovavirus virions. When virions are observed in such specimens, they may be extracted and serotyped with monospecific rabbit sera by immune electron microscopy. FA staining with specific antisera may detect and identify virion antigens in tissue sections and cytologic preparations. Similarly, sera from tumor-bearing hamsters may be employed to detect BKV T antigen, but, as already noted, this test is not virus-specific. Finally, BKV DNA sequences in suspect tissues may be detected by hybridization with radiolabeled BKV DNA probes (Howley, 1980). The HI test has been used extensively to detect and quantitate antibodies to BKV in human serum.

## PATHOGENICITY IN EXPERIMENTAL ANIMALS

### JC Virus

JCV appears to be a strictly human virus with a very restricted host range, and antibodies to it have not been detected in any species of animal except man. Furthermore, with the exception of tumors that arise after the inoculation of newborn hamsters and owl monkeys (see below), no acute or chronic disease attributable to JCV has been found in any of a variety of species inoculated by multiple routes and observed for months to years (Padgett and Walker, 1976). The animals tested include rabbits, guinea pigs, hamsters, mink, and rhesus monkeys. Newborn rhesus monkeys inoculated by several routes apparently became infected because they developed antibody to T antigens, as well as to V antigen. However, no disease or tumors have been recognized during a three-year period of observation (Padgett and Walker, 1976).

JCV is highly oncogenic in newborn Syrian hamsters, especially following intracerebral inoculation, when it produces tumors, which are usually multiple malignant gliomas. Subcutaneous and intraperitoneal inoculation of JCV produces multiple sarcomas in visceral organs (Padgett and Walker, 1976). Recently, malignant astrocytomas have been reported in two owl monkeys inoculated intracerebrally, intravenously, and subcutaneously 16 and 25 months earlier. JCV T antigen was detected in the cells of one of the tumors by FA staining (London et al., 1978). This observation is particularly interesting in the light of a recent report (Castaigne et al., 1974) of multiple gliomas in the brain of an 18-year-old immunodeficient patient with PML.

### BK Virus

Large doses of BKV administered by various routes have produced no recognizable disease or tumors in newborn mice, rats, guinea pigs, or rabbits (Takemoto, 1978). Five newborn rhesus monkeys inoculated intracerebrally and intraperitoneally with large doses of purified BKV remained healthy during a 30-month period of observation, although infection was present, as evidenced by the development of antibodies to both BKV T and V antigens (Takemoto, 1978). In contrast to JCV, BKV is only weakly oncogenic for hamsters.

### Relevance of Human Papovaviruses to Human Disease

Except for the etiologic role of JCV in PML, there is no evidence linking infections with JCV or BKV to human disease. However, the oncogenic potential of these agents and the ubiquity of infections in childhood would appear to justify a careful examination of their potential roles in human cancer. Although several reports concerning the finding of papovavirus virions, antigens, or nucleic acids in human tumors have appeared (Takemoto, 1978), they have not been confirmed by subsequent studies, and there is no convincing evidence in favor of any etiologic role for these agents in human cancer (Howley, 1980). Since none of the members of the polyomavirus genus appears to cause malignancies in their natural hosts under normal conditions, it seems likely that if the human papovaviruses cause any human tumors, the most probable candidates are tumors occurring in immunosuppressed or immunodeficient individuals.

# References

Astrom, K. E., Mancall, E. L., and Richardson, E. P., Jr.: Progressive multifocal leuko-encephalopathy: A hitherto unrecognized complication of chronic lymphatic leukaemia and Hodgkin's disease. Brain 81:93–111, 1958.

Benjamin, T.: Physiological and genetic studies of polyoma virus. Curr Top Microbiol Immunol 59:107, 1972.

Berk, A. J., and Sharp, P. A.: Spliced early mRNAs of simian virus 40. Proc. Natl. Acad. Sci. U.S.A., 75:1274, 1978.

Black, P. H.: The oncogenic DNA viruses. A review of *in vitro* transformation studies. Annu Rev Microbiol 22:391, 1968.

Brown, P., Tsai, T., and Gajdusek, D. C.: Seroepidemiology of human papovaviruses: Discovery of virgin populations and some unusual patterns of antibody prevalence among remote peoples of the world. Am J Epidemiol 102:331, 1975.

Butel, J. S.: Studies with human papilloma virus modeled after known papovavirus systems. J Natl Cancer Inst 48:285, 1972.

Castaigne, P., Rondot, P., Escourolle, R., Dumas, J. L. R., Cathala, F., and Hauw, J. J.: Leucoencephalopathie multifocale progressive et "gliomes" multiples. Rev Neurol 130:379, 1974.

Cavanagh, J. B., Greenbaum, D., Marshall, A. H. E., and Rubinstein, L. J.: Cerebral demyelination associated with disorders of the reticuloendothelial system. Lancet 2:525, 1959.

Ciuffo, G.: Innesto positivo con filtrato di verruca volgare. Giorn Ital Mal Venereol 48:12, 1907.

Coggin, J. R. Jr., and zur Hausen, H.: Workshop on papillomaviruses and cancer. Cancer Res 39:545, 1979.

Coleman, D. V.: The cytodiagnosis of human polyomavirus infection. Acta Cytol 19:93, 1975.

Coleman, D. V., Daniel, R. A., Gardner, S. D., Field, A. M., and Gibson, P. E.: Polyoma virus in urine during pregnancy. Lancet 1:709, 1977.

Coleman, D. V., Gardner, S. D., and Field, A. M.: Human polyomavirus infection in renal allograft recipients. Br Med J 3:371, 1973.

Coleman, D. V., Russell, W. J. I., Hodgson, J., Pe, T., and Mowbray, J. F.: Human papovavirus in Papanicolaou smears of urinary sediment detected by transmission electron microscopy. J Clin Pathol 30:1015, 1977.

Crawford, L. V., Cole, C. N., Smith, A. E., Paucha, E., Tegtmeyer, P., Rundell, K., and Berg, P.: Organization and expression of early genes of simian virus 40. Proc. Natl. Acad. Sci. U.S.A., 75:117, 1978.

Diacumakos, E. G., and Gershey, E. L.: Uncoating and gene expression of simian virus 40 in CV-1 cell nuclei inoculated by microinjection. J Virol 24:903, 1977.

Dougherty, R. M.: A comparison of human papovavirus T antigens. J Gen Virol 33:61, 1976.

Dougherty, R. M., and Di Stefano, H. S.: Isolation and characterization of a papovavirus from human urine. Proc Soc Exp Biol Med 146:481, 1974.

Eckhart, W.: Genetics of polyoma virus and simian virus 40. In Fraenkel-Conrat, H., and Wagner, R. R. (ed.): Comprehensive Virology, vol 9. New York, Plenum Press, 1977, pp. 1–26.

Enders, J. F.: Cell transformation by viruses as illustrated by the response of human and hamster renal cells to simian virus 40. Harvey Lectures 59:113, 1965.

Fareed, G. C., and Davoli, D.: Molecular biology of papovaviruses. Ann Rev Biochem 46:471, 1977.

Favre, M., Breitburd, F., Croissant, O., and Orth, G.: Structural polypeptides of rabbit, bovine, and human papillomaviruses. J Virol 15:1239, 1975.

Fiers, W., Contreras, R., Haegeman, G., Rogiers, R., Van de Voorde, A., Van Heuverswyn, H., Van Herreweghe, J., Volckaert, G., and Ysebaert, M.: Complete nucleotide sequence of SV40 DNA. Nature, 273:113, 1978.

Finch, J. T., and Klug, A.: The structure of viruses of the papilloma-polyoma type. III. Structure of rabbit papilloma virus. J Mol Biol 13:1, 1965.

Fried, M., and Griffin, B. E.: Organization of the genomes of polyoma virus and SV40. Adv Cancer Res 24:67, 1977.

Gardner, S. D.: New human papovaviruses: Their nature and significance. In Waterson, A. P. (ed.): Recent Advances in Clinical Virology, vol 1. Edinburgh, Churchill-Livingstone, 1977, pp. 93–115.

Gardner, S. D., Field, A. M., Coleman, D. V., and Hulme, B.: New human papovavirus (B.K.) isolated from urine after renal transplantation. Lancet 1:1253, 1971.

Gissmann, L., Pfister, H., and zur Hausen, H.: Human papilloma viruses (HPV): Characterization of four different isolates. Virology 76:569, 1977.

Hogan, T. F., Borden, E. C., McBain, J. A., Padgett, B. L., and Walker, D. L.: Human polyomavirus infections with JC virus and BK virus in renal transplant patients. Annals Int Med 92:373, 1980.

Howatson, A. F., Nagal, M., and Zu Rhein, G. M.: Polyoma-like virions in human demyelinating brain disease. Can Med Assoc J 93:379, 1965.

Howley, P. M.: Molecular biology of SV40 and the human polyomaviruses BK and JC. In Klein, G. (ed.): Viral Oncology. New York, Raven Press, 1980, pp. 489–549.

Howley, P. M., and Martin, M. A.: Uniform representation of the human papovavirus BK genome in transformed hamster cells. J Virol 23:205, 1977.

Hsiung, G. D., and Gaylord, W. H., Jr.: The vacuolating virus of monkeys. I. Isolation, growth characteristics, and inclusion body formation. J Exp Med 114:975, 1961.

Ingelfinger, J. R., Grupe, W. E., and Topor, M.: Warts in a pediatric renal transplant population. Dermatologica 155:7, 1977.

Kelly, T. J., Jr., and Nathans, D.: The genome of simian virus 40. Adv Virus Res 21:85, 1977.

Lecatsas, G., Prozesky, O. W., and Scheepers, F.: The cytopathology and development of a human polyoma virus (BK). Arch Ges Virusforsch 44:319, 1974.

Levine, A. J.: The replication of papovavirus DNA. Prog Med Virol 17:1, 1974.

London, W. T., Houff, S. A., Madden, D. L., Fucillo, D. A., Gravell, M., Wallen, W. C., Sever, J. L., Padgett, B. L., Walker, D. L., Zu Rhein, G. M., and Ohashi, T.: Brain tumors in owl monkeys following inoculation with a human polyomavirus (JC virus). Science, 201:1246, 1978.

Mattern, C. F. T., Takemoto, K. K., and DeLeva, A. M.: Electron microscopic observations on multiple polyoma virus-related particles. Virology 32:378, 1967.

Melnick, J. L.: Papova virus group. Science 135:1128, 1962.

Melnick, J. L.: Taxonomy of viruses. Prog Med Virol 23:196, 1977.

Melnick, J. L., Allison, A., Butel, J. S., Eckhart, W., Eddy, B. E., Kit, S., Levine, A. J., Miles, J. A. R., Pagano, J. S., Sachs, L., and Vonka, V.: Papovaviridae. Intervirology 3:106, 1974.

Melnick, J. L., and Stinebaugh, S.: Excretion of vacuolating SV-40 virus (papovavirus group) after ingestion as a contaminant of oral poliovaccine. Proc Soc Exp Biol Med 109:965, 1962.

Narayan, O., Penney, J. B., Jr., Johnson, R. T., Herndon, R. M., and Weiner, L. P.: Etiology of progressive multifocal leukoencephalopathy. N Engl J Med 289:1278, 1973.

Orth, G., Favre, M., and Croissant, O.: Characterization of a new type of human papillomavirus that causes skin warts. J Virol 24:108, 1977.

Orth, G., Jablonska, S., Favre, M., Croissant, O., Jarzabek-Chorzelska, M., and Rzesa, G.: Characterization of two types of human papillomaviruses in lesions of epidermodysplasia verruciformis. Proc Natl Acad Sci USA 75:1537, 1978.

Osborn, J. E., Robertson, S. M., Padgett, B. L., Zu Rhein, G. M., Walker, D. L., and Weisblum, B.: Comparison of JC and BK human papovaviruses with simian virus 40: Restriction endonuclease digestion and gel electrophoresis of result fragments. J Virol 13:614, 1977.

Oxman, M. N.: Some behavioral studies of simian virus 40 (SV40). Arch Ges Virusforsch 22:171, 1967.

Padgett, B. L., Rogers, C. M., and Walker, D. L.: JC virus, a human polyomavirus associated with progressive multifocal leukoencephalopathy: Additional biological characteristics and antigenic relationships. Infect Immun 15:656, 1977.

Padgett, B. L., and Walker, D. L.: New human papovaviruses. Prog Med Virol 22:1, 1976.

Padgett, B. L., and Walker, D. L.: Prevalence of antibodies in human sera against JC virus, an isolate from a case of progressive multifocal leukoencephalopathy. J Infect Dis 127:467, 1973.

Padgett, B. L., Walker, D. L., Zu Rhein, G. M., Eckroade, R. J., and Dessel, B. H.: Cultivation of papova-like virus from human brain with progressive multifocal leucoencephalopathy. Lancet 2:1257, 1971.

Padgett, B. L., Walker, D. L., Zu Rhein, G. M., Hodach, A. E., and Chou, S. M.: JC papovavirus in progressive multifocal leukoencephalopathy. J Infect Dis 133:686, 1976.

Pass, F., and Maizel, J. V., Jr.: Wart-associated antigens. II. Human immunity to viral structural proteins. J Invest Dermatol 60:307, 1973.

Pauca, E., Mellor, A., Harvey, R., Smith, A. E., Hewick, R. M., and Waterfield, M. D.: Large and small tumor antigens from simian virus 40 have identical amino termini mapping at 0.65 map units. Proc Natl Acad Sci USA 75:2165, 1978.

Pitko, V. M., Pyokari, P., Nase, L., and Mantyjarvi, R.: Effect of β-propiolactone on infectivity and haemagglutinin of the BK virus. Acta Pathol Microbiol Scand [B] 83:141, 1975.

Portolani, M., Barbanti-Brodano, B., and La Placa, M.: Malignant transformation of hamster kidney cells by BK virus. J Virol 15:420, 1975.

Rand, K. H., Johnson, K. P., Rubinstein, L. J., Wolinsky, J. S., Penney, J. B., Walter, D. L., Padgett, B. L., and Merigan, T. C.: Adenine arabinoside in the treatment of progressive multifocal leukoencephalopathy: Use of virus-containing cells in the urine to assess response to therapy. Ann Neurol 1:458, 1977.

Reddy, V. B., Thimmappaya, B., Dhar, R., Subramanian, K. N., Zain, B. S., Pan, J., Ghosh, P. K., Celma, M. L., and Weissman, S. M.: The genome of simian virus 40. Science 200:494, 1978.

Richardson, E. P., Jr.: Progressive multifocal leukoencephalopathy. N Engl J Med 265:815, 1961.

Rawson, K. E. K., and Mahy, B. W. J.: Human papova (wart) virus. Bacteriol Rev 31:110, 1967.

Salzman, N. P., and Khoury, S.: Reproduction of papovaviruses. In Fraenkel-Conrat, H., and Wagner, R. R. (eds.): Comprehensive Virology, vol 3. New York, Plenum Press, 1974, pp. 63–141.

Sambrook, J.: Transformation by polyoma virus and simian virus 40. Adv Cancer Res 16:141, 1972.

Shah, K. V.: Evidence for an SV40-related papovavirus infection of man. Am J Epidemiol 95:199, 1972.

Shah, K., and Nathanson, N.: Human exposure to SV40: Review and comment. Am J Epidemiol 103:1, 1976.

Silverman, L., and Rubinstein, L. J.: Electron microscopic observations on a case of progressive multifocal leukoencephalopathy. Acta Neuropathologica 5:215, 1965.

Simmons, D. T., and Martin, M. A.: Common methionine-tryptic peptides near the amino-terminal end of primate papovavirus tumor antigens. Proc Natl Acad Sci USA 75:1131, 1978.

Spencer, E. S., and Anderson, H. K.: Clinically evident, nonterminal infections with herpes viruses and the wart virus in immunosuppressed renal allograft recipients. Br Med J 3:251, 1970.

Sweet, B. H., and Hilleman, M. R.: The vacuolating virus, SV40. Proc Soc Exp Biol 105:420, 1960.

Takemoto, K. K.: Human papovaviruses. Int Rev Exp Pathol 18:281, 1978.

Takemoto, K. K., and Martin, M. A.: Transformation of hamster kidney cells by BK papovavirus DNA. J Virol 17:247, 1976.

Takemoto, K. K., and Mullarkey, M. G.: Human papovavirus. BK strain: Biological studies including antigenic relationship to simian virus 40. J Virol 12:625, 1973.

Takemoto, K. K., Rabson, A. S., Mullarkey, M. F., Blaese, R. M., Garon, C. F., and Nelson, D.: Isolation of papovavirus from brain tumor and urine of a patient with Wiskott-Aldrich syndrome. J Natl Cancer Inst 53:1205, 1974.

van der Noordaa, J.: Infectivity, oncogenicity and transforming ability of BK virus and BK virus DNA. J Gen Virol 30:371, 1976.

Weiner, L. P., Herndon, R. M., Narayan, O., Johnson, R. T., Shah, K., Rubinstein, L. J., Preziosi, T. J., and Conley, F. K.: Isolation of virus related to SV40 from patients with progressive multifocal leukoencephalopathy. N Engl J Med 286:35, 1972.

Weiner, L. P., and Narayan, O.: Virologic studies of progressive multifocal leukoencephalopathy. Prog Med Virol 18:229, 1974.

zur Hausen, H.: Human papillomaviruses and their possible role in squamous cell carcinomas. Curr Top Microbiol Immunol 78:1, 1977.

Zu Rhein, G. M., and Chou, S. M.: Particles resembling papova viruses in human cerebral demyelinating disease. Science 148:1477, 1965.

# RNA Viruses

## ORTHOMYXOVIRUSES AND PARAMYXOVIRUSES **59**

### Douglas D. Richman, M.D.

## MYXOVIRUSES

### DEFINITION

The term myxovirus (*Gr. myxo,* mucus) has been applied to two families of enveloped RNA viruses, the *Orthomyxoviridae* and *Paramyxoviridae* (Table 1). All myxoviruses contain a single-stranded genome enclosed in a helical array of nucleoprotein. The viral RNA polymerase associated with this ribonucleoprotein structure transcribes viral messenger RNA from the virion RNA. Myxovirus virions are pleomorphic ellipsoids or filaments possessing a lipid envelope with surface glycoprotein projections that bind to host cell receptors.

Myxoviruses are transmitted via the respiratory tract, where influenza viruses, parainfluenza

**TABLE 1.  Human Myxoviruses**

| | VIRION DIAMETER (nm) | GENOME SIZE (daltons × 10⁶) | NUMBER OF GENE SEGMENTS | DIAMETER OF RIBONUCLEO-PROTEIN* | NUCLEAR REQUIREMENT FOR REPLICATION | ENZYME ACTIVITIES RNA Polymerase |
|---|---|---|---|---|---|---|
| Orthomyxoviridae | | | | | | |
| Influenza A & B | 80–170 | 5 | 8 | 9 | + | + |
| Influenza C | 80–170 | 5 | 7 (?) | 9 | ? | + |
| Paramyxoviridae | | | | | | |
| Parainfluenza 1–4b | 150–250 | 6 | 1 | 18 | − | + |
| Mumps | 150–250 | 6 | 1 | 18 | − | + |
| Measles (Rubeola) | 150–250 | 6 | 1 | 18 | − | + |
| Respiratory syncytial virus | 90–180 | 6 | 1 | 14 | − | + |

*Three size classes of ribonucleoprotein apparently exist, although their precise measurements vary with techniques of preparation.

viruses, and respiratory syncytial virus produce their predominant disease. Measles, mumps, and the veterinary myxovirus infections also have a respiratory portal of entry, although disease may be manifested primarily in extrarespiratory sites.

In spite of these common myxovirus characteristics, the genome of the orthomyxoviruses is segmented and the genome of the paramyxoviruses is not. These two virus families will be considered separately.

# ORTHOMYXOVIRUSES: THE INFLUENZA VIRUSES

## STRUCTURE AND REPLICATION

Influenza virions are most frequently 80 to 120 nm in diameter (Figs. 1 and 2). Although generally spheroid, the virions may exhibit great variation in length; long filamentous forms are frequently observed. The virions have a bouyant density of 1.23 g/cm³ and a composition of approximately 1 per cent RNA, 73 per cent protein, 20 per cent lipid, and 6 per cent carbohydrate. There are seven structural proteins of the influenza virion. Three large proteins (P1, P2, P3), associated with the virion RNA, have molecular weights between 85,000 and 95,000. Their functions probably include RNA transcription and replication. A 60,000-dalton nucleoprotein (NP) polypeptide is associated with the virion RNA in the ribonucleoprotein structures. The 25,000-dalton membrane or matrix (M) protein underlies the lipid envelope of the virion. The virion surface is studded with numerous glycoprotein projections that consist of two types, the hemagglutinin (H) and the neuraminidase (N). The H is a trimer of a

polypeptide with a molecular weight of 75,000 to 80,000; the N is a tetramer of a 60,000-dalton polypeptide. The most remarkable structural feature of influenza virus is its segmented genome. The genomes of influenza types A and B consist of eight separate segments of single-stranded RNA, each of which is the gene for one viral polypeptide. When a cell is coinfected by two different influenza viruses, gene segments are assembled into progeny virions with an apparently random distribution with regard to parental origin (Fig. 3). This property, termed *genetic reassortment*, permits major single step changes in surface antigens and host susceptibility. This property carries major implications, both for the epidemiology of the disease and for vaccine development.

The total molecular weight of the influenza virion RNA is 5 × 10⁶. The segments of RNA are each associated with NP to form eight separate ribonucleoprotein structures with a diameter of 9 nm and a bouyant density of 1.34 g/cm³. Influenza viruses are "negative stranded" RNA viruses; the virion RNA is complementary to mRNA. A virus

**TABLE 1.  Human Myxoviruses** (Continued)

| ENZYME ACTIVITIES | | | | CULTIVATION OF PRIMARY ISOLATES | | |
|---|---|---|---|---|---|---|
| Hemagglutinin | Neuraminidase | Hemolysin | Membrane Fusion | Embryonated Egg | Primary Human or Monkey Kidney | Continuous Cell Lines |
| + | + | − | − | + | + | MDCK |
| + | − | − | − | + | − | MDCK |
| + | + | + | + | − | + | Some types only: MDCK, HeLa, HEp-2, WI-38 |
| + | + | + | + | + | + | Vero, HeLa, LLC-MK2 |
| + | − | + | + | + | + | HeLa, HEp-2, LLC-MK2 |
| − | − | − | + | − | + | Hep-2, HeLa WI-38 |

coded RNA polymerase is associated with the influenza RNA within the virion and transcribes mRNA from the (−) strand virion RNA. Less than 10 per cent of most influenza virions are infectious, perhaps because they lack a complete set of eight gene segments. Influenza virus C may contain fewer segments, thus differing from types A and B in this characteristic, in the lack of N

activity, and in several other respects. It appears to be medically insignificant and will not be considered further.

A single proteolytic cleavage of the H glycoprotein by a cell or serum protease is necessary to activate the H and thus to render the influenza virion infectious. The replicative cycle of influenza is initiated by attachment of the virion H to an N-

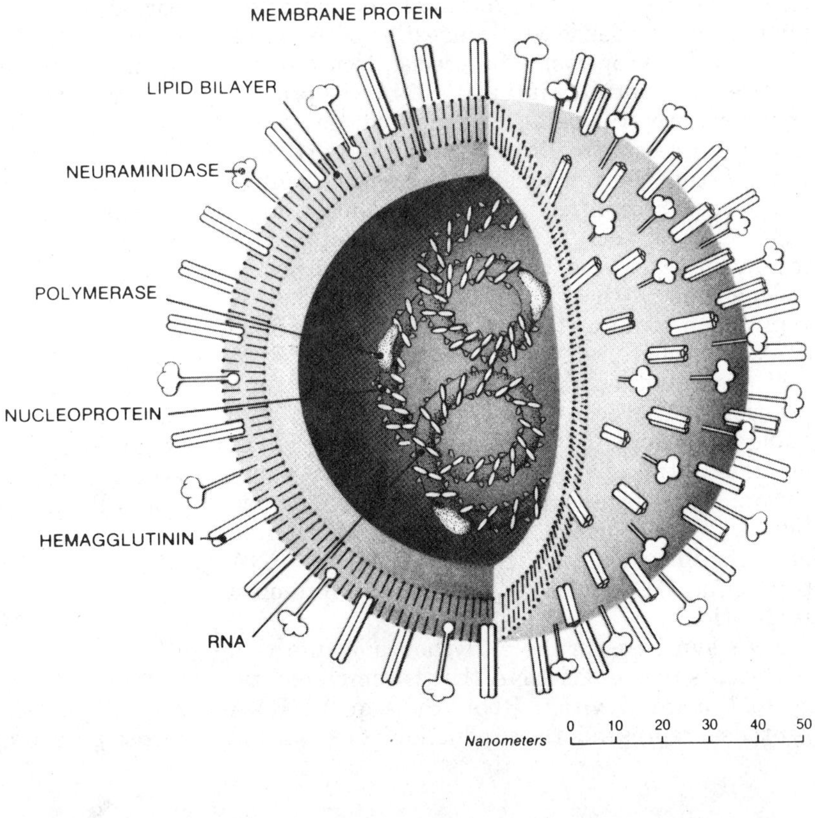

**FIGURE 1.**  *Cutaway diagram of influenza virion structure.*

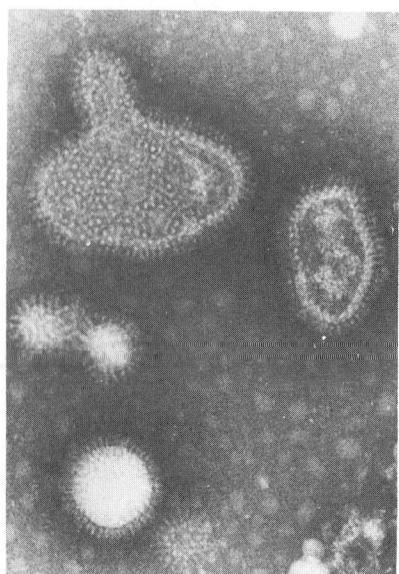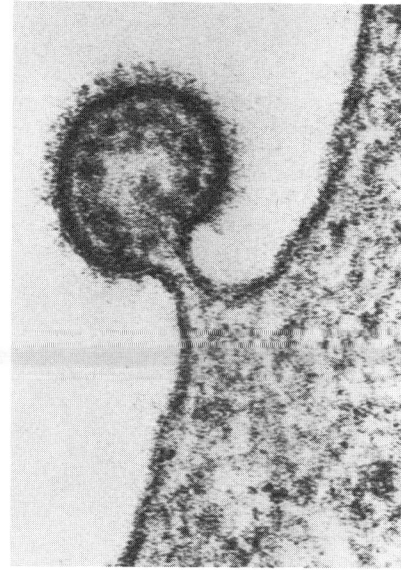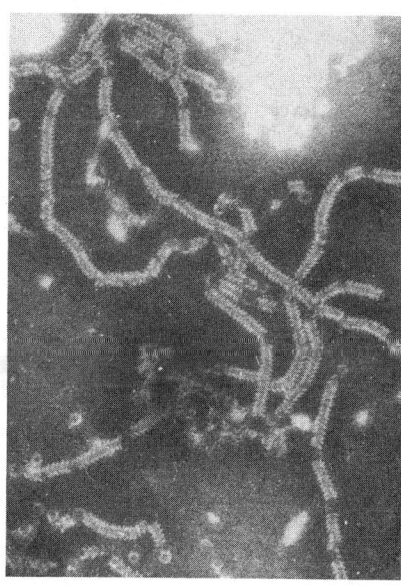

**FIGURE 2.**   Left, *Purified influenza A/Hong Kong/68 (H3N2). Note pleomorphic shapes, variable size, and glyco-protein projections covering the virion surface. Electron-photomicrograph ·kindly provided by A. R. Kalica, Ph.D. Laboratory of Infectious Diseases, NIAID National Institutes of Health, Bethesda, Maryland. (182,000 ×).*

*Center, Respiratory syncytial virus budding from the surface of an infected HeLa cell in culture. Electron-photomi-crograph from Kalica, Wright, Hetrick, and Chanock electron microscopic studies of respiratory syncytial temperature-sensitive mutants. Arch fur die ges Virusf 41:248, 1973, with permission. (132,000 ×).*

*Right, Purified nucleocapsids from mumps virus. Note helical array of ribonucleoproteins to form the nucleocapsid structure with an 18 nm diameter. This nucleocapsid contains an apparent hollow "core," which is apparent on both transverse and end-on views. Electron-photomicrograph from Huppertz, Hall and ter Meulen. Polypeptide composi-tion of mumps virus. Med Microbiol Immunol 163:25, 1977, with permission. (142,025 ×).*

acetylneuraminic acid–containing receptor on a host cell membrane. Two mechanisms of penetra-tion have been proposed: fusion of viral and cell membranes, and endocytotic ingestion of the virus by the cell (viropexis). The precise location, se-quence, and control of influenza RNA and protein synthesis are still being investigated; neverthe-less, the unusual requirement for the participa-tion of the cell nucleus in influenza replica-tion is well recognized. In contrast to most other RNA viruses, such as picornaviruses and para-myxoviruses, whose cytoplasmic replication is independent of the cell nucleus, influenza virus replication requires the presence and function of the cell nucleus, which contains both viral RNA and protein during influenza replication. Enu-cleation of the host cell or treatment of it with sublethal doses of UV irradiation, actinomycin D, or α-amanitin will prevent influenza virus repli-cation. None of these inhibits paramyxovirus rep-lication. Studies using cells resistant to the action of α-amanitin suggest that the host cell RNA polymerase II enzyme is essential for influenza replication.

RNA synthesis in the early hours of infection represents messenger RNA that is complementa-ry to the input virion RNA. Subsequent RNA synthesis represents the production of (−) strand RNA that will be utilized in the assembly of new virions. The viral RNA and proteins are trans-ported to the cell periphery by an undetermined mechanism. Also indefinite are the processes of assembly of these viral components and of bud-ding of virions from the host cell. The first evi-dence of a budding site is the accumulation of the H and N glycoprotein projections in a limited region of the cell outer membrane. A layer of M protein then appears subjacent to the host mem-brane lipid bilayer in this region, which is to be incorporated into the budding virion. Ribonucleo-protein segments can then be seen by electron microscopy attached to these localized regions of altered cell membrane, which then progressively pouch out and finally bud off from the cell surface. Release of new virions from the host cell surface requires hydrolysis by the virion N of the *N*-acetylneuraminic acid–containing receptors that normally are present in the host cell membrane.

## ANTIGENIC COMPOSITION

Two internal structural proteins, the NP and the M protein are used in typing influenza viruses. Each of these two proteins are antigenically identical or highly similar within each of the three influenza types. Moreover, these proteins exhibit no antigenic cross-reactivity among the types. Consequently, whole virus or purified preparations of NP (previously called the soluble [S] antigen) or M protein are used in complement fixation or immunodiffusion tests to type influenza virus isolates as A, B, or C. In addition, these tests are used in the type-specific, but not subtype- or antigenic strain–specific, serodiagnosis of infection. Antibody to the NP or M proteins, which are not exposed on the virion, provides no substantial protection from infection.

The two surface glycoproteins, H and N, are the important antigens for host immunity, for antigenic variation of influenza viruses, and for serodiagnosis of infection. The H binds to $N$-acetylneuraminic acid residues, which are present in all eukaryotic cell membranes. Thus, the virus will probably bind to any cell, including both susceptible host cells and erythrocytes. Attachment to erythrocytes is responsible for hemagglutination, and inhibition of this reaction with antibody, hemagglutination inhibition (HI), constitutes the most utilized assay for measuring antibody against influenza viruses. This technique is also used to characterize antigenic variants of influenza virus. HI antibody neutralizes the infectivity of influenza viruses in vitro and in vivo.

The N enzyme facilitates the release of free virus during the budding process and may also help virions reach the respiratory epithelium, which is protected by mucus and its rich content of glycoproteins containing $N$-acetylneuraminic acid that bind to the virus. N activity is measured by a colorimetric assay of $N$-acetylneuraminic acid released by the enzymatic hydrolysis of a substrate like fetuin. Antibody to N is measured by inhibition of this activity when serum and virus are mixed. This neuraminidase-inhibiting (NI) antibody appears to restrict the spread of virus from infected cells. In monolayer cell cultures infected with influenza virus, HI antibody reduces the number of plaques formed (neutralization of inoculum virus), but the plaques that do appear are of normal size; NI antibody does not reduce plaque number, but does reduce plaque size (restriction of spread of virus from infected to adjacent susceptible cells). In both animal models and in human studies, NI antibody tends to modify the severity of disease expression rather than prevent the acquisition of infection.

Influenza virus has the unique capability of changing the antigenic identity of its H and N. Antigenic changes occur in the H and N polypeptides with a frequency not observed in other viruses or in other influenza virus proteins. The resulting antigenic variants have a selective advantage over the parental antigenic strain in the

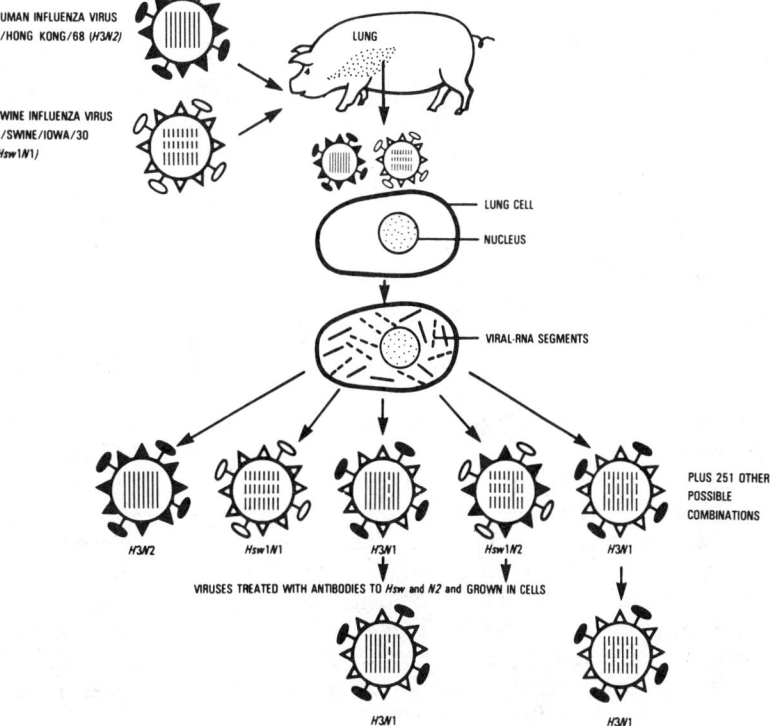

**FIGURE 3.** *Recombination (reassortment) of genetic material from two different type A influenza viruses is represented schematically in this diagram. Here the two influenza viruses, one from man (H3N2) and the other from swine (HswineN1), are shown being inoculated into the nose of a pig. The inoculation results in the simultaneous infection of a single lung cell with the eight separate RNA segments from each virus. Once inside the cell, the viruses multiply, and the 16 different RNA segments can be recombined in many ways during the "packaging" of the new virus particles. In the presence of antibodies to the neuraminidase of the human strain and to the hemagglutination of the swine strain, all the resulting viruses will be neutralized except for those possessing the H3N1 combination of surface antigens. The H3N1 influenza virus may contain many different combinations of RNA that include those coding for the two surface proteins, but their composition with respect to the remaining six segments can vary and some of the recombinants may cause infection in pigs. Such recombination has been demonstrated experimentally to occur in cell culture, in swine, and in fowl. (Adapted from reference 3).*

TABLE 2.   Subtypes of Human Type A Influenza Viruses*

| SUBTYPE | PERIOD OF PREVALENCE | REPRESENTATIVE ANTIGENIC VARIANTS |
|---------|----------------------|-----------------------------------|
| H0N1 | 1933–1947 | A/PR/8/34 |
| H1N1 | 1946–1957<br>1977– | A/FM/1/47<br>A/USSR/90/77 |
| H2N2 | 1957–1968 | A/Japan/305/57 |
| H3N2 | 1968– | A/Hong Kong/1/68<br>A/England/42/72<br>A/Texas/1/77 |
| HswineN1 | None, sporadic infections documented | A/New Jersey/6/76 |

*Table summarizes experience since first isolation in 1933. Prior experience indicated by serologic recapitulation not included.

presence of antibody to the original strain. All three types of influenza virus undergo minor annual changes in their H and N glycoprotein antigens termed *antigenic drift*. These minor changes do not eliminate the basic antigenic relationship to the original strain. When the antigenic change in either H or N is of sufficient magnitude to render them not immunologically cross-reactive, they are given a distinct subtype designation. Such H and N subtypes have been identified only with influenza type A. The appearance of a new subtype is termed *antigenic shift*. Antigenic drift and shift have profound epidemiologic implications as will be considered below.

## NOMENCLATURE

In recognition of the vast array of antigenic variants, combinations of H and N subtypes, and hosts of origin, a World Health Organization committee has devised a systematic classification for influenza viruses. The schema includes *(1) the type; (2) the host species, if not human; (3) geographic origin; (4) strain number for the year; and (5) year of isolation (H and N subtype, if type A)*. Consequently, the human isolate of the swinelike influenza virus was designated A/New Jersey/6/76 (H swine N1). One of the earliest swine isolates of influenza virus is designated A/swine/Wisconsin/15/30 (H swine N1). This nomenclature supercedes the old terminology of $A_0$, $A_1$, and $A_2$, which ignored the independent variation of the H and N proteins. The influenza A subtypes that have circulated since the first human isolation in 1933 by Smith, Laidlaw, and Andrewes are indicated in Table 2. In addition, over two dozen different subtype combinations have been recognized in swine, horses, and fowl.

## PATHOGENESIS AND CLINICAL MANIFESTATIONS

Deposition of droplet nuclei containing influenza virus on almost any portion of the respiratory epithelium can initiate infection. Virus shedding precedes symptoms, which are first noticed one to three days after exposure. Typical symptoms are sneezing, chills, fever, headache, myalgia, nasal obstruction and discharge, sore throat, and nonproductive cough. These symptoms usually subside in two to four days with little residual after a week. Coincident with the onset of symptoms the ciliated epithelium desquamates. Symptoms and local pathology usually lag out of phase with virus shedding, which is usually rapidly diminishing within a day of the onset of symptoms. The involved epithelium regenerates, passing through a series of stages from a transitional basal layer, to stratified squamous to hyperplastic cuboidal until the normal ciliated columnar epithelium is reestablished in one to two weeks.

The pneumonia that can occur in the course of influenza infection can be viral, secondary bacterial, or a mixture of the two. Pure viral pneumonia causes focal alveolar exudation, denuded alveolar walls, capillary thrombosis, and necrosis. The increased susceptibility of lungs infected with influenza virus to secondary bacterial invasion has been well documented and is attributed to loss of ciliary clearance, a rich bacterial growth medium in the alveolar exudate, and injury to leukocytes by influenza. *Staphylococcus aureus*, *Streptococcus pneumoniae*, and *Haemophilus influenzae* are the most frequent secondary pathogens. The bacterial infection may often be difficult to distinguish from the viral on clinical grounds. The course may be biphasic with an interval of partial recovery between the viral syndrome and the bacterial pneumonia, or it may present as a bacterial pneumonia with only epidemiologic, serologic, or cultural evidence to indicate viral infection.

Severe myalgia is common in influenza, and serum creatinine phosphokinase is often elevated. The pathogenesis of this myalgia, which can be severe enough to cause myoglobinuria and renal failure, has not been elucidated. Myocarditis and encephalitis have also been associated with epidemic influenza. In addition, Reye described a syndrome in 1963 of hepatic failure and encephalopathy in children shortly after one of several viral infections—including influenza A on occasion, but most frequently type B. In spite of sporadic claims of virus isolation from blood, there has been as yet no systematic documentation of extrarespiratory viral infection in humans with influenza.

It is important to note that only one half of infected individuals, as determined by antibody responses or viral isolation, develop clinical disease. It is not clear to what extent site of inoculation, inoculum size, and host susceptibility factors contribute to disease severity. Nevertheless, the frequency of lethal complications is significantly increased at the extremes of age, in pregnancy, and by underlying cardiopulmonary disease such as mitral stenosis or emphysema.

## IMMUNITY

Antibody to the H and N prevents reinfection or modifies the severity of the disease. HI antibody plays the major role, although NI antibody alone in high titer can also prevent disease. Protection is correlated with both serum antibodies and IgA secretory antibodies in the respiratory tract. At the same level of serum HI antibody, live respiratory infection provides the greatest degree of protection. Active parenteral immunization with killed virus provides less protection, and passive parenteral immunization provides the least protection of the three methods. Multiple factors are thus important in immunity. The relative contributions of serum antibody, secretory antibody, cell-mediated immunity, and other undefined mechanisms are unknown.

Immunity to a newly emerged antigenic variant is a function both of the degree of immunity to the previously circulating variant and the antigenic relatedness of the two strains. The three types of influenza share no antigenic relatedness and thus induce no cross-protection. Cross-protection becomes more complicated within a type, however. Thus, with a minor antigenic drift a person with immunity sufficient for full protection against the older strain might develop a subclinical infection or mild disease with the newer strain; a person with partial protection against the older strain might develop full-fledged influenza with the newer strain. Antibody levels correlate with protection on a statistical basis in a population, but not with the severity of individual responses to virus infection, which exhibit tremendous variation, in keeping with the multifactorial basis of resistance, including perhaps, nonimmune factors in disease response such as genetics and nutrition. The multiple infections a population experiences with influenza viruses that possess varying antigenic coats often make vaccine studies or immunodiagnosis insecure and difficult to interpret. Many interesting phenomena have been recognized, including cross-reactive and non–cross-reactive antigenic sites on the H and N proteins, and *original antigenic sin,* a term referring to the stronger memory for and the increased responsiveness to the influenza antigen to which an individual was first exposed.

Induction of immunity against mankind's last great infectious plague is a prime goal of modern medicine. Intramuscular injection of the standard vaccine, composed of inactivated egg-grown virus protects 70 per cent of adults against infection with an antigenically identical strain. Children respond with less antibody and more adverse effects to killed vaccine than do adults. With current purification of inactivated vaccine, adverse effects appear to correlate directly with the dose of virion components.

One contribution to influenza vaccine production has been Kilbourne's proposal to recombine high yielding egg-adapted laboratory strains of influenza with each newly circulating epidemic virus. Recombinants possessing the new surface antigens and the high yield growth characteristics have cut cost and increased speed of production of killed vaccines. Nevertheless, the relative inefficacy of the inactivated influenza vaccine, when compared with polio or measles virus vaccines, for example, demands improvement. Among new approaches to immunoprophylaxis is the use of purified glycoprotein subunits. Another proposal is to immunize against the currently circulating N antigen in order to permit a subclinical infection with the circulating strain that would give the complete protection of live virus infection via the respiratory route.

Three approaches to live attenuated vaccine have been pursued. One approach proposed recombination between an older strain attenuated by multiple passages in eggs and an antigenically new epidemic strain. Unfortunately, the recombinants with the new antigens appear to have unpredictable levels of attenuation. A second method that may be combined with the first method selects for mutants that are resistant to nonspecific inhibitors to the H3 hemagglutinin that are present in guinea pig or horse serum, and that, for some reason, correspond to reduced pathogenicity for man.

Chanock has proposed the use of a master strain of donor virus that contains temperature-sensitive mutations that specify a desired level of attenuation and that are not located on the gene segments corresponding to the H and N. An attenuating gene could also be derived from an animal influenza A virus that is not virulent for man. By reassortment, a specified level of attenuation could then be transferred by a rapid, single-step process to a virus containing the prevalent antigens. The precise genetic composition of the recombinant with regard to contribution from the two parental strains can now be ascertained with high resolution electrophoretic or hybridization techniques. The efficacy, safety, and feasibility of producing a live attenuated vaccine virus with the glycoproteins of the most recent strain are being actively investigated.

## LABORATORY DIAGNOSIS

Because the clinical characteristics of viral respiratory syndromes can be produced by dozens of different agents, the diagnosis of influenza requires isolation of the virus from the patient, identification of specific viral antigens in a patient's tissue, or documentation of a specific serologic response by the patient. The standard technique for influenza virus isolation is growth in embryonated hen's eggs after allantoic or amniotic inoculation. Types A and B virus can also be isolated in primary kidney cell cultures, especially those from human embryos and rhesus monkeys. With the diminishing availability of these sources of primary kidney tissue, a reliable tissue culture substrate that can be propagated continuously has been seriously needed. Laboratory strains of virus have been adapted to continuous cell lines; however, as is common with many viruses, the growth requirements of primary isolates are often fastidious. The Madin Darby canine kidney cell line along with trypsin in the culture medium to cleave and activate the H glycoprotein now appears to be a readily available continuous cell line that is as sensitive as eggs or primary kidney cell cultures for the isolation of influenza viruses.

The best specimens for isolation are nasal washings obtained within the first few days of the onset of symptoms. The presence of virus in allantoic or tissue culture fluid is identified by hemagglutinating activity. The viral antigens can then be determined with known antisera in an HI test. Alternatively, known infected tissue culture monolayers can be identified by the hemadsorption of erythrocytes and the antigenic specificity of the agent can be determined by inhibiting the hemadsorption reaction with specific antisera. More recently, specific fluorescent antibody straining has been used to identify infected tissue culture.

The fluorescent antibody method is also showing great promise in the rapid and specific identification of viral antigens in exfoliated nasopharyngeal cells or in expectorated sputum. Caution is warranted, however, because nonspecific staining can lead to false positive diagnoses unless great care has been observed in the preparation of the specific antibody conjugates and in the antigen and serum controls.

Although a fourfold rise in a virus-specific antibody has been used as a diagnostic standard of infection, this approach contains many pitfalls, especially for influenza virus infections. Any of the various influenza antibody measurements available may not reveal a rise in titer in some individuals with documented infection. Consequently, the failure to demonstrate an immune response by using appropriate acute and convalescent sera and a single reliable assay like the HI test does not exclude the diagnosis of influenza.

The complement-fixation test measures antibody to the RNP and M proteins. This antibody usually falls to undetectable levels over a period of months so that an elevated convalescent serum complement-fixation titer has been considered indicative of a recent infection. Unfortunately, children, especially upon primary exposure, usually develop little or no complement-fixing antibody. With repeated influenza exposure this antibody response increases both in magnitude and duration so that elderly adults will often sustain elevated complement-fixation antibody levels for years.

The HI antibody response is generally considered the most reliable serologic indicator of infection. Caution is warranted, however, in using the HI antibody response to determine the antigenic identity of the infecting influenza virus because of the possibility of minor antigenic cross-reactions between sub-types and the existence of immune responses to unrelated subtype antigens based on the phenomenon of original antigenic sin. Consequently, knowledge of the antigenic composition of the prevalent viruses and use of potentially cross-reacting antigens as controls are helpful when performing and interpreting HI tests. Additional and potentially more rapid or less complicated methods, such as radial hemolysis, radial immunodiffusion, radioimmunoassay, indirect immunofluorescence, and immunoenzymatic assays, are continually under investigation.

## EPIDEMIOLOGY

Although structurally similar, the three influenza types vary immensely in epidemiologic impact. Influenza C causes sporadic infections with mild upper respiratory tract disease; it does not cause epidemic influenza. Influenza B causes epidemics and can produce serious pneumonitis in adults. More importantly, it is associated with Reye syndrome in children and is responsible for pneumonitis and croup in infants. The notoriety of influenza A stems from its capacity to produce pandemics.

Because numerous agents can cause similar syndromes, influenza must be detected either by laboratory surveillance for virus isolates and seroconversions, by absenteeism associated with respiratory symptoms, or by excess pneumonia and mortality. By comparing the number of deaths or cases of pneumonia in a selected population with the baseline levels for previous years, the magnitude of the excess can be calculated. This measurement correlates well with the circulation of influenza in the population. Infants, the elderly, and those with underlying cardiopulmonary impairment are most susceptible to the complications of influenza.

The incidence of influenza peaks in the winter months. In tropical climates influenza remains an important disease, but it tends to occur over longer periods with dampened epidemic peaks. The mechanism of "overwintering" — that is, the maintenance of the agent in the population between epidemics has not been completely determined; nevertheless, surveillance of large populations during the summer indicates that the virus remains endemic in the population with sporadic infrequent isolates and subconversions often associated with subclinical infection.

Influenza infection usually induces protective immunity to rechallenge with the homologous virus. The periodic recurrence of influenza in populations with previous experience with the virus results from the capacity of influenza virus to change surface antigens. Both in vitro and in vivo, the presence of partially protective levels of antibody gives a selective advantage to viruses with surface antigens that react less avidly with the antibody. Since a majority of the population develops protective immunity to the circulating influenza strain, an *antigenic drift* occurs in either or in both of the surface antigens, resulting in a relatively more susceptible population. Peptide analysis ("fingerprinting") of the hemagglutinin polypeptide reveals that one or a few amino acid substitutions are responsible for an antigenic drift. Thus, antibody pressure provides a selective advantage for the growth of certain missense mutants.

Although all three types of influenza virus exhibit antigenic drift, influenza A is the most virulent and influenza C the least virulent at given levels of immunity in the population. The progressively increasing sensitivity of the replication of types A, B, and then C to temperatures above body temperature has been proposed as an explanation for the observed gradient in virulence. Regardless of the intrinsic virulence of the different types, one additional property provides influenza A with the capacity to produce pandemic disease. Every 10 to 30 years, one or both of the surface antigens of influenza A changes subtype, rendering a previously immune population completely susceptible. This *antigenic shift* is qualitative rather than the quantitative one characteristic of antigenic drift. Rather than a limited amino acid change typical of antigenic drift, a new subtype polypeptide shows little resemblance to its predecessor on peptide mapping. An accumulating body of circumstantial evidence suggests that antigenic shifts occur as a consequence either of rapid adaptation to man by an animal influenza A virus or of genetic reassortment during coinfection with influenza A viruses derived from man and animal.

Influenza A occurs in animals and man, whereas types B and C appear to be restricted to man. The influenza A strains circulating in animals may provide a source of new antigenic subtypes for human influenza A viruses, thus accounting for antigenic shift. Experimental studies with pigs and turkeys have demonstrated that genetic reassortment occurs in vivo after coinfection with two viruses (Fig. 3). Moreover, the selection of particular combinations of antigenic subtypes can be manipulated by adjusting the preinfection antibody levels present in the animal. These recombinants are then transmissible. One species can transmit its influenza A virus to susceptible members of another species. The phenomenon of influenza virus infection with virus from another host species has been well described on swine farms with the exchange going in either direction between man and pig. Such exchange has also been observed on several occasions between migratory and domestic fowl.

Various combinations of H and N subtypes have been described, suggesting reassortment and interchange. For example, the N1 has been associated with the H0, H1, Hswine, Havian 1, Havian 5, and Havian 6 subtypes. In addition, the human H2 and H3 have been shown by Webster and Laver not only to be antigenically related to several avian and equine subtypes, but to be remarkably similar in their peptide fingerprints to the antigenically related animal hemagglutinins.

Although the first subtype of influenza virus (H0N1) was isolated in 1933, the period of circulation and the antigenic specificity of the three previous subtypes have been deduced with a technique termed *immunologic recapitulation,* by which HI titers against numerous H subtypes are determined in numerous age cohorts. These studies demonstrate that HI antibody to Hswine not based on cross-reaction is present in almost every-

one born before 1918 and disappears in people born after 1927. Thus the 1918–1919 pandemic has been attributed to the Hswine subtype of influenza. This process of immunologic recapitulation indicates that the 1890 epidemic was probably caused by the H3 or related Hequine2 subtypes, and the 1877 pandemic by the H2 subtype. The accumulation of such circumstantial evidence supports the currently accepted working hypothesis that there are a finite number of subtype antigens that recirculate, probably by means of infrequent exchange, between human and animal species.

# PARAMYXOVIRUSES

### CLASSIFICATION

The paramyxoviruses are enveloped, single-stranded, RNA viruses that are transmitted via the respiratory route. They are among the most important respiratory viruses of infants (respiratory syncytial virus and the parainfluenza viruses) and two of the most important contagious diseases of childhood (measles and mumps). Properties of these viruses are delineated in Table 1. The family *Paramyxoviridae* has been divided into three genera. The genus *Paramyxovirus* includes parainfluenza virus types 1, 2, 3, 4a, 4b, and mumps virus. These viruses possess two surface glycoproteins, one with both hemagglutinating and neuramidinase enzyme activities and one with cell fusion and hemolysin activities. These viruses are all antigenically related. Sendai virus (mouse parainfluenza virus type 1), simian virus 5, and Newcastle disease virus of fowl belong to this genus. The genus *Morbillivirus* includes measles, canine distemper, and bovine rinderpest viruses, which are antigenically related, but do not cross-react immunologically with paramyxoviruses of the other two genera. These viruses lack neuramidinase activity and they hemagglutinate only red blood cells of old world monkeys. The genus *Pneumovirus* includes respiratory syncytial virus (RSV) and pneumonia virus of mice. These agents have a smaller nucleocapsid and lack the hemagglutinating, neuramidinase, and hemolysin activities characteristic of the surface glycoproteins of the members of the other two genera.

### STRUCTURE

The most complete biophysical, biochemical, and genetic information regarding the paramyx-

oviruses has been derived from the following animal agents: Sendai virus, simian virus 5, and Newcastle disease virus. Information regarding the human agents will be specified only when it is known and distinctive. *Paramyxovirus* virions are usually spheroids 150 to 250 nm in diameter, although preparations often show variant forms with dimensions ranging from 100 to 700 nm. These virions have a buoyant density of 1.19 to 1.22 $g/cm^3$ and a sedimentation coefficient of 1000 to 1100S. Their genetic material is a linear, single-stranded RNA molecule that has a sedimentation coefficient of 50 to 57S and weighs approximately $6 \times 10^6$ daltons. This RNA represents 0.91 per cent of the total virion weight. The remainder of the virion is composed of 73 per cent protein, 20 per cent lipids, and 6 per cent carbohydrate.

This RNA genome has a coding capacity for one or two more proteins than the slightly smaller influenza virus genome, which codes for seven structural and one nonstructural protein. The protein number and function of the paramyxoviruses have not yet been completely defined. The RNA is surrounded by a helical array of nucleocapsid protein resulting in a ribonucleoprotein structure 18 nm in diameter with a central core 5 nm in diameter (Fig. 2). This structure has a buoyant density of 1.27 to 1.31 $c/cm^3$ and a length of 1 $\mu$m. Associated with the nucleocapsid is the RNA transcriptase, which synthesizes viral messenger RNA with the virion RNA serving as template and host cell providing synthetic machinery and energy. This, the paramyxoviruses, like the influenza viruses, are (−) strand RNA viruses. The ribonucleoprotein is enclosed in an envelope composed of a layer of membrane or matrix (M) protein that underlies the lipid bilayer derived from the host cell during the budding process.

Attached to the envelope are projections consisting of two different glycoproteins, the activities of which distinguish the three genera of the paramyxovirus family. The parainfluenza and mumps viruses possess a glycoprotein (HN) with both hemagglutinin (H) and neuramidinase (N) activities and a glycoprotein (F) with both membrane fusion and hemolysin activities. The HN protein alone presumably serves the two functions of host cell attachment and release served by the two glycoproteins (H and N) of the influenza viruses. As in the case of the influenza viruses, $N$-acetylneuraminic acid present in host cell and red blood cell membranes serves as the receptor and the substrate for the HN activities. This glycoprotein has a molecular weight of 67,000. The F glycoprotein is derived from a precursor polypeptide ($F_o$) with a molecular weight of 65,000. The proteolytic cleavage of an 8000 to 10,000 dalton polypeptide is required to convert the $F_o$ to F and activate the fusion and hemolytic functions. This renders the virion infectious. The cleavage step is accomplished by a host cell protease and that represents one, if not the major, determinant of cell permissiveness in vitro. This host cell characteristic may also represent a critical factor in host range and in tissue tropism in vivo.

Measles virus possesses a similar F glycoprotein; however, the second glycoprotein does not contain the HN activities. Measles virus does, however, agglutinate old world monkey red blood cells. This characteristic has some diagnostic utility, but presumably has no biologic relevance. This glycoprotein is responsible for host cell attachment although the receptor site is not $N$-acetylneuraminic acid. Antibody to this glycoprotein neutralizes measles virus. The glycoproteins of respiratory syncytial virus presumably contribute to host cell attachment and release, but the activities of these proteins have not been delineated.

The replication of the paramyxoviruses is unaffected by inhibitors of cellular DNA synthesis such as actinomycin D or by irradiation or enucleation of the host cell. This requirement only for intact host cell cytoplasmic synthetic machinery is another characteristic that distinguishes the paramyxoviruses from the orthomyxoviruses; however, in other respects, the synthesis and assembly of the virion components closely resemble that of the influenza viruses (Choppin and Compans, 1975). The only recognized difference is the requirement of the orthomyxoviruses to assemble multiple, different ribonucleoprotein structures rather than a large single ribonucleoprotein structure into a virion.

## ANTIGENIC COMPOSITION

### Parainfluenza Viruses and Mumps Virus

There are four serotypes of the human parainfluenza viruses, which are distinct by neutralizing, hemagglutination inhibiting (HI), and complement-fixing antibody (CF) assays. Types 1, 2, and 3 are each antigenically homogeneous and stable as is mumps virus. Type 4 is composed of two subtypes, 4a and 4b, which are distinguishable by neutralization and HI, but not by CF. Antibody to the HN protein has both neutralizing and HI activity. The presence and function of antibody to the F glycoprotein has not been evaluated. CF utilizes the soluble (S) antigen associated with the nucleocapsid. Although these antigens are distinct for each type, hyperimmunization will stimulate cross-reactive antibody to the other types, to mumps virus, and to Newcastle disease virus. This phenomenon occurs with neutralizing, HI, and CF antibody responses. Humans are exposed to most of these agents during childhood and are repeatedly infected with the parainfluenza viruses; this accounts for the heterotypic antibody responses to infection often observed in humans, especially in older people.

### Measles Virus

Measles virus is antigenically homogeneous and stable. It is antigenically related to distemper and rinderpest viruses. CF antibody is detected by utilizing the nucleocapsid protein (soluble [S] antigen). Neutralizing and HI antibody is directed against the monkey red cell hemagglutinating protein. Antibody to the fusion-hemolysin has been rarely studied except in relation to vaccine responses.

### Respiratory Syncytial Virus

Several minor antigenic variants have been detected by neutralization tests with early postinfection sera; however, convalescent human sera appear to be unable to make this distinction. This antigenic variation has no known biologic significance. Analogous to the other paramyxoviruses, CF and neutralizing antibodies can be measured; however, HI is obviously not possible.

## SUSCEPTIBLE HOST CELLS

These agents all initiate their infections on the respiratory epithelium. The susceptibility of epithelial cells to these agents probably accounts for the value of primary human and primate kidney cell cultures for their laboratory isolation (Table 1). The respiratory pathogens (the parainfluenza viruses and RSV) are restricted to the respiratory tract. Measles and mumps disseminate from the respiratory tract via the bloodstream to various target organs as discussed below.

## PATHOGENIC PROPERTIES

All paramyxoviruses are transmitted by inhalation of droplet aerosols or by inoculation of respiratory secretions (by hand, for example) onto the respiratory mucosa. The nature of the resulting infection then depends both on host factors, such as age and immune status, and on the specific agent.

### Parainfluenza Viruses

The replication of these agents is restricted to the respiratory tract. No extrapulmonary replication has been well documented, although viremia has been reported. These agents cause only upper respiratory infections (the common cold syndrome) except in a proportion of infants who develop laryngotracheobronchitis (croup), bronchiolitis or pneumonitis during their primary infection.

### Mumps

Mumps infection causes parotitis after an incubation period of 15 to 18 days after exposure to an infected individual. The incubation period has been reported to range from the extremes of 7 to 23 days. Early in the incubation period, after replication in the respiratory epithelium, viremia disseminates virus throughout the body. Virus is usually detectable in blood, saliva, and parotid duct secretions for two to three days before onset of symptoms. The presence of virus in saliva before symptoms, the variable incubation period, and the numerous asymptomatic but still infectious cases, account for the difficulty in controlling transmission. Fever, malaise, myalgia, and coryza usually initiate the clinical disease. Parotitis usually follows within a day. Virus can be isolated from Stensen's duct or from the saliva for another five to seven days. Parotitis may be bilateral, unilateral, or absent. Other organs are involved, either singly or in a variety of combinations, even in the absence of parotitis. Most frequently recognized is infection of other salivary glands, testes, ovaries, pancreas, breasts, and meninges. Rare reports of thyroiditis and arthri-

tis need confirmation. Myocarditis has been documented but fetal mumps infection as a cause of endocardial fibroelastosis remains controversial. Mumps virus is shed in the urine for ten days or longer after the onset of symptoms, even in the absence of orchitis. In addition, hematuria, proteinuria, and a reversible reduction in creatinine clearance also suggest that nephritis may be common, although neither viral replication in the kidneys nor immune complex disease has been documented.

Mumps meningoencephalitis causes about 10 per cent of all cases of aseptic meningitis, and ranges in presentation from aseptic meningitis to encephalitis. The frequency of subclinical meningitis is unknown; however, an abnormal electroencephalogram (EEG) is uncommon with mumps parotitis in contrast to its frequency in uncomplicated measles. The cerebrospinal fluid in mumps meningitis tends to have lower sugars and higher polymorphonuclear leukocyte counts than in most other viral meningitides. Parotitis is absent in 25 to 50 per cent of cases of mumps meningoencephalitis, but when present, usually occurs three to ten days before CNS symptoms. Although parotitis occurs with equal frequency in both sexes, CNS mumps occurs three times more frequently in males. Sequelae are unusual after CNS mumps; the mortality from encephalitis is 1 per cent. Deafness due to auditory neuritis has been described, and may even occur without encephalitis.

### Measles

After replication in the respiratory mucosa, measles virus is transported to lymphoid tissues, where it multiplies further, and then spreads via the bloodstream in leukocytes. During this asymptomatic incubation period, cytolysis, tissue necrosis, and inflammation are not manifest; the only histologic sign of local replication is multinucleate giant cells with intranuclear inclusions (Warthin-Finkeldey cells). Just before or during the prodrome, these are seen in the lymph nodes, tonsils, appendix, and exfoliated nasal mucosa. The usual incubation period of 10 to 12 days terminates with the onset of coryza, conjunctivitis, dry cough, sore throat, lymphadenopathy, headache, fever, and Koplik's spots. Koplik's spots are tiny erythematous patches with bluish-white apices on the buccal mucosa along the molar bite line. These spots contain the giant cells with eosinophilic intranuclear inclusions that are composed of measles virus-specific proteins as determined by immunofluorescence and viral nucleocapsids as determined by electron microscopy. The exanthem usually appears on the second day, beginning on the head, then spreading to the trunk, and finally to the extremities. The incubation period is usually two to three days shorter when the usual respiratory portal of entry is bypassed by parenteral inoculation with either the wild-type virus experimentally or the live attenuated vaccine. The incubation period is prolonged up to 3 weeks, especially in older people or in recipients of measles antiglobulin.

During the prodrome, virus is present in tears, nasal secretions, throat, urine, and blood. The viremia disappears with the onset of the rash, which is followed within two to three days by the appearance of serum antibody. A causal relationship between the appearance of immunoglobulins and the onset of symptoms has been proposed. Although the cutaneous and upper respiratory involvement is most easily recognized, viremia carries the virus elsewhere throughout the body. Respiratory complications include otitis media, croup, and pneumonitis with or without secondary bacterial pneumonia. An acute abdomen, easily mistaken for appendicitis, may precede the exanthem. Myocarditis and thrombocytopenic purpura are other rare complications.

Although EEG aberrations are detectable in most patients with measles, clinically apparent encephalomyelitis occurs in only one of every 1000 cases. The encephalomyelitis results in a 15 per cent mortality and 25 per cent residual morbidity. Most cases of encephalitis occur on about day six and usually within two weeks of the onset of the rash. Despite its temporal relationship to the rash, the pathology in encephalitis differs from that in other organs, in that inclusion bodies and giant cells are not common. Instead, a perivascular mononuclear infiltrate, demyelination, petechial hemorrhages, and microglial proliferation are seen. The overall mortality from measles can approach 10 per cent in malnourished populations, primarily because of secondary bacterial pneumonia. Infants and the elderly are most susceptible and mortality in them may exceed 25 per cent. In affluent societies the mortality rate approximates 0.1 per cent.

Subacute sclerosing panencephalitis (SSPE) is a rare (1 per 100,000 cases) but intriguing expression of measles infection. It causes an insidious intellectual, behavioral, and motor deterioration, which progresses to convulsions, coma, and death usually within a year of onset. Victims of SSPE manifest a characteristic EEG pattern, markedly elevated serum and CSF measles antibodies, and typical histologic findings distinct from the acute encephalitis of measles. Measles antigen is readily demonstrable in SSPE brains, although virus isolation usually requires extensive effort, including cocultivation techniques. SSPE occurs with a median latent period of 7 years after typical measles in a typical child, but occurring at a younger age and in a more rural area than average. Immune defects and virus variants have been proposed to explain the pathogenesis of SSPE, but documentation for either proposal is inconclusive.

### Respiratory Syncytial Virus

The incubation period of RSV infection is four to five days. RSV replication appears to be restricted to the respiratory mucosa. It produces bronchiolitis, pneumonitis, and, less frequently, croup and apnea. These severe infections usually occur in children less than 6 months old who are experiencing their first RSV infection. The occurrence of severe RSV disease in the first 6 months, when maternal antibodies are still present, or in older children who have received inactivated vaccines suggests an immunopathologic basis. Occurrence of bronchiolitis during primary infection does not correlate with neutralizing or CF antibody levels of either the mother or the infant.

### *IMMUNITY*

### Parainfluenza Viruses

Severe life-threatening infection occurs in infants experiencing their first infection. IgA-neutralizing antibody appears in the nasal secretions after infection. The presence of this secretory antibody correlates well with protection from reinfection but it disappears in one to six months, leaving the child susceptible to reinfection despite substantial levels of serum neutralizing antibody. Past experience with the virus, however, does provide some protection; repeat infections are limited to the upper respiratory tract.

Life-threatening bronchiolitis and pneumonitis due to parainfluenza type 3, as with RSV, occur in infants, many of whom have maternally derived serum antibody. In contrast to RSV, administration of an inactivated vaccine (in one study) did not predispose to more severe disease, although it also failed to provide protection. In contrast to both parainfluenza type 3 and RSV, maternal antibody seems to give some protection from types 1 and 2 infection to infants in their first 4 months. Croup is seen after infection by these two viruses in some infants but also occurs in primary infection of older children.

### Mumps Virus

CF antibody to the nucleocapsid protein (S antigen) is usually apparent at 1 week and peaks at 2 weeks postinfection; it is thus useful for laboratory diagnosis of recent infection. Antibody to the hemagglutinin glycoprotein (V antigen), as measured by hemagglutination inhibition or neutralization of viral infectivity, appears at two to three weeks and peaks at three to four weeks. This antibody is the best indicator of immunity because it is neutralizing antibody and because it is measurable for much longer than CF antibody. Reinfection is extremely rare; however, because asymptomatic infections are common and because other viruses may also cause parotitis, neither a history of parotitis nor its absence is useful in determining previous experience with mumps virus. In addition to mumps virus, parainfluenza viruses, enteroviruses, and influenza A virus have all been implicated as etiologic agents of parotitis.

The live attenuated mumps vaccine is grown in chick embryo cells. The vaccine causes an inapparent infection, seroconversion, and protection from mumps infection in over 95 per cent of seronegative recipients. The vaccine, which is inoculated subcutaneously, stimulates all commonly measured antibody responses but with lower mean titers than does natural infection. This vaccine does not produce detectable virus in saliva, viremia, viruria, or spread to contacts; however, vaccine virus has been isolated from an aborted placenta 10 days postinoculation of the mother. The vaccine was licensed in the United States in 1967, too recent for the long-term duration of immunity to be determined. However, studies to date are very encouraging. Killed mumps vaccines have been shown to protect only for short durations. The efficacy of passive immunization with convalescent serum or pooled γ-globulins has not been demonstrated.

### Measles

Infection confers lifelong protection. The presence of CF, HI, or neutralizing antibody indicates immunity. Passive immunization with pooled IgG is usually effective if given within 1 week of exposure. It is indicated for pregnant women, neonates, and immunosuppressed patients who are exposed and susceptible. Although it prevents reinfection, serum antibody does not appear to be essential for recovery from primary infection or even constitute the sole defense against reinfection because immunoglobulin-deficient patients resolve a measles infection normally and they resist reinfection. In contrast, patients with defective cellular immunity suffer serious complications of measles infection. Enders demonstrated that the syndrome of giant cell pneumonia without the usual morbilliform rash was a consequence of measles infection in such patients.

*Modified measles* is an abbreviated and milder form of ordinary measles, often with a prolonged incubation period. Modified measles is seen in children passively immunized with prophylactic IgG or with transplacental IgG. *Atypical measles* results from infection with either wild type or vaccine measles virus at least 2 years after immunization with formalin-inactivated measles vaccine. It is characterized by fever, pneumonitis, pleural effusion, edema of extremities, and an atypical rash. The rash has a predilection for the extremities and tends to be discrete, often with an urticarial, petechial, or vesicular component in contrast to the typical blanching, erythematous, maculopapular, morbilliform rash of ordinary measles. Norrby has proposed that atypical measles infection is a consequence of the inability of the killed vaccine to stimulate antibody to the F (hemolysin-fusion) protein as does natural or live attenuated vaccine infection.

The live attenuated vaccine, grown in chick embryo fibroblasts at reduced temperature, has supplanted the killed vaccine. The live vaccine is >95 per cent effective. Failures have been attributed to vaccine inactivation and to administration to infants with residual transplacental immunity, usually in infants less than 1 year old. Ten per cent of vaccine recipients have a fever or a mild rash 10 days postinoculation. There is little, if any, vaccine virus excretion and no transmission has been documented. Mean antibody titers tend to be lower after vaccination than with natural infection; however, many vaccinees subsequently exposed to measles appear to have asymptomatic antibody boosts. The measles vaccine is administered in one dose subcutaneously. It can be given in combination with the mumps and rubella live attenuated vaccines with no apparent reduction in the efficacy of any of the three components.

### Respiratory Syncytial Virus

Newborns enjoy relative freedom from infection for two to four weeks, perhaps because exposure is limited or immunity is passed from the mother. For the next six months, with a peak in month two, susceptibility to life-threatening infection increases with no clear relation to levels of passively acquired antibody. Active immunity from primary infection does not prevent reinfection during epidemics, but reinfections are limited to the upper respiratory tract. The role of the secretory immune system has not been evaluated in infants. Adults are all seropositive, and elevated neutralizing antibody in their nasal secretions is correlated with resistance to infection.

Formalin-inactivated virus not only fails to

protect, but places children as old as two years at risk for life-threatening bronchiolitis, a syndrome usually not seen after the sixth month in unimmunized children. Temperature-sensitive mutants of respiratory syncytial virus are being evaluated in the hope of developing an attenuated, live virus vaccine.

## LABORATORY DIAGNOSIS

### Parainfluenza Viruses

When respiratory tissue or secretions are inoculated into cell cultures, the presence of parainfluenza virus may be recognized by cell death or syncytium formation; however, hemadsorption or specific immunofluorescence is more sensitive because isolates in early passage may produce little or no visible cell injury. The parainfluenza virus isolate can be typed by hemadsorption inhibition with type-specific antiserum, by HI or CF characterization of progeny virus from the tissue culture supernatant, or by immunofluorescence of infected tissue culture cells. Rapid diagnosis by identification of specific viral antigen by immunofluorescence in exfoliated nasopharyngeal cells is possible; however, highly specific immune reagents and appropriate controls are required. Persistent infection with simian virus 5 (related to type 2) in simian cell cultures, and of that virus or Sendai virus (related to type 1) in rodent cultures is a common source of error. Primary human embryonic or simian kidney cell cultures are the most sensitive cell lines for isolation of human parainfluenza viruses; HeLa, HEp2, and WI-38 cell lines are also effective for types 2 and 3. Recently a continuous monkey kidney cell line, LLC-MK2, along with trypsin in the culture medium to cleave and activate the F glycoprotein, has been shown to be a sensitive line for the isolation and propagation of parainfluenza viruses. CF antibody responses may not occur in mild disease; consequently, the neutralization or HI tests are more sensitive. In addition, cross-reactive rises in antibody to different types may occur in reinfection.

### Mumps

Although the typical syndrome of parotitis has also been attributed to parainfluenza viruses, coxsackieviruses, and influenza A virus, laboratory diagnosis is indicated when complications occur. Virus can be isolated in the first few days of illness from saliva, parotid duct secretions, urine, or cerebrospinal fluid if meningitis is present. Viruria may persist for over two weeks. Although the virus was originally isolated by inoculation into the amniotic cavity of eight day old embryonated chicken eggs, primary or continuous human and primate cell lines are more sensitive. Cell rounding and syncytia are seen in infected cell monolayers, but hemadsorption and immunofluorescence are more sensitive indicators of infection. Prompt inoculation of a specimen is important because mumps virus infectivity is unstable both at room temperature and at 4° C. As discussed in the section on immunity, the CF antibody response is more prompt but less durable than the HI and neutralization response.

### Measles

Measles usually produces a distinct syndrome even when the typical exanthem cannot be easily recognized — for example, in dark-skinned people. Confirmation is indicated in the atypical or complicated case and can be accomplished by isolation of virus from respiratory secretions, blood, or urine with embryonated eggs or cell culture. The virus is excreted in the respiratory secretions, tears, and urine during the prodrome and for about two days after the appearance of the rash. The virus is also present in blood leukocytes, lymph nodes, spleen, kidney, skin, and lungs. Measles isolation in cell culture, first described by Enders and Peebles in 1954, provided the technology for the most sensitive isolation technique, and thus enabled us to obtain the data that underlie our current concepts of measles immunology, pathogenesis, and epidemiology. Primary human embryo or rhesus monkey kidney cell cultures are the most sensitive; cytopathic effects become apparent in one to two weeks. Isolation may require holding cell cultures for a month with "blind" passaging to permit adaptation of the isolate to cell culture. The classic cytopathology — multinucleate giant cells and intranuclear inclusions — may be apparent only with passaging. Earlier detection of infected cell cultures is possible with specific immunofluorescence or hemadsorption with monkey erythrocytes.

### Respiratory Syncytial Virus

RSV can be isolated from the respiratory secretions by using susceptible host cell cultures, such as primary monkey or bovine kidney, HeLa, HEp-2, or WI-38. Syncytia and eosinophilic cytoplasmic inclusions are produced, but specific confirmation is accomplished by CF of progeny virus or by immunofluorescence of infected cells. Immunofluorescence of exfoliated respiratory epithelial cells is an effective method for the rapid diagnosis of RSV infection. Because RSV is an extremely labile virus, isolation is maximized by collecting good quantities of respiratory secretions — for example, nasopharyngeal washings rather than swabs, and by promptly inoculating cell cultures without prior storage of the specimen. Infants suffering primary infection may shed virus for four to six weeks, even after apparent recovery.

CF is the most readily available and least cumbersome serologic test. However, the neutralization test is more sensitive, with plaque reduction being slightly more sensitive than end-point neutralization of cytopathic effect.

## *EPIDEMIOLOGY*

### Parainfluenza

As with most respiratory agents, the risk of infection increases in those with contact with young children. Thus, high risk situations include large families, child care centers, schools, and pediatric wards of hospitals. Type 3 is the most prevalent of the parainfluenza types. Fifty per cent of children have serologic evidence of infection during their first year and 95 per cent by age six. Type 3 infections occur endemically throughout the year, whereas type 1 and, to a lesser extent, type 2 occur in epidemics during the fall or winter, often in a biannual pattern. Only respiratory syncytial virus exceeds type 3 in frequency as a cause of bronchiolitis and pneumonitis in infants. Type 1 and, to a lesser extent, type 2 are largely responsible for croup (acute laryngo-tracheobronchitis) in infants.

### Mumps

Mumps is not as contagious as measles or varicella; consequently, there is a fair proportion of seronegative young adults, perhaps 10 per cent. This percentage is increased in isolated areas; for example, more than 80 per cent of certain populations of Alaskan Eskimos may be seronegative. Infection is endemic throughout the year with a peak in the late winter and early spring in nontropical climates. Epidemics occur in congregations of children and young adults, especially schools and military situations.

The incidence of encephalitis is 2.5 per 1000 cases of reported mumps; the incidence of fatal mumps is approximately 0.25 cases per 1000 cases of reported mumps. Mumps infections are probably underreported, however, because approximately one third of all infections are subclinical. The age incidence of encephalitis correlates well with the age incidence of parotitis; however, fatalities are disproportionately increased in infants and older adults.

### Measles

Measles represents an ideal subject for epidemiologic study because it is highly contagious, there is a low proportion of subclinical infection, infection confers immunity to reinfection, and there is no evidence to suggest that the virus is heterogeneous with regard to either antigens or virulence. There is no apparent animal reservoir; thus, maintenance requires transmission to susceptible, nonimmune people. Consequently, the virus is best maintained in populous, developing areas, where annual late winter and early spring epidemics are seen, with cases detectable throughout the year. Epidemics occur with lower attack rates and at longer intervals in less populous and more economically developed areas. The virus disappears periodically from sparsely populated and isolated areas, which are subject to outbreaks when the virus is reintroduced from the outside after a critical number of nonimmune individuals have accumulated.

Measles is usually contracted by preschool children in populous, developing areas. In developed countries the disease is most common in elementary school children. In a remote Eskimo village, measles occurs at the age at which the virus is introduced from the outside. Thus, before measles vaccine, children rarely reached adulthood without measles infection except in remote and sparsely populated areas. Since the introduction of measles vaccine — in the United States, for example — the incidence of measles has diminished to 1 per cent of its previous incidence and the disease is occurring in somewhat older individuals. Infection is occurring in older individuals because unvaccinated children tend to be older and because there are fewer susceptibles to maintain annual epidemics.

### Respiratory Syncytial Virus

RSV consistently produces annual winter epidemics between January and March in temperate climates in the northern hemisphere. Epidemics during the rainy summer season have been described in Trinidad. These epidemics attack approximately one third of seronegative children, so that by age five, 95 per cent of children are seropositive. The mechanism of "overwintering," the maintenance of the virus between epidemics, is an enigma. Low rates of endemic infection between epidemics have not been documented as has been done with influenza. In primary infection, viral excretion often persists for one or two months after the resolution of symptoms; however, prolonged excretion after reinfection of either children or adults has not been documented. Reinfection occurs in as many as 20 per cent of children and adolescents annually, diminishing to an annual rate of 3 to 5 per cent in adults. The highest risk of infection occurs in nurseries, institutions, and pediatric wards of hospitals where there are high concentrations of infants.

## References

Stuart-Harris, C. H., and Schild, G. C.: Influenza: The Viruses and the Disease. Littleton, Massachusetts, Publishing Sciences Group, 1976.

Kilbourne, E. D. (ed.): The Influenza Viruses and Influenza. New York, Academic Press, 1975.

Kaplan, M. M., and Webster, R. G.: The epidemiology of influenza. Sci Am 237:88, 1977.

Choppin, P. W., and Compans, R. W.: Reproduction of paramyxoviruses. In Fraenkel-Conrat, H., and Wagner, R. R. (eds.): Comprehensive Virology. New York, Plenum Publishing Corp., p. 95, 1975.

Evans, A. S. (ed.): Viral Infections of Humans, Epidemiology and Control. New York, Plenum Medical Book Company, 1976.

# PICORNAVIRUSES 60

## Nathaniel A. Young, M.D.

### PHYSICAL STRUCTURE AND BIOCHEMICAL PROPERTIES

Picornaviridae is a large family of animal viruses named for their diminutive size, 20 to 30 nm, and nucleic acid type, RNA (Cooper et al., 1978). Picornavirus particles (virions) are icosahedral and consist of two structural moieties: (1) an outer protein shell, or capsid, comprising 70 per cent of the mass, and (2) an inner strand of RNA, which is 30 per cent of the mass. Lacking a lipid envelope, the "naked" virions are not affected by ether, alcohol, or other lipid solvents, although they are readily inactivated by phenol, formaldehyde, or ionizing radiation, which damages the capsid or the enclosed nucleic acid.

The capsid consists of 60 identical subunits, or capsomeres, which are synthesized from equimolar amounts of four different virion polypeptide chains, VP1–4. Three of these polypeptides are large (molecular mass 20,000 to 40,000 daltons, depending on the polypeptide and the particular picornavirus), and the fourth is small (5000 to 10,000 daltons). The capsid not only protects the enclosed viral genetic apparatus but also specifies which cells the virus can infect, since attachment of virus to specific receptors on the cell surface is a consequence of the chemical structure and surface configuration of the capsomeres. This "lock and key" fit of viruses with receptors is probably responsible for the host and tissue tropisms of individual picornaviruses.

The RNA of picornaviruses is linear, single-stranded, and nonsegmented, and has a molecular mass of 2.6 million daltons. After virions adsorb to susceptible cells, the RNA is uncoated and released into the cytoplasm, where it serves as a template for the synthesis of additional RNA. Newly synthesized RNA in turn may be either translated into viral proteins or encapsidated to form progeny virions. A distinctive feature of picornavirus RNA is its function as a monocistronic messenger; protein synthesis on the polyribosome is initiated at a single point on the RNA, from which the entire genome is translated into one large "polyprotein" of molecular mass greater than 200,000 daltons. Nascent chains of the polyprotein are then enzymatically cleaved to form individual polypeptides (Jacobson and Baltimore, 1968).

Also encoded by the viral genome are other noncapsid polypeptides. These include (1) enzyme(s), which catalyze the synthesis of viral RNA, and (2) VPg, a small polypeptide of uncertain function, which is apparently unique to picornaviruses (Cooper et al., 1978). VPg is covalently linked to the 5' end of genomic RNA, but it is not attached to viral messenger RNA. It perhaps functions as a primer for the synthesis of new viral RNA strands, or, alternatively, it may regulate the processing of viral RNA molecules. According to the latter hypothesis, VPg must be removed from RNA molecules before they can be translated into protein and must be added to those RNA molecules destined to become encapsidated as progeny virions (Nomoto et al., 1977).

### CLASSIFICATION OF PICORNAVIRUSES

Picornaviruses are subdivided into four genera* — *Enterovirus, Cardiovirus, Rhinovirus,* and *Aphthovirus* — primarily on the basis of sen-

---

*The four genera have been proposed by the Study Group on Picornaviridae (Cooper et al., 1978) but have not yet been formally recognized by the International Committee on Taxonomy of Viruses.

sitivity to acid, buoyant density of the virion in CsCl, and clinical manifestations (Cooper et al., 1978) (Table 1). Only enteroviruses and rhinoviruses are major human pathogens.

Enteroviruses multiply throughout the alimentary tract and cause a variety of infections, which range in severity from asymptomatic to fatal. Among their distinctive properties are a buoyant density in CsCl of 1.33 to 1.35 g/cm$^3$ and maintenance of infectivity at a pH as low as 3. Because of their acid stability, enteroviruses that have undergone limited replication in the oropharynx survive transit through the stomach and implant in the lower intestinal tract, where they undergo more extensive multiplication. Enteroviruses are also relatively resistant to thermal inactivation at ambient temperatures, especially in the presence of 1 M MgC1$_2$. This chemical is therefore added to live poliovirus vaccines to enhance their stability, especially under field conditions or in tropical regions lacking refrigeration.

Rhinoviruses inhabit the upper respiratory tract and are the principal recognized etiologic agents of the common cold. Unlike enteroviruses, rhinoviruses are acid labile. They begin to lose infectivity at pH 6 and are completely unstable at pH 3. They are further distinguished from enteroviruses by their optimal temperature of replication (33° C) and by their higher buoyant density in CsCl. Preferential replication at lower than body temperature probably reflects their adaptation to the nasal passages.

Cardioviruses, examples of which include encephalomyocarditis virus and Mengo virus, have been recognized only rarely as causes of human diseases (Gajdusek, 1955; Tesh, 1978). Although they have been recovered chiefly from rodents, their natural host(s) is uncertain (Tesh, 1978; Tesh and Wallace, 1978). Their buoyant density and optimal temperature of replication are similar to those of enteroviruses. However, although they are usually stable over the broad range of pH 4 to 10, they differ from enteroviruses in being unstable at pH 6 in the presence of 0.1 M chloride ions.

Aphthoviruses, named for the vesicular lesions that they produce in cloven-footed animals, are an important cause of economic loss in the cattle industry. Their buoyant density is intermediate between those of rhinoviruses and enteroviruses/-cardioviruses. They resemble rhinoviruses in their instability in acid, but at pH 5 to 6 in solutions of high ionic strength they are relatively stable.

Species of the four picornavirus genera are distinguished immunologically, usually by the ability of specific antiserum to neutralize only the

### TABLE 1.   A Classification of the Family Picornaviridae

| GENUS | SUBGENUS[a] | NUMBER OF IMMUNOTYPES (SPECIES) | Infectivity at pH 3 | Infectivity at pH 6 | Density in CsCl g/cm$^3$ | Optimal Growth Temperature |
|---|---|---|---|---|---|---|
| Enterovirus | Poliovirus | 3 | | | | |
| | Coxsackievirus A | 23[b] | | | | |
| | Coxsackievirus B | 6 | + | + | 1.33–1.35 | 37° C |
| | Echovirus | 30[c] | | | | |
| | Enterovirus | 4 | | | | |
| Cardiovirus | — | 1 | + | —[d] | 1.34 | 37° C |
| Rhinovirus | — | >110 | — | ±[e] | 1.38–1.41 | 33° C |
| Aphthovirus | — | 7 | — | ±[f] | 1.43–1.45 | 37° C |

[a]The designation subgenus has not been proposed by the International Committee on Taxonomy of Viruses but is used here for convenience simply to indicate a taxon smaller than a genus but larger than a species.

[b]Coxsackieviruses A1–A24; coxsackievirus A23 has been reclassified as echovirus 9.

[c]Echoviruses 1–34; echoviruses 1 and 8 are identical; echovirus 10 has been reclassified as reovirus 1, and echovirus 28 as rhinovirus 1A; echovirus 34 is a variant of coxsackievirus A24.

[d]Cardioviruses are stable at pH 4–10, but in the presence of chloride ions they are unstable in the region of pH 6.

[e]Rhinoviruses are borderline stable at pH 6 and unstable at lower pH.

[f]Aphthoviruses are unstable below pH 7 at low ionic strength but stable at pH 5–6 in high ionic strength.

homotypic virus. Sixty-six human enterovirus species (immunotypes) and more than 100 human rhinoviruses have been identified. Not included in Table 1 are many immunotypes of simian, porcine, bovine, and insect enteroviruses, as well as bovine, equine, and feline rhinoviruses.

## ANTIGENIC STRUCTURE OF PICORNAVIRUSES

Enteroviruses and rhinoviruses exhibit two distinct antigenic reactivities, C and D, associated with different physical forms of the virus particle (Roizman et al., 1958; Hughes et al., 1974). Empty capsids are C antigenic and give rise to group-specific reactions detectable by complement fixation (CF) or immunoprecipitin reactions. In intact virions, the C antigen is ordinarily masked; instead, the D antigen, which elicits type-specific neutralizing antibodies, is expressed. After infection, serum contains antibodies to both C and D antigens, but when the serum is absorbed with empty capsids it retains only D-specificity. Mild denaturing conditions, such as heating at 50° C or ultraviolet irradiation, convert the reactivity of virions from D to C. When enteroviruses are completely disrupted or when rhinoviruses are subjected to acidity (pH 3), the integrity of both C and D antigens is lost.

D and C antigenic reactivities are explained by changes in the conformation and molecular architecture of the virion. VP4 is essential for D reactivity (Breindl, 1971). When virions are heated, they lose VP4 and RNA and become noninfectious. Empty capsids, consisting of VP1 and VP3 (and some VP2), retain C antigenicity, but this reactivity is also lost when capsids are further disrupted into their constituent capsomeres (Katagiri et al., 1971).

## SUBCLASSIFICATION AND HOST RANGE OF PICORNAVIRUSES

### Enteroviruses

Historically, human enteroviruses have been subclassified into polioviruses, coxsackieviruses, and echoviruses based on antigenic relationships, difference in host range, and types of disease that result. *Polioviruses,* the first to be recognized, produce characteristic lesions when inoculated into the central nervous system of primates (see Chapter 173) and replicate only in primates or primate cell cultures. In contrast, most *coxsackieviruses* are not readily isolated in cell cultures and are only occasionally neuropathogenic for monkeys. However, they cause paralysis and death when inoculated into suckling mice. This property was responsible for their detection and differentiation from polioviruses in 1958, when they were first recovered from the feces of children with a poliomyelitis-like syndrome in the village of Coxsackie, New York (Dalldorf and Sickles, 1948). Shortly after their discovery, it was recognized that some coxsackieviruses, designated group A, produced widespread lesions and flaccid paralysis in skeletal muscle of mice, whereas others, designated group B, produced only focal myositis but more widespread visceral lesions involving the heart, fat, pancreas, and central nervous system, causing spastic paralysis. Moreover, the group B coxsackieviruses, unlike most of those of group A, could be propagated in primate cell cultures (Melnick, 1954). Further attempts to recover viruses from the feces of healthy children led to the discovery in 1949–1950 of still other agents that produced cytopathic effects in primate cell cultures but failed to cause disease in suckling mice or in the central nervous system of primates (Melnick and Agren, 1952; Melnick, 1954; Ramos-Alverez and Sabin, 1954). These agents, initially considered "orphan" viruses because they were unrelated to any disease, were called *echoviruses* (*e*nteric *c*ytopathic *h*uman *o*rphan).

During the quarter century that has elapsed since techniques for detecting enteroviruses were developed, three immunotypes of polioviruses have been recognized, as well as 23 group A coxsackieviruses, 6 group B coxsackieviruses, and 30 echoviruses. Many enteroviruses cannot be subclassified unambiguously. For example, some have the host range of a coxsackievirus but are antigenically related to echoviruses. Therefore, new agents are now designated simply as *enteroviruses* with serial numbers (Rosen et al., 1970). Since adoption of this simplified taxonomic scheme four new immunotypes, enteroviruses 68 to 71, have been recognized. However, because of established precedent, the first 67 immunotypes are still subclassified as polioviruses, coxsackieviruses, or echoviruses.

### Rhinoviruses

There are 89 numbered species of human rhinoviruses. Additional immunotypes awaiting formal recognition have brought the total to at least 110. Human rhinoviruses are infectious only for primates or primate cell cultures, and many can be propagated in vitro only in human embryonic fibroblasts. A few fastidious strains grow only in organ cultures of embryonic human tracheal epithelium. Rhinoviruses have been classified as H or M strains according to their growth in cells of human or monkey origin, but this subdivision has little clinical or epidemiologic significance.

## *RELATIONSHIPS AMONG PICORNAVIRUSES*

Although each immunotype is distinct, human enteroviruses and rhinoviruses are related genetically and immunologically. Genetic relationships among enteroviruses are shown by reciprocal hybridization of their nucleic acids (Young, 1973) or by oligonucleotide "fingerprinting" (Frisby et al., 1976). Different immunotypes within a major group, such as the three species of poliovirus, share 30 to 50 per cent of their nucleotide sequences, whereas homologies among viruses of different groups, such as group A coxsackieviruses and echoviruses, are generally less than 20 per cent. At least 5 per cent of the RNA sequences are common to all human enteroviruses. On the other hand, less than 4 per cent homology has been found among the RNA of three rhinovirus species, suggesting that they are genetically very diverse (Yin et al., 1973).

D antigens of each enterovirus immunotype stimulate type-specific neutralizing antibodies, but immunologic cross-reactions are elicited by the C antigens of related viruses. Heterotypic reactions are most readily demonstrated in the serum of individuals who have previously experienced sequential infections with other enteroviruses. For example, a child whose first coxsackievirus infection is with immunotype B5 usually elaborates neutralizing and CF antibodies that react only or predominantly with homotypic antigens; on the other hand, if he has previously been infected by another group B coxsackievirus, titers of CF antibodies against all six group B coxsackieviruses may rise, even though neutralizing antibody titer rises will be greatest between certain pairs of viruses, such as polioviruses 1 and 2, coxsackieviruses A3 and A8, and echoviruses 6 and 30. Furthermore, a distant immunologic relationship between human enteroviruses and rhinoviruses can be demonstrated in immunoprecipitin reactions or by immune electron microscopy with undiluted human serum (Hughes et al., 1977). The weak cross-reaction of enteroviruses and rhinoviruses probably reflects the broadened antibody response resulting from multiple picornavirus infections, because no cross-reaction can be demonstrated with serum from animals hyperimmunized with a single picornavirus antigen.

## *PATHOGENESIS*

### Enteroviruses

The pathogenesis of poliovirus infections has been extensively studied and is discussed in Chapter 173. Data for other enteroviruses, meager because there are no readily available experimental models, indicate a basic similarity of the major pathogenetic events, excluding those involving the central nervous system. Briefly recapitulated, these events are as follows.

Infection is primarily a result of ingesting fecally contaminated material. In individuals lacking type-specific antibodies, enteroviruses implant and replicate in susceptible tissues of the gut, which probably include mucosal epithelial cells and lymphoid tissue of the lamina propria. Pathologic lesions are not apparent in these sites. Although most enteroviruses multiply in both the oropharynx and the distal small bowel or colon, evidence favors the view that replication in the lower gut is far more efficient (Ogra and Karzon, 1971): (1) Large doses of oral polio vaccines result in virus shedding in both oropharyngeal secretions and feces, whereas with small doses only fecal shedding occurs; (2) virus titers are substantially higher in feces, often $10^6$ infectious units per gram; (3) virus can be recovered from the oropharynx only for several days, rarely as long as three weeks, whereas fecal excretion of virus is more sustained, often five to six weeks or longer; (4) although some enteroviruses — for example, group B coxsackieviruses — are often recovered from both ends of the alimentary canal, echoviruses are commonly recovered only in the feces (Kogon et al., 1969).

After multiplying in the submucosal lymphatic tissues, enteroviruses reach the cervical and mesenteric lymph nodes. From these sites small quantities of virus escape into the bloodstream ("minor viremia") and are disseminated to the reticuloendothelial tissues, such as the liver, spleen, and bone marrow. All the replicative events up to this point produce no symptoms, and in most individuals the infection is contained by host defense mechanisms without further progression. However, in a few infected persons, additional replication in reticuloendothelial tissues produces heavy, sustained shedding of virus into the blood ("major viremia"). This event is temporally associated with the "minor illness" of poliomyelitis and probably the nonspecific febrile illnesses caused by other enteroviruses. Sustained viremia is also responsible for dissemination of virus to target organs, such as the meninges, skin, and heart. In these tissues the virus produces inflammatory lesions, often accompanied by necrosis.

### Rhinoviruses

Rhinoviruses implant and replicate in epithelial cells of the nasal mucosa, producing hyperemia and edema of the mucous membrane and a seromucinous exudate. A scant infiltrate of neutrophils, eosinophils, and mononuclear inflammatory cells is present beneath the epithelium, and mucin secretion by goblet cells is increased. Columnar epithelial cells exhibit impaired mucociliary clearance, become necrotic, and slough. Rhinovirus replication can be detected within 24 hours after implantation, often several days before the onset of symptoms, and reaches a peak in two to three days. Excretion generally ceases by seven days, but in a few individuals it persists up to two weeks (Douglas et al., 1966; Kettler et al., 1969). Rhinoviruses are shed principally from the nose, and the concentration of virus in the nasal mucus is 10- to 100-fold higher than it is in saliva or oropharyngeal secretions (Hendley et al., 1973). The precise anatomic range of infected tissues has not been defined; it has not been established whether infection extends beyond the nose or whether virus in the oropharynx comes principally from contamination from the nose. In normal individuals, as well as in patients with chronic bronchitis, rhinovirus infections have been associated with abnormalities of pulmonary function (Cate et al., 1973), but this may be a consequence of reflex bronchoconstriction rather than of direct viral invasion of the lower respiratory tract.

Although rhinoviruses usually implant in the nose, infection can be initiated experimentally by dropping virus on the conjunctiva. Rhinoviruses introduced into the oropharynx cause infection only with relative difficulty (Hendley et al., 1973), and they are unable to replicate in the lower intestinal tract, even when the acidic environment of the stomach is bypassed and virus is artificially introduced into the small bowel (Cate et al., 1967). Among the possible reasons for failure to replicate in the intestine are lack of appropriate viral receptors on mucosal epithelial cells and the higher temperature at this site compared with the nasal passages. Neither viremia nor dissemination of rhinoviruses beyond the respiratory tract has been documented.

## IMMUNITY

Type-specific neutralizing antibodies in the serum and in mucosal secretions are the factors most responsible for acquired immunity against picornaviruses. Cell-mediated immunity has not been thoroughly studied.

In the nasopharynx and the intestinal tract, secretory IgA antibodies directed against specific immunotypes of polioviruses and rhinoviruses are elicited by the initial infection with these agents (Ogra and Karzon, 1971; Cate et al., 1966; Gwaltney, 1976). Depending on the titer of secretory antibodies, either reinfection by the same immunotype is prevented or the outcome of infection is modified. High titers of IgA antibodies prevent implantation and replication of virus in the gut and pharynx. In contrast, reinfection is possible when antibody titers are low or when the virus challenge is massive. Reinfections are unaccompanied by illness and give rise only to brief excretion of virus (Kogon et al., 1969). IgA antibodies to poliovirus may also be acquired passively in milk by breast-fed infants whose mothers are immune; these antibodies interfere with a "take" by live, oral poliovirus vaccines (OPV) and may also protect against natural infection during early infancy (Warren et al., 1964).

IgM and IgG neutralizing antibodies to enteroviruses begin to appear in the serum as early as one to three days after infection (Ogra and Karzon, 1971). IgA antibodies are usually not detected in serum until two to six weeks; they are generally of low titer and do not develop in all individuals. IgM antibodies usually persist for two to three months, but serum-neutralizing antibodies of the IgG and IgA classes are present for many years, possibly for life. Although serum-neutralizing antibodies do not prevent alimentary infection by enteroviruses, they effectively block viremia and hematogenous dissemination to target organs such as the meninges, skin, and heart. Parenterally administered pooled gamma globulin produces trace levels of serum antibodies to poliovirus that protect against paralysis if given before exposure (Stevens, 1959). Protection against paralytic poliomyelitis is also afforded by either OPV or parenterally administered inactivated polio vaccine (IPV) because both types of vaccine stimulate serum-neutralizing antibodies in a high proportion of recipients. However, OPV has the additional advantage of interrupting the transmission of wild polioviruses in the community, because the attenuated viruses replicate in the alimentary tract and stimulate secretory immunity, thereby preventing subsequent reinfection as well as central nervous system illness (Melnick, 1978).

Rhinoviruses, like enteroviruses, stimulate neutralizing antibodies in both the serum and the nasopharyngeal secretions of up to 80 per cent of infected individuals. Antibody responses at these sites are closely linked, even after nasal or parenteral immunization with inactivated virus. It has not been established unequivocally, therefore, whether secretory or circulating antibodies are more important in type-specific immunity to the common cold (Gwaltney, 1976). Because antibodies in either serum or nasal secretions are not detected until approximately two weeks after infection, when virus shedding has already ceased, it is likely that recovery from acute infection is mediated by other mechanisms, possibly interferon.

Complement-fixing antibodies stimulated by enteroviruses or rhinoviruses are detectable for one to five years after infection. They do not appear in all individuals, and it is unclear whether they are protective.

## LABORATORY DIAGNOSIS

Appropriate specimens for isolation of enteroviruses include, depending on the clinical syndrome, throat washings or swabs, feces, cerebrospinal fluid, vesicle fluid from skin lesions, pericardial fluid, conjunctival swabs (acute hemorrhagic conjunctivitis), and autopsy tissues such as brain, spinal cord, and myocardium. Isolation of an enterovirus from one or more of these sites is usually convincing evidence of an etiologic relationship to illness, but isolation from feces or throat secretions, especially in infants during the summer months when enteroviruses are prevalent, may be only circumstantial evidence of such a relationship because etiologically unrelated intercurrent infection may be present. Isolation of a rhinovirus from nasopharyngeal secretions likewise must be interpreted with regard to the possibility that other, unidentified respiratory pathogens may be present.

Specimens for enterovirus isolation optimally should be transported on wet ice (4° C) to the virus laboratory, where they should be inoculated into human or primate cell cultures, such as rhesus monkey kidney or human embryonic kidney. For the diagnosis of illness due to group A coxsackieviruses, infant mice must also be inoculated. Rhinoviruses can usually be isolated in human diploid fibroblast cell cultures, such as WI 38, although the expense of this procedure is rarely warranted in patients with the common cold. Specimens that cannot be inoculated until many hours after their collection should be frozen, preferably at -70° C or lower. However, the characteristic stability of enteroviruses sometimes permits their recovery even from unrefrigerated specimens that have been mailed to the laboratory. Characteristic cytopathic effects in cell cultures are commonly observed after two to five days and permit a presumptive diagnosis of picornavirus infection. The specific immunotype is identified by the use of polyvalent immune sera in an "intersecting pool" scheme (Lim and Benyesh-Melnick, 1960).

For serodiagnosis, the acute phase serum should be collected as soon after onset of illness as possible, and the convalescent serum should be collected approximately two to three weeks later.

In the individual patient, the diagnosis of enterovirus or rhinovirus infection is made most conveniently by virus isolation. Rising titers of neutralizing antibodies in paired acute and convalescent sera are confirmatory, but serologic diagnosis generally cannot substitute for virus isolation. The reason is that group-reactive antigens encompassing all immunotypes are lacking, and it is not practical to perform serologic tests with type-specific antigens individually for more than 60 enteroviruses or 100 rhinoviruses. The physician should therefore not expect the virus diagnostic laboratory to perform antibody "screens" unless a virus has been isolated from the patient, the particular epidemic immunotype is known or suspected, or the type of clinical illness suggests only a limited number of probable immunotypes. For example, serologic diagnosis of sporadic cases of aseptic meningitis or the common cold is not feasible, but it may be reasonable to measure antibodies to the three poliovirus immunotypes in paralyzed individuals or to coxsackieviruses, B1–B5 in patients with myocarditis.

## EPIDEMIOLOGY

Most enteroviruses and rhinoviruses are distributed worldwide. Seasonal variation in prevalence and patterns of transmission of these two virus groups are dissimilar (Melnick, 1976; Gwaltney, 1976).

### Enteroviruses

In temperate climates, enteroviral infections are most common in the summer and early autumn, whereas in tropical climates infection occurs year round. Virus is spread chiefly by the fecal-oral route directly from person to person or by fomites, although spread by respiratory secretions may play a lesser role. In economically developed countries, usually only one or two immunotypes are prevalent in the community each season; in contrast, children living in urban areas with low standards of sanitation are often multiply infected. Approximately 50 to 80 per cent of enteroviral infections are asymptomatic, and many of the remainder are characterized by undifferentiated febrile illnesses lasting only a few days, often accompanied by upper respiratory tract symptoms. The so-called "characteristic" enterovirus syndromes — such as aseptic meningitis, myopericarditis, and exanthems — are in fact unusual manifestations of infection. Enteroviruses are most efficiently disseminated by infected children less than 2 years old. Introduction of virus into the household by one family member results in high rates of infection among others lacking type-specific neutralizing antibodies; secondary attack rates of approximately 92 per cent for polioviruses, 75 per cent for coxsackieviruses, and 50 per cent for echoviruses have been observed in family surveillance studies in the city of New York (Kogon et al., 1969).

Although the epidemiology of most enteroviruses is basically similar, patterns of infection with some immunotypes are distinctive. Improved standards of hygiene and widespread use of poliovirus vaccines have resulted in striking changes in the epidemiology of poliomyelitis, discussed in Chapter 173. Enterovirus 70 and coxsackievirus A24, the principal etiologic agents of acute hemorrhagic conjunctivitis, are probably transmitted from hand to eye by conjunctival secretions; replication of these viruses in the alimentary tract, if it exists at all, appears to be limited. Coxsackievirus A21 also is shed primarily from the upper respiratory tract, where it produces rhinovirus-like illness.

Control of nonpolio enterovirus infections and illness is best effected by hygienic measures and improvements in sanitation. Isolation of patients with enteroviral illness is generally not helpful in controlling epidemics because simultaneously there is a large reservoir of unidentified, asymptomatically infected individuals who excrete virus. Because nonpolio enteroviral illness is rarely life-threatening and because there are so many immunotypes, control by vaccines is not practical.

### Rhinoviruses

The peak incidence of rhinovirus infections in temperate climates occurs in the colder months, especially the early autumn and spring. In the tropics, peak activity occurs in the rainy season. Crowding indoors and the return of children to school are believed to be among the factors that account for this periodicity. Contrary to popular belief, there is no evidence that susceptibility to the common cold is enhanced by chilling of the body during the winter months. Rhinovirus infections experimentally induced at cold ambient temperatures do not occur with greater frequency of severity (Douglas et al., 1968).

Rhinovirus infections spread primarily in the home and in the classroom. As with enteroviruses, secondary attack rates of 50 to 80 per cent are common among susceptible family members, especially young children. Transmission of the common cold occurs with two to five day intervals between cases and is most efficient when there is close contact between individuals. Although it has long been assumed that rhinoviruses are disseminated by respiratory droplet nuclei, recent data suggest that spread may occur more commonly by transfer of nasal mucus to the hands of infected individuals, who transmit virus via fomites or hand contact to others, who in turn

autoinoculate the nose or conjunctiva (Gwaltney et al., 1978).

Multiple rhinovirus immunotypes often circulate concurrently. Antibody prevalence rates increase with age, beginning in early childhood and peaking in young adults, who commonly have serum antibodies to approximately half of the recognized rhinovirus immunotypes. Most infections are symptomatic, the ratio of apparent to inapparent infections being approximately 3:1.

Practical measures for the control of rhinovirus infections have not been established. If additional studies confirm that transmission occurs primarily from hand to nose rather than by inhalation of respiratory droplets, then handwashing or avoidance of hand contact with individuals with colds may reduce contagion. Prophylaxis with large doses of ascorbic acid is controversial, but this agent appears to be marginal at best in reducing the incidence of severity of colds. Specific chemotherapeutic agents are not available. Control by vaccines is not practical because of the large number of immunotypes.

### References

Breindl, M.: VP4, the D-reactive part of poliovirus. Virology 46:962, 1971.

Cate, T. R., Douglas, R. G., Jr., Johnson, K. M., Couch, R. B., and Knight, V.: Studies on the inability of rhinovirus to survive and replicate in the intestinal tract of volunteers. Proc Soc Exp Biol Med 124:1290, 1967.

Cate, T. R., Roberts, J. S., Russ, M. A., and Pierce, J. A.: Effects of common colds on pulmonary function. Am Rev Respir Dis 108:858, 1973.

Cate, T. R., Rossen, R. D., Douglas, R. G., Jr., Butler, W. T., and Couch, R. B.: The role of nasal secretion and serum antibody in the rhinovirus common cold. Am J Epidemiol 84:352, 1966.

Cooper, P. D., Agol, V. I., Bachrach, H. L., Brown, F., Ghendon, Y., Gibbs, A. J., Gillespie, J. H., Lonberg-Holm, K., Mandel, B., Melnick, J. L., Mohanty, S. B., Povey, R. C., Rueckert, R. R., Schaffer, F. L., and Tyrrell, D. A. J.: Picornaviridae: Second report. Intervirology 10:165, 1978.

Dalldorf, G., and Sickles, G. M.: An unidentified, filtrable agent isolated from the feces of children with paralysis. Science 108:61, 1948.

Douglas, R. G., Jr., Cate, T. R., Gerone, P. J., and Couch, R. B.: Quantitative rhinovirus shedding patterns in volunteers. Am Rev Respir Dis 94:159, 1966.

Douglas, R. G., Jr., Lindgren, K. M., and Couch, R. B.: Exposure to cold environment and rhinovirus common cold: Failure to demonstrate effect. N Engl J Med 279:743, 1968.

Frisby, D. P., Newton, C., Carey, N. H., Fellner, P., Newman, J. F. E., Harris, T. J. R., and Brown, F.: Oligonucleotide mapping of picornavirus RNAs by two-dimensional electrophoresis. Virology 71:379, 1976.

Gajdusek, D. C.: Encephalomyocarditis virus infection in childhood. Pediatrics 16:902, 1955.

Gwaltney, J. M., Jr.: Rhinoviruses. In Evans, A. S. (ed.): Viral Infections of Humans. New York, Plenum Medical Book Company, 1976, pp. 383–408.

Gwaltney, J. M., Jr., Moskalski, P. B., and Hendley, J. O.: Hand-to-hand transmission of rhinovirus colds. Ann Intern Med 88:463, 1978.

Hendley, J. O., Wenzel, R. P., and Gwaltney, J. M., Jr.: Transmission of rhinovirus colds by self-inoculation. N Engl J Med 288:1361, 1973.

Hughes, J. H., Chema, S., Lin, N., Conant, R. M., and Hamparian, V. V.: Acid lability of rhinoviruses: Loss of C and D antigenicity after treatment at pH 3.0. J Immunol 112:919, 1974.

Hughes, J. H., Gnau, J. M., Hilty, M. D., Chema, S., Ottolenghi, A. C., and Hamparian, V. V.: Picornaviruses: Rapid differentiation and identification by immune electronmicroscopy and immunodiffusion. J Med Microbiol 10:203, 1977.

Jacobson, M. F., and Baltimore, D.: Polypeptide cleavages in the formation of poliovirus proteins. Proc Natl Acad Sci USA 61:77, 1968.

Katagiri, S., Aikawa, S., and Hinuma, Y.: Stepwise degradation of poliovirus capsid by alkaline treatment. J Gen Virol 13:101, 1971.

Kettler, A., Hall, C. E., Fox, J. P., Elveback, L., and Cooney, M. K.: The virus watch program: A coninuing surveillance of viral infections in metropolitan New York families. VIII. Rhinovirus infections: Observations of virus excretion, intrafamilial spread and clinical response. Am J Epidemiol 90:244, 1969.

Kogon, A., Spigland, I., Frothingham, T. E., Elveback, L., Williams, C., Hall, C. E., and Fox, J. P.: The virus watch program: A continuing surveillance of viral infections in metropolitan New York families. VII. Observation on viral excretion, seroimmunity, intrafamilial spread and illness association in coxsackievirus and echovirus infections. Am J Epidemiol 89:51, 1969.

Lim, K. A., and Benyesh-Melnick, ML Typing of viruses by combinations of antiserum pools. Applications to typing of enteroviruses (Coxsackie and ECHO). J Immunol 84:309, 1960.

Melnick, J. L.: Application of tissue culture methods to epidemiological studies of poliomyelitis. Am J Public Health 44:571, 1954.

Melnick, J. L.: Enteroviruses. In Evans, A. S. (ed.): Viral Infections of Humans. New York, Plenum Medical Book Company, 1976, pp. 163–207.

Melnick, J. L.: Advantages and disadvantages of killed and live poliomyelitis vaccines. Bull W H O 56:21, 1978.

Melnick, J. L., and Agren, K.: Poliomyelitis and Coxsackie viruses isolated from normal infants in Egypt. Proc Soc Exp Biol Med 81:621, 1952.

Nomoto, A., Kitamura, N., Golini, F., and Wimmer, E.: The 5'-terminal structures of poliovirion RNA and poliovirus mRNA differ only in the genome-linked protein VPg. Proc Natl Acad Sci USA 74:5345, 1977.

Ogra, P. L., and Karzon, D. T.: Formation and function of poliovirus antibody in different tissues. Progr Med Virol 13:157, 1971.

Ramos-Alvarez, M., and Sabin, A. B.: Characteristics of poliomyelitis and other enteric viruses recovered in tissue culture from healthy American children. Proc Soc Exp Biol Med 87:655, 1954.

Roizman, B., Mayer, M. M., and Rapp, H. J.: Immunochemical studies of poliovirus. III. Further studies on the immunological and physical properties of poliovirus particles produced in tissue culture. J Immunol 81:419, 1958.

Rosen, L., Melnick, J. L., Schmidt, N. J., et al.: Subclassification of enteroviruses and ECHO virus type 34. Arch Ges Virusforsch 30:89, 1970.

Stevens, K. M.: Estimate of molecular equivalent of antibody required for prophylaxis and therapy of poliomyelitis. J Hyg (Camb) 57:198, 1959.

Tesh, R. B.: The prevalence of encephalomyocarditis virus neutralizing antibodies among various human populations. Am J Trop Med Hyg 27:144, 1978.

Tesh, R. B., and Wallace, G. D.: Observations on the natural history of encephalomyocarditis virus. Am J Trop Med Hyg 27:133, 1978.

Warren, R. J., Lepow, M. L., Bartsch, G. E., and Robbins, F. C.: The relationship of maternal antibody, breast feeding, and age to the susceptibility of newborn infants to infection with attenuated polioviruses. Pediatrics 34:4, 1964.

Yin, F. F., Lonberg-Holm, K., and Chan, S. P.: Lack of a close relationship between three strains of human rhinoviruses as determined by their RNA sequences. J Virol 12:108, 1973.

Young, N. A.: Polioviruses, coxsackieviruses, and echoviruses. Comparison of the genomes by RNA hybridization. J Virol 11:832, 1973.

# 61 *TOGAVIRUSES*

### *Marian C. Horzinek, D.V.M., Ph.D.*

## DEFINITION

The family Togaviridae includes the genera *Alphavirus, Flavivirus, Rubivirus,* and *Pestivirus.* Members of the family are characterized by spherical virions, 40 to 70 nm in diameter, that consist of a lipoprotein envelope with cellular lipids and virus-specified glycopeptides surrounding a spherical nucleocapsid of icosahedral symmetry. The virus contains a single molecule of single-stranded RNA (molecular weight about 4 $\times$ 10$^6$) with positive polarity that is infectious when extracted and assayed under appropriate conditions. Togaviruses multiply in the cytoplasm and mature by budding (Fenner, 1976).

All species of the genus *Alphavirus* and most flaviviruses multiply in arthropods as well as in vertebrates and constitute the classic arthropod-borne viruses (formerly termed arbo-A and arbo-B viruses, respectively). Arboviruses are viruses that are maintained in nature principally, or to an important extent, through biologic transmission between susceptible vertebrate hosts by hematophagous arthropods (WHO Study Group, 1967). Essential to this ecologic definition is the term "biologic" (as opposed to mechanical) transmission, by which is meant that an "extrinsic incubation period" (5 to 12 days) elapses between the moments when the arthropod vector becomes infected after a blood meal and when it can transmit the virus to a new vertebrate host. Biologic transmission is not confined to the above mentioned togavirus genera: Members of the Reoviridae and Rhabdoviridae families and all Bunyaviridae are also arthropod-borne. On the other hand, members of the Rubivirus (Rubellavirus) and Pestivirus genera (hog cholera, bovine diarrhea viruses) as well as mouse lactic dehydrogenase virus and equine arteritis virus are nonarbotogaviruses (Horzinek, 1973). The following chapters will cover only togaviruses of medical importance—namely, a number of alphaviruses and flaviviruses (Tables 1 and 2) and rubella virus (RUV).

## STRUCTURE

Togaviruses are the smallest enveloped animal viruses; alphaviruses and RUV are about 60 nm in diameter, and flaviviruses are smaller, about

**TABLE 1.  Alphaviruses**

| VIRUS | ABBREVIATION | ISOLATED FROM — Arthropods — Mosq. Culicine | Anopheline | Culicoides | Other | Vertebrates — Man | Other Primates | Rodents | Birds | Bats | Marsupials | Other | Sentinels | ISOLATED IN — Africa | Asia | Australasia | Europe | North America | South America | HUMAN DISEASE — Natural Infection | Lab Infection |
|---|---|---|---|---|---|---|---|---|---|---|---|---|---|---|---|---|---|---|---|---|---|
| Aura | AURA | + | | | | | | | | | | | | | | | | | + | | |
| Bebaru | BEB | + | | | | | | | | | | | | | + | | | | | | |
| Chikungunya | CHIK | + | | | | + | + | | + | + | | | + | + | + | | | | | + | + |
| Eastern equine enc. | EEE | + | + | + | + | + | + | + | + | | + | + | | | + | | | + | + | + | + |
| Everglades | EVE | + | + | | | | | + | | | + | | | | | | | + | | + | |
| Getah | GET | + | + | | | | | | | | | | + | | + | + | | | | | |
| Mayaro | MAY | + | | | + | + | | | | | | | + | | | | | | | + | + |
| Middleburg | MID | + | | | | | | | | | | | | + | | | | | | | |
| Mucambo | MUC | + | | | | + | | + | + | | + | | + | | | | | | | + | + |
| Ndumu | NDU | + | | | | | | | | | | | | + | | | | | | | |
| O'nyong-nyong | ONN | | + | | | + | | | | | | | + | + | | | | | | + | |
| Pixuna | PIX | + | + | | | | | + | | | | | | | | | | | | + | |
| Ross River | RR | + | | | | + | | | + | | + | | | | | | + | | | + | |
| Sagiyama | SAG | + | | | | | | | | | | | + | | | | | | | | |
| Semliki Forest | SFV | + | + | | | | | | + | | | + | + | | | | | | | | + |
| Sindbis | SIN | + | + | + | | + | | | + | | | | + | + | + | + | | | | + | |
| Una | UNA | + | + | | | | | | | | | + | + | | | | | | + | + | |
| Venezuelan equine enc. | VEE | + | + | | | + | | + | | + | + | + | + | | | | | + | + | + | + |
| Western equine enc. | WEE | + | + | + | | + | | + | + | | | + | + | | | | | + | ? | + | + |
| Whataroa | WHA | + | | | | | | | | | | | | | | + | | | | | |

Berge, T. O. (ed.): International Catalogue of Arboviruses. Washington, D.C., U.S. Department of Health, Education, and Welfare, 1975.

45 nm. The size differences as determined by negative staining and thin section electron microscopy are reflected by the sedimentation coefficients, which range between 240 and 300S for the former group and 170 to 220S for the latter group. Gradient analysis has shown that the buoyant densities of infectious virions depend on the substance used for building the gradient; values vary between < 1.18 g/ml for sucrose and 1.24 for cesium chloride and other salts.

In the electron microscope togavirions appear as spherical particles consisting of an envelope and an isometric core. The envelope shows unit membrane characteristics and carries glycoprotein surface projections that are organized in a regular (icosahedral) surface lattice (Fig. 1); they are the substrate for a pH-dependent hemagglutinating activity. Exposure of virions to organic solvents or to detergents inactivates their infectivity by disintegrating the envelope, leading to hemagglutinating membrane fragments and to liberation of the nucleocapsid (30 to 40 nm in diameter for alphaviruses and RUV, and 20 to 30 nm for flaviviruses). The togavirion has a shape and substructure suggestive of icosahedral symmetry. In contrast to naked animal viruses, however, isolated togavirus capsids are nonrigid and sus-

ceptible to RNase, which degrades the viral genome to small fragments. Since this treatment has no effect on intact virions, it is the function of the envelope to protect the viral RNA from enzymatic attack.

Consistent data of overall chemical analysis have been obtained so far only for alphaviruses, since these grow to high titers in tissue culture and can be obtained as suspensions of sufficient purity and concentration. The reported proportions of RNA: protein: lipid: carbohydrate (in glycoprotein) are about 6:61:27:6. The RNA of togaviruses is a single-stranded, colinear molecule that has an average molecular weight of $4.2 \times 10^6$, which corresponds to about 12,000 nucleotides, and sedimentation coefficient of 42 to 49S in sucrose gradients. Studies with alphaviruses have indicated that there is a significant degree of secondary structure in extracted RNA, which is necessary for infectivity. Polyadenylic acid sequences located near the 3′ terminus have been demonstrated; these, together with the absence of a virion-associated polymerase, indicated that togaviral RNA is plus-stranded and might serve as the initial messenger molecule during infection. These assumptions have been confirmed by the demonstration of parental virion RNA in

TABLE 2.  Mosquito-borne Flaviviruses

| Virus | Abbreviation | Culicine | Anopheline | Ixodid | Argasid | Other (arthropod) | Man | Other Primates | Rodents | Birds | Bats | Marsupials | Other (vert.) | Sentinels | Africa | Asia | Australasia | Europe | North America | South America | Natural Infection | Lab Infection |
|---|---|---|---|---|---|---|---|---|---|---|---|---|---|---|---|---|---|---|---|---|---|---|
| Alfuy | ALF | + | | | | | | | | + | | | | | | | + | | | | | |
| Bagaza | BAG | + | | | | | | | | | | | | | + | | | | | | | |
| Banzi | BAN | + | | | | | + | | | | | | | + | + | | | | | | + | |
| Boubyui | BOU | + | + | | | | | + | | | | | | | + | | | | | | | |
| Bussuquara | BSQ | + | | | | | + | | + | | | | | + | | | | | + | + | + | |
| Dengue-1 | DEN-1 | + | | | | | + | | | | | | | | | + | + | | + | | + | + |
| Dengue-2 | DEN-2 | + | | | | | + | + | | | | | | | | + | + | | + | | + | + |
| Dengue-3 | DEN-3 | + | | | | | + | | | | | | | | | + | + | | | | + | + |
| Dengue-4 | DEN-4 | + | | | | | + | | | | | | | | | + | + | | | | + | |
| Edge Hill | EH | + | + | | | | | | | | | | | | | | + | | | | | |
| Ilheus | ILH | + | | | | | + | | | + | | | | + | | | | | + | + | + | + |
| Japanese enceph. | JE | + | + | | | | + | | | + | + | | + | | | + | | | | | + | + |
| Jugra | JUG | + | | | | | | | + | | | | | | | + | | | | | | |
| Kokobera | KOK | + | | | | | | | | | | | | | | | + | | | | | |
| Kunjin | KUN | + | | | | | + | | | + | | | | | | | + | | | | | |
| Murray Valley enceph. | MVE | + | | | | | + | | | | | | | | | | + | | | | + | |
| Ntaya | NTA | + | | | | | | | | | | | | | + | | | | | | | |
| Sepik | SEP | + | | | | | | | | | | | | | | | + | | | | + | |
| St. Louis enceph. | SLE | + | + | | | + | + | | | + | + | | | + | | | | | + | + | + | + |
| Spondweni | SPO | + | | | | | + | | | | | | | | + | | | | | | + | + |
| Stratford | STR | + | | | | | | | | | | | | | | | + | | | | | |
| Tembusu | TMU | + | + | | | | | | | | | | | | | | | | + | + | | |
| Uganda S | UGS | + | | | | | | | | + | | | | + | + | | | | | | | |
| Usutu | USU | + | | | | | | | + | + | | | | | + | | | | | | | |
| Wesselbron | WSL | + | + | | | | + | | + | | | | + | | + | + | | | | | + | + |
| West Nile | WN | + | + | + | + | | + | | + | + | + | | | + | + | + | + | + | | | + | + |
| Yellow fever | YF | + | | | | | + | + | | | | + | | | + | | | | | + | + | + |
| Zika | ZIKA | + | | | | | + | | | | | | | + | + | + | | | | | + | + |

Berge, T. O. (ed.): International Catalogue of Arboviruses. Washington, D.C., U.S. Department of Health, Education, and Welfare, 1975.

polysomes of infected cells and by its translation into virus-specific polypeptides in cell-free systems. Like other mRNAs from eukaryotic systems, viral RNAs contain methylated "capped" structures at their 5′ termini, which in alphaviruses are of the form mG (5′) pppAp.

A minimum of three structural polypeptides has been identified in togaviruses, one of them associated with the nucleocapsid; in alphaviruses and RUV this protein has a molecular weight of 30,000 to 35,000, and in flaviviruses the molecular weight ranges from 13,000 to 14,000. Amino acid analyses have shown that the alphavirus capsid protein has an N-terminal lysine and is relatively hydrophilic, a property consistent with its extensive and rapid interaction with viral RNA.

Two glycosylated envelope proteins have been identified in RUV (50,000 and 63,000 mw) and in most alphaviruses (E1 and E2, 50,000 to 53,000 mw) by SDS polyacrylamide gel electrophoresis. Using chromatographic techniques, three envelope proteins (52,000, 49,000, and 10,000 mw) were isolated from SFV (for abbreviations see Tables 1 and 2). In flaviviruses only one envelope protein (50,000 to 60,000 mw) is glycosylated, whereas the other (8000 to 9000 mw) seems to be buried in the lipid bilayer and may have a bridging function between the peripheral glycoprotein and the capsid. In alphaviruses both the E1 and the E2 proteins occupy a superficial position because they can be stripped away by treatment with proteolytic enzymes and can be demonstrated by enzymatic iodination of undisrupted virions. They probably penetrate the lipid bilayer and interact directly with the capsid.

Togaviral lipid is confined to the envelope; in alphaviruses it has been found that 25 to 31 per

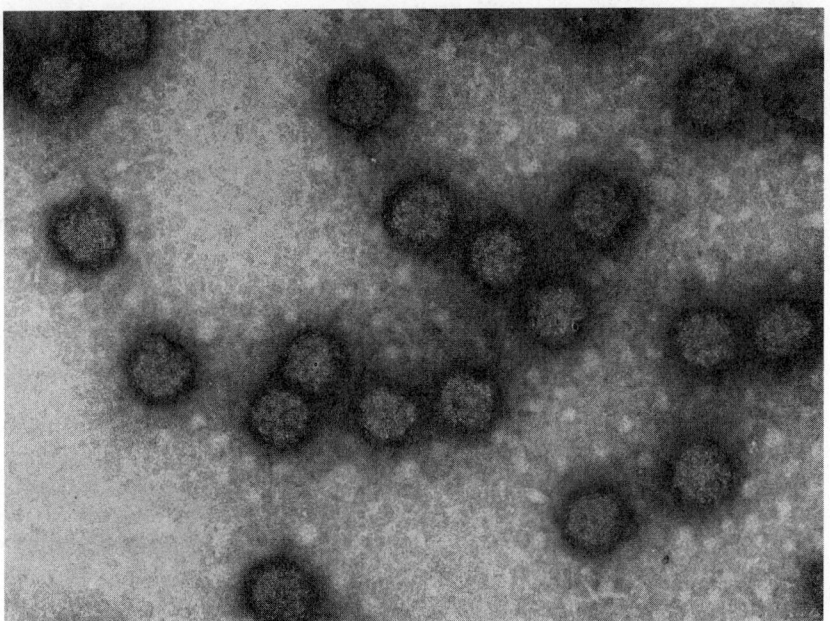

**FIGURE 1.** *Sindbis virus, a member of the genus* Alphavirus *of the* Togaviridae. *Note the regular pattern on the virion surface. Negatively stained preparation (uranyl acetate, after fixation with glutaraldehyde). (Courtesy of Dr. D. J. Ellens, CDI Lelystad, The Netherlands.)*

cent (by weight) is neutral lipid, predominantly cholesterol. Most of the remaining lipids are represented by phosphatidylethanolamine, phosphatidylserine, sphingomyeline, and phosphatidylcholine, which is the principal phosphatide. Of the viral fatty acids, oleic, palmitic, and stearic acids predominate. In general, the composition of togaviral lipids reflects that of the host cell membranes, as shown by a comparative analysis of SFV grown in BHK (baby hamster kidney) and *Aedes albopictus* cells, respectively (Pfefferkorn and Shapiro, 1974).

## ANTIGENIC COMPOSITION

Assignment of a togavirus to the alphagenus or flavigenus is made on the basis of immunologic cross-reactions. Virion surface antigens responsible for adsorption to susceptible cells and erythrocytes can be identified and compared by neutralization (NT) and hemagglutination inhibition (HI) tests. By using solvent-detergent-extracted antigens in complement fixation, gel diffusion, or radioimmunoassays, the total of antigen-antibody reactions can be measured, including those with the capsid protein. Capsid protein has been described as carrying group-reactive determinants, similar to the common nucleoprotein (gs) antigen of the orthomyxoviruses. These capsid determinants may mean that all alphaviruses are related (Dalrymple et al., 1976).

By using sera from animals that have been immunized by one inoculation of virus, it is possible to divide alphaviruses into subgroups and to make specific serologic identifications. Within the alphavirus genus the viruses BEB, CHIK, GET, MAY, ONN, RR, SFV, and UNA form one cluster of antigenically related viruses, AUR, SIN, WEE, and WHA a second one, and MUC, PIX, and VEE a third one. NDU, EEE, and MD are not related to each other nor to any other alphavirus (Casals and Reeves, 1959; Karabatsos, 1975). The following flavivirus subgroups have been recognized by using plaque neutralization: (1) the tick-borne flaviviruses (Table 2) with the exceptions of KAD and POW; (2) APOI, CR, DB, ENT, KAD, MOD, and RB; (3) ALF, JE, KOK, KUN, MVE, SLE, STR, USU, and WN; (4) SPO and ZIKA; (5) IT, NTA, and TMU; (6) BAN, EH, and UGS; and (7) the four DEN type viruses. No relationships to any other flavivirus could be demonstrated with BUS, ILH, MML, POW, WSL, and YF (de Madrid and Porterfield, 1974). RUV is unrelated to any other animal virus and has been classified as a togavirus exclusively for structural reasons. It is the only representative of the rubivirus genus.

It has been possible to determine the antigenic function of the respective alphavirion surface polypeptides. The E1 glycoprotein of SIN carries the complete hemagglutinating activity, whereas E2 appears to be important to infectivity because only antiserum directed against this molecular species effectively neutralized the virus. Glycoprotein E1 appears to be cross-reactive with antiserum to the closely related WEE and may therefore carry the determinant(s) responsible for defining the serologic complexes; E2 appears to be virus-specific (Dalrymple et al., 1976). By studying nucleotide sequence homologies between the nucleic acids of different alphaviruses it was demonstrated that the closely related viruses of CHIK and ONN have only 13 per cent of the base sequences in common, whereas ≤1 per cent of RNA–RNA homologies occur between the other viruses of this genus. These rather low homologies can be reconciled with the established serologic relationship by assuming that the antigenic sites are composed of only a small number of amino acids and/or that the degeneracy of the genetic code allows a much larger homology to be present in the protein sequences than in corresponding RNA base sequences (Wengler et al., 1977).

Because of the simplicity of the test system the hemagglutinating antigen has been studied most extensively (Clarke and Casals, 1958). For diagnostic purposes alkaline aqueous extracts, fluorocarbon, ether-acetone, sucrose-acetone, or Tween 80-ether extracts of infected tissues (mostly mouse brain material for alpha- and flaviviruses) are used. Treatment with protamine sulfate results in precipitation of host material and improvement in the HA patterns. In contrast to most other viruses, the demonstration of HA by togaviruses is dependent on the ionic environment; in general, alphaviruses show optimal activity at pH 5.8 to 6.2 and flaviviruses at 6.2 to 6.4. RUV requires $Ca^{++}$ ions for HA. Dependence on the ionic environment indicates that a specific conformation of the envelope glycoproteins is essential; for example, it has been shown that the isoelectric point of SIN virus E1 protein is the same as the pH that is optimum for HA.

## REPLICATION

Adsorption of alphaviruses to susceptible cells occurs within a few minutes. Because it is dependent on the salt concentration (divalent cations inhibit attachment) and pH but independent of temperature, electrostatic forces are probably involved. The enhancing effect of DEAE-dextran, a polycation, further supports this assumption. Little is known about the requirement for cellular receptors. Since alphaviruses are capable of growing in a variety of cells from phylogenetically unrelated species including mammalian, avian, reptilian, amphibian, piscine, and arthropod, these viruses either have a broad range of receptors or they do not require specific receptors. Penetration of adsorbed virus is dependent on temperature (optimum at 37° C) but independent of the ionic environment and follows first order kinetics. The virion is engulfed by a pinocytotic vacuole and subsequently uncoated.

Replication of viral RNA requires a new protein, a virus-specific RNA-dependent RNA polymerase. For its synthesis, the input parental RNA serves as a messenger. The polymerase is bound to smooth cytoplasmic membranes, where it catalyses the synthesis of so-called replicative intermediates. These consist of partially double-stranded RNA molecules containing one polynucleotide species serving as a template, and a second species of complementary strandedness made up of nascent chains of varying length that are partially base-paired to the template. The major species of alphaviral RNA synthesized in infected cells is not virion RNA ($4.2 \times 10^6$) but a subgenomic RNA species of 26S ($1.6 \times 10^6$) that has the same polarity as virion RNA but contains only one-third of its nucleotide sequences. It serves as the mRNA for the structural proteins of the virion. Studies in SFV-infected cells and with cell-free synthesizing systems have shown that the $5' \rightarrow 3'$ gene order in 26S RNA is C, E3, E2, and E1 and that these proteins are synthesized as a polyprotein of about 130,000 daltons from a single initiation site. By a sequence of nascent and post-translational proteolytic cleavages, this molecule is processed to give the structural virion polypeptides.

The remaining coding capacity corresponding to protein of about 300,000 daltons is used for nonstructural viral polypeptides. Since the 42S RNA is infectious, some, if not all, of these are likely to be components of the viral polymerase. The nucleotide sequence of the 26S RNA is located inward from the 3' end of the 42S RNA, which implies that the genes coding for the nonstructural proteins must be situated in the two thirds of the genome near the 5' terminal. Their synthesis is initiated at a single site near the 5' end and is terminated internally before the structural protein genes. Also, the nonstructural polypeptides are synthesized as a giant precursor molecule that is subsequently processed by proteolytic cleavage.

The alphavirus capsid is assembled in the cytoplasm of the infected cell around the RNA and then attaches to the inner surface of the host cell plasma membrane after that membrane has been modified by the insertion of the virus-specified glycoproteins. The membrane at this stage contains the definite E1 protein and a precursor to the second glycoprotein. The envelopment of the nucleocapsid takes place as it is progressively wrapped into the modified membrane while moving from the cytoplasm to a position physically outside the cell. During the terminal stages of this "budding" process the precursor polypeptide is cleaved to form the E2 glycoprotein.

Intracytoplasmic vacuoles are the first evidence of subcellular alteration associated with virus replication. Alphaviruses and flaviviruses differ with respect to their morphogenesis; the former envelop their capsids by budding preferentially from the marginal membrane, whereas the latter emerge from internal vacuolar membranes. The general picture for RUV resembles that of alphaviruses. Only in alphavirus-infected cells may assembled capsids be detected around cytoplasmic vacuoles.

Different togaviruses vary in the intensity of their cytopathic action, which may depend on the cell species on the one hand and on environmental conditions (medium, pH, temperature, virus dose) on the other. In vertebrate cells growth of alphaviruses is rapid. Only a few hours after infection, newly formed virus is released. Virus production continues at a constant linear rate for up to 10 or 12 hours, approaching 1000 infectious units per cell. Flaviviruses show a latent period of about 12 hours, and a further 10 to 20 hours are required to achieve maximal titers of extracellular virus (Mussgay et al., 1975; Pfefferkorn and Shapiro, 1974).

## PATHOGENIC PROPERTIES

### Alphaviruses and Flaviviruses

The animal classes from which the arthropod-borne togavirus types have been isolated are listed in Tables 1 to 4. Additional information on susceptibility to infection of experimental hosts can be obtained from the *International Catalogue of Arboviruses* (Berge, 1975). In man, infections range in severity from completely subclinical but immunizing ones to rapidly fatal illness. Similar syndromes may be produced by immunologically different viruses, and completely different disease pictures can be caused even by strains of a virus that are immunologically identical.

A tendency to a biphasic temperature curve has been noted, in which the peaks may follow each other without an afebrile interval; this "saddle back" curve is considered typical for YF and DEN infections. However, in infections caused by the tick-borne encephalitis viruses (Table 3) there may be a period of 6 to 14 afebrile days between the two fever peaks. With the first rise in temperature—which may be mild and is often overlooked (in infections with WEE, SLE, and JBE, for example)—systemic infection occurs and virus can be isolated from the blood. The second febrile period is associated with more serious clinical manifestations. During this phase it is often impossible to isolate virus from the blood, and antibodies are usually already demonstrable. During the first febrile attack virus multiplies in the internal organs and leukopenia is usually observed. Leukocytosis is often associated with later, more severe manifestations such as en-

**TABLE 3.  Tick-borne Flaviviruses**

| VIRUS | ABBREVIATION | Ixodid | Argasid | Other | Man | Other Primates | Rodents | Birds | Bats | Marsupials | Other | Sentinels | Africa | Asia | Australasia | Europe | North America | South America | Natural Infection | Lab Infection |
|---|---|---|---|---|---|---|---|---|---|---|---|---|---|---|---|---|---|---|---|---|
| [a]Absettarov | ABS | + | | | + | | | | | | | + | | | | + | | | + | + |
| [a]Hanzalova | HAN | + | | | + | | | | | | | | | | | + | | | + | |
| [a]Hypr | HYPR | + | | | + | | + | + | + | | | + | | | | + | | | + | + |
| Kadam | KAD | + | | | | | | | | | | | + | | | | | | | |
| Karshi | KSI | | + | | | | | | | | | | | + | | | | | | |
| [a]Kumlinge | KUM | + | | | + | | + | + | | | | + | | | | + | | | + | + |
| [a]Kyasanur Forest dis. | KFD | + | + | + | + | + | + | + | + | | | + | | + | | | | | + | + |
| Langat | LGT | + | | | | | | | | | | | | + | | | | | | |
| [a]Louping ill | LI | + | | | + | | + | + | | | | + | | | | + | | | + | + |
| [a]Negishi | NEG | + | | | + | | | | | | | | | + | | | | | + | + |
| [a]Omsk hem. fev. | OMSK | + | | | + | | + | | | | | + | | + | | | ? | | + | + |
| [a]Powassan | POW | + | | | + | | + | | | | | + | | | | | + | | + | |
| Royal Farm | RF | | + | | | | | | | | | | | + | | | | | | |
| [a]Russian spring summer enceph. | RSSE | + | | | + | | + | + | | | | | | + | | + | | | + | + |
| Tyuleniy | TYV | + | | | | | | | | | | | | + | | | + | | | |

[a]Encephalitis in man has been observed after infection with the indicated viruses.

From Berge, T. O. (ed.): International Catalogue of Arboviruses. Washington, D.C., U.S. Department of Health, Education, and Welfare, 1975.

**TABLE 4. Other Flaviviruses, No Arthropod Vector Demonstrated**

| VIRUS | ABBREVIATION | Man | Other Primates | Rodents | Birds | Bats | Marsupials | Other | Sentinels | Africa | Asia | Australasia | Europe | North America | South America | Natural Infection | Lab Infection |
|---|---|---|---|---|---|---|---|---|---|---|---|---|---|---|---|---|---|
| | | ISOLATED FROM (Vertebrates) | | | | | | | | ISOLATED IN | | | | | | HUMAN DISEASE | |
| Apoi | APOI | | | + | | | | | | | + | | | | | | + |
| Batu Cave | BC | | | | | + | | | | | + | | | | | | |
| Carey Island | CI | | | | | + | | | | | + | | | | | | |
| Cowbone Ridge | CR | | | + | | | | | | | | | | + | | | |
| Dakar bat | DB | + | | | | + | | | | + | | | | | | | |
| Entebbe bat | ENT | | | | | + | | | | + | | | | | | | |
| Israel turkey meningo. | IT | | | | + | | | | | | + | | | | | | |
| Jutipa | JUT | | | + | | | | | | | | | | | + | | |
| Koutango | KOU | | | + | | | | | | + | | | | | | | |
| Modoc | MOD | | | + | | | | | | | | | | + | | | |
| Montana myotis leuko. | MML | | | | | + | | | | | | | | + | | | |
| Phnom-Penh bat | PPB | | | | | + | | | | | + | | | | | | |
| Rio Bravo | RB | | | | | + | | | | | | | | + | | + | + |
| Saboya | SAB | | | + | | | | | | + | | | | | | | |
| Sokuluk | SOK | | | | | + | | | | | + | | | | | | |

From Berge, T. O. (ed.): International Catalogue of Arboviruses. Washington, D.C., U.S. Department of Health, Education and Welfare, 1975.

cephalitis. No consistent clinical picture is associated with arbo-togavirus infections. An influenza-like syndrome is observed in mild infections with accompanying headache, nausea, fever, gastrointestinal disturbances, myalgia, and joint pains. Encephalitis in humans and domestic animals is known to be caused by the alphaviruses EEE, VEE, and WEE; the flaviviruses that at times produce central nervous conditions are SLE, JBE, MVE, WN, members of the tick-borne flaviviruses, and possibly ILH. Hepatitis is a typical manifestation of YF in man and has also been observed after infection with KFD. Maculopapular rashes with lymphadenopathy are common in DEN infections and have also been reported for WN, CHIK, and ONN infections. Hemorrhages of varying severity are observed in some DEN epidemics, and in OMSK and KFD infections. The black vomit ("vomito negro") of YF is the result of gastric hemorrhages.

The DEN hemorrhagic fever and a newly recognized DEN shock syndrome (which occurs with significant mortality especially in children in Asia) are known to be immunologic diseases. The four DEN serotypes do not confer a high level of cross-protection; nevertheless, there is a rapid serologic response when an individual who has recovered from an attack of DEN caused by one serotype is infected with another. The secondary antibody response coincides with viremia due to the superinfecting DEN type; circulating immune complexes are then formed, and complement depletion occurs. The immune complexes are deposited in the vessel walls, and hemorrhagic fever and shock result (Theiler and Downs, 1973).

## Rubella Virus

Primates appear to be the natural hosts of RUV; in monkeys (rhesus and African monkeys) infection occasionally causes symptoms but is mostly inapparent. Ferrets, hamsters, guinea pigs, rabbits, and newborn mice also have been found to support multiplication of RUV in vivo and display no clinical signs. Infection in pregnant rats can cause teratogenic damage to the offspring that is similar to that seen in human infants with congenital rubella.

Postnatal infection in adult man frequently starts with mild fever, headache, malaise, and respiratory symptoms some days before the appearance of a maculopapular rash associated with lymphadenopathy. The latter symptom is a prominent feature of the disease, whereas the rash may be absent, especially in younger individuals. Although postnatal infection usually follows a benign course, arthritis, thrombocytopenic purpura, and encephalitis may occur as complications.

The pathogenic significance of RUV lies in its teratogenic properties. About 10 to 15 per cent of living infants born to mothers with apparent or inapparent rubella during the first trimester of pregnancy show evidence of infection that is recognizable at birth or during the first year of life. The consequences of in utero infection include spontaneous abortion, stillbirth, and live birth with moderate to severe abnormalities, as well as completely normal infants. The congenital rubella syndrome consists of neurologic and developmental defects such as hearing loss, eye lesions (pearly cataract, glaucoma, chorioretinitis, microphthalmia, corneal clouding), cardiovascular defects, hepatosplenomegaly, thrombocytopenic purpura, anemia, interstitial pneumonia, metaphyseal bone lesions, and intrauterine growth retardation. Any combination of anomalies may occur in an individual infant.

## IMMUNITY

In infected or vaccinated individuals togaviral antigens cause a pronounced immune response that can be measured in vitro; like most viruses that produce systemic disease with a viremia, togavirus infection is controlled primarily by circulating antibody. Lifelong immunity after a togavirus attack has been observed. For instance, yellow fever antibodies have been found persisting for 75 years in the absence of reexposure. A specific aspect of alphavirus and flavivirus infections is the antibody response of individuals after multiple exposures to antigenically related viruses. In general, with repeated immunizations there is a broadening of the specificity of the antibodies produced and a heightened reaction to the original virus rather than to the virus responsible for reinfection. Thus, sequential infection of humans with two flaviviruses induced neutralizing antibodies that cross-reacted with a third flavivirus to which the subjects had never been exposed. Unfortunately, the existence of cross-reactive antibodies does not necessarily provide resistance to infection. Otherwise, vaccination with a series of carefully selected antigenically related viruses would produce a broad immunity that might be effective against all viruses of this genus. However, this cannot be achieved because of the "original antigenic sin" phenomenon: The immunologic response of a person to a togavirus is dominated throughout his life by his first experience with a virus of that type.

Vaccines against the epidemic and endemic arthropod-borne togavirus infections have been developed for human (medical personnel, laboratory workers, military forces) and veterinary use. Of the inactivated vaccines, formalin-treated TBE virus preparations have been in wide use in the U.S.S.R. Experimental vaccines against other flaviviruses (JBE, SLE, and KFD) have been tested. The accumulated evidence suggests that potent inactivated vaccines can be prepared. The

substrate for virus production must be carefully selected, first for its ability to produce virus in high titer and second for the absence of undesirable components, such as the encephalitogenic factor in brain tissue. A vaccination regime of two initial doses followed by a yearly booster injection has been recommended (Smith, 1969). The immunizing potency of an experimental SFV virion subunit vaccine obtained after different solvent/detergent treatments has been tested in animals. Its efficiency depended on the size of the envelope fragments produced; large fragments (e.g., after Tween 80-ether treatment) offered the best protection (Mussgay et al., 1973).

Of the attenuated live virus vaccines, the YF strains 17D (prepared in chick embryo) and FN (mouse embryo) strains are in common use. The seed virus has to be strictly defined, since loss of immunogenicity has been observed at higher passage levels. The 17D vaccine has been one of the most innocuous and effective vaccines; the first fatality (in a 3-year-old child) was reported after the administration of some 34 million doses and 25 years of use. A number of other live attenuated viruses have given satisfactory antibody responses in human volunteers and experimental animals. Heterotypic immunization using LGT virus, a naturally occurring tick-borne virus from Malaya, against tick-borne viruses highly pathogenic to man (see Table 3) has been successful. When heterotypic vaccinations are used the above-mentioned hazard of immunologic aggravation of diseases must be recognized.

After natural RUV infection, persistent levels of nasopharyngeal-specific IgA, which play an important role in preventing reinfection of adults, have been detected at the portal of entry; cell-mediated immunity has also been demonstrated in tonsillar lymphoid tissue. If fetal infection is to be prevented, adequate and persistent levels of serum antibody, especially IgG, must be present in the mother's plasma. Several attenuated vaccine strains have been developed by serial passages of RUV in vervet monkey kidney cells (HPV 77) followed by passage in primary rabbit kidney (Cendehill) and primary guinea pig kidney cells (the Japanese strain To-336) or in human embryonic kidney cells and W1 38 fibroblasts (RA27/3). Administration of these strains resulted in seroconversion of 95 per cent of susceptible recipients, although antibody levels were often lower than those following naturally acquired disease. Reinfection of reconvalescents or vaccinated individuals does occur and may in fact be responsible for maintaining adequate levels of immunity in a community. In contrast to measles and poliomyelitis, however, the aim of RUV vaccination is not so much to protect the vaccinee herself against a relatively mild disease but to prevent infection of the fetus. Fetal infection is likely to occur only if maternal viremia develops, and viremia has not been observed in immune individuals after either natural or experimental challenge (Banatvala, 1977).

## LABORATORY DIAGNOSIS

### Alphaviruses and Flaviviruses

Suckling mice are considered the universal host system for virus isolation; they are inoculated intracerebrally with sera from patients, post-mortem specimens, or extracts from pools of trapped arthropods. The mice become ill, and frequently have hind limb paralysis, usually two to three days or longer after injection. Affected mice are then sacrificed. Isolation of virus is confirmed by passage of brain suspension material to other suckling mice. For primary isolation, cell cultures of chicken fibroblasts and hamster kidney cells are commonly used; as for continuous lines, Vero (green monkey) and BHK-21 (hamster) cells are routinely employed. Not all cell-virus systems show cytopathic effects after viral multiplication. To isolate virus it is important to inoculate unknown specimens at two or more dilutions, since high concentrations of defective interfering particles may restrict or completely mask the symptoms of infection.

Identification of an isolated agent is usually done by neutralization tests employing mice or cell cultures. The most sensitive animal method is the intraperitoneal inoculation of infant mice with serum-virus mixtures. The reproducibility of this assay is improved by the addition of complement, which in the presence of antibody causes lysis of the viral membrane and inactivation of its genome by RNase. In a neutralization test for virus identification the amount of serum is kept constant and incubated with serial tenfold virus dilutions. By comparing the neutralization indices (the difference in log virus titers in the presence and absence of antibodies) of the virus in question with homologous virus-serum mixtures, type identification can be made. By using this procedure it is also possible to determine the extent of antigenic cross-relationship between viruses within one genus.

In general, cross-reactions between related viruses are more pronounced by hemagglutination inhibition (HI) and complement fixation (CF) tests than by neutralization. From studies on the HI antibody response of experimental animals the following conclusions can be drawn:

1. Each virus, after primary infection, produces a distinctive HI pattern. The reaction may be entirely specific, such that the serum reacts only with the homologous antigen. When cross-reactions occur, they are always significantly lower in titer than the homologous reactions. Cross-reactions are highest with antigens prepared from viruses that are closely related to the immunizing antigen.

2. When animals are inoculated repeatedly with the same virus, the sera are more broadly cross-reactive and titers are higher, but the basic pattern remains the same.

3. Animals immunized to two different viruses of the same genus produce sera that are very widely cross-reactive; their cross-reactivity is always more marked than that observed with sera obtained from animals after two inoculations of the same virus. Anti-flavivirus sera tend to show more pronounced intragenus cross-reactivity than anti-alphavirus sera.

Sera contain nonspecific inhibitors for togavirus HA in high titer; they are lipoproteins and are removed by acetone extraction or adsorption to acid-washed kaolin. In addition, many sera show hemagglutinating activity for goose red blood cells (RBC), which is eliminated by adsorption to erythrocytes before the serum is titrated. Goose RBC are used in many laboratories to test HA, but chicken and pigeon cells (RUV) are also suitable. Optimal temperature is 25° to 37° C for alphaviruses; some flavivirus and RUV require 4° C. Spontaneous elution does not occur.

From the foregoing it is clear that serologic tests for determining the type identity of alphavirus or flavivirus antibodies can be inconclusive, particularly when the sera are collected from patients in endemic areas. In these cases, the mere demonstration of a rise in antibody to a given virus by whatever test is not sufficient evidence that the infection is attributable to the virus used in the test. Only primary infection in individuals not previously exposed to any alphavirus or flavivirus can be reliably diagnosed by means of serology (Theiler and Downs, 1973).

### Rubella Virus

Throat swabs or washings, acute phase blood, cerebrospinal fluid, urine, amniotic fluid, and placental or fetal tissues can be used for isolation in cultures of primary African green monkey kidney, human amnion, RK13 (rabbit), BHK-21 cells, and others. In established cell lines rubella virus may produce a CPE that is markedly influenced by environmental variables (e.g., serum concentration), whereas in primary cells CPE is often absent and virus multiplication must be demonstrated by interference with a challenge virus. For instance, primary African green monkey kidney cells show no evidence of CPE after infection with rubella virus but lose their ability to support growth of added echovirus type 11, coxsackievirus A9, or Newcastle disease virus. From fetal specimens RUV can be best isolated by explanting tissue fragments or trypsinizing fetal tissue; infected cells and media thus obtained can be used for virus identification. Since no antigenic cross-reactions occur between RUV and other togaviruses, unequivocal identification can be made by neutralization of the interfering or cytopathic effect by using a specific antiserum. A more rapid method consists of the application of indirect immunofluorescent antibody staining. In this method, acetone-fixed infected cells on coverslips are incubated with known immune rabbit sera and subsequently with fluorescein-conjugated goat anti-rabbit globulin preparations. The specificity of the cytoplasmic fluorescence must be verified by including preimmune rabbit serum and uninfected cells as controls.

For the determination of RU antibodies, HI, CF, and indirect immunofluorescence are used mostly; the reagents are commercially available. The suggested serologic tests and their interpretations are summarized in Table 5 (Plotkin, 1969). In general, the HI test gives the highest titer levels; CF antibodies tend to fade quickly and are often absent when other tests are still positive. For indirect immunofluorescence a fluorescein isothiocyanate-conjugated anti-human globulin preparation must be used as a second antibody. If this preparation is IgM-specific it can be employed for the diagnosis of congenital infec-

tion (see case E in Table 5). After disease, precipitating antibodies directed against two viral antigens ($\vartheta$ and $\iota$) may be detected in gel double-diffusion tests. Anti-$\vartheta$ antibodies usually parallel those detected by HI, whereas anti-$\iota$ antibodies appear to correlate with resistance to reinfection.

## EPIDEMIOLOGY

For an epidemiologic cycle to occur in nature the following conditions must be met: A critical minimal amount of virus is necessary to establish infection of the arthropod vector. This threshold value is characteristic for every arthropod-virus combination and implies that the virus must circulate in the vertebrate host in sufficient quantities. The susceptibility of a given vector to a given virus can be either inferred from material collected in nature under endemic or epidemic conditions or determined by experimental infection of the arthropod (feeding on or inoculation with virus-containing material). For the virus to be transmitted by the vector, it must pass from the lumen of the arthropod's intestinal tract to susceptible cells, multiply, and reach the salivary glands in quantities adequate to inoculate an infectious dose by bite. This process determines the transmitting efficiency of the vector. Epidemiologically, climate conditions are critical. Thus, the extrinsic incubation period in the vector is shortened by increased temperature. Rainfall

**TABLE 5.  Suggested Testing for Rubella Antibodies in Different Situations**

| | SOURCE OF SERUM | CHOICE OF SEROLOGIC TEST | | | INTERPRETATION |
|---|---|---|---|---|---|
| | | **1st** | **2nd** | **3rd** | |
| A | Patient with rash less than 1 week previously. Convalescent serum 14 to 21 days posteruption | HI | FA | CF | Fourfold rise proves recent infection |
| B | Patient with rash more than 1 week previously. Convalescent serum 21 to 28 days posteruption | CF | FA | HI[a] | Fourfold rise proves recent infection |
| C | Subject in whom immunity is to be determined or pregnant women exposed to rubella | HI | Nt | FA | Presence of antibody at any titer shows immunity |
| D | Possible rubella-syndrome infant older than 6 months | HI | Nt | FA | Presence of antibody suggests congenital infection if child has not been exposed to rubella |
| E | Possible rubella-syndrome infant younger than 6 months | HI | Nt | FA | Presence of antibody suggests congenital infection if titer significantly higher than mother's or if contained in IgM fraction |

[a]Determination of IgM rubella antibody may assist in the diagnosis.

From Plotkin, S. A.: In Lenette, E. H., and Schmidt, N. J. (eds.): Diagnostic Procedures for Viral and Rickettsial Infections. New York, American Public Health Association, 1969.

may favor breeding conditions for mosquitoes. Climate may control the geographic distribution of arboviruses by providing the ecologic conditions for vectors and hosts. Since each species of blood-sucking arthropod has an affinity for a vertebrate species or group of species, detailed knowledge of vector-host preferences or dependencies is essential to the epidemiology and control of arthropod-borne virus diseases. Infection chains and reservoirs (animal species in which virus is maintained and can be disseminated for a prolonged period) have been established for many arthropod-borne togaviruses (Theiler and Downs, 1973).

Rubella virus transmission occurs through droplet infection. The portal of entry is the lymphoid tissue of the pharynx and possibly the conjunctiva. Sources of infection are virus-excreting individuals with or without clinical symptoms. Children with chronic infection are an important source of infection. Rubella has a worldwide distribution. Infections in the northern hemisphere increase during March to May, and more extensive epidemics occur at regular intervals of 5 to 10 years (Norrby, 1969).

## References

Banatvala, J. E.: Rubella vaccines. In Recent Advances in Clinical Virology, Edinburgh, London, New York, Churchill-Livingstone, vol.1, 1977, p. 171.

Berge, T. O. (ed.): International Catalogue of Arboviruses. Washington, D. C., U. S. Department of Health, Education and Welfare, 1975.

Casals, J., and Reeves, W. C.: Arthropod-borne animal viruses. In Rivers, T. M., and Horsfall, F. L. (eds.): Viral and Rickettsial Infections of Man. London, Pitman Medical Publishing Company, 1959, p. 269.

Clarke, D. H., and Casals, J.: Techniques for hemagglutination and hemagglutination-inhibition with arthropod-borne viruses. Am J Trop Med Hyg 7:561, 1958.

Dalrymple, J. M., Schlesinger, S., and Russell, P. K.: Antigenic characterization of two Sindbis envelope glycoproteins separated by isoelectric focusing. Virology 69:93, 1976.

Fenner, F.: Classification and nomenclature of viruses. Intervirology 7:44, 1976.

Horzinek, M. C.; The structure of togaviruses. Progr Med Virol 16:109, 1973.

Karabatsos, N.: Antigenic relationship of group A arboviruses by plaque reduction neutralization testing. Am J Trop Med Hyg 24:527, 1975.

de Madrid, A. T., and Porterfield, J. S.: The flaviviruses (group B arboviruses): A cross-neutralization study. J Gen Virol 23:91, 1974.

Mussgay, M., Weiland, E., Strohmaier, K., Ueberschär, S., and Enzmann, P. J.: Properties of components obtained by treatment of Semliki Forest virus with Tween-80 and tri (N-butyl) phosphate. J Gen Virol 19:89, 1973.

Mussgay, M., Enzmann, P. J., Horzinek, M. C., and Weiland, E.: Growth cycle of arboviruses in vertebrate and arthropod cells. Progr Med Virol 19:257, 1975.

Norrby, E.: Rubella Virus. New York, Springer Verlag, 1969, p. 115.

Pfefferkorn, E. R., and Shapiro, D.: Reproduction of togaviruses. In Fraenkel-Conrat, H., and Wagner, R. R. (eds.): Comprehensive Virology, vol. 2. New York, Plenum Publishing Corporation, 1974, p. 171.

Plotkin, S. A.: Rubella virus. In Lenette, E. H., and Schmidt, N. J. (eds.): Diagnostic Procedures for Viral and Rickettsial Infections. New York, American Public Health Association, 1969, p. 364.

Smith, C. E., Gordon: Arbovirus vaccines. Br Med Bull 25:142, 1969.

Theiler, M., and Downs, W. G.: The Arthropod-Borne Viruses of Vertebrates. New Haven, Yale University Press, 1973.

Wengler, G., Wengler, G., and Filipe, A. R.: A study of nucleotide sequence homology between the nucleic acids of different alphaviruses. Virology 78:124, 1977.

World Health Organizaiton Study Group: Arboviruses and human disease. WHO Technical Report Series No 369, 1967.

# 62  *ARENAVIRUSES*

## *Fritz Lehmann-Grube, M.D.*

### *ARENAVIRUSES*

The group of arenaviruses comprises at present ten members, of which four are pathogenic for man, causing lymphocytic choriomeningitis, Lassa fever, Argentine hemorrhagic fever, and Bolivian hemorrhagic fever. The latter three illnesses are severe and of great public health importance. Arenaviruses are of special interest for investigating virus-host relationships such as pathologic immune phenomena in virus diseases and persistent virus infections.

### *CLASSIFICATION*

The lymphocytic choriomeningitis (LCM) virus was the first arenavirus to be discovered (Table 1).

During serial transfers in monkeys of materials from a fatal case of the 1933 St. Louis epidemic of encephalitis, a virus was encountered that differed from the other isolates of that outbreak. The true origin of this first strain of LCM virus was never determined.

In 1958 the Junin virus was obtained from people suffering from Argentine hemorrhagic fever. The Tacaribe virus was isolated next. Tacaribe virus and Junin virus were antigenically related, as was Machupo virus, recovered from cases of Bolivian hemorrhagic fever in 1965. These three agents formed the Tacaribe complex, soon to be joined by Amapari virus, Tamiami virus, Parana virus, Pichinde virus, and Latino virus.

Similarities between Machupo virus and LCM virus were noted early, but it was their striking

**TABLE 1.** Isolation History and Natural Occurrence of Viruses Presently Recognized as Arenaviruses

| VIRUS | FIRST ISOLATION | | NATURAL OCCURRENCE | |
|---|---|---|---|---|
| | Reference | Source | Principal Host | Geographic Distribution |
| LCM | Armstrong and Lillie (1934) | Monkey (?) | *Mus musculus* | America, Europe |
| Lassa | Buckley and Casals (1970) | Man | *Mastomys natalensis* | Africa (Sierra Leone, Nigeria; other parts) |
| Amapari | Pinheiro et al. (1966) | *Oryzomys* sp. *Neacomys guianae* | *Oryzomys capito Neacomys guianae* | South America (Brazil) |
| Junin | Parodi et al. (1958) | Man | *Calomys laucha\* Akodon azarae* | South America (Argentina) |
| Latino | Webb et al. (1973) | *Calomys callosus* | *Calomys callosus* | South America (Bolivia, Brazil) |
| Machupo | Johnson et al. (1965) | Man | *Calomys callosus* | South America (Boliva) |
| Parana | Webb et al. (1970) | *Oryzomys buccinatus* | *Oryzomys buccinatus* | South America (Paraguay) |
| Pichinde | Trapido and Sanmartin (1971) | *Oryzomys albigularis Thomasomys lugens†* | *Oryzomys albigularis* | South America (Colombia) |
| Tacaribe | Downs et al. (1963) | *Artibeus lituratus‡ Artibeus jamaicensis* Mosquitoes | ?‡ | Central America (Trinidad) |
| Tamiami | Calisher et al. (1970) | *Sigmodon hispidus* | *Sigmodon hispidus* | North America (Florida) |

\*Predominantly *C. laucha musculinus.*
†Subspecies *T. lugens fuscatus.*
‡Isolated between March 1956 and December 1958 from 11 bats and one pool of mosquitoes, but never since.

morphologic resemblance that led to the proposal that the Tacaribe complex viruses and LCM virus should form a taxonomic group. In 1970 the agent causing Lassa fever was isolated from patients with the disease in Nigeria. Its relatedness with the LCM virus was soon recognized, and in the same year a new virus group was defined containing LCM, Lassa, and the Tacaribe complex viruses. The proposed name was arenoviruses (from the Latin word *arenosus*, meaning sandy) — later changed to arenaviruses — which was to reflect the characteristic granules seen by electron microscopy in ultrathin sections of infected cells (Rowe et al., 1970). By approval of the International Committee on Taxonomy of Viruses this virus group has been given the status of a genus named *Arenavirus* belonging to the family *Arenaviridae*; type species is the LCM virus (Fenner, 1976).

## MORPHOLOGY AND BIOCHEMICAL PROPERTIES

Of the many features that the arenaviruses have in common, the morphology of virus particles is salient (Murphy and Whitfield, 1975). Overall shape as well as structural details are identical. Arenavirus particles are round or pleomorphic with diameters of 50 to 300 nm (average 120 nm). In vivo and in vitro they are released from the infected cell by budding (Fig. 1). The viral envelopes are formed from plasma membranes: the density of both layers as well as the width of the intermediary zone increase, and club-shaped surface projections, approximately 10 nm long, are inserted often forming well-delineated margins. In their interior, arenavirus particles characteristically contain variable numbers of electron-dense granules that resemble cellular ribosomes, although morphologic, cytochemical, and functional differences have been noted (Dalton et al., 1968; Mannweiler and Lehmann-Grube, 1973; Welsh et al., 1975). They are usually randomly distributed, but sometimes they are arranged beneath the envelope in a circular pattern. If they are indeed host cell ribosomes, they are not essential for infectivity (Leung and Rawls, 1977). Perhaps they are accidentally incorporated during the budding process as are glycogen granules that have occasionally been observed inside arenavirus particles (Kajima and Majde, 1970).

Nucleocapsids have never been observed in arenavirus particles by thin section electron microscopy of infected cells. Such structures have been visualized, however, in purified preparations after removal of the viral envelopes with detergent (Palmer et al., 1977; Vezza et al., 1977; Gard et al., 1977). Their form varied among different arenaviruses, which may represent dissimilar architectures of individual members but, more likely, resulted from technical differences.

Many determinations of the size of the infec-

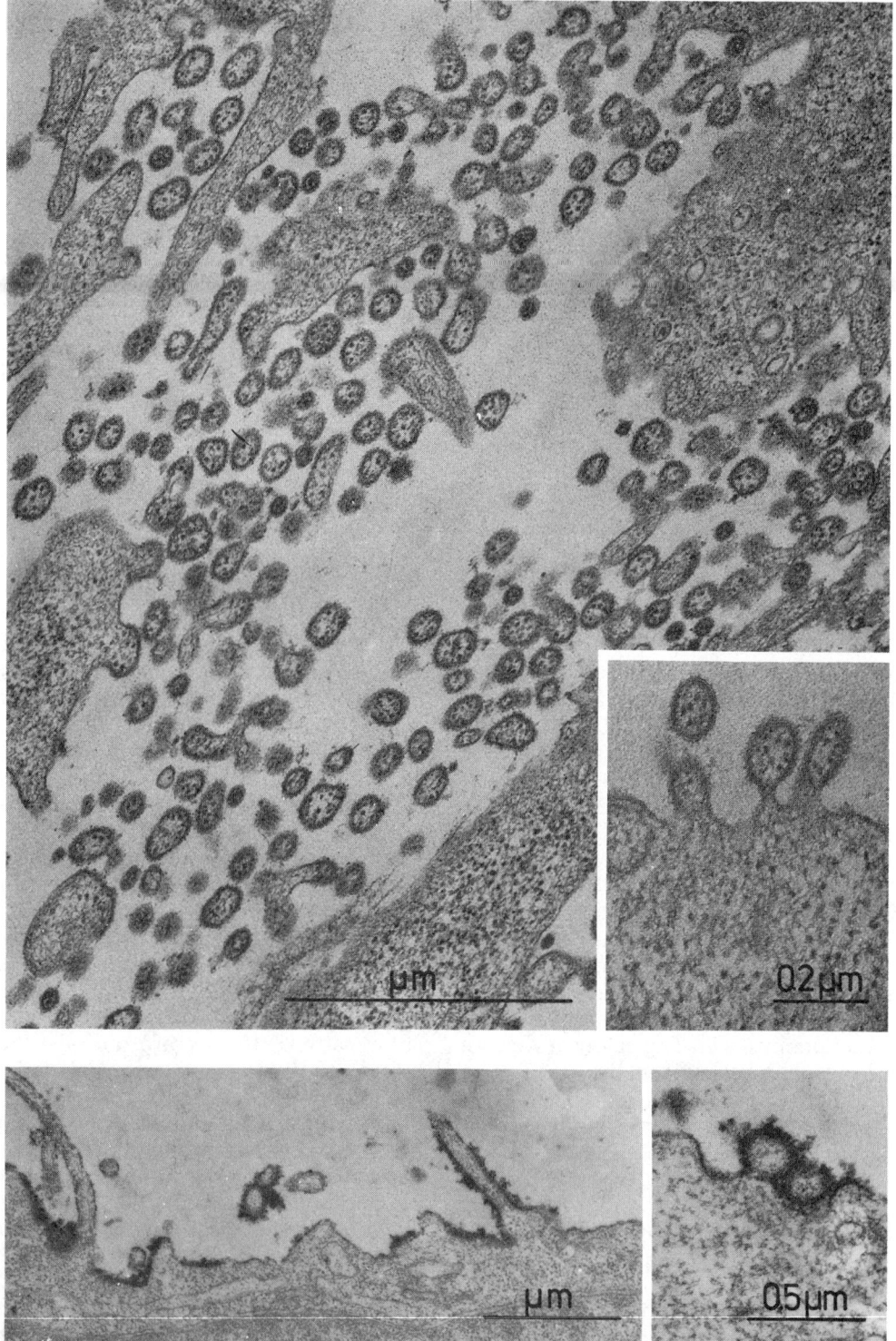

**FIGURE 1.**    *Thin section electron micrographs of LCM virus-infected cultivated mouse (L) cells.*
*Above. Multiple arenavirus particles are seen either released from the plasma membrane or still budding.*
*Below. Demonstration by means of the immunoperoxidase method of LCM virus-specific antigen(s) in association with budding virus particles and in distinct areas of the plasma membrane that are not otherwise visibly altered. Photographs kindly supplied by Dr. K. Mannweiler, Hamburg.*

tious unit by various physical methods have given greatly divergent results, not only between different arenaviruses but also for one virus with different methods. Immuno–electron microscopy has shown (Fig. 1) that the characteristic particles budding from infected cells contain viral antigen(s). However, whether they are all virions and potentially infectious is unknown.

The nucleic acid of arenaviruses is single stranded RNA (Pfau, 1974) consisting of four components that sediment with 31 to 33S, 28S, 22 to 25S, and 18S, respectively. Small molecules with 4 to 6S have also been identified, and a 15S species has been resolved in Pichinde virus, but not yet in other arenaviruses. Present evidence indicates that the 31 to 33S ("L") and the 22 to 25S ("S") RNA classes are coded for by the virus and contain the viral genetic information. In contrast, the 28S and 18S RNA components originate from host cell ribosomes. They probably correspond to the ribosome-like granules seen inside arenavirus particles by electron microscopy (see above). The small RNA species resemble host cell transfer RNA with respect to both size and methylation ratio (Pedersen, 1973; Farber and Rawls, 1975; Vezza et al., 1978).

The virus-specific RNA (L and S) from the virions of Pichinde virus does not have properties of messenger RNA. Polysomal RNA, however, from virus-infected cells does have properties of messenger RNA and, furthermore, is complementary to the virion RNA (Leung et al., 1977). These findings, together with the demonstration of an association of RNA-dependent RNA polymerase with the virion (Carter et al., 1974), strongly suggest that the Pichinde virus RNA — and by analogy the RNA of the other arenaviruses — is negative stranded. This conclusion would explain why attempts to prepare infectious RNA from virions

of LCM virus were unsuccessful (Welsh et al., 1975).

The protein composition of the arenaviruses is less complex than their morphology suggests. Analyses have disclosed three major proteins for LCM and Pichinde virions and only two for Tacaribe and Tamiami virions (Table 2). The place of Junin virus within the two groups is undecided. In view of the divergent results obtained for one virus (Pichinde) by different investigators, the significance of the differences of molecular weights between individual arenaviruses is uncertain. However, the difference of the number of structural polypeptides is real, and is one noteworthy exception to the rule that these viruses possess similar properties. In addition to the (two or three) major proteins, several minor ones have been found associated with the virions (Table 2), but whether all these are of viral origin is not certain.

The arenaviruses disintegrate rapidly in the presence of lipid solvents and detergents, indicating that lipids are needed for their structural integrity. By analogy with other budding viruses, these lipids probably are derived from the host cell membrane forming part of the viral envelope. The glycoproteins are situated on or close to the surface of the virion, probably in the spikes. The one nonglycosylated major protein has always been found in association with the RNA and is probably part of the ribonucleoprotein complex.

The buoyant densities of the infectious units of different arenaviruses vary between 1.17 and 1.18 when determined in sucrose and between 1.18 and 1.20 when determined in CsCl (Pfau, 1974). Gschwender et al. (1975) arrived at values for LCM virus of 1.22 in CsCl and 1.14 in a gradient formed of iodinated organic compounds.

During replication of LCM virus, in addition to

**TABLE 2. Structural Proteins of Arenaviruses**

| | MAJOR PROTEINS | | | | |
| | Glycosylated | | Nonglycosylated | | |
| VIRUS | 1 | 2 | | | REFERENCE |
|---|---|---|---|---|---|
| LCM | "GP-1" 44* | "GP-2" 35 | "NP" 63 | | Buchmeier and Oldstone (1978) |
| Pichinde | "V$_{II}$" 72 | "V$_{III}$" 34 | "V$_I$" 72† | | Ramos et al. (1972) |
| | "G1" 64 | "G2" 38 | "N" 66†,‡ | | Vezza et al. (1977) |
| Tacaribe | None | "G" 42 | "N" 68‡ | | Gard et al. (1977) |
| Tamiami | None | "G" 44 | "N" 66‡ | | Gard et al. (1977) |
| Junin | | "5" 38§ | "3" 64§ | | Martínez Segovia and De Mítri (1977) |

*Designation and approximate molecular weight ($\times 10^3$).

†A minor nonglycosylated protein with molecular weight $12 \times 10^3$ was not reproducibly found.

‡In addition, one minor nonglycosylated protein ("P") with molecular weight $77 \times 10^3$ (Pichinde virus and Tamiami virus) and $79 \times 10^3$ (Tacaribe virus).

§In addition, three minor glycoproteins ("1," "2," "4") with molecular weights $91 \times 10^3$, $72 \times 10^3$, $52 \times 10^3$, and one minor nonglycosylated protein ("6") with molecular weight $25 \times 10^3$.

fully infectious (standard) virus, particles are produced that cannot multiply by themselves but reduce the infectious yield and, if the standard virus is cytolytic, abolish cytopathic effects. These interfering particles are slightly less dense and relatively resistant to ultraviolet light, neutral red, and heat (Welsh et al., 1975; Popescu et al., 1976). Although these properties are characteristic for defective interfering (DI) particles, there is one essential difference. "By definition DI particles are defective virions, which can grow only in the presence of a helper standard virus" (Huang, 1973). In contrast, LCM virus-interfering particles multiply predominantly in cells infected by standard virus alone rather than in cells dually infected with standard virus and interfering particles (Lehmann-Grube et al., 1975). Interfering particles have also been detected in association with several other arenaviruses (Pfau, 1977).

## ANTIGENIC COMPOSITION

Serologic relationships between arenaviruses have been demonstrated by complement-fixation tests (Casals et al., 1975) and immunofluorescence procedures (Wulff et al., 1978). In the case of Tacaribe complex viruses, the viral component responsible for cross-reactivity is the viral nucleoprotein (Buchmeier and Oldstone, personal communication). As a rule, serologic relationships cannot be demonstrated by use of the neutralization test with one notable exception: guinea pigs infected with Tacaribe virus develop protective immunity against Junin virus and also Junin virus-neutralizing antibody (Weissenbacher et al., 1975).

The immunogen that induces complement-fixing antibody has been characterized for LCM and Pichinde viruses (Gschwender et al., 1976; Buchmeier et al., 1977). It is produced in abundance in infected cells and is also a structural component of the virion; it is not, however, represented on the surface of either the virion or the infected cell and is distinct from the antigen combining with neutralizing antibody. Although serologically indistinguishable, the complement-fixing antigen from infected cells differs chemically from the antigen that is associated with the virion. Possibly the cell-associated polypeptides with complement-fixing activity are cleavage products of the nucleocapsid protein, which is the carrier of the complement-fixing activity residing inside the virion.

By necessity, the immunogen leading to the formation of neutralizing antibody is on the surface of the virion, but its chemical nature is unknown; presumably it is a glycoprotein.

In double immunodiffusion tests in agar using extracts of LCM or Pichinde virus-infected cells and the respective antisera one line of precipitation is consistently formed. Its antigenic component is heat-stable and pronase-resistant, and corresponds to the complement-fixing antigen just mentioned. A second line is weaker and less regularly observed; its antigenic component is heat-labile and susceptible to the activity of the enzyme (Bro-Jørgensen, 1971; Buchmeier et al., 1977).

In the cytoplasm of LCM virus infected cells two types of antigens can be distinguished by immunofluorescence (Rutter and Gschwender, 1973). One consists of coarse granules with bright fluorescence; serologically it is identical with the complement-fixing antigen mentioned above. The other antigen has a fine dust-like distribution; its relationship with viral structures is not known.

Several methods detect new antigens on the surfaces of LCM virus-infected cells. Letting the viable cell interact with fluorescein-labeled antibody and inspecting it with an immunofluorescence microscope is one, and incubating the infected cell with antiserum plus complement and watching for lysis is another (Rutter and Gschwender, 1973). New antigens on the surface of LCM virus-infected cells have also been localized by immuno–electron microscopy (Mannweiler and Lehmann-Grube, 1973). Not surprisingly, budding viruses are thus labeled. In addition, virus-specific antigen is found in areas of the plasma membrane where morphologic alterations are not apparent (Fig. 1). Whether they are sites in which budding of virions is imminent or whether some other viral antigen is labeled that is not part of the surface of the viral particles is not known.

The LCM virus does not damage vital tissues of the mouse, at least not enough to impair function (Lehmann-Grube, 1971). Nonetheless, infection of an adult mouse with LCM virus results in severe, sometimes lethal, disease. The explanation is that the immune response may kill the host; the LCM disease of the adult mouse is a pathologic immune response to virus-induced antigens (Hotchin, 1962). The antigens (allergens) that induce the allergic response must be on the surface of infected cells, but whether they are the budding virions or other virus-induced alterations of the cell membrane or a combination of both has not been decided. The immune response of the mouse leading to disease and even death is entirely cell-mediated; T lymphocytes play an essential role (Cole and Nathanson, 1974; Johnson et al., 1978). It is postulated that they damage virus-infected cells of mouse tissues just as the cytotoxic T cells damage virus-infected target cells in vitro (Zinkernagel and Doherty, 1977).

Similar observations have been made with other arenavirus-host combinations — for instance, LCM virus-adult rat, Junin virus-suckling mouse, Tamiami virus-suckling mouse, Lassa fever virus-adult mouse — but in none of these has the immunopathologic nature of the disease been as convincingly demonstrated as in the LCM virus-infected adult mouse.

## VIRUS-HOST RELATIONSHIPS

The host range of LCM virus is so wide that no mammalian species is known to resist infection. Virus strains differ in pathogenic properties. As a rule, disease signs are moderate or not detected; but there are exceptions. One has already been mentioned: the adult mouse responds with a severe illness to infection with LCM virus. Clinical signs also develop in humans and monkeys. One widely employed virus strain ("WE") is absolutely lethal for guinea pigs; in other words, one guinea pig infectious dose of WE strain virus is identical with one lethal dose. In vitro, too, cells from most mammalian species can be infected with LCM virus and respond with replication of infectious virus. Whether virus multiplication is accompanied by cytopathic effects depends on the strain of virus and its previous passage history as much as on origin and properties of the host cells. For instance, passage of LCM virus through mouse brains selects for cytolytic variants, whereas prolonged replication in the mouse spleen results predominantly in noncytopathogenic virus (Popescu and Lehmann-Grube, 1976). Cytopathic effects are blocked by interfering particles (see above).

The principal hosts of the other arenaviruses are listed in Table 1. Infection with Lassa virus of squirrel monkey (*Saimiri scirreus*) and guinea pig (Walker et al., 1975), with Machupo virus of rhesus and cynomolgus monkeys (*Macaca mulatta* and *M. fascicularis*), suckling mouse and suckling hamster, strain C-13 guinea pig, and marmoset (*Saguinus geoffroyi*) (Eddy et al., 1975; Webb et al., 1975), and with Junin virus of guinea pig and suckling mouse (Weissenbacher et al., 1975) leads to disease signs that often resemble human Lassa fever, Bolivian hemorrhagic fever, and Argentine hemorrhagic fever, respectively. Most arenaviruses multiply with cytopathic effects in Vero cells; other cell lines widely employed are L and BHK21.

Arenaviruses have attracted much attention by their propensity to establish prolonged infections in rodents but there is no reason to assume that prolonged infection is restricted to these animals.

The best studied example is the persistent infection of *M. musculus* with LCM virus. When a mouse is infected with LCM virus in utero or shortly after birth, it becomes a lifelong carrier, meaning that the virus is not eliminated and that it multiplies in all organs without causing overt disease (Fig. 2). Although carrier mice respond normally to most antigens, LCM virus-specific antibodies are formed at only low concentrations or cannot be detected (Volkert et al., 1975), and LCM virus-specific cell-mediated immunity is absent (Cihak and Lehmann-Grube, 1978). Since immune elimination of LCM virus is readily accomplished by mice infected as adult animals, failure of virus elimination by a mouse infected congenitally or neonatally is attributed to LCM virus-specific immunologic tolerance (Volkert et al., 1975).

In carrier mice, replication of the virus is regulated so as to replenish losses due to natural decay, but not allow uninhibited increase. The mechanism of virus control is probably very complex (Lehmann-Grube, 1977) and presumably in-

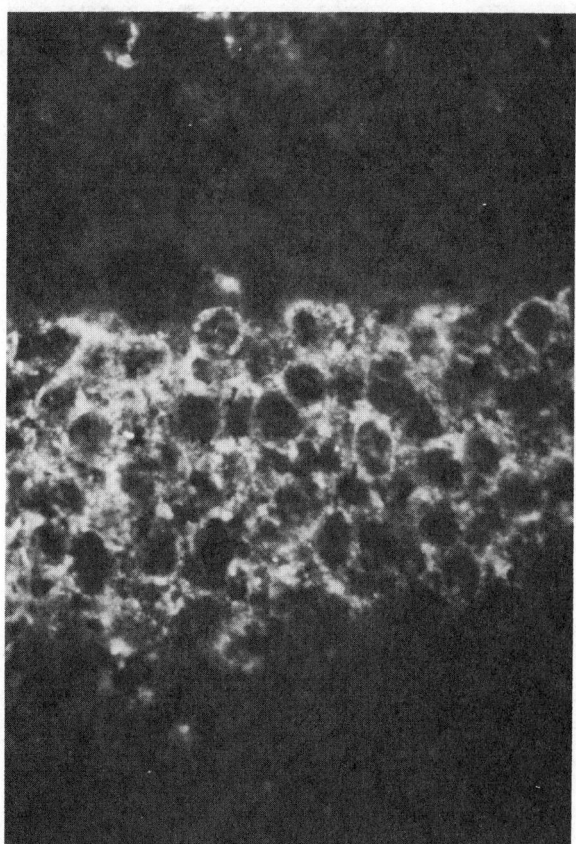

**FIGURE 2.** *Brain of an LCM virus carrier mouse (stratum granulosum areae dentatae of the hippocampal region). Infected cells, primarily neurons, are visualized by immunofluorescence procedure. Photograph kindly supplied by Dr. J. Löhler, Hamburg.*

volves interfering particles that are generated in LCM virus-carrier mice (Popescu and Lehmann-Grube, 1977).

The type of virus-host relationship exemplified by LCM virus *M. musculus* has been termed persistent tolerant infection; its salient features are lifelong duration, lack of a specific immune response, and absence of disease signs. Vertical transmission is also characteristic of the LCM virus-mouse relationship, but not a *conditio sine qua non* for designating an infection persistent tolerant.

The statement that mice persistently infected with LCM virus remain healthy requires qualification. In certain mouse strain-virus strain combinations aging carrier mice develop a "late onset disease" (Hotchin and Collins, 1964) characterized by runting and shortened life span. Many organs are affected, but a mesangioproliferative glomerulonephritis is prominent (Fig. 3). The evidence that the pathogenic mechanism is formation and deposition of immune complexes (Fig. 4) is impressive (Oldstone, 1975). However, the im-

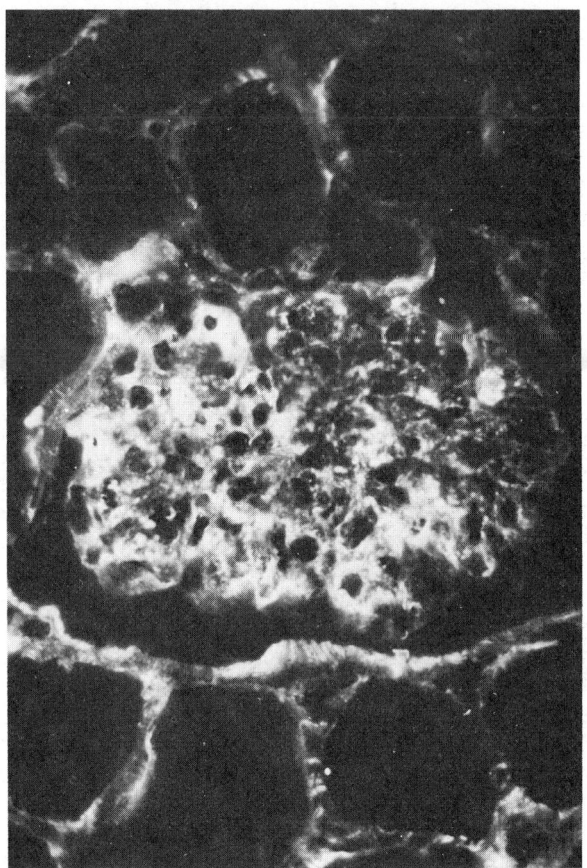

**FIGURE 4.** *Deposition of immune complexes in the kidney of an LCM virus carrier mouse. Host immunoglobulin in the subendothelial space of capillaries and basement membrane of Bowman's capsule of a glomerulus and in the basement membranes of tubuli is visualized by immunofluorescence procedure. Photograph kindly supplied by Dr. J. Löhler, Hamburg.*

munologic specificity of the deposits has not been unequivocally determined.

With the exception of Tacaribe virus all arenaviruses have been isolated from rodents with prolonged infections. However, only for LCM virus *Mus musculus* has the pattern of infection been fully established. Reduced virus-specific immune responsiveness has been documented in several instances, especially well for *C. callosus* infected with Machupo virus (Justines and Johnson, 1969), but it is uncertain whether other arenavirus-host combinations (listed in Table 1) are persistent tolerant infections or merely unusually prolonged, in which case they should be termed chronic.

A better understanding of prolonged infection has been obtained by analyzing persistent infections of cell cultures with LCM virus in L cells and LCM virus, Parana virus, and Pichinde virus in BHK21 cells (Pfau, 1977). It appears that regulation of these infections, which go on for years, depends on an intricate interplay involving cells, virulent standard virus, attenuated standard

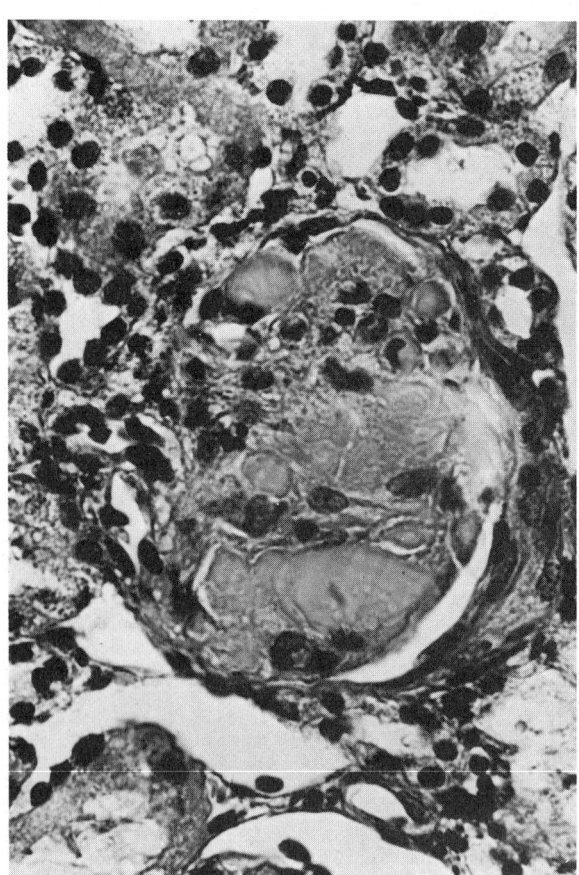

**FIGURE 3.** *Final stage of glomerulonephritis of an LCM virus carrier mouse as part of late onset disease. Note the marked hyalinization of the glomerulum. Photograph kindly supplied by Dr. J. Löhler, Hamburg.*

virus, and interfering particles (Lehmann-Grube et al., 1975).

## EPIDEMIOLOGY

The LCM virus has been found throughout Europe and America; whether it is distributed worldwide, as often stated, is doubtful (Lehmann-Grube, 1971). All other members of this group occur in small areas in South and Central America and in Africa. With the exception of the Tacaribe virus, arenaviruses are maintained in nature by rodents, and rodents are the principal source for infections of other animals and man. The mode of spread is not known with certainty, but the high virus concentrations in nasal secretions, saliva, and urine suggest that the virus is disseminated either by direct contact or via fomites and food. Airborne transmission is a further possibility. Arthropod vectors have never been convincingly incriminated.

The principal host for LCM virus is the persistently infected grey house mouse (*Mus musculus*) (Armstrong et al., 1940). More recently, the Syrian hamster (*Mesocricetus auratus*) has also been identified as an important source for human infections (Ackermann et al., 1972; Gregg, 1975). Probably this animal is not a natural host of LCM virus but is infected from house mice that invade the hamsteries (Skinner et al., 1976). Transmission among members of mammalian species other than *M. musculus* and *M. auratus* are rare. In only one instance has man-to-man infection been documented; the circumstances were unusual (Smadel et al., 1942). Lassa virus is indigenous to certain areas of Africa where it is maintained by *Mastomys natalensis* (Monath, 1975). Unlike infections with other arenaviruses, Lassa virus is easily transmitted from person to person and several hospital-centered outbreaks with usually one index case and secondary infections of medical personnel and visitors have been described. Outbreaks have also occurred in communities. Sources for human infections with Machupo and Junin viruses, etiologic agents of Bolivian and Argentine hemorrhagic fevers, are rodents of the genera *Calomys* and *Akodon* (Johnson et al., 1973; Sabattini et al., 1977). As the names indicate, these diseases occur in Bolivia and Argentina, where they cause considerable health problems.

## References

Ackermann, R., Stille, W., Blumenthal, W., Helm, E.B., Keller, K., und Baldus, O.: Syrische Goldhamster als Uberträger von Lymphozytärer Choriomeningitis. Dtsch med Wsch 97:1725, 1972.

Armstrong, C., and Lillie, R.D.: Experimental lymphocytic choriomeningitis of monkeys and mice produced by a virus encountered in studies of the 1933 St. Louis encephalitis epidemic. Public Health Rep 49:1019, 1934.

Armstrong, C., Wallace, J.J., and Ross, L.: Lymphocytic choriomeningitis. Gray mice, *Mus musculus*, a reservoir for the infection. Public Health Rep 55:1222, 1940.

Bro-Jørgensen, K.: Characterization of virus-specific antigen in cell culture infected with lymphocytic choriomeningitis virus. Acta path microbiol scand, Sect B 79:466, 1971.

Buchmeier, M.J., Gee, S.R., and Rawls, W.E.: Antigens of Pichinde virus. I. Relationship of soluble antigens derived from infected BHK-21 cells to the structural components of the virion. J Virol 22:175, 1977.

Buchmeier, M.J., and Oldstone, M.B.A.: Virus-induced immune complex disease: identification of specific viral antigens and antibodies deposited in complexes during chronic lymphocytic choriomeningitis virus infection. J Immun 120:1297, 1978.

Buckley, S.M., and Casals, J.: Lassa fever, a new virus disease of man from West Africa. III. Isolation and characterization of the virus. Am J Trop Med 19:680, 1970.

Calisher, C.H., Tzianabos, T., Lord, R.D., and Coleman, P.H.: Tamiami virus, a new member of the Tacaribe group. Am J Trop Med 19:520, 1970.

Carter, M.F., Biswal, N., and Rawls, W.E.: Polymerase activity of Pichinde virus. J Virol 13:577, 1974.

Casals, J., Buckley, S.M., and Cedeno, R.: Antigenic properties of the arenaviruses. Bull WHO 52:421, 1975.

Cihak, J., and Lehmann-Grube, F.: Immunological tolerance to lymphocytic choriomeningitis virus in neonatally infected virus carrier mice: evidence supporting a clonal inactivation mechanism. Immunology 34:265, 1978.

Cole, G.A., and Nathanson, N.: Lymphocytic choriomeningitis. Pathogenesis. Progr Med Virol 18:94, 1974.

Dalton, A.J., Rowe, W.P., Smith, G.H., Wilsnack, R.E., and Pugh, W.E.: Morphological and cytochemical studies on lymphocytic choriomeningitis virus. J Virol 2:1465, 1968.

Downs, W.G., Anderson, C.R., Spence, L., Aitken, T.H.G., and Greenhall, A.H.: Tacaribe virus, a new agent isolated from *Artibeus* bats and mosquitoes in Trinidad, West Indies. Am J Trop Med 12:640, 1963.

Eddy, G.A., Scott, S.K., Wagner, F.S., and Brand, O.M.: Pathogenesis of Machupo virus infection in primates. Bull WHO 52:517, 1975.

Farber, F.E., and Rawls, W.E.: Isolation of ribosome-like structures from Pichinde virus. J Gen Virol 26:21, 1975.

Fenner, F.: Classification and nomenclature of viruses. Second report of the International Committee on Taxonomy of Viruses. Intervirology 7:1, 1976.

Gard, G.P., Vezza, A.C., Bishop, D.H.L., and Compans, R.W.: Structural proteins of Tacaribe and Tamiami virions. Virology 83:84, 1977.

Gregg, M.B.: Recent outbreaks of lymphocytic choriomeningitis in the United States of America. Bull WHO 52:549, 1975.

Gschwender, H.H., Rutter, G., and Lehmann-Grube, F.: Lymphocytic choriomeningitis virus. II. Characterization of extractable complement-fixing activity. Med Microbiol Immunol 162:119, 1976.

Gschwender, H.H., Rutter, G., and Popescu, M.: Use of iodinated organic compounds for the density gradient centrifugation of viruses. Arch Virol 49:359, 1975.

Hotchin, J.: The biology of lymphocytic choriomeningitis infection: virus-induced immune disease. Cold Spr Harb Symp Quant Biol 27:479, 1962.

Hotchin, J., and Collins, D.N.: Glomerulonephritis and late onset disease of mice following neonatal virus infection. Nature 203:1357, 1964.

Huang, A.S.: Defective interfering viruses. Ann Rev Microbiol 27:101, 1973.

Johnson, E.D., Monjan, A.A., and Morse, H.C.: Lack of B-cell participation in acute lymphocytic choriomeningitis disease of the central nervous system. Cell Immunol 36:143, 1978.

Johnson, K.M., Webb, P.A., and Justines, G.: Biology of Tacaribe-complex viruses. In Lehmann-Grube, F. (ed.): Lymphocytic Choriomeningitis Virus and Other Arenaviruses. Berlin, Heidelberg, New York, Springer-Verlag, 1973, p. 241.

Johnson, K.M., Wiebenga, N.H., Mackenzie, R.B., Kuns, M.L., Tauraso, N.M., Shelokov, A., Webb, P.A., Justines, G., and Beye, H.K.: Virus isolations from human cases of hemorrhagic fever in Bolivia. Proc Soc Exper Biol Med 118:113, 1965.

Justines, G., and Johnson, K.M.: Immune tolerance in *Calomys callosus* infected with Machupo virus. Nature 222:1090, 1969.

Kajima, M., and Majde, J.: LCM virus as a carrier of non-viral cellular components. Electron microscopic evidence. Naturwissenschaften 57:93, 1970.

Lehmann-Grube, F.: Lymphocytic Choriomeningitis Virus. Virology Monographs Vol. 10. Wien and New York, Springer-Verlag, 1971.

Lehmann-Grube, F.: Lymphocytic choriomeningitis virus carrier mice. Factors determining virus persistence. Medicina (B.A.) 37 Suppl 3:78, 1977.

Lehmann-Grube, F., Popescu, M., Schaefer, H., and Gschwender, H.H.: LCM virus infection of cells in vitro. Bull WHO 52:443, 1975.

Leung, W.C., Ghosh, H.P., and Rawls, W.E.: Strandedness of Pichinde virus RNA. J Virol 22:235, 1977.

Leung, W.C., and Rawls, W.E.: Virion-associated ribosomes are not required for the replication of Pichinde virus. Virology 81:174, 1977.

Mannweiler, K., and Lehmann-Grube, F.: Electron microscopy of LCM virus-infected L cells. In Lehmann-Grube, F. (ed.): Lymphocytic Choriomeningitis Virus and Other Arenaviruses. Berlin, Heidelberg, New York, Springer-Verlag, 1973, p. 37.

Martínez Segovia, Z.M. de, and De Mitri, M.I.: Junin virus structural proteins. J Virol 21:579, 1977.

Monath, T.P.: Lassa fever: review of epidemiology and epizootiology. Bull WHO 52:577, 1975.

Murphy, F.A., and Whitfield, S.G.: Morphology and morphogenesis of arenaviruses. Bull WHO 52:409, 1975.

Oldstone, M.B.A.: Virus neutralization and virus-induced immune complex disease. Progr Med Virol 19:84, 1975.

Palmer, E.L., Obijeski, J.F., Webb, P.A., and Johnson, K.M.: The circular, segmented nucleocapsid of an arenavirus-Tacaribe virus. J Gen Virol 36:541, 1977.

Parodi, A.S., Greenway, D.J., Rugiero, H.R., Frigerio, M., de la Barrera, J.M., Mettler, N., Garzón, F., Boxaca, M., Guerrero, L., y Nota, N.: Sobre la etiología del brote epidémico de Junín. Día méd (B.A.) 30:2300, 1958.

Pedersen, I.R.: LCM virus: its purification and its chemical and physical properties. In Lehmann-Grube, F. (ed.): Lymphocytic Choriomeningitis Virus and Other Arenaviruses. Berlin, Heidelberg, New York, Springer-Verlag, 1973, p. 13.

Pfau, C.J.: Biochemical and biophysical properties of the arenaviruses. Progr Med Virol 18:64, 1974.

Pfau, C.J.: The role of defective interfering (DI) virus in arenavirus infections. Medicina (B.A.) 37 Suppl 3:32, 1977.

Pinheiro, F.P., Shope, R.E., Paes de Andrade, A.H., Bensabath, G., Cacios, G.V., and Casals, J.: Amapari, a new virus of the Tacaribe group from rodents and mites of Amapa Territory, Brazil. Proc Soc Exper Biol Med 122:531, 1966.

Popescu, M., and Lehmann-Grube, F.: Diversity of lymphocytic choriomeningitis virus: variation due to replication of the virus in the mouse. J Gen Virol 30:113, 1976.

Popescu, M., and Lehmann-Grube, F.: Defective interfering particles in mice infected with lymphocytic choriomeningitis virus. Virology 77:78, 1977.

Popescu, M., Schaefer, H., and Lehmann-Grube, F.: Homologous interference of lymphocytic choriomeningitis virus: detection and measurement of interference focus-forming units. J Virol 20:1, 1976.

Ramos, B.A., Courtney, R.J., and Rawls, W.E.: Structural proteins of Pichinde virus. J Virol 10:661, 1972.

Rowe, W.P., Murphy, F.A., Bergold, G.H., Casals, J., Hotchin, J., Johnson, K.M., Lehmann-Grube, F., Mims, C.A., Traub, E., and Webb, P.A.: Arenoviruses: proposed name for a newly defined virus group. J Virol 5:651, 1970.

Rutter, G., and Gschwender, H.H.: Antigenic alteration of cells in vitro infected with LCM virus. In Lehmann-Grube, F. (ed.): Lymphocytic Choriomeningitis Virus and Other Arenaviruses. Berlin, Heidelberg, New York, Springer-Verlag, 1973, p. 51.

Sabattini, M.S., González de Ríos, L.E., Díaz, G., y Vega, V.R.: Infección natural y experimental de roedores con virus Junín. Medicina (B.A.) 37 Suppl 3:149, 1977.

Skinner, H.H., Knight, E.H., and Buckley, L.S.: The hamster as a secondary reservoir host of lymphocytic choriomeningitis virus. J Hyg 76:299, 1976.

Smadel, J.E., Green, R.H., Paltauf, R.M., and Gonzales, T.A.: Lymphocytic choriomeningitis: two human fatalities following an unusual febrile illness. Proc Soc Exper Biol Med 49:683, 1942.

Trapido, H., and Sanmartín, C.: Pichindé virus. A new virus of the Tacaribe group from Colombia. Am J Trop Med 20:631, 1971.

Vezza, A.C., Clewley, J.P., Gard, G.P., Abraham, N.Z., Compans, R.W., and Bishop, D.H.L.: Virion RNA species of the arenaviruses Pichinde, Tacaribe, and Tamiami. J Virol 26:485, 1978.

Vezza, A.C., Gard, G.P., Compans, R.W., and Bishop, D.H.L.: Structural components of the arenavirus Pichinde. J Virol 23:776, 1977.

Volkert, M., Bro-Jørgensen, K., and Marker, O.: Persistent LCM virus infection in the mouse. Immunity and tolerance. Bull WHO 52:471, 1975.

Walker, D.H., Wulff, H., Lange, J.V., and Murphy, F.A.: Comparative pathology of Lassa virus infection in monkeys, guinea-pigs, and Mastomys natalensis. Bull WHO 52:523, 1975.

Webb, P.A., Johnson, K.M., Hibbs, J.B., and Kuns, M.L.: Parana, a new Tacaribe complex virus from Paraguay. Arch ges Virusforsch 32:379, 1970.

Webb, P.A., Johnson, K.M., Peters, C.J., and Justines, G.: Behavior of Machupo and Latino viruses in Calomys callosus from two geographic areas of Bolivia. In Lehmann-Grube, F. (ed.): Lymphocytic Choriomeningitis Virus and Other Arenaviruses. Berlin, Heidelberg, New York, Springer-Verlag, 1973, p. 313.

Webb, P.A., Justines, G., and Johnson, K.M.: Infection of wild and laboratory animals with Machupo and Latino viruses. Bull WHO 52:493, 1975.

Weissenbacher, M.C., de Guerrero, L.B., and Boxaca, M.C.: Experimental biology and pathogenesis of Junin virus infection in animals and man. Bull WHO 52:507, 1975.

Welsh, R.M., Burner, P.A., Holland, J.J., Oldstone, M.B.A., Thompson, H.A., and Villarreal, L.P.: A comparison of biochemical and biological properties of standard and defective lymphocytic choriomeningitis virus. Bull WHO 52:403, 1975.

Wulff, H., Lange, J.V., and Webb, P.A.: Interrelationships among arenaviruses measured by indirect immunofluorescence. Intervirology 9:344, 1978.

Zinkernagel, R.M., and Doherty, P.C.: Major transplantation antigens, viruses, and specificity of surveillance T cells. Cont Top Immunobiol 7:179, 1977.

# **63** *REOVIRIDAE PATHOGENIC FOR MAN*

## *Neville F. Stanley, D. Sc.*

Reoviridae viruses are of interest to molecular biologists because all of them have a double-stranded RNA genome. Because of their great ubiquity in infecting plants, arthropods, and vertebrates, there still exist taxonomic problems that have not yet been resolved owing to paucity of data with some of these viruses. Our concern in this chapter will be with human infections with viruses belonging to three genera within this family. It is convenient on morphologic, biochemical, and biophysical properties to include two recognized (Reovirus and Orbivirus) and two 'tentative' (Rotavirus and Plant-insect) genera within this family (see Table 1) whose nomenclature is still under consideration by an international committee. The table sets out some of the better known viruses that have been sufficiently well described to include them in the family, but only those appropriately marked infect humans and will form the basis for discussion in this brief review.

Most of the orbiviruses and plant-insect viruses replicate in arthropods, whereas there is no evidence to show that reoviruses or rotaviruses replicate in arthropods, although the former have been isolated from mosquitoes (Stanley, 1977).

## REOVIRUSES

The properties, comparative biology, pathogenesis, and diagnostic procedures have been described in a number of reviews (Hassan and Cochran, 1966; Stanley, 1967, 1974, 1977; Rosen, 1968) that are useful for further reference. The viruses were originally discovered by isolation in infant mice when they were called *hepatoencephalomyelitis* viruses (Stanley et al., 1953, 1954). Later these agents were named *reoviruses*, which derives from *r*espiratory *e*nteric *o*rphan (Sabin, 1959). The double-stranded RNA core is surrounded by an inner and an outer protein shell. The outer shell has a diameter of between 60 and 75 nm and is icosahedral (5:3:2 symmetry).

### Antigenic Structure

All mammalian strains of reovirus fall into three serotypes, known as 1, 2, and 3. Hemagglutination-inhibition and neutralization tests have been primarily used for this differentiation, although a common antigen is detected by complement-fixation or by immuno-diffusion. It has not been possible to distinguish antigenic differences between human and animal isolates. All three serotypes produce hemagglutinins to erythrocytes of humans and other animals.

### Susceptible Cell Lines

All three types produce a distinctive cytopathic effect in many cell lines. Those cells that have been used for isolation or replication studies comprise *Macaca* kidney, *Cercopithecus* kidney, primary human kidney, human amnion, HELA and mouse L, as well as cells from marsupials, dogs, cats, guinea pigs, rabbits, dolphins, calves, and chick embryos (Stanley, 1977). The reovirus cytoplasmic inclusions are recognized in the perinuclear areas by staining or electron microscopy. Persistent infection with some cells has been reported and plaques useful for assays and replication studies have been produced with murine and simian cell lines. The main effects on host cell function are inhibition of DNA and protein synthesis and interferon induction.

TABLE 1. Reoviridae

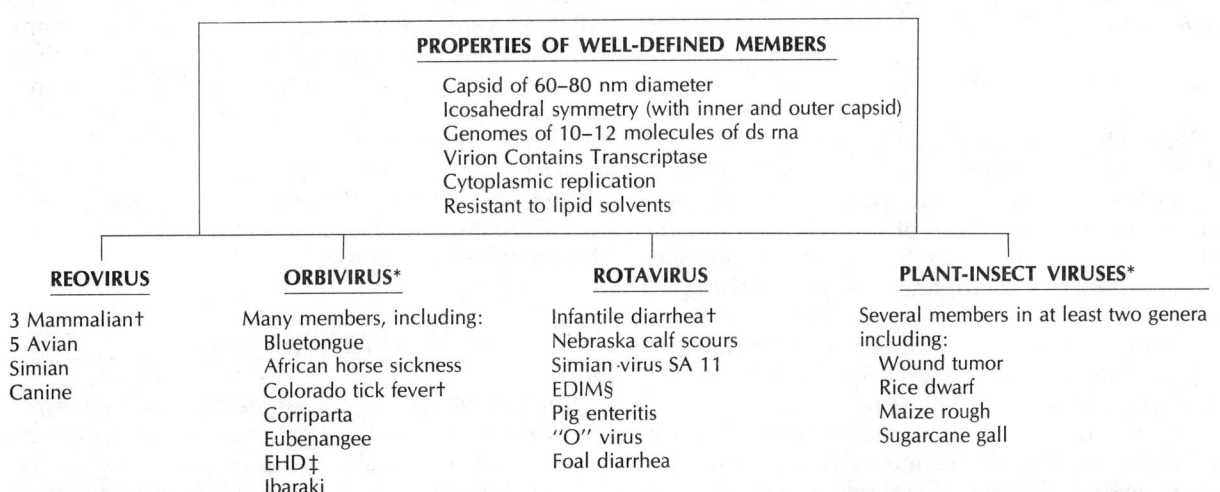

| PROPERTIES OF WELL-DEFINED MEMBERS |
|---|
| Capsid of 60–80 nm diameter |
| Icosahedral symmetry (with inner and outer capsid) |
| Genomes of 10–12 molecules of ds rna |
| Virion Contains Transcriptase |
| Cytoplasmic replication |
| Resistant to lipid solvents |

| REOVIRUS | ORBIVIRUS* | ROTAVIRUS | PLANT-INSECT VIRUSES* |
|---|---|---|---|
| 3 Mammalian† | Many members, including: | Infantile diarrhea† | Several members in at least two genera |
| 5 Avian | Bluetongue | Nebraska calf scours | including: |
| Simian | African horse sickness | Simian virus SA 11 | Wound tumor |
| Canine | Colorado tick fever† | EDIM§ | Rice dwarf |
| | Corriparta | Pig enteritis | Maize rough |
| | Eubenangee | "O" virus | Sugarcane gall |
| | EHD‡ | Foal diarrhea | |
| | Ibaraki | | |

*Natural arthropod transmission.
†Infects humans.
‡Epizootic hemorrhagic disease of deer.
§Epizootic diarrhea of infant mice.

### Clinical Disease

***Human.*** The association of any of three serotypes with disease in man is uncertain because of great virus ubiquity and the absence of clinical manifestations after infection. Outbreaks of mild clinical illness, supported by virus isolation, occur mainly with children with respiratory and gastrointestinal tract involvement. Only four fatal cases have been recorded, and all of these appear to have had a disseminated infection with lesions in brain, heart, lung, or liver (Stanley, 1977). There have been many other associations that need further confirmation — one of particular interest being keratoconjunctivitis (Jarudi et al., 1973).

***Animal.*** Ubiquity of the reoviruses also poses similar difficulties with natural animal infections, although there is little doubt that reovirus 3 produces spontaneous disease in some mouse colonies, and reovirus 2 causes upper respiratory tract infection in laboratory-housed chimpanzees. A considerable amount of useful information has been derived from experimental murine models exploited by Australian workers (Stanley, 1974, 1977). These have developed our knowledge of virus pathogenesis in three areas: reovirus 1 — hydrocephalus; reovirus 3 — active chronic hepatitis and lymphoma; and reovirus 3 — chronic biliary obstruction. In addition to mice, experimental infections have been established in rats, guinea pigs, hamsters, rabbits, ferrets, dogs, swine, cattle, and nonhuman primates. Little is known about humoral or cell-mediated immunity in reovirus infections. Recent studies suggest the association of temperature-sensitive mutants with persistent infection and possibly specific clinicopathologic syndromes (Raine and Fields, 1974).

### Laboratory Diagnosis

This is based on the isolation and identification of the virus by cell cultures or infant mouse inoculation, the detection of the virus or its antigens, the presence of specific cellular changes and/or the development of a specific, significant, serologic response. Standard and detailed techniques have been published (Lennette et al., 1974). When cell cultures are used, primary *Macaca* kidney or human kidney are adequate. Intraperitoneal inoculation of newborn mice is a useful adjunct to cell culture for virus isolation, but the mouse colony should be demonstrated to be free from reovirus. Immunofluorescence and immunoperoxidase techniques have been developed for the detection of reovirus antigens. Serologic diagnosis is not helpful because of the early acquisition of antibody in most populations.

Four serologic tests are currently used for antibody estimation: hemagglutination-inhibition, complement-fixation, neutralization, and immunodiffusion.

### Epidemiology

Antibodies to the three serotypes are widely distributed and antibody conversion rates show that infection is acquired early in life (Stanley et al., 1954, 1964; Stanley, 1961, 1967, 1974, 1977; Stanley and Leak, 1963; Rosen, 1968). The virus is usually isolated from the feces of children. Although the three mammalian types of reovirus have been isolated from large numbers of many vertebrates, an even greater ubiquity is indicated by the widespread occurrence of naturally occurring antibody. It would appear that the following, in addition to man, are frequently infected: nonhuman primates, cattle, horses, sheep, dogs, cats, rats, mice, rabbits, hares, guinea pigs, marsupials, reptiles, poultry, wild birds, and bats (Stanley, 1977).

The epidemiologic patterns indicate fecal-oral transmission, but infection via the respiratory tract has yet to be substantiated. It is possible that animal strains infect man and that human strains may infect animals. Their physical properties enable reoviruses to survive in the environment and they may, therefore, contaminate some ecosystem. It has been suggested (Stanley, 1977) that they be used as a virus marker for bird, animal, or human fecal pollution of water. All types have been isolated from stagnant water, river water, or raw sewage, and sometimes in higher concentrations than entero-viruses. The high rate of isolation from raw sewage (34 per cent) does not correlate with the low isolation rate (0.2 per cent) from human feces. Reoviruses may be recovered more consistently from sewage than most other viruses (England, 1972). Other evidence for gross contamination of the environment is the isolation of reoviruses from mosquitoes.

Although reoviruses then are not to be considered as serious producers of human disease, their involvement in congenital virus infection should be considered (Stanley, 1977).

## ORBIVIRUSES

Borden et al. (1971) suggested the name *orbivirus* (from *orbis* [L], ring or circle) for a distinctive group of viruses equal in hierarchy to the reoviruses. They may be divided into antigenic subgroups, but do not share a common antigen (see Table 1). Although reoviruses are stable at pH 3.0, orbiviruses are inactivated at this pH. By thin section and negative-stain electron microscopy, Murphy et al. (1971) were able to distinguish orbiviruses from togaviruses and reoviruses. The surface architecture of bluetongue virus suggests that this virus with 32 morphologic units has an icosahedral structure, distinct from reoviruses. The virion is smaller than that of reoviruses and possesses large capsomeres with the appearance of rings. The outer layer covering the inner icosahedral capsid is frequently indistinct (see Fig. 1).

Although most members are transmitted by and multiply in arthropods they frequently cause viremia in the vertebrate hosts. The best known and perhaps the most important of the animal pathogens are bluetongue (20 serotypes) and African horse sickness (9 serotypes). The only known human pathogen in this subdivision is Colorado tick fever, which is spread to man through the bite of an infected tick. Only one antigenic type is known and an infection usually produces effective long-lasting immunity. With the exception of one fatal case, the disease is benign with headache, ocular pain, muscle and joint pains, lumbar pains, nausea, and vomiting. The pathogenesis is not clearly understood. Leukopenia is common. Pa-

tients have a persistent circulating erythrocyte-associated viremia and the disease has been transmitted by blood transfusion. Electron microscopy studies suggest that the virus infects early-stage hematopoietic cells with movement of virus to the circulating blood cells (Emmons et al., 1972).

Diagnosis may be made accurately and rapidly by fluorescent antibody staining of peripheral blood smears. The virus can also be isolated from whole blood by inoculation of newborn mice or hamsters, or by cell cultures. Antibodies are usually detected by a complement-fixation test.

The major distribution of the human disease confined to North America has followed the distribution of the wood tick, *Dermacentor andersoni*, which is primarily found in Colorado, Oregon, Utah, Idaho, Montana, and Wyoming. The tick is clearly the true reservoir and the virus may be transmitted transovarially by the adult female. Infected rodents act as reservoirs for the immature tick. Recent studies have indicated endemic areas in California, where 205 cases have occurred since 1954. It has been estimated that more than 2000 cases occur annually in Colorado.

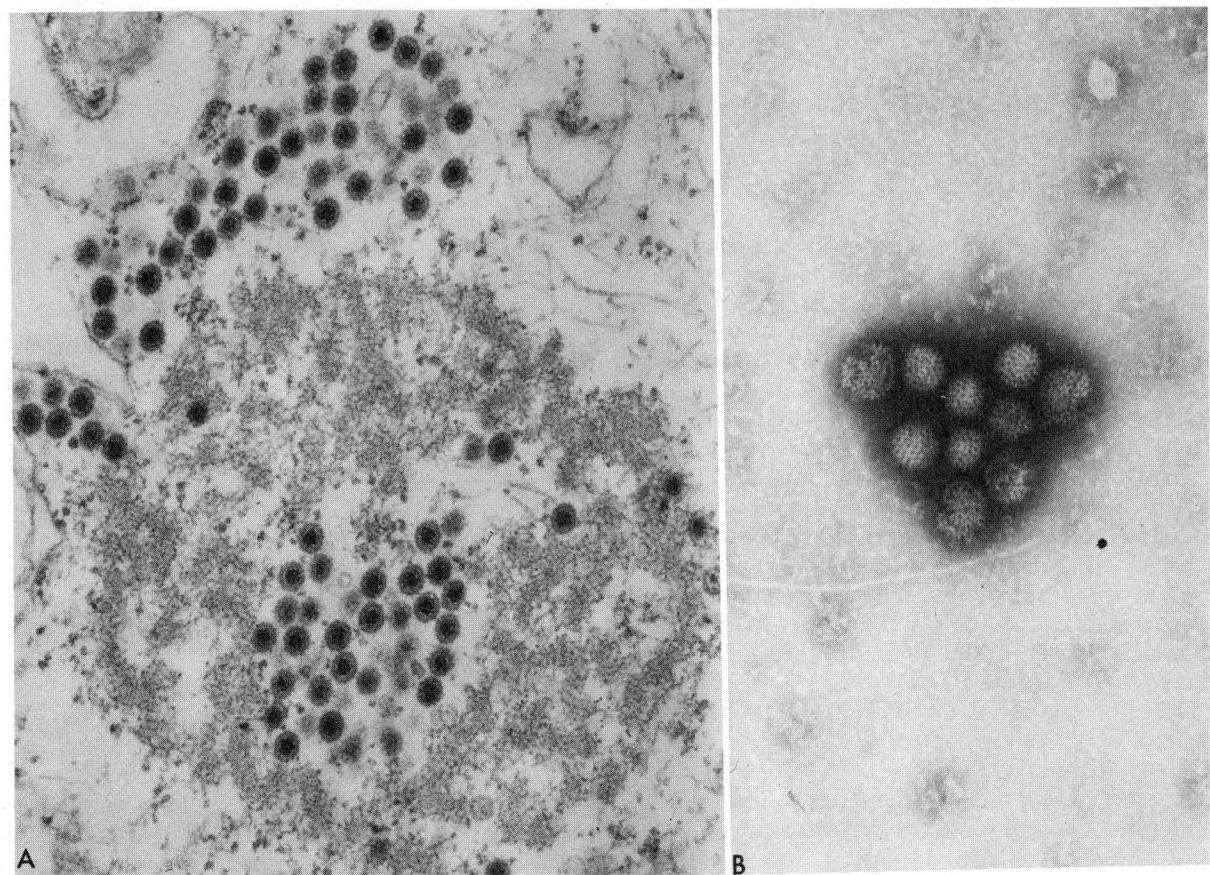

**FIGURE 1.**  *Electron micrographs of bluetongue (an orbivirus) grown in baby hamster kidney cells. (Supplied through the courtesy of Dr. Frederick A. Murphy, Center for Disease Control, Atlanta, Georgia, USA.)*
*(A) × 109,000        (B) × 174,000*

The virus has also been found in an area where *D. andersoni* is absent. This suggests a maintenance cycle different from the chipmunk-ground squirrel *D. andersoni* cycle. The virus has recently been isolated from Ixodid and Argarid ticks (for further reference see Emmons et al., 1972; Oshiro, et al., 1978).

## ROTAVIRUSES

These viruses are the most common cause of infantile enteritis — a disease now known to be widespread throughout the world and usually with a seasonal winter peak. Until agreement has been reached on nomenclature the term *rotavirus* will be used. It is synonymous with *duovirus* used by the Australian workers and some others (Holmes et al., 1975; Davidson et al., 1975). The disease and the virus are currently under extensive study and many of the observations relate to direct electron microscopy of human fecal material. New methods are now being employed and a chapter of this nature will need consistent modification as more precise information becomes available, particularly with the use of antisera against other nonhuman rotaviruses such as calf diarrhea.

### Clinical and Epidemiologic Characteristics

Vomiting and significant dehydration are consistently associated with rotavirus diarrhea. The highest incidence is in children between the ages of 7 and 24 months. Most hospitalized children present with high fever between the second and fifth days after the diarrhea and vomiting. There may be involvement of the upper respiratory tract. The mean duration of uncomplicated cases is between one and two weeks, but coincident pathogenic enterobacterial infection may increase the severity and extend the time of the disease. The incubation period appears to be about two to three days. There is little doubt about the high winter incidence but no completely satisfactory explanation has yet been offered to explain this epidemiology. This epidemiology is not worldwide, since it is not commonly observed in tropical areas. Although adults associated with children with rotavirus diarrhea are usually not infected (serologic estimate), there have been reports of up to 41 per cent of adult contacts being infected (Kim et al., 1977). Nearly all adult contact infections were subclinical. In an interesting epidemiologic study by Murphy et al. (1977), in an examination of 628 newborn babies in Sydney hospitals in Australia, it was found that 49 per cent had rotavirus in their stools. Although none of the one day neonates were positive, many commenced excreting virus within three or four days after birth. Most of these were symptom free. Since there was no seasonal variation observed, it appears that rotaviruses may persist in some Sydney hospital nurseries and are spread between neonates.

### Diagnosis

It is important to differentiate rotavirus infantile diarrhea from enteritis produced by other microorganisms. Although direct electron microscopy, after differential centrifugation, has been the main and initial technique, other effective methods and variations have been introduced. These may be virus or virus antigen detection (by antibody rise) or both. The following methods are currently being explored:

1. Free viral immunofluorescence assay in human stools (Yolken et al., 1977b)

2. Enzyme-linked immunosorbent assay (ELISA) (Yolken et al., 1977a)

3. Fluorescent virus precipitation test (Peterson et al., 1976)

4. Cell culture plus immunofluorescence (Woode et al., 1974; Wyatt et al., 1974, 1976; Banatvala et al., 1975; Albrey and Murphy, 1976; Bryden et al., 1977)

5. Complement-fixation (Kapikian et al., 1975; Tufvesson and Johnsson, 1976a)

6. Electrophoresis:
   a. Immunoelectroosmophoresis (Tufvesson and Johnsson, 1976b)
   b. Polyacrylamide gel (Kalica et al., 1976)
   c. Counter-immunoelectrophoresis (Spence et al., 1977)

### Transmission

Human rotaviruses have been successfully transmitted to lambs, monkeys, dogs, and pigs. This is not surprising in view of the antigenic relationship between rotaviruses of animals and infants.

### Antigenicity

Some of the animal rotaviruses, notably calf rotavirus and the simian SA 11, grow in cell cultures. These viruses cross-react with human rotavirus by complement-fixation, immunofluorescence, and immuno-electron microscopy. In addition the rotaviruses derived from pigs and mice (EDIM) also cross-react with the human strains. So far, all known members share a common antigen, but antigenic differences have yet to be explored. As the simian rotavirus (SA 11) replicates easily in primary cell culture it is being examined for use in the serodiagnosis of human infections (Schoub et al., 1977).

## Morphology

It is impossible to distinguish between rotaviruses from simian, porcine, equine, murine, or human origin by electronmicroscopy. Particles with and without outer capsids have been found in each animal species and their diameter varies between 50 and 68 nm depending on the presence of the outer capsid. When the outer layer is lost the inner capsomeres projecting from the surface give the particles a rough appearance around the edge. Sometimes flattened tubules with hexagonally packed subunits are observed.

For further reading see Flewett et al., 1973; Rodriguez et al., 1977; Middleton, 1977).

## References

Albrey, M. B., and Murphy, A. M.: Rotavirus growth in bovine monolayers. Lancet 1:753, 1976.

Banatvala, J. E., Totterdell, B., Chrystie, I. L., and Woode, G. N.: In-vitro detection of human rotaviruses. Lancet 2:821, 1975.

Borden, E. C., Shope, R. E., and Murphy, F. A.: Physicochemical and morphological relationships of some arthropod-borne viruses to bluetongue virus — a new taxonomic group. Physicochemical and serological studies. J. Gen Virol 13:261, 1971.

Bryden, A. S., Davies, H. A., Thouless, M. E., and Flewett, T. H.: Diagnosis of rotavirus infection by cell culture. J Med Microbiol 10:121, 1977.

Davidson, G. P., Bishop, R. F., Townley, R. R. W., Holmes, I. H., and Ruck, B. J.: Importance of a new virus in acute sporadic enteritis in children. Lancet 1:242, 1975.

Emmons, R. W., Oshiro, L. S., Johnson, H. N., and Lennette, E. H.: Intra-erythrocytic location of Colorado tick fever virus. J Gen Virol 17:185, 1972.

England, E.: Concentration of reovirus and adenovirus from sewage and effluents by protamine sulfate (salmine) treatment. Appl Microbiol 24:510, 1972.

Flewett, T. H., Bryden, A. S., and Davies, H. A.: Virus particles in gastroenteritis. Lancet 2:1947, 1973.

Hassan, S. A., and Cochran, K. W.: Teratogenicity of reo and poliovirus in mice. Bact Proc 42:115, 1966.

Holmes, I. H., Ruck, B. J., Bishop, R. F., and Davidson, G. P.: Infantile enteritis viruses: morphogenesis and morphology. J. Virol 16:937, 1975.

Jarudi, N. I., Huggett, D. O., and Golden, B.: Reovirus keratoconjunctivitis. Canad J Ophthal 8:371, 1973.

Kalica, A. R., Garon, C. F., Wyatt, R. G., Mebus, C. A., van Kirk, D. H., Chanock, R. M., and Kapikian, A. Z.: Differentiation of human and calf reoviruslike agents associated with diarrhea using polyacrylamide gel electrophoresis of RNA. Virology 74:86, 1976.

Kapikian, A. Z., Cline, W. L., Mebus, C. A., Wyatt, R. G., Kalica, A. R., James, H. D., Jr., van Kirk, D., and Chanock, R. M.: New complement-fixation test for the human reovirus-like agent of infantile gastroenteritis. Nebraska calf diarrhea virus used as antigen. Lancet 1:1056, 1975.

Kim, H. W., Brandt, C. D., Kapikian, A. Z., Wyatt, R. G., Arrobio, J. O., Rodriguez, W. J., Chanock, R. M., and Parrott, R. H.: Human reovirus-like agent infection. Occurrence in adult contacts of pediatric patients with gastroenteritis. JAMA 238:404, 1977.

Lennette, E. H., Spaulding, E. H., and Truant, J. P. (eds.): Manual of Clinical Microbiology. 2nd ed. Washington, American Society for Microbiology, 1974.

Middleton, P. J.: Rotavirus: clinical observations and diagnosis of gastroenteritis. In Kurstak, E., and Kurstak, C. (eds.): Comparative Diagnosis of Viral Diseases, vol. 1, Human and Related Viruses,

part A. New York, San Francisco, London, Academic Press, 1977, p. 423.

Murphy, A. M., Albrey, M. B., and Crewe, E. B.: Rotavirus infections of neonates. Lancet 2:1149, 1977.

Murphy, F. A., Borden, E. C., Shope, R. E., and Harrison, A.: Physicochemical and morphological relationships of some arthropod-borne viruses to bluetongue virus — a new taxonomic group. Electron microscopic studies. J Gen Virol 13:273, 1971.

Oshiro, L. S., Dondero, D. V., Emmons, R. W., and Lennette, E. H.: J Gen Virol, 39:73, 1978.

Peterson, M. W., Spendlove, R. S., and Smart, R. A.: Detection of neonatal calf diarrhea virus, infant reovirus-like diarrhea virus, and a coronavirus using the fluorescent virus precipitin test. J Clin Microbiol 3:376, 1976.

Raine, C. S., and Fields, B. N.: Neurotropic-virus host relationship alterations due to variation in viral genome as studied by electron microscopy. Am J Path 75:119, 1974.

Rodriguez, W. J., Kim, H. W., Arrobio, J. O., Brandt, C. D., Chanock, R. M., Kapikian, A. Z., Wyatt, R. G., and Parrott, R. H.: Clinical features of acute gastroenteritis associated with human reovirus-like agent in infants and young children. J Pediat 91:188, 1977.

Rosen, L.: Reoviruses. In Monographs in Virology, 1. Wien, New York, Springer-Verlag, 1968, p. 73.

Sabin, A. B.: Reoviruses. Science 130:1387, 1959.

Schoub, B. D., Lecatsas, G., and Prozesky, O. W.: Antigenic relationship between human and simian rotaviruses. J Med Microbiol 10:1, 1977.

Spence, L., Fauvel, M., Petro, R., and Bloch, S.: Comparison of counterimmunoelectrophoresis and electron microscopy for laboratory diagnosis of human reovirus-like agent-associated infantile gastroenteritis. J Clin Microbiol 5:248, 1977.

Stanley, N. F.: Reovirus — a ubiquitous orphan. Med J Aust 2:815, 1961.

Stanley, N. F.: Reoviruses. Br Med Bull 23:150, 1967.

Stanley, N. F.: The reovirus murine models. In Hotchin, J. (vol. ed.), Melnick, J. L. (ser. ed.): Progress in Medical Virology: Slow Virus Diseases, vol. 18. Basel, Karger, 1974, p. 257.

Stanley, N. F.: Diagnosis of reovirus infections: comparative aspects. In Kurstak, E., and Kurstak, C. (eds.): Comparative Diagnosis of Viral Diseases, vol. 1, Human and Related Viruses, part A. New York, San Francisco, London, Academic Press, 1977, p. 385.

Stanley, N. F., Dorman, D. C., and Ponsford, J.: Studies on the pathogenesis of a hitherto undescribed virus (hepato-encephalomyelitis) producing unusual symptoms in suckling mice. Aust J Exp Biol Med Sci 31:147, 1953.

Stanley, N. F., Dorman, D. C., and Ponsford, J.: Studies on the hepatoencephalomyelitis virus (HEV). Aust J Exp Biol Med Sci 32:543, 1954.

Stanley, N. F., and Leak, P. J.: The serologic epidemiology of reovirus infection with special reference to the Rottnest Island quokka (Setonix brachyurus). Am J Hyg 78:82, 1963.

Stanley, N. F., Leak, P. J., Walters, M.N-I., and Joske, R. A.: Murine infection with reovirus. II. The chronic disease following reovirus type 3 infection. Br J Exp Path 45:142, 1964.

Tufvesson, B., and Johnsson, T.: Occurrence of reo-like calf viruses in young children with acute gastroenteritis. Diagnoses established by electron microscopy and complement fixation, using the reo-like virus as antigen. Acta Path Microbiol Scand(B) 84:22, 1976a.

Tufvesson, B., and Johnsson, T.: Immunoelectroosmophoresis for detection of reo-like virus: methodology and comparison with electron microscopy. Acta Path Microbiol Scand(B) 84:225, 1976b.

Woode, G. N., Bridger, J. C., Hall, G., and Dennis, M. J.: The isolation of a reovirus-like agent associated with diarrhoea in colostrum-deprived calves in Great Britain. Res Vet Sci 16:102, 1974.

Wyatt, G. B., Hocking, B., Bishop, R., and Wyatt, J. L.: Duovirus infection as a cause of infantile gastro-enteritis in Port Moresby. Papua New Guinea Med J 19:134, 1976.

Wyatt, R. G., Kapikian, A. Z., Thornhill, T. S., Sereno, M. M., Kim, H. W., and Chanock, R. M.: In vitro cultivation in human fetal intestinal organ culture of a reovirus-like agent associated with nonbacterial gastroenteritis in infants and children. J Infect Dis 130:523, 1974.

Yolken, R. H., Kim, H. W., Clem, T., Wyatt, R. G., Kalica, A. R., Chanock, R. M., and Kapikian, A. Z.: Enzyme-linked immunosorbent assay (ELISA) for detection of human reovirus-like agent of infantile gastroenteritis. Lancet 2:263, 1977a.

Yolken, R. H., Wyatt, R. G., Kalica, A. R., Kim, H. W., Brandt, C. D., Parrott, R. H., Kapikian, A. Z., and Chanock, R. M.: Use of a free viral immunofluorescence assay to detect human reovirus-like agent in human stools. Infect Immun 16:467, 1977b.

# 64 RHABDOVIRUS

*Bosko Postic, M.D.*
*and Tadeus J. Wiktor, D.V.M.*

The rhabdoviruses are a group of bullet-shaped viruses that infect vertebrates, invertebrates, and plants. An electron micrograph of a rabies virion, a member of the rhabdovirus group, is shown in Figure 1. Most rhabdoviruses measure 180 × 75 nm. Short particles measuring 70 to 100 nm and longer ones measuring up to 400 nm are also seen. Plant rhabdoviruses appear to have a similar conformation but are usually longer and bacilliform in shape.

Out of some twenty animal rhabdoviruses only the vesicular stomatitis virus (VSV) and the rabies virus subgroup are pathogenic for humans and domestic animals. In addition, several rhabdoviruses can cause economically important diseases of fish.

The central helical core of a rhabdovirus consists of a single-stranded RNA genome and various structural proteins forming the nucleocapsid, which is surrounded by a lipid envelope and an outer surface of glycoprotein spikes. The chemical composition of purified rabies virus consists of 22 per cent lipids, 3 per cent carbohydrate, 1 per cent RNA, and 74 per cent protein. Four major polypeptide components of different molecular sizes form the protein moiety of rabies virus; a nucleoprotein, a glycoprotein, and two membrane proteins. Lipid solvents can inactivate the infectivity of rhabdoviruses.

## ANTIGENIC COMPOSITION

Using immunologic techniques (virus neutralization, complement fixation, antibody binding, or fluorescent antibody staining) rhabdoviruses can be classified into several antigenic groups.

In the VSV group containing some seven known strains, two major serotypes (VSV Indiana and VSV New Jersey) can be distinguished; other strains of VSV are related to major serotypes.

The rabies group contains rabies virus and five other viruses that share antigens with rabies virus. These are the Lagos bat, Mokola, Duvenhage, Obodhiang, and Kotonkan viruses, but only two, the Mokola and Duvenhage viruses, may be associated with human disease.

Two antigens of rabies virus have been obtained in pure form: (1) The glycoprotein induces virus-neutralizing antibody and is therefore important in immunity. Antibody to glycoprotein plus complement can produce lysis of cultured cells infected by rabies virus. (2) Antibody stimulated by the viral nucleocapsid does not neutralize virus or cause lysis, but does fix complement (CF). The CF antibody can identify the intracytoplasmic inclusions known as Negri bodies, which consist mostly of rabies virus ribonucleoprotein.

Using cross-neutralization, a limited relationship has been detected between rabies, Mokola, and Lagos bat viruses. In CF tests and fluorescent antibody (FA) assays, there is considerable antigenic similarity between these viruses (Shope et al., 1970). Immunization of mice with Mokola or Lagos virus was not protective against challenge with rabies virus. On the other hand, mice immunized with attenuated rabies virus (high egg passage [HEP], Flury strain) resisted challenge with Lagos bat virus and, to a lesser degree, with Mokola virus (Tignor and Shope, 1972).

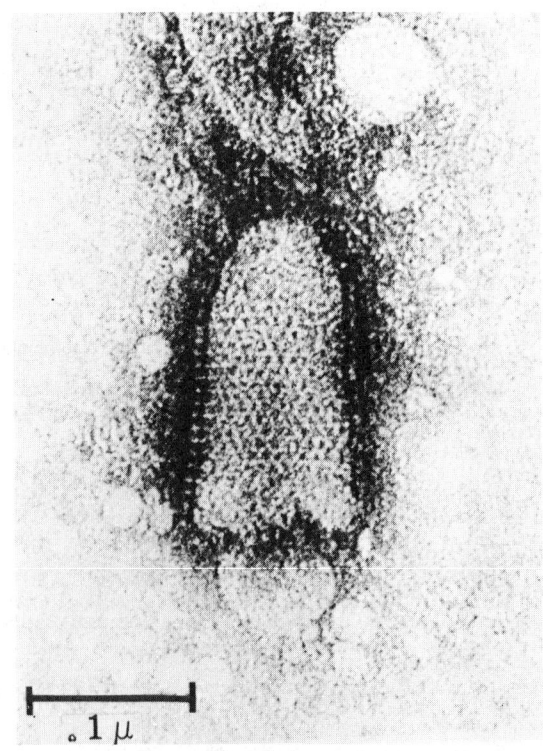

**FIGURE 1.** *Electron micrograph of a rabies virion.*

## SUSCEPTIBLE HOST CELLS

Vesicular stomatitis virus possesses great virulence for many cell cultures, causing a rapid cytopathic effect that is usually complete by 48 hours after infection. Plaques are also formed in cell cultures of several species. This virus is extremely sensitive to the action of interferon and is used for titration of interferon. Under certain experimental conditions, truncated virus particles are produced. These can interfere with the production of standard VSV particles in vivo and in vitro (see the section on Interference in Chapter 12).

In the last century, Louis Pasteur found that the agent of rabies replicates in the nerve tissue. He and his co-workers injected saliva from rabid dogs submeningeally into rabbits (Pasteur et al., 1884). The disease was then serially transmitted with suspensions of brain tissue from inoculated rabbits.

Seventy years later, Kissling and co-workers (Kissling, 1958) propagated rabies virus in cultured cells of non-nervous origin. A wide variety of cells can be infected, but generally no cytotoxicity is observed. The cytoplasm of cultured cells was shown to contain rabies virus antigen by staining with fluorescent antibody. This observation is the basis for diagnostic tests in tissue culture, which replace animal inoculations (see Chapter 167). A continuous line of hamster cells BH-21, is particularly supportive of rabies virus growth and can be used for plaque formation. In the authors' laboratories, rabies virus-infected cell cultures have produced interferon, and conversely, interferon added before inoculation of virus suppressed its replication. In other words, rabies virus not only induces interferon but is also suppressed by it. Interferon also protects laboratory animals from rabies virus (Postic and Fenje, 1971). (See Chapter 12.)

## PATHOGENIC PROPERTIES

Both the Indiana and the New Jersey serotypes of VSV affect many species of animals but have a special predilection for livestock. In these animals vesicular stomatitis is characterized by vesicles on the oral mucosa, especially on the tongue. Vesicles and ulcers may also occur on the udders of cows and mares, and linear necrotic lesions have been observed on the corium and heels of horses and cattle. Over 95 per cent of animals survive the natural infection. The illness in cattle resembles foot-and-mouth disease, but vesicular stomatitis is milder. A related coccal virus was isolated from small rodents but not livestock. This agent is serologically close but not identical with the Indiana strain of VSV. Both types of VSV can produce illness in humans. Most outbreaks occur through professional exposure to animals and are due to the New Jersey serotype. The illness in humans is acute, self-limited, and similar to influenza. Fields and Hawkins (1967) described eight cases of vesicular stomatitis in persons exposed to animals naturally infected with the Indiana serotype. Three of these patients had oral lesions: vesicles on the gum, buccal, and pharyngeal mucosa, or a herpes-like lip lesion. One adult patient experienced a 9-kg weight loss over a period of two weeks. All patients were febrile, and half of them complained of myalgia. Headache, nausea, vomiting, and pharyngitis were also prominent. Recovery occurred in all patients after a course of treatment lasting from two to seven days. In other outbreaks, including those in laboratory workers, most patients became febrile after an incubation period of two to six days, and developed pharyngitis, conjunctivitis, and oral and buccal vesicles with submaxillary and submandibular lymphadenitis. Occasionally, the febrile course was diphasic, and transient leukopenia occurred.

Rabies can affect all warm-blooded animals either naturally or experimentally. It is discussed in Chapter 167. Rabies-related viruses were all isolated in Africa. They appear to play a minor role in human disease. Their pathogenicity for animals is suggested by the sources of isolation. Lagos bat virus was isolated from the pooled brains of an African frugivorous bat. Experimentally, mice, dogs, and monkeys could be infected by the intracerebral route. Negri bodies were not seen in these animals. Mokola virus was isolated from shrews and from two Nigerian patients experiencing a central nervous system infection. One had a fatal poliomyelitis-like disease, and the second patient had a nonfatal febrile illness with convulsions. The pathogenicity of Mokola virus for animals is similar to that of Lagos bat virus. Negri bodies were found in infected monkey brains but not in mice or dogs. Duvenhage virus was isolated in South Africa from the brain of a patient bitten by a bat.

Obodhiang and Kotonkan viruses were isolated from mosquitoes by inoculating homogenized pools into baby mice. According to serologic results, infection by Kotonkan virus may be prevalent in livestock and rodents.

## IMMUNITY

The reader is referred to Chapter 167 for the immunologic aspects of rabies.

Antibodies to VSV appear in infected animals in the 1st week after infection. Antibody determinations to the Indiana or New Jersey serotypes are carried out by a plaque neutralization technique using the homologous virus as indicator. Neutralizing antibodies mediate immunity to the homologous virus in experimental infections.

The immunologic relationship of the rabies-related viruses to rabies virus was discussed previously under Antigenic Composition.

## LABORATORY DIAGNOSIS

As in all virus diseases, the laboratory methods used for rhabdovirus can be subdivided into: (1) tissue diagnosis (see Chapter 167), (2) virus isolation, and (3) serology.

VSV can be cultured from a variety of samples (serum, vesicle fluid, throat swab) by the intracerebral inoculation of baby mice, but only if the time of sampling coincides with viral replication in vivo. Since this event appears to be brief in humans, most cases are diagnosed serologically by the plaque neutralization test.

Rabies-related viruses are isolated by the mouse inoculation method from the sources discussed in Pathogenic Properties. In the brains of infected mice, the effect of these viruses may be hard to distinguish from that produced by rabies virus. Identification of isolates is accomplished by virus neutralization, CF, FA, and vaccination challenge tests. The vaccination challenge appears to be most discriminating; intraperitoneal immunization of mice with Mokola and Lagos bat viruses does not protect against intracerebral challenge with rabies virus. Likewise, immunization with Lagos bat virus does not protect against Mokola virus challenge. Immunization with Mokola virus, however, protects against both homologous and Lagos bat virus challenge. Mice immunized with rabies HEP Flury vaccine resisted challenge with Lagos bat virus and, to a lesser extent, with Mokola virus.

## EPIDEMIOLOGY

VSV has been isolated from a variety of naturally infected animals, mostly livestock. The virus has also been isolated from arthropods, such as *Phlebotomus* sandflies and *Aedes* sp mosquitoes. The role of these arthropods in transmitting the disease is not clear. A prolonged vesicular stomatitis viremia has not been observed naturally or experimentally in a vertebrate. Thus, an infective blood meal for arthropods is probably not readily available in nature.

In humans VSV infection is most commonly acquired in the virus laboratory. Humans who processed animals from an epizootic have also been infected. The route by which VSV infects man is not known in most instances. Inhalation of aerosol, inoculation into the conjunctiva, and entry through abrasions of the skin are equally plausible portals of entry. Human-to-human transmission of vesicular stomatitis is unlikely.

Rabies is primarily a disease of domestic and wild animals. In areas were animal control programs are not extensively developed, dogs or cats account for most rabid animals and cause most human exposures to rabies. In such areas 90 per cent or more of human cases result from exposure to rabid dogs or cats. Effective domestic animal rabies control programs in these areas reduced sharply the numbers of rabid dogs and cats as illustrated by the decrease in the United States in the period 1950 to 1960 (Fig. 2). In the United States since 1960 the vast majority of cases of animal rabies occurred in wild animals, and most of the human rabies cases were secondary to bites by rabid wild animals. Where no wild animal reservoirs exist, as in the United Kingdom, eradication of dog rabies can eliminate rabies.

The epidemiology of human rabies closely follows the epizootiology of animal rabies. Human rabies has been reported from all continents except Australia and the Antarctic, although most cases occur in countries where control of domestic animal rabies has not been well developed. About 700 rabies deaths are reported each year to the World Health Organization, a number that is probably only a fraction of the actual number of cases. Human rabies is most common in persons under age 15, with about 40 per cent of cases occurring in children age 5 to 14. All age groups are susceptible. Most rabies victims are male, since they are more likely to be in contact with infected animals.

Rabies epidemics in humans follow two patterns. In one, a single rabid dog or wolf may attack and bite several people. In the other type of outbreak, human cases result from an increase of rabies in the domestic or wild animal population. Thus Central and Eastern Europe is currently experiencing a threat from rabies "fallout" from a major epizootic of rabies in foxes. The geographic distribution of rabies in wildlife is variable. In the USA, rabies reservoirs are found in wildlife: skunks, foxes, raccoons, and insectivorous bats. In South and Central America, dog and cattle rabies is prevalent; vampire bats there are an important reservoir as well as vectors. In Southeast Asia, dog rabies is enzootic except in Japan and Taiwan, which are rabies-free. European fox rabies has already been noted. North Africa abounds in dog rabies, whereas in sub-Saharan regions other *Canidae* (jackal) and *Felidae* genera also participate in forming the reservoir of enzootic rabies.

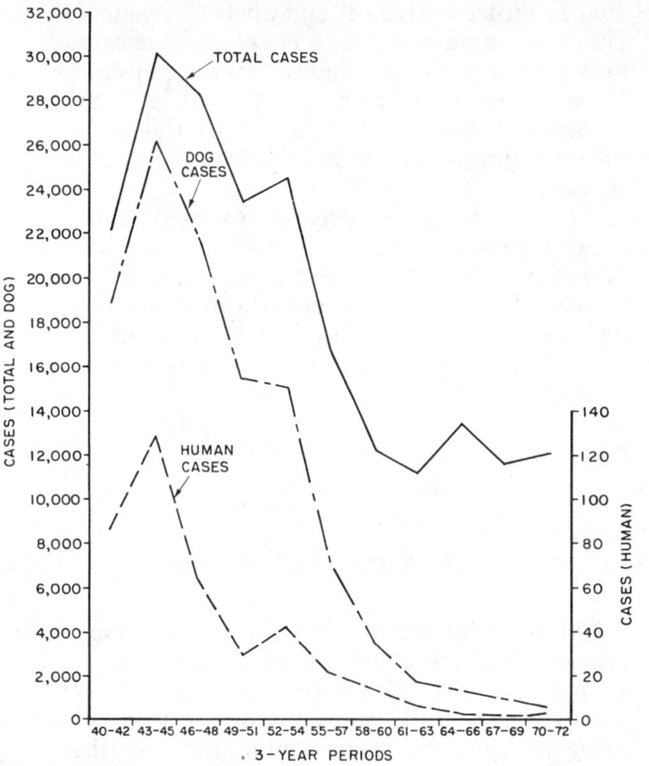

**FIGURE 2.** *Rabies cases by 3-year periods, United States, 1940-1972. (Source: Wiktor and Hattwick, New York, Academic Press, Rhabdoviruses,* In *Kurstak, E. and C., Comparative diagnosis of viral diseases, Vol. I, Part A, p. 775, 1977.)*

The epidemiology of rabies-related viruses is largely unexplored. As noted previously, these viruses only occasionally involve man. Their main medical significance lies in differentiation of them from rabies virus upon isolation from animals, or rarely, a human.

### References

Fields, B. N., and Hawkins, K.: Human infection with the virus of vesicular stomatitis during an epizootic. N Engl J Med 277:989, 1967.

Kissling, R. E.: Growth of rabies virus in non-nervous tissue culture. Proc Soc Exp Biol Med 98:223, 1958.

Pasteur, L., Chamberland, M. M., and Roux, E.: Nouvelle communication sur la rage. C. R. Acad Sci (D) (Paris) 98:457, 1884.

Postic, B., and Fenje, P.: Effect of administered interferon on rabies in rabbits. Appl Microb 22:428, 1971.

Shope, R. E., Murphy, F. A., Harrison, A. K., Causey, O. R., Kemp, G. E., Simpson, D. I. H., and Moore, D. L.: Two African viruses serologically and morphologically related to rabies virus. J Virol 6:690, 1970.

Tignor, G. H., and Shope, R. E.: Vaccination and challenge of mice with viruses of the rabies serogroup. J Infect Dis 125:322, 1972.

Wiktor, T. J,, and Hattwick, M. A. W.: Rhabdoviruses: Rabies and rabies related viruses. In Kurstak, E., and Kurstak, C. (eds.): Comparative Diagnosis of Viral Diseases. New York, Academic Press, Inc., 1977.

# CORONAVIRUS 65

## D. A. J. Tyrrell

The family of viruses known as the coronaviridae affects primarily various species of animals, but there are also coronaviruses that affect humans and cause mild but frequent diseases. Laboratory diagnosis is usually impossible, but it is important for the physician to know about these organisms so that he may understand better the nature of the disease he encounters clinically.

### VIRUS STRUCTURE

The virus particles vary in size and shape (diameter 60 to 200 nm) but are generally spherical. The internal nucleic acid is RNA, which functions as messenger for the translation of protein; this means that the virus is "positive stranded," and thus in the strategy of its multiplication it is quite unlike influenza and parainfluenza viruses, which it superficially resembles. There is a lipid-containing envelope that carries rather widely spaced characteristic projections. These are described as resembling little "petals" or "clubs" and form a ring from which the name of the virus group was derived (Latin, *corona*, crown or halo, Fig. 1).

Virus particles develop in the cytoplasm of infected cells by budding through the membrane into the endoplasmic reticulum. They are released when the cell degenerates and the cytoplasm shatters into many small fragments.

Because of its structure the virus is easily destroyed by detergents and other common antiseptics. It is also easily inactivated by ordinary room temperatures and by drying.

## ANTIGENIC COMPOSITION

Antigenic composition has not been adequately studied, but there are probably three distinct antigens, one of which is the internal nucleoprotein. The surface glycoproteins are apparently the antigens that determine immunity — antibody attaches to them and neutralizes the virus. For technical reasons, mentioned below, we know nothing of the antigens of most human coronaviruses. Some resemble the strain 229E and others OC43 (or OC38) for which antigens are available. Others are apparently distantly related to one or the other of these.

## SUSCEPTIBLE HOST CELLS

The viruses seem to grow in a very limited range of human cells; in fact, many of them were originally isolated only by inoculating them into organ cultures of human fetal trachea or nasal epithelium. Of these viruses, two (OC43 and OC38), which proved to be identical, were found to produce disease in suckling mice and were then adapted to monkey cells in culture, but this has not been done with other viruses. A number of other coronaviruses have been isolated by inoculating clinical specimens into cultures of human embryo fibroblasts; these viruses have all proved to be antigenically related to the first one cultivated in this way, strain 229E. The virus may cause little obvious damage in organ cultures of respiratory epithelium, but it destroys susceptible strains of fibroblasts. It is not as obviously cytopathic as rhinoviruses, which may explain why the type of colds it causes clears up rather quickly.

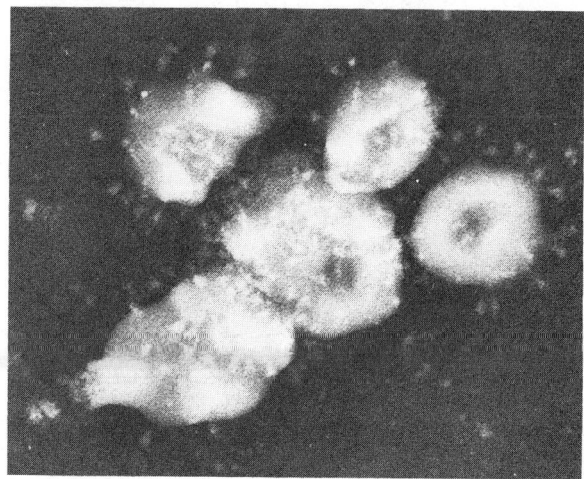

**FIGURE 1.** *A group of five coronavirus particles visualized by negative contrast electron microscope. The particles are pleomorphic and show the typical surface projections. (Courtesy of Mrs. Heather Davies.)*

## PATHOGENIC PROPERTIES

As might be expected, the human coronavirus is infectious when inoculated into the upper respiratory tract. After an incubation period of two to five days it produces a disease characterized by profuse nasal discharge, with nasal obstruction and sneezing. Constitutional upset is mild. There is little or no evidence of an effect on the lower respiratory tract, and the illness clears up rapidly and completely. It may be characterized as a typical streaming cold. In some cases, particularly children, there may be lower respiratory symptoms including wheezing. The virus seems to have no tendency to cause pneumonia or to predispose to bacterial infections.

## IMMUNITY

There is little detailed information on immunity to coronavirus infection. Volunteers may resist infection, in some cases because they possess circulating antibody. Secretory antibody is probably important, but this has not been proved. There is no exact information on the duration of immunity. After infection there may be no detectable antibody response, and it seems likely that reinfection may be possible after a period of months or a few years.

## LABORATORY DIAGNOSIS

The virus is found in respiratory secretions and can be isolated from nasal or throat swabs or from nasal washings. At present the test is strictly a research procedure and requires facilities for organ culture and electron microscopy. Infections can be more easily diagnosed by serologic procedures. There is a complement fixation test for the 229E serotype and a hemagglutination-inhibition test for the OC43 serotype. Paired sera must be collected, the first at onset and the second two to three weeks later; a fourfold rise in titer indicates infection with the virus used in the test or one related to it. The antigens are difficult to obtain, and the antibody titers are often low. Rapid diagnosis by immunofluorescence has been attempted but is not available at the moment.

## EPIDEMIOLOGY

Reliable figures are difficult to obtain, but coronaviruses are probably the second most frequent cause of the common cold, after rhinoviruses, and most likely cause about one case in five. They infrequently precipitate attacks of wheezing and asthma in children. They are usually prevalent during the coldest months of the year, January to April, in the northern temperate zones. There appear to be epidemic waves that can be recognized by laboratory tests but not by any distinctive clinical feature of the disease.

These waves may affect cities and sometimes a whole country in a short period of time.

Although some of the coronaviruses of animals are related antigenically to those that infect man — mouse hepatitis virus is an example — there is no evidence that the viruses actually cross from one species to another.

## HUMAN ENTERIC CORONAVIRUSES

Coronavirus-like particles have been seen by electron microscopy in the feces of patients with diarrheal disease and of others without such symptoms. The virus seems to be extremely difficult to grow but has been propagated in a limited way in organ cultures of human intestine. It has not been proved to cause disease, and nothing is known of its antigens. Future research may show these particles to be important, since there are several coronaviruses that cause significant diarrhea in animals, especially the young.

### References

Bradburne, A. F., and Tyrrell, D. A. J.: Coronaviruses of man. Prog Med Virol 13:373, 1971.
McIntosh, K.: Coronaviruses: A comparative review. Current Topics in Microbiology and Immunology, vol. 63. New York, Springer Verlag, 1974.
Monto, A. S.: Coronaviruses. Yale J Biol Med 47:234, 1974.

# MARBURG VIRUS AND **66** EBOLA VIRUS
### Rudolf Siegert, M.D.

## Marburg Virus

### VIRAL STRUCTURE

Marburg virus is named after a German city in which it was isolated in patients suffering from an unknown hemorrhagic fever (Siegert et al., 1967). Like the closely related Ebola virus, Marburg virus exhibits unique morphologic features, and thus has not yet been classified. Electron microscopy of infected organs and tissue cultures shows cylindrical particles with bizarre shapes, the most frequently found being staffs and long filaments with one rounded end and the other often coiled (Peters et al., 1971; Almeida et al., 1971). In addition, U-shaped, 6-shaped, and annular structures are found (Fig. 1 A-C).

The length of Marburg virus is also unusual. According to electron microscope measurements the average length is 665 nm but can be as much as 12,000 nm. The particles consist of a core with helical symmetry and an envelope with surface projections. The membranous material surrounds the inner cylindrical structure, which is considered to be the nucleocapsid.

The physicochemical composition of Marburg virus is largely unknown; from a few indirect tests, it was concluded that the genetic material is RNA. Experiments with lipid solvents and enzymes indicate that the infectious virion contains lipoprotein.

The morphogenesis of the virus takes place in

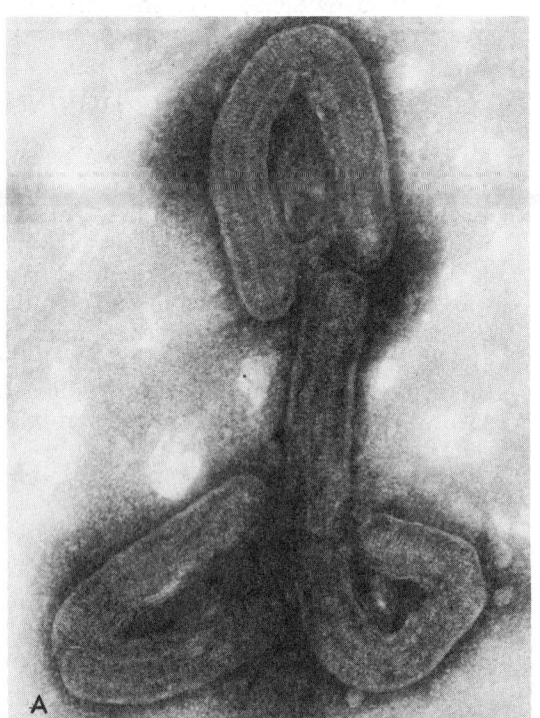

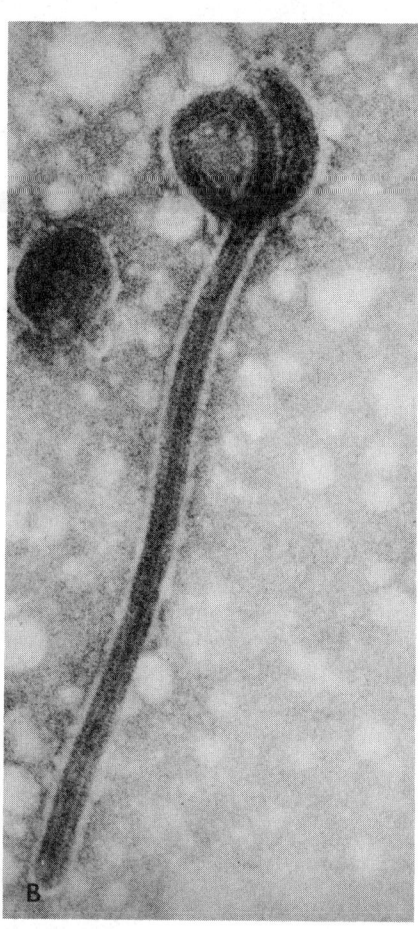

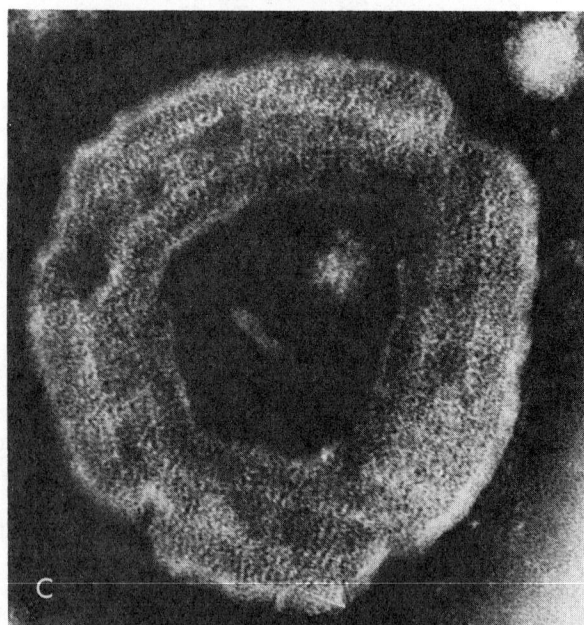

**FIGURE 1.** *Marburg virus, which has been centrifuged directly onto a grid from guinea pig plasma. Fixed in glutaraldehyde and formaldehyde. Negative contrast. A, Three particles — two of normal length and one of longer length. Note membrane, periodicity and central core (× 66,000). B, Particularly long particle (about 2 to 4 μm) (× 46,000). C, Circular form with visible internal component, fixed in formaldehyde, negative contrast (× 300,000). (A and B electron micrographs by D. Peters and G. Müller, Hamburg. In Siegert, R.: The Marburg virus (vervet monkey agent). In Heath, R. B., and Waterson, A. P. (eds.): Modern Trends in Medical Virology. Vol. II. Butterworth Pub. Inc., 1970, p. 204, London. C electron micrograph by Dr. J. D. Almeida, Beckenham, England. In Siegert, R.: Marburgvirus-Krankheit. In Röhrer, H. (ed.): Handbuch der Virusinfektionen bei Tieren, Bd. VI, VEB Gustav Fischer Verlag, Jena 1978, p. 579.)*

cytoplasmic inclusion bodies in the infected cells. They consist of an aggregation of tubular structures (which may be nucleocapsids). These structures are provided with a coat from the cytoplasmic membrane during a budding process.

## ANTIGENIC COMPOSITION

Virus-specific antigen has been demonstrated in infected cells by immunofluorescence and immunoelectron microscopy. Infectiousness can be neutralized by specific antisera. A specific antigen for complement fixation has been prepared from infected Vero-cell cultures. It is antigenically distinct from other viruses.

## SUSCEPTIBLE CELLS

Many cell-culture systems have been examined for their suitability for growing Marburg virus (Siegert, 1972). Primary monkey kidney cells, human amnion, and guinea pig fibroblasts have been found to be most suitable. Although in some cases considerable virus concentrations have been obtained, complete cytopathic effects have developed only in vervet monkey kidney cells after serial passages. In the absence of cell destruction, the propagation of the virus can be recognized by the development of cytoplasmic inclusion bodies as revealed by immunofluorescence (Fig. 2 A, B).

Of the established cell lines examined so far, Vero cells derived from vervet–monkey kidneys and kidney cells from baby hamsters have been best for virus propagation. The cell sheet could not usually be destroyed.

## PATHOGENIC PROPERTIES

Marburg virus is pantropic. Its pathogenicity depends upon virulence and upon the nature of the host (Siegert, 1978).

Experimentally infected monkeys always died, regardless of the virus dose or the route of infection. Observable symptoms are scanty but resemble those found in humans suffering from the same infection (fever, anorexia, petechial exanthema, hemorrhagic diathesis).

Guinea pigs infected intraperitoneally developed fever for several days, as well as certain noncharacteristic symptoms (anorexia, loss of weight, dyspnea, conjunctivitis). The animals almost always survived the first passage, but after several passages they usually died.

We were able to adapt Marburg virus to hamsters and mice, and we found that newborn animals were more susceptible than adults. In contrast, chick embryos were not susceptible.

## IMMUNITY

Infection with Marburg virus induced antibodies in all patients (Slenczka et al., 1970). With

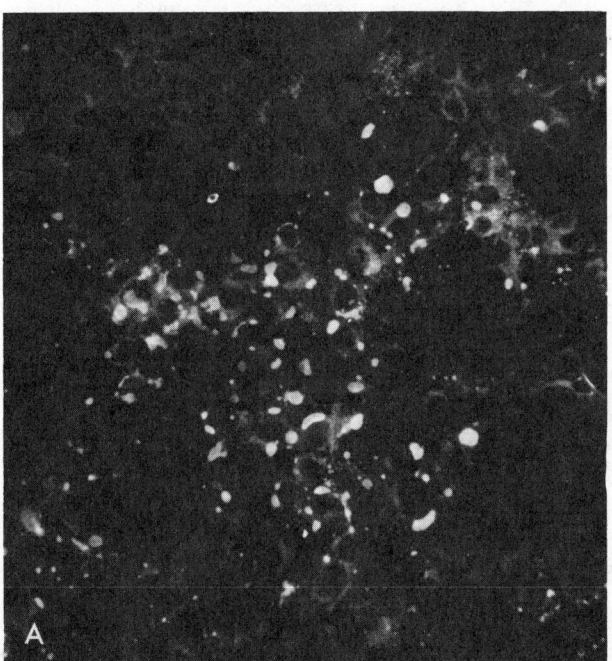

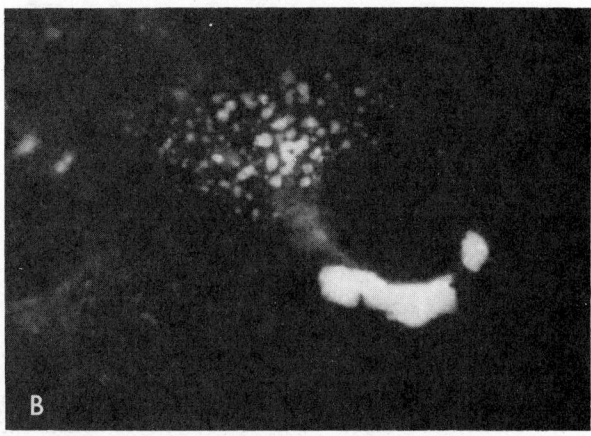

**FIGURE 2.** *Demonstration of viral antigen by direct immunofluorescence in Vero cells four days after infection with Marburg virus. A, Cell culture (× 128), B, Single cell (× 800). (Micrographs by W. Slenczka, Marburg. In Siegert, R.: Marburg virus. In Virology Monographs 11, Springer-Verlag, 1972, p. 97, New York.)*

indirect immunofluorescence, antibodies could be demonstrated during the second week of the disease. They reached a peak one to two weeks later, then declined slowly, and were clearly demonstrable eight years later. Complement-fixing antibodies developed more slowly and declined faster, so that only very low titers were present two years later. The persistence of the antibodies indicates that immunity is long-lasting. Maternal antibodies transmitted transplacentally disappeared within three months in newborn infants. Nothing is known about cellular immunity during the disease.

## LABORATORY DIAGNOSIS

Samples for laboratory examination should be transported in unbreakable plastic containers with screw-on lids. The World Health Organization recommends sending the material to the high-security laboratories (Class III facilities) of the Center for Disease Control in Atlanta, Georgia, or to the Microbiological Research Establishment in Porton, England.

Marburg virus can be demonstrated most reliably in whole blood, serum, and organ specimens obtained during the febrile period (Siegert, 1969). Virus concentrations in throat washes or urine were much lower. In one case the virus was demonstrated in semen, and in another it was found in the anterior chamber of the eye, but all the stool samples were negative.

The high concentrations of virus in the blood and organs in the acute phase of the disease permit rapid demonstration under the electron microscope (Siegert and Slenczka, 1971). Viral particles in serum or plasma can be sedimented directly upon the grid. Their size and shape are sufficiently characteristic to allow a diagnosis. Virus-specific antigen can be demonstrated in autopsy specimens by immunofluorescence.

Virus isolation should always be attempted in case the concentration of virus is too low to be seen by the electron microscope. Vero cells are most suitable for this purpose. Virus multiplication can be recognized a few days after inoculation by the appearance of a virus-specific antigen. Likewise, under an electron microscope, the virus can be demonstrated intracellularly and in the culture fluid. Lassa and yellow fever viruses, which are important for purposes of differential diagnosis, can also be propagated in Vero cells. Antigenic differentiation from Ebola virus is important.

Guinea pigs that become febrile after infection are also suitable for virus isolation. During the febrile phase, the virus can be demonstrated in the serum by electron microscopy and the antigen can be revealed in cell inclusions of organ specimens by immunofluorescence.

For serodiagnosis, blood from the acute and convalescent phases of the disease must be examined in order to detect a decisive rise in the antibody titer. The complement-fixation reaction provides useful results with purified cell-culture antigens. However, the method of choice is immunofluorescence, owing to its greater sensitivity.

## EPIDEMIOLOGY

Only two outbreaks of Marburg virus disease have been reported, with a total of 34 patients. The two episodes differed considerably in basic epidemiology. In 1967, 31 persons in Marburg and Frankfurt (Federal Republic of Germany) and in Belgrad (Yugoslavia) became ill almost simultaneously; seven of them died. The epidemiologic situation was puzzling at first, but it was soon noted that the first victims all worked in institutes in which live poliomyelitis vaccines are produced and tested (Hennessen et al., 1966). It was then learned that all the primary cases had had contact with blood and organs of African green or vervet monkeys (*Cercopithecus aethiops*), which had been imported from Uganda by air freight via London. Those persons who ran the greatest risk were individuals involved in the actual surgical removal of organs from the animals. This is not surprising, since the virus concentrations in the blood and tissues of infected monkeys are particularly high and the measures taken to protect the workers were incomplete. The incidence was lower in persons working with cultures of monkey kidney cells. The remaining cases were persons in contact with patients, either in the family or in hospitals. Later serologic examinations of the environment produced no evidence of inapparent infections.

The most severe courses of the disease were observed in patients with primary infections, and all the fatalities occurred in this group. Patients with secondary infections had a milder course. In these cases, infection took place mainly via lesions of the skin and mucous membranes. In the hospital personnel who contracted the disease while attending infected patients, the infectious medium was blood from the febrile phase. The only infection that occurred in a family was in a woman whose husband was a carrier; she was infected by his semen. As to other possible transmission mechanisms, there is no reason for assuming the existence of oral, aerogenic, or conjunctival portals of entry. The chain of infection ended after at most two human passages.

A second outbreak of the disease, with only three cases, took place in 1975 in Johannesburg

(South Africa) (Gear et al., 1975). The first victim was an Australian who had traveled through Rhodesia shortly before becoming ill. The woman accompanying him then contracted the disease, and the third case was the nurse who had attended the Australian before his death. During the latter's journey, he had had no direct contact with animals. The two women became infected through contact with him while attending him during his illness.

In spite of extensive field studies, the natural reservoir of the virus has not yet been ascertained. Its presence in Uganda and Rhodesia indicates that it is more widespread than was originally assumed. It is probable that monkeys, like humans, were only coincidental hosts. Although Marburg virus has been propagated in intrathoracically inoculated *Aedes aegypti* mosquitoes, no attempt has yet been made to transmit the virus from infected mosquitoes.

# Ebola Virus

## VIRAL STRUCTURE

Ebola virus was isolated in 1976, following an epidemic of hemorrhagic fever in central Africa; it is named after a river in Zaire. In size, shape, and ultrastructure the virus is strikingly analogous to Marburg virus (Bowen et al., 1977; Johnson et al., 1977; Pattyn et al., 1977). At first the two were considered to be identical, but careful comparisons have shown that the normal and double lengths of Ebola virus are 1.25 times those of Marburg virus. Particles with a length of up to 14,000 nm have been found (Slenczka and Peters, 1977). The diameter is listed as being 70 to 100 nm, with an inner helix of 40 nm.

Because of their special morphologic position, these two viruses may be considered the first representatives of an undesignated new group (Simpson and Zuckerman, 1977).

The physicochemical composition of Ebola virus has not yet been examined because it is too dangerous to work with. It is assumed that the genome, like that of Marburg virus, consists of RNA and that the envelope contains lipoprotein.

Ebola virus is constructed of preformed nucleocapsids that develop in the cytoplasm of the host cells and are coated by the plasma membrane during the budding process.

## ANTIGENIC COMPOSITION

The Ebola virus strains from the Sudan and Zaire are identical not only morphologically but also antigenically. They share no antigen with Marburg virus, in spite of their similar structure. Antigens were compared by direct and indirect immunofluorescence.

## SUSCEPTIBLE CELLS

Of the numerous primary and permanent cells of varying origin that have been tested, Vero cells are the most suitable for propagation of Ebola virus. A cytopathic effect develops according to the culture medium used and increases with the number of passages made. The virus can be demonstrated in the cell-culture fluid before the cytopathic effect is apparent. Numerous intracytoplasmic antigen inclusions appear in the infected cells.

## PATHOGENIC PROPERTIES

The range of the natural hosts of Ebola virus is not known. As with Marburg virus, monkeys are highly susceptible in experiments. Rhesus (*Macaca mulatta*) and vervet (*Cercopithecus aethiops*) monkeys become ill a few days after intraperitoneal infection, with symptoms of fever, maculopapular rash, diarrhea, and hemorrhages; they die after a short time.

In addition, Ebola virus is pathogenic for guinea pigs, which develop fever for several days but no other striking symptoms. Mortality is low after the first passages. Newborn and suckling mice die after intracerebral or intraperitoneal infection.

## IMMUNITY

In patients and infected guinea pigs, antibodies were demonstrated by means of indirect immunofluorescence, the complement fixation reaction, and the neutralization test. It is still too early to evaluate the persistence of the antibodies. There is no cross-immunity with Marburg virus.

## LABORATORY DIAGNOSIS

Diagnostic examinations are based on the same principles as those used for diagnosis of Marburg virus (Emond et al., 1977). In every case, a rapid diagnosis should be attempted, with direct electron microscope demonstration of the virus in serum or plasma during the febrile phase and in ultra-thin sections of autopsy liver tissue. In addition, virus isolation should be attempted in Vero cells and guinea pigs. The isolated virus must then be identified by means of immunofluorescence or immunoelectron microscopy, and differentiated from Marburg virus. Ebola virus was found regularly in serum samples taken during the febrile phase and also in the semen of one patient, but could not be demonstrated in throat washings, urine, or feces.

The method of choice for serodiagnosis is immunofluorescence, since it is more sensitive than the complement fixation reaction in demonstrating antibodies.

## EPIDEMIOLOGY

From August to November of 1976 there were epidemics of a hemorrhagic fever with high mortality in the southern Sudan and simultaneously in northern Zaire, around 1000 km away (Brès, 1977). The disease was similar to that caused by Marburg virus. In the Sudanese towns of Nzara and Maridi there were 70 and 229 cases, respectively; of these almost one half died. In Maridi, 76 of 230 hospital employees became ill, and 41 of them died. After transfer of the patients to other hospitals, contact infections occurred in these personnel as well. In Zaire, at least 43 villages within a radius of 50 km around the missionary station at Yambucu were affected; 237 patients were registered, and 211 of them died. Here too there were contact infections among the hospital personnel. In Porton, England, a laboratory technician infected himself accidentally with an injection needle while working with guinea pigs.

The morbidity rates during the two epidemics varied considerably. In the Sudan, the rate was listed as 3.5 to 15.3/1000, and as less than 1 to 8/1000 in Zaire. The number of secondary cases is said to have been approximately 15 per cent in Zaire, whereas in the Sudan there were reports of 13 per cent secondary, 14 per cent tertiary, and 9 per cent quaternary cases. Longer infection chains were rare.

It is still not known how the virus is eliminated from the organism or transmitted. Person-to-person infections require extremely close contact. Exposure was greatest among hospital personnel. In them, contamination with blood and other body fluids played an important part, and transmission was favored by skin and mucous lesions as well as by insufficiently sterilized instruments. Airborne droplet infections appear to play only a minor role, if any.

No arthropods or mammals have been demonstrated to be carriers or hosts.

## References

*Marburg Virus*

Almeida, J. D., Waterson, A. P., and Simpson D. I. H.: Morphology and morphogenesis of the Marburg agent. In Martini, G. A., and Siegert, R. (eds.): Marburg Virus Disease. New York, Springer Verlag, 1971, p. 84.

Gear, J. S. S., Cassel, G. A., Gear, A. J., Trappler, B., Clausen, L., Meyers, A. M., Kew, M. C., Bothwell, T. H., Sher, R., Miller, G. B., Schneider, J., Koornhof, H. J., Gomperts, E. D., Isaacson, M., and Gear, J. H. S.: Outbreak of Marburg virus disease in Johannesburg. Br Med J. 1:489, 1975.

Hennessen, W., Bonin, O., and Mauler, R.: Zur Epidemiologie der Erkrankung von Menschen durch Affen. Dtsch Med Wochenschr 93:582, 1968.

Peters, D., Müller, G., and Slenczka, W.: Morphology, development, and classification of the Marburg virus. In Martini, G. A., and Siegert, R. (eds.): Marburg Virus Disease. New York, Springer Verlag, 1971, p. 68.

Siegert, R.: Probleme der Virusdiagnostik, dargestellt am Beispiel des Marburg-Virus. Verh Dtsch Ges Inn Med 75:565, 1969.

Siegert, R.: Marburg virus. In Virology Monographs 11. New York, Springer Verlag, 1972, p. 97.

Siegert, R.: Marburgvirus-Krankheit. In Röhrer, H. (ed.): Handbuch der Virusinfektionen bei Tieren, Bd. 6. Jena, Gustav Fischer Verlag, 1978, p. 579.

Siegert, R., and Slenczka, W.: Laboratory diagnosis and pathogenesis. In Martini, G. A., and Siegert, R. (eds.): Marburg Virus Disease. New York, Springer Verlag, 1971, p. 157.

Siegert, R., Shu, H. L., Slenczka, W., Peters, D., and Müller, G.: Zur Ätiologie einer unbekannten, von Affen ausgegangenen menschlichen Infektionskrankheit. Dtsch Med Wochenschr 92: 2341, 1967.

Slenczka, W., Siegert, R., and Wolff, G.: Nachweis komplementbindender Antikörper des Marburg-Virus bei 22 Patienten mit einem Zellkultur-Antigen. Arch Virusforsch 31:71, 1970.

*Ebola Virus*

Bowen, E. T. W., Lloyd, G., Harris, W. J., Platt, G. S., Baskerville, A., and Vella, E. E.: Viral haemorrhagic fever in southern Sudan and northern Zaire. Lancet 1:571, 1977.

Brès, P.: Report of the Informal Consultation on the Marburg Virus-like Disease Outbreaks in the Sudan and Zaire in 1976. Held at the London School of Hygiene and Tropical Medicine, 4 and 5 January 1977. New York, World Health Organization, 1977, p. 569.

Emond, R. T. D., Evans, B., Bowen, E. T. W., and Lloyd, G.: A case of Ebola virus infection. Br Med J 2:541, 1977.

Johnson, K. M., Lange, J. V., Webb, P. A., and Murphy, F. A.: Isolation and partial characterisation of a new virus causing acute haemorrhagic fever in Zaire. Lancet 1:569, 1977.

Pattyn, S., van der Groen, G., Jacob, W., Piot, P., and Courteille, G.: Isolation of Marburg-like virus from a case of haemorrhagic fever in Zaire. Lancet 1:573, 1977.

Simpson, I. H., and Zuckerman, A. J.: Marburg and Ebola: Viruses in search of a relation. Nature 266:217, 1977.

Slenczka, W., and Peters, D.: Ebola-Virus, ein neuer Vertreter der Marburg-Virus-Gruppe. Tropenmed Parasitol 28:260, 1977.

# Unclassified Viruses

## *HEPATITIS VIRUSES* **67**

### *Shalom Z. Hirschman, M.D.*

Many viruses, such as cytomegalovirus, measles virus, Epstein-Barr virus, and yellow fever virus, attack the liver during systemic infection. However, in this chapter we will examine the viruses whose only known organ of tropism is the liver. These viruses are the heaptitis A virus, the agent causing infectious hepatitis (short incubation hepatitis), and the hepatitis B virus, the cause of serum hepatitis (transfusion hepatitis, long incubation hepatitis).

Two classic epidemiologic patterns of transmission of viral hepatitis were recognized early and formed the basis for classification of viral hepatitis into two major clinical types. The more common variety of viral hepatitis, which often involved many people and exhibited a shorter incubation period, was termed infectious hepatitis. Hepatitis following blood transfusions or needle wounds, which had a longer incubation period, was called serum hepatitis. Only recently have the virologic differences between these two types of viral hepatitides been established in the laboratory.

The morphologic, biophysical, and biochemical properties of the newly identified hepatitis A and B viruses will be discussed here. The salient characteristics of the two viruses are summarized in Table 1.

**TABLE 1.  Characteristics of Hepatitis A and B Viruses**

| CHARACTERISTIC | VIRUS | | |
| --- | --- | --- | --- |
| | A | B | Non-A, Non-B |
| Epidemiology | Endemic and epidemic, water-borne and food-borne epidemics | Endemic | Endemic |
| Transmission | Fecal-oral | Direct inoculation, ? venereal | Direct inoculation ? other |
| Incubation period | 2–7 weeks | 4 weeks to 6 months | 2–8 weeks |
| Disease | Acute | Acute and chronic | Acute and chronic |
| Size of virus | 27 nm | 42 nm (27 nm core) | ? |
| Coat protein | − | + | ? |
| Nucleic acid | RNA | Circular DNA (mainly double-stranded; molecular weight $\sim 2.1 \times 10^6$) | ? |
| DNA polymerase | − | + | ? |
| Cell culture system | + | − | − |
| Animal infection | Marmosets, chimpanzees | Chimpanzees | Chimpanzees |
| Chronic carrier | − | + | + |
| Vaccine | − | ?Purified coat protein | − |
| Passive immunity with immune globulin | + | + | ?+ |

# HEPATITIS A VIRUS

## *EPIDEMIOLOGY*

Early epidemiologic studies conducted almost three decades ago and studies with stool filtrates fed to human volunteers suggested a fecal-oral route of transmission for the virus causing infectious hepatitis. Indeed, many water- and food-borne outbreaks of disease have been reported. The infection is more common in countries with low standards of living, and in these countries it infects the population at a younger age.

## *ISOLATION AND DETECTION OF VIRUS*

The modern study of hepatitis A virus (HAV) began a decade ago with attempts to transmit this virus to marmosets (*Sanguinus mystax*) (Dienhardt et al., 1967). These studies were only recently brought to practical fruition when strain CR326 of HAV was isolated in Costa Rica from the blood of a child with typical infectious hepatitis by serial passage in marmosets. Neutralizing antibody to CR326 developed in patients with hepatitis A infection. Use of viral antigen (now called hepatitis A antigen [HAAg]) derived from marmoset liver allowed the development of spe-

cific complement fixation, immune adherence, and radioimmunoassay tests for detection of antibody, thus providing sensitive serologic tests for viral infection (Krugman et al., 1975). At the same time, the virus was identified by immune electron microscopy in stool extracts of volunteers infected with virus by the oral route (Feinstone et al., 1973). Viral particles found in stool extracts were clumped by antibody present in convalescent serum.

HAV has been purified from human and chimpanzee stool extracts, from infected marmoset and chimpanzee livers, and from bile of infected chimpanzees (Dienstag et al., 1975). The purification techniques have included precipitation by polyethylene glycol (PEG), gel filtration on Sepharose 2B columns, and isopyknic ultracentrifugation on cesium chloride density gradients in sundry combinations (Bradley et al., 1976).

## *MORPHOLOGY AND BIOCHEMISTRY*

The immunoreactive particles have a diameter of 27 nm (Fig. 1) (Provost et al., 1975). Electron-microscopic observations with positive staining of the particles showed that many particles have a dense core that is presumably composed of nucleo-

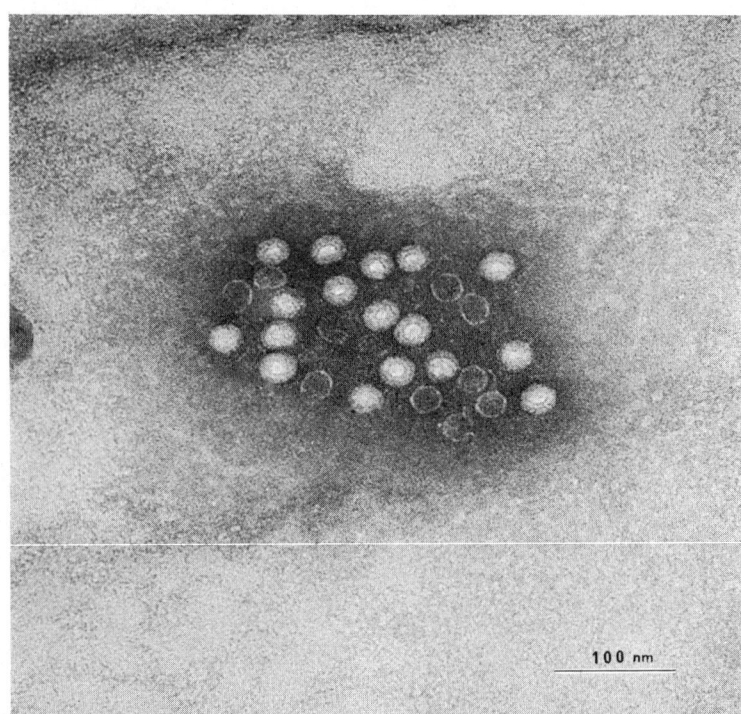

**FIGURE 1.** *Electron micrograph of HAV particles extracted from HAV-infected marmoset liver showing electron dense cores (× 328,600; Prepared by Mr. E.H. Cook, Jr., and provided by courtesy of Dr. Daniel W. Bradley).*

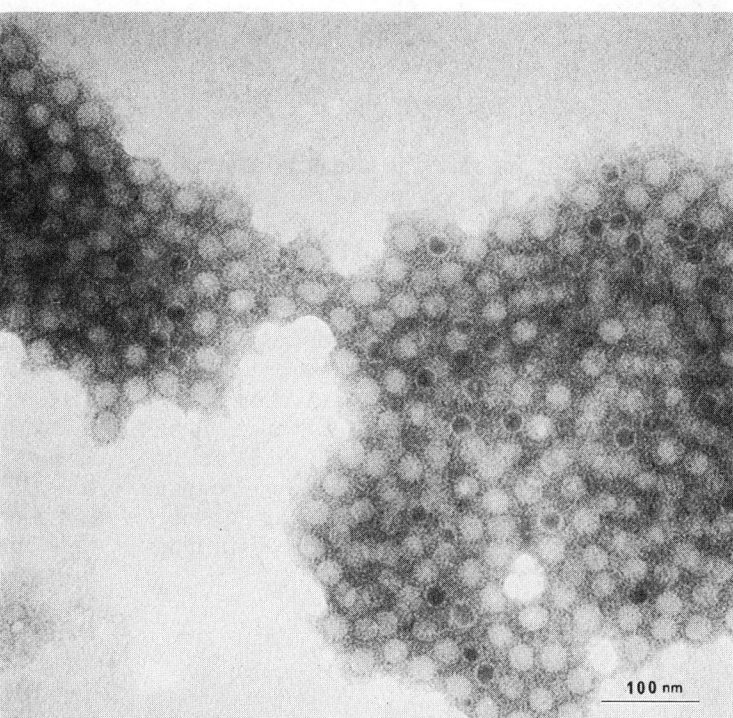

**FIGURE 2.** *Highly purified HAV from pre-acute phase chimpanzee stool aggregated by anti-HAV (× 256,300; Prepared by Mr. E.H. Cook, Jr., and provided by courtesy of Dr. Daniel W. Bradley).*

protein (Fig. 1). The viral particles are clumped by specific antibody (Fig. 2). Infectious virus bands at a density of 1.32 to 1.34 g/ml on cesium chloride density gradients. The infectivity of purified virus is destroyed by heating at 100° C for five minutes but is only partially reduced by heating at 60° C for one hour. Infectivity can be reduced by exposure to ultraviolet light. Purified virus is totally inactivated by treatment with 1:4000 formalin for three days at 37° C. The virus is acid stable. Electronmicroscopic study of marmoset liver showed that the virus was localized in small vesicles in cytoplasm but was absent in the nucleus. Preliminary studies suggested that hepatitis A virus may contain RNA. Acridine orange staining of purified concentrates of CR326 spread on slides gave an orange-red color characteristic of RNA staining, and partial inactivation of viral infectivity, beyond that produced by heat alone, was obtained by reacting the virus with pancreatic RNAse for one hour at 60° C.

## ANIMAL TRANSMISSION AND IMMUNITY

Recently, hepatitis A virus has been successfully transmitted to chimpanzees (Pantroglo- dytes) by fecal extracts from infected patients administered either orally or intravenously. The chimpanzees developed lassitude and anorexia, accompanied by biochemical abnormalities such as elevation of serum glutamic oxaloacetic transaminase (SGOT) within two to five weeks. Viral 27-nm particles appeared in stools during the second week after inoculation and disappeared by the fifth week. Antibody appeared by the third week and remained elevated. Although IgG and IgA immunoglobulins remained unchanged, there was a rise in the level of IgM with the onset of clinical illness. Highly purified HAV derived from extracts of acute phase feces of infected chimpanzees has transmitted typical clinical hepatitis when inoculated into previously uninfected chimpanzees. Thus, it has been established that the 27-nm particles containing HAAg derived from extracts of acute phase feces from both humans and chimpanzees are infectious and provoke a specific antibody response in inoculated chimpanzees. A tissue culture system for propagation of HAV has recently been developed.

Infection with HAV provokes a prolonged antibody response, and immunity appears to be lifelong. Passive protection with immunoglobulin appears to both prevent and ameliorate disease. There is still no vaccine for hepatitis A infection.

# HEPATITIS B VIRUS

## *EPIDEMIOLOGY*

A second form of viral hepatitis is associated with blood transfusions or direct needle inoculation and has a rather prolonged incubation period. In Western Europe and North America cases of serum hepatitis usually appear singly. However, in Asia large segments of the population have been found to be infected. Indeed, infection seems to be acquired even during the neonatal period. Recent evidence has shown that mosquitoes can carry the virus. However, it has not been established whether mosquitoes are important in transmitting the infection. Bedbugs also can harbor the virus and may possibly transmit disease from person to person in close family quarters.

## *BIOCHEMISTRY*

The first biochemical trace of the hepatitis B virus was discovered when a new antigen was found in the blood of an Australian aborigine. This antigen formed a precipitin line with serum from a patient with hemophilia who had received multiple blood transfusions (Blumberg et al., 1967). It was quickly appreciated that this new antigen, termed Australia antigen (also called SH-antigen and hepatitis-associated antigen), was associated with serum hepatitis. The antigen was found to exist in particulate form in the blood of patients with serum hepatitis (Fig. 3) (Bayer et al., 1967). The predominant form was a disk-shaped particle 18 to 20 nm in diameter. Tube forms with diameters of 20 nm and lengths of 50 to 500 nm, and showing cross-striations with a

periodicity of 3 nm also were observed in sera from most patients. A larger particle 40 to 42 nm in diameter, with a double shell and an inner core resembling a viral nucleoid, was also found in sera of patients with antigenemia (Dane et al., 1970). It was suggested that the larger particles represented the complete virion and that the other morphologic forms were excess coat protein. This suggestion was given experimental foundation when the internal component of the larger particle, also called the Dane particle, was released by treating the particles with 0.5 per cent Tween-80 (polysorbate) in phosphate-buffered saline (PBS) (Almeida et al., 1971). The internal component had a diameter of 27 nm and seemed to be morphologically identical to particles found in the nuclei of hepatocytes of patients with serum hepatitis. Thus, the coat protein of the Dane particle was called hepatitis B surface antigen (HBsAg), and the core particle was called hepatitis B core antigen (HBcAg). The long tube forms of HBsAg could be converted to the disk forms by exposure to mildly acidic buffers. Antibody directed against the internal component of the Dane particle, which was different from antibody to HBsAg, was found during acute attacks of hepatitis.

DNA polymerase is present in preparations of hepatitis B antigen containing Dane particles. The enzyme is associated with the core of the Dane particle. The core of the Dane particle contains covalently closed, open circular, mainly double-stranded DNA (Robinson et al., 1974), but has single-stranded regions comprising 30 to 60 per cent of the nucleotides, of molecular weight of $2.1 \times 10^6$ (Fig. 4). The base composition of this DNA is approximately 49 per cent guano-

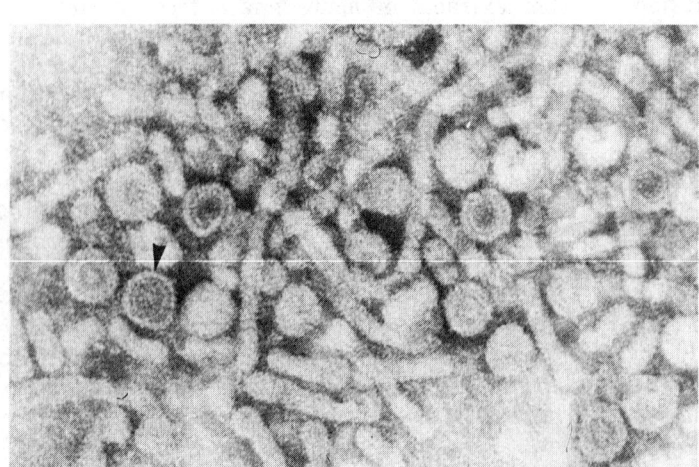

**FIGURE 3.** *Electron micrograph of particulate Australia antigen (hepatitis B surface antigen) showing 18 to 20 nm discs, long tubular forms and 42 nm Dane particles (arrow) (× 250,000; electron micrograph taken by Dr. Michael Gerber).*

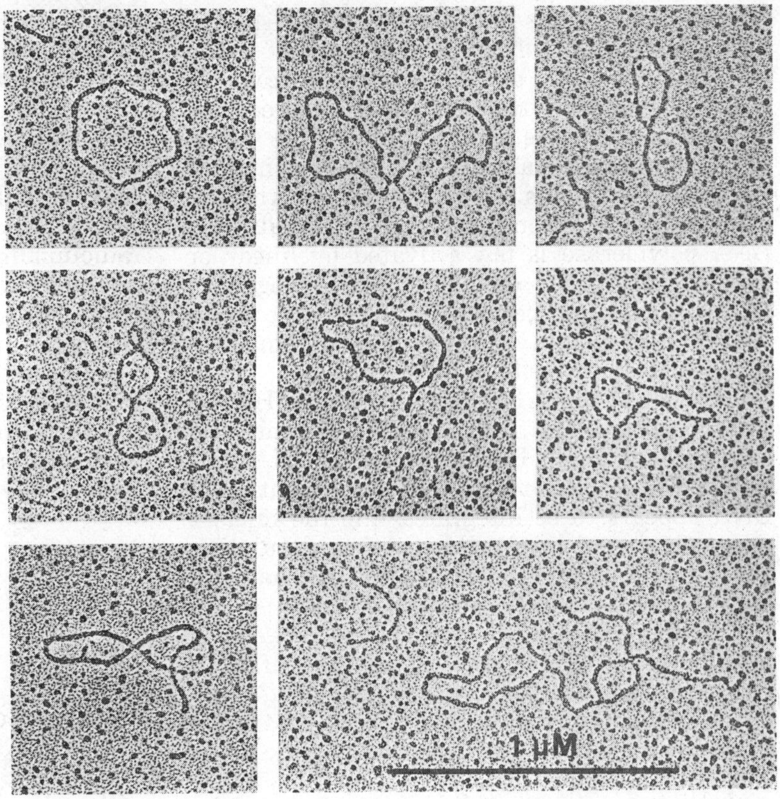

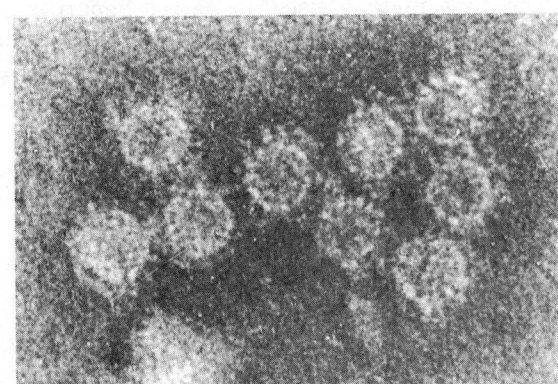

**FIGURE 4.** *Electron micrograph of DNA extracted from Dane particles purified from human plasma showing open circles. (Provided by courtesy of Dr. Lacy R. Overby.)*

sine plus cytosine. In the test tube, the DNA polymerase appears to function as a repair enzyme for the region of single-stranded DNA.

Two populations of Dane particles can be identified in the electron microscope by using positive stains. One population, usually the minor one, shows densely staining cores, whereas the other population, usually the major one, shows lightly staining cores. The densely staining population of Dane particles contains very high DNA polymerase activity, while much less enzyme activity is found in the lightly staining particles. The densely staining particles sediment faster in sucrose. Core particles isolated from the heavier Dane particles band at densities of 1.36 to 1.34 gm/ml in cesium chloride, while core particles from the lighter Dane particles band at 1.33 to 1.30 gm/ml. It has been suggested that the densely staining core particles are complete, containing a full complement of both DNA and DNA polymerase, while the lightly staining core particles may not contain DNA. Core particles of density 1.30 to 1.32 gm/ml have been isolated from purified nuclei of hepatocytes infected by HBV (Fig. 5); although they contained linear double-stranded DNA, these particles did not show DNA polymerase activity. Core particles with DNA polymerase activity have been isolated from total homogenates of both human and chimpanzee liver infected with HBV.

The core particle-associated DNA polymerase is active in very high concentrations of both salts of monovalent cations and magnesium chloride in which other known bacterial, mammalian, and viral DNA polymerases are inhibited (Hirschman and Garfinkel, 1977). This singular property of the core particle DNA polymerase forms the basis for a differential assay of the hepatitis B enzyme in reaction mixtures with $\geq 0.4$ M KCl and $\geq 0.04$ M $MgCl_2$. Hepatitis B DNA polymerase is inhibited by $MnCl_2$ and most other divalent cations.

**FIGURE 5.** *Core particles of HBV isolated from purified nuclei of infected human liver. The diameter of the core particle is 27 nm and the particle contains HBcAg ($\times$ 286,000; electron micrograph taken by Dr. Michael Gerber).*

Nonionic detergents such as Nonidet P-40 enhance the DNA polymerase reaction of Dane particles, perhaps by removing the coat of HBsAg, thus allowing freer access of precursor deoxyribonucleotides to the viral core. The activity of core particle-associated DNA polymerase increases with rising concentrations of both salts of monovalent cations and $MgCl_2$. Hepatitis B DNA polymerase is not activated by linear or circular single- or double-stranded exogenous DNAs, suggesting specificity of the enzyme for its own DNA or inability of the exogenous templates to reach the active site of the enzyme.

Particles 27 nm in diameter containing HBcAg have been purified from infected human and chimpanzee liver. Double-stranded DNA has been isolated from these particles. Hepatitis B DNA appears to be integrated into the nuclear DNA of infected liver cells, and free circulating DNA hybridizing to Dane particle DNA has also been found in plasma of infected patients.

A soluble antigen, called e antigen (HBeAg), is also found in sera of patients with hepatitis B virus infection. The antigen appears during acute infection and then usually disappears, but can be carried chronically in patients with chronic hepatitis B antigenemia and chronic hepatitis. The e antigen appears to be a protein of approximately $17 \times 10^3$ daltons, but the exact nature of this antigen is unknown. At present, three major antigenic subtypes, $HBe_1Ag$, $HBe_2Ag$, and $HBe_3Ag$ are recognized. The presence of e antigen appears to be associated with the presence of Dane particles. Along with hepatitis B core antigen, persistence of HBeAg usually portends chronic hepatitis. HBeAg also appears to be a marker for infectivity of HBsAg positive blood. The major component antigens of HBV are summarized in Table 2.

## ASSAY OF HBAg

The first method used to detect hepatitis B surface antigen in the laboratory was the rather insensitive method of immunodiffusion; this test was followed by the more sensitive counterimmunoelectrophoresis. Newer, more sensitive procedures for detecting HBsAg include the techniques of complement fixation, hemagglutination, and radioimmunoassay. The most commonly used test is the radioimmunoassay, which is now commercially available. Hepatitis B core antigen can be detected both by complement fixation and radioimmunoassay, but the latter is the preferred and more widely used technique. Unfortunately, HBeAg is still determined by immunodiffusion although radioimmunoassays have recently been developed. The wide use of radioimmunoassay, with its greater accuracy in detecting HBsAg, has certainly contributed to the great decrease of transmission of hepatitis B from the blood of commercial donors.

## SUBTYPES OF HBsAg

HBsAg contains a common immunologic determinant, a, and several major subdeterminants that are specified by the viral genome (LeBouvier, 1971). The subdeterminants can be detected by the presence of spurs in immunodiffusion tests with various antisera. Eight distinct categories and two of mixed subtype have been recognized (Table 3). These consist of various combinations of the subdeterminants d/y and w/r. The subdeterminants appear to comprise two groups composed of d/y on the one hand and w1, w2, w3, w4, and r on the other. The two mixed subtypes are very rare and may have been due to phenotypic or genotypic mixing of immunologic markers during simultaneous infection with viruses associated with more than one subtype of HBsAg. Several minor antigenic subdeterminants have been described, including q, x, f, p, j, n, and g; g has been found with w2. Antigenic types ayw2 and ayw3 appear to be more common in Africa and the Middle East. The subdeterminant r appears to predominate in the Far East and is very common in Japan. The antigenic type adw2 is common in the United States. In experiments in which chimpanzees were infected with different strains of HBV carrying distinct antigenic determinants it was found that the viral strains breed true with respect to the antigenic determinants. Purified hepatitis B surface antigen appears to share cross-antigenicity with some normal human proteins. Both lipid and carbohydrates are associated with purified HBsAg. The carbohydrate content appears to vary from 3.6 to 6.5 per cent, and antigenic activity is lost after mild periodate oxidation. The lipids associated with HBsAg include phosphatidylcholine, sphingomyelin, lysophosphatidylcholine, and glycosphingolipid.

TABLE 2.   Major Antigens Comprising
Hepatitis B Virus

| ANTIGEN | CHARACTERISTIC |
| --- | --- |
| Surface; HBsAg | Particulate; viral coat protein; has major and minor antigenic subdeterminants; found in cytoplasm |
| Core; HBcAg | Particulate; viral nucleoid; found in nucleus |
| e; HBeAg | Soluble; present in viral core several subtypes |

**TABLE 3.** Antigenic Subdeterminants
of Hepatitis B Surface Antigen

| MAJOR | MINOR |
|-------|-------|
| aywl  | q |
| ayw2  | x |
| ayw3  | f |
| ayw4  | t |
| ayr   | j |
| adw2  | n |
| adw4  | g |
| adr   |   |
| adwy  |   |
| adyr  |   |

HBsAg of adw and ayw subtypes appears to differ in both biophysical and biochemical characteristics. The buoyant density of HBsAg in cesium chloride is 1.21 g/cc. The molecular weight of adw preparations of HBsAg is $3.7 \times 10^6$. HBsAg of ayw subtype has an average molecular weight of $4.6 \times 10^6$. The acidic isoelectric point (pI) of HBsAg is due to a high proportion of acidic amino acid residues relative to basic amino acids. HBsAg contains high levels of cysteine, proline, leucine, and phenylalanine. Reduction and alkylation destroy the antigenic activity of HBsAg. Nine separate polypeptides have been found in preparations of the ayw subtype of HBsAg and only seven in the preparations of the adw subtype. The polypeptides appear to vary in antigenic activity. Much less is known about the chemical composition of hepatitis B core antigen, but preliminary studies indicate that this antigen has a much simpler composition than that of the surface antigen.

It is thus evident that HBV is a unique virion that contains not only partly single-stranded circular DNA but also a DNA polymerase. The virus contains many antigens that may not all be coded for by the small DNA in the virus (unless one postulates proteins composed of similar subunits and perhaps also overlapping DNA codons). Much further work will be required to delineate the replicative cycle, especially the role of the curious DNA polymerase, of this fascinating virus in the hepatocyte.

## ANTIBODIES TO HBAg

After infection with hepatitis B virus, antibodies to HBcAg (anti-HBc) usually appear when liver disease becomes evident. Antibodies to HBsAg (anti-HBs) usually appear during convalescence and coincide with disappearance of circulating HBsAg. Both animal and human studies indicate that anti-HBc tends to decrease gradually and may become undetectable after one to two years. Anti-HBs lasts much longer and indeed may be present throughout life. Antibody to HBsAg seems to bestow immunity to further infection with HBV. In the chronic carrier state, with persistence of HBsAg, a high level of anti-HBc, but not anti-HBs, is usually found in serum. Anti-HBe appears with onset of overt liver disease in acute hepatitis and is considered a good prognostic sign.

## VACCINES

The thesis that HBsAg represents excess coat protein of the complete hepatitis B virion led to the conclusion that vaccines of purified HBsAg would be protective but not infectious. Preliminary studies with such vaccines composed of purified HBsAg appear to bear out this hypothesis (Melnick et al., 1976). In attempts to avoid possible cross-reactions of HBsAg vaccines with normal human proteins, much effort is being expended on the study of protein subunit vaccines. Small antigenic peptides have been purified from HBsAg.

# OTHER HEPATITIS VIRUSES

Evidence has been accumulating from epidemiologic studies that there may be at least two hitherto unrecognized viral agents causing acute hepatitis. The first such evidence came from epidemiologic and serologic studies of transfusion-associated hepatitis. In these studies it was found that half of the cases that occurred following transfusion were not due to either hepatitis A or B virus and were not caused by other recognizable viral agents such as Epstein-Barr virus or cytomegalovirus. Similar evidence for the presence of other hepatitis viruses has been deduced from a study of patients with multiple attacks of acute viral hepatitis. Some of the patients had four attacks of acute hepatitis, two of which could be accounted for by hepatitis A and hepatitis B infection. Thus it was presumed that the other two attacks may have been caused by other hitherto unrecognized hepatitis viruses. Now that infections of HAV and HBV can be determined serologically, much evidence is accumulating that non-A, non-B hepatitis is a prevalent infection (Feinstone et al., 1975).

## References

Almeida, J. D., Rubinstein, D., and Stott, E. J.: New antigen-antibody system in Australia-antigen-positive hepatitis. Lancet 2:1225, 1971.

Barker, L. F., Chisari, F. V., McGrath, P. P., Dalgard, D. W., Kirschstein, R. L., Almeida, J. D., Edgington, T. S., Sharp, D. G., and Peterson, M. R.: Transmission of type B viral hepatitis to chimpanzees. J Infect Dis 127:648, 1973.

Bayer, M. E., Blumberg, B. S., and Werner, B.: Particles associated with Australia antigen in the sera of patients with leukemia, Down's syndrome and hepatitis. Nature 318:1057, 1968.

Blumberg, B. S., Gerstley, B. J. S., Hungerford, D. A., London, W. T., and Sutnick, A. I.: A serum antigen (Australia antigen) in Down's syndrome, leukemia and hepatitis. Ann Int Med 66:924, 1967.

Bradley, D. W., Hollinger, F. B., Hornbeck, C. L., and Maynard, J. E.: Isolation and characterization of hepatitis A virus. Am J Clin Pathol 65:876, 1976.

Dane, D. S., Cameron, C. H., and Briggs, M.: Virus-like particles in serum of patients with Australia antigen associated hepatitis. Lancet 1:695, 1970.

Dienhardt, F., Holmes, A. W., Capps, R. B., and Popper, H.: Studies on the transmission of human viral hepatitis to marmoset monkeys. J Exp Med 125:673, 1967.

Dienstag, J. L., Feinstone, S. M., Purcell, R. H., Hoofnagle, J. H., Barker, L. E., London, W. T., Popper, H., Peterson, J. M., and

Kapikian, A. Z.: Experimental infection of chimpanzees with hepatitis A virus. J Infect Dis 132:532, 1975.

Feinstone, S. M., Kapikian, A. Z., and Purcell, R. H.: Hepatitis A: Detection by immune electron microscopy of a viruslike antigen associated with acute illness. Science 182:1026, 1973.

Feinstone, S. M., Kapikian, A. Z., Purcell, R. H., Alter, H. J., and Holland, P. V.: Transfusion-associated hepatitis not due to viral hepatitis type A or B. N Engl J Med 292:767, 1975.

Hirschman, S. Z.: Integrator enzyme hypothesis for replication of hepatitis B virus. Lancet 2:436, 1975.

Hirschman, S. Z., and Garfinkel, E.: Ionic requirements of the DNA polymerase associated with serum hepatitis B antigen. J Infect Dis 135:897, 1977.

Krugman, S., Friedman, H., and Lattimer, C.: Viral hepatitis, type A. Identification by specific complement fixation and immune adherence tests. N Engl J Med 292:1141, 1975.

LeBouvier, G. L.: The heterogeneity of Australia antigen. J Infect Dis 123:671, 1971.

Melnick, J. N., Dreesman, G. R., and Hollinger, F. B.: Approaching the control of viral hepatitis type B. J Infect Dis 133:210, 1976.

Provost, P. J., Wolanski, B. S., Miller, W. J., Ittensohn, O. L., McAleer, W. J., and Hilleman, M. R.: Physical, chemical and morphologic dimensions of human hepatitis. A virus strain. Proc Soc Exp Biol Med 148:532, 1975.

Robinson, W. S., Clayton, D. A., and Greenman, R. L.: DNA of a human hepatitis B virus candidate. J Virol 14:384, 1974.

# 6  FUNGI

# 68  *CRYPTOCOCCUS*

## Charles E. Davis, M.D.

*Cryptocoecus neoformans* is a round, yeast-like fungus that produces urease and forms a large heteropolysaccharide capsule in infected tissues. It is abundant in the feces of healthy pigeons but occurs throughout the world, even in areas where pigeons are rare or absent. While it is ordinarily a saprophyte, *C. neoformans* is an important cause of fatal meningitis in certain susceptible individuals. It was classified for many years as an asporogenous yeast in the Cryptococcaceae family of the Fungi Imperfecti, but Kwon-Chung (1975, 1976) has recently demonstrated two perfect (sexual) states among different serotypes of *C. neoformans*. The perfect forms, which appear to be related to the rust and smut pathogens of higher plants, were named *Filobasidiella neoformans* and *F. bacillospora.*

Several other species of encapsulated, round, yeast-like fungi that produce urease also belong to the cryptococcal genus. They look and behave biochemically like *C. neoformans,* except that they grow poorly or not at all at 37° C. This growth limitation probably explains why they cannot cause natural or experimental disease in mammals. Little is known about their activities in the environment, but they are important to the

medical mycologist, who must differentiate them from *C. neoformans.*

## *MORPHOLOGY*

Colors of cryptococci are white or creamy and typical of yeasts. They become yellowish or light tan with age. The colonies are entire without pseudomycelia, and convex and mucoid because of the capsular polysaccharide. Colonies that produce abundant capsule on artificial media may flow to the bottom of agar slants. All strains of *C. neoformans* form capsules in mammalian tissue, but some produce little or no capsule on artificial media. Others lose part or all of their capsule on serial passage in culture. Colonies of unencapsulated cryptococci are dry and glabrous.

Individual cryptococci are round and 3.5 to 7 $\mu$ in diameter. They are surrounded by a capsule of 1 to 30 $\mu$. Reproduction is accomplished by the formation of one or two daughter cells connected to the parental cell by a narrow isthmus. Buds may break off when quite small and cause considerable variation in the size of these round yeasts. Part of the parental wall is broken by the emerging bud.

The cell wall of *C. neoformans* has at least two layers (Fig. 1): an outer, electron-transparent layer and an inner electron-dense, lamellar layer (Cassone et al., 1974). The capsule is just outside the electron-transparent layer, which contains 20-nm particles (Takeo et al., 1973). These particles, which have not been observed in unencapsulated yeast, are excreted into the capsule when cryptococci are grown in vivo (Fig. 2) and are thought to be involved in assembly and transport of capsular polysaccharide (Takeo et al., 1973; Edwards et al., 1967).

When *C. neoformans* reproduces, part of the bud wall (the electron-transparent layer) is synthesized in the parental cell wall, while the electron-dense, lamellar wall is a direct continuation of the parental wall. This process breaks up the parental wall, which is repaired by formation of a septum (Fig. 3). Shadomy (1971) has shown clamp connections between the parental and daughter cells in two strains of *C. neoformans*.

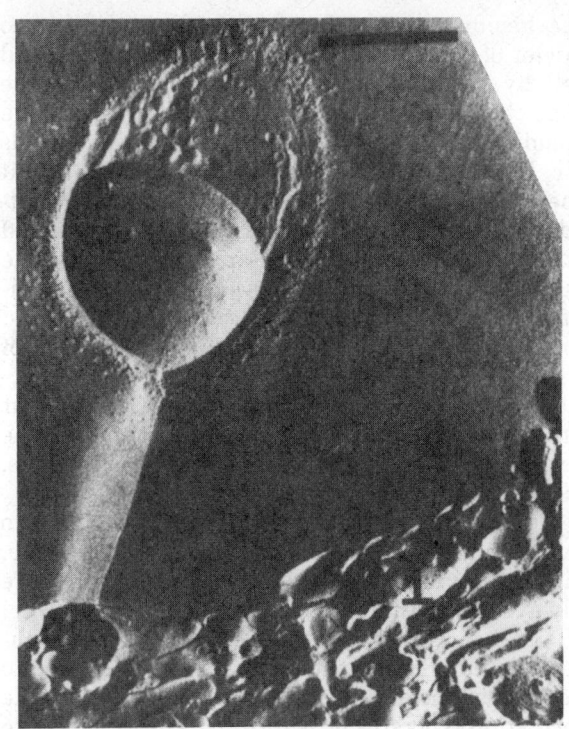

**FIGURE 2.** Cryptococcus *in brain tissue. Wall particles appear to be excreted into inner portion of capsule. Bar corresponds to 1 μm. (From Takeo, K., Ueasaka, I., Uehina, K., and Nishiura, M.: J Bacteriol 113:1449, 1973.)*

The electron-dense wall structure, the rupture of the parental wall by the newly emerging bud, and the presence of clamp connections all support the classification of the cryptococci among

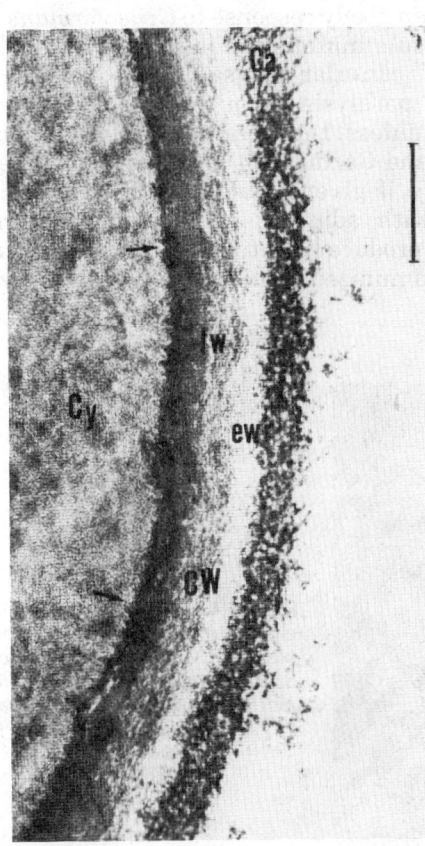

**FIGURE 1.** *Cell wall of* C. neoformans. *Ca, capsule; CW, cell wall; Cy, cytoplasm; ew, electron-transparent layer; lw, electron-dense lamellar layer. The arrows point to the cytoplasmic membrane. The bar corresponds to 0.2 μ. (From Cassone, A., Simonetti, N., and Strippoli, V.: Arch Microbiol 95:205, 1974.)*

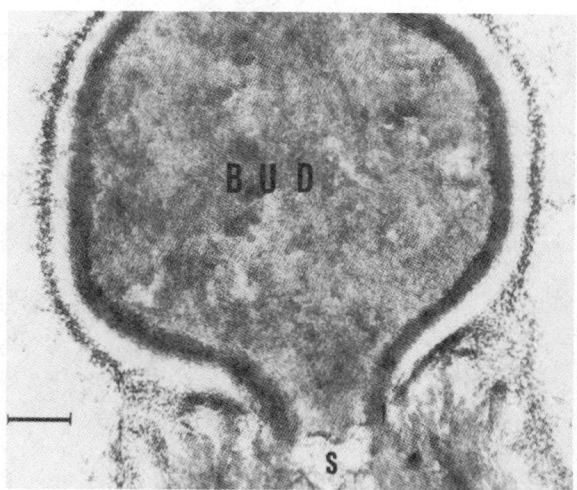

**FIGURE 3.** *Late cryptococcal bud with septum. Note the broken remnants of the electron-dense layer of the parental wall covered by the electron transparent layer and the capsule. S, septum; bar, 0.2 μ. (From Cassone, A., Simonetti, N., and Strippoli, V.: Arch Microbiol 95:205, 1974.)*

the basidiomycetes. In the basidiomycetes, two nuclei of mated cells travel to the newly formed cell by different routes, fuse, and form hyphae that bear a club-shaped structure called a basidium. These characteristics were the basis for Kwon-Chung's discovery (1975, 1976) that the sexual stage of *C. neoformans* was related to the rust and smut pathogens of plants and strengthened the suspected analogy between the budding of basidiomycetous yeasts and the germination of some fungal spores (Marchant and Smith, 1968). Figure 4 shows the hyphal form of *C. neoformans* (*Filobasidiella*) with clamp connections and a basidium. Basidiospores (Fig. 5) that are produced from the basidium complete the sexual cycle and become budding yeasts (Erke, 1976).

During the yeast (asexual) cycle, cryptococci do not form germ tubes, chlamydospores, or hyphae, either in vitro or in vivo. Although they are always encapsulated during infection, cryptococci in the environment are often shrunken and unencapsulated. Hyperosmolarity has been shown to be at least one of the factors that suppress capsule formation (Dykstra et al., 1977). There appear to be surface receptors for capsular polysaccharide in the outer wall of *C. neoformans,* since purified capsule adheres to unencapsulated *C. neoformans* but not to other yeasts or to heat-killed *C. neoformans* (Kozel, 1977).

The nonpathogenic species of cryptococci cannot grow at or above 37° C because an apparent imbalance of growth develops between the cytoplasmic contents and the cell wall. Growth of the cell wall is inhibited and bizarre-shaped spheroplasts and protoplasts emerge, probably from the site of bud formation (Dabbagh et al., 1974). These cells lyse almost immediately unless the experiment is carried out in hypertonic media.

## ANTIGENIC COMPOSITION

The capsule of *C. neoformans,* which is a polymer of mannose, xylose, and glucuronic acid, can be divided into four serotypes (A, B, C, or D) by agglutination or fluorescent antibody testing with hyperimmune sera. The capsular polysaccharide usually elicits only a minimal humoral antibody response in man or experimental animals during infection, possibly because most of the antibody is adsorbed by the abundant capsular polysaccharide in the tissues. During the treatment of cryptococcosis, a good prognosis is associated with falling levels of cryptococcal polysaccharide in the serum; these falling levels are sometimes accompanied by rising levels of cryptococcal antibody (Bardana et al., 1968).

Another possible explanation for the poor or absent antibody response to *C. neoformans* is that the capsule inhibits the immune response. Cryptococcal capsular polysaccharide causes immunologic paralysis in mice (Murphy and Cozad, 1972), unless the dose is carefully monitored (Kozel and Cazin, 1974). Mice form good levels of antibody if given small doses of polysaccharide along with adjuvants or protein carriers, and rabbits produce high titers of antibody if they are hyperimmunized. Antisera to *C. neoformans* cap-

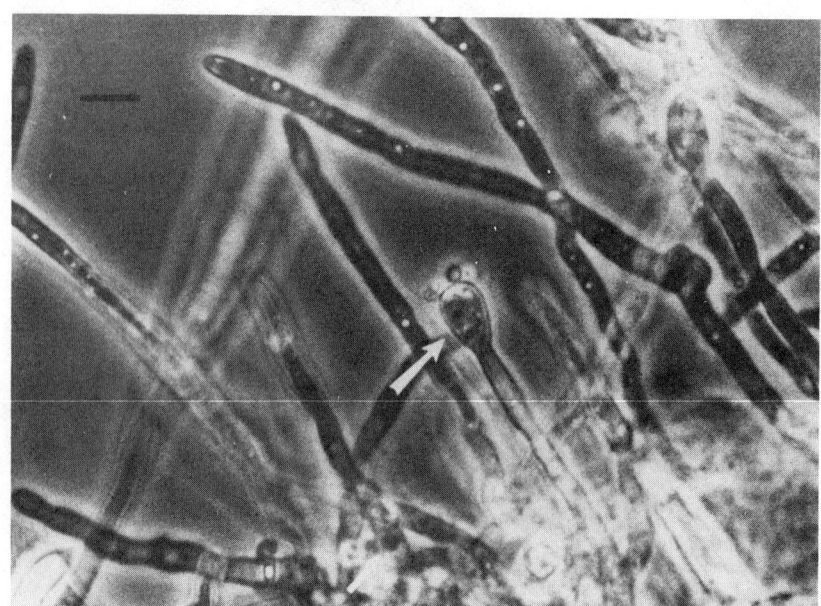

**FIGURE 4.** *Sexual stage of C. (Filobasidiella) neoformans. The arrow points to a basidium with four basidiospores still attached. A clamp connection can be seen four bar lengths to the right bar length 12 μm. (From Erke, K. H.: J Bacteriol 128:445, 1976.)*

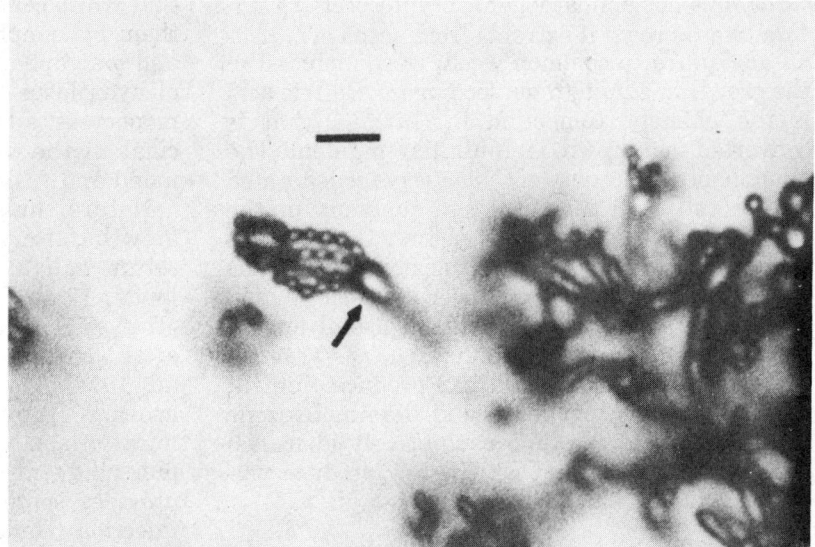

**FIGURE 5.** *Basidium of F. neoformans with four chains of basidiospores. Bar 16 μm. (From Erke, K. H.: J Bacteriol 128:445, 1976.)*

sule cross-reacts with the capsule of Types 2 and 14 pneumococci. Like bacteria, cryptococci undergo a Quellung reaction (capsular swelling) when suspended in homologous antiserum.

The physicochemical differences responsible for the antigenic variations in the four capsular serotypes are unknown, but this grouping appears to have important taxonomic implications. Kwon-Chung (1976) noted that *Filobasidiella neoformans* was produced only by mating Serotype A or D strains, and *F. bacillospora* only by mating Serotypes B and C. The serotypes differ in geographic distribution, rate of isolation from pigeon droppings, and biochemical activities (Bennett et al., 1977, 1978). These differences suggest that *C. neoformans* may consist of two species, *C. neoformans* of Serotypes A and D and *C. neoformans* of Serotypes B and C. There is no evidence that these two "species" differ in pathogenicity.

Because of the prominence of the cryptococcal capsule, the cell-wall glycopeptides of cryptococci have received little attention. Most of the work has been done with *C. laurentii,* a nonpathogenic *Cryptococcus* species. Raizada et al. (1975) have isolated a glycopeptide that consists of three oligosaccharide side chains bound by O-glycosidic linkages to threonyl and seryl residues in a common polypeptide core. The oligosaccharides are $\alpha$ and $\beta$ linked polymers of mannose, galactose, and xylose. Like *Candida* species, cryptococci also contain glucans in their cell wall (Meyer and Phaff, 1977). *C. neoformans* can be converted to protoplasts or spheroplasts by the action of certain glucanases. These polymers of mannose, glucose, and other sugars in the cell wall of cryptococci may be responsible for protective antibody

that can be raised in mice by immunization with either live or killed unencapsulated *C. neoformans.*

## PHYSIOLOGY

Cryptococci are nonfermentative aerobes that attack carbohydrates and other substrates oxidatively. Components of the electron-transport chain (Yamada and Kondo, 1973) and alpha-keto components of the Krebs cycle (Norkrans and Tumblad-Johannson, 1977) have been demonstrated in cryptococci. The complete electron-transport chain has not been worked out, but detailed studies of the benzoquinone coenzymes (coenzyme Q) have been used as taxonomic keys.

The type of coenzyme (categorized according to the number of isoprene units attached to the benzoquinone nucleus) in cryptococci is homogeneous and differs from *Candida.* All species of cryptococci except one saprophytic variant contain coenzyme $Q_{10}$ (Yamada and Kondo, 1973). This coenzyme generally occurs in urease-positive yeasts with a high guanine plus cytosine content.

*C. neoformans* can acquire nitrogen from peptones, urea, and creatinine but cannot reduce nitrate. Among the saprophytic species, only *C. albidus* and *C. terreus* can obtain nitrogen from nitrate, but all can utilize peptones and urea as nitrogen sources.

*C. neoformans* synthesizes phenol oxidases that produce melanin-like pigments from phenols. The color of the pigment depends on the substrate. Staub (1962) found that colonies of *C. neofor-*

*mans,* but not nonpathogenic cryptococci or *Candida,* were brown if extracts from seeds of *Guizotia abyssinica,* a common weed, were included in the growth medium (nigerseed agar). Caffeic acid is the phenolic compound in *Guizotia* that is converted to a brown, melanin-like pigment. The phenoloxidase activity of *C. neoformans* is located in the cell wall and produces pigment in the colonies that does not diffuse into the medium (Shaw and Kapica, 1972). This observation has led to the production of several selective and differential media that have been useful for the isolation and identification of *C. neoformans.* Other species of cryptococci can produce pigment from certain aminophenol and diaminobenzene compounds, and can be presumptively identified by the substrates from which they produce pigment (Chaskes and Tyndall, 1978).

## *Immunity*

The natural resistance of people to *Cryptococcus neoformans* is so strong that cryptococcosis is sometimes referred to in Europe as "malade signal" because it is frequently a sign of underlying disease. About 50 per cent of patients with cryptococcal meningitis are found to have another disease, most frequently a lymphoid malignancy such as Hodgkin's disease. This association and the persistence of abnormal cell-mediated immunity to the cryptococcus in otherwise normal individuals after successful treatment suggests that cell-mediated immunity is the critical line of defense against cryptococcosis. Skin reactivity, lymphocyte transformation, and production of migratory-inhibition factor often show impaired response to cryptococcal antigens and sometimes to other antigens as well (Graybill and Alford, 1974; Schimpff and Bennett, 1975).

Abnormal phagocytes and humoral reactions have not been definitely linked to susceptibility to cryptococcosis. There is no question, however, that human neutrophils and macrophages can ingest and kill *C. neoformans* in vitro (Diamond et al., 1972). In pulmonary infections of mice and other experimental animals, neutrophils clear most of the cryptococci from early infiltrates, and monocytes remove the remainder in the later stages. Although human macrophages do not kill *C. neoformans* very efficiently (Diamond and Bennett, 1973), macrophages that have been activated by sensitized lymphocytes appear to make experimental animals resistant to cryptococcosis. However, two observations suggest that the quantity of the inflammatory response may be more important than the capacity of individual cells to ingest and kill cryptococci. First, many encapsulated cryptococci are probably too large for phagocytes to ingest. Second, there is evidence

that white cells can surround cryptococci and kill them by nonphagocytic mechanisms. Monocytes and macrophages may kill cryptococci by release of hydrolases (Kalina et al., 1974); neutrophils, monocytes, and lymphocytes may be cryptococcicidal in the presence of specific antibody (Diamond and Allison, 1976).

Natural humoral substances that inhibit the growth of cryptococci are present in normal serum, saliva, and spinal fluid (Howard and Bolande, 1966; Reiss et al., 1975). Estrogens and other steroids may damage *C. neoformans* (Mohr et al., 1972) and promote phagocytosis (Mohr et al., 1974). There is little evidence that acquired antibody prevents infection. Immunization of mice with an appropriate concentration of capsule plus adjuvant or live unencapsulated cryptococci provides some protection against experimental infection (Gadebusch and Johnson, 1966; Abrahams, 1966), but the mechanism of this resistance is unknown.

It is surprising that the relative importance of the various aspects of immunity against *C. neoformans* have not been defined because it is the only fungus with a definite pathogenic factor. The capsule is essential to the pathogenicity of *C. neoformans.* Strains of *C. neoformans* that cannot form a capsule do not cause disease. When the capsule of cryptococci is lost through manipulation of growth media, they apparently regain the capsule after inoculation because they kill mice and have capsules in the tissues (Dykstra et al., 1977). The capsular polysaccharide has so many effects on the immune response that it is hard to determine the most important. It suppresses antibody-forming cells (Murphy and Cozad, 1972; inhibits phagocytosis (Bulmer and Sans, 1972) and leukocyte migration (Drouhet and Segretan, 1951); decomplements serum by activation of the alternative pathway (Diamond et al., 1974; Macher et al., 1978); and adsorbs or neutralizes opsonins and other protective antibodies. These various effects of the capsule and the numerous immune responses that are activated by experimental cryptococcosis suggest that a normal person has several lines of resistance against the cryptococcus. Nevertheless, the great predilection for cryptococcal infections in patients with depressed cell-mediated immunity implies that this immunologic defense is of critical value in resisting this infection.

The other property of *C. neoformans* that enables it to infect humans and other animals is its ability to grow at 37° C. The other encapsulated cryptococci grow poorly if at all at 37° C and do not cause disease. Rabbits with a body temperature of 39.6° C are much more resistant than mice to infection, and the only recorded infection of a pigeon (body temperature 42° C) was in superficial tissues that were cooler than the core temperature (Ensley et al., 1979). Cryptococci do not grow above 39° C in vitro but survive temperatures up to 44° C. A fascinating and important corollary to these observations is that cryptococcal meningitis does not cause fever.

## LABORATORY DIAGNOSIS

Identification of *C. neoformans* in wet mounts and smears of infected material and cultivation from these specimens are the cornerstones of the diagnosis of cryptococcal infection. This large, round, encapsulated yeast is most easily identified in gram-stained smears of spinal fluid, respiratory secretions, or other infected material. The yeast cell (3.5 to 7.0 $\mu$) retains the crystal violet and is easily differentiated from surrounding leukocytes because of the large (up to 30 $\mu$), lightly safranin-stained capsular halo (Fig. 6). Virtually the entire slide can be examined under $\times$ 100 power, and suspicious structures can be visualized in more detail under the oil immersion lens. The India ink preparation, prepared by mixing a few drops of the spinal fluid, spinal fluid sediment, or other specimens with a drop of India ink, is also a popular means of detecting cryptococci (Chapter 155), but there is a danger of confusing lymphocytes, tissue cells, fat droplets, aggregated particles of India ink, or even yeast contaminants of the India ink with cryptococci. If CSF (cerebrospinal fluid) is to be examined by India ink, the presumptive diagnosis of cryptococcosis should not be made without observing the typical small single or double bud and confirming the presence of the organism by Gram stain. Specimens of body fluids may be sedimented by centrifugation at 5,000 g or more before microscopic examination and cultivation, but care must be taken to avoid contamination during the process.

Alternatively, a small portion of the fluid can be sedimented for microscopic examination and the remainder cultivated on as many different slants of media as required. Either a portion of the whole fluid or the supernatant from the sedimented fluid should be retained for antigen detection. The larger the volume of spinal fluid cultivated, the greater the chance of isolating the organism, and clinicians should be encouraged to submit as much spinal fluid as possible. We request 15 to 20 ml if the patient does not have increased CSF pressure.

If pulmonary or brain tissue is submitted for culture, impression smears should be made for Gram and special stains and the tissue carefully macerated with a scalpel. Before culture, smears should be made from the macerated tissue, and a portion should be mixed with 1 or 2 ml of 15 per cent potassium hydroxide and incubated at 37° C for 30 minutes before examination as a wet mount with and without India ink. The potassium hydroxide digests cells and artifacts that could be confused with cryptococci.

The histologic examination of tissue should include special stains as well as the routine hematoxylin and eosin stain. Cryptococci can be readily seen on hematoxylin and eosin stain, but the capsule does not stain and can be confused with a space containing a round yeast. Periodic-acid Schiff and Gomori methenamine silver stains are excellent screening stains and often permit visualization of the capsule as an unstained halo surrounding the round budding yeast, but Mayer's mucicarmine technique is the definitive stain because it stains the cryptococcal capsule. In addition to their large capsule, cryptococci differ from *Blastomyces* because the cryptococcal wall is thinner, and the buds are attached to the parent cell by a narrow isthmus. They can be

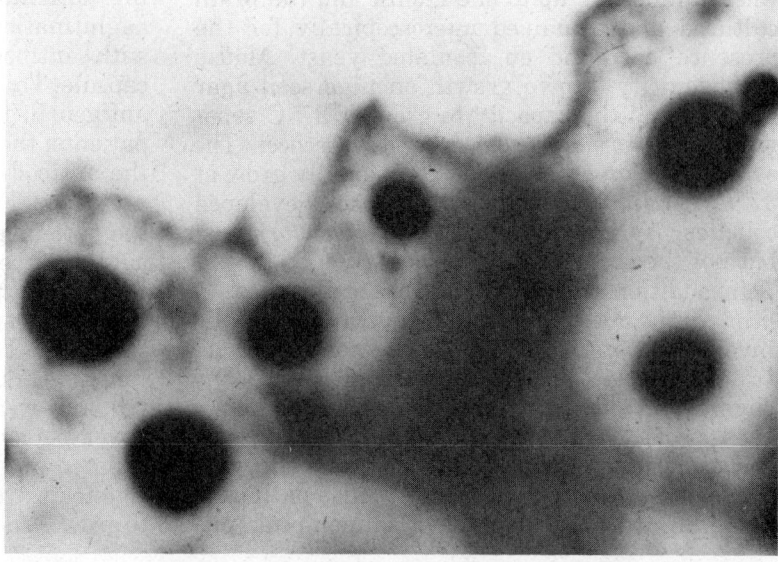

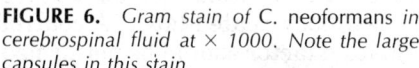

**FIGURE 6.** *Gram stain of C. neoformans in cerebrospinal fluid at $\times$ 1000. Note the large capsules in this stain.*

distinguished from *Candida* because cryptococci are round instead of oval and form no pseudohyphae or hyphae. The spherules of *Coccidioides immitis* contain endospores and do not bud.

In patients with meningitis, the respiratory secretions, CSF, urine, blood, and any tissue obtained by biopsy should be examined microscopically and cultured, at least on Sabouraud's agar. It is helpful, especially if the specimen is contaminated, to cultivate a portion of the specimen on nigerseed agar and on media that contain antibacterial antibiotics. Cryptococci are sensitive to cycloheximide (Actidione), and media containing this antibiotic should be avoided. As many slants as possible should be inoculated and incubated at room temperature or 25 to 30° C. Some tubes may also be placed at 37° C for quick differentiation from saphrophytic cryptococci. Growth often appears within 48 to 72 hours but may be delayed for seven days or more if the inoculum is small. For this reason, cultures should be kept for six weeks before being discarded as negative, and tubed media should be used to avoid drying.

When colonies appear, they are usually convex, mucoid, cream-colored to light tan, or very rarely a light pink. Individual cells are more round than oval, have at least a small capsule in India ink, and do not produce hyphae. In practice, every round yeast, encapsulated yeast, or urease-producing yeast should be subjected to a complete work-up to exclude *C. neoformans.* The cultural identification of *C. neoformans* can be definitely established by three properties: growth of subcultures at 37°C, mouse pathogenicity, and urease production. If mice are inoculated intracerebrally, intravenously, or intraperitoneally with $10^5$ to $10^7$ *C. neoformans,* a rapid, progressively fatal infection follows within one to three weeks. One or two mice should be sacrificed at weekly intervals up to one month and the brain cultured and examined microscopically for the presence of round encapsulated yeast. Mouse pathogenicity, brown growth on nigerseed agar (Fig. 7), and the capacity to grow at 37° C separate *C. neoformans* from other cryptococci. The saprophytic cryptococci that occasionally grow at 37° C usually produce small, poorly developed colonies. We have also found the *C. neoformans,* but not the saprophytes, grows at 39° C.

In addition to these major characteristics, *C. neoformans* does not produce pseudohyphae, chlamydospores, or germ tubes; does not reduce nitrate; does not ferment (produce gas from) any sugars; and always assimilates inositol. Although these properties can separate *C. neoformans* from any other fungus, the assimilation tests shown in Table 1 are usually performed. Mouse pathogenicity, failure to produce deep salmon-pink pig-

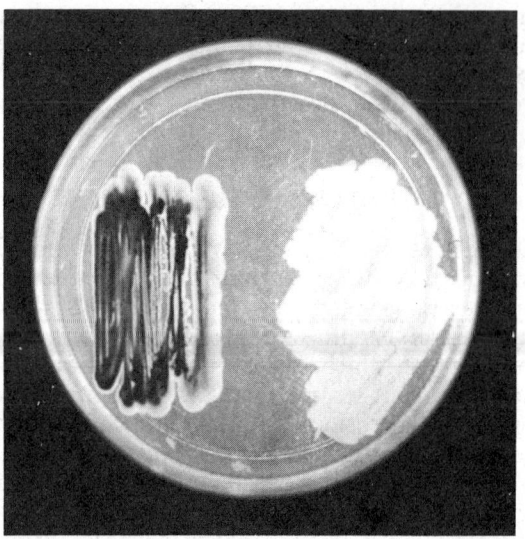

**FIGURE 7.** *The darkly pigmented growth of* C. neoformans *on nigerseed agar clearly differentiates it from the white or cream-colored growth of* Candida albicans *on the other half of the agar plate.*

ment, and assimilation of inositol separate *C. neoformans* from *Rhodotorula* species, which have similar sugar assimilation patterns.

Although the perfect state of *C. neoformans* has been described (see earlier sections on Morphology and Epidemiology), and several strains have produced hyphae in the laboratory, this is an unusual phenomenon and does not ordinarily occur without special techniques and media (Kwon-Chung, 1975, 1976). If hyphae are observed, they resemble the forms shown in Figures 4 and 5. *Filobasidiella* (*Cryptococcus*) *bacillospora* (Serotypes B and C) assimilates malic, fumaric, and succinic acids, while *F.* (*Cryptococcus*) *neoformans* (Serotypes A and D) does not (Bennett et al., 1978).

The only useful serologic technique for identifying patients with cryptococcal infection is the agglutination of latex particles that are coated with antibody raised against the cryptococcal capsule. This test measures cryptococcal capsular antigen in the serum or spinal fluid of infected patients; the capsular polysaccharide reacts with the antibody on the latex particle and agglutinates them. False-positive tests are unusual unless the patient produces rheumatoid factor that also agglutinates the antibody-coated latex. A control to rule out rheumatoid factor should be performed in every test and is provided in the commercial test kits. The latex-agglutination test is very sensitive and is positive in the spinal fluid of most patients with cryptococcal meningitis but in a lower percentage of the serum of patients with isolated pulmonary disease. Although false-positive tests are rare, *C. neoformans* is usually easy to grow, and the diagnosis of cryptococcal infection

**TABLE 1.** Characteristics of *Cryptococcus neoformans**

| SPECIES | MOUSE VIRULENCE | GROWTH AT 37° C | PIGMENT ON NIGERSEED AGAR | UREASE ACTIVITY | KNO₃ | ASSIMILATIONS | | | | | |
|---|---|---|---|---|---|---|---|---|---|---|---|
| | | | | | | Inositol | Sucrose | Lactose | Melibiose | Cellobiose | Raffinose |
| C. neoformans | + | + | + | + | − | + | + | − | − | + | + |
| C. laurentii | − | + or − | − | + | − | + | + | + | + | + | + |
| C. terreus | − | + or − | − | + | + | + | − | rare | − | + | − |
| C. gastricus | − | − | − | + | − | + | − | − | − | + | − |
| C. uniguttulatus | − | − | − | + | − | + | + | − | − | − or + | + |
| C. luteolus | − | − | − | + | − | + | + | − | + | + | − |
| C. albidus var. albidus | − | rare | − | + | + | + | + | + or − | − or + | + | + |
| C. albidus var. diffluens | − | − or + | − | + | + | + | + | − | + or − | + | + |

*Modified from Widra and Long, 1970, and Bennett et al., 1978.

should always be confirmed by culture. Tests for detection of cryptococcal antibody are not useful in the diagnosis of cryptococcal infection because some normal people have antibody and most patients with cryptococcal infection do not. During the course of successful treatment, the titer of cryptococcal polysaccharide should fall, but this may or may not be accompanied by the development of cryptococcal antibody. While this combination of serologic events is probably a good prognostic sign, some patients recover without developing antibody. Furthermore, dead cryptococci may be seen by microscopic examination of the spinal fluid for many weeks or months after successful treatment. If these organisms cannot be cultivated, their presence should not be taken as a bad prognostic sign.

Cryptococcal skin test preparations are useful for epidemiologic surveys but are of no value for diagnosis.

## EPIDEMIOLOGY

Unlike many other fungi that can cause life-threatening infections in apparently normal, non-hospitalized patients, *C. neoformans* is widely distributed throughout the world. It can be isolated from fruit skins and juice, milk, and soil but is most often associated with pigeon dung. It is not part of the normal flora of man or other animals. Although the most common manifestation of cryptococcal infection is meningitis, the primary lesion almost certainly occurs in the lung from inhalation of infective particles. Only 200 to 300 cases of cryptococcal meningitis are reported each year in the United States, but it is estimated that more than 15,000 subclinical respiratory infections occur annually in New York City alone (Ajello, 1969; Littman and Walter, 1968).

Although the capsule of *C. neoformans* is an essential virulence factor, its large size would appear to prevent cryptococci from reaching the terminal bronchioles and causing parenchymal disease. This paradox has probably been solved by two observations. First, in the hyperosmolar, al-

kaline environment of pigeon feces, *C. neoformans* is unencapsulated and shrunken in size, so that a small percentage of the yeast population has a diameter of 1 μ or less and could easily reach the alveoli (Powell et al., 1972). Second, the sexual stage of *C. neoformans, Filobasidiella*, produces basidiospores that are also about 1 μ in diameter. A role for the sexual stage in dissemination of cryptococci has not been proven but is an attractive possibility.

Cryptococci can reach numbers as high as 5 × 10⁷ in pigeon feces and can be recovered in large numbers from the accumulated filth of pigeon roosts, attics, barn lofts, and cornices. It is often the predominant organism in this alkaline, hyperosmolar environment, with its rich content of creatinine and other nitrogen-containing compounds, but may disappear when the bird droppings are mixed with soil. It is infrequently isolated from organically enriched soil (Emmons, 1960). Direct exposure to sunlight also inhibits its growth. In shaded, moist, or desiccated pigeon feces, it may persist for as long as two years or more. It survives better if relative humidity is increased (Ishaq, et al., 1968).

Since *Cryptococcus neoformans* is a stable, soil-dwelling organism in its sexual stage, it is possible that *C. neoformans* was infrequently isolated from soil because it converted to *Filobasidiella* and was not recognized. In fact, only *C. neoformans* Serotypes A and D are isolated from pigeon droppings. The ecologic site of Types B and C is unknown. Almost all clinical infections in the United States are caused by Serotype A strains except in southern California, where 51 per cent of infections are caused by Serotypes B and C (Bennett et al., 1977). The ecologic characteristics of the organism undoubtedly explain this interesting difference in the geographic distribution of infections.

*C. neoformans* infects many animals, but transmission from animal to man or man to man has never been documented. Although Green and Bulmer (1979) have shown that a small number of mice could be infected by gastrointestinal inoculation, ingestion of cryptococci has never been implicated as the portal of entry in human infection, even after exposure to large numbers of cryptococci in unpasteurized milk from cows with cryptococcal mastitis.

The reasons why cryptococci do not compete well with other organisms in the soil are unknown but may involve biological control mechanisms. Bunting et al. (1979) have shown that *Acanthamoeba polyphaga*, a free-living ameba, can phagocytose and kill up to 99 per cent of *C. neoformans* in mixed cultures. One ameba can ingest and kill as many as 84 cryptococci per day. Interestingly, some of the surviving yeast cells developed into colonies containing hyphae. These forms may be a biological "escape hatch" and suggest the possibility that *C. neoformans* survives the hostile environment of the soil by conversion into the sexual stage.

## References

Abrahams, J.: Further studies on acquired resistance to murine cryptococcosis. Enhancing effect of *Bordetella pertussis*. J Immunol 98:914, 1966.

Ajello, L.: A comparative study of the pulmonary mycosis of Canada and the United States. Publ Health Rep 84:869, 1969.

Bardana, E. J., Kauffman, L., and Benner, E. J.: Amphotericin B and cryptococcal infections. Arch Intern Med 122:517, 1968.

Bennett, J. E., Kwon-Chung, K. J., and Howard, D. H.: Epidemiological differences among serotypes of *Cryptococcus neoformans*. Am. J. Epidemiol 10:582, 1977.

Bennett, J. E., Kwon-Chung, J. K., and Theodore, T. S.: Biochemical. differences between serotypes of *Cryptococcus neoformans*. Sabouraudia 16:167, 1978.

Bulmer, G. S., and Sans, M. D.: *Cryptococcus neoformans*. III. Inhibition of phagocytosis. J Bacteriol 95:5, 1968.

Bunting, L. A., Neilson, J. B., and Bulmer, G. S.: *Cryptococcus neoformans*: Gastronomic delight of a soil amoeba. Sabouraudia 17:225, 1979.

Cassone, A., Simonetti, N., and Strippoli, V.: Wall structure and bud formation in *Cryptococcus neoformans*. Arch Microbiol 95:205, 1974.

Chaskes, S., and Tyndall, R. L.: Pigment production by *Cryptococcus neoformans* and other cryptococcus species from aminophenols and diaminobenzenes. J Clin Microbiol 7:146, 1978.

Dabbagh, R., Conant, N. F., Nielsen, H. S., and Burns, R. O.: Effect of temperature on saprophytic cryptococci: Temperature-induced lysis and protoplast formation. J Gen Microbiol 85:177, 1974.

Diamond, R. D., Root, R. K., and Bennett, J. E.: Factors influencing killing of *Cryptococcus neoformans* by human leukocytes *in vitro*. J Infect Dis 125:367, 1972.

Diamond, R. D., and Bennett, J. E.: Growth of *Cryptococcus neoformans* within human macrophages *in vitro*. Infect Immun 7:231, 1973.

Diamond, R. D., May, J. E., Kane, M. A., Frank, M. M., and Bennett, J. E.: The role of the classic and alternate complement pathways in host defenses against *Cryptococcus neoformans* infection. J Immunol 112:2260, 1974.

Diamond, R. D., and Allison, A. C.: Nature of the effector cells responsible for antibody-dependent cell-mediated killing of *Cryptococcus neoformans*. Infect Immun 14:716, 1976.

Drouhet, E., and Segretain, G.: Inhibition de la migration leukocytaire in vitro par un polyoside capsulaire de *Torulopsis* (*Cryptococcus*) *neoformans*. Ann Inst Pasteur 81:674, 1951.

Dykstra, M. A., Friedman, L., and Murphy, J. W.: Capsule size of *Cryptococcus neoformans*: Control and relationship to virulence. Infect Immun 16:129, 1977.

Edwards, M. R., Gordon, M. A., Lapa, E. W., and Ghiorse, W. C.: Micromorphology of *Cryptococcus neoformans*. J Bacteriol 94:766, 1967.

Emmons, C. W.: Prevalence of *Cryptococcus neoformans* in pigeon habitats. Publ Health Rep 75:362, 1960.

Ensley, P. K., Davis, C. E., Anderson, M. P., and Fletcher, K. C.: Cryptococcosis in a male Beccari's Crowned Pigeon. J Am Vet Med Assoc 175:992, 1979.

Erke, K. H.: Light microscopy of basidia, basidiospores, and nuclei in spores and hyphae of *Filabasidiella neoformans* (*Cryptococcus neoformans*). J Bacteriol 128:445, 1976.

Gadebusch, H. H., and Johnson, A. G.: Natural host resistance to infection with *Cryptococcus neoformans*. J Infect Dis 116:551, 1966.

Graybill, J. R., and Alford, R. H.: Cell-mediated immunity in cryptococcosis. Cell Immunol 14:12, 1974.

Green, J. R., and Bulmer, G. S.: Gastrointestinal incubation of *Cryptococcus neoformans* in mice. Sabouraudia 17:233, 1979.

Howard, J. I., and Bolande, R. P.: Humoral defense mechanisms in cryptococcosis. Substances in normal human serum, saliva, and cerebral spinal fluid affecting the growth of *Cryptococcus neoformans*. J Infect Dis 116:75, 1966.

Ishaq, C. M., Bulmer, G. S., and Felton, F. G.: An evaluation of various environmental factors affecting the propagation of *Cryptococcus neoformans*. Mycopathol Mycol Appl 35:81, 1968.

Kalina, M., Kletter, Y., and Aronson, M.: The interaction of phagocytes and the large-sized parasite *Cryptococcus neoformans*: Cytochemical and ultrastructural study. Cell Tiss Res 152:165, 1974.

Kozel, T. R., and Cazin, J., Jr.: Induction of humoral antibody response by soluble polysaccharide of *Cryptococcus neoformans*. Mycopathol Mycol Appl 54:21, 1974.

Kozel, T. R.: Non-encapsulated variant of *Cryptococcus neoformans* II. Surface receptors for cryptococcal polysaccharide and their role in inhibition of phagocytosis by polysaccharide. Infect Immun 16:99, 1977.

Kwon-Chung, J. K.: A new genus, *Filobasidiella*, the perfect state of *Cryptococcus neoformans*. Mycologia 67:1197, 1975.

Kwon-Chung, J. K.: A new species of *Filobasidiella*, the sexual state of *Cryptococcus neoformans* B and C serotypes. Mycologia 68:942, 1976.

Littman, M. L., and Walter, J. E.: Cryptococcosis. Current issues. Am. J. Med. 45:922, 1968.

Macher, A., Bennett, J., Gadek, J., and Frank, M. M.: Complement depletion in cryptococcal sepsis. J Immunol 120:1686, 1978.

Marchant, R., and Smith, D. G.: Bud formation in *Saccharomyces cerevisiae* and a comparison with the mechanism of cell division in other yeasts. J Gen Microbiol 53:163, 1968.

Meyer, M. T., and Phaff, H. J.: Survey for alpha-(1–3) glucanase activity among yeasts. J Bacteriol 131:702, 1977.

Mohr, J. A., Long, H., McKown, B. A., et al.: *In vitro* susceptibility of *Cryptococcus neoformans* to steroids. Sabouraudia 10:171, 1972.

Mohr, J. A., Muchmore, H. G., and Tacker, R.: Stimulation of phagocytosis of *Cryptococcus neoformans* in human cryptococcal meningitis. J. Reticuloendothel Soc 15:149, 1974.

Murphy, J. W., and Cozad, G. C.: Immunological unresponsiveness induced by cryptococcal capsular polysaccharide assayed by the hemolytic plaque technique. Infect Immun 5:896, 1972.

Norkrans, B., and Tumblad-Johannson, I.: Cellular contents of the Krebs cycle keto acids in yeasts grown on different nitrogen sources including hydroxylamine. Arch Microbiol 115:127, 1977.

Powell, K. E., Bernhoff, A., Dahl, A., Weeks, R. J., and Tosh, F. E.: Airborne *Cryptococcus neoformans*: Particles from pigeon excreta compatible with alveolar deposition. J Infect Dis 125:412, 1972.

Raizada, M. K., Schutzbach, J. S., and Ankel, H.: *Cryptococcus laurentii* cell envelope glyco-protein. J Biol Chem 250:3310, 1975.

Reiss, F., Szilagyi, G., and Mayer, E.: Immunological studies of the anti-cryptococcal factor of normal human serum. Mycopathologia 55:175, 1975.

Schimpff, S. C., and Bennett, J. E.: Abnormalities in cell-mediated immunity in patients with *Cryptococcus neoformans* infection. J Allergy Clin Immunol 43:430, 1975.

Shadomy, H. J.: Clamp connections in two strains of *Cryptococcus neoformans*. Recent trends of yeast research. Atlanta Research Articles, School of Arts and Sciences, Georgia State University, 1971.

Shaw, C. E., and Kapica, L.: Production of diagnostic pigment by phenoloxidase activity of *Cryptococcus neoformans*. Appl Microbiol 24:824, 830, 1972.

Staub, F.: *Cryptococcus neoformans* and *Guizotia abyssinica* (syn. *G. oleifera* D.C.( Z Hyg 148:446, 1962.

Takeo, K., Ueasaka, I., Uehina, K., and Nishiura, M.: Fine structure of *Cryptococcus neoformans* grown *in vivo* as observed by freeze etching. J Bacteriol 113:1449, 1973.

Widra, A., and Long, I.: Taxonomic studies on cryptococci and related yeasts. Mycopathol Mycol Appl 40:89, 1970.

Yamada, Y., and Kondo, K.: Coenzyme Q system in the classification of the yeast genera *Rhodotorula* and *Cryptococcus*, and the yeast-like genera *Sporobolomyces* and *Rhodosporidium*. J Gen Appl Microbiol 19:59, 1973.

# CANDIDA AND 69
## TORULOPSIS

### Abraham I. Braude, M.D., Ph.D.

Members of the genera *Candida* and *Torulopsis* are indigenous human yeasts that colonize the skin and mucous membranes of normal people but produce infection only when natural resistance is compromised. The two genera resemble each other morphologically and are related antigenically, but only members of the genus *Candida* commonly cause serious human illness. The genus comprises seven species of medical interest.

The most important of these is *Candida albicans*, but *Candida tropicalis* has become a serious cause of disseminated infection in patients undergoing treatment for hematologic malignancies or receiving bone marrow transplantation (Table 1) (Wingard et al., 1979). The other five species encountered in human disease are designated *C. krusei, C. guilliermondi, C. parapsilosis, C. pseudotropicalis,* and *C. stellatoidea.*

## CANDIDA

### MORPHOLOGY

Members of the genus *Candida* characteristically develop both as yeast cells and as pseudohyphae. *C. albicans,* the principal pathogenic member of the genus, also produces true hyphae. Pseudohyphae are chains of budding cells that fail to detach, so that they develop into a branching network that resembles true hyphae. Colonies composed of pseudohyphae have the soft, white character of yeasts in contrast to the cottony or woolly growth of true mycelia. The yeast cells of *C. albicans* are oval and gram-positive; they vary in size from $2 \times 3\ \mu$ to $8.5 \times 14\ \mu$. Less frequently, elongated cells may be seen after incubation at room temperature. On cornmeal agar, a nutritionally deficient medium composed only of cornmeal and water, *C. albicans* reproduces in four different forms: (1) true mycelia, (2) pseudomycelia, (3) blastospores, and (4) chlamydospores. The blastospores grow in round clusters at intervals along the pseudomycelia. Terminal chlamydospores (macroconidia) growing at the end of the hyphae are the most distinctive feature of *C. albicans* and are rarely produced by any other

species of *Candida.* The chlamydospores are large (8 to 12 $\mu$) and round and have a thick wall (Fig. 1). They are particularly adapted for maintaining vitality during starvation and other adverse conditions. Their large size is due to the storage of

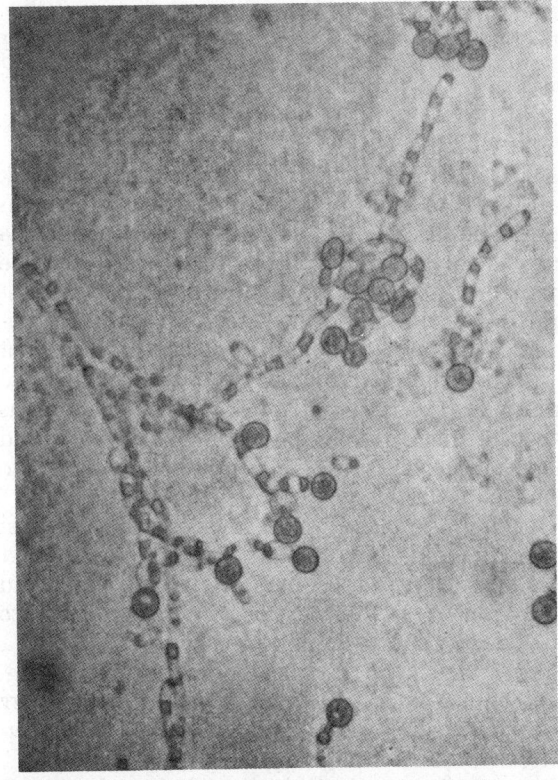

**FIGURE 1.** *Chlamydospores of* C. albicans *after growth on cornmeal agar. The chlamydospores are the sharply defined large round bodies at the tips of the hyphae.*

**TABLE 1.** **Frequency of Isolation of Different Species of *Candida* and *Torulopsis* from Blood Cultures**

| SPECIES | NUMBER OF PATIENTS WITH POSITIVE BLOOD CULTURES |
|---|---|
| C. albicans | 68 |
| C. tropicalis | 18 |
| C. parapsilosis | 12 |
| Torulopsis glabrata | 2 |

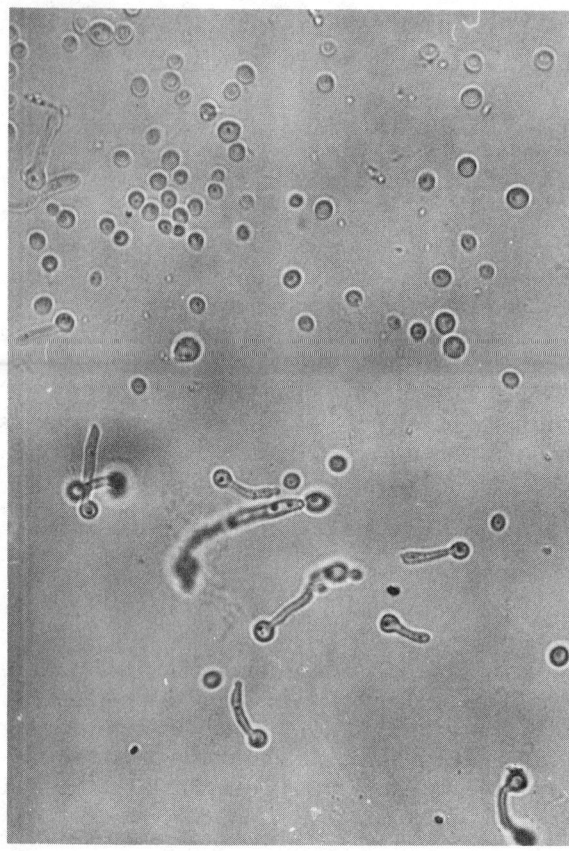

**FIGURE 2.** *Germ-tube formation in C. albicans. Germ tubes are short filaments that protrude from yeast cells within two to four hours after incubation in serum at 37° C. (Reynolds, R., and Braude, A. I.: Clin Res Proc 4:40, 1956.)*

reserve nutritional substance, and their thick wall protects them from an unfavorable environment. The thick wall has two layers, of which the outer is polysaccharide (beta 1:3 glucan) and the inner, protein. There is also a high lipid content (Jansons and Nickerson, 1970). The poor nutritional quality of cornmeal agar causes the yeast cells to differentiate into the well-provisioned chlamydospores. Formation of chlamydospores is a test for distinguishing between *C. albicans* and those species of *Candida* that do not develop into these forms.

Perhaps the most interesting form is the germ tube (Reynolds and Braude, 1956). When yeast cells of *C. albicans* are suspended in serum and incubated at 37° C, they produce within two to four hours a short filament measuring $1.5 \times 15 \mu$ and having the appearance of a bean sprout (Fig. 2). Because germ tubes develop so quickly, they are also used as a rapid test for *C. albicans*. Some of the morphologic features of *C. albicans* are sometimes seen with *C. stellatoidea*, which can also produce blastospores, pseudohyphae, germ tubes, and rarely, chlamydospores.

Since the two are also similar in antigenic structure, *C. stellatoidea* is regarded by some students of yeast taxonomy as an avirulent variant of *C. albicans* (Pollack and Benham, 1957). *C. tropicalis* also produces pseudohyphae, true mycelia and chlamydospores rarely, but not germ tubes. In broth cultures, *C. tropicalis* tends to form a thin film that can trap gas bubbles. The film of *C. tropicalis* is in contrast to that of *C. krusei,* which is much thicker and crawls up the side of the broth culture tube. The flat, dry, dull colonies of *C. krusei* on agar and its cylindrical cell morphology in broth are additional distinctive characteristics. These cells vary considerably in size, and elongated forms may look like crossed matchsticks. The cells of *C. pseudotropicalis* are also elongated in broth cultures but fall apart and lie parallel to each other.

The morphologic differences and species of *Candida* are summarized in Table 2.

## ANTIGENIC COMPOSITION

The various species of *Candida* have been classified into six antigenic groups on the basis of slide agglutination tests with monospecific absorbed rabbit sera (Table 3). Each of 22 species of *Candida* were grouped according to their content of seven heat-stable and three heat-labile antigens. In this system of classification, both *C. stellatoidea* and *C. tropicalis* are closely related antigenically to *C. albicans*. Although all *Candida* species share a common antigen, the antigenic structures of *C. pseudotropicalis, C. krusei, C. parapsilosis,* and *C. guilliermondi* are distinctly different from *C. albicans*. These antigenic relationships have been largely substantiated by means of immunoelectrophoresis of soluble yeast extracts (Biguet et al., 1965). The important antigenic determinants in *Candida* appear to be surface polysaccharides, such as mannans and glucans. Mannan forms the outer layer and glucan the inner layer of the cell wall of *C. albicans*. The two sugars appear to occur naturally as complexes of polysaccharide-protein linked together by *N*-acetylglucosamine. The antigenic specificity of the mannans depends on the lengths of the polysaccharide side branches and the type of glycosidic linkages present in them. The mannans are polymers of mannose that, in the main chain or backbone of *C. albicans,* are connected by alpha 1 to 6 linkages. In the side chains, the linkages are alpha 1 to 2 or rarely, alpha 1 to 3, and there are six mannose units or less. Two serotypes of *C. albicans* have been described whose antigenic distinction may depend on the number and position of the linkages.

**TABLE 2.  Gross and Microscopic Appearance of the Different
Species of *Candida***

| SPECIES | COLONIES ON AGAR[a] | FILM[b] | YEAST CELL MORPHOLOGY | GERM TUBES | CHLAMYDOSPORES |
|---|---|---|---|---|---|
| *C. albicans* | Creamy | 0 | Ovoid | + | + |
| *C. stellatoidea* | Creamy | 0 | Ovoid | ± | Rare |
| *C. tropicalis* | Creamy | Thin, traps bubbles | Ovoid | 0 | 0 |
| *C. krusei* | Flat, dull, dry | Thick, climbs tube | Cylindrical, elongated cells arranged as crossed matchsticks | 0 | 0 |
| *C. pseudotropicalis* | Soft, smooth, white | 0 | Elongated cells lying parallel like logs in a stream | 0 | 0 |
| *C. guilliermondi* | Thin, flat, glossy | 0 | Ovoid or cylindrical | 0 | 0 |
| *C. parapsilosis* | Creamy | 0 | Ovoid, sometimes giant cells | 0 | 0 |

[a]Three days' growth on Sabouraud's dextrose agar at 25° C.
[b]Three days' growth on Sabouraud's dextrose broth at 25° C.

## PHYSIOLOGY

The metabolism of *Candida* cells is the same as that of other aerobic eukaryotic cells. They are capable of both aerobic glycolysis via the hexose monophosphate pathway and of anaerobic glycolysis through the Embden-Meyerhof pathway. They also have Krebs cycle enzymes and the mitochondrial enzymes for oxidative phosphorylation. Oxidative phosphorylation in *Candida* involves mainly cytochromes a, $a_3$, b, c, and $c_1$.

Protein synthesis also resembles that in eukaryotes. *C. albicans* has 80S ribosomes, which dissociate into 60S and 38S subunits (Yamaguchi and Iwata, 1970).

Little is known of the physiologic changes associated with or responsible for the development of hyphae or chlamydospores. Temperature is one important factor; relatively high temperatures (37° C) promote hyphae and blastospores, whereas lower temperatures (<25° C) seem to favor chlamydospores. Mycelial formation is accompanied by a suppression of the pentose phosphate pathway and the diversion of hexoses for cell wall biosynthesis.

**TABLE 3.  Antigenic Grouping of *Candida* Species
of Medical Importance**

| GROUP | SPECIES | THERMOSTABLE ANTIGENS | THERMOLABILE ANTIGENS |
|---|---|---|---|
| I | *C. albicans* | 1, 2, 3, 4, 5, 6, 7 | |
| | *C. tropicalis* | 1, 2, 3, 4, 5, 6 | |
| II | *C. stellatoidea* | 1, 8, 10 | a |
| | *C. pseudotropicalis* | 1, 2, 3, 4, 5, 10 | |
| III | *C. krusei* | 1, 2, 5, 11 | b |
| IV | *C. parapsilosis* | 1, 2, 3, 5, 13, 14, 15 | c |
| V | *C. guilliermondi* | 1, 2, 3, 4, 9 | |
| VI | None of medical importance | | |

## IMMUNITY

Cell-mediated immunity is thought to be more important than humoral immunity in resistance to *Candida* infection. At least in chronic infections of the skin due to *C. albicans*, there are often disturbances of T-cell function. Since there is a familial tendency for mucocutaneous candidiasis to occur in children who have abnormal T lymphocytes it would seem that the disturbance in these cells may sometimes be genetic in origin (see Chapter 211). There is some evidence that candidiasis occurs because the T cell cannot recognize the antigen or produce migration inhibition factor (MIF). There is also suggestive evidence that macrophage chemotaxis is depressed. Despite universal delayed sensitivity to *Candida* antigens in healthy people, those with chronic candidiasis are often anergic to its antigens, and transformation of their lymphocytes by *Candida* antigen is sometimes depressed. B lymphocytes and circulating antibodies, on the other hand, are normal. The importance of abnormal T cells in the cause of impaired immunity to *Candida* is also suggested by the tendency of mucocutaneous candidiasis to occur in patients who have frank thymic disorders such as thymomas and congenital thymic aplasia (DiGeorge syndrome).

Abnormalities in humoral immunity, such as agammaglobulinemia, hypogammaglobulinemia, and multiple myeloma have not displayed a special susceptibility to *Candida* infection. Furthermore, the ability of humoral antibody to prevent experimental candidiasis after active or passive immunization has been inconsistent and unimpressive (Hurd and Drake, 1953).

The natural immunity of healthy persons to *Candida* infection is probably generated early in life when the alimentary tract becomes colonized with *C. albicans*. The surface glycoproteins (mannoproteins and glucoproteins) are thought to stimulate both humoral and cellular immunity.

Thus, normal people develop antibodies and delayed hypersensitivity to *Candida* culture filtrates, which contain glycoprotein and polysaccharide antigens.

## LABORATORY DIAGNOSIS

### Morphologic and Cultural Methods.

*C. albicans* infection of the skin, urinary tract, mouth, vagina, esophagus, and other tissues is easily recognized by microscopic examination of wet mounts (Fig. 3) or Gram stains (Fig. 4) of the lesions. The material is taken for examination by scraping the skin or mucous patches (thrush) and smearing the infected scrapings on a microscope slide for Gram staining. Yeast and mycelial forms of *Candida* are strongly gram-positive. Both superficial and deeper hematogenous *Candida* infections of the skin can be recognized by microscopic examination of smears made from skin scrapings. *C. albicans* is also cultured without difficulty from lesions on any conventional-

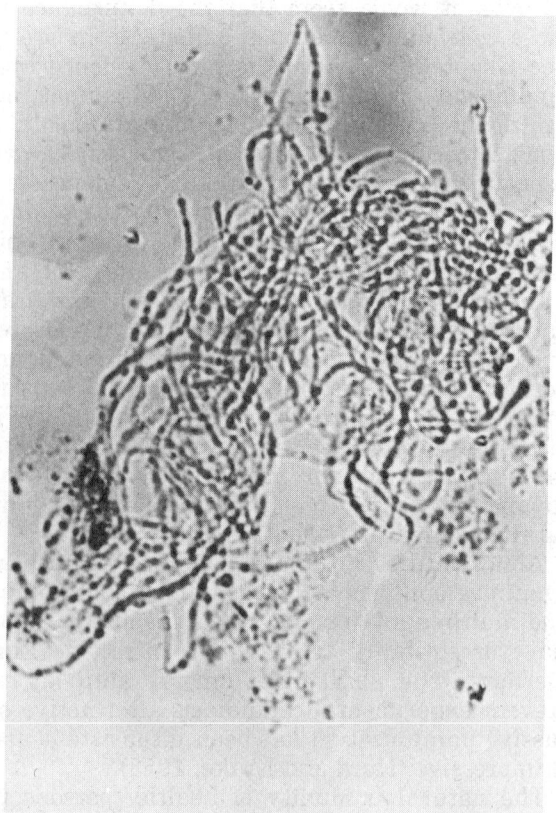

**FIGURE 3.** *Wet mount of* C. albicans *in skin lesion from girl with chronic mucocutaneous candidiasis. The skin scraping had been treated with potassium hydroxide to digest away the epithelial cells and debris before microscopic examination. Note predominance of hyphae.*

al solid or liquid medium. It may appear overnight at 37° C on blood agar or nutrient agar and seldom needs more than 48 hours to grow out. Although less important for diagnosis than smears, culture is necessary for identifying the species of *Candida* and for testing sensitivity to 5-fluorocytosine, a drug to which *C. albicans* can become resistant.

Culture of *Candida* from blood is more difficult than direct culture from infected tissues. The organism may not appear in culture for several days after onset of candidemia, if at all. Blood must be cultured aerobically to get an optimum recovery of *Candida* organisms. The speed of cultural isolation is also accelerated if blood is cultured in pour plates (1.0 ml heparinized blood added to 9 ml warm molten nutrient agar). If candidemia is secondary to contaminated intravenous lines, the diagnosis can also be made by smear and culture of the catheter tip after it is removed from the vein.

The first step in species identification is to test for germ tubes by suspending the yeast in serum and incubating it at 37° C for two to four hours. A presumptive diagnosis of *C. albicans* can be made if germ tubes are produced, and a final diagnosis is made by sucrose assimilation. *C. stellatoidea,* which can also produce germ tubes, can be excluded if sucrose is fermented and assimilated. The other species of *Candida* are also identified by fermentation and assimilation tests.

Assimilation tests are used to determine the ability of a yeast to use a given substance as the sole source of carbon or nitrogen. The test can be done either with solid or liquid media. In the test on solid medium, organisms are dispersed throughout warm agar, which is then poured into a plate before it solidifies. The seeded agar is prepared so that it lacks the specific sugar or nitrogen source under test, and small amounts of the test substance are placed at various points on the surface. The ability to assimilate a given substance is determined by the presence of growth at room temperature in the region where the test substance is applied. The test can also be done by streaking the surface and applying filter paper disks containing test substrate, or by inoculating the surface of agar slants containing each of the individual sugars to be examined. Bromcresyl blue is used as a pH indicator, and each tube is watched for growth and for a change in color from blue to yellow as acid is produced by fermentation. The same media can be used in liquid form for broth assimilation tests. Each broth tube contains one sugar as the test substrate and is inoculated with a suspension of organisms grown for 48 hours in the basal medium to deplete the cells of stored substrate. The tubes are incubated at room temperature, and

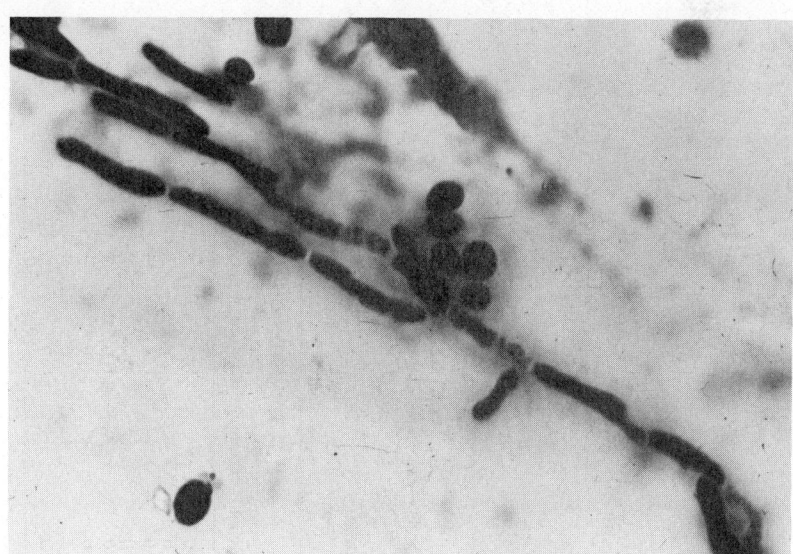

**FIGURE 4.** *Gram stain of smear made from embolus to femoral artery in a patient with* Candida *endocarditis.* C. albicans *is strongly gram-positive. Both hyphae and blastospores appear to be growing in the embolus.*

growth is determined by the development of turbidity. In the nitrate assimilation test, a carbon base is inoculated with 0.078 per cent potassium nitrate in order to determine if this substrate can be used as the sole source of nitrogen.

Fermentation tests determine the ability of yeasts to ferment individual sugars in media that support their growth even in the absence of the test sugar. These media contain peptone, yeast extract (the water-soluble portion of autolyzed bakers' or brewers' yeast that is rich in B vitamins), and a pH indicator. Observations are made on production of both acid and gas. As recorded in Table 4, the yeasts cannot ferment to gas all sugars that they can assimilate. Examples of sugars that are assimilated but not fermented to gas are galactose by *C. stellatoidea* and sucrose by *C. parapsilosis*. It should also be noted that all species of *Candida* of medical importance assimilate and ferment glucose, and all except *C. krusei* assimilate galactose and xylose. Lactose, on the other hand, is assimilated and fermented only by *C. pseudotropicalis*, and inositol by none of them.

In contrast to certain cryptococci, no species of *Candida* in Table 4 can use nitrate as a sole source of nitrogen. Even more important, no species of *Candida*, except certain strains of *C. krusei*, has urease activity. The urease test is thus important for distinguishing *C. albicans* and other species of *Candida* from *Cryptococcus neoformans*, which does have urease activity.

### Serologic Methods

Attempts to diagnose candidiasis by tests for antibody or circulating antigen are not yet reliable. Attempts have been made to find antibody in sera from patients by testing them for their ability to agglutinate *C. albicans* yeast cells, or to precipitate antigens from disrupted *C. albicans* in tubes or in gel diffusion plates. These tests have seldom been useful clinically because patients who develop disseminated candidiasis are often suppressed immunologically and cannot generate a specific immune response. Moreover, disseminated candidiasis is a disorder that requires recognition long before antibody can make its appearance. For this reason, efforts are being made to detect circulating *Candida* antigens by immunologic or chemical methods in order to make a diagnosis of systemic candidiasis in patients with negative blood cultures (Miller et al., 1974).

### EPIDEMIOLOGY

In contrast to the other fungi that cause human infection, members of the genus *Candida* are not inhabitants of the soil but rather indigenous members of the normal flora of the human alimentary tract and skin. *C. albicans* is also widely distributed among animals and is responsible for oral, esophageal, genital, skin, and disseminated hematogenous infections in domesticated mammals or fowl. For example, *C. albicans* has caused epidemic venereal disease among geese and many cases of esophagitis in pigs (Beemer et al., 1973; Kadel et al., 1969). Despite its wide prevalence in these animal reservoirs, the source of human infections by *C. albicans* is endogenous, arising from carriage sites on the patient himself. About 10 per cent of healthy people carry *C. albicans* in their mouth, and 15 per cent carry it in the

## TABLE 4. Assimilation and Fermentation Reactions of Different Species of *Candida* and *T. glabrata*

| | ASSIMILATION RESULTS | | | | | | | | | | | | FERMENTATION (GAS PRODUCTION) | | | | |
| --- | --- | --- | --- | --- | --- | --- | --- | --- | --- | --- | --- | --- | --- | --- | --- | --- | --- |
| | Glucose | Maltose | Sucrose | Lactose | Galactose | Melibiose | Cellobiose | Inositol | Xylose | Raffinose | Trehalose | Dulcitol | Glucose | Maltose | Sucrose | Lactose | Galactose |
| C. albicans | + | + | + | 0 | + | 0 | 0 | 0 | + | 0 | + | 0 | + | + | A* | 0 | + |
| C. stellatoidea | + | + | 0 | 0 | + | 0 | 0 | 0 | + | 0 | + | 0 | + | + | 0 | 0 | 0 |
| C. tropicalis | + | + | + | 0 | + | 0 | + | 0 | + | 0 | + | 0 | + | + | + | 0 | + |
| C. parapsilosis | + | + | + | 0 | + | 0 | 0 | 0 | + | 0 | + | 0 | + | 0 | 0 | 0 | 0 |
| C. krusei | + | 0 | 0 | 0 | 0 | 0 | 0 | 0 | 0 | 0 | 0 | 0 | + | 0 | 0 | 0 | 0 |
| C. pseudotropicalis | + | 0 | + | + | + | 0 | + | 0 | + | + | 0 | 0 | + | 0 | + | + | + |
| C. guilliermondi | + | + | + | 0 | + | + | + | 0 | + | + | + | + | + | 0 | + | 0 | + |
| T. glabrata | + | 0 | 0 | 0 | + | 0 | 0 | 0 | 0 | 0 | + | 0 | + | 0 | 0 | 0 | 0 |

*A, acid, no gas

rectum. Carriage in the mouth and rectum can reach 40 per cent or more in patients and tends to increase with age and antibiotic treatment (Berdon and Seita, 1971; Chitale and Bhende, 1965). Vaginal carriage is highest normally in the childbearing age, when it may reach 10 per cent. *C. albicans* is found less frequently on the skin than on mucous membranes; the skin isolation rate seldom exceeds 5 to 8 per cent even in hospitalized patients. *C. tropicalis* is found occasionally in the mouth and feces, and *C. parapsilosis* in feces but in much fewer numbers than *C. albicans.*

The normal residence of *C. albicans* in the vagina, bowel, mouth, and skin is significant in at least two respects. First, cultural isolation of this yeast from materials passing through the mouth or vagina does not constitute proof of infection. This must be kept in mind especially in the case of sputum, because pulmonary infection due to *C.*

*albicans* is extremely rare, if it ever occurs, and positive candidal cultures of sputum almost always represent contamination of pulmonary secretions by the oral resident yeast flora. The second significant point about the normal carriage sites of *C. albicans* is that they represent foci for transmission. For example, *C. albicans* can spread from the vagina or rectum to cause intertrigenous candidiasis of the groin in diabetics; from the vagina to the infant during passage through the birth canal to cause oral thrush in the newborn; and from the skin via intravenous catheters or from the gut via mucosal ulcers to the circulating blood. Transmission of infection from environmental sources of *C. albicans* occurs in exceptional circumstances but is far less important than transmission from normal carriage sites in the patient (Malmatinis et al., 1968; Cremer and DeGroot, 1967).

# TORULOPSIS

The yeast *Torulopsis glabrata* shares with *C. albicans* all of the first seven heat-stable antigens of Tsuchiya except antigen 4. Like *C. albicans,* it is also a member of the resident flora and forms ovoid cells. In contrast to members of the genus *Candida, T. glabrata* does not form mycelia or pseudomycelia. In this respect, it resembles four other yeasts (*Torulopsis pintolopesii, Saccharomyces tellustris, Candida bovina,* and *Candida sloofii*), from which it can be differentiated by the fact that *T. glabrata* can ferment trehalose, whereas the other four yeasts cannot. This one fermentation is important because all five species have otherwise identical fermentation and assimilation patterns.

It is also important to differentiate this yeast from *Cryptococcus neoformans,* which also forms no mycelia. The quickest way to differentiate them is to test for urease activity, which is present in *C. neoformans* but not in *T. glabrata.* Two other differential points are that *T. glabrata* grows at room temperature (25° C) but *C. neoformans* does not, and *C. neoformans* has a capsule but *T. glabrata* has none. Failure to assimilate inositol distinguishes *T. glabrata* from other cryptococci. The most common clinical source of *T. glabrata* is the urine, but occasionally it has been cultured from the blood (Table 1) and spinal fluid. When inoculated intraperitoneally in mice, it produces small granulomas and has an intracellular appearance in them that resembles that of *Histoplasma capsulatum.*

*T. glabrata* is sensitive to nystatin, amphotericin B, and 5-fluorocytosine in concentrations that can be achieved in human infections.

## References

Beemer, A., Kutten, E., and Katz, Z.: Epidemic venereal disease due to *Candida albicans* in geese in Israel. Avian Dis 17:639, 1973.

Berdon, J., and Seita, C.: The incidence of *Candida albicans* in hospital patients. J Oral Med 26:123, 1971.

Biquet, J., Tran Van Ky, P., Andrieu, S., and Degaey, R.: Étude immunoelectrophorétique de la nature et de l'ordre d'apparition des anticorps précipitants du sérum de lapins en fonction de leur mode d'immunisation contre *Candida albicans.* Sabouraudia 4:148, 1965.

Chitale, A., and Bhende, Y.: The incidence of *Candida albicans* in throat and feces of healthy persons and patients on antibiotic therapy. J Postgrad Med 11:30, 1965.

Cremer, G., and DeGroot,: An epidemic of thrush in a premature nursery. Dermatologia 135:107, 1967.

Hurd, R., and Drake, C.: *Candida albicans* infections in actively and passively immunized animals. Mycopathologia 6:290, 1953.

Jansons, V., and Nickerson, W.: Chemical composition of chlamydospores of *Candida albicans.* J Bacteriol 104:922, 1970.

Kadel, W., Kelly, D., and Coles, E.: Survey of yeastlike fungi and tissue changes in esophagogastric region of stomachs of swine. Am J Vet Res 30:401, 1969.

Malamatinis, J., Mattniller, E., and Westphal, J.: Cutaneous moniliasis affecting varsity athletes. J Am Coll Health Assoc 16:294, 1968.

Miller, G., Witwer, M., Braude, A., and Davis, C.: Rapid identification of *Candida albicans* septicemia by gas-liquid chromatography. J Clin Invest 54:1235, 1974.

Pollack, J., and Benham, R.: The chlamydospores of *Candida albicans*: Comparison of three media for their induction. J Lab Clin Med 50:313, 1957.

Reynolds, R., and Braude, A. I.: The filament-inducing property of blood for *Candida albicans*: Its nature and significance. Clin Res Proc 4:40, 1956.

Rippon, J. W.: Medical Mycology, 1st ed. Philadelphia, W. B. Saunders Co., 1974.

Tsuchiya, T., Fukazawa, Y., and Kawakita, S.: Serologic classification of the genus *Candida.* In Tokyo Research Committee of Candidiasis: Studies of Candidiasis in Japan. Tokyo, Education Ministry of Japan, 1961, p. 34.

Wingard, J., Nierz, W., and Sarah, R.: *Candida tropicalis*: A major pathogen in immunocompromised patients. Ann Intern Med 91:539, 1979.

Yamaguchi, H., and Iwata, K.: *In vitro* and *in vivo* protein synthesis in *Candida albicans.* 2. Dissociation properties in ribosomes. Sabouraudia 8:189, 1970.

# 70 SPOROTHRIX SCHENCKII

## F. Mariat, Dr. ès Sciences; and R.G. Garrison, Ph.D.

*Sporothrix schenckii* is the etiologic agent of sporotrichosis, a chronic mycotic disease of man and animals. The fungus is a dimorphic, pathogenic hyphomycete that occurs naturally on vegetation or as a soil saprophyte. The disease develops after the traumatic introduction of the fungus into the dermis. Classic clinical sporotrichosis usually is seen as an ascending lymphangitis of the extremities after development of the primary lesion at the site of inoculation. Sporotrichosis may occur in other diverse clinical forms and at times it may be severe.

The morphologic and cultural characteristics of this fungal pathogen were first described by Schenck in 1898. In the same publication, E.F. Smith suggested its inclusion in the genus *Sporotrichum*. In 1900, Hektoen and Perkins described a new human case of sporotrichosis and proposed the name *S. schenckii*. A black variety of the fungus was isolated in Europe in 1903 by de Beurmann and Ramond and was described under the name *Sporotrichum beurmanni*. In less than ten years, these authors observed more than 200 cases of sporotrichosis in France and published two classic studies: "Les sporotrichum pathogènes" in 1911 and "Les sporotrichoses" in 1912. Other interesting studies of the fungus were those describing epidemics of sporotrichosis in South Africa in 1927 and especially that of 1941 to 1943. Extensive literature reviews on *S. schenckii* are quoted by Nicot and Mariat (1973), Rippon (1974), and Mariat (1977).

## *TAXONOMY*

For a long time the binomial *Sporothrix schenckii*, as proposed by Hektoen and Perkins, was ignored and the fungus was classified in the genus *Sporotrichum*. At first, two species were recognized on the basis of pigment production: *Sprotorichum beurmanni* (brown to black colonies) and *S. schenckii* (non-pigmented colonies). Other species were created on the basis of differences in cultural characteristics. Later, these species were consolidated into a single taxon, *S. schenckii*. The observations of Carmichael and Nicot and Mariat have established the validity of the binomial *S. schenckii*. The fungus is provisionally classed as

Deuteromycotina (Fungi Imperfecti), Hyphomycetes, sympodulosporae, amerosporae.

The perfect state of *S. schenckii* has not yet been precisely established. On the basis of ecologic, morphologic, physiologic, immunologic, and biochemical properties, it has been speculated that *S. schenckii* is closely related to the ascomycetous fungi of the genus *Ceratocystis*. Mariat (1977) has reviewed the taxonomic problems concerned with the *Sporothrix-Ceratocystis* complex and pointed out the possible phylogenetic relationship of *S. schenckii* to *C. stenoceras* as well as other species of *Ceratocystis*.

### Synonymy

*Sporothrix schenckii* Hektoen and Perkins 1900 = Sporotrichum sp. = *Sporotrichum beurmanni* = *Sporotrichum asteroides* = *Sporotrichum equi* = *Sporotrichum jeanselmei* = *Sporotrichum councilmani* = *Sporotrichum grigsby* = *Sporotrichum oculare* = *Sporotrichum biparasiticus* = *Sporotrichum tropicale* = *Rhinocladium beurmanni*.

Possible perfect stage: *Ceratocystis stenoceras* (Robak) Moreau or another *Ceratocystis* species with a *Sporothrix* mode of conidiogenesis.

## *MORPHOLOGY*

### The Saprophytic Mycelial Phase

The colonial morphology of *S. schenckii* varies with the strain when grown at 20 to 30°C on Sabouraud dextrose agar. It may be smooth, glabrous or velvety, folded or wrinkled, and sometimes moist with or without erect coremia. The color of the colony varies from yellowish white to black. The consistency is always membranous and resistant. Sectorial variation is frequently observed.

The microscopic characters are relatively constant (Fig. 1). The thin, septate, mycelial filaments (1.5 $\mu$m in diameter) branch and bear mononucleate, hyaline conidia, which measure 1.5 to 2.5 by 2.5 to 5.5 $\mu$m. The ovoid to elongate conidia are borne directly on the vegetative filament by short sterigmata (radulaspores), or in clusters or

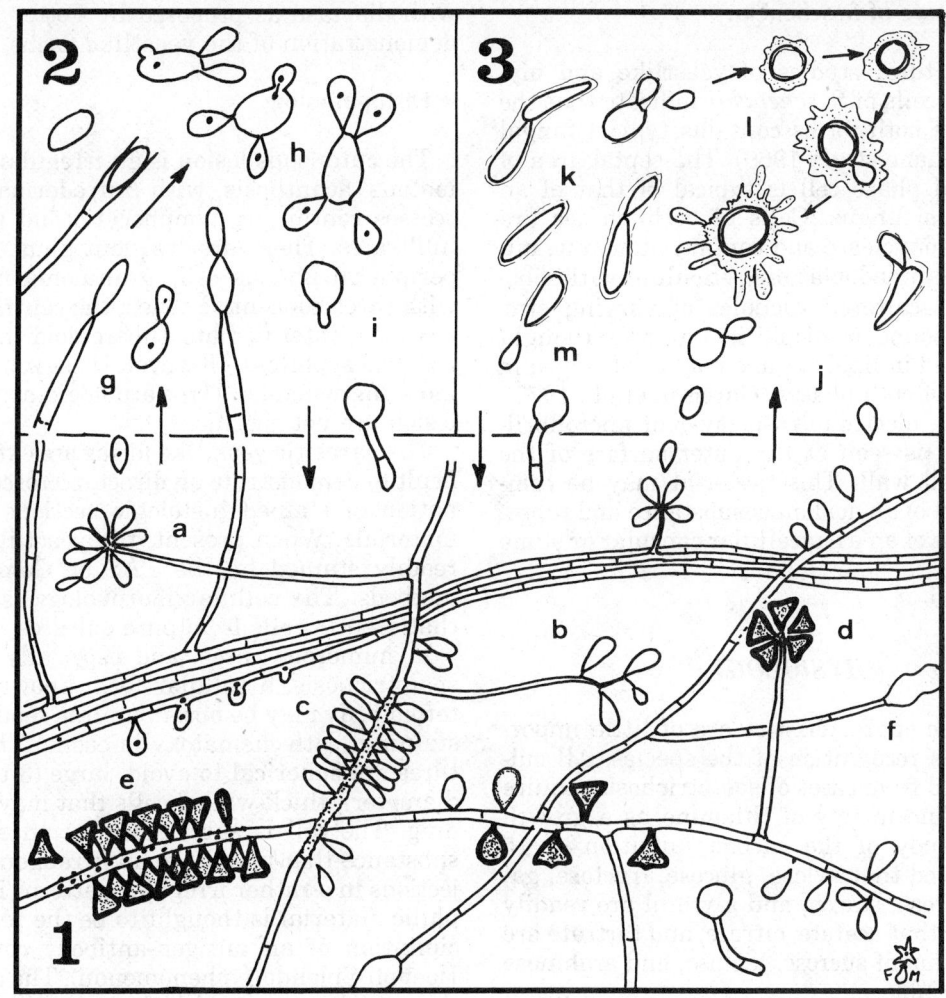

**FIGURE 1.** *Diagrammatic representation of the life cycle of* Sporothrix schenckii. *1, Saprophytic mycelial phase. 2, Yeastlike phase in vitro. 3, Parasitic yeastlike phase in vivo. a, Hyaline conidia in clusters. b, Conidia in sympodium. c, Conidia in radula. d, Triangular pigmented macrospores in clusters. e, Macrospores in radula. f, Chlamydospores. g, Mycelial (M) to yeast (Y) transformation in vitro. h, Yeastlike budding cells in vitro. i, Y→M transformation. j, M→Y transformation in vivo. k, Yeastlike budding cells in vivo. l, Asteroid bodies. m, Y→M transformation.*

bouquets at the top of fertile erect branches. In the latter case, the spores appear successive (sympodulospores). In addition, many strains of *S. schenckii* produce a thick-walled, pigmented spore that is spherical to conical and characteristically triangular in contour. These spores measure from 2.5 to 4.0 μm in diameter. They are borne on the filament in the same fashion as the hyaline conidia but the sterigmata are larger. These conidia may be interpreted as "macrospores" and are considered specific for *S. schenckii*.

### Yeast Phase in vitro

*S. schenckii* is a dimorphic fungus. The saprophytic state is filamentous when grown at 20 to 30°C, whereas the parasitic form is yeastlike when grown under special conditions at 37° C. The unicellular yeastlike form is obtained when grown at 37°C under $CO_2$ on a blood agar base (brain heart infusion agar, for instance) or in liquid shaker culture. Yeastlike colonies grown on a blood agar base appear similar to bacterial colonies and are of a creamy consistency. The surface is moist, smooth, and off-white in color.

Yeastlike cells obtained from in vitro cultures differ in morphology from those seen in vivo. The cells are ovoid to globose to elongate and measure 2.5 to 5.0 by 3.5 to 6.5 μm. Mycelial to yeast transformation occurs by direct budding from the mycelium or by the formation of oidial yeastlike cells within the interior of the same filament (Garrison et al., 1975).

## Ultrastructure of S. schenckii

Ultrastructural studies of yeastlike and mycelial phase cells of *S. schenckii* indicate that the cytoplasm of both forms contains typical fungal organelles (Lane *et al.*, 1969). The septal area of the mycelial phase cell is typical of that of an ascomycetous fungus. Cells of both phases are usually mononucleate and contain numerous mitochondria, an endoplasmic reticulum with ribosomes, and scattered vacuoles of varying size. Membrane-bound, osmiophilic structures thought to be involved in lipid storage may be observed in young cells of both phases (Garrison et al., 1977). A thickened, electron-dense layer of microfibrillar material is seen at the outer surface of the yeastlike cell wall. This material may be composed in part of an acid mucosubstance and represent portions of an extracellular capsular or slime layer.

## *PHYSIOLOGY*

Physiologic characteristics are of little importance for the recognition of the species. All cultures isolated from cases of sporotrichosis require the pyrimidine moiety of thiamine as a growth factor. A study of the carbon nutrition of 15 strains showed that xylose, glucose, fructose, galactose, maltose, starch, and glycerol are readily utilized, but that acetate, citrate, and tartrate are not. Utilization of sucrose, lactose, and arabinose is strain variable.

The precise physiologic conditions necessary for the development of the yeastlike form are not known, although the presence of $CO_2$ appears important. It is interesting that the RNA/DNA ratio of mycelial phase cells is significantly higher than that of yeastlike cells.

## *LABORATORY DIAGNOSIS*

### Direct Examination

Smears of pus or sputum may be examined by the Gram stain or Giemsa stain. In most cases of sporotrichosis, the parasitic yeastlike form of *S. schenckii* is observed very rarely or only with difficulty on staining of clinical materials. However, in some cases they may be abundant. The yeastlike cells are small (2 to 3 by 3 to 6 $\mu$m) and spherical to ovoid to cigar-shaped, and may possess one or two buds. The cells are gram variable and are often surrounded by a clear halo. Staining by the fluorescent antibody method of Kaplan and González Ochoa or pretreatment of smears with diastase as proposed by Fetter may aid in demonstration of the yeastlike forms.

### Histopathology

The cutaneous lesion is an irregular or papillomatous acanthosis with intradermal microabscesses containing lymphocytic and plasmocytic infiltrates. There are frequent giant cells and a peripheral fibrosis. The granuloma may appear with three concentric zones: the central suppurative, the intermediate tuberculoid, and the peripheral syphiloid. However, these zones are often indistinguishable. The pathologic aspects of the lesion are not specific.

The parasitic yeastlike forms are extremely difficult to demonstrate on direct microscopic examination of stained histologic sections of clinical materials. When present, the yeastlike cells are readily stained by the PAS or Gomori-Grocott methods. The cellular morphology is similar to that seen in cells from pure cultures.

In numerous cases, and especially in chronic sporotrichosis, a cellular form known as an asteroid body may be observed. It is readily seen on staining with hematoxylin-eosin. These structures are spherical to ovoid, large (3 to 10 $\mu$m in diameter), thick-walled cells that may show budding. The cell is surrounded by an eosinophilic substance that may have an arrangement of projections in a rather irregular pattern. This eosinophilic material is thought to be the result of precipitation of an antigen-antibody complex (the Hoeppli-Splendore phenomenon). The diameter of the complete asteroid body may reach about 30 $\mu$m.

### Cultures

*S. schenckii* may be isolated readily from clinical materials on a variety of routine culture media. The mycelial phase of the fungus is obtained in three to five days when grown on Sabouraud dextrose agar at room temperature. The fungus is resistant to both cycloheximide and chloramphenicol. Thus, the addition of 0.5 g/liter cycloheximide and 0.1 g/liter chloramphenicol to the isolation medium before sterilization aids the isolation of the fungus in pure culture. The yeastlike form may be obtained by inoculation on brain-heart infusion blood agar and then incubating at 37°C under $CO_2$. Mycelial to yeastlike cell transformation is important for the specific identification of *S. schenckii*.

### Laboratory Animal Inoculations

Intraperitoneal inoculations may be made in male mice or male rats, although male hamsters are the animals of choice. Characteristic disease is produced in two to three weeks, with involvement of the spleen, liver, and testes as target organs. Sections of these organs stained by the PAS, Gomori-Grocott or Gram method reveal abundant intracellular yeastlike forms. Asteroid bodies are usually frequent in histologic sections taken from the testes. It is interesting to note that yeastlike forms are much easier to demonstrate in experimental animal infections than in naturally acquired disease. They are gram positive and resemble large gram-positive rods.

## ANTIGENIC COMPOSITION

Protein and lipid fractions from extracts of *S. schenckii* have been studied, but cell-wall glycoproteins are the most active antigenic components.

Comparative studies done by Toriello and Mariat have shown that polysaccharides synthesized by *S. schenckii* contain mannose and rhamnose as the main sugars, although appreciable amounts of galactose and traces of glucose and hexosamine occur. It is noteworthy that rhamnose is not frequently found in fungi. A protein moiety containing 1.1 to 1.9 per cent nitrogen is bound strongly to the polysaccharides.

The structure of the polysaccharides as peptido-rhamno-mannans has been defined by Lloyd et al., Travassos et al., and Gorin et al., quoted by Mariat (1977).

## IMMUNITY

*S. schenckii* is ubiquitous in the environment, and natural resistance to infection is high. In endemic areas, hypersensitivity is noted in individuals with no clinical signs of disease. In such individuals, this state of hypersensitivity may affect the course of the infection.

Hypersensitivity may be determined by intradermal skin tests with cellular sporotrichin (a suspension of heat and/or chemically killed spores or yeastlike cells containing about $5 \times 10^7$ cells/ml). A positive skin test to cellular sporotrichin occurs in persons having immunosensitizing contact with *S. schenckii*. Clinical signs may or may not occur. Sporotrichin prepared from crude polysaccharide or purified peptido-rhamno-mannan extracts from the culture fluid of yeastlike phase *S. schenckii* is epidemiologically less interesting, but has significant diagnostic value. It is strongly reactive and highly specific.

Humoral immunity in sporotrichosis is not easily detected, the possible reason being the insufficient quality of the antigens employed. Even in cases demonstrated by culture of *S. schenckii*, the titers of the reactions are often very low and are not diagnostic.

Whole yeastlike cell and latex particle agglutination tests seem the most sensitive serologic reactions for study of the disease. Fresh or lyophilized yeastlike cells, crude cultural extracts, or purified polysaccharide extracts of the yeastlike cultural medium may be employed as antigens (Rippon, 1974). Immunodiffusion tests using the same antigens and complement-fixation tests using disrupted yeastlike cell suspensions are diagnostically equivocal.

## ECOLOGY AND EPIDEMIOLOGY

### Ecology of the Fungus

*S. schenckii* is a normal inhabitant of the soil. The fungus occurs in soils rich in organic matter or vegetable debris. It is frequently associated with wood fragments or the bark of trees such as the eucalyptus or pine. It occurs often in association with *Ceratocystis stenoceras*, which *S. schenckii* closely resembles. Thus, both plants and soil may be considered as the natural reservoir of *S. schenckii*. At the same time, the fungus has been isolated from apparently healthy animals, air, water, and a variety of other substrates; these should be considered as possible vectors of the disease. Mammals may develop sporotrichotic infections comparable to that of the human and occasionally are active vectors of the disease.

Mycelial phase elements of the fungus may infect man by inhalation, thereby initiating a primary pulmonary complex that is no longer considered rare. However, the most frequent mode of contamination is through trauma of the skin. Various forms of trauma have been implicated. The most common is a prick from a thorn or plant fragment. Other types of trauma are animal bites, pecks from chickens or other birds, and stings of insects. The handling of fish from a volcanic lake in Guatemala resulted in 43.3 per cent of 53 infections reported from this endemic area of sporotrichosis.

The presence of *S. schenckii* and *C. stenoceras* in the same ecologic site is to be emphasized. *C. stenoceras* is widespread in nature, and its morphologic, biochemical, and antigenic characteristics are very similar, if not identical, to those of *S. schenckii*. It may play an important role in the epidemiology of sporotrichosis.

### Epidemiology of Sporotrichosis

The disease occurs worldwide, but it is found mainly in warm temperate and tropical zones.

The majority of patients are under 30 years of age, and children under 10 years of age are frequently affected. Infection is equally distributed between the sexes. Sporotrichosis is found mainly in persons who are in active contact with plants or soil. It is an occupational disease of nursery workers, florists, potters, workers packing earthenware, and masons working with raw bricks.

*S. schenckii* is only slightly pathogenic, and healthy individuals generally resist infection. The absence of direct contagion from man to man, even under conditions most favorable for the fungus, is indicative of low virulence. To produce lethal sporotrichosis experimentally, male hamsters must receive at least $5 \times 10^6$ cells of a known pathogenic strain by intraperitoneal injection. This number is far higher than that introduced spontaneously by accidental trauma. If traumatic inoculation of a few infecting particles is to induce spontaneous sporotrichosis, then favorable host conditions must be present. Dietary deficiencies, primary pathologic defects, and resensitization are believed to be predisposing factors.

## References

Garrison, R.G., Boyd, K.S., and Mariat, F.: Ultrastructural studies of the mycelial to yeast transformation of *Sporothrix schenckii*. J Bact 124:959, 1975.

Garrison, R.G., Mariat, F., Boyd, K.S., and Fromentin, H.: Ultrastructural observations of an unusual osmiophilic body in the hyphae of *Sporothrix schenckii* and *Ceratocystis stenoceras*. Ann Microbiol (Inst Pasteur) 128B:275, 1977.

Lane, J.W., Garrison, R.G., and Field, M.F.: Ultrastructural studies of the yeast-like and mycelial phases of *Sporotrichum schenckii*. J Bact 100:1010, 1969.

Mariat, F.: Taxonomic problems related to the fungal complex *Sporothrix schenckii/Ceratocystis spp*. In Iwata, K. (ed.): Recent Advances in Medical and Veterinary Mycology. Baltimore, University Park Press, 1977, p. 265.

Nicot, J., and Mariat, F.: Caractères morphologiques et position systématique de *Sporothrix schenckii*, agent de la sporotrichose humaine. Mycopath Mycol Applic 49:53, 1973.

Rippon, J.W.: Medical Mycology. The Pathogenic Fungi and the Pathogenic Actinomycetes. Philadelphia, W.B. Saunders Company, 1974.

# 71 *HISTOPLASMA CAPSULATUM*

*Howard W. Larsh, Ph.D.
and Nancy K. Hall, Ph.D.*

## MORPHOLOGY

*Histoplasma capsulatum* is a dimorphic fungus. In its natural habitat in soils and at room temperature on agar, it grows as a mold. The colony on agar is usually fluffy and either white or buff-brown. Two types of spores are formed by most strains: small spherical aleuriospores (microconidia) that are 2 to 4 $\mu$ in diameter and larger macroaleuriospores (macroconidia) that measure 8 to 14 $\mu$ in diameter. Both types of spores are found at the end of narrow aleuriophores that arise at right angles from vegetative mycelia. With time, the surface of the macroaleuriospores may become covered with evenly spaced spines ("tubercles"), which gives them a characteristic appearance (Fig. 1). These structures are not absolutely diagnostic, however, since a saprophytic mold *Sepedonium* also produces macroaleuriospores.

When *H. capsulatum* grows in tissue, it transforms into a small oval yeast. The yeast phase can also be propagated in vitro on blood agar media. Colonies are white and moist. Individual yeast are 2 to 4 $\mu$ long and reproduce by budding at their narrow end (Fig. 2). The pore that connects mother and daughter cells is narrow and fragile and therefore may break prematurely, producing marked variation in the size of individual cells. The cell wall is thin. When stained, the cytoplasm shrinks away from the cell wall, creating a halo that has been mistaken for a capsule. Each cell contains only one nucleus, which may be hard to see in stained preparations.

The perfect stage of *H. capsulatum* has been described. It is heterothallic and is therefore classified in the family Gymnoascaceae of the Ascomycetes.

The etiologic agent of histoplasmosis, *H. capsulatum,* was identified in 1906 by Darling as a protozoan (*Leishmania*). Later, the infectious agent was proved to be a diphasic fungus with a pathogenic yeast stage and a saprophytic mycelial stage.

## ANTIGENIC COMPOSITION

Four major antigenic preparations are now used for investigative, clinical, and epidemiologic

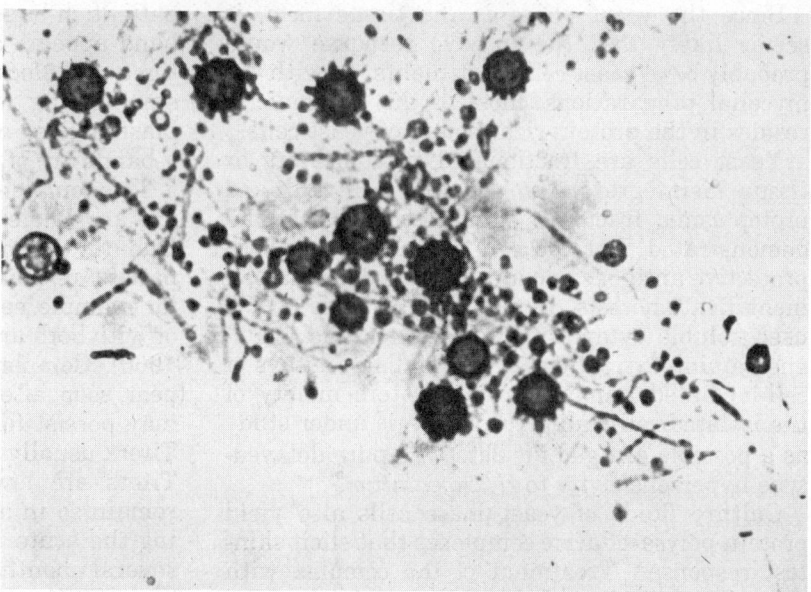

**FIGURE 1.** *Macroaleuriospores (macro-conidia) of* Histoplasma capsulatum *covered with spines or "tubercles."*

studies of histoplasmosis: extracts of mycelial and yeast-phase cells of *H. capsulatum* and culture filtrates of the two morphologic types. The classic mycelial culture filtrate antigen (histoplasmin) is prepared from a synthetic broth culture incubated at room temperature. Filtration of the broth after a period of growth and standardization of the activity by intradermal injection is required. Comparison of potency with that of a standard histoplasmin is also necessary (Goodman et al., 1968).

The active components of mycelial culture filtrates have been identified by using column chromatography and polyacrylamide disk gel electrophoresis (Sprouse et al., 1969). Two antigenic fractions were found in a five-month asparagine medium preparation, the more potent being a high molecular weight protein that elicits a skin-test reaction in guinea pigs with experimental histoplasmosis.

By using an ammonium sulfate precipitation and Pevikon block electrophoresis, crude histoplasmin has also been separated into two main fractions, a protein that elicits a positive skin test and a less reactive fraction rich in polysaccharide (O'Connell et al., 1967). No increase in skin sensitivity was observed with either fraction.

Many techniques have been used to isolate and characterize a reactive component from the mycelial phase cells themselves. Alkali-extracted mycelium yielded a galactomannan protein complex that is separable into polysaccharide and glycoprotein complexes by ion-exchange chromatography (Reiss et al., 1974). The galactomannan did not elicit a skin-test response, but it elicited a cell-mediated reaction (production of migration-inhibition factor) from sensitized lymphocytes.

Polysaccharide antigens of mycelial *H. capsulatum* have been studied after using enzymatic digests to eliminate protein antigens (Kobayashi, 1971). The mannose-glucose polysaccharide was active in serologic tests but was not tested for its ability to elicit skin responses.

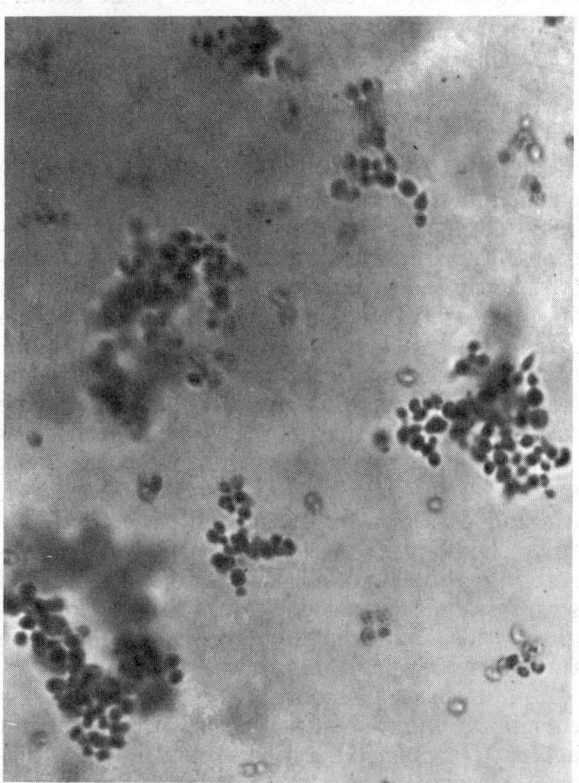

**FIGURE 2.** *Yeast phase of* H. capsulatum *grown in vitro. Individual yeast are 2 to 4 μ long and reproduce by budding.*

Since the yeast phase is the tissue form, it seems likely that the in vivo response would probably be to yeast-cell constituents. As with the mycelial preparations, most of the antigenicity resides in the protein-rich moiety of yeast cells.

Yeast cells are fractionated in sonicators or tissue disintegrators to separate cell-wall and protoplasmic fractions. Salvin and Ribi (1955) demonstrated that the cell wall contained both protective antigens and antigens used for complement fixation tests. Domer and Ichinose (1977) used soluble cytoplasmic substances and ethyl-enediamine extractions of cell walls in assays of cell-mediated immunity. The protein moiety of the isolated cell-wall glycoprotein is under study as a possible antigen for detecting pure delayed-type hypersensitivity to *H. capsulatum*.

Culture fluids of yeast-phase cells also yield protein-polysaccharide complexes that elicit skin-test responses. Treatment of the complex with chloroform eliminated the skin reactivity of the antigen (Dyson and Evans, 1955). An antigen from yeast-phase filtrates was isolated and shown by electrophoresis to be composed of two components, a skin-test reactive protein and a less reactive polysaccharide. Increased specificity has not been achieved.

A purified, specific antigen capable of standardization is being sought in mycelium, mycelial culture filtrates, yeast, and yeast-phase culture filtrates.

## IMMUNITY

Immunity to *H. capsulatum* correlates with the development of delayed hypersensitivity. Antibody to the fungus is produced regularly in response to infection but does not result in immunity. The antibody response is of limited value in the diagnosis of histoplasmosis, because available antigens cross-react with antibodies to other fungi. To maximize the usefulness of serologic testing, two or more samples of sera should be taken for examination during the acute, convalescent, and recovery stages of the infection. Also, tests with a battery of antigens should be used (Campbell, 1960). Interpretation of serologic results should take into account not only cross-reacting antibodies but also antibodies induced with intradermal histoplasmin. Precipitation, agglutination, and complement fixation are the three basic serologic procedures.

The antibody response to *H. capsulatum* is complex. Immunodiffusion of histoplasmin against *Histoplasma* antisera results in six distinct precipitin bands (Heiner, 1958). These bands correlate with the clinical condition of the patient: h-band is associated with infection; m-band appears after skin tests with mycelial antigen or infection; c-band indicates exposure to skin testing with histoplasmin, coccidioidin, or blastomycin; n-band is nonspecific, and x- and y-bands are of unknown significance.

The complement fixation antigens in common use are whole yeast-phase cells or histoplasmin. Due to the unpredictability of the individual patient response, both antigens should be used; for example, sera may react with only one antigen or with both antigens in variable titer (Campbell, 1960). Complement fixation titers normally appear soon after onset of clinical symptoms and may persist for months or years after infection. Titers usually parallel the course of the disease. Titers are low or negative at first (and may remain so in asymptomatic infections), rise during the acute illness, and disappear slowly after several months. In the progressive form of the disease, titers remain high for a long time.

A particulate agglutination test is also used to demonstrate antibodies to *H. capsulatum*. Histoplasmin is adsorbed to collodion particles, to sheep erythrocytes, or to latex particles to serve as antigen. Whole yeast-phase cells can also be used successfully (Cozad and Larsh, 1960).

## LABORATORY DIAGNOSIS

A definitive diagnosis of histoplasmosis can be made by culturing the fungus from tissue secretions or excretions, or by demonstrating the yeast cells histologically. *H. capsulatum* stains very poorly with hematoxylin-eosin and is usually evident only as a protoplasmic mass surrounded by a halo. The yeast cell walls stain red with periodic acid-Schiff stains, although the cytoplasm stains poorly. With silver stains (e.g., Gomori) the cell wall is black. Organisms appear larger with cell-wall stains because the artifactual shrinkage of the cell cytoplasm that occurs during fixation is not evident.

In primary histoplasmosis, sputum is often not produced for culture, but *H. capsulatum* may be cultured from urine. In cavitary pneumonias, sputum or gastric lavage specimens should be submitted for culture. In disseminated disease, scrapings from surface lesions, tissue biopsies (especially liver, bone marrow, and lymph nodes), blood, urine, and sputum may yield positive cultures.

Specimens for microscopic examination of secretions are fixed and air-dried on a microscope slide and then stained using either the Giemsa or Wright method. The yeast appear in histiocytes and macrophages as small oval cells, 2 to 5 $\mu$ in diameter. If rupture of the phagocytic cells occurs, it may be difficult to differentiate the extracellular *H. capsulatum* from other yeasts. Nevertheless, their small size, the budding from the narrow end, and the narrow attachment to the mother cells are distinguishing characteristics.

In pulmonary histoplasmosis, an early morning specimen of sputum should be collected in a sterile glass jar and transported to the laboratory within an hour. A delay in processing sputum increases the degree of contamination by faster growing bacteria and fungi.

The use of test tubes or Petri dishes for inoculation of sputum is debatable. The organism is an obligate aerobe, and Petri dishes allow more inoculum to be spread on the surface of the medium, but unsealed Petri dishes may present a hazard to laboratory personnel. The specimens suspected of harboring pathogenic fungi should be cultured in a bacteriologic safety hood.

Sputum as well as all other secretions and excretions should be treated with antibiotics to suppress contaminating bacteria. To ensure that the specimens are well homogenized, they may be diluted with sterile cysteine-saline and shaken in a mechanical shaker for 30 minutes to an hour. One-half milliliter of sputum, urine, gastric, or bronchial lavage is added to the following media, and the plates incubated for at least four weeks: (1) Emmon's modified Sabouraud's agar pH 7 without antibiotics; (2) Emmon's modified Sabouraud's agar (1 per cent Neopeptone, 2 per cent glucose, 2 per cent agar) pH 7 with penicillin, streptomycin, and Actidione or the same medium with chloramphenicol and Actidione; (3) blood agar base with 5 per cent defibrinated blood with gentamicin and Actidione, or blood agar base with 5 per cent defibrinated blood with gentamicin, carbenicillin, and Actidione. At least one medium should contain no Actidione, since *Cryptococcus neoformans, Petriellidium boydii, Aspergillus* sp., and other fungi that may cause pulmonary disease are inhibited by the antifungal agent.

Sterile tissue grinders are used to prepare tissues for plating. The homogenates are diluted and one-half milliliter is spread on the media listed above. Spinal fluids and other aseptic specimens are plated directly on the media without addition of antibiotics.

A policy of not incubating specimens at 37° C has been followed successfully in our laboratory for years. Most isolates of *H. capsulatum* do not grow well at this temperature , since it is near the maximal growth range of this fungus. If the yeast stage is to be obtained from infected tissue, an enriched medium containing blood should be used and incubated at 30° C. Mycelium can be converted without difficulty to the pathogenic yeast stage by inoculating tissue cultures (e.g., Hela cells).

Periodic examination of the cultures after 7 to 10 days usually reveals growth. From "typical" cultures, lactophenol preparations can be made of the mycelia that reveal microaleuriospores and macroaleuriospores. The former are spherical conidia 2 to 4 $\mu$m in diameter that are borne singly at the tip of short conidiophores. The walls of these spores may be smooth or have small spines. The macroaleuriospores are spherical but on occasion may be pear-shaped. These spores may be 8 to 15 $\mu$m in diameter and are firmly attached to narrow conidiophores. They may have smooth walls, but characteristically there are evenly spaced spines or finger-like appendages.

In the patient with chronic histoplasmosis, an isolate of *H. capsulatum* frequently is "atypical." Neither microaleuriospores nor macroaleuriospores are produced, and the cultures may be neither white nor brown. These isolates must be inoculated into experimental animals or tissue culture to obtain the yeast form of the fungus. Mice are useful for this purpose. Mice often survive the infection and should be autopsied two to four weeks after inoculation to demonstrate the yeast cells in liver and spleen. Sputum, or other material contaminated with bacteria, should be treated with antibiotics before injection.

In ecologic studies, mice are usually used to isolate *H. capsulatum* from soils, bird feces, and other highly contaminated specimens. The samples must be treated with antibiotics before inoculation intraperitoneally. In addition, antibiotics may be added to the drinking water and a second injection of antibiotic after 24 hours administered.

## *EPIDEMIOLOGY*

The growth of *H. capsulatum* in soils enriched with bird or bat droppings is the source of human and animal exposure. Disturbances of the environment in which the fungus is growing produce aerosols containing aleuriospores that may be inhaled and cause primary infections. The specific role of feces in large bird roosts in the epidemiology of the disease is clear. The birds themselves do not contact histoplasmosis as a natural infection, since the blood temperature of birds is too high to support growth of the fungus. The fungus is not communicable from person to person, animal to person, or animal to animal. Each species acquires a natural infection by inhalation of spores. The fungus is also associated with bat guano, and some caves are heavily contaminated. Bats can develop histoplasmosis. The urban brown bat may be another source of histoplasmosis in urban areas.

*H. capsulatum* is an aerobic organism that grows in the upper 1 to 3 centimeters of soil or other enriched materials. Although there is controversy about whether or not this fungus has been isolated from dry pigeon droppings, it is conceded that pigeon droppings will enrich the ability of the soil to support the growth of *H. capsulatum* (Ajello, 1964). It is important to understand that although birds are not naturally infected, their droppings provide an enriched medium for the growth of *H. capsulatum,* whereas certain bats have the disease and their droppings can likewise support the growth of the fungus (Emmons, 1958).

The distribution of *H. capsulatum* in the soil is not uniform, even in highly endemic areas. Frequently *H. capsulatum* can be isolated from soil at the site of a point-source epidemic, but the soil only a few inches away will be negative. It is very difficult to disinfect contaminated soil.

The fungus has a worldwide distribution. Highly endemic areas have been identified by serologic and skin-test surveys with histoplasmin. In highly endemic areas such as the Ohio and Mississippi River valleys in the United States, up to 90 per cent of residents react to histoplasmin. However, the fungus does exist outside these areas where it can be cultured from soil and from native animals (Ajello, 1958; Edwards, 1971). In these areas, such as the eastern seaboard of the United States, skin-test surveys do not reveal the presence of the fungus because only isolated areas of soil are contaminated, and the rate of infection is consequently low.

## References

Ajello, L.: Geographic distribution of *Histoplasma capsulatum.* Mykosen 1:147, 1958.

Ajello, L.: Relationship of *Histoplasma capsulatum* to avian habitats. Pub Health Rep 79:266, 1964.

Campbell, C. C.: The accuracy of serologic methods in diagnosis. Ann NY Acad Sci 89:163, 1960.

Cozad, G. C., and Larsh, H. W.: A capillary tube agglutination test for histoplasmosis. J Immunol 85:387, 1960.

Darling, S. T. A.: A protozoon general infection producing pseudotubercles in the lungs and focal necroses in the liver. JAMA 46:1283, 1906.

Domer, J. E., and Ichinose, H.: Cellular immune responses in guinea pigs immunized with cell walls of *Histoplasma capsulatum* prepared by several different procedures. Infect Immun 16:293, 1977.

Dyson, J. E., and Evans, E. E.: Delayed hypersensitivity in experimental fungus infection. J Lab Clin Med 45:449, 1955.

Edwards, P. Q.: Histoplasmin sensitivity patterns around the world. In Histoplasmos. Proceedings of the Second National Conference. Springfield, Ill., Charles C Thomas, 1971.

Emmons, C. W.: Association of bats with histoplasmosis. Pub Hlth Rept 73:590, 1958.

Goodman, N. L., Sprouse, R. F., and Larsh, H. W.: Histoplasmin potency as affected by culture age. Sabouraudia 6:273, 1968.

Heiner, D. C.: Diagnosis of histoplasmosis using precipitin reactions in agar gel. Pediatrics 22:616, 1958.

Kobayashi, G. S.: Isolation and characterization of polysaccharide of *Histoplasma capsulatum.* In Histoplasmosis Proceedings of the Second National Conference. Springfield, Ill., Charles C Thomas, 1971.

O'Connell, E. J., Hermans, P. E., and Markowitz, H.: Skin reactive antigens of *Histoplasma capsulatum.* Proc Soc Exp Biol Med 124:1015, 1967.

Reiss, E., Mitchell, W. O., Stone, S. H., and Hasenclever, H. F.: Cellular immune activity of a galactomannan-protein complex from mycelia of *Histoplasma capsulatum.* Infect Immun 10:802, 1974.

Salvin, S. B., and Ribi, E.: Antigens from yeast phase of *Histoplasma capsulatum.* Proc Soc Exp Biol Med 108:498, 1955.

Sprouse, R. F., Goodman, N. L., and Larsh, H. W.: Fractionation, isolation and chemical characterization of skin test active components of histoplasmin. Sabouraudia 7:1, 1969.

Thor, D. E., and Dray, S.: A correlation of human delayed hypersensitivity: Specific inhibition of capillary tube migration of sensitized human lymph node cells by tuberculin and histoplasmin. J Immunol 101:51, 1968.

# 72  COCCIDIOIDES IMMITIS

## Henry A. Walch, Ph.D.

### *MORPHOLOGY*

#### Dimorphic Growth Cycle

*Coccidioides immitis* is a fungus that is a part of the microbial population of the soil in certain geographic regions. In the soil it grows as a mycelium, and from branches and strands of hyphae forms square to rectangular arthrospores about 2 to 4 $\mu$ in width and 3 to 10 $\mu$ in length. These chains of arthrospores are arranged with intervening cytoplasmically empty cells and are easily detached and dispersed into the air (Figs. 1 and 2).

Infection of man and other animals usually occurs through inhalation of arthrospores into the lungs. Fungus growth in the body occurs as a rounding up of the arthrospores (Fig. 3) to form spherules that may enlarge to 20 to 100 $\mu$ in diameter (Fig. 4). The one to several nuclei originally present in the arthrospore undergo division and the multinucleate cytoplasm becomes differentiated into numerous, predominantly uninucleate 2 to 3 $\mu$ diameter endospores (Fig. 5), each of which can develop into a mature spherule and continue the parasitic cycle. A clinical specimen containing spherules and endospores that is cultured to a routine isolation medium will pro-

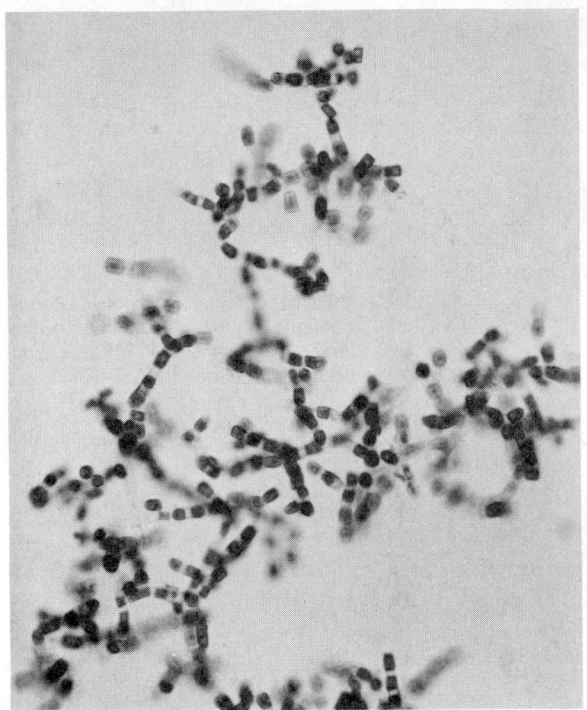

**FIGURE 1.** *Arthrospores of* Coccidioides immitis *(approximately 600 ×).*

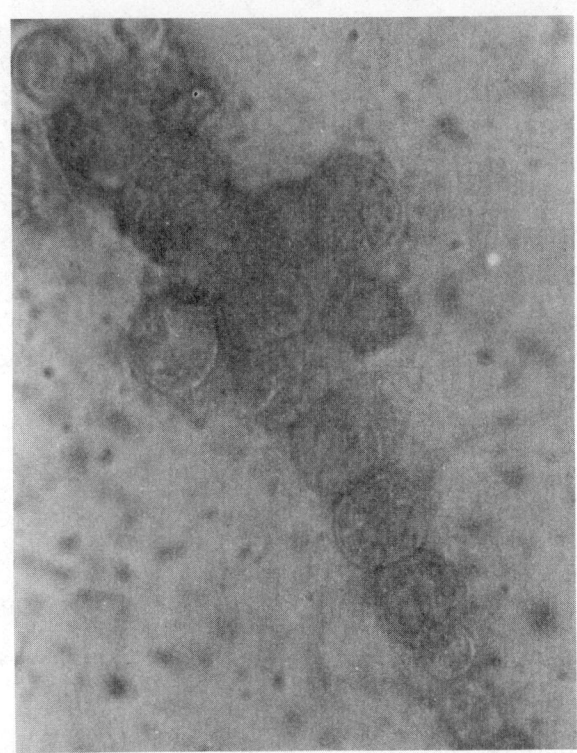

**FIGURE 3.** *Chain of arthrospores of* Coccidioides immitis *undergoing spherulation* in vitro *(approximately 1200 ×).*

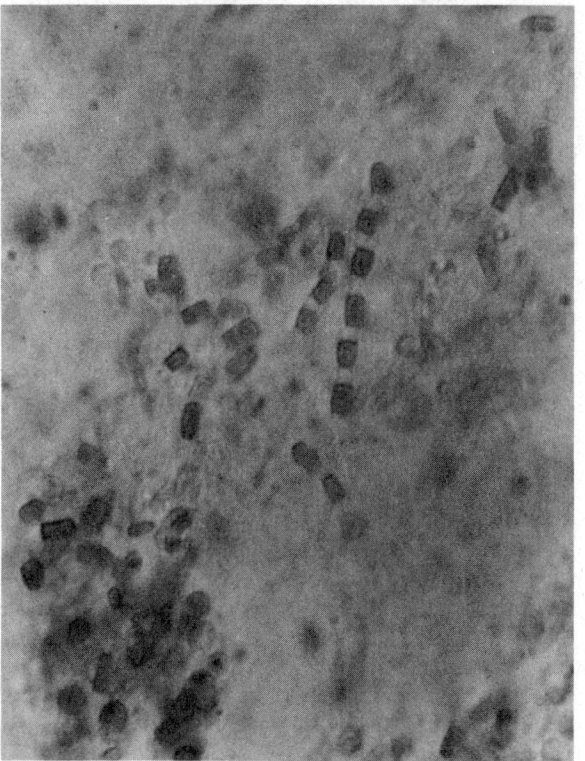

**FIGURE 2.** *Arthrospores of* Coccidioides immitis *(approximately 1200 ×).*

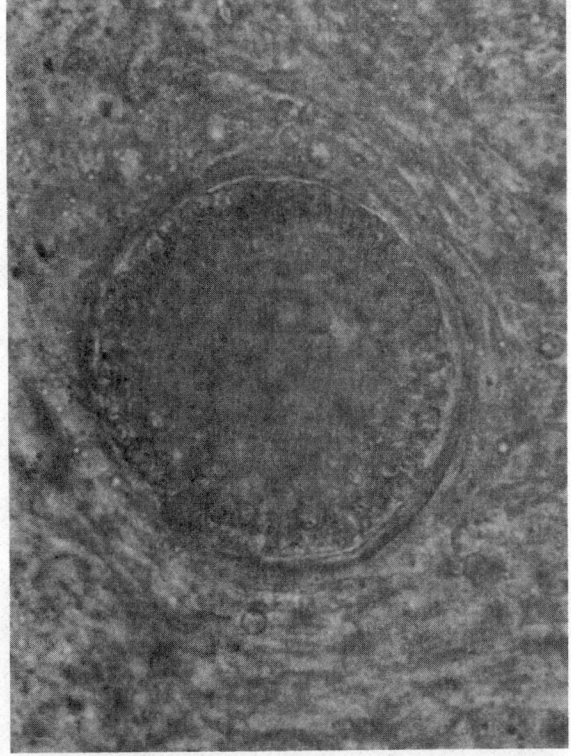

**FIGURE 4.** *Large, mature spherule of* Coccidioides immitis, *unstained in tissue cleared with sodium hydroxide solution (approximately 1200 X).*

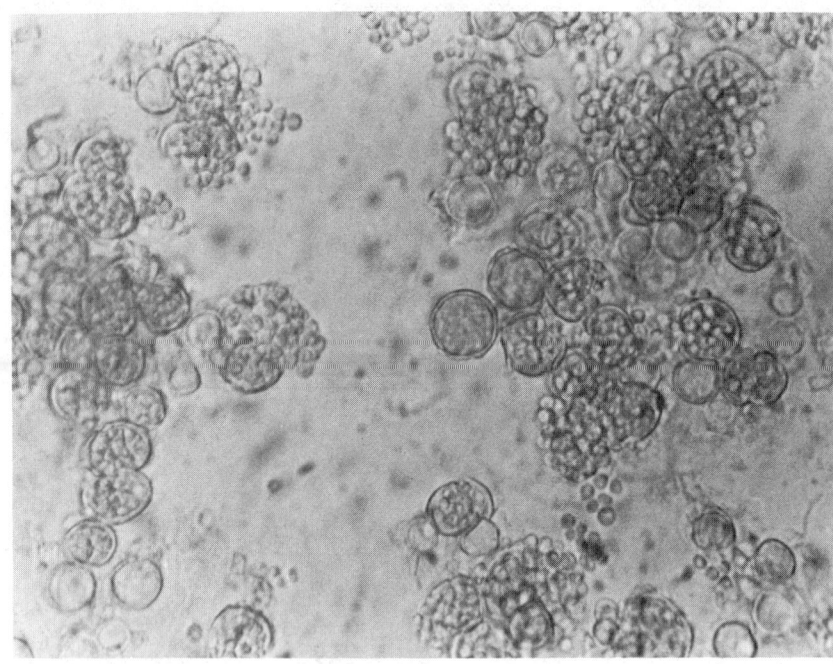

**FIGURE 5.** *Mature* in vitro *formed spherules of* Coccidioides immitis *showing large numbers of released endospores (approximately 1200 X).*

duce the mycelium-arthrospore colony stage (Fig. 6) through the germination and growth of endospores and immature spherules.

It is historically pertinent to note that the spherule-endospore tissue form led the original students of this disease (1892–1896) to conclude that it was of protozoan (coccidioidal) etiology and

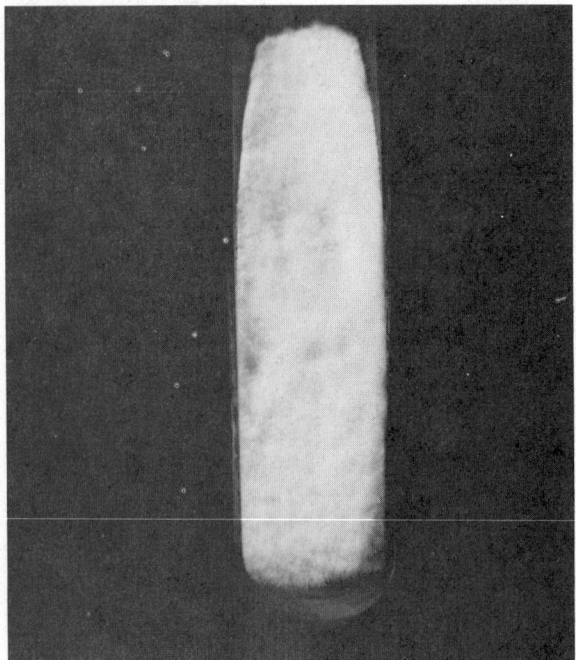

**FIGURE 6.** *Mature culture of* Coccidioides immitis *showing typical aerial mycelium.*

to speciate it as *Coccidioides immitis* (not mild), since the few known human cases were all fatal.

## Classification

The classification of the fungus is still to be resolved, since no sexual stage of growth has been demonstrated. However, cytologic studies of the formation of arthrospores and the ultrastructural characteristics of hyphae (Kwon-Chung, 1969) and studies of arthrospore to spherule morphogenesis (Sun et al., 1976), are mutually supportive of a tentative classification as an ascomycete.

## Cell Wall Composition

The chemical composition of the cell wall is apparently similar to that of other fungi. Analysis of the cell wall has shown chitin to be present in the wall of the three morphologic forms. Other carbohydrate polymers are also present such as B 1–3 glucans, mannans, or possible glucomannans as major cell wall components. Protein is present also, and differences in amino acid composition have been found in the different morphologic forms (Wheat et al., 1977). The cell wall of the mature spherule has five times more chitin than that of the endospore. The spherule wall also differs from the endospore in containing considerable glucose, which may be present as a B 1–3 glucan. Such results, as noted by Collins (1977), indicate that major differences occur in the polysaccharide composition of the wall during endospore to spherule maturation.

## ANTIGENIC COMPOSITION

### Immunologic Test Antigens

Antigens that are used in testing for humoral antibodies or cellular reactivity are called coccidioidins. Two kinds of coccidioidins are available — mycelial and spherule derived.

Mycelial coccidioidin is made from a filtrate of an aging (two months) and autolyzing stationary broth culture, or a pool of broth cultures of different strains to allow for possible antigenic variability. This type of coccidioidin was originally used as a successful serologic and skin test antigen beginning in the early 1940 period (Smith et al., 1950). Because of the extensive past and continued record of use, it serves as a standard of comparison for test antigens. Another type of mycelial coccidioidin is a toluene-induced lysate of a young (two to three day) shaken culture (Pappagianis et al., 1961a). This has been used in immunodiffusion testing and in experimental applications. These coccidioidins can be dialyzed without loss of activity. Heat treatment by autoclaving does not impair the activity of antigens involved in precipitin testing or skin test reactivity. Complement-fixing antigen activity is destroyed, however, by heating at 60° C for 30 minutes.

Spherule coccidioidin (spherulin) is a lysate of a washed, water suspension of in vitro cultured, mature, endosporulating spherules (Levine et al., 1969). In common with the mycelial coccidioidins, the active portion is nondialyzable. In contrast to mycelial coccidioidin, its skin testing potency is definitely impaired by heating at 60° C for 20 minutes.

Analysis of these two complex test antigens by two-dimensional immunoelectrophoresis methods demonstrated at least 26 antigens for mycelial coccidioidin and 12 for spherulin. Ten antigens were in common, two were unique to the spherule, and 16 to the mycelial derived antigens (Huppert et al., 1978).

Spherulin has only recently become available for use as a routine test antigen. It is more reactive and sensitive for cutaneous hypersensitivity testing than is mycelial coccidioidin, and probably more specific (Levine et al., 1973; Stevens, 1974; Levine et al., 1975). It has also been more effective as an antigen when used in the lymphocyte transformation test (Deresinski et al., 1974). Use as a complement-fixing antigen, in comparison with the mycelial coccidioidin, has shown that both were equally sensitive. The results of comparing the reactivity of the two antigens with sera from noncoccidioidal mycoses, however, showed that spherulin was considerably less specific (Huppert et al., 1977).

### Antigen Standardization

Coccidioidins, as mixtures of antigens, are subject to variability of reactivity between different lots produced at different times even though conditions of culture are uniformly maintained. Because of this antigenic heterogeneity and variability, standardization by weight or chemical analysis is not useful. Also, no comparative laboratory animal testing system for biologic reactivity and potency testing is available. Therefore, standardization for serologic or cutaneous hypersensitivity testing must be done by different procedures. Details of these procedures are considered by Huppert (1970), Kobayashi and Pappagianis (1970) and Huppert et al. (1974). In summary, skin test standardization requires human subjects of known cutaneous hypersensitivity and a reference antigen. Serologic standardization requires both a reference serum and antigen and strict adherence to the prescribed test procedure.

### Chemical Composition

Various attempts have been made to chemically separate antigenically active components from mycelial coccidioidin. Ethanol precipitation was used to separate out a skin test reactive and precipitating polysaccharide composed primarily of mannose, which was associated with three to four per cent nitrogen in amino acids. Immunodiffusion and quantitative tube precipitin testing, however, showed that it contained different antigens (Pappagianis et al., 1961b).

Gel molecular filtration and ultrafiltration techniques were used in the course of later studies of the chemical composition. These results showed mannose, 3-O-methylmannose, and peptide components to be consistently present in skin test active fractions (Anderson et al., 1971).

## IMMUNITY

### Infection and Immunity

The extensive human case studies of Smith and his associates (1957) provided evidence that immunity resulted from primary coccidioidomycosis. In addition, asymptomatic infection with conversion to skin test reactivity also seems to result in immunity.

Infection with C. immitis begins with a transitory exposure to the infecting arthrospores, which, after a period of days, begin a transformation to the spherule form. The resulting spherule-to-endospores-to-spherules parasitic cycle involves a continuing multiple antigenic experience for the host. Incidental exposure to the cytoplasm of these structures, in turn, provides additional antigenic stimulation. Some of these antigens will engender the formation of humoral antibodies and others will be active in stimulating a protective cell-mediated immune response.

## Cell-Mediated Immunity

Immunity to *C. immitis* is of the cell-mediated type. Infection is accompanied by cutaneous delayed hypersensitivity, lymphocyte transformation, and macrophage migration inhibition through the use of mycelial and spherule coccidioidins. The role of T cells is implied by the resistance of normal mice to infection after receiving an intravenous inoculation of spleen cells from spherule-vaccinated mice (Beaman et al., 1977), and transfer of delayed hypersensitivity in mice (Rifkind et al., 1976).

In disseminated coccidioidomycosis, the skin test is frequently negative and coccidioidin does not stimulate lymphocyte transformation. Whether this condition represents a nonspecific, preexisting and predisposing immune deficiency, or specific anergy induced by disseminated fungus growth is unsettled.

## Immunization

Formalin-killed vaccines consisting of either mycelium-arthrospores or mature spherules have been compared in mice. The mycelium-arthrospore vaccine provided some protection, whereas the spherule-vaccinated group showed notably better survival and reduced pathologic involvement (Levine et al., 1960).

After mechanical fractionation of ruptured spherules, the spherule wall was an effective immunogen in mice but the soluble cell lysate and the prematurely released endospores were not (Kong et al., 1963). Optimum protection followed immunization with the intact, mature spherule and naturally released endospores were immunogenic, but less so (Levine et al., 1965). Thus, a cycle of immunogen development and decline is associated with the morphogenetic alterations of the parasitic phase of growth.

The monotype spherule-endospore vaccine protects against heterologous strains. When groups of vaccinated mice were subsequently challenged with typical and atypical strains of established virulence, equal protection was demonstrated among all groups, indicating a similarity of immunogenic antigens among different isolates of the fungus (Huppert et al., 1967).

## LABORATORY DIAGNOSIS

### Fungus Growth and Confirmation

*C. immitis* will grow on a wide range of culture media. Commercially available glucose-peptone based selective media containing cycloheximide and antibacterial antibiotics will, generally, provide better growth and sporulation if supplemented with about 0.5 per cent yeast extract. Incubation temperatures of 25 to 30° C are recommended. Although the fungus will grow as the mycelial form on these media at 37° C, the sporulation of some strains is inhibited.

In general, methods that are used for preparation of clinical specimens for bacterial culture will not be inhibitory for *C. immitis* isolation. The processing of sputum, however, must not employ methods designed for isolation of the tubercle bacillus. If it is desirable to digest sputum for fungus culture, equal volumes of either of the mucolytic agents, N-acetyl-l-cysteine or dithiothreitol at a 0.5 per cent concentration made up in 2.94 per cent sodium citrate solution, as per the method of Reep and Kaplan (1972), is suitable.

Confirmation of the presumptively identified culture can be done by spherule demonstration in animals or by in vitro methods. Mice are commonly inoculated intraperitoneally, guinea pigs intratesticularly, in order to demonstrate spherules in tissues. Virulence varies markedly in mice for different strains of the fungus. Also, the mere culture of a fungus from the tissues of an injected animal is not confirmatory since many nonpathogenic fungi will persist without any pathologic effect.

Two convenient in vitro confirmatory identification methods are available. With the method of Sun et al. (1976) arthrospores convert to spherules in three to five days. The method of Standard and Kaufman (1977) uses immunodiffusion for detecting antigens in a fluid culture supernatant and is particularly useful for atypical nonsporulating cultures.

### Immunologic Diagnosis

The two serologic tests that have been most extensively documented and serve as the standards for comparison with other methods are the tube precipitin and the complement-fixation tests. Strict adherence to prescribed procedures and the use of a standardized antigen are required for diagnostic use. Details for the performance of the precipitin test are provided by Kaufman (1976). The complement-fixation procedure using the full volume test is described in the Pan American Health Organization Manual, part II (1974); for the micro complement-fixation test technique consult the United States Public Health Service Publication Number 1228 (1965). Critical evaluations of these complement-fixation methods are contained in the publications of Huppert et al. (1970) and of Kaufman et al. (1970).

Precipitating antibodies occur transiently in the serum and may appear as early as the first week of illness during primary disease. Serum complement-fixing antibodies generally are not evident as early as precipitin antibodies, but they remain detectable for a longer period of time.

Serologic diagnosis and prognosis depends on the testing of subsequent serum samples to determine changes of the complement-fixing antibody titer. The titer usually rises in proportion to severity of disease and declines with improvement of the patient. The generally accepted interpretation of these titers in relation to the disease process is based on the studies of Smith and his associates (1950, 1956). Titers above 1:16 indicate possible dissemination. Lower titers, 1:8 or less, may indicate early, stable residual or meningeal coccidioidomycosis or may be false positives. Negative results do not exclude disease, however, since about 40 per cent of chronic residual pulmonary disease cases are nonreactive. About 25 per cent of patients with coccidioidal meningitis give negative results when the spinal fluid is used for complement fixation but a positive complement-fixation test of cerebrospinal fluid is a valid test for the diagnosis of coccidioidal meningitis. If, however, the spinal fluid is allowed to bind complement overnight in the cold (4° C), only 5 per cent of the meningitis cases tend to be negative (Pappagianis and Crane, 1977).

Alternate immunologic procedures have been studied for routine screening or supplementary test systems. Huppert and his associates (1968) have recommended a combination of the latex particle agglutination test (in place of the tube precipitin test) and the immunodiffusion test that correlates with the complement-fixation test) (IDCF) as a rapid and reliable primary test system. The IDCF test in conjunction with the microcomplement-fixation test is recommended by Kaufman and Clark (1974), since a positive immunodiffusion test and a low complement-fixation titer indicates active or recent disease.

## EPIDEMIOLOGY

### Geographic Distribution

Coccidioidomycosis is endemic only in limited areas of North, Central, and South America. In Southwestern United States, annual infection rates have been estimated at 35,000 to 100,000. These have been predominantly from Arizona and California, with fewer from Texas. New Mexico is of low endemicity and in Nevada and Utah skin test surveys give the only indication of the disease.

Mayorga and Espinoza (1970) reviewed the distribution of coccidioidomycosis in Mexico and Central America. Although most of the reported cases in Mexico are from hospitals in the states of Sonora, Neuvo Leon, and Coahuila, a more extensive occurrence of the disease is indicated by the skin test surveys of Gonzalez-Ochoa (1967). In Central America disease has been reported only from Guatemala, with eight, and Honduras, with two cases. The Guatemala endemic area, however, has a skin test reactor rate of 42.5 per cent.

At the time of Campins' report (1970) Argentina and Venezuela had 27 and 35 cases respectively, and Paraguay and Colombia 2 each. Recent soil isolations have been reported from Argentina (Borghi et al., 1977).

### Transmission to Humans

The incidence of infection is directly related to occupations that break up soil. Incidental infection in an endemic area depends on proximity to areas of soil disturbance, prevailing and seasonal wind conditions, and weather patterns affecting growth of the fungus in the soil.

About 60 per cent of humans infected will be asymptomatic and the remainder will have symptoms ranging from those of a mild respiratory condition to prolonged severe illness. A small number of the primary infections will disseminate to bones, joints, internal organs, or meninges. Disseminated disease occurs in approximately 0.5 to 1.0 per cent of white males, 5 to 10 per cent of black males, and in an even higher percentage of Filipinos.

### Ecology

In the United States and elsewhere the fungus has been most frequently isolated from the soil in semiarid areas from sea level to a few hundred feet elevation, which have mild winters and hot summers, with a yearly rainfall total of 5 to 20 inches occurring in one or two seasonal periods. There are exceptions to these usual geographic areas of disease endemicity. In Mexico, two small tropical areas are apparently endemic. One of these, comprising Colima and Michoacan border areas, has recorded two disseminated cases in children. The other is a limited area in the state of Guerrero where skin test reactivity indicates low endemicity (González Ochoa, 1967). In the United States, from California, soil isolations have been made from a mediterranean woodland region, from areas as high as 3200 feet and from sites where occasional snow and freezing temperatures occur during winter months (Swatek, 1975).

There is no association with the macroflora (Lacy and Swatek, 1974). The fungus has been isolated from the environs and even the burrows of rodents, but there is no evidence that such sites are regular ecologic niches. The chemical and physical conditions in the soil that favor the fungus are not known beyond the general association with alkaline, sandy soil types with a high content of salts.

## References

Anderson, K.L., Wheat, R.W. and Conant, N.F.: Fractionation and composition studies of skin test active components of sensitins from *Coccidioides immitis*. Appl Microbiol 22:294, 1971.

Beaman, L., Pappagianis, D., and Benjamini, E.: Significance of T cells in resistance to experimental murine coccidioidomycosis. Infect Immun 17:580, 1977.

Borghi, A.L., Rossi de Benetti, M.S., and Corallini de Bracalenti, B.J.: *Coccidioides immitis:* Su Aislamiento de Muestras de Suelos de las Provincias de San Luis Y Mendoza. Sabouraudia 15:51, 1977.

Campins, H.: Coccidioidomycosis in South America. A review of its epidemiology and geographic distribution. Mycopath et Mycologia Appl 40:1, 1970.

Collins, M.S., Pappagianis, D., and Yee, J.: Enzymatic solubilization of precipitin and complement fixing antigen from endospores, spherules and spherule fraction of *Coccidioides immitis*. In Ajello, L. (ed.): Coccidiomycosis. Miami, Symposia Specialists, 1977, p. 429.

Deresinksi, S.C., Levine, H.B., and Stevens, D.A.: Soluble antigens of mycelia and spherules in the in vitro detection of immunity to *Coccidioides immitis*. Infect Immun 10:700, 1974.

González Ochoa, A. Coccidioidomycosis in Mexico. In Ajello, L. (ed.): Proceedings of Second Coccidioidomycosis Symposium. Phoenix, The University of Arizona Press, 1967, p. 293.

Huppert, M.: Standardization of immunological reagents. Proceedings — International Symposium on Mycoses. Scientific Publication PAHO No. 205, 1970, p. 243.

Huppert, M., Chitjian, P.A., and Gross, A.J.: Comparison of methods for coccidioidomycosis complement fixation. Appl Microbiol 20:328, 1970.

Huppert, M., Krushow, I., Vukovich, K.R., Sun, S.H., Rice, E.H., and Kutner, L.J.: Comparison of coccidioidin and spherulin in complement fixation tests for coccidioidomycosis. J Clin Microbiol 6:33, 1977.

Huppert, M., Levine, H.B., Sun, S.H., and Peterson, E.T.: Resistance of vaccinated mice to typical and atypical strains of *Coccidioides immitis*. J Bact 94:924, 1967.

Huppert, M., Peterson, E.T., Sun, S.H., Chitjian, P.A., and Derrevere, W.J.: Evaluation of a latex particle agglutination test for coccidioidomycosis. The Am J Clin Path 49:96, 1968.

Huppert, M., Spratt, N.S., Vukovich, K.R., Sun, S.H., and Rice, E.H.: Antigenic analysis of coccidioidin and spherulin determined by two-dimensional immunoelectrophoresis. Infect Immun 20:541, 1978.

Huppert, M., Sun, S.H., and Vukovich, K.R.: Standardization of mycological reagents. Proceedings: International Conference on Standardization of Diagnostic Materials. U.S. Dept. HEW, CDC, Atlanta, 1974, p. 187.

Kaufman, L.: Serodiagnosis of fungal diseases. In Manual of Clinical Microbiology. American Society of Microbiology, 1976, p. 363.

Kaufman, L., and Clark, M.J.: Value of the concomitant use of complement fixation and immunodiffusion tests in the diagnosis of coccidioidomycosis. Appl Microbiol 28:641, 1974.

Kaufman, L., Hall, E.C., Clark, M.J., and McLaughlin, D.: Comparison of macrocomplement and microcomplement fixation techniques used in fungus serology. Appl Microbiol 20:579, 1970.

Kobayashi, G.S., and Pappagianis, D.: Preparation and standardization of antigens of *Histoplasma capsulatum* and *Coccidioides immitis*. Mycopath et Mycolog Appl 41:139, 1970.

Kong, Y.M., Levine, H.B., and Smith, C.E.: Immunogenic properties of undisrupted and disrupted spherules of *Coccidioides immitis* in mice. Sabouraudia 2:131, 1963.

Kwon-Chung, K.J.: *Coccidioides immitis*: Cytological study on the formation of the arthrospores. Canad J Genet Cytol 11:43, 1969.

Lacy, G.H., and Swatek, F.E.: Soil ecology of *Coccidioides immitis* at Amerindian middens in California. Appl Microbiol 27:379, 1974.

Levine, H.B., Cobb, J.M., and Scalarone, G.M.: Spherule coccidioidin in delayed dermal sensitivity reaction of experimental animals. Sabouraudia 7:20, 1969.

Levine, H.B., Cobb, J.M., and Smith, C.E.: Immunity to coccidioidomycosis induced in mice by purified spherule, arthrospore and mycelial vaccines. Trans N Y Acad Sci 22:436, 1960.

Levine, H.B., González-Ochoa, A., and Ten Eyck, D.: Dermal sensitivity to *Coccidioides immitis*. Am Rev Resp Dis 107:379, 1973.

Levine, H.B., Kong, Y.M., and Smith, C.E.: Immunization of mice to *Coccidioides immitis*: dose regimen and spherulation stage of killed spherule vaccines. The J Immun 94:132, 1965.

Levine, H.B., Restrepo, M.A., Ten Eyck, D.R., and Stevens, D.A.: Spherulin and coccidioidin: cross reactions in dermal sensitivity to histoplasmin and paracoccidioidin. Am J Epidem 101:512, 1975.

Mayorga, R.P., and Espinoza, H.: Coccidioidomycosis in Mexico and Central America. Mycopath et Mycologia Appl 40:13, 1970.

Pan American Health Organization. Manual of standardized serodiagnostic procedures for systemic mycoses. Part II. Complement fixation tests. Washington, D.C., Pan American Health Organization, 1974.

Pappagianis, D., and Crane, R.: Survival in coccidioidal meningitis since introduction of amphotericin B. In Ajello, L. (ed.) Coccidioidomycosis. Miami, Symposia Specialists, 1977, p. 223.

Pappagianis, D., Smith, C.E., Kobayashi, G.S., and Saito, M.T.: Studies of antigens from young mycelia of *Coccidioides immitis*. J Infect Dis 108:35, 1961a.

Pappagianis, D., Putman, E.W., and Kobayashi, G.S.: Polysaccharide of *Coccidioides immitis*. J Bact 82:714, 1961b.

Reep, B.R., and Kaplan, W.: The use of N-acetyl-L-cysteine and dithiothreitol to process sputa for mycological and fluorescent antibody examinations. Health Lab Sci 9:118, 1972.

Rifkind, D., Frey, J.A., Davis, J.R., and Petersen, E.A.: Delayed hypersensitivity to fungal antigens in mice. I. Use of the intradermal skin and foot pad swelling tests as assays of active and passive sensitization. J Infect Dis 133:50, 1976.

Smith, C.E., Pappagianis, D., and Saito, M.: The public health significance of coccidioidomycosis. U.S. Public Health Service Publication No. 575, 1957, p. 3.

Smith, C.E., Saito, M.T., Beard, R.R., Kepp, R.M., Clark, R.W., and Eddie, B.V.: Serological tests in the diagnosis and prognosis of coccidioidomycosis. The Amer J Hyg 52:1, 1950.

Smith, C.E., Saito, M.T., and Simons, S.A.: Pattern of 39,500 serologic tests in coccidioidomycosis. JAMA 160:546, 1956.

Standard, P.G., and Kaufman, L.: Immunological procedure for the rapid and specific identification of *Coccidioides immitis* cultures. J Clin Microbial 5:149, 1977.

Stevens, D.A., Levine, H.B., and Ten Eyck, D.R.: Dermal sensitivity to different doses of spherulin and coccidioidin. Chest 65:530, 1974.

Sun, S.H., and Huppert, M.: A cytological study of morphogenesis in *Coccidioides immitis*. Sabouraudia 14:185, 1976.

Sun, S.H., Huppert, M., and Vukovich, K.R.: Rapid in vitro conversion and identification of *Coccidioides immitis*. J Clin Microbiol 3:186, 1976.

Swatek, F.E.: The epidemiology of coccidioidomycosis. In Al-Doory (ed.): The Epidemiology of Human Mycotic Diseases. Springfield, Charles C Thomas Publishers, 1975, p. 74.

United States Public Health Service. Standardized diagnostic complement fixation method and adaption to micro test. U.S. Public Health Service Publication No. 1228, 1965.

Wheat, R.W., Tritschler, C., Conant, N.F., and Lowe, E.P.: Comparison of *Coccidioides immitis* arthrospore, mycelium and spherule cell walls, and influence of growth medium on mycelial cell wall composition. Infect Immun 17:91, 1977.

# BLASTOMYCES AND PARACOCCIDIOIDES **73**

## Smith Shadomy, Ph.D., and Dennis M. Dixon, Ph.D.

### *MORPHOLOGY*

*Blastomyces (Ajellomyces) dermatitidis* and *Paracoccidioides brasiliensis* are dimorphic fungi that grow in tissue as budding yeasts and in culture at room temperature as molds. The two fungi are morphologically similar and share antigens. Despite its name, *P. brasiliensis* is now considered to be in the genus *Blastomyces*.

Yeast cells of *B. dermatitidis* range from 8 to 15μ in size. In wet mounts or when stained with lactophenol cotton blue, the cell wall appears as a highly refractile structure (Fig. 1). The thick nature of the cell wall has led various authors to describe the fungus as doubly rounded or doubly contoured as if delimited by two cell walls. Yeast

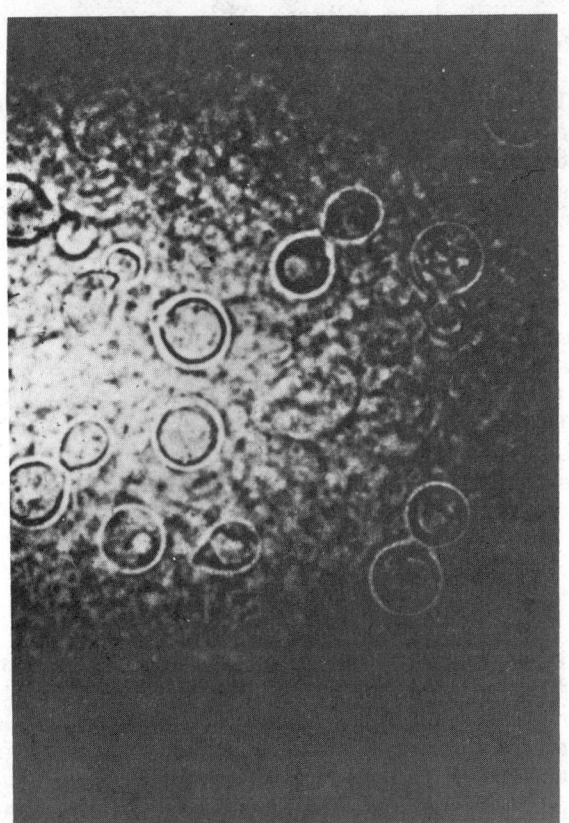

**FIGURE 1.** *Yeast cells of* Blastomyces dermatitidis *in pus. Note thick cell wall and single buds. Compare with multiple buds of* Paracoccidioides brasiliensis *in Figure 2. (× 1200)*

phase cells of *B. dermatitidis* produce single buds that are characterized by a wide pore, approximately one-half the width of the parent cell, between the parent cell and bud. The wall of the bud is initially thinner than that of the parent cell. These features distinguish *B. dermatitidis* from the other human fungal pathogens.

Yeast cells of *P. brasiliensis* are from 2 to 30μ in diameter and have thinner cell walls than *B. dermatitidis*. Additionally, *P. brasiliensis* is differentiated by the production of multiple buds from a single cell. This gives rise to the familiar "Mickey Mouse hat" appearance when three such buds are involved, or the "pilot's wheel" when multiple buds are produced around the circumference of the parent cell (Fig. 2). Also, pores between the parent cell and buds are narrower than those with *B. dermatitidis*.

In culture, *B. dermatitidis* grows as a whitish buff-colored mold with a yellow-brown underside. Colonies may be floccose or glabrous, furrowed or smooth. Microscopically, one sees fine, septate hyphae that have characteristic pyriform conidia measuring 2 to 10μ. The conidia are borne on short lateral or terminal branches (conidiophores) and typically have a truncated base that can be more clearly seen after their separation from the parent conidiophore. Such conidia are commonly termed aleurioconidia or aleuriospores and may be confused with the smooth-walled conidia of *Histoplasma capsulatum* and certain saprophytic *Chrysosporium* species. *B. dermatitidis* and *H. capsulatum* can be differentiated on the basis of yeast phase morphology. *Chrysosporium* species do not grow as a yeast in vitro.

*P. brasiliensis* is essentially indistinguishable from *B. dermatitidis* in the mycelial phase and often does not produce conidia. When present, the conidia are aleurioconidia measuring 2 to 4μ in diameter. Arthroconidia, produced by disarticulation of the vegetative hyphae, and intercolony chlamydospores, or thick-walled swollen cells, have been reported. For both fungi, media such as potato dextrose agar or yeast extract agar usually enhance the production of conidia while limiting the growth of vegetative hyphae.

On Sabouraud's agar at room temperature, both *B. dermatitidis* and *P. brasiliensis* appear as

**665**

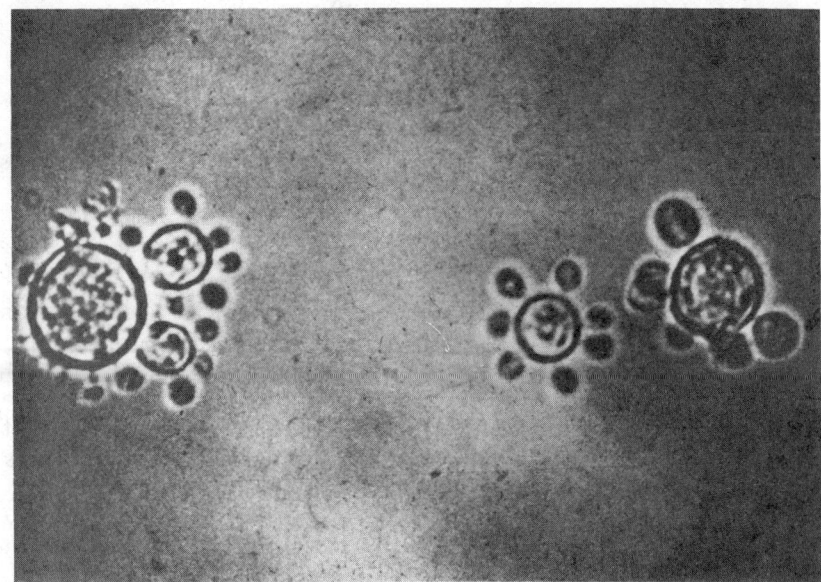

**FIGURE 2.** *Yeast cells of* Paracocci-dioides brasiliensis. *Note thinner cell wall than those of* B. dermatitidis *in Figure 1, and multiple buds in a single cell (pilot's wheel).* (×1500)

slow-growing molds and are indistinguishable from each other. Colonies are generally apparent after one week of incubation, but maximum growth may not be attained for three or more weeks. Colonies typically are white-buff to brown with a yellow-brown reverse and may be floccose to glabrous, furrowed or smooth. *B. dermatitidis* and *P. brasiliensis* occasionally produce tufts of aerial hyphae (coremia) that are most distinctive in young cultures; otherwise, the colonies are similar in appearance to *H. capsulatum*. Microscopically, *B. dermatitidis* consists of fine, septate hyphae and characteristic pyriform conidia measuring from 2 to 10$\mu$.

On brain-heart infusion blood agar at 37° C, both *B. dermatitidis* and *P. brasiliensis* grow as cream-colored, wrinkled, heaped colonies. Growth rates are similar to those of mycelial phase cultures, but the colonial growth is more restricted than the mycelial growth that may cover the agar surface.

*B. dermatitidis* has a sexual stage, *Ajellomyces dermatitidis*. The sexes are separate (heterothallism), and opposite mating types (+ and −) are required to obtain fertile cultures of *A. dermatitidis*. When the two mating types are cultured at 25° C on appropriate media, specialized rounded structures (cleistothecia) are produced. Within these are sac-like structures, or asci, each of which contains eight ascospores. The fungus is therefore classified as an *Ascomycete*. The ascospores are somewhat smaller than the asexual conidia and are infectious. A sexual stage has not been described for *P. brasiliensis*.

## ANTIGENIC STRUCTURE

Blastomycin and paracoccidioidin are concentrates that have been prepared from filtrates of mycelial phase cultures. They are used as the antigens for serodiagnosis of infection with these fungi as well as antigens for in vivo skin tests. These materials are heterogenous mixtures of antigens that lack both sensitivity and specificity, and, to compound the problem, they are poorly standardized. Work is under way to isolate antigens that will be both specific and sensitive for serodiagnosis (Cox and Larsh, 1974a, b). Cell-wall proteins are believed to be the antigens responsible for skin-test reactions. An alkaline-stable, water-soluble extract of yeast cell walls appears to contain a skin-test antigen that is both sensitive and specific (Lancaster and Sprouse, 1976). Restrepo and others have isolated specific antigens from yeast cells that can be used for serodiagnosis of paracoccidioidomycosis (Restrepo, 1966; Kaufman, 1972).

## IMMUNITY

Cell-mediated immunity is a more significant factor than humoral immunity in most of the mycoses, and blastomycosis and paracoccidioidomycosis are no exceptions. Although circulating antibodies can generally be detected at some point in the course of the diseases, they do not appear to be protective. In contrast, cell-mediated immune responses show a positive correlation with the host's ability to overcome the infections. Poor clinical progress is generally correlated with impairment in some aspect of cell-mediated immunity (Mok and Greer, 1977; Musatti et al., 1976). Whether there is a causal relationship between lymphocyte responses and immunity remains to be determined; however, it has been suggested that paracoccidioidomycosis leads to impairments in cell-mediated immunity. Various parameters of cell-mediated immunity need be examined closely in order to assess their roles in determining the clinical manifestations and outcome in these and other systemic fungal infections.

## LABORATORY DIAGNOSIS

*B. dermatitidis* and *P. brasiliensis* bear striking mycologic similarities. Both are dimorphic, existing as molds at room temperature and as yeasts in infected tissues and in vitro at 37° C on enriched media. While *B. dermatitidis* and *P. brasiliensis* are virtually indistinguishable in the mycelial phase, both have certain characteristic morphologic differences in the yeast phase.

While unequivocal diagnosis of any mycosis requires isolation of the causative fungus in vitro, a presumptive diagnosis can be made by direct microscopic observation of the fungus in clinical materials. Samples of cerebrospinal fluid and urine are first sedimented by centrifugation and the sediment taken for direct examination and culture. Tissue must be homogenized using a small amount of physiologic saline and a glass tissue grinder or mortar and pestle. The tissue homogenate is then subject to both culture and direct microscopic examination. Viscous materials are digested by adding a drop of 10 per cent KOH to the material on a microscope slide and covering it with a coverslip while still wet.

The morphologies of *B. dermatitidis* and *P. brasiliensis* in infected tissues are the same as those of the yeast phases when grown in vitro. Histopathologic staining of infected tissue can therefore be a useful adjunct to laboratory diagnosis. Sections of involved tissue should be stained with methenamine silver, periodic-acid Schiff (PAS), and hematoxylin and eosin (H & E). Yeasts that were viable at the time of fixation are discernible with H & E stain, but they are most easily located with methenamine silver, which stains them black. With the Gomeri stain, they appear slightly enlarged due to the impregnation effect of the silver. More details of cell morphology can be resolved with PAS and H & E.

The presence of thick-walled cells producing single buds with a broad base of attachment represents presumptive histopathologic evidence of infection with *B. dermatitidis*. There may be superficial resemblance to *Histoplasma duboisii* (the etiologic agent of African histoplasmosis), but this latter fungus buds with narrow pores. Also, *H. duboisii* is uninucleate, whereas *B. dermatitidis* is typically multinucleate. With PAS and H & E stain, the cytoplasm of *B. dermatitidis* shrinks away from the cell wall, leaving a clear space. This appearance should not be confused with the capsule of *Cryptococcus neoformans*, which stains red with both PAS and Mayer's mucicarmine stains and which produces buds through narrow pores. (*B. dermatitidis* stains poorly at best with mucicarmine.) Single cells of *B. dermatitidis* have been mistaken for spherules of *Coccidioides immitis*. In some cases, it may be difficult to distinguish small intracellular yeast cells of *B. dermatitidis* from *H. capsulatum*. The former may have multiple nuclei that are visible with H & E stain, while the latter has only a single nucleus per yeast cell. In some cases, it may not be possible to exclude a dual infection by histologic criteria alone.

The morphology of *P. brasiliensis* in tissues is like that of the yeasts grown in vitro. Small forms of *P. brasiliensis* with single buds can be differentiated from *B. dermatitidis* on the basis of pore size. Single yeast cells of *P. brasiliensis* can be differentiated from *C. neoformans* and *C. immitis* by using the same criteria that are used for *B. dermatitidis*.

Materials for culture are prepared as described above for direct observation and are streaked in duplicate on both Sabouraud's agar and brain-heart infusion blood agar. Agar media may be used that contain both chloramphenicol, to inhibit bacterial contaminants, and cycloheximide (Actidione), to inhibit saprophytic fungal contaminants. However, such media should not be the sole media employed because certain opportunistic fungal pathogens as well as *Cryptococcus neoformans* are also inhibited by cycloheximide. One set of plates should be incubated at room temperature, or 30° C if possible, and one set at 37° C. Plates should be kept for four weeks before discarding, but growth should be observable after one week of incubation.

*B. dermatitidis* and *P. brasiliensis* can be grown in vitro on a variety of media. The nutritional requirements of both fungi are quite similar, and no special growth factors or vitamins are required. Both fungi are slow growing, with mean generation times of 12 hours or more, and both fungi grow as molds at room temperature as well as at 30° C. Temperature is the primary stimulus

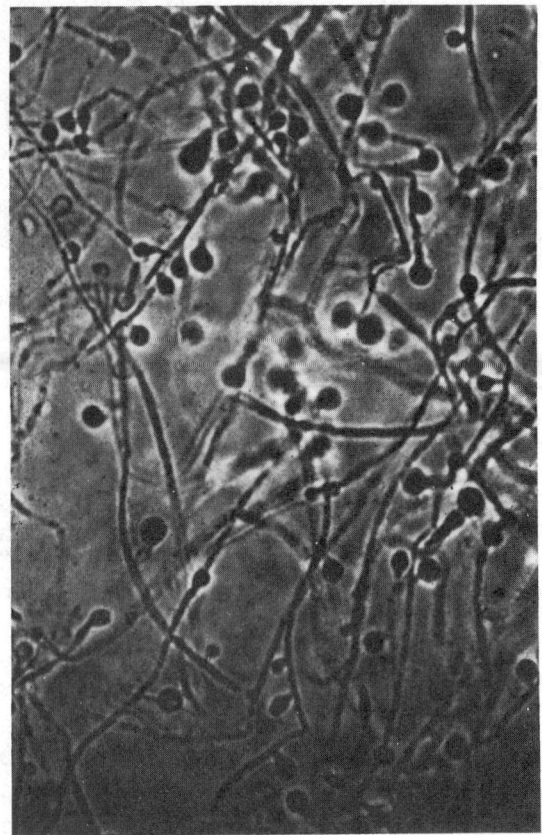

**FIGURE 3.** *Filamentous growth of* Blastomyces dermatitidis *showing spherical or pyriform spores. Note short pedicles that attach spores to hyphae.*

for dimorphism, and culturing on an enriched medium such as brain-heart infusion blood agar with incubation at 35° or 37° C will result in conversion of the fungi to their parasitic yeast phases. Colonies of yeast cells should appear within five days; if they do not, subsequent transfers may be necessary.

The preparations are stained with lactophenol cotton blue and examined microscopically for the charactistic aleurioconidia. For confirmation, yeast phase conversion should be demonstrated. Production of the characteristic budding yeasts differentiate *B. dermatitidis* from *P. brasiliensis* and from the saprophytic *Chrysoporium* species. Cottonseed agar may be more efficient for conversion of *B. dermatitidis* mold to its yeast phase than is brain-heart infusion blood agar. Not all isolates convert to the yeast phase. Inoculation of mice intraperitoneally with mycelia of *B. dermatitidis* produces (after four weeks) local infection that will contain yeasts.

## *EPIDEMIOLOGY*

Recent studies of the epidemiology of blastomycosis have shown that the disease is not limited to North America as believed earlier. Rather, autochthonous infections have been reported in Europe and throughout Africa. The majority of cases, however, do come directly or indirectly from North America, where the disease is endemic to several geographic regions, including the Mississippi, Ohio, and Missouri River basins, as well as the Great Lakes region on the western shore of Lake Michigan.

Paracoccidioidomycosis is limited to Central and South America. In the case of infections reported from other countries, travel to known endemic areas usually can be documented. Highly endemic regions include both humid tropical forests and humid or very humid subtropical forest zones. Most cases have been reported from the state of São Paulo, Brazil.

Both blastomycosis and paracoccidiodomycosis are reported more commonly from rural than from urban areas. With both infections, similar occupational patterns are seen among the patients who are often laborers, farmers, and tree cutters. A unique epidemic of blastomycosis occurred in Bigfork, Minnesota, where members of four families were infected during the clearing of forest undergrowth and construction of a cabin (Tosh et al., 1974).

Neither blastomycosis nor paracoccidioidomycosis is naturally transmissible from man to man or from animal to man. The infections are acquired from some as yet poorly defined sources in nature, probably by inhalation of infectious conidia. The natural habitats of these fungi are assumed to be soil; however, only a few reports of isolation of these organisms from soil have been recorded. Isolation studies employing bird and bat manure have ruled out these materials as natural sources.

Blastomycosis and paracoccidioidomycosis occur in all age groups, but the preponderance of cases occurs in the 20- to 50-year-old age group. Males are more commonly affected than females in ratios of approximately 9 to 1. This is probably a reflection of hormonal as well as sociologic and occupational differences. There is no clear-cut predilection with respect to race as is seen in coccidioidomycosis.

## REFERENCES

Cox, R. A., and Larsh, H. W.: Isolation of skin test-active preparations from yeast-phase cells of *Blastomyces dermatitidis*. Infect Immun 10:42, 1974a.

Cox, R. A., and Larsh, H. W.: Yeast and mycelial-phase antigens of *Blastomyces dermatitidis*: Comparison using disc gel electrophoresis. Infect Immun 10:48, 1974b.

Kaufman, L.: Evaluation of serological tests for paracoccidioidomycosis: Preliminary report. In Pan American Health Organization: Paracoccidioidomycosis. Proceedings of the First Pan American Symposium. Geneva, World Health Organization, 1972, pp. 221–223.

Lancaster, M. V., and Sprouse, R. F.: Isolation of a purified skin test antigen from *Blastomyces dermatitidis* yeast-phase cell wall. Infect Immun 14:623, 1976.
Mok, P. W. Y., and Greer, D. L.: Cell-mediated immune responses in patients with paracoccidioidomycosis. Clin Exp Immunol 28:89, 1977.
Musatti, C. C., Rezkallah, M. T., Mendes, E., and Mendes, N. F.: *In vivo* and *in vitro* evaluation of cell-mediated immunity in patients with paracoccidioidomycosis. Cell Immunol 24:365, 1976.
Restrepo, A.: La prueba de immunodiffusion en el diagnostico de la paracoccidioidomicosis. Sabouraudia 4:223, 1966.
Tosh, F. E., Hammerman, K. J., Weeks, R. J., and Sarosi, G. A.: A common source epidemic of North American blastomycosis. Am Rev Resp Dis 109:525, 1974.

# THE ASPERGILLI 74

## Abraham I. Braude, M.D., Ph.D.

The aspergilli are a group of versatile fungi belonging to the class Hyphomycetes and the family Moniliaceae. As noted in Chapter 14, *Aspergillus fumigatus* and *Aspergillus flavus* are unique in being the only nonzygomycete fungi that grow deep in tissue in mycelial form rather than in yeast form.

The name for this group of fungi is taken from the word aspergillum, which means a brush used for sprinkling holy water. This brush has a remarkable resemblance to the microscopic appearance of the fungus *Aspergillus niger* (Fig. 1).

### MORPHOLOGY

In order to appreciate the structure of the brushlike portion of the aspergilli, it is necessary to be familiar with *four* components: the co-nidiophore, the vesicle, the sterigmata, and the spores. These are identified in Figure 2, where it can be seen that the handle of the brush consists of the unbranched conidiophore, which has a swollen end, the vesicle. A number of little stalks, shaped like a bottle, radiate from the vesicle and are arranged in one or two rows (Fig. 2A or 2B). Chains of spores arise from the tips of these stalks, or sterigmata, in the outer row.

The spores (or conidia) develop from the tips of the fertile sterigmata. The first stage in spore formation is a constriction of an elongated portion of the sterigma; the second stage is the develop-

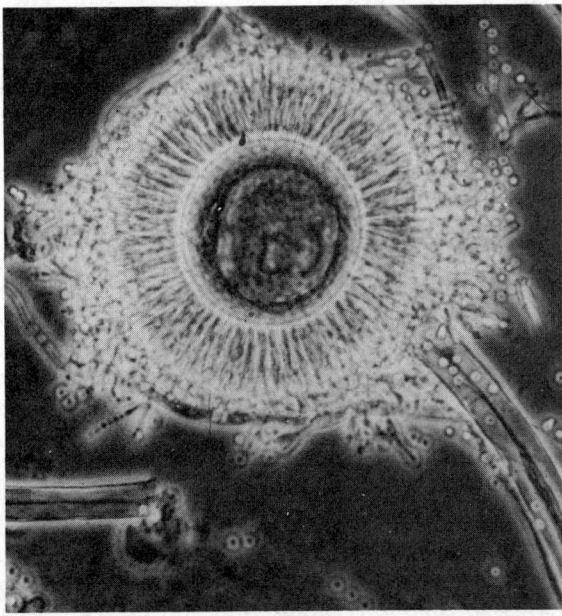

**FIGURE 1.** *Aspergillus niger bears a remarkable resemblance to the aspergillum, a brush used for sprinkling holy water.*

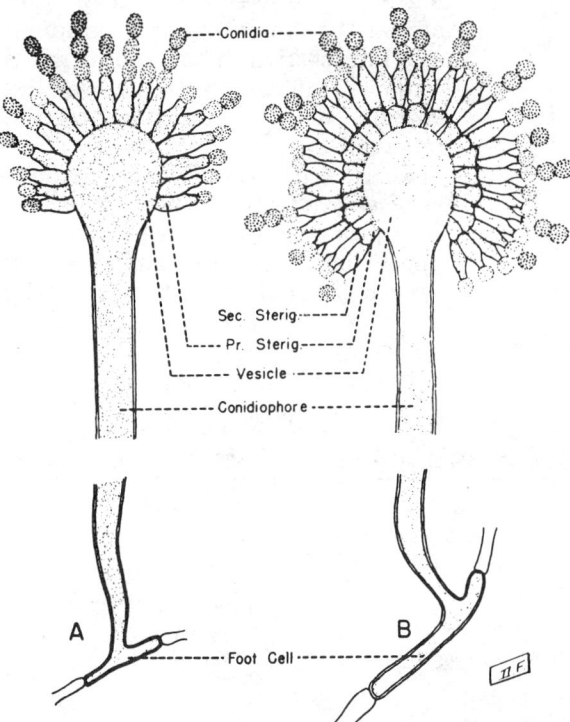

**FIGURE 2.** *Diagram of two different morphologic types of aspergilli showing one row of sterigmata (uniseriate) in A and two rows (biseriate) in B. (From Roper, K. B., and Fennel, D. I.: The Genus Aspergillus. Baltimore, The Williams & Wilkins Company, 1965.)*

ment of a septum that separates the spore from the sterigma. Chains of attached spores evolve as the cutting process continues at the tip of the sterigma. The compact mass of spores around the vesicle is called a conidial head and corresponds to the portion of a brush in which the bristles are set.

At its opposite end, the conidiophore arises from a foot cell, an enlarged thick-walled cell of the segmented mycelium. The conidiophore is borne as a stalk perpendicular to the long axis of the foot cell (Fig. 2).

The morphologic classification of all species of the genus *Aspergillus* is enormously complex and is beyond the scope of this chapter. Those members of medical importance, however, are relatively few and can generally be recognized by their color, the shape of their vesicle, and the arrangement of their sterigmata and spores. The groups of *Aspergillus* species that cause human disease are listed in Table 1 and can be arranged according to the following classification.

I. Green colonies

   A. Sterigmata arranged in single rows (uniseriate)

      1. *Conidial heads are split* (clavate) into two or more divergent columns of compact chains of spores; they have swollen ends. Vesicles are also split and appear as an elongated, gradually swelling portion of the end of the conidiophore. They are fertile over their entire surface and are blue-green (*A. clavatus*).

      2. *Conidial heads are compact, not split*; vesicles are fertile in their upper half so that sterigmata arise from the upper half only. Sterigmata are arranged parallel to each other and to the long axis of the conidiophore, pointing upward; they are green to dark green in color (*A. fumigatus* Fig. 3).

      3. *Conidial heads are not split*; interspersed among the green conidial heads are abundant bright yellow cleistothecia (round bodies containing multiple asci, which are sacs of sexual spores). Cleistothecia are about equal in size to conidial heads (*A. glaucus*).

   B. Sterigmata are arranged in two rows (biseriate): purple cleistothecia and orange-red ascospores (*A. nidulans*).

II. Black colonies. Sterigmata are in either one row or two rows, depending on the species, and arise from the entire surface of the globular vesicle (*A. niger*, Fig. 1).

III. Yellow colonies. A mixture of uniseriate or biseriate sterigmata occur in the same culture or even on the same vesicle; vesicles are globular and are sometimes split. They are fertile over most of their surface (*A. flavus*).

IV. Orange-brown or cinnamon colonies. There are two rows of sterigmata; the vesicles are hemispherical (*A. terreus*).

## ANTIGENIC COMPOSITION

Most immunologic reactions in *Aspergillus* infections have been studied with crude filtrates of *Aspergillus* cultures grown for several weeks at room temperature in Sabouraud broth. These contain countless unidentified antigens that can give up to 20 precipitin lines when examined by immunodiffusion against hyperimmune rabbit serum. Both protein and carbohydrate antigens have been identified in these *Aspergillus* culture filtrates, and some of the proteins have been characterized as enzymes (oxoreductases, hydrolases, proteases). One of the polysaccharides reacts with C-reactive protein. C-reactive protein appears during the acute phase of various infections and other inflammatory processes and reacts with the somatic polysaccharide (C substance) of the pneumococcus. Its reaction with an antigen from *Aspergillus* suggests that this fungal polysaccharide may have properties that are similar to the pneumococcal C polysaccharide. Since the reaction with C-reactive protein clouds the specificity of immunodiffusion reactions with *Aspergillus* filtrates, it is necessary to eliminate the C-reative substance by incorporating sodium citrate in the gel (Longbottom and Pepys, 1964).

The antigens in different species of *Aspergillus* cross-react in serologic tests with each other and

**TABLE 1.** Diseases Caused by Different Species of Aspergilli

| TYPE OF ASPERGILLOSIS | SPECIES OF ASPERGILLUS |
| --- | --- |
| Invasive pulmonary | *fumigatus* |
| Allergic bronchopulmonary | *fumigatus* |
| | *flavus* |
| | *niger* |
| | *terreus* |
| | *clavatus* |
| Pulmonary aspergilloma | *fumigatus* |
| | *niger* |
| Otomycosis | *niger* |
| Sinusitis | *flavus* |
| Disseminated | *fumigatus* |
| | *flavus* |
| Mycetoma | *glaucus* |
| | *nidulans* |

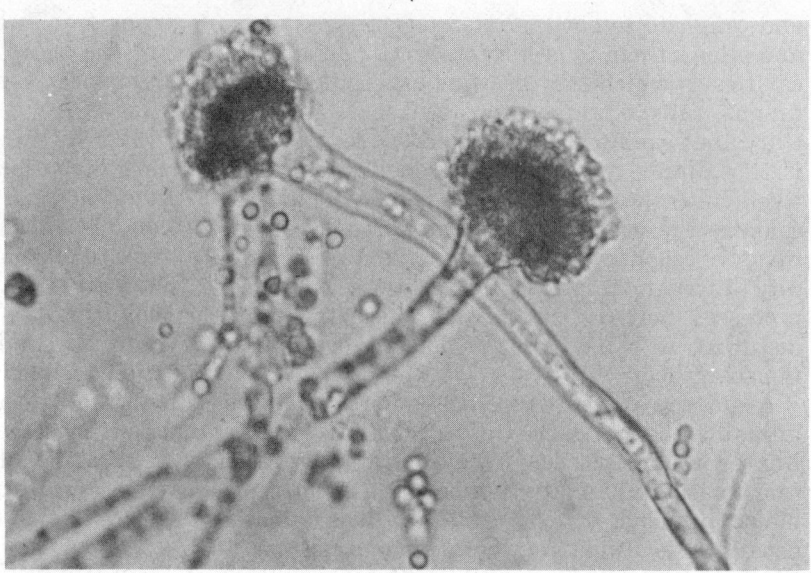

**FIGURE 3.** *Wet mount of* Aspergillus fumigatus *cultured from ethmoid sinus (× 400). Note following diagnostic features typical of A. fumigatus: (1) compact (unsplit) conidial head; (2) single row of sterigmata; (3) sterigmata arise from upper half only; (4) sterigmata are arranged parallel to each other and to the long axis of the conidiophore.*

with antigens of other fungi. These cross-reactions occur mainly between polysaccharide antigens and may occur not only with dermatophytes and *Cladosporium* but also with nematodes, trematodes, cestodes, and vegetable dusts. All of these cause immediate reactions to skin tests in patients with *Aspergillus* hypersensitivity and precipitin reactions with sera from some patients with pulmonary aspergilloma (Pepys, 1969). Galactomannans are prominent polysaccharide antigens in aspergilli as in other fungi, and they may be partly responsible for the cross reactions observed between different species of *Aspergillus* and between aspergilli and other fungi.

## IMMUNITY

At least two types of antibody are important in the pathogenesis of aspergillosis. IgE antibody is responsible for bronchospasm and asthma, whereas IgG seems to cause Arthus-type reactions in the walls of bronchi that progress to bronchiectasis. If the respiratory tract becomes colonized with aspergilli, it releases the multiple antigens described in the previous section, and these sensitize certain patients with inherited hypersensitivity to aspergilli. These atopic patients respond by producing IgE antibody to *Aspergillus* antigens and immediate hypersensitivity reactions in the respiratory tree when they are re-exposed to inhaled *Aspergillus* spores. They also develop high serum levels of IgG antibody, which precipitates *Aspergillus* antigens around the vessels in the alveoli and bronchial walls. The ensuing Arthus inflammatory reaction (Chapter 83) is thought to cause transient pneu-

monitis and a progressive injury to the bronchial wall that culminates in the characteristic bronchiectasis of allergic bronchopulmonary aspergillosis (Golbert and Patterson, 1970).

There is no evidence that antibody can protect against aspergillosis; on the contrary, passive transfer of antibody can reproduce allergic bronchopulmonary aspergillosis (Golbert and Patterson, 1970). There are also no concrete data to indicate that cellular immunity is involved in resistance to *Aspergillus*. From observations of patients and experimental animals, it would appear that neutropenia, steroid administration, and loss of mechanical antimicrobial clearance mechanisms are factors in lowering resistance to aspergillosis. In patients who become neutropenic from leukemia or drugs, aspergilli invade pulmonary vessels and spread unopposed to the brain, kidney, liver, thyroid, and other organs (Young et al., 1970).

Some patients who develop aspergillosis do so while receiving adrenal steroids, but their importance in causing loss of immunity is obscured because many other debilitating factors are associated with steroid use in these cases. In mice, however, the ability of steroids to lower resistance to *Aspergillus* is dramatic; one injection of cortisone allows fatal aspergillosis to develop in animals that are otherwise completely resistant to aspergilli (Sidransky and Friedman, 1959). The importance of mechanical clearing processes, which prevent colonization of the respiratory or alimentary tract by pathogenic organisms, is illustrated by the types of aspergillosis that develop in the lung and esophagus when these mechanisms are lost. Structural damage to the lung and bronchopulmonary tree by any form of bronchiectasis or lung cavity interferes with the ability of cilia and cough to remove inhaled aspergillus spores and allows them to proliferate in the defenseless cavities in which they grow as aspergillomas (or fungus balls). Similarly, when esophageal motility and swallowing is disturbed by severe debilitating illness, aspergilli are propelled less effectively into the acid gastric juice. Instead, they colonize the esophagus and can produce severe invasive esophagitis. Thus, loss of natural immunity through impaired protective mechanical processes may be among the most important disturbances responsible for defective resistance to aspergillosis.

Acquired resistance after infection with aspergillus has been observed experimentally only in limited studies in mice. Mice are normally resistant to aspergillus infection but become susceptible to pulmonary, renal, and fatal disseminated aspergillosis after treatment with cortisone. If they are injected first with viable aspergillosis but not cortisone, they are no longer susceptible to progressive aspergillosis when rechallenged with aspergilli plus cortisone. The mechanism or specificity of this immunity is unknown; neither antibodies nor cellular immunity has been examined carefully enough to indicate its relative contribution to this important phenomenon. Although patients with disseminated aspergillosis have no antibodies to *A. fumigatus* antigens, a loss of humoral immunity cannot be blamed for susceptibility to this infection because the patients are also subject to suppression of cellular immunity by the chemotherapy given for their hematologic malignancies (Young and Bennett, 1971).

## *LABORATORY DIAGNOSIS*

### Mycologic Examination

In spite of the fact that aspergilli are frequently cultured as contaminants in specimens from patients, they may be difficult to recover from patients with certain forms of invasive aspergillosis. Thus, it is unusual to recover aspergilli from the sputum of patients with pulmonary aspergilloma or invasive *Aspergillus* pneumonias, and the fungus is rarely found in blood cultures of patients with disseminated aspergillosis. The organism can be isolated most readily in invasive disease of the lung, brain, sinuses, orbit, or skin when the infected tissue is obtained by biopsy (Fig. 4). In such tissues, the mycelial elements are usually found easily in histologic sections stained with hematoxylin and eosin or the methenamine-silver method; they appear in 24 to 48 hours in culture after aerobic incubation at 35° C on any standard medium. The only nonbiopsied speci-

mens from which aspergilli are easily cultured are the sputa of patients with allergic bronchopulmonary aspergillosis, the pleural fluids in *Aspergillus* empyema, the exudates of burns infected with aspergilli, and the discharges from ears of patients with *A. niger* infection of the external auditory canal. Characteristic hyphae can also be seen in these specimens but may require special treatment before microscopic examination. Such treatment usually consists of mounting the material in 20 per cent potassium hydroxide under a coverslip and incubating at 37 or 56° C until there is dissolution of the organic material in the bronchial plug, ear wax, or burn crust. In some materials, the conidial head may be recognizable and will allow identification of *A. fumigatus*. For the most part, however, exact identification depends on cultural isolation.

### Serologic Tests

Serologic tests for antibodies to aspergilli are valuable in certain forms of aspergillosis that cannot easily be identified by culture. Antibody determinations are also useful in determining whether or not the isolation of the fungus from specimens represents contamination or infection with aspergilli. Although antibodies against *Aspergillus* can be found by immunodiffusion, complement fixation, immunoelectrophoresis, and indirect immunofluorescence, the most widely used test is immunodiffusion (ID) because of its simplicity, sensitivity, and relative reliability. The ID test is most useful for the diagnosis of fungus ball and allergic bronchopulmonary aspergillosis. Patients with fungus balls due to one of the aspergilli have positive reactions. The diagnosis of fungus ball is suspected by characteristic lesions in chest radiographs in patients with underlying cavitary lung disease due to healed tuberculosis, sarcoidosis, bronchiectasis, or bronchogenic carcinoma, and an ID test should be done regardless of a negative sputum culture for aspergilli. Standardized antigen separations should be made from *A. fumigatus, A. niger*, and *A. flavus*. Each of these three species is grown separately in Sabouraud broth cultures at 31° C for five weeks. Reproducible test antigens can be obtained by precipitating them out of culture with acetone, concentrating them eightfold and adjusting the carbohydrate content to 1000 $\mu$g/ml by the anthrone test (Coleman and Kaufman, 1972). If simultaneous ID tests are done in separate plates with each of the three antigens, precipitins will be found in over 90 per cent of patients with fungus balls and 70 per cent of those with allergic bronchopulmonary aspergillosis. The test is controlled with positive reference sera, and the diagnostic precipitin lines are recog-

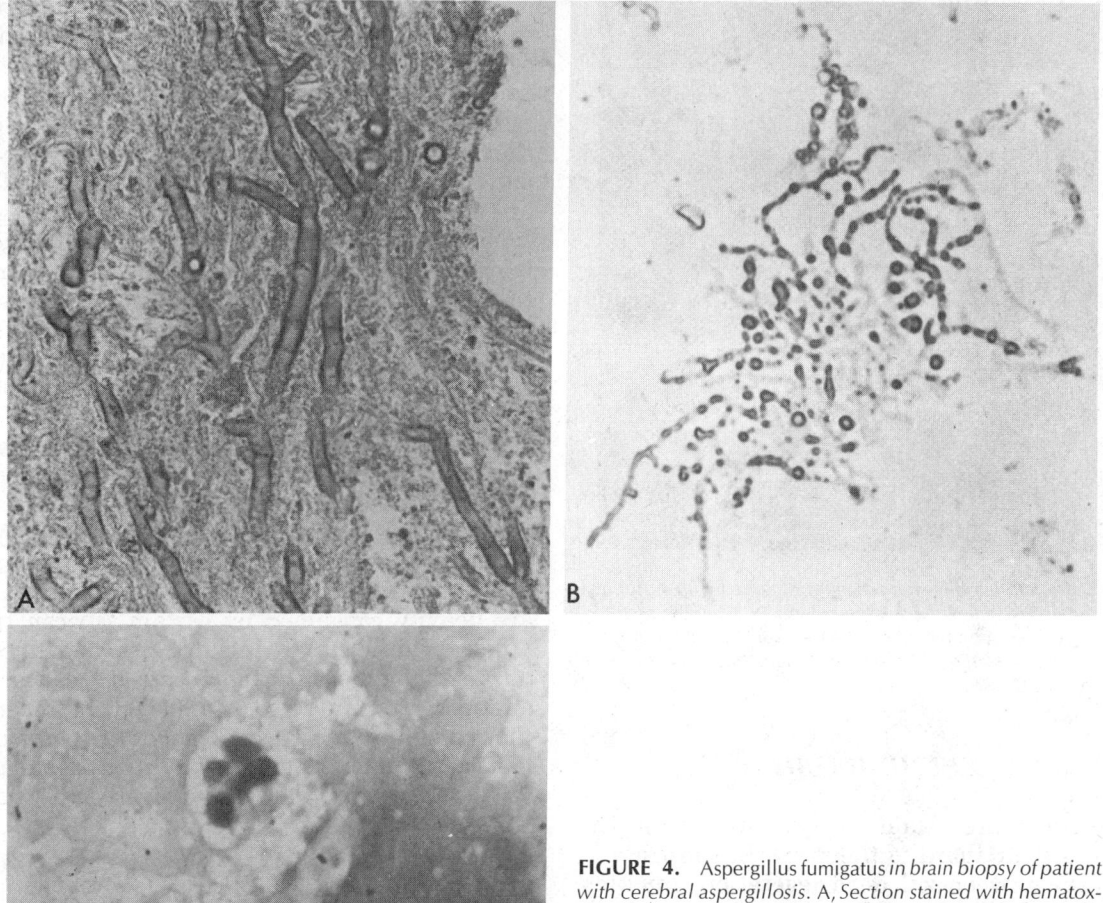

**FIGURE 4.** *Aspergillus fumigatus in brain biopsy of patient with cerebral aspergillosis. A, Section stained with hematoxylin and eosin (×400). Note segmented hyphae, acute angle of branches, and absence of conidial head. (B), Wet mount showing hyphae after cerebral tissue has been digested with KOH. (C), Gram stain of smeared brain tissue. Note that hyphae do not take the Gram stain and appear negatively stained against the background material.*

nized by their fusion with the reference lines (Fig. 5). Nonspecific lines produced by C-reactive substance are identified by their failure to fuse with the reference lines and their fuzzy appearance. They are greatly minimized by using antigens prepared from five week old cultures and eliminated by soaking the agar with 5 per cent sodium citrate for 45 minutes before reading the test. At least three specific precipitin bands are produced by antibody to *A. fumigatus* and one or more by antibody to *A. niger* or *A. flavus*. The precipitat-

ing antibodies belong to the IgG class of immunoglobulin (Warnock and Eldred, 1975). When multiple lines of identity occur with those of reference sera, a diagnosis of *Aspergillus* infection should be very seriously considered. Cross-reactions with antibody to fungi other than aspergilli are not likely to give multiple lines of identity, and clinical experience indicates that precipitins against *Aspergillus* antigens do not occur in normal sera or in those from other systemic fungus infections, bacterial infections, or cancer.

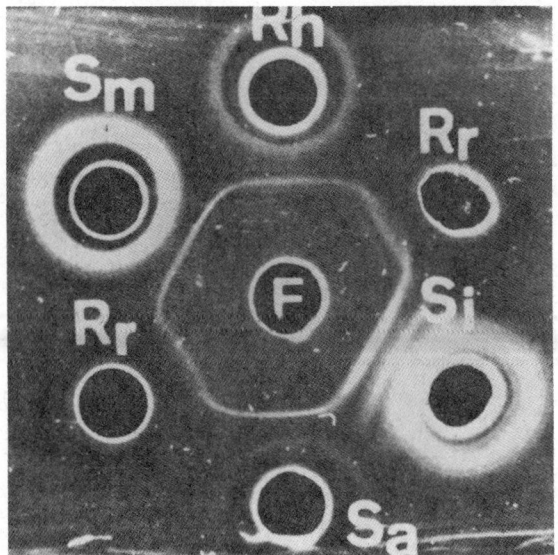

**FIGURE 5.** *Immunodiffusion reactions obtained with* A. fumigatus *against sera of patients with aspergilloma (S$_m$) and invasive (S$_i$)
and allergic bronchopulmonary disease (S$_a$). Reference positive
human serum is R$_r$ (From Coleman, R., and Kaufman, L.: Appl.
Microbiol 23:301, 1972.)*

## EPIDEMIOLOGY

Aspergilli are found everywhere "from the
winds of the Sahara to the snows of the Antarctic." They grow on soil, dead vegetation, any kind
of organic debris, and laboratory reagents. They
are extremely hardy and can withstand extremes
of temperature, pH, and salt concentration. They
are frequently encountered in farm houses,
stables, barns, and grains, and infections have
been acquired through inhalation of spores by
farmers, millers, and gardeners. The most pathogenic species, *A. fumigatus*, is thermophilic —i.e.,
it can grow at the high temperatures that develop
in compost piles from bacterial decomposition of
wet leaves and wood chips. Enormous numbers of
spores are produced, and, if inhaled by susceptible
gardeners, they can produce pulmonary aspergillosis. The same phenomenon accounts for the
heavy growth of *A. fumigatus* in stored hay or
grains. Grain is an important source of infection
in herds and livestock. Epidemics of aspergillosis
involving the air sacs or lungs of birds have been
traced to feeding on moldy grain. Horses, cattle,
and sheep also get pulmonary aspergillosis by
inhaling spores from their feed. Many years ago,
infected squabs were thought to be a source of
human aspergillosis. These pigeons were fattened
by persons known as "gaveurs de pigeons" who
used their tongues to force chewed grain into the
bird's esophagi (Renon, 1897). It is also possible
that the infection was acquired from the grain
rather than from the squab.

Among patients newly admitted to sanitariums
in the south central United States, the incidence
of aspergillosis was reported in 1970 to be nearly
as great as that of chronic pulmonary histoplasmosis (Parker et al., 1970). Since then, it is likely
that more cases of aspergillosis have developed in
patients after admission to the hospital. These
are debilitated patients who have been given
immunosuppressive drugs for treatment of hematologic malignancy or for prevention of renal
transplant rejection. Air ducts contaminated by
bird droppings have been incriminated as a
source of exposure for immunosuppressed patients (Kyriakides et al., 1976), and some observations suggest that the acquisition of pulmonary
aspergillosis in the hospital might be eliminated
if all incoming hospital air were filtered, properly
vented, and not recirculated (Rose, 1972).

Aflatoxins, the mycotoxins produced by *A.
flavus*, are a potential epidemiologic problem because they are found in the ground peanuts that
are heavily consumed by certain African tribes
afflicted with a high incidence of hepatoma. A
direct etiologic relationship between cancer and
aflatoxin has not been established, however, although aflatoxin can cause hepatomas in experimental animals. The epidemiologic problems related to mycotoxin are fully covered in Chapter
15.

## REFERENCES

Coleman, R., and Kaufman, L.: Use of the immunodiffusion test in the
    serodiagnosis of aspergillosis. Appl Microbiol 23:301, 1972.
Golbert, T., and Patterson, R.: Pulmonary allergic aspergillosis. Ann
    Intern Med 72:395, 1970.
Kaufman, L.: Value of immunodiffusion tests in the diagnosis of
    systemic mycotic diseases. Ann Clin Lab Sci 3:141, 1973.
Kyriakides, G., Zinneman, H., Hall, W., Arora, V., Lifton, J., Dewolf,
    W., and Miller, J.: Immunologic monitoring and aspergillosis in
    renal transplant patients. Am J Surg 131:246, 1976.
Longbottom, J. L., and Pepys, J.: Pulmonary aspergillosis: Diagnostic
    and immunologic significance of antigens and C-substance in
    *Aspergillus fumigatus*. J Pathol Bacteriol 88:141, 1964.
Parker, J., Sarosi, G, Doto, I., and Tosh, F.: Pulmonary aspergillosis in
    sanitoriums in the South Central United States. Am Rev Resp Dis
    101:551, 1970.
Pepys, J.: Hypersensitivity diseases of the lung due to fungi and
    organic dusts. In Kallos, P., Goodman, H., Hasek, M., Inderbitzin,
    T., and Waksman, B. (eds.): Monographs in Allergy, Vol. 4. Basel,
    S. Karger, 1969.
Renon, L.: Étude sur l'Aspergillose Chez les Animaux et Chez l'homme.
    Paris, Masson et cie, 1897.
Rose, H. D.: Mechanical control of hospital ventilation and aspergillus
    infections. Am Rev Resp Dis 105:306, 1972.
Sidransky, H., and Friedman, L.: The effect of cortisone and antibiotic
    agents on experimental pulmonary aspergillosis. Am J Pathol
    35:169, 1959.
Warnock, D., and Eldred, G.: Immunoglobulin classes of antibodies to
    *Aspergillus fumigatus* in patients with pulmonary aspergillosis.
    Sabouraudia 13:204, 1975.
Young, R., Bennett, J., Vogel, C., Carbone, P., and DeVita, V.:
    Aspergillosis. The spectrum of the disease in 98 patients. Medicine
    49:147, 1970.
Young, R., and Bennett, J.: Invasive aspergillosis. Absence of detect-
    able antibody response. Am Rev Resp Dis 104:710, 1971.

# THE ZYGOMYCETES 75

## Abraham I. Braude, M.D., Ph.D.

The Zygomycetes are the only medically important class belonging to the group of primitive fungi known as Phycomycetes. The various members of the class Zygomycetes have in common the production of sexual spores known as zygospores. The Zygomycetes produce two entirely different human infections: (1) Mucormycosis is a malignant infection of cerebral, pulmonary, and abdominal blood vessels due to Mucorales, the bread molds. The Mucorales are unique among the pathogenic fungi because they have no septa in their hyphae. (2) Tropical subcutaneous phycomycosis and nasal phycomycosis (or rhinoentomophthoromycosis) are benign chronic infections due to the insect fungi known as Entomophthorales. These curious fungi can shoot off their conidia forcibly.

### MORPHOLOGY

The three pathogenic genera of the order Mucorales are known as *Mucor*, *Rhizopus*, and *Absidia*. All three are characterized by a white or gray woolly growth on food or agar. Under the microscope, the woolly growth consists of mycelium that is not divided into individual cells by septa, so that the entire mass of mycelium forms one large cell containing multiple nuclei. This nonseptate mycelium is called coenocytic, which means *common cell* in Greek.* In all genera of Mucorales, the mycelia give rise to specialized branches known as conidiophores. At the tip of the conidiophores are sacs filled with asexual spores. These sacs, called sporangia, measure 20 to 115 $\mu$ and are seen with the naked eye as dark dots scattered throughout the woolly colony (Fig. 1). In *Rhizopus* and *Absidia*, other specialized branches arise from the mycelium that allow them to spread rapidly over the surface of the agar, climb the sides of the culture plate, and fill it with aerial mycelium. One of these structures is the stolon (or "runner"). It is a filament of mycelium that extends out into the air from the point at which the sporangiophore branches from the mycelium. The newly extended runner then produces a "hold-fast," or rhizoid, which anchors the filament to the surface of the agar, the side of

the plate, or its cover. In *Rhizopus*, the rhizoid is found at a node opposite the origin of the conidiophore. In *Absidia*, on the other hand, the sporangiophore arises from the arch of the stolon at a point between the nodes where the rhizoids branch off. In contrast to *Rhizopus* and *Absidia*, *Mucor* has neither stolons nor rhizoids and consequently fills the culture dish less rapidly and does not adhere to the lid. These relationships are shown in Figures 2, 3, and 4.

In addition to the asexual spores in the sporangia, the Mucorales also produce sexual spores, but they are rarely seen on routine agar cultures. The sexual spores are designated zygospores and result from the fusion of hyphae from two neighboring thalli, a process known as heterothallous conjugation. Despite the implication that two different sexes participate in this conjugation, the conjugating hyphae cannot be distinguished from each other. When two hyphae conjugate, their tips come together and become separated from the rest of the mycelium by a cross-wall, the only septum that characteristically occurs in these

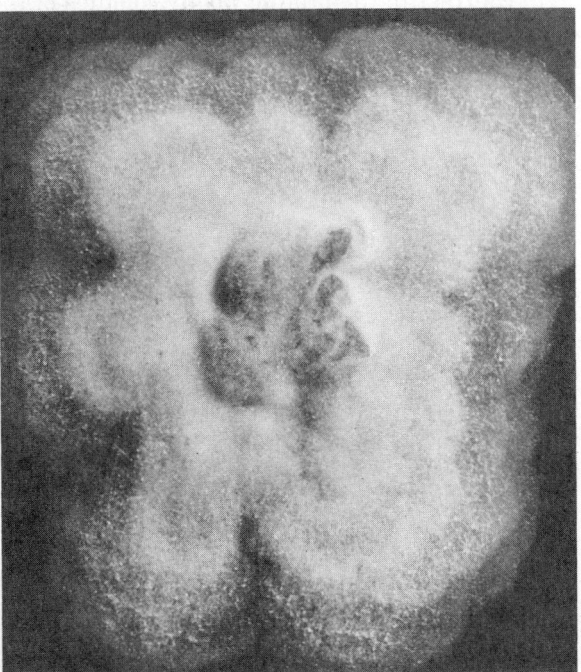

**FIGURE 1.** Mucor pusillus *isolated from blood of patient. Note dots scattered throughout the woolly colony. These dots represent sporangia.*

---

*Since certain green algae are also coenocytic, these nonseptate fungi are also called Phycomycetes, or algae-like fungi.

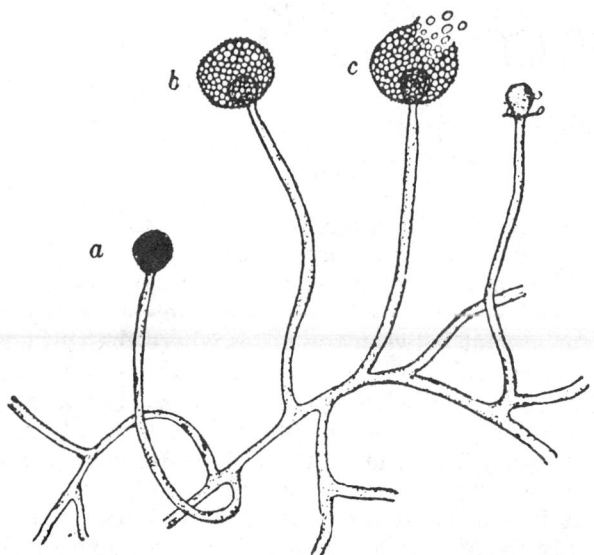

**FIGURE 2.** *Diagram of Mucor sp showing young sporulating head (a), mature sporangium (b and c), and columella after scattering of spores (d). Note that in contrast to Rhizopus and Absidia (Fig. 4) the sporangiophores arise from all parts of the thallus, and no stolons or rhizoids are produced. (From Waksman, S. A., and Starkey, R. L.: The Soil and the Microbe. New York, John Wiley and Sons, 1931.)*

otherwise nonseptate fungi. As the tips fuse, the walls separating them dissolve, so that the multinucleated masses of protoplasm in the two cells can run together, and the nuclei fuse. The wall of the fused cell becomes very thick.

In contrast to the prolific woolly colonies of the Mucorales, those of the Entomophthorales are flat and are covered by short, white mycelial fuzz. In further contrast, the mycelia of the Ento-

mophthorales are septate. The two main pathogenic genera of Entomophthorales are known as *Entomophthora* and *Basidiobolus*.

*Basidiobolus haptosporus*, the organism that causes tropical subcutaneous phycomycosis, grows rapidly at room temperature and produces three kinds of spores: conidia, zygospores, and chlamydospores. The conidia are actually uninucleate sporangia that are carried at the end of a short sporangiophore. These sporangia (or conidia) are discharged forcibly onto the glass surface of the culture tube or lid of the petri dish. The fragment of sporangiophore (or "basidium") immediately adjacent to the ejected sporangium is carried along with it. The sporangium is a smooth, globular structure measuring 16 to 45 $\mu$ in length. The zygospores are the most distinctive spores. They are spherical, have a thick, smooth wall, and measure 20 to 40 $\mu$ in diameter. Two "conjugation breaks" protrude from the zygospore (Fig. 5) as remnants of the hyphal ends (copulation tubes) that fuse during conjugation. The third spore, the chlamydospore, differentiates from other cells within the septate mycelium by developing a markedly thickened cell wall. Production of chlamydospores continues to increase as the culture ages and the relative number of zygospores and sporangia declines.

*Entomophthora coronata*, which causes African nasal phycomycosis (rhinoentomophthoromycosis), also produces many chlamydospores. In contrast to *Basidiobolus*, however, *E. coronata* rarely has any zygospores and has only sparse septa in the mycelium. The organisms contain numerous conidia, which are shot off from their short individual conidiophores, but the expelled conidia do

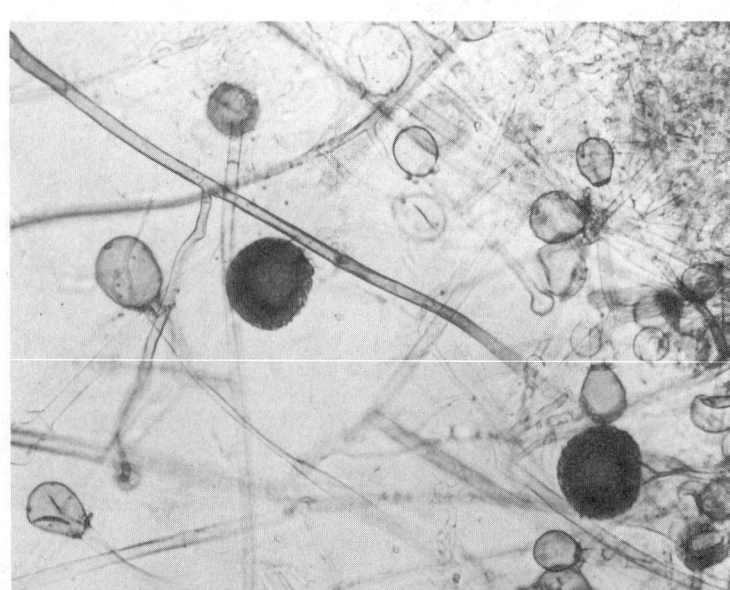

**FIGURE 3.** *Culture mount of Mucor pusillus from blood of fatal case of pulmonary mucormycosis. Note nonseptate mycelium, sporangiophore, and sporangium filled with asexual spores. The tip of the sporangiophore appears within the sporangium as a round swelling known as the columella. (Identification confirmed by J. J. Ellis, Research Mycologist, United States Department of Agriculture Research Service, Peoria, Illinois, Accession #NRRLA 12, 299.)*

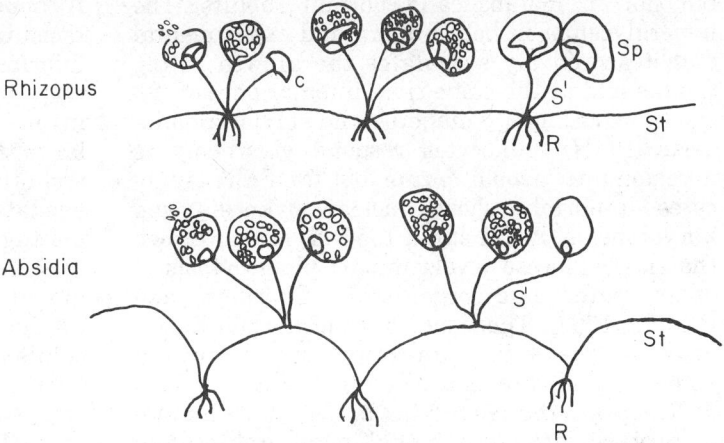

**FIGURE 4.** *Diagram of structural relationships of stolons (ST), rhizoids (R), sporangiophore (S), columella (C), and sporangium (SP) in* Rhizopus *and Absidia. Note that the sporangiophores of* Rhizopus *arise from the point at which the rhizoids are formed, whereas in* Absidia *the sporangiophores come off from the arched stolons. Also note the hemispherical shape of the columella in* Rhizopus *and the pear-shaped columella in* Absidia.

not carry a fragment of conidiophore (or "basidium") as do the conidia of *Basidiobolus*. The discharged conidia of *E. coronata* have the unique property of producing small secondary conidia that may form a crown around the parent (hence the name "coronata"). These secondary conidia are carried on short conidiophores that emerge

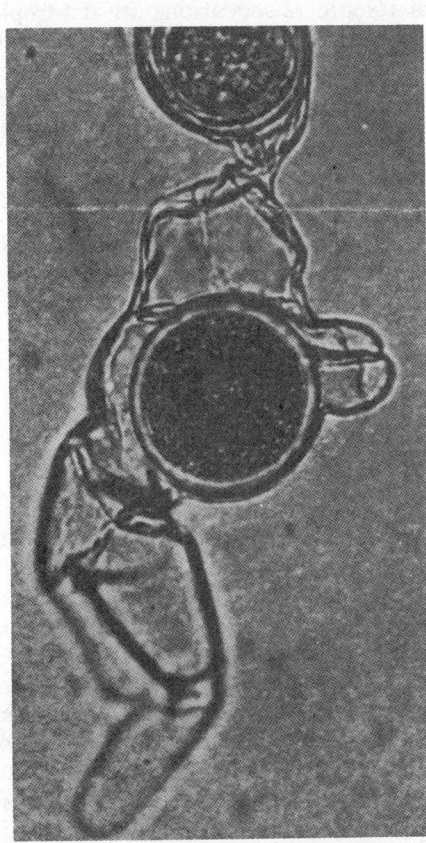

**FIGURE 5.** *Zygospore of* Basidiobolus haptosporus. *The two conjugation beaks that protrude from the zygospore are remnants of the hyphal ends that fuse during conjugation. (From Burkitt, D. P., Wilson, A., and Jelliffe, D.: Br Med J 1:1669, 1964.)*

from the primary conidium. Instead of secondary conidia, degenerating conidia may produce at their periphery many hair-like appendages that resemble flagella.

## ANTIGENIC COMPOSITION

The Zygomycetes have not been subject to the extensive antigenic analysis carried out with other pathogenic fungi, and no serologic test has been standardized for the diagnosis of mucormycosis, subcutaneous phycomycosis, or rhinoentomophthoromycosis. In preliminary studies using immunodiffusion, common antigens shared by *Absidia*, *Mucor*, and *Rhizopus* have been found in culture filtrates, and antigens specific for each of these genera were found in mycelial homogenates (Jones and Kaufman, 1978). The homogenate antigens showed some diagnostic promise when used in tests with sera from patients with zygomycosis, but a great deal of study is needed with this technique before it can be introduced for clinical purposes.

Limited analyses of the Entomophthorales have also found evidence of both common and specific antigens in species belonging to this order (Greer and Friedman, 1966).

## IMMUNITY

Mucormycosis does not characteristically occur in patients who have normal immunity to infection. Instead, it is a disease of severely ill patients who lose their resistance because of hematologic malignancies, immunosuppressive drugs, or metabolic disorders. Uncontrolled diabetes mellitus is often the underlying disease, and an infection closely resembling the disease in man can be produced in rabbits with acute alloxan diabetes, but not in metabolically normal rabbits. The hyperglycemia in both human and experimental diabetes probably stimulates the growth of the fungus and at the same time impairs phagocytosis. In experimental diabetes, the polymorphonuclear (PMN) leukocytes respond vigorously to invasion by *Rhizopus oryzae*, but the PMN leukocytes uniformly show nuclear pyknosis and karyorrhexis (Bauer et al., 1956). It is also known that high glucose levels impair phagocytosis of other pathogenic organisms (Chernew and Braude, 1962). The importance of normal leukocytes in preventing mucormycosis is evident when normal rabbits are inoculated with spores of *R. oryzae*; the leukocytes in the acute inflammatory exudate restrain the fungal proliferation and destroy the spores. Moreover, in neutropenic animals or patients, there is less resistance to mucormycosis. Most reported cases of phycomycosis in nondiabetics have occurred in leukemic patients with severe neutropenia (Parkhurst and Vlahides, 1967; Meyer et al., 1972; McBride et al., 1960). Other cases have occurred in burn wounds in which phagocytosis is impaired.

If leukocytes and other immune factors cannot restrain the fungus, it invades vessels and infarcts tissues. The usual portal of entry appears to be the nasal turbinates or paranasal sinuses; from there, the organism extends along the invaded vessels to the retroorbital tissues and cerebrum. Thrombosis of arteries and veins causes multiple infarcts throughout the brain, but only a minimal inflammatory response is found because the inflammatory cells are depleted or their function is impaired. If spores of the Mucorales are inhaled or ingested, they may invade the walls and vessels of bronchi, stomach, or intestine of neutropenic patients.

In contrast to the Mucorales, the Entomophthorales produce infection in apparently normal people. Like mucormycosis, rhinoentomophthoromycosis also invades the nasal mucosa but stops short of the vessels, and there is no tendency to infarct the tissues. The affinity of spores from both Mucorales and Entomophthorales for the human nasal mucosa is a striking phenomenon, but its mechanism is mysterious. Normally, the cilia of the nose carry foreign particles to the posterior pharynx, where they are swallowed. Since other fungal spores are not arrested in the nose, it is possible that those of the Zygomycetes can impair ciliary action and inactivate this important means of natural resistance to nasal infection. A second possibility is that the nasal mucosa has receptors that hold the spores to the cell surfaces. Finally, it has been suggested that the *N*-acetyl neuraminic acid in nasal mucin has a specific affinity for spores of the Zygomycetes.

Although none of these speculations on natural resistance has been verified, there is more solid information on the mechanism of acquired immunity. It appears that immunity to *E. coronata* involves eosinophils through a mechanism similar to that operating in schistosomiasis, filariasis, and other parasitic infections. The inflammatory exudate around the fungi may be composed almost entirely of eosinophils, and eosinophil granules are aggregated in close apposition to the fungal cell walls (Williams et al., 1969). Charcot-Leyden crystals, which are derived from eosinophils, are also present. In addition to the eosinophil granules and crystals, lysosomes, mitochondria, vacuoles, and pinocytic vesicles are released by cell necrosis. For this reason it has been proposed that the fungi lyse the eosinophils and other inflammatory cells so that their cytoplasmic and nuclear contents are released. These form an eosinophilic precipitate or "sleeve" around the fungus, called the Splendore-Hoeppli phenomenon, like that seen around schistosome ova. The adjacent granulomatous infiltrate is composed of macrophages, lymphocytes, and plasma cells. If current concepts on cellular immunity to worms can be translated into immunity against fungi, these histologic observations in enterophthoromycosis imply that IgE interacts with macrophages and eosinophils so that both cells can kill *E. coronata*. The tissue reaction in subcutaneous phycomycosis due to *Basiliobolus haptosporus* is identical, producing an eosinophilic sheath around the hyphae and showing no invasion of vessels. The cellular immune reaction of eosinophils and macrophages appears to be effective because both infections are benign and may even regress spontaneously (Burkitt et al., 1964). Since the infection by *B. haptosporus* occurs almost exclusively in childhood, it would seem that immunity acquired then protects adults.

## LABORATORY DIAGNOSIS

In cerebral mucormycosis, the fungus can be found in sections and cultures of the infarcted nasal turbinate or paranasal sinus. In pulmonary mucormycosis, it can be found in lung biopsies or in metastatic skin lesions. For mysterious reasons, the etiologic agent of cerebral mucormycosis has rarely if ever been cultured from the brain or spinal fluid, even when fresh tissues known to harbor the characteristic mycelium were subjected to expert mycologic techniques. The fungus most frequently isolated in mucormycosis is *Rhizopus oryzae*. Other species have been identified as *Rhizopus arrhizus*, *Rhizopus rhizopodiformis*, *Absidia corymbifera*, and *Mucor pusillus*. Two other Mucorales, *Cunninghamella elegans* and *C. mortierella*, have also caused human infection on rare occasions. These are easily separated from the other Mucorales because they have no columellas. In addition, *C. elegans* has no sporangium and its conidia arise from a vesicle like that found in *Aspergillus*.

It is impossible to distinguish among the species of Mucorales in the tissues of patients with mucormycosis, but they can be differentiated from the fungi that produce hyphae in tissues. In contrast to the hyphae of *Aspergillus* and *Candida*, those of the Mucorales are nonseptate, branch irregularly, and stain deeply with hematoxylin and eosin or silver-methenamine but poorly with the periodic acid-Schiff (PAS) stain. *Aspergillus* is septate, stains better with PAS than hematoxylin, and branches with great regularity. The various genera of Mucorales are identified by the characteristics in Figures 2, 3, and 4. Special guides must be consulted for identification of species (Ellis and Hesseltine, 1966; Zycha, 1935).

The Entomophthorales, *B. haptosporus* and *E. coronata*, are also identified by biopsy and culture. As noted in the previous section, the two produce identical histologic changes that strongly suggest the diagnosis without culture. In contrast to those of the Mucorales, the hyphae of the Entomophthorales take up hematoxylin poorly and are usually septate. The poorly stained hyphae may appear as circular spaces surrounded by a cuff of amorphous eosinophilic material representing the Splendore-Hoeppli phenomenon. Large numbers of eosinophils are also present in acute exudates. The hyphae may be surrounded by epithelioid cells and ingested by giant cells. The poorly staining walls of the hyphae and the absence of cytoplasm in subcutaneous phycomycosis give the impression of tunnels through subcutaneous inflammatory tissue. Because of the prominent eosinophils, these tunnels were thought at one time to be the track of an unidentified worm larva (Burkitt et al., 1964).

If tiny fragments of tissue are incubated on Sabouraud's medium at 37° C, the fungi grow rapidly, and the characteristic radially folded, wax-colored colonies appear in three days. The diagnostic zygospores are seen after one or two weeks in cultures of *B. haptosporus* but do not develop in *E. coronata*.

## EPIDEMIOLOGY

The Mucorales are ubiquitous thermotolerant molds that thrive in any organic material. *Rhizopus* is an important cause of spoilage in fruits and sweet potatoes. The disease in strawberries is known as leak because of drippings from the softened fruit. The mucors are also found frequently on stale, moist breads ("bread molds") and can hydrolyze starch to sugar. Yet despite their wide prevalence in food and other organic materials, the Mucorales are not commonly encountered in hospital environments where susceptible diabetics, leukemics, and burn patients are likely to be exposed. Recent outbreaks of skin and subcutaneous mucormycosis were reported in hospitals using contaminated commercial elastic dressings (Elastoplast tapes), but cultures of the environment over a ten year period in the same institution have not grown Mucorales (Gartenberg et al., 1978). Their absence in the hospital despite their frequent presence in food is puzzling and might indicate the Mucorales in food can infect debilitated patients without spreading to the hospital environment. This puzzle, and the mysterious failure to culture the fungus from the brains of patients with histologically proven cases of mucormycosis, imply that pathogenic Mucorales may sometimes lose their ability to grow on environmental or laboratory substrates but not in certain tissues.

The epidemiology of infection by the Entomophthorales is also puzzling because infections by these fungi are remarkably infrequent for such ubiquitous fungi. It has been suggested that environmental temperatures limit the period during which *B. haptosporus* can be infectious. The fungus grows poorly at 15° C, so that in temperate climates it can be disseminated only during the few warm months from its reservoir in the gastrointestinal tracts of insectivorous reptiles (Clark, 1968). This factor also explains why nearly all cases of subcutaneous phycomycosis occur in tropical areas such as Uganda, Kenya, Sudan, the Cameroons, Indonesia, India, and parts of Southeast Asia. It has not been reported from the western hemisphere. Infections with *B. haptosporus* occur mainly in children, who probably acquire them from minor trauma or insect bites. It is a fungus of low pathogenicity and is seldom able to cause infection in adults, who seem to acquire immunity from clinical or subclinical exposure earlier in life.

The epidemiology of rhinoentomophthoromycosis due to *E. coronata* differs in two main respects from that of subcutaneous phycomycosis caused by *B. haptosporus*. First, *E. coronata* infections are probably transmitted by spore inhalation rather than insect bites, since the portal of entry is the nose. Second, it is a disease of adult agricultural workers, especially men exposed to the fungus growing in the soil or vegetation of tropical rain forests in Africa. It has also been reported from similar regions such as Columbia, Brazil, India, and Puerto Rico.

## References

Bauer, H., Flanagan, J., and Sheldon, W.: The effects of metabolic alterations on experimental *Rhizopus oryzae* (mucormycosis) infection. Yale J Biol Med 29:23, 1956.

Burkitt, D. P., Wilson, A., and Jelliffe, D.: Subcutaneous phycomycosis: A review of 31 cases seen in Uganda. Br Med J 1:1669, 1964.

Chernew, I., and Braude, A.: Depression of phagocytosis by solutes in concentrations found in the kidney and urine. J Clin Invest 41:1945, 1962.

Clark, B.: The epidemiology of phycomycosis. In Wolstenholme, G., and Porter, R. (eds.): Symposium on Systemic Mycoses. Boston, Little, Brown & Company, 1968, p. 179.

Ellis, J., and Hesseltine, C.: Species of *Absidia* with ovoid sporangiospores. Sabouraudia 5:59, 1966.

Gartenberg, G., Bottone, E., Keusch, G., and Weitzman, I.: Hospital-acquired mucormycosis (*Rhizopus rhizopodiformis*) of skin and subcutaneous tissues: Epidemiology, mycology and treatment. N Engl J Med 299:1115, 1978.

Greer, D, and Friedman, L.: Antigenic relationships between the fungus causing subcutaneous phycomycosis and saprophytic isolates of *Basidiobolus meristosporus* and *B. ranarum*. Sabouraudia 5:7, 1966.

Jones, K., and Kaufman, L.: Development and evaluation of an immunodiffusion test for diagnosis of systemic zygomycosis (mucormycosis): Preliminary report. J Clin Microbiol 7:97, 1978.

McBride, R., Corson, J., and Dammin, G.: Mucormycosis: Two cases of disseminated disease with cultural identification of *Rhizopus*: Review of literature. Am J Med 28:832, 1960.

Meyer, R., Rosen, P., and Armstrong, D.: Phycomycosis complicating leukemia and lymphoma. Ann Intern Med 77:871, 1972.

Parkhurst, G., and Vlahides, G.: Fatal opportunistic diesase. JAMA 202:279, 1967.

Waksman, S. A., and Starkey, R. L.: The Soil and the Microbe. New York, John Wiley and Sons, 1931.

Williams, A., Lichtenberg, F., Smith, J., and Martinson, F.: Ultrastructure of phycomycosis due to entomophthora, basiodiobolus, and associated "Splendore-Hoeppli" phenomenon. Arch Pathol 87:495, 1969.

Zycha, H.: Mucorineae, Kryptogamenflora. Leipzig, Mark Brandenberg, Berlin, Gebrüder Borntraeger, 1935.

# 76 DEMATIACEAE: AGENTS OF CHROMOMYCOSIS

## Yousef Al-Doory, Ph.D.

The dematiaceous fungal agents of chromomycosis comprise a group of genetically related fungi. Five species have been isolated repeatedly from confirmed cases of this disease. The clinical appearance of this chronic disease of the skin and subcutaneous tissues does not indicate which species is the causative agent.

The five fungi can be classified into two types: as a group, *Fonsecaea pedrosoi*, *F. compactum*, *Phialophora verrucosa*, and *Cladosporium carrionii* are characterized by a moldy appearance and an abundance of dry aerial hyphae on culture media; whereas *F. dermatiditis*, the other type, has soft, dark, moist colonies that undergo a yeastlike phase during the course of development.

A few other dematiaceous fungi have been reported occasionally as causative agents of chromomycosis. As an example, *Cladosporium bantianum* has been reported to be the agent for cladosporiosis, which is considered by some workers as cerebral chromomycosis (Al-Doory, 1972).

### MORPHOLOGY

All of the fungi of chromomycosis are slow growing and have dark-colored colonies that show black color through the reverse of the agar. How-ever, individual strains do reveal great variations in color, rates of growth, and gross colony characteristics. *F. pedrosoi* colonies are flat, covered with feltlike, short, aerial hyphae that are dark green to brown or black. *F. compactum* colonies are heaped, brittle, and covered with a coarse aerial hyphae. Colonies of *C. carrionii* may appear smooth or irregular with a defined margin bordered by a darker submerged hyphae. *P. verrucosa* shows dark brown to black colonies with olive to gray aerial hyphae. *F. dermatitidis* colonies mature from moist, glistening, olive to black colonies to those showing feathery strands of submerged, tightly compressed hyphae radiating outward from the margin. These hyphae eventually give rise to olive-gray aerial mycelia (Fig. 1).

Microscopically, these five species of fungi show dark conidia and mycelia with three types of conidiophores (Fig. 2). The phialophora-type is found mainly in *P. verrucosa*. A distinct conidiophore is formed terminally or along the mycelium. It is generally flask-shaped with a rounded oval or elongated base, a constricted neck, and an opening with or without a flaring collarette and lip. The conidia are formed semiendogenously and extrude through the neck.

The second type of conidiophore is the cladosporium-type that is found mainly in *C.*

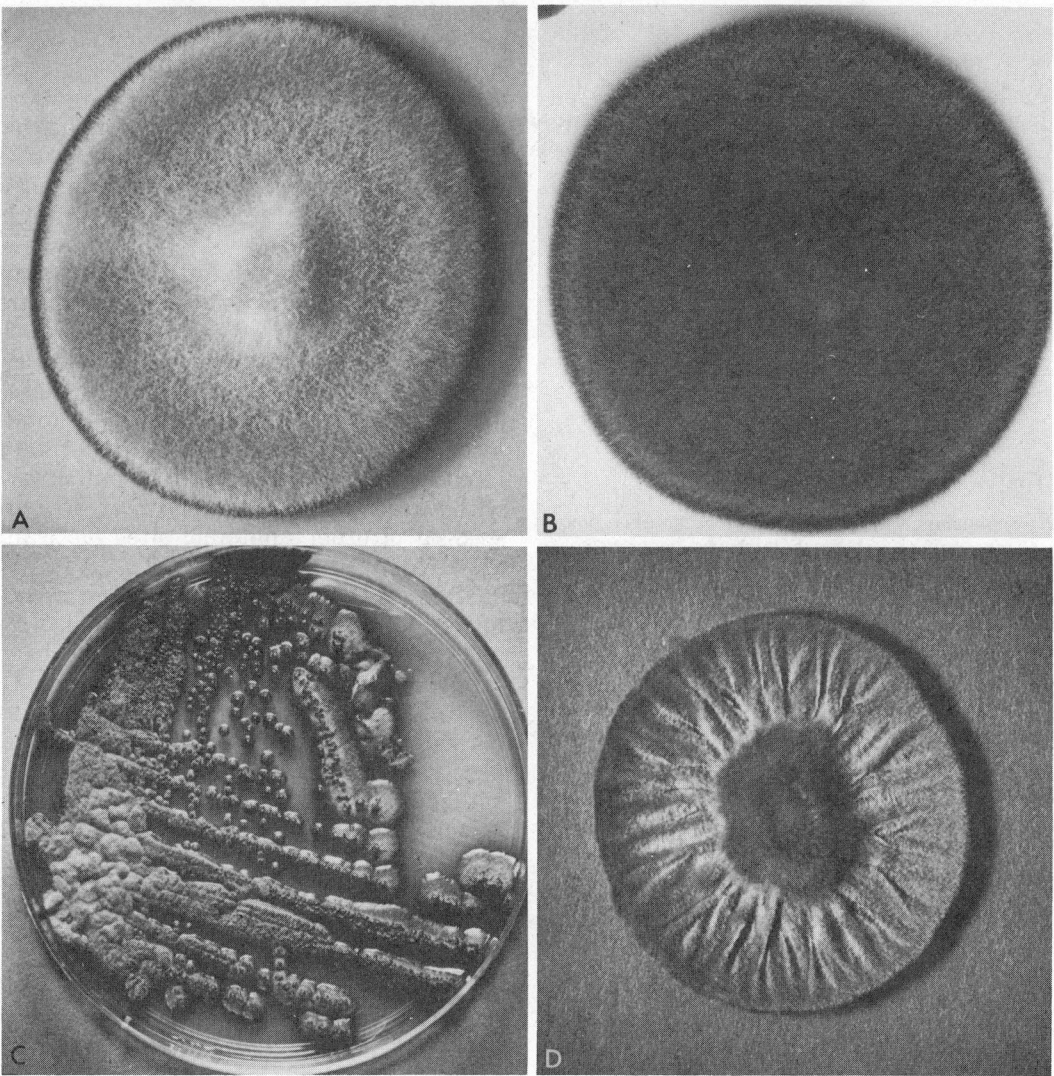

**FIGURE 1.** *Colonies of three causative agents of chromomycosis:* A, *Fluffy, black-gray colony of* Fonsecaea pedrosoi. B, *Fuzzy, black colony of* F. compactum. C,D, *Glistening, yeast colony (C) transferring to fuzzy, mycelial form (D) of* F. dermatitidis. *(Courtesy of Rippon, J. W.: Medical Mycology. W. B. Saunders Co., 1975.)*

*carrionii.* The conidia in this type are formed at the tip of a simple conidiophore that is slightly enlarged at the distal end. A few conidia are formed first at the tip and then bud, forming secondary conidia at their distal poles, and the process continues. This produces long branching chains of conidia.

The third type of conidiophore is the fonsecaea-type (acrotheca-type) found in the three species of *Fonsecaea* in addition to the previous two types. The conidiophore is similar to the vegetative hyphae, in which conidia are formed irregularly at the tip and along the sides of the conidiophore.

## ANTIGENIC COMPOSITION

Few studies of the antigenic composition and relationships of the various etiologic agents of chromomycosis have been reported. Chemical analysis of the cell walls of *F. pedrosoi, P. verrucosa,* and *C. carrionii* reveals a composition of 17 to 31 per cent glucose, 29 to 42 per cent protein components, 8 to 14 per cent mannose, and 6 to 8 per cent glucosamine (Szaniszlo et al., 1972).

Complement fixation, agglutination, agglutination-absorption, and precipitation tests have been used and described (Martin et al., 1936; Seeliger, 1959, 1968). Furthermore, patients with

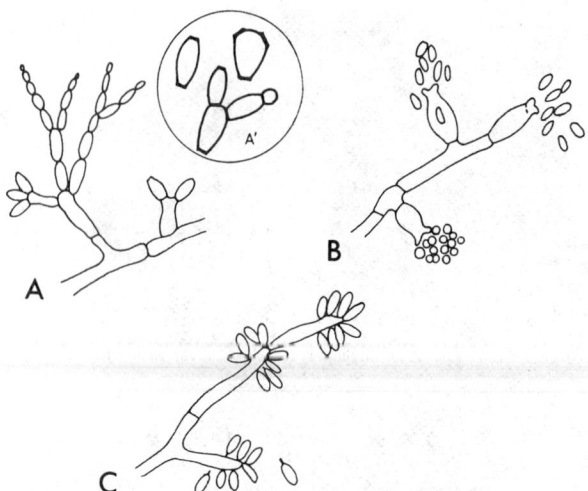

FIGURE 2.  *Sporulation types in the causative agents of chromomycosis. A, Cladosporium-type. Note the thickened sacs or disjunctors (A'). B, Phialophora type. C, Acrotheca type. (Courtesy of Rippon, J. W.: Medical Mycology. W. B. Saunders Co., 1975.)*

chromomycosis were found to have circulating antibodies (Buckley and Murray, 1966; Smith et al., 1968). By cross-precipitation tests, it was shown that *F. pedrosoi, F. compactum,* and *P. verrucosa* are closely related and are antigenically distinct from *C. carrionii* (Buckley and Murray, 1966). By the use of the fluorescent antibody technique, it was shown that *C. carrionii* can be differentiated from *C. bantianum,* which is the causative agent of cerebral chromomycosis (Al-Doory and Gordon, 1963; Gordon and Al-Doory, 1965).

So far, no consistent antigenic patterns have been found to describe firmly and delineate antigenically the various species of chromomycotic fungi. Similarly, there is no serologic test with diagnostic significance for patients in whom the disease is suspected.

## METABOLISM

There are no major studies on the metabolism of chromomycotic fungi in the literature. It is known that these fungi produce neither exotoxins nor endotoxins. At the same time, these fungi lack any of the proteolytic enzymes, which liquify Loeffler's coagulated serum medium or gelatin, or which peptonize milk (Fuentes and Bosch, 1960).

## PATHOGENIC PROPERTIES

The chromomycotic fungi are found in soil, certain plants, and debris. Therefore, infection

from these fungi is exogenous, and actual implantation of the fungus occurs through a break in the skin and/or subcutaneous tissues. It is believed that these fungi are not highly pathogenic because they require repeated exposure to overcome the normal resistance of the human body. Accordingly, chromomycosis is a noncontagious disease, and transfer from man to man has never been reported.

The chromomycotic fungi can infect tissues and organs beyond the portal subcutaneous tissues to cause dissemination or cerebral involvement (Al-Doory, 1972). From the medical histories in the available cases of chromomycosis, there is evidence that, in addition to foci of infection in localized extremity lesions, an aerosol-type of infection may cause a primary pulmonary focus, with subsequent lymphangitic or hematogenous seeding of other anatomic sites (Jotisankasa et al., 1970).

The pathogenicity of the chromomycotic fungi has been tested in various animals (Al-Doory, 1972; Wilson et al., 1933) and has been found capable of producing lesions. The clinical appearance of infected animals was not similar to that of chromomycotic patients, and histopathologically, abscesses in animals contained mycelial elements rather than the regular round sclerotic bodies (MacKinnon, 1934).

## IMMUNITY

Natural resistance to infection with agents of chromomycosis is normally high. It is higher both in preteen individuals than in adults and in females than in males.

No race seems immune. However, a review of 124 patient histories revealed the following: 60 per cent were Caucasian, 30 per cent were black, and 10 per cent were of mixed racial background; among these: six cases were Mongolian; two were Malayan; two were Hindu, and one was a Mexician and one a Jamaican (Carrion and Silva, 1947).

Hypersensitivity has been demonstrated in chromomycotic patients and is diminished following clinical recovery. The relationship of this finding to resistance against reinfection is not known, however (Rippon, 1974).

## LABORATORY DIAGNOSIS

The appearance of the chromomycotic fungi in pus as round, thick-walled, chestnut-brown, sclerotic cells is a significant diagnostic feature in histopathology (Fig. 3). Microscopically, the

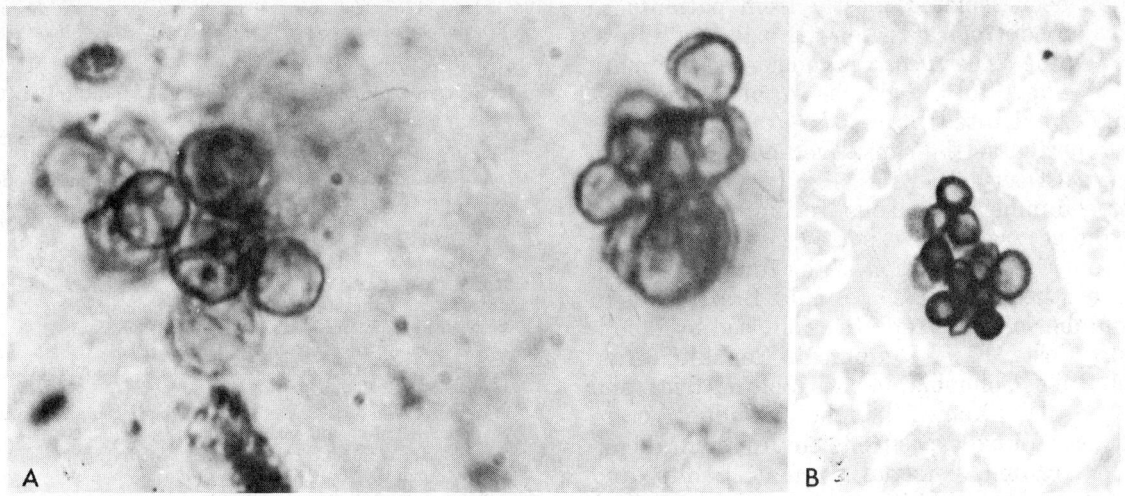

**FIGURE 3.** *Clusters of sclerotic fungal cells from skin of patients with chromomycosis. Note internal septa in* A *and thick walls in* B. *(Courtesy of Al-Doory: Chromomycosis. The Mountain Press.)*

presence of the three types of conidiophore formation is an important feature of the culture of the three species of *Fonsecaea* (conidiophores show various ratios depending on species, strain, and growth environment). In addition, the appearance of the moist, glistening yeast-like colonies is an indication of *F. dermatitidis,* while the appearance of subspherical conidia borne tightly in a compact chain is an indication of *F. compactum.* The presence of only phialophora-type conidiophores in the culture is the characteristic of *P. verrucosa,* while the cladosporium-type conidiophore with its extralong chains of conidia is indicative of *C. carrionii.*

Aging cultures of most strains of these fungi develop masses of pigmented chlamydospores, which have characteristic coarse, dark walls surrounding yellowish-brown, granular protoplasm.

Macroscopically, these fungi feature slow growth of colonies compared with the relatively fast growth of the saprophytic *Cladosporium sp.,* and they are unable to hydrolyze starch, coagulate milk, or liquify gelatin, Loeffler's medium, or any substrate containing protein. The saprophytic species are proteolytic (Fuentes and Bosch, 1960).

## DRUG SENSITIVITY

Chromomycotic fungi are insensitive to various bacterial antibiotics. However, they show various degrees of sensitivity to other chemotherapeutic agents in vitro. The fungal growth of these fungi was found to be inhibited with 0.75 μg/ml of thiabendazole (2-[4'-thiazolyl]benzimidazole) (Blank and Rebell, 1965). The growth of *F. pedro-*

soi was inhibited by sodium sulfamerazine (Keeney et al., 1944), stilbamidine, propamidine, and pentamidine (Bocobo et al., 1953), and deamidines (Al-Doory, 1972).

Amphotericin B is the drug of choice in most mycotic diseases. Chromomycotic fungi are killed by huge doses of this drug in vitro — i.e., a culture of *F. dermatitidis* containing 5 μg/ml of amphotericin B was nonviable at the end of 24 hours; with 2.5 μg/ml of the drug, it was nonviable after 48 hours. Even 0.5 μg/ml caused a reduction in the colony count (Keeney et al., 1944). These fungi are too resistant for use of amphotericin in patients, however. The MIC is greater than 40 μg/ml in vitro, while the maximum dose tolerated by humans is 1 to 1.5 mg per kg per day, which produces a blood level of the drug no greater than 1.8 μg/ml (Littman et al., 1958).

In vivo these fungi show sensitivity to potassium iodide, sodium iodide, copper sulfate, and 5-fluorocytosine. However, currently no drug can be considered the drug of choice for these fungi, either in vitro or in vivo.

## EPIDEMIOLOGY

Although chromomycosis has been reported from every continent and is therefore, of worldwide distribution, the fungi of this disease are more abundant in the tropical and subtropical regions.

It appears that certain species are localized more in certain geographic areas than others. *C. carrionii* has been isolated only from patients in South Africa, Venezuela, and Australia. *F. pedro-*

*soi* has been isolated mostly from patients in tropical or subtropical regions (Brazil, Costa Rica, Cuba), while *P. verrucosa* is considered the main causative agent of the disease in colder climates, mainly the United States. *F. dermatitidis* has been reported as the causative agent of cases in Japan (Al-Doory, 1972).

For a number of reasons, including completeness and accuracy, the reported cases do not fully represent the distribution of the fungi; they are, however, the only guide available. Brazil leads in the number of cases reported, followed by Madagascar, Costa Rica, Dominican Republic, Australia, Cuba, Colombia, Mexico, South Africa, and Paraguay. It is known that the individual's occupation, continued exposure to environmental hazards or trauma, personal hygienic habits, and nutritional and environmental conditions are among the major factors in the infectivity of these fungi. Therefore, these factors play a large role in the distribution of reported cases and may influence the geographic distribution of the fungal agents.

### References

Al-Doory, Y.: Chromomycosis. Missoula, Mont., Mountain Press, 1972.

Al-Doory, Y.: The Epidemiology of Human Mycotic Diseases. Springfield, Ill., Charles C Thomas, 1975.

Al-Doory, Y., and Gordon, M.: Application of fluorescent-antibody procedures to the study of pathogenic dematiaceous fungi. I. Differentiation of *Cladosporium carrionii* and *Cladosporium bantianum.* J Bacteriol 86:332, 1963.

Blank, H., and Rebell, G.: Thiabendazole activity against the fungi of dermatophytosis, mycetomas and chromomycosis. J Invest Dermatol 44:219, 1965.

Bocobo, F. C., et al.: *In vitro* fungistatic activity of stilbamidine, propamidine, pentamidine and diethylstilbestrol. J Invest Dermatol 21:149, 1953.

Buckley, H. R., and Murray, I. G.: Precipitating antibodies in chromomycosis. Sabouraudia 5:78, 1966.

Carrion, A. L., and Silva, M.: Chromoblastomycosis and its etiologic fungi. Ann Cryptogamici Phytopathol 6:20, 1947.

Fuentes, C. A., and Bosch, Z. E.: Biochemical differentiation of the etiological agents of chromoblastomycosis from nonpathogenic *Cladosporium* species. J Invest Dermatol 34:419, 1960.

Gordon, M. A., and Al-Doory, Y.: Application of fluorescent-antibody procedures to the study of pathogenic dematiaceous fungi. II. Serological relationships of the genus *Fonsecaea.* J Bacteriol 89:551, 1965.

Jotisankasa, V., et al.: *Phialophore dermatitidis:* Its morphology and biology. Sabouraudia 8:98, 1970.

Keeney, E. I., et al.: Studies on common pathogenic fungi and on *Actinomyces bovis.* Bull Johns Hopkins Hosp 75:393, 1944.

Littman, M. L., et al.: Coccidioidomycosis and its treatment with amphotericin B. Am J Med 24:568, 1958.

MacKinnon, J. E.: Estudio del primer casa Uruguayo de chromoblastomycosis y revista critica sobra el enfermedad. Arch Urug Med Cir Esep 5:201, 1934.

Martin, D. S., et al.: A case of verrucous dermatitis caused by *Hormodendrum pedrosoi* (chromoblastomycosis) in North Carolina. Am J Trop Med 16:593, 1936.

Rippon, J. W.: Medical Mycology: The Pathogenic Fungi and the Pathogenic Actinomycetes. Philadelphia, W. B. Saunders Company, 1974.

Seeliger, H. P. R.: In The Fungi, vol. 3. New York, Academic Press, 1968.

Seeliger, H. P. R., et al.: Identification of fungi by serologic tests. Further serologic studies with dematiaceous fungi. Proceedings of the Sixth International Congress of Tropical Medicine. Malaria 4:636, 1959.

Smith, D. T., et al. (eds.): Zinsser's Microbiology, 14th ed. New York, Appleton-Century-Crofts, 1968.

Szaniszlo, P. J., et al.: Chemical composition of the hyphal walls of three chromomycosis agents. Sabouraudia 10:94, 1972.

Wilson, S. J., et al.: Chromoblastomycosis in Texas. Arch Dermatol 27:107, 1933.

# *77* MISCELLANEOUS FUNGI: THE AGENTS OF MYCETOMA AND RHINOSPORIDIUM

*Abraham I. Braude, M.D., Ph.D.*

### AGENTS OF MYCETOMA

Mycetoma is a clinical syndrome (Chapter 238) produced either by soil bacteria, the *Actinomycetes,* or by certain soil fungi that enter the tissues after trauma to the skin. The most common site of infection is the foot (Taralakshmi et al., 1977; Reddy et al., 1972), and the most common fungi causing mycetoma are *Petriellidium boydii, Madurella mycetomi* and *Acremonium* sp. Among the less common causes are *Madurella*

*grisea, Leptosphaeria senegalensis, Pyenochaeta rosneroi, Phialophora jeanselmei,* and *Neotestudina rosatti.* Descriptions are provided here of *P. boydii, M. mycetomi,* and *Acremonium* sp. The properties of the others are summarized in Chapter 237.

### Petriellidium boydii

This fungus, also known as *Al1escheria boydii,* is the most common cause of mycetoma in the United States and Europe. It produces on any

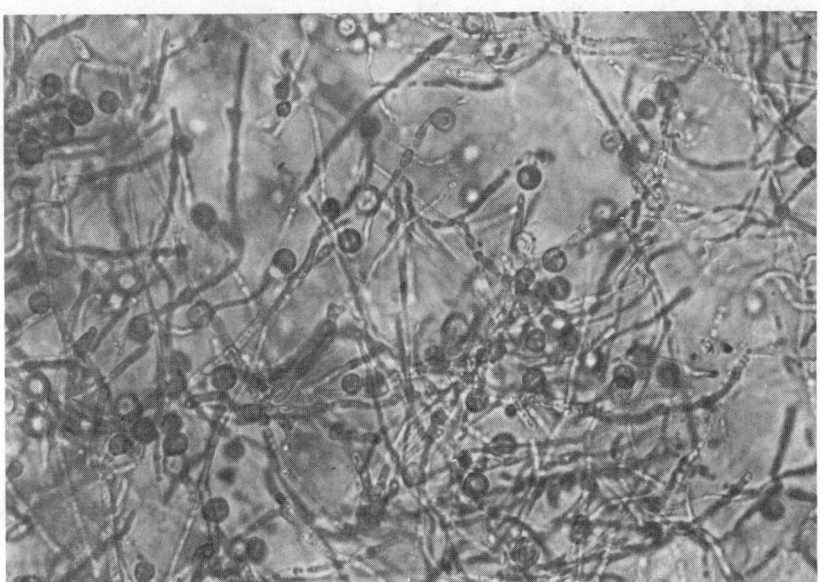

**FIGURE 1.** *Hyphae and asexual spores of* Petriellidium boydii. *The asexual spores are borne singly at the tips and sides of single conidiophores.*

medium a rapidly spreading, fluffy white colony that turns gray and resembles the fur of mice. The most distinctive feature is the manner in which the conidia are attached to the mycelium. These asexual spores are usually borne singly at the tips and sides of single conidiophores but may sometimes occur in small groups (Fig. 1). The spores are egg- or lemon-shaped, measure 4 to 8 by 5 to 15 $\mu$, and have a brown color.

Sexual reproduction is homothallic, i.e., the sexual spores, or ascospores, result from the fusion of cells from the same mycelial mat or thallus. Groups of eight ascospores are contained in sacs known as asci, which measure 8 to 20 $\mu$ in diameter. After a couple of weeks, the asci become enclosed in a protective hollow globe known as an ascocarp or perithecium. The ascocarps are dark brown and have a thin wall composed of one layer of modified hyphal cells. Ascocarps are not seen in many cultures but when present can be found in the agar or in the mycelium near the edge of the colony. When they reach maturity, the thin wall of the ascocarp ruptures and releases the ascospores (Fig. 2).

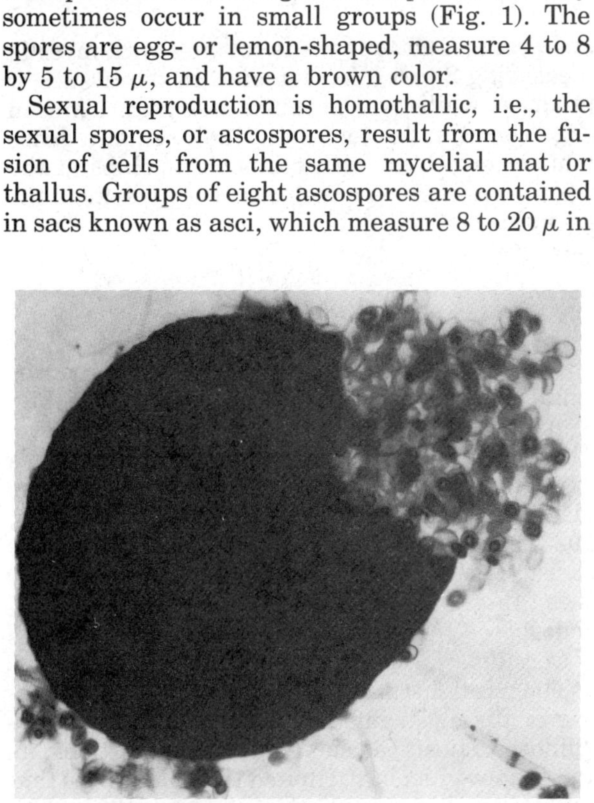

In infected fistulas, colonies of the fungus take the form of white or yellow grains. In wet preparations or stained smears of crushed granules, a mycelial mass is seen. The mycelium measures 2 to 4 $\mu$ in diameter and swells peripherally to 10 $\mu$. The periodic acid-Schiff stain or the Gomori methenamine silver stain may sometimes bring out details of the organism that are not visible in wet mounts.

In addition to mycetomas, the fungus can sometimes be cultured from *Petriellidium* infections of the lung, cornea, ear, and meninges. The infection can be introduced or disseminated by surgery and other invasive therapeutic procedures. Thus, chronic meningitis due to *P. boydii* has followed spinal anesthesia (Benham and George, 1948), and disseminated infection to the spine and long bones has occurred after lung biopsy performed at the time of heart surgery. The fungus is usually but not always resistant to amphotericin B and may be sensitive (<1.0 $\mu$g/ml) to miconazole and ketoconazole.

### M. mycetomi

This fungus is probably the most common cause of eumycotic mycetoma and is found in Asia, Africa, and South America. In India, for example,

**FIGURE 2.** *Ascospores of* P. boydii *escaping from perithecium (ascoscarp). (From Parker, J. C., and Klintworth, G. F.: In Baker R. D. (ed.): Human Infections with Fungi, Actinomycetes, and Algae. New York, Springer-Verlag, 1971.)*

it is isolated at least ten times more often from mycetoma than *P. boydii* (Taralakshmi et al., 1977). *M. mycetomi* varies in colonial appearance from strain to strain, from case to case, and from one geographic area to another. In general, *M. mycetomi* grows well at 37° C, producing in several days a white mycelium that soon turns brown. The growth is compact and has a wrinkled leathery surface, which becomes covered with a powdery down. Diffusible brown pigments stain the reverse side of the agar.

The hyphae are 3 to 4 $\mu$ in width and segmented. Spores are rare but, when present, take two forms: pyriform conidia and phialospores. The pyriform conidia are carried on short conidiophores, and the phialospores are extruded from short bottle-shaped stalks known as phialides.

In tissues, the hyphae form round masses that issue from draining fistulas as hard, black granules measuring 0.5 to 5 mm. The hyphal mass in the dense type is held together by a brownish cement that is homogenously distributed throughout the granule. In the vesicular type of granule, the cement is located around its periphery.

## Acremonium Species (Cephalosporium Species)

The characteristic feature of this genus is the balls of conidia (Fig. 3). The conidia are borne one at a time at the tips of short erect conidiophores that branch from the aerial hyphae. Successive conidia push the others aside so that they form clusters or small balls held together by a sticky exudate. The conidia are nonpigmented and elongated.

The fungus grows rapidly at room temperature

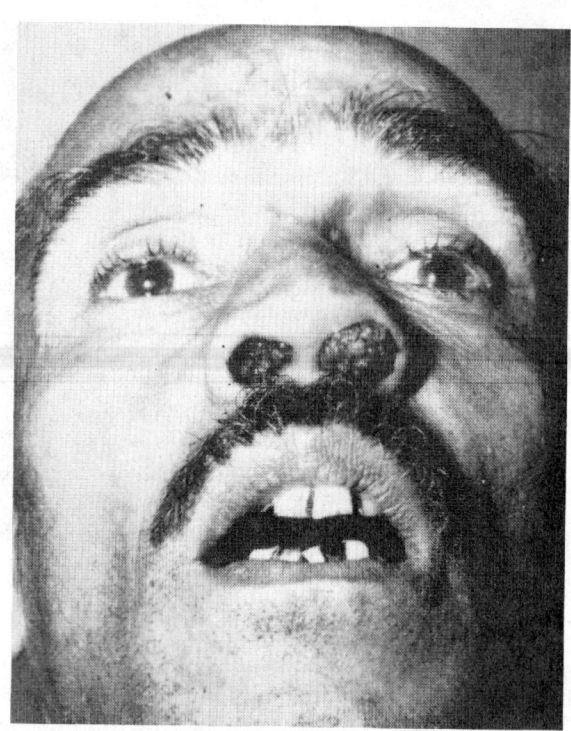

**FIGURE 4.** *Rhinosporidiosis with tumor-like masses in nares. (From Karunaratne, W. A. E.: Rhinosporidiosis in Man. London, The Athlone Press, 1964.)*

and produces cottony white colonies with mycelia measuring 2 to 3 $\mu$ in diameter. In the tissues, it produces white oval granules less than 1 mm in size. The granules contain in their center a dense matt of mycelium with eosinophilic clubs at the periphery. There is no cement. They resemble the granules of *A. boydii*.

## *RHINOSPORIDIUM*

The fungus *Rhinosporidium seeberi* produces small tumor-like masses usually in the nose (Fig. 4) and nasopharynx, but sometimes in the eye. The endosporulating fungus is seen in the tissues but cannot be cultured on laboratory media. It is placed in the class Phycomycetes (Ashworth, 1923) and in the family Coccidioidaceae because characteristic giant sporangia develop in the tissues (Figs. 4 and 5). These thick-walled, endospore-filled sporangia resemble the spherules of *Coccidioides immitis*.

The nasal disease is probably acquired by bathing or diving in infected water. In India, where rhinosporidiosis reaches epidemic proportions, its rarity in women is attributed to social taboos that prohibit women from bathing in open places. The characteristic lesion is a vascularized papillomatous proliferation of the nasal or pharyngeal mucous membrane containing sporangia in vari-

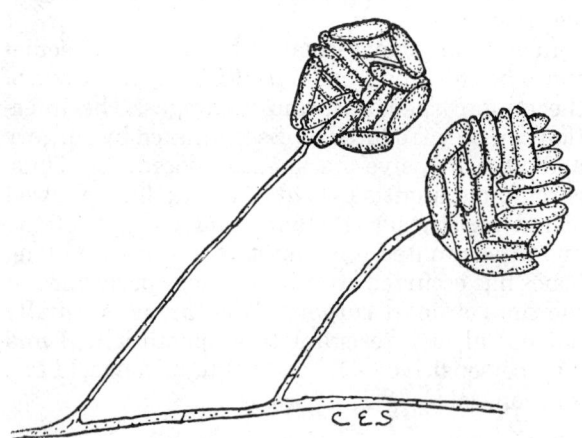

**FIGURE 3.** *Cephalosporium species. The conidia form small balls at the tips of the conidiophores. (Drawing by C. E. Skinner from Skinner, C. E., Emmons, C. W., and Tsachiya, H. M.: Molds, Yeasts, and Actinomycetes. New York, John Wiley and Sons, 1947.)*

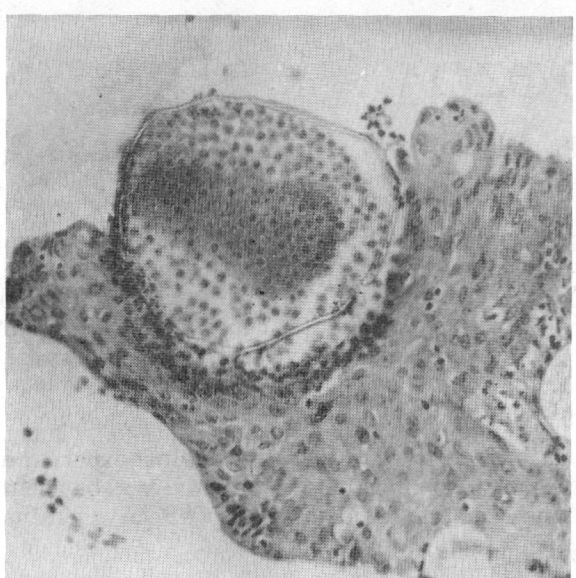

**FIGURE 5.** *A sporangium is embedded in the epithelium, which is attempting to encircle it; sporangium is filled with endospores. (From Karunaratne, W. A. E.: Rhinosporidiosis in Man. London, The Athlone Press, 1964.)*

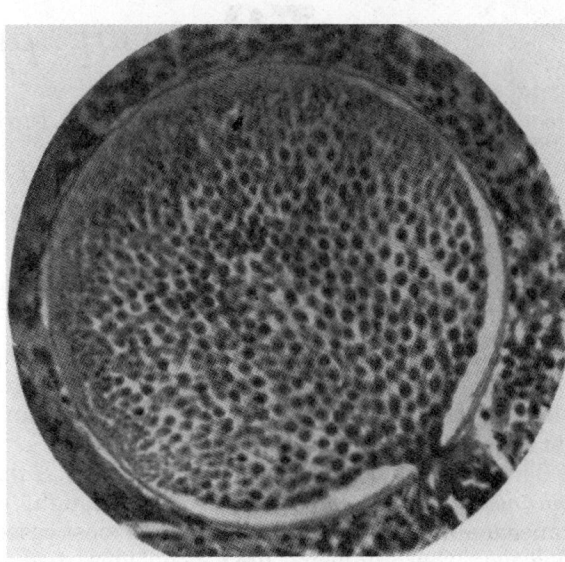

**FIGURE 6.** *Giant sporangium bursting and releasing endospores. (From Karunaratne, W. A. E.: Rhinosporidiosis in Man. London, The Athlone Press, 1964.)*

ous stages of maturity. Red blood cells, inflammatory pus cells, and extruded endospores fill the interstitial tissues. As sporangia enlarge, they compress the columnar epithelium of the pharynx and allow endospores to escape and reinoculate the adjacent tissue. Ocular infection occurs in dry, dusty regions and may be transmitted in dust storms. In Texas, half the cases of rhinosporidiosis are ocular.

The vascularized papillomas produce single or multiple pedunculated, fleshy, red masses in the nares or pharynx and cause rhinitis, epistaxis, and nasal obstruction. In exceptional cases, hoarseness may develop from laryngeal infection. The conjunctiva of the lids is predominantly affected in the ocular form, which tends to be unilateral and remarkably free of pain. Although usually confined to the eye or nose, the infection may infrequently be seen in the vagina, rectum, male urethra, and bronchi. Generalized rhinosporidiosis and visceral involvement have also been reported.

The lesions can be completely removed by surgery or electrocautery. Electrocautery is preferred, because surgery leaves open incisions in which spores can be implanted and produce recurrences.

## References

Ashworth, J. H.: On *Rhinosporidium seeberi* (Wernicke, 1903) with special reference to its sporulation and affinities. Trans R Soc Edin 53:301, 1923.

Benham, R., and George, L.: *Allescheria boydii,* causative agent of a meningitis. J Invest Dermatol 10:99, 1948.

Karunaratne, W. A. E.: Rhinosporidiosis in Man. London, The Athlone Press, 1964.

Parker, J. C., and Klintworth, G. K.: Miscellaneous uncommon diseases attributed to fungi and actinomycetes. In Baker, R. D. (ed.): Human Infections with Fungi, Actinomycetes, and Algae. New York, Springer-Verlag, 1971, p. 958.

Reddy, C., Sundareschwar, B., Pattabni Rama Rao, A., and Reddy, S.: Mycetoma: Histopathologic diagnosis of causal agents in 50 cases. Indian J Med Sci 26:733, 1972.

Skinner, C. E., Emmons, C. W., and Tsuchiya, H. M.: Molds, Yeasts, and Actinomycetes. New York, John Wiley and Sons, 1947, p. 109.

Taralakshmi, V. V., Pankajalakshmi, V. V., Paramaswan, C. N., Shetty, B. M. V., and Subramanian, S.: Mycetomas in Madras. Sabouraudia 15:17, 1977.

# 7 PARASITES
# 78 *THE PROTOZOA*

*Joseph H. Miller, M.S., Ph.D.*

## THE INTESTINAL AND ATRIAL PROTOZOA OF MAN

### Parasitic Amebas of Man

Members of this group include free-living soil/water amebas that are opportunistic parasites of man and the amebic parasites of man's large intestine and mouth.

Three genera of soil amebas — *Naegleria*, *Hartmannella*, and *Acanthamoeba* — are thought to cause meningoencephalitis in man. In most cases, however, the organisms have been identified in fixed tissue specimens from necropsy and exact identification could have been confused by morphologic similarity. When culture was possible, *Naegleria fowleri* was isolated.

The intestinal amebas, on the other hand, are a well-defined group and consist of five species: (1) *Entamoeba histolytica*, (2) *Entamoeba coli*, (3) *Dientamoeba fragilis*, (4) *Endolimax nana*, and (5) *Iodamoeba bütschlii*. Another species, *Entamoeba gingivalis*, is found in the mouth. Only *Entamoeba histolytica* is an important pathogenic species, although *Dientamoeba fragilis* may cause chronic but mild intestinal symptoms. The comparative morphology of these six parasitic species in humans is presented in Figure 1.

### *Soil/Water Amebas*

#### Morphology

*Naegleria fowleri*, the species most often associated with disease in man, is distributed worldwide in water and moist soil. In an ameboid stage, pseudopodia form eruptively. The endoplasm and ectoplasm are well defined, and there is one contractile vacuole. The nucleus has a large central karyosome. A biflagellate form develops in water. A cystic stage may also occur.

#### Epidemiology

Most cases have occurred in young adults after vigorous swimming, leading to the theory that these water-borne amebas may traverse the nasal mucosa, penetrate the cribriform plate, and multiply in the gray matter of the brain.

#### Laboratory Diagnosis

The cerebral spinal fluid should be examined for the presence of motile amebas. Stained preparations will show the characteristic large central karyosome. The organism may also be cultured. *Naegleria* grow out from a central inoculum of *Escherichia coli* on plates containing 1.5 per cent agar without added nutrient or sodium chloride.

#### Drug Susceptibility

Amphotericin B is effective against experimental *Naegleria* infections of mice and may be useful in humans. Sulfadiazine is very effective against experimental acanthamebiasis.

#### Immunity

Experimental animals seem to be immune to reinfection, but these studies are preliminary and incomplete. Most natural infections have occurred in young, healthy individuals.

### *Entamoeba histolytica*

#### Morphology

*E. histolytica* may exist as a trophozoite, precyst, or cyst in feces (Fig. 2). The trophozoite is usually 15 to 25 $\mu$ in length. The clear ectoplasm is sharply demarcated from the granular endoplasm, which may contain ingested red cells. Its single nucleus appears ringlike when stained with iodine in fresh feces. Iron hematoxylin or other permanent staining techniques demonstrate a fine nuclear membrane encrusted with a layer of minute chromatin granules. A small punctiform karyosome is centrally located. The trophozoite is usually extremely active and exhibits progressive motility until it is cooled below the temperature of the human body. The precystic stage is a rounded, nonmotile trophozoite, devoid of inclusions. It is smaller than a trophozoite but usually larger than a cyst. The cysts are round-to-oval hyaline bodies, 5 to 20 $\mu$ in size, with smooth, refractile walls. Immature cysts are uninucleate with a large ringlike nucleus. As nuclear division occurs, individual nuclei decrease in size until the quadrinucleate mature cyst forms. In immature cysts glycogen is usually diffuse, and sausage-shaped chromatoid bodies may be seen. In unstained preparations chromatoid bodies are highly refractile, whereas in iron hematoxylin stains, they are uniformly dark. The chromatoid bodies, which contain ribonucleic acid, disappear as nuclear division occurs in the cyst.

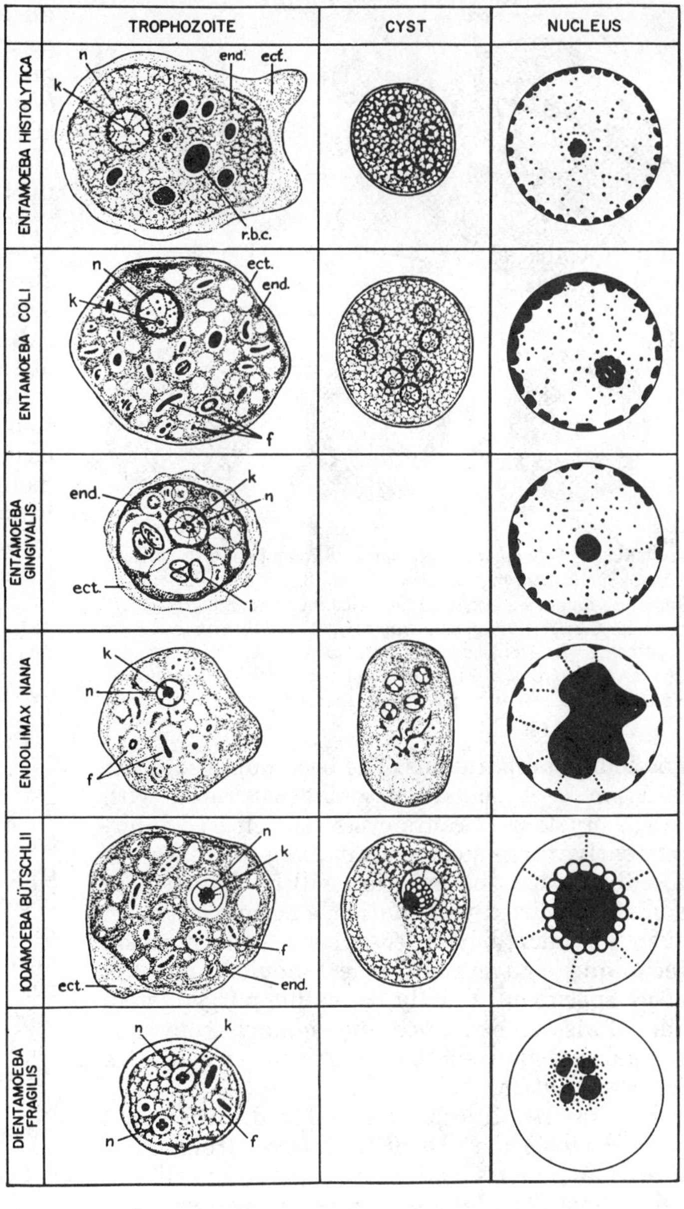

**FIGURE 1.** *Comparative morphology of the amebae of man and schematic representation of their nuclei as seen in iron-hematoxylin stains. ect., ectoplasm; end., endoplasm; f, food vacuoles; i, inclusions; k, karyosome; n, nucleus; r.b.c., red blood cells. (From Brown, H. W.: Basic Clinical Parasitology. Appleton-Century-Crofts, New York, 1975.)*

## Life Cycle/Epidemiology

Cysts in feces are the infective stage. Persons are infected through food or drink contaminated by infective feces, flies, or the unwashed hands of food handlers. Cross-connections between sewage and water lines have been responsible for waterborne epidemics. Excystation occurs when the mature cyst reaches the lower small intestine. A four-nucleate ameba is released, which ultimately divides into eight small trophozoites. These amebas move downward and establish themselves at areas of stasis in the large intestine. They may feed in the lumen and invade the mucosa. Multiplication occurs by binary fission. Cysts are produced and passed in the feces. Tro-

phozoites are seen in diarrheic and dysenteric stools, but they are not resistant to environmental conditions and do not spread the infection. Man is the principal host and source of infection, although natural infections of monkeys, dogs, hogs, and rats with amebas indistinguishable from *E. histolytica* have been reported.

### Laboratory Diagnosis

The laboratory diagnosis rests on the identification of the parasite in the feces or tissues and on serologic studies.

*Intestinal Amebiasis.* Three naturally passed stools over a one-week period should be examined by the direct smear technique, using fresh saline

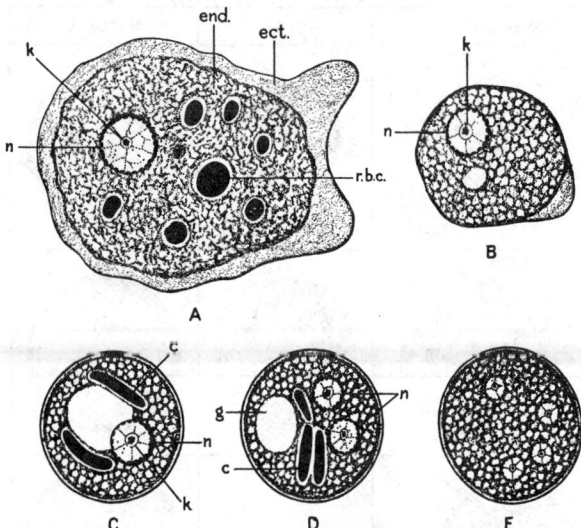

**FIGURE 2.** *Schematic representation of* Entamoeba histolytica. *A, trophozoite containing red blood cells; B, precystic ameba; C, immature uninucleate cyst; D, binucleate cyst; E, mature quadrinucleate cyst; c, chromatoid bodies; ect., ectoplasm; end., endoplasm; g, glycogen vacuole; k, karyosome; n, nucleus; r.b.c., red blood cells. (From Brown, H. W.: Basic Clinical Parasitology. Appleton-Century-Crofts, New York, 1975.)*

and iodine preparations. The best iodine solution is 1 per cent potassium iodide saturated with iodine crystals. Because cysts are released intermittently, three stool examinations increase the likelihood that the infection will be detected. In addition to direct examination, a permanent stain such as hematoxylin eosin and concentration technique (e.g., formalin-ether) should be done on each specimen. Finally, a saline-purged stool should also be examined and sigmoidoscopy performed to visualize lesions and to obtain aspirates for examination.

Trophozoites in aspirates and in diarrheic and purged stools may be distinguished from other intestinal amebas by their progressive motility in saline mounts (Table 1) or their characteristic nuclear morphology in iron hematoxylin or other permanent stain (Figs. 1 and 2). Formed stools are examined for typical cysts. The cysts of *E. histolytica* can be differentiated from the cysts of other intestinal amebas by the presence of typical chromatoid bodies and the type and number of nuclei (Fig. 3 and Table 2).

Several strains of *E. histolytica* have been recognized. *E. hartmanni*, a strain in which the cyst size is less than 10 $\mu$, is considered by some to be a separate, nonpathogenic species.

*Extraintestinal Amebiasis.* All extraintestinal amebiasis originates from a primary intestinal infection, and evidence of such infection should be sought. Extraintestinal amebiasis without demonstrable concurrent intestinal infection is common, however. Serologic methods (complement fixation, immunodiffusion, and indirect hemagglutination) are sensitive and important diagnostic aids for confirming the clinical diagnosis of extraintestinal amebiasis. Many tests are available commercially in kit form. Microscopic examination of aspirates for motile trophozoites as well as cultural procedures are helpful.

### Drug Susceptibility

Although *E. histolytica* is susceptible to many drugs, metronidazole has revolutionized the treatment of amebiasis. Metronidazole is now the treatment of choice for all forms of amebiasis, but it can be given only orally. Patients with severe intestinal amebiasis who are too ill to take oral medication may be successfully treated with emetine. The combination of emetine and chloroquine may also be needed for treatment of the occasional liver abscess caused by a metronidazole-resistant *E. histolytica*.

### Immunity

Invasive amebiasis elicits the production of antibody to many different antigens of *E. histoly-*

**TABLE 1.   Key for the Differentiation of Amebic Trophozoites**

| | |
|---|---|
| I. Iodine-stained smear of fresh feces | |
|   A. Presence of a ring-like nucleus | II A |
|   B. Absence of a ring-like nucleus | II B |
| II. Unstained saline smear of fresh feces | |
|   A. Trophozoites usually medium or large sized (except for small strains of *Entamoeba histolytica*) | |
|     1. Progressive motility with cytoplasm flowing into pseudopod; motile forms have slug-like shape; may or may not contain ingested red cells; nucleus usually not visible without stain | *E. histolytica* |
|     2. No progressive motility; cytoplasm does not flow into pseudopod; blunt pseudopodia extended and retracted; ring-like nucleus frequently visible unstained | *Entamoeba coli* |
|   B. Trophozoites usually small or medium sized; ordinarily motility is sluggish | |
|     1. Pseudopodia often blunt or round, resembling a yeast budding | *Endolimax nana* |
|     2. Pseudopodia angular (triangular or tent-like), rectangular or lobulated; outline of non-motile trophozoites perfectly round or cyst-like | *Dientamoeba fragilis* |
|     3. Pseudopodia blunt; resemble small *E. coli* trophozoites | *Iodamoeba bütschlii* |

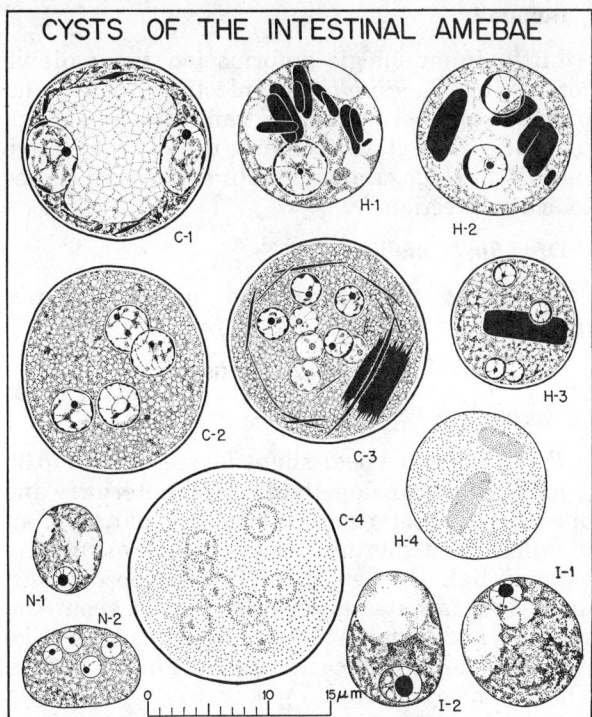

CYSTS OF THE INTESTINAL AMEBAE

**FIGURE 3.** *C-1, Iron-hematoxylin-stained immature binucleate cyst of* Entamoeba coli. *C-2, Iron-hematoxylin-stained immature quadrinucleate cyst of* E. coli. *C-3, Iron-hematoxylin-stained mature cyst of* E. coli. *C-4, Unstained mature cyst of* E. coli. *H-1, Iron-hematoxylin-stained immature uninucleate cyst of* Entamoeba histolytica. *H-2, Iron-hematoxylin-stained immature binucleate cyst of* E. histolytica. *H-3, Iron-hematoxylin-stained mature cyst of* E. histolytica. *H-4, Unstained cyst of* E. histolytica *with chromatoid bodies. N-1, Iron-hematoxylin-stained uninucleate cyst of* Endolimax nana. *N-2, Iron-hematoxylin-stained mature cysts of* E. nana. *I-1, I-2, Iron-hematoxylin-stained mature cysts of* Iodamoeba bütschlii. *(From Hunter, G. W., Swartzwelder J. C., and Clyde, D. F.: Tropical Medicine. W. B. Saunders Co., Philadelphia, 1976.)*

include *Chilomastix mesnili* and *Trichomonas hominis* of the intestine and *Trichomonas tenax* of the mouth. *Giardia lamblia* in the small intestine and *Trichomonas vaginalis* in the urogenital tract of humans are the pathogenic species. The species can be differentiated on the basis of habitat and by the morphologic comparison shown in Figure 4. *Blastocystis hominis*, a commensal yeast found in the intestine of humans, may be confused with the cysts of these flagellates.

### *Giardia lamblia*

#### Morphology

*Giardia lamblia* is a worldwide parasite of the upper small intestine of humans. It has two stages in its life cycle: the trophozoite, which multiplies by binary fission, and the infective cyst, which is passed in the feces (Fig. 4). The trophozoite is a pear-shaped, bilaterally symmetrical flagellate, 12 to 15 $\mu$ long, with a broad rounded anterior surface and a tapering posterior extremity. The dorsal surface is convex. Most of the anterior ventral surface assumes a rigid bilobed concavity (ventral disk) in which a negative pressure is created by the beating of a pair of specialized ventral flagella. The organism is thus able to adhere to the brush border of the duodenal mucosa. Anteriorly, two large nuclei contain karyosomes. Two axostyles between the nuclei pass into the posterior extremity. Three pairs of trailing flagella are located dorsally. The ellipsoid cyst is 9 to 12 $\mu$ long and has a well-defined wall. The mature cyst contains four nuclei and the remnants of organelles found in the trophozoite. Because mitosis occurs in the cyst, two trophozoites are produced during excystation.

#### Life Cycle/Epidemiology

Infected persons, children more frequently than adults, pass cysts in the feces intermittently. Watery stools occasionally contain trophozoites, but they are not infective. Excystation of cysts ingested through fecal contamination of food or drink occurs in the small intestine and establishes the infection. Water-borne epidemics have

*tica*. Neither these antibodies nor other immune mechanisms are known to prevent either extraintestinal invasion or reinfection.

## Intestinal and Atrial Flagellates of Man

Three intestinal and two atrial flagellates are common in humans. The nonpathogenic species

---

**TABLE 2.  Key for the Differentiation of Amebic Cysts**

| | |
|---|---|
| I. Unstained saline smear of fresh feces | |
|   A. Presence of rod-like or sausage-shaped chromatoid bars (in some but not in all infections) | *Entamoeba histolytica* |
|   B. Absence of chromatoid bars | II |
| II. Iodine-stained smear of fresh feces (and of formalin-ether concentrate) | |
|   A. Presence of ring-like nuclei | 1 |
|     1. Medium sized or small cyst with one to four nuclei | *E. histolytica* |
|     2. Large cyst with five or more nuclei | *Entamoeba coli* |
|   B. Absence of ring-like nuclei | 3 |
|     3. Small, round, or oval cyst with nuclei appearing as vacuole-like areas | *Endolimax nana* |
|     4. Medium sized cyst with large dark brown mass sharply delimited from cytoplasm | *Iodamoeba bütschlii* |

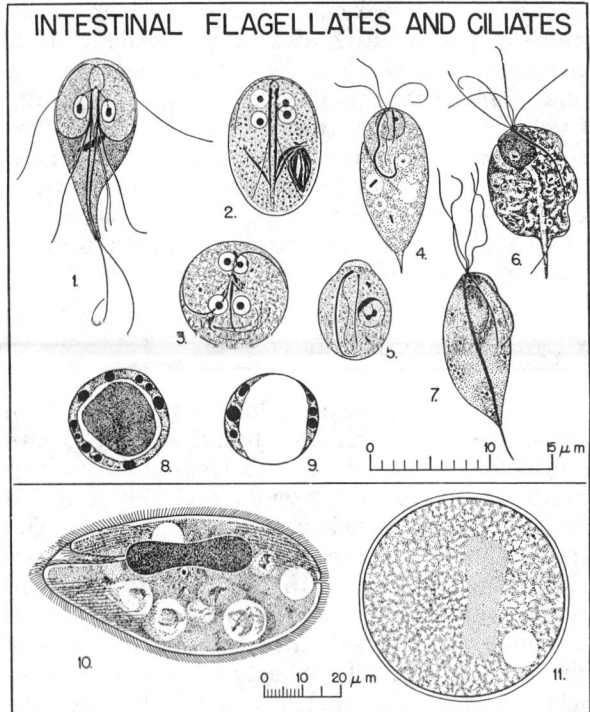

## INTESTINAL FLAGELLATES AND CILIATES

**FIGURE 4.** *1, Iron-hematoxylin-stained trophozoite of* Giardia lamblia. *2, Iron-hematoxylin-stained cyst of* G. lamblia. *3, Iron-hematoxylin-stained cyst of* G. lamblia, *end-view. 4, Iron-hematoxylin-stained trophozoite of* Chilomastix mesnili. *5, Iron-hematoxylin-stained cyst of* C. mesnili. *6, Iron-hematoxylin-stained trophozoite of* Trichomonas hominis. *7, Iron-hematoxylin-stained trophozoite of* Trichomonas vaginalis. *8, Iron-hematoxylin-stained* Blastocystis hominis. *9, Unstained* B. hominis. *10, Trophozoite of* Balantidium coli. *11, Unstained cyst of* B. coli. *(From Hunter, G. W., Swartzwelder, J. C., and Clyde, D. F.: Tropical Medicine. W. B. Saunders Co., Philadelphia, 1976.)*

occurred when drinking water was contaminated by feces containing cysts from human and possibly animal sources. The cysts are resistant to normal chlorination but seem to be destroyed by iodine compounds in concentrations recommended for water purification (Wolfe, 1975).

### Laboratory Diagnosis

The diagnosis may be made by finding the characteristic cysts in iodine and saline mounts of fresh feces (Fig. 4). Motile trophozoites may also be distinguished by their characteristic morphology and jerky motility in watery stools. Permanently stained fecal smears are also used to distinguish *G. lamblia*. Concentration techniques should always be used. The string method (Entero-Test) of recovering trophozoites from duodenal samples is simple and useful when stool findings are negative and symptoms persist.

### Immunity

Little immunologic information is available concerning *G. lamblia*. Reinfection occurs, and immunosuppressive therapy can cause an asymptomatic carrier state to change rapidly into active infection. Hypogammaglobulinemia predisposes to acute infection.

### Drug Susceptibility

*G. lamblia* is sensitive to atabrine, metronidazole, and furazolidone.

## *Trichomonas vaginalis*

### Morphology

*T. vaginalis* is a pear-shaped flagellate, 10 to 30 $\mu$ long, with four flagella directed anteriorly and one directed posteriorly to form the margin of an undulating membrane (Fig. 4). The membrane extends half the length of the trophozoite. An axostyle originates anteriorly, curves about the nucleus, and terminates posteriorly as a tail-like appendage. Multiplication is by binary fission. There is no cyst stage.

### Epidemiology/Life Cycle

*T. vaginalis* inhabits the vagina and the male urethra, epididymis, and prostate. The incidence of infection is higher in females than in males. Coitus is probably the most frequent mode of infection, but the exchange between women of toilet articles contaminated with vaginal discharge is also a common cause of infection.

### Laboratory Diagnosis

The examination of fresh infected vaginal discharge in a drop of saline will disclose motile *T. vaginalis*. The erratic jerky motility of the organism is characteristic. The rippling wave-like motion of the undulating membrane can be visualized clearly when specimens begin to dry. Permanently stained specimens may also be prepared and examined for the undulating membrane and flagella.

Examination of prostatic secretions obtained by prostate massage is the best method for diagnosing infections of men. The secretion should be examined for motile trophozoites with undulating membranes. Smaller numbers of trophozoites may also be found in the urine.

For practical purposes, *Trichomonas* spp may be differentiated on the basis of the source of infected material: *T. tenax* is found in material from the oral cavity, *T. hominis* from feces, and *T. vaginalis* from vaginal discharge, prostatic fluid, or urine.

### Drug Susceptibility

Oral metronidazole is highly effective in eliminating the infection in either sex. No other systemic drug is effective.

## A Parasitic Ciliate of Humans:
### *Balantidium coli*

### Morphology

*B. coli* is the only ciliated pathogen of man (Fig. 4). The large ovoid trophozoite, measuring 50 to 70 μ by 30 to 60 μ, is enclosed by a pellicle covered with longitudinal spiral rows of cilia. The beating cilia account for the smooth gliding motility of the organism in fresh fecal preparations. At the anterior end is a funnel-shaped peristome lined by long cilia. A large kidney-shaped macronucleus with a small rounded micronucleus lying in its concavity is usually centrally located. There are two contractile vacuoles. At the posterior end is a cytopyge for the discharge of solid waste material. The rounded trophozoites secrete a double cyst wall. Cysts measure 50 to 65 μ. The macronucleus, contractile vacuoles, and cilia are visible within the cyst.

### Epidemiology/Life Cycle

*B. coli* trophozoites inhabit the lower ileum and large intestine, where they penetrate the mucosa and multiply by binary fission. Conjugation has been observed in this species. Infective cysts are passed in the feces. Trophozoites do not survive the extracorporeal environment. Cysts ingested in fecally contaminated food or drink produce a single trophozoite. Cysts do not multiply.

Morphologically identical forms of *B. coli* in monkeys, hogs, guinea pigs, and rats do not seem to play a major role in human infections. Instead, infection seems to result primarily from man-to-man transmission via fecal contamination.

### Laboratory Diagnosis

A number of fecal specimens should be examined because the number of parasites may vary from specimen to specimen. Large, motile trophozoites with gliding motility may be found in diarrheic stools. Less frequently, typical large cysts are found in formed stools (Fig. 4). Sigmoidoscopy with aspiration of visible lesions may be helpful.

### Drug Susceptibility

*B. coli* is most sensitive to tetracycline or Diodoquin.

## BLOOD AND TISSUE PROTOZOA OF HUMANS
### Parasitic Trypanosomes of Humans

Three species of hemoflagellates of the genus *Trypanosoma*, family Trypanosomatidae, are pathogenic for man: *Trypanosoma gambiense* and *T. rhodesiense* in Africa and *T. cruzi* in America. The life cycle of each is carried out partly in humans or another mammal and partly in an insect intermediate host, in which cyclic development occurs. *T. gambiense* and *T. rhodesiense* are extracellular trypomastigote parasites of the blood, lymph, or cerebrospinal fluid, whereas *T. cruzi* occurs in trypomastigote forms in the blood and amastigote forms in the tissue.

### *Trypanosoma gambiense*
### Morphology

*T. gambiense* trypomastigotes in the blood of humans are polymorphic. They may be either typical slender flagellates with a pointed anterior end, a blunt posterior extremity, and a long flagellum, or short stumpy forms with or without a short flagellum. The flagellum of the slender form, 8 to 30 μ in length, projects from the anterior end after passing along the edge of the undulating membrane (Fig. 5). A large, oval nucleus is centrally located. A kinetoplast is located posteriorly at the base of the flagellum. The cytoplasm contains minute refractile volutin granules. Motility is wavy and spiraling.

### Life Cycle/Epidemiology

Although *T. gambiense* and *T. brucei* are morphologically identical, they are very different organisms. *T. brucei* is a parasite of wild animals that usually does not infect man, whereas *T. gambiense* is primarily a human parasite, without an important reservoir in wild or domestic animals. *T. gambiense* is transmitted from man to man by tsetse flies of the *Glossina palpalis* group. It is limited by the habitat of its vectors to forest belts, especially along rivers in tropical West and Central Africa. Trypanosomes that have been ingested by the fly during a blood meal undergo reproduction in the midgut. Long slender forms finally appear and move anteriorly through the proventriculus to the salivary glands and ducts, where epimastigote forms are produced. Eventually, short stumpy metacyclic trypanosomes are derived and pass through the channel in the hypopharynx into the bite wound when the fly feeds. During epidemics, a tsetse fly may transmit trypanosomes directly ("flying needle") from an

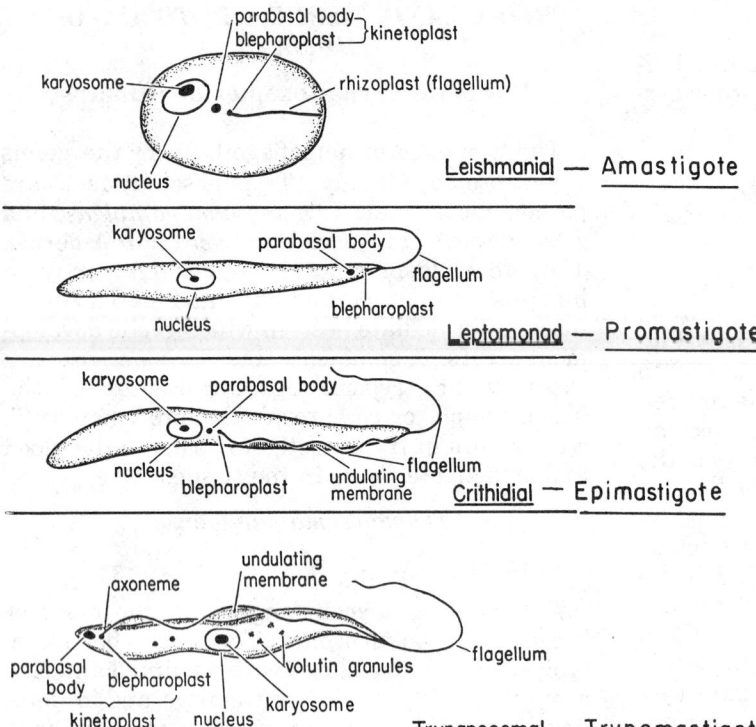

FIGURE 5. *The developmental stages in the family Trypanosomidae. (From Hunter, G. W., Swartzwelder, J. C., and Clyde, D. F., Tropical Medicine. W. B. Saunders Co., Philadelphia, 1976.)*

infected person, if the blood meal is interrupted. Congenital infections and transmission during coitus are rare.

### Laboratory Diagnosis

Diagnosis is made by finding trypanosomes in the blood, lymph node aspirates, or bone marrow in early disease, and in centrifuged cerebrospinal fluid in late disease. Preparations are examined wet for motile organisms or stained with Romanowsky stains. The hematocrit tube-centrifuge technique is valuable in the diagnosis of *T. gambiense* infections (Lumsden, 1977). Small laboratory animals are less susceptible to *T. gambiense* than to the Rhodesian form. Culture of *T. gambiense* is difficult and not useful in diagnosis. Presumptive diagnosis is possible by monitoring serum IgM levels, which are greatly elevated during trypanosomiasis. Serologic techniques include the complement fixation and indirect immunofluorescent tests.

### Drug Susceptibility

*T. gambiense* is sensitive to suramin sodium, pentamidine isethionate, and lomidine methanesulfonate. These drugs are effective in the treatment of the early stages of infection before the central nervous system is involved. In the late stages, synthetic arsenicals or antimony analogs of the melarsen group, which cross the blood-

brain barrier, are used for treatment. Of these drugs, *T. gambiense* is most sensitive to tryparsamide, melarsoprol (Mel B), and MSbB. *T. gambiense* may become resistant to these compounds, which are frequently used in combination with suramin.

### Immunity

*T. gambiense* can escape the immune response of the host by antigenic variation. The variant antigens are glycoproteins, which are the major components of the surface coat (glycocalyx) of the trypanosome. This phenomenon has delayed immunologic approaches to prevention (Doyle, 1977).

### *Trypanosoma rhodesiense*

### Morphology

The morphology of this species is identical with that of *T. gambiense* (Fig. 5).

### Life Cycle/Epidemiology

*T. rhodesiense* is confined to East Africa in savannah areas in which cattle are raised. Its incidence and the occurrence of epidemics are lower than those for *T. gambiense*. *T. rhodesiense* has a large reservoir in wild animals, and the vectors *Glossina morsitans*, *G. pallidipes*, and *G. swynnertoni* feed primarily on ungulates and only infrequently on man. The life cycle is the same as that of *T. gambiense*.

### Laboratory Diagnosis

The same procedures for *T. gambiense* infections are used for *T. rhodesiense* infections. Parasites are usually more numerous in the blood during Rhodesian trypanosomiasis, and small laboratory rodents are easily infected by intraperitoneal inoculation of whole blood that contains trypanosomes.

### Drug Susceptibility

The same drugs used to treat *T. gambiense* infections are used against *T. rhodesiense*.

### Immunity

Immunologic response is the same as that of *T. gambiense*.

### *Trypanosoma cruzi*

### Morphology

*T. cruzi* is a pleomorphic hemoflagellate that infects the blood and tissue of mammals in most countries of the Western Hemisphere. Man is less frequently infected than smaller mammals. The trypomastigote in the blood is about 20 $\mu$ long. In some cases, stumpy forms about 15 $\mu$ long may be observed. In stained blood smears the organism is usually U- or S-shaped and has a large kinetoplast near its posterior end. A flagellum arises in this area, passes through the margin of the undulating membrane, and proceeds free anteriorly for about one third of the body length. The organism does not multiply in the trypomastigote form. The amastigote form is found in various tissue cells. It is a small oval body 3 to 5 $\mu$ in diameter, containing a nucleus and a small rodlike kinetoplast (Fig. 5). In this stage the parasite divides rapidly and forms many amastigotes.

### Life Cycle/Epidemiology

*T. cruzi* is transmitted to small mammals by various species of blood-feeding triatomids that serve as intermediate hosts. Man becomes infected when susceptible species of triatomids become domesticated. Human infections are common in South America and rare in the United States, because domestic triatomes usually live in thatched roofs or cracks in adobe walls in the former location. Trypomastigotes are ingested by triatomids during a blood meal and undergo cyclic development in the gut of the insect. Amastigotes form in the foregut, epimastigotes in the midgut, and infective trypomastigotes in the hindgut. Trypomastigote forms are deposited on the skin with the feces during feeding. The feces is rubbed either into the bite wound or onto the conjunctiva, because the insect usually feeds on the human face while a person is sleeping. Trypomastigotes invade local reticuloendothelial cells and multiply rapidly as amastigotes. Trypomastigote forms are produced and appear in the blood. They circulate to various tissues, where amastigote forms are again produced intracellularly. After an acute phase in man, the parasitemia subsides, but amastigotes may continue to multiply and may lead to serious consequences years later in the chronic stage of the infection.

Nondomestic species of triatomids live in the nests of various mammals and carry on the cycle in nature by fecal contamination or by being eaten by certain mammals. In the latter case, infective stages may be passed across the mucous membranes of the mouth. Various modifications of the life cycle are presented in Figure 6.

Significant human disease is found only in areas in which the triatomid is domesticated and defecates while feeding. Dogs and cats may be important reservoirs in endemic areas. Asymptomatic infections with *T. cruzi* occur and have been documented primarily in geographic areas in which triatomid species do not live in close association with humans. Nonpathogenic strains of *T. cruzi* may be responsible for some of these cases.

Congenital transmission has been reported.

### Laboratory Diagnosis

The laboratory diagnosis depends on finding the organism in blood or tissue. Thick and thin blood films prepared during the acute stage, stained and unstained, may exhibit trypanoform stages. Parasites are never plentiful, however, because they do not multiply in peripheral blood. Concentration of large volumes of blood is helpful. Biopsies may reveal amastigote forms. Blood and bone marrow aspirates cultivated on diphasic blood agar media yield epimastigote forms in about 30 per cent of patients with positive serology. In xenodiagnosis, parasite-free triatomids are allowed to feed on the patient. Two weeks later, the intestinal contents of the triatomids are examined for hemoflagellates. This method of detecting the acute and chronic stages of the disease is not used outside of Latin America. Finally, sensitive serologic techniques (complement fixation, indirect hemagglutination, and indirect fluorescent antibody) are available for establishing a presumptive diagnosis. Many are available commercially as kits (Kagan and Norman, 1974).

*T. rangeli*, a nonpathogenic species of trypanosome, is found in Central and South America in humans and other mammals. It can be differentiated from *T. cruzi* by its smaller kinetoplast and

WILD CYCLES                                                      DOMICILIARY CYCLES

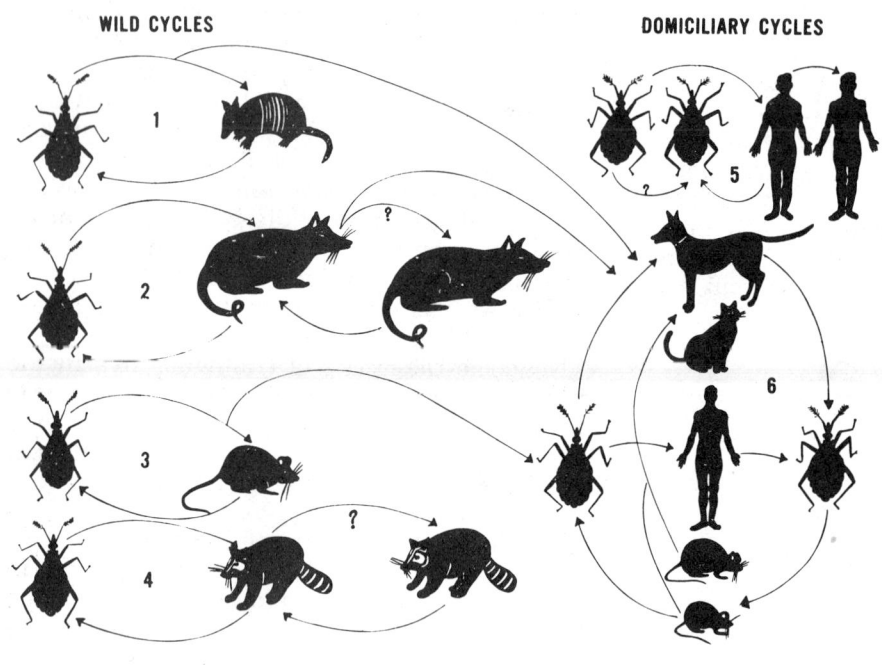

**FIGURE 6.** *Wild and domestic cycles of Chagas' disease — modalities and relationships. 1,* Panstrongylus geniculatus *is often associated with armadillos: adults enter houses, attracted by lights. 2, Opossums (*Didelphis *spp.) are associated with several triatomines and both marsupials and insects visit human dwellings. 3, Rats and other rodents are associated with insects that also fly to houses. 4, Raccoons may be associated with triatomines but, as with opossums, they may transmit T. cruzi among themselves without participation of the insect. 5, In the absence of domestic animals there is a cycle between the insect and man. Transmission from one insect to another has been suggested, and transmission from man to man is a fact, both transplacentally and transfusionally. 6, Other domestic animals might participate in the cycle and some of them may become infected by eating small rodents. (From Zeledón, R. In Trypanosomiasis and Leishmaniasis with special reference to Chagas' disease. Ciba Foundation Symposium 20, new series, 1974. Published by Elsevier. Excerpta Medica. North-Holland, Associated Scientific Publishers, Amsterdam.)*

by the presence of dividing forms in stained blood smears.

### Drug Susceptibility

No known drug will cure *T. cruzi* infections. *T. cruzi* is probably sensitive to the delta-amine quinolines that eradicate the majority of blood forms during acute disease. No known agent is effective against the intracellular leishmanial stage.

### Immunity

*T. cruzi* is strongly immunogenic. The highest titers of antibodies are found during the acute stage. When the parasitemia drops, the titers also decrease. Cell-mediated immunity plays an important role in resistance to *T. cruzi* but may also be responsible for the tissue damage in chronic infections.

Antigenic variation does not occur with *T. cruzi*, and there is cross-immunity between heterologous strains. Vaccination confers only partial protection.

## Parasitic Leishmania of Man

The genus *Leishmania*, family Trypanosomatidae, includes four species — *Leishmania donovani*, *L. tropica*, *L. mexicana*, and *L. braziliensis* —all of which occur as intracellular

amastigotes in man and promastigotes in phlebotomine sandfly intermediate hosts and in cultures (Fig. 5). All species are morphologically identical, and serologic separation has not been entirely satisfactory. They have been separated primarily by their tendency to cause visceral, cutaneous, or mucocutaneous involvement in humans.

### *Leishmania donovani*

#### Morphology

In this species the organism is located in the viscera, in the reticuloendothelial cells of the spleen, liver, bone marrow, and lymph glands. *L. donovani* is a small, round, or ovoid intracellular amastigote, 2 to 5 $\mu$ in diameter. It contains a rodlike kinetoplast and a peripheral nucleus.

#### Life Cycle/Epidemiology

Various species of phlebotomine sandflies, depending on locality, serve as intermediate hosts. Human cells containing amastigote forms are ingested by the fly. The amastigotes are liberated in the insect's gut, transformed into promastigotes, multiply by binary fission, and move to an anterior station in the pharynx of the insect. When the insect bites, these forms pass out of the insect, enter the host's local reticuloendothelial cells, and are then distributed to the viscera.

Human infections occur in India, the Mediterranean countries, Africa, China, Middle Asia, and

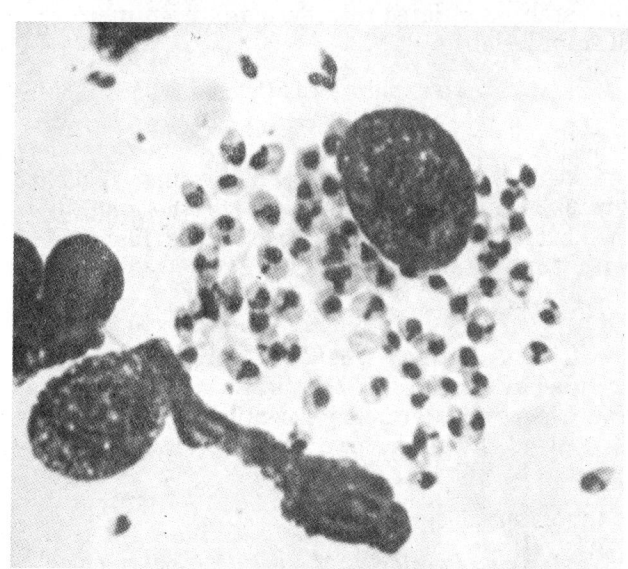

**FIGURE 7.** Leishmania donovani *in stained smear from spleen puncture. (From Hunter, G. W., Swartzwelder, J. C., and Clyde, D. F., Tropical Medicine. W. B. Saunders Co., Philadelphia, 1976.)*

Central and South America. In certain geographic areas man-to-man transmission is the sole method of spread of disease. In other areas, jackals, foxes, and domestic dogs may serve as reservoirs. Animals may acquire leishmaniasis by eating infected carcasses, thus perpetuating an animal reservoir.

### Laboratory Diagnosis

The definitive diagnosis depends on the demonstration of *L. donovani* amastigotes in stained smears from material collected by splenic, liver, or sternal puncture (Fig. 7). Culture of the material on NNN medium is also valuable. Blood culture and examination of stained films of the buffy coat for macrophages containing amastigote forms will yield positive results in most cases. The complement fixation test is usually positive. The formol-gel test is a useful screening technique. When 1 drop of commercial formalin is added to 1 milliliter of serum from a patient with kala-azar, the serum solidifies and becomes opaque within 3 to 30 minutes.

### Drug Susceptibility

*L. donovani* is sensitive to two groups of compounds: (1) pentavalent antimony derivatives, including sodium antimony gluconate, neostibosan, and urea stibamine; and (2) certain aromatic diamidines, including hydroxystilbamidine and pentamidine isethionate.

### Immunity

*Leishmania* organisms are protected from antibodies by their location inside macrophages. Humans have been successfully vaccinated with promastigotes from a rodent strain.

## *Leishmania tropica*

### Morphology

*L. tropica* invades mononuclear and polymorphonuclear leukocytes and epithelial cells of the skin. The intracellular amastigote forms are identical to those of *L. donovani*.

### Life Cycle/Epidemiology

Infection is prevalent in large areas of Asia, the countries around the Mediterranean, and the north and west coasts of Africa. Transmission is the same as for *L. donovani*. Two subspecies have been recognized: *L. tropica major*, which causes "moist" or rural leishmaniasis, and *L. tropica minor*, the cause of "dry" or urban leishmaniasis. Gerbils are a primary extrahuman reservoir of rural leishmaniasis, and dogs are a primary extrahuman reservoir of urban leishmaniasis.

### Laboratory Diagnosis

Diagnosis is made by demonstrating *L. tropica* amastigotes in cells of stained smears obtained from curettage or needle aspiration of the indurated margin of the dermal lesion. Culture of aspirates on NNN medium, with bacterial growth controlled, yields promastigotes. The leishmanial skin test becomes positive early in the infection and remains positive for life.

### Drug Susceptibility

Neostibosan is the most effective drug.

### Immunity

Infection results in life-long immunity to homologous strains. Therefore, children are often deliberately inoculated intradermally with material from lesions.

## Leishmania braziliensis

### Morphology

Like *L. tropica*, *L. braziliensis* invades cells of the skin but may also spread to the mucous membranes. The amastigote stage is identical with that of *L. donovani*.

### Life Cycle/Epidemiology

Infections with *L. braziliensis* are widely distributed as a zoonosis in the forests of Central and South America, with the exception of Chile and Argentina. Rodents serve as reservoirs. Man is infected by phlebotomine sandflies.

### Laboratory Diagnosis

The demonstration of *T. braziliensis* amastigotes from skin lesions (see *L. tropica*) is comparatively easy in early infections because the parasites are numerous. In older infections, culture on NNN medium may be successful. The Montenegro skin test is specific and sensitive, and remains positive for life.

### Drug Susceptibility

*L. braziliensis* is sensitive to pentavalent antimonials, cycloguanil pamoate, and amphotericin B.

### Immunity

Infection produces only strain specific immunity. Experimental work suggests that immunity may be induced by vaccination with epimastigotes from culture.

## Leishmania mexicana

### Morphology

*L. mexicana* amastigotes invade cells of the skin and are identical with those of *L. donovani*.

### Life Cycle/Epidemiology

Infections occur in Mexico, Belize, and northern Guatemala. However, the organism is believed to be present throughout the forests of Central and northern South America. Like *L. braziliensis*, it is also a forest zoonosis maintained in wild rodents with phlebotomine sandflies as vectors.

### Laboratory Diagnosis

Amastigote forms of *L. mexicana* are easy to find in smears of early lesions. In late infections they are difficult to find and isolate. A skin test using refined antigen is helpful (Zeledón and Ponce, 1974).

### Drug Susceptibility

*L. mexicana* is sensitive to pentavalent antimonials and cycloguanil pamoate.

### Immunity

Immunity against reinfection occurs with *L. mexicana*, but little cross-immunity occurs between strains.

# Parasites of Uncertain Taxonomic Status

## Toxoplasma gondii

### Morphology

*T. gondii* is an obligate intracellular sporozoan parasite of man and animals with worldwide distribution. Recent studies of its life cycle suggest a taxonomic relationship to the Eimeriidae, order Coccidia. Tachyzoites, the rapidly multiplying forms in acute infection, are cresent shaped, 6 to 7 $\mu$ long by 2 to 4 $\mu$ wide, and contain an oval nucleus (Fig. 8). Electron microscopy has revealed many organelles in common with the coccidia. Intracellular multiplication occurs by endodyogeny, with two daughter cells forming within the pellicle of the parent. Cysts formed in chronic infections are 200 to 1000 $\mu$ in diameter, oval to round, and contain numerous bradyzoites, the slowly multiplying forms. Oocysts containing eight sporozoites are passed in the feces of infected felines, primarily the domestic cat.

### Life Cycle/Epidemiology

Many animals, both wild and domestic, are infected with *T. gondii*. Man becomes infected primarily by eating poorly cooked or raw meat containing cysts. Contamination of food or drink with oocysts from cat feces also occurs but probably plays only a minor role in human transmission. The ingestion of cysts or oocysts by humans gives rise to a schizogonic or proliferative phase with rapidly multiplying tachyzoites in many tissues. Eventually, as a resting stage, cysts containing many bradyzoites develop. A schizogonic and gametogenic cycle occurs in the intestinal epithelium of felines with production of oocysts. In the acute stage in humans, the organisms may be transferred transplacentally. The life cycle is presented in Figure 9.

### Laboratory Diagnosis

The demonstration of cysts via biopsy specimens does not establish a causal relationship for clinical illness because cysts are found in both acute and chronic infections. Demonstration of organisms in brain impression smears of a new-

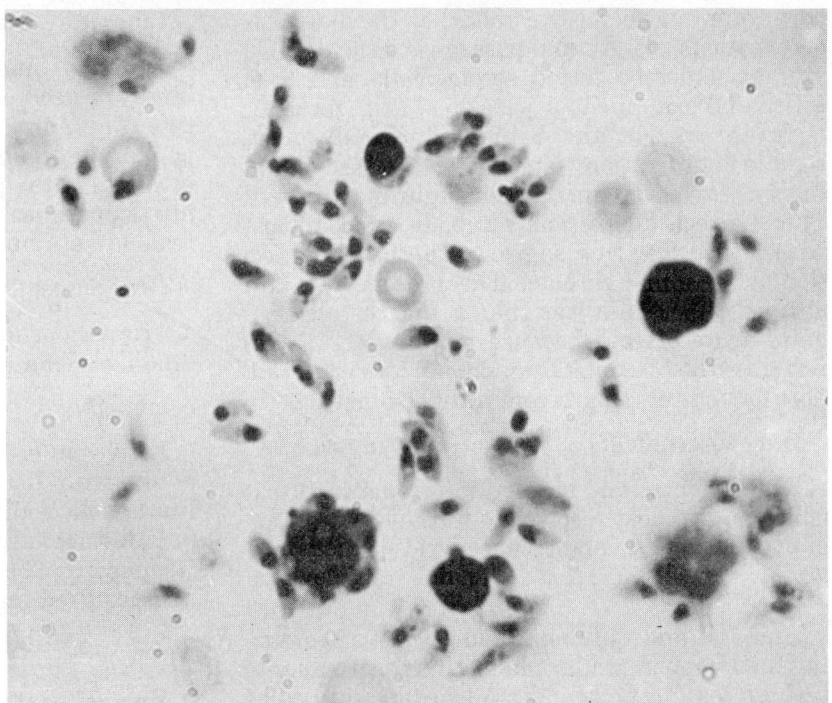

**FIGURE 8.** *Mouse peritoneal fluid demonstrating tachyzoites freed from cells (1000 ×). (From Hunter, G. W., Swartzwelder, J. C., and Clyde, D. F.: Tropical Medicine. W. B. Saunders Co., Philadelphia, 1976.)*

POSTULATED TRANSMISSION OF TOXOPLASMOSIS

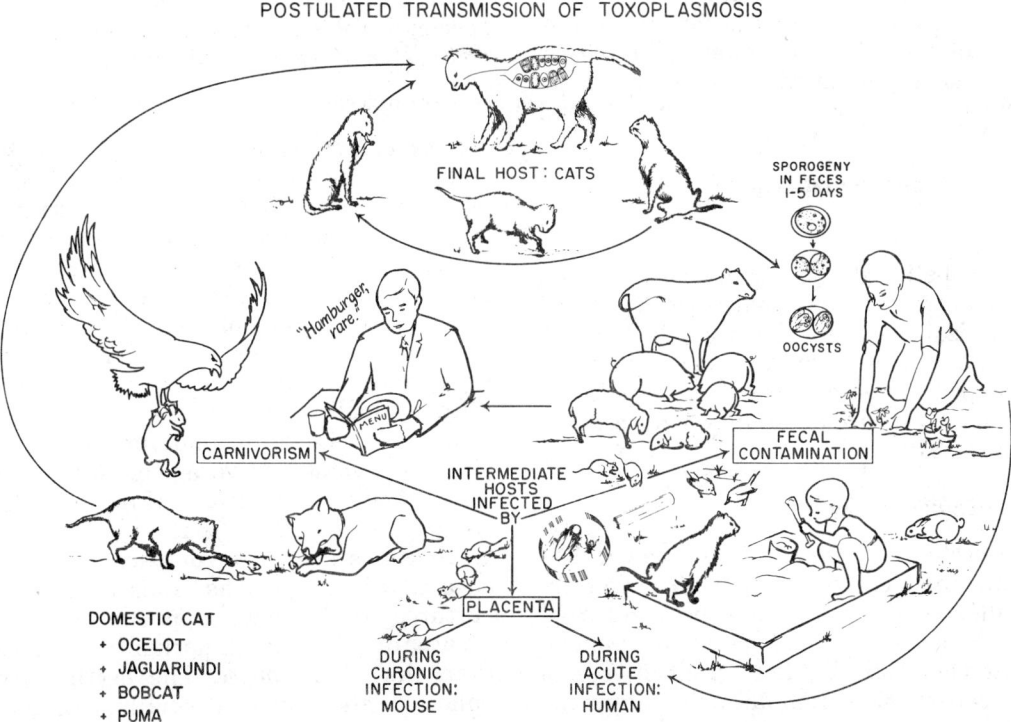

**FIGURE 9.** *Postulated life cycle and transmission of Toxoplasma. Cats and certain other felines are shown as final hosts, and other animals and humans as intermediate hosts. Flies and cockroaches can serve as transport hosts. At right, infection with oocysts is shown. At left, transmission by carnivorism is indicated. Below, the transplacental route of transmission is indicated. (Modified slightly from Frenkel, J. K.: Toxoplasmosis. In Marcial-Rojas, R. A. (ed.): Pathology of Protozoal and Helminthic Diseases. Williams & Wilkins, Baltimore, 1971.)*

born infant at necropsy establishes the diagnosis of toxoplasmosis. Animal passage is difficult. Test animals must be tested serologically and then killed and examined for parasites. Four serologic tests are in use: the Sabin-Feldman dye test, complement fixation test, indirect fluorescent antibody test, and indirect hemagglutination test. The indirect fluorescent antibody test is most widely used. The titer suggests whether the infection is acute or chronic. The presence of IgM antibody in a child less than 6 months old suggests acute disease because maternal IgM does not cross the placenta. Commercial kits are available for indirect fluorescent antibody testing.

### Drug Susceptibility

Experimental and natural infections with toxoplasma are most responsive to the combination of pyrimethamine and trisulfapyridine.

### Immunity

Humoral and cellular immunity develops during the lymphoreticular phase, and the number of tachyzoites rapidly diminishes. Antibodies against several antigens of toxoplasma can be demonstrated, and immune mononuclear cells no longer support the intracellular multiplication of *Toxoplasma* organisms. The development of immunity coincides with the transformation of toxoplasmosis into the chronic, cyst-forming stage. Cysts are isolated from the immune processes, and reactivation can occur when immunosuppression is induced by either natural or artificial means.

## *Pneumocystis carinii*

### Morphology

*P. carinii* is believed by some to be a coccidian. Its exact taxonomic status is unknown. The most easily recognizable stage is the cyst, which is 5 to 12 $\mu$ in diameter and contains eight ovoid or crescent-shaped parasites (sporozoites?) with eccentric nuclei. Cysts are found in a honeycombed exudate in the alveoli.

### Life Cycle/Epidemiology

The life cycle of *P. carinii* is unknown. The infection was first reported in endemic form from Europe, but sporadic cases have been reported worldwide. *P. carinii* is widespread in animals, both wild and domestic, but host specificity seems high, and transmission from animals to humans seems unlikely. Aerosol dispersion of respiratory tract secretions may be involved in epidemics. Sporadic cases are thought to result from latent infections that become activated by immunosuppression.

### Laboratory Diagnosis

Silver or Giemsa stains of tissue from open lung biopsy or needle aspirates have been most productive (Fig. 10). Sputum, tracheal smears, and hypopharyngeal material do not routinely show evidence of the parasite, but bronchial brushings are sometimes useful. Experimental serologic tests are of unproven value.

### Drug Susceptibility

Trimethoprim-sulfamethoxazole and pentamidine isethionate are the only useful drugs.

### Immunity

Active infection occurs in neonates and in adults with disturbances of either immunoglobulins or cell-mediated immunity. Normal adults do not develop disease but are probably infected frequently. The relative importance of natural and acquired immunity is unknown.

## Malarial Parasites of Man

The malarial parasites of man are species of the genus *Plasmodium* in which schizogony (asexual cycle) takes place in human erythrocytes and sporogony (sexual cycle) takes place in mosquitoes of the genus *Anopheles*. All species have similar life cycles and morphology (Fig. 11). The species involved are *Plasmodium falciparum, P. vivax, P. malariae,* and *P. ovale.*

### Morphology

*Plasmodium vivax* (Fig. 12). Young trophozoites appear in Giemsa-stained blood films as delicate rings of blue cytoplasm. Each contains one red nucleus and is about one third the size of the red cell. As the trophozoite grows, it becomes actively motile and its outline becomes extremely irregular. Granules of yellowish-brown pigment develop in the cytoplasm of the parasite. The erythrocyte becomes enlarged, and a bright red diffuse stippling, Schüffner's dots, may be seen in some cases. Large trophozoites undergo schizogony, producing an average of 16 merozoites.

*Plasmodium malariae* (Fig. 13). The ring stage is identical to that of *P. vivax.* Mature trophozoites are more compact than those of *P. vivax* and may extend as bands across the infected erythrocyte. Pigment appears earlier and in greater quantity and is darker brown and coarser than that in *P. vivax.* The erythrocyte is not enlarged and stains normally. An average of eight merozoites is produced by schizogony. The merozoites are arranged in a rosette around a centrally collected pigment mass.

*Plasmodium ovale.* This species resembles *P. malariae* in many ways but the infected erythro-

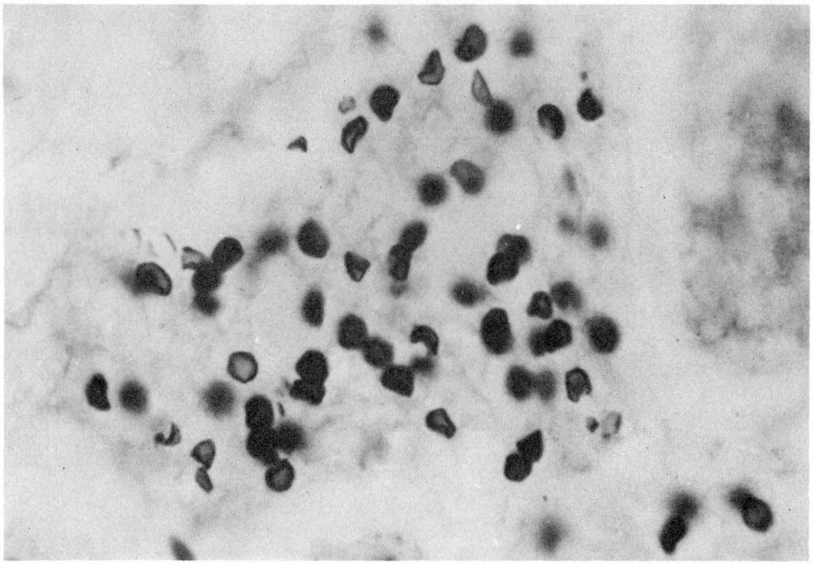

**FIGURE 10.** *Cysts of* Pneumocystis carinii *in alveolar exudate. Note round, crescentic, and other-shaped cysts with collapsed walls; silver methenamine-fast green stain, 1000 ×. (From Hunter, G. W., Swartzwelder, J. C., and Clyde, D. F.: Tropical Medicine. W. B. Saunders Co., Philadelphia, 1976.)*

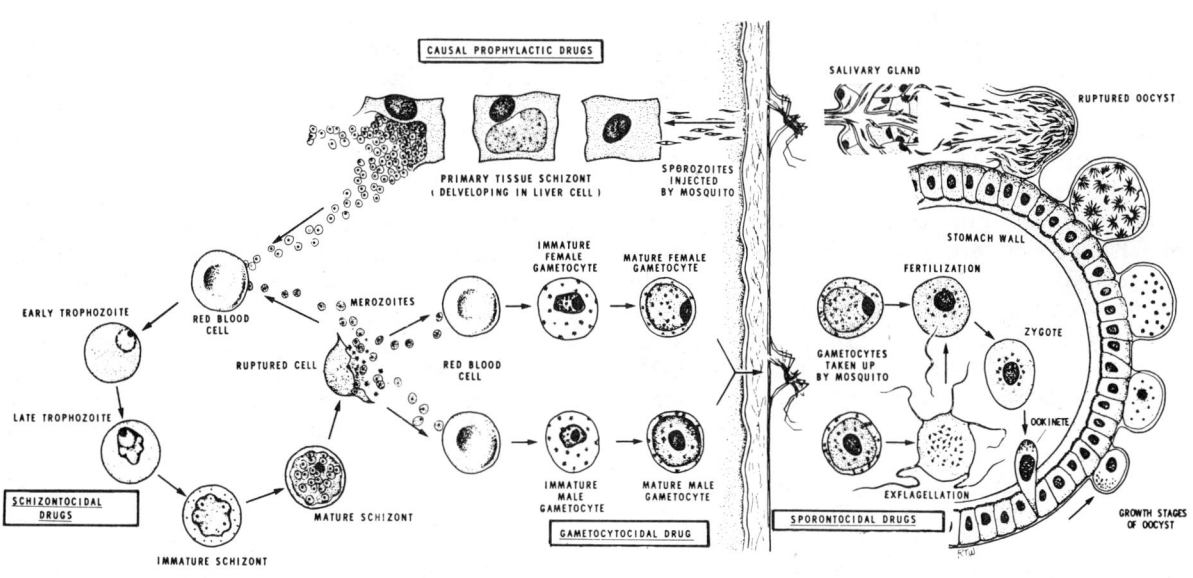

**CYCLE IN MAN**          **CYCLE IN MOSQUITO**

**FIGURE 11.** *Schematic representation of typical malaria life cycle. (Modified from Hunter, G. W., Swartzwelder, J. C., and Clyde, D. F., Tropical Medicine. W. B. Saunders Co., Philadelphia, 1976.)*

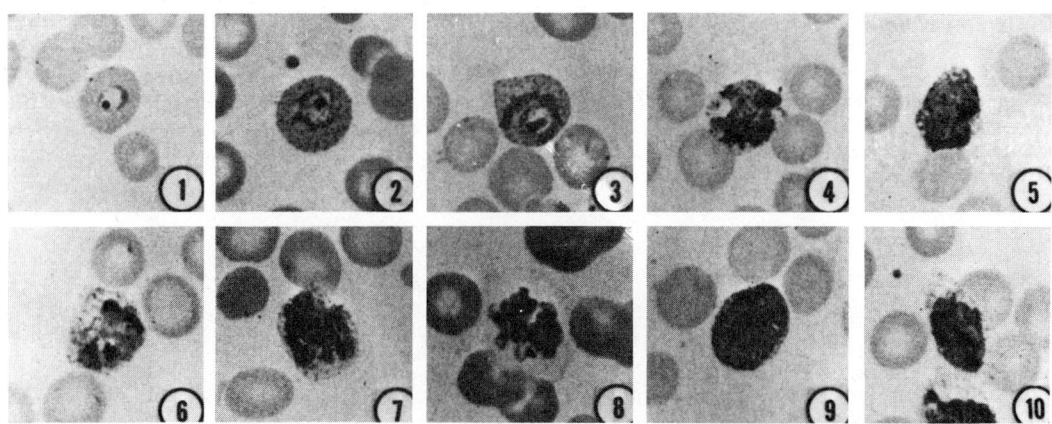

**FIGURE 12.** *Developmental stages of* Plasmodium vivax *in erythrocytes. 1, Young trophozoite, ring stage. 2, Developing trophozoite in enlarged erythrocyte with Schüffner's dots. 3, Older trophozoite with pseudopod. 4, Mature trophozoite with irregular margin. 5, Schizont showing initial division of nucleus. 6, Older schizont with four nuclei. 7, More mature schizont. 8, Mature schizont with 16 nuclei and clumped pigment. 9, Macrogametocyte. 10, Microgametocyte. (From Wilcox, A.: Manual for the Microscopical Diagnosis of Malaria in Man. National Institute of Health Bulletin No. 180, U.S. Government Printing Office, Washington, D.C., 1942.)*

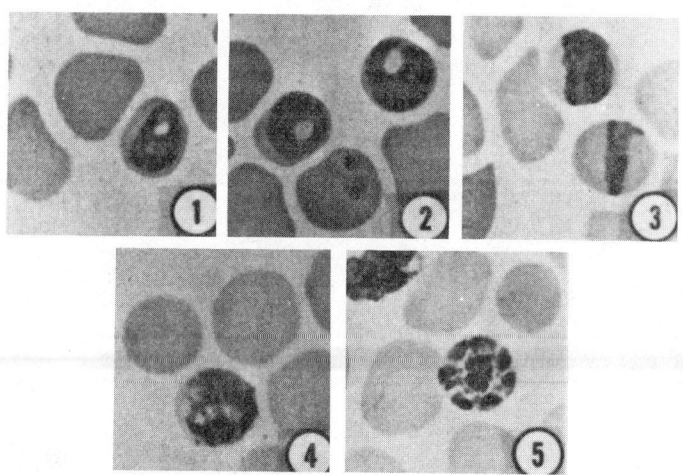

**FIGURE 13.** *Developmental stages of* Plasmodium malariae *in erythrocytes. 1, Maturing trophozoite. 2, One ring form with pseudopod and two mature trophozoites with heavy pigment. 3, Two trophozoites in band form. 4, A schizont with three nuclei. 5, Mature schizont in "rosette' form. (From Wilcox, A.: Manual for the Microscopical Diagnosis of Malaria in Man. National Institute of Health Bulletin No. 180, U.S. Government Printing Office, Washington, D.C., 1942.)*

cytes behave like those infected with *P. vivax*. Erythrocytes, which may show Schüffner's dots, are oval, slightly enlarged, and pale. The margin is often crenated. The trophozoite of *P. ovale* is compact and band forms may appear. An average of eight merozoites is produced by schizogony.

**Plasmodium falciparum** (Figs. 14 and 15). Ring forms are smaller and more delicate than those of *P. vivax* and may have double nuclei. Multiple infection of erythrocytes is common. Infected erythrocytes are not enlarged but may have comma-like red markings, called Maurer's clefts, in the cytoplasm. Infected erythrocytes are removed from the peripheral circulation, and further development and schizogony are accomplished in the capillaries of the viscera. Therefore, intermediate and mature forms of the schizogonic cycle are not seen. Crescentic gametocytes, however, may be seen in the peripheral circulation. Their shape differs from that of the rounded gametocytes of *P. vivax*, *P. malariae*, and *P. ovale*.

### Life Cycle/Epidemiology

Malaria generally occurs between the latitudes 45 degrees north and 40 degrees south. *P. vivax* infections are the most widely distributed; *P. malariae* infections are comparatively rare. *P.*

*falciparum* occurs predominantly in tropical regions, and *P. ovale* is mostly limited to Africa.

The sexual cycle in certain anopheline mosquitoes begins with the ingestion of mature gametocytes (Fig. 11). In the mosquito stomach the microgametocyte produces microgametes (flagella-like structures) that detach (exflagellation) and migrate to the macrogamete (female cell), which was formed by maturation of the macrogametocyte. Fertilization takes place, and the zygote elongates and becomes motile (ookinete). It penetrates the mosquito stomach wall and grows into an oocyst beneath the outer layer. Many filamentous sporozoites are produced by rapid multiplication, which results finally in rupture of the oocyst. Sporozoites move to the salivary glands and are injected at the next feeding.

The asexual cycle begins with the entry of sporozoites into human hosts. They rapidly enter the parenchymal cells of the liver and undergo rapid multiplication (exoerythrocytic stage). The rate of development and certain morphologic characteristics vary with the species of *Plasmodium*. Finally, infected parenchymal cells rupture, releasing myriads of merozoites that invade erythrocytes, producing ring stages. Schizogony occurs in parasitized erythrocytes, and their

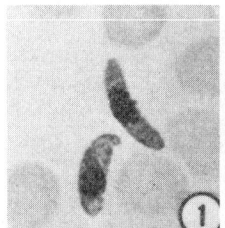 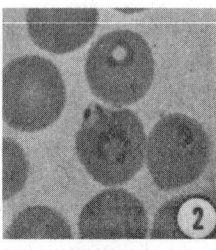 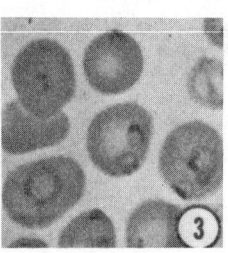

**FIGURE 14.** *Developmental stages of* Plasmodium falciparum *in erythrocytes. 1, Two crescent-shaped macrogametocytes. 2, Ring stages showing double nuclei and marginal forms. 3, Heavy infection showing multiple infection. (From Wilcox, A.: Manual for the Microscopical Diagnosis of Malaria in Man. National Institute of Health Bulletin No. 180, U.S. Government Printing Office, Washington, D.C., 1942.)*

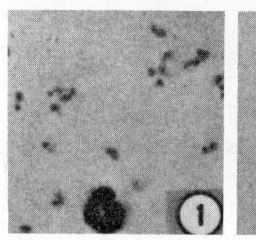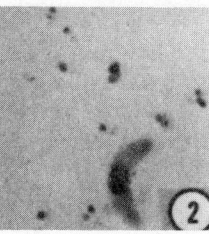

**FIGURE 15.** *Thick blood films of a Plasmodium* falciparum *infection. 1, Ring stage trophozoites appearing as "commas," "exclamation marks," etc. 2, Ring stages and a crescent-shaped gametocyte. (From Wilcox, A.: Manual for the Microscopical Diagnosis of Malaria in Man. National Institute of Health Bulletin No. 180, U.S. Government Printing Office, Washington, D.C., 1942.)*

eventual rupture frees merozoites to invade other erythrocytes and repeat the cycle. The schizogony is usually synchronous in all species except *P. falciparum*. Eventually gametocytes are produced to perpetuate the cycle.

### Laboratory Diagnosis

Definitive diagnosis depends on identifying plasmodia in thick and thin blood smears stained with Giemsa stain (Table 3). Serologic techniques are available and are useful as an aid to diagnosis.

### Drug Susceptibility

The susceptibility of plasmodia to drugs varies with their stage in the life cycle. Plasmodia in the erythrocytic stage are most sensitive to the 4-aminoquinoline drugs, chloroquine and amodiaquine. Chloroquine-resistant strains of *P. falciparum* from Southeast Asia and South America have retained their sensitivity to quinine. Nei-

ther quinine nor the 4-aminoquinolines eradicate the exoerythrocytic stage of malaria. Primaquine is the most active drug against this stage of the life cycle. The dihydrofolate reductase inhibitors, proquanil, pyrimethamine, and trimethoprim, show only weak activity against the erythrocytic stage but are sporontocidal; that is, they prevent development of sporozoites in the mosquito and in humans inoculated with sporozoites by an infected mosquito. Trimethoprim, however, acts synergistically with sulfonamides and sulfones against the erythrocytic stage. *Plasmodium* organisms become resistant to the sulfones, sulfonamides, and dihydrofolate reductase group if they are used alone.

The variation in sensitivity of different stages in the *Plasmodium* life cycle and the tendency of *Plasmodium* organisms to become resistant to a single drug has been countered by treating most forms of malaria with two or more drugs. The combination of chloroquine and primaquine results in radical cure of all forms of malaria except chloroquine-resistant *P. falciparum* malaria. Infections with chloroquine-sensitive *P. falciparum* are eradicated by chloroquine alone, since there is no persistent exoerythrocyte cycle. Chloroquine-resistant *P. falciparum* is treated with two or more schizontocides; the combination of quinine, pyrimethamine, and either a sulfonamide or sulfone is especially effective.

### Immunity

*P. vivax* and *P. falciparum* produce partial homologous immunity that is strain-specific. There is no cross-immunity between species. Man has been immunized with irradiated sporozoites of *P. falciparum* and *P. vivax*, but immunity was

**TABLE 3.  Key for the Differentiation of the Three Common Malaria Species in Peripheral Blood Films**

**THIN FILMS**

1. No intermediate stages present (no late trophozoites or schizonts). Usually only characteristic rings (rod-like nucleus; rings located at periphery of red cell; binucleate rings; small rings; frequently multiple rings in a red cell) and/or cresent-shaped gametocytes present — *P. falciparum*
2. Intermediate stages present (late trophozoites and schizonts) — *P. vivax* or *P. malariae*
   A. Parasitized red cells enlarged and pale; trophozoites with irregular outlines; pigment fine; Schüffner's dots may be present — *P. vivax*
   B. Parasitized red cells normal in size and color; growing forms compact or "band" forms; pigment coarse; no stippling of the red cells — *P. malariae*

**THICK FILMS**

1. No intermediate stages present. Usually only characteristic *rings* (rings, exclamation marks, swallows, comets, etc.) and/or cresent-shaped gametocytes present — *P. falciparum*
2. Intermediate stages present — *P vivax* or *P. malariae*
   A. Trophozoites with irregular cytoplasmic outline — *P. vivax*
   B. Trophozoites with compact cytoplasm or "band" forms — *P. malariae*
   Note: Schüffner's dots are not always present in *P. vivax* infection.
   Crescents are not always present in *P. falciparum* infection.
   Band forms are not always present in *P. malariae* infection.

short-lived. Stages in the erythrocytic cycle produce antibodies, and these forms of the parasite are currently being examined for possible use in vaccines.

## Babesia

Various species of the genus *Babesia* are parasitic in the erythrocytes of many domestic and wild mammals. Ixodid ticks serve as intermediate hosts. Infected ticks may inoculate sporozoites when they feed on man. Only *Babesia bovis* was known to infect man until recent case reports appeared of human infections with *Babesia microti*, a strain found in rodents.

### Morphology

*Babesia* spp form tiny (1.5 to 5 $\mu$) pear-shaped, ovoid, ellipsoid, ring- or rod-shaped bodies in erythrocytes. The number, shape, and size vary with each species. No pigment is produced. Their staining characteristics are the same as those of *Plasmodium*.

### Life Cycle/Epidemiology

*Babesia* species reproduce by binary fission in infected erythrocytes. During division, the erythrocyte ruptures and new erythrocytes are invaded. Sexual development takes place in the arthropod. When sporozoites are finally produced, they invade all the tissues of the tick, including the developing eggs and salivary glands.

Babesiosis is a rare infection in man, but it may be fatal in splenectomized patients or those who are otherwise immunologically compromised. A recent epidemic involving *Babesia microti* occurred on Nantucket Island off the northeast coast of the United States (Spielman, 1976).

### Laboratory Diagnosis

Definitive diagnosis is achieved by the identification of parasites in Giemsa-stained thick and thin blood smears. Differentiation of species is difficult, and the species are easily confused with malaria organisms.

### Drug Susceptibility

The antimalarial drugs have no effect on *Babesia* strains, but the organisms show some sensitivity to the antitrypanosomal drugs 4,4′-diazoaminobenzamidine and pentamidine isethionate, but parasitemia recurs after treatment. Despite the limited response, these three drugs should be used in the immunocompromised patient because infections under these circumstances are often fatal (Miller et al., 1978).

### Immunity

There is serologic cross-reactivity between *B. bovis*, *Plasmodium falciparum*, and *P. vivax*, but cross-immunity between *Babesia* and *Plasmodium* has not been investigated.

### References

Doyle, J. J.: Antigenic variation in the salivarian trypanosomes. In Miller, L. H., Pinto, J. A., and McKelvey, Jr., J. J. (eds.): Immunity to Blood Parasites of Animals and Man. (Advances in Experimental Medical Biology, vol. 93.) New York, Plenum Press, 1977, p. 321.

Kagan, I. G., and Norman, L.: Serodiagnosis of parasitic diseases. In Lennette, E. H., Spaulding, E. H., and Truant, J. P. (eds.): Manual of Clinical Microbiology, 2nd ed. Washington, D. C., American Society of Microbiology, 1974, p. 970.

Lumsden, W. H. R.: Field diagnosis of trypanosomiasis. Trans R Soc Trop Med Hyg 71.8, 1977.

Miller, L H., Neva, F. A., and Gill, F.: Failure of chloroquine in human babesiosis (*Babesia microti*). Ann Intern Med 88:200, 1978.

Spielman, A.: Human babesiosis on Nantucket Island: Transmission by nymphal Ixodes ticks. Am J Trop Med 25:784, 1976.

Wolfe, M. S.: Giardiasis. JAMA 233:1362, 1975.

Zeledón, R., and Ponce, D.: Parasitological and immunological diagnosis of cutaneous leishmaniasis. Proceedings of the Third International Congress of Parasitology 3:239, 1974.

# 79 *NEMATHELMINTHES (Roundworms)*

## A. O. Anya, Ph.D.

The name Nemathelminthes was first used by Gegenbaur in 1859 to describe the roundworms. In his conception, the roundworms included three zoologically distinct groups of animals: the acanthocephalans, the nematodes, and the gordiaceans (nematomorphs). Vejdowsky in 1866 used the term to refer only to the nematodes and the nematomorphs. In most zoology texts, the term includes rotifers, gastrotrichs, kinorhynchs, nematodes, and nematomorphs, which are by implication related. However, the zoologic affinities of these groups are not as clear as their categorization as nemathelminthes would suggest, and Hyman (1951) prefers to regard each as an inde-

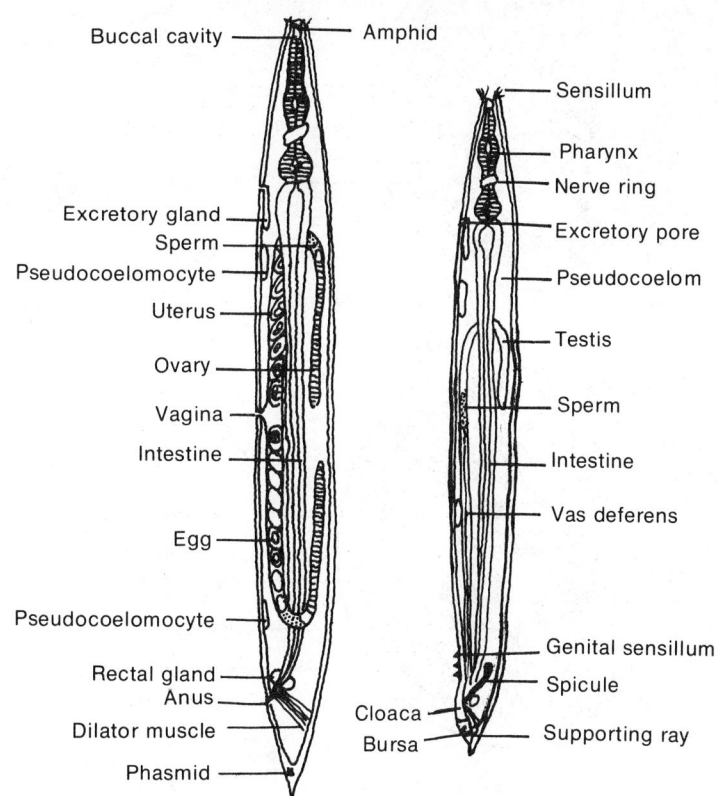

**FIGURES 1 and 2.** *Diagram of a hypothetical nematode: female (left) and male (right).*

pendent entity of phyletic status. Most modern authors have preferred this arrangement (Maggenti, 1976). Because the nematodes are the only Nemathelminthes of medical importance, the following discussion will concentrate on this group.

## *FUNCTIONAL MORPHOLOGY*

Nematodes are generally small, spindle-shaped, unsegmented, bilaterally symmetric organisms. The digestive and reproductive systems lie more or less freely in the fluid-filled body cavity, which is a pseudocoelom (Figs. 1 and 2).

Within the body cavity may also be found two, four, or six ovoid or many-branched cells called pseudocoelomocytes of unknown function. Organs of respiration and circulation are absent, and the "excretory" organs are unlike those of other invertebrates. An often-quoted characteristic of nematodes is the absence of cilia or flagella. The electron microscope, which has opened up a new era in nematode morphology and anatomy, has demonstrated typical flagella in the intestine of a free-living nematode *Eudorylaimus* sp and modified flagella in the sense organs of many nematodes including parasitic species (Zmoray and Guttekova, 1972; McLaren, 1976).

The body surface is covered by a living, thin, relatively inelastic but flexible cuticle made of modified collagen (Anya, 1966). The cuticle lines part of the inner surface of the main body openings of the digestive and reproductive systems. Fine striations and annuli may be present on the cuticular surface.

The cuticle, which is a three-layered structure consisting of cortical, median, and basal layers, is often delimited by a basement lamella from the hypodermis. The latter may be either syncytial or cellular tissue. It projects into the body cavity along the middorsal, midventral, and lateral lines, giving rise to four ridges or chords (Fig. 3). When excretory canals are present, they are embedded in the tissues of the lateral chords. The main nerves run in the middorsal and midventral hypodermal chords.

The muscle layer lies beneath the hypodermis and consists of unique, spindle-shaped, and elongated cells oriented only in the longitudinal direction. There are no circular muscles. The muscle cells are characteristically divided into contractile and noncontractile portions (Fig. 4) and are obliquely striated with the filaments of actin and myosin restricted to the basal contractile portion of the cell. The noncontractile part of the muscle cell contains the main cell organelles, such as the nucleus and mitochondria, as well as stores of

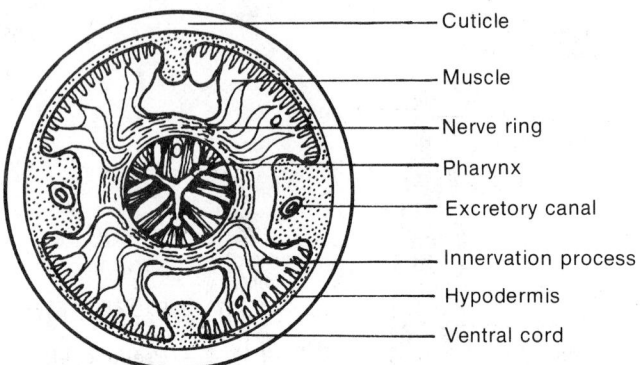

Cuticle

Muscle

Nerve ring

Pharynx

Excretory canal

Innervation process

Hypodermis

Ventral cord

**FIGURE 3.** *Transverse sections through a female nematode in the pharyngeal region (above) and in the midregion (below).*

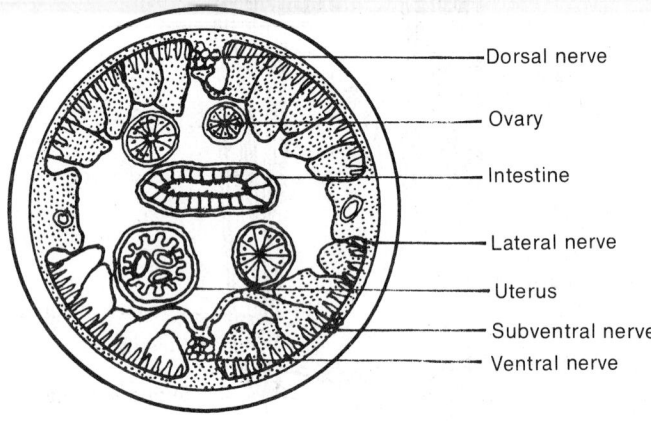

Dorsal nerve

Ovary

Intestine

Lateral nerve

Uterus

Subventral nerve

Ventral nerve

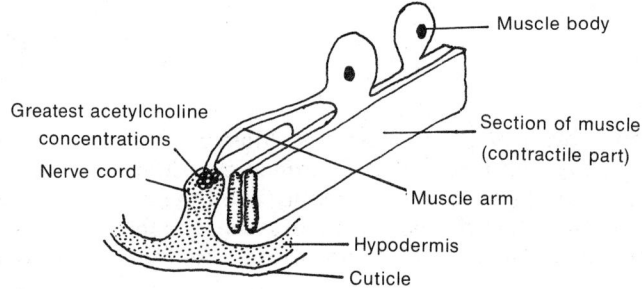

Muscle body

Greatest acetylcholine concentrations

Nerve cord

Section of muscle (contractile part)

Muscle arm

Hypodermis

Cuticle

**FIGURE 4.** *The muscle cells in nematodes. Longitudinal aspect of two muscle cells (above) and muscle cells at myoneural junction, transverse section (below).*

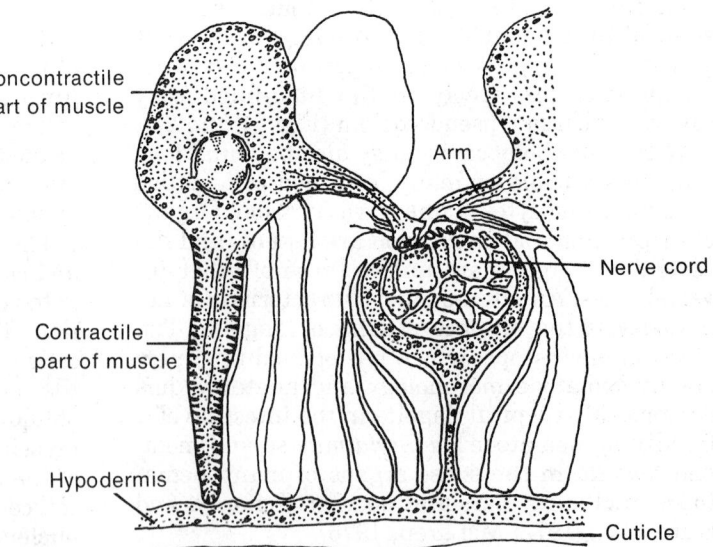

Noncontractile part of muscle

Arm

Nerve cord

Contractile part of muscle

Hypodermis

Cuticle

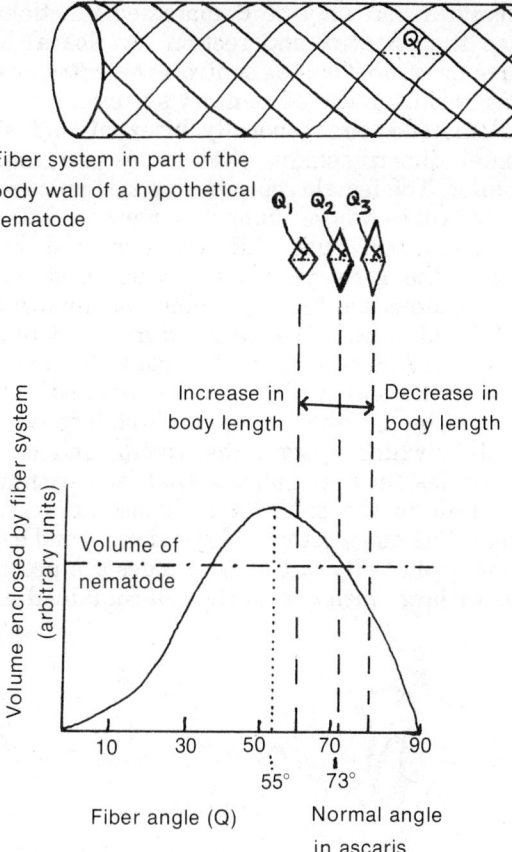

Fiber system in part of the body wall of a hypothetical nematode

**FIGURE 5.** *Arrangement of fibers in cuticle of a nematode (above) and the relationship between the volume enclosed by the fiber system in the cuticle and the angle Q (after Lee and Atkinson, 1976).*

glycogen and fat. The nerve processes extend from the muscle cells to make synaptic contact with the longitudinally oriented nerve trunks in the middorsal and midventral hypodermal chords. Thus, unlike the situation in other organisms, the muscle cells transmit innervation impulses to the nerve tissue.

The fluid-filled body cavity is notable for its high but variable turgor pressure, which ensures that its incompressible fluid content acts as a hydrostatic skeleton that is antagonistic to the longitudinal muscle layer. The efficiency of this arrangement is assured by the special arrangement of the fibers in the nematode cuticle. In *Ascaris lumbricoides,* for example, the fiber layers consist of a meshwork of spiral and relatively inelastic fibers that run counter to one another in a trellis or lattice fashion. This may best be visualized as a series of parallelograms subtending an angle (Q) that will vary within defined limits (Fig. 5). Anisometric extension of the cuticle is thus possible, and the angle Q defines the critical position from which the length and diameter of the cylindrical nematode can change without altering the volume. It has been shown mathematically that as long as Q is larger than 55 degrees, an increase in length of the

worm compensates for a slight decrease in diameter, and, in such an arrangement, the muscles must be oriented longitudinally. Measurements of fixed preparations of the cuticle of *Ascaris* give a value of 75 degrees 30′ for Q (Harris and Crofton, 1957). The interaction of pressure changes with the cuticle and the muscle maintain static equilibrium during variations in body volume, permitting the ingestion or expulsion of fluid despite the high pressure in the body cavity. This system may explain the relative invariability of nematode structure.

The alimentary system includes a mouth, buccal cavity, pharynx (esophagus), intestine, rectum, and anus (Fig. 1). The mouth is usually surrounded by lips arranged according to a hexamerous triradiate arrangement. In the male nematode, the distal section of the reproductive system also opens into the rectal region, converting the rectum into a cloaca. The buccal cavity, like the pharynx, is lined by cuticle, which may be modified into teeth or cutting plates. The triradiate pharynx is a highly muscular organ that may be divisible into muscular and glandular regions. Alternatively, it may contain three glands that open into the lumen at different points along its length. The intestine is lined by microvilli and may be demarcated functionally from the pharynx and rectum (or cloaca) by a valve or sphincter that controls the entry or exit of materials in the alimentary system.

Nematodes are generally bisexual and show sexual dimorphism in that males are usually smaller. The female reproductive system consists of two tubes whose diameters vary in different regions. Each tube differentiates into ovary (where the germinal cells at various stages of development are found), oviduct, seminal receptacle, and uterus. The two uteri may be joined to form a vagina uterina that leads to the exterior through the vulva (Fig. 6). The nematode egg is covered by a highly resistant three-layered eggshell in which lipoproteins, chitin, and certain glycosides form complexes that are extremely resistant to the entry of all substances except gases. The noteworthy ecologic success and evolutionary plasticity of the nematodes are probably due in large measure to the self-contained envi-

ronment of the embryo provided by the eggshell, as well as to the structural stability of the adult that is provided by the unique interacting system of body fluid turgor pressure, muscle, and cuticle.

The male system consists usually of a single tube differentiated into testes, seminal vesicle, and vas deferens (Fig. 7). The vas deferens, which may consist of glandular and ejaculatory portions, opens into the cloaca. The nematode spermatozoon is generally ameboid, but recent work has indicated that the shapes, sizes, and structures of this cell vary in different groups of nematodes (Anya, 1976). However, none has flagella that are characteristic of the sperm cells of other animal groups.

Some nematodes release sex attractants, and the vas deferens secretes substances that may aid the ascent of the sperm cell prior to fertilization (Green, 1967; Anya, 1973). The availability of food in the environment is an important factor

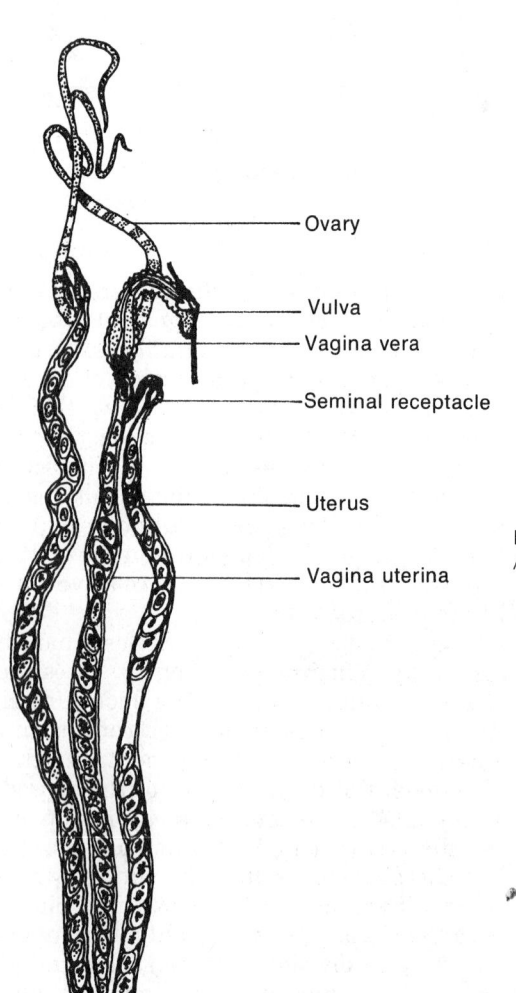

**FIGURE 6.** *Female reproductive system of a parasitic nematode,* Aspiculuris tetraptera.

Ovary

Vulva

Vagina vera

Seminal receptacle

Uterus

Vagina uterina

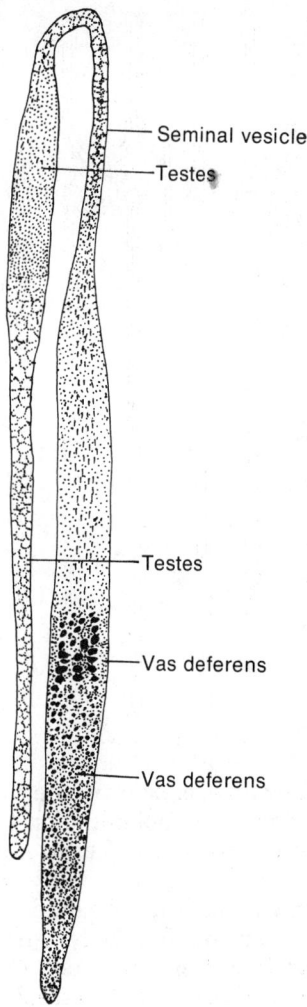

**FIGURE 7.** *Male reproductive system of the parasitic nematode, Aspiculuris tetraptera.*

determining the sex ratio of nematodes; more males are usually found in situations of nutritional stress (Anya, 1976).

What has often been called the "excretory" system in many nematodes has been so regarded purely on morphologic grounds. It is structurally variable, as it is absent in some nematodes and replaced by a pair of glandular cells, the renette cells, in others. The best known representative of the system, however, is the H type seen in *Rhabditis* sp, in which the main (longitudinal) trunks of the H are located in the lateral chords (Fig. 8). The cross-bar of the H is formed by transverse branches that traverse the pseudocoelom in the anterior region. These join before opening to the exterior through the ventrally located "excretory" pore. In some nematodes, the anterior arms of the H-shaped system may be lost, and the excretory system is therefore an inverted U structure. In others, such as the juvenile *Ancylostoma* sp, the inverted U type of "excretory" system may be associated with a pair of glandular renette cells.

The sense organs of nematodes may be associated with the mouth or with the genital or anal openings (and in some nematodes with the caudal region). There are, then, three main groups of sense organs in a nematode: the anteriorly located amphids, the posteriorly located phasmids, and the various papillae associated with the mouth, the genital opening, or the caudal region.

In the primitive state, according to De Conick (1942), the nematode mouth is surrounded by six lips, each of which bears a variable number of papillae (Fig. 9). Generally, 16 such papillae are supposed to be arranged in three concentric circles as follows: an inner and an outer labial papilla on each lip and four cephalic papillae situated behind the lips. The amphids are located on either side of the head region. The pair of phasmids is located posteriorly one on either side of the ventral median line, behind the anal opening in the female. The male nematode may bear (also in the posterior region) several pairs of genital or caudal papillae. The papillae are usual-

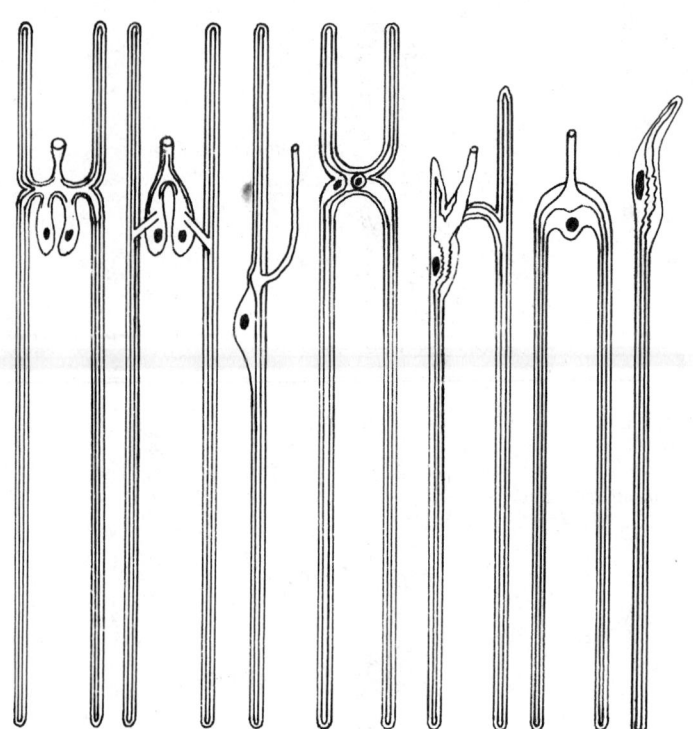

**FIGURE 8.** *Diagrammatic representation of the various types of excretory systems in nematodes.*

ly supported by an expansion of the caudal cuticle called alae or bursae, depending on the structure or the degree of cuticular inflation and the nematode group.

The amphids and the phasmids are cuticle-lined depressions on the body surface. Recent ultrastructural work has revealed that these depressions are associated with receptor and glandular cells with ciliated nerve axons (McLaren, 1976). Nerve processes from these cells have been traced to the circumpharyngeal nerve ring. This association suggests that amphids and phasmids may have a chemosensory and possibly a neurosecretory function, essential perhaps in monitoring the external environment.

The amphid of *Necator americanus* has been studied in greater detail, and the associated secretory cell is most active in the production of

choline-esterase during the period of the life cycle when the change from the lung environment to the intestinal environment takes place. The papillae also have associated ciliated nerve axons, but do not have direct access to the external environment because they are generally covered by a rather thin cuticle. This suggests a possible role as mechanoreceptors.

### LIFE CYCLES

Harris and Crofton (1957), in drawing attention to the relative invariability of nematode structure, had observed that "the elementary student may be forgiven at times for thinking that there is only one nematode but that the model comes in different sizes and with a great

**FIGURE 9.** *En-face view of the hypothetical primitive nematode (after De Conick, 1942).*

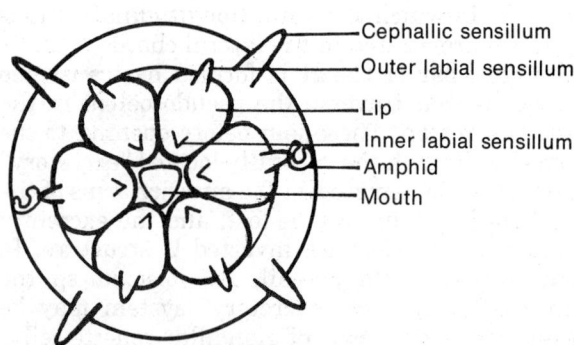

Cephallic sensillum
Outer labial sensillum
Lip
Inner labial sensillum
Amphid
Mouth

variety of life histories." As we saw in the preceding section, the apparent uniformity of nematode structure is meaningful if interpreted in the context of the unique structural relations of cuticle, muscle, and body pressure changes. The apparent variety of life cycle patterns is equally logical (and reducible to basic types) if it is seen as an ecologic adaptive strategy for parasitic life and against the background of the evolutionary history of parasitism among the nematodes. For parasitism as a way of life has evolved independently several times among these organisms. The general pattern of a particular life cycle often reflects, therefore, the ecologic associations in the original habitat where the parasitic relationship first emerged; for example, the mode of entry into the final host and the migratory route in the tissues often reflect the acquisition of the first infection through food or through contact.

Moreover, it must be remembered that parasites occur as a population of organisms within an *individual* member of a host population. The regular infection of *other* members of the host population is a necessary condition for the survival of the parasite species. Successful infection of another host often dictates a period of sojourn in the environment outside the host, and an ability to survive these obviously different conditions of life outside the host is essential to continued existence as a parasitic population. A parasite must therefore be capable of surviving in the very different environments *within* and *outside* a host; alternatively, it must develop a stage or stages in its life cycle adapted to survive best in each of these environments. Nematodes have chosen the latter strategy, and the dispersive phase of the life cycle, which "runs the gauntlet of the improvident external environment," is either the resistant egg, in which a developing embryo or larva is often enclosed, or a specially adapted, hardy, and resistant infective larval stage, generally the third stage larva.

It is best to begin a consideration of the life cycle of the parasitic nematodes from the basic patterns of the nonparasitic, free-living members in the aquatic and soil environment. In these, there are an egg and five stages of growth and development: the first, second, third, and fourth larval stages and the fifth stage, in which the organism attains final maturity or adulthood with fully developed and functional reproductive organs. The six stages in this cycle are represented in Fig. 10 as E (egg), 1, 2, 3, 4 (larval), and A (adult) stages. The transition from one larval stage to the next is marked by a molt: there are four molts in the life cycle of a nematode.

The host in which a parasite attains full development and production is called the *definitive* or *final* host. Earlier stages of development take place in the *intermediate* host, which may also serve as a vector. Temporary hosts that transport the infective stage of the parasite to a suitable environment are often called the *transport* host. Life cycles that involve direct contact between the infective agent (whether egg or infective larva) and the definitive host are called *direct*. If development of any of the stages occurs in a host other than the definitive host, the life cycle is said to be *indirect*.

In the parasitic species, there are five main variations in this basic life cycle. In the first variation, exemplified by the direct life cycle of *Ascaris lumbricoides* and *Trichocephalus trichiurus (Trichuris trichiura)*, the egg is the infective agent. The mature eggs are expelled in the feces of the host. The first-stage larva develops within the *Ascaris* egg and subsequently molts. The $L_2$ enclosed within the eggshell is the infective stage, and it is in this stage that the parasites are commonly encountered in contaminated soils. When the infective egg with the enclosed larva is swallowed in either contaminated food or water by a potential definitive host, man, the larva hatches in the small intestine. The hatching process in the gastrointestinal tract depends upon the interplay of physicochemical factors, chiefly the presence of dissolved carbon dioxide, reducing agents, and an appropriate range of pH (Rogers and Sommerville, 1968). Under appropriate conditions, the larva hatches after digestion of the eggshell by the enzymes chitinase, lipase, and leucine aminopeptidase, which are produced within the egg. The second-stage larva now molts and penetrates the intestinal mucosa as a third-stage larva, which is carried through the lymphatics to the liver, heart, and finally to the lungs within one to three days. During these wanderings (the histotrophic phase), it molts two more times to transform itself into the young adult that breaks through the lung alveoli, ascends the trachea, migrates to the esophagus, and finally descends to the ileum, where the young adult worm reaches egg-producing maturity in about 65 days from the original infection. When evacuated in the feces, the eggs repeat the cycle.

The life cycle is similar in *Trichocephalus trichiurus (Trichuris trichiura)*. The only difference is that the first-stage larvae do not wander as extensively as *Ascaris* larvae. They merely penetrate the villi for a brief sojourn of about a week before returning to the lumen of the cecum to continue their development to full maturity, which takes about three months.

The second pattern, an indirect life cycle, is characteristic of the order Spirurida and is exemplified by the filarial worm of the subcutaneous tissues of man, *Onchocerca volvulus*. Adult females produce eggs that give rise to microfi-

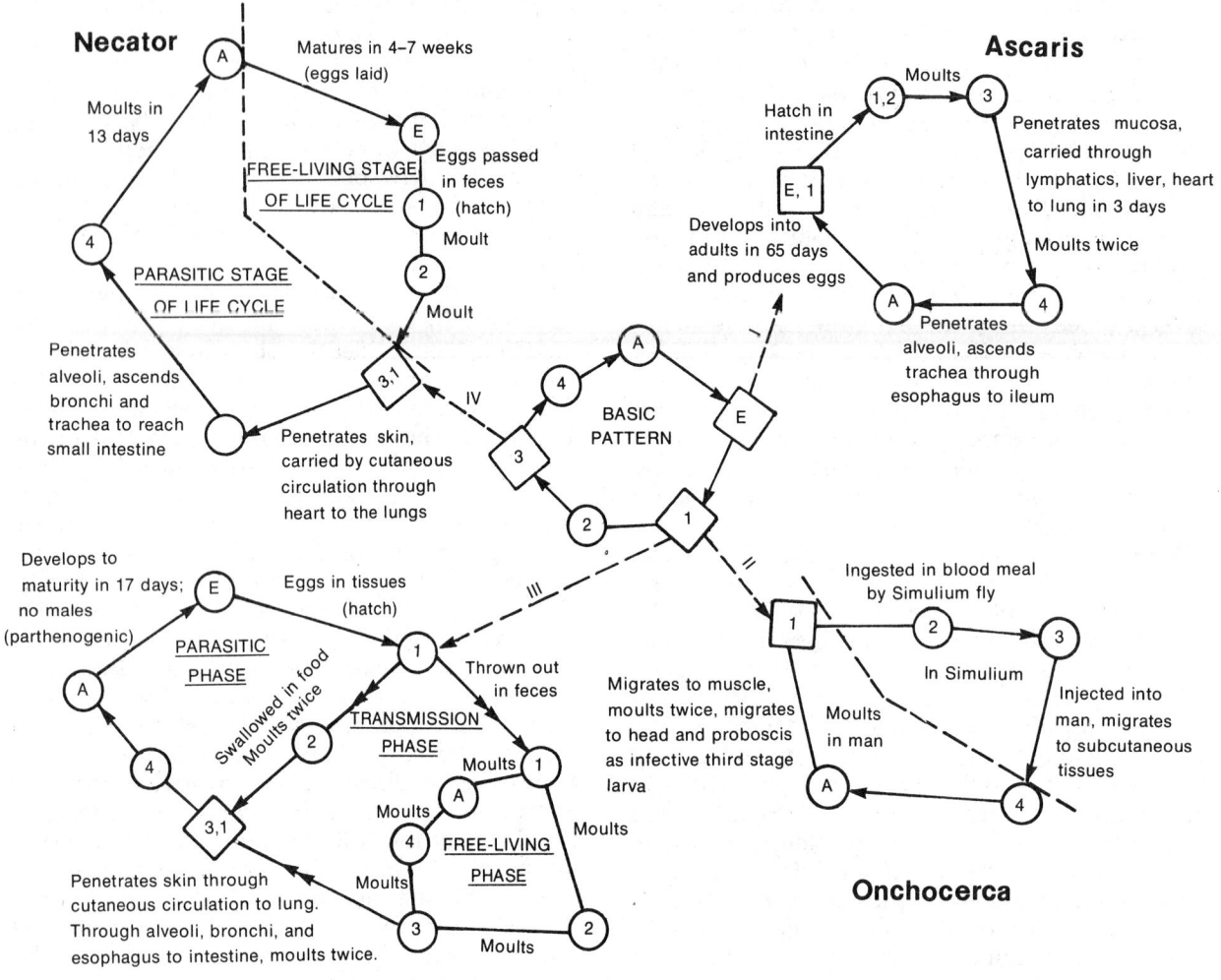

**FIGURE 10.** *Diagrammatic representation of the basic pattern and four of the five variations of life cycle patterns in nematodes (see text).*

lariae enclosed in the inner membrane of the egg while still within the adult females. When released into the cutaneous circulation, these microfilariae reinitiate the cycle with the next insect bite.

The sequence, summarized in Figure 10, II, is as follows. When an insect vector, usually *Simulium damnosum* in the West African region, bites an infected human, the microfilariae are ingested with the blood meal. The microfilariae migrate to the thoracic muscles of the insect, molt twice, and, as the third-stage larvae, finally come to rest in the head and proboscis region of the insect. When an infected *Simulium* fly bites the next human victim, the infective larva is reinjected into the cutaneous circulation. This larva molts, migrates to the subcutaneous tissues of the host, and molts

once more before reaching maturity. Thus, the infective stage for human infection is the third-stage larva, but the first-stage larva is infective for the *Simulium* intermediate host.

The life cycle is essentially the same in all the spirurids with minor variations in the intermediate host or vector that influence the mode of entry into the human host. The intermediate hosts of *Wuchereria bancrofti* are mosquitoes of the genera *Anopheles, Aedes,* and *Culex. Anopheles* is the major vector in West Africa, while *Culex pipiens fatigans* is predominant in Southeast Asia. The vector of *Loa loa* is the day-biting tabanid fly, *Chrysops* sp. Aquatic crustaceans of the genus *Cyclops* are the intermediate hosts of *Dracunculus medinensis.* Man is infected by drinking contaminated water. *Culicoides* sp is the vector of *Dipetalonema streptocerca* in Africa and *Mansonella ozzardi* in South America, where *Simulium* sp may also transmit mansonelliasis.

The third variation that may be considered unique is found in the Rhabditida and exemplified by *Strongyloides stercoralis*. Adult female worms live in the small intestine of the definitive host. Eggs are released in the intestine, where they hatch and give rise to first-stage larvae that reach the soil in the feces. In the soil, two paths of development are open to these larvae. They may follow a free-living, nonparasitic pattern of development in which adult males and females develop from four molts, which give rise to four larval stages and finally adult males and females. The females produce eggs that repeat the cycle.

Alternatively, the first-stage larvae can undergo two successive molts and produce infective third-stage larvae that penetrate the skin of humans, reach the cutaneous circulation, migrate to the lungs, break through the alveoli, ascend the bronchi and trachea to the esophagus, and descend to the intestine. During migration, the parasitic larvae molt twice and reach maturity in about 17 days. There are no males, and egg production is through parthenogenesis. The essential elements of this cycle are summarized in Figure 10, III. The parasitic phase is an example of a direct life cycle, although a free-living phase regularly alternates with this parasitic phase. During the free-living phase, some third stage larvae may also become infective and participate in the parasitic phase by penetrating into the definitive host (Nigon, 1947).

The fourth pattern of the life cycle is exemplified by *Trichinella spiralis* (Fig. 11, I). First-stage larvae are encysted in the muscles of pigs or carnivores such as foxes and wolves. When infected meat is eaten raw or undercooked by another carnivore or human, the cyst walls are digested in the stomach, and the first-stage larvae are released. These larvae invade the mucosa of the duodenum and jejunum and undergo four molts. Some authorities insist that each larva undergoes only three molts within the mucosa, an earlier molt having taken place in the cyst. According to this view, the encysted larva is a second-stage larva.

Immature worms are found in the intestinal lumen within 24 hours of the ingestion of cysts. Adult females are ovoviviparous — i.e., first-stage larvae are released from the uterus rather than eggs. These larvae penetrate the intestinal mucosa, migrate through lymphatics and blood vessels to the skeletal muscles, penetrate the sarcolemma, and form the cyst. The life cycle is completed when the host is eaten by another carnivore (Fig. 11, I). Under normal circumstances, human infections represent a biologic dead end for the parasite. Transmission of the parasite is made possible by the zoonotic maintenance of reservoir hosts in wild carnivores. The nature of the available reservoir host in each locality introduces local variations in the life cycle in different geographic regions (Fig. 11, II to IV).

The final pattern that is also direct is characteristic of most of the Strongylidae, including *Necator americanus*. When eggs are passed out in the feces of the host, the first-stage larvae emerge, feed, and molt into second-stage larvae, which develop into infective third-stage larvae. The latter do not feed. They are enclosed in the uncast sheaths derived from the molted cuticle of the second-stage larva. The survival of third-stage larvae depends upon the reserves of lipids built up in their tissues during the feeding phase of seond-stage larvae. Recent work in our laboratories has shown that the infectivity of *Necator americanus* varies with the lipid level, activity, and age of the larva. Under the tropical conditions of Nsukka, the viability and infectivity of the larva in contaminated fields are maintained for up to 21 days (Udonsi, unpublished observations).

On contact with a human host, infective larvae penetrate the skin, are carried in the circulation through the heart to the lungs, molt within 24 hours, break through the alveoli, ascend the bronchi and trachea, and descend the esophagus to arrive at the small intestine. Here they molt again, usually within 13 days, and the female adults produce eggs in four to seven weeks. There are thus a free-living and a parasitic stage in the life cycle of each *Necator* nematode. The pattern is summarized in Figure 10, IV.

This pattern is essentially the same in other members of the Strongylidae except that most of the trichostrongylids do not infect the host by penetrating the skin. Infective larvae are swallowed with food or water. *Ancylostoma* may also develop by an identical life cycle.

## IMMUNITY

The relationship between a helminth and its host is complex and influenced by physiologic, biochemical, genetic, nutritional, immunologic, and other biologic mechanisms. Host specificity, which is often observed in vertebrate-helminth interactions, may arise from natural host resistance mediated by any of these factors. Acquired immunity, on the other hand, follows the general principles elucidated in studies of viral and bacterial infections. Progress in our understanding of

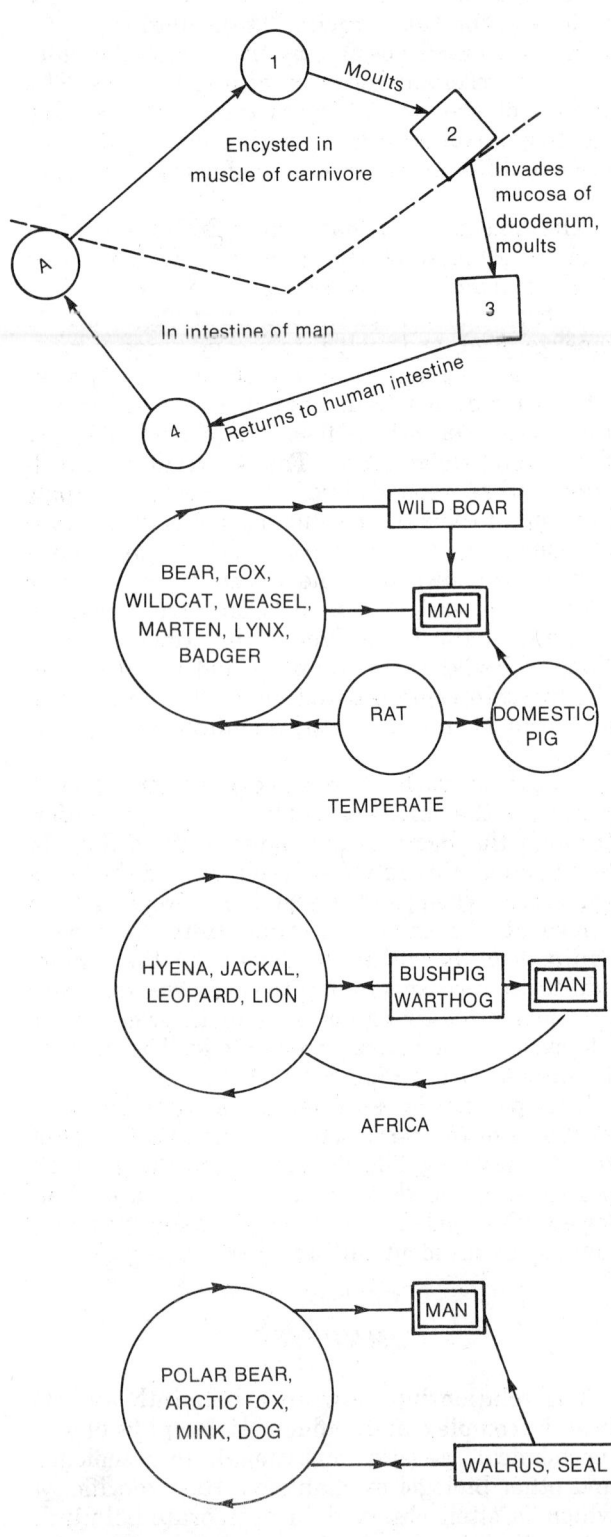

**FIGURE 11.** *The life cycle pattern of* Trichinella spiralis *(the fifth pattern) and the pattern of zoonotic relationship in different geographic regions: temperate, tropical (Africa), and arctic.*

the principles of immunity to helminths was relatively slow until recently.

One explanation for the complexity of helminth immunology is the fact that helminths are collections of different populations of cells with different biochemical, metabolic, and antigenic characteristics. Nevertheless, studies of various experimental systems such as *Nippostrongylus braziliensis* and *Trichuris muris* in mice (Ogilvie and Jones, 1973; Selby and Wakelin, 1973; Wakelin and Lloyd, 1976), *Ascaris suum* and *Toxocara cati* in rats and mice (Larsh and Race, 1975), *Ancylostoma caninum* in dogs (Miller, 1964), and *Onchocerca volvulus* in man (WHO, 1976) have shed considerable light on the essential features and mechanisms of helminth immunogenicity.

The immune response to helminth infections can be mediated through either circulating antibodies or delayed hypersensitivity (cell-mediated immunity) involving lymphoid cells (Larsh and Race, 1975; Muller, 1975). For example, circulating antibodies of the complement-fixing IgG and IgM classes have been detected in onchocerciasis, while *Ascaris* has stimulated the production of IgM, IgA, and IgG. *Trichinella spiralis* elicits predominantly reaginic IgE antibodies. An increase in the serum level of IgE from about 100 ng/ml to 1000 ng/ml encourages the view that IgE is an important line of immunologic defense in these infections. Indeed, a generalized eosinophilia, whose significance is at present uncertain, and these reaginic antibodies are becoming the characteristic indicators of vertebrate host-helminth interactions, especially when the association of parasite with host tissue can be regarded as close, e.g., with *Trichinella spiralis* and *Nippostrongylus braziliensis*.

A feature of helminth immunity is the inability of killed helminth material or purified extracts of helminth excretions or secretions to afford long-lasting protection. Rather, protection has been secured in some cases by the regular and persistent release of antigens. Thus, live vaccines of larvae irradiated by x-rays have provided significant protection in the veterinary field against *Dictyocaulus viviparus* bronchitis in cattle and the canine hookworm. Understandably, live vaccines have not been used in humans.

It is now generally accepted that any of the typical host reactions associated with the immune response, namely anaphylaxis, immune complex disease, and delayed hypersensitivity (cell-mediated immunity), may be manifest in nematode infections. For example, the so-called self-cure phenomenon observed in *Haemonchus contortus*, characterized by the expulsion of pre-existing adult worms on the entry of new infective larvae, is explicable on the basis of anaphylaxis. It is suggested that the release of molting fluid (and thus antigens) by third-stage infective larvae results in an anaphylactic reaction brought about by the production of pharmacologically active substances such as histamine, serotonin (5-HT), and kinins, which render the intestinal mucosa unsuitable for the continued existence of the adult worms. However, recent studies in Kenya have attempted to explain the self-cure phenomenon, not on the basis of local intestinal anaphylaxis but on nutritionally induced unsuitability of the intestine for the adult worms. In *Nippostrongylus braziliensis* (infections of rats) and *Haemonchus placei* (infections of cattle), on the other hand, it has been shown that the immune reaction leads to structural changes in the intestinal cells of the nematodes, characterized by extreme vacuolation and the accumulation of lipids. These nematodes are unable to maintain their normal position in the hosts' intestine because of this interference with their normal metabolism.

After treatment for *Onchocerca volvulus* infections the histologic appearance of tissues suggests that antigens released from dying larvae form complexes with circulating antibodies in and around blood vessels. These immune complexes induce infiltration and degranulation of polymorphonuclear leukocytes. Immune complex formation in the eye or the testes may lead to blindness or infertility, respectively (WHO, 1976).

The importance of cell-mediated immunity in infections with *Trichinella, Nippostrongylus, Trichostrongylus, Trichocephalus (Trichuris),* and *Capillaria* has been demonstrated by protecting animals with immune cells from lymph nodes, spleen, and previously sensitized thymic lymphocytes.

Thus immune phenomena are associated with nematode infections, but the manifestations and modulation of the host responses are complicated by the biologic and functional complexity of the parasites. This complexity limits the effectiveness of helminth-induced antibodies and increases the helminth's chances of adaptation to immunologically induced changes in its environment (Ogilvie and Jones, 1973). Progress in the utilization of immunologic mechanisms for the control of nematode infections has been limited and may remain so, but continued research should provide additional approaches, such as the regulation of parasite reproduction.

## SYSTEMATICS AND LABORATORY DIAGNOSIS

The Nematoda are broadly divided into two taxonomic classes depending upon whether or not they possess the ventrally and posteriorly located female sense organ, the phasmid. Nematodes that possess the phasmid belong to the class Phasmidia (Secernentea) and those without it belong to the class Aphasmidia (Adenophorea). Because the phasmid is not an easy structure to identify, other characteristics such as the structure of the pharynx and excretory system or the life history have often been utilized. The assignment of nematodes into the various orders varies from authority to authority and is of little practical use to the nonspecialist. For example, nematodes may be divided into 11, 16, or 18 orders depending upon the classification scheme adopted (Chabaud, 1974; Crofton, 1966; Maggenti, 1976). Nematodes parasitic in vertebrates and hence of potential medical significance are found in the following orders:

Phylum:   Nematoda (Cobb, 1919)

Class:    Phasmidia (Secernentea) (Dougherty, 1958)

1. Order: Rhabditida (Chitwood, 1933)—e.g., *Strongyloides*

2. Order: Ascaridida (Railliet and Henry, 1925) —e.g., *Ascaris, Enterobius, Toxocara, Anisakis, Toxoascaris*

3. Order: Strongylida (Diesing, 1815)—e.g., *Ancylostoma, Necator, Syngamus, Oesophagostomum, Trichostrongylus, Angiostrongylus*

4. Order: Spirurida (Chitwood, 1933)—e.g., *Wuchereria, Brugia, Loa, Onchocerca, Dracunculus, Dipetalonema, Mansonella, Dirofilaria, Gnathostoma, Habronema*

Class:    Adenophorea (Aphasmidia) (Chitwood, 1958)

5. Order: Trichocephalida (Skryabin and Schultts, 1938)—e.g., *Trichocephalus (Trichuris), Trichinella, Dioctophyma, Capillaria*

The important and obligate parasites of man are summarized in Table 1. An outline of the life cycles with characteristics of diagnostic relevance is presented in Table 2, while an identification key generally based on the features of the life cycle, morphology, and anatomy is presented in Table 3. Table 4 and Figure 12 present aids for the identification of nematodes in tissue sections.

In addition to the adult characteristics indicated in Tables 1 through 4, three main methods are used to identify parasitic nematodes in the laboratory. These are: (1) fecal examination for eggs

**TABLE 1.   Summary of Obligate Parasites of Man Belonging to the Nematoda**

| PHYLUM | CLASS | ORDER | SUPERFAMILY | GENUS AND SPECIES |
|---|---|---|---|---|
| Nematoda | Phasmidia (Secernentea) | Rhabditida | Rhabditoidea | 1. *Strongyloides stercoralis* |
| | | Ascaridida | Ascaridoidea | 2. *Ascaris lumbricoides* |
| | | | Oxyuroidea | 3. *Enterobius vermicularis* |
| | | Strongylida | Strongyloidea | 4. *Ancylostoma duodenale*<br>5. *Necator americanus*<br>6. *Syngamus*[a] sp |
| | | | Trichostrongyloidea | 7. *Trichostrongylus*[a] sp<br>8. *Oesophagostomum*[a] sp |
| | | | Metastrongyloidea | 9. *Angiostrongylus*[a] sp |
| | | Spirurida | Spiruroidea | 10. *Habronema*[a] sp<br>11. *Gnathostoma spinigerum* |
| | | | Dracunculoidea | 12. *Dracunculus medinensis* |
| | | | Filarioidea | 13. *Brugia*[a] sp<br>14. *Wuchereria bancrofti*<br>15. *Dipetalonema perstans*<br>16. *Onchocerca volvulus*<br>17. *Dirofilaria immitis* |
| | Aphasmidia (Adenophorea) | Trichocephalida | Trichuroidea | 18. *Trichocephalus* sp (*Trichuris*)<br>19. *Capillaria phillipensis* |
| | | | Trichinelloidea | 20. *Trichinella spiralis* |
| | | | Dioctophymoidea | 21. *Dioctophyma*[a] renale |

[a]Not obligate parasites of man but of other vertebrates; these have, however, been found often enough in man to deserve consideration as human parasites.

**TABLE 2.    Summary Outline of Nematode Life Cycles of Diagnostic Relevance**

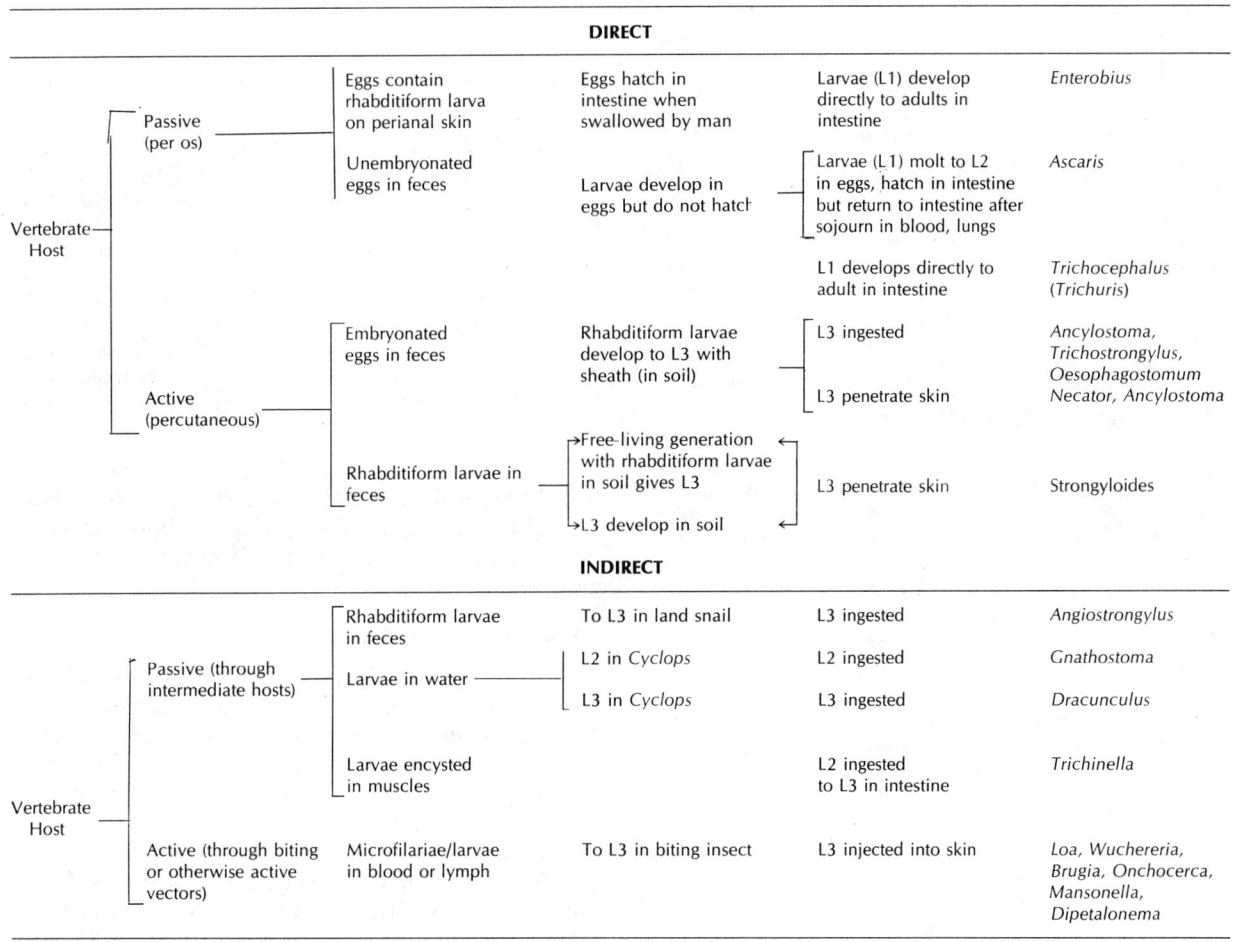

| | | DIRECT | | |
|---|---|---|---|---|
| Vertebrate Host | Passive (per os) | Eggs contain rhabditiform larva on perianal skin | Eggs hatch in intestine when swallowed by man | Larvae (L1) develop directly to adults in intestine | *Enterobius* |
| | | Unembryonated eggs in feces | Larvae develop in eggs but do not hatch | Larvae (L1) molt to L2 in eggs, hatch in intestine but return to intestine after sojourn in blood, lungs | *Ascaris* |
| | | | | L1 develops directly to adult in intestine | *Trichocephalus* (*Trichuris*) |
| | Active (percutaneous) | Embryonated eggs in feces | Rhabditiform larvae develop to L3 with sheath (in soil) | L3 ingested | *Ancylostoma, Trichostrongylus, Oesophagostomum* |
| | | | | L3 penetrate skin | *Necator, Ancylostoma* |
| | | Rhabditiform larvae in feces | Free-living generation with rhabditiform larvae in soil gives L3  →  L3 develop in soil | L3 penetrate skin | *Strongyloides* |

| | | INDIRECT | | |
|---|---|---|---|---|
| Vertebrate Host | Passive (through intermediate hosts) | Rhabditiform larvae in feces | To L3 in land snail | L3 ingested | *Angiostrongylus* |
| | | Larvae in water | L2 in *Cyclops* | L2 ingested | *Gnathostoma* |
| | | | L3 in *Cyclops* | L3 ingested | *Dracunculus* |
| | | Larvae encysted in muscles | | L2 ingested to L3 in intestine | *Trichinella* |
| | Active (through biting or otherwise active vectors) | Microfilariae/larvae in blood or lymph | To L3 in biting insect | L3 injected into skin | *Loa, Wuchereria, Brugia, Onchocerca, Mansonella, Dipetalonema* |

Modified from Muller, 1975.

## TABLE 3.  Key to Nematodes Parasitic in Man

| | |
|---|---|
| 1. Filiform anterior and spindle-shaped posterior; pharynx is either a stichosome that consists of a single row of cells with a centrally located fine tube or a long and narrow structure slightly dilated posteriorly; male with or without copulatory bursa | **2** |
| Regular spindle-shaped, relatively stout or filiform worms with muscular pharynx that may be cylindrical or rhabditiform—i.e., having a posterior bulb that has a valvular apparatus | **3** |
| 2. Male has muscular copulatory bursa without supporting rays; pharynx is long and narrow, not a stichosome; vulva is located anteriorly | Trichocephalida (Dioctophymoidea) *Dioctophyma* sp |
| Filiform anterior and spindle-shaped posterior; male without bursa; pharynx a stichosome; female vulva located at junction of anterior and posterior positions; eggs with characteristic opercular (polar) plug | Trichocephalida (Trichuroidea) *Trichocephalus (Trichuris) trichiurus* |
| Filiform anterior; male without bursa; pharynx a stichosome; female ovoviviparous with larvae in uterus | Trichocephalida (Trichinelloidea) *Trichinella spiralis* **4** |
| 3. Relatively stout round worms with muscular pharynx; cylindrical or with valvular posterior bulb | |
| Filiform worms with cylindrical pharynx | **5** |
| 4. Relatively stout but small worms; muscular pharynx with valvular posterior bulb; male with genital papillae; female with pointed tail; eggs embryonated and slightly flattened on one side | Ascaridida (Oxyuroidea) *Enterobius vermicularis* |
| Relatively stout large worms; mouth usually with three lips; muscular pharynx more or less cylindrical, not dilated posteriorly and without valvular apparatus | Ascaridida (Ascaridoidea) *Ascaris, Toxocara* |
| 5. Filiform worm with cylindrical pharynx; no parasitic males; parasitic female parthenogenetic; small buccal capsule without teeth; larvae always found alongside adult females | Rhabditida (Rhabditoidea) *Strongyloides stercoralis* |
| Filiform worm with cylindrical pharynx that is muscular anteriorly and glandular posteriorly; not usually intestinal | **6** |
| Filiform worm with cylindrical pharynx, muscular throughout its length; copulatory bursa in males with muscular rays | **7** |
| 6. Usually two lateral lips; cuticle of buccal capsule particularly toughened; vulva in middle of female body or posterior; characteristic and spiny head bulb; parasite of alimentary canal, respiratory system, or orbital, nasal, or oral cavity | Spirurida (Spiruroidea) *Gnathostoma* sp |
| Usually without lips; no buccal capsule; vulva in region of pharynx; parasites of circulatory, lymphatic, or serous cavities, not intestinal; females not more than three times longer than males | Spirurida (Filarioidea) *Loa, Wuchereria, Onchocerca, Mansonella, Dipetalonema* |

## TABLE 3.  Key to Nematodes Parasitic in Man *(Continued)*

| | |
|---|---|
| Females much longer than males; atrophied vulva in gravid female | Spirurida (Dracunculoidea) *Dracunculus* sp |
| 7. Parasites of alimentary canal, very rarely found in kidney tissue | **8** |
| Parasites of respiratory system | **9** |
| 8. Buccal capsule very feebly developed or absent; thread-like worms | Strongylida (Trichostrongyloidea) *Trichostrongylus* sp |
| Buccal capsule well developed with ventral teeth; anterior end more or less straight | Strongylida (Ancylostomoidea) *Ancylostoma duodenale* |
| Buccal capsule well-developed with cutting plates; anterior end characteristically recurved | Strongylida (Ancylostomoidea) *Necator americanus* |
| 9. Buccal capsule without teeth or cutting plates but mouth surrounded by characteristic leaf crown | Strongylida (Trichostrongyloidea) *Oesophagostomum* sp |
| 9. Well-developed, toughened, and cuticular buccal capsule; male often attached to female | Strongylida (Strongyloidea) *Syngamus laryngeus* |
| Buccal capsule rudimentary or absent; filiform | Strongylida (Metastrongyloidea) *Angiostrongylus* sp |

or culture of feces for the infective larval stages; (2) examination of blood, tissue fluid, or skin snips for microfilariae; and (3) immunologic techniques.

### Fecal Examination

The simplest method for the detection of helminth eggs in feces is direct examination under the microscope of about 5 mg of feces diluted with tap water or saline and smeared on a slide with a coverslip. Only heavy infections are usually detected by this method.

Modifications of this simple method such as Kato's thick smear technique are also useful. In this method, about 50 mg of a fecal sample is placed on a microscope slide, and a $30 \times 22$ mm piece of cellophane soaked in a mixture of 100 ml of glycerine, 100 ml of water, and 1 ml of 3 per cent aqueous malachite green is placed over it. The specimen is pressed down and examined after 20 to 30 minutes at $37°$ C. The feces has cleared by this time, and the relatively uncleared eggs are seen in bolder relief.

Various methods for the estimation of the intensity of infection by egg counts have been developed. The best known is the Stoll dilution egg counting technique and the McMaster tech-

## TABLE 4. Identification Key For Sections of Nematodes

1. A. Hypodermal chords (few to many) arranged asymmetrically. Lateral excretory canals absent. In the ovaries and testes the germinal region extends the entire length of the gonad, and gametes at various stages of development can be found at any level. Esophagus nonmuscular. — Trichurids (Trichinella, Trichocephalus (Trichuris) (Capillaria)

   B. Hypodermal chords (two to four) arranged symmetrically. Excretory canals in lateral chords except at extremities. In the ovaries and testes the germinal region is confined to the proximal extremity of the gonad, and gametes at uniform stage of development can be found at any one level. — 2

2. A. Intestine composed of a few large multinucleate cells, rarely with more than two cells in a cross-section. Anterior paired excretory gland cells present. — Strongylids (hookworms, Trichostrongylus, Ternidens, Oesophagostomum)

   B. Intestine composed of few to many, small, uninucleate cells; excretory glands single, paired, or absent. — 3

3. A. Somatic muscle cells few, large and flat. Lateral alae present or absent. — 4

   B. Many somatic muscle cells, U-shaped in cross-section. Lateral alae usually absent. — 5

4. A. Lateral alae present. Vagina long and muscular. Esophagus has posterior bulb. Many eggs in uterus. Excretory gland cells absent — Enterobius

   B. Lateral alae absent. Vagina very short. Ova large. Viviparous, with eggs developing into larvae. Excretory cells single or paired. Very small and often larvae (or eggs) in tissues. — Strongyloides

5. A. Somatic musculature divided by large lateral chords (often very wide and flattened) into two crescent-shaped folds. — 6

   B. Somatic musculature divided into four fields — 7

6. A. Females often contain microfilariae and uterus double. Diameter less than 0.5 mm. — Filarids (Wuchereria, Brugia, Dipetalonema, Dirofilaria, Onchocerca, Loa)

   B. Females contain larvae with long pointed tails, uterus single, diameter more than 1 mm. — Dracunculus

7. A. Lateral chords very large and stalked and project into body cavity; frequently unequal in size. — Spirurids (Thelazia, Gnathostoma)

   B. Lateral chords large and project into body cavity but not stalked; usually equal in size. — Ascarids (Ascaris, Toxocara, Toxascaris, Anisakis)

nique. These methods rely upon concentration techniques such as the formol-ether method or the zinc-sulfate centrifugal flotation technique (Muller, 1975). Unfortunately, efforts to relate the egg production of a female worm to the number of eggs recovered from feces have so far proved unreliable. For example, it is becoming increasingly clear that while the number of eggs laid by an individual female worm may vary from time to time and may also vary between individuals, the total egg output of a given worm population is fairly constant and is related to the nutritional status of the host (Michel, 1974). Thus, until we understand the biology of egg production in nematodes, predictions of population size from egg counts continue to be of doubtful validity.

The best known method for the differential diagnosis of nematode infections by culturing larvae in fecal matter is the Harada-Mori test tube and filter paper method (Muller, 1975). Larvae can be identified by the characteristics summarized in Table 5.

### Examination of Blood, Tissue, or Skin Snips for Microfilariae

The easiest method for the diagnosis of the various filariae is to make a wet preparation from a drop of blood with a coverslip. Microfilariae can be easily detected moving under low-power magnification. Light infections are often missed by this method. However, diethylcarbamazine has improved the sensitivity of wet preparations immeasurably, especially in periodic filariasis. When this drug is administered, the microfilariae may be found with ease in the peripheral and cutaneous circulation. When microfilariae are identified, thick blood smears should be stained with hematoxylin or Giemsa stain. Differential diagnosis of the various microfilariae such as Onchocerca, Brugia, Loa, Dirofilaria, Wuchereria, Dipetalonema, and Mansonella is then possible. Finally, membrane filtration techniques using nucleopore or millipore membrane filters (pore size 5 μm) fitted to hypodermic syringes with an adaptor have considerably improved diagnostic accuracy in filariasis.

In tropical Africa, the most important filarial nematode is Onchocerca volvulus, whose microfilariae are easily recognized by their larger size (270 to 320 μm long compared with Dipetalonema or Mansonella) and their characteristic head and pointed tail. The most common diagnostic procedure in Onchocerca infections is examination of skin snip biopsies for emerging larvae. Alternatively, dermal juices obtained after scarification of the skin can be examined after staining. This procedure may pick up not only Onchocerca but also Dipetalonema and even malarial parasites.

The best site for obtaining skin snips may depend upon the geographic strain of the parasite. Skin snips can be taken with a razor blade, sharp scissors, or a scleral punch such as the Holth model. The snips are then examined for living microfilariae in water or saline, with or without teasing. The number of emerging microfilariae is usually counted after 10 to 30 minutes. Examination of emerging larvae in water is preferred, especially under dry conditions, although emergence tends to take longer.

In large-scale epidemiologic surveys, reasonably good results can be obtained by placing

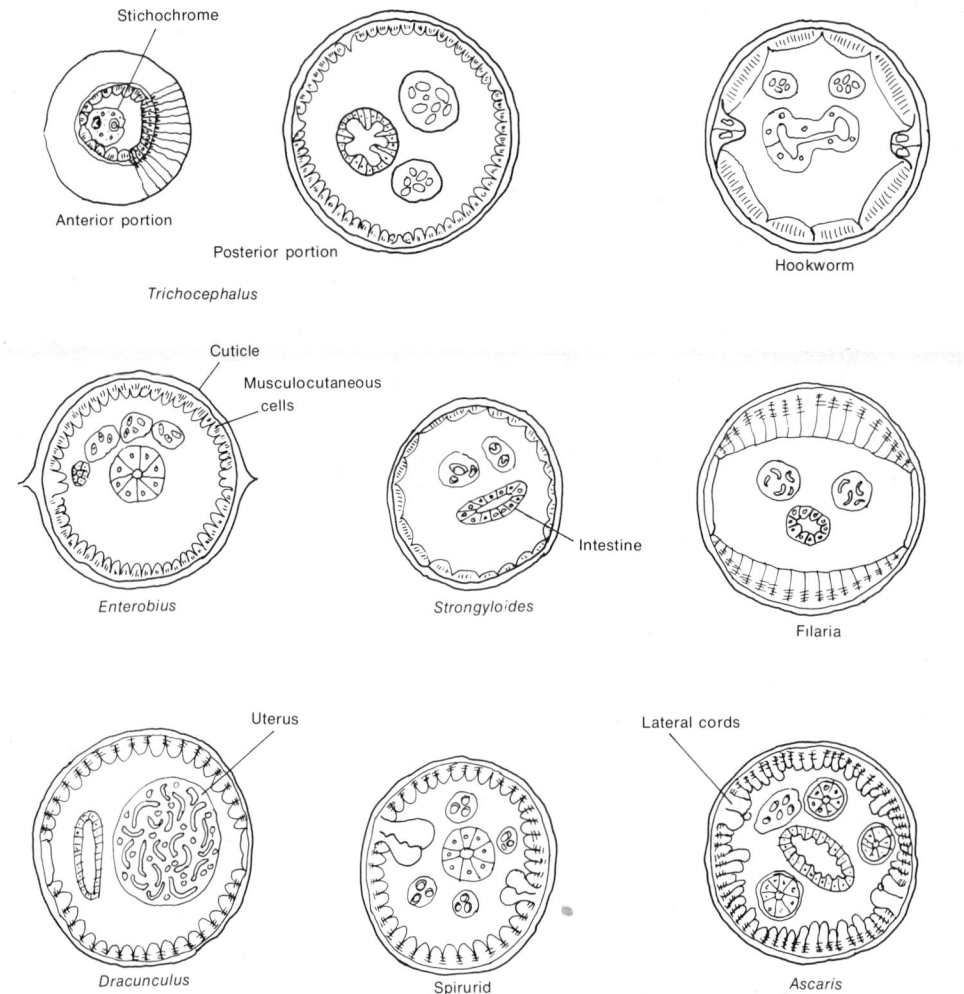

**FIGURE 12.**  *Transverse sections of females of various nematodes (from Muller, 1975; after Chitwood and Lichtenfels, 1972).*

individual snips in a drop or two of saline in wells of an agglutination tray. The microfilariae emerge over a 24-hour period and are then preserved in the wells by the addition of a drop of 10 per cent formol-saline. The trays are sealed with a transparent plastic sealer, and the preserved material can then be examined at leisure.

### Immunodiagnostic Techniques

As emphasized earlier, an individual nematode is a complex population of cells and the source of a complex assortment of antigens. This fact is the source of the two main problems with immunodiagnostic detection of nematode infections. These problems are the lack of specific, well-characterized antigens (this introduces an element of uncertainty in diagnosis) and the high level of cross-reactivity that confuses many positive results. Except in such situations as visceral larva migrans, in which the absence of adult parasites precludes easy detection of the causative agent, parasitologic diagnosis is more reliable at the present time. Nevertheless, many standard immunologic techniques have been used with good, variable, or indifferent results.

Standard serologic procedures such as precipitation tests have been used for the detection of a wide variety of nematodes and other helminths. Serologic procedures have been useful in diagnosing hookworm and *Trichinella* infections, but success often depends on a continuing challenge of the immune system with living parasites. For example, in hookworm infections, there is a lack of correlation between immunologic reactions and the presence of eggs in the feces.

Complement fixation tests (CFT) have been used for the detection of many nematode infections but particularly for visceral larva migrans. Its reproducibility and sensitivity for some nematode infections are questioned, and anticomple-

**TABLE 5    The Differentiation of Infective Filariform Larvae Found in Cultures from Human Fecal Specimens**

| | STRONGY-LOIDES[a] | TRICHO-STRONGYLUS | ANCYLOSTOMA | NECATOR | TERNIDENS |
|---|---|---|---|---|---|
| Length (microns) | 500 | 750 | 660 | 590 | 680 (630–730) |
| Sheath | Absent | Present | Sheath 720 microns, striations not clear | Sheath 660 microns, striations clear at tail end | Present |
| Length of esophagus as proportion of total body length | 1:2 | 1:4 | 1:3 | 1·3 | 1:3 |
| Intestine | Straight | Intestinal lumen zigzagged | Anterior end narrower in diameter than esophageal bulb. No gap between the esophagus and the intestine. | Anterior end as wide as the esophageal bulb. Gap between the esophagus and the intestine. | Following esophagus is a pair of sphincter cells Intestinal lumen somewhat zigzagged. |
| Tail | Divided into three at the tip | End of tail knob-like | Blunt | Sharply pointed | Pointed |
| Head | — | — | Blunt | Rounded | — |
| Mouth | — | — | Mouth spears not very clear and parallel | Mouth spears clear and divergent | — |

[a]Free-living adults and first-stage (rhabditiform) larvae likely to be present as well.

**TABLE 6.    Summary of Drugs of Choice with Nematode Parasites of Man**

| NEMATODE SPECIES | 1 THIABENDAZOLE (MINTEZOL) | 2 MEBENDAZOLE (TELMIN) | 3 LEVAMISOLE (KETRAX) | 4 PIPERAZINE ADIPATE (ANTEPAR) | 5 BEPHENIUM HYDROXYNAPHTHOATE (ALCOPAR) | 6 PYRANTEL EMBONATE (COMBANTRIN) | 7 PYRVINIUM EMBONATE (VANQUIN) | 8 DICHLORVOS | 9 BITOSCANATE | 10 DIETHYLCARBAMAZINE (HETRAZAN) | 11 DITHIAZANINE IODIDE |
|---|---|---|---|---|---|---|---|---|---|---|---|
| Ascaris lumbricoides | | ++++ | ++++ | ++++ | | ++++ | | | | | ++ |
| Trichocephalus (Trichuris trichiura) | ++ | +++ | | | | | | ++ | | | ++ |
| Ancylostoma duodenale | | +++ | | | +++ | ++ | | | | | |
| Necator americanus | | +++ | | | | +++ | | | | | |
| Strongyloides stercoralis | ++++ | ++ | | | | | ++ | | | | +++ |
| Enterobius vermicularis | +++ | +++ | | +++ | | ++++ | | | | | ++ |
| Trichostrongylus | +++ | | | | +++ | +++ | | | | | |
| Larva migrans | ++ | ++ | | | ++ | | | | + | | |
| Dracunculus | ++ | | | | | | | | | +++(mf) | |
| Trichinella | ++ | +++ | | | | | | | | | + |
| Wuchereria (mf) | | | | | | | | | | +++ | |
| Brugia (mf) | | | | | | | | | | +++ | |
| Onchocerca (mf) | | | | | | | | | | +++ | |
| Loa | | | | | | | | | | ++ | |

Also diphetarson, suramin, metriphonate.

mentary activity in sera collected in field studies of onchocerciasis has been a problem (WHO, 1976).

The immunofluorescent antibody test (IFA) has gained wide support, especially for the diagnosis of onchocerciasis. Using frozen sections of the adult worm as antigen, up to 90 per cent of positive cases can be identified by this procedure. Titers of between 1:20 and 1:40 are considered significant. There is good correlation between this test and the results of skin biopsies in surveys of onchocerciasis.

The latest addition to the serologic diagnosis of helminth infections is the enzyme-linked immunosorbent assay (ELISA). This test utilizes the enzymes alkaline phosphatase or peroxidase, labeled with anti-immunoglobulin, in antigen-coated tubes or microtiter plates. This promising technique is as sensitive as the IFA test and is easier to perform.

Other serologic and immunologic diagnostic procedures have been attempted, but results have been so variable that no further consideration will be given to them here.

## DRUG SUSCEPTIBILITY

The search for new and effective drugs against human helminthiasis has underscored the need for a greater understanding of the physiologic basis of anthelmintic action. An ideal anthelmintic should combine extreme toxicity against the parasite with complete inaction against the host tissue. Generally, action is directed against a target tissue or physiologic process whose special position in the overall physiology of the organism guarantees that if the target is rendered nonoperational, the parasite will die. With nematodes, four main targets have been identified: neuromuscular function, energy metabolism, lipoproteins, and hemoproteins. Effective anthelmintics presently in use affect one or the other of these targets.

Table 6 summarizes the anthelmintics of choice for the various human nematodes. The twelve anthelmintics listed represent the best of the newer drugs, many of which have come into use in the last decade or so. In addition to these twelve, diphetarsone (an arsenical), suramin (a urea derivative), and metriphonate (an organophosphorus compound) are also used, particularly for the treatment of filariasis. Of the older drugs, such as carbon tetrachloride and tetrachloroethylene, the latter is still used occasionally for the treatment of hookworms.

Of the newer drugs, the *piperazine* derivatives, piperazine adipate or citrate and diethylcarbamazine citrate, have been particularly popular for the treatment of ascariasis and filariasis, respectively. These drugs are anticholinergic and cause hyperpolarization of the neuromuscular junction. The parasite is expelled as a result of the consequent paralysis. *Thiabendazole* is an effective broad-spectrum anthelmintic that is active against *Ascaris, Strongyloides, Enterobius, Dracunculus, Trichinella,* and larva migrans, among others. It is an inhibitor of fumarate reductase, an important enzyme of energy metabolism in nematodes. *Tetramisole* and *Levamisole* among the newer drugs also act by selective enzyme inhibition. In this case, succinic dehydrogenase, which acts as a fumarate reductase in nematode mitochondria, is also inhibited (Davis, 1973).

*Bephenium,* which is often given as the hydroxynaphthoate, is active against hookworms, *Trichostrongylus,* and larva migrans. The mode of drug action is not well understood, but it is assumed to have a blocking action on the neuromuscular junction. It is more effective against mucosal than luminal helminths.

## EPIDEMIOLOGY

Epidemiologic techniques may be expected to provide the basis for planning and evaluating preventive health care, defining the major patterns and distribution of parasitic disease, and describing and classifying these conditions. The determinants of the distribution and maintenance of human parasitic disease, especially in the tropics, have received scant attention. Ultimate control of the major nematodes such as the hookworms and filariae, however, depends on our understanding of these factors.

The maintenance of a parasitic population in a community depends upon a complex series of interrelated factors (including host behavior) that regulate the number of parasites within individuals as well as the population size of the community. These factors may determine the level and frequency of contact between individual members of the two populations and thus the incidence and intensity of infection. The life cycle of the parasite is important in these considerations because it indicates whether one or two hosts (as distinct populations) are involved, as well as whether one or more parasitic stages should be considered in the total epidemiologic situation. It is usual to express the dynamics of such a host-parasite system in a flow chart such as that indicated in Figure 13 for *Ascaris* and *Trichuris* (direct life cycle) and the hookworms (direct life cycle with a stage consisting of free-living organisms). Although these life cycles of *Ascaris* and *Trichuris* are fairly simple, they involve three distinct populations of organisms, namely, the host, the adult

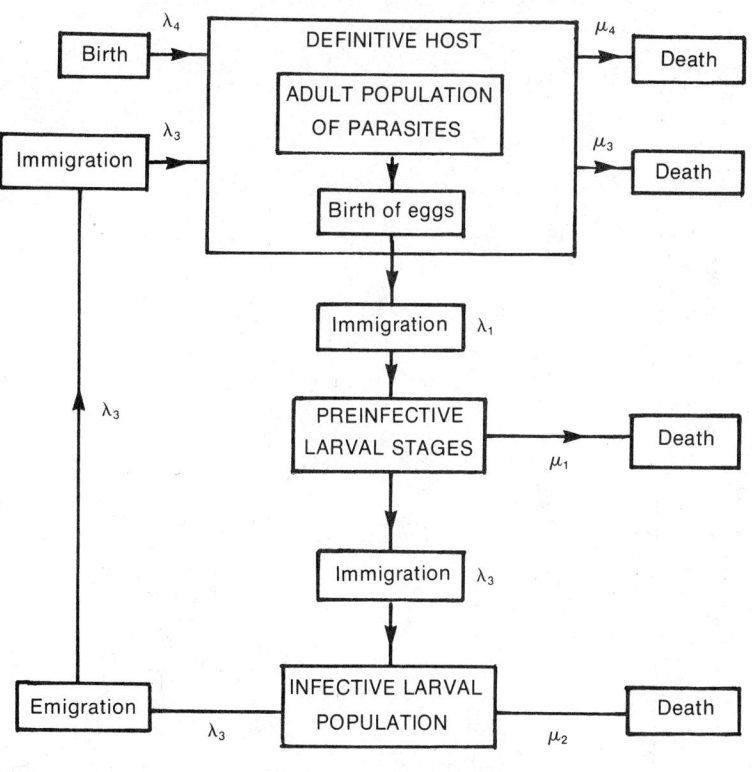

ASCARIS-TRICHURIS FLOW-CHART

**FIGURE 13.** *Diagrammatic representation (as a flow-chart) of the direct life cycle of Ascaris/Trichuris (A) and the Hookworm (B). The population (rate) parameters indicated in the charts determine the flow of parasites through the system and are defined as rates per parasite per unit of time (based on Anderson, 1976).*

HOOKWORM FLOW-CHART

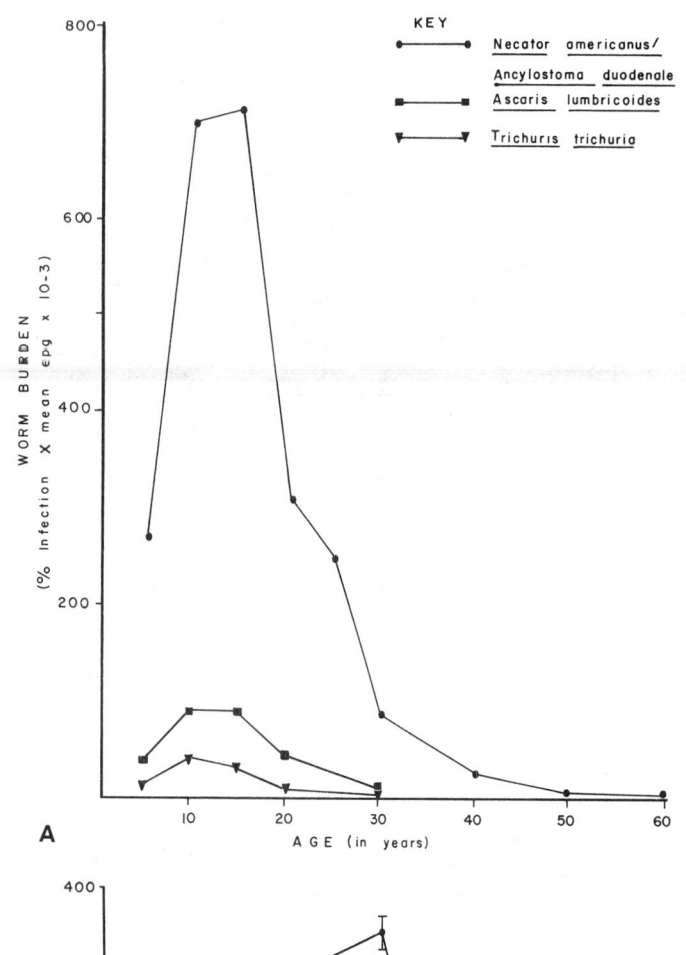

A

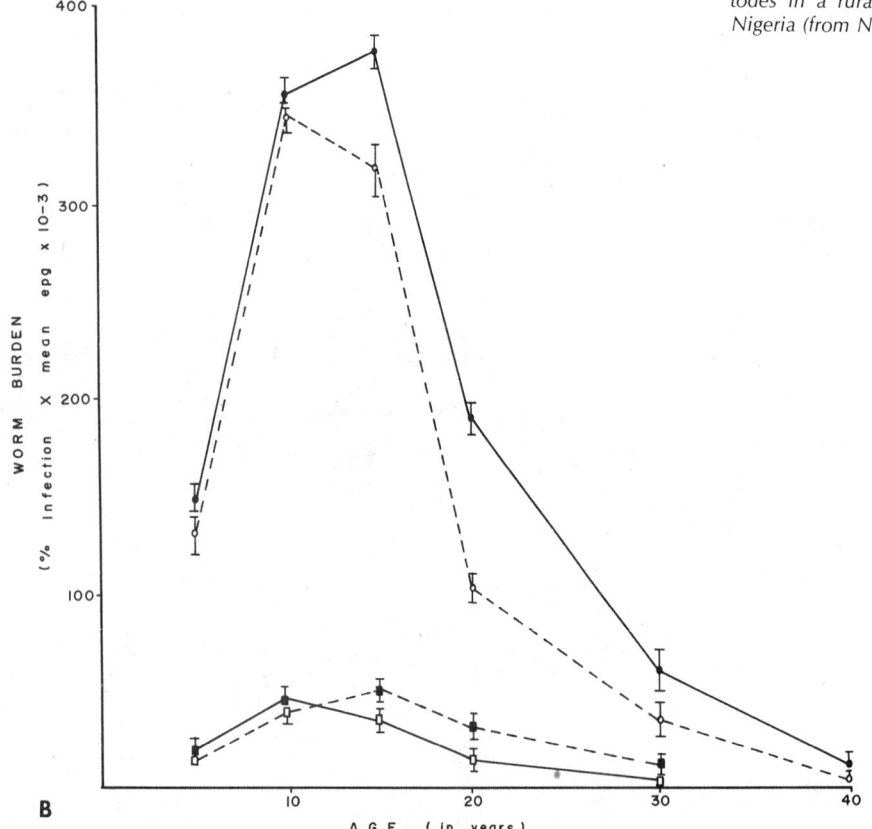

B

**FIGURE 14.** *Graphs summarizing (A) the incidence and (B) the worm burden within age cohorts of three parasitic nematodes in a rural community in Nsukka, Nigeria (from Nwosu and Anya, 1980).*

DEGREE OF HELMINTH INFESTATION

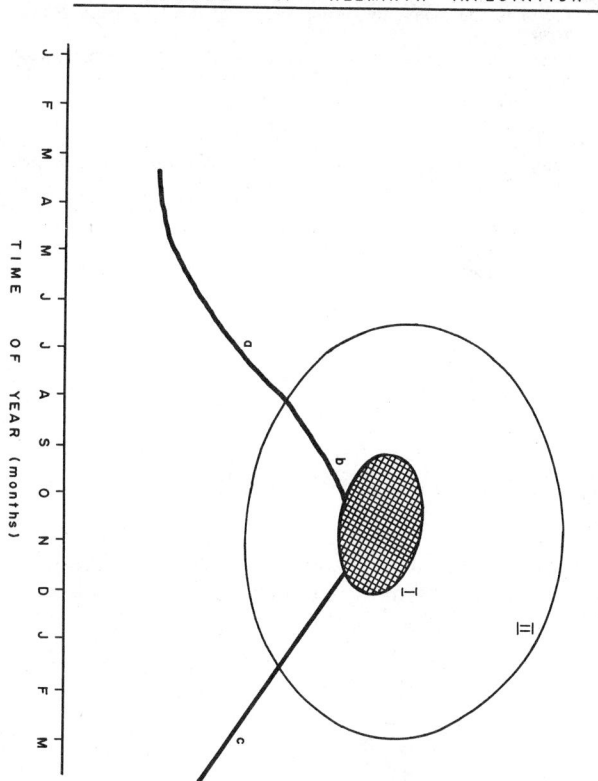

**FIGURE 15.** *Diagrammatic representation of the relationship between infection pressure, season, and distribution within a community of nematode infections and the exploitation of this relationship in control procedures (see text – from Nwosu and Anya, 1980).*

This has given rise to the concept of a target time/target population approach to the control of these helminths. The basic idea is to concentrate mass chemotherapy efforts on that segment of the population with the preponderance of the worm burden during those months that are unfavorable to transmission of the parasites. Thus, the worm population would be depressed below the threshold level for maintenance of the parasite population (within the host population) at a fraction of the normal cost. The concept is summarized in Figure 15. The circles represent the total population (I) and the segmental population (II) with the high worm burden, while a, b, and c represent the periods of normal, high, and depressed infection rates during the year. Concentration of control efforts on II and c is the strategy of choice.

Some of the original work reported in this chapter has been supported by grants from the British Medical Research Council (ODM Research Scheme R2836) and the Senate Research Grant Committee of the University of Nigeria to whom grateful acknowledgment is made. I would also like to acknowledge helpful discussions with my colleagues of the Parasitic Nematodes Research Group, especially Drs. Nwosu and Anubogu.

parasite, and the protected but free-living egg population. Any factor that changes the numbers of any of these populations will alter the infection rate and hence the epidemiologic parameters of the equilibrium between host and parasite. For the hookworm, four distinct populations are involved. In each population, such factors as age, physiology, and ecology will determine population size, contact between the populations, and, ultimately, the infection pressure (Udonsi, 1980). In recent years, the introduction of mathematical models in the analysis of host-parasite systems has increased our understanding of the epidemiologic characteristics of some parasitic diseases (Bradley, 1974; Anderson, 1976).

In our laboratories in Nsukka, this approach has been used in an epidemiologic study of parasitic infections, particularly hookworms. As can be seen from Figure 14, which represents a study of a defined rural community, a small proportion of the population (the 5- to 20-year-olds, 19.5 per cent of the population) harbors a major proportion of the community worm burden. A notable seasonality in the pattern of these hookworm infections has been observed (Nwosu and Anya, 1980).

## References

Anderson, R. M.: Dynamic aspects of parasite population ecology. In Kennedy, C. R. (ed.): Ecological Aspects of Parasitology. Amsterdam, North-Holland Publishing Company, 1976.

Anya, A. O.: Studies on the structure and chemical composition of the nematode cuticle. Observations on some oxyuroids and *Ascaris*. Parasitology 56:179, 1966.

Anya, A. O.: Serotonin (5-hydroxytryptamine) and other indolealkylamines in the male reproductive tract of a nematode. Int J Parasitol 3:573, 1973.

Anya, A. O.: Physiological aspects of reproduction in nematodes. Adv Parasitol 14:267, 1976.

Bradley, D. J.: Stability in host-parasite systems. In Usherand, M. B., and Williamson, M. H., (eds.): Ecological Stability. London, Chapman and Hall, 1974.

Chabaud, A. G.: CIH keys to the nematode parasites of vertebrates. Commonwealth Agricultural Bureau, No. 1. Slough, Buckinghamshire, England, 1974.

Crofton, H. D.: Nematodes. London, Hutchinson, 1966.

Davis, A.: Drug Treatment in Intestinal Helminthiasis. Geneva, World Health Organization, 1973.

De Conick, L.: De symmetrie — verhoudingen aan het vooreinde der vrijlevende Nematoden. Natuurwetench. Tijdschr (Ghent) 24:29, 1942.

Green, C. D.: The attraction of male cyst nematodes by their females. Nematologica 13:172, 1967.

Harris, J. E., and Crofton, H. D.: Structure and function in the nematodes: Internal pressure and cuticular structure in *Ascaris*. J Exp Biol 34:116, 1957.

Hyman, L. H.: The Invertebrates, Vol. 3. New York, McGraw-Hill Book Company, 1951.

Larsh, J. E., Jr., and Race, G. J.: Allergic inflammation as a hypothesis for the expulsion of worms from tissues: A review. Exp Parasitol 37:251, 1975.

Maggenti, A. R.: Taxonomic position of nematoda among the pseudocoelomate bilateria. In Croll, N. A. (ed.): The Organization of Nematodes. New York, Academic Press, 1976.

McLaren, D.: Nematode sense organs. Adv Parasitol 14:195, 1976.

Michel, J. F.: Arrested development of nematodes and some related phenomena. Adv Parasitol 12:279, 1974.

Miller, T. A.: Effect of x-irradiation upon the infective larvae of *Ancylostoma caninum* and the immunogenic effect in dogs of a single infection with 40 kr-irradiated larvae. J Parasitol 50:735, 1964.

Muller, R.: Worms and Disease. London, William Heinemann Medical Books Ltd., 1975.

Nigon, V.: Le determinisme du sex et la pseudogamie chez un nematode parthenogenetique. Bull Biol Fr Belg 81:1947.

Nwosu, A. B. C., and Anya, A. O.: Seasonality in Human Hookworm infection in an endemic area of Nigeria, and its relationship to rainfall. Tropenmed Parasit 31:(1980).

Ogilvie, B. M., and Jones, V. E.: Immunity in the parasitic relationship between helminths and hosts. Prog Allergy 17:93, 1973.

Rogers, W. P., and Sommerville, R. I.: The infectious process and its relationship to the development of early parasitic stages of nematodes. Adv Parasitol 6:327, 1968.

Selby, G. R., and Wakelin, D.: Transfer of immunity against *Trichuris muris* in the mouse by serum and cells. Int J Parasitol 3:717, 1973.

Udonsi, J. K.: Studies on the ecology of the infective larvae of *Necator americanus* (Stiles, 1902) in relation to the epidemiology of human hookworm infections. Ph.D. Thesis, University of Nigeria, 1980.

Wakelin, D., and Lloyd, M.: Accelerated expulsion of adult *Trichinella spiralis* in mice given lymphoid cells and serum from infected donors. Parasitology 72:307, 1976.

World Health Organization: Epidemiology of Onchocerciasis. Technical Report Series No. 597. Geneva, 1976.

Zmoray, I., and Guttekova, A.: Ecological aspect of the study of the intestinal structure of nematodes. Z Parasitenk 39:127, 1972.

# 80 *PLATYHELMINTHES*

## Zbigniew S. Pawlowski, M.D.

Some of the platyhelminthes (flat worms) are free-living animals (for example, Turbellaria), but most are exclusively parasitic and belong to the classes Trematoda (flukes) and Cestoda (tapeworms). Only a few of the Trematoda and Cestoda are parasites of man; the others are parasites of other vertebrates (Tables 1 and 7).

# TREMATODA (FLUKE WORMS)

The trematodes parasitizing man can be classified according to morphologic criteria, localization in the human host, and specificity for the human host (Table 1).

Trematodes are usually classified by their anatomic location, because each family largely localizes in a certain anatomic site of the body; for example: (1) blood flukes — family Schistosomatidae; (2) liver flukes — family Opisthorchiidae and Dicrocoeliidae, Fasciolidae, except Fasciolopsis; (3) intestinal flukes — Fasciolopsis and family Heterophyidae, Echinostomatidae; and (4) lung flukes — family Troglotrematidae.

The host-specificity of trematodes correlates well with their prevalence and medical importance. For example, there are four different degrees of specificity for man among the Schistosoma: (1) man is the main definitive host of *Schistosoma haematobium, Schistosoma intercalatum,* and *Schistosoma mansoni;* (2) man shares *Schistosoma japonicum* with a wide range of animals; (3) man is only an occasional definitive host of *Schistosoma matthei* and *Schistosoma rhodhaini;* and (4) man can be invaded by other trematodes, such as Gigantobilharzia and Trichobilharzia, which cannot complete their development in man and can cause only skin lesions. The trematodes of groups 1 and 2 are of greater medical importance than the occasional or atypical parasites of groups 3 and 4 (Table 1).

## *MORPHOLOGY AND LIFE CYCLES*

### Blood Flukes — Schistosomatidae

Schistosomatidae are exceptional among trematodes in that they are dioecious (sexes separated). The female worm has a cylindric body and the male a canoe-shaped body with a gynecophoral canal in which the adult female spends most of her time. The main species of the schistosomes of man are morphologically distinct (Figs. 1 and 4).

The life cycle of *S. haematobium* is shown in Table 2. *S. mansoni* requires a shorter time of development in the snail (four to five weeks) and in man (25 to 28 days) before first egg production. *S. japonicum* has a shorter time of development in man, but a longer one in the snail (over seven weeks). It is also produces many more eggs (3500 per day per female).

### Liver Flukes

*Clonorchis (Opisthorchis) sinensis, Opisthorchis felineus,* and *Opisthorchis viverrini* are common liver flukes (Komiya, 1966). All have a flat lanceolate body between 10 and 20 mm in length. The testes of *Opisthorchis* spp. are lobed, whereas those of *C. sinensis* are in a dendritic arrangement. The differences between *O. felineus* and *O. viverrini* are biologic rather than morphologic.

**TABLE 1.  Trematodes Parasitizing Man: Habitat and Hosts**

| SPECIES | HABITAT IN MAN | DEFINITIVE HOSTS OTHER THAN MAN | SNAILS AS FIRST INTERMEDIATE HOSTS | OTHER INTERMEDIATE HOSTS (OR PLANTS INVOLVED IN TRANSMISSION) |
|---|---|---|---|---|
| *Schistosoma haematobium* | Vesical and pelvic venous plexuses | — | *Bulinus* | — |
| *S. intercalatum* | Mesenteric veins | — | *Bulinus* | — |
| *S. mansoni* | Mesenteric veins | Baboon, rodents | *Biomphalaria* | — |
| *S. japonicum* | Mesenteric veins | Many domesticated and wild animals | *Oncomelania* | — |
| *Clonorchis* (*Opisthorchis*) *sinensis* | Bile ducts | Dog, cat, pig | *Bulinus, Paraphossalurus* | Cyprinid fishes |
| *Opisthorchis felineus* | Bile ducts | Cat, dog, pig, fox | *Bithynia* | Cyprinid fishes |
| *Opisthorchis viverrini* | Bile ducts | Civet cat | *Bithynia* | Cyprinid fishes |
| *Fasciola hepatica, Fasciola gigantica* | Bile ducts | Sheep and other herbivores | *Lymnaea* | Watercress and grass |
| *Fasciolopsis buski* | Small intestine | Pig | *Segmentina, Planorbis* | Water caltrop and water chestnut |
| *Heterophyes heterophyes* | Small intestine | Dog, cat, fish-eating wild carnivores | *Pirenella, Cerithidia* | Mullet and tilapia fishes |
| *Metagonimus yokogawai* | Small intestine | Dog, cat, pig, fish-eating birds | *Semisulcospira* | Different fresh water fishes |
| *Gastrodiscoides hominis* | Coecum, colon | Pig | *Helicorbis* | Water caltrop |
| *Paragonimus westermani* | Lungs | Cat, tiger, leopard, dog, pig, monkey | *Semisulcospira, Thiara, Oncomelania* | Fresh water crabs and crayfish |

The life cycles of *C. sinensis, O. felineus,* and *O. viverrini* are similar, but the snail and fish hosts and the geographic distribution differ (Tables 1 and 3, Fig. 3).

*Dicrocoelium dendriticum,* an unusual parasite of man, completes its strange life cycle on the ground by using terrestrial snails and ants as hosts. *Fasciola hepatica* is not uncommon in some countries (France, Algeria, Peru, and Cuba). It has a life cycle similar to that of Fasciolopsis (see below), but encysts on watercress, lettuce, and radishes.

### Intestinal Flukes

The most important intestinal fluke is *Fasciolopsis buski,* the largest fluke of man (up to 70 mm long and 20 mm wide). It has no second intermediate host (Table 4, Figs. 2 and 3).

The remaining intestinal flukes (*Heterophyes, Metagonimus,* and *Echinostoma*) are small parasites, 2 to 8 mm long. Fish are the second intermediate hosts (Table 1, Figs. 2 and 3).

### Lung Flukes

*Paragonimus westermani* is the common representative of the family of Troglotrematidae (Yokogawa, 1965). Unlike other trematodes, it has an oval, thick body with a ventral sucker in the middle. Its life cycle includes two intermediate hosts (Table 5, Figs. 2 and 3).

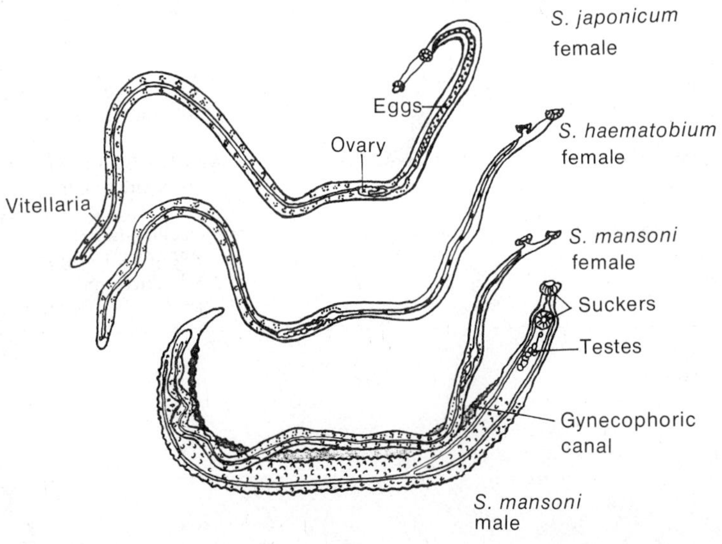

**FIGURE 1.** *Adult schistosomes. Diagram of morphologic characteristics.*

**TABLE 2. Schistosoma haematobium: Life Cycle**

| HOST AND HABITAT | TIME | STAGE AND ACTIVITY | NUMBER |
|---|---|---|---|
| Man | 2–25 years | EGGS fully embryonated expelled in urine (and feces) | 20–260 per worm per day |
| Water | 16–32 hrs | MIRACIDIUM hatches in water and penetrates snail | 1 |
| Snails<br>*Bulinus* spp. | 5–6 weeks | PRIMARY SPOROCYST produces<br>SECONDARY SPOROCYSTS, which produce<br>CERCARIAE, which leave the snail host for months | 1<br>n<br>$n^m$ = ca 250,000 |
| Water | Up to 8 hrs | cercaria swimming in water and penetrating skin | 1 |
| Man<br>lungs, liver,<br>venous plexuses | 6–12 weeks | preadult SCHISTOSOMULA migrating and<br>developing in lungs and liver into<br>ADULT worm situated finally in pelvic and<br>vesical venous plexuses and producing eggs | 1<br>1 |

**TABLE 3. Clonorchis (Opisthorchis) sinensis: Life Cycle**

| HOST AND HABITAT | TIME | STAGE AND ACTIVITY | NUMBER |
|---|---|---|---|
| Man, dog, cat, pig | Up to 20–30 years | EGGS fully embryonated in bile and feces | 1000 per worm per day |
| Water | Up to 3 months | Eggs survive in water | |
| Snail<br>*Bulimus* spp.<br>*Parafossalurus* spp.<br>*Semisulcospira* spp. | 3–4 weeks | MIRACIDIUM hatches from egg ingested by snail<br>SPOROCYST produces<br>REDIAE, which produce<br>CERCARIAE; these actively leave<br>snail-host for months | 1<br>1<br>n<br>$n^m$ |
| Water | 1–2 days | cercaria, free-swimming, penetrate second<br>intermediate host | 1 |
| Cyprinid fish | 3 weeks | METACERCARIA encysts in tissue and survives<br>for many months | 1 |
| Man, dog, cat, pig | 3–4 weeks | Metacercaria excysts in duodenum and<br>PREADULT migrates through ampulla of Vater to<br>bile ducts and develops into<br>an ADULT worm, producing eggs | 1<br><br>1 |

**TABLE 4.   Fasciolopsis buski: Life Cycle**

| HOST AND HABITAT | TIME | STAGE AND ACTIVITY | NUMBER |
|---|---|---|---|
| Man, pig | 6 months | EGGS undeveloped, expelled in feces | 21,000–28,000 per worm per day |
| Water | 3–7 weeks<br>Few hours | egg embryonates in water and hatches as<br>MIRACIDIUM which penetrates snail | 1<br>1 |
| Snail<br>*Segmentina* spp.<br>*Planorbis* spp. | Few weeks | SPOROCYST produces<br>REDIAE of first generation, which produce<br>REDIAE of second generation; these produce<br>CERCARIAE, which actively leave snail | 1<br>$n$<br>$n^m$<br>$(n^m)^p$ |
| Water<br>(Water chestnut)<br>(Water caltrop) | Several months | cercaria shortly encysts on water vegetation<br>and becomes METACERCARIA, which survives<br>several months | 1<br>1 |
| Man, pig | 3–4 months | Metacercaria excysts in duodenum and<br>PREADULT develops into<br>an ADULT worm | 1<br>1 |

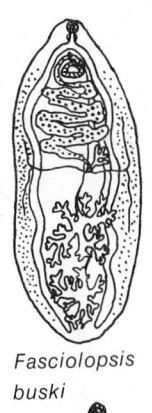
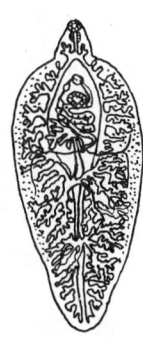
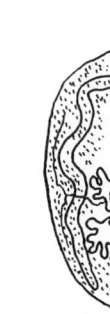

*Fasciolopsis buski*    *Fasciola hepatica*    *Paragonimus westermani*

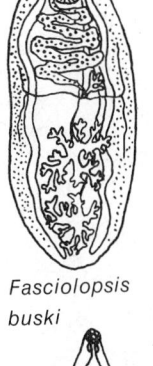
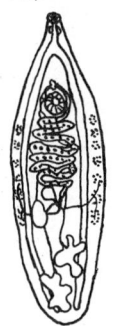
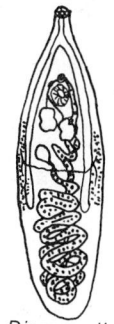

*Clonorchis sinensis*    *Opisthorchis felineus*    *Dicrocoelium dendriticum*

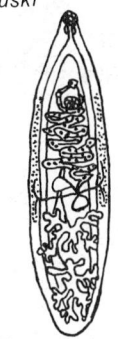
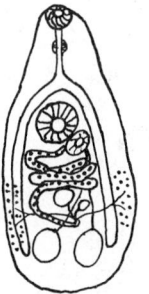
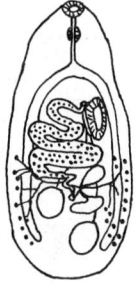
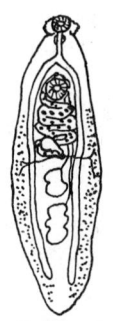

*Gastrodiscoides hominis*    *Heterophyes heterophyes*    *Metagonimus yokogawai*    *Echinostoma ilocanum*

**FIGURE 2.** *Adult trematodes (except the schistosomes). Diagram of morphologic characteristics.*

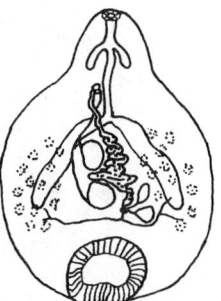

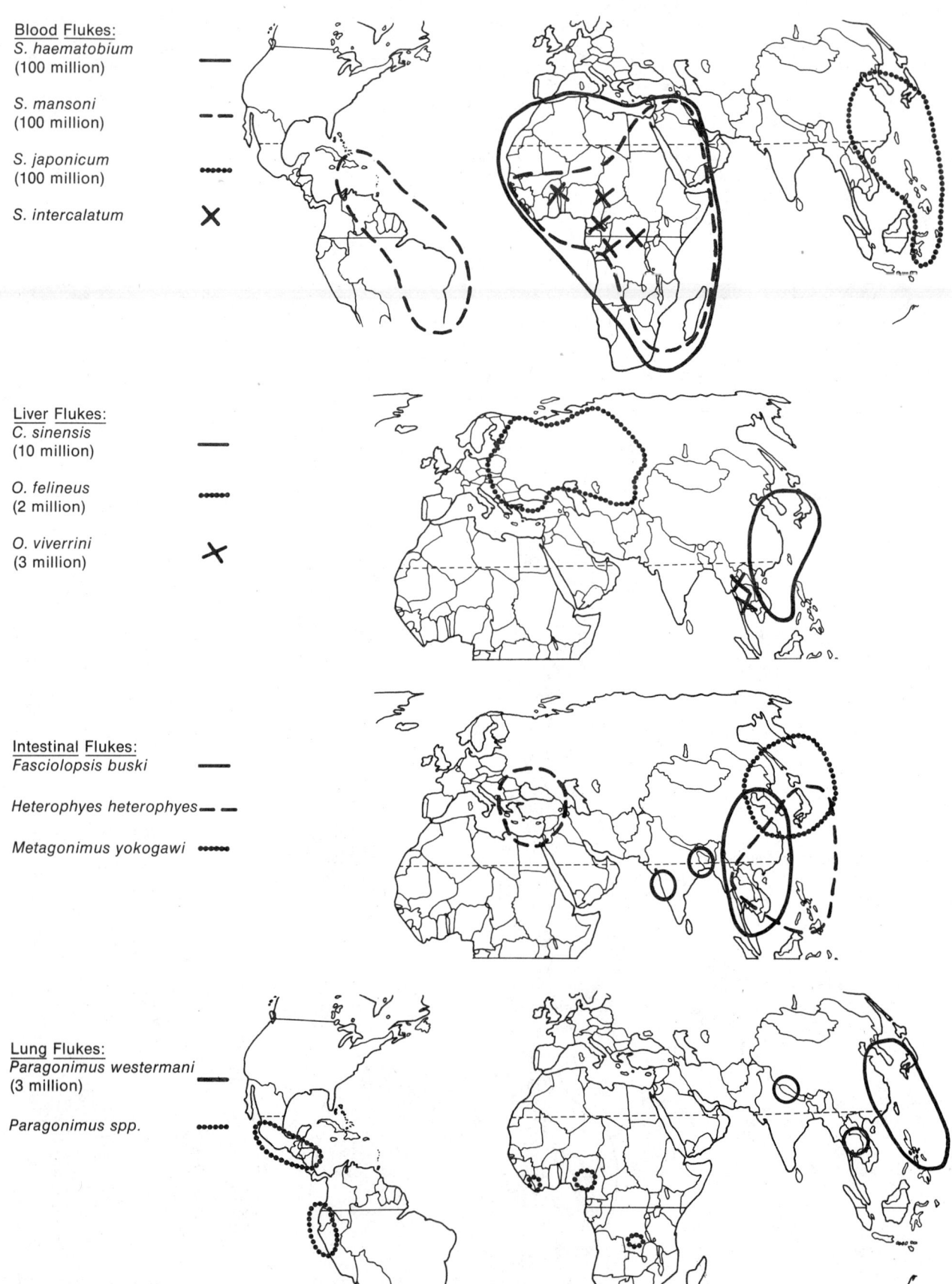

**FIGURE 3.** *Geographic distribution of flukes.*

**TABLE 5.  Paragonimus westermani: Life Cycle**

| HOST AND HABITAT | TIME | STAGE AND ACTIVITY | NUMBER |
|---|---|---|---|
| Man, various mammals | 6–20 years | EGGS expelled in sputum or feces | ? |
| Water | 3 weeks | egg develops into<br>MIRACIDIUM, which hatches in water<br>and penetrates snail in 24 hrs. | 1<br>1 |
| Snail<br>  *Semisulcospira* spp.<br>  *Thiara* spp.<br>  *Oncomelania* spp. | 3 months | SPOROCYST in snail tissue produces<br>  REDIAE I generation, which emerges as<br>  REDIAE II generation; Rediae II produce<br>  CERCARIAE, which actively leave snail | 1<br>$n$<br>$n^m$<br>$(n^m)^p$ |
| Water | 24–48 hrs | cercaria, free-swimming and penetrating crabs | 1 |
| Crabs | Several months | METACERCARIA encysted in crab tissue | 1 |
| Man | | Ingested by definitive host; hatches in duodenum, as | |
| | 20 days |   PREADULT migrates through gut wall, abdominal and<br>  pleural cavities, and lung tissue | 1 |
| | 5–6 weeks |   ADULT, produces eggs in lung cysts | 1 |

## IMMUNOLOGY

Natural resistance to trematodes depends on many biochemical, physiologic, genetic, and nutritional factors, and is low in man. Acquired immunity against trematodes rarely prevents infection but can limit its intensity. For example, new invading schistosomulae are rapidly destroyed by hosts who are already infected with adult worms. However, seven days after infection, preadult schistosomulae are no longer recognized by the host as foreign, probably owing to the incorporation of host antigens into the integument of the trematode. Living adult worms are usually not attacked by immunologic reactions but provoke a reaginic (IgE) response, releasing pharmacologic mediators of anaphylaxis. These hypersensitivity reactions are stage-specific and are intensive against eggs and cercariae. For example, schistosome eggs swept back from the mesenteric veins into the liver cause antibody-mediated reactions (Hoeppli phenomenon) first, and then a cell-mediated delayed hypersensitivity reaction producing eosinophilic granulomas. The skin reaction against penetrating cercariae is also of the cell-mediated type. Antigen-antibody complex diseases occur in schistosomiasis as glomerulonephritis (*S. mansoni*) or Katayama syndrome (*S. japonicum*), which resembles serum sickness with gastroenteritis.

There is no immunization against trematode infection. It is possible, however, that infection or immunization with some less pathogenic, but highly immunogenic, animal schistosomes might partially protect man against human schistosomes.

## LABORATORY DIAGNOSIS

The symptoms or signs of human infections with trematodes are rarely pathognomonic. Therefore, the diagnosis is usually made by finding the eggs (Fig. 4) of the trematode in feces (most species), urine (*S. haematobium*), duodenal contents (*Clonorchis, Opisthorchis, Fasciola*), liver and rectal biopsies (*Schistosoma*), or sputum (*Paragonimus*). The flotation coprologic techniques are less effective than sedimentation or thick smear because the eggs are relatively heavy. Before eggs are produced it is difficult to make the diagnosis. The intradermal test, as well as the complement fixation, indirect hemagglutination, indirect fluorescent antibody, and precipitin tests, is of limited help in the early stages of infection with *Schistosoma, Clonorchis, Opisthorchis,* and *Paragonimus*.

## DRUG SUSCEPTIBILITY

The intestinal flukes are susceptible to many antihelminthics. Liver, blood, and lung flukes are less susceptible, and the drugs are toxic and only partially effective. Recently some effective and less toxic drugs have been developed (praziquantel, amoscanate).

The blood flukes (Schistosomes) are susceptible to antimony compounds, which are rarely used now. The nonmetallic drugs niridazole and hycanthone are active against *S. haematobium*. Metrifonate, the organophosphorus cholinesterase inhibitor of insects, is also a potent inhibitor of nematode cholinesterase; as little as 0.1 $\mu$m

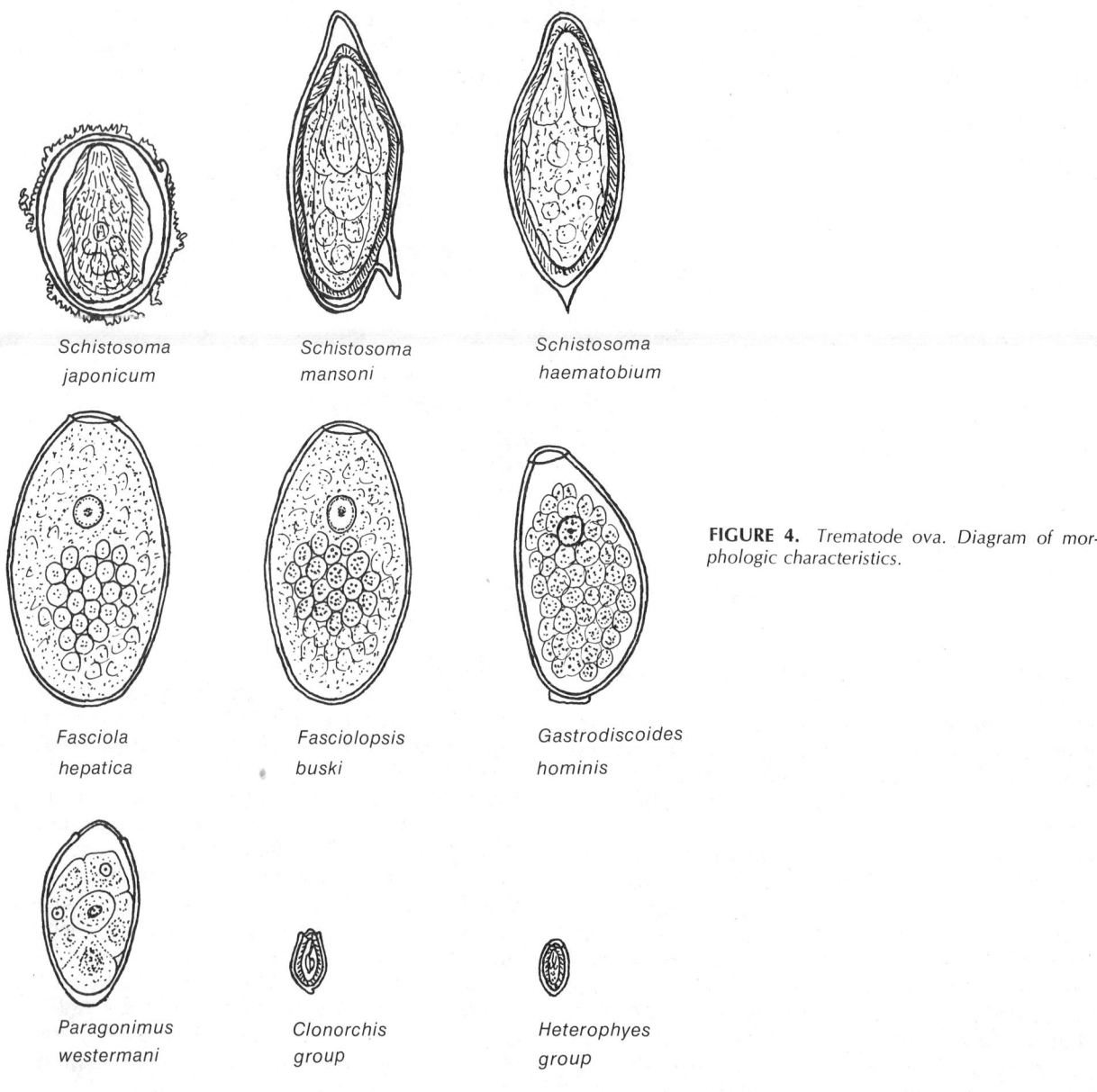

Schistosoma
japonicum

Schistosoma
mansoni

Schistosoma
haematobium

Fasciola
hepatica

Fasciolopsis
buski

Gastrodiscoides
hominis

**FIGURE 4.** *Trematode ova. Diagram of morphologic characteristics.*

Paragonimus
westermani

Clonorchis
group

Heterophyes
group

metrifonate inhibits the *S. haematobium* enzyme by 50 per cent, and lower concentrations inhibit *S. mansoni* cholinesterase. Oxamniquine is effective against *S. mansoni* only. Lung flukes and liver flukes are inhibited by bithionol or chloroquine and intestinal flukes by hexylresorcinol or tetrachlorethylene.

## EPIDEMIOLOGY

Schistosomiasis is a worldwide problem second only to malaria in frequency (about 250 million people; Fig. 3). Some other trematode infections (paragonimiasis, clonorchiasis, fasciolopsiasis) are of serious, but primarily local, medical impor-

tance. Their distribution in the world is focal (Fig. 3) and depends on the presence of a suitable species of snail and certain local behavior factors, such as agricultural practices and ingestion of raw fish, crabs, or snails. In endemic areas, the transmission is usually continuous and results in frequent infection of rather low intensity, due to either infrequent exposure or some degree of concomitant immunity, or both. Epidemics of trematode infection are usually caused by changes in environmental or social factors. Thus, epidemics of *S. haematobium* occur around man-made lakes or in new irrigation systems that introduce the parasite or intermediate host into susceptible areas (Ansari, 1973).

The rise of schistosomiasis in human populations after the introduction of this fluke and its decline after the institution of control programs can be roughly predicted by using mathematical models (Fig. 5), (Macdonald, 1965).

Many of the trematodes parasitizing man are zoonotic in origin; however, the role of animal reservoirs differs and depends partly on human behavior. For example, *Paragonimus africanus* is a zoonotic infection in Nigeria and Cameroon, whereas the transmission of *P. westermani* in China, Japan, and Korea is probably independent of that in animals. In Indonesia, Malaysia, and Ceylon, the infections occur exclusively in animals.

Community control measures require education about transmission, sanitary disposal of feces and urine, and installation of safe water supplies. Mass-control programs are based primarily on improved irrigation and agricultural practices, on using molluscacides, and on mass treatment of infected people (schistosomiasis).

Personal protection is enhanced by using cercarial repellents; avoiding contaminated water for bathing, washing, and drinking (schistosomiasis); cooking fish, crabs, and crayfish (clonorchiasis, opisthorchiasis, heterophyiasis, paragonimiasis); and immersing water plants in boiling water before ingestion (fasciolopsiasis).

# CESTODA (TAPEWORMS)

Tapeworms parasitizing man belong to the order Cyclophyllidea (families Taeniidae and Hymenolepididae) and Pseudophyllidea (*Diphyllobothrium* spp. and *Spirometra* spp.). All the adult tapeworms are intestinal parasites of their definitive vertebrate host; some are human tissue parasites in their larval stage (Table 6).

For some tapeworms (*T. saginata, T. solium*) man is the only definitive host. For a few species (*Diphyllobothrium* spp.) man is one of many vertebrate definitive hosts. For a larger number, man is an occasional definitive or an intermediate host (Pawlowski and Schultz, 1972) (Table 6).

## MORPHOLOGY AND LIFE CYCLE

There are three large (4 to 15 m) tapeworms parasitizing man: *Taenia solium, T. saginata*, and *Diphyllobothrium latum*. Their morphologic characteristics are listed in Table 7 and Figure 6. *Hymenolepis diminuta* and *Dipylidium caninum* are of medium size (20 to 60 cm) and only *Hymenolepis nana* (dwarf tapeworm) is small (15 to 40

mm). The morphology and life cycle of *H. nana* is presented in Figure 7.

The larval stages of the tapeworms parasitizing man are as follows: (1) cysticercus (*T. solium*); (2) cysticercoid (*H. nana*); (3) coenurus (*T. multiceps*); (4) echinococcus (*Echinococcus granulosus* and *Echinococcus multilocularis*); and (5) sparganum, a plerocercoid-type larva (*Diphyllobothrium erinacei, Spirometra mansoni*). The first four are bladderworms of different sizes and different macroscopic and microscopic structures (Table 8, Fig. 8).

Human tapeworms have three basic types of life cycles: (1) The first type has water as an environment, aquatic copepoda (crustaceans) as the first intermediate hosts, fish as the second, and many vertebrates as definitive hosts (*Diphyllobothrium*, Table 9); (2) The second type uses various herbivorous vertebrates as intermediate hosts and carnivorous vertebrates as definitive hosts (*Taenia, Echinococcus*, Table 10); (3) The third type requires only one host because the larval stages develop in the intestinal villi of the definitive host (*H. nana*) (Fig. 7). Those tape-

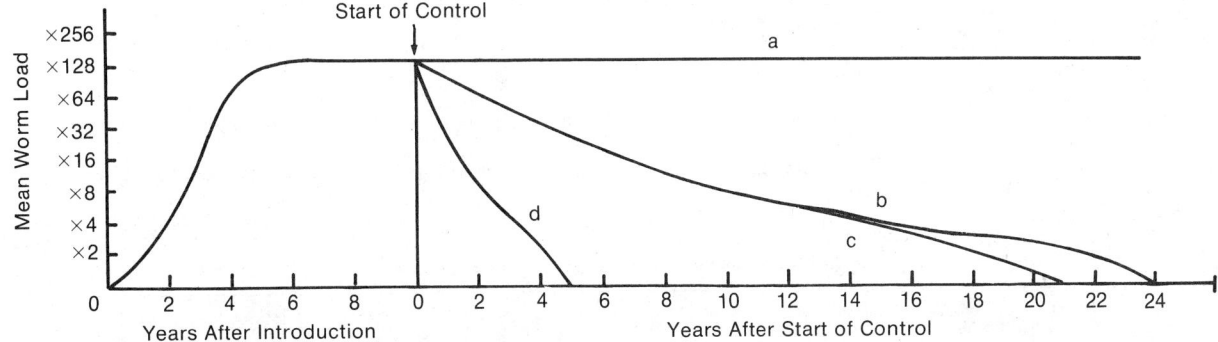

**FIGURE 5.** *Diagram of the rise and fall of the mean load of schistosomes in human populations as predicted by the mathematical model of Macdonald (1965). a = reduction of water contamination to ¹/₁₅ of the original by improvement of sanitation; b = reduction of snail population to ¹/₁₅ original; c = reduction of exposure to water to ¹/₁₅ by public education; d = reduction of longevity of worms to ¹/₁₅ by chemotherapy plus reducing b and c to ¹/₃ of their original values.*

**TABLE 6.   Cestodes Parasitizing Man: Hosts, Habitat, and Distribution**

| TAXONOMIC CLASSIFICATION | HABITAT IN MAN Adult Worm | Larval Stage | DEFINITIVE HOSTS OTHER THAN MAN | INTERMEDIATE HOSTS | WORLD DISTRIBUTION |
|---|---|---|---|---|---|
| Order Cyclophyllidea* Taeniidae | | | | | |
| *Taenia saginata* | Small intestine (jejunum) | No | No | Cattle and other Boviidae | Cosmopolitan |
| *Taenia solium* | Small intestine (jejunum) | CYSTICERCUS in muscle and internal organs (brain, eye) | No | Pig, man, and many other mammals | Central and South America, Mexico, South Africa, India, USSR |
| *Taenia multiceps* | — | COENURUS in brain, eye, skin | Dog and wild canidae | Sheep, other ruminants, and rabbits | Several areas in the world |
| *Echinococcus granulosus* | — | ECHINOCOCCUS in liver, lungs, brain | Dog and wild carnivora | Sheep, cattle, pig, horse, camel, goat, and many wild mammals | Cosmopolitan |
| *E. multilocularis* | — | Alveolar ECHINOCOCCUS in liver | Fox, domestic cat, and wild canidae | Wild rodents | Northern hemisphere |
| Hymenolepididae | | | | | |
| *Hymenolepis nana* | Ileum | Intestinal villi | Full development in man only | | Cosmopolitan, warm countries |
| *H. diminuta* | Small intestine (jejunum) | No | Rats, mice, wild rodents | Fleas, flour beetles | Cosmopolitan |
| Order Pseudophyllidea | | | | | |
| *Diphyllobothrium latum†* | Small intestine (jejunum) | — | Cat, dog, and fish-eating carnivora | Planktonic copepoda (*Cyclops* and *Diaptomus*) and freshwater fish | Lakes, rivers, and deltas in Finland, Siberia, Canada, USA, Chile, Argentina |

*Some other Cyclophyllidea occasionally invade man: e.g., the common dog tapeworm *Dipylidium caninum.*
†Several other species of Diphyllobothrium have been found in man in Alaska. Occasionally in the Far East plerocercoid larvae of *Sparganum proliferum* or *Spirometra mansoni* invade human tissues.

**TABLE 7.   Morphologic Differences Between Large Tapeworms in Man**

| | *Taenia solium* | *Taenia saginata* | *Diphyllobothrium latum* |
|---|---|---|---|
| ENTIRE BODY | | | |
| Length (m) | 1,5–8 | 4–12 | 3–15 |
| Maximal breadth (mm) | 7–10 | 12–14 | 10–12 |
| Proglottids (number) | 700–1000 | ca 2000 | 3000–4000 |
| SCOLEX | | | |
| Diameter (mm) | 0,6–1 | 1,5–2 | Elongate 2–3 mm long |
| Suckers (number) | 4 | 4 | 2 sucking grooves |
| Rostellum | Present | Absent | Absent |
| Hooks (number) | 22–32 | Absent | Absent |
| MATURE PROGLOTTIDS | | | |
| Testes (number) | 375–575 | 800–1200 | ? |
| Ovary (number of lobes) | 3 | 2 | 2 |
| Uterus as | Blind tube | Blind tube | Coiled with a pore |
| Vaginal sphincter | Absent | Present | ? |
| Genital atrium at | Lateral margin | Lateral margin | Ventral surface |
| GRAVID PROGLOTTIDS | | | |
| Uterus (number of branches each side) | 7–12 | 18–32 | None |
| Way of leaving host | In groups, passively | Single, spontaneously | |

| | Taenia solium | Taenia saginata | Diphyllo—bothrium latum | Hymenolepis diminuta | Dipylidium caninum | Hymenolepis nana |
|---|---|---|---|---|---|---|
| Scolex | 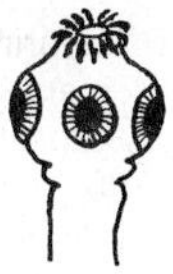 | 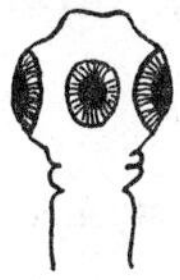 | 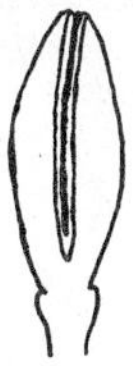 | 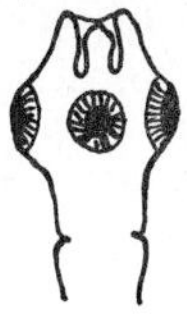 | 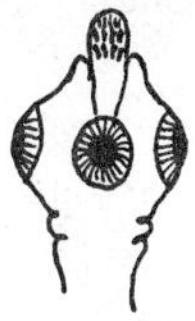 | 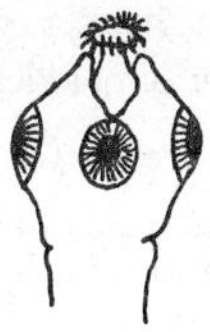 |
| Gravid proglottid | 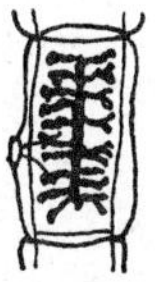 | 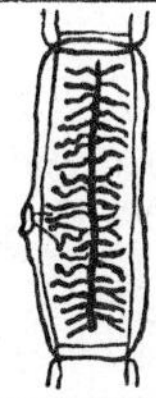 | 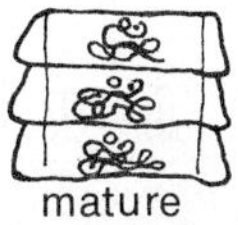 mature proglottids only | 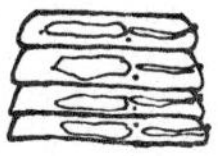 | 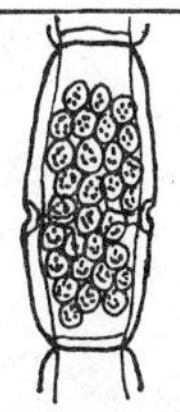 | 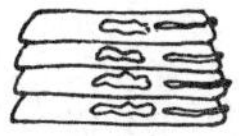 |
| Number of proglottids | 700–1000 | ca 2000 | 3000–4000 | 800–1000 | 60–175 | ca 200 |
| Length of strobila (cm) | 150–800 | 400–1200 | 300–1500 | 30–60 | 20–40 | 1½–4 |

**FIGURE 6.** *Cestodes of man. Diagram of morphologic characteristics.*

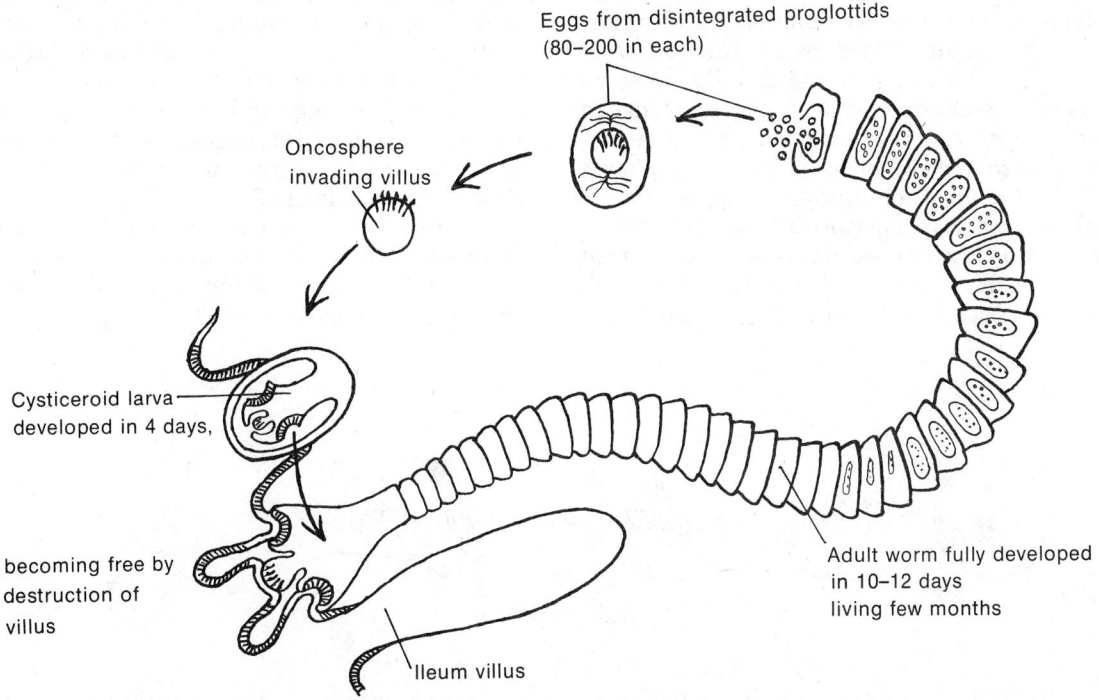

Eggs from disintegrated proglottids (80–200 in each)

Oncosphere invading villus

Cysticeroid larva developed in 4 days,

becoming free by destruction of villus

Ileum villus

Adult worm fully developed in 10–12 days living few months

**FIGURE 7.** *Hymenolepis nana. Diagram of life cycle.*

**Table 8.   Morphologic Differences Between Teniid Larvae Parasitizing Man**

|  | Taenia solium | Taenia saginata | Taenia multiceps | Echinococcus granulosus | Echinococcus multilocularis |
|---|---|---|---|---|---|
| TYPE OF BLADDER | Cysticercus | Cysticercus | Coenurus | Echinococcus | Alveolar Echinococcus |
| MACROSCOPIC STRUCTURE |  |  |  |  |  |
| number of bladders | 1 | 1 | 1 | One primary cyst, many brood capsules | Many |
| maximum size (mm) | 10 | 8 | 30 | 200 | 2 |
| number of scolices in a bladder | 1 | 1 | 100 if fertile | Many thousands if fertile | Few or none |
| MICROSCOPIC STRUCTURE |  |  |  |  |  |
| hooks on scolex | Present | Absent | Present | Present | Present |
| surface | Cuticle | Cuticle | Cuticle | Stratified hyaline membrane | Thin membrane |
| make-up of wall | Wortlike processes | Rugae | Smooth and also rugae | Smooth | Smooth |
| superficial protuberances |  |  |  |  |  |
| height (µm) | 15–27 | 23–27 | 15–22 | No | No |
| width at base | 27–38 | 50–70 | 28–46 | No | No |

worms (*H. diminuta, Dipylidium*) with insects (fleas, beetles) as intermediate hosts rarely parasitize the intestine of man.

## IMMUNOLOGY

The natural resistance of man against cestodes is low. Acquired immunity has been confirmed only in experimental *H. nana* infections. Adults are more resistant than children to human hymenolepiasis, and general immunity and nutrition are the major influences on the course of infection. Living taeniid larvae usually cause no local cellular reaction, but dead parasites invoke a strong response that produces a certain degree of resistance to reinfection. Migrating oncospheres seem to be the most immunogenic stage.

Adult *T. saginata* tapeworms frequently cause a rise in blood IgE but allergic reactions are rare in taeniasis. However, fatal anaphylactic shock may follow rupture of a cyst of *E. granulosus*.

## LABORATORY DIAGNOSIS

Stool examination is useful in the diagnosis of diphyllobothriasis and hymenolepiasis, but has some limitations in taeniasis. Eggs occur in the feces irregularly and those of *T. solium* and *T. saginata* are identical (Fig. 9). The correct differential diagnosis between *T. solium* and *T. saginata* is based on the morphology of scolices (hooks), mature segments (ovarian lobes), and gravid segments (vaginal sphincter, uterine branches) (Table 7). Laboratory identification of intestinal tapeworms is not possible until they start producing eggs and/or excreting proglottids. Differentiation of larval stages usually requires macroscopic and microscopic examination (hooks, protuberances; Table 9).

Immunodiagnostic tests are useful in cysticercosis and echinococcosis. Biopsy is of diagnostic value in the identification of subcutaneously localized larvae (cysticercosis, sparganosis).

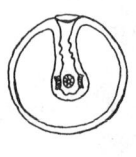 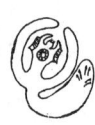 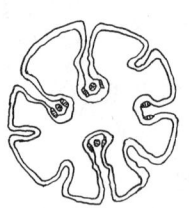 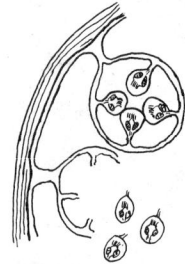 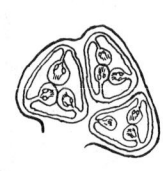

| Cysticerus | Cysticeroid | Coenurus | Echinococcus | Alveolar echinococcus |
|---|---|---|---|---|
| *(T. solium)* | *(H. nana)* | *(T. multiceps)* | *(E. granulosus)* | *(E. multilocularis)* |

**FIGURE 8.** *Larval cestodes. Diagram of morphologic characteristics.*

**TABLE 9.  Diphyllobothrium latum: Life Cycle**

| HOST AND HABITAT | TIME | STAGE AND ACTIVITY | NUMBER |
|---|---|---|---|
| Man and many mammals | Up to 30 years | EGGS undeveloped, expelled in feces | Up to 1,000,000 per day |
| Water | at least 12 days<br>1–2 days | egg embryonates in water, and hatches<br>    free-swimming;<br>    CORACIDIUM is ingested by copepoda | 1<br>1 |
| Fresh water copepoda (crustaceans)<br>    *Diaptomus* spp.<br>    *Cyclops* spp. | 2–3 weeks | PROCERCOID develops in body cavity;<br>    ingested by fish transforms into<br>    plerocercoid | 1 |
| Fresh-water plankton-eating fish<br>    (lota, perch) | 4 weeks | PLEROCERCOID, which develops in muscle<br>    or connective tissues, invades mammals<br>    or fish when ingested | 1 |
| Fresh-water carnivorous fish (pike) as<br>    transport host | Months | plerocercoid | 1 |
| Man and many fish-eating mammals<br>    (dog, cat, bear) | 3–5 weeks | PREADULT and<br>    ADULT tapeworm in small intestine,<br>    produces eggs | 1<br>1 |

**TABLE 10.  Taenia solium: Life Cycle**

| HOST AND HABITAT | TIME | STAGE AND ACTIVITY | NUMBER |
|---|---|---|---|
| Man only | Up to 30 years | EGGS, fully developed, expelled in feces | 500 per one proglottid |
| External environment | Months (years ?) | egg survives in water or soil | 1 |
| Pig; rarely in sheep, dog,<br>cat, and man | 30 minutes<br>60–75 days | ONCOSPHERE hatches in small intestine,<br>    migrates mainly to muscle tissue, and<br>    develops into<br>    CYSTICERCUS, a bladder larva,<br>    which lives for months | 1<br><br>1 |
| Man only | 5–12 weeks | Ingested cysticercus evaginates and transforms<br>    into ADULT worm, which produces<br>    proglottids and eggs | 1 |

T. saginata develops slower in cattle (10–12 weeks) and in man (12 weeks) and produces more proglottids (6–9 per day) and eggs (80,000) per one proglottid.

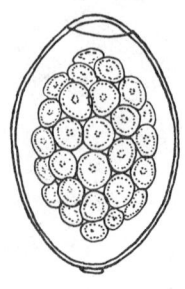
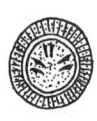
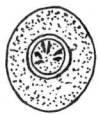
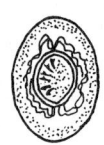
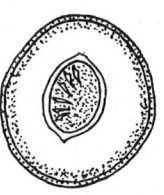

| *Diphyllobothrium latum* | *Taenia solium Taenia saginata* | *Dipylidium caninum* | *Hymenolepis nana* | *Hymenolepis diminuta* |

**FIGURE 9.** *Cestode ova.*

## DRUG SUSCEPTIBILITY

The intestinal tapeworms are susceptible to several taeniacides (niclosamide, paramomycin, Atabrine). Recently, some drugs (praziquantel, mebendazole) have been found that are effective against the larval stages of cestodes.

## EPIDEMIOLOGY

Except for hymenolepiasis, cestode infections are zoonoses involving mainly domesticated animals. Their distribution depends chiefly on agricultural and pastoral practices (taeniasis, echinococcosis, coenurosis). When man is the only definitive host (*T. solium*, *T. saginata*), he is responsible for contamination of the environment with teniid eggs and proglottids of species invasive for the intermediate host (pig, cattle). Man rarely acquires infection from tapeworms circulating in feral (wild animal) cycles (*D. latum*, *E. multilocularis*, *T. multiceps*, *H. diminuta*).

Hands and food contaminated with cestode eggs play an essential role in transmission of infections with *E. multilocularis*, *T. solium* (cysticercosis), and *H. nana*. Autoinfection is rare in *T. solium* taeniasis, but is common in hymenolepiasis and is responsible for the continuation of infection for many years. National programs for the control of echinococcosis in Ireland, Cyprus, and New Zealand were based on education, control of the dog population, mass diagnosis and treatment of dogs, and sanitary practices of sheep slaughter and carcass inspection.

*T. solium* infections usually disappear spontaneously with improved sanitation and modern pig husbandry (Europe). Contamination of the environment by increased numbers of human *T. saginata* carriers makes the control of this taeniasis difficult, in spite of meat inspection that helps to identify and destroy many of the cysticerci.

Personal protection against cestode infections is effected by personal hygiene and avoiding the consumption of raw meat.

## References

Ansari, N. (ed.): Epidemiology and Control of Schistosomiasis (bilharziasis). Basel, S. Karger, 1973.

Komiya, Y.: Clonorchis and clonorchiasis. In Ben Dawes (ed.): Advances in Parasitology. New York and London, Academic Press, 1966, vol. 4, pp. 53.

Macdonald, G.: The dynamics of helminth infections with special reference to schistosomes. Trans R Soc Trop Med Hyg 59:489, 1965.

Pawlowski, Z., and Schultz, M. G.: Taeniasis and cysticercosis (Taenia saginata). In Ben Dawes (ed.): Advances in Parasitology. New York and London, Academic Press, 1972, vol. 10, p. 269.

Yokogawa, M.: Paragonimus and paragonimiasis. In Ben Dawes (ed.): Advances in Parasitology, New York and London, Academic Press, 1965, vol. 3 p. 99, and 1969, vol. 7, p. 375.

# C  GENERAL RESPONSE TO INFECTION

## Immunologic

### MECHANISMS OF NATURAL RESISTANCE TO INFECTION  81

Abraham I. Braude, M.D., Ph.D.

Infectious agents must break through four lines of defense before they can establish themselves in the tissues, namely, the body surfaces, the circulating body fluids, the connective tissue matrix, and the cells. Resistance to infection depends on the joint activity of the processes that operate at these four levels. After recovery from an infection these processes function much more effectively, and resistance may become so great that an individual can withstand heavy exposure to the same infection with no sign of illness. This enhanced resistance is designated acquired immunity, as distinguished from the weaker native resistance or natural immunity.

## AT BODY SURFACES

### Mechanical Factors

The mechanical barrier offered by the epithelial surface of the skin and mucous membranes is probably the most important natural means of preventing infection.

Squamous epithelium is a more effective barrier because several layers of cells connected by desmosomes block the route of invading organisms. Not only is the single layer of columnar epithelium a weaker barrier but also the cells ingest bacteria and thus facilitate their progress to the underlying tissue. Intracytoplasmic microbes have been observed in many studies on the columnar intestinal epithelium. These consist of protozoa, *Escherichia coli, Salmonella, Shigella,* and enteroviruses. Most of these organisms penetrate the epithelial cell through the microvilli on its brush border, but *Entameba histolytica* tropho-

zoites pass through the intracellular junctions between two adjoining cells (Takeuchi, 1975). Rupture of the dermal epithelium by trauma, ischemia, or viruses (especially varicella) is complicated by infection with *Staphylococcus aureus,* group A or B streptococci, and anaerobic bacteria. *S. aureus* and group A streptococci are carried in the nose by many healthy people and readily spread to establish infections of the face if the epidermis is injured. Group A streptococci may also colonize the extremities and trunk and produce impetigo, erysipelas, and cellulitis after the epithelium has been ruptured by insect or animal bites, scratches, accidental injury, or surgical incisions. If the epidermis breaks down after ischemia caused by pressure (bed sores) or vascular insufficiency, anaerobic streptococci and *Bacteroides fragilis* invade the tissues and produce ischemic ulcers.

The bacteria of the mouth and colon also invade broken epithelium but less readily than after injury to the skin. In the mouth, the anaerobic streptococci, *Bacteroides,* and fusobacteria frequently produce infection of necrotic gums and adjacent mucous membranes in persons suffering from poor oral hygiene. The fetid odor of these mouth infections reflects the activity of these anaerobes.

In addition to the epithelial barrier, other mechanical factors enable the body surfaces to resist infection. In the mouth, infectious particles are drawn backward by suction currents that converge at the base of the tongue and bypass the tonsils and posterior pharynx (Bloomfield, 1922). Bacteria transported through the mouth in this fashion are swallowed and exposed to the bactericidal gastric juice. Resident bacteria, however, remain firmly entrenched. These suction currents are set up by movements of the lips and tongue and by swallowing, and are mediated by saliva. Normally they remove particles in 15 to 30 minutes but weaken or disappear if saliva dries up from dehydration or if swallowing is disturbed by paralysis or weakness. Thrush and other oral infections occur in weak or paralyzed patients who lose these oral suction currents.

Cilia provide another means of sweeping mucous membranes free of pathogenic organisms. The bacteria and viruses that are carried on dust particles into the nose may be arrested by the hairs in the nares, but if the particles penetrate beyond this barrier, they are carried backward by cilia to the posterior nasopharynx and then join the oral bacteria swept to the base of the tongue. In the trachea and bronchi, currents of mucus are moved at a rate of 1 to 3 cm/hour by the ciliated epithelium and carry inspired bacteria from the small bronchioles back up to the pharynx where they can be swallowed. The cilia beat at a rate of approximately 1000 per minute and receive their energy from ATP or ADP. The cilia can be bypassed when infectious agents are carried on small particles. Thus particles carrying tubercle bacilli cause more infection experimentally if they are only 3 $\mu$ in diameter than those measuring 10 to 12 $\mu$ even though there are more bacilli on the larger particles. The larger particles are preferentially deposited in the upper airway where they are removed by cilia, whereas the smaller particles are able to pass beyond the cilia.

Particle size is also important in carrying viruses beyond the cilia. Those hygroscopic particles that are discharged in coughs shrink to 1.5 $\mu$ after they leave the nose or mouth and lose moisture, and then swell to 2 $\mu$ in the nose. These particles are small enough to pass beyond the cilia and reach the alveolar ducts, where they swell more by absorption of water from the moist air of the lung and become trapped in the narrow (0.6 $\mu$) alveolar ducts. Larger particles will land on the ciliated respiratory epithelial cells, which have receptors for rhinoviruses, influenza viruses, and *Mycoplasma pneumoniae*. These agents may then initiate infection in the bronchial epithelium. Both influenza and *M. pneumoniae* impair mucociliary transport, so that increased susceptibility to secondary bacterial infection would be expected. Such secondary infection is prominent in influenza but does not occur in *Mycoplasma* infections, possibly because the impaired clearance is more severe in influenza.

Ciliary motion can also be reduced by cigarette smoke and alcohol. The amount of alcohol required for ciliary inhibition approaches the lethal dose and is not the important factor responsible for increased susceptibility of alcoholics to pneumonia. Formaldehyde, cyanide, and acetone are the ingredients in cigarette smoke that retard ciliary movement. When ciliary activity is damaged, the impaired ciliary clearance can be replaced by coughing. Patients with mucoviscidosis, for example, clear radioactive aerosols normally because their cough can compensate for the loss of mucociliary clearance. On the other hand, patients who suffer from congenital immotility of cilia are victims of chronic airway infections despite adequate coughs (Eliasson et al., 1977).

In the small intestine, bacteria are moved along by the action of mucosal villi, which free themselves of adherent particles by causing them to stick to the extensive lacy film of mucus that lines the bowel. The mucus is propelled along in the form of small balls by peristalsis. The absence of this protective mechanism may explain the greater tendency for *Shigella* and enteropathogenic *E. coli* to attack the colon, which has no villi. Peristalsis may be even more important than villous movement in protecting the small bowel from disease. In disorders of small bowel motility in which peristalsis is deficient, as in scleroderma, neurogenic disorders, or surgical blind loops, the colonic bacteria ascend and overgrow the small bowel. A major consequence of this bacterial overgrowth in the small bowel is deconjugation of bile salts by *B. fragilis*, the most populous member of the intestinal flora. The fall in concentration of conjugated bile salts and the corresponding rise in free bile acids (cholic, deoxycholic, and chemodeoxycholic) interfere with fat absorption and produce steatorrhea. Antibiotics that are active against *B. fragilis* will overcome the malabsorption problem. Further evidence of the importance of peristalsis is found in experiments that show that in order to infect guinea pigs with *Shigella,* it is necessary to inhibit intestinal motility with opiates. Opiates or belladonna drugs also impair resistance to human shigellosis. By restricting intestinal motility, these drugs produce more severe infection of the bowel.

Expectoration is a key process for transporting pathogenic bacteria from the respiratory tract, and the flushing action of tears, saliva, and urine removes infectious materials. Flushing the urethra by urinating after coitus will prevent cystitis in women. A sneeze or cough may contain 40,000 or more particles carrying bacteria. This reflex, as well as the epiglottis reflex, which prevents gross aspiration from reaching the pharynx, may be less efficient in adults than in children. If a contrast medium (iodized oil) is placed in the mouth of sleeping patients, chest x-rays will show the medium in the lungs of adults but not in children the following morning (Amberson, 1954). Alcohol, deep anesthesia, and exposure to cold all prevent closure of the glottis and allow aspiration pneumonia to occur.

### Chemical Factors

Body surfaces also owe their freedom from infection to nonmechanical processes. Some of these depend on the action of mucin, a disaccharide of acetylneuraminil-acetylglucosamine attached to a peptide. Because these disaccharides are hydrophilic the mucin is hydrated. The negatively charged neuraminil residues repel each other and expand the hydrated molecule to form a moist lubricating blanket that moves on the surface of cilia and intestinal villi. Mucin granules can adsorb myxoviruses in mucus cells and reexcrete them as unincorporated virus into the moving mucus sheet. Susceptible cells are protected by this mechanism from infection. In a similar process, the mucin-secreting goblet cells of intestinal crypts repond to an inflammatory stimulus by rapidly discharging organisms that could infect the bowel. The N-acetyl neuraminic acid residue on mucin is a receptor for the hemagglutinins on myxoviruses and theoretically, at least, may prevent attachment of myxoviruses to cells by acting as a competitor for cell receptors. Should this occur, however, the viral neuraminidase could still free the virus from the mucin.

Acid kills most bacteria that reach the stomach and is the most important natural barrier to infection by intestinal pathogens (Garrod, 1937). *Brucella, Salmonella, Shigella,* and *Vibrio cholera* die quickly on exposure to gastric juice. In patients whose stomachs have been removed, the incidence of salmonellosis rises 3.3-fold, and the disease is more severe. The same applies to cholera; in a small epidemic in 1971 it was found that 25 per cent of cholera victims had had gastric resections. This association was predictable from the early experiments in 1885 of Robert Koch, who could produce infection in guinea pigs only if cholera organisms were given orally with sodium bicarbonate to neutralize the gastric juice. Bacteria are not the only agents affected by gastric acid. Although many viruses are killed by acid, the acid resistance of enteroviruses, hepatitis viruses, reoviruses, and adenoviruses is important in their ability to infect the bowel and be excreted in the feces. Among patients who get giardiasis, 42 per cent have achlorhydria. Normally the acid pH keeps the stomach and small bowel sterile or nearly so. Not until the pH approaches neutrality in the ileum does the intestinal flora assume a rich and varied character.

The low pH of normal urine may also be important in killing bacteria. Urines of pH 6 or below inhibit growth of *E. coli* and kill gonococci. This phenomenon may help prevent *E. coli* urinary infections and may also explain why the urethras of most men resist infection after exposure to gonorrhea, and why gonorrhea never spreads to the bladder or kidney (McCutchan et al., 1977).

Peroxide ($H_2O_2$) is another bactericidal factor found on mucous membranes. Alone or in conjunction with salivary peroxidase and thiocyanate, $H_2O_2$ kills various pathogenic bacteria, presumably through its powerful oxidizing ability. Peroxidase catalyzes the oxidation of thiocyanate to produce hypothiocyanite ion, which inhibits or kills bacteria (Thomas and Aune, 1978):

$$SCN^- + H_2O_2 \xrightarrow{\text{peroxidase}}$$
Thiocyanate Peroxide

$$OSCN^- + H_2O_2$$
Hypothiocyanite

The $OSCN^-$ radical appears to kill bacteria by oxidation of their sulfhydryls to sulfenyl thiocyanate. The thiocyanate-peroxidase-$H_2O_2$ system is found both in the mouth and in milk.

Peroxide is elaborated by streptococci and other catalase-deficient bacteria in the mouth, bowel, and vagina. $H_2O_2$ from mouth bacteria correlates well with the ability of these normal resident flora to inhibit the diphtheria bacillus. These and other resident bacteria undoubtedly defend the body surfaces against infection by various mechanisms. In addition to $H_2O_2$, *Streptococcus mitis, Streptococcus salivarius,* and *Streptococcus mutans* elaborate antibiotics that range in molecular weight from 200 to 12 million and inhibit growth of most gram-negative and gram-positive cocci, including the pneumococcus and meningococcus (Sanders, 1975). On the other hand, pneumococci that are carried in the throat are usually not inhibited by the resident streptococcal flora, possibly because resistant pneumococci are selected for implantation or acquire resistance afterwards (Johanson et al., 1970). The normal pharyngeal flora also prevent colonization by the gram-negative bacilli that overgrow the pharnyx of persons given penicillin and other antibiotics. These antibiotics can suppress the streptococci that predominate among inhibitory strains in the pharyngeal flora.

### Normal Flora

In the bowel, *E. coli* is antagonistic to enteric pathogens. *Shigella,* for example, cannot be implanted in germ-free guinea pigs if *E. coli* is introduced first, but can cause experimental shigellosis more readily in conventional animals after suppression of the normal bowel flora by antibiotics. Similarly, the infective dose of *Salmonella typhosa* was reduced from 100,000 to 1000 bacteria in volunteers who swallowed streptomycin, a drug that inhibits intestinal *E. coli* but not the anaerobic bacteria of the bowel (Hornick et al., 1970). Colicines, the peptide antibiotics elaborated by *E. coli*, can kill *Salmonella* and *Shigella* and may help prevent intestinal infection by these bacteria. There is also evidence that colicines contribute to recover from shigellosis. *E. coli* and other intestinal bacteria also produce acetic and butyric acids, which can inhibit growth of virulent enteric pathogens.

Antagonists of potential clinical significance have also been found among vaginal flora. *Candida albicans*, a common inhabitant of the vagina, inhibits most gonococci. *Staphylococcus epidermidis*, nonhemolytic streptococci, and *Pseudomonas* are also potent inhibitors of gonococci among vaginal flora. Other bacteria in the vagina can stimulate growth of the gonococcus; the stimulators are gram-positive and predominantly lactobacilli. The inhibition, which is thought to enhance natural resistance to gonorrhea in women, is mediated by acid production (killing of gonococci progressively increases as pH falls below 7.0), and by antibiotics produced by the normal flora. Stimulation of gonococci, which occurs by unknown mechanisms, might be important in promoting infection (Braude et al., 1977).

### Surface Immunoglobulins

Immunoglobulins (Ig) A, M, G, and E all appear on normal mucous membranes and probably contribute to natural resistance. Secretory IgA is probably the most important of these because it is not only most abundant but also resistant to denaturation and hydrolysis by enzymes and chemicals in intestinal and other external secretions. Secretory IgA is a dimer of IgA molecules with a sedimentation coefficient of 11S. Secretory IgA is produced in submucosal plasma cells in close contact with the overlying glandular epithelium. The IgA monomers appear to be linked together by the glycopeptide J chains into stable dimers within the plasma cells. After secretion by the plasma cell, the IgA dimer forms a complex with a protein known as secretory-component. This secretory-component is manufactured by epithelial cells and from its position on the cell membrane is believed to function as a receptor protein that carries the IgA dimer into the cell and then out onto the surface of the mucous membrane (Hauptman and Tomasi, 1978). Secretory piece also appears to facilitate transport of locally synthesized IgM onto mucous membranes.

Local production of all immunoglobulins is stimulated on mucous surfaces by direct contact of B lymphocytes with microbial antigens during subclinical infection or with cross-reacting antigens present in food or in the normal microbial flora. Secretory IgA and other immunoglobulins seem to adhere to epithelial cell surfaces by sticking to the overlying mucus and provide an "antiseptic paint" that can block adherence of pathogenic agents to epithelial cells and neutralize their toxins. IgA has a limited ability, if any, to participate in reactions involving complement and, therefore, in promoting lysis or phagocytosis of bacteria. Furthermore, gonococci, meningococci, and certain streptococci produce a proteolytic enzyme that inactivates IgA1, which constitutes approximately 40 per cent of secretory IgA. Despite these limitations, the surface immunoglobulins undoubtedly contribute to natural resistance by preventing the initial attachment stage of infection by *Salmonella*, *Shigella*, pathogenic *E. coli*, gonococci, meningococci, *V. cholera*, group A streptococci, polio and other enteric viruses, various respiratory viruses, and certain protozoa. The importance of IgA in preventing intestinal infection is emphasized by the unique susceptibility of patients with hypogammaglobulinemia and selective IgA deficiency to giardiasis. Similarly, the presence of secretory IgA in colostrum and human milk may explain the lower incidence of gastrointestinal infections in infants, and their resistance to infection with polioviruses (Winberg and Wessner, 1971). In the respiratory tract, the IgA in mucus can inhibit the neuraminidase activity of influenza virus on the neuraminic acid moiety of mucin and thereby block penetration of the mucin barrier by the virus.

## IN EXTRACELLULAR FLUIDS

After infectious organisms pass beyond the body surfaces into the subepithelial tissues, their survival depends on their ability to withstand the environment of the extracellular fluids until taken up by phagocytic cells. They may elicit inflammatory reactions that confine them to the point of invasion, or they may pass into the lymphatic channels, travel to the lymph nodes, and eventually enter the general circulation. After phagocytosis they may escape from the cells and reappear in the body fluids.

Extracellular fluids are an ideal culture medium for certain organisms, as shown by the value of human blood, serum, and ascitic fluid for the isolation and growth of some organisms in the diagnostic laboratory. On the other hand, fresh human blood may inhibit the growth of meningococci, gonococci, coliform bacteria, *Brucella*, *Haemophilus influenzae*, and coagulase-negative staphylococci. Survival of an infectious agent in the body fluids depends on the temperature, pH, Eh (oxidation-reduction potential), osmolality, antibodies, complement, enzymes, electrolytes, and other metabolically active substances of the given fluid.

### Temperature

The oral temperature of the normal human is about 37° C; that of the internal organs is 1 to 2° C higher. Most pathogenic organisms grow well in this temperature range, but *Sporothrix schenckii* and *Mycobacterium marinum* are exceptions. These do not grow well at 37° C or higher and are the cause of infections that usually remain confined to the extremities, where the temperature is lower. As might be expected from these temperature restrictions, external heat is useful for treating sporotrichosis and *M. marinum* infections. Among viruses, rhinovirus often grows best at 33° C on primary isolation, a property that fits with the reported prevalence of rhinovirus infections in colder weather when the temperature of the nasopharynx might be lowered by cold air. Yet rhinoviruses cause widespread infection in the warm temperatures of the tropics. In any case, the failure of rhinoviruses to replicate well at body temperature probably confines them to the respiratory tract and prevents infection of the warmer internal organs.

The normal body temperature has been important in recovery from transfusion reactions with blood contaminated by psychrophilic ("cold-loving") bacteria that grow well in the refrigerator but die at 37° C. Among cryptococci, only *Cryptococcus neoformans* can grow at 37° C, and it is the only cryptococcus that is pathogenic. *C. neoformans* cannot, however, withstand temperatures above 39° C, a fact that might explain clinical improvement during malaria and other febrile disorders in patients with cryptococcosis (Kligman and Weidman, 1949). On the other hand, artificial fever therapy has been useless in the treatment of cryptococcosis. Experiments in rabbits infected with *Pasteurella multocida* suggest that fever may help control infection by lowering the plasma iron level below that needed for survival of infecting bacteria (Kluger and Rothenburg, 1979).

### Acidity

Homeostatic mechanisms maintain pH of extracellular fluids within such a narrow range that even under the most extreme conditions there is not enough change to influence the reproduction of pathogenic microbes. The only exception is urine, which can become sufficiently acid (pH 4.9 to 5.8) to inhibit or kill *E. coli,* gonococci, and other bacteria (McCutchan et al., 1977).

### Redox Potential

The relatively high oxidation-reduction potential (Eh) of the extracellular fluids helps prevent infection by anaerobic bacteria. Eh is a measure in millivolts of the tendency to give up electrons, or the potential that would exist between the body fluids and a hydrogen half-cell at pH O. Eh of extracellular fluids is a function not only of their inherent reducing tendency but also of their hydrogen ion concentration, and it becomes more negative as hydrogen ion concentration diminishes. The importance of Eh was first brought out in the case of tetanus by Fildes (1929), who showed that tetanus spores will not germinate readily at an Eh more oxidizing than +10 millivolts (mv) at pH 7.0 to 7.6. In living animal tissues he found the Eh to be approximately 120 mv at the prevailing pH 7.4. If the Eh is kept down by electrical methods, clostridia will grow even if a stream of air is passed through the culture (Hanke and Bailey, 1945). If the pH is kept in the acid range (6.4 to 6.8), *Clostridium perfringens* will grow at an Eh of 160 or more. In ischemic tissues, the anoxia lowers the Eh and lactic acid accumulation lowers the pH, so that anaerobic bacteria proliferate at Eh levels that are too high for their growth at the normal pH of 7.4. Since acidosis enhances proteolysis and accumulation of amino acids, the pH falls even more. Anaerobic infections do not occur unless the redox potential is lowered by one of the following disorders: (1) impairment of local blood supply by arterial occlusion; (2) pressure of foreign bodies such as sutures, clothing, dirt, and metal; (3) contamination of wounds with ionized calcium salts commonly present in fertile soil from farmlands, a powerful cause of tissue necrosis; (4) destruction of tissue by trauma, infection, or injection of quinine or epinephrine; (5) growth of aerobic or facultative bacteria in the tissues. The aerobic growth of the group A *Streptococcus* in a medium having an initial Eh of 300 mv induces a fall in redox potential to 150 to 200 mv.

### Natural Antibodies and Complement

In the absence of any detectable previous antigenic stimulus, immunoglobulins appear in human sera that destroy pathogenic organisms in the presence of complement, promote their phagocytosis, or neutralize their toxins. These "natural" immunoglobulins, or antibodies, have been examined mainly for their action against meningococci, *E. coli., Salmonella, H. influenzae,* pneumococci, staphylococci, and diphtheria bacilli. The importance of natural antibody in preventing disease was first appreciated in diphtheria. By demonstrating antitoxin with the Schick test, it has been possible to show a good correlation between resistance to diphtheria and the presence of anti-toxin in people who have had no clinical history of diphtheria or active immunization. The most like-ly stimulus for natural antitoxin is inapparent infection.

The importance of inapparent infection in natu-ral resistance has also been established for the meningococcus. Natural immunity against me-ningococci can result from antibodies that are stimulated by asymptomatic colonization of the throat with these bacteria (Goldschneider et al., 1969). The protective antibody appears to be directed against the meningococcal capsule. Nat-ural antibodies against the capsule also prevent infection by *H. influenzae* and the pneumococcus, but these antibodies are more likely generated by stimuli from antigenically related organisms than from subclinical infection with the specific agents of influenzal and pneumococcal disease. Infants and children develop natural anticap-sular antibody and immunity to *H. influenzae* type b, despite a very low colonization rate of their nasopharynx with *H. influenzae* type b. The same is true in laboratory animals that have high levels of serum antibodies to type b without having been colonized by that organism. *E. coli* K100 appears to be one of the important cross-reacting bacteria for producing *H. influenzae* type b immunity. The K100 antigen is a potent an-tigen for stimulating type b antibody when the whole bacteria are fed to children, and *E. coli* K100 colonizes their bowel naturally. The acidic polysaccharides in the K100 capsule appear to have the cross-reacting determinants for the type b capsule. Various other bacteria of the bowel cross-react with the *H. influenzae* type b capsule, including gram-positive bacteria with polyribitol phosphate in their cell wall teichoic acid. Ribitol is a component of the type b capsular polysaccha-ride antigen of *H. influenzae*.

The production of natural protective antibody against the pneumococcus is more complicated because many types of pneumococci are virulent, whereas only type b is virulent among *H. influen-zae*. Nevertheless, there is enough exposure to cross-reacting antigens in bacteria and foodstuffs to provide good protection against pneumococcal infection by an early age. This is illustrated by the fact that 80 per cent of babies at the age of 1 year have antibody to type 7 pneumococcus, even though the carrier rate is only 1 per cent. The type 7 antibody response results from exposure to cross-reacting surface antigens in *S. viridans*. A partial list of other important cross-reactions with pneumococci is shown in Tables 1 and 2. These cross-reactions help explain how a broad spectrum of natural antibodies against pneumo-coccal infection is acquired early in life, long before subclinical infection with each of these types would be possible. Children with congenital hypogammaglobulinemia who are unable to make this natural antibody suffer from repeated pneumococcal infections of the same or different types (Bruton, 1952). The attacks of pneumococ-cal pneumonia and septicemia begin at 6 months after disappearance of the maternal immunoglob-ulins derived by transplacental passage, and af-fect mainly boys because the disorder is usually X-linked. The protective value of natural IgG antibody against pneumococcal infections in in-fancy and childhood is demonstrated by the effec-tiveness of commercial gamma globulin when given prophylactically to boys with hypogam-maglobulinemia. Commercial gamma globulin is prepared from the blood of healthy people who have not been given pneumococcal vaccines, so that the protective IgG is naturally acquired antibody. The same susceptibility to overwhelm-ing recurrent pneumococcal infections is seen in adults who lose their natural antibody when they develop the specific immunoglobulin disorders of multiple myeloma or acquired hypogammaglobu-linemia.

Although natural antibody seems to be impor-tant against both pneumococci and *H. influenzae*, its mode of action against the two is different. Natural antibody against the pneumococcus (and other gram-positive bacteria) acts exclusively as

**TABLE 1.  Cross-Reactions Between Pneumococci and Various Microorganisms or Plants**

| PNEUMOCOCCUS TYPE | SOURCE OF CROSS-REACTING ANTIGENS |
|---|---|
| 1 | Coliform bacilli<br>Plant hemicelluloses (Felton et al., 1955) |
| 2 | Yeast polysaccharides<br>Gum arabic (Heidelberger et al., 1929)<br>Gum acacia (Marrack and Carpenter, 1938)<br>Cherry gums<br>*K. pneumoniae* polysaccharide B<br>*S. typhi*<br>*S. paratyphi* B<br>Plant hemicelluloses |
| 3 | Gum arabic (Heidelberger et al., 1929)<br>Gum acacia<br>Cherry gums (Marrack and Carpenter, 1938)<br>Meningococcus<br>Gonococcus<br>Plant hemicelluloses |
| 14 | Group A human red cells (Beeson and Goebel, 1939)<br>Anthrax bacillus somatic polysaccharide |
| 29,34,35 | *H. influenzae* type b |

**TABLE 2.   Distribution of Immunizing Antigen Against Pneumococcal Infection in Mice Among Hemicelluloses from Commonly "Edible" and "Inedible" Plants**[a]

| "EDIBLE" PLANTS | | | | "INEDIBLE" PLANTS | | | |
| --- | --- | --- | --- | --- | --- | --- | --- |
| | Immunity Against $10^3$ LD | | | | Immunity Against $10^3$ LD | | |
| Source of Hemicellulose | Pn I | Pn II | Pn III | Source of Hemicellulose | Pn I | Pn II | Pn III |
| Melon, honeydew (rind) | +++ | +++ | +++ | Tomato greens (roots) | +++ | ++ | ++ |
| Collard greens | +++ | +++ | ++ | Pumpkin (skin) | +++ | ++ | + |
| Sunflower seed | +++ | +++ | + | Mosses | +++ | ++ | 0 |
| Pumpkin pulp | +++ | ++ | + | Nightshade | +++ | 0 | 0 |
| Squash (fruit) | +++ | +++ | 0 | Grass, lawn | ++ | ++ | ++ |
| Peanut meal | +++ | ++ | 0 | Cotton, nonabsorbent | + | +++ | 0 |
| Tomato (fruit) | ++ | ++ | +++ | Wood, maple | + | ++ | 0 |
| Watermelon rind | ++ | ++ | ++ | Wood, pine | ++ | ++ | ++ |
| Green bean (fruit) | ++ | ++ | ++ | Squash seed | + | +++ | 0 |
| Parsnip greens | ++ | ++ | + | Ageratum plant | + | ++ | 0 |
| Pomegranate (fruit) | ++ | + | ++ | Cottonseed meal | + | + | 0 |
| Wheat germ | ++ | +++ | 0 | Lupine seed | + | + | 0 |
| Cucumber | ++ | ++ | 0 | Mullen plant | + | + | 0 |
| Kale greens | ++ | ++ | 0 | Iris plant | 0 | ++ | 0 |
| Soybean meal | ++ | ++ | 0 | Spider lily | 0 | ++ | 0 |
| Rape greens | ++ | + | 0 | Gladioli (leaves and bulbs) | 0 | ++ | 0 |
| Lettuce | ++ | 0 | 0 | Corn husks | 0 | ++ | 0 |
| Rutabaga (root) | ++ | 0 | 0 | Nasturtium plant | 0 | 0 | ++ |
| Nutmeg powder | + | +++ | ++ | | | | |
| Onion bulb | + | +++ | 0 | Chickweed plant | 0 | 0 | 0 |
| Lima bean | + | ++ | 0 | Geranium plant | 0 | 0 | 0 |
| Potato, white | + | + | + | Hydrangea plant (leaves and | 0 | 0 | 0 |
| Barley | + | 0 | 0 | small stems) | | | |
| Sugar cane | + | 0 | 0 | Ivy, English | 0 | 0 | 0 |
| Yeast (baker's) | + | 0 | 0 | Japonica plant | 0 | 0 | 0 |
| Apple, Winesap | 0 | +++ | 0 | Marigold | 0 | 0 | 0 |
| Grapefruit rind | 0 | +++ | 0 | Morning glory plant | 0 | 0 | 0 |
| Irish moss (carrageen) | 0 | +++ | 0 | Nicotiana plant | 0 | 0 | 0 |
| Oatmeal | 0 | +++ | 0 | Rose | 0 | 0 | 0 |
| Rhubarb, leaves | 0 | +++ | 0 | Spiderwort | 0 | 0 | 0 |
| Green pepper (fruit) | 0 | ++ | ++ | Sedum plant | 0 | 0 | 0 |
| Cabbage | 0 | ++ | 0 | Vetch seed | 0 | 0 | 0 |
| Coconut | 0 | + | ++ | | | | |
| Cinnamon powder | 0 | 0 | ++ | | | | |
| Carrot | 0 | 0 | + | | | | |
| | | | | | | | |
| Broccoli greens | 0 | 0 | 0 | | | | |
| Swiss chard greens | 0 | 0 | 0 | | | | |
| Eggplant (fruit) | 0 | 0 | 0 | | | | |
| Orange (rind) | 0 | 0 | 0 | | | | |
| Pear (fruit) | 0 | 0 | 0 | | | | |
| Pectin | 0 | 0 | 0 | | | | |
| Radish root | 0 | 0 | 0 | | | | |
| Rice (polished) | 0 | 0 | 0 | | | | |

[a]+++ indicates immunity with 0.0005 mg or 0.005 mg of hemicellulose; ++ indicates immunity with 0.05 or 0.5 mg; + indicates immunity with 1.0 or 5.0 mg.
From Felton, L., et al.: J Bacteriol 69:519, 1955.
Pn indicates pneumococcus type, I, II, or III.

an opsonin to promote phagocytosis, whereas natural antibody to *H. influenzae* can be both opsonic and bacteriolytic. Both IgM and IgG participate in opsonization, but IgM requires complement. The Fc portion of IgG attaches to the neutrophils and the Fab portion to the pneumococcal capsule. This opsonic bridge between leukocyte and pneumococcus does not require complement for phagocytosis to proceed. Complement becomes involved in a different opsonic process when Fab of either

IgG or IgM reacts with capsular polysaccharide to form a complex that activates the classic complement pathway through the sequence C1, C4, C2, and C3. Activation of C3 makes it opsonic, so that it becomes the bridge between the pneumococcus and the phagocytic cell. Complement can also be opsonic for the pneumococcus when the cell wall activates C3 through the alternative pathway, which does not involve the participation of antibody. The generation of pneumococcal opsonins by the alternative pathway does not seem to be important in clinical medicine because it does not protect patients who lack gamma globulin from developing overwhelming pneumococcal infections. On the other hand, complement activation via the classic pathway is important for the opsonic activity of nonimmune human serum because most natural antibody against the pneumococcus is IgM. Because C1 and C2 are inactivated by heating at 56° C, the opsonic activity of nonimmune serum is often referred to as heat labile to distinguish it from the heat-stable, complement-independent, opsonic activity of hyperimmune antipneumococcal serum whose opsonins are IgG.

The natural antibodies against the meningococcus and *H. influenzae* are also opsonic, but in addition, they kill these two gram-negative bacteria by lysis in the absence of phagocytes. Bacteriolysis by natural antibody is a reaction between the bacterial surface antigens (polysaccharide capsules), IgM, and complement. As in opsonization, the reaction may follow either the classic or the alternative pathway of complement. After IgM attaches via the Fab to the capsular polysaccharide antigen, the first step in the classic pathway is attachment of C1 through its subunit C1q to a binding site on the Fc portion of IgM. This interaction with antibody globulin activates C1 and catalyzes the assembly of C4 and C2. Together (C$\overline{42}$) they function as the enzyme C3 convertase. This enzyme cleaves C3 into two fragments, C3a and C3b. The C3a fragment is responsible for opsonization (as described for the pneumococcus), and C3b attaches to receptors on the bacterial cell. After attachment, C3b combines with neighboring

C$\overline{42}$ and apparently modifies the specificity of the latter enzyme so that it can now cleave C5 into C5a and C5b. The large fragment C5b then attaches to the cell membrane, binding in turn C6 and C7 to form the trimolecular complex C$\overline{567}$, which then becomes tetramolecular when C8 is incorporated. The terminal complex of C activation becomes complete when C9 fixes to binding sites on C$\overline{5678}$. The large complex of the five individual terminal C proteins is essential for killing susceptible gram-negative bacteria. This bactericidal activity is far more effective when it is generated via the classic pathway, but it can operate through the alternative pathway (also known as the properdin pathway). The lipopolysaccharide (LPS) in gram-negative bacteria can activate the alternative pathway by reacting directly with a noncomplement protein, C3 proactivator (properdin B) (C3PA). Upon reacting with LPS, C3PA splits into at least two fragments: One has the electrophoretic mobility of gamma globulin (mw 60,000), and a second consists of an acidic peptide (mw 20,000). The larger fragment, known as C3 activator, splits C3 into C3a and C3b (properdin A), and thereby initiates the terminal sequences of complement activation.

In addition to complement, lysozyme, calcium, and magnesium are important components of extracellular fluids that are required for killing gram-negative bacteria. $Ca^{++}$ and $Mg^{++}$ ions are essential for initiation of the classic complement sequence, and lysozyme is needed for disrupting the cell wall peptidoglycan. Lysozyme splits the 1–4 glycosidic linkages between *N*-acetyl muramic acid and *N*-acetylglucosamine in the peptidoglycan so that complement may have greater

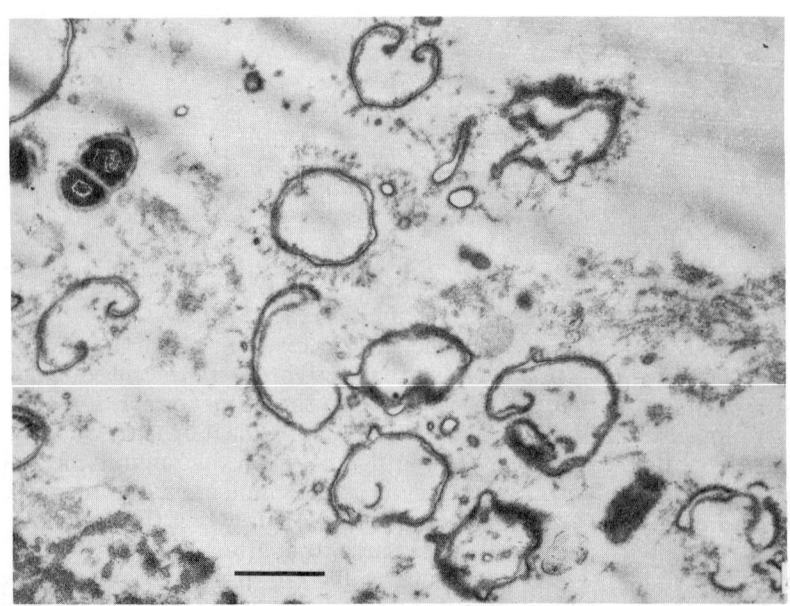

**FIGURE 1.** *Representative electron micrographs of markedly serum-sensitive E. coli bacteria incubated with undiluted fresh normal serum. Note that both cell walls and cytoplasmic membrane are ruptured by the bactericidal action of fresh serum. Compare this with Figure 2, which shows appearance of same bacteria in serum after inactivation of complement. × 16,000 (From Olling, S.: Scand J Infect Dis (Suppl), 1977.)*

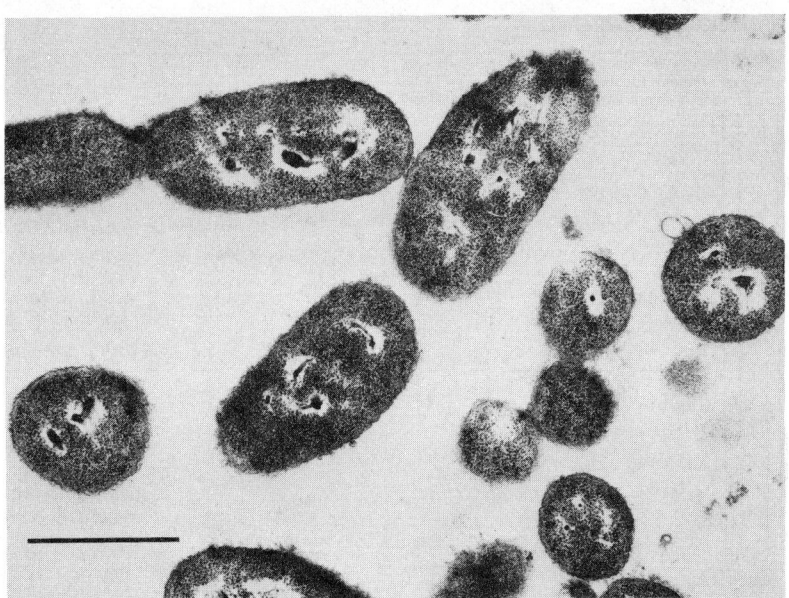

**FIGURE 2.** *Same as Figure 1 except that serum has been heated to inactivate complement. In the absence of complement the bactericidal system is inoperative and does not injure the bacterial cell. × 16,000 (From Olling, S.: Scand J Infect Dis (Suppl), 1977.)*

access for its attack on the cytoplasmic membrane. The electron microscope (Figs. 1 and 2) discloses dramatic disturbances of bacterial morphology in cells that have been killed by serum. Both cell walls and cytoplasmic membranes are ruptured.

In contrast to gram-positive bacteria, which are all resistant to lysis by complement, all species of gram-negative bacteria are susceptible to lysis by the classic or alternative pathway. This difference in susceptibility to killing by complement is best explained by the concept that the cell wall of gram-positive bacteria is a barrier that hinders access of complement to the cytoplasmic membrane. This concept is reinforced by the fact that protoplasts of gram-positive bacteria whose cell walls are removed are killed by complement. The thicker peptidoglycan and the absence of LPS could explain how the cytoplasmic membrane enjoys a sanctuary in gram-positive bacteria from complement. In many gram-negative bacteria, LPS is the key intermediate factor in killing because it activates complement by either pathway. Each of the three primary structural components of LPS — O antigens, core sugars, and lipid A — can activate the classic pathway by reacting with natural antibody (Fig. 3). In the absence of antibody, lipid A can activate either the classic pathway by direct reaction with C1q or the alternate pathway. For unknown reasons, virulent enteric gram-negative bacteria often resist complement-mediated bacteriolysis, survive in the extracellular fluids, and cause bacteremia. The importance of complement in natural resistance to infection is also seen in patients who share a familial deficiency of C6, C7, and C8 and

are subject to severe recurrent attacks of bacteremia due to gonococci and meningococci. Phagocytosis of these bacteria is normal because opsonins can be generated through C3, but the serum of these patients cannot kill pathogenic *Neisseria* because the terminal complex of complement is not formed.

Aside from gram-negative bacteria, certain protozoa, trematodes, and leptospiras undergo lysis in nonimmune serum in the presence of complement. Resistance to such lysis seems to be correlated with virulence. For example, the blood from nearly every person kills members of the *Trypanosoma brucei* group in vitro and protects experimental animals. The only trypanosomes of the *T. brucei* group that resist being killed by human serum are *T. gambiense* and *T. rhodesiense*, which can infect human beings and cause sleeping sickness. *Trypansoma cruzi*, the cause of Chagas' disease, also resists killing by human serum. Such a relationship also seems to exist for highly pathogenic *Schistosoma mansoni*. High dilutions of human serum will lyse cercaria of many trematodes within a few minutes but not those of *S. mansoni* unless the serum is from a patient infected with *S. mansoni* (Culbertson, 1951). Similarly, virulent leptospiras resist killing by normal human serum, which destroys nonpathogenic leptospiras and some avirulent lines of pathogenic leptospiras (Johnson and Harris, 1967).

### Beta-lysin

Although not killed by antibody and complement, most gram-positive bacteria are killed by beta-lysin, a relatively heat-stable cationic pro-

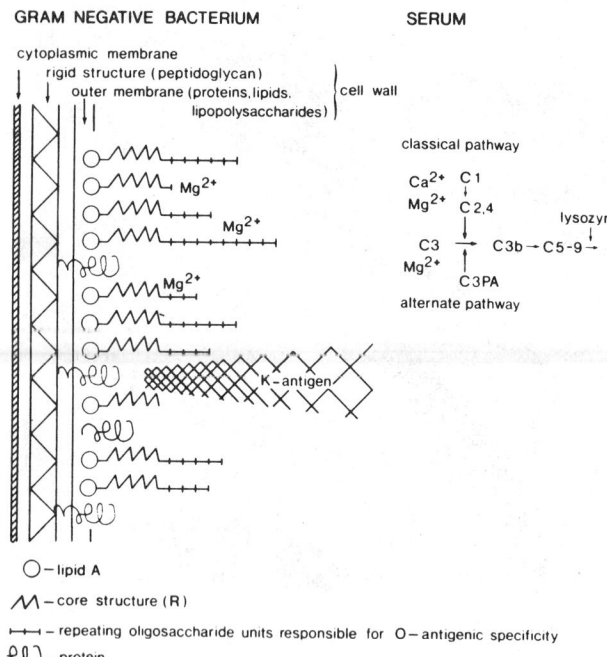

GRAM NEGATIVE BACTERIUM                    SERUM

**FIGURE 3.** *Proposed model for the structure of the surface layers of gram-negative bacteria and the serum factors involved in bacterial killing. Each of the three primary structural components of LPS—O antigens, core sugars, and lipid A—can activate the classic pathway by reacting with natural antibody. Reactions between K antigen or other capsular antigens and antibody can probably also activate the classic pathway. In the absence of antibody lipid A can activate either the classic or the alternate pathway. Activation of complement by either pathway kills the cell. This may occur either because holes are punched in the outer membrane so that lysozyme can hydrolyze the mucopeptide and produce spheroplasts that rupture from osmotic forces, or because activated complement may impose lethal damage to the cytoplasmic membrane. (From Olling, S.: Scand J Infect Dis (Suppl), 1977.)*

tein with a molecular weight of 6,000 (Donaldson, 1975). With the exception of streptococci, most gram-positive bacteria are killed by beta-lysin, but gram-negative bacteria, molds, yeasts, viruses, and mycoplasmas are not killed. Beta-lysin does not require complement to kill and, unlike bactericidal antibody, is present in higher concentrations in serum than in plasma because it is released from platelets when blood clots. It is also present in inflammatory exudates. The bacterial cell membrane is thought to be the primary site of action of beta-lysin.

### Acute Phase Substances

During a variety of unrelated acute illnesses, substances suddenly and promptly appear that react with streptococci. One of these kills group A streptococci, and the other combines with the group-specific polysaccharide C-substance of *S. pneumoniae* (C-reactive protein). Neither is an antibody. The C-reactive protein (CRP) is normally present in trace amounts in human serum but increases rapidly in infection and inflammation as a consequence of increased synthesis in hepatocytes (Kushner and Feldmann, 1978). It was first discovered in pneumococcal pneumonia but later observed in other acute infections, rheumatic fever, cancer, arthritis, serum sickness, ulcerative colitis, myocardial infarction, and various forms of tissue injury. CRP is composed of five subunits in cyclic symmetry and its chemical structure is similar to that of C1t, a serum protein that may be involved in regulation of complement

(C1) function. Despite the ability to react with pneumococcal C polysaccharide and to fix complement with it, CRP has no demonstrable antimicrobial activity except for weak opsonic properties for various pathogenic bacteria. Its protective properties seem to depend instead on its ability to modulate inflammatory and immune responses by inhibiting platelet aggregation and mediator release and by suppressing lymphocyte stimulation and lymphokine production after binding to t-cells (Mortenson et al., 1977).

Both acute-phase substances were discovered by W. S. Tillett (1937), and the bactericidal factor is known as Tillett factor. Its ability to kill streptococci separates it from beta-lysin; Tillett factor is also unusual in that its activity is abolished under anaerobic conditions or in the presence of reducing agents. Both CRP and Tillett factor differ from antibody in their time of appearance and the nonspecificity of their stimuli. The two acute-phase substances are most active in the most active periods of disease, and disappear during convalescence when specific antibody usually begins to increase. For this reason, it has been suggested that acute-phase substances provide a means of body defense against bacterial invasion that is uniquely different from that of the complement-antibody apparatus and the phagocytic system.

### Interferons

Various tissues can react with viruses to elaborate proteins that inhibit infection by the same or different viruses. These inhibitors, designated interferons by Isaacs and Lindenmann (1957), enhance the resistance of cells to infection by viruses. Interferon produced by one type of cell is active against a wide variety of viruses; for example, an interferon produced by treatment of cells with influenza virus will prevent infection not only by various influenza viruses but also by vaccinia viruses, togaviruses, and others. Moreover, interferon produced in cells of different organs show no tissue specificity, so that interferon produced during a pulmonary infection, for example, might inhibit viral growth in the brain. Because interferon has been found in tissues during recovery from viral infection, it has been suggested that this viral inhibitor might depress viral multiplication before specific antibody reaches effective levels. (Interferon is fully discussed in Chapter 12).

### Tuftsin

This tetrapeptide of splenic origin stimulates phagocytosis by a hormonal action on the cell. Its formula is L-threonyl-L-lysyl-L-prolyl-L-arginine. It has a high positive charge that allows it to bind to negatively charged groups (e.g., sialic acid) on the neutrophil surface. An enzyme in the membrane of neutrophils splits tuftsin from a gamma globulin known as leukokinin. Deficiencies of tuftsin occur as a rare familial disorder (Constantopoulos et al., 1972) and apparently

after splenectomy. The susceptibility to overwhelming pneumococcal infection in splenectomized patients is thought by some to be a consequence of tuftsin deficiency.

### Enzymes, Electrolytes, and Other Metabolites

Table 3 summarizes the reaction of bacteria to various substances in normal body fluids that may affect their growth or their ability to counter the mechanisms used to withstand infection.

The peculiar susceptibility of the poorly controlled diabetic to infections by *Klebsiella pneumoniae*, tubercle bacilli, *Mucor, Rhizopus*, and *Candida albicans* suggests that chemical abnormalities of the extracellular fluids may enhance the capacity of these microorganisms to establish infection. At least 0.3 per cent glucose is necessary in culture media for the formation of well-encapsulated *K. pneumoniae* (Hoogerheide, 1939). This concentration of glucose in the tissue fluids in poorly controlled diabetes might enable these bacteria to produce larger capsules and enhance their virulence by enabling them to resist phagocytosis. High concentrations of glucose also favor growth of *Mucor, Rhizopus*, and *C. albicans*. Although there is no evidence that variations in the concentration of glucose in vivo affect the survival of tubercle bacilli, the stimulating effect of keto acids at the acid pH of inflammatory exudates may enhance the growth of these bac-

**TABLE 3.  Factors of Body Fluids that May Affect the Survival of Pathogenic Bacteria or Their Capacity to Injure the Host**

| | MICROORGANISMS | POSSIBLE INFLUENCE ON DEVELOPMENT OF INFECTION |
|---|---|---|
| Glucose | Friedländer's bacillus | Increased production of capsular polysaccharide at levels >0.3 per cent |
| Keto acids | Staphylococci, tubercle bacillus | Stimulate growth at acid pH |
| $CO_2$ | Tubercle bacillus | Inhibits growth |
| $CO_2$ | Pneumococci, gonococci, *Brucella abortus* | Stimulates growth |
| $CO_2$ | Staphylococci | Increases production of toxin |
| Ca, Mg | *Clostridium perfringens* | Required for hemolytic activity |
| Iron | Diphtheria bacillus, *Cl. perfringens, Cl. tetani*, and *Sh. dysenteriae* | Inhibits production of toxin |
| Iron | Staphylococci, clostridia, *Listeria*, mycobacteria | Stimulates growth and virulence |
| Cholesterol | Streptococci | Inhibits streptolysin S |
| Nucleotides | Streptococci | Required for high concentrations of streptolysin O |
| Hematin | Staphylococci | Bactericidal |
| Hematin | *H. influenzae* | Essential for growth |
| Cysteine | *H. influenzae* | Can replace hematin |
| Cysteine or cystine | *Francisella tularensis* | Essential for growth |
| NAD or NADP | *H. influenzae* | Essential for growth |
| Oleic acid | Streptococci, pneumococci | Inhibits growth |
| Glutamine | Streptococci, pneumococci | Required for good growth |
| Spermine | Tubercle bacillus | Bactericidal after activation by spermine oxidase |
| Plasminogen | Streptococci, staphylococci | Converted to active fibrinolysin by streptokinase and staphylokinase |
| Coagulase factor | Staphylococci | Required for the production of fibrinogen by staphylococcal coagulase |

teria in human tuberculosis during uncontrolled diabetes (Dubos, 1954).

In normal persons, the body fluids are well suited to meet the special growth requirements of such organisms as *H. influenzae, B. abortus,* meningococci, gonococci, *Francisella tularensis,* and *Streptobacillus moniliformis.* These bacteria grow better when carbon dioxide is present, and the physically dissolved carbon dioxide in extracellular fluid (about 3 volumes per cent) is optimum for their growth. The requirement of cysteine for growth of *F. tularensis* and *H. influenzae* is also met by body fluids during infection, and human blood can provide the requirement of *H. influenzae* for NAD, NADP, or hematin.

The same constituents of extracellular fluids may also inhibit bacterial growth or activity of toxins. Growth of the tubercle bacilli, for example, may be completely suppressed by excessive concentrations of carbon dioxide, and the beneficial effects in tuberculosis of lung collapse from therapeutic pneumothorax may be related to the high concentration of carbon dioxide in the poorly ventilated lung. Tubercle bacilli are also inhibited by low oxygen tension, and their disappearance from closed caseous areas is attributed in part to local anoxia. In sharp contrast, where an open bronchus permits good oxygenation of the cavity, tubercle bacilli flourish, and conditions are optimal for growth of drug-resistant mutants.

Iron and iron-containing compounds appear to have an important influence on virulence of bacteria. Although hematin is essential for the growth of *H. influenzae,* it may be toxic for certain gram-positive bacteria even in minute amounts. Heme is lethal for staphylococci in concentrations of 0.0003 per cent at pH 7.0 (Dubos, 1954). For the most part, however, iron or heme compounds promote virulence and growth in vivo. Virulence for mice is markedly enhanced, and disseminated lethal infections occur when gonococci are suspended in a mixture of hemoglobin and mucin, the same menstruum in which they exist during menstruation when they most commonly disseminate hematogenously in women. If elemental iron is used in place of hemoglobin the virulence of gonococci is not increased. Under other circumstances, however, iron alone will enhance and iron deprivation will lower bacterial virulence. This correlation of virulence with available iron seems to parallel the ability of iron to stimulate microbial growth. Staphylococci, clostridia, listeria, mycobacteria, various enteric bacteria, *Pseudomonas, Pasteurella, Yersinia, Vibrio, Aeromonas, Candida,* and plasmodia are among the genera of bacteria, fungi, and protozoa whose members are stimulated by excess iron to grow in body fluids (Weinberg, 1978). This growth stimulation by iron in serum and other body fluids is

thought to depend on saturation of transferrin, a nonheme iron-binding protein with a molecular weight in the range of 75,000 to 80,000. It binds reversibly two ferric ions/molecule through tyrosyl and histidyl residues. Under normal conditions human transferrin is only 25 to 35 per cent saturated, so that the amount of free ionic iron in plasma is at least 100 million-fold less than that required for bacterial growth (0.4 to 4.0 $\mu$M). If circulating transferrin is saturated by injecting iron intravenously, intraperitoneally, or intramuscularly, there is an increased mortality rate of animals with experimental candidiasis, tuberculosis, staphylococcal infections, salmonellosis, and meningococcal infections. By saturating transferrin, the injection of iron makes available enough free iron to meet microbial growth requirements. Impaired resistance to infection is not limited to experimental animals treated with iron, since impaired resistance has been reported in human beings after exposure to excess iron. Thus, the incidence of serious gram-negative infections has increased in newborn infants after intramuscular injection of iron (Barry and Reeve, 1977). It should be noted that transferrin can also be saturated if its concentration falls in relation to iron, as occurs in patients with kwashiorkor whose nutritional disorder damages their ability to make iron-binding proteins. The plasma obtained from kwashiorkor victims supports growth of *S. aureus* and is bacteriostatic upon addition of transferrin. Lactoferrin, an iron-binding protein in human milk, has been given credit, along with antibodies, for the lower incidence of gastroenteritis in breast-fed compared with formula-fed infants (Weinberg, 1977). For this reason the practice of supplementing infant formulas with iron has been questioned.

Constituents of body fluids can further influence pathogenicity by affecting bacterial toxins. The virulence of staphylococci is correlated, for example, with coagulase production. Coagulase is generated from staphylococcal procoagulase by an activator in the body fluids, and coagulase converts fibrinogen to fibrin. The tendency for staphylococci to produce extensive thrombosis in the lung and other tissues and to cause severe intravascular coagulation suggests that coagulase activator has an important place in the pathogenesis of staphylococcal infection. Its importance is further implied by the greater resistance to staphylococcal infections among certain animals whose plasma lacks coagulase activator. Staphylokinase, another staphylococcal toxin, acts through plasminogen, a constituent of normal plasma. Both staphylokinase and streptokinase convert plasminogen to plasmin, which can digest fibrin clots and prevent clotting. Both enzymes are elaborated in human infections and stimulate antibodies that neutralize their activity. Staphylokinase is thought to initiate lysis of infected thrombi and the release of septic emboli to the lung during staphylococcal septicemia; streptokinase could explain the poor localization of streptococcal cellulitis by preventing fibrin deposition around an infected focus.

The chemical environment of body fluids may also disturb normal immune processes, especially in the renal medulla. Within the range found in the normal kidney and urine, high concentrations of sodium, urea, and hydrogen ion inhibit phagocytosis of human leukocytes (Chernew and Braude, 1962). These observations help explain why the kidney is uniquely susceptible to invasion by *E. coli, Proteus,* and other bacteria that possess little capacity to establish infection elsewhere.

## IN CELLS

### Transport by Lymphatics

When organisms reach the tissue fluids they may be phagocytized by neutrophils or macrophages, or carried by the lymphatics to the right or left subclavian vein. During the course of this passage to the general circulation they may be trapped in lymph nodes and phagocytized by macrophages. If they get beyond the lymph nodes and into the blood they will then be ingested by circulating neutrophils or by histiocytes in the liver, spleen, bone marrow, adrenal, or pituitary. It is unlikely that any microorganism can enter blood capillaries directly because these vessels are impermeable to substances with a molecular weight of greater than 20,000. Lymph capillaries, on the other hand, easily become permeable to particles as large as red cells, even though they appear to be closed completely by endothelium and have no direct opening into the tissues. Passage through the lymph vessels is an important process in natural immunity because infectious particles are carried to potent fixed phagocytic cells. By itself, however, the lymph has limited protective ability because it contains almost no phagocytic cells and its content of antibodies is less than that of the blood (Braude and Carlson, 1908). The impotence of lymph against gram-positive bacteria can be observed when type III pneumococci are injected intravenously. These bacteria can be cultured promptly from the lymph after intravenous injection because they migrate passively through the walls of blood capillaries into tissue fluid and then through the lymphatic capillaries. Upon intravenous injection of type III pneumococcal antiserum, the blood becomes sterile but pneumococci are still found in the

lymph seven hours later (Field et al., 1937). In the absence of phagocytic cells, pneumococci can multiply in the lymph even in the presence of antibody. The meningococcus, *H. influenzae,* and other gram-negative bacteria, on the other hand, would not survive in lymph because antibody and complement can kill these bacteria without phagocytic cells. This difference accounts for the tendency of certain gram-positive bacteria to remain dormant in the lymphatics and produce recurrent infection. The best known example of this phenomenon is recurrent erysipelas, an infection in which the lymph vessels of the skin are filled with streptococci (Fehleisen, 1886).

The flow of lymph depends on body movement, massage, or the increase in tissue pressure that occurs during inflammation. The network of fibers attached to the outer wall of the lymphatic vessels is stretched by increased tissue pressure so that the lymphatics are opened and can accommodate the larger volumes of lymph that flow during inflammation (Pullinger and Florey, 1935). The importance of adequate lymph flow in the removal of organisms for the prevention of infection is obvious after the lymphatics become obstructed, when the resulting elephantiasis becomes the focus of repeated infections. The remarkable filtering capacity of lymph nodes depends for its efficiency on a network of trabeculae that fills the sinusoids. The histiocytes lining the sinuses can then ingest and destroy the trapped organisms.

### Transport by Blood

Microorganisms carried by the lymphatics to the subclavian veins may be phagocytized in the blood by neutrophilic leukocytes, which are then sequestered in the capillaries of the lung and liver. Many organisms are also removed by the Küpffer cells of the liver and the macrophages in the spleen. Bacteria, fungi, protozoa, and viruses can be taken out of the circulation by both the circulating phagocytes and the macrophage (reticuloendothelial) system. The route of viruses is illustrated by mousepox (Fenner, 1949). After multiplying in the skin, mousepox virus passes within eight hours to the regional lymph node. After multiplication in the node, the virus is carried into the blood and removed by phagocytes in the liver and spleen. Multiplication in the liver may lead to another viremia with secondary spread to the skin, where the characteristic eruption appears. During viremia, pox virus is associated with lymphocytes and monocytes; in lymphocytic choriomeningitis, Rift Valley fever, and Colorado tick fever the virus is adsorbed to erythrocytes. Others, like the togaviruses and the enteroviruses, circulate free in the plasma. After removal by the macrophages in the liver, some viruses (poxviruses, yellow fever virus) multiply in these cells and then infect the hepatic cells. Some pass directly into hepatic cells without multiplication in Küpffer cells (Rift Valley fever virus), and others, such as vaccinia and influenza viruses, are rapidly destroyed within the Küpffer cells (Fenner et al., 1974).

Virulent bacteria may also multiply in the liver and spleen and reenter the circulation to cause bacteremia or fungemia. The ability of the human liver to clear some, but not all, bacteria was discovered in patients with endocarditis when it was shown that hepatic venous blood always contained many fewer colonies of streptococci than blood from arteries or other veins (Beeson et al., 1945). Bacteria may also establish a sustained bacteremia by penetrating the wall of a capillary or venule and producing an infected thrombus. This thrombus may discharge a continuous stream of organisms at a rate that exceeds the ability of phagocytic cells to remove them. Such a bacteremia, often observed with staphylococci and *Bacteroides,* is dominated by lung abscesses.

Fungi and protozoa are no exceptions to the clearance of circulating organisms by the reticuloendothelial system. Perhaps the most dramatic example of phagocytosis by tissue macrophages is the tremendous number of *Histoplasma* organisms present in these phagocytes during human infection. Similarly, malaria illustrates the prominent phagocytosis of protozoa by the reticuloendothelial cells in liver, spleen, and bone marrow. Malaria is unique, however, in that the parasitized red cells are phagocytized but not the parasite alone.

## Mode of Entry

The contact between phagocytic cell and infectious particle in the blood and tissue is made either through chance collision or through a positive attraction between phagocytes and microorganisms known as chemotaxis. In chemotaxis experiments in vitro, phagocytes can be seen to crawl by ameboid motions toward the particle to be ingested. Chemotaxis in vivo has often been difficult to demonstrate, but a striking example can be found in coccidioidomycosis. In the infected tissues, the fungus *Coccidioides immitis* has the form of a thick-walled spherule containing numerous endospores. The intact spherule is surrounded by mononuclear cells, but when it begins to rupture and release its endospores, there is a chemotactic rush of neutrophilic leukocytes to the point on the spherule where the endospores will emerge (Fig. 4). The attraction by the contents of the spherule is so great that neutrophils pour into the empty shell and seem to attack the inner wall even after the endospores are gone. The mechanism of this chemotaxis is not known, but in other infections chemotaxis results from the activation of complement by microbial antigens. This activation may occur via the classic or alternative pathway and generates chemotactic properties in the small peptides C3a and C5a, and in the trimolecular complex $C\overline{567}$. Bacterial proteases and proteases released from neutrophil granules can also attack C3 and C5 to produce chemotactic derivatives. In addition to complement factors, chemotactic products of a low molecular weight

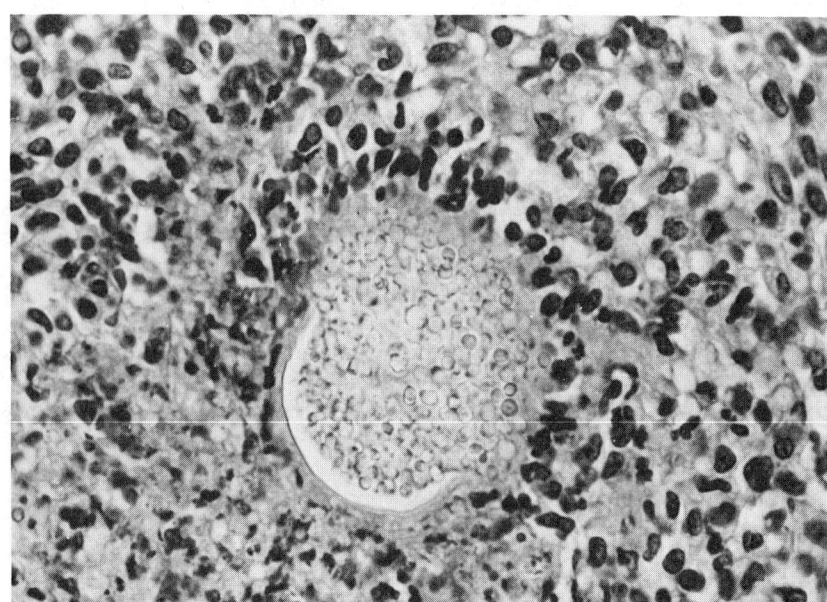

**FIGURE 4.** *Chemotactic rush of neutrophilic leukocytes to the point where the endospores emerge from the rupturing spherule of* Coccidioides immitis. *Notice absence of neutrophils at lower left margin of spherule where its cell wall is intact.*

are elaborated by certain bacteria. Chemotactic factors, regardless of origin, probably create a concentration gradient that directs the phagocyte to its target. It is also possible that chemotactic factors bind to specific receptors on neutrophil or monocyte membranes and activate their contractile apparatus. Anaerobic glycolysis appears to be the major energy source for chemotaxis in neutrophils because inhibitors of the glycolytic pathway depress chemotaxis but inhibitors of oxidative metabolism do not. Chemotaxis of leukocytes probably results from movements of actin and myosin, the contractile proteins of muscle, which are also present in phagocytes Actin polymers in phagocytes form a tangled meshwork whose filaments are cross-linked by myosin and by actin-binding protein. It has been suggested that the cross-linked meshwork forms a rigid gel at the periphery of the cell ("cortical gel"), which provides the conditions for firm contractility that would be needed in pseudopods during chemotaxis and phagocytosis. This theory of phagocytic motility would take into account glycolysis as the energy source for chemotaxis, since ATP is required for movements of myosin and actin during contraction. It would also fit with the observation that cytochalasin B, which dissolves actin gels, inhibits phagocytosis by polymorphonuclear leukocytes and macrophages (Stossel, 1978).

After phagocytes reach their target and make contact, a microbe will be taken into the cell if their surfaces are properly attached. This attachment may depend partly on the hydrophobic character of the organism (Van Oss, 1978). Among the gram-negative bacteria, for example, smooth organisms with complete hydrophilic O polysaccharides are more resistant to phagocytosis than their rough hydrophilic mutants that are deficient in these surface sugars. Similarly, the hydrophobic polysaccharide capsules of pneumococci, *H. influenzae,* and *Klebsiella pneumoniae* make these bacteria more difficult for phagocytes to ingest than their unencapsulated variants. The opsonic activity of complement and specific antibody may also depend on their ability to make hydrophilic bacteria more hydrophobic. The Fc portion of IgG, which protrudes from the opsonized bacterial cell, is reported to be hydrophobic so that it can attach to the surface of the phagocytic cell. The surface protein (protein A) of *Staphylococcus aureus,* on the other hand, binds IgG by attaching to its Fc portion so that the hydrophilic Fab fragment protrudes. As a result, the opsonic property of IgG is subverted by virulent staphylococci and used instead to enhance their virulence by opposing phagocytosis.

Phagocytosis by both neutrophils and macrophages begins when proper contact is made with the microbial agent. The ingested particle is encircled by the phagocytic cell membrane through a process that combines invagination of the membrane and extrusion of pseudopods around the particle. The encirclement of the particle probably requires the participation of the contractile proteins (actin and myosin) and energy from ATP, as well as close adherence between particle and cell membrane and a sticky surface (Stossel, 1977). The sticky surface helps explain particle ingestion as well as why leukocytes stick to each other in clumps during phagocytosis and how the ends of pseudopods fuse to complete the encirclement. In neutrophils, the energy for engulfment comes primarily from anaerobic glycolysis. There are very few mitochondria in polymorphonuclear leukocytes, and Krebs cycle activity provides less than 20 per cent of ATP during glucose catabolism. Peritoneal and lung macrophages, on the other hand, have numerous mitochondria, and ATP is produced mainly from oxidative phosphorylation. Thus, inhibitors of oxidative metabolism (cyanide, dinitrophenol) inhibit ingestion by macrophages but not neutrophils, whereas inhibitors of glycolysis (iodoacetate, NaF) block phagocytosis by neutrophils but not macrophages.

Fusion of the pseudopods at their poles completes the encirclement of the particle by neutrophils and creates a phagocytic pouch, or vacuole, which separates from the cell membrane and moves centrally, accumulating cytoplasmic granules at its periphery (Fig. 5). The granules fuse to the membrane of the phagocytic vacuole and dissolve so that their contents empty into the vacuole. The azurophilic granules (purple color in Wright's stain), which have a dense appearance in the electron microscope, are actually lysosomes and release nucleases, lipases, acid phosphatase, elastase, collagenase, proteases, and other hydrolytic enzymes that digest dead organisms but are not bactericidal. The heme protein, myeloperoxidase (mw 150,000), and the mucopeptidase known as lysozyme are the important bactericidal enzymes released from azurophilic granules Although neither kills pathogenic bacteria by itself, both help in such killing, as described elsewhere. A second group of granules of lower density is known as secondary granules because they appear second in granulocyte maturation. They contain lactoferrin, a bacteriostatic iron-binding protein that resembles transferrin in depriving bacteria of iron. Another group of antibacterial proteins, known as cationic proteins because of their basic charge, is also present in secondary granules. These basic proteins attach to the negatively charged surface of bacteria and kill them through unknown mechanisms.

Four Stages of Phagocytosis of a Bacillus

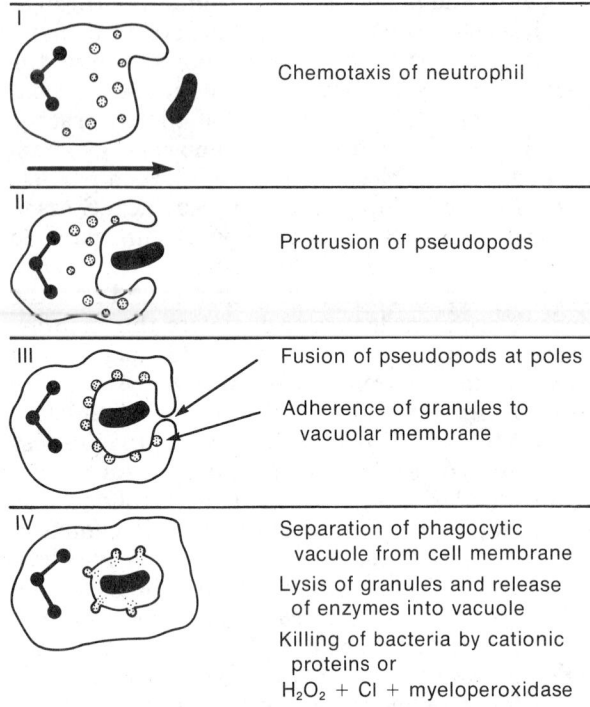

I  Chemotaxis of neutrophil

II  Protrusion of pseudopods

III  Fusion of pseudopods at poles

Adherence of granules to vacuolar membrane

IV  Separation of phagocytic vacuole from cell membrane

Lysis of granules and release of enzymes into vacuole

Killing of bacteria by cationic proteins or $H_2O_2$ + Cl + myeloperoxidase

**FIGURE 5.**  *Phagocytosis.*

Another group of bactericidal substances is produced through a series of metabolic phenomena known as the "respiratory burst" (Babior, 1978). Phagocytosis is undiminished in the absence of oxygen, but killing of the ingested organism does not occur unless there is a sharp increase in oxygen uptake, which is the first event in the respiratory burst. This rise in leukocyte oxygen uptake is stimulated by opsonized bacteria and other particles and by C5a within 30 to 60 seconds after contact with the cell membrane. The immediate consequence of this sudden utilization of oxygen is the production of superoxide ($O_2^-$) by the one-electron reduction of oxygen in the following reaction involving reduced nicotinamide adenine dinucleotide (NADPH):

$$2O_2 + NADPH \longrightarrow 2O_2^- + NADP^+ + H^+$$

The enzyme superoxide dismutase then converts superoxide to hydrogen peroxide ($H_2O_2$):

$$2O_2^- + 2H^+ \xrightarrow[\text{dismutase}]{\text{superoxide}} O_2 + H_2O_2$$

The hydrogen peroxide then acts with myeloperoxidase and a halide to kill the bacteria in the phagocytic vesicle where the myeloperoxidase

has been released upon lysis of the azurophilic granules. Although hydrogen peroxide can kill bacteria, its bactericidal activity is greatly increased in the presence of myeloperoxidase (Klebanoff, 1973). Myeloperoxidase, like other peroxidases, catalyzes oxidation by hydrogen peroxide. In the bactericidal reaction, $Cl^-$ appears to be the main substrate; it is oxidized to hypochlorite as follows:

$$Cl^- + H_2O_2 \xrightarrow[\text{myeloperoxidase}]{} ClO^- + H_2O$$

$I^-$ and $Br^-$ can also be oxidized in this reaction, which incorporates the halide in the bacterial cell. Halogenation of the bacteria is not entirely responsible for their death, however, and other unknown mechanisms must also be involved in the bactericidal effect of myeloperoxidase.

One of the key reactions in the metabolic burst is the hexose monophosphate shunt (HMP), which is the major source of NADPH, the reducing agent needed for production of superoxide. The first step in the shunt produces NADPH by the following reaction:

$$\text{Glucose-6-phosphate} + NADP^+ \xrightarrow[\text{G-6-PD}]{} $$
$$6 \text{ phosphogluconic acid} + NADPH$$

The reaction is catalyzed by G-6-PD (glucose-6-phosphate dehydrogenase). In the second HMP reaction more NADPH is produced as follows:

$$6 \text{ phosphogluconic acid} + NADP^+ \xrightarrow[\substack{\text{6-phosphogluconate} \\ \text{dehydrogenase}}]{} $$
$$NADPH + CO_2 + \text{ribulose-5-phosphate}$$

In patients whose leukocytes are deficient in G-6-PD, inadequate amounts of NADPH are generated after phagocytosis. The deficiency in NADPH results in less production of superoxide and, in turn, insufficient hydrogen peroxide for killing certain bacteria. This metabolic disturbance gives rise to increased susceptibility to pyogenic infections by *E. coli, K. pneumoniae,* and *S. aureus.*

The importance of hydrogen peroxide in killing bacteria is also evident from infections encountered in boys with chronic granulomatous disease (CGD), a disorder in which the respiratory burst and the production of hydrogen peroxide in leukocytes are selectively deficient. Their leukocytes kill streptococci but not staphylococci, so that they are prone to severe staphylococcal but not streptococcal infections. This difference is explained by the absence of catalase in streptococci and its presence in staphylococci. Catalase is needed to destroy hydrogen peroxide, so that

## TABLE 4. Deficiency Diseases and Other Disorders of Natural Resistance to Infection

| DISORDER | IMMUNE DEFECT | PREDOMINANT TYPE OF INFECTION |
|---|---|---|
| Immotile cilia | Loss of respiratory mucociliary clearance | Chronic airway infection |
| Achlorhydria | Loss of gastric bactericidal activity | Cholera, salmonellosis, shigellosis, giardiasis |
| Intestinal blind loop syndrome | Loss of small bowel motility | Overgrowth of small bowel with *B. fragilis* and deconjugation of bile salts causing malabsorption |
| Bruton's disease | Sex-linked agammaglobulinemia | Recurrent sinusitis, otitis, pneumonia, septicemia, and meningitis due to *Pneumococcus* and *H. influenzae;* also echovirus infections and encephalomyelitis |
| Acquired hypogammaglobulinema (adult men and women) | Deficient specific antibody responses | Pneumococcal and *H. influenzae* sinusitis, conjunctivitis, pneumonia, and bacteremia; giardiasis |
| Selective IgA deficiency | IgA less than 5 mg per cent | Recurrent infections of sinuses, bronchi, and lung (esp. middle lobe) with viruses and bacteria; giardiasis |
| Multiple myeloma | Absence of specific antibody globulin | Pneumococcal pneumonia and bacteremia |
| Wiskott-Aldrich syndrome | Low serum IgM; inability to respond to immunization with polysaccharide antigens | Meningitis, otitis media, pneumonia, and septicemia due to pneumococcus, *H. influenza,* and meningococcus |
| Tuftsin deficiency (congenital or after splenectomy) | Defective phagocytosis | Overwhelming pneumococcal septicemia and meningitis |
| Hodgkin's disease | Depressed cellular immunity | Cryptococcosis, listeriosis, herpes zoster |
| Chronic granulomatous disease | Inability to generate $H_2O_2$ in leukocytes | Fatal infections with staphylococci or gram-negative bacilli; normal resistance to pneumococci and other streptococci |
| Congenital thymic aplasia or hypoplasia | Absent T-cell function | Chronic candidiasis; disseminated mycobacterial, cryptococcal, aspergillus, pneumocystis, toxoplasma, strongyloides, and herpes infections |
| Chronic mucocutaneous candidiasis | Defective T-cell function | *Candida albicans* infection of skin and mucous membranes |
| Combined immunodeficiency (including Swiss-type, X-linked, or adenosine deaminase deficiency) | Complete absence of T and B cells | Candidiasis; cytomegalovirus, pneumocystis, and vaccinia infection; poliomyelitis (attenuated vaccine strains); pneumonia and chronic otitis media due to various gram-negative and gram-positive bacteria |
| Familial complement deficiency (C6, C8) | Loss of serum bactericidal power | Severe recurrent meningococcal and gonococcal septicemia |
| Cyanotic congenital heart disease | Polycythemia and cerebral thrombosis | Anaerobic brain abscess |
| Arteriosclerosis obliterans | Low redox potential of leg muscles | Clostridial myonecrosis |

hydrogen peroxide accumulates in streptococci and replaces the deficiency in peroxide within CGD neutrophils. In other words, streptococci provide the missing reagent that is needed for their own destruction by the bactericidal effect of myeloperoxidase-C1-$H_2O_2$. Staphylococci possess catalase and thus protect themselves against this reaction by destroying the peroxide component.

It must be emphasized that other systems for microbial killing exist within phagocytes and that the absence of peroxide-mediated killing does not necessarily promote infection. Alveolar macrophages, for example, have no peroxidase but kill ingested bacteria. Chickens and other birds have no peroxidase in their PMN leukocytes, but these cells kill bacteria and the birds are as resistant to infection as other animals. More important, patients with myeloperoxidase deficiency, in striking contrast to those with chronic granulomatous disease, are rarely troubled by infections (Babior, 1978).

## DISEASES SECONDARY TO DISTURBANCES IN NATURAL RESISTANCE

A number of infections have been discussed in this chapter in relation to specific disturbances in natural resistance. These are summarized in Table 4. The disturbances in acquired cellular immunity described in the next chapter are also listed.

### References

Amberson, J. B.: A clinical consideration of abscesses and cavities of the lung. Bull Johns Hopkins Hosp 94:227, 1954.

Babior, B.: Oxygen-dependent microbial killing by phagocytes. N Engl J Med 298:659, 1978.

Barry, D., and Reeve, A.: Increased incidence of gram-negative neonatal sepsis with intramuscular iron administration. Pediatrics 60:908, 1977.

Beeson, P., and Goebel, W.: The immunological relationship of the capsular polysaccharide of type XIV pneumococcus to the blood group A substance. J Exp Med 70:239, 1939.

Beeson, P., Brannon, E. S., and Warren, J. V.: Observations on the sites of removal of bacteria from the blood of patients with bacterial endocarditis. J Exp Med 81:9, 1945.

Bloomfield, A. L.: The dissemination of bacteria in the upper air passages. I. The circulation of foreign particles in the mouth. Am Rev Tuberc 5:903, 1922.

Braude, B., and Carlson, A. J.: The influence of lymphagogues on the relative concentration of bacterioagglutinins in serum and lymph. Am J Physiol 21:221, 1908.

Braude, A., Corbeil, L., Levine, S., Ito, J., and McCutchan, J.: Possible influence of cyclic menstrual changes on resistance to the gonococcus. In Brooks, G., Gotschlich, E., Holmes, K., Sawyer, W., and Young, F. (eds.): Immunobiology of Neisseria Gonorrhoeae. Washington, D.C., American Society of Microbiology, 1978, p. 328.

Bruton, O.: Agammaglobulinemia. Pediatrics 9:722, 1952.

Chernew, I., and Braude, A.: Depression of phagocytosis by solutes in concentrations found in the kidneys and urine. J Clin Invest 41:1945, 1962.

Constantopoulos, A., Najjar, V., and Smith, J.: Tuftsin deficiency: A new syndrome with defective phagocytosis. J Pediatr 80:564, 1972.

Culbertson, J. T.: Immunologic mechanisms in parasitic infections. In Most, H. (ed.): Parasitic Infections in Man. New York, Columbia University Press, 1951.

Donaldson, D.: Beta-lysin. In Schlesinger, D. (ed.): Microbiology, 1975. Washington, D.C., American Society of Microbiology, 1975, p. 223.

Dubos, R. J.: Biochemical Determinants of Microbial Diseases. Cambridge, Mass., Harvard University Press, 1954.

Eliasson, R., Mossberg, B., Camner, P., and Afzelius, B.: A congenital ciliary abnormality as an etiologic factor in chronic airway infections and male sterility. N Engl J Med 297:1, 1977.

Fehleisen, F.: On erysipelas. In Cheyne, W. W. (ed.): Microparasites in Disease. London, New Sydenham Society, 1886, p. 261.

Felton, L., Prescott, B., Kauffmann, G., and Ottinger, B.: Antigens of vegetable origin active in pneumococcus infections. J Bacteriol 69:519, 1955.

Fenner, F.: Mouse-pox (infectious etromelia of mice): A review. J Immunol 63:341, 1949.

Fenner, F., McAuslan, B., Mims, C., Sambrook, J., and White, D.: The Biology of Animal Viruses, 2nd ed. New York, Academic Press, 1974, p. 363.

Field, M. E., Shaffer, M. F., Enders, J. F., and Drinker, C. K.: The distribution in the blood and lymph of pneumococcus type III injected intravenously into rabbits, and the effect of treatment with specific antiserum on the infection of the lymph. J Exp Med 65:469, 1937.

Fildes, P.: Tetanus: IX. The oxidation-reduction potential of the subcutaneous tissue fluid of the guinea pig: Its effect on infection. Br J Exp Pathol 10:197, 1929.

Garrod, L. P.: The susceptibility of different bacteria to destruction in the stomach. J Pathol Bacteriol 45:473, 1937.

Goldschneider, I., Gotschlich, E., and Artenstein, M.: Human immunity to the meningococcus. II. Development of natural immunity. J Exp Med 129:1385, 1969.

Hanke, M., and Bailey, J.: Oxidation-reduction potential requirements of C. welchii and other clostridia. Proc Soc Exp Biol Med 59:163, 1945.

Hauptman, S., and Tomasi, B.: The secretory immune system. In Fudenberg, H., Stites, D., Caldwell, J., and Wells, J. (eds.): Basic and Clinical Immunology, 2nd ed. Los Altos, Lange, 1978, p. 205.

Heidelberger, M., Avery, O., and Goebel, W.: A "soluble specific substance" derived from gum arabic. J Exp Med 49:847, 1929.

which Klebsiella pneumoniae (Friedländer's bacteria) forms capsules. J Bacteriol 38:367, 1939.

Hornick, R., Greisman, S., Woodward, T., DuPont, H., Dawkins, A., and Snyder, M.: Typhoid fever. I. Pathogenesis and immunologic control. N Engl J Med 283:686, 1970.

Isaacs, A., and Lindenmann, J.: Virus interference. I. The interferons. Proc R Soc B147:258, 1957.

Johanson, W., Blackstock, R., Pierce, A., and Sanford, J.: The role of bacterial antagonism in pneumococcal colonization of the human pharynx. J Lab Clin Med 75:946, 1970.

Johnson, R., and Harris, V.: Antileptospiral activity of serum. II. Leptospiral virulence factors. J Bacteriol 93:513, 1967.

Klebanoff, S.: Myeloperoxidase-halide-hydrogen peroxide antibacterial system. J Bacteriol 95:2131, 1968.

Kligman, A., and Weidman, F.: Experimental studies on treatment of human torulosis. Arch Dermatol Syph 60:726, 1949.

Kluger, M., and Rothenburg, B.: Fever and reduced iron. Their interactions as a host defense response to bacterial infections. Science 203:374, 1979.

Kushner, I., and Feldman, G.: Control of the acute phase response: Demonstration of C-reactive protein synthesis and secretion by hepatocytes during acute inflammation in the rabbit. J Exp Med 148:466, 1978.

McCutchan, J., Wunderlich, A., and Braude, A.: The role of urinary solutes in natural immunity to gonorrhea. Infect Immun 15:149, 1977.

Marrack, J., and Carpenter, B.: The cross-reactions of vegetable gums with type II antipneumococcal serum. Br J Exp Pathol 19:53, 1938.

Mortenson, R., Braun, D., and Gewurz, H.: Effects of C-reactive protein on lymphocyte functions. III. Inhibition of antigen-induced lymphocyte stimulation and lymphokine production. Cell Immunol 28:59, 1977.

Olling, S.: Sensitivity of Gram-negative bacilli to the serum bactericidal activity: A marker of the host-parasite relationship in acute and persisting infections. Scand J Infect Dis (Suppl), p. 8, 1977.

Pullinger, B. D., and Florey, H. W.: Some observations on the structure and functions of lymphatics: Their behaviour in local edema. Br J Exp Pathol 16:49, 1935.

Sanders, W. E.: Interactions between streptococci and other bacteria in the throat. In Schlesinger, D. (ed.): Microbiology, 1975. Washington, D.C., American Society of Microbiology, 1975.

Stossel, T.: How do phagocytes eat? Ann Int Med 89:398, 1978.

Stossel, T.: Phagocytosis. In Greenwalt, T., and Jamieson, G. (eds.): The Granulocyte in Function and Clinical Utilization. New York, Alan R. Liss, Inc., 1977, p. 87.

Takeuchi, A.: Electronmicroscope observations on penetration of the gut epithelial barrier by Salmonella typhimurium. In Schlesinger, D. (ed.): Microbiology, 1975. Washington, D.C., American Society of Microbiology, 1975, p. 174.

Thomas, E., and Aune, T.: Lactoperoxidase, peroxide, thiocyanate antimicrobial system: Correlation of sulfhydril oxidation with antimicrobial action. Infect Immun 20:456, 1978.

Tillitt, W. S.: The bactericidal action of human serum on hemolytic streptococci. I. Observations made with serum from patients with acute infections and from normal individuals. J Exp Med 65:147, 1937.

Van Oss, C.: Phagocytosis as a surface phenomenon. Ann Rev Microbiol 32:19, 1978.

Weinberg, E.: Iron and infection. Microbiol Rev 42:45, 1978.

Winberg, J., and Wessner, G.: Does breast milk protect against septicemia in the newborn? Lancet 1:1091, 1971.

# MECHANISMS OF **82** ACQUIRED RESISTANCE TO INFECTION

## Abraham I. Braude, M.D., Ph.D.

Untreated patients do not recover from an infection unless their resistance increases enough to overcome the infecting agent or its toxins. This state of increased resistance may be manifested in the following ways:

1. The person remains well upon re-exposure to the same pathogenic organism during epidemics with high attack rates. The solid life-long immunity to measles, chickenpox, rubella, and mumps illustrates the permanence of this acquired resistance against highly contagious viral infections.

2. The patient's blood inhibits the growth of the corresponding organism in vitro. This characteristic is typical of blood from patients who have recovered from streptococcal sore throats or pneumococcal pneumonia.

3. The patient's serum will protect laboratory animals from the infectious agent. This protection is found with serum obtained after infections by bacteria (Group A streptococci, pneumococci, diphtheria bacilli, *Klebsiella pneumoniae,* leptospiral organisms, and *Treponema pallidum*), all rickettsiae, all viruses, and certain parasites (*Toxoplasma gondii*).

4. The patient's serum will prevent infection of tissue cultures by the virus that caused his disease.

5. His serum will damage the responsible microorganism (lysis of leptospira, meningococci, and *Haemophilus influenzae*; immobilization of *T. pallidum*; capsular swelling of pneumococci, *K. pneumoniae*, and *H. influenzae*; and distortion of toxoplasmas).

These signs of resistance are specific: The activity of the serum or blood and the resistance of the patient are directed only against the species or serologic type of infectious agent responsible for the illness. They are mediated by specific antibodies that are generated during the early stages of infection and increase as the patient recovers from the illness. In some infections lymphocytes and macrophages are also thought to be involved in acquired immunity to infection.

## ACQUIRED HUMORAL IMMUNITY

As in any type of primary immune response, whether to living or dead antigens, the early humoral response to infection is predominantly IgM. Within ten days, however, IgG begins to appear and thereafter exceeds and outlasts IgM. IgM, which is heavier (M.W. 900,000, sedimentation coefficient 19S), tends to remain within the blood vessels and does not cross the placenta. IgG is smaller (M.W. 146,000, sedimentation coefficient 1S) and is actively transported across the placenta. Thus, IgG is responsible for the long-term immunity against many systemic infections and prevents many bacterial and viral infections in the newborn, whose immune system is undeveloped.

### Opsonins

The mechanism of protection by IgG varies with the organism. As noted in the previous chapter, IgG is opsonic and protects against infections by pneumococci, *H. influenzae, K. pneumoniae,* group B *Streptococcus, Escherichia coli,* and certain other gram-negative bacilli by combining through its Fab portion with the capsular or K antigens. The Fc portion of the IgG attaches at the same time to surface receptors on neutrophilic leukocytes, so that an opsonic bridge occurs between bacterial cell and phagocyte. IgG, as well as IgM, can also promote phagocytosis after combining with bacterial antigens by activating complement via the classic pathway, so that opsonin is generated in the form of activated C3. Opsonins are also important in acquired resistance to *Streptococcus* group A, but they do not react with the streptococcal capsule. The reason for this is that the capsule of group A streptococci is composed of hyaluronic acid, a normal constituent of connective tissues, so that antibody is not produced against it. Instead, opsonins for the group A *Streptococcus* are directed against its M protein, which is carried on fimbria. Since the fimbria extend beyond the capsule, the overlying M protein antigen can react with specific anti-M IgG and thwart the antiphagocytic effect of the capsule.

### Antitoxins

Most bacteria are pathogenic by virtue of their exotoxins, and antibody must neutralize these toxins to provide protection. Recovery from diphtheria is accompanied by the production of anti-

757

toxin, which appears to prevent the attachment of toxin to cells. The evidence supporting this mode of protection by antitoxin comes from observations with fragments A and B of diphtheria toxin. Fragment A has the enzymatic (or toxic) activity and fragment B is necessary for attachment and transport into the susceptible cell. When separate antisera that are specific for either the A or the B fragment are prepared, only the antibody against the B fragment will neutralize the toxin, apparently by interfering with its attachment to cells. In addition to blocking the attachment of toxin to substrate, antibody can accelerate the clearance of the toxic antigen from the circulation before it reaches susceptible cells. Recovery from diphtheria is accompanied by the production of antitoxin, which protects against toxin elaborated in the later stages of infection. Early in the infection, toxin combines with cells before antibody is produced and probably becomes inaccessible to neutralization. After recovery from diphtheria, the active production of diphtheria antitoxin gives protection for years, and its concentration in the body is probably increased periodically as a result of subclinical exposure to the diphtheria bacillus. With the Schick test, antitoxin can be demonstrated by its ability to neutralize the small amount of toxin that is injected into the skin.

Recovery from streptococcal infections is likewise accompanied by the development of antibodies against streptococcal toxins, but none of these antitoxins are known to bring about recovery. Antibodies against streptococcal hemolysin (streptolysin O), fibrinolysin (streptokinase), deoxyribonuclease (streptodornase), and hyaluronidase may all rise in titer as the streptococcal infection subsides but contribute little if anything to protection against the diseases caused by group A streptococci. Thus, sera containing high titers of antistreptolysin O cannot protect animals against *Streptococcus* group A unless antibody to M protein is also present. Antibody to streptococcal erythrogenic toxin will prevent the rash of scarlet fever but not streptococcal infections.

Aside from diphtheria there is no evidence that infection by toxin-producing bacteria produces a protective antitoxin or subsequent immunity. Second attacks of tetanus have occurred because the disease is produced by quantities of toxin that are too small to be antigenic. The lethal dose of botulinus toxin, which is even more potent than tetanus toxin, is also less than the antigenic dose. Protective antisera against the clostridial toxins can be prepared, however, by immunizing with toxoids made from the toxins of *C. botulinus, C. tetani,* and *C. perfringens.*

The endotoxins of gram-negative bacteria also produce protective antitoxins (i.e., antiendotoxins) after immunization with the lipopolysaccharide (LPS) or the whole bacterial cell. The LPS from smooth bacteria stimulates primarily antibody to the O antigenic side chains, and LPS from rough bacteria stimulates antibody to the core (see Chapter 6). Antibody to either O or core antigens of endotoxin can prevent all toxic manifestations of endotoxin, including the local Shwartzman reaction, generalized Shwartzman reaction, and death. Antibody to endotoxin can also protect experimental animals from bacteremias due to gram-negative bacteria. The protection by O antibody is specific and is limited to homologous endotoxins or bacteria, whereas that by core antibody gives broad protection against a wide range of different bacteria and their endotoxins (Braude et al., 1977). The importance of antibody against endotoxin in human disease is still under study.

### Lysins

In addition to preparing the pathogen for phagocytosis or neutralizing its toxin, antibody may destroy it by uniting with its antigens. Destruction of a microorganism, however, is not a universal feature of antibody activity; it is observed with certain gram-negative bacteria, spirochetes, leptospiras, protozoa, and viruses but not with gram-positive bacteria or fungi. Even when antibodies protect against infection by gram-positive bacteria, the antibodies are not lethal to them in vitro.

As noted in the preceding chapter, lysis of gram-negative bacteria by IgG or IgM requires the participation of complement. Perhaps the most important examples of protection by *acquired* bacteriolytic antibodies are those against the meningococcus and *H. influenzae*. In both cases, the bacteriolytic antibody acquired through infection is specifically directed against the capsules. In addition to bacteria, trypanosomes are susceptible to immune lysis. In studying this phenomenon in rats infected with *T. lewisi,* Taliaferro (1938) noted that the infected animal resorts to three mechanisms for disposing of the parasite: lysis, phagocytosis, and inhibition of reproduction. The power of reproduction was lost near the sixth day of infection, and soon afterward the parasites were killed by lysis and phagocytosis. The lysis was caused by the action of antibody plus complement, and was manifested by a precipitous fall in the number of trypanosomes in the blood after the tenth day. Despite these dramatic effects of antibodies, they soon become impotent because the surface antigens of trypanosomes are changed at each succeeding cycle of infection. Although these new antigenic variants are removed by the specific antibody they later stimulate, the next cycle of trypanosomal variants will not be susceptible to existing antibody. As many as 20 successive variants may occur, thus enabling the trypanosome to keep one step ahead of the antibody response. This phenomenon could explain why large amounts of IgM are produced in the serum and cerebrospinal fluid of patients with trypanosomiasis. Most of this immunoglobulin does not react with the trypanosome, possibly because it was stimulated by variants with different antigenic specificities.

## OTHER MECHANISMS OF HUMORAL IMMUNITY

### Antiparasitic

In malaria a different mechanism seems to bring recovery from infection. In this disease, recovery and protection are best correlated with antimerozoite IgG, which probably blocks the invasion of red cells by the parasite. The antibody is primarily strain-specific but also offers some protection against other strains of the same species. The antimalarial IgG persists for relatively long periods and protects newborns and infants by passing the placental barrier and by appearing in breast milk. These antibodies develop slowly, and several infections are sometimes required before immunity to malaria occurs. There are at least three reasons for this sluggish immune response: (1) Malaria suppresses immunity (Williamson and Greenwood, 1978). Humoral immunity is affected more than cellular immunity, probably because macrophages no longer process antigens normally. Immunity to both malaria and other infections is probably suppressed. (2) Immunity is probably stage-specific, so that different antigens determine immunity for each stage in the cycle of parasitic development. (3) In certain forms of malaria, variation can occur among surface antigens as in trypanosomiasis (Brown and Brown, 1965).

Immunity also develops to worms. A study by Taliaferro and Sarles (1939) of immunity to nematodes in rats demonstrated that *Nippostrongylyus muris* may become exposed to lethal antibody by penetrating the intestinal wall and feeding on blood and tissue fluids. Antibody in these fluids forms a precipitate around the mouth of the parasite and seals the genital pore so that egg production is prevented. Unable to obtain nourishment or reproduce, the adult worm may be dislodged by peristalsis. Humoral antibody is probably involved in immunity to other nematodes also. Antibodies act in conjunction with

eosinophils to protect against *Trichinella spiralis* by attacking adult worms in the gut and larvae en route or in the muscle. The immune response, which is elicited by products secreted by both larvae and adults, can reduce fertility of the adult, eliminate the adult before it engages in maximum production of larvae, or prevent the establishment of larvae in muscle. In other words, immunity reduces the number of larvae that can reach muscle and thus reduces the severity of the disease (Despommier, 1977).

Antibody and eosinophils also operate together in killing schistosomules, the first stage in development of *Schistosoma mansoni* infection after penetration of the skin by cercariae. In the presence of IgG antibody from infected patients, both eosinophils and macrophages kill schistosomules. This process, called *antibody-dependent cell-mediated cytotoxicity*, works differently for different cells and immunoglobulins. For example, IgG can behave like any opsonin, attaching via the Fab portion to the target and via Fc to the killer cell. IgE, on the other hand, can bind to the surface of macrophages and activate them so that they kill schistosomules. This type of macrophage activation may involve complexes composed of schistosome antigens with IgE antibody and is specific; that is, other parasites are not injured by these macrophages. Immune serum containing high levels of IgE-immune complexes can protect against experimental schistosomiasis (Capron et al., 1977).

### Antiviral

Opsonization and immune-lysis are also involved in acquired resistance to virus infections after intravenous injection. Opsonic activity was demonstrated by Mims (1964), who injected complexes of mousepox virus and antibody intravenously and found that they were taken up by macrophages in the liver. Virus alone entered hepatic parenchymal cells and multiplied there, whereas virus injected with antibody disappeared after ingestion by macrophages. Immune lysis by antiviral antibody plus complement has been observed with enveloped viruses such as rubella and influenza viruses. Under electronmicroscopy, holes have been seen that appear to be punched through the envelope by complement (Almeida and Lawrence, 1969). Other structural changes have been identified in viruses after neutralization and exposure to complement. For example, studies with equine enteritis virus have shown that ribonucleases can penetrate the injured virus membrane after neutralization by antibody plus complement, and release the RNA from within the nucleocapsid (Radwan and Crawford, 1974). Although antibody on the surface of a virus

particle can simply block viral attachment and
penetration of susceptible cells, many exceptions
to this process have been noted. There is good
evidence, in fact, that the reverse may sometimes
occur — namely, that antibody may help entry of
virus particles into such cells. When particles of
certain viruses such as vaccinia, poliovirus, and
Newcastle disease virus are taken into cells in the
presence of neutralizing antibody, the cells may
not be infected and the virus is degraded (Doles
and Kajiola, 1964; Silverstein and Marcus, 1964).
Even though the target cells are not "professional" phagocytes (such as polymorphonuclears or
macrophages), they confine the ingested virus to
the phagocytic vesicle where nucleases and other
lysosomal enzymes can degrade it. Thus, under
some circumstances antibody seems to prevent
the type of penetration by viruses that would
enable them to appropriate the biosynthetic apparatus of the cell, and instead produces opsonization, phagocytosis, and destruction of virus particles by cells that are not customarily regarded as
phagocytic.

Antibody may also prevent attachment of
viruses to susceptible target cells by changing the
viral surface charge and shape, by blocking critical sites for attachment of virus to cell, and by
clumping virus particles so that many are sequestered within the aggregate. Autoaggregation, or
clumping, of virus particles in the absence of
antibody may have the reverse effect, that is,
prevention of neutralization because the virus in
the center of the clump is protected from antibody. Neutralization also depends on the
number of immunoglobulin molecules and the
fractions of complement. Many immunoglobulin
molecules must attach to each virus particle to
neutralize its infectivity; one antibody molecule is not enough. Complement is an important
accessory factor in neutralization of viruses and
can help to coat the virus surface, agglutinate the
particles, or induce lysis of the virion. Studies
with herpes simplex virus show that C1 is ineffective but sequential incubation with C4, C2, and
C3 contributes to neutralization by coating the
viral surface rather than by virolysis (Daniels,
1975). The lysis of enveloped viruses described
earlier requires the terminal components (C5
through C9). Antibodies on the viral surface may
not be able to neutralize infectivity if they are too
few or are bound to sites that are not critical for
infection. These antibody-viral complexes may
circulate and remain infectious, as in experimental infection with lymphocytic choriomeningitis
virus. Viral-antibody complexes can be neutralized, however, through the participation of antiglobulins such as rheumatoid factor. One of the
rheumatoid factors is a large globulin (M.W.
900,000) of the IgM class that attaches to the Fc
portion of IgG. Upon combining with IgG-virus
complexes, rheumatoid factor itself does not reduce infectivity but allows complement to do so.
Since antiglobulins appear during convalescence
from cytomegalovirus, Epstein-Barr, hepatitis B,
rubella, and influenza virus infection, it is possible that they contribute to recovery by participating in viral neutralization.

### Acquired Secretory Immunity

The agents of most infectious diseases enter the
body through mucous surfaces where secretory
rather than humoral antibody may be important
in recovery from and protection against infection.
The importance of secretory IgA in natural resistance to infection is discussed in the preceding
chapter. Its role in acquired resistance was discovered by Burrows in studies with experimental
cholera (Burrows et al., 1947). He demonstrated
that protection against infection after cholera
vaccination was correlated with fecal antibody
rather than with serum antibody. The ability of
cholera vaccine to protect as many as 60 per cent
of humans against cholera shows the significance
of Burrow's experimental findings in clinical
medicine. Furthermore, protection by vaccines
that contain killed vibrios shows that antibacterial rather than antitoxic immunity can produce acquired resistance. Much evidence suggests
that secretory immunity against cholera vibrios
is mediated primarily by antibody that blocks
their attachment to the intestinal mucosa rather
than by complement-mediated reactions such as
bacteriolysis or opsonization by neutrophils. IgA
cannot fix C1 (Ishizaka et al., 1966), and its
bactericidal activity via the alternative complement pathway has been observed only under
special conditions that would not exist in the
anticomplementary milieu of the gut. The idea
that IgA blocks attachment of vibrios is supported
by Freter's report (1969) that coproantibodies
(fecal antibodies) sharply reduced the number of
vibrios that adhered either to the mucosa in
isolated loops of rabbit intestine or to viable slices
of rabbit ileum. Coproantibody also inhibited the
growth of V. cholera in the presence of viable
mucosal cells, but the mechanism of such growth
inhibition is unknown.

Other pathogenic bacteria adhere selectively to
certain mucosal surfaces. Thus group A streptococci attach to human pharyngeal cells much
better than E. coli, whereas E. coli adhere to
bladder mucosa much better than group A streptococci (Gibbons, 1977). Similarly, gonococci and
group B streptococci adhere to vaginal epithelial
cells in larger numbers than E. coli, Bacteroides
fragilis, fusobacteria, and lactobacilli (Mardh and

Westrom, 1976). Adherence to intestinal epithelium likewise appears to determine the virulence of various enteric pathogens such as *Shigella* and enteropathogenic *E. coli*. This selective adherence of bacteria to certain epithelial cells seems to parallel their relative ability to produce infection in tissues or organs covered by these cells. The surface components of bacteria that are responsible for adherence seem to vary with the organisms and the mucosal surface. There is evidence, for example, that the following surface components are involved in adherence: lipoteichoic acid and surface fibrils for group A streptococci (Beachey, 1975); pili for gonococci, *E. coli,* and *Proteus*; and flagella for *V. cholerae* (Jones and Freter, 1972). The surface components of epithelial cells responsible for adherence seem to be primarily glycoproteins (Gibbons, 1977). Similar glycoproteins are abundant in the mucus that bathes these cells and can apparently block adherence of pathogenic bacteria by competing for attachment sites on the surface of these organisms. The increased flow of mucus during respiratory, intestinal, and genital infections could thus interrupt their spread by delivering two proteins, IgA and glycoprotein, that might block further adherence of pathogenic bacteria to the diseased mucosa. Because secretory IgA is also antitoxic it may contribute to recovery from diphtheria, cholera, and diarrhea caused by the enterotoxins of *E. coli* (Stoliar et al., 1976). Thus, acquired secretory immunity might be both antitoxic and antibacterial. These attractive hypotheses, however, need more critical experimental support.

There is more convincing evidence that immunity against virus infections is acquired by the local production of secretory IgA on mucosal surfaces. This antibody, however, may be more important in providing immunity against reinfection than in recovery from infection. In influenza, for example, IgA appears in nasal washings early during the infection, but its antiviral activity is directed against strains of influenza virus that produced outbreaks in the past. This early IgA seems to be antibody stored in epithelial cells and has been found in both the respiratory and the intestinal mucosa (Kaur et al., 1972). It has no activity against the virus causing the infection and contributes nothing to recovery. Specific secretory IgA with activity against the infecting virus does not appear until two to three weeks after the onset of infection and long after the infection has ended (Alford et al., 1967). For this reason, other processes such as interferon production or cell-mediated immunity are thought to bring about recovery.

The presence of secretory antibody on mucous surfaces acquired after local infection or local inoculation of vaccines can be correlated with resistance to infection by rhinovirus, influenza virus, parainfluenza virus, and polioviruses. The IgA response to local inoculation of living viruses is better than the response to inactivated viruses, and live virus may also produce a systemic humoral immune response. The ability of local antibody to protect against mucosal viral infection was shown by studies in which local inoculation of inactivated viruses succeeded in giving protection when local but not systemic antibody was elaborated. Two striking differences have been noted between local and systemic immunization. For one thing, local immunization of mucous membranes tends to produce a very localized IgA response, which is restricted to the immunized or infected site and does not appear on other mucous membranes. Second, local immunization does not seem to evoke a secondary or booster type of secretory IgA response. Studies on the secondary IgA response are limited, but local vaccination by intranasal instillation of inactivated poliovaccine produced no difference in the quantity or duration of poliovirus antibody after primary and secondary immunization. The absence of a booster effect indicates that the secretory IgA response to poliovirus may be devoid of immunologic memory, and that long-lasting protection after primary immunization may result from continued local antibody synthesis in response to prolonged stimulation by persistent antigen (Ogra et al., 1975).

## NONPROTECTIVE ANTIBODY ACQUIRED DURING INFECTION

Not all antibodies acquired after infection or vaccination can protect against infection, despite their specificity for antigens in the infectious agent. These nonprotective antibodies react with antigens that are not responsible for virulence and are often released from beneath the surface of the infecting agent. The C polysaccharide of streptococci, the structural components of virions, the teichoic acids of staphylococci, the nucleoprotein of *Brucella,* the cell-wall polysaccharide of *B. anthracis,* and the polysaccharides of mycobacteria are examples of antigens that generate specific but nonprotective antibodies during infection. Nonprotective antibodies also develop to viral enzymes that participate in the manufacture of structural proteins and nucleic acids. In fact, antibodies that develop during viral infection may be directed against antigens that are elaborated during viral synthesis but are never incorporated into the virion. The various antibodies that have no role in protection are identified by complement fixation, agglutination, or precipitation and are often useful for diagnosis.

## ACQUIRED CELLULAR IMMUNITY

The increased resistance observed after certain infections, such as those caused by mycobacteria and fungi, is not always accompanied by protective antibody in the blood or body fluids. Persons who have overcome the infection are more resistant to exogenous infection than previously uninfected persons. Although precipitins and complement-fixing antibodies may be present at some stage in these infections, many healthy persons who have recovered from all clinical signs of the disease possess no detectable antibodies for the infectious agent. This type of acquired resistance without demonstrable antibody is manifested by an intense local inflammatory response to the living organisms or to their products. The local reaction is more intense and appears more rapidly than that in the nonimmune individual and prevents the extension of the organism to the regional lymph nodes. Because this reaction is marked by an intense infiltration of inflammatory cells, it is sometimes spoken of as *cellular immunity*, a term that implies a specific increase in the capacity of the cells themselves to resist infection.

Although cellular immunity has been regarded as the basis of acquired resistance to infection in various bacterial, fungal, viral, and parasitic infections, the most important original discoveries in this field were made by Robert Koch (1891) in his studies of experimental tuberculosis. Koch described his discovery of the altered response to tuberculous reinfection in the following manner:

If a normal guinea pig is inoculated with a pure culture of tubercle bacilli, the wound, as a rule, closes and in the first few days seemingly heals. After ten to fourteen days, however, there appears a firm nodule which soon opens, forming an ulcer that persists until the animal dies. Quite different is the result if a tuberculous guinea pig is inoculated with tubercle bacilli. For this purpose it is best to use animals that have been infected four to six weeks previously. In such an animal, also, the little inoculation wound closes at first, but in this case no nodule is formed, On the next, or second day, however, a peculiar change occurs at the inoculation site. The area becomes indurated and assumes a dark color, and these changes do not remain limited to the inoculation point, but spread to involve an area 0.5 to 1.0 cm in diameter. In the succeeding days it becomes evident that the altered skin is necrotic. It finally sloughs, leaving a shallow ulcer which usually heals quickly and permanently, and the regional lymph nodes do not become infected. The action of tubercle bacilli upon the skin of a normal guinea pig is thus entirely different from their action upon the skin of a tuberculous one. This striking effect is produced not only by living tubercle bacilli but also by dead bacilli, whether killed by prolonged low temperature, by boiling, or by certain chemicals.

This remarkable observation by Koch brought out two essential features of the immune response in tuberculosis:

1. *A hypersensitivity reaction to the tubercle bacillus.* The effect of hypersensitivity is to produce an accelerated inflammatory response upon reinfection. This accelerated reaction was actually first described by Jenner with cowpox when he vaccinated people who had recovered from smallpox.

2. *Increased resistance to tuberculosis.* The bacteria are confined to the site of inoculation. In contrast to primary infection, they do not spread to the regional lymph nodes or beyond.

The hypersenstivity reaction in tuberculosis is called "delayed" hypersensitivity because it is not noticed until after 24 hours. It differs from the immediate type of hypersensitivity in anaphylaxis, which elicits tissue reactions within minutes after the antigen is injected. Delayed hypersensitivity is also different from the Arthus reaction, which begins in a few hours after challenge with antigen. These two rapid forms of hypersensitivity require a reaction between antigen and antibody, but delayed hypersensitivity does not. Delayed hypersensitivity is seen in all forms of infection but has special significance in those diseases in which immunity is not acquired through circulating antibody. This is true in all fungus infections; in such bacterial infections as leprosy, brucellosis, tularemia, lymphopathia venereum, and syphilis; in smallpox and certain other virus infections; and in various parasitic infections, including cutaneous leishmaniasis and schistosomiasis.

Because acquired immunity develops simultaneously with hypersensitivity in these diseases, because the two phenomena share the same inflammatory reaction, and because humoral antibody provides no resistance against these infections, it is generally assumed that delayed hypersensitivity can produce this form of acquired resistance. The inflammatory cells in delayed hypersensitivity are those that are important in resistance to infection. When a moderate or large dose of organisms or their antigens are injected into an infected individual, many polymorphonuclear cells appear, followed by mononuclear phagocytes (macrophages), which tend to arrange themselves in sheet-like aggregates and in tubercles. When a very small concentration of organisms is inoculated, only mononuclear phagocytes may appear. These polymorphonuclear and mononuclear cells can kill bacteria and other organisms, and their accelerated delivery to the site of infection in delayed hypersensitivity is associated with a more rapid disappearance of organisms than in controls.

In addition to this accelerated migration, reinfection stimulates macrophages to greater phagocytosis and killing. Because of these increased activities, they have been designated "activated" macrophages. Activation generally occurs after infection by organisms that reside within macrophages. Once activated by such infection, macrophages provide increased resistance against infections caused by other unrelated organisms. This increase in nonspecific resistance is accompanied by greater nonspecific killing of injected organisms. For example, macrophages from animals infected with *Listeria monocytogenes* or *Salmonella typhimurium* can kill *S. typhimurium* equally well (Blanden et al., 1966). The increased antimicrobial properties of activated macrophages are accompanied by other functional and morphologic changes. They are larger than normal macrophages, spread out more and adhere better to glass, and have more cytoplasmic granules. They also utilize more glucose through the hexose monophosphate shunt and have more activity of certain enzymes, such as the membrane enzyme adenylate cyclase and the cytoplasmic enzyme lactic dehydrogenase. They also have more lysosomes with their hydrolytic enzymes.

Lymphocytes also play an important part in cellular immunity by regulating macrophage activity. Soon after reinfection occurs with the intracellular bacteria that induce delayed hypersensitivity, specifically sensitized T lymphocytes react with the bacterial antigens and release substances, known as lymphokines, into the infected tissues. These lymphokines, which are chemotactic, attract macrophages to the infection and activate them. The specifically sensitized T lymphocytes have long lives and can provide long-lasting specific resistance to reinfection by reactivating macrophages. The macrophages, on the other hand, lose their activation within a few weeks. Generally speaking, humoral antibody is involved in these reactions only under exceptional circumstances such as trichinosis and schistosomiasis. Experimental studies indicate that acquired immunity in these parasitic infections results from a form of cellular immunity that is dependent on antibody. The role of humoral antibody in rejecting the invading larvae (schistosomules) has been established by passive transfer of immunity with immune serum. The antibody involved is IgE, which interacts with both macrophages and eosinophils, so that both cells then kill the parasite (Capron et al., 1977).

The mechanisms of cellular immunity in virus infections are still obscure, even though delayed hypersensitivity was first described with inoculation of vaccinia virus by Jenner in 1798. One reason for the difficulty in identifying the cell-mediated component of antiviral immunity is that humoral antibody usually affords prominent protection and may overshadow cellular immune processes. According to current evidence, antibody functions mainly by preventing viral infection and limiting its extracellular spread, and cell-mediated immunity functions by eliminating virus-infected cells. In patients suffering from diseases or receiving drugs that would be expected to lower cellular immunity, there is a predilection for infection with four viruses that acquire their envelope from nuclear or cytoplasmic membranes of infected cells: measles, cytomegalovirus, varicella-zoster, and herpes simplex. These viruses cause severe recurrent infections in patients given immunosuppressive therapy, and children with congenital immunodeficiencies. Since the antigens of these membrane-associated viruses are incorporated in the membrane of the infected cell, they are available on the cell surface for reactions with the inflammatory cells involved in delayed hypersensitivity. This idea gains support from the fact that infections by all membrane-associated viruses are followed by delayed hypersensitivity reactions to the specific viral antigens (Bloom and Rager-Zisman, 1975).

At least three mechanisms have been postulated to explain how cell-mediated reactions could work against virus infections. One is by a reaction of T cells against virus-infected cells. Purified T lymphocytes can lyse target cells containing specific membrane antigens (Henney, 1973). A second potential mechanism involves interferon production by activated lymphocytes. Viral antigens can cause blast cell transformation of specifically immune lymphocytes and the secretion of lymphokines, including interferon. The secretion of lymphokines with chemotactic activity could attract macrophages that can inactivate viruses, including viruses that have combined with antibody. Because macrophages have receptors for the Fc portion of IgG molecules, virus-antibody complexes can be attacked, ingested, and degraded. In the third mechanism, infected cells containing viral antigens in their membranes would be recognized as foreign and rejected by a cell-mediated reaction.

Each of these theoretical processes for mediating cellular immunity in virus infections has been demonstrated in systems examined in vitro. Until these have been found to operate in vivo as well, the role of cell-mediated immunity in human viral infections will continue to be speculative.

## References

Alford, R., Rossen, R., Butler, W., and Kasel, J.: Neutralizing and hemagglutination-inhibiting activity of nasal secretions following experimental human infection with $A_2$ influenza virus. J Immunol 98:724, 1967.

Almeida, J., and Lawrence, G.: Heated and unheated antiserum on rubella virus. Am J Dis Child 118:101, 1969.

Beachey, E.: Binding of group A streptococci to human oral mucosal cells by lipoteichoic acid. Trans Assoc Am Phys 88:285, 1975.

Blarden, R., Mackaness, G., and Collins, F.: Mechanisms of acquired resistance in mouse typhoid. J Exp Med 124:585, 1966.

Bloom, B., and Rager-Zisman, B.: Cell-mediated immunity in viral infections. In Notkins, A. (ed.): Viral Immunology and Immunopathology. New York, Academic Press, 1975, p. 113.

Braude, A., Ziegler, E., Douglas, H., and McCutchen, J.: Protective properties of antisera to R core. In Schlesinger, D. (ed.): Microbiology-1977. Washington, D.C., American Society for Microbiology, 1977, p. 253.

Brown, K., and Brown, I.: Immunity to malaria: Antigenic variation to chronic infections of Plasmodium knowlesi. Nature 208:1286, 1965.

Burrows, W., Elliott, M., and Havens, I.: Studies on immunity to asiatic cholera. IV. The excretion of coproantibody in experimental enteric cholera in the guinea pig. J Infect Dis 81:261, 1947.

Capron, A., Dessaint, J., Joseph, M., Torpier, G., Capron, M., Rousseaux, R., Santoro, F., and Bazin, H.: IgE and cells in schistosomiasis. Am J Trop Med Hyg 26:39, 1977.

Daniels, C.: Mechanism of viral neutralization. In Notkins, A. (eds.): Viral Immunology and Immunopathology. New York, Academic Press, 1975, p. 79.

Despommier, D.: Immunity to Trichinella spiralis. Am J Trop Med (Suppl.) 26:part 2, 68, 1977.

Dales, S., and Kajioka, R.: The cycle of multiplication of vaccinia virus in Earle's strain L cells. 1. Uptake and penetration. Virology 24:278, 1964.

Freter, R.: Studies of the mechanism of action of intestinal antibody in experimental cholera. Tex Rep Exp Biol Med 27 (Suppl 1):299, 1969.

Gibbons, R.: Adherence of bacteria to host tissue. In Schlesinger, D. (ed.): Microbiology, 1977. Washington, D.C., American Society for Microbiology, 1977, p. 395.

Henney, C.: On the mechanics of T cell mediated cytolysis. Transplant Rev 17:37, 1973.

Ishizaka, T., Ishizaka, K., Borsos, T., and Rapp, H.: C'1 fixation by human isoagglutinins: Fixation of C'1 by γG and γM but not γA antibody. J Immunol 97:711, 1966.

Jones, G., and Freter, R.: Adhesive properties of Vibrio cholerae: Nature of the interaction with isolated rabbit brush border membranes and human erythrocytes. Infect Immunol 6:918, 1972.

Kaur, J., McGhee, J., and Burrows, W.: Immunity to cholera: The occurrence and nature of antibody-active immunoglobulins in the lower ileum of the rabbit. J Immunol 108:387, 1972.

Koch, R.: Further communication on a remedy for tuberculosis. Dtsch Med Wochenschr 17:101, 1891

Mardh, P., and Westrom, L.: Adherence of bacteria to vaginal epithelial cells. Infect Immunol 13:661, 1976.

Mims, C.: Aspects of the pathogenesis of virus diseases. Bacteriol Rev 28:30, 1964.

Ogra, P., Morag, A., and Motti, L.: Humoral immune response to viral infections. In Notkins, A. (ed.): Viral Immunology and Immunopathology. New York, Academic Press, 1975, p. 57.

Radwan, A., and Crawford, T.: The mechanism of neutralization of sensitized equine arteritis virus by complement components. J Gen Virol 25:229, 1974.

Silverstein, S., and Marcus, P.: Early stages of Newcastle disease virus–Hela cell interaction: An electron microscopic study. Virology 23:370, 1964.

Stoliar, O., Kaniecki-Green, E., Pelley, R., Klaus, M., and Carpenter, C.: Secretory IgA against enterotoxins in breast milk. Lancet 1:1258, 1976.

Taliaferro, W. H.: Ablastic and trypanocidal antibodies against Trypanosoma dultoni. J Immunol 35:303, 1938.

Taliaferro, W. H., and Sarles, M.: The cellular reactions in the skin, lungs, and intestine of normal and immune rats after infection with Nippostrongylus muris. J Infect Dis 64:157, 1939.

Williamson, W., and Greenwood, B.: Impairment of the immune response to vaccination after acute malaria. Lancet 1:1328, 1978.

# 83  MECHANISMS OF IMMUNOLOGIC INJURY IN INFECTIOUS DISEASES

## Abraham I. Braude, M.D., Ph.D.

Microbial antigens may injure cells or tissues during infection by the seven mechanisms listed in Table 1.

These mechanisms may operate independently or simultaneously, and some may involve both antibodies and mononuclear cells (lymphocytes and macrophages).

### ANTIBODY-MEDIATED CYTOLYSIS

Lysis of cells may result from the interaction of antibody, complement, and microbial antigens on the surface of infected cells (Porter, 1971). This type of injury has been observed almost exclusively in cells infected with viruses that have envelopes such as poxviruses, herpesviruses, paramyxoviruses, arenavirus, togavirus, and rhabdovirus (Rawls and Tompkins, 1975). Viral antigens appear on the surface of infected cells after RNA viruses pass through the cellular cytoplasmic membrane during the release of the nucleocapsid from the infected cell by the process of "budding." The virus picks up its envelope from the cytoplasmic membrane and at the same time deposits viral antigen in the surface of the membrane (Rawls and Tompkins, 1975). A DNA virus such as herpes simplex picks up its envelope by budding through the nuclear membrane, but herpes antigens also appear at the cell surface. The union of IgG or IgM antibodies with viral antigen on the cell surface activates complement via the classic pathway, and cell lysis ensues through the same mechanism as that described for bacterial lysis in Chapter 81. After reacting with antibody and antigenic sites on the cell

**TABLE 1.** Mechanisms of Immunologic Injury in Infections

| MECHANISM | EXAMPLE OF INFECTIOUS AGENTS |
|---|---|
| Antibody-mediated cytolysis | Enveloped virus |
| Complement-mediated chemotaxis | Pyogenic bacteria |
| Immune complex vasculitis | Agents of endocarditis, viral hepatitis, leprosy, and quartan malaria |
| Intravascular coagulation | Meningococcus and other gram-negative bacteria |
| Anaphylaxis | Worms and aspergilli |
| T cell-mediated cytolysis | Lymphocytic choriomeningitis virus |
| Delayed hypersensitivity | *M. tuberculosis, Brucella, Histoplasma,* vaccinia virus |

membrane, C1 is activated to react with C4 and C2. This generates C3 convertase, which splits C3 into two fragments, the larger (C3b) remaining attached to the cell membrane. The protease activity of C3b binds C5, 6, and 7, thus building a complex on the cell surface composed of C1 through C7. Damage to the cell membrane is initiated when C8 is bound to the C1 through C7 complex. Cytolysis is accelerated when C9 becomes incorporated (Kolb and Müller-Eberhardt, 1975). This type of cytolysis is a theoretical mechanism not only for eliminating virus infections but also for injuring the infected organ. The effectiveness of the process in producing cytolysis depends on the type of cell and on the number of antigenic sites that appear on the cell surface (Kibler and Ter Meulen, 1975). For example, during persistent infection in tissue culture by measles virus, relatively few surface antigens appear compared with acute measles infections, and few if any cells undergo lysis. This finding correlates with the absence of necrotic foci in subacute sclerosing panencephalitis, a form of persistent measles infection of the brain.

## COMPLEMENT-MEDIATED CHEMOTAXIS AND SUPPURATION

When the classic complement pathway is activated by union of antibody with microbial antigen, or the alternate pathway by bacterial lipopolysaccharides, the chemotactic factors C3a and C5a are produced. These chemotactic factors attract inflammatory cells that not only attack microbial cells and virus-infected cells but also injure the infected tissues. The chemotactic factors C3a and C5a can also stimulate the release from mast cells of histamine, which in turn increases the permeability of vessels for leukocytes. The heavy influx of granulocytes during inflammation causes the characteristic tissue damage of suppuration by release of proteolytic enzymes from neutrophil granules. These enzymes can destroy both connective tissue proteins (collagen-

ase and elastase) and cells (Williams et al., 1977).

## IMMUNE COMPLEX VASCULITIS (ARTHUS REACTION)

When microbial antigens unite with antibody, the infectivity of the organism may be inactivated so that the infection is terminated. But if the antigen is discharged from organisms protected within a "privileged sanctuary" that cannot be eliminated by immune processes, the steady supply of antigen may form soluble complexes with its antibody. Such complexes can develop from antigens released upon microbial lysis by antibody and complement or as a by-product of microbial growth. These soluble complexes can circulate in the blood until they are deposited in the tissues by phagocytosis or trapping. Phagocytosis by reticuloendothelial (RES) cells removes large complexes preferentially so that the small complexes formed in antigen excess remain in the circulation. If the large complexes contain infectious virus or toxic microbial antigens that persist within the Küpffer cells, they may impair phagocytic clearance by the RES and promote the circulation of complexes (Oldstone and Dixon, 1975). As RES clearance fails and the concentration of complexes mounts in the circulation, the complexes pass through permeable vessels and are deposited in the tissues. The permeability of these vessels is apparently increased when the antigen in the complexes reacts with IgE that is adherent to basophils or mast cells. The antigen thus causes mast cell or basophilic granules to release certain factors that can increase vascular permeability and others that cause platelets to clump and in turn release vasoactive amines. The combined effect of such basophilic and platelet permeability factors on blood vessels permits the leakage of immune complexes and their deposition in the tissue along the vessel walls (Cochrane and Koffler, 1973). In addition, glomerular capillaries have normal endothelial fenestrations that

TABLE 2.   Infectious Diseases Underlying the Production of Immune Complex Glomerulonephritis

| UNDERLYING DISEASE | ORGANISMS |
| --- | --- |
| Subacute bacterial endocarditis | *Staphylococcus aureus, Streptococcus viridans,* enterococcus, *Coxiella burnetii* |
| Ventriculoatrial shunt infections | *S. epidermidis* |
| Malaria | *Plasmodiuim malariae* and *falciparum* |
| Lepromatous leprosy | *Mycobacterium leprae* |
| Syphilis | *Treponema pallidum* |
| Hepatitis | Hepatitis B virus |
| Pneumococcal pneumonia | Type 14 pneumococcus |
| Streptococcal pyoderma or pharyngitis | Group A streptococci |
| Typhoid fever | *Salmonella typhosa* |
| Shistosomiasis | *Schistosoma mansoni* |
| Toxoplasmosis | *Toxoplasma gondii* |

favor leakage of complexes and help explain the unique susceptibility of glomeruli to immune-complex deposition. Immune complexes with a density in the range of 19S or larger are most likely to be deposited along vessels and damage them (Cochrane and Koffler, 1973); complexes with a density of less than 19S not only fix complement poorly but are also cleared slowly from the blood.

One important mechanism for vessel injury requires fixation of complement by the immune complexes (Cochrane and Koffler, 1973). Activation of the complement system generates C3a and C5a, which increase permeability of vessels and attract granulocytes. The accumulation of granulocytes (neutrophilic leukocytes) is followed by the release of their lysosomal enzymes, which destroy the elastic laminae of small arteries and injure the basement membrane of glomerular capillaries. The consumption of complement by these complexes is reflected in the diminished concentration of C3 and other complement components in the serum and by the presence of complement components at the site of immune complex deposition. If complement and polymorphonuclear leukocytes are depleted in experimental animals with immune complex disease, the arterial lesions are prevented, but glomerular injury can still occur (McCluskey and Klassen, 1974) through mediators other than complement.

In bacterial endocarditis, quartan malaria, lepromatous leprosy, syphilis, and viral hepatitis B, the occurrence of immune complex disease is well established (Bayer et al., 1976; Kohler et al., 1974; Gamble and Reardon, 1975). Each of these is a subacute or chronic infection in which a bacterial, protozoan, or viral antigen is released constantly into the bloodstream at a time when high levels of antibody are already present. The immune complexes that result from the union of circulating antigen with antibody produce granular deposits along the glomerular basement membrane. These complexes, containing immunoglobulin plus antigen plus complement, produce electron-dense deposits in the glomerular basement membrane and diffuse proliferative glomerulonephritis. Those infections that have been implicated in the production of immune complex glomerulonephritis are listed in Table 2. In most of these, the specific microbial antigens have been demonstrated in the glomerular deposit. In the immune complex glomerulonephritis of syphilis, schistosomiasis, infected ventriculoatrial shunts, and quartan malaria, the clinical syndrome has usually been that of the nephrotic syndrome.

In viral hepatitis B and lepromatous leprosy there have been prominent clinical features attributed to immune complex deposition outside the kidney. In chronic carriers of hepatitis B virus, for example, hepatitis B surface antigen immune complexes were identified in vascular lesions in periarteritis nodosa. In other cases of viral hepatitis B, immune complexes do not necessarily contain viral antigens. In these immune complexes the antigen is usually IgG and the antibody is IgM (Levo et al., 1977). It appears that some of the IgG generated in various chronic infections can become antigenic itself and stimulate a form of autoimmunity to the patient's own immunoglobulin. Perhaps the antigenic groups of IgG that react with IgM antibody are normally buried within the IgG molecule and become exposed when IgG molecules unfold after union with the specific microbial antigen. Activation of the classic complement pathway by these complexes of IgG and IgM results in systemic vasculitis involving the skin, kidneys, and joints and producing vascular purpura, glomerulonephritis, and arthritis. These immune complexes composed of IgG and IgM have the distinctive property of precipitating at cold temperatures and are known as cryoglobulins.* They occur in leprosy, endocar-

*These cryoglobulins in chronic infections are composed of polyclonal IgM and IgG. They are designated Type III cryoglobulins and must be distinguished from Type I and Type II (mixed monoclonal-polyclonal) cryoglobulins that are produced in certain noninfectious diseases.

ditis, cytomegalovirus infections, and infectious mononucleosis, and can produce vascular lesions in these conditions. The most dramatic of these occur in lepromatous leprosy and take the form of painful red papules known as erythema nodosum leprosum. They may be accompanied by arthritis and glomerulonephritis.

## INTRAVASCULAR COAGULATION

Tissue injury from intravascular coagulation in human infection is best illustrated by the hemorrhagic skin necrosis and renal cortical necrosis of meningococcemia. The hemorrhagic skin necrosis in meningococcemia is an example of the dermal Shwartzman reaction (Davis and Arnold, 1974), and renal cortical necrosis is typical of the generalized Shwartzman reaction. As noted in Chapter 6, either phenomenon can be produced experimentally by giving rabbits two injections of the lipopolysaccharide (LPS) antigen from any gram-negative bacteria. Two intravenous injections of LPS, given 24 hours apart, invariably produce severe disseminated intravascular coagulation (DIC) culminating in bilateral renal cortical necrosis. This dramatic form of kidney damage (Sanarelli-Schwartzman reaction) results from glomerular deposits of fibrin. The dermal Shwartzman reaction is also produced by two separate injections of LPS, the first intradermally and the second intravenously 24 hours later. Soon after the cutaneous dose, the site of the intradermal injection undergoes hemorrhagic necrosis secondary to local thrombosis and infarction. The first injection causes an Arthus-like inflammation about the skin vessels, and the intravenous dose initiates coagulation and thrombosis that are limited to the inflamed vessel.

The essential role of coagulation is illustrated by the prevention of both reactions by heparin and other anticoagulants. In the generalized Shwartzman reaction, the first dose of LPS triggers intravascular conversion of fibrinogen to fibrin by the mechanisms discussed in Chapter 6, but the reticuloendothelial system (RES) clears the fibrin before it can be deposited in the glomerular capillaries and other vessels (Lee and Stetson, 1965). The first dose of LPS seems to condition the RES so that its clearance activity is blocked by the second dose. As a result, the fibrin aggregates produced by the second dose are no longer cleared from the blood; instead, they are filtered out by the glomeruli, where they occlude the capillaries and produce infarction of the renal cortex. DIC consumes clotting factors such as fibrinogen, platelets, and prothrombin. In addition, DIC activates fibrinolysis so that fibrin degradation products are released. These fragments prevent clotting by inhibiting proteolysis of fibrinogen by thrombin and blocking polymerization of fibrin monomer to form a clot. The anticoagulant effect of these degradation products can cause serious bleeding in patients whose clotting factors are depleted by DIC, not only aggravating hemorrhages into the necrotic lesions of the skin and kidneys but also producing hemorrhages in other tissues not affected by the Shwartzman lesions.

Although meningococcemia is the most dramatic and consistent example of the two Shwartzman reactions, severe bacteremias with any gram-negative bacteria can cause DIC. One of the most devastating examples is the DIC that occurs in *E. coli* bacteremia of pregnancy. This condition is characterized by hemorrhagic lesions in the skin and by fatal renal cortical necrosis. For obscure reasons, pregnancy appears to prepare for the generalized Shwartzman reaction so that only one intravenous dose of LPS is required to evoke DIC and renal cortical necrosis.

Although gram-negative bacteria, including rickettsiae, are the primary cause of DIC because of their LPS, infections by gram-positive bacteria, viruses, fungi, and protozoa can also cause intravascular coagulation. These organisms can initiate clotting by various mechanisms such as the release of tissue factor, a lipoprotein contained in the plasma membrane of endothelial cells and monocytes. When tissue factor is liberated by damage of these cells, it can initiate clotting by complexing with Factor VII and calcium ions to activate Factor X. Bacteria can also initiate clotting through their proteolytic enzymes that break down fibrinogen. But the most relevant immunologic mechanism is the initiation of coagulation or of platelet aggregation by circulating immune complexes composed of microbial antigens and antibody. Such complexes can accelerate fibrin formation in vitro, but only in cell-rich plasma, presumably because tissue-factor is released. Similarly, soluble antigen-antibody complexes can initiate clotting in vivo by substituting for the provocative injection of LPS in the dermal Shwartzman reaction. The intravenous injection of antigen into specifically immunized rabbits also produces DIC and the generalized Shwartzman reaction (Lee, 1963).

## ANAPHYLAXIS

Anaphylactic antibodies occur primarily in worm and fungus infections. These antibodies belong mainly to the IgE class and act through attachment via the Fc position to the surface of tissue mast cells and basophils. When a divalent antigen from worms or fungi combines with two

IgE molecules to form a bridge, the antibody becomes distorted. This distortion of IgE on the cell surface causes the discharge of intracellular granules, which release histamine and serotonin. In the lung, histamine and serotonin cause smooth muscle contraction and endothelial injury, resulting in bronchospasm and edema. The eosinophil chemotactic factor of anaphylaxis is released from mast cell granules and attracts eosinophils to the site of anaphylaxis. Eosinophils appear to check the allergic reaction by ingesting the antigen-antibody complexes and by inactivating histamine through the release of histaminase (Goetzl and Austen, 1977). Worms induce very high levels of IgE and eosinophils and various manifestations of anaphylaxis. *Ascaris* worms are especially potent causes of anaphylactic hypersensitivity when they invade the tissues and especially when they migrate through the lungs. They produce the syndrome of eosinophilic pneumonia, an allergic pneumonitis with a prominent asthmatic component. Eosinophilia is also prominent in strongyloidiasis, visceral larva migrans, trichinosis, certain types of filariasis, and acute schistosomiasis. *Angiostrongylus cantonensis*, a nematode that invades the central nervous system, causes eosinophilic meningitis. Systemic fatal anaphylactic shock can occur in echinococcosis upon rupture of a hydatid cyst and release of echinococcal antigen into the peritoneum, where high levels of IgE are delivered from the circulation. A more benign systemic reaction, known as Katayama fever, occurs at the onset of egg production in schistosomiasis, but the role of IgE is debatable in the induction of this reaction.

Among fungus diseases, pulmonary allergic aspergillosis is the most important example of a hypersensitivity disorder mediated by IgE (Golbert and Patterson, 1970). After colonization of the bronchial mucous secretions with aspergilli, these patients develop asthma, eosinophilia, and migratory pulmonary infiltrates suggestive of allergic pneumonitis. IgG also participates in the allergic bronchial reaction by producing an Arthus-type reaction.

### CYTOLYSIS MEDIATED BY T LYMPHOCYTES

T lymphocytes can kill infected cells in the absence of antibody if three requirements are met: (1) antigen of the infecting virus must appear on the surface of the cell; (2) the T-cells must have immune-specificity for the virus; and (3) the T cells must be histocompatible with the target cell. In other words, virus-immune T lymphocytes can cause lysis of infected cells only if the T cell

reacts with the viral antigen on the surface of a cell that is recognized as nonforeign. The recognition of a cell as nonforeign, or "self," is thought to involve a reaction between the lymphocyte and the histocompatibility antigen on the target cell. Thus, the attacking T lymphocyte would require two receptors to kill the infected cells: one for the viral antigen and the other for the histocompatibility antigen (Zinkernagel, 1978). T cell-mediated cytolysis may be important in infections by viruses that do not themselves destroy the infected cell. One example is lymphocytic choriomeningitis (LCM) virus. In intracerebral LCM virus infection of mice, the disease is caused by T cells rather than by the virus. The severity of this infection depends on when the T cells reach the target cells: if they reach the target cells early, they can eliminate the virus infection by destroying the cells before the virus replicates and spreads. At this point the damage to cells would be relatively insignificant. On the other hand, a cytolytic attack by T cells on advanced infections could kill the animal. In lymphocytic choriomeningitis, the choroid plexus is heavily infected, and cytolytic damage to this structure destroys the blood-brain barrier so that lethal cerebral edema occurs. A similar attack by T lymphocytes on liver tissue has been postulated as a mechanism for liver injury in viral hepatitis because the virus is assumed not to be cytotoxic. Hepatitis B surface antigen (HBsAg) can be found in the membrane of liver cells, and T cell-mediated cytotoxicity against $HB_SAg$ has been demonstrated in both acute and chronic hepatitis B (Hirschman, 1979).

From these observations and others, it has been suggested that killer lymphocytes can be beneficial only in infections with highly cytopathic viruses, because the infected cells must be sacrificed to ward off more extensive damage by the virus itself. In infections by viruses with slight cytopathic potential, on the other hand, the onslaught of T cells may cause more tissue injury than the virus (Zinkernagel, 1978).

### DELAYED HYPERSENSITIVITY

This form of hypersensitivity has been most extensively studied in tuberculosis and is also known as the "tuberculin" type of hypersensitivity. When living or dead tubercle bacilli are injected into the tissues of an animal or patient with tuberculosis, the inflammatory reaction does not begin until after a few hours; it progresses to its maximum size and intensity within 24 to 48 hours. This delay in onset and peak intensity of the reaction, compared with the anaphylactic and

Arthus types of inflammatory response, is responsible for the term *delayed hypersensitivity*. The concept that this reaction represents hypersensitivity is based on the fact that in nontuberculous animals, the injection of living bacilli produces no reaction for a week or more (until sensitization has time to develop), and dead bacilli may produce no reaction at any time. The intact bacillus is not required because antigenic tuberculous proteins can also elicit the phenomenon. The same delayed response to antigenic fractions of the infecting organism is seen in many other infections. The response is specific, occurring only when the organisms or antigens causing the infection are injected.

Because delayed hypersensitivity is characterized by necrosis at the injection site if large doses of dead organisms or antigen are used, this reaction is considered to be responsible for necrosis of tissues in natural infection after immune hypersensitivity has developed. In pulmonary tuberculosis, for example, the bacilli multiply slowly in mononuclear phagocytes that aggregate undamaged at the portal of entry until hypersensitivity develops. Then the cells are killed, the tissues undergo necrosis, and tubercle bacilli are discharged by the ulcerating focus into the lumen of the bronchioles (Canetti, 1954, 1958).

Necrosis is thought to be mediated by the lymphocytes that dominate the inflammatory reaction. A few lymphocytes and monocytes first accumulate around vessels in the area into which antigen or bacteria are injected. These specifically sensitized T lymphocytes react with the antigen to release mediators that attract and hold other mononuclear cells in the inflammatory focus. One of these mediators is a chemotactic factor, which attracts macrophages, and the other is migratory inhibitory factor (MIF), which holds them in place. In the meantime, lymphocytes themselves proliferate in situ upon stimulation by specific antigen and release a mitosis-stimulating factor that causes other lymphocytes to multiply. These reactions and others amplify the cellular response and produce the characteristic heavy infiltration of mononuclear cells that is the hallmark of delayed hypersensitivity. Polymorphonuclear leukocytes are seen very early in the inflammatory response but soon disappear before the delayed response is underway. Antibody also seems to be unimportant, because delayed hypersensitivity can be transferred by the mononuclear cells but not by serum.

At least three mechanisms have been proposed to explain cell necrosis by mononuclear cells. First, T lymphocytes attack target cells directly. They can be seen to kill cells in tissue culture, and the amount of killing can be measured by the radioactivity released from target cells labeled with $^{51}$Cr. The second mechanism of killing by lymphocytes is lymphocytotoxin, a mediator released from lymphocytes after reaction with specific antigen. This cytotoxic factor is a protein-like substance with a molecular weight in the range of 85,000 and the capacity to kill a wide variety of different cells (Williams and Granger, 1973). A third process of possible importance in the production of necrosis involves macrophages. In response to lymphocyte mediators and other stimuli, macrophages release hydrolytic enzymes such as cathepsins, hyaluronidase, and collagenases, which can injure the matrix that supports the cells, the vessels that supply them, and the cells themselves.

Killing of cells by T lymphocytes can be specific or nonspecific. Specific cytolysis is carried out by T lymphocytes that have immune specificity for the antigens on the surface of the target cell, as described in the preceding section on cytolysis by T lymphocytes. The surface antigens can be derived from the viruses infecting the cells or from other microbial antigens that adhere to the cytoplasmic membrane of the target cell. Cytolysis is nonspecific when the killer lymphocytes are a product of the mitosis that follows blast transformation. This blast transformation in T cells may be induced either by specific antigen or by lymphocytic mediators released from other lymphocytes.

## References

Bayer, A., Theofilopoulos, A., Eisenberg, R., Dixon, F., and Guze, L.: Circulating immune complexes in infective endocarditis. N Engl J Med 295:1500, 1976.

Canetti, G.: The Tubercle Bacillus in the Pulmonary Lesion of Man. New York, Springer Publishing Company, 1954.

Canetti, G.: Pathogenesis of tuberculosis in man. Ann NY Acad Sci 154:13, 1968.

Cochrane, C., and Koffler, D.: Immune complex disease in experimental animals and man. Adv Immunol 16:186, 1973.

Davis, C., and Arnold, K.: Role of meningococcal endotoxin in meningococcal purpura. J Exp Med 140:159, 1974.

Gamble, C., and Reardon, J.: Immunopathogenesis of syphilitic glomerulonephritis. N Engl J Med 292:449, 1975.

Goetzl, E., and Austen, K.: Cellular characteristics of the eosinophil compatible with a dual role in host defense in parasitic infections. Am J Trop Med Hyg 26:142, 1977.

Golbert, T., and Patterson, R.: Pulmonary allergic aspergillosis. Ann Int Med 72:395, 1970.

Hirschman, S.: Virologic, immunologic, and clinical correlations in viral hepatitis. Seminars Infect Dis 2:48, 1979.

Kibler, R., and Ter Meulen, V.: Antibody-mediated cytotoxicity after measles virus infection. J Immunol 114:93, 1975.

Kohler, P., Cronin, R., Hammond, W., Olen, D., and Carr, R.: Chronic membranous glomerulonephritis caused by hepatitis B antigen-antibody immune complexes. Ann Intern Med 81:448, 1974.

Kolb, W., and Müller-Eberhard, H.: The membrane attack mechanism of complement. J Exp Med 141:724, 1975.

Lee, L.: Antigen-antibody reaction in the pathogenesis of bilateral renal cortical necrosis. J Exp Med 117:365, 1963.

Lee, L., and Stetson, C.: The local and generalized Shwartzman phenomenon. In Zweifach, B., Grant, L., and McClusky, R. (eds.): The Inflammatory Process. New York, Academic Press, 1965, p. 791.

Levo, Y., Gorevic, P., Kassab, H., Zucker-Franklin, D., Gigli, I., and

Franklin, E.: Mixed cryoglobulinemia: Immune complex disease often associated with hepatitis B virus infection. Trans Assoc Am Phys 90:167, 1977.

McCluskey, R., and Klassen, J.: Immunologically mediated glomerular, tubular, and interstitial renal disease. N Engl J Med 288:564, 1973.

Odstone, M., and Dixon, F.: Immune complex disease associated with viral infections. In Notkins, A. (ed.): Viral Immunology and Immunopathology. New York, Academic Press, 1975, p. 341.

Porter, D. D.: Destruction of virus-infected cells by immunological mechanisms. Ann Rev Microbiol 25:283, 1971.

Rawls, W., and Tompkins, A.: Destruction of virus-infected cells by antibody and complement. In Notkins, A. (ed.): Viral Immunology and Immunopathology. New York, Academic Press, 1975, p. 99.

Williams, T., and Granger, G.: Lymphocyte in vitro cytotoxicity: Mechanism of human lymphotoxin-induced target cell destruction. Cell Immunol 6:171, 1973.

Williams, T., Lyons, J., and Braude, A.: In vitro lysis of target cells by rat polymorphonuclear leukocytes isolated from acute pyelonephritic exudates. J Immunol 119:671, 1977.

Zinkernagel, R. M.: Major transplantation antigens in host responses to infection. Hospital Practice 13(7):83, 1978.

# 84 IMMUNOPROPHYLAXIS AND IMMUNOTHERAPY

## Stephen A. Spector, M.D.

In the spring of 1796, Edward Jenner took some fluid from a large cowpox vesicle on the hand of dairymaid Sarah Nelmes and inoculated it at two sites on the arms of 8-year-old James Phipps (Creighton, 1889; Parish, 1965, 1968). The boy developed typical cowpox lesions, and 2 months later, when Jenner inoculated him with smallpox, no disease developed. Less than 200 years later, on October 26, 1977, Ali Maow Maalin, a cook in Merka, Somalia, became the "last reported case" of endemic variola. The global eradication of smallpox must be considered a major accomplishment of modern science and a triumph for immunizations. The elimination of this dreaded disease, as with most immunization programs, was not without setbacks and risks to vaccinees. Prophylactic inoculation against variola (variolation) was practiced in China, India, Persia, and elsewhere for centuries before it was popularized in England by Lady Mary Wortley Montagu in the early 18th century. The practice of variolation was far from safe, and possibly 2 to 3 per cent so vaccinated died of smallpox. This fatality rate was tenfold less than that from naturally occurring smallpox, and the artificial inoculation of variola was widely practiced until Jenner developed his "improved vaccine." The concept of intentionally exposing an individual to either live or killed immunogens to prevent disease, combined with the princple of passive transfer of antibody to prevent and ameliorate infections, serves as the cornerstone of present day immunoprophylaxis.

## PRINCIPLES OF PASSIVE IMMUNIZATION

Short-term immunity to many infections may be conferred by administering preformed antibody as immune serum or gamma globulin prepared from it (Stiehm, 1979). Two types of gamma globulin preparations are available: standard human immune serum globulin (ISG) for general use, and special human immune serum globulins with known antibody content for specific illnesses. Certain diseases may also be ameliorated or prevented by the use of animal sera and antitoxins.

IgG is produced primarily in plasma cells that have evolved from B-lymphocytes. Destruction of IgG-coated bacteria occurs following phagocytosis in the granulocytes of the reticuloendothelial system and in the gastrointestinal tract. IgG crosses the placenta and provides passive protection to the newborn infant for approximately six months. These passively acquired IgG antibodies may inhibit an infant's immune system and prevent an adequate response to certain vaccines.

ISG is prepared by alcohol fractionation of pooled human sera by Cohn's alcohol fractionation procedure, which removes most other serum proteins and hepatitis viruses. ISG is composed of 95 per cent IgG at 165 mg per ml (16.5 per cent solution), along with trace quantities of IgM and IgA globulins and other serum proteins. IgG has a mean half-life of 25 days. Metabolism of IgG is directly controlled by its level in serum; there is an increase in the breakdown of IgG with elevated plasma levels and a decrease in catabolism with decreased levels.

ISG is available only for intramuscular injection. In vitro, it has been shown to aggregate into large molecular weight complexes that can activate spontaneously the complement system. These aggregates are probably responsible for the occasional systemic reactions to ISG that occur in approximately 2 per 1000 injections (Ellis and Henney, 1969). The incidence of reactions is increased with repeated injection of ISG and with intravenous administration. Approximately 20 per cent of patients receiving repeated intramuscular doses of gamma globulin can be expected to experience mild reactions including dyspnea, tightness in chest, faintness, hypotension, flushing, facial swelling, and anxiety (Squire et al., 1969).

Human gamma globulin is frequently used without proven indications. Patients with certain defined immune defects or with documented exposure to one of the infections listed in Table 1 are good candidates for passive prophylaxis. There is no evidence suggesting that the child with an apparent overabundance of upper respiratory infections without documented immunologic deficits benefits from short or prolonged treatment with gamma globulin. Similarly, special human immune serum globulins are in limited supply and should be administered only when patients are likely to benefit from their use (Table 2). Animal antisera and antitoxins particularly should be used only when there are definite indications (Table 2). Refined and concentrated horse sera are still the only effective prophylaxis for diphtheria, gas gangrene, and botulism once exposure has occurred. Animal serum against tetanus and rabies should only be used when special human gamma globulin is unavailable. The use of animal sera may be associated with acute febrile reactions, serum sickness, or anaphylaxis. Febrile reactions following injections of animal serum are usually mild but may be severe, requiring vigorous antipyretic therapy. Serum sickness occurs in from 10 to 40

per cent of recipients of some animal sera and consists of rash, urticaria, arthritis, adenopathy, and fever appearing hours or several days after a second injection, or 7 to 12 days after a first injection. Anaphylaxis occurs in approximately 1 per cent of individuals receiving animal antisera. Since anaphylactic reactions are life-threatening, an intracutaneous skin test, preceded by a scratch or eye test, should be performed on every patient before any injection of animal serum. Since intradermal skin tests have resulted in fatal reactions, a skin test should never be performed unless a syringe containing 1 ml of 1:1000 epinephrine is immediately available. If the skin test is positive or a patient has a strong allergic history, desensitization of the patient should be carried out under close medical supervision if the prophylactic use of animal antiserum is strongly indicated.

A new human antiserum has been developed which attempts to protect patients from death due to gram-negative bacteremia. The antiserum is made by immunizing volunteers against a stable mutant of *Escherichia coli* that lacks the ability to form the O antigenic side chains. The antibody thus formed is against the common lipopolysaccharide core of gram-negative bacteria and in animal studies has been highly effective in protecting against lethal gram-negative bacteremic shock and disseminated intravascular coagulation (Braude et al., 1977). Preliminary human trials have been promising, but further studies are required to establish its effectiveness and value (Ziegler et al., 1978).

**TABLE 1.　Indications for the Use of Standard Immune Serum Globulin (Human)**

| DISORDER | PURPOSE | DOSE (I.M.) | COMMENT |
|---|---|---|---|
| **Proved Value** | | | |
| Antibody deficiency disease (agammaglobulinemia, hypogammaglobulinemia) | Treatment | 0.66 ml/kg every 3–4 wk | Maximum dose is 20–30 ml; double dose at onset of therapy |
| Measles | Modification, prevention | 0.05 ml/kg 0.25 ml/kg | Rarely indicated; give immediately after exposure |
| Viral hepatitis type A (HAV) | Prevention: single exposure continuous exposure | 0.02–0.04 ml/kg 0.06 ml/kg, repeat in 5–6 mo | Give as soon as possible after exposure |
| Viral hepatitis type B (HBV) | Prevention | 0.12 ml/kg | Use when hepatitis B immune serum globulin is not available |
| **Limited Value** | | | |
| Varicella | Modification | 0.06–0.12 ml/kg | Give immediately after exposure; indicated only in serious underlying illness when VZIG or VZIP is not available |
| Rubella | Prevention | 20 ml | For pregnant women in the first trimester |

From American Academy of Pediatrics: Report of the Committee on Infectious Diseases, 18th ed., 1977.

**TABLE 2.** Passive Immunization

| DISEASE | SOURCE OF ANTIBODY | INDICATION | DOSE | ADVERSE REACTIONS | COMMENT |
|---|---|---|---|---|---|
| *Bacterial* | | | | | |
| Diphtheria | Horse serum (antitoxin) | Prevention and treatment | 10,000–80,000 units (I.M. and I.V.) depending on type of involvement and age of patient | Hypersensitivity, serum sickness, anaphylaxis | |
| Pertussis | Human pertussis immune globulin (PIG) | Treatment | <1 year old; 1.25 ml >1 year old; 2.5 ml I.M. | Pain and tenderness at injection site | Doubtful efficacy |
| Botulism | Horse serum against types A, B, and E | Treatment | 1 vial I.V.; 1 vial I.M. Repeat in 2–4 hours if symptoms continue | Hypersensitivity, serum sickness, anaphylaxis | Has not been helpful in infantile botulism Effectiveness uncertain |
| Tetanus | Human tetanus immune globulin (TIG) | Prevention and treatment | Prevention: 250–500 U—half I.M., half locally Treatment: 3000–6000 U—half I.M., half locally | Pain and tenderness at injection site | If TIG unavailable, tetanus antisera from horse serum (TAT) may be used |
| *Viral* | | | | | |
| Hepatitis B | Human hepatitis B immune globulin (HBIG) | Prevention (see text) | 0.06 ml/kg I.M.; repeat after 28 days | Pain and tenderness at injection site | See text |
| Varicella-zoster | Human varicella-zoster immune globulin (VZIG) | Prevention (see text); should be given within 72 hours of exposure | Newborn, 2.0 ml; others, 3–5 ml I.M. | Pain and tenderness at injection site | If VZIG unavailable, VZIP 10 ml/kg I.V. may be used Not indicated for active chickenpox or zoster |
| Rabies | Human rabies immune globulin (RIG) | Prevention | 20 units/kg, half into wound and half I.M. | Pain and tenderness at injection site | If RIG not available, equine rabies immune serum should be used |
| Mumps | Human mumps immune globulin | Prevention and treatment in adult men | 20 ml I.M. | Pain and tenderness at injection site | Questionable efficacy in preventing orchitis in postpubertal males |
| Smallpox | Human vaccinia immune globulin (VIG) | Within 24 hours after known exposure | 0.3 ml/kg I.M. | Pain and tenderness at injection site | Not indicated with active infection |

I.V., intravenous
I.M., intramuscular

## ACTIVE IMMUNIZATION

Active immunization is the induction of immunity by inoculation of a specific organism or some fragment or toxin associated with that organism. Although passive immunizations have prevented some disease, there are clearly many advantages to active vaccination. Some active immunizations give lifelong protection and thus do not require recognition of exposure to be effective. Additionally, the immunity conferred during active immunizations frequently approaches 100 per cent, whereas passive protection is often substantially less successful. The cost of preparing immune sera is more expensive than preparing vaccines.

Most immunogens used for active immunizations are crude fractions of an organism, or killed or live whole bacteria or viruses. The most notable exceptions to this are the vaccines against tetanus and diphtheria, which contain preformed inactivated toxins as immunogens.

Inactivated "killed" vaccines may be produced by three techniques. The first of these consists of whole organisms that are killed by heat or chemicals (e.g., formaldehyde). Examples of such killed vaccines are pertussis, typhoid, cholera, inactivated poliomyelitis, and influenza. These vaccines generally do not confer lasting immunity and frequently are only partially effective. Killed measles vaccine is no longer licensed because it not only offers less protection than does the attenuated live measles vaccine but also sensitizes individuals to future challenge with live measles so that infections are more severe. The killed poliomyelitis vaccine, however, has been extremely useful. Although it has been generally replaced by the attenuated Sabin vaccine, the killed Salk vaccine was effective in substantially reducing the number of clinical cases of paralytic polio in the United States before the introduction of the live polio vaccine. The killed vaccine has virtually eradicated the disease in Scandinavia, where the live vaccine has not been used.

The second method of preparing inactivated vaccines is by using extracted cellular fractions that have been shown to induce immunity in man. Vaccines prepared from the polysaccharide contained in the cell wall of the meningococcus and the capsule of the pneumococcus appear to be effective and safe in adults and children above the age of two years (Lepow et al., 1977; Peltola et al., 1977; Klein and Mortimer, 1978; Cowan et al., 1978; Center for Disease Control, 1978; Wilkins and Wehrle, 1979).

Immunizations with toxoids are prepared by inactivating large amounts of toxin with formalin rather than acting against the organisms themselves. The antibodies induced by these vaccines are active in neutralizing the toxin produced during infection. This third method of preparing inactivated vaccines has been extremely useful in the prevention of diphtheria and tetanus.

The major disadvantages of inactivated vaccines lie in their inability to confer lasting and local immunity. Multiple doses and boosters are required for continued protection, and local IgA fails to develop from the parenteral injection. As a result, protection against respiratory and gastrointestinal infections is suboptimal.

Live attenuated vaccines are prepared by serial passage of organisms in tissue culture or embryos so that the vaccine strain organism loses virulence. Local secretory IgA production may be stimulated by administration of the vaccine at the site of entry in the gut or the respiratory tract (Rothberg et al., 1973). This method of immunization produces the strongest and most durable immunity.

Active immunization may also be achieved by inducing an infection with a nonpathogenic organism that cross-reacts with a virulent organism. For example, Bacillus Calmette-Guérin (BCG), a strain of bovine tuberculosis, is used to induce immunity to human tuberculosis (Eickhoff, 1977). Similarly, protection against smallpox has been achieved by immunization with cowpox or vaccinia (Creighton, 1889).

## PROBLEMS ASSOCIATED WITH IMMUNIZATIONS

Associated with the desired benefits of vaccines are many real and potential problems. Live attenuated viral vaccines may revert to more virulent viruses and result in severe disease. In general, however, reversion has not been a problem, and serious reactions usually reflect abnormal host response rather than virus alteration. Contacts of vaccinees given live viruses may be at risk of developing an infection with the vaccine strain organism. Unfortunate cases of paralytic poliomyelitis have been well documented to occur rarely in both normal and immunosuppressed individuals following immunization or exposure to a recently immunized family member (Davis et al., 1977). Contaminating viruses or other organisms undetected in continuous cultures may lead to acute or chronic diseases and conceivably could result in malignancies in vaccine recipients (Fraumeni et al., 1963). Since many viruses cause latent or persistent infections and may produce slow viral diseases, concern has been expressed that certain vaccines may promote the development of these infections. To date, these concerns have not been substantiated. In fact, the incidence of subacute sclerosing panencephalitis (SSPE) in children following measles vaccine is nine times less common than in children with a history of naturally acquired measles (Modlin et al., 1977). The presence of unsuspected passenger viruses has been found in both live and killed vaccines. Simian viruses 40 (SV40), present in monkey cells, contaminated the polio cultures of both the Salk and Sabin vaccines and were injected with many of the original polio as well as adenovirus vaccines. Avian leukosis viruses are present in most flocks of chickens and their eggs and are subsequent contaminants of any virus grown in chick embryo cells.

Sensitization of individuals either to the organism to which immunity is desired or to the cellular antigens or antibiotics used to grow the organism has been observed. Severe reactions to vaccine prepared with chick or duck embryos are well described. In addition, repeated immunization of experimental animals with large doses of antigen has resulted in conditions similar to amyloidosis and multiple myeloma in man (White et al., 1974).

**TABLE 3.   Transplacental Transfer of Maternal Antibody
in Newborn Infants**

| GOOD PASSIVE TRANSFER | POOR PASSIVE TRANSFER | NO PASSIVE TRANSFER |
|---|---|---|
| Diphtheria antitoxin<br>Tetanus antitoxin<br>Antierythrogenic toxin<br>Antistaphylococcal antibody<br>*Salmonella flagella* (H) antibody<br>Antistreptolysin<br>All the antiviral antibodies present in maternal<br>  circulation (rubeola, rubella, mumps, poliovirus)<br>VDRL antibodies | *Haemophilus influenzae,*<br>*Bordetella pertussis,*<br>*Shigella flexneri,*<br>*Streptococcus* | Enteric somatic (O)<br>  antibodies (*Salmonella,*<br>  *Shigella, E. coli*)<br><br>Heterophile antibody |

## NATURALLY ACQUIRED PASSIVE IMMUNITY

Newborn infants receive many antibodies from the mother. Placental transfer of antibody depends on the quantity of antibodies in the maternal circulation, as well as the molecular size. Only IgG with its low molecular weight passes readily. IgA and IgM are not placentally transmitted. Viral antibodies present in high amounts are equally present in maternal and infant serum, while macroglobulins (e.g., heterophil antibody) are excluded (Table 3). Passively acquired antibody clearly protects against some diseases. Neonatal tetanus, for example, may be completely eliminated by administering at least two doses of tetanus toxoid to pregnant women. Previously immune pregnant women provide sufficient antibodies to their infants to protect them from neonatal tetanus.

Passively acquired antibody may interfere with a newborn's ability to respond adequately to immunizations. Several studies have confirmed that maternally acquired antibody to diphtheria and pertussis may actually inhibit antibody formation following active immunization. Placentally transmitted antibody may neutralize the virus in live vaccines, thus rendering the vaccine ineffective. How long passively acquired antibody may interfere with an infant's ability to respond to certain vaccines is uncertain. Low levels of maternal antibody to measles have been found to persist beyond the twelfth month of life (Albrecht et al., 1977). Several studies have shown that children vaccinated before 12 months of age have a lower seroconversion rate than those immunized after 1 year (Shelton et al., 1978; Wilkins and Wehrle, 1979). Until this question is resolved, it is recommended that children be immunized against measles at 15 months of age. Prolonged acquisition of passive antibody through breast feeding may play a role in those 5 to 10 per cent of normal children who fail to respond adequately to one dose of the live measles vaccine, and certainly may interfere with the success of live polio virus immunization.

## CURRENT IMMUNIZATION SCHEDULES

At present, seven immunizations are recommended for routine use in the United States. The schedule outlined in Table 4 is the suggested sequence outlined in the Red Book, 1977, as recommended by the Committee of Infectious Diseases (American Academy of Pediatrics, 1977). The American Public Health Association and the Advisory Committee on Immunization Practices (ACIP) of the United States Public Health Service also published recommended immunization schedules. Although there is usually consistency among the three organizations, occasionally recommendations may vary slightly.

The combined vaccines recommended for routine use have been shown to be just as efficacious without increased side effects when given concomitantly as when given individually (Center for Disease Control, 1980). Single live virus vaccines should be given one month apart, since interference with the immune response to the

**TABLE 4.   Recommended Schedule for Active
Immunization of Normal Infants and Children**

| | | |
|---|---|---|
| 2 mo | DTP | TOPV |
| 4 mo | DTP | TOPV |
| 6 mo | DTP | TOPV (optional) |
| 1 yr | | Tuberculin test |
| 15 mo | Measles, rubella | Mumps |
| 1½ yr | DTP | TOPV |
| 4–6 yr | DTP | TOPV |
| 14–16 yr | Td—repeat every<br>10 years | |

DPT, diphtheria-tetanus-pertussis vaccine
Td, tetanus-diphtheria vaccine
TOPV, trivalent oral polio vaccine

From American Academy of Pediatrics: Report of the Committee on Infectious Diseases, 18th ed., 1977.

second vaccine has been demonstrated with some immunizations. Two weeks and preferably four weeks should separate administration of killed vaccines with another inactivated or live virus vaccine.

Most immunizations may be associated with various side effects. Local reactions consist of mild induration and tenderness at the injection site. Repeat dosages of tetanus toxoid or typhoid vaccine have been associated with severe local reactions including marked edema, induration, erythema, and tenderness. If there is a severe reaction, subsequent immunization with the offending antigen should be avoided unless there are extremely compelling reasons for repeating the immunization. In such cases, fractional doses should be administered under close medical supervision.

Severe febrile reactions associated with irritability, malaise, headaches, and chills may follow the use of inactivated vaccines and usually subside within 48 hours. Mild febrile reactions are much more common and are easily controlled with antipyretics. Fever and rashes associated with the measles and rubella vaccines usually appear one to several weeks after immunization and persist for one to three days. Arthralgias associated with attenuated rubella vaccines follow a similar time sequence. The persistent arthritic symptoms occasionally associated with rubella vaccines have not been shown to represent vaccine complications and at present are felt to represent coincidental disease.

## IMMUNIZATIONS FOR INDIVIDUALS OUT OF STEP

Interruption of the recommended immunization schedule does not interfere with the final immunologic outcome (Phillips, 1975). It is not necessary to resume the series regardless of the time between discontinuation and reinstitution of immunizations. The schedule for primary immunization of children not immunized in infancy is shown in Table 5. Children less than 7 years old are immunized with the standard DTP triple antigens by using three dosages at intervals of four to eight weeks. Pertussis vaccine is not recommended for children older than 6 years. In addition, children older than 6 years should receive the adult-type diphtheria-tetanus toxoid. The standard DT preparation contains 7 to 25 Lf (flocculating units) and may cause severe reactions in older children and adults. The adult type of combined diphtheria-tetanus toxoid (Td) with adjuvant contains, at most, 2 Lf of diphtheria toxoid and is recommended for all adults and children older than 6 years.

**TABLE 5. Primary Immunization for Children Not Immunized in Early Infancy[a]**

| UNDER 6 YEARS OF AGE | |
|---|---|
| First visit | DTP, TOPV, tuberculin test |
| Interval after first visit | |
|   1 mo | Measles,[b] mumps, rubella |
|   2 mo | DTP, TOPV |
|   4 mo | DTP, TOPV[c] |
|   10 to 16 mo or preschool | DTP, TOPV |
| Age 14–16 yr | Td—repeat every 10 years |

| 6 YEARS OF AGE AND OVER | |
|---|---|
| First visit | Td, TOPV, tuberculin test |
| Interval after first visit | |
|   1 mo | Measles, mumps, rubella |
|   2 mo | Td. TOPV |
|   8 to 14 mo | Td, TOPV |
| Age 14–16 yr | Td—repeat every 10 years |

[a]Physicians may choose to alter the sequence of these schedules if specific infections are prevalent at the time. For example, measles vaccine might be given on the first visit if an epidemic is under way in the community.

[b]Measles vaccine is not routinely given before 15 months of age (see Table 4).

[c]Optional

DTP, diphtheria-tetanus-pertussis vaccine
TOPV, trivalent oral polio vaccine
Td, tetanus-diphtheria vaccine

From American Academy of Pediatrics: Report of the Committee on Infectious Diseases, 18th ed., 1977.

## CONTRAINDICATIONS TO IMMUNIZATIONS

The decision to immunize an individual with a given vaccine should be based on the belief that the benefits accrued by that person and society outweigh the potential risks of vaccination. During the acute febrile phase of an illness, immunization should be deferred. Minor illnesses without fever, however, should not be considered contraindications. Patients with malignancies or receiving immunosuppressive therapy including chemotherapy, radiation therapy, and corticosteroids should not receive live vaccines. Similarly, individuals with immunodeficiency disorders may develop overwhelming infections when immunized with live vaccines and should not be vaccinated. Individuals allergic to eggs, chickens, or ducks should not receive vaccines grown in duck or chick embryos. Vaccines grown in fibroblast cultures derived from chicks or ducks do not contain egg albumin or yolk components and are not contraindicated in individuals with known hypersensitivity to ducks and chickens.

Individuals with neurologic disorders present considerable controversy regarding immunization. Current recommendations are that children with static neurologic disorders should generally be immunized following the usual vaccine schedules. But the child with an evolving neurologic problem should not receive immunizations likely to cause fever or to be associated with central nervous system (CNS) complications.

## PREGNANCY AND IMMUNIZATIONS

In general, the use of attenuated vaccines should be avoided during pregnancy (Levine, 1974). Theoretically, immunization with live virus may be harmless to the pregnant woman and yet be hazardous to her unborn child. Rubella virus is a well-known teratogen for which live attenuated vaccines are used specifically to prevent fetal damage. There is increasing evidence that the attenuated viruses used in rubella vaccines can cause intrauterine infection (Fleet et al., 1974; Wyll and Hermann, 1973). The extent to which the attenuated virus is teratogenic is unknown. It is strongly recommended, therefore, that before any woman of childbearing potential is vaccinated, she should be shown to be serosusceptible and not pregnant. In addition, adequate contraception should be provided for three months following immunization.

It occasionally becomes necessary, because of plans to travel, to immunize a pregnant woman against anticipated high-risk exposures. Under these unavoidable circumstances immunization against yellow fever and poliomyelitis may be warranted. Since in these settings immediate prophylaxis is required for protection against polio, the live oral vaccine is recommended. Generally, all other live vaccines are discouraged during pregnancy. At present, there is no indication for any pregnant woman to be immunized against smallpox. Inactivated vaccines, however, may be used when specifically indicated. Tetanus and diphtheria toxoids (adult Td) may be given routinely to update pregnant women during their antepartum care.

A pregnancy in the family should not alter the immunization schedules of any family members or contacts of the pregnant woman. Specifically, rubella vaccination of children need not be avoided when their mother is pregnant. A woman who is seronegative for rubella during pregnancy should be given the attenuated rubella vaccine postpartum. Similarly, breastfeeding is not a contraindication to the immunization of a mother or her baby.

## IMMUNIZATION FOR TRAVELERS

With increased foreign travel, it has become important that physicians be able to recommend proper immunizations to their patients to protect their health while traveling (Barrett-Connor, 1979; Medical Letter on Drugs and Therapeutics, 1979). Necessary vaccinations include not only those recommended for protection of the traveler but also those required specifically by individual nations. Detailed information is available in *Health Information For International Travel*, prepared by the Center for Disease Control and obtainable from the Superintendent of Documents, US Government Printing Office, Washington, D.C. 20402. Table 6 summarizes some of the present recommendations for foreign travelers. More detailed and up-to-date information can be obtained from the above CDC publication. Other prophylactic measures should be explored as well before the trip is begun, with particular emphasis on medications for the prevention of gastroenteritis and malaria. When children or adolescents travel, their immunization records should be reviewed and routine immunizations updated if necessary. International travelers must have their vaccinations against smallpox, yellow fever, and cholera documented on an approved version of the International Certificate of Vaccination or Revaccination. These certificates, approved by the World Health Organization, are usually available at local health departments and passport offices.

## CONTROVERSIES IN IMMUNIZATIONS

Many of the vaccines currently available are widely accepted as effective and worthwhile (Table 7). Virtually no vaccine, however, has been developed and used without eliciting controversy as to its efficacy, indications, target population, and side effects (Fulginity, 1976). Some of the major controversies involving passive and active immunizations are discussed below. The reader is encouraged to review specific chapters for more detailed descriptions of immunizations available and those currently being developed for individual infectious diseases (Table 8).

### Meningococcal Disease

Group A and group C meningococcal polysaccharide vaccines are currently licensed in the United States (Center for Disease Control, 1978). They are prepared as monovalent and bivalent antigens in lyophilized form requiring rehydration with diluent before use. As with all polysaccharide vaccines, they are type-specific and offer little protection against other serotypes. The recommended dosage of each polysaccharide is 50 $\mu$g administered subcutaneously. The vaccines are safe but of variable efficacy. Field trials in Egypt, the Sudan, and Finland have demonstrated that group A vaccine results in protection against group A meningococcal disease in 90 per cent of individuals, and suggest that children as young as 3 months of age may be immunized successfully. The group C vaccine has also been successful in protecting 90 per cent of adults against disease. Young children, however, do not fare as well, since the C vaccine is only 65 per cent protective in children 2 to 3 years old and provides virtually no protection to children less than 2 years of age. Persistence of antibody is also superior for the type A vaccine. Eighty per cent of children older than 2 years of age when immunized against group A have protective antibody against A disease after four years, while only 40 per cent of children immunized with group C polysaccharide will have antibody against C disease (Lepow et al., 1977; Peltola et al., 1977; Wilkins and Wehrle, 1979). Two flaws of the combined vaccine against serotypes A and C limit its usefulness. First, the highest attack rate for meningococcal disease is in infants less than 2 years old, in whom the vaccine is least effec-

tive. Second, in the United States, serogroup B presently accounts for the great majority of disease due to *Neisseria meningitidis,* and at present an adequately immunogenic preparation of the group B meningococcus is not available. In addition, in the United States meningococcal disease in civilians has tended recently to occur as single isolates or infrequently as clusters, and antibiotic prophylaxis has been successful in reducing the risk of secondary cases in close contacts.

The current meningococcal vaccines are not recommended for routine use in civilians unless an epidemic of meningococcal disease due to serogroups A or C necessitates immunizing susceptible individuals. The vaccine should be considered for travelers visiting countries having an epidemic caused by strains A or C, or as an adjunct to antibiotic prophylaxis for household contacts of cases infected with susceptible strains. A highly immunogenic meningococcal polysaccharide vaccine against group Y is currently being extensively studied and may be available shortly (Farquhar et al., 1978). In addition, a vaccine against a major outer membrane protein of meningococ-

*Text continued on page 782*

### TABLE 6. Immunization for Foreign Travel

| DISEASE | AREAS WHERE INDICATED OR REQUIRED | COMMENTS |
|---|---|---|
| *Bacterial* | | |
| Cholera | Only where required | Risk to tourist small, vaccine of limited efficacy |
| Plague | Southeast Asia or frequent contact with rodents in S. America, Asia, Africa | For most tourists not necessary |
| Tetanus, diphtheria | All persons every 10 years regardless of travel | |
| Tuberculosis | Developing countries | BCG or INH prophylaxis in areas with high risk; otherwise skin test every six months |
| Typhoid | Countries with poor sanitation | Frequently associated with sore arm for one to two days with fever. Requires two doses four weeks apart |
| *Rickettsial* | | |
| Typhus | Mountainous, highland, or cold areas with louse infestation in Ethiopia, Rwanda, Burundi, Mexico, Ecuador, Bolivia, Peru, and Asia | |
| *Viral* | | |
| Hepatitis A | ≥3 months in tropical areas and developing countries | ISG immunization close to departure |
| Poliomyelitis | Rural developing countries | If previously immunized: one dose of TOPV; if no previous immunization: primary series of TOPV or inactivated vaccine; altered immune status: inactivated vaccine |
| Rabies | Only where exposure to rabid animals is a constant threat | Only DEV immunization available presently. When available HDCV is immunization of choice |
| Smallpox | Only where required and then questionable | At present there is no indication, and a physician's letter indicating that vaccination is contraindicated on medical grounds should be seriously considered |
| Yellow fever | Rural S. America, tropical Africa; most countries require vaccine if traveler is coming from area with reported case of yellow fever within six days of arrival. | Should be included by traveler who might change itinerary to include areas with endemic yellow fever. Immunocompromised persons should not be vaccinated |

**TABLE 7. Currently Available Immunizations**

| DISEASE | IMMUNIZING AGENT | INDICATION | ADMINISTRATION Primary | Booster | Route | EFFICACY[a] | ADVERSE REACTIONS | COMMENTS |
|---|---|---|---|---|---|---|---|---|
| *Bacterial* | | | | | | | | |
| Anthrax | Cell-free, alum-concentrated inactivated protein antigen of *Bacillus anthracis* | High-risk >6 mo old | 0.5 ml for three doses given two to three weeks apart | 0.5 ml annually | S.Q.[b] | ++++ | Local erythema, induration; fever | |
| Cholera | Phenol-inactivated *Vibrio cholerae* | Travel to or residence in countries with cholera | Intradermal >5 yr, 0.2 ml; S.Q. or I.M. 6 mo–4 yr, 0.2 ml; 5–10 yr, 0.3 ml; >10 yr, 0.5 ml in two doses at least one wk apart | Every 6 mo or just before cholera season | As indicated | + | Pain, erythema, and induration at injection site; fever, malaise, and headache | |
| Diphtheria, tetanus, pertussis (DTP) | Alum-precipitated or absorbed toxoids of diphtheria and tetanus D 7 to 25 LF killed *B. pertussis* | All persons <7 yr old | See tables 4 and 5 | | | ++++ ++–+++ | See text | See text |
| Tetanus, diphtheria (Td) | T – as above d – ≤2 LF | All persons >7 yr old | See tables 4 and 5; booster every 10 yr for life | | | ++++ | Local pain and induration and mild fever | |
| Meningococcus types A and C | Capsular polysaccharide of *Neisseria meningitidis* types A and C | >2 yr old in epidemic or high-risk setting | 50 µg of each polysaccharide 0.5 ml of vaccine | | S.Q. | +++ | Local erythema and pain | Vaccine ineffective against other types of *N. meningitidis* |
| Plague | Formaldehyde-inactivated *Yersinia pestis* | High-risk | Three doses: first two doses 0.5 ml at least 4 wk apart; third dose 0.2 ml 4 to 12 wk after second dose (see comments) | Same amount as third dose at 6-month intervals to total of five doses (3 primary and two boosters) | I.M.[c] | ++++ | Mild pain, erythema, and local induration with repeated doses; headache, malaise | Adjust dosage for age: <1 yr, one fifth adult dose; 1–4 yr, two fifths adult dose; 5–10 yr, three fifths adult dose |
| Pneumococcus | Capsular polysaccharide to types 1–4, 6, 8, 9, 12, 14, 19, 23, 25, 51, 56 | Persons >2 yr old with high risk of pneumococcal infections | 50 µg of each polysaccharide 0.5 ml of vaccine | Unknown | S.Q. | +++ | Local erythema, induration and pain; fever | See text |

| Disease | Vaccine | Indications | Primary Dose | Booster | Route | Efficacy[a] | Adverse Reactions | Comments |
|---|---|---|---|---|---|---|---|---|
| Tuberculosis | BCG (an attenuated strain of *Mycobacterium bovis*) | Any age: (1) high risk for continued exposure; (2) populations where skin test conversion >1% per yr | Newborns: 0.05 ml; >1 mo old: 0.1 ml | Give full dose to newborn at 1 yr if risk still present; all others not recommended (see comments) | S.Q. or multiple percutaneous | + - ++ | Ulceration, lymphadenitis, osteomyelitis, dissemination, and death | Vaccine should be repeated at two to three months after vaccination if skin test is negative |
| Typhoid | Acetone-killed *Salmonella typhi* | Close contact to typhoid carrier or traveler to high-risk areas | 6 mo–10 yr old: 0.25 ml; >10 yr old: 0.5 ml Two doses divided by four or more weeks | Every three years | S.Q. | ++ - +++ | Local erythema and pain; fever, malaise, headache | See text |
| *Rickettsiae* Typhus | Formaldehyde-inactivated *Rickettsia prowazekii* grown in chick embryos | Travel to or residence in area with known typhus and medical personnel and laboratory workers in frequent contact with *R. prowazekii* | Two doses four or more weeks apart | Every 6–12 months | S.Q. | Unknown | Local pain, induration and erythema; fever and malaise | See text |
| *Viruses* Influenza | Formalin-inactivated influenza virus grown in chick embryos; usually trivalent preparations of influenza viruses expected to be prevalent | All persons ≥6 mo old at increased risk of adverse consequences from infections of lower respiratory tract | One to two doses depending on age and past exposure; doses four or more weeks apart 6–35 mo old, 0.25 ml; ≥3 yr old, 0.5 ml | Annually | S.Q. | ++ - +++ | Local pain, induration and erythema; fever, malaise, allergic hypersensitivity Guillain-Barré syndrome <1/100,000 doses | Live vaccine currently being extensively studied |
| Measles | Live attenuated Edmonston B measles virus from chick embryos | All persons >15 mo old | One dose 0.5 ml | Unknown | S.Q. | ++++ | Fever, rare encephalitis and encephalopathy | See text |

[a]Efficacy:
50–65% = +
65–80% = ++
80–90% = +++
>90% = ++++

[b]S.Q., subcutaneous

[c]I.M., intramuscularly

*Table continued on following page*

**TABLE 7.  Currently Available Immunizations** (Continued)

| DISEASE | IMMUNIZING AGENT | INDICATION | ADMINISTRATION | | | EFFICACY[a] | ADVERSE REACTIONS | COMMENTS |
|---|---|---|---|---|---|---|---|---|
| | | | Primary | Booster | Route | | | |
| Mumps | Live attenuated Jeryl-Lynn strain of mumps virus grown in chick embryo cells | All children >15 mo old (see text) | One dose 0.5 ml | Unknown | S.Q. | ++++ | Uncommon parotitis, allergic reactions, rash, pruritus, purpura | See text |
| Poliomyelitis | OPV (oral polio vaccine)—live attenuated poliovirus to types 1, 2, and 3 | All children ≥6 wk to 18 yr; adults when indicated | Two doses at least 6 weeks apart followed by dose 8 to 12 months later | At 4 to 6 years old or before travel to endemic areas | Oral | ++++ | Rare paralysis in normal individuals | Absolutely contraindicated in any immunocompromised person (see text) |
| | IPV (formalin inactivated polio vaccine) of three serotypes grown in monkey cell cultures | ≥6 wk old in selected instances (see text) | Three doses 4 to 8 weeks apart with fourth dose 6 to 12 months following third dose | Every 5 yr until age 18 yr | S.Q. | ++++ | Local pain | See text |
| Rabies | DEV (duck embryo vaccine) rabies virus grown in duck embryos killed by exposure to B-propiolactone. | Persons at high-risk of rabies virus exposure or following wild animal bites except rodents | Pre-exposure: either two 1 ml injections 1 month apart followed by 3rd injection 6–7 months later; or three 1 ml injections 1 wk apart followed by 4th—3 months later<br><br>Post-exposure: Schedule 1: 21 daily doses; or Schedule 2: 2 daily doses first 7 days, then 7 daily doses | If no antibody response 2 booster doses 1 week apart<br><br>Schedule 1: boosters on day 31 and 41; Schedule 2: boosters on day 24 and 34 | S.Q. | Unknown but probably +++−++++ | Local pain, pruritus, and erythema, fever, malaise, serum sickness, rare anaphylaxis; neuroparalysis 1/24,400 recipients | Inactivated nerve tissue vaccines (NTV) or inactivated suckling rodent brain vaccine (SRBV) are not recommended, since they have an incidence of neuroparalytic reactions in 1/2,000 and 1/8,000 vaccinees respectively |

| Type | Indications | Primary dose | Booster | Route | Efficacy | Adverse reactions | Comments |
|---|---|---|---|---|---|---|---|
| HDCV (human diploid cell vaccine) rabies virus grown in human diploid cell cultures and inactivated by N-tributyl phosphate | As above (preferred vaccine when available) | Pre-exposure: Two 1 ml doses 1 wk apart followed by 3rd dose 2–3 wks later. Post-exposure: Five 1 ml doses on days 0,3, 7,14 and 28 (6th dose on day 90 recommended by WHO) | If no antibody response 1 booster (pre-exposure); If no antibody response 1 booster (post-exposure) | I.M. | Unknown but probably ++++ | Local pain, erythema, pruritus, and swelling, mild headache, malaise, nausea, abdominal pain, myalgias, and dizziness | Post-exposure prophylaxis should always include 1 dose of RIG 20 IU/Kg given ½ into wound and ½ I.M. except in individuals previously vaccinated |
| Rubella | Live attenuated rubella virus RA 27/3 grown in human diploid fibroblast cells | See text | One dose 0.5 ml | Unknown (see text) | S.Q. | ++++ | Rash, lymphadenopathy, joint pain | See text |
| Smallpox | Live attenuated vaccinia virus in lyophilized or glycerinated vaccine | Laboratory workers studying smallpox (see text) | 1 drop | 1 drop every three years | Multiple pressure, multiple puncture, jet injection | ++++ | Fever, pain, malaise, lymphadenopathy, rare dissemination, encephalitis | Chemical agent should not be used to prepare skin |
| Yellow fever | Live attenuated yellow fever virus strain 17D grown in chick embryo cells | Traveling or residing in high-risk area or laboratory worker studying yellow fever | 0.5 ml | Every 10 years | S.Q. | ++++ | Headache, myalgia, and fever | Dakar strain associated with 0.5% incidence of meningoencephalitis and is not recommended |

TABLE 8. Diseases for Which Immunizations
Are Currently Being Investigated or Are of
Limited Availability

Adenovirus
Botulism
Cytomegalovirus
Gonorrhea
*Haemophilus influenzae* type B
Hepatitis A and B
Herpes simplex 1 and 2
Influenza
*Mycoplasma pneumoniae*
*Neisseria meningitidis* types B and Y
Parainfluenza 1–3
*Pseudomonas*
Q fever
Respiratory syncytial virus
Rotavirus
Syphilis
Trachoma
Tularemia
Varicella

cus has shown promise for protection against group B disease.

## Pertussis

In the United States, immunization against pertussis is routinely begun at 2 months of age along with vaccination against diphtheria and tetanus (Center for Disease Control, 1977). Although some physicians in the United States have expressed doubts about the efficacy and overall benefits of the current pertussis vaccine, the raging debate occurring in Europe has been largely avoided (Grady and Wetterlow, 1978; Manclark, 1979; Mathias, 1978; Pittman, 1979). In England, the major reservation to the pertussis vaccine is the high incidence of severe reactions (Enrengut, 1978; Stewart, 1977; Lister, 1977). Reactions to the vaccine have been reported in the United States, but they have not been of the frequency or the severity of the British experience. Estimates of severe neurologic reaction to the pertussis vaccine have ranged from 1:2500 to 1:500,000 children. The adverse reactions described include: high fever; collapse sometimes associated with a shock-like state; prolonged periods of screaming during which the infant cannot be comforted; convulsions with or without fever; frank encephalopathy with changes in the level of consciousness, focal neurologic signs, and convulsions; and thrombocytopenic purpura. Although the incidence of these severe reactions is uncertain, mild reactions including low grade fever and pain and induration at the injection site may occur in as high as 90 per cent of vaccine recipients. Rarely, permanent neurologic sequelae have been described.

The true risk-benefit ratio remains to be established (Koplan et al., 1979). Many British physicians have argued that the current risk of contracting a serious pertussis infection is less than the risk of acquiring permanent neurologic sequelae including mental retardation from the vaccine. Proponents of the vaccine contend that the severe complications and high mortality from pertussis in infancy are major reasons for immunization early in life. They point to the dramatic decline in pertussis since routine vaccination was begun. Opponents of the vaccine, however, vehemently emphasize that the incidence of pertussis was decreasing before routine immunization was begun, and that overall cases with subsequently lower morbidity could have been predicted without the use of pertussis vaccine. The most convincing evidence for vaccine efficacy has come recently from Japan and England, where immunization rates have dropped to 10 per cent and 40 per cent, respectively. Both countries have encountered serious outbreaks of pertussis, and interest has renewed in immunizing children. In underdeveloped nations, pertussis remains a serious health problem, and immunization is the only currently viable method for control of disease.

Over the past 40 years, studies of vaccine efficacy have given results varying from 0 to 90 per cent protection. The full series of pertussis vaccinations presently confers immunity in 80 per cent of recipients. Protection is not long-lasting, however, and after 10 years only approximately 50 per cent of vaccinees have detectable protective antibody. Pertussis immunization is recommended for children from age 6 weeks up to their seventh birthday. Since most cases occur in infants and young children, and two thirds of pertussis deaths occur in infants less than 1 year of age, immunization should be instituted in infancy as part of the DPT vaccine.

Children who have experienced severe reactions following pertussis-containing vaccines should not receive further pertussis immunizations. Static neurologic conditions in infants are not reasons for deferring immunizations against pertussis. In evolving neurologic conditions, however, pertussis immunization should not be used because of the theoretical concern of exacerbating the disorder. There is no convincing evidence that pertussis immune globulin is effective in preventing or treating pertussis, and its use is not recommended.

## Pneumococcus

*Streptococcus pneumoniae* (pneumococcus) remains the most common bacterial cause of otitis media, pneumonia, and meningitis in infants and children. Patients who have undergone splenectomy and individuals with sickle-cell disease, nephrotic syndrome, chronic liver disease, malignancy, or primary immunodeficiency are at increased risk of developing severe pneumococcal infections. A 14-valent polysaccharide vaccine is now licensed for use in the United States (Center for Disease Control, 1978). The vaccine contains purified capsular material of pneumococci extracted separately from American types 1, 2, 3, 4, 6, 8, 9, 12, 14, 19, 23, 25, 51, and 56. Each dose of vaccine contains 50 $\mu$g of each of the 14 polysaccharides that account for 80 per cent of all bacteremic pneumococcal disease in the United States. Similar vaccines have been tried successfully in Europe and South Africa. Field trials have shown that vaccination reduces by 80 per cent the incidence of bacteremic pneumococcal pneumonia caused by the bacterial types included in the vaccine. Nasopharyngeal acquisition of the pneumococcal types included in the vaccine is reduced in vaccinees, and there is no evidence that immunized individuals have any greater risk of acquiring diseases caused by other microorganisms. The duration of protection is unknown, but elevated antibody has been found to persist for at least two years.

Despite the promising findings with the presently licensed pneumococcal vaccine, several problems remain (Artenstein, 1973). A vaccine that is protective against 80 per cent of the disease-causing pneumococci and that is 80 per cent effective is capable of reducing pneumococcal disease by at most approximately 65 per cent. In addition, the current vaccine is ineffective in children less than 2 years old (Klein and Mortimer, 1978). This is particularly unfortunate for children with sickle-cell disease, who are at greatest risk of pneumococcal infection during infancy (Ammann et al., 1977; Ahonkhai et al., 1979).

Pneumococcal vaccine is not currently recommended for healthy individuals. Special populations including residents of nursing homes and institutions, and localized populations experiencing outbreaks may be considered for pneumococcal vaccination. Persons over 2 years of age with sickle-cell disease or other splenic dysfunction including splenectomy, or with chronic illnesses or conditions including diabetes mellitus, chronic cardiorespiratory disease, renal disease, hepatic dysfunction, or old age, may all benefit from pneumococcal vaccination. Caution must be advised, however, against totally relying on the present pneumococcal vaccine to prevent serious *Streptococcus pneumoniae* infections, particularly in children with sickle-cell disease (Ahonkhai, 1979; Ammann et al., 1977). Since the vaccine at best can be expected to prevent 65 per cent of pneumococcal disease, penicillin prophylaxis of

children with sickle-cell disease should be continued despite vaccination until the children are 6 years old, when the risk of pneumococcal infection is markedly decreased and prophylaxis may not be necessary.

## Tuberculosis

The World Health Organization has credited the BCG vaccine with playing a major role in reducing worldwide morbidity owing to tuberculosis (Eickhoff, 1977). Controlled trials, however, have found extremely variable immunity in vaccine recipients. In fact, despite the use of BCG since 1921, there is still debate about whether the vaccine is effective.

BCG is derived from a strain of *Mycobacterium bovis* that was attenuated at the Pasteur Institute in Lille, France, by Calmette and Guérin. All BCG vaccines available today were derived from the original strain. Differences in production, methods and routes of vaccination, and characteristics of the populations and environments in which the vaccine has been used have resulted in great variation in immunogenicity, efficacy, and reactogenicity among the daughter strains. At present, most laboratories producing BCG vaccine maintain production strains in a lyophilized state in an attempt to minimize genetic variation. The production strains are usually named by the city in which they are produced (e.g., BCG-London, BCG-Copenhagen). In the United States, the Bureau of Biologics, Food and Drug Administration, has specified that each freeze-dried BCG strain used for vaccination must have specified characteristics of safety and potency and be capable of inducing tuberculin sensitivity in the guinea pigs and humans (Center for Disease Control, 1979). Unfortunately, induced tuberculin sensitivity has never been proved to be related to immunity.

The rationale behind the use of the BCG vaccine to prevent tuberculosis is to confer cell-mediated immunity against an attenuated, immunologically similar strain of mycobacteria. It is known that most hosts, upon primary infection with tubercle bacilli, are able to mount an immunologic response sufficient to localize the infection and thus establish a latent or dormant infectious state. The inactive infection may continue for life or may reactivate frequently but not invariably during times of altered host cell-mediated immunity. There is evidence that the BCG vaccine prevents the establishment of a latent infection when the vaccinee is challenged with live tubercle bacilli, thus preventing not only primary tuberculosis but also the breakdown or reactivation disease.

The current lyophilized vaccines have demonstrated substantial protection in animals and are currently being tested in India. The most recent field trials, all conducted before 1955 with liquid vaccines, showed protection ranging from 0 to 80 per cent. Some argue that the potencies of the BCG strains used in these studies were sufficiently different to account for the contradictory findings. Another possibility is that populations showing little protection from BCG had a large prior exposure to atypical mycobacterial infections. These previous infections may have induced sufficient immunity to tuberculosis to mask any contribution made by BCG immunization. Interestingly, field trials performed where there is a relatively high incidence of tuberculosis in the control group have tended to show a high efficacy for the BCG vaccine, whereas areas with a low incidence of tuberculosis in the unvaccinated group have shown little benefit from BCG. Continual mycobacterial challenges may be necessary, therefore, to maintain the immunity conferred by BCG vaccination.

In the United States, it is recommended that BCG should be "seriously considered" for patients such as infants who are tuberculin skin-test-negative but who can be expected to have repeated exposure to individuals with sputum-positive pulmonary tuberculosis. In addition, BCG vaccination should be considered for groups in which the skin-test conversion rates exceed 1 per cent annually and in which the usual surveillance and treatment programs have failed or are not feasible. In developing countries where tuberculosis is epidemic and short-term INH prophylaxis or skin-test screening is not possible, BCG is indicated to attempt tuberculosis control.

In the United States, where the current annual infection rate among 6-year-olds is approximately 0.03 per cent, BCG is rarely indicated. Infants tolerate two to three months of INH prophylaxis extremely well and thus can allow time for sufficient screening and treatment of family contacts, eliminating the need for BCG vaccination. In addition, tuberculin skin tests are rendered less valuable, since it is usually impossible to distinguish between a tuberculin reaction caused by a virulent supra-infection and one resulting from persistent postvaccination sensitivity. After the immediate postvaccination period, however, caution is advised in attributing a positive skin test to BCG, and tuberculosis should always be considered a possible diagnosis.

BCG should be used only in individuals who are skin-test-negative to 5 tuberculin units of tuberculin purified protein derivative (PPD). The dosage is indicated by the manufacturer in the package insert. Infants less than 28 days old should receive one half the usual dose. If the need for immunization persists, these children should re-ceive a full dose at 1 year of age. The World Health Organization recommends that BCG be given by intradermal injection to provide for a uniform and reliable dose. In the United States, however, both intradermal and percutaneous vaccines are licensed, and vaccination should only be by the route indicated in the package labeling (Center for Disease Control, 1979). Individuals receiving BCG should have a tuberculin skin test two to three months after immunization. If that skin test is negative and the indications for BCG remain, a second dose of vaccine should be administered.

Adverse reactions to BCG have included severe or prolonged ulceration at the vaccination site, lymphadenitis, osteomyelitis, lupoid reactions, disseminated BCG infection, and death (Passwell et al., 1976). Ulceration and lymphadenitis occur in 1 to 10 per cent of vaccinees; osteomyelitis may occur in 1 per million vaccine recipients but may be as high as 5 per 100,000 in newborns. Disseminated BCG infection and death occur in 1 to 10 per 10 million vaccinees and are seen almost exclusively in children with impaired immunity. BCG should, therefore, not be given to anyone with impaired immune status. Although no harmful effects of BCG on the fetus have been observed, immunization should be avoided during pregnancy unless there is an immediate excessive and unavoidable exposure to infectious tuberculosis.

## Typhoid

Typhoid fever remains a major world health problem, particularly in developing countries, where poor sanitation and ingestion of inadequately cooked food are common. Killed typhoid vaccines have been used since the late 19th century, although their efficacy was not established until the 1960s. The Yugoslav Typhoid Commission in 1962 showed that a heat-killed, phenol-preserved vaccine gave considerable protection against typhoid fever for at least three years, whereas an alcohol-killed, alcohol-preserved vaccine was ineffective. Subsequent field trials in Guyana showed the heat-phenol and acetone-inactivated vaccines to be 65 to 90 per cent effective in preventing typhoid fever (Ashcroft et al., 1967). Although typhoid fever usually confers lifelong immunity, the nature of protection is unknown. The titers of antibodies against O, H, and Vi antigens have not been connected with protection. Naturally occurring sources of *Salmonella typhosa* usually contain $10^5$ or less organisms, resulting in infection of 25 per cent of unvaccinated individuals. Following typhoid fever or immunization, most individuals are protected against a challenge of $10^5$ organisms. Volunteer studies indicate, however, that vaccine-acquired immunity can be easily overcome with a challenge of 50 per cent infectious dose ($10^7$) of *S. typhosa* organisms (Hornick et al., 1970). The effectiveness of paratyphoid A and B vaccines has never been established, and they are not recommended for use either individually or in combination with typhoid vaccine.

Typhoid vaccine in the United States is not recommended for general use (Center for Disease Control, 1978). Persons with intimate exposure to a documented typhoid carrier or travelers to areas where there is a high risk of exposure to typhoid because of poor food or water sanitation should receive typhoid vaccine. In the United states vaccination is not indicated for use in controlling outbreaks from a common source or natural disasters such as floods.

Primary immunizations in adults and children 10 years or older consist of two doses of 0.5 ml of vaccine injected subcutaneously, three or more weeks apart, or three doses at weekly intervals. Children 6 months to 10 years old should receive 0.25 ml of vaccine following one of the same schedules. Revaccinations are recommended every three years if there is continuing exposure, with a single booster given intradermally (0.1 ml of vaccine into the flexor surface of the forearm) or subcutaneously (0.5 ml of vaccine in individuals older than 10 years or 0.25 ml in children less than 10 years old). The acetone-killed vaccine should not be given intradermally. If more than three years have elapsed since the last vaccination only one booster is still required. Reactions including local pain, malaise, headache, and fever are common.

A new live attenuated oral typhoid vaccine is currently being tested. This vaccine uses a mutant (Ty 21a) of *Salmonella typhi* that lacks the enzyme uridine 5'-diphosphate-glucose-4-epimerase. The vaccine, when grown in brain-heart infusion broth in the presence of 0.1 per cent galactose, has shown great promise in early investigations (Gilman et al., 1977).

## Cytomegalovirus

Cytomegalovirus (CMV) is the most common congenital infection resulting in mental retardation and deafness. Primary CMV infection and reactivation disease are often responsible for severe illness and the death of immunocompromised patients; they may also be associated with renal allograft rejection. Pneumonia, hepatitis, encephalitis, atypical lymphocytosis, and leukopenia are all clinical manifestations of CMV infections.

It is likely that everyone develops a persistent CMV infection after primary exposure. Immun-ization against CMV ideally, therefore, would prevent primary as well as reactivated disease. In order to prevent transplacental transmission of CMV, a vaccine should also prevent reinfection viremia. Several theoretical problems must be faced before people are immunized against CMV. The capability of CMV to transform normal cells has stimulated concern that a vaccine might be oncogenic. Additionally, if a persistent infection is established after CMV immunization, reactivation of the vaccine virus may result in more severe disease than natural infection. Moreover, CMV strains are so heterogeneous that it is unclear if enough cross-reactivity exists for a vaccine made from one strain to establish broad protection.

Two live attenuated CMV vaccines are currently being investigated in renal transplant patients. Preliminary studies indicate that both the Towne-125 strain vaccine and the AD-169 strain vaccine can induce CMV-specific cellular immunity in previously seronegative recipients (Just et al., 1975; Plotkin et al., 1976; Glazer et al., 1979). The vaccines, however, have not been able to prevent CMV infections, but reactivation of the vaccine strain virus has not been demonstrated. The effect of immunization of seronegative women with the CMV vaccines and the subsequent incidence of infants born with congenital CMV is unknown. Additional work is being done on a specific CMV immune globulin in an attempt to ameliorate or possibly prevent primary CMV infections. Cautious investigation seems warranted to determine the risks and benefits of these approaches to immunoprophylaxis of CMV infections in selected populations.

## Hepatitis

Standard ISG is effective for the prevention or modification of hepatitis A infection (Krugman et al, 1960; Center for Disease Control, 1977; Woodson and Clinton, 1969). When administered within one to two weeks after exposure to hepatitis A, it prevents illness in 80 to 90 per cent of individuals exposed. ISG should be given as soon after close contact with an infected person as possible and is not indicated if more than 2 weeks have elapsed since exposure or if clinical illness is present. Preexposure prophylaxis should be used for those at high risk of hepatitis A exposure and repeated every four to six months when risk continues. Frequently it is not necessary to continue prophylaxis in individuals with continued high contact over one year, since subclinical disease will often develop within that time.

The benefit of passive immunization against hepatitis B has been less clear. Early studies found that standard ISG was of little or no value in the prevention of post-transfusion hepatitis.

Subsequent studies, however, found that ISG was beneficial and was as useful as the newer hepatitis B immune globulin (HBIG). Initial studies of the two immune globulins suffered from the lack of standardization of the HBIG distributed by various manufacturers. At present, immune globulins with an anti-HBs titer greater than 1:100,000 by passive hemagglutination are designated HBIG.

Other explanations for disparate findings when ISG was compared with HBIG are beginning to be clarified. The original findings of the Veterans Administration Cooperative Study suggested that HBIG was superior to ISG for prophylaxis against hepatitis B following needle-stick exposure (Seeff et al., 1978). Reanalysis of their data in the light of radioimmunoassays for antibody to hepatitis core antigen (anti-HBc) and anti-HBs, however, showed no difference in serologic evidence of hepatitis B infection in exposed individuals. In fact, 12 per cent of individuals in both groups showed serologic evidence of hepatitis B infection. HBIG, however, apparently modified infection, since only 2 per cent of HBIG-treated patients had clinical disease, while 8 per cent of ISG-treated patients were symptomatic. An interesting phenomenon of passive-active immunity is postulated to be responsible for these findings. In the case of HBIG, the passive immunity transmitted is sufficient to ameliorate disease but permits infection and thus active immunity to occur also (Hoofnagle et al., 1979). Passive-active immunity has also been considered important with many special immune globulins.

Individuals with documented exposure to hepatitis B should receive HBIG. If HBIG is not available, ISG should be substituted. The indications for use of HBIG following exposure are: (1) needle-stick or mucosal contact with blood known to contain HBsAg; (2) inadvertent administration of HBsAg-positive blood; (3) sexual exposure to acute disease; and (4) infants born to mothers with acute hepatitis B (Mosley, 1979; Redeker et al., 1975; Szmuness et al., 1974). Preexposure prophylaxis may be indicated in hemodialysis units for patients and staff if adequate prevention and control are not possible and in custodial institutions under conditions of documented reported hepatitis B transmission.

Hepatitis B vaccines are currently under investation (Gerety et al., 1979; Krugman, 1975). These vaccines are prepared by plasmapheresis of suitable persons with high titers of HbsAg. Possible live virus is either heat- or formalin-inactivated during vaccine preparation. Preliminary studies are promising, but several important questions remain. The risk of inducing partial immunity in certain people and creating a pool of individuals more likely to develop chronic hepatitis must be assessed. In addition, since hepatitis B has been associated with an increased rate of hepatocellular carcinomas, there is a possibility that the vaccine might increase the incidence of hepatic cancer.

## Measles (Rubeola)

Measles is a frequently severe illness associated with encephalitis in 1 of 1000 cases and commonly resulting in permanent neurologic sequelae including mental retardation. Respiratory or neurologic complications result in death in approximately 1 of 1000 cases. At present, a highly effective live vaccine is available (Center for Disease Control, 1978). The degree of measles control depends primarily on the extent to which a given population is immunized. The current further-attenuated Edmonston B strain vaccine has been so effective that the major controversies revolve around how best to immunize as many susceptible persons as possible. It is available in monovalent form (measles only) and in combination with rubella (MR) and mumps and rubella (MMR) vaccines. Follow-up studies indicate that durable immunity is achieved in 95 per cent of individuals older than 15 months of age given the live measles vaccine. Children immunized before 12 months of age have significantly lower seroconversion rates following immunization (Wilkins and Wehrle, 1978). Conflicting data exist for children between 12 and 14 months old, but it appears that these children respond adequately to measles immunization. However, because of this uncertainty, it is currently recommended that children receive their primary measles immunization at 15 months of age. Whenever there is high risk of exposure to natural measles, infants should be immunized at 6 months of age and then revaccinated when they are 15 months old.

Despite the widespread use of measles vaccine in the United States, epidemics have continued to occur, albeit to a much lesser extent than in prevaccine years (Orenstein et al., 1978; Weiner et al., 1977; Shasby et al., 1977; McCormick et al., 1977; Modlin et al., 1977). The effects of revaccination have become important with the increasing number of public schools requiring all children to have documented immunization histories before entrance (Deseda-Tous et al., 1978). Fortunately, revaccination has not been associated with any increase in complications in children who have previously received live measles vaccines or who have had natural measles. Increased reactions including local induration, pain, edema, and fever have occurred in over 50 per cent of individuals given live measles vaccine who had previously received killed vaccine (Krause et al., 1978). The risk of atypical measles in these young adults is sufficient, however, to warrant vaccination.

Exposure to measles is not a contraindication to vaccination (Ruuskanen et al., 1978). If given within 72 hours of exposure, evidence suggests that immunization may provide protection. Measles may be prevented or modified by administration of ISG within six days of exposure. Live measles vaccine should not be given until three months after administration of ISG. Measles outbreaks are best controlled by vaccination of susceptible individuals. Widespread use of ISG in these situations is not recommended.

## Mumps

Clinical mumps is generally a benign disease associated with parotid swelling, tenderness, and fever. Meningoencephalitis or meningitis occurs in 0.5 to 10 per cent of all mumps cases. Although death is rare, morbidity may be severe. Bilateral orchitis occurs in approximately 2 per cent of cases in men, but sterility is uncommon. Unilateral deafness following endolymphatic labyrinthitis occurs in 2 per 10,000 cases. Arthritis, nephritis, subacute thyroiditis, pancreatitis, myocarditis, and hepatitis are all uncommon complications of mumps infections.

A highly effective, live attenuated mumps vaccine has been available in the United States since 1967 (Center for Disease Control, 1980; Hayden et al., 1978). The Jeryl-Lynn strain of mumps virus is used for immunization following attenuation of virulence in embryonated hens' eggs, and in tissue culture. Antibody appears in 95 per cent of vaccine recipients older than 12 months of age, and protection lasts for at least 9.5 years. Critics of the vaccine have argued that mumps is not severe enough to warrant widespread immunization. Others have emphasized that the vaccine was licensed before sufficient human trials were completed. The development of the combined measles-mumps-rubella (MMR) vaccine has greatly accelerated the rate of mumps immunization. Well over 30 million doses of mumps vaccine have been administered since it was licensed and have clearly shown the vaccine to be efficacious with few side effects. Uncommon adverse reactions include parotitis, low-grade fever, rash, and pruritus. Severe CNS complications following immunization are rare, occurring in 1 per million individuals immunized.

Mumps vaccine is recommended for all children over 12 months of age. As part of general well-child care, it is best given to a child as the MMR at 15 months. Mumps vaccination is of particular value to susceptible preadolescent males who have no evidence of previous infection, and they should be the target population in countries where the vaccine is not widely available.

## Poliomyelitis

Poliovirus vaccines have been widely used for over 25 years. From 1955 to 1965, the inactivated vaccine was the only widely available polio immunization, and it dramatically reduced the incidence of paralytic poliomyelitis in countries where it was extensively used. Although both the IPV (formalin-inactivated polio vaccine) and the OPV (oral polio vaccine) are effective, the OPV has become the vaccine of choice in the United States (Center for Disease Control, 1979). Countries that prevent poliomyelitis with IPV are generally homogeneous populations that are able to maintain very high vaccination rates. In Sweden and Finland, where only IPV is used, intensive poliovirus surveillance has shown that not only is paralytic disease rare but circulation of the virus is virtually absent. This and animal studies suggest that blocking antibodies produced by IPV can prevent virus implantation despite failure to produce local IgA. In areas with endemic or epidemic poliovirus, however, the populations are best immunized with the live virus vaccine. OPV not only provides intestinal immunity with subsequent prevention of fecal growth of wild virus and decrease in circulating virus in the community but also establishes active infections in the nasopharynx and gastrointestinal tract of vaccinees. The virus that is shed following immunization with OPV spreads to susceptible contacts, resulting in inapparent immunizing infections. Additionally, individuals who have received IPV should be reimmunized every five years until the age of 18 years, whereas over 90 per cent of those receiving OPV have neutralizing antibodies to the three types of poliovirus after eight years. It should be noted that problems have occurred in attempting to immunize effectively some populations in tropical and semitropical areas. Viral interference of infection by other enteroviruses at the time of vaccination with OPV may play some role in reducing "take" rates to 50 per cent in these areas. There is also some evidence that 10 to 20 per cent of children in these populations have an inhibitory substance in their saliva that may prevent poliovirus replication. Probably most important in these vaccine failures is inadequate storage of the OPV, which results in inactivation of virus and decreased response rates. Repeated immunization of target populations, however, can eliminate paralytic disease, as has been demonstrated in Cuba and Puerto Rico.

In countries such as the United States where the use of OPV has made paralytic poliomyelitis uncommon, the use of IPV in certain specific situations is warranted. Current estimates indicate that less than one in three million doses of OPV distributed has been associated with paralytic disease in vaccine recipients or their close contacts. Administration of IPV should be oriented toward minimizing the chance of high-risk individuals developing paralytic poliomyelitis from OPV. IPV should be provided to persons with increased susceptibility to infections, including immunodeficient children, and other immunocompromised individuals and their household contacts. Adults undergoing initial vaccination who have the time and are committed to a full course of inoculations are also candidates for IPV since they have a slightly higher risk of developing paralysis. Adults should receive OPV if possible poliomyelitis exposure is to occur before two doses of IPV four weeks apart can be administered. If OPV is inadvertently administered to a household contact of an immunocompromised person, the patient should be isolated from the immunized person for at least two to three weeks after vaccination. Any child born to a family with a history of immunodeficiency disorders should not be given OPV until the immune status of the child is found to be normal.

Regardless of which immunization is used, the goal of polio immunization programs should be to immunize over 90 per cent of the population. When this is achieved, virtual elimination of paralytic poliomyelitis can be expected.

## Rubella

Rubella is usually a mild childhood disease with rare complications. It was not until 1964, when a major epidemic in the United States resulted in more than 20,000 damaged children born of pregnancies complicated by rubella infection, that the need for a rubella vaccine was clearly established. Control of rubella by vaccination presents a unique problem, since it is the only immunization program that attempts to protect a distant fetus by preventing maternal infection during pregnancy. Two immunization strategies have been used in an attempt to decrease the number of congenitally infected infants. The "United States Program" has instituted routine immunization of all prepubertal children, boys and girls, and the selective immunization of postpubertal girls and women of childbearing age documented to be susceptible to rubella infection (Center for Disease Control, 1978; Modlin et al., 1975). The goal is to induce a high degree of herd immunity, which will prevent circulation of the agent and thus prevent susceptible pregnant women from acquiring rubella. By immunizing young children, the most likely sources of disseminating the infection are in theory eliminated. The "British Program" is directed toward the routine immunization of girls 11 to 14 years of age and selective immunization of women of

childbearing potential. Thus, it attempts to prevent maternal infection without reducing circulation of the wild-type virus in the remainder of the population.

The two immunization strategies presently appear to have yielded different results. In the United States, the incidence of rubella has declined fourfold. Proponents argue that the expected epidemic in the mid-1970s was avoided by massive immunization. Along with the reduction in disease, more importantly, the number of reported cases of congenital rubella in the United States has also declined. In England, on the other hand, only approximately 70 per cent of girls have received the rubella vaccine, and the incidence of congenital rubella has not changed. It is estimated that at least 90 per cent of prepubertal girls would need to be immunized for the incidence of congenital rubella to decline using the "British Program." This approach at best would require a 10-year lag period before the immunized girls became the major portion of the women of childbearing potential, thus affecting the occurrence of congenital rubella.

Although it would appear that the "United States Program" has been more successful than the "British Program," several major problems still exist (Horstmann, 1975). It is estimated that in the United States approximately 450,000 cases of rubella occur yearly. In addition, immunization levels in women are between 85 and 90 per cent, which is essentially unchanged from prevaccine periods. The risk of fetal infection, therefore, is still very real.

Further questions have been raised concerning the duration of immunity to the rubella vaccines (Wilkins and Wehrle, 1979; Fogel et al., 1978). Of youngsters immunized with the HPV77 DE5 vaccine, between 4 and 36 per cent lack HAI antibodies three to five years after immunization. In addition, children immunized before 12 months of age have significantly lower antibody responses to rubella as well as to measles, probably secondary to persistence of passively transferred maternal antibody. Two other rubella vaccines previously licensed in the United States but now withdrawn had lower overall failure rates. The HPV77 DK12 vaccine, available from 1969 to 1973, had a failure rate of less than 1 per cent, and a 1 to 11 per cent serologic failure rate had been noted for the Cendehill vaccine, which was available from 1970 to 1976. The RA27/3 vaccine, which has been extensively used in Europe and since 1979 has been the only rubella vaccine licensed for use in the United States, is highly immunogenic (Plotkin et al., 1973) and has primary and secondary failure rates of less than 3 per cent.

Rubella reinfection is typically an inapparent

infection characterized by the absence of viremia, no or minimal transient pharyngeal virus shedding, and a prompt fourfold or greater rise in rubella HAI antibody. Subclinical reinfection has occurred more frequently after HPV77 or Cendehill immunizations than has been observed with the RA27/3 vaccine or following natural immunity. The potential risks of these subclinical reinfections are unknown but are probably small.

What to do about children, particularly girls, who were immunized with the HPV77 or Cendehill vaccines remains controversial. Revaccination of all prepubertal girls who have previously received these vaccines has been suggested by some (Balfour, 1979). Another approach is premarital screening of all women and immunization with RA27/3 of all seronegative women once adequate precautions are taken to ascertain that they are not pregnant and will not conceive for at least three months after immunization.

### Smallpox

Live vaccinia virus vaccine, which is a stable hybrid of both smallpox and cowpox, is available in both glycerinated and lyophilized forms for immunization against smallpox. Both are equally protective when stored and administered properly. The glycerinated vaccine requires constant refrigeration, whereas the lyophilized vaccine is more stable until it is reconstituted. Protection lasts for approximately three years.

Smallpox vaccine may be administered either by multiple pressure, multiple puncture, or jet injection; all methods are equally effective (Center for Disease Control, 1978). The vaccine site should be examined after six to eight days to ascertain a successful result. Following primary vaccination, a typical Jennerian vesicle should be present. If a vesicle does not develop, the vaccination should be considered a failure. Following revaccination, a major reaction consisting of a vesicular or pustular lesion or an area of definite palpable induration or constant congestion surrounding a central lesion, which may be a crust or an ulcer, should be observed. All other reactions are considered equivocal and suggest vaccine failures. All primary or revaccinated persons without adequate responses should be reimmunized from another vaccine lot until a successful response is achieved.

Despite apparent global eradication of smallpox, more than 4.4 million doses of the vaccine were distributed in the United States in 1978. Severe reactions still develop in at least 1 per 100,000 vaccinees, and death occurs in 6 per 10 million doses administered (Center for Disease Control, 1979a). Any morbidity or mortality caused by smallpox vaccination seems unnecessary. Although some countries still require smallpox vaccination for arriving travelers, there seems little justification for this practice. The World Health Organization's International Regulations provide for smallpox vaccination waiver letters to be issued to travelers for whom vaccination is contraindicated for health reasons. It is the view of many physicians that such letters should be given to all travelers, unless there is a major change in the current world status of smallpox. At present, only the few individuals actively involved in doing research using the smallpox virus should be immunized. The vaccine at any time is strongly contraindicated in individuals with any impairment of immunity or persons with eczema; individuals with active skin lesions including burns, poison ivy, and impetigo; and pregnant women.

### Varicella-Zoster

While varicella has a low incidence of serious complications and sequelae in normal individuals, immunocompromised patients are at high risk of developing serious and potentially fatal infections. These high-risk individuals have been the impetus for the development of means to prevent or ameliorate varicella infections. Varicella-zoster immune globulin (VZIG) prepared from outdated donor blood, or zoster immune globulin (ZIG) obtained from individuals with varicella-zoster infections has been shown to modify or prevent varicella in susceptible children when given within 72 hours of exposure (Brunell and Gershon, 1973; Center for Disease Control, 1979; Gershon et al., 1974; Judelsohn et al., 1974). At present, VZIG is available in the United States through the Division of Clinical Microbiology, Sidney Farber Cancer Institute, 44 Binney Street, Boston, Massachusetts (617-732-3121) for those meeting the criteria outlined in Table 9. Varicella-zoster immune plasma (VZIP), obtained from patients with active zoster, has also been shown to modify varicella infections in high-risk individuals (Balfour and Groth, 1979; Balfour et al., 1977; Geiser et al., 1975). There is no evidence that VZIG or VZIP has any benefit in individuals with active chickenpox or zoster and neither should be used in these situations. A recent study using dialyzable transfer factor has suggested that this method of passive immunization may be useful in preventing varicella in children with leukemia (Steele et al., 1980). The limited availability of specific varicella transfer factor at present makes this preventive approach impractical for wide use.

An experimental varicella vaccine has been extensively studied in Japan and is currently under investigation in the United States (Asano

**TABLE 9.   Five Criteria for Release of Varicella-Zoster Immune Globulin (VZIG) for the Prophylaxis of Varicella**

I. One of the following underlying illnesses or conditions
   A. Leukemia or lymphoma
   B. Congenital or acquired immunodeficiency
   C. Under immunosuppressive medication
   D. Newly born of mother with varicella
II. One of the following types of exposure to varicella or zoster patient
   A. Household contact
   B. Playmate contact (>1 hour play indoors)
   C. Hospital contact (in same two- to four-room bedroom or adjacent beds in a large ward)
   D. Newborn contact (newborn whose mother contracted varicella less than five days before delivery or within 48 hours after delivery)
III. Negative or unknown prior disease history
IV. Age of less than 15 years
V. The request for treatment must be initiated within 72 hours of exposure

From Center for Disease Control: Varicella-zoster immune globulin. Morbid Mortal Weekly Rep 28:589, 1979.

et al., 1977; Takahashi et al., 1974). The potential of preventing varicella and its complications in childhood and the misery of herpes zoster in adult life has made some researchers believe that the varicella vaccine may be widely used. Controversy remains, however, about the eventual target population for such a vaccine. Some argue that normal children are at little risk from chickenpox and are not suitable candidates. The risk that more frequent or serious herpes zoster infections will follow vaccination, or that initial infection with varicella will be postponed from childhood when it is mild to adulthood when it is more often severe makes routine immunization against varicella potentially unattractive. High-risk, immunocompromised children are considered to be the group most likely to benefit from a varicella vaccine. This population, however, is the group in which live vaccines are usually avoided and which is most likely to respond inadequately to immunizations. Preliminary studies in Japan have indicated that children with leukemia, neuroblastoma, retinoblastoma, and others with chronic illnesses receiving steroid therapy can be successfully immunized. Clearly, further research will be necessary before benefits and risks of the live varicella vaccines are fully evaluated.

### Rickettsial Diseases

The incidence of Rocky Mountain spotted fever (RMSF) continues to increase in the United States. Laboratory workers are at high risk of developing disease while working with *Rickettsia rickettsii,* the causative agent in RMSF. The first

RMSF vaccine developed in 1924 was a phenol and formalin–inactivated preparation obtained from infected tick tissue. Since the 1940s, a killed vaccine produced in infected yolk sacs of embryonated eggs had been used. Although early findings in guinea pigs and human field trials suggested vaccine efficacy, after over 30 years of use studies have clearly shown the yolk sac vaccine to be ineffective in preventing infections in humans after laboratory exposure or direct challenge. Since 1970, a new formalin-inactivated vaccine, prepared from *R. rickettsii* grown in tissue culture of chick embryo fibroblasts and purified by sucrose density gradient, has been studied (Kenyon and Pedersen, 1975; Kenyon et al., 1975). The vaccine has proved to be highly immunogenic and protective in guinea pigs and rhesus monkeys and has been encouraging in preliminary human trials (Ascher et al., 1978). At present, however, no effective vaccine for RMSF is available.

Louse-borne typhus remains a major problem in rural or remote highland areas of Ethiopia, Rwanda, Burundi, Mexico, Guatemala, Ecuador, Bolivia, Peru, and the mountanous areas of Asia. A formalin-inactivated vaccine prepared from *Rickettsia prowazekii* grown in embryonated eggs is currently available (Center for Disease Center, 1978). Although no controlled studies of typhus vaccine have been carried out in humans, field and laboratory experiences suggest that the incidence and severity of typhus cases are diminished following vaccination, particularly if booster doses have been received. The vaccine protects against louse-borne (epidemic) typhus only and not against murine or scrub typhus. Typhus vaccine is recommended only for those individuals who live or visit areas where typhus cases actually occur and who will be in constant contact with the indigenous population. Medical personnel who provide care for patients in areas in which louse-borne (epidemic) typhus occurs or researchers working with *R. prowazekii* should be immunized.

At present, there is no effective vaccine against Q fever. A formalin-inactivated preparation prepared from *Coxiella burnetii* is relatively effective in eliciting an immunogenic response and providing protection in humans but is associated with an unacceptably high incidence of sterile abscesses at injection sites. A live attenuated vaccine utilizing *C. burnetii* strain M-44 initially appeared promising, but recent guinea pig studies showing microscopic evidence of myocarditis and hepatitis following vaccination suggest that the vaccine will require further attenuation before human use can be recommended (Johnson et al., 1976, 1977; Robinson and Hasty, 1974).

## IMMUNIZATIONS FOR DEVELOPING COUNTRIES

Issues concerning immunizations in developed industrial countries often have little relevance for the over three billion people living in less developed nations who suffer from a multitude of infectious diseases. Preventing congenital rubella, avoiding mumps, meningoencephalitis, and orchitis, and protecting immunocompromised individuals from overwhelming varicella infections are medical luxuries shared only by inhabitants of wealthy developed nations. The collective state of ill health in these underdeveloped countries at present, unfortunately, makes comprehensive primary health care an impossibility. Selective primary health care that chooses priorities for disease control is currently the only reasonable goal (Walsh and Warren, 1979). Water and sanitation programs associated with vector control and improved nutrition must be combined with educational campaigns if infectious diseases are to be controlled. Selective immunization for children up to 3 years old and women of childbearing age should at least include vaccination against measles, diphtheria, pertussis, and tetanus. Further immunizations including those against poliomyelitis, tuberculosis, and typhoid could make a large impact on the general state of health in developing countries. The cost of these programs would be substantial and would require a worldwide commitment in order to be successful.

## References

### General

Artenstein, M. S.: The current status of bacterial vaccines. Hosp Prac 8:49, 1973.

Barrett-Connor, E.: Advice for young travelers. Pediatr Rev 1:25, 1979.

Center for Disease Control: Recommendation of the Immunization Practices Advisory Committee (ACIP): General recommendations on immunization. Morbid Mortal Weekly Rep 29:83, 1980.

Collins, F. M.: Vaccines and cell-mediated immunity. Bacteriol Rev 38:371, 1974.

Fraumeni, J. F., Ederer, F., and Miller, R. W.: An evaluation of the carcinogenicity of simian virus 40 in man. JAMA 185:713, 1963.

Fulginiti, V. A.: Controversies in current immunization policy and practices: One physician's viewpoint. Curr Probl Pediatr 66:3, 1976.

Harrison, H. R., and Fulginiti, V. A.: Bacterial immunizations. Am J Dis Child 134:184, 1980.

Krugman, S., and Katz, S. L.: Childhood immunization procedures. JAMA 237:2228, 1977.

Levine, M. M.: Live-virus vaccines in pregnancy risks and recommendations. Lancet 2:34, 1974.

Marks, J. S., Halpin, T. J., Irvin, J. J., Johnson, D. A., and Keller, J. R.: Risk factors associated with failure to receive vaccinations. Pediatrics 64:304, 1979.

Medical Letter on Drugs and Therapeutics: Immunizations for travelers. 21:57, 1979.

Mortimer, E. A.: Immunization against infectious disease. Science 200:902, 1978.

Phillips, C. F.: Children out of step with immunization. Pediatrics 55:877, 1975.

Rand, K. H., and Merigan, T. C.: Can immunization eradicate viral diseases?: Arch Intern Med 137:723, 1977.

Rothberg, R. M., Sumner, C. K., and Michalek, S. M.: Systemic immunity after local antigenic stimulation of the lymphoid tissue of the gastrointestinal tract. J Immunol 111:1906, 1973.

Walsh, J. A., and Warren, K. S.: Selective primary health care: An interim strategy for disease control in developing countries. N Engl J Med 301:967, 1979.

White, C. S., Adler, W. H., and McGann, V. G.: Repeated immunization: Possible adverse effects. Ann Intern Med 81:594, 1974.

### Passive Immunization

Braude, A. I., Ziegler, E. J., Douglas, H., and McCutchan, J. A.: Antibody to cell wall glycolipid of gram-negative bacteria: Induction of immunity to bacteremia and endotoxemia. J Infect Dis 136:S167, 1977.

Ellis, E. F., and Henney, C. S.: Adverse reactions following administration of human gamma globulin. J Allergy 43:45, 1969.

Squire, J. R., et al.: Hypogammaglobulinaemia in the United Kingdom. Lancet 1:163, 1969.

Stiehm, E. R.: Standard and special human immune serum globulins as therapeutic agents. Pediatrics 63:301, 1979.

Stiehm, E. R., and Fudenberg, H. H.: Antibodies to gamma-globulin in infants and children exposed to isologous gamma-globulin. Pediatrics 35:229, 1965.

Ziegler, E. J., McCutchan, J. A., and Braude, A. I.: Clinical trial of core glycolipid antibody in gram-negative bacteremia. Trans Assoc Am Physicians 91:253, 1978.

### Cytomegalovirus

Glazer, J. P., et al.: Live cytomegalovirus vaccination of renal transplant candidates. Ann Intern Med 91:676, 1979.

Just, M., Buergin-Wolff, A., Emoedi, G., and Hernandez, R.: Immunization trials with live attenuated cytomegalovirus, Towne 125. Infection 3:111, 1975.

Plotkin, S. A., Farquhar, J., and Hornberger, E.: Clinical trials of immunization with the Towne 125 strain of human cytomegalovirus. J Infect Dis 134:470, 1976.

### Diphtheria, Pertussis, Tetanus

Barkin, R. M., and Pichichero, M. E.: Diphtheria-pertussis-tetanus vaccine: Reactogenicity of commercial products. Pediatrics 63:256, 1979.

Center for Disease Control: Diphtheria and tetanus toxoids and pertussis vaccine. Morbid Mortal Weekly Rep 26:401, 1977.

Enrengut, W.: Whooping cough vaccination. Lancet 1:370, 1978.

Grady, G. F., and Wetterlow, L. H.: Pertussis vaccine: Reasonable doubt. N Engl J Med 298:966, 1978.

Kendrick, P. L.: Can whooping cough be eradicated? J Infect Dis 132:707, 1975.

Koplan, J. P., et al.: Pertussis vaccine — An analysis of benefits, risks, and costs. N Engl J Med 301:906, 1979.

Linneman, C. C., et al.: Use of pertussis vaccine in an epidemic involving hospital staff. Lancet 2:540, 1975.

Lister, J.: The care of children — Pertussis vaccination. N Engl J Med 296:984, 1977.

Manclark, C. R.: Summary of an international symposium on pertussis. J Infect Dis 140:129, 1979.

Mathias, R. G.: Whooping cough in spite of immunization. Can J Public Health 69:130, 1978.

Peebles, T. C., et al.: Tetanus-toxoid emergency boosters. N Engl J Med 280:575, 1969.

Pittman, M.: Pertussis toxin: The cause of the harmful effects and prolonged immunity of whooping cough. Rev Infect Dis 1:401, 1979.

Stewart, G. T.: Vaccination against whooping cough. Lancet 1:234, 1977.

White, W. G., et al.: Duration of immunity after active immunization against tetanus. Lancet 2:95, 1969.

### Hepatitis

Center for Disease Control: Immune globulins for protection against viral hepatitis. Morbid Mortal Weekly Rep 26:415, 1977.

Gerety, R. J., Tabor, E., Purcell, R. H., and Tyeryar, F. J.: Summary of an international workshop on hepatitis B vaccines. J Infect Dis 140:642, 1979.

Hoofnagle, J. H., et al.: Passive-active immunity from hepatitis B immune globulin. Ann Intern Med 91:813, 1979.

Krugman, S.: Viral hepatitis: Recent developments and prospects for prevention. J Pediatr 87:1067, 1975.

Krugman, S., Ward, R., Giles, J. P. and Jacobs, A. M.: Infectious hepatitis: Studies on the effect of gamma globulin and on the incidence of inapparent infection. JAMA 174:823, 1960.

Mosley, J. W.: Hepatitis B immune globulin: Some progress and some problems. Ann Intern Med 91:914, 1979.

Redeker, A. G., et al.: Hepatitis B immune globulin as a prophylactic measure for spouses exposed to acute type B hepatitis. N Engl J Med 293:1055, 1975.

Seeff, L. B., et al.: Type B hepatitis after needle-stick exposure: Prevention with hepatitis B immune globulin. Ann Intern Med 88:285, 1978.

Szmuness, W., et al.: Hepatitis B immune serum globulin in prevention of nonparenterally transmitted hepatitis B. N Engl J Med 290:701, 1974.

Woodson, R. D., and Clinton, J. J.: Hepatitis prophylaxis abroad. JAMA 209:1053, 1969.

### Measles

Albrecht, P., Ennis, F. A., Saltzman, E. J., and Krugman, S.: Persistence of maternal antibody in infants beyond 12 months: Mechanism of measles vaccine failure. J Pediatr 91:715, 1977.

Center for Disease Control: Measles prevention. Morbid Mortal Weekly Rep 27:427, 1978.

Deseda-Tous, J., et al.: Measles revaccination. Am J Dis Child 132:287, 1978.

Krause, P. J., et al.: Revaccination of previous recipients of killed measles vaccine: Clinical and immunologic studies. J. Pediatr 93:565, 1978.

Landrigan, P. J., and Witte, J. J.: Neurologic disorders following live measles-virus vaccination. JAMA 223:1459, 1973.

Marks, J. S., Halpin, T. J., and Orenstein, W. A.: Measles vaccine efficacy in children previously vaccinated at 12 months of age. Pediatrics 62:955, 1978.

McCormick, J. B., Halsey, N., and Rosenberg, R.: Measles vaccine efficacy determined from secondary attack rates during a severe epidemic. J Pediatr 90:13, 1977.

Modlin, J. F., Jabbour, J. T., Witte, J. J., and Halsey, N. A.: Epidemiologic studies of measles, measles vaccine, and subacute sclerosing panencephalitis. Pediatrics 59:505, 1977.

Orenstein, W. A., et al.: Current status of measles in the United States, 1973–1977. J Infect Dis 137:847, 1978.

Ruuskanen, O., Salmi, T. T., and Halonen, P.: Measles vaccination after exposure to natural measles. J Pediatr 93:43, 1978.

Shasby, D. M., et al.: Epidemic measles in a highly vaccinated population. N Engl J Med 296:585, 1977.

Shelton, J. D., et al.: Measles vaccine efficacy: Influence of age at vaccination vs duration of time since vaccination. Pediatrics 62:961, 1978.

Weiner, L. B., et al.: A measles outbreak among adolescents. J Pediatr 90:17, 1977.

Wilkins, J., and Wehrle, P. F.: Additional evidence against measles vaccine administration to infants less than 12 months of age: Altered immune response following active/passive immunization. J Pediatr 94:865, 1979.

Wilkins, J., and Wehrle, P. F.: Evidence for reinstatement of infants 12 to 14 months of age into routine measles immunization programs. Am J Dis Child 132:162, 1978.

### Meningococcus

Center for Disease Control: Meningococcal polysaccharide vaccines. Morbid Mortal Weekly Rep 27:327, 1978.

Farquhar, J. D., et al.: Clinical and serological evaluation of meningococcal polysaccharide vaccine groups A, C, and Y. Proc Soc Exp Biol Med 157:79, 1978.

Lepow, M. L., et al.: Persistence of antibody following immunization of children with groups A and C meningococcal polysaccharide vaccines. Pediatrics 60:673, 1977.

Peltola, H., et al.: Clinical efficacy of meningococcus group A capsular polysaccharide vaccine in children three months to five years of age. N Engl J Med 297:686, 1977.

Wilkins, J., and Wehrle, P. F.: Further characterization of responses of infants and children to meningococcal A polysaccharide vaccine. J Pediatr 94:828, 1979.

### Mumps

Biedel, C. W.: Recurrent mumps parotitis following natural infection and immunization. Am J Dis Child 132:678, 1978.

Center for Disease Control: Mumps vaccine. Morbid Mortal Weekly Rep 29:87, 1980.

Hayden, G. F., Preblud, S. R., Orenstein, W. A., and Conrad, J. L.: Current status of mumps and mumps vaccine in the United States. Pediatrics 62:965, 1978.

Hosai, H., et al.: Studies on live attenuated mumps virus vaccine. Biken J 13:121, 1970.

Lerner, A. M.: Guide to immunization against mumps. J Infect Dis 122:116, 1970.

Yamanishi, K., et al.: Studies of live attenuated mumps virus vaccine: Biological characteristics of the strains adapted to the amniotic and chorioallantoic cavity of developing chick embryos. Biken J 13:127, 1970.

Yamauchi, T., Wilson, C., and St. Geme, J. W.: Transmission of live, attenuated mumps virus to the human placenta. N Engl J Med 290:710, 1974.

### Pneumococcus

Ahonkhai, V. I., et al.: Failure of pneumococcal vaccine in children with sickle-cell disease. N Engl J Med 301:26, 1979.

Ammann, A. J., et al.: Polyvalent pneumococcal-polysaccharide immunization of patients with sickle-cell anemia and patients with splenectomy. N Engl J Med 297:897, 1977.

Center for Disease Control: Pneumococcal polysaccharide vaccine. Morbid Mortal Weekly Rep 27:25, 1978.

Cowan, M. J., et al.: Pneumococcal polysaccharide immunization in infants and children. Pediatrics 62:721, 1978.

Fikrig, S. M., et al.: Antibody response to capsular polysaccharide vaccine of Streptococcus pneumoniae in patients with nephrotic syndrome. J Infect Dis 137:818, 1978.

Klein, J. O., and Mortimer, E. A.: Use of pneumococcal vaccine in children. Pediatrics 61:321, 1978.

Minor, D. R., Schiffman, G., and McIntosh, L. S.: Response of patients with Hodgkin's disease to pneumococcal vaccine. Ann Intern Med 90:887, 1979.

### Poliomyelitis

Center for Disease Control: Poliomyelitis — United States, Canada. Morbid Mortal Weekly Rep 28:229, 1979.

Davis, L. E., et al.: Chronic progressive poliomyelitis secondary to vaccination of an immunodeficient child. N Engl J Med 297:241, 1977.

John, T. J., et al.: Effect of breast-feeding on seroresponse of infants to oral poliovirus vaccination. Pediatrics 57:47, 1976.

Krugman, R. D., et al.: Antibody persistence after primary immunization with trivalent oral poliovirus vaccine. Pediatrics 60:80, 1977.

Melnick, J. L.: Vaccines and vaccine policy: The poliomyelitis example. Hosp Pract 13:41, 1978.

Nightingale, E. O.: Recommendations for a national policy on poliomyelitis vaccination. N Engl J Med 297:249, 1977.

Rousseau, W. E.: Persistence of poliovirus neutralizing antibodies eight years after immunization with live, attenuated-virus vaccine. N Engl J Med 289:1357, 1973.

### Rabies

Center for Disease Control: Rabies prevention. Morbid Mortal Weekly Rep 29:265, 1980.

Nicholson, K. G., Turner, G. S., and Aoki, F. Y.: Immunization with a human diploid cell strain of rabies virus vaccine: Two year results. J Infect Dis 137:783, 1978.

Plotkin, S. A., and Wiktor, T.: Vaccination of children with human cell culture rabies vaccine. Pediatrics 63:219, 1979.

### Rickettsial Diseases

Ascher, M. S., et al.: Initial clinical evaluation of a new Rocky Mountain spotted fever vaccine of tissue culture origin. J Infect Dis 138:217, 1978.

Center for Disease Control: Typhus vaccine. Morbid Mortal Weekly Rep 27:189, 1978.

Johnson, J. W., Eddy, G. A., and Pedersen, C. E.: Biological properties of the M-44 strain of *Coxiella burnetii.* J Infect Dis 133:334,
1976.
Johnson, J. W., et al.: Lesions in guinea pigs infected with *Coxiella
burnetii* strain M-44. J Infect Dis 135:995, 1977.
Kenyon, R. H., and Pedersen, C. E.: Preparation of Rocky Mountain
spotted fever vaccine suitable for human immunization. J Clin
Microbiol 1:500, 1975.
Kenyon, R. E., Sammons, L. C., and Pedersen, C. E.: Comparison of
three Rocky Mountain spotted fever vaccines. J Clin Microbiol
2:300, 1975.
Robinson, D. M., and Hasty, S. E.: Production of a potent vaccine
from the attenuated M-44 strain of *Coxiella burnetii.* Appl Microbiol 27:777, 1974.

*Rubella*

Balfour, H. H.: Rubella reimmunization now. Am J Dis Child
133:1231, 1979.
Boue, A., Nicolas, A., and Montagnon, B.: Reinfection with rubella in
pregnant women. Lancet 1:7712, 1971.
Center for Disease Control: Rubella vaccine. Morbid Mortal Weekly
Rep 27:451, 1978.
Fleet, W. F., et al.: Fetal consequences of maternal rubella immun-
ization. JAMA 227:621, 1974.
Fogel, A., et al.: Response to experimental challenge in persons
immunized with different rubella vaccines. J Pediatr 92:26,
1978.
Horstmann, D.: Controlling rubella: Problems and perspectives. Ann
Intern Med 83:412, 1975.
Medical Letter on Drugs and Therapeutics: The new rubella vaccine.
21:53, 1979.
Modlin, J. F., et al.: A review of five years' experience with rubella
vaccine in the United States. Pediatrics 55:20, 1975.
Plotkin, S. A., Farquhar, J. D., and Ogra, P. L.: Immunologic properties of RA27/3 rubella virus vaccine. JAMA 225:585, 1973.
Schoenbaum, S. C., et al.: Benefit-cost analysis of rubella vaccination
policy. N Engl J Med 294:306, 1976.
Wilkins, J., and Wehrle, P. F.: Further evaulation of the optimum
age for rubella vaccine administration. Am J Dis Child
133:1237, 1979.
Wyll, S. A., and Herrmann, K. L.: Inadvertent rubella vaccination of
pregnant women. JAMA 225:1472, 1973.

*Smallpox*

Center for Disease Control: Adverse reactions to smallpox vaccina-
tion, 1978. Morbid Mortal Weekly Rep 28:265, 1979a.
Center for Disease Control: Smallpox certification — East Africa.
Morbid Mortal Weekly Rep 28:497, 1979b.
Center for Disease Control: Smallpox vaccine. Morbid Mortal Weekly
Rep 27:156, 1978.
De Vries, R. P., Kreeftenberg, M., Loggen, H., and Van Rood, J. J.:
In vitro immune responsiveness to vaccinia virus and HLA. N
Engl J Med 297:692, 1977.

*Tuberculosis*

Center for Disease Control: BCG vaccines. Morbid Mortal Weekly
Rep 28:241, 1979.
Eickhoff, T. C.: The current status of BCG immunization against
tuberculosis. Annu Rev Med 28:411, 1977.
Passwell, J., et al.: Fatal disseminated BCG infection. Am J Dis
Child 130:433, 1976.

*Typhoid*

Ashcroft, M. T., et al.: A seven year field trial of two typhoid vaccines in Guyana. Lancet 2:1056, 1967.
Center for Disease Control: Typhoid vaccine. Morbid Mortal Weekly
Rep 27:231, 1978.
Gilman, R. H., et al.: Evaluation of a UDP-glucose-4-epimeraseless
mutant of *Salmonella typhi* as a live oral vaccine. J Infect Dis
136:717, 1977.

Hornick, R. B., et al.: Typhoid fever: Pathogenesis and immunologic
control. N Engl J Med 283:686, 739, 1970.

*Varicella*

Asano, Y., et al.: Protection against varicella in family contacts by
immediate inoculation with live varicella vaccine. Pediatrics
59:3, 1977.
Balfour, H. H., and Groth, K. E.: Zoster immune plasma prophylaxis
of varicella: A follow-up report. J Pediatr 94:743, 1979.
Balfour, H. H., Groth, K., McCullough, J., Kallis, J., Marker, S.,
Nesbit, M., Summons, R., and Najarian, J.: Prevention or modification of varicella using zoster immune plasma. Am J Dis Child
131:693, 1977.
Brunell, P. A., and Gershon, A. A.: Passive immunization against
varicella-zoster infections and other modes of therapy. J Infect
Dis 127:415, 1973.
Center for Disease Control: Varicella-zoster immune globulin. Morbid Mortal Weekly Rep 28:589, 1979.
Geiser, C. F., et al.: Prophylaxis of varicella in children with neo-
plastic disease: Comparative results with zoster immune plasma
and gamma globulin. Cancer 35:1027, 1975.
Gershon, A. A., Steinberg, S., and Brunell, P. A.: Zoster immune
globulin. N Engl J Med 290:243, 1974.
Judelsohn, R. G., et al.: Efficacy of zoster immune globulin. Pediatrics 53:476, 1974.
Steele, R. W., Myers, M. G., and Vincent, M. M.: Transfer factor for
the prevention of varicella-zoster infection in childhood leukemia.
N Engl J Med 303:355, 1980.
Takahashi, M. Otsuka, T., and Okuno, Y.: Live vaccine used to
prevent the spread of varicella in children in hospital. Lancet
2:1288, 1974.
Uduman, S. A., Gershon, A. A., and Brunell, P. A.: Should patients
with zoster receive zoster immune globulin? JAMA 234:1049,
1975.

*Other Articles*

Balfour, H. H., and Amren, D. P.: Rubella, measles and mumps
antibodies following vaccination of children. Am J Dis Child
132:573, 1978.
Beachey, E. H., Stollerman, G. H., and Bisno, A. L.: A strep vaccine:
How close? Hosp Pract 14:49, 1979.
Center for Disease Control: Plague vaccine. Morbid Mortal Weekly
Rep 27:255, 1978.
Center for Disease Control: Cholera vaccine. Morbid Mortal Weekly
Rep 27:173, 1978.
Center for Disease Control: Yellow fever vaccine. Morbid Mortal
Weekly Rep 27:268, 1978.
Horstmann, D. M.: Viral vaccines and their ways. Rev Infect Dis
1:502, 1979.
Krugman, S.: Present status of measles and rubella immunization in
the United States: A medical progress report. J Pediatr 90:1,
1977.
Melnick, J. L.: Viral vaccines: New problems and prospects. Hosp
Pract 13:104, 1978.
Sato, H., et al.: Transfer of measles, mumps and rubella antibodies
from mother to infant. Am J Dis Child 133:1240, 1979.
Stumpf, D. A., and Frost, M.: Immunity after rubella and measles
viral vaccines. Am J Dis Child 132:748, 1978.
Weibel, R. E., et al.: Long-term follow-up for immunity after monovalent or combined live measles, mumps and rubella virus
vaccines. Pediatrics 56:380, 1975.

*Books*

American Academy of Pediatrics: Report of the Committee on Infec-
tious Disease, 18th ed., Evanston, Illinois, 1977.
Creighton, C.: Jenner and Vaccination: A Strange Chapter of Medi-
cal History. London, Suvan Sonnen Schein & Company, 1889.
Parish, H. J.: A History of Immunization. London, E. & S. Living-
stone Ltd., 1965.
Parish, H. J.: Victory with Vaccines. London, E. & S. Livingstone
Ltd., 1968.
Voller, A., and Friedman, H.: New Trends and Developments in
Vaccines, Baltimore, University Park Press, 1978.

# Metabolic

# 85 *FEVER*

*Sheldon M. Wolff, M.D.*

Fever has been recognized as a major manifestation of a large variety of diseases since antiquity. Although clinicians and investigators have been interested in the mechanisms of production of fever in the intact human for decades, it has been only during the past 15 years that significant progress has been made. It is not known if this commonest of all clinical symptoms is of any value in host defenses or whether it is a nonspecific response.

Normal body temperature follows a very reproducible circadian rhythm, with the maximum temperature ordinarily occurring in the late afternoon or early evening and then gradually falling to its low point in the morning. Normal temperature can be influenced by a variety of stimuli such as exercise, menstrual cycle, and environmental temperature changes, but it generally follows the same circadian pattern in a given individual. Thirty-seven degrees centigrade (98.6° F) is generally accepted as the "normal" temperature. These are mean values derived from old studies. When interpreting a temperature reading, there are a number of variables to be considered. Among these are how it was obtained (i.e., from which orifice), time of day, and whether the subject had just participated in strenuous physical activity. An isolated temperature reading in a patient is usually of little value, since so many factors can influence body temperature. Fever is a symptom of disease, and it is rare for it to be the sole sign or symptom of an illness. Normal individuals may have temperatures that occasionally rise above 38° C in the evening, and, unless multiple readings are taken, or a careful history obtained and a physical examination done, one would be incorrect in calling such an isolated reading a fever. All of the preceding facts emphasize that a temperature reading may be of no value unless it is considered merely as part of a more detailed evaluation of the patient as a whole.

Regardless of the cause of fever, most of the physiologic processes that occur when body temperature rises follow similar patterns. It is well established that the thermoregulatory center resides in the anterior hypothalamus in the floor of the third ventricle. The development of fever depends upon an intricate set of interrelated events involving heat loss, heat production, and peripheral vasoconstriction. Some of these events are mediated by neurohumoral agents such as norepinephrine and serotonin, but the exact role of such substances in the febrile response in human beings is unclear. When a patient first develops a fever, he or she may have a chill, which is accompanied by an increase in metabolic activity as measured by such things as oxygen consumption. The severity and length of the chill depend on the stimulus. Concomitant with or shortly after the increased metabolic activity, core temperature begins to rise. Peripheral vasoconstriction occurs with the chill and is associated with a decrease in heat loss, which is maximal over the more peripheral areas of the body. The increase in metabolic activity persists during the fever. With the dissipation of the fever, peripheral vasodilatation occurs, and heat loss ensues. Depending on the height of the fever, the rate of heat loss, and the rapidity of the lowering of the temperature, sweating (i.e., diaphoresis) that can be marked may occur.

Certain clinical findings accompany fever in human beings regardless of the cause. The presence or absence and the magnitude of such findings depend on the severity and duration of the febrile reaction. Headache, myalgias, arthralgias, nausea, vomiting, backache, and feelings of warmth are some of the more common complaints heard from patients with fever. Tachycardia is usual, although in certain infectious diseases a relative bradycardia may be seen. Tachypnea, widening of the pulse pressure, and flushing are additional signs that are usually noted in febrile human beings.

Fever can be a prominent symptom of all infectious and inflammatory diseases. It is also seen in a wide variety of neoplastic and metabolic illnesses. The agents that cause fever are called pyrogens, and the list of pyrogenic substances continues to increase. For example, most bacteria, viruses, and fungi are pyrogenic. Exogenous pyrogens also include the endotoxins of gram-negative bacteria, antigens in previously sensitized subjects (Root and Wolff, 1968), antigen-antibody complexes (formed either in vivo or in vitro), and some synthetic polynucleotides. Certain C-19, C-21, and C-24 steroids of endogenous human origin that share the 5-$\beta$-H configuration are potent pyrogens. The best known of these is etiocholanolone (Wolff et al., 1967). Some hormones, such as progesterone, have also been shown to be pyrogenic. What role, if any, is played by these pyrogenic steroids in human disease is not known.

It is generally accepted that the basic series of events put into motion by any exogenous pyrogen is the same. In addition, as noted above, the febrile response is similar. In other words, there is a "final common pathway" that results in fever regardless of the cause. The basic hypothesis states that pyrogens interact with host cells, which in turn release an endogenous pyrogen (or leukocytic pyrogen); this endogenously produced substance then stimulates the thermoregulatory centers in the brain, resulting in fever. Much of the information that resulted in this hypothesis has been obtained from experimental animals, but during the past few years information gained from investigations on human cells has become available. Despite the recent rapid advances, considerably more work needs to be done before we can define in exact terms the pathogenesis of fever in man (Dinarello and Wolff, 1978).

It was originally suggested that the neutrophil was the blood leukocyte that was solely responsible for endogenous pyrogen production (Wood, 1958). However, it was later demonstrated that blood leukocytes from patients with severe granulocytopenia or monocytic leukemia produced large quantities of endogenous pyrogens when stimulated in vitro. Thus, the blood monocyte was established as a potent source of endogenous pyrogen, and this finding provided an explanation for the presence of fever in patients without circulating granulocytes. The human eosinophil is also a source of endogenous pyrogen. Certain tumors, namely hypernephromas, which are often associated with febrile episodes, have been shown to release endogenous pyrogens spontaneously in vitro. Kupffer cells in the liver, splenic macrophages, alveolar macrophages, and peritoneal lining cells are sources of endogenous pyrogen in rabbits and most likely are potent producers of this mediator substance in humans. Clinically, it is important to recognize sources of endogenous pyrogen other than peripheral neutrophils or monocytes, since patients without circulating or marrow phagocytes often have marked febrile responses to infection. Kupffer and other fixed phagocytic cells are probably sources of endogenous pyrogen in such patients. It is clear that only phagocytic cells derived from bone marrow precursors produce endogenous pyrogen. Lymphocytes are not a source of endogenous pyrogen.

When blood leukocytes are incubated with inhibitors of protein synthesis such as puromycin or cycloheximide during the activation process, the subsequent production of endogenous pyrogen is prevented (Nordlund et al., 1970). Neither cycloheximide nor puromycin prevents phagocytosis. Hence, the activation process is unaffected by these drugs. Actinomycin, which prevents the transcription of DNA into messenger RNA, also prevents the production of endogenous pyrogen in vitro. It is clear that the process of activation of leukocytes to make endogenous pyrogen begins with the repression of the genome for endogenous pyrogen and that new messenger RNA must be synthesized.

Considerable progress has been made recently in the characterization of human leukocytic pyrogen. The major portion of human leukocytic pyrogen is a protein with a molecular weight of 15,000 and an isoelectric point of 6.9. A second molecule with a molecular weight of 45,000 and an isoelectric point of 5.1 is also produced. Antibodies to these molecules have been produced and a radioimmunoassay developed (Dinarello et al., 1977). These advances should lead to the measurement of this mediator protein in various disease states. Such measurements will undoubtedly improve our ability to diagnose and to treat specifically febrile states.

The preoptic region of the anterior hypothalamus appears to control body temperature. The hypothalamus also contains the monoamines that are critical for normal thermoregulation. When tumors or vascular accidents have involved this center in patients, hypothermia or, rarely, hyperthermia has occurred. Moreover, the circadian temperature rhythm may be lost in such patients.

The preoptic anterior hypothalamus contains the neurons that respond when endogenous pyrogen is injected in animals, and it seems likely that the same area contains pyrogen-sensitive neurons in man. The mechanism by which endogenous pyrogen causes thermosensitive neurons to increase their firing rate is unknown; however, it has been suggested during the past five years that prostaglandins have a critical role in the production of fever. Mounting evidence suggests that endogenous pyrogen induces synthesis of prostaglandins in the hypothalamus, in which they function as central transmitters in initiation of fever; furthermore, the well-known ability of aspirin and similar drugs to reduce fever appears to be directly related to their ability to block prostaglandin synthesis. Aspirin and other salicylate-like antipyretics do not affect either the production of endogenous pyrogen by leukocytes or the pyrogenicity of the endogenous-pyrogen molecule. The ability of an antipyretic to reduce fever is proportional to its ability to inhibit prostaglandin synthesis. In addition, antipyretics do not lower body temperature in human beings unless fever is present; thus, they do not affect the body temperature of subjects in whom the normal daily temperature is above the mean or exhibits a wide circadian range.

## References

Dinarello, C. A., Renfer, L, and Wolff, S. M.: Human leukocytic pyrogen: Purification and development of a radioimmunoassay. Proc Natl Acad Sci USA 74:4624, 1977.

Dinarello, C. A., and Wolff, S. M.: Pathogenesis of fever in man. N Engl J Med 298:607, 1978.

Nordlund, J. J., Root, R. K., and Wolff, S. M.: Studies on the origin of human leukocytic pyrogen. J Exp Med 131:727, 1970.

Root, R. K., and Wolff, S. M.: Pathogenetic mechanisms in experimental immune fever. J Exp Med 128:309, 1968.

Wolff, S. M., Kimball, H. R., Perry, S., Root, R. K., and Kappas, A.: The biological properties of etiocholanolone. Ann Intern Med 67:1268, 1967.

Wood, W. B., Jr.: Studies on the cause of fever. N Engl J Med 258:1023, 1958.

# 86 SHOCK IN INFECTIOUS DISEASES

## Herbert S. Heineman, M.D.

### DEFINITION

Shock is a syndrome of generalized metabolic failure resulting from prolonged inadequacy of tissue perfusion. Its early clinical manifestations reflect malfunction of those organs most dependent on uninterrupted blood flow, particularly the brain, as well as compensatory adjustments designed to maintain adequate arterial pressure. As these adjustments fail, urinary output decreases and biochemical indices of distorted metabolism, specifically nonoxidative glycolysis with low yield of high energy chemical bonds, are detectable, testifying to the widespread nature of the disorder. In the end, it is the failure of energy production rather than damage to a particular organ that leads to death.

Other terms, such as "circulatory collapse," "circulatory failure," and "hypoperfusion," have been substituted for "shock" in an attempt to pinpoint the specific nature of the derangement. When it occurs as a specific complication of infection, it is referred to as "infectious shock," "septic shock," "bacteremic shock," and even "endotoxin shock." The last three terms specifically implicate bacterial infection and are therefore too restrictive. Because "infectious shock" is sufficiently broad as well as concise, this term will be used in the present chapter.

### ETIOLOGY

Shock may occur in the course of almost any severe infection, but it is particularly characteristic of bacteremia due to gram-negative bacilli. In fact, although gram-negative bacteremia is a common event in seriously ill patients, shock occurs in only a small minority, and the proximate factors leading to this complication have not been identified. The importance of endotoxin, the lipopolysaccharide composing part of all gram-negative cell walls, is readily apparent because it produces a similar syndrome in experimental animals. Partly because of the extensive use of endotoxin as an investigative tool, endotoxin shock is commonly regarded as the prototype of infectious shock. Care must be taken not to use the terms interchangeably, because to do so could lead to incorrect therapy for shock of other causes.

Besides gram-negative bacilli, some of the better known etiologic agents associated with circulatory collapse are meningococci, clostridia, and staphylococci. Shock in meningococcemia is unique because of the hemorrhagic syndrome so commonly associated with it. In the case of clostridia and staphylococci, which contain no endotoxin, protein exotoxins that produce the syndrome in animals and may play an important role in human shock have been identified. The issue is complicated by the production of numerous distinct exotoxins by the same organism. For example, clostridial alpha-toxin, or phospholipase C, appears to be implicated in both hemolysis and progressive tissue destruction and has been identified in the blood during clostridial septicemia (Moore et al., 1976); however, vascular collapse does not correlate with hemolysis, and a role for other exotoxins seems likely.

Shock also occurs in infections due to fungi, rickettsiae, and viruses. Fungal endotoxins with varying effects in experimental animals have been described, but their role in humans is speculative. No shock-producing substances of microbial origin have been identified in rickettsial or viral infections.

## PATHOGENESIS AND PATHOLOGY

The feature that distinguishes infectious shock from shock of other causes (cardiac, hemorrhagic, neurogenic) is the occurrence of widespread circulatory collapse without preceding loss of intravascular fluid or identifiable damage to a critical organ. In this connection, it must be emphasized that many infections do cause damage to specific organs, and this may result in vascular collapse just as if the damage had been inflicted by a noninfectious agent. The detailed mechanisms of shock in such cases will not be described here, but their various causes are listed in Table 1. Recognition of the many distinct mechanisms that produce shock is essential for proper patient evaluation because of the different therapeutic measures appropriate to each.

Understanding of the pathogenesis of true infectious shock in humans has been hampered, first, by the absence of any characteristic pathologic changes that could localize the primary insult; second, by interspecies differences among animals that make extrapolation of experimental observations to humans hazardous; and third, by overlapping but apparently distinct syndromes associated with different infections.

Common to all forms of infectious shock is a maldistribution of blood. Repeated observations and measurements have shown that hypotension and diminished tissue perfusion occur in the presence of normal blood volume. Furthermore, central venous pressure is typically low at the onset, and fluid overloading is often well tolerated, indicating that cardiac decompensation does not play a primary role. By exclusion, this places the functional deficit in the vascular system. On the basis of cardiac output measurements, two kinds of infectious shock have been described, low resistance ("hot dry") and high resistance ("cold clammy"), with features shown in Table 2. Terminally, all patients pass through the cold clammy stage, which represents compensatory sympathetic vasomotor activity.

Low resistance dynamics may be seen in the early stages of shock caused by any bacterial infection, but they are particularly characteristic of shock due to gram-positive cocci. In this stage, hot dry skin is evidence of hyperkinetic circulation, and hemodynamic measurements may reveal a markedly lowered peripheral resistance and a cardiac output well above normal. Despite this, the patient is hypotensive and obtunded, and oxygen extraction by the cells is disproportionately decreased. For a given cardiac index, variation in arteriovenous oxygen difference has been found to reflect the severity of shock and to correlate with ultimate survival (Nishijima et al., 1973). This finding suggests a specific defect in oxygen extraction at the tissue level independent of central hemodynamics. The most widely proposed mechanism is arteriovenous shunting, al-

**TABLE 1.    Classification of Shock Associated with Infection**

| MECHANISM OF SHOCK | DISEASES IN WHICH MECHANISM IS OPERATIVE |
| --- | --- |
| I. Shock Secondary to Identifiable Factors | |
| A. Loss of blood volume | |
| 1. Fluid loss due to capillary damage | Gas gangrene; anthrax; hemorrhagic fever; allergic reaction to antibiotic |
| 2. Fluid loss due to malfunction in fluid regulation | |
| a. Severe diarrhea | Cholera; staphylococcal enteritis |
| b. Adrenal insufficiency | Tuberculosis; histoplasmosis |
| c. Uncontrolled diuresis | Salt-losing pyelonephritis |
| d. Peritoneal exudation | Peritonitis |
| B. Impaired cardiac function | |
| 1. Myocardial failure | |
| a. Myocarditis | Diphtheria; infective endocarditis; influenza; rickettsial infections; trichinosis; toxoplasmosis; trypanosomiasis (Chagas' disease) |
| b. Myocardial infarction | Coronary embolism in infective endocarditis |
| c. Myocardial abscess | Infective endocarditis; septicemia |
| d. Acute valvular insufficiency | Infective endocarditis |
| 2. Cardiac tamponade | |
| a. Pericardial effusion | Pericarditis |
| b. Hemopericardium | Ventricular rupture, as in tuberculous myocarditis |
| 3. Mechanical outflow obstruction | |
| a. Intraventricular blockage | Intraventricular rupture of echinococcus cyst |
| b. Pulmonary embolism | Myocarditis with mural thrombosis |
| C. Loss of arteriolar tone | |
| 1. Destruction of vasomotor center | Bulbar poliomyelitis |
| 2. Anaphylaxis | Rupture of echinococcus cyst; allergic reaction to antibiotic |
| II. True Infectious Shock | |
| Maldistribution of blood | Gram-negative bacillary infection; meningococcemia; clostridial infections; staphylococcal and other gram-positive coccal septicemia; influenza; rickettsial infection; systemic candidiasis |

**TABLE 2.  Two Types of Infectious Shock**

| CHARACTERISTIC | LOW RESISTANCE | HIGH RESISTANCE |
|---|---|---|
| Arterial blood pressure | Low | Low |
| Tissue oxygenation | Decreased | Decreased |
| Cardiac output | High | Low |
| Peripheral vascular resistance | Low | High |
| Venous sequestration | Absent | Present |
| Arteriovenous shunting | Present | Absent |
| Arteriovenous oxygen difference | Low | High |

though it is not clear whether such shunting is truly anatomic or whether normal gas exchange in the capillary bed simply does not take place, thus creating a purely physiologic shunt (Archie, 1976; Seyfer et al., 1977).

High resistance dynamics eventually supervenes in patients dying in shock. In this stage, there is a marked increase in peripheral resistance on the arterial (resistance) side of the circulation, but central venous pressure remains low until cardiac decompensation sets in, indicating pooling of blood in a dilated venous (capacitance) bed. In different animal species, particular venous beds (for example, splanchnic or pulmonary) have been implicated. In humans, specific localization has not been demonstrated, and the defect is believed to be generalized. Venous pooling leads in turn to diminished venous return to the heart, diminished cardiac output, and compensatory arteriolar constriction. Resembling hemorrhagic shock, it is manifested by cold clammy skin, tachycardia, thready pulse, mental obtundation, and oliguria.

In addition to measurable parameters of altered circulatory dynamics, several indices of altered metabolism can be detected. One of these is disseminated intravascular coagulation, most dramatically seen in meningococcemia, in which widespread deposition of fibrin thrombi may occur in small vessels. Because coagulation factors are consumed faster than they can be replaced, the blood may become virtually incoagulable, and this results in hemorrhages into the skin (ecchymoses) and viscera. The adrenal glands are frequently the site of visceral hemorrhage, which results in the so-called Waterhouse-Friderichsen syndrome. Adrenal hemorrhage was originally thought to explain infectious shock on the basis of adrenal insufficiency. However, this explanation is rendered invalid by the inconsistency of pathologic findings in patients dying of infectious shock, the presence of a normal concentration of adrenocortical steroids in the blood, and the failure of physiologic doses of steroids to reverse the course.

The mechanism of disseminated intravascular coagulation is poorly understood. Endotoxins from gram-negative bacteria are capable of activating Factor XII (Hageman factor), which could initiate the clotting cascade. However, this leaves unexplained the occurrence of the same phenomenon in infections due to organisms that do not contain endotoxin.

Whether intravascular coagulation actually plays a role in circulatory collapse is debatable. Although the fibrin thrombi are capable of causing mechanical vascular obstruction, the extent of thrombosis seen at autopsy is highly variable, and in many cases of shock studied during life it is not possible to demonstrate significant consumption of coagulation factors. Finally, even though abnormal coagulation can be arrested by the administration of heparin, clinical trials have failed to show improvement in prognosis as a result. Rather than being part of the fundamental process of shock, intravascular coagulation may be only one of its complications.

Along similar lines, several vasoactive substances appear in the blood of endotoxin-shocked animals — for example, catecholamines, histamine, serotonin, and prostaglandins. Also, animals may become abnormally reactive to adrenalin. However, from all these observations it has not been possible to construct a comprehensive sequence of events that explains exactly how endotoxin or any other microbial product leads to circulatory collapse in infection.

Recent work suggests a possible role for endorphins in shock due to endotoxin (and other causes). In shocked animals, hypotension was dramatically reversed by naloxone, an opiate antagonist (Faden and Holaday, 1980).

Whatever the mechanism of infectious shock, the end result is metabolic failure at the cellular level. It is usually assumed that the critical substance of which cells are deprived is oxygen, and indeed, one of the universal consequences of shock is anaerobic metabolism, which can be demonstrated by increased concentrations of lactate in the blood. However, other metabolic effects not readily linked to oxygen utilization have been described — for example, failure of gluconeogenesis in the face of increased glucose utilization (Archer et al., 1976; Garcia-Barreno and Balibrea, 1978). The basic biochemical lesion has been traced to the inner mitochondrial membrane, whose transport function is believed to be inhibited by products of lipolysis (Jones, 1977).

## CLINICAL MANIFESTATIONS

### History and Physical Findings

In most patients suffering from infectious shock, this complication occurs in a setting in which the infection is already recognized. However, vascular collapse may be the first or only sign of severe infection, especially in elderly debilitated patients who may not demonstrate fever or local symptoms.

Gram-negative bacillary (endotoxin) shock is seen most frequently in patients with urinary infection, when trauma to the infected tissues (for example, cystoscopy) induces a sudden burst of bacteremia. The effects closely resemble those in experimental animals infused with endotoxin. Within a few hours of the traumatic event, the patient suddenly has shaking chills followed by a steep rise in temperature to 39° C or higher with corresponding tachycardia. The blood pressure may begin to fall within less than an hour or several hours later, and this is accompanied by prostration, apprehension, vomiting, and confusion. Examination at first may reveal hot dry skin, systolic pressure of less than 80 mm Hg, and diastolic pressure that is barely recordable. Hyperventilation to the point of respiratory alkalosis is typical of this stage. If the condition is untreated or unresponsive to treatment, peripheral vasoconstriction sets in with cold clammy cyanotic extremities, further diminution in pulse pressure, continued hyperventilation as metabolic acidosis ensues, and oliguria. Various therapeutic measures may prolong life for several days without reversal of shock, until death supervenes.

A similar sequence of events, likewise associated with gram-negative bacteremia, occurs following septic delivery or abortion. It has been observed that, except for pregnant women, patients under 40 infrequently develop shock from gram-negative bacillary infections (Weil, 1977). On the other hand, shock due to meningococcemia is typically a syndrome of children and young adults, because of the age distribution of meningococcal infection. The full-blown syndrome of meningococcemia is easily recognized, but this infection should be suspected even in the absence of meningitis or cutaneous manifestations whenever fever and shock occur in a previously healthy young person.

The clinical syndromes of shock in gram-positive infections differ chiefly in the settings in which they occur. The best recognized pathogens are the histotoxic clostridia — that is, those with the capacity for progressive and destructive tissue invasion — and coagulase-positive staphylococci. Shock is a typical concomitant of clostridial myonecrosis (gas gangrene), a syndrome easily recognized by the presence of large areas of edematous, often crepitant, discolored, and exquisitely tender muscle tissue. Invasion of muscle appears to be a prerequisite, as clostridial cellulitis sparing the muscle is generally not associated with

this degree of systemic toxicity (MacLennan, 1962). However, shock does occur in the absence of myonecrosis when clostridia invade the blood stream from such foci as the large intestine and the uterus. In the latter cases, jaundice, hemoglobinemia, and hemoglobinuria may develop because of intravascular hemolysis, a feature that is usually absent in clostridial myonecrosis.

Shock may occur in staphylococcal septicemia with or without evidence of focal infection. The prototype of shock without focal infection was manifested in a disastrous outbreak in Bundaberg, Australia (Kellaway et al., 1928), following injection of a contaminated diphtheria toxin-antitoxin mixture. Shock and death occurred too rapidly to be explained by widespread staphylococcal infection and was probably caused by exotoxin. In more typical situations, shock occurs during the course of severe staphylococcal infection, such as pneumonia.

A wide variety of other inections may be complicated by shock (Heineman and Braude, 1961), with clinical manifestations basically reflecting the underlying cause. Finally, it must be remembered that shock may be caused by damage or malfunction of specific organs (see Table 1) — for example, myocarditis, adrenal insufficiency, pulmonary embolism, and massive diarrhea. Alertness to these possibilities is especially important because of their unique therapeutic implications.

### Laboratory Tests

Hematologic findings are variable, more often reflecting the underlying infection than any characteristic of shock as such. Depending on the state of endotoxemia, for example, either leukopenia or leukocytosis may be present. Hemoglobin concentration may be normal, elevated (for example, hemoconcentration in cholera), or depressed (for example, intravascular hemolysis in clostridial septicemia). More specifically associated with shock is thrombocytopenia, which is one of the manifestations of disseminated intravascular coagulation. In such a case, other evidence of coagulopathy is also found, such as prolongation of prothrombin time and partial thromboplastin time and the presence of fibrin split products in the blood (Hardaway, 1976).

Findings specific for shock regardless of its cause relate to the deterioration of oxidative metabolism by the tissues — for example, decreased arteriovenous oxygen gradient, metabolic acidosis, and increased serum lactate concentration.

In shock due to bacterial or fungal sepsis, the causal organisms can usually be recovered from the blood. However, blood cultures are more often negative than positive in clostridial myonecrosis and may be so even in gram-negative bacillary shock, emphasizing the role of bacterial toxins apart from the presence of replicating organisms.

Arterial hypoxia has been noted in some patients with infectious shock. Radiologically visible pulmonary infiltrates may be present that resemble those of pulmonary edema. However, they occur in the absence of heart failure and are generally ascribed to "shock lung" or "adult respiratory distress syndrome." In this condition, increased capillary permeability leads to interstitial edema and eventually hyaline membrane formation, with resultant block of alveolocapillary oxygen diffusion.

### COMPLICATIONS AND SEQUELAE

The mortality in infectious shock is high, its incidence generally being quoted at about 70 per cent. A lower incidence is found in series involving predominantly younger patients, specifically women with complications of pregnancy, for in this age group the prognosis is better than in elderly debilitated patients, in whom infectious shock occurs most frequently.

The road to recovery may be marked by acute renal failure due to shock or hemoglobinuria, or by infarction of organs rendered vulnerable to ischemia through occlusive arterial disease of old age, such as the myocardium or brain. Peripheral gangrene may be seen even in young subjects with shock-related coagulative disorders, as in meningococcemia.

In addition, there may be sequelae related to damage done by the infection itself or by heroic therapeutic measures, such as surgery, corticosteroids, and toxic antibiotics.

### DIAGNOSIS

The diagnosis of infectious shock is easy in the typical case, and it can be made by an alert observer before serious damage is done. There are two diagnostic signs: (1) presence of infection, and (2) falling blood pressure without hemorrhage or cardiac failure. These easily recognized signs are emphasized because if a patient has already been in shock for several hours before his hypotensive state is noticed, damage to cellular metabolic functions may have already been done and such damage will be progressively harder to reverse. On the other hand, since hypotension occurs very early in the course, close monitoring of vital signs in patients with severe infections, and especially in those who have just undergone manipulation of infected pelvic organs, is the key to early diagnosis and eventual recovery.

Besides hypotension, patients in shock may exhibit hyperventilation, confusion, apprehension, prostration, and vomiting. Depending on the type of circulatory derangment, the skin may be hot and dry or cold and clammy.

Circulatory insufficiency at the tissue level is recognized most easily by oliguria (hourly urine output of less than 20 ml) and subsequent increases in concentrations of blood urea and creatinine and a decrease in bicarbonate. If laboratory facilities for its determination are available, excess lactate will be found in the serum (more than 16 mg/dl), specifically indicating inadequate tissue oxygenation.

### TREATMENT

The aims of treatment in infectious shock are control of the infection and correction of the circulatory disturbance. On the basis of the relative roles of the infecting organism and the circulatory disturbance, patients may be divided into five groups.

*Group 1:* Specific antibiotic treatment for the infection is available; for example, shock cases due to bacteria, rickettsiae, and fungi. Infection and shock must be treated simultaneously.

*Group 2:* Specific antibiotics are available to combat the organism but not its effects; for example, gas gangrene and diphtheria. Surgery and administration of antitoxin may be indicated, although the value of antitoxin in the treatment of shock has not been proved in either gas gangrene or diphtheria.

*Group 3:* No specific antibiotic treatment for the infection is available; for example, shock cases due to viruses. The objective of therapy is to sustain life long enough to allow the host to control the infection.

*Group 4:* Specific antibiotic treatment is available but not critical, since invasion of tissues by the infecting organism is not a significant feature of the illness; for example, cholera.

*Group 5:* The potential for shock continues to exist even after the infection is under control; for example, pulmonary embolism from myocarditis, coronary embolism from endocarditis, chronic sequelae of poliomyelitis, and tuberculous adrenal insufficiency.

When it is recalled that, in addition to the foregoing possibilities, some infections can cause shock in more than one manner, the necessity for an accurate appraisal of the situation becomes obvious.

### TREATMENT OF INFECTION

The urgency of treatment of patients in shock necessarily will modify the approach to selection of antibiotics. However, since the object of antibiotic therapy should always be to eliminate the infection, the guiding principle here, as in less desperate situations, should be to identify the etiologic organism as soon as possible and to prescribe an optimal antibiotic regimen to which it is sensitive. Unfortunately, there is no time to withhold treatment, so that other guides to the selection of the proper drugs must be employed. The history is often helpful in this regard. For example, a sudden temperature elevation and shock occurring in a patient with an indwelling urethral catheter is presumptive evidence of bloodstream invasion by an organism originating in the urinary tract. If the results of a recent urine culture are available, one may assume that the same organism is responsible for infection of both urine and blood. Physical examination occasionally is so typical of a specific infection that antibiotic therapy can be chosen on this basis alone. A good example is the child or young adult with an acute illness characterized by fever, nuchal rigidity, purpura, and shock. Meningococcemia should be suspected and treated with large intravenous doses of potassium penicillin G or, in the case of penicillin allergy, chloramphenicol sodium succinate.

Sometimes the smear from a lesion is sufficiently characteristic to allow positive identification, as in gas gangrene, meningococcal infection (spinal fluid or exudate from a punctured petechia), and staphylococcal pneumonia. In the infrequent cases of septicemia that occur without an obvious focus of infection, it is wise to use a combination of antibiotics that can be expected to cover most possibilities, such as a cephalosporin and an aminoglycoside. An anti-*Pseudomonas* beta-lactam antibiotic may be indicated in patients susceptible to *Pseudomonas* infection, as in leukemia, severe burns, or following long hospitalization.

When shock is due to mechanical factors, as in pulmonary embolism from a mural thrombus, myocardial infarction from coronary embolism in bacterial endocarditis, or Addisonian crisis in tuberculosis of the adrenals, the infection itself generally demands less urgent treatment, since it is not the immediate presence of the bacteria that causes circulatory collapse.

## TREATMENT OF SHOCK

The prognosis in shock could probably be improved if it were possible to address the basic cellular lesions that underlie collapse of normal energy metabolism. Unfortunately, these lesions are only beginning to be understood, so that there is still no foundation for the development of a specific therapeutic strategy. Based on present knowledge, the only rational objective of therapy can be to restore the circulation. The agents employed, listed in order of importance, are (1) fluids, (2) vasoactive drugs, (3) adrenal corticosteroids, and (4) digitalis. Additional measures include assisted ventilation and, questionably, anticoagulation.

### Fluids

Replenishment of the venous bed is always the first consideration and is frequently all that is needed. It is understood, of course, that the need for extra fluid is created not by dehydration (except in fluid-losing conditions such as cholera) but by an abnormal increase in the capacity of the vascular bed owing to loss of venous tone. In the early stages, simply ensuring an adequate venous return to the right atrium will result in adequate cardiac output. However, myocardial depression may limit the ability of the heart to handle the volume of fluid necessary to reverse shock, at which point further fluid loading would result in pulmonary edema. To avoid this, the pre-load of the heart should be carefully monitored. The simplest measurement is that of central venous pressure, which is done by means of a catheter opening in the superior vena cava just outside the right atrium. As long as the pressure does not exceed 10 cm saline, infusion of fluids can safely be continued; above 15 cm saline, there is danger of overloading the heart. However, since the real danger to life is pulmonary edema, many authorities feel that a more appropriate measurement is that of the left atrial filling pressure, which can be closely approximated by the pulmonary wedge pressure. The latter is obtained through a balloon-tipped catheter passed through the right cardiac chambers and pulmonary artery as far as it will go, at which point the pulmonary venous pressure is reflected back into it. Continued infusion is safe as long as the pulmonary wedge pressure is less than 15 mm Hg; above 20 mm Hg, there is danger of pulmonary edema.

The fluid most commonly used for replenishment, when there has been no extravascular fluid loss, is normal saline. If there has been exudation of fluids through capillary leakage, as in gas gangrene or peritonitis, or through inflammatory diarrhea, as in shigella dysentery, it is rational to use a colloid such as 5 per cent human serum albumin.

If the maximum tolerated amount of fluid does not reverse the shock state, the rate of infusion must be reduced to the minimum necessary to maintain patency of the access line, and therapeutic efforts are continued with vasoactive agents.

## Vasoactive Drugs

In contrast to fluid loading, which simply fills the vascular bed to its exaggerated capacity, the aim of vasoactive drugs is to alter the capacity of the vessels selectively to overcome specific abnormalities of blood distribution. In theory, this should be the obvious first line of approach, but the fact is that no drug with the right selectivity has been identified. It must be remembered that the two recognized defects of distribution are dilatation of the venous bed and arteriovenous shunting. Defects in cardiac output and arteriolar tone are not primary in most cases, yet all vasoactive drugs in use affect cardiac performance and arteriolar tone predominantly. The only advance made in the past several decades has been identification of effective beta-adrenergic drugs, such as isoproterenol and dopamine, that raise the blood pressure by increasing the cardiac output while decreasing peripheral resistance, thereby increasing total blood flow. Their vasomotor effect is opposite from that of alpha-adrenergic drugs, such as noradrenalin and metaraminol, whose antihypotensive action is based primarily on increase in peripheral resistance; these drugs may actually decrease tissue perfusion, so that the metabolic insult is aggravated at the same time that central arterial pressure is increased.

Isoproterenol has been used successfully but nowadays is not favored because of its tendency to increase ventricular irritability and bring about potentially dangerous arrhythmias, to increase myocardial oxygen demand, and to shunt blood from the viscera to skeletal muscle. Dopamine lacks these adverse cardiac effects and shunts blood to the viscera, a specific distributive effect aptly termed "dopaminergic" (Reid and Thompson, 1975). This drug is administered by intravenous drip at an initial rate of 2 to 20 $\mu$g/kg body weight/minute, then titrated to the desired response (see Monitoring section below).

## Adrenal Corticosteroids

Steriods are considered by many to be useful therapeutic agents in treatment of infectious shock, although their action, unlike that of fluids and vasoactive drugs, is not immediately reflected in hemodynamic measurements. It is not clear whether their mechanisms of action involve their anti-inflammatory effect (Cline and Melmon, 1966), a direct effect on the circulation (Sambhi et al., 1965), or some as yet undetected property, although the need for superpharmacologic doses suggests mechanisms distinct from those involved in other applications of these agents. Methylprednisolone and dexamethasone in respective loading doses of 30 mg/kg and 3 mg/kg, followed by fractional doses every 4 to 6 hours for up to 48 hours, illustrate the order of magnitude of the dosage used. Significant reduction in mortality was found in a prospective double-blind, controlled study with these drugs (Schumer, 1976). The possibility that steroids might impair resistance to infections is generally considered of secondary importance in these desperate situations, especially since antibiotic coverage is provided. Because their effect is delayed by several hours, the loading dose of steroids should be given as soon as it is clear that fluid loading alone is insufficient.

## Digitalis

Myocardial depression can occur in sepsis, and failure of cardiac output to increase in response to increasing pulmonary wedge pressure has been shown to correlate with mortality (Weisel et al., 1977). It seems appropriate, therefore, to digitalize a patient in whom central venous or pulmonary wedge pressure rises rapidly during fluid infusion without satisfactory clinical response. Caution is necessary in patients with myocarditis or myocardial anoxia because these states heighten susceptibility to the toxic effects of digitalis, and dangerous arrhythmias may result.

## Assisted Ventilation

In certain patients, arterial hypoxemia complicates shock, possibly because of intrapulmonary arteriovenous shunting or alveolocapillary block due to "shock lung." In these patients, oxygen administered by intermittent positive pressure or positive end-expiratory pressure may be helpful (Ledingham and McArdle, 1978).

Oxygen under pressure has been advocated for the treatment of severe clostridial infections because of its proposed inhibition of toxin production. Although opinion regarding its true value and potential hazards is divided, it is commonly used in centers equipped with hyperbaric chambers (Darke et al., 1977).

## Anticoagulants

The abnormal measurements of coagulation factors in disseminated intravascular coagulation (prothrombin time, partial thromboplastin time, fibrin split products) can frequently be reversed by heparin. However, several clinical trials have failed to convince investigators that anticoagulation significantly affects the outcome. As a result, this measure is not recommended in infectious shock.

## MONITORING THERAPY IN THE SHOCK PATIENT

Since the two most important therapeutic measures, namely, fluids and vasoactive drugs, are titrated on an hour-to-hour or minute-to-minute basis, and overtreatment may have serious adverse effects, it is important to monitor the response accurately and quantitatively. Measurement of blood pressure, which is so useful in the initial diagnosis, has only limited usefulness once vasoactive drugs are used, since central arterial pressure may correlate very poorly with tissue blood flow. A more relevant criterion of response is one that measures end-organ performance. The most readily available is urine output, increase in which is usually taken as indicative of increased renal perfusion. Less readily measured on a continuing basis but valuable as an indicator of anaerobic metabolism is serum lactate, which should decrease as the shock state is reversed.

## PROPHYLAXIS

Since shock is a complication of severe infection, its prevention lies in the timely and effective treatment of infection when this is possible. One approach is carefully selected antibiotic prophylaxis for invasive procedures likely to be complicated by local infection or bacteremia, for example, surgery on the urinary tract (Sullivan et al., 1973), gastrointestinal and biliary tracts (Stone et al., 1976), and pelvic organs (Roberts and Homesley, 1978).

### References

Archer, L., Benjamin B., Lane, M. D., and Hinshaw, L. B.: Renal gluconeogenesis and increased glucose utilization in shock. Am J Physiol 231:872, 1976.

Archie, J. P., Jr.: Systemic and regional arteriovenous shunting in endotoxic and septic shock in dogs. Surg Forum 27:55, 1976.

Cline, M. J., and Melmon, K. L.: A possible explanation of the anti-inflammatory action of cortisol. Science 153:1135, 1966.

Darke, S. G., King, A. M., and Slack, W. K.: Gas gangrene and related infection: Classification, clinical features and aetiology, management and mortality. A report of 88 cases. Br J Surg 64:104, 1977.

Faden, A., and Holaday, J.: Experimental endotoxin shock: The pathophysiologic function of endorphins and treatment with opiate antagonists. J Infect Dis 124:229, 1980.

Garcia-Barreno, P., and Balibrea, J. L.: Metabolic responses in shock. Surg Gynecol Obstet 146:182, 1978.

Hardaway, R. M., III: Gram-negative shock. Antibiot Chemother 21:208, 1976.

Heineman, H. S., and Braude, A. I.: Shock in infectious diseases. Disease-a-Month, October, 1961.

Jones, G. R. N.: The basic biochemical lesion in shock. Biochem Soc Trans 5:213, 1977.

Kellaway, C. H., MacCallum, P., and Tebbutt, A. H.: Report of the Royal Commission of Enquiry into the Fatalities at Bundaberg. Med J Austral 2:2, 38, 1928.

Ledingham, I., and McArdle, C. S.: Prospective study of the treatment of septic shock. Lancet 1:1194, 1978.

MacLennan, J. D.: The histotoxic clostridial infections in man. Bacteriol Rev 26:177, 1962.

Moore, A., Gottfried, E. L., Stone, P. H., and Coleman, M.: Clostridium perfringens septicemia with detection of phospholipase C activity in the serum. Am J Med Sci 271:59, 1976.

Nishijima, H., Weil, M. H., Shubin, H., and Cavanilles, J.: Hemodynamic and metabolic studies on shock associated with Gram negative bacteremia. Medicine 52:287, 1973.

Reid, P. R., and Thompson, W. L.: The clinical use of dopamine in the treatment of shock. Bull Johns Hopkins Hosp 137:276, 1975.

Roberts, J. M., and Homesley, H. D.: Low-dose carbenicillin prophylaxis for vaginal and abdominal hysterectomy. Obstet Gynecol 52:83, 1978.

Sambhi, M. P., Weil, M. H., and Udhoji, V. N.: Acute pharmacodynamic effects of glucocorticoids. Cardiac output and related hemodynamic changes in normal subjects and patients in shock. Circulation 31:523, 1965.

Schumer, W.: Steroids in the treatment of clinical septic shock. Ann Surg 184:333, 1976.

Seyfer, A. E., Zajtchuk, R., Hazlett, D. R., and Mologne, L. A.: Systemic vascular performance in endotoxic shock. Surg Gynecol Obstet 145:401, 1977.

Stone, H. H., Hooper, C. A., Kolb, L. D., Geheber, C. E., and Dawkins, E. J.: Antibiotic prophylaxis in gastric, biliary and colonic surgery. Am Surg 184:443, 1976.

Sullivan, N. M., Sutter, V. L., Mims, M. M., Marsh, V. H., and Finegold, S. M.: Clinical aspects of bacteremia after manipulation of the genitourinary tract. J Infect Dis 127:49, 1973.

Weil, M. H.: Current understanding of mechanisms and treatment of circulatory shock caused by bacterial infections. Ann Clin Rev 9:181, 1977.

Weisel, R. D., Vito, L., Dennis, R. C., Valeri, C. R., and Hechtman, H. B.: Myocardial depression during sepsis. Am J Surg 133:512, 1977.

# METABOLIC EFFECTS OF **87** INFECTION

## William R. Beisel, M.D.

Defensive mechanisms that protect the host against invading microorganisms include the inflammatory, phagocytic, and immunologic responses. In addition, cells throughout the body undergo a variety of predictable changes in their metabolic function during a generalized infection. These metabolic responses account for some of the clinical features of infectious illness.

The predictable metabolic changes during infection can be considered physiologic or homeostatic responses, since they appear to contribute to survival. Because similar metabolic responses occur during infections caused by widely different microorganisms, the responses are said to be generalized or nonspecific. The magnitude and duration of generalized metabolic responses are governed by the severity and persistence of an infectious process rather than by its cause. Thus, generalized infectious illnesses are accompanied by fever, increased oxygen consumption, the need to generate additional carbohydrate fuels, redistribution within the body of amino acids, lipids, electrolytes, and minerals, increased utilization of vitamins, and hepatic synthesis of enzymes and "acute phase" serum proteins.

Other metabolic changes may be superimposed upon the broad group of physiologic ones. These additional changes are secondary to localization of an infectious process within a major organ. For example, pneumonia can interfere with gas exchange in the lungs, pyelonephritis can cause uremia, and diarrhea can cause a loss of intestinal fluids and electrolytes. Localized infections can thus produce both generalized illness and single organ dysfunction. In some instances, the metabolic consequences of these combinations can become life-threatening in their severity.

## METABOLIC COSTS OF INFECTION

Certain daily costs must be met in order to maintain host resistance mechanisms. These costs can be expressed in metabolic terms, since they are based on the need for energy-producing substrates to manufacture cells, precursor components, and molecules important to host resistance. For example, new phagocytes, lymphocytes, and epithelial cells must be produced each day; immunoglobulins and other molecules with unique roles in host defense must also be synthesized. As discussed in the next chapter, malnourished patients become increasingly susceptible to infection if they cannot meet the daily nutritional requirements for maintaining resistance mechanisms.

Because fever causes metabolic rates to increase, additional costs are incurred by the patient with fever. These costs must be met either by using fuels already present in body stores or by increasing the intake of calories and other nutrients.

Because a loss of appetite is common during acute febrile illness, metabolic costs are generally met by mobilizing substrates from tissue stores. This mobilization process can be recognized by measurable losses from the body of nitrogen and the other principal intracellular elements (potassium, phosphorus, magnesium, sulfur, and zinc), and by a loss of body weight and muscle mass. Other metabolic costs are met by changing the patterns of cellular metabolism by using biochemical pathways already available within different tissues. Some of these pathways must be augmented by manufacturing additional enzymes. If an infection is not rapidly controlled, its metabolic costs can deplete body stores of vital nutrients.

Metabolic costs of a curable infection continue to increase until after fever has disappeared, and complete recovery from the metabolic consequences of an infection may require several additional weeks or even months. Depleted nutritional stores make the convalescing patient extremely susceptible to a secondary or superimposed infection by new microorganisms. Until stores can be replenished, it is possible for metabolic losses to initiate a vicious cycle of recurring infections and progressive malnutrition.

## IMPORTANCE OF HOST METABOLIC RESPONSES DURING INFECTION

Infectious illness occurs at all ages and is managed by medical practitioners in all specialty fields. Clinicians should understand the biochemical, metabolic, and hormonal events that lead to loss of body nutrients and altered cellular functions. If the clinician can predict the most likely time of onset, magnitude, and duration of important metabolic responses, he should be able to plan optimal supportive care as an adjunct to antimicrobial drug therapy. It is important to anticipate and recognize the special metabolic complications of infection that are immediate threats to survival.

## INCREASED DEMANDS FOR METABOLIZABLE ENERGY

One of the principal metabolic effects of a febrile infection is the increase in oxygen consumption. The basal metabolic rate increases about 13 per cent for each degree (Centigrade) rise in body temperature. The increased demand for cellular energy develops at the same time that anorexia causes a decline in food intake.

During simple starvation in the absence of infection, the energy needs of the tissues are met chiefly by lipids. These include free fatty acids obtained from adipose tissue and ketones synthesized from fatty acid precursors within the mitochondria of liver cells. Because the use of glucose is curtailed, less is manufactured. These metabolic adjustments to simple starvation allow the body to conserve protein and amino acid stores and to minimize nitrogen losses.

Infectious illnesses are generally accompanied by a reduction in food intake, but the usual metabolic adjustments to simple starvation are not made. Rather, glucose production is stimulated and ketone body production is inhibited. During infection, readjustments take place in metabolic pathways of individual cells and tissues, especially in muscle and liver cells. The endogenous metabolism of body fats, carbohydrates, and proteins are all involved in this process. While free fatty acids continue to be used as major sources of fuel, most of the extra requirements for cellular energy are supplied by glucose. Glucose production is speeded up within the liver by using amino acids as major additional substrates. Amino acids move more rapidly than usual from serum into liver cells. At the same time, large quantities of additional glucose-producing free amino acids, namely, alanine and glutamine, are manufactured and released by skeletal muscle for transport via plasma into the liver. Skeletal muscle contains the largest source of "labile" body protein — protein that can be degraded rapidly during an infection to yield free amino acids for use in other tissues. Some of the newly released branched-chain amino acids (leucine, isoleucine, and valine) are oxidized in situ and used for fuel in muscle cells. Nitrogen groups released by this process are used within muscle for the synthesis of alanine and glutamine. The body thus seems willing to degrade the proteins in skeletal muscle and other somatic tissues to produce amino acids that maintain visceral organ functions, generate energy, and manufacture new cells and proteins.

All the sugar-regulating hormones help stimulate or modulate the increased production and release of glucose by the liver. Plasma concentrations of glucagon, insulin, glucocorticoids, catecholamines, and growth hormone increase. Thyroid hormones are also used more rapidly.

The increased hepatic output of glucose leads to high blood glucose values and a larger glucose pool. A speedier turnover of glucose within this larger pool is caused by its increased use as a cellular fuel.

Severe hypoglycemia, accompanied by a fall of body temperature to subnormal values, can occur if the liver fails to maintain its output of glucose. Failure of hepatic glucose production is generally due to one of two basic mechanisms: (1) depletion of the supply of substrates or (2) failure of the molecular mechanisms required for producing glucose (hepatic cell failure).

Substrate depletion accounts for severe hypoglycemia during bacterial sepsis in newborns. Because infants are born with little skeletal muscle, their stores of "labile" protein are too limited to support a prolonged need for glucose production.

Failure of hepatic cells is usually caused by direct injury to the cells by viruses, such as hepatitis or yellow fever viruses, or by bacterial products such as endotoxin. Liver cells may also fail to synthesize glucose during the terminal stages of overwhelming infections.

## ALTERATIONS IN LIPID METABOLISM

In addition to producing more glucose during acute infections, liver cells accelerate lipid metabolism. The hepatocellular uptake of plasma free fatty acids is increased. Production of triglycerides within liver cells is accelerated and more triglycerides move into the plasma. Some triglycerides may also accumulate as droplets in liver cells and cause fatty metamorphosis.

On the other hand, less free fatty acids are used for the synthesis of ketone bodies than would normally be expected during fasting. Increased release of insulin from the pancreas, a common secondary manifestation of generalized infection, and the lipogenic action of insulin on hepatic cells account for this curtailment in production of ketone bodies. As a result, ketone bodies are not made available to meet body energy requirements. Curtailment of ketone body production is thus a physiologic hormonal response during infection rather than a pathologic breakdown of biochemical pathways.

According to evidence obtained with isotope tracers, the liver, in addition to increasing its output of triglycerides, produces and releases more cholesterol and phospholipids during infection. Since these lipids are all released into plasma as lipoproteins, the liver must produce lipid transport proteins, but little is known about the mechanisms that regulate the rates of lipid release into plasma. However, changes in plasma lipid concentrations are controlled by the rates of lipid removal (or utilization) as well as by changes in the rates of lipid production. Plasma cholesterol, phospholipid, free fatty acid, and triglyceride values vary individually during different infections or even during different stages of a single infection. A massive accumulation of triglycerides is consistently observed during gram-negative sepsis and may give the plasma a milky appearance. Triglycerides accumulate because of increased hepatic production and decreased activity of the lipolytic enzymes that initiate cellular removal of triglycerides from plasma.

## CHANGES IN PROTEIN AND AMINO ACID METABOLISM

All aspects of protein metabolism are affected by infection. Every host defense mechanism depends on the presence or function of some kind of body protein, whether it is a cellular enzyme, a structural protein, a cell membrane receptor, an immunoglobulin, a transport protein, a component of the complement, kinin, or coagulation systems, or some other plasma protein. Infection causes cells to speed up the production of some proteins, to slow the production of others and at the same time to break down "labile" body proteins into free amino acids.

During acute infections, plasma albumin values decline. The catabolism of skeletal muscle proteins exceeds their rate of production, and increased quantities of free amino acids are released into plasma. Despite the entry of more free amino acids into plasma, there is a still greater increase in uptake of amino acid by the liver. As a result, plasma concentrations of most free amino acids decline, especially the branched-chain group.

Free amino acids are used to produce phagocytic and lymphoid cells and to maintain the functional and structural integrity of other tissues. The liver also increases production of certain enzymes and the "acute phase" plasma proteins. These include C-reactive protein, haptoglobin, alpha$_1$-antitrypsin, ceruloplasmin, fibrinogen, and others.

Before amino acids are used for producing glucose, their amino nitrogen must be removed from the carbon skeleton. This nitrogen is converted into urea within the hepatic cells and excreted in the urine. Increased free tryptophan in liver cells is shunted into the serotonin pathway or degraded via the kynurenine pathway for excretion as urinary diazo-positive reactants.

Because of the increased use of amino acids to produce glucose and urea, losses of nitrogen in the urine are high during the acute stages of most febrile infections. Additional nitrogen is lost by sweating, by vomiting or diarrhea, or by nasal secretion and sputum production during respiratory tract infections. The diminished intake of nitrogen-containing foods in combination with continued losses causes negative nitrogen balance.

Nitrogen balance does not become negative during the incubation period of an infection, but begins to be negative soon after the onset of fever. Losses of body nitrogen may reach 10 to 15 g per day if fever is high; cumulative total losses may exceed 100 g during the course of an acute illness. Large daily losses of nitrogen cannot be sustained indefinitely. If an infection becomes subacute or chronic, the body again approaches a state of nitrogen equilibrium, but at a cachectic level.

After recovery, nitrogen balance should become strongly positive as degraded proteins are resynthesized. The process of rebuilding nitrogen stores can be speeded up by increasing the dietary intake of high quality protein foods, especially during early convalescence.

## CHANGES IN MINERAL METABOLISM

Principal body minerals undergo a complex variety of changes during acute infection. Large amounts of some minerals are lost from the body, while others show either a physiologic redistribution or a sequestration in certain tissues. Minerals of soft tissue are lost during acute infections roughly in parallel with the losses of body nitrogen. The negative balances are caused by the combination of diminished dietary intake plus losses in the urine or feces of magnesium, phosphorus, potassium, sulfur, and zinc. Change in calcium stores is generally minimal unless long-term immobilization is a component of the illness, as in paralytic poliomyelitis. Similarly, deficits of body phosphorus appear to reflect losses from soft tissue rather than bone.

Although negative phosphorus balance generally parallels that of nitrogen, phosphorus losses during the period of early symptoms are also influenced by changes in acid-base balance. When fever occurs, respiratory rates become faster. The increased loss of carbon dioxide causes respiratory alkalosis accompanied by a transient disappearance of phosphorus through sweat and urine. During infections characterized by severe or protracted diarrhea, potassium ions escape by way of the intestine. This loss of potassium from the tissues may be large enough to produce the vacuolar changes in kidney tubules and myocardial cells characteristic of potassium deficiency.

Each of the three most widely studied essential trace minerals—iron, zinc, and copper—undergoes an abrupt redistribution within the body during infectious illnesses. These changes are under physiologic control mechanisms and are stimulated by inflammatory responses and activation of phagocytic cells. The concentrations of iron and zinc abruptly decline in the plasma as they are taken up by the liver. These two minerals become physiologically "sequestered" within cellular storage sites. Iron is held as hemosiderin or ferritin, while zinc is bound within liver cells to newly synthesized metallothionein. Copper, on the other hand, is secreted by the liver into plasma as a component of newly synthesized ceruloplasmin.

A rapid decline in plasma iron and zinc concentrations may precede the onset of fever, while the increase in plasma copper follows soon afterward. Since only the "loosely bound" fractions of plasma zinc move into the liver, plasma values of zinc rarely fall more than 50 per cent. In contrast, plasma iron may fall to undetectable values, leaving the iron-binding capacity of plasma almost entirely unsaturated. At the same time, plasma copper and ceruloplasmin values may double or triple.

Physiologic sequestration inhibits the incorporation of iron into hemoglobin and eventually causes the "anemia of infection." This process cannot be reversed by oral or parenteral iron. In addition to its temporary sequestration within the liver, appreciable quantities of zinc may be lost in the urine. The redistribution of iron, zinc, and copper are reversed after recovery from infection. Little is known about the responses of other trace minerals.

## CHANGES IN ELECTROLYTE AND WATER METABOLISM

Fluid and electrolyte responses vary greatly during different infectious diseases. Imbalances can cause death, either from severe dehydration or from fluid overload.

In most acute infections, an increased adrenal output of aldosterone during fever causes renal tubular cells to reabsorb sodium and chloride. This mechanism accounts for the virtual disappearance of these electrolytes from urine and their retention in body fluids, and for a secondary increase in the extracellular fluid volume. Recovery from an acute period of fever may be followed by diuresis in early convalescence.

Retention of body water can also be caused by "inappropriate" secretion of antidiuretic hormone from the posterior pituitary. This phenomenon is common in infections of the central nervous system and may occur during severe generalized infections. Some severe infections may also be complicated by the accumulation and sequestration of sodium within cells that results in declining plasma sodium concentrations. Attempts to correct low sodium values with saline may lead to acute cardiac failure or cerebral edema. If low plasma sodium values during severe infections cannot be explained by losses from the body, the patient should be managed by careful restriction of fluid and sodium intake until the total daily urine volume consistently increases.

On the other hand, diarrhea may produce massive loss of extracellular fluids and electrolytes. In cholera or severe enterotoxic diarrhea, fluid loss may lead to hypovolemic shock and death. Therapy requires prompt resuscitation with isoosmotic saline and correction of concomitant acidosis and potassium deficiency.

## ACID-BASE DISTURBANCES

Pathogenic mechanisms may produce a wide variety of acid-base abnormalities during dif-

ferent kinds of infections. Rapid breathing during fever causes excessive loss of dissolved carbon dioxide from the blood and a transient period of uncompensated respiratory alkalosis. In contrast, pneumonia that prevents ventilatory exchange of pulmonary gases leads to oxygen deficits and carbon dioxide retention with respiratory acidosis. Respiratory acidosis can also result from acute poliomyelitis or tetanus, both of which can cause neuromuscular abnormalities that prevent the thoracic movements required for breathing.

Increased cellular generation of organic acids may produce metabolic acidosis. Septic shock or localized capillary-bed stasis can lead to cellular hypoxia, which increases lactic acid production and the severity of metabolic acidosis. Acute intestinal loss of bicarbonate during severe diarrhea can also produce acute metabolic acidosis. On the other hand, the cumulative loss of body potassium that accompanies protracted diarrhea can lead to secondary chronic metabolic alkalosis.

## ENDOCRINE RESPONSES

As alluded to above, certain hormonal actions help to modulate salt and water metabolism and energy-generating responses during infection. In contrast, several major hormones, including thyroid and parathyroid hormones, certain pituitary trophic hormones, and the gonadal steroids have no clearly defined role.

The adrenal glucocorticoid hormones serve a central but largely "permissive" role. These steroids are necessary to allow some molecular mechanisms to function in hepatic cells. The adrenal secretion of cortisol increases several fold early in the course of fever. This increase in cortisol secretion is accompanied by smaller increases in the adrenal output of ketosteroids and pregnanetriol. These increases do not persist beyond the onset of recovery. Increased adrenal output is never of sufficient magnitude or duration to produce negative nitrogen balances or the other physiologic changes known to accompany the administration of pharmacologic doses of synthetic glucocorticoid hormones.

Failure of hepatic enzyme systems during overwhelming infections may permit the plasma concentration of cortisol to reach unusually high levels. Conversely, destruction of the adrenals by infection prevents steroid production and leads to death unless this complication is recognized and treated. If an infection becomes subacute or chronic, steroid output also falls into a subnormal range.

Substances released by phagocytes and lymphocytes also have hormone-like functions that can stimulate both local and generalized physiologic responses. These biologically active products include prostaglandins, lymphokines, enzymes, and endogenous mediators such as those that initiate fever, mobilize neutrophils, or cause trace mineral redistribution.

### SUMMARY

Generalized infectious illnesses are accompanied by a broad group of metabolic, biochemical, and endocrinal responses. Although caused by many different molecular mechanisms, generalized metabolic changes occur in relatively predictable patterns related to the onset, severity, and duration of fever. These changes include the catabolism of skeletal muscle proteins, acceleration of hepatic gluconeogenesis, ureagenesis and lipogenesis, inhibition of ketogenesis, retention of extracellular salt and water, loss of major intra-

cellular elements, and redistribution within the body of certain trace minerals. Other metabolic changes develop if an infection becomes localized in a predominant organ system. Some metabolic consequences of infection, which include hypoglycemia, hypovolemia, fluid overload, and failure of various key organs, are life-threatening.

The views of the author do not purport to reflect the positions of the Department of the Army or the Department of Defense. (Para. 4-3, AR 360-5.)

### References

Beisel, W. R.: Effect of infection on nutritional needs. In Rechcigl, M. (ed.): Handbook of Nutrition and Food: Nutritional Requirements. Cleveland, CRC Press, Inc., 1980.

Beisel, W. R., Blackburn, G. L., Feigin, R. D., Keusch, G. T., Long, C. L., and Nichols, B. L. (eds.): Symposium on Impact of Infection on Nutritional Status of the Host. Am J Clin Nutr 30:1203, 1439, 1977.

Suskind, R. M. (ed.): Malnutrition and the Immune Response. New York, Raven Press, 1977.

# 88 MALNUTRITION AND INFECTION

## Gerald T. Keusch, M.D.

*Sorrow may be fated, but to survive and grow is an achievement all its own.*

R. COLES
*Children of Crisis, 1964*

Malnutrition of the affluent as well as the poor, whether because of excess, insufficiency, or inappropriate choice of foods, is a common malady throughout the world. In developing countries the most common clinical forms of malnutrition are due either to insufficiency of food per se, resulting in marasmus, or to inadequacy of specific nutrients in the diet including protein, vitamin A, or iron, resulting in kwashiorkor, xerophthalmia, and anemia, respectively. However, such "pure" inadequacies rarely exist, and it is reasonable to suggest that most malnutrition is caused by a lack of both protein and calories, for which the term protein-calorie malnutrition (PCM) will be used. Upon this base of PCM are engrafted specific nutrient inadequacies that differ in type from one country to the next.

In developing nations the youngest in society are the principal targets of PCM. In industrialized nations adults are at greatest risk, developing PCM secondary to debilitating chronic dis-

eases, neoplasms, alcoholism, inflammatory bowel disease, or renal failure. Recently, adult PCM has also been recognized in hospitalized patients who are maintained on the routine, semistarvation regimens of parenteral fluid and electrolytes during the treatment of many acute medical and surgical illnesses. In both situations malnutrition greatly exaggerates both the susceptibility to infectious agents and the severity of the illnesses they produce. Because infection itself causes losses of nutrients by a number of mechanisms, the interaction of infection and malnutrition may lead to progressive debilitation and increased mortality. This interaction has been termed "synergistic," but it is difficult to define this synergism precisely. The minimum consequence in young children is impaired growth that may result in permanent stunting and failure to achieve optimal intellectual potential. In adult PCM, the analogous end of the spectrum may be impaired wound healing or infection that prolongs hospitalization. In both age groups, the other end of the spectrum is death. In developing countries the overall mortality in childhood from birth to age 7 often reaches 50 per cent, primarily because of the combined forces of infection and malnutrition.

Several important points have emerged from recent studies in developing countries. First, malnutrition and infectious diseases must be understood as ecologic problems that are interrelated, not only to each other but also to cultural, sociological, political, and economic factors, for which long-term corrective measures are required. The ultimate solution to these problems lies neither in a simple nutritional supplement nor in a vaccine, for example, but in the complex and difficult process of national development. Second, PCM is usually caused by a succession of insults, most often infections, over an extended period of time rather than by a single event or even multiple events at a particular time. Third, intrauterine events, both nutritional and infectious, may alter in utero development, birth weight, and postnatal growth, and postnatal morbidity and mortality from infectious agents.

The purpose of this chapter is to examine the interaction between malnutrition and infection in sufficient detail to permit the physician to make rational medical decisions for his patients in the short term. The important interactions between nutrition and infection may be broadly classified as effects of infections on nutrition and effects of nutrition on infections.

## EFFECT OF INFECTIONS ON NUTRITION

It has long been known that both acute and chronic infections can cause marked debilitation; for example, acute typhoid fever can result in severe loss of muscle mass and body weight, and tuberculosis was so commonly associated with chronic wasting that it was called consumption. More recent observations, largely by Beisel and colleagues, have shown that even mild infections of well-nourished individuals cause a stereotyped metabolic response with nutritional consequences. The extent of these changes is determined in part by the severity and duration of infection, the nutritional status of the affected person at the time, and cultural responses to illness including alterations in diet and the administration of foods and drugs believed to have medicinal benefits, but which may in fact be harmful. One of the earliest physiologic responses to infection is anorexia. Neither the mechanism nor the purpose of this loss of appetite is known. Many dietary practices, including imposed star-

vation to "rest the bowel" or the provision of bland, poorly nutritious foods that are "easy to digest," probably originated as responses to this anorexia. However, the practices often continue long after the anorexia is past. At this time, young children will voluntarily increase food intake several-fold and achieve positive metabolic balance and "catch-up growth" that will return them to the growth curve they were following when the infection occurred. At precisely this time in early convalescence, cumulative losses of nitrogen, energy stores, trace metals, and other tissue components are at their maximum, and must be restored for the original state of health to be regained.

Fever is another early manifestation of infection. Although some have claimed that the fever response in the malnourished patient is blunted, there are no convincing data to support this anecdotal claim. On the contrary, I have observed that, except in the most severely malnourished subjects, the fever response appears to be intact. While the mechanism of fever production is largely known, its purpose is not. The clearest experiments have been performed with cold blooded lizards challenged with a natural bacterial pathogen, *Aeromonas hydrophila*. Significant increases in survival occur if the animals are allowed to raise their core body temperature (i.e., develop fever) by behavioral modifications when placed in a thermal gradient. Whatever its purpose, fever is a primitive response that would not have withstood the forces of natural selection if it did not have survival value.

Whatever the benefit, fever is not without cost. The extra heat to produce fever comes largely from involuntary work by muscles — the shivering response. It costs the febrile, septic patient an increase in caloric consumption equivalent to 25 to 40 per cent of the resting metabolic expenditure to produce fever, and the source of these extra calories is ultimately his own tissue proteins. Body stores of energy in carbohydrates (glucose and glycogen) are limited and amount to a reserve sufficient for only 12 to 24 hours of survival. Because ketones are not efficiently utilized by the septic patient, perhaps because of hyperinsulinemia, fat reserves are not useful sources of calories. Gluconeogenesis in the liver utilizing amino acids, principally alanine, from muscle is the source of the emergency energy required. Thus, infected patients literally consume themselves as muscle protein is mobilized and transported to the liver for gluconeogenesis and for new protein synthesis as well (vide infra). Alanine used for gluconeogenesis is ultimately wasted because the nitrogen removed during deamination is excreted as urea and the carbon skeleton is oxidized to carbon dioxide and re-

TABLE 1.   Possible Role in Infection of
Certain Acute Phase Plasma Proteins

| ACUTE PHASE PROTEIN | KNOWN OR PRESUMED FUNCTION | POSSIBLE ROLE IN INFECTION |
|---|---|---|
| $\alpha_1$-Acid glycoprotein | Increases platelet adherence to collagen and affects spacing of collagen fibrils | ?Improved wound healing |
| $\alpha_1$-Antitrypsin | Protease inhibitor; inhibition of plasmin and Hageman cofactor | Control of inflammation, induced tissue destruction, and DIC |
| $\alpha_2$-Macroglobulin | Formation of complex with proteases to facilitate their removal | Increased granulocytopoiesis and activation of macrophages |
| C-reactive protein | Binds to phosphocholine groups in cell membranes | Activation of complement system |
| Ceruloplasmin | Copper transport | ? |
| Haptoglobin | Complexes with free plasma hemoglobin to facilitate uptake by mononuclear phagocytes and regulate urinary losses | Reduces iron available to pathogenic bacteria for growth and production of toxins |

moved by respiration. In addition, feedback control of hepatic gluconeogenesis is abrogated so that glucose infusion does not stop the process as it does in starved, noninfected volunteers. Glucose synthesis and oxidation are both increased during sepsis, the former more than the latter, accounting for an increase in the glucose pool size and fasting hyperglycemia. The glucose tolerance test curve becomes abnormal and diabetic in shape, but glucose oxidation is not diminished.

Fever is also the clinically apparent trigger for a number of diverse metabolic effects of infection including: (1) negative metabolic balances for nitrogen, magnesium, potassium, and phosphate; (2) loss of water and electrolytes through sweating and respiratory insensible losses; (3) tachypnea and respiratory alkalosis; (4) increased secretion of adrenocorticosteroids, glucagon, and insulin with numerous secondary metabolic effects. Fever itself is caused by production of a small polypeptide mediator called endogenous pyrogen (EP) that is made and released into the bloodstream by stimulated leukocytes. When EP reaches the hypothalamus it causes an upward resetting of the setpoint in the thermoregulatory center, and body temperature is raised accordingly. The apparent relationship between fever and altered metabolism, however, is not caused by EP activity but by a possibly distinct but analogous mediator (or group of mediators), also produced by white blood cells, called leukocyte endogenous mediator (LEM). Thus, stimulation of leukocytes results in both EP and LEM release, and fever and metabolic changes are therefore parallel phenomena. Administration of EP causes fever; administration of LEM causes release of amino acids from muscle, increased uptake of amino acids by the liver, synthesis of acute phase globulins in the liver, uptake and sequestration of iron, zinc, and other trace metals into hepatic macrophages, and elevations of serum insulin and glucagon. It appears that LEM plays a role in both catabolic and anabolic events during infection.

Although these changes in metabolism may serve body defense mechanisms, they are a form of nutrient wastage when there is no compensatory increase in intake. In fact, anorexia would interfere with increased intake, even if food were available. The synthesis of acute phase proteins, immunoglobulins, and complement and the production of phagocytic and lymphoid cells by the infected child deplete the available precursor materials and interfere with the synthesis of visceral protein. Hypoalbuminemia and cessation of linear growth are the result. Such wastage has been termed "functional," although many of the events, like fever itself, have no well-established beneficial function. Table 1 lists some of the postulated benefits of acute phase plasma proteins. Absolute losses, sequestration of nutrients, and diversion of nutrients to new pathways combine to produce broad disturbances in host nutriture.

## EFFECTS OF MALNUTRITION ON HOST DEFENSES AND RESPONSES TO INFECTIOUS AGENTS

The key feature of the cyclical interaction of nutrition and infection is the adverse effect each has on the other. Thus, many host defense mechanisms are exquisitely sensitive to nutritional deprivation, and this nutritionally induced immunodeficiency plays an important role in increasing the susceptibility to a given inoculum of an infectious agent, as well as the severity of the disease it produces. As already noted, frequent and severe infections may preclude nutritional rehabilitation, because there is insufficient time between episodes to replace cumulative losses.

Specific host defenses can be classified into cellular (phagocytosis and cell-mediated immunity) and humoral (antibody and complement) mechanisms. Normal resistance to infection requires adequate function of all these components because they work in an integrated manner against some infectious agents, and one element of the immune response may be the critical defense against other agents. Although many functional defects can be detected in these four biologic systems in the severely malnourished host, these deficiencies may simply represent end-stage disease and anabolic failure. Developing malnutrition undoubtedly exerts selective influences on host metabolism, so that some pathways are preserved and others are curtailed. Selective changes such as these directly influence the clinical features and manifestations of malnutrition. Therefore, it is the less severely malnourished host who must be understood physiologically in order to identify critical adverse factors amenable to therapy. The limited data available at present suggest early malnutrition significantly impairs cell-mediated immunity, functioning through the T lymphocyte, and synthesis of complement. The function of phagocytes and antibody synthesis are not significantly impaired, although they may be reduced in efficiency and antigen-binding avidity, respectively (Table 2).

With increasing malnutrition, the number and function of circulating T cells diminishes, and the T-cell areas of central (i.e., thymus) and peripheral (i.e., spleen and lymph node) lymphoid organs become depleted of cells. Therefore, reactions dependent upon intact T-cell function may become impaired. This is easily demonstrated by skin test reactivity to tuberculin or other antigens that provoke delayed hypersensitivity. Malnourished individuals do not develop a positive skin test to new antigens nor do they respond normally to previously encountered ones (the recall response). Nutritional rehabilitation restores both recall and normal reactivity to new antigens. Skin responses to tuberculin are more than a diagnostic test for *Mycobacterium tuberculosis* infection. They are a cutaneous example of granuloma formation, the host defense responsible for containing tuberculosis. Thus tuberculosis is highly prevalent in the malnourished and also tends to be widespread and severe because of this failure of the host defenses.

Cell-mediated immunity (CMI) may also be responsible for immunopathology in some diseases such as schistosomiasis or even tuberculosis. Theoretically, deficiency of CMI might lessen the severity of such diseases, and malnutrition might be protective. This is difficult to document in human populations. When a clear-cut decrease in host defenses is balanced against the theoretical benefits from diminished CMI, it is the former that stands out; the adverse consequences far outweigh the possible benefits. For example, the measles rash, a manifestation of cell-mediated immunopathology, may be atypical in the child with malnutrition; however, he may die of giant cell pneumonia because of inadequate CMI in the lung.

The extensive role of complement in host defenses has become clear only in the past few years. Complement-mediated chemotaxis, opsonization, and vascular changes during the inflammatory response may be the critical early defense in pyogenic infections. The alternative pathway of activation of the complement effector sequence is now known to be markedly affected by malnutrition. Serial studies have documented a reversible deficiency in the concentration and functioning of most complement components during malnutrition and nutritional rehabilitation. This repair requires time, and in the interval death from infection may be the ultimate consequence.

Recent investigations have pointed to an ad-

TABLE 2.    Effects of Malnutrition on Host Defense Mechanisms

| MECHANISM | USUAL FUNCTION IN HOST DEFENSE | EFFECT OF MALNUTRITION | |
| | | Severe | Moderate |
| --- | --- | --- | --- |
| Phagotosis | | | |
| Neutrophil | Ingestion and destruction of pyogenic bacteria | Impairment | None |
| Mononuclear phagocyte | Ingestion and destruction of facultative intracellular bacteria and fungi, virus | Impairment | None |
| | Processing of antigen of B-cell and T-cell responses | ? | ? |
| Cell-mediated immunity (T lymphocyte) | Activation of macrophage recruitment, scavenger and bactericidal functions, granuloma formation and delayed hypersensitivity. Killer-cell function for virus-infected cells, or helper function for antibody synthesis to certain antigens | Impairment | Impairment |
| Antibody synthesis (B lymphocyte) | Neutralization or killing of bacteria and other pathogens; neutralization of biologically active products and toxins | Impairment | None ?Decreased antigen-binding affinity for some antigens. |
| Complement | Opsonization, chemotaxis, increased vascular permeability and bacteriolysis. Participation in destruction of virus-infected cells. | Impairment | Impairment |

verse effect of both iron and vitamin A deficiencies on host defense mechanisms. Additional animal and human study is needed to document the extent of this effect and its mechanism. It is likely that a combination of multiple, minor abnormalities in immune defense systems can produce a major defect in the host. Similarly, multiple nutrient deficiencies of minor to moderate degree may interact to produce a significant nutritional impairment.

## THE ARENA OF THE INTERACTION

From the foregoing discussion it is evident that the problems of malnutrition and infection must be considered together because each affects the other significantly. When malnutrition is common, the cure and prevention of infectious diseases must be undertaken with this fact in mind. Traditional preventive medicine intervention such as the use of vaccines may be fraught with failure (polio) or danger (measles) in the malnourished host. A vaccination campaign should not be started without considering the impact of the nutritional state on immune responses. In addition, the problems of containment of the immunization strain of live vaccines, on the one hand, and the development of latent infections with late pathology, on the other hand, become crucial. The same reasoning process tells us that attempts to improve nutrition will be analagous to filling leaky buckets if the problem of infections is not engaged directly. Thus, whether dealing with individual patients or with large populations, whether concerned prinicipally with nutritional status or with the morbidity and mortality of infections, the physician must learn to think of nutrition and infection as interrelated processes. Concern for convalescent care and total nutritional rehabilitation becomes a part of proper therapy when this approach is taken, and the physician becomes a promoter of health as well as an alleviator of disease.

## References

Beisel, W. R., Blackburn, G. L., Feigin, R. D., et al. (eds.): Symposium on Impact of Infection on Nutritional Status of the Host. Am J Clin Nutr 30:1203, 1439, 1977.

Keusch, G. T., and Katz, M.: Malnutrition and infection. In Winick, M. (ed.): Nutrition and Development. New York, Plenum Publishing Corporation, 1978.

Scrimshaw, N. S., Taylor, C. E., and Gordon, J. E.: Interactions of nutrition and infection. WHO Monograph Series No. 57, Geneva, 1968.

Suskind, R. (ed.): Malnutrition and the Immune Response. New York, Raven Press, 1977.

# II Clinical Infectious Diseases

## A UPPER RESPIRATORY AND ORAL INFECTIONS

### PHARYNGITIS AND TONSILLITIS 89

Hans A. Valkenburg, M.D., Ph.D.

### DEFINITION

Pharyngitis and tonsillitis ("sore throat") are usually acute infections that may be limited to those anatomic locations, part of a more generalized respiratory infection, or a manifestation of a systemic illness such as infectious mononucleosis (see Chapter 203). In all cases, tonsillar inflammation is a major manifestation. Usually this syndrome is divided into exudative (membranous) and non-exudative pharyngitis, based on the presence or absence of a tonsillar exudate.

### ETIOLOGY

The most important cause of sore throat, because of the possibility of serious suppurative and nonsuppurative sequelae, is *Streptococcus pyogenes* (group A beta-hemolytic streptococcus; see Chapter 24). Occasionally, groups C and G beta-hemolytic streptococci are responsible, particularly in tropical areas. *Corynebacterium diphtheriae* (see Chapter 90) is still an important cause of pharyngitis in some countries. These bacterial pathogens typically cause an infection that is characterized by tonsillar exudate or a membrane. *Neisseria gonorrhoeae* can also cause exudative pharyngitis. Other bacteria, such as *Neisseria meningitidis* and *Haemophilus influenzae* type B, undoubtedly cause nasopharyngeal infections, but these are either asymptomatic or too nondescript to be recognized as clinical entities.

The majority of pharyngeal infections are non-bacterial. Of patients with nonbacterial pharyngitis, adenovirus can be recovered from about 25 per cent. Other viruses that are often isolated include herpes simplex, coxsackie virus A, and the echovirus group. Primary herpes infection is often manifest as pharyngitis associated with gingivitis; otherwise herpes does not cause pharyngitis. Coxsackieviruses usually cause herpangina (Chapter 100); echovirus pharyngitis may be associated with exanthems, which can simulate rubeola, rubella, or even meningococcemia. Epstein-Barr virus, the agent of infectious mononucleosis, often causes a sort throat. Unlike most other viral infections, it is typically exudative. *Mycoplasma pneumoniae* may also cause a sore throat, although this is usually only one manifestation of a more generalized respiratory infection. Isolated pharyngitis has been produced in volunteers.

### PATHOGENESIS AND PATHOLOGY

#### Streptococcal Pharyngitis

Infection is usually spread by droplets sprayed from air passages, but the organism can also be transmitted by dust or fomites or from skin lesions. Epidemics of tonsillitis or scarlet fever can also originate from contaminated milk or food. The source of infection can be either a carrier or a patient; children are more likely to transmit infection than adults. Nasal carriers are less common than throat carriers but shed large numbers of bacteria and are more infectious (Holmes and Williams, 1958). Convalescent carriers are more likely to harbor M-typable group A streptococci than chronic carriers. M protein confers virulence to the organism (see Chapter 24).

The outcome of streptococcal infection depends on the virulence of the organism and the resistance of the host. Organisms harboring M protein are more virulent, and most epidemic strains are M-typable. In the presence of high antibacterial immunity, that is, antibody to the particular M protein, the streptococcus may fail to become established or may be confined to the surface of the mucosa or skin of the host. When antibacterial resistance is low or the streptococcus is highly virulent, colonization results in tonsillitis or impetigo and suppurative complications, such as lymphadenitis or septicemia. If the invading organism produces large amounts of erythrogenic toxin and antitoxic immunity is also low, the patient may develop scarlet fever. Eradication of a streptococcal infection by antibiotics may permit reinfection with the same M type at a later time owing to insufficient development of type-specific antibodies (Valkenburg et al., 1963). Children who have had tonsillectomies have a lower incidence of symptomatic streptococcal pharyngitis but not of asymptomatic infection nor of nonstreptococcal pharyngitis.

Little information is available about the pathology of streptococcal pharyngitis and tonsillitis. Generalized pharyngeal erythema and edema is characteristic, and a discrete or patchy exudate due to polymorphonuclear cell infiltrates that appears after 12 to 36 hours is common. Deep-seated cellulitis in streptococcal upper respiratory tract infections involves tonsillar and peritonsillar tissues. Spread to regional (cervical) lymph nodes with suppurative lymphadenitis is common. In young children the lymphadenitis may be confused with mumps.

Nonbacterial pharyngitis is usually caused by respiratory viruses that are spread by droplet or direct contact. The viruses multiply locally in the respiratory epithelium. Adenovirus is remarkable because it apparently can remain latent within lymphoid tissue in the oropharynx. Coxsackievirus A is primarily an enterovirus, but large numbers of virus particles can be found in nasal and pharyngeal secretions of patients with herpangina.

## CLINICAL MANIFESTATIONS

The clinical manifestations of streptococcal pharyngitis are determined by the patient's age,

immune status, the virulence of the organism, and the presence of tonsils. In infants there is usually only a mucopurulent nasal discharge and fever. This illness, which lasts about one week, cannot be distinguished from a common cold except by culture. Older children, up to the age of about 3 years, react to infection with mild constitutional symptoms including anorexia, vomiting, fever to 103° F, and listlessness. Purulent coryza is characteristic but nonspecific. Anterior cervical adenitis is usual, and the subacute illness may persist for as long as four to eight weeks.

In older children and adults, streptococcal pharyngitis characteristically begins abruptly with fever, sore throat, vomiting (sometimes with abdominal pain), headache, and malaise. Throat symptoms may not appear for up to 24 hours from onset. If the infectious organism produces erythrogenic toxin and the patient lacks antitoxin, the erythematous punctiform exanthem of scarlet fever develops 12 to 48 hours later.

It must be recognized, however, that a definitive diagnosis of streptococcal pharyngitis cannot be made on clinical grounds. No single characteristic, tonsillar exudate, for example, has a diagnostic sensitivity of greater than 50 per cent. The combination of fever, moderate to marked pharyngeal erythema, and anterior cervical adenitis (with or without tonsillar exudate) is associated with a positive throat culture for group A streptococci in 75 per cent of cases. If there are also palatal petechiae, the diagnostic accuracy approaches 90 per cent. Unfortunately, only a minority of patients with streptococcal pharyngitis have these specific signs. (Stollerman and Bernstein, 1961). The remainder of patients have an illness that cannot be differentiated from nonbacterial pharyngitis. In fact, close to 90 per cent of patients with sore throats have so few complaints that they do not even consult physicians. Many of these sore throats are due to streptococcal infections. Both streptococcal and nonstreptococcal sore throats are self-limited infections that resolve within four to five days. Therefore, the response to empiric therapy does not differ either. Even the most severe streptococcal sore throat resolves by 10 days without treatment.

Diphtheria, when it involves the tonsils and pharynx, usually begins insidiously. The membrane develops after 24 hours and varies in extent from a small patch to a complete tonsillar blanket. It is smooth, white or gray, and adherent. The underlying tissues bleed if the membrane is removed. There is a variable amount of reactive adenitis, which may be dramatic ("bull neck"). In mild cases the membrane sloughs in 7 to 10 days, and the patient recovers. In severe cases, the fever and toxemia increase and progress to stupor, coma, and death within 7 to 10 days.

Viral pharyngitis can mimic streptococcal pharyngitis, including the presence of a tonsillar exudate. There are a few distinct syndromes, however. The punctate vesicles in the soft palate, anterior tonsillar pillars, and uvula are typical and characteristic of herpangina (coxsackievirus A). Infectious mononucleosis is usually associated with generalized lymphadenopathy, splenomegaly, and atypical lymphocytosis. Other viral infections are less characteristic.

## COMPLICATIONS AND SEQUELAE

### Suppurative Complications

The most common suppurative complication of pharyngitis or tonsillitis is peritonsillar abscess. The incidence varies between 1.5 and 4 per cent of all cases of pharyngitis, increases with age, and occurs in men 1.5 times more often than in women. The incubation period is between two and nine days after the onset of the sore throat. Retropharyngeal abscess and otitis media are less frequent complications (each occurs in less than 0.5 per cent of cases); otitis occurs in children. In about half the cases with peritonsillar abscess or otitis, the condition is already present at the time of the first visit to the doctor and therefore could not have been prevented. Tonsillectomy reduces the risk of peritonsillar abscess by approximately 90 per cent.

Erysipelas is now a rare suppurative complication of streptococcal upper respiratory tract infection (see Chapter 206). It is more common in older people with degenerative skin changes in whom it usually involves the face or legs. Erysipelas starts abruptly after an incubation period of about a week with generalized symptoms. Sensations of burning and tightness develop at the site of invasion, and are followed by rapidly spreading erythema. The spreading edge is sharply defined and elevated. There is a marked tendency for recurrences in the same location.

Suppurative lymphadenitis, sinusitis, osteomyelitis of the frontal bone, and thrombophlebitis are rare complications due to local spread of streptococci. Bacteremia is extremely rare.

### Nonsuppurative Sequelae

The most prominent complications of streptococcal pharyngitis and pyoderma are rheumatic fever and glomerulonephritis. Acute rheumatic fever never follows impetigo, but acute glomerulonephritis can be preceded by either streptococcal pharyngitis or pyoderma.

The attack rates for rheumatic fever during an epidemic of a rheumatogenic strain can be as high as 3 per cent in a closed (e.g., school) population but are considerably lower in sample studies of open populations. The attack rates of acute nephritis after infection with a known nephritogenic strain are around 10 to 15 per cent, regardless of the site of the primary infection. The stricter the definition one uses for streptococcal infection, the higher the attack rates for the late sequelae. In patients with characteristic clinical signs and symptoms from whom group A streptococci are isolated and who develop antibodies to streptolysin O, the attack rate for rheumatic fever is 0.95 to 1.70 per cent. For glomerulonephritis, it is 0.19 to 3.40 per cent.

### Scarlet Fever

Scarlet fever results when an erythrogenic strain of streptococcus invades a susceptible host. This complication may follow either throat or skin infections. The onset occurs suddenly with fever, sore throat, and vomiting, although the latter two symptoms may be absent. The exanthem follows within 24 to 36 hours and evolves from above downwards. During the first days, the tongue is covered with a thick white "fur," which peels from the tip and edges in a few days to develop into the typical strawberry tongue. Enanthems and petechiae may be found on the palate. Desquamation of the rash begins four to five days after onset and may persist for weeks if the rash is severe.

## GEOGRAPHIC VARIATION IN DISEASE

In temperate climates more than 60 per cent of all people have at least one attack of sore throat annually, but only 2 per cent of the total population consult their doctor for this complaint. In half of these patients, S. pyogenes is isolated. Based on sample studies, 14 per cent of the general population suffers from a streptococcal sore throat annually. Twenty to 25 per cent of people over 5 years of age carry group A streptococci in their throat, but only 10 per cent of these have a simultaneous sore throat.

In subtropical and tropical areas the incidence of pharyngitis and tonsillitis is not known. However, scarlet fever is rarely observed, and tonsillectomy is seldom performed. On the other hand, skin infections are common and are probably the major source of epidemics of acute nephritis. Carrier studies in schoolchildren suggest that streptococcal infections are about as common in subtropical climates as in temperate zones. This finding corresponds with the high attack rate of rheumatic fever among children in North America.

In tropical Africa, carriage of group A streptococci in the throat is low (about 2 per cent) but is three times higher in the skin. Streptococcal pharyngitis is rare (occurring in less than 0.5 per cent of young schoolchildren), but skin infections occur in more than 7 per cent. Ninety per cent of these skin infections are caused by S. pyogenes.

Crowding and poor socioeconomic conditions contribute to the spread of streptococci, regardless of race or the site of infection. Tonsillectomy reduces carrier rates for streptococci but not the incidence of clinical upper respiratory tract disease (Matanoski, 1972).

Although the attack rates for rheumatic fever and glomerulonephritis are still high in some developing areas of the world, this problem has decreased considerably in the more developed countries over the past 30 years. The reason for this is not the disappearance of streptococcal infections or even the liberal application of antibiotics. More likely explanations are that the virulence of the streptococcus has changed or that the relation between the organism, host, and environment has changed as a result of improved socioeconomic, hygienic, and nutritional conditions.

Available data suggest that in any country 10 to 15 serotypes of S. pyogenes circulate. According to hospital admissions records, rheumatic fever and rheumatic heart disease are still common in poor countries (Strasser, 1978), but the course of streptococcal pharyngitis and diphtheria may be modified by immunity acquired during previous skin infections with these bacteria (Franz et al., 1964).

### DIAGNOSIS

Because streptococcal pharyngitis and tonsillitis cannot be diagnosed from clinical signs and symptoms only, a throat culture has to be done to establish the cause. A single throat culture is about 90 per cent sensitive in diagnosing streptococcal pharyngitis if it is obtained by vigorously swabbing the tonsils and pharynx, inoculating onto a rich agar base with 5 per cent sheep red blood cells, and incubating in a 5 per cent carbon dioxide atmosphere. More than a twofold rise or fall in antibody titers between two serum samples taken at least 3 weeks apart is also absolute evidence for a recent infection. One should be cautious in interpreting titers from a single specimen. In children high ASO titers (e.g., over 1:400 Todd units) may be observed long after a strepto-

coccal infection has occurred. The most common antibodies measured are those against streptolysin O (ASO), DNAase-B, and hyaluronidase. Both ASO and anti-DNAase-B antibodies can be found after uncomplicated streptococcal pharyngitis. Leukocytosis is usually present in streptococcal pharyngitis but is often absent in streptococcal pyoderma and impetigo.

### TREATMENT

Controlled trials of streptococcal pharyngitis have shown that clinical recovery is similar in cases with and without antibiotic treatment (Haverkorn et al., 1971). Eradication of S. pyogenes is most successful after parenteral administration of penicillin. Oral penicillin is less effective because the patients do not take the drug for the obligatory period of 10 days. Persistent carriage of the same type of streptococcus in over 70 per cent of the patients is observed after treatment with sulfonamides or aspirin.

Eradication of group A streptococci from the throat can be achieved by one injection of long-acting benzathine benzylpenicillin G (1.2 million units in persons over 12 years; 600,000 units in children). When treatment is started within a few days after the onset of symptoms, the frequency of secondary infections such as acute otitis and peritonsillar abscess is reduced. Penicillin instituted within the first week is effective prophylaxis for rheumatic fever but reduces the incidence of acute nephritis by only about 50 per cent. Patients who are allergic to penicillin can be treated successfully with oral erythromycin (40 mg/kg/day). Tetracyclines should not be used because some group A streptococci are resistant to them.

Most of the questions about treatment of streptococcal pharyngitis and pyoderma are related to identifying subclinical infection, differentiating true infection from the carrier state, and defining the risk of rheumatic fever and acute nephritis. Scarlet fever and suppurative complications should be treated with adequate doses of penicillin.

### PROPHYLAXIS

In developed countries with a moderate or cold climate, most patients with (mild) pharyngitis and tonsillitis do not consult the doctor and hence cannot be protected from the complications of streptococcal infection. However, the risk of contracting rheumatic fever or acute nephritis is low in these countries under nonepidemic conditions.

In general, penicillin should be given to patients with suspected streptococcal infection, especially if there is a history of rheumatic fever, chorea, or acute glomerulonephritis. If a throat culture can be obtained, it is justified to await the results of the culture before instituting antibiotic therapy. Sequelae can be prevented even if treatment is delayed for one week.

In epidemic situations, contacts of patients with scarlet fever, rheumatic fever, or acute nephritis should be treated with penicillin. In closed communities, such as boarding schools, outbreaks of streptococcal infections should be aborted by the administration of benzathine penicillin to the entire community. Immunization against group A streptococci is not yet possible.

Recurrent attacks of rheumatic fever can be prevented successfully by monthly injections of long-acting penicillin. This prophylaxis should be continued as long as contacts with streptococcal reservoirs are likely to occur. Prophylaxis for recurrences of acute nephritis is less successful, probably because of differences in the pathogenesis of this (auto)immunologic disease.

## References

Franz, K. H., Muller, A. S., Rienmeijer, B. J., Bynum, G., and Nolan, G.: Results of Dick and Schick tests in Liberian children. Trans R Soc Trop Med Hyg 58:68, 1964.
Haverkorn, M. J., Valkenburg, H. A., and Goslings, W. R. O.: Streptococcal pharyngitis in the general population. I. A controlled study of streptococcal pharyngitis and its complications in the Netherlands. J Infect Dis 124:339, 1971.
Holmes, M. C., and Williams, R. E. O.: Streptococcal infections among children in a residential home. I. Introduction and definitions; the incidence of infection. J Hyg 56:43, 1958.
Matanoski, G. M.: The role of the tonsils in streptococcal infections: A comparison of tonsillectomized children and sibling controls. Am J Epidemiol 95:278, 1972.
Maxted, W. R., and Potter, E. V.: The presence of Type 12 M-protein antigen in Group G streptococci. J Gen Microbiol 49:119, 1967.
Moffet, H. L., Siegel, A. C., and Doyle, H. K.: Nonstreptococcal pharyngitis. J Pediat 73:51, 1968.
Stollerman, M., and Bernstein, S. H.: Streptococcal pharyngitis: Evaluation of clinical syndromes in diagnosis. Am J Dis Child 101:476, 1961.
Strasser, T.: Rheumatic fever and rheumatic heart disease in the 1970s. WHO Chronicle 32:18, 1978.
Valkenburg, H. A., Goslings, W. R. O., Bots, A. W., De Moor, C. E., and Lorrier, J. C.: Attack rate of streptococcal pharyngitis, rheumatic fever and glomerulonephritis in the general population. II. The epidemiology of streptococcal pharyngitis in one village during a two-year period. N Engl J Med 268:694, 1963.
Valkenburg, H. A., Haverkorn, M. J., Goslings, W. R. O., Lorrier, J. C., De Moor, C. E., and Maxted, W. R.: Streptococcal pharyngitis in the general population. II. The attack rate of rheumatic fever and acute glomerulonephritis in patients not treated with penicillin. J Infect Dis 124:348, 1971.

# *DIPHTHERIA* **90**

## *Richard V. McCloskey, M.S., M.D.*

Diphtheria is one of the best understood of all infectious diseases. Much is known about the bacterium, *Corynebacterium diphtheriae,* which causes the disease. The organism's unique toxin and its biochemical action have been identified. Recent experiments have shown that very small numbers of molecules of toxin can kill mammalian cells. Uchida demonstrated that synthesis of diphtheria toxin is determined by a structural gene of bacteriophage virus present in toxin-producing *C. diphtheriae.* The molecular events that lead to inhibition of protein synthesis after initial interaction between cell and toxin have been clarified by Collier, Gill, and Pappenheimer and their colleagues between 1960 and 1970. It is not yet clear how the inhibition of protein synthesis relates to the signs and symptoms of diphtheria and to death due to diphtheritic intoxication (Bonventre, 1975). Unfortunately, the promise of control of diphtheria by widespread prophylactic immunization with toxoid has been dimmed by failure to immunize successfully many populations, even in those countries where toxoid and the funds to administer it are in generous supply.

## *DEFINITION*

Diphtheria is an acute communicable disease caused by *C. diphtheriae,* which infects the upper respiratory tract and skin. The cardinal signs and symptoms are a membrane in the pharynx, sore throat, fever, nausea, vomiting, headache, and chills. Death results from respiratory obstruction or myocarditis. Myocarditis is caused by an exotoxin elaborated only by strains of *C. diphtheriae* lysogenic for specific bacteriophages (Barksdale and Arden, 1974; Groman, 1955).

## *EPIDEMIOLOGY AND GEOGRAPHIC VARIATIONS*

Modern epidemics of diphtheria disrupt community life in every respect. Morbidity and death from diphtheria may exhaust the community's medical resources and disorganize its facilities for delivering health care. Intimate contact with infected persons is required for the spread of diphtheria, usually by way of infected droplets or nasopharyngeal secretions. Infective skin exudate is also involved in man-to-man spread. Transmission may also occur by way of animals, fomites, or milk. Carriers are persons harboring a toxinogenic strain of *C. diphtheriae* in the nasopharynx or skin. If the carrier remains asymptomatic he can be detected only by culture of the nasopharynx or skin. Attention is often directed toward these persons when their close associates, siblings, or marital partners develop diphtheria. A carrier state may exist for several days before onset of symptoms. A convalescent carrier state occurs after symptoms subside. The duration of a convalescent carrier state is greatly shortened by treatment of diphtheria with penicillin or erythromycin. These carriers constitute the reservoir from which the disease spreads to susceptible patients. Recent surveys of diphtheria carriers show that 88 per cent have completed or partially completed a course of diphtheria immunization. In the past decade, diphtheria in the United States has been a disease of urban populations rather than of rural populations.

In developing countries, for example, India, the highest death rate occurs in infancy and between 5 and 14 years of age (Udani et al., 1975). Tonsillar and pharyngeal localizations are the most common presentations of diphtheria in India, the United States, Canada, Iran, and Gambia (Heyworth et al., 1973; Zamiri et al., 1972). The disease may be more often manifest as a skin disease in tropical and subtropical areas than as a respiratory tract infection in those areas. It has been suggested that skin infections are important in maintaining endemicity of *C. diphtheriae* infections in tropical and subtropical areas. Skin infections, because of greater contagiousness, result in higher environmental carrier levels of *C. diphtheriae* than respiratory tract diphtheria (Koopman and Campbell, 1975; Belsey and Le Blanc, 1975). As the incidence of skin infections increases, so do the reservoir, acquisition, and transmission of *C. diphtheriae*. Such mechanisms have been thought to be important in instituting respiratory tract diphtheria in tropical and, more recently, in temperate climates (Belsey, 1969; Zalma et al., 1970).

Diphtheria affects mainly poor persons living under crowded conditions and having poor access to health care (Heath and Zusman, 1962; McLeod, 1950). The tragedy of such outbreaks is that morbidity and mortality are highest in children under 14 years. In the United States, attack rates are highest in blacks and Mexican Americans between 5 and 14 years old (Brooks, 1969). Attack rates among unimmunized household members and contacts are higher than in fully immunized persons. More people develop diphtheria when susceptible children congregate in schools and households.

Epidemiologists use several techniques to classify toxin-producing *C. diphtheriae* in order to identify the epidemic strain and disrupt its method of spread. Three types, *mitis, intermedius,* and *gravis,* are identified by colony morphology and a number of biochemical properties (McLeod, 1943). The clinician should understand that this classification does not necessarily imply that disease caused by an *intermedius* strain is invariably less severe than that produced by a *gravis* strain. *Mitis* strains, however, have produced less severe disease than that caused by the other two biotypes. *Gravis* types have produced epidemics in populations of unimmunized persons previously experiencing disease due to *mitis* or *intermedius* strains. Well-immunized populations more often experience disease caused by *mitis* types. Each type can cause epidemic diphtheria.

*C. diphtheriae* strains can be classified by patterns of bacteriophage lysis into at least 35 types (Saragea and Maximescu, 1966). Each bacteriophage type is stable and specific. This powerful epidemiologic tool has revealed that a particular lysotype may persist in the throats of healthy carriers for years and that in a given geographical area a single lysotype may be obtained from both patients and asymptomatic carriers. Some bacteriophage types are confined to or more frequently found in certain countries, suggesting that the lysotyping scheme may reflect the adaptability of *C. diphtheriae* to selected populations. The ease with which a strain of *C. diphtheriae* can be induced to liberate the identifying bacteriophage virus into the surrounding medium (lysogenicity) may be directly correlated with high toxin production and high capacity to spread among a population.

Recent urban epidemics of diphtheria in the United States have been difficult to control, even though hundreds of thousands of persons completed diphtheria immunization. Immunization with diphtheria toxoid of susceptible persons must be combined with a program that identifies carriers of diphtheria and terminates the carrier state by antibiotic treatment. Quarantine is not effective in an open urban society.

## ETIOLOGY

The only organism causing diphtheria is *C. diphtheriae,* a gram-positive bacillus that is pleomorphic, unencapsulated, and nonmotile. Smears prepared with differential stains (Albert's stain) may reveal metachromatic granules. The organism may be arranged in palisades, L or V forms, or in groups resembling "Chinese characters" when examined in stained preparations. Growth is aerobic on ordinary media, although media containing potassium tellurite, or coagulated serum (Loeffler's medium) promote growth. Colonies of *Corynebacterium* species (as well as streptococci and staphylococci) growing on tellurite-containing media develop a grayish black color. *C. diphtheriae* characteristically produces both a brown-gray halo and a garlic odor when growing on Tinsdale's agar. *C. diphtheriae* cohabitates the mucous membranes of man with other morphologically similar saprophytic diphtheroids from which it must be distinguished (see Chapter 25).

## BIOCHEMISTRY OF DIPHTHERIA TOXIN

Myocarditis and neuritis are caused by the toxin elaborated by *C. diphtheriae* and absorbed by the infected patient. The toxin is an acidic globular protein with a gram-molecular weight of 62,000 to 63,000 (Gill and Pappenheimer, 1973). It is characterized by extreme potency, a cellular site of activity, and a latent period before inhibition of cellular protein synthesis is manifest. Strains of *C. diphtheriae* infected by a lysogenic bacteriophage virus produce the toxin in the presence of a critical concentration range of iron in the surrounding medium. Protein synthesis is terminated by a unique chain of events (Bowman, 1970; Collier, 1967; and Gill et al., 1973). Toxin gains access to cytoplasmic portions of the cell by bypassing normal cellular digestive mechanisms. After crossing the cell membrane, toxin inactivates a factor (called elongation factor), which is one of several soluble proteins needed for the translocation step of protein synthesis. The toxin catalyzes the reaction: nicotine adeninedinucleotide + elongation factor ⇌ adenosine diphosphoribose − elongation factor complex + nicotinamide + hydrogen. When the elongation factor is linked with adenosine diphosphoribose, it is inactive. Translocation of peptidyl-tRNA from acceptor to donor sites on the ribosome is disrupted, and protein synthesis stops. The whole toxin itself is actually a proenzyme. The reaction with adenosine diphosphoribose (ribosylation reaction) is actually caused by a proteolytic fragment of the whole toxin (fragment A). Nontoxinogenic *C. diphtheriae* elaborates a physicochemically similar but immunochemically dissimilar and biologically innocuous protein. Therefore, identification of toxin production in vitro by *C. diphtheriae* (toxinogenicity) is of paramount importance. This is usually accomplished by demonstrating immunoprecipitation lines produced by a strain of *C. diphtheriae* growing on agar upon which is placed a filter paper strip containing a diluted, highly purified diphtheria antitoxin (Elek's test) (see Chapter 25). Spreading factor (substance B or hyaluronidase) (O'Meara et al., 1947) contributes to local edema, necrosis, and hemorrhage. It was produced by essentially all *C. diphtheriae* organisms isolated from clinical infections in Ireland during 1947 and may be of importance in producing "hypertoxic" diphtheria (see below) and diphtheria occurring among immunized persons. Other biologically active extracellular products of *C. diphtheriae* play some role in the production of diphtheria because nontoxinogenic *C. diphtheriae* may cause clinical diphtheria, although of a milder variety than that produced by toxinogenic organisms.

## SYMPTOMS AND CLINICAL MANIFESTATIONS

Diphtheria may be symptomless or a rapidly fatal hypertoxic disease that devastates the heart and lungs (Boyer and Weinstein, 1948; Fisher and Cobb, 1948; McCloskey et al., 1969). The primary determinants of diphtheria are the patients' immunity toward diphtheria toxin, the virulence and toxinogenicity of the infecting strain of *C. diphtheriae,* and the anatomic location of the infection (Edward and Allison, 1951). Additional characteristics that may influence the symptoms elicited are age, co-existing systemic disease, and pre-existing local nasopharyngeal disease. The incubation period is usually two to six days. Most of the patients, excluding those with the mildest of nasal or skin infections, present to the physician after several days of systemic illness. The speed of onset is variable. Some authors describe an abrupt onset. More often there is no dramatic deterioration in health. Younger patients may be desperately ill in the face of deceptively modest malaise and fatigue. The temperature gradually rises, seldom exceeding 102° F except in those most severely ill. Children are less likely than adults to complain of sore throat, which at any age is not usually the initial complaint. Other signs and symptoms depend on the extent of the local diphtheritic lesion.

### Anterior Nasal Diphtheria

These patients may be minimally inconvenienced while producing a thick mucopurulent nasal discharge which may irritate the external nares and upper lips. A creamy yellowish membrane, with or without crusting, may be seen in

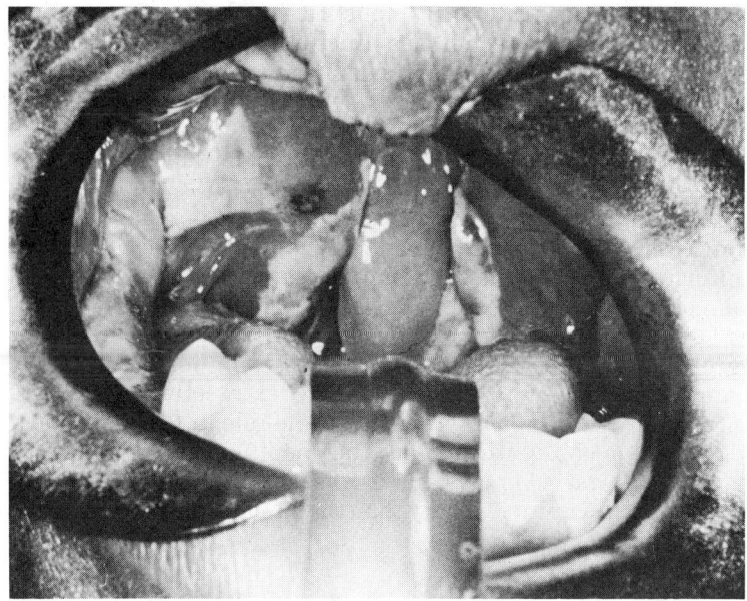

**FIGURE 1.** *Pharynx of a 39 year old woman with bacteriologically confirmed diphtheria. Photograph taken four days after the onset of fever, malaise, and sore throat. Hemorrhage is apparent in one area where membrane was removed by swabbing.*

the nose. Severe intoxication from nasal diphtheria is not common.

### Tonsillar (Faucial) Diphtheria

The membrane begins as a glary thin mucilaginous structure on one or both tonsils. It is not confined to tonsillar crypts. By the time medical advice is sought, usually there is a characteristic graying green color of some area of the membrane. The membrane, which is several millimeters thick, may be difficult to dislodge with a swab and often leaves a bleeding surface on the tonsil when torn off (Fig. 1). Sometimes the membrane crosses anatomic borders and may spill over the anterior pillar of the tonsil, which is often enlarged. The five most common complaints during a recent outbreak in Texas were sore throat (85 per cent), pain on swallowing (23 per cent), nausea and vomiting (25 per cent), and headache (18 per cent) (McCloskey et al., 1971). The most common sign was fever (85 per cent). Moderately tender lymph nodes 1 to 2 cm in diameter can usually be palpated in the anterior triangle of the neck.

### Pharyngeal Diphtheria

Outside the palatine tonsil the membrane spreads to the uvula, the soft palate, and the pharyngeal wall. The marked swelling of the tonsils at this point often obscures large areas of membrane on the posterior aspect of the tonsil. The nasal mucosa may be involved and may bleed profusely. The greenish character of the membrane is more prominent. There may be necrotic black patches in older areas of the membrane. The so-called diphtheritic fetor is of little diagnos-

tic value because it is also observed in infectious mononucleosis and Vincent's infection. A hot tender edema (bull neck) of the anterior part of the neck may obscure the angle of the jaw, the border of the sternocleidomastoid muscle, the clavicle, and enlarged lymph nodes, which become more prominent as the edema subsides. The child with pharyngeal diphtheria is pathetically weak, limp, unresisting, pale, and exhausted. Bleeding from the upper airway is a grave prognostic sign.

### Laryngeal and Bronchial Diphtheria

The membrane may extend downward or involve the larynx exclusively and cause hoarseness, inspiratory and expiratory stridor, dyspnea, and cyanosis. The accessory muscles of respiration are used. Casts of the major bronchi can be formed by the membrane (Fig. 2). If not removed by bronchoscopy, this membrane may cause death by hypoxia.

## DIFFERENTIAL DIAGNOSIS

The diagnosis must rest on clinical grounds alone, since treatment cannot await bacteriologic confirmation. Diphtheria must be considered whenever a membrane is present in the throat, especially if the uvula is involved. In infectious mononucleosis the membrane is confined to the tonsils and remains creamy white without necrotic patches for a longer time than the diphtheritic membrane. Streptococcal pharyngitis causes fiery redness of the throat and white exudate. Severe throat pain and faucial distortion are not seen in

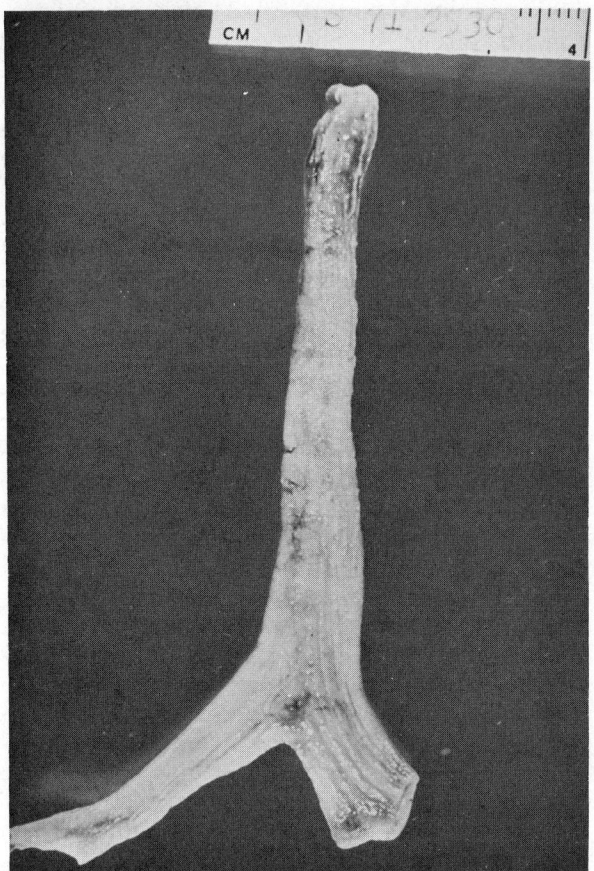

**FIGURE 2.** *Diphtheritic membrane forming a cast of the trachea and main bronchi. This membrane could not be removed at bronchoscopy and eventually caused death by hypoxia.*

uncomplicated diphtheria. The foul necrotic exudate complicating leukemia may be impossible to distinguish from that of diphtheria. Vincent's angina may involve the gums and is identified by Gram's stain of the exudate. Simultaneous infection with streptococci (32 per cent in a recent outbreak) does not alter the physical findings suggestive of diphtheria. The laboratory findings in diphtheria are nonspecific and include moderate leukocytosis, mild fever, and transient albuminuria.

## PROGNOSIS AND COMPLICATIONS

The outcome depends on (1) the location and extent of the membrane; (2) amount of toxin absorbed; and (3) patient's immunity status. Myocarditis and cardiac arrhythmia may be seen from the second to the sixth week. ST-T wave changes and abnormalities occur in 40 per cent of the electrocardiograms but are not always accompanied by signs of congestive heart failure.

### Myocardial Complications

There is a correlation between delayed conduction velocity of the median, ulnar, and common peroneal nerves and myocardial conduction system disturbances (Burkhardt et al., 1938; Kazemi et al., 1973). Moreover, the delayed peripheral nerve conduction velocity precedes clinical evidence of myocarditis and myocardial conduction system abnormalities. The determination of peripheral nerve conduction delay may be used to predict the appearance of myocarditis and cardiac arrhythmias.

Most of the electrocardiographic abnormalities appear during the first week of illness. ST-T wave changes that are destined to improve usually do so within 10 days of appearance of the abnormalities. The severity of the illness and the toxemia are roughly related to the incidence of EKG abnormalities and acute circulatory failure. Acute circulatory failure is practically never seen with nasal diphtheria but may occur in 9 per cent of patients with pharyngeal-laryngeal infection, largely a consequence of the greater amount of toxin that is produced by the more extensive deeper respiratory infections. Acute circulatory failure appears with a sudden onset of pallor, hypotension, collapsed peripheral pulses, and profuse perspiration. The EKG in acute failure may be normal. Muffled heart sounds, murmurs, embryocardia, pulse rate, and pulse pressure are not always associated with well-defined electrocardiographic abnormalities.

Nevertheless, diphtheria with ST-T wave changes has a significantly higher mortality rate (28 per cent) than diphtheria without EKG changes (6 to 10 per cent). Serial tests of serum glutamic oxalacetic transaminase (SGOT) levels will identify most patients with myocarditis (Naiditch and Bower, 1954).

Early identification of diphtheritic myocarditis is important in reducing morbidity and mortality. Since clinical examination of the heart is not reliable for diagnosis of myocarditis, patients with EKG abnormalities during diphtheria should be monitored in specialized units equipped with all support facilities, which can offer effective treatment of the more serious arrhythmias and conduction disturbances that may occur. Atrioventricular (AV) block and left bundle branch block (LBBB) are ominous signs, associated with mortality of 60 to 100 per cent. Recent case reports have shown that electrical pacing with temporary transvenous pacing electrodes or myocardial demand pacemakers can resolve AV block and LBBB produced by diphtheritic myocarditis (Matisonn et al., 1972). Treatment regimens usually include salt restriction, careful fluid balance, and short-acting digitalis preparations if congestive heart failure is marked. Antiarrhythmic agents, such as procaine amide, Xylocaine, and isoprenaline are used when indicated to suppress or control specific arrhythmias. High doses of adrenal steroids are often given with the aim of reducing edema and fibrosis of the myocardium or conducting system, but there is no firm evidence that steroids accomplish these objectives.

Since myocarditis represents severe intoxication, the physician should expect to encounter other toxic manifestations. Intensive nursing care may be needed to support respiration and to prevent permanent complications of peripheral neuritis. Thrombocytopenia also occurs in malignant diphtheria. Active platelet destruction may complicate the myocarditis and warrant platelet transfusions.

A rare cardiac complication of diphtheria is infective endocarditis due to *C. diphtheriae* (Davidson et al., 1976). Blood cultures may contain toxinogenic or nontoxinogenic *C. diphtheriae*. The infection can be established on normal or previously deformed valves. This unusual complication may occur in the absence of clinical diphtheria when signs of endocarditis are present. Treatment is long-term antibiotic therapy (see *Treatment*). The reported mortality rate is 70 per cent.

Patients with hypertoxic diphtheria may develop peripheral circulatory failure, hypotension, thrombocytopenia, and skin hemorrhages in the first week (Fisher and Cobb, 1948). They usually die with evidence of bleeding into the vascular endothelium, tracheobronchial mucosa, and adrenals. Palatal paralysis, the most common and often the only paralysis, appears in the third week, often after myocarditis. Paralysis of respiratory muscles, pharynx, and larynx appears six to eight weeks after onset. There may be a deceptively symptom-free interval before the patient is unable to swallow and develops aspiration pneumonia. Late-appearing tachycardias may cause death at this time. A Guillain-Barré-like peripheral neuritis may also appear as a late complication.

## TREATMENT

A patient with tonsillar or nasopharyngeal diphtheria requires isolation in the hospital at bed rest for 10 to 14 days. The early use of adequate amounts of diphtheria antitoxin (DAT) remains the most important specific mode of treatment. Every patient with diphtheria merits DAT therapy, even though a week or more may have passed since the onset. Since DAT is composed of horse serum, intradermal and/or conjunc-

tival tests should be performed before administration. If either is positive, desensitization is justifiable even though it is time-consuming and hazardous because DAT is the only specific treatment available. DAT prepared from human serum would obviate some of these problems. The dose of DAT need not be complicated. If the membrane does not extend beyond the tonsil it may be treated by intramuscular administration of 20,000 units if there is no thrombocytopenia. More extensive membrane requires 80,000 to 100,000 units, preferably intravenously. The minimum amount of DAT necessary to prevent complications is unknown. Penicillin or erythromycin is used to eliminate the organism from the upper respiratory tract and to terminate the carrier state. If the patient cannot swallow, treatment with parenteral penicillin produces less pain upon injection than does parenteral erythromycin. Tetracycline, rifampin, clindamycin, and ampicillin are effective in vitro against *C. diphtheriae* but cephalexin, oxacillin, and lincomycin are not. Both benzathine penicillin and erythromycin therapy can terminate the carrier state (McCloskey et al., 1974). Myocarditis, congestive failure, and arrhythmias require intensive cardiac care and strict bed rest. Cardiac pacemakers can control arrhythmia. Unless congestive heart failure appears, digitalization is unnecessary. Airway obstruction requires tracheostomy. Bronchoscopy may be performed to remove membrane from the larger bronchi. Careful nursing care is necessary to prevent pneumonia caused by gram-negative bacilli acquired in the hospital. Therapy is always expensive and not always successful.

## PREVENTION

The complications of diphtheria can be prevented by active immunization beginning in childhood, with booster immunizations every 10 years thereafter. Active immunization and early treatment of carriers are both necessary for control of the disease. Immunization with DPT (diphtheria-pertussis-tetanus vaccine) should be administered to infants at 6 weeks of age. Three 0.5-ml injections of DPT are given at monthly intervals, with a booster dose of 0.5 ml at 6 months or 1 year. Children who have received this primary series should receive a booster dose before entering school. For older children, primary immunization may be accomplished by two doses of pediatric diphtheria-tetanus (DT) vaccine of 0.5 ml each, six weeks apart with a booster dose six months to one year later. Persons over 12 years should be primarily immunized on the same schedule, but adult-type diphtheria-tetanus vaccine (dT) should be used. Schick tests are unnecessary before adult immunizations. Persons who are heavily exposed (physicians, nurses, hospital workers) to diphtheria should receive a booster 0.5 ml dose of dT every five years (McCloskey, 1969). All others should receive 0.5 ml of dT at 10-year intervals. Exposure to a suspected case dictates administration of a 0.5 ml dT booster dose to those exposed who have been immunized previously but have not had a recent booster.

## References

Altshuler, S. S., Hoffman, K. M., and Fitzgerald, P. J.: Electrocardiographic changes in diphtheria. Am J Med 29:294, 1948.

Barksdale, L., and Arden, S. B.: Persisting bacteriophage infections, lysogeny, and phage conversions. Ann Rev Microbiol 28:265, 1974.

Belsey, M.A.: *Corynebacterium diphtheriae* skin infections in Alabama and Louisiana. A factor in the epidemiology of diphtheria. N Engl J Med 280:135, 1969.

Belsey, M. A., and LeBlanc, D. R.: Skin infections and the epidemiology of diphtheria. Am J Epidemiol 102:179, 1975.

Bonventre, P. F.: Diphtheria Microbiology, 1975. Washington, D.C., American Society of Microbiology. 1975, pp. 272–277.

Bowman, G. C.: Studies on the mode of action of diphtheria toxin III. Effect on subcellular components of protein synthesis from the tissues of intoxicated guinea pigs and rats. J Exp Med 131:659, 1970.

Boyer, N. H., and Weinstein, L.: Diphtheritic myocarditis. N Engl J Med 239:913, 1948.

Brooks, G. F.: Recent trends in diphtheria in the United States. J Infect Dis 120:500, 1969.

Burkhardt, E. A., Eggleston, C., and Smith, L. W.: Electrocardiographic changes and peripheral nerve palsies in toxic diphtheria. Am J Med Sci 195:301, 1938.

Collier, R. J.: Effect of diphtheria toxin on protein synthesis: Inactivation of transfer factors. J Mol Biol 25:83, 1967.

Collier, R. J.: Diphtheria toxin: Mode of action and structure. Bacteriol Rev 39:54, 1975.

Davidson, S., Rotem, Y., Bozkowski, B., and Rubenstein, E.: *Corynebacterium diphtheriae* endocarditis. Am J Med Sci 271:351 1976.

Edward, D. G., and Allison, V. D.: Diphtheria in the immunized with observations on diphtheria-like disease associated with nontoxinogenic strains of *Corynebacterium diphtheriae*. J Hyg 49:205, 1951.

Fisher, A. M., and Cobb, S.: The clinical manifestations of the severe form of diphtheria. Bull Johns Hopkins Hosp 83:297, 1948.

Gill, D. M., Pappenheimer, A. M., Jr., and Uchida, T.: Diphtheria toxin protein synthesis and the cell. Fed Proc 32:1508, 1973.

Groman, N. B.: Evidence for the active role of bacteriophage in the conversion of nontoxinogenic *Corynebacterium diphtheriae* to toxin production. J Bacteriol 69:9, 1955.

Heath, C. W., and Zusman, J.: An outbreak of diphtheria among skid-row men. N Engl J Med 267:809, 1962.

Heyworth, B., and Ropp, M.: Diphtheria in the Gambia. J Trop Med Hyg 76:61, 1973.

Kazemi, B., Tahernia, A. C., and Zandian, K.: Motor nerve conduction in diphtheria and diphtheritic myocarditis. Arch Neurol 29:104, 1973.

Koopman, J. S., and Campbell, J.: The role of cutaneous diphtheria infections in a diphtheria epidemic. J Infect Dis 131:239, 1975.

Matisonn, R. E., Mitha, A. S., and Chesler, E.: Successful electrical pacing for complete heart block complicating diphtheritic myocarditis. Br Heart J 38:423, 1976.

McCloskey, R. V.: Diphtheria antitoxin titers in hospital workers after a single dose of adult type diphtheria tetanus toxoid. Am J Med Sci 258:209, 1969.

McCloskey, R. V., Eller, J. J., Green, M., Mauney, C. U., and Richards, S. E. M.: The 1970 epidemic of diphtheria in San Antonio. Ann Intern Med 75:495, 1971.

McCloskey, R. V., Green, M. J., Eller, J., and Smilack, J.: Treatment of diptheria carriers: Benzathine penicillin, erythromycin, and clindamycin. Ann Intern Med 81:788, 1974.

McLeod, J. W.: The types mitis, intermedius, and gravis of *Corynebacterium diphtheriae*. Bacteriol Rev 7:1, 1943.

McLeod, J. W.: A survey of the epidemiology of diphtheria in northwest Europe and North America in the period of 1920–1946. J Pathol Bacteriol 62:137, 1950.

Moffat, R. C.: Diphtheritic heart block. Angiology 10:609, 1972.

O'Meara, R. A. Q., Baker, R. S. W., and Balch, H. H.: Production of substance B by *Corynebacterium diphtheriae*. Lancet 1:212, 1947.

Saragea, A., and Maximescu, P.: Phage typing of *Corynebacterium diphtheriae*. Bull WHO 35:681, 1966.

Tahernia, A. C.: Electrocardiographic abnormalities and serum transaminase levels in diphtheritic myocarditis. J Pediatr 75:1008, 1969.

Udani, P. M., and Kumbhat, M. M., Bhat, U. S., Nadkarni, M. S., Bhave, S. K., Ezuthachan, S. G., and Kamath, B.: Diphtheria. Some epidemiological observations in Bombay: A clinical and bacteriological study of 320 and autopsy study of 5 children. Prog Drug Res 19:423, 1975.

Zalma, V. M., Older, J. J., and Brooks, G. F.: The Austin, Texas diphtheria outbreak. Clinical and epidemiological aspects. JAMA 211:2125, 1970.

Zamiri, I., McEntegart, M. G., and Saragea, A.: Diphtheria in Iran. J Hyg (Camb) 70:619, 1972.

# *VINCENT'S INFECTION* **91**

## *Howard Robert Attebery, D.D.S.*

### *DEFINITION*

Acute necrotizing ulcerative gingivitis (ANUG) is an ulcerative necrosis of the interdental papillae and the marginal gingivae. The acute stage is characterized by sudden onset and severe pain. The chronic form shows interproximal destruction of the periodontal tissues with alveolar bone loss.

The term ANUG is restricted to disease of the gingivae. If the disease spreads to other oral structures the term acute necrotizing ulcerative mucositis (ANUM) or Vincent's stomatitis is used. Vincent's angina is an acute pseudomembranous involvement of the pharynx or tonsils. ANUG, ANUM, or Vincent's angina is classified as Vincent's disease or Vincent's infection. ANUG is also known as trench mouth, Plaut-Vincent's infection, fusospirochetosis, and ulceromembranous gingivitis.

### *ETIOLOGY*

The suspected etiology is complicated, consisting of a bacterial fusospirochetal complex and a group of predisposing factors. Poor oral hygiene, local irritation from food impaction or poor dental restoration, excessive smoking, erupting teeth, and third molar tissue flaps are important local factors. Malnutrition, fatigue, emotional or physical stress, endocrine dysfunctions, and metabolic disturbances are among the predisposing systemic factors. Since the lesions of ANUG always contain a predominantly gram-negative fusospirochetal complex, and since the disease is rapidly brought under control with antibiotics, the consensus reigns that the disease is bacterial. However, it is not clear whether the bacteria initiate the disease or are secondary invaders. No single organism or combination of organisms has yet proved to be the causative factor. The fusiform most often identified from the necrotic material is *Fusobacterium nucleatum,* an anaerobic member of the normal oral flora.

## PATHOGENESIS AND PATHOLOGY

Electron microscopic studies show that ANUG lesions have four distinct strata all occupied by spirochetes. Spirochete invasion of normal tissue occurs below the necrotic zone (Listgarten, 1965; Heylings, 1967). These spirochetes have not been cultured. Listgarten (1967) also showed by electron microscopy that necrotic areas form around these large spirochetes.

Since a large number of gram-negative bacteria are present in the ANUG lesion, endotoxin may be involved in this inflammatory disease. One investigation, using biopsied specimens, showed negative results for immune complex participation (Dolby, 1972).

Kardachi and Clark in 1974 postulated that the disease starts as an aseptic necrosis secondary to capillary stasis, due largely to stress, smoking, and poor oral hygiene. Stress and smoking stimulate epinephrine and norepinephrine release. Poor oral hygiene might contribute to the stasis through bacterial products from the accumulating dental plaque.

## CLINICAL MANIFESTATIONS

The disease may begin suddenly with gingival bleeding, fetid odor, and pain. These symptoms are accompanied by necrosis of interproximal papillae, pseudomembranes, lymphadenopathy, and excess salivation. The incidence of gingival bleeding is 96 per cent, pain 86 per cent, and fetid odor 84 per cent (Barnes, Bowles, and Carter, 1973). Patients often complain of a metallic taste and loss of the tactile sense in their teeth. Fever, anorexia, and other gastrointestinal symptoms may also occur.

## COMPLICATIONS AND SEQUELAE FROM ANUG

The disease may spread to other mucosae from the gingivae to cause stomatitis and tonsillitis or gangrenous stomatitis or angina. The most serious oral complication is noma. Noma usually begins in the corner of the mouth or cheek and rapidly involves the entire thickness of the lips and cheeks, with conspicuous necrosis and complete sloughing of tissue. The disease may also spread to the lungs and produce pulmonary fusospirochetosis. Transient bacteremia or septicemia may occur from the mass of bacteria at bleeding sites. Meningitis has been reported after Vincent's disease. Genital fusospirochetosis follows contact with infected saliva (Von Hamm, 1938). Oral surgical procedures or any other gingival manipulations should be postponed until the disease has subsided.

## GEOGRAPHIC VARIATIONS IN THE DISEASE

ANUG afflicts adolescents and adults throughout the world. Few data are available on comparative prevalences for vast areas of the world. Vincent's disease is severe in populations in which protein and calorie malnutrition is common in children (Russell, 1967).

ANUG is rarely seen in children in the United States, Canada, or Europe, but is common in children in other parts of the world (Jiminez, 1969). The children affected are usually from the lower socioeconomic groups who are suffering from lack of protein. In Nigerian villages ANUG is seen in children as young as three or four years and noma is also common (Emslie, 1963; Sheiham, 1965).

## DIAGNOSIS

A gingival disease with sudden onset accompanied by pain, blunted papillae, and fetid odor is ANUG. Herpetic gingivitis does not start at the papillae and there is no fetid odor. The lymphadenopathy of herpes appears before the oral lesions and with ANUG the lymphadenopathy occurs after the lesions are present.

ANUG will not be confused with secondary syphilis of the mouth if the characteristics described above are kept in mind. Oral lesions from leukemia, infectious mononucleosis, granulocytopenia, and other blood dyscrasias may be a diagnostic problem, and warrant blood counts and differential smears.

It was once a common procedure to stain a smear of the oral lesion with 2 per cent methyl violet or with carbol fuchsin for microscopic examination; large numbers of fusiform bacteria and spirochetes were seen in Vincent's disease. The clinical symptoms are so widely appreciated today that microscopic examinations are seldom used to confirm the clinical picture. Without the clinical picture a positive smear is meaningless because fusobacteria and spirochetes are present in every mouth.

## TREATMENT

For severe infections antibiotics should be used. Procaine penicillin, 600,000 units, is given intramuscularly twice daily for three to seven days. Metronidazole is given orally, 200 mg, three times daily for three to seven days. The alternate drug of choice is tetracycline, given orally 250 mg every four hours (Braude, 1976).

Oral rinses of a 3 per cent hydrogen peroxide solution diluted 1 part to 3 parts of water should be used at least every two hours while awake. If possible the diet should be rich in protein and calories and contain soft or liquid nonirritating foods. Three days after starting treatment, when the mouth is comfortable, the dentist can debride the lesions, curette, do minor scaling, and clean the teeth. Instructions should now be given on oral hygiene procedures so that the patient can institute an effective home treatment program. In addition, a list of predisposing factors should be discussed with a view to removing or avoiding them.

ANUG tends to recur if treatment and oral hygiene are stopped and if predisposing factors are neglected. If severe ANUG does not improve rapidly with treatment a blood dyscrasia should be investigated.

When the necrotizing ulcerative gingivitis has subsided, and the gingivae have stabilized, a dentist should be consulted to determine if a recontouring surgical procedure is needed.

The treatment of ANUM is the same as for ANUG. However, for noma (gangrenous stomatitis) the antibiotic treatment should be prolonged, nutrition restored, and the underlying disease corrected (Uohara, 1967).

## PROPHYLAXIS

ANUG is no longer considered to be contagious. The high incidence of disease among individuals living in close proximity is thought to be due not to contagiousness but rather to a common environmental predisposing factor or factors. Many of the large outbreaks attributed to ANUG have been in reality due to herpetic gingivostomatitis, which is contagious.

To prevent the initial encounter with ANUG or to prevent its recurrence, the predisposing factors listed previously have to be eliminated or diminished. The avoidance of stress, smoking, and fatigue, keeping the mouth as clean as possible, and the use of good nutritional practices are the major factors in the prevention of Vincent's infection.

### References

Barnes, P. B., Bowles, W. F., III, and Carter, H. G.: Acute necrotizing ulcerative gingivitis: a survey of 218 cases. J Perio 44:35, 1973.
Braude, A. I.: Antimicrobial Drug Therapy. Philadelphia, W. B. Saunders Company, 1976.
Dolby, A. E.: Acute ulcerative gingivitis: Immune complex. J Dent Res 51:1639, 1972.
Emslie, R.: Cancrum oris. Dent Practit 13:481, 1963.
Heylings, R. T.: Electron microscopy of acute ulcerative gingivitis (Vincent's type) Br Dent J 122:51, 1967.
Jiminez, L. M., Ramos, J., Garrington, G., and Baer, P.: The familial occurrence of acute necrotizing gingivitis in children in Colombia, South America. J Perio 40:414, 1969.
Kardachi, B. J., and Clarke, N. G.: Aetiology of acute necrotising ulcerative gingivitis: a hypothetical explanation. J Perio 45:830, 1974.
Listgarten, M. A.: Electron microscopic observations on the bacterial flora of acute necrotizing ulcerative gingivits. J Perio 36:328, 1965.
Listgarten, M. A., and Lewis, D. W.: The distribution of spirochetes in the lesion of acute necrotizing ulcerative gingivitis: An electron microscopic and statistical survey. J Perio 38:379, 1967.
Russell, A. L.: Epidemiology of periodontal disease. Int Dent J 17:282, 1967.
Sheiham, A.: An epidemiological study of oral diseases in Nigerians. J. Dent Res 44:184, 1965.
Uohara, G. I., and Knapp, M. J.: Oral fusospirochetosis and associated lesions. Oral Surg Oral Med and Oral Path 24:113, 1967.
Von Hamm, E.: Venereal fuso-spirochetosis. Am J Trop Med 18:595, 1938.

# SINUSITIS 92

## Paul B. van Cauwenberge, M.D.

### DEFINITION

Sinusitis is an inflammation of the mucous membranes of the paranasal sinus cavities. Acute sinusitis is defined as an inflammatory response of less than 3 weeks' duration. Subacute sinusitis has a duration of 3 weeks to 3 months, and chronic sinusitis lasts longer than 3 months. This subdivision is important because of the different histopathology and consequently different treatment of acute, subacute, and chronic sinusitis.

## *ETIOLOGY*

Sinusitis results from the spread of an infection in the surrounding tissues, especially nasal and dental infections, but also from an obstruction of the ostium of the sinus. This ostium plays a crucial role because the ventilation of the sinuses depends on the ostial function. Closure or narrowing of the natural ostium impairs ventilation and causes transudation from the mucous membrane. Because of the obstructed ostium, fluid stagnates in the sinus and provides a rich bacterial culture medium.

In cases of dentogenous sinusitis, infection starts at the floor of the maxillary sinus and results from the spread or rupture of an apical abscess, a granuloma, or a dental cyst. This is the origin of an ascending inflammation of the mucosal lining. Infrequently, the ostium is completely closed by this type of infection.

A brief review of anatomy is necessary to understand the etiology and natural history of paranasal sinusitis. The nasal sinuses are cavities of varying sizes that develop from the nasal chambers. They consist of four paired structures: the maxillary, frontal, ethmoidal, and sphenoidal sinuses (Figs. 1 and 2). Only the maxillary and ethmoidal sinuses are present at birth, while the sphenoidal sinus is very small and the frontal sinus is absent at birth.

The ostia of the frontal, ethmoidal, and maxil-

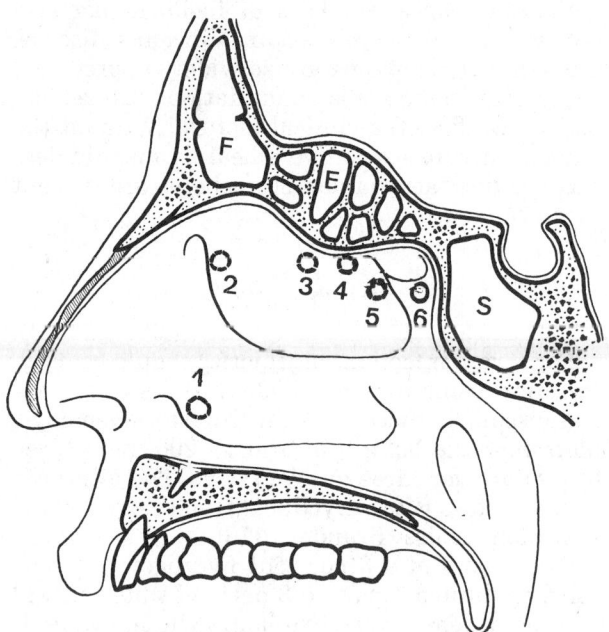

**FIGURE 2.** *Diagram of a sagittal cross-section of the skull, showing the frontal (F), ethmoidal (E), and sphenoidal (S) sinuses with projection of their ostia: (1) distal end of the nasolacrimal duct, (2) frontal sinus ostium, (3) ostium of the anterior ethmoidal cells, (4) maxillary sinus ostium, (5) ostium of the posterior ethmoidal cells, and (6) sphenoidal sinus ostium.*

lary sinuses are situated at the lateral nasal wall, under the insertion of the middle turbinate. The sphenoidal ostium is found at the anterior wall of this sinus.

## *MICROBIOLOGY*

Whereas infectious rhinitis is generally caused by viruses (rhinoviruses, respiratory syncytial virus, and others), bacteria are found in sinusitis. However, studies dealing with bacteriologic findings in sinusitis are characterized by a diversity of results depending on the regions, the date, and the laboratories concerned.

### Aerobes

Our examination of secretions obtained by antral puncture in adults disclosed that 84 per cent of the cultures in acute sinusitis and 83 per cent in chronic sinusitis contain aerobes. *Streptococcus pneumoniae, Hemophilus influenzae,* and *Staphylococcus aureus* are the most frequently encountered bacteria (Van Cauwenberge et al., 1976). *Branhamella catarrhalis (Neisseria catarrhalis)* is thought to play a role in "starting" the infection (Brorson et al., 1976). During antimicrobial treatment, bacteria may turn into L-forms.

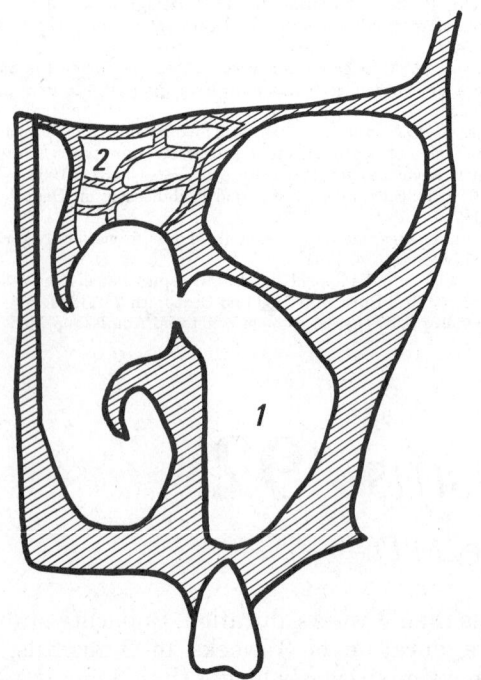

**FIGURE 1.** *Diagram of a frontal cross-section of the skull, showing the left maxillary sinus (1) with its ostium and the ethmoidal cells (2).*

### Anaerobes

A high incidence of anaerobic sinusitis is reported by Frederick and Braude (1974) and Van Cauwenberge et al. (1977). They found, respectively, 28 per cent (heavy growth) and 33 per cent of the secretions contained anaerobes. Dentogenous sinusitis, putrid secretions, and unilateral infections are likely to contain anaerobes. The most frequently encountered microorganisms are *Peptostreptococcus* and *Bacteroides* spp. In view of the histopathologic changes in sinusitis, it is not surprising to find this high occurrence of anaerobes. The decreased mucosal blood flow, the increased intrasinal pressure, the occasional angiitis, and the viscid secretions provoke a low oxygen tension and a low pH, providing the optimal oxidation-reduction potential that is necessary for anaerobic proliferation.

### Yeasts and Molds

These are rarely reported as etiologic agents in sinusitis. Occasionally, aspergillosis and mucormycosis (see below) of the sinuses occur.

## *PREDISPOSING FACTORS*

### Intranasal

Any condition impairing the ostial function and thus impairing ventilation of the sinus can give rise to sinusitis. The most important factors are septal deviation, a narrow bony sinus ostium, choanal atresia, cleft palate, nasal infection, allergic and vasomotor rhinopathy, benign and malignant tumors, adenoidal hypertrophy, and intranasal foreign bodies.

### Systemic Diseases

The production of abnormal sinus secretions as in cystic fibrosis facilitates bacterial growth. Immune deficiencies, such as hypo- or agammaglobulinemia and neutropenia, also promote sinusitis. In the immotile cilia syndrome, sinusitis is nearly always present.

## *PATHOGENESIS AND PATHOLOGY*

The tissue pathology of sinusitis is divided into acute, subacute, and chronic sinusitis.

In acute sinusitis (Fig. 3), a vasodilation of the vascular bed allows serum, red blood cells, and polymorphonucleocytes to penetrate into the sinus cavity. This material, together with epithelial debris, constitutes pus. The submucosa is edematous and shows a polymorphonuclear infiltrate, while the periosteum and bone remain intact.

In subacute sinusitis there is a striking proliferation of young connective tissue.

Chronic sinusitis should be considered to be the result of an unhealed acute form. Histopathologic examinations show two important findings: proliferation and necrosis (Figs. 4 and 5). The mucosal lining undergoes polypoid changes, metaplasia into a pseudostratified squamous form, and necrosis of the epithelium. In the submucosa, proliferation of young, well-vascularized connective tissue is noted, together with infiltration by lymphocytes, plasmocytes, macrophages, and eosinophils. Edema also occurs as a result of angiitis, with secondary venous and lymphatic obstruction. Occasionally, the bone and its periosteum become necrotic and proliferate.

**FIGURE 3.** *Artist's impression of the histopathologic changes in acute sinusitis. A vasodilation in submucosa allows serum, polymorphonucleocytes (P), and erythrocytes (E) to penetrate into the sinus cavity.*

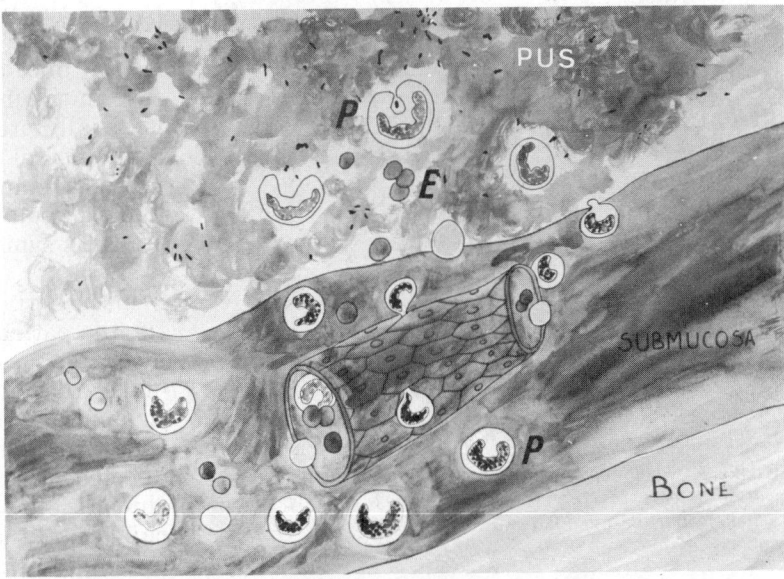

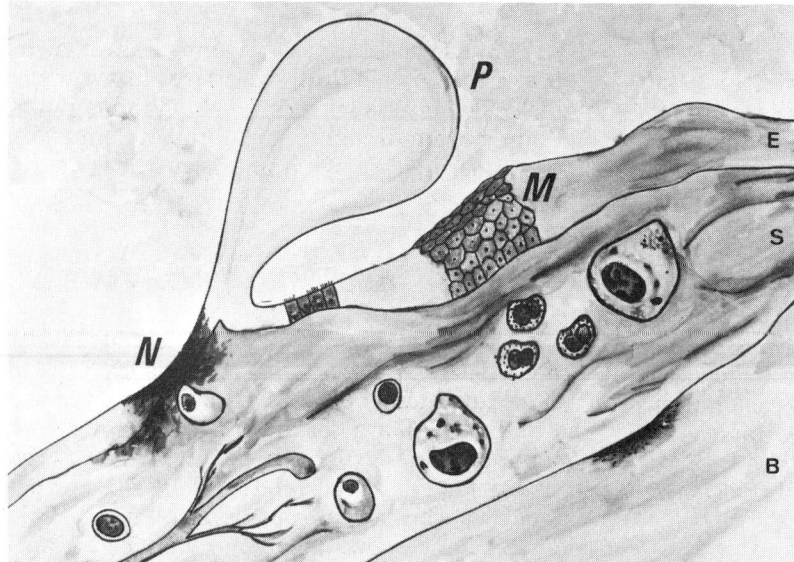

**FIGURE 4.** *Artist's impression of the histopathologic changes in chronic sinusitis. Epithelial (E) changes are: polypoid formations (P), hyperplasia and metaplasia (M), and necrosis (N). In the submucosa (S), note proliferation of young, well-vascularized connective tissue with infiltration by various cells. The bone (B) with its periosteum may become necrotic and proliferate.*

## CLINICAL MANIFESTATIONS

In acute sinusitis, pain is the most important symptom. It is mostly intense, gnawing, and compressing, and increases on stooping and jarring. It localizes to the involved sinuses. Nasal obstruction, mucoid or mucopurulent discharge, disturbed smell, and epistaxis may also be present. There may be fever, but other symptoms of systemic illness are seldom found. The ascent or descent of the sinus infection may lead to hearing problems, because of involvement of the eustachian tube, and to sore throat, coughing, and hoarseness.

In acute maxillary sinusitis, pain is intense and referred to the area overlying the nasal sinus, the root of the nose, and the upper premolars and molars. Because of the obstruction of the nasofrontal duct and the consequent negative pressure in the frontal sinus, vacuum headache pain is usually present. The pain may also spread to the temporal and retroauricular regions. In dentogenous sinusitis, the characteristic symptomatology of pulpitis or dental abscess is added to the sinusitis symptoms. Nasal obstruction is always present.

In the early stages of an acute maxillary sinusitis, the patient complains of a seromucous nasal discharge, associated with a viral infection. Secondary bacterial invasion transforms the secretions into a mucopurulent or purulent nasal discharge or postnasal drip. A swelling over the affected cheek is rare in uncomplicated maxillary sinusitis of nasal origin, although it may occur in children. It is, on the other hand, a common finding in dentogenous sinusitis.

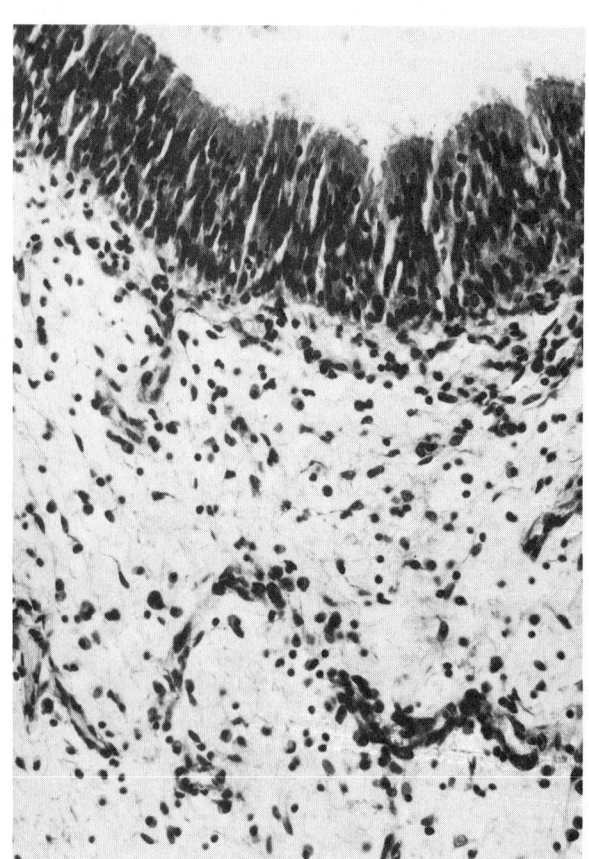

**FIGURE 5.** *Photomicrograph of the epithelial and subepithelial layer in a case of chronic sinusitis. Notice the hyperplastic epithelum and the infiltration of the edematous submucosa by lymphocytes and plasmocytes.*

Acute frontal sinusitis is mostly associated with ethmoidal or maxillary sinusitis. It is very rare as an isolated infection. A very intense, sharp pain is felt in the supraorbital region. Nasal obstruction and discharge are usually present. Because of the intimate relationship with the orbit, edema of the upper eyelid often accompanies an acute frontal sinusitis.

Acute ethmoidal sinusitis, like frontal sinusitis, is seldom found as an isolated phenomenon but usually accompanies maxillary and frontal sinusitis. The ethmoidal cells are the best developed sinuses at birth and are the most frequently involved sinuses in acute sinusitis in children.

Because the ethmoidal cells are separated from the orbital contents only by an extremely thin bony lamella (the lamina papyracea), orbital symptoms and complications are common. The orbital symptoms may be lacrimation, edema of the eyelids, and even impairment of visual acuity. Pain is severe, is located along the inner canthus of the eye, and may spread to the infraorbital and temporal region. Nasal obstruction and discharge are usually present.

Acute sphenoidal sinusitis is unusual as a separate entity but may accompany acute ethmoidal and maxillary sinusitis. The symptoms of infection in other sinuses tend to overshadow any specific symptomatology of the sphenoiditis. The only outstanding feature of acute sphenoidal sinusitis is distinct pain at the occipital and parietal regions.

In chronic sinusitis nasal discharge is the most common symptom. The secretions may be mucoid or mucopurulent, blown from the nose, or appearing as a postnasal drip. Nasal obstruction often occurs because of the edematous nasal mucous membranes and the presence of nasal polyps and viscid secretions. Pain is rare in chronic sinusitis, except in acute exacerbations. As in acute sinusitis, disorders of smell may occur, and infections may extend to the ear, throat, larynx, and bronchi. The symptoms of chronic sinusitis are extremely variable. They may be severe enough to prevent the patient from working, or so mild that he is hardly aware of any problem.

In chronic ethmoidal sinusitis, nasal polyps are very common, while in chronic frontal sinusitis, the formation of a mucocele may lead to orbital swelling and destruction of the surrounding tissues. Chronic sphenoidal sinusitis gives rise to unilateral facial pain and pain behind the eye, while headaches referred to the occipital and parietal regions are also characteristic.

### Sinusitis in Children

Because of the marked fall in the incidence of sinusitis in children in the antibiotic era and the improvement in public health, there is no longer a special problem with sinusitis in children (Bernstein, 1971). It is of interest, however, that the nasal sinuses are evaginations of the mucous membrane of the nasal cavities, so that sinusitis often accompanies rhinitis in children. The symptoms are identical to acute rhinitis in the early stages of infection, e.g., purulent nasal secretions, nasal obstruction, cough, and sneezing. As the disease advances, local and systemic symptoms become more evident, because the infected secretions are trapped within the sinus cavity. It is extremely difficult to elicit symptoms referable to any particular sinus in small children, unless there are complications like those in acute ethmoiditis.

## COMPLICATIONS AND SEQUELAE

Ascending infection of the eustachian tube and middle ear and descending infection of the pharynx, larynx, and bronchi often accompany sinusitis. These complications are usually not dangerous and disappear with proper treatment of the infection. More serious complications arise when infections spread from the paranasal sinuses to adjacent intracranial structures or to the orbit (Litton, 1971).

Maxillary sinusitis seldom leads to severe complications, but all the other sinuses have walls contiguous with the dura.

Acute ethmoiditis may progress to acute meningitis in children. Before the era of antibiotics, this infection was often a fatal one. In adults, frontal, ethmoidal, and sphenoidal sinusitis may be complicated not only by meningitis, but also by epidural and subdural abscesses, brain abscesses, and cavernous sinus thrombosis. Orbital cellulitis and abscesses are common as a complication of ethmoiditis in children, and of ethmoidal and frontal sinusitis in adults, especially in cases of frontal mucocele. Osteomyelitis of the walls of the sinus may develop in chronic sinusitis and less often in acute sinusitis, and occasionally it may produce fistulas.

## GEOGRAPHIC VARIATIONS

These depend on nutrition, air pollution, and access to antibiotics. Poor standards of public health and general living conditions, along with nutritional deficiencies, favor the development of sinusitis, especially in children (Takahashi, 1977). In areas of air pollution, the occurrence of sinusitis is much higher than in rural areas. Hot, dry or cold, moist climates also promote sinusitis. It must be stressed that in areas deprived of antibiotics, the incidence of sinusitis and its com-

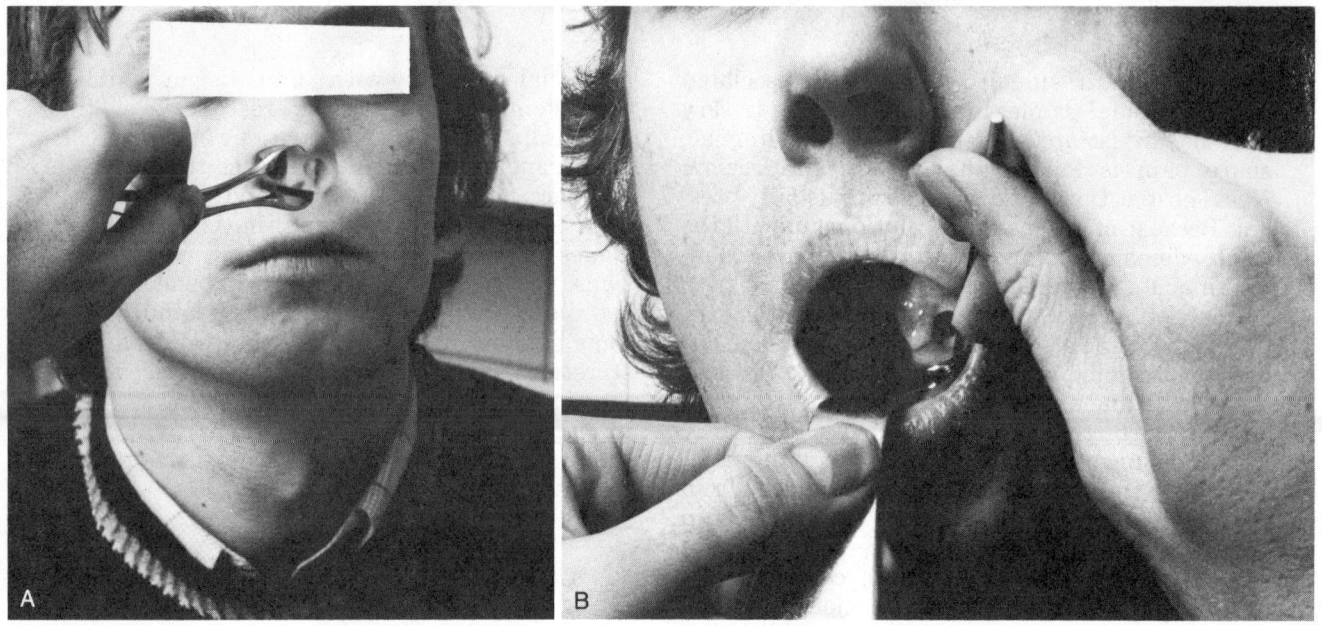

**FIGURE 6.** *Demonstration of anterior (A) and posterior (B) rhinoscopy.*

plications is higher than in the more privileged countries.

### DIAGNOSIS

A careful history of the present complaints, their treatment, past illness, and therapy must be obtained. Details of the pain and the character of the nasal obstruction and discharge are important. It is also essential to know the exact surgical procedures employed for patients who have had operations for sinusitis.

Inspection of the nose and pharynx is the most important examination (Fig. 6). Anterior rhinoscopy may reveal edema and erythema of the

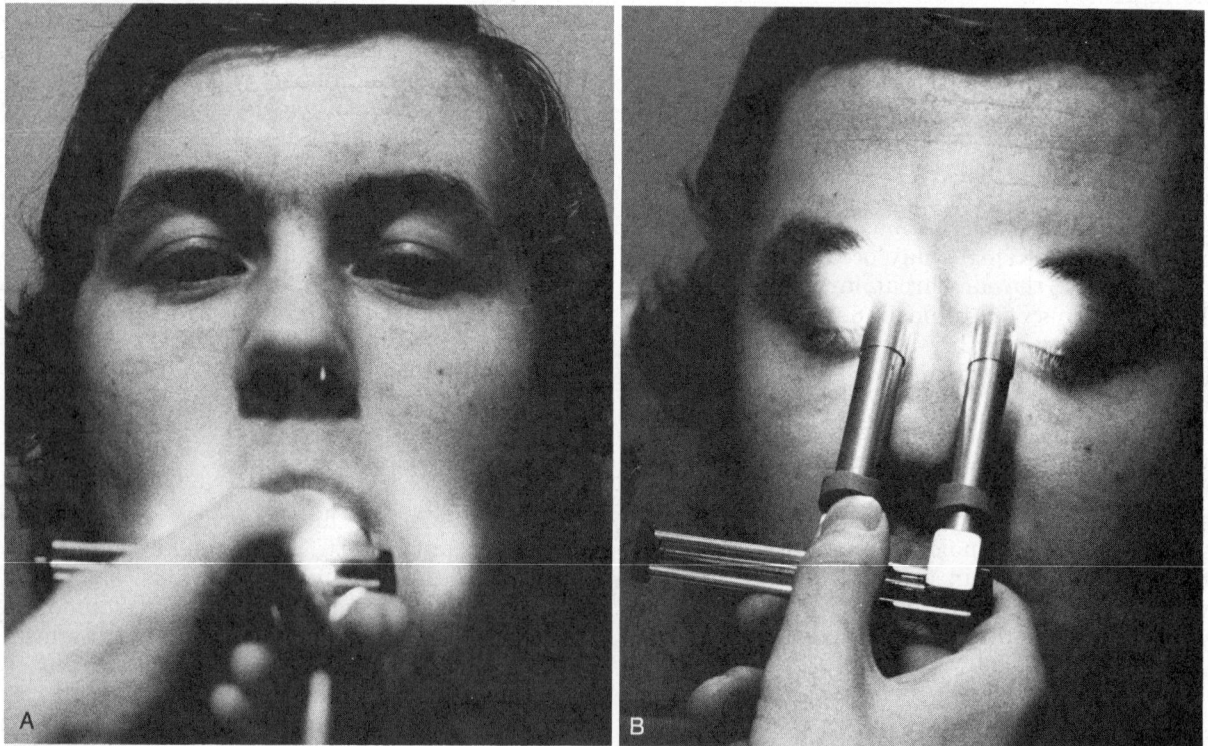

**FIGURE 7.** *Transillumination of the maxillary (A) and frontal (B) sinuses.*

nasal mucosa, especially of the inferior turbinate. In suppurative sinusitis, mucoid and mucopurulent secretions are noticed. The localization of these secretions aids in the determination of which sinuses are involved. While in frontal sinusitis secretions are visible anteriorly at the inferior turbinate, maxillary and ethmoidal secretions appear over the posterior end of the inferior turbinate. One must also look for nasal polyps, nasal septum deviations, and malignant processes. A posterior rhinoscopy and inspection of the oropharynx may also reveal redness, edema, and drainage of mucoid and mucopurulent secretions. In cases of sphenoidal sinusitis, the pus is mainly visible at the posterior wall of the nasopharynx. Palpation may reveal tenderness over the involved sinuses, and the condition of the teeth should be inspected.

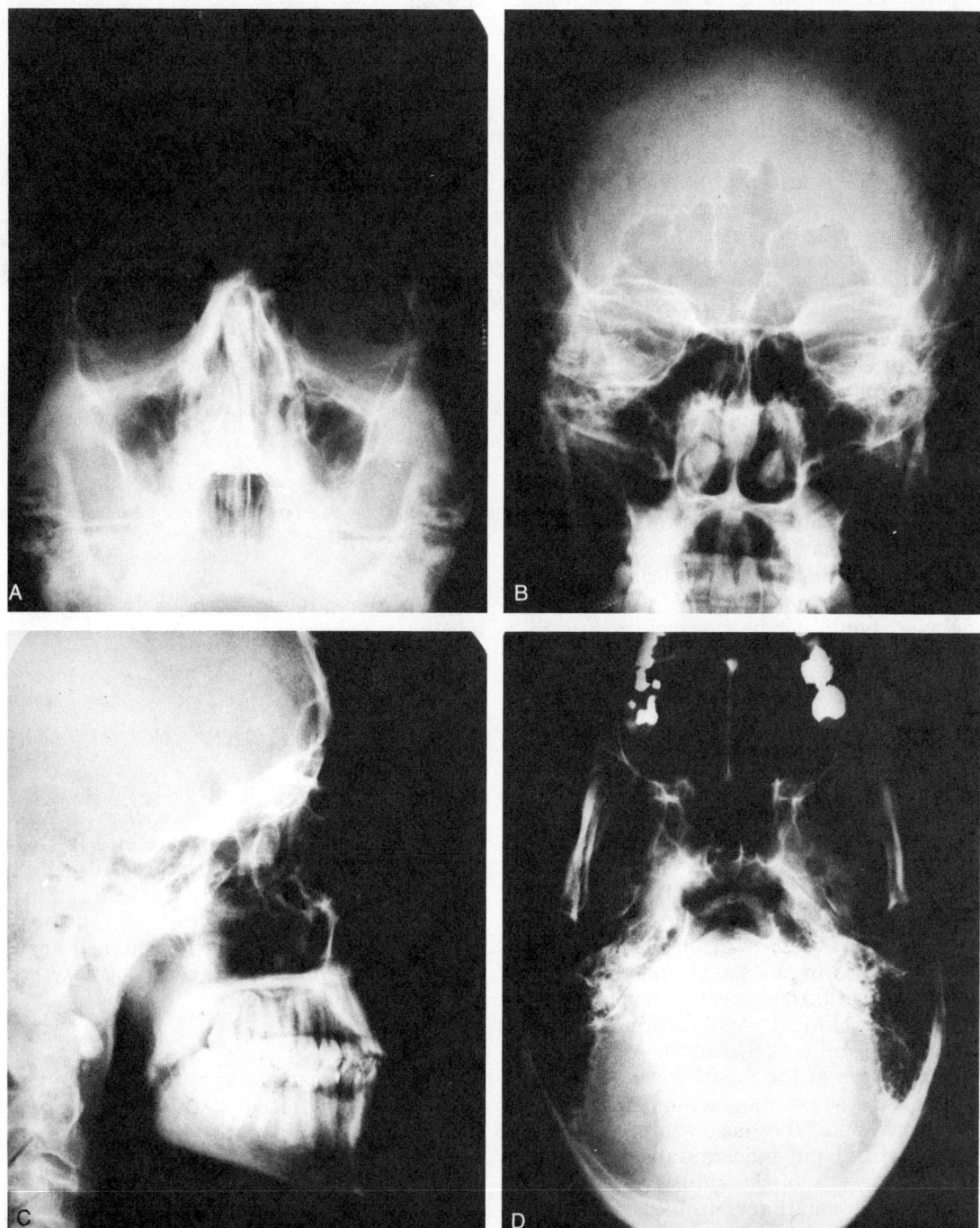

**FIGURE 8.**   *The standard paranasal sinus X-rays: (A) Waters view; (B) Caldwell view; (C) profile; and (D) Hirz view.*

Transillumination (Fig. 7) can be useful in the diagnosis of everyday acute sinusitis. It requires a completely darkened room and a bright light source. The maxillary sinuses are illuminated by placing the light in the patient's mouth. The patient is asked to close his lips tightly around the covered light source. In normal maxillary sinuses, the light is transmitted to the anterior wall of the antrum so that a bright crescent zone is seen in the infraorbital region. The pupil is also lighted. Another method is to place the light source on the maxillary sinus roof. It can then be seen through its floor, the palate. Illumination of the frontal sinus is obtained by placing a covered light source against the frontal sinus floor. The diagnostic value of transillumination has considerable limitation, however. It is much less accurate than x-ray, especially in bilateral sinusitis, in patients with a dense bony structure, in children, and after previous operation upon the sinuses.

Radiography is an indispensable examination in the exact diagnosis of sinusitis. The standard paranasal sinus examination consists of the Waters view (occipitomental position), the Caldwell view (occipitomental position), the profile view (lateral position), and the basal view (Bowen, Hirz, submentovertical position). Observations are made on the presence of thickening of the mucous membrane, an air-fluid level, polypoid tumors, and bony destruction. Complete sinus opacification may be the result of a marked mucous membrane thickening or a complete filling of the sinus by transudate, exudate, or blood, and neoplasia should not be overlooked (Fig. 9). Special techniques are x-ray examination with radiopaque substances and tomography. Panoramic tomography is a very useful examination in sinusitis of dental origin (Fig. 10).

Endoscopic examination of the maxillary sinus permits direct vision of the antral mucosa. With this method, biopsy of the lesions is also possible.

### Diagnosis of Mucormycosis

This rare sinus infection occurring in diabetic patients in acidosis is caused by phycomycetes. It leads to an angiitis in the nasal and paranasal regions resulting in thrombosis and hemorrhagic infarction. Early clinical manifestations are a black and bloody unilateral rhinorrhea. Rhinoscopy and inspection of the mouth reveal a black inferior turbinate sometimes accompanied by a necrotic perforation of the nasal septum and the hard palate. Orbital and endocranial extension is common. Radiography of the sinuses reveals involvement of the maxillary, frontal, and ethmoidal sinuses, showing a homogeneous sinus opacification. Mucormycosis of the sinuses is a

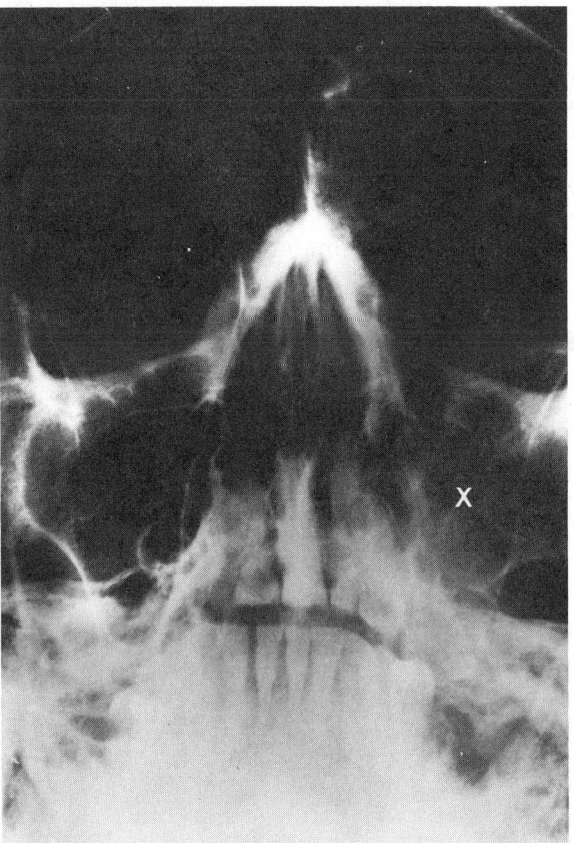

**FIGURE 9.** Complete opacification of the left maxillary sinus and partial opacification of the left frontal sinus (Waters view).

lethal disease. Only with early diagnosis and adequate treatment do some patients survive (Chapter 97).

## TREATMENT AND PROPHYLAXIS

"Given the correct diagnosis and management, sinus disorders are as amenable to successful treatment as disease anywhere else in the body" (Bernstein, 1971). There are three difficult factors in sinusitis treatment: (1) the sinuses are contained within rigid bony walls, (2) the clearance of the secretions depends on normal ciliary activity, and (3) drainage for the sinus cavity requires an unobstructed orifice.

### Acute Sinusitis

An uncomplicated acute sinusitis can be cured without surgery, because the tissue changes are still reversible. With appropriate treatment, the purulent exudate is evacuated through the opened sinus ostium, the edema is resorbed, and the sinus epithelium can regrow over the submucosa. Drainage of the secretions is achieved by the administration of local shrinking agents and/or

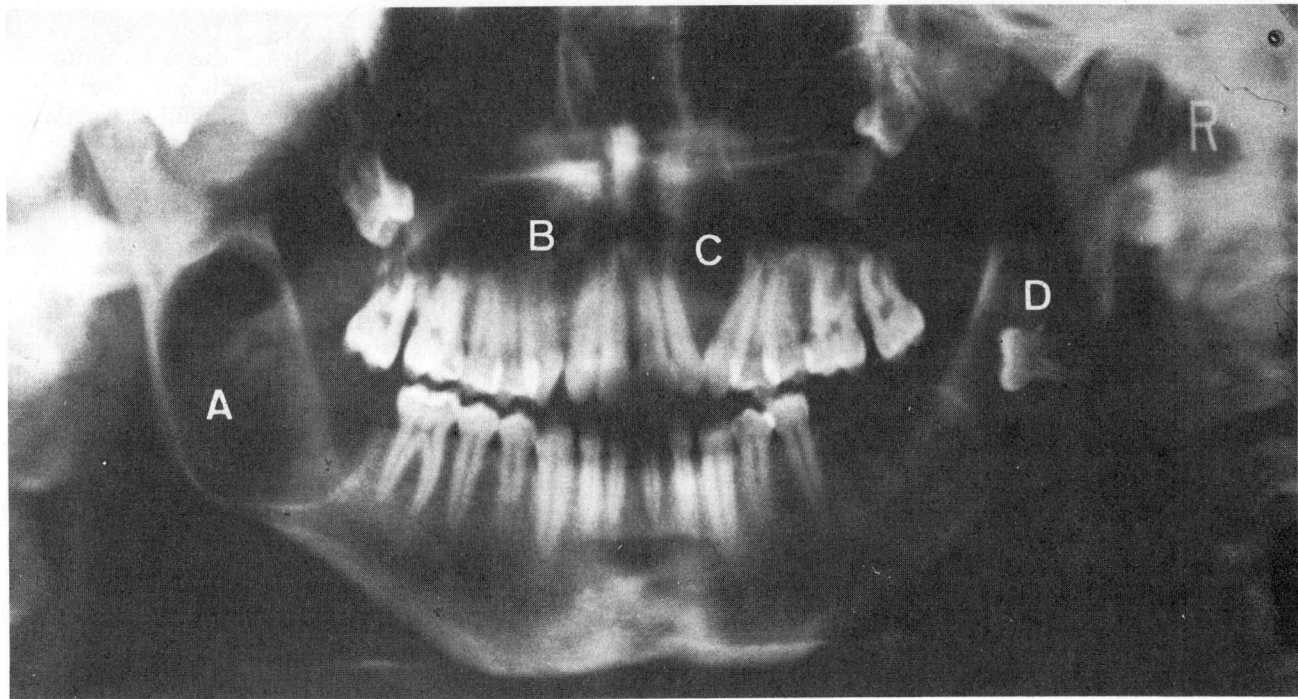

**FIGURE 10.** *Panoramic tomography showing two dental cysts (B, C) causing maxillary sinusitis. Note also two mandibular cysts (A, D). (Courtesy of Dr. R. van Clooster.)*

oral decongestant preparations: antihistamines, and sympathomimetic drugs. In purulent acute sinusitis, an antimicrobial drug is effective. It is active against *H. influenzae, S. pneumoniae,* and the anaerobic *Peptostreptococcus.* Also, the antibiotic must penetrate sufficiently into the infected mucous membrane and produce few side effects. Accordingly, the following drugs are recommended in the treatment of uncomplicated sinusitis (peroral administration): amoxycillin (500 mg four times daily in adults), bacampicillin (400 mg two or three times daily), doxycycline (100 mg once or twice daily), cotrimoxazol (160 mg trimethoprim and 800 mg sulfamethoxazole twice daily), and cefaclor (250 mg four times daily). In severe or complicated cases intravenous administration of antibiotics is recommended: 4 g ampicillin + 2 g dicloxacillin or doxycycline (200 mg daily). If the complicated sinusitis is caused by betalactamase-producing *Hemophilus influenzae,* chloramphenicol should be given intravenously (4 g daily).

### Subacute Sinusitis

The suppuration in these cases may be reversible with medical treatment alone, or with simple repetitive irrigation; or it may go on to chronicity, with irreversible tissue damage. In cases of maxillary sinusitis, an antral irrigation is performed. After administration of a local anesthetic, the puncture needle penetrates the medial wall of the maxillary sinus (lateral nasal wall) under the inferior turbinate (Fig. 11).

The sinus is washed out with sterile water at body temperature; and antibiotics with corticosteroids may be introduced. This irrigation is repeated every 2 to 4 days until the rinsing water is free of pus.

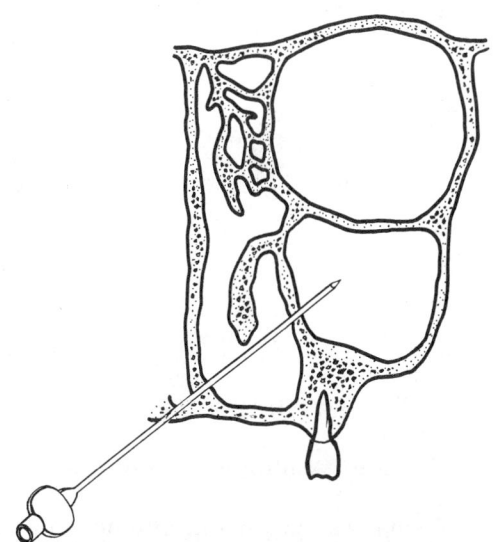

**FIGURE 11.** *Puncture of the maxillary sinus.*

## Chronic Sinusitis

In many cases, patients with chronic sinusitis do not have many complaints and are sometimes not aware of their disease. In these cases, no medical interference is warranted. On the contrary, when the patient is suffering from severe mucopurulent or purulent nasal discharge or nasal obstruction, or when complications are likely to occur or are already present, surgery must be performed in order to drain pus, ventilate air-containing cavities, and remove irreversibly damaged mucoperiosteum.

In cases of maxillary sinusitis, an intranasal antrostomy or the Caldwell-Luc procedure can be performed. Ethmoidal sinusitis can be approached by transantral, intranasal, or external ethmoidectomy, of which the last is the most effective and safe technique. Subacute frontal sinusitis can be cured by trephination, while chronic frontal sinusitis requires definitive frontal surgery in the form of a nonobliterative or an obliterative procedure. The sphenoid sinus may be approached through the ethmoidal labyrinth after an external ethmoidectomy, through the nasal septum, or transantrally.

### Sinusitis in Children

Sinusitis in children should be handled in a very conservative manner, much more so than in adults. A supplementary aid in treatment is the Proetz displacement (aspiration and irrigation of the nose and sinuses). It is imperative, prior to undertaking a sinus irrigation, to have adequate radiographs to show the size of the sinus, its position, and its relationhip to other structures. If surgical intervention is necessary, it should be minimal; e.g., in chronic maxillary sinusitis, the Caldwell-Luc procedure should be avoided if possible, and the intranasal antrostomy is recommended.

## Mucormycosis

First, it is necessary to treat the underlying disease, usually diabetes. In addition, surgical debridement of the affected tissues, and drainage and curettage of the sinus, orbit, and nasal fossa should be performed. Amphotericin B is given intravenously in doses of 50 mg daily for a total of 2.2 g.

## PROPHYLAXIS

Predisposing factors, such as nasal septal deviation and allergy, should be treated. Adequate treatment of acute and subacute sinusitis should prevent the development of a chronic form. Complications of sinusitis have become rare since the era of antibiotics. Proper surgical management of chronic sinusitis, with restoration of normal sinus ventilation and removal of all irreversibly damaged tissues, should prevent relapses.

### References

Bernstein, L.: Pediatric sinus problems. Otolaryngol Clin North Am 4:127, 1971.
Brorson, J. E., Axelsson, A., and Holm, S. E.: Studies on Branhamella catarrhalis with special reference to maxillary sinusitis. Scand J Infect Dis 8:151, 1976.
Van Cauwenberge, P., Verschraegen, G., and Van Renterghem, L.: Bacteriologic findings in sinusitis (1963–1975). Scand J Infect Dis Suppl 9:72, 1976.
Van Cauwenberge, P., Van Renterghem, L., Verschraegen, G., and Kluyskens, P.: Bacteriology in sinusitis with special reference to the role of the anaerobes. In Proceedings of the International Symposium of Infection and Allergy of the Nose and Paranasal Sinuses. Tokyo, Scimed Publications, Inc., 1977, pp. 151–155.
Frederick, J., and Braude, A. I.: Anaerobic infection of the paranasal sinuses. New Engl J Med 290:135, 1974.
Litton, W. B.: Acute and chronic sinusitis. Otolaryngol Clin North Am 4:25, 1971.
Takahashi, R.: Environmental factors in the development of infection and allergy of the nose and paranasal sinuses. In Proceedings of the International Symposium of Infection and Allergy of the Nose and Paranasal Sinuses. Tokyo, Scimed Publications, Inc., 1977, pp. 21–26.

# 93 OTITIS MEDIA AND OTITIS EXTERNA

Burt R. Meyers, M.D., and William Lawson, M.D., D.D.S.

## OTITIS MEDIA

### Definition; Etiology; Pathogenesis

Otitis media is an acute and chronic inflammatory state of the middle ear which may be suppurative or nonsuppurative. Acute otitis media is primarily a disease of infants and children, whereas the chronic form and its complications generally arise in later life. Although the majority of infections are bacterial, other agents (including viruses and mycoplasma) may produce an acute syndrome with serous effusion.

The eustachian tube has a cardinal role in the

development of otitis media. In acute suppurative otitis media the occurrence of a viral upper respiratory tract infection produces hyperemia and edema of the nose and nasopharynx with partial occlusion of the eustachian tube orifice. This impairment of middle ear ventilation results in the transudation of fluid from the negative pressure produced by the continuous resorption of gases by the hyperemic middle ear mucosa. This, coupled with copious mucoid secretions and frequent sneezing, coughing, and swallowing, permits pathogenic organisms such as *Streptococcus pneumoniae* and *Hemophilus influenzae*, which normally colonize the nasopharynx, to enter the eustachian tube and middle ear, where they produce inflammation, exudation, and finally suppuration. Many of the viral exanthems are often followed by middle ear infections, probably as a result of the same mechanisms. Certain systemic bacterial infections, such as pneumococcal pneumonia and meningococcal meningitis, may be associated with otitis media; however, it is not clear if these represent local extension from the oropharynx or are secondary to hematologic seeding.

Epidemiologic data seem to support this concept of the pathogenesis of acute bacterial otitis media. First, there is a seasonal variation in its incidence; it is more common during the winter months when viral respiratory infections are frequent. Attacks accompany or follow viral infections and the offending bacteria are those normally found in the nasopharynx. Anatomic predisposing factors in young children include the configuration of the eustachian tube and lymphoid hyperplasia of Waldeyer's ring. The great frequency of acute otitis media in infants and young children may be related to the relatively short and straight course of the eustachian tube in this age group, permitting direct access from the nasopharynx to the middle ear.

The role of immunologic factors in the etiology of otitis media is unclear. In chronic serous and acute purulent otitis media the fluid present in the middle ear space contains antibodies of all immunoglobulin classes. However, the high titer of secretory IgA in serous otitis indicates that the fluid is not entirely produced by transudation but contains constituents produced locally. Patients with either hypo- or agammaglobulinemia are prone to bacterial infections including otitis media. Opsonification is necessary for phagocytosis of the microorganisms most responsible for this infection, and the lack of globulins may account for their increased virulence in this group of patients.

There may be ethnic and social factors operative in the susceptibility to otitis. There appears to be a propensity for otitis media in certain races;

both American Indians and Asians have a higher incidence of infection. It has been suggested but not proven that economically depressed groups may be more prone to infection.

In chronic otitis media there is persistent obstruction of the eustachian tube, produced by a variety of factors such as chronic nasal and pharyngeal infection, lymphoid hyperplasia, allergy, or cleft palate. With recurrent infection the middle ear mucosa may undergo alterations with metaplasia and an increase in goblet cells or irreversible changes with the formation of polyps, granulations, and tympanosclerosis. The tympanic membrane may become atrophic, sclerotic, or perforated, with ingrowth of epithelium and formation of a secondary cholesteatoma. Persistent infection may also result in destruction of the ossicles. Extension of the infection into the mastoid may cause sclerosis with limited pneumatization, osteitis, or osteomyelitis of the bone, possibly with the formation of a sequestrum. The hyaline submucosal plaques of tympanosclerosis may calcify, producing immobility of the tympanic membrane, fixation of the ossicles, and partial obliteration of the tympanic cavity. From persistent negative pressure due to eustachian tube dysfunction, fluid may accumulate and thicken, producing an adhesive otitis. This may result in immobilization of the ossicular chain and retraction of the tympanic membrane, with progressive conductive hearing loss. In some cases, continuous retraction of the pars flaccida produces a primary acquired cholesteatoma.

## Bacteriology

Bacteriologic studies on the etiology of acute otitis media have been best described in children. When tympanocentesis was performed and the fluid examined it was noted that *S. pneumoniae*, *H. influenzae* (nontypable strains), and *Streptococcus pyogenes* were responsible for 90 per cent of positive culture specimens. Though studies vary, most find rates of 50 per cent *S. pneumoniae* and 20 to 30 per cent *H. influenzae*, and *S. pyogenes* in those isolates remaining. *H. influenzae* type B isolates may accompany cellulitis secondary to this pathogen. Since anaerobic cultures are less frequently performed, it appears they are not responsible for acute infection.

*S. pneumoniae* is the most common cause of otitis media in the adult, accounting for more than 80 to 90 per cent of the isolates. *S. pyogenes*, *Staphylococcus aureus*, and *H. influenzae* comprise the other pathogens. In the adult with chronic otitis media, with a history of acute exacerbation, the usual pathogens are *S. pneumoniae*, *H. influenzae*, and *S. aureus*. In chronic otitis media associated with aural drainage, gram-negative microorganisms including *Proteus* sp., *Pseudomonas* sp., *Escherichia coli*, or *S. aureus* have been isolated. Recent reports have found anaerobes in mixed cultures from 50 per cent of isolates obtained by tympanocentesis. Bacterial isolates from the complications of chronic otitis, such as brain abscesses, are often anaerobic, suggesting a causal relation.

*Mycoplasma pneumoniae*, adenovirus, influenza virus, and respiratory syncytial virus have been isolated from middle ear aspirates.

## Clinical Features; Diagnosis

In acute bacterial otitis media the presenting symptom is pain. In infants this may be communicated by crying and tugging at the ears. It may be accompanied by high fever. Otoscopy may reveal only injection over the handle of the malleus, or diffuse redness and loss of anatomic landmarks, or even bulging of the entire eardrum. Insufflation with a pneumatic otoscope may help in revealing a bulging drum by its immobility. If a significant amount of a fluid accumulates in the middle ear there is also a decrease in hearing acuity. With continued suppuration there may be spontaneous perforation of the tympanic membrane with the development of a purulent discharge and lessening of the pain. These perforations tend to heal with resolution of the infection. However, in a small number of cases, infection with β-hemolytic streptococci produces an early and extensive necrotizing otitis with loss of the pars tensa and portions of the ossicular chain.

Viral otitis media may also accompany upper respiratory infections. In this condition the dominant symptom is fullness and mild hearing loss; pain is uncommon and generally signifies secondary bacterial infection. Otoscopy usually reveals only dullness and either mild retraction or fullness of the drumhead, depending on the quantity of fluid produced. Impedance audiometry may reveal a persistent negative pressure in the middle ear space or a pattern of decreased compliance suggestive of fluid. Treatment is directed toward improvement of eustachian tube function and aeration of the middle ear space by the use of decongestants and the Valsalva maneuver. Viral infections, especially influenza and occasionally mycoplasma, may attack the tympanic membrane itself, causing bullous myringitis. The syndrome produces intense pain lasting 1 or 2 days. Otoscopy reveals hemorrhagic blebs over the drumhead, which often spontaneously rupture, producing bleeding in the ear canal or fullness in the tympanic cavity. This condition is self-limiting, requiring only analgesics or anodyne eardrops for a few days. Persistent pain signifies secondary bacterial infection and requires systemic antibiotics.

## Complications

Acute mastoiditis is now an uncommon complication of acute suppurative otitis media and results from incomplete or inappropriate antibiotic coverage or an immunologically deficient host. It usually is associated with chronic otitis media and cholesteatoma. Severe inflammation in the middle ear space may result in attic block with accumulation of pus in the mastoid air cells and the dissolution of the bony septa between them. The patient may then develop fever and mastoid pain. Otoscopy may reveal an intact eardrum with sagging of the posterosuperior canal wall or an actively draining perforation. The mastoid area may show tenderness or swelling or outward displacement of the pinna if a subperiosteal abscess develops. Radiographs will show clouding and coalescence of the mastoid air cells and blurring of the bony margins. Simple mastoidectomy may be required if infection does not resolve after a few days of systemic antibiotic therapy.

Acute petrositis classically is characterized by Gradenigo's syndrome, in which diplopia caused by a sixth cranial nerve palsy and ocular pain accompany aural discharge. It occurs most commonly in patients with chronic otitis media, some of whom have undergone a prior simple mastoidectomy. Failure of resolution with high-dose intravenous antibiotic therapy requires surgical drainage of the petrous apex.

Serous or suppurative labyrinthitis may complicate acute otitis media, producing vestibular (vertigo, nystagmus, nausea, vomiting) or cochlear (neurosensory hearing loss) symptoms. Inflammation of the labyrinth may occur through the middle ear (round or oval window) or secondary to meningitis. With serous labyrinthitis the symptoms are generally mild and self-limiting and respond to intravenous antibiotics and drainage of the middle ear space by myringotomy. With suppurative labyrinthitis, there is complete loss of hearing, severe vertigo, absent caloric response, and the danger of intracranial extension. If meningeal symptoms develop and cerebrospinal fluid abnormalities are found, surgical drainage of the labyrinth is necessary; otherwise intravenous antibiotics are usually adequate to control the infection.

Facial nerve paralysis may occur in acute or chronic otitis media from edema of the nerve in response to suppuration extending through a dehiscence in the tympanic portion of its bony canal. It almost invariably responds completely to high-dose antibiotic therapy and prompt myringotomy. Some authors also advocate steroid therapy (prednisone, 60 to 80 mg daily) and surgical decompression, which is reserved for only those few cases that go on to show evidence of degeneration of the nerve.

### Intracranial Complications

The development of meningitis, epidural or brain abscess, otitic hydrocephalus, and lateral sinus thrombosis may follow middle ear infection. These may extend intracranially directly through a bony dehiscence or surgical defect, or by thrombophlebitis of emissary veins or Haversian systems, or via the labyrinth. Continued fever, pain, toxicity, the development of headache, somnolence, irritability, or nausea and vomiting despite antibiotic therapy signal extension of the infection. There may be continued aural drainage through a perforation, or an intact inflamed or even normal eardrum found on otoscopy. Radiographs may or may not reveal bone destruction. Examination of the cerebrospinal fluid, ophthalmoscopy for the detection of papilledema, and blood cultures are mandatory with this clinical picture. These patients should also have a detailed neurologic examination and be observed closely for the development of signs of meningeal irritation. If a brain abscess is suspected, bone and brain scanning and computerized axial tomography may define the lesion. Management includes intense antibiotic therapy initially and, when the patient's condition warrants, definitive surgery. Surgery is generally required since these complications usually accompany chronic otitis media and mastoiditis, often with cholesteatoma. Meningitis can be managed primarily with antibiotics, but recurrent otogenic meningitis suggests chronic mastoiditis, a condition that often requires radical mastoidectomy for exploration and removal of diseased bone and granulation tissue. Craniotomy may be needed for drainage of a brain abscess.

### Treatment

Studies in children have been carried out to determine the level of antibiotic present in the middle ear during an infection. Antibiotic levels have been calculated by tympanocentesis and comparisons to the serum level, minimum inhibitory concentration (the least amount of antibiotic which inhibits growth in the test tube), and response of the patient determined. The following compounds have been found in concentrations adequate to inhibit *S. pneumoniae* strains isolated: penicillins G and V, amoxicillin, erythromycin estolate, triple sulfonamide, cefaclor, trimethoprim, sulfamethoxazole, and others. The levels of penicillin found in one study would not have inhibited 75 per cent of *H. influenzae* isolated.

In other studies, levels of 4 $\mu$g/ml were found after penicillin V and these were inhibitory and efficacious. Erythromycin estolate would have been effective against only 60 per cent of these strains.

The treatment of choice for an adult with uncomplicated otitis media is penicillin. This may be administered orally as phenoxymethyl penicillin, or may be given once intramuscularly in a dose of 1.2 million units. Procaine and benzathine penicillin (Bicillin), 1.2 million units, is especially effective. In adults allergic to penicillin, erythromycin, 250 mg, should be given orally every 6 hours for 7 to 10 days. Oral cephalosporins have also been proven effective but their cost may be prohibitive for developing nations. Tetracycline hydrochloride may be used, but resistant *S. pneumoniae*, *S. pyogenes*, and *S. aureus* strains have been reported. The use of tetracycline in children under 8 years is contraindicated because of staining of the permanent dentition.

In the patient with a history of chronic suppurative otitis with exacerbations, treatment directed against *S. aureus* (presumed penicillin-resistant) and *H. influenzae* is necessary if material for culture is unavailable. A penicillinase-resistant penicillin like dicloxacillin is recommended for *S. aureus* infection and ampicillin for *H. influenzae*, both at a dose of 250 mg every 6 hours. Increasing numbers of *H. influenzae* strains are being isolated that are resistant to ampicillin because of $\beta$-lactamase production. In those patients, trimethoprim-sulfamethoxazole or an oral cephalosporin such as cefaclor would be efficacious.

The use of an antihistamine or decongestant should accompany antibiotic therapy for acute otitis media. For an acute episode in which severe pain is accompanied by a bulging tympanic membrane, myringotomy will provide rapid relief. In prolonged or repeated episodes of acute otitis media or hearing loss accompanied by an abnormal eardrum, fluid in the middle ear space must be presumed and myringotomy, generally with the insertion of a ventilating tube, is indicated. In young children with recurrent otitis media, adenoidectomy may also be performed in an attempt to clear the eustachian tube orifices of the obstructing lymphoid tissue. Attention must also be directed to the elimination of other etiologic factors such as chronic nasal or sinus infection and allergy.

The treatment of chronic otitis media in the adult requires not only a systemic but also a topical antibiotic in order to control the otorrhea. A variety of otic preparations have been devised that are directed primarily against the offending gram-negative flora (e.g., gentamicin, colimycin, chloromycetin, and polymyxin eardrops). The definitive management of chronic otitis media and its complications, including tympanic membrane perforation, cholesteatoma, conductive hearing loss, and mastoiditis, are primarily surgical and are detailed in standard textbooks of otology (e.g., Shambaugh and Glasscock: *Surgery of the Ear*).

### Tuberculous Otitis

Tuberculous involvement of the middle ear occurs in both adults and children, although more commonly in the latter. Congenital cases have been reported. The human strain is generally the causative organism, producing secondary involvement of the temporal bone. The proposed routes of infection are via the eustachian tube, by hematogenous spread, or, on rare occasions, directly through the auditory canal.

Characteristically, there is painless aural discharge through multiple tympanic membrane perforations. Later in the disease these coalesce into one large opening with exuberant granulations and extensive destruction in the middle ear space. There is also severe hearing loss (generally conductive) early in the disease. Occasionally there is bilateral involvement. Unlike other forms of chronic otitis media in which x-rays of the mastoid bones reveal sclerosis, in tuberculous otitis they are generally extensively pneumatized. The middle ear infection rapidly involves the mastoid, and complications develop, including facial paralysis, labyrinthine fistula, subperiosteal and cervical abscess, meningitis, cutaneous fistula, and formation of a sequestration of bone.

Diagnosis may be established by biopsy of middle ear tissue revealing caseating epithelioid granulomas. Cultures are positive in only a small number of cases. Tuberculin skin tests are usually positive and chest x-rays may reveal old or acute tuberculous changes. Tuberculous mastoiditis should be suspected in any patient with painless otitis media accompanied by severe hearing loss, profuse granulations in the middle ear space, and evidence of coalescent mastoiditis in a well-pneumatized mastoid.

The treatment of this condition is primarily with antituberculous therapy, principally isoniazid and ethambutol. Surgery, primarily radical mastoidectomy, is reserved for those cases that are refractory to treatment or develop the complications of otitis media.

### Prophylaxis

Since viral syndromes of the upper respiratory tract often precede otitis media, their prevention might decrease bacterial invasion. At present immunization is effective against the viral ex-anthems but a "cold" vaccine is not available. The use of prophylactic antibiotics in proved viral infections has not been of value and is not recommended. Intermittent administration of antibiotics to patients with a history of chronic suppurative or serous otitis has been carried out but proof of its efficacy is lacking. $\gamma$-Globulin should be administered to patients with either congenital or acquired agammaglobulinemia.

## OTITIS EXTERNA

### Definition; Etiology; Pathogenesis

Otitis externa is an inflammatory condition of any portion of the skin of the external auditory canal. It has been classified by Senturia and Marcus (1967) as an infectious disease, neurogenic eruption, allergic dermatosis, traumatic lesion, and disease of unknown etiology. This reflects the multiplicity of causative factors in the pathogenesis of this condition. The most important factors are high humidity and temperature, trauma or excoriation of the skin, and allergy to hair sprays and dyes. The significance of climatic conditions is seen in the popular names used for description, such as swimmer's ear, hot-weather ear, or Hong Kong or Singapore ear. The incidence of this disease has been estimated at 3 to 10 per cent of the general population, and as high as 50 per cent of otologic cases. This increased prevalence is especially notable in tropical and subtropical zones.

The most commonly encountered form of this condition is diffuse otitis externa, either acute or chronic, arising from bacterial infection. Otitis externa results from disruption of the physiologic defense mechanisms operative in the external auditory canal. The most important of these is the local pH, whereby the acidity of the secretions of the skin, sweat, and sebaceous glands is bacteriostatic or bactericidal to organisms that would flourish in an alkaline medium (Goffin, 1963). Other protective factors include the secretion of lysozyme by sweat glands. The antimicrobial action of unsaturated fatty acids derived from lipids secreted by sebaceous glands may be active against gram-negative bacteria and certain fungi. The water-repellent coating of waxes secreted by the apocrine glands and the clearing action of the lateral migration of keratin through the ear canal also play a protective role (Cassisi et al., 1977).

While the sigmoid configuration of the external canal limits the entry of exogenous material, it also promotes the entrapment of water to form a skin-lined culture tube. The presence of exostoses, whose growth is encouraged by cold-water swimming, further enhances the retention of moisture. Prolonged exposure to moisture produces maceration of the epithelial lining with swelling of the surface keratin and blockage of the ducts of the glands, which in turn are penetrated by endogenous nonpathogenic organisms. This produces a low-grade inflammation and promotes the invasion by exogenous, primarily gram-negative organisms (Senturia, 1957). This is further aggravated by the development of an itch-scratch cycle.

### Bacteriology

Studies of the flora of the normal external auditory canal show that *Staphylococcus epidermidis* and diphtheroids are the predominant organisms. *S. aureus* is only occasionally and *Pseudomonas* sp. rarely isolated. However, in chronic otitis externa *Pseudomonas* sp. becomes the predominant organism cultured, followed by *S. aureus*. Cassisi et al. (1977) found, on study of 232 ears with a positive culture, a single organism in 63 per cent, two organisms in 31 per cent, and three organisms in 5 per cent. Of these, 59 per cent were gram-negative and 41 per cent were gram-positive. *Pseudomonas* sp. constituted 66 per cent of the first group; the remainder were primarily *Proteus, Enterobacter, Klebsiella*, and *E. coli*. Of the gram-positive organisms, *S. aureus* comprised 30 per cent and *Streptococcus* strains only 12 per cent. Fungal forms were isolated in a very small number of the cases with acute diffuse otitis externa.

### Clinical Features; Diagnosis

The clinical manifestations of the commonly encountered acute diffuse form of otitis externa vary widely in intensity. The dominant symptoms are itching and pain. The pain may be mild to extremely severe because of progressive swelling in a confined space. There may be an accompanying exudate which may be thin and watery or purulent. With continued swelling and exudate in the canal the patient may describe or present with hearing loss. On clinical examination canal wall edema and erythema are the most common findings. The swelling may progress to the point of total closure of the canal, preventing visualization of the eardrum. Examination of the tympanic membrane is mandatory since otitis externa may be secondary to suppurative middle ear disease. Aural drainage and excoriation of the canal lining also occur frequently. Pain on manipulation of the pinna, periauricular edema, and regional lymphadenopathy accompany severe attacks. Constitutional symptoms are unusual and represent bacterial invasion of the surrounding soft tissues. The chronic diffuse form, common in humid climates, is characterized also by itching and fullness of the ears. In this condition, *Aspergillus niger, Actinomyces*, or yeasts produce a chronic superficial infection. Otoscopy reveals erosion and desquamation of the epithelial lining, with formation of a membrane and a musty-smelling exudate. Occasionally a fungus ball may fill the canal. Eczematoid and seborrheic changes in the external auditory canal, meatus, concha, or remainder of the pinna represent allergic and dermatologic conditions, respectively, rather than infectious processes. Rarely, in uncontrolled chronic otitis externa, extensive hyperkeratosis and subcutaneous fibrosis produce stenosis of the external auditory canal.

### Treatment

Treatment is directed to symptomatic relief and control of the infectious organisms. A topical preparation containing antibiotics effective against *Pseudomonas* (e.g., polymyxin B or colistin) and staphylococci (e.g., neomycin) in a mildly acidified hygroscopic vehicle (e.g., propylene glycol) along with an anti-inflammatory agent (hydrocortisone) produces relief in the vast majority of cases of acute diffuse otitis externa. The skin swelling may be so severe that a small gauze wick may have to be inserted to permit entry of the drops into the canal. This may be combined with the use of an astringent such as Thiersch's solution. Supplemental analgesics may also be required for the control of pain until the edema subsides. Systemic antibiotics directed against gram-positive cocci (penicillin, ampicillin, cephalosporin, erythromycin) are indicated only when there is evidence of perichondritis or periauricular swelling or regional lymphadenopathy. With chronic otitis externa and after the severe inflammation has subsided in the acute form, cleansing, drying, and acidification of the canal are necessary. Debris may be removed by irrigation or aspiration, followed by the use of Burow's solution or acidified alcohol (2 to 4 per cent boric or acetic acid in 70 per cent ethanol). These latter agents are also very effective against fungal organisms commonly present in the chronic form. Systemic antifungal therapy has no role in the treatment of chronic otitis externa or otomycosis. When stenosis of the external auditory canal occurs, treatment consists of total excision of the hypertrophic lining, widening of the bony canal, and skin grafting of the defect.

### Prophylaxis

Patients with recurrent and chronic otitis externa must keep the external auditory canal dry.

This includes the exclusion of moisture by earplugs when swimming or bathing and the periodic use of alcohol eardrops if water enters or itching occurs.

## MALIGNANT OTITIS EXTERNA

Malignant otitis externa is an infection caused by *Pseudomonas aeruginosa* which begins in the external auditory canal and extends into the temporal bone; it may invade the base of the skull, contiguous soft tissues, and the brain. It occurs primarily in elderly diabetics but has also been reported with blood dyscrasias (e.g., chronic lymphocytic leukemia, granulocytopenia). In a series of 72 patients, all but 4 patients were diabetic. Of these 68 cases, 6 had only chemical diabetes and 27 were insulin-dependent. The pathogenicity of the *Pseudomonas* organism appears to be its ability to produce a vasculitis, with accompanying thrombosis and ischemic necrosis of tissue; however, the reason for its invasiveness in this select group is unclear.

The infection spreads through skin and cartilage to cause mastoiditis or osteomyelitis of the skull, cranial nerve palsies, sinus thrombosis, meningitis, and death. The mastoid may be destroyed by direct extension without middle ear involvement. One of the most characteristic symptoms of this condition is intense local pain. Facial nerve paralysis generally results from infection of the nerve within the soft tissues and is a poor prognostic sign. In one series, this occurred in 32 per cent of patients; half of the survivors were left with permanent nerve damage. The development of paralysis of the cranial nerves that pass through the jugular foramen generally signifies thrombosis of the jugular bulb and sigmoid sinus.

The disease should be suspected in any case of a refractory otitis externa, especially if granulations are present in the canal along with persistent purulent discharge, particularly in a diabetic. If there is no history of diabetes a glucose tolerance test should be performed. Fever may or may not be prominent, but the erythrocyte sedimentation rate is generally elevated. Cultures of the aural discharge will reveal *Pseudomonas* sp. Cerebrospinal fluid (CSF) analysis reveals mild pleocytosis, with normal glucose and a negative Gram stain. When meningitis develops, polymorphonuclear leukocytes will increase and a low CSF sugar will be found. Radionuclide scanning and computerized axial tomography may be used to define the areas of the involvement.

After appropriate cultures are taken, initial therapy with either carbenicillin, ticarcillin, or piperacillin coupled with an aminoglycoside should be instituted. This combination has produced synergistic effects in the laboratory. Carbenicillin in a dose of 5 g every 4 to 6 hours, or ticarcillin at one half the dose should be given intravenously. Both drugs have approximately 5 meq of sodium per gram, and in the elderly who may be in congestive heart failure, the amount of sodium delivered is a limiting factor. For the aminoglycoside, tobramycin 1 mg/kg given every 8 hours is a more logical choice than gentamicin because of its greater effect in vitro against *Pseudomonas* sp. and the smaller dose necessary to achieve synergism with carbenicillin or ticarcillin. We have cautiously administered these drugs parenterally for 4 to 6 weeks to four patients. None has needed surgery and all have recovered, though in one patient cranial nerve deficits improved only slightly. Monitoring of the eighth nerve and renal function is mandatory in patients receiving parenteral aminoglycosides for a prolonged time. Treatment of concomitant infections if they occur, adequate fluid replacement, and nutritional balance hasten recovery.

Antibiotic treatment should be continued for as long as improvement continues, usually 6 weeks. Surgery should be reserved until symptoms progress; intervention consists of radical mastoidectomy with debridement of all necrotic soft tissue and bone. Sinus thrombosis may be an indication for mandatory surgery.

## References

Cassisi, N., Cohn, A., Davidson, T., and Witten, B. R.: Diffuse otitis externa. Clinical and microbiologic findings in the course of a multicenter study on a new otic solution. Ann Otol Suppl 39:1–16, 1977.

Chandler, J. R.: Malignant external otitis: Further considerations. Ann Otol 86:417–428, 1977.

Goffin, F. B.: pH as a factor in external otitis. New Engl J Med 268:287–289, 1963.

Senturia, B. H.: Diseases of the External Ear. Springfield, Ill., Charles C Thomas, 1957.

Senturia, B. H., and Marcus, M. D.: Diseases of the external ear. Minn Med 50:837–838, 1967.

Shambaugh, G. E., and Glasscock, M. E., III: Surgery of the Ear. 3rd ed. Philadelphia, W. B. Saunders Co., 1980.

# EPIGLOTTITIS AND PSEUDOCROUP

## 94

### P. Branefors, M.D., Ph.D.

## DEFINITION

In the laryngeal region there are two diseases caused by infections: acute epiglottitis and pseudocroup (laryngitis subglottica). Both processes affect mainly children. Acute epiglottitis is a rare disease. Pseudocroup is more than 10 times as common. Because they have some clinical signs in common, acute epiglottitis is often mistaken for pseudocroup. It is, however, of the utmost importance to differentiate these two entities, since epiglottitis is a hyperacute and potentially fatal bacterial infection. Pseudocroup is generally of viral origin and only rarely constitutes a threat to life.

Acute epiglottitis is an inflammation of the supraglottic region and may affect not only the epiglottis, but also the aryepiglottic folds and even the prevertebral soft tissue. The pharynx is usually only slightly affected, and the true vocal cords and the subglottic tissue are seldom involved.

Pseudocroup is characterized by marked swelling of the tissue just below the vocal cords — the subglottic region — which is the narrowest part of the upper airway in small children.

## ETIOLOGY

As already mentioned, acute epiglottitis is of bacterial origin. The most common cause is *Haemophilus influenzae* type b. In children, blood cultures are nearly always positive for *H. influenzae* type b, and nose and throat cultures also yield *H. influenzae* in most cases. Blood cultures from adults are less likely to be positive. A greater proportion of adults than children have infections due to bacteria other than *H. influenzae*. Betahemolytic group A streptococci, *S. pneumoniae, Staphylococcus aureus,* and nonencapsulated *H. influenzae* have been isolated from pharyngeal swabs and on occasion from blood cultures. In a substantial number of pediatric and adult patients, throat cultures yield only a mixed flora of commensal bacteria.

Pseudocroup, on the other hand, is caused most commonly by parainfluenzae types 1, 2, and 3. Other viruses that are isolated less often are influenza A, respiratory syncytical virus, and, occasionally, members of the enterovirus group such as coxsackie and echoviruses. Allergy may predipose to pseudocroup in certain children.

The incidence of pseudocroup is highest in children from the age of 6 months to 3 years, while acute epiglottitis is most common in children 2 to 7 years old. It is important, however, to be aware of the fact that acute epiglottitis may occur at any age, in newborns as well as in old people. Some individuals may have a hereditary predisposition for pseudocroup, which is twice as common in boys as in girls. A child may have several attacks of pseudocroup before age 3.

## PATHOGENESIS AND PATHOLOGY

The generally clear-cut distinction between the manifestations of supraglottic and subglottic infections (epiglottitis and psueodcroup) is due to differences in the anatomy of the two regions. At the level of the true vocal cords, the mucosa is firmly attached to the underlying cartilage. In contrast, the supra- and subglottic mucosa and submucosa are quite loosely connected to the underlying tissue. Therefore, when infected, these tissues tend to become very swollen, which may lead to a life-threatening obstruction of the air passages (Fig. 1). In most cases of acute epiglottitis, the inflammatory edema is most pronounced in the epiglottis, which may become several times larger than normal. Occasionally the epiglottis is only slightly inflamed, while other parts of the supraglottic region show more pronounced inflammatory edema.

In acute epiglottitis, the submucosa is edematous and enormously infiltrated with polymorphonuclear and mononuclear cells. Interstitial hemorrhage and thrombosis of the small vessels in the submucosa are prominent. The mucosa, especially over the epiglottis, is markedly edematous, hemorrhagic, and sometimes even necrotic (Kissane and Smith, 1967). Abscesses may also develop.

The pathogenesis of the intense inflammatory changes that occur in acute epiglottitis, especially when they are caused by *H. influenzae* type b, has not yet been clarified. The epiglottic region is

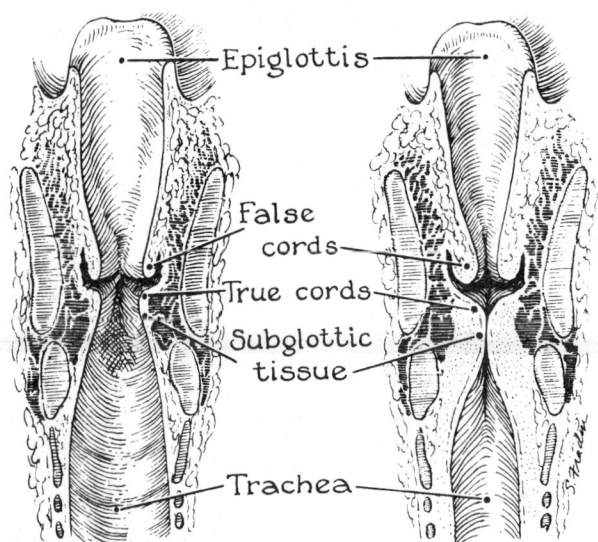

**FIGURE 1.** *Larynx and trachea. Compare the normal anatomy on the left with the typical changes of pseudocroup on the right. (From Krugman and Ward: Infectious Diseases of Children. 4th ed. St. Louis, C. V. Mosby Company 1968.)*

probably the route of entry for the bacteria. As such, there may be local accumulation of *H. influenzae* endotoxin with induction of the local Shwartzman phenomenon. In addition, it may be that sensitization to the causative organism must be present before the clinical picture of acute epiglottitis can develop, since patients with acute epiglottitis are in an age group in which specific antibodies against *H. influenzae* capsular antigens can be demonstrated in most individuals. In acute epiglottitis, an allergic reaction of the Arthus type might also contribute to the pronounced pathologic changes (Branefors-Helander and Jeppsson, 1975).

The pathogenesis of the respiratory obstruction associated with epiglottitis appears to be related to the anatomy of the area. The considerable edema swells the epiglottis, which curls posteriorly and inferiorly. In combination with the edema of the other supraglottic tissues, the airway is narrowed, especially during inspiration when the tissues are forced downward, creating a ball-valve effect. As a result, hypoxia ensues but not hypercarbia, since expiration can continue normally. Sitting up, leaning forward, and breathing slowly appear to maximize the airway lumen.

The pathologic findings in fatal cases of pseudocroup are edema and a predominantly mononuclear infiltrate. The bronchi may be plugged with a thick, gummy exudate that accumulates as a result of the inflammation and the ineffectual cough. This exudate can cause atelectasis and further respiratory distress.

## CLINICAL MANIFESTATIONS

Acute epiglottitis is a true medical emergency because in children, sudden respiratory obstruction may occur without warning at any time, even during early stages of the infection. The onset is usually sudden, although slight symptoms such as a sore throat and vomiting may have preceded the symptoms of croup for one or two days. In children, the interval from apparent health to severe symptoms may be as short as 2 to 3 hours and is usually less than 24 hours. In adults, the onset is often more insidious and the symptoms less severe, but hyperacute courses may also occur. Children have a high fever (around 39° to 40° C) more commonly than adults. Throat pain is often severe. High fever accompanies *H. influenzae* type b septicemia. Patients, especially children, often have a toxic appearance; a pale, ashen color is more typical than true cyanosis. Patients with advanced illness have respiratory distress with slow, difficult breathing, and they may have inspiratory stridor (a harsh, rasping sound on respiration). Accessory respiratory muscles may be used, and there is retraction of the suprasternal notch and intercostal muscles. Because of pain, patients refuse to eat and drink and may even have difficulty swallowing saliva. Therefore, drooling is a common characteristic sign of acute epiglottitis. Older children often sit up, lean forward on their arms, and open their mouths. Small children may be in a state of complete fatigue and lie down quietly (an ominous sign). In acute epiglottitis, the voice is muffled (as if there were a hot potato in the mouth) but is not typically hoarse. There may be some cough.

An attack of pseudocroup is usually preceded by symptoms of a slight upper respiratory tract infection. In some cases, however, the child is apparently healthy when he goes to sleep but awakens in the night with stridor; a hollow, barking cough; and a hoarse voice. In severe cases the patient displays marked dyspnea and loud inspiratory stridor. The child uses the accessory respiratory muscles, and breathes with intercostal, supraclavicular, and epigastric retractions. The temperature in pseudocroup is normal or only slightly elevated, rarely above 38.5° C. An attack may last for only a few hours, although a duration of one or two days is more common. Some children may have several attacks of pseudocroup during the winter months.

## COMPLICATIONS

Most patients with acute epiglottitis have an uneventful recovery, provided that the correct diagnosis is made early and adequate treatment is started immediately. The severest course of acute epiglottitis involves sudden respiratory obstruction leading to cardiac arrest and death. The respiratory obstruction may be caused either by secretions or by the edematous epiglottis. A relatively common complication of acute epiglottitis is pneumonia. A more unusual complication is acute *H. influenzae* type b meningitis, a consequence of the septicemia.

## DIAGNOSIS

Patients with acute epiglottitis are often admitted to the hospital with an incorrect diagnosis, most commonly pseudocroup. The diagnosis of acute epiglottitis is established by the clinical symptoms. Dysphagia with refusal to eat and drink and inability to swallow the saliva is pathognomonic. The diagnosis may sometimes be confirmed by rapid direct inspection of the pharynx. A bright red cherry-like epiglottis may be seen. Inspection by a physician at home should be done without depression of the tongue, since this maneuver can cause laryngeal spasm leading to total obstruction of the air passage and cardiac arrest. Further, the patient should be in a sitting position when examined. Respiratory distress is a late sign in acute epiglottitis and necessitates urgent action. In all cases of suspected epiglottitis, the patient should immediately be sent to the nearest emergency unit or ENT department. If possible, the physician should accompany the patient to the hospital and be prepared to try mouth-to-mouth resuscitation if respiration ceases.

At the hospital, the diagnosis may be confirmed by indirect laryngoscopy if equipment for immediate intubation is available. In some centers, soft tissue air-contrast radiographs have been used to establish the diagnosis. The contour of the epiglottis is larger and more rounded than normal. In pseudocroup, a narrowed air passage below the larynx is visible. Radiographs may also help to exclude the possibility of a foreign body in the air passages or the esophagus. A foreign object is one of the common causes of sudden respiratory distress with cough in small children and must be excluded before intubation is performed.

Another differential diagnosis to bear in mind in patients with respiratory distress and stridor is allergic edema of the larynx (angioneurotic edema). In these cases, a history of previous allergic manifestations is generally obtained. Although it is now a rare disease, diphtheritic croup must also be considered. The onset in diphtheria is generally more insidious, and the diphtheritic membranes may be seen on the pharynx as well. A peritonsillar abscess may cause severe pain,

dysphagia, and a muffled voice, but does not usually cause rapidly developing airway obstruction. Retropharyngeal abscess must also be considered, but pain is not usually as severe. Tonsillar and retropharyngeal infections are usually accompanied by cervical swelling due to edema and adenitis, while patients with epiglottitis usually have normal cervical nodes, probably because of the hyperacute onset. In adults, the possibility of a laryngeal tumor should also be considered.

## GEOGRAPHIC VARIATIONS

Both diseases are illnesses of the temperate zones of the world. There are great variations in the frequency of acute epiglottitis from year to year as well as from season to season. Cases may occur any time of the year, although they are most common during the winter months. In areas where acute epiglottitis is comparatively common (e.g., Scandinavia), cases tend to occur in small groups, probably reflecting the epidemiologic situation in the community. Pseudocroup is most common during the cold season.

## TREATMENT

At the hospital, ENT department, or Intensive Care Unit, equipment for securing a safe air passage should be ready. All children with epiglottitis should be intubated. During the last decade, nasotracheal intubation has replaced the tracheostomy (Battaglia and Lockhart, 1975). In most cases of epiglottitis, less than 48 hours of intubation is required. In pseudocroup, intubation is rarely necessary.

In addition to intubation, patients with epiglottitis should be given antibiotics parenterally (after blood cultures are performed). Ampicillin, 200 to 400 mg/kg/day, is the drug of choice, except in areas where penicillin-resistant *H. influenzae* is prevalent, in which case chloramphenicol, 100 mg/kg/day, should be employed. Antibiotics are not usually indicated in pseudocroup, but steroids may be efficacious. A humid atmosphere with increased oxygen is beneficial for patients with either acute epiglottitis or pseudocroup. Dehydration should be avoided by the administration of parenteral fluids.

### References

Battaglia, J. D., and Lockhart, C. H.: Management of acute epiglottitis by nasotracheal intubation. Am J Dis Child 129:334, 1975.
Branefors-Helander, P., and Jeppsson, P.-H.: Acute epiglottitis. A clinical, bacteriological and serological study. Scand J Infect Dis 7:103, 1975.
Kissane, J. M., and Smith, M. G.: Pathology of Infancy and Childhood. 2nd ed. St. Louis, C. V. Mosby Company, 1967.

# 95 *LUDWIG'S ANGINA*

*Burt R. Meyers, M.D.*

In 1836, Wilhelm Frederick von Ludwig, a Stuttgart physician, read a detailed report to the medical society describing five cases of infections involving the floor of the mouth (von Ludwig, 1836). This clinical condition was known as morbus strangulatorius, garotillo (Spanish after the hangman's loop), angina maligne, and cynanche (dog choking), all referring to the respiratory obstruction so prominent in this syndrome. Ludwig's original description of a rapidly spreading cellulitis or phlegmon, brawny in character, originating in the area of the submaxillary gland and extending by continuity without involving the lymph nodes, has been only slightly modified by subsequent investigators. The infection may start in either the sublingual or the submaxillary space (Fig. 1), but must involve both in order to meet the criteria of Ludwig's syndrome. Involvement of only the submaxillary space with suppuration has been called pseudo-Ludwig's angina.

## ETIOLOGY

From 51 to 90 per cent of the cases are related to a dental extraction. Ludwig's angina has also followed lacerations of the floor of the mouth, mandibular fractures, foreign bodies, and peritonsillar abscess. Systemic disease may play a role because cases have occurred in patients with acute and chronic glomerulonephritis, systemic lupus erythematosus, diabetes mellitus, hypersensitivity states, malnutrition, and aplastic anemia, and in those who are immunosuppressed. In the author's experience, patients are frequently chronic alcoholics who engage in a drinking bout after dental extraction.

The bacteria responsible for the infection are believed to originate from the oral flora. The earlier investigators found predominantly streptococci, both hemolytic and nonhemolytic. Staphylococci, including *S. aureus* and *S. epidermidis,* have also been isolated, although the role of the latter is not clear. Fusiform bacillae and spiralla-like forms have been seen on smear, and in some cases foul-smelling pus has been described. Although references were made earlier to the possibility that anaerobes were involved, no anaerobic cultures were obtained until recently, when case reports of anaerobic infection have appeared (Maki and Agger, 1977; Gross, 1976).

Gram-negative aerobic bacteria, including *Escherichia coli, Pseudomonas aeruginosa,* and *Haemophilus in/uenzae,* have been noted. In many cases, however, mixed cultures were recovered.

## PATHOLOGY AND PATHOGENESIS

Infection primarily occurs in the submandibular space, an area that extends from the mucous membranes of the floor of the mouth superiorly to the muscle and facial attachment of the hyoid bone below. The mylohyoid muscles divide the

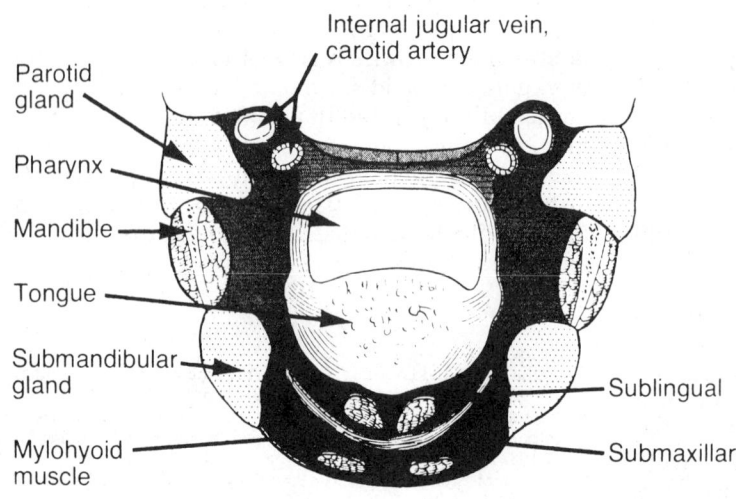

Parotid gland

Internal jugular vein, carotid artery

Pharynx

Mandible

Tongue

Submandibular gland

Mylohyoid muscle

Sublingual

Submaxillary

**FIGURE 1.** *Oblique section of top of neck shows continuity of sublingual and submaxillary spaces and potential for spread of infection from one to another. (From Johnson and Tucker, 1976.)*

space horizontally into the sublingual space superiorly and the submaxillary space inferiorly.

Extractions of the second and third molar teeth are implicated in the pathogenesis of this syndrome because the position of their root apices beneath the mylohyoid ridge and the relative thinness of the mandibular alveolar bone lingually give dental infections ready access to the submaxillary space (Fig. 2). Following extraction, hairline fractures may occur in the lingual cortex of the mandible, and these, coupled with pulp infections, may explain the egress of bacteria. The apices of the premolars and often the first molar are superior to the mylohyoid ridge, and when infections occur, they enter the sublingual space. When the sublingual space is infected, edema, swelling, and elevation of the tongue develop. As this space becomes progressively involved, the tongue is displaced, and the supraglottic larynx becomes edematous and distorted, compromising the airway.

Following the facial planes, the infection may dissect into the parapharyngeal or pharyngeomaxillary space, giving it access to the carotid sheath. The internal carotid may form a mycotic aneurysm and be eroded with massive hemorrhage. Further extension may result in thromboses of the internal jugular vein or cavernous sinus thrombosis. Dissection into the superior mediastinum, involving the pericardium and pleural space, has been observed by the author.

In most cases the involved areas are brawny, indurated, and edematous and are involved with a spreading cellulitis that may be gangrenous. The salivary glands and lymph nodes are usually spared. However, in some cases drainage of the tooth sockets or abscess formation in the neck has been described.

## CLINICAL MANIFESTATIONS

Most patients present with painful swelling of the face and neck. There is usually a history of dental extraction, recent dental pain, infection, or some intraoral problem such as gingivitis (Maki and Agger, 1977). Fever and tachycardia are usually present. Depending on the extent of tongue involvement, the patient will complain of dysphagia, drooling, and dyspnea. Signs of dehydration may be present. Trismus develops when the internal pterygoid muscles are involved, and this implies that the infection has spread to the pharyngomaxillary space.

Oral, facial, cervical, and even supraclavicular swelling may be found on examination. The neck may have a bull-like appearance. The involved areas are indurated, painful and usually not fluctuant. Enlargement of the tongue and protrusion from the oral cavity may be found. The tongue is often edematous and elevated, touching the roof of the mouth. There is swelling of the submental and submaxillary spaces, often bilaterally. The lymph nodes and submaxillary glands are not involved. A recent extraction site or carious tooth may be noted. Respiratory obstruction causes stridor and cyanosis. Massive hemoptysis may follow vascular erosion. When the mediastinum is involved, anterior chest pain signifies pericarditis. Pleuritic chest pain and pleural effusion suggest mediastinal extension. Patients may have patchy aspiration pneumonia.

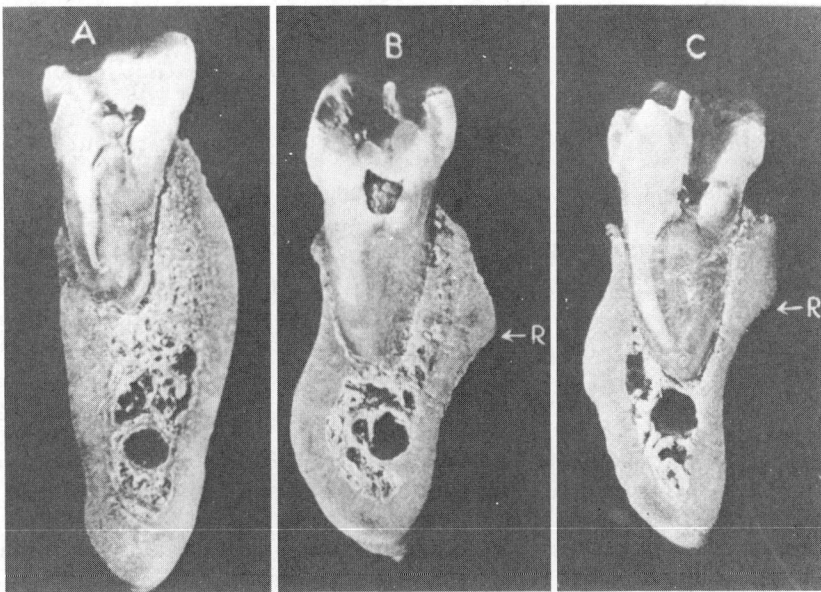

FIGURE 2. *Cross-sections through to mandible: A, first molar tooth; B, second molar tooth; C, third molar. Note the difference in the relation of the mylohyoid ridge (R) to the apices of the teeth. The second and third molar teeth have roots below the mylohyoid ridge and are more likely to cause submaxillary cellulitis. The first molar is more likely to cause sublingual infection. (From Tschiassny, K., 1943.)*

## DIAGNOSIS

Facial swelling, a swollen tongue, and thickening of the floor of the mouth suggest the diagnosis of Ludwig's angina. The patient may present with respiratory distress (Meyers, 1972). The oral cavity must be examined and any areas of suppuration aspirated for Gram stain and culture, both aerobically and anaerobically. Gram stain of the aspirate may reveal mixed flora, and a fetid odor indicates anaerobic infection. Blood cultures should also be performed.

## TREATMENT

The mainstay of therapy is to ensure an adequate airway. Since respiratory obstruction occurs very rapidly, patients must be constantly observed for this development. At the first signs of respiratory embarrassment, early tracheostomy under local anesthesia is mandatory. Since swallowing is often impaired and aspiration a possibility, a cuffed tracheostomy tube is recommended. Because of the distortion of the upper airway, direct laryngoscopy and intubation are extremely dangerous, for they may result in laryngospasm and sudden death. Fiberoptic laryngoscopy has been performed to secure an airway and avoid tracheostomy.

In the severely ill patient, antibiotic coverage at first should be directed at four possible groups of bacteria: (1) penicillinase-producing staphylococci, (2) gram-negative enteric organisms, (3) streptococci, and (4) anaerobes. Though most oral anaerobes are sensitive to penicillin, recent isolates of *Bacteroides melaninogenicus* that produce a beta lactamase have been reported (Murray, 1977). A dose of clindamycin 600 mg every six hours I.V. and oxacillin 2.0 g every three hours I.V. should be given along with gentamicin or tobramycin in doses adjusted for age and renal function. When culture and sensitivity reports are available, therapy may be altered accordingly.

In the pre-antibiotic era various drainage procedures through submandibular and intraoral incisions were performed. The rationale was to decompress the submandibular space; however, in one report suppuration was found in only 1 of 51 cases. Incision and drainage should be performed only in the presence of fluctuation. If the infection extends into the parapharyngeal space, drainage of this deep neck infection is usually required by an external approach.

### References

Gross, B. D.: Ludwig's angina due to bacteroides. J Oral Surg 34:456, 1976.

Johnson, J. T., and Tucker, H. M.: Recognizing and treating deep neck infection. Postgrad Med 59:95, 1976.

Maki, D., and Agger, W. A.: Morbid Mortal Weekly Report 26:199, 1977.

Meyers, B. R., Lawson, W., and Hirschman, S. Z.: Ludwig's angina. Case report, with review of bacteriology and current therapy. Am J Med 53:257, 1972.

Murray, P. R., and Rosenblatt, J. E.: Penicillin resistance and penicillinase production in clinical isolates of Bacteroides melaninogenicus. Antimicrob Agents Chemother 11:605, 1977.

Tschiassny, K.: Ludwig's angina. An anatomic study of the role of the lower molar teeth in its pathogenesis. Arch Otolaryngol 38:485,

von Ludwig, F. W.: Eine neue Art von Halsentzeundung. Med Cor B1 Württemb arztl Ver 6:21, 1836.

# 96 ACTINOMYCOSIS

## Abraham I. Braude, M.D., Ph.D.

## DEFINITION

Actinomycosis is a noncontagious infection produced by an anaerobic organism normally resident in the mouth. The disease is characterized by chronic inflammatory induration and sinus formation.

## ETIOLOGY

The causative agent is *Actinomyces israelii,* a branching gram-positive filamentous organism. Another actinomycete, *Arachnia propionica,* may produce chronic abscesses and draining sinuses. Intolerance of free oxygen and failure to grow on Sabouraud's medium distinguish *A. israelii* from *Nocardia* and other actinomycetes. On blood agar, colonies require 4 to 6 days of anaerobic incubation at 37° C to reach a size of 1 to 2 mm. Although most strains require anaerobic conditions for isolation, some can be subcultured aerobically in 10 to 20 per cent carbon dioxide. *Actinomyces israelii* has never been found outside human beings or animals, and case-to-case transmission is unknown. *Ar. propionica* resembles *A. israelii* in oxygen requirements, colonial morphology, and microscopic appearance. Distinction is based on the ability of *Ar. propionica* to produce large amounts of propionic acid and the presence of diaminopimelic acid in its cell wall (Brock et al., 1973).

## PATHOGENESIS

The oxidation-reduction potential of normal tissues is probably too high for multiplication of *A. israelii* but dead tissues allow it to reproduce and spread. The frequency of actinomycosis of the face and neck may be explained by the greater population of *A. israelii* on teeth, in carious teeth, and in tonsillar crypts, and by trauma from eating, dental procedures, or infection with oral bacteria. Anaerobic conditions also prevail in atelectatic areas of the lung after aspiration of *A. israelii* so that pulmonary actinomycosis can develop. It is also conceivable that pulmonary actinomycosis may arise hematogenously from an infected focus in the mouth. Mediastinal actinomycosis probably spreads from the esophagus into the superior or posterior mediastinum, quickly involving the pleura to produce early pleural effusion or empyema, and then tending to attack the adjacent ribs and vertebral bodies. Eventually mediastinal actinomycosis produces abscesses that point in the paravertebral region. Ileocecal actinomycosis is the most common intestinal form, occurring after appendiceal rupture and the escape of actinomycetes to form an inflammatory mass in the right iliac fossa. The liver is the solid abdominal viscus most frequently attacked by actinomycosis. Grossly the lesions resemble large metastatic tumor masses, which undergo necrosis and abscess formation. The abscesses become loculated and the liver takes on a honeycombed appearance (Cope, 1952).

From foci in the jaw, lung, or intestine, actinomycosis may spread by contiguity or through the bloodstream to the liver, spine, brain, kidneys, genitalia, spleen, and subcutaneous tissues. Lymphatic spread is rare and actinomycosis of lymph nodes probably never occurs (Colebrook, 1921).

The inflammatory reaction to *A. israelii* is characterized by three features: (1) chronic suppuration, (2) extensive necrosis, and (3) intense fibrosis. The so-called "sulfur granules" in the inflammatory lesion are composed of intertwined mycelial filaments, or colonies, of *A. israelii*.

## CLINICAL MANIFESTATIONS

The essential feature of actinomycosis is a painful, indurated swelling. This lesion may appear over the jaw a week or more after such trauma as tooth extraction or compound fracture of the mandible. As it increases in size, points of suppuration — the openings of fistulas — appear on the bluish red surface of the edematous skin. Trismus is prominent early. Cervical lymphadenopathy is rare.

The lower lobes of the lung are frequently affected, and the disease suddenly becomes evident when the pleura and chest wall are involved by direct extension from the lung. Physical examination at this time reveals a diffuse, tender, indurated swelling of the chest wall with pulmonary consolidation and empyema. Until then the patient may notice only fever, cough, and expectoration. In fact, the symptoms may be so mild that they are thought to be those of mild bronchitis. When fever and severe cough occur, a chest x-ray may be taken and consolidation found (Fig. 1), but frequently no diagnosis is made until the chest wall is invaded.

Abdominal actinomycosis is often mistaken for appendicitis, carcinoma of the cecum, tuberculosis, or amebiasis. Patients with abdominal actinomycosis are subjected to surgery for drainage of a supposed appendiceal abscess, and the true nature of the disease is recognized only when an indurated draining sinus stubbornly refuses to heal.

Actinomycosis may also be mistaken for tumor of the reproductive organs in women or for tuberculous psoas abscess. The ovary and fallopian tube have frequently been the seat of actinomycosis after extension from an appendiceal focus. Lately tubo-ovarian actinomycosis has been associated with intrauterine devices (Hager and Majmudar, 1979). There is nothing pathognomonic that would distinguish the clinical features of genital actinomycosis in women from those of chronic pelvic inflammatory disease, and the diagnosis is often made by examination of a tube or ovary after surgical removal. Sometimes diagnostic pus can be obtained from an abscess pointing through the skin of the groin or buttock, or bulging into the posterior vagina. Rarely, peritonitis develops. Actinomycosis involving the perianal region can cause recurrent multiple draining sinuses and fistulas in ano (Brewer et al., 1974).

Spread to the liver can occur from any abdominal focus via the portal vein. Sometimes the primary focus is inapparent clinically and hepatic actinomycosis appears as an isolated disease. It begins then with fever, sweats, weight loss, and hepatomegaly with or without palpable nodules on the liver surface.

In the rare case of hematogenously disseminated actinomycosis, lesions appear in all parts of the body. Painful indurated nodules under the skin of the legs, arms, back, and scalp are prominent, and nonsuppurative effusions of the pleura or pericardium develop. The primary focus for dissemination is usually the lung (Varkey et al., 1974).

The kidneys may be infected during the course of disseminated actinomycosis, or may be the only

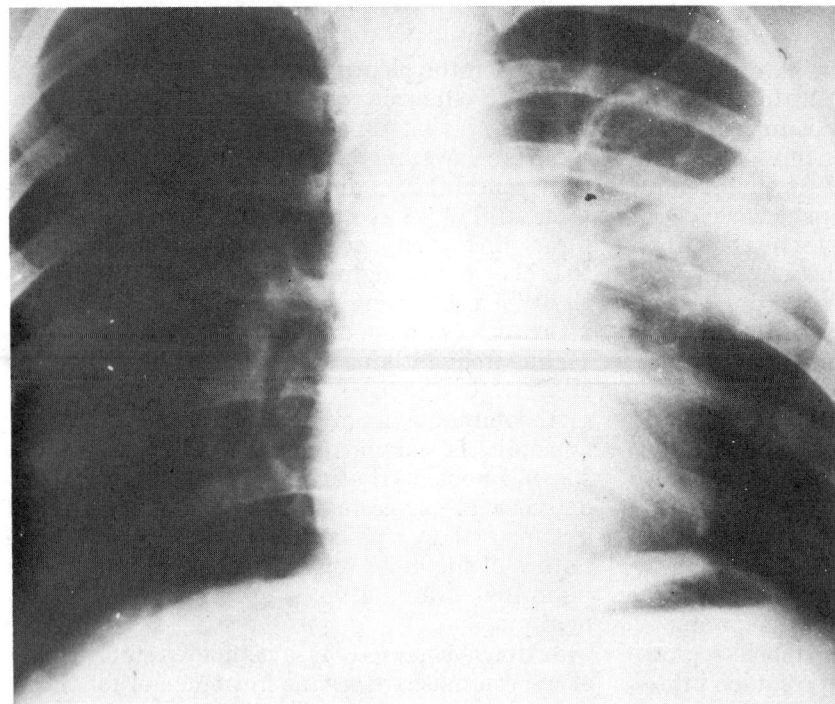

**FIGURE 1.** *Actinomycosis of the lung. The diagnosis was made when the infection broke through the chest wall and A. israelii was found in the pus by Gram stain and culture (Fig. 2).*

detectable site of disease. Solitary actinomycosis of the kidney is usually a chronic suppurative process resembling a renal carbuncle. Fever, sweats, and weight loss may precede any sign of renal disease, so that actinomycosis of the kidney may be the source of an unexplained (or cryptic) fever. Eventually tenderness and pain over the kidney and a palpable renal mass will develop.

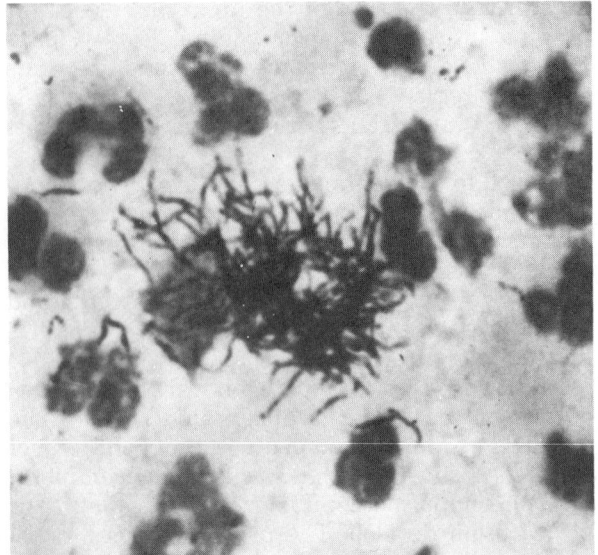

**FIGURE 2.** *Gram stain of pus from sinus in chest wall of patient in Figure 1. The gram-positive branching filaments were found to be A. israelii on culture.*

## COMPLICATIONS

The chief complications of all forms of actinomycosis result from direct invasion by contiguous spread into neighboring structures. Thoracic actinomycosis may extend retroperitoneally upward through the diaphragm, medially through the psoas to the vertebrae, or down into the pelvis (Cope, 1952). Hepatic actinomycosis may also rupture through the diaphragm into the lung or through the anterior abdominal wall. Mediastinal actinomycosis attacks adjacent ribs, pericardium, or vertebrae. Actinomycotic osteomyelitis almost always results from contiguous, rather than hematogenous, spread.

The most serious hematogenous complication is actinomycotic brain abscess, which usually spreads from pulmonary actinomycosis.

## GEOGRAPHIC VARIATIONS IN DISEASE

Actinomycosis occurs everywhere and anyone may have *A. israelii* as a normal inhabitant of the mouth or bowel. Variations in frequency of actinomycosis will depend on geographic differences in dental hygiene. The old idea that actinomycosis was a disease of farmers because they chewed straws is absurd. The reason some farmers get actinomycosis is that they have bad teeth.

## DIAGNOSIS

The disease is easily recognized by detecting *A. israelii* in pus obtained from sinuses, empyema fluid, or abscess cavities. The significance of actinomycetes in sputum is difficult to interpret because the organisms are normal inhabitants of the mouth. Sulfur granules vary in size from several microns to 3 mm in diameter. Large granules are found if a thorough search is made by diluting the pus with saline solution and filtering through gauze. They are white, yellow, or brown and stand out sharply against the background of blood-tinged pus. Gram-positive branching filaments or bacilli that fail to grow aerobically are key findings (Fig. 2). Granules of other organisms (staphylococci, nocardias, monosporia), fragments of caseous material, and clumps of pus cells or fibrin may be confused with actinomycotic granules. Sabouraud's medium will not support the growth of *A. israelii*. Cultural isolation of *A. israelii* is not difficult if anaerobic methods are used. A small, microaerophilic gram-negative bacillus, *Actinobacillus actinomycetemcomitans,* is often associated with *A. israelii* in actinomycosis. Anaerobic streptococci, *Bacteroides,* and other anaerobes are also present frequently. Hence actinomycosis is characteristically a mixed anaerobic infection.

Biopsy may help establish the diagnosis if the actinomycotic colony ("ray fungus") is observed microscopically. Demonstration of the organism may be difficult, requiring careful search of many sections.

Intradermal or serologic tests with *A. israelii* or its fractions are of no diagnostic aid. Radiologic examination may suggest actinomycosis if consolidation of the lungs and periosteal proliferation of the ribs are found, because this combination rarely occurs in other conditions (Flynn and Felson, 1970). The appearance of the spine in lateral veiws may be almost pathognomonic, because the areas of absorption and newly formed bone give a picture of a coarse sieve not seen in any other vertebral disease (Fig. 3).

## TREATMENT

Penicillin and the tetracycline antibiotics are so effective that the disease is disappearing through the wide use of these drugs prophylactically after dental extraction and in other conditions that might evolve into actinomycosis. When either is administered in large doses over long periods of time, remarkable improvement may be expected even when the purulent foci are inaccessible to surgical drainage (Nichols, 1970). Many reports indicate that tetracycline is superior to penicillin. When tetracycline is given in doses of 500 mg every 6 hours there is a reduction in pain and swelling within a few days as well as gain in strength, increase in weight, and prompt defervescence. In view of the tendency for actinomycosis to relapse, treatment should be continued for several weeks after the patient appears cured. Because penicillin is no more effective than the tetracyclines and because it requires repeated intramuscular or intravenous injection of large doses for long periods of time, it should be reserved for patients who cannot tolerate tetracycline drugs. The optimum dose of penicillin is not known, but at least 4 million units daily should be given parenterally.

Surgical drainage is a valuable adjunct to chemotherapy and may occasionally lead to spontaneous cure (Colebrook, 1921). Older treatments such as iodides, irradiation, and the sulfonamides have no place in the treatment of actinomycosis, and amphotericin B is of no value.

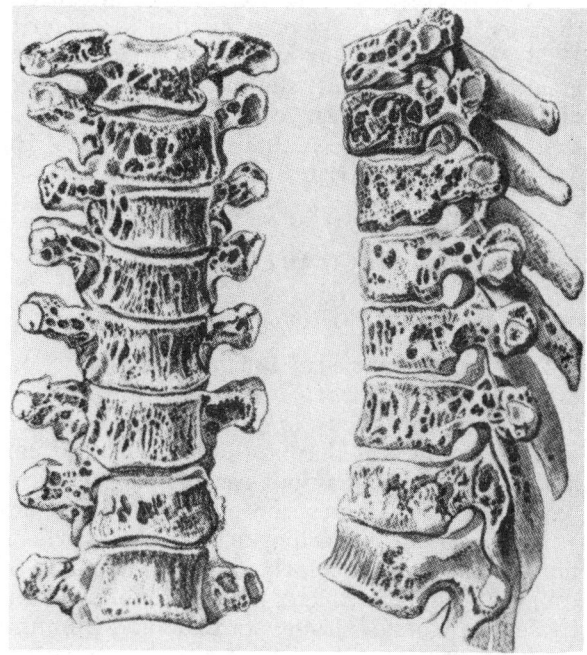

**FIGURE 3.** *Effect of actinomycosis on the vertebrae. The slow absorption and formation of new bone allows the vertebral body to retain its strength so that vertebral collapse is rare. The intervertebral disks are also spared, for the most part. Thus spinal actinomycosis differs markedly from tuberculosis which causes vertebral collapse and disk destruction. In actinomycosis the spine takes on the appearance of a coarse sieve. (From Cope, V.Z.: Human Actinomycosis. London, William Heinemann, Ltd., 1952.)*

## References

Brewer, N., Spencer, R., and Nichols, D.: Primary anorectal actinomycosis. JAMA 228:1397, 1974.

Brock, D. W., George, L., Brown, J., and Hicklin, M.: Actinomycosis caused by *Arachnia propionica*. Am J Clin Pathol 59:66, 1973.

Colebrook, L.: A report on 25 cases of actinomycosis with special reference to vaccine therapy. Lancet T:893, 1921.

Cope, V. Z.: Human Actinomycosis. London, William Heinemann, Ltd., 1952.

Flynn, M. W., and Felson, B.: The roentgen manifestations of thoracic actinomycosis. Am J Roentgenol 110:707, 1970.

Hager, W., and Majmudar, B.: Pelvic actinomycosis in women using intrauterine devices. Am J Obst Gynecol 156:60, 1979.

Nichols, D.: Actinomycosis: Results in 156 patients. *In* Progress in Antimicrobial and Anticancer Chemotherapy. Proc. 6th Internat. Cong. Chemother., Univ. Tokyo Press 11:8, 1970.

Varkey, B., Landis, F., Tang, T., and Rose, H.: Thoracic actinomycosis: Dissemination to skin, subcutaneous tissue, and muscle. Arch Int Med 134:689, 1974.

# 97 PHYCOMYCOSIS (ZYGOMYCOSIS)

## Francis D. Martinson, M.D., Ch.B. (Ed), F.R.C.S. (Eng & Ed)

### DEFINITION

The term phycomycosis should refer to all infections caused by fungi of the large group Phycomycetes, but it has, by clinical usage, been restricted to those caused by species of two orders, Mucorales and Entomophthorales. Since both belong to Zygomycetes, one of the six classes into which the Phycomycetes have been divided (Ainsworth, 1973), "zygomycosis" is considered a more appropriate collective name, the infections being subdivided into "mucormycosis" and "entomophthoromycosis" (Clark, 1968) according to the order of fungi involved (Fig. 1).

### MUCORMYCOSIS

#### Etiology

The fungi identified so far in human infections are species of *Rhizopus, Absidia, Mucor, Mortierella, Cunninghamella,* and *Saksenaea.* Like other Zygomycetes they are ubiquitous and normally saprobic to man but become pathogenic in patients with diabetes and other prolonged acidoses, leukemia, kwashiorkor, severe diarrheas, malignancies, particularly the lymphomas, and congenital defects of IgA production and also in those on cytotoxic drugs, steroids, and immunosuppressives.

Very occasionally the predisposing factor eludes detection.

#### Pathogenesis and Pathology

The fungi penetrate the mucosa of the respiratory or digestive tract or gain entry through lacerations, burns, and occasionally surgical incisions, inducing a granulomatous reaction. They have a propensity for penetrating blood vessels, thereby causing thromboses, infarcts, and hemorrhages, and being disseminated to all organs. Secondary infection often supervenes.

On microscopy large numbers of neutrophils but very few eosinophils are seen; very occasionally lymphocytes and plasma cells may predominate. There are scattered areas of infarcts and hemorrhages. Fungi are easily identified with hematoxylin-eosin stains but less so with Grocott's methenamine silver. They are often seen penetrating vascular walls. Fibrosis is rarely present except in those granulomas occasionally seen at the site of prolonged intravenous infusion lines, or in the rare sclerosing orbital lesion in which the tuberculoid giant cell granuloma may also be present. Also rare is the circumfungal eosinophilic mantle often seen in entomophthoromycosis (vide infra).

#### Clinical Manifestations

The disease affects any age and either sex. The clinical features vary according to the sites of commencement or main activity of the granuloma. These sites are the head and neck, bronchopulmonary region, digestive tract, superficial tissues, and other deep-seated foci. Infection from any of these may at any stage become disseminated.

#### Head and Neck Infection

Various self-explanatory names such as rhino-orbital, rhinocerebral, orbital, orbitocerebral, facial and nasal, and rhinomucormycosis have been used to indicate the site of involvement. The infection almost invariably starts in the nose or

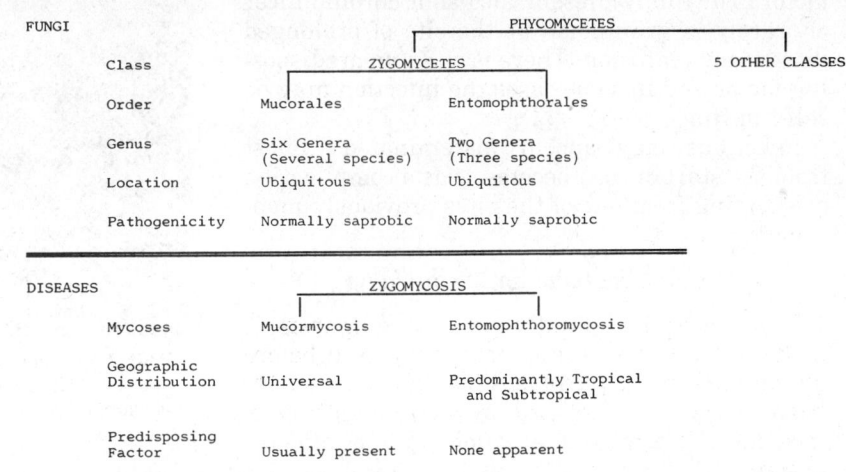

**FIGURE 1.** *Classification of Phyco-mycetes and human zygomycoses.*

HUMAN PHYCOMYCOSES

| | | PHYCOMYCETES | | |
|---|---|---|---|---|
| FUNGI | | | | |
| Class | | ZYGOMYCETES | | 5 OTHER CLASSES |
| Order | Mucorales | | Entomophthorales | |
| Genus | Six Genera (Several species) | | Two Genera (Three species) | |
| Location | Ubiquitous | | Ubiquitous | |
| Pathogenicity | Normally saprobic | | Normally saprobic | |

| | | ZYGOMYCOSIS | |
|---|---|---|---|
| DISEASES | | | |
| Mycoses | Mucormycosis | | Entomophthoromycosis |
| Geographic Distribution | Universal | | Predominantly Tropical and Subtropical |
| Predisposing Factor | Usually present | | None apparent |
| Course of Infection | Usually acute | | Chronic |

paranasal sinuses. On inspection the granuloma is covered by black or brown crusts and foul, blood-stained discharge. Subsequent progress depends on the direction and rate of local or vascular spread. There may be swelling of the nose and cheek, followed by ulceration through to the face or palate. Spread to the orbit produces orbital edema, proptosis, ophthalmoplegia, loss of vision, deep pain, and anesthesia of the face around the eye. Intracranial spread direct from the nose or via the orbit produces evidence of meningitis, cerebral infarct or hemorrhage, or cavernous sinus thrombosis. Vascular dissemination may be early or late, commonly spreading to the lung first.

*Diagnosis.* Radiographic appearances are nonspecific and may resemble those of sinusitis or malignancy.

Biopsy is taken for both histopathologic examination and mycologic culture. Existence of one of the predisposing factors or a history of administration of immunosuppressives should arouse suspicion.

Conditions simulated are acute sinusitis, osteomyelitis, carbuncle, rhinitis caseosa, malignant tumors, cancrum (noma), orbitoethmoidal aspergilloma, midline lethal granuloma, and Burkitt's lymphoma.

### Bronchopulmonary Infection

This is due to inhalation of infected material from the upper respiratory tract or to vascular dissemination from another site. Symptoms consist of dyspnea, cough, hemoptysis, and sometimes progressive or sudden chest pain. Later the lesions may spread to the mediastinal viscera (esophagus or pericardium) or outward to the chest wall or may also disseminate further afield.

*Diagnosis.* Here also radiologic features are not specific and, like the symptoms, may suggest pneumonia, tuberculosis (with or without cavitation), neoplasm, or pulmonary embolism. Examination of the sputum often does not reveal the fungus. The true diagnosis is usually made after pneumonectomy and histopathologic examination of the specimen, and at this stage it is often too late.

### Digestive Tract Lesions

These may be due to ingestion of infected material, direct spread to the esophagus from the lungs, or vascular spread. Ulcers, usually multiple in the stomach, form in the wall of the viscus, or a nutrient vessel may be thrombosed, leading to local gangrene. Hematemesis, melena, and perforation with peritonitis are late signs which also suggest various intra-abdominal emergencies; hence the correct diagnosis is made occasionally after laparotomy but more often at necropsy.

### Focal Infection

This may, uncommonly, occur in other intra-abdominal organs, for example, the kidney, spleen, or liver, sometimes without evidence of the mode of entry; hence diagnosis is made only after surgical intervention and histopathologic examination of the diseased viscus.

### Superficial Lesions

Superficial lesions may be acute, presenting as a spreading necrosis from a deep-seated lesion or commencing in a laceration, burn, or surgical wound. There is usually an obvious predisposing factor. They may present also as a chronic ulcer or, rarely, a granuloma at the site of prolonged intravenous infusion. There is often no predisposing factor and in some cases the infection may be self-limiting.

Infections may appear disseminated almost from the start or may become so as a complication originating from one of the sites previously mentioned.

### Complications and Sequelae

Most cases end fatally because diagnosis is made too late, but a few cases, diagnosed before dissemination or irreversible damage, have been successfully treated by a combination of medical therapy and excision of the affected organ.

Occasionally early infection may resolve spontaneously after cure or control of the underlying disease, especially diabetes; however, it usually does not respond to treatment if the predisposing factor is not first eliminated.

### Treatment

Wherever the lesion may be, the predisposing disease must first be identified and controlled or cured if treatment is to succeed. In a diabetic, for example, the hyperglycemia and acidosis must be corrected rapidly. Second, the organ or the part of it affected must be excised if possible, or surgical drainage carried out. Third, medical therapy consisting of intravenous amphotericin B, the specific drug for this infection, should be given in doses of 50 mg intravenously daily for a total dose of approximately 2.2 g.

## ENTOMOPHTHOROMYCOSIS

There are three known clinical syndromes caused by fungi that are normally saprobic yet become pathogenic without apparent predisposing adverse host conditions.

### Basidiobolomycosis

This name was coined by Vanbreuseghem (1966) for the disease first described by Lie Kian Joe and his colleagues in 1956 under the name subcutaneous phycomycosis.

#### Etiology

The disease is caused by *Basidiobolus haptosporus (meristosporus)*.

#### Pathogenesis and Pathology

The infection follows traumatic implantation of the fungus. It begins and spreads as a subcutane-

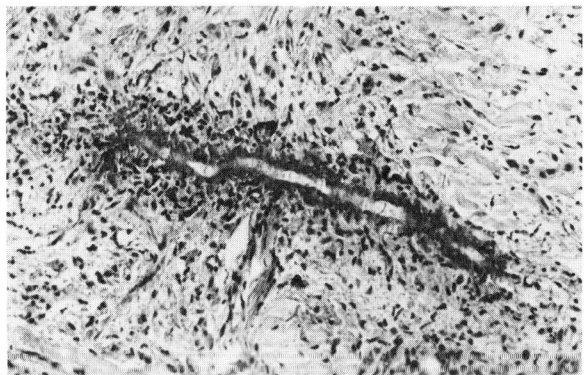

**FIGURE 2.** *Fungus cut longitudinally surrounded by amorphous mantle, the "Hoeppli-Splendore phenomenon," and chronic inflammatory reaction.*

ous granuloma, often infiltrating muscle but never involving bone. Regional lymph glands may occasionally undergo reactive hyperplasia but do not become infected except occasionally when engulfed and infiltrated by the advancing granuloma. The blood picture is not affected.

The granuloma is tough and creamy pink. Its cut surface is homogeneous or streaky and studded with occasional small abscesses. If cut up, digested in potassium hydroxide, teased out, and examined microscopically, the hyphae are easily recognized. They usually show up poorly in sections stained with hematoxylin and eosin but well with Grocott's methanamine silver. In the former they often exhibit the "Hoeppli-Splendore phenomenon" (Fig. 2), a strongly eosinophilic mantle considered by Williams and colleagues (1969) to be antigen-antibody reaction. Eosinophils are numerous but fibrosis predominates in older areas. Microabscesses may be seen with fungi in them or within multinucleate giant cells (Fig. 3). Tuberculoid giant cell granulomas are present. Reported vascular penetration is atypical and very rarely observed.

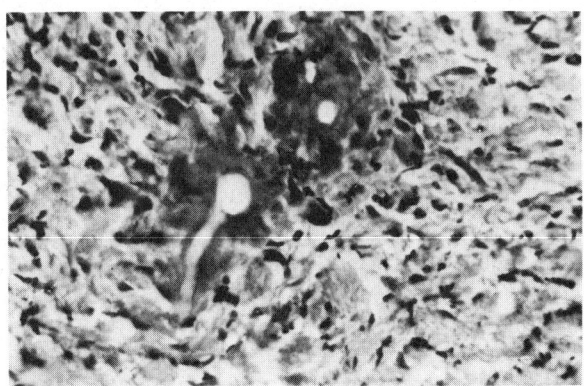

**FIGURE 3.** *Hyphae cut across and longitudinally, lying in microabscess. (From Martinson, F. D.: Rhinophycomycosis. J Laryng 77:691, 1963.)*

## Clinical Manifestations

About 80 per cent of all patients are under 10 years old. Males outnumber females by about 3:1. The lesion commences anywhere on the body but commonly the lower half and sometimes simultaneously at more than one site. It enlarges slowly to become a painless smooth or lobulated mass, characteristically very firm with palpably discrete borders — a diagnostic feature — and is freely movable over underlying muscles until it invades them. It may become enormous after several months and cross anatomic regional boundaries. The penis, vulva, and scrotum are not spared. There are no constitutional disturbances. The overlying skin does not usually ulcerate unless traumatized, and then secondary bacterial or other fungal infection may occur.

## Complications and Sequelae

Infiltrating perineal muscles, the granuloma enters the pelvis and obstructs the rectum, ureter, or sometimes the iliac vessels, or in the neck may involve the perilaryngeal muscles, causing obstruction. Very extensive and long-standing involvement of an arm has been followed by muscle atrophy. Deaths are rare and usually due to secondary fungal or bacterial infection including tetanus. Also rare are totally resistant lesions that eventually require amputation of the affected part. Spontaneous arrest of spread is uncommon and spontaneous resolution is even less frequent. Complete cure can be achieved but extensive fibrosis and disfigurement may sometimes persist. It is uncertain whether reinfection can occur after cure.

## Diagnosis

Radiography will rule out upper respiratory tract involvement, bony lesions, and calcified parasitic infections. Biopsy should be taken from the growing edges where the typical granuloma and viable culturable fungi are usually found. Mycologic culture is imperative for accurate diagnosis.

## Differential Diagnosis

In the head and neck, cervical adenitis, neoplasm, facial onchocerciasis, and rhinoentomophthoromycosis should be excluded. In the foot the absence of discharging sinuses and bony involvement rules out mycetoma. Lymphedema is much less firm, has no discrete edge, and usually extends distally to the toes.

## Treatment

Between 1.5 and 3.5 g of potassium iodide, depending on the age of the patient, is given three times a day. The combination of trimethoprim, 160 mg and sulfamethoxazole, 800 mg, orally twice a day is usually more effective and should be given first trial. Treatment should continue for at least a month after the swellings have completely subsided because one cannot judge exactly when the fungi have been adequately controlled or eliminated, and inadequate treatment leads to resistance and apparent recurrence. As long as treatment is adequate in dosage and duration, a successful outcome can be anticipated in cases that are uncomplicated by secondary infection or not unduly neglected before treatment is sought.

## Rhinoentomophthoromycosis

Various names have been given to this disease but this one coined by Clark (1968) is generally accepted.

## Etiology

The causative organism, *Entomophthora coronata (Conidiobolus coronatus),* was first identified in nasal granulomas in horses by Emmons and Bridges in 1961, and in human infection by Bras and co-workers in 1965. Infection follows traumatic implantation of the spores by an insect or the fingernail.

## Pathogenesis and Pathology

The granuloma commences in the submucosa, usually of the inferior turbinate, and spreads without ulcerating to the nasopharynx or paranasal sinuses and externally through interosseous sutures and foramina without eroding bone (Fig. 4). In the face it soon invades muscle and becomes closely applied to the skin but does not ulcerate it.

Histopathologic features are identical to those of basidiobolomycosis previously described. Differentiation is therefore by mycologic culture.

## Clinical Manifestations

About 80 per cent of all cases occur in adolescents or adults, with a male to female ratio of about 8:1. The inferior turbinate is large and nonulcerated. There is nasal obstruction and occasionally epistaxis. Externally the firm granuloma spreads over the dorsum to the glabella, forehead, cheek, eyelids, alae nasi, and upper lip and, unlike basidiobolomycosis, usually restricts itself to the central part of the face above the level of the angle of the mouth. It rarely spreads further unless there has been trauma or surgical intervention at these limits (Figs. 5A and 6). There is no pain, pyrexia, or glandular infection, and no constitutional upset unless caused by secondary infection.

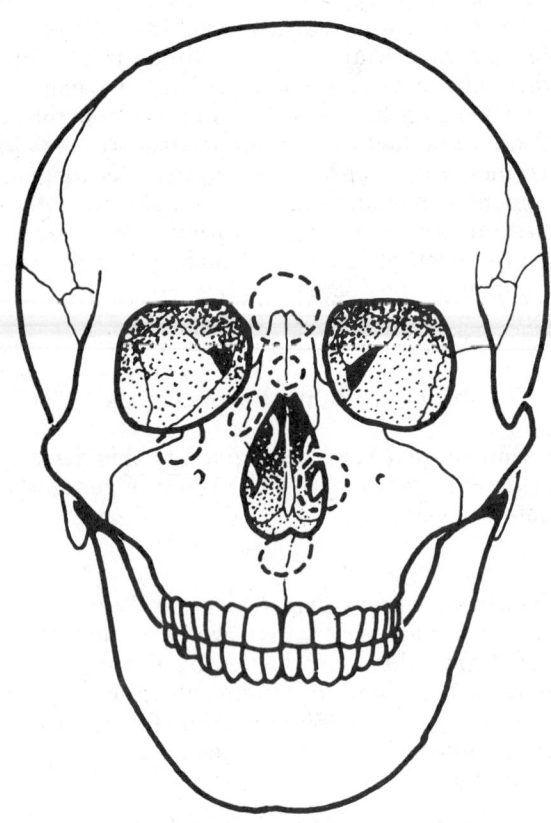

**FIGURE 4.** *Dotted circles indicate sites through which granulomas usually emerge from nasal cavity. (From Martinson, F. D.: Rhinophycomycosis. J Laryng 77:691, 1963.)*

**FIGURE 5.** A, *Involvement of dorsum of nose, glabella, upper lid, cheek, and upper lip before treatment. B, Same patient after treatment. (From Martinson, F. D.: Clinical, epidemiological and therapeutic aspects of entomophthoromycosis. Ann Soc Belg Med Trop 52:339, 1972.)*

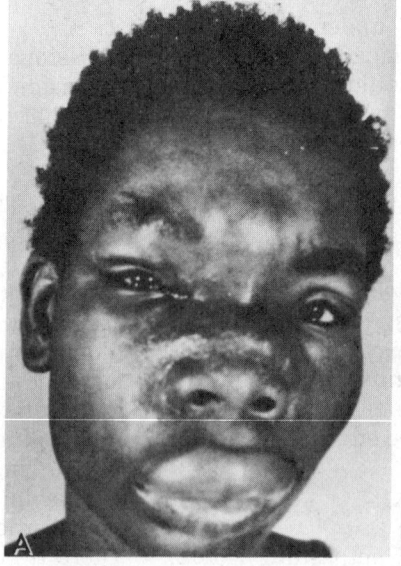
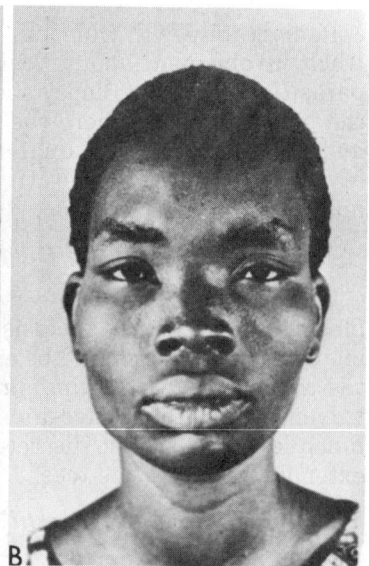

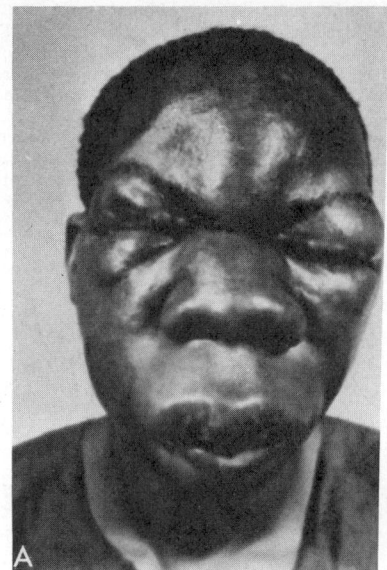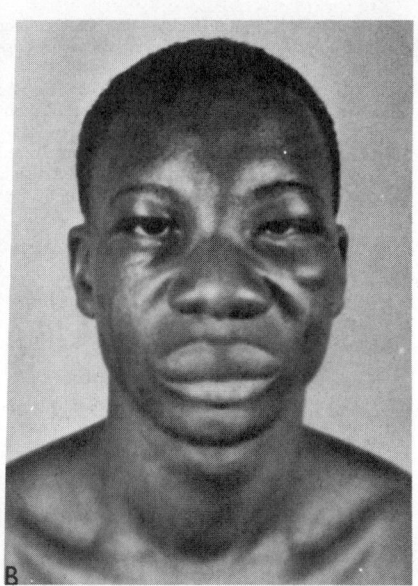

**FIGURE 6.** A, *Severe extensive lesion involving eyelids, glabella, dorsum of nasal alae, and upper lip (lower lip not involved). B, Same patient halfway through treatment. (From Martinson, F. D.: Upper respiratory infection due to Conidiobolus coronatus: "Rhino-entomophthoromycosis" ISIAN 170–174: 1976.)*

### Diagnosis

Radiography excludes bony disease and shows the extent of sinus and pharyngeal involvement (Cockshott et al., 1968). Biopsy should be taken from the nasal cavity or through the buccal sulcus if possible to avoid a visible facial scar. Culture should be performed to confirm the diagnosis.

Pharyngeal and nasal neoplasms, hypertrophic rhinitis, rhinoscleroma, fibrous dysplasia, dental cyst, angioneurotic edema, nodular leprosy, goundou, facial onchocerciasis and African histoplasmosis, and chronic forms of mucormycosis must be excluded.

### Complications and Sequelae

Secondary bacterial paranasal sinus infection is not a serious problem. Rarely the pharyngeal granuloma may spread downward to obstruct the larynx. Spontaneous arrest of spread may occur but spontaneous resolution is rare or nonexistent. Complete cure can be achieved and the face returns to its normal appearance and texture (Fig. 5B). No deaths due to proven infection have been recorded.

Treatment is identical with that of basidiobolomycosis.

### Pulmonary Infection by *Conidiobolus incongruus*

Only one case of this, the third entomophthoromycosis, has been reported. It occurred in the United States in 1970. Unlike previously described infections, it affected the lung of a previously healthy 15-month-old child and caused signs of respiratory obstruction and later heart failure. Radiography showed areas of increased density in one lung and the mediastinum. The diagnosis of Entomophthorales infection was made following thoracotomy and biopsy of the granuloma, which involved the lung, mediastinum, and pericardium. Inhalation of an insect was considered the probable mode of infection.

Treatment with amphotericin B led to complete recovery and no apparent sequelae. Culture by King and Jong in 1976 showed the fungus to be *Conidiobolus incongruus*. In this sole case, as in other entomophthoromycoses, there was no tissue destruction. But one cannot assess from an isolated case whether the pattern of the disease is representative.

### References

Ainsworth, G. C.: Introduction and keys to higher taxa. In Ainsworth, G. C., Sparow, F. K., and Sussman, A. S. (eds.): The Fungi: An Advanced Treatise. Vol. IVA New York, Academic Press, 1973, pp. 1–7.

Bras, G., Gordon, C. C., Emmons, C. W., Prendegast, K. M., and Sugar, M.: A case of phycomycosis in Jamaica. Infection with Entomophthora coronata. Am J Trop Med 14:141, 1965.

Clark, B. M.: Epidemiology of phycomycosis. In Wolstenholme, G. E. W., and Porter, R. (eds.): Systemic Mycoses. London, J. & A. Churchill, Ltd., 1968, pp. 179–192.

Cockshott, W. P., Clark, B. M., and Martinson, F. D.: Upper respiratory infection due to Entomophthora coronata. Rhinoentomophthoromycosis. Radiology 90:1016, 1968.

Emmons, C W., and Bridges, C. H.: Entomophthora coronata, the etiological agent of a Phycomycosis in horses. Mycologia 53:307, 1961.

King, D S., and Jong, S. O.: Identity of the etiological agent of the first deep entomophthoraceous infection of man in the United States. Mycologia 68.181, 1976.

Lie Kian Joe, Njo-Injo Tjoel Eng, Pohan, A. and van der Meulen, H.: Basidiobolus ranarum as a cause of a subcutaneous phycomycosis in Indonesia. Arch Derm 74:378, 1956.

Martinson, F. D.: Rhinophycomycosis. J Laryngol 77:691, 1963.

Martinson, F. D.: Clinical epidemiological and therapeutic aspects of entomophthoromycosis. Ann Soc Belge Med Trop 52:329, 1972.

Vanbreuseghem, R.: Guide pratique de mycologie médical et vétérinaire. Paris, Masson et Cie, 1966.

Williams, A. O., Lightenberg, F. Von, Smith, J. H., and Martinson, F. D.: Ultrastructure of phycomycosis due to Entomophthora and Basidiobolus species and associated "Splendore-Hoeppli" phenomenon. Arch Path 87:459, 1969.

# 98 THRUSH OF THE MOUTH AND ESOPHAGUS

## John E. Edwards, Jr., M.D.

## DEFINITION

Although the term thrush has been used to refer to infection caused by organisms of the genus *Candida* in any anatomic site (usually mucosal), the word thrush is most appropriately applied to a specific form of oral candidiasis classified by Lehner (1966) as acute pseudomembranous moniliasis. The condition is characterized by creamy-white, curd-like patches on the tongue or other oral mucosal surfaces. The patches are removable by scraping, which leaves a bleeding, raw, and painful surface.

Lehner, in 1966, expanded upon his classification of the several forms of oral candidiasis; this classification serves as an excellent framework for organization and discussion of these diseases (Table 1).

In esophageal candidiasis, recognized with increased frequency in recent years, the esophageal mucosa is invaded by *Candida* hyphae, usually in the distal two-thirds of the esophagus. The patchy plaque formation can be visualized at endoscopy.

**TABLE 1. Classification of Oral Candidiasis***

**ACUTE**
  Acute Pseudomembranous Moniliasis (Thrush)
  Acute Atrophic Moniliasis (Antibiotic Sore Mouth)

**CHRONIC**
  Chronic Atrophic Moniliasis (Denture Sore Mouth)
  Chronic Hyperplastic Moniliasis
    Chronic Oral Candidosis (*Candida* Leukoplakia)
    Endocrine Candidosis Syndrome
    Chronic Localized Mucocutaneous Candidosis
    Chronic Diffuse Candidosis

*(From Lehner, 1966)

## ETIOLOGY

Thrush of the mouth and esophagus is caused by yeasts of the genus *Candida*, constituents of the flora of normal young individuals (Nolte, 1977). The clinical and pathologic manifestations are a result of direct tissue invasion by the yeasts and the ensuing inflammatory response.

Among the numerous species of Candida, only seven have been recovered commonly from man, including patients with thrush. These species are *C. albicans, C. guilliermondi, C. krusei, C. parapsilosis, C. stellatoidea, C. tropicalis*, and *C. pseudotropicalis*. They vary in pathogenicity in the mouth and elsewhere, but *C. albicans* is considered the most pathogenic (Howlett, 1976). To date, *C. krusei* is the only species other than *albicans* that has been associated with esophageal candidiasis (single case, Holt, 1968).

## PATHOGENESIS AND PATHOLOGY

Since *Candida* organisms are normal commensals of low pathogenicity, the normal defense mechanisms must be compromised for the organism to invade the tissues and cause disease. The compromise may be at a local or systemic level, or both. An example of local level compromise is the mucosal damage associated with ill-fitting dentures and the resultant trauma to the oral mucosa. A second example is oral candidiasis associated with inhalation of steroid beclomethasone dipropionate in the treatment of asthma. Topical antibiotics, xerostomia, heavy smoking, cessation of smoking (acute period), and radiation of the head and neck also lower local resistance to thrush.

The same factors that compromise systemic immunity and predispose to oral and esophageal candidiasis also predispose to disseminated candidiasis. They include systemic antibiotics, immunosuppressive agents, hyperalimentation fluids, polyethylene catheters, pressure monitoring devices, heroin abuse, organ transplantation, extensive abdominal surgery, and placement of prosthetic cardiac valves.

In newborns, thrush has been related to maternal vaginal candidiasis during delivery.

Approximately 50 per cent of esophageal candidiasis occurs without oral candidiasis (Grieve, 1964). Although *Candida* esophagitis has been reported without underlying illnesses, it is much more commonly associated with hematopoietic or lymphatic malignancy.

Discussion of the pathology of oral and esophageal candidiasis is facilitated through the classification of Lehner, found in Table 1.

### Acute Pseudomembranous Candidiasis

A pseudomembrane composed of desquamated epithelial cells, keratin and necrotic tissue, food debris, leukocytes, and bacteria forms the curd-like patches visualized clinically. The membrane is attached to the epithelium by *Candida* hyphae. Although the inflammatory reaction in the epithelium is usually minor, microabscesses may be present.

### Acute Atrophic Candidiasis

The epithelium of the tongue undergoes atrophy, presumably as a sequel to acute pseudomembranous candidiasis and detachment of the pseudomembrane. Lehner has also suggested that the condition occurs de novo and that some cases of "antibiotic sensitive tongue" are this form of candidiasis. An inflammatory edema is the predominant reaction and is responsible for the smooth appearance of the tongue.

Median rhomboid glossitis may be a result of *Candida* infection rather than a congenital anomaly as previously thought (Cook, 1975). Although "black hairy tongue" was once considered to be due to *Candida*, it is now thought to be secondary to changes in oral bacterial flora that cause hypertrophy of the tongue papillae. The role of *Candida* in tongue fissures is doubtful because invasion of tissue has not been established by biopsy.

### Chronic Atrophic Candidiasis

This condition is "denture sore mouth" and is characterized by chronic inflammation, edema, and thinning of the epithelium in areas under the dental plate. The masses of hyphae recovered from the involved area do not generally invade the tissue. Inflammation occurs predominantly under the maxillary denture and is rare under the mandibular plate. An interesting postulate for the maxillary localization is that the negative pressure caused by the weight of the maxillary denture keeps the area dry and deficient in salivary antibodies. Since individuals without denture stomatitis may also have hyphae in large numbers under the denture plate (Olsen and Birkeland (1977) and Budtz-Jorgensen et al. (1975)), the specificity of *Candida* as the agent causing denture sore mouth has been questioned. Yeasts were found in 98 per cent of individuals with denture sore mouth. *C. albicans* was isolated in pure or mixed culture with other yeast species in 86.5 per cent and other yeast species such as *Trichosporon, Torula, Saccharomyces,* and *Rhodotrula*, were isolated in pure culture in 6.5 per cent.

Angular chelitis is frequently associated with denture stomatis. *Candida* has been considered the specific cause of this chronic inflammatory reaction at the corners of the mouth. However, in patients with angular cheilitis, an infective etiology has been found in only 68 per cent, *Staphylococcus aureus* in pure or mixed culture in 79 per cent, *Candida* species alone in 44 per cent, and beta-hemolytic streptococci alone in 15 per cent. Thus, *Candida* species were not the most common, nor the only significant infective agent causing angular cheilitis. Noninfective factors also appear responsible for angular cheilitis; these are loss of vertical dimension of mouth, drooling of saliva, vitamin deficiencies, and allergy to denture-base materials or cleansing agents.

### Chronic Hyperplastic Candidiasis

***Chronic Oral Candidiasis (Candida leukoplakia).*** This condition is a firm white plaque of the cheek, lips, and tongue. The lesion consists of parakeratosis, acanthosis, pseudoepitheliomatous hyperplasia, microabscess formation, edema of the superficial layers of epithelium and chronic inflammatory cell infiltration of varying intensity of the cornium. Hyphae are always present, but only in the superficial part of the epithelium.

***Endocrine Candidiasis Syndrome – Chronic Localized Mucocutaneous Candidiasis and Chronic Diffuse Candidiasis.*** These syndromes are discussed in Chapter 210. The histopathology is not different from other forms of chronic *Candida* infection.

### Candida Esophagitis

Both acute and chronic inflammation are present. There is associated hyperkeratosis, pseudo-keratosis, acanthosis, proliferation of the rete ridges, ductal squamous metaplasia, lymphoid nodule and lymphoid follicle formation, ductal dilatation, and focal oncocytic hyperplasia. In addition, a pseudomembrane may form similar to that of thrush, which can cause intraluminal protrusions and result in partial esophageal obstruction. Intraluminal diverticulosis may also be present; however, these diverticulae may more frequently be related to mucosal hyperplasia, and pseudodiverticulae may be a more accurate term. *Candida* esophagitis usually affects the lower two-thirds of the esophagus. As a result of a chronic inflammation and/or abscess formation, segmental narrowing may occur with shoulder defects. Fistulas may form and achalasia may occur.

## CLINICAL MANIFESTATIONS

*Acute pseudomembranous candidiasis* (thrush) is characterized by bluish-white to white, adherent, milk curd-like patches on the oral mucosa (Fig. 1). They are relatively nonpainful and are not easily removed. When freed from their base, however, the exposed surface is painfully raw and bleeds easily. The patient may be relatively asymptomatic despite extensive involvement. A metallic taste or loss of taste may precede the infection. In contrast, *acute atrophic candidiasis* is characterized by considerable pain, smoothness of the tongue, and a generalized glossitis. *Chronic atrophic candidiasis* (denture stomatitis) causes inflammation of the denture-bearing area. These lesions may be white and cause a burning sensation. There is a high incidence of angular cheilitis. *Chronic hyperplastic candidiasis (Candida leukoplakia)* is characterized by white, firm, and persistent plaques, most commonly involving the cheek, tongue, palate, and lips and resembles leukoplakia. These lesions may have a protracted course, lasting for years.

The most common symptoms of *Candida* eso-

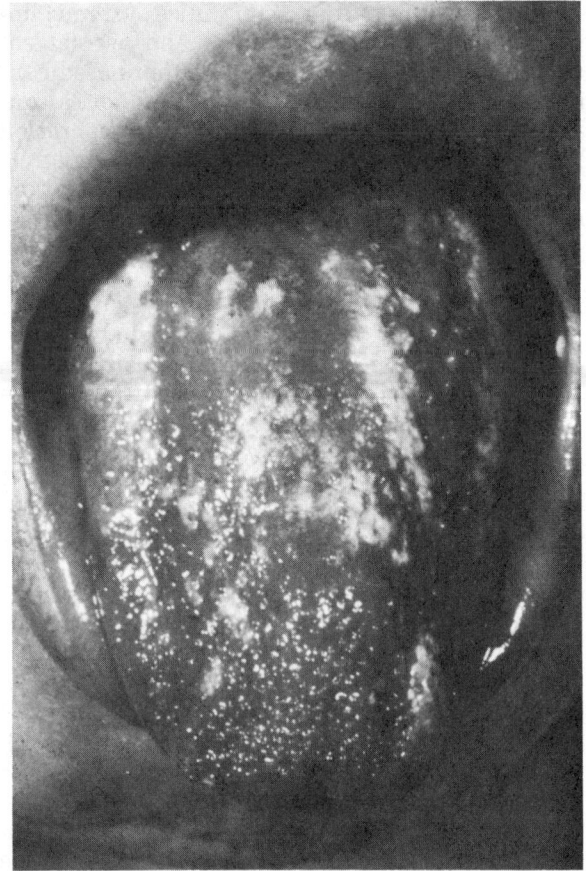

**FIGURE 1.** *Typical mild to moderate oral thrush with white, mild-curd patches over tongue surface.*

phagitis are painful difficult swallowing, substernal chest pain, nausea, and vomiting. Lack of normal peristalsis may result in aspiration. The denervation, in its most extensive form, may result in true achalasia. On the other hand, some patients have had extensive disease with minimal or no symptoms. Some forms of *Candida* esophagitis may resemble thrush in appearance with white patches over the esophageal mucosa (Fig. 2).

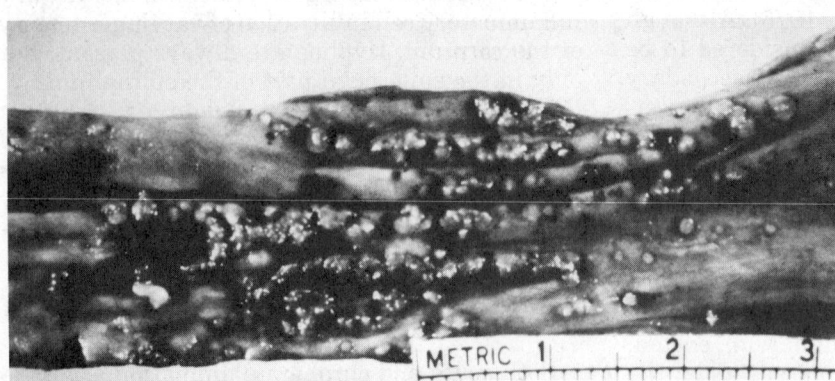

**FIGURE 2.** Candida *esophagitis visualized at autopsy. Note resemblance to oral thrush.*

## COMPLICATIONS AND SEQUELAE

In the neonate, elderly, or immunocompromised host, pain during eating may interfere with nutrition. Thrush may extend contiguously from the mouth to the bronchopulmonary tree (including larynx) into the esophagus or into bone and cause osteomyelitis of the palate. Limited data suggest that *Candida* leukoplakia may rarely be precancerous. Although it would seem that esophageal candidiasis results from extension of oral candidiasis, only half of the cases have been associated with oral disease. Generalized hematogenous dissemination of candidiasis may also occur from the mouth.

The complications of esophageal candidiasis are fistula formation, ulceration, luminal obstruction, loss of peristalsis, achalasia, diverticulae, aspiration, pneumonia, bleeding, and presumably dissemination. Esophageal perforation secondary to *Candida* esophagitis is rare.

## DIAGNOSIS

The only method to diagnose definitively any form of *Candida* infection is by biopsy of the involved tissue and demonstration of *Candida* invasion by hyphae or pseudohyphae. Because of the presence of *Candida* as part of the normal oral flora, simply recovering the organism from saliva or from a swab does not prove *Candida* infection. However, it is not always necessary to make a tissue-proven diagnosis of oral or esophageal *Candida* infection in order to manage patients. For instance, the typical milk curd, white exudate that shows multiple pseudohyphae or hyphae on either Gram stain or potassium hydroxide preparation can be presumed to be thrush and the appropriate therapy should be instituted. More aggressive biopsy procedures should be reserved for refractory or atypical situations.

Oral infections with several different bacteria, including staphylococci, streptococci, lactobacilli, neisseria, and coliforms may occur in immunocompromised patients and may resemble candidiasis. Efforts should be made to rule out other organisms causing lesions resembling thrush (Tyldesley et al., 1976).

The diagnosis of esophageal candidiasis can be made by biopsy during endoscopy. The cobblestone appearance of the esophageal mucosa and the x-ray appearance with contrast studies are helpful in the presumptive diagnosis. X-ray of the esophagus shows a shaggy outline of the mucosa (Fig. 3), loss of mucosal folds, deep ulceration, and nodular filling defects that may be secondary to either mucosal edema, ulceration, or pseudomem-

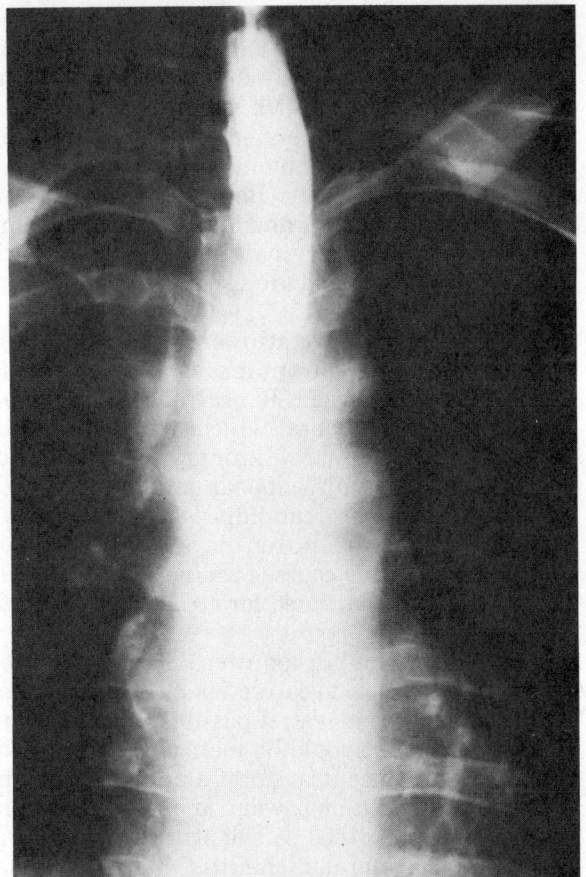

**FIGURE 3.** *X-ray appearance of Candida esophagitis. Note irregularity of right border of esophagus compared with normal-appearing left border.*

brane formation. On fluoroscopy, peristalsis is diminished or absent and contrast media may be seen entering the lungs. Segmental narrowing may occur and contrast media may adhere to the esophageal wall. Large filling defects may resemble esophageal varices. It is important to point out that radiologic examination may be negative in cases of *Candida* esophagitis proved at endoscopy or postmortem examination.

## TREATMENT

The most important facet of the treatment of any *Candida* infection is elimination of predisposing factors, including antibiotics, steroids, cytotoxic agents, ill-fitting dentures or any of the others listed under *Pathogenesis*.

The main drug for thrush is nystatin, which is available in oral suspension at concentration of 100,000 units per cc; as vaginal suppositories containing 100,000 units of nystatin with lactose, ethyl cellulose, stearic acid, and starch; or as tablets containing 500,000 units. The dose of the suspension for infants is 1 ml in each side of the mouth, four times per day (one-half that amount in premature and low birth weight infants) and 4 to 6 ml, four times per day, in adults with half the dose in each side of the mouth. The tablets can be sucked four times daily. Because of the unpleasant taste of the tablets and oral suspension, some patients prefer the vaginal suppositories, which are more palatable and are used identically to the oral tablets.

Alternatives to nystatin are gentian violet, which may be disadvantageous because of its staining, amphotericin B oral suspension, and amphotericin B troches, which are available in the United Kingdom. Preliminary trials with clotrimazole troches also appear promising. Acute pseudomembranous candidiasis generally resolves within seven to ten days of therapy but occasionally longer courses are necessary. Treatment should be continued for 48 hours after clinical resolution.

Denture sore mouth requires the treatment for thrush, in addition to correction of ill-fitting dentures and their removal, if possible, until healing occurs. Dentures should be meticulously cleaned. A 2 per cent concentration of amphotericin B in an adhesive paste or powder or incorporation of nystatin into modified soft denture liners is also effective. The angular cheilitis associated with denture sore mouth is treated with topical nystatin or 3 per cent amphotericin B cream or ointment applied four times per day. In addition, defects in the denture design, which may help cause skin folds at the mouth corners, must be corrected. Management of the chronic hyperplastic candidiasis syndromes will be discussed in Chapter 210.

*Candida* leukoplakia is treated with a longer course of nystatin and surgical removal in refractory cases.

*Candida* esophagitis is usually more difficult to treat than oral thrush. In some patients, pain or swallowing may be so severe that oral nystatin cannot be delivered to the esophagus and amphotericin B must be given intravenously in doses of 30 mg on alternate days for a total of 750 to 1000 mg (or less if there is rapid clinical improvement). Clotrimazole, 5-fluorocytosine, and intravenous miconazole may also prove useful.

## References

Budtz-Jörgensen, E., Stenderup, A., and Gabrowsky, M.: An epidemiologic study of yeasts in elderly denture wearers. Community Dent-Oral Epidemiol 3:115, 1976.
Cooke, B. E. D.: Median rhomboid glossitis. Candidiasis and not a developmental anomaly. Brit J Dermatol 93:399, 1975.
Grieve, N. W. T.: Monilial oesophagitis. Brit J Radiol 37:551, 1964.
Holt, J. M.: Candida infection of the oesophagus. Gut 9:227, 1968.
Howlett, J. A.: The infection of rat tongue mucosa in vitro with five species of Candida. J Med Microbiol 9:309, 1976.
Lehner, T.: Classification and clinico-pathological features of Candida infections in the mouth. In Winner, H. I., and Hurley, R. (eds.): Symposium on Candida Infections. Edinburgh and London, E & S. Livingstone, Ltd., 1966, p. 119.
MacFarlane, T. W., and Helnarska, S. J.: The microbiology of angular cheilitis. Brit Dent J 140:403, 1976.
Nolte, W. A.: The oral microflora. In Nolte, W. A. (ed.): Oral Microbiology with Basic Microbiology and Immunology. 3rd ed. St. Louis, C. V. Mosby Company, 1977, p. 220.
Olsen, I., and Birkeland, J. M.: Denture stomatitis — yeast occurrence and the pH of saliva and denture plaque. Scand J Dent Res 85:130, 1977.
Tyldesley, W. R., Rotter, E., and Sells, R. A.: Bacterial thrush-like lesions of the mouth in renal transplant patients. Lancet 1:485, 1976.

*General References*

Cawson, R. A.: Chronic oral candidiasis, denture stomatitis and chronic hyperplastic candidiasis. In Winner, H. I., and Hurley, R. (eds.): Symposium on Candida Infections. London, E. & S. Livingstone, Ltd., 1966, p. 138.
Kods, B. E., Wickremesinghe, P. C., Kozinn, P. J., Iswara, K., and Goldberg, P. K.: Candida esophagitis. A prospective study of 27 cases. Gastro 71:715, 1976.
Kozinn, P. J., Taschdjian, C. L., and Wiener, H.: Incidence and pathogenesis of neonatal candidiasis. Pediatrics 21:421, 1955.
Sheft, D. J., and Shrago, G.: Esophageal moniliasis. The spectrum of the disease. JAMA 213:1859, 1970.
Sherlock, P., Goldstein, M. J., and Eras, P.: Esophageal moniliasis. Mod Treat 7(6):1250, 1970.

# 99 *HERPES STOMATITIS*

## Michael N. Oxman, M.D.

### DEFINITION

Herpes stomatitis (acute herpetic gingivostomatitis) is an acute inflammatory infection of the mucous membranes of the mouth due to herpes simplex virus (HSV). It is the result of primary HSV infection of a susceptible person and occurs mainly in children under 5 years of age. The disease is normally self-limited, and symptoms generally disappear in 12 to 14 days. In the newborn or immunosuppressed patient, infection may disseminate to the liver, lungs, adrenal glands, and other viscera. In young adults, primary oropharyngeal HSV infections more often produce acute pharyngitis and tonsillitis, without lesions in the anterior part of the mouth. In this age group, primary HSV infection is an important cause of acute pharyngotonsillitis, and its clinical manifestations are often indistinguishable from those of Group A streptococcal infection.

Although gingivostomatitis and pharyngotonsillitis are the most common clinical manifestations of symptomatic primary infection, they are seen in only a small minority of infected individuals. Most primary oropharyngeal HSV infections do not produce overt disease. This is in contrast to the occurrence of clinically apparent varicella in over 95 per cent of those infected with varicella-zoster virus. However, HSV does resemble varicella-zoster virus and other members of the herpesvirus family in its remarkable propensity for causing latent infections. Thus, whether symptomatic or not, primary HSV infection of the oropharyngeal mucosa is followed by an infection that lasts a lifetime. For the most part, the virus remains latent, but it may be reactivated by various stimuli (for example, fever, trauma, sunlight), causing recurrent infections. These usually present as herpes labialis, the well-known "cold sore" or "fever blister" that occurs on or adjacent to the vermillion border of the lip. Herpes labialis is far more common than acute herpetic gingivostomatitis or pharyngotonsillitis; it afflicts 30 to 50 per cent of the world's adult population.

## ETIOLOGY

Herpes simplex virus is one of the most ancient and widely disseminated infectious agents of man, but its ubiquity is not generally appreciated because the initial infection only rarely results in overt disease. The term *herpes* is derived from the Greek word meaning "to creep," and clinical descriptions of herpes labialis date from the time of Hippocrates (Juel-Jensen and MacCallum, 1972). The infectious nature of herpes labialis was established as early as 1912, when Grüter produced keratitis in rabbits with material from human herpetic lesions (Grüter, 1920). Several investigators reasoned that herpes labialis must represent the reactivation of a latent HSV infection previously initiated by an earlier primary infection of the oral mucosa (Goodpasture, 1929), but the nature of that primary infection was not recognized until 1938. In the United States, Dodd et al. (1938) showed that HSV was the cause of acute gingivostomatitis in infants and young children. Burnet and Williams (1939), in Australia, confirmed that observation and, in addition, showed that acute herpetic gingivostomatitis was always a manifestation of primary HSV infection.

Herpes simplex virus (herpesvirus hominis) is a member of the herpesvirus group (Chapter 56), which includes three other human herpesviruses (varicella-zoster virus, cytomegalovirus, and Epstein-Barr virus). These herpesviruses are morphologically indistinguishable and share a number of properties, including a remarkable propensity for establishing lifelong latent infections. The HSV virion has an internal core that contains the viral genome, a linear molecule of double-stranded DNA with a molecular weight of 100 million. The core is enclosed within an icosahedral capsid 100 nm in diameter and is composed of 162 identical protein subunits (capsomers). This nucleocapsid is surrounded by one or two additional layers of protein and, finally, by a loose lipoprotein envelope derived from the nuclear membrane of the infected host cell. The complete virion is roughly spherical with a diameter of 150 to 200 nm. The virus envelope contains radially-oriented viral glycoproteins that mediate the attachment of the virion to susceptible host cells. Only enveloped virions are fully infectious, and this accounts for the lability of HSV; infectivity is rapidly destroyed by organic solvents, detergents, proteolytic enzymes, heat, and extremes of pH. The envelope glycoproteins are antigenic and elicit neutralizing antibodies. The appearance of these viral glycoproteins on nuclear and cytoplasmic membranes early in the course of HSV infection provides a mechanism for host-immune recognition and lysis of HSV-infected cells. In addition to structural components of the virion, certain enzymes essential for virus replication are synthesized in HSV-infected cells. These include a virus-specified DNA polymerase and a deoxypyrimidine kinase (thymidine kinase), both of which are important targets for antiviral chemotherapy.

There are two distinct serotypes of HSV, HSV Type 1 (HSV-1) and HSV Type 2 (HSV-2), which differ in their clinical and epidemiologic behavior (Nahmias and Roizman, 1973) and can be distinguished on the basis of antigenic, biologic, and biochemical differences (Table 1). The two serotypes of HSV also differ in their mode of transmission (Nahmias and Josey, 1976). HSV-1 is transmitted primarily by nonvenereal routes, usually involving contact with infected saliva. HSV-2 is transmitted venereally or from a maternal genital infection to the newborn. Acute herpetic gingivostomatitis is caused by HSV-1, which is also the serotype responsible for most cases of HSV pharyngitis and tonsillitis, and for most cutaneous lesions above the waist. HSV-1 is also responsible for herpes simplex keratitis (Chapter 232) and for herpes simplex encephalitis (Chapter 168). HSV-2 is the serotype responsible for most cases of herpes genitalis and for cutaneous lesions below the waist. HSV-2 also causes the majority of neonatal HSV infections and is associated epidemiologically with carcinoma of the cervix.

**TABLE 1.  Differences Between Herpes Simplex Virus Type 1 (HSV-1) and Type 2 (HSV-2)**

| CHARACTERISTICS | HSV-1 | HSV-2 |
|---|---|---|
| **Clinical** | | |
| *Manifestations of Primary Infection* | | |
| Acute herpetic gingivostomatitis | +[a] | −[b] |
| Acute herpetic pharyngotonsillitis | + | −[c] |
| Acute herpetic keratoconjunctivitis | + | − |
| Neonatal herpes simplex infections | ±[d] | + |
| *Manifestations of Recurrent Infection* | | |
| Herpes labialis | + | − |
| Herpes keratitis | + | − |
| *Manifestations of Primary or Recurrent Infection* | | |
| Cutaneous herpes | | |
| Skin above waist | + | − |
| Skin below waist | − | + |
| Hands or Arms | + | + |
| Herpetic whitlow | + | + |
| Eczema herpeticum | + | − |
| Herpes genitalis | −[e] | + |
| Herpes simplex encephalitis | + | − |
| Herpes simplex meningitis | ±[f] | + |
| **Epidemiologic** | | |
| Transmission | Non-venereal | Venereal |
| Epidemiologic association with carcinoma of the cervix | − | + |
| **Latency** | | |
| Trigeminal and cervical sensory ganglia | + | − |
| Sacral ganglia | − | + |
| **Biochemical** | | |
| DNA guanine + cytosine | 67% | 69% |
| Homology between viral DNAs | approximately 40% | |
| Stability of virus-specific thymidine kinase at 40° C | + | − |
| **Biologic** | | |
| Neurotropism in mice on peripheral inoculation | less neurotropic | more neurotropic |
| Pock size on chick chorioallantoic membrane | small | large |
| Plaque formation in chick embryo cell monolayer culture | − | + |
| Temperature sensitivity of replication (40° C) | − | + |
| Heparin sensitivity | + | − |
| Inhibition of replication by thymidine | − | + |

**Other**
HSV-1 and HSV-2 can be unequivocally differentiated by serologic techniques, by DNA:DNA hybridization, by restriction endonuclease fingerprinting of viral DNA, and by electrophoretic analysis of virus-specified proteins.

[a] + = frequent or predominant cause.
[b] − = infrequent cause (except under special epidemiologic circumstances).
[c] HSV-2 is frequently isolated when pharyngotonsillitis is associated with orogenital sexual contact.
[d] HSV-1 is isolated from 20 to 30 per cent of cases, reflecting the increasing frequency with which HSV-1 causes genital herpes (in the mother), as well as some cases of postnatal infection acquired from individuals shedding HSV-1.

Although HSV-1 and HSV-2 have many common antigens and share about 40 per cent of their DNA base sequences, they each have type-specific antigenic determinants that permit them to be differentiated unequivocally by a variety of serologic techniques (Rawls, 1979). In addition, HSV-1 and HSV-2 can be readily distinguished by nucleic acid hybridization, by electrophoretic analysis of virus-specified proteins, and by restriction endonuclease fingerprinting of the viral DNA (Honess and Watson, 1977). The latter technique, which can also distinguish between different strains of the same serotype, has been particularly useful for epidemiologic studies (Linneman et al., 1978; Buchman et al., 1978, 1979).

Unlike other human herpesviruses, HSV has a wide host range. HSV can infect many experimental animals, including rats, mice, hamsters, guinea pigs, rabbits, nonhuman primates, chick embryos, and a wide variety of cell cultures from human and animal tissues. In cell cultures, HSV causes cytoplasmic edema (so that cells become enlarged and round), acidophilic Cowdry Type A intranuclear inclusion bodies, and fusion of cells into multinucleated giant cells. The same cytopathology is seen in cutaneous and visceral lesions in vivo. These changes are the same as those produced by varicella-zoster virus. The cytopathic effect of varicella-zoster virus in tissue culture, however, remains focal because progeny virus is cell associated, whereas HSV is released into the medium and rapidly spreads to infect cells throughout the culture.

## PATHOLOGY AND PATHOGENESIS

HSV infection is usually cytolytic, and the resulting pathology is a consequence of necrosis of infected cells together with local inflammation. In immunosuppressed patients, the herpetic lesions may be atypical and difficult to recognize clinically. The skin and mucous membrane lesions of HSV-1 and HSV-2 are the same and resemble those produced by varicella-zoster virus. The characteristic cytopathology, which can be observed in vivo as well as in tissue culture, consists of "ballooning degeneration" of individual infected cells, the production of Cowdry Type A intranuclear inclusion bodies, and the formation of multinucleated giant cells. Individual infected cells become greatly enlarged with pale, vacuolat-

[e] HSV-1 is now being isolated from 5 to 30 per cent of patients with genital herpes, primarily from individuals with a history of orogenital sexual contact. In addition, herpetic vulvovaginitis in infants is generally caused by HSV-1, acquired from adults or by autoinoculation of infected saliva.
[f] Some cases reported, but insufficient data to estimate frequency.

ed cytoplasm. The nuclei exhibit margination of chromatin and contain inclusion bodies. These are initially homogeneous and slightly basophilic, and often fill the nucleus. However, they rapidly condense and evolve into sharply demarcated acidophilic inclusion bodies that are separated from the deeply basophilic ring of marginated chromatin at the nuclear membrane by a clear zone or halo (Fig. 1). Multinucleated giant cells are formed primarily by cell fusion, a process associated with the appearance of HSV-specified glycoproteins on the membranes of infected cells.

HSV infection of the skin and mucous membranes causes intraepidermal vesicles. The virus, usually acquired by contact with infected saliva, replicates locally in the cells of the stratum spinosum. Infected cells undergo ballooning degeneration with loss of intercellular bridges, and are soon separated by intercellular edema. At this early stage, the lesions are papular and contain a few small multinucleated giant cells. Typical intranuclear inclusion bodies are already present. The papular lesions rapidly evolve into intraepidermal vesicles as a result of the infection and

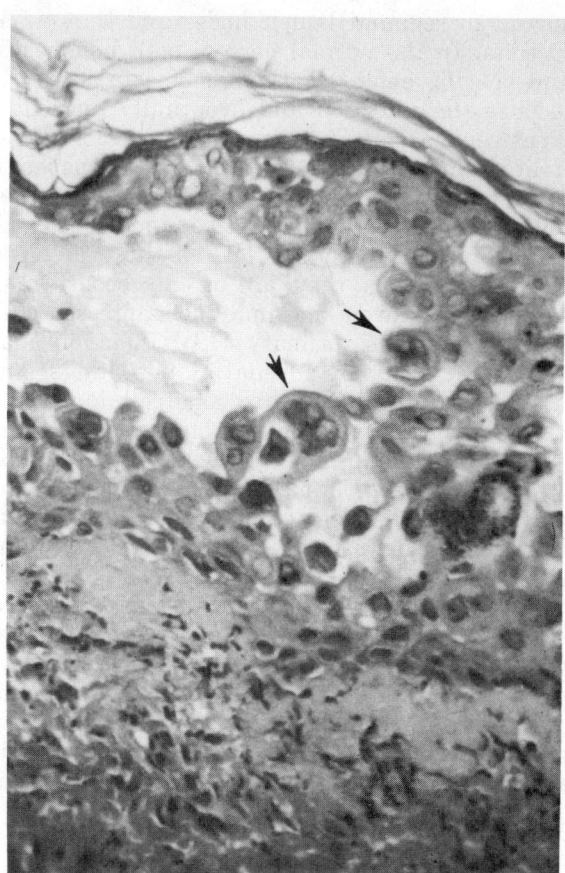

**FIGURE 2.** *Herpes simplex, early vesicle. Intraepidermal vesicle produced by herpes simplex virus infection of the skin. Infected epithelial cells show "ballooning degeneration" with the formation of multinucleated giant cells (arrows). Edema fluid has elevated the overlying stratum corneum. The underlying dermis shows edema and mononuclear cell infiltration. Hematoxylin and eosin. Magnification 200 ×. (Courtesy Dr. P. J. Barr.)*

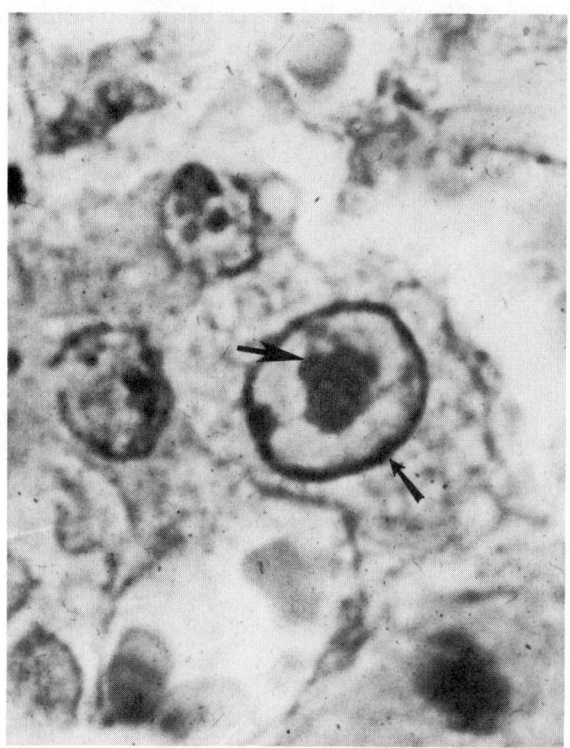

**FIGURE 1.** *Herpes simplex, intranuclear inclusion body. A section of liver from a malnourished child who died with disseminated herpes simplex virus infection. A parenchymal cell shows a typical eosinophilic Cowdry type A intranuclear inclusion body (large arrow), which is separated from the basophilic ring of marginated chromatin at the nuclear membrane (small arrow) by a clear zone or halo. Hematoxylin and eosin. Magnification 2,000 ×.*

degeneration of more epithelial cells and the continuing influx of edema fluid, which elevates the uninvolved stratum corneum to form a delicate clear vesicle (Fig. 2). The vesicle fluid contains fibrin, degenerating epithelial cells, multinucleated giant cells, and a large amount of cell-free virus. In the underlying dermis or lamina propria capillary dilatation and infiltration of inflammatory cells is pronounced, but necrosis is absent. The inflammatory cells soon invade the vesicle, and the fluid becomes cloudy. When the vesicle is in the skin, the fluid is absorbed, leaving a flat adherent crust that becomes detached when subjacent epithelial cells grow back. The lesions heal without scars. Lesions in the mucous membranes develop in the same way, but the thin roof of the vesicle quickly breaks down, and a shallow ulcer remains.

During primary infection (for example, acute herpetic gingivostomatitis) there is usually spread to regional lymph nodes and sometimes viremia. In the normal person, both nonspecific and specific defense mechanisms join forces to localize the infection and eventually terminate virus replication. These mechanisms include activated macrophages, interferons, nonspecific killer lymphocytes, sensitized killer lymphocytes, antiviral antibody, and antibody-mediated cell cytotoxicity (Chapter 83). When these defenses are deficient, as they are in newborns, malnourished children, and immunosuppressed children and adults, primary HSV infection may spread to the liver, adrenal glands, lungs, and brain. Individuals with abnormal cellular immunity are particularly vulnerable. In visceral lesions (for example, in the liver) there is usually coagulation necrosis of parenchymal cells, stroma, and blood vessels. Cells containing typical intranuclear inclusion bodies are generally found at the periphery of the necrotic areas.

Early in the course of acute herpetic gingivostomatitis or asymptomatic primary oropharyngeal HSV-1 infection, virus invades local nerve endings in the mucous membranes of the mouth and ascends within axons to reach the trigeminal ganglion. There it establishes a latent infection in sensory neurons that persists for the life of the host (Goodpasture, 1929; Stevens, 1975). Despite the host's immunity, this latent virus can be reactivated by various stimuli. The reactivated HSV may then travel within axons from the neuronal soma to the periphery and infect the perioral skin or mucous membranes. Replication and cell-to-cell spread in epithelial cells produce an intraepidermal vesicle indistinguishable from that produced by primary HSV infection. It is noteworthy that, during recurrent HSV infections, there are inflammatory changes in the portion of the corresponding sensory ganglion that contains neurons that provide sensation to the skin at the site of the recurrent lesion (Howard, 1905). Humoral and cellular immune mechanisms normally limit this local virus replication and spread, so that recurrent HSV infections are generally less severe, less extensive, and of shorter duration than primary infections. In fact, many recurrences are asymptomatic, resulting only in the shedding of virus in saliva.

HSV-1 is a remarkably successful parasite. Primary infection usually occurs during childhood but rarely causes severe disease. In fact, it is most often asymptomatic (Fig. 3). After primary infection, HSV, in contrast to many other viruses, does not disappear and leave behind a solid im-

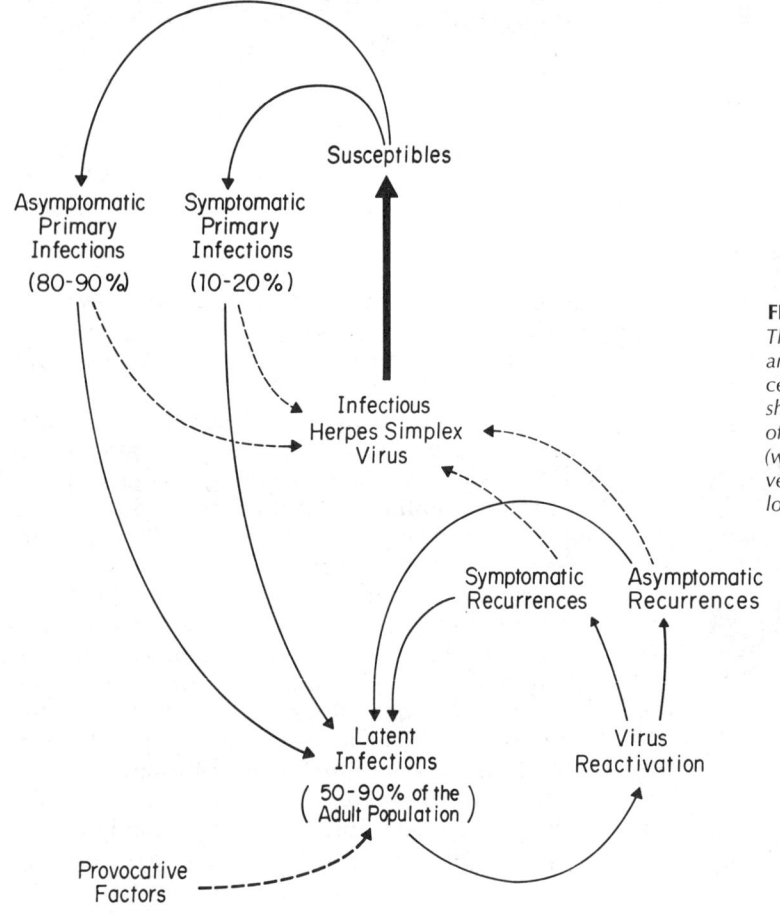

**FIGURE 3.** *The ecology of herpes simplex virus. The 50 to 90 per cent of adults with latent infections are the reservoir of herpes simplex virus. New susceptibles (usually children) are infected when adults shed virus during recurrences (for example, episodes of herpes labialis). After their primary infection (which is usually asymptomatic), the children develop latent infections and join the pool of lifelong virus carriers.*

munity to reinfection. Instead, it persists for the life of the host, who, in spite of the presence of HSV-specific humoral and cellular immunity, is subject to recurrent attacks of HSV infection. This persistence of HSV is in the form of a latent infection that is completely asymptomatic most of the time. However, a variety of provocative factors, such as fever, emotional stress, sunlight, menstruation, or trauma, can reactivate the virus and produce a brief, self-limited episode of recurrent infection, during which HSV is shed into the environment. When symptomatic, these episodes of recurrent HSV-1 infection generally present as herpes labialis. But they are often asymptomatic and detectable only by the presence of HSV-1 in the saliva. HSV-1 infections rarely produce severe disease in the normal host, and persistence of the virus does not interfere with long-term survival. Thus most infected individuals remain in the community as lifelong carriers of HSV. The periodic reactivation of latent HSV infection provides ample opportunity for the transmission of HSV to susceptible children before the adult carriers succumb to old age or to other diseases. In this regard, it is probably no accident that herpes labialis is frequently brought on by the fever associated with severe and life-threatening bacterial infections. The remarkable degree to which HSV is adapted to man, its natural host, is underlined by its behavior in other species. For example, in rabbits or mice, HSV-1 infections are generally severe and often fatal. Similarly, *Herpesvirus simiae* causes severe and generally fatal encephalitis in man, whereas, in its natural host, it produces a mild or asymptomatic infection that is followed by lifelong latency (Chapter 169).

It is clear from studies in humans and experimentally infected animals that latent HSV is harbored in sensory ganglia innervating the site of primary HSV infection (Baringer, 1975; Stevens, 1975). Thus, lesions of recurrent HSV-1 are usually within the distribution of the second or third division of the trigeminal nerve, and only rarely in areas of skin innervated by the first division. This implies that latent HSV infections in neurons have little tendency for horizontal spread to other neurons within the ganglion. Recurrent infections — that is, herpes labialis or asymptomatic shedding of HSV-1 in saliva — are regularly induced by section or manipulation of the sensory root of the trigeminal ganglion (Carton and Kilbourne, 1952; Pazin et al., 1978). The appearance of recurrent herpetic lesions in the skin depends upon the integrity of the peripheral sensory nerve. Local denervation by section of the branches of the sensory nerve prevents the recurrence of HSV in the denervated skin but not in adjacent skin with intact sensation. Latent infection has not been demonstrated in the skin at sites of recurrent lesions (Rustigian et al., 1966), but HSV-1 has been detected by explantation and cocultivation techniques in human trigeminal, superior cervical, and vagus ganglia (Bastian et al., 1972; Baringer and Swoveland, 1973; Warren et al., 1978). Similarly, latent infection with HSV-2 has been detected in human sacral ganglia (Baringer, 1974).

Elegant studies in experimentally infected animals indicate that within latently infected sensory ganglia it is the sensory neurons rather than the supporting cells that harbor the virus (Stevens, 1975). However, the nature of the latent neuronal infection is not clear. Perhaps, the viral genome persists in some nonreplicating form, with infectious virus being produced only during episodes of reactivation. Alternatively, the persistence of HSV might be maintained by a very low level of virus replication within the neurons. In either case, the neuron appears to be unique in its ability to produce infectious HSV (either constantly or only during recurrences) without undergoing lysis. Immune reactions determine the course and outcome of each phase of HSV infection. Antiviral antibody, cellular immunity, and nonspecific factors that limit virus replication (for example, interferon, antiviral drugs) can limit the severity of primary infection and reduce the incidence of latency. In latently infected animals and humans, immunosuppression increases both the frequency and the severity of recurrent infections (Rand et al., 1976). Both humoral and cellular immunity also seem to be important in maintaining latency, but the mechanisms involved are unclear. Perhaps the capacity of the latently infected neuron to replicate HSV is modulated by the interaction of antibody or sensitized cells with virus-induced antigens on the cell membrane (Lehner et al., 1975). Even more obscure, at present, is the mechanism by which such diverse stimuli as fever, sunlight, emotional stress, physical trauma, and menstruation can induce the reactivation of latent HSV infection.

## CLINICAL MANIFESTATIONS

The manifestations of HSV infection are determined by the nature of the HSV infection itself — that is, whether it is a primary or a recurrent infection; the portal of entry of the virus; the serotype and the amount of virus initiating the infection; and by such host factors as age, immune status, nutritional status, and the presence or absence of conditions like eczema or burns that alter the resistance of the skin. The major clinical syndromes produced by HSV infection are listed in Table 1. Herpes simplex encephalitis and meningitis are discussed in Chapter 168, and HSV infections of the eye are discussed in Chapter 232. Genital herpes and neonatal HSV infection, which are caused predominantly by HSV-2, are discussed in Chapter 151. The remaining syndromes, which are caused most often by HSV-1, are discussed below. Because they often differ, the clinical manifestations of primary and recurrent HSV-1 infections are discussed separately.

The distinction between primary and recurrent HSV infections is complex because HSV-1 and HSV-2, though antigenically distinct, have common antigenic determinants that can induce cross-reactive humoral and cellular immune responses. These immune responses provide some protection against heterotypic infection in vivo. Thus, HSV infection in someone who has never been infected with either HSV serotype (for example, genital herpes in a patient with no antibody to HSV-1 or HSV-2) is not equivalent to infection with the same HSV serotype in an individual previously infected with the heterologous serotype (for example, genital herpes in a patient with a history of herpes labialis and preexisting antibody to HSV-1). The initial HSV-2 infection is usually less severe in a person already immune to HSV-1 than in someone without prior HSV-1 infection. Nevertheless, both types of initial HSV-2 infection are ordinarily described as *primary* genital herpes (primary HSV-2 infections). The distinction may be relevant among people living under better socioeconomic conditions in whom the acquisition of HSV-1 infection is delayed so that most children reach sexual maturity without having been infected with HSV-1. The term recurrent infection, as generally used, refers to the recurrence of infection by the same serotype. The source of virus responsible for the recurrence may be endogenous (for example, in the case of herpes labialis) or exogenous (for example, a herpetic whitlow caused by HSV-1 in a respiratory therapist with a history of herpes labialis and preexisting antibody to HSV-1). It is clear from restriction endonuclease fingerprinting of viral DNA, that while most episodes of recurrent genital herpes are due to the reactivation of endogenous HSV-2 latent in sacral ganglia, some recurrences represent venereally acquired exogenous reinfection with a new HSV-2 strain (Buchman et al., 1979).

## Primary Infections

### Acute Herpetic Gingivostomatitis

Acute herpetic gingivostomatitis is the most common herpetic infection of childhood. It occurs primarily in children between 6 months and 5 years of age, but it may also be seen in older children and adults (Black, 1938; Dodd et al., 1938; Burnet and Williams, 1939; Scott et al., 1941; Buddingh et al., 1953). The source of infection is usually an adult with herpes labialis or an asymptomatic recurrence who is shedding HSV-1, but it may be another infected child, especially in a household or institutional epidemic (Juretić, 1966). The incubation period is usually 4 to 6 days, with a range of 2 days to 2 weeks. The illness begins with the abrupt onset of fever (usually to 102° to 104° F), anorexia, and listlessness; the infant soon becomes restless, irritable, and unwilling to eat or drink. The mouth usually becomes sore 12 to 96 hours after the onset of constitutional symptoms, but before oral lesions appear. Gingivitis is the most constant and striking lesion of the disease, occurring in every case. The gums are first hyperemic and then become markedly swollen (sometimes almost covering the teeth), reddened, friable, and exquisitely tender. They bleed easily and sometimes spontaneously, and there is a bright red line along the dental margin (Fig. 4). In most patients, vesicular lesions also develop on the oral mucous membranes. They first appear as tiny vesicles on an erythematous base, but these quickly rupture, leaving very tender, round, 1 to 3 mm, shallow, yellowish-gray, indurated ulcers or plaques. They often run together and are surrounded by a thin red halo. These lesions may occur anywhere on the mucous membranes of the mouth or pharynx, but they are most common on the tongue, the inner surface of the lips, and the buccal and sublingual mucosa. Lesions occur less frequently on the soft palate and on the gums themselves, occasionally in the pharynx, and rarely in the larynx. The submandibular and anterior cervical lymph nodes are almost always enlarged and tender. The breath is usually fetid

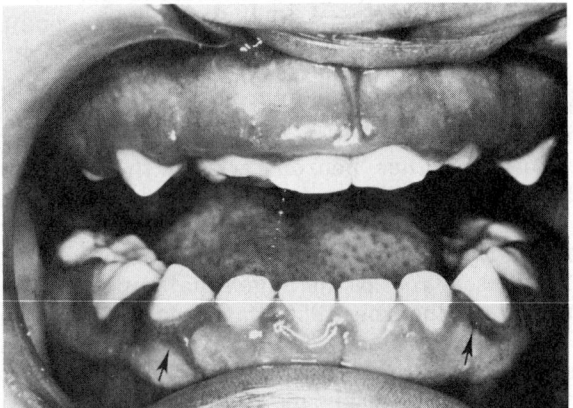

**FIGURE 4.** *Acute herpetic gingivostomatitis. Gingivitis in a child with acute herpetic gingivostomatitis. The gums are tender, swollen, and hyperemic, and there is a bright red line along the dental margin (arrows).*

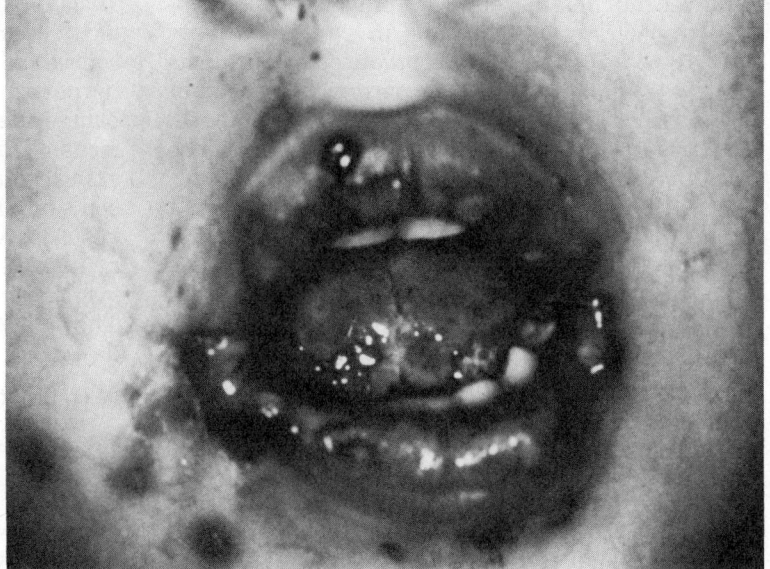

**FIGURE 5.** *Acute herpetic gingivostomatitis. In addition to vesicles on the oral mucosa, palate, and tongue, this child with acute herpetic gingivostomatitis has herpetic vesicles on the lips and perioral skin.*

due to the overgrowth of oral anaerobic bacteria. Salivation and drooling are marked. Herpetic lesions readily develop in areas of skin contaminated with infected saliva. Thus, many patients develop herpetic vesicles in the perioral skin (Fig. 5), and herpetic paronychia are seen in finger suckers. Cutaneous vesicles may also appear at more distant sites, and autoinoculation occasionally results in herpetic vulvovaginitis and HSV infection of the eye.

Acute herpetic gingivostomatitis is self-limited in normal children, and there are no sequelae, but the disease varies considerably in severity and duration. An occasional infant may be extremely ill with high fever; systemic toxicity; and severe and extensive mucosal lesions that prevent adequate drinking. Fortunately, most symptomatic cases are mild, and, of course, most primary HSV-1 infections are asymptomatic. Symptoms subside after an average of 12 to 14 days. The acute phase generally lasts for 5 to 7 days, after which the temperature returns to normal, the soreness in the mouth disappears, and the oral lesions begin to heal. The herpetic ulcers generally heal in 4 to 5 days, but the gingivitis often resolves more slowly, and the adenopathy may persist for several weeks.

HSV-1 can be readily isolated from saliva and stool during the active disease. Furthermore, althoughout neutralizing antibody appears in the first week of illness and reaches maximum levels by the third week, most of the children continue to excrete virus for many weeks after recovery, without any clinical evidence of infection (Scott et al., 1941; Buddingh et al., 1953). Eventually, shedding of HSV-1 in the saliva becomes inter-

mittent, but this intermittent shedding continues indefinitely, both in those who are and who are not subject to recurrent herpes labialis (Cesario et al., 1969; Douglas and Couch, 1970).

Although most primary HSV-1 infections are asymptomatic, the incidence of symptoms varies markedly from one study to another. Surveillance of many normal children indicates that primary HSV-1 infection causes manifest disease in anywhere from approximately 1 per cent to over 15 per cent (Scott, 1957; Juretić, 1966). The most thorough study has yielded the highest incidence (Juretić, 1966). In family and orphanage epidemics, the incidence of overt disease is higher, often approaching 100 per cent (Hale et al., 1963; Juretić, 1966). Among the possible reasons for these variations are differences in the dose of virus transmitted, the age of the infected children, the general health and nutritional status of the children studied, the intensity of surveillance, and the diagnostic criteria.

HSV-1 causes primary acute herpetic gingivostomatitis in adults as well as children. In adults, the disease begins with malaise; soreness in the mouth and throat; pain on swallowing; swollen, tender, bleeding gums; and anterior cervical and submandibular lymphadenopathy. Pharyngitis is much more prominent in adults than in children, occurring in nearly every case. About 1 to 3 days after onset, small, discrete, round vesicles appear on the oral and pharyngeal mucosa, the tongue, the inner surface of the lips, and the palate. These are identical in their appearance and evolution to those seen in children (Rogers et al., 1949; Farmer, 1956; Sheridan and Herrmann, 1971). The course of the disease in adults is like that in children but less severe. Drooling is not a problem, and perioral skin lesions are rare in patients over 16 years of age. Lesions produced by autoinoculation — namely, herpetic paronychia or whitlows, skin lesions at sites distant from the mouth, ocular infections, and vulvovaginitis — are also rare in adults.

## Acute Herpetic Pharyngotonsillitis

In adults, primary oropharyngeal HSV-1 infection causes pharyngitis and tonsillitis much more frequently than gingivostomatitis. The illness begins with fever, malaise, headache and sore throat. Tiny vesicles appear on the tonsils and posterior pharynx and quickly break down to form shallow ulcers that run together. A grayish-yellow exudate forms on the tonsils and posterior pharynx in over one-half of the patients. Lesions of the anterior mouth or lips are seen in only 10 per cent of adults with herpetic pharyngitis and tonsillitis, and the disease is usually indistinguishable from the pharyngitis and tonsillitis caused by the Group A streptococcus (Evans and Dick, 1964; Glezen et al., 1975). In a 6-year study, 10 per cent of susceptible college and graduate students got primary HSV infection each year. Although fewer than 3 per cent of these infections resulted in clinically recognized disease, primary HSV infections accounted for 12 per cent of the acute respiratory illness in students admitted to the student infirmary (Glezen et al., 1975). In this age group, HSV caused more cases of pharyngitis and tonsillitis than did the Group A streptococcus.

## Acute Herpetic Vulvovaginitis

In infants, acute herpetic vulvovaginitis may result from autoinoculation during primary oropharyngeal HSV-1 infection or from contact with an adult shedding HSV. It is a rare manifestation of primary HSV infection. There is fever and malaise, and the perineal area is red, edematous, and studded with tiny vesicles that rapidly evolve into shallow, yellowish-white ulcers 2 to 4 mm in diameter. These are extremely painful, and dysuria may lead to urinary retention. Lesions coalesce to form larger ulcers, and the inguinal lymph nodes are enlarged and tender. Fever and constitutional symptoms subside in a week, and healing is complete without scarring in 12 to 18 days.

## Primary Herpetic Infections of the Skin

In contrast to mucous membranes, the intact skin is resistant to HSV infection. Consequently, primary cutaneous HSV infections are relatively uncommon in healthy individuals. When they do occur, they are usually associated with heavy virus exposure and trauma to the skin. The majority of primary cutaneous infections occur in the course of acute herpetic gingivostomatitis or herpes genitalis. Sometimes it is viremia that brings the virus from the primary oral or genital focus of infection to the skin, but more often the skin lesions result from autoinoculation. The lesions begin as erythematous papules, develop into vesicles, and progress through pustules to crusts over several days. In primary infections, the vesicles tend to be discrete rather than grouped. They generally heal without scarring in 7 to 14 days.

## Traumatic Herpes

On occasion, primary cutaneous herpes appears in a normal person without oropharyngeal or genital infection. Such lesions result from the direct exogenous infection of skin rendered susceptible by trauma. This can occur when a parent who is shedding HSV-1 in saliva "kisses away" the pain of a child's abrasion. A diaper rash can be the site of primary cutaneous HSV-1 infection in infants (Juel-Jensen and MacCallum, 1972). Primary cutaneous herpes has also been reported among wrestlers ("herpes gladiatorum"). Presumably, traumatized skin is infected with virus shed in saliva (Selling and Kibrick, 1964). In addition to the local lesions, which are generally confined to the area of traumatized skin, there is usually regional lymphadenopathy and often symptoms of systemic illness. Cutaneous HSV infections are often severe and life-threatening when they occur in patients with disorders of the skin, such as eczema or burns, which permit more extensive local virus replication and spread, and facilitate visceral dissemination.

## Herpetic Whitlow (Herpetic Paronychia)

Primary HSV infections of the fingers are relatively uncommon except when susceptible individuals are heavily exposed to the virus. As noted above, this may occur in acute herpetic gingivostomatitis as a result of finger sucking. It also occurs in primary herpes genitalis, presumably as a result of a similar exposure to infected vaginal secretions. However, the most common form of herpetic whitlow is that which occurs among physicians, nurses, respiratory therapists, and dental personnel. Stern et al. (1959) reported a series of 54 cases of herpetic whitlow occurring in nurses, most of whom were caring for tracheostomy patients in a neurosurgical unit. HSV was present in the saliva of only 1.2 per cent of patients on hospital admission, but it could be isolated from the bronchial secretions of 6.5 per cent of tracheostomy patients. Only nurses without antibody to HSV were afflicted. The whitlow

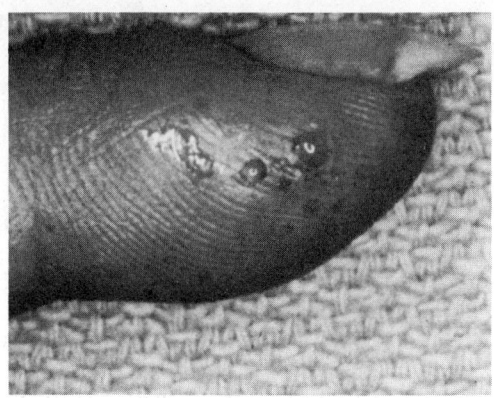

**FIGURE 6.** *Herpetic whitlow. The terminal segment of the index finger of a respiratory therapist is exquisitely painful, swollen, and erythematous, with multiple deep and superficial herpetic vesicles. Herpes simplex virus type 1 was isolated from vesicle fluid.*

begins with intense itching and pain in the infected finger. Within a day, a deep vesicle appears, usually in the terminal segment of one digit. Soon other vesicles appear (Fig. 6) and then coalesce. The process continues, destroying considerable tissue. Many cases seem to have pus under the cuticle, but incision discloses only a little clear fluid or, at a later stage, thick, yellow, necrotic debris. Intense local pain is always present. Systemic symptoms and epitrochlear or axillary lymphadenopathy are common, and neuralgia may occur. The lesions tend to progress for about 10 days, during which time pain continues unabated. There is then abrupt improvement, and the lesions begin to dry. Resolution is usually complete by 18 to 20 days. If the lesion is incised, secondary bacterial infection may occur, prolonging the period of disability. Subsequent recurrences at the same site are common, but they are less severe than the primary infection and are not accompanied by constitutional symptoms. Most of the herpetic whitlows that occur in medical and paramedical personnel are caused by HSV-1. A history of trauma is uncommon, but contact with oral or respiratory secretions is almost universal. The thumb or index finger is most often affected, and involvement of more than one finger is uncommon.

### Herpetic Infections of the Eye

Primary herpetic infection of the eye may occur alone or by autoinoculation during acute herpetic gingivostomatitis. It is usually manifest as a unilateral follicular conjunctivitis with preauricular adenopathy and is often accompanied by fever and constitutional symptoms. Blepharitis with vesicles on the lid margin is common, and vesicles may also occur on the periorbital skin. Superficial corneal involvement, if present, is

characterized by dendritic ulcers. Healing is spontaneous and is usually complete in 2 to 3 weeks. Ocular herpetic infections are discussed in detail in Chapter 232.

### Recurrent Infections

#### Herpes Labialis

Herpes labialis (cold sore, fever blister) is the most common manifestation of recurrent HSV-1 infection. It occurs in 30 to 50 per cent of adults (Embil et al., 1975; Grout and Barber, 1976; Young et al., 1976b). In most patients (60 to 80 per cent), the recurrence has a prodrome of pain, burning, tingling, or itching at the site of the subsequent eruption. This usually lasts for 6 hours or less (but occasionally for 24 to 48 hours) and is followed by a small cluster of raised erythematous papules that rapidly develop into tiny, thin-walled intraepidermal vesicles (Fig. 7). These quickly become pustular and then either burst or dry, with the formation of a scab. If the scab is removed shortly after its formation, it leaves a shallow ulcer. Left undisturbed, the scab is soon displaced by the regrowth of epidermis. The evolution of the lesion is generally rapid, with the papular stage lasting for only a few hours and vesicles crusting within 2 days (Spruance et al., 1977). Lesion area (usually < 100 mm$^2$) and pain are maximal during the vesicular stage and decline rapidly thereafter. Healing is completed, with loss of the scab and without scarring, within 6 to 10 days. Patients sometimes have local lymphadenopathy but not constitutional symptoms.

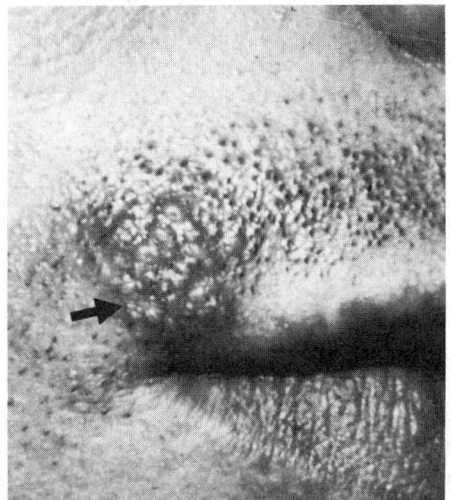

**FIGURE 7.** *Herpes labialis. Following a 12-hour prodrome of localized itching and burning, this medical student developed a small group of erythematous papules that quickly evolved into a typical cluster of tiny vesicles on an erythematous base (arrow).*

The most common site of herpes labialis is the vermillion border of the lip (95 per cent), usually the outer third, and more often the lower lip than the upper. Other sites are the nose, the chin, the cheek, and, rarely, the oral mucosa. HSV is not the cause of recurrent aphthous ulcers (Blank et al., 1950). Most people subject to herpes labialis suffer 1 to 2 episodes per year, but some have recurrences at intervals of a month or less. In a given person, the lesion generally recurs at the same site, and the provoking factor may also be stereotyped. In some, it is exposure to sunlight; in others, menses; and in others, emotional stress induced by school examinations.

The virus titer is highest ($>10^5$ infectious doses per ml of vesicle fluid) during the first 24 hours, when the lesions are vesicular, and it decreases steadily thereafter. HSV is rarely recovered after 5 days. HSV is usually present in the saliva during episodes of herpes labialis; it has been recovered from the saliva of 25 to 85 per cent of patients tested while lesions of herpes labialis were present (Douglas and Couch, 1970; Spruance et al., 1977; Pazin et al., 1978). HSV can also be recovered from 1 to 5 per cent of saliva samples obtained from adults when they are free of herpes labialis, but the concentration of virus is considerably lower. Repeated sampling reveals asymptomatic salivary shedding of HSV-1 at some time by most seropositive individuals. Intraoral lesions are rarely present, and virus is not recovered from parotid secretions. Thus, the source of HSV in the saliva is a mystery.

### Recurrent Ocular Herpes

Ocular herpes may recur in the form of keratitis, blepharitis, or keratoconjunctivitis, as discussed in detail in Chapter 232. Many patients suffer multiple recurrences of herpes keratitis, and this may cause considerable disability and even permanent visual loss. Asymptomatic virus shedding also occurs, and HSV can be isolated from the conjunctivae in the absence of clinical disease.

### Recurrent Cutaneous Herpes

Primary herpes results in a latent infection in the corresponding sensory ganglia. Thus, it is often followed by recurrent herpetic infections at or near the site of the initial lesion. Because the virus originates in sensory ganglia and is transported to the skin by sensory nerves, the lesions of recurrent cutaneous herpes may assume a segmental or dermatomal distribution that resembles herpes zoster (Slavin and Ferguson, 1950). However, the lesions of recurrent herpes simplex are usually confined to a smaller area of the skin within the dermatome than is herpes zoster; per-

haps because the primary cutaneous infection is more circumscribed in herpes simplex than in varicella, HSV establishes latency in fewer sensory neurons within the ganglion. The lesions of recurrent herpes simplex occur most often on the face, on the hands and arms, and on skin innervated by the sacral ganglia. They generally appear as grouped vesicles rather than the individual vesicles seen in primary infections (Fig. 8). They also tend to recur repeatedly, usually at the same site. In contrast, herpes zoster rarely recurs, and when it does, it almost never involves the same dermatome. Nevertheless, the appearance, evolution, and histopathology of the skin lesions are the same in herpes zoster and recurrent herpes simplex, and it is often totally impossible to distinguish between these two entities without laboratory identification of the etiologic agent. A prodrome of pain, burning, itching, or tingling often precedes the herpetic lesions by 1 to 3 days. The lesions begin as grouped erythematous papules that progress to vesicles, pustules, and crusts over several days. They heal without scarring in 6 to 10 days. Regional lymphadenopathy is sometimes present, but there are no constitutional symptoms. Recurrent cutaneous herpes is sometimes associated with severe local neuralgia, and recurrences on extremities may be accompanied by local edema and lymphangitis (Nicolau and Poincloux, 1924; Slavin and Ferguson, 1950; Behrman and Knight, 1954; Juel-Jensen and MacCallum, 1972; Layzer and Conant, 1974).

### Recurrent Herpetic Whitlow

Primary herpetic whitlows are frequently followed by multiple recurrences. While unaccompanied by constitutional symptoms and of somewhat shorter duration, the recurrent whitlow is often as painful as the primary lesion. It is frequently accompanied by swelling and edema of

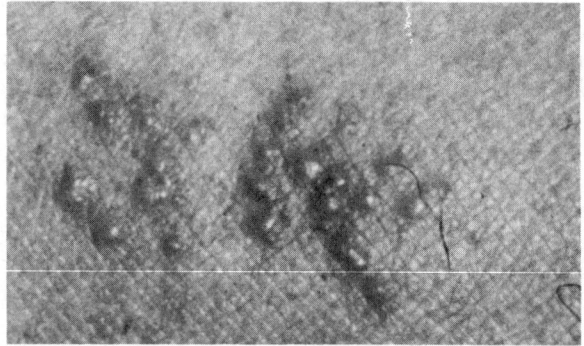

**FIGURE 8.** *Recurrent cutaneous herpes simplex. A young woman who had cutaneous lesions on her arm during an episode of primary herpetic gingivostomatitis (the results of autoinoculation) has subsequently suffered periodic recurrences. They appear as a typical patch of grouped vesicles on an erythematous base.*

the hand, by regional adenopathy, and by severe neuralgic pain in the arm (Nicolau and Poincloux, 1924; Juel-Jensen and MacCallum, 1972). It may also be accompanied by lymphangitis.

## COMPLICATIONS AND SEQUELAE

In the normal person (beyond the neonatal period), HSV infections are usually asymptomatic. Even symptomatic infections are almost always benign and self-limited. The only major exception is herpes simplex encephalitis, a rare complication of primary and recurrent HSV-1 infection that is responsible for the majority of cases of sporadic acute necrotizing encephalitis in the Western World. Herpes simplex encephalitis is discussed in Chapter 168.

The newborn infant seems unable to limit the replication and spread of HSV. Consequently, neonatal HSV infections have a mortality of over 60 per cent, with severe sequelae in many survivors. Most infections are acquired during passage through the birth canal of a mother with genital herpes and, accordingly, are caused by HSV-2. A minority may be acquired postpartum by nosocomial spread from other infants in the nursery or by contact with an adult shedding HSV-1 in saliva. Although the oropharynx is probably an important portal of entry, the infected neonate rarely has gingivostomatitis.

Acute herpetic gingivostomatitis is rarely complicated by bacterial infection. In severe cases, the painful lesions in the mouth may prevent drinking and cause dehydration and acidosis. Occasionally, oropharyngeal or genital herpes in adults is complicated by clinically significant viremia with extensive cutaneous dissemination. This results in a varicelliform eruption that may be difficult to distinguish from chickenpox (Naraqi et al., 1976; Long et al., 1978). While most of these patients have some underlying immunosuppressive disease or are receiving immunosuppressive drugs, such as prednisone, this complication also occurs in individuals who on careful examination appear to be normal. Other manifestations of virus dissemination are occasionally seen during primary oropharyngeal or genital herpes in apparently normal individuals. These include herpes simplex esophagitis, cystitis, hepatitis, and meningitis. Moreover, the complication may occur during an otherwise asymptomatic infection — that is, in the absence of signs or symptoms of disease at the portal of entry.

A variety of compromised hosts are at increased risk of developing severe, even fatal, HSV infections. These are malnourished children, pregnant women, patients who are immunosuppressed by disease or therapy (especially patients with deficient cellular immunity) and patients with disorders of the skin such as eczema or burns. Severe and fatal disseminated HSV infections are frequent in malnourished children (Becker et al., 1968). The disease begins with acute herpetic gingivostomatitis, which is followed by a sustained viremia with dissemination of infection to the liver, adrenal glands, lungs, and other viscera. There is also extensive infection of the esophagus and intestinal mucosa, due either to viremia or to large amounts of swallowed virus. Disseminated HSV infection with fatal hepatitis and encephalitis has also been observed in pregnant women with primary oropharyngeal or genital herpes, and in older adults, often in association with corticosteroid therapy (Juel-Jensen and MacCallum, 1972; Goyette et al., 1974; Young et al., 1976a; Keane et al., 1976). Both the frequency and the severity of HSV infections are markedly increased in patients with hematologic malignancies, and in renal and cardiac transplant recipients, particularly in the first 2 to 3 months after transplantation, when immunosuppression is greatest (Logan et al., 1971; Muller et al., 1972; Montgomerie et al., 1969; Korsager et al., 1975; Rand et al., 1976; Schneidman et al., 1979; Arvin et al., 1980). These infections occur mainly in patients with pre-existing antibody to HSV and thus generally reflect the reactivation of latent infection. Most seropositive transplant recipients shed HSV, and, while this is sometimes asymptomatic, it is often associated with severe and persistent disease. The clinical manifestations are chronic, deep, mucocutaneous ulceration; keratoconjunctivitis; and fatal herpetic hepatitis or meningoencephalitis. Also common are herpetic tracheobronchitis, pneumonia, and esophagitis, complications that may result from either local extension or viremic spread. Herpes esophagitis, in particular, is a common but generally unrecognized manifestation of HSV infection in immunologically compromised and debilitated patients, especially in the presence of a nasogastric tube (Nash and Ross, 1974). There are typical herpetic ulcers of the esophageal mucosa that may become confluent in the lower third. *Candida* esophagitis may coexist and further obscure the diagnosis. Herpetic esophagitis is generally thought to result from the direct extension of infection from the oropharynx. However, it may also be a recurrent infection resulting from reactivation of virus latent in the vagus ganglia (Warren et al., 1978).

In patients with atopic eczema, the skin is especially susceptible to HSV infection and appears deficient in its capacity to limit virus replication and spread. When they (or patients with certain other skin disorders, such as Darier's disease, Sézary syndrome, pemphigus, and burns) are exposed to HSV, they develop a severe and sometimes fatal infection (eczema herpeticum, Kaposi's varicelliform eruption), which was initially described by Kaposi as a complication of eczema in children (Brain, 1956; Wenner, 1944; Ruchman et al., 1947). Eczema herpeticum is usually a primary infection in which the eczematous skin is the portal of entry. The source of virus is most often an adult with herpes labialis. The disease begins acutely with high fever (104 to 105° F), irritability, and restlessness, and with the appearance of numerous small vesicles, primarily on the eczematous skin (Fig. 9). Individual lesions resemble those of varicella and quickly become umbilicated. They may appear in crops, with new lesions continuing to appear for a week or more. Individual lesions evolve from vesicle to pustule to crust over a few days. The largest numbers are found in the eczematous skin, where they may be confluent, but smaller numbers also appear on adjacent intact skin. The affected skin is edematous, and there is always regional or general lymphadenopathy. Fever and constitutional symptoms usually subside by the tenth day, and lesions heal in 2 to 3 weeks. Eczema herpeticum varies in severity from a mild disease to a rapidly fatal fulminant infection. When the cutaneous lesions are extensive, large areas of skin may be denuded of epithelium, with severe loss of fluid, electrolytes, and protein and marked susceptibility to bacterial superinfection. Mortality in children may be as high as 10 to 15 per cent, and is often associated with visceral dissemina-

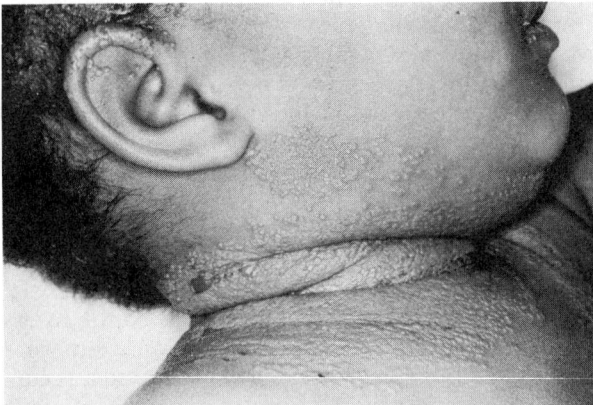

**FIGURE 9.** *Eczema herpeticum. An infant with atopic eczema developed fever, irritability, and numerous tiny vesicles that quickly became umbilicated. His mother had developed herpes labialis four days earlier. A Tzanck smear from the base of a vesicle showed multinucleated giant cells and eosinophilic intranuclear inclusion bodies. Herpes simplex virus type 1 was isolated from vesicle fluid.*

tion and infection of the liver, lungs, adrenal glands, gastrointestinal tract, and brain. Recurrences are common, and, while they are generally less severe and of shorter duration than primary infections, they may still result in severe, even fatal, disease. Enormous quantities of virus are present in the skin of patients with eczema herpeticum, and care must be taken lest they be the source of hospital epidemics and infections — for example, herpetic whitlows — in hospital personnel.

Burned patients resemble patients with eczema in their vulnerability to HSV infection (Foley et al., 1970). Areas of healing second-degree burns are easily infected and appear to provide ideal conditions for HSV replication. The resulting infection resembles eczema herpeticum, with multiple small vesicles and erosive lesions in areas of healing partial-thickness injury. The HSV infection may contribute to mortality by interfering with healing, increasing the extent of cutaneous damage, promoting bacterial superinfection, and disseminating to produce infection of the liver, lungs, adrenal glands, gastrointestinal tract, urinary bladder, and other viscera.

The intimate association of HSV with neurons has led many observers to implicate this virus in the pathogenesis of various neurologic syndromes of unknown etiology, including trigeminal neuralgia, atypical pain syndromes, idiopathic facial paralysis (Bell's palsy), temporal lobe epilepsy, recurrent psychosis, and multiple sclerosis (Juel-Jensen and MacCallum, 1972; Nahmias and Roizman, 1973; Finelli, 1975). However, the ubiquity of HSV, its lifelong latent residence in seropositive individuals, and its frequent reactivation by a variety of stimuli minimize the etiologic significance of any temporal association between the occurrence or recurrence of HSV infection and the onset of another disease. Of all of these associations, the best supported is that of HSV with atypical pain syndromes, including trigeminal neuralgia. Recurrent cutaneous HSV infections are sometimes associated with a prodrome of severe neuralgic pain that may continue for several days after the eruption has appeared (Slavin and Ferguson, 1950; Layzer and Conant, 1974). However, the pain almost never persists after the cutaneous lesions have healed, and, in spite of numerous recurrences in the same site, there is rarely any evidence of permanent neurologic impairment. This is in marked contrast to herpes zoster, which almost never recurs in the same site, but which may often be associated with prolonged postherpetic neuralgia, as well as sensory loss and signs of lower motor neuron damage. These sequelae may be explained by the pathologic changes observed in herpes zoster; there is acute inflammation and subsequent fibrosis of the sensory nerve and ganglion corresponding to the involved area of skin. This process, the direct result of virus infection, may extend centrally to involve the corresponding segment of the spinal cord. Similar changes have been observed in the sensory nerve and ganglion in cases of recurrent herpes simplex (Howard, 1905). Thus, it is not surprising that in some cases in which cutaneous herpes simplex is associated with severe neuralgia, repeated attacks over a period of years have resulted in the development of chronic pain and permanent sensory and motor deficits (Behrman and Knight, 1954; Juel-Jensen and MacCallum, 1972; Krohel et al., 1976). Furthermore, the well-documented occurrence of zoster sine herpete (that is, the reactivation of latent varicella-zoster virus in a dorsal root ganglion with associated neuralgic pain but without the development of skin lesions) provides a model for the association of HSV with unilateral pain syndromes that occur in the absence of a rash. The leading candidate here is trigeminal neuralgia, which almost always involves pain in the distribution of the second and third divisions of the trigeminal nerve, the same region involved in most cases of recurrent facial or labial herpes simplex. The association is supported by serologic studies (Juel-Jensen and Mac-Callum, 1972), by the association of some cases of trigeminal neuralgia with recurrent cutaneous herpes in the same area (Behrman and Knight, 1954), and by the almost invariable occurrence of facial herpes in the denervated skin following section of the trigeminal sensory root for the relief of trigeminal neuralgia (Carton and Kilbourne, 1952). These observations indicate that sensory neurons in the trigeminal ganglion, which mediate the pain of trigeminal neuralgia, may also harbor latent HSV, but they do not prove that the virus is responsible for the recur-

rent episodes of pain. Moreover, the absence of antibody to HSV in some patients with trigeminal neuralgia indicates that even if HSV does cause this syndrome, it is not the only cause. The association of HSV with idiopathic facial paralysis (Bell's palsy) is based primarily upon serologic studies and is tenuous at best (Adour et al., 1975; Finelli, 1975). The association of HSV with the other neurologic syndromes may only be coincidental, for it is based upon virus isolations, serologic studies, and observed temporal relationships between attacks of recurrent herpes and the neurologic syndrome in a very small number of cases.

Recurrent HSV infections may be associated with allergic cutaneous and mucocutaneous disorders, especially erythema multiforme (Nasemann, 1964; Shelley, 1967; Britz and Sibulkin, 1975). In 10 to 15 per cent of cases, erythema multiforme is preceded by a symptomatic attack of recurrent herpes simplex. Furthermore, the disease has been induced by the intradermal inoculation of inactivated HSV antigen in patients who suffer erythema multiforme in association with recurrent herpes simplex, whereas the same inoculation did not induce erythema multiforme in individuals with a history of uncomplicated recurrent herpes simplex (Nasemann, 1964; Shelley, 1967). The erythema multiforme usually begins 3 to 10 days after the appearance of the herpetic lesions and varies in severity from mild disease with typical target (iris) lesions on the extremities (erythema multiforme minor) to severe and extensive disease with lesions over the entire body, including the palms and soles (Fig. 10), and painful bullous-erosive lesions on the mucous membranes of the eyes, nose, oropharynx, genitalia, and anus (erythema multiforme major, Stevens-Johnson syndrome). Although the mucosal lesions may be

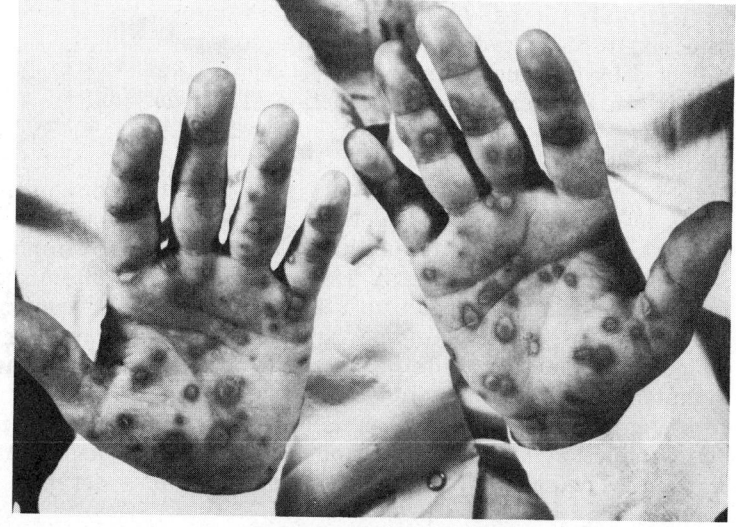

**FIGURE 10.** *Recurrent erythema multiforme associated with recurrent herpes simplex. A young man with recurrent herpes simplex involving a small patch of skin over the left scapula regularly develops erythema multiforme 3 to 5 days after the onset of each herpetic recurrence. The rash, which consists of characteristic target (iris) lesions, involves primarily the skin of the trunk and extremities, including the palms and soles. Herpes simplex virus type 1 is regularly isolated from the herpes lesion, but it is not present in the target lesions, and no inclusion bodies or multinucleated giant cells were detected when the lesions of erythema multiforme were biopsied.*

confused with lesions caused directly by HSV infection, their histopathology is quite distinct (Lever, 1975). They are vasculitic in origin, and vesicles, when present, are subepidermal. Their formation represents an allergic response, presumably to circulating HSV antigens or HSV antigen-antibody complexes, and is not the result of virus replication in the skin. Thus, they do not contain inclusion bodies or multinucleated giant cells and almost never yield HSV when cultured.

## GEOGRAPHIC VARIATION IN DISEASE AND EPIDEMIOLOGY

Herpes simplex viruses are ubiquitous and highly successful parasites of man. They are worldwide in distribution and, although many experimental animals can be infected, humans are the only natural reservoir, and no vectors are involved in transmission. The principal mode of transmission is by contact with infected secretions.

Geographic variations in the pattern of diseases caused by HSV (for example, the occurrence of fatal disseminated HSV-1 infections in African children) reflect differences in the conditions of host populations and in the age of acquisition of infection, and not variations in the parasite. There is no evidence of differing racial or sexual susceptibility to HSV.

There are two distinct serotypes of HSV, HSV-1 and HSV-2, which can be distinguished on the basis of antigenic, biologic, and biochemical differences (Nahmias and Dowdle, 1968; Nahmias and Roizman, 1973; Honess and Watson, 1977). However, the greatest difference between HSV-1 and HSV-2 is probably their epidemiology. HSV-1 is transmitted mainly by nonvenereal routes, as a result of contact with infected saliva. HSV-2 is transmitted venereally or from a mother's genital infection to her newborn. These differences are reflected by differences in the age of acquisition and in the anatomic sites of infection (Table 1). Since transmission of HSV-2 is directly related to sexual activity, most primary HSV-2 infections occur after puberty and involve the genitals and other body sites below the waist. The epidemiology of HSV-2 infection is discussed in Chapter 151.

Primary infection with HSV-1 occurs most frequently in children, causing acute herpetic gingivostomatitis in a few, and asymptomatic infections in the majority. Whether or not it produces symptoms, the primary infection results in a latent infection that persists indefinitely, and in the production of antibodies and cell-mediated immunity, which help to keep the endogenous HSV-1 in the latent state and render the host moderately resistant to exogenous reinfection. The presence of antibody is evidence of prior HSV-1 infection and identifies carriers of HSV-1. These antibody-positive individuals are subject to periodic reactivation of their latent HSV-1, and this results in symptomatic disease (herpes labialis) or asymptomatic shedding of HSV-1 in saliva (Fig. 3). It is the latently infected adults, 1 to 5 per cent of whom are shedding virus in their saliva at any given time, who are the major source of the virus that produces primary infections in susceptible children. This pattern of lifelong latent infection with periodic reactivation and virus shedding ensures the survival of HSV, even in populations too small and isolated to support the continuous circulation of such epidemic diseases, as measles and influenza (Black, 1975). Thus, HSV-1 is endemic in every human society throughout the world. However, the rate of infection is related to the degree of exposure, and this is greatly influenced by population density, housing conditions, and hygiene. Crowding and poor hygiene promote the transmission of HSV-1, and, accordingly, the frequency of HSV-1 infection is inversely related to socioeconomic status (Burnet and Williams, 1939; Juel-Jensen and MacCallum, 1972; Nahmias and Josey, 1976). Thus, while nearly 100 per cent of Bantu children in Cape Town acquire antibody to HSV-1 by the age of 4 years, only about one-third of English and American university students have antibody to the virus. Age-specific differences in the response to HSV-1 infection (for example, gingivostomatitis in young children vs. pharyngitis and tonsillitis in adults) and the increased severity of HSV-2 infections in persons without prior HSV-1 infection result in different patterns of symptomatic HSV infection in different societies or even in the same society at different stages in its development.

## DIAGNOSIS

HSV infections are identified by their characteristic clinical picture and a positive laboratory diagnosis. Although a presumptive diagnosis can often be made on clinical grounds alone (for example, herpes labialis), HSV infections are often confused with other diseases, and laboratory confirmation of the clinical diagnosis is usually necessary. This is especially true now that specific antiviral chemotherapy is becoming available. For example, diagnostic studies have revealed that many herpetic eruptions on the buttocks and legs that were thought to be herpes zoster are actually zosteriform herpes simplex. They have also demonstrated that some cases of typical eczema herpeticum are actually caused by varicella-zoster virus.

The differential diagnosis of HSV infection depends upon the anatomic site involved. Acute herpetic gingivostomatitis can usually be recognized clinically, but it may sometimes be confused with herpangina (caused by Coxsackie A viruses), Stevens-Johnson syndrome, aphthous ulcers, or oral candidiasis. The vesicular lesions of herpangina are clinically indistinguishable from those caused by HSV, but they are usually confined to the soft palate and posterior pharynx. Gingivitis, which is invariably present in acute herpetic gingivostomatitis, does not occur in herpangina. The oral lesions of Stevens-Johnson syndrome may look the same as those of acute herpetic gingivostomatitis, but the rash is characteristic (Fig. 10). The histopathology of the lesions of Stevens-Johnson syndrome (and of herpangina and aphthous ulcers) is totally different from that of the lesions induced by HSV. Varicella usually produces a few lesions in the mouth, but the typical rash on the trunk develops rapidly, making the diagnosis obvious.

Acute herpetic pharyngotonsillitis may be confused with acute exudative tonsillitis caused by Group A streptococci, diphtheria, or infectious mononucleosis. When vesicular lesions are absent, microbiologic cultures, blood smears, serologic tests, and virus isolation may be required to make the diagnosis.

Acute herpetic vulvovaginitis may sometimes be confused with ammoniacal dermatitis (diaper rash), impetigo, candidiasis, or gonococcal infection. The diseases may be differentiated by smears and cultures. Autoinoculation with vaccinia may be hard to distinguish from herpetic vulvovaginitis, but this can be done by histopathologic examination and confirmed by immunologic studies or virus isolation. The eradication of smallpox and cessation of routine vaccination should eliminate this complication.

Eczema herpeticum must be differentiated from eczema vaccinatum, varicella-zoster virus infection of the eczematous skin, and from secondary bacterial infection. A careful epidemiologic history is often helpful, but the diagnosis must be established by histopathologic and immunofluorescent examination of the involved tissue and by virus isolation. The herpetic lesions may be very atypical and are often superinfected with bacteria. This is especially true in burn patients, in whom the diagnosis often depends upon a high index of suspicion and laboratory examination of suspect tissues.

Traumatic herpes may be confused with herpes zoster, contact dermatitis, and bacterial super-

infection of the traumatized site. Immunofluorescent examination of the involved tissue or virus isolation is required to establish the diagnosis.

Herpetic whitlow is often mistaken for a bacterial infection, treated with antibiotics, and, when there is no improvement, incised. The presence of vesicles (Fig. 6) may suggest herpetic infection, but the diagnosis is made by aspiration, with immunofluorescent staining of the exfoliated cells and virus isolation.

Herpetic keratoconjunctivitis may be confused with infections of the eye caused by adenoviruses and enteroviruses, and also with bacterial and mycobacterial conjunctivitis. Histopathologic and immunofluorescent examination of conjunctival scrapings, and virus or bacterial isolation, are required for diagnosis.

Recurrent cutaneous herpes simplex may be confused with herpes zoster. However, herpes simplex characteristically recurs repeatedly at the same site, whereas herpes zoster almost never recurs in the same dermatome. The lesions caused by the two viruses are indistinguishable histologically, but they may be easily differentiated by immunofluorescent staining and virus isolation. The lesions may also be confused with contact dermatitis.

Disseminated cutaneous lesions occurring in the course of primary or recurrent HSV infections cannot be distinguished from the lesions of varicella or disseminated herpes zoster, except by virus isolation or immunofluorescent staining.

The histopathology of the skin and mucous membrane lesions caused by HSV provides a rapid and practical means of diagnosis. Multinucleated giant cells and epithelial cells containing eosinophilic intranuclear inclusion bodies distinguish the lesions of HSV from those produced by almost all other agents. Only measles and varicella-zoster virus produce multinucleated giant cells and eosinophilic intranuclear inclusion bodies. The rash of measles is normally not vesicular, the disease does not resemble HSV infection clinically or epidemiologically, and the skin lesions of measles are histopathologically distinct from those of HSV. The characteristic cytologic changes induced by HSV (and varicella-zoster virus) can be easily demonstrated in Tzanck smears prepared at the bedside (Fig. 11). Cells are scraped from the base of an early vesicle in the skin (mucous membranes, conjunctivae), spread gently on a glass microscope slide, and stained with hematoxylin-eosin, Giemsa's, Papanicolaou's, or Paragon Multiple stain (Blank et al., 1951; Barr et al., 1977; Rawls, 1979). Punch biopsies provide more reliable material for histologic examination and also facilitate diagnosis in the prevesicular stage. Tissue for histopatho-

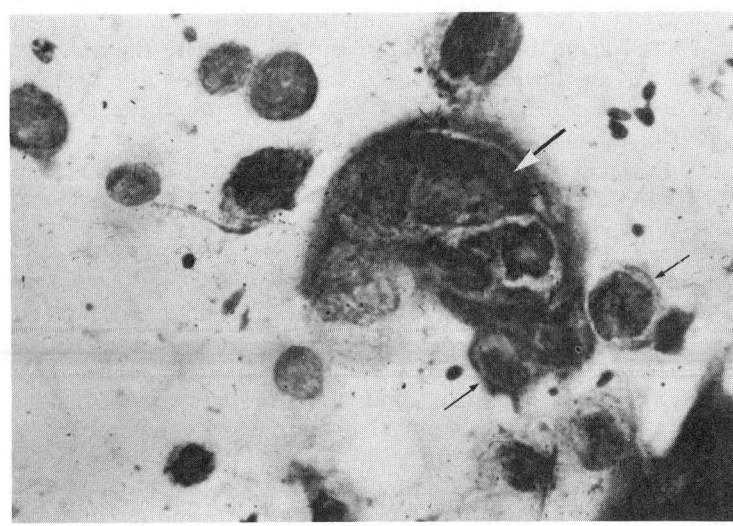

**FIGURE 11.** *Tzanck smear. Cells scraped from the base of a herpetic vesicle were smeared on a glass slide and Giemsa stained. The multinucleated giant cell contains a dense clump of nuclei (large arrow). Two adherent cells (small arrows) are probably in the process of fusing with the giant cell.*

logic examination should be fixed in Bouin's or another acid fixative to best demonstrate intranuclear inclusion bodies. Scrapings, vesicle fluid, and biopsy specimens can also be examined for virus particles by electronmicroscopy. However, neither electronmicroscopy nor histopathologic examination can distinguish HSV from varicella-zoster virus infection. This can only be done by virus isolation or by immunologic techniques that can detect specific virus antigens in tissue or vesicle fluid.

The application of immunofluorescent staining techniques to cellular material obtained by scraping or biopsy gives a rapid and specific diagnosis. Highly specific antiserum differentiates HSV from varicella-zoster virus and can even distinguish between HSV-1 and HSV-2 (Olding-Stenkvist and Grandien, 1976; Rawls, 1979). A number of other approaches to the rapid detection and identification of virus antigens are under study, including enzyme-linked immunosorbent assays (ELISA) and solid-phase radioimmunoassays. Nucleic acid hybridization techniques can detect viral genetic information in tissue. However, the most sensitive and definitive diagnostic method is virus isolation (Cho and Feng, 1978).

Experimental animals and embryonated eggs have now been replaced in most laboratories by tissue cultures of mammalian cells for isolation of HSV (Rawls, 1979). The most sensitive cells for HSV isolation are primary human embryonic kidney, primary human amnion, and primary rabbit-kidney cells, and diploid human lung and foreskin fibroblasts. Tissue for virus isolation should be finely minced and/or dispersed with collagenase or trypsin, washed with tissue culture medium, and inoculated into tissue cultures. The inoculation of viable cells rather than a clarified

suspension of homogenized tissue will increase the likelihood of isolating HSV from specimens containing small amounts of virus, especially if antibody is also present. Vesicle fluid should be aspirated from fresh vesicles and inoculated directly into tissue cultures. Since the titer of virus in vesicle fluid is usually maximal during the first 24 to 48 hours (Spruance et al., 1977), every effort should be made to culture patients as soon after the onset of their disease as possible. Other tissues and body fluids should also be cultured when suspect. These include blood, spinal fluid, urine, stool, saliva, throat washings or swabs, urethral swabs, seminal fluid, and vaginal and cervical secretions. Many require special preparation before inoculation (Rawls, 1979). All specimens for virus isolation should be carried to the virology laboratory on ice and processed immediately. They may be held at 0° C for several hours, but if tissue cultures cannot be inoculated within 12 to 18 hours, specimens should be stored at −70° C or lower. Typical cytopathic effects are usually apparent within 24 to 48 hours if the specimen contains much virus, but cultures should be observed for at least 2 weeks before being considered negative. Virus isolates can be identified as HSV and typed as HSV-1 or HSV-2 by a variety of serologic techniques (Nahmias and Dowdle, 1968; Plummer, 1973; Plummer et al., 1974; Rawls, 1979) or by nucleic acid hybridization (Brautigam et al., 1980). When the virus isolate has been identified as HSV, it can also be typed as HSV-1 or HSV-2 by restriction endonuclease cleavage and electrophoretic analysis of the viral DNA (Lonsdale, 1979; Linnemann et al., 1978; Buchman et al., 1979) or electrophoretic analysis of the virus proteins (Cassai et al., 1975). Both techniques can also distinguish between different strains of the same HSV serotype. HSV-1 and HSV-2 can also be differentiated by biologic and biochemical differences (Table 1; Kelman et al., 1975; Marks-Hellman and Ho, 1976; Nordlund et al., 1977), but these methods are less definitive than serotyping or analysis of viral DNA.

A number of serologic assays have been developed to detect and quantitate antibodies to HSV (Nahmias and Dowdle, 1968; Plummer, 1973; Nahmias and Josey, 1976; Rawls, 1979). They have been valuable for epidemiologic surveys and can give a retrospective diagnosis of primary HSV infection. However, their diagnostic value is limited by the need to obtain a convalescent serum in order to demonstrate seroconversion. A rising titer (as opposed to the acquisition of antibody by a seronegative individual) is not diagnostic of primary infection because recurrent herpes simplex infections may also occasionally be associated with a fourfold or greater increase in antibody titer. The diagnostic value of serologic assays is also limited by the antigenic cross-reactivity of HSV-1 and HSV-2. Antibodies produced in response to infection by either of the two serotypes react with both HSV-1 and HSV-2, although the response to the homologous virus is generally greater. A number of techniques have been developed to detect type-specific responses (Plummer, 1973; Plummer et al., 1974), but they often fail to give clear-cut results. The isolation of type-specific HSV antigens (Chen et al., 1978) should permit the development of truly type-specific serologic assays.

## TREATMENT

In a normal person, primary infections with HSV-1 are usually asymptomatic. Most symptomatic infections are self-limited and relatively brief, so that treatment is chiefly supportive. Attempts at specific therapy have focused upon severe infections, such as herpes simplex encephalitis (Chapter 168), and recurrent infections, which account for significant morbidity because of their frequency and ubiquity.

Acute herpetic gingivostomatitis, even when severe, is self-limited. Therapy should reduce pain and maintain nutrition. Cold, bland liquids and semisolids (for example, ice cream) are usually well tolerated. Frequent bland mouthwashes (for example, with a solution of sodium bicarbonate) may reduce pain and improve oral hygiene. Systemic analgesics also help. A topical anesthetic (for example, viscous xylocaine) relieves pain and promotes eating and drinking. Infants must be carefully observed for dehydration and acidosis, and if oral intake cannot be maintained, they should receive parenteral fluids and electrolytes in the hospital. Antibiotics have no effect, and corticosteroids are contraindicated.

Acute herpetic pharyngitis and tonsillitis are also treated symptomatically with systemic analgesics and warm saline or tap water gargles. The local pain of acute herpetic vulvovaginitis may be relieved by warm sitz baths and systemic analgesics. Pain and local edema may cause urinary retention, and this may require catheterization. Herpetic whitlows are treated with systemic analgesics. Elevation of the affected hand often helps to reduce pain. The lesion should not be incised.

In eczema herpeticum and HSV infections of burns, the major concerns are bacterial superinfection and fluid and electrolyte balance. Silver nitrate (0.5 per cent), aluminum acetate, sulfamylon, silver sulfadiazine, or povidone-iodine dressings may be employed, and frequent surveillance for bacterial infection by gram-stain and culture is essential. If bacterial superinfection ensues, systemic antibiotic therapy should be initiated with drugs selected on the basis of sensitivity studies of the infecting organisms. Because of their severity and propensity for dissemination, these HSV infections are candidates for specific antiviral therapy.

Human immune serum globulin contains significant levels of antibody to HSV-1 and HSV-2. Although of unproven efficacy, it seems reasonable to administer it in relatively large amounts (10 to 40 ml) to patients early in primary eczema herpeticum, to HSV-infected burn patients, and to other compromised hosts with primary HSV infections.

Severe cases of erythema multiforme or Stevens-Johnson syndrome, which usually begin as the lesions of recurrent herpes with which they are associated are resolving, may respond to a short, tapering course of parenteral corticosteroids. However, care must be taken that the skin and mucosal lesions do not represent HSV dissemination. Steroids in any form are contraindicated in active HSV infections.

Herpetic infections of the eye should be treated by an ophthalmologist. Corticosteroids (local or systemic) are contraindicated. They facilitate progression and local extension of infection and should be avoided in undiagnosed conditions that might prove to be herpetic. HSV infections in the eye are amenable to topical treatment with several different nucleoside derivatives that interfere with viral DNA replication. Human interferon is also effective. Active nucleoside derivatives include 5-iodo-2'-deoxyuridine (idoxuridine or IDU), 9-$\beta$-arabinofuranosyladenine (adenine arabinoside, vidarabine, or ara-A), and trifluorothymidine (Richman and Oxman, 1978). Corneal infections are uniquely susceptible to antiviral therapy, and responses in the eye are easily evaluated. Therefore, it was no accident that herpes keratitis was the first infection for which the efficacy of antiviral chemotherapy was established (Chapter 232).

Significant progress has been made in the development of specific antiviral therapy for severe HSV infections, especially for herpes simplex encephalitis (Chapter 168), and many important lessons have been learned (Richman and Oxman, 1978). These include the realization that anecdotal experience, case reports, and uncontrolled trials can lead to the false impression of efficacy and can encourage both physicians and patients to use remedies that are ineffective and harmful. Also clear is that the efficacy and toxicity of an antiviral agent can be evaluated only by means of a randomized, double-blind, placebo-controlled study involving proven cases of the disease. The most promising chemotherapeutic agents for severe HSV infections are nucleoside derivatives which interfere with HSV DNA synthesis, and interferon. Two of the former, iododeoxyuridine and 1-$\beta$-D-arabinofuranosylcytosine (cytosine arabinoside or ara-C), are too toxic and have too low a therapeutic index for systemic administration. A third, adenine arabinoside (vidarabine), has proved to be effective for therapy of herpes simplex encephalitis (Whitley et al., 1977) and for neonatal HSV infections (Whitley et al., 1980). It is also being evaluated for the treatment of severe mucocutaneous HSV infections in compromised patients. Also being evaluated is a more soluble (and thus more easily administered) monophosphate derivative of ara-A. More encouraging still is the advent of a new generation of antiviral drugs specifically designed to take advantage of the presence of HSV-specific enzymes. The first of these, 9-(2-hydroxyethoxymethyl) guanine (acycloguanosine or acyclovir), is phosphorylated by the HSV-specified deoxypyrimidine kinase but not by the comparable host-cell enzyme. Thus, it is taken up and converted to its active form by HSV-infected cells but not by uninfected host cells. In addition, the active intracellular form of the drug, acyclovir triphosphate, inhibits the HSV-specified DNA polymerase to a far greater extent than host-cell DNA polymerases (Elion et al., 1977). Consequently, acyclovir is a highly effective and nontoxic inhibitor of HSV in tissue culture and in animal models of HSV infection. It is being evaluated in patients with HSV encephalitis and other severe HSV infections, and in patients with primary and recurrent mucocutaneous herpes simplex.

Though generally regarded by the unafflicted as little more than a common nuisance, herpes labialis and other recurrent mucocutaneous HSV infections frequently cause physical and emotional distress. Furthermore, they may produce severe and progressive disease in immunologically compromised patients. Thus, many patients with recurrent herpes seek medical advice and generally receive some form of treatment. Over the years, these treatments have ranged from psychotherapy and vitamins to smallpox vaccinations, the local application of corticosteroids, X-irradiation, and photodynamic inactivation with neutral red and light. The rapidity with which each new therapy is generally embraced by physicians and their patients testifies to the lack of efficacy of the methods previously in vogue. Because many of these forms of therapy are hazardous, as well as ineffective (for example, X-irradiation, corticosteroids, smallpox vaccinations), it is important that any new treatment be carefully evaluated before being accepted for general use.

A number of therapeutic regimens involving the topical application of agents designed to limit virus replication have been advocated for the treatment of recurrent mucocutaneous herpes simplex. However, controlled studies have shown them all to be ineffective (Overall, 1979). They include iododeoxyuridine (Kibrick and Katz, 1970); ara-A (Adams et al., 1976); ara-A monophosphate (Spruance et al., 1979); photodynamic inactivation with neutral red and light (Myers et al., 1975); and ether (Corey et al., 1978). Several problems are encountered in attempting to treat recurrent herpes simplex topically with agents capable of inhibiting HSV multiplication. During recurrent infections, HSV multiplication usually reaches its peak shortly after the onset of visible lesions, and, thus, unless therapy is initiated very early, the drug may be applied too late to have much impact on the course of the disease. The cornified layer of the epidermis is impenetrable and prevents most drugs that are applied to the surface from reaching the deeper layers of the epidermis in which HSV replicates. Thus, it is noteworthy that when iododeoxyuridine was applied in dimethyl sulfoxide to increase skin penetration, it shortened the duration of recurrent herpetic lesions (MacCallum and Juel-Jensen, 1966; Juel-Jensen and MacCallum, 1972). Recurrent herpes simplex results from the reactivation of HSV that is latent in the corresponding sensory ganglion. It seems unlikely that local therapy applied to the skin will alter the latent HSV infection at this distant ganglionic site. Thus, topical therapy may succeed in decreasing the duration and severity of an individual recurrence, but it probably will not alter the frequency of subsequent recurrences (Myers et al., 1975). This is, however, not true for primary infections. By reducing the replication of HSV at the portal of entry, topical therapy may reduce the quantity of virus reaching the sensory ganglion and thereby reduce the number of latently infected neurons. This, in turn, may reduce the frequency of subsequent attacks of recurrent herpes simplex.

Patients have been treated with a variety of substances in an attempt to increase their immune responses to HSV and thereby reduce the frequency and severity of herpetic recurrences. These have included smallpox vaccinations (Kern and Schiff, 1959); levamisole (Mehr and Albano, 1977); Bacillus Calmette-Guerin [BCG] (Bierman, 1976); and a variety of live and inactivated HSV "vaccines" (Wise et al., 1977). When subjected to controlled trials, none of these treatments have altered the frequency or severity of herpetic recurrences.

Recently, Pazin et al. (1979) have demonstrated that parenteral human leukocyte interferon administered perioperatively reduces the frequency of reactivation of latent HSV infection that is induced by surgical manipulation of the trigeminal sensory root. In this placebo-controlled study, the incidence and severity of herpetic lesions and the frequency of asymptomatic salivary shedding of HSV were both reduced in recipients of interferon.

It appears that we are just entering a new era characterized by the rational development and evaluation of antiviral agents effective against HSV infections. Although the cold sore may be with us for some time to come, we can expect that such agents as interferon and acyclovir, used separately and in combination, will markedly reduce the mortality and morbidity of the more serious HSV infections.

## PROPHYLAXIS

There is no effective specific prophylaxis for HSV infection. HSV-induced disease can theoretically be prevented by avoiding exposure to virus or by modifying host resistance so that exposure produces either no infection or an attenuated infection unaccompanied by disease. Since much of the morbidity associated with HSV is the result of recurrent infections, prophylaxis, to be effective, would have to prevent the establishment of latent infections or at least greatly reduce the frequency and severity of their subsequent reactivation.

The ubiquity of HSV infection and the frequency of asymptomatic virus shedding make avoidance of exposure impractical except under very special circumstances. Medical and dental personnel can reduce the risk of acquiring herpetic whitlows by wearing gloves when using tracheal catheters or when working with their fingers in patients' mouths. Patients with eczema herpeticum (who shed enormous quantities of HSV) should be isolated. Individuals with symptomatic herpes labialis (who shed virus in saliva more frequently and in larger quantities than they do when they are asymptomatic) should avoid contact with particularly vulnerable individuals — for example, newborns or children with eczema. Men with active genital herpes should use condoms. The incidence of neonatal herpes may be reduced by delivering infants whose mothers have genital herpes at term by cesarean section, in order to avoid exposure to virus during passage through the infected birth canal.

We do not understand the mechanisms by which such provocative factors as fever, sunlight, emotional stress, and menstruation induce the reactivation of latent HSV. Thus it is not surprising that no means has yet been developed that is effective for the prevention of recurrent herpes simplex. Some individuals whose episodes of recurrent herpes simplex regularly follow specific provocative events (for example, herpes labialis following exposure to sunlight) are convinced that they can prevent the recurrent episodes by avoiding the provocative events (for example, by the local application of a sunscreen containing derivatives of para amino benzoic acid). However, the efficacy of this approach is still unproven.

Immunization represents the usual method by which individuals can be rendered immune to specific infectious agents without suffering the consequences of natural infection. This is generally accomplished by means of live attenuated vaccines or the administration of appropriate viral antigens (either in the form of inactivated virus particles or virus proteins that have been separated from the virus nucleic acid). Successful immunization induces in the host virus-specific neutralizing antibody and cell-mediated immunity. Although live and inactivated HSV vaccines (including nucleic acid–free vaccines) can protect experimental animals from lethal primary HSV infections and can reduce the incidence of ganglionic infection in animal models, there are many problems that remain before an HSV vaccine can be employed in people.

We do not presently understand the nature of immunity to HSV infection. Recurrent infections occur in the presence of high titers of neutralizing antibody. In fact, it appears that the level of antibody to HSV reflects the level of continuing antigenic stimulus. Thus, most HSV reactivation occurs in those renal transplant recipients with the highest pretransplantation titers of antibody to HSV (Pass et al., 1979). Moreover, while an increased frequency of HSV reactivation is associated with the period of maximal immunosuppression in organ transplant recipients and is correlated with a depressed lymphocyte response to HSV antigens (Rand et al., 1976), many normal individuals with recurrent herpes have cell-mediated immunity to HSV that appears normal when assayed by presently available techniques. Thus, there are serious questions as to the biologic relevance of presently available assays of cell-mediated immunity to HSV. In addition, concerns about the possible consequences of latent infection and the oncogenic potential of HSV make it unlikely that a live attenuated HSV vaccine, or even a killed vaccine that contains HSV DNA, will be acceptable for use in humans. Further developments will require a clearer understanding of latency and of host resistance to HSV infection.

## References

Adams, H. G., Benson, E. A., Alexander, E. R., Vontver, L. A., Remington, M. A., and Holmes, K. K. Genital herpetic infection in men and women: Clinical course and effect of topical application of adenine arabinoside. Infect Dis 133:Suppl.:A151, 1976.

Adour, K. K., Bell, D. N., Hilsinger, R. L.: Herpes simplex virus in idiopathic facial paralysis (Bell palsy). JAMA 233:527, 1975.

Arvin, A. M., Pollard, R. B., Rasmussen, L. E., and Merigan, T. C.: Cellular and humoral immunity in the pathogenesis of recurrent herpes viral infections in patients with lymphoma. J Clin Invest 65:869, 1980.

Baringer, J. R.: Recovery of herpes simplex virus from human sacral ganglions. N Engl J Med 291:828, 1974.

Baringer, J. R.: Herpes simplex virus infection of nervous tissue in animals and man. Prog Med Virol 20:1, 1975.

Baringer, J. R., and Swoveland, P.: Recovery of herpes-simplex virus from human trigeminal ganglions. N Engl J Med 288:648, 1973.

Barr, R. J., Herten, R. J., and Graham, J. H.: Rapid method for Tzanck preparations. JAMA 237:1119, 1977.

Bastian, F. O., Rabson, A. S., Yee, C. L., and Tralka, T. S.: Herpesvirus hominis: Isolation from human trigeminal ganglion. Science 178:306, 1972.

Becker, W. B., Kipps, A., and McKenzie, D.: Disseminated herpes simplex virus infection. Am J Dis Child 115:1, 1968.

Behrman, S., and Knight, G.: Herpes simplex associated with trigeminal neuralgia. Neurology 4:525, 1954.

Bierman, S. M.: BCG immunoprophylaxis of recurrent herpes progenitalis. Arch Dermatol 112:1410, 1976.

Black, W. C.: Acute infectious gingivostomatitis ("Vincent's stomatitis"). Am J Dis. Child 56:126, 1938.

Black, F. L.: Infectious diseases in primitive societies. Science 187:515, 1975.

Blank, H., Burgoon, C. F., Coriell, L. L., and Scott, T. F. M.: Recurrent aphthous ulcers. JAMA 142:125, 1950.

Brain, R. T.: The clinical vagaries of the herpes virus. Br Med J 1:1061, 1956.

Brautigam, A. R., Richman, D. D., and Oxman, M. N.: Rapid typing of herpes simplex virus isolates by DNA: DNA hybridization. J Clin Microbiol. 12:226, 1980.

Britz, M., and Sibulkin, D.: Recurrent erythema multiforme and herpes genitalis (Type 2). JAMA 233:812, 1975.

Buchman, T. G., Roizman, B., Adams, G., and Stover, B. H.: Restriction endonuclease fingerprinting of herpes simplex virus DNA: A novel epidemiological tool applied to a nosocomial outbreak. J Infect Dis 138:488, 1978.

Buchman, T. G., Roizman, B., and Nahmias, A. J.: Demonstration of exogenous genital reinfection with herpes simplex virus type 2 by restriction endonuclease fingerprinting of viral DNA. J Infect Dis 140:295, 1979.

Buddingh, G. J., Schrum, D. I., Lanier, J. C., and Guidry, D. J.: Studies of the natural history of herpes simplex infections. Pediatrics 11:595, 1953.

Burnet, F. M., and Williams, S. W.: Herpes simplex: a new point of view. Med J Aust 17:637, 1939.

Carton, C. A., and Kilbourne, E. D.: Activation of latent herpes simplex by trigeminal sensory-root section. N Engl J Med 246:172, 1952.

Cassai, E. N., Sarmiento, M., and Spear, P. G.: Comparison of the virion proteins specified by herpes simplex virus types 1 and 2. J Virol 16:1327, 1975.

Cesario, T. C., Poland, J. D., Wulff, H., Chin, T. D. Y., and Wenner, H. A.: Six years experience with herpes simplex virus in a children's home. Am J Epidemiol 90:416, 1969.

Chen, A. B., Ben-Porot, T., Whitley, R. J., and Kaplan, A. L.: Purification and characterization of proteins excreted by cells infected with herpes simplex virus and their use in diagnosis. Virology 91:234, 1978.

Cho, C. T., and Feng, K. K.: Sensitivity of the virus isolation and immunofluorescent staining methods in diagnosis of infections with herpes simplex virus. J Infect Dis 138:536, 1978.

Corey, L., Reeves, W. C., Chiang, W. T., Vontver, L. A., Remington, M., Winter, C., and Holmes, K. K.: Ineffectiveness of topical ether for the treatment of genital herpes simplex virus infection. Medical Intelligence 299:237, 1978.

Dodd, K., Johnston, L. M., and Buddingh, G. J.: Herpetic stomatitis. J Pediatr 12:95, 1938.

Douglas, R. G., and Couch, R. B.: A prospective study of chronic herpes simplex virus infection and recurrent herpes labialis in humans. J Immunol 104:289, 1970.

Elion, G. B., Furman, P A., Fyfe, J. A., de Miranda, P., Beauchamp, L., and Schaeffer, H. J.: Selectivity of action of an antiherpetic agent, 9-(2-hydroxyethoxymethyl) guanine. Proc Natl Acad Sci USA 74:5716, 1977.

Embil, J. A., Stephens, R. G., and Manuel, F. R.: Prevalence of recurrent herpes labialis and aphthous ulcers among young adults on six continents. CMA J 113:627, 1975.

Evans, A. S., and Dick, E. C.: Acute pharyngitis and tonsillitis in University of Wisconsin students. JAMA 190:699, 1964.

Farmer, E. D.: Diseases of the mouth caused by the herpes simplex virus. Proc R Soc Med 49:640, 1956.

Finelli, P. F.: Herpes simplex virus and the human nervous system: Current concepts and review. Milit Med 140:765, 1975.

Foley, F. D., Greenawald, K. A., Nash, G., and Pruitt, B. A.: Herpesvirus infection in burned patients. N Engl J Med 282:652, 1970.

Glezen, W. P., Fernald, G. W., and Lohr, J. A.: Acute respiratory disease of university students with special reference to the etiologic role of herpesvirus hominis. Am J Epidemiol 101:111, 1975.

Goodpasture, E. W.: Herpetic infection, with especial reference to involvement of the nervous system. Medicine 8:223, 1929.

Goyette, R. E., Donowho, E. M., Hieger, L. R., and Plunkett, G. D.: Fulminant herpesvirus hominis hepatitis during pregnancy. Obstet Gynecol 43:191, 1974.

Grout, P., and Barber, V. E.: Cold sores — an epidemiological survey. J R Coll Gen Pract 26:428, 1976.

Grüter, W.: Experimentelle und klinische untersuchungen über den sogenannten Herpes corneae. Ber Dtsch Ophthalmol Ges 42:162, 1920.

Hale, B. D., Rendtorff, R. C., Walker, L. C., and Roberts, A. N.: Epidemic herpetic stomatitis in an orphanage nursery. JAMA 183:1068, 1963.

Honess, R. W., and Watson, D. H.: Unity and diversity in the herpesviruses. J Gen Virol 37:15, 1977.

Howard, W. T.: Further observations on the relation of lesions of the gasserian and posterior root ganglia to herpes, occurring in pneumonia and cerebrospinal meningitis. Am J Med Sci 136:165, 1905.

Juel-Jensen, B. E., and MacCallum, F. O.: Herpes Simplex Varicella and Zoster. Philadelphia, Lippincott, 1972.

Juretić, M.: Natural history of herpetic infection. Helv Paediatr Acta 4:356, 1966.

Keane, J. T., Malkinson, F. D., Bryant, J., and Levin, S.: Herpesvirus hominis hepatitis and disseminated intravascular coagulation. Arch Intern Med 136:1312, 1976.

Kelman, A. D., Capozza, F., and Kibrick, S.: Differential action of deoxynucleosides on mammalian cell cultures infected with herpes simplex virus types 1 and 2. J Infect Dis 131:452, 1975.

Kern, A. B., and Schiff, B. L.: Smallpox vaccinations in the management of recurrent herpes simplex: A controlled evaluation. J Invest Derm 33:99, 1959.

Kibrick, S., and Katz, A. S.: Topical idoxuridine in recurrent herpes simplex. Ann NY Acad Sci 173:83, 1970.

Korsager, B., Spencer, E. S., Mordhorst, C.-H., and Andersen, H. K.: Herpesvirus hominis infections in renal transplant patients. Scand J Infect Dis 7:11, 1975.

Krohel, G. B., Richardson, J. R., and Farrell, D. F.: Herpes simplex neuropathy. Neurology 26:596, 1976.

Layzer, R. B., and Conant, M. A.: Neuralgia in recurrent herpes simplex. Arch Neurol 31:233, 1974.

Lehner, T., Wilton, J. M. A., and Schillitoe, E. J.: Immunological basis for latency, recurrences, and putative oncogenicity of herpes simplex virus. Lancet 2:60, 1975.

Lever, W. F.: Histopathology of the Skin, 5th ed., Philadelphia, Lippincott, 1975.

Linnemann, C. C., Buchman, T. G., Light, I. J., Ballard, J. L., and Roizman, B.: Transmission of herpes-simplex virus type 1 in a nursery for the newborn: Identification of viral isolates by D.N.A. "fingerprinting." Lancet 1:964, 1978.

Logan, W. S., Tindall, J. P., and Elson, M. I.: Chronic cutaneous herpes simplex. Arch Dermatol 103:606, 1971.

Long, J. C., Wheeler, C. E., and Briggaman, R. A.: Varicella-like infection due to herpes simplex. Arch Dermatol 114:406, 1978.

Lonsdale, D. M.: A rapid technique for distinguishing herpes-simplex virus type 1 from the type 2 by restriction-enzyme technology. Lancer 1:849, 1979.

MacCallum, F. O., and Juel-Jensen, B. E.: Herpes simplex virus skin infection in men treated with idoxuridine in dimethyl sulphoxide: Results of a double-blind controlled trial. Br Med J 2:805, 1966.

Marks-Hellman, S., and Ho, M: Use of biological characteristics to type herpesvirus hominis types 1 and 2 in diagnostic laboratories. J Clin Microbiol 3:277, 1976.

Mehr, K. A., and Albano, L.: Failure of levamisole in herpes simplex. Lancet 2:773, 1977.

Montgomerie, J. Z., Becroft, D. M. O., Croxson, M. C., Doak, P. B., and North, J. D. K.: Herpes-simplex-virus infection after renal transplantation. Lancet 2:867, 1969.

Muller, S. A., Herrmann, E. C., and Winkilmann, R. K.: Herpes simplex infections in hematologic malignancies. Am J Med 52:102, 1972.

Myers, M. G., Oxman, M. N., Clark, J. E., and Arndt, K. A.: Failure of neutral-red photodynamic inactivation in recurrent herpes simplex virus infections. N. Engl J Med 293:945, 1975.

Nahmias, A. J., and Dowdle, W. R.: Antigenic and biologic differences in herpesvirus hominis. Prog Med Virol 10:110, 1968.

Nahmias, A. J., and Josey, W. E.: Epidemiology of herpes simplex viruses 1 and 2. In Evans, A. S. (ed.): Viral Infections of Humans. New York, Plenum Medical Book Co., 1976.

Nahmias, A. J., and Roizman, B.: Infection with herpes simplex viruses 1 and 2. N Engl J Med 289:667, 719, 781, 1973.

Naraqi, W., Jackson, G. G., and Jonasson, O. M.: Viremia with herpes simplex type 1 in adults: Four nonfatal cases, one with features of chicken pox. Ann Intern Med 85:165, 1976.

Nasemann, T.: Ueber das postherpetische erythema exsudativum multiforme. Hautarzt 15:346, 1964.

Nash, G., and Ross, J. S.: Herpetic esophagitis: A common cause of esophageal ulceration. Hum Pathol 5:339, 1974.

Nicolau, S., and Poincloux, P.: Etude clinique et experimentale d'un cas d'herpès récividant du doigt. Ann Inst Pasteur 38:977, 1924.

Nordlund, J. J., Anderson, C., Hsiung, G. D., and Tenser, R. B.: The use of temperature sensitivity and selective cell culture systems for differentiation of herpes simplex virus types 1 and 2 in a clinical laboratory. Proc Soc Exp Biol Med 155:118, 1977.

Olding-Stenkvist, E., and Grandien, M.: Early diagnosis of virus-caused vesicular rashes by immunofluorescence on skin biopsies. Scand J Infect Dis 8:27, 1976.

Overall, J. C., Jr.: Dermatologic diseases. In Galasso, G. J., Merigan, T. C., and Buchanan R. A. (eds.): Antivirals in Man. New York, Raven Press, 1979.

Pass, R. F., Whitley, R. J., Whelchel, J. D., Diethelm, A. G., Reynolds, D. W., and Alford, C. A.: Identification of patients with increased risk of infection with herpes simplex virus after renal transplantation. J Infect Dis 140:487, 1979.

Pazin, G. J., Ho, M., and Jannetta, P. J.: Reactivation of herpes simplex virus after decompression of the trigeminal nerve root. J Infect Dis 138:405, 1978.

Pazin, G. J., Armstrong, J. A., Tai Lam, M., Tarr, G. C., Jannetta, P. J., and Ho, M.: Prevention of reactivated herpes simplex infection by human leukocyte interferon after operation on the trigeminal root. N Engl J Med 301:225, 1979.

Plummer, G.: A review of the identification and titration of antibodies

to herpes simplex viruses type 1 and type 2 in human sera. Cancer Res 33:1469, 1973.

Plummer, G., Goodheart, C. R., Miyagi, M., Skinner, G. R. B., Thouless, M. E., and Wildy, P.: Herpes simplex viruses: discrimination of types and correlation between different characteristics. Virology 60:206, 1974.

Rand, K. H., Rasmussen, L. E., Pollard, R. B., Arvin, A., and Merigan, T. C.: Cellular immunity and herpesvirus infections in cardiac-transplant patients. N Engl J Med 296:1372, 1976.

Rawls, W. E.: Herpes simplex virus types 1 and 2 and herpesvirus simiae. In Lennette, E. H., and Schmidt, N. J. (eds.): Diagnostic Procedures for Viral, Rickettsial and Chlamydial Infections, Washington, D.C., American Public Health Association, p. 309, 1979.

Rogers, A. M., Coriell, L. L., Blank, H., and Scott, T. F. M.: Acute herpetic gingivostomatitis in the adult. N Engl J Med 241:330, 1949.

Richman, D. D., and Oxman, M. N.: Antiviral Agents. In Weinstein, L., and Fields, B. N. (eds.): Seminars in Infectious Disease, Vol. 1. New York, Stratton Intercontinental Book Corp., 1978.

Ruchman, I., Welsh, A. L., and Dodd, K.: Kaposi's varicelliform eruption: Isolation of the virus of herpes simplex from the cutaneous lesions of three adults and one infant. Arch Derm & Syph 56:846. 1947.

Rustigian, R., Smulow, J. B., Tye, M., Gibson, W. A., and Shindell, E.: Studies on latent infection of skin and oral mucosa in individuals with recurrent herpes simplex. J Invest Dermatol 47:218, 1966.

Schneidman, D. W., Barr, R. J., and Graham, J. H.: Chronic cutaneous herpes simplex. JAMA 241:592, 1979.

Scott, T. F. M.: Epidemiology of herpetic infections. Am J Ophthalmol 43:134, 1957.

Scott, T. F., Steigman, A. J., and Convey, J. H.: Acute infectious gingivostomatitis. JAMA 117:999, 1941.

Selling, B., and Kibrick, S.: An outbreak of herpes simplex among wrestlers (herpes gladiatorum). N Engl J Med 270:979, 1064.

Shelly, W. B.: Herpes simplex virus as a cause of erythema multiforme. JAMA 201:153, 1967.

Sheridan, P. J., and Herrmann, E. C.: Intraoral lesions of adults associated with herpes simplex virus. Oral Surg Oral Path 32:390, 1971.

Slavin, H. B., and Ferguson, J. J.: Zoster-like eruptions caused by the virus of herpes simplex. Am. J. Med 8:456, 1950.

Spruance, S. L., Overall, J. C., Kern, E. R., Krueger, G. G., Pliam, V., and Miller, W.: The natural history of recurrent herpes simplex labialis: Implications for antiviral therapy. N Engl J Med 297:69, 1977.

Spruance, S. L., Crumpacker, C. S., Haines, H. H., Bader, C., Mehr, K., MacCalman, J., Schnipper, L. E., Klauber, M. R., Overall, J. C., and the Collaborative Study Group: Ineffectiveness of topical adenine arabinoside 5'-monophosphate in the treatment of recurrent herpes simplex labialis. N Engl J Med 300:1180, 1979.

Stern, H., Elek, S. D., Millar, D. M., and Anderson, H. F.: Herpetic whitlow: A form of cross-infection in hospitals. Lancet 2:871, 1959.

Stevens, J. G.: Latent herpes simplex virus and the nervous system. Curr Top Microbiol Immunol 70:31, 1975.

Warren, K. G., Brown, S. M., Wroblewska, Z., Gilden, D., Koprowski, H., and Subak-Sharpe, J.: Isolation of latent herpes simplex virus from the superior cervical and vagus ganglions of human beings. N Engl J Med 298:1068, 1978.

Wenner, H. A.: Complications of infantile eczema caused by the virus of herpes simplex: Description of the clinical characteristics of an unusual eruption and (b) identification of an associated filtrable virus. Am. J. Dis Child 67:247, 1944.

Whitley, R. J., Soong, S-J., Dolin, R., Galasso, G. J., Ch'ien, L. T., Alford, C. A., and the Collaborative Study Group: Adenine arabinoside therapy of biopsy-proved herpes simplex encephalitis. N Engl J Med 297:289, 1977.

Whitley, R. J., Nahmias, A., Soong, S. J., Galasso, G. J., Fleming, C. L., and Alford, C. A.: Vidarabine therapy of neonatal herpes simplex virus infections. Pediatrics 66:495, 1980.

Wise, T. G., Pavan, P. R., and Ennis, F. A.: Herpes simplex virus vaccines. J Infect Dis 136:706, 1977.

Young, E. J., Killam, A. P., and Greene, J. F.: Disseminated herpes-virus infection: Association with primary genital herpes in pregnancy. JAMA 235:2731, 1976a.

Young, S. K., Rowe, N. H., and Buchanan, R. A.: A clinical study for the control of facial mucocutaneous herpes virus infections. Oral Surg 41:498, 1976b.

# 100 HERPANGINA

*James Connor, M.D.*

## DEFINITION

Herpangina was first defined as a clinical entity by Zahorsky in 1920 when he described an acute febrile disease in children characterized by vesicular and ulcerative lesions on the anterior tonsillar pillars, tonsils, soft palate, and posterior buccal mucosa (Zahorsky, 1924). His description of the illness in 82 patients referred to "herpetic sore throat" but he later renamed the clinical complex "herpangina" in his 1924 report.

## ETIOLOGY

The viral etiology of herpangina was first established in 1951 by Huebner and his co-workers. In children with the clinical syndrome, H3 virus (Coxsackie A) was isolated from stool cultures, and serum neutralizing antibody rise to H3 virus was demonstrated. Since that time the clinical syndrome has been associated with a number of different viral serotypes, including Coxsackie A viruses 1 through 10, 16, and 22, Coxsackie B 1 through 5, and ECHO 9, 16, and 17 (Cherry and Jahn, 1965).

## CLINICAL MANIFESTATIONS

The original clinical description of herpangina by Zahorsky remains accurate today:

The disease begins suddenly as an acute febrile movement. The temperature often rises to 104° F. A convulsion may occur. Vomiting is often present. Anorexia and prostration are marked. The throat and posterior part of the mouth show minute vesicles, or if these have ruptured, small punched-out ulcers. They occur on the anterior pillar of the fauces, the tonsils, the pharynx, and the edges of the soft palate. The number of lesions varies from two to twenty. Dysphagia is often marked. The general and local symptoms disappear in a few days. The disease may be easily confused with ulcerative stomatitis which sometimes begins in the throat. The disease usually occurs in the summer months, in an epidemic manner, and children are most frequently affected.

After an incubation period of 4 to 10 days the enanthem begins as small papules and progresses to vesicles within 24 hours. They rupture, leaving ulcers surrounded by an inflammatory areola ranging in size from 1 to 5 mm with erythematous borders. These ulcers then become covered by a thin gray-white membrane. The appearance is quite different from erosions of ulcerative stomatitis. Although clinical symptoms diminish in 2 to 3 days, the ulcers persist 4 to 6 days, leaving a slight hypopigmented scar at the site.

Since multiple types of Coxsackie A, B, and ECHO viruses have been associated with the clinical entity herpangina, some patients have had additional signs common to enterovirus infection, including parotitis, aseptic meningitis, paralytic poliolike illness, exanthem, and pleurodynia.

## EPIDEMIOLOGY

As stated by Zahorsky, the disease tends to be epidemic in nature during the summer months. Its highest incidence is in the 3- to 10-year age group and occurs only in persons without preexisting, type-specific neutralizing antibody. The prevalent strains produce clinical illness in 30 to 50 per cent of infected persons. Epidemiologic data based on viral isolations from stool show an 85 per cent recovery rate from patients, 60 per cent from neighborhood contacts, 40 per cent from family contacts, and 3.5 per cent from others. The disease has only recently been reported in newborn infants.

## DIAGNOSIS

The laboratory may confirm a specific virologic diagnosis, but the clinical syndrome is usually obvious. The white blood counts tend to be normal with a relative lymphocytosis. Stool is the richest source of virus and is positive in 85 per cent of cases; anal (57 per cent) and throat swabs (58 per cent) also have good yield.

The differential diagnosis must rule out herpes gingivostomatitis. A diagnosis of herpes is favored if there are fetor oris; hyperemia, hypertrophy, and/or hemorrhage of gingivae; cervical adenopathy; or involvement of tongue, lip, and eye. These are common in herpes and rare to unheard of in herpangina. Another distinguishing feature is that most Coxsackie virus enanthemata occur in the posterior half of the oropharynx, and herpangina lesions are mainly anterior.

## TREATMENT

There is no specific treatment. Symptoms are mild and all patients recover.

## References

Cherry, J. D., and Jahn, C. L.: Herpangina: the etiologic spectrum. Pediatr 36:632, 1965.
Huebner, R. J., Cole, R. M., Beeman, E. M., et al.: Herpangina: etiologic studies of a specific infectious disease. JAMA 145:628, 1951.
Zahorsky, J.: Herpangina (a specific disease). Arch Pediatr 41:181, 1924.

# BACTERIAL PAROTITIS 101

## Donald L. Leake, A.B., M.A., D.M.D., M.D.

### DEFINITION

Bacterial parotitis is an acute or chronic inflammation of bacterial origin of one or both parotid salivary glands. Suppurative parotitis, pyogenic parotitis, and septic parotitis are synonyms. In postoperative surgical patients, it is sometimes described as surgical parotitis.

### ETIOLOGY

Bacterial parotitis is most often caused by *Staphylococcus aureus* (Petersdorf, 1958), although the infecting organisms may be quite varied, reflecting the oral flora (Burnett and Scherp, 1968; Speirs and Mason, 1972; Spratt, 1961). There may be a single organism, or an infection may be mixed. The bacteriology may be undefined.

In the newborn period, staphylococci are most commonly implicated (Leake and Leake, 1970). *Pseudomonas aeruginosa,* streptococci, especially *S. viridans,* pneumococci, and *Escherichia coli* occasionally are found. In a study of suppurative parotitis in older children, one third of the infections were caused by *S. aureus,* approximately one third resulted from streptococci, and the final third were distributed among *Haemophilus,* beta-hemolytic streptococci, and combinations of alpha-hemolytic streptococci, and *S. aureus* or pneumococci.

In another series of still older patients, studied in the 1950s, *Streptococcus viridans* accounted for 65 per cent of the cases and pneumococci for another 20 per cent. Streptococci, *Proteus, E. coli,* and diptheroids may be either normally or transiently found in the oral cavity.

### PATHOGENESIS AND PATHOLOGY

#### Acute Bacterial Parotitis

Acute bacterial parotitis usually occurs in debilitated patients, and dehydration is typically a common predisposing condition (Petersdorf et al., 1958). In the very young patient, only a moderate degree of dehydration is necessary to produce salivary stasis (Leake and Leake, 1970; Leake et al., 1971). Infection may then take place by bacteria ascending the duct. Infection of the gland also may be the result of septicemia. Occasionally caused by staphylococci, hematogenous parotitis is more often caused by gram-negative organisms such as *E. coli* or *Pseudomonas.*

The parotid is almost purely a serous gland and is very susceptible to infection secondary to stasis. By contrast, the submaxillary gland is a mixed gland that produces both mucous and serous secretions. It is thought that mucus is bacteriostatic and that the submaxillary salivary glands tend to become infected only when the duct is occluded as by a sialolith.

Decreased host resistance, dehydration, and poor oral hygiene predispose to acute bacterial parotitis. With dehydration from any cause, commonly diarrhea or vomiting, inadequate fluid replacement, or severe diaphoresis, there may be a concomitant reduction of salivary flow. Anticholinergics, antihistamines, some tranquilizers, and diuretics also may decrease salivary flow.

Bacterial parotitis occasionally occurs in patients who are otherwise healthy (Leake and Leake, 1970). Obstruction from a sialolith, stricture, or a mucous plug should be sought. While rare in the parotid gland, stones do occur and may occlude or partially obstruct Stensen's duct. This causes stasis of salivary flow and predisposes the gland to infection. Palpation with thumb and index finger usually suffices to establish the presence of a stone in the duct. It can be confirmed by x-ray in most cases. Mucous plugs sometimes can be expressed in the course of palpation. Strictures can be determined by gentle probing with a lacrimal duct probe or by sialography.

Obstruction of the salivary flow may result in irreversible tissue damage to the gland parenchyma. The inflammatory response causes a marked polymorphonuclear leukocyte infiltration in the stroma, the parenchyma, and the ducts. The progression to the chronic stage of the inflammatory process is marked by increasing numbers of lymphocytes and plasma cells. Fibrosis may replace portions of the gland or, if the inflammatory process is reversed, there may be regeneration of glandular and ductal elements.

### Recurrent Parotitis

The pathogenesis of recurrent parotitis in children is unknown. It has been proposed that the episodes are the sequelae of acute infections, congenital sialoangiectasis with some degree of stasis, or autoimmune disease. Boys are affected more often than girls.

In adults, recurrent parotitis occurs more commonly in women than in men and seems often to be associated with Sjögren's syndrome. This symptom complex includes keratoconjunctivitis sicca, xerostomia, and a collagen disease, particularly rheumatoid arthritis.

The histopathology of chronic parotitis is better known than is the pathogenesis. Hyperplasia of the duct epithelium, periductal lymphocytic infiltration, acinar atrophy, and fibrosis ultimately progress to loss of acini and replacement by fibroadipose tissue.

## CLINICAL MANIFESTATIONS

In acute parotitis there is a sudden onset of swelling with purulent drainage from Stensen's duct (Krippaehne et al., 1962; Leake and Leake, 1970; Leake et al., 1971; Petersdorf et al., 1958). It is usually unilateral, although as many as 25 per cent of the cases may be bilateral. The swelling is diffuse and involves the whole gland. The area is firm, smooth, and extremely tender to palpation. The entire side of the face may be swollen. Often there is trismus. Generally, there is a low-grade fever and moderate leukocytosis. Malaise and loss of appetite are common. With antibiotic therapy and adequate hydration, the swelling subsides over a period of a week.

The course of recurrent parotitis is variable

(Pearson, 1961; Rose, 1954). Painful attacks are often intensified by eating. Secretions are generally flocculent and turbid in appearance in contrast to the free-flowing saliva of the normal parotid. Attacks last from two to seven days and may occur as often as every few months. Usually the onset is unilateral, but it may become bilateral. Occasionally both sides are involved simultaneously. The gland may be somewhat more prominent than normal between attacks. In many patients, the recurring painful swellings ultimately resolve, undoubtedly because of the replacement of functioning acini by fibrosis. Chronic recurrent parotitis in children usually subsides by the middle teens, suggesting the possibility of a hormonal association.

### Complications and Sequelae

In the pre-antibiotic era, bacterial parotitis was a serious and often fatal postoperative complication, particularly in elderly patients. Bacterial parotitis also poses a threat, notably in patients with severe underlying diseases such as poorly controlled diabetes mellitus, carcinoma, leukemia, Hodgkin's disease, or renal failure, and in those who have just experienced cerebral vascular accidents. Septicemia, resulting in septic shock, may be the terminal event. In children as in adults, underlying diseases contribute to susceptibility. Myelogenous leukemia, dysautonomia (Riley-Day syndrome), acute glomerulonephritis, hypothyroidism with immunologic deficiency, cystic hygroma, and hemangiomas have been implicated. The occurrence of bacterial parotitis in a sick, hospitalized patient is a poor portent, but many mild cases are treated successfully without hospitalization.

Adequate antibiotic therapy based on culture and sensitivity findings and attention to fluid and electrolyte balance have decreased the mortality figures reported from 90 per cent in 1920 to approximately 20 per cent since the 1960s. Bacterial parotitis may be an incidental feature of a terminal disease.

As the inflammatory process invades the parenchyma, multiple abscesses form and sometimes coalesce. If the pus penetrates the capsule and invades the surrounding tissue, it may dissect into the deep fascial planes of the neck, flow posteriorly to the external auditory canal, or drain from the fistulae through the overlying skin.

Sialography (the instillation of radiopaque contrast material via Stensen's duct) in recurrent parotitis will show sialoangiectasis, a dilation of the ducts and a decrease in their number. Small, cystic dilatation of the terminal radicals reflects loss of acini. Sialography is contraindicated in acute phases of parotitis.

## DIAGNOSIS

The diagnosis of bacterial parotitis is usually made readily on the basis of visible suppuration at the parotid duct orifice (Krippaehne et al., 1962; Leake and Leake, 1970; Leake et al., 1971; Petersdorf et al., 1958). If pus is not spontaneously draining from the duct, it can be expressed by placing the thumb of the examining hand just inside the mouth anterior to the parotid orifice and the fingers of the same hand placed externally over the parotid gland anterior to the ear. A gentle milking of the gland by moving the fingers forward will produce a specimen. Inspissated saliva may form a plug in the duct and obstruct the flow of saliva in the patient with a dry mouth. After expelling an inspissated plug, the character of the pus can be determined. In acute parotitis the flow generally is copious. In chronic or recurrent parotitis, the appearance of the pus may be somewhat turbid or flocculent (Pearson, 1961). A specimen should be used to prepare a stained smear, and bacteriologic culture and antibiotic sensitivity should be determined. When no exudate can be expressed, it is possible to cannulate the duct with a fine catheter or a blunt-end abscess needle to irrigate the gland and thus obtain a specimen for culture.

In the history, the onset of swelling, the duration and frequency, particularly if recurrent, and precipitating factors such as food or juice should be noted. Acute swelling, secondary to an obstruction, may occur immediately after eating or drinking. A stone or calculus in the parotid salivary duct often can be palpated. When a sialolith is suspected, a periapical dental film can be placed intraorally under the suspected area and an x-ray taken with a dental x-ray machine.

There is a moderate to marked polymorphonucleocytosis and low grade fever (100° to 101°F). The gland is swollen and tender. The patient may be dehydrated or may be receiving medications that contribute to dryness.

The differential diagnosis of salivary gland swelling includes tumors that often involve only a part of the gland. Lymphadenopathy in the parotid and buccinator area may be due to an inflammatory process in the adjacent anatomy including the oral cavity, teeth, facial skin, eyes, or external auditory canal, or it may be caused by neoplastic disease (Banks, 1968). Cat scratch fever may produce lymphadenopathy in the parotid or buccinator node areas. Other causes of salivary gland swellings include mumps, amyloidosis, sarcoidosis (Heerfordt's syndrome), disseminated lupus erythematosus, lymphoma, leukemia, and such granulomatous diseases as tuberculosis, atypical mycobacteria, and actinomycosis. Asymptomatic or slightly tender swellings of the parotids may occur after ingesting iodine, for example, supersaturated potassium iodide (SSKI), with the thiouracils or following intravenous urography (Alexander et al., 1968; Nakadar and Harris-Jones, 1971). Guanethidine, an antihypertensive agent, may result in salivary gland enlargement also. Toxic parotitis has also been reported, secondary to copper, lead, or mercury poisoning.

Bilateral, nontender parotid swelling may be found in patients with chronic alcoholism and malnutrition as in Laennec's cirrhosis.

In older women Sjögren's syndrome, a symptom complex composed of keratoconjunctivitis sicca, xerostomia, and rheumatoid arthritis or other collagen disease, is commonly associated with bacterial parotitis (Bloch et al., 1965).

Parotid swelling and fever, sometimes associated with lacrimal adenitis and uveitis (Mikulicz's syndrome), occurs in patients with chronic disease such as tuberculosis, leukemia, Hodgkin's disease, or lupus erythematosus (Morgan and Castleman, 1953). The onset often is sudden, although the course is long and usually painless. Salivary gland enlargement has also been observed in Waldenström's macroglobulinemia.

Benign bilateral hypertrophy of the masseter muscles due to habitual clenching of teeth may be confused with painless parotid swelling.

The differential diagnosis of acute facial swellings, aside from intrinsic salivary gland disease, includes cellulitis, sometimes associated with unerupted third molars and mandibular cysts.

A rare cause of parotitis is that associated with Reiter's syndrome (a triad of arthritis, conjunctivitis, and urethritis). Rarer still is the parotitis secondary to lipoidproteinosis infiltrating the parotid duct and causing stenosis.

In areas of the world where hydatid disease is endemic, cysts in the parotid area due to *Echinococcus granulosa* may cause swelling that simulates parotitis. Other exotic causes of parotitis include yaws and aspergillosis.

Sialography may be helpful in distinguishing tumors from other chronic parotid swellings. With tumors, the parotid gland tends to be displaced laterally. Sjögren's syndrome almost always reveals sialoangiectasis by sialographic examination and may present parotid swelling without suppuration. Recurrent sialoadenitis also shows sialoangiectasis when studied by sialography.

A patient may very occasionally present with a history of recurrent swelling in the parotid or submaxillary area. Radiographs may show small radiopacities suggesting sialolithiasis. These small concretions in vessel walls are phleboliths. Sialography will reveal them to be outside the parotid gland (Dempsey and Murley, 1970).

Sialography may be therapeutic for recurrent parotitis. Sialoadenitis often is improved after sialography.

Because as many as 20 per cent of sialoliths are radiolucent, standard radiographic examinations may fail to reveal their presence. Sialography usually shows the point of obstruction when there is a sialolith.

Radionuclide scans may provide useful information in the differential diagnosis of swellings of the parotid area (Grove and DiChiro, 1968). Warthin's tumors are noteworthy in that the rate of radioisotope uptake by them is greater than by normal parotid tissue.

## TREATMENT

Bacteriologic culture and sensitivity studies dictate the proper antibiotic therapy. Antibiotics and adequate hydration are essential to the treatment of acute bacterial parotitis. Good oral hygiene and other supportive measures are appropriate. Analgesics often are necessary in acute phases of parotitis.

Staphylococcal parotitis is treated with 1.0 g oxacillin intravenously every six hours in the adult if the organism produces penicillinase; otherwise, 1.0 million units of benzylpenicillin is given every six hours intravenously. After the infection is brought under control, dicloxacillin is prescribed orally in place of intravenous drugs. It is given in a dose of 500 mg every six hours.

Patients with recurrent parotitis should be given antibiotics, although it has been reported that many patients do equally well without treatment, and recovery occurs over a period of a week.

In the presence of confirmed abscess formation, incision and drainage may be helpful, although the parotid duct provides a built-in mechanism for drainage. In acute parotitis, irradiation has

been used, but most organisms are sensitive to one or more antibiotics, and irradiation is no longer recommended. Chronic parotitis is less responsive to radiation, and it is mentioned only to be condemned.

For chronic recurrent painful parotitis, ligation of the parotid duct will produce autoparotidectomy without associated hazard to the facial nerve (Diamont, 1958).

## PROPHYLAXIS

Protection against bacterial parotitis depends on adequate hydration, hygiene, and appropriate supportive measures including avoidance of drugs that decrease salivary flow.

### References

Alexander, W. D., Harden, R. M., and Shimmins, J.: The concentration of iodide, pertechnetate and bromide in human saliva and gastric juice. J Physiol 194:89, 1968.

Banks, P.: Nonneoplastic parotid swellings: A review. Oral Surg Oral Med Oral Pathol 25:732, 1968.

Bloch, K. S., Buchanan, W. W., Wohl, M. J., and Bunim, J. J.: Sjögren's syndrome, a clinical, pathological, and serological study of sixty-two cases. Medicine 44:187, 1965.

Burnett, G. W., and Scherp, H. W.: The microbial flora of the oral cavity. In Oral Microbiology and Infectious Disease. Baltimore, The Williams & Wilkins Company, 1968, p. 273.

Dempsey, E. F., and Murley, R. S.: Vascular malformations simulating salivary disease. Br J Plast Surg 23:77, 1970.

Diamont, H.: Ligation of the parotid duct in chronic recurrent parotitis. Acta Otolaryngol 49:375, 1958.

Grove, A. S., and Di Chiro, G.: Salivary gland scanning with technetium-99M pertechnetate. Am J Roentgenol 102:109, 1968.

Krippaehne, W. W., Hunt, T. K., and Dunphy, J. E.: Acute suppurative parotitis. Ann Surg 156:251, 1962.

Leake, D. L., and Leake, R. C.: Neonatal suppurative parotitis. Pediatrics 46:203, 1970.

Leake, D. L., Krakowiak, F. J., and Leake, R. C.: Suppurative parotitis in children. Oral Surg Oral Med Oral Pathol 31:174, 1971.

Morgan, W. S., and Castleman, B.: A clinicopathologic study of "Mikulicz's disease."Am J Pathol 29:471, 1953.

Nakadar, A. S., and Harrison-Jones, J. N.: Sialadenitis after intravenous pyelography. Br Med J 3:351, 1971.

Petersdorf, R. G., Forsyth, B. R., and Bernanke, D.: Staphylococcal parotitis. N Engl J Med 259:1250, 1958.

Pearson, R. S. B.: Recurrent swellings of the parotid gland. Gut 2:210, 1961.

Rose, S. S.: A clinical and radiological survey of 192 cases of recurrent swellings of the salivary glands. R Coll Surg Engl Ann 15:374, 1954.

Speirs, C. F., and Mason, D. K.: Acute septic parotitis: Incidence, aetiology and management. Scot Med J 17:62, 1972.

Spratt, J. S., Jr.: The etiology and therapy of acute pyogenic parotitis. Surg Gynecol Obstet 112:391, 1961.

*Melvin I. Marks, M.D.*

## DEFINITION

Mumps is an acute, communicable viral infection most commonly manifest as parotitis. Mumps virus may also infect the central nervous system, other salivary glands (i.e., submandibular, sublingual), the pancreas, the testes, and the ovaries. Although often occurring together, parotitis or infection of one or more of the other organs may be present independently. As many as one-half of mumps infections may be asymptomatic.

## ETIOLOGY

Mumps was first described as a clinical entity in the 5th century BC by Hippocrates. The condition, characterized by nonsuppurative swelling of the parotid glands, was successfully reproduced in monkeys in 1934 by Johnson and Goodpasture. These experiments provided evidence that the syndrome was caused by a filterable (i.e., viruslike) agent that could be passed from human to animal and produced in monkeys by injection of infected saliva. In 1945, the virus was successfully grown in hens' eggs, and the viral property of hemagglutination described. Some of the host's responses were also defined, including the development of complement-fixing antibody and the acquisition of dermal hypersensitivity. Attenuation of the virus was achieved in the 1960's, and the contemporary live attenuated mumps virus vaccine was prepared in chick embryo tissue culture by Bunyak and Hilleman in 1966.

Mumps virus is a member of the paramyxovirus group, which also includes influenza, parainfluenza, and measles viruses (Chapter 59). These viruses share properties of hemagglutination, hemadsorption (often employed for identification of these agents), and infection via the respiratory route. Mumps virus is neurotropic in experimental animal infections. Influenza and parainfluenza viruses can cause infections resembling mumps.

## PATHOGENESIS AND PATHOLOGY

Man is apparently the only reservoir for mumps virus, and person-to-person contact is essential for spread. Prospective study of normal subjects with respiratory infections and appropriate controls has provided evidence that mumps virus is often associated with upper (e.g., common cold syndrome and pharyngitis) and lower (e.g., bronchopneumonia, croup, and bronchiolitis) respiratory symptoms. These clinical findings attest to the initial respiratory colonization in mumps infection. Virus attaches to and invades respiratory epithelial cells and elicits local host immune responses, including secretory IgA, edema, lymphocytic infiltration, and increased vascular permeability. The manifestations of mumps virus infection at this site and throughout the body are extremely variable and reflect many viral and host factors and their interactions. Although strain differences other than attenuation have not been described for mumps viruses, these may exist and thereby account for the neurotropism and other selective features of infection that occur. The immune subject has no symptoms or may have some respiratory discomfort associated with the successful containment of mumps virus infection to the surface epithelium. This is most likely achieved by neutralization of the virus or interference with viral attachment by secretory immunoglobulin (IgA). Nonspecific host defenses, such as mucus, ciliary movement, temperature, and interferon, may also play roles.

In susceptible hosts, virus multiplies in the upper respiratory tract, and occasionally in the conjunctiva, before entering the circulation. Viremia is followed by infection of many glands and the central nervous system. The determinants of clinical expression of infection are unknown. It is probable that most salivary glands, other secretory organs, and the nervous system are infected, although this may not be clinically apparent. Variability in the incubation period may relate to the inoculum of virus and the age and immune responsiveness of the host. The timing and clinical expression of disease may also be determined by host genetic factors.

Infection with mumps virus stimulates humoral and secretory antibody, as well as cell-mediated immune responses. The latter can be measured by cutaneous hypersensitivity, lymphocyte proliferation in response to mumps antigen, and the specific immune release of radioactivity from mumps-infected tissue culture cells (Chiba et al., 1976). Thus, the immunopathogenesis of mumps infection in humans involves direct virus infection, interaction of virus with local IgA antibodies, cell-mediated immune responses systemically and in infected tissues (acting alone or in combination with humoral antibody), and neutralization of virus by circulating antibody. Interferon has also been demonstrated in the cerebrospinal fluid and saliva in the first 3 days of infection. Postinfectious tissue injury, manifest as recurrent encephalomyelitis or orchitis, is occasionally observed and may be mediated by antigen-antibody complexes and/or complement.

Parotid swelling is caused by interstitial edema secondary to increased capillary permeability. There are varying degrees of degeneration of duct epithelium and polymorphonuclear cell infiltration in the early stages of parotitis. A periductal and perivascular mononuclear cell infiltrate follows. There is usually minimal necrosis and scarring (Fig. 1).

Changes in the brain may be those characteristic of postinfectious encephalomyelitis or, more commonly, of acute viral meningoencephalitis. These include neuronal destruction by intracellular virus and inflammation. Postinfectious perivascular demyelinization, lymphocytic infiltration, and gliosis may occur later. The pathogenesis in these cases is likely due to antigen-antibody and complement complexes or sensitization of the host to circulating breakdown products of neuronal degeneration. These findings are based on relatively few examinations. It is assumed, therefore, that most cases of mumps meningoencephalitis have a transient inflammatory response secondary to vasculitis, perivascular edema, and glial reaction followed by complete recovery. Only rare cases progress to more severe perivascular edema, hemorrhage, and anoxia secondary to the vasculopathy. Encephalomyelitic changes and/or hypoxic damage may contribute to the clinical observations of late-onset encephalitis and prolonged cerebrospinal fluid pleocytosis.

Certain pathologic features suggest that mumps meningoencephalitis may cause aqueductal stenosis and hydrocephalus in rare instances. Viral nucleocapsid-like material is present in ependymal cells in the cerebrospinal fluid of patients with mumps meningitis but not in enteroviral meningitis (Herndon et al., 1974). It is postulated that scarring occurs after ependymal cell necrosis and leads to narrowing and obstruction of the aqueduct of Sylvius. These changes have been reproduced in hamsters experimentally infected with mumps virus.

The pathologic features of orchitis consist of massive interstitial edema and perivascular lymphocytic exudate, which may progress to focal hemorrhage and destruction of germinal epithelial cells. The spermatic cord and tunica vaginalis are usually involved as well. Epithelial breakdown products, cellular inflammatory debris, and fibrin may obstruct the tubules. There are also focal tubular lesions and deposition of collagen in areas of hemorrhage and necrosis. These lead to

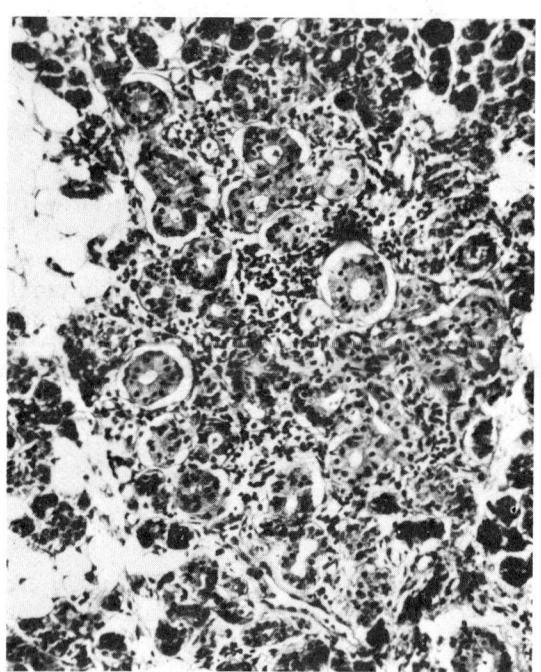

**FIGURE 1.** *Mumps parotitis. There is marked periductular infiltration of mononuclear cells. These inflammatory cells extend outward between acini. This is associated with atrophy, degeneration, and necrosis of acinar cells. H & E. 100 ×. (Courtesy of Robert P. Bolande, M.D.)*

scarring and atrophy in the final stages. It must be emphasized that these changes are focal in nature, involve both testes in only 10 to 20 per cent of cases, and are extremely variable in degree. Complete destruction of germinal tissue and/or loss of tubular function is very rare. Epididymitis accompanies orchitis in approximately 85 per cent of cases and is characterized by dense lymphocytic inflammation of the connective tissue, usually with sparing of the epithelial components. Occasionally, a hydrocele may develop (Fig. 2).

Less common pathologic features of mumps infection include acute interstitial (occasionally necrotizing) pancreatitis (Fig. 3) and thyroiditis. Endolymphatic labyrinthitis is an extremely rare but serious form of mumps infection. Clinical features of tinnitus, vertigo, vomiting, and deafness are caused by inflammation of the stria vascularis with subsequent permanent degeneration of the involved cochlear receptors.

The consequences of intrauterine mumps infections have been the subject of much investigation and speculation. It has been suggested that endocardial fibroelastosis, a myocardiopathy of young infants, and aqueductal stenosis with subsequent hydrocephalus are conditions closely related to intrauterine mumps infection. There are several immunologic, epidemiologic, and animal studies

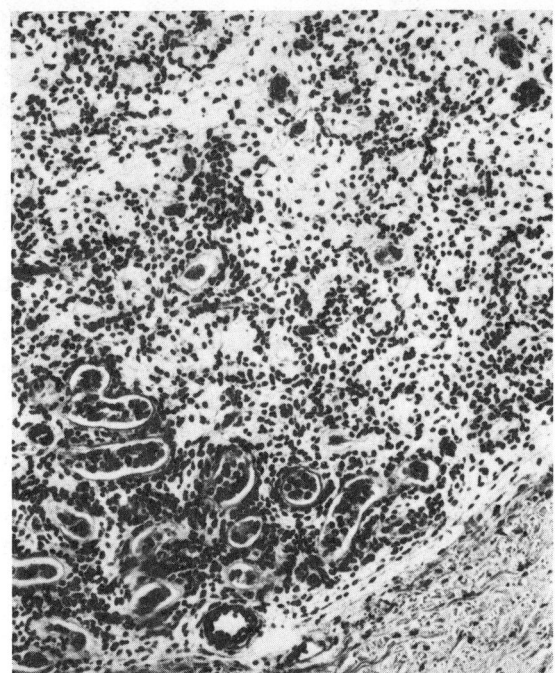

**FIGURE 2.** *Mumps orchitis. There is marked interstitial edema and mononuclear cell infiltrate of the testis obliterating many seminiferous tubules. A few can be still identified at the bottom adjacent to the tunica albuginea. H & E. 100 ×. (Courtesy of Robert P. Bolande, M.D.)*

that support these contentions. Mumps virus is particularly destructive to myocardial tissue in chick embryos and is also neurotropic in suckling hamsters. Patients with endocardial fibroelastosis usually have cutaneous hypersensitivity to mumps antigen but do not have circulating mumps antibody. Experimental infections in chick embryo and clinical observations in the offspring of patients with documented intragestational mumps suggest that this "split immune response" is also characteristic of intrauterine mumps infection (Aase et al., 1972). The absence of humoral antibody in the presence of lymphocyte sensitization and cutaneous mumps hypersensitivity persists well into childhood.

## CLINICAL MANIFESTATIONS

The most common form of mumps infection is parotitis (Fig. 4). Swelling of the parotid gland is usually unilateral in the first 2 days of infection but then becomes bilateral in approximately 70 per cent of cases. The incubation period is frequently 17 to 21 days; however, cases have been reported as early as 12 days after exposure and as late as 35 days. In more severe cases, a mild prodrome of fever, malaise, headache, chills, sore

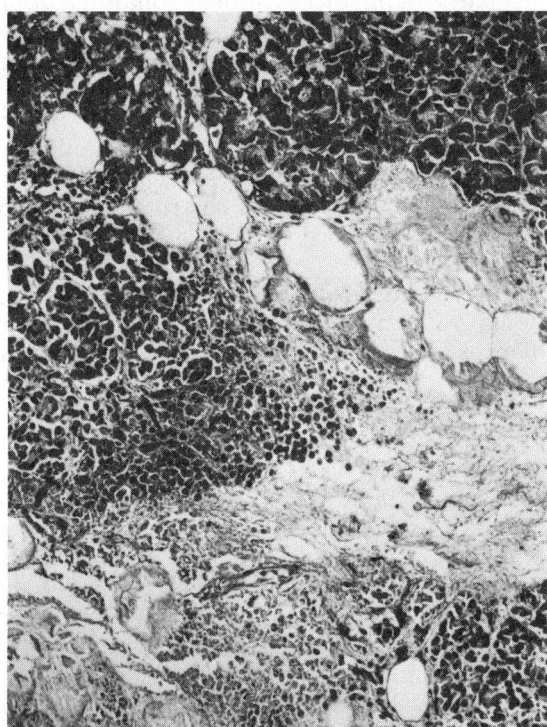

**FIGURE 3.** *Mumps pancreatitis. This shows a section of an acute fatal necrotizing mumps pancreatitis. The periphery of this pancreatic lobule shows extensive necrosis and inflammatory exudate. The interlobular and peripancreatic adipose tissue show the saponification type of fat necrosis, typical of pancreatitis. H & E. 100 ×. (Courtesy of Robert P. Bolande, M.D.)*

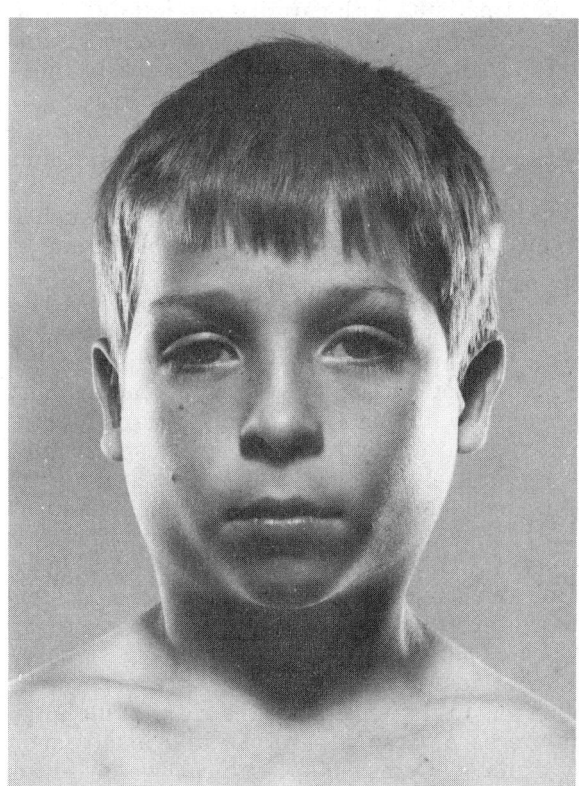

**FIGURE 4.** *Mumps parotitis. Bilateral parotid enlargement in an 8-year-old boy, more marked on right side. (Courtesy of G. Ahronheim, M.D.)*

throat, earache, and parotid tenderness may precede parotid swelling by 2 to 3 days. Exanthems and enanthems have also been described. There is considerable variability in the relationship of parotitis to the other manifestations of mumps infection. For example, orchitis and/or meningitis may precede the appearance of parotitis or may occur as the sole manifestations of mumps infection. As many as one-half of children under the age of 5 years are asymptomatic; others may have a respiratory syndrome. These children are important in the spread of mumps to susceptible contacts.

The parotid gland is variably enlarged, tense, and tender, and there may be pain on movement of the jaw. Local heat and erythema are absent. Swelling, which often obliterates the hollow between the mastoid process and the ascending ramus of the lower jaw, is usually maximal over a 2- to 3-day period and disappears by 7 to 10 days. Swelling of the sublingual and submaxillary salivary glands is frequently present as well. Stensen's duct may be partly occluded by inflammation. Parotid and salivary gland pain can be experienced upon exposure to acid drinks and stimulation of the secretory mechanism of the parotid gland. The papillae at the opening of Stensen's or Wharton's duct may be reddened, but this is an inconsistent finding.

Most patients with parotitis are mildly febrile, but this rarely lasts longer than 5 days. Symptoms are mild in children and often absent in the youngest patients. The disease is usually not seen in infants under 6 to 9 months of age owing to the presence of passively acquired (maternal) immunity. Adults are more likely to develop constitutional symptoms and extraparotid lesions such as orchitis. They commonly have a prodrome of fever, headache, and chills as well.

Although sometimes considered complications of mumps, central nervous system (CNS) involvement, orchitis, and ocular manifestations can occur without parotitis and represent primary infection by mumps virus. As many as one-half of patients with mumps have cerebrospinal fluid pleocytosis, and one-quarter have signs of meningeal involvement. Mumps is the most common cause of endemic aseptic meningitis in North American children. Wilfert (1969) reviewed the clinical features of 45 children with mumps meningoencephalitis and found that 13 had no evidence of parotitis. In most cases, CNS signs became evident 1 to 6 days after the onset of parotitis; however, in three patients, the signs of meningitis preceded those of parotid gland involvement by 3 days. Occasionally, several weeks ensue between the onset of parotitis and the appearance of meningoencephalitis. The majority of patients with CNS involvement have meningoencephali-

tis; nevertheless, the clinical syndrome may be predominantly that of aseptic meningitis or, alternatively, encephalitis. Although the criteria for encephalitis are arbitrary, pure mumps encephalitis has been estimated to occur in approximately 8 per cent of patients with CNS involvement. Meningoencephalitis is more frequent in males (3:1); however, mumps infection shows no sex predilection.

Other manifestations of mumps infection include conjunctivitis, dacryoadenitis, pancreatitis, oophoritis, thyroiditis, and arthritis. These are discussed in more detail under complications. Approximately 6 per cent of patients develop presternal pitting edema, probably due to obstruction of anterior chest wall lymphatics by swollen lymph nodes and salivary glands. This complication requires no treatment and is most commonly seen between days 5 and 8 after the onset of parotitis.

## COMPLICATIONS

An outline of some of the reported complications of mumps infection is presented in Table 1. Many of these have been associated with mumps and have not been proven to be due to the virus. It is not surprising to see protean manifestations of an infection characterized by widespread organ involvement and complex host-parasite interactions.

Recurrent idiopathic parotitis may follow mumps parotitis. Inflammation of Stensen's duct may lead to sialectasis and a predisposition to abnormal flow of saliva and obstruction. Secondary infections and/or stricture of the duct may ensue.

Seizures occur in as many as 18 per cent of patients with mumps encephalitis. Coma, disturbances of sensorium, ataxia, and transient or, rarely, permanent paralysis of ocular or facial muscles have also been described. Labyrinthitis and nerve deafness, complications of CNS mumps infection, may be preceded by tinnitus, vertigo, nausea, and vomiting. A rare complication of mumps is a paralytic poliomyelitis-like syndrome of transient asymmetric flaccid paralysis of the lower extremities, frequently accompanied by myalgia and intact sensation. Urinary sphincter dysfunction and extensor plantar responses may also be present.

Atrophy occurs in as many as one-half of patients with mumps orchitis, but this is focal in nature, and sterility after mumps is extremely rare. In a study of 132 men with orchitis, 47 developed some degree of atrophy, but this was bilateral in only 2 (Beard et al., 1977). One of these men subsequently fathered a child, and the

## TABLE 1.   Complications of Mumps

**Neurologic:**
  Meningoencephalitis
  Guillain-Barré syndrome
  Myelitis
  Neuropathies
  Deafness
  Labyrinthitis
  Hydrocephalus
  Diabetes insipidus

**Ocular:**
  Conjunctivitis
  Scleritis
  Keratitis
  Optic neuritis
  Iritis
  Iridocyclitis
  Dacryoadenitis

**Genitourinary:**
  Orchitis (testicular or atrophy)
  Epididymitis
  Oophoritis
  Nephritis
  Priapism
  Bartholinitis
  Prostatitis

**Hematologic:**
  Thrombocytopenia
  Hemolysis
  Leukemoid reaction
  Paroxysmal cold hemoglobinuria
  Splenomegaly

**Other:**
  Pancreatitis
  Thyroiditis
  Mastitis
  Hepatitis
  Polyarthritis
  Myocarditis
  Pericarditis
  Laryngitis
  Psychosis
  Teratogenicity (microcephaly, hydrocephalus,
    endocardial fibroelastosis, abortion)

with vomiting and severe epigastric pain. Abdominal muscular spasm may be present and the clinical syndrome may suggest appendicitis. This is also true of patients with mumps of the right ovary. Epidemiologic and serologic correlations between mumps pancreatitis and juvenile diabetes mellitus have been reported. Genetic predisposition and other factors are also important.

The virus has been isolated from the thyroid during acute mumps thyroiditis. It has been estimated that as many as one-half of the patients with subacute thyroiditis have a history of recent mumps infection.

Arthritis has been reported in approximately 0.4 per cent of patients with mumps. Knees, ankles, shoulders, and wrists are most frequently involved, but any joint in the body may be affected. Most patients with the polyarthritis syndrome are adults, and the condition usually has its onset 10 days to 2 weeks after the onset of parotitis. Arthritis usually lasts only a few days, although several cases have persisted for as long as 3 months. The migratory nature of the disease may confuse the differential diagnosis.

Thrombocytopenic purpura may occur in children after natural disease and with mumps vaccination. Other hematologic changes are outlined in Table 1.

In addition to endocardial fibroelastosis and aqueductal stenosis, mumps virus infection in the first trimester of pregnancy has also been associated with imperforate anus; spina bifida; microcephaly; and auditory, optic, and urogenital deformities, although a cause-and-effect relationship has not been demonstrated. In addition, lenticular cataracts have been produced in chick embryos infected early in embryonic development.

Approximately 15 to 50 deaths per year occur in the United States in patients with mumps infection. The case fatality ratio is approximately 0.1 to 0.4 per 100,000 cases of mumps. There is no sex predilection among those fatally infected, and 38 per cent of the deaths occur in patients over the age of 40 years.

## GEOGRAPHIC VARIATIONS IN DISEASE

Mumps infections occur throughout the world and in all seasons, although there is some increase in incidence during the winter and spring months. The majority (85 to 90 per cent) of infections occur in children under 14 years of age. Epidemics of mumps affecting all ages occur in populations with little exposure to the virus. Such "virgin" populations have been described in the St. Lawrence and St. George Islands in Alaska (Reed et al., 1967). High attack rates for clinical

other was lost to follow-up. Two patients in this cohort subsequently developed testicular neoplasms. The association of testicular or mammary neoplasia with mumps has been noted in the past, although the etiologic significance is unknown. There has been no evidence of congenital malformations in any children fathered by men with a history of mumps orchitis.

Oophoritis is difficult to diagnose, although ovarian enlargement may be palpable in some patients. It occurs in approximately 7 per cent of patients with mumps and is manifest by lower quadrant or back pain. Sterility after oophoritis has not been reported.

Pancreatitis occurs in less than 10 per cent of patients with mumps and is usually associated

(65 per cent) and subclinical (20 per cent) disease were noted in these islands. The clinical manifestations of mumps were similar to those seen with endemic infection. Evidence of life-long immunity was provided by 13 patients in these communities who had their previous exposure to mumps 58 years before the reported epidemics. None of these patients developed clinical illness, although 6 of the 10 tested seroconverted upon reexposure to the virus.

Public health surveys of mumps infection in the continental United States report an incidence of approximately 20 to 30 cases per 100,000 population per year. A prospective study performed in 1968 revealed approximately 2000 cases per 100,000 population per year (Levitt and Casey, 1970). The difficulty of frequency estimates in this disease is compounded by the frequent occurrence of subclinical infection and by the fact that physicians rarely see more than 40 per cent of clinical cases. Secondary attack rates in families of children with mumps range from 14 to 46 per cent.

## DIAGNOSIS

The diagnosis of mumps is usually based on the presence of parotitis and a history of contact with the illness. Other viral causes of mumps include parainfluenza and influenza viruses (Brill and Gilfillan, 1977). A differential diagnosis of parotid swelling is included in Table 2 and should be considered when a history of exposure is not provided or the illness is atypical.

Unlike bacterial parotitis, there is little heat and redness over the parotid in mumps (see Chapter 101). The pathogenesis of many parotid swellings involves xerostomia with retrograde infection by normal oral flora, cellular metaplasia in the duct walls, and some degree of obstruction. Chronic changes include stricture, calculus formation, and sialectasis. Approximately 6 per cent of patients with sarcoidosis have chronic parotid swelling due to granulomatous changes.

Parotid and, occasionally, submandibular swelling may represent an allergic response to drugs. Eosinophils in the glandular secretions support this diagnosis. Iodides are commonly responsible, and isoprenaline parotitis has been reproduced in rats; other drugs are listed in Table 2. Adrenal corticosteroid therapy may be of benefit in this condition.

Malnutrition, alcoholism, and diabetes mellitus all may be associated with parotid enlargement. The term "nutritional mumps" has been used in these cases and suggests a common pathogenesis that is related to fatty infiltration of the

**TABLE 2. Parotid Swelling — Differential Diagnosis**

**Infectious:**
Mumps
Parainfluenza
Influenza
Cytomegalovirus
Coxsackie virus
Lymphocytic choriomeningitis
Echovirus
Suppurative (bacterial)
Actinomyces
Mycobacteria
Cat scratch disease

**Noninfectious:**
Drug hypersensitivity
  (thiouracil, phenothiazines, thiocyanate, iodides, copper,
  isoprenaline, lead, mercury, phenylbutazone)
Sarcoidosis
Tumors, mixed
Hemangioma, lymphangioma
Sialectasis
Sjögren's syndrome
Mikulicz's syndrome
  (scleroderma, mixed connective tissue disease,
  systemic lupus erythematosis)
Recurrent idiopathic parotitis
Pneumoparotitis
Trauma
Sialolithiasis
Foreign body
Cystic fibrosis
Malnutrition (marasmus, alcoholic cirrhosis)
Dehydration
Diabetes mellitus
Waldenström's macroglobulinemia
Reiter's syndrome
Amyloidosis

**Nonparotid Swelling:**
Hypertrophy of masseter muscle
Lymphadenopathy
Rheumatoid mandibular joint swelling
Tumors of jaw
Infantile cortical hyperostosis

gland, acinar swelling, and increase in zymogen granules. Parotitis has also been produced in rats by protein deprivation.

Curious noninfectious etiologies for parotid swelling include papillary hypertrophy secondary to cheek biting and the trauma of poorly fitting dentures. "Wind parotitis," also called pneumoparotitis, is the name given to parotid swelling due to the introduction of air into the gland. This may be secondary to trauma or surgery or self-induced. It has also been reported in musicians playing wind instruments, glassblowers, and persons who have performed strenuous inflation of rubber balloons. Occasionally, crepitation may be detected along the course of Stenson's duct in these patients.

Laboratory findings are nonspecific in uncomplicated mumps parotitis. The white blood cell count is usually within the normal range although there may be a relative lymphocytosis. A polymorphonuclear leukocytosis (15,000 to 20,000/mm³) is common with extraparotid manifestations. This is also true of the erythrocyte sedimentation rate, which, normal or slightly elevated with mumps parotitis, is markedly elevated with arthritis and orchitis. The serum amylase is above normal in mumps and can be used to differentiate nonparotid from parotid swelling. It cannot be relied upon to differentiate pancreatitis from parotitis.

Cerebrospinal fluid (CSF) pleocytosis is usually in the order of 100 to 500 cells/mm³. This may be predominantly polymorphonuclear in the early stages; however, a mononuclear cell reaction is characteristic thereafter. The CSF protein is normal or slightly elevated, and the glucose concentration may be down in 2 to 20 per cent of cases. Persistence of pleocytosis for 3 to 4 days in the majority of cases, and for as long as 15 weeks in occasional cases, has been reported. Similarly, increased CSF protein concentration has been observed for as long as 29 days. Late inflammatory changes in the CSF may be the hallmark of postinfectious encephalomyelitis.

A specific viral diagnosis can be made by inoculation of primary Rhesus monkey (or other appropriate cell line) with saliva, urine, blood, or CSF from patients with mumps and/or mumps meningoencephalitis. Saliva may contain virus from 7 days before the onset of parotitis to 8 days after. In exceptional cases, virus has been cultured up to 14 days after the onset of parotitis despite the absence of clinical disease at the time. The virus has also been isolated directly from parotid, testicular, and thyroid tissue. A characteristic cytopathic effect appears in tissue culture 5 to 7 days after inoculation, and the hemadsorption test with guinea-pig red blood cells is positive. The virus is further identified by neutralization of this hemadsorption with specific antisera. More rapid experimental approaches have been used for the diagnosis of mumps infection, including direct fluorescent antibody staining of epithelial cells in the saliva and hemagglutination by saliva, urine, and CSF.

Serologic diagnosis of mumps infection is based upon demonstration of one of several humoral antibody responses. Two complement-fixing mumps antigens have been described. The viral (V) antigen is found on the surface and the soluble (S) antigen in the core. Antibody directed against the soluble antigen rises significantly over the first 2 to 6 weeks of illness and then begins to fall. Viral-associated antigen stimulates a slower antibody response that persists for 6 months to a year. Because of the earlier rise and fall of the antibody against soluble antigen, a high S/V ratio of complement-fixing antibody may indicate recent infection. Similarly, complement-fixation titers greater than 1/200 suggest recent infection because such antibody concentrations are present in less than 2 per cent of the adult population. The short duration of these antibodies makes the complement-fixation test less satisfactory for detection of long-term immunity. Hemagglutination inhibition or, preferably, neutralizing antibody is a more sensitive test for this purpose. Neutralizing-antibody titers of greater than ½ correlate with immunity. At least a fourfold antibody titer rise accompanies acute infection. Heterologous serologic responses to parainfluenza virus have been documented with mumps infection as well.

The mumps skin test has occasionally been used as an indicator of immunity. Preparations of this material are extremely variable in their antigenic potency, and false-positive and false-negative results are common. If the test is done, a tissue-culture control antigen should be administered intradermally in the contralateral forearm. One-tenth milliliter of the test and control antigen materials is administered intradermally, and the results are recorded at 24 and 48 hours. A transverse diameter of erythema around the test antigen of 10 mm or more than around the control is used to define positivity. The skin test may boost humoral antibody in patients with preexisting titers.

The differential diagnosis of meningoencephalitis in the absence of parotitis is usually dependent on laboratory and epidemiologic findings. Causes other than mumps include enteroviral, herpes simplex, and tuberculous infections. The low CSF sugar concentration in the presence of a lymphocytic cellular reaction may suggest meningeal tuberculosis. Orchitis in the absence of parotitis may be due to Coxsackie viruses types A and B, echoviruses, and lymphocytic choriomeningitis virus. Noninfectious causes of testicular hypertrophy need to be excluded as well.

## TREATMENT AND PROPHYLAXIS

Mumps is usually a benign and self-limited infection that requires little treatment. Antipyretics and rest may be used, but there is no specific antiviral therapy.

Patients with mumps meningoencephalitis may have severe headache and require aspirin or codeine. This should be used with caution in patients with encephalitis, in which masking of the symptoms and signs may be dangerous. The headache in this condition is often relieved by lumbar puncture.

Patients with orchitis may require more potent analgesics such as meperidine or morphine. Support for the scrotum and warm or cold compresses are often useful. The patient's subjective response to this treatment can be used as a guide. A controlled study demonstrated no benefit from adrenocorticosteroid therapy in orchitis. Knowledge that the incidence of sterility after orchitis is extremely rare should assist the physician in providing the reassurance and sympathy that these patients often require. Other modalities such as diethylstilbestrol, injection of the spermatic cord with local anesthetics, incision of the tunica albuginea, and oxyphenbutazone have no proven usefulness.

Mumps vaccine (5000 $TCID_{50}$/dose) is immunogenic in 93 to 98 per cent of subjects and has a protective efficacy of about 95 per cent. Neutralizing antibody has been shown to persist for at least 9½ years. Immunity is also durable after mumps immunization combined with measles and rubella vaccines (Weibel et al., 1978). Although antibody titers are lower than after natural infection, they are still protective. Adverse effects after vaccination are mild and extremely rare. These include parotitis, low-grade fever, rash, pruritus, and purpura; serum amylase concentrations are not usually elevated. Central nervous system problems have been temporarily related to vaccination but usually not with greater incidence than expected in the normal population. Thus, approximately one case of CNS illness per million doses of vaccine has been reported in the United States. These problems include cranial neuropathies (diplopia, Bell's palsy) that usually occur within 8 days after vaccination and encephalopathy (meningoencephalitis, febrile convulsions) most often noted 3 weeks after immunization.

The live attenuated virus vaccine (Jeryl Lynn strain) produces a noncommunicable, subclinical infection, and the virus has been isolated from vaccinees only in rare instances. The vaccine is contraindicated in patients allergic to egg protein or neomycin, which are present in the preparation. In view of possible teratogenicity, it is also contraindicated in pregnancy. The vaccine virus has infected the placenta of susceptible women (although viremia has not been demonstrated after vaccination). As with other live virus vaccines, administration to immunosuppressed and/or debilitated patients is contraindicated.

The vaccine should be used to prevent mumps in all children over the age of 13 months. It is probable that seroconversion rates will be highest after this age. Simultaneous administration of mumps and measles virus vaccines at 13 to 15 months of age is safe and effective. Mumps and mumps vaccination is followed by a period of diminished cutaneous tuberculin sensitivity. Skin testing should, therefore, be carried out before, or simultaneous with, vaccination.

Prophylaxis for family contacts and containment of epidemic spread are difficult to achieve via isolation or vaccination procedures. Isolation is ineffective because the virus is present in the saliva for as long as a week before the onset of symptoms, and many patients are asymptomatic with infection. Use of respiratory droplet isolation procedures (mask and handwashing) may be indicated in certain situations (e.g., admission of a patient with mumps to hospital). Materials in contact with patient secretions and urine should be disinfected. Vaccine-induced antibody may develop slowly (14 to 28 days) and may, therefore, not prevent infection during the first few weeks following vaccination. Skin tests cannot be relied upon to predict susceptibility. There is no contraindication to vaccination of seropositive individuals with mumps vaccine, and indeed, this procedure often boosts humoral antibody without adverse effects.

In an effort to study the efficacy of mumps hyperimmune globulin, 56 serologically susceptible subjects received this material during a mumps epidemic. The attack and complication rates were not altered (Reed et al., 1967). Use of immunoglobulin to prevent mumps orchitis in adult males is also not supported by these data.

Although mumps is generally a mild and self-limited illness, there are occasional deaths from it. Patients with severe parotitis and neurologic or testicular involvement may also suffer greatly. Now that an effective vaccine is available, such severe or fatal cases need no longer occur.

## References

Aase, J. M., Noren, G., Reddy, D., and St. Geme, J., Jr.: Mumps-virus infection in pregnant women and the immunologic response of their offspring. New Engl J Med 286:1379, 1972.

Beard, C. M., Benson, R. C., Kelalis, P. P., Elveback, L. R., and Kurland, L. T.: The incidence and outcome of mumps orchitis in Rochester, Minnesota, 1935 to 1974. Mayo Clin Proc 52:3, 1977.

Brill, S. J., and Gilfillan, R. F.: Acute parotitis associated with influenza Type A. New Engl J Med 296:1391, 1977.

Chiba, Y., Dzierba, J. J., Morag, A., and Ogra, P. L.: Cell-mediated immune response to mumps virus infection in man. J Immunol 116:12, 1976.

Herndon, R. M., Johnson, R. T., Davis, L. E., and Descalgi, L. R.: Ependymitis in mumps virus meningitis. Arch Neurol 30:475, 1974.

Levitt, L. P., and Casey, H. L.: Mumps in General Population. Am J Dis Child 120:134, 1970.

Reed, D., Brown, G., Merrick, R., Sever, J., and Feltz, E.: A mumps epidemic on St. George Island, Alaska. JAMA 199:113, 1967.

Weibel, R. E., Buynak, E. B., McLean, A. A., and Hilleman, M. R.: Persistence of antibody after administration of monovalent and combined live attenuated measles, mumps, and rubella virus vaccines. Pediatrics 61:5, 1978.

Wilfert, C. M.: Mumps meningoencephalitis with low cerebrospinal fluid glucose, prolonged pleocytosis, and elevation of protein. New Engl J Med 280:855, 1969.

# INFLUENZA 103

*R. Gordon Douglas, Jr., M.D.*

## DEFINITION

Influenza is an acute infectious disease caused by influenza A or B virus. It occurs in outbreaks, usually in the winter months in temperate climates, and produces symptoms of fever, cough, headache, and myalgias. The disease is usually self-limited, but pulmonary complications develop in a few cases. Infection with influenza viruses may also produce pharyngitis, croup, tracheobronchitis, bronchiolitis, pneumonia, or even common colds. Conversely, other respiratory viruses such as rhinoviruses, adenoviruses, or enteroviruses may produce sporadic cases of acute, self-limited, febrile illness that mimic those produced by influenza viruses.

## ETIOLOGY

Influenza viruses are members of the Orthomyxoviridae family. Influenza virus type A and influenza virus type B are two genera within this family. The third type of influenza virus, type C, probably represents another genus, although it has not been officially so classified. Influenza viruses are medium-sized (80 to 100 nm) enveloped viruses containing a helical nucleocapsid that is segmented into eight separate pieces. A total of eight gene products (proteins) has been identified. The most important antigenic determinants are the two surface glycoproteins known as the hemagglutinin (H) and the neuraminidase (N), named after certain biological functions possessed by these proteins. The H and N project as spikes from a lipid envelope that is derived from host cell membrane. Changes in the antigenicity of these surface proteins are thought to be important determinants of the unusual epidemiologic behavior of influenza virus. Both surface proteins undergo relatively minor changes that occur frequently, that is, almost every year. These are referred to as "antigenic drift," and they probably result from point mutations resulting in alterations of one or more amino acids. More dramatic changes in the antigenicity of either or both proteins are referred to as "antigenic shift." Antigenic shift is thought to occur most often from genetic reassortment (recombination) that occurs when two influenza viruses simultaneously infect a single cell (Webster et al., 1971). As a result of the presence of a segmented genome, random reassortment of the eight RNA segments from each parent results in creation of new virions with varying characteristics of either parent. In this way, progeny virus that retain the virulence factors of one parent but also contain "new" H or N or both develop. To date, four hemagglutinins (H0, H1, H2, H3) and two neuraminidases (N1, N2) have been recognized.

Influenza A viruses are named by their H and N to identify the subtype (e.g., H3N2, H1N1), and by site of origin and year to recognize strain variation within a subtype (e.g., A/Hong Kong/68 H3N2, A/England/42/72 H3N2, A/Texas/77 H3N2 [Table 1]).

## EPIDEMIOLOGY

Influenza A and B virus infections characteristically occur in epidemics (Kilbourne, 1975). In a given community or region they begin rather abruptly, reach a sharp peak in two to three weeks, and last five to six weeks. During these epidemics, the number of people with febrile respiratory disease increases, school and industrial absenteeism rises, and hospital admissions for pneumonia, chronic obstructive pulmonary disease, croup, and congestive heart failure all increase. There are also more deaths.

Such epidemics may be localized to a community or region, or they may involve countries or continents or occur worldwide, in which case they are called pandemics. Epidemics do not occur everywhere simultaneously; rather, sequential spread from one area to another over several months is usual. Epidemics occur during October through April in the northern hemisphere and May through September in the southern hemisphere.

## PATHOGENESIS AND PATHOLOGY

Influenza viruses are transmitted from person to person via the respiratory route, predominantly by small particle aerosols ($<10\mu$ mass median

**TABLE 1.** Antigenic Shift of Influenza A

| YEAR | SUBTYPE DESIGNATION | COMMON NAME |
|------|---------------------|-------------|
| 1889 | H3N2 | — |
| 1918 | Hsw1N1 | Swine |
| 1929 | H0N1 | A$_0$ |
| 1946 | H1N1 | A' |
| 1957 | H2N2 | A$_2$, Asian |
| 1968 | H3N2 | Hong Kong |
| 1977 | H1N1 | Russian |

diameter). It is also possible that some spread occurs from closer contact transmission including hand-to-hand contact or fomites or by direct deposition of large droplets of respiratory secretions containing infectious virus.

Virus is deposited on the mucosal epithelium of the respiratory tract where it may be neutralized by specific secretory IgA antibody and nonspecific mucoproteins or removed by the mucociliary blanket or cough reflex. If it is not neutralized or removed, virus adsorbs to and penetrates a columnar epithelial cell, where it initiates the viral replication cycle. As infectious virus is released from cells, it spreads to adjacent cells where the replication cycle is repeated. Within a relatively short time many cells in the respiratory tract are infected. Such replication eventually kills the cell. The incubation period from deposition of virus to onset of illness (usually one to two days) varies from 18 to 72 hours, depending in part on the size of the inoculum dose. Virus is shed from the respiratory tract just before the onset of illness. Virus titers in nasal or tracheal secretions peak within 24 hours, remain elevated for 24 to 48 hours, and then rapidly decrease. As virus titers fall, interferon is detected in the respiratory secretions and may be responsible for recovery from illness. Viral replication is the major determinant of illness, since neither antibody nor cell-mediated responses can be detected at this time in unprimed subjects. The occurrence of systemic symptoms and fever suggests that virus disseminates hematogenously, but infectious virus has only rarely been recovered from blood.

During acute uncomplicated influenza ciliated columnar epithelial cells commonly desquamate into the lumen of the bronchus. Individual cells show shrinkage, pyknotic nuclei, and loss of cilia. In fatal influenza viral pneumonia, extensive hemorrhage, hyaline membrane formation, and few polymorphonuclear cells are found in the lung.

Neutralizing, hemagglutination-inhibiting (HAI), neuraminidase-inhibiting (NI), and complement-fixing (CF) antibodies develop in the serum of patients experiencing primary infection with influenza virus. They are first detected the second week after exposure and reach peak titers by four weeks. In patients who have been primed by previous infection, the antibody response is more brisk. HAI, NI, and neutralizing antibodies persist for months to years and gradually decline thereafter. Neutralizing and HAI tests distinguish among strains as well as among subtypes of influenza. CF antibody is directed against the ribonucleoprotein and is type-specific, so that all strains and subtypes within the influenza A type cross-react in CF tests.

Secretory antibodies, predominantly IgA, develop in the respiratory tract after influenza infection. Their peak titers are reached 14 days after the onset of infection. They are found in saliva, nasal secretions, sputum, and tracheal washings by neutralization tests. Secretory antibodies do not persist as long as serum antibodies, usually only several months.

Substantial levels of antibody protect against infection. Serum HAI titers of 1:40 or greater or neutralizing titers of 1:8 or greater are commonly associated with protection against infection. Similarly, most persons with nasal neutralizing antibody titers of 1:4 or greater are protected against infection.

Antibody also modifies the course of illness. That is, if antibody is present in lower titers in serum, or is present in serum and not in nasal secretions, the subject may become infected but will experience a milder illness than someone who has no antibody. In addition, antibody that is directed against neuraminidase or against a heterotypic strain may prevent severe illness but not infection.

## CLINICAL FINDINGS IN UNCOMPLICATED INFLUENZA

Influenza characteristically starts abruptly. Many patients can pinpoint the hour of onset. At first systemic symptoms such as feverishness, chilliness or frank shaking chills, headache, myalgias, malaise, and anorexia predominate. The temperature usually rises rapidly to a peak of 38 to 40° C or higher within 12 hours of onset. Usually myalgias and headache are the most troublesome symptoms, and their severity is related to the height of the fever. Myalgias may involve the extremities or the long muscles of the back, and arthralgias are commonly observed. Systemic symptoms usually persist for three days, the usual duration of fever.

When present, ocular symptoms such as photophobia, tearing, burning, and pain on moving the eyes are helpful diagnostically. Respiratory symptoms, particularly dry cough and nasal discharge, are usually present also at the onset but are overshadowed by the systemic symptoms. Nasal obstruction, hoarseness, and dry or sore throat may also be present. These symptoms tend to become more prominent as the disease progresses.

Fever is usually continuous but may be intermittent, especially if antipyretics are administered. On the second and third days of illness, the temperature elevation is usually 0.5 to 1.0 degree lower than on the first day. The duration of fever is three days commonly, but it may last from one to five or more days.

Early in the illness the patient appears toxic with flushed face and hot moist skin. The eyes are watery and reddened and clear nasal discharge is common. The mucous membranes of the nose and throat are hyperemic, but exudate is not observed. Small, tender cervical lymph nodes are often present. Transient scattered ronchi or localized areas of rales are found in less than 20 per cent of cases.

Respiratory symptoms and signs usually persist for three to four days after fever subsides. Cough, lassitude, and malaise commonly persist for one to two or more weeks.

The above description of illness occurs with any type, subtype, or strain of influenza A or B virus (Douglas, 1975). In contrast, influenza C infection causes afebrile common colds and rarely if ever produces the influenza syndrome. It also does not occur in epidemics.

Maximal temperatures tend to be higher among children, and cervical adenopathy is more frequent among children than adults. Among elderly persons, fever remains a frequent finding, although the height of the febrile response may be lower than among children and young adults.

## COMPLICATIONS AND SEQUELAE

### Pulmonary Complications

Three pulmonary complications of influenza are well recognized: primary influenza viral pneumonia, secondary bacterial infection, and mixed viral and bacterial pneumonias.

*Primary Influenza Viral Pneumonia.* This complication has occurred primarily in persons with underlying cardiovascular, pulmonary, renal, or other chronic disease, although cases occur in every large outbreak in young healthy adults. Pregnancy has been implicated as a risk factor in some epidemics. Following a typical onset of influenza there is rapid progression of fever, cough, dyspnea, and cyanosis. Physical examination and chest x-ray reveal bilateral findings but no consolidation. Blood gas studies show marked anoxia. Sputum culture reveals normal flora, whereas viral cultures yield high titers of influenza A virus. Such patients do not respond to antibiotics and mortality is high.

Milder forms of influenza viral pneumonia involving only one lobe or segment have been described. They are not invariably lethal and are more likely to be confused with pneumonia due to *Streptococcus pneumoniae* than with pneumonia produced by viral infection. Pneumonia and/or bronchiolitis occurs in children but is less common than in adults.

*Secondary Bacterial Pneumonia.* Patients who are elderly or have chronic pulmonary, cardiac, metabolic, or other diseases have a classic influenza illness followed by a period of improvement lasting one to four days. Recrudescence of fever is associated with symptoms and signs of bacterial pneumonia such as cough, sputum production, chest pain, and an area of consolidation seen on physical examination and chest roentgenogram (Schwarzmann et al., 1971). Gram stain and culture of sputum reveal predominance of a bacterial pathogen, most often *S. pneumoniae, Staphylococcus aureus,* or *Haemophilus influenzae.* Such patients usually respond to specific antibiotic therapy.

*Mixed Viral-Bacterial Pneumonias.* During an outbreak of influenza many cases are observed that do not clearly fit the description of primary influenza or secondary bacterial pneumonias. The disease does not progress relentlessly, yet the fever pattern is not biphasic. These patients may have primary viral, secondary bacterial, or mixed viral and bacterial infection of the lung and many respond to antibiotics.

*Croup.* Significant numbers of cases of croup occur in influenza A and B outbreaks. Such cases associated with influenza A virus are more severe but less frequent than those associated with parainfluenza virus types 1, 2, or 3, or respiratory syncytial virus.

*Exacerbation of Chronic Obstructive Pulmonary Disease.* In adults with chronic obstructive pulmonary disease, infection with influenza A or B virus may result in acute exacerbation of chronic bronchitis, a syndrome associated with other respiratory viruses and bacteria as well. Such infections may result in permanent loss of pulmonary function.

Although the majority of patients with influenza do not have clinically detectable pneumonia, abnormalities in gas exchange and peripheral airway resistance frequently occur in nonpneumonic influenza infections and persist well beyond the period of clinical illness (Little et al., 1978). These findings suggest that viral invasion of the lower respiratory tract is common in influenza and may help to explain the relatively long convalescence. Lower respiratory tract disease is found by auscultation or roentgenogram in about 10 per cent of patients. The rate is lower in children and young adults but rises rapidly after age 50.

### Nonpulmonary Complications

*Myositis.* Myositis and myoglobinuria with tender leg muscles and elevated serum creatinine phosphokinase (CPK) levels have been reported in children after influenza B and less commonly influenza A infection. The pain may be severe enough to prevent walking.

**Cardiac Complications.** Both myocarditis and pericarditis have been associated with influenza A and B virus infections. However, neither myocarditis nor pericarditis is observed commonly at autopsy among those dying of primary influenza viral pneumonia.

**Central Nervous System Complications.** Guillain-Barré syndrome has been reported to occur after influenza A infection, as it has after numerous other infections, but no definite etiologic relationship has been established. In addition, cases of transverse myelitis and encephalitis have occurred rarely.

**Reye's Syndrome.** Reye's syndrome, first described in 1963, is now a frequently recognized hepatic and central nervous system complication of influenza B and, less commonly, influenza A infection. Pathologic examination reveals a liver that is pale yellow due to the presence of multiple small droplets of lipids uniformly distributed throughout hepatocytes. Neither the brain nor the liver shows inflammatory changes. The virus infection may act merely as a triggering mechanism for a toxin. However, no such toxin has yet been found. The urea-cycle mitochondrial enzymes in the liver are transiently abnormal.

The syndrome occurs only in children between the ages of 2 and 16 years, and its mortality is 10 to 40 per cent. Because of the epidemic nature of influenza, Reye's syndrome also occurs epidemically as well as endemically. Most of the large outbreaks have resulted from influenza B virus infection. However, a number of cases of Reye's syndrome have followed chickenpox and have been associated with other viruses in individual cases.

Reye's syndrome usually starts with nausea and vomiting several days after a typical upper respiratory, gastrointestinal, or chickenpox infection. Within one or two days mental changes are noted. The manifestations range from lethargy to delirium, obtundation, seizures, and respiratory arrest. The children are usually afebrile and have hepatomegaly but not jaundice. Mortality is related to stage of coma on admission to the hospital, and appears to be decreasing with earlier recognition and hospitalization. Lumbar puncture reveals increased intracranial pressure and normal protein values and cell counts, confirming the presence of encephalopathy rather than meningoencephalitis. The most frequent laboratory abnormality is elevation of the blood ammonia value, which occurs in almost all patients. Hypoglycemia is present more often in patients with antecedent varicella or gastrointestinal illness than in those with upper respiratory illness. Serum glutamic oxaloacetic transaminase (SGOT), serum glutamic pyruvic transaminase (SGPT), bilirubin, and prothrombin values are commonly elevated, as are CPK and lactic dehydrogenase (LDH) levels.

## DIAGNOSIS

Specific viral diagnosis is made by virus isolation, serology, and epidemiology. Detection of infectious virus or viral antigen in respiratory secretions is optimal for clinical purposes, since serologic tests, although sensitive and specific, are still negative during the acute illness. Virus can be isolated readily from nasal swab specimens, throat swab specimens, nasal washes, and sputum. Sputum is the best specimen, but if it is not produced, a combined nose and throat swab specimen or a nasal wash is ideal. Such swabs should be thrust into containers of viral transport medium and brought to the laboratory at once. Specimens for diagnosis of influenza are inoculated onto Madin-Darby canine kidney (MDCK) or cynomologous kidney cell cultures, and virus replication is detected by hemadsorption. About two thirds of the positive cultures can be detected within three days of inoculation and the remainder by seven days. Many hospital or regional viral diagnostic laboratories can recover influenza virus by these cell culture techniques or by inoculation of embryonated hens' eggs.

Complement-fixing antibody tests are most commonly used for serologic diagnosis. Serum specimens from the acute and convalescent periods (obtained 10 to 20 days after the acute phase serum) should be submitted for testing. Fourfold or greater rises or falls in titer are considered diagnostic of infection, and a high convalescent titer, when only one convalescent specimen is available, suggests recent infection.

Diagnosis can also be made on epidemiologic grounds, for example, influenza virus is confirmed in a region or community by the local or by the state or national health department, persons presenting with fever, muscle aches, and cough most likely have influenza (Marine et al., 1976).

## TREATMENT

### Uncomplicated Influenza

Amantadine is approved in the United States for treatment of influenza. It shortens the duration of signs and symptoms of clinical influenza by approximately 50 per cent. Its major drawback is minor reversible central nervous system side effects such as insomnia, dizziness, and difficulty in concentrating, which occur in about 5 per cent of subjects. However, in controlled studies the reduction of influenza symptoms is greater than the occurrence of drug side effects, resulting in net benefit to patients. The usual dose is 200 mg orally for the first dose and then 100 mg twice daily for three to five days.

Acutely ill, febrile patients should rest in bed and take enough fluids. Acetylsalicylic acid 0.6 to 0.9 g every three to four hours reduces headache, fever, and myalgias. Nasal obstruction may be relieved by phenylephrine or oxymetazoline hydrochloride nasal sprays or drops, and cough may be reduced by cold water vaporization or guaifenesin cough syrup containing dextromethorphan, 1 to 3 teaspoons every three to four hours.

### Pulmonary Complications

Because there have been no controlled studies of amantadine treatment of influenza viral pneumonia, its use in this condition is based on extrapolation from cases of uncomplicated influenza, anecdotal case reports of benefit, and the effect of amantadine on peripheral airway resistance in uncomplicated influenza. Supportive care is important, including fluid and electrolyte management, supplemental oxygen, intubation, tracheostomy, assisted ventilation, and use of positive end expiratory pressure. For patients with proven or suspected bacterial superinfection, antibiotics should be administered. Because of the rapidly advancing nature of many cases of pneumonia that occur during an influenza epidemic, therapy to cover the potential pathogens, most importantly *S. aureus, S. pneumoniae,* and *H. influenzae,* is indicated if a clearcut diagnosis cannot be made from Gram stain of the sputum or transtracheal aspirate. Cephamandole, 12 g/day I.V. in divided doses, might be a reasonable choice in this situation because it has good in vitro activity against the three most common organisms, including ampicillin-resistant *H. influenzae.* Alternatively, a semisynthetic penicillinase-resistant penicillin such as methicillin or nafcillin, 12 g/day I.V. in divided doses, and ampicillin, 8 to 12 g/day I.V. in divided doses, could be used. If ampicillin-resistant *H. influenzae* is suspected, chloramphenicol may be substituted for ampicillin. If there is a suspicion of gram-negative rod pneumonia due to organisms other than *H. influenzae,* cephamandole, cefazolin, or an aminoglycoside such as gentamicin, tobramycin, or amikacin could be considered. For penicillin-allergic patients, vancomycin for *S. aureus,* chloramphenicol for *H. influenzae* and *S. pneumoniae,* or clindamycin for *S. aureus* and *S. pneumoniae* may be considered.

### Other Complications

There is no specific therapy for cardiac, central nervous system, or other complications, including Reye's syndrome.

## *PREVENTION*

The mainstay for prevention of influenza in the United States is inactivated virus vaccines. In some other countries, live virus vaccines are used. Vaccines are safe and effective in preventing influenza, but several problems are worthy of mention. Most studies indicate that vaccines have a protective efficacy of only about 70 per cent. Mild local side effects occur in 25 per cent of vaccine recipients, and systemic side effects, including fever, occur in 1 to 2 per cent. Guillain-Barré syndrome (GBS) occurred in 1 in 100,000 patients, and 5 per cent of those with GBS died during the 1976 Swine Influenza Immunization Program in the United States. Although a potential risk, GBS has not occurred with other influenza vaccines.

The Public Health Advisory Committee on Immunization Practices in the United States, the World Health Organization, and other government bodies make recommendations annually with regard to the composition of the vaccine. In general, the vaccines have contained both an A type and a B type virus (bivalent), usually the types isolated in the previous winter's influenza season. In some years, two A types have been included in addition to a B type (thus, trivalent) because both A types have circulated in the previous winter and because the type of influenza to be encountered cannot be reliably predicted.

Inactivated vaccines have recently been purified and their antigenic mass standardized. One dose of 7 $\mu$g of antigen is enough to elicit serum HAI titers of 1:40 or greater in 90 per cent of persons who have previously been exposed to the antigen. Two doses are necessary to achieve comparable levels in unprimed subjects.

The only contraindication to vaccination is hypersensitivity to hens' eggs. If an individual can eat eggs or egg-containing products, the vaccine is safe. In the United States and Great Britain, vaccine is recommended for persons at increased risks of dying from pulmonary complications of influenza. These include anyone with a chronic disease. Antibody responses are usually good or only slightly diminished in these chronic conditions and additional harmful effects have not been observed in groups of patients with renal disease, systemic lupus erythematosus, or multiple sclerosis. Pregnancy is not a contraindication to vaccination. Priority for vaccination should be given to persons who provide essential community services (e.g., policemen, firemen) and to hospital workers to prevent nosocomial spread.

### Chemoprophylaxis

Amantadine is an approved prophylactic agent against influenza (Monto et al., 1979). It is as effective as vaccine and adds to vaccine efficacy. Because two 100 mg capsules are required each day for five to six weeks, and because of cost, side effects, and the need for a surveillance program to detect the onset of an epidemic, vaccine is preferred to amantadine for routine prophylaxis. However, there are certain situations in which the prophylactic use of amantadine may be important. Persons who have not received vaccine at the time of an influenza outbreak should be given vaccine together with amantadine 100 mg twice daily for 10 to 14 days. Persons with egg hypersensitivity, who cannot receive influenza vaccine, may be given amantadine for the duration of the outbreak. Household contacts of an index case may be given amantadine. Staff and patients in hospitals or institutions may be given amantadine to prevent an outbreak.

## References

Douglas, R. G., Jr.: Influenza in man. In Kilbourne, E. D. (ed.): Influenza Viruses and Influenza. New York, Academic Press, 1975, p. 395.

Dowdle, W. R., Noble, G. R., and Kendal, A. P.: Orthomyxovirus-influenza: Comparative diagnosis unifying concept. In Kurstak, E., and Kurstak, C. (eds.): Comparative Diagnosis of Viral Diseases. New York, Academic Press, 1977, p. 447.

Glezen, W. P., and Couch, R. B.: Interpandemic influenza in the Houston area, 1974–76. N Engl J Med 298:587, 1978.

Kilbourne, E. D.: Epidemiology of influenza. In Kilbourne, E. D. (ed.): Influenza Viruses and Influenza. New York, Academic Press, 1975, p. 483.

Little, J. W., Hall, W. J., Douglas, R. G., et al.: Airway hyperreactivity and peripheral airway dysfunction in influenza A infection. Am Rev Resp Dis 118:295, 1978.

Marine, W. M., McGowan, J. E., Jr., and Thomas, J. E.: Influenza detection: A prospective comparison of surveillance methods and analysis of isolates. Am J Epidemiol 104:248, 1976.

Masurel, N., and Marine, W. M.: Recycling of Asian and Hong Kong influenza A virus hemagglutinins in man. Am J Epidemiol 97:44, 1973.

Monto, A. S., Gunn, R. A., Bandyk, M. G., et al.: Prevention of Russian influenza by amantadine. JAMA 241:1003, 1979.

Schwarzmann, S. W., Adler, J. L., Sullivan, R. J., et al.: Bacterial pneumonia during the Hong Kong influenza epidemic of 1968–1969. Arch Intern Med 127:1037, 1971.

Webster, R. G., Campbell, C. H., and Granoff, A.: The "in vivo" production of "new" influenza A viruses. I. Genetic recombination between avian and mammalian influenza viruses. Virology 44:317, 1971.

# 104 *PERTUSSIS*

## *James D. Connor, M.D.*

### *DEFINITION*

Pertussis is an acute disease of the respiratory tract usually characterized by progressive, repetitive, paroxysmal coughing, mild systemic complaints, and lymphocytosis. Because the hallmark of the clinical disease is an inspiratory whoop, it is commonly referred to as whooping cough. Pertussis occurs throughout the world in immunized and unimmunized populations, usually causing sharp outbreaks or epidemics of disease in cycles of two to four years. The disease is caused by *Bordetella pertussis,* a minute bacillus that was first isolated from children with the disease by Bordet and Gengou in 1906. Although infection may occur at any age, the clinical disease is most frequently recognized in older infants and children with typical paroxysms and the characteristic inspiratory whoop. The morbidity is associated with the severity of coughing paroxysms and is especially marked in infants under 1 year of age (Buchanan and Broohn, 1970). The incidence has continued to decline throughout the era of active immunization, and the mortality rate has declined markedly in both immunized and unimmunized populations in developed countries.

### *ETIOLOGY*

*B. pertussis*, originally known as the Bordet-Gengou bacillus, was assigned to the genus *Haemophilus* along with *Haemophilus influenzae*. After it was recognized that the pertussis bacillus did not require hemin and DPN (see Chapter 36) for growth, it was placed in a separate genus (see Chapter 35) that now also includes *B. parapertussis* and *B. bronchiseptica* (formerly *Brucella bronchiseptica*). In optimal liquid or semisolid medium, *B. pertussis* is a highly uniform, minute coccobacillus measuring approximately 0.5 $\mu$ in length. It stains faintly eosinophilic with the Gram stain. The bacilli are encapsulated but nonmotile. Under suboptimal conditions, the bacilli become pleomorphic and produce long rod forms mixed with *coccoid* and *ovoid* organisms. This change in appearance is accompanied by defects in the antigenic structure, including the loss of the antigen that induces protection in animals and humans. *B. pertussis* produces several other antigens, including agglutinogens, which are used to identify different antigenic types in the genus *Bordetella* as well as individual clinical strains of *B. pertussis*. Eldering and Kendrick

(1957) identified agglutinogen Types 1 through 6 among various strains of *B. pertussis*, with Types 2, 3, and 5 being major agglutinogens for *B. pertussis* while Types 4 and 6 were minor. Type 7 is common to the genus; Type 12 is species-specific for *B. bronchiseptica* and Type 14 for *B. parapertussis* (Eldering et al., 1957). Therefore, it is possible to differentiate the three members of the genus antigenically by agglutination with immune sera. Although there are common antigens among the genus, no cross-immunity has been recognized. Other antigens of *B. pertussis* include heat-labile and heat-stable toxins, histamine-sensitizing factor, hemagglutinins, and lymphocyte-promoting factor (Munoz, 1963; Pittman, 1970). The last is the factor responsible for the characteristic lymphocytosis that appears during the paroxysmal stage of the disease and after immunization with whole killed bacilli (Welsh et al., 1959). Lymphocytosis may be induced specifically in laboratory animals by injection of purified lymphocyte-producing factor. The role of these antigens in the pathogenesis of the disease is unknown (Pittman, 1970).

## INCIDENCE

In relatively isolated, unimmunized populations, pertussis occurs in sharp outbreaks and epidemics. During epidemics the incidence of the characteristic acute disease is highest among infants and young children. This age group is at highest risk because it was born after the preceding epidemic. The primary attack rate in this group may be as high as 40 to 60 per cent, with a secondary attack rate among family members of 70 to 90 per cent. In immunized populations, the attack rate varies between 16 and 50 per cent in different countries, probably depending on the type of surveillance, the potency of the vaccine, and the age of the immunized. Very young infants as well as older children and adults may account for the majority of cases in outbreaks among well-immunized populations, since older infants and younger children have relatively greater protection from more recent immunization. There is no recognized carrier state; infants that are considered index cases in families may actually have been infected by an adult family member with unrecognized disease. The manner in which the endemic reservoir of infection is maintained is unknown. The disease usually occurs in late spring or summer and persists throughout the fall and early winter. Outbreaks among susceptible hospital personnel may be particularly inconvenient and have been known to jeopardize critical health care services (Kurt et al., 1972).

The mortality rate has fallen remarkably over the last three decades, even among the youngest infants, in whom it has always been highest (Buchanan and Broohn, 1970). A great reduction in the incidence of protein-calorie malnutrition may be the most important reason for this decline. Since antibiotics do not alter the morbidity or duration of the primary disease, it is unlikely that they influence the mortality of the primary disease. However, the mortality from secondary infectious complications, such as bacterial pneumonia, probably has been reduced by antibiotics. Primary nursing care and supportive measures may also be responsible for reduced mortality.

The reduction in incidence clearly began before the introduction of general immunization in the United States but the wide use of potent killed bacillary vaccines has certainly contributed to the continuing fall in incidence. The diagnosis is also often missed or uncomfirmed because most general diagnostic laboratories have never developed the methods necessary for isolating and identifying *B. pertussis*, and young graduating physicians may never have seen the clinical disease. The present low incidence among highly immunized populations is unlikely to fall further unless effective methods are found to immunize susceptible adults and infants under 3 to 4 months of age.

The marked susceptibility to the disease during the early weeks or months of life attests to the lack of protection provided by maternally transmitted antibody and predicts that biologic means of inducing passive protection are ineffective. In contrast to most childhood infections, the mortality of pertussis is significantly higher among females than among males at all ages. At one time, 90 per cent of cases with characteristic clinical disease occurred in children under the age of 9 years (Ipsen and Bowen, 1955). In recent years, there has been a considerable shift downward in age, with a predominance of cases among the very young who are either unimmunized or incompletely immunized.

## PATHOLOGY AND PATHOGENESIS

Three types of lesions predominate in the respiratory tract. In early paroxysmal and mid-paroxysmal stages of the disease, peribronchitis and peribronchiolitis may develop. These lesions consist of moderate to dense accumulations of lymphocytes, mast cells, and plasmocytes that infiltrate the supporting tissues of smaller bronchi and bronchioles. At either this stage or later, endobronchiolitis and endobronchitis may occur. These lesions are characterized by accumulation of debris within the bronchial lumen and infiltration of the bronchial wall by mononuclear cells.

Clusters of bacilli may be found either on the ciliated epithelial cells or mixed with debris, but they are not found in peribronchial tissues. Atelectasis may accompany these changes. In prolonged or severe disease, alveolar lesions consisting of thickening of the wall, mononuclear cell infiltration, and accumulation of fibrinous debris have been described. Peribronchial lymphadenopathy commonly accompanies the peribronchial lesion. In late disease, dysplasia and thickening of the bronchial epithelium is associated with replacement of columnar cells by squamous cells. Although the pathology of the disease is well established, the pathogenesis of the changes has not been determined. During infection, bacterial replication is essentially confined to the respiratory mucous membrane, with no bacillemia. The induction of lymphocytosis by the lymphocyte-promoting factor demonstrates that antigenemia occurs; thus, the immune response of the host is probably generated both through local and humoral mechanisms.

## CLINICAL MANIFESTATIONS

The clinical syndrome of pertussis has been divided into several stages, beginning with the early and most communicable period called the catarrhal or preparoxysmal stage. The catarrhal stage begins at the end of the incubation period, or about five to ten days after exposure. Generally, the manifestations are those of any early upper respiratory infection, with irritation of the mucous membranes, hacking cough, and fever. The duration of the catarrhal stage is usually seven to ten days, and it is generally not recognized as pertussis.

The paroxysmal stage begins at the end of the catarrhal stage; if there was fever during the catarrhal stage, it usually subsides. The disease is usually first recognized during the paroxysmal stage. Particularly in older infants and children, this stage is marked by crescendo development of inexorable paroxysmal coughing. Ultimately, the paroxysms may be induced by any stimulus (e.g., speech, swallowing, movement, tracheal pressure), and they occur with increasing frequency, severity, and duration as the paroxysmal stage progresses. Each paroxysm may consist of several bouts separated by momentary intervals insufficient for inspiration, until hypoxia and partial asphyxia occur. The end of the paroxysmal episode may be marked by a massive single inspiratory stroke causing the whoop of inspiratory stridor. During severe paroxysms, the patient may become plethoric or cyanotic, with bulging eyes and anxious or frantic countenance; it may appear that the patient's life is threatened. After severe episodes, the immediate post-tussive period may be marked by apparent respiratory arrest. In infants, the post-tussive period may also be marked by a state of exhaustion and lethargy during which the usual environmental stimuli fail to bring about a typical response. In the most severely affected infants, this state may merge into the next paroxysm on awakening. Vomiting occurs frequently at the end of a paroxysm. Paroxysmal coughing may last from seven days to a month and may vary from mild uncomplicated episodes to severe protracted episodes requiring hospitalization and acute supportive care.

The greatest morbidity of the disease is due to repetitive paroxysmal coughing that is inexorable, fatiguing, and at times pernicious. In the very young, individual paroxysms may present with frightening signs of hypoxia (cyanosis), asphyxia (pallor, limpness, post-tussive cyanosis), recurrent vomiting, and overt signs of mucous impaction of the trachea or larynx. These cases require intensive supportive care for a minimum of five to seven days.

During the most severe period, fatigue, weakness, pallor, anorexia, and somnolence may characterize the intervals between paroxysms. As the frequency, duration, and severity of attacks decrease, the morbidity is recognized only during an attack. Following the early paroxysmal stage, nighttime attacks may continue to occur over a prolonged period, sometimes for one to five months following the acute illness, with significant disruption of the rest patterns of adult members of the household. Bacilli are recovered from the nasopharynx most frequently during the catarrhal (preparoxysmal) and early paroxysmal stages. This correlates with the period of highest communicability. In rare cases, it is possible to transmit the infection during the later stages and to isolate bacilli for prolonged periods.

Infants, particularly those under 6 months of age, may not develop typical paroxysms and thus may go undiagnosed. The typical whoop may not be a part of the clinical syndrome in young infants. Instead, recurrent periods of apparent strangling and asphyxia may occur and lead to a variety of presumptive diagnoses other than pertussis.

Between attacks, quiet breathing usually occurs without abnormal auscultatory findings. The abnormal chest x-ray shows minimal peribronchial inflammatory changes (Barnhard, 1960), but chest x-ray is frequently normal. Pertussis pneumonia rarely occurs; it is characterized by an unusual course with fever, auscultatory rales, and a "shaggy cardiac border" indicative of intense interstitial pneumonitis.

In a majority of cases (estimated to be 80 per

cent in unimmunized older infants and children) hyperleukocytosis and lymphocytosis develop during the paroxysmal stage; their presence is helpful in making the diagnosis. The total white blood cell count may rise to greater than 100,000/mm³; commonly the count is in the range of 25,000 to 40,000/mm³ with a predominance of small mature lymphocytes. These cells appear in the circulation as a result of discharge of the marginal pool under the influence of the lymphocyte-promoting factor of *B. pertussis*. Again, hyperleukocytosis may not be present in infants under 6 months of age, but relative lymphocytosis usually is present (Brooksaler and Nelson, 1967).

The convalescent stage is usually characterized by a return to normal activity and development without complications. In a majority of patients, immunity is conferred by a single attack.

## COMPLICATIONS AND SEQUELAE

Complications and sequelae are steadily declining among infants and children in developed countries (White et al., 1964). Bronchiectasis is no longer a complication of pertussis in the United States. Likewise, central nervous system complications, such as seizures or encephalopathy, are very uncommon even in severe outbreaks. Less serious complications include epistaxis and hemorrhage into the conjunctivae and soft tissues about the eyes due to the high venous pressure that accompanies paroxysms. Occasionally, hemorrhage from the tracheobronchial tract may accompany or follow the paroxysm; usually these hemorrhagic episodes do not cause serious complications or marked blood loss. Rarely, intracranial hemorrhage may occur, causing neurologic damage, but the symptoms and signs of intracranial hemorrhage commonly resolve during the decline of the paroxysmal stage. Otitis media and purulent pneumonia were once recognized as important and frequent complications. The use of antibiotics to eradicate *B. pertussis* from the tracheobronchial tree is probably responsible for the disappearance of these complications. Other mechanical complications include anal prolapse, hernia, and trauma to the frenulum of the tongue (Zamora et al., 1962).

## GEOGRAPHIC VARIATION

Before the great increase in international travel, isolated populations such as those in the Faroe Islands and Iceland responded to the introduction of pertussis with isolated epidemics that occurred at intervals of five to seven years, with no cases between epidemics. All susceptibles were infected within a moderate period of time (usually about one year), and the infection disappeared until a new generation of susceptibles appeared and pertussis was reintroduced. With the new ease of movement within urban societies and across international boundaries, the characteristics of the epidemics have changed to that of waves that occur on a base of relative subepidemic or endemic infection. Thus, it is likely that cases will occur throughout a given outbreak period with relative frequency, then subside to a lower endemic frequency and recur seasonally each year.

In most recent outbreaks in the United States, the great majority of cases have occurred in children under 5 years of age, and more than 50 per cent have occurred in infants less than 1 year of age. In other countries in which general immunization is practiced, most cases also occur within the first 10 years of life, and the majority within the first 5 years. The morbidity rate (cases reported per 100,000 population) has continued to decline throughout most of the world; in the United States, it had declined to 4.2 cases per 100,000 population by 1970. In other countries in which immunization is the rule, the morbidity rate is also declining. However, it still reaches more than 80 per 100,000 population in some countries. These differences probably relate to the percentage of susceptibles that are vaccinated and to the reliability of the vaccines. In countries yet to establish effective vaccine programs, the morbidity rate varies from 100 to 500 per 100,000 population.

The mortality rate among immunized and unimmunized populations has continued to decline more rapidly than the morbidity rate. The decline in mortality is probably related to adequate nutrition, the literacy rate, and the accessibility of medical care for acute cases. The case-fatality ratio in the United States for all cases fell to 0.3 per cent or less during the 1960s and may be below 0.1 per cent in the 1970s. In some countries in continental Europe, England, and Scandinavia, mortality has reached a nadir, with no calculable rate. Thus, various factors have provided satisfactory solutions to the problems of mortality in those countries. The incidence of disease may not decline further until more effective means of inducing and maintaining immunity are found. In contrast, in Central America the case-fatality rate was 18 per cent in the 1960s, and it continues to be high in other countries in which the populations are predominantly rural, the literacy rates are low, and access to emergency medical care is limited.

## DIAGNOSIS

It is easy to make a clinical diagnosis of pertussis in an infant or young child who presents in the paroxysmal stage with an antecedent history that is compatible with the catarrhal stage. Other causes of paroxysmal cough must be considered, however.

The differential diagnosis includes other infections that give rise to tracheobronchial lymphadenopathy, a foreign body in the bronchial airway, necrotizing bronchiolitis caused by adenovirus, interstitial pneumonitis caused by respiratory syncytial virus, parainfluenza virus, and *H. influenzae* Type B bronchitis; any of these may cause a cough of paroxysmal nature. Some of the viral infections result in frequent vomiting with the paroxysms. Both *B. parapertussis* and *B. bronchiseptica* infections may cause a mild clinical syndrome (parapertussis) that is indistinguishable from mild to moderate pertussis. Recently, adenoviruses have been isolated from a pertussis syndrome in patients without other demonstrable infectious agents.

The specific diagnosis of pertussis is established by isolating the bacillus from the nasopharynx or identifying it in smears of the nasopharynx by immunofluorescence techniques. The medium and the principles that are important in the isolation and identification of *B. pertussis* were originally described by Bordet and Gengou. Bordet-Gengou (B-G) culture medium, with minor modifications, is still the preferred medium. Commercial preparations from which a final complete medium is prepared are usually satisfactory. If properly prepared, adequately stored, and appropriately used, B-G medium will result in frequent isolations of *B. pertussis* from nasopharyngeal swabs of individuals with clinical disease (Miller et al., 1943). The isolation rate depends upon a concentration of whole blood in the final medium higher than that usually utilized in diagnostic bacteriology. For that reason, 20 to 30 per cent whole, defibrinated sheep blood is incorporated into appropriately prepared Bordet-Gengou medium. The medium may be stored in sealed plastic sleeves for two weeks or longer. The agar surface should be glistening, moist, and cherry-red.

After inoculation with material from nasopharyngeal swabs, B-G plates should be incubated in a humidified environment at 35° C for five to seven days. Minute, milky-white, convex colonies may be found as early as 72 hours or as late as five to six days. The isolation rate may be improved by inoculating two B-G plates, one containing 0.25 IU of penicillin G per milliliter of agar and the other containing no penicillin (Bradford et al., 1946). Overgrowth of nasopharyngeal microflora may be controlled by the penicillin, but some strains of *B. pertussis* are also sensitive to this concentration. Microscopic examination of a Gram stain of a single colony from the isolation plate reveals minute, lightly stained, gram-negative coccoid and ovoid bacteria. If the medium is inadequate, pleomorphism may be noted, with long rod forms mixed with coccobacillary forms. Final identification is established immunologically. Macroscopic agglutination occurs when a moderate suspension of bacteria mixed with specific immune serum against *B. pertussis*. The suspension is prepared by swabbing the surface of a plate with confluent growth and immersing the swab in several drops of saline on a glass slide or plate; diluted serum is added to the slide suspension. With slow agitation and mixing, agglutination occurs in five to ten minutes. Macroscopic agglutination firmly establishes a final identification of the *Bordetella* genus. Alternatively, a similar slide preparation of the bacilli may be air-dried and reacted with fluorescein-conjugated immune globulin specific against *B. pertussis*. Bright specific fluorescence under the ultraviolet microscope establishes the identification of *B. pertussis*. *B. pertussis* and *B. parapertussis* can be differentiated by using commercially prepared immunofluorescence reagents against each bacillus.

The immunofluorescence technique can also be used to obtain an immediate specific diagnosis by examining nasopharyngeal swabs for *B. pertussis* (Holwerda and Eldering, 1963). Nasopharyngeal swabs are used to make several smears on clean glass slides. After air-drying, the fluorescent globulin is applied to the smears and the excess stain is removed by appropriate washing. Under the ultraviolet microscope, the minute coccoid or ovoid bacteria are highly fluorescent. Properly applied, the direct immunofluorescence method results in a frequency of bacteriologic diagnosis that equals or exceeds that of the culture method. By either method, study of unimmunized cases in the paroxysmal stage of the disease should result in a specific diagnosis in 70 to 90 per cent of cases. In contact cases and immunized cases, a laboratory diagnosis is established less frequently.

Differentiation by bacteriologic characteristics is also practical. In contrast to *B. pertussis*, both *B. parapertussis* and *B. bronchiseptica* will form colonies on infusion agar, without blood, during subcultivation. *B. parapertussis* colonies have a characteristic light chocolate pigment (Bradford and Slavin, 1937), whereas *B. pertussis* colonies remain pearly white. Biochemical differences are also found among the species and may also be used in differentiation.

Some of the serologic methods used to make a retrospective diagnosis of pertussis are used in public health laboratories; none is in general use (Ross et al., 1970). The agglutination test has been the most widely applied, but it has been used most commonly to evaluate responses to immunization, not to the natural infection, since agglutinating antibody may be absent in human or animal serum that has protective antibody. Thus, after natural infections of infants, agglutinins may be present in only 30 to 50 per cent of cases, in contrast to protective antibody, which is present in 90 to 100 per cent of cases.

Recently, a simple, inexpensive gel precipitin method has been developed that demonstrates precipitating antibody against extracted *B. pertussis* antigens (Aftandelians and Connor, 1973). Between 80 and 90 per cent of patients with the clinical syndrome develop gel precipitins during convalescence; 25 to 30 per cent of immunized patients also develop these antibodies. The gel precipitin test may have application in the routine diagnosis of an infection in an unimmunized patient or in the identification of an outbreak. In the latter case, it has been found that 80 to 90 per cent of clinical cases will have precipitin antibody in convalescent serum, in contrast to 25 to 30 per cent of newborns, immunized children, and healthy adults.

## IMMUNITY

Immunity is probably conferred through a variety of host factors, but none has been identified as being of singular importance in solid protection (Pittman, 1970). Agglutinins and complement-fixing antibody correlate with the immune state when they are present in high serum concentrations after immunization or unrecognized infection, but immunity may be present in their absence. Bactericidal antibody develops after infection or immunization of animals without the development of protective antigen. Mouse-protecting antibody correlates best with protective immunity. It is considered to be present when convalescent serum protects the mouse against a lethal intracerebral infection with a mouse-virulent strain of pertussis. However, the presence of protective antibody in serum correlates with immunity only after active infection or intensive (complete) immunization. In the latter case, immunity wanes rapidly, so that adults or children who are five years of more away from the last immunizing injection, even if they have detectable mouse-protective antibody, are liable to an attack rate of 35 to 95 per cent when they are exposed in families in which there is an index case. On the other hand, naturally acquired immunity is highly effective, with an estimated recurrence rate of approximately 2 per cent. Undoubtedly, there are factors of importance other than protective antibody, and these are probably present on surface membranes as well as at the initial site of infection within the respiratory tract. Immune serum enhances phagocytosis and also contains antiadherence factors. These and other factors limit or control the loci of early infection. When inflammation develops at the site of infection on the respiratory membranes, the organisms may also be exposed to immune serum containing protective antibody and the complement-dependent bactericidal antibody. Much work is still required to define clearly the mechanisms of immunity to pertussis.

## TREATMENT

Small infants with frequent, severe paroxysms, especially if complicated by post-tussive exhaustion and spells of unresponsiveness, should be hospitalized for supportive care. In well-nourished, well-developed infants, the height of the paroxysmal stage may be reached and passed in a period of five to seven days, and the need for hospitalization then declines. Intravenous hydration is infrequently required. Oxygenation is usually not required because the inspiratory volume is ineffectve during a paroxysm, and the respiratory exchange is adequate between paroxysms. When seizures develop, they may be repetitive, requiring both anticonvulsive therapy and strong supportive measures. In the most severe cases in infants, transient respiratory arrest following an extensive paroxysm may require resuscitation. Endotracheal suction by direct or indirect methods is infrequently required, since compacted endobronchial mucus is usually expelled at the end of a paroxysm. However, during episodes of post-tussive cyanosis, moderate suctioning may be required to remove incompletely expelled mucus from the upper airway as well as from the trachea. Antitussive medications and heavy sedation are to be avoided.

Malnourishment may develop in severe, prolonged cases due to exhaustion, lack of intake, and frequent vomiting. Small, repetitive feedings are usually tolerated immediately after paroxysm (or after vomiting), when the cough reflex is suppressed. Likewise, a feeding may be repeated directly after the loss of the previous meal. In the hospital, strict isolation is required to reduce contact with susceptible children, visiting adults, and hospital employees.

As measured by clinical response, the benefit of

antibiotic chemotherapy has never been proved in comparison with placebo controls. However, erythromycin for five to seven days in appropriate dosage eradicates infection on the tracheobronchial membrane and reduces contact spread of the infection. Ampicillin has been recommended, but in some cases pure cultures of pertussis bacilli have been found on nasopharyngeal swabs after ampicillin therapy. Several reports show that corticosteroids modify the clinical course compared with placebo controls. Therefore, severe cases may benefit from cortisone at an appropriate pharmacologic dosage for five to seven days. Corticosteroids are not recommended for mild or moderate cases. Like antibiotics, pertussis hyperimmune globulin has not proved to be effective when used during the paroxysmal stage. Nevertheless, some physicians recommend hyperimmune globulin for severely affected infants under 6 months of age, since earlier studies reported moderate benefit.

## PROPHYLAXIS

The standard method of active immunization against pertussis utilized three primary injections of a highly concentrated suspension of killed whole *B. pertussis* organisms in a repository vehicle combined with diphtheria and tetanus toxoids (DPT) (Felton, 1957). Slow absorption from the repository injection site provides an adjuvant effect on the immune response; thus, the combined form of immunization against the three diseases is preferable to injections of solitary antigens. Since there is no effective immunity against pertussis in the newborn period, immunization is started as soon as the immune response mounted by the infant is adequate to provide protection. For this reason, the primary injection series usually begins at 2 to 3 months of age and is completed by 4 to 5 months of age. Immunity against pertussis is not developed until some time after the second injection; the magnitude of protection is extended by the third injection. In order to extend protection further, a booster is given at 1 year of age and is repeated one or two times before school age. Studies of fully immunized children who have had intimate contact with the naturally occurring disease (Preston, 1972) and other studies indicate that 12 to 50 per cent of immunized children may develop pertussis. The greatest protection is observed during the first 36 months after completion of the series or after a booster. Immunity wanes remarkably after three years. Lambert's study of an epidemic in Kent County, Michigan, indicated that seven years after the last immunization the attack rate was

47 per cent. After 12 years or more, the rate was 95 per cent among contacts exposed to index cases in families (Lambert, 1965).

Up to 25 per cent of infants receiving second or third injections of DPT vaccine may have a local or systemic response, or both, consisting of swelling and tenderness at the injection site and moderate fever beginning 12 to 24 hours after the injection and declining sharply within 24 hours. Earlier in the vaccine era, evidence of encephalitis following second or third injections of DPT in infants was seen with a frequency of 1 case per 200,000 vaccine doses; however, this complication is now rare (1 case in 1 million doses in the United States). Latest statistics comparing the morbidity of immunization with the morbidity of disease continue to demonstrate the benefit of general immunization against pertussis.

Another type of pertussis vaccine is commercially available; it contains a soluble protective antigen derived from *B. pertussis* combined with diphtheria and tetanus toxoids. This vaccine also induces mouse-protective antibody and agglutinins in recipients, but its protective value has not been compared in the field with that of standard killed bacillary vaccine.

A booster injection may reestablish immunity in a previously immunized family contact, but active immunization during the incubation period or during active disease is neither effective nor desirable. The effectiveness of commercially prepared hyperimmune globulin for preventing pertussis in contacts has not been proved. However, it is sometimes used for attempted prophylaxis, particularly in small infants for whom the risk of moderate or severe morbidity is high. Chemoprophylaxis should be attempted in infant or child contacts, preferably with erythromycin for five to seven days. If the disease does not develop after the full incubation period, the exposed individual should then be immunized appropriately. Disease in exposed adults is usually moderate, and it may be either mild or uncharacteristic. Since the attack rate is very high in adults of families with index cases, it may be appropriate in the future to consider prophylactic treatment and immunization of the older age group as well as infants and children.

## PERTUSSIS SYNDROME

Pertussis syndrome is the name given to a syndrome that is clinically indistinguishable from pertussis but in which no evidence of infection with *B. pertussis* or *B. parapertussis* can be detected, while evidence of other infectious agents, including viruses, can be demonstrated

(Olson et al., 1964; Nelson et al., 1975). Pertussis syndrome is a relatively new term. It first occurred in the 1960s and has been frequently used in the last ten years. *Adenoviruses* are the infectious agents most frequently associated with the pertussis syndrome; Types 1, 2, 3, 5, and 6 have been isolated from nasopharyngeal and pharyngeal swabs, and some of these serotypes have been isolated from the urine and stools of patients during the paroxysmal stage (Connor, 1970). Likewise, rises in viral antibody have been demonstrated in the convalescent serum. Evidence of adenoviral infection in infants and children with the syndrome exceeds the combined rate of viral isolation and serologic titer rise in a matched control population, indicating a strong association between the viral infection and the disease. However, there is a parodox involved; among those patients in whom a bacteriologic diagnosis of pertussis infection can be established, there is also a marked increase in the relative frequency of adenoviral infection. In addition, the frequency of pertussis antibody rises in those with demonstrable viral infection is high, a further indication of an association between the viral infection and infection with pertussis bacilli. Recent reports (Collier et al., 1966) correlate with observations made earlier in the century by pathologists who frequently found intranuclear inclusions in the lungs of patients dying of pertussis (McCordock and Smith, 1934). To date, no proof exists of a solitary viral infection causing the typical pertussis syndrome, since primates infected with adenoviruses or filtered secretions of patients fail to develop a pertussis syndrome. Neither is there enough evidence to date to exclude adenoviruses as the causes of endemic or sporadic cases. It is clear that the relative frequency of adenoviral infection among bacteriologically proven cases is very high. In the combined infection, it is yet to be determined whether the viral infection is reactivated from a latent state or whether host susceptibility for one or the other is enhanced by the primary agent.

## *PARAPERTUSSIS*

Parapertussis is an acute disease of the respiratory tract caused by infection with *B. parapertussis* (Miller et al., 1941). The characteristics of the clinical syndrome are indistinguishable from those of a mild or moderate case of pertussis. During an outbreak, the diagnosis is evident clinically in only 5 per cent of infected persons. *B. parapertussis* organisms are coccobacillary, gram-negative, nonmotile bacilli that are usually indistinguishable from *B. pertussis* on primary isolation. They were first described by Eldering and Kendrick in the United States in 1937 and later during the same year by Bradford and Slavin, who called attention to pigment changes that are useful in the laboratory differentiation of *B. parapertussis* and *B. pertussis*. On Bordet-Gengou medium, *B. parapertussis* grows more rapidly than *B. pertussis*. Otherwise, the colonies may be identical until a pigment change occurs that lends a light chocolate hue to the colonies of the parapertussis bacilli. Transfer to regular infusion agar can usually be accomplished from the isolation plate, which quickly distinguishes it from *B. pertussis*. *B. parapertussis* shares antigens (agglutinogens) with both *B. pertussis* and *B. bronchiseptica* and reacts lightly with immunofluorescent serum against *B. pertussis* owing to common antigen or antigens.

The incidence of parapertussis is estimated to be 2 to 10 per cent that of pertussis (Eldering and Kendrick, 1952). In Denmark, parapertussis occurs in four-year cycles. A distinct wave or outbreak rising above the endemic level of disease in urban environments occurs between pertussis outbreaks (Lautrop, 1971). As with pertussis, it is assumed that the most contagious period is during the catarrhal stage, before the onset of paroxysms. Single cases can be moderately severe, but the infection is usually mild. Mortality is certainly rare; however, fatal cases have been reported in which *B. parapertussis* was isolated from the trachea at postmortem examination (Zuelzer and Wheeler, 1946). Most cases are unrecognized, even during an outbreak, because the clinical course is mild compared to pertussis. More severe cases are often misdiagnosed as pertussis. It is presumed that the infection proceeds in the same manner as pertussis, but it is more difficult to distinguish clearly separate stages because the total period of the clinical disease is usually shorter and the severity less than in pertussis. However, when paroxysms develop they are characteristic of pertussis, and typical whoops may be heard.

The pathology of parapertussis in the human has not been well described because of the mildness of the disease. In animals, mononuclear cell inflammation surrounding and within bronchi and bronchioles closely resembles the pathologic pattern seen in pertussis. There is no cross-immunity between parapertussis and pertussis. As with pertussis, immunity following disease is solid, and a second attack is rare. Immunization against pertussis does not protect against parapertussis. The disease is not preventable by any currently available means. Treatment is usually not required, although supportive care may be justified in moderately severe cases.

## References

*Pertussis*

Aftandelians, R., and Connor, J. D.: Immunologic studies of pertussis. Development of precipitins. J Pediatr 83:206, 1973.
Barnhard, H. J., and Kniker, W. T.: Roentgen findings in pertussis. Am J Roentgenol Radium Ther Nucl Med 84:445, 1960.
Bradford, W. L., Day, E., and Bery, G. P.: Improvement of the nasopharyngeal swab method of diagnosis in pertussis by the use of penicillin. Am J Public Health 36:468, 1946.
Brooksaler, F., and Nelson, J. D.: A re-appraisal and report of 190 confirmed cases. Am J Dis Child 114:389, 1967.
Buchanan, T. M., and Broohn, G. F.: Pertussis in the US. J Infect Dis 122.129, 1970.
Eldering, G., Hornbeck, C., and Baker, J.: Serological study of *Bordetella pertussis* and related species. J Bacteriol 74.133, 1957.
Felton, H. M.: Pertussis: Current status of prevention and treatment. Pediatr Clin North Am 4:271, 1957.
Holwerda, J., and Eldering, G. D.: Culture and fluorescent antibody methods in the diagnosis of whooping cough. J Bacteriol 86:449, 1963.
Ipsen, J., and Bowen, H. E., Whooping cough trends in age-specific attack rates. Am J Public Health, 45:312, 1955.
Kurt, T. L., Yeager, A. S., Guerette, S., and Dunlop, S.: Spread of pertussis by hospital staff. JAMA 221:264, 1972.
Lambert, H. J.: Epidemiology of a small pertussis outbreak in Kent County, Michigan. Pub Health Rep 80:365, 1965.
Miller, J. J., Jr., Leach, C. W., Saito, R. M., et al.: Comparison of the nasopharyngeal swab and the cough plate in the diagnosis of whooping cough and *Hemophilus* pertussis carriers. Am J Public Health 33:839, 1943.
Munoz, J. J.: Symposium on relationship of structure of microorganisms to the immunological properties. I. Immunological and other biological activities of *Bordetella pertussis* antigens. Bacterial Rev 27:325, 1963.
Pittman, M.: *Bordetella pertussis* — bacterial and host factors in the pathogenesis and prevention of whooping cough. In Mudd, S. (ed.): Infectious Agents and Host Reactions. Philadelphia, W. B. Saunders Company, 1970, p. 239.
Preston, N. W., and Stanbridge, T. N.: Efficacy of pertussis vaccines: A brighter horizon. Br Med J 3:448, 1972.
Ross, C. A., Calder, M. C., Cruickshank, R., et al.: Diagnosis of whooping cough: Comparison of serological tests with isolation of *Bordetella pertussis*. A combined Scottish study. Br Med J 4:637, 1970.
Welsh, J. D., Denny, W. F., and Bird, R. M.: The incidence and significance of the leukemoid reaction in patients hospitalized with pertussis. South Med J 52:643, 1959.
White, R., Finberg, L., and Tramer, A.: The modern morbidity of pertussis in infants. Pediatrics 33:705, 1964.
Zamora, A. F., Chiozza, A., and Alonso, A. T.: Complications of whooping cough in 500 cases. Rev Assoc Med Argent 76:121, 1962.

*Pertussis Syndrome*

Collier, A. M., Connor, J. D., and Irving, W. R., Jr.: Generalized Type 5 adenovirus infection associated with the pertussis syndrome. J Pediatr 69:1073, 1966.
Connor, J. D.: Evidence for an etiological role of adenoviral infection in pertussis syndrome. N Engl J Med 283:390, 1970.
McCordock, H. A., and Smith, M. G.: Intranuclear inclusions: Incidence and possible significance in whooping cough and in a variety of other conditions. Am J Dis Child 47:771, 1934.
Nelson, K. F., Gavitt, F., Batt, M. D., et al.: The role of adenoviruses in the pertussis syndrome. J Pediatr 86:335, 1975.
Olson, L. D., Miller, G., and Hanshaw, J. B.: Acute infectious lymphocytosis presenting as a pertussis-like illness; its association with adenovirus Type 12. Lancet 1:200, 1964.

*Parapertussis*

Bradford, W. L., and Slavin, B.: An organism resembling *Hemophilus pertussis*: With special reference to color changes produced by its growth upon certain media. Am J Public Health 27:1277, 1937.
Bradford, W. L., and Slavin, B.: Parapertussis. Lancet 75:232, 1955.
Eldering, G., and Kendrick, P. L.: Incidence of parapertussis in Grand Rapids area as indicated by 16 years' experience with diagnostic culture. Am J Public Health 42:27, 1952.
Lautrop, H.: Epidemics of parapertussis. Lancet 1:1195, 1971.
Miller, J. J., Jr., Saito, T. M., and Silverberg, R. J.: Parapertussis: Clinical and serological observations. J Pediatr 19:229, 1941.
Zuelzer, W. W., and Wheeler, W. E.: Parapertussis pneumonia. Report of two fatal cases. J Pediatr 29:493, 1946.

# B PLEUROPULMONARY INFECTIONS

# 105 *COMMON PNEUMONIAS DUE TO PYOGENIC COCCI*

*W. G. Johanson, Jr., M.D.*
*Junji H. Higuchi, M.D.*

## DEFINITION

Bacterial pneumonia is an inflammatory process of the lung characterized by alveolar consolidation due to the presence of pathogenic bacteria. It is almost always acute and abrupt in onset.

## ETIOLOGY

The "pyogenic cocci," *Streptococcus pneumoniae* (pneumococcus), *Streptococcus hemolyticus*, and *Staphylococcus aureus*, are the most common etiologic agents of bacterial pneumonia. The pneumococcus is by far the most important, causing perhaps 80 per cent of all bacterial pneumonias. Of the many types of pneumococci (over 80), only 14 capsular types (1, 2, 3, 4, 6, 8, 9, 12, 14, 19, 23, 25, 51, and 56) are responsible for about 80 per cent of bacteremic pneumococcal pneumonias (Center for Disease Control, 1978), a fact that makes preventive vaccination against pneumococcal infection feasible.

# PNEUMOCOCCAL PNEUMONIA

## *PATHOGENESIS AND PATHOLOGY*

Pneumococci enter the body via the respiratory tract. Although 30 to 40 per cent of healthy persons may harbor pneumococci in their upper respiratory secretions, such carrier organisms are usually not the capsular types that produce pneumonia. Highly virulent strains are passed from person to person, including both asymptomatic carriers and persons with evident infection. Nonhuman reservoirs of the organism are not important in the epidemiology of human pneumococcal infections. Whether transmission among humans occurs by airborne means or by personal contact is not settled; however, pneumococcal pneumonia is probably due not to direct inhalation of the organism into the lungs but to aspiration of upper respiratory secretions. Several observations support this view. The lung possesses remarkably effective defenses against airborne bacteria (Green, 1970). Large ($>10 \mu$m) airborne particles impinge on the mucosa of the upper respiratory tract by inertial impaction, are carried to the oropharynx by ciliary action, and are swallowed. Smaller particles may land on ciliated airways; the cross-section of the branching airway system expands markedly so that flow becomes progressively slower as inhaled particles pass into the airways, causing them to be deposited by gravitational settling. Particles that land on ciliated airways are rapidly removed by ciliary action; the time needed for removal depends on the site of deposition but may be as rapid as 30 minutes for particles deposited in major airways. Particles that reach the alveolar spaces are cleared from the lung much more slowly, and, in the case of infectious agents, phagocytosis and in situ killing of the organisms become the critical elements of host defense. The alveolar macrophage normally performs this function without the participation of either polymorphonuclear leukocytes or serum factors. This process is so efficient that normal lungs contain no bacteria and few or no PMNs, despite the daily inhalation and aspiration of infectious agents. Early investigators were unable to cause pneumonia in normal experimental animals by exposing them to airborne bacteria despite demonstrated deposition of organisms in the lungs. Infection could be produced only if the animals were manipulated, for example, by the administration of alcohol. More recent studies using quantitative bacteriologic techniques have shown that most bacterial species, including the pyogenic cocci, are rapidly killed in the lungs of normal animals following exposure to contaminated aerosols and that an initial inoculum of as many as $10^5$ bacteria causes no disease.

In contrast to the lower airways, organisms are present in enormous numbers in upper respiratory secretions. Saliva may contain $10^8$ to $10^9$ aerobic bacteria per ml. Bacteria that persist following inoculation into the upper respiratory tract multiply and may subsequently gain access to the lungs via aspiration; even normal persons have been shown to aspirate oropharyngeal secretions during sleep (Huxley et al., 1978). Aspiration of only small quantities can infect the lung. As little as 0.01 ml would deliver a large bacterial load to a small region of lung, in contrast to the diffuse deposition that occurs with airborne organisms. Pneumococci implanted in the noses of experimental animals reach the lungs within a few minutes, and pneumonia can be readily produced in experimental animals by an inoculum of $10^4$ pneumococci delivered in a small fluid bolus into the airways.

These experimental observations illustrate several important features of the pathogenesis of pneumococcal pneumonia. First, pneumococcal pneumonia is uncommon among healthy people; at least 75 per cent of patients with pneumococcal pneumonia have underlying diseases (Sullivan et al., 1972). Second, pneumonia is likely to occur in people who handle upper respiratory secretions poorly, owing to either increased volume of secretions as with viral infection or impaired laryngeal reflexes during sleep or coma. Third, pneumonia is likely to occur in patients whose pulmonary antibacterial defenses are impaired, as in patients with chronic obstructive lung disease or congestive heart failure (Winterbauer et al., 1969).

Pneumococcal pneumonia develops in the absence of swift phagocytosis of organisms on the alveolar surface. The pneumonic process is initiated by bacterial multiplication and an outpouring of protein-rich edematous fluid and erythrocytes into alveolar spaces secondary to increased permeability of the alveolocapillary membrane. Edema is followed by an influx of neutrophils that phagocytose bacteria and eventually fill the alveolar spaces. Pneumococcal pneumonia is thus a spreading process characterized by capillary congestion, alveolar hemorrhage, edema, and rapid bacterial proliferation at the leading edge ("red hepatization"), and dense consolidation due to leukocytes and organizing exudates ("gray hepatization") at the center. Pneumococci invade the pulmonary lymphatics early, presumably in the edematous regions; bacteremia occurs when the hilar lymph nodes do not remove enough bacteria from the lymph draining the lung.

The inflammatory process spreads from acinus to acinus via the pores of Kohn and from lobe to lobe by spilling of contaminated materials into the airways. Its progress tends to be checked by the pleura or its interlobular extensions, although involvement of the pleura itself may cause pleural effusion. Empyema results if organisms pass through the pleura.

Despite the intense inflammation and the enormous number of bacteria present, necrosis of lung tissue rarely occurs in pneumococcal pneumonia. Healing is initiated by an influx of macrophages, probably derived in large part from circulating blood monocytes. These cells ingest alveolar debris, consisting of dead organisms and PMNs, strands of fibrin, and erythrocytes, and the architecture of the lung is preserved. Normal function returns within a few weeks. The lack of tissue destruction is apparently due to two factors. Pneumococci, with the possible exception of type 3, do not possess necrotizing extracellular enzymes. Destruction of lung tissue by leukocytic proteases is apparently prevented by the abundant exudation of plasma, containing the protease inhibitors alpha-1-antitrypsin and alpha-2-macroglobulin, into the lung.

## CLINICAL MANIFESTATIONS

Most patients report symptoms of rhinorrhea, pharyngitis, and cough for several days before the onset of pneumococcal pneumonia. Although these symptoms suggest a preceding viral illness, proof of this association has been scanty except in the case of influenza A. These prodromal symptoms are overshadowed by the abrupt occurrence of fever, typically 102° F, pleuritic chest pain, and at least one shaking chill. Repeated rigors are uncommon in pneumococcal pneumonia and sug-

gest another bacterial cause. Cough may intensify, although sputum production is frequently scant in the first few days. The sputum is typically "rusty" in color due to alveolar hemorrhage. The severity of these symptoms and the accompanying prostration cause most patients to seek medical attention within 48 hours of onset. In elderly patients, the presenting complaints may include only fever and depressed consciousness. In patients with chronic heart or lung disease, the principal symptom may be only worsening dyspnea, although signs of infection can also be found.

On physical examination the patient is warm to touch, perspiring, tachycardic, and tachypneic. Cool vasoconstricted skin, with or without hypotension, is a manifestation of impending cardiovascular collapse and is an ominous sign. The signs of pneumonia will vary with its stage. The earliest sign consists of fine, inspiratory crackles (rales) that appear before consolidation is evident by x-ray or by auscultation as altered breath sounds with increased transmission of tracheal sounds to the chest wall. The intensity of the breath sounds may be increased, normal, or decreased. Over consolidated lung served by a patent bronchus, breath sounds are "tubular." In tubular breathing, the inspiratory and expiratory phases are nearly equal in intensity, mimicking the breath sounds heard normally over the trachea. Breath sounds are normally tubular over the interscapular portion of the chest, especially in thin persons and in people with narrow anteroposterior thoraces. Altered transmission of sound to the chest wall should be sought with several techniques. Increased transmission of the whispered voice ("whispered pectoriloquy") is easiest for most examiners to appreciate and is elicited by having the patient whisper "one, two, three." Increased tactile fremitus can be detected by placing the palm over the consolidated area while the patient says loudly "ninety-nine." "Egophony," or the "E to A" sign, is more difficult to detect, although it is striking when present. Each sign depends upon the presence of two factors: consolidated lung and a patent bronchus in the immediate vicinity. Dullness on percussion will be present if the volume of consolidated lung is sufficient and is adjacent to the region of chest wall being percussed. The major value of percussion and examination for fremitus is detection of the flatness and diminished fremitus of pleural effusion. It is important to remember that bronchial obstruction with distal pneumonia or atelectasis may produce exactly the same signs as a pleural effusion.

During treatment, fine rales may disappear while signs of consolidation increase. This stage is followed by the appearance of coarse rales and even rhonchi, usually associated with abundant sputum production as the alveolar process begins to resolve.

Dense consolidation extending from one pleural surface to another, the pattern of lobar consolidation, is distinctly uncommon on radiography. Most often the areas of increased roentgenographic density are patchy and frequently multiple, with lack of respect for segmental boundaries. An air bronchogram is usually present, a finding that confirms that the abnormal shadow is due to consolidation, at least in part. With preexisting lung disease, especially emphysema, the pattern of radiographic abnormality may be markedly altered, varying from multiple cavitary infiltrates to poorly defined, hazy peribronchial densities (Ziskind et al., 1970). Pleural effusions, usually small, are present in 10 per cent of patients with pneumococcal pneumonia at the time of initial presentation.

The blood leukocyte count is most often 15,000 to 30,000 per mm³, although very high or very low values may be found; either extreme augurs a poorer prognosis. Regardless of the total count, an increased percentage of PMNs is immature. The BUN may be slightly elevated, usually due to prerenal factors. A BUN of more than 50 mg/100 ml has been associated with a lower rate of survival in patients with pneumococcal pneumonia. Evidence of glomerulitis, including protein, casts, and erythrocytes in the urine, is uncommon. These findings are usually transient and appear to be caused by circulating pneumococcal capsular material, possibly complexed to immunoglobulin. Jaundice may occur as a result of hepatocellular damage or hemolysis, the latter particularly in G-6-PD-deficient patients.

Arterial blood gas analysis is an important facet of the evaluation of many patients with pneumococcal pneumonia. Cyanosis is unreliable, and its apparent absence should not dissuade the examiner from obtaining arterial blood for study. Patients with extensive disease, respiratory distress, compromised cardiopulmonary function, or an altered mental state should have such studies. Patients with pneumonia are typically hypoxemic with hypocarbia and acute respiratory alkalosis. The degree of hypoxemia does not correlate well with the extent of disease as judged radiographically in that some patients with apparently small and usually scattered infiltrates will be severely hypoxemic. The mechanism of hypoxemia is the continued perfusion of regions of lung in which ventilation has been impaired by alveolar filling. This abnormality leads to regions with low ventilation-to-perfusion ratios and intrapulmonary shunts; to the extent that the latter is responsible, the arterial oxygen tension will fail to rise with supplemental oxygen therapy. Hypocarbia and respiratory alkalosis are due to tachypnea and increased alveolar ventilation.

## DIAGNOSIS

The diagnosis of pneumococcal pneumonia depends on the establishment of two facts: that the patient's symptoms are the result of pneumonia and that the pneumonia is due to the pneumococcus. The former is usually straightforward, while the latter finding is frequently difficult to establish with certainty. Purulent sputum and a radiographic infiltrate are found in conjunction with an appropriate history and physical findings. Common sense will help sort out most of the more difficult problems in differential diagnosis. For example, patients with congestive heart failure may have infiltrates, leukocytosis, and perhaps even low-grade fever, but they certainly do not have chills or purulent sputum unless a complicating infection is present.

Confirmation of the etiologic role of the pneumococcus in pneumonia may require examination of several types of specimens. By far the most valuable specimen for culture is the blood, because contaminating organisms are not present and the results can be readily interpreted. About one third of patients with pneumococcal pneumonia have demonstrable bacteremia (Austrian and Gold, 1964; Tilghman and Finland, 1937). Since a similar fraction of patients with other common bacterial pneumonias are bacteremic, blood cultures should be obtained on all patients suspected of having bacterial pneumonia. Pleural fluid is present in few patients with pneumococcal pneumonia on admission, but the organism can be demonstrated in about one half of such fluids. Since the presence of pleural fluid strongly suggests other bacterial causes for the pneumonia, specimens of such fluid should always be obtained and examined by stain and culture before therapy is instituted.

Cultures of expectorated nasopharyngeal sputum and swabs may be seriously misleading in the evaluation of patients with pneumococcal pneumonia because many sputum or pharyngeal cultures contain other bacteria than pneumococcus. Further, since pneumococci can be recovered from sputum in at least 30 per cent of patients without pneumonia, its presence in sputum does not confirm the diagnosis of pneumococcal pneumonia (Barrett-Connor, 1971). Microscopic examination of Gram-stained, expectorated sputum is more useful than culture in establishing the diagnosis of pneumococcal pneumonia (Heineman et al., 1977). The cellular content of the smear should be determined first, since specimens that contain numerous squamous epithelial cells are not representative of lower respiratory tract flora. The finding of typical lancet-shaped, encapsulated, gram-positive diplococci in association with macrophages or PMNs and in the absence of other bacteria strongly supports the diagnosis.

A technique devised to minimize contamination by the oropharyngeal flora is transtracheal aspiration, in which a specimen is collected via a catheter passed through the cricothyroid membrane into the trachea. This technique increases the yield of pneumococci from patients with pneumonia and tends to reduce the number of contaminating agents. False-positive cultures are obtained in 20 to 30 per cent of patients, but false-negative results occur in less than 1 per cent of patients in the absence of antimicrobial therapy (Bartlett, 1977). In chronic lung disease with persistent colonization of the lower airways, the specificity of transtracheal aspirates is diminished. Complications of the procedure, consisting principally of hemorrhage and subcutaneous emphysema, are infrequent, but fatalities have occurred. Transtracheal aspiration should not be performed in small children, in patients with hemorrhagic diathesis, or in uncooperative patients. Performed carefully by experienced personnel, this technique may provide valuable diagnostic information in patients with pneumonia.

Specimens for smear and culture may be obtained from the distal lung by bronchoscopy, using either flexible or rigid instruments. The former are better tolerated by acutely ill patients and allow sampling of more peripheral regions under direct vision. Unless special precautions are taken, bronchoscopically obtained specimens are routinely contaminated by oropharyngeal organisms. However, it is possible to collect secretions with sterile bronchial brushes that are protected from contamination during introduction by encasement within a sterile catheter. This procedure is useful in patients with complicated pneumonias or in whom the diagnosis is uncertain and unlikely to be resolved by simpler techniques.

Material may be aspirated directly from the lung with a thin (20-gauge) needle inserted through the chest wall. Although the needle track crosses the pleural space, empyema following transthoracic aspiration of pneumonia is exceedingly uncommon. Pneumothorax occurs in 5 to 22 per cent of patients but rarely requires treatment. This procedure has been used widely in children but relatively infrequently in adult patients. The rate of false-negative results is reported to range from 16 to 28 per cent. Transthoracic aspiration of the lung is probably underutilized as a technique of obtaining diagnostic material in patients with pneumonia and may be especially useful when fiberoptic bronchoscopy is not readily available. However, the procedure should not be performed by inexperienced operators or when complete resuscitative support is not available.

To summarize the foregoing, the diagnosis of pneumococcal pneumonia is assured when pneumococci are recovered from the blood, pleural fluid, or transthoracic lung aspirate. Isolation from a sterile swabbing of the involved lung segment or from a transtracheal aspirate is strong supporting evidence, while isolation of pneumococci from culture of expectorated sputum has less diagnostic value, although it may support a diagnosis of pneumococcal pneumonia made on clinical grounds.

Using these bacteriologic criteria, including recovery of pneumococci from expectorated sputum in conjunction with an illness and response to therapy that are compatible with pneumococcal pneumonia, recent investigators have found that S. pneumoniae is responsible for 60 to 70 per cent of bacterial pneumonias among adults (Dorff et al., 1973; Sullivan et al., 1972). If patients are included in whom no bacterial agent was recovered but who responded to penicillin therapy, the proportion of adult pneumonias that are probably due to pneumococci approaches 80 per cent.

## DIFFERENTIAL DIAGNOSIS

Both infectious and noninfectious processes must be considered in the differential diagnosis of fever and infiltration of the lung. Pneumonias caused by other pyogenic cocci or by aerobic bacilli may closely mimic pneumococcal pneumonia clinically, and their differentiation depends largely on bacteriologic findings. Lung abscess due to anaerobic bacteria may simulate pneumococcal pneumonia, although the typical illness associated with abscess formation is subacute and protracted; cavitation is rare with pneumococcal infection, and putrid sputum does not occur. Mycoplasma pneumonia is usually associated with a prominent cough, but sputum production is scanty and organisms are infrequent in tracheobronchial secretions; typically, patients with mycoplasmal infection complain of headache, myalgias, and malaise for several days, while the patient with pneumococcal pneumonia experiences an abrupt onset of fever, cough, and sputum production.

Pulmonary embolism may cause difficulty in differential diagnosis. Such patients rarely have temperatures exceeding 101° F or leukocyte counts over 12,000/mm³. Arterial blood gases show similar changes in pneumonia and embolism, namely, hypoxemia and hypocarbia. The hemoptysis of pneumococcal pneumonia usually consists of rusty sputum or streaks of blood within purulent sputum, whereas that associated with embolism is often gross blood without purulent sputum. However, in some patients, the distinction between pulmonary embolism and pneumococcal pneumonia cannot be made with confidence on clinical findings alone, and additional studies are required. In most cases, a perfusion (or ventilation and perfusion) lung scan will suffice. It must be remembered that perfusion will always be diminished in the region of lung consolidation, and no useful information will be gained in this area. However, if the scan fails to demonstrate perfusion defects in other lung regions, pulmonary embolism is highly unlikely, since nearly all such patients demonstrate multiple perfusion defects.

Carcinoma of the lung may present as pneumococcal pneumonia. In some patients, associated symptoms of weight loss, hoarseness, or prior hemoptysis may suggest the proper diagnosis. In others, the chest radiograph reveals a mass lesion or hilar adenopathy that can never be attributed to pneumococcal pneumonia in an adult. In some patients, the only clue to the presence of a tumor is the failure of the pneumonic process to resolve with therapy. All patients with pneumonia should be followed until resolution is complete clinically and radiographically.

## TREATMENT

Penicillin is the treatment of choice for pneumococcal pneumonia. There is no evidence that the dose of penicillin should be titered against the severity of the pneumonia. Administration of more than 2.4 million units per day increases the incidence of superinfection, usually by gram-negative bacilli, and does not reduce the mortality or morbidity of the initial infection. For hospitalized patients, treatment should be initiated with procaine penicillin, 600,000 units intramuscularly every eight hours. Ambulatory patients can be treated with an oral penicillin such as phenoxymethyl penicillin, 250 mg every six hours. Patients who are allergic to penicillin can be effectively treated with erythromycin or clindamycin. Tetracycline is contraindicated in certain localities where as many as 25 per cent of isolates of *S. pneumoniae* have been resistant to it. Such resistance is usually found in less than 5 per cent of isolates. Antimicrobial treatment should be continued for seven days.

Unfortunately, these recommendations for therapy may need modification in the near future. Penicillin-resistant pneumococci have caused recent outbreaks of serious disease in several hospitals in South Africa (Jacobs et al., 1978) and have been isolated from humans in many parts of the world. Although the emergence of resistant strains appears to follow antibiotic usage, these strains do not produce beta-lactamase, and the mechanism of microbial resistance is unknown.

Supplemental oxygen, intravenous fluids, and analgesics for relief of pleuritic pain may also be required. Evacuation of tracheobronchial secretions is best ensured by maintaining systemic hydration, and parenteral fluids should be used if needed. Inhalation of bland aerosol mists and positive pressure breathing treatments are unnecessary in most patients but may be of benefit in patients with underlying airway obstruction and in those with an ineffective cough for other reasons. Postural drainage may assist in the evacuation of secretions from involved regions of the lung.

## COMPLICATIONS AND SEQUELAE

### Initial Complications

Shock is present in 5 to 10 per cent of patients admitted with pneumococcal pneumonia. Circulatory collapse is more likely to occur in bacteremic patients and in patients who show dense lobar consolidation radiographically. Not surprisingly, these findings are more common among patients who delay seeking medical attention for several days after the onset of symptoms. Hypotension usually responds promptly to intravenous fluids; dopamine may be used initially as a temporary measure but is usually unnecessary when the intravascular volume has been repleted with isotonic solutions. Cardiac output in patients with sepsis due to gram-positive organisms is usually high, and myocardial-stimulating drugs are not required. In patients with underlying heart disease, diffuse pulmonary infiltrates, or physical findings suggesting left ventricular failure, the treatment of shock can be undertaken safely only when left ventricular performance is monitored via a balloon catheter positioned in a pulmonary artery. Volume expansion of patients in left ventricular failure is obviously catastrophic.

Empyema is present in about 5 per cent of patients with pneumococcal pneumonia. Pleural disease should be sought as a part of the initial evaluation of all patients with pneumonia. Of the 10 per cent of patients with pneumococcal pneumonia who have effusions, half will have sterile exudates while in the others the fluid will contain organisms. The nature of these fluids varies from mild exudates to gross pus. Untreated empyemas always become grossly purulent and entrap the lung with an extensive pleural "peel" consisting of organizing proteinaceous exudate and loculated abscesses. This reaction is much more common with pleural infection due to gram-negative bacilli, hemolytic streptococci, *S. aureus*, and anaerobic bacteria but occurs following pneumococcal infection if untreated. Although penicillin in the usual doses sterilizes the pleural space, the pleural reaction may continue. Therefore, the key principle underlying treatment of pleural effusion in association with pneumonia is drainage. In the presence of pneumococcal infection, fluid that is clear or slightly turbid should be aspirated at the time of the initial thoracentesis; recurrence is usually slight in the presence of penicillin therapy. If the initial fluid is grossly purulent, chest tube drainage should be instituted promptly to prevent loculation. Young children have a greater propensity to clear extensive pleural reactions and require mechanical drainage less often.

Extrapulmonary pneumococcal infections occur rarely in patients with pneumonia and are usually evident shortly after admission. Meningitis must be considered in any patient with pneumonia who manifests depressed consciousness, stiff neck, or severe headache. Endocarditis, pericarditis, and septic arthritis are rare complications of pneumococcal pneumonia.

### Late Complications

Effusion during treatment occurs typically on the third or fourth day of illness and is associated with pleural pain and continuing fever. Thoracentesis reveals slightly turbid fluid with 5000 to 10,000 leukocytes per mm³, predominantly PMNs. The organisms cannot be seen by Gram stain or recovered in culture. Treatment consists of needle aspiration of the bulk of the fluid. Such "sterile empyemas" are by far the most common cause of persistent fevers beyond three or four days of starting penicillin therapy. Some patients present in this stage of illness, i.e., pleural effusion, chest pain, and fever, usually after having taken antimicrobial agents. Since the underlying pneumonia may no longer be readily apparent radiographically or on physical examination, the diagnosis may be obscure; examination of the pleural fluid for pneumococcal capsular polysaccharides by counterimmunoelectrophoresis may identify the cause of such parapneumonic effusions.

Lung abscess does not follow pneumococcal pneumonia, except possibly with infection due to type 3 organisms. Occasionally, air-fluid levels appear in one or more areas on the chest radio-

graph during resolution of the illness. Such cavities are usually pre-existing lesions, the result of emphysema or remote chronic infection, which have filled with fluid during the course of pneumonia. Treatment should be gauged by the patient's clinical course, and endobronchial drainage should be encouraged. No treatment may be indicated if the patient has become afebrile and is steadily improving.

Pneumococcal pneumonia should resolve completely radiographically (Jay et al., 1975). The rate of resolution is much slower in elderly patients and in those with chronic lung disease or alcoholism (Fig. 1). Consolidative changes should disappear in all patients within ten weeks; evidence of volume loss may persist somewhat longer. There is no reason, as a general rule, to follow patients with weekly radiographs after discharge from the hospital; however, all patients

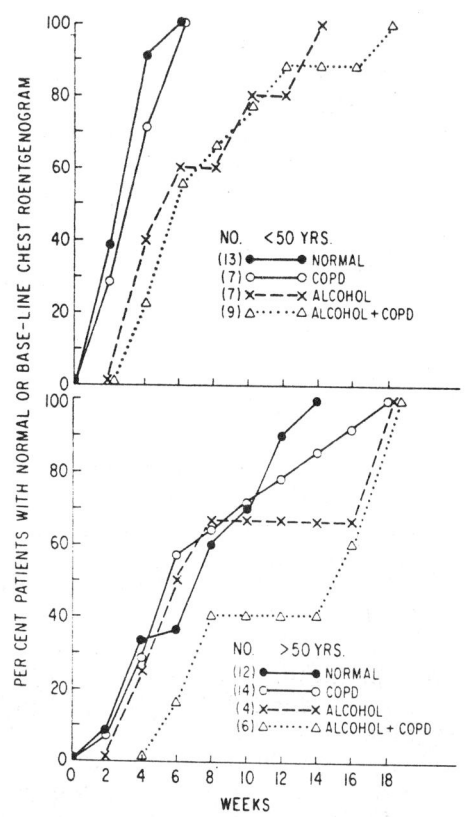

**FIGURE 1.** *Effects of age on the radiographic resolution of* Streptococcus pneumoniae *pneumonia in patients without underlying disease (normal), with chronic obstructive pulmonary disease (COPD), with acute alcoholism (Alcohol), and with both (Alcohol + COPD).*

*Note that radiographic resolution was more rapid in patients less than 50 years of age in all groups. The presence of COPD or alcoholism prolonged resolution in patients under and over 50 years of age. The presence of COPD and alcoholism resulted in markedly delayed radiographic resolution, especially in patients over 50 years of age (Jay et al., 1975).*

should have a radiograph ten weeks after discharge, and patients with persistent abnormalities should undergo more extensive evaluation to rule out bronchial obstruction or other regional lung dysfunction.

## PREVENTION

Immunization with polyvalent pneumococcal vaccines reduces the occurrence of pneumococcal disease in susceptible populations (Austrian et al., 1976). The feasibility of this approach rests on the continued demonstration that only a few of the over 80 pneumococcal types are responsible for the majority of clinical infections. A commercial vaccine contains purified capsular polysaccharides from 14 types (types 1, 2, 3, 4, 6, 8, 9, 12, 14, 19, 23, 25, 51 and 56) that account for 80 per cent of bacteremic pneumococcal infections in the United States. Immunization is recommended for patients with sickle cell anemia, azotemia, chronic cardiopulmonary disease, diabetes, liver disease, and the aged, especially those confined to institutions. Mild pain and erythema may occur at the injection site for a day.

# PNEUMONIA DUE TO STAPHYLOCOCCI

## PATHOGENESIS AND PATHOLOGY

Staphylococcal pneumonia tends to occur in three situations: following epidemic influenza, among hospitalized patients, and in persons who inject unsterile materials into their veins. In the first two circumstances, colonization of the upper respiratory tract by *Staphylococcus aureus* usually precedes the development of pneumonia. About one third of healthy adults harbor *S. aureus* in their upper respiratory tracts; the anterior nares is the most common site, but the organism is frequently present in the posterior pharynx as well. In experimental animals, influenza causes a marked impairment in the ability of lung defenses to inactivate *S. aureus*. In this setting *S. aureus* presumably proliferates in the virus-injured upper tract and enters the lung, and pneumonia results. Among hospitalized patients, colonization may occur with nosocomial strains of *S. aureus* acquired from personnel who are nasal carriers or from other patients via the hands of hospital personnel. Staphylococcal pneumonia occurs principally in certain high-risk groups of hospitalized patients including newborn infants and postoperative patients. The injection of unsterile materials intravenously allows *S. aureus* to enter the bloodstream.

The sequence of events in the lungs during staphylococcal pneumonia has not been studied closely. Specimens observed at autopsy show confluent areas of consolidation characterized by intense PMN infiltration, edema, and hemorrhage. Clumps of cocci are demonstrable by special stains. Tissue necrosis and the formation of abscesses ranging in size from microscopic foci to enormous cavities are regular features. Airways may be occluded by accumulation of sloughed epithelium, inflammatory exudate, and mucus.

## CLINICAL MANIFESTATIONS

Staphylococcal pneumonia usually starts with shaking chills and high fever. Hematogenous staphylococcal pneumonia has characteristic radiographic features, including multiple 1 to 2 cm nodules, which undergo cavitation rapidly, and early development of pleural effusion. Pneumatoceles, which are expanding thin-walled cysts, develop rarely in adults but are common in children. Nosocomial staphylococcal pneumonia does not have distinguishing characteristics but presents with a nonspecific pulmonary infiltrate, increasing fever, leukocytosis, and purulent tracheobronchial secretions. Bacterial pneumonia complicating influenza tends to occur in two forms: as a lobar or segmental process occurring five to seven days after the onset of influenza symptoms or as a diffuse process that appears virtually concurrently with the onset of influenza (Louria et al., 1959). The diffuse form may be difficult to distinguish from viral pneumonia, and its mortality approaches 70 per cent. The mortality of localized forms of bacterial pneumonia after influenza is equal to that of similar pneumonias that occur in the absence of influenza. *S. aureus* may cause either form.

## DIAGNOSIS

As with pneumococcal pneumonia, the diagnosis of staphylococcal pneumonia depends on culture from blood, pleural fluid, or, least reliably, tracheobronchial secretions. The presence of staphylococci in Gram-stained specimens of tracheobronchial secretions in one of the above clinical settings strongly suggests the diagnosis of staphylococcal pneumonia and demands prompt treatment with an agent resistant to penicillinase. In the hematogenous form, Gram stains of cerebrospinal fluid or urine sediment also may reveal gram-positive cocci and lead to a rapid presumptive diagnosis.

### TREATMENT

Since the majority of isolates of *S. aureus* are resistant to penicillin, initial treatment should be with a penicillinase-resistant drug such as methicillin, oxacillin, or cephalothin intravenously until the patient is afebrile and stable for

five days. Parenteral or oral therapy should be continued for at least 10 to 14 days.

### COMPLICATIONS

Staphylococci pneumonia may be complicated by abscess, empyema, pyopneumothorax, and obstruction of major airways by intensely purulent exudate and sloughed epithelium. These complications occur so often that each must be considered in all patients with staphylococcal pneumonia to prevent delay of their recognition and treatment.

# PNEUMONIA DUE TO STREPTOCOCCUS (PYOGENES)

### CLINICAL

Pneumonia due to *Streptococcus pyogenes* is rare, accounting for less than 5 per cent of bacterial pneumonias, and pneumonia due to other streptococci is even less common. Streptococcal pneumonia has occurred in near-epidemic proportions as a complication of viral infection in closed populations. High rates of upper respiratory streptococcal carriage and an epidemic viral illness, usually influenza or measles, provide the necessary conditions for such an outbreak. Streptococcal pneumonia now occurs sporadically, principally among young people.

The infection starts abruptly with shaking chills, fever, and frequently pleural pain. Radiographs of the chest reveal consolidation of varying extent and, in 30 to 50 per cent of cases, pleural effusion. The tendency to cause early and frequently extensive pleural disease is the only feature that distinguishes this pneumonia from that due to the pneumococcus.

### DIAGNOSIS AND TREATMENT

Isolation of *S. pyogenes* from blood or pleural fluid establishes the diagnosis, but isolation from expectorated sputum alone is of less certain significance because this organism may be carried in the upper respiratory tracts of healthy individuals. Treatment with procaine penicillin, 600,000 units twice daily intramuscularly for seven days, is effective. Erythromycin stearate, 500 mg orally four times daily for seven days, is a suitable alternative for penicillin-sensitive patients.

The major complication is empyema, which may result in a patient with an extensive exudative pleural reaction. In adults prompt drainage of the empyema via a thoracostomy tube will usually avoid the need for later decortication; procrastination in effecting adequate drainage frequently leads to a long and complicated hospital course. Because pleural disease in children more often resolves with antibiotics and needle aspiration of the pleural space, placement of intercostal drainage tubes can be postponed.

# PNEUMONIA DUE TO NEISSERIA MENINGITIDIS

Meningococcal pneumonia occurs as an occasional consequence of meningococcemia, usually with meningitis, and as a primary pneumonia without extrathoracic disease. The latter type of pneumonia may follow influenza and perhaps

adenoviral respiratory infection (Ellenbogen et al., 1974). Meningococcal pneumonias have been documented most often in groups in which there is a high proportion of upper respiratory tract carriage of the organism, such as military populations (Irwin et al., 1975). It seems likely that the incidence of meningococcal pneumonia has been underestimated in the past, at least in certain populations. Because the meningococcus is an encapsulated organism, the pathogenesis of meningococcal pneumonia is presumably similar to that described for the pneumococcus.

## CLINICAL MANIFESTATIONS AND DIAGNOSIS

The clinical features of meningococcal pneumonia do not differentiate it from other bacterial pneumonias. The occasionally positive blood culture confirms the diagnosis. *N. meningitidis* has been difficult to recover from expectorated sputum in many reported cases, whereas transtracheal aspirates or transthoracic lung aspiration reveals the organism (Ellenbogen et al., 1974; Irwin et al., 1975). These observations suggest that the meningococcus fares poorly in competition with other organisms during cultivation on artificial media and, further, that *N. meningitidis* might be incriminated more often in pneumonia if invasive culturing techniques were employed routinely.

## TREATMENT

Procaine penicillin in a dose of 600,000 units every 12 hours for seven days is given for meningococcal pneumonia not complicated by meningitis. Chloramphenicol (500 mg orally or 1.0 g intravenously every six hours) is a suitable alternative for penicillin-sensitive individuals.

## References

Austrian, R., Douglas, R. M., Schiffman, G., Coetzee, A. M., Koornhof, H. J., Hayden-Smith, S., and Reid, R. D. W.: Prevention of pneumococcal pneumonia by vaccination. Trans Assoc Am Physicians 89:184, 1976.

Austrian, R., and Gold, J: Pneumococcal bacteremia with special reference to bacteremic pneumococcal pneumonia. Ann Intern Med 60:759, 1964.

Barrett-Connor, E.: The nonvalue of sputum culture in the diagnosis of pneumococcal pneumonia. Am Rev Resp Dis 103:845, 1971.

Bartlett, J. G.: Diagnostic accuracy of transtracheal aspiration bacteriologic studies. Am Rev Respir Dis 115:777, 1977.

Dorff, G. J., Rytel, W., Farmer, S. G., and Scanlon, G.: Etiologies and characteristic features of pneumonias in a municipal hospital. Am J Med Sci 266:349, 1973.

Ellenbogen, C., Graybill, J. R., Silva, J., Jr., and Homme, P. J.: Bacterial pneumonia complicating adenoviral pneumonia: A comparison of respiratory tract bacterial culture sources and effectiveness of chemoprophylaxis against bacterial pneumonia. Am J Med 56:169, 1974.

Green, G. M.: The Amberson Lecture: In defense of the lung. Am Rev Respir Dis 102:691, 1970.

Heineman, H. S., Chawla, J. K., and Lofton, W. M.: Misinformation from sputum cultures without microscopic examination. J Clin Microbiol 6:518, 1977.

Huxley, E. J., Viroslav, J., Gray, W. B., and Pierce, A. K.: Pharyngeal aspiration in normal adults and patients with depressed consciousness. Am J Med 64:564, 1978.

Irwin, R. S., Woelk, W. K., and Coudon, W. L., III: Primary meningococcal pneumonia. Ann Intern Med 82:493, 1975.

Jacobs, M. R., Koornhof, H. J., Robins-Browne, R. M., et al.: Emergence of multiple resistant pneumococci. N Engl J Med 299:735, 1978.

Jay, S. J., Johanson, W. G., Jr., and Pierce, A. K.: Radiographic resolution of *Streptococcus pneumoniae* pneumonia. N Engl J Med 293:798, 1975.

Louria, D. B., Blumenfeld, H. L., Ellis, J. T., et al.: Studies on influenza in the pandemic of 1957-1958. II. Pulmonary complications of influenza. J Clin Invest 38:213, 1959.

Center for Disease Control: Morbidity and Mortality Weekly Report 27 (4), January 27, 1978.

Sullivan, R. J., Jr., Dowdle, W. R., Marine, W. M., and Hierholzer, J. C.: Adult pneumonia in a general hospital: Etiology and host risk factors. Arch Intern Med 129:935, 1972.

Tilghman, R. C., and Finland, M.: Clinical significance of bacteremia in pneumococci pneumonia. Arch Intern Med 59:602, 1937.

Winterbauer, R. H., Bedon, G. A., and Ball, S. W. C., Jr.: Recurrent pneumonia: Predisposing illness and clinical patterns in 158 patients. Ann Intern Med 70:689, 1969.

Ziskind, M. M., Schwarz, M. I., George, R. B., et al.: Incomplete consolidation in pneumococcal lobar pneumonia complicating pulmonary emphysema. Ann Intern Med 72:835, 1970.

# 106 *COMMON GRAM-NEGATIVE BACILLARY PNEUMONIAS*

*W. G. Johanson, Jr., M.D.*
*Junji H. Higuchi, M.D.*

## DEFINITION

Gram-negative bacillary pneumonia is an inflammatory process of the alveolar portions of the lung due to the presence of gram-negative bacilli.

## ETIOLOGY

The gram-negative bacilli that produce pneumonia in humans are principally *Klebsiella pneumoniae, Escherichia coli,* and *Pseudomonas aeruginosa* (Tillotson and Lerner, 1966). A variety of other gram-negative organisms produce pneumonia occasionally. Neither the epidemiology of infection nor the clinical illness produced by the less common bacilli differs importantly from that associated with more common organisms.

## PATHOGENESIS AND PATHOLOGY

Bacterial pneumonia of all types is uncommon among healthy individuals; this is especially true of pneumonias due to gram-negative bacilli. Only about 10 per cent of bacterial pneumonias acquired in the community are due to these organisms, and affected patients virtually always have serious underlying diseases. *K. pneumoniae* is responsible for most community-acquired bacillary pneumonias, followed by *E. coli, Proteus,* and other organisms. *P. aeruginosa* is rarely the cause of pneumonia acquired outside the hospital but is a common cause of nosocomial pneumonia.

In Chapter 105 the concept that bacterial pneumonia results from aspiration of upper respiratory secretions was developed. This concept applies particularly well to pneumonia due to gram-negative bacilli. These organisms are found in the oropharynx of only 2 to 6 per cent of healthy people. Hospital personnel who are exposed to patients with infections due to bacilli may acquire these hospital strains in their gas-

trointestinal tracts, but the organisms are excluded from their upper respiratory tracts. Gram-negative bacilli instilled into the upper respiratory tracts of healthy subjects are rapidly removed, and persistent colonization does not occur. Thus, it appears that highly effective mechanisms prevent colonization of the upper respiratory tracts of healthy individuals by gram-negative bacilli (Johanson et al., 1969).

The incidence of oropharyngeal colonization with gram-negative bacilli rises dramatically in patients with acute or chronic illness, approaching 50 per cent of subjects in most studies. The organisms that colonize are those that cause pneumonia. Colonization of the upper respiratory tract with gram-negative bacilli markedly increases the risk of subsequent pneumonia among seriously ill hospitalized patients; in one study of 213 patients admitted to an intensive care unit, pneumonia occurred in 23 per cent of colonized patients compared to 3 per cent of noncolonized patients (Johanson et al., 1972). Thus, patients who are already ill with other diseases are most likely to develop oropharyngeal colonization with gram-negative bacilli; the organisms probably reach the lungs by aspiration of small quantities of oropharyngeal secretions, and pneumonia develops when the organisms multiply more rapidly than they are killed by intrinsic defenses.

The sequence of histologic changes that take place during the development of pneumonia due to aerobic bacilli has not been well characterized. Broth culture filtrates of several species contain substances that are chemotactic for PMNs. In experimental animals exposed to aerosolized bacilli or to purified endotoxin, PMNs appear promptly in the walls of airways and alveoli and, to a lesser degree, in alveolar spaces. On the other hand, the cellular reaction of patients dying of bacillary pneumonia is occasionally only mononuclear, suggesting that failure of the PMN response may have played a critical role in the outcome.

Microscopically, in bacillary pneumonias necrosis of lung tissue and, especially with *P. aeruginosa* infections, fibrinoid necrosis of pulmonary arteries and veins are characteristic. It is not clear whether lung necrosis results from these vascular lesions or from destruction of alveolar walls by bacterial collagenases and elastases. Bacillary pneumonia may be peribronchial initially but may coalesce to a lobar consolidation and extensive abscess formation. Resolution usually leaves persistent disturbances in lung structure and function.

## CLINICAL MANIFESTATIONS

Pneumonia due to aerobic bacilli, when community-acquired, is usually a catastrophic, prostrating, acute infection. The pneumonia may be somewhat obscured by the underlying disease. However, chills, fever, cough productive of purulent or bloody sputum, and chest pain are common symptoms. Excessively mucoid sputum containing blood ("currant jelly sputum") is occasionally seen with *K. pneumoniae* pneumonia but is a nonspecific finding. Hypotension, frank shock, and delirium are more common with this type of pneumonia than with pneumococcal pneumonia.

Rales and signs of consolidation may be present, depending on the extent of involvement and the stage of the process. Pleural effusion and empyema are much more common than with pneumococcal pneumonia, and evidence of pleural disease must be sought carefully by clinical and radiographic techniques. Cavitation of the lung parenchyma is common but can rarely be detected on physical examination.

Radiographic changes are nonspecific. Infiltrates range from scattered peribronchial disease to dense unilobar consolidation, most often involving an upper lobe. Edema, hemorrhage, and tissue necrosis of the involved lobe may increase its volume so that fissures bulge in pneumonia due to *K. pneumoniae*. Pleural disease is frequent. Air-fluid levels may be seen with abscess formation, varying from multiple nodular lesions to entire lobes or even one lung; demonstration of air-fluid levels, of course, requires that radiographs be obtained with the patient upright, a procedure that may be difficult in seriously ill patients.

Nosocomial (hospital-acquired) pneumonia may be difficult to detect. At least 75 per cent of such pneumonias are due to gram-negative bacilli. However, the patients usually have complicated illnesses or are postoperative, and the signs and symptoms of their underlying processes obscure the onset of nosocomial pneumonia. The combination of leukocytosis, fever, new or progressing infiltrates on radiographs and the presence of purulent secretions are reliable signs of pulmonary infection in this setting.

## DIAGNOSIS

As with pneumococcal pneumonia, the problem of diagnosis is twofold: it must be determined that pneumonia is present and that it is due to gram-negative bacilli. The presence of pneumonia is usually readily apparent in nonhospitalized patients but may be difficult to ascertain among critically ill patients who may have radiographic infiltrates due to other causes. About 25 per cent of patients with gram-negative bacillary pneumonias have positive blood cultures that establish the bacteriologic etiology of the pulmonary disease. Pleural fluid, when present, usually contains the responsible bacteria and should always be aspirated for diagnostic purposes. A major diagnostic problem is presented by patients whose upper respiratory tracts have been colonized by gram-negative bacilli and who then develop signs and symptoms of lower respiratory infection. Several approaches have been proposed to distinguish colonization from significant infection, including washing of sputum to remove surface contaminants and quantitative cultures of the sputum. Neither technique clearly distinguishes colonization from infection in our experience. Transtracheal aspiration may be helpful, although in this patient population multiple pathogenic species are frequently recovered from the trachea. Gram stain of material recovered by this technique is far more valuable than culture in determining whether or not infection is present. In especially difficult situations, transthoracic lung aspiration or transbronchoscopic lung biopsy is indicated to determine the cause of progressing lung infiltrates.

## COMPLICATIONS AND SEQUELAE

Overall, about 50 per cent of patients with pneumonia due to gram-negative bacilli die (Pierce and Sanford, 1974). Among intensive care patients, the mortality of nosocomial *P. aeruginosa* pneumonia approaches 80 per cent. The causes of death are multifactorial, including the underlying disease, shock, lung necrosis, and acute respiratory failure. Lung abscess and empyema are early complications. Lung abscess may require repeated bronchoscopy to promote endobronchial drainage; the temptation to aspirate intrapulmonary collections of pus transthoracically via needle or chest tube should be resisted, since such procedures violate the pleural space and may add the complication of bronchopleural fistula to an already desperate situation. Massive hemoptysis and pyopneumothorax secondary to pleural rupture are major complications.

Pleural effusions developing during bacillary pneumonia usually contain infecting bacteria. At first the fluid is free-flowing and easily aspirated, but it loculates if removal is delayed, and adequate drainage via needle or chest tube may not be possible. Decortication, the débridement of the pleural space, should be considered in patients with extensive pleural disease who still have fever after seven days of tube drainage and adequate antimicrobial therapy.

## TREATMENT

Antimicrobial therapy of these infections must be guided by in vitro susceptibility testing. Community-acquired infections with *K. pneumoniae* may respond well to treatment with single agents such as cephalothin in doses of 1.0 g intravenously every three hours or 80 mg of gentamicin intravenously three times daily. However, seriously ill patients or patients who acquire gram-negative bacillary pneumonia in the hospital should receive a combination of agents such as cephalothin and kanamycin or carbenicillin and gentamicin until the drug susceptibility of the organism is known. The adult dose of kanamycin when used with cephalothin is 0.5 g intramuscularly every six hours. Supportive care, including the use of parenteral fluids, oxygen, and clearing of secretions from the tracheobronchial tree, is particularly important in the treatment of these infections. Respiratory failure is a common cause of death and may be due to obstruction of airways by tenacious secretions.

## PROPHYLAXIS

Contaminated respiratory therapy equipment has been responsible for many nosocomial bacillary pneumonias, and continued awareness of this potential hazard and rigorous enforcement of preventive measures are indicated (Pierce et al., 1970). Medications, parenteral solutions, and even hand lotions are also potential sources of contamination. Further, it is likely that colonization occurs in many patients following transport of the organisms from other patients on the hands of their attendants. This mode of transmission is especially common in critical care areas where susceptible patients are concentrated in relatively small spaces.

Attempts to reduce the susceptibility of the patient to colonization by gram-negative bacilli have not been highly successful. Topical instillation of bactericidal agents into the oropharynx tends to promote drug resistance and does not lower the incidence of pneumonia. Systemic antibacterial therapy increases the tendency of sick people to sustain colonization with gram-negative bacilli. Active or passive immunization against gram-negative bacilli has met with some success in certain patient groups at high risk for *P. aeruginosa* infection. Immunization appears to reduce somewhat the severity of subsequent infections; however, the specificity of the protection afforded is too narrow to permit the use of immunization for other than highly selected patient groups.

## PNEUMONIA DUE TO HAEMOPHILUS INFLUENZAE

Although serious infection with *Haemophilus influenzae* occurs predominantly among children less than 3 years of age, pneumonia due to *H. influenzae* may also occur in adults (Quintiliani and Hymans, 1971; Tillotson and Lerner, 1968). These pneumonias appear to consist of either a localized (lobar or segmental) consolidation or a diffuse bronchopneumonia. Both types occur mainly in patients with serious underlying illnesses, especially chronic obstructive lung disease. Patients with localized consolidation have an illness similar to pneumococcal pneumonia; and upper respiratory tract illness usually precedes the onset of chills, pleuritic chest pain, and purulent sputum. Pleural effusion is common. Chest radiography reveals a consolidating process, most often in the right lower lobe, with or without evidence of effusion. Cavitation may develop but is not common at first.

Patients with the bronchopneumonia form of *H. influenzae* pneumonia usually have a less acute illness; increased cough, sputum production, and low-grade or intermittent fever may have been present for days or even weeks. Radiographs of the chest reveal multiple, small, ill-defined densities scattered throughout both lungs. Pleural effusion is rare with this type of illness.

In both types of pneumonia numerous small, pleomorphic gram-negative bacilli and many polymorphonuclear leukocytes are seen in smears of the sputum. Culture of *H. influenzae* requires special attention. Heat-labile inhibitors in fresh human and sheep blood agar interfere with isolation, but these are inactivated by the heating process that is used for making chocolate agar. Both chocolate agar and Fildes peptid digest agar provide the X factor (heme) and the V factor (nicotinamide adenine nucleotide) required for growth and primary isolation of *Haemophilus* organisms. Blood cultures and demonstration of capsular antigen by counterimmunoelectrophoresis are also important for diagnosis.

Encapsulated strains, especially Type b, cause most if not all pneumonias due to *H. influenzae*. The pathogenicity of nonencapsulated and nontypable strains is controversial. These organisms may be found in the upper respiratory tracts of healthy individuals and are commonly present in the tracheobronchial secretions of persons with chronic bronchitis. Evidence of the pathogenicity of the nontypable strains in chronic bronchitis rests largely on the higher frequency of its isolation in purulent secretions compared with nonpurulent secretions; however, many investigators have found nontypable strains of *H. influenzae* in the sputum of as many as 25 to 50 per cent of bronchitic patients during stable periods without purulent exacerbations, and the role of this organism in causing episodes of purulent bronchitis is uncertain.

The treatment of choice for pneumonia due to *H. influenzae* is ampicillin, 0.5 g intravenously every four to six hours. Chloramphenicol in doses of 500 mg orally every four hours or 1.0 g intravenously every six hours is used in patients who are allergic to penicillin or from whom penicillinase-producing *H. influenzae* are recovered. A rapid penicillinase test permits the choice of antibiotics upon isolation of the organism. If the diagnosis is seriously suspected before the culture is positive, both antibiotics can be used until the penicillinase test is completed, and then one of the drugs is stopped. Treatment of the underlying chronic pulmonary disease usually expedites symptomatic recovery.

### References

Johanson, W. G., Jr., Pierce, A. K., and Sanford, J. P.: Changing pharyngeal bacterial flora of hospitalized patients: Emergence of gram-negative bacilli. N Engl J Med 281:1137, 1969.

Johanson, W. G., Jr., Pierce, A. K., Sanford, J. P., and Thomas, G. D.: Nosocomial respiratory infections with gram-negative bacilli. Ann Intern Med 77:701, 1972.

Pierce, A. K., and Sanford, J. P.: Aerobic gram-negative bacillary pneumonias. Am Rev Respir Dis 110:647, 1974.

Pierce, A. K., Sanford, J. P., Thomas, G. D., and Leonard, J. S.: Long-term evaluation of decontamination of inhalation therapy equipment and occurrence of necrotizing pneumonia. N Engl J Med 282:528, 1970.

Quintiliani, R., and Hymans, P. J.: The association of bacteremic *Haemophilus influenzae* pneumonia in adults with typable strains. Am J Med 50:781, 1951.

Tillotson, J. R., and Lerner, A. M.: Pneumonias caused by gram-negative bacilli. Medicine 45:625, 1966.

Tillotson, J. R., and Lerner, A. M.: *Hemophilus influenzae* bronchopneumonia in adults. Arch Intern Med 121:428, 1968.

# *MELIOIDOSIS* 107

## Robert Nicol Thin, M.D. FRCPE

### DEFINITION

Melioidosis is a rare disease that is due to the gram-negative bacillus *Pseudomonas pseudomallei*. The main endemic areas of the world are Southeast Asia and Northern Australia, and a few cases have originated in other places between the 20° north and south parallels of latitude, such as Ecuador and Panama (Howe, et al., 1971). The disease may be acute (and frequently fulminating and fatal), less acute, or chronic; it may also be subacute, mild, or subclinical (diagnosed only by the results of serologic tests).

### ETIOLOGY

Melioidosis was first recognized in 1911 by Whitmore in Rangoon at an autopsy examination. The causative organism, *P. pseudomallei*, has been called by a variety of names, including *Pfeifferella whitmori*, *Loefflerella whitmori*, and *Malleomyces pseudomallei*. Surveys have shown that this organism occurs naturally in the soil and surface water in Northern Australia, East and West Malaysia, Singapore, and Vietnam.

*P. pseudomallei* is a small, motile, gram-negative, non–acid-fast, non-spore-bearing bacillus that shows characteristic bipolar staining. It grows on ordinary media, although it may be overgrown by other organisms. In suspected cases, specimens from all septic lesions, and blood in acute cases, should be cultured. Nutrient agar, incorporating 3 per cent glycerol and 1:200,000 crystal violet, is a useful selective medium on which smooth colonies, deeply tinted by the dye, are visible after 24 hours incubation. They enlarge to a maximum diameter of 7 mm after 14 days incubation when they have a dry, wrinkled, beaten aluminium appearance. A characteristic pungent, yeasty odor is given off by fresh cultures, and this may be a useful clue to the presence of this organism. Twenty-four hours incubation in nutrient broth produces an even turbidity and surface pellicle. The organism is pathogenic for most laboratory animals, and in animals, melioidosis resembles glanders. In male guinea pigs a characteristic acute orchitis is produced

(Strauss reaction); a similar reaction occurs in guinea pigs infected with *Actinobacillus mallei* (the glanders bacillus). Serologic tests assist in diagnosis; the polysaccharide hemagglutination test is more sensitive and specific than the simple agglutination, or complement-fixation, tests, which are limited by cross-reactions with *A. mallei, Escherichia, Aerobacter, Klebsiella,* and *Salmonella* species (Alexander et al., 1970; Strauss et al., 1969).

## PATHOGENESIS AND PATHOLOGY

In the published reports, men are infected more than women, but this is because most cases described in the world literature have been reported among nonindigenous servicemen serving in areas of conflict in Southeast Asia. The local population in this area has been less carefully studied.

*P. pseudomallei* is found in a wide variety of animals, including rats, rabbits, guinea pigs, sheep, goats, pigs, and horses. At one time, it was thought that man was infected by direct contact with diseased animals or by ingestion or inhalation of infected material from them. Although the route of infection is not definitely known, it is now believed that the organism is usually acquired directly from infected soil and surface water. *P. pseudomallei* enters the body either through open skin lesions or by inhalation (Editorial, *Lancet,* 1975). A high incidence of pulmonary infection was noted in helicopter crewmen in Vietnam; this was probably due to organisms in the dust and spray raised by helicopter rotors. A high incidence of preceding superficial trauma in which lesions were exposed to surface water has been reported, and there have also been cases in which the initial lesion was a burn. It is possible that organisms enter the body by ingestion, but it seems unlikely that they survive in the normal stomach. One case of probable sexual transmission of melioidosis has been reported and this is the only well-documented case of person to person transmission (McCormick et al., 1975).

Unrecognized chronic infections may flare up after sudden reduction in host resistance, as in patients suffering from trauma or burns. Other predisposing causes appear important in the development of acute melioidosis. These include chronic debilitating conditions, such as diabetes, chronic renal and liver disease, and pregnancy. Previously healthy individuals are more likely to develop subacute or chronic melioidosis.

The lesions of melioidosis occur most commonly in the lungs, and they are also found in the joints, liver, spleen, kidney, and bone marrow. Less often, lesions occur in the adrenal glands and lymph nodes, but any organ can be affected, including the heart and brain. Patients with acute illness of short duration have small abscesses, whereas those with longer illnesses tend to have larger abscesses.

Lesions start as microscopic foci that develop into inflammatory nodules, and multiple nodules coalesce to form abscesses. The lesions have a characteristic histology (Piggot and Hochholzer, 1970). They start as collections of polymorphonuclear neutrophils surrounded by zones of congestion. When larger, they have centers of necrotic caseous material containing nuclear debris, surrounded by a narrow zone of lymphocytes and histiocytes, and outside this a thin layer of fibrous tissue may form. At the periphery, intensely congested dilated capillaries form a distinctive collar, sharply demarcating the lesion from the surrounding tissue.

At autopsy in fulminating cases, *P. pseudomallei* may be cultured from the heart blood and abscesses (Thin et al., 1970) and can be seen in histologic sections, stained by the Gram method or by immunofluorescence.

## CLINICAL MANIFESTATIONS

The incubation period is unknown, but is almost certainly very variable. The clinical manifestations of melioidosis vary greatly and there are no specific diagnostic features (Editorial, *Lancet*, 1975).

The acutely ill patient has a high fever, chills, a cough often productive of blood-stained mucopurulent sputum, diarrhea, and abdominal pain. Physical examination may reveal signs of pneumonia, empyema, and lung abscess, mild jaundice, hepatomegaly, splenomegaly, acute or subacute arthritis, and septic pustules. There may be overwhelming septicemia and the patient's condition can rapidly worsen with increased confusion, tremor, profuse watery diarrhea that may resemble cholera, and a pustular rash, until he becomes comatose and dies in septicemic shock.

In the subacute case, pulmonary features often predominate. There is fever, cough productive of mucopurulent sputum that may be streaked with blood, signs of pneumonia, lung abscess, and, occasionally, pleural involvement. Joint pains may occur; there may also be a sparse pustular rash and hepatosplenomegaly. Subacute or chronic illness may precede or follow the acute disease, or may develop in the absence of acute illness. Pneumonitis may occur alone and the clinical features may resemble tuberculosis.

Chronic forms are very variable. Osteomyelitis, lung abscess, psoas or subcutaneous abscesses, liver or spleen abscesses, and lymphadenopathy occur (Prevatt and Hunt, 1957). Fistulas may appear. There may be a long latent period (up to 24 years has been recorded) between exposure and the diagnosis of melioidosis. Chronic melioidosis may persist for many months.

Melioidosis may also take the form of a mild, self-limiting febrile illness without any specific features. It must be considered among the many causes for short-term "fever of undetermined origin" among people who are in or who have visited endemic areas. This form of melioidosis will be diagnosed only by serologic tests. Surveys have shown raised serum antibody titers among those living in, and those who have visited, endemic areas. Raised antibody titers have been found in a higher proportion of those surveyed than would be expected from the comparatively few recorded clinical cases. Unsuspected or subclinical infection is therefore more prevalent than was realized at one time.

Cases have been reported in which, initially, there has been an unremarkable skin lesion, often traumatic in origin, with or without localized infection, lymphangitis or lymphadenitis, followed by progression to systemic melioidosis. Such cases occurring in endemic areas must be carefully investigated and vigorously treated.

## COMPLICATIONS AND SEQUELAE

The main problem with melioidosis is that however mild the condition is at first, there may be rapid progression to a severe fulminating illness in which the patient's condition deteriorates until he dies. Therefore, it is vital that all suspicious cases be carefully investigated. Occasional chronic cases may be left with deformities, such as flexion contractures, which are probably more common in local populations than is generally realized. Residual pulmonary changes may persist, including linear radiologic scars, cavities, and emphysema.

In adequately treated cases, there will be no sequelae but prolonged treatment is vital, as will be emphasized later, and a long, careful, follow-up after treatment is important.

## GEOGRAPHICAL VARIATIONS

As already noted, melioidosis takes many forms, but no relation has been reported between the place where the organism was acquired and the course of the disease.

## DIAGNOSIS

Melioidosis may be suspected at the bedside, but the diagnosis can be confirmed only in the microbiologic laboratory (Editorial, *Lancet*, 1975). Simple laboratory investigations are of little value; some cases have a polymorphonuclear leukocytosis and a high erythrocyte sedimentation rate. The chest radiograph frequently shows infiltration resembling pulmonary tuberculosis and cavities are common. Like tuberculosis, pulmonary melioidosis usually affects the upper lobes and this may cause confusion. Sometimes, many cavities are present, resembling staphylococcal pneumonia, and segmental consolidation may also occur.

As already mentioned, *P. pseudomallei* can be easily cultured. In acute cases, blood should always be cultured and the presence of bipolar rods in blood cultures from these patients, after 24 hours incubation, may be the first microbiologic indication of the diagnosis. The organism is easily isolated from pus and has been found in almost all body fluids except feces. It is vitally important for physicians to be acutely aware of the possibility of melioidosis and to send specimens to the laboratory from all septic lesions. The laboratory staff should be informed that melioidosis is a possible diagnosis so that appropriate culture media may be used from the beginning. The diagnosis of melioidosis should be considered in all patients who are in, or who have returned from, endemic areas with fever of undetermined origin, pulmonary disease, or pyogenic lesions, and in all patients in whom the diagnosis is obscure. It must be remembered that in some reported cases there has been a very long latent period between return from endemic areas and the development of melioidosis.

This condition must be differentiated from a wide variety of other diseases. The acute fulminating form must be distinguished from other causes of septicemia, typhoid fever, malaria, leptospirosis, typhus, plague, and mycoses. Pulmonary forms must be differentiated from tuberculosis, lung abscess, and pneumonia, particularly staphylococcal pneumonia, and pulmonary mycoses. Confusion with pulmonary tuberculosis has often occurred in the past. Jaundice and hepatomegaly, due to melioidosis, may mimic hepatitis A and B, infectious mononucleosis, and cytomegalovirus disease. Chronic forms resemble osteomyelitis due to other causes, and tuberculous and other chronic abscesses. Simple febrile illness must be differentiated from other causes of fever of undetermined origin.

## TREATMENT

Antibiotics are vital for treating melioidosis. Simple disk sensitivity tests usually indicate that *P. pseudomallei* is sensitive to tetracycline, chloramphenicol, sulfadiazine, and novobiocin, and resistant to the penicillins. Quantitative assays show more complex patterns; colonies from one specimen may show different sensitivities, and sensitivity may vary between consecutive specimens taken from one patient. Careful laboratory investigations are essential for good antibiotic treatment; the ideal regimen for treating acute melioidosis has yet to be established. Huge intravenous doses of chloramphenicol and novobiocin, plus intramuscular kanamycin have cured such cases; but more recently it has been shown that combinations of drugs may shown antagonism in vitro. Such antagonism has been shown between kanamycin and chloramphenicol, tetracycline and kanamycin, and sulfadiazine and chloramphenicol. The clinical significance of such antagonism remains to be assessed. It appears probable that tetracycline is, at present, the drug of choice in all but the most severe cases; the daily dosage should be 3 g, which should be continued until serial cultures give negative results for at least one month and chest radiographs have cleared or stabilized with minimal residual change. If the patient is extremely toxic, chloramphenicol 3 g daily should also be given, and, in the severe septicemic cases, tetracycline 3 g and chloramphenicol 4 to 6 g, should be given intravenously. Prolonged treatment is most important; three to six months may be necessary in some cases (Howe, et al., 1971). Serial cultures should be sent for microbiologic examination; if therapy is stopped prematurely, relapse is likely to follow. The patient should therefore be followed after treatment to ensure that remission is maintained.

In vitro *P. pseudomallei* is sensitive to co-trimoxazole and this has been used successfully in several cases (John, 1976). Co-trimoxazole offers theoretical advantages: it is bactericidal, whereas tetracycline and chloramphenicol are bacteriostatic agents; but some isolates are resistant to lower concentrations of trimethoprim or sulphamethoxazole. During the acute stages, the patient's vital functions should be carefully monitored, and supportive measures may be important. Accessible abscesses should be drained surgically.

## PROPHYLAXIS

At present, no artificial immunization is available against melioidosis. The best method of prevention is to avoid undue exposure to soil and surface water in endemic areas, especially after the start of heavy rain since organisms are particularly prevalent in surface water at this time. Improved drainage for poorly drained areas will also help to reduce exposure.

## CONCLUSIONS

Melioidosis is more prevalent in endemic areas than is generally realized. The main endemic area, Southeast Asia, is an important tourist and trading area; with air travel, patients suffering from melioidosis may present anywhere in the world, with any clinical form of melioidosis, but a long latent period may elapse between exposure and illness. A large number of United States servicemen, and servicemen of other countries, were exposed to infection in endemic areas in the late 1960s and early 1970s. This form of delayed melioidosis may continue to be a problem in such individuals for some years to come. To make a rapid diagnosis, physicians must be alert to the possibility of this condition, take appropriate specimens for microbiologic examination, and inform their laboratory colleagues if they suspect melioidosis. Antibiotic treatment should be vigorous and prolonged, and careful follow-up is important to ensure a satisfactory cure.

## References

Alexander, A. D., Huxsoll, D. L., Warner, A. R., Shepler, V., and Dorsey, A.: Serological diagnosis of human melioidosis with indirect hemagglutination and complement fixation tests. Appl Microbiol 20:825, 1970.

Editorial: Melioidosis. Lancet 2:962, 1975.

Howe, C., Sampath, A., and Spotnitz M.: The pseudomallei group, a review. J Infect Dis 124:598, 1971.

John, J. F.: Trimethoprim-sulphamethoxazole therapy of pulmonary melioidosis. Am Rev Respir Dis 114:1021, 1976.

McCormick, J. B., Sexton, D. J., McMurray, J. G., Carey, E., Hayes, P., and Feldman, R. A.: Human to human transmission of *Pseudomonas pseudomallei*. Ann Intern Med 83:512, 1975.

Piggot, J. A., and Hochholzer, L.: Human melioidosis. A histopathologic study of acute and chronic melioidosis. Arch Pathol 90:101, 1970.

Prevatt, A. L., and Hunt, J. S.: Chronic systemic melioidosis. Review of literature and report of a case, with a note of visual disturbance due to chloramphenicol. Am J Med 23:810, 1957.

Strauss, J. M., Alexander, A. D., Rapmund, G., Gan, E., and Dorsey, A. E.: Melioidosis in Malaysia III. Antibodies to *Pseudomonas pseudomallei* in the human population. Am J Trop Med Hyg 18:703, 1969.

Thin, R. N. T., Brown, M., Stewart, J. B., and Garrett, C. J.: Melioidosis — a report of ten cases. Q J Med 153:115, 1970.

Thin, R. N. T., Groves, M., Rapmund, G., and Mariappan, M.: *Pseudomonas pseudomallei* in the surface water of Singapore. Singapore Medical Journal 12:181, 1971.

# MYCOPLASMA PNEUMONIA 108

## Maurice A. Mufson, M.D.

### DEFINITION

Mycoplasma pneumonia (formerly atypical or Eaton agent pneumonia), caused by *Mycoplasma pneumoniae*, is an acute infection of the lower respiratory tract that exhibits the following characteristics: (1) usually involves the dependent lobes of the lung, (2) lasts 14 to 21 days in untreated cases, (3) stimulates the formation of specific antibodies during convalescence, (4) stimulates the production of cold agglutinins or other nonspecific antibodies in more severely ill individuals, (5) responds to treatment with erythromycin or tetracycline and its analogues, and (6) almost always heals without sequelae.

### ETIOLOGY

*Mycoplasma pneumoniae* (formerly known as PPLO or the Eaton agent organism), which belongs to the class Mollicutes, order Mycoplasmatales, family Mycoplasmataceae, and genus Mycoplasma, is the etiologic agent of mycoplasma pneumonia (syn. *Mycoplasma pneumoniae* pneumonia) (Tully, 1978). Mycoplasmas are the smallest (0.3 nm in diameter) free-living microorganisms capable of replicating on cell-free media. On appropriate media they form microscopic colonies of 50 to 250 nm in diameter (see Fig. 2, Chapter 53). Individual mycoplasmas may be coccobacillary or filamentous. They contain DNA and RNA and possess a lipophilic, triple-layered limiting membrane, but they lack a cell wall. *M. pneumoniae* ferments glucose, produces peroxide, and hemolyzes erythrocytes layered over colonies on agar media. These characteristics differentiate it from other mycoplasmas (see Table 3, Chapter 53). Unlike bacteria, *M. pneumoniae* incorporates, although it does not synthesize, sterols into its cell membrane.

### PATHOGENESIS AND PATHOLOGY

The respiratory tract is the primary target of *M. pneumoniae*; infections occur at all anatomic levels including the oropharynx, trachea, bronchi, and lungs. Clinical pneumonia develops in 3 to 10 per cent of infected individuals in "open" populations and in 50 per cent of infected individuals in the family environment. Mycoplasma infection is endemic throughout the world, but superimposed epidemics occur every four or five years. Infrequently, *M. pneumoniae* may infect other organs such as the central nervous system, pancreas, joints, skin, heart, and pericardium. Although the mode of spread to these other organs is probably hematogenous, this has not been documented.

*M. pneumoniae* spreads by infectious droplets from person to person. Aerosol particles less than 5 nm in diameter reach the lower respiratory tract directly, but larger particles deposit on the nasal and upper respiratory tract passages. Colonization of the respiratory tract occurs readily and persists for days or weeks.

The effect of *M. pneumoniae* infection on the respiratory tract seems to involve diverse and multiple factors whose importance and interrelations are unresolved (Archer, 1979). *M. pneumoniae* attaches to neuraminic acid residues on ciliated epithelial cells and stops ciliary activity with subsequent destruction of cilia and cell surfaces. Attachment may be mediated by glycoproteins in the membrane of the mycoplasma. The infection is superficial (see Fig. 1 in Chapter 53); intracellular organisms have not been observed by electron microscopy. *M. pneumoniae* does not produce endotoxin or exotoxins; it produces hydrogen peroxide, which may be toxic to cells if a sufficient concentration of peroxide is maintained at the cell surface by close association of the mycoplasma and the cell. The organism is motile, although it lacks flagella, and this property may enhance its pathogenic potential. An actin-like protein, which has been extracted from *M. pneumoniae*, may be involved in motility of this organism.

While antibody to *M. pneumoniae* appears to mediate recovery from infection and resistance to reinfection, cellular immune responses also may be involved, since *M. pneumoniae* stimulates lymphocyte transformation and production of macrophage migration inhibition factor (Whittlestone, 1976). Peribronchial mononuclear infiltrates that characterize *M. pneumoniae* infection support this thesis. IgA secretory antibody in nasal secretions and complement-mediated lysis may play a prominent role in preventing infection. C1 is membrane-bound by *M. pneumoniae*. Circulating antibody to *M. pneumoniae* correlates with protection from infection, but this protection wanes and reinfections can occur five years after the first infection.

Multiple autoantibodies develop during *M. pneumoniae* infections including anti-red cell (cold agglutinins), antibrain, antilung, and antiliver antibodies. Antibodies also develop to other bacteria including streptococcus MG and reagin-like antibody that yields false-positive tests for syphilis. These nonspecific, that is, nonmycoplasma-reactive, antibodies may contribute to the pathogenicity of disease through autoimmune mechanisms. The pneumonia caused by *M. pneumoniae* may be influenced by antigen-antibody reactions in the lung. Infection in childhood may sensitize the child so that subsequent infections with *M. pneumoniae* are more severe. Circulating immune complexes have been detected and may contribute to some of the extrapulmonary manifestations of this infection.

*M. pneumoniae* causes a patchy, interstitial pneumonia with acute and chronic inflammation and swollen alveolar lining cells. The bronchiolar walls are thickened by congestion and edema. There is an intraluminal exudate of polymorphonuclear leukocytes, epithelial cells, and proteinaceous debris. Perivascular and peribronchial cuffing by lymphocytes may be prominent (see Fig. 3A, Chapter 53). In experimental infections of hamsters, the histopathologic changes develop slowly in primary infections and rapidly in reinfection.

## CLINICAL MANIFESTATIONS

Characteristically, the onset of *M. pneumoniae* pneumonia is insidious. A nonproductive cough is the most common first symptom (Mufson and Zollar, 1975). As the illness progresses, the cough produces white and watery or mucoid sputum. Blood-tinged or blood-streaked sputum is infrequent and frank hemoptysis is rare. Fever of 100 to 103° F develops in nearly all patients. Fever and the physical findings of pneumonia last for one to two weeks in untreated individuals. Headache is a prominent feature of the illness and may be intensified during high fever.

Other common findings include chills, malaise, rhinorrhea, chest pain, and generalized myalgia. Most of these symptoms develop in at least half of the patients. Rales and rhonchi can be detected in three fourths of the patients with pneumonia but often are not evident until after the first few days of illness. Early in the course of the illness, the patient frequently appears much more ill than the physical findings indicate, but the pulmonary findings increase after a few days. Although these clinical features are characteristic of mycoplasma pneumonia, they do not serve to differentiate it from other nonbacterial pneumonias.

Tympanitis occurs in 10 per cent of patients with mycoplasma pneumonia. Bullous myringitis, which develops less often, is characterized by large hemorrhagic bullae on the tympanic membrane that heal without scarring. *M. pneumoniae* can be isolated from the bullae.

Mycoplasma pneumonia usually occurs unilaterally in the lower lobe. Bilateral infiltration occurs in about one fourth of cases; upper lobe involvement is less frequent. The radiographic appearance of mycoplasma pneumonia (Fig. 1) is diffusely reticulonodular, segmental, or lobar (Putnam et al., 1975). The infiltrate often radiates from the hilum to the base of the lung. Radiographically, mycoplasma pneumonia cannot be distinguished from other nonbacterial pneumonias. Unilateral or bilateral pleural effusions occasionally occur, but they are usually very small and almost always resolve completely.

Routine laboratory examinations do not contribute to a definitive diagnosis of mycoplasma pneumonia. They are consistent with any nonbacterial infection. An elevated peripheral white blood cell count occurs in only 15 per cent of the clinically evident cases, and an elevated erythrocyte sedimentation rate occurs in only about one third of cases.

Cold agglutinins develop in one half of all patients with mycoplasma pneumonia, but in a higher percentage of severely ill individuals. A titer greater than 1:40 can be detected in a single serum specimen obtained early in the course of the illness, and a fourfold or greater rise in cold agglutinin antibodies develops during convalescence. Cold agglutinins represent a nonspecific antibody response, and this finding by itself is not diagnostic of *M. pneumoniae* infection. Rising titers of type-specific *M. pneumoniae* antibodies appear during convalescence (see Diagnosis).

## COMPLICATIONS AND SEQUELAE

Most patients with mycoplasma pneumonia recover without sequelae or complications. Symptoms and signs of pneumonia usually abate within 10 to 14 days. Antibiotics hasten recovery. Radiographic findings usually resolve within three to four weeks in untreated patients, but nearly one in five may have persistent infiltrates for as long as four months. Even these late-resolving pneumonias usually heal without sequelae.

Lung abscess occurs rarely in mycoplasma pneumonia (Cherry and Welliver, 1976). In these exceptional cases of cavity formation, which have been recognized in both adults and children, one or several small cavities form in areas of segmen-

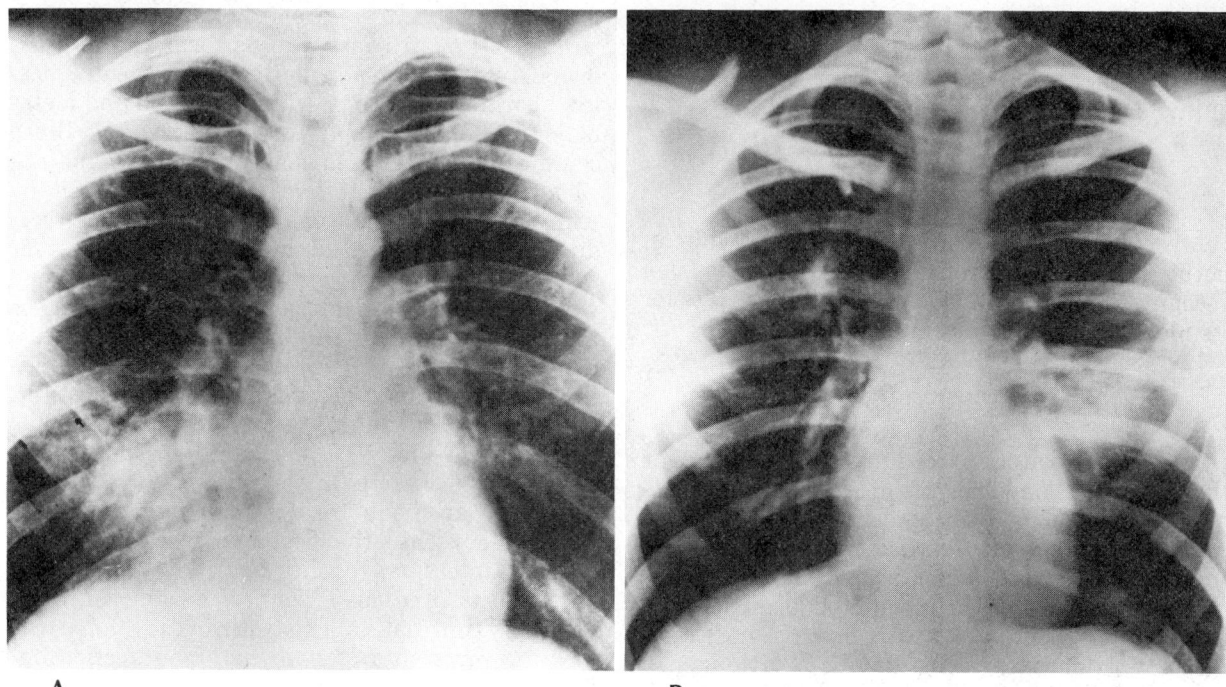

**FIGURE 1A and 1B.** *Mycoplasma pneumonia in two patients illustrating segmental infiltrate radiating from hilum.*

tal consolidation and heal completely or with minimal scarring.

Although an occasional pleural effusion develops in patients with mycoplasma pneumonia, residual pleural abnormalities are rare. Other rare sequelae include severe respiratory failure, adult respiratory distress syndrome, and disseminated pulmonary disease. Widespread pulmonary involvement is more common in children and adolescents. More severe pneumonia occurs in individuals with underlying autoimmune disorders.

In a small number of cases the course of mycoplasma pneumonia is complicated by involvement of other organs. These complications include myocarditis or pericarditis or both, the Stevens-Johnson syndrome, nonspecific exanthems, hemolytic anemia, arthritis, and central nervous system manifestations (Murray et al., 1975). The number of cases described with each of these complications is fewer than 200. No reliable data are available that permit calculation of complication rates. Considering the high incidence of *M. pneumoniae* infection (and pneumonia) and the few reports of cases with other manifestations, the rate of complications in mycoplasma pneumonia is probably less than one in several thousand cases.

Clinical signs of myocarditis, pericarditis, or perimyocarditis include fever, chest pain, pericardial friction rub, and an enlarged heart. Electro-

cardiographic examination indicates epicardial injury, nonspecific ST-T wave abnormalities, and various arrhythmias. Deaths are rare.

Hemolytic anemia, another uncommon complication of mycoplasma pneumonia, is accompanied by cold agglutinin titers of 1:1000 or higher. The hemolytic anemia frequently occurs late in the course of the illness, when the cold agglutinin titers reach peak levels and the pneumonia begins to resolve. The severity of the hemolysis can vary from mild to marked. It is self-limiting, and complete recovery ensues in several weeks. The pathogenesis of the hemolytic anemia is autoimmune; 19S cold agglutinins formed in response to *M. pneumoniae* infection are specific antibodies to the I antigen of the red blood cell membrane as demonstrated by their failure to react with cord blood or fetal erythrocytes, which lack the I antigen. Anti-I cold agglutinins might be expected to form if *M. pneumoniae* contains antigens that cross-react with red blood cells. Although direct evidence that *M. pneumoniae* contains an I antigen (or an antigenic configuration similar to I antigen) is lacking, absorption experiments with antibody to this organism and I red blood cells suggest that possibility.

The central nervous system manifestations of *M. pneumoniae* infection span the spectrum of possible nervous tissue infection: aseptic meningitis, meningoencephalitis, cerebellar ataxia, hemiplegia, transverse myelitis, polyradiculitis, and psychosis. More than half of patients with central nervous system disease caused by *M. pneumoniae* also have had prior or simultaneous pulmonary involvement.

## GEOGRAPHIC VARIATIONS

Mycoplasma pneumonia occurs worldwide in both temperate and tropical climates. It has been recognized in all countries where specific tests for its identification have been employed.

## DIAGNOSIS

Specific laboratory procedures must be used for the definitive diagnosis of mycoplasma pneumonia (Clyde, 1979). The organism can be recovered on special supplemented media (see Chapter 53) from sputa, throat swabs, pleural fluids, or tissues. The specimen is inoculated directly onto agar plates or into a diphasic broth. Small colonies appear on the agar in 10 to 12 days (longer in some instances). They can be identified as *M. pneumoniae* by metabolic characteristics and by growth neutralization tests using antibody-impregnated disks. Similarly, in 10 to 12 days spherules and acid production appear in the diphasic medium. Growth in diphasic media can be confirmed by subculturing the organism onto agar, and specific identification can be established by disk neutralization tests. A rapid means of differentiating the colonies of *M. pneumoniae* from other *Mycoplasma* organisms is by hemadsorption and hemolysis of guinea pig erythrocytes. Erythrocytes suspended in buffer will hemadsorb to colonies of *M. pneumoniae* but not to other *Mycoplasma* organisms. If the red cells are added in an agar overlay, hemolysis around the colonies can be seen with the naked eye within one to two days.

The development of a fourfold or greater rise in specific antibody during convalescence is also diagnostic of mycoplasma infection. By contrast, IgM cold agglutinins typically develop in only half of all cases but in a greater percentage of the more severely ill.

Antibody responses to *M. pneumoniae* can be measured by any of several procedures: indirect immunofluorescence, complement fixation, metabolic inhibition, tetrazolium reduction inhibition, indirect hemagglutination, mycoplasmacidal assay, and radioimmunoprecipitation. The individual antibody assays differ significantly in sensitivity, ease of performance, and cost. Immunofluorescence, mycoplasmacidal assay, and radioimmunoprecipitation tests provide a high to very high degree of sensitivity, but they are complex and are used mainly for research pur-

poses. The other tests are only moderately sensitive, but they are easier to perform and are less expensive. Of the tests applicable for the diagnostic laboratory, the complement fixation and metabolic inhibition tests are used most widely. Since complement fixation is easily performed and antibody to *M. pneumoniae* can be measured by using the standard complement fixation procedure, most diagnostic laboratories use this test for antibody determinations. The test can be done with either the lipid antigen of *M. pneumoniae* or the whole organism. The lipid antigen provides a more sensitive antigen and yields higher antibody levels. However, it shares similarities with galactolipids of plants (vegetables), and nonspecific antibody may be measured in individuals sensitized to these galactolipids.

Specific antibody to *M. pneumoniae* becomes detectable within the first two weeks after the onset of infection, reaches peak levels in two to six months, and may persist for four or more years. By contrast, cold agglutinins develop in the first few days after *M. pneumoniae* infection but usually disappear within six months, as is generally true of IgM antibodies. There is no cross-relationship between specific *M. pneumoniae* antibody and cold agglutinin antibody. If tests for specific *M. pneumoniae* antibody are not available, the demonstration of high titers of cold agglutinins provides strong presumptive evidence of infection with *M. pneumoniae* and justifies the initiation of effective broad spectrum antibiotic treatment.

## TREATMENT

Tetracycline, 2 g daily in four divided doses, or erythromycin, 1 to 2 g daily in four divided doses, for 10 days will effectively treat the disease, lessen the severity of symptoms and signs, and shorten the course of the illness (Mufson and Zollar, 1975). (The analogues of tetracycline are also effective in appropriate dosages.) Although the severity and duration of disease are reduced by treatment with effective antibiotics, the organism is not immediately eradicated from the respiratory tract. Shedding of the organism usually continues for some time after therapy has been discontinued. In addition to antibiotic treatment, the usual supportive measures for pneumonia are helpful: bed rest, adequate diet, abundant liquids, antipyretics for fever, antitussives, and bronchodilators.

## PROPHYLAXIS

Immunoprophylaxis for high-risk populations is under investigation. Inactivated and live attenuated vaccines have been tested experimentally in volunteers. Inactivated vaccines that were tested for efficacy in large groups of volunteers proved only marginally effective. Although they stimulated antibody production, their protective efficacy was relatively low. Live attenuated *M. pneumoniae* vaccines may provide a better means of protection, but they are still being developed. Temperature-sensitive mutants and organisms attenuated by multiple passages are currently under investigation.

## References

Archer, D. B.: Pathogenic mechanisms of mycoplasmas. Nature 277:268, 1979.

Cherry, J. D., and Welliver, R. C.: *Mycoplasma pneumoniae* infections of adults and children (medical progress). West J Med 125:47, 1976.

Clyde, W. A., Jr.: *Mycoplasma pneumoniae* infections of man. In Tully, J. G., and Whitcomb, R. F. (eds.): The Mycoplasmas. Vol. II, Human and Animal Mycoplasmas. New York, Academic Press, 1979, p. 275.

Mufson, M. A., and Zollar, L. M.: Non-bacterial respiratory infections. DM November, 1975.

Murray, H. W., Masur, H., Senterfit, L. B., and Roberts, R. B.: The protean manifestations of *Mycoplasma pneumoniae* infection in adults. Am J Med 58:229, 1975.

Putnam, C. E., Curtis, A. M., Simeone, J. F., and Jensen, P.: Mycoplasma pneumonia. Clinical and roentgenographic patterns. Am J Roentgenol 91:560, 1975.

Tully, J. G.: Biology of the mycoplasmas. In McGarrity, G. J., Murphy, D. G., and Nichols, W. W. (eds.): Mycoplasma infection of cell cultures. New York, Plenum Publishing Company, 1978, p. 1.

Whittlestone, P.: Immunity to mycoplasmas causing respiratory diseases in man and animals. Adv Vet Sci Comp Med 20:277, 1976.

# *PSITTACOSIS* **109**

## *Stanley D. Freedman, M.D.*

### *DEFINITION*

Psittacosis is a disease of birds that is transmissible to humans. There is a variable pattern of disease in the avian species, either a minor illness but prolonged excretion of the causative agent, or a severe infection, rapidly evolving, with mortality rates of over 60 per cent. Similarly, in humans the disease ranges from subclinical cases to fulminant infections with mortality rates in some epidemics of 20 per cent. At first only psittacine birds (parrots, parakeets, cockatiels, macaws, and other birds of the order Psittaciformis) were regarded as sources of human infection, but now the disease is known to affect many other species of birds such as pigeons, turkeys, chickens, ducks, canaries, sea gulls, egrets, and chaparral birds. Thus the more inclusive term ornithosis was suggested for this disease. The causative agent is *Chlamydia psittaci*; therefore, the generic term psittacosis is preferred for human disease.

### *ETIOLOGY*

The agent responsible for psittacosis belongs to the genus *Chlamydia*, formerly called *Bedsonia*. The chlamydiae have been placed in their own order, the Chlamydiales, because of a unique developmental cycle described in Chapter 52. Earlier, they were considered to be large viruses because of their size and obligatory intracellular parasitism. Over the years the differences from viruses and the similarities to bacteria have been delineated (Moulder, 1964; Manire, 1977). Chlamydiae contain both DNA and RNA, and divide by binary fission. They appear on light microscopy as gram-negative bacilli about one third the size of *E. coli*, and, in fact, their cell walls are structurally and chemically analogous to those of gram-negative bacteria. They have ribosomes that are similar in size to those of bacteria. There may be multiple serotypes of *C. psittaci* because multiple infections in individual patients have been documented.

### *PATHOGENESIS*

Psittacosis in humans develops after exposure to discharges of infected birds and is therefore a true zoonosis. Affected birds demonstrate nonspecific signs of disease. Chlamydiae infect most of the organs and are shed in secretions from the eyes and nostrils as well as in the feces. In addition, the organism remains viable in dried feces, and can be cultured from bird feathers and dust in the vicinity of the infected birds. The agent can be shed for prolonged periods by asymptomatic birds or by birds who have recovered from infection. One should consider all avian species as potential sources. Human-to-human transmission is rare but has occurred and is a problem for hospital personnel. Disease acquired by this route is considered more severe than that acquired directly from an avian source.

Latent infections and the carrier state are recognized in birds (Manire, 1977). In parrots and parakeets persistently high antibody levels are associated with latent psittacosis infection (usually in the spleen). These birds show some degree of resistance to reinfection, but they are prone to relapses when environmental conditions are adverse. Australian budgerigars, a common host, excrete large amounts of chlamydiae through the alimentary canal during egg laying and hatching. Their nestlings are then infected, and a chain of latent infection is established. When infected birds are introduced into aviaries, susceptible contacts more frequently develop latent or subclinical infections with repeated relapses rather than lethal infections. These features explain the persistence of *C. psittaci* in birds.

The route of entry into humans is the respiratory tract in nearly all cases, but infection may occur after a bite from an infected bird. After inhalation, the organism spreads hematogenously to the reticuloendothelial system, where it matures before clinical illness develops. It is unclear if the subsequent pulmonary involvement represents progressive pneumonitis originating at the site of implantation of the droplet nuclei or if the lung is infected hematogenously as are the other organ systems.

Antibody develops between the third and fifth week of infection and gradually wanes thereafter. Cellular immunity is thought to be important, since reinfection is rare. However, prolonged illness and carrier states with shedding of the agent in the respiratory secretions have been described.

## PATHOLOGY

The initial inflammatory reaction in the lungs begins with a polymorphonuclear infiltrate, and this intra-alveolar cellular exudative process resembles a bacterial infection. Later this changes to a lymphocytic and mononuclear cell reaction in the alveoli and interstitium. Both prominent alveolar pneumocytic hyperplasia with slough and erythroleukophagocytosis have been noted. Abundant fibrin is present. Varying degrees of edema, necrosis, and hemorrhage occur. Pulmonary macrophages containing basophilic cytoplasmic inclusion bodies, if present, characterize the disease as psittacosis. These inclusion bodies have been called LCL bodies after the independent discoverers, Levinthal, Coles, and Lillie (Coles, 1930; Levinthal, 1930). Unlike influenza, the tracheobronchial epithelium is spared (Yow, 1959). Grossly, lobular pneumonia is most commonly seen. Hepatic inflammation with intralobular focal necrosis occurs, and elementary bodies can be found in Küpffer cells. Inflammatory changes in other organ systems, notably the peri-

cardium and myocardium, have been described, and the basophilic inclusion bodies may be seen in these tissues as well. Direct central nervous system involvement is distinctly unusual; meningeal exudate containing the inclusions has been reported (Walton, 1954). In turkeys, interestingly, the disease is predominantly a myocarditis.

## CLINICAL MANIFESTATIONS

It is important to stress that the signs and symptoms of psittacosis vary greatly, and this accounts for the difficulties of diagnosis. The clinical course ranges from subclinical to fatal infections. The incubation period is 7 to 14 days but may be longer. The early symptoms are sore throat, anorexia, weakness, malaise, myalgia, and headache. Photophobia, nausea, and vomiting are less often reported. Chills are common; true rigors are not. A nonproductive cough is characteristic of the disease but, rarely, may be absent. Hemoptysis is unusual, and chest pain due to pleuritis or pericardial inflammation is infrequent. Epistaxis occurs in up to one fourth of the cases. Confusion and mild disorientation are the most common sensorial changes. Of the many symptoms, diffuse headache is almost always present and is so intense that it may dominate the clinical picture. In fact, the presentation of profound headache and weakness with only minimal pulmonary signs or symptoms is typical for psittacosis.

Fever is the most constant sign, reaching 39 to 41° C at the height of illness, and is sometimes accompanied by a relative bradycardia. A faint macular eruption reminiscent of rose spots is described. Pharyngitis and cervical adenopathy may be present. Tachypnea and fine crepitant rales are the usual pulmonary findings and often occur late in the course of the disease. Percussion flatness, altered tactile fremitus, egophony, and whispered pectoriloquy are frequently absent, although consolidation can occur. Hepatosplenomegaly is common, not unexpectedly, considering the pathogenesis of this infection. The finding of splenomegaly with pneumonia should alert one to the diagnosis of psittacosis. Signs of meningeal irritation and focal central nervous system findings are not part of this disease. Icterus, cyanosis, signs of congestive heart failure, and coma are manifestations of fulminant infections and fortunately are uncommon.

The similarity of these signs and symptoms with those of other diseases is evident. The differential diagnosis includes encephalitis, influenza, typhoid fever, mycoplasmal pneumonia, Q fever, bacterial pneumonia, and tuberculosis. A history of bird exposure is obviously important.

Psittacosis acquired from parrots or parakeets is usually more serious than that from pigeons or turkeys. Mild disease, if not treated, usually subsides within two to three weeks with the fever and pneumonia running a parallel course. More chronic illness is recognized. With therapy, there is prompt clinical response within 24 to 72 hours.

## COMPLICATIONS AND SEQUELAE

Clinical relapse is recognized but is quite unusual. Thrombophlebitis of the lower extremities occurs during convalescence, and pulmonary infarction is feared (Jörgensen and Steffensen, 1956). Psittacosis does not predispose to secondary bacterial infections (Yow, 1959). Sequelae due to permanently altered organ systems are not recognized. Chlamydial infections have been implicated as a cause of myocarditis (which occurs in avian infections) on the basis of serologic tests. There is no direct evidence of *C. psittaci* infection in these cases.

## GEOGRAPHIC VARIATIONS IN DISEASE

Since this is a true zoonosis acquired from birds, the distribution of cases is widespread. It was first recognized as a disease in Switzerland and later in France and Germany. Soon thereafter cases were reported in many different countries. Psittacine birds everywhere have been recognized as the source. When they are shipped from one country to another there are outbreaks of infection among the birds. High rates of infection among birds are associated with the adverse conditions that occur during shipping. Some variations in incidence and severity are noted in the disease transmitted from other species of birds. In the United States psittacosis is an occupational disease seen most commonly in processing plants; the reservoir is the turkey. In eastern Europe the duck is an important source.

## DIAGNOSIS

Clinical signs and symptoms are not diagnostic. The importance of the epidemiologic history has been stressed. Similarly, routine laboratory studies are not helpful. Leukopenia may be present early in the disease in about 25 per cent of patients. Leukocytosis develops during convalescence. The sedimentation rate is usually normal.

Mild proteinuria may be present early. Cold agglutinins are absent. Although headache and mild sensorial changes may dominate the clinical picture, the cerebrospinal fluid is normal (mild pleocytosis is the exception). The x-ray findings vary widely; the most common pattern is a patchy infiltrate in the lower lobes. Pleural effusions are very uncommon, although there is pleural involvement pathologically.

Early in the disease *C. psittaci* can be isolated from the blood and sputum, and it persists in the sputum during convalescence (Meyer and Eddie, 1951). The chlamydiae are isolated from infected material by inoculating the material intraperitoneally into mice, into the yolk sac of embryonated hen's eggs, or into tissue cultures. A tissue culture technique using irradiated or IUDR-treated McCoy cells has recently been reported to increase the yield of chlamydiae. Such isolation procedures are not generally available, and the yield remains low in human infections.

The serologic test most widely used is the complement fixation test. This uses a heat-stable chlamydial group antigen prepared from infected chick embryos. With this antigen, the complement fixation antibody reaches a maximum titer that ranges from 1:32 to 1:256 during the third to fifth week of illness, and slowly diminishes thereafter. A fourfold rise in titer can be demonstrated between acute and convalescent serum specimens. The rise in titer may be delayed by therapy. Problems with anticomplementary sera and the presence of chlamydial antibodies in certain lots of normal guinea pig complement have led to some of the difficulties with this technique. The antigen used for CF tests is a group-specific antigen that measures antibody response to all chlamydiae and is therefore not specific for psittacosis. A radioisotope precipitation technique and an indirect fluorescent antibody test have been used in special laboratories. Recently, the enzyme-linked immunosorbent assay method has been adopted for chlamydial infections and may become the preferred serologic procedure.

## TREATMENT

Tetracycline is a highly effective treatment of choice. The usual adult dose is 500 mg orally every six hours; it is usually continued for 12 to 14 days to prevent relapse. This treatment causes defervescence and clinical improvement within 24 to 72 hours. Intravenous fluids, oxygen, and other supportive measures may be necessary. Intravenous penicillin in a dose of one million units every four hours can be used as an alternate form of therapy. The mortality rate may reach 20 per cent with no treatment.

## PROPHYLAXIS

There is no human vaccine, and vaccines for psittacine birds have not been generally effective. However, chlamydial infections in psittacines and poultry are effectively controlled by the incorporation of chlortetracycline in the feed during quarantine. Properly administered and supervised programs should eliminate the reservoir for human psittacosis, but this treatment program does not always eliminate the infection in birds. Unfortunately, the disease remains an important occupational hazard of poultry workers (Schacter, 1978).

## References

Coles, A. C.: Micro-organisms in psittacosis. Lancet 1:1011, 1930.

Jörgensen, M., and Steffensen, K.: Ornithosis: An analysis of 44 human cases with positive complement fixation tests. Dan Med Bull 3:20, 1956.

Levinthal, W.: Die Ätiologie der Psittacosis. Klin Wochen schr 9:654, 1930.

Manire, G. P.: Biologic characteristics of chlamydiae. In Hobson, D., and Holmes, K. (eds.): Nongonococcal Arthritis and Related Infections. Washington, D. C., American Society of Microbiology, 1977, p. 167.

Meyer, K., and Eddie, B.: Human carrier of the psittacosis virus. J Infect Dis 88:109, 1951.

Moulder, J. W.: The psittacosis group as bacteria. In Ciba Lectures in Microbial Biochemistry, New York, John Wiley & Sons, 1964.

Schacter, J.: Psittacosis: The reservoir persists. J Infect Dis 137:44, 1978.

Walton, K. W.: The pathology of a fatal case of psittacosis showing intracytoplasmic inclusions in the meninges. J Pathol Bacteriol 68:565, 1954.

Yow, E.: The pathology of psittacosis: A report of two cases with hepatitis. Am J Med 27:739, 1959.

# 110 Q FEVER

*Walter P. G. Turck, M.B.*

## DEFINITION

Q fever is a rickettsial zoonosis of sudden onset with influenza-like symptoms of fever, sweating, and severe headache. Over half the patients have a pneumonitis resembling that found in viral pneumonias. Usually a self-limited acute disease, it may be subacute or chronic (see Chapter 193). In the United States it is considered to be one of the three rickettsial diseases of greatest importance (Woodward, 1973).

It differs from other rickettsial diseases as follows: a rash may occur but does not form part of the typical picture; propagation of the disease does not depend on an arthropod vector; the etiological agent is filterable, more resistant to physical and chemical factors, and does not produce agglutinins against the X strains of *Proteus vulgaris* that are responsible for the Weil-Felix reaction. For these reasons the organism was assigned to a separate genus, *Coxiella*, in honor of Cox, who had described it in the United States, with the qualification *burneti* retained for Burnet, who had recognized it almost simultaneously in Australia. The name "Q (for query) fever," adopted by Derrick as a temporary expedient until further knowledge allowed a better name, has persisted. In the French literature the name "la maladie de Derrick et Burnet" exists as an alternative.

## ETIOLOGY

The etiologic agent is *Coxiella burneti*, a pleomorphic rod that is between 0.3 and 0.7 $\mu$ long and occasionally plump or coccoid in shape — an appearance consistent with that of rickettsiae. It is an obligate, intracellular parasite that grows in the cytoplasm but not in the nuclei of endothelial and serosal cells, where it may be present in large, closely packed masses. It is transmissible to guinea pigs and mice, and may be grown and maintained in the yolk sac of the chick embryo by serial passage. In the guinea pig it induces a fever that lasts for four to six days when it circulates in the blood, but it does not cause a tunica or scrotal reaction. Guinea pigs that develop fever become immune to further infection. Large numbers of the organisms are found in the liver and spleen of infected mice.

*C. burneti* can undergo a host-controlled variation (phase variation) that is in many ways similar to the rough-smooth variations of *Diplococcus pneumoniae*. Rickettsial suspensions prepared from the yolk sac of chick embryos infected with recent isolates from patients, animals, or arthropods will not fix complement with convalescent-phase sera from patients with Q fever. After serial passage in the chick embryo most strains alter and will then fix complement with these sera. The original nonreactive state and the reactive state induced by passage in the chick embryo are called, respectively, phase I and phase II. Rickettsiae in phase II can be made to revert to phase I by passage through guinea pigs, mice, or hamsters (Stoker and Fiset, 1956). This definition of phase variation by complement fixation has recently been questioned, and other serologic methods of determining the phase of *C. burneti*, have been proposed. Since a transition phase, similar to a pure phase II serologically but more virulent, has been recognized, the phase state of a strain may be determined by other criteria based on its physicochemical characteristics, susceptibility to nonspecific phagocytosis by polymorphonuclear leukocytes, and ability to multiply in the mouse spleen and in cell cultures (Brezina, 1978).

Strains of *C. burneti* also vary in virulence and sensitivity in detecting antibody in human and guinea pig sera.

## EPIDEMIOLOGY

### Incidence and Distribution

Q fever is a disease of men rather than of women because of occupational exposure, and usually affects those between 20 and 60 years of age. Symptomatic infection in childhood is rare, but subclinical infection, which is usually acquired by ingestion of milk, is not uncommon. In areas of high Q fever endemicity human fetal infection has been demonstrated, but whether such fetal infection has any later effect on the developing child is unknown.

Abattoir workers, farm workers, shepherds, dairy workers, veterinary personnel, wool sorters, and tanners are particularly liable to infection, as are newcomers to any community that has already acquired immunity from previous exposure.

In many regions a seasonal variation in incidence occurs, related in most cases to farming activity. Higher incidences are to be expected at times of calving, lambing, or shearing. Dry summers encourage airborne propagation.

Q fever is found throughout the world with the exception of Sweden, Norway, Iceland, and New Zealand. The few reported Scandinavian patients were probably infected while traveling or working in the Mediterranean region, where Q fever is common.

### Transmission

One reason for the success of *C. burneti* has been its ability to grow equally well in the intestine of ticks, the reproductive tract of cows or sheep, and the respiratory tract of humans (Marmion 1953).

The organism has been found in at least 30 species of ticks, and since transovarian transmission occurs in many of these, an arthropod reservoir may be recognized (Fig. 1). The tick facilitates a wildlife cycle in which the participating animal varies in different parts of the world. The bandicoot and kangaroo in Australia and the merion in North Africa are typical examples. A

similar relationship may exist between some argasid ticks and birds. Although these reservoirs maintain *C. burneti* in the world, they are of little direct relevance to Q fever in man, for whom livestock represents a more important reservoir. However, on rare occasions a connection between the two cycles may be established, as when the infection is transmitted to sheep by ticks that have previously fed on kangaroos, or when infectious tick feces are inhaled by man. Man rarely gets Q fever from a tick bite.

*C. burneti* infection is widespread among cattle, sheep, and goats. The organism may be present in high concentrations in the placental and birth fluids and in the feces and urine of these animals.

Human Q fever is acquired by inhalation of infected aerosols. *C. burneti* may be disseminated as a primary aerosol after parturition by an infected animal. Alternatively, because the organism is resistant to heat, drying, and sunlight, a *C. burneti* laden dust often forms from contaminated birth fluids, blood, feces, or urine. Such dusts may be disseminated by dry and windy weather or carried on fomites such as wool, hides, farmworkers' clothing, straw, and packing materials, to be released later as secondary aerosols in other environments. Farm dogs, particularly if fed on infected placentas, and farmyard chickens may contribute their own excreta to this part of the cycle.

Lower but significant concentrations of the organism are found in the udders and milk of infected cows. Drinking infected raw milk accounts for most sporadic cases. The protective or neutralizing properties of whey antibody in infected milk are a possible explanation for the low incidence of clinical Q fever arising from this mode of transmission.

Within the herd or flock the infection is probably maintained by inhalation of infected dusts and aerosols. In some herds the organism may be transferred from udder to udder by the milking process or by animal bedding.

Man-to-man infection is extremely uncommon, but in rare instances patients with *C. burneti* in their sputum, urine, or placenta have been identified as sources of infection. A high incidence of infection has been reported among laboratory workers handling infected tissues, specimens, and laboratory animals, and among medical and paramedical personnel attending autopsies on cases of Q fever.

## PATHOGENESIS AND PATHOLOGY

The organism has a predilection for the vascular endothelium of arteries, veins, and capillaries,

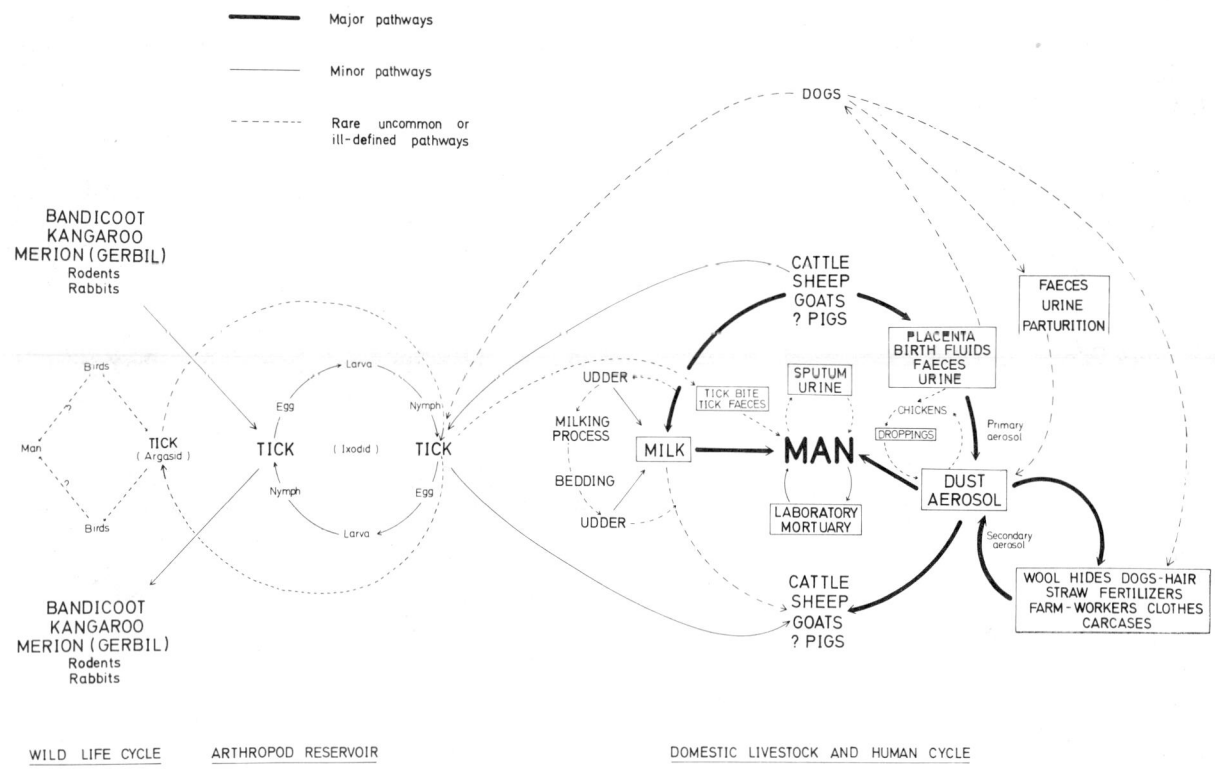

**FIGURE 1.** *Transmission cycles for* Coxiella burneti *infection.*

the epithelium of the respiratory tract and renal tubules, and serosal cells. Man usually acquires the infection by the inhalation of contaminated aerosols or dusts or by the ingestion of infected milk or food. Milk is usually the vehicle for only mild clinical infections unless the strain contained is very virulent, but milk is responsible for many subclinical infections. Contrary to earlier opinions that inhalation of *C. burneti* was invariably associated with pneumonia there is now strong circumstantial evidence that the lungs serve mainly as a portal of direct entry to the systemic circulation (Tiggert et al., 1961). In Q fever the mean incubation period is longer than that of other rickettsioses. During this period, the length of which is inversely proportional to the amount of infected material inhaled, the rickettsiae are multiplying and spreading within the body. Rickettsemia persists during the period of primary fever. These facts, coupled with the observation that pneumonia may occur as a late complication, indicate that Q fever is essentially a systemic infection (Derrick, 1973).

Acute Q fever is seldom fatal in otherwise healthy persons, but rare deaths have occurred from fulminating pneumonia or massive hepatic

necrosis. Histopathologic studies of pneumonia in man are scarce because of limited autopsy material, but the hepatic lesion has become clarified through biopsies.

In fatal cases of severe pneumonia the consolidated areas may contain foci of suppuration and hemorrhage. The interlobar fissures and pleural surfaces may contain fibropurulent exudate and be associated with pleural effusions. The bronchi may be hyperemic and edematous. Microscopically, there has been severe focal necrotizing hemorrhagic intra-alveolar pneumonia with associated necrotizing bronchitis and bronchiolitis (Urso, 1975). The intra-alveolar infiltrate is fibrinous, and histiocytes, lymphocytes, and plasma cells predominate. Alveolar septa are swollen with monocytic infiltrates, but hyaline membranes are absent. A peribronchial interstitial infiltrate is often seen. The bronchi contain a similar fibrinocellular exudate with necrosis in the mucosa and desquamation of epithelium in the bronchioles. Pneumonitis of such severity is never seen in other rickettsial disease — apart from the more florid cases of scrub typhus (Allen and Spitz, 1945).

In the liver abnormalities may be observed

microscopically as early as the late incubation period (Dupont et al., 1971) and are invariably present once the disease is fully established (Powell, 1961). The earliest lesions are numerous small foci of histiocytes with fewer lymphocytes, polymorphonuclear leukocytes, and eosinophils, and no reticulin. Small areas of liver cell necrosis also occur as in viral hepatitis. A nonspecific progressive inflammatory infiltrate is seen in the portal triads. The histiocytic foci enlarge to form granulomata with central necrosis surrounded by epithelioid cells and a few Langhans' giant cells. Such granulomata may occasionally surround a hepatocyte showing fatty change (Bouzakoura and Cox, 1974). Uninvolved hepatic cells may undergo mild to moderate focal cytoplasmic fatty change. Thickening and eosinophilia of the sinusoid walls with patchy necrosis are occasionally noted (Bernstein et al., 1965). Most cases heal completely, but persistence of abnormalities is highly variable. The granulomata heal by absorption and fibrosis in several weeks or months, but fatty change may persist for a long time. In the sole fatal case reported with hepatic lesions, the main findings were a panlobular necrosis with marked perilobular infiltration of polymorphonuclear leukocytes, plasma cells, and lymphocytes, and no liver regeneration (Tonge and Derrick, 1959).

Perivascular hemorrhages, cellular infiltration, and a slight increase in neuroglial cells have been observed in the brain. The capillaries may show swelling of the endothelium and may contain thrombi.

The spleen and lymph nodes show histiocytic hyperplasia. Focal hypoplasia, vasculitis, and granulomata with peripheral fibrinoid deposits have been seen in bone marrow, and focal interstitial nephritis with tubular degeneration has been seen in the kidney. Lesions of the testis have also been reported.

With appropriate tinctorial or fluorescent antibody techniques C. burneti has been seen in the cytoplasm of endothelial cells of alveolar and intracerebral capillaries, in arterial walls, in histiocytes in the liver, lungs, spleen, and testes, and in neuroglial cells of the brain.

There may be a relative lymphocytosis in the blood and elevation of the sedimentation rate. Rarely, an absolute lymphocytosis mimicking infectious mononucleosis may occur. Thrombocytopenia with increased numbers of megakaryocytes in the marrow smear has also been reported. Abnormal cephalin-cholesterol flocculation and thymol turbidity tests reflect increases in serum gamma globulin and IgM. Elevations of serum alkaline phosphatase and aminotransferases are common, but increases in the latter are invariably moderate.

## CLINICAL FEATURES

The incubation period ranges from 11 to 26 days but is usually 18 to 20 days. Massive doses, as may be acquired in laboratory infections, may be associated with much shorter periods, whereas prolonged incubation probably represents minimal dosage.

The onset is sudden, with fever that rises progressively over two to four days to 39 to 40° C. At this point there may be marked prostration and delirium. High fever persists for another four to seven days and then falls by lysis to normal temperature within 15 days. Accompanying the fever is a severe retro-orbital or occipital headache. Arthralgias and muscular aches and pains in the calves and lumbar region are usual. Profuse sweats, chills, and occasional rigors also occur. There is general malaise, often accompanied by anorexia, nausea, diarrhea, or constipation. In milder cases the fever may occur in the evening only and be accompanied by no other symptoms.

The most striking physical finding is a relative bradycardia. The pharynx and tonsils may be hyperemic. The constant rash seen in other rickettsial diseases does not occur, but evanescent exanthems resembling those of measles, rubella, scarlet fever, or urticaria, and distributed over the shoulders, thorax, or trunk, have been described in 5 to 10 per cent of cases. Purpura is rare.

As described so far the infection resembles influenza, and in many patients no further symptoms develop. In others there is pulmonary or hepatic involvement. Pneumonia occurs in just over half the patients. Cough due to bronchitis is common. On the third to fifth day there may be moderate dyspnea and a sense of constriction around the chest. The sputum may become purulent or slightly blood-stained. The physical signs vary from those of consolidation to small patches of basal crepitant roles. Poorly defined lobar or segmental infiltrates are seen in the x-ray. These infiltrates have hazy outlines and a ground glass appearance, are frequently multiple, and are usually in the lower lobes, often in association with linear atelectasis. They persist for 10 to 30 days and may recur.

Liver involvement is more common than originally thought. Moderate hepatomegaly may be detected in up to two thirds of patients, but jaundice is uncommon (Powell, 1961). Clinically, the picture may be very similar to that of viral hepatitis (Alkan et al., 1965).

Headache with neck stiffness is common and the cerebrospinal fluid findings may be those of a mild aseptic meningitis. Febrile convulsions and encephalitis have occurred in childhood Q fever, but usually the infection is mild or inapparent at this age.

## COMPLICATIONS AND SEQUELAE

In most patients the illness lasts up to 15 days, but fever may be prolonged in a continuous or intermittent form with persistent malaise for as long as eight weeks (Derrick, 1973). The more severe forms, found mostly in patients over the age of 40 or in those with liver involvement or impaired immune mechanisms, have a slow convalescence.

Complications are not rare. Thrombophlebitis, sometimes with pulmonary embolism or infarction, has been noted. Intermittent claudication has been attributed to Q fever arteritis. Myocarditis and pericarditis may occur separately or together and pericardial pain may dominate the clinical picture. Orchitis, epididymitis, parotitis, thyroiditis, and pancreatitis may be associated with Q fever. Pleural effusions are not uncommon, but ascites is rare. Arthritis, acute nephritis, and thrombocytopenia have been reported as separate complications. Encephalitis and encephalomyelitis may occur late in the disease. Other neurologic complications include extrapyramidal disease, dementia, toxic confusional states, and manic psychosis. Visual disturbances may be caused by retinal vasculitis, chorioretinitis, or uveitis. Abortion may have been a complication of Q fever infection in a few instances.

Recovery from acute Q fever is the rule, but infection with *C. burneti* may become latent and persist for long periods. For fuller discussion of this subject and the clinical manifestations of the whole spectrum of chronic Q fever, including endocarditis, the reader is referred to Chapter 193.

Death from acute Q fever is extremely rare and usually occurs only in elderly and diseased patients.

Following recovery from acute Q fever, most patients enjoy life-long immunity, but rare cases of reinfection have been reported.

## GEOGRAPHIC VARIATIONS IN DISEASE

Although the influenza-like symptoms are found in most outbreaks throughout the world, the pneumonic form of Q fever has been particularly common in Europe and America. In Australia, most cases have had evidence of hepatic involvement. Significant variations have occurred within smaller geographic limits. In California, hepatic complications were rare in the

south but relatively frequent in the north. A difference in the infecting strain possibly accounts for this phenomenon.

## DIAGNOSIS

The diagnosis of Q fever should be considered whenever a patient with a fever of unknown origin, especially if accompanied by severe headache, is discovered to have the appropriate epidemiologic background. Such a background includes veterinary work; employment in an abattoir; laboratory work with infected material; contact with wool, hides, or farm products; work or home near farms or in areas where sheep, cattle, or goats graze; or military deployment in areas with primitive animal husbandry. The diagnosis should be suspected in patients with hepatitis, particularly if the serum alkaline phosphatase is elevated and a liver biopsy shows granulomata. If pneumonitis is present, Q fever must be considered along with virus and primary atypical pneumonias and psittacosis.

Serologic tests confirm the diagnosis. The complement fixation test with the phase II antigen is the most frequently used test and gives clear results. Complement-fixing antibodies rise in the second week of illness, reach their peak at the end of the third week, and may persist for many months. Two specimens of serum are required, an early one and another after 12 to 20 days. A four-fold rise in antibody titer is taken as evidence of recent infection. For retrospective diagnosis in the convalescent period, an isolated titer of at least 1:32 strongly suggests recent acute Q fever (Murphy and Field, 1970), but strain variation in virulence and ability to detect antibody must be taken into account. Early effective antibiotic treatment may slow the rise in titer.

Failure to recognize a prozone phenomenon may allow false negative results to be recorded in the complement-fixation test in sera with high antibody titers. Positive sera for Q fever may give false-positive serologic tests for syphilis. Q fever complement-fixing antibody has been found in adenovirus 7 and 27 infections, psittacosis, and Rocky Mountain spotted fever, but the Q fever titers have been low and have not risen significantly. Anamnestic response have been recorded in *Mycoplasma pneumoniae* infection.

Agglutination tests have also been used in Q fever. Agglutinins rise and peak approximately one week earlier than complement-fixing antibody. Microagglutination and the radioisotope precipitation techniques are more sensitive and useful for population surveys.

*C. burneti* may be isolated from blood by guinea pig inoculation during the febrile period, and also from sputum, urine, cerebrospinal fluid, milk, placenta, and postmortem tissues. Frequent infections among laboratory staff make serologic methods preferable in routine situations.

## TREATMENT

The only drugs of proven value for acute Q fever are tetracycline and chloramphenicol. Neither is rickettsiocidal. The small but definite risk of marrow toxicity from chloramphenicol makes tetracycline the drug of choice. Tetracycline should be given in a dose of 2 grams per day in divided doses for at least two weeks. On this regimen the fever falls within two days in most cases, but if fever is slow to respond, the antibiotic must be continued until 48 hours after fever disappears. Premature withdrawal of the antibiotic is usually followed by relapse. If fever recurs after the standard regimen, a second course of tetracycline should be given.

## PROPHYLAXIS

Ideally all workers in occupations where the risk of Q fever is high should be immunized. Vaccines are prepared from *C. burneti* grown in the yolk sac. The protective polysaccharide antigen seems to be present in the rickettsial cell wall, and is present in larger amounts in extracts of *C. burneti* in phase I than in phase II. A killed Q fever vaccine, injected subcutaneously and capable of protecting man against airborne infection, has been available for many years but has been associated with severe local and general reactions. Russian investigators have developed a living vaccine from an attenuated (M-44) strain and report encouraging results. In Czechoslovakia and Romania, vaccines prepared from a trichloracetic acid extract of soluble phase I antigenic component produced a satisfactory antibody response with minimal local or systemic reactions (Brezina et al., 1974). Further evaluation is necessary. In high risk groups skin testing with a small phase I vaccine dose can be used to identify those needing an immediate vaccination schedule (Peacock et al., 1979).

Vaccination can reduce infection rates in cattle and sheep (Sádecký and Brezina, 1977) but it is an expensive procedure, and since Q fever causes little or no illness in livestock, there is little economic incentive for this type of control.

In endemic areas milk from cattle or goats should be pasteurized or boiled. A change in location and timing of lambing and calving, in housing and density of animals, and in other conditions of animal husbandry may alter the pattern of human infection. In cases admitted to hospital, sputum and urine should be disinfected by autoclaving. Persons attending postmortem examinations of cases of Q fever, and undertakers handling such cases, should wear masks and protective clothing and take specimens with precautions to minimize aerosol formation (Andrews and Marmion, 1959). In institutions in which sheep are used as experimental animals similarly strict precautions are recommended (Curet and Paust, 1972).

## References

Alkan, W. J., Evenchik, Z., and Eshchar, J.: Q fever and infectious hepatitis. Am J Med 38:54, 1965.

Allen, A. C., and Spitz, S.: A comparative study of the pathology of scrub typhus (tsutsugamushi disease) and the other rickettsial diseases. Am J Pathol 21:603, 1945.

Andrews, P. S., and Marmion, B. P.: Chronic Q fever. 2. Morbid anatomical and bacteriological findings in a patient with endocarditis. Br Med J 2:983, 1959.

Bernstein, M., Edmondson, H. A., and Barbour, B. H.: The liver lesion in Q fever. Arch Intern Med 116:491, 1965.

Bouzakoura, C., and Cox, J. N.: Granulomatous hepatitis in Q fever. Schweiz Med Wochenschr 104:796, 1974.

Brezina, R.: Phase variation phenomenon in *Coxiella burneti*. In Kazár, J., Ormsbee, R. A., and Tarasèvich, I. N. (eds.): Rickettsiae and Rickettsial Diseases. Bratislava, Veda, 1978, p. 221.

Brezina, R., Schramek, Š., Kazár, J., and Urvölgyi, J.: Q fever chemo-vaccine for human use. Acta Virol (Praha) 18:269, 1974.

Curet, L. B., and Paust, J. C.: Transmission of Q fever from experimental sheep to laboratory personnel. Am J Obstet Gynecol 114:566. 1972.

Derrick, E. H.: The course of infection with *Coxiella burneti*. Med J Aust 1:1051, 1973.

Dupont, H. L., Hornick, R. B., Levin, H. S., Rapoport, M. I., and Woodward, T. E.: Q fever hepatitis. Ann Intern Med 74:198, 1971.

Marmion, B. P.: World-wide Q fever. Lancet 2:616, 1953.

Murphy, A. M., and Field, P. R.: The persistence of complement-fixing antibodies to Q fever *(Coxiella burneti)* after infection. Med J Aust 1:1148, 1970.

Peacock, M. G., Fiset, P., Ormsbee, R. A., and Wisseman, C. L.: Antibody response in man following a small intradermal inoculation with *Coxiella burneti* phase I vaccine. Acta Virol (Praha) 23:73, 1979.

Powell, O. W.: Liver involvement in Q fever. Aust Ann Med 10:52, 1961.

Sádecký, E., and Brezina, R.: Vaccination of naturally infected ewes against Q fever. Acta Virol (Praha) 21:89, 1977.

Stoker, M. G. P., and Fiset, P.: Phase variation of the Nine Mile and other strains of *Rickettsia burneti*. Can J Microbiol 2:310, 1956.

Tiggert, W. D., Benenson, A. S., and Gochenour, W. S.: Airborne Q fever. Bacteriol Rev 25:285, 1961.

Tonge, J. I., and Derrick, E. H.: A fatal case of Q fever associated with hepatic necrosis. Med J Aust 1:594, 1959.

Urso, F. P.: The pathologic findings in rickettsial pneumonia. Am J Clin Pathol 64:335, 1975.

Woodward, T. E.: A historical account of the rickettsial diseases with a discussion of unsolved problems. J Infect Dis 127:583, 1973.

# 111 *VIRAL PNEUMONIA*

*Richard E. Bryant, M.D.*

## DEFINITION

Viral pneumonia is an inflammation of lung parenchyma caused by a virus. Diagnosis is proved by microscopic or cultural evidence of virus in lung tissue without concomitant microbial infection. For practical purposes, however, the diagnosis of viral pneumonia is made by viral isolation and/or serologic evidence of viral infection in a patient with a nonbacterial pneumonia. Patients may develop bacterial pneumonia as a complication of a viral respiratory infection or may have viral pneumonia as a component of polymicrobic pulmonary infection.

## ETIOLOGY

The incidence of viral pneumonia is dependent on the age, immunologic status, and environmental circumstances of the population being considered. During an eight-year period, Foy and co-workers (1973) documented pneumonia in a large prepaid medical group at a rate of 10 cases/1000 patient years. Children under 5 had a rate of 42 cases/1000 patient years. Infection rates of viral pneumonia per 1000 patient years were as follows: influenza A, 0.2; influenza B, 0.2; parainfluenza, 0.8; respiratory syncytial virus, 1.2; and adenovirus, 0.4. Less common causes of viral pneumonia include herpesviruses, rhinoviruses, rubeola, echoviruses, coronaviruses and coxsackieviruses. Rare cases have been reported with reovirus type 3, lymphocytic choriomeningitis, variola, vaccinia, and rabies viruses.

Respiratory syncytial virus is the most common cause of viral pneumonia in children under 5 years of age and causes infection most frequently in midwinter to spring. Respiratory syncytial virus can also cause pneumonia in the elderly.

Influenza A and adenovirus deserve special consideration because of their epidemic potential and the mortality, morbidity, and long-term sequelae associated with these infections. Adenoviruses are a common cause of pneumonia in military recruits and have been recognized as an important cause of chronic pulmonary disease in infants and young children.

Pneumonia caused by herpesviruses often represents a complication of altered host defenses. Primary varicella pneumonia rarely occurs in normal children. However, 90 per cent of cases of varicella pneumonia occur in adults or in patients with depressed resistance. Varicella pneumonia is a dreaded complication of pregnancy, or of disseminated zoster following chemotherapy of leukemia or lymphoma. Cytomegalovirus infection is usually recognized as a secondary event in patients with impaired defenses. This virus may cause primary pneumonia or may be associated with polymicrobic pulmonary infection.

Bacterial superinfection has been characteristically associated with influenza A virus infection during the third trimester of pregnancy, in the elderly, and in patients with rheumatic heart disease, mitral stenosis, or chronic bronchopulmonary disease. There is an increased frequency of bacterial superinfection in children with measles or chickenpox and in recruits with adenoviral infection.

## PATHOLOGY

Bronchiolitis, interstitial pneumonitis, and exudation of fluid into alveoli are present to a variable degree in all forms of viral pneumonia.

Influenza viral pneumonia is characterized by ulcerative and destructive bronchitis and by development of diffuse hemorrhagic necrotizing pneumonitis.

Respiratory syncytial virus, parainfluenza virus, and adenovirus cause necrotizing bronchitis, bronchiolitis, and interstitial pneumonia. Intranuclear inclusions may be seen in tissues of patients with varicella-zoster pneumonia, cytomegalovirus pneumonia, *Herpesvirus hominis* pneumonia, and early in the course of adenoviral pneumonia. Multinucleated giant cells, intranuclear inclusions, intracytoplasmic inclusions, and hyperplasia of distal bronchial cells are pathologic features of rubeola pneumonia.

## EPIDEMIOLOGY AND PATHOPHYSIOLOGY

Many respiratory viruses are spread from person to person by inhalation of material aerosolized during coughing or sneezing (Knight, 1973). This is probably the primary mechanism of transmission of adenovirus and influenza virus infection. Rhinovirus infection may be transmitted primarily by direct contact with infected secretions. It is likely that both mechanisms are responsible for transmission of many viral respiratory infections. After implantation and replication in the respiratory cells, viruses are released and spread down the respiratory tract in mucus, by cell-to-cell transmission, or by lymphatic or systemic routes.

A number of defense mechanisms are impaired during viral infection. Ciliated cells are destroyed and bronchial clearance mechanisms disrupted during influenza. Increased mucous secretion and post-nasal discharge help deliver both virus and bacteria to the lower respiratory tract. Influenza A and adenoviral infection may cause dysfunction of phagocytic cells. Impairment of delayed hypersensitivity during viral pneumonia has been attributed to virus-mediated lymphocyte dysfunction. Structural damage of bronchi, bronchioles, and alveolar epithelium, direct toxicity of viruses to alveolar macrophages, and the presence of increased alveolar fluid during a viral infection probably all enhance susceptibility of patients to bacterial superinfection.

Pulmonary function may be severely impaired in viral pneumonia. Injury to type 2 alveolar epithelial cells can cause loss of surfactant and collapse of alveoli. Alternatively, bronchiolitis can trap air and cause hyperinflation of involved segments. The pathologic findings of increased tissue fluid, capillary thickening and induration, and exudation of fluid into alveoli may present clinically as decreased lung compliance, increased work of breathing, dyspnea, and cyanosis. Hypoxia results primarily from abnormalities of ventilation and perfusion. The acute changes of viral pneumonia, which include increased tissue fluid with minimal alveolar exudation, account for the discrepancy between the radiologic and the auscultatory findings. There is rarely enough alveolar fluid to produce auscultatory signs of pulmonary consolidation.

Varicella pneumonia is usually more severe than other forms of primary viral pneumonia. This infection frequently involves both upper and lower lobes bilaterally. Nodular lesions throughout the lung coalesce and cause severe hypoxia. Vesicular lesions on the pleura appear to cause the pleuritic pain that is frequent in varicella pneumonia.

## CLINICAL PRESENTATION

Viral pneumonia usually starts insidiously with a prodrome of nasal stuffiness, rhinorrhea, coryza, eye discomfort, and a variable degree of sore throat, pain on swallowing, or hoarseness. Headache, malaise, chills, fever, myalgia, and nonproductive cough may appear next. With extensive pneumonitis, symptoms of fever, severe dyspnea, cough, and prostration may occur abruptly (Louria, 1959). The latter presentation is seen in patients with acute pulmonary insuffi-

ciency from a variety of causes and has been referred to as the adult respiratory distress syndrome (ARDS).

There are few clinical presentations of lower respiratory infection that are distinctive. Incubation periods for most viral respiratory infections vary from one to six days. Symptoms of patients with viral pneumonia overlap with those of patients with viral upper respiratory disease.

Physical examination of the patient with viral pneumonia is rarely diagnostic. In patients without cutaneous manifestations, upper respiratory tract findings are usually limited to nonspecific rhinitis, conjunctivitis, pharyngitis, or myringitis. A pharyngeal exudate suggests adenoviral infection. Cytomegalovirus infection is suggested by fundoscopic findings of chorioretinitis. Otitis media may be present in patients with respiratory syncytial virus or adenovirus infection. Auscultation of the chest usually reveals relatively few rales and rhonchi. Physical findings are usually less prominent than infiltrates seen on chest x-ray. Breath sounds are frequently reduced, but physical findings of consolidation are rare. Hyperresonance to percussion and the presence of sternal or intercostal retraction due to labored breathing or pleural effusion are unusual findings in viral pneumonia.

### Influenza A Viral Pneumonia

This is the most common cause of viral pneumonia in adults. Symptoms of influenza usually begin abruptly with severe headache, myalgia, prostration, chills, and fever of 39 to 40° C. Many patients are dizzy. Rhinorrhea, nasal congestion, and sore throat are frequent complaints. Hoarseness and photophobia occur less commonly. Gastrointestinal symptoms are rare.

Cough, tachypnea, dyspnea, and persistently high fever are prominent features of primary influenza viral pneumonia. Sputum is usually scanty but may become bloody as the disease progresses. Chest pain is substernal and nonpleuritic. Auscultatory findings are usually limited to rales and rhonchi. Chest x-rays show diffuse, often bilateral, bronchopneumonia.

The white blood cell count is frequently greater than 10,000 per mm$^3$ during the acute phase of infection and does not distinguish between primary viral pneumonia and secondary bacterial infection. Differential counts of the peripheral blood smear may reveal a marked "left shift." A mild leukopenia and lymphocytosis may occur late in the course of infection. Although of little value clinically, the sedimentation rate is more likely to be normal in patients with primary viral pneumonia than in those with bacterial superinfection. Changes in $pO_2$, $pCO_2$, and pH provide important but nonspecific evidence of the severity of infection. Hypoxemia ($pO_2 < 60$ mm Hg) and hypercarbia are ominous prognostic signs.

Diagnosis is established by culture and/or demonstration of a fourfold rise in complement fixation titer. Patients with viral influenza during the third trimester of pregnancy or in association with mitral stenosis, chronic lung disease, or immunodeficient or immunosuppressed states are especially susceptible to secondary bacterial pneumonia. Bacterial superinfection characteristically occurs one to five days after onset of viral illness when the patient appears to be getting well. Alternatively, patients may present with a concomitant viral pneumonia and bacterial pneumonia caused by *Staphylococcus aureus, Streptococcus pneumoniae, Haemophilus influenzae,* or *Streptococcus pyogenes* (Louria, 1959). Purulent sputum or physical findings of consolidation suggest the presence of bacterial superinfection.

The place of amantadine in therapy of influenza A viral pneumonia is promising but unproved. Pulmonary function test abnormalities associated with influenza A viral disease of the lower respiratory tract have been shown to improve with amantadine (Little et al., 1976). Unfortunately, there are no controlled studies documenting the beneficial effects of amantadine in naturally occurring influenza viral pneumonia. For the present, it seems advisable to use amantadine as an adjunct to therapy of patients thought to have pneumonia caused by, or associated with, influenza. This is especially appropriate in patients with severe viral pneumonia during an influenza A epidemic. Amantadine may be given orally to adults in doses of 100 mg every six to eight hours (Knight and Kasel, 1973).

Pathologic changes associated with influenza A viral pneumonia include destruction of ciliated epithelial cells and disruption of goblet cells and mucous glands that may extend to the basement membrane. Bronchioles become thickened, distended, and infiltrated with mononuclear cells with resultant interstitial edema that extends into interlobular septa. Necrotizing bronchiolitis and ulceration may be marked, and capillary thrombosis and necrosis may lead to necrotizing hemorrhagic pneumonitis. Exudation of fluid into the alveolar spaces may have a hyaline appearance and a variable composition of fibrin, red blood cells, or white blood cells, depending on the extent of hemorrhagic pulmonary edema.

### Adenoviral Pneumonia

Adenoviral pneumonia is usually seen in military recruits and is caused by type 3, 4, or 7. Adenoviral pneumonia is rare in civilian adults. Children may have severe or fatal pneumonia caused by type 1, 2, 3, or 7. Complications of bronchiectasis or chronic pulmonary disease after adenoviral infection are seen only in children. Symptoms and physical findings of patients with adenoviral pneumonia are shown in Tables 1 and 2.

As shown by comparison with patients with pneumococcal pneumonia, there are few features that help to distinguish adenoviral pneumonia from pneumococcal pneumonia. Sore throat, nausea, or vomiting occurs more frequently in patients with adenoviral infection. Physical findings of pharyngitis, rhinitis, and auscultatory rales occur commonly in patients with adenoviral infection (Bryant and Rhoades, 1967). Bronchophony and egophony have been observed almost exclusively in patients with pneumococcal pneumonia. Myringitis and conjunctivitis occur infrequently. Herpes labialis was present in only one patient with adenoviral infection. There are few laboratory findings suggestive of adenoviral pneumonia. Leukocyte counts may range from 5000 to 30,000 cells per mm.[3] Two thirds of patients will have less than 10,000 cells per mm[3]. When present, leukocytosis usually declines rapidly during the first week. Sputum is scanty, but may be purulent or bloody. Skin test reactivity

**TABLE 1.  Symptoms of Patients with Pneumonia**

|  | ADENOVIRAL— 12 PATIENTS (%) | PNEUMOCOCCAL— 25 PATIENTS (%) |
|---|---|---|
| Cough | 100 | 96 |
| Sore throat | 92 | 28 |
| Nausea | 75 | 28 |
| Vomiting | 58 | 28 |
| Diarrhea | 25 | 8 |
| Rhinorrhea | 75 | 48 |
| Chest pain | 67 | 80 |
| Chills | 33 | 52 |
| Headaches | 33 | 56 |
| Myalgia | 33 | 28 |

**TABLE 2.  Physical Findings of Patients with Pneumonia**

|  | ADENOVIRAL— 12 PATIENTS (%) | PNEUMOCOCCAL— 25 PATIENTS (%) |
|---|---|---|
| Pharyngitis | 92 | 64 |
| Rhinitis | 75 | 44 |
| Conjunctivitis | 33 | 44 |
| Myringitis | 25 | 28 |
| Herpes labialis | 8 | 12 |
| Rales and rhonchi | 92 | 96 |
| Bronchophony and/or egophony | 8 | 48 |

may be transiently suppressed. Characteristic roentgenographic features of adenoviral pneumonia may include: (1) irregular reticular infiltrates that may appear mottled or may coalesce in some areas; (2) indistinct segmental margins; (3) predilection for lower lobes; (4) occasional hilar enlargement (Fig. 1). Infiltrates may decrease in some segments while increasing in others. Pleural effusions are very rare. Roentgenograms usually clear by the second or third week. There is no effective therapy for adenoviral pneumonia. Diagnosis is usually established by sequential complement-fixation testing or by culture. Pathologic lesions of adenoviral pneumonia consist of bronchiolitis, interstitial pneumonitis, and intranuclear inclusions in alveolar cells in necrotic areas.

### Rubeola (Measles) Pneumonia

Pneumonia is said to occur in 7 to 50 per cent of patients with rubeola. It is usually observed in children under 6 years of age and occurs within five days of the development of the rash. The signs and symptoms of patients with rubeola pneumonia differ little from those of patients without pneumonia except for findings of rales and rhonchi on chest examination and x-ray evidence of an interstitial pneumonia. Lower lobes are frequently involved, and signs of consolida-

tion or pleural effusions occur rarely unless secondary bacterial infection is present.

Exacerbation or persistence of fever or leukocytosis suggests the presence of bacterial superinfection. *S. pneumoniae, S. pyogenes, S. aureus,* and *H. influenzae* are the most common bacterial pathogens causing superinfection. Secondary bacterial pneumonia occurs more often in immature or debilitated children and accounts for most severe or fatal complications of measles. Bacterial superinfection can also occur in healthy young adults. Olson and Hodges (1975) identified secondary bacterial infection in 10 of 16 naval recruits. Diagnosis was established by transtracheal aspiration culture and prompt response to antibiotic therapy. *Neisseria meningitidis,* serogroup Y, was the only species of bacteria isolated from six patients.

Primary measles pneumonia is an interstitial pneumonia characterized by multinucleated giant cells with nuclear and cytoplasmic inclusions. Measles pneumonia in the immunocompromised patient is an especially virulent disease. It may occur without rash and is usually fatal. Since live attenuated measles vaccine can cause giant cell pneumonia in immunodeficient patients, it should not be given to them.

When people who are partially immunized against rubeola acquire measles naturally, they

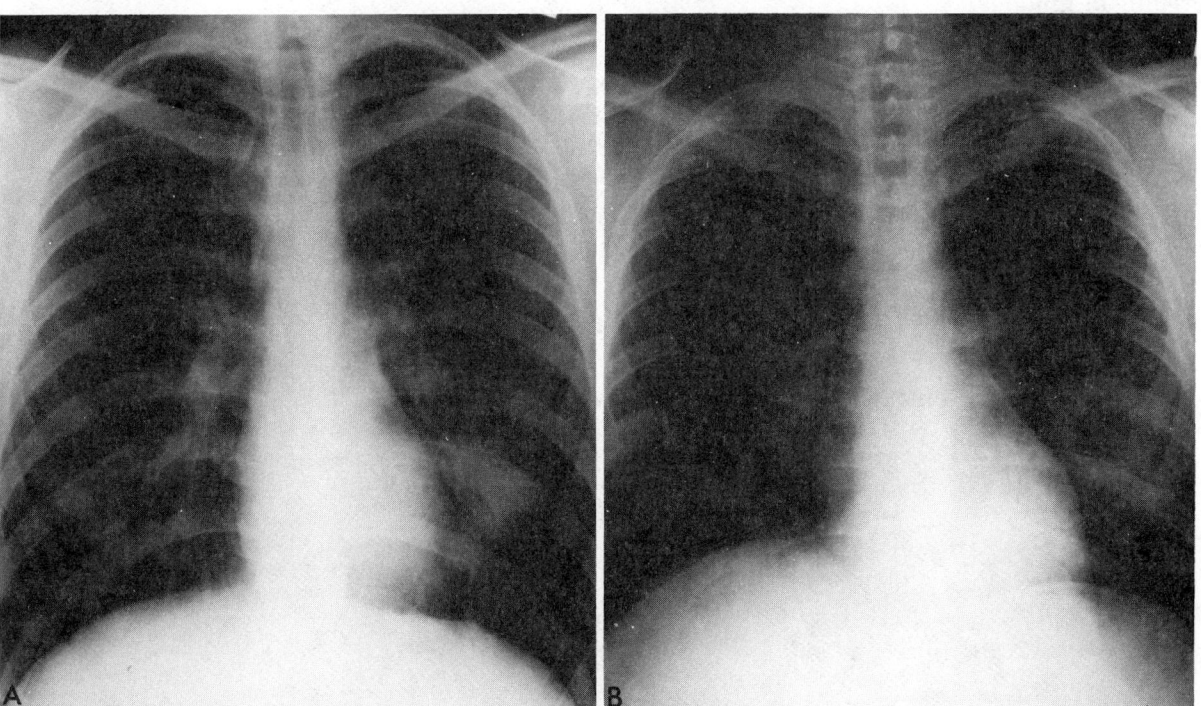

**FIGURE 1.**  A, *Patchy infiltrates with indistinct segmental margins most prominent in lingula.* B, *Left lower lobe pneumonia with reticular infiltrates.*
   *Right hilar enlargement subsided after parenchymal lesion began to clear on left. Both patients were young healthy adults who recovered promptly from their adenoviral pneumonia.*

may have an atypical rash and pneumonia characterized by hilar adenopathy, pleural effusion, and peripheral eosinophilia. Nodular infiltrates may persist after this disease subsides.

### Varicella (Chickenpox) Pneumonia

Primary varicella pneumonia is largely an adult disease. Ninety per cent of patients are more than 20 years of age. In children, primary varicella pneumonia usually represents a complication of neonatal infection, immunodeficiency, debilitation, or drug-induced suppression of host defenses. Varicella pneumonia usually occurs within one to six days after onset of the typical vesicular rash. Symptoms frequently increase in severity over a one- to three-day period with severe cough, pleuritic chest pain, dyspnea, tachypnea, and hemoptysis.

Adults with varicella pneumonia characteristically have a nonproductive cough and dyspnea. Approximately 40 per cent of patients are cyanotic and 20 per cent complain of chest pain.

The characteristic generalized papulovesicular eruption of chickenpox is present in all patients with varicella pneumonia. Mucosal lesions occur in 26 per cent of patients with pneumonia. Auscultation of the chest reveals rales and rhonchi in only 50 to 60 per cent of patients. Hyperresonance or decreased breath sounds may be present. Tachypnea and labored breathing may be the most prominent findings.

Roentgenographic characteristics of varicella pneumonia are diffuse bilateral nodular infiltrates with peribronchial distribution. Nodules rarely exceed 5 mm but may coalesce in the hilus or lung bases. Nodular and reticular infiltrates may become dense enough to obscure the lung markings (Fig. 2).

Laboratory tests are rarely helpful. Intranuclear inclusions may be seen in skin scrapings or in sputum cytologic examination. Leukocytosis is present in one third of patients. Thrombocytopenia is rare. Hypoxia is common in patients with varicella pneumonia who have the adult respiratory distress syndrome.

Sputum examination is especially important in children with varicella pneumonia because of their susceptibility to superinfection. Criteria for distinguishing bacterial superinfection from primary varicella pneumonia are shown in Table 3.

There is controversy over the value of zoster immune globulin or plasma, and of adenine arabinoside in therapy of varicella pneumonia. Both may be of value in the critically ill patient with severe immunodeficiency. Exogenous interferon and transfer factor have been considered as possible modes of therapy, but their value is unproved.

Immunoprophylaxis with zoster-immune globulin (ZIG) or varicella-zoster immune globulin (VZIG) is beneficial to the nonimmune patient with compromised host defenses who is treated

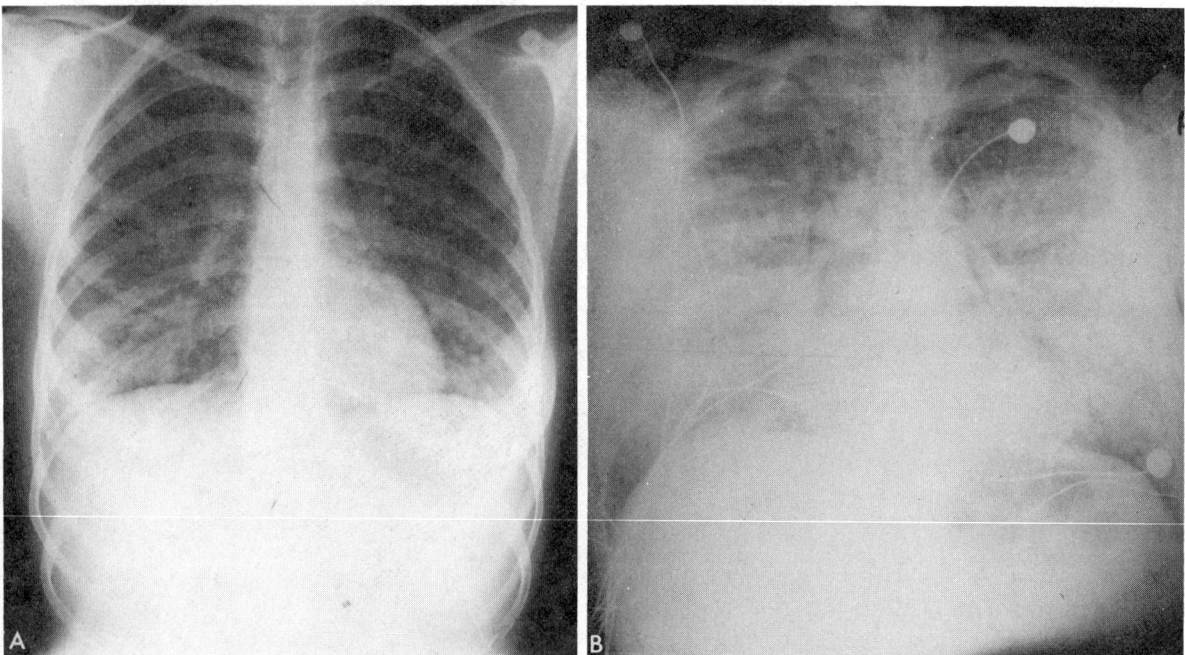

**FIGURE 2.** *Roentgenographic changes associated with varicella pneumonia. The fine nodular infiltrates shown in A are characteristic of the diffuse bilateral changes seen in early varicella pneumonia. More extensive involvement with coalescence of nodular densities is shown in B. Both patients were adults without secondary infection.*

**TABLE 3.   Differential Characteristics Between Primary Varicella Pneumonia and Varicella with Secondary Bacterial Pneumonia**

| VARICELLA PNEUMONIA | BACTERIAL PNEUMONIA |
| --- | --- |
| Adults | Usually children less than 7 years of age |
| Usually early in course with marked paucity of physical findings | Late in course with secondary rise in temperature |
| Normal to slightly increased white blood cell count | Elevated white blood cell count and "left shift" of differential |
| Negative blood and sputum cultures | Positive blood and sputum cultures |
| Diffuse nodular infiltration, usually without true consolidation | Symmetric distribution on x-ray with segmental or lobar consolidation |

From Triebwasser. J. H. et al.: Medicine 46:409, 1967.

within 72 hours of exposure to infection. Circumstances or disease states appropriate for ZIG immunoprophylaxis include: leukemia, lymphoma, congenital or acquired immunodeficiency, immunosuppression or steroid therapy, and the newborn of mothers with varicella. Inquiries concerning acquisition or use of ZIG should be made to the Massachusetts State Biologic Laboratories, 617-522-3700. Consultation concerning alternate modes of therapy can be obtained from the Communicable Disease Center in Atlanta, Georgia, 404-329-3745 (day) or 404-326-3644 (night).

The pathology of varicella pneumonia is characterized by vesicles on pleural and tracheobronchial surfaces and by interstitial pneumonitis that extends in a peribronchiolar distribution. Focal areas of hemorrhagic consolidation occur in the lung parenchyma. Alveoli and bronchi are filled with hyaline material containing fibrin, red blood cells, and monocytes. Capillary endothelium undergoes swelling, cell necrosis, and mononuclear perivascular infiltration. Intranuclear inclusions may be found in septal cells, giant cells, fibroblasts, capillary endothelium, and tracheobronchial epithelial cells. Healing of focal areas of necrosis associated with varicella can lead to a miliary pattern of pulmonary calcification.

### Cytomegalovirus (CMV Pneumonia)

This infection often occurs in patients with leukemia, lymphoma, or tissue transplantation. The virus may cause primary pneumonia in the neonate or immune deficient adult or may occur as part of a mixed pulmonary infection (Abdallah et al., 1976). It is often difficult to identify the precise role that CMV plays in a patient's illness.

There are few distinguishing features of CMV pneumonia. The best clue is a slowly progressive viral pneumonia syndrome in an immunosuppressed patient. Cytomegalovirus infection is further suggested by a finding of chorioretinitis. Roentgenograms usually show reticular, bilateral, and ill-defined densities. There is no specific therapy for CMV pneumonia.

Two forms of CMV infection occur in transplant patients. The first is reactivation of CMV infection, which causes a relatively mild disease with brisk antibody response. The second is primary CMV pneumonia, which in immunodeficient patients is often fatal. The primary CMV infection syndrome begins with spiking fever, leukopenia, prostration, and orthostatic hypotension and hypoxemia without initial x-ray evidence of pneumonia (Simmons et al., 1977). Patients have dyspnea and nonproductive cough. Hypoalbuminemia, thrombocytopenia, and lymphopenia are often present. Antibody response to CMV is minimal as the disease progresses with worsening of pulmonary, hepatic, and cerebral function. Myalgia, arthralgia, muscle wasting, abdominal distention, and tenderness are prominent features of the relentless three- to four-week course of this disease.

Chest radiographs usually show diffuse bilateral interstitial or alveolar infiltrates. Despite extensive viremia, viruria, and high titers of virus in most tissues, acute rejection is not seen on renal biopsy. Most patients with hypoxia due to CMV pneumonia die.

Successful therapy requires recognition of this disorder and rapid reduction of immunosuppressive therapy. Preliminary studies suggest that use of a live attenuated CMV vaccine before tissue transplantation may protect patients from lethal primary CMV pneumonia after transplantation (Glazer et al., 1978).

Isolation of CMV lung from tissue of patients with pneumonia is clearly a more sensitive means of detecting virus than is the morphologic demonstration of intranuclear inclusions (Abdallah et al., 1976). Lung biopsy will show interstitial pneumonia in most instances, but only a third of culture-positive biopsies will show intranuclear inclusions. Specific immunofluorescent stains of biopsy tissue for CMV may be especially useful as a diagnostic method in the future. Serologic evidence of CMV or herpesvirus infection is not an acceptable criterion for diagnosing viral pneumonia because of the variability of such titers and the ubiquity of the viruses. However, positive viral cultures from blood, urine or sputum or demonstration of multinucleated giant cells in urine or sputum is strong circumstantial evidence that CMV is one of the pathogens causing pneumonia in the compromised patient. Patients with CMV pneumonia may have concomitant infection with *Pneumocystis carinii,* fungi, mycobacteria, gram-negative bacilli, or a variety of bacteria or viruses.

### Respiratory Syncytial Virus Pneumonia

This infection may occur in the elderly but is most serious in the very young. Bronchiolitis occurs most frequently in children less than 1 year old and bronchopneumonia most often in 4- to 5-year-old children. Bronchiolitis and pneumonia may be present in the same patient. Dyspnea, fever, and wheezing are prominent symptoms. Intercostal retraction with wheezing respiration may be marked. Cough may or may not be present. Sputum is scanty. Affected children are usually irritable and tachypneic. Rales and rhonchi are present on auscultation. Chest radiographs show bilateral bronchopneumonia. Hyperlucency from air trapping may be present in bronchiolitic areas. Leukocyte counts are nondiagnostic. Needle aspiration culture may be necessary to establish the diagnosis of viral disease and exclude bacterial superinfection in the severely ill child. Use of immunofluorescent microscopic techniques to demonstrate virus in respiratory secretions will become more important when effective chemotherapeutic agents are discovered in the future. At present, therapy of respiratory syncytial viral pneumonia is limited to supportive measures, maintenance of ventilation, and removal of secretions interfering with respiration.

Immunization against respiratory syncytial (RS) virus is harmful because the vaccinated children get a more severe disease.

## COMPLICATIONS AND ADVERSE SEQUELAE OF VIRAL PNEUMONIA

Complications of viral pneumonia may be immediate or delayed. Patients with fulminant infection may develop acute respiratory insufficiency indistinguishable from the adult respiratory distress syndrome. Concomitant encephalitis, myocarditis, hepatitis, nephritis, or a hemorrhagic diathesis may be unusual clinical features of viral pneumonia. Abortion or fetal wastage has been documented best in association with varicella pneumonia in the third trimester of pregnancy.

Mortality from viral pneumonia depends on the adequacy of host defenses, the presence of complications, and the extent of the inflammatory process. A high mortality occurs at the extremes of age or with pre-existing heart disease, lung disease, or immunodeficiency. Adenoviral pneumonia in the very young has been reported to have an 8 to 10 per cent mortality. Varicella pneumonia in the adult is lethal in 10 to 30 per cent of patients but the death rate may reach 40 per cent in pregnant women (Triebwasser et al., 1967).

Respiratory syncytial virus infection in the elderly can be complicated by bacterial superinfection. This complication may also occur in children who have a lower respiratory tract infection with rubeola or varicella. *S. aureus* frequently causes infection under these circumstances.

There is little information about the extent or frequency of delayed complications of viral pneumonia. Pulmonary function defects will probably persist in most patients with severe varicella pneumonia or with viral infection presenting as the adult respiratory distress syndrome. Subtle changes in pulmonary function attributable to less severe involvement will continue to elude detection until prospective studies are done.

The most severe delayed complications of viral pneumonia in children follow adenoviral infection. These consist of obliterative bronchiolitis, severe bronchiectasis, lobar collapse, unilateral hyperlucent lung, post-inflammatory vascular disease, and residual pulmonary fibrosis. Long-term complications associated with respiratory syncytial viral disease may be more subtle than those with adenovirus. Kattan and co-workers (1977) observed a high frequency of hyperinflation, abnormal gas exchange, and small airway disease in patients examined 10 years after an episode of bronchiolitis during their first 18 months of life. The high incidence of wheezing observed in patients with a history of respiratory syncytial virus infection in childhood raises the possibility of a participatory role of respiratory syncytial virus in the pathogenesis of asthma in some patients.

## GEOGRAPHIC VARIATION IN DISEASE

There are few studies documenting a racial predisposition to the adverse sequelae of viral pneumonia despite recognition of excess mortality associated with rubeola or varicella infection in certain countries. Age-specific death rate of rubeola in Greenland was three- to fivefold higher than that in the United States in a comparable period. Developing nations in Africa may have an even higher mortality. Most deaths from rubeola in children less than 2 years old are associated with pneumonia. Varicella pneumonia also has a high mortality in such populations, but it is not clear whether primary viral pneumonia or a greater frequency of bacterial superinfection is responsible for the excess mortality. Similarly, it is not known whether age, malnutrition, anemia, lack of herd immunity, underlying disease, or genetic or environmental factors affect the adverse course of such populations.

Excess mortality and morbidity have been reported with adenoviral pneumonia in Polynesian, Auckland, and Manitoba Eskimo populations. Lang and co-workers (1969) reported a 20 per cent incidence of bronchiectasis and a 40 per cent incidence of other types of chronic pulmonary disease in New Zealand children convalescing from severe adenoviral pneumonia.

## DIAGNOSIS

With the exceptions noted for certain entities, the clinical presentation and roentgenographic findings of viral pneumonia are not specific (Table 4). Primary influenza A viral pneumonia, varicella pneumonia, and rubeola pneumonia usually present with bilateral involvement. Infants with respiratory syncytial infection may have bilateral disease or involvement of the right upper lobe. Most patients with viral pneumonia have involvement of lower lobes. Infiltrates are usually reticular, feathery, or mottled. Segmental margins are indistinct. Late in the course of infection, exudation of fluid into alveoli is associated with development of an acinar pattern of radiodensity in addition to an overall reticular pattern. Segmental atelectasis may occur in a small percentage of cases. During the course of infection, hilar adenopathy may develop and new reticular infiltrates may appear as infiltrates in other areas of the lungs disappear. With more severe involvement, the infiltrates may coalesce. Pleural effusions are uncommon, and lobar consolidation is so rare that when it does occur it suggests the presence of bacterial superinfection. Similarly, rapid progression of pneumonia over a few hours suggests the presence of bacterial infection. Radiographic differentiation of bacterial and viral pneumonia is accurate in only two thirds of cases (Tew et al., 1977).

Laboratory proof of viral infection is obtained by culture of nasal or oropharyngeal swabs, gargle, or sputum and demonstration of a fourfold rise in antibody titers to the specific virus in the absence of evidence of bacterial infection. Rigorous proof of viral pneumonia is provided by cultural or ultramicroscopic demonstration of virus in diseased lung tissue obtained by biopsy or needle aspiration. Strict criteria for demonstrating viral growth from pulmonary tissue that is sterile by conventional bacterial cultures are rarely met. Diagnosis may be suggested by demonstration of viral antigens in exfoliated cells from the nose or oropharynx by immunofluorescent microscopic techniques. This method has been used with respiratory syncytial virus, parainfluenza virus, influenza A virus, and cytomegalovirus.

It is important to differentiate viral pneumonia from the primary atypical pneumonia syndrome caused by *Mycoplasma pneumoniae,* psittacosis, Q fever, tularemia, or *Legionella pneumophila.* A careful history, physical examination demonstrating splenomegaly due to psittacosis, or a skin lesion of tularemia may be helpful, but most often it is necessary to treat the patient empirically on the basis of epidemiologic, clinical, and laboratory evidence that is imprecise.

It is mandatory that the physician distinguish viral pneumonia from bacterial pneumonia or bacterial superinfection of viral disease. The diagnosis of bacterial infection is favored by recurrent chills, abrupt onset of hypotension, physical or radiologic evidence of pulmonary consolidation, and compromised defense mechanisms that predispose to bacterial infection. Diagnosis is confirmed by microscopic demonstration of bacteria in purulent sputum obtained by having the patient cough, or by performing fiberoptic bronchoscopy, endotracheal aspiration, or transtracheal aspiration techniques. The former may be misleading because of contamination of sputum by bacteria in the mouth. Transtracheal aspiration specimens are less apt to be contaminated, but the procedure is contraindicated in the presence of severe hypoxia or bleeding diathesis, or in uncooperative patients. Thoracotomy may be required for diagnosis in special circumstances. X-ray evidence of lobar infiltrates, pneumatoceles, cavitation, or pleural effusion is evidence of bacterial infection. Pleural fluid should be examined and cultures of blood and other body fluids should be performed. Direct needle aspiration of infected lung tissue has been used extensively to document bacterial pneumonia in children.

## TREATMENT

With the exceptions discussed previously under influenza A and varicella pneumonia, treatment of viral pneumonia is for the most part nonspecific. Most patients have minimal involvement and require only supportive therapy. Patients with fulminant infection presenting as the adult respiratory distress syndrome (ARDS) require heroic efforts to improve oxygenation. It has been suggested that alveolar exudation of fluid, decreased lung compliance, and increase in interstitial fluid can be managed best by use of positive end expiratory pressure (PEEP) or continuous

TABLE 4. Clinical Findings Suggesting Cause of Pneumonia

| CAUSE | EPIDEMIOLOGIC | SYMPTOMS | PHYSICAL EXAMINATION | LABORATORY | CHEST X-RAY |
|---|---|---|---|---|---|
| Influenza A | Epidemic or pandemic period, history of exposure, susceptible host | "Flu"-like symptoms, chills, fever, myalgia, headache, rhinorrhea photophobia, sore throat, scanty sputum may become bloody | Prostration, rhinitis, conjunctivitis, pharyngitis, rales, and rhonchi | WBC is nondiagnostic. lymphocytosis late, few bacteria or neutrophils in sputum. Hypoxia or hypercarbia is an ominous prognostic sign | Bilateral bronchopneumonia with reticular pattern. Effusions rare |
| Adenovirus | Increased risk of exposure—military recruits, children, nursery epidemic | Relatively nonproductive cough, sore throat, nausea, vomiting, rhinorrhea | Rhinitis, pharyngitis, rales, and rhonchi. Otitis in children | Leukocytosis early, scanty sputum, rarely purulent or bloody | Interstitial bronchopneumonia of lower lobes |
| Respiratory syncytial virus | Extremes of age. Peak age 4 to 5 years old | Dyspnea, wheezing, and cough | Fever, tachypnea, cyanosis, wheezing respiration, rales, and rhonchi | Scanty sputum | Interstitial pneumonia may have hyperinflation in some areas |
| Cytomegalovirus | Compromised host | Depends on immune status | Chorioretinitis otherwise dependent on secondary pathogens | Demonstration of CMV in tissue or sputum by immunofluorescent microscopy or culture. Presence of giant cells on lung biopsy | Interstitial pneumonia |
| Varicella-zoster (chickenpox) | History of exposure of a susceptible patient (see Table 3) | Rash followed by cough, dyspnea, and pleurisy | Papulovesicular rash. Tachypnea cyanosis, rales, and rhonchi | Intranuclear inclusion in skin scraping or sputum | Diffuse bilateral nodular infiltrates. Infiltrates may coalesce |
| Rubeola (measles) | History of exposure of susceptible patient | Measles prodrome, cough, and sputum production usually within first five days of rash | Persistence of exacerbation of fever exanthem of measles. Rales and rhonchi | Leukocytosis suggests bacterial superinfection | Lower lobe interstitial pneumonia |
| Bacterial superinfection of viral respiratory disease | More frequent in children with varicella or lung disease, compromised host with CMV pneumonia | Exacerbation of fever, cough and hypoxia. Purulent sputum | Pleural effusion. Signs of pulmonary consolidation. Rapidly worsening course | Leukocytosis. Purulent sputum | Lobar pneumonia. Pleural effusion, coalescence of infiltrates |
| Chlamydia (in infants) | Neonates | Progressive increase in respiratory symptoms from 2 to 6 weeks. Protracted course | Afebrile-mucoid nasal discharge, tachypnea. Conjunctivitis (50 per cent). Middle ear abnormalities (50 per cent). Distinctive staccato cough. Good breath sounds. Rales | Eosinophilia, two- to four-fold rise in serum IgG, IgM, and IgA levels. Culture and/or serology | Hyperexpansion with diffuse interstitial and patchy alveolar infiltrates. Clears slowly |

positive airway pressure (CPAP) (Taylor et al., 1976). Either method is usually performed in an intensive care unit in association with intubation, mechanical control of ventilation, and high concentrations of oxygen. Airway pressure must be regulated to optimize ventilation and minimize impairment of venous return. This frequently permits reduction of the concentration of inspired oxygen to a level less likely to be harmful to the lung (i.e., $\leq 50$ per cent $FiO_2$). Additional measures for treating patients with ARDS include corticosteroids, intentional dehydration with diuretics, and other methods that attempt to reduce lung water (O'Brien and Sweeney, 1973). Severe hypoxia in patients with ARDS has been treated with hyperbaric oxygen or extracorporeal membrane oxygenation devices. Both procedures are still experimental and results have been surprisingly poor.

In seriously ill patients with pneumonia, therapy must be started before the diagnosis is proved conclusively. Differentiation of primary viral pneumonia from antibiotic responsive pneumonia may be difficult. Bacterial pneumonia or superinfection requires precise diagnosis and appropriate antimicrobial therapy. In critically ill patients with pneumonia of undetermined origin, it is usually wisest to perform appropriate diagnostic procedures, treat appropriately for suspected microbial pathogens and stop antibiotics when the clinical course, cultures, biopsy, or serologic studies confirm the absence of antibiotic responsive pathogens.

## PROPHYLAXIS

The need for isolation of patients with viral pneumonia due to varicella-zoster, rubeola, or influenza is discussed elsewhere. Chemoprophylaxis with amantadine hydrochloride is currently available only for influenza A infection and is discussed in Chapters 59 and 103 of this book. The recommended regimen of this drug for a susceptible adult is 100 mg twice daily during the epidemic period. Adverse side effects include agitation, dizziness, lethargy, drowsiness, insomnia, and nightmares, but these occur rarely. Patients may describe livido reticularis or ankle edema. Even less commonly, patients may develop congestive

heart failure, orthostatic hypotension, or convulsions as complications of amantadine therapy. Amantadine is contraindicated during pregnancy.

Vaccination to prevent viral infection is well established for influenza. Recent reports of Guillain-Barré syndrome complicating "swine flu" immunization should not preclude immunization of patients with increased risk of complications from influenza. Incomplete immunization against rubeola can predispose patients to development of an atypical rubeola pneumonia syndrome. Use of live virus vaccine should reduce this problem.

## References

Abdallah, P. S., Mark, J. B. D., and Merigan, T. C.: Diagnosis of cytomegalovirus pneumonia in compromised hosts. Am J Med 61:326, 1976.

Bryant, R. E., and Rhoades, E. R.: Clinical features of adenoviral pneumonia in Air Force recruits. Am Rev Resp Dis 96:717, 1967.

Foy, H. M., Cooney, M. K., McMahan, R., and Grayston, J. T.: Viral and mycoplasma pneumonia in a prepaid medical care group during an eight year period. Am J Epidemiol 97:93, 1973.

Glazer, J. P., Friedman, H. M., Grossman, R. A., et al.: Cytomegalovirus vaccination and renal transplantation. Lancet 1:90, 1978.

Kattan, M., Keens, T. G., Lapierre, et al.: Pulmonary function abnormalities in symptom-free children after bronchiolitis. Pediatrics 59:683, 1977.

Knight, V.: Airborne transmission and pulmonary deposition of respiratory viruses. In Knight, V. (ed.): Viral and Mycoplasma Infections of the Respiratory Tract. Philadelphia, Lea & Febiger, 1973, p. 1.

Knight, V., and Kasel, J. A.: Influenza viruses. In Knight, V. (ed.): Viral Mycoplasma Infections of the Respiratory Tract. Philadelphia, Lea & Febiger, 1973, p. 108.

Lang, W. R., Howden, C. W., Laws, J., et al.: Bronchopneumonia with serious sequelae in children with evidence of adenovirus type infection. Br Med J 1:73, 1969.

Little, J. W., Hall, W. J., et al.: Amantadine effect of peripheral airways abnormalities in influenza. Ann Intern Med 85:117, 1976.

Louria, D. B., Blumenfeld, H. L., Ellis, J. T., et al.: Studies on influenza in the pandemic of 1957–1958. II. Pulmonary complications of influenza. J Clin Invest 38:213, 1959.

O'Brien, T. G., and Sweeney, D. F.: Interstitial viral pneumonitis complicated by severe respiratory failure. Successful management using intensive dehydration and steroids. Chest 63:314, 1973.

Olson, R. W., and Hodges, G. R.: Measles pneumonia, bacterial superinfection as a complicating factor. JAMA 232:363, 1975.

Simmons, R. L., Motas, A. J., Rattazzii, L. C., et al.: Clinical characteristics of the lethal cytomegalovirus infection following renal transplantation. Surgery 82:537, 1977.

Taylor, G. J., Brenner, W., and Summer, W. R.: Severe viral pneumonia in young adults. Therapy with continuous positive airway pressure. Chest 69:6, 1976.

Tew, J., Calenoff, L., and Berlin, B. S.: Bacterial or nonbacterial pneumonia: Accuracy of radiographic diagnosis. Diag. Radiol. 124:607, 1977.

Triebwasser, J. H., Harris, R. E., Bryant, R. E., and Rhoades, E. R.: Varicella pneumonia in adults. Medicine 46:409, 1967.

# 112 BACTERIAL LUNG ABSCESS (INCLUDING NOCARDIOSIS)

## S.J.D. Brooks, M.D.
## and Abraham I. Braude, M.D., Ph.D.

### DEFINITION

A lung abscess results when necrosis and lique-faction occur in an area of suppurative pneumonitis. When the liquefied material is discharged into a bronchus, air enters, and a cavity with an air-fluid level remains.

### ETIOLOGY

Aspiration lung abscess is due to a mixed anaerobic infection (Bartlett et al., 1973). The anaerobic bacteria that cause lung abscess are listed in Table 1. Anaerobes outnumber aerobes 10 to 1 in the mouth, and the ratio is greatly increased in dental or gum disease. A concentration of $10^{11}$ bacteria/ml of saliva occurs in these diseases. They proliferate in tonsillar crypts, chronic sinusitis, and dead tissues of the mouth, all of which can be foci for delivering infection to the lungs by aspiration. Aspiration abscess acquired outside the hospital is caused by a mixed anaerobic infection, whereas in hospitals it is invariably a mixed infection with aerobes plus anaerobes (Lorber and Swenson, 1974). Among the anaerobic organisms isolated from lung abscesses are the gram-negative bacteria *Bacteroides melaninogenicus*, *Bacteroides fragilis*, *Fusobacteria* sp, *Bacteroides corrodens*, and *Veillonea* sp.

The anaerobic gram-positive organisms are the *Peptococcus* and *Peptostreptococcus* sp, *Eubacterium*, and *Propionobacterium* sp. *Actinomyces israelii* and *Arachnia propionica* are also anaerobic gram-positive bacilli that can cause lung abscess. These are discussed in Chapter 96.

The aerobic organisms most commonly isolated from lung abscess are *Staphylococcus aureus* and the gram-negative bacilli *Klebsiella pneumoniae*, *Escherichia coli*, *Pseudomonas aeruginosa*, and *Pseudomonas pseudomallei*.

*Legionella pneumophila* (Chapter 113) and *Francisella tularensis* (Chapter 243) are fastidious organisms that cause severe pulmonary suppuration. *Streptococcus pyogenes*, *Neisseria meningitidis*, *Pasteurella multocida*, *Yersinia enterocolitica*, *Bacillus cereus*, *Listeria monocy-togenes*, *Haemophilus influenzae*, *Campylobacter fetus*, and *Corynebacterium equi* are occasionally reported in association with lung abscess. The bacteriology of aerobic lung abscesses is summarized in Table 2.

### PATHOGENESIS

Bacteria reach the lung either by aspiration from the upper respiratory tract, hematogenous spread, inhalation, or contiguous spread from infected adjacent organs. Pus may spread from one site to another within the lung via the bronchi, a process known as internal bronchoembolism.

Aspiration is prevented by the cough and gag reflexes. Although some aspiration occurs at night, these reflexes protect the lung from large or frequent aspirations. They are compromised in patients whose level of consciousness is depressed by alcoholic stupor, narcotics, overdose, fits, anesthesia, or brain injury; in patients with neuromuscular diseases such as bulbar or pseudobulbar palsy, laryngeal palsy, or myasthenia gravis patients with esophageal diseases in which there is abnormal peristalsis, obstruction, or a fistula into the lungs; and in patients with gastrointestinal lesions that cause vomiting and reflux or disturb the integrity of the gastroesophageal junction.

Aspirated material carries with it the bacterial flora of the oropharynx. Solid materials such as pus, dental tartar, tissue fragments (from tonsils, adenoids, or malignant tissue), and food particles are especially hazardous because they cause areas of atelectasis in which bacteria can multiply. Brock (1952) called this aspirated, infected material a bronchoembolus and showed that its destination in the lung varied according to its size, the posture of the patient, and the direction of gravitational flow at the time of aspiration (Figs. 1 and 2). If the patient is lying on his back, the bronchoembolus lodges more frequently in the right lung because the right bronchus is wider and at a lesser angle to the trachea (Flavell, 1966). The first dependent bronchial orifice on its floor is that leading to the apical segment of the lower lobe of the right lung, which turns out to be the most common location for an aspiration abscess. If the patient is lying on his right side, the embolus enters the bronchus to the right superior lobe and then, according to the degree of anterior or posterior tilt of the body, the anterior, apical, or posterior branches of the bronchus. The posterior segment is most commonly affected. With the patient in the left lateral position, the apicoposterior is favored. When the patient is upright, the embolus enters the lower lobe branches. A similar course of events occurs if it enters the left lung. The middle lobe and lingula are rarely affected, because aspiration must take place in the prone or semiprone positions, as when someone vomits in the bent-forward position or after near drowning. The latter is more common in males because they float in the prone position.

Septic emboli from the heart or peripheral veins may also cause a lung abscess. Endocarditis of the right side, due to infection of a congenitally deformed valve or to intravenous drug addition, showers emboli into the lungs. *S. aureus* is responsible in 85 per cent of cases, but a wide range of organisms comprise the remaining 15 per cent. Septic emboli may come also from phlebitis in the pelvic veins or in more peripheral veins after intravenous cannulation. Pelvic thrombophlebitis results from colonic or gynecologic disease and follows surgery, childbirth, and abortions. *Bacteroides* spp. are especially likely to invade these

**TABLE 1.   Anaerobic Organisms Found in Lung Abscess**

| ORGANISM | GRAM STAIN | COLONY CHARACTER | OTHER CHARACTERISTICS |
|---|---|---|---|
| *Bacteroides* sp | Uniform or pleomorphic gram-negative rods | Nonhemolytic. *B. melaninogenicus* produces brown or black pigment darkening with age | Some strains motile. *B. fragilis* growth enhanced by 20 per cent bile and is penicillin-resistant. *B. melaninogenicus*, *B. oralis*, and *B. fragilis* are most often isolated |
| *Fusobacteria* sp | Slender, gram-negative rods with pointed ends | | Produces lactic acid from peptone or glucose, where *Bacteroides* produces butyric acid. *F. nucleatum* most often isolated |
| *Peptostreptococcus* | Small cocci in pairs. Gram-positive | Translucent pearly gray colonies | Fetid odor from some species. Capnophilic |
| *Peptococcus* | Small cocci in singles, pairs, or tetrads, never in chains. Gram-positive | Tiny black pearl colonies on blood agar | Capnophilic |
| *Veillonella* | Gram-negative tiny cocci in pairs or short chains | | Capnophilic |
| *Bifidobacterium* | Gram-positive bacillus. Has Y or V forms. Club or spatulate endings. Stains irregularly | | Primary pathogen |
| *Eubacterium* | Gram-positive bacillus | | Most frequently isolated, but probably not a primary pathogen |
| *Propionibacterium* | Gram-positive bacillus. Pleomorphic. Branched rods or filaments. Club-shaped. One end rounded, other tapered single, or paired cells in V or Y configuration | Occasionally beta-hemolytic | |
| *Clostridium* sp | Thick, gram-positive bacilli with spores | | Rarely found in lung abscesses but often associated with chest trauma |
| *Bacteroides corrodens* | Gram-negative rod | Very fastidious, slow growing. Grows in depressions in the agar. Thin-spreading edges | Capnophilic |
| *Actinomyces israelii* | Gram-positive filamentous actinomycete | 1 to 2 mm after four to six days | Intolerant of $O_2$. Cannot grow on Sabouraud's medium. Some strains grow in 10 to 20 per cent $CO_2$. Often found with *Actinobacillus actinomycetemcomitans* and other anaerobes |
| *Arachnia propionica* | Identical to *A. israelii* | Identical to *A. israelii* | Differs from *A. israelii* because it produces large amounts of propionic acid and has diaminopimelic acid in cell wall |

venous channels, but streptococci, staphylococci, and gram-negative organisms have been isolated from abscesses caused by such emboli. Intravenous cannulation is an important iatrogenic cause of phlebitis, and lung abscess has been reported in association with intravenous drips, cardiac pacemakers, ventriculovenous shunts, hemodialysis shunts, and hyperalimentation. *S. aureus* causes 50 per cent of these infections, and the rest are caused by a great variety of opportunistic organisms. A fibrin clot forms where the vein is pierced, and this acts as a bacterial trap. Inflammation causes the clot to enlarge, and septic emboli

result from clot fragmentation. Burn patients develop *Pseudomonas* thrombophlebitis. Septic emboli may also come from inflammatory areas in bone, pharynx, or kidney. Infected particulate matter may pass directly into the lungs after intravenous injection by addicts. Less than 5 per cent of bland infarcts become infected from within the lung.

When bacteria reach the lung, the infection is controlled or arrested by polymorphonuclear leukocytes, macrophages, and IgG, unless there is neutropenia, neutrophil dysfunction, or any breach in the integrity of the T and B cell system,

**TABLE 2.   Aerobic Bacteria Found in Lung Abscesses**

| ORGANISM | GRAM STAIN | COLONY CHARACTER | OTHER CHARACTERISTICS |
|---|---|---|---|
| **A. Gram-Negative Bacteria** | | | |
| *Klebsiella pneumoniae* | Gram-negative encapsulated rods. Singles, pairs, chains | Large, moist mucoid | Subtyped according to capsular antigens. Its sensitivity to cephalothin and immotility distinguish it from *Enterobacter* |
| *Pseudomonas* sp | Straight or curved gram-negative rods | Diffusible fluorescent pigments. Sticky mucoid colonies | Motile by polar flagella. *P. aeruginosa* the most common. No capsule. Oxidase-positive |
| *P. pseudomallei* | Short gram-negative rod | Cream to bright orange colonies. Wrinkled colonies at 72 hours. Grows on EMB and McConkey | Motile. Wright's stain shows bipolar "safety pin" appearance |
| *P. mallei* | Small, slender rod, gram-negative | | Nonmotile. Staining irregularities with methylene blue. Needs glycerol for optimum growth. Giemsa stain best |
| *Escherichia coli* | Gram-negative rod | Mucoid, gray-white colonies. Sometimes hemolytic. Characteristic green sheen on EMB agar | Motile, lactose fermenter. Encapsulated |
| *Proteus* sp | Gram-negative rods. No capsule | Swarms on media. Strong putrefactive odor with *P. vulgaris* | Motile. Lactose-negative. Urease-positive. *P. mirabilis* most common. *P. vulgaris* produces penicillinase; *P. mirabilis* does not |
| *Salmonella* sp | Gram-negative rod | | Motile. Nonfermenter of lactose |
| *Legionella pneumophila* | Gram-negative on direct tissue stain | Very fastidious and difficult to grow. Propagated in yolk sacs of embryonated eggs | Best seen with modified Dieterle silver impregnation stain. Direct fluorescent antibody test on infected tissue |
| *Francisella tularensis* (tularemia) | Gram-negative. Tiny coccoid to ellipsoid pleomorphic rods | Minute, transparent droplike colonies | Nonmotile. Requires cysteine or cystine compounds in the media. Hazardous to bacteriologists |
| *Pasteurella multocida* | Gram-negative coccobacillus. Bipolar staining capsules best seen on Giemsa stain | Nonhemolytic. Produces brown discoloration of media. Characteristic smell | Very sensitive to penicillin. Extremely pathogenic in mice and other laboratory animals |
| **B. Gram-Positive Bacteria** | | | |
| *Staphylococcus aureus* | Gram-positive cocci. Singles, pairs, or clusters | Hemolytic. Round, raised shiny opaque colonies | Produces coagulase, hemolysins, fibrinolysin, and hyaluronidase |
| *Nocardia asteroides* | Gram-positive actinomycete. Long, branched mycelial form in exudates | | Relatively acid-fast. Grows rapidly on Sabouraud's media or 10 per cent blood agar |
| *Streptococcus pyogenes* | Gram-positive cocci in chains | Beta-hemolytic. Sensitive to bacitracin disk | Produces large number of extracellular toxins |
| *Streptococcus pneumoniae* | Lancet-shaped gram-positive cocci in pairs or short chains | Alpha-hemolytic. Sensitive to optochin disk and soluble in bile | Nonmotile encapsulated. Only type III causes lung abscess |

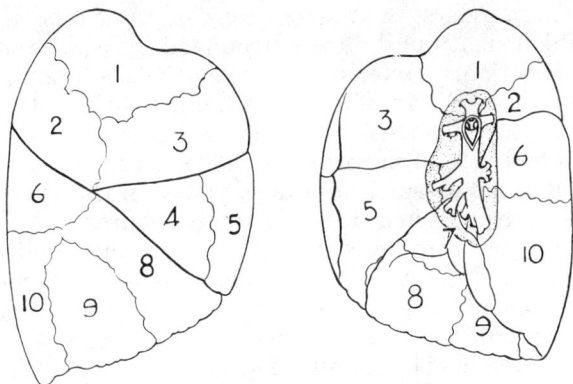

**FIGURE 1.** *The segments of the right lung. The posterior segment (No. 2) of the upper lobe is most vulnerable to bronchoembolism when patient is on his right side, and the apical segment (No. 6) of the lower lobe is most vulnerable when he is on his back. (From Brock, R. C.: Lung Abscess. Springfield, Ill., Charles C Thomas, 1952.)*

which is essential to the formation and efficient function of IgA, IgG, and macrophages. This occurs in congenital agammaglobulinemia, Hodgkin's disease, multiple myeloma, and chronic lymphatic and lymphocytic leukemias. Steroids, immunosuppressives, and antineoplastic drugs increase susceptibility. Chronic disease of the heart, lung, kidney, and liver depress immunity in the lung, as do diabetes mellitus, hypoxia, alcohol, and hypothermia.

Many who develop pneumonia with abscess formation have their lung defenses compromised by one or more of these disturbances. The most common organisms responsible for these pneumonias are *S. aureus* and the gram-negative *bacilli*. They colonize the oropharynx in long-stay hospital inpatients, and they reach the lung by inhalation or aspiration.

*S. aureus* infections may follow influenza. Infants under 1 year old and pregnant women are also vulnerable to staphylococcal pneumonia. Alcoholism, chronic lung disease, immunosuppression, and diabetes mellitus play an important debilitating role in gram-negative infections. *Pseudomonas* spp. proliferate in antiseptic solutions and creams and in the nebulizers of ventilators. This organism is a particular hazard to those on ventilators, to burn patients, and to infants with congenital heart disease.

Abscesses can also be formed in or from existing pathology. Anaerobic abscesses may develop from aspirated material trapped distally to an obstructing bronchial carcinoma (Fig. 3). Bronchogenic cysts are infected via the bronchus or the bloodstream, but dermoid cysts and sequestered lobes are always infected hematogenously. Bronchiectasis, bronchogenic cysts, and infected carcinomas may spread by internal bronchoembolism to set up secondary abscesses. Rarely, infections may spread from the spine, the esophagus, or beneath the diaphragm to invade the lung.

## PATHOLOGY

### Aspiration Lung Abscess

When the aspirated bronchoembolus obstructs the bronchus, it causes atelectasis, which provides the ideal environment for anaerobes. The infection is usually confined to the bronchopulmonary segment served by that bronchus so the abscess is unilobar and unilateral. A localized pneumonitis and consolidation is followed 10 to 14 days later by necrosis. The affected segment or subsegment always extends to the visceral pleura, but the pleura itself, along with a small layer of subjacent lung, does not become necrotic because its blood supply is from a subpleural vascular plexus. As a result, pleurisy and effusion occur, but empyema is unusual. Granulation tissue lines the cavity, which contains liquefied pus, tissue sloughs, debris, and organisms. Pneumonitis surrounds the granulation tissue. Ultimately, the abscess ruptures into a bronchus, pus drains into the bronchial tree, air enters the cavity, and an air-fluid level results. The slough prevents complete emptying by exerting a ball-valve effect. Without treatment, the abscess becomes chronic and is filled with thick gluelike material. Satellite abscesses are scattered through its thick fibrous walls, which become adherent to the pleura. Chronic pneumonitis is present, and the lung becomes honeycombed by fistulous tracks. Erosion of large blood vessels may cause hemoptysis, and septic thrombosis of the pulmonary veins results in septic emboli to the brain.

**FIGURE 2.** *Influence of position on segmental localization of lung abscess. A, With the patient on his back, the apical segment of the lower lobe is the most dependent site for localization of bronchoemboli. B, The posterior segment of the upper lobe is most vulnerable when the patient is lying on his side. (From Brock, R. C.: Lung Abscess. Springfield, Ill., Charles C Thomas, 1952.)*

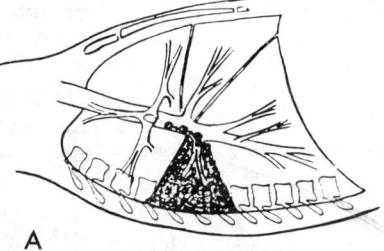

A

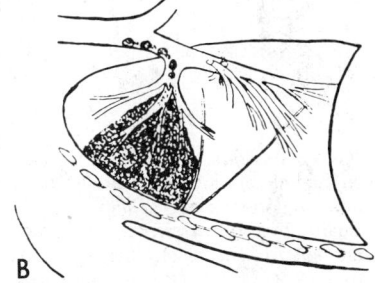

B

## Inhalational Lung Abscess

Staphylococcal pneumonia begins in the airways following inhalation. There is an intense granulocyte response. The alveoli are destroyed and peritracheal abscesses form. Because air can enter these abscesses but cannot escape, the weakened tissue becomes distended, and thin-walled cavities are created that contain a small amount of pus. These pneumatoceles may become very large. They occur especially in children and are virtually pathognomonic of staphylococcal pneumonia. The alveoli are filled with proteinaceous material, bacteria, debris, and neutrophils. Multiple thick-walled abscesses occur as well, and bronchopleural fistulas and empyema result. A fulminant hemorrhagic *Staphylococcus* pneumonia follows influenza A. The lungs are plum-colored, engorged, and heavy. The cut surfaces show multiple tiny abscesses.

*Pseudomonas* pneumonia is characterized by peribronchial abscesses and alveolar necrosis (Fetzer et al., 1967). Yellow-brown, necrotic, umbilicated nodules form that contain myriads of bacteria arranged around large blood vessels. The alveolar septa are intact, and there is a minimal inflammatory response in which lymphocytes and monocytes predominate. *E. coli* causes a hemorrhagic pneumonia. Mononuclear cells infiltrate the interstitium, and proteinaceous exudate fills the alveoli. Areas of atelectasis and emphysema are prominent.

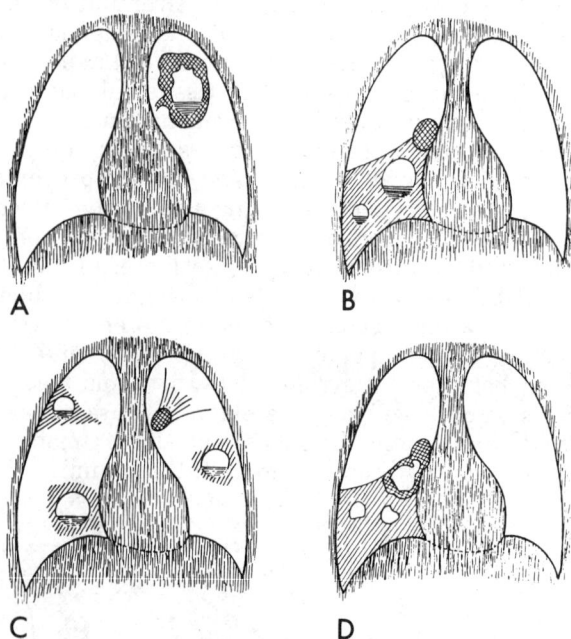

**FIGURE 3.** *Formation of lung abscess in patients with bronchogenic carcinoma. A, Abscess after necrosis of central portion of tumor. B, Abscess due to infection of lobe obstructed by tumor (usually two or more). C, Spillover abscesses from primary carcinoma in left upper lobe. D, Combination of A and B. (From Brock, R. C.: Lung Abscess. Springfield, Ill. Charles C Thomas, 1952.)*

In glanders, the abscess consists of nodules in which neutrophils are surrounded by a zone of congestion. Extensive nuclear degeneration causes small foci of deeply staining debris. Later, the abscess consists of epithelioid cells around a central core of necrosis. Melioidosis causes thin-walled abscesses in the upper lobes; if the lower lobes are affected, it is via the bloodstream. The abscesses contain a core of debris and multinucleated giant cells surrounded first by a layer of neutrophils and then by a layer of hemorrhage. In chronic infections, a core of caseation necrosis is surrounded by granulation tissue, plasma cells, and mononuclear cells.

### Hematogenous Lung Abscess

Septic emboli (in contrast to bronchoemboli) occlude branches of the pulmonary artery and cause gangrenous infarction. The infarction progresses rapidly to cavity formation, pleural effusion, and empyema. *S. aureus* is by far the most common organism isolated, but *B. fragilis,* other *Bacteroides,* and gram-negative organisms are also responsible.

## *CLINICAL MANIFESTATIONS*

### The Clinical Setting

An accurate diagnosis can be made on the basis of the history, clinical findings, and setting in which the infection occurred. In aspiration lung abscess, there may be a history of alcoholic stupor or an epileptic fit in a patient with gingival disease; the symptoms of pulmonary infection have a subacute onset with the production of copious foul sputum. In hospitals, the precipitating event is likely to be a neurologic illness, esophageal disease, or anesthesia; and a mixed aerobic/anaerobic infection is present.

Septic emboli typically occur in a young male addict and cause a disease of dramatic suddenness because of pulmonary infarction and fulminant pulmonary infection. Occasionally, it occurs among patients hospitalized for intestinal or gynecologic disease (Griffith et al., 1977) or in those given intravenous cannulation.

Gram-negative bacterial pneumonia and lung abscesses may occur outside the hospital, but most are nosocomial infections in patients already very ill with chronic debilitating illnesses or immunosuppression. Superinfection with *Klebsiella* and other gram-negative bacteria may cause lung abscess in patients receiving penicillin therapy for pneumococcal pneumonia (Fig. 4). *Pseudomonas* spp. have a propensity to attack patients with burns or in ventilators.

Staphylococcal pneumonia occurs after influen-

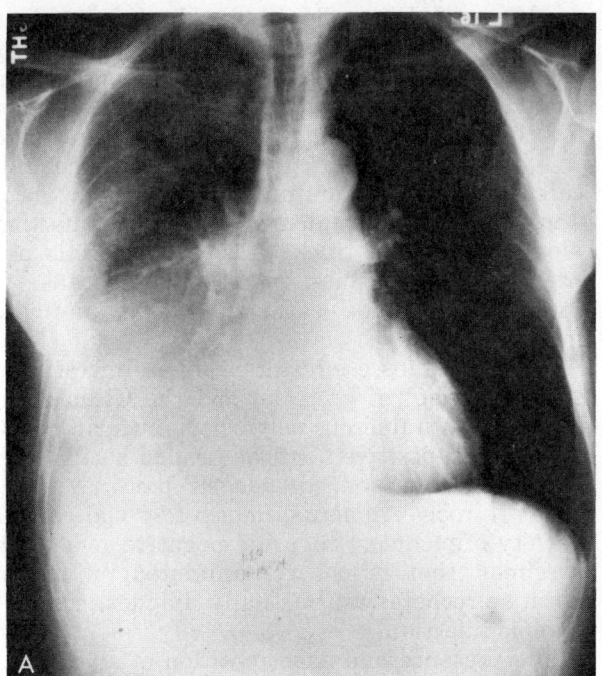 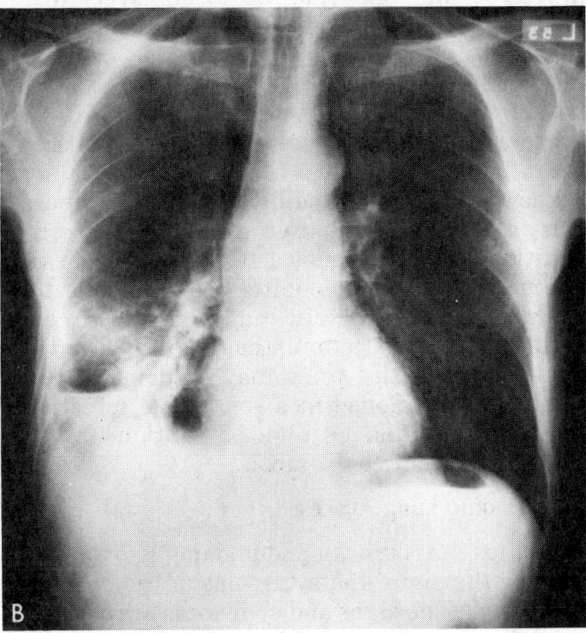

**FIGURE 4.** *Superinfection lung abscess due to* Klebsiella pneumoniae *in patient treated with 800,000 units penicillin G daily for pneumococcal pneumonia. A, Chest x-ray showing pneumonia before lung abscess. B, Chest x-ray showing* Klebsiella *lung abscess.*

za A and is a common cause of sepsis in infants. Pneumatoceles and empyema are pathognomonic of staphylococcal disease at that age. It may also occur in the same context as the gram-negative pneumonias and is a leading cause of septicemia, endocarditis, pneumonia, and lung abscess in patients with intravenous catheters.

### Aspiration Abscess

Occasionally, a patient may willfully conceal part of the history, especially when it concerns alcoholic stupor, epilepsy, or criminal head injuries. Men outnumber women at least 4 to 1 among patients with aspiration abscesses. It is virtually unknown in edentulous patients unless there is a previous history of stupor. Malaise, fever, nonproductive dry cough, chills, and pleuritic pain or a dull, deep-seated ache in the chest begin three to four days after aspiration. After bronchial communication occurs, the contents of the entire abscess may be expectorated, but usually the amount of sputum steadily increases, and the abscess is only partially drained. The pus is foul in about 50 per cent of cases; only certain obligate anaerobes produce the foul odor, which takes about one week to develop and is quickly abolished by penicillin. Physical signs are minimal before and after abscess formation. There may be dullness, reduced breath sounds, and fremitus, and few rales, if any. These findings differ from those of lobar pneumonia because in

lung abscess the lobe does not have the firmness of pneumococcal hepatization. Instead, it is a poorly ventilated, wet, sodden spongy lobe, heavy with pus and undergoing disintegration (Amberson, 1954). A pleural effusion may be found. Spontaneous cure is rare without treatment. If clubbing of the fingers is found in a patient with an acute abscess, bronchogenic carcinoma should be suspected.

With chronic abscess, the patient becomes wasted, ill, and toxic; and he has a persistent cough and sputum. His fingers are clubbed, and there is weight loss, anemia, and low-grade fever. Brain abscess and severe hemoptysis may occur. Rarely, a chronic abscess can be clinically silent.

### Embolic Lung Abscess

When lung abscess is due to septic emboli, the signs and symptoms are tachypnea, tachycardia, dyspnea, chest pain, hemoptysis, and syncope (MacMillan et al., 1978). They may be preceded by chills, fever, and rigors. Less than 20 per cent of cases of tricuspid endocarditis have cardiac signs and must be suspected on the basis of intravenous drug addiction, septicemia, and pulmonary infarction. Drug addiction is recognized by the needle tracks and microabscesses in the skin. Emboli from the heart cause multiple lesions in the lower lobes with pleural effusion. Cavitation occurs in 25 per cent of lesions, but empyema is rare. Positive blood cultures in endocarditis of the right side are to be expected, in contrast to aspiration abscesses in which positive blood cultures are rare.

Emboli from peripheral veins are larger than those from endocarditis, and approximately 50 per cent of lesions cavitate. A solitary abscess occurs in half the cases. Over 80 per cent have leukocytosis and positive blood cultures. Pleural effusion and empyema are common. The external condition of a vein is not a reliable guide to the presence of thrombophlebitis even though it is inflamed, because a vein may be the source of emboli long after a cannula has been removed. In women, thrombosed veins may be palpated in a vaginal fornix. Sometimes soft tissue infections have resolved, and an infected contiguous vein remains as a source of emboli.

### Pneumonic Lung Abscess

Cavities that occur in pneumonia are overshadowed by the signs and symptoms of the pneumonia. Many of the signs and symptoms are common to all the pneumonias (Chapters 105 and 106), including fever, breathlessness, pleurisy, tachypnea, and purulent, blood-stained sputum. Cavitation occurs in approximately 50 per cent of pneumonias due to gram-negative bacteria. Staphylococcal pneumonia carries a high mortality after influenza A and in infancy. Pneumatocele may be associated with mediastinal shift and symptoms of lung compression. Empyema occurs early and in 90 per cent of children, and metastatic infections of the skin occur in 15 per cent of cases.

## *DIAGNOSIS*

A provisional diagnosis can often be made on the basis of the history and clinical findings. Severe alcoholism is prominent in 70 per cent and dental caries in nearly 100 per cent of aspiration abscesses. A putrid sputum is diagnostic of an anaerobic infection. Culture of bronchial secretions accurately reflects the responsible organisms, but when expectorated, such secretions are contaminated by mouth organisms. Because of this, specimens should also be taken from blood, pleural fluid, empyema fluid, discharging sinuses, and the tips of intravenous cannulas, which are less likely to be contaminated. When this is not possible, transtracheal aspiration should be considered for obtaining a specimen (Bartlett and Finegold, 1972). The front of the neck is cleaned, and local anesthetic is infiltrated in the area of the thyroid cartilage. With the neck hyperextended, a 16-gauge intracatheter is passed through the cricothyroid membrane and threaded into the

trachea, and the needle is pulled back. Secretions are sucked into a syringe or into a Lukens trap by a constant suction apparatus. This procedure should not be done on anyone with bleeding disorders, cardiac arrhythmias, uncontrolled cough, or hypoxia. The procedure may be complicated by bleeding from an aberrant artery, local and mediastinal emphysema, and an infection along the needle track. If squamous cells are present, the specimen is discarded because it indicates that the catheter passed into the mouth.

Aspiration abscess results from an infection by several species of bacteria; and the Gram stain should show numerous polymorphonuclear leukocytes, gram-positive fusiform beaded bacilli with tapered or cigar-shaped ends, streptococci, gram-negative rods resembling *Bacteroides* spp., and a variety of pleomorphic gram-negative rods. In a specimen that is not contaminated by mouth flora, spirochetes are virtually diagnostic of anaerobic infection.

The presence and exact position of an abscess can only be determined by examining both posteroanterior and lateral chest x-rays. Aspiration abscesses almost always occur in the apical segment of a lower lobe or the posterior segment of an upper lobe. They are usually solitary and have thick walls with a ragged lining. Empyema occurs with 30 per cent of all embolic abscesses. Their walls are also thick and their lining ragged. Staphyloccal pneumonia has no lobe predilection; and in children, pneumatoceles, pneumothorax, and pyopneumothorax are diagnostic. *Klebsiella*, and occasionally *Pseudomonas*, cause pneumonias that affect predominantly the upper lobes. All cause thick-walled abscess with ragged linings. The lower lobes are affected by *Pseudomonas*, *E. coli*, *N. asteroides*, and *A. israelii* infection. *Proteus*, *Klebsiella*, *Nocardia*, and *F. tularensis* all cause radiographic appearances that can mimic *M. tuberculosis*.

Ordinary lung abscesses must be differentiated from carcinomatous abscesses, which are thick-walled and have eccentric cavities. They should be suspected if the abscess is located in a segment that is not dependent during aspiration; in other words, abscesses in the anterior segment, lingula, or middle lobe should raise the question of carcinoma. Sputum cytology makes the diagnosis in 90 per cent of cases (Wallace et al., 1979). It should be kept in mind that one third of lung cavities are due to underlying bronchogenic carcinoma in patients over 45 (Brock, 1952). Bronchogenic cysts are thin-walled, occur in the medial third of the lower lobes, and remain after the infection has been cured. Sequestrated segments have thin walls also and usually occur in the lower lobes. Dermoid cysts are found in the anterior mediastinum. *Entamoeba hystolytica* and *Echinococcus granulosus* affect the lower lobes. In the latter, air between the endocyst and ectocyst creates a halo effect, and, where the lining membrane falls into the cavity fluid, the "water lily" sign results.

Tuberculosis, atypical mycobacterial infections, cryptococcosis, histoplasmosis, and blastomycosis produce cavitary disease and are important in the differential diagnosis in endemic areas. All may be acquired by visitors to these areas.

## COMPLICATIONS AND SEQUELAE

Aspiration abscess has few complications or sequelae, surgery is rarely required, and mortality is low. With any large abscess there is a risk of asphyxiation from sudden rupture and discharge of pus through both lungs. Since chronic abscesses are unusual, severe hemoptysis, bronchopleural fistulas, and empyemas are not common. After successful treatment, the cavity may persist for one or more years, but eventually it closes spontaneously. A bronchogram may reveal residual asymptomatic bronchiectasis.

Septic emboli cause infarction, septicemia, and fulminant pulmonary infection, any of which may be lethal. Empyema occurs with 30 per cent of emboli from peripheral sites. If the primary source is promptly and adequately treated, there should be few sequelae.

Bacteremia and shock are important complications in staphylococcal and gram-negative pneumonias. Often the prognosis is that of the underlying disease, but it is difficult to control infections in those with marked neutropenia. Pleural effusion and empyema are common. Dissemination of abscesses to other organs may occur in staphylococcal pneumonia. There is a high mortality when the pneumonia complicates influenza or occurs in infancy. Pneumatoceles may cause mediastinal compression, but usually the air spontaneously reabsorbs. Gram-negative organisms may cause fibrosis, shrinkage, and chronic cavitation.

## GEOGRAPHIC VARIATION

In Nigeria, aspiration abscess is still a dangerous disease with a high mortality (Adebonojo et al., 1979; Atherstone and Gelfant, 1972; Sofowora and Onadeko, 1971). It often presents in the chronic stage, and hemoptysis is frequent and requires immediate surgery. The maximum incidence is in the fourth decade of life when bronchiectasis, lobar pneumonia, and esophageal stricture are common causes. Its severity is attributed to late presentation for medical care, sickle cell disease, and poor nutrition. In Zimbabwe, there is also a high incidence in the fourth decade of life. However, it is a much milder disease and has a low mortality. Again, lobar pneumonia figures prominently in the etiology. The incidence and pattern of the disease in India and Japan seem to mirror those in Western countries (Shinoi, 1960; Kaltreider, 1976).

Glanders is seen only in Africa, Asia, and South America. Melioidosis is endemic in Southeast Asia and occurs sporadically in the surrounding nations. Tularemia is endemic in Europe, Asia, Texas, Oklahoma, Louisiana, and Arkansas. All these diseases may affect travelers to endemic areas.

## TREATMENT

### Aspiration Lung Abscess

Penicillin is the treatment of choice in aspiration abscess even in the presence of penicillin-resistant *B. fragilis* (Abernathy, 1968; Bartlett and Gorbach, 1975). Penicillin is equally effective whether given orally, intramuscularly, or intravenously. Clindamycin is used in patients allergic to penicillin. It kills *B. fragilis* but can cause life-threatening colitis, neutropenia, and liver function disturbance. Postural drainage of the abscesses is important conjunctive therapy. Surgical resection is used only for severe hemoptysis (Thoms and Arbulu, 1970) or for the few abscesses that do not respond to the antibiotic schedules listed in Table 3. With adequate treatment, all patients are afebrile, and cavities shrink by 10 days. At six weeks, 70 per cent are healed. Clinical recovery is accompanied by decreased production and less purulence of sputum, an increae of weight and appetite, a fall in leukocyte count, and disappearance of fever. Failure of response raises the question of bronchogenic carcinoma.

### Embolic Lung Abscess

The source of septic emboli must be identified early and treated vigorously in order to minimize the need for heparin and to prevent a fatal embolus. All intravenous cannulas should be removed and abscesses drained. Veins suspected of being the source of emboli may need exploration, ligation, or excision. Because a wide variety of organisms cause phlebitis at intravenous drip sites, the initial antimicrobial drug therapy may have to be based on Gram stain of the cannula tip. Clindamycin or metronidazole should be used for septic emboli of pelvic origin because *B. fragilis* is likely to be involved there. If tricuspid endocarditis cannot be controlled with high doses of antimi-

TABLE 3.   Treatment of Lung Abscess

| ORGANISM | TREATMENT OF CHOICE | ALTERNATE |
| --- | --- | --- |
| Anaerobic bacteria (aspiration) | Penicillin G, 1 megaunit every six hours. Penicillin V, 750 mg orally every six hours | Clindamycin, 300 mg intravenously every four hours or 450 mg orally every six hours |
| S. aureus (penicillinase-negative) | Penicillin G, 2 mega units every six hours intravenously until cured | Cefazolin, 1 g every six hours intramuscularly or intravenously |
| S. aureus (penicillinase-positive) | Methicillin or oxacillin, 1.0 g intravenously every three hours | Cefazolin, 1 g every six hours intramuscularly or intravenously |
| K. pneumoniae | Gentamicin, 80 mg intravenously three times daily plus chloramphenicol. Succinate, 1.0 g intravenously every six hours | Kanamycin, 0.5 g intramuscularly (or amikacin, 250 mg intravenously) every six hours plus chloramphenicol succinate, 1.0 g intravenously every six hours |
| P. aeruginosa | Carbenicillin, 2.0 g intravenously every two hours plus gentamicin, 80 mg intravenously every eight hours | Polymyxin B or colistin, 80 mg intramuscularly every eight hours |
| Proteus sp | Gentamicin, 80 mg intravenously | Amikacin, 50 mg every 12 hours intramuscularly or chloramphenicol succinate, 1.0 g every six hours |
| A. israelii | Penicillin G, 4 mega units daily intramuscularly | Tetracycline, 500 mg orally every six hours |
| N. asteroides | Trisulfapyrimidines, 500 mg (167 mg each of sulfadiazine sulfamerazine and sulfamethazine), two tablets orally every two hours | Cycloserine, 250 mg orally twice daily |
| F. tularensis | Streptomycin, 0.5 g every six hours for three days, then 0.5 g every eight hours for three days | Tetracycline or chloramphenicol, 500 mg orally every four hours for ten days |
| P. pseudomallei | Tetracycline, 0.5 g every four hours plus sulfisoxazole, 1.0 g orally every six hours | Chloramphenicol, 0.5 g every three hours plus sulfisoxazole, 1.0 g orally every six hours |
| P. mallei | Sulfadiazine, 2 g orally every six hours | |
| L. pneumophila | Erythromycin, 2.0 to 4.0 g intravenously every day | |

crobials because of drug resistance, it should have early excision.

Staphylococcal pneumonia is treated with methicillin or cefazolin, and if pneumatoceles cause respiratory embarrassment, they should be aspirated. Pneumothorax and pyopneumothorax must be drained. Gram-negative organisms are treated with the antibiotics listed in Table 3. Immunosuppressive drugs may be reduced in dosage, if necessary, until the infection can be controlled.

## PREVENTION

Lung abscesses will continue to be a problem among intravenous drug addicts and alcoholics. In all vulnerable groups, oropharyngeal sepsis should be eradicated before surgery or dental procedures and after fracture of the jaw in order to reduce the risk of aspiration abscess. Staphylococcus lung abscess can be minimized by influenza vaccination because primary Staphylococcus lung abscess in adults is almost exclusively a complication of influenza. The development of a pneumococcal vaccine that reflects African serotypes may have an important role to play in Nigeria, since abscess commonly follows lobar pneumonia there.

The biggest reduction may occur as a result of better control of iatrogenic nosocomial infection (Stein and Pruitt, 1970). Intravenous cannulation should be kept to the absolute minimum. Intravenous drip sites and the delivery tubing should be changed frequently. In hemodialysis, those shunts with the lowest infection rate, such as the Cimino shunt, should be used. An awareness of the importance of nosocomial infections and the need for constant monitoring of the prevalent pathogens and their antibiotic sensitivities are essential. Respirator ventilators should be sterilized and constantly monitored for Pseudomonas sp. L. pneumophila should be eradicated from the cooling towers of air conditioning systems, especially in hotels and hospitals (Dondero, 1980). Patients with dangerous organisms resistant to many antibiotics should be isolated from debilitated or immunosuppressed individuals.

# NOCARDIOSIS

### DEFINITION

Nocardiosis, an infection caused by an aerobic actinomycete, may produce lung abscesses and spread to the brain and elsewhere, or it may appear as a chronic deforming granulomatous infection limited to the foot (mycetoma, Chap 238).

### ETIOLOGY

Pulmonary and disseminated nocardiosis usually results from infection with *Nocardia asteroides*. This organism is relatively acid-fast, and its bacillary form resembles the tubercle bacillus, but *N. asteroides* is easily differentiated from the tubercle bacillus by rapid growth on Sabouraud's medium or 10 per cent blood agar at room temperature, and by the presence in exudates of long-branched, gram-positive mycelial forms.

### PATHOGENESIS

*Nocardia asteroides* can be recovered readily from soil. Nocardiosis appears, therefore, to be an exogenous infection usually having its portal of entry in the lungs. In almost every patient with nocardiosis (other than maduromycosis), the earliest and most extensive lesions are acute pulmonary suppurative foci (Weed et al., 1955). A well-defined wall is absent, a fact that probably accounts for the marked tendency of nocardial abscesses to spread to the brain and to a lesser extent to the spleen, skin, peritoneum, and kidney. Occasionally, noncaseating granulomas are found. Susceptibility to nocardiosis is increased in Cushing's syndrome, in pulmonary alveolar proteinosis, and in some patients with lymphomas or leukemia after antitumor chemotherapy (Andriole et al., 1964; Danowski et al., 1962).

### CLINICAL MANIFESTATIONS

The chief symptom is cough, usually productive of a thick, sometimes bloody, sputum. Chest pain and dyspnea are common, as are fever, sweats, chills, leukocytosis, weakness, anorexia, and weight loss. The illness may be prolonged and present the picture of chronic pulmonary tuberculosis, lung abscess (Fig. 5), or unresolved suppurative pneumonia. This syndrome can be interrupted suddenly by the acute neurologic changes of metastatic brain abscess. At this time, the patient may have severe headache and focal sensory or motor disturbances. The protein concentration, cells, and pressure of the spinal fluid are increased, but the concentration of glucose is not

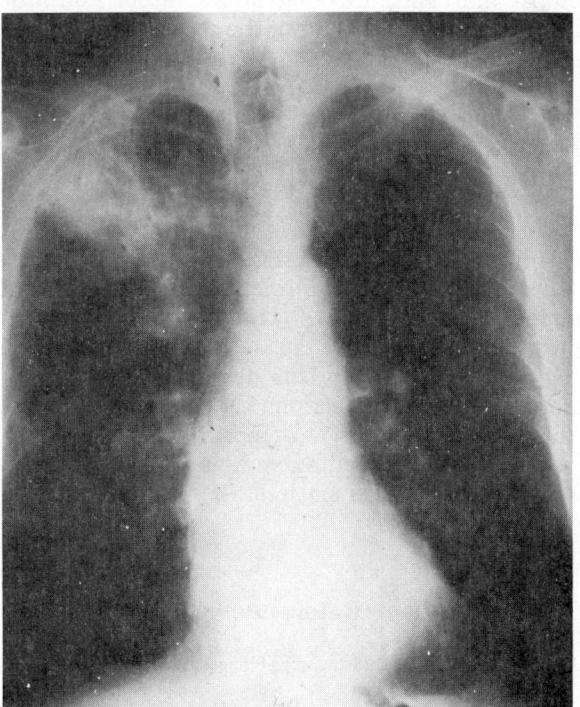

**FIGURE 5.** *Nocardial lung abscess resembling tuberculosis.*

reduced unless the meninges are also infected. Occasionally, abscess is the first clinical manifestation of nocardiosis, especially in Cushing's syndrome secondary to adrenal steroid therapy. Infection of the skin is frequent and produces numerous scattered abscesses or single draining sinuses of the hand, chest wall, or buttocks.

The disease is usually fatal after months to years, if not treated.

### DIAGNOSIS

Because patients with nocardiosis are suspected of having tuberculosis, their sputa are examined for tubercle bacilli. The usual methods for concentrating tubercle bacilli often kill *N. asteroides*; *N. asteroides* may also be overlooked in smears stained by the Ziehl-Neelsen method because it is less resistant than the tubercle bacillus to decolorizing by alcohol. Killing the organism can be avoided by concentrating with trisodium phosphate, and overdecolorizing can be avoided by using 1 per cent sulfuric acid.

Although sulfur granules are not found in pulmonary or disseminated nocardiosis, the gram-positive filamentous organisms in nocardial exudates often resemble *Actinomyces israelii*. The two pathogens can be distinguished, however, by the ease with which *N. asteroides* is cultivated on

Sabouraud's medium or blood agar aerobically and by its acid-fast staining characteristics. In biopsy material, the nongranulomatous and minimally fibrotic character of the nocardial suppurative reaction also helps to distinguish it from infections due to *A. israelii*. The absence of tubercles is valuable in differential diagnosis from tuberculosis.

## TREATMENT

Administration of sulfadiazine is sometimes successful treatment. Penicillin and tetracycline appear to be ineffective, and resistance of nocardiosis to these drugs may be used in distinguishing it from actinomycosis due to *A. israelii* and from pulmonary infections that respond to these antibiotics. Patients with nocardiosis should receive 8 to 12 g of sulfadiazine daily. Cycloserine shows promise for patients allergic to sulfonamides.

## References

Abernathy, R. S.: Antibiotic therapy of lung abscess. Dis Chest 53:292, 1968.
Adebonojo, S. A., Osinowo, O., and Adebo, O.: Lung abscess. A review of three years' experience at the University College Hospital, Ibadan. J Nat Med Assoc 71:39, 1979.
Amberson, J. B.: A clinical consideration of abscesses and cavities of the lung. Bull Johns Hopkins Hosp 94:227, 1954.
Andriole, V. T., et al.: The association of nocardiosis and pulmonary alveolar proteinosis. Ann Intern Med 60:266, 1964.
Atherstone, N., and Gelfand, M.: Lung abscess in Africans admitted to the Medical Unit, Harare Hospital. Cent Afr J Med 18:49, 1972.
Bartlett, J. G., and Finegold, S. M.: Anaerobic pleuropulmonary infections. Medicine 51:413, 1972.
Bartlett, J. G., and Gorbach, S. L.: Treatment of aspiration pneumonia and primary lung abscess. Penicillin G vs clindamycin. JAMA 234:935, 1975.
Bartlett, J. G., Rosenblatt, J. E., and Finegold, S. M.: Percutaneous transtracheal aspiration in the diagnosis of anaerobic pulmonary infection. Ann Intern Med 79:535, 1973.
Brock, R. C.: Lung Abscess. Springfield, Ill., Charles C Thomas, 1952.
Danowski, T. S., et al.: Cushing's syndrome in conjunction with *Nocardia asteroides* infection. Metabolism 11:2, 1962.
Dondero, T. J., et al.: An outbreak of Legionnaire's disease associated with a contaminated air conditioning cooling tower. N Engl J Med 302:365, 1980.
Fetzer, A. E., Werner, A. S., and Hagstrom, J. W. C.: Pathologic features of pseudomonal pneumonia. Am Rev Resp Dis 96:1121, 1967.
Flavell, G.: Lung abscess. Br Med J 1:1032, 1966.
Griffith, G. L., Maull, K. I., and Sachatello, C. R.: Septic pulmonary embolization. Surg Gynecol Obstet 144:105, 1977.
Kaltreider, H. B.: Expression of the immune mechanism in the lung. Am Rev Resp Dis 113:347, 1976.
Lorber, B., and Swenson, R. M.: Bacteriology of aspiration pneumonia. Ann Intern Med 81:329, 1974.
MacMillan, J. C., Milstein, S. M., Samson, P. C.: Clinical spectrum of septic pulmonary embolism and infarction. J Thorac Cardiovasc Surg 75:670, 1978.
Shinoi, K.: Lung abscess in Japan. J Thorac Cardiovasc Surg 40:461, 1960.
Sofowora, E. O., and Onadeko, B. O.: Lung abscess in Nigerians. Trop Geogr. Med 23:126, 1971.
Stein, J. M., and Pruitt, B. A.: Suppurative thrombophlebitis. A lethal iatrogenic disease. N Engl J Med 282:1452, 1970.
Thoms, N. W., and Arbulu, A.: Significance of hemoptysis in lung abscess. J Thorac Cardiovasc Surg 59:5, 1970.
Wallace, R., Cohen, A., Aeve, R., Greenberg, D., Hadlock, F., and Park, S.: Carcinomatous lung abscess. Diagnosis by bronchoscopy and cytopathology. JAMA 242:521, 1979.
Weed, L. A., et al.: Nocardiosis: Clinical, bacteriologic, and pathologic aspects. N Engl J Med 253:1138, 1955.

# 113 LEGIONELLOSIS (LEGIONNAIRES' DISEASE AND PONTIAC FEVER)

Jeffrey D. Band, M.D.
David W. Fraser, M.D.

## DEFINITION

Legionellosis is an acute bacterial infection of humans caused by *Legionella pneumophila*, a fastidious gram-negative bacillus. Two distinct clinicoepidemiologic syndromes have been observed: Legionnaires' disease, a multisystem illness characterized by pneumonia and a high case-fatality ratio, and Pontiac fever, a nonpneumonic, self-limited, acute febrile illness without associated deaths. Legionellosis occurs both sporadically and in explosive clusters such as the epidemic at the American Legion Convention in Philadelphia in 1976 (Fraser et al., 1977). Although the organism was initially identified by McDade in late 1976, subsequent investigation has shown that the disease is not new. The earliest documented case occurred in 1947, and at least five outbreaks of respiratory illness of previously undefined etiology that preceded the 1976 Philadelphia outbreak have now been shown to have been caused by *L. pneumophila*. Search for *L. pneumophila* in cases of pneumonia of uncertain cause has recently led to the discovery of other fastidious pneumonia-causing bacteria, including the Pittsburgh pneumonia agent and atypical *Legionella*-like organisms.

## *ETIOLOGY*

*L. pneumophila* is a faintly staining, thin, pleomorphic gram-negative bacillus measuring 0.3 to 0.9 $\mu$m by 2 to 3 $\mu$m, although filamentous forms have also been observed (McDade et al., 1977) (Fig. 1). Ultrastructurally, the organism resembles a typical gram-negative bacillus with a double envelope of unit membrane and an extremely thin cell wall (Fig. 2). Vacuoles may be seen within the organism that stain with Sudan black B. *L. pneumophila* can be stained with the Wolbach modification of the Giemsa stain or a modification of the Dieterle silver impregnation stain, although neither reaction is specific (Chandler et al., 1977). In tissue, the organism is typically found within macrophages or free in the alveoli. Direct immunofluorescent staining with conjugated rabbit antiserum is a more specific method of identification (Cherry et al., 1978). The organism has been isolated from respiratory secretions, pleural fluid, lung tissue, and blood of patients with Legionnaires' disease as well as from several environmental sites, such as water within heat rejection systems (cooling towers, evaporative condensers), rivers, lakes, ponds, and riparian soil. Successful isolation techniques include intraperitoneal inoculation of guinea pigs with subsequent culturing of infected tissue in embryonic hens' eggs and on solid agar medium and, more recently, direct plating of specimens on solid agar medium that contains supplementary L-cysteine and ferric salts. Examples of media used for isolation are Mueller-Hinton agar base with 1 per cent Isovitalex and 1 per cent hemoglobin (MH-IH agar) or with 0.04 per cent L-cysteine and 0.25 per cent ferric pyrophosphate (FG agar) and charcoal yeast-extract (CYE) agar. The organism does not grow on most conventional media.

*L. pneumophila* grows slowly (3 to 10 days) on MH-IH or FG agar, producing small, glistening gray colonies with discoloration of the surrounding agar by brown soluble pigment. A yellow fluorescence of both the colonies and the surrounding medium is demonstrable under longwave (366 $\mu$m) ultraviolet light. The presence of sufficient L-tyrosine or L-phenylalanine seems to be important for production of the brown soluble pigment. On CYE agar, colonies appear earlier (2 to 4 days) and are more numerous than on MH-IH or FG agar. Growth appears optimal at pH 6.0 to 7.0 and at 35 to 37° C. The organism is a strict aerobe, but growth on FG and MH-IH media may be stimulated by the addition of 2.5 per cent carbon dioxide.

Biochemically, *L. pneumophila* is catalase-positive and weakly oxidase-positive. It has not been shown to ferment carbohydrates other than starch, to reduce nitrate, or to degrade urea, although it does elaborate a gelatinase. The organism also produces a cephalosporinase. Gas-liquid chromatographic measurements have shown that more than 80 per cent of the organism's fatty acids have branched chains, a distinctively unusual pattern for a gram negative bacterium. Further studies of the biochemical characteristics, molecular weight of the genome ($\sim 2.5 \times 10^9$), guanine-cytosine content (39 per cent), and DNA homology have not demonstrated relatedness with any known family of bacteria; a new family (Legionellaceae), genus, and species have been proposed for *L. pneumophila* (Brenner et al., 1979).

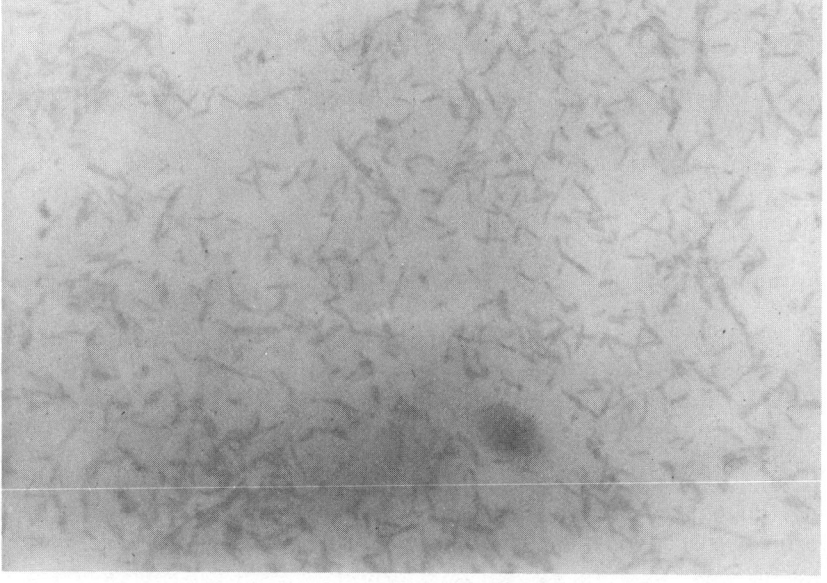

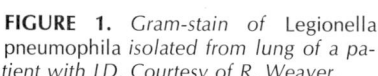
**FIGURE 1.** *Gram-stain of* Legionella pneumophila *isolated from lung of a patient with LD. Courtesy of R. Weaver.*

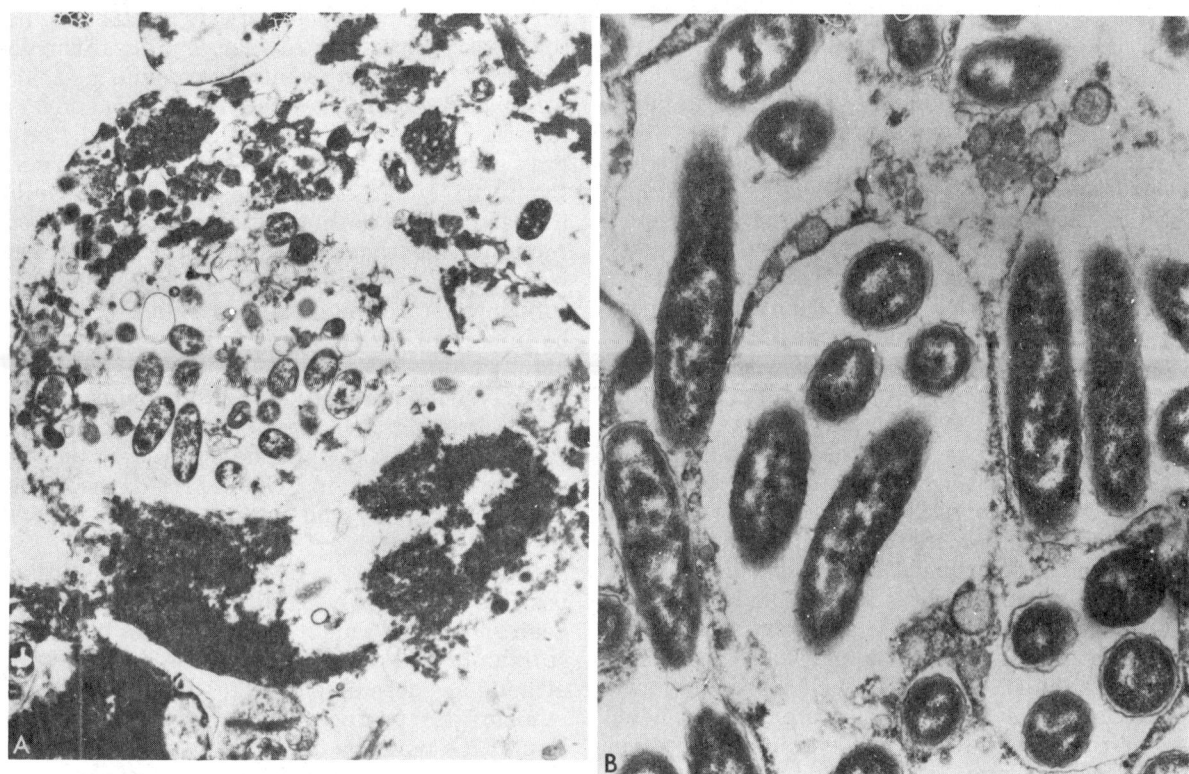

**FIGURE 2.** *Electron micrograph of* L. pneumophila. A, *Within phagosome of alveolar macrophage from patient. Note both intact and degenerating organisms are present. 21,300× B, In yolk-sac membrane of embryonic hen's egg organisms are intracellular and enclosed by a double envelope, each composed of a triple-layered unit membrane. 47,400× Courtesy of F. W. Chandler.*

At least four distinct serogroups of *L. pneumophila* have been identified by immunofluorescence studies (McKinney et al., 1979). Most of the clinical isolates belong to serogroup 1 (type strain Philadelphia 1). The other serogroups are serogroup 2) (type strain Togus 1), serogroup 3 (type strain Bloomington 2), and serogroup 4 (type strain Los Angeles 1). Serogroup-specific antigens from strains of *L. pneumophila* have been isolated and partially characterized. Other antigens seem to be shared by all four serogroups. Strains have been isolated that do not stain with existing antisera, suggesting the probability that there are additional serogroups.

*L. pneumophila* can survive for months in distilled water and for over a year in tap water. The organism has not been isolated from natural animal reservoirs.

## EPIDEMIOLOGY

Legionnaires' disease occurs sporadically, endemically, and in explosive point-source outbreaks that last for several days to a few weeks. An incubation period of 2 to 10 days has generally been observed (mean of 5.5 days). Attack rates have ranged between 0.1 per cent and 4.0 per cent of those exposed. In sharp contrast, Pontiac fever (nonpneumonic short-incubation-period legionellosis) has been recognized only in epidemic form and is characterized by an incubation period of 5 to 66 hours (mean of 36 hours), and attack rates of 95 to 100 per cent have been seen in the two reported outbreaks. Outbreaks of legionellosis have occurred in the United States and among Scottish tourists returning from vacation in Spain (Table 1) and have ranged in size from 8 to 221 cases. Most of the outbreaks have been associated with buildings or institutions such as hotels, hospitals, and a health department building. Recurrent outbreaks at the same institution and continuing occurrence of endemic disease at high rates have been reported.

Sporadic cases have been identified in nearly every state in the United States (approximately 500 reported cases in the United States in 1978) and also in Great Britain, the Netherlands, Switzerland, Sweden, Spain, Italy, Austria, Israel, Australia, and Canada. Cases will certainly be identified from additional countries as the disease is more widely sought. Data from several serologic surveys in the United States suggest that exposure to the organism may vary widely from region to region. In most studies, the prevalence of antibody titers of ≥128 to serogroup 1 by immunofluorescence testing is 1 to 4 per cent. However, in some areas considered hyperendemic for *L. pneumophila* serogroup 1, antibody titers of ≥128 have been found in 5 to 25 per cent. The incidence of Legionnaires' disease in the United States or other countries is unknown. Between 0.5 and 4.5 per cent of otherwise undiagnosed pneumonia cases have now been confirmed as Legionnaires' disease (LD) by immunofluorescence testing, suggesting an incidence of 2 to 16 cases/100,000 population per year in the United States. In a study of the incidence of community-acquired LD in Seattle, Washington, 1 per cent of

the patients with pneumonia of uncertain etiology had a fourfold rise in antibody titer to *L. pneumophila*, representing an incidence of 12 cases/100,000 population per year (Foy et al., 1979). Legionellosis may also occur as a sporadic nosocomial infection.

A summer seasonality has been observed both for point-source outbreaks and for sporadic cases, although cases occur in all months of the year. The majority of cases have occurred in middle-aged or elderly persons; the mean age of patients is about 55 years. Few cases have been identified in children. Persons with the nonpneumonic form of legionellosis are generally younger than persons with Legionnaires' disease. The distribution

**TABLE 1.  Summary of 16 Outbreaks of Legionellosis**

| LOCATION | DATE | NO. OF CASES | ESTIMATED ATTACK RATE (%) | INCUBATION PERIOD | SYNDROME | CASE-FATALITY RATIO (%) | SOURCE OF ORGANISM |
|---|---|---|---|---|---|---|---|
| 1. St. Elizabeth Hospital Washington, D. C. | July–Aug 1965 | 81 | 1.4 | — | LD | 17 | Suspect excavation site |
| 2. Oakland County Health Department Pontiac, Michigan | July–Aug 1968 | 144 | 95 | 5–66 hours (mean 36 hours) | Pontiac fever | 0 | Evaporative condenser |
| 3. Hotel Benidorm, Spain | July 1973 | 8 | — | — | LD | 38 | — |
| 4. James River, Virginia | July 1973 | 10 | 100 | 17–43 hours (mean 37 hours) | Pontiac fever | 0 | Suspect turbine condenser |
| 5. Odd Fellow Convention Philadelphia, Pennsylvania | Sept 1974 | 11 | 2.9 | 1–9 days | LD | 10 | Associated with grand ballroom of hotel |
| 6. American Legion Convention Philadelphia, Pennsylvania | July–Aug 1976 | 221 | 4.0 | 2–10 days | LD | 15 | Associated with lobby of hotel and street in front of hotel |
| 7. Hospitals Columbus, Ohio | July–Sept 1977 | 15 | — | — | LD | 13 | — |
| 8. Community and Hospital Kingsport, Tennessee | Aug–Sept 1977 | 33 | 0.2 | — | LD | 19 | — |
| 9. Community and Hospital Burlington, Vermont | May–Dec (Aug–Sept peak) 1977 | 69 | — | — | LD | 25 | Hyperendemic |
| 10. Hospital Los Angeles, California | 1977 → (peak, late fall) | 106 | 0.5 | — | LD | 26 | Nosocomial outbreak |
| 11. Hotel Bloomington, Indiana | 1978 → (peak, summer–fall) | 56 | 0.1–0.2 | 4–12 days | LD | 12 | Hyperendemic |
| 12. Country Club Atlanta, Georgia | July 1978 | 8 | 1.5 | — | LD | 0 | Evaporative condenser? |
| 13. Garment district New York, New York | Aug–Sept 1978 | 38 | — | — | LD | 8 | — |
| 14. Hospital Memphis, Tennessee | Aug–Sept 1978 | 39 | 2.8 | 2–10 days | LD | 13 | Cooling tower condenser |
| 15. Veterans of Foreign Wars Convention Dallas, Texas | Aug–Sept 1978 | 18 | 0.2 | 2–10 days | LD | 6 | — |
| 16. Community and Hospital Norwalk, Connecticut | 1978 (peak, summer–fall) | 28 | 0.7 | — | LD | 36 | Hyperendemic area |

by sex of cases of Legionnaires' disease demonstrates a striking male predominance in outbreaks and for sporadic cases (male: female ratio of 2 to 3:1). Other risk factors for illness are underlying chronic disease states such as renal insufficiency or malignancy, use of corticosteroids or immunosuppressive agents, cigarette smoking, heavy alcohol consumption, construction work, living near ongoing excavation or construction, and recent travel (Tables 2 and 3).

Airborne transmission *L. pneumophila* has been the only documented natural mode of spread of legionellosis, although in most outbreaks and in sporadic cases the mode of spread has not been proved. Secondary cases of Legionnaires' disease have never been identified, and to date there has been no documented instance of person-to-person spread. In four outbreaks, heat-rejection systems (cooling tower, 1; evaporative condensers, 2; steam-turbine condenser, 1) have been epidemiologically implicated as the vehicles of spread. Water in these systems is commonly contaminated with bacteria and as heat is exchanged from water to air through evaporation, as in cooling towers or evaporative condensers, an aerosol is generated that may contain microorganisms that are thereby disseminated. It is likely that infection occurs through inhalation of these bacteria as droplet nuclei.

In the 1968 outbreak of Pontiac fever in Pontiac, Michigan, only those persons who were in the health department building when the central air-conditioning system was in operation became ill. Guinea pigs exposed to unfiltered air in the building became ill with pneumonia, while most of those exposed to filtered air were spared. Aerosols of water from the evaporative condenser in the health department building also produced pneumonia in guinea pigs. *L. pneumophila* was isolated from the frozen stored lungs of these guinea pigs 10 years later, and seroconversion to *L. pneumophila* was documented for 31 of 37 workers from whom paired sera were still available. Two defects were found in the central air-conditioning system: (1) cracks permitted aerosol from the evaporative condenser to accumulate in an adjacent supply air duct, and (2) air exhausted from the evaporative condenser contaminated the independent circulation of conditioned air because of the proximity of exhaust and intake vents on the roof.

In a 1973 outbreak of Pontiac fever in Virginia, workers who cleaned the inside of a condenser with compressed air became ill. It is postulated that these men inhaled contaminated aerosols and droplet nuclei generated in the cleaning process. Nine of the 10 workers had either demonstrable seroconversion to *L. pneumophila* or single elevated titers. In 1978, two outbreaks of Legionnaires' disease were linked to heat-rejection systems. At an Atlanta country club, illness was associated with increased golfing activity in the 2 to 10 days before onset; *L. pneumophila* was isolated from an evaporative condenser at the clubhouse. Exhaust from this condenser projected toward the practice green and the 10th and 16th tees.

At a Memphis hospital, disease occurred within days after an unused auxiliary cooling tower was turned on and ceased within nine days after this system was shut down. A significant association was noted between acquisition of Legionnaires' disease and hospitalization in rooms that received air from intake vents located near the auxiliary cooling tower.

Other outbreaks have occurred at sites without

**TABLE 2.  Summary of Factors that Predispose to Legionellosis**

| RISK FACTOR | ASSOCIATED WITH OUTBREAKS | ASSOCIATED WITH SPORADIC CASES |
|---|:---:|:---:|
| Advancing age | + | + |
| Male sex | + | + |
| Underlying chronic diseases | | |
|    Renal insufficiency | + | + |
|    Malignancy | | |
| Immunosuppressive therapy | + | + |
| Cigarette smoking | + | + |
| Heavy alcohol consumption | + | + |
| Construction work | − | + |
| Residence near ongoing construction | | |
|    or excavation | +/− | + |
| Recent travel | +/− | + |
| Time spent in epicenter | + | − |

+, yes
−, no

air-conditioning or heat-rejection systems — in Spain in 1973 and in Washington, D. C. in 1965. At a hospital in Washington, D. C. in 1965, 81 persons developed Legionnaires' disease in the summer. Illness was significantly associated with exposure to the hospital grounds or sleeping by open windows. During the summer, extensive excavation had been undertaken to install a water-sprinkling system. It is postulated that organisms became airborne and disseminated during excavation or backfilling. In a large study of sporadic cases, no association was observed between acquisition of disease and the use of air conditioning, heating, humidifying, or dehumidifying systems, although disease did occur more frequently in construction workers and in individuals living near ongoing construction or excavation sites (Storch et al., 1979).

*L. pneumophila* has been recovered from numerous environmental sites, with or without demonstrated association with cases of legionellosis. Person-to-person spread has not been documented, but in one study, hospital staff caring for patients with Legionnaires' disease had a higher proportion of seropositivity to *L. pneumophila* as measured by an indirect hemagglutination assay compared with hospital staff not caring for Legionnaires' disease patients (Saravolatz et al., 1979). However, increased amounts of patient contact did not correlate with higher rates of seroreactivity, and the specificity of the hemagglutination assay has not been established. Furthermore, this observation has not been documented at other hospitals.

## PATHOGENESIS AND PATHOLOGY

Studies on the pathogenesis of legionellosis are limited. The portal of entry appears to be the respiratory tract, since the only consistent changes observed in patients with Legionnaires' disease are in the lungs (Fig. 3). Characteristically, the lesion produced is an acute fibrinopurulent bronchopneumonia with acute diffuse alveolar damage (Blackmon et al., 1978). The intra-alveolar infiltrate consists of large numbers of neutrophils admixed with macrophages and fibrin (Fig. 4). Desquamation of alveolar epithelium may be prominent, and small focal areas of necrosis may be observed. Necrosis with cavity formation is uncommon and, when observed, is frequently either in an immunocompromised patient or in a person with a concomitant gram-negative bacterial superinfection. Pathologic changes are observed in the terminal bronchioles, but the large airways are spared. Bacilli can be demonstrated in the exudate with a modification of Dieterle silver impregnation stain or the Wol-

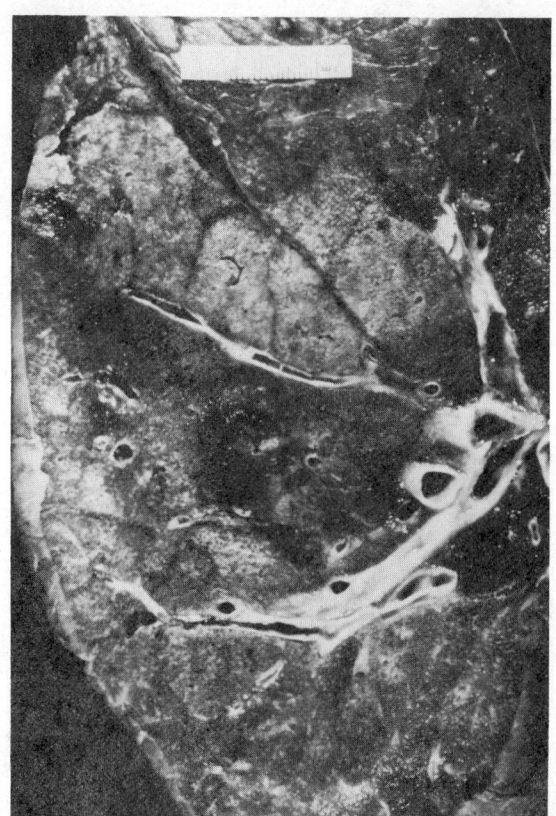

**FIGURE 3.** *Macroscopic appearance of lung tissue obtained from a fatal case of Legionnaires' disease pneumonia. Note circumscribed peripheral nodular pneumonia. Several similar nodules were present in other lobes. From Winn, W. C., Jr.: Arch Pathol 102:347, 1978.*

bach modification of the Giesma stain, but rarely with the Brown-Benn or Brown-Hopps modification of the Gram stain. Organisms may be seen within macrophages and neutrophils and extracellularly. Hilar lymph nodes are rarely enlarged, but the organism has been observed within the hilar lymphatic tissue by direct immunofluorescent staining techniques. The direct immunofluorescent stain (DFA) is more sensitive and specific for *L. pneumophila*, with the highest yield observed in lung tissue scrapings. The Gimenez stain is useful for impression smears and frozen sections but not for paraffin-embedded tissue. In some patients pneumonia does not resolve completely; varying degrees of interstitial inflammation and fibrosis may be found months to years later.

Bacteremia has been documented in Legionnaires' disease, but whether the multisystem manifestations frequently observed in these patients are due to direct bacterial invasion or to other mechanisms is unknown. *L. pneumophila* has rarely been identified in other organ systems, and no consistent histopathologic findings have been noted. Although the organism can lyse guin-

**TABLE 3. Comparative Epidemiologic and Clinical Features of the Atypical Pneumonias**

| EPIDEMIOLOGIC FEATURES | LEGIONNAIRES' DISEASE | MYCOPLASMA PNEUMONIA | PSITTACOSIS | Q FEVER | TULAREMIA | VIRAL PNEUMONIA[a] | HISTOPLASMOSIS | COCCIDIOIDOMYCOSIS |
|---|---|---|---|---|---|---|---|---|
| Incubation period (days) | 2–10 | 12–21 | 7–14 | 14–38 | 1–8 | 1–3 | 3–21 | 7–28 |
| Seasonality | Summer | Fall-winter | Year-round ? summer peak | Year-round ? spring peak | Year-round ? summer peak | Fall-winter | ? Winter nadir | Summer-fall |
| Patient age | Middle-age, elderly | Children and young adults | Adult | Adult | Adult | Children, young adult, elderly | All | All |
| Sex ratio | M>F | M=F | M≥F | M≥F | M>F | M=F | M=F | M=F |
| Exposure to animals | 0 | 0 | Psittacine birds, turkeys pigeons | Livestock | Rodents, rabbits, ticks | 0 | Starlings, chickens, bats | 0 |
| Exposure to other infective sources | Construction sites/recent travel | 0 | Pet shop | Contaminated milk fomites (hay) | 0 | 0 | Great river valleys — N. America, S. America, Africa, and S. Asia; construction sites and river valleys in U.S.A. | Southwest U.S. and Chaco district of Argentina; construction sites in these areas |
| Person-to-person transmission | 0 | + | rare | 0 | 0 | + | 0 | 0 |
| Underlying chronic diseases | + | 0 | 0 | 0 | 0 | +/- | +/- | 0 |
| Smoking/alcohol abuse | + | 0 | 0 | 0 | 0 | +/- | +/- | 0 |
| **CLINICAL FEATURES** | | | | | | | | |
| Rapidity of onset | Abrupt or insidious | Insidious | Abrupt or insidious | Abrupt | Abrupt | Abrupt | Abrupt | Abrupt |
| Myalgias, malaise, headache | + | + | + | + | + | + | + | + |
| Unproductive to minimally productive cough | + | + | + | + | + | + | + | + |
| Upper respiratory symptoms | 0 | + | +/- | 0 | +/- | + | +/- | +/- |

| | | | | | | | | |
|---|---|---|---|---|---|---|---|---|
| Rigors | + (Recurrent) | Rare | Rare | Rare | | Rare | Rare | + |
| Diarrhea | + | Infrequent | Infrequent | Infrequent | Infrequent | Infrequent | 0 | 0 |
| Temperature ≥39° C | + | + | + | Rare | + | + | + | + |
| Other focal signs | Confusion | Bullous myringitis, rash, pharyngitis, arthritis, myocarditis, various neurologic signs | Hepatosplenomegaly, rash, myopericarditis | Hepatomegaly, tender liver, endocarditis | Lymphadenopathy, hepatosplenomegaly, rash, ocular findings | Pharyngitis, conjunctivitis | Mucous membrane lesions, rash (erythema-nodosum), lymphadenopathy | Rash (erythema nodosum), meningitis, lymphadenopathy |
| WBC per mm³ | 5,000–20,000 | 5,000–20,000 | 10,000–20,000 | 10,000–20,000 | 15,000–20,000 | 10,000–25,000 | 10,000–20,000 | 10,000–20,000 |
| Unexplained hematuria | + | Rare | 0 | 0 | 0 | Rare | Rare | 0 |
| Abnormal liver and renal function | + | Occasional liver abnormalities | Occasional | Occasional | | Occasional | Occasional | Occasional |
| Chest radiographs<br>Character of infiltrate | Patchy bronchopneumonia | Perihilar bronchopneumonia | Interstitial pneumonia or lobar pneumonia | Interstitial pneumonia | Diffuse bronchopneumonia or lobar pneumonia | Perihilar bronchopneumonia | Patchy bronchopneumonia | Patchy bronchopneumonia |
| Hilar adenopathy | 0 | Rare | Rare | Rare | + | Rare | + | Rare |
| Pleural effusion | 20–30% (small) | 10–25% (small) | Rare | Rare | + | Rare | Rare | Common |
| Cavitation/calcification | Rare/0 | 0/0 | 0/0 | 0/0 | 0/0 | 0/0 | Occasional/+ | +/+ |
| Diagnostic serologic tests | IFA[b] | Cold agglutinins CF[c] | CF | CF | Agglutinins | HI[d] CF | CF ID[e] | CF ID |
| Case-fatality ratio (%) | 15–20 | <0.1 | 15–20 (untreated) 5 (treated) | <1 | 30–40 (untreated) | ? | <1 | <1 |
| Treatment | Erythromycin | Erythromycin or tetracycline | Tetracycline | Tetracycline | Streptomycin | — | Amphotericin B — if progressive disseminative, or cavitary | |

[a] Influenza, parainfluenza, adenovirus
[b] IFA, indirect fluorescent antibody
[c] CF, complement fixation
[d] HI, hemagglutination inhibition
[e] ID, immunodiffusion

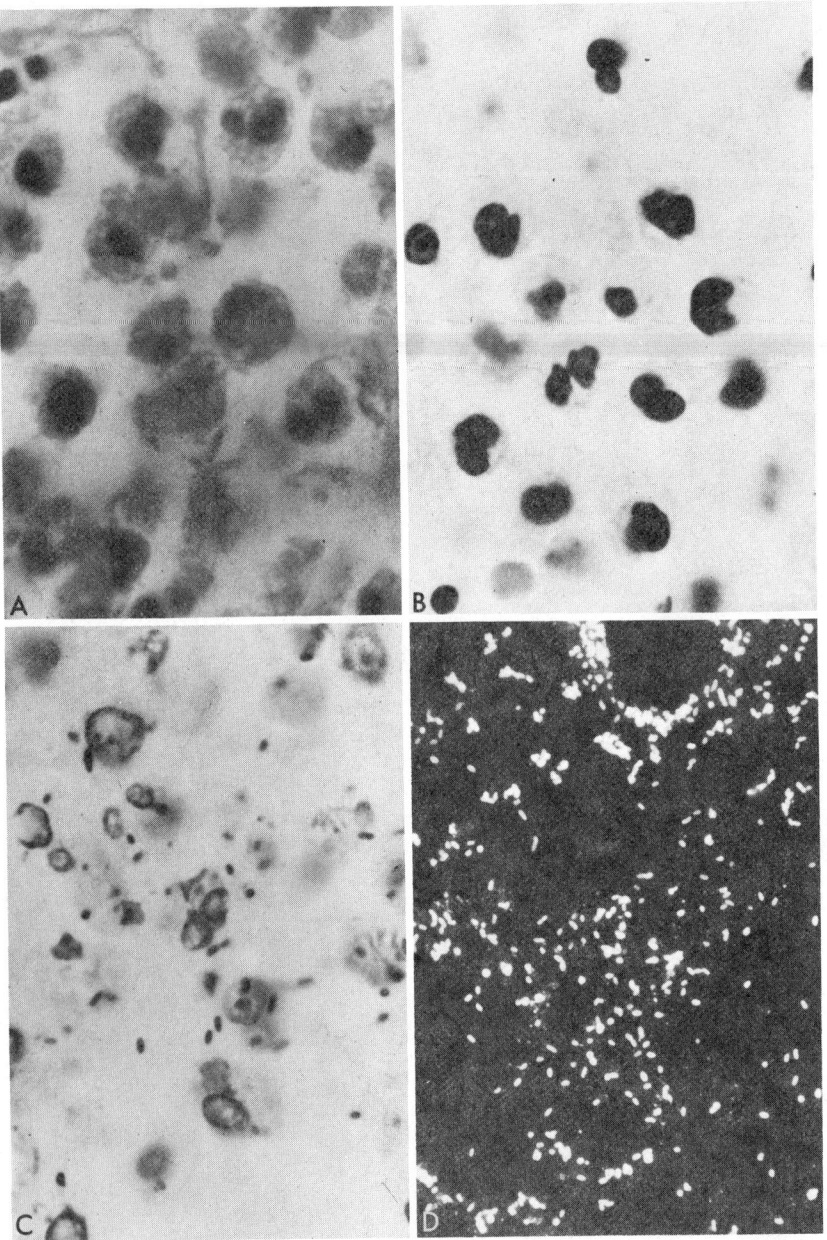

**FIGURE 4.** *Microscopic appearance of Legionnaires' disease pneumonia. A, Intra-alveolar exudate consisting of fibrin, polymorphonuclear leukocytes, and macrophages. Note necrosis of inflammatory exudate. Hematoxylin and eosin, 600 × B, Gram-stained smear of lung tissue. Note paucity of visualized organisms. C, Myriads of small pleomorphic intracellular and extracellular bacilli. Dieterle silver impregnation stain, 600× D, Fluorescent-antibody stains of scraping of formalin-fixed lung tissue from a patient with fatal pneumonia caused by L. pneumophila. Courtesy of F. W. Chandler and W. B. Cherry.*

ea pig red cells and has certain properties of endotoxin (cell suspensions induce gelation of *Limulus* amebocyte lysate and are pyrogenic to rabbits), the role of toxins or enzymes in producing human disease is not known.

The pathogenesis of Pontiac fever is not known. No histopathologic studies have been done to date in humans because the disease is uniformly benign and self-limited. Mechanisms of immunity to *L. pneumophila* are currently being investigated. Humoral immunity may be important in humans. A cell membrane fraction containing protein, carbohydrate, and lipid induces an antibody response in experimental animals and pro-

tects them against subsequent challenge with homologous live organisms (Wong et al., 1979). Complement and bactericidal antibodies appear to play important roles in mediating resistance. The role of the cell-mediated immune system has not been studied.

## CLINICAL MANIFESTATIONS

### Legionnaires' Disease

Legionnaires' disease has a broad range of manifestations from a mild grippe to a fulminant multisystem disease (Tsai et al., 1979). After an incubation period of 2 to 10 days (mean of 5.5 days), the patient may have a prodrome of malaise, diffuse myalgias, headache, and fever often accompanied by rigors. Cough, dyspnea, and chest pain are also common early manifestations. Upper respiratory symptoms including sore throat, nasal congestion, and coryza are infrequently reported. Chest pain is usually pleuritic rather than musculoskeletal in nature and at times may be incapacitating. Other common presenting problems include diarrhea (without mucus, blood, or pus), which may be present in up to 40 per cent of the patients, and mental confusion or delirium. Over the next several days, the fever usually persists unremittingly (up to 41° C), and the patient may continue to have recurrent rigors. Respiratory symptoms may progress, and in nearly 50 per cent of the patients the cough becomes productive usually of a small amount of mucoid rather than mucopurulent sputum. On examination the patient often appears severely ill, tachypneic, and diaphoretic, and in respiratory distress. The temperature is above 38.9° C in half of the patients, and respiratory rates are over 25/min in 40 per cent, and although tachycardia is frequently observed, the heart rate is often slower than would be expected for the amount of fever. Additional findings have been largely confined to the lungs and include moist inspiratory rales, rhonchi, and, for <25 per cent of the patients, evidence of consolidation. Skin rash, mucous membrane lesions, lymphadenopathy, and hepatosplenomegaly are not typical of Legionnaires' disease. On occasion, transient neurologic deficits have been observed. Laboratory findings include a normal or moderately elevated white blood cell count ($\leq$20,000 wbc/mm$^3$) with an increase in band cells, an elevated erythrocyte sedimentation rate, and mild abnormalities in liver and renal function. Significant proteinuria and microscopic hematuria may be present. Thrombocytopenia and disseminated intravascular coagulation have been observed. Hyponatremia, possibly due to the syndrome of inappropriate antidiuretic hormone secretion and hypophosphatemia, may also be seen in some patients. Sputum, if obtainable, is generally characterized by few polmorphonuclear cells and no predominant bacterial species. Pleural fluid, which may be seen in up to 40 per cent of the patients, is usually scant and may be characterized as a transudate or exudate. Radiographic findings include poorly defined infiltrates that may initially be unilateral but generally progress to bilateral patchy or nodular alveolar involvement (Fig. 5). Lobar consolidation is seen in less than 25 per cent of those patients with pneumonia. Cavitation and abscess formation are uncommon (Fig. 6). Serologic tests such as cold and febrile agglutinins are either negative or not found in significant titers.

### Pontiac Fever

Pontiac fever is an acute, self-limited, febrile illness with an incubation period of 5 to 66 hours (mean of 36 hours) (Glick et al., 1978). The illness is also characterized by an abrupt onset of malaise, diffuse myalgias, headache, and fever. Upper respiratory symptoms may be present. A mild unproductive cough, nausea, and dizziness are additional features. Physical findings include temperature of up to 41° C, tachypnea, and tachycardia. Examination of the chest is unremarkable. Leukocyte counts have ranged from normal levels to 25,000 wbc/mm$^3$. Chest x-rays do not reveal pulmonary infiltrates.

### Other Infections

Infection with *L. pneumophila* may be associated with clinical syndromes other than those typical of Legionnaires' disease and Pontiac fever. Patients with serologically confirmed legionellosis have had only diarrhea and fever without any evidence of pneumonia, prolonged fever alone, or pneumonia accompanied by culture-negative endocarditis. Not all patients with confirmed infection require hospitalization, and asymptomatic seroconverters have been documented. Mild illness without radiographic evidence of pneumonia occurred in 28 of 142 patients who had chest x-rays in the 1976 Philadelphia outbreak. The total clincial spectrum of infection with *L. pneumophila* has not yet been defined.

## COMPLICATIONS AND SEQUELAE

Patients with the syndrome of Pontiac fever recover spontaneously in two to five days without treatment. No deaths or long-term sequelae have been noted with this syndrome. Patients with Legionnaires' disease, however, may suffer respiratory failure. During the 1976 Philadelphia outbreak, 16 per cent of hospitalized patients needed assisted ventilation. Acute renal failure, disseminated intravascular coagulation, and shock may also complicate the illness. The overall case-fatality ratios observed for outbreak settings and for sporadic cases are between 14 per cent and 18 per cent. These rates are higher for older individuals and for individuals with underlying disease problems or receiving immunosuppressants (Beaty et al., 1978). Death usually is a result of pulmonary insufficiency or shock. The fever continues until the institution of appropriate antimicrobial therapy or until spontaneous resolution of the infection on the seventh to twelfth day of illness. Roentgenographically, the

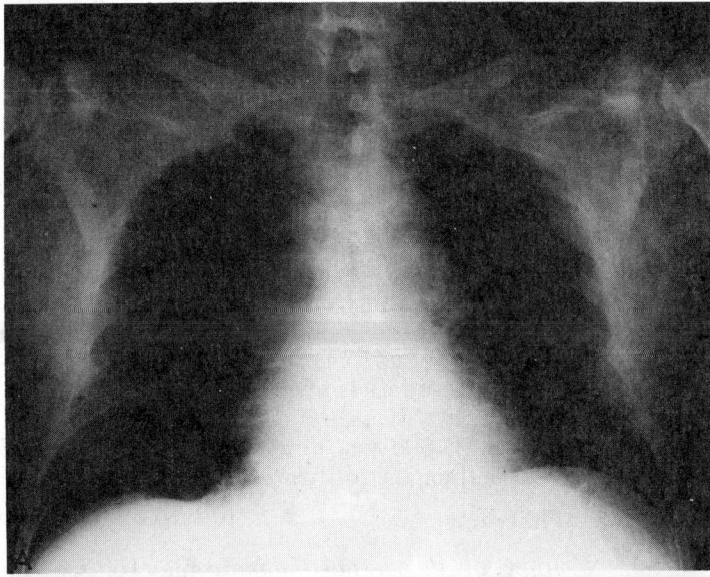

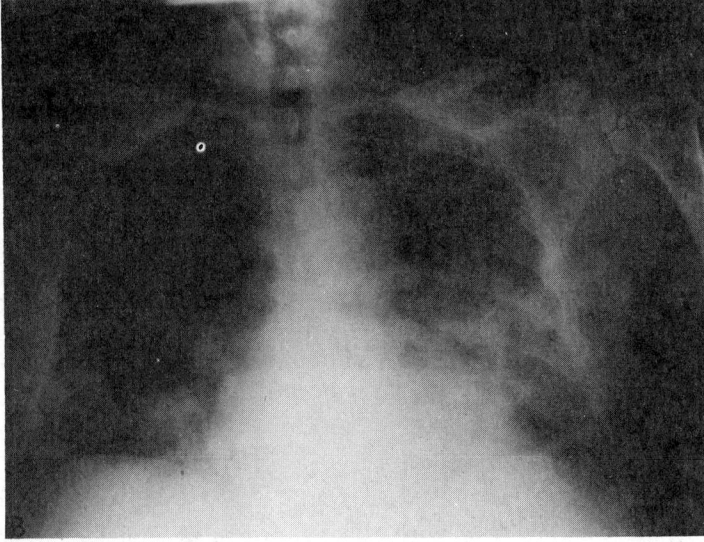

**FIGURE 5.** *Legionnaires' disease in a middle-age male with cough and fever. A, Note stringy, poorly defined left perihilar infiltrate on admission. B, Five days after admission. Note progression of bronchopneumonia with bilateral patchy involvement. From Tsai, T. F.: Ann Intern Med 90:510, 1979.*

pneumonia resolves slowly and can take several months to do so. Recovery is usually complete, although impairment of pulmonary diffusion capacity has been documented two years after the acute illness (Lattimer et al., 1979). Whether patients with documented *L. pneumophila* infection are protected from reinfection or whether there is the possibility of reactivation of infection during immunosuppressant therapy is not yet known.

## DIAGNOSIS

Clinical diagnosis of Legionnaires' disease may be difficult because it can resemble other common bacterial pneumonias or infections caused by a wide variety of organisms including *Mycoplasma*

*pneumoniae, Chlamydia psittaci* (psittacosis), *Coxiella burnetti* (Q fever), *Francisella tularensis* (tularemia), influenza and other respiratory viruses, cytomegalovirus, *Histoplasma capsulatum, Coccidioides immitis, Toxoplasma gondii,* and *Pneumocystis carinii.* Other noninfectious illnesses that may at times resemble Legionnaires' disease include the hypersensitivity pneumonitides, collagen vascular disorders with pulmonic involvement, drug reactions, and a few types of toxins. Careful microscopy and culture of respiratory secretions should help to distinguish Legionnaires' disease from other bacterial pneumonias. Epidemiologic features that can assist in the diagnosis of Legionnaires' disease include the occurrence predominantly in middle-aged and elderly men, peak incidence in the summer, incubation period of 2 to 10 days, lack of history of exposure to animals, lack of person-to-person spread, occurrence in individuals with a history of underlying chronic disease states, a history of heavy cigarette smoking or alcohol use, and a recent history of travel or exposure to construction or excavation sites. An explosive common-source outbreak of pneumonia in the summer within 10 days of suspected exposure and with no evident person-to-person spread would be highly suggestive of Legionnaires' disease. Specific clinical features that may also assist in the diagnosis are the presence of watery diarrhea, altered states of consciousness, high unremitting fever with repeated rigors, relative bradycardia, lack of preceding upper respiratory symptoms, abnormal liver and renal function, including an active urinary sediment, and negative sputum and blood cultures on conventional media. Significant negative features directly attributable to Legionnaires' disease are the absence of an exanthem or enanthem, pharyngitis, lymphadenopathy, and hepatosplenomegaly.

Definitive diagnosis requires the isolation of *L. pneumophila* from clinical specimens, demonstration of the organism or its antigens in tissue or body fluids, or documentation of ≥ fourfold rise in specific antibodies. *L. pneumophila* has been recovered from respiratory secretions, pleural fluid, blood, and lung tissue by using special culture media. However, growth may take several days.

The organism has been visualized in respiratory secretions (both expectorated and obtained by transtracheal aspiration), pleural fluid, and lung tissue with various staining procedures. Direct immunofluorescent staining (using a polyvalent conjugate) appears to be specific, although *Mycobacteria* and an occasional strain of *Pseudomonas fluorescens* may also stain brightly. Recent experience suggests that positive direct immunofluorescent smears can be found in up to 71 per cent of the cases if multiple samples of sputum are obtained from the same patient (Gump et al., 1979). *L. pneumophila* antigen can be demonstrated in urine of patients with Legionnaires' disease by an enzyme-linked immunosorbent assay (ELISA). The most commonly used method for the diagnosis of Legionnaires' disease is serologic measurement of antibodies specific to *L. pneumophila*. These methods include indirect immunofluorescent (IFA) staining, hemagglutination, hemagglutination inhibition, microagglutination, and ELISA. The IFA test has been the serologic method most widely applied to date. A ≥ fourfold increase of antibody (to a titer of ≥128) during convalescence is considered diagnostic; this increase is usually observed within three weeks of onset of illness but may not occur until the sixth week of illness (Kirby et al., 1978). The sensitivity of the IFA can be estimated from

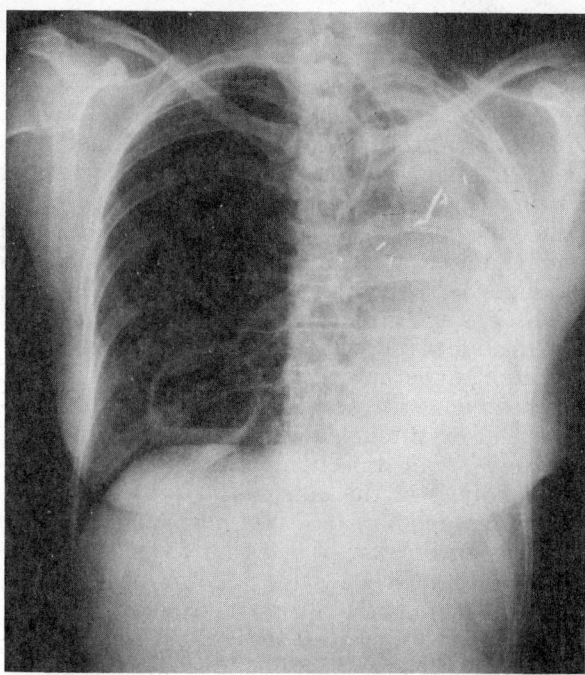

**FIGURE 6.** *Large pulmonary abscess that developed in the right lung of a patient with Legionnaires' disease who had previously had left pneumonectomy for carcinoma. Gump, D. W.: Ann Intern Med 90:539, 1979.*

well-defined outbreaks that have shown 75 to 85 per cent of persons with clinical and epidemiologic compatible illness to have ≥ fourfold increase of antibody to a titer of ≥128 (McDade et al., 1977). Antibody is generally specific for the serogroup causing infection, but patients with broadly reacting sera have been observed (Wilkinson et al., 1979). Rising titers to *L. pneumophila* have been seen in patients with culture-proved plague and tularemia, and concomitant increases in antibody to other pathogens including *M. pneumoniae, C. psittaci,* and influenza virus have been documented. Improvement of the specificity of IFA for *L. pneumophila* may occur when sera are mixed with the supernatant of a culture of *E. coli* 013, apparently through the adsorption of antibodies to common gram-negative bacterial antigens. Elevated titers to *L. pneumophila* may be demonstrable for more than 10 years, but typically, after a peak in early convalescence, titers drop 1 to 2 dilutions after 6 months and 2 dilutions after 18 months.

The diagnosis of Pontiac fever is made on clinical, epidemiologic, and serologic grounds and has thus far been recognized only in epidemic form.

## THERAPY

*L. pneumophila* is susceptible to a wide variety of antimicrobial agents according to in vitro tests.

On the basis of minimal inhibitory concentrations observed in agar dilution testing, the organisms were susceptible to erythromycin, rifampin, the aminoglycosides, the penicillins, cefoxitin, chloramphenicol, trimethoprim-sulfamethoxazole, and doxycycline. The organism was not susceptible to other cephalosporins, tetracycline, clindamycin, or vancomycin. Only erythromycin and rifampin were markedly effective in prophylaxis and in treatment of infected embryonic hens' eggs and guinea pigs.

Although a randomized prospective trial of antimicrobial therapy of Legionnaires' disease has not been done, several clinical observations suggest that erythromycin may be effective against *L. pneumophila* infection in humans. Retrospective analysis of the outcome in patients in the 1976 Philadelphia, 1977 Vermont, and 1977 Los Angeles outbreaks showed that case-fatality ratios were lowest for those patients treated with erythromycin. In the Vermont outbreak, the case-fatality ratio for patients treated with erythromycin was 5 per cent, significantly lower than the ratio of 17 per cent for patients not treated with erythromycin (Broome et al., 1979). The dose, route, and duration of the most effective therapy are not known. For seriously ill patients and for patients who cannot tolerate oral therapy, 500 to 1000 mg of erythromycin intravenously every six hours (15 mg/kg every six hours for children other than neonates) for at least 14 days is recommended. Less seriously ill patients have been treated with 500 mg of erythromycin orally every six hours for a minimum of 14 days. Occasionally patients may relapse after therapy is discontinued (usually these patients had received less than 14 days' therapy), but they have generally improved when erythromycin therapy was resumed. There is little clinical experience with rifampin as therapy for Legionnaires' disease. It is recommended that rifampin be reserved for combined therapy with erythromycin for those patients not responding to high-dose intravenous erythromycin therapy alone and possibly for those patients with documented lung abscess. For patients with severe hepatic insufficiency, although few data are available, it is generally recommended that the dose of erythromycin be decreased by 25 to 50 per cent. Intravenous erythromycin is extremely irritating to the veins and needs to be diluted (1 to 2 mg/ml) and administered slowly. Either the lactobionate or the glucceptate salt is recommended for intravenous use. For oral administration, either the stearate salt or base is recommended; the estolate ester has been associated with cholestatic jaundice.

Supportive therapeutic measures are of major importance in the treatment of seriously ill patients with respiratory failure, shock, or acute renal failure. Mechanical ventilation, fluid management, vasoactive drugs, and dialysis may be required for these clinical problems.

Specific therapy is probably not needed for the Pontiac fever syndrome.

## PREVENTION AND CONTROL

The environmental reservoir and distribution in nature of *L. pneumophila* have not been defined nor has the mode of spread in sporadic cases and most outbreaks of legionellosis. In settings in which spread has been demonstrated to be due to aerosolized droplet nuclei from heat-rejection devices, stopping the production of the aerosols and eliminating the organism from the contaminated system may prevent further cases. Whether chemical treatment and other preventive maintenance of these systems can prevent some outbreaks is not yet known. A vaccine is currently being tested in animal models. The value of respiratory isolation and secretion precautions is untested; secondary person-to-person spread, if it occurs, must be rare. However, laboratory workers should exercise care in handling cultures and potentially contaminated specimens so as not to generate aerosols. Work with the organism should be done in a biologic safety cabinet.

## OTHER FASTIDIOUS BACTERIA ASSOCIATED WITH PNEUMONIA

Several cases of pneumonia that clinically resemble Legionnaires' disease have recently been shown to be caused by previously uncharacterized gram-negative bacilli. These share several phenotypic characteristics with *L. pneumophila,* including ability to grow on charcoal yeast extract agar but not on the more commonly used bacteriologic media. Pneumonia caused by Pittsburgh pneumonia PPA) (=TATLOCK) has been recognized as a nosocomial infection in immunosuppressed patients (Pasculle 1979). Atypical *Legionella*-like organisms (=WIGA) have been found to cause community-acquired cases perhaps from water sources (Cordes 1979). One case of pneumonia in a patient with oat-cell carcinoma was shown to be caused by TEX-KL (=NY-23) (Lewallen 1979). How cases caused by these organisms can be differentiated from Legionnaires' disease clinically, and how infection is acquired have not been defined. Diagnosis can be made by a culture of lung tissue directly on charcoal yeast extract agar or after passage in guinea pigs and embryonated eggs; detection of organisms in lung tissue by direct immunofluorescence; or, in the case of PPA and WIGA, by demonstration of rising titers to the organisms by indirect immuno-fluorescence. The specificity and sensitivity of the diagnostic tests have not been measured. The paucity of documented cases caused by these bacteria does not permit assessment of optimal antibiotic therapy; however, unlike *L. pneumophila,* PPA has not been found to produce a cephalosporinase, so beta-lactam antibiotics might be expected to be effective in PPA pneumonia.

## References

Balows, A., Fraser, D. W. (eds.): International Symposium on Legionnaires' disease. Ann Intern Med 90:491, 1979.

Beaty, H. N., Miller, A. A., Broome, C. V., Goings, S. A. J., and Phillips, C. A.: Legionnaires' disease in Vermont, May to October 1977. JAMA 240:127, 1978.

Brenner, D. J., Steigerwalt, A. G., and McDade, J. E.: Classification of the Legionnaires' disease bacterium: *Legionella pneumophila,* genus novum, species nova, of the family *Legionellaceae,* family nova. Ann Intern Med 90:656, 1979.

Broome, C. V., Goings, S. A. J., Thacker, S. B., Vogt, R. L., Beaty, H. N., Fraser, D. W., and the Field Investigation Team: The Vermont epidemic of Legionnaires' disease. Ann Intern Med 90:573, 1979.

Chandler, F. W., Hicklin, M. D., and Blackmon, J. A.: Demonstration of the agent of Legionnaires' disease in tissue. N Engl J Med 297:1218, 1977.

Cherry, W. B., Pittman, B., Harris, P. P., Hebert, G. A., Thomason, B. M., Thacker, L., and Weaver, R. E.: Detection of Legionnaires' disease bacteria by direct immunofluorescent staining. J Clin Microbiol 8:329, 1978.

Cordes, L. G., Wilkenson, H. W., Gorman, G. W., Fikes, B. J., and Fraser, D. W.: Atypical *Legionella*-like organisms: Fastidious water-associated bacteria pathogenic for man. Lancet 2:927, 1979.

Foy, H. M., Broome, C. V., Hayes, P. S., Allan, I., Cooney, M. K., and Tobe, R.: Legionnaires' disease in a prepaid medical-care group in Seattle 1963–1975. Lancet 1:767, 1979.

Fraser, D. W., Tsai, T. F., Orenstein, W., Parkin, W. E., Beecham, H. J., Sharrar, R. G., Harris, J., Mallison, G. F., Martin, S. M., McDade, J. E., Shepard, C. C., Brachman, P. S., and The Field Investigation Team: Legionnaires' disease: A description of an epidemic of pneumonia. N Engl J Med 297:1189, 1977.

Glick, T. H., Gregg, M. B., Berman, B., Mallison, G. F., Rhodes, W. W., Jr., and Kassanoff, I.: Pontiac fever: An epidemic of unknown etiology in a health department. I. Clinical and epidemiologic aspects. Am J Epidemiol 107:149, 1978.

Gump, D. W., Frank, R. O., Winn, W. C., Jr., Foster, R. S., Jr., Broome, C. V., and Cherry, W. B.: Legionnaires' disease in patients with associated serious disease. Ann Intern Med 90:538, 1979.

Hebert, G. A., Thomason, B. M., Harris, P. P., Hicklin, M. D., and McKinney, R. M.: "Pittsburgh pneumonia agent": a bacterium phenotypically similar to *Legionella pneumophila* and identical to the TATLOCK bacterium. Ann Intern Med 92:53, 1980.

Jones, G. L., Herbert, G. A. (eds.): Legionnaires': The Disease, the Bacterium and Methodology. Center for Disease Control Laboratory Manual. Atlanta, Center for Disease Control, 1979.

Kirby, B. D., Snyder, K. M., Meyer, R. D., and Finegold, S. M.: Legionnaires' disease: Clinical features of 24 cases. Ann Intern Med 89:297, 1978.

Lattimer, G. L., Rhodes, L. V., III, Slaventi, J. S., Galgon, J. P., Stonebraker, V., Boley, S., and Haas, G.: The Philadelphia epidemic of Legionnaires' disease: Clinical, pulmonary, and serologic findings two years later. Ann Intern Med 90:522, 1979.

Lewallen, K. R., McKinney, R. M., Brenner, D. J., Moss, C. W., Dail, H. H., Thomason, B. M., and Bright, R. A.: A newly identified bacterium phenotypically resembling, but genetically distinct from *Legionella pneumophila*: an isolate in a case of pneumonia. Ann Intern Med 91:834, 1979.

McDade, J. E., Shepard, C. C., Fraser, D. W., Tsai, T. F., Redus, M. A., Dowdle, W. R., and the Laboratory Investigation Team: Legionnaires' disease: Isolation of a bacterium and demonstration of its role in other respiratory disease. N Engl J Med 297:1197, 1977.

McKinney, R. M., Thacker, L., Harris, P. P., Lewallen, K. R., Herbert, G. A., Edelstein, P. H., and Thomason, B. M.: Four serogroups of Legionnaires' disease bacteria defined by direct immunofluorescence. Ann Intern Med 90:490, 1979.

Pasculle, A. W., Myerowitz, R. L., and Rinaldo, C. R., Jr.: New bacterial agent of pneumonia isolated from renal-transplant recipients. Lancet 2:58, 1979.

Saravolatz, L. D., Arking, L., Wentworth, B., and Quinn, E.: Prevalence of antibody to Legionnaires' disease bacterium in hospital employees. Ann Intern Med 90:601, 1979.

Storch, G., Baine, W. B., Fraser, D. W., Broome, C. V., Clegg, H. W., II, Cohen, M. L., Goings, S. A. J., Politi, B. D., Terranova, W. A., Tsai, T. F., Plikaytis, B. D., Shepard, C. C., and Bennett, J. V.: Sporadic community Legionnaires' disease in the United States. A case-control study. Ann Intern Med 90:596, 1979.

Tsai, T. F., Finn, D. R., Plikaytis, B. D., McCauley, W., Martin, S. M., and Fraser, D. W.: Legionnaires' disease: Clinical features of the epidemic in Philadelphia. Ann Intern Med 90:509, 1979.

Wilkinson, H. M., Fikes, B. J., and Cruce, D. D.: Indirect immunofluorescence test for serodiagnosis of Legionnaires' disease: Evidence for serogroup diversity of Legionnaires' disease bacterial antigens and for multiple specificity of human antibodies. J Clin Microbiol 9:379, 1979.

Wong, K. H., Schalla, W. O., Arko, R. J., Bullard, J. C., and Feeley, J. C.: Immunochemical, serologic, and immunologic properties of major antigens isolated from the Legionnaires' disease bacterium. Observations bearing on the feasibility of a vaccine. Ann Intern Med 90:634, 1979.

# *TUBERCULOSIS* **114**

## *William Lester, M.D.*

### *DEFINITION*

Tuberculosis is an infectious disease usually acquired by inhalation of *Mycobacterium tuberculosis* and characterized by nodular, caseating granulomas (called tubercles) that fibrose, ulcerate, or calcify. The disease remains localized to the lungs in most patients but may involve almost any part of the body, especially the meninges, kidneys, bones, and lymph nodes. It may also be disseminated. Sensitized T-cell lymphocytes participate in the development of delayed hypersensitivity and the formation of caseating granulomas, whereas humoral antibodies play a minimal role in the disease. Clinical manifestations of the disease may appear shortly after the start of infection upon the development of tuberculin sensitivity, and especially if the inoculum is large; or they may arise after a variable period of dormancy (years to decades), particularly when immunity has been compromised. Tuberculosis has an inverse relationship to the standard of living within a society and increases dramatically during times of social catastrophe. Tuberculosis invariably decreases as the standard of living and nutrition improve.

## *ETIOLOGY*

Tuberculosis is defined as that disease caused by *M. tuberculosis.* Popular convention also has included disease caused by *M. bovis* but not by other mycobacteria. This produces confusion, since other mycobacteria produce disease that clinically, roentgenographically, and pathologically is identical to that produced by *M. tuberculosis.* Infections caused by *M. kansasii* and the *M. avium-intracellular complex* are examples and can be recognized only upon the cultural recovery of the organism. Thus, if cultures are unavailable, for whatever reason, the term tuberculosis is applied to all cases of mycobacterial disease except that caused by *M. leprae.*

The tubercle bacillus *(M. tuberculosis)* is aerobic or microaerophilic, nonmotile, non–sporeforming, high in lipid content, and acid- and alcohol-fast (Barksdale and Kim, 1977). It grows slowly and differs from other myobacteria by its ability to produce niacin. Unless modified by drug resistance, tubercle bacilli are virulent for man and most laboratory animals, especially guinea pigs. Colonies of tubercle bacilli are slow-growing, buff in color, rough and eugonic in appearance, and they usually require 10 to 21 days' incubation on complex media for their recognition and identification.

## *PATHOGENESIS AND PATHOLOGY*

The clinical manifestations and pathologic findings in patients with tuberculosis are the result of the interplay between delayed hypersensitivity and cellular immunity, on the one hand, and the extent and virulence of the tuberculous infection on the other. The complexity of this interaction can explain the fact that the pathologic findings can vary from acute to subacute to chronic, depending upon the immune state of the patient and the extent and nature of disease, as well as the time in the natural history of the disease (Youmans, 1979).

In most cases of tuberculosis, the infection is acquired by the inhalation of tubercle bacilli dispensed into the air from an active case by coughing, singing, and similar activities. Airborne particles measuring 1 to 5 $\mu$ and containing tubercle bacilli are inhaled into the airways and deposited in the alveoli. The tubercle bacilli are ingested by the alveolar macrophages and multiply intracellularly, and an acute exudative reaction results. At this time, delayed hypersensitivity has not yet been developed, and the multiplying tubercle bacilli spread by lymphohematogenous routes to other parts of the lung, to draining lymph nodes, and, ultimately, to such remote locations as bone marrow, meninges, and kidneys. However, shortly after the initiation of infection, cellular immunity and delayed hypersensitivity begin to develop and become manifest 4 to 6 weeks later. The macrophages are then increasingly lethal for tubercle bacilli and the tuberculoprotein released into the tissue causes platelet thrombi and vascular occlusion, so that local lesions become necrotic and caseation necrosis is seen in its classic form. This phenomenon greatly diminishes the risk of dissemination, but at the cost of irreversible damage to the lung.

Thus, in the previously uninfected patient, the initial lesions of tuberculosis are those of an acute pneumonitis that spreads to the hilar lymph nodes, and the combined process is called a Ghon complex. At this time necrosis is minimal, the tubercle bacilli multiply without restraint, and they may disseminate either scantily or in large numbers, depending on the size of the original inoculum and the patient's resistance. This is a period of great risk to the patient, because fatal dissemination may occur either as a consequence of impaired immunity, overwhelming infection, or a combination of the two factors.

Under ordinary circumstances, most patients infected with tubercle bacilli never have clinical manifestations of the disease but show delayed hypersensitivity to tuberculoprotein and are designated positive tuberculin reactors. However, tubercle bacilli survive in the tissues of such patients for the rest of their lives and become capable of multiplying and spreading whenever immunity decreases as a result of malnutrition, diabetes mellitus, and immunosuppression. Most of these reactivated cases show only pulmonary involvement, but in about 10 per cent, their disease appears in extrapulmonary sites, such as the lymphatics, kidneys, pleura, bones, and meninges. This small proportion of extrapulmonary cases is important because, if not diagnosed and treated, the meningeal, miliary, and renal forms of the disease are invariably fatal.

The pathogenesis of tuberculosis depends on the socioeconomic environment in which the disease occurs. In populations living in very primitive and crowded conditions, tuberculosis causes a high infant and child mortality, and a second peak in early adult years. In societies with better nutritional support and higher standards of living, the disease becomes more common in older individuals, as more and more children grow up without ever being exposed to tuberculosis. By the same token, the pathologic manifestations of tuberculosis are more acute, and dissemination more likely, when the disease is epidemic in an undeveloped society than when encountered in such societies as Western Europe or much of North America.

The site of major involvement obviously is important in transmission because it depends on the excretion of large numbers of viable tubercle bacilli in the sputum. Thus, most extrapulmonary foci are dangerous only to the patient and do not disseminate viable and infectious tubercle bacilli into the environment. However, once an area of caseating granulomatous disease erodes into a bronchus and sloughs its liquid contents into the air passage, the classic tuberculous cavity is developed. At this time, the growth rate of tubercle bacilli located in the necrotic wall of the cavity is greatly stimulated, and large numbers of virulent tubercle bacilli are discharged into the draining bronchus. These tubercle bacilli spread through the bronchi to other parts of the lung, causing an acute tuberculous pneumonia and, at the same time, spread by coughing into the environment, where they infect others. The extending necrotizing inflammation can cause a pulmonary hemorrhage by eroding a blood vessel. Thus, the presence of cavitary pulmonary tuberculosis increases the risk of infection for other patients and also impairs the prognosis for the individual patient. For these reasons, early identification and treatment of sputum-positive patients is an important element in the control of tuberculosis.

## CLINICAL MANIFESTATIONS

Although many clinical manifestations of tuberculosis are possible, most patients present as cases of pulmonary tuberculosis with varying degrees of fever, asthenia, cough, weight loss, and pulmonary hemorrhage. These symptoms vary, depending on the stage at which the patient's condition is first diagnosed. Thus, in patients encountered early in the course of their disease, clinical findings and evidences of toxicity are few; such patients have little fever or constitutional signs and their disease is evident only in a chest roentgenogram, a positive tuberculin reaction, and low bacillary counts in their sputum. However, in patients identified late in the course of their disease, constitutional signs are pronounced: high, hectic fever; weight loss; cachexia; advanced findings on physical examination; anemia and hemoptysis; and high bacillary counts in their sputum. Once a patient becomes symptomatic, the disease is in an advanced state, so that

every effort should be made to recognize the disease at the earliest possible stage when it can be treated most effectively and before irreversible tissue damage can occur.

As already indicated, tuberculosis may involve areas of the body other than the lungs. Miliary tuberculosis is caused by the discharge of variable numbers of viable tubercle bacilli into the bloodstream and dissemination of the infection throughout the body. Untreated, it is invariably fatal. It occurs most commonly shortly after initial infection with an overwhelming inoculum, or late in life with decline in immunologic competence. In both instances, the patient cannot resist infection, and the prognosis is very poor unless promptly recognized and vigorously treated.

As might be expected, the clinical manifestations of miliary tuberculosis are extremely variable, since they depend on the stage at which the process is recognized. The very early case, most often seen in infants, may have only low-grade fever, fail to thrive, and show little or no roentgenographic abnormalities. At the other end of the scale, the disease is most extensive, giving rise to extreme dyspnea that is unresponsive to oxygen therapy and producing massive roentgenographic abnormalities that represent the replacement of alveoli with innumerable tubercles. The diagnosis usually is easy in the advanced case but can be made only by biopsies in the early stages of miliary tuberculosis.

Meningeal tuberculosis may occur as part of a miliary or hematogenous process or may develop after a tuberculoma erodes into the meningeal space. Again, this is a process that can vary widely in its clinical manifestations, ranging from only low-grade fever and headache in the early case to extreme wasting, fever, opisthotonus, and massive neurologic findings in the patient with advanced disease. In the early stages, treatment is quite effective, and irreversible neurologic damage is minimal. In the advanced stages, even though antituberculosis chemotherapy may be effective, irreversible neurologic damage is inevitable, as manifested by epilepsy, cortical atrophy, or residual cranial nerve or hypothalamic injury. Here again, the disease may indicate the loss of immunologic competence, and early diagnosis is important because the process invariably is fatal if not treated. The spinal fluid should be examined and cultured in all suspect cases, and the usual findings are lymphocytic preponderance with elevated protein and decreased sugar content. (See Chapter 154.)

Renal tuberculosis is also fatal, if it is not recognized and is allowed to progress. It may occur in conjunction with other forms of tuberculosis, or it may be the only manifestation of the

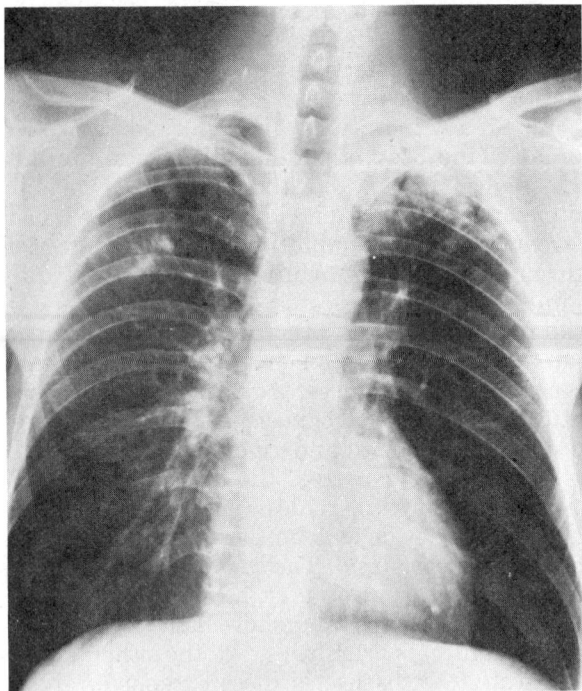

**FIGURE 1.** *Typical roentgenographic findings in adult pulmonary tuberculosis. The cardinal features are caseonodular granulomatous disease with necrosis and cavitation, fibrosis and volume loss, and hilar retraction to the affected area. Note left upper lobe fibrocavitary disease with nodular spread to anterior segment right upper lobe.*

disease. Renal tuberculosis usually arises from the erosion of a tuberculoma through a papilla into the renal pelvis, so that viable tubercle bacilli are discharged into the urinary tract. The infection tends to spread to other parts of the kidney, ureters, bladder, and testicles. Healing often causes ureteral obstruction and obstructive nephropathy. Far-advanced cases are complicated by renal calculi, and in the end-stages, multiple perineal and inguinal urinary fistulae create a life of torture. Therefore, it is important to diagnose renal tuberculosis as early as possible in order to minimize irreversible tissue damage and preserve as much renal function as possible. In the early stages, the only finding is a persistent, low-grade pyuria, and the lesions are too small to demonstrate by pyelography. It can be diagnosed only by cultures of urine on medium appropriate for the growth of tubercle bacilli.

Other extrapulmonary manifestations of tuberculosis are less threatening to life but still represent extensive spread of the disease; these result from pleural, osseous, lymph node, pericardial, intestinal, or peritoneal involvement. Biopsy and culture are the only means for making an exact diagnosis and should be done whenever a chronic granulomatous process involves one of these locations. Patients who have extrapulmonary mani-

festations of tuberculosis have demonstrated their inability to localize the infection and, therefore, are at greater risk of having other lesions develop as time goes on unless they are vigorously and effectively treated.

Since the clinical manifestations of pulmonary tuberculosis are quite variable, it is important to emphasize that in many cases the diagnosis will be first suspected from abnormal roentgenographic findings in patients who have nondescript or ill-defined complaints. The essential roentgenographic features of tuberculosis are granulomas with varying degrees of calcification, pneumonic areas undergoing necrosis; cavity formation, often with air-fluid levels; and usually significant volume loss in the lobe or segment involved. All of these are superimposed upon fibrosis. The roentgenographic findings of pulmonary tuberculosis vary as widely as the clinical findings. They range from small or large closed lesions with or without calcification (tuberculomas) to fibrocavitary involvement. The fibrocavitary disease is usually in the apical posterior segments of the upper lobe or the superior segment of the lower lobe. All of these lesions may be accompanied by pleural fibrosis, and they may occur singly or together. As can be seen in Figures 1 and 2, the usual upper lobe fibrocavitary process is highly suggestive of granulomatous infection but may not be pathognomonic of tuberculosis, since histoplasmosis and other fungal diseases may produce a similar process. In addition, although less commonly seen, acute tuberculous pneumonia

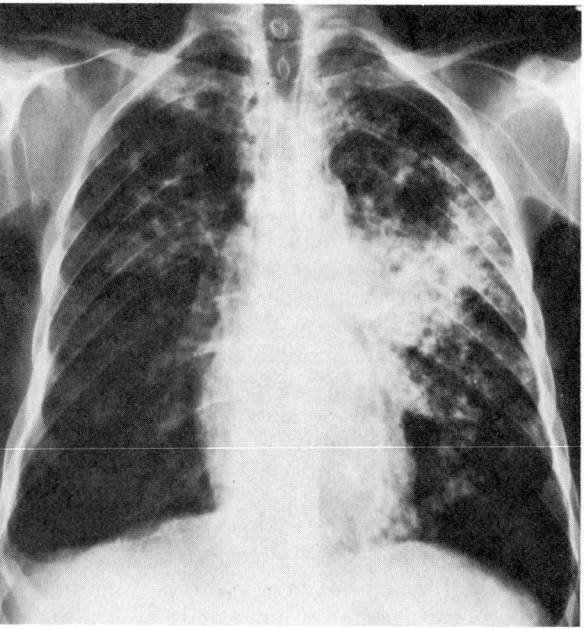

**FIGURE 2.** *Bilateral upper lobe fibrocavitary tuberculosis with extensive bronchogenic spill.*

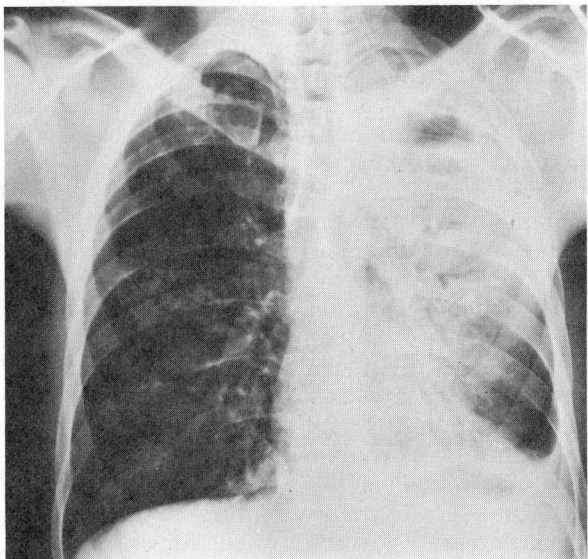

**FIGURE 3.** *Destroyed left lung with large apical tuberculous cavity and air-fluid level.*

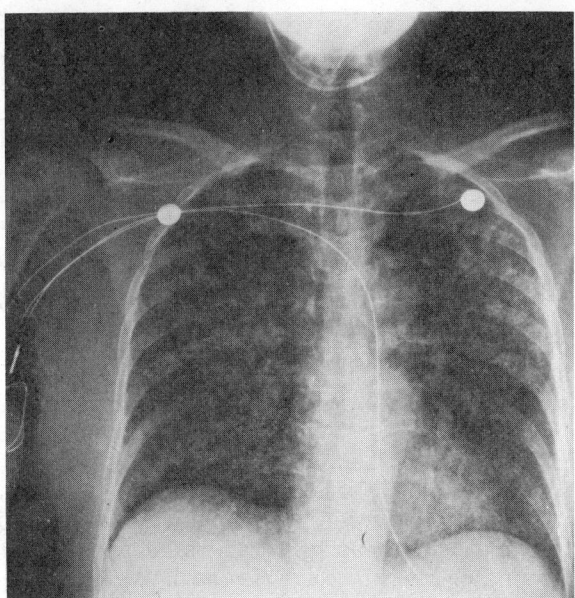

**FIGURE 4.** *Fatal case of massive miliary tuberculosis.*

may resemble a pneumococcal or *Klebsiella* infection roentgenographically.

Far-advanced cases of pulmonary tuberculosis often present with the picture of a destroyed lung (Fig. 3), usually the left, bronchopleural fistula, and empyema. This finding is highly suggestive of tuberculosis, especially in a young person.

Ideally, the diagnosis of miliary tuberculosis should be made before significant roentgenographic findings appear, since chemotherapy is most effective at the early stage. However, in practice, many patients are not seen until the process is well established. In such cases, the earliest roentgenographic finding is a ground-glass haziness of definition in the chest film that is best recognized by comparison with earlier films. Later, innumerable pinpoint alveolar densities appear uniformly distributed throughout the chest, go on to coalesce, and terminally become confluent (Fig. 4). By the time the process has become confluent and massive, it usually is irreversible and the prognosis is poor, in spite of vigorous antituberculosis chemotherapy.

## COMPLICATIONS AND SEQUELAE

Most people infected with tubercle bacilli never develop clinical disease but only demonstrate delayed hypersensitivity to tuberculoprotein in the form of a positive tuberculin reaction. Among the minority who develop clinical disease, it may become apparent shortly after infection has started, especially if the infecting dose is massive or the patient has impaired immunity. In others, the

disease may become clinically apparent at any later time because tubercle bacilli can survive in infected tissue for a lifetime, and, if the general health of the individual is impaired, the subclinical stable lesions may break down and the infection spread. Thus, the most common complication of tuberculous infection is activation whenever the patient's resistance is decreased. For this reason, the development frequently of pulmonary tuberculosis in older patients, known to be positive tuberculin reactors, can be regarded as a late complication of tuberculous infection. The same can be said for extrapulmonary manifestations.

If diagnosis is made late in the course of the disease, there is massive destruction of organs such as lung or kidney by necrosis and fibrosis. If diagnosis is made in the early stages of involvement, tissue destruction is minimal if effective treatment is started promptly. Thus, in one sense, significant organ destruction from tuberculosis can be considered a sequel of the disease, which can be avoided with proper treatment.

## GEOGRAPHIC VARIATIONS

There are wide geographic variations in the incidence of tuberculosis throughout the world. In Western Europe in the 18th and 19th centuries A.D., tuberculosis was so common and severe that it was called "The Captain of the Men of Death," and the disease came close to destroying Western society. Today, the disease has decreased markedly in incidence and severity in developed societies but remains a major problem in many areas of the world, especially those in which malnutrition, overcrowding, and poverty are common denominators. Wars and social upheavals only accentuate this difference. It is clear that the impact of tuberculosis on the Western World was decreasing markedly before any effective treatment was available. Hence, the decline in incidence and severity occurred as a result of improvements in diet, living condition, and personal hygiene. Similar improvement can be anticipated if the standard of living can be raised in those areas of the world today in which tuberculosis remains a major threat. In addition, the decline in the disease today should become even more rapid because of effective antituberculosis chemotherapy.

Tuberculosis also has been called a disease of social pathology, because it tends to be a disease of the poor and underprivileged within any society and is increasingly rare among the more fortunate. Even in countries such as the United States, tuberculosis remains a significant problem in the inner-city ghettos and among the poor. Since this is a worldwide phenomenon, it means that case-finding and treatment facilities must be made available for everybody, but especially for those populations who are least exposed to modern medical practice and have the greatest difficulty in understanding what it comprises.

### DIAGNOSIS

The key to the diagnosis of tuberculosis is a high index of suspicion for the disease and the prompt utilization of appropriate diagnostic procedures. Ideally, all cases should be confirmed by culturing tubercle bacilli. In practice, however, this is not possible for much of the world, and simpler procedures are all that can be used. Thus, sputum specimens should be obtained and stained for acid-fast bacilli by the Ziehl-Neelsen, Kinyoun, or fluorochrome techniques. The latter technique has the advantage of greater sensitivity and speed but requires a fluorescence microscope.

Because most cases of tuberculosis present as pulmonary disease, which is the most infectious, diagnostic efforts should be concentrated on patients with active pulmonary tuberculosis. Mass radiography helps identify suspect cases, and all symptomatic patients should be sent for chest roentgenograms. At the same time, appropriate sputum specimens should be obtained for smear and, if possible, culture. Sputum induction by inhaled saline aerosols is of value for patients who cannot produce adequate sputum specimens, but such procedures should not be done in nonventilated areas. Bronchial brushing and lavage to obtain secretions for smear and culture is effective in many patients with low bacillary output, but should only be done if conventional sputum studies have been negative.

Many different media are available throughout the world for the cultivation of tubercle bacilli, and the choice of one or several depends, to an extent, on the resources of each facility. The most commonly used medium in the United States today is the Middlebrook-Cohn 7H11. This has the advantage of being transparent, thus permitting earlier recognition of colonies, but it has the disadvantage of requiring 5 per cent $CO_2$ in the incubator. A significant advantage of the 7H11 medium is that it is easily adapted to drug susceptibility studies. Traditional Lowenstein-Jensen medium also is commonly used for initial isolation of tubercle bacilli.

Because of the great variability of the extrapulmonary manifestations of tuberculosis, all biopsy specimens of chronic inflammatory or suppurative disease should be submitted for culture of tubercle bacilli in addition to histologic examination. A common error is for a biopsy specimen such as necrotic lymph node or fistula tract to be excised, not cultured, and placed in formalin for fixation. This renders the procedure valueless for the diagnosis of tuberculosis.

The tuberculin test should be a definite part of the evaluation of all suspect cases of tuberculosis. As with any biological test, 100 per cent correlation with disease does not occur, but a positive tuberculin reaction is demonstrated in more than 95 per cent of patients with tuberculosis. Thus, a negative tuberculin test makes the diagnosis of tuberculosis unlikely, but does not rule it out in any absolute sense. Tuberculin testing for diagnostic purposes should be done by the intradermal or Mantoux technique. Only carefully standardized tuberculin, such as PPD-S or its equivalent, should be used at a concentration of 5 tuberculin units injected intradermally into the medial aspect of the skin of the forearm and read at 48 to 72 hrs. The reading consists of the measurement of the greatest diameter of induration recorded in millimeters. Thus, a properly recorded tuberculin test specifies the material injected (PPD-S), its strength in tuberculin units, and the millimeters of induration observed at 48 to 72 hrs. The result should not be recorded as positive or negative because these standards have changed from time to time; if recorded in millimeters, the result can always be interpreted in terms of current standards. At present, induration 10 mm or greater in diameter is considered a positive reaction, while that between 6 and 10 mm is deemed indeterminate, and less than 6 mm is negative.

Tuberculin testing is of great value in identifying the people at risk of breaking down with tuberculosis within a population. Present experience in the United States today shows that more than 90 per cent of all new active cases come from known positive tuberculin reactors, even though they comprise less than 8 per cent of the total population. Thus, tuberculin testing provides a means of detecting potential cases that can be protected by chemoprophylaxis. It is prudent to tuberculin test all patients with diseases that in the future might require steroid therapy or immunosuppression before such treatment is initiated. Such therapy depresses tuberculin hypersensitivity and therefore gives rise to a false negative response, and it is well known that patients with positive tuberculin reactions are at risk of developing active tuberculosis when they are immunosuppressed.

Pleural effusion is a fairly common manifestation of tuberculosis and is often misdiagnosed if the proper studies are not initiated at the time of diagnostic thoracentesis. It arises most commonly in the early months or years after infection has occurred and hypersensitivity is at its peak. The pathogenesis of tuberculosis pleural effusion involves a subpleural focus of active infection that erodes into the pleural space and actively seeds it with tubercles, or the leakage of tuberculoprotein into adjacent tissues so that an exudative inflammatory response is evoked. The fluid that is produced usually is serofibrinous in nature and has the characteristics of an exudate. Early in its formation, acute inflammatory cells (polymorphonuclear leukocytes) prevail; as the process matures, round cell pleocytosis becomes apparent. The fluid usually resolves with treatment but may produce pleural fibrosis and restriction of thoracic movement. For this reason, as much of the fluids as possible should be removed at the time of thoracentesis.

Today, in most parts of the world, tuberculosis is a diminishing cause of pleural effusion; lung cancer, viral infections, congestive heart failure, and pulmonary embolism are more common causes. Therefore, at the time the thoracentesis is done, proper diagnostic studies should be initiated on the pleural fluid. These include determinations of specific gravity, protein concentration, glucose, and lactic dehydrogenase (LDH). At the same time, serum determinations should be obtained for glucose and LDH. In addition, the cells in the pleural fluid should be counted and a cell block made for cytologic study. Whenever practicable and when there are no contraindications (low or absent platelets, prolonged bleeding time), pleural biopsy should be done at the time of initial thoracentesis and appropriate sections stained for acid-fast bacilli. If an adequate pleural specimen is obtained, caseating tubercles are often seen. In addition, pleural fluid always

should be cultured for tubercle bacilli. If these procedures are done routinely at the time of diagnostic thoracentesis, the role of tuberculosis is accurately delineated. If they are not done, and the pleural fluid is examined casually, many cases of tuberculosis pleurisy are missed.

## TREATMENT

Modern antituberculosis chemotherapy is so effective today that no patient should die of the disease if they can survive the first 30 days of treatment (Johnston and Wildrick, 1974). The problem is to identify the patients needing treatment and make certain that they actually take their medications as ordered. Because of the way in which tuberculosis remains endemic in the lower social strata, many of the patients are poorly motivated to cooperate in their treatment. However, the important thing is to deliver the most effective treatment possible rather than wasting time denigrating the patients. More ingenuity is needed to provide effective rewards for cooperative patients.

The ultimate aim of antituberculosis chemotherapy is *tissue sterilization* (the elimination of all viable tubercle bacilli in the body of the infected patient). Twenty years ago, attainment of this aim was thought unlikely; today, it is a reality. There are now at least 12 drugs of varying efficacy being used throughout the world, and it is not practical to make recommendations in specific terms that are applicable worldwide. However, the basic principles of antituberculosis chemotherapy are universal.

Tissue sterilization is best achieved by an early intensive treatment regimen utilizing the best three drugs available followed by a longer period of maintenance therapy comprising the two most effective drugs of the initial program. In this way, the early intensive period reduces the bacterial population most rapidly and thereby renders the emergence of drug resistance least likely. The longer period of maintenance therapy ensures the ultimate destruction of any of the persisting, slowly metabolizing tubercle bacilli.

The 12 antituberculosis drugs available are listed in Table 1 with their recommended dosages and major toxic reactions. It should be emphasized that hypersensitivity varying from mild symptoms to major anaphylactic reaction can occur from any of these drugs. Practical considerations dictate specific choices as to drug regimens because of factors of cost and availability. For a variety of reasons, the best oral drugs are isoniazid (INH), rifampin (RM), ethambutol (EM), and pyrazinamide (PZA). The best aminoglycoside is streptomycin (SM). Thus, these five drugs provide

**TABLE 1.   Drug Treatment of Tuberculosis**

| MAJOR ORAL DRUGS | DOSAGE | MAJOR TOXIC EFFECTS |
|---|---|---|
| Isoniazid | 300 mg daily | Hepatotoxicity, polyneuritis |
| Ethambutol | 15 mg/kg daily | Decrease in visual acuity |
| Rifampin | 600 mg daily | Hepatotoxicity |
| Pyrazinamide | 2 to 3 g daily | Hepatotoxicity, hyperuricemia |
| Ethionamide | 1.0 g daily | Gastrointestinal intolerance |
| **LESS EFFECTIVE ORAL DRUGS** | | |
| Cycloserine | 1.0 g daily | Convulsion, depression |
| Aminosalicylic acid | 12 to 15 g daily | Gastrointestinal intolerance, hepatotoxicity |
| Thiacetazone | 150 mg daily | Hepatotoxicity |
| Aminoglycosides (parenteral administration) in order of preference<br>   Streptomycin<br>   Kanamycin<br>   Capreomycin<br>   Viomycin | 1.0 g or 15 mg/kg daily during initial phase of therapy | Audiovestibular injury, renal damage |

the basis for modern chemotherapy regimens. The remaining seven drugs should be used only in special situations.

At the time antituberculosis chemotherapy is initiated, the status of the patient should be carefully evaluated. Every effort should be made to determine whether or not the patient has undergone any previous antituberculosis treatment. If so, the possibility of drug resistance should be considered, and an initial four-drug regimen set up until the results of drug susceptibility studies are available. If there is no history of previous treatment, the patient can be committed to the usual initial triple-drug regimen, unless the patient comes from an area known to have significant rates of drug resistance, in which case a four-drug regimen might well be justified.

The basic regimen recommended consists of daily SM for 30 to 60 days, plus INH, EM, RM, or PZA in a double oral drug program for 10 to 12 months. Current studies are being reported that indicate that the previous recommendations for duration of therapy for 18 to 24 months are no longer justified. It may well be that 12 months is unnecessarily long. It is very probable that the most effective regimen is SM-INH-RM; however, the other possible combinations are so effective that it would require controlled studies involving many thousands of patients to get a satisfactory answer as to which is best.

In addition to changing concepts as to the duration of treatment, it now is clear that, after the early initial intensive period of treatment, twice-weekly intermittent administration of drugs is highly effective and can be maintained within a framework of 6 to 12 months. Such programs have been shown to be comparable in efficacy to programs based on daily drug adminis-

tration of equal duration, and they obviously produce great economies in terms of time and effort (Fox and Mitchison, 1974; Dutt et al., 1979). It is hoped that such savings can be invested in greater care in making certain that the drugs are taken as prescribed and, in many instances, supervised administration becomes quite practical. The drug dosages for the twice-weekly regimens are determined by multiplying the daily dose by seven and dividing by two, except for RM, which is best given in a dose of 600 mg twice weekly.

As antituberculosis chemotherapy was developing 20 to 25 years ago, surgery was thought to be a valuable adjunct in treatment. Collapse procedures were developed for control of disease in drug-resistant, therapy-failure cases, and pulmonary resections were recommended for the removal of irreversibly damaged tissue (cavities, destroyed lobes or segments, and areas of bronchiectasis). However, with the passing of time and the improvement of the efficacy of antituberculosis chemotherapy, these indications for surgical treatment of tuberculosis have become obsolete and no longer applicable. Today, there is one remaining problem in tuberculosis for which a skilled and experienced thoracic surgeon can be helpful, and that is in the management of bronchopleural fistula and empyema. Open drainage in such cases in conjunction with optimal chemotherapy may be life-saving but requires careful teamwork; fortunately, such cases are rare. Therefore, the investment of money, facilities, and personnel required to support an active surgical program for tuberculosis treatment is unjustified, and such resources are used much better if they are put into the support of the chemotherapy program and appropriate public health facilities.

The addition of steroid therapy to effective

antituberculosis chemotherapy is of little or no value in the usual case of tuberculosis and has some risk, especially if drug-resistant infection is a possibility. However, the combination of prednisone 30 to 40 mg daily for 4 to 6 weeks plus intensive antituberculosis chemotherapy is justified by the following cases: (1) hypertoxic patients who may otherwise not survive long enough for chemotherapy to become effective (usually 3 weeks), (2) patients with meningeal tuberculosis who appear to be developing acute cerebral edema or spinal block and (3) patients with massive miliary disease who have major diffusion defects and cannot maintain adequate oxygen levels. Fortunately, the latter two categories are not common; therefore, steroids are most frequently used in patients of the first category.

One of the valuable by-products of the lengthy chemotherapy trials evaluated in the treatment of tuberculosis was an experience and understanding of the role of adverse drug reactions in the outcome of chemotherapy. The commonly used antituberculosis drugs (SM, INH, EMB, and RM) fortunately have few adverse reactions, although, when they occur, they may be highly significant. On the other hand, the less commonly used antituberculosis drugs have a wide variety of adverse side effects, some of which can be life-threatening. Therefore, when a physician assumes responsibility for antituberculosis chemotherapy, he should acquaint himself in detail with the pharmacology of the drugs he is using and adequately monitor his patients in order to protect them against serious adverse drug reactions.

In general, there are four major types of adverse drug reactions: hypersensitivity, toxic action, side effects, and idiosyncrasy. Of these, only hypersensitivity is life-threatening, and its recognition is of paramount importance. Any patient receiving antituberculosis chemotherapy who unexpectedly develops fever, rash, purpura, or marked vasomotor reactions after parenteral injections should be considered as possibly developing hypersensitivity to one or more of the drugs included in the regimen. These findings should lead to a cessation of the treatment program until all have disappeared. The continuance of drugs and in the presence of developing hypersensitivity is dangerous and may lead to a life-threatening reaction. Hypersensitivity may develop to any drug.

Toxic effects are dose-related and are a reflection of the molecular nature of the drug. If ignored, they can be dangerous but can usually be controlled easily by the experienced physician by appropriate reductions in dosage. An example is the neurotoxicity of isoniazid.

Side effects are related to the nature of the drug and the size of the dose. The usual effect is nausea and vomiting, as seen when paraaminosalicylic acid is prescribed. Although a nuisance factor, side effects rarely are dangerous and usually can be controlled by the competent physician.

Idiosyncratic reactions are unpredictable and represent peculiar and illogical responses to any particular drug. They rarely are dangerous but may produce sufficient symptoms to warrant replacement of the offending drug.

Today, there exist at least 11 major antituberculosis drugs. Therefore, if any one produces major problems, an appropriate alternative usually can be found. If a drug must be stopped because of adverse reactions in the early weeks of treatment, it usually can be replaced by another drug. If, however, a drug must be stopped in the third or later months of treatment, it should be replaced with two other drugs until it is certain that the patient has acquired negative culture status and drug resistance has not emerged.

## PROPHYLAXIS

With the advent of INH, chemoprophylaxis of tuberculosis became feasible, and many studies confirmed its value. The drug was safe, economical, and effective when given for 1 year in a daily dose of 300 mg to known positive tuberculin reactors. Since most cases of tuberculosis arise in patients with positive tuberculin reactions, it was easy to identify the population at risk by tuberculin testing.

Carefully designed double-blind studies have shown that the use of INH chemoprophylaxis in positive tuberculin reactors with no evidence of disease for 1 year reduces the rate of tuberculous disease by 70 to 80 per cent during the year of drug ingestion, and the long-term reduction remains in the 60 to 70 per cent range. It also is clear that certain positive tuberculin reactors obviously are at greater risk than others. Infants, known recent converters, silicotics, diabetics, and immunosuppressed patients are at greater risk than adult or elderly patients with no associated risk factors. Therefore, each facility should evaluate its population in terms of priority. Hepatotoxicity of INH is strongly age-dependent, occurring in about 0.2 per cent of children below the age of 15 and 2.0 per cent or more of individuals over 55. Therefore, each patient should be evaluated individually in terms of the risk-benefit ratio. When properly used, INH chemoprophylaxis is very valuable for the reduction of tuberculosis.

Vaccination with BCG (Bacille Calmette-Guérin) has significant value in control of tuberculosis, especially in areas of the world in which case rates are high and tuberculosis mortality is centered on the very young. The vaccine is made from a strain of bovine tubercle bacilli that was made avirulent over a period of years by Calmette and Guérin. It has been grown all over the world and is very difficult to standardize. For these and other reasons, controversy exists as to the overall efficacy of BCG vaccination. As previously indicated, at this time, BCG vaccination is worthy of consideration in a society with high and unchanging rates of tuberculosis, especially when the infant mortality for the disease remains elevated. It markedly reduces the early infant mortality if done on newborn infants. However, for much of the world, BCG vaccination no longer is recommended.

Tuberculosis is an infectious disease of major public health significance for much of the world today. Therefore, it is of critical importance to find the patients capable of spreading the infection, eliminate their infectiousness by effective treatment, and, at the same time, identify the persons whom they have infected. Those individuals capable of transmitting tuberculosis, for all practical purposes, are those patients with active pulmonary disease excreting large numbers of viable tubercle bacilli in their sputum; patients with extrapulmonary tuberculosis are not disseminators of the disease but are victims of it.

The individuals at risk of acquiring tuberculosis are the household and occupational contacts of the infectious or "index" case. Such contacts ideally should be evaluated by tuberculin testing, chest radiography of all positive reactors, and initiation of either curative or prophylactic antituberculosis treatment. If no disease is detectable, prophylactic drug therapy is given, but full chemotherapy is indicated for the positive tuberculin reactor contact who has detectable pulmonary disease. It should be emphasized that among household contacts, infants and small children are most likely to be the first and most seriously infected. However, as the standard of living improves, the age distribution of tuberculosis shifts increasingly to the older age groups, and, in this circumstance, the identification and prophylactic treatment of positive tuberculin reactors becomes an important element in the prevention of late breakdowns of the disease. Mass radiography is not a practical solution for this problem.

## References

Barksdale, L., and Kim, K.-S.: Mycobacterium. Bacteriol Rev 41:217, 1977.
Dutt, A. K., Jones L., and Stead, W.: Short-course chemotherapy for tuberculosis with largely twice-weekly isoniazid-rifampin. Chest 75:441, 1979.
Fox, W., and Mitchison, D. A.: Short-course chemotherapy for tuberculosis. Lung Disease: State of the Art 1974-75. American Lung Association, p. 176.
Johnston, R. F., and Wildrick, K. H.: The impact of chemotherapy on the care of patients with tuberculosis. Lung Disease: State of the Art 1974-75. American Lung Association, p. 147.
Youmans, G. P.: Tuberculosis. Philadelphia, W.B. Saunders Company, 1979.

# 115 *NONTUBERCULOUS MYCOBACTERIAL INFECTIONS*

*William Lester, M.D.*

## DEFINITION

Nontuberculous mycobacterial infections may be clinically, pathologically, and radiologically identical to tuberculosis but are caused by mycobacteria that have primary drug resistance, diminished virulence for guinea pigs, and distinct cellular and colonial morphologic differences from tubercle bacilli. At first these organisms were classified as atypical, anonymous, or unclassified mycobacteria, but now they have achieved species designation, and the term nontuberculous mycobacteria is more appropriate.

The genus *Mycobacterium* is one of the most widely distributed bacterial genera in nature and ranges from saprophytes to such important pathogens as *M. tuberculosis* and *M. leprae*. Classically, the term tuberculosis long has been applied to infections caused by *M. tuberculosis* and *M. bovis*. This discussion will be restricted to human mycobacterial infections caused by bacteria other than *M. tuberculosis, M. bovis,* or *M. leprae*.

Nontuberculous mycobacterial infections may present clinical manifestations that are indistinguishable from those of tuberculosis and can be recognized only by cultural recovery of the etiologic agent. Such infections may disseminate to many organs, especially in patients with impaired immunity. At the other extreme, they may cause only self-limited, localized lymph node suppuration. In many other instances, however, they may produce pulmonary involvement that is indistinguishable from that seen in classic tuberculosis. Finally, they may produce isolated extrapulmonary lesions — bone and joint, renal, or skin lesions — somewhat like those seen in tuberculosis (Chapman, 1977; Lester, 1966; Lincoln and Gilbert, 1972).

## ETIOLOGY

It is convenient to separate the nontuberculous mycobacteria into the four groups originally proposed by Runyon (1959) on the basis of simple morphologic characteristics that usually are easily recognized in initial cultures. These four groups are:

I. Photochromogens. These form a yellow carotene pigment on exposure to light. Colonies grown in the dark are buff colored and become yellow on exposure to light.
II. Scotochromogens. Colonies are pigmented when grown in the dark.
III. Nonphotochromogens. The buff or yellow color of these colonies does not change on exposure to light.
IV. Rapid growers. The rapid growth of these organisms makes mature colonies visible in four to six days when they are incubated at 37° C, whereas most other mycobacteria require one to two weeks.

All four groups are resistant to drugs on initial isolation (primary resistance). However, photochromogens are less resistant to routine antituberculosis agents — isoniazid, ethambutol, and rifampin — than the mycobacteria in groups II, III, and IV.

Table 1 is a general summary of the taxonomy and characteristics of mycobacteria, especially those considered to be nontuberculous. Although this classification is by no means final, it is noteworthy that the original classification proposed by Runyon, which was based on simple colonizing characteristics of the mycobacteria, has held up in the face of biochemical studies, serologic analysis, and patterns of mycobacteriophage susceptibility.

Certain generalizations are suggested from Table 1 that should alert the clinician to the

**TABLE 1.** Nomenclature and Characteristics of Mycobacteria

| ORGANISM | RELATIVE PATHOGENICITY FOR MAN | CLINICAL MANIFESTATIONS | NIACIN PRODUCTION | CATALASE PRODUCTION |
|---|---|---|---|---|
| M. tuberculosis | + + + + | Human tuberculosis | + | + + |
| M. bovis | + + + + | Human tuberculosis | Variable | + |
| M. africanum | + + + | Pulmonary | Variable | + |
| M. ulcerans | + + + + | Cutaneous | − | + + + + |
| **Group I** | | | | |
| M. kansasii | + + + | Pulmonary, extrapulmonary, disseminated | − | + + + + |
| M. marinum | + + + | Extrapulmonary, cutaneous | Variable | + |
| M. simiae | + + | Pulmonary | + | + + + + |
| **Group II** | | | | |
| M. flavescens | 0 | None | − | + + + + |
| M. gordonae | 0 | None | − | + + + + |
| M. scrofulaceum | + + | Pulmonary, extrapulmonary, lymphadenitis | − | + + + + |
| **Group III** | | | | |
| M. avium | + + + | Pulmonary, extrapulmonary, disseminated | | + |
| M. gastri | 0 | None | − | + |
| M. terrae | Rare | Extrapulmonary, disseminated | − | + + + + |
| M. triviale | | Extrapulmonary, arthritis | − | + + + + |
| M. intracellulare | + + + | Pulmonary, extrapulmonary, lymphadenitis, disseminated | − | + + + |
| M. xenopi | + | Cutaneous | − | + |
| **Group IV** | | | | |
| M. chelonei | | Pulmonary, extrapulmonary, abscesses, lymphadenitis | − | + + + + |
| M. fortuitum | | Pulmonary, extrapulmonary, disseminated, abscesses | − | + + + + |

possibility of nontuberculous mycobacterial infection. First, as mentioned previously, all the mycobacteria in the four Runyon groups are characterized by significant primary drug resistance. Thus, any resistant isolate obtained from a patient with a clear history of *no* prior antituberculosis treatment should be viewed as a potential nontuberculous mycobacterium. Second, a negative niacin test on a drug-resistant mycobacterium greatly enhances the likelihood that it is nontuberculous. Finally, a resistant culture with a negative niacin test and a strong catalase reaction almost certainly will be a nontuberculous mycobacterium.

Table 1 also emphasizes that the nontuberculous mycobacteria produce syndromes that are indistinguishable from classic tuberculosis. Since there is no evidence that these infections are transmitted from one case to another, they will most likely not diminish in frequency in the future as has tuberculosis. Thus, the proportion of nontuberculous mycobacterial infections will probably increase as infections due to *M. tuberculosis* decline.

Since these organisms are widespread and many can occur as contaminants, a single isolation may have no etiologic significance. Multiple specimens should be obtained for culture, and these will usually be positive if the patient has a nontuberculous mycobacterial disease. The isolation of nontuberculous mycobacteria from a single specimen, especially if the colony count is low, is not diagnostic, and treatment should not be started until further efforts to recover the organism succeed and confirm the diagnosis.

## PATHOGENESIS

The pathogenesis and epidemiology of nontuberculous mycobacterial disease are poorly understood. Transmission from one patient to another has not been demonstrated, and all authorities agree that individual cases represent no public health threat. Many of the etiologic organisms can be recovered from soil, water, or organic debris and may be ingested or inhaled in dust particles or, like *M. marinum,* introduced into the skin through abrasions.

Since the nontuberculous mycobacteria have diminished virulence and cause a low rate of disease among infected patients, those individuals who have severe disseminated infections with these organisms may well have abnormal immune responses. Thus, these infections are being recognized more frequently in immunosuppressed patients who have organ transplants or are being treated for leukemia and cancer, and they should

be kept in mind in all patients undergoing immunosuppressive therapy for any reason.

Skin test preparations similar to PPD-S (tuberculin from *M. tuberculosis*) have been prepared from various nontuberculous mycobacteria. PPD-Y, prepared from *M. kansasii,* and PPD-B, prepared from *M. intracellulare,* are the most useful. These preparations, applied and read like PPD-S, have demonstrated striking epidemiologic differences in reactivity. In areas where *M. kansasii* and *M. intracellulare* are endemic, many positive reactions to PPD-Y and PPD-B will be found. Such studies also indicate that the disease-infection ratio for such organisms is low. However, because of common or shared antigens with other mycobacteria, the results of such skin tests alone are not diagnostic in any individual case. PPD-Y and PPD-S are closely related antigenically, whereas PPD-B is less likely to cross-react with PPD-Y. Thus, a patient with a large reaction to PPD-B and little or no reaction to PPD-S has probably been infected with *M. intracellulare.* Results of differential skin tests may therefore be of epidemiologic importance, but the exact diagnosis in any individual case depends on the recovery of the specific organism in cultures.

Among nontuberculous mycobacterial infections, most reported cases of pulmonary disease have been caused by *M. kansasii* or *M. intracellulare-avium* complex. Both infections are concentrated in relatively small geographic areas with sharp differences in local frequency. Comparative skin-testing with mycobacterial sensitins also shows sharp differences in frequency of reactions in adjacent areas. Such differences cannot be explained on the basis of climatic or environmental factors and raise the possibility that food, water, milk, or other routes of transmission may be responsible. Although the role of these latter possibilities has not been established, it is likely that different mechanisms of transmission apply to various environments, since these organisms are largely ubiquitous.

Another unexplained feature of pulmonary disease caused by *M. kansasii* or the *M. intracellulare-avium* complex is that approximately two-thirds of cases occur in males. There is no documented occupational exposure related to these infections. However, *M. kansasii* disease is more common in urban patients, whereas that caused by *M. intracellulare-avium* complex is more frequent in rural areas.

Isolated cervical lymph node disease is a very common manifestation of nontuberculous mycobacterial infection, especially in young children; it suggests that the oropharyngeal route may be a major portal of infection. The striking infrequency with which pleural effusions are caused by these organisms suggests that inhalation may not be a common route of infection.

## PATHOLOGY

The gross and microscopic features of nontuberculous mycobacterial disease are identical to those characteristic of *M. tuberculosis*. The most characteristic finding is that of caseating granulomas with varying proportions of Langhans' giant cells, epithelioid cells, and acid-fast bacilli. The amount of fibrosis and caseation necrosis is related to the chronicity and extent of the lesion. Disseminated infections in immunosuppressed patients often do not show the classic caseating granulomas, usually because the lesions have not had time to mature. Because the granulomas are not diagnostic, the diagnosis depends on the cultural isolation and identification of the organism.

## CLINICAL MANIFESTATIONS

Nontuberculous mycobacterial infection varies widely in its manifestations. It can be an isolated, self-limited, lymph node infection, usually cervical, which improves spontaneously or after resection of the infected tissue. On the other hand, it may be a rapidly progressive, overwhelming disseminated infection with massive lymphohematogenous invasion of all major organs and little chance for survival. Fortunately, such disseminated cases are rare. They usually are associated with massive infection, very poor host resistance, or both.

A significant number of patients have a fibrotic, fibrocavitary, or pneumonic pulmonary disease that is roentgenographically indistinguishable from tuberculosis. The disease often progresses more slowly than tuberculosis, but fresh pneumonic lesions and acute toxicity are encountered in some individuals. The pulmonary disease will show progression, fever, toxicity, hemorrhage, weight loss, and cachexia similar to tuberculosis. Most patients with pulmonary disease due to nontuberculous mycobacteria will have infections caused by either *M. kansasii* or *M. intracellulare-avium* complex. In both instances, but especially in the latter, primary drug resistance is prominent. If it is not recognized and the patient is erroneously given drugs of minimal efficacy, therapy will fail and the probability of response to a retreatment regimen will be diminished. Thus, although the disease in general may be more indolent than tuberculosis, it is more refractory to treatment and requires meticulous attention to the selection of an optimally effective chemotherapeutic regimen. Failure is associated with progression of the disease, and spontaneous remissions do *not* occur.

Pulmonary disease due to groups II and IV mycobacteria is rare. Unfortunately, no one has encountered more than a few such cases, and little is known of their natural history or prognosis. They are usually infections superimposed on old pulmonary processes — bullous or cystic disease, fibrosis, bronchiectasis, or old tuberculosis. Therefore, the role of these organisms as primary pathogens is obscure. Patients excreting either group II or group IV organisms must be carefully studied to determine if the organism isolated is a commensal or a pathogen.

## COMPLICATIONS AND SEQUELAE

Rapid progression of obstructive lung disease occurs in adult patients who may at the time of initial diagnosis show relatively limited lung involvement and good overall pulmonary function. The condition of such patients, even though effectively treated so that infection is controlled, may deteriorate rapidly and may progress to incapacitating obstructive lung disease. Thus, whenever pulmonary disease caused by nontuberculous mycobacteria is encountered, all possible measures should be introduced to diminish the progression of obstructive lung disease. The one measure that may be most helpful in diminishing the progress of obstructive lung disease is the elimination of cigarette smoking. The reason for this association between pulmonary infection with nontuberculous myocbacteria and obstructive lung disease is unknown. More than 50 per cent of patients with pulmonary disease caused by *M. kansasii* or *M. intracellulare-avium* complex will have coexisting obstructive pulmonary disease. It is possible that defects in alveolar and mucociliary clearance may play a role.

## GEOGRAPHIC VARIATIONS IN DISEASE

It is difficult to discuss the geographic variations in disease caused by nontuberculous mycobacteria because facilities for their proper recognition and identification are not available in much of the world. Despite limited facilities and the tentative state of classification, these mycobacteria are known to be worldwide in distribution. If all biopsy specimens were cultured appropriately for mycobacteria as well as for bacteria and fungi, our understanding of the regional or local basis of these infections would be greatly augmented.

Human disease due to *M. kansasii* is often strikingly localized within a large community, suggesting a focal exposure. However, evidence of case-to-case transmission, including household contact spread, is absent.

Human disease due to *M. intracellulare-avium* complex also tends to show certain focal epidemiologic characteristics. Although it is more common in the southeastern area of the United States, isolated cases are seen throughout the world. Human cases of *M. avium* infection are seen more frequently in farming populations of central Europe, but little is known of their distribution elsewhere.

There is a well-known association of *M. marinum* infection with swimming pool granulomas in patients who swim in hot springs.

The extent to which nontuberculous mycobacteria are responsible for chronic skin ulcers in humid tropical countries is not well known or understood. Probably they are more closely related than is presently recognized. Once again, the availability of reliable facilities for culturing appropriate specimens would help to increase our knowledge of these organisms.

## DIAGNOSIS

Because the clinical spectrum of disease caused by these organisms is nonspecific, it has not been possible to develop reliable clinical, pathologic, or radiologic criteria for specific diagnosis. Only bacteriologic diagnosis is reliable, and cultures from sputum, gastric contents, purulent secretions, tissue biopsy, and urine must be planted on Loewenstein-Jensen or Middlebrook-Cohn 7 H 10 or 7 H 11 culture media. The demonstration of acid-fast organisms in stained preparations of the specimens is not adequate for diagnosis but should alert the physician to the necessity of culturing on such media. The isolation of nontuberculous mycobacteria in only a single specimen or with a very sparse colony count should be viewed with suspicion. In patients afflicted with nontuberculous mycobacterial disease the organ-

isms are usually found in multiple cultures and in large numbers.

In many instances nontuberculous mycobacteria produce such lesions as suppurative adenitis, skin ulcers, or a localized nodule. A common error is to overlook culturing the excised specimen and do only histologic studies, resulting in a report to the clinician of caseating granulomas with demonstrable acid-fast organisms that have not been cultured. Once the node is fixed in formalin, the only opportunity to make a specific diagnosis is lost.

Relatively simple routine laboratory studies and procedures will lead to recognition of most cases of nontuberculous mycobacterial infections. Incubators should be dark, and cultures should be checked weekly and examined under a dissecting microscope. If drug susceptibility studies and catalase and niacin tests were done on all initial isolates, the finding of primary drug resistance in niacin-negative, highly positive catalase cultures would almost certainly identify the organisms as one of the nontuberculous mycobacteria. Whenever possible all questionable cultures should be sent to an appropriate reference laboratory for full evaluation.

## TREATMENT

Isolated lymph node involvement without dissemination probably is handled best by excision and does not require intensive chemotherapy unless the patient has impaired immunity. Such lymph node involvement is seen most commonly in the neck, and by deep extension may encroach upon vital structures such as the jugular vein and facial nerve. Since the extent and depth of the involvement cannot be determined accurately before biopsy-excision, the procedure should be done by a surgeon who is experienced in the anatomic relationships of the area. Whenever possible it is best to remove the involved tissue as completely as possible.

Disseminated infection and pulmonary disease require chemotherapy (Tables 2 and 3). *M. kansasii* is resistant to the conventional antituberculosis drugs streptomycin, isoniazid, and etham-

TABLE 2.  Parenteral Antituberculosis Drugs

| | NORMAL ADULT DAILY DOSE | DURATION OF ADMINISTRATION | TOXICITY |
|---|---|---|---|
| Streptomycin | 1.0 gm 15 mg/kg body weight | 30–90 days | Vestibular, auditory, renal |
| Viomycin | 1.0 gm | 30–90 days | Vestibular, auditory, renal |
| Kanamycin | 1.0 gm | 30–90 days | Auditory, vestibular, renal |
| Capreomycin | 1.0 gm | 30–90 days | Vestibular, auditory, renal |

**TABLE 3.   Oral Antituberculosis Drugs**

| | NORMAL ADULT DAILY DOSE | DURATION OF ADMINISTRATION | TOXICITY |
|---|---|---|---|
| Isoniazid | 300 mg | 18–24 months | Neuropathy, hepatic signs |
| Ethambutol | 15 mg/kg body weight | 18–24 months | Optic signs |
| Rifampin | 600 mg | 18–24 months | Hepatic signs |
| Pyrazinamide | 2–3 gm | 18–24 months | Hepatic signs, hyperuricemia |
| Ethionamide | 1.0 gm | 18–24 months | Gastrointestinal discomfort, depression, hypothyroidism |
| Cycloserine | 1.0 gm | 18–24 months | Depression, convulsions, psychosis |
| Para-aminosalicylic acid | 12. gm | 18–24 months | Hepatic signs, cutaneous reactions |
| Thiacetazone | 150 mg | 18–24 months | Hepatic signs |

butol but usually only to low concentrations of these agents. The organism is very sensitive to rifampin. Thus, adult patients with pulmonary or disseminated *M. kansasii* infection are best treated with an intensive drug regimen consisting of streptomycin, isoniazid, and rifampin daily. If rifampin is not available, ethambutol or para-aminosalicylic acid can be substituted. The streptomycin should be continued daily until there is a satisfactory clinical response and cultures become negative. The two oral drugs should then be continued for 24 months. Such a program, especially if rifampin is included, should result in success rates approaching 100 per cent. If this therapy fails or if the patient had been inadequately treated in the past, a triple drug retreatment regimen based on another aminoglycoside such as capreomycin, viomycin, or kanamycin may be used plus two oral drugs selected from pyrazinamide, ethionamide, or cycloserine.

The results of chemotherapy in patients with *M. intracellulare-avium* infections are not as good as those in disease caused by *M. kansasii*. The *M. intracellulare-avium* complex is characterized by primary drug resistance to all of the available antituberculosis drugs and to higher concentrations of these agents than are readily attainable in the body on the usual dosages. For this reason, only 20 to 30 per cent of patients with *M. intracellulare* infections respond to the conventional drug regimens used in the treatment of tuberculosis. If untreated, the pulmonary or disseminated form of this infection is fatal; therefore, every effort should be made to treat these cases effectively and in specialized facilities.

Although it is not ideal, the most effective treatment for *M. intracellulare* infections consists of a six-drug regimen — one given parenterally, selected from among streptomycin, capreomycin, viomycin, or kanamycin, and five oral agents, chosen from among isoniazid, rifampin, ethambutol, pyrazinamide, ethionamide, cycloserine, or para-aminosalicylic acid. Such a regimen obviously requires expert and intensive monitoring for side effects and adverse reactions and should be used only in patients with life-threatening disease who have no other therapeutic options. Every effort should be made to continue the six-drug regimen until satisfactory clinical response and negative culture status have been obtained. Thereafter, the parenteral drug can be stopped, and every effort is made to continue the five-drug oral program for a total of 24 months. Such a regimen will succeed in approximately 80 per cent of cases, except in elderly or debilitated patients, who respond less well. It should not be used casually or without careful evaluation of each patient.

Usually pulmonary disease caused by *M. intracellulare-avium* complex is not recognized until it has become extensive and multifocal. In such cases surgical treatment is not practical. However, occasional patients will be encountered in whom the disease is circumscribed and limited to one lobe or one lung. Pulmonary resection can be curative in such cases even though their sputa are positive at the time of surgery. Thus, although such patients are uncommon, they should be identified early in the course of their disease and should undergo resection at the earliest opportunity after chemotherapy has been initiated.

Experience is lacking in the treatment of disease caused by nontuberculous mycobacteria other than *M. kansasii* and *M. intracellulare-avium* complex. Therefore, although it is impossible to recommend specific regimens for these other infections, certain general principles can be stated. Skin ulcers may heal spontaneously; if they do not, they may require block excision and skin grafting. If lymph node involvement is progressive or disfiguring, it is best treated by excision by a surgeon experienced in dissecting an extensive process involving the deep structures of the neck or axilla. Although a palpable node is the only clinical sign of infection, the adjacent area may be deeply infiltrated by underlying disease.

### References

Barksdale, L., and Kim, K.: Mycobacterium. Bact Rev 41:217, 1977.
Chapman, J. S.: The Atypical Mycobacteria and Human Mycobacteriosis. New York, Plenum Medical Book Comparny, 1977.

Lester, W.: Unclassified mycobacterial diseases. Ann Res Microbiol 17:351, 1966.
Lincoln, E. M., and Gilbert, L. A.: Disease in children due to myobacteria other than *Mycobacterium tuberculosis*. Am Rev Respir Dis 105:683, 1972.
Runyon, E. H.: Anonymous mycobacteria in pulmonary disease. Med Clin North Am 43:273, 1959.

# 116 PULMONARY CRYPTOCOCCOSIS

*Gerald Medoff, M.D.*

## DEFINITION

Pulmonary cryptococcal infection has been known for many years, but its true incidence, clinical manifestations, and course have come to light very slowly. It was not until 1968 (Tynes et al., 1968; Warr et al., 1968) that it was shown that the organism could be cultured from sputum frequently and that a saprophytic form of cryptococcosis that was distinct from the invasive form of the disease could exist.

## ETIOLOGY

Pulmonary cryptococcal infection is caused by the single species *Cryptococcus neoformans*. It is an encapsulated yeast-like fungus, pathogenic for animals and man. Four serotypes, A, B, C, and D, have been described. Serotypes A and D appear to be most frequently associated with human disease. The organism is ubiquitous and is commonly found in nature.

## PATHOGENESIS AND PATHOLOGY

The presence of *C. neoformans* in bird dung is well documented, but this association is best known in regard to pigeon droppings. Concentrations of fungi as high as $5 \times 10^7/g$ of feces have been found in some samples. In most cases of cryptococcal infection the source can not be discerned. The presence of the fungus in bird droppings and the great numbers of birds found in the environment suggest this route of transmission. However, direct epidemiologic evidence for this is lacking. Man-to-man transmission or direct animal transmission to man has not been documented.

Cryptococcal infection comes to medical attention most frequently as a central nervous system disease (see Chapter 155), but in almost all human infections the fungus enters the body through the respiratory tract by inhalation of infectious particles. Until recently, it was not clear how a heavily encapsulated yeast 3 to 10 $\mu$ in diameter could be aerosolized and reach the alveolar spaces in the lung. However, in laboratory studies yeasts with decreased capsules 0.5 to 2 $\mu$ in diameter have been described and shown to be capable of colonizing the alveoli and thereby initiating the disease. More recently, a description of the perfect states of the organism *Filobasidiella neoformans* (Kwon-chung, 1975) has implicated inhalation of the small, light basidiospores as another mode of contracting the infection.

Phagocytosis is important in the killing of *C. neoformans*, and both the classic and alternative complement pathways are required for optimal ingestion of the fungi (*Diamond* et al., 1974). It also seems that nonphagocytic mononuclear cells can kill *C. neoformans*, but only if anticryptococcal antibody is present (Diamond, 1974). In most cases the normal host response can deal with the infection, and only a small granulomatous cryptococcoma and perhaps minimal granulomatous cryptococcal lymphadenitis occur. However, in a few cases the infection produces diffuse cryptococcal pneumonia and lymphadenitis. Unlike other forms of cryptococcal infection, pneumonia occurs commonly in patients without apparent immune deficiency, although most patients with pulmonary cryptococcal infection appear to have underlying pulmonary disease of various types.

In routine hematoxylin and eosin stains, the organism is poorly demarcated. In tissue sections stained by the periodic acid-Schiff or Gomori methenamine silver method, round to oval budding cells are easily seen. The capsular polysaccharide stains a brilliant pink with Mayer's mucicarmine stain, which differentiates this organism from other yeasts that do not possess a capsule. The yeast cell also takes the gram stain (Fig. 1).

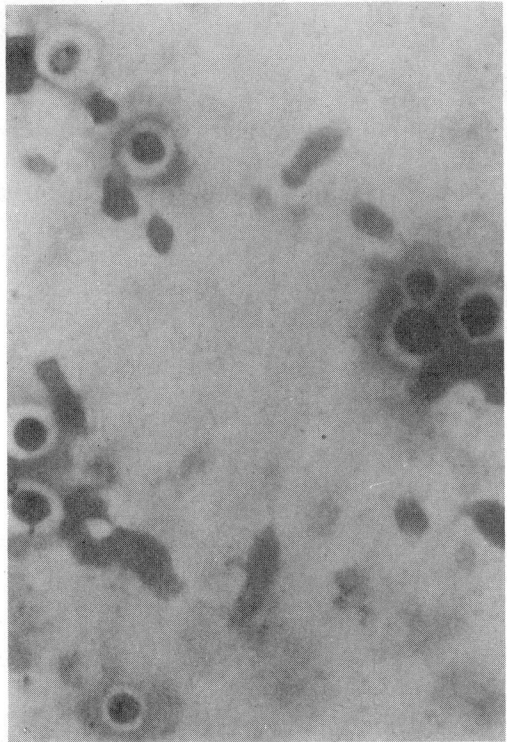

**FIGURE 1.** *Cryptococci in bronchial brushings from patient with lingular cryptococcosis. Note budding and encapsulation. The yeast cells are gram positive (Gram stain ×500).*

## CLINICAL MANIFESTATIONS

The cryptococcus seems to be considerably more prevalent in human sputum than is generally appreciated, but most of these infected people have no cryptococcal disease; hence, colonization with *C. neoformans* is probably the most common form of infection (Hammerman et al., 1973). De-

spite this, isolation of *C. neoformans* from respiratory secretions is rare enough to be taken seriously and pursued until localized or disseminated cryptococcosis is excluded.

Pulmonary cryptococcal infection presents no characteristic clinical picture. It appears to have a marked predilection for the white male and may start like influenza with cough and minimal pleuritic chest pain. Frequently patients have a history of prolonged respiratory infection with cough, low-grade fever, easy fatigability, and weight loss. An asymptomatic coin lesion on the chest radiograph may be the only manifestation of disease.

The cryptococcal lesions in the lungs may be solitary, multiple (Fig. 2), or disseminated, or may take the form of a tumor mass or diffuse pneumonitis. Cavities or mediastinal adenopathy are rare, but pleural effusion is not uncommon. The typical clinical course of pulmonary cryptococcal infection has not been well defined, but from a review of the accumulated experience of patients with cryptococcal pneumonia, it appears that most patients will recover without treatment. Cellular reactions may not occur, and large discrete cryptococcal masses may give the impression of a myxoma.

## COMPLICATIONS AND SEQUELAE

Complications and sequelae of cryptococcal pulmonary infections are unusual. Pneumonia or diffuse pulmonary infection may be fatal or may damage the lung with permanent impairment of pulmonary function. Local lesions (a coin lesion or a mass) may require a thoracotomy to rule out a neoplasm. In a few patients pulmonary infec-

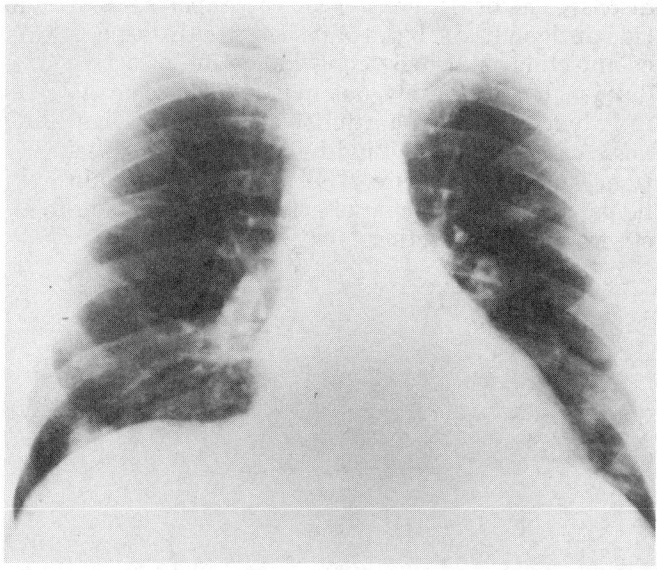

**FIGURE 2.** *Cryptococcal infection of lung. There are multiple nodular lesions in both lungs.*

tion may disseminate to the central nervous system especially, but rarely to the bone, skin, eye, adrenals, spleen, or kidney.

## GEOGRAPHIC VARIATIONS IN DISEASE

Cryptococcal infection in general occurs sporadically in all parts of the world without any significant geographic variation. Evidence from skin test surveys suggests that it probably has a higher incidence in people who have a significant exposure to birds. However, standardized skin test reagents are not available, and epidemiologic studies are limited in this regard.

There are four serotypes of *C. neoformans* labeled A through D. In a recent epidemiologic study, the most prevalent serotype isolated from the environment and from cases of clinical infection was serotype A. Serotypes B and C were infrequent causes of infection except in southern California. Interestingly, these serotypes were not isolated at all from environmental sources, indicating that the site or sites in nature where serotypes B and C exist are currently unknown and differ from those of serotypes A and D. Serotype D may be unusually prevalent both in the environment and in patients from Denmark and Italy (Bennett et al., 1977).

## DIAGNOSIS

The presence of *C. neoformans* in the sputum or bronchial washings (Fig. 1) in the presence of an active pulmonary process is strong evidence of disease. The detection of cryptococcal polysaccharide antigen in the blood of patients with suspected infection is also a strong indication of active disease. Unfortunately, one may have to resort to lung biopsy to make a definitive diagnosis. Diagnosis can be made by finding cryptococci in sections and upon culture. The mucicarmine stain helps identify the characteristic capsular substance in biopsy sections.

## TREATMENT AND PROPHYLAXIS

The treatment of pulmonary cryptococcal infection has not been defined. Total excision of localized lesions, which are usually removed to rule out a tumor, requires no medical therapy. Most patients with cryptococcal pneumonia apparently recover without treatment, and dissemination to the CNS is quite rare. The following management of patients whose sputum or lungs contain cryptococci is recommended by Hammerman et al. (1973) and appears reasonable:

1. Close observation for one to two months. If there is evidence of progression or if there is failure of the chest lesion to resolve, treatment should be instituted.

2. Evidence of dissemination from the lungs justifies a full course of therapy.

As with CNS infection, amphotericin B at a dosage of 0.3 to 1.0 mg/kg/day for six to ten weeks is recommended. A good index of response is the serum antigen, which should be negative when therapy is stopped. Some investigators use 5-fluorocytosine 150 mg/kg/day alone or added to the amphotericin B (see Chapter 154 for a further discussion of the combined regimen).

No prophylaxis is necessary for this disease except avoidance of unnecessary exposure to bird droppings.

### References

Bennett, J. E., Kwon-Chung, K. J., and Howard, D. H.: Epidemiologic differences among serotypes of *Cryptococcus neoformans.* Am J Epidemiol 105:582, 1977.
Diamond, R. D.: Antibody-dependent killing of *Cryptococcus neoformans* by human peripheral blood mononuclear cells. Nature 247:148, 1974.
Diamond, R. D., May, J. E., Kane, M. A., Frank, M. M., and Bennett, J. E.: The role of the classical and alternate complement pathways in host defenses against *Cryptococcus neoformans* infection. J Immunol 112:2260, 1974.
Hammerman, K. J., Powell, K. E., Christianson, C. S., Huggin, P. M., Larsh, H. W., Vivas, J. R., and Tosh, F. E.: Pulmonary cryptococcosis: Clinical forms and treatment. A Center for Disease Control mycoses study. Am Rev Resp Dis 108:1116, 1973.
Kwon-Chung, K. J.: Description of a new genus *Filobasidiella*, the perfect state of *Cryptococcus neoformans.* Mycologia 67:1197, 1975.
Tynes, B., Mason, K. N., Jennings, A. E., and Bennett, J. E.: Variant forms of pulmonary cryptococcosis. Ann Intern Med 69:1117, 1968.
Warr, W., Bates, J. H., and Stone, A.: The spectrum of pulmonary cryptococcosis. Ann Intern Med 69:1109, 1968.

# NORTH AMERICAN BLASTOMYCOSIS 117

Abraham I. Braude, M.D., Ph.D.

## DEFINITION

Blastomycosis is a fungus infection of the skin, lungs, and other viscera caused by *Blastomyces dermatitidis*. It occurs primarily in North America. A similar disease is caused by *Paracoccidioides brasiliensis* in South America. Paracoccidioidomycosis is described in Chapter 118.

## ETIOLOGY

In infected tissues, *B. dermatitidis* has the appearance of a yeast, forming single buds from 3 to 24 $\mu$ in diameter. Two features aid in recognition: (1) its thick wall, spoken of as "double-contoured," because the inner and outer margins can be seen; and (2) the wide opening between parent cell and bud at the base of attachment.

In culture, *B. dermatitidis* is dimorphic and appears as a wrinkled, waxy yeast form on blood agar incubated at 37° C or as a mold with branching hyphae on Sabouraud's agar at room temperature. On microscopic examination, the cultured yeast may be identical with that in the infected lesions or may have abortive mycelia. The mycelia give rise to oval or pear-shaped spores.

## PATHOGENESIS AND PATHOLOGY

Although *B. dermatitidis* has seldom been cultured from the soil and soon disappears after inoculation into natural soil, soil is the most likely source of the fungus. Most infections occur in people who are in close contact with soil, especially in the Mississippi and Ohio River Valleys. Bird droppings must also be considered as a possible source of human infection because *B. dermatitidis* has been recovered from pigeon manure. A strong association between canine and human blastomycosis has been observed, but it is unlikely that the infection was transmitted from dogs to man; rather, both were probably exposed together to the same source in nature (Sarosi et al., 1979).

The lung is the major portal of entry for blastomycosis. Because of strong natural resistance to *B. dermatitidis,* most persons develop subclinical pulmonary infections recognizable only by skin tests. Heavy infection in healthy persons can cause multiple benign pulmonary lesions that heal spontaneously. Primary lesions may give rise to progressive disease, with or without a variable latent interval. The pulmonary lesion may enlarge and spread to other parts of the lung before dissemination to skin and bones; or systemic dissemination may occur from a small stationary pulmonary focus, sometimes after reactivation from a dormant stage. In patients with leukemia or other forms of depressed immunity, the infection can cause fulminant pulmonary dissemination (Onal et al., 1976).

The basic lesion in blastomycosis is the suppurative granuloma with Langhans and foreign-body giant cells. In the skin and mucous membranes, this combination of abscesses and epithelioid cell granulomas occurs in the midst of pseudoepitheliomatous hyperplasia. Characteristic cells of *B. dermatitidis,* with its single broad-based bud, can be seen in these lesions.

## CLINICAL MANIFESTATIONS

The rare acute pulmonary form of North American blastomycosis varies from asymptomatic infection to a severe illness resembling acute histoplasmosis. Two clinical types of acute infection have been recognized. The first consists of fever, productive cough, and joint and muscle pains, with multiple nodular pulmonary densities in roentgenograms and budding yeast in the sputum. In the second type, pleuritic chest pain of variable severity and lasting only a few hours is the distinctive feature, but chest x-rays reveal no pleural effusions despite multiple pulmonary nodules. Both forms are benign, and the patient recovers without specific treatment.

In the typical case of progressive North American blastomycosis, the onset is insidious. The patient may seek medical attention because of a persistent "chest cold," low-grade fever, weight loss, or progressive disability. Physical examination and a roentgenogram of the chest disclose evidence of pneumonia, which may involve any segment or lobe of the lung. Cavitation is frequent, and mediastinal lymph nodes may be prominent. Hemoptysis, purulent sputum, chest pain, and dyspnea appear as the disease progresses. Although the pulmonary infection may subside spontaneously, extrapulmonary lesions of the skin, bones, joints, and viscera eventually call attention to dissemination. These metastatic suppurative lesions are accompanied by an increase in fever, sweats, chills, and weakness. Death in the untreated infection sometimes occurs in less than 6 months, but most patients live for 1 or 2 years. The overall mortality rate in systemic blastomycosis is said to be 92 per cent in patients whose cases have been followed for 2 years or longer without specific therapy.

## COMPLICATIONS

Metastatic infections of the skin, bone, and genitourinary tract are the chief complications of pulmonary blastomycosis. The adrenal may also be infected.

Infection of the skin by *B. dermatitidis* is the most common form of extrapulmonary disease, occurring in as many as 80 per cent of patients with blastomycosis. It first appears on unclothed areas such as the hands, face, forearm, or lower leg (Fig. 1), but not the scalp, palms, or soles. The infection begins as a firm nodule surrounded by similar lesions that tend to coalesce. Suppuration in the center of the nodule is followed by partial healing and fibrosis as extension occurs peripherally. The hyperplastic epithelium gives these lesions a hard, raised, wartlike margin. When fully developed, blastomycosis of the skin presents the appearance of one or more ragged ulcers with partially healed centers and thick, raised margins.

Because blastomycosis of the skin is often the first clinical sign of the disease, it was previously thought to result from direct inoculation of the fungus into the site of the lesion. According to present concepts, direct inoculation is an extremely rare cause of cutaneous blastomycosis and produces an entirely different lesion than that seen in hematogenous infection of the skin. The primary cutaneous lesion resembles a chancre with its indurated ulcer and regional adenopathy (Wilson et al., 1955). It tends to appear on the fingers and remain there until it heals. It does not disseminate.

Osteomyelitis is the next most common hematogenous complication of pulmonary blastomycosis. As many as half the patients with blastomycosis have osteolytic skeletal lesions, sometimes as the only sign of the disease. Almost any bone may show hematogenous infection, but the verte-

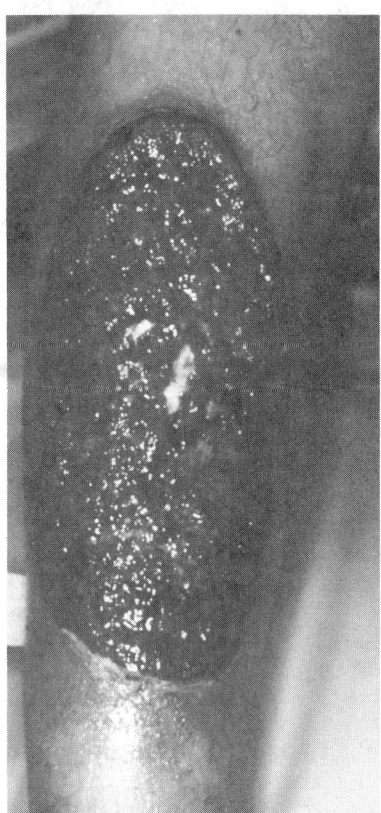

**FIGURE 1.** *Blastomycosis of leg acquired in Arkansas by an engineer working for the telephone company in the Arkansas wilderness. The lesion healed completely with 30 mg amphotericin B daily.*

brae and ribs do so most frequently. Blastomycosis of the vertebrae may be indistinguishable from tuberculosis of the spine. In both diseases, the infection begins in the vertebral body, destroys the disk, and produces paraspinal or epidural abscesses that cause paraplegia by compressing the spinal cord (Greenwood and Voris, 1950). The brain may also suffer compression from intracranial extradural abscesses secondary to osteomyelitis of the skull (Fig. 2).

Direct hematogenous spread to the brain is less common than to bone. Primary blastomycosis of the nervous system may take the form of meningitis, single or multiple brain abscesses, and brain or cord granuloma (Fig. 3) (Fetter et al., 1967). In blastomycotic meningitis, there is headache, vomiting, confusion, and a stiff neck. The cerebrospinal fluid shows pleocytosis with either lymphocytes or neutrophils predominating, an elevation of the protein to 300 mg/ml or more, and a reduction in glucose. The meningitis causes a fibrinopurulent exudate that may spread diffusely through the subarachnoid space or become localized at the base of the brain, so that an obstructive hydrocephalus develops.

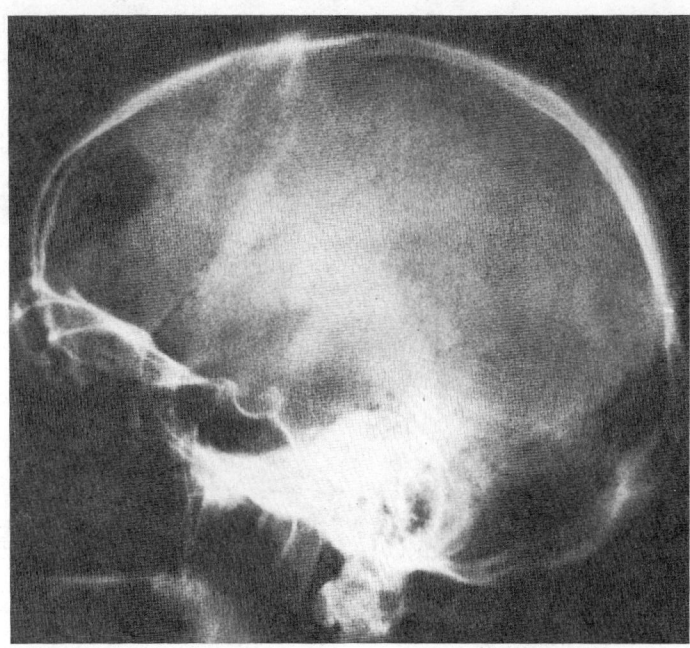

**FIGURE 2.** *Osteomyelitis of the skull due to Blasto-myces dermatiditis. Osteolytic lesion with irregular margins of the frontal bone is secondary to dissemination from the lungs. (From Bell, W., and McCormick, W.: Neurologic Infections in Children. Philadelphia, W. B. Saunders Company, 1975, p. 334.)*

The third most common hematogenous complication is blastomycosis of the prostate, epididymis, and testis. The kidney and female genitalia, on the other hand, are rarely affected.

## GEOGRAPHIC DISTRIBUTION

Most cases of blastomycosis have been reported from the Mississippi and Ohio River Valleys and the Southeastern United States. The infection also occurs in Canada, Mexico, Central America, South America, and Africa. African cases were found in Zaire, Uganda, Tanzania, Gambia, Zambia, Rhodesia, Tunisia, Morocco, and South Africa (Bregant et al., 1973). The identity of the strains isolated from American and African cases of blastomycosis has not been established.

## DIAGNOSIS

Pulmonary blastomycosis closely resembles tuberculosis, carcinoma of the lung, aspiration pneumonitis, and other fungus infections, including coccidioidomycosis, actinomycosis, nocardiosis, and histoplasmosis. Differentiation must be based on the recovery of the etiologic agent, because neither clinical nor epidemiologic features are specific.

It is usually possible to find *B. dermatitidis* by microscopic examination of biopsied material, sputum, or pus. The yeastlike forms can be observed if a drop of purulent material is first mixed on a slide with a drop of 10 per cent potassium

hydroxide and kept at room temperature for 30 minutes. Buds of *B. dermatitidis* are connected to the parent cell by a wide communication. *Blastomyces dermatitidis* is isolated by culturing pus on Sabouraud's agar at room temperature and on blood agar at 37° C.

The diagnostic value of the skin test for blastomycosis is limited. The complement-fixation test in North American blastomycosis is positive in high titer with serums of patients who have

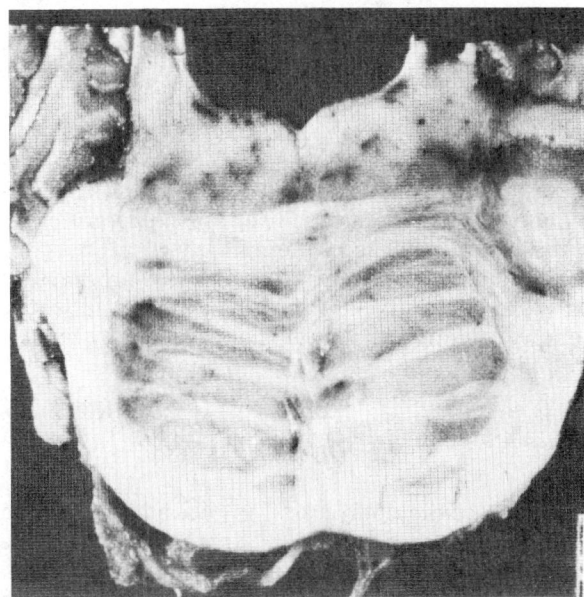

**FIGURE 3.** *Blastomycosis of the brain. A solitary solid granuloma of the pons is located at the level of the trigeminal nerves. (From Bell, W., and McCormick, W.: Neurologic Infections in Children. Philadelphia, W. B. Saunders Company, 1975, p. 335.)*

systemic infections but has limited diagnostic value, because the antigens are neither specific or sensitive (Kaufman, 1976). The immunodiffusion test, on the other hand, is specific and has a sensitivity of 80 per cent. Negative tests with either method do not exclude a diagnosis of blastomycosis (Kaufman et al., 1973). The results of intradermal and serologic tests may be of prognostic value. Patients with marked dermal hypersensitivity and low serum titers of complement-fixing antibody are said to have a better prognosis in North American blastomycosis than those with negative skin tests and high complement-fixation titers.

## TREATMENT

Amphotericin B can cure blastomycosis. Blastomycosis also responds but less favorably to 2-hydroxystilbamidine. Either drug is given daily or every other day by slow intravenous drip in increasing doses. The maximum adult daily dose of amphotericin B is 40 mg, and that of 2-hydroxystilbamidine is 250 mg. Blastomycosis should be treated with a total of 1.5 g amphoteri-cin B; 7 to 8 g of 2-hydroxystilbamidine may be required. Anesthesia over the distribution of the trigeminal nerve is the main untoward reaction from 2-hydroxystilbamidine; it persists after treatment. Surgical excision of pulmonary cavities or destroyed tissues is sometimes necessary in addition to chemotherapy.

### References

Bregant, S., Gigase, P., Bastin, J. P., and VanDePitte, J.: La blastomy-cose Norde-Américaine en République du Zaire. Bul Soc Path Exot 66:77, 1973.
Fetter, B., Klintworth, G., and Wilson, S.: Mycoses of the central nervous system. Baltimore, Williams & Wilkins Company, 1967.
Greenwood, R. C., and Voris, H. C.: Systemic blastomycosis with spinal cord involvement. J Neurosurg 7:450, 1950.
Kaufman, L.: Serodiagnosis of fungal diseases. In Rose, N., and Friedman, H. (eds): Manual of Clinical Immunology. Washington, D.C., Am. Soc. Microbiol., 1976, p. 366.
Kaufman, L., McLaughlin, D., Clark, M., and Blumer, S.: Specific immunodiffusion test for blastomycosis. Appl Microbiol 26:244, 1973.
Onal, E., Lopata, M., and Lourenco, R.: Disseminated pulmonary blastomycosis in an immunosuppressed patient. Am Rev Resp Dis 113:83, 1976.
Sarosi, G., Echman, M., Davies, S., and Laskey, W.: Canine blastomycosis as a harbinger of human disease. Ann Int Med 91:733, 1979.
Wilson, J., Cawley, E., Weidman, F., and Gilmer, W.: Primary cutaneous North American blastomycosis. AMA Arch Dermat Syph 71:39, 1955.

# 118 PARACOCCIDIOIDOMYCOSIS (SOUTH AMERICAN BLASTOMYCOSIS)

Alberto Thomaz Londero, M.D.

## DEFINITION AND ETIOLOGY

Paracoccidioidomycosis is a systemic mycosis caused by the dimorphic fungus *Paracoccidioides brasiliensis*. Paracoccidioidal infection may be benign and self-limiting or it may progress to involve virtually any organ. As a result, the clinical manifestations of the disease may be protean.

## EPIDEMIOLOGY

Paracoccidioidomycosis is found in Latin America from Mexico to Argentina, with the exception of Chile, Nicaragua, and the Caribbean Islands. Cases reported in countries outside Latin America have involved patients who lived for some time in the endemic areas.

The infection primarily affects rural inhabi-tants and is acquired mostly between the ages of 15 and 19 years. Both sexes are infected at the same rate. Fifty-two per cent of cases of the progressive form of the disease are seen in patients between 30 and 50 years of age, with a male/female ratio of 14.7 to 1. The disease is rare in children. All races are susceptible, although European and Asian immigrants present very severe clinical pictures.

## PATHOGENESIS AND PATHOLOGY

Like other agents of systemic mycosis, *P. brasiliensis* enters the human body by inhalation and causes a primary lymph node complex in the lung (Severo et al., 1979a). Hematogenous dissemination to other organs can occur simultaneously. These disseminated lesions usually heal or become latent if immunity is normal. Rarely, the primary lesion progresses, disseminates, and causes very severe disease. This is presumed to occur in patients under 20 years of age (Restrepo, 1978).

The latent primary lesions may be reactivated many years later and may occur in patients seen in nonendemic countries (Balabanov et al., 1964; Murray et al., 1974). The reactivation may be brought on by a deficiency in cell-mediated immunity and may occur spontaneously without apparent cause or secondary to immunosuppressive disease and/or therapy (Severo et al., 1979b). The reactivation of a latent lesion in the lung may cause a progressive pulmonary infection that sometimes disseminates hematogenously to other organs.

Mucocutaneous ulcers are the most common disseminated manifestation. These ulcers are secondary to inflammation of the underlying skeletal muscles. (Mackinnon, 1961). When *P. brasiliensis* is inoculated into the skin, a chancriform or sporotrichoid lesion is produced (Castro et al., 1975).

The gross pathology is similar to that of other systemic mycoses or tuberculosis. The most common reaction to *P. brasiliensis* is granulomatous. When there is no secondary infection, the granulomas are composed of epithelial cells and Langhans' foreign-body giant cells. Necrosis can occur in the center of the nodule. When the epithelioid nodule is not necrotic, it resembles a sarcoid. Regressing nodules become fibrotic or hyalinized. A mixed granulomatous and pyogenic reaction with microabscesses also occurs. Diffuse or extensive inflammation is rare.

Paracoccidioidal lesions show variable suppuration, macrophages, giant cells, caseous necrosis, and fibrosis as in other systemic mycotic lesions. Only the presence of *P. brasiliensis* allows the identification of the lesions.

## CLINICAL MANIFESTATIONS

Clinical manifestations are so protean that the mycosis may simulate an enormous number of diseases. These manifestations may be grouped into four clinical forms: (1) primary pulmonary, (2) progressive pulmonary, (3) disseminated, and (4) acute juvenile.

### Primary Pulmonary Form

The primary lesion in the lung is similar to Ghon's complex in tuberculosis. In the early stages, the disease is thought to be either asymptomatic or too mild to be differentiated from a slight bacterial or viral infection. The infection is not recognizable except for the immunologic response to *P. brasiliensis,* as shown by the skin test and precipitin test. Primary lesions usually heal but rarely with calcification (Angulo-Ortega, 1972). A radiologic picture of these lesions has not yet been characterized. Early hematogenous spread may occur to other organs, where asymptomatic lesions develop. The metastatic foci usually heal but are rarely calcified, so that they are seldom found. Some foci of infection may remain quiescent (latent) in the lung and perhaps in other organs as well. Their reactivation would explain progressive cases diagnosed outside endemic areas.

### Progressive Pulmonary Form

Approximately 30 per cent of patients manifest this form of the disease. The progressive pulmonary form results from a reactivation of a quiescent lesion or, rarely, the progression of a primary focus (Londero et al., 1978). Early progressive lung lesions may be asymptomatic. More rarely, patients present nonspecific respiratory symptoms. A small nodule or one or more small apical infiltrations are seen in radiographs. After months or years, the lesions may spread throughout the lungs, and then symptoms appear (Fig. 1). Patients present a history of a subacute or chronic (rarely acute) respiratory infection with a prolonged or recurrent course. A cough is always present that produces mucoid or mucopurulent sputum, later becoming bloody. Dyspnea and, less frequently, fever, thoracic pain, and weight loss are subsequent complaints. Physical signs vary according to the extent and localization of the lung lesions, but they are not specific. In the early stage of the disease radiologic pictures are often not characteristic of paracoccidioidomycosis (Fig. 2), but in advanced stages they show suggestive bilateral, symmetric and polymorphic lesions. Patients with localized paracoccidioidal lesions have been observed for as long as 15 years without dissemination (Fig. 3). On the other hand, it has been reported that 7.6 per cent of these patients develop disseminated lesions (usually oral) within a short time.

### Disseminated Form

About 65 to 70 per cent of patients present the disseminated form of the mycosis. Most of them have pulmonary lesions as well as disease elsewhere. The lung lesions may be overlooked because respiratory symptoms and physical signs are scarce, although radiologic lesions are extensive. More rarely, lesions are not evident on the chest radiograph. When there are no mucocutaneous manifestations, the pulmonary lesions may be misdiagnosed as tuberculosis. Extrapulmonary lesions in disseminated paracoccidioidomycosis are found most frequently in the mucous membranes, lymph nodes, skin, spleen, adrenal glands, intestine, and liver, and less frequently in

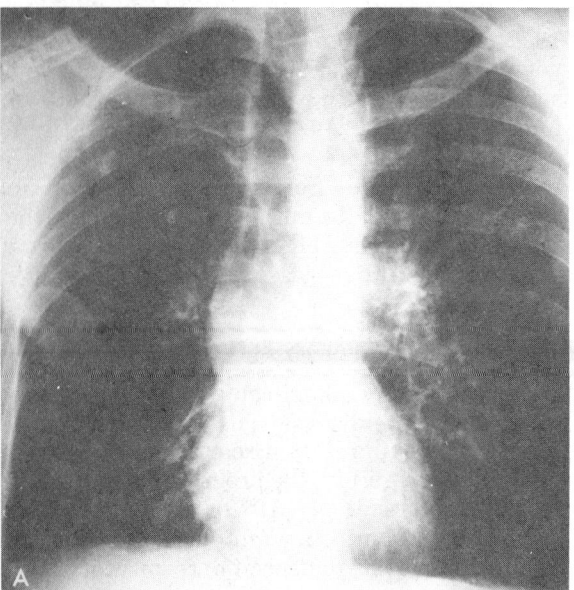
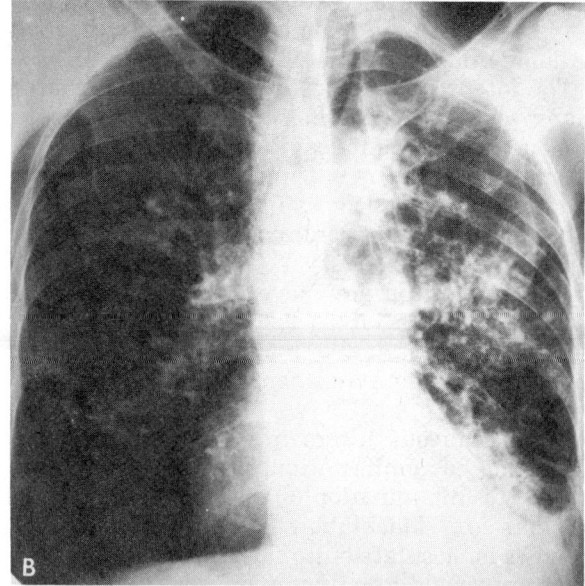

**FIGURE 1.** *Chest radiographs showing (A) small infiltrations in the upper right lobe (April, 1976) and (B) generalization of the infection to both lungs (May, 1977).*

the arteries, bones, brain, meninges, genitals, heart, kidney, and endocrine glands. The clinical presentation of the disseminated form is variable, depending on the site or sites and extent of involvement. The lesions may be generalized (affecting many organs or systems) or they may be confined to one organ.

Mucocutaneous and lymphatic lesions are the most frequent manifestations of hematogenous dissemination. They are the most obvious lesions and sometimes may be the presenting symptoms.

Lesions are found most often on the mucosal surfaces of the lips, gums, palate, and tongue (Fig. 4) and may extend to the skin around the mouth. Sometimes the lesions originate in the pharynx or the larynx. They appear as ulcers with a granulomatous mulberry-like base. Painful ulcers are usually superficial and enlarge slowly at the periphery. In advanced cases they deepen and destroy the buccal structures. Sometimes a peculiar hard, deep infiltration of the lips may occur. Ulcerative gingivitis may cause loss of

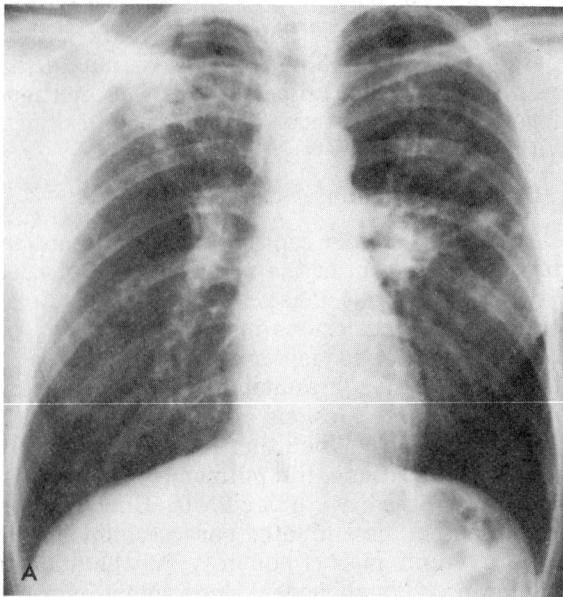
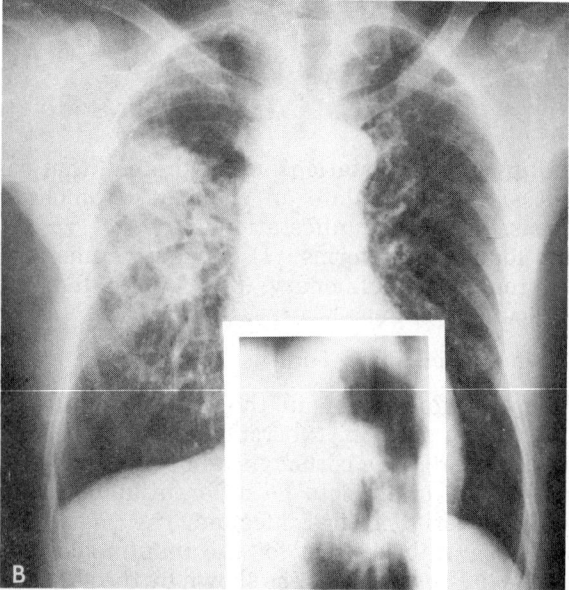

**FIGURE 2.** *Chest radiographs showing consolidations and necrotic cavities simulating (A) tuberculosis and (B) bacterial abscess (insert: tomogram).*

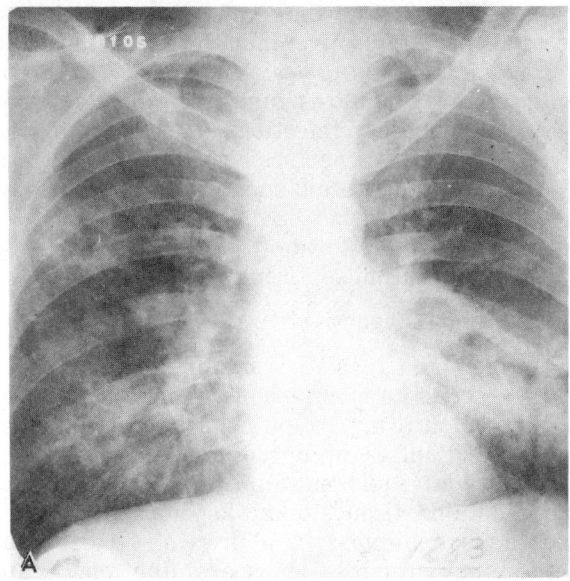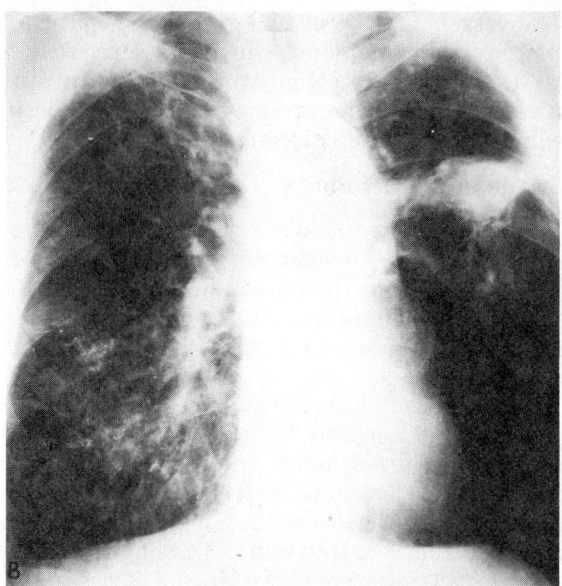

**FIGURE 3.** *Chest roentgenograms of same patient in 1963 (A) and in 1978 (B). On both occasions he was referred for mycologic examination. From 1963 through 1964, he was treated with sulfa drugs. From 1965 to 1978 the disease relapsed, and the patient presented recurrent respiratory undifferentiated infections, which were treated as tuberculosis.*

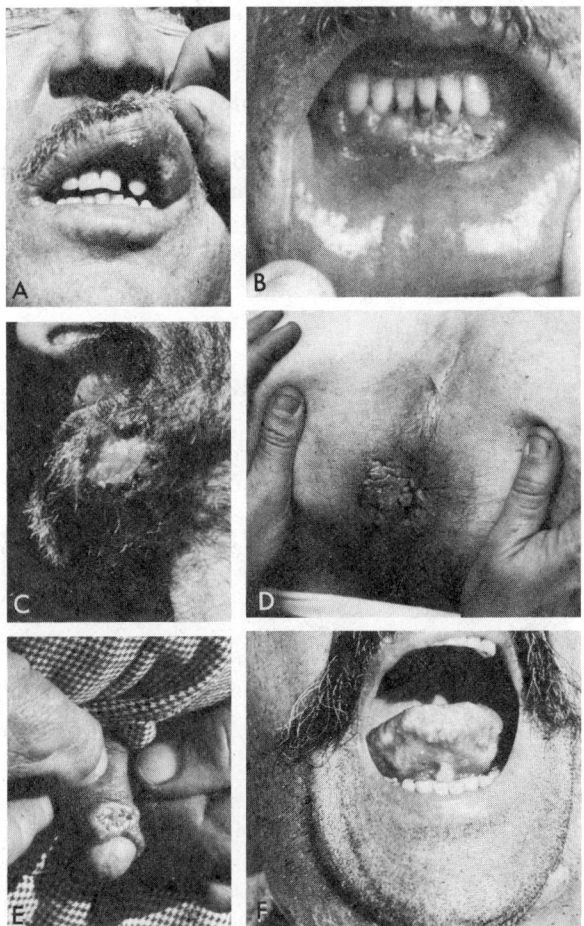

**FIGURE 4.** *Mucocutaneous and lymphatic lesions: Ulcerations of the lips (A), gums (B), jaw (C), and penis (E). Granulomatous lesion of the perineum (D). Lesion of the tongue and a right submaxillary adenopathy (F).*

teeth. Extensive disease of the oropharynx can interfere with eating, and destruction of the vocal cords may cause dysphonia or aphonia.

A great variety of skin lesions has been described. The crusting ulcer of the skin usually results from the extension of the buccal lesions at the mucocutaneous border of the lips. Solitary ulcerative or granulomatous lesions may occur in the anorectal region and elsewhere rarely (Fig. 4). Generalized polymorphic skin lesions are also rare.

Cervical lymph nodes are involved early and are discrete, firm, and hard. They may enlarge, become painful, suppurate, and drain. Massive cervical lymph nodes may be the only abnormality on physical examination.

When no mucocutaneous lesion or superficial lymph node involvement is present (in 5 to 20 per cent of the patients with disseminated form), the clinical picture of the mycosis may take many forms that vary according to the type of organ involved, the sequence of organ involvement, the severity of destruction, and the chronicity of the disease.

Visceral lymph node enlargements may cause intestinal obstruction or cholestatic jaundice. Intestinal paracoccidioidal lesions may produce symptoms of a mild enteritis, bowel tumor, or an acute abdomen. Lesions of the adrenal glands may be asymptomatic, but when they are severe, they may cause Addison's disease (Marsiglia and Pinto, 1966). Signs of brain tumor or leptomeningitis are the most common manifestation of central nervous system involvement (Raphael, 1966). Mild paracoccidiodal arteritis is very common, and aortitis or thrombotic occlusion of the mesenteric vessels may occur. All grades of hepatic and splenic involvement may develop. Paracoccidioidal osteomyelitis, epididymitis, and prostatitis have been reported. Cardiac, renal, and endocrine lesions (other than adrenal) are rare.

### Acute Juvenile Form

In highly endemic areas this syndrome occurs in children and adolescents, probably soon after the primary lung infection. Reticuloendothelial infection predominates, whereas pulmonary and mucosal lesions are very rare. The disease runs an acute course.

Patients complain of malaise, fever, weight loss, and widespread lymphadenopathy. Sometimes generalized pain and hemorrhages are present. The liver and spleen enlarge, and the mesenteric lymph nodes may become so big that they obstruct the intestine. Disseminated skin lesions (acneiform) or subcutaneous abscesses are sometimes present. Chest x-ray may show disseminated miliary foci. Osteolytic lesions are not uncommon. The clinical picture may simulate that of septicemia, leukemia, or lymphoma.

## COMPLICATIONS AND SEQUELAE

The most frequent sequelae result from therapeutic measures. Pulmonary fibrosis may cause "cor pulmonale." Aphonia and dysphonia may result from destructive lesions of the vocal cords. Tracheal or glottic stenosis and microstomy are complications of scar retraction.

## GEOGRAPHIC VARIATIONS

Paracoccidioidomycosis is not uniformly distributed in Latin America. Climatic conditions help determine the extent of this disease throughout a geographic area.

Clinical manifestations of the mycosis present interesting geographic variations in Brazil. Cutaneous and lymphatic lesions are uncommon in the south but very frequent in the central and eastern parts of the country. Gastrointestinal manifestations of the disease are frequently reported in patients from the central Brazilian plateau, but they are very rare in the southern area. The reverse is true for the pulmonary lesions. The juvenile form of the disease and the osseous manifestations are almost entirely confined to patients in the states of Minas Gerais, Rio de Janeiro, and São Paulo.

## DIAGNOSIS

The diagnosis must be based on the demonstration of P. brasiliensis in specimens taken from the lesions. The clinical diagnosis can only be suspected from suggestive mucocutaneous lesions. Paracoccidioidal lung lesions must be differentiated from tuberculosis, histoplasmosis, and nonspecific respiratory infections. The disseminated forms, especially when lesions are confined to a system or organ, present such variable manifestations that differential diagnosis is almost impossible. The juvenile form of the infection must be differentiated from septicemias and lymphomas.

### Laboratory Diagnosis

Mycologic diagnosis is very simple when there is easy access to such lesions as mucocutaneous ulcers, suppurating lymph nodes, and productive lung infection. Scrapings of mucocutaneous lesions, exudate, pus, sputum, bronchial washing, organic fluids, tissues taken for biopsy, and feces should be examined in a drop of 10 per cent potassium hydroxide. Before examination, organic fluids and sodium hydroxide-treated sputum can be centrifuged (Lopes, 1955). P. brasiliensis is a large, 10 to 40 $\mu$, double-walled, round organism with multiple buds (Fig. 5).

### Cultures

Pus, exudate, centrifugal body fluids, and tissues used in biopsies should be incubated on Mycosel agar at both 25 and 35° C. Isolates of this fastidious fungus should be identified on the basis of the dimorphic forms seen at 25 and 35° C. Sputum and feces should be inoculated intratesticularly into guinea pigs, and the aspirated pus from the animal should then be cultured.

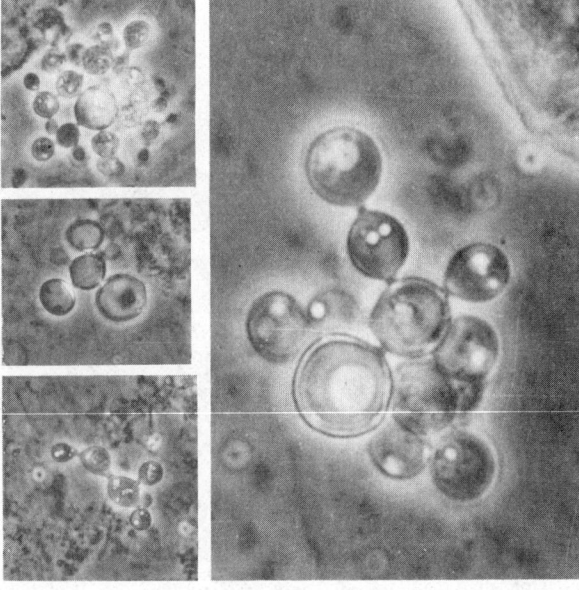

**FIGURE 5.** *Multibudding forms of* P. brasiliensis *in sputum.* ×250 *and* ×60

### Serologic Diagnosis

Serologic tests are helpful in patients whose lesions are difficult to approach. The immunodiffusion test is the most useful test because of its simplicity and specificity (Yarzabal et al., 1978; Restrepo, 1966). Immunoelectrophoresis and counterimmunoelectrophoresis give quicker results than immunodiffusion but are used in only a few laboratories. All these tests have high sensitivity and specificity when a good antigen is used. Recently, Restrepo and Moncada (1978) introduced the latex agglutination test. It can be used more widely, but its sensitivity is 70 per cent, and it gives cross-reactions with sera of patients with histoplasmosis. The complement fixation test is more useful for prognostic purposes.

## TREATMENT

Three drugs are used in the treatment of paracoccidioidomycosis — sulfonamides, amphotericin B, and miconazole (Stevens, 1977).

Among the sulfonamides, sulfadiazine, sulfamethoxypiridazine, and sulfamethoxine are used most often. Sulfadoxine and sulfamethoxazol plus trimethoprim have also been used. They are administered in the usual dosage for bacterial infections. Treatment is given for one or more months, and then the dose is reduced by half and continued for two to five years more. Amphotericin B has been used less often. It is given in a dose of 0.5 mg per kg intravenously every other day for a total dose of 1.5 to 2.0 g. A combination of sulfonamides with amphotericin B has also been recommended. Miconazole was introduced more recently. It is administered intravenously in a dose of 200 mg (diluted in 5 per cent glucose solution) and orally at the same time in a dose of 3 g daily for 20 days. Then oral treatment is continued in a dose of 3 g daily for 40 days, and finally half of this dose is used for two years or more.

The criteria of cure cannot be based on the clinical and radiologic disappearance of the lesions, because relapses are the rule when treatment is stopped. Serologic criteria of cure are based on a fall in titer to zero or to low stable levels (serologic scar). It is important to note that clinical, radiologic, or serologic cure does not mean mycologic cure.

## PROPHYLAXIS

Paracoccidioidomycosis is acquired by inhalation of the spores of *P. brasiliensis,* which lives in soil (Albornoz, 1971). Environmental conditions associated with its presence are still unknown; for that reason, prophylactic measures cannot be suggested.

### References

Albornoz, M. B.: Isolation of *Paracoccidioides brasiliensis* from rural soil in Venezuela. Sabouraudia 9:248, 1971.

Angulo-Ortega, A.: Calcifications in paracoccidioidomycosis. Are they the morphological manifestations of subclinical infection. *In* Pan American Health Organization: Paracoccidioidomycosis. Scientific Publication No. 254. Washington, D.C., 1972, p. 129.

Balabanov, K., Balabanoff, V. A., and Angelov, N.: Blastomycose sud-americaine chez un laboureur bulgare revenu depuis 30 ans de Brésil. Mycopathologia 24:265, 1964.

Castro, R. M., Cucé, L., and Fava-Netto, C.: Paracoccidioidomicose: Inoculação acidental in "anima nobili." Relato de um caso. Med Cutan Iber Lat Am 4:289, 1975.

Londero, A. T., Ramos, C. D., and Lopes, J. O.: Progressive pulmonary paracoccidioidomycosis. A study of 34 cases observed in Rio Grande do Sul (Brazil). Mycopathologia 63:53, 1978.

Lopes, O. S. S.: Descrição de uma técnica de concentração para pesquisa do *Paracoccidioides brasiliensis* no escarro. Hospital (Rio) 47:557, 1955.

Mackinnon, J. E.: Miositis en la blastomicosis suramericana y en la histoplasmosis. Mycopathologia 15:171, 1961.

Marsiglia, I., and Pinto, J.: Adrenal cortical insufficiency associated with paracoccidioidomycosis (South American blastomycosis). J Clin Endocrinol 26:1109, 1966.

Murray, H. W., Littman, M. L., and Roberts, R. B.: Disseminated paracoccidioidomycosis (South American blastomycosis) in the United States. Am J Med 56:209, 1974.

Raphael, A.: Localização nervosa na blastomicose sul-americana. Arq Neuropsiquiatr 24:69, 1966.

Restrepo, A.: La prueba de immunodiffusion en el diagnostico de la paracoccidioidomicosis. Sabouraudia 4:223, 1966.

Restrepo, A.: Paracoccidioidomicosis. Acta Med Colombiana 3:33, 1978.

Restrepo, A., and Moncada, L. H.: Una prueba de latex en lamina para el diagnostico de la paracoccidioidomicosis. Bol Panam 84:520, 1978.

Severo, L. C., Geyer, G. R., Londero, A. T., Porto, N. S., and Rizzon, C. F. C.: The primary pulmonary lymph node complex in paracoccidioidomycosis. Mycopathologia 67:115, 1979a.

Severo, L. C., Londero, A. T., Geyer, G. R., and Porto, N. S.: Acute pulmonary paracoccidioidomycosis in an immunosuppressed patient. Mycopathologia 68:171, 1979b.

Stevens, D. A.: Miconazole in the treatment of systemic fungal infections (editorial). Am Rev Resp Dis 116:801, 1977.

Yarzabal, L. A., Albornoz, M., Cabral, M., and Santiago, A. R.: Specific double diffusion microtechnique for the diagnosis of aspergillosis and paracoccidioidomycosis using monospecific antisera. Sabouraudia 16:55, 1978.

# 119 HISTOPLASMOSIS

George A. Sarosi, M.D., F.A.C.P.
Scott F. Davies, M.D.

## DEFINITION

Histoplasmosis refers to infection by the pathogenic fungus *Histoplasma capsulatum*. Exposure occurs by inhalation of organisms living in the soil. Although the primary infection is in the lung, *Histoplasma* may cause a wide variety of clinical manifestations because of its tendency to invade the bloodstream during the primary infection and its capacity under favorable conditions to cause progressive disease in one or multiple sites.

Infection by the related fungus *Histoplasma duboisii* (African histoplasmosis) also probably occurs via respiratory exposure to the organism in the soil. The yeast form is much larger than that of *Histoplasma capsulatum*. Spread to bone and skin is common. The clinical features of this illness resemble North American blastomycosis more than histoplasmosis caused by *Histoplasma capsulatum* (Williams et al., 1971).

## ETIOLOGY

*Histoplasma capsulatum* is a dimorphic fungus that grows on Sabouraud's medium at 25° C as a fluffy white mycelium bearing characteristic macroconidia ("tuberculate chlamydospores"). The organism is free-living in nature in this mycelial phase. In contrast, at 37° C on blood agar and in infected mammalian tissue, the fungus grows as an oval budding yeast 2 to 4 microns in diameter. The organism is identified in the laboratory by conversion of the isolate from the mycelial to the yeast phase and by demonstration of typical tuberculate chlamydospores in microscopic mounts of the mycelial phase. Small laboratory animals can be infected by intraperitoneal injections of either clinical specimens (treated with penicillin) or suspensions of culture. The organism can be isolated from the spleen or liver of infected animals after sacrifice three to four weeks after infection.

## PATHOGENESIS AND PATHOLOGY

The concentration of *Histoplasma* in the soil varies widely from site to site even within a highly endemic area. Excrement of chickens, starlings, pigeons, and other wild birds provides an excellent growth medium, although birds are

protected from infection by their high body temperature. Bat droppings also support the growth of *Histoplasma*.

In highly endemic areas infection is nearly universal in humans and is common in wild and domestic animals. A minor disturbance of contaminated soil is enough to scatter spores in the air. Inhalation of spores may cause patchy areas of interstitial pneumonitis. The spores undergo metamorphosis to yeast cells, which are engulfed by macrophages and multiply intracellularly with a generation time of 11 hours (Howard, 1965). The regional lymph nodes are quickly involved, and hematogenous spread occurs. The fungus is cleared from the blood by reticuloendothelial cells throughout the body. Specific lymphocyte-mediated cellular immunity develops within 7 to 14 days and rapidly limits the infection both in the lung and at distant sites (Howard et al., 1971). Necrosis and granuloma formation occur at sites of infection. Humoral antibody also develops but is of little importance in limiting infection. Hyperimmune serum is of no benefit in experimental infection; hypogammaglobulinemic patients are not more prone to progressive infection.

The histology of the individual lesions depends on the adequacy of the immune response. In overwhelming infections, macrophages are crowded with organisms with little surrounding tissue reaction. In contrast, when the primary disease is limited by normal defenses, pulmonary and reticuloendothelial granulomas are well developed with only rare organisms, central necrosis, and dense surrounding fibrosis (Straub and Schwarz, 1955). Multinucleated giant cells may be seen. Eventual calcification of individual foci may lead to characteristic small scattered calcifications in the liver, spleen, and lung (Fig. 1). Although organisms are routinely seen on histopathologic examination of healed granulomas, organisms can only rarely be cultivated from these lesions.

## CLINICAL MANIFESTATIONS

Infection with *Histoplasma capsulatum* was first described in 1906 by Samuel Darling, who found a disseminated infection of the reticuloendothelial organs with an organism that he thought to be protozoan at autopsy of a laborer working on the Panama Canal. Sporadic autopsy

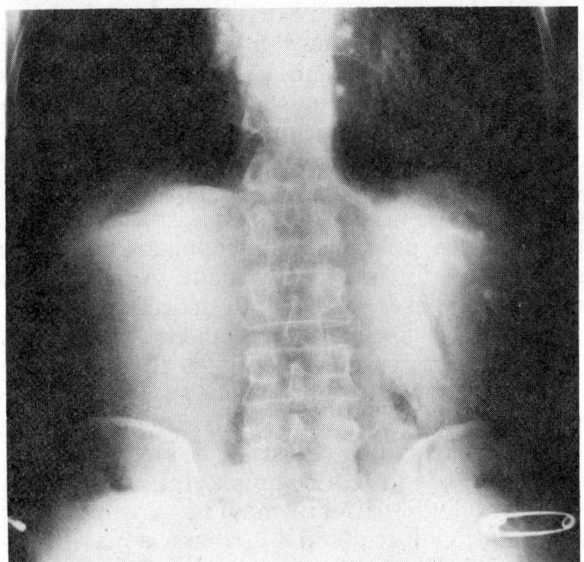

**FIGURE 1.** *The abdominal flat film of a patient from an area endemic for* Histoplasma capsulatum *shows scattered calcifications in the liver, lung, and spleen. There was no history of previous symptomatic pulmonary or systemic infection. The calcifications reflect healing of primary lesions that were associated with a benign fungemia. They are not indicators of true dissemination.*

reports of similar cases followed. In 1934 the first premortem diagnosis of such a patient was made by finding the characteristic intracellular organisms on a peripheral blood smear. DeMonbreun isolated the infecting agent from this patient and proved that it was a fungus. In 1945 Christie and Peterson and Palmer, using antigen derived from this first isolate, demonstrated the totally unexpected finding that great numbers of asymptomatic people in the central United States had been previously infected with the fungus. Skin test reactions to the antigen correlated with the presence of pulmonary calcifications in individuals who did not respond to tuberculin skin tests.

Most of the histoplasmin skin test reactors in these early surveys had had asymptomatic primary infections. However, the retrospective discovery of a highly symptomatic but also self-limited form of pulmonary histoplasmosis soon followed. Small groups of patients exposed to high concentrations of organisms at a variety of point sources had been described in the earlier literature as victims of an unknown epidemic pulmonary illness. An epidemiologic investigation of one such outbreak in a military camp in 1944 demonstrated convincingly that *Histoplasma capsulatum* had been the offending pathogen. Follow-up six years after the outbreak revealed that 16 of 21 men had scattered punctate pulmonary calcifications on chest radiographs and that all had positive histoplasmin skin tests (Grayston and Furcolow, 1953). Furthermore, *Histoplasma capsulatum* was cultured from the storm cellar where the soldiers

initially had been infected. Epidemiologic investigations of other outbreaks were similarly successful.

It had been believed for 40 years that histoplasmosis was a universally fatal illness. The discovery that it was a very common, usually benign, and remarkably self-limited infection opened the way for further understanding of its varied clinical manifestations. The known forms of the disease (Goodwin and Des Prez, 1973) are discussed below.

### Primary Pulmonary Histoplasmosis

If exposure is light, pulmonary histoplasmosis may be totally asymptomatic. Nevertheless, chest roentgenograms, even in asymptomatic cases, may show patchy, nonsegmental areas of pneumonitis mainly involving the lower lobes. Hilar adenopathy is common and tends to be more prominent than in primary tuberculosis. Pleural effusions are distinctly uncommon.

A heavier exposure may cause a nonspecific influenza-like illness with fever, chills, myalgias, headache, and a nonproductive cough. Pleuritic pain occurs in a minority of patients. Symptoms, if present, follow exposure by one to two weeks. Regardless of the presence or absence of symptoms, it is at this time that primary fungemia generally occurs. Organisms can on occasion be recovered from the blood and bone marrow at this stage of infection without implying that there will be progressive dissemination. Following heavy exposure, more diffuse pulmonary involvement may occur, with an extensive micronodular infiltrate on the roentgenogram. In a normal person, the entire process usually resolves quickly. Rarely it may continue for weeks to months with a remitting and relapsing course. Calcified granulomas, the residue of the primary fungemia, are commonly demonstrated postmortem in spleens and livers of patients from endemic areas.

The chest roentgenogram usually returns to normal after the primary pulmonary infection. However, a variety of benign residual abnormalities can be seen. The initial infiltrates may "harden" and leave one or several nodules. These "histoplasmomas" may grow slowly over a period of months to years. Central necrosis may lead to a dense core of calcium (a "target" lesion), but this is not universal. Infrequently, alternate periods of activity followed by healing may result in characteristic concentric rings of calcium as the lesion slowly enlarges. Lymph node calcification, either in association with a histoplasmoma or as a solitary finding, is common. Finally, small, punctate, "buckshot" calcifications may be scattered over both lung fields, a pattern very characteristic of healed primary histoplasmosis (Fig. 2).

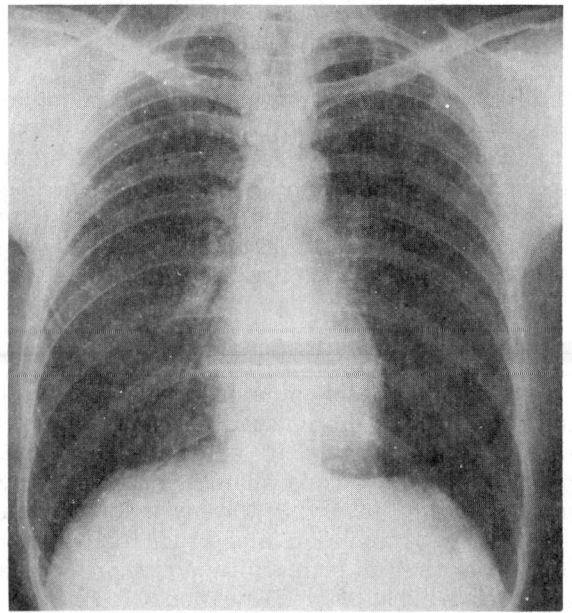

**FIGURE 2.** *The chest roentgenogram of a patient from an endemic area shows extensive calcifications characteristic of old primary histoplasmosis. The exact time of the primary infection could not be determined by history, despite the striking residual roentgenographic abnormality.*

Large epidemics have been associated with excavation of infected soil for construction of roads or buildings. The association of erythema nodosum and erythema multiforme with acute histoplasmosis was first appreciated during investigations of these epidemics. Careful follow-up studies of these patients have revealed that progressive dissemination after a primary respiratory infection is exceedingly rare. Only one case of disseminated disease was seen among more than 6000 cases in an urban epidemic. In one more recent urban epidemic, however, nearly 10 per cent of infections resulted in dissemination (Ajello et al., 1971).

Immunity is incomplete. Heavy exposure at a later date can result in a second illness with an earlier onset and a shorter symptomatic period. There has been some speculation that this shorter illness may have an allergic component. Serial studies of individuals in endemic areas demonstrate waxing and waning of both skin test positivity and the serologic titers, which suggests that periodic re-exposure to the organism results in asymptomatic immunogenic infections.

### Chronic Cavitary Histoplasmosis

Upper lobe cavitary histoplasmosis closely resembles reinfection tuberculosis in roentgenographic appearance. In fact, it was first described among sanitorium patients being treated for pre-

sumed tuberculosis (Furcolow and Brasher, 1956). However, the mechanism of infection is not endogenous reactivation, as it is in tuberculosis. Rather, cavitary histoplasmosis is the direct result of a progressive primary infection.

Cavitary histoplasmosis usually occurs in middle-aged male smokers with structural changes of centrilobular emphysema. In most cases, acute pulmonary histoplasmosis in this setting usually resolves without sequelae. In a minority of cases, infected air spaces persist and lead to a progressive, fibrosing cavitary process, which requires specific antifungal chemotherapy. Although bilateral upper lobe involvement is most characteristic, cavitary disease may occur in any part of the lung (Goodwin et al., 1976).

Chronic cough is a common clinical presentation, although patients may be asymptomatic. Constitutional symptoms increase as the illness progresses. Weight loss is usual in far advanced disease. Fever may not be present.

The coexistence of cavitary histoplasmosis with either tuberculosis or bronchogenic carcinoma is common. In one large retrospective study of cavitary histoplasmosis, 20 per cent of the cases simultaneously also had one of these other diseases (Parker et al., 1970).

### Disseminated Histoplasmosis

Disseminated histoplasmosis refers to any progressive extrapulmonary infection with *Histoplasma capsulatum*. It may occur as an overwhelming postprimary spread with very little cellular inflammatory reaction despite the presence of massive numbers of organisms. This pattern has been seen most often in very young children and is called the infantile form. Among adults, dissemination is most common in the elderly. Adults usually demonstrate more of an inflammatory reaction with fewer organisms and definite granuloma formation. The disease in adults may follow a smoldering subacute course.

Disseminated histoplasmosis can present as an opportunistic infection in the immunosuppressed patient. High-dose glucocorticoid therapy is an important predisposing factor (Davies et al., 1977). In the immunosuppressed child, dissemination usually follows a primary pulmonary infection. In the immunosuppressed adult, there is usually no history of a preceding respiratory illness, and the mechanism of infection may be an endogenous reactivation. The degree of granulomatous response in the immunosuppressed patient may vary from almost none (the "infantile" form) to a considerable amount.

Glucocorticoids may also limit the ability of a normal patient to control a primary pulmonary infection. Patients who are not immunosuppressed initially but who are given glucocorticoids during an undiagnosed primary *Histoplasma* infection (often for a presumed diagnosis of sarcoidosis) may develop progressive systemic illness.

Only about half of patients with disseminated histoplasmosis present with cough, dyspnea, or other pulmonary symptoms. The chest roentgenogram may be normal or may show a diffuse interstitial infiltrate that suggests a hematogenous process. Although at least a third of patients with normal immunity will have a localized interstitial infiltrate on chest roentgenogram, such a finding is unusual in the immunosuppressed adult.

Other clinical features of disseminated histoplasmosis include high fever, hepatosplenomegaly, and lymphadenopathy. Skin lesions include mucocutaneous ulcerations that are often painful and subcutaneous nodules. Ulcerative lesions of the tongue, palate, epiglottis, and larynx are particularly characteristic. Since primary inoculation of the skin is most unusual, skin lesions nearly always imply dissemination.

Involvement of the adrenal glands in disseminated histoplasmosis must be emphasized; adrenal hypofunction is a significant cause of mortality (Sarosi et al., 1971). Adrenal granulomas are regularly found at autopsy in the more reactive forms of disseminated histoplasmosis.

Diarrhea secondary to involvement of the gastrointestinal tract is uncommon but can be a prominent symptom. Hemorrhage and perforation have occurred. The infection can mimic granulomatous colitis.

The clinical picture of disseminated histoplasmosis is extremely variable and quite nonspecific. Fever is the only constant finding. Diagnosis depends on demonstration of the organism in histopathologic material or on culture from clinical specimens. Early diagnosis is important because specific therapy is generally effective if the patient survives long enough to receive an adequate course.

Laboratory findings may include anemia, leucopenia, and thrombocytopenia. Liver function tests may be abnormal; an elevated alkaline phosphatase is most characteristic. Disseminated intravascular coagulation occurs rarely.

Other cases of progressive extrapulmonary histoplasmosis present with a more localized infection. These include central nervous system histoplasmoma, endocarditis, pericarditis, and isolated gastrointestinal histoplasmosis, usually involving the terminal ileum. These cases may represent instances of endogenous reactivation in which the inability to contain the organism is more focal.

## GEOGRAPHIC VARIATIONS IN DISEASE

*Histoplasma capsulatum* has been isolated from the soil in more than 50 countries. It is most common in temperate climates along river valleys and has been found in North, Central, and South America, India, and Southeast Asia. It is rare in Europe and practically nonexistent in Australia.

However, it must be noted that despite a worldwide distribution, the Ohio and Mississippi River valleys in the central United States represent a unique area of heavy concentration of the fungus. In this region there are 500,000 pulmonary infections annually and a total of perhaps 40,000,000 persons with previous infection. More than 90 per cent of adults are skin-test positive, and the organism can be demonstrated at autopsy in more than 70 per cent of cases. A similar situation has not been demonstrated in any other area.

*Histoplasma duboisii* is apparently limited to Africa. Most reports have been from the West African nations of Nigeria, Zaire, and Senegal. *Histoplasma capsulatum* has also been found in Africa, but isolates have been very uncommon.

## COMPLICATIONS AND SEQUELAE

A common sequela of primary histoplasmosis is the presence on chest roentgenogram of a "coin lesion," which must be differentiated from bronchogenic carcinoma. Central calcification or concentric rings of calcium are helpful; if present, these findings exclude malignancy. If there is no calcification, thoracotomy may be necessary, especially if old roentgenograms are not available or the lesion is enlarging.

Uncommon local complications within the chest due to direct extension of the active inflammatory process include fibrosing mediastinitis, which can cause the superior vena cava syndrome, and pericarditis, which can lead to pericardial calcification. The esophagus can also be involved by direct extension of the inflammatory process from adjacent lymph nodes causing dysphagia, traction diverticula, or even frank abscess.

Rarely, old inactive histoplasmosis can also lead to complications. Broncholiths may develop when calcified nodes erode into the bronchial tree. Hemoptysis is common in this setting.

Focal areas of posterior uveitis known as "histospots" are a significant ophthalmologic problem and may lead to blindness. They occur in areas endemic for histoplasmosis, but their precise pathogenesis is uncertain.

In the absence of active dissemination, healed granulomas involving the adrenals may be the cause of Addison's disease in some cases. The presentation is that of primary adrenal insufficiency, not infection.

## DIAGNOSIS

The diagnosis of acute pulmonary histoplasmosis in an endemic area is suggested by a history of exposure to an aerosol of contaminated soil in a patient with compatible clinical and roentgenologic findings. A positive skin test and rising complement-fixing antibodies against yeast and mycelial antigens are confirmatory. Skin testing is performed with histoplasmin, a mycelial antigen. The skin test is generally positive two weeks after initial exposure and remains positive for years. Serologic titers against yeast and mycelial antigens are elevated at three to four weeks in most cases. They usually decrease over 3 to 12 months but occasionally remain high for many years. Nonetheless, titers against the yeast antigen of 1:16 or greater in the appropriate clinical setting are highly suggestive of recent infection. A rising titer is diagnostic. Unlike the situation in coccidioidomycosis (see Chapter 120), a high titer during primary infection is not a bad prognostic sign.

Chronic cavitary histoplasmosis is easier to diagnose. Skin tests and serologic titers are almost invariably positive, and the organism is routinely found in the sputum. However, the coexistence of tuberculosis or carcinoma is not uncommon.

Diagnosis of disseminated histoplasmosis depends on a high index of suspicion. Adult cases are not limited to endemic areas, suggesting endogenous reactivation as the mechanism of some infections. Skin tests and the complement fixation titers are negative in more than half the patients. Histoplasmosis must be included in the differential diagnosis of illnesses with hectic fever in immunosuppressed patients and of progressive systemic infections in infants who live in endemic areas. Organisms may be seen on smears of peripheral blood or grown from routine blood cultures if they are incubated for 10 to 15 days. Bone marrow aspirates yield organisms on direct smear or by culture in almost 70 per cent of patients. Liver biopsy is helpful. Biopsies of mucosal and skin lesions should be performed. Urine cultures are occasionally positive. All tissue obtained should be stained specifically for fungus with Gomori's methenamine silver or the periodic acid-Schiff techniques. Yeast forms can be missed on routine hematoxylin and eosin sections.

Several diagnostic pitfalls must be noted. A histoplasmin skin test can stimulate the formation of antibody to histoplasma antigens, especially if the patient had unrecognized primary histoplasmosis in the past. This booster response peaks by the end of the second week following the skin test. The titer rise is greater to the mycelial antigen than to the yeast phase antigen. Although the titer is usually higher to the yeast phase in primary pulmonary infection, blood for serologic tests should be obtained before the skin test is placed.

Another significant problem is that of cross-reactivity between the antigens for *Histoplasma capsulatum*, *Blastomyces dermatitidis*, *Coccidioides immitis*, and other common fungi. Although the antibody response to the specific etiologic agent is usually more marked than the response to cross-reacting organisms, positive skin tests and serologic titers against other fungi can be expected.

## THERAPY AND PROPHYLAXIS

No treatment is required for the usual primary pulmonary infection. Amphotericin B may be used for severe primary infections in which exposure is unusually heavy or patients are febrile for longer than three weeks. A total course of 500 mg (given as 1 mg/kg every other day) may be adequate, but this has not been well studied. Very rarely, a massive primary exposure may result in acute respiratory failure with marked hypoxia. Oxygenation and ventilatory support may be required; the use of amphotericin B is mandatory. Isolation of patients with histoplasmosis is not necessary because human-to-human transmission does not occur.

No therapy is required after excision of a solitary pulmonary nodule that proves to be a histoplasmoma.

Progressive chronic cavitary histoplasmosis requires full therapy with amphotericin B. This can be given in a dose of 1 mg/kg (not to exceed 50 mg) every other day for a total dose of 35 to 40 mg/kg. It may be necessary to treat some patients longer (Parker et al., 1970).

Disseminated histoplasmosis must also be treated with a minimum dose of 40 mg/kg of amphotericin B over many weeks. The response is gratifying if therapy is started early (Sarosi et al., 1971).

There is no effective immunization against histoplasmosis. Efforts to decontaminate the soil are too expensive to be practical on a widespread basis. However, 3 per cent formaldehyde spray has been used successfully to sterilize localized areas.

## References

Ajello, L., Chick, E. W., and Furcolow, M. L. (eds.): Histoplasmosis. Proceedings of the Second National Conference. Springfield, Ill., Charles C Thomas, 1971.

Christie, A., and Peterson, J. C.: Pulmonary calcification in negative reactors to tuberculin. Am J Pub Health 35:1131, 1945.

Darling, S. T.: Protozoan general infection producing pseudotubercles in the lungs and focal necrosis in liver, spleen and lymph nodes. JAMA 46:1283, 1906.

Davies, S. F., Khan, M., and Sarosi, G. A.: Histoplasmosis in immunologically suppressed patients. Occurrence in a non-endemic area. Am J Med 64:94, 1978.

DeMonbreun, W. A.: The cultivation and cultural characteristics of Darling's *H. capsulatum*. Am J Trop Med 14:93, 1934.

Furcolow, M. L., and Brasher, C. A.: Chronic progressive (cavitary) histoplasmosis as a problem in tuberculosis sanitoriums. Am Rev Tuberc Pul Dis 73:609, 1956.

Goodwin, R. A., and DesPrez, R. M.: Pathogenesis and clinical spectrum of histoplasmosis. South Med J 66:13, 1973.

Goodwin, R. A., Owens, F. T., Snell, J. D., Hubbard, W. W., Buchanan, R. D., Terry, R. T., and DesPrez, R. M.: Chronic pulmonary histoplasmosis. Medicine 55:413, 1976.

Grayston, J. T., and Furcolow, M. L.: Occurrence of histoplasmosis in epidemics: Epidemiological studies. Am J Pub Health 43:665, 1953.

Howard, D. H.: Intracellular growth of *Histoplasma capsulatum*. J Bacteriol 89:518, 1965.

Howard, D. H., Otto, V., Guptka, R. K.: Lymphocyte-mediated cellular immunity in histoplasmosis. Infect Immun 4:605, 1971.

Palmer, C. E.: Non-tuberculosis pulmonary calcification and sensitivity to histoplasmin. Pub Health Rep 60:513, 1945.

Parker, J. D., Sarosi, G. A., Doto, I. L., Bailey, R. E., and Tosh, F. E.: Treatment of chronic pulmonary histoplasmosis. A National Communicable Disease Center cooperative mycoses study. N Engl J Med 283:225, 1970.

Sarosi, G. A., Voth, D. W., Dahl, B. A., Doto, I. L., and Tosh, F. E.: Disseminated histoplasmosis: Results of a long-term follow-up. A center for Disease Control cooperative mycoses study. Ann Intern Med 75:511, 1971.

Silverman, R. N., Schwarz, J., Lahey, M. E., and Carson, R. P.: Histoplasmosis. Am J Med 19:410, 1955.

Straub, M., and Schwarz, J.: The healed primary complex in histoplasmosis. Am J Clin Pathol 25:727, 1955.

Williams, A. O., Lawson, E. A., and Lucas, A. O.: African histoplasmosis due to *Histoplasma duboisii*. Arch Pathol 92:306, 1971.

# *COCCIDIOIDOMYCOSIS* **120**

## *Abraham I. Braude, Ph.D., M.D.*

### *DEFINITION*

Coccidioidomycosis is a pulmonary and disseminated infection of respiratory origin caused by the soil-resident fungus *Coccidioides immitis*. The infection occurs in man and animals and is endemic in arid regions of the Americas.

### *ETIOLOGY*

The etiologic agent is the pathogenic fungus *C. immitis*, which occurs in the soil in the Lower Sonoran life zone of the Southwestern United States and in similar desert regions of Mexico (Gonzales-Ochoa, 1967), and Central and South America (Negroni, 1967). These geographic areas are characterized botanically by the presence of the creosote bush. *C. immitis* is adapted to the high salinity and alkaline pH in these soil areas.

The fungus is dimorphic, replicating in the soil in the mycelial phase and in tissue in the spherule phase. In the soil, the mycelium is composed of long hyphae 2 to 4 $\mu$ in diameter, which subsequently fragment into highly resistant barrel-shaped arthrospores.

During the summer months, the intensely hot air sterilizes the surface soil of *C. immitis*, but the fungus remains viable in the subsurface layer and in rodent burrows. After rainfall, surface growth of *C. immitis* is stimulated, and numerous arthrospores are formed. These arthrospores become airborne with winds or when the soil is disturbed during excavation or construction.

The airborne arthrospores are the infectious units of the fungus, and inhalation initiates the infection. Each arthrospore develops into a spherule, or sporangium, which may reach a diameter of 36 to 60 $\mu$ (Fig. 1). Within the spherule numerous sporangiospores 2 to 5 $\mu$ in diameter are formed. These spores are released when the spherules rupture, resulting in spread of infection within the host.

### *PATHOGENESIS AND PATHOLOGY*

Infection is almost invariably the result of inhalation of the arthrospores from soil. The organisms are phagocytosed by pulmonary macrophages and replicate within these host cells in the form of spherules. A few cases of percutaneous inoculation coccidioidomycosis, usually laboratory acquired, have been reported.

The basic host defense against *C. immitis* is cell-mediated immunity in the form of delayed hypersensitivity. In the majority of patients, such immunity appears within a few weeks of the onset of symptoms. During the early phase of the infection, the fungus replicates unrestricted in the macrophages. However, with the development of cell-mediated immunity, the macrophages become activated and kill the ingested fungi. This acquired immunity is reflected in a positive delayed hypersensitivity skin test to coccidioides skin-test reagent.

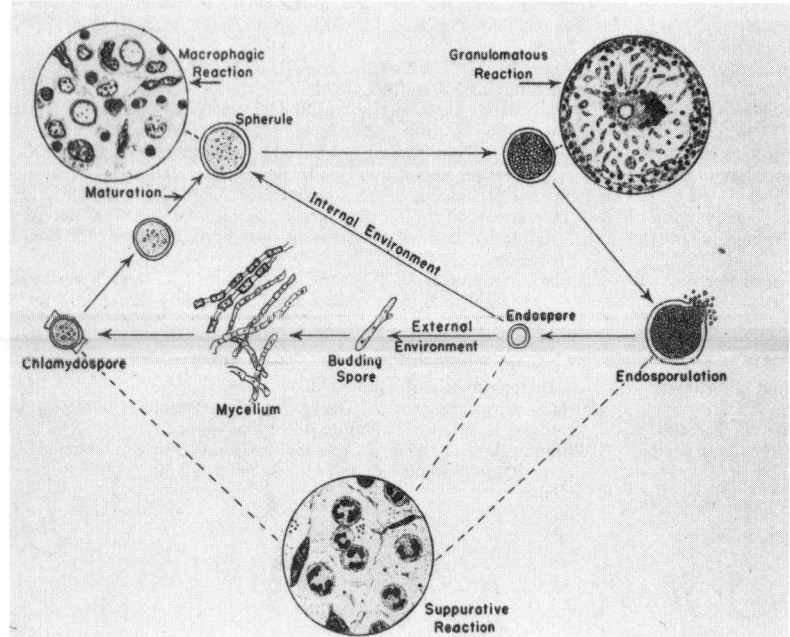

**FIGURE 1.** *Life cycle of Coccidioides immitis and related histologic response (from Forbus and Bestebreurtje, 1946).*

In a minority of patients, cell-mediated immunity to the fungus appears to be defective, delayed, or absent. In such cases, either active chronic pulmonary lesions persist, or hematogenous dissemination to other organs occurs. In patients with either of these two progressive forms of infection, the basic host defect is cell-mediated anergy specifically to *C. immitis* antigens. This defect appears to involve the thymus-dependent (T) lymphocyte. The skin-test response, lymphocyte-transformation test, and macrophage-immobilizing factor test to coccidioidin are all negative. In addition, histologic examination of coccidioidin skin-test sites in these patients show only polymorphonuclear leukocytes and macrophages but not the lymphocyte response seen in skin-test-positive patients. In contrast to the specific anergy to coccidioidin that accompanies progressive coccidioidomycosis, the thymus-dependent immune system is otherwise intact, as evidenced by normal in vitro lymphocyte responses to the nonspecific lymphocyte mitogen phytohemagglutinin and positive in vitro lymphocyte transformation and delayed hypersensitivity skin-test responses to other antigens. In some patients who are particularly ill with progressive disseminated coccidioidomycosis, there is also a depression in cell-mediated immune response to noncoccidioidal antigens, which probably reflects a nonspecific effect of overwhelming illness and is of a different mechanism from the basic *Coccidioides*-specific immune defect. In the minority of patients with disseminated infection that recover, cell-mediated immunity to coccidioidin develops, and in those patients who demonstrate nonspecific depression of thymus-dependent reactivity to other antigens, such reactivity reappears.

The basic pathologic response to coccidioidomycosis is the granuloma (Forbus and Bestebreurtje, 1946). Initially, polymorphonuclear leukocytes enter the site of infection, followed by monocytes and lymphocytes and occasional plasma cells. In lesions, the characteristic *C. immitis* spherules, both intact and ruptured, can be seen. As the spherule ruptures, polymorphonuclear cells swarm around the extruded endospores but are usually ineffectual and are replaced by the granuloma (Baker and Braude, 1956).

The disease is not contagious because the spherule and endospores released from lesions apparently cannot survive in the external environment. For this reason, isolation procedures during the treatment of patients with coccidioidomycosis are not required. However, transmission to hospital personnel via organisms that had reverted to the mycelial phase on a plaster cast in a patient with draining osteomyelitis was reported.

## CLINICAL MANIFESTATIONS

Coccidioidomycosis usually presents as an acute to subacute pneumonia, which may be complicated by chronic pulmonary infection or dissemination to other sites and organs. The incubation period is one to four weeks. Studies undertaken in military populations in endemic areas have shown that approximately 60 per cent of *C. immitis* infections are asymptomatic. Of the remaining 40 per cent, the clinical manifestations range from mild undifferentiated respiratory illness to severe pneumonia. The pulmonary infiltrate is usually found in one lower lobe, although multilobar disease also occurs. Fever is invariably present. Cough is frequent although mild, and sputum is scanty and white. Hemoptysis is not common. Pleurisy is also a manifestation of the disease and can be the presenting symptom.

In Caucasians, approximately 5 per cent of males and 24 per cent of females present with allergic manifestations such as rash and arthralgia. The rash ranges in character from a mild pruritic maculopapular eruption, most commonly on the chest and trunk, to erythema nodosum, usually on the lower extremities. The arthralgia was originally termed "desert rheumatism," and the erythema nodosum was called "bumps" before their relation to coccidioidomycosis was discovered. These manifestations are probably based upon *Coccidioides* antigen-antibody reactions.

The course of the primary infection may be protracted, with several weeks to months of debility in varying degrees. The pneumonia usually heals without residual effects, although characteristic thin-walled cavities or small nodules may persist.

## COMPLICATIONS AND SEQUELAE

In those cases in which the primary pulmonary infection fails to heal, either chronic pulmonary lesions or dissemination supervenes.

The pulmonary complications occur in approximately 5 per cent of patients and include cavities and nodules. These lesions may be either inactive or active and resemble chronic pulmonary tuberculosis (Sarosi et al., 1970). These patients have a long history of cough, weight loss, fever, chest pain, and dyspnea, and their sputum is filled with spherules. In most cases, activity is associated with a diminished or absent cell-mediated immune response to the fungus as reflected in the delayed hypersensitivity skin test.

Dissemination via the bloodstream occurs in 0.1 per cent of Caucasians and in up to 1 per cent of blacks and 10 per cent of Filipinos and Orientals. Dissemination in most cases is probably an early event, although it may not be recognized until several months after the onset of pulmonary infection. Dissemination is more common in men than in women. It is a particular hazard in those receiving cytotoxins, immunosuppressants, and corticosteroids. Renal transplant recipients who have diabetes mellitus have a uniquely high incidence of dissemination. Pregnancy also increases the risk of dissemination, although the fetus is usually unaffected (Smale and Waechter, 1970).

Dissemination to the central nervous system is the most ominous form of disease and carries a mortality rate of nearly 100 per cent in untreated patients. The infection presents with the insidious onset of fever, headache, and meningeal signs and runs a course of months to years. The leptomeninges are primarily involved, and only rarely are cerebral lesions such as pituitary abscesses produced. With extensive disease, the ventricles may also be infected.

The spinal fluid is under increased pressure and shows an elevated protein content of about 300 mg per 100 ml. The glucose concentration is usually but not invariably depressed to a level below 40 mg per 100 ml. Leukocytes are present in counts of several hundred/mm$^3$. The cells are usually mononuclear, although polymorphonuclear leukocytes may temporarily predominate with acute or exacerbated disease. The infecting organisms are only rarely seen or cultured in the cerebrospinal fluid.

Hematogenous dissemination may also affect the lungs and may closely resemble miliary tuberculosis. The course may be chronic and progressively downhill or acute, fulminating, and rapidly fatal. Radiography shows diffuse nodular densities in both lungs, and hypoxia may be severe (Fig. 2). Diagnosis can be made in 60 per cent of the cases by liver biopsy, even though the liver is not enlarged and function tests are normal. Transbronchial biopsy may also produce diagnostic material.

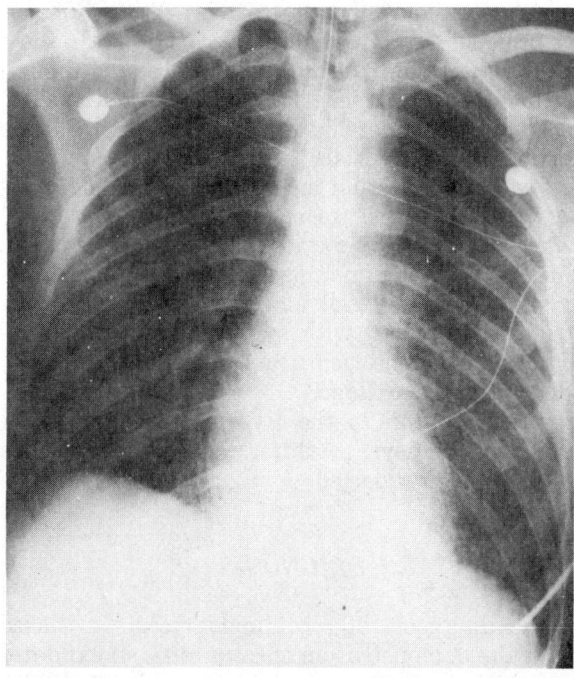

**FIGURE 2.** *Fatal miliary coccidioidomycosis of lung.*

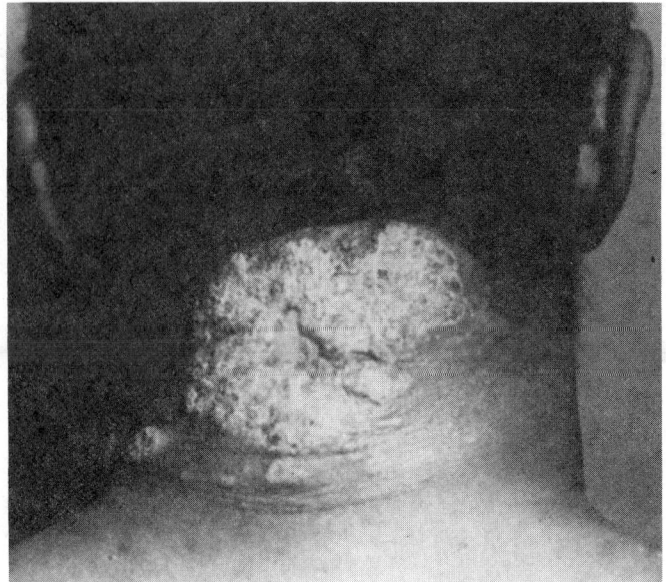

**FIGURE 3.**  *Verrucous skin lesion of coccidioidomycosis.*

Dissemination to the subcutaneous tissue produces large, fluctuant, usually cool, and painless nodules. These lesions are frequently multiple, occur on all parts of the body, and spontaneously drain a whitish, blood-tinged purulent exudate without a distinctive odor. Spherules are abundant in these exudates. Another characteristic skin lesion is the verrucous granuloma resembling that of blastomycosis (Fig. 3).

Osteomyelitis and arthritis also are relatively frequent. All bones are involved, most frequently the spine. The lesions are usually painless and may be associated with overlying subcutaneous lesions. Radiographically, osteomyelitis appears as punched-out areas of rarification with some reactive new bone formation if there is a healing component. Multiple lytic lesions of ribs and skull may resemble metastatic carcinoma or multiple myeloma (Bayer et al., 1976).

The joint infection may cause a chronic monoarticular arthritis (most frequently in the knee) without evidence of coccidioidomycosis elsewhere. The radiographic findings are minimal and usually show no bone involvement. Unless it is recognized and treated with synovectomy and intra-articular amphotericin, the disease will destroy the articular cartilage.

Dissemination to the liver, spleen, adrenals, pituitary, kidneys, prostate, and seminal vesicles have all been reported.

## DIAGNOSIS

The diagnosis of coccidioidomycosis is based upon the demonstration of *C. immitis* in exudates and tissues and measurement of the antibody and delayed hypersensitivity responses of the patient to the fungus.

The infecting spherules and endospores can be seen in simple wet mount preparations of sputum and exudates. In biopsy material the organisms are well stained by PAS and silver stains.

Culture of the organism can be accomplished on routine fungal media such as Sabouraud's agar, but growth is also abundant on blood agar and other routine bacteriologic media. Growth usually requires 5 to 10 days and occurs in the mycelial and arthrospore phase. Culture of *C. immitis* from the urine may be the first clue of disseminated infection and indicates involvement of the kidney, prostate, or epididymis. Culture of the fungus in the spherule phase has been described with Converse medium at 40° C, but the procedure is not used in routine diagnosis. Because arthrospores develop on laboratory media, this organism poses a significant infection risk to laboratory personnel, and cultures must be manipulated with caution and in appropriate isolation equipment.

The delayed hypersensitivity skin-test response is useful in both the diagnosis and the assessment of the prognosis in coccidioidomycosis. The skin-test antigen, coccidioidin, is derived from a filtrate of the mycelial arthrospore phase-grown organisms. The standard dilution is 1:100. Also available is a 1:10 dilution, although this is of use primarily in patients with chronic pulmonary disease who may be anergic to the 1:100 dilution. In addition, a skin-test reagent prepared from spherule-phase organisms is available; however, the role of this material is yet to be defined (Levine et al., 1973).

In patients with self-limiting pulmonary infection, a positive delayed hypersensitivity skin-test response to coccidioidin develops within one to three weeks of the onset of symptoms and persists for life. A positive skin-test response on initial testing is of limited use because it may represent past asymptomatic infection; however, a negative skin-test response followed a short time later by conversion to positivity is diagnostic. The skin-test response and immunity are of lifelong duration.

In patients with dissemination or progressive pulmonary infection, the skin-test response to coccidioidin remains negative. In the minority of patients who recover from the severe complications of disseminated coccidioidomycosis, a positive skin test develops.

In patients with coccidioidomycosis precipitating 19S and complement-fixing 7S antibodies may develop. In about 75 per cent of patients with the self-limiting pulmonary infection, precipitating antibody is detectable. This antibody appears within the first two weeks of symptoms and persists for only three to six months. Complement-fixing antibody, however, appears in only about 25 per cent of patients with self-limiting infection, and when it occurs it is present in titers of less than 1:32. This antibody declines over a period of months to a few years.

In the disseminated disease, precipitating antibody develops in about 50 per cent of patients and wanes within a few months. The complement-fixing antibody develops in the majority of patients with disseminated disease and is present in titers of greater than 1:32. This antibody indicates the status of dissemination because it persists and rises with progressive infection and declines with quiescence or response to treatment.

The cerebrospinal fluid complement-fixing antibody titer is of particular use both in diagnosing meningitis and in monitoring its course. This antibody is produced locally within the central nervous system and is not serum antibody that has passively diffused into the spinal fluid. The spinal fluid complement-fixing antibody may be the first laboratory sign of meningitis, appearing before any other marked abnormality in the spinal fluid. Sequential titers will reflect the natural course of the infection or the response to treatment, a decline being associated with a favorable course.

## TREATMENT

Amphotericin B remains, after 20 years of availability, the mainstay of antifungal chemotherapy in coccidioidomycosis. All strains of *C.* *immitis* are inhibited by amphotericin B, but the drug is not fungicidal in clinically achievable concentrations. In most cases of acute pulmonary infection, amphotericin B is not given because its side effects, particularly nephrotoxicity, are more severe than the self-limiting disease itself. Whether or not early treatment of pulmonary infection might decrease the incidence of chronic pulmonary disease or dissemination has not been evaluated. Nonetheless, it might be prudent to treat pulmonary infection in patients who have a high risk of progressive disease, such as those with dark skin, diabetes mellitus, or underlying lymphoma or leukemia, or those who are receiving cytotoxic or corticosteroid drug therapy. The drug might also be indicated in pregnancy but only after the first trimester, because the effect of amphotericin on the fetus is unknown.

Amphotericin B is frequently used in patients with chronic active pulmonary infection, although this treatment usually only ameliorates symptoms, and repeated courses are required to maintain remission.

Amphotericin B is most clearly indicated in patients with disseminated infection, but unfortunately it is in just such patients that the response to treatment is poorest. In patients with osteomyelitis with multiple lesions, intravenous amphotericin B may be helpful, while in those with single lesions, excision should be performed if possible. Subcutaneous lesions do not usually need surgical drainage because they frequently drain spontaneously.

In chronic pulmonary disease, surgery may be employed, the usual criteria for such intervention being hemoptysis or an enlarging cavity with impending rupture. Because of the presence of occult satellite lesions, lobectomy rather than segmental resection is frequently necessary. Surgery may be complicated by bronchopleural fistulae with empyema and the appearance of new pulmonary lesions in contiguous segments. The use of amphotericin B in the intraoperative period for preventing surgical complications is debatable.

## PROPHYLAXIS

Prevention is based upon avoiding exposure to dust containing arthrospores. Planting fields with grass prevents aerosolization of arthrospores, as does wetting the soil with water or commercial dust retardants.

There is no commercial vaccine, although an experimental vaccine composed of inactivated in vitro cultured spherules is undergoing evaluation (Pappaganis and Levine, 1975).

## References

Baker, O. and Braude, A.: A study of stimuli leading to the production of spherules in coccidioidomycosis. J Lab and Clin Med 47:169, 1956.

Bayer, A., Yoshikawa, T., Galkin, J., and Guze, L.: Unusual syndromes of coccidioidomycosis: Diagnostic and therapeutic considerations. Medicine 55:131, 1976.

Forbus, W., and Bestebreurtje, A.: Coccidioidomycosis: A Study of 95 Cases of the Disseminated Type with Special Reference to the Pathogenesis of the Disease. Mil Surgeon 99:653, 1946.

Gonzales-Ochoa, A.: Coccidioidomycosis in Mexico. In Coccidioidomycosis: Proceedings of Second Coccidioidomycosis Symposium. Tucson, University of Arizona Press, 1967.

Levine, H., Gonzales-Ochoa, A., and Ten Eyck, D.: Dermal hypersensitivity to *Coccidioides* immunity. A comparison of responses elicited in man by spherulum and coccidioidin. Am Rev Resp Dis 107:379, 1973.

Negroni, P.: Coccidioidomycosis in Argentina. In Coccidioidomycosis: Proceedings of Second Coccidioidomycosis Symposium. Tucson, University of Arizona Press, 1967.

Pappagianis, D., and Levine, H.: The present status of vaccination against coccidioidomycosis in man. Am J Epidemiol 102:30, 1975.

Petersen, E., Friedman, B., Crowder, E., and Rifkind, D.: Coccidioiduria: Clinical significance. Ann Intern Med 85:34, 1976.

Sarosi, G., Parker, J., Doto, I., and Tosh, F.: Chronic Pulmonary Coccidioidomycosis: A National Communicable Disease Center Cooperative Mycosis Study. N Engl J Med 283:326, 1970.

Smale, L., and Waechter, K.: Disseminated coccidioidomycosis in pregnancy. Am J Obstet Gynecol 107:356, 1970.

# 121 ASPERGILLOSIS

## George A. Sarosi, M.D., F.A.C.P.

## DEFINITION

Aspergillosis refers to any infectious process caused by one of the numerous members of the genus *Aspergillus*. The vast majority of these human infections are caused by *Aspergillus fumigatus*; occasionally infections are caused by *Aspergillus niger, Aspergillus clavatus, Aspergillus flavus*, or *Aspergillus nidulans*. These fungi have low pathogenicity for immunologically intact humans and will not invade them unless the normal defense mechanisms are weakened by illness or medication. Common sites of infection are the lung, external ear, orbit, and paranasal sinuses. In severely immunocompromised patients dissemination can occur.

## ETIOLOGY

Members of the genus *Aspergillus* are ubiquitous in nature. In addition to their pathogenicity for man and other mammals, some species are infectious for birds, insects, or, more commonly, plants. In nature the fungus grows as an aerial mycelium that releases spores. When these are inhaled, they reach the lung or the upper airway. In the laboratory the fungus will grow well on most media, including Sabouraud's agar, and equally well at room temperature or 35° C. The colonies are fast growing and appear first as white filamentous surface growth on solid media. They quickly become green to dark green as spores are produced. These colonies are composed of segmented mycelia. Expanded, knob-like swellings called conidiophores are located on the ends of specialized mycelia. These conidiophores, or spore-heads, are covered by multiple spores that become airborne when the mycelium is disturbed. Identification of the species of *Aspergillus* that is present is often a difficult task and is usually done on the basis of the morphology of the conidiophores and their spore-bearing surfaces.

## PATHOGENESIS AND PATHOLOGY

After becoming airborne, the infecting spore may settle on some external surface or may be inhaled into the lung. In external otitis caused by *Aspergillus*, there is no tissue invasion. On histopathologic examination the organism is seen in the superficial keratinized layer of the skin, evoking little or no inflammatory response. Occasionally, and usually in debilitated patients, superficial lesions invade the middle ear, paranasal sinuses, and orbit, evoking a mixed polymorphonuclear-macrophage inflammatory exudate with giant cells. Hyphae are scarce in routine hematoxylin-eosin stained sections, but are readily seen in silver stains. Speciation is difficult unless well-preserved conidiophores are seen in the section. Clinically significant involvement of the gastrointestinal tract below the oropharynx is rare, although isolation of *Aspergillus* species from the gut is not. *Aspergillus* may produce multiple deep esophageal or gastrointestinal ulcers that invade the muscularis and occasionally perforate.

In disseminated (or pyemic) aspergillosis, there is widespread necrosis of various organs. Multiple areas of bronchopneumonia occur in the lung where invasion of blood vessels causes thrombosis, infarction, and cavitation. Metastatic abscesses are common in the brain, liver, and heart. Despite this evidence of hematogenous spread, recovery of the organism from blood culture is rare.

*Aspergillus* endocarditis also occurs, usually after cardiac surgery. The vegetations are large, bulky, and friable, and frequently cause distant emboli in major arteries.

Perhaps the most distinctive lesion produced by *Aspergillus* species is the intracavitary fungus ball that is often referred to erroneously as a "mycetoma." These matted masses of aspergilli grow in pre-existing cavities that communicate with bronchi. The fungus ball is composed of mycelia as well as necrotic debris, and the entire mass is often attached at one place to the underlying cavity. The cavity is lined by respiratory epithelium, but outside the fibrous capsule there is a varying amount of mononuclear cell infiltrate, liberally sprinkled with eosinophils. The cavity colonized by the fungus may be an inactive residual lesion that is secondary to tuberculosis, another fungal disease (such as histoplasmosis), sarcoidosis, carcinoma, or bronchiectasis (British Tuberculosis Association, 1968, 1970). The first sign of colonization by *Aspergillus* is usually thickening of the cavity wall, which can be seen in the chest roentgenogram.

*Aspergillus* is also a secondary invader in the pleural cavity. Thus, pleural aspergillosis occurs almost exclusively in established cases of empyema, usually tuberculosis, with a bronchopleural fistula (Krakowka et al., 1970). This form of aspergillosis is more common than the scarcity of publications on it would indicate.

In bronchial allergic aspergillosis the expectorated mucus plugs contain mycelia that are visible to the naked eye in the form of brown or tan flecks interspersed throughout the thick tenacious mucus. When these specks of mycelia are examined as a wet preparation, the characteristic septate hyphae are seen but not the spore-bearing conidiophores. The dilated bronchi contain inspissated mucus in the lumen. The hyphae in the mucus do not invade the bronchial wall. In addition to fungal elements the mucus also contains much eosinophilic debris. The walls of the bronchi are heavily infiltrated by eosinophils as well. In the surrounding pulmonary tissue some of the smaller bronchioles are obliterated by masses of granulation tissue, and the alveoli show focal eosinophilic pneumonia. A special feature of the bronchiectasis in allergic aspergillosis is the normal pattern of many small bronchi and bronchioles beyond the grossly dilated proximal bronchi (Scadding, 1967). Most other diseases causing bronchiectasis produce obliteration of the bronchioles so that the dilated bronchi end blindly and no longer communicate with their alveoli (Fig. 1). There is evidence that the bronchi are damaged by an Arthus-type reaction in which antigen-antibody precipitates are involved. The antigens are derived from the *Aspergillus* mycelium in the mucus plugs. The eosinophilic pneumonia is thought to depend on both reaginic and precipitating antibody for its development.

## CLINICAL MANIFESTATIONS

External otitis usually causes pain, redness, and swelling of the ear. Invasion of a paranasal sinus produces local swelling and redness in the involved area. Marked tenderness in the area of induration suggests osteomyelitis. In the sinuses, nose, and palate the fungus grows as a large, bulky, soft tissue mass that can bleed profusely when touched.

In the syndrome of allergic bronchopulmonary aspergillosis, most of the early symptoms are

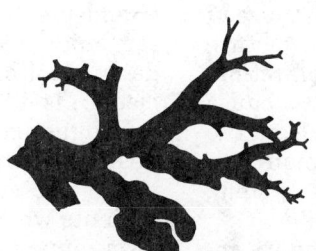

ALLERGIC ASPERGILLOSIS

**FIGURE 1.** *Comparison of bronchograms in different forms of bronchiectasis. In allergic aspergillosis, the dilated bronchi characteristically communicate with normal small bronchi and bronchioles beyond the grossly dilated primary bronchi. Conversely, in postpneumonic staphylococcal and post-tuberculous bronchiectasis, the dilated bronchi usually end blindly. (From Scadding, J. G.: Scand J Resp Dis 48:372, 1967.)*

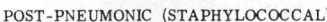

POST-PNEUMONIC (STAPHYLOCOCCAL)

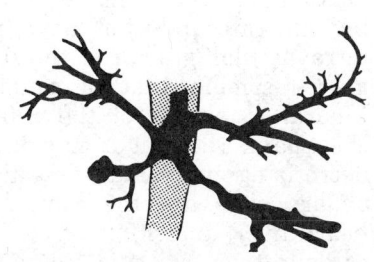

POST-TUBERCULOUS

related to underlying chronic asthma (Henderson, 1968; Hinson et al., 1952). Episodic dyspnea is common. Whereas not all patients with the syndrome have a distinct history of asthma, all have evidence of airway obstruction when carefully tested. As fungi proliferate in the thick asthmatic mucus, they bring on intermittent bouts of increased bronchial obstruction. When this happens, fever and cough are common, and active infiltrates are seen on the chest x-ray. Mucus plugs are frequently expectorated, and pleuritic chest pain and peripheral blood eosinophilia are common. Despite these episodes in the early stages of disease, the patients are relatively asymptomatic between acute exacerbations of bronchial plugging except for the symptoms of underlying asthma. Later, however, repeated attacks of bronchial plugging may result in gradual destruction of the bronchial mucosa, and saccular bronchiectasis may develop. If this occurs, the symptoms of infective bronchiectasis may dominate the clinical picture, with continuous production of purulent sputum even during the intervals between episodes of bronchial plugging. Hemoptysis occurs in about half of the patients and is almost always scanty; the blood comes from the bronchiectatic lesions.

The major clinical feature of intracavitary fungus balls is hemoptysis. Hemoptysis may sometimes be profuse and even life-threatening; aspiration of the blood into the uninvolved lung may occur, and exsanguination is possible. Otherwise, the main symptoms are related to the underlying chronic cavitary disease and are determined by the extent of pulmonary destruction that was present before the fungus ball appeared.

With the advent of antineoplastic drugs and organ transplantation, the pyemic or septicemic form of aspergillosis has become common in medical centers. Patients under treatment with large doses of glucocorticoids and cytotoxic agents are at risk. Frequently, the patients have been rendered granulocytopenic with therapy and have been ill and under treatment with antimicrobial agents for previous infections. The symptoms of this form of invasive aspergillosis are those of an acute pulmonary infection, with fever, cough, and tachypnea. Hemoptysis is common but seldom massive. The chest film may show rapidly cavitating infiltrates in any of the lung fields; because of intravascular growth of the fungus, the picture may resemble that of pulmonary infarction. Pleural extension of the infiltrate may cause chest pain. The fungus may disseminate from the necrotizing pulmonary infection. Common secondary sites are the central nervous system, heart, liver, and skin.

Pleural aspergillosis occurs as a secondary invader in empyema with a bronchopleural fistula.

It is difficult to distinguish the symptoms of pleural aspergillosis from those of the preexisting chest disease. The symptoms of aspergillosis infection are usually recognized when they cause worsening of the existing illness; they consist of fever, cough, and systemic toxicity, which all subside when the fungi are sterilized by treatment.

## COMPLICATIONS AND SEQUELAE

Once *Aspergillus* infection becomes established in paranasal sinuses, extension to the orbit and the central nervous system may occur. When the orbit is invaded, proptosis and ophthalmoplegia may be the dominant signs. A stroke indicates invasion of an intracranial vessel and hemorrhagic infarction. If the patient survives long enough, abscesses form.

The most important late complication of allergic bronchopulmonary aspergillosis is bronchiectasis, predominantly in the upper lobe, with resultant bronchial obstruction and fibrosis. Occasionally, the fungus will persist in the lumen of these dilated bronchi and produce an aspergilloma in situ.

Intracavitary fungus balls produce few late sequelae as a rule. Progressive breathlessness secondary to the underlying cavitary disease will continue, but the fungus ball will not invade to cause disseminated disease. Continuous low-grade hemoptysis is the main late complication, but exsanguination or fatal aspiration of blood can occur.

Septicemic aspergillosis carries a very poor prognosis. Very few patients will survive long enough to develop late sequelae. Occasionally, however, patients survive the acute necrotizing pneumonia and develop fungus balls in the residual necrotic cavities.

## GEOGRAPHIC VARIATION IN DISEASE

Allergic bronchopulmonary aspergillosis is common in Great Britain and northern Europe and considerably less common in North America (Henderson, 1968; Hinson et al., 1952; Longbottom and Pepys, 1964). The syndrome has been described from other continents, but its true incidence is difficult to ascertain.

Fungus balls appear to be common wherever healed cavitary tuberculosis is common; one would expect to find a high incidence of these patients where the incidence of cavitary tuberculosis remains high.

Invasive septicemic aspergillosis seldom occurs

in immunologically normal people. Its frequency is highest in countries where aggressive cytotoxic and glucocorticoid therapy for the treatment of neoplastic disease is common and where organ transplantations occur frequently. Most cases have been reported from specialized centers in the United States dealing with neoplastic disease and renal transplantation.

Orbital aspergillosis predominates in localities with a warm and humid climate and most cases have been reported from Sudan, India, and the southern United States (Hedges and Leung, 1976).

## DIAGNOSIS

Diagnosis of allergic bronchopulmonary aspergillosis requires the following criteria (Henderson, 1968; Hinson et al., 1952; Longbottom and Pepys, 1964):

1. Chronic asthma, or evidence of chronic airway obstruction.

2. More than two distinct episodes of transient pulmonary infiltration, separated by an asymptomatic interval confirmed by chest x-ray.

3. Precipitins to *A. fumigatus* antigens in serum.

4. Peripheral blood eosinophilia in excess of 500 eosinophils per cubic millimeter when the infiltrates are present.

5. Demonstration of *A. fumigatus* in sputum at least twice by culture or direct visualization of the fungus.

6. Dual skin-test results; immediate wheal and flare (type I) reaction, followed in five to six hours by a type III (Arthus) reaction after injection of *Aspergillus* antigens.

Recent work has revealed that patients with allergic bronchopulmonary aspergillosis (ABPA) can be reliably separated from asthmatics without ABPA (who may meet many of the above criteria) by virtue of much higher levels of specific IgE and IgG antibodies directed against *Aspergillus fumigatus* (Wang, et al., 1978).

An important diagnostic feature is the discrepancy between the relatively mild clinical symptoms and the extensive pulmonary consolidation. This relationship helps in differentiating allergic aspergillosis from bacterial pneumonia in which a similar area of consolidation would produce severe symptoms. In the late stages of bronchopulmonary aspergillosis, when cavitation occurs or the upper lobes shrink, a diagnosis of pulmonary tuberculosis is often made erroneously.

Diagnosis of the other forms of aspergillosis is

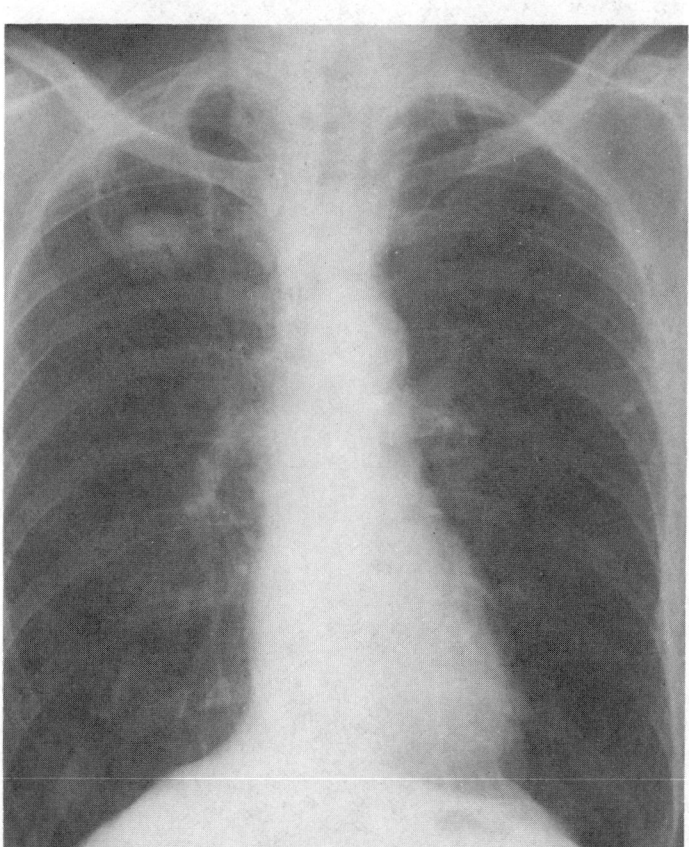

**FIGURE 2.** *Fungus ball* (Aspergillus fumigatus) *in a residual old tuberculous cavity (upright position).*

complicated by the fact that recovery of the fungus from expectorated sputum is often difficult in patient's with aspergillosis and common in patients without aspergillosis because aspergilli may colonize the normal mouth and upper airways. Hence, the most reliable diagnostic method is direct sampling of infected tissues.

In sino-orbital disease direct biopsies of the large friable masses of fungus should be performed, and care must be taken not to contaminate the instruments by passing them through the mouth and oropharynx.

The diagnosis of pleural aspergillosis is easily made by finding brown clumps of hyphae in the pleural pus (Young et al., 1970).

In invasive pulmonary aspergillosis the chest roentgenogram is not diagnostic and may mimic lung abscess, carcinoma, pneumonia, or pulmonary infarction. In suspicious cases, fiberoptic bronchoscopy may be used to obtain biopsy material and brushings for culture and to show invasive fungal elements histopathologically. If bronchoscopy fails to confirm the diagnosis, early open biopsy should be done.

The chest radiograph helps in the diagnosis of intracavitary fungus balls. The appearance of a crescentic radiolucency surrounding a mass is highly suggestive (Monod's sign) (Figs. 2 and 3). Although other fungi, notably *Allescheria boydii*, may produce a similar x-ray picture, the majority of such lesions indicates *Aspergillus* sp.

Agar diffusion tests for precipitins are positive in patients with allergic bronchopulmonary aspergillosis, fungus balls, and pleural aspergillosis. In contrast, positive serologic tests are infrequent in invasive disseminated aspergillosis.

## *TREATMENT*

Prednisone in a dose of 7.5 mg/day has been used successfully to treat allergic bronchopulmonary aspergillosis and to prevent recurrences. Nebulized amphotericin B and nystatin have also been used but are difficult to evaluate.

Surgical excision with wide débridement of the margins can be successful in sino-orbital disease.

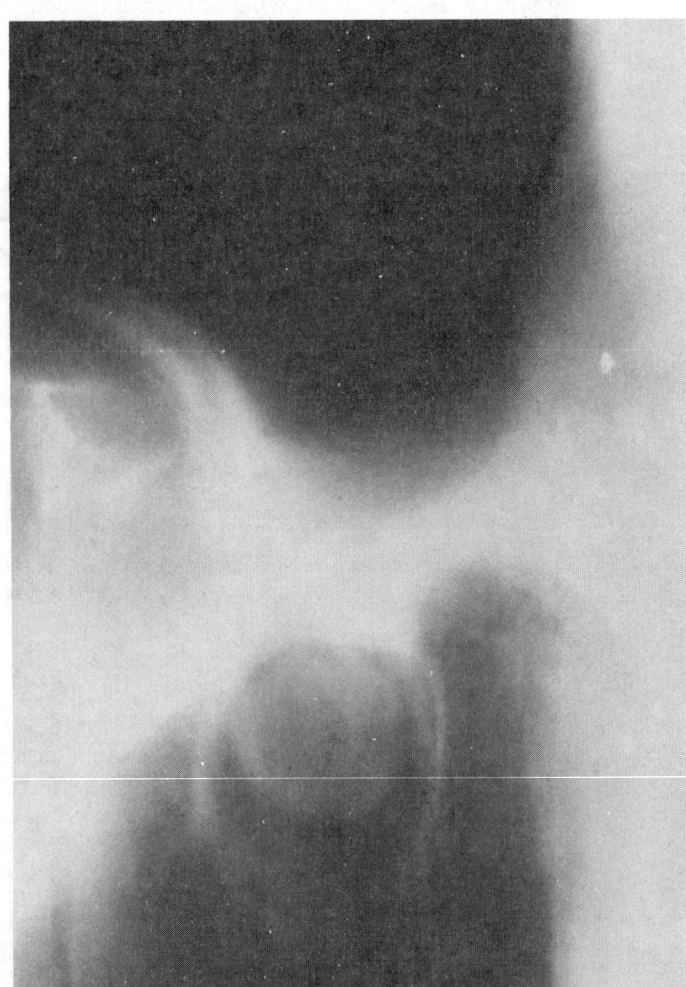

**FIGURE 3.** *Tomogram of the same fungus ball seen in Figure 2. Patient is now lying down — note different position of the fungus ball.*

In patients with aspergilloma, resection of the involved lobe has been curative when the underlying chronic pulmonary disease has not been too severe to prohibit such intervention. The fungus ball must be resected when hemoptysis threatens to kill the patient. Intravenous amphotericin B is probably of no value (Hammerman et al., 1974; Varkey and Rose, 1976). Successful treatment with endobronchial and intracavitary amphotericin B has been reported only in isolated cases and should be regarded as anecdotal, especially since fungus balls may lyse spontaneously or be expectorated.

In disseminated invasive aspergillosis intravenous amphotericin B is the treatment of choice. Even though such treatment often fails because of the severe underlying illness, it may be effective when used early in the course of the disease in an average daily dose of 0.6 mg/kg (Aisner et al., 1977; Pennington, 1976).

In pleural aspergillosis, the local instillation of nystatin sometimes sterilizes the infection within a few weeks.

### PROPHYLAXIS

Since the fungus is ubiquitous in nature it is impossible to avoid exposure to it during everyday living. Protection of immunologically incompetent patients in a hospital setting should include careful environmental monitoring and elimination of recognized foci of fungal growth. In the winter, when *A. fumigatus* spores are most prevalent, prednisone (7.5 mg/day) can prevent recurrent attacks of pulmonary consolidation and eosinophilia in patients with allergic bronchopulmonary aspergillosis (Safirstein et al., 1973).

### References

Aisner, J., Schimpff, S. C., and Wiernik, P. H.: Treatment of invasive aspergillosis: Relation of early diagnosis and treatment to response. Ann Intern Med 86:539, 1977.

British Tuberculosis Association: Aspergillus in persistent lung cavities after tuberculosis. Tubercle 49:1, 1968.

British Tuberculosis Association: Aspergilloma and residual tuberculous cavities — the results of a resurvey. Tubercle 51:227, 1970.

Hammerman, K. J., Sarosi, G. A., and Tosh, F. E.: Amphotericin B in the treatment of saprophytic forms of pulmonary aspergillosis. Am Rev Resp Dis 109:57, 1974.

Hedges, T., and Leung, L.: Parasellar and orbital apex syndrome caused by aspergillosis. Neurology 26:117, 1976.

Henderson, A. H.: Allergic aspergillosis: Review of 32 cases. Thorax 23:501, 1968.

Hinson, K. F. W., Moon, A. J., and Plummer, N. S.: Bronchopulmonary aspergillosis. A review and a report of eight new cases. Thorax 7:317, 1952.

Krakowka, P., Rowenska, E., and Holweg, H.: Infection of the pleura by *Aspergillus fumigatus*. Thorax 25:245, 1970.

Longbottom, J. L., and Pepys, J.: Pulmonary aspergillosis: Diagnostic and immunological significance of antigens and C-substance in *Aspergillus fumigatus*. J Pathol Bacteriol 88:141, 1964.

Pennington, J. E.: Successful treatment of Aspergillus pneumonia in hematologic neoplasia. N Engl J Med 295:426, 1976.

Safirstein, B., D'Souza, M., Simon, G., Tai, E., and Pepys, J.: Five-year follow-up of allergic bronchopulmonary aspergillosis. Am Rev Resp Dis 108:450, 1973.

Scadding, J. G.: The bronchi in allergic aspergillosis. Scand J Resp Dis 48:372, 1967.

Varkey, B., and Rose, H. D.: Pulmonary aspergilloma. A rational approach to treatment. Am J Med 61:626, 1976.

Wang, J. L. F., Patterson, R., Rosenberg, M., Roberts, M., and Cooper, B. J.: Serum IgE and IgG antibody activity against *Aspergillus fumigatus* as a diagnostic aid in allergic bronchopulmonary aspergillosis. Am Rev Respir Dis 117:917, 1978.

Young, R. C., Bennett, J. E., Vogel, C. L., Carbone, P. P., and DeVita, V. T.: Aspergillosis. The spectrum of the disease in 98 patients. Medicine 49:147, 1970.

# PULMONARY 122
# MUCORMYCOSIS
## Burt R. Meyers, M.D.

### DEFINITION

Pulmonary mucormycosis is an infection of the lung by the nonseptate fungi known as *Phycomycetes*. The disease is characterized by pneumonia, invasion of pulmonary vessels, and infarction of the lung (Baker, 1956). It usually occurs in patients with diabetes, leukemia, or lymphoma.

### ETIOLOGY

*Phycomycetes* are ubiquitous fungi of soil, fruits, vegetables, and moldy bread but have been isolated only rarely from the air in hospitals. Members of the order Mucorales, belonging to the genera *Mucor, Rhizopus*, and *Absidia*, have been isolated from rhinocerebral mucormycosis and other forms of human infection, but the exact genera causing most cases of pulmonary mucormycosis have not been identified. This is because diagnosis has been made not from culture but rather from the appearance of the nonseptate fungi in histologic sections of biopsies or postmortem tissues. In the few cases with positive cultures, the fungi have been identified as *Mucor pusillus* (see Chapter 75; Meyer et al., 1973), *Rhizopus* sp. (Record and Ginder, 1976) and *Absidia* sp. (Lombardi et al., 1970).

## PATHOGENESIS AND PATHOLOGY

The spores of the Mucorales are inhaled through the nares into the nasal sinuses, bronchial tree, and lung parenchyma. An ulcer of the skin has also been proposed as a rare portal of entry from which the infection spreads to the lung. The hyphae invade blood vessels and cause pulmonary infarction, pulmonary hemorrhage, and gangrene of the lung. The bronchial walls and lymphatics may also be invaded. Pulmonary infarction may be secondary to thrombi that develop in the region of the fungus or to vascular occlusion by the mass of hyphal elements. The infarct may be large and fatal or small and nonprogressive; in the latter instance, it may produce a solitary nodule in the chest x-ray. The Mucorales also produce acute inflammation with a polymorphonuclear reaction unless the patient is severely neutropenic. The broad (4 to $20\mu$) nonseptate hyphae are surrounded by neutrophilic leukocytes. This inflammatory reaction gives a clinical picture of pneumonia or lung abscess. Thus, mucormycosis may be characterized by infarct, pneumonia, lung abscess, or a combination of the three processes.

Infection with *Phycomycetes* commonly occurs in compromised patients, including those with acute leukemia and lymphomas or recipients of kidney transplants. In most cases, the patients are receiving either corticosteroids, Cytoxan, or immunosuppressive agents. Diabetic patients, especially those in ketoacidosis, are also prone to mucormycosis.

## CLINICAL PRESENTATION

Pulmonary mucormycosis may be acute and fulminant or subacute and slowly progressive. In the patient who is immunosuppressed or has an underlying malignancy, especially leukemia or lymphoma, the presence of chills, fever, and pulmonary infiltrates should rouse suspicion of infection with the Mucorales. Whereas bacterial, especially gram-negative, pneumonias are much more likely to cause this syndrome, the sudden development of chest pain (mainly pleuritic in nature), bloody sputum, and pleural friction rub and the roentgenographic appearance of a pulmonary infarction should suggest mucormycosis. The usual picture, however, is that of a patchy, nonhomogeneous infiltrate that may progress despite antibiotic therapy to lobar consolidation with the development of a cavity. A hemorrhagic pleural effusion may also be found. In diabetics, the disease may be less fulminant and produce a subacute pneumonitis with cavitation. Solitary pulmonary nodules, composed of a small mycotic infarct, have also been described (Gale and Kleitsch, 1972).

## COMPLICATIONS

The three major complications of pulmonary mucormycosis are fatal hemorrhage, dissemination, and bacterial superinfection. Abrupt, massive, and fatal hemoptysis can occur if the pulmonary artery is eroded by the hyphae (Murray, 1975). Hematogenous dissemination reaches nearly every organ, including the heart, brain, kidney, thyroid, bone, pancreas, bowel and spleen (Meyer et al., 1973). Severe bacterial infections, especially with *Pseudomonas* or *Staphylococcus aureus*, may aggravate and obscure the fungus infection (Meyer et al., 1972).

## DIAGNOSIS

The diagnosis must be suspected in a compromised patient with fever, pulmonary infarct, and an acute pneumonitis that does not respond to antibiotics (Fig. 1). *Phycomycetes* are rarely observed on Gram stain or isolated in sputum culture, and the specific diagnosis has most often been made post mortem or following open lung biopsy. Transbronchial biopsy of the lung parenchyma to obtain tissue for smears, culture, and pathologic section may be useful if not contraindicated by thrombocytopenia. Platelet transfusions should be given before the procedure in a thrombocytopenic patient. The presence of large, broad, nonseptate hyphae, sometimes with hyperacute, even right-angle, branching suggest that Mucorales are present. These fungi may be confused with aspergilli, though the latter are narrower and septate.

Clinical isolates should be grown on blood or Sabouraud's agar at 37° C. Growth usually appears at 1 to 2 days, though cultures should be kept for 10 to 14 days. The direct plating of biopsy material on agar has increased the yield of positive cultures. There are no reliable serologic tests for mucormycosis.

Differential diagnosis must take into account other fungi and parasites that produce pulmonary disease in the compromised patient. *Nocardia asteroides* may produce an acute necrotizing pneumonia, with a tendency to spread to the brain. The branching, gram-positive, partially acid-fast filamentous rods of *N. asteroides* are often seen in sputum smears of patients with pulmonary nocardiosis. *Pneumocystis carinii* infection and cytomegalic inclusion disease produce acute pneumonia in immunosuppressed patients, but often present as acute respiratory distress

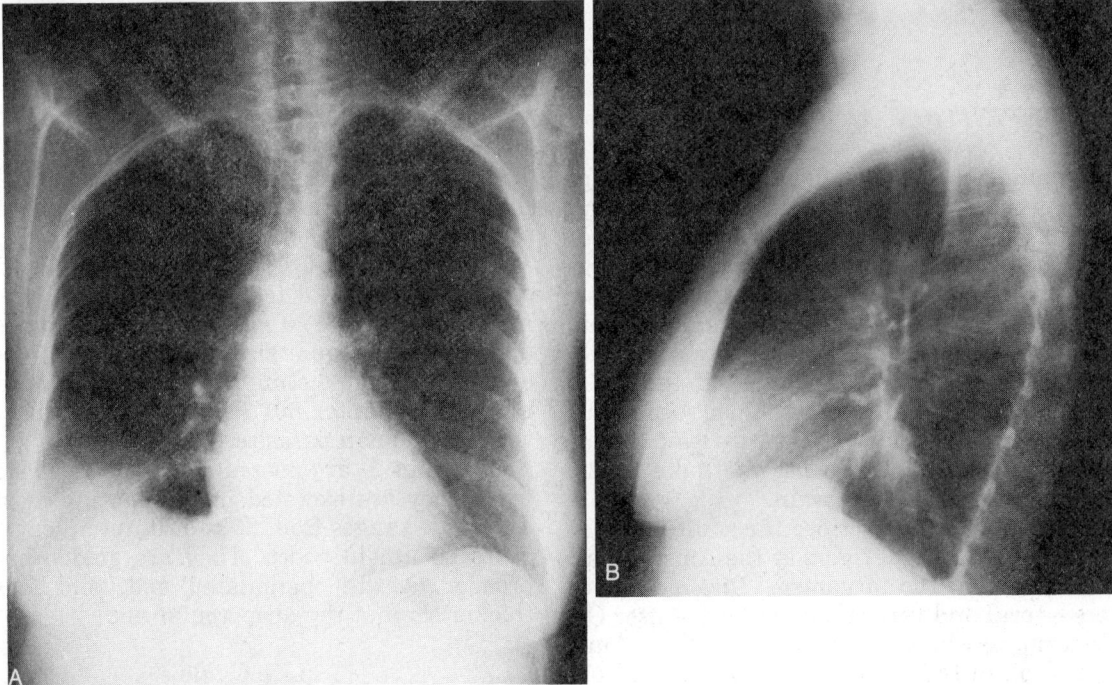

**FIGURE 1.** *Mucormycosis of right lower lobe in patient with idiopathic pancytopenia. At autopsy there was invasion of the pulmonary artery and mediastinum by mucor. A, mycotic mural thrombus, 6 cm in length, of the abdominal aorta extended into the left renal artery where it produced necrotizing enteritis. Mucor was also isolated from skin lesions of the feet. The increased iron stores from transfusion for pancytopenia may have contributed to infection by saturating transferrin and thus making available adequate iron for growth of mucor in the tissues.*

syndromes. The patients are dyspneic and hypoxic, and the roentgenogram reveals a diffuse interstitial pattern. Fiberoptic bronchoscopy with brushing and/or biopsy is necessary for the diagnosis of *Pneumocystis* infection. Cytomegalic inclusion disease may be diagnosed by serology or lung biopsy. The pulmonary vasculature is not invaded in either *Pneumocystis* or cytomegalovirus infections, and cavitation and pulmonary infarction are not found.

Aspergilli invade blood vessels and can produce a clinical picture identical to that of mucormycosis. *Aspergillus* pneumonia is more common in immunosuppressed patients, and aspergilli are the most common infectious agents found post mortem in patients with leukemia. Differentiation from mucormycosis must usually be made by transbronchial or open lung biopsy because aspergilli do not often appear in the sputum. If biopsy is impossible, amphotericin *B* therapy is warranted for patients who present the picture of mycotic pulmonary pneumonia with infarction.

## TREATMENT

Prompt therapy is essential. Antileukemic and cancer chemotherapy should be regulated, if pos-

sible, to permit the neutrophil count to rise. Most cases of pulmonary mucormycosis have been terminal infections in debilitated patients with leukemia or lymphoma. Survival from pulmonary phycomycosis has been obtained, however, by treatment with Amphotericin B in a total intravenous dose of 1200 mg over 12 weeks in a patient with acute lymphocytic leukemia (Medoff and Kobayashi, 1972). Surgical resection of infarcted lung has been performed successfully in some cases. The role of white blood cell transfusion in the leukopenic patient with these infections has not been determined. Without treatment, the infection is almost always lethal.

## References

Baker, R. D.: Pulmonary mucormycosis. Am J Path 32:287, 1956.

Gale, A. M., and Kleitsch, W. E.: Solitary pulmonary nodule due to phycomycosis (mucormycosis). Chest 62:752, 1972.

Lombardi, D. L., Mason, J. O., and Hughes, R. K.: Pneumocystis and mucormycosis pneumonitis. Chest 57:318, 1970.

Medoff, G., and Kobayashi, G.: Pulmonary Mucormycosis. N Engl J Med 286:86, 1972.

Meyer, R., Kaplan, M., Ong, M., and Armstrong, D.: Cutaneous lesions in disseminated mucormycosis. JAMA 225:737, 1973.

Meyer, R., Rosen, P., and Armstrong, D.: Phycomycosis complicating leukemia and lymphoma. Ann Int Med 77:871, 1972.

Murray, H. W.: Pulmonary mucormycosis with massive fatal hemoptysis. Chest 68:65, 1975.

Record, N. B., Jr., and Ginder, D. R.: Pulmonary phycomycosis without obvious predisposing factors. JAMA 235:1256, 1976.

# 123 *PARAGONIMIASIS*
## Charles E. Davis, M.D.

## DEFINITION AND HISTORY

Paragonimiasis (endemic hemoptysis) is a lung infection of man and other mammals acquired by ingestion of fresh water crabs or crayfish infested with larvae of *Paragonimus*, the trematode lung fluke. Although it is widely distributed, the most important foci are in Southeast Asia and the Far East. It is often confused with tuberculosis because the adult worms are walled off in cystic cavities or "burrows" that cause hemoptysis when they erode into a bronchus. Nevertheless, it is a relatively benign disease unless the fluke localizes in ectopic foci like the brain.

Kerbert (1878) first described the adult fluke in the lungs of two Bengal tigers at the Amsterdam Zoo. He named the organism *Distoma* (two suckers — oral and ventral) *westermani* (after G. F. Westerman, who was the Director of the Amsterdam Zoo). In 1880, Ringer discovered an adult worm in the lung of a Formosan man at autopsy and forwarded it to Manson, who realized that its ova were identical to those in the bloody sputum of a Chinese patient that he was attending at the time. He also recognized that it was a distome and published these cases as human infections with *Distoma ringeri* (Manson, 1881). Manson subsequently studied the disease in Formosa while Baelz (1880) was making independent observations in Japan. When they exchanged specimens, they realized that "endemic hemoptysis" of Formosa and Japan were caused by the same parasite (Manson, 1883).

In 1889, Leuckhart concluded that the tiger and human lung flukes were identical. Braun (1899) first suggested the genus name of *Paragonimus,* but *Distoma* persisted for many years as an alternative name for *Paragonimus* and as the name for the Fasciola group of trematodes. "Pulmonary distomiasis" is still used occasionally as a synonym for paragonimiasis.

The life cycle of *Paragonimus* was worked out by Nakagawa (1916), who demonstrated larvae in the freshwater crab, S. Yokogawa (1915), who traced the migration of the fluke from the intestine to the lungs of the definitive host, and Ameel (1934), who described the developmental stages of *Paragonimus.*

Paragonimiasis is a major health problem in many parts of the world but is of far greater importance in Korea than in any other country. For this reason, the Korean War in the 1950s, which involved personnel from many countries, thrust this disease into international prominence.

## ETIOLOGY

*Paragonimus* is a typical, hermaphroditic, leaf-like fluke that is thicker, broader, and more opaque than other flukes. It belongs to the family Troglotrematidae. The adult is red to brown and 7 to 12 mm long by 4 to 7 mm in width. External microscopic spines, a ventral and oral sucker of approximately equal size, and its ovoid, "fleshy" appearance help distinguish it from other trematodes (see Chapter 80). *P. westermani* (Fig. 1) is the chief human parasite.

Ova (Fig. 2) are operculated and undeveloped when they are excreted in the sputum or stool. Their size ranges from 80 to 120 $\mu$m in length by 50 to 60 $\mu$m in width. They are golden brown, broader at the operculated end, and form a thicker shell at the abopercular end.

### Life Cycle

Ova are passed in the sputum or feces of the infected mammal. If they reach fresh water, they hatch within 17 to 28 days. The operculum opens to allow the free-swimming first larval stage (miracidium) to emerge. The miracidium pene-

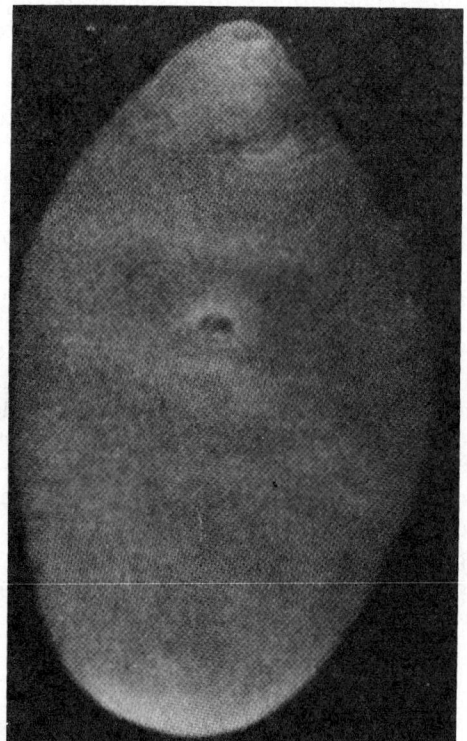

**FIGURE 1.** *Adult* Paragonimus westermani. ×5 *(From Mitsuno et al.: J Nerv Ment Dis 116:685, 1952.)*

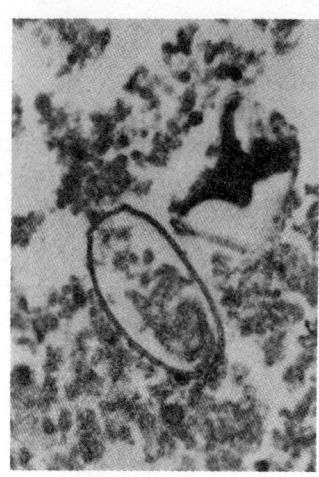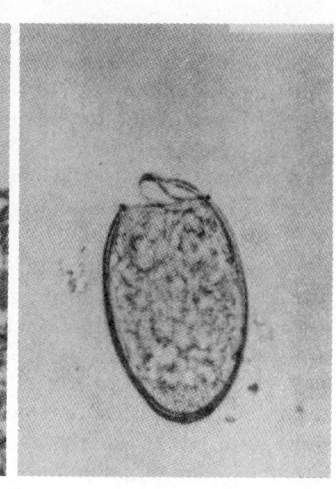

**FIGURE 2.** *Ova of* P. westermani. Left, *typical appearance of egg in tissue section. The operculum is often missed because the section does not pass through the center of the ovum along its long axis.* Right, *typical ova with the operculum partly open. (From Mitsuno et al.: J Nerv Ment Dis 116:685, 1952.)*

trates various species of snails within 24 hours. The most important snail hosts in Asia are the species of *Semisulcospira* (Kobayashi, 1918), but other species serve as the first intermediate host in other geographic areas. During a three- to five-month developmental period in the snail, the larvae develop through two rediae stages to produce a stumpy-tailed, second larval stage called a cercaria. Freshwater crabs or crayfish either eat the digestive gland of the snails or are penetrated by free-swimming cercaria that have emerged from the tissues of the snail (Yokogawa, 1965). More than 11 different species of crayfish and crabs have been reported as second intermediate hosts of *P. westermani* alone. The distribution of *P. westermani* and the other species of *Paragonimus* is clearly dependent on the presence of the appropriate snail and freshwater crustacean.

Man is infected by eating raw, salted, or wine-soaked (drunken) fresh water crabs or crayfish. The disease is limited to areas where these crustaceans are eaten in this manner. Heating the crustaceans to 55° C kills the cercariae. However, Yokagawa (1965) has shown that infectious metacercariae that adhere to knives and strainers during the preparation of crabs for inclusion in soups and other cooked dishes can be transferred by these utensils and by hands to salads and other uncooked dishes. He suggests that this is probably the route of infection in geographic areas of Japan where crabs or crayfish are not ordinarily eaten raw. Another way that *Paragonimus* may be transmitted to people that do not ordinarily eat raw freshwater crustaceans is in folk medicines. Yun (1960) reported seven cases of paragonimiasis in children whose only exposure to raw crustaceans was the liquid from crushed, strained crayfish, which is a common folk remedy for measles in rural Korea.

More recently, it has been demonstrated that when wild boars ingest the metacercariae of *P.*

*westermani*, the larvae do not migrate to the lungs. Instead, they encyst in the muscle. These encysted forms are immature and infectious for experimental animals and are probably the source of infection in some areas of Japan where raw freshwater crustaceans are not eaten (Miyazaki and Habe, 1976).

After man or other mammalian hosts ingest infected raw crabs or crayfish, the metacercariae encyst in the duodenum and migrate through the wall of the small intestine into the peritoneal cavity. Most reach the lungs by penetrating the diaphragm. Abnormal migration routes to ectopic sites are responsible for many of the bizarre and severe complications of paragonimiasis. The parasites are encapsulated by the host, develop into adults, and produce ova within four to six weeks. When the cyst erodes into a bronchus, ova are expectorated along with blood and purulent sputum. Swallowed ova are also excreted in the feces. When these ova reach fresh water, the life cycle begins again. The life span of adult *Paragonimus* varies, but some have lived at least 20 years (Yokogawa, 1965).

## Speciation

For many years, the major issue in the speciation of *Paragonimus* was whether *P. westermani* was the only species that infected man. The criteria for speciation of *Paragonimus* progressed through two stages before the modern era. At first, each isolation of *Paragonimus* from a new host or a new geographic region was considered to be a new species. Later, most species were thought to be identical to *P. westermani*, which was assumed to be the only *Paragonimus* that infected man. Among the reasons for this confusion are the variation in the shape and size of ova produced by a single lung fluke and the fleshiness of adult flukes that makes it difficult to work out their internal morphology. Now species are usually determined by the arrangement of the spines, the shape of the ovary and testes, the relative size of the oral and ventral suckers, and the properties of the ova. A lung fluke is usually not accepted as a new species, however, until the entire life cycle and each larval stage are described and characterized.

Between 15 and 25 lung flukes from different mammalian hosts and geographic areas are thought to be distinct species by some investigators (Yokogawa, 1969). Of these, only about six have been isolated from man. *P. westermani* causes virtually all paragonimiasis in Asia and the Far East. *P. africanus* is a newly recognized species that is probably responsible for West African paragonimiasis. *P. mexicanus* has caused autochthonous cases of human paragonimiasis in Mexico, Central America, and Peru. *P. kellicotti* is a well-defined species that has been isolated from many wild and domestic animals in the western hemisphere and has probably caused rare autochthonous human cases in the United States. *P. heterotremus* and *P. skrjabini* are rare causes of human paragonimiasis in China.

*P. westermani* is by far the most important cause of paragonimiasis in humans and may coexist with the other valid species in Central America, South America, and Africa. All species require snails as the first intermediate host and utilize crabs or crayfish as the normal second intermediate host. The species of snail or freshwater crustacean may differ. The six species that have been isolated from man are thought to cause identical diseases.

### Geographic Distribution and Host Range

The human species of *Paragonimus* are widely distributed over three land masses: Asia, Africa, and the western hemisphere. The most important foci of infection in Asia and the Far East are in China, Japan, Taiwan, Korea, the Philippines, Thailand, Laos, and Vietnam. The major foci in Africa are in the West African countries of Nigeria, the Republic of Dahomey, Cameroon, and the Zaire Republic. Paragonimiasis occurs in Mexico and all of Central America, but Costa Rica has the highest prevalence. Cases have been documented from Peru, Ecuador, Venezuela, Brazil, and Colombia in South America (Yokogawa, 1969). The other species of *Paragonimus* that usually infect only wild and domestic animals are even more widely distributed. It is likely that the geographic distribution of human paragonimiasis is limited primarily by the eating habits of the population. Civil war in Nigeria from 1967 to 1970 caused massive population movements and

short food and cooking supplies. As a result large numbers of people turned to improperly cooked freshwater crabs as a source of protein. This change in eating habits caused a hundred-fold increase in the number of recognized cases of paragonimiasis in some areas of Nigeria after the civil war (Nwokolo, 1972).

All species of *Paragonimus,* including *P. westermani,* infect wild and domestic animals. Paragonimiasis has been reported to infect almost every carnivorous animal, but members of the cat family, dog family, and pigs are among the most common hosts. Minks are commonly infected with *P. kellicotti* in the United States.

### PATHOGENESIS AND PATHOLOGY

The pathologic manifestations of paragonimiasis are related to the migratory route of the larvae and the inflammatory response stimulated by the larvae and adult worms. In experimental infections, only a small percentage of ingested worms reach the lungs. Mild inflammatory changes occur at the site of penetration through the small intestine, but some young flukes do not penetrate. Instead, they encyst in the intestinal mucosa, develop into adults, and produce ova. Inflammation may progress to ulceration and excretion of ova in the stool. Parasites that localize in the abdominal cavity may provoke an abscess that simulates an intra-abdominal bacterial infection. Eosinophilia occurs during the migratory phase but usually subsides after the worms have encysted in the lung.

The typical manifestations of paragonimiasis occur in the lungs. Migration of the larvae across the pleural space into the lung parenchyma from the diaphragm can cause pneumothorax and pleural effusion. Intrapulmonary migration causes transient eosinophilia and polymorphonuclear infiltration that may resemble Löeffler's syndrome. After migration, the developing parasite elicits a polymorphonuclear response, necrosis of the parenchyma, and formation of a fibrous tissue capsule (Fig. 3). The necrosis in the center of the cyst or capsule is supplemented by the polymorphonuclear enzymes but may also be formed by arteriolar obstruction and infarction (Diaconita and Goldis, 1964). These cavities or "burrows" become walled off by fibrous transformation that is partly contributed by foreign body granulomas. These granulomas usually surround the cavity and encircle ova or egg shells. The egg tubercles consist of lymphocytes, plasma cells, eosinophils, fibroblasts, and histiocytes. Langhan's giant cells and multinuclear foreign body cells sometimes engulf the ova (Fig. 4). Calcification of old lesions is usually in the vicinity of the

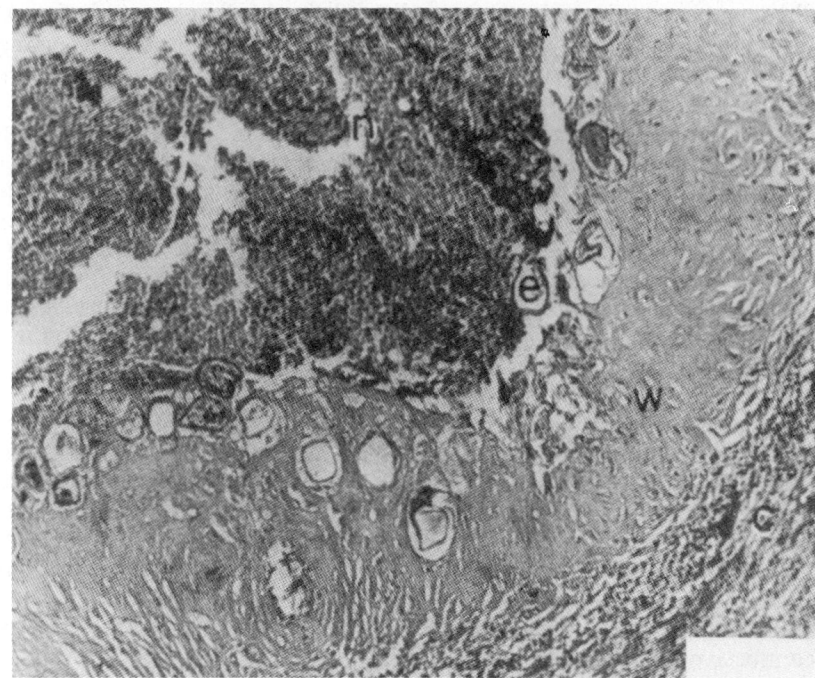

**FIGURE 3.** Paragonimus *cyst. n = necrotic debris, e = ova, which are most concentrated along the inner aspect of the cyst wall, w = cyst wall composed of a dense layer of collagenous connective tissue and chronic inflammation. (From Mitsuno et al.: J Nerv Ment Dis 116:685, 1952.)*

eggs in these egg granulomas. Interstitial pneumonia and bronchopneumonia with peribronchitis and endobronchitis may occur during migration but also often accompany erosion of the cavities into bronchioles. After the rupture, the sputum consists of mixtures of polymorphonuclear leukocytes, lymphocytes, ova, and blood.

Grossly, the cavities are grayish-white nodules that vary from grape to plum size. On section they are irregular or uneven in shape. The cyst walls are thick and fibrosclerotic (Yokogawa, 1965). Microscopically, they consist of the egg granulomas described above. The adult fluke may be seen either grossly or microscopically within the cavities.

Hyperplasia of the bronchial epithelium and bronchial erosion and ulceration occur in the area of the cysts. The bronchiectasis that complicates

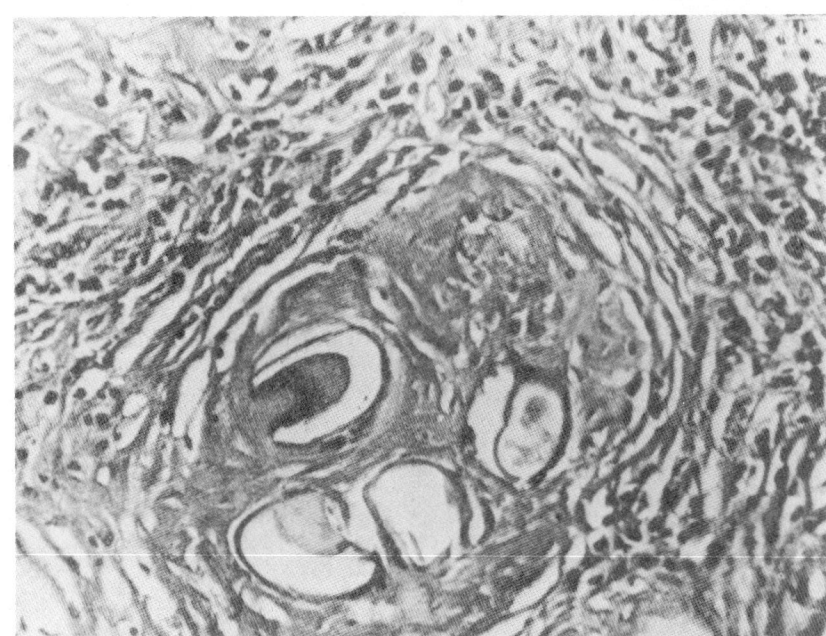

**FIGURE 4.** *Foreign body giant cell engulfing egg shells. (From Mitsuno et al.: J Nerv Ment Dis 116:685, 1952.)*

chronic paragonimiasis is caused by bronchial obstruction secondary to *Paragonimus* cavities and bronchial inflammation and hyperplasia.

Toxins have not been isolated from *Paragonimus* and it seems likely that arteriolar inflammation and egg granulomas are elicited mechanically and by hypersensitivity. The gamma-globulin concentrations are high during this stage of the disease (Sadun and Buck, 1960), and fully developed tubercles develop alongside foreign body granulomas.

Ectopic paragonimiasis in the brain and other organs causes "burrows" or cavities and granulomas similar to those in the lung (Fig. 5) (Mitsuno et al., 1952). The lesions enlarge during the process of liquefaction, probably because fluid is imbibed, and cause brain damage and atrophy. Calcification of the abundant granulomas is common. Adult flukes are found less commonly in cavities in the brain than the lung. The reasons for this difference are not known, but it is possible that adult flukes migrate out of this abnormal site. Yokogawa (1921) found larvae in the loose connective tissue of the neck and suggested that the larvae migrate through the loose connective tissue along the blood vessels and nerve trunks through the jugular foramen into the brain. Experimentally, flukes migrated out of the brain into the pleural cavity by way of the cerebral sinuses, the internal jugular veins, and the pulmonary arteries (Yokogawa, 1921).

## CLINICAL MANIFESTATIONS

The typical patient with pulmonary paragonimiasis presents to the physician with a history of chronic bronchitis and blood-tinged or reddish-brown sputum. In spite of a long history of disease, the general health is often unimpaired. Cough occurs predominantly in the early morning and produces gelatinous or blood-tinged sputum that is either streaked with blood or is a reddish-brown color. Among 270 Koreans who did not seek medical advice but had *Paragonimus* ova in their sputum, almost 25 per cent were asymptomatic (Sadun and Buck, 1960). The percentage of asymptomatic patients decreased with advancing years. Almost all patients over 30 years of age had pulmonary symptoms, and 72 per cent of the 270 had hemoptysis.

Hemoptysis occurs in 65 to 100 per cent of hospitalized patients. If blood-tinged sputum, brownish or red sputum, and frank hemoptysis are included in the definition of hemoptysis, 80 to 100 per cent of patients are affected (Table 1). Chest pain, occurring in about a third of patients, is usually pleuritic in nature and may be accompanied by pleural effusion or empyema. Fever at the time of admission to the hospital is common but may subside on bed rest. Loss of appetite and weight loss occur in about 10 per cent of patients.

Physical findings are sparse. Dullness and rales are distinctly uncommon and suggest the possibility of coexisting pulmonary tuberculosis or bacterial pneumonia. Clubbing of the fingers is uncommon unless the patient has developed full-blown bronchiectasis.

The white blood cell count may be slightly elevated early in the course of pulmonary involvement but returns to normal after the first year. Low-grade, peripheral eosinophilia is a uniform finding. Eosinophilia to 50 per cent may occur during the migratory phase of early infec-

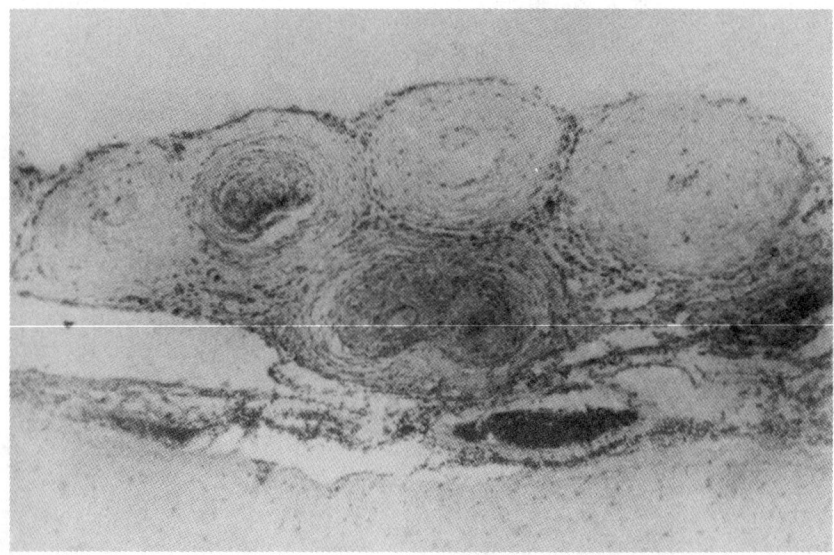

**FIGURE 5.** *Meningeal tubercle in cerebral paragonimiasis. (From Mitsuno et al.: J Nerv Ment Dis 116:685, 1952.)*

TABLE 1. Symptoms and Signs of
Pulmonary Paragonimiasis in
Hospitalized Patients[a]

| SYMPTOM OR SIGN | PER CENT | COMMENT |
|---|---|---|
| Cough | 95 | |
| Hemoptysis | 80–100 | blood-tinged, reddish-brown, and frank hemorrhage |
| Chest pain | 36 | |
| Fever and night sweats | 33 | |
| Weight loss | 11 | |
| *Physical examination* | | |
| Dullness and rales | — | unusual |
| *Laboratory examination* | | |
| Leukocytosis above 10,000/mm³ | 20 | early infections |
| Eosinophilia 10 to 20 per cent | 100 | |
| Hypergamma-globulinemia | — | statistically significant difference between patients and controls |
| *X-ray* | | |
| Abnormal chest x-ray | 76–100 | |
| Pleural effusion or empyema | 13 | |

[a]Number of patients evaluated range from 63 to more than 250 depending on the symptom or sign. Data from series published by Sadun and Buck, 1960; Nwokolo, 1972; Iwasaki, 1955.

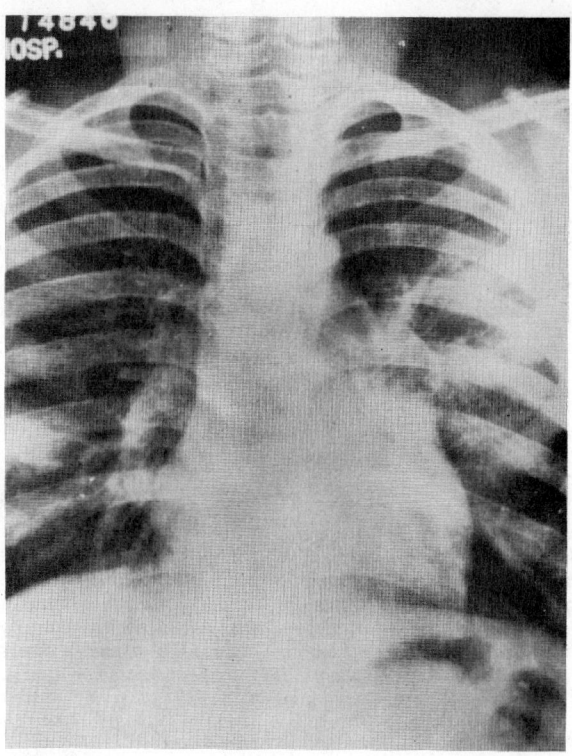

**FIGURE 6.** *Infiltrative form of pulmonary paragonimiasis. No cysts or cavities could be detected on tomograms. (From Sadun, E., and Buck, A.: Am J Trop Med Hyg 9:562, 1960.)*

tion. Elevation of the serum globulin with a reduction in albumin and other globulins is a common finding.

Most patients have abnormal chest x-rays. Chien (1955) and Sadun and Buck (1960) described a typical pattern of changes progressing from the early active stages to late residual stages after the parasites have died. A pulmonary infiltrate with the appearance of localized pneumonitis occurs in response to parenchymal migration. Cysts may or may not be present (Figs. 6 and 7). The infiltrate is replaced by isolated nodules that may cavitate because of air that has entered the nodules from the bronchioles. These nodules may be infraclavicular, basal, or disseminated (Fig. 8). One or two basal, round or elliptical nodules are easy to diagnose as possible paragonimiasis, but the disseminated form in which nodules of various densities are found in x-rays of both lungs is frequently confused with tuberculosis. The fact that the apex is usually spared, however, should cast doubt on the diagnosis of tuberculosis. The late stages of the disease are characterized by fibrosis and calcification that occur after the parasite dies. Fibrosis also occurs outside the nodular areas and may be extensive. Round or oval spots of calcification represent areas where cysts have been absorbed and replaced by calcification. Individuals who live in endemic areas are reinfected frequently and may have lesions in all stages.

Pleural reactions are common and are often bilateral. They range from small effusions to thickened, fibrotic pleura. The fibrotic tissue examined after decortication frequently contains ova.

## COMPLICATIONS AND SEQUELAE

The major pulmonary complications include bronchiectasis, fibrosis, and chronic obstructive bronchopulmonary disease. Right heart failure occurs rarely. Superimposed pulmonary tuberculosis and pyogenic pneumonia are common complications.

The most dramatic complications of paragonimiasis occur, however, when the young flukes fail to reach the lung or migrate into ectopic foci. The worm often encysts widely in the abdomen and pelvis. The retroperitoneum, scrotum, kidneys, mediastinum, lymph nodes, and orbit are less frequently invaded (Mitsuno et al., 1952). By far the most common and most threatening ex-

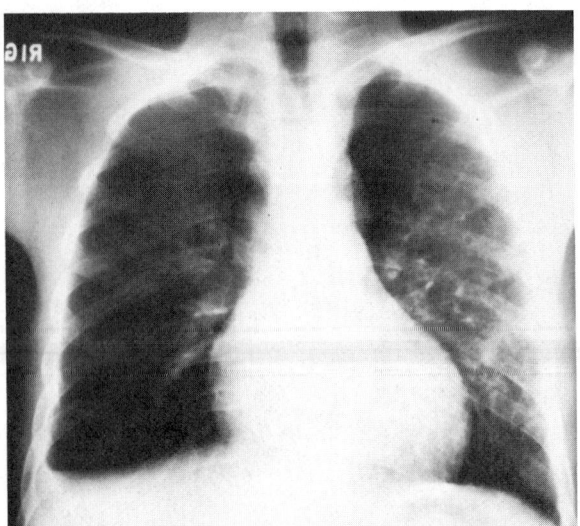

**FIGURE 7.** *A 14-year-old Laotian with hemoptysis and Paragonimus ova in sputum and stool. Extensive reticular infiltrates with loss of volume are most prominent in the superior segment of the left lower lobe. There are no large cavities but lucencies within the infiltrate may represent Paragonimus cysts. Bilateral pleural disease is more prominent on the right. (From University of California at San Diego Medical Center, Case number 751728-G.)*

most patients with cerebral paragonimiasis die before age 20. The frequency of reported cerebral foci in paragonimiasis varies from 0.8 per cent to 26 per cent (Oh, 1968; Yokogawa, 1965). Since 50 per cent of the population of some areas of Korea were estimated to have paragonimiasis in the 1950s and 1960s, it is very possible that 0.5 per cent or more of the population had cerebral paragonimiasis.

In the acute stage or in spinal cord localization, meningitis may be the presenting syndrome. More commonly, patients present with epilepsy, tumor syndromes, or organic brain syndromes. Headache, seizures, visual disturbances, and motor and sensory disorders are the most common symptoms. Mental deterioration, hemiplegia, hemihypesthesia, homonymous hemianopsia, and optic atrophy are the most common signs (Oh, 1968). Lumbar puncture reveals a pleocytosis of 3 to 125 leukocytes per $mm^3$, an elevated protein concentration, and a normal sugar level. More than 50 per cent of patients have calcifications on skull x-rays (Fig. 9) (Oh, 1968). Calcifications are usually found in clusters of a few to more than 50 more or less spherical elements ranging in size from a few to more than 30 mm (Galatius-Jensen and Uhm, 1965). Calcifications are most common in the occipital and parietal areas, slightly less common in the temporal lobes, and unusual in the

trathoracic localization, however, is in the brain. Of 143 patients with paragonimiasis studied by Sadun and Buck (1960), 22 (15 per cent) had extrathoracic lesions. The brain was invaded in 12 (8 per cent). Thus, in this series as well as in many others (Yokogawa, 1965), cerebral paragonimiasis accounts for about half the ectopic foci. It is more common in men than women and usually occurs in children and young adults (76 per cent under age 20) (Misuno et al., 1952). The age distribution probably represents the fact that

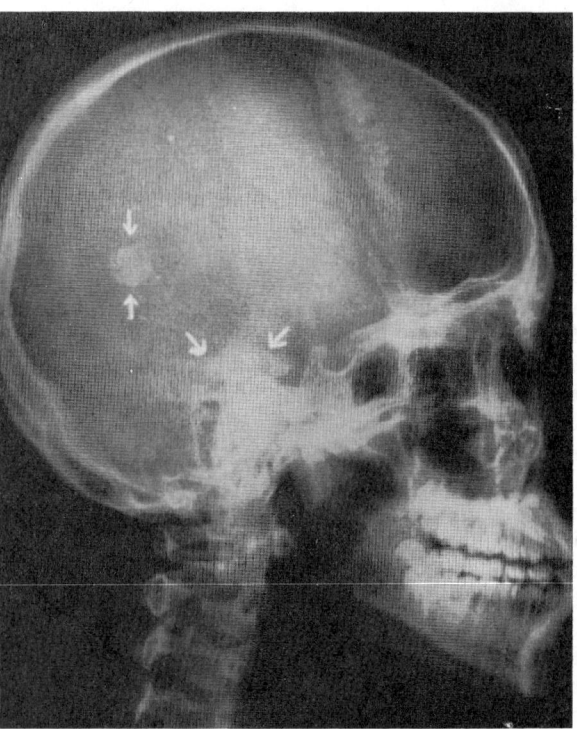

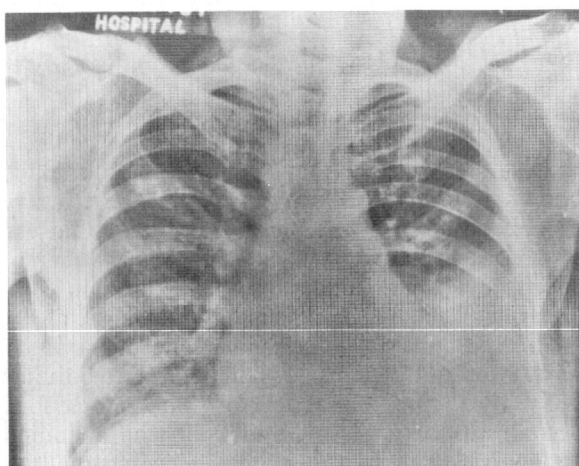

**FIGURE 8.** *Disseminated nodular-cystic paragonimiasis with left empyema. (From Sadun, E., and Buck, A.: Am J Trop Med Hyg 9:562, 1960.)*

**FIGURE 9.** *Intracerebral calcification of paragonimus cysts in 18-year-old with Jacksonian epilepsy. (From Sadun, E., and Buck, A.: Am J Trop Med Hyg 9:562, 1960.)*

frontal lobe. Without surgical intervention, the time from onset of symptoms to death varies from one to four years.

Ectopic lesions in other organs usually cause the symptoms of either abscess or tumor. Hematuria is a common presenting symptom of renal paragonimiasis. Paragonimiasis of the abdominal wall has simulated appendicitis (Kay, 1955).

## GEOGRAPHIC VARIATIONS IN DISEASE

Oriental paragonimiasis caused predominantly by *P. westermani* has been more extensively studied than American infections with *P. mexicanus* or African infections with *P. africanus*. To date, there is no evidence that the syndromes caused by these major human parasites are different. *P. heterotremus* and *P. skrjabini* are rare causes of pulmonary paragonimiasis in China. Most patients have had subcutaneous swellings with or without pulmonary involvement. This high incidence of ectopic subcutaneous localization may indicate that these species are not well adapted to man, since the major human parasite, *P. westermani,* seems to localize in the muscle and subcutaneous tissue of unusual hosts like the hog, rat, and chicken (Miyazaki and Habe, 1976).

## · DIAGNOSIS

Paragonimiasis is most often confused with pulmonary tuberculosis but may be misdiagnosed as aspiration lung abscess or, in the early infiltrative stage, as bacterial or viral pneumonia. Pulmonary fungal infections, like histoplasmosis and blastomycosis, could also be mistaken for paragonimiasis in areas where these diseases coexist. A history of exposure to uncooked freshwater crabs or crayfish should alert the physician to the possibility of paragonimiasis. If the patient also has hemoptysis or reddish-brown sputum, paragonimiasis must be carefully considered. Aspiration lung abscess should be preceded by an episode of unconsciousness and be accompanied by foul-smelling and tasting (fetid) sputum. The color of the sputum, frequent absence of fever (especially on bed rest), and the usual relative well-being of the patient with paragonimiasis help differentiate it from bacterial and viral pneumonias. Serologies and skin tests for pulmonary fungal infections and the color and nature of the sputum in paragonimiasis aid in the differentiation between these diseases.

Except for miliary lesions and extensive bronchopneumonia, almost all of the roentgenographic features of pulmonary tuberculosis may be mimicked by paragonimiasis. Furthermore, as many as 30 to 100 per cent of patients in areas endemic for paragonimiasis may have positive tuberculin tests (Nwokolo, 1972; Sadun and Buck, 1960). In these areas, patients may also have active disease with both organisms. There are several major radiologic differences, however, (Ogakwu and Nwokolo, 1973). Paragonimiasis usually affects the midzones of the lungs instead of the apices and causes "bubble" cavities, smooth-edged translucencies within an area of consolidation. Fluid levels are rare. The lesions of paragonimiasis are often poorly defined shadows of low density that are not very extensive. Finally, the appearance of early paragonimiasis may undergo marked changes within a relatively short period in the absence of treatment.

The nature of the pleural effusion in the two diseases also differs. The pleural fluid of patients with paragonimiasis often contains 80 to 90 per cent eosinophils instead of the predominance of lymphocytes in tuberculous effusions.

The definitive diagnosis of paragonimiasis is made by demonstrating *Paragonimus* ova (see Fig. 2) in the sputum. If three specimens are examined, the direct sputum is positive in about 80 per cent of patients with pulmonary paragonimiasis and pigmented sputum. Concentration of 24-hour sputum collection by techniques like those used for acid-fast bacilli will identify ova in an additional 12 to 15 per cent. Direct and concentrated stools will also reveal ova in a high percentage of patients because of the habit of swallowing sputum. Finally, surgical specimens should be examined grossly for the adult fluke (see Fig.1) and sections carefully examined for the ova.

In patients with extrapulmonary paragonimiasis and some patients with pulmonary disease, ova may not be detected. In these cases the skin test and serologic tests are particularly valuable. The complement fixation test performed with a fractionated antigen from the adult worm (Sawada et al., 1968) is usually positive only in active disease. The skin test with purified antigens standardized to contain 10 mg of protein/100 ml was first widely used by Sadun and Buck (1960). It produces a wheal within 15 to 20 minutes that is at least twice the size of a control injection of buffered saline in virtually 100 per cent of patients with paragonimiasis. It also cross-reacts strongly with *Clonorchis sinensis* and remains positive after successful treatment or self-cure. Yokogawa (1969) found that in patients without demonstrable ova in the sputum, a positive complement fixation test correlated with improvement after specific treatment. Patients with a positive skin test and a negative complement fixation test did not improve.

## TREATMENT

Bithionol, 2,2′ thiobis (4,6-dichlorophenol), is the treatment of choice for paragonimiasis. This drug has several actions on metabolic pathways in the parasite and has recently been convincingly shown to interfere with fumarate utilization by inhibiting fumarate reductase (Hamajima et al., 1979). Morphologic changes that correlated with the metabolic effect included separation of the tegument from the basement membrane and deterioration of structures beneath the membrane.

A daily dosage of 30 to 40 mg/kg orally every other day for 10 to 15 doses cures more than 90 per cent of patients with paragonimiasis (Yokogawa et al., 1963). Ova usually disappear within ten days and the chest x-ray improves within two weeks. Only a few chest x-rays remain abnormal after 6 to 12 months. If symptoms recur or ova reappear in the sputum, the patients should be retreated.

Bithionol also acts on flukes in ectopic foci. Good results have been obtained in several patients with cerebral paragonimiasis (Yokogawa et al., 1961; Chu, 1962). This is an important advance because surgical management is difficult and often disappointing.

Side effects are troublesome, but treatment seldom has to be discontinued (Yim, 1970). Diarrhea is the most common side effect. It may occur in as many as 50 per cent of patients but is usually transient and subsides within a few days after treatment is completed. Skin rashes occur in about 15 per cent of patients about one to two weeks after beginning therapy. The rash is a generalized urticarial or papular eruption that is severely pruritic. It is probably stimulated by allergic reactions to destroyed worms because it occurs most frequently in patients with very heavy infections. Headache and giddiness occur in about 10 per cent of patients.

Several new agents are being tested against paragonimiasis but no effective alternate therapy is available yet.

## PROPHYLAXIS

Ova in the excreta of people with paragonimiasis are the major source of contamination of freshwater crustaceans. Wild and domestic animals are a minor reservoir (Yokogawa, 1965). Accordingly, Yokogawa (1965) and Kim (1970) have shown that mass therapy with bithionol is effective and causes the disease to die out slowly in the tested area. At the present time, this seems to be the prophylactic technique of choice. Eradication of the snail host is impractical, and hungry populations cannot be educated to avoid the use of night soil on their crops or to stop eating the abundant crustaceans. Efforts to teach the people to cook crayfish and crabs should be continued even though they have not been well accepted.

### References

Ameel, D. J.: *Paragonimus,* its life history and distribution in North America and its taxonomy (Trematoda: Troglotrematidae). Am J Hyg 19:279, 1934.

Baelz, E.: Über parasitäre Häemoptoë (Gregarinosis pulmonum). Zentralbl Med Wissensch 18:721, 1880.

Braun, M.: Über clinostomum Leidy. Zool Anz 22:484, 1899.

Chien, M. H.: Roentgenological diagnosis of paragonimiasis. Chin M J 73:37, 1955.

Chu, D. S.: Clinical observations on chemotherapy of cerebral paragonimiasis with bithionol. Korean Cent J Med 7:1, 1962.

Diaconita, G. H., and Goldis, G. H.: Investigations on pathomorphology and pathogenesis of pulmonary paragonimiasis. Acta Turberc Scand 44:51, 1964.

Galatius-Jensen, F., and Uhm, I. K.: Radiological aspects of cerebral paragonimiasis. Br J Radiol 38:404, 1965.

Hamajima, F., Fujino, T., Yamagami, K., and Eriguchi, N.: Studies of the *in vitro* effects of bithionol and menicholopholan on flukes of *Clonorchis sinensis, Metagonimus takahashii* and *Paragonimus miyazakii.* Int J Parasitol 9:241, 1979.

Iwasaki, M.: Clinical studies of paragonimiasis (in Japanese). Rinshō Naiko Shōnika 10:207, 1955.

Kay, S.: *Paragonimus westermani* infestation involving the anterior abdominal wall. Report of a case simulating acute appendicitis. JAMA 159:1734, 1955.

Kerbert, C.: Zur trematoden Kenntnis. Zool Anz 1:271, 1878.

Kim, J.: Treatment of *Paragonimus westermani* infections with bithionol. Am J Trop Med Hyg 19:940, 1970.

Kobayashi, H.: Studies on the lung fluke in Korea. I. On the life history and morphology of the lung fluke. Mil Med Hochs Keijo 2:95, 1918.

Leuckhart, R.: Die parasiten des Menschen und die von ihnen herrührendra Krankheiten, 2nd ed. Leipzig, C. F. Winter, 1889.

Manason, P.: On endemic hemoptysis. Lancet I:532, 1883.

Manson, P.: *Distoma ringeri.* M Times Gaz 2:8, 1881.

Mitsuno, T., Siko, T., Inanaga, K., and Zimmerman, L. E.: Cerebral paragonimiasis, a neurosurgical problem in the Far East. J Nerv Ment Dis 116:685, 1952.

Miyazaki, I., and Habe, S.: A newly recognized mode of human infection with the lung fluke, *Paragonimus westermani* (Kerbert, 1878). J Parasitol 62:646, 1976.

Nakagawa, K.: The mode of infection in pulmonary distomiasis. Certain fresh water crabs as intermediate hosts of *Paragonimus westermani.* J Infect Dis 18:131, 1916.

Nwokolo. C.: Endemic paragonimiasis in Eastern Nigeria. Clinical features of the recent outbreak following the Nigerian civil war. Trop Geogr Med 24:138, 1972.

Ogakwu, M., and Nwokolo, C.: Radiological findings in pulmonary paragonimiasis as seen in Nigeria: A review based on one hundred cases. Br J Radiol 46:699, 1973.

Oh, S. J.: Paragonimus meningitis. J Neurol Sci 6:419, 1968.

Sadun, E., and Buck, A.: Paragonimiasis in South Korea — immunodiagnostic, epidemiologic, clinical, roentgenologic and therapeutic studies. Am J Trop Med Hyg 9:562, 1960.

Sawada, T., Takei, K., Sato, S., and Matsuyama, S.: Studies on the immunodiagnosis of paragonimiasis. 3. Intradermal skin tests with fractionated antigens. J Infect Dis 118:235, 1968.

Yokogawa, M.: Paragonimus and paragonimiasis. Adv Parasitol 3:99, 1965.

Yokogawa, M.: Paragonimus and paragonimiasis. Adv Parasitol 7:375, 1969.

Yokogawa, M., Iwasaki, M., Shigeyasu, M., Hirose, H., Okura, T., and Tsuji, M.: Chemotherapy of paragonimiasis with bithionol. V. Studies on the minimum effective dose and changes in abnormal x-ray shadows in chest after treatment. Am J Trop Med Hyg 12:859, 1963.

Yokogawa, M., Yoshimura, H., Okura, T., Tsuji, M., Sano, M., Iwasaki, M., and Hirose, H.: Chemotherapy of paragonimiasis with bithionol. II. Clinical observations on the treatment of bithionol. Jap J Parasitol 10:317, 1961.

Yokogawa, S.: On the migratory course of the human lung fluke in the final host (in Japanese). Taiwan Igakkwai Zasshi 152–153:685–728, 1915.
Yokogawa, S.: An experimental study of the intracranial parasitism of

the human lung fluid, *Paragonimus westermani.* Am J Hyg 1:63, 1921.
Yun, D. J.: Paragonimiasis in children in Korea. J. Pediatr 56:736, 1960.

# INFECTION WITH **124** PNEUMOCYSTIS CARINII
### Stephen N. Cohen, M.D.

## DEFINITION

*Pneumocystis carinii* is an organism of uncertain taxonomy. Infection with *Pneumocystis* is clinically recognized as interstitial pneumonia. It occurs as an endemic and intermittently epidemic illness of premature or malnourished infants clustered in nurseries and foundling homes, or sporadically in patients with defective immunity. It is particularly likely to affect patients who have received prolonged corticosteroid therapy for lymphoreticular malignancy, organ transplantation, or collagen-vascular disease. Ruskin (1976) has authoritatively reviewed our current knowledge of this infection.

## ETIOLOGY

*Pneumocystis* was first detected in the lungs of guinea pigs and rats by the Brazilian investigators Chagas (1909) and Carini (1910), who considered it an unusual variant of the trypanosomes with which they had experimentally infected the rodents. Shortly thereafter, the Delanoes at the Institut Pasteur in Paris demonstrated these structures in the lungs of ordinary sewer rats and appreciated that they were a unique new microorganism, which they named *P. carinii* (Delanoe and Delanoe, 1912). Thirty years then elapsed before *Pneumocystis* was definitely associated with human disease by Van der Meer and Brug in 1942, who described three cases of pneumonia caused by this organism.

Our inability until recently to propagate *Pneumocystis* in vitro has prevented the fulfillment of Koch's postulates and seriously hampered the study of *P. carinii.* Many wild and domestic animals are naturally infected with *Pneumocystis,* but the organisms are ordinarily sparse and difficult to detect. Corticosteroids activate latent *Pneumocystis* infection of rodents, providing a model infection with a large number of organisms (Weller, 1956; Frenkel et al., 1966). Electronmicroscopic investigation of the organism's life cycle

in animals (Campbell, 1972) and the response of experimental infection to treatment with classic antiprotozoal chemotherapy suggest that *P. carinii* is a protozoan. The trophozoite is probably motile, may reproduce by binary fission, and invades the lung parenchyma. The trophozoite wall then thickens, and the organisms encyst. The cyst matures with the development of eight intracystic merozoites or "daughter" bodies, which are liberated when the cyst wall ruptures and, in turn, develop into trophozoites (Fig. 1). Serologic comparisons of morphologically identical human and animal strains of *P. carinii* have been inconclusive. Cross-infection studies suggest species-specificity, but the histologic features of the infections are similar.

## PATHOGENESIS

Any hypothesis of the pathogenesis of *Pneumocystis* infection must take into account certain epidemiologic and experimental observations.

Most infants involved in nursery epidemics are about 4 months old, an age that allows little environmental contact and coincides with the physiologic nadir of serum immune globulin levels. However, most infected infants are not hypogammaglobulinemic, and there is no consistent correlation between immunoglobulin levels per se and *Pneumocystis* infection in either infants or adults.

Serologic studies suggest that unrecognized infection with *P. carinii* must be extremely common in infancy, one survey finding immunofluorescent antibody in 100 per cent of children two years of age (Meuwissen et al., 1977).

Sporadic *Pneumocystis* pneumonia is five times more common in the first year of life than at any other age, and over 25 per cent of sporadic illness occurs before age 5 years. Nursery outbreaks, which were common in Europe during the early post-World War II years, have become unusual there, but outbreaks have subsequently been reported from Korea, Vietnam, and Iran under

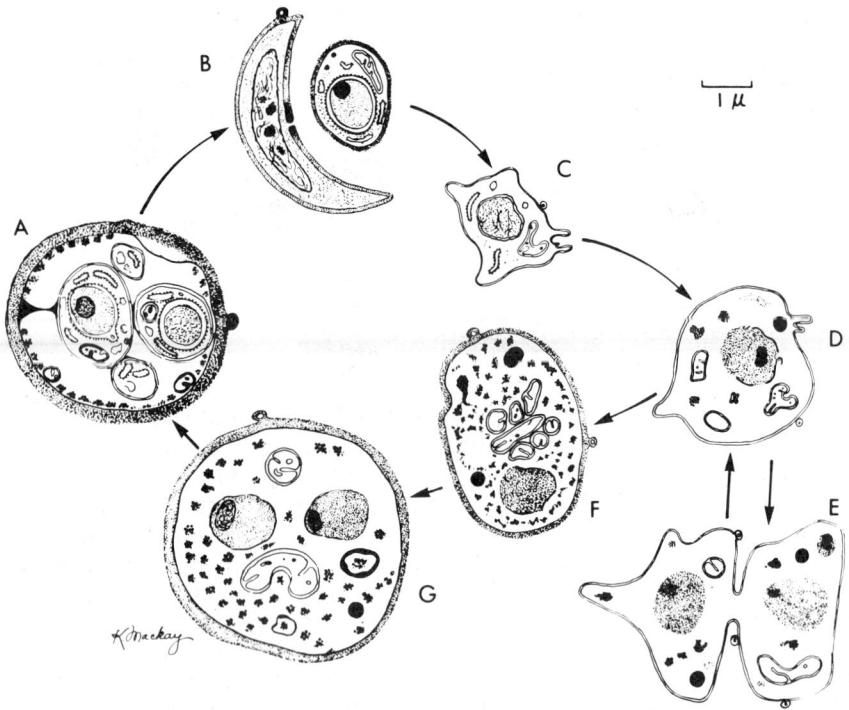

**FIGURE 1.** *Probable life cycle of* Pneumocystis *within pulmonary alveoli. A, Mature cyst with intracystic bodies; B, empty cyst and recently escaped intracystic body; C, small trophozoite; D, larger trophozoite; E, possible budding or conjugating form; F, large trophozoite undergoing thickening of pellicle; G, precyst. (From Campbell, W. G., Jr.: Ultrastructure of pneumocystis in human lung. Arch Pathol 93:312, 1972.)*

similar conditions of crowding and malnutrition. Adult patients who suffer a high incidence of *Pneumocystis* infection also are subject to frequent reactivation of latent infections (tuberculosis, cryptococcosis, varicella-zoster infection, cytomegalovirus, toxoplasmosis). Cell-mediated immune mechanisms are probably more important than humoral defenses for all of these infections, and such mechanisms are impaired in these patients. Latent *Pneumocystis* infection is present in many animal species and is activated readily by starvation or by corticosteroid administration.

A number of case reports, as well as serologic studies showing a greater prevalence of antibody to *Pneumocystis* in contacts of infected patients than in healthy adults, suggest that person-to-person spread of infection in hospital among immunosuppressed patients or in the family is possible, and airborne transmission of experimental infection has been unequivocally demonstrated (Hendley and Weller, 1971).

A reasonable speculation on the pathogenesis of *Pneumocystis* infection begins with the excretion of trophozoites of *P. carinii* (or perhaps cysts, which might be hardier) in the fomites of individuals whose pulmonary infection is mild. The organisms are then aspirated and transformed, if initially encysted, into invasive trophozoites upon reaching the alveoli, whereupon the normal host's leukocytes, primarily macrophages, rapidly phagocytize and destroy most of them. Antibody

and complement may facilitate the phagocytosis and killing of ingested organisms but are probably not critical in determining the outcome of infection. Clinical disease may be absent but is otherwise mild. A small proportion of organisms encyst and escape destruction by the host defenses. These organisms persist in the tissues, possibly for the life of the host, but they may be intermittently released, like the periodic excretion of EB virus or cytomegalovirus by the normal host, perhaps during intercurrent viral infection. In infants and children with defective cell-mediated immunity due to malnutrition, congenital deficiencies (usually lymphopenic hypogammaglobulinemias) or immunosuppression due to chemotherapy such as cyclophosphamide and/or corticosteroids, and very rarely in apparently normal persons, the primary infection develops into a severe interstitial pneumonia. Primary infection may also cause *Pneumocystis* pneumonia in immunologically depressed adults who will usually have been receiving corticosteroid therapy, but it is more likely that pneumonia in the adult arises from the uncontrolled reactivation of latent infection. If the infection is not limited by the immune defenses, the organisms proliferate and attach to and occlude the alveolar surfaces, causing an alveolar-capillary block with hypoxia. Many episodes of *Pneumocystis* pneumonia arise as steroid therapy is being reduced, suggesting that the inflammatory reaction to infection contributes to the pulmonary disease; the attendant exudation of serum proteins into the alveolus and within the alveolar walls further impairs gas exchange.

## PATHOLOGY

The lungs of a patient with severe, diffuse, interstitial pneumonia resemble liver tissue, are heavy, and are usually dark bluish-purple. Only the marginal areas may be aerated. Subpleural air blebs may rupture and presumably cause occasional spontaneous pneumothorax. There is rarely a pleural reaction or necrosis of the lung unless *Pneumocystis* infection is complicated by infection with other organisms. Less extensively involved lungs do not have so characteristic an appearance.

Microscopically, the alveoli of hematoxylin-eosin stained sections are filled with pinkish, foamy, honeycombed, or vacuolated material, the clear areas often containing small dots (Figs. 2 and 3). The alveolar content is PAS-positive and consists largely of coalesced, desquamated microphages whose digestive vacuoles contain degenerating organisms. Hyaline membranes may or may not be present. Giant cells and hypertrophied lining cells are often seen in the alveolar walls, sometimes with some lymphoid cells. Plasma cells have been prominent in the interstitial infiltrates of the infantile pneumonias seen in nursery outbreaks, and fluorescence studies demonstrate immunoglobulins bound to the intra-alveolar masses of *Pneumocystis* organisms. Plasma cells and globulins are not usually seen in

tissues taken from immunosuppressed or congenitally lymphopenic patients. There are rare reports in which the dominant histologic elements are epithelioid-giant cell granulomas in the alveolar spaces. In cases of long duration, organization of the alveolar exudate with an appearance of fibroblasts, macrophages, and calcification may occur.

Cysts clumped within alveoli are best visualized with the methenamine silver stain (Grocott, 1955) (Fig. 4). They have thin, black capsules that are round or slightly wrinkled but often appear folded into a cup or crescent shape. The cysts are approximately 4 to 6 $\mu$ in diameter, or half the width of a red blood cell, with which they can be confused. The unfolded cysts often "contain" a pair of darkly staining structures 1 to 2 $\mu$ long and shaped like opposed parentheses; these structures (actually thickenings in the wall) are pathognomonic of the parasite. Budding is not seen. Cysts may also be visualized in tissue, though with less contrast against the background, by using the modified toluidine blue O stain (Chalvardjian and Grawe, 1963). Giemsa, Gridley, and Gram-Weigert stains also have their enthusiasts. Cysts rapidly lose their "internal" structure, and organisms usually fragment and disappear from the sections within a few days of starting treatment, but may persist for 10 to 14 days or even longer, despite an apparent clinical response.

Although *Pneumocystis* infection seldom extends beyond the lung, local lymph nodes may be involved, and in rare instances organisms spread hematogenously and proliferate in the liver, spleen, marrow, myocardium, kidney, adrenal,

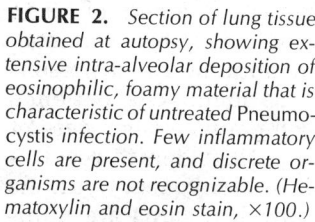

**FIGURE 2.** *Section of lung tissue obtained at autopsy, showing extensive intra-alveolar deposition of eosinophilic, foamy material that is characteristic of untreated* Pneumocystis *infection. Few inflammatory cells are present, and discrete organisms are not recognizable. (Hematoxylin and eosin stain, ×100.)*

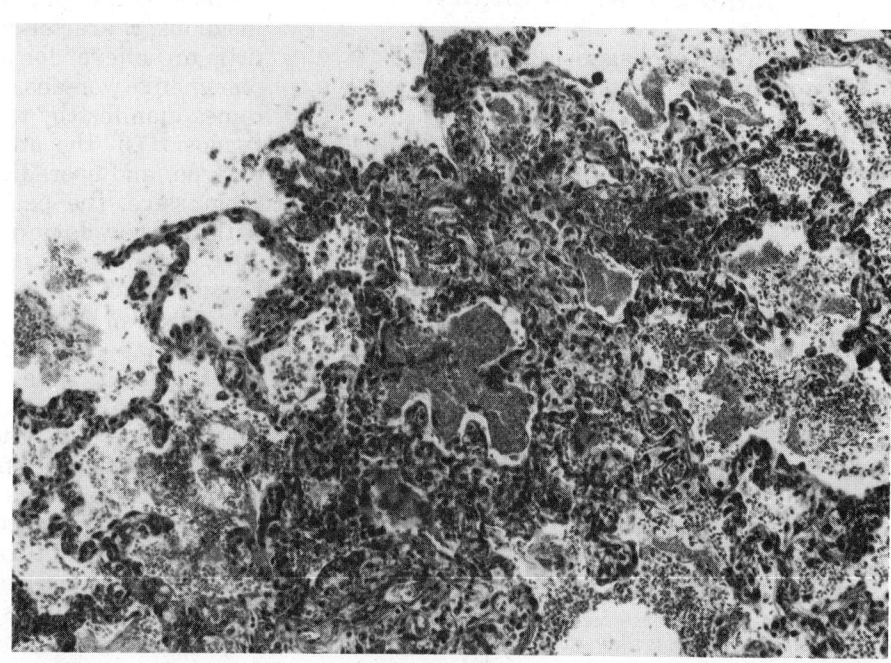

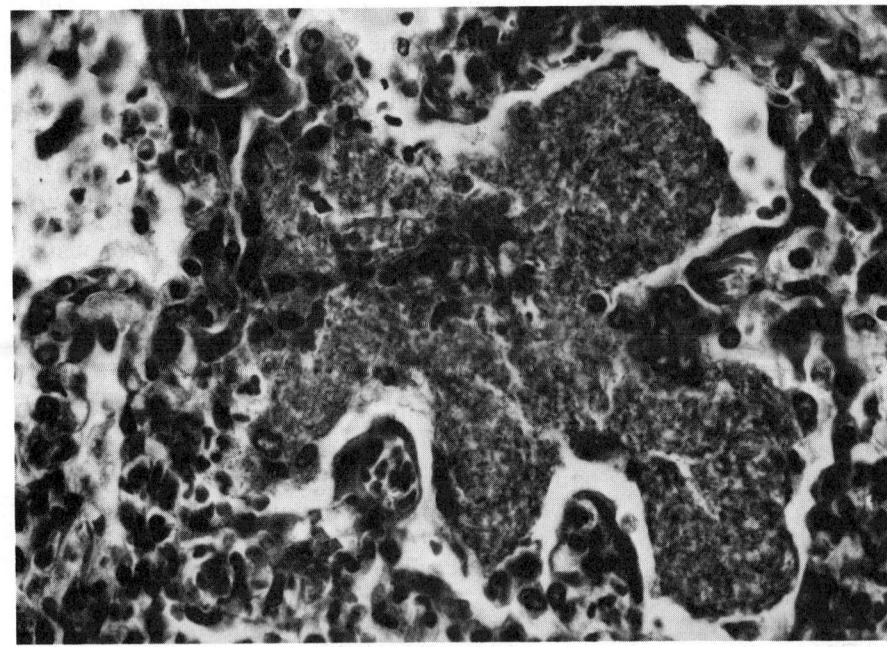

**FIGURE 3.** *High-power view of the lung tissue of Figure 2. The eosinophilic intra-alveolar material may appear completely amorphous, but often closely packed vacuoles in this matrix contain a single off-center granule, which is highly suggestive of* P. carinii. *(Hematoxylin and eosin stain, ×400.)*

thyroid, pancreas, colon, and other tissues, often with abscess formation.

In addition to the widespread histologic involvement in clinically severe *Pneumocystis* disease, similar microscopic findings may be restricted to focal areas in patients with inapparent *Pneumocystis* infections that are often associated with depressed immunity, radiation therapy, and malignancy.

## CLINICAL MANIFESTATIONS AND LABORATORY FINDINGS

The mainstay of diagnosis is a high index of suspicion in the susceptible parent population,

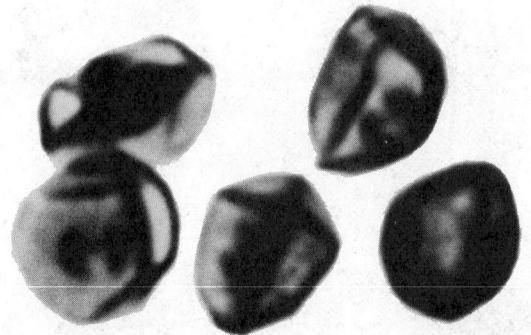

**FIGURE 4.** *Biopsy imprint smear stained with methenamine silver from lung of patient with* Pneumocystis pneumonia. *The clustering, the slightly folded edges, and the cyst wall components, which appear as comma-shaped structures within the cysts, are characteristic. The organisms have a similar appearance in tissue sections, as well as in imprints or sections stained with toluidine blue O. (Grocott's methenamine silver stain, ×1000.)*

since there are no reliable indicators of the presence of *Pneumocystis* infection. *P. carinii* is responsible for one fourth to one half of all interstitial pneumonia in immunosuppressed patients and affects at least 1 per cent of all children with acute lymphocytic leukemia each year (Walzer et al., 1974). Illness tends to occur as corticosteroid dosage is reduced. The clinical presentation of *Pneumocystis* infection is highly variable and may depend upon the coexistence of infection with other organisms, which occurs in as many as 25 per cent of sporadic cases. Endemic and epidemic illness among nursery infants may often be insidious, characterized only by poor feeding and little or no fever for a few weeks. Gradually, the pneumonia worsens, and respiratory distress becomes manifest by tachypnea and eventually by cyanosis. On the other hand, illness in infants may be, and sporadic cases usually are, rapidly progressive, the patient appearing in extremis within a few days during which fevers of 39 to 40° C, often with shaking chills, are common. Cough, which is usually nonproductive, is present in less than half of the patients. The patient's earliest and often only complaint is shortness of breath, but at times the patient denies respiratory distress despite obvious tachypnea. Cyanosis may develop, but other physical signs are minimal, and auscultation of the chest is remarkable only for the absence of findings.

Chest radiographs usually reveal diffuse, bilateral granular infiltrates that spread from the hilus in a pattern similar to that of pulmonary edema and initially spare the periphery (Fig. 5). This picture may progress over several hours to

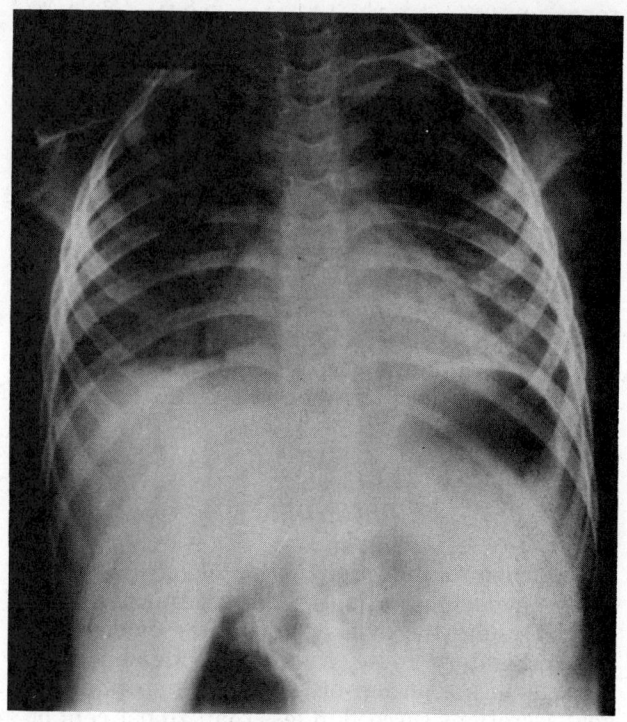

**FIGURE 5.** *Chest X-ray of patient with bilateral, interstitial pneumonia due to* Pneumocystis *infection. The granular infiltrates are most prominent centrally and at the bases, with relative sparing of the periphery and apices. Air bronchograms are seen in the consolidated areas behind the cardiac shadow.*

complete opacification of the lungs with air bronchograms. An occasional patient with extreme dyspnea has a normal chest film, but extensive changes usually develop within the next 24 to 48 hours. The radiographs of clinically severe, biopsy-confirmed illness may rarely show lobar pneumonia, focal bronchopneumonia, or even pulmonary nodules.

Most laboratory studies are unrewarding. Lymphopenia and hypoalbuminemia are often present, but only irregularly is hypogammaglobulinemia evident. The most consistent and diagnostically useful laboratory abnormality is arterial hypoxemia, with $pAO_2$ commonly in the range of 35 to 45 mm Hg.

## COMPLICATIONS AND SEQUELAE

The mortality of untreated *Pneumocystis* infection in nursery outbreaks before the introduction of specific chemotherapy was about 50 per cent, while that of sporadic cases was close to 100 per cent, there being only one report documenting recovery of an untreated patient with a predisposing illness. Death results from pulmonary insufficiency due to *Pneumocystis* infection or to the local and systemic effects of associated infection.

The pulmonary insufficiency resulting from the pneumonic process may be aggravated by pneumothorax or pneumomediastinum arising from the infection itself, from respiratory therapy at

high inspiratory pressures, or from diagnostic sampling of the lung.

Patients who recover from acute *Pneumocystis* pneumonia generally have little or no clinically significant residua of pulmonary damage. However, pulmonary fibrosis has been described late in the acute stage of illness in fatal cases and in at least two long-term survivors. The frequency of this complication is difficult to ascertain because of a paucity of published reports with adequate follow-up, and because many of these patients also receive irradiation, potentially pneumotoxic drugs such as methotrexate, and prolonged high tension oxygen therapy.

Involvement of organs other than the lung has not been recognized before death, possibly because it is overshadowed by overwhelming hypoxia.

## GEOGRAPHIC VARIATIONS

Sporadic *Pneumocystis* infections in immunosuppressed patients are worldwide in distribution. Nursery outbreaks, in contrast, are reported primarily in developing countries or impoverished areas of wealthy countries.

The identification of *Pneumocystis* infection in European nurseries after World War II may well have reflected the availability of antibiotics, which prevented the death of these malnourished children from acute bacterial infection (Dutz,

1970). As the nutritional status of Europe improved markedly in the decade following World War II, reports of illness in nurseries became uncommon. Episodes subsequently reported from Asia and Africa probably reflect similar socioeconomic conditions that provide antibiotic therapy and adequate diagnostic facilities in institutions but inadequate nutrition for many people. Malnutrition is the only experimental manipulation that activates latent *Pneumocystis* infection in animals as effectively as corticosteroid administration and has been unequivocally shown to impair the immune response, particularly cell-mediated reactions (Smythe et al., 1971; Hughes et al., 1974).

## DIAGNOSIS

Diagnosis of infection with *Pneumocystis* requires a demonstration of the organism in the lung. Despite the evidence of contagiousness by the respiratory route, attempts to demonstrate organisms in sputum or aspirated hypopharyngeal secretions succeed in less than 10 per cent of biopsy-proven cases and usually only serve to delay diagnosis. Bronchial brushing succeeds in 80 to 85 per cent of cases (Repsher et al., 1972). Brushing has occasionally been associated with hemorrhage and with pneumothorax, but the latter complication occurs spontaneously in other infected patients. Bronchopulmonary lavage, which is potentially hazardous in hypoxic patients, has also been reported to yield positive smears in a high proportion of cases.

*Pneumocystis* may be present in the respiratory secretions of healthy infants living in endemic areas (Dutz, 1970). Thus, finding *Pneumocystis* organisms in sputum or brushings is not synonymous with their presence in the lung parenchyma, just as the isolation of pneumococcus from sputum cannot be taken as conclusive proof of pneumococcal pneumonia. Techniques that sample the substance of the lung are not only definitive but best reveal alternative or concomitant infectious processes. The procedure of choice is open lung biopsy, which, despite the risks of hypoxia, postoperative pneumothorax, and (particularly in thrombocytopenic patients) hemorrhage, has proved remarkably safe. Platelet transfusions can be administered preoperatively if needed. The area of maximal involvement can be readily identified, adequate amounts of tissue can be obtained for both histologic and microbiologic studies, bleeding is easily controlled under direct inspection, and a chest tube prevents the accumulation of intrapleural air.

Other popular invasive techniques include needle aspiration with a 22-gauge, 1-inch needle through the chest wall, usually in the right axilla (Johnson and Johnson, 1970) or transbronchial biopsy with a flexible forceps. The disease is commonly diffuse, and these techniques are very often successful; occasionally inadequate sampling may be a problem. Pneumothorax occurs in about one third of cases, and half of these require a chest tube. Transthoracic Vim-Silverman needle biopsy has been largely abandoned because of an apparently high incidence of severe postbiopsy pneumothorax and uncontrolled bleeding.

The cut surface of the material obtained by biopsy should be rubbed firmly on several clean glass slides to prepare imprint smears or scraped with a scalpel blade and smears made of the scrapings. If aspirates have been obtained, a drop of the aspirate is placed on each slide. The air-dried slides are then stained. A portion of the tissue should also be fixed and submitted for histologic examination, including specimens prepared with PAS and methenamine silver stains. Smears are first examined with the toluidine blue O stain, which demonstrates the cyst wall and, usually, the comma-like internal structures. If organisms are not found, additional slides can be prepared by using the more tedious methenamine silver stain, in which the gray-black organisms stand out most clearly against the counterstained green background. However, it is unusual for the silver stain to detect organisms missed by toluidine blue O. Experience is necessary for the proper interpretation of these smears, particularly from samples taken through the bronchi in which debris often stains artifactually. Particular confusion may arise with silver stains from red blood cells (which, however, usually stain yellow-orange), less often with the grayish nuclei of polymorphonuclear leukocytes or with yeast, both of which pick up both toluidine blue O and silver stains but lack the characteristic internal structure. The limitations of these and other stains are well discussed in recent reviews by Kim and Hughes (1973) and by Kagan and Norman (1977). Experimental fluorescent antibody (FA) reagents for direct staining have been developed and promise greater sensitivity, but false-positive results have also been reported with FA, which is no more rapid than the toluidine blue O method.

Specimens examined for *Pneumocystis* should also be cultured and stained for bacteria, fungi, and mycobacteria. Viral cultures are desirable, although no useful therapy is presently available, and the recovery of an agent such as cytomegalovirus from the lung may be difficult to interpret.

*Pneumocystis* has recently been serially propagated in the widely available Vero cell line (Latorre et al., 1977), suggesting that diagnostic specimens might be routinely cultured with this method. Culture is almost always a more sensitive diagnostic technique than microscopic examination, however, and may prove to identify *Pneumocystis* in a number of carriers or individuals with inconsequential or latent infections that do not require therapy.

Serologic diagnosis has been used in Europe and Asia, particularly in evaluating nursery outbreaks. Crude antigens are prepared from the infected lungs of patients or steroid-treated rats and are usually employed in a complement fixation test. Titers of ≥ 1:4 are usually considered positive, although each laboratory must standardize its own test procedure. Immunofluorescent tests upon fixed sections of human lung have also been studied extensively. European investigators found elevated CF titers in 75 to 100 per cent of nursery cases, but American investigators have found only about 15 per cent of sporadic cases positive for CF antibody. This discrepancy is probably not due to antigenic differences between strains nor to technique; similar results are obtained in all laboratories when the same sera are examined. The likely explanation for the seronegative American cases is the overwhelming preponderance in the U.S.A. of immunosuppressed patients, who fail to develop a normal antibody response. Serologic diagnosis is in any case only possible in retrospect, as antibody is absent during the acute onset of disease and requires several weeks to develop.

The absence of antibody during the acute stage of illness may be due to its reaction with an excess of circulating antigen. The prospect of employing antigen detection as a diagnostic test, however, is discouraged by a report that although antigen is not found in control patients, it is detected as frequently in marrow-transplant patients who remain asymptomatic as in those who are acutely ill with *Pneumocystis* pneumonia (Meyers et al., 1979).

## TREATMENT

Two antimicrobial agents have found wide acceptance in the therapy of *Pneumocystis* pneumonia: pentamidine, a drug long employed in both treatment and prophylaxis of Gambian sleeping sickness, and cotrimoxazole, or trimethoprim-sulfamethoxazole, a widely used antibacterial combination.

### Pentamidine

Pentamidine is an aromatic diamidine that was originally developed as a hypoglycemic agent. Since the discovery of its effectiveness against the early stages of *Trypanosoma gambiense* infection in 1941, the drug has been administered to mil-

lions of Africans with minimal toxicity. Successful treatment of *Pneumocystis* pneumonia was first reported by Ivady and Paldy in 1958, who employed pentamidine in nursery epidemics. Numerous investigators have subsequently confirmed their results. Pentamidine is supplied as the isethionate salt, a white powder that should be kept in a cool location until use and that must be dissolved in sterile distilled water for parenteral administration. The drug is poorly soluble in saline, which should not be used. If contamination is avoided, the solution can be kept refrigerated for five to seven days, when slight turbidity or crystalline deposits may develop. These do not denote a loss of activity, and the solution remains suitable for intramuscular, but not intravenous, injection. Pentamidine is not absorbed orally. The usual dosage is 4 mg of the salt per kg (or 100 to 150 mg/m² body surface area), given in a volume of no more than 3 ml, and administered intramuscularly once daily for 12 to 14 days. The anterior thigh is a useful injection site for pediatric patients with little muscle mass. Intravenous (IV) administration is not recommended unless the patient is severely thrombocytopenic; in that case, the drug should be diluted to 5 to 10 ml and given over a 5 to 10 minute interval, during which the IV fluid is kept running and blood pressure is monitored. Plasma levels are low; pentamidine is concentrated primarily in the kidneys and to a lesser extent in the liver. Excretion is prolonged, with most of the drug being recovered unchanged in the urine over a six- to eight-week period. It has been suggested from animal studies that the lungs may concentrate pentamidine that has been slowly released from other tissues.

A wide spectrum of complications has been reported in recipients of pentamidine, but many reports are difficult to assess because of severe underlying illness (Western et al., 1970). Side effects do not usually prevent completion of a full course of therapy. The most serious problem is pain and/or abscess formation at the injection site, which occurs in nearly 20 per cent of patients and may result in lethal superinfection. Azotemia develops during therapy in a similar proportion of patients but is generally mild and reversible when the drug is discontinued. Depression of blood glucose or of serum calcium is less common and usually asymptomatic, but should be considered in any patient who deteriorates neurologically. Elevation of liver enzymes or bilirubin has also been reported but is usually slight and transient. Rare individuals develop rashes, and fatal erythema multiforme and toxic epidermal necrolysis with renal failure have been described. Thrombocytopenic purpura occurs uncommonly. "Herxheimer-like" reactions (exacerbation of illness with treatment) have been recognized in trypanosome-infected Africans but are very unusual with *Pneumocystis*. There is no evidence that the pulmonary fibrosis occasionally seen following *Pneumocystis* pneumonia is related to pentamidine treatment.

### Trimethoprim-Sulfamethoxazole

Combination therapy with the antifolates pyrimethamine and sulfadiazine for the protozoan infections malaria and toxoplasmosis is well accepted. In 1966, Frenkel et al. reported that pentamidine and pyrimethamine-sulfadiazine were about equally potent in treating cortisone-induced *Pneumocystis* infection of rats. The slightly more rapid clearing of parasites by the diamidine was balanced by its greater toxicity, especially necrosis at the injection site. Subsequent uncontrolled clinical trials of pyrimethamine-sulfadiazine in *Pneumocystis*-infected humans gave mixed results.

A new antifolate combination, trimethoprim-sulfamethoxazole (TMP-SMX), was superior to pentamidine in treating *Pneumocystis* pneumonia induced in cortisone-fed rats. Accordingly, Hughes et al. (1975) administered TMP-SMX to immunosuppressed children who were moderately ill with *Pneumocystis* infection and obtained results equal to those expected with pentamidine. Adult cases have also responded well (Lau and Young, 1976).

The combination of trimethoprim-sulfamethoxazole is available as tablets containing 80 mg TMP and 400 mg SMX and also as double-strength tablets containing 160 mg TMP and 800 mg SMX, or as a suspension containing 40 mg TMP and 200 mg SMX per 5 ml. A parenteral preparation is presently available only on an experimental basis. Doses have ranged as high as 20 mg TMP and 100 mg SMX/kg per day, divided into two to four doses and administered for 14 days. Side effects of the antifolate combination are largely limited to occasional skin rashes and other allergic responses well known for sulfonamides. Folate deficiency should be uncommon because of the short duration of therapy. Furthermore, TMP has a poor affinity for mammalian dihydrofolate reductase, and sulfonamides cannot function as antifolates in mammals. If chronic antifolate administration does lead to deficiency, the patient should be given intramuscular folinic acid, a form of the vitamin that man can utilize but protozoans cannot.

In a carefully controlled clinical comparison of pentamidine versus TMP-SMX, the drugs were found equally effective in treating *Pneumocystis* pneumonia, but TMP-SMX caused substantially fewer undesirable side effects (Hughes et al., 1978). Combined therapy with both pentamidine and

TMP-SMX has not been evaluated in man but offered no significant advantage over administration of TMP-SMX in experimental infection of rats (Kluge et al., 1978).

Treatment other than antimicrobial chemotherapy is limited to respiratory support and oxygen therapy. Elevated levels of inspiratory oxygen are extremely important to the hypoxic patient in the few days before histologic improvement can occur. An occasional patient may survive only with the aid of a membrane oxygenator during this critical period. The clinician must follow these seriously ill patients closely for signs of the reactivation of other latent infections or of bacterial or fungal superinfection of their poorly aerated lungs. Acute pulmonary deterioration should also suggest the possibility of unrecognized pneumothorax or some mechanical complication of respiratory therapy. Although tapering of steroid dosage is often temporally associated with the onset of symptomatic *Pneumocystis* pneumonia, the administration of steroids does not appear to improve the outcome. Injections of immune serum globulin have also been without obvious effect in controlling *Pneumocystis* infection of immunosuppressed children.

Antimicrobial therapy has improved the survival rate of patients with *Pneumocystis* pneumonia. If the patient's pneumonia is due only to *Pneumocystis,* he usually becomes afebrile within one or two days and, within that time, notes first a halt to the progression of his shortness of breath, and then an improvement in this symptom. The chest film does not clear as rapidly but lags several days to weeks behind the symptoms except in the mildest cases. Although only 10 per cent or fewer patients fail to clear the infecting parasite from their tissues within a few days of instituting treatment, the mortality for sporadic cases remains in the range of 30 to 50 per cent. Deaths may result from associated pulmonary infections as well as from nonpulmonary complications in the immunosuppressed patient but are most frequently due to respiratory failure, particularly in the presence of pre-existing pulmonary disease or a delay in diagnosis. In contrast, the introduction of pentamidine therapy has reduced the mortality of nursery epidemic disease, admittedly not always biopsy-proven, from about 50 per cent to 3 per cent. Improved survival from *Pneumocystis* pneumonia probably requires earlier diagnosis and better respiratory support rather than new antimicrobials.

It has not been possible to study the antimicrobial resistance of *Pneumocystis* strains from the small proportion of patients who fail to clear the organisms despite an appropriate dose and duration of treatment. Perhaps the organisms in these patients are not unusual but persist because the immune defect prevents a critical response of which recovered patients are capable. Furthermore, successful control of one clinical episode of *Pneumocystis* infection apparently cannot be relied upon to immunize or to eradicate organisms from the host. As noted earlier, asymptomatic infants in endemic surroundings carry *Pneumocystis* in their respiratory secretions for prolonged periods, and recurrent bouts of *Pneumocystis* are known to occur in both immunosuppressed patients and animals.

## PROPHYLAXIS

The evidence for respiratory transmission of *Pneumocystis* infection is sufficient to suggest that any patient with acute *Pneumocystis* pneumonia should be segregated from individuals known to be highly susceptible to severe *Pneumocystis* disease, i.e., malnourished, steroid-treated, or otherwise immunologically incompetent patients.

Chemoprophylaxis against *Pneumocystis* pneumonia is effective. Hughes et al. (1977) protected cancer patients, mainly children with lymphatic leukemia, with 150 mg trimethoprim plus 750 mg sulfamethoxazole/M²/day, given as two divided doses 12 hours apart. Prophylaxis was continued for two years, and the only untoward effect was a moderate increase in oral candidiasis. They recommend screening of blacks for glucose-6-phosphate dehydrogenase deficiency before employing this treatment. Unfortunately, prophylaxis does not eradicate carriage of latent infection (Hughes, 1979), which develops at the same rate as in untreated control patients after prophylaxis has been discontinued (Wolff and Baehner, 1978). The available evidence suggests that prophylaxis is necessary as long as the predisposing conditions exist. For example, Western et al. (1975) administered pentamidine for 14 days to cortisone-treated rats and delayed their death from *Pneumocystis* pneumonia for a mean of 13 days in comparison with controls, and Hughes et al. (1974) completely protected cortisone-injected rats by chronic administration of TMP-SMX.

Clinical reports from Hungary and Iran report similar success with pentamidine and with pyrimethamine-sulfadiazine. The toxicity of pentamidine excludes chronic administration, but the ease and safety of oral antifolate therapy is well suited to prophylaxis.

An effective vaccine might appear to be an even more attractive means of preventing *Pneumocystis* infection. One attempt to immunize rats against infection failed despite the development

of high antibody titers before cortisone administration. Since a deficient immune response seems to be the sine qua non for clinically significant *Pneumocystis* infection, any vaccine may be doomed to failure. The passive administration of immune serum globulin is ineffective in preventing the development of *Pneumocystis* pneumonia in children with congenital hypogammaglobulinemia (although the product administered is deficient in IgM and IgA). Transfer of cell-mediated immunity with living cells cannot be attempted because of the hazard of graft-versus-host reaction in this population.

## References

Campbell, W. G., Jr.: Ultrastructure of pneumocystis in human lung. Arch Pathol 93:312, 1972.
Carini, A.: Formas de eschizogonia do *Trypanosoma lewisii*. Soc Med Cir Sao Paolo, 16 Aout 1910.
Chagas, C.: Nova tripanozomiaze humana. Mem Inst Oswaldo Cruz 1:159, 1909.
Chalvardjian, A. M., and Grawe, L. A.: A new procedure for the identification of *Pneumocystis carinii* in tissue sections and smears. J Clin Pathol 16:383, 1963.
Delanoe, P., and Delanoe, M.: Sur les rapports des kystes de Carini du poumon des rats avec le *Trypanosoma lewisii*. C R Acad Sci (Paris) 155:658, 1912.
Dutz, W.: *Pneumocystis carinii* pneumonia. Pathol Annu 5:309, 1970.
Frenkel, J. K., Good, J. T., and Shultz, J. A.: Latent pneumocystis infection of rats, relapse and chemotherapy. Lab Invest 15:1559, 1966.
Grocott, R. G.: A stain for fungi in tissue sections and smears. Am J Clin Pathol 25:975, 1955.
Hendley, J. O., and Weller, T. H.: Activation and transmission in rats of infection with pneumocystis. Proc Soc Exp Biol Med 137:1401, 1971.
Hughes, W. T.: Limited effect of trimethoprim-sulfamethoxazole on *Pneumocystis carinii*. Antimicrob Agents Chemother 16:33, 1979.
Hughes, W. T., Feldman, S., Chaudhary, S. C., Ossi, M. J., Cox, F., and Sanyal, S. K.: Comparison of pentamidine isethionate with trimethoprim-sulfamethoxazole in the treatment of *Pneumocystis carinii* pneumonia. J Pediatr 92:285, 1978.
Hughes, W. T., Feldman, S., and Sanyal, S. K.: Treatment of *Pneumocystis carinii* pneumonitis with trimethoprim-sulfamethoxazole. Can Med Assoc J 112:475, 1975.
Hughes, W. T., Kuhn, S., Chaudhary, S., Feldman, S., Verzosa, M., Aur, R. J. A., Pratt, C., and George, S. L.: Successful chemoprophylaxis for *Pneumocystis carinii* pneumonia. N Engl J Med 297:1419, 1977.
Hughes, W. T., McNabb, P. C., Makres, T. D., and Feldman, S.: Efficacy of trimethoprim and sulfamethoxazole in the prevention and treatment of *Pneumocystis carinii* pneumonitis. Antimicrob Agents Chemother 5:289, 1974.
Hughes, W. T., Price, R. A., Sisko, F., Havron, W. S., Kafatos, A. G., Schonland, M., and Smythe, P. M.: Protein-calorie malnutrition. A host determinant for *Pneumocystis carinii* infection. Am J Dis Child 128:44, 1974.
Ivady, G., and Paldy, L.: Ein neues Behandlungsverfahren der interstitiellen plasmazelligen Pneumonie Frühgeborener mit fünfwertigen Stibium und aromatishen Diamidinen. Monatsschr Kinderheilkd 106:10, 1958.
Johnson, H. D., and Johnson, W. W.: *Pneumocystis carinii* pneumonia in children with cancer. JAMA 214:1067, 1970.
Kagan, I. G., and Norman, L.: The laboratory diagnosis of *Pneumocystis carinii* pneumonia. Health Lab Sci 14:155, 1977.
Kim, H., and Hughes, W. T.: Comparison of methods for identification of *Pneumocystis carinii* in pulmonary aspirates. Am J Clin Pathol 60:462, 1973.
Kluge, R. M., Spaulding, D. M., and Spain, A. J.: Combination of pentamidine and trimethoprim-sulfamethoxazole in the therapy of *Pneumocystis carinii* pneumonia in rats. Antimicrob Agents Chemother 13:975, 1978.

Latorre, C. K., Sulzer, A. J., and Norman, L. G.: Serial propagation of *Pneumocystis carinii* in cell line cultures. Appl Environ Microbiol 33:1204, 1977.

Lau, W. K., and Young, L. S.: Trimethoprim-sulfamethoxazole treatment of *Pneumocystis carinii* pneumonia in adults. N Engl J Med 295:716, 1976.

Meuwissen, J. H. E., Tauber, I., Leeuwenberg, A. D. E. M., Beckers, P. T. A., and Sieben, M.: Parasitologic and serologic observations of infection with *Pneumocystis* in humans. J Infect Dis 136:43, 1977.

Meyers, J. D., Pifer, L. L., Sale, G. E., and Thomas, E. D.: The value of *Pneumocystis carinii* antibody detection for diagnosis of *Pneumocystis carinii* pneumonia after marrow transplantation. Amer Rev Respir Dis 120:1283, 1979.

Repsher, L. H., Schroter, G., and Hammond, W. S.: Diagnosis of *Pneumocystis carinii* pneumonitis by means of endobronchial brush biospy. N Engl J Med 287:340, 1972.

Ruskin, J.: Pneumocystis carinii. In Remington, J. S., and Klein, J. O. (eds.): Infectious Diseases of the Fetus and Newborn Infant. Philadelphia, W. B. Saunders Company, 1976.

Smythe, P. M., Schonland, M., Brereton-Stiles, G. G., Coovadia, C. C., Grace, H. J., Loening, W. E. K., Mafoyane, A., Parent, M. A., and

Vos, G. H.: Thymolymphatic deficiency and depression of cell-mediated immunity in protein-calorie malnutrition. Lancet 2:939, 1971.

Van der Meer, G., and Brug, S. L.: Infection par pneumocystis chez l'homme et chez les animaux. Ann Soc Belg Med Trop 22:301, 1942.

Walzer, P. D., Perl, D. P., Krogstad, D. J., Rawson, P. G., and Schultz, M. G.: *Pneumocystis carinii* pneumonia in the United States. Ann Intern Med 80:83, 1974.

Weller, R.: Weitere Untersuchungen über experimentele. Ratten-pneumocystose in Hinblick auf die interstitielle Pneumonie der Frühgeborenen. Z Kinderheilkd 78:166, 1956.

Western, K. A., Norman, L., and Kaufmann, A. F.: Failure of pentamidine isethionate to provide chemoprophylaxis against *Pneumocystis carinii* infection in rats. J Infect Dis 131:273, 1975.

Western, K. A., Perera, D. R., and Schultz, M. G.: Pentamidine isethionate in the treatment of *Pneumocystis carinii* pneumonia. Ann Intern Med 73:695, 1970.

Wolff, L. J., and Baehner, R. L.: Delayed development of *Pneumocystis* pneumonia following administration of short-term high-dose trimethoprim-sulfamethoxazole. Am J Dis Child 132:525, 1978.

# C ABDOMINAL INFECTIONS

# 125 *FOOD POISONING*

## Sam T. Donta, M.D.

## INTRODUCTION

This chapter deals with diseases caused by bacterial toxins that are ingested preformed or are elaborated in the intestine by bacteria ingested in contaminated food. Most of the toxins affect the gastrointestinal tract directly. These intoxications are to be contrasted with gastrointestinal infections by bacteria ingested in contaminated food (Chapter 126). The distinction between infections and intoxications is somewhat arbitrary, since the pathogenesis of many enteric infections requires the elaboration of enterotoxins.

Approximately three fourths of cases of food poisoning are due to microbes or their products. The three leading causes of bacterial food poisoning throughout the world are *Staphylococcus aureus*, *Clostridium perfringens*, and *Salmonella* sp. *Salmonella* causes a direct infection of the intestine, as does *Vibrio parahemolyticus*, which is the major etiologic agent in certain coastal areas. Less frequent causes include *Shigella* sp., *Bacillus cereus*, *Escherichia coli*, and *Clostridium botulinum*. Although other bacteria have been implicated in sporadic cases, their pathogenetic roles remain uncertain.

## PATHOGENESIS

The pathogenesis of the clinical disorders depends on the outcome of interactions between ingested bacteria, their toxins, and host defense mechanisms. In general, bacteria cause illness because they are toxigenic or because they can invade tissues and cause inflammation. Some resistance to enteric bacteria or their toxins is provided by gastric acid, proteolytic enzymes, intestinal motility, secretory and humoral immune mechanisms, and the resident microflora itself; the role of cellular immunity has not been assessed.

Gastric acid is ineffective against the acid-stable enterotoxins of *Staphylococcus aureus* and the neurotoxins of *Clostridium botulinum*. In the case of acid-labile toxins and susceptible organisms, disease may result if either the amount of toxin or the number of bacteria ingested exceeds the inactivation potential of gastric acid, or if gastric acidity is reduced or absent. Patients who have a gastrectomy or who have achlorhydria are more susceptible to enteric diseases. Neutralization of gastric acid with food or with antacids probably enhances the potential to develop enteric disease (Donta, 1975).

# STAPHYLOCOCCAL FOOD POISONING

## *ETIOLOGY*

With rare exceptions, coagulase-positive strains of *Staphylococcus aureus* are responsible for this clinical syndrome. *Staphylococcus epidermidis* has also been incriminated, but most of the implicated strains are not enterotoxigenic.

## *PATHOGENESIS*

People are the major reservoir of the organism; as much as 50 per cent of the population are carriers of *S. aureus,* but not all strains are enterotoxigenic.

Following inoculation of food with staphylococci, the organisms begin to multiply at rates that are temperature-dependent. At between 10 and 45° C, cell division can occur as rapidly as every 20 minutes and, depending on the initial inoculum, total counts per gram of food can reach levels of $10^5$ to $10^8$ in a few hours.

As organisms reach their stationary phase of growth, enterotoxin is produced. Although the stimulus to enterotoxin synthesis is not known, toxin is probably elaborated in response to a still unidentified nutritional stimulus, and its synthesis is under some degree of catabolite repression. The ingestion of food contaminated with enterotoxin is responsible for staphylococcal food poisoning. In contrast, staphylococcal enterocolitis results from hematogenous seeding of the intestine during bacteremia or from intestinal overgrowth of staphylococci after administration of certain antibiotics or after abdominal surgery.

A variety of foods have been implicated in epidemics of *S. aureus* food poisoning; ham products, cold meats, salads, and cream-filled desserts are commonly involved. Contaminated foods do not usually have altered odor or taste properties. Outbreaks are more common during the summer.

Five antigenically-distinct enterotoxins (A through E) have been identified. Most strains of *S. aureus* can produce one or more types of enterotoxin. All types have been implicated in outbreaks of food poisoning, although types A, B, and D are most common. The purified enterotoxins are single polypeptide chains of ~30,000 daltons and are stable to heat, acid, and several proteolytic enzymes. A plasmid coding for enterotoxin production has been found, but recent evidence suggests that the genetic determinants may be chromosomal in nature (Shafer and Iandolo, 1978).

Once 1 $\mu$g or more of toxin is ingested, a neural response is initiated that results in centrally activated, vagal-mediated emesis and hypermotility of the bowel (Elwell et al., 1975). There are no direct local effects of the toxin on the upper or lower small bowel, and no fluid accumulates in experimentally ligated intestinal loops, in contrast to the effects seen with other enterotoxins. The delta-toxin of *S. aureus* is an exception; it does induce fluid secretion in small intestinal segments that may be of pathogenetic significance in staphylococcal enterocolitis (Kapral et al., 1976).

## *CLINICAL MANIFESTATIONS*

One to six hours after the ingestion of enterotoxin-containing food, nausea and vomiting begin. Emesis continues at 15 to 30 minute intervals until the illness subsides. The illness lasts no longer than 24 hours and usually no more than a few hours after the onset of clinical symptoms. Abdominal cramping and diarrhea occur and can occasionally be severe enough to cause dehydration and prostration. Other symptoms are excessive salivation, sweating, headache, and chills. Fever is notably absent.

There are no complications or sequelae except those related to dehydration. In the very old and very young, circulatory collapse may ensue.

## *GEOGRAPHIC VARIATION*

Staphylococcal food poisoning is a cosmopolitan disease. There are no reliable statistics about its incidence in most of the world, but since toxigenic *S. aureus* is distributed worldwide, the incidence of food poisoning is influenced primarily by the patterns of food preparation and storage, and food hygiene.

## *DIAGNOSIS*

The sudden onset and short incubation period of the clinical illness suggests a staphylococcal etiology. Involvement of other persons and an incriminated food source lend further support to the diagnosis. The short incubation period and short duration of illness distinguish it from most other forms of bacterial food poisoning; chemical food poisoning has an even shorter incubation period.

Diagnosis is made by the detection of staphylococcal enterotoxin and/or $\geq 10^5$ staphylococci per g in food. Immunologic assays have replaced bioassays for the detection of toxin in foods but are not sufficiently sensitive to detect the toxin in body fluids. An antitoxin response can be found two to six weeks following the clinical illness.

### TREATMENT

No specific therapy is available. Because the illness is not an infection, no antibiotics are needed. Supportive therapy should consist of bed rest and an abdominal heating pad to relieve cramping. Food and oral fluids should be avoided during the acute attack; they may only increase the possibility of aspiration pneumonitis. Occasionally, intravenous fluids may be indicated if dehydration develops, and phenothiazines may be needed to help control vomiting.

### PROPHYLAXIS

Since the enterotoxins are very stable, all preventive measures must be directed toward the circumstances that permit contamination of food with staphylococci and subsequent multiplication of the organism. Food handlers with skin infections should not be permitted to work, and effective hand washing techniques should be encouraged. Disposable gloves should probably be worn by all commercial food handlers. Perishable items, especially those frequently implicated in staphylococcal food poisoning, should be kept under constant refrigeration at temperatures of less than 7° C.

Although an antitoxin response has been noted in experimental animals and in patients, its protective value for preventing future attacks is not known.

# BOTULISM

### ETIOLOGY

The causative agent is *Clostridium botulinum*, a spore-forming bacillus that can produce one of seven types of neurotoxins (A through G). The organism is widely distributed in nature, and, although a strict anaerobe, it grows well on a variety of media. Neutral or slightly alkaline conditions favor spore formation. The spores withstand boiling for up to 20 hours but are inactivated by autoclaving temperatures (120° C) after exposure for 20 or more minutes. The toxin is destroyed by temperatures of 100° C for 10 minutes or 80° C for 30 minutes, but is resistant to acid and proteolytic enzymes.

### PATHOGENESIS

The ubiquitous organism and its spores are found in animals and soil, so that a variety of foods are often contaminated. Because toxin formation requires strict anaerobic conditions, however, only rarely do people ingest food with toxin. The vast majority of exposures involve raw, smoked, and fermented fish products and preserved foods or meat (especially home-cured ham) that has been standing at room temperature for several days. Improperly home-canned foods, especially vegetables, are responsible for more than 75 per cent of food-borne botulism. Whereas acidic vegetables (e.g., tomatoes) do not generally support the growth of *C. botulinum*, some tomatoes have a low content of acid and overripe tomatoes can lose their acidity.

Botulism can also result from contamination of wounds with the spores of *C. botulinum*, with subsequent germination, multiplication of organisms, and elaboration of toxin (Merson and Dowell, 1973). Types A and B have been recovered from patients with this form of botulism.

Infants between 3 and 26 weeks of age may develop botulism secondary to ingestion of *C. botulinum* spores and intestinal infection with *C. botulinum*. Honey has been implicated as a contaminated food source, but it is likely that there are other sources of the bacteria. In California, where this syndrome was first identified, Types A and B organisms and toxin have been recovered from the stools of affected infants (Arnon et al., 1977).

Following the ingestion of food containing nanogram quantities of toxin, the toxin is absorbed from the upper small bowel, eventually reaching its target tissue, cholinergic nerve endings. There the toxin binds to membrane receptors yet to be identified and inhibits the release (exocytosis) of acetylcholine. Neither the storage of acetylcholine nor the entry of calcium into the nerve terminals during depolarization is affected by the toxin.

The toxin is a large molecular weight complex (900,000 daltons) which, in type A toxin, contains hemagglutinin activity. Type B and E toxins are secreted as inert protoxins that are activated by proteolysis. A component of the toxin with a molecular weight of 150,000 has been isolated; the active fragment may be as small as 10,000 daltons (see Chapter 5).

## CLINICAL MANIFESTATIONS

Symptoms begin as early as two hours or as late as three to eight days after the ingestion of toxin, with the usual interval being 12 to 36 hours. Earlier onset of symptoms is usually associated with more severe disease and a worse prognosis. Symmetric involvement of cranial nerves and a descending pattern of weakness or paralysis are the hallmarks of botulism. Diplopia, dysarthria, and dysphagia are the most common symptoms; in severe cases, respiratory paralysis occurs. Cranial nerve involvement, especially nerve VI, may be the only neurologic manifestation. Cognitive, cortical motor, and sensory functions remain intact. Symptoms referable to the autonomic nervous system include mucous membrane dryness (dry mouth) and constipation. Nausea, vomiting, and diarrhea can occur early in the disease, and are probably the result of disturbances mediated by factors other than neurotoxin. There are cranial nerve palsies and abnormal pupils in botulism but no sensory deficits. As more cranial nerves become affected, the more likely a patient is to develop respiratory insufficiency.

Type A disease is usually more severe than type B or E disease, although all three have been fatal. Type E botulism seems to cause more gastrointestinal symptoms than others, and the recurrent neurologic symptoms seen with this type are apparently due to intestinal infection with *C. botulinum,* so that production and absorption of toxin are continuous. It is conceivable that the prolonged paralysis (weeks to months) that can occur in type A or B disease is also the result of continued infection and absorption of toxin from the colon.

The incubation period of 4 to 14 days in wound botulism probably reflects the length of time needed for infection to become established. Early gastrointestinal symptoms are not observed, but this form of botulism is otherwise identical to food-borne botulism.

The infant form of botulism is characterized by acute hypotonia, generalized muscle weakness, and a "floppy" appearance. Constipation and weak sucking are prominent, and ptosis, loss of neck muscle strength, and diminished gag reflex are common.

## COMPLICATIONS AND SEQUELAE

Mortality in classic botulism varies from outbreak to outbreak. Case/fatality ratios vary from 2:1 to 25:1 in recent years. Ventilatory insufficiency is the most life-threatening aspect of botulism. There are no long-term sequelae in patients who survive.

## GEOGRAPHIC VARIATION

Botulism occurs worldwide. The varying incidence is undoubtedly a function of the eating habits of populations and the control exercised over commercial food processors rather than the distribution of *C. botulinum.* Cases due to ingestion of raw or lightly smoked fish are usually caused by Type E toxin and occur more commonly in the U.S.S.R., Scandinavia, Japan, and the Great Lakes region of the United States than elsewhere because of dietary preferences. In the United States, Types A and B poisoning are more common and are usually associated with home-canned vegetables, fruits, or prepared meats. In France, most cases occur after the patients have eaten home-cured hams and are usually due to Type B toxin.

Most cases of infant botulism have been diagnosed in California. Now that the syndrome has been publicized, cases are being recognized outside California and the United States.

## DIAGNOSIS

Awareness of the possibility that botulism may be responsible for symptoms and signs of a predominantly neurologic disorder is the key to early diagnosis. Since it may not be possible to incriminate a food source, the diagnosis should be made on the clinical presentation of a symmetric descending paralysis of the cranial nerves, extremities, and trunk.

The differential diagnosis includes a variety of disorders, although myasthenia gravis and the Guillain-Barré syndrome are confused with botulism most frequently. In myasthenia gravis, weakness may not be symmetric and is accentuated by repetitive muscle use; the improvement in strength in myasthenia after injection of edrophonium chloride (tensilon) distinguishes it from botulism. The Guillain-Barré syndrome is distinguished by its ascending form of paralysis, frequent sparing of cranial nerves, sensory abnormalities, and abnormal cerebrospinal fluid. Other important disorders to be considered include poliomyelitis, drug toxicity (methylalcohol, atropine, aminocyclitols), cerebrovascular accidents, multiple sclerosis, and diabetic neuropathy. The definitive diagnosis is made by the detection of toxin in the serum of affected individuals. Toxin can be detected in serum for up to several weeks after the onset of symptoms. The finding of toxin and/or *C. botulinum* in patient feces or in a suspected food strongly supports the diagnosis. Immunologic assays are apparently less sensitive than the mouse toxin-neutralization test. Electromyographic studies are often helpful and demonstrate potentiation (facilitation) of the action potential upon rapid repetitive stimulation and a depressed response to a single supramaximal stimulus. These findings most closely resemble those found in the myasthenic syndrome of Lambert and Eaton (carcinomatous neuropathy) and help to distinguish botulism from the Guillain-Barré syndrome.

### TREATMENT

The mainstay of therapy is trivalent (A, B, E) antitoxin, available in the United States from the Center for Disease Control. Each vial of equine antiserum contains 7500 IU Type A, 5500 IU of Type B, and 8500 IU of Type E antitoxin. Two vials are administered intravenously, and two more are injected four hours later. Desensitization may be necessary if the patient is allergic to horse serum. Repeated injections of antiserum may be needed if symptoms recur, as can happen in Type E botulism.

Supportive treatment, especially of respiration, can help reduce morbidity and mortality. Tracheostomy and mechanically assisted respiration should be employed early when indicated.

Emetics and cathartics for cleansing the gastrointestinal tract of toxin and organisms are probably of little value if antiserum is available and may precipitate aspiration pneumonia in patients who have dysphagia.

Although penicillin is probably not helpful in most patients with food-borne botulism, it should be strongly considered for patients with Type E botulism who appear to have concomitant intestinal infection. Penicillin is indicated in the management of infant botulism and patients with wound botulism, because these two forms of the disease are the result of active infection with *C. botulinum*. Antibiotic therapy need not be continued longer than one week. In wound botulism, aggressive débridement is necessary.

The use of guanidine hydrochloride to counteract the neurotoxic effects has been generally unsuccessful and is not routinely recommended, especially if antiserum and supportive therapy are available.

Without antitoxin therapy, the overall mortality can be as high as 70 per cent. With therapy, the mortality rate has been reduced to about 25 per cent.

### PROPHYLAXIS

Education of the public on the dangers of home canning and processing (aging, smoking) of meat and fish should help to decrease the incidence of botulism. Pressure cooking should be used for all vegetables, including tomatoes, because reliance on acidity alone to inhibit toxin production is undependable. In the absence of pressure cooking, citric acid should be added to home-canned tomatoes.

Canned commercial products that are damaged or are under increased air pressure should not be consumed. Public health officials should be notified whenever botulism is suspected.

Although a formalinized toxoid is used to produce protective immunity in research workers, immunization of the public is not recommended because of the low incidence of botulism. Protective immunity apparently does not develop from botulism, probably because of the small quantities of toxin present.

# CLOSTRIDIUM PERFRINGENS FOOD POISONING

### ETIOLOGY

*Clostridium perfringens* is a spore-forming bacillus that is classified into five types (A through E) on the basis of its ability to produce various toxins. Only types A and C have been associated with food-borne disease, although type D has recently been shown to elaborate an enterotoxin that is immunologically and biologically identical to that produced by the other two types. *C. perfringens* causes approximately one third of cases of food poisoning throughout the world. Type C organisms produce a beta-toxin that may be responsible for an endemic necrotizing enteritis ("pig bel") of the New Guinea highlands.

### PATHOGENESIS

The organism is ubiquitous and can be isolated from soil and the intestinal tracts of man and other animals. Contaminated meat products, especially beef and gravy, constitute the majority of implicated food sources.

Several characteristics of *C. perfringens* are important in relation to food poisoning. Optimal temperature for growth in meat is 43 to 47° C, a temperature range that is frequently maintained inside a large piece of meat that is slowly cooling. The spores are sometimes quite heat-resistant and are activated at 75 to 80° C. Heat resistance, heat activation, and rapid multiplication predispose to contamination. Furthermore, heating the meat drives out sufficient air to make the meat anaerobic. Although these conditions promote growth of *C. perfringens,* they are not conducive to sporulation. Since toxin is produced during sporulation, it is unlikely that significant amounts of preformed toxin are absorbed from meat under most circumstances. Instead, sporulation and toxin production occur after the ingested bacteria reach the intestine. Administration of enterotoxin to volunteers causes diarrhea when gastric acid is neutralized (Skjelkvale and Vemura, 1977).

All the symptoms and signs of the illness can be attributed to an enterotoxin produced by *C. perfringens* types A, C, and D. The purified 35,000-dalton protein is heat-labile and acid-labile, and is inactivated by some proteolytic enzymes but not by trypsin. In ligated rabbit ileal loops, the absorption of glucose is inhibited, and the toxin induces a reversal of net transport, with resultant secretion of water, sodium, and chloride (Duncan and Strong, 1969). In addition, the epithelium of villous tips is denuded in the presence of toxin. This cytotoxic effect of the *C. perfringens* enterotoxin resembles that noted with *Shigella dysenteriae* toxin in tissue cultures and contrasts with the noncytotoxic effects of *V. cholerae* and *E. coli* enterotoxins (Keusch and Donta, 1975). The effects of the clostridial enterotoxin are not mediated through adenylate cyclase, although an intermediary role of prostaglandins has not been excluded. The ileum appears to be most sensitive to the toxin's effects (McDonel, 1974).

Pig-bel (necrotizing enteritis), which occurs in the highlands of New Guinea is due to *C. perfringens* type C infection. Bacteria ingested with a high consumption of protein ("pork feasting") proliferate in the intestine and elaborate beta toxin, which is responsible for patchy gangrene of the jejunum and ileum. The natives may be deficient in intestinal proteases, since the beta toxin is very sensitive to proteolysis.

## CLINICAL MANIFESTATIONS

The incubation period can be as short as two to four hours, but most affected individuals have symptoms that begin 8 to 12 hours following the ingestion of contaminated food. Frequent episodes of watery diarrhea and cramping abdominal pain are the major complaints. Blood or mucus in the feces does not occur, except in the necrotizing enteritis form of type C disease. Fever is absent, and vomiting or nausea is rare. The illness is usually over in 24 hours.

Pig-bel is characterized by anorexia, severe abdominal pain, and bloody diarrhea. There can be intestinal obstruction due to sequential necrosis of the small intestine.

## GEOGRAPHIC VARIATION

Clostridial food poisoning occurs worldwide. There are no reliable incidence figures for most of the world. Pig-bel is limited to the highlands of Papua New Guinea.

## DIAGNOSIS

The diagnosis is based on the clinical picture, an implicated food source, and the recovery of *C. perfringens* from the food source and the patient. As *C. perfringens* is normally found in feces, large numbers ($>10^5$ organisms/g) must be isolated from feces and food to confirm the diagnosis. Immunologic assays are used to detect enterotoxin in food but are not sensitive enough to detect toxin in body fluids. Staphylococcal food poisoning causes more frequent and severe vomiting, and other enteric disorders can usually be distinguished by their longer duration of illness and the inflammatory signs and symptoms of invasive organisms such as *Salmonella* and *Shigella*.

## TREATMENT

Because the illness is short, no treatment is needed. On occasion, oral or intravenous fluid replacement may prevent dehydration in the elderly or newborn. Antibiotics are not indicated, and there are no known agents to counteract the effects of the enterotoxin. There is no effective therapy for pig-bel enteritis.

## PROPHYLAXIS

Because it is nearly impossible to eradicate spores without pressure cooking, the public needs education on the dangers of allowing meat dishes to be kept at room temperature. Food should be served hot or kept refrigerated. Reheating of food destroys the heat-labile enterotoxin but may not destroy the organisms and spores themselves.

The role of humoral or local immunity is unknown. Repeat episodes of clostridial food poisoning have been reported. Pig-bel enteritis can be prevented by active immunization with beta toxoid from *C. perfringens* type C (Lawrence et al., 1979).

# BACILLUS CEREUS FOOD POISONING

## ETIOLOGY

Most strains of *Bacillus cereus* can elaborate an enterotoxin that appears to be responsible for the clinical picture. The organism is a gram-positive, spore-forming rod, but, unlike the clostridia, it grows best under aerobic conditions.

## PATHOGENESIS

The spores of *B. cereus* are heat-resistant, and, after the germination and multiplication process that occurs at temperatures of between 15 and 50° C, enterotoxin can be elaborated by the organisms. Typically, fried or boiled food has been allowed to stand at room temperature and is then reheated at temperatures too low to destroy the organisms or spores. The enterotoxin is destroyed by heating and is inactivated by acid pH. Enterotoxic activity appears to be distinct from the hemolysin and phospholipase produced by *B. cereus* and can elicit fluid accumulation in ligated rabbit ileal loops (Spira and Goepfert, 1975). Although the molecular mechanisms mediating enterotoxicity are unknown, it appears that direct stimulation of the adenylate cyclase system is not involved. The enterotoxin can cause cytotoxic changes in certain tissue cultures, but the relationship between these two activities has not been established.

It is likely that two disease phases, or even two syndromes, are possible: a short incubation illness associated with the ingestion of preformed toxin, and a larger incubation illness due to in vivo production of enterotoxin. Some authors have suggested the existence of two separate enterotoxins — one that is similar to staphylococcal enterotoxin and induces vomiting primarily, and the other a diarrheagenic toxin. In volunteer studies in the mid 1950s, Hauge demonstrated that ingestion of approximately $10^{10}$ organisms in a vanilla sauce could reproduce the clinical disease.

## CLINICAL MANIFESTATIONS

The incubation period can be as short as 30 to 120 minutes after the ingestion of preformed toxin that has escaped inactivation by gastric acid. An incubation period of 8 to 12 hours is also common, as was the case in Hauge's volunteer studies, and probably represents the period of time needed for in vivo production of enterotoxin. Watery diarrhea that is devoid of blood or mucus occurs at 15- to 30-minute intervals and is accompanied by abdominal cramping but not by fever. Nausea and vomiting can occur, especially in association with a shorter incubation period. The entire illness lasts 12 to 24 hours and usually leaves no sequelae.

## GEOGRAPHIC VARIATION

The organism is common in soil and on vegetation, but no animal reservoir is known. It has been most commonly associated with starches and grain products, especially rice, instant mashed potatoes, and pasta, but other foods such as milk products, meat loaf, vegetable sprouts, green bean salad, and soups have been implicated as well. Although currently *B. cereus* accounts for less than 5 per cent of all cases of food poisoning in the United States, increasing awareness of the disorder and improved methods of detection may place its true incidence at a higher level. The illness occurs worldwide.

## DIAGNOSIS

The diagnosis primarily rests on the clinical picture and an implicated food source. Demonstration of more than $10^5$ organisms per g of food or feces lends strong support to the diagnosis. The enterotoxin has not yet been demonstrated in food or body fluids. Differentiation from staphylococcal or clostridial food poisoning may be difficult on clinical and epidemiologic grounds alone.

## TREATMENT

As the disease is of short duration and is primarily an intoxication, no specific therapy is warranted. Rarely, parenteral fluid replacement and antiemetics may be needed.

## PROPHYLAXIS

Public awareness of the epidemiology and pathogenesis of the disease is the most important preventive measure. Special attention needs to be given to the storage of rice after it is fried or boiled. Food processing firms, especially those concerned with grain products, must be made aware of the potential problems, and inspection procedures designed to minimize contamination are needed.

## References

Arnon, S. S., Midura, T. F., Clay, S. A., Wood, R. M., and Chin, J.: Infant botulism, epidemiological, clinical, and laboratory aspects. JAMA 237:1946, 1977.

Donta, S. T.: Changing concepts of infectious diseases. Geriatrics 30:123, 1975.

Duncan, C. L., and Strong, D. H.: Ileal loop fluid accumulation and production of diarrhea in rabbits by cell-free products of *Clostridium perfringens*. J Bacteriol 100:86, 1969.

Elwell, M. R., Liu, C. T., Spertzel, R. O., and Beisel, W. R.: Mechanisms of oral staphylococcal enterotoxin B-induced emesis in the monkey. Pro Soc Exp Biol Med 148:424, 1975.

Kapral, F. A., O'Brien, A. D., Ruff, P. D., and Drugan, W. J., Jr.: Inhibition of water absorption in the intestine by *Staphylococcus aureus* delta-toxin. Infect Immun 13:140, 1976.

Keusch, G. T., and Donta, S. T.: Classification of enterotoxins on the basis of activity in cell culture. J Infect Dis 131:58, 1975.

Lawrence, T., Shaun, F., Freestone, D. S., and Walker, P. D.: Prevention of necrotizing enteritis in Papua New Guinea by active immunization. Lancet 1:227, 1979.

McDonel, J. L.: In vivo effects of *Clostridium perfringens* enteropathogenic factors on the rat ileum. Infect Immun 10:1156, 1974.

Merson, M. H., and Dowell, V. R., Jr.: Epidemiologic, clinical, and laboratory aspects of wound botulism. N Engl J Med 289:1005, 1973.

Shafer, W. M., and Iandolo, J. J.: Chromosomal locus for staphylococcal enterotoxin B. Infect Immun 20:273, 1978.

Skjelkvale, R., and Uemura, T.: Experimental diarrhoeae in human volunteers following oral administration of *Clostridium perfringens* enterotoxin. J Appl Bacteriol 43:281, 1977.

Spira, W. M., and Goepfert, J. M.: Biological characteristics of an enterotoxin produced by *Bacillus cereus*. Can J Microbiol 21:1236, 1975.

# BACTERIAL ENTERITIS **126**

## Harvey S. Kantor, M.D.

*I am poured out like water and all my bones are out of joint: my heart is like wax; it is melted in the midst of my bowels.*

Psalms 22:14

## INTRODUCTION

Inflammatory disease of the small intestine and colon as a consequence of bacterial infection is one of the most common afflictions of man throughout history. It is a worldwide problem and no population or individual is spared. In areas where malnutrition and crowded living conditions exist, enteric disease represents a striking cause not only of morbidity but also of mortality. In most instances enteric infection is self-limiting, but in some cases appropriate specific therapy can shorten the illness, and in a smaller number, similar treatment may be life-saving.

## SHIGELLOSIS

### Definition

Shigellosis (bacillary dysentery) is an acute, self-limited infection of the intestinal tract caused by bacteria of the genus *Shigella*. The spectrum of disease varies from the asymptomatic carrier to diarrhea or to frank dysentery characterized by fever, tenesmus, abdominal cramps, and diarrhea with stools containing mucus and blood. Man is the principal host of shigellae, and the infection is usually transmitted by the oral-fecal route.

### Etiology

*Shigella* species belong to the family Enterobacteriacea and are gram-negative, nonmotile organisms. Strains of *Shigella* can be characterized by specific cell wall antigens, and there are four serologic groups responsible for disease in man. The clinically important species within the respective groups are *Sh. dysenteriae* (Shiga bacillus), *Sh. flexneri*, *Sh. boydii*, and *Sh. sonnei*. The organisms are distinguished from *Escherichia coli* by their failure to ferment lactose (*Sh. sonnei* ferments lactose slowly), from salmonellae by their inability to produce gas in glucose, and from *Salmonella typhi* by their lack of motility.

### Pathogenesis and Pathology

*Shigella* must adhere to the mucosal surface, penetrate epithelial cells, and multiply within the mucosa to cause disease. Otherwise, these organisms are rapidly cleared from the gut. The number (10 to 100) of invasive organisms needed to cause disease is much smaller than that required for the noninvasive toxigenic pathogens such as *Vibrio cholerae* and *E. coli* ($10^8$ organisms). Since shigellae invade the colon but not the jejunum, it may be necessary to postulate a site-specific receptor mechanism that selectively recognizes virulent bacteria and mediates bacterial penetration of the bowel.

After multiplication within epithelial cells, the bacteria may spread from cell to cell. In acute shigellosis, there is a distinct gradation of inflammation, diminishing from the luminal surface of the colon to the submucosa, which shows little reaction. The number of bacteria sharply decreases toward the submucosa and this may explain why bloodstream invasion is infrequent. In contrast, the luminal concentration of shigellae may reach $10^6$ to $10^{10}$ organisms per gram of stool. The severe inflammation probably is an important factor in limiting the disease to the bowel wall and causes fever, cramps, tenesmus, inflammation, mucosal ulceration, microabscess formation, and fluid and electrolyte loss into the intestinal lumen.

Shigellosis may cause three patterns of diarrhea: (1) classic dysentery, with multiple small liquid stools containing blood, mucus, or pus; (2) uncomplicated watery diarrhea; or (3) a combination of watery diarrhea and dysentery. Watery diarrhea frequently precedes the dysentery, signifying early involvement of the small intestine. The mechanisms of diarrhea are unknown but may involve an enterotoxin with effects like those of *V. cholerae* and *E. coli. Shigella dysenteriae* 1 elaborates a protein exotoxin that causes enterotoxicity (intestinal fluid-secreting activity) and stimulation of adenylate cyclase, resulting in increased intracellular cyclic AMP levels in the ligated rabbit ileal loop model, neurotoxicity in mice, cytotoxicity for HeLa cells, and inhibition of mammalian and bacterial protein synthesis. A toxin with similar biologic and antigenic properties has been found in *Shigella flexneri* 2a, and a cell-free cytotoxin has been isolated from *Shigella sonnei.*

The significance of toxin in the pathogenesis of shigellosis is unclear. Studies of Shiga dysentery using live bacterial challenge in humans and monkeys reemphasize the importance of tissue invasion, since nonpenetrating mutants that were toxin-producing failed to elicit overt signs of illness. These findings do not exclude a function for the toxins of these three species of Shigella. It is conceivable that toxin elaborated after penetration could be a virulence factor. Sera from patients with shigellosis due to *Sh. flexneri* and *Sh. sonnei,* as well as *Sh. dysenteriae* 1 develop antibodies that neutralized *Sh. dysenteriae* 1 toxin in vitro, thus suggesting that toxin is produced in vivo.

## Clinical Manifestations

The most frequent presenting symptoms in patients with shigellosis are diarrhea, abdominal pain, and fever. The incubation period is about two to four days but may be as long as a week.

Occasionally diarrhea is absent at the onset of illness but will develop within 24 hours. Bloody diarrhea occurs in 25 to 50 per cent of cases. Abdominal tenderness, most pronounced in the lower quadrants, is found, and hyperactive bowel sounds are common, but there is no peritoneal irritation.

## Complications and Sequelae

In most cases the shigellosis seen in well-nourished populations is a mild illness that terminates without complications in a few days.

In severe infections, which occur especially in young children and elderly individuals, dehydration, acid-base disturbances, and shock may supervene early because of excessive loss of fluid and electrolytes; these are the most frequent serious complications of *Shigella* gastroenteritis. Other complications of shigellosis, found most often in children, are seizures, meningism, pneumonia and, rarely, agranulocytosis. *Shigella* bacteremia may occur rarely and produces metastatic septic foci. Reiter's syndrome — urethritis, conjunctivitis, and arthritis — may develop two to four weeks after the onset of *Shigella* dysentery; individuals with a specific histocompatibility antigen (HL-A B27) appear to be at much higher risk of this complication. Perforation of the intestine is rare despite considerable ulceration. Pyelonephritis, empyema, glomerulonephritis, and otitis media may develop (Barrett-Connor, 1970). A complication that apparently is peculiar to one strain of *Shigella* is peripheral neuropathy, which occasionally occurs after *Sh. dysenteriae* infections. Chronic bacillary dysentery may mimic the anatomic and clinical features of ulcerative colitis. Mucosal ulceration produced by *Shigella* occasionally provides a portal of entry for other enteric bacteria to the bloodstream.

Shigellae, like other bacterial enteric pathogens, cause more subclinical than clinical cases, and short-term fecal excretion of organisms may persist for days to weeks. An asymptomatic carrier state beyond one year has been reported for *Sh. sonnei* and *Sh. flexneri* 2a (Levine et al., 1973).

## Geographic Variations in Disease

Shigellosis is worldwide in distribution, occurring in arctic, temperate, and tropical climates. Wherever acute diarrheal diseases are a major health problem, *Shigella* organisms cause most of the more severe diarrheal illnesses.

Over the past 10 years *Sh. sonnei* has accounted for most of the *Shigella* isolations in the United States, with *Sh. flexneri* second. A similar trend has been observed in Great Britain, Western Europe, Japan, and Korea. It has been suggested that the predominance of *Sh. sonnei* within a particular country is associated with increasing industrialization, economic development, and a higher standard of living. In the United States, *Sh. flexneri* has predominated in states that are largely rural, sparsely populated, poorly industrialized, or that have a large American Indian population.

*Sh. dysenteriae* 1 has never been a frequent cause of diarrhea and dysentery in the Western Hemisphere. Shiga dysentery has been consistently present primarily in the Middle and Far East. After an absence of several decades, *Sh. dysenteriae* 1 reappeared in Central America and caused a dysentery pandemic from 1968 to 1972 that encompassed five countries and was responsible for unusually severe cases of dysentery.

### Diagnosis

*Shigella* infections should be considered in anyone with diarrhea, with or without fever. A positive diagnosis depends on isolating shigellae from the stools. Since a small percentage of initial stool cultures may not yield shigellae, more than one stool sample during the first 24 hours may increase the chances for isolating this organism. Although many shigellae bacilli are usually excreted during active disease, they often remain alive in the feces only briefly and must be cultured without delay. A rectal swab is an excellent method of obtaining specimens for culture. Specimens from intestinal ulcers, taken under direct vision through a sigmoidoscope, are most likely to contain the organisms.

*Shigella* dysentery has a more acute onset than amebic dysentery and is usually self-limited, whereas amebic dysentery may have spontaneous remissions and frequent relapses. Sigmoidoscopic examination of the colon may provide a further distinction — diffuse mucosal involvement with multiple, very superficial ulcers is characteristic of shigellosis, whereas undermined ulcers with raised edges and normal intervening mucosa are the typical finding in amebiasis. Microscopic examination of stool in shigellosis shows discrete red cells, numerous intact polymorphonuclear leukocytes, scanty nonmotile microorganisms, and numerous macrophages; that of amebic infection contains clumped red cells, degenerate leukocytes, numerous motile microorganisms, and trophozoites of *Entamoeba histolytica*. The presence of fecal leukocytes appears to indicate a colitis with disruption of the distal intestinal mucosa. Fecal leukocytes may also be found in patients with salmonellosis, invasive *E. coli* colitis, and ulcerative colitis, but they are not seen in diarrheas caused by enterotoxins or in viral diarrhea.

Other causes of diarrhea considered in the differential diagnosis include *Giardia lamblia*, viral agents, and staphylococcal and clostridial enterotoxins, none of which usually cause clinical dysentery. Shigellosis can be distinguished with certainty from acute ulcerative colitis only by bacteriologic studies.

Serologic tests have not been very useful for diagnosis of shigellosis.

### Treatment

The role of specific antimicrobial therapy in the treatment of shigellosis is uncertain. In some studies, antibiotics shortened the duration of symptoms and the excretion of organisms in the stool. In other studies, these differences were not found between the treated and untreated groups. Furthermore, the repeated emergence of *Shigella* strains that are resistant to whatever antibiotics had been in common use at the time has made it difficult to choose a drug that is both effective and safe. The spread of resistance transfer factor may be accelerated by selective pressures exerted on intestinal flora by the administration of broad spectrum drugs.

The primary treatment of shigellosis is supportive; in patients who are acutely ill, particularly young children or elderly persons, the main goal is restoration of fluids and electrolytes. It is reasonable to withhold antibiotics from patients who are moderately ill. In severe dysentery, antibiotics should be selected on the basis of sensitivity tests and the prevailing pattern of sensitivity in each community. Sulfonamides, formerly the drugs of choice, are no longer reliable. Ampicillin is the current drug of choice; it should be administered orally as 50 (adult) to 100 (children) mg/kg body weight/day given in four equal doses for three to five days. When shigellae are resistant to ampicillin, they usually have multiple antibiotic resistance to tetracyclines, sulfonamides, and chloramphenicol. Under these circumstances, trimethoprim-sulfamethoxazole is the best choice; it is administered for 5 days in two divided oral doses of 20 to 25 mg/kg/dose of sulfamethoxazole and 4 to 5 mg/kg/dose of trimethoprim (Chang et al., 1977).

Drugs that retard intestinal motility, such as paregoric or diphenoxylate hydrochloride with atropine (Lomotil), may prolong the clinical illness, the duration of the diarrhea, and excretion of shigellae and should therefore be avoided (Dupont and Hornick, 1973).

### Prophylaxis

Sanitary disposal of human feces so that they cannot contaminate water or food supplies is basic to prophylaxis in shigellosis. Attempts to develop a safe, effective vaccine are under investigation, but progress has been hampered by the numerous serotypes of these organisms, the need for booster vaccinations, and the brief period of immunity.

## SALMONELLOSIS

### Definition

The term salmonellosis refers to infections caused by bacteria of the genus *Salmonella*, which consists of more than 1400 serotypes. The clinical manifestations of human salmonellosis can be divided into four syndromes: gastroenteritis ("food poisoning"), enteric fever (typhoid-like disease), bacteremia with and without focal extra-intestinal infection, and asymptomatic carrier state. Infection caused by *Salmonella typhi* (typhoid fever) is considered separately in Chapter 31.

### Etiology

Salmonellae are gram-negative, facultatively anaerobic, and generally motile bacilli that do not ferment lactose and, with the exception of *S. typhi*, produce acid and gas from glucose. They are classified in three primary species: *S. typhi, S. choleraesuis,* and *S. enteritidis. S. typhi* and *S. choleraesuis* each consist of a single serotype. In contrast, over 1400 antigenically distinct serotypes of *S. enteritidis* have been defined. The serotype of each *Salmonella* organism depends both on its somatic or O antigens and on its H or flagellar antigens.

The salmonellae fall into divisions according to their host preference and the clinical syndromes they produce (Table 1). It should be noted that *Salmonella* serotypes that are not adapted to specific hosts constitute the vast majority of *Salmonella* species. These species cause over 80 per cent of current *Salmonella* infections in the United States, generally taking the form of acute gastroenteritis.

### Pathogenesis and Pathology

As long as fifty years ago, salmonellae species were suspected of having the ability to invade and pass through or between the intact epithelial cells of intestinal mucosa from the gut lumen. Recent studies show that only *Salmonella* strains that invade the ileal epithelium can cause enteritis or intestinal fluid secretion and subsequent diarrhea. Strains that do not penetrate cause no

**TABLE 1.    Relation of Salmonella Species and Representative Serotypes to Human Disease**

| SPECIES | REPRESENTATIVE SEROTYPE | NATURAL HOST | HUMAN DISEASE |
|---|---|---|---|
| *S. typhi* | — | Man | Enteric fever |
| *S. choleraesuis* | — | Swine | Bacteremia or focal infection |
| *S. enteritidis* | | | |
| | paratyphi[a] schottumulleri[a] hirschfeldi[a] | Man | Enteric fever |
| | typhimurium | | Gastroenteritis, bacteremia, and focal infection |
| | newport enteritidis and hundreds of related serotypes | No host specificity | Gastroenteritis |
| | dublin | Cattle | |
| | pullorum gallinarium | fowl | None |
| | abortusequi abortusovis | horses sheep | |

[a]These three salmonella serotypes were formerly designated *S. paratyphi* A, *S. paratyphi* B, and *S. paratyphi* C, respectively.

Adapted from Grady, G. F., and Keusch, G. T.; N Engl J Med. 285:831, 1971.

disease. These organism have a predilection for villous epithelium, tend to spare crypt cells, and inflict far less damage on epithelium than do shigellae. The preferential attachment of these salmonellae to the tips of villi suggests a specific receptor on villi. Salmonellae do not multiply in epithelial cells as shigellae do. Because the number of salmonellae in the epithelial lining rapidly decreases, ulcer formation is salmonellosis is infrequent.

The biochemical lesion underlying intestinal fluid secretion and diarrhea in *Salmonella* enteritis remains elusive. In animal models infected with *S. typhimurium,* changes in ileal water and electrolyte transport, stimulation of adenylate cyclase, and elevation of intracellular cyclic AMP levels have been found to be qualitatively similar to those described in cholera and enterotoxigenic *E. coli* diarrhea. Pretreatment with indomethacin, an inhibitor of prostaglandin synthesis, abolishes both fluid secretion and adenylate cyclase activation. In cholera toxin–stimulated intestinal loops, pretreatment with indomethacin partially inhibits intestinal secretion but does not alter the activation of adenylate cyclase. This difference in response to indomethacin suggests that *Salmonella* and cholera toxin modulate intestinal adenylate cyclase by different mechanisms. Giannella and his colleagues (1975) have suggested that local prostaglandins, produced as a consequence of the acute inflammatory reaction attending *Salmonella* infection, result in adenylate cyclase activation and cyclic AMP-mediated fluid secretion. The significance of these findings in the pathogenesis of salmonellosis is unclear; indomethacin causes a striking enhancement of intestinal water absorption in the absence of tissue inflammation, and direct measurements of elevated small intestinal intracellular prostaglandin concentrations during salmonellosis have not been reported.

Mucosal invasion alone appears not to be a sufficient stimulus to cause transport abnormalities. It has been found that when infection occurred with strains of *S. typhimurium* that invade intestinal mucosa without causing associated secretion of intestinal fluid, sodium and choloride transport and adenylate cyclase activity were unchanged.

A heat-labile enterotoxin from cultures of *S. enteritidis* and *S. typhimurium* has recently been found in the bacterial cell wall or outer membrane. There is, however, no evidence that the *Salmonella* enterotoxin has a role in the enteric disease produced by the organism.

Within 24 hours most of the bacteria have passed through the epithelium into the lamina propria, where an intense infiltration with inflammatory cells is evoked by the infection. It has

been suggested (Sprinz, 1969) that the tissue response determines the clinical features. *Salmonella* species other than *S. typhi* and *S. paratyphi* elicit a polymorphonuclear leukocyte response that quickly eliminates the organisms and is generally limited to gastroenteritis, although metastatic abscesses can occur. In typhoid and paratyphoid infections the predominant response is mononuclear, and the clinical syndrome is enteric fever. The Peyer's patches of the distal ileum are the primary site of bacterial penetration with infection spreading to the regional lymph nodes. Many *Salmonella* species will be successfully contained by mucosal and lymphatic barriers and restricted to the intestine. The more virulent serotypes spill into the thoracic lymph from the intestinal lymph nodes, reach the systemic circulation, and disseminate to the liver, spleen and other parts of the reticuloendothelial system.

Between $10^5$ and $10^6$ viable salmonellae must be swallowed by volunteers for clinical disease to occur, whereas a transient carrier state will follow ingestion of 10- to 100-fold fewer organisms. Salmonellosis occurs most frequently in infants and the aged. It also occurs frequently as a second illness in persons whose resistance has been lowered by another infection, neoplastic disease, or malnutrition. *Salmonella* infections complicate malaria, sickle cell anemia, and bartonellosis at a significantly higher frequency than that of other pathogens. Hemolysis is the common feature of the three diseases, and the free hemoglobin may block killing of *Salmonella* organisms by macrophages.

### Clinical Manifestations, Complications, and Sequelae

Two thirds of all recognized diseases caused by *Salmonella* in man take the form of enteritis. Certain *Salmonella* serotypes are consistently associated with specific clinical syndromes (see Table 1). Despite this, every serotype can produce any of the varied clinical patterns of salmonellosis. The separation of human salmonellosis into four syndromes is useful for classification, but in practice the syndromes overlap.

*Gastroenteritis.* Although referred to as *Salmonella* food poisoning, the disease is actually an intestinal infection. No preformed toxin is involved as in staphylococcal food poisoning (see Chapter 125). In 1976 salmonellae were responsible for more cases (33 per cent) of food-borne acute gastroenteritis of confirmed etiology in the United States than any other cause. The incubation period is 12 to 48 hours or longer. The first symptoms are nausea and vomiting, which subside within a few hours, followed rapidly by gripping abdominal pain. The most prominent symptom is usually diarrhea of variable severity, ranging from only one or two loose stools in mild cases to profuse, bloody diarrhea in severe cases. The temperature is moderately elevated (less than 102° F) for 24 to 48 hours in most cases. In uncomplicated gastroenteritis in adults, bacteremia occurs in less than 4 per cent of patients. Bowel sounds are hyperactive and abdominal tenderness is moderate. In some patients the abdominal findings are severe enough to be confused with acute appendicitis or cholecystitis. The illness often subsides within five days but may last only one day or persist for weeks. If simultaneous infection by more than one serotype occurs, the clinical picture does not differ from that produced by a single strain. Microscopic stool examinations may disclose many polymorphonuclear leukocytes.

*Enteric Fevers.* Although enteric fever is most often produced by *S. typhi* and the paratyphoid bacilli (*S. enteritidis,* serotypes *S. paratyphi, S. schottmuller,* and *S. hirschfeldi*), it may be caused by any serotype of *Salmonella.* Regardless of serotype, the manifestations of enteric fever are similar. When caused by serotypes other than *S. typhi,* the clinical picture is usually milder, but otherwise it is indistinguishable from typhoid fever. The clinical features of typhoid fever are described in Chapter 179.

*Salmonella Bacteremia (Septicemia).* Bacteremia is continuous in enteric fever. Cherubin and his co-workers (1974) have described another syndrome caused by nontyphoidal *Salmonella,* characterized primarily by prolonged fever and intermittent bacteremia. It occurs in about 5 to 10 per cent of all infections. It has a bimodal age distribution that divides the cases into two etiologic and prognostic groups. The first and largest group consists of children who present with fever and gastroenteritis. The bacteremia in this group is brief and is often discovered after the patient has become asymptomatic. The second group is composed of adults who have either a transient bacteremia during an episode of gastroenteritis or an underlying disease such as cancer, hemolytic anemia, or liver disease with symptoms of septicemia and no gastroenteritis. The significance of *Salmonella* in the blood in persons with no other illness is the high risk of development of metastatic infections. This risk is more important than the bacteremia, which has a low mortality compared with that of bacteremias due to other gramnegative organisms. *S. typhimurium* most often causes *Salmonella* bacteremia and is followed in frequency by *S. enteritidis* and *S. choleraesuis.*

Chronic *Salmonella* bacteremia has been associated with concomitant *Schistosoma mansoni* infection. Colonization of the ceca of the schistosomes by *Salmonella* may provide a continuing reservoir of *Salmonella* organisms.

*Focal Infections.* *Salmonella* bacteremia frequently causes metastatic abscesses. Osteomyelitis, meningitis, and pneumonia are more common than *Salmonella* pyelonephritis, endocarditis, and suppurative arthritis. Diseased tissues such as aneurysms, hematomas, and infarcts are at higher risk for localization of *Salmonella* infections.

*Carrier State.* The transient asymptomatic carrier may be even more common than patients with gastroenteritis. All individuals with *Salmonella* infections excrete the organisms for varying time periods and are referred to as convalescent carriers. In the early period of acute gastroenteritis as many as $10^6$ to $10^9$ salmonellae per gram of feces may be present. With recovery, the number of bacteria that can be recovered from stools gradually diminishes. By the third month, approximately 90 per cent of patients will have stopped excreting organisms. Individuals who excrete salmonellae for one year or more are considered to be chronic carriers. The incidence of chronic carriers of *S. paratyphi* is about 3 per cent and of nontyphoidal serotypes less than 1 per cent. The severity of the initial infection has no relation to the duration of Salmonella carriage. Gallbladder disease predisposes to chronic carriage.

### Geographic Variations

Salmonellosis is a common worldwide disease and is reported most extensively in North American and European countries. Ingestion of food contaminated directly or indirectly with *Salmonella*-infected feces of man and wild or domesticated vertebrates is the primary source of infection or disease. In the United States it is estimated that salmonellae are the causal agent of two million cases of human gastroenteritis annually but that only 1 per cent of the total is reported. Some *Salmonella* serotypes tend to demonstrate geographic patterns. *S. typhimurium* is an example of a serotype with a widespread distribution; it is the most common cause of human salmonella infections in the United States and Europe. Other species may have such a limited distribution in nature that their isolation from an infected person may be used to determine the source of infection. For instance, in 1976, *Salmonella* surveillance in the United States revealed that 98 per cent of isolates of *S. weltrevreden* were reported from Hawaii. However, mass production of foods coupled with a rapid transportation system can spread *Salmonella*-contaminated food great distances.

## Diagnosis

The diagnosis of salmonellosis on clinical grounds is difficult and must be considered in every case of diarrhea. The diagnosis can be established only by isolation of *Salmonella* from blood, stool, urine, or elsewhere. Agglutination tests are of little value.

## Treatment

*Salmonella* gastroenteritis is usually a mild, self-limited illness. With careful attention to the management of fluids and electrolytes, recovery is generally uneventful. Antibiotic therapy does not shorten or help the illness. In fact, specific antimicrobial therapy prolongs rather than shortens postconvalescent fecal excretion of *Salmonella* species, thus increasing spread of infection (Aserkoff and Bennett, 1969). Drug therapy also promotes the acquisition of antibiotic-resistant strains. Occasionally antibiotics appear to convert gastroenteritis or simple carrier states to systemic disease with bacteremia. Antibiotics are indicated only for patients with *Salmonella* gastroenteritis with bacteremia or in neonates, the elderly, patients with lymphoproliferative, cardiovascular, or bone and joint disorders, and those with chronic hemolytic anemia. These are patients who are at high risk of developing bacteremia or metastatic infection. Agents that impair intestinal motility such as opiates and diphenoxylate hydrochloride with atropine (Lomotil) are often administered for symptomatic relief of abdominal cramps and diarrhea. When used excessively, they seem to delay convalescence, prolong fecal carriage of *Salmonella,* and rarely cause bacteremia.

For the treatment of the enteric fevers and *Salmonella* bacteremia, the drug of choice is chloramphenicol given only intravenously* in a dose of 4 gm/day (in four equally divided doses every six hours) for three to four weeks. Ampicillin should be reserved for chloramphenicol-resistant, ampicillin-sensitive organisms and should be given intravenously in the range of 8 to 12 g/day. The trimethoprim-sulfamethoxazole combination is effective and should be given orally in doses of 160 mg trimethoprim and 800 mg sulfamethoxazole every 12 hours. Metastatic abscesses must be drained.

Antibiotic therapy is ineffective for eradication of salmonellae in the convalescent carrier. Chronic carriers with normal gallbladders are treated with 1.5 g ampicillin plus 0.5 g probenecid orally every six hours for 30 days. If cholelithiasis is present, cholecystectomy may also be necessary.

## Prophylaxis

The prevention and control of *Salmonella* infections is complicated by the ubiquitous distribution of these organisms in nature. They infect many species of animals and can survive for prolonged periods in the inanimate environment.

Man acquires salmonellosis primarily by ingestion of contaminated water, milk, and food. Food production, food processing, water supplies, and sewage systems must maintain a high level of sanitation. Acutely ill individuals who are excreting Salmonella organisms should be isolated. Asymptomatic carriers should practice high standards of personal hygiene and should not be employed as food handlers.

No effective immunization is available against nontyphoidal Salmonella species.

# *ESCHERICHIA COLI DIARRHEA*

## Definition

Certain strains of *Escherichia coli* can produce acute diarrhea. Two clinical syndromes are recognized: an acute watery diarrhea varying in severity from mild disease to a serious dehydrating cholera-like illness, and a shigellosis-like illness characterized by tenesmus, bloody diarrhea, and fever. As an enteric pathogen, *E. coli* has been commonly associated with acute "nonspecific" diarrhea of infants and children. *E. coli* is also the most common cause of acute diarrhea in travelers (Merson et al., 1976). The mode of transmission of this illness is probably the fecal-oral route.

### Etiology

*E. coli* are gram-negative, nonspore-forming rods of the family Enterobacteriaceae. Those causing gastroenteritis are indistinguishable by conventional criteria from the *E. coli* of the normal intestinal flora.

### Pathogenesis and Pathology

Strains of *E. coli* can cause diarrhea in man by at least two mechanisms: certain strains elaborate an enterotoxin, while others penetrate the intestinal mucosa.

***Enterotoxins.*** Heat-labile and heat-stable enterotoxins have been described for *E. coli* (Kantor, 1975). The heat-labile toxin is of large molecular weight and appears to be similar to cholera toxin

---

*Chloramphenicol sodium succinate, when given by the intramuscular route, is of little value because of its slow rate of conversion to the active compound; oral adminstration of chloramphenicol should be avoided because almost all cases of bone marrow aplasia that have been recorded have occurred in patients receiving the drug by mouth.

both antigenically and in its mechanism of action. Both cholera toxin and the heat-labile toxin give rise to a noninflammatory secretory diarrhea by first binding to a ganglioside receptor on the intestinal mucosal cell surface, and then activating adenylate cyclase so that intracellular cyclic AMP is elevated. This results in anion hypersecretion, inhibition of sodium absorption, and ultimately, an outpouring of fluid from the gut and watery diarrhea. Major pathologic changes and tissue invasion of intestinal mucosa do not occur.

The mechanism by which cyclic AMP mediates enhanced intestinal secretion is unknown. It has been proposed that cyclic AMP-dependent protein kinases are the molecular receptors for cyclic AMP and mediate the biologic effects of cyclic AMP by regulating phosphorylation of membrane protein. This hypothesis is supported by the recent finding that there is a direct correlation between intestinal secretion and activation of cyclic AMP-dependent protein kinase by cholera toxin.

In contrast to the heat-labile toxin, the stable toxin is of low molecular weight and is antigenically unrelated to either the heat-labile toxin or to cholera toxin; it neither stimulates intestinal adenylate cyclase nor alters intracellular cyclic AMP levels. Recent work suggests that the diarrheagenic effect of the heat-stable toxin is mediated by way of guanylate cyclase stimulation and increased intestinal mucosal concentrations of cyclic GMP (Field et al., 1978; Hughes et al., 1978).

The first step in the pathogenesis of disease produced by enterotoxigenic *E. coli* is colonization of the small intestine. A surface-associated antigen that determines adhesiveness to the human intestinal mucosal surface and subsequent colonization has been identified on *E. coli*. When seen by electron microscopy, this colonization factor possesses a unique pilus-like structure that can be distinguished immunologically from the common pili of *E. coli*. Both of the essential virulence factors for enterotoxigenic *E. coli*, enterotoxin production and the presence of a colonization factor, are controlled by plasmids, the transmissible extrachromosomal genetic elements. In contrast, the gene for toxin production in *V. cholerae* is located on the bacterial chromosome and can also be conjugally transmitted. This raises an interesting evolutionary question of whether there may once have been an exchange of genetic information between these two organisms for toxin production.

***Invasion.*** Certain strains of *E. coli* may penetrate the cells of the intestinal epithelium and cause a syndrome similar to shigellosis. These strains do not produce an enterotoxin, and pili are not required to attach to and invade the mucosa. Some of the invasive strains may possess somatic antigens related to one of the various *Shigella* serotypes. Like shigellae, the invasive *E. coli* strains multiply predominantly in the colon. The number of invasive *E. coli* necessary to produce diarrheal disease in volunteers is at least 10,000 times higher than the infectious dose for *Sh. flexneri* 2a. The massive infecting dose may be one of the reasons these organisms have been overlooked in the past.

*E. coli* species responsible for nosocomial urinary tract infections and bacteremias have rarely invaded the bowel or produced enterotoxin.

***Another Mechanism of Action.*** A third mechanism for *E. coli* diarrhea that is distinct from the cholera-like or shigella-like mechanisms has been recently proposed. Certain strains of *E. coli* do not produce enterotoxin or penetrate intestinal epithelial cells. The diarrheal disease appears to result from penetration of the glycolyx, adherence to the mucosal cell surface with subsequent disruption of the microvillus brush border, followed by a moderate inflammatory response and intense edema of the lamina propria (Ulshen and Rollo, 1980).

### Clinical Manifestations

Diarrheal disease caused by enterotoxigenic *E. coli* may vary in severity from a mild one-day illness consisting of abdominal cramps, vomiting, loose stools, and a low-grade fever, to a severe secretory diarrhea resembling cholera. Profuse rice-water stools may cause hypovolemic shock. The illness caused by *E. coli* that produces heat-labile toxin cannot usually be distinguished from that due to heat-stable toxin producers. The incubation period in volunteers varies from 24 to 48 hours. Occasionally asymptomatic pharyngeal colonization occurs in patients with diarrhea.

Most persons will stop shedding enterotoxigenic *E. coli* within four to five days after recovery from diarrhea. However, in some individuals, particularly those living in endemic areas, asymptomatic excretion may be more persistent.

The clinical picture of invasive *E. coli* infection is indistinguishable from shigellosis: high fever, chills, headache, myalgia, and abdominal cramps, followed by diarrhea and dysentery. Spontaneous recovery occurs with no specific antibiotic therapy.

### Geographic Variation

Although evidence suggests that *E. coli* diarrheal disease is worldwide, accurate statistics come from only a few areas. As an added difficulty, there is a striking variability in the severity of the illness due to enterotoxigenic *E. coli.* The diarrhea caused by these organisms in children in the United States appears less severe than that in infected adults in Central America, Calcutta, or Vietnam. This observation can be explained by the higher mortality and morbidity of diarrheal disease associated with malnutrition, poor sanitation, and crowding; however, strains do vary in their toxin activity. A similar variation in enterotoxigenicity has been described for *V. cholerae.*

In developing countries and in the tropics and subtropics, these organisms account for a significant proportion of endemic diarrhea and are present in 20 to 50 per cent of cases in natives and in travelers to such areas.

### Diagnosis

*E. coli* diarrheal disease should be a primary diagnostic consideration in two clinical settings: (1) in any acute gastroenteritis in which a recognized enteric pathogen cannot be isolated, and (2) in an acute cholera-like dehydrating diarrhea in patients who have not been to an area endemic or epidemic for *V. cholerae* and in whom this organism cannot be recovered.

Laboratory identification of toxigenic and invasive *E. coli* is difficult. Stool cultures are of little value because *E. coli* normally inhabit the bowel. There are no assays for either type of *E. coli* that are readily adapted for routine diagnosis. The selection of *E. coli* colonies for virulence testing is random and insensitive; about $10^6$ bacteria per gram of feces must be present for detection. Serum antitoxin titers to heat-labile toxins do not regularly rise after diarrheal illness except in heavily endemic areas, and serum antibodies to the heat-stable variety have not been recognized. A significant rise in titer of serum antibody to the somatic antigen of invasive *E. coli* has been documented in animal models. The application of this technique as a diagnostic tool in human infection has not yet been determined. The routine serogrouping of *E. coli* for "enteropathogenic" serotypes has been unreliable for predicting if a strain is toxin-producing or invasive (Gangarosa and Merton, 1973).

Enterotoxin is demonstrated by inducing diarrhea in the gut of laboratory animals such as the rabbit or suckling mouse. The rabbit test will detect both heat-labile and heat-stable toxin, while the mouse test is specific for the stable toxin. Another approach, which allows multiple specimens to be examined, is the use of tissue culture assays. Chinese hamster ovary cells or adrenal tumor cells will show characteristic morphologic changes only when exposed to the heat-labile toxin.

The detection of invasive *E. coli* relies on the development of keratoconjunctivitis in the eyes of guinea pigs inoculated with the test organism (Sereny test).

It should be noted that occasionally infection with toxigenic *E. coli* may simultaneously coexist with viral gastroenteritis.

### Treatment

Rehydration is the main treatment of disease caused by enterotoxigenic *E. coli.* Oral glucose in a balanced electrolyte solution is a simple and effective alternative to intravenous fluid replacement. Antibiotics do not shorten the illness, and may cause harm. A single conjugative plasmid in *E. coli* carries the genes for both drug resistance and enterotoxin production, so that the indiscriminate use of antibiotics for enterotoxic diarrhea, which promotes antibiotic resistance in Enterobacteriaceae, may also promote the acquisition of plasmids mediating the production of enterotoxin. A nontoxic agent, bismuth subsalicylate,* rapidly relieves diarrhea, nausea, and abdominal pain when given orally in 30 to 60 ml amounts every 30 minutes for eight doses (Dupont et al., 1977).

Neither antibiotics nor drugs that retard intestinal motility have any established value for treatment of disease caused by invasive E. coli.

### Prophylaxis

No vaccine is available for use in man. Both food and water may be the vehicles for transmission of this disease. Accordingly, protection will be afforded by eating only cooked food that is held at proper temperatures, and boiling inadequately treated water before drinking.

Healthy transient carriers are probably an important reservoir for the spread of these organisms, but they will remain undetected until a simple method for detecting these organisms becomes available.

### *CLOSTRIDIUM PERFRINGENS ENTERITIS*

### Definition

*Clostridium perfringens* is a major cause of intestinal disease. In 1976, *C. perfringens* was responsible for 4.5 per cent of the confirmed food-borne disease outbreaks in the United States. The illness is principally associated with the ingestion of meat and poultry that has been improperly stored after cooking. It is a self-

---

*Commercially available as Pepto Bismol.

limited gastroenteritis without constitutional symptoms.

### Etiology

*C. perfringens* organisms are anaerobic spore-forming bacilli. Their natural habitat is the soil and the intestinal tracts of animals and man. This organism is considered to be more widely distributed over the surface of the earth than any other pathogenic bacterium.

### Pathogenesis and Pathology

Enteritis caused by *C. perfringens* has been correlated with the ingestion of strains that produce a heat-labile enterotoxin. The enterotoxin has been purified and is a protein with a molecular weight of 35,000. Like cholera and *E. coli* enterotoxins, the enterotoxin of *C. perifringens* reverses net water and salt transport from absorption to secretion in the terminal ileum. It differs from cholera and *E. coli* toxins in several respects: (1) the abnormal intestinal transport does not appear to be mediated by cyclic AMP; (2) glucose absorption, which is undisturbed by cholera and *E. coli* toxins, is markedly inhibited by *C. perfringens* enterotoxin; and (3) extensive intestinal mucosal damage that predominantly affects villus tips is caused by exposure to the enterotoxin of *C. perfringens*.

The enterotoxin of *C. perfringens* is produced in an unusual manner. Most enterotoxins are synthesized during the phase of vegetative growth. *C. perfringens* enterotoxin is elaborated only during sporulation. Furthermore, the toxin is a structural protein in the bacterial spore coat (Ducan, 1975).

The sequence of events leading to the clinical expression of enteritis are ingestion of the viable organisms, passage to the intestine, and sporulation followed by lysis and release of the enterotoxin. The role of preformed toxin in food is unknown.

### Clinical Manifestations and Complications

Manifestations of *C. perfringens* enteritis occur 8 to 14 hours after the ingestion of the contaminated food. Moderate to severe cramping abdominal pain and watery diarrhea are the most prominent symptoms. Mild malaise may be present, but there is no fever or prostration. Nausea and vomiting are rare. Recovery is rapid, often within 24 hours.

A rare type of necrotizing inflammatory disease of the small bowel, enteritis necroticans, has been frequently associated with foods heavily contaminated with beta-toxin-producing, type C strains of *C. perfringens* (Murrell et al., 1966). There is severe upper abdominal pain, bloody diarrhea,

vomiting, segmental gangrene of the small intestine, and often a high mortality. The beta-toxin is thought to be responsible for the extensive mucosal injury in this disease.

### Diagnosis

The etiology is established by the isolation of $\geq 10^5$ *C. perfringens* per gram of incriminated food and the recovery of an organism with the same serotype from the stool of the patient.

### Treatment and Prophylaxis

In most cases, *C. perfringens* enteritis is a self-limited disease of short duration. No specific treatment is required. It is best prevented by prompt refrigeration of cooked foods, particularly meat and poultry.

## VIBRIO PARAHAEMOLYTICUS GASTROENTERITIS

### Definition

*Vibrio parahaemolyticus* is a leading cause of acute, self-limited, food-borne gastroenteritis acquired by consumption of raw or processed seafood, usually in the summer (Barker and Gangarosa, 1974).

### Etiology

*V. parahaemolyticus* is a halophilic (salt-loving) anaerobic gram-negative rod found in marine life and coastal water throughout the world. The organism can be serotyped with specific somatic antisera. Serologic testing, although useful for epidemiologic purposes, has limited diagnostic value because of extensive cross-reactivity with other marine vibrios. *V. parahaemolyticus* will not grow on most routine laboratory enteric media unless these media have a high salt content.

### Pathogenesis and Pathology

The mechanism by which *V. parahaemolyticus* causes an acute enteritis is not completely resolved. Using animal models and human volunteers, a strong correlation has been found between enteropathogenicity and a positive Kanagawa reaction (the production of a hemolysin by this organism on special high salt agar). Paradoxically, *V. parahaemolyticus* strains isolated from seafood that is epidemiologically linked with specific outbreaks of acute gastroenteritis are almost invariably Kanagawa-negative. The Kanagawa hemolysin has been purified but has not been demonstrated to be clearly enterotoxic. Direct bacterial invasion of ileal mucosa has been observed in some experimental models, whereas in others the viable organisms produce rapid cytotoxicity to epithelial cells without cellular invasion. Like toxigenic *E. coli,* enteropathogenic strains of *V. parahaemolyticus* adhere to epithelial cell surfaces, but nonvirulent strains do not.

### Clinical Manifestations

*V. parahaemolyticus* gastroenteritis most commonly resembles *Salmonella* enterocolitis; explosive watery diarrhea is the cardinal manifestation, followed less frequently by abdominal cramps, nausea, and vomiting. Occasionally, some patients have chills or fever. The median incubation period ranges from 14 to 23 hours, and the illness lasts about three days.

Another *V. parahaemolyticus* syndrome resembles *Shigella* dysentery and is characterized by fever, abdominal pain, and bloody, mucoid stools.

Bacteremia and localized tissue infections are rare.

### Geographic Variation

This disease has a world wide distribution, appears primarily in areas adjacent to marine waters, and occurs exclusively in warm weather.

### Diagnosis, Treatment, and Prophylaxis

The diagnosis should be suspected when acute diarrhea develops following the ingestion of seafood. Confirmation depends on the recovery of the organism from stool and incriminated food.

Specific antimicrobial therapy is not indicated in most cases because of the limited severity and duration of the illness.

Prevention is best achieved through measures that ensure adequate cooking, hygienic preparation, and rapid refrigeration of seafood.

# CAMPYLOBACTER ENTERITIS

### *DEFINITION*

*Campylobacter fetus* (formerly known as *Vibrio fetus*), long recognized as a commensal and a pathogen of various domestic animals, has been increasingly implicated as an enteric pathogen of man over the past 30 years. *C. fetus* may also be responsible for a wide variety of clinical syndromes, including bacteremia, phlebitis, arthritis, septic abortion, and meningitis.

### *ETIOLOGY*

*Campylobacter* are gram-negative, motile, nonsporing, curved, spiral rods. All are microaerophilic and do not grow under aerobic or strict anaerobic conditions. They do not ferment carbohydrates and are distinguished from true vibrio species by differences in their DNA base-pair ratios. Three subspecies (sspp) of *C. fetus* have been identified: *fetus, intestinalis,* and *jejuni.* To date, only *C. fetus* sspp *intestinalis* and *jejuni* have been reported as pathogenic for man; *C. fetus* sspp *fetus* is found associated only with bovine abortion.

### *PATHOGENESIS AND PATHOLOGY*

The pathogenesis and mode of transmission of human campylobacteriosis is poorly understood. Although the infection is a recognized zoonosis, there is no evidence that exposure to *C. fetus* in its natural habitat—that is, the intestinal tract of domestic animals—immediately precedes human

campylobacteriosis. That this pathogen of animals is a human enteric pathogen is based on the following observations: *C. fetus* sspp *jejuni* has been simultaneously recovered from feces and blood cultures of patients with diarrhea; the organism disappears from the stools during convalescence; significant specific rising serum antibody titers develop in patients with campylobacter enteritis; clustering of symptomatic cases occurs; a human volunteer ingested *C. fetus* sspp *jejuni*, developed a typical clinical illness, and the organism was recovered from his feces; and treatment with an antibiotic to which the organism is sensitive in vitro leads to rapid disappearance of *C. fetus* sspp *jejuni* from feces and prompt resolution of symptoms.

The pathology of *C. fetus* infections suggests that the disease should be considered in enterocolitis. Acute hemorrhagic necrosis of the jejunum and ileum has been observed at autopsy. The organism has been recovered from aspirates taken from different levels of the small bowel. The frequent occurrence of blood and polymorphonuclear leukocytes in the feces of affected individuals (Blaser et al., 1979) suggests that the large bowel is also commonly involved. Histologic sections show an acute colitis with inflammatory infiltrates of the lamina propria and crypt abscesses. These pathologic features are nonspecific and may also be seen in shigellosis, *Salmonella* colitis, amebiasis, Crohn's disease, and ulcerative colitis.

*C. fetus* neither produces an identifiable enterotoxin nor is cytotoxic for gut mucosa; the microorganism appears to penetrate the intestinal wall by an as yet undefined mechanism, perhaps similar to that observed with other pathogens, such as nontyphoidal salmonellae and yersiniae, which may cause similar clinical illnesses.

The survival of the organism in the bloodstream may be associated with the presence of a glycoprotein cell surface antigen that has antiphagocytic properties. This virulence factor renders the organism resistant to phagocytosis by macrophages and may allow it to persist.

## CLINICAL MANIFESTATIONS, COMPLICATIONS, AND SEQUELAE

Three reasonably distinct patterns of human *C. fetus* infection can be delineated that correlate the bacterial subspecies with the age, sex, underlying health of the host, the clinical presentation, and the outcome (Torphy and Bond, 1979).

The first, most frequent pattern of disease is enteritis. It is usually uncomplicated and due to *C. fetus* sspp *jejuni*. A typical incubation period is about 2 to 5 days. Although campylobacter enteritis affects all age groups, the incidence is highest in young children. The male:female ratio is about 3:2. The most common clinical features are fever, bloody diarrhea, and abdominal pain. Vomiting and dehydration are not common. Fever may be accompanied by several constitutional symptoms, such as malaise, headache, musculoskeletal pain, and occasionally rigors and delirium. The severity of the illness is quite variable; in most cases it is brief, self-limiting, and will subside within a week. In some cases, mild abdominal pain may persist for several weeks after the onset of symptoms and occasionally the illness is persistent or relapsing. The incidence of asymptomatic fecal excretion of *C. fetus* sspp *jejuni* has been estimated at 1.3 per cent in Belgian children and 13 per cent in black South African children. Untreated children continue to excrete *C. fetus* sspp *jejuni* for about 4 to 5 weeks after the onset of symptoms.

A second form of disease consists of focal infections, often associated with vasculitis and/or chronic bacteremia. These infections are most often due to *C. fetus* sspp *intestinalis* and occur in older, debilitated, or chronically ill adults, particularly males. To date, over 100 varieties of human infection caused by *C. fetus* have been described, including meningitis, septic arthritis, pneumonia, empyema, peritonitis, hepatitis, pericarditis, endocarditis, mycotic aneurysm, and thrombophlebitis. In addition, *C. fetus* infection has been associated with Reiter's syndrome as well as a reactive arthritis in an HLA-B27 positive patient. A vascular tropism has been proposed in that vascular sites are frequently infected by *C. fetus,* vascular necrosis has been frequently reported in cases of endocarditis and pericarditis, and thrombophlebitis is commonly associated with *C. fetus* bactere-

mia. In some, febrile episodes were prolonged and relapsing, reminiscent of brucellosis or malaria. The patient's age and underlying diseases appear to determine the severity of *C. fetus* sspp *intestinalis* infections. Thus, these infections have been more common in patients with diabetes, malignancy, hepatorenal disease, and severe cardiovascular disease. In this respect, this organism can be considered an opportunistic pathogen.

A third pattern, perinatal infections, causing abortion, prematurity, neonatal sepsis, and meningitis, is the least frequent and usually due to *C. fetus* sspp *intestinalis*. These infections are usually fatal to the fetus or infant, whereas the mothers survive the illness. Venereal transmission, a common mode of spread of *Campylobacter* species in cattle, has been proposed but not proved in human perinatal infections.

## GEOGRAPHIC VARIATIONS IN DISEASE

*Campylobacter* enteritis is widely distributed in tropical as well as temperate areas of the world. *C. fetus* sspp *jejuni* can be isolated in from 1.3 to 11 per cent of persons with diarrhea (when using selective culturing techniques). It appears to be one of the most common bacterial causes of enteritis in some areas of the world, such as the United Kingdom, The Netherlands, and Canada; *C. fetus* sspp *jejuni* is a common cosmopolitan enteric pathogen. The geographic distribution of *C. fetus* sspp *intestinalis* is not yet known. In a serologic survey, antibody titers to *C. fetus* sspp *intestinalis* were 4 times higher in preparations of commercial human γ-globulin obtained from South Africa than in batches from other parts of the world.

## DIAGNOSIS

Diarrhea, abdominal pain, and constitutional symptoms, especially fever, are the predominant clinical features of *Campylobacter* enteritis. From the symptoms and natural history, the diagnosis may easily be confused with viral or other bacterial gastroenteritis, such as salmonellosis, shigellosis, or yersinia. The frequent occurrence of either gross or occult blood and leukocytes in the stools is an important diagnostic feature. The acute colitis that may be present can mimic acute ulcerative colitis.

A rapid presumptive diagnosis can be made by direct phase-contrast microscopy of stools and visualization of the motile curved spiral rods, resembling treponemes. Confirmation of the diagnosis is made by isolation of *C. fetus* from stools cultured on selective medium containing antibiotics and grown under microaerophilic conditions. Cultures are usually positive after 48 hours. Serologic diagnosis has not proved useful in *Campylobacter* infections.

## TREATMENT

Most patients with *Campylobacter* enteritis will have a mild self-limited illness and do not require antimicrobial therapy. Fluid replacement may be needed in more severely ill patients. Uncontrolled reports suggest that antimotility agents, such as diphenoxylate hydrochloride (Lomotil), should be avoided in *Campylobacter* enteritis. A premature return to solid foods may precipitate a recurrence of symptoms. Although controlled clinical trials have not yet been carried out, erythromycin has been recommended as the preferred antibiotic for the treatment of severe enteritis given as 25 to 50 mg/kg/day in three divided doses for 7 to 10 days. Occasional reports of erythromycin-resistant strains of *C. fetus* warrant determination of antibiotic sensitivities of clinical isolates. Extraintestinal disease has been treated successfully with various antimicrobial agents depending on the site of infection. Gentamicin is the drug of choice for the treatment of septicemia, endocarditis, and other nonenteric *Campylobacter* diseases when the antibiotic sensitivity is not known. For infections of the central nervous system, chloramphenicol is recommended. Treatment of systemic infections for 4 weeks has been suggested because relapse has occurred in a few cases after shorter treatment.

## PROPHYLAXIS

The epidemiology of *C. fetus* infection in man remains obscure. At least six routes of transmission have been suggested: (1) direct contact with infected animals, (2) ingestion of contaminated food, (3) ingestion of contaminated water, (4) venereal transmission, (5) placental transfer or exposure at delivery, and (6) person-to-person spread by fecal-oral route (Taylor et al., 1979). Additionally, *C. fetus* has been suggested to be part of the normal indigenous flora. Attempts at preventing this disease will be more likely to succeed when the modes of transmission are better resolved.

# References

*Shigellosis*

Barrett-Connor, E., and Connor, J. D.: Extraintestinal manifestations of shigellosis. Am J Gastroenterol 53:234, 1970.
Chang, M. J., et al.: Trimethoprim-sulfamethoxazole compared to ampicillin in the treatment of shigellosis. Pediatrics 59:726, 1977.
Dupont, H. L., and Hornick, R. B.: Adverse effect of lomotil therapy in shigellosis. JAMA, 226:1525, 1973.
Levine, M. M., et al.: Long-term shigella-carrier state. N Engl J Med 228:1169, 1973.

*Salmonella Enteritis*

Askeroff, B., and Bennett, J. V.: Effect of antibiotic therapy in acute salmonellosis on the fecal excretion of salmonellae. N Engl J Med 281:636, 1969.
Cherubin, C. E., et al.: Septicemia with non-typhoid salmonella. Medicine 53:365, 1974.
Giannella, R. A., et al.: Pathogenesis of salmonella-mediated intestinal fluid secretion. Gastroenterology 69:1238, 1975.
Sprinz, H.: Pathogenesis of intestinal infections. Arch Pathol 87:566, 1969.

*E. coli Diarrhea*

Dupont, H. L., et al.: Symptomatic treatment of diarrhea with bismuth subsalicylate among students attending a Mexican University. Gastroenterology 73:715, 1977.
Field, M., et al.: Heat-stable enterotoxin of *Escherichia coli:* In vitro effects on guanylate cyclase activity, cyclic GMP concentration and ion transport in small intestine. Proc Natl Acad Sci 75:2800, 1978.
Gangarosa, E. J., and Merson, M. H.: Epidemiological assessment of the relevance of so-called enteropathogenic serogroups of *Escherichia coli* diarrhea. N Eng J Med 296:1210, 1977.
Kantor, H. S.: Enterotoxins of *Escherichia coli* and *Vibrio cholerae:* Tools for the molecular biologist. J Infect Dis 131:S22, 1975.
Merson, M. H., et al.: Traveler's diarrhea in Mexico. A prospective study of physicians and their family members attending a congress. N Engl J Med 294:1299, 1976.
Ulshen, M. H., and Rollo, J. L.: Pathogenesis of *Escherichia coli* gastroenteritis in man—another mechanism. N Engl J Med 302:99, 1980.

*Clostridium perfringens Enteritis*

Duncan, C. L.: Role of clostridial toxins in pathogenesis. In Schlessinger, D. (ed.): Microbiology, 1975. Washington, D.C., American Society for Microbiology, 1975, pp. 283–291.

*Vibrio parahaemolyticus Gastroenteritis*

Barker, W. H., and Gangarosa, E. J.: Food poisoning due to *Vibrio parahaemolyticus.* Ann Rev Med 25:75, 1974.

*Campylobacter Enteritis*

Blaser, M. J., et al.: Campylobacter enteritis: clinical and epidemiologic features. Ann Intern Med 91:179, 1979.
Taylor, P. R., et al.: *Campylobacter fetus* infection in human subjects: association with raw milk. Am J Med 66:779, 1979.
Torphey, D. E., and Bond, W. W.: *Campylobacter fetus* infections in children. Pediatrics 64:898, 1979.

# 127 APPENDICITIS AND DIVERTICULITIS

## O. J. A. Gilmore, M.S., F.R.C.S.(ENG.), F.R.C.S.(ED.)

## *DEFINITIONS*

### Appendicitis

The word appendicitis refers to inflammation occurring in the vermiform appendix. In infants, the appendix is a conical outpouching or diverticulum at the apex of the cecum. With differential growth of the cecum, the appendix eventually comes to arise medially and slightly posteriorly, just below the ileocecal valve. The base of the appendix lies where the teniae of the cecum converge, thus enabling the surgeon to find it at operation.

### Diverticulitis

The word diverticulum is derived from the Latin and literally means a wayside house of ill-repute. Diverticula are of two types: *congenital* (in which all three coats of the bowel are present in the wall of the diverticulum) and *acquired* (in which the muscular wall is absent). Diverticula occur in many parts of the alimentary tract from the esophagus to the rectum but are most common in the colon.

"Diverticulitis" refers to inflammation in an acquired colonic diverticulum. "Diverticulosis" implies that colonic diverticulae are present but are not inflamed. The term diverticular disease of the colon should now be used instead of diverticulosis or diverticulitis, which are misleading. Diverticula tend to develop where blood vessels penetrate the muscle and therefore are more common on the mesenteric border. They vary from a few millimeters to several centimeters in diameter, and their necks may be narrow or wide.

## *ETIOLOGY*

There is no specific microbial cause of appendicitis or diverticulitis. Infection is caused by the bacteria that make up the autochthonous microflora. Since anaerobes make up 90 per cent of the fecal flora, these infections are polymicrobial and have the characteristics of anerobic infections. *Bacteroides* species, *Clostridia*, and peptostreptococci are the most frequently isolated anaerobes; *E. coli*, and enterococci are the most commonly isolated aerobic bacteria either from the inflamed serosa or from an associated abscess.

## *PATHOGENESIS*

The incidence of both appendicitis and diverticular disease appears to be closely linked both historically and geographically with a low fiber diet and its associated excess of refined carbohydrates in the form of white flour and sugar (Cleave and Campbell, 1966; Burkitt, 1973). Such a diet results in an increase in inspissated feces and fecoliths, which may enter the appendix or a diverticulum and cause obstruction. In addition, the bacterial flora of the colon and the appendix change with such a diet. The number of *Bacteroides* and lactobacilli tend to increase, while the enterococci and Enterobacteriaceae decrease.

Pressure studies of the colon indicate that segmentation occurs, narrowing the colonic lumen at intervals. Thus, the colon acts not as a tube but as a series of "little bladders" whose outflow is temporarily obstructed at both ends. When this occurs, high pressures develop, sometimes in excess of 90 mm Hg, which can produce "blow-outs" or diverticula. People who throughout their lives take a high residue diet and produce a bulky stool have a colon of wide diameter and tend not to develop such high intracolonic pressures.

### Appendicitis

Acute appendicitis results from obstruction of the lumen followed by infection. In children and teen-agers obstruction is usually associated with hyperplasia of the lymphoid follicles, and in adults with inspissated feces or a fecolith. Other less common causes of obstruction are foreign bodies, strictures, worms, and tumors. The rate at which the inflammation proceeds depends upon the degree of obstruction and the virulence and number of the bacteria present. The most common aerobic organisms found in the appendix are *Escherichia coli* and the most common anaerobes are *Bacteroides* species.

The inflammatory process advances through catarrhal inflammation to acute inflammation with pus in the lumen and then to gangrene and perforation due to increasing intraluminal pressure that occludes the mural blood supply. Approximately 30 per cent of patients with acute appendicitis are found to have a gangrenous or perforated appendix at operation (Gilmore and Martin, 1974). If the pathologic process is relatively slow, adhesions form around the appendix between loops of bowel, the greater omentum, and the parietal peritoneum, thereby localizing the peritonitis should perforation occur. If appendicitis progresses rapidly to perforation and adhesions have not formed, general peritonitis then ensues, increasing both the morbidity and mortality of the disease.

### Diverticulitis

Acute inflammation in a diverticulum, like appendicitis, is associated with obstruction that is usually due to a hard concretion or fecolith. In these cases acute diverticulitis may progress in a manner similar to that of appendicitis, and gangrene and perforation may result, causing local or generalized peritonitis depending on whether or not the inflamed area has become walled off by the adhesions. As in appendicitis, *E. coli* and *Bacteroides* species are the dominant organisms. Unlike appendicitis, however, the acute inflammatory process is not usually limited to a single diverticulum. This is because the adjacent bowel wall becomes inflamed and edematous, and thus neighboring diverticula become occluded so that the process spreads along the colon.

Chronic inflammation is much more common in diverticular disease. Bacteria cross the thin diverticulum wall and induce extramucosal inflammation. Granulation tissue forms, and this later becomes converted into fibrous tissue; as a result, a palpable mass may form, or the bowel lumen may become narrowed or obstructed.

## CLINICAL MANIFESTATIONS

### Appendicitis

***Symptoms.*** Acute appendicitis has varied manifestations and may mimic many other acute abdominal conditions (Gilmore et al., 1975). In a typical case, the initial symptoms are central abdominal pain and anorexia. Some patients complain of nausea, and others vomit once or twice but not persistently. The initial pain is visceral and usually consists of a central ache but may be colicky, depending upon the degree of appendicular obstruction. Later, when the inflamed appendix irritates the parietal peritoneum, the pain increases and moves to the right iliac fossa. If the appendix is retrocecal or lying between loops of small bowel (retroileal) or in the pelvis, this localization may not occur or may be less marked. Some patients admit to constipation and others, especially young children and those with a pelvic appendix, to diarrhea.

***Physical Signs.*** In classic acute appendicitis, the face is flushed, the tongue furred, and the patient has a temperature of about 38° C and an oral fetor. The temperature rarely goes much above 38° C unless perforation has occurred. The pulse rate is often normal, but there may be a mild tachycardia. After examination of the head and neck, the chest must be examined to exclude pneumonia. Inspection of the abdomen may reveal reduced respiratory movements in the lower half if the symptoms have been present for more than a few hours. Gentle palpation reveals tenderness in the right iliac fossa that is often maximal around McBurney's point. Guarding is present and, in advanced cases, rigidity and rebound tenderness. Rebound tenderness should be elicited by gentle percussion, not by pressing the hands in at the site of maximum tenderness and suddenly removing them. This method only causes the patient unnecessary distress. Rovsing's sign (pain in the right iliac fossa when the left iliac fossa is pressed) is sometimes helpful, as is the psoas stretch sign. This consists of turning the patient on the left side and extending the right hip; if this causes increased discomfort it suggests that the appendix is retrocecal.

If symptoms have been present for more than 48 hours, the patient may have a mass in the right iliac fossa representing adherent ilium and omentum around the inflamed appendix.

Rectal examination is mandatory in every patient, and in women, when the diagnosis is doubtful, a vaginal examination is also necessary. Pelvic examination is undertaken to elicit tenderness in pelvic appendicitis and to exclude other lesions such as salpingitis or an ovarian cyst.

***Laboratory Diagnosis.*** Acute appendicitis is a clinical diagnosis. Laboratory investigations are of secondary importance. A patient with the symptoms and signs of appendicitis deserves an appendectomy as soon as possible. In case of doubt, a raised leukocyte count with a shift to the left suggests appendicitis, but a normal count does not exclude the diagnosis. In appendicitis, there are no pathognomonic radiologic signs except for the presence of a fecolith. The urine should always be examined to exclude infection.

### Diverticulitis

***Symptoms.*** Uncomplicated diverticular disease is symptomless, but diverticulitis, like appendicitis, presents with pain. The initial pain consists either of a suprapubic ache or, more often, due to parietal peritoneal irritation, a left lower quadrant pain. Such patients often complain of alternating diarrhea and constipation. Nausea and anorexia are relatively uncommon and vomiting even less so. In very loose terms, diverticulitis can be considered as a left-sided appendicitis occurring in an older patient.

Some patients present with peritonitis after perforation of a diverticulum. A few complain of pneumaturia due to a ruptured diverticulum that causes a vesicocolic fistula. Massive rectal bleeding is an unusual presentation.

**Physical Signs.** In diverticulitis, like appendicitis, the patient may have a mild fever and tachycardia. The tongue may be furred, and there may be an oral fetor. Often, however, physical signs are limited to the abdomen. Examination reveals tenderness and guarding in the left iliac fossa. Rigidity and rebound tenderness indicate advanced pathology. The presence of a mass in diverticulitis, owing to the slower advancement of the inflammatory process, is much more common than in appendicitis. There may also be pelvic tenderness or even a pelvic mass.

In both conditions, when perforation occurs without localization, generalized peritonitis ensues, and the patient usually presents with fever of 39° C or more, a pulse rate of over 100, and a rigid abdomen.

**Laboratory Investigations.** In diverticulitis the leukocyte count is similar to that in appendicitis. Full sigmoidoscopy without anesthesia and with limited air insufflation should be undertaken. Sometimes a diverticulum is seen, but more commonly narrowing of the colon, spasm, or rigidity with increased mucus is noted. Perforation of a diverticulum may result in collections of extraluminal gas that can be seen on a plain film of the abdomen. Definitive diagnosis is based on barium enema examination but this must not be undertaken in patients with an acute attack because of the risk of causing perforation. In case of doubt, fiberoptic colonoscopy may be helpful but should not be undertaken if the patient is acutely ill.

## DIFFERENTIAL DIAGNOSIS

### Appendicitis

In children nonspecific mesenteric adenitis is the condition that most frequently mimics appendicitis. Constipation and tubo-ovarian disorders such as ruptured, twisted, or bleeding ovarian cysts and salpingitis constitute the main differential diagnoses in women (Gilmore, 1978). Other confusing conditions include acute pyelonephritis, ureteric colic, ectopic pregnancy, Meckel's diverticulitis, Crohn's disease, tuberculous ileitis, small bowel obstruction, intussusception, carcinoma of the cecum, gastroenteritis, acute pancreatitis, torsion of the omentum, perforated peptic ulcer, and, very occasionally, basal pneumonia and myocardial ischemia.

### Diverticulitis

Acute diverticulitis, in which a long sigmoid loop comes to lie in the right iliac fossa, may also present as appendicitis. The most common differential diagnosis to diverticulitis, however, is carcinoma of the colon.

## COMPLICATIONS

### Appendicitis

The most common complications of appendicitis are perforation, peritonitis, and abscess formation. Perforation may result in local or generalized peritonitis or in local abscess formation. General peritonitis in turn may result in a pelvic or subphrenic abscess. Portal pyemia, a suppurative thrombophlebitis of the portal system, is an unusual complication. Liver abscess can result.

### Diverticulitis

Acute diverticulitis may result in similar complications. In addition, fistulous communications may develop between the colon and the bladder or between the colon and the small bowel. Intestinal obstruction occurs, usually because of excessive peridiverticular fibrosis and occasionally because of adhesions.

Both appendicitis and diverticulitis may kill the patient, especially the very young and the very old. The most common postoperative complication in both diseases is wound infection, and its likelihood increases if the appendix ruptures. Abdominal actinomycosis is a rare complication of both conditions.

## GEOGRAPHIC VARIATION

Appendicitis and diverticulitis appear to be diseases of western civilization. Both are more common in Europe and North America than in Asia and Africa. In western countries, about 5 to 8 per cent of people develop appendicitis, usually before age 20. Diverticular disease is the most common colonic pathology in developed countries. It is estimated that 10 per cent of people in their fifth decade and 60 per cent of people in their ninth decade have diverticula. In parts of Africa in which people still adhere to a traditional diet of grain, maize, and fruit, both appendicitis and diverticulitis are rarities. Like appendicitis, the incidence of diverticulitis is increasing in urban areas of developing countries (Archampong et al., 1978).

## TREATMENT

### Appendicitis

The treatment of appendicitis is appendectomy. Conservative treatment with antibiotics and intravenous fluid should be used only in the absence of anesthesia or a competent surgeon, or when the patient presents with an appendiceal mass. An aminoglycoside such as kanamycin or gentamicin for coliforms, and clindamycin or metronidazole for anaerobes are the antimicrobials of choice. If the mass increases in size or the patient's general condition deteriorates, the appendiceal abscess must be drained. In those patients with a mass who stabilize, an appendectomy is done two to three months later.

In the remainder, appendectomy should be carried out as soon as possible after adequate preoperative preparation and under general anesthesia. A right iliac fossa skin crease incision over the site of maximum tenderness is employed. The muscles are then split in the direction of their fibers. This gridiron incision is the incision of choice, since it is less liable to complications, including sepsis, than the paramedian incision (Gilmore and Sanderson, 1975). The appendix is then located at the base of the cecum, delivered into the incision, and removed. The mesentery of the appendix is divided between clamps, and the base of the appendix is then crushed, ligated, and inverted into the cecum by means of a purse-string suture.

Intravenous antibiotics as described above are indicated if the appendix is gangrenous or perforated or if there is an abscess. The first dose should be given at the time of operation and the course continued for two to three days. Drainage, preferably through the wound, is necessary if there is an abscess or excessive soiling of the peritoneum. In generalized peritonitis, the peritoneal cavity should be lavaged with 1 to 2 liters of warm normal saline until the effluent is clear. Postoperatively, the patient may start drinking as soon as the bowel sounds return and eat following the passage of flatus. In case of peritonitis, progress is slower, and the patient requires nasogastric aspiration and intravenous fluids until borborygmi are heard.

### Diverticulitis

In contrast to appendicitis, diverticulitis is usually treated conservatively. In mild cases, an antispasmodic and a high residue diet suffice. In patients with signs of peritoneal irritation, nasogastric aspiration, intravenous (I.V.) fluids, and parenteral antibiotics—kanamycin (twice daily) or gentamicin (every 8 hours) with clindamycin (every 8 hours) or metronidazole (every 8 hours)—are indicated.

Surgery is reserved for patients with complications and for those with recurrent attacks that do not respond to medical treatment. The complications of diverticular disease often require urgent surgery and are associated with some morbidity and a significant mortality.

Perforation (30 to 40 per cent) is the most common complication and results in local or generalized peritonitis or abscess formation. These patients used to be treated by performing a transverse colostomy as the first stage of a three-stage procedure. This, however, is inadequate. One must also drain the perforation site or, preferably, exteriorize the colon at the site of perforation so that a stream of fecal material above the hole in the colon is avoided. Some surgeons advocate primary resection and anastomosis, even in the presence of pus, and claim a lower mortality. If this is done, it is prudent to carry out a covering transverse colostomy. The same antibiotics are given in perforations of the colon as in perforations of the appendix since the bacterial flora are similar.

Fistula formation, usually to the bladder and sometimes to the small bowel, vagina, skin, or hip joint, is the second most common complication (10 to 15 per cent). Barium enema examination shows diverticular disease, but the fistula is rarely demonstrated. Colovesical fistulas are best diagnosed from the symptoms of pneumaturia, foul-smelling urine, and a persistent or recurrent urinary tract infection due to mixed fecal organisms. The diagnosis is confirmed by cytoscopy. The majority of fistulas can be dealt with by a one-stage resection and anastomosis after careful preoperative preparation. Complex fistulas may require a three-stage procedure consisting of (1) performance of a transverse colostomy, (2) resection and anastomosis of the fistula(s), and (3) closure of the colostomy.

Obstruction (5 to 10 per cent) in diverticular disease is rarer than in carcinoma. Relief of obstruction from diverticular disease may require a one-, two-, or three-stage procedure, depending on the general condition of the patient and the severity of the obstruction.

Massive hemorrhage is an unusual but well-recognized complication of diverticular disease. Depending on the site and speed of the bleed, the blood presenting at the anus varies from brown to bright red in color. Selective mesenteric arteriography may locate the site of hemorrhage, and, if the bleeding does not cease, urgent resection is required. Local resection is adequate if the site of hemorrhage is known; if not, the patient should have a total colectomy. Ileorectal anastomosis can be done then or at a later stage, depending on the condition of the patient and the experience of the surgeon.

Patients with diverticulitis who have repeated attacks of pain and fail to respond to medical treatment should always be considered for elective surgery. Resection in these patients need not be as extensive as in carcinoma, since only the involved segment needs excision. Although anastomotic complications are common in diverticulitis, a one-stage procedure can be done. Many surgeons prefer a three-stage procedure.

### PROPHYLAXIS

Africans who still adhere to their traditional way of life and consume a high residue diet containing a mininum of carbohydrates rarely develop either appendicitis or diverticulitis. If the rest of us adopted a similar diet from childhood, we would be less likely to develop appendicitis and very unlikely to get diverticulitis.

Postoperative wound infection after appendectomy and colon resection can be prevented by a short course of systemic metronidazole and kanamycin.

### References

Archampong, E. Q., et al.: Third world diverticular disease. Ann R Coll Surg Engl 60:464, 1978.

Burkitt, D. P.: Some diseases characteristic of modern western civilization. Br Med J 1:274, 1973.

Cleave, T. L., and Campbell, G. D.: Diabetes, Coronary Thrombosis and the Saccharine Disease. Bristol, John Wright & Sons Ltd., 1966.

Gilmore, O. J. A.: Diagnostic error in acute appendicitis. Med Annual 1978. Bristol, John Wright & Sons Ltd., 1978.

Gilmore, O. J. A., Brodribb, A. J. M., Browett, J. P., Cooke, T. J. C., Griffin, P. H., Higgs, M. J., Ross, I. K., and Williamson, R. C. N.: Appendicitis and mimicking conditions. A prospective study. Lancet 2:421, 1975.

Gilmore, O. J. A., and Martin, T. D. M.: The aetiology and prevention of wound infection after appendectomy. Br J Surg 61:281, 1974.

Gilmore, O. J. A., and Sanderson, P. J.: Prophylactic interparietal povidone iodine in abdominal surgery. Br J Surg 62:792, 1975.

# 128 *CHOLERA*

*Craig K. Wallace, M.D.*

### DEFINITION

Cholera is an acute infectious disease resulting from an enterotoxin elaborated by *Vibrio cholerae* in the small intestine, generally occurring in epidemics and causing rapid massive gastrointestinal fluid loss, extreme saline depletion, acidosis, and shock. A mortality rate of over 60 per cent in untreated patients is completely reversed by the prompt replacement of fluid and electrolytes (Barua and Burrows, 1974).

### ETIOLOGY

The *V. cholerae* is a short, slightly curved, rod-shaped, gram-negative staining bacterium that is rapidly motile by means of a single polar flagellum (see Chapter 32, Fig. 2). It grows aerobically on nutrient media at 37° C, preferably at an alkaline pH. It possesses both O and H antigens and serologic identification is based upon differences in the polysaccharide O antigens.

The common delta of the Ganges and Brahmaputra Rivers of India and Bangladesh has been a known focus of cholera since first described in European literature by a Portuguese observer early in the 16th Century. Until the 19th century, cholera was confined to Asia, almost exclusively to India; however, cholera extended beyond this area, spreading along the trade routes over most of the globe in six pandemics between 1817 and 1923. Subsequently, cholera was again confined to the endemic regions of Southeast Asia except for one isolated epidemic in Egypt during 1947. The present seventh pandemic spread of disease extended from the Celebes in 1961 northward to Korea and westward to the whole of Africa and southern Europe.

Since the discovery of the cholera vibrio by Robert Koch in 1884, a wide variety of hemolytic vibrios have been found in nature; true cholera vibrios were not hemolytic. This distinction seemed valid until 1906, when Gotschlich isolated hemolytic strains of cholera vibrios from the dead pilgrims at the El Tor quarantine station in Egypt. There was no cholera epidemic at that time and the pathogenicity of this hemolytic (El Tor) cholera vibrio was not ascertained. In 1939, DeMoor described cholera in Sulawesi (Celebes), Indonesia that was due to the El Tor biotype of *V. cholerae*. This El Tor vibrio is the etiologic agent in the seventh pandemic. Interestingly, the El Tor biotype of *V. cholerae* has lost its hemolytic characteristic in recent years and is now distinguished from the classical vibrio by resistance to Murkerjee's phage IV, resistance to polymyxin, and the ability to agglutinate chicken red blood cells (Wallace, 1969).

### PATHOGENESIS AND PATHOLOGY

The cholera patient ingests viable *V. cholerae*. The organisms multiply in the small bowel and produce an enterotoxin, which stimulates the mucosal cells to secrete large quantities of isotonic fluid faster than the colon can reabsorb, so that a watery, isotonic diarrhea results. All strains of *V. cholerae* can produce in the same stool fluid-electrolyte losses that cause the physical findings and laboratory abnormalities of cholera. There is no evidence that the vibrio invades any tissue or that the enterotoxin directly affects any organ other than the small intestine. Cholera has the shortest incubation period of any infection; grave symptoms may occur within a few hours of infection.

Vibrio enterotoxin has a molecular weight of 84,000 and stimulates adenyl cyclase in the intestinal epithelial cells. The resultant increase in intracellular cyclic adenosine $3',5'$-monophosphate leads to the secretion of isotonic fluids by all of the small intestine. This enterotoxin-induced electrolyte secretion occurs with no demonstrable histologic damage to intestinal epithelial cells or capillary endothelial cells of the lamina propria.

The cholera stool has little protein and is isotonic, with plasma having a remarkably predictable composition of approximately 135 mEq sodium, 15 mEq potassium, 105 mEq chloride, and 45 mEq bicarbonate per liter in adults (Watten et al., 1959). In children the electrolyte composition of the diarrheal fluid is different and contains on the average 100 mEq sodium, 25 mEq potassium, 75 mEq chloride, and 32 mEq bicarbonate per liter.

## CLINICAL MANIFESTATIONS

Most infections with *V. cholerae* are asymptomatic or mild. The ratio of severe disease to mild and inapparent infections has been from 1:5 to 1:10 in classic cholera and only about 1:25 to 1:100 for El Tor cholera. The hospitalized cases of both forms of disease, therefore, represent extreme manifestation of disease, with most infections going undetected unless intensive bacteriologic or serologic studies are made.

The sudden onset of profuse, effortless diarrhea is the *sine qua non* of symptomatic cholera. The diarrheal stool initially may contain fecal particles or be bile-tinged, but shortly a "rice water stool" is seen. This is a continuous, light-gray, water diarrhea with flecks of mucous material but no pus or blood, and an odor like amniotic fluid. A rare patient may have pooling in the gut without diarrhea (*cholera sicca*). Most patients, soon after the onset of diarrhea, have copious effortless vomiting that is precipitous but not persistent. Severe muscular cramps, most frequently located in the fingers, toes, and lower extremities, but which may be generalized, are present in 75 per cent of patients. Patients usually are not seen by a physician until 8 to 16 hours after onset of diarrhea. If not moribund, the patient is hoarse, reasonably alert, and oriented. Marked dehydration causes sunken eyes and cheeks, dry tongue and mucous membranes, poor skin turgor, shriveled feet, and "washer-woman's hands." The lips are cyanotic, skin is cold and clammy, temperature is subnormal, and respirations are rapid and shallow.

There is a tachycardia and hypotension or an imperceptible pulse and blood pressure. The abdomen is scaphoid, nontender, and the bowel sounds are not remarkable.

Children do not respond as do adults. They frequently have fever, tetany or generalized convulsions, and pulmonary edema.

Laboratory studies reveal a metabolic acidosis and confirm the clinical findings of dehydration and hemoconcentration (Watten et al., 1959). The plasma electrolytes (mEq/liter of plasma water), are normal except for a low bicarbonate that averages from 7 to 18 mEq/liter.

Prompt fluid, electrolyte, and base replacement rapidly ameliorates all signs and symptoms except diarrhea. The illness may last from 12 hours to 7 days (Carpenter et al., 1966).

## COMPLICATIONS AND SEQUELAE

There should be no complications or sequelae if cholera is treated promptly and correctly.

Cholera may, of course, be superimposed upon preexisting disease. Persistent circulatory failure will cause hypotensive shock, cyanosis, and anuria. Most patients are anuric upon admission and may remain oliguric for several days. If rehydration is not achieved rapidly and maintained, acute renal failure may ensue. Prolonged acidosis may cause persistent cramps and vomiting, increased dyspnea, rales, and pulmonary-myocardial failure. Acidosis is often intensified by infusion of abundant saline without alkali. Untreated hypokalemia may cause muscle weakness, ileus, cardiac arrhythmia, abdominal distention, and occasional central nervous system disturbances. The patient must be carefully monitored for overhydration. If it does occur, the hepatojugular reflux and slow full pulse usually give adequate warning before pulmonary edema.

Fetal mortality and abortion, especially in the third trimester, are frequent in pregnant women with cholera.

Pediatric cholera is especially severe; water exchange in proportion to body weight is far greater than in adults and fluid balances are more readily disturbed. A few children with prolonged diarrhea and impaired oral intake have premonitory drowsiness or convulsions as a result of hypoglycemia.

Under ideal conditions and with prompt and adequate fluid replacement, mortality and significant sequelae approach zero. Oral glucose-electrolyte therapy can be effective even under the most primitive conditions. Unfortunately, death rates as high as 60 per cent are still being reported especially at the start of an epidemic. This reflects the lack of pyrogen-free intravenous fluids in remote areas and the difficulties of initiating prompt treatment to large numbers of patients under emergency conditions.

## GEOGRAPHIC VARIATIONS IN DISEASE

The spectrum of illness is identical throughout the world: most infections are asymptomatic, and relatively few are in typical patients with shock from marked dehydration, who respond rapidly to fluid therapy.

Koch's discovery of the vibrio, although elucidating the etiology of cholera, did not lead to clarification of the epidemiology and ecology of the disease. Why the cluster of infection has remained in the delta of the Ganges and Brahmaputra Rivers is unknown. With the exception of the present pandemic, all epidemics have originated from this endemic focus. We do not know why that from time to time at irregular intervals the disease spreads from country to country and from continent to continent (Pollitzer, 1959). These widespread epidemics last several years and then inexplicably abate.

What factors favor a new cholera epidemic and continent migration? As suggested by Jusatz (1977) the initial spread of disease continued only very slowly *overland*, not reaching central European countries and Great Britain until 1831. Since 1865, cholera has moved more rapidly by *sea*; pilgrims making their way to and from Mecca, especially, have carried cholera far and wide. A third phase became evident during the present, or seventh, cholera pandemic when *air* passengers provided a particularly fast transit mode for the vibrio to cholera-free areas in the space of hours. *Water* is the most frequent transport medium of the cholera vibrios outside the human body. The type of water supply, the velocity of the rivers, as well as the quality of water, especially its acidity or alkalinity, are considered of great significance in accounting for the movement and distribution of cholera in different geographic areas. Deserts and water poor areas are largely circumvented during cholera migrations. The influence of the *seasons* indicates that cold, snow, and frost are inhibiting factors. Other seasonal variations are seen, such as, those in India and Bangladesh. In Calcutta, cholera always decreases with the onset of the annual monsoon; whereas in Dacca, less than 200 miles distant, the onset of the monsoon is coincident with an increase of cholera infections. Another predisposing factor is the *mass movement of people*, such as for religious and military events.

Of note, the classic *V. cholera* has not been involved in the post-1961 migrations, but rather the biotype El Tor has been identified in all countries invaded during the seventh pandemic. This variant causes disease identical to that caused by the so-called classic vibrio, but there are marked epidemiologic differences. The infection-to-case ratio is higher with El Tor cholera. It is excreted over a longer period of time. The El Tor vibrio is generally hardier, surviving longer in the environment on infected foodstuffs and in water and feces, which makes it more easily detectable in surveys of water and night soil. The few chronic carriers of *V. cholerae* described in the literature have all been infected with the El Tor biotype.

## DIAGNOSIS

The clinical impression of typical cholera needs no laboratory confirmation for treatment purposes. Laboratory confirmation, however, is necessary to differentiate the sporadic case from other diarrheal diseases and to alert public health personnel. Although the epidemiologic and fulminant characteristics of cholera are suggestive, past experience has shown that diagnoses of the first few cases usually take too long because the laboratory is unprepared.

Direct plating of a cholera stool on bile salt, gelatin-tellurite-taurocholate (GTT), or thiosulfate-citrate-bile salt-sucrose (TCBS) agar is optimal for cultural diagnosis. On the first two media, *V. cholerae* appear as typical translucent colonies in 18 hours (See Chapter 32); oblique lighting makes it possible to identify one vibrio colony from among several hundred colonies of other organisms. On TCBS agar, *V. cholerae* appear at 24 hours as large, discrete yellow colonies. Cultural identification of large numbers of vibrios ($10^7$ to $10^9$/ml) in the stools is relatively simple. In the patient with fewer vibrios, as in convalescence, recovery can be enhanced by enrichment for six hours in alkaline peptone water before subculture to solid media.

Rapid identification of vibrios in stools or primary culture is possible by observing immobilization of vibrios by type-specific antisera, by darkfield or phase microscopy, or by immunofluorescent methods.

Serologic diagnosis requires demonstration of rises in agglutinating or vibriocidal antibody titers. Significant rises in both titers are present by the seventh to tenth day of illness in over 90 per cent of patients with bacteriologically proven *V. cholerae* infection.

## TREATMENT

Replacement of water and electrolytes lost in stool and vomitus is the basis of cholera therapy.

This regimen has been used in many parts of the world with a mortality of less than 1 per cent.

## Oral and Intravenous Fluids

A supply of preweighed salts and glucose for the preparation of an oral replacement solution should be available, preferably stored in double plastic bags, to be added to a specified volume of ordinary water before use. An acceptable composition is glucose 20 g/liter, sodium chloride 4 g/liter, sodium bicarbonate 4 g/liter, and potassium chloride 1 g/liter of drinking water.

An intravenous solution containing approximately 140 mEq/liter sodium, 10 mEq/liter potassium, 100 mEq/liter chloride, and 50 mEq/liter bicarbonate is simple to use but generally not available. Ringer's lactate is recommended as a single intravenous rehydration fluid by the World Health Organization and is readily available. This is especially satisfactory for children. Effective and available are two solutions given in a 2:1 ratio as isotonic saline: isotonic sodium lactate (1/6 molar) or isotonic sodium bicarbonate.

If potassium is not given intravenously it may be given orally and will be absorbed regardless of the stool volume or intestinal transit time. Ten milliliters of a solution containing 100 g each of potassium citrate, potassium acetate, and potassium bicarbonate in 1 liter of water given three times a day orally will balance the potassium losses in the average patient.

## Treatment Centers

Predetermined treatment areas should be available to any potential patient within three hours after the onset of symptoms. Adequate glucose and salts for making up oral solution, plastic oro- or nasogastric tubes, pyrogen-free intravenous fluids, intravenous administration tubing, large-gauge needles, scalp vein sets, and a scale should be available.

Cholera beds, a simple cot with a reinforced hole located in the center for the patient's buttocks, should be available. These can be made of canvas on a wooden frame or even boards elevated upon supports. Any 2 to 3 gallon receptacle can be easily calibrated and when placed under the hole in the cot will be effective for collecting and measuring excreta. The time and amount of all infusions or oral fluids when initiated and the output when discarded must be carefully recorded at the bedside.

## Management

The patient should be weighed; if a scale is not available, this may be estimated. The degree of dehydration may be assessed by clinical observation to determine the amount of replacement fluid needed. *Mild* dehydration (5 per cent body weight deficit) is indicated by only a slightly decreased skin turgor and tachycardia. *Moderate* dehydration (8 per cent body weight deficit) is indicated by markedly decreased skin turgor, tachycardia, and hypotension. *Severe dehydration* (10 per cent body weight deficit) has all the above plus cyanosis, stupor, or coma. By knowing the weight and approximating the volume deficit, the amount of fluid necessary for rehydration can be determined.

In the comatose patient administer intravenous fluid through an 18-gauge needle. A smaller-gauge needle or a scalp vein set is usually necessary for children. The femoral vein in adults or the external jugular vein in children may be utilized in patients with severe vascular collapse. Fluids may be given by holding the needle in place until the plasma volume expands sufficiently so that superficial veins become visible and the infusion can be easily transferred to a more suitable vein. Intravenous fluid should be started rapidly by giving at least 100 ml per minute to the collapsed adult patient until blood pressure is restored. After rehydration a slower rate of infusion should balance the measured diarrheal output and estimated insensible loss. An adult's insensible water loss is approximately 1 ml/kg per hour and should be replaced. The oral administration of this amount of water contributes to the patient's state of well being. During the acute phase of disease, the vital signs should be checked at two-hour intervals. There can be no substitute for careful, constant clinical observation.

Initial rehydration and maintenance therapy solely by the administration of oral fluids is encouraged because of its safety, ease of administration, and general availability. The solution should be warmed to about 45° C before administration. Some prefer to give the solution through a thin plastic oro- or nasogastric tube connected to an infusion bottle. From 750 to 1500 ml per hour is given for the first four hours, depending upon the degree of admission dehydration. Thereafter, the measured output plus the calculated insensible loss during the preceding four-hour period indicates the volume of oral solution to be given. Allow further oral fluids upon demand and a soft diet as tolerated. Vomiting does not occur after initial correction of the dehydration and acidosis (Pierce and Hirschhorn, 1977).

Treatment of pediatric cholera is difficult in respect to initiating and maintaining intravenous fluids. Water loss in proportion to body weight is far greater than in adults, fluid balances are more readily disturbed, and the electrolyte losses are different from those in adults. Children should be closely followed with frequent clinical observations, including weight, to avoid overhydration. Children should never gain more than 10 per cent of their admission body weight. If possible, children should be treated in a separate pediatric area. Intravenous fluids as outlined above have been used with success, and particular attention is advised to replacing insensible losses with oral glucose water. Children with prolonged diarrhea and impaired oral intake can have drowsiness or convulsions as a result of hypoglycemia. They respond dramatically to 50 per cent intravenous glucose solution, although fruit juice suffices in the conscious patient. Convulsions and coma unrelated to fever, hypoglycemia, hypocalcemia, hypernatremia, or overhydration may be seen. Intravenous magnesium sulfate succeeds occasionally when other methods fail to control convulsions.

Although adequate intravenous saline and alkali replacement alone results in rapid recovery of virtually all cholera patients, a dramatic reduction in duration and volume of diarrhea, and early eradication of vibrios from the stool may be effected by antibiotic therapy. Oral tetracycline, 500 mg every six hours for adults and 10 mg/kg body weight every six hours for children for the first 48 hours has been most successful. Other antibiotics, including chloramphenicol and furazolidone, are slightly less effective than tetracycline (Wallace et al., 1968).

Additional adjuncts of therapy (oxygen, cardiorespiratory stimulants, vasopressors, and antidiarrheal compounds) are not indicated and divert essential medical and financial resources.

Therapy is continued until the diarrhea has practically ceased and fluid electrolyte requirements can be met by oral fluids and a soft diet. Patients may be discharged as soon as they are ambulatory, eating, without diarrhea, and putting out adequate urine. The public health problems of unsuspected carriers and convalescents who excrete vibrios are unsolved.

## PROPHYLAXIS

The current cholera vaccines composed of classic or El Tor strains are of limited value. In field trials in endemic areas, vaccines have been only about 50 per cent effective in reducing incidence of clinical illness for a period of three to six months. They do not prevent transmission of infection.

Primary immunization with commercial vaccines, containing 10 billion organisms per millimeter, is given in two doses one week to one month or more apart, either subcutaneously or intramuscularly as follows: 0.2 ml from six months to four years of age, 0.3 ml five to ten years, and 0.5 ml over ten years. A booster immunization in a similar dosage may be given every six months for travel or to residents in highly endemic, unsanitary areas. When cholera occurs in an annual two or three month "season," protection is best if the booster dose is given at the beginning of the season. The primary series need not be repeated.

Field trials have shown that antibiotics like tetracycline and chloramphenicol prevent the transmission of infection among close contacts of cholera patients, but giving these drugs to both close and community contacts has not controlled cholera outbreaks. In any circumstance, the indiscriminate use of antimicrobial drugs is to be avoided. If chemoprophylaxis is considered at all the drug chosen should be administered only with close supervision for contraindications and for follow-up of reactions.

Cholera can be eliminated only by improved standards of living, public health, and sanitation. In those parts of the world where water supply and sewage disposal are adequate, cholera no longer poses a problem.

## References

Barua, D., and Burrows, W.: Cholera. Philadelphia, W. B. Saunders Company, 1974.

Carpenter, C. C. J. et al.: Clinical studies in Asiatic cholera, I–VI. Bull Johns Hopkins Hosp 118:165, 1966.

Jusatz, H.: Cholera. In Howe, G. M. (ed.): A World Geography of Human Diseases. London, New York, and San Francisco, Academic Press, 1977, p. 131.

Pierce, N. F., and Hirschhorn, N.: Oral fluid — a simple weapon against dehydration in diarrhoea. WHO Chronicle 31:87, 1977.

Pollitzer, R.: Cholera. Geneva, WHO Monograph Series, No. 43, 1959.

Wallace, C. K. et al.: Optimal antibiotic therapy in cholera. Bull WHO 39:239, 1968.

Wallace, C. K.: Cholera: A Continuing Threat and Challenge. In Lincicome, D. R., and Woodruff, D. W. (eds.): International Review of Tropical Medicine. New York and London, Academic Press, 1969, p. 159.

Watten, R. H. et al.: Water and electrolyte studies in cholera. J Clin Invest 38:1879, 1959.

# YERSINIA ENTERITIS 129

## Gerald T. Keusch, M.D.

### DEFINITIONS AND HISTORY

Abdominal infections of man with *Yersinia enterocolitica* and *Y. pseudotuberculosis* cause a variety of syndromes, but enteritis (enterocolitis) and mesenteric adenitis are by far the most common. Enterocolitis is an acute, febrile dysentery that usually occurs in children under 5 years of age infected with *Y. enterocolitica*. Mesenteric adenitis, which may imitate appendicitis, is most common in 5- to 15-year-olds and may be caused by either species of *Yersinia*. Reactive polyarticular arthritis is a late, noninfectious complication of *Yersinia* enteritis in adults. It occurs most commonly among those with a certain HLA type in Scandinavia.

*Yersinia* is a new genus that was created to accommodate *Y. pestis* (the plague bacillus, Chapter 243), *Y. enterocolitica,* and *Y. pseudotuberculosis*. Although *Yersinia* organisms share many characteristics with *Francisella* and *Pasteurella* and were formerly classified with these bacteria, they fit the definition of Enterobacteriaceae (Chapter 31) and are now included in this family.

*Y. pseudotuberculosis* was first isolated in 1883 from necrotizing granulomas in the livers, spleens, and lymph nodes of various mammals and birds. The disease was called pseudotuberculosis because of the nature of the lesions. Occasional cases of human septicemia were described early in this century. but acute mesenteric adenitis, the chief form of intestinal disease caused by this bacterium, was not reported until 1954. *Y. enterocolitica* was unknown until 1939 and was not recognized as a human pathogen until 1964. Since then, there has been a spectacular rise in the reported incidence of *Y. enterocolitica* enteritis. This has been due principally to heightened interest in the organism rather than recent pandemic spread.

### ETIOLOGY

Members of the genus *Yersinia* have been reclassified into the Enterobacteriaceae family because they are facultatively anaerobic, oxidase-negative, gram-negative bacilli that ferment glucose and reduce nitrate. Motile species synthesize peritrichous flagella. *Y. enterocolitica* and *Y. pseudotuberculosis* may be coccobacillary but are usually relatively large bacilli, 0.5 to 1.0 by 1 to 2 $\mu$m. They must be differentiated from *Proteus* on the one hand and the plague bacillus *(Y. pestis)* on the other (Table 1). They may also be difficult to isolate from cultures of the stool.

When first recovered from the stool, *Y. pseudotuberculosis* is likely to be discarded as a *Proteus* species, a normal member of the fecal flora, because both are lactose-negative and urease-positive, and both produce an alkaline slant/acid butt reaction on triple sugar iron agar (TSI). *Y. enterocolitica* can ferment both sucrose and glucose in TSI and therefore produces the acid slant/acid butt characteristic of *Escherichia coli*. Because this pattern is typical of the nonpathogens, the organism is likely to be discarded. Once selected for further study, however, identification is quite straightforward. Failure to produce $H_2S$ or deaminate phenylalanine and the absence of motility at 37° C are among the important reactions that differentiate *Yersinia* from the indole-negative *Proteus* spp (Delorme et al., 1974). Motility when grown at 22° C but not at 37° C, and urease activity are important properties of the

**TABLE 1.** Selected Microbiologic Characteristics of *Yersinia*

| PROPERTY | Y. PSEUDOTUBERCULOSIS | Y. ENTEROCOLITICA | Y. PESTIS |
|---|---|---|---|
| TSI[a] reaction (slant/butt) | Alkaline/acid | Acid/acid | Alkaline/acid |
| H₂S production (TSI) | − | − | − |
| Indole | − | + (except serotype 0:3) | − |
| Urease production (Christensen's) | + | + | − |
| Ornithine decarboxylase | − | + | − |
| Rhamnose fermentation | + | − | − |
| Sucrose fermentation | − | + | − |
| Lactose fermentation | − | − | − |
| Motility  22° C | + | + | − |
|          37° C | − | − | − |
| Esculin hydrolysis | + | − | + |

[a]TSI, Triple sugar iron agar. *Y. enterocolitica* produces an acid slant because it ferments sucrose.

two organisms that distinguish them from *Y. pestis*. Ornithine decarboxylase activity, indole production, and sucrose fermentation are seen with *Y. pseudotuberculosis* but not *Y. enterocolitica* (Table 1). The biochemical identification can be confirmed by agglutination with specific typing sera.

Isolation of both organisms is enhanced by the cold enrichment technique, in which a 10 per cent suspension of feces (or other sample) in phosphate-buffered saline, pH 7.6, is maintained at 4° C for serial subculture to enriched media for 7 to 28 days. *Yersinia*, but not other Enterobacteriaceae, preferentially multiply at this low temperature to give progressive enrichment of *Yersinia* in the buffer. Cultures should be incubated always at both room temperature and 37° C because primary isolation from clinical material may be achieved only at the lower temperature. Certain characteristics, such as the synthesis of peritrichous flagella and surface O antigens, are expressed only at temperatures less than 30° C.

*Yersinia* organisms are sensitive to several different bacteriophages, and one phage has been used to differentiate *Y. pestis* from *Y. pseudotuberculosis* (Gunnison et al., 1951).

On the basis of somatic O antigens, 34 serogroups of *Y. enterocolitica* and six types designated by Roman numerals (with four subtypes) of *Y. pseudotuberculosis* can be distinguished. Antibodies to these antigens develop during disease, acutely rising and falling in several weeks for *Y. pseudotuberculosis,* and increasing and regressing more slowly over several months for *Y. enterocolitica*. Most human *Y. pseudotuberculosis* infections are due to type I. Agglutinins to type II are frequently found in apparently healthy individuals in Finland (see Geographic Variations), while type IV is rarely obtained from human sources.

Most human illness due to *Y. enterocolitica* has been caused by a few serogroups, including 0:3, 0:5, 0:8, and 0:9. With the exception of serogroup 0:3, which is often found in pigs, these strains are apparently adapted to people; the other strains appear to be adapted to animals. Recently, attempts have been made to classify the organism into two groups. One comprises the human-adapted strains, which are uniform and typical with regard to microbiologic growth characteristics and biochemical, serologic and phage-typing patterns. These strains tend to produce certain "classic" clinical syndromes, including acute enteritis, mesenteric adenitis, terminal ileitis, and septicemia. The second group contains organisms usually recovered from the environment, a wide range of animal hosts, or foods. They are of different serotypes than the first group and tend to be biochemically atypical. They ferment rhamnose (and usually raffinose and melibiose) at 22° C, and they fail to ferment sucrose. These organisms have been responsible for less typical syndromes in people, including urinary tract infection, wound infection, localized skin abscesses, conjunctivitis, and mild diarrhea.

## PATHOGENESIS AND PATHOLOGY

*Y. pseudotuberculosis* and *Y. enterocolitica* cause pseudotuberculosis in mammals and birds. Current evidence suggests that they are zoonotic bacteria that are transferred between human beings and animals, primarily through fecal contamination of food or water. Pseudotuberculosis is therefore not quasituberculosis nor is it transmitted like mycobacterial infection.

In all geographic areas, the organisms are isolated during the coldest months of the year. This seasonal incidence may partly reflect a cold enrichment phenomenon but probably also occurs because *Y. enterocolitica* and *Y. pseudotuberculosis* require low temperatures for the synthesis of virulence factors. When grown at 37° C, these organisms are often rough and avirulent for animals, whereas the same strain grown at 22° C may produce lethal disease.

*Y. enterocolitica* and *Y. pseudotuberculosis* both synthesize endotoxins (O antigens) with biologic properties similar to those of the endotoxins of other gram-negative bacteria, but there is no evidence that these lipopolysaccharides contribute to the unique abdominal disease syndromes caused by *Yersinia*. *Y. enterocolitica* seems to produce a heat-stable enterotoxin (Feeley et al., 1977) that could contribute to the symptoms of *Yersinia* enteritis.

However, both *Yersinia* can invade mammalian cells. Some strains of *Y. enterocolitica* can penetrate the conjunctiva of guinea pigs and penetrate the lamina propria of the rabbit ileum (Une, 1977; Feeley et al., 1977). *Y. pseudotuberculosis* penetrates and survives for at least 3 days inside HeLa cells (Feeley et al., 1977).

Cellular penetration correlates better than enterotoxicity with the pathology in animals and people. Enteric infections cause ulcerations in the terminal ileum, involvement of Peyer's patches, and suppurative granulomatous lesions in the ileocecal lymph nodes. Pseudotuberculosis in animals and septicemia in man causes similar lesions in the liver, spleen, and other organs.

The reactive polyarthritis that may follow infection with *Yersinia* is immunologic rather than infectious, although septic arthritis may develop during the course of septicemia (Spira and Kabins, 1976). The occurrence of reactive arthritis, most commonly in Scandinavia, suggests that strain specificity is responsible for joint localization. Arthritis also occurs most commonly in patients with histocompatibility antigen HLA-B27, which strongly supports an immunologic mechanism for this manifestation.

## CLINICAL MANIFESTATIONS

*Y. pseudotuberculosis* and *Y. enterocolitica* both cause a variety of enteric illnesses. The frequency of each clinical syndrome varies with the agent (Table 2). The most common clinical presentation of infection with *Y. pseudotuberculosis* is acute mesenteric adenitis (pseudoappendicitis). Acute enteritis (watery diarrhea) is the most common presentation of infection with *Y. enterocolitica,* which is a more common cause of all the clinical syndromes than *Y. pseudotuberculosis.* The portal of entry of both species is presumed to be the alimentary tract. Differences in the clinical manifestations are probably due to the degree of penetration of the organism into or through the intestinal mucosa, which is related to strain and inoculum size. In experimental oral infection of mice, *Y. enterocolitica* grown at room temperature and given in very large numbers causes septicemia, whereas lower inocula of the same organism cause only intestinal disease. The clinical manifestations of *Y. enterocolitica* are more protean than *Y. pseudotuberculosis* and are generally related to the age of the patient (Table 3). The reasons for these associations are not understood, and exceptions certainly occur.

Acute enteritis from *Y. enterocolitica* in a child less than 5 years old usually presents as acute, watery diarrhea without blood or mucus (Delorme et al., 1974). There is nothing to distinguish this illness from the many other causes of watery diarrhea in children. It is not known if this illness is mediated by the heat-stable enterotoxin produced by the organism. The manifestations of this disease are generally self-limited within 5 to 10 days. Recently, it has been recognized that *Y. enterocolitica* can also cause epidemic gastroenteritis, probably water- or food-borne. This illness may affect either children or adults

**TABLE 3. Age-Related Clinical Presentations of *Y. enterocolitica* Infection (Leino and Kalliomaki, 1974)**

| AGE GROUP (Years) | CLINICAL PRESENTATION |
|---|---|
| <5 | Acute diarrhea |
| 5 to 15 | Acute mesenteric adenitis ("pseudoappendicitis") |
| 10 to 20 | Acute terminal ileitis ("pseudo Crohn's disease") |
| Adults | Acute diarrhea and nongastrointestinal manifestations |

**NONGASTROINTESTINAL MANIFESTATIONS**

| | |
|---|---|
| Infants and adults more than 60 years | Septicemia |
| Compromised hosts | Septicemia |
| Adults (especially females) | Erythema nodosum |
| Adults | Polyarthritis |

and may resemble staphylococcal "food poisoning" (abrupt onset of nausea, vomiting, abdominal cramps, and watery diarrhea) except that one half to two thirds of patients with *Y. enterocolitica* gastroenteritis also have fever. The other syndrome associated with acute epidemic gastroenteritis is a self-limited, 24-hour febrile diarrheal illness. The presence of blood, mucus, and large numbers of leukocytes in the stools of many of these patients suggests that this illness is an invasive inflammatory enteritis.

In children from 5 to 15 years of age, both *Y. pseudotuberculosis* and *Y. enterocolitica* are most likely to cause acute mesenteric adenitis, sometimes called "pseudoappendicitis." The illness often begins nonspecifically with headache, arthralgia, and fever but may begin with diarrhea when *Y. enterocolitica* is the etiologic agent. After a few days, the patient develops diffuse abdominal pain that localizes to the right lower quadrant after a variable interval of hours to days. There is often tenderness, particularly over McBurney's point, located about 5 cm medial to the right anterior iliac spine along the line connecting the iliac spine and the umbilicus. There is usually localized rebound tenderness in this area and tenderness to the right on rectal examination, but these signs are ordinarily less impressive than would be expected from the other clinical findings. Unless the patient has had an appendectomy or the examiner detects a mass, the diagnosis of acute appendicitis is made, and a laparotomy is performed. The appendix is either normal or only slightly reddened, but the mesenteric lymph nodes overlying the terminal ileum are markedly enlarged (2 to 8 cm in diameter), intensely inflamed, and usually matted together. The mesentery surrounding the nodes and the serosa of the adjacent terminal ileum and cecum

**TABLE 2. Intestinal Manifestations of Yersiniosis**

| CLINICAL PRESENTATION | INFECTING ORGANISM | |
|---|---|---|
| | *Y. pseudotuberculosis* | *Y. enterocolitica* |
| Mesenteric adenitis | + + + +[a] | + + |
| Terminal ileitis | + | + |
| Acute enteritis | ± | + + + + |

[a]Frequency of the manifestation from rare (±) to common (+ + + +).

are also inflamed. There is ordinarily a small quantity of free fluid in the peritoneal cavity. The surgeon usually performs an appendectomy and should also perform a biopsy on the involved nodes for culture and histology. The illness resolves after a few days to two weeks.

In older adolescents and young adults, the inflammatory process may be mostly limited to the terminal ileum, with only minimal suppurative adenitis of the mesenteric nodes. This acute ileitis may be caused by either species of *Yersinia*. The clinical features may resemble acute mesenteric adenitis, but it can progress occasionally to a fatal hemorrhagic necrosis of the ileocecal area or even of the entire bowel. In some individuals, the illness begins with acute diarrhea and abdominal pain, which either persists or remits and exacerbates for weeks to months. Radiologic examination uniformly shows abnormalities of the terminal ileum that range from thickening of the mucosal folds or distortion of the mucosal pattern to nodular filling defects or even solitary or multiple ulcerations (Vantrappen et al., 1977). Barium enema is usually normal, but there may be spasm of the terminal ileum due to inflammation.

In adults, acute self-limited dysentery may be followed in one to six weeks by acute polyarthritis of the knees, ankles, and small joints of the hands or feet. The joint symptoms are usually polyarticular, migratory, and bilateral. Persistent activity in one or more joints for several months is common, and some patients may experience chronic rheumatoid arthritis-like symptoms for over a year. Joint manifestations have been noted principally in Scandinavia and are associated with the presence of histocompatibility locus HLA-27.

## GEOGRAPHIC VARIATIONS

*Yersinia pseudotuberculosis* and *Y. enterocolitica* are probably distributed worldwide, but the majority of cases have been identified in a few Scandinavian countries, France, South Africa,

and Canada, and more recently in the United States and Japan. The incidence is much higher in Scandinavia and other parts of Europe than in the rest of the world. The high prevalence in temperate and cold climates could be related to cold selection or enhancement of virulence, but *Yersinia* can generally be found in any country if it is carefully sought clinically and bacteriologically.

In addition to this high prevalence of *Yersinia* in certain geographic areas, some specific serotypes exhibit a limited geographic range and association with specific clinical syndromes (Table 4). The high prevalence of certain serologic types in Scandinavia and the susceptibility of histocompatibility type HLA-27 strongly suggest a role for genetic predisposition to infection.

## DIAGNOSIS AND DIFFERENTIAL DIAGNOSIS

Acute yersinial diarrhea can only be differentiated from diarrhea caused by other agents by culture and/or serology. The cold enrichment technique is particularly valuable, but the diligence of the laboratory in seeking this microorganism is equally important. Plates for primary culture and subculture should always be held at 22 to 25° C, as well as at 37° C, to enhance recovery. Serologic diagnosis is useful but less reliable, because titers may either not develop (certain serotypes) or disappear rapidly during convalescence. Furthermore, although *Y. pseudotuberculosis* and *Y. enterocolitica* are easily separated serologically, these organisms cross-react with other bacteria (Table 5). In regions in which *Brucella abortus* infections are prevalent, absorptions of serum are necessary for the serodiagnosis of *Y. enterocolitica* 0:9. Fortunately, the seroreaction to *Y. pseudotuberculosis* type I, which accounts for 90 per cent of human infections with this organism, is quite specific. The cross-reactive type IV *Y. pseudotuberculosis* is rarely isolated from human sources.

TABLE 4.   Seroepidemiologic and Clinical Classification of
*Y. enterocolitica*

| SEROTYPE | DISTRIBUTION | CLINICAL PATTERN[a] |
|---|---|---|
| 0:3/Biotype 4/phage type 8 | Europe, Japan | Classic; also polyarthritis |
| 0:3/Biotype 4/phage type 9A | South Africa | Classic; ?polyarthritis |
| 0:3/Biotype 4/phage type 9B | Canada | Classic |
| 0:5,27/Biotype 2/phage type 10 | United States | Classic |
| 0:8/Biotype 1/phage type 10[b] | United States | Classic |
| 0:9/Biotype 2/phage type 10 | Scandinavia | Classic; also erythema nodosum |
| 0:12, 0:14, 0:16, NAG[c] | Worldwide | Diverse, atypical |
| 0:17/Biotype 1/phage type 10 | United States, worldwide | Diverse, atypical |

[a]See text.
[b]Phage type 10 includes all nontypable strains.
[c]Nonagglutinable with the 34 antisera currently available.

**TABLE 5. Serologic Cross-Reactions Between Yersinia Species and Other Bacteria**

| ORGANISM | CROSS-REACTING ANTIGENS |
|---|---|
| Y. enterocolitica 0:9 | Brucella (smooth)<br>Salmonella group N |
| Y. pseudotuberculosis type II | Salmonella group B |
| Y. pseudotuberculosis type IV<br>type IV_A | Salmonella group D<br>E. coli 0:17, 0:77<br>Enterobacter cloacae |
| Y. pseudotuberculosis type VI | E. coli 0:55 |

Because acute mesenteric adenitis mimics appendicitis, the diagnosis is usually made at surgery. *Y. pseudotuberculosis* has a marked predilection for young boys, however, and the agglutinin titer may already be elevated on admission to the hospital. Therefore, for *Y. pseudotuberculosis*, but not *Y. enterocolitica*, which takes longer to cause an antibody response, it is at least theoretically possible to make a specific serodiagnosis shortly after admission and avert unnecessary surgery. When postpubertal females are affected, an important preoperative differential diagnosis is gynecologic disease, including ruptured or bleeding ovarian cysts, salpingitis, retrograde menstrual bleeding, or fibroid uterus. Diverticulitis, acute cholecystitis, and even urinary tract infection can also mimic this condition and should be considered, especially in adults.

*Staphylococcus aureus* and *Streptococcus pyogenes*, coxsackie viruses, and echoviruses have also been isolated from inflamed mesenteric nodes. The specific diagnosis can be made by isolation of the organism directly from the biopsied node. Therefore, resected tissues should be subjected to routine cultures, as well as cold enrichment and periodic subculture at 22° C and 37° C. The histologic changes of *Yersinia* adenitis are characterized by suppurative granulomas that resemble those of cat-scratch disease and lymphogranuloma venereum.

*Brucella, Francisella, Salmonella typhi, Entamoeba histolytica,* and *Mycobacterium tuberculosis* can cause terminal ileitis like *Yersinia*. Microbiologic diagnosis is required. Initially, the illness may be indistinguishable from Crohn's disease. For this reason, ileal biopsy is not suggested because the development of fistulae is a common complication of Crohn's disease. Biopsy and culture of the mesenteric nodes in *Yersinia* infection does not cause fistulae and establishes the correct diagnosis. Subsequent radiologic study may be helpful if the patient does not improve because late fistulae, stenosis, pseudodiverticula, skip lesions, or marked persistent thickening of the bowel or mesentery do not occur following *Yersinia* infections.

## THERAPY

*Y. enterocolitica*, especially serotypes 0:3 and 0:9, and *Y. pseudotuberculosis* exhibit similar antimicrobial sensitivity patterns. They are usually quite sensitive to the aminoglycosides, chloramphenicol, colistin, sulfonamides, tetracycline, and the combination of trimethoprim-sulfamethoxazole. Because it synthesizes broad-spectrum, constitutive and/or inducible beta-lactamases, *Y. enterocolitica* is resistant to penicillin, ampicillin, amoxicillin, and the cephalosporins, including cefamandole. *Y. pseudotuberculosis* is usually quite sensitive to penicillin, ampicillin, and the cephalosporins. Strains of either organism may become resistant to almost any antimicrobial due to acquisition of a transferable drug-resistant plasmid.

There is, however, no evidence yet that antibiotics are useful in the therapy of any of the enteric *Yersinia* infections. These infections appear to run their course independent of surgery or antimicrobial therapy. Controlled clinical trials will be required to determine whether antimicrobials can shorten the usual course. The important measures are to rule out the presence of true surgical emergencies, replace fluids, and allow sufficient time for recovery. Antidiarrheal mixtures of any sort are not helpful in enteric infections and should be avoided.

When *Yersinia* septicemia develops, however, the situation is markedly altered. This is not a benign, self-limited condition. Many of these patients are immunocompromised, and the mortality is high. Correct antimicrobial therapy is essential. A parenteral aminoglycoside such as gentamicin at 3 to 5 mg per kg is a good initial choice while awaiting the results of sensitivities. Some septicemic patients may develop hepatic or splenic abscesses. Surgical drainage is desirable but may be impossible in the face of multiple lesions.

## References

Delorme, J., Laverdiere, M., Martineau, B., and Lafleur, L.: Yersiniosis in children. Can Med Assoc J 110:281, 1974.

Feeley, J. C., Wells, J. G., and Tsai, T. F.: Enterotoxin detection in *Yersinia enterocolitica*. In Third International Symposium on *Yersinia*. Montreal, Basel-Karger, 1977.

Gunnison, J. B., Larson, A., and Lazarus, A. S.: Rapid differentiation between *Pasteurella pestis* and *Pasteurella pseudotuberculosis* by action of bacteriophage. J Infect Dis 88:254, 1951.

Leino, R., and Kalliomaki, J. L.: Yersiniosis as an internal disease. Ann Intern Med 81:458, 1974.

Spira, T. J., and Kabins, S. A.: *Yersinia enterocolitica* septicemia with septic arthritis. Arch Intern Med 136:1305, 1976.

Une, T.: Studies on the pathogenicity of *Yersinia enterocolitica*. I. Experimental infection of rabbits. Microbiol Immunol 21:349, 1977.

Vantrappen, G., Agg, H. O., Ponette, E., Geboes, K., and Bertrand, P. H.: *Yersinia* enteritis and enterocolitis: Gastroenterological aspects. Gastroenterology 72:220, 1977.

# 130 AMEBIC DYSENTERY (INTESTINAL AMEBIASIS)

## Francisco Biagi, M.D.

### DEFINITION

Amebic dysentery is a form of acute intestinal amebiasis characterized by a severe picture of tenesmus with passage of mucus and bloody stools; diarrhea (abundant liquid stools) usually accompanies the dysentery. Tenesmus is the sensation of urgent evacuation against resistance from spasm of the sphincter ani secondary to rectal ulcers. The evacuation is small and painful and leaves the feeling of a full rectum; in infants, tenesmus causes spasmodic bowel movements with mild rectal prolapse and is detected by inspection of the perineal region when the child cries.

If infections by *Naegleria* and *Acanthamoeba* are excluded, amebiasis is defined as infection by *Entamoeba histolytica*. According to epidemiologic, clinical, and autopsy observations, we may differentiate nine basic anatomoclinical types of amebiasis (Table 1). The term intestinal amebiasis comprises five different types.

### ETIOLOGY

*E. histolytica* is a Sarcodina protozoan that moves and phagocytoses by pseudopods and reproduces as a trophozoite by binary fission. It has a nucleus with fine peripheral chromatin and a central endosome (Fig. 1). Within the intestinal lumen and under ill-defined conditions, it may become encysted and is excreted. The mature cysts have four nuclei.

In view of the limitations of most medical laboratories, the name *E. histolytica* is used here in the broad sense and includes *E. hartmanii*, small or large race, Laredo type, and other forms, which may be differentiated only through subtle features by a few experts. *E. histolytica* can be differentiated from *Entamoeba coli, Iodamoeba bütschlii, Endolimax nana,* and *Dientamoeba fragilis* in any clinical laboratory (Biagi, 1976).

### EPIDEMIOLOGY

The great majority of cases are caused by the ingestion of cysts and only rarely by direct implantation of trophozoites into the skin. The source of infection is the stool of human carriers. Since the cyst is killed by desiccation, fecal contamination must be recent in order for transmission to occur. The process of cyst transmission from carriers is called fecalism and involves dissemination of stools in the environment and transmission of cysts to the new host mainly by food handlers. Dissemination occurs by means of open

### TABLE 1. Clinical Types of Amebiasis

| LOCATION OF PARASITE[a] | CLINICAL TYPE OF AMEBIASIS | FORMS OF AMEBIASIS | | DIAGNOSIS | |
|---|---|---|---|---|---|
| | | | | PE[c] | Serology |
| Colonization of intestinal lumen | 1. Carrier[b] | Intestinal | Luminal | | — |
| Invasion of intestinal wall | 2. Asymptomatic<br>3. Chronic intestinal<br>4. Acute intestinal<br>5. Ameboma | Intestinal | Invasive | + | + |
| Invasion of liver | 6. Hepatitis<br>7. Liver abscess | Extraintestinal | Invasive | — | + |
| Invasion of other organs and tissues | 8. Cutaneous<br>9. Other locations | Extraintestinal | | | |

[a]A patient may present with disease in several locations at the same time.
[b]A patient of this type may later suffer an invasion of tissues by the parasite. Carriers can also result from satisfactory clinical treatment that does not include parasitologic cure, in which case serology might be positive for a period of time.
[c]PE, Parasitologic examination of feces.

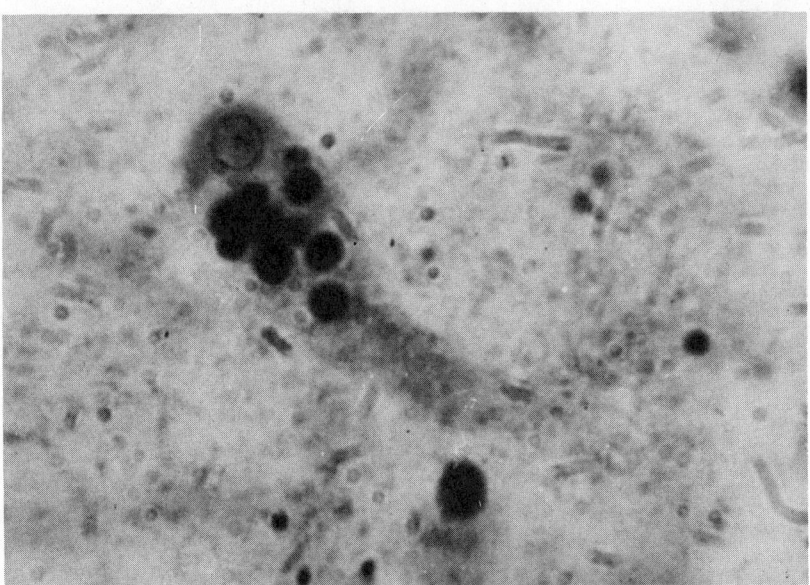

**FIGURE 1.** *Trophozoite of* Entamoeba histolytica *in the feces; iron hematoxylin stain showing erythrocytes and the typical nucleolus.*

air defecation, defective sewage disposal, irrigation with contaminated water and filthy personal sanitation.

Once the cyst has arrived in the intestine, schizogony ends with hatching of eight trophozoites, and these establish a colony of trophozoites in the lumen of the bowel. This luminal colony disappears spontaneously in 50 per cent of cases within six months, but reinfections maintain the prevalence rate. The monthly incidence is about one twelfth of the prevalence rate. The larger number of clinical cases during the hot season suggests that the incidence of infection may be variable throughout the year. Prevalence rates usually are between 0 and 10 per cent in temperate and developed areas of the world and 5 to 60 per cent in tropical developing areas. Within the same city, prevalence rates show big differences in diverse sociocultural groups. Generally speaking, prevalence is higher in communities with poor housing, inadequate excreta disposal, high population density, improper personal hygienic habits, and a tropical climate. The infection is seldom found during the first two weeks of life. Prevalence increases slowly throughout the first year, and then rapidly from the second to fourth year of age; thereafter it is sustained through adulthood with no sex difference. An infection does not generate protection against reinfections.

Serologic tests are the basis for estimating the frequency of invasive amebiasis. In the United States, positive serologic tests for amebiasis are found in 0.4 to 3.6 per cent of the population, so there may be approximately five million people with invasive amebiasis at a given time. In Mexico the average figure is 5 per cent. Amebiasis has

been demonstrated to be a cause of death in 5 to 11 per cent of autopsies in different hospitals in Mexico City. In other Latin American countries, the figure ranges from 2 to 4 per cent. In the United States and Europe, only a few cases have been found at autopsy.

## PATHOGENESIS AND PATHOLOGY

The basic pathogenic mechanism is the production of tissue lysis by enzymes of *E. histolytica*. In the intestine and the skin, this lysis results in ulcers; in the liver, brain, and other organs it causes necrosis like that of abscesses, with the necrotic material resembling pus.

After the infection has been established in the bowel lumen (luminal amebiasis), trophozoites sometimes invade the intestinal wall to the submucosa, where they produce necrosis and initiate invasive amebiasis (Biagi and Beltran, 1969). First, a small ulcer opens into the lumen, forming a lesion known as a "bouton de chemise" because the large circular submucosal necrosis, with its small opening onto the surface, has the configuration of a button (Fig. 2). This early lesion quickly ulcerates the overlying mucosa and produces ulcers of variable form, size, and number (Fig. 3), ranging from a few tiny ulcers to ulceration of the whole colon. The size of the ulcers determines the severity and clinical type of intestinal amebiasis.

The parasite seems to reach the liver frequently but rarely colonizes it. The necrotic foci in the liver are too small at first to be detected unless a careful autopsy examination is done at the proper time. This very early stage is called amebic hepa-

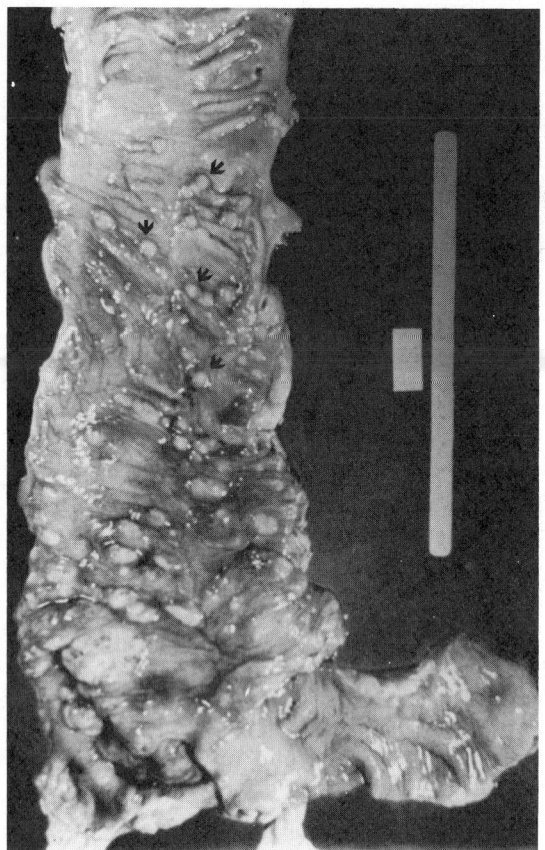

**FIGURE 2.** *Small amebic ulcers (arrows) in "bouton de chemise" at the cecum.*

chemotaxis is absent, and leukocytes making chance contact with *E. histolytica* are immediately lysed.

Intestinal amebiasis is more severe in infants than in adults. Intestinal amebiasis progresses faster in infants and preschool children, and intestinal perforation is the most common cause of death. The most common cause of death from amebiasis in adults is an amebic liver abscess; 90 per cent of the cases are found in men and 10 per cent in women. There is an equal sex distribution of liver abscess in children, and 90 per cent of the cases have concurrent, usually severe, intestinal involvement. Among adults with liver abscess, only 30 per cent have intestinal involvement, and it is usually mild.

Geographic areas also show differences. Areas with a low transmission rate have few reinfections, low prevalence, few clinical cases, and very infrequent fatalities. In areas with high prevalence, by contrast, reinfections are frequent, clinical amebiasis is abundant, and large numbers of fatal cases are seen at autopsy.

titis, in contrast to the large necrotic lesions of amebic liver abscesses. Less frequently, the amebae may continue migrating through the blood stream to the lungs, spleen, kidneys, and brain (Fig. 4).

It is estimated in Mexico that of every 1000 persons with luminal amebiasis, 200 have invasion of the intestinal wall, and one develops liver abscess (Biagi, 1976; Brandt and Pérez-Tamayo, 1970). Each of these three stages is the result of multifactorial interactions. The establishment of *E. histolytica* in the gut lumen is favored by the presence of the normal intestinal flora, by ingestion of many cysts, and by a starch diet. Migration to the intestinal wall and the liver is promoted by cholesterol, steroid hormones, large numbers of trophozoites, and high virulence of the strain. According to experimental evidence, previous infections may also favor invasion because the trophozoites can digest antiameba immunoglobulin attached to their surface and thus use them for nutrition.

Another pathologic feature is the very mild or absent inflammatory reaction. It appears that

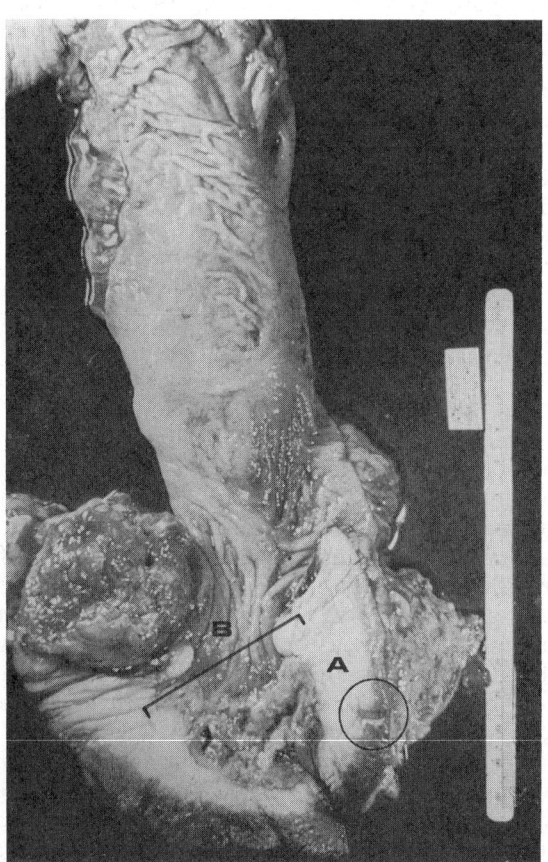

**FIGURE 3.** *Larger amebic ulcer at the rectum (A) with a small cutaneous lesion (B) by fistula formation.*

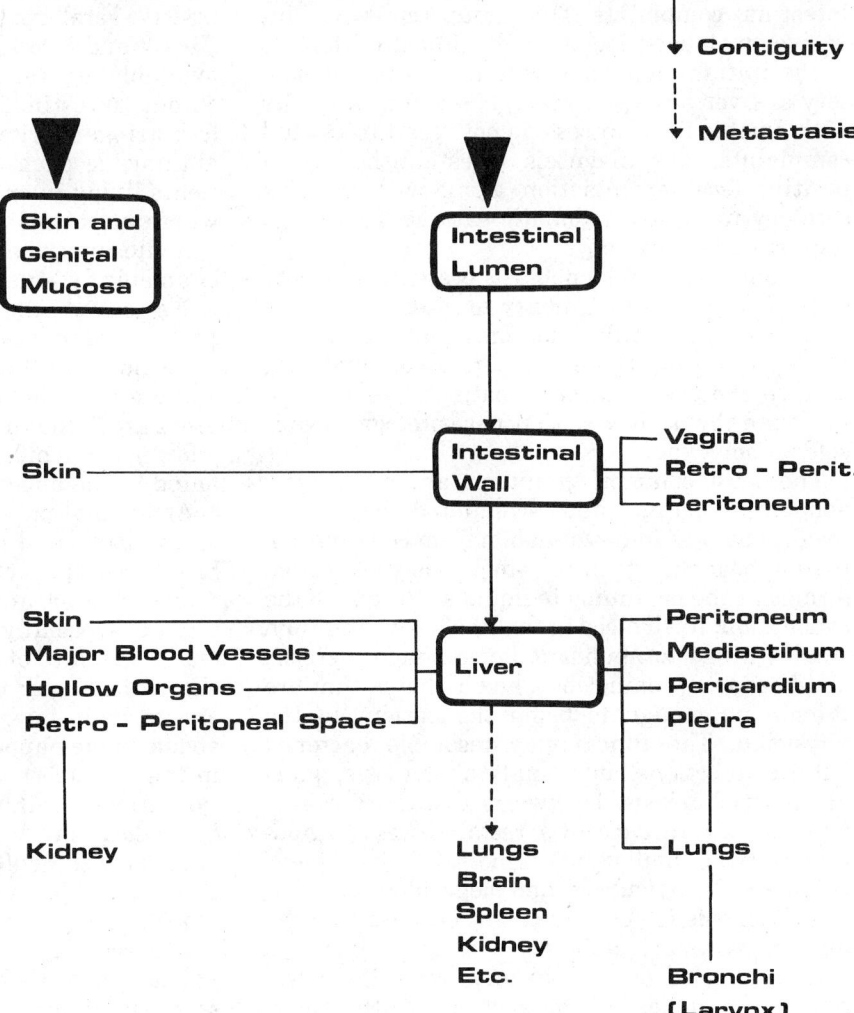

**FIGURE 4.** *Migratory pattern of Entamoeba histolytica in man. (From Biagi, F.: Enfermedades Parasitarias. 2nd ed. Prensa Medica Mexicana, 1976.)*

## CLINICAL MANIFESTATIONS AND DIAGNOSIS

The clinical picture of intestinal amebiasis is related to the size of the ulcers. The incubation period is not well known; it appears to be as short as two days in the newborn and may be as long as a few months. The prepatent period is equal to or shorter than the incubation period. Five clinical forms of intestinal amebiasis are recognized, as indicated in Table 2.

Amebiasis carrier state has neither symptoms nor antibody response because it is only a luminal infection. It accounts for 80 per cent of the cases and is the most common type of infection. Diagnosis can be made by positive fecal examinations with negative serology. It is the least dangerous clinical form because chemotherapy is very effective, and the prognosis is best.

Asymptomatic amebiasis, in contrast to the previous type, has tissue invasion and antibody formation. Small ulcers are found in the bowel at autopsy or rectosigmoidoscopy in persons with no intestinal complaints. This group represents invasive amebiasis; even though clinically silent, it is the initial stage for severe illness like dysentery or liver abscess. In fact, two thirds of adults with amebic liver abscess do not recall intestinal complaints. The diagnosis is established by a positive fecal examination along with positive serology in an asymptomatic patient. This stage requires chemotherapy.

Chronic intestinal amebiasis presents a variety of clinical pictures secondary to intestinal ulcers that give rise to mild symptoms that the patient tends to ignore. There are periods of remission and recrudescence. These patients very often medicate themselves so that parasitologic cure is seldom achieved.

The most common symptoms are meteorism; abdominal pain, often stimulated by eating meals; changes in bowel habits from constipation to diarrhea; change in the stool consistency from formed at the beginning to liquid at the end of the evacuation; fresh blood in the stools, varying from small strings to abundant hemorrhage; pyrosis; and headache, somnolence, and asthenia that are prominent enough to bring the patient to the physician. The illness may resemble bacterial enteric infections, intestinal tuberculosis, giardiasis, trichuriasis, hookworm disease, strongyloidiasis, ulcerative colitis, rectal abscess, regional enteritis, malignant tumors of the bowel, polyposis, diverticulosis, and megacolon. The precise diagnosis is very important because therapy and prognosis are different.

After a good clinical history, rectosigmoidoscopy is desirable, but the absence of ulcerations does not exclude the diagnosis because lesions may be present only in the cecum. When ulcers are found, they permit sampling of the edge for parasites. Rectoscopy alone is helpful and can be done with a simple plastic tube 2 × 15 cm attached to an otoscope.

Stool examinations must be done properly and by competent personnel to demonstrate *E. histolytica*. If cysts are sought by a concentration method on three consecutive daily samples of formed stool, they are found in 85 per cent of the cases. Six examinations give 95 per cent accuracy. Diarrhea stools require examination while fresh if trophozoites are to be found. Serologic tests, such as indirect hemagglutination and immunodiffusion, are positive in approximately 98 per cent of the cases and at moderate titers (1:32 to 1:2048) (Healy and Kraft, 1972).

A patient who is only a carrier may have positive stool examinations for amebae when the intestinal complaints have another cause. In order to establish the diagnosis of intestinal amebiasis, it is helpful to find ulcers in the bowel, *E.*

*histolytica* in stools (cysts or trophozoites), and positive serologic tests with *E. histolytica* antigen (Healy and Kraft, 1972). If these studies are not available or reliable, a working diagnosis of chronic intestinal amebiasis may be made with less stringent criteria and a therapeutic trial with antiamebic drugs carried out, especially in patients living in or having traveled through areas where amebiasis is common and severe.

Acute intestinal amebiasis may take the form of amebic dysentery, episodes of bloody diarrhea, and so-called fulminant amebiasis. It may also be only a severe case of diarrhea with no blood or tenesmus. In all cases, the patient is severely ill and often needs hospitalization. Large ulcerated areas are found in the bowel, mainly at the cecum and rectosigmoid; in a few cases, ulcers are also found in the appendix or the terminal ileum.

Abdominal pain is prominent, and evacuations are multiple and usually scanty with mucus and blood. Tenesmus characterizes the dysentery syndrome. Water and electrolyte balance may be altered, especially in children, and fever is present in one third of the cases. The general status of the patient may undergo marked deterioration, and toxemia may be present. Signs of an acute abdomen may appear, due either to severe lesions in the wall of the colon or to intestinal perforation. Among children living in endemic areas, *E. histolytica* may be found in the stool in 5 per cent of cases with acute simple diarrhea, one third of cases with bloody diarrhea, and the majority of those with dysenteric syndrome. In children, severe cases may develop without previous intestinal complaints while in adults they are usually severe recrudescences.

Rectosigmoidoscopy is hazardous in severe cases because the colon may be very fragile. Fresh blood on the stools suggests bowel ulcers. Flat x-ray of the abdomen is done to detect evidence of peritonitis. If there is hepatomegaly, which is found in nearly 40 per cent of children with acute intestinal amebiasis, a liver scan or ultrasound examination should be done to look for abscesses.

Examinations of freshly passed stool demonstrate trophozoites, often with phagocytosed erythrocytes, in 90 per cent of the cases on the first examination; if a second stool sample is taken from the next evacuation, the diagnosis can be confirmed in almost all cases. Microscopic stool examinations should be performed before any specific therapy, because the first dose of an antiamebic drug or even an antibiotic may turn them negative, even though the parasite is still present and causing disease. Diagnosis is established after the finding of parasites in a patient with the clinical picture described above. If a reliable parasitologic examination is not available, or some therapy has been started and the patient is living in, or has traveled through, an area where amebiasis is common and severe, it is wise to complete full therapy because acute intestinal amebiasis is life-threatening. In contrast to bacterial or viral diarrheas, in children in whom correction of fluid and electrolyte disturbances is usually sufficient therapy, amebiasis might go on to perforation with such treatment unless specific antiamebic therapy is given also.

Serologic tests are usually positive in adults with acute intestinal amebiasis but take more time to perform than fresh stool examination. In infants, the picture progresses so rapidly that one third do not have time to develop positive serology before hospitalization.

Acute intestinal amebiasis can resemble enteric bacterial or viral infections, balantidiasis, trichuriasis, rectal stenosis with ulcerations, malignant tumors of the bowel, and ulcerative colitis. A culture for enteric bacteria should always be performed, since differentiation on clinical grounds is not reliable. Fever, hepatomegaly, tenesmus, meteorism, or blood in the stools may be present in both parasitic and bacterial diarrhea. A few patients have a double etiology.

Ameboma, an uncommon inflammatory pseudotumor of the bowel wall, produces chronic changes in intestinal habits, bloody stools, meteorism, and abdominal pain. An abdominal mass is palpated and demonstrated by barium enema. It is rare in adults and almost never seen in children.

The finding of the parasite on fecal examination and a positive serology confirms the diagnosis of ameboma but does not exclude neoplasm; diagnostic error in both directions has been confirmed at autopsy. The treatment consists of partial colectomy and antiamebic drugs.

## COMPLICATIONS

As shown in Figure 4, the complications of intestinal amebiasis result from extension into surrounding organs and are life-threatening. If peritoneal and retroperitoneal extension occurs, bacterial infection becomes the most important problem. Fistula formation to the female genitalia usually involves invasion by the parasite. Cutaneous amebiasis is discussed in Chapter 219. Hepatic amebiasis is not considered to be a complication because spread to the liver is part of the natural history of the infection along the regular pathway of migration.

## TREATMENT

The dichloroaocetamides and oxyquinolines, which act only within the lumen of the bowel because their absorption is small, are useful in treating intestinal amebiasis (Welling and Monro, 1970). The imidazoles, emetines and chloroquines can act systemically against invasive amebiasis because they can be given parenterally or are fully absorbed from the small intestine. No drug can act against *E. histolytica* in all sites; some patients have luminal amebiasis only or tissue invasion alone, but others have parasites in the tissues and the lumen. Table 2 is presented as a guide to help select the type of drugs for an individual case. The objective is to achieve both clinical and parasitologic cure. Sometimes a patient with intestinal amebiasis may achieve clinical cure after imidazol or emetine therapy and may require dichloroacetamides or oxyquinolines for parasitologic cure.

The imidazoles are important because they are active in patients with chronic intestinal amebia-

**TABLE 2.  Drugs of Choice in Amebiasis**

| LOCATION OF PARASITES[a] | CLINICAL TYPES OF AMEBIASIS | DRUGS AND AMEBICIDAL CONCENTRATION ($\mu$g/ml) | | | | | |
|---|---|---|---|---|---|---|---|
| | | Oxyquinolines (8) | Arsenicals (8) | Emetine (3) | Chloroquine (300) | Imidazoles (3) | Dichloroacetamides (0.04–0.6) |
| Intestinal lumen | 1. Carrier | × | × | | | | × |
| Intestinal wall | 2. Asymptomatic | × | × | | | | × |
| | 3. Chronic intestinal | × | × | | | × | × |
| | 4. Acute intestinal | | × | | | × | × |
| | 5. Ameboma | | × | | | × | × |
| Liver | 6. Amebic hepatitis | | × | × | | × | |
| | 7. Amebic liver abscess | | × | × | | × | |
| Others | 8. Cutaneous | | × | | | × | |
| | 9. Other locations | | × | | | × | |

[a]A patient may have infection in several locations.

sis and amebic liver abscess. Metronidazol is the most important of the imidazoles; tinidazole has the longest and nimorazole the shortest half-life. All can produce pyrosis, nausea, and vomiting; all have antabuse effect; and all are potentially mutagenic. Although there is no evidence of teratogeny, use in the first trimester of pregnancy is not recommended. They cause a problem in nursing mothers because they pass into the milk and produce anorexia in the infant. In spite of these limitations, they are widely used and effective. Their dosage is 20 to 40 mg/kg body weight per day for 5 to 15 days (usually 10). Timidazole may be used for 2 to 5 days.

Emetines are cardiotoxic on overdosage, but with careful administration are safe to use; their injection is painful. The dosage is 1 mg/kg body weight (not more than 60 mg) per day for 10 days.

Dichloroacetamides are very active and are almost nonabsorbed. Meteorism and loose stools are the most important side effects. Etichlordifene is ten times more active than teclozan. Dosage is 20 mg/kg body weight (up to one g) per day for 5 days.

Oxyquinolines have been in use for many years. In patients under very prolonged therapy, a few cases of optic neuritis have been described; mutagenic activity has also been found. Dosage is 30 mg/kg body weight for 10 to 20 days.

Acute intestinal amebiasis demands bed rest and proper control of fluids and electrolytes. Partial colectomy is sometimes necessary when the intestinal wall is extensively damaged or perforation has occurred; these cases have a high mortality. Diet should be bland during the first days; afterwards, vegetables should be introduced to regulate the bowel. In endemic areas in which patients have reinfections, the repeated episodes of amebiasis may leave in their wake a prolonged irregularity of bowel movements.

With proper treatment tenesmus should disappear and diarrhea should improve in 48 hours. The physician should be familiar with drug side effects in order to differentiate them from a persistence of the disease. About one week after treatment, all symptoms should have disap-peared. Rectosigmoidoscopy shows improvement of ulcers on the third day and the healing of most of them by the seventh day of treatment. In all cases, three examinations for amebae should be done by a concentration method two weeks after treatment to assess parasitologic cure. Quantitative serology two months later is also useful to demonstrate a drop in titer; tests become negative in 2 to 24 months, depending on the initial titer. Thus, serology is not always diagnostic because a positive test may also represent a past infection.

## PROPHYLAXIS

Good standards of urbanization, housing, personal hygiene, and food handling have no substitute; these require a good level of economic productivity and may be the result of individual attitudes and a positive community structure. In endemic areas, patients should be instructed to avoid food handled after cooking or uncooked food, such as fruit cocktails, hard-boiled eggs, and salads. Unfortunately, the most popular and tasty food in endemic areas is handled extensively. It is important to do fecal examinations and serologic tests as soon as intestinal complaints start, or every year in endemic areas.

Chemotherapy for control or prophylaxis has been documented as useful, even in open communities, on the basis of repeated mass therapy. It is effective, less expensive, and less dangerous than amebiasis; for this purpose, the best choice is the dichloracetamides because they act in the lumen of the intestine and are effective against diverse types of intestinal amebiasis, including carriers.

### References

Biagi, F.: Enfermedades Parasitarias. 2nd ed. Prensa Medica Mexicana, 1976.
Biagi, F., and Beltrán, F.: The challenge of amoebiasis; Understanding pathogenic mechanisms. Int Rev Trop Med 3:219, 1969.
Brandt, H., and Pérez-Tamayo, R.: Amebiasis. Prensa Med Mex, 1970.
Healy, G. R., and Kraft, S. C.: The indirect hemagglutination test for amebiasis in patients with inflammatory bowel disease. Am J Digest Dis 17:97, 1972.
Welling, P. G., and Monro, A. M.: The pharmacological basis of therapeutics. 4th ed. New York, Macmillan Publishing Company, 1970, p. 1151.

# GIARDIASIS AND 131 BALANTIDIASIS

## Liisa Jokipii, M.D.,
## and Anssi M. M. Jokipii, M.D.

### *GIARDIASIS*

#### Definition

Infestation of the upper small intestine by *Giardia lamblia* may be asymptomatic or may cause giardiasis. In acute giardiasis abdominal symptoms usually appear within 2 weeks after infestation. The patient may recover spontaneously or the disease may continue for several years as chronic giardiasis. Endemic giardiasis differs in some features from travelers' giardiasis.

#### Etiology

Several other names have been used for *G. lamblia*, such as *Lamblia intestinalis*, *G. intestinalis*, *G. enterica*, *Megastoma enterica*, and *Cercomonas intestinalis*. *G. lamblia* is a worldwide flagellated protozoon, and its closest relatives are the Giardia parasites of other animals and the genus Trichomonas. Despite morphologic similarity, the giardiae of various species seem host specific. *G. lamblia* is an obligate parasite of man, and its vegetative form, the trophozoite, proliferates in the human small intestine. It has the stable shape of a split pear, two nuclei, four pairs of flagella, and a ventral sucking disk (Fig. 1), and it multiplies by binary fission. For unknown reasons, the motile trophozoites transform into oval immobile cysts, which means that the protozoon is surrounded by a wall (Fig. 2). *G. lamblia* divides once within the cyst, which thus usually contains four nuclei. The cysts are excreted in feces and they are the infective stage of the parasite. They are resistant to environmental factors, except drying and heating; for example, they survive many usual disinfectants and possibly the chlorination of drinking water. The mode of transmission is the ingestion of fecally contaminated material, either through a vehicle, such as water, food, toys, or insects, through direct contact from one person to another, or as autoinfection. *G. lamblia* is highly contagious: 10 or 100 cysts may be enough to infect all recipients (Rendtorff, 1954).

#### Pathogenesis and Pathology

Ingested cysts of *G. lamblia* are carried through the stomach and liberate trophozoites, which settle in the small intestine and attach to the epithelium. The parasite inhabits the duodenum and the upper parts of the jejunum, but the caudal extent of its residence is unknown. It has been

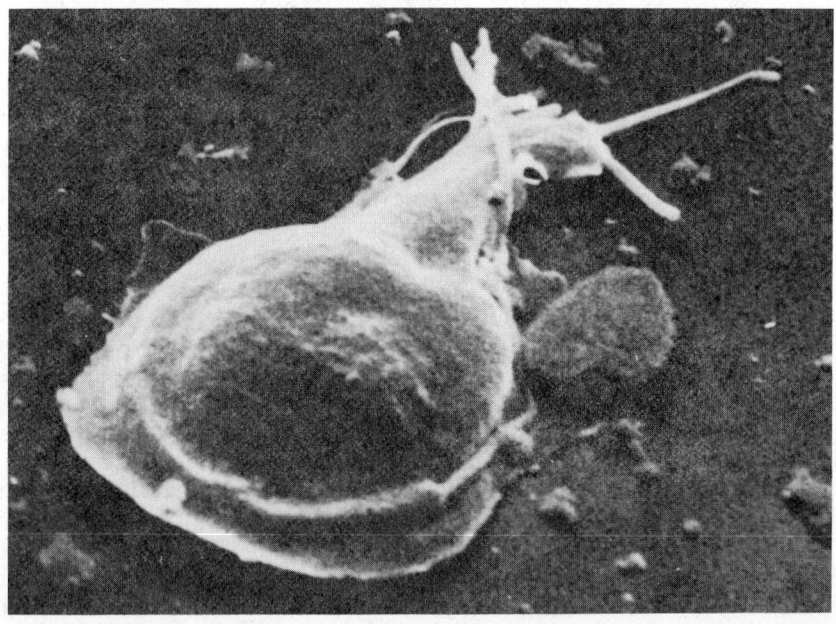

**FIGURE 1.** *Trophozoite of G. lamblia (5000×; scanning electron microscopy by Dr. Ismo Virtanen).*

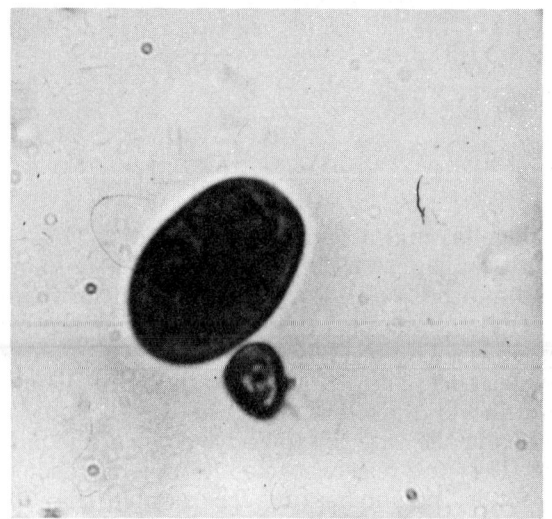

**FIGURE 2.** *Iodine-stained cyst of G. lamblia (2000×).*

found in the gallbladder. Most *G. lamblia* trophozoites lie freely in the intestinal mucus, many adhere to the epithelial surface, and some may invade epithelial cells and penetrate as far as the lamina propria (Saha and Ghosh, 1977).

Giardiasis may present without detectable lesions of the small intestine, but either acute or chronic giardiasis may cause morphologic changes in the mucosa. Microvilli may be shortened and epithelial mitoses increased. Inflammation of the epithelium and lamina propria, edema, and infiltration by neutrophils, eosinophils, lymphocytes, and plasma cells may be seen, and in advanced cases there may be elongation of crypts and changes in villous architecture, varying from mild blunting of the villi to subtotal villous atrophy. Parasitic tissue invasion or accelerated mucin production leading to plugging of crypts has been proposed as the explanation for the pathogenesis of giardiasis, but it remains obscure because the described pathologic changes are found in only some giardiasis patients. The mucosal abnormalities are reversible upon eradication of the parasite.

A correlation between the degree of mucosal changes and the severity of illness has been reported (Hoskins et al., 1967). In asymptomatic *G. lamblia* infestations, mononuclear cells may be increased in the mucosa, and microvilli may be injured (Barbieri et al., 1970). In acute infections polymorphonuclear leukocytes predominate, and in chronic cases the cellular infiltrate is mainly mononuclear. The morphologic changes in children are the same as those in adults, although less severe and less common. In patients with immunodeficiency the mucosal changes of giardiasis are more severe, and are characterized by nodular lymphoid hyperplasia and the virtual lack of plasma cells.

*G. lamblia* infestation causes malabsorption of fat, vitamin A, folic acid, vitamin $B_{12}$, and xylose and disaccharidase deficiency. The ensuing steatorrhea and lactose intolerance may resemble those of celiac disease. Although more severe malabsorption is associated with greater morphologic changes (Wright et al., 1977), the latter are seldom sufficient to explain the malabsorption. The mechanical barrier created by numerous parasites adhering to the epithelium and competition for nutrients between the parasite and the patient may contribute to malabsorption.

## Clinical Manifestations

At least every fourth healthy individual exposed to *G. lamblia* by visiting an endemic area may become infected (Jokipii and Jokipii, 1974; Brodsky et al., 1974). The incidence depends on the number of cysts ingested (Rendtorff, 1954) and on the duration of exposure. Most healthy children entering an infected nursery acquire the parasite in a few months (Black et al., 1977). Immunodeficiency and reduced gastric acidity predispose to giardiasis, but explain only a minority of cases. In outbreaks of giardiasis overt illness occurs in 50 to 90 per cent of persons with parasitic infestation after an incubation period of 1 to 2 weeks (Jokipii and Jokipii, 1974; Brodsky et al., 1974). Serum immunoglobulin levels are not below normal in unselected giardiasis patients, and information about intestinal fluid immunoglobulins is contradictory.

The symptoms of giardiasis are predominantly abdominal, and those listed in Table 1 can occur alone or in various combinations. There are statistical differences between epidemic and chronic or endemic giardiasis, and children differ because of their growing and limited ability to describe symptoms. Asymptomatic intervals are typical of giardiasis. The disease is not life threatening, but a few deaths have been reported in infants (Ormiston et al., 1942).

The severity of acute giardiasis ranges widely from mild malaise to profuse watery diarrhea. It often begins with watery diarrhea that lasts for a few days and gives way to frequent loose stools. There is an urgency to defecate in the mornings and after meals. The stools may be offensive, frothy, and yellow or pale gray in color, and with prolonged diarrhea the patient loses considerable weight. A second group of patients suffer from abdominal pains without change in defecation. These vary from colicky cramps to mere discomfort, most frequently epigastric. In a third type of patient, giardiasis may present with flatulence in the absence of diarrhea or pain; in Table 1, flatus, borborygmus, belching, and abdominal distention are included in flatulence. Even small meals pre

**TABLE 1.** **Symptomatology of Parasitologically Confirmed Giardiasis**

| SYMPTOM | FREQUENCY OF SYMPTOM (Per cent) | | |
| --- | --- | --- | --- |
| | Outbreaks* (acute) | Endemic* (chronic) | Children* |
| Diarrhea | 84 | 55 | 53 |
| Constipation | 8 | 18 | 31 |
| Blood in stool | 0 | 6 | 7 |
| Abdominal pain | 72 | 61 | 37 |
| Flatulence | 65 | 44 | NR† |
| Nausea | 56 | 20 | NR |
| Vomiting | 24 | 16 | 30 |
| Anorexia | 69 | 16 | 28 |
| Loss of weight | 63 | 32 | 7 |
| Failure to thrive | NR | NR | 49 |
| Anemia | NR | NR | 23 |
| Weakness | 76 | 12 | 31 |
| Fever | 15 | 8 | 6 |
| Nervousness | NR | 31 | 18 |
| Urticaria | NR | 5 | NR |
| No symptoms | 9 | 12 | 17 |

*Based on 402 (outbreaks), 1548 (endemic), or 492 (children) patients from the literature.
†NR, not recorded sufficiently.

cipitate fullness and other symptoms leading to anorexia despite hunger. Acute giardiasis may be self-limited or may last for 2 to 3 months, whereas more prolonged cases fit in with the description of chronic giardiasis.

The intermittent symptomatology of chronic giardiasis, or of repeated infections in endemic areas, is indistinguishable from, and is as nonspecific as, that of acute giardiasis in individual cases, but the average patients differ (Table 1). Chronic giardiasis may last for years or even decades, and intestinal malabsorption develops in many of the patients.

### Complications and Sequelae

Irreversible sequelae have not been associated with giardiasis, most complications are rare, and their causal relationship with giardiasis has not been proved. Aside from nonspecific symptoms, the malabsorption syndrome may include milk intolerance, meat intolerance, anemia, and steatorrhea. In a few instances *G. lamblia* has caused cholecystitis (Calder and Rigdon, 1935; Hartman et al., 1942), but the frequency of this association is not known. Infrequent manifestations suggesting immunologic sensitization, such as urticaria, arthritis, and uveitis, are probably caused by *G. lamblia,* since they subside with specific treatment.

### Geographic Variations in Disease

Heterogeneity in *G. lamblia* from various parts of the world has not been described, and each human race is susceptible to the infection. The parasite is worldwide, but owing to social conditions some aspects of giardiasis vary between countries. Its prevalence seems inversely related to the hygienic standard; in Scandinavia, for instance, persons with a history of traveling to endemic areas account for the 1 per cent prevalence of infestation. In such countries most cases of giardiasis are of the acute type, described as travelers' giardiasis, and occur in young adults. In endemic areas asymptomatic infestations are more common, the infections are of the chronic or recurrent type, and the prevalence is highest in children. Relatively high figures come from Eastern European countries and former colonial powers like Great Britain and the Netherlands, and the highest from tropical or subtropical areas in India, Southeast Asia, South America, and Africa. In travelers' epidemics a high proportion of persons from nonendemic areas may acquire clinical giardiasis, whereas those coming from other endemic areas may be protected. Also, residents of the endemic area that has become the site of an epidemic are less susceptible to the giardiasis than nonresidents (Wright and Vernon, 1976). Diet may affect the clinical picture, and the pathologic changes are more common and more severe in connection with strongly spiced food, as in India.

### Diagnosis

Giardiasis should be suspected in all cases of prolonged abdominal illness. Although in some geographic areas clinical history and epidemiologic information may reveal most cases of giardiasis, the demonstration of *G. lamblia* is the only way to establish the diagnosis. The usual procedure is to examine feces either immediately after defecation for cysts and trophozoites or after the concentration of a formalin-preserved specimen for cysts. In parasitologically confirmed cases of giardiasis, stool examination often gives a negative result during the first 3 weeks after infection — that is, there is a period of prepatency (Rendtorff, 1954; Jokipii and Jokipii, 1977)—and, later, cyst-passing is intermittent. Repeated examinations are therefore advisable. Trophozoites of *G. lamblia* should be looked for in duodenal or jejunal biopsy or aspirate when abdominal disease persists without diagnosis and fecal examinations have not been helpful. Simpler methods of duodenal sampling, such as swallowing and pulling back a nylon thread, are being developed.

### Treatment and Prophylaxis

Nitroimidazoles are the drugs of choice in giardiasis. Metronidazole, 200 or 250 mg thrice daily, or tinidazole, 150 mg twice daily, for seven to ten days produces cure rates of about 75 per cent. Repeating the course after a week's pause will cure more than 90 per cent. Tinidazole as a single dose of 2 g or a three-day course of metronidazole, 2 g once daily, will cure more than 90 per cent. The oldest specific treatment, quinacrine (mepacrine), 100 mg thrice daily for seven to ten days, is also effective. The one-week courses of metronidazole or quinacrine have been used in infants at one-third the adult dosage. Since asymptomatic carriers are potential sources of epidemics, and since they may become ill later, it is advisable to treat them.

The drugs relieve the symptoms and eradicate the parasite from the feces in a few days in almost all cases. The success of therapy should be controlled clinically and by stool examination at 2, 4, and 8 weeks, since late relapses may occur. Treatment failures are more frequent in acute than in chronic giardiasis, and light infestations are more readily cured than heavy ones. After the eradication of *G. lamblia*, symptoms indistinguishable from giardiasis may continue in 10 per cent of the patients for up to a year (Jaremin et al., 1976; Jokipii and Jokipii, 1978). This has been termed postgiardiac syndrome.

No specific prophylaxis is available, and the way to escape giardiasis is to avoid all forms of unboiled water in endemic areas.

### *BALANTIDIASIS*

*Balantidium coli* in the human colon causes intestinal balantidiasis and may lead to extraintestinal balantidiasis. The infestation may be asymptomatic and the disease may be acute or chronic. The parasite is worldwide, it is the only ciliated protozoon infecting man, and *B. coli* from primates, pigs, and rats may cause human disease. It is rare in man, and pig feces have been the obvious source of most infections; its infective form is the cyst, which may survive for weeks outside the host. The dimensions of both the trophozoite and the cyst of *B. coli* are approximately five times those of *G. lamblia*.

After the ingestion of cysts, trophozoites are liberated in the small intestine, settle in the large bowel, and start lysing the epithelium. They may cause ulcerations and rarely penetrate into the peritoneal cavity to cause peritonitis. Ulcers and hemorrhages of the mucosa are scattered, and the tissue reactions consist mainly of edema and mononuclear cell infiltration. Neutrophils predominate after secondary bacterial invasion. A few cases of vaginitis have been caused by *B. coli*.

Man is generally resistant to *B. coli*, the infections are often asymptomatic, and most cases of overt balantidiasis are of the chronic, intermittent type, resembling chronic giardiasis (Table 1) without malabsorption or flatulence and with blood in feces more frequently. In acute balantidiasis, dysentery, colicky pains, nausea, anorexia, and vomiting predominate; the patients lose weight, and anemia may develop. In compromised patients fulminating balantidiasis may be fatal in a few days.

Balantidiasis is diagnosed by stool examination: direct smears may reveal trophozoites, sometimes visible to the naked eye, in dysenteric stools or cysts in formed stools. Concentration techniques do not increase the number of isolations (Walzer et al., 1973), and although *B. coli* can be cultured in vitro, the method is not used for diagnosis. Tetracycline, 500 mg thrice daily for 10 days, is an effective therapy. There is no specific prophylaxis, and prevention consists of recognizing and avoiding sources of infection.

### References

Barbieri, D., DeBrito, T., Hoshino, S., Nascimento F[a], O. B., Martins Campos, J. V., Quarentei, G., and Marcondes, E.: Giardiasis in childhood. Absorption tests and biochemistry, histochemistry, light, and electron microscopy of jejunal mucosa. Arch Dis Child 45:466, 1970.

Black, R. E., Dykes, A. C., Sinclair, S. P., and Wells, J. G.: Giardiasis in day-care centers: evidence of person-to-person transmission. Pediatrics 60:486, 1977.

Brodsky, R. E., Spencer, H. C., Jr., and Schultz, M. G.: Giardiasis in American travelers to the Soviet Union. J Infect Dis 130:319, 1974.

Calder, R. M., and Rigdon, R. H.: Giardia infestation of gall bladder and intestinal tract. Am J Med Sci 100:82, 1935.

Hartman, H. R., Kyser, F. A., and Comfort, M. W.: Infection of the gallbladder by Giardia lamblia. JAMA 118:608, 1942.

Hoskins, L. C., Winawer, S. J., Broitman, S. A., Gottlieb, L. S., and Zamcheck, N.: Clinical giardiasis and intestinal malabsorption. Gastroenterology 53:265, 1967.

Jaremin, B., Chmielewski, J., Zwierz, C., and Spiralska, I.: A "postgiar-diac syndrome" (an analysis of the observed cases). Bull Inst Marit Trop Med Gdynia 27:93, 1976.

Jokipii, A. M. M., and Jokipii, L.: Prepatency of giardiasis. Lancet 1:1095, 1977.

Jokipii, A. M. M., and Jokipii, L.: Comparative evaluation of two dosages of tinidazole in the treatment of giardiasis. Am J Trop Med 27:758, 1978.

Jokipii, L., and Jokipii, A. M. M.: Giardiasis in travelers: a prospective study. J Infect Dis 130:295, 1974.

Ormiston, G., Taylor, J., and Wilson, G. S.: Enteritis in a nursery home associated with Giardia lamblia. Br Med J 2:151, 1942.

Rendtorff, R. C.: The experimental transmission of human intestinal protozoan parasites. II. Giardia lamblia cysts given in capsules. Am J Hyg 59;209, 1954.

Saha, T. K., and Ghosh, T. K.: Invasion of small intestinal mucosa by Giardia lamblia in man. Gastroenterology 72:402, 1977.

Walzer, P. D., Judson, F. M., Murphy, K. B., Healy, G. R., English, D. K., and Schultz, M. G.: Balantidiasis outbreak in Truk. Am J Trop Med 22:33, 1973.

Wright, R. A., and Vernon, T. M.: Epidemic giardiasis at a resort lodge. Rocky Mt Med J 73:208, 1976.

Wright, S. G., Tomkins, A. M., and Ridley, D. S.: Giardiasis: clinical and therapeutic aspects. Gut 18:343, 1977.

# INTESTINAL 132 ROUNDWORMS

## Elizabeth Barrett-Connor, M.D., D.C.M.T. (London)

### ASCARIASIS

Ascariasis, caused by the largest and most common roundworm of man, *Ascaris lumbricoides,* is found throughout temperate and tropical climates in most parts of the world.

#### Etiology

Infective eggs are chiefly transmitted from hand to mouth by children who have touched or eaten contaminated soil, or by ingestion of raw vegetables grown in infected soil. Larvae are released, penetrate the intestinal blood vessels, and are carried to the lungs. The larvae break out of the alveolar capillaries, migrate up the pulmonary tree, and are swallowed. They mature in the lumen of the small intestine, where they maintain their position by propulsive muscular activity. The adults produce eggs two to three months after infection is acquired and live an average of one year. They do not multiply in man. In soil, fertilized eggs become infective in about three weeks and can survive for years under appropriate conditions. Where sanitation is inadequate or where human feces are used as fertilizer, virtually everyone is infected. It is believed that one fourth of the world population has ascariasis.

#### Pathogenesis and Pathology

Larvae migrating through the lung can cause a patchy pneumonia, with focal hemorrhage, consolidation, and eosinophilia. Adult ascarids in the human intestine cause no lesions unless they produce obstruction. The changes that occur then are secondary to mechanical obstruction of a hollow viscus. For example, obstruction of the biliary tree can cause obstructive jaundice or ascending cholangitis. Obstruction of the pancre-atic duct can cause pancreatitis. Obstruction of the upper airway can cause death from suffocation. Partial or complete small bowel obstruction, and occasionally volvulus or intussusception, may be caused by a mass of worms. Rarely, adults or ova are found outside the intestine in the liver, lung, or peritoneum, usually surrounded by granulomatous reaction.

#### Clinical Manifestations

The pulmonary phase of larval migration, in the second week after ingestion of ova, usually passes unnoticed. However, in some cases migrating larvae cause Loeffler's syndrome; indeed, *Ascaris* is the commonest helminth reported as a cause of this disease (Spillman, 1975). Loeffler's syndrome is typically a one-week illness characterized by symptoms of tracheobronchitis and rapidly changing pulmonary infiltrates, followed by marked peripheral eosinophilia. The presence of a papular or urticarial rash in 15 per cent of cases, the greater frequency of the syndrome in adults rather than children in areas where *Ascaris* is acquired seasonally, the presence of eosinophilia, and studies of IgE all suggest that the pulmonary disease is due to a hypersensitivity reaction.

Most patients with ascariasis are asymptomatic. The spontaneous passage of large worms from the mouth, nose, or anus may be the first indication of infection. The most serious consequence, which occurs in perhaps 2 in 1000 infections is obstruction caused by one or more adult *Ascaris*. Obstructive complications are observed primarily in preschool children. Complications include obstruction of the biliary or pancreatic ducts, appendicitis, volvulus, intussusception, intestinal perforation, and, most commonly, intesti-

**TABLE 1.  Intestinal Roundworms**

| ROUNDWORM | DISTRIBUTION | ACQUISITION | DIAGNOSTIC FORM | COMPLICATIONS AND SEQUELAE | TREATMENT |
|---|---|---|---|---|---|
| *Ascaris lumbricoides* | Worldwide in temperate and tropical areas | Ingestion of ova in contaminated soil or vegetables | Ova in stool; adult worm in stool, mouth, or nose | Obstruction of intestine, biliary tract, pancreatic duct or airway, Loeffler's syndrome | Piperazine, pyrante pamoate |
| Hookworms (*Ancylostoma* and *Necator*) | Worldwide | Filariform larvae in soil penetrate skin of feet | Ova in stool | Anemia | Tetrachlorethylene, pyrantel pamoate, levamisole, or mebendazole |
| Trichostrongylus | Japan, Korea, Indonesia, Iran, and other parts of Asia and Africa | Ingestion (most common) and skin penetration | Ova in stool | ? | Unnecessary (see text) |
| *Strongyloides stercoralis* | Worldwide, patchy | Larvae in soil penetrate skin of feet and perianal region (auto-infection) | Rhabditiform larvae in stool | Malabsorption with immunoglobulin deficiencies, severe disseminated disease in immunocompromised host | Thiabendazole |
| *Capillaria philippinensis* | Philippines, Thailand | ? Ingestion of larvae in raw fish | Ova in stool | May cause severe, fatal disease with steatorrhea, wasting, cardiopathy | Mebendazole |
| *Enterobius vermicularis* | Worldwide | Fecal-oral transmission of ova | Ova demonstrated on perianal skin by cellophane-tape test | Migration of female worm to ectopic sites | Often unnecessary, mebendazole, pyrvinium pamoate, pyrantel pamoate |
| *Trichuris trichiura* | Worldwide | Ingestion of embryonated ova from soil | Ova in stool | Rectal prolapse and dysentery in children | Only if symptomatic; mebendazole effective |

nal obstruction caused by a bolus of worms. Signs and symptoms of the obstructive complications are not specific for ascariasis. On occasion, an abdominal mass that contains a visible or palpable moving bolus of worms affords a preoperative diagnosis, but often the diagnosis is first made at surgery.

A common and insidious complication of ascariasis is malnutrition. This is a consequence of competition of parasites and host for limited nutrients, and occurs in children who have a borderline diet and a heavy worm burden. Repeated worming results in a significant improvement in growth and development as compared with untreated infected controls.

### Diagnosis

Except for a past history of worm passage, there are no diagnostic signs or symptoms of ascariasis. Diagnosis at the stage of larval migration is rarely possible, although transient patchy infiltrates and eosinophilia are suggestive. Occasionally, a diagnostic third-stage larva can be found in the sputum. Normal stools at the time of migration followed by the appearance of ova in

the stools within three months establishes a probable retrospective diagnosis. (Serologic tests do not distinguish this illness from other larval migrations.) During the intestinal phase eosinophilia is usually absent. Diagnosis is made by microscopic examination of unconcentrated stool. A few patients harbor only male *Ascaris*, no eggs are excreted, and the diagnosis is made after passage of a worm or by demonstration of ascarids on roentgenographic examination of the abdomen.

### Treatment

Because a single ascarid sometimes causes a serious complication, the goal of therapy is cure. Many drugs are effective for the treatment of ascariasis. The choice depends on availability, cost, and the necessity for single dose treatment in a given patient population. Piperazine citrate is an effective and inexpensive ascaricide used extensively over the years. A single oral dose of 75 to 100 mg/kg/body weight to a maximum of 3.5 g gives a cure rate of about 75 per cent, and a two-day course cures over 90 per cent of patients. Levamisole in a single dose of 2.5 mg/kg is as effective as piperazine. Pyrantel pamoate is more efficient, curing 90 to 100 per cent of patients after a single oral dose of 10 mg/kg. Other broad spectrum antihelmintics such as bephenium hydroxynaphthoate, thiabendazole, and mebendazole are also ascaricidal but are rarely as effective as pyrantel pamoate in a single dose.

Intestinal obstruction is treated by nasogastric suction. After vomiting is controlled, piperazine is given in the standard dosage by nasogastric tube and flushed through with saline, and the tube is then clamped for one or two hours. This process can be repeated every 8 to 12 hours for up to six doses until the obstruction is relieved. The symptoms usually improve in one or two days, but *Ascaris* organisms may not appear in the stool until four days after the initiation of therapy. In about one fifth of cases obstruction cannot be relieved and surgery is necessary.

### Prophylaxis

Improved sanitation, the building and use of latrines, and the prohibition of the use of untreated human wastes as fertilizer all reduce the prevalence of ascariasis. In communities where such programs are not yet available, periodic mass worming of children has been recommended to prevent malnutrition and possibly reduce the risk of surgical complications of infection. (Gupta et al., 1977).

## HOOKWORM INFECTION AND DISEASE

Hookworm infection is the presence of adult hookworms, *Ancylostoma duodenale* or *Necator americanus,* in the human intestine; hookworm disease occurs when the worms are present in sufficient numbers to cause iron deficiency anemia. Both *A. duodenale* and *N. americanus* are found in most parts of the world, although *N. americanus* is the predominant species in the Americas and Central Africa, and *A. duodenale* the prevailing species in coastal North Africa.

### Etiology

Man is the principal host of *A. duodenale* and *N. americanus.* Hookworms are found wherever people go without shoes and defecate promiscuously into a warm, moist, and shaded soil suitable for the maturation of larvae. When eggs in feces are deposited on soil under optimal conditions, the ova hatch to rhabditiform larvae in one to two days, and molt to become infective filariform larvae within one week. Infective larvae may survive for as long as one year. On contact, the larvae penetrate skin or buccal mucosa, enter the circulation, and are carried to the lungs, where they pass from the capillaries to the alveoli. They ascend the respiratory tree, are swallowed, and mature to adults in the small intestine four to seven weeks after infection. Infection may also be established by ingestion of *A. duodenale* larvae. The organisms may remain dormant in the intestine or tissues for as long as nine months before ova are found in the stool (Banwell and Schad, 1978). The adult worms attach to the mucosa by buccal capsules and suck blood. Hookworms do not multiply in man. They survive two to ten years (average four years), although egg production decreases after two years. It is estimated that one fourth of the world population has hookworm infection, but most have a light infection, unassociated with disease.

### Pathogenesis and Pathology

Migration of larvae through the lungs may produce changes similar to those caused by *Ascaris* larvae. The attachment of worms to the wall of the small intestine results in digestion of the distal villi. The intestinal mucosa between parasites appears normal. The major disorder produced by the hookworm is iron deficiency anemia, which is caused by the leeching of blood from the host. Bone marrow examination reveals absent iron stores. In advanced cases, cardiovascular changes consistent with severe anemia are seen.

### Clinical Manifestations

Skin penetration usually goes unnoticed but may cause "ground itch," with intense pruritus and papulovesicular rash at the site of larval entry. Larval migration through the lungs infrequently causes Loeffler's syndrome, as described under Ascariasis. Although massive infections can cause abdominal pain, diarrhea, and weight loss, intestinal symptoms are rare. The only significant consequence of hookworm infestation occurs when a heavy worm burden is coupled with an iron-poor diet. In this setting hookworm anemia, also called hookworm disease, is seen (Roche and Layrisse, 1966). Anemia is most apt to occur in women and children, owing to their greater iron needs. Anemia is also more common with *A. duodenale* infestation because it is a more efficient blood leech than *N. americanus.* A single *A. duodenale* sucks 0.15 ml per day compared with 0.03 ml by *N. americanus.* The signs and symptoms of anemia due to hookworm disease are those of any iron deficiency anemia. As in patients with iron deficiency of other causes, malabsorption has been reported in children with hookworm disease.

### Diagnosis

Diagnosis is rarely possible during the larval migration phase preceding the appearance of ova in the feces. Iron deficiency anemia and a slight eosinophilia in an individual with a history of soil contact in an endemic area should suggest hookworm disease, but eosinophilia may be absent. Occult blood is often found in the stool. In severe cases the serum albumin level may be low.

The diagnosis is confirmed by the demonstration of hookworm eggs in the feces. Any infestation that can produce anemia is readily found on microscopic examination of a fecal smear without concentration. Unconcentrated smears will demonstrate eggs if the counts are greater than 1200 eggs/ml. (Egg counts of at least 2000/ml in feces in women and children and 5000/ml in men are usual in patients whose anemia is due to hookworm infestation.) Quantitative techniques can be used to confirm the cause of anemia in patients with other possible causes of iron deficiency.

### Treatment

Light infestations do not cause disease and require no treatment. For patients requiring treatment, a significant reduction in worm burden is an acceptable goal of therapy. Eradication of every worm is not necessary to prevent anemia and is impractical in populations with a high probability of reinfection.

A variety of agents has been used successfully. Cure rates may differ according to hookworm species and geographic areas, in part related to criteria for cure. The choice of agent should depend on the experience in a given area, the cost and availability of the drug, the likelihood of population compliance if multidose regimens are selected, the potential benefit of broad spectrum agents, and the frequency and severity of side effects. Tetrachlorethylene in a single dose of 0.12 ml/kg (maximum, 5 ml) cures approximately half of all patients and reduces the worm burden in most of the remainder. It is dependable and cheap. Purgatives are not required and indeed reduce the effectiveness and increase the toxicity of tetrachlorethylene. One dose of any of the following is also effective: 5 mg of bephenium hydroxynapthoate, 10 mg of pyrantel pamoate, or 25 mg/kg/body weight of levamisole. Mebendazole requires 100 mg twice a day for three days for effective treatment.

None of these anthelmintics are recommended for pregnant women, who should delay specific therapy until completion of pregnancy. Any patient with severe anemia should be treated first with iron therapy, which will promptly correct the anemia without affecting the worm load. Some authorities treat all patients who have hookworm anemia with iron as well as a vermifuge to hasten recovery from anemia.

### Prophylaxis

Shoes and latrines prevent hookworm infestation. Public health education must be coupled with attempts to improve sanitation. Otherwise, the newly built latrines are not used, and shoes are saved for special occasions.

## TRICHOSTRONGYLIASIS

There are at least seven species of the genus *Trichostrongylus,* all of which are parasites of mammals, that occasionally infect the intestinal tract of man. Human infection with *Trichostrongylus* is most common in Japan, Korea, Indonesia, and Iran, but is also found in other parts of Asia and in Africa (Ghadirian and Arfaa, 1975).

### Etiology

Adult nematodes in the small intestine of ruminants lay eggs that are passed in feces. Infective larvae develop in suitable soil and infect man by skin penetration and pulmonary migration as in hookworm infection or, more often, by mouth as a result of ingestion of infected vegetation. When infection occurs by the oral route there is apparently no pulmonary migration, and the larvae mature to adults directly in the small intestine. Man usually acquires the infection from eating larvae on green vegetables or chewing contaminated grasses. Although human infections from this nematode are much less common than those caused by other intestinal nematodes, over two thirds of the population of some areas are infected.

### Pathogenesis and Pathology

Very little is known about this infection in man. Larvae are believed to mature while burrowed in the intestinal mucosa. The adults live attached to the duodenum and jejunum and suck blood in the manner of hookworms.

### Clinical Manifestations

*Trichostrongylus* infections are usually light, transient, and asymptomatic. Because most patients who have trichostrongyliasis also have other intestinal parasites, it is not possible to attribute symptoms directly to this infection.

### Diagnosis

Eggs are readily found in the stool and are easily confused with hookworm ova. Because *Trichostrongylus* infection is refractory to the usual anthelmintics, the discovery of ova in feces is not infrequently attributed to intractable hookworm infection.

### Treatment

*Trichostrongylus* infection rarely, if ever, requires treatment. Because these nematodes lie protected in the intestinal mucosa, they are not eradicated by most of the broad spectrum anthelmintics. Thiabendazole and, less frequently, bephenium hydroxynapthoate have been used successfully. Thiabendazole, 25 mg/kg twice daily for two days, affords good cure rates but often causes nausea, dizziness, vomiting, and anorexia.

### Prophylaxis

Theoretically, prevention can be achieved by avoiding the consumption of raw plants grown in contaminated soil.

## *STRONGYLOIDIASIS*

Strongyloidiasis, which is caused by the intestinal nematode *Strongyloides stercoralis,* has a patchy worldwide distribution. It often coexists with but is less common than hookworm.

### Etiology

Like hookworm, *S. stercoralis* infects man by skin penetration. Within 48 hours the larvae migrate through the pulmonary capillaries. Some larvae may develop into adult worms in the lungs, but most pass from the respiratory tract to the duodenum and jejunum, where the females invade the mucosa and deposit eggs about one month after the initial infection. The larvae ordinarily hatch in the mucosa and bore into the intestinal lumen. Rhabditiform larvae are usually found in the feces. At times, the larvae may develop into the infective filariform stage in the intestine and penetrate the intestinal mucosa or perianal skin. This autoinfection is responsible for the heavy parasitism seen in some patients and for the persistence of infection long after the host has left an endemic area.

*Strongyloides* also has a free-living cycle. After leaving the host, rhabditiform larvae may develop into infective larvae either directly or indirectly through a generation of free-living males and females. Under appropriate conditions, the free-living cycle can be continued indefinitely.

### Pathogenesis and Pathology

Migration of larvae through the lungs may produce changes similar to those caused by *Ascaris.* The severity of the pulmonary process in strongyloidiasis is proportional to the number of parasites in the tissues, which reflects the level of autoinfection. Mechanical, lytic, and allergic mechanisms of lung damage have been proposed.

In the small intestine adult females are anchored to the epithelium or deep in the mucosa. Small bowel biopsy usually shows eggs in crypts and submucosa, little inflammatory reaction, and flattening or atrophy of the villi. In patients with autoinfection, larvae may be seen migrating through the intestinal wall.

In fatal cases, adult worms, larvae, and eggs are found widely disseminated throughout the body. The heaviest parasitism occurs in the intestine and lungs. Hemorrhage, eosinophilia, and consolidation are seen in the alveoli. In the intestines, there is a variable amount of mucosal edema, necrosis, ulceration, and pseudopolyposis. A diffuse enteritis may progress to hemorrhagic enterocolitis and fibrosis. Dead and dying larvae presumably cause the most marked inflammatory response, which may be primarily granulomatous, lymphocytic, or eosinophilic. Other changes compatible with secondary bacterial infection are common.

### Clinical Manifestations

Most infections are asymptomatic. An itchy, maculoerythematous rash is sometimes noted at the site of skin penetration. Persons sensitized by prior infection show a more marked cutaneous reaction. Acute pneumonitis is sometimes seen during the primary passage of the larvae through the lungs, but this is probably more often a consequence of autoinfection when larger numbers of larvae are migrating through the lungs. The most common complaints are watery, rarely bloody, diarrhea or symptoms suggestive of duodenal ulcer. In some patients, particularly, but not always, those with immunoglobulin deficiencies, a malabsorption syndrome may be seen.

Disseminated strongyloidiasis is a serious and potentially fatal complication of massive autoinfection. This type of hyperinfection can occur in apparently healthy hosts but is much more common in patients who are immunocompromised owing to disease (malignancy, malnutrition, burns, chronic renal failure, tuberculosis, leprosy) or drugs (chemotherapy and corticosteroids) (Purtilo et al., 1974). Symptoms and signs reflect the involved organ systems and are nonspecific. Clinical pictures suggestive of miliary tuberculosis, an acute abdomen, paralytic ileus, and granulomatous or ulcerative bowel disease have been observed. Secondary bacterial infection may result in gram-negative sepsis with fever, abdominal pain, and shock.

### Diagnosis

Patients with pneumonia and eosinophilia should have a sputum examination for larvae. At the time of pulmonary migration, *Strongyloides* filariform larvae, each with a characteristic forked tail, often can be demonstrated in unstained or Papanicolaou-stained sputum.

The initial diagnosis of strongyloidiasis is usually attempted by stool examination. *Strongyloides* larvae can be found in only one-fourth of stool specimens from infected patients. (*Strongyloides* ova are rarely found in the stool, and hookworm larvae, which differ morphologically from those of *Strongyloides,* are not seen in stool unless there is a long interval between passage and examination.) The yield from stool examination can be increased by suspending approximately 100 g of fresh stool in fine surgical gauze over a glass, adding lukewarm water to the level of suspended stool, and waiting one hour for the larvae to migrate through the gauze to the bottom of the glass. The sediment is examined for larvae.

A duodenal or jejunal specimen yields the diagnosis in approximately 90 per cent of cases. Similar results can be achieved by examination of the bile-stained mucus that adheres to a nylon yarn, which is withdrawn several hours after being swallowed in a weighted gelatin capsule.

Peripheral eosinophilia is found in over 90 per cent of persons with strongyloidiasis. Unfortunately, only 20 per cent of patients with massive autoinfection and disseminated strongyloidiasis have peripheral eosinophilia as a clue to diagnosis.

Roentgenograms of the chest may show a miliary pattern, a lobular or lobar infiltrate, or cavities. Not infrequently, active tuberculosis coexists with pulmonary strongyloidiasis and may be responsible for part of the clinical and radiographic picture. Barium examination of the small intestine sometimes demonstrates duodenitis or a tubular rigid deformity of the small bowel; the latter is said to be strongly suggestive of chronic strongyloidiasis.

### Treatment

The potential for autoinfection, illness, and even death supports the need for curative treatment. Patients who are candidates for immunosuppressive therapy should be systematically studied for strongyloidiasis and should receive specific therapy before corticosteroids or immunosuppressives are begun. Thiabendazole, 25 mg/kg twice daily for two days, is the preferred drug. Approximately 10 per cent of patients will require a second course of therapy for cure. In disseminated strongyloidiasis, thiabendazole should be continued for at least five days. Total doses of as high as 50 g have been required for cure. Disseminated strongyloidiasis is fatal despite treatment in 50 per cent of patients. When

possible, immunosuppressives should be discontinued until the parasite is eradicated.

### Prophylaxis

Preventive measures are the same as those used to control hookworm infection.

## *INTESTINAL CAPILLARIASIS*

Human intestinal capillariasis is a new disease caused by the intestinal nematode *Capillaria philippinensis*. It is presently limited to specific coastal areas of the Philippines and one small focus in Thailand. Although there are over 200 nematodes of the genus *Capillaria,* only a few have been found in man and only *C. philippinensis* is an important cause of disease.

### Etiology

Human intestinal capillariasis was first noted in the intestine of a severely wasted man who died in a Manila hospital in 1963. Three years later an epidemic of disease caused by this parasite affected over 1500 persons in northern Luzon, Philippines.

All stages of the parasite can be found in humans. Autoinfection and parasite multiplication are believed to be responsible for the very heavy infections seen in some patients. The high morbidity and mortality indicate that this parasite is new to humans. How this new infection was introduced remains a mystery. Although a marine fish or mammal is the suspected natural host, examinations of thousands of fish and other aquatic specimens have been negative. Infective larvae develop in the intestines of lagoon fish that are eaten raw in the affected communities; however, ingestion of raw fish is not new to this area. Feeding embryonated eggs to a variety of animals and humans in transmission experiments has failed to produce infection.

### Pathogenesis and Pathology

Unlike most intestinal nematodes, *C. philippinensis* can multiply within the intestinal tract of man. Dissemination of parasites may occur, but usually, even in fatal cases, the parasites are limited to the small intestine. At autopsy the small bowel is indurated, edematous, and distended with watery fluid. In some cases the ileal fluid contains from 10,000 to 200,000 larvae and adults per liter. Eggs, larvae, and adult worms are found in enormous numbers in the glands and lamina propria of the small intestine, particularly the jejunum. The flattened or obliterated villi of malabsorption may be seen. There is a modest increase in the number of lymphocytes in the lamina propria, but no acute inflammatory reaction is present, nor is eosinophilia a consistent finding.

Altered absorption and intestinal protein loss result in chronic diarrhea and wasting. The cause of this effect is unknown; overwhelming numbers of parasites, a parasite-toxin, a parasite-allergin, or a parasite-induced deficiency of digestive enzyme(s) has been postulated as the pathogenic factor.

### Clinical Manifestations

The first symptoms are very characteristic loud gurglings in the stomach and diffuse abdominal pain. Two to three weeks later diarrhea, which is at first watery and then bulky and foul, appears. Severe muscle wasting, weakness, edema, and cardiopathy follow in the majority of cases. Early in the epidemic in 1966, virtually every person who had eggs in their stools became symptomatic, and nearly one quarter died two weeks to two months after the onset of illness, usually of heart failure or bacterial infection (Watten et al., 1972). Recently, there have been increasing numbers of asymptomatic persons with ova in their stools, and the severe form of the disease is less common. The reason for the lower pathogenicity of the disease is unknown. It may be that early recognition of the characteristic symptoms leads to earlier treatment.

### Diagnosis

In residents of an endemic area, the characteristic noisy stomach is practically diagnostic. Later steatorrhea, wasting, and eosinophilia suggest the diagnosis. Diagnosis is confirmed by stool examination. Eggs resemble those of *Trichuris trichiura* and are usually plentiful.

Other laboratory studies show anemia, hypoalbuminemia (with high values of alpha-2 and gamma-globulins compared with controls), and high IgE levels. Eosinophilia may be present. Marked electrolyte derangements, particularly hypokalemia, are usual. Increased fecal fat, impaired vitamin $B_{12}$ absorption (Shilling test), and an abnormal D-xylose test are all characteristic of symptomatic intestinal infection with *C. philippinensis*. A severe protein-losing enteropathy can be demonstrated in persons with either symptomatic or asymptomatic infection.

### Treatment

Until recently, thiabendazole for 30 to 40 days was the best treatment, but some patients relapsed and many had gastrointestinal side effects, dizziness, and weakness. Recently mebendazole has become the treatment of choice. Four hundred milligrams daily in divided doses for 20 to 30 days gives good cure rates without side effects. Diarrhea usually decreases and the patient feels better within 48 hours of initiation of treatment; in the interim, fluid and electrolyte replacement is important.

### Prophylaxis

No methods of control are known, although the avoidance of uncooked fish is recommended.

## ENTEROBIASIS

Enterobiasis is infection of the intestinal tract of man with the pinworm *Enterobius vermicularis*. Pinworm infection is worldwide in distribution and vies with *Ascaris* for first place as the most common nematode of man. Unlike *Ascaris*, pinworm is equally common in developed and developing countries.

### Etiology

This small roundworm lives in the cecum and adjacent portions of the gastrointestinal tract. Adult worms seldom live more than two months and do not multiply in man. The male is smaller than the female and is rarely seen. At night, the gravid female migrates from the anus to deposit thousands of eggs on the perianal or perineal skin. The embryonated ova are infective within a few hours and are transferred to the mouth of the same or another host by way of hands, bedclothes, and possibly aerosols. Man is the only known host. Owing to their personal hygienic habits, children are most often infected and reinfected. However, when a child brings the infection into a household, other members of all ages are often infected. It is estimated that 30 per cent of children and 15 per cent of adults have pinworm (Weller and Sorenson, 1941). For unknown reasons, enterobiasis is less prevalent in blacks.

### Pathogenesis and Pathology

Pinworms cause no recognized intestinal pathologic signs. Some patients experience pruritus ani. This symptom leads to scratching and thus to direct anus-finger-mouth transmission, a highly efficient mechanism for parasite survival. Why some infected persons have severe pruritus ani and most have none is not known.

Occasionally adults, larvae, or ova are reported from unusual ectopic sites (Chandrasoma and Mendis, 1977). For example, pinworm migration into the female genital tract is a rare cause of pelvic granulomas. Although it is not infrequently found in the appendix, the association of pinworm infection with appendicitis seems to be coincidental rather than causal.

## Clinical Manifestations

The symptoms attributed to pinworm are legion and include anorexia, enuresis, masturbation, nausea, vomiting, abdominal pain, diarrhea, weight loss, and irritability. In controlled studies none of these symptoms, not even the single symptom generally attributed to pinworm infection—pruritus ani—are more common in infected than in uninfected children. Pruritus ani does, however, disappear with pinworm treatment and reappear with reinfection (Weller and Sorenson, 1941). Migration into the female urethra may be a cause of "night cries" in little girls and possibly of cystitis.

## Diagnosis

Pinworm is a noninvasive infection, and therefore neither eosinophilia nor elevations in serum IgE are found. Adult pinworms can be seen with the naked eye and may be brought to the physician for diagnosis. Under the microscope, the egg-laden female can be differentiated easily from artifacts and fibers. Pinworm eggs are not often found in the stool but can be demonstrated by the cellophane-tape test. In this procedure, the adhesive side of cellophane tape is pressed repeatedly against the perianal skin as soon as the patient awakens in the morning and before bathing. The tape is placed adhesive side down on a glass slide, with or without a drop of toluene, and the slide is examined microscopically for adherent ova. A single test will detect approximately half of all infections, three tests will diagnose 90 per cent of cases, and five tests are diagnostic of 100 per cent.

## Treatment

In the absence of symptoms, there is no reason to treat this infection. Once the diagnosis is made, parents should be educated about the high prevalence and low pathogenic potential of pinworms. In societies in which worms are equated with a lack of personal cleanliness, parents should be advised that pinworm carries no such stigma and that the most rigidly applied sanitary measures, such as sterilization of bedclothes and two showers daily, have failed to control enterobiasis.

A high cure rate can be achieved with a variety of agents, several in single oral dose regimens. A single oral dose of mebendazole, 100 mg independent of body weight, or pyrantel pamoate, 11 mg/kg, or pyrvinium pamoate, 5 mg/kg to a maximum of 250 mg, will cure about 90 per cent of cases. A second course two weeks later is usually recommended. To prevent reinfection, some experts suggest that all other infected household members be treated, although there is no evidence that this measure significantly reduces reinfection.

## Prophylaxis

No effective control measures are known.

## TRICHURIASIS

Trichuriasis, caused by the intestinal whipworm *Trichuris trichiura*, is worldwide in distribution, and is found particularly in rural areas with poor sanitation.

## Etiology

Man, the principal host of *T. trichiura*, is infected by the ingestion of embryonated ova. Larvae hatch in the small intestine, and young worms develop to mature, egg-producing adults in one to three months. In very heavy infections whipworms may be found throughout the large intestine, but usually they remain in the cecum and ascending colon. Adult worms do not multiply in man but live for several years, producing characteristic eggs that embryonate in two to four weeks when deposited in most shaded soil.

## Pathogenesis and Pathology

Adult *Trichuris* live with their thin anterior end inserted into the mucosa of the large bowel. The parasites are readily visible; rectal prolapse or sigmoidoscopy may disclose myriads of white worms on the mucosa. Manual detachment of the parasite leaves a small petechial hemorrhage at the site. In light infections there is remarkably little cellular response. In heavy infections the unparasitized mucosa is hyperemic, friable, and edematous. The mechanism of these changes and of the diarrhea or dysentery attributed to this nematode is unknown. Whipworm infection may coexist with amebic or balantidial dysentery.

## Clinical Manifestations

Most persons with trichuriasis have light infections of no medical importance. Heavy infections occur primarily in young children. Diarrhea, dysentery, and rectal prolapse are the only diseases attributable to heavy *T. trichiura* infection. In some cases dysentery is a consequence of amebiasis, which often coexists with trichuriasis.

## Diagnosis

The diagnosis is readily made by microscopic stool examination. A single unconcentrated stool specimen can lead to identification of as few as five worm pairs. Indeed, the prolific production of readily identifiable eggs ensures that this diagnosis is rarely missed by the laboratory.

## Treatment

It is unnecessary to treat asymptomatic patients. When therapy is indicated, reduction in worm burden rather than cure is an acceptable goal. Until recently no safe, effective, and nontoxic oral drugs were available for treatment of trichuriasis. Now mebendazole in a dose of 100 mg twice a day for three days regardless of body weight yields a cure in over 75 per cent of cases and a reduction in worm burden in over 90 per cent, with no untoward effects (Peña Chavarría et al., 1973). Because mebendazole acts on contact with the worms, some patients with diarrhea may receive no benefit. The same treatment regimen can be repeated in three weeks, if necessary.

## Prophylaxis

The same control measures as those used for ascariasis are recommended.

## References

Spillman, R. K.: Pulmonary ascariasis in tropical communities. Am J Trop Med Hyg 24:791, 1975.

Gupta, M. C., Arora, K. L., Mithal, S., and Tandon, B. N.: Effect of periodic deworming on nutritional status of ascaris-infested preschool children receiving supplementary food. Lancet 2:108, 1977.

Banwell, J. G., and Schad, G. A.: Hookworm. Clinics in Gastroenterology 7:129, 1978.

Roche, M., and Layrisse, M.: The nature and causes of "hookworm anemia." Am J Trop Med 15 (pt 2): 1031, 1966.

Ghadirian, E., and Arfaa, F.: Present status of trichostrongyliasis in Iran. Am J Trop Med Hyg 24:935, 1975.

Purtilo, D. T., Meyers, W. M., and Connor, D. H.: Fatal strongyloidiasis in immunosuppressed patients. Am J Med 56:488, 1974.

Watten, R. H., Beckner, W. M., Cross, J. H., Gunning, J. J., and Jarimillo, J.: Clinical studies of capillariasis philippinensis. Trans R Soc Trop Med Hyg 66:828, 1972.

Weller, T. H., and Sorenson, C. W.: Enterobiasis: Its incidence and symptomatology in a group of 505 children. N Engl J Med 224:143, 1941.

Chandrasoma, P. T., and Mendis, K. N.: *Enterobius vermicularis* in ectopic sites. Am J Trop Med Hyg 26:644, 1977.

Peña Chavarría, A., Swartzwelder, J. C., Villarejos, M., and Zeledón, R.: Mebendazole, an effective broad-spectrum anthelmintic. Am J Trop Med Hyg 22:592, 1973.

# *CESTODIASIS* **133**

## *Z. S. Pawlowski, M.D.*

Man can be infected with two classes of flatworms, the cestodes (tapeworms) and the trematodes (flukes). Adult tapeworms possess a scolex or head, a neck, and multiple hermaphroditic segments, or proglottids, that produce ova. Adults attach to the intestine of the definitive host by suckers or hooklets on the scolex; adult tapeworms only rarely cause serious disease. Larval forms are released from ingested ova and develop into bladderworms in the tissues of intermediate hosts, where they frequently produce severe and fatal diseases. The definitive host becomes infected after ingesting the larvae contained in the raw or rare flesh of the intermediate host. Man is thus the definitive host for tapeworms whose larval forms encyst in the flesh of the animals that comprise his sources of meat. He can be the intermediate host of other tapeworms when he accidentally ingests ova excreted in the feces of domesticated or wild animals. Abdominal or intestinal cestodiasis refers to tapeworm infections for which man is the definitive host. Somatic or tissue cestodiasis refers to the severe diseases that occur when man is the intermediate host of a cestode.

The most common causes of abdominal cestodiasis are *Hymenolepis nana*, the dwarf tapeworm; *Taenia saginata*, the beef tapeworm; and *Taenia solium*, the pork tapeworm. Less frequent causes are *Diphyllobothrium latum*, the broad or fish tapeworm; *Dipylidium caninum*, a dog tapeworm; and *Hymenolepis diminuta*, the rat tapeworm. Some other *Diphyllobothrium* spp, *Bertiella* spp, *Inermicapsifer* spp, *Raillietina* spp, and *Multiceps* spp are exceptionally rare and focally distributed causes of abdominal cestodiasis.

Somatic or tissue infections with the larval stages of cestodes may be caused by *T. solium*, *T. multiceps*, *Echinococcus granulosus*, *E. multilocularis*, *Diphyllobothrium erinacei*, *Sparganum proliferum*, *Mesocestoides* spp, and *Spirometra mansoni*.

## *HYMENOLEPIS NANA (HYMENOLEPIDOSIS)*

### Definition

*H. nana*, which mainly affects children, is the most common cause of intestinal cestodiasis in the world. Hymenolepidosis infections are chronic and greatly modified by immunity. Although widespread, these infections are mild and self-limited.

### Etiology

Children are infected by ingesting *H. nana* eggs from the feces of human carriers. *H. nana* is a dwarf tapeworm that can grow to 4 cm and localizes in the ileum of man. Although the lifespan of adult tapeworms is only a few weeks, the intestinal population of tapeworms stays at hun-

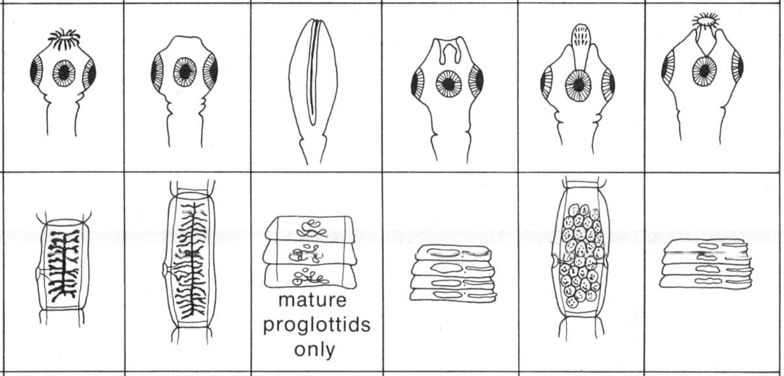

| | Taenia solium | Taenia saginata | Diphyllo-bothrium latum | Hymenolepis diminuta | Dipylidium caninum | Hymenolepis nana |
|---|---|---|---|---|---|---|
| Scolex | | | | | | |
| Gravid proglottid | | | mature proglottids only | | | |
| Number of proglottids | 700–1000 | ca 2000 | 3000–4000 | 800–1000 | 60–175 | ca 200 |
| Length of strobila (cm) | 150–800 | 400–1200 | 300–1500 | 30–60 | 20–40 | 1½–4 |

**FIGURE 1.** *Cestodes of man. Diagram of morphologic characteristics.*

dreds to thousands for many years because *H. nana* can complete its life cycle in humans, who continually reinfect themselves with ova from their own feces and with larvae developing in their intestines.

Larvae hatch from ingested ova in the small intestine, penetrate a villus, and develop into small cysticercoids. After a few days, the parasites break out of the cysticercoid back into the intestinal lumen, attach to the mucosa, and develop into maturity (Fig. 1).

### Pathogenesis and Pathology

Mechanical and toxic irritation of the intestinal mucosa by larval and adult worms causes enteritis in heavy infections. Lysis, desquamation, or necrosis of epithelial cells of the intestinal mucosa is caused by adult parasites and invading larvae. Larval stages may produce complete destruction of the invaded villi. Intestinal absorption, especially in the ileum, may be disturbed.

### Clinical Manifestations

Symptoms depend on the intensity of the infection as modified by the individual's general nutrition and immunity. Most patients are asymptomatic. Abdominal discomfort, diarrhea, inanition, irritability, and urticaria have been ascribed to hymenolepidosis. Evaluation of sequelae is difficult because *H. nana* infection frequently coexists with malnutrition, protein deficiency, and other parasitic or bacterial infections of the intestine.

### Geographic Variations

In arid and warm climates in populations with low standards of sanitation, 5 to 20 per cent of children may be infected with *H. nana*. Infection is especially common in Latin America, the Mediterranean countries, and the Indian subcontinent but occurs throughout the world. In adults infection either disappears spontaneously or continues at very low levels. Epidemics may occur in orphanages and other closed communities where fecal transmission is likely.

### Diagnosis

Infection is recognized by finding typical ova (Fig. 2) in the feces. Ova can usually be detected by direct examination, but repeated examinations by flotation methods may be necessary after treatment or in light infections when the output of eggs is inconstant.

### Treatment

Niclosamide (Yomesan) is the drug of choice. A dose of 60 to 80 mg/kg, but not more than 2 g daily, given for five to seven days cures 90 per cent of infections. Heavy infections may require another course of treatment after two weeks. Paromomycin (45 mg/kg for five to seven days) and praziquantel are alternative drugs. Adolescents and adults are usually asymptomatic but should probably be treated to reduce the prevalence of *H. nana*.

### Prophylaxis

Good personal hygiene and high levels of general sanitation diminish the exposure to infection.

In epidemic situations mass treatment of the infected, isolation of the uninfected, long-term surveillance, and improvement of sanitation are important control measures.

## TAENIA SAGINATA (TAENIASIS)

### Definition

Man is the definitive host for *T. saginata*, the beef tapeworm, which causes a benign intestinal infection. When man ingests the larval form of *T. saginata*, the cysticercus, in raw beef, the larva excysts, attaches to the small intestine, and matures into an adult.

### Etiology

The adult beef tapeworm is between 4 and 12 meters long. Its scolex is usually localized in the upper jejunum, but its strobila may extend down to the terminal ileum. The parasite can live as long as its host and not uncommonly persists for 30 to 40 years.

### Pathogenesis and Pathology

*T. saginata* may cause subacute inflammation of the small intestinal mucosa but usually causes no pathologic change. Intestinal transit time and gastric acidity may decrease. Moderate eosinophilia may occur but is not correlated with a rise in serum IgE.

### Clinical Manifestations

Ninety-eight per cent of carriers feel some sensation in the perianal area when proglottids migrate or are discharged out of the anus. Other symptoms are present in 76 per cent of patients, but many of these complaints may be related to the patients' knowledge that they harbor a large worm in their intestine. Abdominal pain, nausea, anorexia, weight loss, weakness, globus hystericus, vomiting, diarrhea or constipation, increased appetite, increased body weight, and allergic symptoms have all been reported. In fact, most patients are probably asymptomatic until they discover that they are parasitized. Tissue infection, or cysticercosis, of man has never been sufficiently documented as a complication of *T. saginata* infection.

Appendicitis or cholecystitis may be caused by motile proglottids of *T. saginata* that stray into the appendix or gallbladder.

### Geographic Variations

Geographic variations in the disease may occur; the natural transmission of *T. saginata* in the Philippines and Taiwan is not clear. Infections are common both in urban (Europe and the United States) and pastoral communities. East and central Africa, the south-central Asian republics of the U.S.S.R., and the Near East countries are areas with a high prevalence of infection.

### Diagnosis

*T. saginata* must be differentiated from *T. solium*, which causes cysticercosis. Finding *Taenia* eggs on anal swabs or during fecal examination confirms the diagnosis of taeniasis but does not differentiate *T. saginata* from *T. solium* because the ova are indistinguishable (Fig. 2). Final species determination requires examination of either the scolex (unarmed in *T. saginata*) or the gravid proglottids (more than 15 uterine branches per side in *T. saginata*) (Fig. 1). Differentiation of *T. saginata* from *T. solium* is of critical clinical and epidemiologic importance.

### Treatment

The drug of choice is niclosamide. An early morning single dose of 2 g in adults is effective in 90 per cent of cases. Purgation is usually not necessary. The only contraindication to treatment with niclosamide is the first trimester of pregnancy, when any anthelmintic treatment is undesirable. Alternative drugs are paromomycin in a single dose of 4 g, metallic tin compounds (five-day treatment), mepacrine, bithionol, and pumpkin seeds. The efficacy of the treatment is evaluated either by finding the scolex (which is

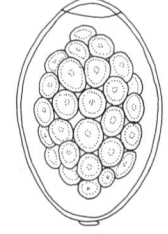 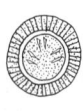 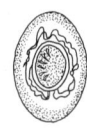 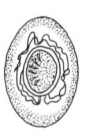 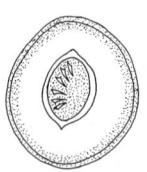

| Diphyllobothrium latum | Taenia solium Taenia saginata | Dipylidium caninum | Hymenolepis nana | Hymenolepis diminuta |

**FIGURE 2.** *Ova of cestodes that are parasites of man (cm = 30 μ).*

unnecessary with niclosamide), or by negative examination for eggs and proglottids four months after treatment.

### Prophylaxis

For personal prophylaxis one should avoid eating raw or semiraw beef. Lightly infected beef carcasses may pass the routine meat inspection. Prophylaxis at the national level requires proper disposal of sewage, meat inspection, and freezing of lightly infected carcasses.

## TAENIA SOLIUM

### Definition

*Taenia solium* taeniasis is a human intestinal infection caused by the adult pork tapeworm. *T. solium* cysticercosis is an infection with the larval stage, the cysticercus. *T. solium* cysticercosis is often fatal because the larvae frequently localize in the brain.

### Etiology

Adult pork tapeworms do not differ very much from *T. saginata*, but they can be differentiated. The pork tapeworm is smaller ($1\frac{1}{2}$ to 8 m), the scolex is armed with hooks, and the proglottids have a three-lobed ovary and less than 15 lateral uterine branches on the side (Fig. 1). The proglottids do not move actively and are usually expelled passively with feces in groups of three to five. The ova of *T. solium* are indistinguishable from those of *T. saginata*. The cysticercus is a larva, 5 to 20 mm in diameter, that consists of a bladder filled with fluid surrounding a scolex armed with hooks. Man acquires intestinal infection by ingesting undercooked pork infected with cysticerci (taeniasis) or *T. solium* ova disseminated by a human carrier (cysticercosis). Autoinfection with *T. solium* eggs can cause cysticercosis. Although *T. solium* occurs focally throughout the world, it is highly prevalent in areas with poor sanitation where raw, uninspected pork is eaten. In seven countries of Central and South America cysticercosis is found in over 1 per cent of the pigs slaughtered. Other endemic foci include central and southern Africa as well as some countries of Southeast Asia. *T. solium* is nearly eradicated from Europe and North America.

## T. SOLIUM TAENIASIS

The pathogenesis, pathology, and clinical manifestations of *T. solium* taeniasis are similar to those of *T. saginata*. Because cysticercosis may complicate *T. solium* infections, however, early treatment is important for clinical and epidemiologic reasons. *T. solium* taeniasis usually responds better than *T. saginata* to niclosamide or other taeniacides. The success of treatment should be evaluated by periodic examination of the feces by the laboratory and visual inspection of the feces for proglottids by the patient. Proglottids usually reappear within two months if treatment is unsuccessful.

## T. SOLIUM CYSTICERCOSIS

### Pathogenesis and Pathology

Man may be parasitized by one to more than 1000 cysticerci. Muscular localization of cysticerci is frequently unnoticed unless calcified cysticerci are incidentally recognized by x-ray examination. Subcutaneous cysticerci produce detectable nodules that are easy to obtain for biopsy. Ocular and cerebral localizations of cysticerci cause the most serious damage, and cysticerci seem to have a predilection for the central nervous system. Localization in the brain parenchyma and the subarachnoid space are most common. Less frequently, cysticerci localize in the ventricles, brain stem, cerebellum, and spinal cord. Meningitis, meningoencephalitis, ependymitis, and/or signs of focal damage occur, depending on the site of localization. Living cysticerci usually provoke a mild cellular response. Dead ones cause a foreign body granuloma and may become calcified.

### Clinical Manifestations

Injury from cysticercosis is mechanical rather than toxic, and the localization and number of cysticerci determine the symptoms and signs. There are four syndromes of cerebral cysticercosis: (1) Symptoms of a slow-growing intracranial tumor with focal neurologic deficits, epileptic seizures, and increased intracranial pressure. This presentation occurs mainly in adults with a single or few cysticerci. (2) Rapid development of increased intracranial pressure, loss of vision, and organic brain syndrome (occurs mainly in children with heavy infections). (3) Symptoms of leptomeningitis, ependymitis, and internal hydrocephalus; these symptoms occur when cysticerci localize at the base of the brain. (4) Sudden unexpected death when cysticerci affect vital centers of the brain.

The symptoms of ocular cysticercosis vary according to the part of the eye affected. Cysticercosis often remains asymptomatic in other internal organs and tissues.

### Diagnosis

The diagnosis of cysticercosis is made by identification of the scolex and hooks or other micro-

scopic structures of the cysticercus wall in biopsied or autopsied material. Differentiation from
other bladder larvae that invade humans more
rarely may be difficult.

The presumptive diagnosis of cysticercosis may
be based on the clinical findings of subcutaneous
nodules, a cysticercus-like body in the eye, calcified cysticerci on radiographs, and/or a high
antibody titer against *Taenia* antigens by indirect hemagglutination, immunofluorescence, or
bentonite flocculation.

The detection of *Taenia* eggs or proglottids from
the patient or a close relative make the possibility
of cysticercosis more likely.

### Treatment

Until recently, the only effective treatment for
cerebral or ocular cysticercosis has been surgery.
The neurosurgical fatality rate is between 24 and
67 per cent, depending on the localization and
number of parasites. Furthermore, successful surgery may not result in cure but only in clinical
improvement. There is now a good prospect for
successful chemotherapy of some cases of human
cysticercosis because mebendazole and praziquantel kill cysticerci in vivo, but adjunctive
surgery will probably also be necessary in some
cases.

### Prophylaxis

*T. solium* infections are controlled by meat
inspection, improvement of general sanitation,
health education, and early treatment of human
taeniasis. Personal prophylactic measures
against cysticercosis are the same as those used
in other fecal-borne infections.

## DIPHYLLOBOTHRIASIS

*Diphyllobothrium latum*, the fish tapeworm, is
the longest tapeworm of man (3 to 15 m). The
strobila of *D. latum* resides in the small intestine
and absorbs large quantities of vitamin $B_{12}$. If the
parasite is located in the proximal portion of the
jejunum, hyperchromic changes and even frank
pernicious anemia may occur.

*D. latum* infection is easy to diagnose by fecal
examination; a large number of characteristic
operculated ova (Fig. 2) are produced as early as
three to five weeks after ingestion of an invasive
plerocercoid larva in fish. Proglottids are also
distinctive because of the rosette-shaped uterus
that lies medially in each segment (Fig. 1). Diphyllobothriasis is easily cured with niclosamide
or other taeniacides.

The infection is common in communities where
freshwater fish are eaten raw or partly cooked, for
example, among fishermen at river deltas or

lakes in Finland, Siberia, Canada, United States,
Chile, and Argentina. Infection can be prevented
by avoiding raw or undercooked fish in endemic
areas. Control of endemic diphyllobothriasis is
difficult because of the traditional eating habits of
the local population and the large reservoir of
infection in wild, fish-eating animals.

## OTHER INTESTINAL CESTODIASES

At least seven other species of *Diphyllobothria*
have been reported as sporadic causes of human
disease in Alaska, Greenland, and Peru. Clinical
and epidemiologic aspects of these are the same
as those for *D. latum*.

Hymenolepidosis due to *H. diminuta* (the rat
tapeworm) is not as rare in the world as was once
believed. More than 1 per cent of children are
infected in the New Guinea highlands and some
villages in Iran, where human population have
close contact with the parasite in rodents and the
insects (fleas, beetles, *Myriapoda*) that serve as
intermediate hosts. Clinical manifestations of *H.
diminuta* infection are usually mild. The diagnosis is made by finding typical eggs in the feces.
Infection can be easily eradicated by treatment
with niclosamide or other taenicides.

*Dipylidium caninum* is a common tapeworm of
dogs and cats and incidentally of man. Most
infections occur in children, who ingest fleas and
flour beetles that are infected with cysticercoid
larvae. Dipylidiasis only rarely causes diarrhea
or allergic reactions. The diagnosis is made by
finding the characteristic pumpkin seed-shaped
proglottids (Fig. 1) or ova (Fig. 2) in the feces.
Taenicides are very effective, and many infections probably clear spontaneously.

Rarely, man may be parasitized by the common
rat tapeworm *Raillietina* spp, the monkey tapeworm *Bertiella studeri*, and *Inermicapsifer cuben-
sis*, whose primary host is unknown. Little is
known about the clinical, epidemiologic, and taxonomic features of these parasites.

## ECHINOCOCCOSIS (HYDATID DISEASE)

### Definition

Echinococcosis is a zoonotic human infection
caused by the larval form, or hydatid, of *Echinococcus granulosus*. Man acquires the infection by
ingesting ova shed in the feces of infected dogs.
The clinical course is that of a chronic, space-
occupying lesion mainly in the liver or lungs. Patients may remain asymptomatic or die of complications, depending on the size and location of the
hydatid cyst.

## Etiology

In the traditional, pastoral life cycle, man is infected by close contact with his sheep dogs. In the natural cycle, the hydatid occurs in the organs of sheep (intermediate host), which, like man, are infected by ova disseminated in the feces of dogs. Dogs are infected when they eat the hydatids in the tissue of sheep. In the sylvatic cycle, man is infected by ova from his hunting dogs, who are infected by eating larvae in the tissues of wild herbivores. *E. granulosus* larvae in man consist of a primary cyst, which can continue to develop for years to a size of over 20 cm in diameter. Secondary (daughter) cysts are produced in the primary cysts or, rarely, outside the hydatid. Brood capsules containing tens to hundreds of invaginated protoscolices may develop inside the primary and daughter cysts. Protoscolices that are liberated from a cyst may develop into secondary cysts, for example, in the abdominal cavity.

## Pathogenesis and Pathology

Hydatid cysts develop most frequently in the liver (60 per cent) and lungs (20 per cent), rarely in the brain (3 per cent), eye, heart, bone, and other internal organs. The primary cyst is usually surrounded by a thick fibrous capsule produced by the host. Pathologic changes depend largely on the location and size of the cyst and are mainly due to pressure from the enlarging cyst. Complications include anaphylaxis from sudden rupture of a cyst, pyogenic abscesses in secondarily infected cysts, spontaneous fractures of infected bones, respiratory distress, liver damage, and severe ocular or CNS damage. Anaphylaxis can occur when cysts rupture spontaneously or at surgery because many individuals have become sensitized by leakage of small amounts of material from the intact cyst.

## Clinical Manifestations

Symptoms depend on the location and size of the cyst. Hepatic echinococcosis is usually asymptomatic until the cyst has become large. Even then, the symptoms are usually vague unless secondary pyogenic infection or pressure on blood vessels or bile ducts causes obstructive jaundice and portal hypertension. Echinococcosis of the lung may remain asymptomatic for years. Rupture into the pleural cavity or the bronchi, bacterial infection, or pressure on pulmonary vessels or bronchi may cause lung abscesses, bronchopleural fistulae, atelectasis, or pulmonary hypertension. Cerebral echinococcosis is often fatal because of the size of the growing cyst. In other internal organs, echinococcosis produces symptoms characteristic of slow-growing, benign tumors. Calcified cysts in the spleen or kidney, for example, may be found without any symptoms or other signs of disease.

## Geographic Variation

Each strain of *E. granulosus* circulating in definite natural cycles (dog-sheep-dog, dog-pig-dog, dog-horse-dog, domesticated herbivora-wild carnivora-man) shows its own growth pattern in in vitro culture and different degrees of invasiveness for man. These differences may explain the occurrence of outbreaks of human echinococcosis in certain regions of the world; e.g., in the Turkana tribe in Kenya. Echinococcosis is endemic in many countries throughout the world where sheep, sheep dogs, and man live in close contact.

## Diagnosis

The definitive diagnosis of *E. granulosus* depends on the identification of typical hooklets and brood cysts on microscopic examination of the excised cyst. Rarely, hooks are present in the sputum, duodenal contents, feces, urine, or peritoneal or pleural fluid. Radiographic examination that shows a pulmonary cyst or a subdiaphragmatic calcified cyst and positive serologic (hemagglutination, complement fixation, flocculation, and immunofluorescent antibody) and positive skin tests strongly support the diagnosis.

## Treatment

Some cases of human echinococcosis need no treatment (old calcified cysts, small hepatic cysts, some pulmonary cysts). Various surgical techniques such as total extirpation, marsupialization, and removal after opening have been developed to remove symptomatic hydatid cysts. The success of surgical intervention depends on proper diagnosis of the number, localization, and size of the cysts, as well as on the skill of the surgical team. Surgical rupture of the cyst may cause anaphylactic shock or secondary echinococcosis unless its contents are sterilized with 15 or 20 per cent hypertonic saline. Chemotherapeutic and immunologic methods of treatment are being investigated.

## Prophylaxis

Personal prophylaxis in endemic areas is based on avoiding contact with infected dogs and their feces. Some countries have developed public health programs for control of echinococcosis.

## *OTHER TISSUE CESTODIASES*

Alveolar echinococcosis, caused by *Echinococcus multilocularis,* differs from *E. granulosus* infection in many respects. The distribution of *E.*

*multilocularis* is limited to the northern hemisphere (southern Germany, Switzerland, Siberia, and Alaska). The parasite circulates naturally in wild Canidae and wild rodents. Man is incidentally infected when he ingests ova on the fur or in the feces of infected foxes or other Canidae. Domestic cats that catch and eat the flesh of wild rodents have recently been implicated as a source of human infection. *E. multilocularis* larvae usually develop in the liver. The larvae are alveolar and consist of hundreds or thousands of small vesicles (0.5 to 2 mm in diameter). Some develop a scolex. Alveolar echinococcus may be necrotic in its center but may also spread, either by producing new vesicles peripherally or by metastasizing to other organs. The clinical manifestations of alveolar echinococcosis are similar to those of liver neoplasm, including protracted jaundice and emaciation. The prognosis is poor. Serologic (immunofluorescent antibody and hemagglutination) tests and the patient's history (possibility of exposure) are helpful. The final diagnosis is established at surgery or at autopsy by parasitologic and histopathologic examination of the cysts. Surgical treatment is sometimes successful. Recently, high doses of mebendazole have been used in human cases of alveolar echinococcosis with promising results.

Coenurosis in man is caused by bladder larvae of *T. multiceps,* a tapeworm that parasitizes dogs and sheep. Cerebral and ocular coenurosis produces symptoms similar to those of cerebral or ocular cysticercosis. The definitive diagnosis is usually possible only by parasitologic examination of larvae removed at surgery or autopsy.

Other tapeworm larvae that invade man include *Sparganum proliferum, Diphyllobothrium erinacei,* and *Spirometra mansoni,* which occur in the Far East and South America. The larvae usually invade the subcutaneous tissue or the eye, causing the disease called sparganosis. The infection is acquired by ingestion of raw frog or snake or by the use of their raw tissues as poultices. Treatment is surgical.

## References

Muller, R.: Worms and Disease. London, W. Heinemann Medical Books, 1975, p. 38.

Pawlowski, Z., and Schultz, M. G.: Taeniasis and cysticercosis (*Taenia saginata*). Adv Parasitol 10:269, 1972.

Slais, J.: The morphology and pathogenicity of the bladder worms *Cysticercus cellulosae* and *Cysticercus bovis.* Prague, Academia, 1970.

Smyth, J. D., and Heath, D. D.: Pathogenesis of larval cestodes in mammals. Helm Abstr 39:1, 1970.

# SCHISTOSOMIASIS **134**

## Gunther Dennert, Ph.D.

### DEFINITION

Human schistosomiasis is a water-borne, parasitic disease that presently afflicts at least 200 million people in Asia, Africa, the Caribbean, and Latin America. It was first recorded in Egypt about 4000 years ago. Schistosomiasis is caused by schistosomes or bloodflukes — digenetic trematodes from the superfamily of Schistosomatoidea. Unlike other trematodes, they are elongated and resemble roundworms, apparently as an adaptation to living in blood vessels. They have oral and ventral suckers and a nonmuscular pharynx. The female worm is held in the gynaecophoric canal of the male (the schist) and lays nonoperculate eggs. The eggs are excreted with human waste and release a free-swimming form that infects and multiplies in the intermediate host, a snail. A second free-swimming form is released from the snail and infects the definitive vertebrate host. Their geographic distribution (see Chapter 80) is limited by the availability of a suitable snail host.

### ETIOLOGY AND LIFE CYCLE

Schistosomiasis is caused by one of three parasitic worms that live in one of several sets of veins. *S. mansoni* inhabits the inferior mesenteric veins and causes intestinal schistosomiasis. The eggs have a large lateral spine. The principal molluscan hosts are snails of the genus *Biomphalaria.* Among vertebrates besides man, rodents, insectivores, marsupials, and cattle can be infected, providing an animal reservoir for this parasite. *S. mansoni* occurs in most African countries, Saudi Arabia, the northern and eastern parts of South America, and some Caribbean islands. *S. haematobium* lives in the vesical venous plexus and causes urinary schistosomiasis. It is less adaptable to nonhuman hosts, but other primates and even some rodents can be infected. This species lays eggs with a large terminal spine and is endemic in Africa and some Middle Eastern countries. *S. japonicum* is found mostly in the superior mesenteric veins and causes intestinal schistosomiasis like that of *S. mansoni.* Its eggs have a tiny lateral spine. The principal snail host is the genus *Oncomelania*. *S. japonicum* is the least host-specific of the three schistosomes and infects many different domestic animals. It is found in the Philippines, Japan, the Chinese mainland, Thailand, Indonesia, and the Mekong Delta.

The life cycle of schistosomes (Chapter 80) (Ansari, 1973; Jordan and Webbe, 1969) alternates between two generations. The sexual generation lives in the vertebrate and lays eggs from which a short lived, free-swimming form (miracidium) hatches. The miracidium infects a freshwater snail and establishes the second, asexual generation. It becomes a mother sporocyst that gives rise to daughter sporocysts, which in turn produce numerous cercariae. The cercariae leave the snail, infect the vertebrate by skin penetration, migrate as schistosomula to the target tissue, and mature into adult worms.

The function of the spine on the eggs may be to anchor them so as to resist the flow of blood and to penetrate venules. Eggs release histiolytic substances as they pass through the tissues and during maturation of the miracidium. Most eggs (about 50 per cent) do not reach the lumen of the bladder or intestine but are trapped in tissues and cause serious tissue damage. Excreted eggs hatch at low osmotic pressure in water at temperatures of between 10 and 30° C. The miracidium (about 0.16 mm in length) is propelled by cilia on four rows of epidermal plates. It has a bilobed, probably nonfunctional gut and four flame cells that serve as the excretory system. The miracidium shows positive phototaxis and negative geotaxis and swims to the snail to which it attaches. Penetration is aided by glands that secrete lytic substances. The miracidium loses its ciliated coat after penetration and reforms into a nonmotile sac, the mother sporocyst, in which germinal cells differentiate to daughter sporocysts. This process takes about 10 to 15 days. The daughter sporocysts are motile and migrate to the hepatic and gonadal tissues while they grow. Cercariae differentiate from germinal cells in the daughter sporocysts, pass through the blood sinuses and tissues, and leave from the edge of the snail's mantle. The sporocysts regenerate and produce more cercariae. The output of cercariae is variable, but up to 100,000 cercariae can be released per snail. The life cycle in the snail takes about four to seven weeks.

The cercariae have a discrete head and a bifurcated tail that allows locomotion. The head carries small oral and ventral suckers, a nonfunctional gut, flame cells, and a primitive nervous system. Three or four pairs of unicellular glands close to the ventral sucker (posterior postacetabular glands) secrete mucilage that assists in

attachment. The other glands (preacetabular glands) empty during penetration. If the cercariae fail to find a vertebrate host they will die after about 8 to 12 hours because their glycogen reserve is exhausted. After penetration, the cercaria, having emptied its glands and shed its tail and cercarial glycocalyx, is now called a schistosomulum (about 0.1 mm in length). The trilaminate tegument is replaced within a few hours by a multilaminate one that is characteristic of the adult worm. There is some evidence that the schistosomula take up host antigens, which may prevent immune attack by masking the foreign antigens. Within the next 48 hours the schistosomula penetrate the subcutaneous tissue and enter the venous blood vessels and peripheral lymphatics. During the next five to seven days, they are transported via the heart to the lungs.

The next stage of the migration is not well understood. The schistosomula either migrate via the blood vessels to the portal system or directly through the diaphragm, which takes about 10 to 20 days. The parasites mature and mate in the liver and then migrate to the veins of the vesical plexus or to the mesenteric veins, where egg production begins. The worms migrate as a pair with the female held in the schist of the male. When the caliber of the venules becomes small enough to restrict migration, the female often leaves the male and continues to migrate as far as the size of the smallest venules will permit. Between 300 and 3000 eggs can be released per day per worm and are found in the stool or urine as early as 30 to 40 days after infection. Schistosomes usually live 5 to 10 years but have also been reported to survive for more than 30 years. Adult parasites (Chapter 80) are between 6 and 28 mm long. Their most important energy source is carbohydrate that is incompletely degraded to organic acids such as lactic acid, acetic acid, and propionic acid. Erythrocytes are ingested, and a hematin-like pigment that is regurgitated by the parasites is phagocytosed by reticuloendothelial cells.

## PATHOGENESIS AND PATHOLOGY

The pathology of schistosomiasis (Warren, 1973; Lichtenberg et al., 1971; Sadun et al., 1970) can be divided into stages that are associated with the life cycle of the schistosome in the infected individual. The pathogenesis of most of the lesions and clinical manifestations are related to the host response to the invading cercariae, the migrating adult worms, and the ova. The fundamental lesion of schistosomiasis, the granuloma, is formed around the ova in response to antigens contained in the hatching fluid. The cercariae, schistosomula, and adult worms also sensitize the host not only to their own antigens but also to cross-reactive antigens in the ova. Although many ova are excreted in the body fluids of the patients, a large number remain in the mucosa of the bowel and bladder. Others are "swept back" in the portal circulation to the liver or to ectopic localization in the lungs or central nervous system (CNS). Granuloma formation around these retained ova account for the manifestations of established, chronic schistosomiasis.

## Schistosome Dermatitis

Schistosome dermatitis occurs in response to cercarial skin penetration and migration. The cercaria cause minute areas of necrosis during penetration and early migration, but these mechanical effects cause no signs or symptoms. The dermatitis, which may range from transient urticaria to macules to a papular rash, is uncommon in natives of endemic areas. It occurs more commonly in visitors who have been sensitized recently but lack the relative immunity of local inhabitants with low-grade, established schistosomiasis. Penetration of cercariae disorganizes the squamous cells, and migration damages the transitional cells of the granular layer beneath the squames. Experimental studies suggest that unsensitized individuals develop edema and a polymorphonuclear infiltrate that is replaced by mononuclear cells within 48 hours. Sensitized individuals develop a more rapid and more intense polymorphonuclear response with more tissue damage. The accelerated reaction can be provoked either by serum or lymphoid cells (Colley et al., 1972; Stirewalt and Dorsey, 1974).

## Acute Schistosomiasis (Katayama Syndrome)

Schistosomula migration usually causes no symptoms, but inflammatory reactions in the lungs and liver may occasionally produce fever and cough. Maturation, migration of adults, and early egg production may cause an acute febrile illness called Katayama fever. It can occur in any form of schistosomiasis but is most common in infections with *S. japonicum,* probably because this schistosome produces the most ova. The majority of patients with schistosomiasis, however, never experience the acute phase of the disease. The acute syndrome is caused by local reactions to young schistosomes and ova and consists of local and general symptoms including abdominal pain, diarrhea, fever, weakness, myalgia, and headache. The pathogenesis is similar to that of serum sickness — that is, it appears to be an immune complex disease elicited by antibody production to the antigenic stimulus of cercariae, adult worms, and ova.

## Established and Chronic Schistosomiasis

In established infections intensive ova production by adult worms and excretion of large numbers of ova by the patient has commenced. In late infections egg output is often decreased as the disease becomes chronic with portal hypertension or obstructive uropathy. The pathologic reaction of established and late schistosomiasis is essentially a series of chronic inflammatory lesions elicited primarily by ova but also by dead worms. Therefore, the severity of the disease is proportional to the severity of the infection — the relative burden of worms and ova. A heavy burden of worms and ova is necessary to produce significant disease because small vascular lesions are easily repaired. The pathologic manifestations of significant disease consist of progressive tissue destruction and formation of fibrous tissue in various organs, depending on the species of schistosome.

## The Egg Granuloma

Severe pathologic manifestations of schistosomiasis (Warren, 1972) are to a large extent the result of an immunologic response of the host to the eggs. The eggs start eliciting a reaction when the encased miracidium matures (day 6). Histiolytic substances are secreted, leading to a focal granulomatous reaction (day 12). In acute schistosomiasis, a periovular area of necrosis is seen with or without deposition of a hyaline eosinophilic band (Hoeppli phenomenon), surrounded by an exudative cellular reaction consisting of many polymorphonuclear leukocytes, lymphocytes, and eosinophils. Later, the central necrosis and the perivascular eosinophilic material disappear, and the leukocytes are replaced by epithelioid cells (Fig. 1). Foreign body giant cells surround and invade the dead egg, completing the formation of the pseudotubercle, which is the classic lesion of schistosomiasis (Fig. 2). The egg may become calcified or may disappear entirely. Healing may be complete or scarring may occur with thickening of the wall of the intestine or bladder or obstruction of the portal venules. Thus, the most serious lesions occur during early infection, so that a massive primary infection may lead later to severe clinical symptoms.

The pathogenesis of the egg granuloma has been studied mostly in mice. Eggs are isolated from mouse tissue and injected into the tail vein of recipient mice. Mice previously sensitized by intraperitoneal injection of eggs show an accelerated and augmented inflammatory response around eggs in the lungs. The ability to respond in this fashion can be transferred to recipient mice by injecting lymphoid cells but not serum and can be inhibited in presensitized mice by antilymphocyte serum. This is in agreement

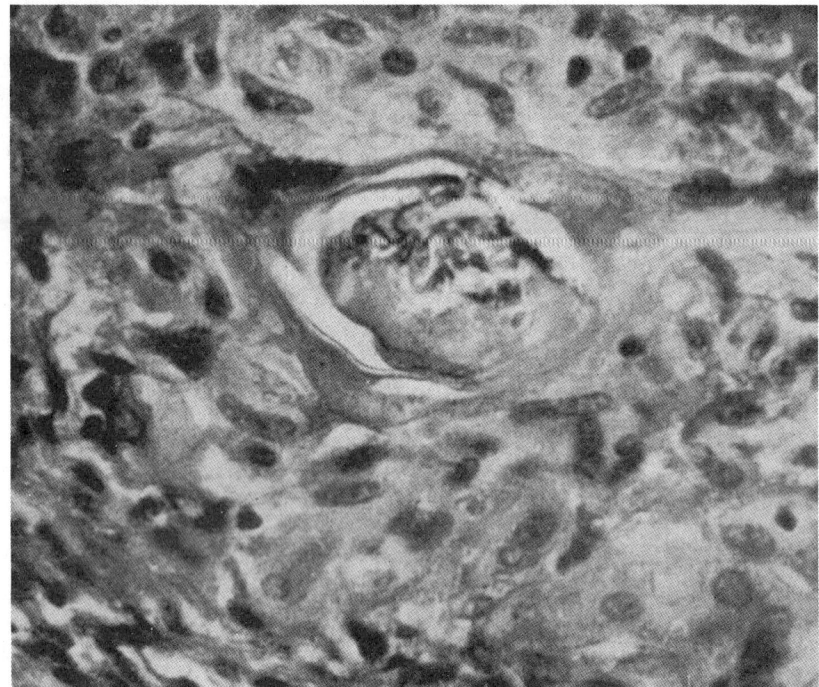

**FIGURE 1.** *Biopsy of liver showing a schistosome egg surrounded by epithelial cells (×480) (From Diaz-Rivera, R. S. et al.: Ann Intern Med 47:1082, 1957.)*

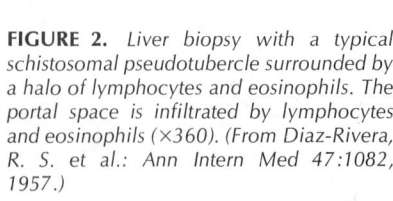

**FIGURE 2.** *Liver biopsy with a typical schistosomal pseudotubercle surrounded by a halo of lymphocytes and eosinophils. The portal space is infiltrated by lymphocytes and eosinophils (×360). (From Diaz-Rivera, R. S. et al.: Ann Intern Med 47:1082, 1957.)*

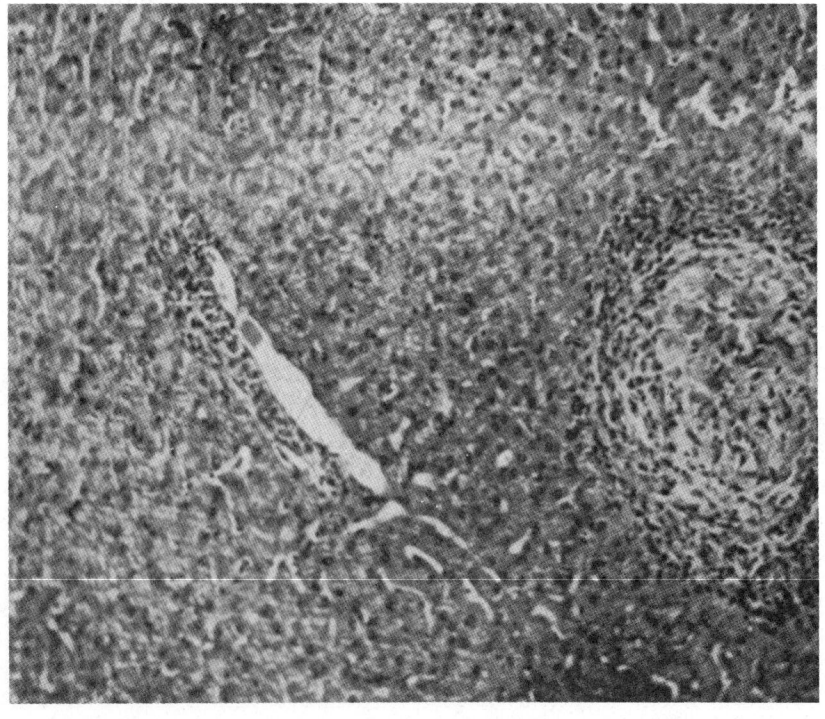

with the contention that the granuloma formation is a kind of delayed type hypersensitivity (DTH) reaction. Sensitization can also be achieved by a cell-free extract from eggs (SEA), and granuloma formation can be induced by SEA-coated bentonite particles. Eggs depleted of SEA by incubation in tissue culture do not induce granulomas. Granuloma formation is inhibited by substances that inhibit DTH but not by humoral antibody synthesis. It is also suppressed in thymectomized, immuno-incompetent animals. The egg granuloma may benefit the infected animal to some degree by curtailing the diffusion of antigens. As mentioned above, mice that have passed the acute stage of infection regularly modulate their granulomas, so that lesions become smaller during the chronic phase of the disease. Similar reactions may occur in man.

## S. mansoni and S. japonicum

Both schistosomes live in the mesenteric veins and therefore affect primarily the gastrointestinal tract and the liver. There is generalized lymphadenopathy, soft hepatomegaly, and soft splenomegaly in established infections. Eggs in the mucosa and submucosa of the colon and small intestine give rise to granulomas. The intestinal mucosa is reddened and edematous with yellowish papules, small hemorrhages, and occasional small ulcerations. Acute changes in the colon are confined to the lumen. Later, massive oviposition causes progression from the pseudotubercular stage to a diffuse transmural fibrosis. Massive intraluminal polypoid lesions are frequent in Egypt. Ova that are "swept back" by the portal venous current cause liver inflammation and damage. Hepatic granulomas induced by these ova may totally occlude the intrahepatic radials of the portal venules. Acute endophlebitis results in occlusion of other vessels by organized thrombi. Recanalized, newly formed blood vessels communicate through the wall of the vein with other vessels (Garcia-Palmieri and Marcial-Rojas,

1962). There is also a great increase in thin, straight arterial branches without evidence of obstruction. As shown in Figure 3, this increase in arterial branches is responsible for a large periportal vascular network that maintains normal blood flow to hepatic cells but contributes to portal hypertension. Eventually, there is a marked increase in fibrous tissue in the portal fields that surrounds and compresses the hepatic venules. These vascular and fibrotic changes in the portal areas cause them to be markedly broadened and lengthened, so that they stand out in cross-section. This appearance has given rise to the term "pipestem" fibrosis to describe this condition. The liver is enlarged, slightly nodular, and not hobnailed. The gross appearance is altogether different from that seen in Laennec's cirrhosis. The hepatic parenchymal cells do not show the degenerative or necrotic changes of Laennec's or post-hepatitis cirrhosis.

This unique type of liver pathology explains the development of severe portal hypertension with preservation of the function of hepatic parenchymal cells. Maintenance of liver cell function may contribute to the capacity of patients with schistosomal portal hypertension to tolerate multiple episodes of bleeding from esophageal varices. Massive varices develop in patients with severe illness at a much younger age than is characteristic of patients with Laennec's cirrhosis.

Most patients do not develop severe hepatosplenic schistosomiasis. The pathologic findings vary from a few hepatic granulomas to fully developed pipestem fibrosis. Severely infected individuals may develop portal hypertension within a few months, but the pathologic process more commonly develops over a period of many years.

Embolization of ova into the pulmonary vasculature may result in multiple intravascular granulomas and arteritis, pulmonary hypertension, and cor pulmonale. The pathognomonic lesions are intra-arterial and para-arterial granulomas that form a dumbbell shape (Fig. 4). Pulmonary localization occurs much more fre-

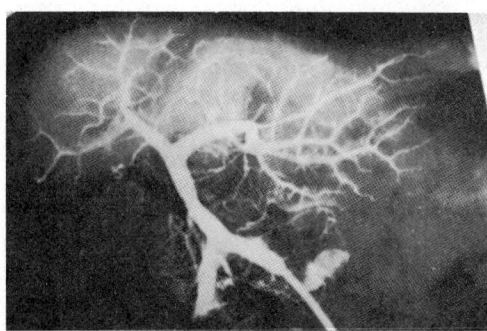 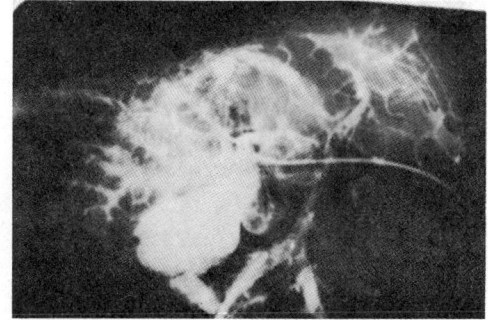

**FIGURE 3.** *Radiographs of postmortem liver of patient with hepatosplenic schistosomiasis after radiopaque medium was injected into portal system (left) and hepatic artery (right). Note that the fine periportal vascular network is visible on the right after arterial injection but not on the left after portal vein injection. (From Andrade, Z. A., and Cheever, A. W.: Am J Trop Med Hyg 20:425, 1971.)*

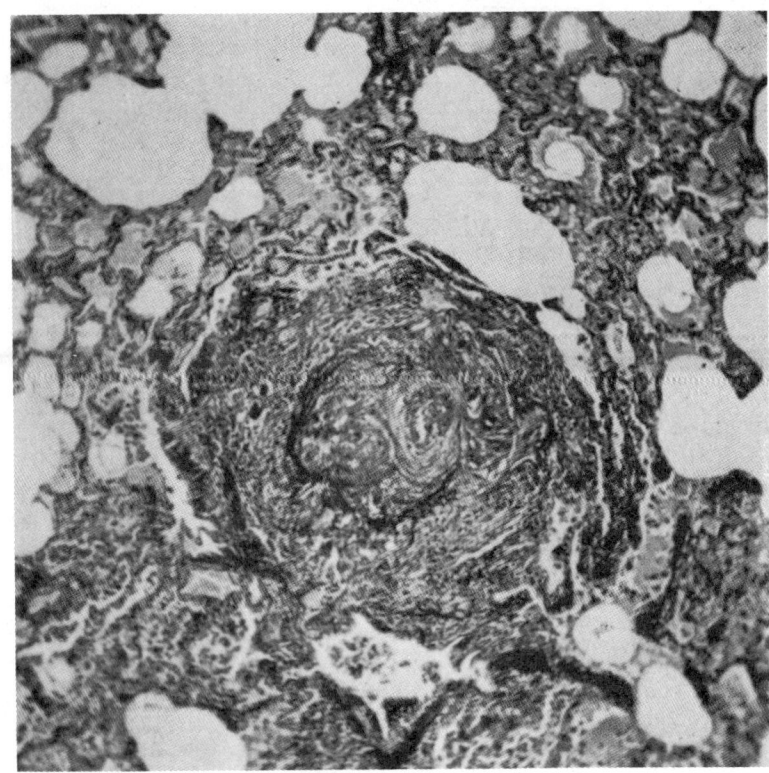

**FIGURE 4.** *Pulmonary schistosomiasis with intra-arterial and para-arterial granulomas, forming a dumbbell shape (elastic stain ×80). (From Marchand, E. J. et al.: Arch Intern Med 100:965, 1957.)*

quently in patients with portal hypertension secondary to severe hepatosplenic disease. Significant, isolated pulmonary schistosomiasis is rare.

*S. japonicum* affects the same organs as *S. mansoni*, but there are pathologic differences. *S. japonicum* lays about 10 times more eggs than *S. mansoni*. These eggs are found in aggregates and tend to calcify. There is more infiltration of neutrophils and a larger, more exudative granuloma. *S. japonicum* pairs tend to stay in one location and produce large masses of eggs that cause intestinal obstruction and a higher frequency of ectopic localization.

Splenomegaly occurs in all patients with severe hepatosplenic schistosomiasis. At least two factors contribute to splenic enlargement, namely, passive congestion and cellular proliferation. In early infection, cell proliferation is prevalent in the red pulp and germinal centers of the lymphoid follicles. Later, a multifocal basophil proliferation is observed that coincides with elevated immunoglobulin levels in the serum. Distended venous sinuses and dense splenic cords are caused by portal hypertension. Giant follicular lymphoma may develop in affected spleens.

In addition to pipestem fibrosis, chronic parenchymal hepatitis occurs in some patients with hepatosplenic schistosomiasis. In this condition, inflammatory cells infiltrate the liver and destroy liver cells at the limiting plate. In early infection, even before oviposition, a diffuse infiltration of

eosinophils can be seen. Later, this infiltration becomes more patchy and perivascular. In patients with decompensated hepatosplenic schistosomiasis, chronic hepatitis, which is characterized by septal fibrosis, active periportal inflammation, and bile duct proliferation, is more prominent than it is in patients with compensated hepatosplenic schistosomiasis. These histologic manifestations of the disease and their progression do not appear to be related to the intensity of the infection and egg production. Hepatitis B antigen has been reported in 4 per cent of the patients with hepatosplenic schistosomiasis compared with less than 1 per cent of uninfected controls.

### S. haematobium

*S. haematobium* organisms lay as many eggs as *S. mansoni*, but they are released in aggregates and tend to calcify. Since the adult worms live in the veins of the vesical plexus, they affect primarily the urinary tract, and secondarily the lungs. The eggs are found in the mucosa and submucosa of the bladder and the lower part of the ureters. They give rise to granulomas that initially are very cellular and large (polypoid lesions) and may block the flow of urine and lead to hydronephrosis, a condition often seen in schoolage children. Later, the lesions, now called sandy patches, become relatively acellular and fibrous and contain calcified eggs. Calcified eggs may cause bladder calcification and deformation. Although sloughing of necrotic polypoid patches is detectable in the early active phases of the disease, chronic ulceration of the bladder occurs later at sites of very heavy egg burdens. Some active lesions may persist as polyps in the later, inactive stages of disease if the antecedent active infection was heavy. The rectum, seminal vesicles, prostate, ureter, and urethra may be involved. Eggs can be found in the lung and less often in the liver. If the CNS is involved, lesions are usually found in the spinal cord. In some geographic areas, mixed infections with *S. mansoni* are frequent.

## CLINICAL MANIFESTATIONS

The host-parasite relationship is well balanced in schistosomiasis. The majority of infected people are asymptomatic or have mild, nonspecific symptoms. Only 5 to 10 per cent of infected populations have severe clinical symptoms, and the life expectancy of persons in an infected population is not significantly different from that of individuals in an uninfected one.

### Acute Schistosomiasis Due to *S. mansoni* and *S. japonicum*

The disease is recognized infrequently at this stage because most patients are asymptomatic. This phase of the illness usually follows exposure to heavily contaminated streams or bodies of water. Immediate itching and urticaria occur in a small percentage of patients and may begin as soon as the film of water on the skin begins to dry. Schistosome dermatitis may develop into papular lesions that persist for approximately five to seven days. Papular dermatitis is more common, however, when the skin is penetrated by avian schistosomes (see sections on Pathogenesis and Pathology and Geographic Variations).

During the migration of the schistosomula, fever and cough may be experienced in association with mechanical and inflammatory changes in the lung and liver, but this stage is usually asymptomatic. In acute schistosomiasis the worms mature in the liver, migrate to the small venules, and begin egg production. The acute disease is similar in all three forms of schistosomiasis and has an explosive onset about 20 to 40 days after heavy exposure. Major symptoms include chills, spiking fever with afternoon elevations to 105° F, generalized weakness, myalgia, headache, anorexia, profuse diarrhea, and weight loss. Extensive urticaria may occur in large patches on various parts of the body. Nausea and vomiting are common and cough may be prominent. The fever usually lyses spontaneously 2 to 10 weeks after onset.

Physical findings are usually minimal but may include urticaria, patches of moist rales over both lung fields, generalized lymphadenopathy, and hepatosplenomegaly. Edema and purpura of the eyelids may occur.

On sigmoidoscopic examination the rectal mucosa is hyperemic and edematous with pinpoint yellowish elevations, minute hemorrhages, and shallow ulcerations (Garcia-Palmieri and Marcial-Rojas, 1962).

The leukocyte count may be normal or elevated, but eosinophilia, which may approach 70 per cent is always present. Levels of immunoglobulins E and G are elevated.

In Asia this disease is called Katayama fever. This syndrome, which resembles serum-sickness, occurs more frequently during acute infection with *S. japonicum,* which produces about 10 times more ova per female worm than *S. mansoni* or *S. haematobium.*

### Chronic Schistosomiasis Due to *S. mansoni* and *S. japonicum*

Most patients with chronic schistosomiasis never experience acute symptoms. The classic pseudotubercle may be found in liver biopsies as early as 80 days after exposure, but symptoms or signs of chronic schistosomiasis usually take from months to many years after initial contact to appear. Multiple exposures are probably necessary to acquire enough egg granulomas to produce severe chronic disease.

Patients with chronic schistosomiasis usually go to the doctor because of gastrointestinal bleeding or hepatosplenomegaly. The most striking symptoms are melena and hematemesis. Abdominal discomfort and intermittent diarrhea may be prominent. Patients with schistosomal portal hypertension tolerate multiple episodes of esophageal bleeding better than patients with intrahepatic portal hypertension (Garcia-Palmieri and Marcial-Rojas, 1961). Jaundice is characteristically absent except in terminal illness.

The liver is usually large, firm, and nontender. The spleen is greatly enlarged in virtually all cases of severe schistosomiasis due to *S. mansoni* and *S. japonicum.* Other findings that accompany Laennec's cirrhosis such as ascites, spider nevi, peripheral edema, testicular atrophy, and feminization are characteristically absent. The healthy appearance and absence of the stigmata of liver disease in the usual patient with hepatosplenic schistosomiasis are shown in Figure 5. In contrast, the patient in Figure 6 shows the signs of decompensated hepatosplenic schistosomiasis, which is present in only a small minority of cases.

Thrombocytopenia accompanies the severe hypersplenism. There is also blood-loss anemia, reduced hepatic clearance, hyperglobulinemia, hy-the suprapubic or perineal region. Bladder distention and hydronephrosis result from granulomas in the bladder wall, ureters, urethra, and prostate. Recurrent pyogenic urinary tract infections are common.

Cystoscopy discloses bleeding points, minute ulcers, and calcified sand-like excrescences in chronic cases. Pyelography reveals hydronephrosis, often with acute and chronic pyelonephritis, bladder calcification, and bladder-filling defects (Fig. 7).

## COMPLICATIONS AND SEQUELAE

The most common cause of death in hepatosplenic schistosomiasis is exsanguination from bleeding esophageal varices. Although rare, hepatic coma may occur after hemorrhage. In decompensated hepatosplenic schistosomiasis, chronic hepatitis with periportal inflammation

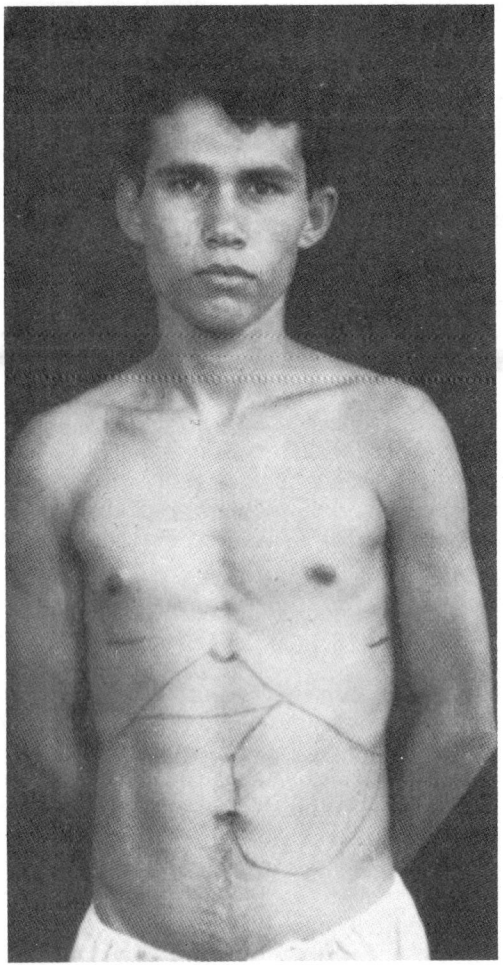

**FIGURE 5.** *Typical patient with compensated hepatosplenic schistosomiasis. Despite major hepatosplenomegaly, the patient appears healthy and shows none of the secondary manifestations of severe liver disease. (From Reboucas, G.: Yale J Biol Med 48:369, 1975.)*

poalbuminemia in 25 per cent of cases, elevated serum alkaline phosphatase, and diminished prothrombin. The serum bilirubin and pyruvic and oxalacetic transaminases are normal or slightly elevated. Varices can usually be demonstrated by esophagram, esophagoscopy, or splenoportography.

### Schistosomiasis Due to *S. haematobium*

All manifestations of acute schistosomiasis described above may occur during infections with *S. haematobium*. Although most worms migrate from the mesenteric to the pelvic veins and discharge their ova in the wall of the bladder, some ova are also deposited in the rectal mucosa.

Urinary frequency and dysuria are common early symptoms, but hematuria may be the first symptom. Microscopic hematuria progresses to frank bloody urine as the bladder mucosa ulcerates. Intermittent pain is usually referred to

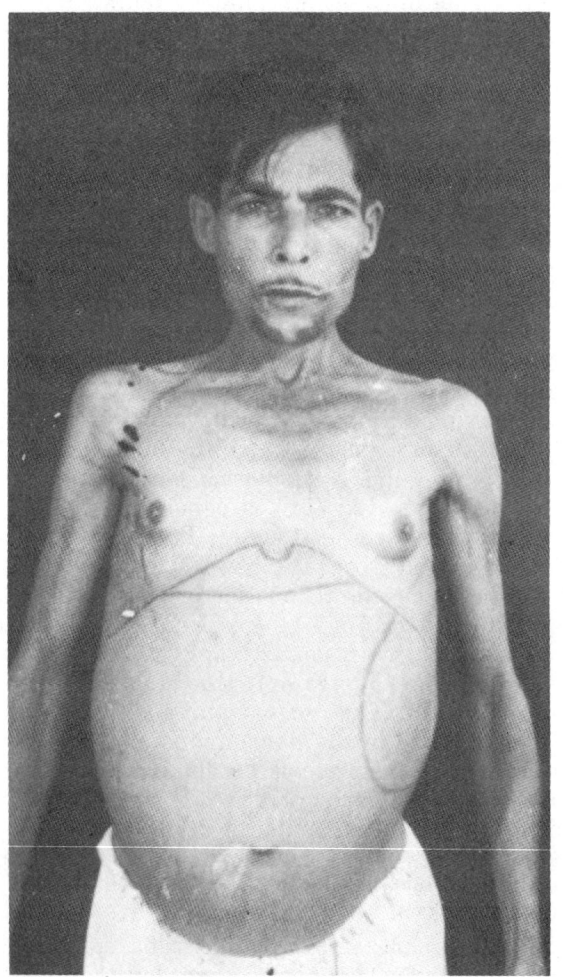

**FIGURE 6.** *Unusual patient with decompensated hepatosplenic schistosomiasis. This patient has gross ascites, gynecomastia, and emaciation. (From Reboucas, G.: Yale J Biol Med 48:369, 1975.)*

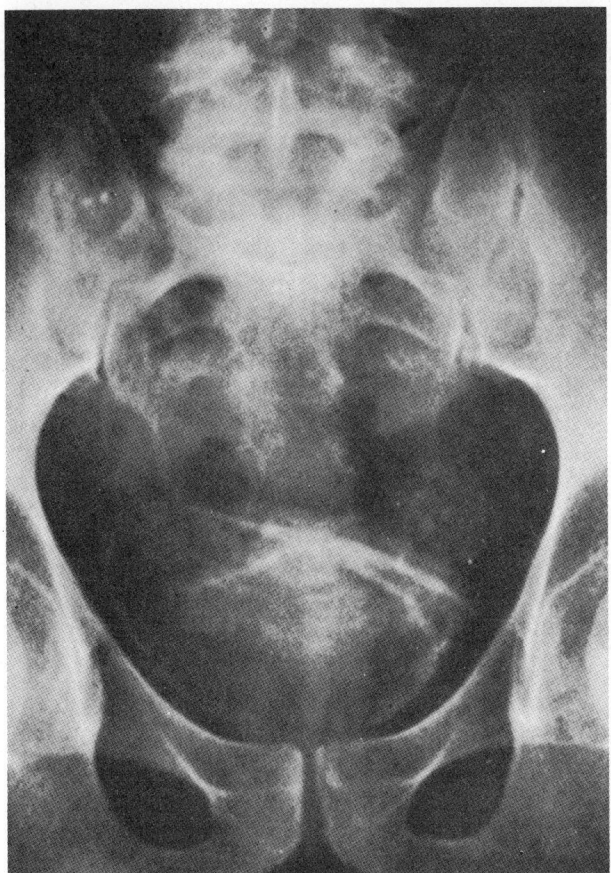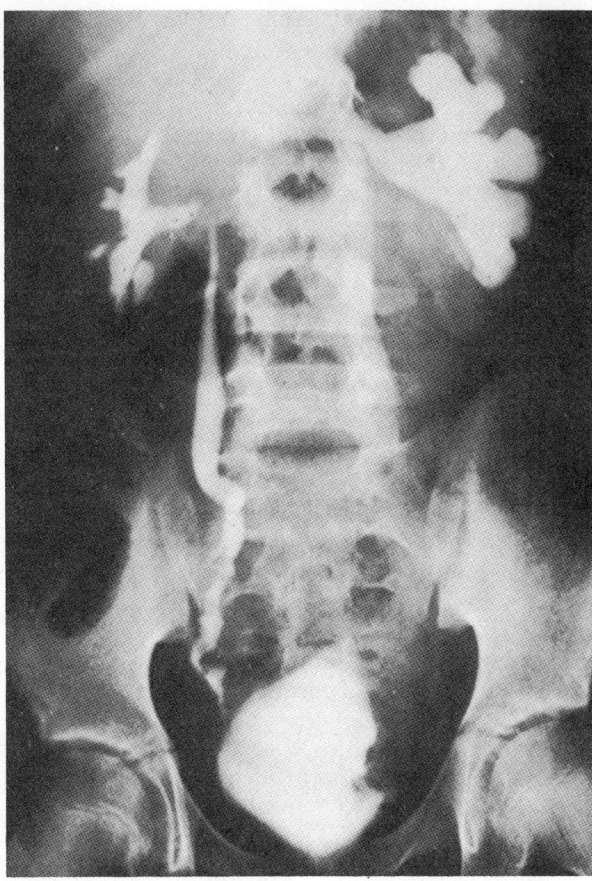

**FIGURE 7.** *Plain film of the abdomen (left), showing calcification of the bladder, and intravenous pyelogram (right), showing left hydroureter and hydronephrosis, right ureteral deformity, and bladder filling defects. (From Lehman, J. et al.: Ann Intern Med 75:49, 1971.)*

and bile duct proliferation is more prominent than in compensated schistosomiasis. In Brazil 1 per cent of spleens removed contain giant follicular lymphoma.

Mesangioproliferative glomerulonephritis with immune complexes has been demonstrated in renal biopsies. Chronic glomerulonephritis unrelated to the granulomas of urinary schistosomiasis has been reported in as many as 12 per cent of severe, postmortem cases.

Obstructive uropathy, chronic pyelonephritis, and renal failure are major complications of urinary schistosomiasis. The association of bladder carcinoma and *S. haematobium* is well-known. A causal role has been ascribed to beta-glucuronidase, which is increased in the urine of infected patients and is known to hydrolyze inactive glucuronides into carcinogenic substances (Norden and Gelfand, 1972).

Ectopic deposition of ova is a common and potentially severe complication of schistosomiasis. Pulmonary lesions may vary from scattered, asymptomatic granulomas to massive perivascular fibrosis with secondary cor pulmonale. Ectopic granulomas may occur in the spinal cord or brain.

Localization of *S. japonicum* in the brain is a major cause of epileptiform seizures.

Salmonellosis is common in patients infected with *S. mansoni* and *S. haematobium*. Reduced hepatic clearance and urinary obstruction probably contribute to the occurrence and persistence of these infections, but salmonellae also infect the tegument and tissues of schistosomes (Young et al., 1973).

## GEOGRAPHIC VARIATIONS

The manifestations of schistosomiasis vary with the geographic distribution of the different schistosomes. *S. japonicum* females produce about 10 times as many ova as the other schistosomes. Consequently, ectopic lesions and the early hypersensitivity manifestations of Katayama fever occur more commonly in Oriental schistosomiasis. Furthermore, the ova are deposited in aggregates, induce a more exudative response, and tend to calcify. For these reasons, and because of the greater number of ova, infections with *S. japonicum* are more fulminating and may progress to lethal pipestem cirrhosis within a year.

Within the geographic distribution of *S. mansoni,* severe hepatosplenic pathology is more common in Brazil, Egypt, and Puerto Rico than it is in the eastern, western, and southern parts of Africa. This difference has been ascribed to diet, but it is difficult to be certain that the differences are not due primarily to the degree of exposure and relative burden of ova and adult worms. Giant follicular lymphoma was found in 1 per cent of spleens removed from patients in Brazil, but further studies are necessary to establish the true comparative frequency of this complication.

Free-swimming cercariae of more than 20 non-human schistosomes are prevalent in many parts of the world. These parasites of birds and small mammals are distributed throughout the Americas, Europe, Australia, and New Zealand as well as Africa and Asia. Like the human schistosomes, they are limited by the distribution of a suitable snail host. Although these nonhuman schistosomes can penetrate human skin, the cercariae die in the skin or subcutaneous tissue. Unsensitized individuals may experience only a fleeting macular rash, but the sensitized patient can develop a papular eruption that persists for 7 to 10 days. The disease is self-limited and treatment is symptomatic.

A fourth species of schistosome, *S. intercalatum,* is found only in limited foci in West Central Africa and differs from *S. mansoni* in that the lateral spine is bent, the ova are acid-fast by Ziehl-Neelsen stain, and symptomatic disease is limited to the gastrointestinal tract (Wright, 1973). It is uncertain whether *S. intercalatum* is a separate species or a subspecies of *S. mansoni* or whether the morphology of the ova and the disease are merely altered by host defenses or other local environmental influences.

## IMMUNITY

Protective immunity (Allison et al., 1974; Smithers and Terry, 1975) has been demonstrated only in experimental animals, and only after infection with the living schistosomes. Good evidence indicates that the adults, not the eggs, provide the main stimulus for immunity in the rhesus monkey. Transfer of worms into rhesus monkeys induces protection to reinfection that is directed against the migrating schistosomula in the lungs. It is important to note that adult worms are protected from the immunity they provoke. Smithers and Terry call this phenomenon "concomitant immunity" and explain it on the basis of absorption of host antigens onto the surface of the worm, so that the worm antigens are concealed. Immunization of mice or rhesus monkeys with one schistosome species may convey immunity to another because of cross-reacting antigens. Unfortunately, immunity in animals that are good hosts for schistosomes, like man, is relatively weak, perhaps because the parasite and host share antigens or because the parasite surface is coated with host antigens. In contrast to man, animals that develop protective immunity can eliminate worms; for example, immunoincompetent rats show a delayed, yet efficient, elimination of the parasite.

The evidence for immunity in man (Bradley and McCullough, 1973; Warren, 1973b) is circumstantial. In most endemic areas, most infections occur in the second decade of life, as reflected by peak egg output. This age prevalence could be due to a combination of two factors. One is the more frequent water contact in early life and the other is the spontaneous death of worms. Several studies support the importance of these factors. The prevalence in women in Sierra Leone, who have more water contact than men throughout life, falls only a little from the peak, as compared with the greater fall in men. However, a group of men in Brazil who moved from a nonendemic to an endemic area showed the highest prevalence and intensity of infection 15 to 19 years after they moved. Also, in areas of very high transmission in Sierra Leone and southern Rhodesia, the prevalence peak is reached before age 10, whereas it occurs in the second decade of life in nearby areas with low transmission rates. Furthermore, in areas of high transmission rates in southern Rhodesia and St. Lucia (West Indies), children show a much higher egg output than do children in areas of low transmission rates. Among adults from these two areas, however, the egg output is similar and reduced. All these findings may point to some regulatory suppressive mechanisms, possibly acquired concomitant immunity 10 to 20 years after the initial infection. But these mechanisms, whatever their basis, are inefficient.

## DIAGNOSIS

Schistosomiasis must be suspected in any patient with a possible exposure history who presents with any of the following symptoms: fever, eosinophilia, hepatosplenomegaly, hematuria, obstructive uropathy, urinary tract infection, pulmonary granulomas, melena, or cor pulmonale. Patients may even present with granulomatous lesions of the skin or convulsions secondary to ectopic localization of ova.

Demonstration of the parasite is still the only reliable way to diagnose schistosomiasis. Ova of *S. mansoni* and *S. japonicum* (Chapter 80) may be demonstrated directly by examination of fecal smears, but this technique is not very sensitive, and negative stools must be examined by a concentration technique. For concentration, stools are suspended in 0.5 per cent glycerol in water and the suspension washed, sieved, and either centrifuged or allowed to yield sediment. The formol-ether and merthiolate-iodine-formol methods (Allen and Ridley, 1970; Beer, 1972) may be used either directly or on the sediment to remove detritus, mucus, and fats. The Bell filtration method uses ninhydrin as the stain (Bell, 1963), and the Kato technique (Martin and Beaver, 1969) uses a solution of glycerol malachite green.

After collecting urine near midday, S. haematobium ova are identified by sedimenting, filtering and examining the residue microscopically, with or without staining. The proportion of live eggs may be determined by suspending the ova in water, exposing them to light, and counting hatched miracidia. The number of viable ova measures the effectiveness of treatment.

Ova in stools must be repeatedly washed and concentrated before reliable viability tests may be performed. Rectal biopsy is the most successful method of diagnosing schistosomiasis when the stools are negative and the best way to assess the effectiveness of chemotherapy (Figs. 8 and 9). Biopsy material may be sectioned and processed like other tissue, but a squash preparation of the fresh tissue should always be examined as well. The viability of eggs can be tested by incubating the squashed biopsy material for 15 minutes in water.

Routine immunodiagnostic tests are either nonspecific, too insensitive, or both. Complement fixation, cholesterol-lecithin-flocculation, and immunofluorescent procedures are usually positive in heavy infections, but none are reliable in light infections. Recently, Pelley (1977) and his colleagues have described a promising radioimmunoassay in which they used radiolabeled egg antigen to detect 98 per cent of heavily infected adults and 83 per cent of lightly infected adolescents. This test was also specific.

## TREATMENT

Until recently, the only drug treatment for schistosomiasis has been the antimonials. Although fairly efficient, they are too toxic and frequently require supplemental surgical treatment. Their toxicity prevents their use for mass chemotherapy. Stibophen is available as a solution of 8.5 mg/ml of antimony and is given over two to three weeks to an accumulated dose of 80 ml. Antimony potassium tartrate is injected intravenously in a 0.5 per cent solution on alternate

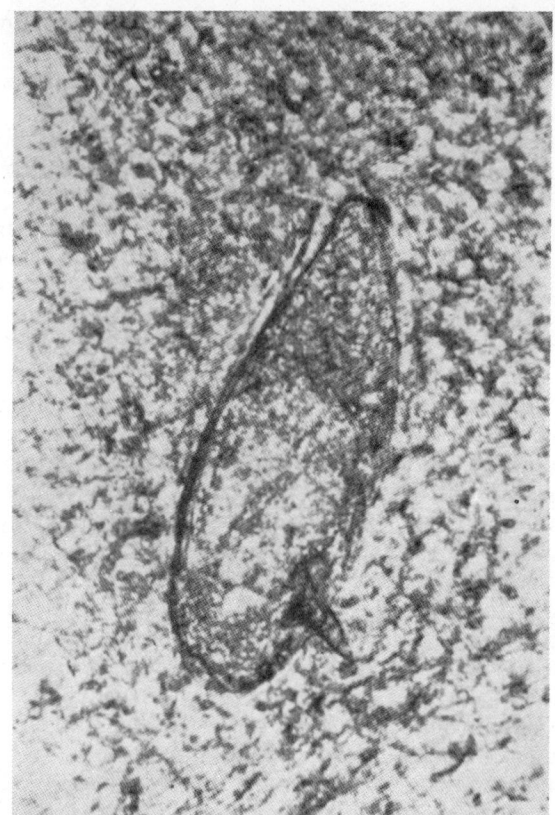

**FIGURE 8.** *Rectal biopsy containing a mature, viable ovum of* S. mansoni *(× 425). (From Spingarn, C. L. et al.: New Engl J Med 256:290, 1957.)*

days to a total of 360 ml. S. haematobium is the most sensitive to antimonials and S. japonicum the most resistant. Under the influence of antimonials, the schistosomes lose their hold in the blood vessels and are swept into the liver (hepatic shift). The observation that schistosomes are subject to a hepatic shift has popularized the use of an operation in which an extracorporeal filter is connected between a portal vein and a cutdown to

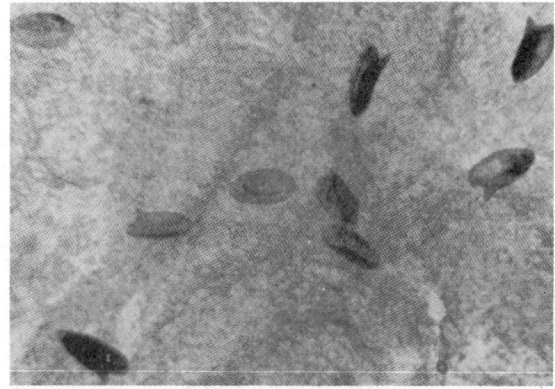

**FIGURE 9.** *Rectal biopsy showing degenerating ova of* S. mansoni *after treatment (× 75). (From Spingarn, C. L. et al.: New Engl J Med 256:290, 1957.)*

a peripheral vein in order to filter out parasites (Goldsmith et al., 1967).

The two newer drugs, niridazole and hycanthone, are not free from side effects, and there is concern about mutagenicity and carcinogenicity (Batzinger and Bueding, 1977), but they are more effective and less toxic than the antimonials.

Niridazole, a nitrothiazole derivative, can be given orally and is therefore useful for mass therapy, particularly for children. The recommended dose is 25 mg/kg in two daily doses for one week. The drug is very effective against *S. haematobium*, but less so against *S. mansoni* and produces cure in 20 to 100 per cent of patients depending on the dose. Vomiting, nausea, and diarrhea are common, and mental disturbances may occur. Experimentally, niridazole is anti-inflammatory (Riesterer et al., 1971) and suppresses delayed hypersensitivity as manifested by skin tests (Daniels et al., 1975) or formation of the egg granuloma (Mahmoud et al., 1975). This anti-inflammatory property may contribute to the effectiveness of niridazole against schistosomiasis.

Hycanthone is also suitable for mass therapy, since the total dose can be given in a single injection. The recommended dose has been 2.5 ± 0.5 mg/kg in one intramuscular injection. No deaths have been reported from the use of this drug, but vomiting and diarrhea are common. Ninety-seven per cent of patients with *S. mansoni* infections have been cured and the results with *S. haematobium* are probably equally as good. Several studies have indicated that half the recommended dose (1.5 mg/kg) achieves high cure rates. These studies (Warren et al., 1978; Rees et al., 1975) were based on the premise that elimination of all worms is not necessary for arresting the disease and that the preimmunity achieved by retaining a very low level of egg production may be useful in endemic areas.

Metrifonate, which is still under trial, arrests egg production in *S. haematobium* but is not useful for *S. mansoni*. Oxamniquine can be given orally and is effective against *S. mansoni*. Drowsiness, hallucinations, and excitability may be experienced, and very high doses are required for children.

Surgical treatment of schistosomiasis involves the correction of obstructive uropathy, resection of bladder polyps, resection of colonic polyps, and partial colectomy for severe gastrointestinal polyposis and fibrosis. Portal hypertension can be reversed by a distal splenorenal shunt (Wilson, 1976).

### *PROPHYLAXIS*

Visitors to endemic areas can escape schistosomiasis by avoiding contact with fresh water. Because this is difficult or impossible for the local population, extermination of the intermediate snail host is the most practical method of control. Niclosamide appears to be the best molluscicide and has an excellent record in Rhodesia, the Philippines, Egypt, Tanzania, and South Africa. It is used in a concentration of 4 to 8 parts per million per hour (ppm/hr) in flowing water. The most active molluscicide is *N*-trityl-morpholine, which is used at 0.1 to 0.5 ppm/hr. Sodium pentachlorophenate has been relatively reliable in Japan, Egypt, Rhodesia, and Venezuela when used at 50 to 80 ppm/hr. Copper sulfate (20 to 30 ppm/hr) is used in Egypt and the Sudan.

The snail habitat should be destroyed by clearing weeds from waterways, increasing the flow of water in irrigation ditches, and lining ditches with concrete. Clean water must be provided for household use in endemic areas. Safe sewage disposal is needed to prevent live eggs from reaching fresh water.

Mass chemotherapy with niridazole or hycanthone is another important method of control. The erection of new dams, extension of irrigation, and the use of freshwater ponds for commercial fish farming have complicated control efforts.

### References

Allen, A. V. H., and Ridley, D. S.: Further observations on the formol-ether concentration technique for faecal parasites. J Clin Pathol 23:545, 1970.

Allison, A. C., et al.: Immunology of schistosomiasis. Bull WHO 51:533, 1974.

Andrade, Z. A., and Cheever, A. W.: Alterations of the intrahepatic vasculature in hepatosplenic schistosomiasis mansoni. Am J Trop Med Hyg 20:425, 1971.

Ansari, N.: Epidemiology and control of schistosomiasis (bilharziasis). Basel, S. Karger, 1973.

Batzinger, R. P., and Bueding, E.: Mutagenic activities of five antischistosomal compounds. J Pharmacol Exp Ther 200:1, 1977.

Beer, R. J. S.: A rapid technique for the concentration and collection of helminth eggs from large quantities of faeces. Parasitology 65:343, 1972.

Bell, D. R.: A new method for counting *Schistosoma mansoni* eggs in faeces, with special reference to therapeutic trials. Bull WHO 29: 525, 1963.

Bradley, D. J., and McCullough, F. S.: Egg output stability and the epidemiology of *Schistosoma haematobium*. II. An analysis of the epidemiology of endemic *S. haematobium*. Trans R Soc Trop Med Hyg 67:491, 1973.

Colley, D. G., Magalhaes-Filho, A., and Barros Coelho, R.: Immunopathology of dermal reactions induced by *Schistosoma mansoni* cercariae and cercarial extract. J Trop Med Hyg 21:558, 1972.

Daniels, J. C., Warren, K. S., and David, J. R.: Studies on the mechanism of suppression of delayed hypersensitivity by the antischistosomal compound niridazole. J Immunol 115:1414, 1975.

Diaz-Rivera, R. S., Ramos Morales, F., Sotomayer, Z. R., Lichtenberg, F., Garcia-Palmieri, M. R., Cintron-Rivera, A. A., and Marchand, E. J.: The pathogenesis of Manson's schistosomiasis. Ann Intern Med 47:1082, 1957.

Garcia-Palmieri, M. R., and Marcial-Rojas, R. A.: The protean manifestations of schistosomiasis mansoni. A clinicopathological correlation. Ann Intern Med 57:763, 1962.

Goldsmith, E. I., et al.: Surgical recovery of schistosomes from the portal blood. JAMA 199:235, 1967.

Jordan, P., and Webbe, G.: Human schistosomiasis. London, Heinemann, 1969.

Katz, M.: Anthelminthics. Drugs 13:124, 1977.

Lehman, J., Stauffer, Z. F., Bassily, S., and Kent, D. C.: Hydronephrosis, bacteriuria, and maximal urine concentration in urinary schistosomiasis. Ann Intern Med 75:49, 1971.

von Lichtenberg, F., et al.: Experimental infection with *Schistosoma japonicum* in chimpanzees: Parasitologic, clinical, serologic and pathological observations. Am J Trop Med Hyg 20:850, 1971.

Mahmoud, A. A. F., Mandel, M. A., Warren, K. S., and Webster, L. T.: Niridazole. II. A potent, long-acting suppressant of cellular hypersensitivity. J Immunol 114:279, 1975.

Marchand, E. J., Marcial-Rojas, R. A., Rodriguez, R., Polanco, G., and Diaz-Rivera, R. S.: The pulmonary obstruction syndrome in *Schistosoma mansoni* pulmonary endarteritis. Arch Intern Med 100:965, 1957.

Martin, L. K., and Beaver, P. C.: Evaluation of Kato thick-smear technique for quantitative diagnosis of helminth infections. Am J Trop Med Hyg 17:382, 1969.

Norden, D. A., and Gelfand, M.: Bilharzia and bladder cancer. An investigation of urinary glucuronidase associated with *S. haematobium* infection. Trans R Soc Trop Med Hyg 66:865, 1972.

Pelley, R. P., Warren, K. S., and Jordan, P.: Purified antigen radioimmunoassay in serological diagnosis of schistosomiasis mansoni. Lancet 2:781, 1977.

Reboucas, G.: Clinical aspects of hepatosplenic schistosomiasis: A contrast with cirrhosis. Yale J Biol Med 48:369, 1975.

Rees, P. H., Bowny, H. N., Robert, J. M. D., and Thuku, J. J.: The treatment of schistosomiasis mansoni in Murang'a District, Kenya: A double blind controlled trial of three hycanthone regimens and oxamniquine. Am J Trop Med Hyg 24:823, 1975.

Riesterer, L., Majer, H., and Jaques, R.: On the anti-inflammatory properties of the schistosomicide niridazole (Ambilhar). Experientia 27:546, 1971.

Sadun, E. H., et al.: Experimental infection with *Schistosoma haematobium* in chimpanzees: Parasitologic, clinical, serologic and pathological observations. Am J Trop Med Hyg 19:427, 1970.

Smithers, S. R., and Terry, R. J.: The immunology of schistosomiasis. Adv Parasitol 13:41, 1975.

Spingarn, C. L., Edelman, M. H., Gold, T., Yarnis, H., and Turell, R.: Value of rectal biopsies in the diagnosis and treatment of *Schistosoma mansoni* infections. N Engl J Med 256:290, 1957.

Stirewalt, M. A., and Dorsey, C. H.: *Schistosoma mansoni:* Cercarial penetration of host epidermis at the ultrastructural level. Exp. Parasitol 35:1, 1974.

Warren, K. S.: The immunopathogenesis of schistosomiasis: A multidisciplinary approach. Trans R Soc Trop Med Hyg 66:417, 1972.

Warren, K. S.: The pathology of schistosome infections. Helminth abstracts series A 42:591, 1973a.

Warren, K. S.: Regulation of the prevalence and intensity of schistosomiasis in man: Immunity or ecology? J Infect Dis 127:595, 1973b.

Warren, K. S., Ouma, J. H., Arap Siongok, T. K., and Houser, H. B.: Hycanthone dose-response in *Schistosoma mansoni* infection in Kenya. Lancet 1:352, 1978.

Wilson, R. B.: Surgical implications of *Schistosoma mansoni* infestation. Mt Sinai J Med 43:657, 1976.

Wright, W. H.: Geographic distribution of schistosomas and their intermediate hosts. In Ansari, N. (ed.): Epidemiology and Control of Schistosomiasis (Bilharziasis). Baltimore, University Park Press, 1973, pp. 32–249.

Young, C. W., Higashi, G., Kamel, R., El-Abdin, A. Z., and Mikhail, I. A.: Interaction of salmonellae and schistosomes in host-parasite relations. Trans R Soc Trop Med Hyg 67:797, 1973.

# *VIRAL GASTROENTERITIS* **135**

## Ruth Bishop, D.Sc.

Gastroenteritis is a common illness that occurs in epidemic and sporadic form throughout the world. The disease is most severe in infants and young children, and is one of the major causes of death in childhood, particularly in malnourished children. Gastroenteritis results from infection of the gastrointestinal tract by a variety of microorganisms, including viruses, and clinical symptoms are not a reliable guide to the identity of the microbial pathogen.

### DEFINITION

Viral gastroenteritis is an infection of the gastrointestinal tract by a recognized viral enteric pathogen resulting in mucosal inflammation and altered transport of water and electrolytes.

### ETIOLOGY

Electron microscopy has identified two types of viral particles that do not grow readily in cell culture but are undoubtedly responsible for gastroenteritis in humans (Leading Article, 1975). Advances in knowledge of these agents are reviewed in detail by Schreiber et al., (1977).

### Human Parvovirus-like Agents

This is a heterogeneous group of viruses (27 to 30 nm in diameter) associated with epidemics of gastroenteritis in children and adults. The particles have a variety of names, which usually indicate the geographic location of the outbreak and include Norwalk agent (Kapikian et al., 1972), Hawaii agent, Montgomery County agent (Thornhill et al., 1977), and W agent (Appleton et al., 1977). These particles have been only partially characterized. They have similar morphologies but are antigenically distinct, and are thought to be parvoviruses or picornaviruses. Norwalk agent is representative of this group.

*Norwalk Agent.* This agent was first seen by immune electron microscopy of diarrheal feces from an experimentally infected adult volunteer (Fig. 1). Extracts of diarrheal feces, processed to remove contaminating bacteria and larger viruses, regularly produce acute gastroenteritis in 50 per cent of adult volunteers after oral ingestion. The incubation period is 18 to 48 hours, and symptoms last for 24 to 48 hours. Virus-like particles are detectable in feces for 72 hours from onset of symptoms and are absent from stools during convalescence. Seroconversion occurs during infection, but immunity is not lasting.

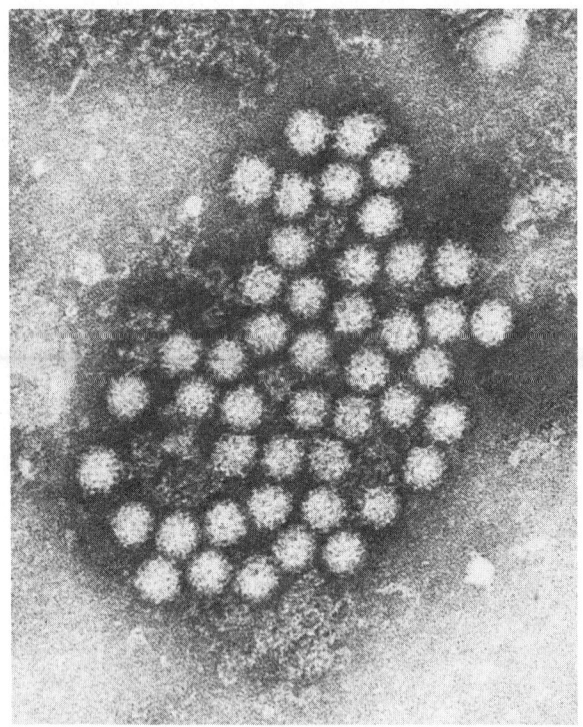

**FIGURE 1.** *Immune aggregate of Norwalk agent in stool filtrate. (×156,000) (From Kapikian, A. Z. et al.: J Virol 10:1075, 1972.)*

The extent to which this and related agents are responsible for sporadic and epidemic diarrhea in children and adults throughout the world is not known. Antibodies detected in a commercial preparation of immune serum globulin indicate that this or a related particle commonly infects the general population in the United States.

### Rotaviruses

First described in 1973 in epithelial cells of duodenal mucosa from children with acute gastroenteritis (Bishop et al., 1973), this virus has since been given several names, including duovirus, rotavirus, orbivirus, infantile gastroenteritis virus (IGV), and human reovirus-like agent (HRVL). The name rotavirus has been most widely accepted.

Rotavirus particles seen in diarrheal feces (Fig. 2) are double-stranded RNA viruses, to be classified as members of a new genus within the family Reoviridae. This new genus includes other rotaviruses that cause diarrhea in the young of many mammalian species, including calves, pigs, lambs, foals, mice, and rabbits. These animal viruses are morphologically identical with human rotaviruses but differ antigenically from them and from each other.

Rotaviruses cause sporadic and epidemic disease in all age groups, but severity of disease and serologic response to infection differ.

***Newborn Babies.*** Rotaviruses infect many newborn babies in obstetric hospital nurseries during the first week of life. Diarrhea can be severe but is often asymptomatic because of passive protection by maternal antibodies acquired transplacentally or through breast milk. Breast milk contains rotavirus antibodies during the first week of lactation; however, not all breast-fed babies are protected against symptomatic infection.

Virus particles are shed in feces before onset of symptoms, so isolating only symptomatic babies is unlikely to control spread of infection in a communal nursery. Seroconversion, measured by complement fixation or indirect immunofluorescence, seldom occurs after infection in the newborn. It is not known whether infection in the neonatal period results in immunity to disease in later childhood.

***Infants and Young Children.*** In temperate climates, most children aged three months to five years who require hospitalization for acute gastroenteritis shed rotaviruses in their feces, often in enormous numbers. Rotavirus infection is seasonal with a peak incidence during winter months (Davidson et al., 1975). The incubation period of the disease is 24 to 48 hours. Virus particles are usually shed in feces in detectable numbers for four to eight days after onset of symptoms. Nosocomial infection is common in children less than three years of age admitted to

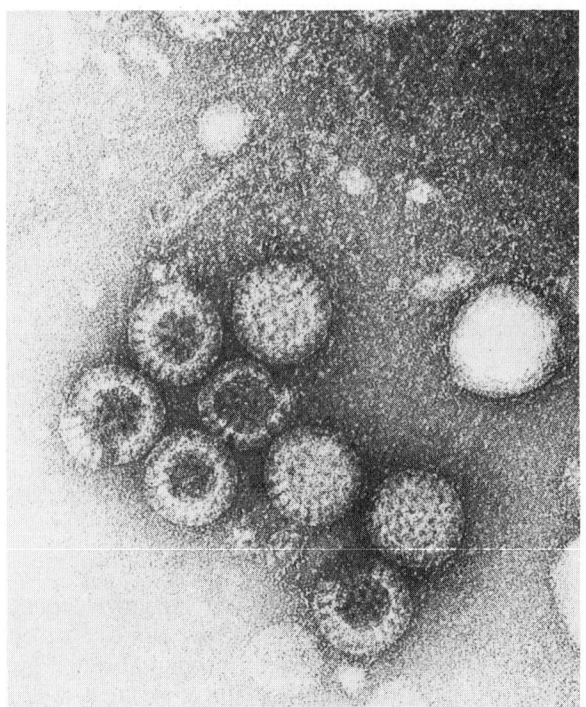

**FIGURE 2.** *Rotavirus particles in extract of diarrheal stool. (× 132,000).*

hospital with other illnesses. Most infants and young children with rotavirus diarrhea show no detectable levels of complement-fixing antibody at the onset of symptoms, and seroconversion occurs during the disease. The duration of immunity is not known. Symptomatic reinfection has been recorded.

Rotaviruses are an important cause of diarrhea in tropical climates, but their seasonality and importance as an etiologic agent relative to enterotoxigenic *Escherichia coli* is not known.

***Older Children and Adults.*** By the age of three to five years, most children possess CF antibodies to rotavirus (Blacklow et al., 1976; Gust et al., 1977), and infection is often asymptomatic. Epidemics of diarrhea have been documented in school children 6 to 12 years old and in adults. Fourfold or greater rises in CF rotavirus antibody occur in some adults with diarrhea, but rotavirus particles are not usually shed in feces in sufficient numbers to be detected by electron microscopy.

### Other Viruses

A variety of virus particles has been observed by electron microscopy in diarrheal feces from newborn babies, children, and adults. Their relation to the etiology of diarrhea is uncertain, but some may prove to be pathogens following satisfaction of Koch's postulates as applied to viruses (Rivers, 1937).

***Astroviruses.*** These viruses were first described in the United Kingdom in the stools of newborn babies with mild diarrhea and later associated with nosocomial gastroenteritis (Kurtz et al., 1977). The particles are 28 to 30 nm in diameter, exhibit a star-like appearance, and grow poorly, producing no cytopathogenic effects in human embryo kidney cells. The geographic distribution throughout the world is unknown.

***Coronaviruses.*** These agents may be enteric pathogens in man as they are in pigs, dogs, and calves (Kapikian, 1977). Coronavirus-like particles have been seen in an outbreak of gastroenteritis in the United Kingdom and in feces from Indian villagers, Australian aborigines, and residents of a training center for the intellectually retarded. They may not be associated with any specific disease but may contribute to intestinal morphologic abnormalities and malabsorption.

***Adenoviruses.*** Electron microscopy has revealed adenoviruses that are not cultivable by the usual cell culture techniques in 5 to 10 per cent of children with gastroenteritis and in nosocomial gastroenteritis. Their etiologic association with development of disease is uncertain.

Adenoviruses and echoviruses cultivable by routine cell culture have been isolated from occasional epidemics of diarrhea. Calicivirus particles

have been described in the gut mucosa obtained at postmortem from one child with acute gastroenteritis. A variety of small virus-like particles 22 nm in diameter have been seen in human feces (Flewett et al., 1974). They may be bacteriophages or nonpathogenic viruses that infect human gut cells or are shed into the gut lumen from other tissues.

## PATHOGENESIS AND PATHOLOGY

Infection with rotaviruses, Norwalk agent, and Hawaii agent results in similar nonspecific and reversible inflammatory changes in human gut mucosa.

The viruses multiply in mature epithelial cells lining the villi of the small intestine (Fig. 3). These cells show vacuolation of the endoplasmic reticulum, swollen mitochondria, increased numbers of cell lysosomes, and multivesicular bodies. Microvilli are irregular and shortened. The cells undergo lysis, leaving the villi denuded. The villi rapidly collapse and are covered by immature epithelial cells that migrate from the crypts.

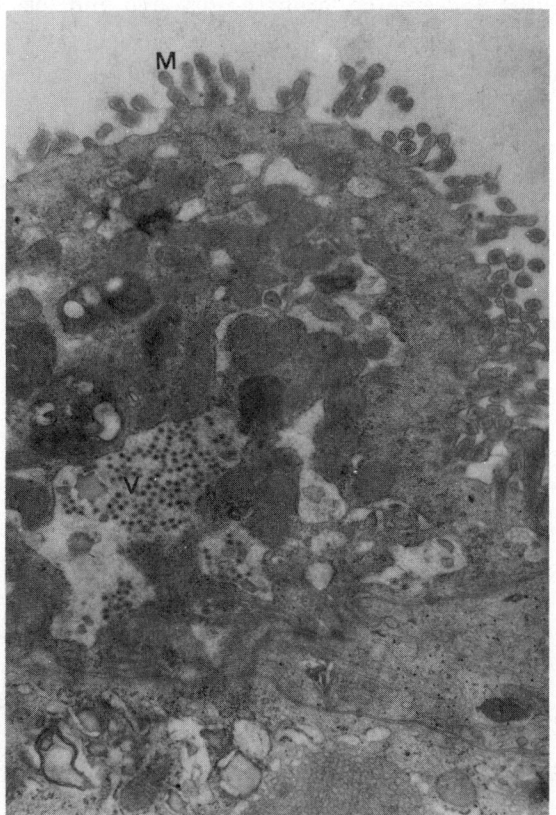

**FIGURE 3.** *Portion of an epithelial cell of a duodenal villus infected with rotavirus. M, microvilli; V, rotavirus particles. (× 16,000)*

The pathogenesis of diarrhea probably involves two stages. Initially, denudation of villi allows leakage of fluid and electrolytes into the gut lumen. Later, contraction of the denuded villi and replacement of mature epithelial cells by enzymatically immature cells are associated with the more severe stage of diarrhea (Davidson et al., 1977). This severe stage is probably due to a combination of factors that may include a decrease in the total absorptive surface of the small intestine, a decrease in activity of epithelial cell brush border enzymes including disaccharidases, and secretion by crypt-type cells. Glucose-coupled sodium transport is decreased during viral enteritis compared with infection due to enterotoxigenic bacteria (for example, *Vibrio cholerae* or *E. coli*), in which it is unaffected.

Infection with viral enteric pathogens seems to be restricted to the mucosa of the small intestine, although the stomach and rectal mucosa are mildly inflamed in some children. There is no proof of viremia. Histologically, the gut mucosa shows mild to moderate patchy inflammatory change in most patients (Figs. 4, 5, and 6). Villi appear shorter and blunter and are lined by epithelial cells that are cuboidal and irregular in shape. The lamina propria is infiltrated with mononuclear cells and polymorphonuclear leukocytes. In some children the damage and loss of

villi are severe enough to resemble celiac disease (Fig. 7).

It is not known to what extent the severity of clinical symptoms is correlated with the extent of infection along the small intestine. Infection in fatal cases has been seen to extend along the length of the small bowel.

Persistent histologic damage and depression of disaccharidase levels occur in some children, particularly those less than six months old, and may account for sugar intolerance after the symptoms of acute gastroenteritis have subsided. In most children and adults diarrhea is of short duration (one to three days), and the gut mucosa is histologically normal three to four weeks from onset of symptoms.

The bacterial flora of the upper small intestine remains normal in well-nourished children and adults during acute viral gastroenteritis, although increased numbers of *Candida albicans* are present in some children and may prolong gut damage and exacerbate sugar intolerance. Colonization of the stomach and small intestine may be a consequence of acute gastroenteritis in malnourished children.

### CLINICAL MANIFESTATIONS

Viral gastroenteritis has a sudden onset. The symptoms are watery diarrhea, fever, nausea and vomiting, and colicky abdominal pain. Vomiting and fever often precede diarrhea. Stools contain excess electrolytes and may also contain excess sugar (> 0.5 per cent) but blood or leukocytes are uncommon. An apparent upper respiratory tract infection with pharyngeal and tympanic membrane erythema may be present.

Loss of salt and water in stools has little systemic effect in older children and adults. In infants and children less than five years old such losses can lead rapidly to dehydration, electrolyte imbalance, acidosis, shock, and death. Early signs of dehydration are often difficult to detect, particularly in obese or malnourished children. The detectable signs of dehydration are dry mouth, sunken eyes, poor peripheral circulation, and sunken fontanelles. The child may be either irritable or lethargic. The skin loses its elasticity and, if pinched up on the abdominal wall, does not immediately spring back. Decreased urine output is often difficult to detect because movements may be very watery.

The best guide to the degree of dehydration in well-nourished children is measured weight loss. Loss of 5 per cent of body weight (5 per cent dehydration) can just be detected clinically. Severe dehydration occurs when 10 per cent or more

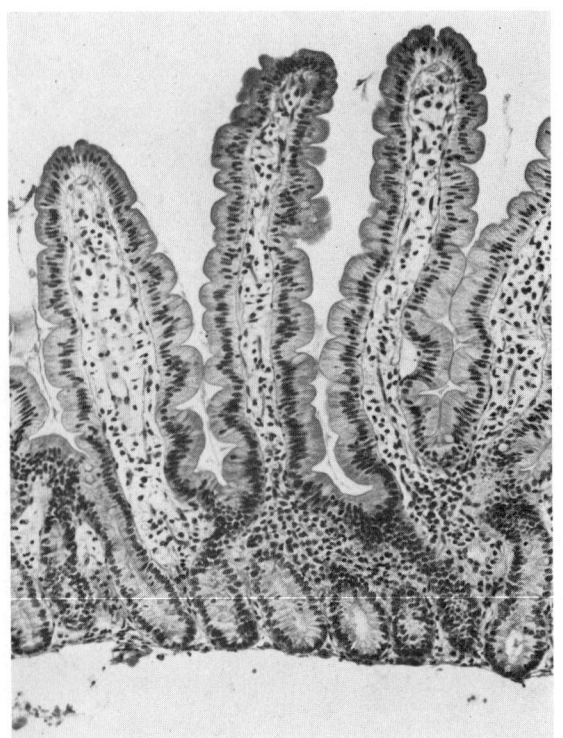

**FIGURE 4.** *Normal duodenal mucosa from a 4-year-old child.* (*Hematoxylin and eosin,* ×125)

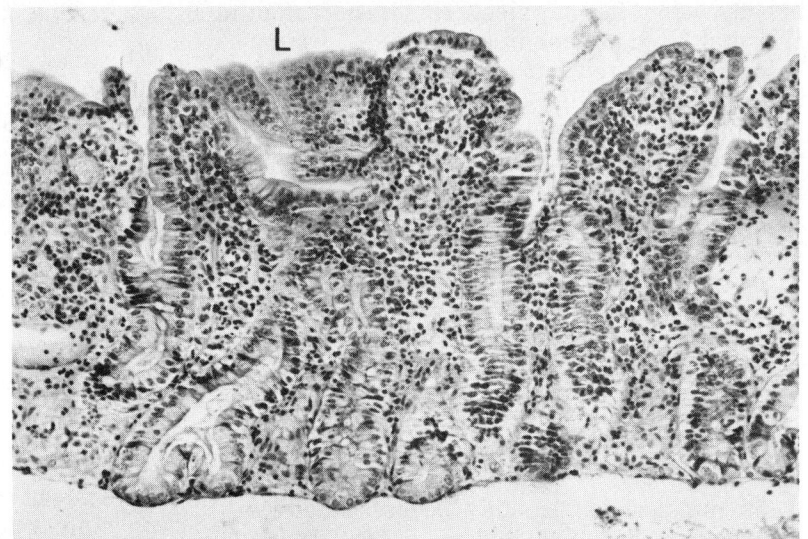

**FIGURE 5.** *Moderately damaged duodenal mucosa from a 19-month-old child with rotavirus enteritis after two days of illness. Villi are shortened. There is cellular infiltration of the lamina propria and patchy epithelial damage. L, lumen. (Hematoxylin and eosin, ×125)*

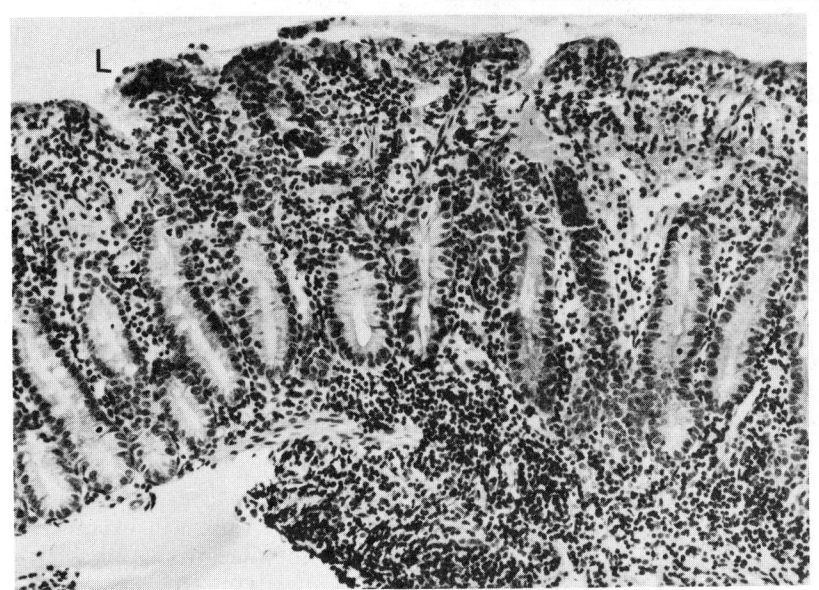

**FIGURE 6.** *Severely damaged duodenal mucosa from a 31-month-old child with rotavirus enteritis after two days of illness. (Hematoxylin and eosin, ×125)*

**FIGURE 7.** *Duodenal mucosa from a 13-month-old child with celiac disease. (Hematoxylin and eosin, ×125)*

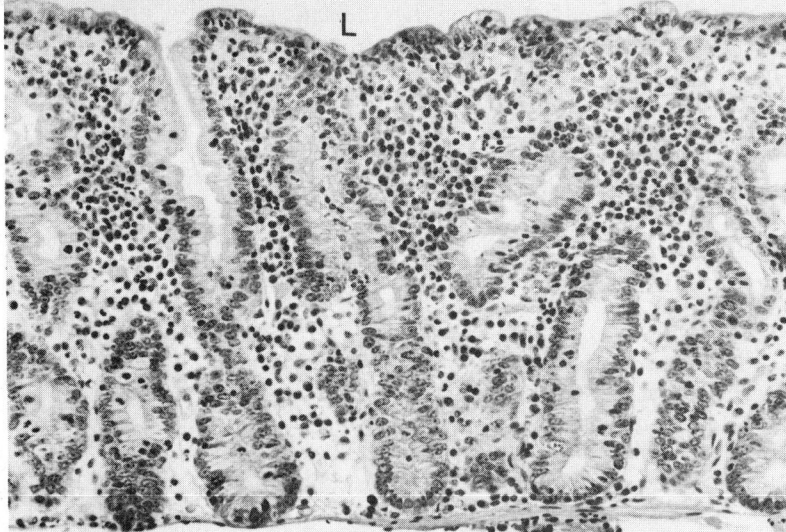

of body weight has been lost. This is equivalent to the total blood volume in an infant.

In most children salt losses equal water losses so that serum sodium levels change little. Some patients lose more water than salt and develop hypernatremia. Others become hyponatremic, a special problem in malnourished children. Severe hypokalemia may occur in enteritis associated with malnutrition.

## COMPLICATIONS AND SEQUELAE

Viral gastroenteritis is usually self-limited, lasting less than a week. The complications are dehydration with peripheral circulatory failure and death, and hypernatremia (serum sodium >150 mmol/L), which may be associated with convulsions. Sequelae include a persistence of diarrhea, which is associated with sugar intolerance, exacerbation of existing malnutrition, and protracted diarrhea of infancy.

Approximately 1 per cent of children admitted to hospital in urban developed communities die from dehydration and fluid-electrolyte imbalance. Mortality rates among malnourished children for whom medical attention is not readily available can be as high as 30 per cent (Rohde and Northrup, 1976). The severity of diarrhea increases with the degree of malnutrition. Deaths due to viral gastroenteritis in India alone may approach 350,000 per year (Maiya et al., 1977).

Sequelae of viral gastroenteritis differ according to age and nutritional state. Well-nourished older children and adults usually recover quickly with no sequelae. In young children, particularly those less than six months old, diarrhea due to sugar intolerance, which is caused by depression of disaccharidase enzymes, can persist for months.

In malnourished children, the diarrheal episode leads to further malnutrition owing to decreased appetite and restriction of calorie intake. An infant or child given no food will lose approximately 1 per cent of his body weight per day. If the child is already on the borderline of malnutrition this weight loss is serious and can contribute to growth retardation.

## DIAGNOSIS

Viral gastroenteritis cannot reliably be distinguished from gastroenteritis caused by other infectious agents on clinical evidence alone. Diagnosis is based on finding viral particles in stool or gut contents, or demonstration of a seroresponse to a viral antigen during infection.

### Detection of Viral Particles

A variety of techniques of locating noncultivable viruses in diarrheal stools are available. These techniques vary in efficiency and in practicality. Most have been used only to detect rotaviruses. Feces should be obtained no later than four days after onset of symptoms and can be stored, preferably at +4° C or −70° C, until tested. All techniques are relatively insensitive compared with cell culture for isolation of cultivable viruses.

*Electron Microscopy.* This technique is simple, rapid, and efficient. It permits detection of a wide variety of morphologically different particles but is impractical for large-scale surveys. Fluid feces can be screened for virus particles after negative staining with sodium phosphotungstate or ammonium molybdate. Extracts free of cell debris can also be prepared by differential centrifugation in an ultracentrifuge (Bishop et al., 1974). Norwalk agent and similar parvovirus-like agents require immune electron microscopy for detection, whereby fecal extracts are reacted with convalescent serum from a patient recently infected with the appropriate viral agent (Kapikian et al., 1975b).

*Counter Immunoelectro-osmophoresis.* Stool suspensions and rotavirus antisera are placed in adjacent wells on an agarose slide and examined for precipitin lines after incubation and application of an electric current (Middleton et al., 1976). The technique is less sensitive and less specific than electron microscopy but easy to perform, inexpensive, and suitable for rapid screening of many specimens.

*Enzyme-Linked Immunosorbent Assay (ELISA).* Rotavirus antigen in stool extracts is detected by incubation in microtiter trays with rotavirus antisera, followed by the addition of enzyme-conjugated anti-immunoglobulins (Yolken et al., 1977a). The test is sensitive and specific and applicable to large-scale epidemiologic surveys.

*Radioimmunoassay (RIA).* After the reaction of crude unfiltered fecal suspensions with rotavirus antisera in microtiter trays [125]I-labeled globulin is added (Kalica et al., 1977).

*Fluorescent Virus Precipitation Test.* This test is described by Yolken and his co-workers (1977b). It detects virus-antibody complexes by fluorescent microscopy of stool extracts.

*Cell Culture Methods.* Use of fetal intestinal organ culture or monolayers of fetal epithelial cells is inefficient. A technique described by Banatvala et al. (1975) in which 20 per cent fecal filtrate is inoculated onto monolayers of pig kidney cells (IBRS-2) and then centrifuged, incubated, and stained by indirect immunofluorescence is relatively efficient in detecting rotavirus but impractical for large-scale surveys.

### Detection of Antibodies

The in vitro techniques for detection of rotavirus antibodies include complement fixation (Kapikian et al., 1975a), indirect immunofluorescence with sections of infected gut or cell cultures, RIA, and ELISA. Most of these techniques have been adapted for use as antigen the readily available animal rotaviruses (NCDV, SA11, or O agent) that are antigenically related to human rotavirus.

Antibody response to infection with Norwalk agent and related agents is demonstrated by immune electron microscopy.

*Rotavirus treatment*

## *TREATMENT*

Antidiarrheal preparations and antispasmodics are of little value in treatment of viral gastroenteritis and may be dangerous for young children. Antiemetics may give relief in older children and adults when the main symptom is vomiting. Antibiotics are of no value in treatment of viral enteritis and in fact may cause further mucosal damage. When the etiologic agent is unknown, antibiotics are indicated only if there is clinical suspicion of septicemia or meningitis.

Childhood diarrhea is initially treated by oral rehydration at home. Although glucose-stimulated $Na^+$ absorption is decreased in viral gastroenteritis, it is possible that sufficient uninfected gut remains to allow some absorption of water, electrolytes, and glucose. It is extremely important to start rehydration early, because dehydration begins with the first diarrheal stool. The measures adopted for oral rehydration vary according to the state of nutrition of the child. Well-nourished children in developed countries are treated by temporary withdrawal of regular feeds, and oral feeding with isotonic carbohydrate solutions, such as soft drinks exhausted of carbonation, glucose, or corn syrup in boiled water (one tablespoon/liter). It is important not to give solutions containing large amounts of sodium since they may lead to, or worsen, hypernatremia.

In developing countries, rehydration is begun at home by using Oralyte packets (UNICEF), containing NaCl 3.5 g, $NaHCO_3$ 2.5 g, KCl 1.5 g, and glucose 20 g. These are available at village stores or are distributed by local health workers. Contents of the package are diluted in one liter of clean water and given initially to assuage thirst. This is followed by one glass of prepared fluid for each stool passed (Rohde and Northrup, 1976). If the UNICEF packages are not available, a simple rehydration kit can be assembled locally (Cut-

ting, 1976). Breast feeding, if established, should be continued.

Once moderate dehydration is evident, the patient should be hospitalized. Electrolyte and acid-base studies are not required routinely but are indicated if there is severe dehydration, disturbance of the conscious state, twitching, or convulsions. Intravenous fluid volumes are adjusted to replace fluid and electrolyte *deficit* with saline (40 mmol/L of sodium chloride and dextrose, 5 per cent). Once urine output is established, 40 mmol/L of potassium chloride is added. The deficit of fluid and electrolytes is usually replaced during the first 24 hours in the absence of hypernatremic dehydration. During the first 24 hours it is also necessary to administer *maintenance* fluid requirements and to replace *continuing losses* due to vomiting, diarrhea, and insensible losses. Maintenance fluid requirements adjusted for age are then continued until an oral diet is established.

Hypernatremic dehydration has special hazards including convulsions and other neurologic sequelae. Intravenous rehydration should be slow (e.g., replacement of deficit over 48 hours or more). This allows more time for electrolyte and water transport across cell membranes and decreases the likelihood of cerebral edema.

Peripheral circulatory failure occurs in severe dehydration (>10 per cent body weight loss). It is characterized by tachycardia, weak pulse, low blood pressure, and cold mottled skin over the extremities. The first priority is to restore circulation with isotonic fluids. In otherwise healthy children isotonic electrolyte solutions containing some bicarbonate (20 to 25 ml/kg given in 30 minutes) will suffice. In malnourished children hypoproteinemia may be present, so plasma or whole blood may be more appropriate. After circulation has been restored, rehydration and maintenance fluids are given as above.

Within 24 to 48 hours of the start of intravenous therapy, oral fluids can usually be reintroduced. Initially, glucose-electrolyte solutions are given as described above. In most patients the previous diet can be resumed a day or two later, but fruits and other foods that may cause loose movements in healthy children should be avoided. If diarrhea persists, stools should be checked for sugar content by the Clinitest method (Kerry and Anderson, 1964). A sugar concentration of greater than 0.5 per cent is abnormal. Glucose-containing milk substitutes can be used when available. Many children with lactose intolerance can tolerate sucrose feeds. It may be necessary to stop breast feeding temporarily; the mother should express breast milk meantime to maintain the flow. In malnourished children and infants under three months the primary concern after 48 to 72 hours should be reestablishment of an adequate nutrient intake, even at the expense of an increase in fecal output. If oral feeding cannot be resumed within three or four days, the use of parenteral nutrition should be considered.

## PROPHYLAXIS

Improvements in housing, environmental sanitation, and purity of water supplies should reduce the incidence of enteric disease in developing countries but may have little impact on viral gastroenteritis, since this remains a major health problem even in wealthy, developed, urban communities. Control of viral enteritis awaits understanding of the mechanisms of immunity and may be achieved eventually by oral vaccination, particularly against rotavirus; however, more immediate prophylactic measures against viral gastroenteritis are available and should be used.

### Prevention of Gastroenteritis in Infants

Infection with rotaviruses in babies is often asymptomatic, probably due to passive protection by maternal antibody acquired transplacentally or in breast milk. In countries where nutrition of the small child is threatened by poverty and inadequate diet, breast feeding may be vital in protecting against viral enteric infection.

### Prevention of Nosocomial Infection

This should be possible by attention to strict standards of hygiene in hospital wards. Design and staffing of wards must take into account the highly infectious nature of viral enteric pathogens.

### Prevention of Dehydration

This is of major importance in reducing deaths due to viral gastroenteritis and may be a key factor in preventing onset or exacerbation of malnutrition in infants in poor communities (Rohde and Northrup, 1976). It is necessary first to inform mothers that diarrhea is not a normal phase of growth but a life-threatening disease. Through health education, parents can be made to understand the need for early oral rehydration and can be given the means to do so with readily available cheap sources of glucose and electrolytes.

## References

Appleton, H., Buckley, M., Thom, B. T., Cotton, T. L., and Henderson, S.: Virus-like particles in winter vomiting disease. Lancet 1:409, 1977.

Banatvala, J. E., Totterdell, B., Chrystie, I. L., and Woode, G. N.: *In vitro* detection of human rotaviruses. Lancet 2:821, 1975.

Bishop, R. F., Davidson, G. P., Holmes, I. H., and Ruck, B. J.: Virus particles in epithelial cells of duodenal mucosa from children with acute non-bacterial gastroenteritis. Lancet 2:1281, 1973.

Bishop, R. F., Davidson, G. P., Holmes, I. H., and Ruck, B. J.: Detection of a new virus by electron microscopy of faecal extracts from children with acute gastroenteritis. Lancet 1:149, 1974.

Backlow, N. R., Echeverria, P., and Smith, P. H. Serological studies with reovirus-like enteritis agent. Infect Immun 13:1563, 1976.

Cutting, W. A. M.: In Acute Diarrhoea in Childhood. Ciba Foundation Symposium 42 (new series). Amsterdam, Elsevier Publishing Company, 1976, p. 361.

Davidson, G. P., Bishop, R. F., Townley, R. R. W., Holmes, I. H., and Ruck, B. J.: Importance of a new virus in acute sporadic enteritis in children. Lancet 1:242, 1975.

Davidson, G. P., Gall, D. G., Butler, D. G., Petric, M., and Hamilton, J. R.: Human rotavirus enteritis induced in conventional piglets: Intestinal structure and transport. J Clin Invest 60:1402, 1977.

Flewett, T. H., Bryden, A. S., and Davies, H.: Diagnostic electron microscopy of faeces. I. The viral flora of faeces as seen by electron microscopy. J Clin Pathol 27:603, 1974.

Gust, I. D., Pringle, R. C., Barnes, G. L., Davidson, G. P., and Bishop, R. F.: Complement-fixing antibody response to rotavirus infection. J Clin Microbiol 5:125, 1977.

Kalica, A. R., Purcell, R. H., Sereno, M. M., Wyatt, R. G., Kim, H. W., Chanock, R. M., and Kapikian, A. Z.: A microtitre solid phase radioimmunoassay for detection of the human reovirus-like agent in stools. J Immunol 118:1275, 1977.

Kapikian, A. Z., Wyatt, R. G., Dolin, R., Thornhill, T. S., Kalica, A. R., and Chanock, R. M.: Visualization by immune electron-microscopy of a 27 nm particle associated with acute infectious non-bacterial gastroenteritis. J Virol 10:1075, 1972.

Kapikian, A. Z., Cline, W. L., Mebus, C. A., Wyatt, R. G., Kalica, A. R., James, H. D., Jr., Van Kirk, D., Chanock, R. M., and Kim, H. W.: New complement-fixation test for the human reovirus-like agent of infantile gastroenteritis. Nebraska calf diarrhoea virus used as antigen. Lancet 1:1056, 1975a.

Kapikian, A. Z., Feinstone, S. M., Purcell, R. H., Wyatt, R. G., Thornhill, T. S., Kalica, A. R., and Chanock, R. M.: Detection and identification by immune electron microscopy of fastidious agents associated with respiratory illness, acute non-bacterial gastroenteritis and hepatitis A. In Pollard, M. (ed.): The Gustav Stern Symposium, Antiviral Mechanisms. Perspectives in Virology, Vol. 9. New York, Academic Press, 1975b, p. 9.

Kapikian, A. Z.: The Coronaviruses. In Oxford, J. S. (ed.): Chemoprophylaxis and Virus Infections of the Respiratory Tract, Vol. 2. CRC Press, 1977, p. 95.

Kerry, K. R., and Anderson, C. M.: A ward test for sugars in faeces. Lancet 1:981, 1964.

Kurtz, J. B., Lee, T. W., and Pickering D.: Astrovirus associated gastroenteritis in a children's ward. J Clin Pathol 30:948, 1977.

Leading article: Rotaviruses of man and animals. Lancet 1:257, 1975.

Maiya, P. P., Pereira, S. M., Mathan, M., Bhat, P., Albert, M. J., and Baker, S. J. Aetiology of acute gastroenteritis in infancy and early childhood in Southern India. Arch Dis Child 52:482, 1977.

Middleton, P. J., Petric, M., Hewitt, C. M., Szymanski, M. T., and Tam, J. S.: Counter-immunoelectro-osmophoresis for the detection of infantile gastroenteritis virus (orbi-group) antigen and antibody. J Clin Pathol 29:191, 1976.

Rivers, T. M.: Viruses and Koch's postulates. J Bacteriol 33:1, 1937.

Rohde, J. E., and Northrup, R. S.: Taking science where the diarrhoea is. In Acute Diarrhoea in Childhood. Ciba Foundation Symposium 42 (new series). Amsterdam, Elsevier Publishing Company 1976, p. 339.

Schreiber, D. S., Trier, J. S., and Blacklow, N. R.: Recent advances in viral gastroenteritis. Gastroenterology 73:174, 1977.

Thornhill, T. S., Wyatt, R. G., Kalica, A. R., Dolin, R., Chanock, R. M., and Kapikian, A. Z.: Detection by immune electron-microscopy of 26- to 27-nm virus-like particles associated with two family outbreaks of gastroenteritis. J Infect Dis 135:20, 1977.

Yolken, R. H., Kim, H. W., Clem, T., Wyatt, R. G., Kalica, A. R., Chanock, R. M., and Kapikian, A. Z.: Enzyme linked immunosorbent assay (ELISA) for detection of human reovirus-like agent of infantile gastroenteritis. Lancet 2:263, 1977a.

Yolken, R. H., Wyatt, R. G., Kalica, A. R., Kim, H. W., Brandt, C. D., Parrott, R. H., Kapikian, A. Z., and Chanock, R. M.: Use of a free viral immunofluorescence assay to detect human reovirus-like agent in human stools. Infect Immunol 16:467, 1977b.

# CHOLECYSTITIS AND CHOLANGITIS  136

## Kaoru Shimada, M.D.

### CHOLECYSTITIS

#### Definition

Cholecystitis, inflammation of the gallbladder, may be acute or chronic. Over 90 per cent of cases are associated with gallstones. Acute cholecystitis is usually superimposed on a chronic process, and is precipitated by obstruction of the cystic duct by a stone (or rarely, by invasion of resident organisms or edema in the absence of calculus).

#### Etiology

Gallbladder outlet obstruction is the common factor in the vast majority of cases of acute cholecystitis. The impacted calculus is the commonest cause for obstruction. Other possible causes of obstruction are malformation of the cystic duct; mucosal edema and fibrosis secondary to inflammatory changes at duct orifice; kinking and torsion of the cystic duct; stasis bile plugs; compression by adhesions or by enlarged lymph nodes; infiltration by neoplasm; and parasites, particularly *Ascaris lumbricoides*. Outlet obstruction by itself does not evoke acute cholecystitis, and one or more additional factors are required to initiate the inflammatory process. Bacterial infection was once regarded as the principal etiologic factor, but was not consistent with the fact that patients without cholecystitis sometimes had bacteria in the gallbladder and that, in the early stage of acute cholecystitis, sterile cultures were obtained by surgery from the bile or gallbladder wall. Experimentally bacteria alone cannot produce acute cholecystitis unless there is damage to the gallbladder or interference with its blood supply. From these findings the idea evolved that cholecystitis is caused by chemical action and that infection is superimposed upon the damaged gallbladder. Acute cholecystitis has been reproduced experimentally by injecting pancreatic juice or concentrated bile into the obstructed gallbladder. Lecithin, a phospholipid normally present in bile, is converted to lysolecithin by phospholipase, an enzyme in the pancreatic juice and liver. The toxicity of lysolecithin for membranes may be implicated, at least experimentally, in acute cholecystitis in the obstructed gallbladder. Thus, in some cases it is possible that reflux of pancreatic juice is responsible for the development of acute cholecystitis. Bile acids are found conjugated with glycine or taurine in bile. The major human bile acids are cholic, chenodeoxycholic, and deoxycholic acids. Unconjugated bile acids are much more toxic than conjugated and deoxycholic acid produces the most marked reaction. Deconjugation of bile salts by bacteria may enhance the inflammatory reaction that the bile salts are thought to trigger. The infecting organisms most often recovered from acute cholecystitis are primarily enteric bacteria, such as *Escherichia coli, Klebsiella, Enterobacter, Proteus,* and streptococci, including the enterococcus. Little information is available on anaerobic organisms in the biliary tract. The anaerobic bacteria usually described are clostridia, gram-positive cocci, gram-positive nonsporulating bacilli, and *Bacteroides fragilis* (Shimada et al., 1977). Since *B. fragilis,* clostridia and *Streptococcus fecalis* can hydrolyze bile acid conjugates, it is possible that these bacteria produce more toxic bile salts in the gallbladder, and play a role in the etiology of cholecystitis.

Infecting bacteria may reach the gallbladder via bile duct, blood, or lymphatics, or by direct extension from neighboring organs. Severe systemic infection may be accompanied by cholecystitis. Salmonella infection of the gallbladder is frequently observed in patients who have a history of typhoid fever. Other possible factors are vascular (arteritis, arteriolitis, venous or lymphatic stasis), neural (imbalance between sympathetic and vagal action), and humoral (cholecystokinin). The etiologic factors of chronic cholecystitis are believed to be the same as those involved in acute cholecystitis. However, the details of its evolution remain obscure.

#### Pathologic Anatomy and Pathogenesis

In acute cholecystitis, the gallbladder is hyperemic, edematous, and enlarged. The lumen is tensely filled with a mixture of turbid bile, inflammatory exudate, and pus. The cystic duct may be obstructed owing to stone incarceration and/or dyskinesia of Oddi muscles or cell debris. Microscopically, inflammatory changes consist of vascular congestion, interstitial edema, and cellular infiltration. In severe cases, the mucosa may be gangrenous and frequently have ulceration that penetrates the wall of the bladder. The morphologic features of chronic cholecystitis vary with the stage of inflammation. The gallbladder is sometimes contracted and scarred, or normal in size, or enlarged, and may develop inflammatory adhesions to the surrounding tissues. Commonly, the wall shows fibrous thickening, or may be severely distended by obstruction. The contents are clear, turbid, or composed of mucoid bile and multiple gallstones. Histologically, the herniation of the epithelium into the smooth musculature, known as Rokitansky-Aschoff's sinuses, is recognized in up to 90 per cent of cases. Acute inflammatory changes are often superimposed on the chronically inflamed gallbladder.

Autopsy studies revealed that more than half of all adults have incidental evidence of inflammatory changes in the gallbladder, of no clinical significance.

### Clinical Manifestations

Cholecystitis is prominent in those who are "female, fat, and forty." It occurs about three times as often in women as in men, and especially in obese persons. Although cholecystitis is seen at all ages, it is uncommon until the thirties, and most common in the fifth and sixth decades. Acute cholecystitis is frequently precipitated by overwork or a heavy meal. The most prominent symptom is severe right upper quadrant pain, which usually radiates to the right shoulder or infrascapular region. It may start with discomfort in the midepigastrium, increase in intensity as biliary colic develops, and soon becomes a continuous and unbearable pain in the right hypochondrium, accentuated by movement or deep inspiration. Breathing may be shallow and rapid to prevent intensifying the pain. The patients writhe or lie in a jackknife position. Nausea and vomiting are frequent. Fever (38° C to 39° C) and chills occur regularly. Most patients exhibit tenderness and muscle spasm in the right upper quadrant and epigastrium. An acutely inflamed gallbladder is palpable only at times. If the patient takes a deep, slow breath while the physician's fingers are hooked up deep beneath the right costal arch, there may be momentary interruption of breathing because of pain (Murphy's sign). The clinical manifestations of acute cholecystitis depend on the severity of inflammation. As inflammation progresses from serous to seropurulent, purulent, and phlegmonogangrenous, the manifestations become worse. Rebound tenderness in the right hypochondrium and midepigastrium occurs in suppurative cholecystitis with peritoneal inflammation. Persistent vomiting, the spread of tenderness, and rebound tenderness over the abdomen commonly indicate either perforation of the gallbladder or associated pancreatitis.

Leukocytosis is usually moderate. Leukocytosis over 20,000 raises the suspicion of gangrene or perforation. The serum bilirubin and alkaline phosphatase may be elevated mildly even in the absence of common duct obstruction, probably owing to inflammatory edema of the extrahepatic bile duct. Serum bilirubin over 5 mg/100 ml suggests concomitant common duct stone. Rise of serum amylase level reflects associated pancreatitis. Urobilinogen is usually increased in the urine, and decreases rapidly after the inflammation subsides.

Bile may be collected by duodenal intubation (Meltzer-Lyon test) but only after acute inflammation has fully subsided to avoid gallbladder contraction. Many pus cells and epithelial cells are observed. If concentrated gallbladder bile (B-bile) does not appear the cystic duct may be obstructed or the gallbladder nonfunctioning. A carefully collected specimen can be used for bacteriologic examination.

A plain film of the abdomen frequently shows gallstones. Intravenous cholecystocholangiography by drip infusion will not opacify the gallbladder if the cystic duct is obstructed or the gallbladder is unable to concentrate the dye. Excretion of contrast media may also fail in acute hepatitis or acute pancreatitis. Thus, a negative cholecystogram should be interpreted with caution. On the other hand, visualization of a gallbladder with normal shape and contractive properties rules out acute cholecystitis. Gallbladder scanning with either [131]I-rose bengal or [99m]Tc-Diethyl IDA (diethyl-acetoamilide-iminodiacetic acid) is also used in the evaluation of cholecystitis. If no radioactivity accumulates in the gallbladder, usually within 90 minutes after injection, the bile duct may not be patent and inflammation is likely. [131]I-rose bengal accumulates in the gallbladder despite moderate liver injury if the bile duct is patent.

Chronic cholecystitis is almost invariably associated with gallstones. The manifestations of chronic cholecystitis fall into two categories: vague digestive complaints and recurrent biliary colic. The digestive complaints include postprandial belching and intolerance of fat. Although occasionally the attacks may not be clear-cut, the diagnosis is suggested by right hypochrondrium tenderness, indigestion after a fat meal, and inflammatory signs such as slight fever and positive test for C-reactive protein. On cholecystography, calculi are frequently demonstrated. The gallbladder is not visualized, or is opacified very faintly without contracting. Hydrops of the gallbladder or limy bile are radiologic findings compatible with chronic cholecystitis. Duodenal drainage may provide important information if the diagnosis is in doubt. Since chronic cholecystitis may cause a wide variety of nonspecific symptoms, the diagnosis is often misused as a wastebasket for functional indigestion in patients with no gallbladder disease. The term should be reserved for patients with recurrent attacks of acute cholecystitis in whom gallbladder function is abnormal on x-ray or in whom chronic inflammation is seen in the gallbladder on peritoneoscopy.

Many attacks of acute cholecystitis subside within one to three days, but in a few cases the inflammatory process does not abate and is progressive. Septicemia, cholangitis, pancreatitis, pylephlebitis, and perforation are complications of acute cholecystitis. Chronic cholecystitis with cholelithiasis is prone to relapse and recurrence.

### Diagnosis

Differential diagnosis includes perforated peptic ulcer, acute pancreatitis, appendicitis, mesenteric arterial occlusion, bowel strangulation, pyelonephritis, urolithiasis, acute salpingitis, pleurisy, right lower lobe pneumonia, and myocardial infarction. In cases with jaundice, one must also exclude acute hepatitis, hemolytic crisis, and malignancy of the extrahepatic biliary system. These diseases are easily differentiated from acute cholecystitis. Most errors in diagnosis occur in patients with pyelonephritis, urolithiasis, or pyonephrosis. In general back tenderness is more severe, fever is higher, leukocytosis is greater with an infected kidney, but none of these is specific or pathognomonic. Urinalysis will usually exclude renal infections. Intravenous pyelography, cholecystocholangiography and ultrasound examination of the biliary system should be done before surgical exploration for unexplained right upper quadrant pain.

A particularly difficult diagnostic problem is presented by acute pancreatitis, which tends to occur in alcoholic patients. Elevated levels of lipase in serum, and amylase level in both serum and urine suggest pancreatitis. However, it should be remembered that pancreatitis and cholelithiasis often occur together. Patients with hepatic problems (acute hepatitis, hepatic congestion, or metastatic disease) may have severe pain and a mass in the right hypochondrium. Liver function studies and scan may be useful for differential diagnosis.

### Treatment

It is generally accepted that symptomatic cholelithiasis is a surgical disease. The same applies to most patients with cholecystitis, since over 90 per cent have gallstones, but the time for operation is controversial. Some surgeons prefer early surgical treatment within 24 to 48 hours after the onset to avoid rupture of the gallbladder during the attack. The collected experiences indicate that for the acute attack, operative and nonoperative measures are equally effective in patients without coincident serious disease such as diabetes mellitus. It should be emphasized, however, that the patient must be managed medically if suitable operating facilities and experienced personnel are not available. Most patients, especially those under 50 can be treated conservatively until recovery from the acute attack. Elective cholecystectomy is recommended after several weeks.

Parenteral fluids, nasogastric suction, antispasmodics, analgesics, and antibiotics are used in acute cholecystitis. Nasogastric suction not only decompresses the stomach, but also reduces the stimulus to gallbladder contraction from gastrointestinal hormones. Meperidine 0.1 g and atropine sulfate 0.5 g every 4 to 6 hours, as needed, is given subcutaneously for moderate pain. For severe pain, a combination of opium and atropine sulfate may prove satisfactory. Antibiotics are an essential part of therapy. One should choose a drug excreted in bile in high concentration and effective against coliform bacteria. Cefazolin in doses of 1 g intravenously every eight hours fulfils these requirements. Ampicillin (1 g intravenously every six hours) or tetracycline (250 mg intravenously every six hours) is also recommended, but ampicillin is not effective against *Klebsiella* or *Enterobacter,* which are the next most common organisms in bile. The efficacy of the aminoglycosides in biliary tract infection is in doubt, since their biliary excretion is negligible. Over 80 to 90 per cent of patients respond to these medical measures within one to three days. Failure to improve would indicate a complication requiring emergency operation.

Aged patients with acute cholecystitis are less likely to respond to conservative therapy, especially when diabetic. Advanced age, arteriosclerosis and decreased resistance to infection together cause a high incidence of perforation with consequent infection. There is no place for prolonged medical treatment of acute cholecystitis in diabetics, and old age is no longer a contraindication for biliary surgery, even as an emergency operation. In a desperate situation, cholecystostomy may be life-saving.

Cholecystectomy is indicated for chronic cholecystitis if patients have biliary stones, or convincing evidence of gallbladder nonfunction. For patients whose diagnosis is questionable, who have minimal symptoms, or who refuse surgery, medical management is composed of a low fat diet and antispasmodics. Patients who complain of vague gastrointestinal symptoms with minor abnormalities on cholecystogram — that is, faint opacification and impaired contraction — are a difficult problem. Conservative treatment and repeated evaluation of upper GI and biliary tract is better for these patients than surgery, since those who have a normal biliary tract at surgery are not relieved by cholecystectomy. Operation should be reserved for surgically correctable biliary disease.

## CHOLANGITIS
### Definition and Etiology

Cholangitis is an inflammation of intra- and extrahepatic bile ducts usually associated with bacterial infection, and characterized by the triad of Charcot (1877): spiking fever with chills, jaundice, and pain in the right upper abdominal quadrant. Obstruction of the common duct is an important etiologic factor. Cholangitis occurs primarily in elderly patients with choledocolithiasis or scarring at the choledochoduodenal junction. The incidence of cholangitis is low with biliary neoplasms. The same bacteria are found in the bile as in cholecystitis, and two or more organisms are often cultured.

Cholangitis comprises a variety of clinical syndromes depending on the degree of obstruction. The nonsuppurative form is most common. At the other extreme is the catastrophic picture of acute suppurative obstructive cholangitis (Welch and Donaldson, 1976). Nonsuppurative cholangitis subsides promptly after antibiotics without surgical therapy, probably because the obstruction is transient. Acute suppurative cholangitis appears to be related to complete obstruction of bile flow within the common duct in the presence of pathogenic bacteria. Its development after transhepatic or retrograde cholangiography, suggests that these procedures can elevate pressure in the bile duct and simulate sudden obstruction.

### Pathology

Above the obstruction, the bile duct becomes distended and its wall shows inflammatory thickening. The liver is enlarged and in suppurative cholangitis there may be multiple microabscesses. There is the neutrophil infiltration within small ducts in periductal and portal areas, proliferation of ducts, and centrilobular bile stasis.

### Manifestations and Treatment

Acute suppurative cholangitis starts abruptly, progresses rapidly, and is often fatal in a few hours or days. Patients suffer agonizing right upper quadrant pains, progressive obstructive jaundice, unremitting high fever, and circulatory collapse. Septicemia, shock, and mental confusion or delirium are common. Septic shock is thought to be the common cause of death. Antibiotics have no effect unless biliary obstruction is relieved.

Only surgical decompression of the pus-filled duct is life-saving. Operative mortality approximates 40 to 50 per cent in patients with hypotension and septicemia, but is much lower if surgery is performed before septic shock develops. Therefore, surgery should be considered as an emergency procedure if patients deteriorate rapidly or do not improve within 24 to 36 hours. Fluid and electrolyte replacement is essential both pre- and postoperatively to prevent renal failure. It is also important to administer intravenously antibiotics effective against gram-negative bacteria and anaerobes, such as cefazolin and clindamycin in combination. A dose of 1 g cefazolin and 600 mg clindamycin can be given every six hours.

## ORIENTAL CHOLANGIOHEPATITIS

Oriental cholangiohepatitis, or recurrent pyogenic cholangitis, is found almost exclusively in Hong Kong and in Southeast Asia, where infestation of bile ducts with *Clonorchis sinensis* is endemic (Stock and Fung, 1962). In clonorchiasis, the bile ducts become thickened and dilated, and there is pericholangitis and atrophy of liver parenchyma. These pathologic changes in biliary trees may predispose to further infection. Characteristic "earthy" stones of Aschoff, the bilirubin stones with low cholesterol content, frequently contain the clonorchis ova or disintegrated adult worm as nidi. Manifestations are almost the same as those of other types of cholangitis. The clinical course is acute, chronic, or relapsing, and, in some cases, terminates in hepatic failure. Antibiotics achieve temporary control of acute exacerbation, but recurrence is common. Surgical intervention for removal of stones is not entirely satisfactory, since intrahepatic stones cannot usually be extirpated. However, considerable relief for long periods of time is achieved by establishment of external biliary drainage or by postcholelithotomy management such as duodenal intubation with administration of cholagogues and choleretics.

### References

Charcot, J. M.: Lecon sur les maladies due Foie des Voies Filiares et des Reins, Paris, Faculte de Medecine de Paris, 1877.
Du Plessis, D. J., and Jersky, J.: The management of acute cholecystitis. Surg Clin North Am 53:1071, 1973.
Halasz, N. A.: Counterfeit cholecystitis, a common diagnostic dilemma. Am J Surg 130:189, 1975.
Salk, R. P., Greenburg, A. G., Farris, J. M., and Peskin, G. W.: Spectrum of cholangitis. Am J Surg 130:143, 1975.
Schein, C. J.: Acute Cholecystitis. New York, Harper & Row, 1972.
Shimada, K., Inamatsu, T., and Yamashiro, M.: Anaerobic bacteria in biliary disease in elderly patients. J Infect Dis 135:850, 1977.
Stock, F. E., and Fung, J. H.: Oriental cholangiohepatitis. Arch Surg 84:47, 1962.
Welch, J. P., and Donaldson, G. A.: The urgency and surgical treatment of acute suppurative cholangitis. Am J Surg 131:527, 1976.

# LIVER AND 137
# SUBPHRENIC ABSCESS

*Edward Brook Rotheram, Jr., M.D.*

## DEFINITION AND ETIOLOGY

Liquefactive or suppurative lesions of the liver and subphrenic spaces are caused by *Entamoeba histolytica* or by a variety of bacterial species of which a few are well-known pathogens but most are poorly virulent members of the normal intestinal flora. The latter are often recovered in mixed culture and many are strict anaerobes (Sabbaj et al., 1972).

## PATHOGENESIS AND PATHOLOGY

Amebic liver abscess is secondary to amebic colitis, spread to the liver by way of the portal vein. Although a diffuse hepatitis often accompanies severe amebic colitis, three-quarters of amebic liver abscesses occur as solitary lesions and many develop in the absence of symptomatic colitis. Inexplicably, men are afflicted far more often than women. As with all solitary abscesses of portal venous origin, the right hepatic lobe is involved eight to nine times more often than the left lobe. Since blood from the splenic vein streams preferentially into the left lobe, the right lobe, already six times larger, receives an even larger proportion of the blood coming from the heavily colonized lower intestine.

Named for their ability to lyse living tissue, *E. histolytica* organisms alone do not incite a local granulocytic inflammatory response. Although strict anaerobes, they do not produce a foul odor. Thus, amebic abscess fluid, in the absence of bacterial superinfection, consists of liquefied liver tissue containing few if any granulocytes and no bacteria on gram stain or culture. Motile trophozoites are confined largely to the abscess wall, and their demonstration in the abscess fluid is difficult. The classic "anchovy paste" results from hemorrhage into the abscess cavity. If bleeding has not occurred, the fluid is yellow or green rather than red or chocolate brown. Since bacteria produce cavities filled with granulocytes, the adjective "pyogenic" is applied to all liver abscesses of bacterial etiology. If the pus has a fetid odor, the presence of anaerobic bacteria is ensured whether or not aerobes are also recovered.

Bacteria can reach the liver by way of the biliary tree, the portal vein, the hepatic artery, a contiguous infection, or a penetrating wound. Bacterial colonization of the unobstructed biliary tract is well tolerated as illustrated by the chronic typhoid carrier. However, partial obstruction of the common bile duct by stone, benign stricture, or periampullary carcinoma leads to ascending cholangitis if the bile is infected. Abscesses secondary to ascending cholangitis are often multiple and caused by those bacteria associated with cholelithiasis (Table 1). Although strict anaerobes are relatively infrequent in ascending cholangitis, *Clostridium perfringens* must be considered. Since cholelithiasis and prior operations upon the biliary tract are associated with a high incidence of biliary tract infection, the obstructing lesion is often not neoplastic and prompt diagnosis can be rewarded by a full recovery.

Bacteremia of the portal vein (pylephlebitis) results from septic thrombophlebitis in tributary veins draining foci of infection in the gastrointestinal tract. (Thrombosis of the portal vein itself is rare.) Resulting liver abscesses are usually single, but two or three large abscesses or even multiple small abscesses can occur. Their bacterial flora is of lower intestinal origin and, hence, often polymicrobial and predominantly or exclusively anaerobic (Table 1). The failure to recover these anaerobic bacteria because of unsatisfactory culture methods accounts for the high incidence of sterile pyogenic liver abscesses reported in many series. Most liver abscesses for which no source can be found (cryptogenic abscesses) are presumed to arise from subclinical self-limited infections within the portal system, such as a colonic diverticular abscess. Blunt trauma to the abdomen can disrupt the bowel mucosa and allow bacterial seeding of a simultaneously induced hepatic hematoma. A liver abscess may present several weeks after the trauma. Although portal bacteremia is thought to be common in uncomplicated Crohn's disease and ulcerative colitis, liver abscess rarely occurs in the absence of intestinal perforation and local abscess formation. The liver's defense against infection is not easily breached by the portal route.

Invasion of the liver via the hepatic artery implies a systemic bacteremia often due to virulent bacteria, such as *Staphylococcus aureus* and *Streptococcus pyogenes*. The range of invasive microorganisms is greater in granulocytopenic and immunosuppressed patients and includes *Pseudomonas aeruginosa* and fungal species such as *Candida albicans*. Resulting liver abscesses are usually multiple and small or microscopic in size,

**TABLE 1.  Bacterial Etiology of Liver and Subphrenic Abscesses**

A. Abscesses secondary to ascending cholangitis, bilary and upper intestinal tract surgery, and penetrating trauma. *

| MICROORGANISM | APPROXIMATE INCIDENCE (%) |
|---|---|
| *Escherichia coli* | 40 |
| *Klebsiella pneumoniae* | 20 |
| Other Enterobacteriaceae | 15 |
|    *Enterobacter* spp. | |
|    *Proteus* spp. | |
|    *Citrobacter* spp. | |
|    *Salmonella* spp. | |
| *Staphylococcus aureus* | 15 |
| *Clostridium* spp. | 10 |
| *Pseudomonas* spp. | 10 |
| Enterococcal spp. | 10 |
| Other streptococcal spp. | 10 |
| *Bacteroides fragilis* | 5 |

B. Fetid abscesses secondary to pylephlebitis, appendiceal, colonic, and pelvic foci.†

| MICROORGANISM | APPROXIMATE INCIDENCE (%) |
|---|---|
| Anaerobic streptococcal spp. | 30 |
| Microaerophilic streptococcal spp. | 30 |
| *Bacteroides fragilis* | 25 |
| Other *Bacteroides* spp. | 15 |
| *Sphaerophorus* spp. | 10 |
| *Fusobacterium* spp. | 10 |
| *Actinomyces* spp. | 10 |
| *Escherichia coli* | 10 |
| Other Enterobacteriaceae spp. | 10 |
| Enterococcal spp. | 10 |
| Other aerobic streptococcal spp. | 10 |

*More than 25 per cent of cultures will yield two or more microbial species. The streptococci are particularly likely to appear in mixed culture.
†More than 50 per cent of cultures will yield two and often more microbial species.

and similar abscesses are present in other organs. Foci of infection contiguous with the liver result from natural catastrophes such as a perforated peptic ulcer or from surgical procedures. The invading bacterial flora may be simple or complex and of high or low intrinsic virulence. Careful examination of pus from an associated wound infection may permit identification of the bacteria involved. Liver abscesses resulting from penetrating trauma have much in common with those resulting from contiguous infection.

The term subphrenic abscess is applied to any intraperitoneal or retroperitoneal collection of pus occurring in the zone bounded by the diaphragm above and the transverse colon below. The massive right lobe of the liver suspended from the posterior aspect of the diaphragm (not from the dome as commonly taught) creates two large potential peritoneal spaces, one above the liver in contact with the diaphragm and one below the liver excluded from such contact. Both spaces easily become divided by pyogenic membranes, and abscesses are usually loculated anteriorly, posteriorly, or laterally, rather than occupying the entire potential space. The small left

lobe of the liver creates no effective division of the left subphrenic space, in which only the lesser omental sac is a distinct anatomic subdivision. Abscesses in either of these two left-sided spaces are likely to produce diaphragmatic irritation.

Bacteria reach the subphrenic spaces by rupture of an underlying hepatic abscess or by spread of infected material within the peritoneal cavity. Venous and lymphatic channels play no direct role. Natural or surgical injury to organs within the subphrenic zone, such as the gallbladder, stomach, duodenum, and pancreas, is a common antecedent, and abscesses of the left lateral subphrenic space are often due to infection of a hematoma after splenectomy. However, subphrenic abscesses may also result from remote intra-abdominal foci, such as a perforated appendix. The potential spaces of the upper abdomen exhibit negative pressures characteristic of the intrapleural space above and so tend to aspirate peritoneal exudates. This mechanism is thought to explain the formation of subphrenic abscesses in the absence of a contiguous route of infection. The occurrence of isolated abscesses in remote recesses suggests that bacteria spread widely

LIVER AND SUBPHRENIC ABSCESS — 137

through the peritoneum after focal contamination. Since abscess formation is comparatively rare, the peritoneum must possess a high natural resistance to infection.

Retroperitoneal subphrenic abscesses may be secondary to infection in or around the kidneys, pancreas, duodenum, or vertebrae. Such abscesses usually point below the subphrenic zone, since the retroperitoneal pathway of least resistance leads inferiorly along the psoas muscle.

Inflammatory edema from infection in the upper abdomen is cleared cephalad through a rich lymphatic network in the diaphragm. Overload of this system results in a sterile pleural effusion with the characteristics of an exudate. Lymphatic spread does not account for infected pus within the pleural space, since a direct communication through the diaphragm can almost always be demonstrated when pleural empyema complicates a subphrenic infection.

## CLINICAL MANIFESTATIONS

The clinical manifestations of liver abscesses vary with respect to their microbial etiology, to their anatomic location in the liver, and to the type and pace of their underlying pathogenic mechanism (Barbour and Juniper, 1972; Rubin et al., 1974). Historical details, depending heavily upon the events that have led to the abscess, may be rich or meager. If the onset is insidious, weight loss and debility are prominent. Nausea and vomiting are unusual except in biliary tract obstruction. Fever is almost always present but may be low grade in an indolent process or high and spiking with chills in the presence of bacteremia or rapidly enlarging abscesses. Right subcostal pain, aggravated by percussion over the lower ribs, and a palpable tender liver are common, but many other findings depend upon the location of the abscess. Abscesses in the right or left lobes adjacent to the diaphragm mimic intrathoracic infection. The patient may complain of cough and pleuritic pain in the chest or shoulder. Protracted episodes of hiccough may occur. The involved hemidiaphragm may be elevated and fixed on inspiration, with rales and bronchial breathing heard in the adjacent lung as a result of compressive atelectasis. Abscesses in the posterior or lateral portions of the right hepatic lobe may produce a tender fullness with localized subcutaneous edema in the overlying rib spaces or in the costovertebral angle. An abscess in the left hepatic lobe often presents as a tender epigastric mass.

The clinical manifestations of the small abscesses associated with septicemia are overwhelmed by those of the systemic infection. Fortunately, treatment of the septicemia constitutes treatment of the liver infection. However, a liver abscess may also be obscured when a contiguous or remote intra-abdominal infection dominates the physician's attention. Prompt diagnosis in this circumstance is often life-saving.

Subphrenic abscess may be indistinguishable, clinically, from liver abscess, and indeed the two conditions may coincide (Harley, 1949). A common presentation is a low-grade or episodic fever in a patient recovering slowly and incompletely from abdominal surgery. An obvious infection elsewhere in the wound or abdomen may distract attention from the subphrenic zone. Thoracic symptoms and signs, as described for liver abscess, may occur when the infection contacts the diaphragm. Subhepatic abscesses tend to produce few or no localizing manifestations. Abscesses beneath the left hemidiaphragm may be missed by physicians unaware that one-quarter of subphrenic abscesses are on the left side.

Patients with isolated subphrenic abscesses have suffered vague pains, debility, fever, and anemia for more than ten years before diagnosis. Such indolence has given rise to an oft repeated paraphrase: "Pus somewhere, pus nowhere, pus under the diaphragm."

## COMPLICATIONS AND SEQUELAE

Both amebic and pyogenic liver abscess may rupture to produce subphrenic abscesses and, occasionally, generalized peritonitis. Liver abscesses or subphrenic abscesses of either etiology may rupture through the diaphragm to produce empyema, pericardial effusion and tamponade, lung abscess, and bronchobiliary fistula. Interestingly, decompression through the bronchial tree is associated with a mortality rate lower than that observed in abscesses that do not drain spontaneously. Rarely, an abscess may point and drain through the skin. Bacteremia may be complicated by hypotensive shock and by metastatic abscesses in other organs. A persisting focus of infection may become reactivated months to years after apparent cure.

## GEOGRAPHIC VARIATIONS IN DISEASE

Since one in ten patients with clinical amebiasis presents a liver abscess, *E. histolytica* is by far the most common cause of liver abscess in endemic areas. Conversely, amebae account for a small fraction of liver abscesses in economically advanced countries of the temperate zones where a breakdown in sanitation produces epidemic amebiasis. The increasing travel to and from endemic regions, the existence of endemic foci within countries largely free of the disease, and the latency for which amebiasis is notorious are further reasons to consider an amebic etiology regardless of the patient's current residence.

Within any one geographic area, referral centers are more likely to see abscess resulting from biliary tract obstruction or contiguous infection in older patients suffering from cancer. Abscesses secondary to pylephlebitis in younger patients are likely to predominate in hospitals giving largely primary care.

## DIAGNOSIS

A polymorphonuclear leukocytosis of over 15,000/mm³ is characteristic of both amebic and pyogenic liver abscesses. Leukemoid reactions may be seen. The degree of anemia correlates with the duration of the inflammatory process or with the amount of blood loss from associated lesions, such as amebic colitis or diverticulitis. The serum alkaline phosphatase is elevated in more than 90 per cent of all liver abscesses. The elevation may be slight and the accompanying bilirubin concentration normal when liver abscesses arise via the portal venous or hepatic arterial routes. In ascending cholangitis there is often a marked rise in the alkaline phosphatase and clinical jaundice. Other tests of liver function are variable and of little help in diagnosis.

Blood cultures are positive in at least 50 per cent of pyogenic liver abscesses. The high frequency of bacteremia in ascending cholangitis has long been known, but the renewed interest in anaerobic infections has led to an appreciation that systemic bacteremia is also common in pylephlebitis. A patient presenting with fever, chills, elevated alkaline phosphatase, and a continuous anaerobic bacteremia must be suspected of having pylephlebitis even though no evidence of a gastrointestinal focus can be found. An associated liver abscess must be ruled out. A liver or subphrenic abscess is also one cause of an obscure intermittent bacteremia.

Roentgenographic studies are often abnormal in hepatic and subphrenic abscesses. Either hemidiaphragm may be elevated and relatively immobile, often with a pleural effusion or pulmonary infiltrates above. A left subphrenic abscess may separate the gastric air bubble from the diaphragm in the erect posteroanterior view of the chest. An abscess in or around the left lobe of the liver may produce pressure deformities in the barium- or gas-filled stomach or colon. An air-fluid level proved to be outside the bowel and hence within liver tissue or a subphrenic space is virtually diagnostic of a pyogenic abscess. It must

be remembered that free air within an uninfected peritoneum may be observed up to three weeks after surgery.

Hepatic photoscans using technetium-99m sulfur colloid performed in anterior, posterior, and lateral projections will detect most liver abscesses larger than 2 cm in diameter. They appear as defects in an otherwise homogeneous uptake of radioactivity by the liver. Conversely, gallium-67 citrate is concentrated in a pyogenic abscess to produce an area of increased uptake on photoscan. Neither isotope will differentiate an abscess from primary or metastatic cancer. Although small abscesses are easily missed on hepatic angiography, this technique may show vessels or a venous blush within neoplastic lesions. Radioisotope scans are also valuable in demonstrating subphrenic abscesses. A combined liver-lung scan may show a cold area between the two organs when the abscess is suprahepatic. Large collections of pus within the abdomen can usually be demonstrated on gallium-67 scans but interpretation of the uptake may be difficult, especially in the postoperative patient, since the isotope collects in recent wounds, hematomas, and colonic feces as well as in abscesses and neoplasms.

Scanning with ultrasound does not require the expense and availability of radioisotopes, but it does require careful and conservative interpretation. The interposition of fatty or air-filled organs between the transducer and the area of interest may prevent study of certain portions of the subphrenic zone. Vascular and biliary structures, especially when distorted by disease, may be misinterpreted. Nevertheless, the technique can be helpful, since it tends to show best those abscesses most accessible to needle aspiration. Needle exploration is in disfavor not because of fear of disseminating infection but because false negative results are common. A successful ultrasound study will give the precise location and depth of a fluid-filled cavity and even identify the tissues through which the exploring needle must pass to reach it.

Computerized axial tomography (CAT) offers no advantage over the combined use of the nuclear scan with ultrasound. Moreover, CAT scan is more expensive and carries a greater risk of radiation exposure.

In the absence of amebic colitis, clinical differentiation between amebic and pyogenic abscess may be difficult. More than 90 per cent of patients with an amebic abscess have high antibody titers to E. histolytica as measured by indirect hemagglutination, indirect immunofluorescence, immunodiffusion, or countercurrent immunoelectrophoresis. Similarly, low or absent antibody titers to Echinococcus granulosus are helpful in excluding hydatid cyst of the liver. As discussed under *Pathogenesis and Pathology,* fluid obtained by percutaneous needle aspiration will usually distinguish amebic from pyogenic abscesses. Amebae are so difficult to demonstrate in the face of pyogenic inflammation that the incidence of bacterial superinfection of amebic abscesses (before drainage) is not known. If new techniques, such as the enzyme-linked immunosorbent assay can detect amebic antigens in abscess fluid, the question of dual etiology will be more easily resolved.

## TREATMENT AND PROPHYLAXIS

Surgical decompression of the biliary tract is mandatory for liver abscesses secondary to ascending cholangitis. Large pyogenic liver abscesses, whether single or multiple, usually require surgical drainage for cure. Many abscesses in the right lobe of the liver are best drained posteriorly through the bed of the twelfth rib, but other patients require an abdominal exploration and do well with transperitoneal drainage (Block et al., 1964). Noninvasive methods for locating abscesses and for following their response to treatment have improved greatly in the past few years. It may be possible to cure more pyogenic abscesses through a combination of percutaneous aspiration and vigorous antibiotic treatment. Multiple small liver abscesses have been healed by antibiotics alone, whether or not surgery is needed for a primary intra-abdominal lesion.

Metronidazole has revolutionized the treatment of amebic liver abscess by eliminating the need for surgical drainage in most cases. The dose of metronidazole is 750 mg orally three times daily for five days. For the occasional amebic abscess that appears resistant to metronidazole (Griffin, 1973) it may be necessary to give 65 mg emetine hydrochloride IM daily for ten days in combination with 250 mg chloroquine orally twice daily. Chloroquine is continued for at least 28 days or longer if clinical signs or ultrasound give evidence of incomplete resolution.

The vast majority of demonstrable subphrenic abscesses require surgical drainage. Abscesses loculated posteriorly in the suprahepatic or infrahepatic spaces may be drained by a transthoracic or posterior extraperitoneal approach. However, transabdominal exploration of the subphrenic zone may detect loculated extensions or separate collections of pus easily missed by techniques giving limited exposure. Antibiotics have reduced the danger of spreading infection during transperitoneal drainage.

Regardless of the surgical approach to hepatic and subphrenic abscesses, antibiotics must be given in full doses for three weeks or longer. Empirical treatment of all the bacteria implicated in abscesses of biliary, upper intestinal, and traumatic origin is unwieldy. Cephalothin, 12 to 15 gm daily intravenously, plus gentamicin, 80 to 100 mg every eight hours intramuscularly, provides broad coverage but may not be adequate for *C. perfringens, Bacteroides fragilis, P. aeruginosa,* or the enterococci. Antibiotic therapy tailored to the microbes actually identified in culture is obviously superior to an empirical approach. Fetid anaerobic abscesses of colonic and pelvic origin are well treated by penicillin G, 20 million units a day intravenously, and clindamycin, 600 mg every six hours intravenously. Clindamycin is effective against *B. fragilis,* which is routinely resistant to beta-lactam antibiotics and sometimes resistant to the tetracyclines. An aminoglycoside such as kanamycin or gentamicin is also indicated until *Escherichia coli* and other facultative gram-negative rods are excluded by aerobic culture of the pus.

These abscesses produce prolonged, expensive illnesses, and overall mortality rates continue to approach 50 per cent. However, the prompt diagnosis and treatment of patients without underlying neoplastic disease shifts the odds strongly in favor of survival. Antibiotics have not decreased the overall incidence of these infections. Here again, the gross statistics may be misleading, since these abscesses now occur less frequently in young people with benign underlying disease and more frequently in older people after extensive surgery for malignant disease. Given the high natural resistance of the liver and peritoneum to infection, appropriate antibiotic therapy of a primary contamination or overt infection must prevent the complication of hepatic and subphrenic abscess in many instances. When antibiotics fail to prevent such a complication, they are accused, with some justification, of suppressing its clinical manifestations and delaying its diagnosis. Successful prophylaxis goes unnoted.

## References

Barbour, G. L., and Juniper, K., Jr.: A clinical comparison of amebic and pyogenic abscess of the liver in sixty-six patients. Am J Med 53:323, 1972.

Block, M. A., Schuman, B. M., Eyler, W. R., Truant, J. P., and DuSault, L. A.: Surgery of liver abscess. Arch Surg 88:602, 1964.

Griffin, F. M., Jr.: Failure of metronidazole to cure hepatic amebic abscess. N Engl J Med 288:1397, 1973.

Harley, H. R. S.: Subphrenic abscess. Thorax 4:1, 1949.

Rubin, R. H., Swartz, M. N., and Malt, R.: Hepatic abscess: Changes in clinical, bacteriologic and therapeutic aspects. Am J Med 57:601, 1974.

Sabbaj, J., Sutter, V. L., and Finegold, S. M.: Anaerobic pyogenic liver abscess. Ann Int Med 77:629, 1972.

# 138 *GRANULOMATOUS HEPATITIS*

*Steve Kohl, M.D.*
*Herbert L. DuPont, M.D.*

## DEFINITION

Granulomatous hepatitis is the development of multiple granulomas in liver tissue. Granulomas are defined as "microscopic focal vascularized aggregation of histiocytes and hypertrophied fibroblasts that assume a round to oval shape" (Robbins, 1979).

Granulomatous hepatitis is a pathologic description, not an etiologic diagnosis. This condition is a nonspecific reaction of the liver to a large number of stimuli, many specifically treatable. Discovery of a granulomatous reaction in hepatic tissue of a patient with systemic illness demands an orderly, extensive diagnostic evaluation. In many cases this will be long and expensive, but it is justified by the probability of discovering a cause that can be specifically treated.

## PATHOGENESIS

Granuloma formation appears to be a normal response to certain indolent but persistent agents that are not readily degraded by phagocytic cells. Common etiologic agents include fungi, intracellular bacteria, mycobacteria, foreign bodies, and protozoa. It also appears to be a response of immune suppressed and immune deficient patients as in chronic granulomatous disease. Viral hepatitis is granulomatous in renal dialysis patients who are receiving immunosuppressant therapy, and *Listeria monocytogenes* elicits a granulomatous response in neonates and debilitated adults. Alteration of antigens or bacterial virulence can convert a stimulus that ordinarily produces a purulent response (such as that of live streptococci in mice) to one that produces a granulomatous response (live streptococci plus penicillin or heat-killed streptococci in mice). Antigen-antibody complexes can also induce granuloma formation.

The basic understanding of granuloma formation and classification has been advanced by animal experiments demonstrating that granulomas are a mononuclear cell (lymphocyte and macrophage) response to both inflammatory (agent-specific) and immunologic (host-specific) stimuli. An inflammatory granuloma is associated with a uniform, dose-dependent response that is independent of previous challenge. Granulo-

mas generated by immunologic factors display an amnestic immunologic response when rechallenged with the sensitizing antigen, so that granuloma cells accumulate more rapidly (Warren, 1976). This is presumably due to previously sensitized memory lymphocytes (probably T cells) responding to antigens phagocytized by the liver macrophages (Kupffer cells). These lymphocytes begin the inflammatory cascade, recruiting other lymphocytes, monocytes, and macrophages to the site and orchestrating a complex combination of cellular and humoral responses that result in a granuloma formation with containment of the antigen. Identification of the various agents and mechanisms that cause an inflammatory and/or immunologic granulomatous response in man may eventually help facilitate the diagnosis and specific therapy.

In general, hepatic granulomas, though often numerous, have minor effects on liver function. These effects are usually manifested as mild obstructive signs (slight increase in bilirubin and serum transaminases and a greater elevation in serum alkaline phosphatase levels). There is often prolonged Bromsulphalein (BSP) retention, hypergammaglobulinemia, low serum albumin values, and elevated serum cholesterol levels. Occasionally, strategically located granulomas will produce striking abnormalities as a result of hepatic obstruction. A radionuclide liver scan in granulomatous hepatitis tends to reveal a patchy, mottled uptake or a normal liver. In one patient subjected to angiographic study there was a rich arterial supply and patchy patterns of increased vascularization on the arterial, parenchymal, and venous phases. This pattern is the same as that seen with metastatic lesions, regenerating nodular hyperplasia, and multiple small liver abscesses.

## PATHOLOGY

A granuloma is a collection of mononuclear inflammatory cells (lymphocytes and macrophages) and epithelial cells (mononuclear inflammatory cells) usually arranged in an oval to round structure and often containing giant cells (formed by fusion of macrophages) and variable degrees of central necrosis. There may also be a minor infiltration of fibroblasts, plasma cells, eosinophils, and polymorphonuclear leukocytes. Active granulomas tend to contain more inflammatory cells, while older, more quiescent granulomas may be partially or entirely replaced by hyaline and calcified material, with or without a peripheral rim of mononuclear leukocytes. Despite the common notion that histologic variations have etiologic significance, there are few features that differentiate hepatic granulomas and relate them to etiologic agents. Caseous necrosis, classically linked to tuberculosis, is not diagnostic of the condition and can also be seen with tularemia, brucellosis, syphilis, fungal infection, Q fever, Wegener's granulomatosis, and chronic granulomatous disease of childhood. Although tuberculosis often produces less sharply defined granulomas with more inflammatory cells and necrosis, and sarcoidosis generally causes more circumscribed and compact masses of epithelial cells and giant cells without necrosis and surrounding inflammation, exceptions are frequently encountered. Other differences between the granulomatous reaction of tuberculosis and sarcoidosis have been suggested. The reticulum network tends to be damaged by tuberculosis, whereas in sarcoidosis it is generally well maintained. In one study, multiple granulomas were more typically associated with miliary tuberculosis (95 per cent) than with sarcoidosis (65 per cent) (Alexander and Galambos, 1973), although the opposite was found in another series (Hughes and Fox, 1972). Such generalities may influence a pathologist's opinion, yet the definitive etiologic diagnosis rests upon demonstration of the agent

in the pathologic specimen, growth of the agent from the specimen, or ancillary clinical and laboratory data.

## INCIDENCE

The incidence and etiology of granulomatous hepatitis depends on the patient population, geographic location, underlying disease state, reasons for pathologic examination of liver tissue (e.g., liver abnormalities, fever, incidental operative biopsy), and the method of tissue sampling. Granulomas have been identified in 0.7 to 9 per cent of more than 13,000 liver biopsies performed in published studies, with a mean of 4 per cent (Bunim et al., 1962; Guckian and Perry, 1966; Alexander and Galambos, 1973; Hughes and Fox, 1972; Klatskin and Yesner, 1950; Iverson et al., 1970; Wagoner et al., 1953; Pequignot et al., 1973; Bain et al., 1973; Mir-Madjlessi et al., 1973). In studies of patients with fever of undetermined origin, the diagnosis of granulomatous hepatitis was made in 2 to 11 per cent. Hepatic granulomas are found more often in cases of confirmed brucellosis or miliary tuberculosis. Results agree whether liver tissue is obtained through operative, autopsy, or needle biopsy procedures. The diffuse nature of the process is obvious when it is considered that a needle biopsy specimen represents approximately 1/50,000 of the liver (Klatskin and Yesner, 1950).

Tables 1 through 3 list the various etiologic agents and conditions associated with hepatic

---

**TABLE 1. Infections Associated with Granulomatous Hepatitis**

| BACTERIAL | VIRAL |
|---|---|
| Syphilis | Influenza |
| Tularemia | Viral hepatitis |
| Brucellosis | Cytomegalovirus disease |
| Meliodosis | Epstein-Barr virus infection |
| Listeriosis | |
| Tuberculosis | **FUNGAL** |
| Atypical mycobacterial disease | |
| Leprosy | Histoplasmosis |
| BCG infection | Coccidioidomycosis |
| Granuloma inguinale infection | Aspergillosis |
| Actinomycosis | Cryptococcosis |
| Nocardiosis | Candidiasis |
| **RICKETTSIA** | **PROTOZOAN-PARASITIC** |
| Q fever | Ascariasis |
| | Schistosomiasis |
| **CHLAMYDIA** | Ancylostomiasis |
| | Amoebiasis |
| Psittacosis | Strongyloidiasis |
| Lymphogranuloma venereum infection | Toxoplasmosis |
| | Tongue worm infection |
| | Visceral larval migrans |

## TABLE 2.   Drugs and Toxins Associated with Granulomatous Hepatitis

Sulfonamides
Phenylbutazone
Allopurinol
Halothane
Methyldopa
Quinidine
Chlorpropamide
Penicillin
Hydralazine
Beryllium
Corn starch
Copper
Talc
Tolbutamide

granulomas. Extrapulmonary tuberculosis and sarcoidosis are among the more common causes of granulomatous hepatitis. Other conditions such as brucellosis, though rare, are almost invariably associated with hepatic granulomas.

Table 4 summarizes the relative incidence of etiologic agents from a review of ten published series containing 586 cases of granulomatous hepatitis (Bunim et al., 1962; Guckian and Perry, 1966; Alexander and Galambos, 1973; Hughes and Fox, 1972; Iverson et al., 1970; Wagoner et al., 1953; Pequignot et al., 1973; Bain et al., 1973; Mir-Madjlessi et al., 1973; Terplan, 1971). A search for recently discovered causes of granulomatous hepatitis not represented in these series, such as cytomegalovirus and certain

## TABLE 3.   Miscellaneous Conditions Associated with Granulomatous Hepatitis

### CANCER

Hodgkin's disease
Others

### IMMUNE DEFECTS

Chronic granulomatous
   disease of childhood
Hypogammaglobulinemia

### LIVER DISEASE

Biliary cirrhosis
Chronic active hepatitis

### OTHERS

Sarcoid
Wegener's granulomatosis
Allergic granulomatosis
Inflammatory bowel disease
Whipple's disease
Collagen vascular disease
Systemic sclerosis

## TABLE 4.   Etiology of 586 Cases of Granulomatous Hepatitis

| | |
|---|---|
| Sarcoidosis | 191 (34%) |
| Tuberculosis | 173 (30%) |
| Hodgkin's disease | 9 |
| Viral hepatitis | 8 |
| Schistosomiasis | 8 |
| Histoplasmosis | 8 |
| Brucellosis | 6 |
| Syphilis | 6 |
| Berylliosis | 3 |
| Liver disease | |
|    Cirrhosis | 23 |
|    Fatty infiltration | 13 |
|    First and second degree biliary cirrhosis | 11 |
|    Hepatitis, nonviral | 7 |
| Unknown | 102 (17%) |

2 cases each:  Lymphopathia venereum, infectious mononucleosis, cancer, erythema nodosum, fungal
(unspecified)

1 case each:  Q fever, visceral larval migrans, actinomycosis,
systemic sclerosis, collagen vascular disease,
blastomycosis, influenza B, viral (unspecified)

Bunim et al., 1962; Guckian and Perry, 1968; Alexander and Galambos, 1973; Hughes and Fox, 1972; Iverson et al., 1970; Wagoner et al., 1953; Pequignot et al., 1973; Bain et al., 1973; Mir-Madjlessi et al., 1973; Terplan, 1971.

drugs, will reduce the relative number of cases without diagnosis. Prospective studies have demonstrated that, with careful reevaluation, it is possible to increase the percentage of etiologic diagnoses (Guckian and Perry, 1968).

## ETIOLOGY AND CLINICAL MANIFESTATIONS

### Infections

*Tuberculosis.* Infections are the most commonly diagnosed causes of granulomatous hepatitis, and tuberculosis is the most common infectious cause, accounting for nearly one third of all cases of granulomatous hepatitis (Table 4). The frequency of developing tuberculous hepatic granulomas is related directly to the extent and duration of the infection. In active pulmonary tuberculosis granulomas are found in 25 to 42 per cent of cases; in extrapulmonary nonmiliary disease they occur in 80 per cent; and in fatal, miliary, or chronic untreated tuberculosis granulomas are seen in nearly all cases (Alexander and Galambos, 1973; Frank and Raffensperger, 1965).

Patients with tuberculous granulomas of the liver are generally febrile, and 50 per cent have hepatomegaly. Liver function testing often reveals increased bilirubin, transaminase, alkaline phosphatase, and retention of BSP dye, particularly in miliary disease. Increased serum immunoglobulin levels are also common. Other than demonstrating the causative agent in a granuloma, the most helpful laboratory procedure is the tuberculin skin test. Most patients with tuberculosis, unless moribund, will respond to an intermediate or second strength PPD (purified protein derivative) skin test with Tween stabilized antigen, applied correctly and read at the appropriate time.

The characteristic granuloma of tuberculosis containing caseous necrosis (Fig. 1) is present in 15 to 50 per cent of cases showing a granulomatous reaction. As previously mentioned, granulomas of other causes may also show caseous necrosis, although the finding of caseation should lead to a suspicion of tuberculosis. Acid-fast bacilli are found in the liver with varying frequency in different series, although it is agreed that they are difficult to visualize. The frequency of positive acid-fast smears ranges from 0 to 45 per cent with the higher frequency seen among patients with miliary tuberculosis. The use of fluorescent-staining procedures may increase this low yield.

Culture of the bacillus from hepatic granulomas has been generally unrewarding except in miliary tuberculosis, where as many as 60 per cent of cultures may be positive (Alexander and Galambos, 1973). Other mycobacteria, including the leprosy bacilli in lepromatous leprosy, atypical mycobacteria (usually group III) in immune-suppressed patients, and bacille Calmette-Guérin (BCG) in patients receiving intralesional anticancer therapy, also cause granulomas.

The overall low incidence of positive cultures from lesions associated with mycobacteria supports the hypothesis that the granulomas are in large part hypersensitivity reactions to components of these organisms and not necessarily to the live bacillus.

The close association between mycobacterial infection and granulomatous hepatitis has led to the frequent empiric institution of antituberculous therapy in patients with granulomatous hepatitis when the diagnosis is not etiologically established. However, spontaneous remission of granulomatous hepatitis is common, making it difficult to ascribe etiologic significance to a satisfactory response to empiric tuberculosis therapy.

The presence of liver granulomas in a person with tuberculosis implies extrapulmonic mycobacterium infection, and the reader is referred to Chapter 114 for guidelines of specific therapy.

**Syphilis.** Syphilis involves the liver in 5 per cent of inadequately treated cases. Before 1941, approximately 5 in 1000 routine autopsies performed in the United States had evidence of syphilitic liver involvement. The granuloma (syphiloma) is found both in the second and third stages of disease. The granulomas often caseate and coalesce to form liver gummas, although at times no necrosis is found, and the histologic reaction is similar to that found in tuberculosis or sarcoid. Spirochetes have been found by careful darkfield examination of liver tissue, but diagnosis is most easily approached by serologic means. The finding of a positive serologic response for syphilis in a patient with hepatic granuloma is of course not diagnostic of syphilitic involvement of the liver, and the strength of the association relies on the incidence of positive serologic tests in the population from which the individual is drawn and exclusion of other causes of granulomatous liver reaction.

**Brucellosis.** Brucellosis, particularly that due to *Brucella abortus*, almost always involves the liver. *Br. suis* also may involve the liver. Granulomas are often found in the absence of hepatomegaly or altered liver function tests. The likelihood of finding granulomas in inactive cases is much lower. The histopathologic signs are nonspecific and may include caseous necrosis. Diagnosis of brucellosis is made by culturing the causative organism from blood, marrow, or biopsy material or by a positive agglutination test with *Brucella* antigens in a significant titer (usually >1:100). Special culture techniques employing

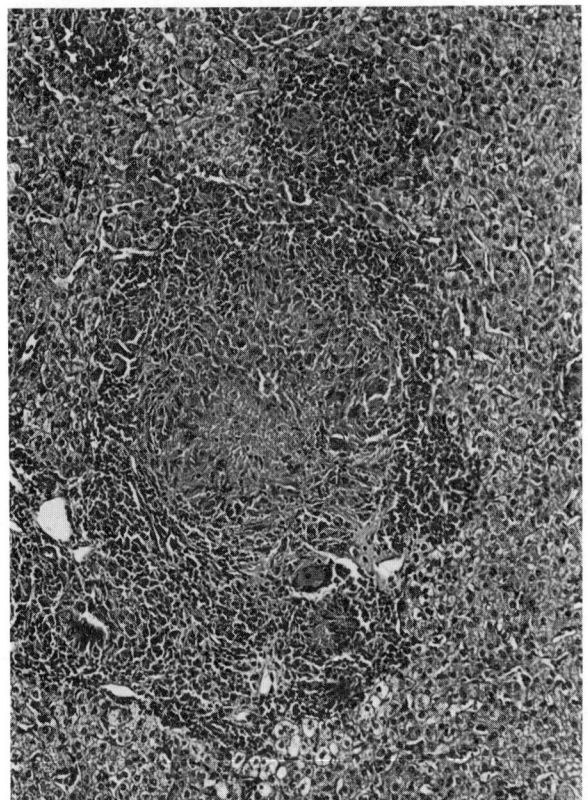

**FIGURE 1.** *Tuberculous granuloma of the liver.*

Castaneda media or *Brucella* agar are required. Brucella involvement of the liver rarely progresses to cirrhosis.

***Tularemia.*** Although clinical liver manifestations are not common in tularemia, in one series 10 of 12 autopsy cases had hepatic lesions, and in another series of 21 cases, the majority had granulomas and caseous necrosis (Schiff, 1956). The agglutination test for tularemia is the most valuable for establishing the diagnosis. Cultivation of *Francisella tularensis* from tissues or blood is difficult and hazardous for laboratory technicians.

***Listeriosis.*** *Listeria monocytogenes* infection occurs in immune-suppressed hosts, postpartum women, and neonates, as well as otherwise healthy people. Disseminated listeriosis in neonates can occur both prenatally and peripartum. The infant often has skin granulomas as well as granulomas in almost any organ, including the liver. The organism is easily cultured from the blood and granulomas. Mortality is high in the immunosuppressed patient or neonate with infection even though the organism is sensitive to readily available antimicrobials such as ampicillin and penicillin.

***Viral Agents.*** Viral causes of liver granulomas are more difficult to verify. Although granulomatous hepatitis has been found in association with documented viral infection, the growth of virus from a granuloma has not been achieved. Infectious mononucleosis often involves the liver, with 85 per cent of affected individuals demonstrating altered liver enzymes. Focal round cell infiltrations occur but are not diagnostic of granulomatous hepatitis. One patient in each of two large series was felt to have liver granulomas associated with infectious mononucleosis.

Cytomegalovirus hepatitis resulted in a granulomatous reaction in three well-documented cases in two published series (Reller, 1973; Bonkowsky et al., 1975). In these cases no giant cells or viral inclusions were noted in the liver. Diagnosis was made by a fourfold or greater rise or fall in serologic titer and, in two patients, by concomitant isolation of cytomegalovirus from cervix or saliva. Influenza B virus infection has been associated with granulomatous hepatitis in one case (Klatskin and Yesner, 1950). Two series of small clusters of mononucleosis-like illness with granulomatous liver involvement involving five cases in Israel (Eliakim et al., 1968) and two cases in New York (Gelb et al., 1970) have been reported. Each series consisted of young to middle-aged people (16 to 52 years) with self-limited febrile illness, lymphocytosis, atypical lymphocytes seen on peripheral blood smear, and liver biopsies containing multiple granulomas without caseation or giant cells. In one of the series cytomegalo-

virus antibody titers were not obtained, and in both series heterophils were negative but Epstein-Barr virus antibody titers were not done.

Chronic active hepatitis has rarely been associated with granuloma formation, which may reflect a dysfunctional host response to persistent hepatitis B virus infection. During an outbreak of B-antigen-negative hepatitis in a renal dialysis unit, two patients showed changes of chronic persistent hepatitis on liver biopsy specimens and two had grade IV sclerosis, all with caseating granulomas present (Galbraith et al., 1975). The etiology of hepatitis that commonly occurs in patients undergoing renal hemodialysis is not always established and may be multifactoral. In a study of long-term dialysis patients, six of seven had mild focal hepatitis. One of these patients had severe involvement with noncaseating granuloma formation. Changes of viral hepatitis were not present (Bergman et al., 1972). Many of these patients had been treated with drugs that have been associated with hepatic granuloma formation, such as methyldopa, and many had had blood transfusions, increasing the risk of viral infections associated with granulomas. In addition, dialysis produces red cell sludging and offers opportunities for antigen challenge of patients who may be immunosuppressed for a variety of reasons.

It is probable that as we become more sophisticated in our methods of diagnosing viral disease, we will find a closer association between certain viral diseases and granulomatous hepatitis.

***Q Fever.*** The only rickettsial agent clearly associated with granulomatous hepatitis is *Coxiella burnetii*, the causative agent of Q fever. Common clinical manifestations of the disease are fever, severe headache, pneumonitis, and chemical hepatitis. In one case, granulomas containing fluorescent antibody-positive organisms have been identified. The liver also was diffusely infiltrated with lymphocytes, polymorphonuclear leukocytes, eosinophils, plasma cells, and histiocytes (DuPont et al., 1971). In the same report, two volunteers experimentally infected with an aerosol challenge of *Coxiella burnetii* showed laboratory evidence of hepatitis 8 to 12 days after inoculation (during the late incubation period). Liver biopsy revealed foci of mononuclear cell inflammation and Councilman-like bodies, although rickettsiae were not seen.

***Psittacosis.*** Psittacosis, an avian-acquired cause of interstitial pneumonitis, has been associated with a hepatitic granulomatous response.

***Fungal Agents.*** A wide variety of fungal diseases can cause granulomas of the liver (Table 1). Histoplasma is the most common fungal agent identified, and its incidence is related to geographic location. In a large series of patients with granulomatous hepatitis reported from the United States, histoplasmosis accounted for 12 per cent of the cases, the second most frequent diagnosis after sarcoid (Mir-Madjlessi et al., 1973). In this series, 80 per cent of the patients with histoplasmosis had fever while a third had hepatomegaly and/or splenomegaly. Laboratory and pathologic findings were nonspecific, with only 16 per cent having altered liver function tests. In a prospective evaluation of 26 patients with progressive disseminated histoplasmosis, 21 had liver abnormalities. Granulomas were present in five of eight undergoing liver biopsy, fungal cultures were positive in four, and fungi were visible in three culture-positive liver specimens (Fauci and Wolff, 1976). The diagnosis can be suspected by a positive serologic reaction (false-negative results are common) and can be confirmed only by direct visualization or by growth of the organism from liver or bone marrow. The skin test is of little clinical use and may confuse the serologic evaluation. Cryptococcosis can also produce a hepatitis, and encapsulated yeast may appear in the liver. The presence of fungus in liver signifies visceral dissemination and mandates careful search for other foci in the bone marrow, lung, or central nervous system.

*Parasitic Agents.* Table 1 enumerates the many parasitic diseases that may elicit a granulomatous reaction. In one series of 214 cases reported from the United States, schistosomiasis accounted for eight (4 per cent) (Bunim et al., 1962). Although the parasitic etiologies are less common in urban centers, it can be anticipated that with increasing international travel, infections with these agents will become more common. In countries like Uganda, schistosomiasis is one of the most common causes of liver granuloma. Careful histopathologic examination of granulomas in certain cases may disclose eggs or migrating larvae such as those occurring in infection due to *Strongyloides stercoralis. Toxocara canis* and *T. cati,* which cause visceral larval migrans, may elicit a granulomatous reaction with eosinophilic infiltrates. In this situation, eosinophilia, high levels of isohemagglutinin antibody, and newly available serologic tests are diagnostically helpful.

## Drugs

A variety of drugs have been associated with hepatic granuloma formation (Table 2). An early report of penicillin-associated granulomatous hepatitis in a patient also treated with sulfadiazine has not been substantiated by other similar cases. Recent drug associations have included allopurinol, methyldopa, and chlorpropamide as well as phenylbutazone, halothane, hydralazine,

sulfonamides, and phenytoin. Quinidine is estimated to result in a hypersensitivity reaction in 6 per cent of individuals receiving it. In 32 patients (of 487) receiving quinidine who developed hypersensitivity reactions, 10 had clinical and biochemical evidence of hepatic abnormalities. Liver biopsy of four of these revealed granulomas upon rechallenge with quinidine (Geltner et al., 1976). In most instances, discontinuation of the offending drug has resulted in resolution of the clinical and histopathologic findings.

### Chemical Agents

Table 2 enumerates the various chemicals that have been associated with liver granulomas. Many of these represent single case reports, and the patients may have had other underlying conditions, making it difficult to be sure of the association. Beryllium dust may result in an acute pneumonitis after only a brief exposure, but long-term exposure to beryllium oxide has been associated with diffuse hepatic granulomas that are histopathologically indistinguishable from sarcoid. Copper, particularly as Bordeaux mixture, which is copper sulfate neutralized with hydrated lime, has been associated with a syndrome of fever, pneumonitis, hypergammaglobulinemia, and lung or liver granulomas. This has occurred in vineyard sprayers using the copper solution for 3 to 15 years. Rubeanic acid stain has demonstrated the presence of copper in the liver and lungs of these individuals. The Kupffer cells often reveal yellow-brown copper containing inclusions.

### Sarcoidosis

Sarcoidosis and tuberculosis are the two most commonly diagnosed causes of granulomatous hepatitis. In more recent series from the United States and Europe, sarcoidosis is the leading cause, presumably because of the decreasing incidence of tuberculosis, especially the extrapulmonary form. In patients with liver granulomas from hospitals serving poor urban populations in the United States, however, the incidence of tuberculous liver involvement continues to exceed that of sarcoidosis. In our review of approximately 600 published cases of granulomatous hepatitis, sarcoidosis was the most common single diagnosis, accounting for approximately one third of all cases and 40 per cent of all diagnosed cases (Table 4). Two thirds of patients dying of sarcoid have liver lesions at postmortem examination. This figure agrees with the 75 to 85 per cent incidence of liver granulomas that are found when biopsies of the liver are made antemortem in patients with sarcoid (Bunim et al., 1962; Klatskin and Yesner, 1950; Wagoner et al., 1953; Frank and Raffensperger, 1965), although there is a selection factor here because liver biopsy is the primary method of diagnosis of the condition.

The clinical presentation of sarcoidosis with hepatic granuloma is not unlike that of other conditions causing granulomatous hepatitis. There is no sex predilection, and most patients are under the age of 50. From 13 to 50 per cent have fever, while 30 to 80 per cent or more have hepatomegaly. The associated findings of sarcoidosis — splenomegaly, weight loss, abnormal chest radiograph, cutaneous and ocular signs — are present with varying frequency, depending on how the patients reported are selected (that is, those referred to a sarcoid clinic versus those with fever of undetermined origin or those having a liver biopsy for a variety of reasons). Chemical analysis for liver abnormalities generally reveals increases in alkaline phosphatase and BSP retention, and decreased prothrombin levels in half of the patients. The bilirubin level is less commonly elevated. The calcium, globulin, and eosinophil counts are often increased. The tuberculin test is usually negative in sarcoidosis, and the usefulness of the Kveim test remains highly controversial. In some hands Kveim antigen testing appears to have diagnostic value, but others find it negative in 80 per cent of patients diagnosed as having sarcoidosis (Israel and Goldstein, 1973). Whether these results depend on the antigen, the location of the series, multicausality of sarcoid, or other factors is unknown.

The diagnosis of sarcoid is made by demonstrating granulomas in more than one organ and excluding other causes of granulomatous disease. The diagnosis at times may be made only after an extensive search for granulomas in the bone marrow, mediastinal or abdominal lymph nodes, spleen, and conjunctival tissue. The use of invasive procedures to establish the diagnosis is justified only in the patient in whom another diagnosis has not been made and who remains symptomatic with fever or liver abnormalities.

Steroids are the cornerstone of therapy for sarcoidosis. They are indicated in patients with unrelenting fever or progressive liver abnormalities. Although granulomas may be present for years, progression to fibrosis and cirrhosis occurs only rarely and does not appear to be related to type of treatment administered.

### Neoplastic, Immune Disorder, and Liver Disease

Neoplastic diseases, in particular Hodgkin's disease, have been associated with granulomatous hepatitis. Liver biopsy obtained at staging laparotomy has shown granulomas in 5 per cent of patients with Hodgkin's disease. It is unclear if this represents a normal immunologic or inflammatory response to tumor products or whether it is the response of an immunologically abnormal host to an agent or agents that would ordinarily not elicit a granulomatous reaction. It is important to search carefully for infectious causes of granuloma formation in these patients, especially mycobacterial and fungal agents, in view of the high rate of infectious complications. The presence of Reed-Sternberg cells in liver granulomas indicates stage 4 Hodgkin's disease. Ovarian cancer and malignant melanoma have been associated rarely with a granulomatous reaction in the liver.

Several immune deficiency states have been associated with liver granuloma formation. Chronic granulomatous disease is a condition in which phagocytic leukocytes (polymorphonuclear leukocytes and monocyte-macrophages) can ingest certain organisms normally but fail to kill them. The basic biochemical defect appears to involve an inability by the host leukocyte to generate certain bactericidal chemicals (superoxide, hydrogen peroxide, and perhaps others). The condition is typically manifested as a sex-linked, early onset (within the first 5 years of life) increase in susceptibility to infections. Although most commonly a pediatric disease, a milder form of this disease has been described in older individuals. The sites most commonly involved are the skin, lungs, liver, and lymph nodes. The common infecting organisms include *Staphylococcus aureus,* gram-negative bacilli, and fungi. The typical histologic picture is a granulomatous response with polymorphonuclear leukocyte infiltration. Bacteria that would cause abscess formation in a normal person produce granulomas instead, presumably because the leukocytes in chronic granulomatous disease cannot degrade or remove bacterial antigens. Diagnosis of chronic granulomatous disease is confirmed by assay of leukocyte function. Polymorphonuclear leukocytes from affected patients are unable to reduce nitro-blue tetrazolium dye, do not produce the oxygen burst or chemiluminescence that normally accompanies phagocytosis, and are unable to kill *S. aureus* in vitro.

Although hypogammaglobulinemia (a B cell defect) has been linked with granulomatous hepatitis, other concomitant defects of T cell function have not been defined in this syndrome. Collagen vascular diseases, vasculitides, and diseases of unknown etiology that are associated with autoimmune responses and immune alterations have been associated with granulomatous hepatitis (Table 3).

Primary liver abnormalities have been associated with granulomas. It is difficult to show clearly an association between granulomatous hepatic response and progressive liver fibrosis. It is evident that granulomatous hepatitis associated with a variety of causes can occasionally progress to cirrhosis (sarcoid, drugs, toxins). Also, when liver biopsy is performed on patients with cirrhosis, granulomatous reactions are encountered occasionally. Whether immune alterations that accompany cirrhosis predispose to granuloma formation when the host is challenged with various antigens, whether in cirrhotic patients an autoimmune phenomenon is initiated whereby the immune response is directed against liver tissue and leads to granuloma formation, or whether the occasional coexistence of cirrhosis and granulomatous reaction is merely a random phenomenon are unknown.

Biliary cirrhosis, in which there are characteristic lymphoid follicles, destructive lesions of small bile ducts, and antimitochondrial antibody, has been associated with granulomatous hepatitis. Biliary cirrhosis tends to be less of a diagnostic enigma owing to the characteristic histopathologic picture of the surrounding liver tissue.

### Granulomatous Hepatitis of Unknown Etiology

The etiology of granulomatous hepatitis is often not identified. In most large studies, this group of patients is the second or third most common (after sarcoid and tuberculous liver disease). More intensive and thorough diagnostic evaluation has been shown to improve the frequency of establishing a diagnosis (Guckian and Perry, 1968). The use of serologic tests, biopsy of other tissues (peritoneal nodes, skin, bone marrow, spleen), the Kveim test if a reliable antigen is available, and judicious long-term observation have led to diagnoses that are not apparent on initial evaluation of the patient. The eventual diagnoses of these cases are similar to those of granulomatous hepatitis as a whole; sarcoid and tuberculosis are most common, followed by less commonly implicated infectious agents, malignancies, and hypersensitivity reactions.

Despite careful evaluation, however, there still remains a large portion (10 to 40 per cent) of cases in which no etiologic diagnosis is reached. In most series males outnumber females. The age range is usually older than that seen in the entire group of patients with liver granulomas. The clinical presentation is similar to that of cases of proven etiology, with common occurrence of high and prolonged fever, hepatomegaly, weight loss, and mildly elevated liver enzyme levels.

Associated laboratory abnormalities of undiagnosed granulomatous hepatitis often include increased erythrocyte sedimentation reaction and hypergammaglobulinemia. The histopathology is completely nonspecific and may include giant cells or caseous necrosis.

Although most of the available studies were published before certain infectious agents (cytomegalovirus, Epstein-Barr virus) and drugs were associated with granulomatous hepatitis, the chronicity of some of these cases (4 to 20 years in some series) would seem to exclude many of these causes (Terplan, 1971; Farrell and Powell, 1976; Simon and Wolff, 1973; Mir-Madjlessi et al., 1974). The granulomatous involvement of one organ system alone is not consistent with our current diagnostic criteria for sarcoidosis.

Management of these cases, after extensive evaluation, may include a trial of empiric therapy. Since the diagnosis of tuberculosis is often not excluded, the empiric use of antituberculous drugs is warranted in the patient with symptomatic or progressive disease. Response to antituberculous therapy may reflect an appropriate response in the patient with tuberculosis or it may be due to spontaneous remission of granulomatous hepatitis of unknown etiology. In addition, the use of certain antituberculous drugs such as streptomycin may affect other infections causing granulomatous hepatitis such as tularemia. If symptoms continue after two to four months' therapy with antituberculous medications in conjunction with attempts to exclude additional infectious diseases through appropriate serologic, histopathologic, and cultural studies, then corticosteroid therapy, which appears to be useful in controlling the symptoms if not the histopathology, is indicated. Antituberculous therapy should be continued in patients with positive skin tests for tuberculosis who are treated with corticosteroids. The prognosis of patients with this perplexing disease is good, and there is usually good to excellent response to empiric therapy as outlined above (Israel and Goldstein, 1973; Farrell and Powell, 1976; Neville et al., 1975; Simon and Wolff, 1973). It is expected that as newer causes of granulomatous hepatitis are identified and improved laboratory testing becomes available, the percentage of patients without confirmation of an etiologic diagnosis will decrease.

### References

Alexander, J. F., and Galambos, J. T.: Granulomatous hepatitis. The usefulness of liver biopsy in the diagnosis of tuberculosis and sarcoidosis. Am J Gastroenterol 59:23, 1973.

Bain, B. J., Harris, O. D., and Quinn, R. L.: The contribution of percutaneous liver biopsy to the management of liver disease. Med J Aust 2:160, 1973.

Bergman, L. A., Thomas, W., Jr., Reddy, C. R., Ellison, M. R., Smith, E. C., and Dunae, G.: Nonviral hepatitis in patients maintained by long-term dialysis. Arch Intern Med 130:96, 1972.

Bonkowsky, H. L., Lee, R. V., and Klatskin, G.: Acute granulomatous hepatitis. Occurrence in cytomegalovirus mononucleosis. JAMA 233:1284, 1975.

Bunim, J. J., Kimberg, D. V., Thomas, L. B., VanScott, J., and Klatskin, G.: The syndrome of sarcoidosis, psoriasis and gout. Ann Intern Med 57:1018, 1962.

DuPont, H. L., Hornick, R. B., Levin, H. S., Rapoport, M. I., and Woodward, T. E.: Q fever hepatitis. Ann Intern Med 74:198, 1971.

Eliakim, M., Eisenberg, S., Levij, I. S., and Sacks, T. G.: Granulomatous hepatitis accompanying a self-limited febrile disease. Lancet 1:1348, 1968.

Farrell, G. C., and Powell, L. W.: Chronic granulomatous hepatitis. Aust NZ J Med 6:474, 1976.

Fauci, A. S., and Wolff, S. M.: Granulomatous hepatitis. In Progress in Liver Disease, New York, Grune and Stratton, 1976.

Fitzgerald, M. X., Fitzgerald, O., and Towers, R. P.: Granulomatous hepatitis of obscure aetiology. Q J Med 150:371, 1971.

Frank, B. B., and Raffensperger, E. C.: Hepatic granulomata. Report of a case with jaundice improving on antituberculous therapy and review of the literature. Arch Intern Med 115:223, 1965.

Galbraith, R. M., Portmann, B., Eddleston, A. L., and Williams, R.: Chronic liver disease developing after outbreak of HBsAg-negative hepatitis in haemodialysis unit. Lancet 2:886, 1975.

Gelb, A. M., Brazenas, N., Sussman, H., and Wallach, R.: Acute granulomatous disease of the liver. Digest Dis 15:842, 1970.

Geltner, D., Chajek, T., Rubinger, D., and Levij, I. S.: Quinidine hypersensitivity and liver involvement. A survey of 32 patients. Gastroenterology 70:650, 1976.

Guckian, J. C., and Perry, J. E.: Granulomatous hepatitis. An analysis of 63 cases and review of the literature. Ann Intern Med 65:1081, 1966.

Guckian, J. C., and Perry, J. E.: Granulomatous hepatitis of unknown etiology. Am J Med 44:207, 1968.

Hughes, M., and Fox, H.: A histological analysis of granulomatous hepatitis. J Clin Pathol 25:817, 1972.

Israel, H. L., and Goldstein, R. A.: Hepatic granulomatosis and sarcoidosis. Ann Intern Med 79:669, 1973.

Iverson, K., Christoffersen, P., and Poulsen, H.: Epithelioid cell granulomas in liver biopsies. Scand J Gastroenterol (Suppl) 7:61, 1970.

Klatskin, G., and Yesner, R.: Hepatic manifestations of sarcoidosis and other granulomatous diseases. Yale J Biol Med 23:207, 1950.

Mir-Madjlessi, S. H., Farmer, R. G., and Hawk, W. A.: Granulomatous hepatitis. A review of 50 cases. Am J Gastroenterol 60:122, 1973.

Mir-Madjlessi, S. H., Farmer, R. G., and Hawk, W. A.: Spectrum of hepatic manifestations of granulomatous hepatitis of unknown etiology. Am J Gastroenterol 62:221, 1974.

Neville, E., Piyasena, K. H. G., and Geraint James, D.: Granulomas of the liver. Postgrad Med J 51:361, 1975.

Pequignot, H., Cocheton, J., Christorofov, B., and Louvel, A.: Transparietal puncture biopsy of the liver. A review of 464 cases. Mater Med Pol 5:99, 1973.

Robbins, S. L.: Inflammation and repair. In Pathologic Basis of Disease. Philadelphia, W. B. Saunders Company, 1979, p. 55.

Schiff, L.: Diseases of the Liver. Philadelphia, J. B. Lippincott Company, 1956.

Simon, H. B., and Wolff, S. M.: Granulomatous hepatitis and prolonged fever of unknown origin. A study of 13 patients. Medicine 52:1, 1973.

Terplan, M.: Hepatic granulomas of unknown cause presenting with fever. Am J Gastroenterol 55:43, 1971.

Wagoner, G. P., Anton, A. T., Gall, E. A., and Schiff, L.: Needle biopsy of the liver. VIII. Experiences with hepatic granulomas. Gastroenterology 25:487, 1953.

Warren, K. S.: A functional classification of granulomatous inflammation. Ann N Y Acad Sci 278:7, 1976.

# **139** *FLUKE INFECTIONS*

## *Elizabeth Barrett-Connor, M.D.*

### *FASCIOLIASIS*

#### Definition

Fascioliasis is a zoonosis caused by the liver fluke, *Fasciola hepatica*. Human infection occurs sporadically on a worldwide basis.

#### Etiology

Man is an accidental host. Fascioliasis is essentially a disease of sheep, goats, and cattle, in which it produces liver rot and therefore assumes economic importance. *F. hepatica* is enzootic in many wild animals, including rabbits and deer. Operculated eggs are passed in the feces of infected animals and hatch a ciliated miracidium into water. Larval development takes place in a fresh water snail, ultimately releasing cercaria that encyst on aquatic vegetation. When ingested by a suitable host, the parasites excyst and migrate through the intestinal wall into the peritoneal cavity. After penetrating the liver capsule, immature flukes migrate through the liver for several weeks and finally reach the bile ducts where they mature three months after infection and release eggs into the

feces. Human infection is usually acquired by eating wild watercress grown in meadows frequented by sheep or other naturally infected herbivores. The use of casually gathered watercress to decorate food or drink has been followed by infection. Man can also be infected by chewing grasses containing metacercariae, and possibly by drinking contaminated water, since metacercariae can form on minute particles on surface water.

#### Pathogenesis and Pathology

Migration of the immature flukes through the liver causes hepatitis, with parenchymal cell necrosis and an inflammatory and eosinophilic cellular response. Liver biopsy after recovery from this phase of illness shows no persistent hepatocellular pathology. The other characteristic finding is hyperplasia of the main bile duct with a thickened duct wall and an infolded endothelium surrounding an enlarged duct lumen. This process is probably essential for the establishment of the mature flukes, which are too large to be accommodated by unaltered bile ducts. Hyperplasia of the main bile duct occurs while immature *Fasciola* are still in the liver parenchyma, long before they enter the duct, and may be due to the stimulus of proline elaborated by the flukes (Isserhoff et al., 1977). Experimentally, bile duct hyperplasia can be induced either by flukes maintained in the peritoneum without access to the liver, or by intraperitoneal proline.

## Clinical Manifestations

There are two phases of illness, the first caused by migration of young flukes through the liver, and a second caused by mature flukes in the biliary ducts. Infected patients may experience both phases, only the first phase, only the second phase, relapses of either phase, or may remain asymptomatic indefinitely.

Early symptoms due to transhepatic migration of flukes begin two to three months after ingestion of metacercariae; symptoms include intermittent fever, malaise, night sweats, weight loss, and pain in the right upper quadrant. Urticaria with dermatographia or persistent nonproductive cough may be the most prominent symptoms in some cases. Relapses of the acute phase may occur, possibly owing to flukes reentering the liver. This illness may last several weeks.

The adult flukes are established in the biliary tract three or four months after infection, where they may survive for over ten years and cause no symptoms. In some cases obstructive jaundice occurs months or years later. Most patients with *Fasciola* bile duct obstruction are diagnosed at surgery, when one or more large flukes are found obstructing the biliary tract. *F. hepatica* has also been recovered from many ectopic sites, including skin, brain, and lung.

## Geographic Variations in Disease

Most reported cases have originated in Latin America, particularly in Chile and Cuba, but the largest single outbreak occurred in France with 500 cases in 1956. *Fasciola gigantica,* closely related to *F. hepatica,* is a trematode infection of domestic stock, and occasionally man, in tropical and subtropical areas of Africa, Asia, Europe, Hawaii, and Russia.

In some parts of the mideast, notably Syria, Lebanon, and Armenia, raw sheep or goat liver is eaten. Flukes of *F. hepatica* become attached to the mucosa of the epiglottis or posterior pharynx and cause edema and suffocation. This condition is called halzoun.

## Diagnosis

Only a history of contact with a sheep-growing area and fondness for wild watercress offer clues to the diagnosis of the sporadic case. Eosinophilia, often exceeding 50 per cent, is common in the first phase, and liver function tests suggest hepatitis. During the first three months serologic tests are usually positive, but stools are negative for ova because the fluke is not yet mature in the biliary tract.

During the obstructive phase eosinophilia may persist, but is most often absent. A history of recent hepatitis may suggest the etiology of biliary tract disease to the astute clinician, but often hepatitis is denied or its significance is missed. Large operculate eggs, which must be differentiated from those of *F. buski,* are found in the stool of two-thirds of cases (Fig. 4, Chapter 80). Ova are not found in the stools at any time in nearly one-third of cases. Diagnosis in stool-negative cases can usually be made by demonstrating ova in duodenal aspirate or by serologic tests. False-positive diagnosis may be a problem in areas where raw liver is eaten and ingested *F. hepatica* are passed in the feces. This possibility can be excluded by examining the stool after several days on a liver-free diet.

On occasion, *F. gigantica* has induced an abscess or a tumor-like reaction in the liver, which can be seen as a low density, irregular calcification on abdominal roentgenogram. The appearance of this hepatic calcification is considered to be virtually diagnostic.

## Treatment

No effective treatment is known for the migratory phase of illness. Symptomatic improvement may occur with chloroquine, emetine, or metronidazole therapy, leading to the mistaken diagnosis of amebic liver disease. Bithionol is the preferred treatment for preoperative or postoperative patients with ova in the stool. The recommended dose is 30 to 50 mg/kg on alternate days for 10 to 15 doses.

## Prophylaxis

Avoiding watercress, unless known to be grown commercially under specific regulations, is the best way to prevent fascioliasis. Control measures aimed at reducing infection in domestic animals, including drainage of pastures and application of molluscicides, may be helpful.

## *OPISTHORCHIASIS*

### Definition

Opisthorchiasis is a common liver fluke infection of the dog, cat, fox, and pig. Although man is an incidental host, millions of people are infected. *Opisthorchis sinensis, Opisthorchis felineus,* and *Opisthorchis viverrini* are the major pathogens.

## Etiology

In some endemic areas over 80 per cent of the population is infected. Infection rates increase with age. Man is infected by eating raw, pickled, or smoked fish containing encysted metacercariae. After ingestion the parasites excyst and attach themselves to the duodenal wall. Subsequently they migrate through the ampulla of Vater into the biliary tree or, less often, up the pancreatic duct, and attach themselves to the epithelial lining. The flukes mature in 1 month. Flukes do not multiply in man but may persist for many years, producing eggs that are passed in the feces. The life cycle requires two intermediate hosts. Ova released in feces are ingested by snails, which in time release cercaria. These infect freshwater fish, often of the carp family.

## Pathology and Pathogenesis

In the bile ducts adult flukes initially induce epithelial proliferation and adenomatous hyperplasia with the formation of new glands and goblet cells. Proliferation is gradually replaced by fibrosis around a dilated duct. These changes are irreversible. At autopsy, the dilated fibrosed ducts can be seen on the cut surface of the liver. The pancreatic duct, the only other structure affected by opisthorchiasis, may show hyperplasia, squamous metaplasia, or fibrosis. Cholangitis, cholangiohepatitis, liver abscess, and pancreatitis are complications of obstruction and secondary infection. Intrahepatic gallstone formation is not unusual. Cirrhosis, at one time attributed to chronic liver fluke infection, is probably coincidental. Similarly, hepatocellular carcinoma does not seem to be causally related to opisthorchiasis. Opisthorchiasis does, however, predispose to cholangiocarcinoma. In Hong Kong, about 15 per cent of all primary liver cancers are cholangiocarcinomas attributed to opisthorchiasis (Belamaric, 1973).

## Clinical Manifestations

Prolonged exposure is required to achieve a heavy worm burden, so that flukes and disease attributed to them are not common in children. In general, the severity of liver fluke disease is probably proportional to the number of parasites, but there are patients with heavy infections (over 1000 flukes) who appear perfectly well, and others with few flukes who suffer complications.

As with other intestinal parasites, most of those infected have no illness. Symptoms commonly attributed to moderate infection, such as low grade fever, anorexia, nausea, diarrhea, bloating, flatulence, and abdominal or back pain, have been equally common in uninfected controls; such symptoms are reported more often by nonAsians than Asians, whether or not they have opisthorchiasis (Strauss, 1962). Some manifestations clearly reflect the effect of worms on bile or pancreatic duct function; these include hepatomegaly, jaundice, pyogenic cholangitis, liver abscess, and pancreatitis.

## Complications and Sequelae

Either opisthorchis ova or adults may form a nidus for gallstones. When worms obstruct the cystic or common bile duct, the enlarged gallbladder may simulate carcinoma of the pancreas. As noted above, cholangiocarcinoma of the liver is a late complication of opisthorchiasis.

The prognosis is uncertain. Patients may go for years excreting eggs without symptoms and then rather abruptly deteriorate and die of liver or pancreatic disease.

## Geographic Variations

*Opisthorchis sinensis (Clonorchis sinensis)* is found in Indochina, Hong Kong, Japan, Korea, North Vietnam, and Taiwan. *Opisthorchis felineus* is found primarily in India, Vietnam, the Philippines, Korea, and Japan. *O. viverrini* is most common in northern Thailand, Laos, and West Malaysia. These flukes are morphologically and pathologically very similar, although *O. viverrini* may be less pathogenic than *O. sinensis.*

## Diagnosis

Opisthorchiasis should be suspected in a patient from an endemic area who presents with abdominal pain, jaundice, hepatomegaly, an enlarged gallbladder, or obscure liver disease (How and Pang, 1964). The peripheral white blood cell count may show eosinophilia, a polymorphonuclear leukocytosis, or be normal. Liver function tests are usually moderately deranged, even in patients who are completely asymptomatic. The diagnosis is made by identification of small operculate eggs (see Fig. 4 in Chapter 80) in unconcentrated feces. A direct smear should be positive in any patient with ten or more adult flukes, because the flukes are prolific egg producers. If stool examination is negative, diagnosis requires microscopic examination of a duodenal or bile duct aspirate. Serologic and intradermal tests can be used to confirm the diagnosis, but are rarely necessary and are not available in most areas.

Liver scan often shows hepatomegaly with diffusely poor uptake, a nonspecific finding. Intravenous cholangiography may show filling defects in the common bile duct and gall bladder. Percutaneous transhepatic cholangiogram may show multiple cystic ectasias of the intrahepatic bile ducts or mulberry-like dilatation. These findings are nearly pathognomonic of opisthorchiasis.

## Treatment

Until recently, medical treatment has been unsatisfactory. Chloroquine, dehydroemetine or bithionol usually suppress ova production, but do not cure the patient. Investigational drugs, such as Toluene-2, 4 diisothiocyanate (an analogue of Jonit), menichloropholan (Bayer 9015, a dihydroxy biphenyl compound), Praziquantel (Merck-Bayer), and Bilevon (Bayer) are said to be more effective in preliminary trial. Data are insufficient to evaluate their potential toxicity, which must be weighed against the often benign course of opisthorchiasis. In advanced cases surgery can sometimes relieve biliary obstruction.

## Prophylaxis

Populations at risk should be taught about the route of infection and warned to avoid raw fish. Destruction of the intermediate snail host is an attractive idea but impractical.

## *FASCIOLOPSIASIS*

### Definition

Fasciolopsiasis is an intestinal infection of man and pigs caused by *Fasciolopis buski.*

### Etiology

*F. buski* normally lives in the small intestine of man and hogs. Large operculated eggs are excreted in the stool. The two intermediate hosts are freshwater snails and water plants. Water chestnuts, water lily shoots, water caltrops and other water plants may have hundreds of metacercariae on their outer coverings. Man becomes infected by placing one of these plants in the mouth either for eating, peeling, or holding during collection. Excysted metacercariae attach to the mucosa in the duodenum. Each fluke matures and releases eggs in one to three months. *F. buski* does not multiply in the intestine. In some endemic areas over two-thirds of the population is infected. Overt infection is most common in poor and malnourished children.

## Pathogenesis and Pathology

Very little has been written about the pathogenesis or pathology of *F. buski* infection. The large flukes apparently damage the mucosa of the intestine at the site of attachment, causing local ulceration, inflammation, and diarrhea. Abscess formation, hemorrhage from erosion of mucosal vessels, and local bowel obstruction have been described. Edema of the face and legs and ascites are usually attributed to an unidentified toxic metabolite of the parasite.

## Clinical Manifestations

Most adults and approximately one-third of infected children are asymptomatic. The onset of illness coincides with the maturation of flukes in the intestine. Typically many flukes are present before symptoms attributable to *F. buski* occur: the usual worm burden of 10 to 20 flukes is probably of little clinical significance. At least 100 worms have been required to produce illness in an adult and in fatal cases 1000 to 3000 flukes may be recovered at autopsy. Many reported symptoms are nonspecific ones common in endemic areas, and, except in massive infections, are no more common in fasciolopsiasis than in uninfected controls. Typical symptoms attributed to *F. buski* infections are abdominal pain, often relieved by food and simulating peptic ulcer disease, intermittent nondysenteric diarrhea, flatus, excessive appetite, or anorexia.

## Complications and Sequelae

In heavily infected children, the disease may simulate protein-calorie malnutrition with massive edema, including facial edema and ascites, pallor, and hepatomegaly. Edema may occur because of competition by the flukes for limited nutrients in the malnourished, or it may occur because the infestation precipitates Kwashiorkor; however, edema can precede severe malnutrition or diarrhea. Heavily infected children often pass flukes per rectum and vomit flukes. Generally, the younger the patient, the larger the worm burden and the more inadequate the nutrition, the more severe the symptoms, and the greater the potential for a fatal outcome.

## Geographic Variations

Fasciolopsiasis is found in rural parts of Central and South China, India, Bangladesh, Vietnam, Thailand, and Taiwan.

## Diagnosis

The clinical picture is not specific, unless the patient is passing worms, but is sufficiently characteristic to arouse suspicion in endemic areas (Plaut et al., 1969). Anemia, leukocytosis, and eosinophilia (5 to 30 per cent) are common. Diagnosis is based on finding the characteristic ova (Fig. 4, Chapter 80) in the stool.

## Treatment

The traditional treatment has been hexylresorcinol (Crystoids anthelmintic). The dose is 0.4 g for patients less than seven years old and 1 g if older. Tetrachlorethylene, given in one dose of 0.12 cc/kg of body weight (maximum 5 cc dose), is equally effective and now preferred (Suntharasamai et al., 1974). Up to half of persons treated with tetrachlorethylene may have transient side effects, usually nausea and dizziness.

## Prophylaxis

Prevention of *F. buski* infection would require public health education, improved sanitation, prohibition of swine access to areas where water plants are grown, and warning against consumption of raw water plants. Which, if any, of these measures are practical will depend on the endemic area under consideration.

## *HETEROPHYDIASIS*

### Definition

Heterophydiasis is infection caused by the *Heterophyidae* parasites of mammals and fish-eating birds. *Heterophyes heterophyes, Metagonimus yokogawai, Haplorchis yokogawai* and *H. pumilio* are the heterophyids most commonly recovered from man.

### Etiology

The parasite life cycle requires both a fresh or brackish water snail and a fish, often of the mullet family, as intermediate hosts. Infection is acquired by the ingestion of uncooked fish. The adult parasite is found in the small intestine of man and a variety of fish-eating mammals and birds. Growth is rapid; mature ova are found in the stools less than two weeks after ingestion of metacercariae. Each fluke lives only about two months. In some areas the prevalence in young people exceeds 80 per cent.

## Pathology and Pathogenesis

The adult flukes are attached deep in the crypts of Lieberkühn of the small intestine. Infection may cause inflammation and increased mucous production, or there may be little tissue reaction. Ova or dying flukes in the bowel wall cause a granulomatous reaction. Rarely, ova embolize to distant sites, most notably the nervous system and heart. In some cases, eggs reach the mitral valve, eventually causing fibrosis and calcification.

### Clinical Manifestations

These parasites usually produce no symptoms unless present in large numbers. The most typical symptoms are abdominal pain simulating peptic ulcer disease or diarrhea (Sheir and El-Shabrawy, 1970). Diarrhea is usually nondysenteric, although bloody diarrhea has been reported. Diarrhea may persist for months.

### Complications and Sequelae

In the Philippines, heterophyid myocarditis is said to be an important cause of death. The clinical picture may be that of myocardial or valvular disease.

### Geographic Variations

Human infection with *Heterophyes heterophyes* is found in Japan, China, the Philippines, Egypt, Israel, Greece, and Western India. A similar small fluke, *Metagonimus yokogawai,* is common in the Orient and is also found in the Balkans, Spain, Russia, and Israel.

### Diagnosis

Diagnosis is based on finding small operculated ova (Fig. 4, Chapter 80) in the feces. *Heterophyes* ova cannot be differentiated readily from *Metagonimus* ova, and both resemble those of *Opisthorchis.* Adult worms are not seen in the feces except after appropriate treatment.

### Treatment

A 50 to 70 per cent cure rate can be achieved with the standard hookworm doses of tetrachlorethylene or bephenium hydroxynaphthoate, with the standard ascaris dose of piperazine, or with a three-day course of niclosamide. A single dose of piperazine, 50 mg/kg the evening preceding the first of two doses of niclosamide improves the cure rate.

## Prophylaxis

Eradication of heterophydiasis is precluded by the multiple reservoir hosts. Mollusciciding with present techniques also is not feasible. The only method of prevention is to avoid eating uncooked fish in endemic areas.

## References

Belamaric, J: Intrahepatic bile duct carcinoma and C. sinensis infection in Hong Kong. Cancer 31:468, 1973.

Hammond, J. A.: Human infection with the liver fluke Fasciola gigantica. Trans Roy Soc Trop Med Hyg 68:253, 1974.

Hardman, E. W., Jones, R. L. H., and Davies, A. H.: Fascioliasis — a large outbreak. Br Med J 3:502, 1970.

Harinasuta, C. (ed.): Proceedings of the Fourth Southeast Asian Seminar on Parasitology and Tropical Medicine, Schistosomiasis and Other Snail-Transmitted Helminthiasis. Bangkok, Thai Watana Panich Press Co., Ltd., 1969.

Hou, P. C., and Pang, L. C. S.: Clonorchis sinensis infestation in man in Hong Kong. J Pathol Bacteriol 87:245, 1964.

Isseroff, H., Sawma, J. T., and Reino, D.: Fascioliasis: Role of proline in bile duct hyperplasia. Science 198:1157, 1977.

Koompirochana, C., Sonakul, D., Chinda, K., Stitnimankarn, T.: Opisthorchiasis: A clinicopathologic study of 154 autopsy cases. Southeast Asian J Trop Med Public Health 9:60, 1978.

Plaut, A. G., Kampanart-Sanyakorn, C., and Manning, G. S.: A clinical study of Fasciolopsis buski infection in Thailand. Trans R Soc Trop Med Hyg 63:470, 1969.

Sheir, Z. M., and El-Shabrawy, Aboul-Enein M: Demographic, clinical and therapeutic appraisal of heterophydiasis. J Trop Med Hyg 73:148, 1970.

Suntharasamai, P., Bunnag, D., Tejavanij, S., Harinasuta, T., Migasena, S., Vutikes, S., and Chindanond, D.: Comparative clinical trials of niclosamide and tetrachlorethylene in the treatment of Fasciolopsis buski infection. Southeast Asian J Trop Med Public Health 5:556, 1974.

Strauss, W. G.: Clinical manifestations of clonorchiasis: a controlled study of 105 cases. Am J Trop Med 11:625, 1962.

# VISCERAL LEISHMANIASIS **140**
## Anthony D. M. Bryceson, M.D.

### DEFINITION

Visceral leishmaniasis (kala-azar, ponos) is an infection with one of the viscerotropic species of parasites of the genus *Leishmania*, *L. donovani*, *L. infantum*, or *L. chagasi*. The disease is usually a zoonosis, transmitted by phlebotomine sandflies between wild or peridomestic animals. Man is infected when he interrupts the natural cycle, so that human disease is usually sporadic. Epidemics in which man is the only reservoir arise from time to time in the Indian subcontinent.

The disease is a severe chronic infection of the reticuloendothelial system, characterized by fever, chills, weight loss, splenomegaly, leukopenia, anemia, and a high natural mortality.

### ETIOLOGY

*Leishmania* exist in two forms, one in the vertebrate host, including man, and the other in the sandfly and in artificial culture (Hommel, 1978). In the vertebrate host the parasite is in the amastigote (Leishman-Donovan body) stage, so called because it has no free flagellum. It is a round or oval body 2 to 3 $\mu$ across containing a nucleus and a smaller kinetoplast, which stain, respectively, red and purple with Geimsa, Wright's, or Leishman's stain, and stand out against the pale blue cytoplasm. *Leishmania* are strict intracellular parasites and are found in macrophages in which they multiply by binary fission. Heavily parasi-tized host cells rupture, and fresh cells are invaded. Sandflies become infected when they feed on an infected person or animal and take up parasites from blood or skin. In the sandfly the parasite is in the promastigote (leptomonad) stage, so called because of the anterior origin of its flagellum. Promastigotes are supple, highly motile, spindle-shaped organisms, 15 to 25 $\mu$ long and 1.5 to 3.5 $\mu$ broad. They are found in the hindgut or midgut of the sandfly, where they divide and migrate forward into the pharynx and buccal cavity, rendering the sandfly infective. The cycle of development in the sandfly takes about seven days. Once inoculated into man, the promastigotes rapidly penetrate macrophages, flagellum first, and transform into amastigotes.

Biochemical taxonomy of *Leishmania* (isoenzymes, DNA analysis) has proved a valuable adjunct to the traditional epidemiologic and serologic methods of species differentiation (Chance et al., 1977).

It has been suggested that the zoonotic origin of *L. donovani* was among jackals in the steppes of Central Asia, where sporadic cases of visceral leishmaniasis are still seen among nomads and in settlers in the outskirts of rapidly expanding towns. From here the disease spread and developed three distinct epidemiologic patterns.

#### Visceral Leishmaniasis with a Canine Reservoir

This is the pattern in a belt that stretches from Portugal to Peking between latitudes 30 and 48 degrees North, the most important areas being the Mediterranean littoral, including North Africa, the shores of the Caspian Sea, central Soviet Asia, and northeast China. The main vectors are *Phlebotomus perniciosus* and *P. ariasi* in Western Europe, *P. major* in Eastern Europe, *P. papatasii* in the Middle East, and *P. chinensis* in China. In the Mediterranean and Chinese foci, the host-parasite relationship is relatively stable, and the disease is most common among children between one and four years of age. For this reason the parasite has been designated *L. infantum*, although adults in areas into which the disease has newly been introduced or visitors of any age are highly susceptible. Domestic dogs and foxes are the reservoir.

Portuguese and Spanish settlers possibly introduced *L. donovani* into the New World and initiated a zoonosis among foxes and dogs, although man may still be an occasional reservoir. The New World parasite has been designated *L. chagasi*. The likely vector is *Lutzomyia longipalpis*. Visceral leishmaniasis is epidemic in northeast Brazil and sporadic in Amazonia, northern Argentina, and Paraguay. It extends up through Venezuela and Colombia as far as Guatemala and Mexico. It is a disease of towns and villages rather than of the forest. In Brazil male children are most commonly affected.

### Visceral Leishmaniasis with Rodent Vector

This is the pattern in Africa south of the Sahara from Lake Chad in the west to Somalia in the east, sparing the highlands of Ethiopia. The apparent absence of the disease in West Africa and south of the equator is unexplained. In the Sudan the zoonosis is between the Nile rat (*Arvicanthus niloticus*) and *P. orientalis* on the flood plains of the Nile and its tributaries. Visceral leishmaniasis is found among nomads who occupy temporary villages in riverine acacia woodland and migrant workers from adjoining countries.

In Kenya the disease is associated with termite hills where the vector *P. martini* rests and round which village men gather in the evenings. The reservoir is probably the gerbil *Tatara vicina*. The disease is usually sporadic, but epidemics have occurred. Males are affected four times as often as females, and the disease is most common in teenagers.

### Visceral Leishmaniasis with a Human Reservoir

This is true epidemic kala-azar and is the pattern of the disease in northeast India, Bangla-

desh, Assam, and Burma. Classically, the disease spreads along the Brahmaputra valley every 20 years or so. Transmission is by the highly anthropophilic, domestic sandfly *P. argentipes*. Often, many cases are found to have originated from one house. The disease is commonest in young adults. Man is the only reservoir, and *P. argentipes* is readily infected from blood or from the lesions of post-kala-azar dermal leishmaniasis. The disease virtually disappeared over large areas as a result of DDT spraying for malaria control, but returned to Bihar in 1975, killing many thousands.

### Factors Affecting Transmission

Opportunities for contact with infected sandflies largely determine the pattern of disease in a given area. The pattern is modified by the level of immunity of the population or individual. An attack of visceral leishmaniasis confers lifelong immunity, which determines the periodicity of epidemics. Subclinical infections with *L. donovani* or possibly even lizard and rodent species of *Leishmania* affect the pattern of spread in Africa.

## *PATHOGENESIS*

Parasites inoculated by the infective sandfly are taken up by macrophages in which they multiply. The site of early multiplication may be in the skin or possibly in the viscera to which parasites have been carried by the blood stream.

### Susceptibility and Resistance

Evidence from skin testing, serology, and liver biopsy suggests that subclinical cases outnumber clinical cases by about 30:1 during outbreaks of visceral leishmaniasis in the Mediterranean and in Africa. The situation in India is not known, but may be similar. Susceptibility of mice to *L. donovani* is genetically determined (Bradley, 1974), but genetic markers for human susceptibility have not yet been identified. Resistance to infection depends upon the development of specific cell-mediated immunity. When this response is efficient, the illness is mild or symptomless and pathology is limited to small self-healing tuberculoid granulomas in the liver, and possibly other organs. The leishmanin skin test becomes positive and antibodies appear in the serum.

### The Established Disease

Cell-mediated immunity fails to develop or is suppressed early in the infection and parasites spread through the blood stream to spleen, liver, bone marrow, lymph nodes, intestinal lymphatic tissue, and skin and multiply freely in macrophages or other reticuloendothelial cells. Damage and hyperplasia of these organs cause reticuloendothelial blockade and chronic parasitemia. Enlargement of the spleen causes sequestration of erythrocytes, granulocytes, and platelets, all of whose half-lives are reduced. Increased plasma volume and immune lysis of erythrocytes due to complement activation also contribute to anemia. Leukopenia, and possibly immunosuppression due to lymph node derangement, predispose to secondary infection. Reticuloendothelial bombardment leads to overproduction of globulin, especially IgG, little of which is specific antibody and none of which is protective. Some of it is autoantibody. It has been suggested that this hyperglobulinemia may contribute to the pathogenesis of hemolytic anemia, nephritis, and amyloidosis. Bleeding, late in the disease, may be due to thrombocytopenia and clotting defects secondary to hepatocellular damage.

## PATHOLOGY

Histologically the disease is characterized by massive proliferation of parasitized macrophages with little or no lymphocytic response (Winslow, 1971). The spleen is grossly enlarged, smooth, and firm, and the capsule is thick. The pulp is friable and infarcts are usual. There is massive hyperplasia of reticuloendothelial cells that are heavily parasitized. In the liver, Kupffer cells are hyperplastic and contain parasites. Occasionally, parenchymal cells are parasitized. In chronic untreated cases there is parenchymal cell degeneration, which may be followed after several years by fibrosis and even cirrhosis with clinical and biochemical evidence of hepatic dysfunction.

The bone marrow is heavily infiltrated with parasitized macrophages. Erythropoiesis and granulopoiesis are normal in the early stages of the disease, but may be depressed later. The peripheral blood shows anemia and leukopenia. Lymph nodes and lymphoid tissue of the nasopharynx and gut are enlarged and contain many parasitized cells.

Immunoglobulin and complement are deposited in the glomerular basement membrane. In fatal cases, hyaline thickening of the glomerular mesangium has been found. Amyloidosis may develop in chronic cases. The skin, although normal in appearance, contains many intracellular parasites. In post-kala-azar dermal leishmaniasis, there is variable infiltration with lymphocytes, histiocytes, and parasites.

## CLINICAL MANIFESTATIONS

The incubation period is normally two to six months, but may be as short as ten days or as long as nine years. The onset is usually insidious, especially in indigenous peoples who may feel well and have a good appetite despite daily bouts of fever; however, in the poorly nourished with several underlying parasitic infections, the disease may progress rapidly. In Africa a primary cutaneous nodule may be noticed for a few months before there are any systemic symptoms. The earliest symptom is fever, usually gradual in onset and accompanied by sweats, often without preceding chills. Alternatively, the onset is sudden with high fever and chills. This is common in Americans and Europeans who have contracted the disease while visiting an endemic area. Associated with fever there may be dizziness, weakness, and weight loss. Other common early symptoms include cough, diarrhea, pain or discomfort in the left hypochondrium, and symptoms of complicating secondary infections.

The important physical findings are fever, splenomegaly, lymphadenopathy, and skin changes. At first fever is often inconstant, with apyrexial periods of several days or weeks. In over 80 per cent of cases, however, the fever eventually develops a characteristic pattern with twice daily elevations reaching 38 to 40° C, and may then undulate as in brucellosis. In the most acute cases, fever and toxemia may be the only signs. Splenic enlargement is not necessarily rapidly progressive, nor does the size of the spleen correlate with the duration of the disease. In many instances, however, it reaches the right iliac fossa (Fig. 1). It is firm and not tender, unless there has been a subcapsular infarct. The liver enlarges more slowly and becomes palpable in about 20 per cent of cases and is also firm and not tender. Generalized lymphadenopathy is common in patients from Mediterranean countries, Africa, or China. Various changes have been reported in the skin. Classically, there is hyperpigmentation of hands, feet, and abdomen. This may be missed in black Africans; in lighter-skinned Indians it looks gray or black (kala-azar means black sickness). In Africans warty eruptions or ulcers of the skin and oronasal lesions are occasionally seen (Abdalla et al., 1975).

## COMPLICATIONS

As the disease progresses, anemia becomes clinically apparent. There may be bleeding from the nose or gums. In long-standing cases jaundice and signs of hypoalbuminemia may develop,

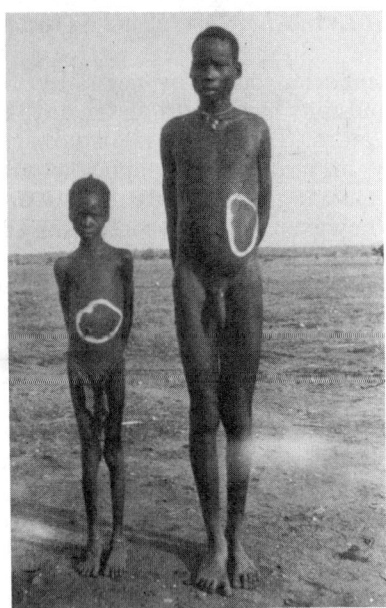

**FIGURE 1.** *Marked splenomegaly of visceral leishmaniasis.*

namely, brittle hair, opaque nails, subcutaneous edema, and ascites. Finally, after a course that may run for a few months or for as long as five years, the patient becomes emaciated and exhausted. Intercurrent infections are the cause of death in 90 per cent of fatal cases. The most common are cancrum oris, pneumonia, pulmonary tuberculosis, bacillary dysentery, amebic dysentery, and, in Africa, brucellosis. Massive gastrointestinal hemorrhage accounts for another 1 to 2 per cent.

Untreated, 75 to 90 per cent of patients with established disease die. Treated patients should recover. The mortality of late or severe disease in malnourished patients treated under difficult conditions can be over 25 per cent. Bad prognostic signs include extreme emaciation and toxemia, agranulocytosis, and the absence of the lymphocytosis, which usually appears during treatment.

### SEQUELAE

A small, unknown proportion of recovered patients develop cirrhosis later. Another proportion may relapse. In the great majority, however, recovery, if it takes place, is complete, and the patient is immune against reinfection, probably for life.

#### Post-Kala-azar Dermal Leishmaniasis

About 20 per cent of Indian patients develop a rash one to two years after treatment or sponta-

neous recovery. The lesions develop slowly and may last for several, even 20, years. In Africa the rash develops in 2 per cent of cases, usually during treatment, and does not persist. It commonly starts as hypopigmented or erythematous macules on the face and sometimes on the arms, legs, and trunk. On the face, the rash gradually becomes papular or nodular, especially on the forehead, cheeks, and earlobes, and closely resembles lepromatous leprosy (Fig. 2). In 25 per cent of cases the lesions resolve spontaneously.

### GEOGRAPHIC VARIATIONS IN DISEASE

Despite the extremely varied epidemiology of the disease, and despite the enormous opportunity for variation that the parasite is offered by continuous fly and animal passage, there is surprisingly little variation of the disease in man. Differences in age and sex patterns, due to endemicity, epidemicity, and opportunity for contact have been considered under *ETIOLOGY*.

In Africa, the primary leishmanioma is a common feature, and in the Sudan mucocutaneous lesions are seen, but it is not established whether they are due to *L. donovani* or to *L. tropica*. In Kenya lymphadenopathy may be the only sign of visceral disease. Spontaneous recovery is more common, up to 80 per cent, in Sudan than elsewhere.

Post-kala-azar dermal leishmaniasis is charac-

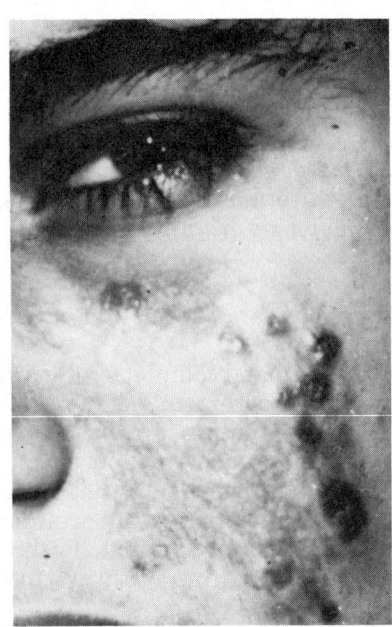

**FIGURE 2.** *Post-kala-azar dermal leishmaniasis.*

teristic of Indian Kala-azar, but rare elsewhere. For differences in response to treatment, see *TREATMENT*.

## DIAGNOSIS

The diagnosis must be suspected in any person living in, or having visited, an endemic area who has a prolonged fever. The diagnosis is likely in the presence of splenomegaly, granulocytopenia, anemia, and hyperglobulinemia and is made by isolation of the parasite or by characteristic im- munologic changes.

### Isolation of Parasite

This is best done by needle aspiration of bone marrow, spleen, liver, or lymph nodes. Material obtained is:

1. Used to make a thin film on a glass microscope slide, stained, and examined under oil immer- sion for amastigotes, which must be distin- guished from platelets. Parasitized macro- phages usually rupture on smearing and free parasites must be looked for. Bone marrow as- piration is the procedure of choice. However, splenic puncture is safe so long as the tip of the spleen is well below the costal margin and the prothrombin and bleeding times are normal. A hypodermic needle on a syringe is inserted into the spleen, allowed to rest a moment, and withdrawn without suction. Organisms are seen in about 90 per cent of splenic aspirates and rather less often from other tissues. Buffy coat preparations show parasites in over 90 per cent of cases in India, but in only about 1 per cent in Africa.

2. Inoculated onto NMN (Novy-MacNeal-Nicolle) medium overlaid with balanced salt solution, containing streptomycin and penicillin (but not amphotericin). Cultures are kept in the dark at 22 to 25° C (not at 37° C), and every three to four days a drop of fluid is examined wet for promastigotes. If after four weeks no parasites are seen, the fluid overlay is reino- culated onto a fresh NMN slope. Culture great- ly improves the chances of making a diagnosis. Blood culture is commonly positive and is a simple method of assessing treatment.

3. Inoculated intraperitoneally into hamsters, which are susceptible to a single amastigote. Although sensitive, this method is slow and seldom valuable.

### Immunologic Tests

Anti-leishmanial antibodies can be demon- strated by indirect immunofluorescence of pro-

mastigotes in over 90 per cent of cases and by precipitation in gel in 95 per cent (Ranque et al., 1975). Cross-reactions with *Trypanosoma cruzi* antibodies can be absorbed out. Complement fixa- tion is positive in 65 per cent, but if the older antigen made from Kedrowsky's bacillus is used, reactions may be expected in some patients with mycobacterial disease. Serum obtained by eluting blood dried onto filter paper in the field can be used satisfactorily in all these techniques. The leishmanin test is negative in cases of active vis- ceral leishmaniasis, but becomes positive after recovery (Pampiglione, 1975). It is most intense after one to two years, and slowly fades.

Total serum proteins are raised up to and over 10 g per 100 ml. This increase is due almost en- tirely to the IgG fraction of γ-globulin. On im- munoelectrophoresis the IgG pattern is charac- teristically skewed. In some cases IgM is also slightly increased, but this is said to be transient and to revert rapidly to normal on treatment. In advanced cases serum albumin levels fall. This disturbed globulin pattern underlies the older diagnostic aldehyde test, which is also positive in other diseases with a grossly disturbed globulin pattern.

### Other Laboratory Findings

Leukopenia is the most characteristic finding. The total count is below 2000 cells/mm$^2$ in 75 per cent of cases with absolute neutropenia and eo- sinopenia and relative lymphocytosis and mono- cytosis. Agranulocytosis occasionally develops. Anemia is slower in onset but becomes severe. It is normocytic and normochromic unless compli- cated by bleeding or deficiency states. There is often a mild reticulocytosis, and erythrocyte half- life is reduced. Thrombocytopenia is usual and progresses with the disease. Early on, tests of clotting are normal but later the prothrombin, partial thromboplastin, bleeding, and clotting times are prolonged. There are no characteristic findings in the urine.

### Differential Diagnosis

In Europeans, Americans, and others who are not immune, malaria must be excluded by exami- nation of thick and thin blood films. In immunes, the presence of malarial parasites in the blood film does not exclude leishmaniasis. In many parts of the tropics where malaria and schisto- somiasis are endemic, a palpable spleen is com- monplace and is usually unrelated to a recent febrile illness. Diseases that can be confused with visceral leishmaniasis include aleukemic leuke- mia and lymphomas, tropical splenomegaly syn- drome, cirrhosis of the liver with portal hyperten- sion and hypersplenism, miliary tuberculosis, histoplasmosis, acute schistosomiasis, brucellosis, typhoid, and other septicemias, including bacterial endocarditis.

## TREATMENT

### Chemotherapy

Pentavalent antimony is the drug of choice. Of the available preparations, sodium stibogluconate (pentostam, Solustibostam) is probably the best. This is marketed as a solution containing 100 mg Sb/ml. The dose is 0.1 to 0.2 ml/kg of body weight daily by intravenous or intramuscular injection, not exceeding 10 ml per dose. In India six injections are usually adequate, but elsewhere 30 are considered necessary. Alternative preparations include the following: 1) Meglumine antimoniate (Glucantime, 30 mg/ml), 0.4 ml/kg of body weight daily for 14 days. 2) Ethyl stibamine (Neostibosan), which must be freshly prepared as a 5 per cent solution. The adult dose is 2 ml the first day, 3 ml the second day, and 4 ml daily thereafter for 8 to 16 doses by intravenous injection. 3) Urea stibamine, 100 to 200 mg intravenously on alternate days for 15 doses. Side effects of pentavalent antimony are cumulative but rare. They are nausea, vomiting, urticaria, bradycardia, and electrocardiographic changes. The response to antimonial treatment varies in kala-azar from different parts of the world. It is excellent in India and Brazil but less satisfactory in East Africa and the Mediterranean. Poor response may be due to inadequate dosage or duration of treatment. If antimony is unsuccessful, the choice then lies between two toxic drugs, pentamidine isethionate (Lomidine, 40 mg/ml) and amphotericin B (Fungizone). The dose of pentamidine is 0.1 ml/kg of body weight by intramuscular injection every three to four days for 10 doses, or less frequently if side effects develop. If the drug is accidentally injected intravenously, the patient will collapse, but recovers quickly if the feet are raised. Cumulative side effects include fatigue, anorexia, nausea, abdominal pain and, in 2 per cent of cases, prolonged hypoglycemia. Ten per cent of patients develop diabetes, whose onset is not related to the duration of treatment. If this drug has to be used, a glucose tolerance test should be performed weekly. Amphotericin B is given by slow intravenous infusion in 5 per cent dextrose in a dose of 1 mg/kg of body weight on alternate days to a total of 2 g for a 50-kg adult. Side effects include rigors, thrombophlebitis, nausea, vomiting, fatigue, anemia, and uremia. This drug is more difficult to administer than pentamidine but is preferable.

### Supportive Treatment

Bed rest, good nursing care, oral hygiene, an adequate fluid intake, and sufficient food are all desirable. Complicating infections must be sought and treated. Anemia responds as the patient recovers; but if severe, and especially if there is bleeding, blood transfusion should be given. Deficiencies of iron, folate, and other vitamins should be corrected.

### Response to Treatment

Little improvement may be seen until the course of treatment is nearly over. The patient then continues to improve steadily. Lymphocytosis and reticulocytosis are good signs. No criterion of cure has been established. The patient should be seen monthly for six months and at one year. At each visit blood is cultured for *Leishmania,* spleen size is measured, and hemoglobin and serum IgG are estimated. Complement-fixing antibody should not be detectable after six months. The spleen does not always become impalpable, and may indicate cirrhosis.

### Relapses and Post-Kala-azar Dermal Leishmaniasis

These usually respond to a further course or courses of antimony. If not, one of the other drugs may be used. One month should elapse before treatment is repeated. Rarely, if repeated courses of drugs fail to eliminate the parasite, the spleen remains huge, and the patient suffers from hypersplenism. Splenectomy may be indicated. It must be followed by a course of chemotherapy, and in malarial areas by antimalarial prophylaxis for life.

## PROPHYLAXIS

On a mass scale the detailed epidemiology of the local disease must be known. This will permit reservoir control (destruction of stray dogs, early detection and treatment of cases) and vector control (insecticide spraying in the right places) to be carried out, and people may be able to avoid contact with infected flies, e.g., Kenyan termite hills. In some areas insecticide spraying against malarial mosquitoes reduced or eliminated kala-azar. Personal prophylaxis depends on wearing protective clothing in the evenings, the use of insect repellents, and sleeping under fine mesh netting.

## References

Abdalla, R. E., El Hadi, A., Ahmed, M. A., and El Hassan, A. M.: Sudan mucosal leishmaniasis. Trans Roy Soc Trop Med Hyg 69:443, 1975.

Bradley, D. J.: Genetic control of natural resistance to *Leishmania donovani*. Nature (Lond.) 250:353, 1974.

Chance, M. L., Gardener, P. J., and Peters, W.: Biochemical Taxonomy of *Leishmania* as an ecological test. Colloques Internationaux du C.N.R.S. No. 329, p. 53, 1977.

Hommel, M.: The genus *Leishmania*: biology of the parasites and clinical aspects. Bulletin de l'Institut Pasteur 76:5, 1978.

Pampiglione, S., Manson-Bahr, P. E. C., La Placa, M., Borgatti, M. A., and Musumeci, S.: Studies in Mediterranean leishmaniasis 3: The Leishmanin test in kala-azar. Trans Roy Soc Trop Med Hyg 69:60, 1975.

Ranque, J., Quillici, M., Dunan, S., and Ranque, Ph.: Diagnostic immunologique de la leishmaniose viscerale (10 années d'expérience). Ann Soc Belge Méd Trop 55:579, 1975.

Sen Gupta, P. C., and Mukherjee, A. M. Indian Med Ass 50:1, 1968.

Winslow, D. J.: Visceral leishmaniasis. In Marcel-Rojas, R. A. (ed.): Pathology of Rickettsial and Helminthic Diseases. Baltimore, Williams and Wilkins Company, 1971, p. 86.

# SPIROCHETAL HEPATITIS 141

### János Fehér, M.D., C.Sc.

Two main types of inflammatory liver diseases are caused by microorganisms of the family *Spirochetaceae*. These are syphilitic hepatitis and leptospiral hepatitis. The two entities are discussed separately.

## SYPHILITIC HEPATITIS

### DEFINITION

Syphilitic hepatitis is an inflammatory disease of the liver that may develop either early or late in the course of syphilis and may occur in congenital syphilis and in lues congenita tarda.

### ETIOLOGY

The pathogenic agent of syphilitic hepatitis is *Treponema pallidum*, a thin, delicate, spiral organism with 6 to 14 spirals and tapered ends, measuring 5 to 15 μm in total length and 0.2 to 0.3 μm in width. The depth and amplitude of the spirals is about 1 μm. In histologic preparations *T. pallidum* in barely stainable. It can be impregnated with silver because it reduces silver nitrate to metallic silver. In wet preparations it can be examined under the darkfield microscope. It also can be demonstrated by direct and indirect immunofluorescence (Al-Sammarrai, 1977) and by electronmicroscopic techniques (Ovcinnikov and Delektorskij, 1972). None of the pathogenic treponemes has yet been cultured in vitro. After drying in air and after oxidation, it perishes very quickly. Its virulence in humans is extremely high, and artificial infection has been successful in apes. Lesions can be regularly produced in rabbits, and virulent strains of *T. pallidum* are usually maintained in that species.

### PATHOGENESIS AND PATHOLOGY

At the site of inoculation *T. pallidum* rapidly penetrates intact mucous membranes or abraded skin and enters the lymphatics and blood vessels within a few hours to produce systemic infection and metastatic foci long before the appearance of the primary lesion. The mean incubation period is 20 to 25 days, but it may range from 10 to 90 days. *T. pallidum* is, as a rule, demonstrable at the inoculation site. The *primary lesion* persists for two to six weeks, then heals spontaneously. In the *secondary phase* of syphilis, within 2 to 12 weeks after the initial lesion, maculopapular exanthems develop in most patients. Metastatic foci may arise in widely differing forms on the skin and mucous membranes and in internal organs. The progression is intermittent with different manifestations and latent cycles. The lesions are a function not only of the treponemes but also of the immune reaction of the host. In many cases, lesions may develop in a number of different organs.

Symptomatologically, three stages can be differentiated in syphilis: (1) *primary syphilis*, primary chancre and regional lymphadenopathy; (2) *secondary syphilis*, symptoms of hematogenous dissemination, (3) *tertiary syphilis*, chronic organ diseases.

From the point of view of immunity, syphilis can be divided into *early* and *late* stages. Changes in the immune reaction and termination of hematogenous dissemination demarcate the two forms. Early syphilis has two phases, seronegative and seropositive.

As a result of hematogenous dissemination, the treponemes may enter the liver and, in the early phase, may produce the characteristic early syphilitic hepatitis. In our syphilitic material we found early syphilitic hepatitis in about 10 per cent of early syphilitic patients. The liver is enlarged, and jaundice may occur (Fehér et al., 1975).

Early syphilitic hepatitis shows varying degrees of histologic abnormality. In the patients that show minimal changes, there is proliferation of sinus endothelial cells and Kupffer cells, together with many granulocytes, eosinophils, and lymphocytes in the sinusoids. The periportal region is swollen, and the walls of the arteries and portal vein branches are thickened and infiltrated with inflammatory cells. In these cases, the architecture of the liver is not altered, and there is no evidence of cholestasis. In more severe cases focal liver necrosis occurs. Only one or two liver cells may become necrotic in some cases, whereas necrosis is more extensive in others. In the necrotic areas, neutrophil and eosinophil granulocytes, lymphocytes, and mast cells are found, and the reticulin structure is destroyed (Fig. 1). In some areas of necrosis, fibroblasts and epithelioid cells are seen, as well as an acute inflammatory infiltrate. Necrotic foci are found in all parts of the lobules but are more common in the periportal region and around the central vein (Fig. 2). The necrotic inflammatory foci around the central vein appear to be characteristic of syphilitic hepatitis, as they were present in all of our patients

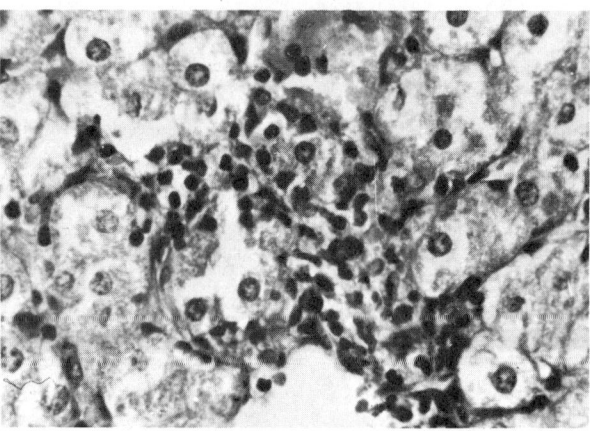

**FIGURE 2.**   *Light micrograph of liver tissue from patient with early syphilis, showing lymphocytic infiltration of region around vena centralis. (Hematoxylin and eosin, ×400.)*

with liver damage. The walls of the branches of the central vein are thickened with increased reticulin and collagen fibers. Glycogen content is markedly reduced in the necrotic areas and in their immediate neighborhood. In half of our cases, treponemes were demonstrated in liver biopsy material. They were found in the inflammatory necrotic foci, in the sinus endothelial cells, in the Disse spaces and sometimes in the intrahepatic bile capillaries (Fig. 3).

After penicillin treatment, syphilitic hepatitis heals with accumulation of collagen in the walls of sinusoids and in the spaces between the liver cells.

## CLINICAL MANIFESTATIONS

The *latent form* of syphilitic hepatitis can be detected only by liver function tests. It does not

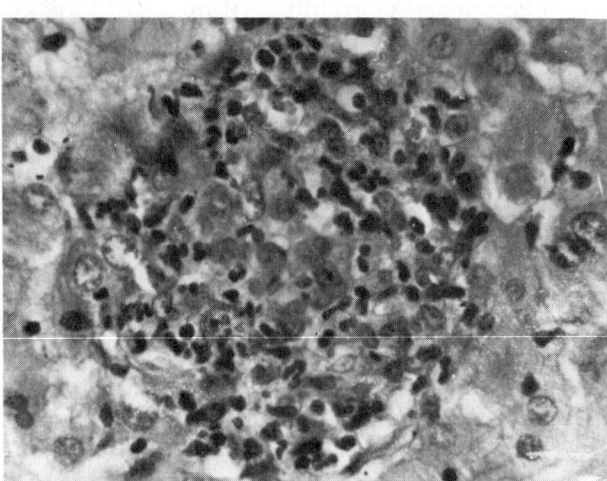

**FIGURE 1.**   *Light micrograph of liver tissue from patient with early syphilis, showing focal inflammatory reaction. (Hematoxylin and eosin, ×400.)*

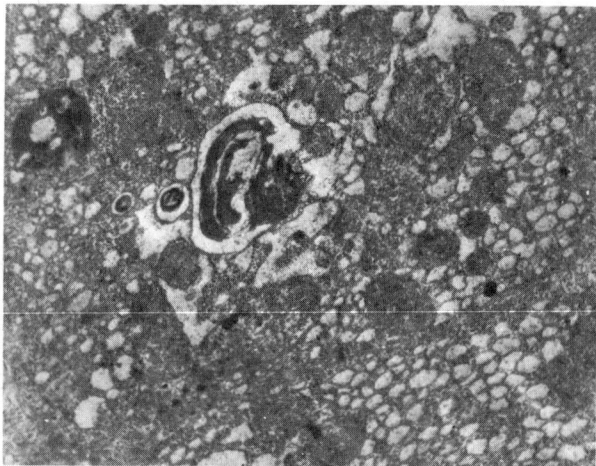

**FIGURE 3.**   *Electron micrograph of liver cell, showing tubularization of endoplasmic reticulum and intracellular treponema. (×9200.)*

cause any clinical symptoms and develops after the primary infection.

*Early syphilitic hepatitis* occurs in the secondary stage of syphilis. The liver is enlarged, but there is no pain, and subicterus or icterus develops. Hepatitis often coincides with the appearance of luetic exanthems. It usually heals within a few weeks, but in some rare cases it undergoes yellow atrophy (Leonard, 1944).

*Late luetic hepatitis* is characterized by pain, fever, and sometimes splenomegaly. The pain is colicky owing to tension of the liver capsule and to liver swelling. The fever is irregular and may be accompanied by chills. It is impossible to differentiate this interstitial form of hepatitis from luetic liver cirrhosis.

Some forms of *luetic liver cirrhosis* may arise from syphilitic hepatitis. We have observed the development of chronic aggressive hepatitis in certain cases of early syphilitic hepatitis. Luetic liver cirrhosis is thought to evolve from such chronic syphilitic liver lesions.

*Hepatic gumma* is the most frequent form of luetic liver disease. It is characterized by sudden sharp pain. The spleen is usually enlarged and irregular, and intermittent fever is a constant symptom. Without treatment, the patients become cachectic. The gummas are palpable as knots or lumps of various sizes, and occasionally liver tumor is suspected. Round masses are often palpable below the liver margin. Some patients present signs of cholangitis, while in others the symptoms are those of gallstones. The cicatrized contraction of gummas causes a lobular distortion of the liver known as *hepar lobatum*.

The *hepatitis of congenital lues* (brimstone liver) is not encountered in adults. Only its late form, the hepatomegaly of lues congenita tarda, occurs in adults.

## COMPLICATIONS

With adequate penicillin therapy, the latent and early forms of syphilitic hepatitis usually heal completely. In some cases the picture of chronic aggressive hepatitis may develop and may progress to cirrhosis. Very rarely, acute hepatitis may undergo yellow atrophy. Cirrhosis, frequently in the company of hepatic gummas,

may also develop from the hepatitis of late syphilis. Gummas in the portal region cause obstructive jaundice, and portal obstruction leads to the development of ascites.

Hepatitis B virus may be inoculated simultaneously with syphilis because the hepatitis B virus may be sexually transmitted (Papaevangelou et al., 1974). The $HB_sAg$ can be demonstrated in the sera of some patients with syphilitic hepatitis in early syphilis only.

## GEOGRAPHIC VARIATIONS IN DISEASE

Syphilis and syphilitic hepatitis is endemic all over the world. There is no essential difference in the clinical symptoms and in the course of the disease, unless it is associated with another infection or combined with malnutrition. More severe cases are found in less developed countries and in populations living under poor hygienic conditions.

## DIAGNOSIS

The diagnosis of syphilis is based on serologic tests (VDRL, FABS, Kolmer) and on demonstration of treponemes in local lesions of the skin and mucous membranes. In syphilitic hepatitis, hepatomegaly and an increase in the serum bilirubin concentration are common. The SGOT and SGPT activity is increased, the prothrombin time and BSP value are abnormal, and serum protein levels are altered. The changes in serum immunoglobulins, especially IgG and IgM concentrations, resemble those found in viral hepatitis. The diagnosis can be established histologically by liver biopsy; treponemes can be demonstrated occasionally (Fehér et al., 1975).

## TREATMENT

Syphilitic hepatitis should be differentiated from other forms of hepatitis. The specific therapy is penicillin treatment. For these patients, some weeks rest can be recommended. Patients with syphilitic hepatitis must be treated in hospital.

# LEPTOSPIRAL HEPATITIS

## DEFINITION

Leptospiral hepatitis (Weil's disease) is the most important manifestation of leptospirosis. It

is a zooanthroponosis, i.e., an acute infectious disease that can be transmitted from animals to humans. The typical course is biphasic. In the initial phase, which lasts about one week, there are septicemic symptoms of headache, nausea, fever, conjunctivitis, and myalgia. The second phase is called the toxic or immune phase and coincides with the appearance of circulating IgM antibodies. The symptoms of organ involvement (i.e., of hepatitis, nephritis, meningitis, and combinations of these syndromes) arise in this phase.

### ETIOLOGY

The genus *Leptospira* contains only one species, *L. interrogans*, which may be subdivided into two complexes, the parasitic *L. interrogans* and the saprophitic *L. biflexa* strains. *L. interrogans* is a delicate undulant microorganism 0.1 to 0.2 $\mu$m in width and, as a rule, 6 to 9 $\mu$m in length; it has some forms that are 2 to 3 $\mu$m in length or as much as 30 $\mu$m. These microorganisms grow vigorously in egg albumin broth and in the chorioallantoic membrane of the chick embryo. On the basis of antigenic variations, about 130 serotypes (actually subserotypes) can be differentiated, which are classed into 16 serogroups according to their common antigens. *L. icterohaemorrhagiae*, which has 13 serotypes, is the most important serogroup. Other serogroups are: *L. australis, L. autumnalis, L. bataviae, L. bellum, L. canicola, L. celledoni, L. cynopteri, L. grippotyphosa, L. hebdomidis, L. hyos, L. javanica, L. panama, L. pomona, L. pyrogenese,* and *L. shermani.*

### PATHOGENESIS AND PATHOLOGY

There is an incubation period of one to two weeks before leptospiremia develops, with the general syndrome of septicemia lasting for about one week. Then, when immunity develops, leptospiremia disappears and is followed by the second phase, the appearance of acute lesions in different organs; it is characterized by leptospiral hepatitis, nephritis, meningitis, and hemorrhages. Mild cases do not progress beyond the first phase. In more severe cases, jaundice, hemorrhagic lesions, and renal disease may develop. The severity of the disease depends on the antigenic type of the invading leptospirae and on the immune reaction of the patient.

The jaundice in leptospiral hepatitis may be hepatocellular after liver cell necrosis, obstructive if cholangitis occurs, hemolytic, or a combination of the three (Bruns, 1967).

Necrosis in the liver is minimal and focal. Dissociation of cells from one another is prominent but is probably a postmortem phenomenon for the most part. The centrizonal necrosis of

acute hepatitis is absent. Active hepatocellular regeneration, shown by mitoses and nuclear polyploidy, is out of proportion to cell damage. There is proliferation of Kupffer cells (Sherlock, 1975). Periportal infiltration with leukocytes is a constant finding, and centrizonal bile is prominent if the patient is deeply jaundiced. The bile capillaries are dilated; occasionally bile thrombi occur. The liver sinusoids are full of blood, and focal hemorrhages can be observed in the parenchyma.

The histologic demonstration of leptospirae is rarely possible except in patients with massive infection and in the earliest stage. Leptospirae are found in liver cells and in necrotic foci.

In patients who have died with either hepatic involvement, renal involvement, or both, the significant gross changes include hemorrhages and bile pigmentation of the hepatic tissue. The hemorrhages, which vary from petechial to ecchymotic, are widespread and are most prominent in the skeletal muscle, kidneys, adrenals, liver, stomach, spleen, and lungs (Sanford, 1974).

### CLINICAL MANIFESATATIONS

The incubation period following immersion or laboratory exposure is usually 7 to 14 days, but ranges from 2 to 20 days and averages 10 days.

Two extremes of leptospirosis can be differentiated — *benign* and *malignant* forms, with several transitional forms. The malignant icterohemorrhagic form is also called Weil's disease after the first description (Weil, 1886). Hepatitis occurs rarely in anicteric (benign) cases but frequently in icteric (malignant) forms.

Leptospirosis is typically a biphasic disease. In the *first or septicemic phase* leptospirae are present in the blood and cerebrospinal fluid. The onset is abrupt with prostration, high fever, and rigors. The temperature rises rapidly to 39 to 41° C and falls by lysis within 5 to 10 days. Characteristic symptoms are frontal headache, less often retroorbital, bitemporal, or occipital headache, and conjunctival suffusion. Anorexia, nausea, vomiting, and abdominal pain simulate an acute abdominal emergency. Severe muscular pains, especially in the back or calves, are common (Sherlock, 1975). After five days, the symptoms of meningism or slight meningitis appear. On days 4 to 8, macular, maculopapular, or urticarial exanthems sometimes develop on the trunk and extremities. This septicemic stage without manifestations of visceral disease lasts five to eight days, and then fever falls by lysis. Patients who recover at this point (benign, anicteric form) exhibit only slight hepatorenal manifestations. Transition into hepato-nephritis is rare. The first phase terminates after four to nine days, usually with defervescence and improvement of the symptoms. This coincides with the disappearance of leptospirae from the blood and cerebrospinal fluid.

The *second, toxic or immune, phase* is marked by circulating IgM antibodies and by disease of the liver, kidney, and meninges. The concentration of $C_3$ in the serum remains normal during this phase. After a relatively asymptomatic period of one to three days, the fever and earlier symptoms recur, and the signs of malignant leptospirosis, hepatitis, nephritis, and meningitis, alone or in combination, may develop. Hemorrhagic symptoms include epistaxis, conjunctival suffusion, petechiae, hematemesis, and melena. Cough accompanies pneumonitis.

Leptospiral hepatitis occurs in icteric, icterohemorrhagic, and icterouremic forms. Jaundice is the most conspicuous finding, and the prognosis depends on the degree of renal failure. Bleeding and splenomegaly are common.

This phase is characterized by low blood pressure and cardiac dilatation. There may be transient arrhythmias and electrocardiographic abnormalities. Death may be due to circulatory failure.

During this phase leptospirae can be found in the urine, and rising antibody titers are demonstrated in the serum.

Some clinicians distinguish a *third or convalescent phase* (Sherlock, 1975). During this period, usually between the second and fourth weeks, both fever and pain may recur. The pathogenesis of this stage is poorly understood (Sanford, 1974).

## GEOGRAPHIC VARIATIONS IN DISEASE

The individual forms of leptospiral hepatitis produced by different serotypes are essentially the same from the points of view of epidemiology, symptoms, and pathogenesis. Some variations due to differences between the serotypes that occur on different continents are found. *L. bataviae* causes the Indonesian form of Weil's disease with severe jaundice. One of its variants has been observed in northern Italy. *L. icterohaemoglobinurica* produces the leptospiral blackwater fever of Africa and Indonesia. *L. autumnalis* is the pathogenic agent of Japanese autumn fever. Hemorrhages, lymphadenopathy, and disturbances of vision are characteristic of this disease, in addition to the signs characteristic of Weil's disease. *L. pyrogenes* is found in Indonesia, Australia, and Italy. At least 22 serotypes of leptospirae occur naturally in the United States (Sanford, 1974).

Within the serogroup *L. bovis* special serotypes have been described in the Soviet Union, United States, Japan, Israel, and Switzerland. A few cases in which *L. bovis* was the pathogenic agent of human disease have been reported (Bruns, 1967).

## DIAGNOSIS

Leptospirae may be isolated readily during the septicemic phase from blood and cerebrospinal fluid or during the second phase from urine. After five to eight days they disappear from the blood into the internal organs. Darkfield microscopy or stained preparations of blood or urine are unreliable. Conclusive evidence may be obtained by culture and inoculation into guinea pigs or hamster. Whole blood should be inoculated immediately into tubes containing semisolid medium such as Fletcher's medium (Füzi, 1961; Sanford, 1974).

Specific antibodies appear in the serum during the second phase, and diagnosis requires a fourfold or greater rise in complement-fixing or microscopic agglutination titers. Cross-agglutination reaction between various serotypes commonly occurs. Serotype-specific antigens are required in the microscopic agglutination for precise identification of the infecting leptospiral organism. Early antibiotic treatment may prevent an antibody response.

Leukocytosis with neutrophilia and the erythrocyte sedimentation rate are increased. The findings in the cerebrospinal fluid resemble those encountered in aseptic meningitis. Platelet count and bleeding, coagulation, and prothrombin times are normal in spite of the hemorrhagic diathesis (its cause may be capillary damage).

Liver function tests are abnormal. GOT, GPT, LDH, and alkaline phosphatase levels are only moderately elevated. Dysproteinemia and increased gammaglobulin and bilirubin levels may also be found.

## TREATMENT

Penicillin, streptomycin, chloramphenicol, tetracycline, and erythromycin are effective against leptospirae in vitro. They control guinea pig infection if given within 24 hours. Although large doses of penicillin G have been recommended, there is no conclusive evidence of its value in man. It would certainly be useless after the first four days (Sherlock, 1975). The usual dose is 1,000,000 units penicillin G, intravenously, four times daily for seven days. For patients who are allergic to penicillin, tetracycline may be used in doses of 0.5 g orally four times daily for seven days. If oliguria or anuria supervene, peritoneal or hemedialysis should be available for the treatment of acute tubular necrosis.

### PROPHYLAXIS

Bathing in stagnant water should be avoided. Protective clothing (rubber boots and gloves) should be provided for workers exposed to leptospirae. Specific immune serum has been effective in exposed laboratory workers but is limited in availability. In cases of probable infection, chemoprophylaxis with therapeutic doses of penicillin or tetracycline is recommended. Human vaccines are not available, but animal vaccines are effective.

### References

Al-Sammarrai, H. T., and Henderson, W. G.: Immunofluorescent staining of *Treponema pallidum* and *Treponema pertenue* in tissues fixed by formalin and embedded in paraffin wax. Br J Vener Dis 53:1, 1977.

Bruns, G.: Vergleichende pathologische Anatomie der Leptospirosen. In Kathe, J., and Mochmann, H. (eds.): Leptospiren und Leptospirosen. Jena, Gustav Fischer Verlag, 1967, p. 151.

Fehér, J., Somogyi, T., Timmer, M., and Józsa, L.: Early syphilitic hepatitis. Lancet 2:896, 1975.

Füzi, M.: Physiologie der Leptospirosen. In Kathe, J., and Mochmann, H. (eds.): Leptospiren und Leptospirosen. Jena, Gustav Fischer Verlag, 1967, p. 351.

Leonard, M. F.: Acute yellow atrophy of the liver in early syphilis: A case report with summary of the literature. Am J Med Sci 208:461, 1944.

Papaevangeolu, G., Trichopoulos, D., Papoutsakis, G., Kremastinou, T., and Pavlides, E.: Hepatitis B antigen in prostitutes. Br J Vener Dis 50:228, 1974.

Ovcinnikov, N. M., and Delektorskij, V. V.: Effect of crystalline penicillin and bicillin-1 on experimental syphilis in the rabbit. Electronmicroscopic study. Br J Vener Dis 48:327, 1972.

Sanford, J. P.: Leptospirosis. In Wintrope, M. M., et al. (eds.): Harrison's Principles of Internal Medicine. 7th ed. New York, McGraw-Hill Book Company, 1974, p. 887.

Sherlock, S.: Diseases of the Liver and Biliary System. 5th ed. Oxford, Blackwell Scientific Publications, 1975.

Weil, A.: Über eine eigentümliche, mit Milzschwellung, Ikterus und Nephritis einhergehende akute Infektionskrankheit. Dtsch Arch Klin Med 39:209, 1886.

# 142 VIRAL HEPATITIS

### Shalom Z. Hirschman, M.D.
### Fenton Schaffner, M.D.

### INTRODUCTION

Viral hepatitis is a common infectious disease throughout the world. During the decade of 1966 to 1976 the case rate of viral hepatitis per 1000 population was at a low of 18.56 in 1966, reached a high of 33.64 in 1971, and declined to 26.46 in 1976. However, the case rate for hepatitis B virus infection has steadily increased from 1.79 in 1966 to 6.92 in 1976. The case rates for hepatitis A infection appeared to be declining during the six years from 1971 to 1976.

In Chapter 67, the properties of the hepatitis A and B viruses, including epidemiology and geographic distribution, were considered. In this chapter the pathogenesis, clinical manifestations, and untoward sequelae of infections with these viruses will be detailed.

### HEPATITIS A

#### Transmission

The distribution of hepatitis A is worldwide, and disease is more prevalent in areas of poor hygiene and low socioeconomic standards (Murray, 1955). The infection appears to be spread by the fecal-oral route. Although sporadic cases of the disease develop from close person-to-person contact, many food- and water-borne epidemics have been reported (Dienstag et al., 1975). Occasionally, hepatitis A virus (HAV) infection is transmitted by parenteral injection. This route of infection may be more common in drug addicts. One of the most explosive water-borne outbreaks of hepatitis, presumed to be Type A, occurred in 1955 and 1956, when 29,000 people were infected within a six-week period in Delhi, India.

The incubation period of hepatitis A virus infection is usually about 30 days with a range of 15 to 50 days (Table 1). Hepatitis A antigen (HAAg) is found in the stool at least five days before the activities of transaminases in serum begin to increase and one to two weeks before the onset of clinical symptoms. The maximal fecal excretion of HAAg occurs at about the time of peak transaminase activity and then rapidly falls as jaundice ensues. The feces of patients with hepatitis A contain virus for about one to two weeks before, and about one week after, the appearance of jaundice. The total infectious period for the stool is about three weeks. When HAAg is no longer detectable in the stool, anti-HA is found in serum. The level of antibody rises quickly and remains elevated for at least ten years after recovery. The persistence of antibody may explain the long-lasting immunity of patients to reinfection with

**TABLE 1.  Clinical Presentations of Hepatitis A and B**

|  | HEPATITIS A | HEPATITIS B |
|---|---|---|
| Incubation period | 15 to 50 days | 40 to 180 days |
| Prodrome | Malaise, fever, gastroenteritis | Malaise, fever, urticaria, and arthritis |
| Onset | Acute | Gradual except in infancy |
| Clinical course | Usually mild with complete resolution in two to four weeks; fatal hepatic necrosis uncommon | Patient moderately ill; most recover; some develop chronic hepatitis; fatal hepatic necrosis uncommon |
| Chronic carrier | No | Yes |
| Chronic active hepatitis | No | Yes |
| Immunologic sequelae | None known | Glomerulonephritis, periarteritis nodosa |

HAV. Recent serologic surveys have shown that only about 25 to 30 per cent of adults in the United States have anti-HA antibody. Where hepatitis A is endemic, 90 per cent of individuals acquire antibody by the age of 15. Thus, in underdeveloped areas, infection with HAV occurs mainly in the young.

### Clinical Presentation

Jaundice may be the first sign of hepatitis A virus infection, but most patients have symptoms for several days before jaundice becomes apparent. The most common prodromal symptoms are anorexia and malaise, often with abdominal discomfort and nausea. At times the abdominal pain may be acute and may suggest an acute abdomen. Although nausea is common, few patients vomit. Many patients also report losing their taste for cigarettes. Constipation may be as common as diarrhea. Patients in the pre-icteric stage also may complain of headaches and generalized myalgia. The headache is rarely severe but at times may suggest meningitis. The patient may have fever to 104° F and may even have chills. Rash, either papular, macular, or petechial, is uncommon. In general, children have much milder symptoms than adults. The prodromal or pre-icteric stage usually lasts less than one week, although some patients feel ill for as long as two weeks. The true nature of the illness becomes apparent with the onset of jaundice. Just before the jaundice, the patient usually notices dark urine and pale feces. As the jaundice appears, the patient becomes afebrile. The liver is often not enlarged but is usually tender. Hepatomegaly is often present in patients with severe illness unless massive necrosis develops, in which case the liver rapidly shrinks. Splenomegaly is present in

less than 20 per cent of patients. The main symptom during the icteric phase is extreme fatigability. In milder cases, the patient feels well in a few days. However, many patients may feel tired and anorectic for one to two weeks. After two weeks, in most patients, the jaundice begins to recede and disappears by the end of the month. Some patients continue to complain of fatigability for many months after acute illness. In a few patients, especially women between 30 and 50 years of age, the jaundice may deepen and persist for two to three months before clearing. Pruritus may be a bothersome symptom, yet the patient remains relatively well. This type of illness, jaundice with cholestasis, always clears, although the duration of jaundice may be many weeks, especially in patients near puberty and in older individuals.

### Patterns of Illness

The types of clinical illness caused by hepatitis A virus can be categorized as follows: anicteric hepatitis, icteric hepatitis, and fulminant hepatitis. Chronic hepatitis does not seem to occur. Many cases of hepatitis A are anicteric, and the patient may have very mild vague symptoms or none at all. Rarely, patients may suffer from a fulminant form of illness in which jaundice deepens rapidly, and the patient has frequent bouts of vomiting and rapidly falls into coma. Signs of hepatic failure are present. Such patients usually die within ten days of onset.

### Diagnosis

The activity of the aminotransferases in serum, aspartate aminotransferase or glutamic oxaloacetic transaminase (SGOT), and alanine aminotransferase or serum glutamic pyruvic transaminase (SGPT), begins to rise several days before clinical jaundice becomes apparent. The final peak level of transaminase activity found in serum is quite variable in patients with hepatitis. The activity of the transaminases usually peaks within one week and then begins to decline. As it declines, the activity of alkaline phosphatase is usually rising, reaching a peak several days to one week after the transaminase peak; gamma glutamyl transpeptidase activity is also elevated at this time. The bilirubin level rises as jaundice appears, preceded by bilirubinuria, and conjugated bilirubin predominates. Leukopenia is seen in the early stages of acute hepatitis, and atypical lymphocytes may be present in about 25 per cent of cases. Patients with fulminant hepatitis may have leukocytosis. The erythrocyte sedimentation rate (ESR) is often less than normal when jaundice appears. Elevation of the ESR later in illness may indicate persisting inflammatory changes in the liver. In most patients with acute hepatitis, the serum albumin and globulin remain normal. Prolongation of the prothrombin time and depletion of other clotting factors manufactured in the liver may be present during the acute phase of hepatitis. Hypoalbuminemia, acidosis, and hyperammonemia with encephalopathy are seen only in fulminant hepatitis.

Diagnosis and prognosis have been facilitated by needle biopsy. Pathologically, viral hepatitis is characterized by a combination of morphologic components that include (1) acute cytologic damage, (2) inflammation, and (3) hepatocellular necrosis (Schaffner, 1970). In acute hepatitis, single hepatocytes, or small groups of them, undergo necrosis that elicits both focal and portal inflammation (Fig. 1). The necrosis is located anywhere in the lobule but may be accentuated in the central zone. The inflammatory reaction consists of leukocytes, lymphocytes, and macrophages. The portal inflammation may vary from minimal to marked. The walls of the central veins are edematous and contain scattered macrophages and other inflammatory cells. Acidophilic or Councilman-like bodies are hepatocytes that have undergone coagulation necrosis (Fig. 2). Regeneration begins in the early stages of viral hepatitis and is more prominent in the periportal region. Fulminant hepatitis causes massive necrosis of hepatocytes (Fig. 3).

All patients (except those few who die of massive necrosis) recover completely. However, in some patients the activity of the transaminases may be elevated for months. Liver biopsy of such patients may show minimal nonspecific inflammation or may be normal. Recent serologic evidence indicates that patients with hepatitis A do not develop chronic aggressive hepatitis. Aplastic anemia, usually fatal, may follow acute hepatitis on rare occasions.

### Differential Diagnosis of Acute Hepatitis

The differential diagnosis of acute hepatitis commonly focuses on infectious mononucleosis and cytomegalovirus infection. Infectious mononucleosis is usually accompanied by sore throat and lymphadenopathy; the heterophil agglutinins are positive by the second to fourth week of illness. Although the results of liver function tests are often mildly abnormal, jaundice is uncommon. Cytomegalovirus infection in adults usually involves the liver, but jaundice, when present, is mild; the diagnosis can be suggested by a fourfold rise in complement-fixing antibody. Leptospiral infection may also mimic acute hepatitis. The kidneys are often involved, and menin-

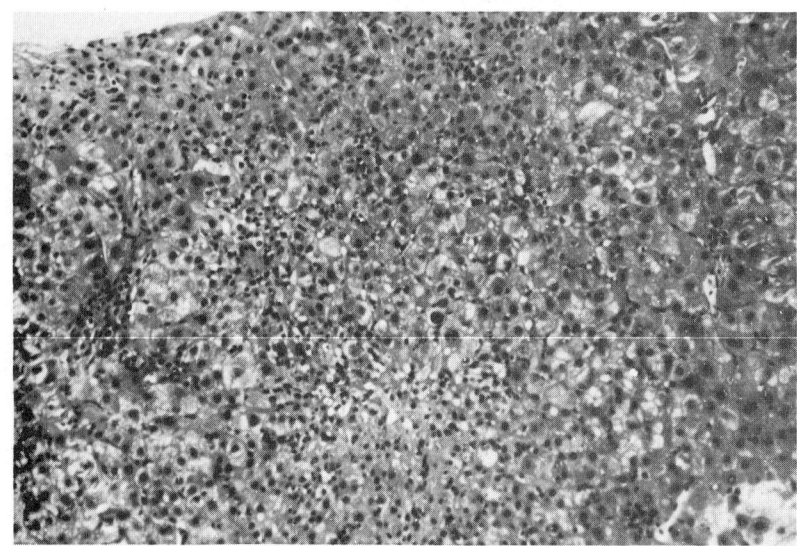

**FIGURE 1.**  *Liver biopsy specimen from patient with acute viral hepatitis showing diffuse spotty necrosis. Hematoxylin and eosin, × 40.*

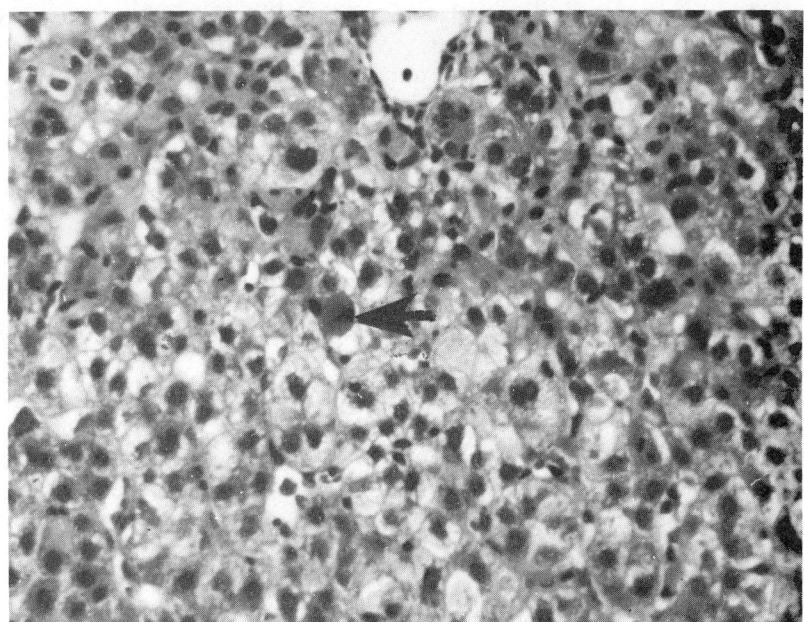

**FIGURE 2.** *Acidophilic "Councilman-like" body (arrow) and diffuse inflammation with variation in size and staining of hepatocytes. A central vein in the center of the top edge shows inflammation in its walls (central phlebitis). Hematoxylin and eosin, × 100.*

gitis may be present. Serologic tests are most often used to establish a diagnosis. Yellow fever, the hemorrhagic fevers, and various other arbovirus infections must be considered in areas of endemicity. Parasitic diseases such as malaria, schistosomiasis, kala-azar, and clonorchiasis must also be considered in geographic areas of prevalence. Adverse reactions to drugs such as isoniazid, methyldopa, and chlorpromazine also cause acute and chronic hepatitis, which often cannot be separated from viral hepatitis.

### Treatment

There is no specific treatment for hepatitis A virus infection. The patient's sense of well-being is the best guide for the amount of bed rest required; a simple guide is avoidance of fatigue. The patient in the acute stages of the illness usually does not feel like being up and around, and therefore should stay at reasonable rest. Simple exercises during convalescence may help restore a sense of well-being and forestall development of muscle weakness that accompanies

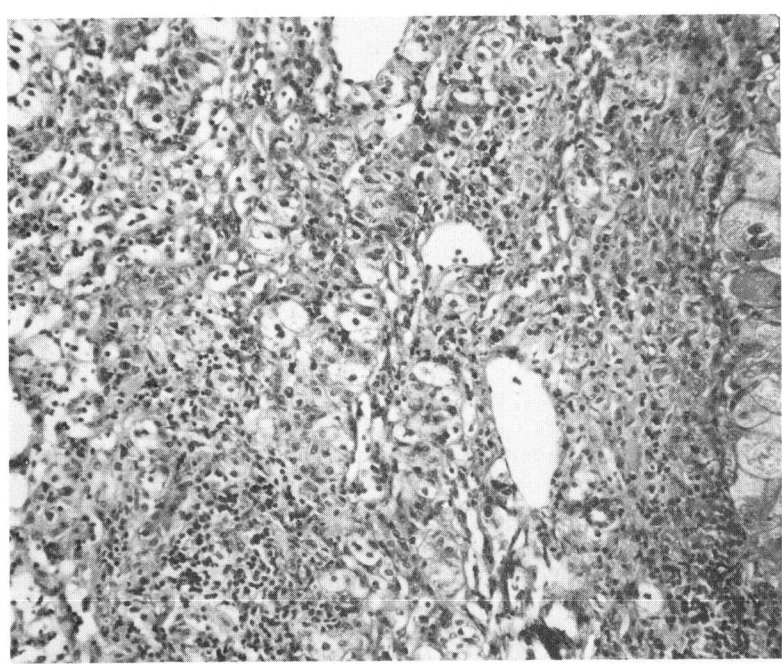

**FIGURE 3.** *Early massive necrosis and beginning collapse in acute hepatitis. A row of surviving hepatocytes is seen at right border. Hematoxylin and eosin, × 100.*

protracted illness. In the early part of the illness, when anorexia is prominent, frequent small, light, and attractive feedings appear to be best tolerated. Intravenous fluid should be avoided if possible because overhydration and electrolyte imbalances are easily produced. A normal balanced diet should be prescribed. There is no rational basis for a low fat diet. Corticosteroids have no benefit in treatment of acute viral hepatitis and should be avoided. The treatment of acute fulminant hepatitis leaves much to be desired. A low protein diet, lactulose or neomycin, and bowel cleansing help reduce the intensity of encephalopathy. Exchange transfusions, parabiotic filtration, or in vitro filtration systems to remove toxic circulating substances are experimental and so far have been disappointing. A chronic carrier state for hepatitis A virus is not apparent.

Patients should exercise good personal hygiene to prevent spread of disease to other patients and staff in hospital and to family members at home. In hospital, the usual enteric precautions should be used in handling materials from patients with acute viral hepatitis A. Good sanitation and high standards of hygiene among food handlers should help to prevent water–borne outbreaks. Many studies have substantiated the fact that gamma globulin offers good protection against hepatitis A (Krugman, 1976). It may be given to close contacts who are at special risk. Even if gamma globulin does not prevent infection, it may attenuate the disease. Conventional immune serum globulin (ISG) appears to be effective. Gamma globulin should be administered in doses of between 0.03 ml and 0.06 ml per pound of body weight. It is most effective if given during the first few days following contact with a patient with hepatitis A. Efforts to prepare an active vaccine against hepatitis A infection are hampered by lack of a tissue culture system for propagation of the virus.

## HEPATITIS B

### Transmission

Hepatitis B virus (HBV) infection is endemic throughout the world (Mosley, 1975). The virus can be transmitted from mother to child during delivery but rarely transplacentally. The rise in the use of blood transfusions has probably contributed to the increasing recognition of the disease in the western hemisphere. The increased use of donor blood in renal hemodialysis and in cardiovascular surgery also has increased the risk of transmission of HBV infection. Furthermore, the increase in drug addiction with intravenously used drugs such as heroin has led to the spread of HBV infection. Hepatitis B surface antigen (HBsAg) may also be found in the saliva and urine of infected patients, and there is much epidemiologic evidence for nonparenteral routes of transmission, especially from one sexual partner to the other. HBsAg has been detected in semen. Recent studies have shown that HBV infection can be reactivated in patients who are treated with immunosuppressive agents.

### Clinical Presentation

The incubation period of HBV infection averages about 90 days, with a range of 40 to 180 days. Symptoms during the prodromal period that occur about one to three weeks before the appearance of jaundice are similar to those described for hepatitis A virus infection but are more gradual in onset. In addition, a symptom complex that includes urticarial skin eruption with arthritis has been described during the prodromal period of HBV infection. This prodrome seems to have an immunologic basis, and the complement levels in the synovial fluid of affected joints are low. Slowly increasing jaundice may be the first sign. Hepatitis B is considered to be a more severe disease than hepatitis A and causes more deaths. The greater severity is probably related to the older age of the patients and the frequent presence of some underlying disease. Patients may have anicteric disease, acute hepatitis with recovery, subacute fatal hepatitis, fulminant hepatitis, and chronic active or persistent hepatitis. The differences in clincial presentation of hepatitis A and hepatitis B are summarized in Table 1.

There are also several differences between HBV infection in adults and infection in children (Table 2). Hepatitis B in the neonatal period is rare and is usually transmitted from the mother during birth. However, the mortality rate is highest in infants, being 4 to 5/100,000 population under 1 year of age. Mortality drops greatly after 1 year of age and rises again slowly in later years, reaching a high level after age 60. In children, the onset of clinical symptoms is more abrupt, and the icteric phase is short. Gastrointestinal symptoms, particularly vomiting and abdominal pain often with ketoacidosis, are usual; urticaria and arthritis are rare in children in contrast to adults. Immune complex phenomena such as glomerulonephritis and papular acrodermatitis are more common in children, while arthritis is more common in adults. Tender hepatomegaly with splenomegaly early in the course of disease is more frequent in children. Fever in children is high but brief, and is moderate but protracted in adults. The duration of hepatitis is usually short in children but is protracted in adults.

**TABLE 2.** Comparison of Hepatitis B Infection in Children and Adults

| CLINICAL PRESENTATION | CHILDREN | ADULTS |
|---|---|---|
| Susceptibility | High | Low |
| Peak incidence | Infants | Young adults |
| Onset | Acute | Gradual |
| Fever | High but brief | Moderate but protracted |
| Duration | Short | Often protracted |
| Mortality | High in infants | High in elderly |
| Carrier state | Frequent | Uncommon |
| Chronic hepatitis | Mainly infants | Mainly elderly |

## Antigenic Markers of HBV Infection

HBsAg usually appears in the serum several weeks after exposure before the onset of clinical symptoms and even before the activity of the transaminases in serum begin to rise (Krugman et al., 1974). Hepatitis B core antigen (HBcAg), DNA polymerase activity, and hepatitis Be antigen (HBeAg) usually appear when HBsAg is detected. In some patients, HBeAg, HBcAg, and DNA polymerase activity may precede the appearance of HBsAg. Anti-HBc appears in serum usually with the onset of acute illness (Hoofnagle et al., 1977). Anti-HBs usually appears during convalescence when circulating HBsAg has disappeared. Anti-HBe usually appears when anti-HBc is present.

Abnormalities in the results of biochemical tests of liver function in HBV infection are similar to those found in hepatitis A infection. About 10 per cent of patients who have acute hepatitis B will become chronic carriers of HBsAg. The presence of HBeAg without anti-HBe, and the persistence of high levels of anti-HBc without anti-HBs are correlated with development of the carrier state. Hepatitis B surface antigenemia is found in approximately 0.1 to 0.4 per cent of apparently healthy volunteer blood donors in the United States. Anti-HBs is found in about 15 per cent of adults in the United States. The vast majority of these antibody-positive individuals had subclinical or anicteric hepatitis. The carrier state for HBsAg seems to develop more frequently in children after hepatitis B infection.

## Pathology

Hepatocytes containing HBsAg can be recognized in liver biopsy specimens (Fig. 4). They are larger than normal, and the bulky cytoplasm has

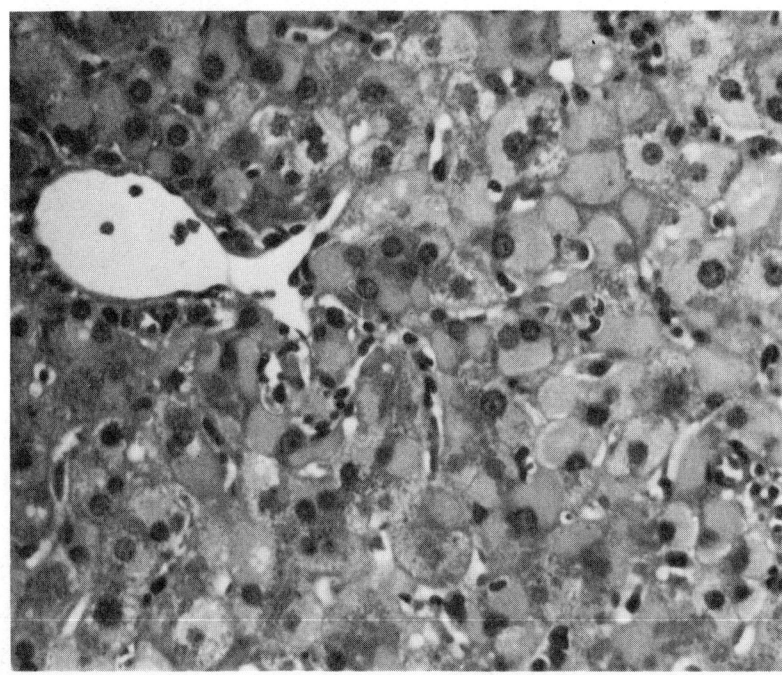

**FIGURE 4.** *Ground glass hepatocytes near central vein on upper left in an HBsAg carrier. Hematoxylin and eosin, ×250.*

a smudged appearance similar to ground or frost-ed glass. These cells are usually present in small groups with no zonal predilection. Ground glass hepatocytes were first noted in asymptomatic carriers of HBsAg; they also have been seen in HBsAg-positive chronic hepatitis when diffuse liver cell injury is not severe. Electron microscop-ic studies have shown that HBsAg is associated with the endoplasmic reticulum of the cytoplasm of the hepatocyte. Naked core particles contain-ing HBcAg are found in the nucleus of infected cells, especially in immunosuppressed individu-als. Immunofluorescent studies have shown that anti-HBs attaches to particles in cytoplasm and anti-HBc attaches to particles in the cell nuclei of infected livers. Cytoplasmic HBsAg can also be detected by staining methods with paraffin sec-tions. Due to the large antigenic load in hepato-cytes and in serum of patients with hepatitis B virus infection, it has been hypothesized that the liver cell injury in this infection is caused by immunologic mechanisms.

Necrosis of hepatocytes in acute hepatitis B results in a focal scattered centrolobularly accen-tuated inflammatory response, portal inflamma-tion, and endophlebitis of the central veins. In more severe cases, necrosis extends in a line from the portal tract to the central vein. This bridging necrosis often presages chronic hepatitis and cir-rhosis (Fig. 5).

Most patients with hepatitis B virus infection survive the acute illness. Patients who become chronic carriers of HBsAg may be asymptomatic or symptomatic. Microscopic examinations of the liver in asymptomatic carriers of HBsAg may be normal or may show chronic portal hepatitis that is recognized clinically as chronic persistent hep-atitis. In this entity, the inflammation that had extended from the parenchyma into the portal tracts in the acute state regresses until it is within the portal tracts, allowing the limiting plates of hepatocytes to restore themselves. This lesion will heal in most cases over a period of several years. However, progression to more serious disease does occur in a small percentage of patients. Some patients with HBV infection de-velop chronic periportal hepatitis known clini-cally as chronic aggressive or chronic active hep-atitis. The portal and periportal inflammation in these patients does not subside, and the loss of hepatocytes in the limiting plates associated with inflammation and subsequent fibrosis is a process of piecemeal necrosis, the hallmark of chronic active hepatitis (Fig. 6). The bridging necrosis and collapse seen in acute hepatitis may persist or may develop anew from the chronic periportal hepatitis. Although this form of hepatitis may heal spontaneously in a minority of cases, it is more likely to progress to cirrhosis.

### Immunologic Sequelae

HBV infection has several immunologic seque-lae, the manifestations of which differ in children and adults. The lack of arthritis and urticaria in the early stages of the disease in children has already been mentioned. Papular acrodermatitis is found mainly in children in association with lymphadenitis and mild hepatitis. The skin dis-ease is the major manifestation in these children, and virus antigen has been found in the skin. Papular acrodermatitis may be recurrent in young adults with persistent hepatitis B surface

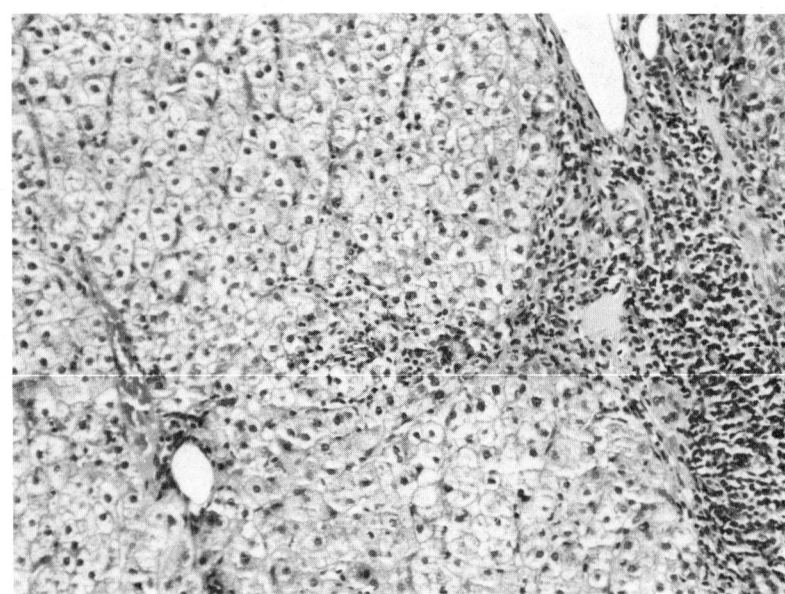

**FIGURE 5.** *Beginning bridging necrosis in acute hepatitis from large portal tract on right to central area on left. Hematoxylin and eosin, ×40.*

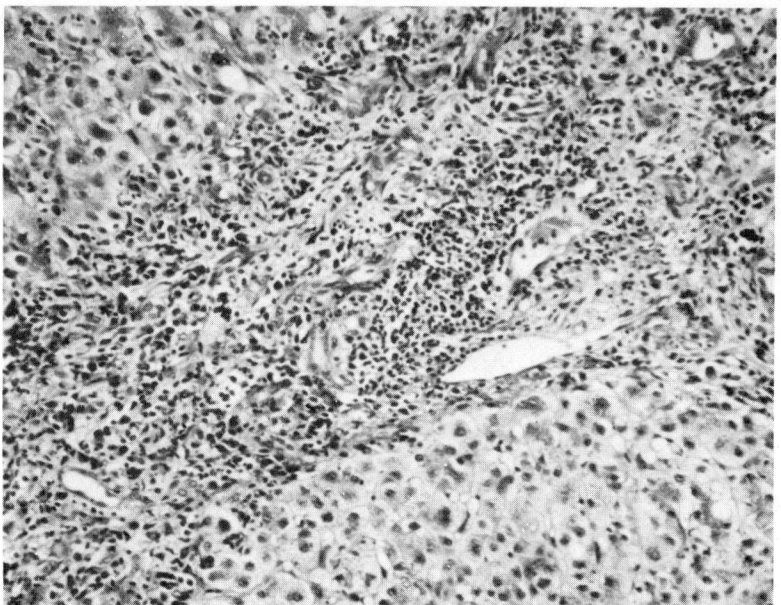

**FIGURE 6.** *Large fibrotic and inflamed portal tract with piecemeal necrosis on upper left in patient with chronic active hepatitis. Hematoxylin and eosin, ×40.*

antigenemia. Glomerulonephritis, which is more common in children than in adults, results from the deposition of antigen-antibody complexes. Endocapillary proliferative, membrane proliferative, and membranous types of glomerulonephritis have been associated with hepatitis B infection. Aplastic anemia has been reported following hepatitis B infection in children and young adults. Periarteritis nodosa is another immunologic complication of HBV infection seen mainly in adults.

### Hepatitis B and Hepatic Cancer

There is a relationship among HBV infection, cirrhosis, and primary hepatocellular carcinoma in many areas of the world such as the Far East, where HBV is highly endemic and carriers of HBsAg are common. In these areas, primary hepatocellular carcinoma is one of the most common neoplasms. The exact role of HBV as an oncogenic agent in the liver has not yet been defined.

### Prevention of HBV Infection

The primary need is to eradicate the carrier state of hepatitis B. For the present, personal hygiene, control of drug abuse, and public education remain the mainstays of prevention. The most effective way of decreasing the incidence of hepatitis B virus infection in countries where the virus is spread mainly by blood transfusion is to test all donor blood by sensitive techniques such as radioimmunoassay for the presence of HBsAg. Such routine testing of all donors and all blood, combined with decreased use of commercial

donors, has already lessened the incidence of hepatitis B following blood transfusion. Recent studies have shown that dentists with chronic hepatitis B surface antigenemia may spread disease to their patients. Hyperimmune globulin containing high titers of anti-HBs may be effective in reducing the incidence of hepatitis B infection in persons accidentally inoculated with infected blood, in patients and staff in renal dialysis units, and in spouses of patients with acute HBV infection. The protection is temporary, generally lasting from four to six months. Recently, some lots of immune serum globulin (ISG) were found to contain appreciable titers of anti-HBs, probably reflecting the rising incidence of infection in the general population. Vaccines prepared from purified HBsAg have been reported to be effective in protecting both people at risk and chimpanzees from infection with HBV. Much work is being expended on the development of HBsAg protein subunit vaccines to preclude cross-reaction between vaccines containing purified HBsAg and normal human proteins. Vaccines are needed for groups at special risk of acquiring HBV infection. These include patients requiring repeated transfusions, patients and staff in renal dialysis units, staff in institutions for the mentally retarded, homosexuals, drug addicts, and prostitutes, and persons in endemic areas.

Known antiviral chemotherapeutic agents are not effective in the treatment of HBV infection; the possible role of adenine arabinoside requires further study. However, preliminary studies have shown that injection of human interferon into patients with chronic HBsAg, including Dane particles and DNA polymerase activity, leads to a disappearance of the Dane particle and the surface antigenemia. Concomitantly, the patients did seem to have some symptomatic improvement, and liver function abnormalities returned to normal. Interferon is very expensive, the effect of its long-term administration in man is not known, and the studies were not randomized or controlled; thus, the ability of interferon to cure patients of hepatitis B virus infection remains to be established.

## NON-A, NON-B HEPATITIS

Non-A, non-B hepatitis accounts for 50 per cent or more of post-transfusion hepatitis. The incubation period appears to be prolonged as in hepatitis B. Furthermore, the clinical presentation of non-A, non-B hepatitis, including chronic carriage of virus and risk of developing chronic active hepatitis, also resembles that of hepatitis B. There is no cross-antigenicity between HBV and the non-A, non-B viruses. However, no antigenic markers have been identified for the latter viruses. Non-A, non-B hepatitis is an infection that requires much epidemiologic and laboratory investigation (Hoofnagle et al., 1977).

## CHRONIC ACTIVE HEPATITIS

Chronic active hepatitis is a chronic inflammatory disease of the liver, lasting at least six months without remission and appearing as a sequel to HBV infection or non-A, non-B hepatitis (Boyer, 1976). Chronic active hepatitis does not appear to be a sequel of hepatitis A virus infection. The onset of the disease is usually insidious with extreme fatigue. There may be fluctuating jaundice, anorexia with weight loss, intermittent fever, and amenorrhea. Examination of the patient shows spider nevi and hepatosplenomegaly.

Late in the course of the disease, hepatic encephalopathy, edema, ascites, and bleeding from esophageal varices may develop.

The serum bilirubin level may or may not be increased, but the SGPT and SGOT activities are elevated often to more than five times normal, and there is polyclonal hypergammaglobulinemia. The same disease may occur, however, in congenital or acquired hypogammaglobulinemia. The serum alkaline phosphatase and gamma glutamyl transpeptidase values are also elevated. The prothrombin time may be increased.

Liver biopsy must be done to differentiate this condition from chronic persistent hepatitis and to delineate the extent of damage to the liver and of fibrosis. Microscopically, the liver shows lymphocytic and plasma cell infiltration of the portal areas with inflammation of the liver lobule, including erosion of the limiting plate or piecemeal necrosis, bridging necrosis, and fibrosis (Fig. 6). There is a wide spectrum in the clinical illness and presentation from mildly symptomatic to very ill patients; the clinical presentation often does not correlate with the pathology.

There are three major types of chronic active hepatitis — one associated with hepatitis B antigen, a non-B post-transfusion form, and an autoimmune or lupoid type (Table 3). The first affects mainly men 30 to 50 years old and is especially apt to develop in transfusion recipients, drug addicts, male homosexuals, immunosuppressed patients (such as renal dialysis patients), patients with malignancy, patients with organ transplants, and babies exposed to HBV. The autoimmune type affects mainly women (in a 3:1 ratio) in the second decade and may be associated with a variety of immunologic phenomena including positive LE cells, antinuclear factor, Coombs' positive hemolytic anemia, and particularly, smooth muscle antibody (Table 3).

Differential diagnosis includes granulomatous hepatitis, Wilson's disease, primary biliary cir-

TABLE 3.   Clinical Presentations of Chronic Active Hepatitis

| CLINICAL PRESENTATION | AUTOIMMUNE | ASSOCIATED WITH HBsAg |
|---|---|---|
| Sex | Mainly females | Mainly males |
| Age | Second and fifth decades | Infants and elderly; immunosuppressed patients |
| Increase in serum gammaglobulin | Marked | Moderate |
| Smooth muscle antibody | High | Low |
| LE cells | In 15 per cent | Absent |
| Corticosteroid therapy | Most respond | Few respond |

rhosis, pericholangitis with inflammatory bowel disease, alcoholic liver disease, cytomegalovirus hepatitis, alpha 1-antitrypsin deficiency, and drug-related chronic hepatitis.

The mainstay of therapy is prednisone or prednisolone (Summerskill et al., 1975). Some patients require azathioprine in addition. Patients with non-B chronic active hepatitis respond better to therapy than those with HBsAg. In the individual patient, response to therapy must be weighed against the side effects of the corticosteroids.

### References

Boyer, J. L.: Chronic hepatitis. A perspective on classification and determinants of prognosis. Gastroenterology 70:1161, 1976.

Dienstag, J. L., Routenberg, J. A., Purcell, R. H., Hooper, R. R., and Harrison, W. O.: Foodhandler-associated outbreak of hepatitis A. Ann Intern Med 83:647, 1975.

Hoofnagle, J. H., Gerety, R. J., and Barker, L. F.: Antibody to hepatitis B-virus core in man. Lancet 2:869, 1973.

Hoofnagle, J. H., Gerety, R. J., Tabor, J., Feinstone, S. M., Barker, L. F., and Purcell, R. H.: Transmission of non-A, non-B hepatitis. Ann Intern Med 87:14, 1977.

Krugman, S.: Effect of human immune serum globulin on infectivity of hepatitis A virus. J Infect Dis 134:70, 1976.

Krugman, S., Hoofnagle, J. H., Gerety, R. J., Kaplan, P. M., and Gerin, J. L.: Viral hepatitis type B. DNA polymerase activity and antibody to hepatitis B core antigen. N Engl J Med 290:1331, 1974.

Mosley, J. W.: Hepatitis types B and non-B. Epidemiologic background. JAMA 233:697, 1975.

Murray, R.: Viral hepatitis. Bull NY Acad Med 31:341, 1955.

Schaffner, F.: The structural basis of altered hepatic function in viral hepatitis. Am J Med 49:658, 1970.

Summerskill, W. H. J., Korman, M. G., Ammon, H. V., and Baggenstoss, A. H.: Prednisone for chronic active liver disease: Dose titration, standard dose, and combination with azathioprine compared. Gut 16:876, 1975.

# *YELLOW FEVER* **143**

## *Francisco de Paula Pinheiro, M.D.*

### DEFINITION

Classically, yellow fever is an acute viral illness characterized by jaundice, hemorrhage, and renal damage. Its clinical spectrum varies from fulminant fatal disease to a mild febrile illness. Inapparent infections are frequent. The yellow fever virus is a member of the group B arboviruses, or *Flavivirus* genus of the family Togaviridae. At present, the virus is known to persist enzootically in forests of certain areas of Africa and South America through a cycle that is not yet fully understood. The virus is transmitted to man by infected mosquitoes. In the past, yellow fever was also maintained in urban centers, where the agent was transmitted from man to man by the mosquito *Aedes aegypti*.

### ETIOLOGY

In the older classification system (Casals, 1957), the yellow fever virus is a member of the group B arboviruses. It is now considered to be the type species of the genus *Flavivirus* of the Togaviridae family. The virus particles are spherical and possess a lipid-containing envelope and an icosahedral nucleocapsid. The virions contain an infectious single-stranded RNA genome. Electron microscopy of infected mouse brain and liver reveals that the virus particles exist in the cytoplasm of infected cells and that their diameter is about 38 nm, with a range of 33 to 43 nm (Bergold and Weibel, 1962). In the mouse brain,

the particles are found only in the astrocytes, which are accumulated within the cisterna and ducts of the endoplasmic reticulum. The virus is labile in the absence of protein. It is more stable when suspended in phosphate buffer solution (ph 7.0) containing 10 per cent normal human serum, 10 per cent monkey serum, or 0.75 per cent bovine albumin. Virus infectivity can be preserved for one month in blood kept at 4° C. Viral infectivity is destroyed by heating at 60° C for 10 minutes. The virus is sensitive to the action of ether and sodium deoxycholate and is readily inactivated by common chemical disinfectants. It can be preserved for years when whole infected tissues or tissue suspensions are kept at −60° C or in liquid nitrogen. Lyophilization, followed by cold storage, is the preferred method of preserving infectivity.

The virus possesses a hemagglutinin that is active against erythrocytes of several animal species, particularly those of the goose. The activity of this hemagglutinin is markedly influenced by pH, which optimally should be about 6.2 to 6.6.

Yellow fever virus causes encephalitis and death in suckling mice after intracerebral, intraperitoneal, or subcutaneous inoculation. Many adult mice die when infected intracerebrally but usually not when infected by the other two routes. All primates are susceptible to infection, but mortality depends upon the species, route of inoculation, and strain of virus. Rhesus monkeys and other primates from India, as well as certain monkeys from South America, develop fatal infection. Wild strains are pantropic and affect a variety of the organs and tissues of rhesus monkeys but have a special predilection for the liver, kidneys, and heart. After serial passages in the mouse brain, the virus loses its affinity for monkey viscera and becomes markedly neurotropic. Some marsupials and a few rodents develop viremia without overt disease.

The agent has been propagated in several cell cultures of vertebrate origin such as primary chick embryo, BHK-21, Vero, HeLa, pig kidney, and others. It causes either plaque formation, cytopathic effect, or both. It also replicates and causes cytopathologic signs in the invertebrate cell line derived from *Aedes pseudoscutellaris*. Some strains of the virus multiply in the cell cultures of *Aedes albopictus*, but they do not produce cytopathologic signs (Varma et al., 1975/76).

## PATHOGENESIS AND PATHOLOGY

The pathogenesis of yellow fever is not yet well understood. When rhesus monkeys are experimentally infected with small inocula, the virus cannot be detected for 24 hours (Strano et al., 1975). At the end of this period, Kupffer cells are found to contain intracytoplasmic areas of acidophilic degeneration. Between 24 and 48 hours after the infection, glycogen is reduced in the hepatocytes, and the titer of virus in the blood increases and peaks at about 96 hours postinfection. At 72 hours, many Kupffer cells are degenerating, and the alterations in hepatocytes are more evident. The glycogen gradually disappears, and fatty degeneration characterized by small and large droplets of fat both in the cytoplasm in the nucleus becomes apparent. Migration of chromatin to the nuclear membrane is followed by rupture of the membrane. Intranuclear eosinophilic bodies can also be recognized in the hepatic cells (Torres, 1928). Eosinophilic hyaline degeneration of the hepatocytes also occurs, resulting in the formation of eosinophilic masses, commonly known as Councilman bodies. Between 96 and 120 hours after the infection, the lesions are fully developed. Characteristically, the cells from the midzone of the hepatic lobule are more profoundly affected. At this site, the necrosis may become nearly confluent. Typically, the liver cords are discontinuously involved, so that living and necrotic cells are interspersed. The absence of significant inflammation is a cardinal feature.

The pathology in the liver of rhesus monkeys closely resembles that observed in the infected human liver. In human beings, midzone necrosis is also characteristic but may involve almost the entire lobule. Councilman bodies may be absent if death occurs after the tenth day of illness. In-

terestingly, there is complete reversibility of the lesions in survivors. Classic histologic features of yellow fever are present only in the acute stage. During convalescence, the histologic picture resembles that of persistent, nonspecific hepatitis (Francis et al., 1972). Liver biopsy, however, is contraindicated in the acute phase of the illness.

The kidney, heart, and other organs of man may also be affected (Bugher, 1951). The tubular epithelium of the kidney undergoes changes varying from cloudy swelling and desquamation to simple necrosis. These changes are most severe in the convoluted tubules. The cells lining Bowman's capsule are also damaged, but the glomeruli are affected less than the tubules.

Fatty degeneration of myocardial fibers is a uniform finding when the heart is involved. Lesions may occur in the sinoauricular node and the bundle of His. Involvement of the brain is minimal; perivascular hemorrhage is the most consistent finding. Significant necrosis of the cortical cells of the outer fascicular zone of the adrenals may occur.

## CLINICAL MANIFESTATIONS, COMPLICATIONS, AND SEQUELAE

The incubation period varies from three to six days in naturally acquired yellow fever. It can be as long as ten days, however, in individuals accidentally exposed to infectious blood. Apparently the virus can either penetrate intact skin or areas of minor unnoticed abrasion.

The clinical course varies from benign febrile illness to the classic clinical picture of hepatic failure, albuminuria, hemorrhagic manifestations, coma, and death. During the 1960 to 1962 yellow fever outbreak in Ethiopia, a fulminating form of the disease was observed, characterized by high fever, severe headache, tachycardia, prostration, and death in two to three days (Serié et al., 1968). Little or no hepatic or renal involvement was seen.

The following classification according to the severity of clinical disease has been suggested (Kerr, 1975): (1) Very mild. Patients experience only transient fever and headache that persists from a few hours to one or two days. (2) Mild. The fever and headache are more pronounced and may be accompanied by nausea, epistaxis, Faget's sign (see below), slight albuminuria, and subclinical elevations of bilirubin. The illness usually lasts from two to three days. Findings similar to these have been described among patients infected during outbreaks that occurred near Belem, Brazil (Causey and Maroja, 1959). Some of these patients also complained of epigastric pain, backache, general body pain, vertigo, vomiting, photophobia, and a prolonged period of asthenia. Epistaxis was not observed. (3) Moderately severe. The fever is higher, the headache and backache are more severe, and the nausea and vomiting are more intense. Jaundice and albuminuria are usually present. Black vomitus, melena, or uterine hemorrhage may occur. The fever persists for about one week. (4) Malignant. All the classic signs and symptoms of the disease are present. Patients may die within three to four days.

### Evolution of Severe Forms

Two periods can be recognized during the course of the moderately severe and malignant forms of the disease: the period of infection (viremia) and the period of intoxication.

The period of infection is characterized by the sudden onset of intense chills of short duration followed by fever of 39° to 40° C. There is severe headache, nausea, vomiting, generalized muscle pain, and backache. The face and sometimes the neck and upper part of the thorax are congested. The conjunctivae are suffused. The gums may be swollen and ooze blood on gentle pressure. Epistaxis is common. The patient is uncomfortable, anxious, and unable to sleep. By the second day, the appearance of a pulse-temperature dissociation begins: the temperature is high, and the pulse gradually slows down (Faget's sign). This viremic phase of the illness lasts about three days, and the virus is present in the blood.

This period is followed by a remission that lasts from a few hours to two days. The general symptoms begin to diminish, the fever falls, and the headache decreases. After the remission, the period of intoxication is recognized by the appearance of hemorrhages, jaundice, and albuminuria. The fever rises, and the general symptoms reappear with great intensity.

Hemorrhagic manifestations are a major element of this stage. "Coffee-grounds" hematemesis from a small amount of swallowed blood and capillary hemorrhage into the stomach is followed by black vomitus, which is caused by massive hemorrhage into the stomach and the subsequent action of gastric juice on the blood. Melena, metrorrhagia, bleeding from the gums, and epistaxis also occur. Petechiae and ecchymoses of the skin are accompanied by bleeding from injection sites. Hematuria is rare. The jaundice is usually mild, although it may become pronounced if death is delayed.

Oliguria is common, but complete anuria is very rare. Albuminuria develops and increases rapidly. It is considered one of the most prominent findings in the disease, but it disappears in a few days in patients who recover. There is no hemoglobinuria. Hypotension occurs late in the course and may be accompanied by nonspecific abnormalities in the electrocardiogram. The liver and spleen are not palpable, but palpation of the epigastrium will elicit pain. Paroxysms of hiccoughing may occur, especially in severe cases.

Death occurs after one or two days of coma or suddenly after an attack of hematemesis. Death occurs most commonly between the sixth and eighth days of illness. The overall mortality rate among hospitalized patients may be as high as 40 to 50 per cent. Survivors exhibit long-lasting immunity.

### Laboratory Findings

Leukopenia with a selective depression of polymorphonuclear cells occurs inconsistently. A moderate leukocytosis may be observed before death and during convalescence. The bilirubin level, especially the direct fraction, is increased. The serum glutamic pyruvic transaminase (SGPT) and serum glutamic oxaloacetic transaminase (SGOT) levels and the urea and creatinine concentrations in the blood are markedly increased in severe cases. Thrombocytopenia is also common in severe cases, with platelet counts as low as 30,000 per mm³. The coagulation time and the prothrombin time are prolonged, and the levels of fibrinogen are reduced. Clot retraction may be poor. Coagulation factors II, V, and VII plus X, VIII, IX, X, and XIII may be depressed (Santos, 1973). The albumin concentration in the urine can reach 40 g per liter, but it is absent or shows only a moderate increase in mild cases. Casts may also be observed in the urine.

### Differential Diagnosis

Mild cases of yellow fever cannot readily be distinguished from a number of other febrile conditions, including dengue, influenza, typhoid fever, and malaria. During the period of intoxication, this illness must be differentiated from infectious hepatitis, leptospirosis, malaria, Lassa fever, Bolivian hemorrhagic fever, the effects of certain chemical poisons, and other conditions that can cause jaundice and hemorrhage. A careful clinical history and the epidemiology, considered along with the laboratory findings, will help establish the diagnosis of yellow fever. The definitive diagnosis, however, can be established only by one of the following methods: virus isolation, serologic test, and/or liver histopathologic examination.

Complications that are not a part of the natural course of the disease are uncommon. Parotitis, usually unilateral, has been observed. In spite of marked renal and heart involvement in certain patients, suvivors recover completely without sequelae.

## GEOGRAPHIC VARIATIONS IN DISEASE

Yellow fever is currently maintained enzootically only in certain forested areas of South America and Africa. However, the virus has been historically endemic and even epidemic in several urban centers of the Americas, Africa, and Europe. Thus, two epidemiologic cycles of yellow fever can be recognized: urban and jungle. Each is quite distinct in the New World but less so in Africa.

### Urban Cycle

This cycle is maintained by the transmission of virus from man to man by the bite of the mosquito *Aedes aegypti.* The mosquito can transmit the virus from 9 to 30 days after ingesting blood from a viremic patient and is thought to remain infected for life. Yellow fever transmitted by *Aedes aegypti* occurred in the past in many cities of South America, the Caribbean, the United States, and West Africa. It is also reported to have reached Spain, France, Italy, and England. The last case of urban yellow fever in the Americas was registered at Port-of-Spain in 1954 and in Africa at Luanda, Angola, in 1971.

### Jungle Yellow Fever

The two main foci of jungle yellow fever are considered to be the Amazon and Congo river basins. Although the maintenance of the virus in these regions is not fully understood, monkeys and certain mosquito species play an important role. In South America, mosquitoes of the genus *Haemagogus* are the main vectors. These day-biting mosquitoes are found predominantly in the forest canopy, although they can be captured on the forest floor. They occasionally bit man inside houses located near forests. *Sabethes chloropterus* and *Haemagogus leucocelaenus* are considered to be secondary vectors of the virus in South and Central America. *Sabethes* species may be responsible for the persistence of the virus during dry periods in Central America from 1948 to 1957. Although monkeys are considered to be the main vertebrate hosts for the virus, it is thought that marsupials may also act as hosts in some areas. Experimentally, the three-toed sloth, *Bradypus tridactylus,* develops a heavy, persistent viremia but does not die (Johnson, 1978). There is no direct evidence, however, that *Bradypus* plays a role in the virus cycle.

In Africa, the mosquito *Aedes africanus* is responsible for the transmission of the virus among monkeys. This mosquito can also infect man. *Aedes opok* is also regarded as a sylvatic vector in Central Africa (Cordellier et al., 1977). In East African epidemics, *Aedes simpsoni, Aedes vittatus, Aedes metallicus,* and *Aedes taylori* have been implicated as vectors. The 1960 to 1962 epidemic of yellow fever in Ethiopia was basically rural in nature and was linked to villages harboring *Aedes simpsoni* (Sérié et al., 1968). In West Africa, yellow fever epidemics in rural environments have been associated with *Aedes luteocephalus, Aedes vittatus, Aedes taylori,* and *Aedes aegypti,* with possible mosquito transmission from man to man (Cordellier et al., 1977). Workers at the Institut Pasteur in Dakar have recently isolated three strains of yellow fever virus from *Aedes furcifer* males captured in Sénégal (Cornet et al., 1979).

In the enzootic areas of South America, the virus is believed to move in waves through populations of susceptible monkeys, with periodic invasions of other areas such as Central and Southern Brazil and northern Paraguay and Argentina (Kerr, 1975; Pinheiro et al., 1978). Northward migration of the virus to Central America was documented during 1948 to 1957. In West Africa, the virus spreads in similar wave-like movements (Cordellier et al., 1977). Nevertheless, the precise mechanism of virus persistence is unknown. Transovarial transmission in the mosquito has recently been demonstrated (Aitken et al., 1979) and may play a role in viral persistence.

The number of cases of yellow fever reported to the World Health Organization in the decade 1967 to 1976 was 780 in the Americas and 588 in Africa. Cases reported from the Americas during this period occurred in Brazil, Bolivia, Peru, Paraguay, Venezuela, Argentina, Equador, and Panama. African reports came from Nigeria, Upper Volta, Ghana, Sierra Leone, Cameroon, Togo, Angola, Zaire, and Guinea. The extensive Ethiopian epidemic of yellow fever in 1960 to 1962, in which there was an estimated morbidity of 100,000 and a mortality of 30,000, was especially severe (Sérié et al., 1968). Subsequently, smaller outbreaks have been recorded in both continents, including the countries of Brazil, Bolivia, Peru, Colombia, Venezuela, Nigeria, Upper Volta, Sierra Leone, and Angola.

## DIAGNOSIS

Clinically, yellow fever is relatively easy to diagnose when classic signs are present. The final diagnosis, however, depends upon laboratory methods, which are of particular importance for the recognition of modified cases of the illness. There are three laboratory procedures for the specific diagnosis of yellow fever: (1) Virus isolation. Blood must be drawn within the first three to four days of the infection. Although the virus has been isolated from blood stored for days or even weeks at 4° C, it should be kept at −50° C or below, if the inoculation cannot be performed on the day of collection. The virus has also been isolated from liver specimens collected from fatal cases. Serum, whole blood, or 10 per cent liver suspensions should be inoculated into infant white mice and tissue cultures. It is also desirable to inoculate an additional group of mice with a 1:10 dilution of serum or blood. When the mice sicken, the brain is harvested and used for virus identification by complement fixation or neutralization tests against yellow fever–specific antiserum. Vero and *Aedes pseudoscutellaris* cell lines are even more susceptible to the virus than mice (Varma et al., 1975/76). Virus growth can be detected in these cultures by the appearance of cytopathic effect. (2) Serologic tests. Paired sera should be collected for this purpose. The first sample should be taken as soon as possible after the onset of illness and the second one two to three weeks later. Sera should be tested by hemagglutination-inhibition, complement fixation, and neutralization procedures against yellow fever virus and other flaviviruses known to exist in the area where the case occurred. The convalescent serum should have an antibody titer to yellow fever antigen at least four times greater than the serum from the acute phase. Due to the antigenic cross-reactions between yellow fever and other group B arboviruses, it is sometimes difficult or even impossible to make a diagnosis by serologic tests. In patients who have experienced a previous *Flavivirus* infection of another type, antibody rises to a variety of *Flavivirus* antigens can be observed. (3) Histopathologic examination. This method depends upon the demonstration of councilman bodies and the other characteristic lesions of yellow fever in liver sections. Liver specimens collected postmortem by direct incision of the abdominal wall or through a viscerotome should be preserved in 10 per cent formalin until examination.

## TREATMENT

The treatment of yellow fever is symptomatic. Bed rest is important. The patient should be hospitalized under careful observation in order to avoid harm to the damaged liver. The fever must be controlled and pain may require analgesics. Tranquilizing drugs should be administered if the patient becomes agitated. Antiemetics should be used to control nausea and vomiting. Administration of intravenous fluids such as glucose in physiologic saline and electrolyte solutions are recommended to avoid dehydration and maintain the electrolyte balance. Blood transfusions may be required to replace blood loss by hemorrhage. Disseminated intravascular coagulation (Santos, 1973) may be improved by the intravenous use of 5000 units of heparin every six hours. This treatment, however, may not prevent death, indicating that other factors contribute to a fatal outcome. Dialysis should be performed when there is renal failure. The use of antibiotics is often necessary to combat secondary bacterial infections. New antiviral drugs such as ribavirin (1-$\beta$-D-ribofuranosyl-1,2,3, triazole-3-carboxamide) deserve evaluation through careful trials.

## PROPHYLAXIS

Vaccination is essential for residents and visitors to endemic areas. Two attenuated strains of yellow fever virus are presently used for the protection of susceptible people. One is the 17D strain, derived from a wild strain passaged serially in tissue culture prepared from mouse and chick embryos and then grown in embryonated eggs. The other is the French neurotropic stain, which was attenuated by intracerebral passages in mice.

The 17D vaccine is safe and effective. It has been given to more than 100 million persons with only a few serious complications. Complications attributed to 17D vaccine include 15 nonfatal cases of encephalitis in children under 1 year of age, all of whom recovered without sequelae, and a single fatal case in a 3-year-old child who developed encephalitis. Allergic reactions have also been observed and are probably due to the presence of egg protein in the vaccine. The vaccine is administered by subcutaneous inoculation with syringe or Ped-o-jet. Immunity develops within ten days and may last 18 years or more, although the International Regulations for travelers require booster shots every ten years. The vaccine is heat labile and must be carefully refrigerated. The commonly available 17D vaccine is contaminated with avian leukosis virus; however, a leukosis-free 17D vaccine produced in England is now available. The vaccine is not recommended for children less than 1 year of age.

The French neurotropic vaccine is also very effective, but serious neurologic complications have been associated with its use, especially in children less than 7 years old. It should be given only to those beyond this age. This vaccine is administered by cutaneous scarification. One advantage over the 17D vaccine is that it is much less heat labile.

Eradication of *Aedes aegypti* mosquitoes, the

primary urban vector, is an important measure for control of yellow fever, especially in urban centers located near forests in which jungle yellow fever is present. Protective clothing can be worn, and insect repellents are useful.

## References

Aitken, T. H. G., Tesh, R. B., Beaty, B. J., and Rosen, L.: Transovarial transmission of yellow fever virus by mosquitoes (*Aedes aegypti*). Am J Trop Med Hyg 28(1):119, 1979.

Bergold, G. H., and Weibel, J.: Demonstration of yellow fever virus with the electron microscope. Virology 17:554, 1962.

Bugher, J. C.: The pathology of yellow fever. In Strode, G. K. (ed.): Yellow Fever. New York, McGraw-Hill Book Company, 1951, p. 137.

Casals, J.: The arthropod-borne group of animal viruses. Trans NY Acad Sci Ser 2, 19:219, 1957.

Causey, O. R., and Maroja, O.: Isolation of yellow fever virus from man and mosquitoes in the Amazon region of Brazil. Am J Trop Med 8:368, 1959.

Cordellier, R., Germain, M., Hervy, J. P., and Mouchet, J.: Guide Pratique Pour Étude des Vecteurs de Fièvre Jaune en Afrique et Methodes de Lutte. Office de la Recherche Scientifique et Technique Outre-Mer, Documentations Techniques 33, 1977.

Cornet, M., Robin, Y., Heme, G., Adam, C., Renaudet, J., Valade, M., and Eyraud, M.: Une poussée épizootique de fièvre jaune selva-tique au Sénégal Oriental. Isolement du virus de lots de moustiques adultes mâles et femelles. Médecine et Maladies Infectieuses, 9(2):63, 1979.

Francis, T. L., Moore, D. L., Edington, G. M., and Smith, J. A.: A clinicopathological study of human yellow fever. Bull W H O 46:659, 1972.

Johnson, K. M.: Personal communication, 1978.

Kerr, J. A.: Yellow fever. In Tice: Practice of Medicine, Vol. 4. 1975.

Pinheiro, F. P., Travassos da Rosa, A. P. A., Moraes, M. A. P., Almeida Neto, J. C., Camargo, S., and Filgueiras, J. P.: An epidemic of yellow fever in Central Brazil 1972-1973. 1. Epidemiological studies. Am J Trop Med 27:125, 1978.

Santos, F.: Dosagem dos fatores da coagulação na febre amarela. Tese Faculdade de Medicina, Univ. Federal do Rio de Janeiro, 1973.

Série, C., Lindrec, A., Poirier, A., Andral, L., and Neri, P.: Études sur la fièvre jaune en Ethiopie. 1. Introduction. Symptomatologie clinique amarile. Bull W H O 38:835, 1968.

Série, C., Andral, L., Poirier, A., Lindrec, A., and Neri, P.: Études sur la fièvre jaune en Ethiopie. 6. Étude épidémiologique. Bull W H O 38:879, 1968.

Strano, A. J., Dooley, J. R., and Ishak, K. G.: Manual sobre la fiebre amarilla y su diagnostico diferencial histopatologico. Organizacion PanAmericana de la Salud Publicación Cientifica 299, 1975.

Torres, C. M.: Inclusions nucléaires acidophiles (dégénérescence oxychromatique) dans le foie de *Macacus rhesus*, inoculé avec le virus brésilien de la fièvre jaune. C R Soc Biol 99:1344, 1928.

Varma, M. G. R., Pudney, M., Leake, C. J., and Peralta, P. H.: Isolation in a mosquito (*Aedes pseudoscutellaris*) cell line (Mos. 61) of yellow fever virus strains from original field material. Intervirology 6:50, 1975/76.

# 144 *WHIPPLE'S DISEASE*

## *Stanley D. Freedman, M.D.*

### *DEFINITION*

In 1907, Dr. G. H. Whipple, a pathologist at Johns Hopkins University, described a fatal illness in a 36-year-old man who complained of arthralgias and arthritis for several years before developing cough, fever, weight loss, progressive debility and weakness, and malabsorption (Whipple, 1907). Pallor, wasting, a full abdomen, articular abnormalities, and lymphadenopathy were noted on physical examination. At autopsy, Whipple found enlarged mesenteric nodes, "foamy" mononuclear phagocytic cells especially in the lamina propria of the intestinal mucosa, and rod-shaped organisms in various tissues. The disease, in essence, remains well defined by Whipple's remarkable description.

### *ETIOLOGY*

The foamy material in the macrophages of the lamina propria was shown to consist of periodic acid-Schiff (PAS)-positive particles by Black-Schaffer in 1949. This tinctorial identification of glycoproteins led to further speculation about the metabolic causes of the disease. Nine years later, Sieracki (1958) elaborated upon the morphologic appearance of these cytoplasmic particles, calling them "sickle-form particles" and the cells containing them "sickle-form particle-containing (SPC) cells." SPC cells were soon identified in tissues from all major organ systems and provided histologic confirmation of the systemic nature of Whipple's disease. These tinctorial reactions and morphologic characteristics were found to be present in Whipple's original case when reexamined by the PAS technique by Mendeloff; this histologic picture remains pathognomonic of the disease.

Electronmicroscopic studies suggested that the particles were bacillary bodies that had all the structural features of bacteria (Haubrich et al., 1960; Yardley and Hendrix, 1961; Chears and Ashworth, 1961). These rodlike organisms averaged 1.5 microns in length and 0.15 microns in width and had a three-component cell wall (Fig. 1 A and B). They divided by binary fission. The rods were both intra- and extracellular and disappeared with therapy. Bacterial cell walls remaining after treatment correlated with the PAS-positive material in the remaining macrophages. More recently, immunofluorescent studies of jejunal biopsy tissue demonstrated similar bacterial antigens in the macrophages of different patients and suggested that a single organism was

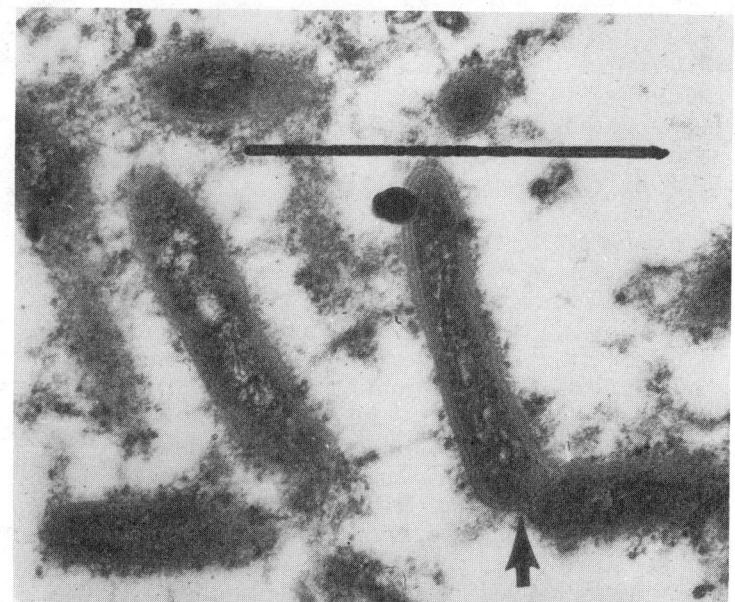

FIGURE 1. *Electron microscopy showing the structure of the bacilliform bodies. (From Haubrich et al.: Gastroenterology 39:454, 1960.) Note 3 component cell wall in A and numerous bacilliform bodies with scanning electronmicroscope in B.*

A

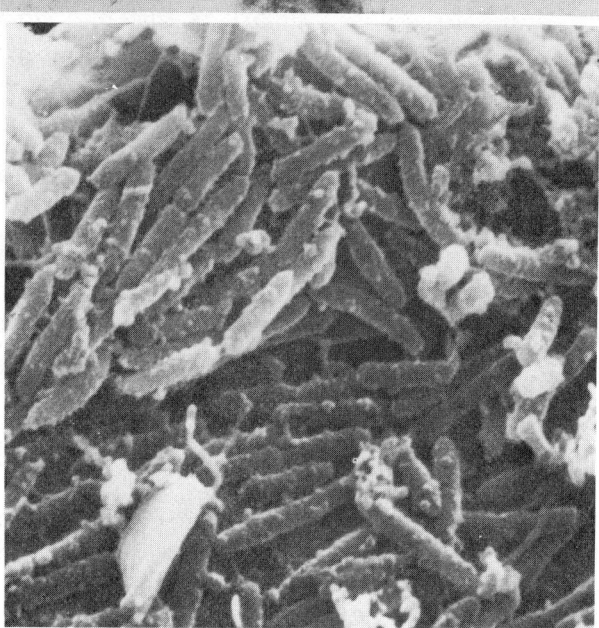

B

responsible for the disease (Keren et al., 1976).

This strong anatomic evidence for a bacterial etiology of Whipple's disease has not been confirmed by culture. Different organisms have been isolated and cell-wall deficient bacteria incriminated, but the identity of these rods is obscure, and Koch's postulates remain unfulfilled.

## PATHOGENESIS AND PATHOLOGY

### Pathogenesis

Disordered fat metabolism was first thought to explain the clinical and pathologic features, and numerous other theories have been proposed, but an infection seems to be the most likely cause. The dramatic clinical response and the disappearance of the bacilli under electron microscopy after antibiotic therapy are compelling arguments in favor of a bacterial etiology.

The portal of entry is unknown, although the most likely route is oral. This is inferred from the demonstration of more organisms in the upper portions of the gastrointestinal tract and a progressive decline as samples are obtained from the jejunum and ileum, and by the observation that the diagnostic morphologic abnormalities in the small intestine are universally present, whether or not other tissues and organs are involved.

Multiplication within the lamina propria and invasion of the absorptive cells and lymphatics with spread to the mesenteric nodes and beyond are the presumed mechanisms for subsequent hematogenous spread. The evidence for such dissemination is found in cases of Whipple's disease involving multiple systems.

Steatorrhea is mainly due to functional and morphologic alterations of the absorptive cells, which are invaded by the bacillary structures. These cells revert to normal and the bacteria disappear soon after treatment, and coincident with this, fat absorption returns to normal. The dense infiltration of the lamina propria by the PAS-positive macrophages, the enlarged and abnormal mesenteric nodes, and the bacteria present in lysosomes within the lymphatic endothelium may impair lipid transport but are not thought to be a major cause of malabsorption.

The impressive predominance of Whipple's disease in middle-aged men, the chronicity and remittent nature of the illness, and the pathologic alterations all suggest that host factors play an important role in the expression of this disease, but these host factors are undefined. Some form of immunologic tolerance is thought to be present, but immunologic studies are inconclusive. Several investigators have demonstrated impaired cell-mediated immunity, mainly on the basis of altered delayed cutaneous hypersensitivity; however, these findings are inconsistent.

### Pathology

The peritoneal and serosal surfaces of the bowel are covered with strands and nodular collections of soft, yellow-white, fibrinous material, and slight oozing occurs when the fibrinous adhesions are removed from the surface of the intestine. The small bowel wall can be thickened and irregular, particularly the proximal third. The colon is usually normal on gross inspection. Enlarged mesenteric nodes are striking (Fig. 2), and retroperitoneal adenopathy is present. Splenomegaly is frequent. Nodular excrescences on the ventricular surfaces in the brain and vegetations on the endothelial surfaces of the heart have been described.

The small bowel villi are blunted and edematous (Fig. 3), and within these villi are large collections of foamy macrophages (Fig. 4). With the PAS stain, the sickle-form cytoplasmic particles and the intra- and extracellular amorphous clumps of PAS-positive material appear as brilliant magenta (Fig. 5). These SPC cells, the hallmark of Whipple's disease, are most abundant in the lamina propria of the small bowel, but are also evident in the mesenteric nodes and have been demonstrated in most organs and tissues of

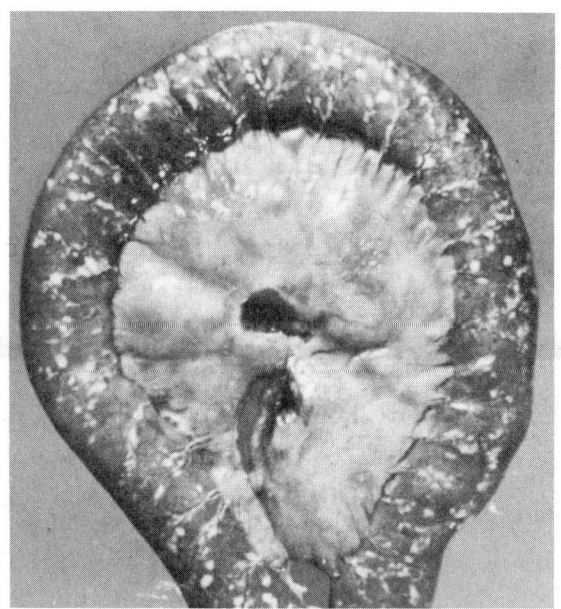

**FIGURE 2.** *Appearance of large mesenteric nodes and fibrinous deposits in a case of Whipple's disease.*

the body. The sickle-form particles are bacilliform bodies, as already mentioned. There may also be an increased number of plasma cells in the affected villi. Accumulations of neutral fat are seen in the intestinal mucosa and lymph nodes ("lipodystrophy"). Inflammation is minimal.

## CLINICAL MANIFESTATIONS

Whipple's disease predominantly affects middle-aged white men, with manifestations usually appearing in the fourth and fifth decades. Exceptions to the usual picture continue to be reported, but the total number of such cases remains small.

Weight loss is almost universal and is sometimes extreme. Diarrhea occurs in over three fourths of the cases and can be watery stools or true steatorrhea. Abdominal pain is less frequent, usually epigastric. Articular manifestations provide the diagnostic clue and are present in at least 65 per cent of the cases (Maizel et al., 1970). The fascinating feature of the arthralgias is that they may precede the other manifestations by many years, frequently five to six. The arthralgia is migratory and involves multiple joints, with the ankles, knees, shoulders, and wrists most commonly involved. Arthritis can be dramatic and is an inflammatory, predominantly large-joint, asymmetric, monoarticular disease. Destructive arthritis is unusual.

Abdominal distention and lymphadenopathy

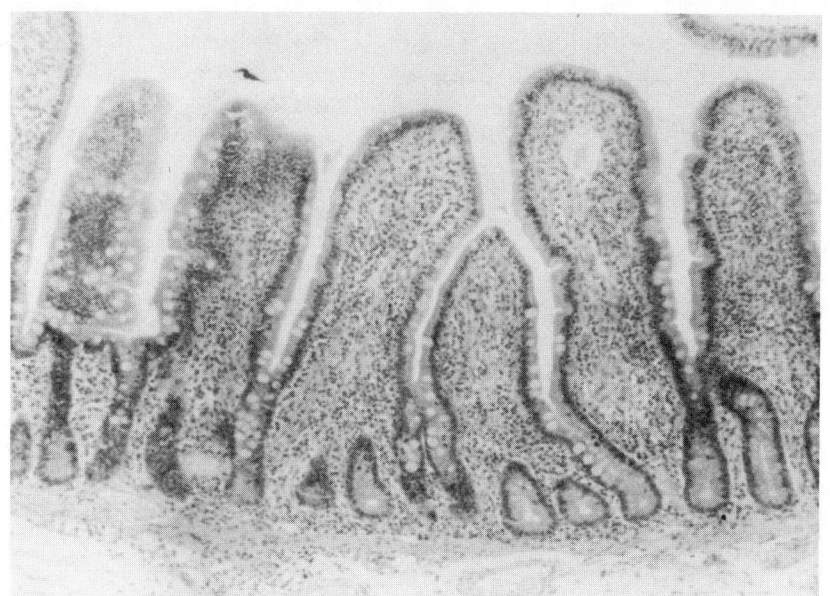

**FIGURE 3.** *Small bowel morphology demonstrating enlarged, blunted villi.*

are the most common signs, occurring in over half of the cases. Hyperpigmentation, especially of the exposed skin, is frequently reported. Edema, glossitis, and splenomegaly are less often found.

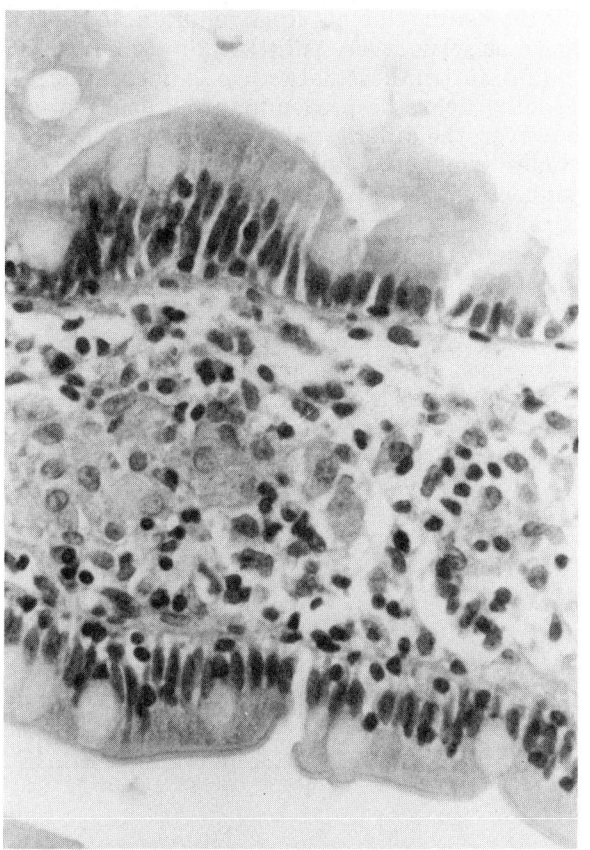

**FIGURE 4.** *Foamy macrophages infiltrating the villi.*

Fever is present in approximately half of the patients reported and can be quite variable, ranging from low-grade pyrexia to intermittent fever with rigor. In fact, it is not uncommon for Whipple's disease to present as a "fever of unknown origin." Further, this illness should be added to the list of diseases associated with relapsing fever, as demonstrated in Figure 6.

There are a number of neurologic signs now reported, and the most common are dementia, myoclonus, supranuclear ophthalmoplegia, and ataxia (Knox et al., 1976). Signs of valvular disease (aortic and mitral) related to endocarditis are noteworthy (Kraunz, 1969; Wright et al., 1978). Ocular inflammation is rare (Font et al., 1978).

Anemia is present in over 90 per cent of the patients and is most often attributed to impaired erythropoiesis due to chronic inflammation. Iron deficiency anemia associated with gastrointestinal blood loss has been documented. Megaloblastic anemia is rare. White blood counts are usually normal, but some eosinophilia occurs. Serum albumin is often reduced, and hypocalcemia occurs secondary to steatorrhea. Malabsorption is manifested by increased stool fat in most cases, impaired D-xylose absorption, and reduced serum carotene. The synovial fluid has an inflammatory character with high viscosity and protein and many leukocytes (predominantly mononuclear). There is roentgenographic evidence of sacroiliitis along with reports of HLA B27 positivity and circulating immune complexes. The cerebrospinal fluid is normal, but SPC cells have been found. Various gastrointestinal roentgenographic signs have been reported, but they are all nonspecific.

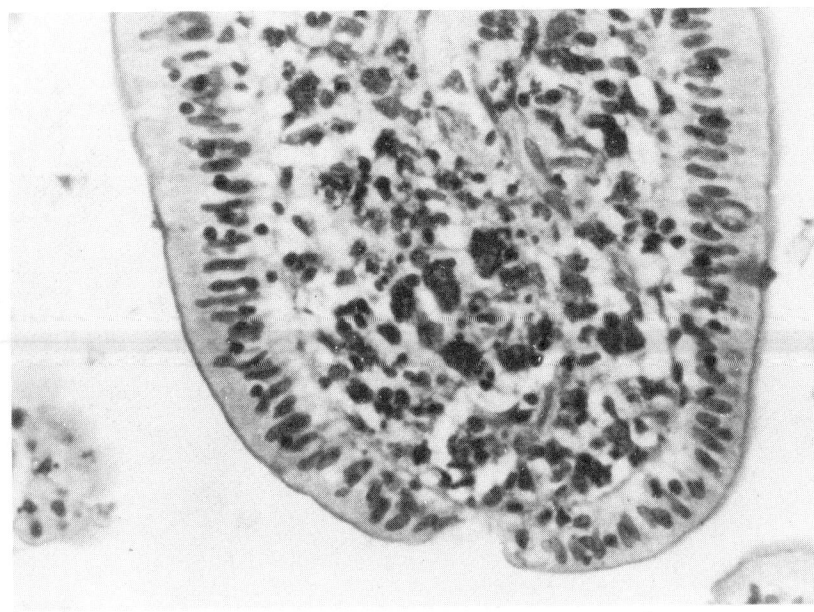

**FIGURE 5.** *Note dark staining PAS-positive material, intra- and extracellular. Higher power necessary to identify SPC cells.*

Computerized scanning can now demonstrate the enlarged mesenteric and retroperitoneal lymph nodes.

## COMPLICATIONS AND SEQUELAE

Whipple's disease is inexorably fatal if not treated. However, even with treatment, some neurologic manifestations may be permanent and even progressive (Feurle et al., 1979; Knox et al., 1976; Bayless and Knox, 1979). Ocular changes may also persist. Stenotic and destructive valvular deformities require individualized study and management. The arthritides are nondeforming, and the vast majority of treated patients have a favorable outcome.

## GEOGRAPHIC VARIATIONS IN DISEASE

Most cases are reported from the United States, Continental Europe, and England, and some from South America. Further, within the United States, there are areas (for example, the Southeast and upper Midwest) where the prevalence seems clearly higher. The reasons for this and for the other epidemiologic characteristics alluded to above remain unknown, but subtle ecologic factors related to the presumed causative agent may be responsible.

## DIAGNOSIS

Recurring asymmetric arthralgias and inflammatory arthritis, involving large joints, in a white man over 35 years of age should suggest the diagnosis of Whipple's disease. The full-blown picture with weight loss and diarrhea is rather characteristic of this disorder. X-rays of the small bowel show mainly thickening of mucosal folds in the duodenum and proximal jejunum. In contrast to celiac sprue, there is little if any small intestinal dilatation, flocculation, or segmentation. Depending upon the predominant clinical features, however, the differential diagnosis frequently includes lymphoma, inflammatory bowel disease, connective tissue disorders, sarcoidosis, and a chronic infection such as tuberculosis (the main consideration in Whipple's original case).

Although the disease may be strongly suggested by a number of the clinical manifestations enumerated, the sine qua non for the diagnosis rests upon the demonstration of the foamy macrophages, which are PAS-positive and diastase-resistant, in the lamina propria of the enlarged and blunted villi. These macrophages have been

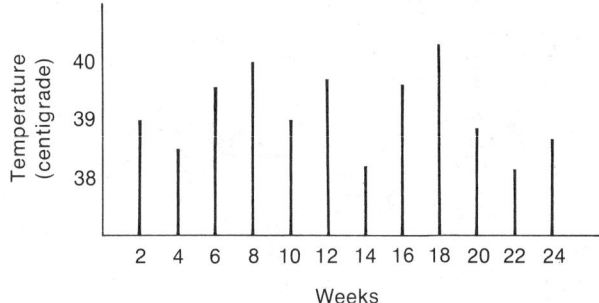

**FIGURE 6.** *Fifty-eight-year-old man with relapsing fever (every two weeks) due to Whipple's disease. Each febrile episode lasted 24 hours.*

found in the intestinal mucosa of patients whether or not gastrointestinal abnormalities were present. The necessary tissue can be obtained by peroral small bowel biopsy. The finding of PAS-positive material in cells from other sources, such as lymph nodes, cannot be considered pathognomonic of Whipple's disease. However, there is a recent, disquieting report of a patient with presumed Whipple's disease who had negative small bowel biopsies and in whom the diagnosis was made by lymph node biopsy revealing PAS-positive cells, which on electron microscopy contained bacilliform bodies morphologically consistent with those seen in Whipple's disease (Mansbach et al., 1978).

## *THERAPY*

It is only since the early 1960's that antibiotics were recognized as being curative (Maizel et al., 1970; Bayless, 1970). In fact, antibiotic treatment produces dramatic improvement in all signs and symptoms during the first few weeks. The optimum therapeutic program is not known. Some have recommended parenteral therapy with procaine penicillin G, 1,200,000 units plus streptomycin, 1 g to be given daily for two weeks. This is followed with tetracycline, 250 mg orally four times per day. It is not known if this regimen is preferable to tetracycline initially. Prolonged therapy is required, and the incidence of relapses is considerably less if such treatment is given for a full year. If relapses occur, indefinite therapy may be indicated, possibly at reduced doses after remission is again achieved. Drugs other than tetracycline have been successfully used orally, and include penicillin, ampicillin, and erythromycin, all in a dose of 1 g per day. Chloramphenicol and, more recently, trimethoprim-sulfamethoxazole (Tauris and Moesner, 1978) can be added to the list, thus providing alternatives for patients who do not respond to or cannot tolerate the tetracyclines.

Whipple's disease involving the central nervous system (CNS) can be more difficult to treat. In part, this may be due to the blood-brain barrier and the inadequate levels of antimicrobial agents in the CNS tissues. In such cases, it may be necessary to use over 12 million units of penicillin I.V. per day and/or chloramphenicol to achieve a response, and to rely upon oral agents that do penetrate the CNS, such as trimethoprim-sulfamethoxazole, given indefinitely.

Obviously, attention to nutritional needs, including vitamin and mineral replacement, and to the possible complications mentioned previously is mandatory. Corticosteroid therapy is no longer appropriate, but some have used it for short periods in severely ill cachectic patients. Further refinements in management await the identification of the still elusive rod-shaped organism.

## References

Bayless, T. M.: Whipple's disease. Newer concepts of therapy. Adv Intern Med 16:171, 1970.

Bayless, T. M., and Knox, D. L.: Whipple's disease: A multisystem infection (editorial). N Engl J Med 300:920, 1979.

Black-Schaffer, B.: The tinctorial demonstration of a glycoprotein in Whipple's disease. Proc Soc Exp Biol Med 72:225, 1949.

Chears, W. C., and Ashworth, C. T.: Electronmicroscopic study of the intestinal mucosa in Whipple's disease. Gastroenterology 41:129, 1961.

Feurle, G. E., Volk, B., and Waldherr, R.: Cerebral Whipple's disease with negative jejunal histology. N Engl J Med 300:907, 1979.

Font Rao, N. A., Issareslu, S., and McEntee, W. J.: Ocular involvement in Whipple's disease. Arch Ophthalmol 96:1431, 1978.

Haubrich, W. S., Watson, J. H. L., and Sieracki, J. C.: Unique morphologic features of Whipple's disease: A study by light and electronmicroscopy. Gastroenterology 39:454, 1960.

Keren, D. F., Weisburger, W. R., Yardley, J. H., et al.: Whipple's disease: Demonstration by immunofluorescence of similar bacterial agents in macrophages from three cases. Johns Hopkins Med J 139:51, 1976.

Knox, D. L., Bayless, T. M., and Pittman, F. E.: Neurologic disease in patients with treated Whipple's disease. Medicine 55:467, 1976.

Krauns, R. F.: Whipple's disease with cardiac and renal abnormalities. Arch Intern Med 123:701, 1969.

Maizel, H., Ruffin, J. M., and Dobbins, W. D.: Whipple's disease: A review of 19 patients from one hospital and a review of the literature since 1950. Medicine 49:175, 1970.

Mansbach, C. M., Shelburne, J. D., Stevens, R. D., and Dobbins, W. O.: Lymph-node bacilliform bodies resembling those of Whipple's disease in a patient without intestinal involvement. Ann Intern Med 89:64, 1978.

Sieracki, J. C.: Whipple's disease — observation on systemic involvement. Arch Pathol 66:464, 1958.

Tauris, P., and Moesner, J.: Whipple's disease. Clinical and histopathologic changes during treatment with sulfamethoxazole-trimethoprim. Acta Med Scand 204:423, 1978.

Whipple, G. H.: A hitherto undescribed disease characterized anatomically by deposits of fat and fatty acids in the intestinal and mesenteric lymphatic tissues. Johns Hopkins Hospital Bull 18:382, 1907.

Wright, C. B., Hiratzka, L. F., Crossland, S., Isner, J., and Snow, J. A.: Insufficiency requiring valve replacement in Whipple's disease. Ann Thorac Surg 25:466, 1978.

Yardley, J. H., and Hendrix, T. R.: Combined electron and light microscopy in Whipple's disease. Demonstration of "bacillary bodies" in the intestine. Bull Johns Hopkins Hosp 109:80, 1961.

# 145 *PERITONITIS*

## *Dennis L. Kasper, M.D.*

### DEFINITION

Peritoneal infections involve the serous membrane that lines the abdominal cavity and covers most of the intra-abdominal viscera. This membrane is divided into a parietal portion that lines the walls of the cavity and a visceral portion that encloses the intraperitoneal organs. In men, the peritoneal cavity is completely closed; however, in women, it communicates with the environment through the genital viscera of the pelvis.

Two major pathologic processes, peritonitis and abscesses, can affect the peritoneum. Peritonitis refers to nearly all inflammatory lesions of infectious etiology in which pus is not localized. Abscesses are localized collections of pus that can involve the abdominal viscera and either the intraperitoneal or retroperitoneal spaces.

### ETIOLOGY

The most common causes of sterile peritonitis are blood, which causes chemical irritation and inflammation; bile from perforation or rupture of the biliary system; pancreatic enzymes, which are released into the peritoneum in acute hemorrhagic pancreatitis; carcinomatosis; and surgically introduced foreign materials, particularly talcum powder.

Bacteria are the most common cause of infectious peritonitis. These infections may be primary or secondary (Table 1). Primary bacterial peritonitis usually occurs in patients with altered susceptibility to infection. It is an acute or subacute infection caused by a single microbe that seeded the peritoneum either during a transient bacteremia or during a bacteremia from a distant site of infection.

In the past, children with the nephrotic syndrome developed primary peritonitis that was usually caused by *Streptococcus pneumoniae* or other species of *Streptococcus*, but this has subsequently become an unusual complication of nephrosis. Now, however, almost 10 per cent of patients with cirrhosis of the liver who also have portal hypertension and overt ascites develop spontaneous primary peritonitis for which there are multiple etiologic agents. *Escherichia coli* (36 per cent) and other enterics cause 60 per cent of these infections. Less frequent enterics and other gram-negative bacteria include *Pseudomonas, Proteus, Klebsiella, Bacteroides,* and *Salmonella* (Conn and Fessel, 1971). *S. pneumoniae* and other strep-

tococci account for approximately 25 per cent of these infections.

Secondary peritonitis, which is more common than primary, is caused by: (1) lesions that damage the integrity of one of the viscera covered by the peritoneum, with leakage of microbes or irritants into the intraperitoneal or retroperitoneal spaces; (2) disruption of the peritoneum from outside the abdomen without actual penetration of the viscera; or (3) surgical contamination (Table 1). These lesions result in bacterial infection of the peritoneum with organisms that are usually part of the normal flora of the violated sites.

*Mycobacterium tuberculosis* is an important cause of chronic infectious peritonitis. Peritoneal inflammation caused by fungi is distinctly uncommon, but *Candida albicans* can cause massive ascites by direct peritoneal involvement. Fungi have also caused secondary peritonitis after the organism has entered the peritoneum from intestinal leakage. Peritonitis occurs in 2 to 4 per cent of patients with disseminated histoplasmosis.

Parasitic infestations can lead to clinical peritoneal disease that can mimic tuberculosis or carcinomatosis. *Schistosoma mansoni* can cause

---

**TABLE 1.    Etiology of Bacterial Peritonitis**

I. Primary peritonitis without disruption of the integrity of the gastrointestinal tract in:
   A. Nephrotics
   B. Cirrhotics
   C. Otherwise healthy young children occasionally
II. Secondary peritonitis
   A. Related to diseases and injuries of the gastrointestinal tract
      1. Appendicitis
      2. Diverticulitis
      3. Perforation due to malignant tumor
      4. Perforated peptic ulcer
      5. Devitalization of intestinal wall by circulatory impairment, volvulus, or intussusception
      6. Perforations caused by trauma such as gunshot or stab wounds
   B. Related to lesions of the biliary system and pancreas
      1. Suppurative cholecystitis
      2. Bile peritonitis
      3. Pancreatitis
   C. Related to lesions of the female genital tract
   D. Related to lesions of the male genitourinary tract, especially injuries or suppurating lesions of the bladder and, rarely, kidneys
   E. Postoperative
      1. Operative contamination of peritoneum
      2. Leaking anastomosis
      3. Retained foreign body
   F. Perforating wounds of abdominal wall only
III. *Mycobacterium tuberculosis*

---

granulomatous peritonitis without extraintestinal involvement. Enterobiasis has been reported to cause granulomatous peritonitis in women, apparently by retrograde migration through the genital tract. Amebiasis of the gastrointestinal tract, liver, or spleen can cause perforation of the involved viscera and secondary bacterial peritonitis. Ectopic *Paragonimus* cysts, as well as migratory *Ascaris*, may localize in the abdominal cavity and produce an acute abdomen. Mechanical irritation of the stroblia and attachment of the scolex of intestinal tapeworms, especially *Taenia solium*, is a rare cause of intestinal perforation and secondary bacterial peritonitis. The hepatic cysts of *Echinococcus granulosus* can rupture into the abdominal cavity. Any of the migrating parasites may carry bacteria with them from the gastrointestinal tract and set up distant bacterial abscesses.

## PATHOLOGY AND PATHOGENESIS

The inflammatory process in bacterial peritonitis is typical of other acute bacterial infections and consists primarily of an infiltration of neutrophils with a fibrinopurulent exudate. The membranes undergo sequential pathologic changes. Two to four hours after involvement, the membrane loses its gray, glistening quality and becomes dull and lusterless. At this time, a small quantity of serous or slightly turbid fluid accumulates. Later, this fluid becomes creamy and suppurative and may either be localized by the omentum and viscera to a small area of the peritoneal cavity or become generalized. Rarely, the exudate resolves without residual fibrosis. Usually, the exudate eventually accumulates into well-loculated collections of pus called abscesses that may develop anywhere in the abdominal cavity, including the subhepatic and subdiaphragmatic spaces, the retroperitoneum, or within the viscera. The exudate may cause adhesions after the formation of abscesses.

The pathogenesis of primary peritonitis has not been well defined, but it is thought that ascites is an ideal culture medium for bacteria that reach the peritoneum by hematogenous spread. This is an attractive hypothesis to explain the development of peritonitis in cirrhotic patients with portal hypertension because their portal-systemic collaterals bypass the liver, a major bacterial filter.

It is probable that some cases of primary peritonitis originate from transmural migration of bacteria. The polymicrobic nature of some of these infections without evidence of a perforated bowel argues strongly for this mechanism of peritoneal contamination. Furthermore, $^{14}$C-labeled *E. coli* have been shown to traverse the intact intestinal wall in dogs after hypertonic irrigations of the peritoneum (Schweinburg et al., 1950). For these reasons, it seems likely that the source of infection in some cirrhotics, and perhaps in a substantial number of patients receiving peritoneal dialysis, is transmural migration of intestinal bacteria.

The pathogenesis of secondary bacterial peritonitis, which has been well defined in the experimental animal, is dependent on the composition of the normal bowel flora. The largest populations of bacteria in the body reside in the gastrointestinal tract. Most of these bacteria are obligate anaerobes, which outnumber aerobic bacteria 100- to 1000-fold. The largest concentrations of bacteria are in the colon, where the number of anaerobes may reach $10^{11}$ per g and may outnumber coliforms 1000-fold. The stomach and upper small bowel support a rather sparse population ($<10^5$) of bacteria that are mainly washed down from the oropharynx. The lower ileum is a transitional area, with up to $10^8$ bacteria per ml. In the upper gastrointestinal tract anaerobes and aerobes are equal in number. This anatomic distribution of bacteria in the gastrointestinal tract explains the fact that perforation of the upper intestine results in lower rates of infection and morbidity than colonic perforation. Because of the high bacterial counts in the lower gastrointestinal tract, careful bacteriology yields an average of five different species, often two aerobes and three anaerobes, from secondary intra-abdominal infections. This high incidence of anaerobic microorganisms and the polymicrobial nature of these infections are characteristic of intra-abdominal infection related to perforation of the lower gastrointestinal tract (Gorbach and Bartlett, 1974).

Careful bacteriologic studies have shown that certain species are predictably isolated from patients with intra-abdominal infection. Of the aerobes the gram-negative enteric bacilli are most common: these include *Escherichia coli*, *Klebsiella, Proteus,* and *Pseudomonas*. Enterococci are the most common gram-positive aerobic bacteria. The major anaerobic isolates are *Bacteroides fragilis* (65 per cent of all cases), *Clostridium* species (60 per cent of cases), and anaerobic cocci (32 per cent). Despite the multiplicity of isolates from intra-abdominal infections, these particular species account for a small proportion of an endless array of bacteria found in the normal bowel. Studies using an animal model of intra-abdominal sepsis have clarified the complex role of these bacteria in the pathogenesis of peritonitis and subsequent abscess formation (Weinstein et al., 1974). These studies, which employed an intraperitoneal implant of fecal contents in rats, showed a two-stage disease. During the first five days, there was acute peritonitis with free-flowing peritoneal exudate. The cumulative natural mortality rate during this stage was 43 per cent; this early stage was caused by aerobic gram-negative bacteria, particularly *E. coli*. The second stage, characterized by the formation of multiple intra-abdominal abscesses in all survivors, was caused by anaerobic bacteria.

Abscess formation in the animal model usually required the synergistic interaction of an aerobe and an anaerobe. This requirement held unless the anaerobe was *Bacteroides fragilis*, which could induce abscesses without the synergistic help of an aerobe (*E. coli* or enterococci). *B. fragilis*, but not other *Bacteroides* species, contains a capsular polysaccharide, which is responsible for abscess formation (Onderdonk et al., 1977).

Anaerobes are also more common in the vagina than aerobes and play a major role in secondary pelvic peritonitis and abscess after septic abortion, postoperative surgery on the reproductive tract, puerperal sepsis, and endometritis. Furthermore, *B. fragilis*, anaerobic streptococci, and other enteric bacteria colonize the vagina in increased numbers postoperatively and after difficult deliveries (Gibbs et al., 1975). For these reasons, the microbiology of secondary peritonitis of pelvic origin is similar to that of intestinal origin, except for group B *Streptococci, Corynebacterium* (Haemophilus) *vaginale*, and rarely gonococci, which are more common in pelvic infections. The prominence in these infections of *Bacteroides* species that are capable of degrading heparin (Gesner and Jenkin, 1961) may explain the tendency toward suppurative pelvic thrombophlebitis and septic pulmonary emboli.

The pathogenesis of tuberculous peritonitis is well understood. It is usually the result of reactivation of latent peritoneal foci that were established at the time of hematogenous spread from the primary pulmonary focus in patients who do not have active pulmonary tuberculosis. Tuberculous peritonitis can occur, however, at the time of hematogenous spread from active pulmonary or miliary tuberculosis.

## CLINICAL MANIFESTATIONS

The clinical symptoms and onset of infectious peritonitis vary with the etiology, the precipitating event, and the population studied. The signs and symptoms may be deceptively absent in the very young or old. The presentation of patients in shock or on corticosteroids may be acute, subacute, chronic, or insidious.

Of the more acute forms, primary spontaneous peritonitis usually occurs in patients with decompensated hepatic function and secondary ascites and jaundice. Portal-systemic collaterals are pres-

ent in 80 per cent and azotemia in 55 per cent of patients. The symptoms or signs may be masked by hepatic failure; 35 per cent of patients have no peritoneal signs, and 5 per cent are completely asymptomatic. Spontaneous primary peritonitis causes abdominal pain in 80 per cent and hypotension in 70 per cent; it is associated with encephalopathy in more than 70 per cent of cases. Sudden deterioration in the condition of a patient with cirrhosis should alert the physician to the possibility of bacterial peritonitis.

In patients with secondary peritonitis, the mode of onset varies with the precipitating event and may be acute or subacute. Abdominal pain and distention are usually prominent. Other findings include diffuse muscle spasm, absence of abdominal respiratory movement, abdominal tenderness, rebound tenderness, rigidity of the abdominal wall, and decreased or absent peristalsis. There may be tenderness or a mass on rectal or vaginal examination as well as fever, toxemia, or shock.

The onset of tuberculous peritonitis is insidious. More than 70 per cent of patients have had symptoms for more than four months before presentation. These signs are nonspecific, and the diagnosis of tuberculous peritonitis must be considered in any patient with ascites, fever, abdominal pain, anorexia, malaise, weakness, and weight loss. Abdominal pain, which is usually vague and dull, is reported by only 50 per cent of patients with tuberculous peritonitis. Some patients complain of vomiting, constipation, and diarrhea. Seventy-five per cent have ascites. Abdominal tenderness is reported by 65 per cent of patients. Despite classic descriptions, the "doughy" abdomen is rare. Twenty-five per cent of patients have hepatomegaly, and 20 per cent have an abdominal mass.

## COMPLICATIONS AND SEQUELAE

The complications and sequelae of peritonitis can be divided into three general categories (Table 2). In the early phase of peritonitis, metabolic alterations place increased demands on the circulatory system. The amount of fluid lost into the peritoneal cavity may approach 50 per cent of the plasma volume. This fluid and electrolyte imbalance is complicated by ileus, which causes loss of fluid into the lumen of the bowel. There may be a large loss of potassium from the intracellular to the extracellular fluid with a shift of sodium into the intracellular compartment. The potassium loss may be masked by hemoconcentration and should be monitored by electrocardiography. Serum levels of glucocorticoids, aldosterone, and catecholamines are usually elevated.

**TABLE 2.   Complications and Sequelae of Peritonitis**

I. Early acute phase
  A. Metabolic
    1. Fluid and electrolyte imbalance
    2. Hypokalemia
    3. Elevated glucocorticoids, aldosterone, catecholamines
    4. Vasoconstriction with decreased renal perfusion and cardiac action
  B. Respiratory embarrassment
  C. Bacteremia
  D. Shock
II. Abscesses
  A. Anatomically dependent areas
  B. Localized near the site of contamination
III. Adhesions

Elevation of catecholamines may contribute to peripheral vasoconstriction and decreased perfusion of vital organs, which can cause declining renal and cardiac function. The evolving ileus and progressive elevation of the diaphragm can interfere with ventilatory capacity and respiratory exchange.

Bacteremia with either aerobes (usually gram-negative rods) and/or anaerobes (most commonly *B. fragilis*) is common during the acute phase of peritonitis. All of these complications can contribute to the development of shock, which is associated with a high mortality rate, even in the face of appropriate therapy.

The major sequelae of peritonitis are abscesses. Intraperitoneal abscesses develop in one of two general patterns. The first is the result of diffuse peritonitis in which loculations of purulent material usually occur in anatomically dependent areas such as the pelvis, the kidney pouch, and the subphrenic or paracolic "gutter" areas. The second results from a localized focus of peritonitis related to some contiguous disease process such as pelvic inflammatory disease, in which the inflammatory response is rapid and effective enough to prevent diffuse peritonitis.

Adhesions may complicate either localized or generalized peritonitis and can cause intestinal, circulatory, or neural compression and obstruction.

## GEOGRAPHIC VARIATIONS IN DISEASE

Spontaneous primary and secondary bacterial peritonitis occur in all geographic areas and are caused by the same bacteria. Studies of human colonic flora have generally shown marked quantitative and qualitative similarities in bacterial species despite variations in race, diet, or geographic locale.

In the United States, tuberculous peritonitis is commonly encountered in cities with large populations of individuals who seem to be socioeconomically predisposed to tuberculosis. This group includes the poorly nourished, debilitated, and cirrhotic patients found in municipal hospitals. There is no age or sex predilection, but from 80 to 90 per cent of people with this disease are black. The predisposition of blacks to tuberculosis is probably due to poverty and crowding, which also influence the relatively high rate of tuberculosis in developing countries.

On a worldwide basis, tuberculosis is a widely distributed disease, and peritonitis is a common manifestation.

Except for infections with *Candida*, which are part of the endogenous flora of patients all over the world, the rare fungal and parasitic infections of the peritoneum occur within the geographic distribution of the particular agent.

## DIAGNOSIS

The differential diagnosis of peritonitis is extensive (Table 3). These etiologies can be grouped into intra-abdominal inflammations (including septic and nonseptic conditions), metabolic processes, intrathoracic conditions, and infections that commonly cause the clinical picture of peritonitis.

**TABLE 3.   Differential Diagnosis of Peritonitis**

I. Intra-abdominal
  A. Septic, but contained within an organ (e.g., biliary)
    1. Primary
    2. Secondary
    3. Contained within an organ (e.g., cholecystitis)
  B. Nonseptic
    1. Intestinal obstruction
    2. Internal hemorrhage
    3. Pancreatitis
    4. Renal disease
II. Metabolic
  A. Porphyria
  B. Diabetic acidosis
  C. Plumbism
  D. Arachnidism
III. Intrathoracic
  A. Myocardial infarction
  B. Pleurisy
  C. Pneumonia
  D. Epidemic pleurodynia
IV. Infections with abdominal manifestations
  A. Tabetic crisis
  B. Malaria
  C. Typhoid fever
  D. Herpes zoster of the lower spinal roots
  E. Osteomyelitis
V. Others
  A. Periarteritis nodosa
  B. Retroperitoneal catastrophes
    1. Rupture of aneurysm
    2. Dissection of aorta
  C. Familial Mediterranean fever

The diagnosis of peritonitis can be additionally complex because of the great variation in the presenting signs and symptoms. Only careful evaluation of the patient, the clinical laboratory data, and the radiologic information can ensure an accurate diagnosis. First, careful attention must be paid to a history of antecedent illnesses, such as diverticulitis, duodenal ulcer, and pancreatitis, that would predispose to peritonitis from intra-abdominal fecal contamination. The characteristics of the abdominal pain can help determine the etiology of the disease. The physician must determine its site of origin, the site of greatest intensity, and the radiation and character of the pain (Cope, 1963).

Most patients with bacterial peritonitis have fever and leukocytosis. Other laboratory abnormalities are related to the involved viscera or the underlying etiology. Therefore, the physician must carefully consider the possible metabolic or intra-abdominal nonseptic conditions that might mimic bacterial peritonitis. Urinalysis and measurement of blood sugar, bilirubin, amylase, alkaline phosphatase, serum ketones, or urinary porphyrins may be helpful, but all laboratory data must be assessed critically. For example, pyuria usually reflects pathology of the genitourinary tract but can be seen when adjacent viscera are inflamed as in diverticulitis or appendicitis. The serum amylase may be very high in acute pancreatitis, but modestly elevated levels can occur in peritonitis owing to many etiologies. Microbiologic studies are extremely important; in particular, aerobic and anaerobic cultures of the blood and peritoneal fluid are essential. Examination of the abdomen by x-ray may reveal displacement of the gastrointestinal tract or ureters, free air in the peritoneal cavity, encapsulated air or gas in an abscess, features of ileus or obstruction, evidence of peritoneal fluid, obliteration of the psoas shadows, calcification within the gallbladder or other organs, or restricted motion of the diaphragm (fluoroscopy). Chest x-ray may show unilateral elevation of the diaphragm and basilar atelectasis or pleural effusions and may help to differentiate peritonitis from an intrathoracic infection. Other radiologic procedures that can be of diagnostic value include radioisotopic scanning procedures for localization of abscesses, arteriography, liver-lung scan (most useful for subdiaphragmatic abscesses), ultrasound, and computerized tomographic scans.

Needle aspiration of the peritoneum can be diagnostic. Typical results of the laboratory examination of ascitic fluid from patients with bacterial and tuberculous peritonitis are outlined in Table 4. Peritoneal biopsy is also a valuable procedure and establishes the diagnosis in 50 to 60 per cent of patients with tuberculous peritoni-

tis and in 25 to 40 per cent of cases of carcinoma.

The diagnosis of abscesses is difficult. Persistence of fever and leukocytosis after abdominal surgery should be regarded as intra-abdominal abscess unless proved otherwise. Laboratory tests are of little aid in the diagnosis of intraperitoneal abscesses that do not involve organs, but roentgenologic examination can be very helpful for locating intra-abdominal abscesses. In subdiaphragmatic abscess, the abnormalities are usually seen on chest x-ray; possible findings include pleural effusion; elevation and decreased mobility of the diaphragm; lower lobe infiltration or atelectasis; a unilateral widening of the angle between the chondral arch and the sternum; and obliteration of the costophrenic angle on lateral examination, all of which may be mistaken for pneumonia postoperatively. Other important radiologic signs that may require contrast studies include gas-fluid levels (33 per cent positive in overpenetrated views) and displacement of the spleen, stomach (in the Trendelenburg position), colon, or left lobe of the liver. Combined liver-lung scan has been very helpful in the diagnosis of subdiaphragmatic abscess.

Abscesses elsewhere in the peritoneum or retroperitoneum may be more difficult to detect than subphrenic abscesses. Here again, an abscess may be demonstrable as a space-occupying lesion displacing loops of intestine or obliterating the intermuscular and subperitoneal fat layers of the adjacent abdominal wall. Perinephric abscesses usually present with fever, unilateral flank pain, abdominal pain, dysuria, and an abdominal or

**TABLE 4.** Typical Laboratory Characteristics of the Peritoneal Fluid from Patients with Bacterial Peritonitis

|  | BACTERIAL PERITONITIS | TUBERCULOUS PERITONITIS | UNINFECTED CIRRHOTIC FLUID |
|---|---|---|---|
| Specific gravity | ↑ | ↑ (↓ [a]) | ↓ (<1.012) |
| Protein | ↑ | ↑ (↓ [a]) | ↓ (<2.5 g per cent) |
| Cell count | ↑ | ↑ (↓ [a]) | ↓ (<250 WBC/mm$^3$) |
| Differential | >50 per cent PMN[b] | <30 per cent PMN | not helpful |
| Amylase | nl | nl | nl |
| Glucose | ↓ | ↓ | nl |
| Gram stain | + | − | − |
| Culture |  |  |  |
|   Anaerobic | + | − | − |
|   Aerobic | + | − | − |
|   Tuberculous | − | +[b] | − |
|   Fungi | − | − | − |
| Cytology | − | − | − |
| Lipid content | − | − | − |

[a] Usually elevated, but can be normal or low in cirrhotic patients with tuberculous peritonitis.
[b] Greater yield if larger volumes are cultured.
↑, increase
↓, decrease
PMN, polymorphonuclear leukocytes
nl, normal

flank mass. Mild leukocytosis, normal or slightly elevated blood urea nitrogen, and pyuria are also common. Three fourths of the patients have abnormalities demonstrable by intravenous pyelogram; calicectasis, caliceal stretching, and stones are common. Fifty per cent of these patients have abnormal chest x-rays with findings similar to those of subdiaphragmatic abscesses. Abscesses of the iliac fossa (psoas abscess) are also retroperitoneal and present with findings similar to those of perinephric abscesses, except that these patients may also have an unexplained limp, pain on walking, and pain on extension of the thigh. A history of recent obstetric or gynecologic procedure, rectal and vaginal examination, positive smear or culture results from culdocentesis, and clinical or roentgenographic evidence of septic pulmonary emboli help to establish the diagnosis of pelvic peritonitis or abscess.

## TREATMENT

The general principles of therapy for peritonitis are: (1) improvement of vascular perfusion to correct fluid and electrolyte imbalances; (2) minimization of the effects of bacteria and their toxic components; (3) reduction of paralytic ileus; (4) elimination of the primary source of infection by excision, closure, or isolation; (5) drainage of the primarily infected site; and (6) treatment of local or distant complications (Finegold, 1977).

The initial treatment of peritonitis is supportive therapy in combination with appropriate antimicrobial agents. The choice of appropriate antimicrobials depends upon the sensitivity patterns of the microorganisms involved in the infectious process and the ability of an antibiotic to penetrate the peritoneum. Primary bacterial peritonitis is best treated with penicillin G if the causative agent is either *S. pneumoniae* or group A *Streptococcus*. If the etiologic agent is *E. coli*, an aminoglycoside (gentamicin or kanamycin) is appropriate until the results of sensitivities are available.

Antimicrobial therapy of peritonitis secondary to a gastrointestinal or vaginal source should be directed at both aerobic and anaerobic gram-negative bacteria, particularly *B. fragilis*, because of the resistance of this organism to the penicillins. There are several commonly accepted alternative forms of therapy. The most widely accepted regimen is clindamycin (25 to 35 mg/kg per day in four divided doses) and gentamicin (4 to 6 mg/kg per day in three divided doses). Clindamycin is very active against all anaerobes, including *B. fragilis*, as well as many gram-positive bacteria. Recent data suggest that metronidazole or cephoxitin may also be effective against the anaerobic bacteria in peritonitis. Gentamicin and other aminoglycosides (e.g., kanamycin, amikacin, tobramycin) are all effective against the enteric aerobic bacteria. Alternative regimens would be either chloramphenicol (succinate derivative) in initial doses of 30 to 60 mg/kg per day, depending on the severity of the illness, or cephoxitin. These latter two antibiotics are active against *B. fragilis*, other anaerobes, and the resident aerobic enteric gram-negative bacterial flora. Therapy of postoperative peritonitis should also include antibiotics that are active against penicillinase-producing staphylococci. Therefore, a penicillinase-resistant penicillin or a cephalosporin may be included. There is no substantial evidence that specific treatment for enterococci is necessary. There is also no substantial evidence that intraperitoneal administration of antimicrobials is helpful; in fact, this form of treatment is not recommended. Infected peritoneal dialysates may be an exception. In pelvic thrombophlebitis, heparin should be given in conjunction with antibiotics, and ligation of the inferior vena cava may be necessary in some patients with multiple episodes of septic pulmonary emboli.

Because tuberculous peritonitis is usually a manifestation of miliary disease or localized intraperitoneal reactivation tuberculosis, it can be treated with isoniazid alone at the usual dose of 300 mg daily. Coexistent renal or cavitary tuberculosis requires the addition of a second drug to prevent the emergence of isoniazid-resistant organisms in these well-aerated tissues.

In virtually all instances of secondary peritonitis or intra-abdominal abscesses, free drainage of pus must be obtained. Antibiotics may be useful in the early stages of abscess formation before the infection is walled off, and some patients can be treated with antimicrobials alone during the period if they can withstand a few days more of illness. Successful treatment with antibiotics may account for the reported cases of abscesses that resolved without drainage. In some patients with appendicitis, diverticulitis, or pancreatitis, a mass, frequently referred to as a phlegmon, is felt on examination of the infected area three to four days after the onset. In general, surgeons feel that this situation does not call for surgery because the phlegmon resolves without intervention. Therefore, conservative therapy is advised in some forms of localized peritonitis, particularly appendiceal abscesses, diverticulitis, pancreatitis, or some cases of perforated peptic ulcers. However, surgical intervention is required in most cases of peritonitis and abscesses. There is no justification for withholding incision and drainage in an extremely ill patient whose only chance for survival is surgical drainage. The overall mortality rate for this disease is extremely high, and early surgery is the only treatment that has been shown to reduce mortality.

## PROPHYLAXIS

The only effective means of preventing peritoneal infections is early, appropriate attention to the primary conditions that cause the problem. Preventive measures for secondary peritonitis include early surgical intervention and appropriate antimicrobial chemoprophylaxis for cases in which there has been gross bacterial contamination of the peritoneal cavity. In such cases, the combination of clindamycin and gentamicin is effective in lowering the incidence of infectious complications. In the animal model of peritonitis discussed above, these two agents had contrasting but important prophylactic effects. Gentamicin reduced mortality, but the survivors had abscesses. Clindamycin failed to reduce mortality rates significantly, but surviving animals did not have abscesses. When the combination of clindamycin and gentamicin was given, the salutary effects of the two drugs were additive.

The short-term use (three doses on the first preoperative day) of oral preoperative neomycin (1 g) and erythromycin (1 g) combined with vigorous purgation has been shown to reduce the incidence of wound infections and other septic complications of elective operations on the colon and rectum (Clark et al., 1977). Evidence is

accumulating that prophylactic preoperative, intraoperative, and short-term postoperative cephalosporins and other antimicrobials may reduce the high incidence of infection after vaginal hysterectomy, radical surgery for gynecologic malignancy, and cesarean section after rupture of the membrane and labor (Veterans Administration Ad Hoc Committee, 1977).

## References

Clarke, J. S., Condon, R.E., Bartlett, J. G., Gorbach, S. L., Nichols, R. L., and Ochi, S.: Preoperative oral antibiotics reduce septic complications of colon operations. Ann Surg 186:251, 1977.

Conn, H. O., and Fessel, M. J.: Spontaneous bacterial peritonitis in cirrhosis: Variations on a theme. Medicine 50:161, 1971.

Cope, F.: The Early Diagnosis of the Acute Abdomen. London, Oxford University Press, 1963, p. 196.

Finegold, S. M.: In Haeprech, P. D. (ed.): Peritonitis in Infectious Diseases. Hagerstown, Md., Harper and Row, 1977, p. 669.

Gesner, B. M., and Jenkin, C. R.: Production of heparinase by Bacteroides. J Bacteriol 81:595, 1961.

Gibbs, R. S., O'Dell, T. N., McGregor, R. R., et al.: Puerperal endometritis: A prospective microbiologic study. Am J Obstet Gynecol 122:820, 1975.

Gorbach, S. L., and Bartlett, J. G.: Management of anaerobic infections. N Engl J Med 290:1177, 1237, 1289, 1974.

Onderdonk, A. B., Kasper, D. L., Cisneros, R. L., and Bartlett, J. G.: The capsular polysaccharide of Bacteroides fragilis as a virulence factor: Comparison of the pathogenic potential of encapsulated and unencapsulated strains. J Inf Dis 136:82, 1977.

Schweinburg, F. B., Seligman, A. M., and Fine, J.: Transmural migration of intestinal bacteria: A study based on the use of radioactive Escherichia coli. N Engl J Med 242:747, 1950.

Veterans Administration Ad Hoc Interdisciplinary Committee on Antimicrobial Drug Usage: Prophylaxis in Surgery. JAMA 237:1003, 1977.

Weinstein, W. M., Onderdonk, A. B., Bartlett, J. G., and Gorbach, S. L.: Experimental intraabdominal abscesses in rats: Development of an experimental model. Infect Immun 10:1250, 1974.

# D UROGENITAL INFECTIONS

# 146 *URINARY TRACT INFECTION AND PYELONEPHRITIS*

## M.P. Glauser, M.D.

Urinary tract infections are among the most common infections in man. They are responsible for considerable morbidity, and when associated with urinary obstruction or renal papillary damage lead to serious kidney damage. This chapter will review the current views on the pathogenesis of urinary tract infections and chronic pyelone-

phritis, as well as their prevention and treatment.

## DEFINITIONS

*Urinary tract infection* (UTI) is the presence of microorganisms in a properly collected specimen of urine (bacteriuria). UTI may be localized to any portion of the urinary tract and may be symptomatic or asymptomatic.

The *urethral syndrome* is the presence of urinary symptoms such as frequency and dysuria without bacteriuria.

*Acute nonobstructive pyelonephritis*, also referred to as acute pyelonephritis, is used *clinically* to describe the syndrome of acute illness with fever, flank pain, and tenderness combined with bacteriuria. Symptoms of lower urinary tract infection, such as frequency and dysuria, may coexist.

*Acute suppurative pyelonephritis* is defined *pathologically* as the presence of acute inflammation, exudation, and suppuration due to bacterial infection in the renal parenchyma. This picture is seen when renal infection occurs during UTI in the presence of urinary tract abnormalities or underlying renal disease. It can lead to scar formation (chronic pyelonephritis).

*Chronic pyelonephritis* is the presence of scarring in the kidney parenchyma believed to be of infectious origin. Occasionally this may be extensive and severe enough to cause renal insufficiency. Interstitial inflammation and scarring caused by infection is indistinguishable from renal inflammation of another origin (interstitial nephritis).

*Interstitial nephritis* is renal interstitial inflammation and scarring from causes other than infection, such as chronic obstruction, analgesic abuse, hyperuricemia, nephrosclerosis, diabetes, and sickle cell anemia.

## ETIOLOGY

The vast majority of urinary tract infections are caused by Enterobacteriaceae originating from the gut. In ambulatory patients, the most common organism causing UTI is *Escherichia coli* (50 to 85 per cent of cases). This predominance is not as marked in patients who have hospital-acquired or repeated urinary tract infections treated with antibiotics, in whom *Proteus, Aerobacter,* and *Pseudomonas* are more frequently observed. Moreover, *Proteus* spp. may predominate in boys with UTI (Hallett et al., 1976). Brucellae and salmonellae may cause UTI, the latter especially in patients with associated urinary schistosomiasis (Hathout et al., 1966). *Streptococcus faecalis* is the only intestinal gram-positive bacterial species found in any significant proportion of infected urine samples. Strict anaerobic bacteria are recovered from only 1 per cent of all cases of bacteriuria documented by suprapubic aspiration (Segura et al., 1972). How-

ever, Maskell and co-workers (1979) have reported recently the isolation in pure culture of $CO_2$-dependent, fastidious gram-positive organisms in patients complaining of frequency and dysuria, suggesting that corynebacteria and lactobacilli might play a pathogenic role in the urethral syndrome.

Gram-positive cocci are rarely the cause of UTI. *Staphylococcus aureus* found repeatedly in the urine may be the manifestation of renal microabscesses secondary to bacteremia, and a primary source of infection (e.g., endocarditis or osteomyelitis) should be sought. The frequency of coagulase-negative staphylococci (*S. saprophyticus*) is reported to be second only to *E. coli* as the cause of UTI in young women (Maskell, 1974; Sellin et al., 1975; Wallmark et al., 1978). Others, however, report much lower rates (Williams et al., 1976).

*Mycoplasma hominis, Chlamydia trachomatis, Ureaplasma urealyticum,* and *Trichomonas vaginalis* commonly cause urethritis but do not appear to be responsible for UTI. *Candida albicans* and other *Candida* spp may be found in diabetic women and in patients with indwelling catheters but usually represents harmless colonization. *Candida* found repeatedly in a properly collected urine specimen could originate from the kidney, a common site for metastatic infections during candidemia (Louria et al., 1962). Ascending *Candida* pyelonephritis is unusual (Tennant et al., 1968).

Viruses are frequently found in the urine during viral infections (Utz, 1974). Except for certain types of immune complex disease in which viruses could be deposited in the glomeruli, the role of viruses in kidney and urinary tract infections is poorly defined. Adenovirus Type 11 has been implicated in acute hemorrhagic cystitis in children (Numazaki et al., 1973), and cytomegaloviruses have been involved in acute rejection of transplanted kidneys (Simmons et al., 1974).

## PATHOGENESIS AND PATHOLOGY

### Incidence

In the first week of life UTI appears to be mainly of hematogenous origin and is more common in boys (Bergstrom et al., 1972). Thereafter, the incidence in girls rises almost linearly with increasing age, but boys are spared. UTI is found in about 1 per cent of school girls (Kunin et al., 1964) and reaches a peak of 10 to 12 per cent of women over 60 (Miall et al., 1962; Freedman et al., 1965). In men, on the other hand, infections are uncommon, with a prevalence of about 1 per cent at the age of 60 (Freedman et al., 1965). In certain areas endemic for urinary schistosomiasis, the prevalence in boys may be as high as 5 per cent (Laughlin et al., 1978).

### Route of Infection and Host Defense Mechanisms

In the vast majority of patients, the microorganisms responsible for UTI originate from the intestinal aerobic gram-negative bacterial flora.

*In women,* the urethral meatus and the urethra normally harbor *Lactobacillus* spp, *S. epidermidis, Corynebacterium* spp, and anaerobes, but no aerobic gram-negative flora (Marrie et al., 1978). On the other hand, enterobacteria are found in the vaginal vestibule of women who are about to develop UTI. This happens sometimes just before the onset of bacteriuria (Stamey et al., 1971). Several factors probably favor the introital colonization by gram-negative aerobic intestinal flora. For instance, women resisting colonization possess vaginal antibodies against the fecal flora that are often lacking in women who become colonized (Stamey et al., 1978). Furthermore, vaginal cells from women with recurrent infections seem to attach to *E. coli* more readily than do the cells from women who resist infection (Fowler and Stamey, 1977), probably through a mannose-like receptor on the cell surface that binds to a mannose-specific substance on the surface of the bacterium (Ofek et al., 1977). This attachment may be prevented by specific competitive inhibition (Aronson et al., 1979).

Whereas the vaginal vestibule is the reservoir for UTI in girls and women, there is evidence that in *boys* the preputial sac and possibly the urethra may play this role (Hallet et al., 1976). In *men* bacterial prostatitis, obstruction, and infection of the kidney are the major causes of UTI.

The short urethra of women favors the ascent of bacteria into the bladder. However, the antibacterial properties of prostatic fluid may also account for the increased resistance to UTI observed in men (Stamey et al., 1968). Mild trauma to the female urethra such as urethral milking (Bran et al., 1972) or sexual intercourse (Buckley et al., 1978) has been shown to increase the probability of finding bacteria in the bladder in women.

Incomplete emptying of the bladder with each voiding (congenital abnormalities, urethral strictures, cystocele, bladder diverticula, prostatic hypertrophy, neurologic disorders) favors UTI because it impedes the clearance of infected urine from the bladder lumen. The frequency of infection of retained urine may be increased in patients whose urine promotes growth of bacteria through factors such as high pH and favorable osmolality (Lees and Osborne, 1979). Furthermore, anatomic abnormalities and retention of urine may interfere with the natural bactericidal properties of the bladder mucosa and with the efficiency of phagocytosis. For these reasons, it may be particularly dangerous to carry vaginal and urethral microorganisms into the bladder with an instrument or indwelling catheter in patients with residual urine.

Urinary antibodies to the infecting microorganisms most probably play a role in UTI. It has been observed that patients successfully treated for asymptomatic bacteriuria more often develop new symptomatic infections than do patients who have received no treatment at all (Asscher et al., 1969). This suggests that acquired antibodies might offer protection against the infecting strain and that treatment permits new virulent strains to infect the urinary tract. This observation is substantiated by the recent findings that specific urinary IgA antibodies prevent bacterial adherence to uroepithelial cells (Svanborg Edén and Svennerholm, 1978).

### Bacterial Virulence

Several factors seem to play a role in the virulence of the *E. coli* strains that cause UTI. In symptomatic bacteriuric patients, the strains isolated from the urine are not necessarily the same as those isolated from a random sample of the fecal flora (Lindin-Janson et al., 1977). There is an increase in frequency and quantity of the $K_1$ capsular antigen on *E. coli* organisms cultured from patients with pyelonephritis (Kaijser, 1973), an observation also made in neonatal *E. coli* meningitis (Robbins et al., 1974). The $K_1$ antigen appears to be related to increased tissue invasiveness (Schiffer et al., 1976) and increased resistance to opsonization (Bortolussi et al., 1978) and phagocytosis (Weinstein et al., 1978). Bacterial adherence to human uroepithelial cells is increased in *E. coli* isolated from symptomatic bacteriuric patients and can be correlated with the presence of pili on their cell surfaces (Svanborg Edén and Hanson, 1978). It has been demonstrated experimentally that in ascending pyelonephritis pili are an important virulence factor and that antipili antibodies can protect against kidney infection (Silverblatt, 1974; Silverblatt and Cohen, 1979).

### UTI in Patients with Indwelling Catheters

The risk of urinary infection in patients undergoing urethral catheterization is small in normal people but increases in hospitalized patients or in patients with urethrovesical abnormalities. In patients with long-term catheterization, infection is almost inevitable. Despite all attempts at sterility when the catheter is inserted, regular cleaning of the meatal-catheter junction, closed drainage systems for collecting the urines, and regular antibiotic irrigations, infection rates increase steadily with the length of time the catheter is in place (Warren et al., 1978). Urethral catheter-associated infections are the most common hospital-acquired infections, cause considerable illness, and can be fatal. The most practical way to minimize this important problem is to use indwelling catheters only when absolutely necessary. When mandatory, the most important aspect of infection prevention is scrupulous aseptic technique in handling the catheter.

### Ascent of Infection to the Renal Pelvis and Parenchyma

Once bladder urine has been infected, bacteria may ascend to reach the kidney. There is no evidence of a lymphatic route of kidney infection. Hematogenous kidney infection occurs with *S. aureus, S. faecalis,* salmonellae and brucellae, fungi, *Mycobacterium tuberculosis,* and viruses. There is also experimental evidence that during severe reflux, *E. coli* may enter the bloodstream through pyelovenous communications and then recirculate to the kidney, producing pyelonephritis (Fierer et al., 1971). However, most infections spread to the kidney by way of the ureter and many factors predispose to it. A normal *vesicoureteral* valve is probably an important mechanism of defense against ascending infection. In children with vesicoureteral reflux, infected urine may reach the kidney freely. Furthermore, infection may cause vesicoureteral valve reflux (Kaveggia et al., 1966). Reflux may not be necessary for bacteria to reach the renal pelvis because motile bacteria are able to ascend the ureter even against a descending flow (Braude, 1973).

Urinary tract obstruction occurring anywhere from the kidney to the urethral meatus predisposes not only to infection within the urinary tract but also to its spread to the renal parenchyma. Calculi produce obstruction and act as a locus of infection where bacteria are protected from host defenses or antibacterial agents. Infection with urease-producing bacteria, such as *Proteus* spp or *Klebsiella,* results in alkaline urine, which favors the production of magnesium ammonium-phosphate stones. Thus, calculi may either cause or result from urinary tract infections.

During pregnancy the incidence of UTI is not increased compared with nonpregnant women, but symptoms are more severe. The normal dilatation of the upper collecting system during pregnancy increases the likelihood that the infection will reach the kidney and produce the clinical syndrome of acute pyelonephritis (Norden and Kass, 1968).

### Significance of Renal Involvement in Uncomplicated Urinary Tract Infections

Many methods for detecting involvement of the kidneys during urinary tract infections have been developed. These include measures of renal function (e.g., decreased urinary concentrating ability), increased serum antibody levels to the infecting organism and increased leukocyte excretion (>20,000/ml) in the urine; culture of urine obtained by catheterization of the ureters; the bladder washout technique; and more recently, antibody coating of bacteria. The incidence of renal involvement during UTI varies depending on the patients selected and the technique used, but it is generally believed that between 30 and 50 per cent of uncomplicated cases of UTI involve the kidney (Stamey et al., 1965; Fairley et al., 1971; Thomas et al., 1974).

The crucial question is: *what is the significance of kidney involvement during urinary tract infections in the absence of obstruction or underlying kidney disease?* Since population studies show that between 2 and 10 per cent of females have bacteriuria, and that between 20 and 50 per cent of women will contract UTI at some time during their lives, it is evident that millions of people have kidney infections during their lifetime. If renal infection destroys kidney function, chronic pyelonephritis should be the leading cause of end-stage renal disease. Fortunately, this is not the case. Renal failure occurs in about 60 people per million population per year and is usually not of infectious origin. Among 173 dialysis candidates, Schechter and colleagues (1971) found that chronic pyelonephritis was the primary cause of end-stage renal failure in only 22 patients (13 per cent) and this condition was almost always associated with urinary tract abnormalities. Murray and Goldberg (1975) found that among 101 patients with end-stage interstitial nephritis, bacterial infection (present in 27 per cent) was found only in the presence of another preceding primary cause of renal damage. This epidemiologic evidence suggests that the bacteria reaching the kidney during uncomplicated UTI do not result in significant functional damage.

*Acute Nonobstructive Pyelonephritis.* This clinical symptom complex probably represents an acute infectious inflammatory episode occurring in the pelvis and/or the renal parenchyma. The evidence for parenchymal inflammation is the presence of white blood cell casts in the urine. However, very little is known about the pathologic features of this syndrome because the overwhelming majority of these patients recover and the kidneys are not examined histologically. Since multiple episodes of acute nonobstructive pyelonephritis do not seem to lead to kidney damage (Freedman and Andriole, 1974), the inflammation is probably not severe enough to cause irreversible necrosis.

*Acute Suppurative Pyelonephritis and Papillary Necrosis.* When kidney infection occurs in the presence of obstruction or renal disease such as chronic interstitial nephritis of various origins, susceptibility to renal damage increases considerably.

Much experimental as well as clinical evidence has shown that the papillae and the kidney medulla are especially susceptible to bacterial infection, particularly in the presence of obstruction (Freedman, 1979). Because antibacterial defenses are severely impaired in this hypertonic environment, the papillae and medulla have been called "an immunological desert" (Braude, 1973). Furthermore, the papilla and the medulla are susceptible to damage by analgesic drugs and probably to many other agents that are concentrated there during the process of excretion in the urine (chronic interstitial nephritis). The mechanism responsible for analgesic nephropathy seems to be mainly vascular insufficiency and secondary papillary and medullary ischemia (Freedman, 1979). When infection complicates obstruction or pre-existing papillary and medullary damage, it is so severe that the ensuing acute inflammation and suppuration cause permanent renal parenchymal damage (chronic pyelonephritis). *Papillary necrosis* may be precipitated and destroy a portion, if not all, of the kidney.

*UTI in Childhood: Vesicoureteral Reflux, Intrarenal Reflux, and Renal Scarring.* The greater part of progressive renal destruction due to infection probably occurs very early in life as a result of vesicoureteral reflux and infection. Most kidney scars develop before the age of 4 years. It has been clearly demonstrated that those radiographic lesions called "chronic atrophic pyelonephritis" or "atrophic pyelonephritic scars" are directly related to severe vesicoureteral reflux and intrarenal backflow of the urine (Hodson, 1969). In fact, the scars are most likely to develop at the very site where intrarenal reflux occurs (Rolleston et al., 1974). This clinical observation has been reproduced experimentally in piglets, in which intrarenal reflux has been shown to occur in those compound papillae whose papillary duct orifices cannot be occluded by a rise in the intracalyceal pressure (Ransley and Risdon, 1974). Recent experimental work suggests that the renal scars develop in relation to refluxing papillae only when the urine is infected (Ransley and Risdon, 1978). Because the scars occur very early in life and because reconstructive surgery in obstructive nephropathy should be performed before 1 year of age if renal function is to be preserved (Mayor et al., 1975), detecting reflux and infection in infancy may be a way of preventing chronic pyelonephritis. Recent prospective studies in girls have failed to show that persistent bacteriuria leads to scarring of the kidney if the kidneys were unscarred at the beginning of the follow-up period (Newcastle Asymptomatic Bacteriuria Research Group, 1975; Lindberg et al., 1978; Cardiff-Oxford Bacteriuria Study Group, 1978; Savage et al., 1978). However, in girls with pre-existing kidney scars, the Cardiff-Oxford Study (1978) showed that progression of the lesions occurred in approximately one-fourth of the subjects, and that most of these children had vesicoureteral reflux and persistent UTI or recurrent bacteriuria.

### The Pathogenesis of Chronic Pyelonephritis

Chronic pyelonephritis may develop after acute infection of the kidney in the presence of obstruction or interstitial nephritis. More often it is the result of vesicoureteral reflux and infection early in childhood.

Because chronic pyelonephritic kidneys are often sterile at autopsy, much experimental work has been performed in order to understand the pathogenesis of the disease. Mechanisms other than bacterial infection have been postulated. These include the persistence of bacterial protoplasts or of large amounts of bacterial antigens within the lesions and the existence of autoimmune mechanisms due to antigen-antibody complexes, altered renal tissue antigenicity, or antibodies cross-reacting with common antigens shared by the infecting bacteria and renal tissue. The evidence is not conclusive, however. Recently, animal observations have suggested that chronic pyelonephritis results from kidney damage, scarring, and shrinkage secondary to suppuration and necrosis during acute obstructive pyelonephritis. These experiments, which were performed in an animal model that mimics human chronic pyelonephritis because the disease developed in the presence of obstruction, showed that residual infection or autoimmune processes were not responsible for the development of the disease (Glauser et al., 1978).

## CLINICAL MANIFESTATIONS

The clinical manifestations of UTI are basically of two types: the symptoms of lower urinary tract infection (urethritis and cystitis) and the symptoms of upper urinary tract infection (acute nonobstructive pyelonephritis).

## Urethritis and Cystitis

Patients with *urethritis* complain of dysuria — that is, pain or burning during urination, as well as urgency and frequency. In women, these manifestations may also be due to vulvitis or vaginitis, both of which are usually accompanied by vaginal discharge. It has been suggested that when the complaint is of pain or burning felt to be inside the body ("internal" dysuria as opposed to "external" dysuria, in which pain or burning is felt to be in the labia) and when vaginal discharge is absent, there is a high probability that the cause is true urethritis due to UTI (Komaroff et al., 1978). Among women complaining of frequency and dysuria, between one-third and one-half do not have bacteriuria (Gallagher et al., 1965, Fairley et al., 1971). These patients are regarded as having the *urethral syndrome*. As already mentioned, fastidious anaerobic organisms from the vaginal flora may cause infection in some of these patients (Maskell et al., 1979; see Etiology).

*Cystitis* produces suprapubic pain, tenderness, and frequency due to diminished bladder capacity. Sometimes there may be hematuria. Urethrocystitis may be asymptomatic, or it may manifest itself, especially in older women, by malodorous urine or urinary incontinence. It is always difficult to be certain in the presence of cystitis symptoms that the infection is limited to the bladder, even in the absence of systemic symptoms such as fever. Their mere presence should alert the physician to possible renal infection and/or prostatitis or infection elsewhere in the body.

By far the most common cause of cystitis is the ascent of bacteria from the urethra in females. In males, it is almost always associated with prostatic or kidney infection. Rarely, cystitis may be due to urinary infections arising from contiguous infection from the bowel (diverticulitis, appendiceal abscess) or to viruses. Acute cystitis may occasionally develop without a demonstrable infectious agent, especially in men and boys (abacterial cystitis). Chronic cystitis may result if treatment of the acute phase has been insufficient or if incomplete voiding (residual urine) occurs. Chronic cystitis may be the manifestation of tuberculosis of the kidney and bladder, or it may be due to parasitic infections such as schistosomiasis or rarely, amebiasis or echinococcosis. Interstitial cystitis affects middle-aged women and is characterized by fibrosis of the bladder wall, thus decreasing the bladder capacity. Affected women present with a long history of progressive frequency and dysuria. Infection is rarely present, and an autoimmune process has been postulated in the pathogenesis of this disease. Hem-orrhagic cystitis may follow radiation therapy on the bladder area or cyclophosphamide treatment.

## Acute Nonobstructive Pyelonephritis ("Acute Pyelonephritis")

The syndrome of "acute pyelonephritis" is less frequently encountered as a manifestation of UTI than the symptoms of urethrocystitis. Acute pyelonephritis is predominantly a disease of young women. When it occurs in men, it is associated with a high incidence of obstruction (mainly prostatic hypertrophy), stones, or other urologic abnormalities (Kent and Braude). During pregnancy there is an increased likelihood of developing acute pyelonephritis from UTI.

The syndrome consists of flank pain, renal tenderness upon palpation, and fever and chills. It usually follows or is concomitant with symptoms of lower urinary tract infection. Nonspecific symptoms such as nausea, vomiting, diarrhea, or constipation may be diagnostically confusing. Furthermore, flank pain and renal tenderness may be absent, or there may be a pain in the right upper abdominal quadrant that simulates acute cholecystitis. The symptoms of acute pyelonephritis may disappear spontaneously. Therefore, improvement of clinical symptoms does not indicate successful treatment once it has been started; improvement must be confirmed by sterility of subsequent urine cultures.

Next to the presence of bacteriuria, the key finding in confirming the presence of infectious inflammation of the kidney is leukocyte casts in the urine. Acute pyelonephritis is also accompanied by leukocytosis, and sometimes the infecting microorganism is recovered from the blood. Bacteremia should always raise the possibility of the presence of obstruction (Kent and Braude).

The prognosis for recovery from an episode of acute nonobstructive pyelonephritis is very good, and most patients respond rapidly to treatment.

## COMPLICATIONS AND SEQUELAE

### Gram-Negative Bacteremia

UTI is the main port of entry into the bloodstream by gram-negative rods and may be responsible for gram-negative septic shock and death (see Chapter 177). Bacteremia is especially likely to occur during UTI in patients who have underlying urologic or renal abnormalities. This is also true for patients who undergo urologic procedures because the instrument has to be introduced through the heavily colonized urethra and, in men, through an infected prostatic region.

Metastatic infection secondary to urinary tract septicemia may localize in the skeleton, endocardium, or other parts of the body (Siroky et al., 1976).

### Kidney Damage

Severe kidney damage has been described after acute pyelonephritis. In most cases, this is probably due to papillary necrosis in patients who had unrecognized or mild diabetes mellitus (Davidson and Talner, 1978) or other factors predisposing to interstitial nephritis.

As already mentioned, kidney infection that is superimposed on chronic interstitial nephritis may cause *papillary necrosis*. The symptoms of acute infectious papillary necrosis are the same as those of acute pyelonephritis, except that the course may be much more severe and may lead either to acute renal insufficiency if the process is bilateral or to death from intractable infection. In rare instances, papillary necrosis may evolve silently in the presence of UTI and may be identified later on pyelography. This is particularly likely to occur in diabetic patients.

*End-stage chronic pyelonephritis,* resulting from single or multiple bouts of exudative and suppurative infectious episodes, probably occurs in approximately 10 individuals per 1,000,000 population per year. It is doubtful if it ever occurs without concomitant urinary tract abnormality or underlying renal disease, either of which predisposes to progressive kidney damage (Schechter et al., 1971; Murray and Goldberg, 1975).

### Renal and Perirenal Abscess, Emphysematous Pyelonephritis, and Xanthogranulomatous Pyelonephritis

Although renal and perirenal abscesses seem to have been caused in the past by the hematogenous spread of staphylococci (renal carbuncle), more recent series show that gram-negative rods predominate as the causative agents (Salvatierra et al., 1967; Thorley et al., 1974). A distinction has been proposed between the renal carbuncle, which is a blood-borne staphylococcal infection localized to the cortex of the kidney, and the gram-negative renal abscess, which originates in the renal medulla from urinary tract pathogens (Schiff et al., 1977). Most gram-negative bacterial *renal abscesses* are due to ascending UTI in association with obstruction, either in the kidney (renal calculi) or in the ureter. Less commonly, renal abscess is secondary to papillary necrosis, carcinoma, or infection of a renal cyst. Renal abscess may spread into the perinephric space, causing a *perinephric abscess*. Patients with renal and/or perirenal abscesses usually present with an insidious history of fever of two to three weeks' duration, flank and/or abdominal pain, leukocyto-

sis, and, most often, pyuria. The long duration of the symptoms seems to distinguish these patients from those with acute nonobstructive pyelonephritis (Thorley et al., 1974). Furthermore, patients with renal and/or perirenal abscesses usually have an abnormal intravenous pyelogram (IVP) with an intrarenal mass, an altered renal silhouette, or a bulge in the renal outline. Perirenal abscess usually produces an absence of motility of the affected kidney during deep inspiration and expiration (fixation of the kidney), a very useful sign that should always be looked for on IVP when abscesses are suspected. Ultrasound scans and computerized axial tomography may also be most helpful in this situation. It is likely that these newer, noninvasive diagnostic techniques will reveal that intrarenal or perirenal abscess is more common in the course of acute pyelonephritis (particularly in the presence of obstruction) than was previously appreciated.

In diabetic patients, renal and perirenal suppuration and necrosis may be accompanied by the production of gas and may cause *emphysematous pyelonephritis* (Carris and Schmidt, 1977). This rare clinical picture is probably due to the bacterial fermentation of glucose by *E. coli* or other gram-negative enteric rods.

In some instances, mostly when obstruction is present, chronic renal infection and suppuration may evolve into *xanthogranulomatous pyelonephritis* (Malek and Elder, 1978; Goodman et al., 1979). In this process, lipid-laden macrophages and epithelioid cells are found in the kidney and surrounding tissues. It occurs most frequently in middle-aged women, who present with nonspecific symptoms such as malaise and fatigue, fever and chills, flank pain, and recurrent episodes of UTI. In most cases there is pyuria, and IVP discloses an enlarged, nonfunctionig kidney, very often with calculi in the pelvis or ureter. The process is usually unilateral and may be localized to a part of the kidney, simulating a tumor. Cure is achieved by nephrectomy.

## DIAGNOSIS

### Collection of the Specimen

The diagnosis of UTI can be made only by finding bacteria in the urine. Because voided bladder urine may be contaminated by the resident microbiota of the urethra and vagina, urine collection must be performed with great care. In men, the glans penis must be cleaned with soap, water, and dried with sterile sponges. In women, while the labia are spread apart, careful washing of the urethral meatus must be performed from front to back with sponges soaked with soap. Disinfectants should not be used for cleaning because they may artifically lower the bacterial count if they get into the urine sample. A specimen of "midstream" urine is then collected during forceful urination after the first 10 to 20 ml of urine have been voided ("urethral specimen"). When collaboration from the patient cannot be obtained, catheterization or suprapubic aspiration may be necessary. The latter technique is safe and requires only a full bladder. After skin disinfection, a needle 10 to 12 cm long with a 0.9-mm diameter (3.5-inch, 20-gauge needle) affixed to a 20-ml syringe is inserted through the skin at the midline, about one-third of the distance from the symphysis pubis to the umbilicus, and directed toward the coccyx. Normal bladder urine is sterile, and microorganisms cultured from urine taken directly from the bladder should not be discarded as contaminants, even if present in low concentration. It is possible, however, that urine obtained by suprapubic aspiration may be contaminated by reversal of flow of urine which has already entered the urethra.

Because urine is a medium in which bacteria grow readily, urine specimens that cannot be examined within one hour after collection should be kept refrigerated before being processed. If this is not possible, the specimen must be discarded and another sample collected.

### Quantitative Cultures

Quantitative cultures of urine have been proposed to distinguish between urinary contaminants and organisms actually infecting the bladder, ureters, or kidneys. *Bacterial contamination* from the external genitalia usually results in less than $10^4$ bacteria/ml of urine, provided the specimen has been properly collected and transported. However, it is not uncommon for even $10^5$ bacteria/ml to be found in voided urine as a result of contamination. Two or more types of bacteria often indicate contamination. Bacterial counts of 100,000 ($10^5$) or more per milliliter of clean-voided urine are usually found in true infections (significant bacteriuria). This large number of bacteria is partly due to bacterial multiplication in the bladder urine between urination. Samples from the ureters, from the renal pelvis, or from renal urine may have many fewer bacteria and yet indicate infection. Furthermore, lower bacterial counts may be found in patients who are undergoing diuresis, have indwelling catheters or ileal conduits, or receive inadequate or insufficient antibacterial drugs. Therefore, any degree of bacteriuria should be evaluated in a patient with urinary tract symptoms. The first morning specimen, which should be examined whenever possible, may give more clear-cut results because it gives bacteria the opportunity to grow overnight in the bladder urine. In patients who have *symptomatic* UTI, one specimen containing $10^5$ or more organisms is probably sufficient to establish the diagnosis. In *asymptomatic* females, one specimen of properly collected urine showing $10^5$ bacteria makes a diagnosis of UTI 80 per cent likely; if two consecutive samples contain the same microorganism in concentrations of at least $10^5$, there is a 95 per cent chance that true infection exists (Kass, 1957). In asymptomatic males, $10^5$ bacteria recovered from a single clean-voided specimen of urine can be considered diagnostic of true UTI (Gleckman et al., 1979).

Quantitative cultures of urine are made by culturing a known amount of urine on a solid medium. The most precise way to do this is probably the pour-plate technique. Quantitative loop plating is a simpler way of culturing urine. However, much experience has been gained in recent years with the dip-slide method, which may allow the nurse to inoculate the urine directly at the bedside. This can also be done at home by cooperative and reliable patients. These plastic slides coated with culture media are sold commercially and have made routine quantitative cultures of urine available in almost every doctor's office.

### Microscopic Examination

Microscopic examination of uncentrifuged urine is a fast and useful test for urinary infection. The fresh urine may be looked at without staining (Barbin et al., 1978), but Gram stain of a drop of urine may also be performed. When the bacteria count is around $10^5$ or more, at least one bacterium per high-power field ($\times$ 1000) is likely to be seen. On the other hand, specimens containing less than $10^4$ organisms usually do not show organisms in several fields. Thus, the microscopic examination of the urine provides rapid and inexpensive clues to the diagnosis of UTI. Pyuria (i.e., leukocytes in the urine) may also be found by microscopic examination of urine, but leukocytes in the urine do not mean that UTI is present. Vaginal infection, prostatitis, urethritis, urinary stones, renal tuberculosis, glomerulitis, interstitial nephritis, and other diseases may produce white blood cells in the urine. However, in most symptomatic cases, both leukocytes and bacteria can be observed on microscopic examination (Fairley et al., 1971; Robins, 1975). Sterile urine samples with pyuria should be cultured for mycobacteria.

Red blood cells in the urine may result from UTI or other causes of inflammation, but red cell casts suggest glomerulitis.

Microscopic examination may also reveal numerous squamous epithelial cells of vaginal origin, indicating improper collection of the specimen and contamination. Squamous epithelial cells may also originate from the trigone; normally, this portion of the bladder is covered by a transitional epithelium, but inflammatory changes may cause squamous metaplasia there, particularly in postmenopausal women. Urinary squamous cells may therefore originate from the bladder urine.

### Radiologic Evaluation

The radiologic findings in infants and children with UTI and reflux is beyond the scope of this chapter (for review, see Ransley and Risdon, 1978). In women, an IVP should be performed only after repeated episodes of urinary infection that may be due to urinary tract abnormalities or stones. However, the vast majority of women with recurrent UTI do not present abnormalities (Fair et al., 1979). In men, on the other hand, because urinary tract infections are relatively rare, one may consider carrying out IVP after the first infectious episode, mainly to detect obstruction.

During acute nonobstructive pyelonephritis, the intravenous urogram is normal in most patients (Little et al., 1965). When involvement is particularly severe, however, there may be enlargement of the kidney as well as a generalized or focal decrease in the nephrographic density, reflecting the patchy distribution of the pyelonephritic process. The ureter and pelvis often show dilatation that may mimic the signs of obstruction. This is due to the absence of peristalsis secondary to infection with gram-negative bacilli (Harrison and Schaffer, 1979).

It seems reasonable to perform an intravenous urogram in patients presenting with symptoms of acute pyelonephritis that do not respond promptly to proper antibiotic treatment in order to rule out obstruction. Obstruction in the presence of acute pyelonephritis must be relieved.

The distinction between localized pyelonephritis and an abscess may be difficult from the radiologic standpoint. Evolution toward perirenal abscess may be indicated by disappearance of the renal outline and by fixation of the kidney (see Complications and Sequelae). Ultrasound examination and computerized axial tomography may be very helpful in this situation to demonstrate the presence of pus in or around the kidney. The presence of gas indicates emphysematous pyelonephritis.

In the rare patient who presents late radiologic sequelae of acute nonobstructive pyelonephritis, wasting of the kidney parenchyma develops a few weeks after the acute episode, with deformities of the papillae and calyces (Davidson and Talner, 1978). This suggests that papillary necrosis may accompany the most severe forms of acute pyelonephritis.

## TREATMENT

### Asymptomatic Urinary Tract Infections

As already suggested in the *Pathogenesis* section, there is no real evidence of a need to treat asymptomatic urinary tract infections in nonpregnant women.

On the other hand, asymptomatic UTI in preschool children with vesicoureteral reflux should be considered for treatment because some of these children are likely to develop kidney scarring and possibly renal failure. Similarly, patients with known urinary tract obstruction or underlying renal disease should be treated in order to prevent severe renal infection. Eradication of asymptomatic bacteriuria in a pregnant woman is mandatory because it will prevent the development of acute pyelonephritis.

### Symptomatic Urinary Infections

In symptomatic patients with infection, most antibacterial drugs that reach adequate urinary concentrations will clear the infection. The real questions — and the subject of controversy — are what dosage and for how long.

In an experimental in vitro model simulating bladder conditions with periodic dilution and discharge, it has been shown that a heavy bacterial population is suppressed when it is exposed to a single dose of many antibacterial drugs (Greenwood and O'Grady, 1977). This experimental observation correlates with the clinical efficacy of a single-dose treatment in patients with urinary infections localized to the bladder (Ronald et al., 1976; Bailey and Abbott, 1977; Fang et al., 1978; Bailey and Abbot, 1978; Källenius and Winberg, 1979; Greenwood et al., 1980).

However, in patients with infection localized to the kidney, early *relapse* (i.e., recurrent infection with the same microorganism) frequently seems to occur after single-dose treatment (Ronald et al. 1976). Even conventional therapy may not prevent relapsing infection in half of the patients treated for ten days (Fang et al., 1978). Nevertheless, since renal involvement during uncomplicated UTI is not an immediate threat to the patient, one can reasonably consider that single-dose treatment is appropriate as initial therapy. If relapse does occur (usually during the days or first weeks following treatment), a more prolonged course of therapy should probably be undertaken such as 10 to 15 days. In fact, there are suggestions that a 6 weeks course of antimicrobial therapy might be more efficient in eradicating relapsing infections than a conventional 10–15 days treatment. This has been shown in women with infection originating from the upper urinary tract (Turck, 1978), in renal transplant patients with UTI (Rubin 1979) and in men with recurrent UTI (Gleckman 1979).

In addition to infectious renal involvement, relapse may also be due to persistent infection within a renal stone, to prostatic hypertrophy, or to infection (chronic bacterial prostatitis). It has been suggested that in some selected patients, a relapse after single-dose therapy may be an indication for radiological urinary tract investigation, since abnormal pyelograms are seen more frequently in relapsing patients treated with single-dose therapy (Fang et al., 1978; Fairley et al., 1978). However, the inconvenience of radiologic investigations as well as their possible side effects and cost should be weighed against the good prognosis of UTI in the long term.

Neither single-dose treatment nor the longer, more conventional treatment will prevent *reinfection* by new microorganisms. In women, reinfection is much more common than relapse. It usually occurs within one month of stopping treatment and increases in frequency with the passage of time.

The next important step after initiating therapy is to monitor its efficacy. Urine cultures performed 24 to 48 hours after starting treatment or at the end of therapy should be sterile. The persistence of microorganisms may represent inadequate drug dosage or, more likely, resistance to the drug.

### Acute Pyelonephritis Syndrome, UTI in the Presence of Obstruction, and Renal Abscess

Acute pyelonephritis should be treated with drugs in dosages large enough to reach adequate concentrations in the renal parenchyma. There are several reasons why this attitude is justified. First, many patients are severely ill and when they are first seen, it is not known whether or not they have obstruction, deformity, or underlying renal disease that may precipitate bacteremia, renal abscess, or papillary necrosis. Experimentally, it has been shown that in acute suppurative pyelonephritis due to obstruction, the sooner treatment is initiated, the greater the protection against renal parenchymal destruction (Glauser et al., 1978). Furthermore, a combination of antibiotics that is synergistic in vitro against the infecting organism, such as beta-lactam antibiotic with an aminoglycoside, has been experimentally shown in vivo to achieve sterility faster and more reliably than either drug alone (Glauser et al., 1979a). Since sterility must be achieved in order to prevent relapse in the presence of obstruction, a combination of synergistic antibiotics should be used whenever possible. In addition to surgical drainage, the same therapeutic considerations apply to the treatment of gram-negative

renal and perirenal abscesses. Renal carbuncles (see Complications and Sequelae) have been successfully treated without drainage with long-term penicillinase-resistant penicillins (Schiff et al., 1977)

### Choice of Drug

Most symptomatic patients with UTI can be treated with orally administered drugs such as a sulfonamide, a combination of sulfonamide and trimethoprim, ampicillin, or amoxycillin, or nitrofurantoin (see Table 1). After microscopic examination has demonstrated the presence of bacteria and leukocytes that make a diagnosis of UTI likely, a dip-slide quantitative culture should be performed. Treatment then can be started without awaiting culture results.

Improvement of clinical symptoms does not correlate with successful treatment, since improvement frequently occurs in the absence of any treatment or in patients who receive ineffective treatment. If the culture performed 24 to 48 hours after starting therapy on ambulatory patients is sterile, the specimen cultured before treatment can be discarded without further identification or antibiotic sensitivity tests. On the other hand, if there is any doubt about the efficacy of treatment, the choice of drug should be adjusted according to sensitivity tests performed from the initial culture.

Patients with acute pyelonephritis should be treated with drugs that achieve serum and tissue bactericidal activity. Ampicillin or amoxycillin is the drug of choice. A cephalosporin agent may be necessary in some instances, depending upon the sensitivity tests. A synergistic combination of a beta-lactam antibiotic with an aminoglycoside may be indicated if suppuration is suspected, especially in the presence of obstruction.

Specific treatment schedules are given in Table 1.

## PROPHYLAXIS

Some patients are so disturbed or incapacitated by recurrent symptomatic episodes of UTI that prolonged therapy or prophylaxis may be necessary. Careful history-taking will often reveal that these symptomatic episodes are related to recent sexual activity. One dose of almost any oral antimicrobial, taken just after sexual intercourse, will help to prevent these episodes (Vosti et al., 1975).

Long-term prophylactic use of low-dose antimicrobial drugs has been shown to reduce the frequency of recurrent symptomatic UTI in children, women, and men. Before such prophylaxis is started, however, sterilization of the urine should be achieved with an appropriate antimicrobial

**TABLE 1.  Treatment of Urinary Tract Infection**

| INFECTION | TREATMENT OF CHOICE | ALTERNATE |
|---|---|---|
| Urethritis or cystitis symptoms, gram-negative bacteria seen on microscope examination, but microorganism not yet identified. | Sulfisoxazole 1.0 g two to four times daily for 5 to 8 days | Amoxycillin (or ampicillin) 250 mg, three to four times daily for 5 to 8 days or amoxycillin 3 g as a single dose or trimethoprim 160 mg and sulfamethoxasole 800 mg for 5 to 8 days or nitrofurantoin 100 mg two to four times daily for 5 to 8 days |
| Urethritis or cystitis symptoms, microorganism identified. | *E. coli*<br>as above<br>*P. mirabilis*[1]<br>Amoxycillin (or ampicillin) 250 mg three to four times daily for 5 to 8 days | As above<br><br>Trimethoprim 160 mg and sulfamethoxazole 800 mg twice daily for 5 to 8 days or cephalexin 250 mg daily four times daily for 5 to 8 days |
| | *K. pneumoniae*[1]<br>Trimethoprim 160 mg and sulfa-methoxazole 800 mg twice daily for 5 to 8 days | Cephalexin 250 mg three to four times daily for 5 to 8 days |
| | *P. aeruginosa*,[1] *E. aerogenes*,[1] *P. vulgaris*[1]<br>Indanyl carbenicillin 1.0 g or tetracycline 250 mg, four times daily for 5 to 8 days | Gentamicin or tobramycin 40 mg I.M. twice daily for 5 to 8 days |
| | *S. fecalis*<br>Amoxycillin (or ampicillin) 250 mg three to four times daily for 5 to 8 days | Tetracycline[2] 250 mg orally four times daily for 5 to 8 days |
| Pyelonephritis, organism not known. | Amoxycillin (or ampicillin) 500 mg to 2.0 g four times daily I.V. (consider adding I.V. gentamicin or tobramycin 1.0 to 1.5 mg/kg three times daily) until evident clinical improvement.<br>Follow with amoxycillin (or ampicillin) 500 mg four times daily, for a total duration treatment of 14 days | Amoxycillin or ampicillin 500 mg to 1.0 gm orally four times daily for 10 to 14 days or trimethoprim 160 mg and sulfamethoxazole 800 mg orally twice daily or cefalothin 1 to 2 g I.V. four times daily, or cefamandole or cefoxitin 1 g I.V. four times daily, until evident clinical improvement.<br>Follow with oral drug according to susceptibility testing |
| Pyelonephritis, microorganism identified. | *E. coli*<br>As above<br>*P. mirabilis*[1]<br>As above | As above<br><br>As above<br>or cephalexin 500 mg four times daily for 14 days |
| | *K. pneumoniae*[1]<br>Cefalothin 1 to 2 g, or cefamandole or cefoxitin 1 g I.V. four times daily (consider adding gentamicin or tobramycin 1.0 to 1.5 mg/kg three times times daily) until evident clinical improvement.<br>Follow with cephalexin 500 mg to 1.0 g four times daily or trimethoprim 160 mg and sulfamethoxazole 800 mg twice daily for a total duration treatment of 14 days | Cephalexin 500 mg 4 times daily or trimethoprim 160 mg and sulfamethoxazole 800 mg orally twice daily for 14 days |
| | *P. aeruginosa*,[1] *P. vulgaris*,[1] *E. aerogenes*[1]<br>Ticarcillin 5.0 g (or carbenicillin 10 gm) I.V. three times daily (consider adding gentamicin[3] or tobramycin[3] 1.0 to 1.5 mg/kg three times daily) for 14 days | Amikacin 7.5 mg/kg I.M. or I.V. twice daily for 14 days or sodium colistimethate 40 mg I.M. three times daily for 14 days or tetracycline[2] 500 mg orally four times daily plus sodium colistimethate 40 mg I.M. three times daily for 14 days. |
| | *S. fecalis*<br>Amoxycillin (or ampicillin) 500 mg to 2.0 g I.V. four times daily plus gentamicin or tobramycin 1.0 to 1.5 mg/kg three times daily for 14 days | Vancomycin 1.0 g I.V. twice daily for 14 days or vancomycin 1.0 g I.V. twice daily plus gentamicin or tobramycin 1.0 to 1.5 mg/kg three times daily for 14 days |
| | *B. suis*<br>Tetracycline[2] 500 mg orally four times daily plus streptomycin 1.0 g I.M. daily, for two to four weeks | Tetracycline[2] 500 mg orally four times daily for two to four days or trimethoprim 160 mg and sulfamethoxazole 800 mg twice daily orally for 2 to 4 weeks |

**TABLE 1.  Treatment of Urinary Tract Infection** (Continued)

| INFECTION | TREATMENT OF CHOICE | ALTERNATE |
|---|---|---|
| *C. albicans* | Amphotericin B 20 to 50 mg I.V. every other day | Amphotericin B 20 to 30 mg I.V. every other day plus 5-fluorocytosine 30 to 40 mg/kg orally three to four times daily |
| *M. tuberculosis* | Isoniazid 300 mg orally, plus ethambutol 1.0 g orally daily | Isoniazid 300 mg orally plus ethambutol 1.0 g orally plus rifampin 600 mg orally daily or streptomycin 1.0 g I.M. daily plus para-aminosalicylic acid 2.0 g orally every 6 hours |

1. Because of inconstant sensitivity to antibiotics, susceptibility testing should be performed.
2. Tetracycline should be avoided in pregnant women, infants, and young children.
3. Gentamicin, tobramycin, and amikacin should *not* be mixed with ticarcillin or carbenicillin in the same solution. They must be injected separately.

drug. Half a tablet of a combination of sulfamethoxazole-trimethoprim (200 mg and 20 mg, respectively), taken at bedtime (so that antibacterial activity will be maintained in the urine during the night) seems to be the best available drug, probably because it inhibits the enterobacteriaceae in the fecal flora and because trimethoprim concentrates in the vaginal secretions and prevents colonization of the periurethral area (Harding and Ronald, 1974; Stamey et al., 1977). In fact, half a tablet at bedtime three times a week seems to be just as effective as every day (Harding et al., 1979). Nitrofurantoin, 50 mg nightly, is also used with success but, at least in men, has not been shown to be as effective as the sulfamethoxazole-trimethoprim combination (Scherwin and Holm, 1977). Similarly, a sulfonamide agent alone or methenamine-mandelate with acidification of the urine is probably less effective (Harding and Ronald, 1974; Vainrub and Muscher, 1977).

Because they accumulate and persist in the kidney parenchyma, from which they are slowly excreted, aminoglycoside antibiotics are promising prophylactic drugs. When used in low doses, they have been shown experimentally to prevent UTI and pyelonephritis, even in the presence of obstruction (Glauser et al., 1979b).

## CONCLUSION

UTI occurs predominantly in females. Except in very young children with vesicourethral reflux, in pregnant women, and in the presence of obstruction or underlying renal disease, it is a self-limiting disease, which most probably does not endanger the patient in the long range. Many possible drugs are available for treatment, but their cost and possible side effects should be weighed against the mildness of the disease. Very effective prophylaxis exists for patients with frequent recurrent symptomatic UTI.

# References

Aronson, M., Medaliz, O., Schori, L. Mirelman, D., Sharon, N., and Ofek, I.: Prevention of colonization of the urinary tract of mice with *Escherichia coli* by blocking of bacterial adherence with methyl α-D-mannopyranoside. J Infect Dis 139:329, 1979.

Asscher, A. W., Sussman, M., Waters, W. E., Evans, J. A. S., Campbell, H., Evans, K. T., and Williams, J. E.: Asymptomatic significant bacteriuria in the non-pregnant woman. II. Response to treatment and follow-up. Br Med J 1:804, 1969.

Bailey, R. R., and Abbott, G. D.: Treatment of urinary tract infection with a single dose of amoxycillin. Nephron 18:316, 1977.

Bailey, R. R., and Abbot, G. D.: Treatment of urinary tract infection with a single dose of trimethoprim-sulfamethoxazole. Can Med Assoc J 118:551, 1978.

Barbin, G. K., Thorley, J. D., and Reinerz, J. A.: Simplified microscopy for rapid detection of significant bacteriuria in random urine specimens. J Clin Microbiol 7:286, 1978.

Bergstrom, T., Larsson, H., Lincoln, K., and Winberg, J.: Studies of urinary tract infections in infancy and childhood. XII. Eighty consecutive patients with neonatal infection. J Pediat 80:858, 1972.

Bortolussi, R., Low, R., Ferrieri, P., and Quie, P. G.: K₁ capsular antigen production in *E. coli* and relationship to opsonization. Proceedings of the 18th Interscience Conference on Antimicrobial Agents and Chemotherapy, Atlanta 1978, abstract 505.

Bran, J. L., Levison, M. E., and Kaye, D.: Entrance of bacteria into the female urinary bladder. N Engl J Med 286:626, 1972.

Braude, A. I.: Current concepts of pyelonephritis. Medicine 52:257, 1973.

Buckley, R. M., McGuckin, M., and MacGregor, R. R.: Urine bacterial counts after sexual intercourse. N Engl J Med 298:321, 1978.

Cardiff-Oxford Bacteriuria Study Group: Sequelae of covert bacteriuria in school girls. A four-year follow-up study. Lancet 1:889, 1978.

Carris, C. K., and Schmidt, J. D.: Emphysematous pyelonephritis. J Urol 118:457, 1977.

Davidson, A. J., and Talner, L. B.: Late sequelae of adult-onset acute bacterial nephritis. Radiology 127:367, 1978.

Fair, W. R., McClennan, B. L., and Gilbert Jost, R.: Are excretory urograms necessary in evaluating women with urinary tract infection? J Urol 121:313, 1979.

Fairley, K. F., Carson, N. E., Gutch, R. C., Leighton, P., Grounds, A. D., Laird, E. C., McCallum, P. H. G., Sleeman, R. L., and O'Keefe, C. M.: Site of infection in acute urinary-tract infection in general practice. Lancet 2:615, 1971.

Fairley, K. F., Whitworth, J. A., Kincaid-Smith, P., and Durman, O.: Single-dose therapy in management of urinary tract infection. Med J Aust 2:75, 1978.

Fang, L. S. T., Tolkoff-Rubin, N. E., and Rubin, R. H.: Efficacy of single-dose and conventional amoxicillin therapy in urinary-tract infection localized by the antibody-coated bacteria technic. N Engl J Med 298:413, 1978.

Fierer, J., Talner, L., and Braude, A. I.: Bacteremia in the pathogenesis of retrograde *E. coli* pyelonephritis in the rat. Am J Pathol 64:443, 1971.

Fowler, J. E., and Stamey, T. A.: Studies on introital colonization in women with recurrent urinary infections. VII. The role of bacterial adherence. J Urol 117:472, 1977.

Freedman, L. R., Phair, J. P., Seki, M., Hamilton, H. B., and Nefzger, M. D.: The epidemiology of urinary tract infections in Hiroshima. Yale J Biol Med 37:262, 1965.

Freedman, L. R.: Interstitial renal inflammation, including pyelonephritis and urinary tract infection. In Earley, L. E., and Gottschalk, C. W. (eds.): Strauss and Welt's Diseases of the Kidney. Boston, Little, Brown & Company, 1979, p. 817.

Freedman, L. R., and Andriole, V.: The long-term follow-up of women with urinary tract infections. Villareal, H. (ed.): Proceedings of the 5th International Congress of Nephrology, Mexico 1972, vol. 3. Basel, S. Karger, 1974, p. 230.

Gallagher, D. J. A., Montgomerie, J. Z., and North, J. D. K.: Acute infections of the urinary tract and the urethral syndrome in general practice. Br Med J 1:622, 1965.

Glauser, M. P., Lyons, J. M., and Braude, A. I.: Prevention of chronic experimental pyelonephritis by suppression of acute suppuration. J Clin Invest 61:403, 1978.

Glauser, M. P., Lyons, J. M., and Braude, A. I.: Synergism of ampicillin and gentamicin against obstructive pyelonephritis due to *Escherichia coli* in rats. J Infect Dis 139:133, 1979a.

Glauser, M. P., Lyons, J. M., and Braude, A. I.: Prevention of pyelonephritis due to *Escherichia coli* in rats with gentamicin stored in the kidney. J Infect Dis 139:172, 1979b.

Gleckman, R., Crowley, M., and Natsios, G. A.: Therapy of recurrent invasive urinary-tract infections of men. N Engl J Med 301:878, 1979.

Gleckman, R., Esposito, A., Crowley, M., and Natsios, G. A.: Reliability of a single urine culture in establishing diagnosis of asymptomatic bacteriuria in adult males. J Clin Microbiol 9:596, 1979.

Goodman, M., Curry, T., and Russel, T.: Xanthogranulomatous pyelonephritis: A local disease with systemic manifestations. Report of 23 patients and review of the literature. Medicine 58:171, 1979.

Greenwood, D., and O'Grady, F.: Is your dosage really necessary? Antibiotic dosage in urinary infection. Br Med J 2:665, 1977.

Greenwood, D., Kawada, Y., and O'Grady, F.: Treatment of acute bacterial cystitis: economy versus efficacy (letter). Lancet 1:197, 1980.

Hallett, R. J., Pead, L., and Maskell, R.: Urinary infection in boys. A three-year prospective study. Lancet 2:1107, 1976.

Harding, G. K. M., and Ronald, A. R.: A controlled study of antimicrobial prophylaxis of recurrent urinary infection in women. N Engl J Med 291:597, 1974.

Harding, G. K. M., Buckwold, F. J., Marrie, T. J., Thompson, L., Light, R. B., and Ronald, A. R.: Prophylaxis of recurrent urinary tract infection in female patients: Efficacy of low-dose, thrice-weekly therapy with trimethoprim-sulfamethoxazole. JAMA 242:1975, 1979.

Harrison, R. B., and Schaffer, H. A.: The roentgenographic findings in acute pyelonephritis. JAMA 241:1718, 1979.

Hathout, S., Ghaffar, Y., Awny, A., and Hassan, K.: Relation between urinary schistosomiasis and chronic enteric carrier state among Egyptians. Am J Trop Med 15:156, 1966.

Hodson, C. J.: The effects of disturbance of flow on the kidney. J Infect Dis 120:54, 1969.

Kaijser, B.: Immunology of *Escherichia coli*: K antigen and its relation to urinary-tract infection. J Infect Dis 127:670, 1973.

Källenius, G., and Winberg, J.: Urinary tract infections treated with single dose of short-acting sulphonamide. Br Med J 1:1175, 1979.

Kass, E. H.: Bacteriuria and diagnosis of infections of the urinary tract. Arch Intern Med 100:709, 1957.

Kaveggia, L., King, L. R., Grana, L., and Idriss, F. S.: Pyelonephritis: A cause of vesicoureteral reflux? J Urol 95:158, 1966.

Kent, R. S., and Braude, A. I.: Unpublished observation.

Komaroff, A. L., Pass, T. M., McCue, J. D., Cohen, A. B., Hendricks, T. M., and Friedland, G.: Management strategies for urinary and vaginal infections. Arch Intern Med 138:1069, 1978.

Kunin, C. M., Deutscher, R., and Paquin, A., Jr.: Urinary tract infection in school children: an epidemiologic, clinical and laboratory study. Medicine 43:91, 1964.

Laughlin, L. W., Farid, Z., Mansour, N., Edman, D. C., and Higashi, G. I.: Bacteriuria in urinary schistosomiasis in Egypt. Am J Trop Med 27:916, 1978.

Lees, G. E., and Osborne, C. A.: Antibacterial properties of urine: A comparative review. J Am Anim Hosp Assoc 15:125, 1979.

Lindin-Janson, G., Hanson, L. A., Kaijser, B., Lincoln, K., Lindberg, U., Olling, S., and Wedel, H.: Comparison of *Escherichia coli* from bacteriuric patients with those from feces of healthy school children. J Infect Dis 136:346, 1977.

Lindberg, U., Claesson, I., Hanson, L. A., and Jodal, U.: Asymptomatic bacteriuria in school girls. VIII. Clinical course during a three-year follow-up. J Pediat 92:194, 1978.

Little, P. J., McPherson, D. R., and de Wardener, H. E.: The appearance of the intravenous pyelogram during and after acute pyelonephritis. Lancet 1:1186, 1965.

Louria, D. B., Stiff, D. P., and Bennet, B.: Disseminated moniliasis in adults. Medicine 41:307, 1962.

Malek, R. S., and Elder, J. S.: Xanthogranulomatous pyelonephritis: A critical analysis of 26 cases and review of the literature. J Urol 119:589, 1978.

Marrie, T. J., Harding, G. K. M., and Ronald, A. R.: Anaerobic and aerobic urethral flora in healthy females. J Clin Microbiol 8:67, 1978.

Maskell, R.: Importance of coagulase-negative staphylococci as pathogens in the urinary tract. Lancet 1:1155, 1974.

Maskell, R., Pead, L., and Allen, J.: The puzzle of "urethral syndrome": a possible answer? Lancet 1:1058, 1979.

Mayor, G., Genton, N., Torrado, A., and Guignard, J. P.: Renal function in obstructive nephropathy: long-term effect of reconstructive surgery. Pediatrics 56:740, 1975.

Miall, W. E., Kass, E. H., Ling, J., and Stuart, K. L.: Factors influencing arterial pressure in the general population in Jamaica. Br Med J 2:497, 1962.

Murray, T., and Goldberg, M.: Chronic interstitial nephritis: Etiologic factors. Ann Intern Med 82:453, 1975.

Newcastle Asymptomatic Bacteriuria Research Group: Asymptomatic bacteriuria in school children in Newcastle upon Tyne. Arch Dis Childh 50:90, 1975.

Norden, C. W., and Kass, E. H.: Bacteriuria of pregnancy — a critical appraisal. Annu Rev Med 19:431, 1968.

Numazaki, Y., Kumasaka, T., Yano, N., Yamanaka, M., Miyazawa, T., Takai, S., and Ishida, N.: Further study on acute hemorrhagic cystitis due to adenovirus type 11. N Engl J Med 289:344, 1973.

Ofek, I., Mirelman, D., and Sharon, N.: Adherence of *Escherichia coli* to human mucosal cells mediated by mannose receptors. Nature 265:623, 1977.

Ransley, P. G., and Risdon, R. A.: Renal papillae and intrarenal reflux in the pig. Lancet 2:1114, 1974.

Ransley, P. G., and Risdon, R. A.: Reflux and renal scarring. Br J Radiol Suppl 14, 1978.

Robbins, J. B., McCracken, G. H., Gotschlich, E. C., Ørskov, F., Ørskov, I., and Hanson, L. A.: *Escherichia coli* $K_1$ capsular polysaccharide associated with neonatal meningitis. N Engl J Med 290, 1216, 1974.

Robins, D. G., Rogers, K. B., White, R. H. R., and Osman, M. S.: Urine microscopy as an aid to detection of bacteriuria. Lancet 1:476, 1975.

Rolleston, G. L., Maling, T. M. J., and Hodson, C. J.: Intrarenal reflux and the scarred kidney. Arch Dis Childh 49:531, 1974.

Ronald, A. R., Boutros, P., and Mourtada, H.: Bacteriuria localization and response to single-dose therapy in women. JAMA 235:1854, 1976.

Rubin, R. H., Fang, L. S. T., Cosimi, A. B., Herrin, J. I., Varga, P. A., Russel, P. S. and Tolkoff-Rubin, N. E.: Usefulness of the antibody coated bacteria assay in the management of urinary tract infection in the renal transplant patient. Transplantation 27:18, 1979.

Salvatierra, O., Buckley, W. B., and Morrow, J. W.: Perinephric abscess: a report of 71 cases. J Urol 98:296, 1967.

Savage, D. C. L., Adler, K., Howie, G., and Wilson, M. I.: Controlled trial of therapy in covert bacteriuria of childhood. Lancet 1:358, 1978.

Schechter, H., Leonard, C. D., and Scribner, B. H.: Chronic pyelonephritis as a cause of renal failure in dialysis candidates. JAMA 216:514, 1971.

Scherwin, J., and Holm, P.: Long-term treatment with sulfamethoxazole-trimethoprim (Bactrim) and nitrofurantoin in chronic urinary tract infections. A controlled clinical trial. Chemotherapy 23:282, 1977.

Schiff, M., Glickman, M., Weiss, R. M., Ahern, M. J., Touloukian, R. J., Lytton, B., and Andriole, V. T.: Antibiotic treatment of renal carbuncle. Ann Intern Med 87:305, 1977.

Schiffer, M. S., Oliveira, E., Glade, M. P., McCracken, G. H., Sarff, L. M., and Robbins, J. B.: A review: Relation between invasiveness and the $K_1$ capsular polysaccharide of *Escherichia coli*. Pediat Res 10:82, 1976.

Segura, J. W., Kelalis, P. P., Martin, W. J., and Smith, L. H.: Anaerobic bacteria in the urinary tract. Mayo Clin Proc 47:30, 1972.

Sellin, M., Gillespie, W. A., Cooke, D. I., Sylvester, D. G. H., and Anderson, J. D.: Micrococcal urinary-tract infections in young women. Lancet 2:570, 1975.

Silverblatt, F. J.: Host-parasite interaction in the rat renal pelvis. A possible role for pili in the pathogenesis of pyelonephritis. J Exp Med 140:1696, 1974.

Silverblatt, F. J., and Cohen, L. S.: Antipili antibody affords protection against experimental ascending pyelonephritis. J Clin Invest 64:333, 1979.

Simmons, R. L., Lopez, C., Balfour, H., Kalis, J., Rattazzi, L. C., and Najarian, J. S.: Cytomegalovirus: Clinical virological correlations in renal transplant recipients. Ann Surg 180:623, 1974.

Siroky, M. B., Moylan, R. A., Austen, G., and Olsson, C. A.: Metastatic infection secondary to genitourinary tract sepsis. Am J Med 61:351, 1976.

Stamey, T. A., Govan, D. E., and Palmer, J. M.: The localization and treatment of urinary tract infections: The role of bactericidal urine levels as opposed to serum levels. Medicine 44:1, 1965.

Stamey, T. A., Fair, W. R., Timothy, M. M., and Chung, H. K.: Antibacterial nature of prostatic fluid. Nature 218:444, 1968.

Stamey, T. A., Timothy, M., Millar, M., and Mihara, G.: Recurrent urinary infections in adult women. The role of introital enterobacteria. Calif Med 115:1, 1971.

Stamey, T. A., Condy, M., and Mihara, G.: Prophylactic efficacy of nitrofurantoin macrocrystals and trimethoprim-sulfamethoxazole in urinary infections. Biologic effects on the vaginal and rectal flora. N Engl J Med 296:780, 1977.

Stamey, T. A., Wehner, N., Mihara, G., and Condy, M.: The immunologic basis of recurrent bacteriuria: role of cervicovaginal antibody in enterobacterial colonization of the introital mucosa. Medicine 57:47, 1978.

Svanborg Edén, C., Jodal, U., Hanson, L. A., Lindberg, U., and Akerlund, A. S.: Variable adherence to normal human urinary-tract epithelial cells of Escherichia coli strains associated with various forms of urinary-tract infection. Lancet 2:490, 1976.

Svanborg Edén, C., and Hanson, L. A.: Escherichia coli pili as possible mediators of attachment of human urinary tract epithelial cells. Infect Immun 21:229, 1978.

Svanborg Edén, C., and Svennerholm, A.-M.: Secretory immunoglobulin A and G antibodies prevent adhesion of Escherichia coli to human urinary tract epithelial cells. Infect Immun 22:790, 1978.

Tennant, F. S., Remmers, A. R., and Perry, J. E.: Primary renal candidiasis. Associated perinephric abscess and passage of fungus balls in the urine. Arch Intern Med 122:435, 1968.

Thomas, V., Shelokov, A., and Forland, M.: Antibody-coated bacteria in the urine and the site of urinary-tract infection. N Engl J Med 290:588, 1974.

Thorley, J. D., Jones, S. R., and Sanford, J. P.: Perinephric abscess. Medicine 53:441, 1974.

Turck, M.: Importance of localization of urinary tract infection in women. In Kass, E. H., and Brumfitt, W. (eds.): Infections of the urinary tract. Proceedings of the third international symposium on pyelonephritis. The University of Chicago Press, 1978, p. 114.

Utz, J. P.: Viruria in man, an update. Prog Med Virol 17:77, 1974.

Vainrub, B., and Muscher, D. M.: Lack of effect of methenamine in suppression of, or prophylaxis against, chronic urinary infection. Antimicrob Agents Chemother 12:625, 1977.

Vosti, K. L.: Recurrent urinary tract infections. Prevention by prophylactic antibiotics after sexual intercourse. JAMA 231:934, 1975.

Wallmark, G., Arremark, I., and Telander, B.: Staphylococcus saprophyticus: a frequent cause of acute urinary tract infection among female outpatients. J Infect Dis 138:791, 1978.

Warren, J. W., Platt, R., Thomas, R. J., Rosner, B., and Kass, E. H.: Antibiotic irrigation and catheter associated urinary-tract infections. N Engl J Med 229:570, 1978.

Weinstein, R., Stevens, P., and Chu, C.: Relationship between resistance to phagocytosis and content of E. coli K₁ capsular antigen. Proc 18th Interscience Conference on Antimicrobial Agents and Chemotherapy, Atlanta 1978, abst 506.

Williams, D. N., Lund, M. E., and Blazevic, D. J.: Significance of urinary isolates of coagulase-negative Micrococcaceae. J Clin Microb 3:556, 1976.

# PROSTATITIS 147

## William R. Fair, M.D.

### DEFINITION

The term prostatitis is often used to describe a symptom complex rather than a specific disease entity. Clinicians frequently make the diagnosis of prostatitis without objective evidence that the patient has an infected prostate. Furthermore, some patients who are said to have prostatitis have normal prostatic secretions, while the secretions of others reveal a marked inflammatory response. In an attempt to bring some order into the confusion surrounding the term prostatitis, a recent classification based on symptoms, urine and prostatic fluid cultures, and microscopic examination of the expressed prostatic secretion (EPS) appears to have decided advantages (Drach et al., 1978). In this classification, prostatitis is divided into four distinct categories. Although the specific symptoms of each entity are discussed in detail below, a general definition of each follows:

### Acute Bacterial Prostatitis

Patients with acute bacterial infection of the prostate are clearly ill and have systemic symptoms and infected urine. Acute bacterial prostatitis is easily diagnosed. It should not present a diagnostic dilemma.

### Chronic Bacterial Prostatitis

This diagnosis should be restricted to patients with chronic infections of the prostate proven to be caused by a specific microbial agent. Between episodes of urinary tract infection, *the patient is usually asymptomatic.* The EPS findings are variable. At times, the secretion may appear normal, but careful microscopic examination often reveals an increased number of leukocytes and fat-laden macrophages (oval fat bodies) and a decrease in or absence of the small, so-called "lecithin bodies" that are characteristically abundant in prostatic fluid.

### Nonbacterial Prostatitis

This description is used when the diagnosis of bacterial prostatitis has been excluded, but examination of the EPS reveals a consistent and prominent inflammatory reaction. Thus, the EPS findings are: (1) greater than 10 to 15 leucocytes per high-power microscopic field; (2) an increase in oval fat bodies (fat-laden macrophages, which are easily recognized as large cells that are partially or completely filled with doubly refractile lipid particles); and (3) a decrease in or total absence of "lecithin granules," the small particles characterized by brownian movement that are abundant in the prostatic secretions of normal men.

### Prostatodynia

Patients with prostatodynia, which simply means "prostatic pain," have the clinical symptoms of "prostatitis" (see below) but no objective evidence of prostatic inflammation. Microscopic examination of the EPS is entirely normal, and bacteriologic culture is negative.

## *ETIOLOGY*

### Bacterial Prostatitis

The bacteria that cause both acute and chronic bacterial prostatitis are the same organisms that are responsible for the majority of urinary tract infections, i.e., gram-negative aerobic enteric bacteria. *Escherichia coli, Pseudomonas, Klebsiella,* and *Proteus* are the most common. *Staphylococcus epidermidis* and *Streptococcus faecalis* (enterococci) are not uncommon but cause prostatitis less frequently than the gram-negative bacilli. The diagnosis of gram-positive bacterial prostatitis is more difficult because gram-positive organisms are part of the normal urethral flora of many men. Consequently, urine and EPS collections are frequently contaminated with these organisms, often in high colony counts. If the patient presents with symptoms suggesting prostatitis, and segmented cultures reveal gram-positive organisms in the EPS specimen, the clinician often assumes that a cause-and-effect relationship exists. Proof of this hypothesis is difficult unless bladder infections with the same organism (as is the case in gram-negative bacterial prostatitis) can be demonstrated. Some authorities feel gram-positive prostatitis is a common entity, however, and that urinary infection is uncommon only because most gram-positive organisms do not grow well in urine and cannot reach colony counts high enough to document a bladder infection (Drach, 1974).

### Nonbacterial Prostatitis

The cause of nonbacterial prostatitis is unknown, although all of the following infectious agents have been suggested:

*Anaerobic Bacteria.* In a careful study of patients with nonbacterial prostatitis Meares (1973a), did not find one case of prostatitis due to anaerobic bacteria.

*Viruses.* To date there is no compelling evidence that viruses can cause prostatitis, although many cases of symptomatic prostatitis seem to develop following viral upper respiratory infections (Austen, 1966).

*Parasites.* *Trichomonas vaginalis* infection of the prostate is difficult to document since the prostatic secretions are readily contaminated if only the urethra is infected. However, I have successfully treated a small number of patients with *T. vaginalis* apparently localized to the prostate. As with urethral infestations, the sexual partner must be treated simultaneously to prevent rapid reinfection.

*Fungi.* Rare cases of fungal prostatic infection have been reported (Meares, 1975). These cases have all been secondary to generalized systemic infection.

*Mycoplasma.* T-strain mycoplasma *(Ureaplasma urealyticum)* have been shown to cause prostatitis in a few patients (Taylor-Robinson, 1977; Brunner et al., 1978). Although the precise incidence is unknown, *Ureaplasma* probably do not account for a significant number of cases. The fact that *Ureaplasma,* like bacteria, are part of the urethral flora of normal, asymptomatic men means that without the use of the segmented lower tract localization technique, it is difficult to establish a definite etiologic relationship.

*Chlamydiae.* Recent reports have implicated *Chlamydia* as the cause of some cases of nonbacterial prostatitis (Bruce et al., 1979), but other investigators doubt, on the basis of the accumulated evidence to date, that chlamydiae are a frequent cause of prostatitis (Mårdh et al., 1978).

*Eosinophilic Granulomas.* These have been found in the prostates of asthmatic patients and have been termed "allergic prostatitis" (Kelalis et al., 1964). A larger number of cases of idiopathic granulomatous prostatitis have been reported (Schmidt, 1965). These appear unrelated to any infectious etiology.

### Prostatodynia

The etiology of this condition is unknown, although a variety of causes, from neurogenic bladder dysfunction to a psychogenic disturbance, have been suggested.

## *DIAGNOSIS*

The diagnosis of acute bacterial prostatitis is easily made from the clinical symptoms and the finding of infected urine. However, the diagnosis of chronic bacterial prostatitis as opposed to nonbacterial prostatitis and prostatodynia is more difficult. In the absence of a urinary tract infection, there are no characteristic symptoms that distinguish men with a chronic bacterial infection of the prostate from those in the latter two categories. The physical examination of the prostate is not particularly helpful. The oft-described "boggy prostate" is an extremely subjective description of the gland that varies from examiner to examiner. Pain on examination is also subjective and varies with the patient. Furthermore, prostatic biopsy is not an easy way to confirm bacterial prostatitis. The problem encountered in making the diagnosis by histologic means is similar to that encountered in diagnosing pyelonephritis (the infection may be focal, in which case a single biopsy may completely miss the lesion, and a great many conditions other than bacterial infection produce an indistinguishable inflammatory reaction).

It is essential, however, that the diagnosis of chronic bacterial prostatitis be completely excluded before the patient can be considered to have either nonbacterial prostatitis or prostatodynia. In summary, the diagnosis of chronic bacterial prostatitis can be made only by the obvious approach of culturing bacteria from the prostatic secretion.

It is difficult, however, to obtain a culture of prostatic secretion uncontaminated by urethral organisms. For this reason, the diagnosis of chronic bacterial prostatitis must be made by a technique that enables the physician to distinguish urethral from prostatic infection. The technique originally described by Meares and Stamey (1968) for localization of lower tract infection is excellent and the only way true bacterial prostatitis can be differentiated from urethral contamination. In this technique, a clean-voided urine and expressed prostatic secretion (EPS) are collected in such a way as to give four specimens: (1) the first-voided 10 ml (VB$_1$ — the symbol for voided bladder No. 1); (2) the midstream aliquot (VB$_2$ — the symbol for voided bladder No. 2); (3) the expressed prostatic secretion (EPS) obtained by prostatic massage; and (4) the first 10 ml of urine obtained immediately after prostatic massage (VB$_3$ — the symbol for voided bladder No. 3).

Great care must be taken in the collection to ensure that possibilities of contamination are minimized. The patient must be well hydrated before the collections are attempted. In a circumcised man, no cleansing of the glans penis is necessary. Uncircumcised men should be instructed to retract the foreskin fully and keep it retracted throughout the entire collection procedure. The glans is cleansed with a detergent soap, all soap removed with a rinse of sterile water, and the glans carefully dried with a sterile sponge. The first-voided 10 ml of urine (VB$_1$) is collected with a sterile culture tube held directly in front of the external meatus by the physician. As the patient continues to void, the physician removes the culture tube from the stream of urine. When the patient has voided approximately 200 ml, the second culture tube is inserted into the stream of urine for collection of the 10-ml midstream aliquot (VB$_2$). Immediately after collection of the second specimen, the patient is instructed to stop voiding and shake off any drops of urine that may still be forming at the urethral meatus. The patient then bends forward while keeping the foreskin retracted with one hand and holds a wide-mouth sterile container beneath the meatus with his other hand. As the physician massages the prostate, the drops of prostatic fluid fall directly into the specimen container. The collection is facilitated by the use of the examiner's thumb to exert intermittent gentle pressure on the bulbar urethra. After the prostatic specimen is collected, the patient voids again. The first 10 ml of urine collected after the prostatic massage is labeled VB$_3$ and is obtained in the same manner as the first-voided specimen. If the foreskin slips back over the meatus at any time during the procedure, it is important that the cleansing and drying be repeated in order to prevent bacterial contamination of the cultures. Gram-negative bacteria are plentiful beneath the foreskin and can easily contaminate the cultures. It is equally important to remove all of the detergent from the glans before collecting any cultures. Contamination of voided urine by even small quantities of the antibacterial detergent solution may invalidate the quantitative bacterial count. It is not necessary to cleanse the glans of the circumcised patient.

The diagnosis of bacterial prostatitis or urethritis is made by comparing the quantitative colony count in the various specimens. If the bladder urine is sterile, comparison of the VB$_1$ and VB$_3$ bacterial counts localizes the infection to either the urethra or the prostate. When the VB$_1$ count exceeds that of the VB$_3$ by a factor of one log (a tenfold increase), the diagnosis is anterior urethritis. If the VB$_3$ count is substantially greater than the VB$_1$, the diagnosis is prostatitis. In acute bacterial prostatitis, the count in the prostatic secretion is much higher than the urethral count. The difference is usually smaller in chronic bacterial prostatitis. When the VB$_1$ and the VB$_3$ counts are approximately equal, the EPS culture is valuable for differentiating prostatitis from anterior urethritis.

If the bladder urine is infected with greater than 100,000 bacteria per milliliter, one cannot differentiate the focus of infection. In these cases, the patient is given an antibacterial drug to sterilize the urine. Either nitrofurantoin, 100 mg every 6 hours, or oral penicillin G, 250 mg every 6 hours, is satisfactory for this purpose. These agents sterilize the urine but have no effect on the bacterial count of the EPS specimen because they do not diffuse into the prostate. With the urine sterilized by one of these antibiotics that reach high levels in the urine, the patient undergoes repeat lower tract localization. The EPS and $VB_3$ cultures are streaked immediately on the agar plate to minimize contact of the prostatic fluid with the antibiotic-containing urine. When the urine is sterilized by antibiotics, even exceedingly low counts of bacteria in the EPS and $VB_3$ specimens establish the diagnosis of bacterial prostatitis. Actual counts obtained from a patient on antibiotics are illustrated in the following case history.

## Clinical Case (Table 1)

The following case illustrates the typical history, culture results, and course of a patient with recurrent episodes of bacterial prostatitis. His symptoms disappeared on antimicrobial therapy. When the antibiotic was stopped, the patient's urine became infected again, and his symptoms recurred. Despite treatment with a full therapeutic course of trimethoprim and sulfamethoxazole followed by long-term suppression with one nightly dose of the same drug, the *E. coli* persisted in the prostatic secretion.

L.N., a 59-year-old white male, first presented with low-grade fever, malaise, urgency, frequency, and dysuria on September 6, 1976. The spun urine sediment was loaded with white blood cells and motile bacilli, and a urine culture grew out greater than 100,000 *E. coli* per milliliter. The patient was given co-trimoxazole (trimethoprim and sulfamethoxazole), 2 tablets twice a day, and quickly became asymptomatic. Although two urine cultures obtained while he was taking the drug were sterile, small numbers of *E. coli* were cultured from the prostatic fluid both times. The antibacterial agent was stopped after completion of a 24-day course. He was asymptomatic for more than 1 month, but returned on November 1 with mild frequency and dysuria. Urine cultures again were positive for *E. coli*. He was treated with co-trimoxazole again, and his symptoms subsided. EPS cultures still grew small numbers of *E. coli* while the patient was on the drug. When last seen, he was asymptomatic on a nightly dose of co-trimoxazole, but EPS cultures remained positive.

Thus, the diagnosis of chronic bacterial prostatitis is reserved for patients with recurrent urinary tract infection associated with bacteria in the prostatic secretions.

As mentioned under "Definition," patients with nonbacterial prostatitis have prostatic symptoms and a consistent, sterile inflammatory response in the prostatic secretions. If the patient has a history of urinary tract infection, lower tract bacterial localization studies, as described earlier, should be performed to ensure that the bacteria are not sequestered in the prostate and periodically seeding the urinary tract. However, the vast majority of patients with nonbacterial prostatitis do not have a history of even one episode of

### TABLE 1. Chronic Bacterial Prostatitis
### L.N., a 59 year old white man

| DATE | DAYS ON (+) OR OFF (−) DRUG | $VB_1$ | COLONIES PER ML $VB_2$ | EPS | $VB_3$ | ORGANISMS |
|---|---|---|---|---|---|---|
| 6 Sept 76 | — | 100,000 | 100,000 | ND | ND | *E. coli* |
| 13 Sept 76 | + 7 TMP-Sx ii b.i.d. | 0 | 0 | 20 | 0 | *E. coli* |
| 27 Sept 76 | + 21 TMP-Sx | 0 | 0 | 50 | 0 | *E. coli* |
| 4 Oct 76 | − 4 TMP-Sx | 100 | 0 | 20 | 200 | *E. coli* |
| 28 Oct 76 | − 28 TMP-Sx | 0 | 0 | 10,000 | 2,000 | *E. coli* |
| 1 Nov 76 | − 32 TMP-Sx | 100,000 | 0 | ND | 100,000 | *E. coli* |
| 8 Nov 76 | + 7 TMP-Sx ii b.i.d. | 0 | 0 | 730 | ND | *E. coli* |
| 15 Nov 76 | + 14 TMP-Sx i nightly | 0 | 0 | 10 | 0 | *E. coli* |
| 7 Jan 77 | + 67 TMP-Sx i nightly | 0 | 0 | 30 | 0 | *E. coli* |
| 7 Feb 77 | + 98 TMP-Sx i nightly | 0 | 0 | 70 | 10 | *E. coli* |

$VB_1$ = The first-voided 10 ml (void bladder No. 1)
$VB_2$ = Midstream specimen (void bladder No. 2)
EPS = Expressed prostatic secretion
$VB_3$ = Post–prostatic massage specimen (void bladder No. 3)
ND = Not done
TMP-Sx = Trimethoprim-sulfamethoxazole

urinary tract infection. The diagnosis can be made from the characteristic symptoms and an inflammatory response in the expressed prostatic secretion; negative cultures confirm the diagnosis.

The diagnosis of prostatodynia is made by finding normal prostatic secretion in a patient with similar symptoms (but with no history of urinary tract infection) and sterile urine and prostatic secretion.

## CLINICAL MANIFESTATIONS

### Acute Bacterial Prostatitis

Acute bacterial prostatitis is easily recognized. Typically the patient presents with sudden onset of fever, chills, and signs of a systemic illness. He usually has irritative voiding symptoms with prominent frequency and dysuria and may also complain of anorexia, malaise, perineal discomfort, arthralgias, and vague myalgias. The prostate is swollen, firm, and indurated; feels warm to the touch; and is exquisitely tender to palpation. Because of the risk of seeding bacteria into the bloodstream from an infected prostate, no attempt should be made to massage the prostate to obtain prostatic secretions. Only a very gentle diagnostic examination of the prostate should be done.

Classically, the urinalysis confirms the diagnosis of an acute urinary tract infection with bacteria and a large number of white cells in the spun urine sediment. Urine culture is invariably positive for bacteria.

### Chronic Bacterial Prostatitis (CBP)

The clinical presentation of the patient with chronic bacterial prostatitis is more subtle. Typically, the patient is a man with a history of recurrent urinary tract infections. Frequently, the symptoms began during or after the patient had an indwelling catheter, but chronic bacterial prostatitis may develop without prior catheterization. The unique feature of chronic bacterial prostatitis is that most men have no specific symptoms until they develop symptoms of a bladder infection. These are most frequently irritative symptoms, like dysuria, frequency, urgency, and nocturia, but fever and signs of systemic illness may herald the onset of the urinary tract infection, and the patient may appear to be quite ill. Although CBP may follow an episode of acute prostatitis in some patients, most men with CBP have no antecedent history of acute prostatitis.

The physical findings are variable. In longstanding bacterial prostatitis the prostate is usually small and may feel firm. Although the gland may be slightly tender during the sympto-

matic phase of the disease, pain on examination is not a common feature. The term "boggy prostate" is often used as a synonym for prostatitis, but there is no typical consistency of the prostate in chronic bacterial prostatitis. The patients sometimes have prostatic calculi that can be palpated as firm areas in the gland.

When symptomatic, the patient invariably has pyuria, bacteriuria, and a positive urine culture. However, from a practical viewpoint, chronic bacterial prostatitis is the diagnosis of virtually every man with a history of recurrent urinary tract infections and an intravenous pyelogram that fails to reveal the source (such as stones or upper tract obstruction) for recurrent bacteriuria. Thus, chronic bacterial prostatitis should be suspected in any man with a history of recurrent bladder or kidney infections. The symptoms typically respond well to antimicrobials, and the patient is usually asymptomatic while he is taking the medication. However, at variable intervals after the antibiotics are stopped, the residual infection in the prostate seeds the bladder urine, and the symptoms recur.

The characteristics of the expressed prostatic secretion in chronic bacterial prostatitis are also variable. The secretion may be inflammatory and contain oval fat bodies on some occasions but, at other times, in the same person, it may be quite benign, particularly if the patient is on suppressive antimicrobials. In the latter situation, neither physical examination nor microscopic examination of the EPS gives any hint of persistent chronic bacterial infection. Cultures of the urine and EPS are mandatory in order to make the diagnosis.

### Nonbacterial Prostatitis (NBP) and Prostatodynia

The symptoms of nonbacterial prostatitis and prostatodynia are indistinguishable. Generally, the symptoms consist of variable degrees of perineal aching; back pain; groin pain that occasionally radiates to the thigh, particularly its inner aspect; musculoskeletal soreness; and irritative voiding symptoms (frequency, urgency, and dysuria). The patients often refer to pain on ejaculation, although this is not always present. Urethral discharge is uncommon. A urethral discharge in a patient with these symptoms is much more likely to be caused by urethritis. There are no specific physical findings in nonbacterial prostatitis and prostatodynia. The term "boggy prostate," which is often used to describe the findings on rectal examination of these patients, is a rather nonspecific term. There is no characteristic consistency of the prostate in either of these conditions. Prostatic calculi can be found in these patients just as they can be in men with otherwise perfectly normal prostates. Thus, it is not possible to distinguish between NBP and prostatodynia on the basis of either symptoms or physical examination. The single distinguishing characteristic is the difference in the microscopic examinaton of the EPS. The EPS of patients with nonbacterial prostatitis consistently contains large numbers of white blood cells, often in clumps or aggregates, an increase in the number of fat-laden macrophages (oval fat bodies), and a decrease in the number of lecithin bodies. In contrast, the EPS of patients with prostatodynia is perfectly normal. These unfortunate individuals simply have "prostatic pain" without any objective evidence of prostatic inflammation. Cultures of urine and prostatic secretion are sterile in both conditions.

## PATHOGENESIS AND PATHOLOGY

The bacteria that infect the prostate probably reach the gland by ascending from the urethra. Although colonic bacteria are the most frequent cause of bacterial prostatitis, there is no strong evidence that the organisms spread to the prostate from the colon or by lymphatics from the rectum. Stamey (1972) has postulated that sexual intercourse may play a role in prostatic infection because the male sex partners of women with vaginal colonization by gram-negative bacilli develop transient urethral colonization with the same bacteria.

The importance of the prostate in the genesis of urinary tract infections appears to be twofold. First, the antibacterial activity of the normal prostatic secretion is a significant defense mechanism against the development of urinary tract infections. This antibacterial activity appears to be related directly to the high concentration of zinc in the prostatic secretion (Fair and Stamey, 1969; Fair et al., 1973; Fair and Wehner, 1971). The prostatic secretion of some men with chronic bacterial prostatitis lacks this antibacterial activity (Fair et al., 1973). If this deficiency preceded the infection, it may have made these men more susceptible to prostatitis. Second, persistent bacteria in the prostate intermittently "seed" the bladder urine with pathogenic organisms and cause most of the cases of recurrent bacteriuria in men. The failure of most antibacterials to diffuse into the gland and concentrate in its secretion accounts for the difficulty in eradicating organisms from the prostate. The gland thus serves as a reservoir of infection that often defies all attempts at cure.

Because of its diverse etiologies, there is no typical pathologic finding in patients with prostatitis. Acute bacterial prostatitis caused edema, capillary engorgement, a diffuse infiltration of

neutrophils, and a few round cells. The infiltration of polymorphonuclear leukocytes is accompanied by profuse desquamation of epithelial cells and leukocytes into the tubular lumen. In severe cases, microabscesses may develop and completely break down prostatic tissue. As the process becomes more chronic, the neutrophils are replaced by plasma cells, lymphocytes, and monocytes, and the degree of fibrosis steadily increases.

There are no characteristic tissue changes noted in patients with nonbacterial prostatitis and prostatodynia. The tissue often appears normal.

## COMPLICATIONS AND SEQUELAE

The complications of acute bacterial prostatitis are the same as those of any other severe urinary tract infection. Pyelonephritis is commonly seen if antibacterial treatment is delayed. If septicemia develops secondary to polynephritis, gram-negative shock and cardiovascular collapse may result. Recurrent bladder and upper tract infections are frequent complications of chronic bacterial prostatitis. Except for complications from secondary bacteriuria, chronic bacterial infection of the prostate does not appear to cause significant sequelae.

There is no documented evidence linking prostatitis to subsequent development of benign prostatic hypertrophy (BPH) or carcinoma of the prostate. True, documented chronic bacterial prostatitis is a relatively uncommon disease, however. The possibility that the more frequent entities of nonbacterial prostatitis and prostatodynia might be associated with BPH and carcinoma of the prostate has not been carefully studied.

## GEOGRAPHIC VARIATIONS IN DISEASE

Prostatitis is a worldwide affliction. Because of the difficulty in establishing the correct etiology of prostatitis, it is not known whether geographic variations in the frequency of bacterial prostatitis, nonbacterial prostatitis, or prostatodynia exist. Certainly, the symptom complex caused by benign inflammatory disease of the prostate occurs in all areas of the world. There are some racial and geographic differences in benign prostatic hypertrophy and carcinoma of the prostate, but, as already discussed, there is no evidence that prostatitis is one of the causative factors of either disease.

## TREATMENT AND PROPHYLAXIS

### Acute Bacterial Prostatitis

In contrast to chronic bacterial prostatitis, patients with acute bacterial prostatitis respond dramatically to therapy with antibacterials that do not diffuse into the normal prostate. It is thought that the intense inflammatory reaction caused by acute infection alters the permeability of the prostatic membrane and permits drugs to penetrate the infected prostate. An appropriate antibiotic selected according to the results of in vitro sensitivity tests should be given to the patient in doses that achieve bactericidal concentrations in the serum. Most patients respond very rapidly if therapy is instituted immediately with trimethoprim-sulfamethoxazole (2 tablets twice daily), ampicillin (250 mg four times daily), or one of the other penicillins or cephalosporins. Patients with pronounced systemic symptoms should be treated parenterally with the combination of gentamicin (3 mg/kg) or another aminoglycoside plus penicillin or ampicillin (3.0 to 6.0 g IV daily) or cefazolin (1.0 g IM twice daily) while awaiting the results of cultures and sensitivity tests.

Systemic supportive measures such as bed rest, adequate hydration, analgesics, antipyretics, and stool softeners should also be used. Urethral instrumentation should *never* be considered. When the occasional instance of acute urinary retention occurs, suprapubic needle aspiration of the bladder is safer, more comfortable for the patient, and less likely to cause future complications than urethral catheterization.

### Chronic Bacterial Prostatitis

The treatment of chronic bacterial prostatitis remains unsatisfactory because most antimicrobials do not diffuse into the prostatic secretion of these patients (Winningham et al., 1968; Reeves and Gilchick, 1970; Stamey et al., 1970). Studies in dogs of the factors influencing the diffusion of antimicrobials into the prostate have shown that the most important characteristics are: (1) lipid solubility and (2) a favorable dissociation constant (pKa). An antibacterial with an alkaline pKa diffuses from serum into an acidic prostatic fluid and, by the mechanisms of "ion-trapping," concentrates in the secretion. In the presence of a highly alkaline secretion, however, the opposite occurs and the concentration in the prostatic fluid never approaches the serum levels. Trimethoprim (TMP) concentrates in prostate of normal dogs and should be highly effective at eradicating chronic bacterial prostatitis. In clinical practice, however, cure remains a formidable task even when the organism is known to be sensitive to drugs that concentrate in uninfected canine prostatic fluid. Meares (1973b) and Drach (1974b) found that only 30 per cent of patients treated with trimethoprim and sulfamethoxazole for CBP were cured after completion of therapy. These findings cast doubt on the applicability of the canine model to drug diffusion into the human prostate. The pH of normal canine prostatic fluid is approximately 6.4. Normal human prostatic fluid has a mean pH of 7.3, and it increases to 8.3 in the presence of CBP (Fair and Cordonnier, 1978). These observations probably explain the discrepancy between the experimental data and the clinical results.

Despite the discouraging results of treatment with trimethoprim-sulfamethoxazole in most series, the results with other agents are even more dismal. Thus, except for prostatitis due to gram-positive organisms or *Pseudomonas aeruginosa,* which are relatively resistant to TMP, TMP-Sx is still the agent of choice. Recent encouraging results with kanamycin suggest that this drug may be useful for sensitive organisms (Pfau and Sacks, 1976). Erythromycin (0.5 g four times daily) is the treatment of choice for gram-positive infections.

Transurethral resection of the prostate (TURP) is no better than treatment with antimicrobials. Only about one-third of patients subjected to TURP are permanently free of infection (Stamey, 1972). Moreover, the almost certain development of retrograde ejaculation and the possible risk of incontinence make most surgeons loath to perform TURP in young men unless the repeated infections cannot be controlled by medication.

Prevention of the symptoms of CBP is more successful than treatment. Men with CBP are asymptomatic between episodes of bladder bacteriuria, which can usually be prevented by a single nightly dose of an appropriate antimicrobial. For example, I have successfully treated several young men for recalcitrant *Pseudomonas* prostatitis for periods exceeding 24 months with a nightly dose of 250 mg of tetracycline.

While the prognosis of acute bacterial prostatitis is excellent, the prospect for cure of CBP is less favorable. However, prevention of bladder infection and control of symptoms in most patients with low-dose suppressive medication is easily accomplished.

### Nonbacterial Prostatitis and Prostatodynia

Since the cause of these entities is unknown, no rational plan of therapy or prophylaxis can be formulated. Some patients respond symptomatically to empiric therapy with tetracycline or one of the long-acting tetracycline derivatives. On the theory that the prostate is "congested," some clinicians recommend periodic prostatic massages or more frequent ejaculations. The relief of pain is presumably the result of mechanical emptying or "drainage" of fluid from the engorged prostatic duct. Other patients seem to respond to anticholinergics, sedatives, muscle relaxants, or analgesics. Sitz baths are also often prescribed. Therapy with phenoxybenzamine has been reported to relieve the symptoms of prostatodynia (Drach, 1979).

Prophylactic recommendations have included prostatic massage, frequent sexual activity, sexual abstinence, vitamins, sunflower seeds, and oral zinc supplementation. To date, there are no data to support any of these measures.

## References

Austen, G., Jr.: The test of time. IX. Prostatitis: acute and chronic. Brit M Q 17:27, 1966.

Bruce, A. W., Willett, W. S., Chadwick, P., and O'Shaughnessy, M.: The role of Chlamydiae in genito-urinary disease. J Urol 1979 (in press).

Brunner, H., Weidner, W., Krause, W., and Rothauge, C. F.: Zur Bedutung von Ureaplasma urealyticum bei unspezificher prostato-urethritis — quantitative Untersuchungen an 312 Patienten. Dtsch Med Wochenschr 103:465, 1978.

Drach, G. W.: Problems in diagnosis of bacterial prostatitis: Gram-negative, gram-positive, and mixed infections. J Urol 111:603, 1974a.

Drach, G. W.: Trimethoprim-sulfamethoxazole therapy of chronic bacterial prostatitis. J Urol 111:637, 1974b.

Drach, G. W.: Personal communication, 1979.

Drach, G. W., Meares, E. M., Jr., Fair, W. R., and Stamey, T. A.: Classification of benign diseases associated with prostatic pain: prostatitis or prostatodynia? (Letter to the Editor) J Urol 120:266, 1978.

Fair, W. R., and Cordonnier, J. J.: The pH of prostatic fluid: a reappraisal and therapeutic implications. J Urol 120:695, 1978.

Fair, W. R., Couch, J., and Wehner, N.: Purification and assay of the prostatic antibacterial factor (PAF). Biochem Med 8:329, 1973.

Fair, W. R., and Stamey, T. A.: Bactericidal properties of prostatic fluid. In Bacterial Infection of Male Genital System (Workshop), October 1967. Warrenton, Va., National Research Council, National Academy of Sciences, 1969.

Fair, W. R., and Wehner, N.: Further observations on the antibacterial nature of prostatic fluid. Infect Immun 3:494, 1971.

Kelalis, P. T., Harrison, E. G., Jr., and Greene, L. F.: Allergic granulomas of the prostate in asthmatics. JAMA 118:963, 1964.

Mårdh, P-A., Ripa, K. T., Colleen, S., Treharne, J. D., and Darougar, N. S.: The role of Chlamydia trichomatis in non-acute prostatitis. Br J Vener Dis 54:330, 1978.

Meares, E. M., Jr.: Bacterial prostatitis versus "prostatosis": a clinical and bacteriological study. JAMA 224:1372, 1973a.

Meares, E. M., Jr.: Observations on the activity of trimethoprim-sulfamethoxazole in the prostate. J Infect Dis (Suppl):S679, 1973b.

Meares, E. M., Jr.: Prostatitis — a review. Urol Clin North Am 2:3, 1975.

Meares, E. M., Jr., and Stamey, T. A.: Bacteriologic localization patterns in bacterial prostatitis and urethritis. Invest Urol 5:492, 1968.

Pfau, A., and Sacks, T.: Chronic bacterial prostatitis: new therapeutic aspects. Brit J Urol 48:245, 1976.

Reeves, D. S., and Gilchick, M. B.: Secretion of the antibacterial substance trimethoprim in the prostatic fluid of dogs. J Urol 42:66, 1970.

Schmidt, J. D.: Non-specific granulomatous prostatitis: classification, review and report of cases. J Urol 94:607, 1965.

Stamey, T. A.: Urinary Infections. Baltimore, Williams & Wilkins Co., 1972, p. 166.

Stamey, T. A., Meares, E. M., Jr., and Winningham, D. J.: Bacterial prostatitis and the diffusion of drugs into prostatic fluid. J Urol 103:187, 1970.

Taylor-Robinson, D.: Possible role of ureaplasmas in non-gonococcal urethritis. In Hobson, D., and Holmes, K. K. (eds.): Non-gonococcal Urethritis and Related Infections. Washington, D.C., American Society of Microbiology, 1977.

Winningham, D. J., Nemoy, N. J., and Stamey, T. A.: Diffusion of antibiotics from plasma into prostatic fluid. Nature 219:139, 1968.

# 148 NONVENEREAL INFECTIONS OF THE FEMALE GENITALIA

*Edward Brook Rotheram, Jr., M.D.*

## DEFINITION AND ETIOLOGY

Deep infections of the female genitalia not acquired or transmitted by sexual contact may be granulomatous (tuberculous) or pyogenic. Exogenous pyogenic infections are produced by single pathogens such as *Streptococcus pyogenes* or *Staphylococcus aureus*, microbes that are rarely recovered from normal vaginal and cervical secre-tions. When these specific infections occur after obstetric and gynecologic procedures, faults in aspetic technique should be suspected, especially if epidemic spread is observed. In endogenous pyogenic infections, the pus contains a mixture of poorly virulent aerobic and anaerobic bacteria that are frequently recovered from normal vaginal and cervical secretions. Most pyogenic infections occurring endemically within the hospital are endogenous.

# PYOGENIC INFECTIONS

## *PATHOGENESIS AND PATHOLOGY*

Nonvenereal pyogenic infections of the female genitalia originate in poorly oxygenated, poorly defended spaces or cavities containing material conducive to rapid bacterial growth. In abortal and postpartum sepsis, the uterine cavity contains dead fetal tissue. Before delivery, the amniotic space and its fluid are available for bacterial growth. Following obstetric and gynecologic surgery, collections of blood or lymph fulfill the criteria for bacterial growth admirably. A fallopian tube partially or totally occluded by inflammatory disease presents another nidus. Infection occurs when such spaces, regardless of their size, are inoculated with a specific pathogen. When large spaces are contaminated by secretions of the adjacent vagina and cervix, certain members of the normal flora may evade the inflammatory response and proliferate. The strict anaerobes and the microaerophilic species of the normal flora usually become numerically dominant in these relatively avascular spaces. *Bacteroides, Peptostreptococcus,* and microaerophilic streptococcal species are often recovered in high concentrations when quantitative anaerobic cultural techniques are employed (Rotheram and Schick, 1969). Less frequently, other fastidious microbes such as *Actinomyces, Proprionibacterium, Clostridia* species, and even *Corynebacterium vaginale (Haemophilus vaginalis)* are recovered in large numbers. Certain facultative anaerobes such as *Escherichia coli, Proteus mirabilis, Staphylococcus epidermidis*, group B streptococci, and the enterococci are also frequently recovered. Although these facultative species are usually present in far smaller concentrations than the strict anaerobes, their importance in endogenous infections was overemphasized before the complete bacteriologic studies of the past 15 years because they grow so readily in air. Although they have now been placed in proper perspective, these facultative species, particularly the gram-negative bacilli, cannot be ignored. Not only may they occasionally dominate the pelvic infection, but also they may produce shock when they enter the bloodstream.

Infection of a pelvic space may spread through lymphatic channels and produce cellulitis and abscesses of the broad ligaments and other retroperitoneal spaces of the pelvic floor. Infection can also extend from the uterine cavity into the fallopian tubes to produce tubal or tubo-ovarian abscesses. These may rupture and cause peritonitis and either local or remote intraperitoneal abscesses.

Many acute pyogenic infections of the female genitalia are accompanied by a bacteremia that reflects the local infection in that it is frequently anaerobic and polymicrobial. Hematogenous abscesses in distant organs show a similar flora. Septic thrombophlebitis explains the paradox of how a mixed infection in an avascular space gains ready access to the bloodstream. Since strict anaerobes induce thrombophlebitis more readily than facultative bacteria, *Escherichia coli* and the enterococci may often owe their access to the bloodstream to vascular lesions induced by the strict anaerobes. When confined to small tributaries, venous thrombosis may seal off the infection with spontaneous resolution of accompanying bacteremia. Conversely, thrombosis may extend to larger veins and produce a severe continuous septicemia.

## *CLINICAL MANIFESTATIONS*

### Septic Abortion (Postabortal Endometritis)

Infection rarely complicates spontaneous abortion but frequently follows an induced incomplete abortion. Within two to five days of uterine instrumentation, the typical patient develops a shaking chill and high fever. An enlarged tender uterus discharges a foul-smelling mixture of blood and pus. Leukocytosis is expected. Bacteremia can be demonstrated in over 50 per cent of cases if the blood is cultured within 24 hours of the chill. Half of the positive blood cultures yield two or more bacterial species, and anaerobic and microaerophilic isolates outnumber facultative isolates 4 to 1. Bacterial species recovered in concentrations of more than $10^6$ colonies/ml of uterine exudate show the same 4:1 ratio of fastidious to rapid-growing bacteria.

Despite early evidence of invasive infection, most patients recover promptly after evacuation of the uterus, a fact well known in the preantibiotic era. However, the complications of septic abortion, discussed separately below, are notoriously severe. The full spectrum of the disease ranges from death within hours of onset to a prolonged, debilitating illness.

The diagnosis of septic abortion is difficult only when local signs of infection develop with uncharacteristic indolence in a patient who falsely denies pregnancy and/or uterine instrumentation.

## Puerperal Sepsis (Postpartum Endometritis)

Chills and fever associated with a large tender uterus and profuse lochial flow begin abruptly two to five days after delivery, which may not have been difficult. Lacerations of the cervix or uterine wall obviously predispose to infection, but retained placental fragments are all that is needed to initiate endometritis. Before the use of aseptic technique, epidemics of puerperal sepsis with high mortality rates were reported from all countries where labor and delivery occurred in hospitals. These epidemics were undoubtedly caused by *Streptococcus pyogenes* transmitted from mother to mother by physicians' hands. This exogenous infection is characterized by the rapid development of intense pelvic cellulitis, and death can occur quickly from an overwhelming bacteremia (blood poisoning). This accelerated course is explained by the ability of *Streptococcus pyogenes* to spread rapidly through lymphatics despite the interposition of lymph nodes, which are ordinarily quite effective in limiting pyogenic infection. Sporadic cases of this specific exogenous infection still occur, although early treatment often results in a mild illness. *Staphylococcus aureus, Neisseria gonorrhea,* and even *Streptococcus pneumoniae* may also be recovered in puerperal cultures, but, as in septic abortion, the great majority of nonepidemic infections are caused by endogenous bacteria such as *E. coli* and anaerobes. The lower the virulence of the invading bacteria, the more important are local disturbances in tissue resistance. Hence, removal of retained tissues from the uterus is the cornerstone of treatment of endogenous infection. The complications of endogenous infection maintain puerperal sepsis as a leading cause of maternal death.

## Subgluteal and Retropsoas Abscess

Although perivaginal tissues are remarkably resistant to infection, pudendal or paracervical block anesthesia during delivery can result in pelvic abscesses. Presumably a hematoma is induced and infected by the needle that must pass through the vagina. From this nidus, pus can dissect along the lumbosacral plexus superiorly to reach the retropsoas space and inferiorly to involve the subgluteal space posterior to the hip joint (Hibbard et al., 1972). Symptoms and signs of infection may develop insidiously after a normal delivery as the patient complains of increasingly severe pain and limitation of motion in the hip, with or without psoal spasm. Paraplegia, muscle destruction, bacteremic shock, and death have resulted from the failure to detect and drain these abscesses.

## Chorioamnionitis

The chorioamniotic space is infected within 24 hours after rupture of the fetal membranes. When rupture is premature, 80 to 90 per cent of women go into spontaneous labor within this period of time. The longer the uterus remains unemptied, the greater the danger of infection to mother and child. Although some mothers may develop fever and bacteremia (with or without shock), others may show little or no evidence of infection while the fetus is suffering irreparable harm. Obviously, the temptation to delay delivery is greatest when the fetus is immature, but if amniocentesis confirms the suspicion of infection, nothing is gained by delay.

## Postoperative Infections

Cesarean section must be considered a contaminated procedure if the fetal membranes have been ruptured for eight hours or longer. Hysterotomy yields an infection rate as high as that for cholecystectomy and bowel resection. Fortunately, many infections are subcutaneous and respond promptly to drainage through the wound. A few involve the uterine wall, adnexa, intraperitoneal spaces, or bowel and may be fatal.

Abdominal and vaginal hysterectomies are also associated with a high incidence of infection with a broad range of morbidity (Ledger, 1969). Premenopausal women undergoing vaginal hysterectomy are at greatest risk: Hemostasis is difficult because their pelvic tissues are more vascular, ovulation exposes the ovarian stroma to infection, and preexisting salpingitis is more common. *Vaginal cuff abscess* is the most frequent and least serious infectious complication. Fever occurs early, usually within five days, symptoms are few, and drainage is followed by rapid recovery. The fever due to *pelvic cellulitis* tends to occur later in the postoperative period but still within the average hospital stay. Fever does not remit if an associated cuff abscess is drained. No other masses are felt, although the pelvis remains tender. The response to antibiotics is usually brisk.

*Adnexal infection* is often discovered after the patient has been discharged. The typical patient is readmitted with fever, lower abdominal pain, and a mass in the pelvis. Partial intestinal obstruction may be present. In *tubo-ovarian abscess*, tubal obstruction occurs when the ovary is caught up in an inflammatory reaction of the fimbria. Ultimately the ovary forms a tiny portion of an abscess within the tube. *Ovarian abscess* is quite distinct pathologically. Bacteria enter the ovary either through a ruptured follicle or by way of a surgical biopsy. The abscess develops within the ovarian tissue and spares the tubal structures.

Although both types of abscesses may rupture, the ovarian abscess is particularly prone to this potentially fatal complication.

### Nonspecific Pelvic Inflammatory Disease (Salpingo-oophoritis)

Not all women who present with fever, lower abdominal pain, peritoneal irritation, cervical discharge, and adnexal masses have gonorrhea. When the syndrome is recurrent, recovery of the gonococcus in culture is unusual. The end stage of the recurrent disease is a fibrotic pelvis containing tubo-ovarian abscesses to which loops of small intestine may adhere. The abscesses typically contain a mixture of endogenous bacteria. The innate resistance of pelvic structures to endogenous bacteria suggests that this infection is superimposed upon a prior inflammatory process: gonorrhea, endometritis associated with pregnancy or contraceptive devices, and an adjacent abscess of intestinal origin. In contrast to most of the infections already discussed, blood cultures are rarely positive.

## COMPLICATIONS

Leakage or rupture of adnexal abscesses produces pelvic and generalized peritonitis, pelvic and remote intraperitoneal abscesses, mechanical intestinal obstruction, and adynamic ileus. Hemorrhage and/or acute bacteremias may produce hypovolemic and/or septic shock with a significant incidence of renal failure. Gram-negative bacteremias occurring in the peripartum period are likely to trigger disseminated intravascular coagulation. Indeed, human equivalents of the local and generalized Senarelli-Shwartzman reactions occur complete with renal cortical necrosis. A rare complication of pregnancy, aptly termed the plasmapheresis syndrome, results from the body's failure to control yet another aspect of the inflammatory response: a global increase in capillary permeability rapidly leads to hypovolemia, hemoconcentration, and shock. Administration of salt and albumen results in more edema and damage to the brain and lungs.

Clostridial myonecrosis, uterine gangrene, and even tetanus can complicate the anaerobic infections. Clostridial septicemia (distinguished from bacteremia by intravascular hemolysis) often originates in the postabortal and postpartum uterus. Suppurative thrombophlebitis in pelvic and ovarian veins produces fever, tachycardia, and multiple pulmonary emboli. This triad does not respond to antibiotics, which may nevertheless prevent hematogenous infection of the lungs, liver, brain, and endocardium.

The youthful organs of most patients suffering

these complications are valuable allies of the physician, who by skillful diagnosis and treatment can salvage most of these patients.

## SEQUELAE

Sterility may follow any severe infection of the female genitalia. Pyogenic infections, however, do not cause the high incidence of sterility and ectopic pregnancy characteristic of tuberculosis. For example, most women who suffer recurrent salpingitis can carry out a successful pregnancy if one fallopian tube remains patent.

## DIAGNOSIS

Diagnosis depends heavily upon a knowledge of the individual infectious entities, predisposing factors, and likely complications. Similarly, the pelvic examination is far more revealing if the mind as well as the fingers are exercised. Sonography aids in the interpretation of the pelvic examination. Blood cultures are indicated not only before antibiotics are started but also when antibiotics do not appear to be working.

Secretions for culture can be obtained on swabs from an operative wound, the cervical os, and the uterine cavity, but the swabs must not dry out before the culture is made. Hematomas and abscesses may be aspirated by both vaginal and abdominal routes. Culdocentesis and amniocentesis are now performed frequently with little morbidity. Secretions are sent to the laboratory in the syringe used for aspiration.

All secretions require careful evaluation if they are not to be misleading. Regardless of the laboratory report, gross pus is rarely sterile and fetid pus is never free of strict anaerobes (Fig. 1). Smears often show an abundant variety of gram-positive and gram-negative bacteria. The aerobic culture identifies most exogenous pathogens. Those bacteria observed on Gram stain but missing in culture are usually fastidious anaerobes. For example, a light growth of enterococci cannot account for myriads of tiny, gram-positive cocci observed on the stain, nor can an abundant growth of *E. coli* explain the observation of many small encapsulated rods. Fortunately, *Bacteroides* and anaerobic streptococci are dependable in their sensitivity to various antibiotics, and patients can be successfully managed without optimal anaerobic bacteriology or sensitivity tests.

*Clostridium perfringens* may be recovered on culture in the absence of myonecrosis or septicemia. The diagnosis of these two complications must be based upon associated clinical manifesta-

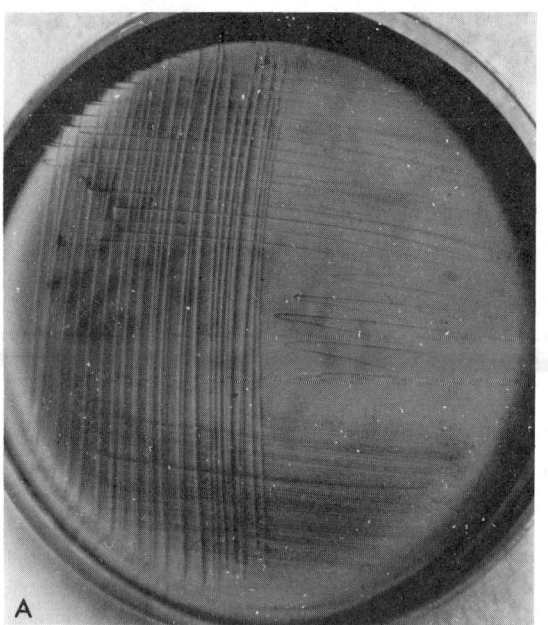
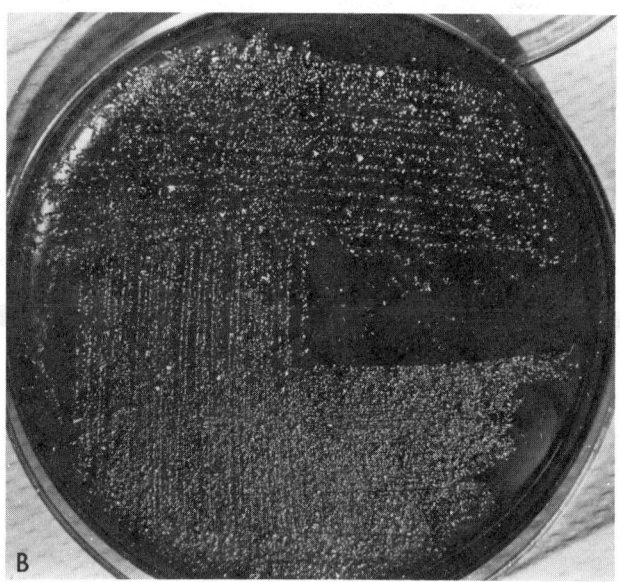

**FIGURE 1.** *Both blood agar plates were inoculated with pus aspirated from a tubo-ovarian abscess. A, This plate was incubated aerobically and remained sterile. The plate shown in B was incubated anaerobically and yielded six bacterial species, three of which were abundant.*

tions if unnecessary surgery is to be avoided. Even at surgery, uterine gangrene may be a difficult diagnosis (Hawkins et al., 1975).

## TREATMENT

Evacuation or excision of infected cavities and any associated abscesses is central to the treatment of pyogenic infections of the female genitalia. Delay in emptying an infected uterus is rarely justified. Vaginal drainage of pelvic abscesses produces less morbidity than transabdominal drainage, provided no major loculations are missed. Some delay to permit abscesses to coalesce and point vaginally may be warranted. However, ovarian abscesses and other well-formed abscesses high in the pelvis are indications for immediate abdominal drainage and excision of damaged genital structures.

Even before the bacteriologic complexity of endogenous infection was fully appreciated, high doses of intravenous penicillin (2.0 million units every three hours) clearly reduced the local and systemic complications of acute pyogenic infections and permitted earlier and less destructive surgery. Intravenous clindamycin in a dose of 600 mg every six hours for *Bacteroides fragilis,* and intramuscular kanamycin (0.5 gm twice daily) or gentamicin (80 mg every eight hours) for *Escherichia coli* provides broader coverage. Tetracyclines should be avoided in pregnancy and the puerperium. The effect of various antibiotic regimens on the final outcome of nonspecific salpingo-oophoritis is not known.

Heparin appears to be a useful adjunct to antibiotics in the treatment of septic thrombophlebitis. Ligation of the inferior vena cava and left ovarian vein is required rarely today. Since pregnancy is associated with low reserves of folic acid, any myelopoietic stress can induce a megaloblastic crisis with leukopenia and thrombocytopenia. All periparturient women who are seriously ill should receive folic acid.

## PROPHYLAXIS

Although the vagina cannot be completely decontaminated, the number of resident bacteria can be reduced by the removal of excessive secretions through treatment of a specific vaginitis (due to *Trichomonas vaginalis* or *Candida albicans*) and by thorough mechanical cleansing before surgery. Conization of the cervix induces bacterial multiplication, and hysterectomy should follow conization within 48 hours or be delayed several weeks to lower the risk of operative infection. To prevent exogenous infection, aseptic technique must be maintained even in the presence of gross contamination with vaginal flora. Hemostasis is a critical element of surgical technique for preventing infection. A biopsy of the ovary should never be made in a contaminated field such as that produced by culpotomy. Any patient at risk of an anaerobic infection should have had previous tetanus immunization.

NONVENEREAL INFECTIONS OF THE FEMALE GENITALIA — 148 **1197**

A single antibiotic such as cephalothin given immediately before and for 24 hours after vaginal hysterectomy strikingly reduces postoperative infections in those (premenopausal) women at greatest risk (Mead, 1974). Apparently the presence of an antibiotic within the hematomas formed at surgery delays bacterial growth and often tips the early inflammatory battle in favor of the host.

# GRANULOMATOUS INFECTIONS

Granulomatous infection would be synonymous with tuberculosis of the female genitalia if it were not for the rare infections with *Histoplasma capsulatum* and *Coccidioides immitis*. Tubercle bacilli reach the fallopian tubes hematogenously during the primary phase of pulmonary or intestinal tuberculosis. If infection is not arrested in one tube, it is rarely arrested in the other. Bacilli then spread upward to produce localized pelvic peritonitis in one half of patients and perioophoritis in one third. Downward spread produces endometritis in almost 60 per cent of cases, but the cervix and vagina are far more resistant. Coincidental renal tuberculosis occurs in less than 5 per cent of cases.

Systemic manifestations of chronic infection are often absent despite many years of involvement. Most patients without progressive pulmonary disease appear healthy, and fever is absent or low grade. However, 85 per cent of patients are nulliparous, and sterility is the chief complaint of 50 per cent. Mild pelvic pain and abnormal vaginal bleeding are the next most frequent complaints. The most common physical finding is an adnexal mass, which is often unilateral despite pathologic involvement of both tubes.

Local complications such as intestinal obstruction and fistula are rare. Generalized peritonitis and hematogenous dissemination develop only rarely from a genital focus. Thus, sterility reigns unchallenged as the major complication. Conception is more likely following treatment, but the risk of ectopic pregnancy is then increased.

If endometritis is present, diagnosis may be made by curettage performed near the end of the menstrual cycle. Endometrial tubercles are hard and contain few bacilli because the regular shedding of the endometrium allows no time for caseation to occur. Culture of the endometrial tissue is usually required for a definitive diagnosis. Peritoneal granulomas may be observed, and biopsies and cultures of them may be made by culdoscopy and peritoneoscopy. In geographic areas in which the disease is infrequently encountered, most cases are discovered unexpectedly at surgery.

Medical treatment is the same as for progressive pulmonary tuberculosis (Schaefer, 1967). Even large cold abscesses will resolve without surgical intervention, which may, however, be undertaken with little fear as long as medical treatment is begun postoperatively.

# VULVOVAGINITIS

Vulvovaginitis is an abnormal increase in vaginal secretions with inflammation of the vaginal mucosa and adjacent vulvar skin. Purulent cervical discharge is a separate entity caused by *Neisseria gonorrhea*, nonspecific salpingo-oophoritis, an intrauterine contraceptive device, or less well established causes such as *Chlamydia trachomatis*.

At menarche, estrogen secretion causes glycogen to accumulate within a thickened vaginal squamous epithelium. The sparse but varied vaginal flora of childhood become dominated by *Lactobacillus* species that are capable of utilizing glycogen and lowering the pH of the secretions to 5 or less. The vagina becomes resistant to pyogenic bacteria such as *Neisseria gonorrhea* and *Strep-*

*tococcus pyogenes*, which cause vaginitis in childhood. *Trichomonas vaginalis* can proliferate in normal adult secretions. A significant proportion of women who acquire this motile protozoan through sexual intercourse promptly develop vaginitis that clears upon elimination of the trichomonads. *Candida albicans*, present in normal feces, has ready access to the vagina. Sexual transmission is not needed, and altered host resistance must play a large role in its ability to establish vaginal moniliasis. Pregnancy, oral contraceptives, cervical discharge, glycosuria, and oral antibiotics are believed to stimulate overgrowth of *C. albicans* through alterations in the volume, glycogen content, and pH of vaginal secretions and the suppression of competing fecal and vaginal bacteria. Vulvitis is partly a result of contact hypersensitivity to the parasite growing on epithelial cells.

Some women have increased vaginal secretions without abundant trichomonads or yeasts (nonspecific vaginitis). These secretions usually show some imbalance among "normal" vaginal microbes. *Corynebacterium vaginale (Haemophilus vaginalis)*, *Ureaplasma urealyticum*, *Mycoplasma hominis*, and strictly anaerobic bacteria are often more numerous than *Lactobacilli* (as they may be in the specific forms of vaginitis). Although the pathogenesis of this mild illness is not understood, some investigators postulate a central role for *C. vaginale* (Pheifer et al., 1978).

Classically, *T. vaginalis* produces a profuse, thin, greenish, malodorous discharge containing many granulocytes and so many motile trichomonads that microscopic examination of fresh wet secretions suffices for diagnosis. *C. albicans* causes a scantier, thicker exudate containing yeasts and granulocytes on wet mount or Gram stain. Epithelial cells scraped from inflamed vulvar skin show the fungus in its hyphal phase on Gram stain. Not infrequently, both agents of specific vaginitis occur simultaneously. Primary or recurrent *Herpes simplex* must be considered in the presence of vulvar vesicles or ulcers.

In nonspecific vaginitis, a scant discharge with a disagreeable odor but few granulocytes is present at the introitus. Vulvar irritation appears minimal, although the patient may complain of itching, burning, and dyspareunia. Diagnosis requires the exclusion of a purulent cervical discharge and the two specific agents.

*T. vaginalis* infection responds promptly to one oral dose of 2 g of metronidazole, which should not, however, be given during pregnancy (Dykers, 1975). To avoid reinfection, sexual partners should be treated simultaneously or they should use condoms for several months until trichomonads are eliminated spontaneously from the male urethra. *C. albicans* infection is treated by vaginal application of nystatin or miconazole daily for 14 days, and severe vulvitis responds promptly to topical corticosteroid cream. Initial results are good, but recurrence is common, even when predisposing factors are eliminated. Then, an attempt to reduce fecal yeast with oral nystatin seems reasonable (Miles et al., 1977).

With the possible exception of metronidazole, there is no evidence that any of the current therapies for nonspecific vaginitis is effective. Probably the less done the better, since local or systemic treatment may perpetuate a floral imbalance or produce inflammation itself.

# TOXIC SHOCK SYNDROME

Toxic shock syndrome (TSS) is an acute febrile illness of previously healthy women who become hypotensive and sometimes die of shock. The disease occurs during a menstrual period and has been attributed to growth of *Staphylococcus aureus* in the vagina during menstruation and to elaboration of a staphylococcal toxin. The use of vaginal tampons has been incriminated as a contributory factor.

*Staphylococcus aureus* has been cultured from the vagina in 98 per cent of women with the toxic shock syndrome (Morbidity-Mortality Weekly Reports, 1980), whereas staphylococci are almost never cultured from the vagina otherwise (Braude et al., 1978). The use of tampons is thought to contribute to the disease by carrying staphylococci from the finger into the vagina upon insertion and by occluding the vaginal canal; thus the trapped menstrual blood secretions would promote growth of staphylococci and toxin production. Trauma to the mucosa during insertion would then allow absorption of toxin into the systemic circulation. It has also been suggested that vaginal occlusion forces retrograde passage of contaminated

menstrual blood through the fallopian tubes into the peritoneal cavity, where staphylococcal toxin can be rapidly absorbed into the general circulation. Although these ideas on pathogenesis are speculative, they get support from the fact that TSS has become prominent only since the incorporation into tampons of synthetic materials that can expand them enough to occlude the vagina. It should also be noted that a significant association has been found between TSS and continuous use of tampons during the menstrual period.

The absence of staphylococcal bacteremia in TSS also supports the idea that elaboration of a toxin or toxins by staphylococci in the menstrual secretions is responsible for the disease. A staphylococcal toxin, designated type A, has been isolated from strains of staphylococci recovered from patients with TSS. This toxin causes fever in rabbits and enhances the ability of endotoxin to cause fatal shock, myocardial necrosis, and hepatic necrosis in animals (Schlievert et al., 1979). Another toxin obtained from staphylococci associated with TSS has produced in newborn mice epidermal lesions that were distinct from those of staphylococcal exfoliative toxin (Todd et al., 1978). The importance of either toxin in the pathogenesis of this disease is not settled. It is possible that a mixture of staphylococcal toxins may be necessary to produce all of the manifestations of TSS. If toxins are involved, they may not be immunogenic in certain cases because the syndrome tends to recur, and second attacks may be more severe than the first. Recurrent attacks of a toxemic disease could be explained in several ways: (1) the toxin is so potent that the effective dose is smaller than the immunogenic dose (as in tetanus, a disease in which second attacks also occur); (2) any of several staphylococcal toxins might cause TSS, so that immunity to one would not protect against another; (3) patients who get TSS are immunodeficient with respect to antitoxin production; (4) the disease requires sensitization to a staphylococcal product and is thus a form of allergic shock.

Whatever the cause of shock, it is accompanied by intravascular coagulation, renal failure, acidosis, fine desquamation or sloughing of the skin, and pulmonary insufficiency. The shock has an oligemic phase, secondary to diarrhea and vomiting, and partly corrected by replacement of fluids. Hemodynamic measurements have demonstrated high cardiac output, low peripheral resistance, normal pulmonary artery wedge pressure, and normal pulmonary resistance (McKenna et al., 1980). Myoglobinuria has been observed and is considered a possible factor in the renal failure. Elevated levels of creatinine-kinase and severe muscle pain are all further evidence of rhabdomyolysis.

Symptoms start abruptly during the menstrual period with fever over 38.9° C (102° F), sore mouth and throat, headache, weakness, severe myalgia, conjunctival burning (or purulent conjunctivitis), vomiting, abdominal pain with severe watery diarrhea, and a rash. The rash may be a generalized diffuse macular erythema covering the trunk and extremities or a localized eruption. Within 2 to 4 days, the patient may become disoriented and lose consciousness. Hypotension develops in most cases and proceeds to severe shock. In addition to shock, the three most serious problems are disseminated intravascular coagulation (DIC), renal failure, and respiratory distress. The DIC is characterized by depressed fibrinogen levels, increased split products, prolonged prothrombin time, and thrombocytopenia. These clotting disturbances may lead to purpura, severe gastrointestinal bleeding, or vaginal hemorrhages. The renal failure is characterized by elevated blood creatinine and urea nitrogen, oliguria, proteinuria, hematuria, and pyruria with sterile urine. Pancreatitis has also been reported, and may be responsible for abdominal pain in some cases (McKenna et al., 1980).

Except for marked desquamation or peeling of the skin and severe hair loss, there are no characteristic complications or sequelae, and full recovery is the rule in those who survive. The desquamation occurs during convalescence on the face, trunk, palms, and soles, but may be limited to the fingertips. Considerable hair may be lost from the scalp several weeks later.

Recurrences are a problem in over half the cases. These can be either mild and cause no shock, or severe and fatal.

Cases of TSS can be expected wherever tampons are used, but have only been reported thus far from the United States and include cases in Wisconsin, Illinois, Oklahoma, Minnesota, Massachusetts, Colorado, and California. By September 1980, 299 cases had been reported to the Center for Disease Control since the first report in 1978 (Todd et al., 1978). The absence of case reports from other countries might be explained by the possibility that distribution of both the more occlusive tampons and the TSS-producing staphylococci are limited to the United States.

TSS should be considered seriously in a young woman who suddenly develops fever, rash, myalgias, and hypotension during menstruation. In the presence of these clinical manifestations, the diagnosis can be strengthened by the isolation of *S. aureus* from the vagina. The Center for Disease Control has formulated 5 criteria for case definition:

1. Fever over 38.9° C
2. Erythematous macular rash with later desquamation
3. Hypotension
4. Involvement of at least 3 organ systems from among the following: gastrointestinal, muscular, mucous membranes, renal, hepatic, hematologic, or central nervous system
5. Negative cultures of blood, throat, or cerebrospinal fluid, and negative serologic tests for Rocky mountain spotted fever, leptospirosis, or measles

Several laboratory results are important for identifying disorders in the various systems. The level of creatinine phosphokinase should be at least twice normal to provide evidence that the muscular system is affected. Renal involvement is evident if the blood urea nitrogen or creatinine is increased or if there are abnormal numbers of white cells in the urine (in the absence of urinary infection). Liver disease is manifested by elevated levels of bilirubin, SGOT, and SGPT. A platelet count below 100,000/mm³ is the chief sign of a hematologic disturbance.

TSS may resemble Rocky Mountain spotted fever, leptospirosis, and measles (including atypical measles) because of the fever, rash, conjunctivitis, myalgia, headache, and depressed sensorium. Hepatic abnormalities in leptospirosis and the clotting disturbances in Rocky Mountain spotted fever also resemble those in TSS. The leukopenia of measles is an important differential point because almost all cases of TSS have a leukocytosis. Rocky Mountain spotted fever is a problem only in endemic areas where it can be suspected from a history of tick bites and finding a tick on the body. The blood leukocyte count is also helpful in nonicteric leptospirosis because it is not elevated as it is in TSS. Aseptic meningitis in most cases of leptospirosis may also distinguish it from TSS.

Two other newly recognized entities have presented diagnostic problems in patients with TSS. One of these is Kawasaki disease (Chapter 201), in which the fever, conjunctival hyperemia, palmar erythema, and skin desquamation are all suggestive of TSS. The two are differentiated by the absence of myalgia, hypotension, renal failure, and thrombocytopenia in Kawasaki disease. Reye's syndrome is the other recently described disease that has been confused with TSS. The combination of a depressed consciousness and liver disease is common to both conditions and is responsible for the problem in differential diagnosis. Shock, however, is terminal and neurogenic in origin only in Reye's syndrome, and the serum ammonia concentration is normal. The mental obtundation in TSS is usually secondary to reduced cerebral perfusion from shock, and the patients become alert when the blood pressure is restored.

Antistaphylococcal beta-lactamase–resistant antibiotics are used for treatment, although their value is dubious. Instead, the chief measures are intravenous fluids and vasopressor drugs for correcting the hypotension and shock. Corticosteroids are probably beneficial also. Blood transfusions are given for severe gastrointestinal or vaginal hemorrhages, and mechanical ventilation is required for treating respiratory distress. Severe thrombocytopenia is treated with platelet transfusions. Hypokalemia (from diarrhea and steroid therapy) requires potassium replacement for 3 to 5 days. Intravenous bicarbonate is given in order to combat the metabolic acidosis that occurs when lactic acid accumulates during hypoperfusion.

The disease can undoubtedly be eliminated if women stop using tampons. Otherwise, the risk can be lowered by intermittent, instead of continuous, use of tampons. Those brands of tampons, such as the Rely brand, which have been used by most victims of TSS, should be avoided. Although antibiotics are of doubtful efficacy in treatment, antistaphylococcal beta-lactamase resistant drugs can prevent recurrences in some cases. The Center for Disease Control advises that tampons not be used by women who have had an attack of TSS until staphylococci are eradicated from the vagina by antibiotics.

## References

Braude, A., Corbeil, L., Levine, S., Ito, J., and McCutchan, J.: Possible influence of cyclic menstrual changes on resistance to the gonococcus. In Immunobiology of Neisseria gonorrhoeae. Brooks, G. (ed.): Am Soc Microbiol 1978, p. 328.

Dykers, J. R.: Single dose metronidazole for trichomonal vaginitis. N Engl J Med 293:23, 1975.

Hawkins, D. F., Sevitt, L. H., and Fairbrother, P. F.: Management of septic chemical abortion with renal failure. Use of a conservative regimen. N Engl J Med 292:722, 1975.

Hibbard, L. T., Snyder, E. N., and McVann, R. M.: Subgluteal and retropsoal infection in obstetrical practice. Obstet Gynecol 39:137, 1972.

Ledger, W. J.: Postoperative pelvic infections. Clin Obstet Gynecol 12:265, 1969.

McKenna, V., Meadows, J., Brewer, N., Wilson, W., and Perrault, J.: Toxic shock syndrome, a newly recognized entity. Mayo Clinic Proc 55:663, 1980.

Mead, P. B.: Practical applications of antibiotics in prevention and treatment of pelvic infections. J Reprod Med 13:135, 1974.

Miles, M. R., Olsen, L., and Rogers, A.: Recurrent vaginal candidiasis. Importance of an intestinal reservoir. JAMA 238:1836, 1977.

Morbidity Mortality Weekly Report — Follow up on Toxic Shock Syndrome 29:441, 1980.

Pheifer, T. A., Forsyth, P. S., Durfee, M. A., Pollock, H. M., and Holmes, K. K.: Nonspecific vaginitis. Role of *Haemophilus vaginalis* and treatment with metronidazole. N Engl J Med 298:1429, 1978.

Rotheram, E. B., and Schick, S. F.: Nonclostridial anaerobic bacteria in septic abortion. Am J Med 46:80, 1969.

Schaefer, G.: Diagnosis and treatment of female genital tuberculosis. Int Surg 48:240, 1967.

Schlievert, P., Schoettle, D., and Watson, D.: Purification and physicochemical and biological characterization of a staphylococcal pyrogenic exotoxin. Infect Immun 23:609, 1979.

Todd, J., Fishout, M., Kapral, F., and Welch, T.: Toxic shock syndrome associated with phage-group-1 staphylococci. Lancet 2:1116, 1978.

# GONORRHEA AND NONGONOCOCCAL URETHRITIS

# 149

## J. Allen McCutchan, M.D.

Gonorrhea (from the Greek *gonos* [seed] and *rhoia* [a flow]) is a sexually transmitted infection of columnar and transitional epithelia by *Neisseria gonorrhoeae*. Genital infections (cervicitis in women and urethritis in men) may spread by ascending the genital tract or by invading the blood. The syndromes of gonococcal bacteremia are discussed in Chapter 180. Gonococci may directly infect extragenital mucous membranes such as the conjunctiva, pharynx, and rectum. Patients without symptoms may be colonized and can infect others.

Nongonococcal urethritis, a syndrome caused by several sexually transmitted agents, is usually less severe than gonorrhea. It may coexist with gonorrhea and make its appearance as postgonococcal urethritis after gonococci are eliminated by antibiotics. *Chlamydia trachomatis,* which appears to be the major cause of the syndrome, also infects the eyes of adults and the eyes and lungs of neonates by way of the maternal cervix. *Ureaplasma urealyticum,* another candidate agent, is less clearly implicated. *Trichomonas, Candida,* and *Herpes simplex* occasionally cause urethritis, and other unidentified agents may cause some cases.

## ETIOLOGY

### Gonorrhea

*Neisseria gonorrhoeae* is an aerobic, gram-negative diplococcus requiring enriched media and elevated levels of carbon dioxide for growth. Cytochrome oxidase distinguishes *Neisseria* from most Enterobacteriaceae. Colony morphology, growth on selective enriched media containing antibiotics, staining with specific fluorescent antibody, and carbohydrate fermentations distinguish the gonococcus from other *Neisseria* organisms (Chapter 29). Pathogenic *Neisseria,* but not nonpathogens, produce an enzyme that cleaves one of the two subtypes of IgA (IgA$_1$) into Fab and Fc fragments. It is possible, but unproved, that inactivation of mucosal IgA is essential for virulence. Nongonococcal *Neisseria* organisms are frequently found in the pharynx and are rarely isolated from anogenital cultures but do not appear to produce local disease. A detailed discus-sion of the microbiology of the gonococcus is presented in Chapter 29.

The cell wall of the gonococcus is similar to that of other gram-negative bacteria. Several components of its outer membrane appear to contribute to virulence. Pili, which are found on fresh isolates but are difficult to demonstrate in vivo, determine colonial morphology on agar and mediate attachment to mammalian cells. The lipopolysaccharide endotoxin can directly damage tissue and enhance the inflammatory response via interactions with cellular and humoral defenses. A capsule, thus far demonstrated only under special conditions in vitro, may be antiphagocytic, but its chemical or immunologic properties are unknown. Leukocyte association factor, a surface protein, enhances attachment of gonococci to polymorphonuclear leukocytes but not to other cells.

Strain-specific nutritional requirements for amino acids, purines, pyrimidines, and vitamins have been used to type gonococci (auxotyping). Dependence on arginine, hypoxanthine, and uracil or on proline characterizes many strains isolated from asymptomatic and bacteremic infections. These strains show a geographic distribution that parallels the incidence of these syndromes. This auxotype may identify a clone of unusual virulence and may help to account for the more frequent development of bacteremia in asymptomatic carriers.

### Nongonococcal Urethritis

*Chlamydia trachomatis* is a strict intracellular bacterium (see Chap. 52). Certain serogroups cause lymphogranuloma venereum (see Chap. 152), and others cause nongonococcal urethritis (NGU). The evidence that *Chlamydia* causes NGU is as follows: (1) *Chlamydia* is more frequently isolated from men with NGU than controls, (2) there is an acute antibody response in men with *Chlamydia*-positive NGU (Holmes et al., 1975), (3) *Chlamydia* causes urethritis in nonhuman primates, and finally, (4) when mixed gonococcal and chlamydial infections are treated with penicillin, *Chlamydia* organisms persist and are associated with a high incidence of postgonococcal urethritis (Bowie et al., 1977). When patients with NGU are treated with sulfisoxazole (active against *Chlamydia* but not *Ureaplasma*), response is common in *Chlamydia*-positive, *Ureaplasma*-negative cases, but is less frequent in *Ureaplasma*-positive, *Chlamydia*-negative cases. Aminocyclitols (active against *Ureaplasma* but not *Chlamydia*) cure *Ureaplasma*-positive, *Chlamydia*-negative cases but not *Chlamydia*-positive, *Ureaplasma*-negative cases. These studies suggest a role for both *Ureaplasma* and *Chlamydia* in NGU, but the role of *Ureaplasma* remains controversial. About 20 per cent of cases are negative for both organisms, do not respond well to antibiotics, and have not yielded a likely pathogen.

## PATHOGENESIS

### Gonorrhea

During transmission, gonococci are deposited with normal flora and genital secretions on the genital mucosa. To survive in the male urethra, they must avoid being washed out or killed by urine. In the cervix and vagina gonococci must survive hydrogen ion and other inhibitory products of the normal flora. The inhibitory effect of vaginal and urethral flora and of urine is well documented, and carriage of inhibitory lactobacilli in the endocervix has been correlated with resistance to gonorrhea (Saigh et al., 1978).

The susceptible columnar epithelium of the urethra, endocervix, or deeper genital tissues is invaded after gonococci penetrate the mucus and attach to epithelial cells. The major inflammatory response in gonorrhea occurs in the submucosa. Organisms apparently penetrate the intact mucosa before much inflammation begins, elicit an intense polymorphonuclear leukocyte response, and then destroy the overlying mucosa (Harkness, 1948). Experimental infection of the isolated human fallopian tube shows that gonococci adhere to specific appendages of the mucus-secreting epithelial cells of women but not females of other species, are phagocytosed by these cells, and are then passed into the submucosa through and between them. They disrupt ciliary activity by means of a soluble toxin but do not attach to ciliated cells, and can severely damage tissues in the absence of an inflammatory response (Ward et al., 1974; McGee et al., 1978).

The mechanism by which gonococci ascend the genital tract is unknown. Their attachment to sperm is one mechanism of transport. The gonococcal toxin (probably endotoxin) rapidly immobilizes cilia, thus preventing them from removing the gonococci from the fallopian tubes.

The intense submucosal inflammation in gonorrhea produces an exudate containing polymorphonuclear leukocytes (PMN) and gonococci. Some PMN concentrate many gonococci in their cytoplasm either within individual phagosomes or, less commonly, as large clusters within a single phagosome. Most gonococci within PMN are rapidly killed, but some may escape destruction or even reproduce within the phagocytes (Veale et al., 1977). Acquired opsonizing antibody that increases phagocytosis of gonococci by human PMNs can be demonstrated in the sera of prostitutes (Bisno et al., 1975).

Despite the antibody response to gonococci, infection does not produce immunity. Treated patients can acquire the same strain from their untreated sexual partners. Before antibiotic treatment became available, men with prolonged untreated infections commonly had multiple episodes of gonorrhea, presumably caused by different strains. Possible reasons for the ineffective immune response in patients with gonorrhea are treatment, antigenic variation among strains, and short-lived immunity. Furthermore, gonococci growing in vivo show a resistance to both phagocytosis and serum bactericidal activity that is not seen when the same strain is grown on agar (Penn et al., 1977).

### Nongonococcal Urethritis

The pathogenesis of chlamydial infections has been extensively studied in the eye but not in the genital tract. The histopathology of experimental urethritis in nonhuman primates resembles that in human conjunctivitis and cervicitis. Follicular lesions in the eye and urethra contain intraepithelial inclusion bodies typical of *Chlamydia* and are composed of subepithelial collections of macrophages and lymphocytes. Human chlamydial urethritis has a similar follicular appearance, which is distinctly different from the deep mucosal erosions of gonorrhea. Local and systemic antibody responses occur, but their role in immunity is not clear. Recurrent infections are common in some men, others remain asymptomatic during prolonged carriage, and still others resist infection. The reasons for this variable response are not known.

## CLINICAL SYNDROMES

### Genital Infection in Men

Urethritis is the most common gonococcal infection in men, but it is exceeded in frequency by nongonococcal urethritis (NGU) in some groups. Gonococcal urethritis can be clinically distinguished from NGU in most cases (Jacobs and Kraus, 1975). After an incubation period of two to five days typical acute anterior gonococcal urethritis presents with severe dysuria, purulent discharge, and a positive gram stain of urethral pus (typical diplococci within polymorphonuclear leukocytes) (Fig. 1). In nongonococcal urethritis, dysuria is usually less severe and more chronic, discharge is mucoid and scant, and the exudate has no diplococci in the Gram stain. Less common symptoms of either form of urethritis are frequency of urination, urgency, genital itching, inguinal adenitis, and fever. Age, marital status, sexual history, and history of gonorrhea or urethritis do not aid in separating these syndromes. In the United States and Britain, NGU is more common in whites than in blacks and in those of high socioeconomic status, but the reason for this difference is unknown.

Despite these differences in typical signs and symptoms, however, in certain patients NGU may be severely painful and purulent, and gonococci may colonize the urethra without producing symptoms. The importance of asymptomatic colonization of the male urethra by gonococci has only recently been appreciated (Handsfield et al., 1974). Asymptomatic men can transmit gonor-

rhea and may become symptomatic after prolonged carriage. For this reason, cultures of male contacts of infected women should be made (negative Gram stain does not exclude asymptomatic colonization), and the men should be treated if the culture is positive or follow-up is not assured.

Gonococcal and nongonococcal urethritis may coexist. When gonorrhea is treated with drugs that do not eliminate *Chlamydia,* about one third of patients develop recurrent urethritis two to three weeks later. Most cases of postgonococcal urethritis occur in men who harbor *Chlamydia* and whose postgonococcal disease responds to antichlamydial antibiotics. Some cases of postgonococcal urethritis are not associated with *Chlamydia.*

Untreated gonococcal anterior urethritis reaches a symptomatic peak in two to three weeks, but it may persist for several months and may relapse. Local extension to the posterior urethra, periurethral glands, prostate, seminal vesicles, and epididymis is common in patients with untreated disease but is rare in promptly treated cases. Complications of ascending infec-

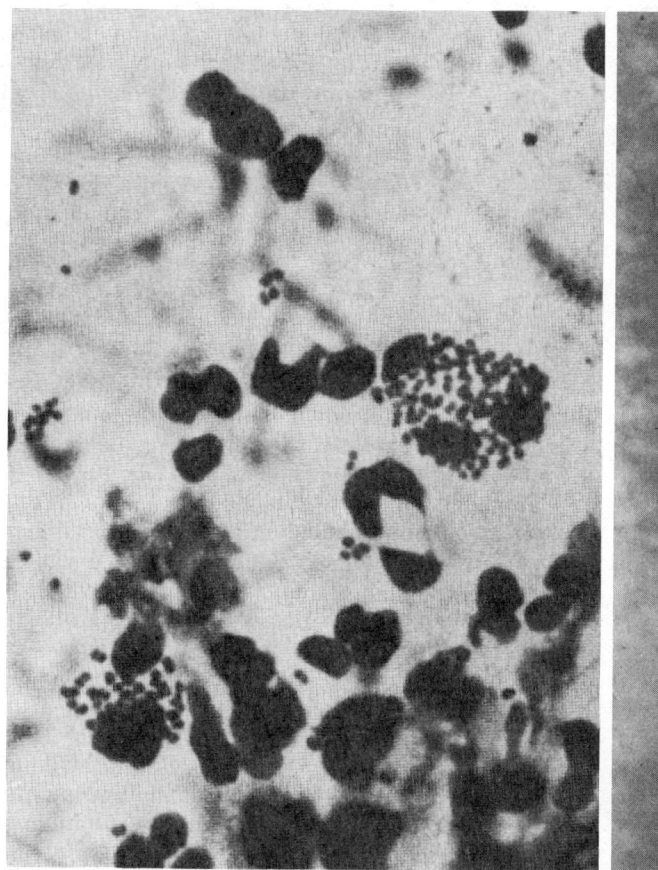 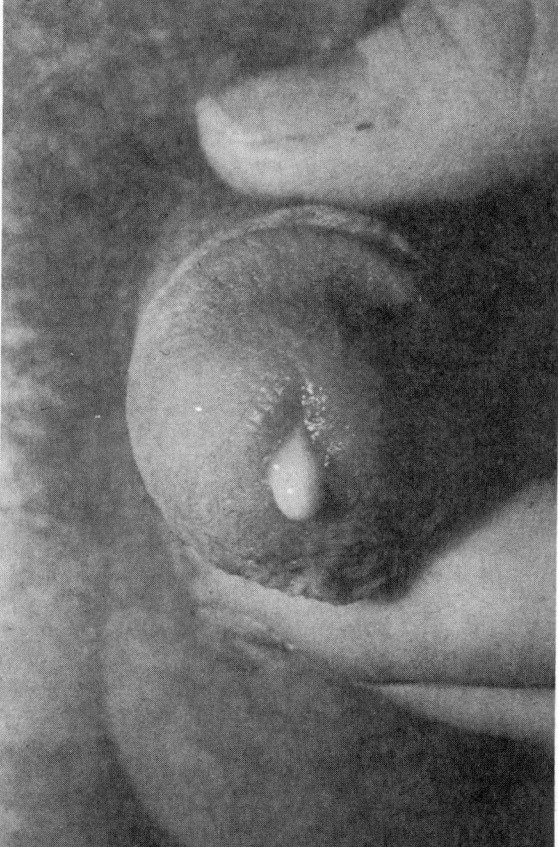

**FIGURE 1.** *Right panel — Spontaneous appearance of thick, purulent exudate at the urethral meatus is characteristic of gonococcal urethritis, but uncommon in nongonococcal urethritis. Left panel — Gram stain of urethral pus from gonorrhea shows many polymorphonuclear neutrophils, some containing ingested gram-negative diplococci. (Reprinted with permission from Wisdom, A.: Color Atlas of Venereology, Chicago, Year Book Medical Publishers, Inc., 1973.)*

tion include urethral stricture and sterility. The role of gonorrhea and the agents of nongonococcal urethritis in epididymitis and prostatitis is not clear. Cultures of epididymal aspirates from young men with acute epididymitis commonly grow chlamydiae but only rarely grow gonococci; those from older men grow coliform bacteria. Acute and chronic prostatitis is rarely associated with viable gonococci in prostatic secretions. Organisms that stain with fluorescent gonococcal antiserum but do not grow in culture are found in the prostatic secretions of 67 per cent of patients with cured gonorrhea long after treatment and in 10 per cent of patients with chronic prostatitis.

## Genital Infections in Women

Although many women with uncomplicated gonorrhea have no symptoms, the majority are symptomatic (McCormick et al., 1977). Undue emphasis on the lack of symptoms in women has probably resulted from studies of women identified by tracing them as contacts or by screening. The primary site of infection is usually the endocervix with secondary infection or colonization of the urethra and rectum. Endocervical gonorrhea may produce increased or purulent vaginal secretions, or menorrhagic or intermenstrual bleeding. Urethritis gives rise to dysuria, urinary frequency, and urgency. Despite frequent colonization of the rectum, symptomatic proctitis is uncommon. Infection of the paraurethral (Skene's) glands simulates urethritis. Acute Bartholin's duct infection usually presents as a unilateral, exquisitely tender mass lateral to the introitus.

Gonococci ascend the genital tract in women to infect the fallopian tubes and pelvic peritoneum. This most common complication (10 to 17 per cent) of gonorrhea (often called pelvic inflammatory disease or salpingitis) occurs more frequently in women who have intrauterine devices or a history of prior attacks, but rarely occurs during pregnancy. Acute salpingitis usually begins with diffuse pelvic pain and tenderness, fever, malaise, and, infrequently, vomiting. Tenderness may be lateralized and simulate appendicitis, ruptured ectopic pregnancy, or ovulation pain. Examination for pain on cervical movement and Gram stain of urethral, endocervical, or rectal smears may help to confirm the diagnosis. Subacute salpingitis causes prolonged or recurrent attacks of pelvic pain and tenderness usually associated with episodic low-grade fever and menstrual disturbances. The intensity of pain and tenderness varies widely with time and among patients. Bilateral enlargement or thickening of the fallopian tubes is characteristic. Symptoms may simulate urinary tract, bowel, or lower back diseases. Chronic salpingitis is usually preceded by acute

or subacute attacks but may appear de novo with sterility, ectopic pregnancy, or as asymptomatic thickening or abscess formation in the adnexal regions.

In any form of salpingitis, gonococci may not be recovered, and mixtures of anaerobic and aerobic vaginal flora may be found instead (Eschenbach et al., 1975). The role of gonococci in cases of pelvic inflammatory disease from which other organisms are cultured is not clear. Experimental infection of human fallopian tubes by gonococci in vitro disrupts the function of the ciliated cells that maintain mucus flow toward the uterus. This damage to cilia could allow the normal vaginal flora to ascend and replace the gonococcus, which would explain why gonococci are most frequently cultured in acute salpingitis and diminish as symptoms continue (Lip and Burgoyne, 1966). Salpingitis causes sterility and ectopic pregnancy by obstructing the fallopian tubes. Sterility occurs in at least 20 per cent of women treated for salpingitis.

Of the agents of nongonococcal urethritis, *Chlamydia trachomatis* and *Herpes simplex* cause cervicitis and *Trichomonas* causes vaginitis. It appears that chlamydial infection is usually asymptomatic in women but may play a role in salpingitis. Six of 20 fallopian tube cultures obtained at laparoscopy in Swedish women with acute salpingitis grew chlamydiae (Mardh, 1977). Definition of the role of *Chlamydia* in salpingitis awaits further histologic and serologic study.

## Anorectal Gonorrhea

Gonococci infect the rectum during penoanal contact in women and male homosexuals or by secondary spread from the endocervix in women (Klein et al., 1977). The stratified squamous epithelium of the anus withstands invasion, but the columnar epithelium of the rectum becomes inflamed and friable. Mucopurulent or bloody discharge may occur, but most patients remain asymptomatic. Acute symptoms of proctitis (severe burning, tenesmus, or purulent discharge) are unusual (2 to 5 per cent) and even mild symptoms (itching, mucoid discharge, painful defecation, and constipation) are uncommon (< 10 per cent).

Proctoscopic examination reveals mucosal pus in more than half of patients, rectal erythema, and friability without ulcerations. Other causes of venereally acquired proctitis include primary and secondary syphilis, lymphogranuloma venereum, granuloma inguinale, and amebiasis. Complications are rare in the postantibiotic era but include strictures, anal fistulas, and perianal abscesses.

## Pharyngeal Gonorrhea

Gonococcal pharyngitis is a disease of women and homosexual men who practice fellatio. Most carriers are asymptomatic, but pharyngitis, tonsillitis, and gingivitis have been ascribed to the gonococcus. Among patients with gonorrhea in other sites, about 20 per cent of homosexual men and 10 per cent of heterosexual women harbor gonococci in the pharynx. Gonococci disseminate in the blood more frequently from the pharynx than from other sites, but gonococci in the throat are rarely a source of transmission to sexual partners (Wiesner et al., 1973).

## Gonococcal Perihepatitis
## (Fitz-Hugh–Curtis syndrome)

The association of acute, severe, pleuritic, right upper abdominal pain with salpingitis or cervical gonorrhea has led clinicians to formulate the concept of gonococcal perihepatitis. This clinical syndrome is accompanied by exudative peritonitis (early) and "violin string" adhesions (late) involving Glisson's capsule, as seen at surgery or laparoscopy. Despite many attempts, however, gonococci have not been cultured from the peritoneum. Although not proven by culture to be caused by gonococci, a diagnosis of perihepatitis may spare the patient an exploratory laparotomy and warrants treatment with penicillin. Perihepatitis simulates a variety of hepatic and biliary tract diseases with hepatomegaly, mild elevation of liver enzymes, leukocytosis, and elevated erythrocyte sedimentation rate (Litt and Cohen, 1978). Pleural effusions, hepatic friction rubs, and even transient nonvisualization of the gallbladder occur infrequently in perihepatitis. Clinical evidence of salpingitis is usually but not invariably present, and rare cases have been reported in men (see Chap. 180). Residual pain after medical therapy has been relieved by lysis of adhesions through the laparoscope (Reichert and Valle, 1976).

## Gonococcal Conjunctivitis

Conjunctivitis in neonates is most often caused by the gonococcus but also by *Chlamydia*, staphylococci, *Haemophilus,* and *Moraxella.* Neonatal gonorrheal ophthalmia appears three to seven days postpartum, usually as a bilateral, profuse, and purulent conjunctivitis. If the conjunctival sac becomes sealed by dried exudate, the trapped pus may invade the cornea to produce keratitis or panophthalmitis (Thatcher and Pettit, 1971). These serious sequelae are responsible for legislation requiring prophylaxis at delivery in many countries. Instillation of 1 per cent silver nitrate after swabbing the eyes (method of Crede) is the safest and most effective prophylactic technique.

Prophylactic local antibiotics or careful surveillance followed by specific diagnosis and treatment of the child and mother have also been successful. The latter method has the advantage of detecting gonorrhea in the mother but risks the vision of children who escape surveillance. Children or adults can be infected by autoinoculation, sexual activity, laboratory accidents, or use of contaminated urine as a folk remedy for other forms of conjunctivitis.

## Gonorrhea in Children

Aside from ophthalmia neonatorum, vulvovaginitis is the most common form of gonorrhea in prepubescent children (Barrett-Connor, 1973). Unlike the stratified squamous epithelium of the adult vagina, the immature vaginal and vulvar epithelium in girls is readily infected. Although fomites and nonsexual intimacy have been implicated, most cases result from sexual abuse by adult relatives. The medicolegal implications of this diagnosis require careful bacteriologic confirmation.

Painful inflammation and purulent or bloody discharge from the vulva and vagina are the most common symptoms, but associated urethritis, pelvic peritonitis, and proctitis also occur. Differential diagnosis includes thread worm (*Enterobius* or *Oxyuris*) infestations, shigellosis, or candidiasis. Boys and girls may also acquire the other syndromes of adult gonorrhea (Nelson et al., 1976). In all such cases other family members should be investigated for gonorrhea and child abuse.

## DIAGNOSIS

Gonococci can be found rapidly in Gram-stained specimens or by fluorescent antibody staining. Positive Gram stains show typical diplococci within polymorphonuclear leukocytes. Results of Gram staining correlate well with cultures from men with urethritis but are often falsely negative in specimens from the endocervix and are of no value in rectal or pharyngeal disease. Fluorescent antibody staining is technically demanding and has been used most successfully to find rare organisms in joint fluids and skin lesions of patients with gonococcemia.

Culture of gonococci requires careful specimen collection and preservation during transport. Specimens should be collected on bacteriologic loops or nontoxic swabs because cotton and other materials may contain inhibitors. Urethritis may be diagnosed by collecting urethral exudate or by culturing urinary sediment. When direct inoculation onto culture media is impossible, swabs should be placed in a transport medium appropriate to the time in transport and the environmental temperature. Cultivation and identification of *N. gonorrhoeae* require enriched and selective media. Because gonococci are inhibited by normal microbial flora, antibiotics should be incorporated into culture media. A combination of vancomycin (for gram-positive bacteria), colistin, and trimethoprim (for gram-negative bacilli), and nystatin (for commensal fungi) have improved the yield from heavily contaminated areas such as the rectum, pharynx, and cervix. Because normal flora and nonpathogenic *Neisseria* organisms are suppressed on chocolate agar containing antibiotics (Thayer-Martin media), the growth of characteristic small translucent colonies that are strongly oxidase-positive and composed of gram-negative diplococci allows presumptive diagnosis of *N. gonorrhoeae*. The need to differentiate the gonococcus from nonpathogenic *Neisseria* strains or meningococci depends on the site cultured and the medicolegal and social consequences of the diagnosis. Other *Neisseria* organisms frequently live in the pharynx but are found only infrequently on other mucosal surfaces. Specific identification of the gonococcus can be made by saccharolytic reactions or by fluorescence with highly absorbed antiserum. The gonococcus produces acid from glucose only and the meningococci does so from both glucose and maltose. Nonpathogenic *Neisseria* organisms have other saccharolytic patterns.

Diagnosis of nongonococcal urethritis can be made clinically but must be supported by negative cultures for gonococci and objective evidence of urethritis. Polymorphonuclear leukocytes in urethral discharge (>5/oil immersion field) or in sediment from the first 10 ml of overnight urine (>15/high-dry [×400] field) supports the diagnosis of urethritis. If there are no gram-negative diplococci on Gram stain and no signs or symptoms of prostatitis, a presumptive diagnosis of NGU can be made. Cultures for *Herpes, Chlamydia,* and *Ureaplasma* and cytology for chlamydial inclusion bodies may be useful but are not widely available. Examination of wet mounts for *Trichomonas* and *Candida* is unnecessary unless antibiotics fail.

## EPIDEMIOLOGY AND GEOGRAPHIC VARIATION

Patients with gonorrhea are typically male, young, urban, and promiscuous. The male predominance (about 3:1) reflects the greater frequency of asymptomatic disease in women, so that fewer infected women are identified. When women are screened thoroughly and contacts are traced carefully, the ratio of men to women falls

dramatically. The relative incidence is also affected by prostitution, which results in a small, highly promiscuous group of women transmitting gonorrhea to a larger group of men, and homosexuality, which allows transfer of infection between men. In the United States, gonorrhea shows a remarkably sharp peak in incidence among those 20 to 24 years old. The increase in cases during the last epidemic (1956–1975) occurred in those under age 24 (Fig. 2). Women tend to contract gonorrhea at a younger age than men (e.g., modal age of 24 in men and 19 in women in Denmark). The higher incidence of gonorrhea reported in cities may reflect better reporting practices in large urban venereal disease clinics as well as real differences in rates. The effect of promiscuity is illustrated by the high rates of gonorrhea among female prostitutes and males with many sex partners.

Gonorrhea and other venereal diseases traditionally increases at times of social upheaval. The two world wars and the wars in Korea, Vietnam, and Bangladesh all resulted in epidemic peaks in those geographic regions. During the past twenty

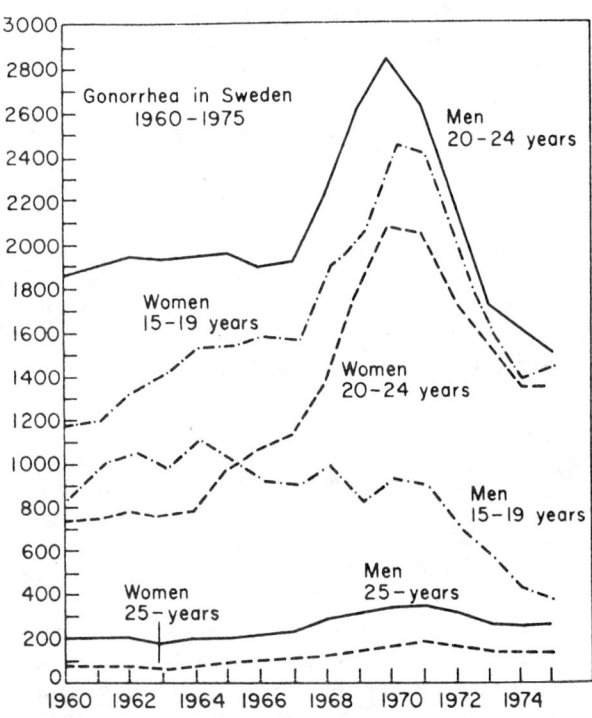

**FIGURE 2.** *Incidence of gonorrhea in Sweden by age groups from 1960 to 1975 (cases per 100,000 population). People under the age of 24 (primarily men 20 to 24 and women 15 to 24) have constituted the major increase in cases. (Reprinted with permission from Kallings, L. O., and Moberg, I.: Gonorrhoea: Epidemiology and Pathogenesis (Skinner, F. A., et al., eds.), London, Academic Press, 1977.)*

years a dramatic increase in gonorrhea has been reported from many countries throughout the world (Fig. 3). There are two causes of this epidemic at a time of relative peace and prosperity: (1) changing sexual mores in the industrialized nations have allowed earlier, more frequent, and more promiscuous sexual activity in young adults, and (2) urbanization and economic immigration in the developing nations have separated people from their spouses and families.

At least two changes in the gonococcus may have contributed to the epidemic. One change is the increased resistance of gonococci to penicillin. This has resulted in increased failure rates with penicillin treatment. The second change is selection of strains that cause asymptomatic disease in men (e.g., AHU auxotypes) by aggressive treatment programs. By remaining asymptomatic and thus untreated, these strains of gonococci continue to spread to female contacts of these colonized men.

The incidence of various forms of gonorrhea, susceptibility to antibiotics, and patterns of spread vary geographically. Physicians must be aware of local factors that could alter diagnosis and therapy. For example, isolates of gonococci from the western Pacific region are less likely to disseminate in the blood, are more resistant to penicillin by two different mechanisms, and are more often acquired from prostitutes than European or American strains (see Chapter 180 for further discussion). The spread of gonococci bearing the plasmid-mediated penicillinase as a marker can be traced to its geographic origin. After two different strains arose simultaneously in West Africa and Southeast Asia in 1976, the West African strain spread to Europe and the Southeast Asian strain spread to the United States. Despite aggressive attempts to control it, the Asian strain appears to be endemic at a low level in the United States, but the West African strain has not become established in Europe. Thus, in the jet age strains acquiring drug resistance may spread rapidly throughout the world but have not replaced conventional strains.

Nongonococcal urethritis (NGU) and gonorrhea (GCU) are found in the same age group and both are frequently carried by asymptomatic female sex partners. Compared to GCU, NGU occurs in men of higher socioeconomic status, in men with fewer sexual partners, and in whites more frequently than in blacks. In the United States NGU is as common as gonorrhea, and in England it is more common. Within the United States there appears to be marked geographic variation in ratios of NGU by region and type of population served by the reporting clinic. In England the number of cases of NGU has increased faster than GCU during the past two decades.

## THERAPY

### Gonococcal Infections

Despite increasing resistance to penicillin over the past 20 years and the recent appearance of plasmid-coded penicillinase conferring high level resistance, penicillins remain the preferred therapy for most gonococcal infections (Table 1). In patients who are allergic to penicillins or harbor penicillinase-producing strains (PPNG), tetracycline, spectinomycin, or cefoxitin are alternatives. Since gonococci are susceptible to many antibiotics, some regimens other than those listed may cure some infections but are not preferred because of efficacy, cost, and side effects.

It is important to consider the reliability of the

**FIGURE 3.** *Incidence per 100,000 population of cases of gonorrhea reported to WHO by 12 European countries and the United States. Problems of reporting make it unlikely that these figures reflect the true incidence. Thus, they cannot be used as a basis for international comparisons but show the increasing incidence in many countries over the past 20 years. (Reprinted with permission — see Figure 2).*

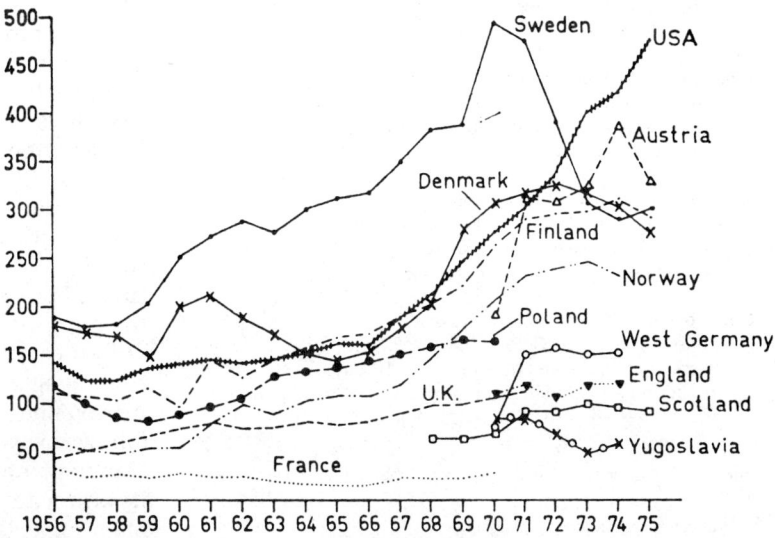

patients, their history of drug intolerance, and the antibiotic susceptibility of the gonococcus in making a selection among the regimens recom-

### TABLE 1.  Therapy of Gonococcal Infections

**UNCOMPLICATED GONOCOCCAL INFECTIONS**
**Single Session, Intramuscular**
A.  Procaine penicillin G 4.8 million units (100,000 units/kg)[a] intramuscularly with probenecid 1.0 g orally
    In patients allergic to penicillin, following treatment failure, or if gonococcus is penicillinase-producing (PPNG), use regimen B or C
B.  Spectinomycin[b] 2 g (40 mg/kg) intramuscularly
C.  Cefoxitin[b] 2 g intramuscularly with probenecid 1.0 g orally

**Single Session, Oral**
D.  Ampicillin[b] 3.5 g (50 mg/kg)[a] or amoxicillin[b] 3.0 g (50 mg/kg)[a] either with probenecid 1.0 g orally

**Multiple Dose, Oral**
E.  Tetracycline 0.5 g (10 mg/kg)[a] orally four times daily for five days (not to be used in pregnancy or in children less than 8 years of age)

**ACUTE SALPINGITIS OR EPIDIDYMITIS**
**Oral**
F.  Tetracycline 0.5 g orally four times daily for ten days
G.  Regimen A or D (above) initially followed by ampicillin or amoxicillin 0.5 g orally four times daily for ten days

**Intravenous**
H.  Aqueous crystalline penicillin G 20 million units intravenously (in six to eight divided doses) until improved followed by regimen G, or
I.  Tetracycline 0.25 g intravenously four times daily (or doxycycline 100 mg every 12 hours) until improved followed by regimen F
    If above regimens are inappropriate because of drug allergy, PPNG, or pregnancy:
J.  Spectinomycin 2 g twice daily for five to seven days
K.  Cefoxitin 1 g intravenously four times daily for ten days

**CONJUNCTIVITIS**
**Prophylaxis in Neonates**
L.  Tetracycline, erythromycin, or 1 per cent silver nitrate ophthalmic preparations in both eyes once immediately postpartum

**Infants Born to Mothers with Gonorrhea**
M.  Aqueous penicillin G 50,000 units intramuscularly or intravenously once postpartum (treat as below if symptoms develop)

**Neonatal Gonococcal Ophthalmia**
N.  Aqueous penicillin G 25,000 units/kg intravenously twice daily for seven days plus saline irrigation of the eyes as needed to maintain drainage

**Gonococcal Conjunctivitis** (child or adult)
O.  Aqueous penicillin G 100,000 units/kg/day intravenously in six to eight divided doses for 7 to 10 days plus irrigation and chloramphenicol (1 per cent ophthalmic) one drop every 5 to 30 minutes initially

---

[a] For children weighing less than 45 kg; larger children can receive adult doses.

[b] Not effective in gonococcal pharyngitis.

mended in Table 1. Tetracycline is cheap and lowers the rate of postgonococcal urethritis, but requires multiple doses and is contraindicated in children under 8 years old and in pregnant women. Since spectinomycin is relatively expensive, it should be reserved for patients with penicillin allergy, treatment failure, or penicillinase-producing gonococci (PPNG). Cefoxitin is painful on intramuscular injection and expensive but, unlike most cephalosporins, is resistant to gonococcal penicillinase and therefore useful in treating strains that are completely resistant to penicillins.

Most patients with gonococcal infections can be treated as outpatients. Patients with salpingitis who appear septicemic, have abscesses, are pregnant, fail to improve, or cannot be treated orally should be hospitalized. Gonococcal conjunctivitis requires hospitalization for intravenous antibiotics and saline lavage to maintain drainage. Patients with perihepatitis are usually hospitalized for observation to rule out more serious liver or biliary tract diseases. Patients with most other infections need no additional therapy, except for epididymitis, which may require scrotal suspension, sitz baths, analgesics, and occasionally bed rest.

The dose of penicillins and tetracyclines used to treat gonorrhea is also adequate for treatment of incubating syphilis, but a serologic test is necessary to exclude older disease that requires more prolonged treatment. All patients treated for gonorrhea should be recultured as a test of cure 7 to 14 days after treatment is completed, and women should be recultured six to eight weeks later. Culture of the rectum, the most likely site of failure in women, as well as the cervix is indicated at follow-up. Proctitis may need longer treatment (three to five days) with oral drugs if the first single-session treatment fails. Symptomatic pharyngitis should not be treated with a single dose of ampicillin, amoxicillin, or spectinomycin, but can be treated with nine tablets of sulfamethoxazole/trimethoprim once daily for five days, if patients are allergic to penicillin. Patients being treated with multiple dose regimens should be warned that they may remain infectious during treatment. Conjunctivitis is highly infectious and requires isolation during the first 24 hours of treatment, frequent irrigation of the eyes, and topical chloramphenicol or tetracycline as well as systemic penicillin.

Two complications of gonococcal therapy aside from drug allergy occasionally occur. Inadvertent intravenous injection of procaine penicillin G is followed by almost immediate development of transient neurologic and cardiorespiratory toxicity (procaine reaction). Patients with syphilis may experience the Herxheimer reaction (see

Chapter 150) after receiving treatment for gonorrhea. Either of these reactions could simulate drug allergy and may produce severe symptoms.

Treatment of asymptomatic sexual contacts of patients with proven or suspected gonorrhea before culture results are known (epidemiologic treatment) is an accepted practice (Judson and Maltz, 1978). This practice is justified by the high likelihood of infection, opportunity for further transmission while awaiting diagnosis, and the inability or unwillingess of patients to return for follow-up. The decision to treat an exposed person should be based not only on the risk of infection as estimated from the nature of and time since last exposure, but also on the certainty of the diagnosis in the contact, the reliability of the patient in abstaining from additional exposures and returning for therapy, and the reliability of cultures. The following patients are usually considered for treatment because of high risk of infection (shown in parentheses): (1) female contacts of men with proven (two thirds) or suspected (one half) gonorrhea, (2) homosexual males with anal exposure to gonococcal urethritis (one half), (3) male contacts of women with suspected or proven gonorrhea (one third), and (4) neonates born to mothers with cervical gonorrhea.

### Nongonococcal Urethritis

The optimal dose and duration of therapy for NGU have not been determined. Tetracyclines give symptomatic relief in doses of 250 mg four times a day for two to three weeks and 500 mg four times a day for one week. Relapse and reinfection occur, and the latter can probably be reduced by simultaneous treatment of sexual partners. Minocycline 100 mg twice a day for one to three weeks appears at least as good as tetracycline at 250 mg four times a day for the same period, but it has vestibular side effects. Erythromycin 500 mg four times a day for 7 to 14 days can be used in pregnancy to treat contacts or in men who cannot take tetracycline. Sulfonamides are active against *C. trachomatis,* and spectinomycin treats *U. urealyticum*, but neither is preferred therapy for NGU or postgonococcal urethritis.

### Undiagnosed Urethritis

Management of men with undiagnosed urethritis depends on Gram stain of urethral exudates. Positive Gram stains warrant treatment of the patients and their contacts for gonorrhea. Patients with negative or equivocal Gram stains should be treated for nongonococcal urethritis. Their sexual partners need culturing and epidemiologic treatment with the same regimen.

### Recurrent Urethritis

Symptoms may recur after standard therapy for urethritis because of treatment failure, reinfection, dual infections, or incorrect diagnosis. Drug-resistant gonococci, failure to complete multiple dose regimens, and reinfection are important causes of recurrent gonococcal urethritis. Postgonococcal urethritis has been discussed in the section on clinical syndromes. If nongonococcal urethritis does not respond, treatment of both the patient and his sexual partner(s) with erythromycin 250 mg every six hours for seven days may be tried. If erythromycin fails to produce a response, prostatitis and other causes of urethritis (*Trichomonas*, condylomas, or urethral strictures or ulcers) should be searched for with smears and urethroscopy. If no other cause is found, a prolonged course of tetracycline (250 mg every six hours for 30 days) cures some patients.

## PREVENTION

Gonorrhea can be prevented by condoms, postcoital antibiotics, or vaginal chemicals, contraceptives, and antibiotics. Because prophylactic antibiotics select for resistant strains, they are self-defeating if applied widely for an extended period, and therefore are not recommended. Most vaginal contraceptives and some intrauterine devices inhibit gonococci and some appear to prevent gonorrhea in women using them, but their impact on the spread of gonorrhea is unknown.

The recent epidemic occurred in several countries where aggressive programs of treatment and contact-tracing were already in operation. For this reason, this traditional approach to prevention needs revision. Immunization of the population at high risk remains attractive and candidate vaccines are being evaluated. Wide use of even a partially effective vaccine could dramatically reduce the high level of disease.

## REFERENCES

Barrett-Connor, E.: Gonorrhea. Curr Probl Pediatr, 3, (11), 1973.

Bisno, A. L., Ofek, I., Beachy, E. H., and Curran, J. W.: Human immunity to *Neisseria gonorrhoeae*: Acquired serum opsonic antibodies. J Lab Clin Med 86:221, 1975.

Bowie, W. R., Wang, S. P., Alexander, E. R., Floyd, J., Forsyth, P. S., Pollock, H. M., Lin, J. L., Buchanan, T. M., and Holmes, K. K.: Etiology of nongonococcal urethritis. J Clin Invest 59:735, 1977.

Eschenbach, D. A., Buchanan, T. M., Polloch, H. M., Forsyth, P. S., Alexander, E. R., Lin, J. S., Wang, S. P., Wentworth, B. B., McCormick, W. M., and Holmes, K. K.: Polymicrobial etiology of active pelvic inflammatory disease. N Engl J. Med 293:166, 1975.

Handsfield, H. H., Lipman, T. O., Harnisch, J. P., Troncha, E., and Holmes, K. K.: Asymptomatic gonorrhea in men. N Engl J Med 290:117, 1974.

Harkness, A. H.: The pathology of gonorrhoeae. Br J Vener Dis 24:137, 1948.

Holmes, K. K., Handsfield, H. H., Wang, S. P., Wentworth, B. B., Turck, M., Anderson, J. B., and Alexander, E. R.: Etiology of non-gonococcal urethritis. N Engl J Med 292:1199, 1975.

Jacobs, N. F., and Kraus, S. J.: Gonococcal and non-gonococcal urethritis in man. Ann Intern Med 82:7, 1975.

Judson, F. M., and Maltz, A. B.: A rational basis for the epidemiological treatment of gonorrhea in a clinic for sexually transmitted diseases. Sex Trans Dis 5:89, 1978.

Klein, E. J., Fisher, L. S., Chow, A. W., and Guze, L. B.: Anorectal gonococcal infection. Ann Intern Med 86:340, 1977.

Lip, J., and Burgoyne, X.: Cervical and peritoneal bacterial flora associated with salpingitis. Obstet Gynecol 28:561, 1966.

Litt, I. F., and Cohen, M. I.: Perihepatitis associated with salpingitis in adolescents. JAMA 240:1253, 1978.

Mardh, P. A., Rīpa, T., Svensson, L., and Westrom, L.: Chlamydia trachomatis infection in patients with acute salpingitis. N Engl J Med 296:1377, 1977.

McCormicK, W. M., Stumacher, R. J., Johnson, K., and Donner, D.: Clinical spectrum of gonococcal infection in women. Lancet 1:1182, 1977.

McGee, Z. A., Melly, M. A., Gregg, G. R., Horn, R. G., Taylor-Robinson, D., Johnson, A. P., and McCutchan, J. A.: Virulence factors of gonococci: Studies using human fallopian tube organ cultures. In

Brooks, G. F., et al. (eds.): Immunobiology of Neisseria gonorrhea. Washington, American Society for Microbiology, 1978, p. 258.

Nelson, J. D., Mohs, E., Dajani, A. S., and Plotkin, S. A.: Gonorrhea in preschool and school-aged children. JAMA 236:1359, 1976.

Penn, C. W., Veale, D. R., and Smith, H.: Selection from gonococci grown in vitro of a colony type with some virulence properties of organisms adapted in vivo. J Gen Microbiol 100:147, 1977.

Reichert, J. A., and Valle, R. F.: Fitz-Hugh-Curtis syndrome. JAMA 236:266, 1976.

Saigh, J. H., Sanders, C. C., and Sanders, W. E.: Inhibition of Neisseria gonorrhoeae by aerobic and facultatively anaerobic components of the endocervical flora: Evidence for a protective effect against infection. Infect Immun 19:704, 1978.

Thatcher, R. W., and Pettit, T. H.: Gonorrheal conjunctivitis. JAMA 215:1494, 1971.

Veale, D. R., Penn, C. W., and Smith, H.: The resistance of gonococci to killing by human phagocytes. In Skinner, F. A., et al. (eds.): Gonorrhea: Epidemiology and Pathogenesis. London, Academic Press, 1977, p. 97.

Ward, M. E., Watt, P. J., and Robertson, J. N.: The human fallopian tube: A laboratory model for gonococcal infection. J Infect Dis 129:650, 1974.

Weisner, P. J., Tronca, E., Bonin, P., Pederson, A. H. B., and Holmes, K. K.: Clinical spectrum of pharyngeal gonococcal infection. N Engl J Med 288:181, 1973.

# 150 SYPHILIS OF THE GENITAL TRACT

## Daniel M. Musher, M.D.

## DEFINITION

Syphilis (originally called the great pox to distinguish it from smallpox, which was then a less frightening disease) is an infection caused by *Treponema pallidum*. The ulcerated papule that arises at the initial site of treponemal inoculation is called a primary syphilitic chancre. Clinically unrecognized dissemination of treponemes from this primary site results in widespread cutaneous lesions that are called "secondary," although they may appear when the initial syphilitic chancre is still present, or develop in patients in whom a primary lesion has gone unrecognized. Disseminated lesions do not progress to form chancres because, by the time of their appearance, the patient has developed some degree of protective immunity. Other organs such as mucous membranes, lymph nodes, bones, joints, eyes, and central nervous system may also be involved. Without treatment, the lesions of secondary syphilis resolve spontaneously, but relapses occur in up to 20 per cent of patients. The resulting asymptomatic state is called early latent syphilis. After 1 year of latency, relapses no longer occur, and late latency is said to be present. The diagnosis of late latent syphilis is made as a matter of public health policy in an asymptomatic person who gives a positive reaction to VDRL and fluo-

rescent treponema antibody (FTA-ABS) tests, whose cerebrospinal fluid is normal (see below), and who has not received definitive treatment for syphilis. Primary and secondary infection and latency that is known to be of less than 1 year's duration together comprise early syphilis. Late syphilis becomes clinically apparent after months or years of latency in about one-third of those who contract early syphilis and do not receive adequate treatment, although a greater percentage have abnormalities at autopsy. Late syphilis is often divided into: (1) "benign" infection, in which the disease is limited to granulomatous involvement of skin, bones, cartilage, soft tissue, and viscera; (2) cardiovascular syphilis; and (3) neurosyphilis. Congenital syphilis is acquired by the fetus when *T. pallidum* crosses the placenta, usually during the second half of pregnancy, although recent evidence suggests that this may occur in the first trimester as well. Endemic syphilis or bejel, a nonvenereally acquired infection caused by *T. pallidum*, occurs in The Middle East, Africa, and rarely in Middle and Eastern Europe. The early age of acquisition of bejel by nonvenereal routes, together with malnutrition and primitive living conditions, is probably responsible for the differences (noted in Chapter 215) between endemic and sporadic syphilis, although actual differences between the pathogenicity of the causative organisms can be demonstrated in laboratory animals.

## ETIOLOGY

*Treponema pallidum* is a highly motile, "spiral" or "coiled" organism in the order Spirochetales, an order that includes *Spirocheta, Treponema, Borrelia,* and *Leptospira. T. pallidum* is a natural pathogen only for man, although infection has been produced experimentally in primates and a few laboratory animals. With the unusual exception of laboratory accidents (including transfusion of blood), all cases are acquired by direct contact among human beings.

## PATHOGENESIS AND PATHOLOGY

*T. pallidum* gains entrance to the body as a result of intimate, usually sexual, contact presumably through tiny breaks in squamous or mucous epithelium. As with other infections, immediately after inoculation, some organisms lodge in the dermis, while others escape to draining lymph nodes. During the ensuing weeks, treponemes proliferate locally in the dermis and continue to escape into the bloodstream; this spirochetemia sets the stage for disseminated and perhaps for late forms of syphilis, as is discussed below. After a 14- to 21-day incubation period, a red painless papule appears at the site of inoculation; within a few days, it ulcerates, producing the typical syphilitic chancre. Histologic examination of the papule reveals a relatively acellular central area rich in mucopolysaccharides, surrounded by an infiltrate consisting of degranulated polymorphonuclear leukocytes and lymphocytes. As the lesion evolves, the central area undergoes necrosis, and plasma cells and macrophages come to predominate at the periphery. Endothelial proliferation and perivascular infiltration by lymphocytes and plasma cells are characteristically present. Syphilitic chancres heal spontaneously within 3 to 6 weeks. The mechanism for healing is obscure; some kind of local immunity probably plays a role since disseminated (secondary) lesions appear and progress while the primary lesion is regressing. These disseminated lesions result from spirochetemia that has occurred during the incubation period and/or pretreatment stage of the chancre. Three or more weeks elapse between deposition of *T. pallidum* in the dermis and emergence of secondary lesions; perhaps their appearance in "crops" results from heavy hematogenous seeding at various times in the course of primary infection or from reseeding during secondary infection. The

curious progression of infection despite the presence of specific antitreponemal antibody and other immunologic aspects of the infection are discussed elsewhere in this textbook and reviewed in depth in Schell and Musher, 1981. The tendency of syphilis to produce skin lesions may relate to heat sensitivity of *T. pallidum* and their preference for cooler areas; in experimental animals, disseminated skin lesions appear only in areas that have been shaved. Although primary infection causes lesions that ulcerate, secondary lesions do not, presumably because some degree of systemic immunity has already developed. Except for this difference, the histology of disseminated lesions is quite similar to that of syphilitic chancres.

Late syphilitic lesions have a granulomatous appearance, often with giant cells, although only infrequently are palisading cells seen at the periphery. Their pathogenesis is unknown; the presence of treponemes has not been conclusively demonstrated. Some authors have stated that late lesions develop because of reinoculation of *T. pallidum* into a person with latent syphilis. This concept is supported by results of experimental studies in syphilitic volunteers. However, lesions occur on the extremities and trunk far more frequently than in genital or oral areas. Moreover, lesions in bones and viscera could not arise in this fashion. Others believe that these granulomas arise as a result of an immune response to treponemal antigen that has persisted since treponemal dissemination, but this hypothesis is unproven. Support is derived from studies that show that delayed hypersensitivity to preparations made from *T. pallidum* begins to appear late in secondary syphilis, just before the onset of latency, and is uniformly present in late syphilitics. However, the question of why one particular area should retain antigen while other areas do not remains unanswered.

## CLINICAL MANIFESTATIONS

### Primary Syphilis

Examination at the time a lesion first appears usually reveals one or more painless papules, 0.5 to 2 cm in diameter. Within a few days, these papules ulcerate, producing syphilitic chancres that are usually round but may be elongated, depending on their relation to tissue lines (Chapel, 1978). Lymph nodes that drain the infected area are enlarged. Most lesions in men occur on the penis (Fig. 1) and in women on the labia, fourchette, and cervix, although lesions frequently occur elsewhere on the genitalia, in the mouth, and in other erogenous zones. Chancres in the anus, which are particularly common in homosex-

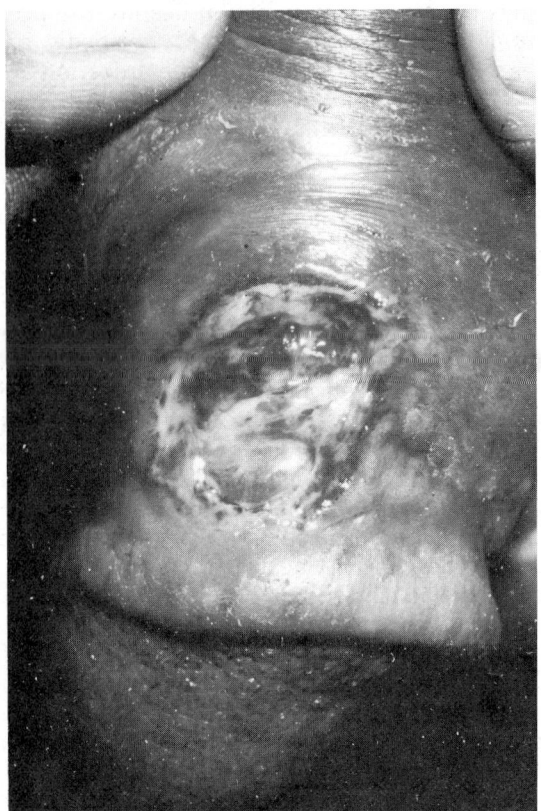

**FIGURE 1.**  *Chancre of penis.*

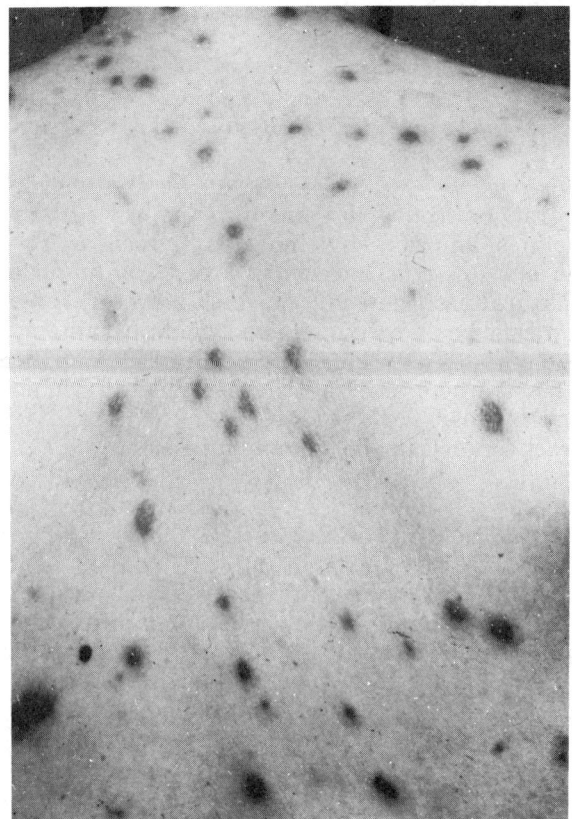

**FIGURE 2.**  *Papular lesions of secondary syphilis.*

ual men, may cause irritation or pain on defecation, and feces may be blood-streaked. Because they are usually nontender, anal chancres may be overlooked, in which case a diagnosis of primary infection is not made at all. In fact, most diagnoses of active syphilis in women and homosexual men are made in the secondary stage.

### Secondary Syphilis

The skin involvement of the secondary stage of syphilis is discussed in greater detail in Chapter 214. The initial finding is usually a diffuse macular eruption that may involve the trunk or occur everywhere except for the face, hands, and feet. This eruption may be evanescent, in which case papulosquamous lesions develop a few days later, or it may progress directly into the papulosquamous stage. The appearance of well-demarcated papules that occur symmetrically nearly everywhere on the body except the face, but involving palms and soles, is characteristic of disseminated syphilis (Fig. 2). The lesions may be smooth, follicular, or scaly in texture and dusky red or brownish in color. Vesicles are said not to occur, although vesicular-pustular lesions may well have been the rule centuries ago when syphilis was called the great pox. Mucosal lesions or

plaques are not uncommon. Circular lesions may appear on the face in dark-skinned individuals. Condylomata are large plaquelike vegetative lesions occurring in warm, moist areas that represent a confluent area of syphilitic infection. These result from local spread of *T. pallidum,* either from primary or secondary lesions. Diffuse lymphadenopathy is often present in patients who have disseminated syphilis. Fever, malaise, headache, sore throat, and arthralgias may occur. Periostitis, which is usually asymptomatic, may be found in one-third of cases if bone scans are routinely done; the skull, tibia, sternum, and ribs are most frequently involved. Radiographs show osteolytic areas without sclerosis (Dismukes et al., 1976). Up to 10 per cent of patients with disseminated syhilis may have abnormal liver function. In the occasional case of clinical hepatitis, it is difficult to exclude the coincidental occurrence of viral hepatitis, especially in a patient who is likely to contract syphilis (Fehér et al., 1975). (See Chapter 141.) Iritis, anterior uveitis, and meningitis also occur in secondary syphilis. The nephrotic syndrome may be seen and is presumably due to glomerular deposits of treponemal antigen and antibody. Rarely, hematuria may be a prominent finding. Patchy alopecia of the scalp results from syphilitic involvement of hair follicles.

### Late Syphilis

Of a large group of patients who were observed with untreated syphilis for many years, clinical findings of late benign syphilis developed in 15 per cent, cardiovascular syphilis in 10 per cent, and neurosyphilis in 7 per cent (Clark and Danbolt, 1964). Cardiovascular syphilis has been present at autopsy in up to half of untreated syphilitics. Most patients with late benign syphilis have only involvement of skin; this subject and neurosyphilis are discussed in Chapters 214 and 161, respectively. Late syphilis of the bone most commonly affects tibia, fibula, clavicle, and skull, although any bone or multiple areas may be involved (Fig. 3) (Kampmeier, 1964). The symptoms of pain and swelling, which are nearly always present, are consistent with the periosteal location of the granulomatous reaction. Roentgenograms reveal periosteal thickening that may be accompanied by erosion and/or an osteoblastic response of the underlying bone. Syphilis of the tibia or fibula with ulceration of overlying soft tissue often causes symptoms and signs suggestive of chronic venous stasis. Destruction of cartilage plays an important part in determining the clinical appearance of the lesions. The bones of the nose and hard palate are often destroyed by subperiosteal gummas. These are localized, dull red tumors that break down in the center and perforate. The entire bridge of the nose is often lost (Fig. 4).

Gummas of the joints are frequently found in the company of syphilitic osteomyelitis as pain-

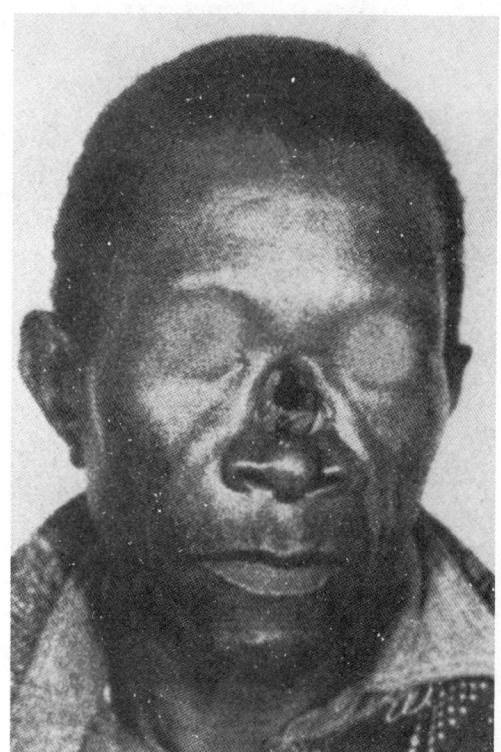

**FIGURE 4.** *Gumma of the nose with perforation and destruction of the septum. (From Howles, J. K.: Synopsis of Clinical Syphilis. St. Louis, C. V. Mosby Co., 1943.)*

less swellings of the knee or sternoclavicular joints. The joint gummas may take the form of single tumors or diffuse infiltrations. A diffuse gummatous synovitis causes thickening of the synovium, extensive effusion, and destruction of the cartilage. Gummas of the joint must be distinguished from Charcot's joint, which is due to neurotropic disturbances following nerve injury in tabes dorsalis, and is not caused by treponemal infection of the joint. The knee is most often affected. It becomes suddenly swollen from serous effusion and bent backward from weight bearing on an unstable joint. Although the bone is destroyed, the patient can walk on it without pain. Charcot's joint may also occur in the hips, shoulders, spine, and elbows (Fig. 5).

Visceral gummas occur mainly in the liver and testes. Single gummas of the liver are usually in the left lobe. Gummas become scars, and multiple gummas produce hepar lobatum, in which the liver is divided into multiple lobes, or partitions, by deep fissures that represent former gummas. Numerous small gummas of the entire liver may cause widespread dense scars, which separate nodular projections that cover the surface of the shrunken organ and resemble Laennec's cirrhosis. Such patients have portal obstruction with ascites. The symptoms depend on the number and

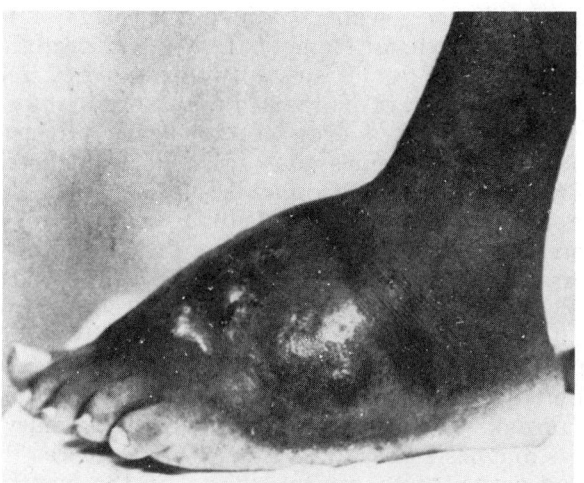

**FIGURE 3.** *Gummas of the bones in the foot resembling mycetoma. (From Howles, J. K.: Synopsis of Clinical Syphilis. St. Louis, C. V. Mosby Co., 1943.)*

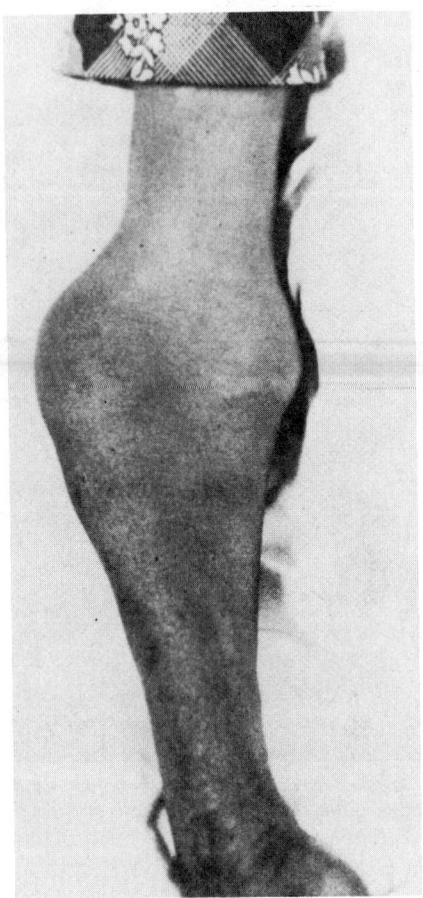

**FIGURE 5.** *Charcot's joint of the elbow. (From Howles, J. K.: Synopsis of Clinical Syphilis. St. Louis, C. V. Mosby Co., 1943.)*

size of the lesions. Fever, pain, and jaundice may occur, and the liver is occasionally enlarged on physical examination.

Syphilis of the testicle usually causes diffuse interstitial fibrosis and is called the "billiard ball" testis because it contracts into a round, hard mass. Lesions of the testes are often accompanied by painful nodules of the spermatic cords and painless gummatous swellings of the epididymis. A hydrocoele may be the first sign of syphilitic epididymitis.

Late syphilis of the uterus, fallopian tubes, and ovaries is so rare, if it ever occurs, that it is of no significance.

In the rectum, gummatous infiltration usually starts just above the anus as smooth, round, submucous lesions that measure up to 2 to 3 cm in diameter. These spread, ulcerate, and rupture, sometimes producing rectovesical or rectovaginal fistulas.

Syphilis of the stomach is rare and may imitate peptic ulcer or carcinoma of the stomach. This variability in clinical syndrome is explained by corresponding differences in the pathologic processes, which vary from one or more gummas to ulcerating nodules and diffuse fibrosis resembling linitis plastica. The pylorus is most frequently involved, and there may be gummas in the liver simultaneously. Acid secretion may be reduced or absent even after injection of histamine. A therapeutic trial of penicillin may be a valuable diagnostic test.

Syphilitic aortitis is most frequently asymptomatic; it may be recognized radiologically by calcifications in the ascending aorta or at autopsy by the shaggy appearance of the proximal aorta (Heggtveit, 1964). Endarteritis of the vasa vasorum with resulting medial necrosis is thought to be responsible. Aneurysm of the ascending aorta used to be relatively common, presenting as a bulging, pulsatile mass in the thorax or neck. Involvement of aortic valve cusps may cause aortic insufficiency, which has to be differentiated from that due to any other cause. The coronary artery ostia may be involved, causing symptoms of ischemia or, rarely, frank infarction. Interestingly, these complications do not occur in patients who contract their infection before the age of 15 years.

## DIAGNOSIS

### Clinical Diagnosis

Genital lesions due to *T. pallidum* need to be differentiated from those due to herpes simplex virus, which are usually multiple, small, painful, vesicular lesions but which may produce one, or a few large, relatively painless erosions. A history of recurring vesicles in the same area may be obtained. The so-called chancre is a painful erosion 1 to 2 cm in diameter that has a necrotic exudate; this lesion is usually attributed to *Hemophilus ducreyi*. Trauma during sexual intercourse or a fixed drug eruption may produce noninfectious lesions that resemble a chancre. Erosions on the cervix may be indistinguishable from syphilitic chancres. Reiter's syndrome may present with genital ulcers in the absence of conjunctivitis or arthritis, and the examiner may overlook oral lesions in Behçet's syndrome; genital lesions in these conditions are usually quite painful. An individual who has had prior infection may develop small, atypical chancres because of some degree of immunity. In summary, the diagnosis of syphilis should be considered in any patient with genital lesions. In the mouth, aphthous ulcers and cancer of the lip or tongue may be confused with primary syphilis. Syphilis of the anus may cause symptoms of hemorrhoidal irritation or proctitis or may be confused with carcinoma (Drusin et al., 1977).

Secondary syphilis causes findings reminiscent of diseases that produce widespread, symmetric skin lesions. These include acute exanthems of any kind (except vesicular), pityriasis rosea, psoriasis, erythema multiforme, and drug eruptions.

The differential diagnosis of late syphilis of the skin is discussed in Chapter 214. Late syphilis of the bone may be confused with osteogenic sarcoma or osteomyelitis, whether pyogenic or mycobacterial. Disfiguring late syphilitic lesions of the nasal septum, palate, or pharynx may simulate leprosy, carcinoma, Wegener's (midline) granuloma, and related conditions or autoimmune vasculitides such as systemic lupus erythematosus. Although syphilitic aortic insufficiency must be differentiated from that due to other causes, an aneurysm of the ascending aorta is relatively specific in suggesting the diagnosis of syphilis.

### Laboratory Diagnosis

In early syphilis, the use of darkfield microscopy to detect *T. pallidum* in exudate obtained directly from suspicious lesions remains the most direct, immediate, and specific way of establishing the diagnosis of syphilis. This examination is positive in most chancres, although bacterial superinfection and/or prior local use of ointments may obscure the treponemes. Darkfield microscopy in secondary lesions is less rewarding, especially if the examiner is not skilled in exposing the base of the ulcer while maintaining a blood-free field prior to aspirating material for examination. The ordinary microbiologic techniques are not helpful because the narrow width of the causative organism precludes visualization by light microscopic examination of stained material, nor has *T. pallidum* yet been cultivated successfully in vitro.

The presence of antibodies to cardiolipin has been used widely since the time of Wassermann to diagnose syphilis. These antibodies are usually detected in reference or city and state health laboratories by the VDRL (Venereal Disease Research Laboratory) test or, increasingly, in hospital and office practices using the RPR (rapid plasma reagin) test or a modification thereof, which gives nearly identical results. Results are reported with dilutions (titers) so that the degree of reactivity can be determined. The VDRL is reactive in about 75 per cent of patients at the time that they seek medical attention for primary syphilis. After treatment, it nearly always reverts to negative over a period of 6 months. It is worthwhile to repeat the VDRL 3, 6, and 12 months after treatment for syphilis in order to avoid problems relating to diagnosis of reinfection at a later date. Disseminated syphilis is always characterized by a reactive VDRL, usually in a dilution $\geq$ 1:16. Persistence of VDRL antibody after appropriate antibiotic therapy is not uncommon; this is sometimes called a serofast state, although repeat VDRL determinations over a 2-year period show that the VDRL usually becomes negative. In the absence of treatment, the VDRL slowly returns to normal and is, in fact, negative in nearly half of patients with late syphilis. It should be stressed, however, that active late benign syphilis with periostitis or gumma is virtually always associated with a positive serologic reaction. One-third of patients with syphilitic aortitis have a negative VDRL; in some of the individuals, the aorta may have been damaged during active infection, but the resulting weakness may lead to aneurysm formation long after the infection and/or immunologic reaction has subsided. The VDRL may be reactive, generally in a low dilution ($\leq$ 1:4), in nonsyphilitic patients who have infections due to viruses (especially infectious mononucleosis and hepatitis), mycoplasma, or protozoa. A positive VDRL is also seen in the absence of syphilis in heroin addicts, elderly subjects, and patients with cirrhosis, malignancy (especially if associated with production of excess globulin), or autoimmune disease. VDRL reactivity in these conditions has acquired the unfortunate designation "biologic false-positive" to indicate that it does not connote infection due to *T. pallidum;* this term is best avoided.

Infection with *T. pallidum* causes the host to produce specific antibodies that are detected clinically by using the FTA-ABS test. FTA-ABS is an acronym for *F*luorescent *T*reponemal *A*ntibody, following *abs*orption with *T. phagedenis (T. reiteri)* to eliminate nonspecific group antibodies that cross-react with other treponemes. About 90 per cent of patients with a primary syphilitic chancre have a positive FTA-ABS by the time they are seen by their physician (Duncan et al., 1974). All patients with disseminated and late infection have a positive FTA-ABS. This test is highly specific as well as being extremely sensitive. A few disease states such as systemic lupus erythematosus, polyarteritis, and related conditions are said to cause a falsely positive FTA-ABS, but the sophisticated observer can often detect a distinctive beaded pattern in these reactions. The FTA-ABS is usually performed only in city health and other reference laboratories. Once positive, the FTA-ABS usually remains so for life. As a result, despite its exquisite sensitivity and specificity, this test may not be helpful diagnostically in an individual patient.

## TREATMENT

Syphilis is generally treated in accord with recommendations by the United States Public Health Service with little, if any, attempts to tailor the therapy to individual cases. Implementation of these pragmatic recommendations generally succeeds in arresting the clinical syndrome for which they are prescribed. The question of ultimate cure will be discussed below. Early syphilis (primary or secondary) is treated with 2.4 million units of benzathine penicillin administered on 1 day or with daily injection of 600,000 units of procaine penicillin for 8 days (Fiumara, 1977). Patients with primary syphilis who are allergic to penicillin should receive tetracyline or erythromycin, 500 mg four times daily for 15 days. Early latent syphilis (defined as the unusual situation in which an asymptomatic individual has had untreated primary or secondary syphilis within the past year or has a positive VDRL that was known to have been negative 1 year ago) is treated in the same fashion. Patients who have a positive VDRL and FTA-ABS that is of indeterminate age or in whom syphilis occurred more than 1 year ago and was treated inadequately are considered to have late latent syphilis. This definition is admittedly arbitrary, since serologic tests may remain positive after adequate treatment for syphilis. A lumbar puncture should be done in such cases to exclude asymptomatic neurosyphilis. If the cerebrospinal fluid is entirely normal, three doses of benzathine penicillin, 2.4 million units 1 week apart, are currently recommended even though a normal cerebrospinal fluid does not necessarily exclude the diagnosis of neurosyphilis, and, there is no evidence to show that the older recommended therapy of one 2.4-million-unit dose of benzathine penicillin failed to arrest progression to tertiary disease. The need to do a lumbar puncture has received new emphasis since failure of neurosyphilis to respond to benzathine penicillin has been documented in some cases. Current recommendations for treating neurosyphilis include 10 daily injections of 1.2 million units procaine penicillin or even larger doses of aqueous penicillin intravenously.

Late benign syphilis usually responds promptly to treatment with procaine penicillin G; 600,000 units should be given each day for 10 days. Symptoms resulting from granulomas of skin, bone, or viscera rapidly disappear, as do the lesions themselves; obviously, cartilaginous structures that have already been destroyed do not regenerate. Three doses of benzathine penicillin, 2.4 million units at weekly intervals, are thought to give equivalent results. Erythromycin or tetra-cycline, 2 g daily for 30 days, is prescribed for patients who cannot take penicillin and appears to be effective although this has not been as well studied as penicillin therapy. Cardiovascular syphilis should be treated similarly. Patients with symptomatic aortic insufficiency should be evaluated for valve replacement (Grabau et al., 1976).

Several investigators have presented evidence that *T. pallidum* persists in the central nervous system, the aqueous humor, and lymph nodes, despite recommended doses of penicillin (Dunlop, 1972; Tramont, 1976). Much of this evidence is thought to represent artifactual finding of treponeme-like structures in darkfield examination of tissues, although infective organisms have been found in some instances. It is not clear that persistence of treponemes is associated with increased morbidity or that therapeutic recommendations need to be changed.

Aside from drug reactions, the only complication of therapy for syphilis is the development of fever that reaches a peak of 39.5° C within 6 to 8 hours and lasts 24 to 48 hours, sometimes associated with increased prominence of skin lesions. This febrile response (called the Jarisch-Herxheimer reaction) may be due to release of treponemal endotoxin or formation of circulating antigen-antibody complexes. During the reaction, there is a fall in serum complement levels (Fulford et al., 1976).

## CONGENITAL SYPHILIS

Congenital syphilis is the main exception to the general rule that syphilis is acquired by venereal contact. The congenital infection is acquired by transplacental passage of *T. pallidum* from an infected pregnant woman to her fetus. Infection is said not to occur until after the fourth month of pregnancy and not to be common until after the sixth month (Dippell, 1944), when atrophy of the Langhans cell layer permits passage of the treponemes. A recent study with the light microscope has shown structures resembling *T. pallidum* in aborted fetuses in the ninth to tenth weeks (Harter and Benirschke, 1976). Hager (1978) has hypothesized that treponemes may regularly be present in the fetus early in pregnancy, but that the search for characteristic syphilitic lesions has been unsuccessful because of the immunologic immaturity of the fetus. Since the fetus acquires infection directly by the hematogenous route, it is not surprising that widespread, disseminated disease occurs.

The fetus may arrive as a stillbirth or be born with a variety of signs and symptoms of disseminated syphilis (Ingall and Norins, 1976). An enlarged liver and spleen and hematologic abnormalities are present in nearly all affected infants, and lymph nodes are enlarged in more than one-half. Radiologic and histologic findings of periostitis and osteochondritis can be found in nearly all patients. Generally, the disease appears in the second to sixth weeks of life. The first symptom is usually snuffles; this resembles a head cold, causes a purulent nasal discharge, and results from disease of the nasal mucous membrane. Skin lesions and mucous patches then appear in the mouth, lips, nose, pharynx, and anogenital region. The infant may also have fever. Ultimately, in the absence of treatment, wasting develops, culminating in marasmus and death. This set of symptoms and signs is rapidly reversed by treatment (Ingall and Norins, 1976).

Late manifestations of congenital syphilis are those that appear after 2 years of age. They are divided into two kinds. (1) "Stigmata" become apparent with the development of structures such as teeth* and long bones† but actually result from early damage to these tissues by the congenital infection. These changes are prevented completely by treatment before the third month of life. (2) Other late manifestations resemble, by analogy, the lesions of late (tertiary) syphilis in the adult in that their pathogenesis is obscure, and continued signs of inflammation are present in involved tissues. These include lesions of the eye (keratitis and uveitis) and skin, gummas of nasal and facial bones, periostitis, and central nervous system disease.

Adequate treatment of the infected pregnant woman prevents congenital syphilis. Infants with active infection should be separated, for the purposes of treatment, into those with normal and those with abnormal cerebrospinal fluid (CSF). If the CSF is normal, definitive therapy is 50,000 units benzathine penicillin per kilogram body weight on a single day. In cases in which the central nervous system is thought to be involved

---

*The syphilitic tooth described by Jonathan Hutchinson is an upper incisor with a tapered, bulbous shape (resembling a pumpkin seed) and a gap or notch in the center of the biting edge.

†Osteochondritis of the femur, tibia, radius, and ulna and dactylitis of the first and second phalanges of the hands are the chief manifestations of long bone disease in early congenital syphilis. These are painful and of short duration and usually disappear without deformity. These lesions, which occur in infancy and early childhood, differ from long bone disease of later childhood and adolescence, which is a relatively painless disease of the diaphysis and does not extend beyond the epiphyseal line. The latter type seems to be activated by trauma and is, therefore, common in the tibias of boys. Saber shin (Fig. 6) is the most characteristic type of bone syphilis.

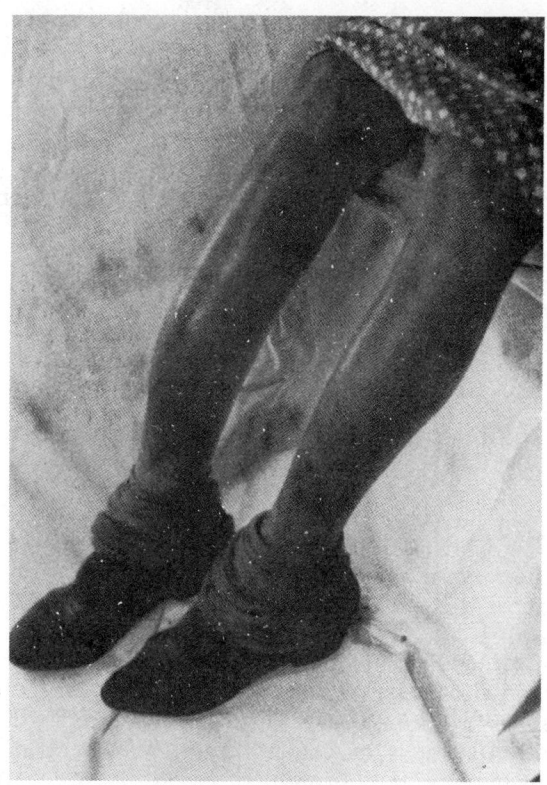

**FIGURE 6.**   *Saber shin of congenital syphilis. (From Howles, J. K.: Synopsis of Clinical Syphilis. St. Louis, C. V. Mosby Co., 1943.)*

because the CSF is abnormal, procaine penicillin G, 50,000 units/kg, should be given daily for 10 days. Antibiotics other than penicillin are not currently recommended for the treatment of congenital syphilis.

## References

Chapel, T. A.: The variability of syphilitic chancres. Sex Transm Dis 5:68–70, 1978.

Clark, E. G., and Danbolt, N.: The Oslo study of the natural course of untreated syphilis. An epidemiologic investigation based on a re-study of the Boeck-Brussgaard material. Med Clin North Amer 48:613–623, 1964.

Dippell, A. L.: The relationship of congenital syphilis to abortion and miscarriage, and the mechanism of intrauterine protection. Am J Obstet Gynecol 47:369–376, 1944.

Dismukes, W. E., Delgado, D. G., Mallernee, S. V., and Myers, T. C.: Destructive bone disease in early syphilis. JAMA 236:2646–2648, 1976.

Drusin, L. M., Singer, C., Valenti, A. J., and Armstrong, D.: Infectious syphilis mimicking neoplastic disease. Arch Intern Med 137:156–160, 1977.

Duncan, W. C., Knox, J. M., and Wende, R. D.: The FTA-ABS test in dark-field-positive primary syphilis. JAMA 228:859–860, 1974.

Dunlop, E. M. C.: Persistence of treponemes after treatment. Brit Med J 2:577–580, 1972.

Fehér, J., Somogyi, T., Timmer, M., and Józsa, L.: Early syphilitic hepatitis. Lancet 2:896–899, 1975.

Fiumara, N. J.: The treatment of seropositive primary syphilis — an evaluation of 196 patients. Sex Transm Dis 4:92–95, 1977.

Fulford, K. W. M., Johnson, N., Loveday, C., Storey, J., and Tedder, R. S.: Changes in intra-vascular complement and anti-treponemal antibody titres preceding the Jarisch-Herxheimer reaction in secondary syphilis. Clin Exp Immunol 24:483–491, 1976.

Grabau, W., Emanuel, R., Ross, D., Parker, J., and Hedge, M.: Syphilitic aortic regurgitation. An appraisal of surgical treatment. Brit J Vener Dis 52:366–373, 1976.

Harter, C. A., and Benirschke, K.: Fetal syphilis in the first trimester. Am J Obstet Gynecol 124:705–711, 1976.

Hager, W. D.: Transplacental transmission of spirochetes in congenital syphilis: a new perspective. Sex Transm Dis 5:122–123, 1978.

Heggtveit, H. A.: Syphilitic aortitis. A clinicopathologic autopsy study of 100 cases, 1950 to 1960. Circulation 29:346–355, 1964.

Howles, J. K.: Synopsis of Clinical Syphilis. St. Louis, C. V. Mosby, 1943.

Ingall, D., and Norins, L.: Syphilis. In Remington, J. S., and Klein, J. O. (eds): Infectious Diseases of the Fetus and Newborn Infant. Philadelphia, W. B. Saunders Co., 1976, pp. 414–463.

Kampmeier, R. H.: The late manifestations of syphilis: skeletal, visceral, and cardiovascular. Med Clin North Amer 48:667–697, 1964.

Schell, R. F., and Musher, D. M. (eds.): The immunology of treponemal infection. New York, Marcel Dekker, 1981.

Tramont, E. C.: Persistence of *Treponema pallidum* following penicillin G therapy. Report of two cases. JAMA 236:2206–2214, 1976.

# 151 GENITAL HERPES

## Michael N. Oxman, M.D.

## DEFINITION

Genital herpes (herpes genitalis) is an acute inflammatory herpes simplex virus (HSV) infection of the male or female genital tract. It may result from either a primary or a recurrent HSV infection. Primary genital herpes is a venereally transmitted exogenous infection that is generally caused by HSV Type 2 (HSV-2). Recurrent genital herpes usually results from the reactivation of endogenous HSV-2, which is latent in sacral sensory ganglia. However, recurrent genital herpes may occasionally represent a sexually transmitted exogenous reinfection (Buchman et al., 1979).

Herpes genitalis in the female causes painful vesicles and ulcers of the vulva and vagina, and these may extend to the skin of the perineum, buttocks, and thighs. The cervix is also usually infected. In the male, painful vesicles and ulcers appear on the glans penis, prepuce, and shaft of the penis, and sometimes extend to the scrotum and adjacent perineal areas. Bilateral inguinal lymphadenopathy is present in both sexes and, in primary infections, it is usually painful and accompanied by constitutional symptoms. The clinical manifestations of primary and recurrent herpes genitalis are similar, although primary episodes are usually more severe and slower to resolve. This is in marked contrast to oropharyngeal infections with HSV-1 (Chapter 99), in which primary and recurrent infections cause totally different syndromes (that is, acute herpetic gingivostomatitis vs herpes labialis).

## ETIOLOGY

Genital herpes simplex has been a recognized clinical entity for more than two centuries and was described as a venereal disease as early as 1883, when Unna observed that it was a "vocational disease" of Hamburg prostitutes (Hutfield, 1966; Unna, 1883). In the 1920's, Lipschütz called attention to the transmission of "venereal herpes" by sexual contact and demonstrated that the viruses of "venereal herpes" and "herpes febrilis" (the fever blister) were biologically and antigenically different (Nahmias and Dowdle, 1968). However, the work of Lipschütz was ignored. Slavin and Gavett (1946) isolated HSV from lesions of the vulva, demonstrated that herpetic vulvovaginitis was a manifestation of primary HSV infection, and described the conjugal transmission of HSV from a husband with penile herpes to his wife. However, genital herpes was not accepted as a sexually transmitted disease until the rediscovery of the two serotypes of HSV in the late 1960's and the development of assays to distinguish between them permitted the different epidemiology of HSV Type 1 (HSV-1) and HSV Type 2 (HSV-2) to be delineated (Nahmias and Dowdle, 1968).

HSV-1 and HSV-2 are very closely related members of the herpesvirus group, which includes three other human herpesviruses, varicella-zoster virus, cytomegalovirus and Epstein-Barr virus. HSV-1 and HSV-2 are morphologically indistinguishable, share approximately 40 per cent of their DNA base sequences, have many antigens in common, and produce identical lesions in the skin and mucous membranes (Chapter 56). Although their similarities are much greater than their differences, HSV-1 and HSV-2 can be distinguished on the basis of certain antigenic, biologic, and biochemical differences (Table 1 in Chapter 99). Furthermore, they differ significantly in their clinical and epidemiologic behavior (Nahmias and Roizman, 1973; Nahmias and Josey, 1976). HSV-2 is transmitted venereally or from a maternal genital infection to the newborn. It is the predominant cause of genital herpes, neonatal herpes, and herpetic infections of the skin below the waist. It is also associated epidemiologically with carcinoma of the cervix. HSV-1 is transmitted primarily by nonvenereal routes, usually involving contact with infected saliva. It is the principal cause of herpetic gingivostomatitis and pharyngotonsillitis, eczema herpeticum, skin infections above the waist, infections of the eye, and herpes simplex encephalitis. HSV replication and the differentiation of HSV-1 from HSV-2 are discussed in Chapters 56 and 99.

## PATHOLOGY AND PATHOGENESIS

The pathology and pathogenesis of genital herpes simplex appears to be analogous to the pathology and pathogenesis of oropharyngeal infections caused by HSV-1 (Chapter 99), and the skin and mucous membrane lesions of HSV-1 and HSV-2 are indistinguishable. The virus is introduced into the genital mucosa by sexual contact with a partner who has a symptomatic or asymptomatic genital infection. It replicates in cells of the stratum spinosum, producing characteristic cytopathic effects that include cell swelling ("ballooning degeneration"), loss of intercellular bridges, the development of Cowdry Type A intranuclear inclusion bodies, and membrane changes that result in cell fusion with the formation of multinucleated giant cells. The infected cells are soon separated by intercellular edema which, together with inflammation and capillary dilatation in the underlying lamina propria, results in the formation of an erythematous papule. The infection and degeneration of additional epithelial cells and the continuing influx of edema fluid elevates the uninvolved stratum corneum to form a delicate, clear, intraepidermal vesicle that contains fibrin, degenerating epithelial cells, multinucleated giant cells, and large amounts of infectious virus. The vesicle is soon invaded by inflammatory cells from below, and the fluid becomes cloudy. Adjacent vesicles may coalesce to form small bullae. In moist areas, such as the cervix, vagina, and labia minora in females and under the foreskin in uncircumcised males, the vesicles are macerated and quickly rupture, liberating infectious virus and leaving very tender, painful, shallow ulcers that are covered with a yellowish-gray exudate and surrounded by a narrow red areola. The virus liberated from ruptured vesicles spreads the infection locally to the cervix, vagina, vulva, and, often, to the surrounding skin. During primary infections, there is also significant involvement of regional lymph nodes and viremia. In the normal patient, a variety of nonspecific and specific immunologic defenses, including local production of interferon, antibody formation, and various forms of cell-mediated immunity combine to localize the infection and eventually terminate virus multiplication (Moller-Larsen et al., 1978; O'Reilly et al., 1977). If these defenses are deficient, as they are in many immunosuppressed patients, primary (or recurrent) infection may result in viremic spread to the skin and visceral organs, or produce chronic progressive local lesions. Although we cannot presently identify those host responses that are critical to the control of HSV infections, studies in animals and experience with compromised human hosts indicate that cell-mediated responses are essential. Interestingly, antigens shared by HSV-1 and HSV-2 must be involved, for prior oropharyngeal infection with HSV-1 reduces the severity of primary herpes genitalis caused by HSV-2 (Nahmias et al., 1970; Rawls et al., 1971).

During the course of primary herpes genitalis, even when it is asymptomatic, virus invades local sensory nerve endings, ascends within axons, and establishes a latent infection in sensory neurons within the corresponding sacral ganglia (Baringer, 1974). Despite the host's immunity, this latent infection persists for life and is periodically reactivated by various stimuli (for example, menses, sexual intercourse). The reactivated HSV then travels within axons from the neuronal soma to the genital skin or mucosa, where it replicates in epithelial cells and produces an intraepidermal vesicle histologically indistinguishable from that observed during primary genital herpes. Preexisting humoral and cellular immunity normally limit this local virus replication so that recurrent infections are generally less severe, more circumscribed, and of shorter duration than primary infections (Yen et al., 1965; Ng et al., 1970; Poste et al., 1972; Kaufman et al., 1973; Adams et al., 1976; Vontver et al., 1979).

## CLINICAL MANIFESTATIONS

In general, primary herpes genitalis is more severe and prolonged than recurrent genital herpes (Yen et al., 1965).

The incubation period following sexual contact ranges from 2 to 7 days (Poste et al., 1972; Kaufman et al., 1973). In the female, primary herpes genitalis often begins with local tenderness or burning involving the labia and vaginal mucosa. This is soon followed by the appearance of typical herpetic vesicles, usually on the labia majora, labia minora, vaginal mucosa, and cervix, and sometimes also on the clitoris, around the urethra, and on the perianal skin, buttocks, and thighs. There is often a profuse watery vaginal discharge. Vesicular lesions within the labia minora rupture quickly, leaving shallow, exquisitely tender ulcers covered with a yellowish-gray exudate and surrounded by a red areola (Fig. 1). Vesicles in drier areas, such as the outer surface

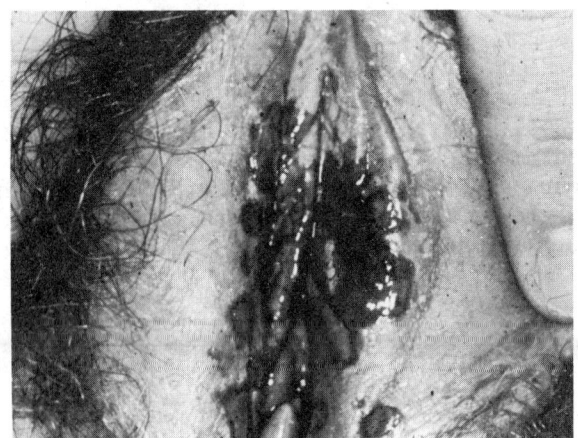

**FIGURE 1.** *Herpes genitalis in the female. This young woman with primary herpetic vulvovaginitis has shallow, exquisitely tender ulcers on the inner surface of the labia majora, the labia minora, and the vaginal mucosa. The ulcers are covered with a yellowish-gray exudate and surrounded by a red areola. Further examination also reveals herpetic cervicitis.*

of the labia majora and adjacent skin, may remain intact and evolve into pustules and then crusts over several days. The lesions are often extensive, and there is usually inflammation and edema of the vaginal mucosa and vulva. New lesions appear for a week or more, and they may coalesce, forming bullae and larger ulcerations. Most patients have severe vulvar pain and tenderness of the affected tissues. Most also have dysuria, and this is sometimes so severe that it results in urinary retention. There is bilateral painful inguinal and pelvic lymphadenopathy, and this is usually accompanied by constitutional symptoms, such as fever, headache, malaise, and myalgias. In spite of its severity, primary herpetic vulvovaginitis is normally self-limited. Virus replication is maximal during the first 3 to 4 days and declines thereafter, although some patients may continue to shed virus for several weeks. Pain begins to remit in 10 to 14 days and healing occurs without residua in 3 to 5 weeks. The cervix, which is involved in almost all women with symptomatic primary genital herpes, appears to be the source of virus which is frequently shed for weeks after visible lesions have healed and symptoms have disappeared (Adams et al., 1976; Overall, 1979; Vontver et al., 1979).

Recurrent herpes genitalis in the female is usually less severe and the lesions more circumscribed than primary infection, although it tends to involve the same sites. Vesicles frequently appear in clusters, usually after a prodrome of pain, burning, tingling, or itching at the site of the impending eruption. They evolve in the same manner as the primary lesions, but somewhat more rapidly, and there are fewer days of new vesicle formation. Lymphadenopathy is usually

present, but fever and constitutional symptoms are uncommon. Virus is present in smaller amounts in recurrent lesions and can almost never be recovered after the seventh day. Pain also disappears during the first week, and the lesions generally resolve within 10 to 14 days.

In the male, the lesions of primary herpes genitalis usually appear on the glans penis, the prepuce, and the shaft of the penis, and less often on the scrotum, thighs, and buttocks. Their evolution is similar to that observed in the female. In dry skin (for example, on the shaft of the penis) they progress from papule to vesicle to pustule to crust and then heal, as described for cutaneous lesions caused by HSV-1 (Chapter 99). In moist areas (for example, under the prepuce), the vesicles are quickly macerated and evolve into ulcers identical to those described above in the female. New lesions continue to appear for a week or more, and there is local pain, tenderness, inflammation, and edema. As in the female, there is bilateral tender inguinal and pelvic lymphadenopathy and usually constitutional symptoms as well. Virus is present in large amounts during the first 3 to 5 days and can usually be recovered for an additional week or more. Pain usually resolves late in the second week, and healing occurs without scarring in 3 to 4 weeks.

Recurrent herpes genitalis in the male usually has a prodrome of pain, burning, itching, or tingling at the site of the impending lesion. One or more small patches of grouped vesicles (Fig. 2) appear, most often on the shaft of the penis or on the prepuce. They begin as papules and, on dry skin, evolve into vesicles, pustules, and crusts in the same manner as in herpes labialis (Chapter 99). When they occur under the prepuce, they are quickly macerated, forming painful ulcers. There is often inguinal lymphadenopathy, but rarely

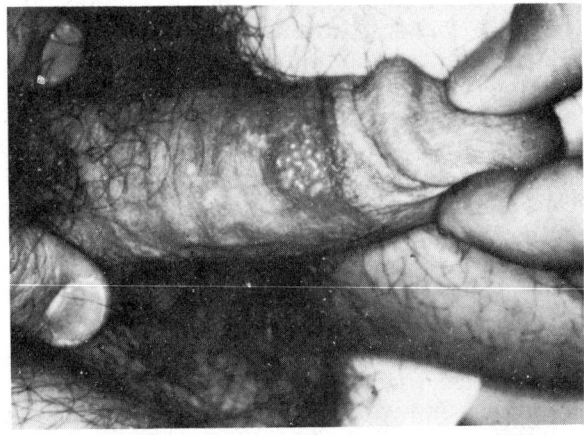

**FIGURE 2.** *Recurrent herpes genitalis in the male. A typical patch of grouped vesicles on an erythematous base is seen on the shaft of the penis. (Courtesy of Dr. M. T. Jarratt.)*

constitutional symptoms. The titer of virus is lower in recurrent lesions, and it can rarely be recovered after 4 to 5 days. Pain is only present in about 60 per cent of recurrent episodes in the male. It disappears with the virus, and the lesions heal in 7 to 10 days.

In approximately 5 per cent of patients, recurrent herpes genitalis may present with a single large, shallow, minimally tender ulcer, up to 1 cm in diameter, with a clean, granular base and sharply demarcated edges. This lesion, which has been called a herpetic chancre (Chang et al., 1974), may be mistaken for a syphilitic chancre. However, both herpes genitalis and syphilis may coexist in the same patient. Thus, laboratory diagnosis is essential.

## COMPLICATIONS AND SEQUELAE

Though often physically and mentally distressing, primary and recurrent genital herpes are self-limited and, in the normal person, almost always resolve spontaneously without complications or sequelae.

Those complications that do occur may be divided into three categories: (1) bacterial or fungal superinfection; (2) extragenital infection or aberrant behavior by the virus in an apparently normal person; and (3) HSV infections in compromised hosts.

Bacterial and fungal superinfection is surprisingly uncommon. Occasionally, balanoposthitis occurs in an uncircumcised male from bacterial superinfection of herpetic ulcers on the prepuce. Ulcerative lesions in moist skin areas may also become superinfected, and *Candida* vaginitis occasionally complicates herpetic vulvovaginitis, especially in patients with diabetes. These complications usually respond to local therapy and rarely require systemic antibiotics.

There are a number of examples of extragenital HSV-2 infections that may result from direct extension of the genital infection, autoinoculation, viremia, or exogenous extragenital infection (Hutfield, 1968). Herpetic urethritis usually occurs in association with primary genital herpes. Typical herpetic lesions may be visible near the urethral meatus or they may be intraurethral. There is usually severe burning pain on micturition, but little or no discharge. Typical intranuclear inclusion bodies and multinucleated giant cells may be demonstrated in urethral smears. The urethritis may recur, with or without recurrent genital lesions. Herpetic cystitis has also been observed in patients with primary herpes genitalis and may account for some instances of dysuria and urinary retention. In many cases, virus may reach the bladder by direct extension from the urethra, but the occurrence of cystitis caused by HSV-1 in adults with oropharyngeal HSV infections suggests that the bladder may also be infected as a result of viremia.

Infection of the cervix occurs in almost every symptomatic case of primary genital herpes, and probably causes much of the profuse watery vaginal discharge that usually begins shortly after the onset of the disease. In addition, the cervix appears to be the site of infection in asymptomatic cases of genital herpes, which actually comprise the majority of genital HSV-2 infections (Ng et al., 1970; Rawls et al., 1971; Poste et al., 1972). On occasion, the cervical infection may be extremely severe, producing necrotic cervicitis. Symptoms include profuse vaginal discharge; dysuria; abdominal, pelvic, or genital pain; and constitutional symptoms. The cervix is extremely tender, bleeds easily, and exhibits extensive superficial necrosis with sloughing of necrotic epithelium. Healing occurs spontaneously in 2 to 3 weeks. One-half of the cases occur in the absence of other genital lesions.

Anal herpes may occur as a complication of genital herpes in the female, the virus spreading from the vulva to the perineum, anus, and anal canal. However, most cases occur in homosexual males as a result of anal intercourse (Jacobs, 1976). Typical herpetic lesions occur on the perianal skin and in the anal canal, where they frequently coalesce, producing an ulcerative cryptitis. Pain is severe, frequently radiating to the groin, buttocks, and thighs. There is often a serous rectal discharge and bilateral inguinal adenopathy, and constitutional symptoms are common. Pain in the anal canal usually results in reflex inhibition of defecation and sometimes tenesmus. In spite of its severity, the disease is self-limited and healing usually occurs without scarring in 2 to 3 weeks. Recurrent attacks of anal herpes are common after primary infection.

Contiguous spread or autoinoculation during primary genital herpes frequently results in cutaneous lesions on the buttocks, thighs, or other areas of skin below the waist. When these lesions subsequently recur (typically in the absence of any genital lesions) they resemble herpes zoster and are often associated with a prodrome of deep neuralgic pain. Autoinoculation of the finger during primary genital herpes results in a herpetic whitlow that is indistinguishable from the whitlows that occur in hospital personnel as a result of contact with HSV-1 in saliva and respiratory secretions (Chapter 99). Most herpetic whitlows in adults (other than hospital personnel) appear to be caused by HSV-2 and to occur in association with primary genital herpes (Glogau et al., 1977). These troublesome lesions tend to recur.

The increasing popularity of oral-genital sexual practices is changing the epidemiology of HSV-1 and HSV-2 infections. HSV-1 is causing disease in territory formerly exclusively inhabited by HSV-2, and vice versa. Consequently, we are now finding that 5 to 30 per cent of genital herpes is caused by HSV-1, and that some cases of herpetic gingivostomatitis and pharyngotonsillitis in adults are caused by HSV-2. There is no detectable difference in these diseases when they are caused by HSV-1 or HSV-2.

Severe disseminated HSV infections are common in immunosuppressed children and adults (see below). Yet, while viremia probably occurs during most primary HSV infections in normal hosts, it is rarely manifest clinically. Occasionally, however, apparently healthy young adults with primary genital herpes develop disseminated infection. This generally involves the skin, rather than internal organs, and produces a disease that is virtually indistinguishable from varicella. The illness is self-limited and usually resolves in 12 to 15 days. However, skin lesions commonly recur at sites of primary cutaneous infection.

Neurons play a critical role in the pathogenesis of HSV infections, and thus it is not surprising that many complications involve the central and peripheral nervous system. An acute aseptic meningitis may occur in the course of primary genital herpes. HSV-2 can be isolated from the spinal fluid, but it is not clear whether the virus reaches the central nervous system by passage in sensory nerves or as a result of viremia. The meningitis usually follows a brief and benign course, although it may sometimes be associated with polyradiculitis or ascending myelitis (Chapter 168). Herpes simplex meningitis recurs in some patients in association with recurrent genital herpes. Recurrent genital herpes and recurrent zosteriform herpes involving the skin below the waist may be associated with severe local neuralgia, usually in a L5-S1 dermatome distribution. When the recurrent herpetic lesions and neuralgia involve the extremities, there may also be local edema and lymphangitis. The neuralgia may precede the eruption by several days and usually resolves along with the cutaneous lesions (Slavin and Ferguson, 1950; Layzer and Conant, 1974; Hinthorn et al., 1976). Although resolution is generally complete and multiple recurrences occur without any permanent residua, repeated attacks over a period of years may sometimes result in chronic pain and permanent sensory and motor deficits. Primary genital or anal herpes is sometimes complicated by urinary retention, and this may be accompanied by neuralgic pain and blunting of sensation over the sacral dermatomes. Patients with this syndrome have hypotonic blad-

ders and spinal fluid pleocytosis, indicating that the urinary retention reflects acute herpetic lumbosacral radiculomyelitis (Caplan et al., 1977; Oates and Greenhouse, 1979). This complication of genital herpes resolves spontaneously without residua in 7 to 10 days.

Recurrent genital herpes may be associated with recurrent episodes of erythema multiforme or Stevens-Johnson syndrome. As is the case with HSV-1 (Chapter 99), this complication appears to be an allergic response to circulating HSV antigens or antigen-antibody complexes. The lesions are not the direct result of replication of HSV-2 in the skin or mucous membranes.

Compromised patients are at increased risk of severe, even fatal, HSV infections. Those at greatest risk appear to have abnormal cellular immunity, eczema, or burns. The risk to the compromised patient and the nature of the pathologic process appear to be the same with HSV-1 and HSV-2. Most reported infections in compromised patients have been with untyped HSV or with HSV-1, but this is mainly a matter of exposure and epidemiology. HSV-2 also causes many severe infections in patients with malignancies undergoing chemotherapy and in organ transplant recipients. Most of these result from local extension or systemic dissemination of herpes genitalis (Logan et al., 1971; Muller et al., 1972; Sutton et al., 1974; Stone et al., 1977; Lopyan et al., 1977; Schneidman et al., 1979). Most episodes of genital herpes in these patients are recurrent infections, and they often evolve normally and resolve without complications. However, in some cases, the local lesions do not resolve but slowly progress to form a gradually enlarging ulcer with a sharp erythematous border and a base covered with purulent exudate. These lesions may last for months and are usually exquisitely tender. In other patients, genital herpes may disseminate, producing widespread cutaneous lesions and fatal involvement of multiple visceral organs.

One of the most important complications of genital herpes occurs when infection in a pregnant woman is transmitted to her newborn infant (Nahmias and Visintine, 1976; Hanshaw and Dudgeon, 1978). The incidence of recognized neonatal HSV infection in the United States is estimated to be about one in 7500 deliveries, but it is probably closer to one in 20,000 deliveries. In most cases, the infant appears to acquire infection perinatally during passage through the birth canal of a mother with genital herpes. In some cases, infection may occur in utero as a result of maternal viremia or ascending infection from the cervix. Rarely, infection may be acquired postpartum from the mother, other family members, or nursery personnel. Primary genital herpes during the first trimester may, rarely, cause viremia and transplacental transmission of HSV-2 to the fetus. This is likely to cause fetal death and abortion, but occasionally the infected fetus survives and is later born with multiple congenital anomalies (Hanshaw and Dudgeon, 1978). The overall risk of neonatal herpes has been estimated to be about 10 per cent in infants born to mothers with symptomatic genital herpes after 32 weeks of gestation, and about 50 per cent if virus is present at delivery (Nahmias and Visintine, 1976). HSV infection in the newborn is almost never asymptomatic. In two thirds of infected infants, there is disseminated visceral infection with severe involvement of the liver, adrenal glands, lungs, brain, and other organs. The initial manifestations usually appear during the first week of life, often at birth, but occasionally as late as 3 weeks postpartum. They are relatively nonspecific, consisting of lethargy, fever or hypothermia, vomiting, and poor feeding. Jaundice, purpuric rash, apneic spells, respiratory distress, and cyanosis may also appear. The clinical picture resembles bacterial sepsis. One-half of these infants have clinical evidence of central nervous system involvement. The disease progresses rapidly, with the frequent development of pneumonia, shock, and disseminated intravascular coagulation. The mortality in this group is 80 per cent, with death usually occurring in the second postpartum week. Most survivors have severe psychomotor and ocular sequelae. About one third of infants with neonatal herpes do not have evidence of disseminated infection. Their symptoms start later, and one-half present with herpetic skin lesions, oropharyngeal lesions, or ocular infection. The remainder present with symptoms of central nervous system infection, but most of these infants also eventually develop lesions of the skin, mouth, or eye. Neurologic disease kills 40 per cent of this group, and most of the survivors have severe neurologic sequelae. The overall mortality in neonatal herpes is 60 to 70 per cent, and fewer than 20 per cent of patients survive without significant sequelae. HSV-2 causes about 70 per cent of the cases, but there is no apparent difference between the nature or severity of the disease produced by HSV-1 and HSV-2.

It has been suggested that HSV-2 may play a role in the etiology of carcinoma of the cervix (Rotkin, 1973; Rawls et al., 1977). This idea is based largely upon the capacity of HSV to induce cell transformation and the observation made in many seroepidemiologic studies that more patients with cervical carcinoma have antibody to HSV-2 than matched controls. In addition, several investigators have found HSV antigens and nucleic acid sequences in cervical carcinoma cells. However, epidemiologic studies indicate only that HSV-2 infection and carcinoma of the cervix are covariable, both linked to an early age of first coitus and multiple sexual consorts. Furthermore, HSV-2 is latent in sacral ganglia and is periodically reactivated, producing recurrent cervical infections that are generally asymptomatic. Thus, it would not be surprising, at least on occasion, to find evidence of HSV-2 in cervical tissues. Thus, much work is still to be done to establish the exact relationship of HSV-2 infection to carcinoma of the cervix.

## GEOGRAPHIC VARIATION IN DISEASE AND EPIDEMIOLOGY

Although it differs from HSV-1 in its epidemiology, HSV-2 appears to be an equally successful and ubiquitous parasite of man (Chapter 99). Except for neonatal infections, which are rare, and, because of their high mortality, contribute nothing to the survival of the virus in the human population, HSV-2 infections do not generally occur before puberty. Thereafter, the acquisition of HSV-2 infection is a function of sexual activity. The prevalence of antibody to the virus exceeds 70 per cent in prostitutes and is only 3 per cent in chaste women (Nahmias and Josey, 1976). As in the case of HSV-1 (Fig. 3 in Chapter 99), latency and asymptomatic virus shedding play a critical role in maintaining HSV-2 in human populations.

Systematic virologic and cytologic surveys have revealed that more than one-half of all genital herpes infections in females are asymptomatic (Nahmias et al., 1969; Nahmias et al., 1970; Ng et al., 1970; Rawls et al., 1971; Dueñas et al., 1972; Poste et al., 1972). Primary HSV-2 infections are more often symptomatic than recurrent infections. In fact, most of the asymptomatic primary infections seem to occur in women who have had a previous HSV-1 infection and who already have humoral and cellular immunity to HSV-1. These women are, presumably, partially immune to HSV-2 because of the antigenic cross-reactivity of the two HSV serotypes. The overall rate of asymptomatic genital excretion of HSV in women varies from 0.03 per cent to 7 per cent, depending upon the population studied (Dueñas et al., 1972; Nahmias and Josey, 1976; Bolognese et al., 1976). The figure is highest in prostitutes and women attending venereal disease clinics, and lowest in private patients. The rate of asymptomatic shedding is two to three times higher in pregnant than nonpregnant women. The principal source of virus in these asymptomatic women appears to be the cervix.

The situation in males is unclear. Centifanto et al. (1972) reported the isolation of HSV-2 from 15 per cent of 190 men with no history of genital herpes. The material sampled consisted of urethral swabs (of which 7.6 per cent were virus-positive), prostatic fluid, prostatic biopsies, and surgical specimens of vas deferens (of which 20 per cent or more yielded virus). Subsequently, the same group reported their failure to isolate HSV from semen obtained during a symptom-free interval from 30 healthy males subject to recurrent genital herpes (Deture et al., 1978). Other workers have only rarely isolated HSV from the urethra in healthy, asymptomatic males. Jeansson and Molin (1974) reported the isolation of HSV from the urethra of 4.4 per cent of males and from the cervix of 5.2 per cent of females attending a Swedish venereal disease clinic. More than 25 per cent of the males and 30 per cent of the females who yielded virus were free of signs and symptoms of either genital herpes or gonorrhea. In contrast, no urethral isolates were obtained from 131 males attending a dermatology clinic, and the cervical isolation rate among females attending gynecology and birth control clinics was 0.5 per cent. Longitudinal studies of individual patients demonstrated intermittent asymptomatic shedding by both males and females. More than 90 per cent of the isolates were HSV-2. Although the risk of infection is unknown when a susceptible individual has sexual intercourse with a partner asymptomatically shedding HSV-2, the rate of transmission during intercourse by a symptomatic male is 75 to 80 per cent (Nahmias et al., 1969; Rawls et al., 1971).

## DIAGNOSIS

The diagnosis of genital herpes is often clinically apparent, especially with recurrent infections, but there are a number of diseases that can cause ulcerative genital lesions that may be confused with those of genital herpes. Moreover, the incidence of dual infections is higher than random (Hutfield, 1968; Young, 1972; Young et al., 1977).

The methods for obtaining specimens for virus isolation, fluorescent antibody staining, and cytologic examination have already been described in detail (Chapter 99). The simplest and most rapid method of diagnosis is the examination of cells scraped from the base of a vesicle or ulcer (Tzanck smear) or scraped from the surface of the cervix or the vaginal mucosa (Papanicolaou smear) and stained by the Papanicolaou or Paragon Multiple stain technique as described in Chapter 99. Eosinophilic intranuclear inclusion bodies and multinucleated giant cells indicate HSV or varicella-zoster virus infection. Fluorescent antibody staining of similar smears can give

a specific diagnosis, although its accuracy depends on the quality of the serologic reagents employed. A punch biopsy taken at the edge of a lesion provides better tissue for cytologic and immunofluorescent diagnosis. As with HSV infections elsewhere, virus isolation is the most sensitive diagnostic technique. It is approximately twice as sensitive as cytology in genital herpes. Specimens are more likely to yield virus if they are obtained from a vesicular lesion early in the course of the disease. This is especially true with recurrent infections.

The diseases to be considered in the differential diagnosis of herpes genitalis are syphilis, chancroid, lymphogranuloma venereum, granuloma inguinale, vaccinia, herpes zoster, erythema multiforme, Behçet's syndrome, contact dermatitis, candidiasis, and impetigo. Multinucleated giant cells and eosinophilic Cowdry Type A intranuclear inclusion bodies indicate the presence of either HSV or varicella-zoster virus, and fluorescent antibody staining and virus isolation can give the specific diagnosis. However, patients are often simultaneously infected by more than one agent, and it is, therefore, important to rule out at least some of the other possibilities (Hutfield, 1968; Young, 1972; Young et al., 1977). Syphilis is the most important of these diseases. The chancre of syphilis may mimic the ulcerative lesions of genital herpes, although it tends to be more indurated, indolent, and painless. The mucous patches of secondary syphilis may also resemble the ulcerated lesions of genital herpes, but are usually accompanied by a generalized rash or other secondary manifestations. The diagnosis should be attempted by dark-field examination and serology. The ulcers of chancroid are soft and painful with ragged undermined margins, and there is prominent, painful, often fluctuant inguinal adenopathy. The demonstration of *Haemophilus ducreyi*, a small gram-negative rod, in smears of the ulcer or by culture, can help establish the diagnosis. The diagnosis of lymphogranuloma venereum and granuloma inguinale are discussed in Chapter 152. Vaccinia, which should rarely be seen now that routine smallpox vaccination has been abandoned, can be differentiated from HSV and varicella-zoster by the presence of cytoplasmic inclusion bodies and the absence of intranuclear inclusion bodies and multinucleated giant cells. The histopathology of erythema multiforme and Behçet's syndrome are very different from that of genital herpes, and both are accompanied by characteristic lesions outside of the genital area. However, erythema multiforme is induced in some patients by genital herpes, and the lesions may therefore coexist. Bacterial and candidal infections may be diagnosed by gram-stained smears and cultures.

The serologic diagnosis of HSV infections is discussed in Chapter 99. The antigenic cross-reactivity of HSV-1 and HSV-2 limits the usefulness of currently available serologic techniques (Rawls, 1979). For example, it may not always be possible to differentiate reliably between an initial and a recurrent HSV-2 infection in a patient with high levels of antibody induced by prior HSV-1 infections. Primary HSV-2 infections, even in persons with preexisting antibody to HSV-1, usually cause an increase in the titer of antibody reacting with HSV-2 and alter the ratio of titers to the two HSV serotypes. Recurrent infections, however, only occasionally elevate the antibody titer significantly. The availability of type-specific HSV antigens should soon result in the development of type-specific serologic tests.

## TREATMENT

Primary genital herpes is a self-limited disease which, in the normal person, resolves spontaneously without sequelae. However, it is followed by a latent HSV-2 infection in sacral ganglia and, in most people, by repeated episodes of recurrent infection. While these, too, are ordinarily self-limited, they produce enough physical and psychological distress to cause most affected persons to seek some form of relief. The desire for relief from this recurrent affliction has been further stimulated by the recognition that genital herpes during pregnancy may cause serious infection of the fetus or newborn infant, and by the widely publicized association between HSV-2 infection and carcinoma of the cervix.

The topical application of a variety of agents designed to limit virus replication has been tried in patients with recurrent genital herpes. Each new regimen has been greeted with enthusiasm on the basis of anecdotal observations and uncontrolled trials, only to be proved ineffective when careful, double-blind, placebo-controlled studies were carried out (Chapter 99; Overall, 1979). Topical therapies that have proved to be ineffective for recurrent genital herpes include iododeoxyuridine ointment, photodynamic inactivation with neutral red or proflavine and light, adenine-arabinoside (which is effective parenterally for herpes simplex encephalitis and neonatal HSV infections), ether (Corey et al., 1978), surfactant (Vontver et al., 1979), and adenine arabinoside monophosphate (Spruance et al., 1979). In addition, BCG vaccine, levamisole, multiple smallpox vaccinations, and live and killed HSV vaccines have also proved to be ineffective. Recently, Blough and Guintoli (1979) reported that the topical application of 2-deoxy-D-glucose, an inhibitor of glycosylation, was effective in the treatment of recurrent genital herpes; however, this has not been confirmed by other investigators.

The theoretical problems of topical therapy in recurrent mucocutaneous HSV infections are discussed in Chapter 99. The same considerations certainly apply to recurrent genital herpes. It seems unlikely that therapy of the skin or mucous membranes will change the latency of HSV-2 in the sacral ganglia. Thus, it is unlikely to alter the frequency of subsequent recurrences. Moreover, if virus replication reaches a peak within 2 to 3 days of onset, antiviral therapy will have to be applied early to have any chance of being effective. However, because of the prolonged period of virus replication that occurs in *primary* genital herpes, topical antiviral therapy, if effective in halting virus replication, might well reduce the number of latently infected neurons and thereby reduce the frequency and severity of subsequent recurrences. The development of a new generation of highly selective (and nontoxic) antiviral agents (Chapter 99) should provide better opportunities for effective topical therapy and also yield drugs with therapeutic indices high enough to warrant their parenteral use in primary and recurrent genital herpes. The availability of adequate amounts of human interferon, which should soon result from the application of recombinant DNA technology, will offer additional therapeutic opportunities. The combined use of interferon and selective inhibitors of HSV DNA synthesis, such as acycloguanosine, should improve efficacy without increasing toxicity.

While little progress has yet been made in the specific treatment of primary and recurrent genital herpes, there have been developments in the therapy of life-threatening HSV infections. Adenine arabinoside, a nucleoside analog that inhibits HSV replication in tissue culture and animal models, is effective when administered parenterally in adults with herpes simplex encephalitis (Whitley et al., 1977) and in newborns with disseminated and localized central nervous system HSV infections (Whitley et al., 1980). The mortality in adult encephalitis was reduced from 70 per cent in placebo recipients to 28 per cent in patients treated with adenine arabinoside. In neonatal HSV infections, mortality was reduced from 74 per cent to 38 per cent, and there was a proportionate increase in the number of infants who survived without significant sequelae.

These results are encouraging, but we can expect even better results in the near future as newer and more selective nucleoside analogs, such as acycloguanosine (Chapter 99) are introduced, and as human interferon becomes more available.

In the newborn, and perhaps also in immunosuppressed patients exposed to HSV-2 infection, the early administration of human HSV immune serum globulin containing high levels of antibody to HSV-2 should be considered.

## PROPHYLAXIS

There is no effective specific prophylaxis for HSV infections and, as discussed in Chapter 99, it will probably be some years before we have an effective vaccine. Thus, prophylaxis is limited to attempts to protect certain particularly vulnerable patients from exposure to HSV.

Since males with symptomatic herpes genitalis appear to transmit infection to 75 per cent or more of susceptible consorts, males with active genital herpes should refrain from intercourse or use condoms.

Because infants born by vaginal delivery to mothers with active genital herpes at term have a high risk of acquiring infection, it seems reasonable that women with active genital herpes at term and intact membranes should be delivered by cesarean section (Nahmias and Visintine, 1976; Hanshaw and Dudgeon, 1978; Kibrick, 1980). It should be noted, however, that the efficacy of this procedure has not been proved. Once the membranes have ruptured, delivery by cesarean section is probably not warranted (Light and Linnemann, 1974). The infant delivered through an infected birth canal should probably be given large doses of immune serum globulin, preferably with a high titer of antibody to HSV-2. Although there is no evidence that passively administered antibody is protective, it reduces the mortality of primary HSV infections in animals, and infants with high titers of transplacentally acquired antibody to HSV-2 have a more favorable outcome than infants with low antibody titers (Yeager et al., 1980). Topical adenine arabinoside eye drops should also be administered, since the eye is one portal of entry for HSV-2 (Nahmias and Visintine, 1976). When new and nontoxic inhibitors of HSV replication become available, their prophylactic administration should also be considered.

## References

Adams, H. G., Renson, E. A., Alexander, E. R., Vontver, L. A., Remington, M. A., and Holmes, K. K.: Genital herpetic infection in men and women: Clinical course and effect of topical application of adenine arabinoside. J. Infect Dis 133 Suppl.: A151, 1976.

Baringer, J. R.: Recovery of herpes simplex virus from human sacral ganglions. N Engl J Med 291:828, 1974.

Blough, H. A., and Guintoli, R. L.: Successful treatment of human genital herpes infections with 2-deoxy-D-glucose. JAMA 241:2798, 1979.

Bolognese, R. J., Corson, S. L., Fuccillo, D. A., Traub, R., Moder, F., and Sever, J. L.: Herpesvirus hominis type II infections in asymptomatic pregnant women. Obstet Gynecol 48:507, 1976.

Buchman, T. G., Roizman, B., and Nahmias, A. J.: Demonstration of

exogenous genital reinfection with herpes simplex virus type 2 by restriction endonuclease fingerprinting of viral DNA. J Infect Dis 140:295, 1979.

Centifano, Y. M., Drylie, D. M., Deardourff, S. L., and Kaufman, H. E.: Herpesvirus type 2 in the male genitourinary tract. Science 178:318, 1972.

Chang, T.-W., Fiumara, N. J., and Weinstein, L.: Genital herpes: Some clinical and laboratory observations. JAMA 229:544, 1974.

Caplan, L. R., Kleeman, F. J., and Berg, S.: Urinary retention probably secondary to herpes genitalis. N Engl J Med 297:920, 1977.

Corey, L., Reeves, W. C., Chiang, W. T., Vontver, L. A., Remington, M., Winter, C., and Holmes, K. K.: Ineffectiveness of topical ether for the treatment of genital herpes simplex virus infection. N Engl J Med 299:237, 1978.

Deture, F. A., Drylie, D. M., Kaufman, H. E., and Centifano, Y. M.: Herpes virus type 2: Study of semen in male subjects with recurrent infections. J Urol 120:449, 1978.

Dueñas, A., Adam, E., Melnick, J. L., and Rawls, W. E.: Herpesvirus type 2 in a prostitute population. Am J Epidemiol 95:483, 1972.

Glogau, R., Hanna, L., and Jawetz, E.: Herpetic whitlow as part of genital virus infection. J Infect Dis 136:689, 1977.

Hanshaw, J. B., and Dudgeon, J. A.: Viral Diseases of the Fetus and Newborn. Vol. 17 in series Major Problems in Clinical Pediatrics, Schaffer, A. J., and Markowitz, M. (eds.). Philadelphia, W. B. Saunders Co., 1978.

Hinthorn, D. R., Baker, L. H., Romig, D. A., and Liu, C.: Recurrent conjugal neuralgia caused by herpesvirus hominis type 2. JAMA 236:587, 1976.

Hutfield, D. C.: History of herpes genitalis. Br J Vener Dis 42:263, 1966.

Hutfield, D. C.: Herpes genitalis. Br J Vener Dis 44:241, 1968.

Jacobs, E.: Anal infections caused by herpes simplex virus. Dis. Colon Rectum 19:151, 1976.

Jeansson, S., and Molin, L.: On the occurrence of genital herpes simplex virus infection: Clinical and virological findings and relation to gonorrhoea. Acta Dermatovener (Stockh) 54:479, 1974.

Kaufman, R. H., Gardner, H. L., Rawls, W. E., Dixon, R. E., and Young, R. L.: Clinical features of herpes genitalis. Cancer Res 33:1446, 1973.

Kibrick, S.: Herpes simplex infection at term: What to do with mother, newborn, and nursery personnel. JAMA 243:157, 1980.

Layzer, R. B., and Conant, M. A.: Neuralgia in recurrent herpes simplex. Arch Neurol 31:233, 1974.

Light, I. J., and Linneman, C. C.: Neonatal herpes simplex infection following delivery by cesarean section. Obstet Gynecol 44:496, 1974.

Logan, W. S., Tindall, J. P., and Elson, M. L.: Chronic cutaneous herpes simplex. Arch Derm 103:606, 1971.

Lopyan, L., Young, A. W., and Menegus, M.: Generalized acute mucocutaneous herpes simplex type 2 with fatal outcome. Arch Derm 113:816, 1977.

Moller-Larsen, A., Haahr, S., and Black, F. T.: Cellular and humoral immune responses to herpes simplex virus during and after primary gingivostomatitis. Infect Immun 22:445, 1978.

Muller, S. A., Herrmann, E. C., and Winkilmann, R. K.: Herpes simplex infections in hematologic malignancies. Am J Med 52:102, 1972.

Nahmias, A. J., and Dowdle, W. R.: Antigenic and biologic differences in herpesvirus hominis. Prog Med Virol 10:110, 1968.

Nahmias, A. J., Dowdle, W. R., Naib, Z. M., Josey, W. E., McLone, D., and Domescik, G.: Genital infection with type 2 herpes virus hominis: A commonly occurring veneral disease. Br J Vener Dis 45:294, 1969.

Nahmias, A. J., and Josey, W. E.: Epidemiology of herpes simplex viruses 1 and 2. In Evans, A. S. (ed.): Viral Infections of Humans. New York, Plenum Medical Book Company, 1976.

Nahmias, A. J., Josey, W. E., Naib, Z. M., Luce, C. F., and Duffey, A.: Antibodies to herpesvirus hominis types 1 and 2 in humans: I. Patients with genital herpetic infections. Am J Epidemiol 91:539, 1970.

Nahmias, A. J., and Roizman, B.: Infection with herpes simplex viruses 1 and 2. N Engl J Med 289:667, 719, 781, 1973.

Nahmias, A. J., and Visintine, A. M.: Herpes simplex. In Remington, J. S., and Klein, J. O. (eds.): Infectious Diseases of the Fetus and Newborn Infant. Philadelphia, W. B. Saunders Company, 1976.

Ng, A. B. P., Reagan, J. W., and Yen, S. S. C.: Herpes genitalis: Clinical and cytopathologic experience with 256 patients. Obstet Gynecol 36:645, 1970.

Oates, J. K., and Greenhouse, P. R. D. H.: Retention of urine in anogenital herpetic infection. Lancet 1:691, 1979.

O'Reilly, R. J., Chibbaro, A., Anger, E., and Lopez, C.: Cell-mediated immune responses in patients with recurrent herpes simplex infections. II. Infection-associated deficiency of lymphokine production in patients with recurrent herpes labialis or herpes progenitalis. J Immunol 118:1095, 1977.

Overall, J. C.: Dermatologic diseases. In Galasso, G. J., et al., (eds.): Antiviral Agents and Viral Diseases of Man. New York, Raven Press, 1979.

Poste, G., Hawkins, D. F., and Thomlinson, J.: Herpesvirus hominis infection of the female genital tract. Obstet Gynecol 40:871, 1972.

Rawls, W. E.: Herpes simplex virus types 1 and 2 and herpesvirus simae. In Lennette, E. H., and Schmidt, N. J. (eds.): Diagnostic Procedures for Viral, Rickettsial and Chlamydial Infections. Washington, D.C., American Public Health Association, p. 309, 1979.

Rawls, W. E., Bacchetti, S., and Graham, F. L.: Relation of herpes simplex viruses to human malignancies. In Arber, W., et al., (eds.): Current Topics in Microbiology and Immunology, Vol. 77. Berlin, Heidelberg, Springer Verlag, 1977.

Rawls, E. W., Gardner, H. L., Flanders, R. W., Lowry, S. P., Kaufman, R. H., and Melnick, J. L.: Genital herpes in two social groups. Am J Obstet Gynecol 110:682, 1971.

Rotkin, I. D.: A comparison review of key epidemiological studies in cervical cancer related to current search for transmissible agents. Cancer Res. 33:1353, 1973.

Schneidman, D. W., Barr, R. J., and Graham, J. H.: Chronic cutaneous herpes simplex. JAMA 241:592, 1979.

Slavin, H. B., and Ferguson, J. J.: Zoster-like eruptions caused by the virus of herpes simplex. Am J Med 8:456, 1950.

Slavin, H. B., and Gavett, E.: Primary Herpetic Vulvovaginitis. Proc Soc Exptl Biol Med 63:343, 1946.

Spruance, S. L., Crumpacker, C. S., Haines, H., Bader, C., Mehr, K., MacCalman, J., Schnipper, L. E., Klauber, M. R., and Overall Jr, J. C.: Ineffectiveness of tropical adenine arabinoside 5'-monophosphate in the treatment of recurrent herpes simplex labialis. N Engl J Med 300:1180, 1979.

Stone, W. J., Scowden, E. B., Spannuth, C. L., Lowry, S. P., and Alford, R. H.: Atypical herpesvirus hominis type 2 infection in uremic patients receiving immunosuppressive therapy. Am J Med 63:511, 1977.

Sutton, A. L., Smithwick, E. M., Seligman, S. J., and Kim, D.-S.: Fatal disseminated herpesvirus hominis type 2 infection in an adult with associated thymic dysplasia. Am J Med 56:545, 1974.

Unna, P. G.: On herpes progenitalis, especially in women. J Cutan Vener Dis 1:321, 1883.

Vontver, L. A., Reeves, W. C., Rattray, M., Corey, L., Remington, M. A., Tolentino, E., Schweid, A., and Holmes, K. K.: Clinical course and diagnosis of genital herpes simplex virus infection and evaluation of topical surfactant therapy. Am J Obstet Gynecol 54:548, 1979.

Whitley, R. J., Soong, S.-J., Dolin, R., Galasso, G. J., Ch'ien, L. T., Alford, C. A., and the Collaborative Study Group: Andenine arabinoside therapy of biopsy-proved herpes simplex encephalitis. N Engl J Med 297:289, 1977.

Whitley, R. J., Nahmia, A., Soong, S.-J., Galasso, G. J., Fleming, C. L., and Alford, C. A.: Vidarabine therapy of neonatal herpes simplex virus infections. Pediatrics 66:495, 1980.

Yeager, A. S., Arvin, A. M., Urbani, L. J. and Kemp III, J. A.: Relationship of antibody to outcome in neonatal herpes simplex virus infections. Infect Immun 29:532, 1980.

Yen, S. S. C., Reagan, J. W., and Rosenthal, M. S.: Herpes simplex infection in female genital tract. Obstet Gynecol 25:479, 1965.

Young, A. W.: Herpes genitalis. Med Clin North Am. 56:1175, 1972.

Young, A. W., Tovell, H. M. M., and Sadri, K.: Erosions and ulcers of the vulva: Diagnosis, incidence and management. Obstet Gynecol 50:35, 1977.

# *LYMPHOGRANULOMA* **152** *VENEREUM, CHANCROID, AND GRANULOMA INGUINALE*

## H. Hunter Handsfield, M. D.

## *LYMPHOGRANULOMA VENEREUM*

### Definition

*Lymphogranuloma venereum* (LGV) is a sexually transmitted infection caused by specific strains of *Chlamydia trachomatis*. It is characterized by a transient and often undiagnosed primary cutaneous or mucosal lesion, with subsequent regional lymphadenitis. Synonyms include lymphopathia venereum, lymphogranuloma inguinale, tropical bubo, and others. Although recognized in the nineteenth century, Nicholas, Durand, and Favre provided the first definitive description in 1913.

### Etiology

The chlamydiae (formerly *Bedsonia*) are bacteria that grow only within eukaryotic cells and require tissue culture for isolation. Two species are pathogenic for man: *C. psittaci*, the cause of psittacosis, and *C. trachomatis*, immunotype variants of which cause trachoma (primarily types A, B, Ba, and C), inclusion conjunctivitis, nongonococcal urethritis, and related syndromes (primarily types D through K), and LGV (types $L_1$, $L_2$, and $L_3$). Compared with types A through K, the LGV strains of *C. trachomatis* cause greater cytopathologic effect in tissue culture, are relatively resistant to neuraminidase, and, except for type

$L_3$, are more lethal to mice after intracerebral inoculation.

## Epidemiology and Geographic Variation

LGV is worldwide in distribution, but is endemic in tropical climates and in areas of economic deprivation. The greatest incidences are seen in Africa, Southeast Asia, and India, and LGV is now uncommon in North America and Europe; 348 cases were reported in the United States in 1978. Although LGV is sexually transmitted in almost all cases, the influence of nonsexual socioeconomic factors is demonstrated by the decrease in incidence that has occurred in areas that have undergone economic improvement, such as the southeast United States.

The age distribution of LGV matches that of all sexually transmitted infections, with most cases in persons aged 18 to 40 years. The diagnosis is established 6 to 20 times more frequently in men, reflecting the greater incidence of minimal symptoms and perhaps asymptomatic carriage of *C. trachomatis* in women. In Europe and North America, LGV is seen predominantly in homosexual males.

Active LGV is rarely documented in sex contacts of infected patients, suggesting that asymptomatic carriage is common. Partners should probably be treated routinely, although there are no firm data on the appropriate antimicrobial agent and dosage for presumed carriers. Since two or more sexually transmitted infections often are present simultaneously, all patients with LGV should be examined for gonorrhea and syphilis.

## Pathogenesis and Pathology

The primary lesion of LGV has been variously described as a small cutaneous papule, pustule, or ulcer with nonspecific histologic features. Patients do not usually notice primary cutaneous lesions, and clinicians identify them only infrequently (20 to 40 per cent in most reports). Moreover LGV strains of *C. trachomatis* have been isolated only rarely from primary cutaneous lesions, and have been isolated from urethras of men with LGV and men with uncomplicated nongonococcal urethritis. These facts suggest that an identifiable primary cutaneous lesion often does not occur, and that chlamydial urethritis (with or without symptoms) may be the primary lesion in some men.

*C. trachomatis* is transported by the lymphatics to regional lymph nodes. At this time, a transient bacteremia may occur, and *C. trachomatis* has been identified in blood, cerebrospinal fluid, and lung tissue of rare patients with LGV. Initially, the lymph node contains stellate microabscesses, with central granulocytes surrounded by palisading mononuclear inflammatory cells. These later coalesce to form the classic fluctuant bubo. Several lymph nodes are usually infected simultaneously, becoming mutually adherent through an intense periadenitis. *C. trachomatis* may be isolated from the inflammatory exudate in 60 to 70 per cent of cases. Fixation to overlying skin is followed by spontaneous rupture and drainage. After a variable course that may include several cycles of partial healing, scarring, and recurrent drainage over months or years, chronic lymphatic obstruction may supervene, leading to the lymphedema, susceptibility to secondary infection, and tissue destruction that constitute the chronic sequelae of LGV.

At the time of bubo formation fever, chills, myalgia, headache, hyperglobulinemia with elevations of IgA, IgG, and IgM, leukocytosis, and elevation of the erythrocyte sedimentation rate are common. Less frequent are keratoconjunctivitis, meningoencephalitis, splenomegaly, erythema nodosum, erythema multiforme, polyarthritis, false-positive reagin tests for syphilis, circulating rheumatoid factor, and cryoglobulinemia.

Antibodies to *C. trachomatis* may be detected in the blood during and after bubo formation by complement fixation, immunofluorescence, neutralization, and other techniques. Cellular immunity may develop, as reflected in the Frei skin test and by species-specific lymphocyte transformation in vitro. Although these responses may be partially protective, reinfection is believed to occur in heavily endemic areas.

## Clinical Manifestations

The painless primary lesion (or urethritis) appears after an incubation period of one to three weeks. Primary lesions are 1 to 4 mm in diameter, have been identified most frequently on the penis of men, and are believed to occur most frequently on the external genitalia, vaginal mucosa, or cervix in women. The primary lesion heals spontaneously after several days; regional lymphadenopathy then develops after a latent period that varies from a few days to several weeks.

The location of the primary lesion in part determines the subsequent manifestations. The lymphatics of the penis, scrotum, female external genitalia, and distal third of the vagina drain primarily into the inguinal and femoral lymph nodes, resulting in the "inguinal syndrome," the most frequently diagnosed form of LGV. Lymphadenopathy is unilateral in approximately one-half to two-thirds of cases and bilateral in the remainder. Over one to four weeks, the nodes gradually become fluctuant, and fixed to the overlying skin with erythema, warmth, and eventual rupture. Occasionally there is spontaneous regression without rupture. In 15 to 30 per cent of patients, both the femoral and inguinal nodes are involved; their separation by the inguinal ligament results in the pathognomonic "groove sign." The adenopathy initially causes little discomfort, but becomes increasingly painful and tender as the nodes enlarge and fluctuance and skin fixation progress.

When primary lesions occur in the upper vagina, cervix, or anorectum, with lymphatic drainage into pelvic and deep iliac lymph nodes, the "genitoanorectal syndrome" may result. Occurring in less than 25 per cent of diagnosed cases of LGV, primarily in women and homosexual men, the acute stage is characterized by proctitis and subsequent perirectal abscesses, presumably due to intraluminal or perirectal rupture of fluctuant nodes. Separation into the two syndromes may be artifactual; up to 75 per cent of women with the inguinal syndrome, for example, may have pelvic or iliac node involvement as well.

In recent years, several cases of cervical, supraclavicular, and mediastinal node involvement have been reported; all have been related to orogenital sexual practices.

The systemic clinical and laboratory manifestations outlined above *(Pathogenesis and Pathology)* occur simultaneously with regional lymphadenitis, but often are mild and may go unnoticed. Occasionally, with iliac or pelvic node infection that does not progress to the overt genitoanorectal syndrome, the systemic manifestations may be the only signs of disease.

### Complications and Sequelae

The majority of patients eventually have complete resolution, with or without antimicrobial therapy. Ten to 20 per cent of untreated patients, however, develop lymphatic obstruction with chronic lymphedema that may result in genital elephantiasis ("esthiomene" in women) and polypoid vulvar or perirectal masses of hypertrophied lymphoid tissue ("lymphorrhoids"). Chronic persistent chlamydial infection (often with bacterial super-infection) may result in draining inguinal sinuses, urethral fistulas and strictures, genital ulcerations, and rectal strictures.

### Diagnosis

The diagnosis of LGV commonly rests on clinical assessment and serologic testing. Isolation of an LGV strain of *C. trachomatis* is the only

incontrovertible proof of the diagnosis, but laboratories with this capability are not widely available. Identification of typical basophilic cytoplasmic inclusions by Giemsa staining of pus aspirated from a bubo is a highly specific but very insensitive test. The histopathology of the lymphadenitis is otherwise nonspecific, and biopsy or excision of involved lymph nodes is contraindicated on clinical grounds.

The complement-fixation (CF) test is the most widely available serologic test, and uses a heat-stable antigen common to all chlamydiae (Schachter et al., 1969). There is controversy regarding the definition of significant CF titers, and there is probably geographic variation; however, a titer of $\geq$ 1:64 is highly specific for LGV and has a sensitivity of about 70 to 80 per cent. In the United States, CF titers of 1:8 to 1:32 occur in 20 to 80 per cent of patrons of public venereal disease clinics, and usually reflect past or present infection with non-LGV strains of *C. trachomatis,* rather than subclinical or previously treated LGV. Even such low titers, however, support the diagnosis if a fourfold rise or fall occurs during a compatible clinical syndrome. A microimmunofluorescence test, not yet widely available, is more sensitive than the CF test and has the advantages of differentiation of strains of *C. trachomatis* and ease of automation.

The Frei test detects delayed hypersensitivity by using intradermal inoculation of material prepared from an LGV organism grown in chick embryo yolk sacs. In most investigators' hands, the Frei test is both insensitive (30 to 50 per cent false negatives) and nonspecific (up to 50 per cent false positives), and is therefore of questionable diagnostic value (Schachter et al. 1969). Because of these problems, the antigen is no longer commercially available in the United States.

The differential diagnosis includes all causes of regional lymphadenopathy. Chancroid and granuloma inguinale are distinguished by the typical skin lesions and absence of systemic symptoms. The acute genitoanorectal syndrome of LGV can be confused with ulcerative colitis, Crohn's disease, amebiasis, and other causes of proctocolitis and perirectal abscess. In areas of low endemicity, rectal stricture is often confused with carcinoma. Confusion with syphilis may occur because of occasional biologic false-positive reagin tests in patients with LGV.

### Treatment

*C. trachomatis* is sensitive in vitro to the tetracyclines, the agents of choice. Tetracycline hydrochloride is given orally in a dose of 500 mg four times daily for four to six weeks. The sulfonamides and erythromycin are effective alternatives. Lymphadenopathy resolves slowly, although systemic signs and symptoms subside promptly. Draining sinus tracts should be examined and treated for bacterial superinfection.

Fluctuant buboes should be aspirated with an 18-gauge needle as often as necessary to prevent rupture, taking care to enter the node through adjacent normal skin in order to avoid establishing a sinus tract. Surgical incision or excision often leads to sinus formation and secondary infection, and is contraindicated.

## Prevention

Condoms may give some protection, but avoidance of sexual contact with infected individuals or carriers is the only sure means of prevention. An effective vaccine is not available and none is anticipated.

## *CHANCROID*

### Definition

Chancroid (soft chancre) is a sexually transmitted infection caused by *Haemophilus ducreyi,* and is characterized by painful genital ulceration, inguinal lymphadenitis, but no systemic symptoms. Chancroid was differentiated from syphilis by Bassereau in 1852, and Ducrey described the causative bacillus in 1889.

### Etiology

*H. ducreyi* is a small, facultatively anarerobic, gram-negative coccobacillus. In liquid media, and to a lesser extent in vivo, it tends to grow end-to-end in chains; two or more chains often lie in parallel. The inclusion of the Ducrey bacillus in the genus *Haemophilus* has recently been reconfirmed (Hammond et al., 1978).

### Epidemiology and Geographic Variation

Chancroid is transmitted almost exclusively by sexual contact. As is true for lymphogranuloma venereum and granuloma inguinale, however, nonsexual socioeconomic factors have greatly influenced the frequency of chancroid in various populations, and the disease is now uncommon in Europe and North America, although it is not as rare as suggested by reported incidences (455 cases in the United States in 1978). The greatest incidences are in tropical and subtropical developing countries.

As for all sexually transmitted infections, most cases of chancroid occur between 15 and 40 years of age. An asymptomatic carrier state in women has been postulated to explain the 80 to 90 per cent dominance of males in most published reports of chancroid, but bacteriologically confirmed asymptomatic carriage of *H. ducreyi* has been reported only rarely. Moreover, recent studies have shown male:female ratios between 1:1 and 2:1 and have documented genital ulcers in the majority of sexual contacts of patients with chancroid. The epidemiology of chancroid therefore requires further study using definitive bacteriologic techniques. Other sexually transmitted infections often are present simultaneously; syphilis was diagnosed in 7 per cent of U.S. military personnel who acquired chancroid in Korea.

### Pathogenesis and Pathology

The primary lesion of chancroid begins as a small papule or vesicle that becomes pustular and ulcerates within one to two days. The ulcer may enlarge for several days or weeks. A mixed bacterial flora is always present, but the role of organisms other than *H. ducreyi* in uncomplicated chancroid is unknown. Three histologic zones have been described: a superficial zone of polymorphonuclear leukocytes, erythrocytes, bacteria, and necrotic debris; a central zone of edema and neovascularization; and a deep zone of macrophages, lymphocytes, and plasma cells. Central necrosis, spontaneous rupture, and drainage occur in the regional lymph nodes of most untreated patients. Fever, leukocytosis, and other signs of systemic illness are rare and suggest another diagnosis or superinfection; bacteremia and pathology distant from regional lymph nodes have not been described.

### Clinical Manifestations

The incubation period of one to five days is followed by the exquisitely painful nonindurated primary lesion, a round, irregular, or serpiginous ulcer of the external genitalia; in men, almost all lesions involve the penis, typically the glans or corona (Fig. 1). Individual lesions vary from 3 to 20 mm in diameter. The edges are undermined, the adjacent skin is inflamed, and the gray-white base bleeds readily when traumatized. Multiple primary lesions occur in up to half the cases, often in the form of "kissing" lesions caused by autoinoculation of normal skin in apposition to the initial lesion.

Regional lymphadenitis occurs in 30 to 50 per cent of cases, appears within a few days of onset of the primary lesion, and involves a single inguinal node unilaterally in about two-thirds of cases. Untreated, the involved node becomes fluctuant

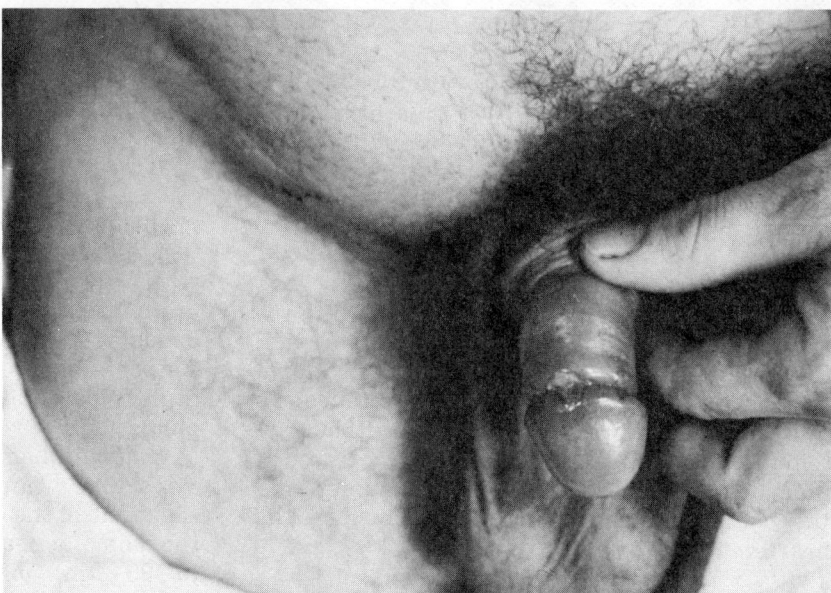

**FIGURE 1.** *A case of chancroid with multiple typical penile ulcers and fluctuant inguinal lymphadenopathy. The small eschars adjacent to the bubo are due to multiple needle aspirations.*

and ruptures spontaneously, followed by gradual healing.

### Complications and Sequelae

"Phagedenic" chancroid, with large undermined ulcers that progress rapidly and cause extensive tissue destruction and scarring, is infrequent and probably results from secondary infection by a mixed aerobic and anaerobic flora. Uncomplicated chancroid usually heals spontaneously over several weeks or months, without significant scarring or lymphatic obstruction (Gaisin and Heaton, 1975).

### Diagnosis

Although the clinical presentation of chancroid often is characteristic, isolation of *H. ducreyi* is the only definitive means of diagnosis. Material from the undermined edge of an ulcer or pus aspirated from an infected lymph node should be inoculated onto chocolate agar containing a nutritional supplement, such as IsoVitalex and 3 µg/ml vancomycin (Hammond et al., 1978); previously reported techniques for isolation in various liquid media are less sensitive. Microscopic examination of material obtained from genital ulcers is both insensitive and nonspecific, but observation of small gram-negative bacilli in pus aspirated from a bubo is helpful. Serologic tests are under investigation but are not generally available.

In geographic areas where genital herpes virus infections are highly prevalent and chancroid is uncommon, most genital ulcers of typical "chancroidal" morphology are, in fact, herpetic. In this setting, cultures for both *Herpes simplex* and *H. ducreyi* are indicated. Primary syphilis is distinguished by the nontender indurated chancre, but darkfield examination and syphilis serology are indicated for any genital ulceration. The systemic symptoms, more chronic course, and lymphadenopathy without prominent genital ulceration all help distinguish LGV from chancroid. Traumatic genital lesions may become secondarily infected and ulcerate, with or without regional lymphadenitis.

### Treatment

*H. ducreyi* is usually susceptible to the sulfonamides and tetracyclines. The majority of clinical isolates in many areas of the world contain plasmids that encode for β-lactamase and are thus resistant to the penicillins. A sulfonamide is the agent of choice; 1 g of sulfisoxazole is given orally four times daily for one to three weeks, or until healing is complete. Tetracycline hydrochloride, 500 mg four times daily for the same duration, is also effective. Some authorities recommend a sulfonamide-tetracycline combination, and sulfamethoxazole with trimethoprim has been effective. Kanamycin, streptomycin, erythromycin, and others have been advocated for cases resistant to sulfonamides or tetracycline, but have not been evaluated in well-controlled studies in which the diagnosis was proved by isolation of *H. ducreyi*. Ampicillin is effective for chancroid caused by strains of *H. ducreyi* that do not produce β-lactamase. Fluctuant lymph nodes should be aspirated through adjacent normal skin as often as necessary to prevent spontaneous rupture.

## Prevention

Avoidance of sexual contact with infected individuals is the only known means of prevention. Condoms may reduce the transmission rate.

## GRANULOMA INGUINALE

### Definition

Granuloma inguinale (donovanosis) is an infection caused by *Calymmatobacterium granulomatis,* and is characterized by indolent cutaneous or mucocutaneous ulceration, usually without systemic symptoms. The disease was recognized by McLeod in India in 1882, and Donovan described the characteristic intracellular inclusions that bear his name in 1905.

### Etiology

*C. granulomatis* is an encapsulated, bipolar-staining, short gram-negative bacillus. It is antigenically related to *Klebsiella* species, and has been cultivated only in yolk sacs of embryonated chicken eggs and on media containing egg yolk. Its biochemical characteristics are unknown, and its antimicrobial susceptibilities have only been surmised on the basis of responses of patients to various drugs. The organism has been isolated from feces, and it is possible that a fecal reservoir plays an epidemiologic role in some populations.

### Epidemiology and Geographic Variation

Granuloma inguinale is the rarest of all sexually transmitted infections in Europe and North America (75 cases were reported in the United States in 1978), but is an endemic problem in tropical and subtropical climates, especially among economically disadvantaged populations. Tropical South America, the West Indies, the Indian subcontinent, Africa, and Southeast Asia apparently have the highest incidences.

The importance of sexual transmission of granuloma inguinale has been debated, but the most recent epidemiologic data and the weight of clinical experience indicate that sexual transmission is the rule (Lal and Nicholas, 1970). The age range reflects the frequency of sexual activity, with most cases occurring between ages 15 and 40. The reported male:female ratio varies from 2:1 to 10:1; in North America, many cases occur in homosexual males. Although most reports suggest that active disease is diagnosed in less than 20 per cent of sex partners of patients, other studies have documented rates of 50 to 65 per cent. Granuloma inguinale does not appear to be highly contagious, and sex partners have been reported free of infection despite several years of repeated intercourse with infected patients.

### Pathogenesis and Pathology

The first identifiable lesion is an indurated papule that ulcerates over several days to weeks, with formation of pink-red hypertrophic granulation-like tissue with little or no purulent exudate or inflammation of the adjacent skin. There is extensive epithelial proliferation and acanthosis, and dense infiltration by macrophages and plasma cells, with variable numbers of polymorphonuclear leukocytes and lymphocytes; true granulomas do not form (Davis, 1970), the name of the disease notwithstanding. The pathognomonic feature is the presence of large (25 to 90 $\mu$m) macrophages that contain large numbers of *C. granulomatis*, identified as Donovan bodies. These cells and the Donovan bodies are difficult to identify in route paraffin-embedded tissue sections, but are easily identified in smears of scrapings or crushed tissue, or in thin (1 $\mu$m) sections of tissue embedded in plastic. With Wright or Giemsa staining, the organisms appear as blue-black bipolar-staining coccobacilli 1 to 2 $\mu$m in length, lying in large cystic vacuoles within the macrophages.

The ulcer may enlarge slowly for months or years, with extensive tissue destruction. Spontaneous resolution and healing may occur in some cases, but are often followed by later relapse. Bacteremia has not been documented, but metastatic systemic infection, manifested primarily by multifocal osteomyelitis, has been reported.

### Clinical Manifestations

The incubation period has been reported to vary between one week and six months, but averages two to four weeks. The primary cutaneous papule and subsequent ulcer are usually painless (Davis, 1970). In women and heterosexual men, over 90 percent of lesions involve the external genitals, perianal skin, and the inguinal region. The anus and perianal skin are the usual sites in homosexual men. Almost any cutaneous or accessible mucous membrane site may be involved, and oral granuloma inguinale may follow orogenital sex.

The ulcers have a characteristic appearance, with heaped-up pink or red granulation-like tissue; "kissing" lesions, due to local autoinoculation, are frequent. Extension, healing, and scarring may be observed simultaneously. Extension of induration and swelling into the inguinal region results in a "pseudobubo," which may subsequently break down into a typical ulcer. True lymph node involvement is uncommon. Fever, leukocytosis, and other signs of systemic illness are infrequent, and suggest secondary infection.

### Complications and Sequelae

When treated before extensive tissue destruction occurs, granuloma inguinale is a benign disease with no known sequelae. Unfortunately, many patients, especially among uneducated and economically disadvantaged populations, have had symptoms for several months when they present for medical care. Extensive local tissue destruction may occur over months or years, resulting in autoamputation of external genitalia, local bone and deep soft tissue destruction, and sepsis and death due to bacterial superinfection. Systemic dissemination with focal visceral or bony involvement is a rare complication. Squamous cell carcinoma has been reported to occur in association with chronic granuloma inguinale more frequently than expected by chance, a situation that is complicated by the clinically similar appearance and local destructiveness of the two conditions.

### Diagnosis

The diagnosis is suspected on the basis of the clinical appearance of the lesions, and is confirmed by identification of Donovan bodies after Wright or Giemsa staining of methanol-fixed smears of scrapings of a fresh ulcer or of crushed tissue obtained by biopsy. The appearance of the ulcers, the lack of suppuration of the pseudo-buboes, and absence of systemic signs all serve to differentiate granuloma inguinale from other genitoulcerative disorders. Advanced disease may be mistaken for carcinoma until histologic examination is complete. Isolation of *C. granulo-*

*matis* is not feasible, and there is no serologic test.

### Treatment

Tetracycline hydrochloride, 500 mg four times daily, is the treatment of choice in most geographic areas, but frequent failure of tetracycline has been documented in New Guinea and Vietnam. Streptomycin, 0.5 to 1.0 g intramuscularly twice daily, is usually successful. Ampicillin, 500 mg four times daily by mouth, is usually successful in tetracycline-resistant cases, although failures have been reported (Kuberski, 1980). Erythromycin and chloramphenicol are other alternatives. In all cases, therapy is given for at least 10 to 14 days, or until healing is complete.

### Prevention

As with all sexually transmitted infections, avoidance of sexual contact with infected individuals is the only sure means of prevention. There is no vaccine.

### References

Davis, C. M.: Granuloma inguinale: A clinical, histological, and ultrastructural study. J Am Med Assoc 211:632, 1970.

Gaisin, A., and Heaton, C. L.: Chancroid: Alias the soft chancre. Int J Dermatol 14:188, 1975.

Hammond, G. W., Lian, C. J., Wilt, J. C., and Ronald, A. R.: Comparison of specimen collection and laboratory techniques for isolation of *Haemophilus ducreyi*. J Clin Microbiol 7:39, 1978.

Kuberski, T.: Granuloma inguinale (Donovanosis). Sex Transm Dis 7:29, 1980.

Lal, S., and Nicholas, C.: Epidemiological and clinical features in 165 cases of granuloma inguinale. Br J Vener Dis 46:461, 1970.

Lykke-Oleson, L., Pedersen, T. G., Larsen, L., and Gaarslev, K.: Epidemic of chancroid in Greenland 1977–78. Lancet 1:654, 1979.

Schachter, J., Smith, D. E., Dawson, C. R., Anderson, W. R., Deller, J. J., Jr., Hoke, A. W., Smart, W. H., and Meyer, K. F.: Lymphogranuloma venereum. I. Comparison of the Frei test, complement fixation test, and isolation of the agent. J Infect Dis 120:372, 1969.

Schachter, J., and Dawson, C. R.: Human Chlamydial Infections. Littleton, Massachusetts, PSG Publishing Company, 1978, pp. 45–62.

# E NEUROLOGIC INFECTIONS

# 153 *PURULENT BACTERIAL MENINGITIS*

*Thomas A. Hoffman, M.D.*

## DEFINITION

Purulent meningitis is an acute life-threatening illness caused by invading bacteria that elicit an inflammatory response in the meninges and cerebrospinal fluid (CSF). The incidence of meningitis varies inversely with age. The age of the patient also affects the relative frequency with which the various organisms cause meningitis. Prompt diagnosis and early institution of specific antibiotic therapy are essential steps in managing this condition. Despite the availability of effective antimicrobial agents, the case fatality rate of bacterial meningitis is approximately 15 per cent. Neurologic sequelae occur in an appreciable number of infants and children.

## ETIOLOGY

### Common Causative Agents

Three encapsulated organisms cause over 80 per cent of the cases of purulent meningitis. The most frequent cause is *Haemophilus influenzae*, a pleomorphic gram-negative rod that has a capsule composed of polyribitol phosphate. This polysaccharide is the specific antigen of type b strains of *H. influenzae* and is present in several other bacteria including those considered normal flora. Subclinical infection by these other bacteria occurs frequently during childhood, resulting in the formation of protective antibodies against *H. influenzae* type b in most individuals within the first five years of life. The attack rate of *H. influenzae* meningitis is highest among infants during the second six months of life. The age-related incidence of *H. influenzae* meningitis decreases with each succeeding year after one year and becomes almost negligible after childhood. Since the overall incidence of *H. influenzae* meningitis is apparently increasing in the antibiotic era, this organism has become an occasional cause of meningitis in adults. *Neisseria meningitidis* is the second most frequent cause of endemic purulent meningitis and is responsible for epidemics of meningitis. Pathogenic strains of this gram-negative diplococcus are, however, subdivided into at least four serologic groups based upon their capsular polysaccharides. The meningococcal polysaccharides of groups A, B, C, and Y organisms can induce the formation of group-specific antibodies. Asymptomatic nasopharyngeal infection by *N. meningitidis* is common and confers group-specific immunity. Immunity is also acquired by a complete cross-reaction between the group B meningococcal polysaccharide and the K1 capsule of *Escherichia coli*. The prevalence of protective antibodies against the various serogroups of *N. meningitidis* increases with age, and the age-related incidence of meningococcal meningitis declines during childhood. The disease occurs in adolescents and in adults at incidence rates that are substantially lower than those in children. *Streptococcus pneumoniae*, the other common cause of bacterial meningitis, and *N. meningitidis* are the principal causes of bacterial meningitis in individuals over ten years of age. All ages are susceptible to *S. pneumoniae* meningitis, since this gram-positive diplococcus has numerous capsular types that cause meningitis. However, 18 serotypes of *S. pneumoniae* cause 90 per cent of the disease (Gotschlich, 1978). Conditions that predispose to acquiring pneumococcal meningitis include sickle cell disease, splenectomy, alcoholism, and head trauma. Pneumococci and meningococci are susceptible to penicillin G at concentrations of 0.1 u/ml or less. Tenfold higher concentrations of ampicillin or penicillin are required for activity against most *H. influenzae*; however, plasmid-mediated penicillinase activity has been noted in approximately 15 per cent of the strains causing meningitis. Chloramphenicol continues to be active against all of the common causative agents.

### Uncommon Causative Agents

A variety of organisms infrequently cause bacterial meningitis. *Listeria monocytogenes* is predominantly a cause of meningitis in neonates or in the elderly; however, this form of meningitis also occurs in adults with lymphoproliferative malignancies and in those receiving immunosuppressive therapy (Lavetter et al., 1971). Ampicillin has greater bactericidal activity against *L. monocytogenes* than does penicillin. *Staphylococcus aureus* meningitis is a rare complication of a suppurative process elsewhere in the body. *Streptococcus pyogenes* bacteremia infrequently results in bacterial meningitis. The principal causes of bacterial meningitis in the neonatal period are *Streptococcus agalactiae* (group B streptococci) and *E. coli*, which are acquired at birth. Prematurity and premature rupture of the membranes are important predisposing factors in neonatal meningitis. Most *E. coli* strains causing neonatal meningitis have the K1 capsular polysaccharide. Meningitis caused by gram-negative bacilli other than *H. influenzae* also occurs in adults, although predominantly as a hospital-acquired complication of severe head trauma or a neurosurgical procedure (Mangi et al., 1975). Contiguous spread of gram-negative bacilli from an adjacent area of suppuration may also occur. Meningitis occurring in association with shunts used for the management of hydrocephalus is frequently caused by *Staphylococcus epidermidis;* however, meningitis caused by *S. aureus* and gram-negative bacilli is also associated with these shunts. Other infrequent causes of meningitis include *Pasteurella multocida*, a penicillin-susceptible organism found in the mouth of domestic animals, and *Acinetobacter calcoaceticus*, which is resistant to penicillin. Since *A. calcoaceticus* is a gram-negative coccobacillary organism, it can be misidentified as meningococci in smears.

## PATHOGENESIS AND PATHOLOGY

Hematogenous spread from the upper respiratory tract is the principal route by which the common causative agents produce meningitis. The sequence of events has been examined in an experimental model of meningitis after intranasal inoculation of organisms (Moxon et al., 1974; Moxon and Ostrow, 1977). Although the size of the inoculum influences the occurrence of bacteremia, the intensity of the bacteremia varies inversely with age and has a direct relationship to the occurrence of meningitis. The severity of the bacteremia occurring within 24 hours after inoculation appears to be a primary determinant in the pathogenesis of meningitis. Invasion of organisms through the meningeal blood vessels apparently occurs in the large venous sinuses of the cranial dura. Organisms pass into the CSF through the delicate arachnoid membrane. CSF flows between this avascular membrane and the pia, another thin membrane that adheres to the surface of and carries the blood vessels to the brain. Diapedesis of polymorphonuclear (PMN) leukocytes occurs in the meningeal blood vessels, which become hyperemic and surrounded by purulent exudates. These inflammatory changes in the leptomeninges precede the appearance of inflammatory cells in the CSF. The inflammatory process increases progressively for 72 hours after the induction of meningitis (McAllister et al., 1975). Bacteria multiply in the CSF to levels that frequently exceed $10^5$/ml, which is the concentration required for organisms to be visualized on Gram-stained smears (Feldman, 1977). As white blood cells (WBC) accumulate in the subarachnoid space, the CSF acquires a turbid appearance and the cortical areas of the brain become edematous. Occasionally, PMN leukocytes infiltrate the cortex, but the pia limits organisms from invading the brain tissue. These inflammatory changes cause increased intracranial pressure, which may eventually cause herniation. The extent to which inflammation progresses is the major determinant of the outcome (McAllister et al., 1975). Meningitis also affects the barrier that limits the entry of substances into the CSF from the blood. Inflammation of the meninges enhances the entry of solutes, serum proteins, and some antibiotics from the CSF from the blood. However, the transport of glucose into the CSF is decreased in bacterial meningitis.

Bacterial meningitis may also result from contiguous spread of infection. Head trauma, even when seemingly minor, can disrupt the normal anatomic barriers and allow organisms in the nasopharynx to enter the meninges. Bacteria in foci of infection in the paranasal sinuses, mastoids, psoas muscles, or brain tissue may spread contiguously to invade the meninges.

## CLINICAL MANIFESTATIONS

Bacterial meningitis in adults has a characteristic clinical pattern, although the progression of symptoms is somewhat variable. It is a febrile illness of short duration with the major symptoms being headache and stiff neck. Lethargy or drowsiness is frequent. Confusion, agitated delirium, and stupor are less frequent presenting findings; however, coma is an ominous prognostic sign. Most patients with bacterial meningitis are febrile, although the height of fever is variable. Pain and resistance to flexion of the neck are the characteristic findings on physical examination. Other signs of meningeal irritation can also be elicited. Kernig's sign is present when the leg cannot be extended more than 135 degrees on the thigh when flexed 90 degrees at the hip. Brudzinski's sign is present when flexion of the neck causes involuntary flexion of the thighs and legs.

Focal neurologic signs are infrequent presenting findings. However, nuchal rigidity may not be elicited in comatose patients who may have signs of focal or diffuse neurologic impairment. Papilledema is not a presenting feature of bacterial meningitis and suggests the presence of an accompanying process (Swartz and Dodge, 1965). A frequent presenting sign in meningococcal meningitis is a petechial rash, which occurs rarely in other kinds of bacterial meningitis. The clinical pattern of bacterial meningitis in young children is often atypical, since headache and nuchal rigidity are frequently absent. Irritability, especially upon movement, is a typical presenting sign of meningitis in a young child. In addition, seizures may be a presenting manifestation of meningitis in infants. Neonatal meningitis has an extremely varied and nonspecific clinical presentation. Bulging of the fontanelle may occur and is a sign of increased intracranial pressure.

Bacterial meningitis produces various changes in the CSF; however, their magnitude depends on the stage of disease in which the CSF is examined. The CSF pressure tends to be moderately elevated, but it may be markedly elevated in severely ill patients. Infected CSF appears turbid, and microscopic evaluation reveals a pleocytosis of PMN leukocytes. Although the number of white blood cells in infected CSF varies widely, counts range from 1000 to 10,000 WBC/ml in the majority of cases. The concentration of total proteins in CSF is increased in proportion to the concentration of white cells present. Reduction of the CSF glucose level to less than 40 per cent of the simultaneous blood glucose level is a feature that suggests bacterial meningitis. However, hypoglycorrhachia is found in only half of the patients with bacterial meningitis. These changes in the CSF reflect the intensity of the inflammatory process but have no prognostic significance.

## COMPLICATIONS AND SEQUELAE

Several life-threatening complications may occur during the acute phase of bacterial meningitis. Marked cerebral edema, which may cause herniation of the temporal lobes or cerebellum, is manifested by coma, oculomotor nerve paralysis, and episodes of respiratory arrest. Coma may also result from diffuse cortical damage. This cortical lesion has a multifactorial etiology including increased intracranial pressure, cerebral vascular occlusions, hypoxia, and other toxic factors (Swartz and Dodge, 1965). Prolonged seizures that are either focal or generalized may also contribute to death. Death may also result from the systemic effects of an overwhelming bacteremia. An example of this is fulminant menin-

gococcemia in which bacteria invade the meninges even though the inflammatory response in the CSF is minimal. Also, acute endocarditis is a frequent finding in fatal cases of pneumococcal meningitis.

Other acute complications of bacterial meningitis include seizures, cranial nerve impairment, focal cerebral deficits, and water retention due to inappropriate secretion of antidiuretic hormone (Kaplan and Feigin, 1978). Generalized brief seizures occur at some stage in approximately 20 per cent of patients with bacterial meningitis. The most frequent cranial nerve dysfunction is impaired ocular movement, which tends to be transient. Damage to the eighth cranial nerve complex, however, may persist. Focal cerebral necrosis resulting from cortical vein thrombosis is an infrequent complication of bacterial meningitis; focal cerebral signs tend to occur within the first few days of illness and often in association with seizures. Delayed thrombosis of the cortical veins is an unusual complication that results in the appearance of focal neurologic deficits after apparent clinical recovery. Another late complication is a subdural effusion that occurs in approximately 15 per cent of infants with bacterial meningitis. Blockade of the aqueduct by the inflammatory exudate causes a loculated infection in the ventricles that impairs the entry of antibiotics into this area. This condition has been termed ventriculitis and is a complication that occurs almost exclusively in infants.

The late sequelae of bacterial meningitis are deafness, mental deficits, and hydrocephalus. Studies indicate that from 5 to 30 per cent of surviving infants and children have one or more of these sequelae (Swartz and Dodge, 1965; Feigin and Dodge, 1976).

## GEOGRAPHIC VARIATION

Bacterial meningitis has a worldwide distribution; however, geographic location is a factor that affects the relative frequency with which the various pathogens cause meningitis. Epidemics of meningococcal disease occur at cyclic intervals in many parts of the world. Meningitis by some of the uncommon causative agents also shows geographic variation. For example, meningitis caused by *Salmonella* species has a tendency to occur in underdeveloped countries where the sanitation is poor. Another consideration relates to the prevalence of antibiotic-resistant organisms in certain areas of the world. The recent emergence of ampicillin-resistant *H. influenzae* in the United States has been observed. Pneumococci that are resistant to penicillin have been identified in South Africa.

## DIAGNOSIS

Examination of the CSF is essential for the definitive diagnosis of bacterial meningitis. A Gram-stained smear provides particularly useful information for acute management, since the organism is likely to be seen and recognized in over 70 per cent of the CSF specimens from which an agent is eventually cultured (Swartz and Dodge, 1965). Other rapid diagnostic tests involve the detection of various bacterial products in CSF. These include the detection of specific capsular antigens by immunologic methods and endotoxin detection by the limulus assay. Although these newer tests have limitations, they may be used as an adjunct to the stained smear. Other changes in the CSF that are characteristic of bacterial meningitis are a brisk pleocytosis by PMN leukocytes, hypoglycorrhachia, and an elevated total protein concentration. The usual means for establishing the diagnosis of bacterial meningitis is culture of CSF. Blood cultures frequently yield the same organisms, but cultures of the nasopharynx are frequently misleading. Prior antibiotic therapy has been implicated as a reason for failure to isolate organisms from the CSF.

Recurrent episodes of bacterial meningitis that are commonly caused by *S. pneumoniae* suggest the presence of a skull defect and associated CSF rhinorrhea. Other causes of recurrent bacterial meningitis are parameningeal foci of infection, immunoglobulin disorders, and complement deficiencies.

Aseptic meningitis occasionally presents with a mild pleocytosis of predominantly PMN leukocytes and must be differentiated from bacterial meningitis. When aseptic meningitis presents in this manner, the proportion of PMN leukocytes in the CSF decreases markedly over the subsequent eight hours. Consequently, reexamination of the CSF after withholding antibiotic therapy for 8 to 12 hours is a useful means for distinguishing between these two syndromes (Feigin and Shackelford, 1973). The magnitude of the CSF pleocytosis as well as the predominance of PMN leukocytes in CSF aids in the rapid differentiation of bacterial meningitis from meningitis caused by other infectious agents except *Naegleria*. Bacterial endocarditis may produce a meningeal inflammatory reaction; however, the CSF is typically sterile in this condition. Meningeal reactions resembling bacterial meningitis also occur in neoplastic meningitis, chemical meningitis, sarcoidosis, and as a hypersensitivity reaction to drugs (e.g., sulfonamides). Parameningeal foci of infection including mastoiditis, sinusitis, brain abscess, subdural empyema, and epidural abscess typically have a mild pleocytosis in the CSF.

Recurrent nonbacterial meningitis occurs in Behçet's syndrome, Mollaret's meningitis, and systemic lupus erythematosus.

## TREATMENT

Specific antibiotic therapy exists for most organisms that cause bacterial meningitis (Table 1). An important objective of this therapy is to obtain an antimicrobial concentration in the CSF at which the causative organism is susceptible. It is essential to begin antibiotic therapy immediately, when changes in the CSF are typical of bacterial meningitis. Examination of the stained smear aids in the initial selection of antibiotic therapy, as does knowing the age of the patient and geographic considerations. Therapy can be adjusted when the organism has been identified and its antimicrobial susceptibility has been determined. Treatment is usually given for ten days. The penetration of the penicillin antibiotics into the CSF decreases as the meningeal reaction subsides. Consequently, sufficiently large doses of these drugs must be given during the entire course of therapy. Penicillin G is the recommended antibiotic for initial treatment of community-acquired bacterial meningitis in adults when the stained smear fails to reveal an organism. Because of its wide antibacterial spectrum and excellent penetration, chloramphenicol is a particularly useful agent for treatment of bacterial meningitis. In addition, this drug appears to have a bactericidal action against the common causative organisms (Rahal and Simberkoff, 1979). Chloramphenicol is recommended for initial treatment of children with bacterial meningitis in areas where ampicillin-resistant *H. influenzae* is known to exist. Neonates should not, however, be treated with chloramphenicol because of its toxic side effects. Since gentamicin and other aminoglycoside antibiotics do not reliably penetrate the blood-CSF barrier, intrathecal or, alternatively, intraventricular administration of these agents is usually necessary (Rahal et al., 1974). The cephalosporins are contraindicated in meningitis, since they are partly inactivated in CSF.

Parenteral fluids should be carefully administered to avoid hyponatremia and water intoxication. Maintenance of adequate ventilation, prevention of aspiration, treatment of seizures with anticonvulsants, and reduction in fever constitute important supportive measures. Treatment of cerebral edema remains controversial. Corticosteroids have no beneficial effect on the outcome of purulent meningitis; repeated drainage of CSF has no therapeutic efficacy. Osmotic diuretics have been used successfully to reduce increased intracranial pressure, even though their adminis-

**TABLE 1. Antimicrobial Treatment of Bacterial Meningitis**

| CAUSATIVE ORGANISM | RECOMMENDED TREATMENT PROGRAM | | | |
| | Antibiotic | Adult Dose | Route[b] | Alternative Drug |
| --- | --- | --- | --- | --- |
| S. pneumoniae, N. meningitidis S. pyogenes, S. agalactica, P. multocida and other penicillin-susceptible organisms | penicillin G | $2 \times 10^6$u every 2h (200,000 to 300,000 u/kg/d in children) | i.v. | chloramphenicol |
| H. influenzae (ampicillin-susceptible), L. monocytogenes, ampicillin-susceptible gram-negative bacilli, neonatal meningitis[a] | ampicillin | 1.5 g every 2 hr (300 to 400 mg/kg/d in children) | i.v. | chloramphenicol |
| H. influenzae (ampicillin-resistant), community-acquired gram-negative bacillary meningitis in adults | chloramphenicol | 1.0 g every 3 to 4 h | i.v. or p.o. | an aminoglycoside antibiotic |
| Hospital-acquired gram-negative bacillary meningitis in adults | gentamicin | 80 mg every 8 h plus 5 mg once daily | i.v. i.t. | depends upon results of susceptibility testing |
| P. aeruginosa, indole-positive Proteus species | pipercillin | 1.5 to 2 g every 2 h | i.v. | carbenicillin (500 mg/kg/d) |
| S. aureus (penicillin-resistant) | methicillin, nafcillin, or oxacillin | 1.0 to 1.5 g every 2 h | i.v. | vancomycin |

[a]Chloramphenicol is contraindicated in neonates.

[b]Intravenously, (i.v.), intrathecal (i.t.), orally (p.o.)

tration may be associated with a late rebound effect.

The definitive treatment for recurrent bacterial meningitis associated with an anatomic defect is surgical correction.

## PROPHYLAXIS

Prevention of bacterial meningitis by immunization is a desirable goal that is actively being pursued. A major problem is the limited immunogenicity of purified polysaccharide vaccines in children under 2 years of age, since this population is highly susceptible to bacterial meningitis (Gotschlich, 1978). A vaccine containing group A and group C meningococcal polysaccharides can be given to the population at risk when these serogroups of N. meningitidis cause epidemic meningitis. The polyvalent pneumococcal vaccine is indicated for children with sickle cell disease because of their high risk of pneumococcal meningitis. Other approaches toward the prevention of neonatal meningitis and endemic meningitis by immunization are being investigated.

Chemoprophylaxis of household contacts effectively reduces the secondary attack rate of meningococcal disease by interrupting the transmission of organisms to other susceptible family members. Chemoprophylaxis of meningococcal disease is described in Chapter 181. The prevention of secondary cases of H. influenzae disease by chemoprophylaxis is presently being studied, since the secondary attack rate in household contacts under 6 years of age is similar to that of meningococcal disease (Ward et al., 1979).

## References

Feigin, R. D., and Dodge, P. R.: Bacterial meningitis: Newer concepts of pathophysiology and neurologic sequelae. Pediatr Clin North Am 23:541, 1976.

Feigin, R. D., and Schackelford, P. G.: Value of repeat lumbar puncture in differential diagnosis of meningitis. N Engl J Med 289:571, 1973.

Feldman, W. E.: Relation of concentrations of bacteria and bacterial antigen in cerebrospinal fluid to prognosis in patients with bacterial meningitis. New Engl J Med 296:433, 1977.

Fraser, D. W., Darby, C. P., Koehler, R. E., et al.: Risk factors in bacterial meningitis. J Infect Dis 127:271, 1973.

Gotschlich, E. C.: Bacterial meningitis: The beginning of the end. Am J Med 65:719, 1978.

Kaplan, S. L., and Feigin, R. D.: The syndrome of inappropriate secretion of antidiuretic hormone in children with bacterial meningitis. J Pediatr 92:758, 1978.

Lavetter, A., Leedom, J. M., Mathies, A. W., Jr., et al.: Meningitis due to Listeria monocytogenes. N Engl J Med 285:598, 1971.

Mangi, R. J., Quintiliani, R., and Andriole, V. T.: Gram-negative bacillary meningitis. Am J Med 59:829, 1975.

McAllister, C. K., O'Donoghue, J. M., and Beaty, H. N.: Experimental pneumococcal meningitis: Characterization and quantitation of the inflammatory process. J Infect Dis 132:355, 1975.

Moxon, E. R., and Ostrow, P. T.: Haemophilus influenzae meningitis in infant rats: Role of bacteremia in pathogenesis of age-dependent inflammatory responses in cerebrospinal fluid. J Infect Dis 135:303, 1977.

Moxon, E. R., Smith, A. L., Averill, D. R., et al.: *Haemophilus influenzae* meningitis in infant rats after intranasal inoculation. J Infect Dis 129:154, 1974.

Rahal, J. J., Jr., Hyams, P. J., Simberkoff, M. S., et al.: Combined intrathecal and intramuscular gentamicin for gram-negative meningitis. N Engl J Med 290:1394, 1974.

Rahal, J. J., Jr., and Simberkoff, M. S.: Bactericidal and bacteriostatic action of chloramphenicol against meningeal pathogens. Antimicrob Agents Chemother 16:13, 1979.

Swartz, M. N., and Dodge, P. R.: Bacterial meningitis — a review of selected aspects. N Engl J Med 272:725, 779, 842, 898, 954, and 1003, 1965.

Ward, J. I., Fraser, D. W., Baraff, L. J., et al.: *Haemophilus influenzae* meningitis: A national study of secondary spread in household contacts. N Engl J Med 301:122, 1979.

# TUBERCULOUS MENINGITIS AND TUBERCULOMA OF THE BRAIN **154**

## TUBERCULOUS MENINGITIS

### Gérard de Crousaz, M.D.

Tuberculous meningitis can occur at any age except in the newborn. It develops in tuberculosis in four particular settings:

1. As a complication of primary infection, with or without miliary spread. The younger the child is, the higher the risk is. In an unprotected population, the primary infection occurs before the age of 5 years in 75 per cent of children. Meningitis complicates 1 in 300 of such cases. It appears mainly within six months after contact and two months after conversion of the tuberculin test.

2. As a complication of end-stage chronic tuberculosis, predominantly of the lungs, with or without miliary spread. This affects mainly the elderly. The tuberculin test often becomes negative.

3. As a concurrent illness together with another localization of tuberculosis, mainly pulmonary or miliary. This affects older children and adults.

4. As an isolated form of tuberculosis. This condition overlaps the previous one because small lesions or even miliary spread found at necropsy are not detectable clinically. This type of meningitis constitutes about 20 per cent of adult cases.

Meningitis developing in each of these circumstances has many common features. It is fatal within one to eight weeks if untreated and carries a high risk of severe sequelae if treatment is delayed. The basal cisterns are principally affected by the exudate, which becomes granulomatous tissue. This can lead to three major complications: damage to cranial nerves, arteritis with cerebral infarction, and obstruction to cerebrospinal fluid (CSF) flow with hydrocephalus. The spinal cord and roots are likewise exposed to arteritis and compression.

The situations defined in paragraphs 1 and 2 above are by far the most common in those areas of the world in which tuberculosis still has a high prevalence, and meningitis affects mainly infants. These same conditions are practically extinct in the developed countries, in which meningitis can have a thousand-fold lower incidence and is nearly restricted to adults.

The patient's history, the clinical findings, and the pattern of CSF abnormalities together support the probability of diagnosis in the majority of cases. A specific therapy then has to be initiated without waiting for positive cultures, because a delay of three to six weeks would ruin the patient's chances of recovery.

### ETIOLOGY

*Mycobacterium tuberculosis* infects the pia and arachnoid layers. The ratio of the human to bovine types differs in urban and rural areas. *Mycobacterium bovis* once caused up to 40 per cent of tuberculosis in children but is now absent in many countries in which bovine tuberculosis has been eradicated.

### PATHOGENESIS AND PATHOLOGY

A hematogenous route is responsible for practically all cases of meningeal tuberculosis, but an intermediate cerebral lesion linking bacteremia to meningeal seeding is considered obligatory because injection of *M. tuberculosis* into the carotids or veins has repeatedly failed to produce meningitis in various animal species. Careful search of brains from patients dead after a short course of disease has revealed older tuberculous nodules, which are considered to be the link in 70 to 90 per cent of cases (Rich and McCordock, 1933). Bacteremia and the development of parenchymal nodules in the brain can be inapparent clinically or masked by some other manifestation of disease.

Release into the leptomeninges of bacilli and tuberculous antigens, hitherto enclosed within the parenchymal brain nodules, may occur early or after a latent period of months or years. A virulent or aggressive acute infection may be responsible for this release from recent lesions. In those nodules that were dormant for months or years, some disturbance in the patient's resistance is required. Immunosuppressive and physical factors are classic triggers of this release: recent measles (reported in 5 to 10 per cent of tuberculous meningitis complicating the primary infection), head trauma, sun exposure, and malnutrition are examples (Illingworth, 1956; Lincoln et al., 1960; Tandon and Pathak, 1973).

Even though older nodules are often located on the convexity of the hemispheres, release of bacilli and antigens gives rise to an inflammation extending along the basal cisterns, the major route of CSF flow.

Direct spread from a site of tuberculous otitis, skull osteitis, or spondylitis is unusual.

The macroscopic appearance of meningeal tuberculosis varies from inconspicuous in acute cases to spectacular in patients whose death has been delayed by therapy. An exudate fills the basal cisterns, mainly interpeduncular and chiasmatic, extending laterally in the sylvian fissures and cisterna ambiens, downward along the prepontine, cisterna magna, and spinal spaces. Fibrocaseous transformation with eventual calcifications develops mainly in cases of long duration.

White tubercles, 1 to 3 mm in size, can be seen within the meningeal exudate on the convexity of the hemispheres (mainly around vessels of the sylvian fissure), on the ependyma and choroidal plexuses, and sometimes on the inner surface of the dura mater. On brain slices, many tubercles have a corticopial distribution, and a few lie deeper in the cortex.

Arteries embedded in the exudate may be occluded. Infarctions, occasionally hemorrhagic, are not uncommon in the basal nuclei and hypothalamus or in the corticosubcortical regions, mainly around the sylvian fissure and the inferior aspect of the frontal lobe. Brain edema is usual when death occurs early. Early hydrocephalus from ependymitis blocking the aqueduct is rare, but it is a common late finding due to atrophy.

Microscopically, lesions are initially exudative with a few tubercles. Tuberculous lesions of different ages are found throughout the evolution of the infection. Underlying parenchymal structures may be invaded, particularly along perforating vessels. Arteritis is more significant than phlebitis. Many small vessels are occluded by thrombosis or a tuberculous granuloma; thrombosis occasionally occludes larger arteries.

Nonspecific features such as infarctions, areas of ischemic changes, and astrocytic proliferation may be found.

Spinal arteritis with infarction, cord or cauda equina compression from arachnoidal adhesions or granulomas, is found mainly in long protracted cases.

Besides the tuberculoma, some rare forms of neurotuberculosis deserve mention: tuberculous encephalopathy without meningitis; spinal meningitis around either an extradural tuberculous abscess with radiculopathy or a spinal cord tuberculoma; and localized meningitis "en plaque." These account for some 5 per cent of meningitides (Udani et al., 1971; Tandon and Pathak, 1973).

## CLINICAL MANIFESTATIONS*

Most cases progress through three stages as defined by the British Medical Research Council (Streptomycin in Tuberculosis Trials Committee, 1948). The prognosis is correlated with the stage reached at the time treatment is initiated.

Stage 1 (early, prodromal): patients have mainly nonspecific symptoms, few or no signs of meningitis, are fully conscious, and have no neurologic defects.

Stage 2 (medium, intermediate): patients usually have signs of meningitis, minor or no neurologic defects, no marked change in the level of consciousness.

Stage 3 (advanced, late, paralytic): patients obviously are very ill, are deeply stuporous or comatose, or have gross pareses.

---

*This description is based upon various large clinical series. Cases that are exclusively or mainly pediatric were found in Western (Illingworth, 1956; Lincoln et al., 1960), African (Freiman and Geefhuysen, 1970; Osuntokur et al., 1971), and Indian sources (Udani et al., 1971). In adults, the author's personal experience was consolidated with other large series (Lepper and Spies, 1963; Falk, 1965; Weiss and Flippin, 1965). More recent reports demonstrate diagnostic problems due to a decline in the frequency of the disease in Western countries (Meyers and Hirschman, 1974; Karandanis and Shulman, 1976; Haas et al., 1977).

The prodromal stage lasts for two weeks to two to three months in 70 per cent of cases, excluding the extreme age groups, in which it is less often detected. Symptoms are nonspecific and misleading, except in cases with known tuberculosis of another organ, known contact, or documented tuberculin test conversion. In young children, a history of exposure to known contacts (mainly household) is nearly diagnostic. In older patients seen at a later stage, a history of this prodromal stage practically rules out a pyogenic or viral meningitis.

Apathy with bursts of irritability, nocturnal wakefulness, and minor headaches form a vague neurologic component. Pain may be localized in one ear or a paranasal sinus, and there is very often a coincident nonspecific upper respiratory infection. Anorexia, loss of weight, nausea and vomiting, abdominal pain (sometimes prominent), and constipation may erroneously point to some abdominal disorder. Myalgia and lumbosacral pain with radicular radiation in one or both lower limbs are frequent complaints in the adult. Transient or intermittent low-grade fever may add to the feeling that the patient has some "flu-like" disorder that fails to resolve.

The intermediate stage of meningitis develops over days or two to three weeks with no clear-cut separation from the prodrome; its onset is usually acute in infants and the elderly but in only 5 per cent of any other age groups (Taylor et al., 1955). Headaches and vomiting are the major complaints in 75 per cent of patients. Neck stiffness and the Kernig and Brudzinski signs are present in two thirds to three fourths of patients, though often inconspicuous; these signs are more often absent in the extreme age groups. Low to moderate fever (not above 39° C or 102° F) is the rule; isolated higher peaks are not unusual. Infants may have a persistent fever of 40° C (104° F) or more at this stage. An afebrile course is recorded in 3 to 5 per cent of pediatric and up to 10 per cent of adult series. At the other extreme, fever is reported as the presenting and only finding for days or weeks in about 10 per cent of cases. This stage may begin without fever in malnourished patients (Tandon and Pathak, 1973).

Apathy and irritability tend to evolve into confusion and lethargy. Psychotic behavior, and alcohol or drug withdrawal syndromes in chronic addicts, can mask the underlying disease. Intracranial hypertension is not impressive at this stage. Choroidal tubercles are found in less than 10 per cent of cases, more often in cases of concomitant miliary tuberculosis. The cranial nerves are involved in some 25 per cent of cases. An early sign that suggests the diagnosis consists of dilated pupils, reacting poorly or not at all to light, in fully awake patients without limitation of eye movements and with no ptosis (Fisher, 1974). External oculomotor paresis, usually incomplete and unilateral, affects mainly the third nerve, then the sixth and fourth nerves. Peripheral facial paresis is less common, and other cranial nerves are rarely affected. Focal or generalized convulsions are a presenting or early symptom in 10 to 15 per cent of children and in fewer adults. Transient or mild paresis can follow the seizure or occur alone in both groups.

The advanced stage is usually reached gradually, but at any age and especially in the extreme age groups, cases can suddenly become advanced with the onset of convulsions, coma, or hemiplegia. This accounts for some 10 per cent of patients with coma and/or gross paresis. A strokelike onset in adults, intracranial hypertension with focal cerebral signs, or poliomyelitis-like flaccid paralysis are some treacherous modes of onset.

Signs of meningeal irritation may disappear in a deep coma, but fever is persistent. Papilledema is seen in some 40 per cent of patients, and over one half have oculomotor or facial nerve involvement. Gross paralysis, mainly hemi-, tetra-, or paraplegia, is seen in up to 40 per cent of cases; these paralyses are reversible and may affect either side alternately. Abnormal movements, particularly ballismus, can occur. Other focal defects, such as aphasia or cerebellar signs, are detected only after improvement of stupor or coma. Over one half of the children have fits.

In the end-stage leading to death, there are decerebrate posture, disturbance in regulation of blood pressure and respiration, and hyperpyrexia followed by hypothermia.

Even successful therapy does not reverse the course of the disease immediately; on the contrary, an acute transient deterioration is actually frequent during the first week of treatment. Subsiding fever and clearing of consciousness occur mainly from the second to the fifth week in patients who are doing well. Some previously undetectable defects can appear, however, while new ones may develop.

Patients treated unsuccessfully or too late may survive in any degree of coma, mental deterioration, mono- to tetraparesis, blindness, or deafness. Later, death from intercurrent disease is frequent in these severely brain- or cord-damaged patients.

Relapses can occur when therapy is discontinued too early. Clear instructions on continuation of drugs must be given to the patient and to his family, and regular follow-up visits are important.

Many series originating from both developed and developing countries report a mortality rate of 5 to 20 per cent and full recovery in up to 60 to 70 per cent. It would seem realistic to expect a less optimistic prognosis, because most patients are not treated in specialized units. A mortality of one third to one half, with survivors distributed equally among those with moderate to severe sequelae and those with full recovery (or, at worst, mild sequelae) is probably closer to a worldwide situation. Unfavorable prognostic factors are a delay in treatment until a late stage, an age below 3 or over 40, the presence of associated diseases, and a very high initial CSF protein level (Lepper and Spies, 1963; Falk, 1965; Weiss and Flippin, 1965).

## COMPLICATIONS AND SEQUELAE

Two major complications, although rare, can induce acute intracranial hypertension early in the course of the disease. Brain edema commonly aggravates the condition of critically ill patients in the first days of treatment. Great amounts of tuberculin released from the killed bacilli are thought to enhance abruptly this inflammatory swelling. Obstructive hydrocephalus due to ependymitis in the aqueduct, or exudative material in the cisterna magna blocking the foramina of Magendie and Luschka, can cause tentorial herniation. This complication is worsened by repeated lumbar punctures and requires ventricular drainage if it is confirmed by neuroradiologic procedures.

Major neurologic complications that arise in Stages 2 and 3 have been described. The leptomeninges are occasionally superinfected by bacteria or fungi. Intracranial hemorrhages occasionally develop within infarcted areas. Both oversecretion and undersecretion of antidiuretic hormone is common in a mild form. Major extracranial complications are pyogenic infections (pneumonia, septicemia, urinary tract infection, infected bedsores) and gastric mucosal erosions with hemorrhage.

Complications can occur later as a result of progressive fibrosis; arachnoidal adhesions can block the pericerebral or spinal CSF flow even after the active phase is controlled by chemotherapy. Compressive-ischemic damage to the optic chiasm, hypothalamo-pituitary structures, spinal cord, or roots (especially of the cauda equina) can appear during convalescence. An increasing protein concentration in the lumbar CSF, with normal cells and glucose, is a warning sign of these spinal blocks. Focal or generalized epilepsy persists or appears in 10 per cent of survivors. Obesity, sexual precocity, Cushing's syndrome, and diabetes insipidus are occasional endocrine sequelae (Udani et al., 1971).

Drug-induced complications should be kept in mind. They were common when streptomycin was the only drug available (deafness, labyrinthine destruction, spinal dermoids or cholesteatomas from daily intrathecal injections). Neurologic side effects of the newer drugs include an occasional acute optic neuropathy (ethambutol) and cerebral dysfunction (cycloserine).

Sequelae range from mild to very severe. Intensive care reduces the mortality but increases the number of disabled survivors. A final assessment can be made only after one to two years, since many abnormalities in the active phase disappear, and a few others appear later.

The most disabled patients are often left with more than one of the following disorders: mental retardation or dementia, hemi- or paraplegia, epilepsy, cerebellar ataxia, blindness, deafness, or strabismus. Moderate sequelae include mild mental retardation, epilepsy, reduced vision, partial deafness, hemiparesis, and mild ataxia. Minor sequelae are more frequent if accurately sought and include some degree of behavioral or learning disorder, visual field defects, paresis of one oculomotor or facial nerve or of the lumbosacral roots, disturbance of micturition and hyperreflexia. Intracranial calcifications, mainly behind the optic chiasm, have been uncommon since isoniazid was introduced. Like diffuse or focal EEG abnormalities, they occur in survivors with or without clinical sequelae.

## GEOGRAPHIC VARIATIONS

In developed countries, three factors account for the considerable decrease in incidence of the disease over the last century: improvement of overcrowded, sub-standard living conditions and personal hygiene; chemotherapy; and, to a lesser degree, public health programs.

Today, many developing countries have instituted public health programs; others have not. In those that have, the incidence of the disease has been rapidly reduced by 50 to 80 per cent or more, even without substantial changes in economic conditions. Mandatory BCG (Bacillus Calmette-Guerin) inoculation in infancy and detection and treatment of pulmonary tuberculosis by mass chest roentgenography have thus proved their effectiveness here. The number of tuberculous meningitides per thousand hospital or pediatric admissions provides the only comparative figures. The highest incidence over the last 20 years have been recorded in South Asia, Africa, and South America and amounted to 10 to 50 cases per 1000 pediatric admissions. This incidence is no doubt similar to that in European and North American areas 80 years ago. Prophylactic measures have reduced this incidence to somewhere between 1 and 25 per 1000. However, tuberculous meningitis remains a major medical problem in developing countries, especially in children.

A steady decline of the disease has been reported in developed countries during the last three decades. In 1947, England and Wales reported about 2000 cases per year, accounting for 10 to 20 per cent of all bacterial meningitides; the annual rate fell to 56 from 1967 through 1971, or 3.9 per cent of all bacterial meningitides (Stevenson, 1973). Pediatric cases have virtually disappeared, and two thirds of cases occur in those aged 20 to 40 years, with a hint of a shift toward older age groups. Thus, 10 of 19 patients seen in 1966 through 1974 were over 40 years old (Haas et al., 1977).

An example of a very low incidence is that at the University Hospital in Lausanne, Switzerland, which serves an area without any economically depressed population group. The incidence was 0.019 per 1000 hospital admissions from 1972 through 1978, a three-fold decrease as compared with the previous decade. Over the last 12 years, the rate was 0.09 per 1000 pediatric hospital admissions. As a contrast, large indigent urban populations provide higher rates locally, especially if composed of immigrants. In Birmingham, England, during the period 1950 to 1960, the ratio of tuberculosis among Indians and Pakistanis versus the local British population was 20 to 1 (Springett, 1964); immigrants from the Mediterranean area to Central Europe had a fairly high ratio of tuberculous meningitis. Rates nowadays should not exceed the 0.5 to 0.8 per 1000 hospital admissions recorded in 1959 in Cleveland, Ohio (Hinman, 1967).

## DIAGNOSIS

Lumbar puncture is mandatory and urgent. It has to be repeated for diagnostic purposes if one or more of the classic abnormalities are lacking, which is more likely to occur in the early stages of the disease. Serial taps should, however, be avoided if the first one discloses a very high initial pressure (above 400 mm).

The CSF may be clear, opalescent, or turbid, and sometimes is xanthochromatic or slightly hemorrhagic. If left to sit for 10 to 20 hours, its surface is often covered with a weblike pellicle that should be examined for acid-fast bacilli.

### CSF Cytology

The classic picture consists of 10 to 500 white blood cells per cmm, predominantly lymphocytic. Higher counts are seen in 10 to 15 per cent of cases, often concomitant with a predominantly polymorphonuclear reaction. On repeated diagnostic punctures within the first days, the marked variability of the total cell count with transient bursts of polymorphonuclears is, by itself, highly suggestive of the disease (Lepper and Spies, 1963). Erythrocytes in varying amounts are commonly found, presumably from traumatic tap.

### Chemistry

Chloride levels are of disputed value. They are often low.

Glucose concentration is below the normal range of 40 mg per 100 ml (or if blood levels are increased, below two fifths to one half of the blood glucose level) in 70 to 85 per cent of initial lumbar punctures. Repeated punctures in an early stage usually demonstrate the suggestive cross of the lowering glucose curve and the increasing protein curve, but this may not occur in adults. A low CSF glucose level should therefore not be required as a diagnostic criterion of tuberculous meningitis.

Protein levels are 60 to 200 mg per 100 ml in the majority of initial samples. Initial values above 300 mg indicate a bad prognosis. Differential protein fractionation is useful if total levels are below 80 mg per 100 ml. Detectable IgM in the early phase of a lymphocytic meningitis without high protein levels argues against a viral infection (Smith et al., 1973). Intrathecal inflammation is more difficult to evaluate if total protein levels exceed 80 mg per 100 ml in the CSF, since above this level, any plasma globulins have free access to CSF.

Some elaborate diagnostic tests of the CSF are not yet widely used. The bromide partition test analyzes the ratio of serum to CSF bromide 48 hours after ingesting bromide. This ratio is below 1.9 in nearly all tuberculous and in a few pyogenic meningitides and is reported normal in all other neurologic diseases (Smith et al., 1955; Da Costa et al, 1977). CSF lactic acid is increased above 3.9 mEq/L in tuberculous meningitis but not in aseptic meningitis; it is also increased in cerebral anoxia and is therefore not discriminating (D'Souza et al., 1978). Measuring the titer of humoral antibodies to PPD tuberculin in CSF and serum appears to be highly specific and deserves a broader trial.

### Bacteriology

If acid-fast bacilli are found on CSF smear, they are immediately diagnostic, but this painstaking procedure was positive in only 10 to 40 per cent of recent series (Barois, 1975; Haas et al., 1977; Mathew et al., 1970). Older positive findings in up to 80 to 90 per cent required the centrifugation of 10 to 20 ml of lumbar CSF (Illingworth, 1956) or serial suboccipital punctures on the admission day.

Cultures are positive in 45 to 85 per cent of cases, according to the amount of samples used and the laboratory's facilities (Haas et al. 1977; Karandanis and Shulman, 1976; Bertoye et al., 1970). Most Asian and African series attain bacteriologic proof in 10 to 15 per cent (Vejjajiva, 1974; Osuntokun et al., 1971). Initiation of treatment should by no means be delayed until the results of cultures are available, since this takes three to six weeks.

Guinea pig inoculation has the same rate of positive results, is more painstaking, and takes more time.

In the course of treatment, control of CSF is advisable once a week for the first month, then every other week for two months, and later once a month. Usually the glucose level is the first parameter to improve, followed by cell count, and later by protein levels. Even in uncomplicated cases, it takes three to six months until CSF abnormalities disappear.

### Neurodiagnostic Procedures

Electroencephalography isotopic brain scan and cisternography, angiography, air encephalography, and computerized tomography (CT) are not diagnostic. Their use on admission should be limited to patients whose first manifestations were focal cerebral or a severe intracranial hypertension. They are very useful once complications occur in the course of treatment; differentiating acute brain edema from obstructive hydrocephalus (with carotid angiogram or the safer and more accurate CT scan); evaluating arteritis as a cause of infarction (angiogram); and detecting and localizing pericerebral or spinal blocks (isotopic cisternogram and myelogram, air encephalogram) (Tandon and Pathak, 1973).

### Blood Studies

The peripheral neutrophil count does not exceed 10,000/cmm, and the total leukocyte count is usually not as high as in the pyogenic meningitides (Karandanis and Shulman, 1976). Hyponatremia is found on admission in 45 to 75 per cent of adults, a finding suggestive of meningeal tuberculosis if the CSF is not purulent and vomiting is not prominent. Hyponatremia is also common in *Herpes simplex* encephalitis. The blood glucose level is often above normal and must be taken into account in evaluating the CSF glucose level.

### Intradermal Tuberculin Reaction (Mantoux)

This test has a limited diagnostic value. It is reported negative in 3 to 15 per cent of tuberculous meningitides in European series (Barois, 1975). African and Indian pediatric series reported a negative Mantoux test in 15 to 37 per cent of cases, possibly due to malnutrition and to the frequency of recent measles (Osuntokun et al., 1971; Da Costa et al., 1977). A positive test in infancy and documented positive conversions are highly informative, while a documented negative conversion suggests sarcoidosis or another disease capable of producing anergy.

### Search for Other Localizations of Tuberculosis

This is imperative and is often more rewarding than CSF investigation. Direct examination and cultures of sputum, gastric washings, and urine should be performed before therapy is started.

Radiologic evidence of pulmonary tuberculosis is very frequent in meningitis following the primary infection: up to 90 per cent present the primary complex in various stages of evolution or a miliary spread. In older patients, the coincidence of meningitis with pulmonary lesions apparently dropped from around 70 per cent in the 1950s (Weiss and Flippin, 1961; Falk, 1965) to some 55 per cent in recent series (Haas et al., 1977), thus adding a further diagnostic problem where the disease is now rare. Meningeal tuberculosis is accompanied by lesions outside the chest in about 10 per cent of cases, and these lesions are mainly genitourinary. Tuberculous meningitis without evidence of tuberculosis elsewhere is found clinically in 20 to 30 per cent of adults and postmortem in 10 per cent (Falk, 1965).

### Differential Diagnosis

The diagnosis is easy when the classic history and findings are present in a patient with known tuberculous infection and characteristic CSF abnormalities. The numerous atypical presentations, however, may raise problems, and the following possibilities should be considered.

Viral meningitis is either acute or the second part of a biphasic febrile disease and has no neurologic signs other than apathy, irritability, and some confusion. The CSF cell count can change from a predominance of polymorphonuclears to lymphocytes, but not the reverse; the CSF glucose is normal in 95 per cent of cases, and even when depressed, it becomes normal again when lymphocytes predominate (Karandanis and Shulman, 1976). The CSF protein level rarely exceeds 120 to 150 mg per 100 ml. All parameters usually improve on the next tap.

Subacute listeriosis with cerebral signs may be difficult to distinguish from tuberculous meningitis until the CSF culture is positive for *Listeria monocytogenes*. Partially treated bacterial meningitis rarely offers a confusing CSF picture (Mandal, 1976). Subarachnoid hemorrhage, in the absence of a history or in case of minimal leak, can resemble tuberculous meningitis. Hemosiderin-containing macrophages in the CSF may help in making the diagnosis.

In neurosyphilis, there may be cranial nerve signs and a CSF pattern like that in tuberculous meningitis, but a normal CSF glucose in syphilis and a positive serologic test for syphilis separate the two conditions. Sarcoid of the nervous system, with its depressed CSF glucose in two thirds of the cases (Gaines et al., 1970), can be indistinguishable from meningeal tuberculosis.

Leukemic meningitis occurs mainly in hematologic remission; the CSF glucose level and often the CSF protein level are within the normal range. Carcinomatous or sarcomatous meningitis can be easily confused with tuberculous meningitis because it may develop without a detectable primary tumor, tends to cause massive involvement of the cranial and spinal nerves and/or severe intracranial hypertension, and lowers the CSF glucose level while elevating the protein level. In all three conditions, the diagnosis depends on cytologic examination of the CSF.

Focal cerebral signs and/or intracranial hypertension with predominantly lymphocytic meningitis can be seen in any viral meningoencephalitis (particularly that due to *Herpes simplex* virus), bacterial brain abscess, fungal infection, parasitic disease, and intracranial venous thrombosis. Necrotic malignant tumors close to the pia or ependyma and benign intraventricular tumors can cause a "meningitis" with occasionally a low glucose level.

Focal neurologic or electroencephalographic findings pointing to temporal lobe disease may be helpful in recognizing Herpes encephalitis. A useful point in diagnosis of cryptococcal meningitis is that there is seldom fever in this fungus infection. In addition, the cryptococci are easily cultured in a week or less from the CSF and may be seen there in Gram stains. Cryptococcal antigen may be found in the CSF by immunologic tests. Brain abscesses can often be recognized because there is usually a chronic focus of infection in the ears, mastoid, sinuses, or lung from which the infection spreads to the brain. Cysticercosis of the brain can be a difficult diagnostic problem and may ultimately depend on cysticercal serology for diagnosis. Occasionally, the telltale subcutaneous cysticercal calcifications can be seen in roentgenograms of the chest or extremities, and a history of residence in an endemic area may be obtained. In Mexico, for example, cysticercosis is the main cause of epilepsy. The characteristic mass lesions of brain abscess and cysticercosis should be found by computerized axial tomography of the brain in countries in which this procedure is available.

The fever with apathy and confusion of typhoid and brucellosis may be easily confused with that of meningeal tuberculosis, especially, if *Brucella* or typhoidal meningitis occurs. Both *S. typhosa* and *Brucella* sp can be cultured from the blood without much trouble, and in brucellosis, the agglutinin test is invariably positive.

## TREATMENT

A combination of several antituberculous drugs for several months, followed by one drug for a total of 18 to 24 months, is the usual therapy.

Isoniazid plus rifampin and ethambutol is one of the favorite combinations now. Isoniazid, 5 to 8 mg/kg in adults and 10 mg/kg in children, can be given in a single daily dose; 50 mg of pyridoxine daily is added to prevent neuropathy. As the single most effective drug, isoniazid is the one to continue for 18 to 24 months. Rifampin, 600 mg daily in adults (10 mg/kg if overweight or underweight) and 15 to 20 mg/kg in children, is given in one dose and for a period of five to six months. Ethambutol, 15 mg/kg in a single daily dose, should be given for three to six months. Feeding by nasogastric tube is often necessary for this combination. In case of intolerance to either drug, ethionamide, 15 to 30 mg/kg per day in children or 500 to 1000 mg in adults as a single dose (or para-aminosalicylic acid and streptomycin, as detailed below) can be substituted. Liver function tests must be made regularly.

The combination of streptomycin and isoniazid, with or without para-aminosalicylic acid, is still advocated in certain countries. Streptomycin, 40 mg/kg per day in children or 2 g daily in adults, is injected for three to four months; it can be reduced later. Isoniazid is recommended at an initial higher dose than in the previous regimen: 8 to 10 mg/kg in adults and 15 to 20 mg/kg in children. Control of renal function and of audiolabyrinthine function is necessary.

Corticosteroids are of debatable value but are widely used in practice. They should be restricted to those patients with early brain edema occurring spontaneously or after onset of treatment (dexamethasone, 4 to 10 mg I.V. every four hours for one or two days, tapered off over the next week). Corticosteroids do not prevent the fibrosis that results from organization of exudate in the subarachnoid spaces and produces cisternal or spinal blocks.

Antiepileptic drugs are given if necessary. A possible interaction with antituberculous drugs should be kept in mind.

Nursing care in severely ill patients may require a nasogastric tube for feeding and drug intake, urinary catheter, pharyngeal aspiration, occasional tracheotomy, and assisted ventilation. Electrolytes must be monitored, and superinfections treated. Changes of posture are needed to prevent bed sores and ankylosis.

Surgical procedures consist mainly of ventricular shunt in case of obstructive hydrocephalus. A sudden blindness may occasionally justify a decompression of the optic chiasm.

### *Prophylaxis*

Pulmonary tuberculosis in one member of the household is the most common cause of tuber-culous meningitis in infants and children. Isoniazid should be given in a daily dose of 10 mg/kg to all children under 5 years old who react to tuberculin. In the United States Public Health Service prophylaxis study of 275 children with positive tuberculin tests, there were no cases of meningeal tuberculosis among those given 4 to 6 mg/kg isoniazid daily for one year, whereas six cases of the disease occurred in the controls given a placebo instead of isoniazid. Mass BCG vaccination of the newborn has probably been the most effective step in dramatically reducing the disease in many developing countries. It confers a protection at best of about 80 per cent, so that a previous vaccination does not rule out the possibility that a case of meningitis is of tuberculous origin.

# TUBERCULOMAS OF THE BRAIN

*Douglas D. Richman, M.D.*

Tuberculomas of the brain are an uncommon extrapulmonary manifestation of tuberculosis. They are focal caseating granulomatous lesions within the substance of the brain that behave clinically as space-occupying lesions. Tuberculomas are important in the differential diagnosis of space-occupying lesions of the brain because they can be cured.

Tuberculomas of the brain are recognized predominantly in populations with a high incidence of tuberculosis, where they may comprise a large proportion of intracranial tumors. They may occur at any age but are most frequent in children and young adults. However, in developed countries, where tuberculin reactivity has shifted largely to older persons, tuberculoma of the brain is also seen more at an older age.

The pathogenesis of brain tuberculomas can be deduced from Rich's studies of the pathogenesis of tuberculous meningitis (Rich, 1951). He demonstrated that tuberculous meningitis was almost always associated with focal caseous lesions that were older than the meningitis and communicated with the meninges. The pathophysiology and the clinical picture of tuberculous meningitis are a consequence of the inflammatory response to the discharge of mycobacteria and their antigens into the cerebrospinal fluid from the local caseous lesion. Such local lesions far exceed in number the cases of meningitis because most do not rupture into the cerebrospinal fluid. A tuberculoma of the brain probably becomes evident clinically in the rare circumstance in which a caseous lesion of the brain grows without rupturing.

Tuberculomas of the brain are usually typical caseating granulomas containing variable microscopic calcification and surrounded by chronic and subacute inflammation. Tuberculomas may range in size from microscopic to those that extend throughout a whole lobe of the brain.

The failure of a tuberculoma to rupture results in a strikingly different clinical presentation from meningitis. A tuberculoma may appear either abruptly with signs of a space-occupying lesion of the brain or as a slowly progressive intracranial tumor with symptoms lasting a year or longer. The patient may have seizures, focal neurologic signs, and, most frequently, signs and symptoms of elevated intracranial pressure such as headache, vomiting, visual disturbances, and papilledema. Without extracranial tuberculosis, which is seldom found, intracranial tuberculosis should be suspected from fever, a positive tuberculin test, an epidemiologic background of tuberculosis, or a past history of tuberculosis. There is nothing to distinguish the clinical manifestations of tuberculomas from other space-occupying lesions of the brain.

Tuberculomas may occur anywhere in the brain; however, they appear to have a slightly increased predilection for infratentorial structures, especially the cerebellum. In the past, the diagnosis of a single lesion has been made as often as multiple lesions; however, with more sensitive and accessible radiographic techniques, including angiography and computerized tomography, multiple lesions are being recognized more frequently. This tendency to multiple lesions makes localization of a tuberculoma by neurologic examination less accurate than localization of a malignancy or another tumor.

The plain roentgenogram of the skull may show signs of increased intracranial pressure, such as increased convolutional markings, erosion of the dorsum sellae, or separation of the sutures in infants. Calcification in the lesion has been visualized only rarely by x-ray.

Radionuclide brain scans have been negative in only a few reports when the lesion was located in the posterior fossa. Cerebral angiography has demonstrated displacement of vessels without the neovascularization seen with many malignancies. In a few published reports, computerized tomography has succeeded in localizing tuberculomas and because of its ease, noninvasiveness, and sensitivity will probably be valuable for their diagnosis.

Tuberculomas of the brain must be recognized early so that antituberculous drugs can be started before elevated intracranial pressure causes irreversible neurologic damage, such as blindness, or kills the patient. Most of the literature on this disease has been written by neurosurgeons who have treated patients for space-occupying lesions. With modern chemotherapy, surgery should be limited to biopsy or decompression; excision or drainage is not necessary except to relieve pressure and can cause complications. The place for excision becomes even more dubious now that multiple tuberculomas are being increasingly recognized. The response to chemotherapy is usually so prompt and clear-cut that a therapeutic trial has diagnostic value. Three hundred milligrams of isoniazid, along with 600 mg of rifampicin, daily in the adult probably constitute the best regimen currently available in view of their efficacy against *M. tuberculosis* and their ability to penetrate the brain. Although tuberculomas are too rare to allow a systematic evaluation of steroids, these drugs are probably indicated initially for a short period to diminish the inflammatory response. Steroids may preclude the need for surgical decompression, and a short course carries little risk in the presence of specific antituberculous chemotherapy. It must be remembered, however, that the nonspecific improvement with steroids will eliminate the diagnostic value of a therapeutic trial of antituberculous drugs.

## References

Anderson, J. M., and Macmillan, J. J.: Intracranial tuberculoma — an increasing problem in Britain. J Neurol Neurosurg Psychiatry 38:194, 1975.

Balaparameswararao, M. S., and Dinakar, I.: Tuberculomas of the brain. Int Surg 57:216, 1972.

Barois, A.: Les méningites tuberculeuses. Rev Prat 25:633, 1975.

Bertoye, A., Garin, J. P., Vincent, P., Monier, P., Bertrand, J. L., Da Costa, H., Borker, A., and Loken, M.: Distribution of orally administered bromine-82 in tubercular meningitis: Concise communication. J Nucl Med 18:123, 1977.

Damergis, J. A., Leftwich, E. I., Curtin, J. A., and Witorsch, P.: Tuberculoma of the brain. JAMA 239:413, 1978.

D'Souza, E., Mandal, B. K., Hooper, J., and Parker, L.: Lactic-acid concentration in cerebrospinal fluid and differential diagnosis of meningitis. Lancet 2:579, 1978.

Falk, A.: Tuberculous meningitis in adults, with special reference to survival, neurologic residuals, and work status. Am Rev Resp Dis 91:823, 1965.

Fisher, C. M.: In Picard, E. H., and Richardson, E. P.: Seizures, hemiparesis and coma with cerebrospinal fluid pleiocytosis. N Engl J Med 290:1130, 1974.

Freiman, I., and Geefhuysen, J.: Evaluation of intrathecal therapy with streptomycin and hydrocortisone in tuberculous meningitis. J Pediatr 76:895, 1970.

Gaines, J. D., Eckman, P. B., and Remington, J. S.: Low CSF glucose level in sarcoidosis involving the central nervous system. Arch Intern Med 125:333, 1970.

Haas, E. J., Madhavan, T., Quinn, E. L., Cox, F., Fisher, E., and Burch, K.: Tuberculous meningitis in an urban general hospital. Arch Intern Med 137:1518, 1977.

Hinman, A. R.: Tuberculous meningitis at Cleveland Metropolitan General Hospital 1959 to 1963. Am Rev Resp Dis 95:670, 1967.

Illingworth, R. S.: Miliary and meningeal tuberculosis. Difficulties in diagnosis. Lancet 2:646, 1956.

Karandanis, D., and Shulman, J. A.: Recent survey of infectious meningitis in adults: Review of laboratory findings in bacterial, tuberculous, and aseptic meningitis. South Med J 69:449, 1976.

Lepper, M. H., and Spies, H. W.: The present status of the treatment of tuberculosis of the central nervous system. Ann NY Acad Sci 106:106, 1963.

Lincoln, E. M., Sordillo, S. V. R., and Davies, P. A.: Tuberculous meningitis in children. A review of 167 untreated and 74 treated patients with special reference to early diagnosis. J Pediatr 57:807, 1960.

Mandal, B. K.: The dilemma of partially treated bacterial meningitis. Scand J Infect Dis 8:185, 1976.

Mathew, N. T., Abraham, J., and Chandy, J.: Cerebral angiographic features in tuberculous meningitis. Neurology 20:1015, 1970.

Mayers, M. M., Kaufman, D. M., and Miller, M. H.: Recent cases of intracranial tuberculomas. Neurology 28:256, 1978.

Meyers, B. R., and Hirschman, S. Z.: Unusual presentations of tuberculous meningitis. Mount Sinai J Med 41:407, 1974.

Osuntokun, B. O., Adeuja, A. O. G., and Familusi, J. B.: Tuberculous meningitis in Nigerians. A study of 194 patients. Trop Geogr Med 23:225, 1971.

Rich, A. R.: The Pathogenesis of Tuberculosis. 2nd ed. Springfield, Ill. Charles C Thomas, 1951, pp. 882–894.

Rich, A. R., and McCordock, H. A.: The pathogenesis of tuberculous meningitis. Bull Johns Hopkins Hosp 52:5, 1933.

Smith, H., Bannister, B., and O'Shea, M. J.: Cerebrospinal-fluid immunoglobulins in meningitis. Lancet 2:591, 1973.

Smith, H. V., Taylor, L. M., and Hunter, G.: The blood-cerebrospinal fluid barrier in tuberculous meningitis and allied conditions. J Neurol Neurosurg Psychiatry 18:237, 1955.

Springett, V. H.: Tuberculosis in immigrants. An analysis of notification rates in Birmingham, 1960–62. Lancet 1:1091, 1964.

Stevenson, J.: Bacterial meningitis and tuberculous meningitis. Br Med J 2:411, 1973.

Streptomycin in Tuberculosis Trials Committee, Medical Research Council: Streptomycin treatment of tuberculous meningitis. Lancet 1:582, 1948.

Tandon, P. N., and Pathak, S. N.: Tuberculosis of the central nervous system. In Spillane, J. D. (ed.): Tropical Neurology. London, Oxford University Press, 1973, p. 37.

Taylor, K. B., Smith, H. V., and Vollum, R. L.: Tuberculous meningitis of acute onset. J Neurol Neurosurg Psychiatry 18:165, 1955.

Udani, P. M., Parekh, U. C., and Dastur, D. K.: Neurological and related syndromes in CNS tuberculosis. Clinical features and pathogenesis. J Neurol Sci 14:341, 1971.

Vejjajiva, A.: Neuro-tuberculosis. An unsolved problem. J Med Assoc Thai 57:89, 1974.

Weiss, W., and Flippin, H. F.: The prognosis of tuberculous meningitis in the isoniazid era. Am J Med Sci 242:423, 1961.

Weiss, W., and Flippin, H. F.: The changing incidence and prognosis of tuberculous meningitis. Am J Med Sci 250:80, 1965.

# 155 CRYPTOCOCCAL MENINGITIS

*Gerald Medoff, M.D.*

## DEFINITION

Cryptococcal meningitis is a chronic, subacute, or rarely, acute, central nervous system infection caused by the yeast *Cryptococcus neoformans*. It is the most familiar and most common manifestation of disease caused by this fungus and is the form that has the highest mortality.

## ETIOLOGY

Cryptococcal meningitis is caused by a single species, *Cryptococcus neoformans*, an encapsulated yeast-like fungus that is pathogenic for animals and man.

## PATHOGENESIS AND PATHOLOGY

The presence of *C. neoformans* in bird droppings is well documented, and, at least in the case of human infection, epidemiologic data imply that the pigeon may be the chief vector of the disease. The organism is recovered in large numbers from pigeon feces and the debris of pigeon roosts in attics and old buildings. The recent discovery of the sexual (perfect) stage of *C. neoformans* and its phylogenetic relationships to various plant pathogens suggests that there may be other forms of this organism in nature that are important in the natural history of the disease (Kwon-chung, 1975).

Necropsy studies indicate that, with rare exceptions, cryptococci enter the body through the lungs by inhalation of the aerosolized infectious particles found in the dried pigeon droppings. The primary pulmonary focus is usually subclinical; if it is symptomatic, the infection usually resolves spontaneously. Cutaneous, skeletal, and visceral lesions may occur during hematogenous dissemination of the disease, but involvement of the central nervous system (CNS) with subacute or chronic meningoencephalitis is the most frequently diagnosed and most familiar form of the mycoses. The reason for the predilection of *C. neoformans* for the CNS has not been explained, but once dissemination to the CNS occurs, the infection is progressive and, in the absence of chemotherapy, death will result. The progressive nature of the infection in the CNS as compared with lung is unexplained but may be related to a less efficient cellular or phagocytic response or a deficiency of other factors important in an adequate host response to the cryptococci (Diamond et al., 1974). In support of this conception, cryptococcal infection of the central nervous system is accompanied by minimal inflammatory reaction. Even in fatal cases of meningitis the gross appearance of the meninges and brain may be almost normal. Meningeal reaction is more pronounced at the base of the brain and in the dorsal area of the cerebellum. In these areas thickening and opacity of the membrane may cause the meninges to adhere to the cortex. If the meningeal disease progresses to encephalitis, the brain may contain numerous cystic spaces. Characteristically, the subarachnoid space contains an adherent mucoid exudate with mononuclear cells and may present the picture of a pure histiocytic granuloma. Many microscopic fields may reveal no other inflammatory cells but a few lymphocytes.

In sections stained with hematoxylin and eosin, fungus cells appear as pale blue, often thin-walled, spherical or oval bodies either without visible internal structure or with a poorly defined, frequently eccentric pink cytoplasmic mass within the cells. The size of the fungi ranges from 3 to 10 $\mu$. In the hematoxylin and eosin sections, there is frequently a clear halo separating the fungus wall from the cytoplasm of the phagocytic cell. When stained with mucicarmine, this clear zone is revealed as a pink capsule.

In active growing cryptococcal lesions, budding cells are found without difficulty. In old lesions or in lesions with a large amount of cellular reaction and few fungi, budding is difficult to demonstrate.

## CLINICAL MANIFESTATIONS

Unlike the pulmonary infection, 50 per cent of patients with cryptococcal meningitis have an underlying disease such as lymphoma, other malignancies, diabetes, or other diseases that primarily affect the immune system or require therapy with immunosuppressive drugs.

Cryptococcal invasion of the central nervous system may produce signs and symptoms of meningitis, meningoencephalitis, or a space-occupying lesion. The clinical findings vary according to the location and extent of involvement of the fungus. The course is usually subacute or chronic and can vary from a few months to years, with periods of spontaneous remission followed by recurrence of progressive disease. A few patients have a fulminant form of the disease with a rapid downhill course that lasts from two days to three weeks. The usual course lasts weeks to months with progressive deterioration. Untreated, about 80 per cent of patients die within six months of the onset of infection.

The most frequent symptom is headache; other common complaints include fever, weight loss, mental aberrations, nausea, and vomiting. On examination, obtundation or confusion, cranial nerve dysfunction, meningeal signs, and signs of increased intracranial pressure are found in varying degrees. Extraneural manifestations such as skin lesions, lymphadenitis, bone lesions, and other visceral involvement may occur in about 10 per cent of the cases of cryptococcal meningitis. The symptoms and physical findings in some patients may be very minimal, and many patients are afebrile and complain only of a slight headache. One must always have a high index of suspicion of this disease in patients who are at high risk, and the appropriate diagnostic tests must be done immediately to rule it out (Spickard, 1973).

The cerebrospinal fluid formula usually provides the first clue to the diagnosis. The white cell count in the spinal fluid generally ranges between 40 and 400 per cubic millimeter with a predominance of lymphocytes. Early in the disease, however, polymorphonuclear leukocytes may be the major cell type. The glucose concentration is often, but not invariably, below 50 mg per 100 ml, or 50 per cent or less than a simultaneously obtained blood glucose value. The protein level is usually elevated, especially in the presence of hydrocephalus, and the CSF pressure may be normal or high. Therefore, the cerebrospinal fluid abnormalities in this infection closely resemble those found in tuberculous meningitis.

## COMPLICATIONS AND SEQUELAE

Cryptococcal meningitis has a mortality of 100 per cent in untreated patients and 30 to 40 per cent in patients who are appropriately treated. The mortality depends on a number of factors, including age, underlying disease, and general physical status of the patient. Those patients who survive may suffer permanent damage to brain tissue as a result of the infection or may require placement of a ventricular shunt owing to hydrocephalus. Permanent deafness or dysfunction of any of the cranial nerves may also occur as a result of the infection.

## GEOGRAPHIC VARIATION

Cryptococcal meningitis occurs sporadically and has a worldwide geographic distribution. It occurs more often than would be expected by chance in white males and in association with Hodgkin's disease, leukemia, lymphoma, diabetes mellitus, and in patients being treated with steroids or other immunosuppressive agents. However, 50 per cent of patients with the infection have no underlying disease and appear to be immunologically normal. The current estimates of the incidence of cryptococcal meningitis range from 200 to 300 cases of meningitis per year in the United States, but this is probably a falsely low figure because the disease is not reportable. Of the four serotypes of C. neoformans, A is most commonly involved in meningitis. Types B and C are more common in southern California, and D may be more common in Europe (Bennett et al., 1977).

## DIAGNOSIS

Routine laboraory studies of blood and urine are usually normal or have no abnormalities that are diagnostic of the infection. When a diagnosis of cryptococcal meningitis is suspected, the cerebrospinal fluid should be examined microscopically with the use of the India ink technique. This test is positive in 50 to 70 per cent of cases. The sensitivity of this test is increased by centrifuging several milliliters of CSF before mixing a drop of the sediment on a microscope slide with an equal volume of India ink reagent. Although typical cryptococci are easy to identify, artifacts can be mistaken for organisms by the inexperienced eye. Obviously, confirmation of positive results of this test by culture is obligatory.

The isolation of C. neoformans by culture remains the single best diagnostic test. Five to 10 ml of CSF should be concentrated by centrifugation. The sediment should be used to inoculate fungal culture media without antibiotics. Incubation at 37° C should be aerobic. Ideally, three to five negative cultures should be obtained before the diagnosis is dismissed. Because cryptococci grow well on routine media such as chocolate agar plates, special fungal media are not an absolute necessity. The specific identification of C. neoformans involves a combination of physiologic and biochemical characteristics and the ability of the organism to cause encephalitis in newborn mice after intracerebral injection. The cultures will be positive in about 95 per cent of cases. Cultures of urine should be done and are positive in about a third of cases. Sputum and blood cultures may also be helpful, although the latter are usually positive only in fulminant disease. In some patients cerebrospinal fluid obtained by cisternal tap is positive when cultures obtained by lumbar puncture are negative.

The development of the latex agglutination test for the detection of cryptococcal antigen in CSF, blood, urine, or other body fluids has been a great advance in the diagnosis of cryptococcal meningitis (Gordon and Vedder, 1966). The polysaccharide antigen can be detected in the cerebrospinal fluid of patients with cryptococcal meningitis in about 94 per cent of cases. Tests for the demonstration of serum antibody to the cryptococcus have been somewhat less useful in diagnosis but may be more helpful in determining the responses of the patient to therapy. It is important to remember that patients with a positive rheumatoid factor may have a falsely positive result when cerebrospinal fluid is examined for cryptococcal antigen.

In a very small number of cases, all of the above tests are negative, and a positive diagnosis can then be made by culturing or seeing the organisms in a biopsy specimen taken from the central nervous system.

## TREATMENT AND PROPHYLAXIS

Before the introduction of amphotericin B in 1957, cryptococcal meningitis was almost uniformly fatal. The intravenous administration of this drug has produced a cure rate of approximately 60 per cent (Diamond and Bennett, 1974). If treated daily, adults are usually given approximately 0.5 mg/kg of body weight, although doses as low as 0.3 mg/kg and as high as 1.0 mg/kg have been used. If the patient is to be treated every other day, twice as much is given per infusion. The duration of therapy has been guided by the rapidity with which the CSF findings become normal (including the antigen determination) and how well the patient does clinically. Generally, patients are treated for six to ten weeks with a total dosage of 1.5 to 3.0 grams of amphotericin B (Bennett, 1974). Occasionally, the India ink test can remain positive for months to years even though cultures are negative. This finding is not an indication for continuation of therapy beyond the usually recommended dosages.

Because intravenously administered amphotericin B does not attain therapeutic concentrations in the CSF, the drug has been injected directly into the subarachnoid space. The value of this procedure is unknown. Probably intrathecal therapy should be reserved for patients who have not responded to an adequate course of systemic therapy or for those who have severe kidney disease and cannot tolerate systemic amphotericin B. If intrathecal treatment is to be used for longer than one or two weeks, it is preferable to administer the drug into a lateral cerebral ventricle through a subcutaneous siliconized rubber reservoir (Ommoya valve) rather than by lumbar or cisternal injection. Using this route, the drug is given two or three times weekly in graded doses up to a maintenance dose of about 0.5 mg per dose.

5-Fluorocytosine (5-FC) is an oral antifungal agent with good in vitro effect against *C. neoformans*. It readily penetrates the CSF, and toxic reactions are uncommon. Its use probably should be restricted in patients with compromised renal function. Unfortunately, at the dosage used (150 mg/kg day), its therapeutic effect appears to be inferior to that obtained with amphotericin B (Bennett, 1974). In addition, drug resistance commonly occurs during therapy with 5-FC; this is not true for amphotericin B. For these reasons 5-FC alone is not recommended for use in cryptococcal meningitis.

Combination therapy of amphotericin B and 5-FC has shown in vitro (Medoff et al., 1972) and in vivo synergism (Block and Bennett, 1973) against *C. neoformans*. Preliminary studies in humans have also been promising (Utz et al., 1975), and this regimen may turn out to be the best treatment for cryptococcal meningitis. The usual dosages are 150 mg 5-FC per kg daily orally and 20 mg amphotericin B intravenously daily. The amphotericin dose is reached gradually by giving 1 mg intravenously on the first day, 5 mg on day 2, 10 mg on day 3, 15 mg on day 4, and 20 mg on day 5 and thereafter. Combined treatment is given for 6 weeks.

Other drugs such as amphotericin B methyl ester and miconazole are under investigation to determine their therapeutic efficacy against cryptococcal meningitis. It is too early to tell whether these will prove to be an improvement over the existing regimens.

In addition to antifungal therapy, patients should be carefully monitored for complications of the infection such as seizures, inappropriate ADH, and hydrocephalus. If hydrocephalus occurs, a ventricular shunt may be necessary.

No prophylactic measures against *C. neoformans* infection are known at present.

## References

Bennett, J. E.: Chemotherapy of systemic mycoses. N Engl J Med 290:30, 1974 and 290:320, 1974.

Bennett, J. E., Kwon-chung, K. J., and Howard, D. H.: Epidemiologic differences among serotypes of *Cryptococcus neoformans*. Am J Epidemiol 105:582, 1977.

Block, E. R., and Bennett, J. E.: Combined effects of 5-fluorocytosine and amphotericin B in therapy of murine cryptococcosis. Proc Soc Exp Biol Med 142:476, 1973.

Diamond, R. D., and Bennett, J. E.: Prognostic factors in cryptococcal meningitis. Ann Intern Med 80:176, 1974.

Diamond, R. D., May, J. E., Kane, M. A., Frank, M. M., and Bennett, J. E.: The role of the classical and alternate complement pathways in host defenses against *Cryptococcus neoformans* infection. J Immunol 112:2260, 1974.

Gordon, M. A., and Vedder, D. K.: Serologic tests in diagnosis and prognosis of cryptococcosis. JAMA 197:961, 1966.

Kwon-chung, K. J.: Description of a new genus Filobasidiella, the perfect state of *Cryptococcus neoformans*. Mycologia 67:1197, 1975.

Medoff, G., Kobayashi, G. S., Kwan, C. N., Schlessinger, D., and Venkov, P.: Potentiation of rifampicin and 5-fluorocytosine as antifungal antibiotics by amphotericin B. Proc Natl Acad Sci USA 69:196, 1972.

Spickard, A.: Diagnosis and treatment of cryptococcal disease. South Med J 66:26, 1973.

Utz, J. P., Garriques, I. L., Sande, M. A., Warner, J. F., Mandell, G. L., McGehee, R. F., Duma, R. J., and Shadomy, D.: Therapy of cryptococcosis with a combination of fluorocytosine and amphotericin B. J Infect Dis 132:368, 1975.

# COCCIDIOIDAL MENINGITIS   **156**

### David A. Stevens, M.D.

## DEFINITION

Coccidioidal meningitis is a granulomatous infection of the central nervous system (CNS) caused by *Coccidioides immitis*, a soil-associated fungus. This disease resembles tuberculous meningitis and is the most severe and ominous complication of disseminated coccidioidomycosis because the mortality rate of untreated cases approaches 100 per cent. Dissemination occurs early after the primary pulmonary infection. The symptoms of meningitis usually appear within six months of primary coccidioidomycosis. Most primary infections are asymptomatic or undiagnosed, so that meningitis may be the first recognized manifestation of coccidioidomycosis (Pappagianis and Crane, 1977). Less than 0.5 per cent of Caucasians with primary coccidioidomycosis develop disseminated disease.

## ETIOLOGY

*C. immitis* is a dimorphic fungus that lives in the soil of the lower Sonoran life zone of the southwestern United States, Mexico, and South America. It is well adapted to the high salinity and alkaline pH of the desert. *C. immitis* replicates in the soil as a mycelium with long hyphae that fragment into hardy barrel-shaped arthrospores. Inhalation of air-borne arthrospores initiates the primary infection in man and animals. In the tissues, each arthrospore develops into a sporangium (spherule) of 30 to 60 $\mu$ in diameter. Sporangiospores (endospores) are relased from the spherule when it ruptures. They spread the infection within the tissues and develop into new spherules. On culture media or in the environment, spherules develop into the mycelial form. (See Chapters 72 and 120.)

## PATHOGENESIS AND PATHOLOGY

The fungus is inhaled into the lung and replicates there, stimulating cell-mediated immunity. If the host defenses fail to contain the infection, it may result in chronic pulmonary disease or hematogenous dissemination. The basilar meninges and sulci are the most common sites of metastatic CNS infection. Chronic basilar meningitis is complicated by hydrocephalus.

The basic tissue response to *C. immitis* is granulomatous, but focal areas of purulence occur, and fibrosis may develop in cases of long duration. Space-occupying lesions in the brain or spinal cord are rare. Intracranial or spinal epidural abscesses are usually secondary to an overlying osteomyelitis. The characteristic tissue form of the fungus, the spherule, can be found in the granulomas. Granulomatous cerebral arteritis and multiple areas of encephalomalacia that are probably caused by ischemia may accompany the meningitis. Granulomatous ependymitis may also be prominent.

## CLINICAL MANIFESTATIONS AND DIAGNOSIS

The florid signs and symptoms of meningeal irritation that are common in bacterial meningitis are usually absent in coccidioidal disease. The most common symptom is headache (Kelly et al., 1977). Fever, weakness, confusion, sluggishness, seizures, abnormal behavior, stiff neck, diplopia, ataxia, vomiting, and focal neurologic defects may occur. Coccidioidal skin lesions at the nasolabial fold are said to frequently accompany meningeal disease. Examination of the cerebrospinal fluid (CSF) reveals a pleocytosis that is usually mononuclear (eosinophils are sometimes seen), but polymorphonuclears may predominate early or during exacerbations. The CSF glucose level is decreased and the protein level is increased. Cultures of the CSF are positive in less than one third of cases, and direct visualization of the organism is extremely rare. Complement-fixing (CF) antibody is present in the serum, but may not be as high as the titers ($\geq$ 1:32) usually associated with other forms of disseminated disease unless other foci are present. Most patients also have CF antibody to *C. immitis* in their CSF (70 per cent on the first examination). In those who do not and who also have low titers in the serum, it is difficult to establish the diagnosis, and repeated assays for antibody in the CSF must be performed. As the disease progresses, almost all patients develop antibody in the CSF. CF antibody can also be detected in the unconcentrated CSF in some patients with parameningeal lesions (e.g., epidural abscesses, bony lesions that abut the dura) but is not seen in other forms of coccidioidal disease without accompanying meningitis. Cisternal or lumbar CSF is a much better indicator of disease activity than ventricular fluid, which commonly has a higher glucose concentration, a lower protein concentration, lower antibody titers, and fewer cells. Thus, the diagnosis should be suspected in a patient with typical CSF findings and either a history or evidence of previous or concurrent coccidioidal disease, including serum CF antibody, culture of *C. immitis* from another site, positive skin test, or appropriate travel or exposure history. Other causes should be excluded by bacterial, viral, and mycobacterial cultures of the CSF. The diagnosis of coccidioidal meningitis is confirmed either by detection of CF antibody in the CSF in the absence of parameningeal disease or by a positive CSF fungal culture. It is important to make the diagnosis early because early treatment appears to correlate with a successful outcome.

The CF titers of the CSF parallel the course of the disease in the same way that serum CF titers follow the course of other systemic disease (see Chapter 120). Rising titers indicate worsening disease, and falling titers indicate improvement. Patients who relapse after a response to therapy usually develop a pleocytosis or chemical abnormalities before the CSF antibody recurs.

## TREATMENT AND COMPLICATIONS

Without treatment, about 90 per cent of patients die within one year. Untreated cases of chronic meningitis are rare but one survived over 10 years. Intrathecal amphotericin B is the accepted treatment. Patients who have only meningitis are also treated with modest courses (0.5 to 1.0 g) of systemic amphotericin. This practice is intended, at least in part, as prophylaxis against other occult disseminated foci since intrathecal therapy is the essential treatment of meningitis (Buchsbaum, 1977). This situation differs from cryptococcal meningitis, which may be successfully treated by intravenous amphotericin alone in many patients. If patients are known to have other foci of coccidioidal infection, the duration of treatment should be altered to that usual for infection of that organ.

Intrathecal therapy can be administered by four routes: lumbar, cisternal, ventricular, and cervical. Corticosteroids (25 mg of hydrocortisone) may be administered simultaneously to reduce local reactions. It is advisable to begin therapy with low doses of amphotericin (0.01 to 0.025 mg) and increase the dose gradually as tolerated. Lumbar delivery is by barbotage or by suspension of the drug in hypertonic (10 per cent) glucose. With the patient on a table tilted head down, the hypertonic solution reaches the basilar area with minimal dilution. The maximum lumbar dose is usually about 0.5 mg, but the dose and frequency may need to be modified because of intolerance. Complications of lumbar therapy include local and radicular pain, headaches, paresthesias, nerve palsies that do not necessarily correspond to the level of injection, bladder dystonia, and impotence. The symptoms are usually transient. These problems have been attributed largely to amphotericin-induced arachnoiditis. However, it has recently been shown that amphotericin can also cause neurotoxic myelopathy, probably on a vascular basis (Carnevale et al., 1977). Transient symptoms may precede more profound deficits. Cisternal therapy has the advantage of placing the drug closest to the site of maximum infection, the basilar meninges. Doses of 0.01 to 1.0 mg have been used; 0.25 mg in a 0.5 ml volume is most common. Complications of cisternal therapy are rare if the injections are given by a physician experienced in cisternal puncture but include headaches, nausea, vomiting, hypertension, bradycardia, arrhythmias, cranial palsies, dysequilibrium and gait problems, and rare instances of upper motor neuron impairment. These complications are caused by arachnoiditis, possibly by direct neurotoxicity, and by hemorrhage. Hemorrhage may cause meningismus, compression of the brain stem, and obstruction of the outflow of the fourth ventricle. Direct puncture of the brain, usually the medulla but occasionally the cerebellar tonsil or pons, causes immediate cough, vomiting, weakness, electric sensations, and respiratory difficulties. Ventricular therapy through an Ommaya reservoir places the drug distant from the usual principal site of infection but is necessary if the ventricles are infected. It is useless in the presence of a ventricular shunt because the drug is diverted out of the central nervous system unless the distal end of the tubing is placed in the cisterna magna. The usual dose is 0.01 to 0.5 mg. Mechanical problems often complicate this form of therapy, and the ventricular end of the catheter may cause damage. Bacterial superinfection is much more common with indwelling catheters (Pappagianis and Crane, 1977). Experience with lateral cervical puncture is limited but is reputedly safe and less troublesome than other methods if the physician is experienced in the technique. Delivery by any route may be obstructed by infection and/or fibrosis. These complications may be detected by myelography, radioisotope flow studies, or computerized tomography.

There are no clear-cut guidelines for the frequency and duration of therapy. Recommendations for duration vary from three months after the CF antibody disappears from the CSF to treatment for life. Holeman had good results with a large, long-term series of patients treated with intrathecal amphotericin three times weekly for three months or until the cells in the CSF are $<10/mm^3$ (whichever is longer), then one to two times weekly for several months tapering to once every one to six weeks. Whenever the cell count exceeds 10, the frequency is increased until the count falls below this level. If frank clinical relapse or marked abnormalities in the CSF recur, the patient is retreated like a new patient. Therapy is discontinued only after the CSF has been completely normal for at least a year on a once every six weeks treatment schedule. After treatment is discontinued, the CSF is examined every six weeks for at least one to two years. This is important because other studies have indicated that relapses occur most commonly one to two years after the end of a course of apparently successful therapy. Holeman has reported at least four patients treated by this regimen who appear to be cured more than 2 years after therapy was discontinued. Winn (1967) achieved comparable results with intrathecal amphotericin two times weekly until the CSF improved, then one to two times weekly until three months after the CF antibody disappeared from the CSF. He also examined the CSF intermittently for at least two years.

A new imidazole, miconazole, offers a possible alternative to amphotericin. Some patients with disease that was unresponsive to amphotericin have responded to intravenous miconazole alone, intrathecal miconazole alone, or a combination of the two (Deresinski et al., 1977; Sung and Grendahl, 1977). Doses of 20 mg intrathecally are well tolerated and produce CSF levels that exceed the minimal inhibitory concentration of *C. immitis* for 24 hours (Devesinski et al., 1977). Patients with meningeal disease of longer duration are less likely to respond, and relapses have occurred after short courses of therapy (Deresinski et al., 1977). The relative efficacy of miconazole and amphotericin B awaits further comparative trials. The ability to treat meningitis by a systemic route of administration would represent a significant advance and is essential for patients with internal obstruction to the flow of CSF.

An important consideration in the management of patients with coccidioidal meningitis is awareness of the possibility of hydrocephalus and ventriculitis. Hydrocephalus is often the basis for deterioration in a patient whose CSF is unchanged or even improving on therapy (Kelly et al., 1977). Patients with ventriculitis are refractory to therapy. Computerized tomography has practically replaced pneumoencephalography, ventriculography, angiography, and brain scans in the detection of these complications. Shunting the flow of the CSF may prevent irreversible brain damage from hydrocephalus. Spread of infection from the distal end of the shunt is an unavoidable risk of this procedure. Concomitant intravenous therapy should be administered as long as ventricular cultures remain positive.

## References

Buchsbaum, H. W.: Clinical management of coccidioidal meningitis. In Ajello, L. (ed.): Coccidioidomycosis: Current Clinical and Diagnostic Status. New York, Stratton, Intercontinental Medical Book Corp., 1977, pp. 191–199.

Carnevale, N. T., Galgiani, J. N., Langston, J. W., and Stevens, D. A.: Myelopathy due to intrathecal amphotericin B. In Ajello, L. (ed.): Coccidioidomycosis: Current Clinical and Diagnostic Status. New York, Stratton, Intercontinental Medical Book Corp., 1977, pp. 259–260.

Deresinski, S. C., Galiani, J. N., and Stevens, D. A.: Miconazole treatment of human coccidioidomycosis: Status report. In Ajello, L. (ed.): Coccidioidomycosis: Current Clinical and Diagnostic Status. New York, Stratton, Intercontinental Medical Book Corp., 1977, pp. 267–292.

Holeman, C. W., and Johnson, P.: Long-term follow up of amphotericin treated coccidioidal meningitis patients. Proceedings of the Twenty-First Annual Coccidioidomycosis Study Group Meeting, Abstract 1, 1976.

Kelly, P. C., Sievers, M. L., Thompson, R., and Echols, C.: Coccidioidal meningitis: Results of treatment in 22 patients. In Ajello, L. (ed.): Coccidioidomycosis: Current Clinical and Diagnostic Status. New York, Stratton, Intercontinental Medical Book Corp., 1977, pp. 239–251.

Pappagianis, D., and Crane, R. Survival in coccidioidal meningitis since introduction of amphotericin B. In Ajello, L. (ed.): Coccidioidomycosis: Current Clinical and Diagnostic Status. New York, Stratton, Intercontinental Medical Book Corp., 1977, pp. 223–237.

Sung, J. P., and Grendahl, J. G.: Clinical experimental therapy with miconazole for human disseminated coccidioidomycosis. In Ajello, L. (ed.): Coccidioidomycosis: Current Clinical and Diagnostic Status. New York, Stratton, Intercontinental Medical Book Corp., 1977, pp. 293–309.

Winn, W. A.: Coccidioidal meningitis: A follow-up report. In Ajello, L. (ed.): Coccidioidomycosis. Tucson, University of Arizona Press, 1967, pp. 55–61.

# 157 LYMPHOCYTIC CHORIOMENINGITIS

*Fritz Lehmann-Grube, M.D.*

## DEFINITION

Lymphocytic choriomeningitis is an illness of animals and man after infection with the lymphocytic choriomeningitis (LCM) virus. The symptomatology of the human disease ranges from a grippe-like syndrome to meningitis and encephalomyelitis. Lymphocytic choriomeningitis is a zoonosis; the principal reservoir in nature of LMC virus is the gray house mouse.

## ETIOLOGY

The LCM virus was discovered independently and at about the same time on three occasions in the United States. Armstrong and Lillie (1934) encountered it when they passaged in monkeys infectious materials from a fatal case of the 1933 St. Louis epidemic of St. Louis encephalitis; Traub (1935) found albino mice from a laboratory colony to be infected; and Rivers and Scott (1935) isolated this agent from two cases of meningitis. The name was chosen to reflect the pathologic picture produced in monkeys and mice by intracerebral inoculation of the virus.

For a long time the LCM virus remained unclassified until other agents with similar properties were revealed, which led to the formation of a taxonomic group with the name arenoviruses (Rowe et al., 1970), later changed to arenaviruses (Fenner, 1976).

The LCM virus is released from the infected cell by a budding process in which the plasma membrane becomes the viral envelope. Size range and mean diameter of the pleomorphic virions are, respectively, 50 to 300 nm and ca 120 nm. The viral envelopes are covered with club-shaped projections that are approximately 10 nm long. In their otherwise unstructured interior, LCM virus particles contain one to several 20- to 25-nm electron-dense particles closely resembling cellular ribosomes (Dalton et al., 1968; Mannweiler and Lehmann-Grube, 1973). Their appearance is so characteristic for all the arenaviruses that they have formed the basis for the name *arenosus* (Latin), meaning sandy.

The virions contain single-stranded RNA consisting of four large and several small pieces with sedimentation coefficients 31, 28, 23, and 18S and 4 to 5.5S, respectively (Pedersen, 1973). The 18 and 28S segments are of host cell ribosomal origin

and probably correspond to the ribosome-like granules seen with the electron microscope. In the case of the related Pichinde virus, host cell ribosomes have been shown not to be essential for infectivity (Leung and Rawls, 1977). Three major viral polypeptides have so far been resolved, two surface glycoproteins with molecular weights of ca $54 \times 10^3$ and $35 \times 10^3$ and one nonglycosylated nucleocapsid protein with molecular weight of ca $63 \times 10^3$ (Buchmeier and Oldstone, 1978).

Two antigenic complexes with distinct specificities are recognized (Gschwender et al., 1976). One complex situated on the surface of the virion and also on the infected cell is identified by the neutralization test or related procedures. The other LCM virus-specific antigen is usually detected by complement fixation. It is produced in large quantities in the infected cell and is also an internal component of the virion, but it is not on the surface of either the virion or the infected cell. Besides the complement-fixation test, this antigen can be detected and measured by immunofluorescence procedures, double immunodiffusion tests, and radioimmunoassays.

## PATHOGENESIS AND PATHOLOGY

The disease of the adult mouse infected with LCM virus is entirely immunopathologic in nature. This well established fact has sometimes led to the assumption that in human lymphocytic choriomeningitis similar mechanisms are involved. There is nothing to indicate that the human illness has an allergic mechanism different from the immunopathologic component assumed to be associated with most viral diseases.

Human lymphocytic choriomeningitis is rarely fatal, and in the few cases with autopsy findings the etiology was not always convincingly revealed. In the case of Mitchell and Klotz (1942), in which the clinical diagnosis was LCM virus meningitis, the brain was swollen, thereby causing a cerebellar pressure cone. The arachnoid was markedly thickened and contained many lymphocytes and monocytes. With the severely altered vessels the inflammation extended into the Virchow-Robin spaces. There was little infiltration of the nervous tissue itself. Scheid et al. (1956b) described hemorrhagic necrotizing meningoencephalitis mainly involving the cortex. The central portions of the brain were less severely affected, showing predominantly perivascular infiltrations and glial proliferations. Capillary hemorrhages were also found in the cerebellar cortex, in the pontine nuclei, and in the nuclei of the cranial nerves with a pattern reminiscent of encephalitis caused by *Rickettsia prowazekii*. Death after meningoencephalitis was described by Warkel et al. (1973). In the brain there was marked meningeal perivascular inflammation, being most extensive in the sulci and over the brain stem and extending into dilated Virchow-Robin spaces. In the pons and medulla there were focal inflammatory nodules, and in the subcortical white matter of the cerebrum, pons, and cerebellum minimal to moderate signs of edema were observed. There was marked perivascular cuffing in the spinal cord and its coverings.

The three fatalities described by Armstrong and the infant that had died after transplacental infection (see below) are not included here because these cases were unusual and probably not representative of human lymphocytic choriomeningitis.

## CLINICAL MANIFESTATIONS

When describing the symptomatology of human lymphocytic choriomeningitis, it is customary to disregard mode of infection and source of the virus. This approach does not appear permissible because the consequences of natural infections, accidental laboratory infections, and infections induced for therapeutic purposes (pyretotherapy) differ markedly. In particular, the history of the virus seems to have profound effects on the clinical picture in man. In the following, a subdivision will be made, and illnesses due to infection under natural conditions will be considered first.

Armstrong (1942) differentiated three major forms: the "grippal or non–nervous system," the "meningeal," and the "meningoencephalitic" types. This classification has been found useful (Scheid, 1957; Lehmann-Grube, 1971) and will be adhered to here. Inapparent infections with LCM virus have been detected occasionally.

The incubation period is 6 to 13 days or longer. The grippal type of lymphocytic choriomeningitis is characterized by malaise, fever, headache, myalgia, and may run a remittent course with two or three phases. The frequency of the grippal type is difficult to assess. Recent hamster-associated outbreaks indicate that it may be more common than previously assumed. Among 47 persons infected with LCM virus after contact with pet hamsters, Ackermann et al. (1972) in Germany observed the grippal type 16 times; under similar conditions Deibel et al. (1975) in New York made the diagnosis 34 times among a total of 60 cases.

The most frequent clinical manifestation of LCM virus infection is the syndrome designated by Wallgren (1925) as acute aseptic meningitis. I shall use the term LCM virus meningitis. Often preceded by a prodromic "grippe," the onset is acute with headache, fever, malaise, and muscular pain soon followed by stiff neck, vomiting, and Brudzinski's and Kernig's signs. The cerebrospinal fluid shows moderate to marked lymphocytic pleocytosis and moderate increase of protein. Hypoglycorrhachia is not a regular finding.

The distinction between meningitic and meningoencephalomyelitic types is not sharp. In meningoencephalomyelitis a multitude of symptoms and signs may be grouped in all possible combinations. Usually the course is mild and may consist solely of clouding of consciousness and fleeting organic signs of involvement of the central nervous system. Sometimes, however, the illness may be severe. Scheid et al. (1968) described in a young man a picture resembling von Economo's encephalitis lethargica. There are also cases with transverse myelitis (Werner and Wolf, 1972), and sometimes an organic type of psychosis develops lasting for a few days (Scheid and Jochheim, 1956).

The LCM virus has been incriminated in recurrent or chronic diseases, but in only one patient (Treusch et al., 1943) was the etiology convincingly established. The case of encephalitis with unilateral orchitis and unilateral parotitis (Lewis and Utz, 1961) has remained a unique observation.

None of these syndromes is pathognomonic for lymphocytic choriomeningitis. Nor may the diagnosis be suspected from other nondescript symptoms associated with the disease, such as pharyngitis, sore throat, pain on moving the eyes, pleural pain, constipation or diarrhea, nausea and vomiting, skin rashes, swelling of lymph nodes, arthritis, coryza, and cough. The blood picture, too, is not very helpful. The erythrocyte sedimentation rate and leukocyte count are normal or slightly increased. Sometimes there is leukopenia.

The LCM virus may affect the unborn child if a pregnant mother becomes infected. Early in pregnancy, abortion seems to be the consequence (Ackermann et al., 1975; Biggar et al., 1975), but later the child may suffer malformations, especially hydrocephalus (Ackermann et al., 1974; Sheinbergas, 1976; Chastel et al., 1978). In one case a pregnant woman fell ill with LCM virus meningitis and the newborn child died at the age of 12 days. LCM virus was recovered from its cerebrospinal fluid obtained one day before death (Komrower et al., 1955).

It has already been pointed out that lymphocytic choriomeningitis may exhibit unusual features if the infecting virus had been maintained under laboratory conditions. The most striking example is the three fatalities described by Armstrong (1942). Of these, two had been manufacturing distemper vaccine (presumably from cultivated dog tissues) and the third had assisted at their autopsy. There was cerebral edema but very little involvement of the meninges or choroid plexus. Rather, general damage to blood vessels was prominent. These unusually virulent isolates were shown to be LCM virus with specific antisera, but differed with respect to host range and pathologic changes in experimentally infected animals.

Another case in point is H.-L. W. described by Scheid et al. (1956a). This physician had worked experimentally with *Toxoplasma gondii,* employing monkeys, hamsters, and mice. He suffered from a severe illness with meningoencephalitis, myocarditis, and involvement of liver and kidneys, and for some time the prognosis was considered unfavorable. Laboratory mice were incriminated at first, but later found free of infection. Instead, the *Toxoplasma* strain with which the patient had been working, and which had been passaged for an unknown number of years in the peritoneal cavity of mice, turned out to be contaminated with LCM virus.

Of 30 persons who worked experimentally with Syrian hamsters in whom the LCM virus was unintentionally passaged together with an infected line of hamster fibrosarcoma, 10 had severe "grippe-like" illness with fever, headache, myalgias, anorexia, and chest pain. None had meningitis. During convalescence, unilateral orchitis developed in three of nine men. Arthralgias were invariably experienced, which, in two cases, progressed to frank arthritis of the hands (Baum et al., 1966).

Another unusual series of LCM virus infections involved personnel at a university medical center engaged in tumor research (Hinman et al., 1975; Vanzee et al., 1975). Again, the virus had come from transplantable tumors and had been passaged in Syrian hamsters from where it had

spread to persons either handling them or working in the animal rooms. Of 48 infected individuals, only 21 had clinically apparent lymphocytic choriomeningitis. Fever, severe myalgias, headache, and chills were prominent. Two patients had LCM virus meningitis. Because leukopenia occurred in 10 of 11 patients and thrombocytopenia in eight of eight, Vanzee et al. (1975) suggested that these signs are characteristic for lymphocytic choriomeningitis. Although leukopenia has frequently been described in cases with unusual passage histories of the virus, the leukocyte counts are often normal when LCM virus comes directly from persistently infected house mice or from hamsters infected after a series of spontaneous transmissions from animal to animal. Death is an extremely rare outcome of LCM virus infection. The nine fatal cases with established etiology are listed in Table 1.

## COMPLICATIONS AND SEQUELAE

Complications have not been described. Sequelae are uncommon even if the illness was initially severe. In a few patients paralyses or muscle weaknesses have remained, and in one person a "flu-like illness" was followed by lasting unilateral sensorineural deafness and labyrinth damage (Hirsch, 1976). The "severe sequelae" in one case of LCM virus encephalitis mentioned by Meyer et al. (1960) were not specified.

## EPIDEMIOLOGY

It is often said that the LCM virus is distributed worldwide. Although this may be true, proof is available only for Europe (including Western Russia) and North and South America.

When Rivers and Scott (1935) demonstrated an association between LCM virus and acute aseptic meningitis, it was thought that this syndrome was in fact a disease entity caused by the LCM

**TABLE 1.   Cases of Fatal Lymphocytic Choriomeningitis**

| SPECIAL FEATURES | AUTHOR |
| --- | --- |
| 1. Laboratory exposure to serially passed virus | Armstrong, 1942 |
| 2. Laboratory exposure to serially passed virus | Armstrong, 1942 |
| 3. Performed autopsies on case 1 or 2 | Armstrong, 1942 |
| 4. LCM virus meningitis, 12-year-old child | Mitchell and Klotz, 1942 |
| 5. 12-day-old infant died of infection acquired transplacentally | Komrower et al., 1955 |
| 6. Bulbar paralysis | Adair et al., 1953 |
| 7. Landry-type ascending paralysis | Adair et al., 1953 |
| 8. Meningoencephalitis | Scheid et al., 1956b |
| 9. Meningoencephalitis | Warkel et al., 1973 |

virus, but it was soon realized that acute aseptic meningitis had numerous causes among which the LCM virus played but a minor role. It should be stressed that under natural conditions lymphocytic choriomeningitis is rare, as illustrated by the longitudinal study begun in 1941 by Rasmussen, continued by Adair et al. (1953), and concluded in 1958 by Meyer et al. (1960). In only concluded in 1958 by Meyer et al. (1960). In only 126 of 1568 patients (8 per cent) was the "acute infectious disease with CNS manifestations of apparent viral etiology" caused by the LCM virus.

The principal source of the LCM virus in nature is the gray house mouse (Armstrong, 1942) which may carry the virus lifelong in high concentrations in all its tissues. In mice the infection is perpetuated by vertical transmission. Carrier mice shed the virus with nasal secretions, saliva, and urine (Traub, 1939). Spread to other animals and man is accomplished either by direct contact, especially by a bite, or by contaminated fomites and possibly aerosols; vectors do not appear to play a role (Lehmann-Grube, 1971). Of the house mice, few are virus carriers and these are unevenly distributed among the mouse population (Ackermann et al., 1964).

As a rule, man is the last link of the infectious chain, and the same may be said about members of other species. There are, however, exceptions, of which the Syrian hamster (*Mesocricetus auratus*) is most noteworthy. This animal is easily infected by contact with carrier mice and produces large quantities of virus. Virus is shed for weeks and even months, predominantly with urine, thereby infecting other hamsters living in the same colony. Eventually, however, the virus is eliminated and, hence, infection of the hamster is not persistent in the way infection of a carrier mouse is (Skinner et al., 1976). Nonetheless, once a hamster colony is infested, it may remain so as long as susceptible young ones are born. Since LCM virus-infected hamsters are usually outwardly free of disease signs, they are not eliminated and, if sold, represent a hazard to their new owners.

Carrier mice and infected pet hamsters are the main sources of the LCM virus for man, and it is their distribution as well as frequency and intimacy of contact with people that determines the epidemiologic pattern of human infections. Infectious spread from mice occurs sporadically over long periods of time in certain rural areas. If looked for, carrier mice have invariably been found living in the same house as the diseased persons or in close proximity. If, on the other hand, the virus comes from freshly purchased hamsters, small or even large outbreaks are observed, mainly among city dwellers and often involving several members of a family.

## DIAGNOSIS

No combination of symptoms or signs of human lymphocytic choriomeningitis is pathognomonic. Hence, confirmation of the etiology in a suspected case requires isolation of the agent and demonstration of a significant increase of specific antibodies. The virus may be detected during the acute stage in blood and cerebrospinal fluid that are inoculated into the brains of *adult* laboratory mice. A tentative diagnosis may be made if these animals exhibit characteristic neurologic disturbances five or more days after inoculation. Confirmation is obtained by protection tests employing LCM virus-immune mice that are challenged by intracerebral inoculation with the new agent.

For obscure reasons, the complement fixation test is often used for serologic diagnosis despite its severe limitations. In human infections LCM virus-specific complement-fixing antibody always remains in low concentration and sometimes is not detectable. Thus, false negative results are often obtained with this test (Lehmann-Grube, 1971; Lewis et al., 1975). For diagnosis of a recent infection, antibody is most reliably determined by indirect immunofluorescent procedures (Cohen et al., 1966; Lewis et al., 1975), and an infection of the more distant past is best verified by demonstrating neutralizing antibody with mice as assay hosts, either as neutralization index (Lehmann-Grube et al., 1960) or as neutralization factor (Lehmann-Grube, 1978). Other methods have also been recommended (Blechschmidt et al., 1977; Thacker et al., 1977; Lehmann-Grube and Ambrassat, 1977), but they require experience and special facilities.

## TREATMENT AND PROPHYLAXIS

Lymphocytic choriomeningitis is treated by supportive measures selected to meet the clinical requirements of each case. No specific antiviral drugs or vaccine for human use have been developed.

### References*

Ackermann, R., Bloedhorn, H., Küpper, B., Winkens, I., and Scheid, W.: Über die Verbreitung des Virus der Lymphozytären Choriomeningitis unter den Mäusen in Westdeutschland. I. Untersuchungen überwiegend an Hausmäusen (Mus musculus). Zbl Bakt, I Orig 194:407, 1964.
Ackermann, R., Körver, G., Turss, R., Wönne, R., and Hochgesand, P.: Pränatale Infektion mit dem Virus der Lymphozytären Choriomeningitis. Bericht über zwei Fälle. Dtsch med Wschr 99:629, 1974.

*See Chapter 62 for References cited in text but not listed here.

Ackermann, R., Stammler, A., and Armbruster, B.: Isolierung von Virus der Lymphozytären Choriomeningitis aus Abrasionsmaterial nach Kontakt der Schwangeren mit einem Syrischen Goldhamster (Mesocricetus auratus). Infection 3:47, 1975.

Adair. C. V., Gauld, R. L., and Smadel, J. E.: Aseptic meningitis, a disease of diverse etiology: clinical and etiologic studies on 854 cases. Ann Intern Med 39:675, 1953.

Armstrong, C.: Some recent research in the field of neurotropic viruses with especial reference to lymphocytic choriomeningitis and herpes simplex. Milit Surgeon, Wash 91:129, 1942.

Baum, S. G., Lewis, A. M., Rowe, W. P., and Huebner, R. J.: Epidemic non-meningitic lymphocytic-choriomeningitis-virus infection. An outbreak in a population of laboratory personnel. N Engl J Med 274:934, 1966.

Biggar, R. J., Woodall, J. P., Walter, P. D., and Haughie, G. E.: Lymphocytic choriomeningitis outbreak associated with pet hamsters. Fifty-seven cases from New York state. JAMA 232:494, 1975.

Blechschmidt, M., Gerlich, W., and Thomssen, R.: Radioimmunoassay for LCM virus antigens and anti-LCM virus antibodies and its application in an epidemiologic survey of people exposed to Syrian hamsters. Med Microbiol Immunol 163:67, 1977.

Chastel, C., Bosshard, S., Le Goff, F., Quillien, M.-C., Gilly, R., and Aymard, M.: Infection transplacentaire par le virus de la chorioméningite lymphocytaire. Résultats d'une enquête sérologique rétrospective en France. Nouv Presse Méd 7:1089, 1978.

Cohen, S. M., Triandaphilli, I. A., Barlow, J. L., and Hotchin, J.: Immunofluorescent detection of antibody to lymphocytic choriomeningitis virus in man. J Immun 96:777, 1966.

Deibel, R., Woodall, J. P., Decher, W. J., and Schryver, G. D.: Lymphocytic choriomeningitis virus in man. Serologic evidence of association with pet hamsters. JAMA 232:501, 1975.

Hinman, A. R., Fraser, D. W., Douglas, R. G., Bowen, G. S., Kraus, A. L., Winkler, W. G., and Rhodes, W. W.: Outbreak of lymphocytic choriomeningitis virus infections in medical center personnel. Am J Epidem 101:103, 1975.

Hirsch, E.: Sensorineural deafness and labyrinth damage due to lymphocytic choriomeningitis. Report of a case. Arch Otolaryng 102:499, 1976.

Komrower, G. M., Williams, B. L., and Stones, P. B.: Lymphocytic choriomeningitis in the newborn. Probable transplacental infection. Lancet I: 697, 1955.

Lehmann-Grube, F.: An improved method for determining neutralizing antibody against lymphocytic choriomeningitis virus in human sera. J Gen Virol 41:377, 1978.

Lehmann-Grube, F., Ackermann, R., Jochheim, K.-A., Liedtke, G., and Scheid, W.: Über die Technik der Neutralisation des Virus der lymphozytären Choriomeningitis in der Maus. Arch ges Virusforsch 9:64, 1960.

Lehmann-Grube, F., and Ambrassat, J.: A new method to detect lymphocytic choriomeningitis virus-specific antibody in human sera. J Gen Virol 37:85, 1977.

Lewis, J. M., and Utz, J. P.: Orchitis, parotitis and meningoencephalitis due to lymphocytic-choriomeningitis virus. N Engl J Med 265:776, 1961.

Lewis, V. J., Walter, P. D., Thacker, W. L., and Winkler, W. G.: Comparison of three tests for the serological diagnosis of lymphocytic choriomeningitis virus infection. J Clin Microbiol 2:193, 1975.

Meyer, H. M., Johnson, R. T., Crawford, I. P., Dascomb, H. E., and Rogers, N. G.: Central nervous system syndromes of "viral" etiology. A study of 713 cases. Am J Med 29:334, 1960.

Mitchell, C. A., and Klotz, M. O.: Lymphocytic choriomeningitis. Canad J Public Health 33:208, 1942.

Rivers, T. M., and Scott, T. F. M.: Meningitis in man caused by a filterable virus. Science 81:439, 1935.

Scheid, W.: Das Virus der lymphozytären Choriomeningitis und seine Bedeutung für die Neurologie. Fortschr Neurol Psychiatr 25:73, 1957.

Scheid, W., Ackermann, R., and Felgenhauer, K.: Lymphozytäre Choriomeningitis unter dem Bild der Encephalitis lethargica. Dtsch med Wschr 93:940, 1968.

Scheid, W., and Jochheim, K.-A.: Akute Encephalomyelitis und Virus der lymphozytären Choriomeningitis. Nervenarzt 27:385, 1956.

Scheid, W., Jochheim, K.-A., and Mohr, W.: Laboratoriumsinfektionen mit dem Virus der lymphozytären Choriomeningitis. Dtsch Arch klin Med 203:88, 1956a.

Scheid, W., Jochheim, K.-A., and Stammler, A.: Tödlicher Verlauf einer Infektion mit dem Virus der lymphocytären Choriomeningitis. Dtsch Zschr Nervenheilk 174:123, 1956b.

Sheinbergas, M. M.: Hydrocephalus due to prenatal infection with the lymphocytic choriomeningitis virus. Infection 4:185, 1976.

Thacker, W. L., Lewis, V. J., Haller, G. J., and Baer, G. M.: A rapid fluorescent focus-inhibition test for determining the neutralizing-antibody response to lymphocytic choriomeningitis virus. Canad J Microbiol 23:522, 1977.

Traub, E.: A filterable virus recovered from white mice. Science 81:298, 1935.

Traub, E.: Epidemiology of lymphocytic choriomeningitis in a mouse stock observed for four years. J Exp Med 69:801, 1939.

Treusch, J. V., Milzer, A., and Levinson, S. O.: Recurrent lymphocytic choriomeningitis. Report of a case in which treatment was with pooled normal adult serum. Arch Intern Med 72:709, 1943.

Vanzee, B. E., Douglas, R. G., Betts, R. F., Bauman, A. W., Fraser, D. W., and Hinman, A. R.: Lymphocytic choriomeningitis in university hospital personnel. Clinical features. Am J Med 58:803, 1975.

Wallgren, A.: Une nouvelle maladie infectieuse du système nerveux central? (Méningite aseptique aiguë). Acta paediat 4:158, 1925.

Warkel, R. L., Rinaldi, C. F., Bancroft, W. H., Cardiff, R. D., Holmes, G. E., and Wilsnack, R. E.: Fatal acute meningoencephalitis due to lymphocytic choriomeningitis virus. Neurology 23:198, 1973.

Werner, W., and Wolf, G.: Akute Querschnittssyndrome bei lymphozytärer Choriomeningitis (LCM). Fortschr Neurol Psychiatr 40:662, 1972.

# 158 *BACTERIAL BRAIN ABSCESS*

## *Herbert S. Heineman, M.D.*

## DEFINITION

A brain abscess, which is a focus of suppuration within the substance of the brain, is one of a group of intracranial suppurative diseases that includes extradural abscess, subdural abscess, and septic cortical thrombophlebitis.

## ETIOLOGY

Nervous tissue appears to be highly resistant to bacterial invasion, in that bacteremia from any cause rarely results in infection of the brain. For example, in subacute endocarditis, where bacteremia may be sustained for weeks, damage to the brain is more likely to result from rupture of a mycotic aneurysm or cerebral infarction. Even the presence of highly virulent organisms in the subarachnoid space, as occurs in most cases of bacterial meningitis, almost never leads to infection of the brain. A brain abscess is most likely to occur in one of the following situations: (1) chronic cerebral anoxia, particularly when associated with a left-to-right intracardiac shunt; (2) chronic suppuration in the bone adjacent to the brain; (3) septic embolization from a chronic suppurative focus in another part of the body; and (4) direct implantation of bacteria by accidental or surgical trauma.

The role of chronic cerebral anoxia is best illustrated by the susceptibility of children with cyanotic congenital heart disease to brain abscess. In these patients, arterial hypoxemia complicated by polycythemia may result in cerebral infarction. Since brain abscess is a rare complication of cerebral infarction due to atherosclerosis, an additional etiologic factor in the children may be the bypassing of the pulmonary bacterial clearance mechanism.

The bacteriology of brain abscess has changed appreciably within the past 40 years. Hemolytic streptococci and pneumococci, leading pathogens in the past, are infrequently found nowadays, probably because the initial respiratory infections caused by them yield so readily to antibiotics. In other respects, the change is more apparent than real. Early descriptions of brain abscess referred to the frequent occurrence of "sterile" pus; from the remainder, hemolytic streptococci, pneumococci, staphylococci, and gram-negative enteric bacilli were recovered. In some cases, pus that yielded negative cultures showed an abundance of gram-positive cocci or gram-negative bacilli on microscopic examination. In the past two decades, the important role of endogenous anaerobic bacteria has been increasingly appreciated (Heineman and Braude, 1963; de Louvois, 1978; Ingham et al., 1978). The actual incidence of the various bacterial species recovered has varied from one report to another. For example, Heineman and Braude found anaerobic gram-positive cocci (streptococci) and gram-negative bacilli (*Bacteroides*) to be the most frequent; de Louvois and colleagues (1977), with equally meticulous attention to bacteriologic technique, noted a high incidence of capnophilic aerotolerant streptococci. In correlating bacteriology with localization (and portal of entry) of an abscess, de Louvois (1978) found that capnophilic streptococci (particularly *Streptococcus milleri*) were particularly associated with frontal lobe abscesses, while mixtures of anaerobic bacteria as well as aerobic enteric bacilli were typical of temporal lobe abscesses. Even allowing for these differences, the following generalizations appear to be justified: (1) hemolytic streptococci and pneumococci are now infrequent causes of intracranial suppurative disease; (2) staphylococci are associated with septicemia and penetrating trauma, including surgery, but are otherwise infrequently found; (3) *Haemophilus influenzae* is more or less limited to the age group showing high susceptibility to this organism (children from 2 to about 7 years), and aerobic enteric bacilli are limited to newborns and elderly debilitated patients; and (4) with the aforementioned exceptions, aerobic gram-negative bacilli are uncommonly found alone, and their importance, if any, is overshadowed by that of the mixture of anaerobes in whose company they occur.

*Actinomyces israelii, Nocardia asteroides,* and *Haemophilus aphrophilus* are occasionally implicated in brain abscess.

## PATHOGENESIS AND PATHOLOGY

It is believed that infection with all but the most virulent bacteria (such as *Nocardia asteroides*) is preceded by damage to the nervous tissue. In the absence of trauma, the usual precipitating factor is infarction. In keeping with this concept, most abscesses originate at the junction of the gray and white matter, the least well perfused area of the brain. Septic embolization provides a mechanism for both infarction and infection. Its source may be distant, for example, the thorax or pelvis; in this case embolization occurs via the arterial blood, and the abscess may occur in any part of the brain but particularly in the distribution of the middle cerebral artery. More commonly, the source is a space in the skull from which sepsis travels via emissary veins to a nearby part of the brain: from the middle ear and mastoid, the temporal lobe and cerebellum are most commonly infected; from the frontal sinus, spread is typically to the frontal lobe.

As in other tissues, abscess formation is preceded by a stage of inflammation characterized by vascular congestion, edema, and infiltration with polymorphonuclear cells. This presuppurative stage, sometimes referred to as focal encephalitis or (when anatomically appropriate) cerebritis, is potentially reversible. The walling-off process begins at the end of the first week with a thin membrane. This is followed by the development of a fibrous capsule, thicker on the cortical than on the ventricular side, which matures after approximately three weeks from onset of infection. At this stage, the so-called acute abscess, the lesion is still surrounded by a varying zone of cerebral edema whose volume may be larger than that of the abscess itself. It is this edema that is largely responsible for persistent or progressive clinical manifestations leading to death or forced surgical intervention. In some cases, encapsulation is functionally complete, surrounding edema subsides spontaneously, and a chronic abscess may be tolerated for months or years with few or no symptoms.

Brain abscess almost never occurs as a consequence of bacterial meningitis. In the unusual cases where both coexist, they are believed to represent either concurrent infection or rupture of the abscess.

## CLINICAL MANIFESTATIONS

Clinical manifestations of intracranial abscess reflect three separate processes: systemic reaction to infection, increased intracranial pressure, and damage or destruction of brain tissue. In addition, most patients will demonstrate a typical primary focus of infection.

Systemic manifestations, such as chills and fever, are most commonly associated with septicemia, acute sinusitis, or acute otitis. When the underlying process is indolent, the presence of a brain abscess may produce low-grade fever, but in some cases systemic reaction is totally absent.

Increased intracranial pressure almost always accompanies intracranial suppurative disease, contributes significantly to morbidity and mortality, and causes the commonest symptom, namely, headache. Nonspecific as headache is in infectious disease, and despite its more specific association with otitis and sinusitis, it has considerable value in the diagnosis of intracranial suppurative disease. This symptom is characterized by progressive severity, intractability, and occasional localization to the affected side of the head. In patients accustomed to headache because of their underlying infection, the change in character of this symptom coincident with intracranial spread should raise the suspicion of brain abscess. In advanced cases, vomiting may occur, consciousness may be clouded until coma supervenes, and funduscopic examination may reveal papilledema. Meningeal irritation is absent unless a subdural abscess is present or a brain abscess has ruptured, a complication that is frequently fatal.

Localizing neurologic signs reflect the particular site of the inflammatory process. For example, temporal lobe abscesses are characterized by expressive aphasia and a homonymous contralateral upper quadrant visual field defect; increased pressure may temporarily paralyze the ipsilateral third and sixth cranial nerves. In cerebellar abscesses, nystagmus with the fast component toward the lesion and ipsilateral incoordination

and hypotonia occur; the ipsilateral sixth and seventh cranial nerves may be temporarily paralyzed by pressure. Parietal lobe abscesses may lead to contralateral hemisensory deficits. In frontal lobe abscesses, typical manifestations are impaired consciousness and contralateral motor deficits; however, lateralizing signs are frequently absent. Occipital lobe lesions may result in contralateral homonymous hemianopia.

Even focal neurologic dysfunction is as often due to inflammation or edema as to destruction of nervous tissue. Focal signs may even appear during antibiotic treatment and then regress as inflammation subsides (Heineman et al., 1971).

Although the clinical picture is dominated by the intracranial process, examination usually reveals evidence of suppuration elsewhere, for example, the middle ear.

The peripheral blood generally shows neutrophilic leukocytosis, but in subacute or chronic abscesses, the blood count may be normal.

## COMPLICATIONS AND SEQUELAE

In a disease as severe as brain abscess, the chief complication is death, which until recently occurred in an average of about 40 per cent of patients. In one of the seeming paradoxes of modern medicine, reviews of several hundred cases of brain abscesses published during the first 30 years of the antibiotic era showed that this infectious disease, caused by bacteria susceptible to a wide range of antibiotics and treated by advanced surgical technique, carried no better a prognosis between 1962 and 1967 (Garfield, 1969) than it did between 1938 and 1951 (Jooma et al., 1951) or, for that matter, in 1893 (MacEwen, 1893). The logical conclusion was that irreversible damage had often occurred before any treatment was instituted, and that the chief obstacle to recovery was late diagnosis. With the availability of noninvasive radiologic techniques such as the technetium brain scan and computerized axial tomography (see section on Diagnosis), a more aggressive yet safer approach to early diagnosis is possible, and the pathologic process can be aborted much earlier, possibly without the need for surgery.

Death is often caused by intracranial hypertension leading to an uncinate or medullary pressure cone. In other cases, the abscess ruptures into a lateral ventricle, exciting a violent inflammatory response. Rupture through the cortex is comparatively infrequent, in keeping with the asymmetry of the abscess capsule (see Pathology section).

Among patients who survive, neurologic recovery on the whole is remarkably good. This discrepancy between severity of the acute illness and paucity of residual dysfunction can be explained by the relative roles of edema and suppuration in giving rise to clinical manifestations. If important motor, visual, or speech areas are actually destroyed, corresponding degrees of paresis, field defect, or speech impairment may result.

The most frequent sequela is focal epilepsy, which is presumably due to the inevitable scar that remains when an abscess is drained or excised. Several reviews have placed the frequency of this complication in the vicinity of 50 per cent. In the majority of affected survivors, seizures begin at some time during the first two years following surgery; in a small number, however, ten or more years may elapse.

## GEOGRAPHIC VARIATIONS

Since intracranial abscesses are essentially complications of respiratory infections, their incidence may be expected to parallel that of otitis, sinusitis, and chronic suppurative lung disease. However, descriptions of clinical features and bacterial etiology do not permit any conclusions regarding geographic variation in the disease itself.

## DIAGNOSIS

### Clinical

A high index of suspicion is necessary to diagnose intracranial suppurative disease at a stage when the prognosis is still favorable. The varied clinical manifestations have been described above. Since symptoms of intracranial hypertension or inflammation usually precede focal neurologic abnormalities by days or even weeks, close attention should be paid to such apparently nonspecific complaints as fever, headache, vomiting, visual disturbances, or drowsiness. When these symptoms occur in a patient with an appropriate portal of entry, a painstaking neurologic examination should be performed, with particular emphasis on visual fields, cognitive function, and coordination. Persistence of unaccustomed headache justifies a neuroradiologic investigation even when the physical examination of the nervous system discloses no abnormalities.

### Radiologic

Routine skull radiographs are of limited value but are readily available. They may show a shift in a calcified pineal gland or, rarely, an air-fluid level in a gas-containing brain abscess. Films should be examined for clouding of the frontal sinuses and sclerosis of the mastoid bones, which support the presence of underlying suppurative disease in those areas.

An excellent screening technique for demonstrating a focal inflammatory process is the technetium-99m pertechnetate brain scan. However, although sensitive, it lacks discrimination, and the picture may be obscured by the underlying inflammatory process in the paranasal sinuses or mastoids or by blood in dilated dural venous sinuses.

The best combination of safety, sensitivity, and specificity is found in the computerized axial tomogram, or CAT scan. This scan has excellent localizing capability and, especially when used with a contrast medium, renders a picture that is quite characteristic of an abscess. When an abscess has not yet formed, that is, in the stage of focal encephalitis, this picture is less specific but its localization value is just as great. Unfortunately, equipment for this test is expensive and is not universally available. Figure 1 shows the appearance of a brain abscess by these techniques.

Other radiologic techniques that previously enjoyed widespread use are arteriography, which is particularly useful for demonstrating avascular mass lesions, and ventriculography, which showed lateral displacement of the ventricular system by a cerebral hemispheric mass or internal hydrocephalus due to an obstructing cerebellar mass. Both these techniques are invasive and because of their inherent hazards have been largely replaced by the CAT scan.

Electroencephalography is useful for lateralizing a cerebral lesion, but the abnormalities are not specific for abscess. Posterior fossa (cerebellar) abscesses cannot be localized by this technique.

Lumbar puncture is contraindicated when a brain abscess is suspected (Garfield, 1969). As in the case of other asymmetrical space-occupying lesions associated with intracranial hypertension such as brain tumors, relief of pressure in the lumbar area may result in herniation of the brain through the tentorium cerebelli or the foramen magnum. Lethal compression of the hippocampal unci or the medulla oblongata may occur immediately or hours later. It should be emphasized that the slow withdrawal of a small amount of cerebrospinal fluid does not protect against this disastrous complication, as seepage continues through the punctured dura long after the needle has been withdrawn. In cases in which spinal fluid was examined, it showed at most a moderate mononuclear pleocytosis with normal glucose concentration; in other cases, no abnormalities were found. Therefore, this examination is not only dangerous but of little help.

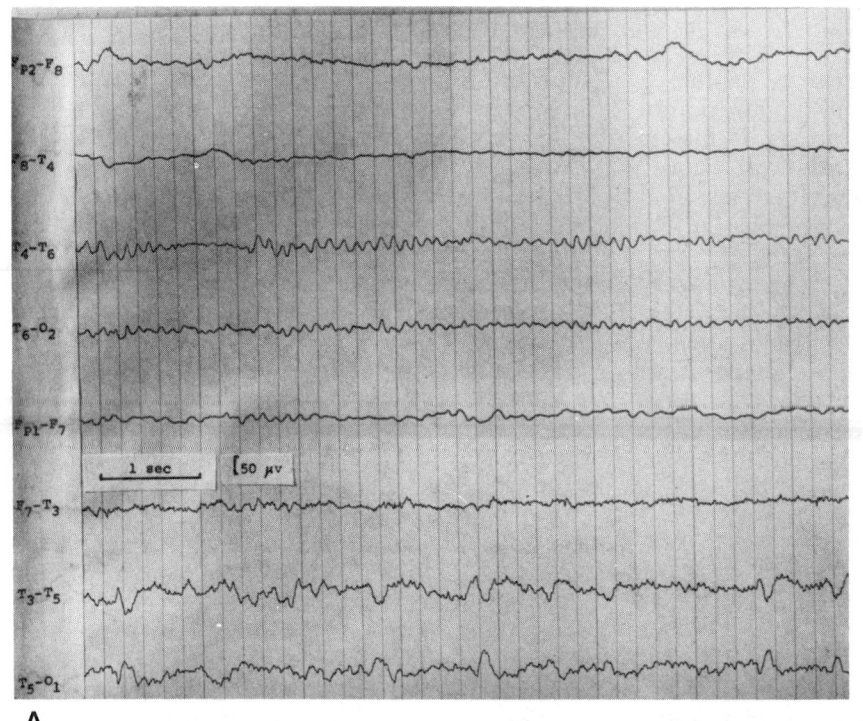

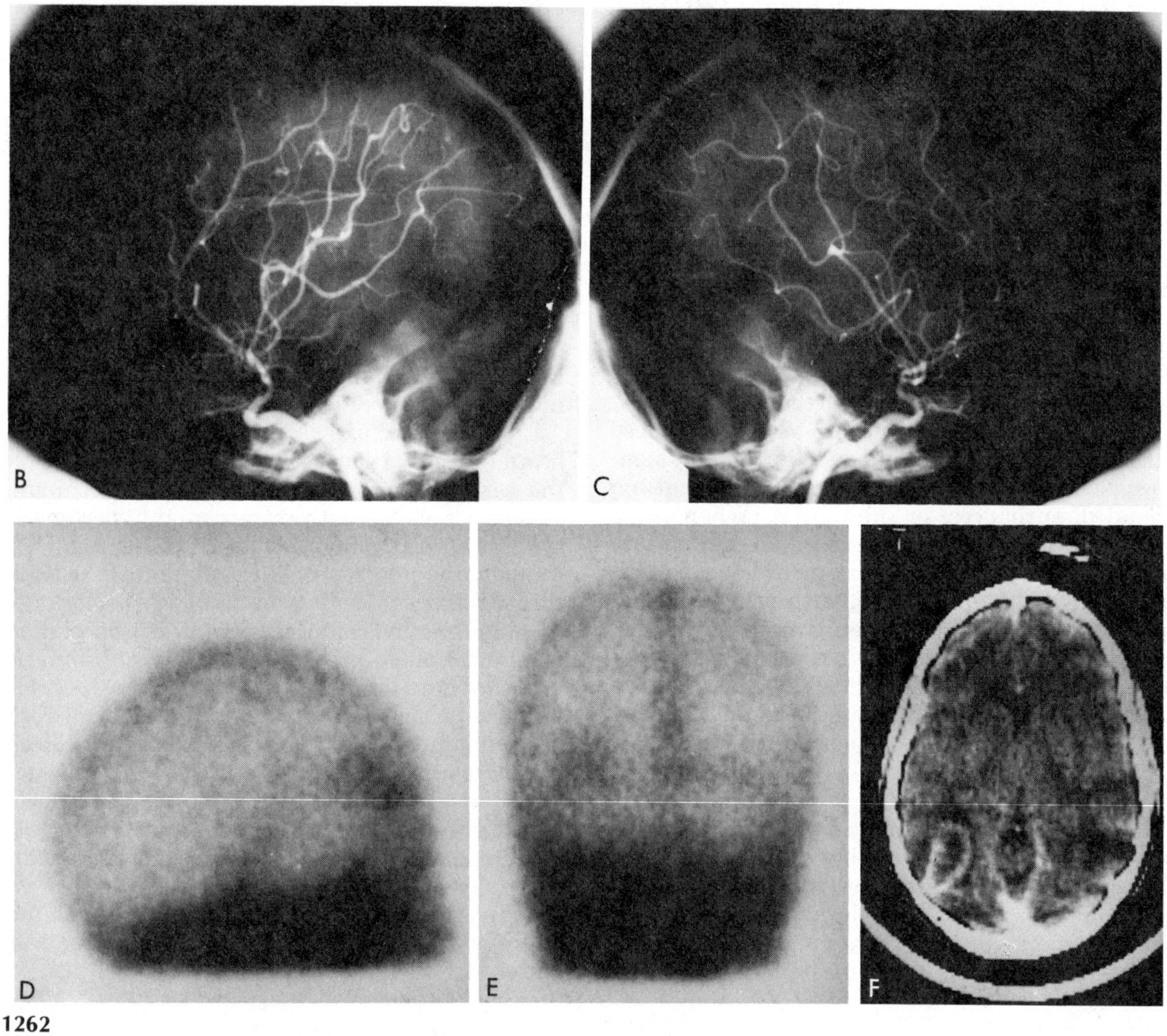

**FIGURE 1.** *Demonstration of a left parieto-occipital abscess in a patient with congenital heart disease by four techniques. A, Electroencephalogram. Note high voltage slow waves in leads $T_3$–$T_5$ and $T_5$–$O_1$ (left) compared with normal alpha rhythm in leads $T_4$–$T_6$ and $T_6$–$O_2$ (right). B and C, Carotid arteriogram. Note straightened (stretched) branches of middle cerebral artery in B compared with normally tortuous branches in C. D and E, Technetium scan. "Hot spot" is visible in both lateral (D) and posterior (E) projections. F, CAT scan. "Doughnut" configuration, with central lucency surrounded by enhanced density, is typical of abscess.*

### Bacteriologic

Some of the bacteria most commonly found in brain abscesses are fastidious in their growth requirements and are killed by undue exposure to atmospheric oxygen. Pus should be submitted to the laboratory immediately upon withdrawal with instructions for prompt anaerobic as well as aerobic culture. Microscopic examination of a Gram-stained smear of the pus should be routine.

## TREATMENT

In theory, treatment of intracranial suppurative disease is straightforward — drainage of pus and administration of antibiotics. In fact, acquired antibiotic resistance is not a serious problem and complications due to the surgical procedure itself are unusual. Yet despite these favorable conditions, the outcome still leaves much to be desired. As mentioned earlier, the chief reason for treatment failure appears to be delay in diagnosis, permitting the development of intolerable intracranial hypertension and, eventually, destruction of brain tissue. This situation can be remedied by clinical awareness and the ready use of safe and sensitive neuroradiologic tests.

The components of therapy are (1) timing and choice of neurosurgical procedure, (2) selection and dosage of antibiotic therapy, and (3) monitoring of the disease during recovery.

### Surgery

There has been considerable debate on the relative merits of aspiration, drainage, and excision of the lesions (Jooma et al., 1951). Under ideal conditions of localization, as may be achieved with a technetium or CAT scan, aspiration and drainage have led to satisfactory results. However, reaccumulation of pus and failure to drain loculated daughter abscesses are potential dangers, and the patient's course must be closely followed by serial scans until the process is completely resolved. To avoid these problems, the prevalent opinion now is that excision is preferable, provided that the condition of the patient permits such surgery and the abscess is not in a vital area. Lesser procedures have been associated with slower convalescence and even relapse. Surgery is ideally performed when the abscess is well encapsulated, which may take three weeks or more to complete. A patient who survives that long without significant deterioration will probably withstand surgery well and recover. Unfortunately, progressive intracranial hypertension often demands surgical intervention at a time when both the poor clinical condition of the patient and the immaturity of the abscess militate against a successful outcome. As an ancillary measure, intracranial pressure can be temporarily lowered by an adrenocorticosteroid, for example, dexamethasone phosphate 4 mg parenterally every six hours. However, this treatment could interfere with the process of encapsulation.

The critical clinical indicator for assessing the urgency of operation is the patient's state of consciousness. More important than the development of new focal signs, progression from alertness to stupor or coma means that pressure must be relieved; the surgeon achieves this objective through the combined effects of craniotomy and removal of pus.

### Antibiotics

The contribution of antibiotics to surgical management so far has been disappointingly small, as judged by the overall lack of improvement in mortality since they were introduced. In part, this result is due to long-standing ignorance about the bacteriology of brain abscess and the pharmacokinetics of antibiotics in central nervous system infections, and in part to the inability to diagnose intracranial infection in a presuppurative stage when antibiotics are most effective.

It is almost axiomatic in the field of infectious diseases that antibiotics are selected on the basis of objective microbiologic data. When pus from a brain abscess is examined by appropriate microscopy, culture, and susceptibility tests, this requirement can be met. However, if the ideal time to treat such infection is before pus is formed, and the objective in fact is to avoid craniotomy altogether, then this crucial selection has to be made without the benefit of any direct examination. Unhappily, organisms cultured from the primary source, such as the middle ear cavity, or even from the blood may not accurately reflect the bacteriology of a brain abscess. On the other hand, published data (see Etiology section) indicate that certain bacterial species are characteristically found in abscesses of different origins. This justifies the general recommendations listed in Table 1. The selections given reflect the best available combination of antibacterial effectiveness and central nervous system penetrability. The penicillins are particularly suitable because of their overall lack of toxicity. Chloramphenicol has a broad antibacterial spectrum and penetrates well into the central nervous system.

Cephalosporins and aminoglycosides, as classes, are not as effective in central nervous system infections.

A drug that has not yet been widely evaluated but shows promise of usefulness is metronidazole (Ingham et al., 1978). Because of its selective

**TABLE 1.  Selection of Antibiotics Based on
Presumed Portal of Entry**

| PORTAL OF ENTRY | ANTIBIOTICS | DOSAGE |
|---|---|---|
| Ear, sinus, chest, mouth, unknown | Potassium penicillin G plus chloramphenicol succinate | 4 million units every four hours IV<br>1 gram every six hours IV |
| Accidental penetrating head trauma | Sodium nafcillin | 2 grams every four hours IV |
| Infected surgical wound[a] | According to results of wound culture | |
| Septicemia, endocarditis | According to results of blood culture | |

[a]If surgery involved chronically infected ear, sinus, or chest, penicillin and chloramphenicol should be included regardless of wound culture.

effectiveness against anaerobes, including *Bacteroides fragilis,* it should be considered for use in abscesses originating from the ear, sinus, or chest. However, it is ineffective against aerotolerant streptococci and, because the latter are especially common in frontal lobe infections (de Louvois, 1978), it should not be used alone. Doses of 400 to 600 mg intravenously every eight hours appear to be effective.

Sulfonamides are the drugs of choice for nocardial brain abscesses. Sulfadiazine can be given orally in a dose of 1 g every two hours. Trisulfapyrimidines have also been used successfully in this dosage.

### Monitoring Recovery

There are no established criteria to determine the proper duration of therapy. The clinical course alone is unreliable as a guide, since patients may not fully recover or may suffer a relapse if antibiotics are discontinued too soon. If the abscess is surgically drained or excised, the cavity may be filled with a radiopaque material such as thorium dioxide or microbarium sulfate, which is taken up by the cells lining the cavity. This allows the progressive diminution of the lesion to be monitored by simple radiographs of the head. In cases managed without surgery, progress can be followed by the same techniques used in diagnosis, namely, technetium brain scans and computerized axial tomography. In the absence of objective indicators of healing, four to six weeks' therapy is recommended. In general, full doses should be administered parenterally for the entire duration of treatment; since subsidence of the inflammatory reaction reestablishes the normal blood-brain barrier, there is no reason for decreasing the dose or using a less reliable route of administration.

## PROPHYLAXIS

Intracranial abscess is essentially a complication of extracranial disease; therefore, timely and effective treatment of the latter constitutes the best preventive measure. The relative decline in abscesses caused by hemolytic streptococci and pneumococci compared with earlier reports may be due in part to the ready susceptibility of these organisms to antibiotics, which are commonly given for acute otitis and sinusitis. Control of chronic infection in these sites, in which most intracranial abscesses in adults are found nowadays, is more difficult and often requires surgery. As an increasing variety of congenital cardiac anomalies yields to surgical correction, the incidence of brain abscess in these patients should diminish.

## INTRACRANIAL SEPTIC THROMBOPHLEBITIS

Aseptic dural sinus or cortical vein thrombosis sometimes occurs as a late complication of bacterial meningitis. In these cases, thrombosis is secondary to a severe inflammatory process, perhaps aggravated by increased tissue pressure but not primarily a septic process. Septic thrombophlebitis, on the other hand, occurs by a mechanism similar to that involved in intracerebral suppuration, namely, direct spread of infection through the veins. The severity of this complication varies with the anatomic site. Among the more critical sites are the cavernous sinus and the superior sagittal sinus.

### Cavernous Sinus Thrombosis

This sinus may be infected from the sphenoid or posterior ethmoid sinus or the mastoid. The most characteristic portal of entry, however, is the upper half of the face, with retrograde thrombosis or venous embolism via the facial, angular, and superior ophthalmic veins. Because cutaneous infections of the face are mostly caused by coagulase-positive staphylococci, these organisms are most commonly implicated in cavernous sinus thrombosis. The initial clinical manifestations of staphylococcal infection, such as rigors, fever, nausea, and lethargy, are predominantly constitutional. Peripheral leukocytosis is the rule, and the etiologic organisms can usually be cultured from the blood. In infections arising from a paranasal sinus or mastoid, the bacteria are those typically involved in infections in those areas and the systemic reaction may be less severe and acute. In either case, localizing signs due to venous obstruction soon evolve, making the diagnosis fairly easy. In typical cases, edema of the eyelids, forehead, and base of the nose is followed by chemosis and proptosis. Venous engorgement may be apparent on the forehead and in the retina. Compression of cranial nerves III to VI in the orbit or cavernous sinus results in pain and hyperesthesia and varying degrees of ophthalmoplegia and cycloplegia.

Although cavernous sinus thrombosis is basically a unilateral process, it may become bilateral if thrombosis extends through the intercavernous sinuses (circular sinus) to the opposite side. A rare complication in these cases is infarction or abscess of the pituitary, which is surrounded by the circular sinus.

### Superior Sagittal (Longitudinal) Sinus Thrombosis

This is a relatively uncommon condition secondary to infection in a cavernous or lateral sinus, vertebral vein, or osteomyelitis of the calvaria. Clinical manifestations depend on the site of occlusion and involvement of tributary cortical veins. Posterior occlusion may lead to intracranial hypertension, engorgement of scalp veins, and edema of the forehead. Anterior occlusion of the sagittal sinus may be largely asymptomatic. However, if cortical veins are likewise occluded, the result may be varying degrees of cerebral infarction, with neurologic signs involving principally the legs, sometimes accompanied by focal seizures of first one and then the other side. The full-blown clinical picture is fairly easy to recognize.

### Lateral Sinus Thrombosis

Involvement of the lateral sinus is usually secondary to infection in the middle ear. Although cerebral infarction is uncommon, increased intracranial pressure may result, especially if the right lateral sinus, which is usually the larger of the two, is involved. A diagnostic feature is edema and venous engorgement behind the ear of the affected side.

### Treatment

The only useful form of therapy is the parenteral administration of large doses of antibiotics. Their selection is based on the known or suspected bacteriology of the initiating focus and the blood (see earlier section on Antibiotics).

## *CRANIAL EPIDURAL ABSCESS*

There is normally no epidural (extradural) space, since the dura closely adheres to the inner table of the skull. A collection of pus creates an artificial epidural space by dissecting between the bone and the dura. This usually results by direct extension from osteomyelitis of the skull, which in turn is an extension of frontal sinusitis or mastoiditis or an infected wound. As long as the dura is not penetrated and no important venous channels are affected, the clinical manifestations are essentially those of the underlying osteomyelitis, with fever, local edema, pain, and tenderness. Neurologic findings may be totally absent, but there may be a low-grade mononuclear pleocytosis of the spinal fluid with all other values normal. Since the diagnosis is usually made at surgery, it can only be speculated that some cases may be aborted by antibiotic therapy directed at the underlying infection.

### References

de Louvois, J.: The bacteriology and chemotherapy of brain abscess. J Antimicrob Chemother 4:395, 1978.

de Louvois, J., Gortvai, P., and Hurley, R.: Bacteriology of abscesses of the central nervous system: A multicentre prospective study. Br Med J 2:981, 1977.

Garfield, J.: Management of supratentorial intracranial abscess: A review of 200 cases. Br Med J 2:7, 1969.

Heineman, H. S., and Braude, A. I.: Anaerobic infection of the brain: Observations on eighteen consecutive cases of brain abscess. Am J Med 35:682, 1963.

Heineman, H. S., Braude, A. I., and Osterholm, J. L.: Intracranial suppurative disease: Early presumptive diagnosis and successful treatment without surgery. JAMA 218:1542, 1971.

Ingham, H. R., Selkon, J. B., and Roxby, C. M.: The bacteriology and chemotherapy of otogenic cerebral abscesses. J Antimicrob Chemother 4 (Suppl C):63, 1978.

Jooma, O. V., Pennybacker, J. B., and Tutton, G. K.: Brain abscess: Aspiration, drainage, or excision. J Neurol Neurosurg Psych 14:308, 1951.

MacEwen, W.: Pyogenic and Infective Diseases of the Brain and Spinal Cord. Glasgow, J. Maclehose and Sons, 1893.

# 159 *CEREBRAL MUCORMYCOSIS*

*Donald Armstrong, M.D.*

## DEFINITION AND ETIOLOGY

Cerebral mucormycosis refers to invasion of the central nervous system by any of the three genera of the family Mucoraceae. Rhinocerebral mucormycosis is the term indicating that the naso pharynx or sinuses are involved as well as the central nervous system. The disease has been intermittently called phycomycosis, but the preferred term is mucormycosis as proposed by Baker (1970, 1971). The reason for this is that the class phycomycetes includes the families Mucoraceae and Entomophthoracae. The Mucoraceae includes the genera *Rhizopus, Mucor,* and *Absidia,* the organisms that cause this disease. In contrast, tropical subcutaneous phycomycosis and rhinoentomophthoromycosis are caused by members of the family Entomophthoracae and are subcutaneous infections characterized by eosinophilic granulomas and geographically limited in most cases to the tropics. Mucormycosis is worldwide in distribution and the cerebral form is the result of deep, invasive infection in immunologically altered patients. The species *Rhizopus arrhizus* and *R. oryzae* occur most commonly, but others such as *Absidia ramosa, A. corymbifera,* and *Mucor pusillus* can also cause disease. It has been estimated that cultural proof is available in less than 10 per cent of cases (Rippon, 1974).

## PATHOLOGY AND PATHOGENESIS

The original cases of cerebral mucormycosis were reported in patients with diabetes mellitus in ketoacidosis (Gregory et al., 1943), but since then patients with other underlying diseases have been described (Baker, 1970, 1971, Rippon, 1974, and Meyer and Armstrong, 1973). Table 1 lists the factors predisposing to and the types of underlying diseases reported in cerebral mucormycosis in the approximate order of frequency. Although almost all of these patients are immunosuppressed in one way or another, there is no unifying defect evident. Acidosis, whether diabetic or due to infantile diarrhea or renal failure, is one of the obvious common denominators, but patients with leukemias, lymphomas, or renal transplants have not been in acidosis or diabetic (Meyer and Armstrong, 1973, Meyer et al., 1972, and Hammer et al., 1975). Corticosteroid therapy has been a common feature in many of the immunosuppressed patients. In another series of patients with lymphoma and leukemia, two common denominators were leukopenia and antibiotic therapy (Meyer et al., 1972). Some of these patients did have chemical diabetes mellitus, but it was usually mild and none were in acidosis. In patients with leukemia the incidence has obviously increased (Meyer et al., 1972) and the reason for this is not evident unless longer periods of leukopenia (and therefore antibiotic therapy) due to more aggressive chemotherapy programs may be responsible. Some large series of renal transplantation patients have not reported mucormycosis and there may be geographic regional or other epidemiologic factors that are not recognized (Schneck, 1971). Invasive disease can be more readily induced in prednisone-treated animals (Baker, 1971) and in one patient reported, this was the only form of immunosuppressive therapy, although the patient had a leukopenia of undetermined etiology (Meyer et al., 1972).

In addition to immunosuppressed patients and those in diabetic acidosis, a rare patient with well-controlled diabetes mellitus seems predisposed to cerebral mucormycosis (Sandler et al., 1971). Intrathecal injection of spores into normal rabbits has not produced disease, but after allox-

**TABLE 1. Predisposing Factors to Cerebral Mucormycosis**

| FACTORS | UNDERLYING DISEASE |
|---|---|
| Acidosis* | Diabetes, renal failure, infantile diarrhea |
| Immunosuppression*†‡ | Leukemia, lymphoma, organ transplantation |
| Diabetes mellitus* | Diabetes mellitus, including prednisone induced |
| Narcotics addiction† | None |
| Postcraniotomy† | None |

*Rhinocerebral form.
†Cerebral form.
‡One patient treated for a dermatologic disease with azathioprine and prednisone has been reported. Prednisone has been common in most patients.

an diabetes the same number of spores resulted in fatal infection (Rippon, 1974). Many immunosuppressed patients have had hyperglycemia although none were in acidosis (Meyer et al., 1972; Hammer et al., 1975). Intravenous inoculation of *Mucor* organisms along with narcotics has caused intracranial mucormycosis in addicts, but injection of *Mucor* spores intravenously into monkeys does not result in disseminated infection unless corticosteroids are given (Baker, 1971). This suggests that immunosuppression results from drug addiction (Louria et al., 1967). Postcraniotomy infections occur in patients with no apparent predisposing factors (Meyer and Armstrong, 1973, Ignelzi and VanderArk, 1975). In one report a normal person developed a mucormycotic brain cyst which showed blood vessel invasion (Murrsan, 1960), but resembled a brain tumor rather than progressive cerebral mucormycosis.

The infection reaches the central nervous system most commonly by direct extension from nasopharynx via the cribriform plate or the paranasal sinuses to the brain. Spread can be by direct extension across tissue planes or along blood vessels, nerves, and lymphatic channels. Invasion of blood vessels with thrombosis and infarction occurs consistently in mucormycosis. The fungus invades the clot and grows into the infarcted tissue. Less often invasion of veins causes thrombosis. Although the ear is also a potential route to the brain, it is not clear that the pathway may instead be from sinuses to brain to ear. All recently documented cases have invaded sinus, orbit, or cerebral vessels as well as middle ear and brain tissue (Bergstrom et al., 1970).

For obscure reasons *Mucor* organisms may be difficult to isolate from biopsy or autopsied tissue. They are common laboratory contaminants and

some species grow readily on bread as well as laboratory medium. The diagnosis may depend on histopathology. The organisms are usually seen easily by hematoxylin and eosin stain, but are distinguished best with the Gomori methenamine silver stain (Fig. 1). The broad hyphae vary in size from 6 to 50 $\mu$ but are usually within 10 to 20 $\mu$. They are only sparsely septate or may appear nonseptate (Rippon, 1974). Haphazard branching at right angles is more apparent in wet mounts than in histopathology sections. They invade vessels, perivascular tissues, and infarcts (Fig. 1). Tissue necrosis and abscesses develop in the central nervous system after direct extension or hematogenous spread. If the lungs are the source for hematogenous spread, pulmonary lesions with typical vessel invasion are usually evident, and the cerebral lesions may be anywhere in the brain. In contrast rhinocerebral mucormycosis spreads from the nasopharynx or paranasal sinuses to the frontal lobes or the base of the cerebrum. Osteomyelitis may result from direct extension. When the sinuses are involved the orbit is frequently invaded. Internal carotid thrombosis secondary to direct extension has been reported in 33 per cent of patients (Rippon, 1974). Cavernous sinus thrombosis is less frequent but one of these vessels is estimated to be invaded in more than 66 per cent of patients with rhinocerebral mucormycosis (Meyer and Armstrong).

### CLINICAL MANIFESTATIONS OF HEMATOGENOUS CEREBRAL MUCORMYCOSIS

The patient usually has a leukemia or a lymphoma or is immunosuppressed following

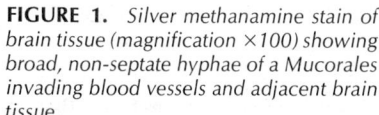

**FIGURE 1.** *Silver methanamine stain of brain tissue (magnification ×100) showing broad, non-septate hyphae of a Mucorales invading blood vessels and adjacent brain tissue.*

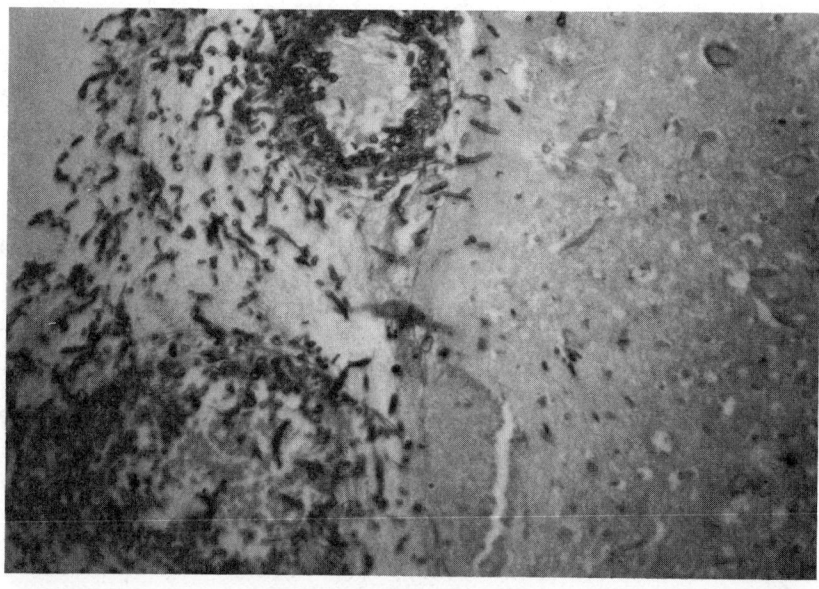

organ transplantation. In rare cases narcotics addiction or cranial surgery have been the predisposing factors (Table 1). The symptoms and signs are those of one or more intracranial expanding lesions and are usually associated with pulmonary lesions and fever. The signs depend on the area of the brain involved and the degree of increased intracranial pressure. Skin lesions may occur in disseminated disease.

## DIAGNOSIS OF HEMATOGENOUS CEREBRAL MUCORMYCOSIS

The blood count is not helpful, leukocytosis is not regular, and many patients are leukopenic. Disseminated disease may be reflected by abnormal liver functions. Chest x-rays vary from patchy bronchopneumonia to large wedge-shaped lesions suggesting pulmonary infarcts. Cerebral angiograms may disclose occlusion of vessels or aneurysms. Radionuclide brain scans help localize lesions for biopsy or extirpation (Meyer, 1977). The organism has not been cultured from the cerebral spinal fluid and the cell counts and chemistries are not diagnostic. The fluid may be xanthochromic and in patients with leukemia it may contain erythrocytes, even in the absence of thrombocytopenia. Specific diagnosis requires biopsy of a brain lesion with wet mount, culture, and histopathology. One argument for a brain biopsy of a single lesion is that extirpative therapy has appeared useful in rhinocerebral mucormycosis and because chemotherapy with amphotericin B has failed (Meyer and Armstrong, 1973). As this syndrome becomes more widely recognized, clinical diagnoses without demonstration of the fungus will allow earlier therapy with amphotericin B especially in patients where bleeding is a contraindication to surgery. The differential diagnosis in such patients includes toxoplasma encephalitis, or brain abscess due to *Aspergillus* spp. or to *Nocardia asteroides*. Toxoplasmosis or aspergillosis may require brain biopsy for documentation, although there are serologic tests that may suggest the diagnosis. In nocardiosis, the organism can frequently be isolated from the sputum or skin lesions, but a brain biopsy may be necessary for both diagnosis and drainage. Serologic tests for antibody or circulating antigen have not been developed for the Mucoraceae.

## CLINICAL MANIFESTATIONS OF RHINOCEREBRAL MUCORMYCOSIS

This disease should be suspected in patients in acidosis or who are immunosuppressed in the treatment of leukemias and lymphomas or organ transplantation and in a rare patient with well-controlled diabetes mellitus (Table 1). The original description (Gregory et al., 1943) stressed the triad of uncontrolled diabetes mellitus, orbital infection, and meningoencephalitis and subsequent descriptions have added little (Meyer and Armstrong, 1973; Ferry, 1961; and Grass, 1961). The patient may give a history of persistent nasal discharge or bleeding. In the more fulminant form he may be first seen in stupor or coma, but even in these cases careful questioning may disclose a history of preceding headache, eye irritation, periorbital numbness or swelling, lacrimation, or nasal symptoms for one to seven days. In diabetic acidosis the onset is usually rapid, and the course fulminant. In some cases the first evidence that the patient had diabetes was concomitant ketoacidosis and rhinocerebral mucormycosis. In patients with other underlying diseases the course may be subacute.

Physical findings are those of the underlying disease and frequently a state of depressed consciousness beyond what might be expected from other findings. Unilateral orbital edema may be striking and periorbital or suprasinus cellulitis prominent. Proptosis or ophthalmoplegia occurred in two-thirds of the cases in one series (Ferry, 1961). Involvement of the second, third, fourth, and sixth cranial nerves along with the first and second divisions of the fifth may cause loss of vision, internal and external ophthalmoplegia, corneal anesthesia, and anhidrosis. Paralysis of the seventh cranial nerve and contralateral hemiplegia have been described in one-third of cases. Less often homolateral jugular tenderness occurs secondary to thrombophlebitis of the internal jugular vein. Nuchal rigidity is not common, nor is involvement of other cranial nerves.

## DIAGNOSIS OF RHINOCEREBRAL MUCORMYCOSIS

Black, necrotic exudate in the nasopharynx or issuing from the sinuses should suggest mucormycosis. There may be bleeding or weeping of a thin, yellowish fluid. The laboratory findings are those of the underlying condition and are not specific for mucormycosis. Sinus x-rays are usually negative and skull x-rays rarely show evidence of bone destruction adjacent to infected sinuses. Angiograms may show partial or complete vascular occlusion, particularly of the internal carotid artery. Brain nucleotide scans may be positive (Meyer, 1977). Cerebrospinal fluid is nondiagnostic. A definitive diagnosis rests on demonstration of the organism on smear or culture, but preferably on biopsy. Since Mucoraceae may be seen or cultured from patients who are colonized but not infected, demonstration of tissue invasion is the most reliable method.

The differential diagnosis includes nasopharyngeal infections due to *Pseudomonas aeruginosa,* which can cause black nasal lesions. Since mixed infections do occur (Meyer, 1973), if there is any suggestion by smear or culture that *P. aeruginosa* is involved, it is prudent to treat for this life-threatening infection until it is excluded. *Aspergillus* organisms may also cause the rhinocerebral syndrome and should be demonstrable on biopsy. A bacterial pathogen in the smears and cultures may be only secondary invaders or noninvasive colonizers. When suspicion is high for mucormycosis, a biopsy should be done. Cavernous sinus thrombosis due to other organisms, such as *Staphylococcus aureus,* in diabetics should be considered. Other conditions that may simulate rhinocerebral mucormycosis are syphilis, tuberculosis, neoplasms, midline lethal granuloma, and rhinosporidiosis. These are almost always far less acute, but a biopsy will decide the diagnosis.

## TREATMENT

In the fulminant form of the disease a biopsy should be obtained and treatment started with amphotericin B pending the results. If the first biopsy is negative, and the clinical picture is convincing, amphotericin B should be continued and a deeper biopsy performed. Surgical exploration and extirpation of nasal or sinus lesions should be considered because the organism may not be found in the superficial necrotic tissue. Strong clinical suspicion and positive smear are also indications for therapy while awaiting results. Even in patients with less fulminant disease, amphotericin B could be started while waiting for culture or biopsy results. Once the diagnosis has been established and treatment with amphotericin B has been instituted, surgery must be considered. Although patients have been cured with amphotericin B alone, many more have been cured with amphotericin B and surgery, and some with surgery alone (Meyer and Armstrong, 1973). The surgical procedure must be left in the hands of the ear, nose, and throat, or ophthalmology specialist, but the internist should encourage removal of as much involved tissue as possible so that only viable tissue is left in order that adequate tissue levels of amphotericin B can be assured. Eye enucleation has been done in some cases. The following schedule is recommended for amphotericin B: 1. Test dose (to see if patient develops anaphylaxis) 1 mg in 250 ml of 5 per cent D/W over one to two hours; 2. follow immediately with 10 mg in 500 ml of 5 per cent D/W over four to six hours; 3. follow immediately with 20 mg in 500 ml of 5 per cent D/W over four to six hours; 4. follow immediately with 30 mg in 500 ml of 5 per cent D/W over four to six hours; then establish an alternate daily dose of 1.2 mg/kg/day intravenously in 1000 ml of 5 per cent D/W over six hours. If severe chills and fever occur at any of the dosage schedules, then the rate of administration should be slowed and the next dose should be the same or decreased by 5 to 10 mg. Most patients will tolerate this type of schedule. An alternate schedule is: 1. the same 1 mg test dose of amphotericin B; 2. follow with 24 mg (the remainder of the vial) in 1000 ml of 5 per cent D/W over six hours; 3. follow with 50 mg in 1000 ml of 5 per cent D/W over six hours; then establish a daily dose of 1 mg/kg/day, and following that with 1.2 mg/kg on alternate days (Meyer and Armstrong, 1973; Battock et al., 1968). The following means of controlling side effects are used: heparin 10 mg in the fluid containing the amphotericin B to decrease thrombophlebitis at the infusion site; aspirin, diphenhydramine, and chlorpromazine one hour before starting the infusion to control chills, fever, nausea, and vomiting; and if this fails hydrocortisone succinate 50 to 100 mg.

Renal function will usually be impaired, and if the creatinine rises to 3.0 mg (or BUN to 30 mg) then the next dose should be decreased by 5 to 10 mg or more until renal function improves. Renal loss of potassium is usually significant and potassium blood levels should be followed and supplemented as necessary. With long term therapy anemia usually develops and may require blood transfusion if the amphotericin B cannot be stopped. The total dose of amphotericin B has varied between 525 mg and 3 g in patients who have been cured (Meyer and Armstrong, 1973). Nasopharyngeal lesions can be irrigated with amphotericin B (1 mg/ml) (Meyer and Armstrong, 1973; Battock et al., 1968) but efficacy has not been tested by control studies. Since patients have been cured with surgery alone, systemic amphotericin B has not been proved necessary, but since other patients have been cured with the drug alone, it seems reasonable to use both treatment modalities in an illness that originally carried a mortality of 90 per cent, and more recently with early diagnosis and therapy, has decreased to at least 50 per cent (Rippon, 1974; Meyer and Armstrong, 1973).

A major consideration in therapy is control of the underlying disease. The acidosis, whatever its cause, should be brought under control. Diabetes mellitus should be carefully controlled. Immunosuppression should be decreased when that appears to be responsible, but in acute leukemia every effort should be made to achieve a remission.

## COMPLICATIONS AND SEQUELAE

Residual neurologic defects, such as hemiparesis, facial palsies, ophthalmoplegia, and blindness are frequent and can be prevented only by early diagnosis and treatment.

## PROPHYLAXIS

Prevention is difficult to achieve, since we do not know why some immunosuppressed or acidotic patients develop cerebral mucormycosis and others do not. Careful control of diabetes mellitus and minimum immunosuppression in all patients seem reasonable. Early control of acidosis is usually achievable. Prevention of narcotic addiction will prevent that form of the disease. Although outbreaks in hospitals caring for immunosuppressed patients have not yet been described for mucormycosis, they have been for *Aspergillus*

species. They can be anticipated for Mucoraceae and prevented by scrupulous housecleaning.

### References

Baker, R. D.: Mucormycosis (opportunistic phycomycosis). In Baker, R. D. (ed.): The Pathologic Anatomy of Mycosis. Human Infection with Fungi, Actinomycetes, and Algae. New York, Springer-Verlag, 1971, Chap. 21.
Baker, R. D.: The phycomycoses. Ann NY Acad Sci 174:592, 1970.
Battock, D. J., Grausz, H., Bobrowsky, M., and Littman, M. L. Alternate-day amphotericin B therapy in the treatment of rhinocerebral phycomycosis (mucormycosis). Ann Intern Med 68:122, 1968.
Forry, A. P.: Cerebral mucormycosis (phycomycosis). Ocular findings and review of literature. Surv Ophthalmol 6:1, 1961.
Gass, J. D. M.: Ocular manifestations of acute mucormycosis. Arch Ophthalmol 65:226, 1961.
Gregory, J. E., Golden, A., Haymaker, W.: Mucormycosis of the central nervous system. A report of three cases. Bull Johns Hopkins Hosp 73:405, 1943.
Hammer, G. S., Bottone, E. J., and Hirschman, S. Z.: Mucormycosis in a transplant recipient. Am J Clin Path 64:389, 1975.
Meyer, R. D.: Scan findings in rhinocerebral mucormycosis. (Letter) J Nucl Med 18:96, 1977.
Meyer, R. D., and Armstrong, D.: Mucormycosis — Changing status. CRC critical reviews in clinical laboratory sciences 4:421, 1973.
Meyer, R. D., Rosen, P. P., and Armstrong, D.: Phycomycosis complicating leukemia and lymphoma. Ann Intern Med 77:871, 1972.
Rippon, J. W.: Mucormycosis. In Medical Mycology. The Pathogenic Fungi and The Pathogenic Actinomycetes. Philadelphia, W. B. Saunders Co., p. 430, 1974.
Schneck, S. A.: Neurology and neuropathology of immunosuppressive therapy and acquired immunological deficiency. Res Publ Assoc Res Nerv Ment Dis 49:293, 1971.

# 160 CEREBRAL ASPERGILLOSIS

## Donald Armstrong, M.D.

### DEFINITION

Cerebral aspergillosis refers to infection of the brain with *Aspergillus*. It may represent the only area of *Aspergillus* infection, it may represent invasion of the brain as part of the general dissemination of aspergillosis, or it may result from direct extension of an infection from a contiguous area such as the sinuses, orbit, or ear.

### ETIOLOGY

The etiologic agent is usually one of seven species of the genus *Aspergillus* (Young et al., 1972). These are *Aspergillus fumigatus, A. flavus, A. glaucus, A. terreus, A. niger, A. nidulans,* and *A. clavatus. A. fumigatus* is the most frequent pathogen and *A. flavus* is more likely to reach the brain via the sinuses or orbit (Rippon, 1974). Others of the more than 300 species of *Aspergillus*

(Raper and Fennel, 1965), can also be pathogenic, but they cause invasive disease less often than the species listed above. Since the diagnosis is frequently made on a histologic basis, the true distribution among the infecting species is uncertain.

Aspergilli grow at temperatures ranging from 27° to 45° C (thermotolerance) and are common laboratory contaminants. They produce fluffy white or variously pigmented colonies. On wet mounts they are seen as dichotomously branching organisms made up of septate hyphae and conidiophores. The configuration of the conidiophores (fruiting heads) and vesicles are used for speciation (see Chapter 74). Since the fungi grow so well on so many media, it is puzzling that they cannot be more readily isolated from autopsy or biopsy material. This may be because of the specimen selection process; the best one seems always to go to the pathology laboratory. Clinical specimens such as a brain biopsy should be examined after digestion with 10 per cent potassium hydroxide. Aspergilli have inconstant Gram-staining properties, but once a microbiologist becomes familiar with their appearance on wet mount, they are easily recognized.

## PATHOGENESIS AND PATHOLOGY

The pathogenesis is *not clear*. The organisms are ubiquitous; many patients develop allergy or heavy colonization, but invasive disease is rare. The early literature stressed occupational and exposure hazards (Rippon, 1974) such as moldy barns, grain, pigeon fanciers, and wig dusters, but in recent analyses of invasive disease, this sort of history is absent. A number of cases have occurred in apparently normal persons with no exposure history (Khoo et al., 1966; Mukoyama et al., 1969), but several large series have been reported more recently from among immunosuppressed patients, usually with leukemias or lymphomas (Young et al., 1970; Meyer et al., 1973; Fisher et al., in press). There has been a documented increase in incidence of disseminated aspergillosis in leukemia patients at risk (Meyer et al., 1973). Almost all of these patients have been on antimetabolites or cytotoxic agents, adrenocorticosteroids, and antibiotics. Frequent bacterial infections, particularly with *Pseudomonas aeruginosa,* have usually preceded the aspergillosis, and patients have survived after effective antibacterial therapy. Similar immunosuppressive factors are present in patients treated for solid tumors or organ transplantation (Young et al., 1970; Meyer et al., 1973; Fisher et al., in press; Burton et al., 1972; Gurwith et al., 1971). In addition, a few cases have been reported in patients with sarcoidosis, collagen-vascular disease, chronic granulomatous disease, tuberculosis, histoplasmosis, congenital heart disease, bacterial pneumonias, alcoholism, and cirrhosis (Rippon et al., 1974; Khoo et al., 1966; Mukoyama et al., 1969). Some patients had been receiving antibiotics for unspecified reasons (Khoo et al., 1966; Mukoyama et al., 1969). Accidental direct inoculation at surgery, intravenously and even intraperitoneally, has resulted in dissemination including cerebral involvement, and intravenous injection is presumably the route of infection among narcotic addicts (Kaufman et al., 1976). Experimental infections in mice have shown that antibiotics alone did not appear to increase susceptibility to invasive disease, but the addition of adrenocorticosteroids did (Sidransky and Friedman, 1959). Chicks with leukemia induced by avian myeloblastosis virus developed invasive aspergillosis more often than normal controls (Chick and Durham, 1963). Leukopenia has been noted in a high percentage of patients who develop invasive aspergillosis (Visudhiphan et al., 1973; Meyer et al., 1973; Fisher et al., in press) and aspergillosis is relatively common in patients with chronic granulomatous disease. These observations suggest that neutrophil function is important in resistance to aspergillosis. Such patients had normal delayed hypersensitivity but did not develop a humoral antibody response to aspergilli (Greenberg et al., 1977) for unexplained reasons. On the other hand, we have seen patients with chronic granulomatous disease develop multiple immunodiffusion bands against an infecting *Aspergillus* species.

The fungus reaches the central nervous system by two main routes (Table 1). Hematogenous spread occurs primarily from the lungs and rarely from the gastrointestinal tract. There may be no evident primary lesion either clinically or histopathologically, but often the lung contains evidence of invasion. In some instances there is no apparent source, while in most others brain involvement clearly represents part of general hematogenous dissemination. Direct extension from infected adjacent tissues occurs from the sinuses, orbit, or ear. On rare occasions a rhinocerebral syndrome is seen (see Chapter 158) in patients with neoplastic disease who are not in acidosis.

The gross pathology reveals abscess formation and infarcts with clotted vessels (Fig. 1), usually in patients with altered immune responses, or granulomatous lesions, usually in patients with intact immune responses. The organisms have a marked tendency to invade arteries, resulting in thrombosis and infarction of brain tissue and secondary invasion of infarcted areas. Invaded arteries range in size from the internal carotid artery to small arterioles. As a result, mycotic aneurysms have occurred (Horten et al., 1976) (Fig. 2). The fungi form septate, acutely branching hyphae that are rather uniform in size (average 3 $\mu$, ranging from 2.2 to 4.5 $\mu$) (see Chapter 74, Fig. 4). Conidiophores are rarely seen in areas of abscess formation; they are more common where air is present as in mycetomas (fungus balls) of the lungs. In granulomatous

**TABLE 1.    Aspergillus Cerebral Infections**

| TYPE OF INFECTION | UNDERLYING DISEASE* OR PROCEDURE |
|---|---|
| Orbit, nasal, sinus route (rhinocerebral syndrome) | None (immunosuppressed) |
| Granulomas | None |
| Abscess, with infarcts | Immunosuppressed, endocarditis |
| Mycotic aneurysm | Endocarditis |
| Direct inoculation | Neurosurgery, lumbar puncture |

*Frequent but not always.

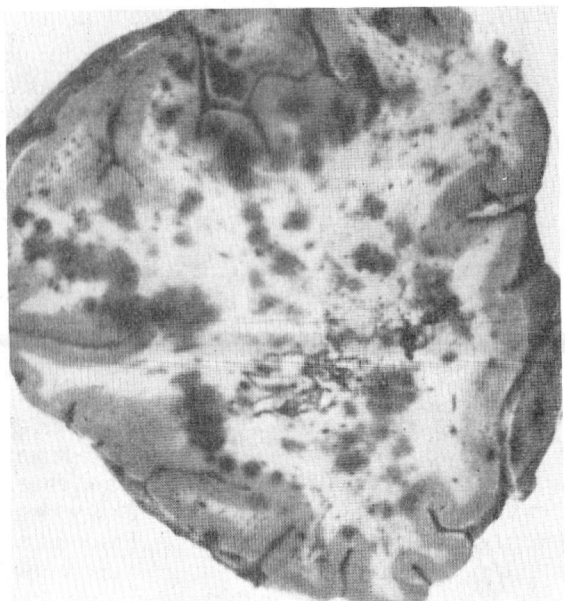

**FIGURE 1.** *Cerebral aspergillosis. Section of right frontal lobe showing the central white matter studded with hemorrhagic and necrotic lesions. Fungal hyphae with the branched septate forms typical of the Aspergillus group are plentiful throughout most of the cortical lesions. (From Burston, J., and Blackwood, W.: J Pathol Bacteriol 86:225, 1963.)*

lesions, vessel invasion is less common, and hyphae may be seen within giant cells. On hematoxylin and eosin stains, spaces where the hyphae were invading tissue may be the only evidence of their presence. Gomori methenamine silver stain distinctly identifies the septate hyphae, and periodic acid-Schiff stain is also effective.

## CLINICAL MANIFESTATIONS

The clinical manifestations vary with the type of syndrome and the area of the brain involved. With orbital invasion blurred vision can progress to blindness along with proptosis, all of which are usually slow in development. Invasion of the brain, when the disease progresses to that, proceeds along the optic nerve or its vessels, the optic chiasm, or through the orbit to the base of the frontal lobes. When the sinuses are involved, persistent sinusitis of gradually increasing severity precedes frontal lobe signs and symptoms that result from direct extension. Likewise, a history of chronic otitis media accompanies invasive spread from the mastoids to the brain. An acute rhinocerebral syndrome simulating cerebral mucormycosis occurs on rare occasions in immunosuppressed patients. Orbital infiltration with proptosis in a patient living in the Sudan or another region with a warm, moist climate should

suggest *A. flavus* as a possible etiology (Hedges and Leung, 1976).

Aspergillus granulomas of the brain may develop in a single focus or multiple foci, and signs and symptoms result from the position of the focus. They are those of a slowly growing lesion such as a tuberculoma or a neoplasm.

Abscesses and vessel invasion also cause signs and symptoms depending on the area or areas of the brain or the artery involved. The patients, who are usually immunosuppressed, have often survived one or more severe bacterial infections and are still receiving antibiotics. Leukopenia is commonly present. Fever may recur or persistent fever may become even higher. Pulmonary lesions may appear on radiographs along with neurologic symptoms and signs, or these may appear without evident disease elsewhere. Both posterior and anterior circulations may be invaded, and hemiplegia may occur if large arteries are thrombosed. Progression of signs and symptoms is acute or subacute. Prompt diagnosis is impera-

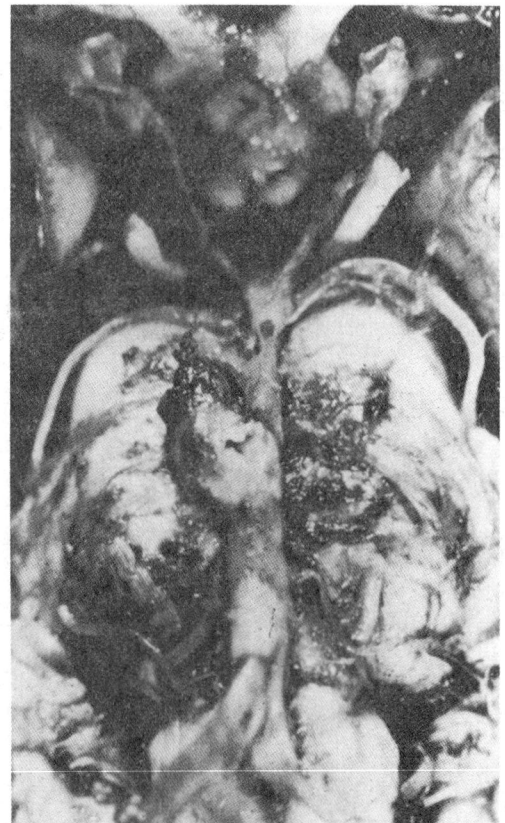

**FIGURE 2.** *Mycotic Aspergillus aneurysm originating near the basilar artery. The aneurysm caused fatal massive subarachnoid hemorrhage in a 75-year-old man. The aneurysm and adjacent basilar artery had necrotic foci with heavy infiltrations of neutrophils (suppurative arteritis) and many Aspergillus hyphae. The probable source of the fungus was the frontal sinus. (From Davidson, P., and Robertson, D.: J Neurosurg 35:71, 1971.)*

tive, and brain biopsy should be considered early. Rarely, the meninges are infected, signs of meningitis appear, and the organisms may be isolated from the cerebrospinal fluid (CSF). Examination of the CSF is usually not helpful, however. From none to a few thousand cells may be found, including erythrocytes, and either mononuclear or polymorphonuclear leukocytes may be predominant. The protein concentration is usually elevated, and the glucose level is normal. Definitive diagnosis usually depends on brain biopsy.

Infections secondary to direct inoculation of aspergilli result in clinical manifestations that depend on the site of inoculation (Visudhiphan et al., 1973; Feely and Steinberg, 1977). Wound abscesses following neurosurgery have been due to aspergillosis. *Aspergillus* meningitis has occurred after lumbar punctures, and the organisms have been isolated on repeat lumbar puncture (Rippon, 1974). *Aspergillus* peritonitis with dissemination to the brain and elsewhere has resulted from contamination of peritoneal dialysis fluid or equipment (Ross et al., 1968).

Metastatic cerebral aspergillosis from endocarditis has been reported following heart surgery, with and without artificial valve implacement (Rippon, 1974; Horten et al., 1976). Blood cultures are most often negative, so this fungus should be considered in patients with blood culture-negative clinical endocarditis. Early surgery for both diagnosis and treatment appears to be the only reasonable approach.

Mycotic aneurysms of intracranial vessels occur rarely without specific signs or symptoms of aspergillosis (Horten et al., 1976). The diagnosis is made at surgery (Fig. 2).

## COMPLICATIONS AND SEQUELAE

Complications and sequelae are the result of destroyed nerve tissue. Blindness, permanent hemiplegia, facial paralysis, and other neurologic deficits have persisted in the few patients who have survived. This further underscores the need for early diagnosis and therapy.

## GEOGRAPHIC VARIATIONS

Cerebral aspergillosis secondary to infection of a paranasal sinus has been reported, especially from the Sudan, but also from other warm, moist climates such as Africa and the southern United States (Hedges and Leung, 1976). Granulomas of the brain have been reported from all over the world, and brain abscesses appear wherever patients are immunosuppressed and autopsies are

done (Linares et al., 1971; Correa et al., 1975; Deshpande et al., 1975).

## DIAGNOSIS

The diagnosis, as outlined above, almost always depends on tissue biopsy or aspiration. Rarely, the CSF is positive on smear and culture; when the culture alone is positive, there is always a question of laboratory contamination. When a biopsy is done, a small portion of the tissue should be used for a wet mount. The tissue can be dissected under a dissecting microscope or it can be macerated in a mortar and pestle, treated with 10 per cent potassium hydroxide, and examined microscopically. If enough tissue is available both procedures can be done along with a Gram stain, which sometimes outlines the hyphae (see Chapter 74, Fig. 4B, C) and can help in detecting bacterial, cryptococcal, or candida infections. There is a modified serum immunodiffusion test that has been helpful in detecting disseminated disease if baseline-negative sera have been available (see Chapter 74, Fig. 5) (Schaefer et al., 1976). False-negative tests have occurred, but when a conversion from a negative to a positive reaction was seen, it was associated with invasive disease (Fisher et al., in press; Schaefer et al., 1976). This test has not, however, been specifically correlated with cerebral aspergillosis.

The differential diagnosis in the immunosuppressed patient includes brain abscess or infection due to various organisms including *Mycobacterium* species, *Nocardia asteroides, Candida* species, *Mucoraceae, Cryptococcus neoformans, Toxoplasma gondii,* and *Herpes simplex.* Mixed anaerobic and aerobic bacterial brain abscesses are also possible. In a recent series from a cancer center, *Aspergillus* species were the most common cause of brain abscess (Chernik et al., 1977). Because of the large number of organisms possibly responsible, requiring many different potentially toxic therapeutic agents, empirical trials should be avoided and a definitive diagnosis sought by brain biopsy.

## TREATMENT

Treatment consists of surgical drainage and, if necessary, extirpation of necrotic, imperfused tissue. Amphotericin B is the treatment of choice and has been curative when associated with surgery. Even the immunosuppressed patient may respond, but attempts to decrease immunosuppressive therapy are probably important (Gurwith et al., 1971). A rapid schedule for amphotericin B therapy is given in Chapter 158 on cerebral mucormycosis. An infected artificial heart valve must be removed. Emetine, 5-fluorocytosine, and estrogens have been advocated, but their efficacy is unproved (Burton et al., 1972). Leukocyte transfusions have been used in patients with chronic granulomatous disease with reports of a dramatic response, but amphotericin B was administered at the same time (Greenberg et al., 1977).

## PROPHYLAXIS

Prevention may be possible in hospitals that care for large numbers of immunosuppressed patients. In such settings there have been reports of multiple cases of aspergillosis in which common sources such as air conditioners and insulation material were implicated (Rose, 1972; Aisner et al., 1976). Precautions should be taken by properly cleaning and monitoring air conditioners and air distribution equipment. Building materials that might harbor *Aspergillus* species should be avoided. Since a few cases have been described following occupational exposure, masks with filters should be used for work in high-risk areas.

### References

Aisner, J., Schimpff, S. C., Bennett, J E., Young, V. M., and Wiernick, P. H.: Aspergillus infections in cancer patients. Association with fireproofing materials in a new hospital. JAMA 235:411, 1976.

Burton, J. R., Zachery, J. B., Bessiu, R., Rathbon, H. K., Greenough, W. B., Sterioff, S., Wright, J. R., Slavin, R. E., and Williams, G. M.: Aspergillosis in four renal transplant recipients. Diagnosis and effective treatment with amphotericin B. Ann Intern Med 77:383, 1972.

Chernik, N., Armstrong, D., and Posner, J. B.: Central nervous system infections in patients with cancer. Changing patterns. Cancer 40:268, 1977.

Chick, E. W., and Durham, N. C.: Enhancement of aspergillosis in leukemic chickens. Arch Pathol 75:81, 1963.

Correa, A. J. E., Brinckhaus, R., Kesler, S., and Martinez, E.: Aspergillosis of the fourth ventricle. Case report. J Neurosurg 43:236, 1975.

Deshpande, D. H., Desai, A. P., and Dastur, H. M.: Aspergillosis of the central nervous system. A clinical and mycopathological study of 9 cases. Neurology India 23:167, 1975.

Feely, M., and Steinberg, M.: Aspergillus infection complicating transsphenoidal yttrium-90 pituitary implant. Report of two cases. J Neurosurg 46:530, 1977.

Fisher, B., Yu, B., and Armstrong, D.: The early diagnosis and treatment of aspergillosis complicating neoplastic disease. In press, 1980.

Greenberg, D., Ammann, A. J., Wara, D. W., and Kaltreider, H. B.: Immunity to aspergillus in patients with chronic granulomatous disease. J Pediatr 90:601, 1977.

Gurwith, M. J., Stinson, E. B., and Remington, J. S.: Aspergillus infection complicating cardiac transplantation. Report of 5 cases. Arch Intern Med 128:541, 1971.

Hedges, T. R., and Leung, L-S. E.: Parasellar and orbital apex syndrome caused by aspergillosis. Neurology 26:117, 1976.

Horten, B. C., Abbott, G. F., and Porro, R. S.: Fungal aneurysms of intracranial vessels. Arch Neurol 33:577, 1976.

Kaufman, D. M., Thal, L. J., and Farmer, P. M.: Central nervous system aspergillosis in two young adults. Neurology 26:484, 1976.

Khoo, T. K., Sugai, K., and Leong, T. K.: Disseminated aspergillosis. Case report and review of the world literature. Am J Clin Pathol 45:697, 1966.

Linares, G., McGarry, P. A., and Baker, R. D.: Solid solitary aspergillotic granuloma of the brain. Report of a case due to *Aspergillus candidus* and review of the literature. Neurology 21:177, 1971.

Meyer, R. D., Young, L. S., Armstrong, D., and Yu, B.: Aspergillosis complicating neoplastic disease. Am J Med 54:6, 1973.

Mukoyama, M., Gimple, K., and Poser, C. M.: Aspergillosis of the central nervous system. Report of a brain abscess due to A. *fumigatus* and review of the literature. Neurology 19:967, 1969.

Raper, K. B., and Fennel, D. I.: The Genus Aspergillus. Baltimore, The Williams & Wilkins Company, 1965.

Rippon, J. W.: Aspergillosis. In Medical Mycology: The Pathogenic Fungi and the Pathogenic Actinomycetes. Philadelphia, W. B. Saunders Company, 1974, p. 406.

Rose, H. D.: Mechanical control of hospital ventilation and aspergillus infections. Am Rev Resp Dis 105:306, 1972.

Ross, D. A., Anderson, D. C., MacNaughton, M. C., and Steward, W. K.: Fulminating disseminated aspergillosis complicating peritoneal dialysis in eclampsia. Arch Intern Med 121:183, 1968.

Schaefer, J. C., Yu, B., and Armstrong, D.: An aspergillus immunodiffusion test in the early diagnosis of aspergillosis in adult leukemia patients. Am Rev Resp Dis 113:325, 1976.

Sidransky, H., and Friedman, L.: The effect of cortisone and antibiotic agents on experimental pulmonary aspergillosis. Am J Pathol 35:169, 1959.

Visudhiphan, P., Bunyaratavej, S., and Khantanaphar, S.: Cerebral aspergillosis. Report of three cases. J Neurosurg 38:472, 1973.

Young, R. C., Jennings, A., and Bennett, J. E.: Species identification of invasive aspergillosis in man. Am J Clin Pathol 58:554, 1972.

Young, R. C., Bennett, J. E., Vogel, C. L., Carbone, P. P., and DeVita, V. T.: Aspergillosis, the spectrum of the disease in 98 patients. Medicine 49:147, 1970.

# 161 *NEUROSYPHILIS*

*Hooshang Hooshmand, M.D.*

The great pandemic of syphilis in Europe and Asia occurred soon after the discovery of the New World by Columbus, but the clinical manifestations of the disease were not distinguished from other venereal diseases until the late 19th century. In 1905, Schaudinn and Hoffmann discovered *Treponema pallidum*; in 1906, Wassermann developed the complement fixation test for the diagnosis of the disease; and in 1913, Naguchi and

Moore identified *Treponema* in the brains of patients with neurosyphilis. Ehrlich discovered the effectiveness of arsenicals for the treatment of syphilis in 1910.

The universal use of penicillin since the Second World War significantly decreased the number of syphilitics. The disease has not disappeared, however. In the past 15 years, the number of syphilitics — and partially treated syphilitics — with late and atypical manifestations of neurosyphilis has increased (Cattrell, 1977; Hooshmand, 1972). This increase has been especially prominent in the young and among homosexual men (Cattrell, 1977; DHSS Report, 1974).

## DEFINITION AND ETIOLOGY

The major forms of symptomatic syphilis of the central nervous system (CNS) are meningovascular neurosyphilis, general paresis of the insane (GPI), and tabes dorsalis. Mixtures of these manifestations of neurosyphilis are common, and atypical presentations are increasing. The frequency of CNS invasion by *T. pallidum* during primary and secondary syphilis is unknown, but 7 to 8 per cent of patients with primary syphilis develop some form of neurosyphilis. Patients are said to have asymptomatic neurosyphilis when an abnormality of the cerebrospinal fluid is the only manifestation of CNS involvement.

*T. pallidum*, a member of the order Spirochetales, is a highly motile, spiral organism that is discussed in Chapter 49.

## PATHOGENESIS AND PATHOLOGY

Spirochetes may invade the CNS during the spirochetemia that accompanies either primary or secondary syphilis. *T. pallidum* has been demonstrated in many tissues, including the CNS and aqueous humor, during the secondary stage.

The basic lesion of meningovascular syphilis is an obliterative endarteritis. *T. pallidum* and the inflammatory infiltrate of monocytes, lymphocytes, and plasma cells invade the intima of arteries of all sizes and cause fibrosis, narrowing of the lumen, inflammation of the adventitia, and perivascular infiltration of the vasa vasorum. In severe infections, the muscle fibers of the intima are separated, and the internal elastic lamina is split by the infiltrate (Heubner's arteritis, Fig. 1). These changes cause reactive intimal hyperplasia and hypertrophy of the endothelium. Obliteration of the blood supply may cause multiple small infarcts. Intermittent healing causes fibroblastic proliferation and fibrosis. A cloudy, gray leptomeningeal exudate accompanies the vascular changes and is most prominent at the base of the brain and along the blood vessels of the cerebral convexities.

GPI is a progressive, chronic cerebral degeneration that is probably caused by the same kinds of vascular changes that occur in meningovascular neurosyphilis, but the inflammatory reaction is not prominent and consists primarily of perivascular cuffing of the smaller vessels. It is especially

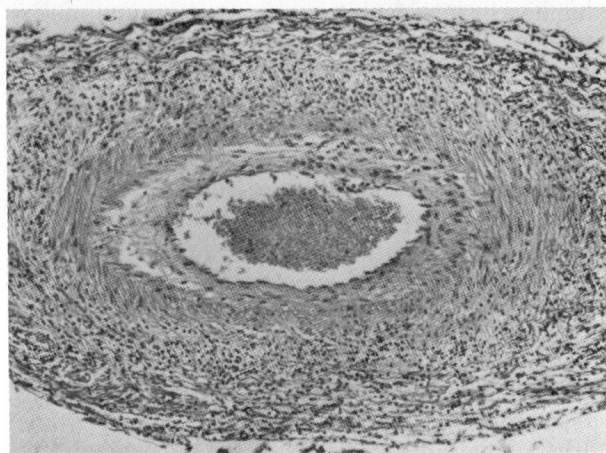

**FIGURE 1.** *Heubner's arteritis of basilar artery. (From Chason, J. L.: In Anderson, W.A.D. (ed): Pathology. Vol. 2. St. Louis, The C. V. Mosby Co., 1971.)*

characterized by widespread atrophy of the ganglion cells, microglial proliferation and elongation, marked astrocytosis, and the presence of iron-laden macrophages in the walls of cortical blood vessels. Leptomeningitis is also prominent in GPI. Its intensity parallels the severity of the vascular changes.

Tabes dorsalis is a degeneration of the dorsal columns of the spinal cord (Fig. 2) probably caused by the effect of the inflammatory response on the dorsal roots. Demyelinization is prominent. The location of the lesion that produces the Argyll-Robertson pupil is unknown.

The gumma is a typical granuloma with a necrotic, coagulated center and obliterative endarteritis of small vessels. Spirochetes are present but scarce. The development of granulomas and polyarteritis suggests that much of the tissue

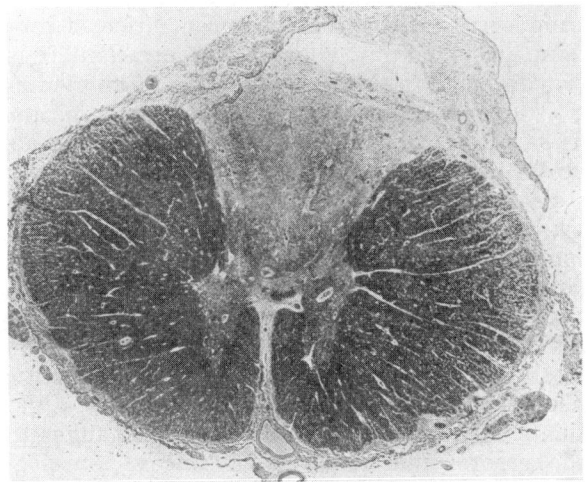

**FIGURE 2.** *Tabes dorsalis with extreme sclerosis of the posterior columns. (From MacCallum, W. G.: A Textbook of Pathology. 6th ed. Philadelphia, W. B. Saunders Co., 1938.)*

damage in late syphilis is due to immune mechanisms. The endarteritis and immune-complex glomerulonephritis (O'Regan et al., 1976) suggest that antigen-antibody complexes contribute to the pathogenesis of typical syphilitic lesions. The tuberculoid nature of the gumma indicates that delayed hypersensitivity and cellular immunity also cause tissue destruction in late syphilis.

## CLINICAL MANIFESTATIONS

Invasion of the CNS by *T. pallidum* during the primary or secondary stage of syphilis results in asymptomatic neurosyphilis in as many as one third of patients (Cattrell, 1977; Hooshmand et al., 1972). Some of these infections probably regress spontaneously because only 7 to 8 per cent of untreated patients with primary syphilis develop signs of neurosyphilis. The classic manifestations of meningovascular syphilis, general paresis, and tabes dorsalis are seen in less than one third of patients with neurosyphilis (Hooshmand et al., 1972); atypical mixed presentations are much more common. The clinical presentations of neurosyphilis can be conveniently divided into early (6 weeks to 6 months) and late (5 to 35 years) manifestations.

### Early Manifestations

Aseptic meningitis is said to occur in 2 per cent of syphilitics, but in my experience and that of others (Cattrell, 1977), it is seen more frequently now than before. It may occur during the secondary stage of infection or be delayed for as long as several months. The manifestations are headache, vomiting, and irritability. Symptoms of encephalitis, seizures, and acute hydrocephalus occur but are unusual. The cerebrospinal fluid contains an average of 500 cells that are mostly lymphocytes, an increased concentration of protein, and a normal glucose concentration. It is easy to make the clinical diagnosis when meningitis accompanies the rash of secondary syphilis. The CSF VDRL (Venereal Disease Research Laboratories) test is positive.

Patients respond promptly to adequate therapy, but partial treatment aimed at treating concomitant diseases such as gonorrhea may cause only partial regression of the treponemal infection of the brain and permit progression to the late manifestations of neurosyphilis several years later (Hooshmand et al., 1972). Asymptomatic neurosyphilis, which occurs in one third of patients with primary syphilis, causes changes in the cerebrospinal fluid in the absence of neurologic symptoms and signs.

### Late Manifestations

When the initial infection goes unnoticed or is lost in secondary amnesia, the disease manifests itself years later in atypical forms with partial pictures of meningovascular syphilis, general paresis, or tabes dorsalis (Cattrell, 1977; Hooshmand et al., 1972). These manifestations include a partial stroke, adult onset seizure, brain tumor secondary to gumma, partial tabetic changes such as abdominal or joint pain, isolated syphilitic optic atrophy, partial or progressive dementia, severe incapacitating facial pain, and a spectrum of almost unlimited manifestations of this great imitator of neurologic diseases.

General paresis occurs most commonly between the ages of 30 and 60 and in men more frequently than in women. Many more patients present with simple dementia than with megalomania, paranoia, and manic behavior. Fine tremors, convulsions, strokes, localizing signs, and symptoms of tabes dorsalis (taboparesis) may accompany the typical presentation of dementia. In some patients, the only symptoms may be poor memory, poor judgment, or a sudden change in personality. Examination of the spinal fluid and electroencephalogram (EEG) is very important because these manifestations of GPI may be very mild and subtle at onset. Only an astute physician with neurosyphilis in mind and the proper laboratory tests can diagnose early general paresis. The patient is usually unaware of his deterioration.

The cerebrospinal fluid is almost always abnormal with 5 to 100 mononuclear cells, an elevated protein concentration, and a positive VDRL test (see Diagnosis). The EEG is usually abnormal.

Isolated meningovascular syphilis usually occurs five to ten years after the primary infection and usually presents as meningitis with meningovascular occlusion, infarction, and encephalomalacia. Patients may be seen first with seizures or the typical manifestations of a cerebrovascular accident. The CSF is abnormal, as discussed above in meningitis, and serum and serologic tests are usually positive.

Overt tabes dorsalis is seen less frequently than GPI. Tabes occurs somewhat earlier in the course (often within the first 10 years) than general paresis, which usually appears after 10 to 20 years or longer. Patients with tabes may complain only of abdominal or joint pain, which may be mistaken for aseptic necrosis of the joint. Careful neurologic examination, however, is likely to show a significant decrease of position and vibration sense and a marked delay in response to pain stimulation in the affected extremity. Deep pain sensation elicited by squeezing the Achilles tendon may be totally absent (Abadie's sign). Areas of hypalgesia, paresthesia, hypesthesia (Hitzig zones), and marked delay of response to deep pain in the involved extremity are common.

Dysfunction of the dorsal roots occurs slowly, and stumbling and difficulty in walking due to impaired joint position sense may be the first symptom of tabes. Patients assume the typical broad-based gait to compensate for this impairment. Paresthesias are often ignored by the patient until they are accompanied by "lightning pains," which occur in at least 75 per cent of patients with typical tabes. Lightning pains are most common in the lower extremities but may occur anywhere in the body. Abdominal or visceral crises from involvement of the thoracoabdominal roots may simulate intra-abdominal disease and provoke unnecessary abdominal surgery.

Overflow urinary incontinence, constipation, and impotence may develop secondary to involvement of the sacral roots. Hydronephrosis and pyelonephritis are common complications of the hypotonic bladder.

Patients with the fully developed picture of tabes have such impairment of position sense that they have marked swaying when they stand with their feet together and their eyes closed (Romberg's sign). Vibratory sensation may be lost, and stretch reflexes, especially of the Achilles tendons, are diminished or absent when the sensory arch is involved. Pain sensation may be so impaired that the patient is unaware of repeated trauma to the feet and weight-bearing joints. Destruction by repeated trauma causes Charcot's joints.

The CSF contains mononuclear cells, an increased protein concentration, and reaginic antibody early in the course of tabes. Later, especially after incomplete treatment, the cerebrospinal fluid may be normal and the VDRL test negative (10 to 20 per cent of patients).

A wide spectrum of neuro-ophthalmologic disease may accompany tabes or occur without any other manifestation of neurosyphilis. These consist of the Argyll-Robertson pupil (poor pupillary responsiveness to light but retained accommodation), progressive unilateral or bilateral optic atrophy, and partial ptosis or external ophthalmoplegia, which may be misdiagnosed as myasthenia. Progressive loss of vision of unknown etiology should raise the suspicion of neurosyphilis. The myotonic pupil of Adie, which also responds very sluggishly to light but normally to accommodation, must be differentiated from the Argyll-Robertson pupil. It is usually found in young women and is almost always unilateral. The pupil is usually larger than the one on the normal side and has a smooth oval outline. The typical Argyll-Robertson pupil has a ragged outline and an irregular shape.

Approximately 5 per cent of the patients thought to have the incurable and fatal disease amyotrophic lateral sclerosis (ALS) actually suffer from curable neurosyphilis. Neurosyphilis can mimic the manifestations of ALS in every respect. It is imperative to examine the CSF (cells, protein, serology, and immunoglobulin) of all patients who are suspected of having ALS.

Gummas of the brain or spinal cord are very rare. The clinical manifestations are indistinguishable from a slowly growing neoplasm. A positive serologic test for syphilis or cerebrospinal fluid abnormalities in a patient with clinical or radiologic evidence of intracranial or spinal cord mass should suggest the correct diagnosis.

Pachymeningitis hypertrophica, which mimics cervical spondylosis, is a rare manifestation of neurosyphilis. A diffusely hypertrophic and ragged meningeal involvement on myelography of the cervical spine, accompanied by a mononuclear pleocytosis and an elevated CSF protein level should raise the possibility of neurosyphilis. If syphilis is not considered and if CSF or serum serology is not tested, the patient may be subjected to unnecessary surgery.

Progressive deafness of unknown etiology should also suggest the possibility of neurosyphilis. Perceptive deafness is one of the most common manifestations of congenital syphilis. The cochlear portion of the eighth nerve is typically involved. These patients usually have seronegative syphilis, and the CSF serology may even be nonreactive.

CNS involvement occurs in approximately 10 per cent of congenitally syphilitic children. The most common manifestations are convulsions, minimal brain damage, mental retardation, communicating hydrocephalus, and a combination of communicating hydrocephalus and microcephaly. Optic atrophy, chorioretinitis, basilar meningitis with multiple involvement of the cranial nerves, acute syphilitic meningitis, and increased intracranial pressure culminating in coma can also occur. After the child reaches the teenage years, the manifestations of general paresis or tabes dorsalis may become prominent and coexist with frequent seizures, progressive dementia, and progressive deafness and optic atrophy. Clinical awareness of the typical manifestations of interstitial keratitis, Hutchinson's teeth, and progressive dementia, deafness, and optic atrophy in the absence of a reactive serology is important. The patient's condition can be improved significantly by treatment with a combination of large doses of penicillin and steroids.

## COMPLICATIONS AND SEQUELAE

Syphilis involves arteries of all sizes, and meningovascular syphilis may cause massive strokes from vascular occlusion. Infarction of the spinal cord may also occur. If this is asymmetric, weakness and diminished touch and position sense on the involved side may be accompanied by diminished pain and temperature sense on the opposite side below the infarction (Brown-Sequard syndrome). Although the onset of symptoms of general paresis is often mild and subtle, the condition progresses rapidly, and untreated patients usually become helpless invalids within three years. Uropathy, impotence, addiction to narcotics because of persistent pain, joint destruction due to trauma (Charcot's joints), and blindness are among the major complications of tabes dorsalis.

## GEOGRAPHIC VARIATIONS

There are no known geographic variations in neurosyphilis, but Caucasians are more prone to the development of neurosyphilis than blacks following untreated primary syphilis.

## DIAGNOSIS

It can be difficult to make the diagnosis of neurosyphilis because of the obscurity of the clinical symptoms, the rising incidence of atypical presentations, and the well-known absence in many cases of antibody in the nontreponemal serologic tests (Smith, 1969). Penicillin therapy in the first and second stages (infectious stages) of syphilis has altered the clinical picture of neurosyphilis (Koffman, 1956); consequently the classic textbook pictures of tabes dorsalis, general paresis of the insane, and meningovascular syphilis are becoming rare and are often replaced by atypical and mixed forms (Hooshmand et al., 1972; Koffman, 1956).

The diagnosis must be suspected on clinical grounds. Strong support can be added by cellular and chemical abnormalities of the CSF. Approximately 70 per cent of all neurosyphilitics may have only 5 to 10 mononuclear leukocytes per $mm^3$ in the CSF, but fewer than 20 per cent have less than 5 leukocytes per $mm^3$. The number of cells in the CSF often increases during therapy. The CSF protein level is elevated to 50 to 100 mg per 100 ml in almost half the patients (Hooshmand et al., 1972). The spinal fluid gamma globulin and serum immunoglobulin levels are elevated in more than two thirds of neurosyphilitics (Hooshmand et al., 1972).

The EEG is abnormal in 60 per cent of all neurosyphilitics and in more than 80 per cent with general paresis (Cattrell, 1977; Hooshmand, 1976). The EEG changes may consist only of generalized slowing of the background or may take the form of PLED (periodic lateralized epileptiform discharges). Angiography of patients with meningovascular syphilis may show irregular disease of the small arteries and angiopathy (Vatz et al., 1974). Computerized tomography may show atrophy of the brain of patients with GPI.

Although the serologic tests for syphilis are of critical importance for confirming the diagnosis, their pitfalls must be recognized. The nontreponemal serum serologic tests (reaginic tests such as the VDRL, abbreviated as STS in this chapter) for syphilis are not sensitive enough and can be nonreactive in the late stages of syphilis (Smith, 1969). In as high as 39 per cent of cases of neurosyphilis, these tests may be nonreactive (Harner et al., 1968). Of the specific treponemal tests, the fluorescent antibody-absorptive (FTA-ABS) test seems to be the most sensitive (Deacon et al., 1966). The serum FTA-ABS test is specific in over 95 per cent of the cases (Deacon et al., 1966; Hooshmand et al., 1972).

The serologic tests of the spinal fluid do not parallel the serologic tests of serum. The STS is more sensitive than the FTA-ABS test in the spinal fluid (Wilner et al., 1968). The FTA-ABS seems to be reactive in the spinal fluid only when the spinal tap has been traumatic and the CSF has been contaminated with peripheral blood (Escobar et al., 1970; Rudolph, 1976; and Wilner et al., 1968).

Falsely reactive serologic tests in collagen diseases such as lupus erythematosus occur in the FTA-ABS test as well as the STS. If lupus erythematosus is suspected, the *Treponema pallidum* immobilization test (TPI), which is not falsely positive (Shore, 1976), should be performed.

In general, the serum FTA-ABS test and the cerebrospinal fluid STS are the most sensitive tests for the diagnosis of neurosyphilis (Hooshmand et al., 1972; Rudolph, 1976). However, a nonreactive serology in either the blood or spinal fluid does not rule out neurosyphilis (Hooshmand et al., 1972). The clinical syndrome, cellular and chemical changes in the CSF, and the serologic tests must all be considered in order to diagnose neurosyphilis accurately. None of these factors alone can prove or disprove neurosyphilis. The serum STS can be reactive in as low as 48.5 per cent of patients diagnosed as having neurosyphilis (Hooshmand et al., 1972). On the other hand, the serum FTA-ABS test seems to be reactive in almost 100 per cent of these patients (Hooshmand et al., 1972). Less than 1 per cent of neurosyphilitics are seronegative for the FTA-ABS test.

## *TREATMENT*

Treatment with penicillin has reduced the total number of syphilitic and neurosyphilitic patients but at the same time has complicated the clinical picture because inadequate therapy has produced partial and atypical syndromes of neurosyphilis. Depending on the dosage and route of administration, the failure rate has been reported to be as high as 30 per cent (Wilner et al., 1968). The high failure rate of some series, which may be even higher than treatment with arsenic or bismuth or fever therapy with malaria, is probably due to two major factors:

1. Late diagnosis of neurosyphilis. This is especially true of general paresis when the disease has advanced to a point of ireversible brain damage. These patients can be identified by CT scan, which shows severe atrophy of the entire brain.

2. Treatment with improper types of penicillin. In this regard, the recommendations of the U.S. Public Health Service and the World Health Organization for treatment of neurosyphilis seem to be inadequate for effective treatment of this disease (Hooshmand et al., 1972; Mohr et al., 1976; Yoder, 1975).

The recommendations of these organizations are treatment with procaine penicillin G or procaine penicillin G in oil with 2 per cent aluminum stearate in 1.2 million-unit doses given intramuscularly at three day intervals for a total of 9 million units, or penicillin G benzathine, 2.4 million units intramuscularly at weekly intervals for three weeks.

However, recent studies (Cattrell, 1977; Hooshmand et al., 1972; Mohr et al., 1976; Tramont, 1976; Yoder, 1975) demonstrate that these forms of treatment are ineffective and are apt to fail. The main reason for failure of treatment with benzathine penicillin is that this form of long-acting penicillin has such a large molecule that it cannot pass through the blood-brain barrier (Hooshmand et al., 1972). As a result, this treatment does not provide a high enough CSF level to destroy all the spirochetes in the CNS. A total of 9 million units of procaine penicillin in doses of 1.2 million units every three days may also provide too low a level of penicillin to eradicate reliably all *T. pallidum* organisms. The doses of penicillin used for the treatment of neurosyphilis have been increasing since 1943 with a corresponding increase in the cure rate. Schirren (1965) and Durel

(1959) demonstrated that treatment with 15 to 20 million units of penicillin killed all the spirochetes. The success of treatment can be increased from the previously reported 30 per cent (Wilner et al., 1968) to as high as 90 per cent (Hooshmand et al., 1972) with adequate doses of penicillin.

Treatment of neurosyphilis with procaine penicillin G intramuscularly in doses of 1 to 2 million units every other day for a total of 20 million units seems to be adequate therapy. The patient must be treated for at least three weeks (Cattrell, 1977; Durel, 1959; Hooshmand et al., 1972; Schirren, 1965) in order to eradicate all of the spirochetes.

Patients with meningovascular syphilis with or without seizure disorders respond best to therapy. They often become practically asymptomatic after treatment. All patients with an incomplete clinical picture of tabes dorsalis have also experienced some degree of recovery.

Even partially treated neurosyphilitics who had continued to deteriorate after the standard recommended treatment improved significantly and cleared the leukocytes from their spinal fluid when re-treated with 20 million units of penicillin over a three-week interval. The prognosis for control of seizure disorders (Hooshmand, 1976) in neurosyphilis is related not only to the administration of adequate penicillin therapy but also depends on the accompanying clinical picture and duration of neurosyphilis. The prognosis is poorest among the cases with a partial picture of GPI and best among patients with cerebrovascular disease. Of 24 patients with adult onset seizure secondary to neurosyphilis, 14 did not need further anticonvulsant therapy after treatment with penicillin. Of the 12 who had partial evidence of tabes dorsalis along with seizure disorder, 4 had experienced only one or two adult onset seizures before therapy and did not need any further anticonvulsants after proper penicillin therapy (Hooshmand, 1976).

The reversal of the abnormal CSF cell count has been used as the main criterion for success in the treatment of neurosyphilis. However, in tabes dorsalis or GPI, a normal CSF can become abnormal after penicillin therapy (Lopez et al., 1953). A normal CSF may change temporarily and develop a pleocytosis of 6 to 19 cells per $mm^3$ one to three weeks after the initiation of penicillin therapy. Active progression of disease may also occur without cells in the spinal fluid either before or after treatment. The deterioration of GPI may continue despite adequate doses of penicillin (Wilner et al., 1968).

Even if the CSF is normal at the beginning of treatment, lumbar puncture should be performed six weeks after treatment is completed and again three months later. The cell count usually returns to normal in one to three months. If abnormalities persist, the CSF should be retested at six-month intervals. If the CSF becomes normal after treatment, there is no need for retreatment. Repetition of treatment is indicated if the CSF fails to become normal within three months or if the cell count increases again after a period of normalcy (Dattner-Thomas concept).

Once the CSF has returned to normal, annual lumbar punctures should be done for at least five years.

### Herxheimer Reaction

This is a systemic and focal reaction that may occur within one to eight hours of antibiotic treatment of syphilis. It occurs more frequently in secondary syphilis than in patients with late neurosyphilis and has been correlated with the release of an endotoxin-like substance from the spirochetes (Gelfand et al., 1976). Only 20 to 30 per cent of the patients with neurosyphilis experience the Herxheimer reaction. The manifestations include temporary fever, headache, meningeal irritation, and, in occasional grave cases, seizures, high fever, and death. Hallucinations, temporary hemiparesis, blindness, and lightning pains can occur.

Large doses of steroids, such as dexamethasone or hydrocortisone, are recommended, but they are of unproven value.

In case of allergy to penicillin, the treatment of choice is erythromycin in doses of 500 mg four times a day for at least 15 days. Tetracyclines in the same dose are also beneficial but are associated with a higher incidence of recurrence.

### *PROPHYLAXIS*

The only prophylaxis for neurosyphilis is the prevention and adequate treatment of primary and secondary syphilis. Condom prophylaxis can be effective if properly utilized, but education, case finding, and treatment is much more effective. Serologic screening in venereal disease clinics, family planning clinics, and hospitals (especially obstetric units) are vital adjuncts to treatment of symptomatic cases. Furthermore, physicians must be educated to report all cases of syphilis to the Public Health Department. Every contact of a patient with infectious syphilis should be treated regardless of serologic results. Finally, physicians must be educated to recognize even the atypical manifestations of neurosyphilis so that the disastrous effects of late untreated general paresis and tabes dorsalis can be prevented by adequate penicillin therapy.

### References

Cattrell, R. D.: Neurosyphilis. Br J Hosp Med 17:585, 1977.
Chason, J. L.: Nervous system and skeletal muscle. In Anderson, W. A. D. (ed.): Pathology. Vol. 2. St. Louis, The C. V. Mosby Co., 1971, p. 1821.
Deacon, W. E., Lucas, J. B., and Price, E. V.: Fluorescent treponemal antibody-absorption (FTA-ABS) test for syphilis. JAMA 198:624, 1966.
DHSS (1974) on the State of Public Health: Annual Report of the Chief Medical Officer. 1974, London, Her Majesty's Stationery Office, 1974.
Durel, P.: La Maladie syphilitique et ses deux phases therapeutiques. Presse Med 67:1575, 1959.
Escobar, M. R., Dalton, H. P., and Allison, M. J.: Fluorescent antibody tests for syphilis using cerebrospinal fluid: Clinical correlation in 150 cases. Am J Clin Pathol 53:886, 1970.
Gelfand, J. A., Elin, R. J., and Berry, F. W.: Endotoxemia associated with the Jarisch-Herxheimer reaction. N Engl J Med 295:211, 1976.
Harner, R. E., Smith, J. L., and Israel, C. W.: The FTA-ABS test in late syphilis: A serological study in 1,985 cases. JAMA 203:545, 1968.
Hooshmand, H., Escobar, M. R., and Kopf, S. W.: Neurosyphilis, a study of 241 patients. JAMA 219:726, 1972.
Hooshmand, H.: Seizure disorders associated with neurosyphilis. Dis Nerv Syst 37:133, 1976.
Koffman, O.: The changing pattern of neurosyphilis. Can Med Assoc J 74:807, 1956.
Lopez, I. J., and Olivares, E.: Methods for the reactivation of negative fluids in neurosyphilis. J Nerv Ment Dis 117:329, 1953.
MacCallum, W. G.: A Textbook of Pathology. 6th ed. Philadelphia, W. B. Saunders Co., 1938, p. 727.
Mohr, J. A., Griffiths, W., Jackson, R., Saadah, H., Bird, P., and Riddle, J.: Neurosyphilis and penicillin levels in cerebrospinal fluid. JAMA 236:2208, 1976.
O'Regan, S., Fong, J. S. C., de Chadarevian, J. P., Rishikof, J. R., and Drummond, K. R.: Treponemal antigens in congenital and acquired syphilitic nephritis. Ann Intern Med 85:325, 1976.
Rudolph, A. H.: Examination of the cerebrospinal fluid in syphilis. Cutis 17:749, 1976.
Schirren, C. G.: Current problems of diagnosis and therapy of gonorrhea and syphilis. München Med Wochenschr 107:1189, 2681, 1965.
Shore, R. N.: Lupus erythematosus and reactive tests for syphilis: Update. Cutis 17:745, 1976.
Smith, J. L.: Spirochetes in Late Seronegative Syphilis, Penicillin Notwithstanding. Springfield, Ill., Charles C Thomas, Publisher, 1969.
Tramont, E. C.: Inadequate treatment of neurosyphilis with penicillin. N Engl J Med 294:1296, 1976.
Vatz, K. A., Scheibel, R. L., Keiffer, S. A., and Anjari, K. A.: Neurosyphilis and diffuse cerebral angiopathy: A case report. Neurology 24:472, 1974.
Wilner, E., and Brody, J. A.: Prognosis of general paresis after treatment. Lancet 2:1370, 1968.
Yoder, F. W.: Penicillin treatment of neurosyphilis. Are recommended doses sufficient? JAMA 232:270, 1975.

Lubor Červa, Dr. Sc.

The term amebic meningoencephalitis may designate any of three different diseases: (1) naegleriasis — primary amebic meningoencepha-litis (PAME); (2) acanthamebiasis; or (3) amebiasis of the brain caused by *Entamoeba histolytica*.

## NAEGLERIASIS

### DEFINITION

This is a primary type of acute purulent meningitis caused by the parasitic ameba *Naegleria fowleri*; it occurs mostly in young persons in robust health. Unless it is treated specifically, its outcome is generally fatal.

### ETIOLOGY

The causative agent of PAME is the ameboflagellate *Naegleria fowleri,* which is free-living in either water or soil. Sessile amebic forms measure from 10 to 20 $\mu$m; mobile amebae produce wide eruptive lobopodia (Fig. 1); and their posterior ends may change into a specific supporting organ, the so-called uroid. They possess pulsating vacuoles and a single spherical nucleus with a characteristically big endosome. In a liquid environment, the amebae are capable of transforming into oval-shaped flagellates that are about 15 $\mu$m in size and have two flagella (Fig. 2). The trans-formation is reversible. The resting stages of the protozoan are spherical to ovoid cysts, and they have a smooth surface measuring roughly 10 $\mu$m in diameter (Fig. 3). They are resistant to desiccation and to prolonged exposure to other nonphysiologic conditions.

### PATHOGENESIS

In man the sole portal of entry of infection is the nasal mucosa and the olfactory nerve. Infection occurs after swimming and washing in infected water. For their critical stage of reproduction pathogenic amebae need a water temperature of more than 20° C. Hitherto either natural water reservoirs in the warm season, artificially heated water of swimming pools, or warm industrial affluent and occasionally warm mineral springs have been identified as the sources of the infectious agent. Amebae inhaled with water attach themselves to the nasal mucosa where they reproduce rapidly. They pass through

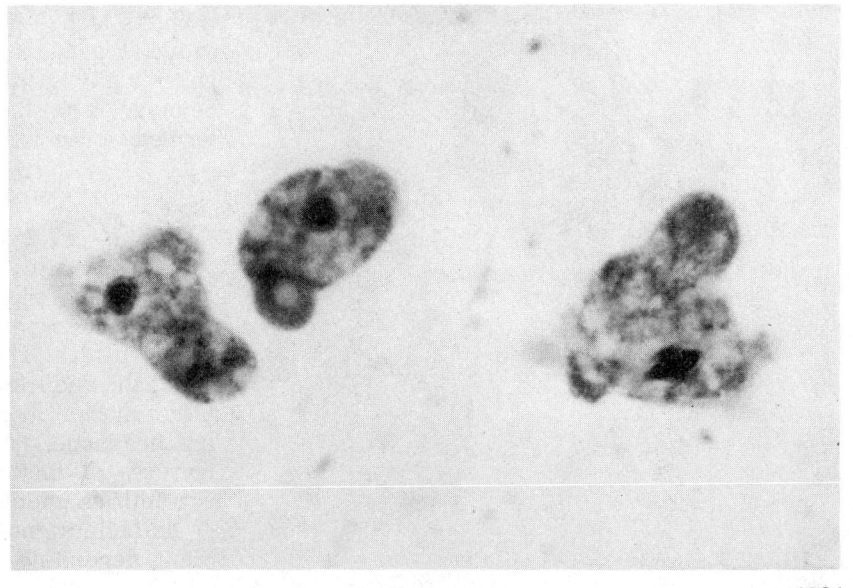

**FIGURE 1.** Naegleria fowleri *in axenic culture. Note the typical rounded lobopodia, the structure of the nucleus, and the promitotic division of the nucleus in one of the amebae. Iron hematoxylin stain after Heidenhain.* ×1300

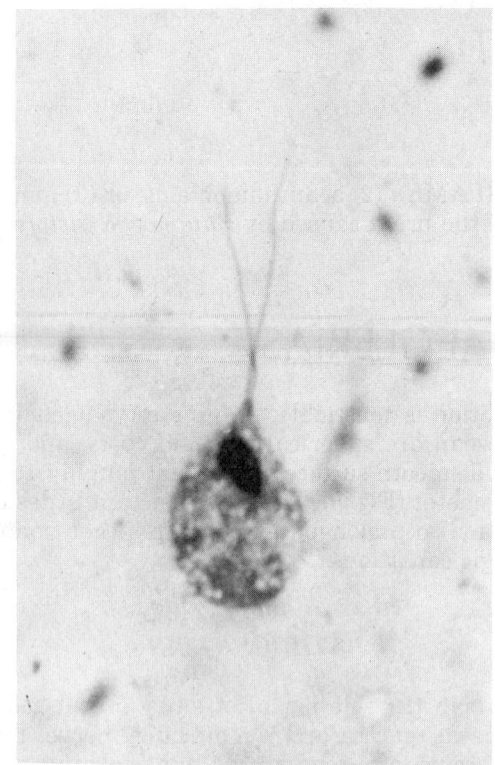

**FIGURE 2.** Naegleria fowleri, *flagellate stage. Giemsa stain.*

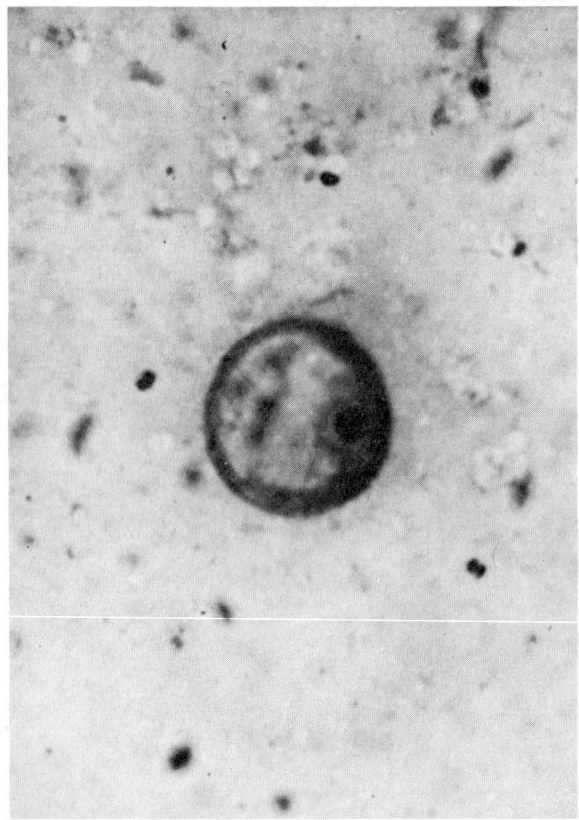

**FIGURE 3.** Naegleria fowleri, *cystic stage. Giemsa stain.*

the mucosa to the filaments of the olfactory nerve and along these to the base of the brain. They then spread actively in the brain or passively in the cerebrospinal fluid. From the meningeal spaces, they penetrate centripetally to the cortical and subcortical tissue of the brain and medulla.

## PATHOLOGY

Brain edema varies from mild to moderate. The leptomeninges are infiltrated to a varying extent with a cellular exudate, which can be best observed at the base of the brain. Either one or both olfactory bulbs become necrotic and adhere to the cortex of the frontal lobes. The ventricular fluid is generally clear, and the choroid plexus shows no gross changes. The cerebellum and the medulla are also the site of edema and meningeal infiltration. Minute foci of softening or petechiae are present in areas of frank meningitis. Terminal changes in other organs (mainly in lungs) are not directly related to the amebic infection. Microscopically, the meninges of both the brain and the medulla are permeated with an infiltrate dominated by polymorphonuclears (PMNs). Among the PMNs, only solitary amebae can be identified, and these are frequently phagocytized. Masses of proliferating protozoans are present in the perivascular spaces of the cortical and subcortical layers of the brain (Fig. 4). These masses develop faster than the inflammatory cell reaction. The base, the frontal, and the temporal lobes tend to be affected most. Multiplication of amebae in the cerebellum is massive in the granular layer and destroys the ganglionic layer.

In histologic preparations, amebae measure 8 to 10 $\mu$. They are spherical, and their nucleus, with its large endosome, is typical of the limax group (Fig. 5). In these preparations, no reliable generic and specific identification of amebae can be made on the basis of morphology. Cysts are not formed in the tissues.

## CLINICAL FEATURES

The clinical picture of PAME is that of an acute purulent meningitis. It affects mostly persons in robust health. The disease begins abruptly with headache and sometimes slight upper respiratory inflammation. It progresses rapidly with increasing headache, fever, and all the accompanying features of meningitis. Spasms of the face or extremities, mental disorders, parosmia (olfactory hallucinations), and other neurologic findings occur, depending on the location and extent of the

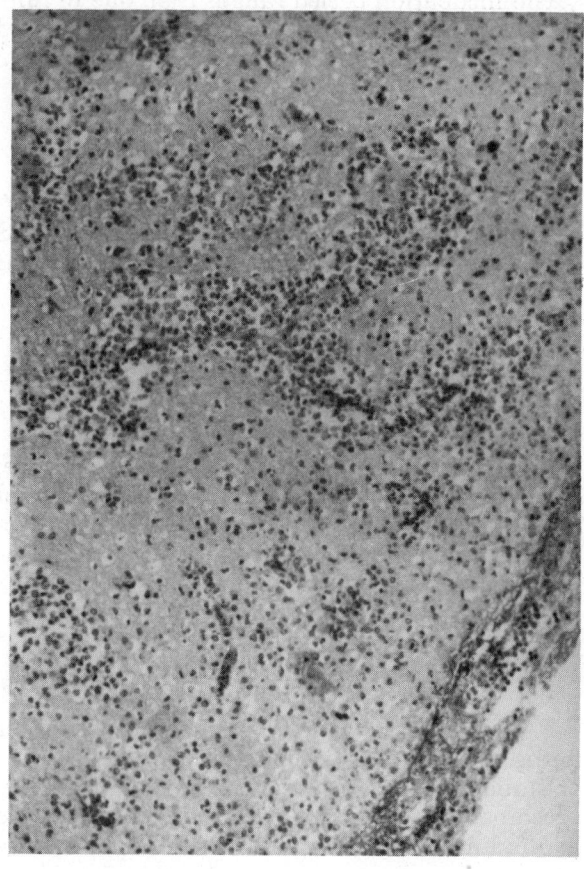

**FIGURE 4.**  *Naegleriasis in man. Heavily invaded cerebral subcortical tissue. Amebae are concentrated in perivascular spaces. Trichrome after Masson. ×200*

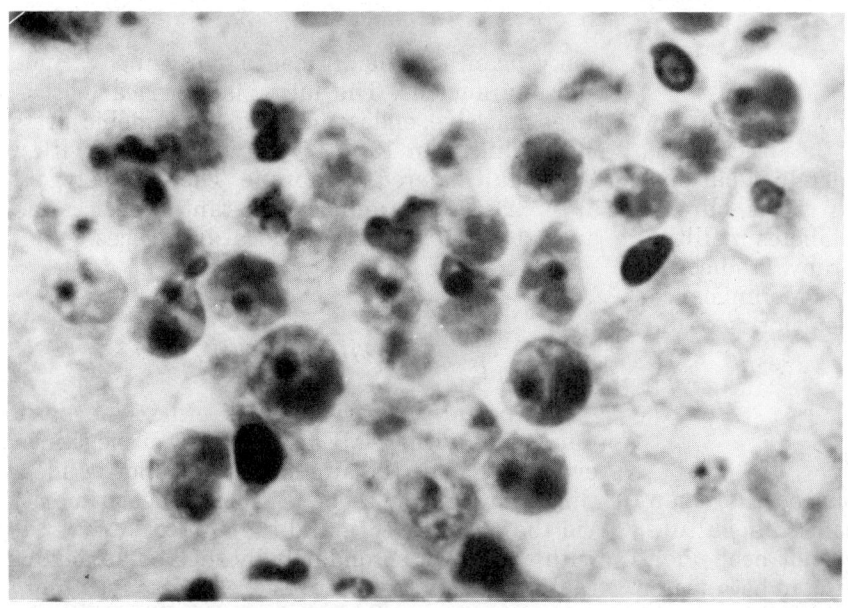

**FIGURE 5.**  *Detail of naegleriae in the cerebral tissue of man showing their typical morphology. Trichrome after Masson. ×1300*

cerebral lesions. Increasing intracranial pressure produces a deep coma and death.

The incubation period ranges from one to nine days (average five) after exposure to infected water. The disease lasts from one to seven days (average five).

### COMPLICATIONS

Amebic infection of other organs than the CNS may occur, but this does not change the clinical picture.

### GEOGRAPHIC DISTRIBUTION AND VARIATIONS

PAME has been reported in Australia, Europe, North America, and New Zealand. The clinical course is remarkably uniform in the various localities. The isolated causative agents are identical both morphologically and serologically.

### DIAGNOSIS

PAME cannot be distinguished from other forms of purulent meningitis by clinical features or standard laboratory examinations of the cerebrospinal fluid (CSF). A specific diagnosis is made by finding naegleriae in fresh CSF either by microscopic examination or by culture. Motile amebae can be readily distinguished from other cellular elements in the purulent CSF. The CSF can be cultivated on both solid and liquid media or in tissue culture. A period of 24 hours at an incubation temperature of 37 to 42° C is the earliest possible time at which positive findings may be expected.

A specific examination for PAME should be made in any patient with purulent meningitis if the patient was in good health before the illness and has a history of swimming, if bacteriologic examination of the CSF is negative, and if the course of the disease has not been influenced by antibiotics or sulfonamides.

### TREATMENT

The only drug that appears promising against *Naegleria fowleri* in vivo is amphotericin B in a dose of 1 mg/kg/day administered intravenously in a slow infusion or in combination with intrathecal injection. Only one case of successful treatment has been reported.

### PROPHYLAXIS

In endemic areas the only means of prophylaxis is to avoid swimming in water potentially contaminated with naegleriae.

# ACANTHAMEBIASIS

### DEFINITION

Acanthamebiasis is a uniformly fatal acute or chronic protozoan infection of the brain, eye, lung, liver, kidney, pancreas, and skin of patients with underlying malnutrition, cirrhosis, chronic alcoholism, Hodgkin's disease, diabetes mellitus, immunosuppression due to therapy or disease, and other debilitating conditions. Meningoencephalitis is one of the most frequent forms of disease.

### ETIOLOGY

Amebae of the genus *Acanthamoeba* (Hartmannella) have been seen but not isolated in culture, and the individual species have not been identified. This type of amebae live free in both water and soil. The living ameba is ovoid and measures from 20 to 50 μm (Fig. 6). The ameba moves by a slow flow of its plasma, which may form typical spiky acanthopodia. It has a pulsating vacuole and one nucleus. The latter is spherical with a large massive endosome (Fig. 7). Amebic cysts measuring from 10 to 25 μm are covered with a thick multilayered membrane. They are polygonal in shape and are most resistant to desiccation and other unfavorable physical influences.

### PATHOGENESIS

The portal of entry may be either the nasal mucosa (as with PAME) or an injury of the skin or eye. Sometimes the site of entry cannot be identified. The brain may be invaded either primarily via the nasal mucosa and the olfactory nerve (as with PAME) or secondarily by the hematogenous route. The clinical features are those of a fulminating meningoencephalitis (like PAME) or a chronic purulent meningitis, in which case the necrotic cerebral foci are smaller.

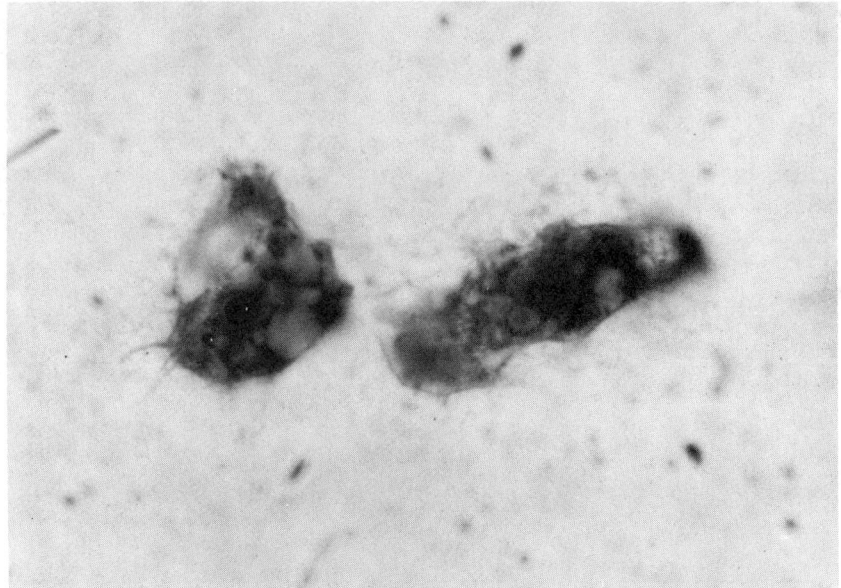

**FIGURE 6.** Acanthameoba culbertsoni *in axenic culture. Note the typical acanthopodia. Trichrome after Masson.* ×1300

## PATHOLOGY

In some cases the macroscopic picture is similar to that of PAME. In others, no cerebral edema and no other severe gross changes occur except necrotic foci that vary in size. Microscopic examination shows foci of necrotizing chronic granulomatous encephalitis in the cerebral cortex, cerebellar cortex, fornix, septal nuclei, thalamus, hypothalamus, pons, and midbrain. The lesions contain Langhans' giant cells. The individual lesions contain anywhere from solitary amebae to massive numbers in the perivascular spaces (Fig. 8), similar to *Naegleria* infection, but cellular reaction is better developed than in PAME. The size of the amebae in histologic preparations ranges from 10 to 50 $\mu$m; their nuclei are typical of the limax group (Fig. 9). An occasional characteristic polygonal cyst may be formed in the tissues.

## CLINICAL FEATURES

Meningeal symptoms are usually preceded by headache and fever. The disease most often devel-

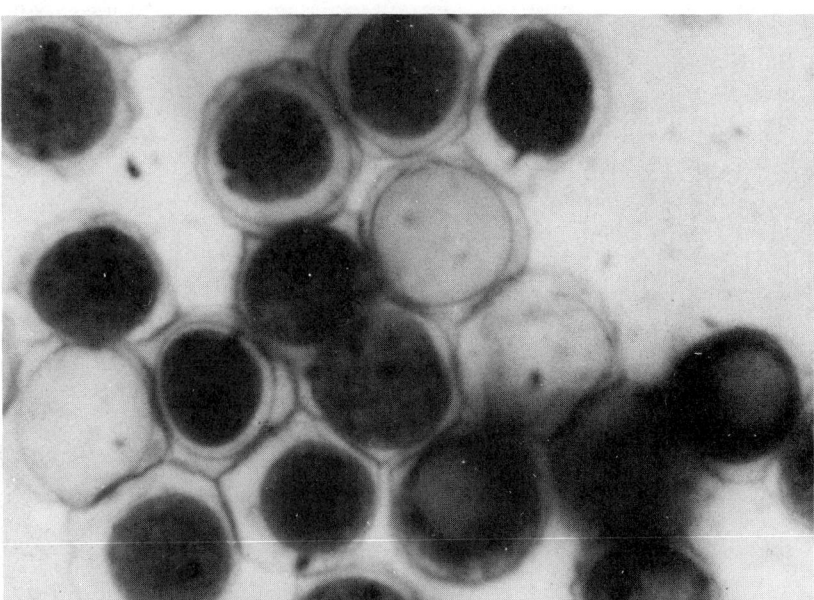

**FIGURE 7.** Acanthamoeba culbertsoni, *cystic stages. Hematoxylin stain after Carazzi.* ×1300

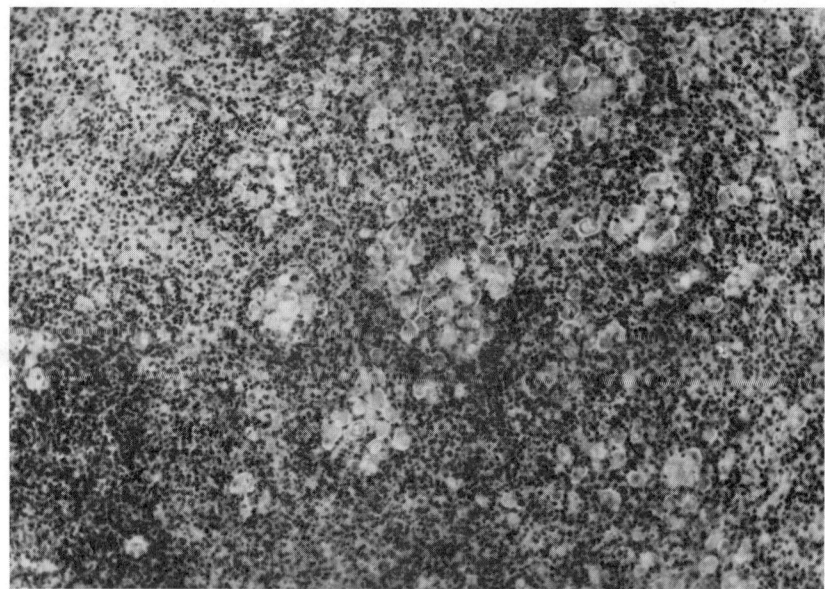

**FIGURE 8.** *Experimental cerebral acanthamebiasis in guinea pig after intracerebral inoculation with A. culbertsoni. Perivascularly located amebae are surrounded by massive leukocytic infiltration. Trichrome after Masson. ×200*

ops more slowly than PAME. Hemiparesis or ataxia follows frequently after the development of meningismus. Death occurs after a deep coma. The immediate cause of death is not necessarily central nervous system failure. If the focal lesions in the CNS are not extensive, the CSF may be clear. The number and type of cells have no relevance to the diagnosis; in some cases, lymphocytes predominate in the CSF. The incubation period may range from roughly ten days to several months. The total duration of the disease from the first symptoms to death is three to seven weeks.

## COMPLICATIONS

The incidence of focal lesions in other organs or generalized disease is frequent. The clinical picture is dominated by neurologic features. Acanthamebiasis may cause isolated keratoconjunctivitis and uveitis.

## GEOGRAPHIC DISTRIBUTION

Cases of meningoencephalitis caused by acanthamebae have been reported from America,

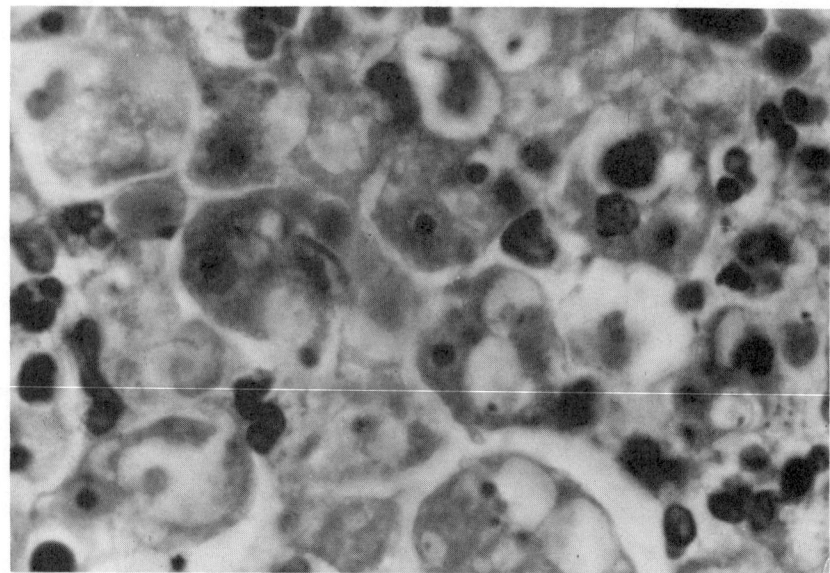

**FIGURE 9.** *Acanthamoeba culbertsoni in cerebral tissue of an experimentally infected guinea pig (detail). Trichrome after Masson. ×1300*

Africa, and Asia. However, the pattern of distribution of pathogenic amebae of the genus *Acanthamoeba* is cosmopolitan and so is the potential incidence of the infection.

### DIAGNOSIS

Like PAME, acanthamebiasis cannot be distinguished by standard clinical or laboratory findings from an acute or chronic meningoencephalitis of bacterial origin. In some cases, no amebae are found in the fresh CSF. However, in the second week of the disease, it may be possible to obtain positive results from a serologic examination with antigens from several acanthamebic strains such as *A. culbertsoni, A. castellanii,* and

*A. rhysodes.* The complement fixation, indirect hemagglutination, indirect fluorescent antibody, and immobilization tests are used for this purpose.

### TREATMENT

Sulfadiazine and other sulfonamides are of doubtful value, and other drugs with a satisfactory amebicidal effect in vitro do not enter the nervous tissue in high enough concentrations.

### PROPHYLAXIS

Prophylaxis is unknown.

# BRAIN AMEBIASIS CAUSED BY *ENTAMOEBA HISTOLYTICA*

### DEFINITION

This is a relatively infrequent form of extraintestinal amebiasis. It presents the picture of a brain abscess without marked meningeal features, and no amebae in the cerebrospinal fluid.

# AFRICAN SLEEPING SICKNESS   **163**

### Elizabeth Barrett-Connor, M.D.

### DEFINITION

Two subspecies of the hemoflagellate *Trypanosoma brucei, T. brucei rhodesiense,* and *T. brucei gambiense,* cause African trypanosomiasis, an infection transmitted only on the African continent between 15°N and 15°S latitude. Although there is considerable overlap, the Rhodesian form occurs primarily in East Africa as far south as Botswana, whereas the Gambian infection is seen primarily in West Africa, the Congo, and Angola.

### ETIOLOGY

The African trypanosomes are transmitted to man by the bite of tsetse flies of the genus *Glossina.* Within two or three days the infective (metacyclic) form is transformed into a long thin form that multiplies in the skin and then, one to

three weeks after inoculation, disseminates to the blood and lymphatic circulation. At this time, infective forms can be obtained by the tsetse fly during a blood meal. Within 15 to 35 days, the salivary glands of the tsetse fly contain metacyclic trypanosomes infective for the human host, and the cycle can repeat itself (Mulligan, 1970).

Human infection caused by *T. brucei rhodesiense* tends to have a short course, thereby reducing the chance for transmission to tsetse flies. Consequently, the main reservoirs of *T. brucei rhodesiense* are bushbuck and hartebeest (Mulligan, 1970). Human infections most often occur when man intrudes on largely uninhabited bush and woodlands. Cases tend to be single or grouped, although occasional epidemics have been reported. In contrast, *T. brucei gambiense* typically causes chronic disease in man, who is the primary reservoir of infection. Infection is usually acquired near river banks where people gather. Disease patterns may be endemic or epidemic. Recent reliable data on the prevalence or incidence of African trypanosomiasis are unavailable.

## PATHOGENESIS AND PATHOLOGY

Trypanosomes can alter their surface antigen every three to eight days. Until near death, the host responds by producing specific IgM for each surface variant (Mulligan, 1970, Whittle et al., 1977). Parasite lysis releases stable internal antigens that stimulate the production of IgG. Immune complexing may follow waves of parasitemia or treatment (Whittle et al., 1977).

Generalized hyperplasia of the reticuloendothelial system reflects the host response to repeated waves of new antigen. Macrophages and plasma cells replace small lymphocytes in the germinal centers of the lymph nodes. Similar changes are seen in the spleen, which is the presumed major site of trypanosome destruction and of IgM production. In late wasting disease, the lymph nodes become atrophic and fibrotic; at this stage immunologic deficiency can be demonstrated.

In some cases, there is cardiac dilatation and hypertrophy. Chronic myocarditis is common. On occasion there is pericarditis, pancarditis, focal valvulitis, a sclerotic endocardium, or lesions of the conducting system (Poltera, et al., 1976). Histologic examination shows interstitial hemorrhage and a marked interstitial and perivascular mononuclear cell infiltration. Trypanosomes can sometimes be demonstrated in pericardial fluid, but the parasite is rarely demonstrable in tissues.

The most characteristic lesions are found in the brain of patients who die with chronic disease. (Patients who die with the acute form often have no central nervous system pathology.) The more chronic the infection the more intense and widespread the meningeal inflammatory reaction. Lesions tend to be most marked at the base of the brain and in the lateral cisternae. The pia-arachnoid is thickened and attached to the brain surface; histology shows an increase in lymphocytes, plasma, and morular cells. Morular cells are altered plasma cells up to 20 $\mu$ in diameter; the cytoplasm is filled with large droplets resembling a raspberry. As the disease progresses, more remote parts of the meninges are involved and morular cells predominate. Later, mononuclear cells infiltrate the perivascular area at the site of entry into the brain. Vessels then are surrounded by 1 to 20 layers of cells. Morular cells in the perivascular cuff are virtually pathognomonic of sleeping sickness (Mulligan, 1970). Trypanosomes are rarely seen. Unlike other chronic brain diseases, there is little cortical damage in sleep-

ing sickness, although chromatolysis of neurons near cuffed blood vessels may be seen in some advanced cases.

The pathogenesis of the vascular lesions of trypanosomiasis is unknown, but it has been postulated that they are caused by the release of kinins by antigen-antibody complexes. This hypothesis is supported by the elevated levels of IgM, by the nature of the vascular lesions in rabbits experimentally infected with *T. brucei*, and by the fact that kinin concentrations are increased in experimental infections of laboratory animals (Richards, 1965) and human volunteers (Boreham, 1970). The possibility of direct damage of blood vessels and platelets by trypanosomes has not been ruled out, and recent studies have documented the occurrence of thrombocytopenia in naturally occurring infections of human beings (Barrett-Connor et al., 1973) and experimental infections of rats (Davis et al. 1974) and macaques. Furthermore, there is some evidence that *T. rhodesiense* can cause platelet lysis by a mechanism independent of immune complexes as mediated by immune adherence, complement-mediated lysis, and kinins (Davis et al., 1974).

## CLINICAL MANIFESTATIONS

In both Rhodesian and Gambian trypanosomiasis there may be a nodule or chancre at the site of the tsetse bite. Four to ten days after inoculation the area becomes hard and painful and surrounded by a zone of erythema that may undergo patchy desquamation. These lesions are usually accompanied by regional lymphadenopathy, rarely ulcerate, and characteristically disappear spontaneously in two weeks. Trypanosome chancres are more common in Europeans than in Africans, and in Rhodesian than in Gambian infection.

Fever begins five days to two weeks after inoculation and may precede parasitemia by several days. The temperature curve is typically high and irregular. Febrile episodes last for one day to one week, separated by intervals of days or weeks, and tend gradually to become less severe. Fever may clear spontaneously before the next phase of illness begins. During the early febrile period there may be hepatomegaly, splenomegaly, transient edemas, and, most commonly, generalized painless lymphadenopathy. The last is most prominent in the posterior cervical nodes in patients with Gambian infection (Winterbottom's sign). A faint erythematous blotchy or circinate rash sometimes seen on the trunk of patients with light skin is the most specific early sign of sleeping sickness.

During this stage nonspecific neurologic manifestations may include severe headache, deep muscle pain, insomnia, poor concentration, and excessive hunger (Mulligan, 1970; Basson et al., 1977). Personality changes — particularly a change from a responsible to an irresponsible behavior pattern — are described by those who know the patient. Examination may show delayed pain and delayed deep hyperesthesia (Kerandel's sign); striking or squeezing the tibia causes a delayed and disproportionate pain response. A certain sad staring appearance of the face, impossible to describe but unmistakable when seen, has been reported by several workers.

In Rhodesian trypanosomiasis the central nervous system is invaded within three to six weeks of inoculation (Mulligan, 1970, Basson et al, 1977). Fever, weakness, and headache persist or recur. Pallor, jaundice, and purpura or petechiae, signs of anemia and thrombocytemia, are seen in some cases. Tachycardia out of proportion to fever and other signs of cardiac dysfunction, including heart failure, also are noted, and the patient may die of myocarditis before more neurologic signs and symptoms appear (Poltera et al., 1976). If the patient survives the first few weeks, irritability, insomnia, sluggish mental responses, and personality changes usually become marked, but true somnolence is rare. Most untreated patients die from heart failure or bacterial infection in less than six months (Mulligan, 1970; Basson et al. 1977).

In the Gambian form of infection, months or years may elapse before the typical disease known as sleeping sickness ensues. Drowsiness and an uncontrollable urge to sleep appear in all untreated patients at some time during the course of illness. Tremors, rigidity, and cerebellar ataxia may precede or follow somnolence. The gait is said to be more ataxic and the tremor coarser than in Parkinsonism. Some patients present primarily with psychosis, which may be mistakenly attributed to viral encephalitis, neurosyphilis, mental illness, or brain tumor. In other cases the picture may simulate tuberculous meningitis. Neurologic examination rarely demonstrates localizing abnormalities other than those suggesting involvement of the basal ganglia. Unless treated, the patient usually dies of bacterial infection and malnutrition less than one year after the onset of neurologic signs.

## COMPLICATIONS AND SEQUELAE

Patients with Rhodesian trypanosomiasis may die of myocarditis or hemorrhage associated with thrombocytopenia and disseminated intravascular coagulation before neurologic signs and symp-

toms appear. After the central nervous system is invaded by either parasite, most untreated patients die of bacterial pneumonia, malnutrition, or dehydration.

Once illness develops, the case-fatality rate of either type of untreated disease exceeds 90 per cent, which places African trypanosomiasis among the most lethal of infectious diseases. However, not all of those infected become ill. Screening surveys demonstrate asymptomatic parasitemias in some persons living in areas endemic for either Rhodesian or Gambian trypanosomiasis (Mulligan, 1970; Whittle, 1977; WHO Bull, 1976).

## GEOGRAPHIC VARIATIONS IN DISEASE

It should be noted that although the signs and symptoms of Rhodesian and Gambian disease have been presented separately, persons infected in East Africa may actually have an indolent course, and persons infected in West Africa may have the acute fulminating picture of Rhodesian disease. Non-Africans, in particular, are apt to have an acute illness, even when acquired in areas where natives experience disease of insidious onset and chronic course.

## DIAGNOSIS

A history of sojourn in an endemic area is the first prerequisite for a diagnosis of African trypanosomiasis. The shortest route to diagnosis is microscopic identification of the parasite. *T. brucei rhodesiense* cannot be differentiated morphologically from *T. brucei gambiense*.

Diagnosis before bloodstream invasion is possible if the aspirate from the erythematous border of the chancre is stained and examined microscopically. More often diagnosis is made later when the peripheral blood (usually in Rhodesian disease), or a lymph node aspirate (usually in Gambian disease) reveals the parasite. Blood or node aspirates can be examined unstained for motile trypanosomes, or with Giemsa stain. The yield from blood is enhanced by using thick films, in the manner for malaria, or by examination of the buffy coat. There are also several concentration techniques. In one simple method, 10 ml of heparinized blood is lysed by the addition of 30 ml of 0.87 per cent $NH_4Cl$ (870 mg of $NH_4Cl$ in 100 ml of water), and centrifuged for 15 minutes. The sediment is then examined in the same fashion as the blood smear. In sophisticated laboratory facilities, trypanosomes can be separated from blood on DEAE cellulose columns and concentrated by

Millipore filtration; this method is 100 to 1000 times more sensitive than examination of unconcentrated blood. Material obtained from lymph node aspiration rarely requires concentration techniques. Small, rather unimpressive posterior cervical nodes often yield the diagnosis. When trypanosomes cannot be demonstrated directly, they can usually be found in the blood of laboratory rodents dying of trypanosomiasis days or weeks after intraperitoneal inoculation of blood from infected patients. Standard tissue section techniques are not a practical route to diagnosis.

Serodiagnosis is used occasionally, but serologic tests are most valuable for epidemiologic studies and mass screening programs. A variety of techniques have been applied to the study of African trypanosomiasis, most notably indirect fluorescent antibody, immunodiffusion, IgM antibody, capillary passive hemagglutination, and enzyme-linked immunosorbent assay (ELISA) (Whittle et al., 1977; WHO Bull., 1976). Although data on the specificity (ability to correctly identify persons without trypanosomiasis) of ELISA are not complete, this technique appears to be the most sensitive, identifying more than 95 per cent of persons with demonstrable trypanosomes (WHO Bull., 1976). ELISA can be carried out with simple equipment and read visually, permitting its use under field conditions.

Because appropriate treatment differs in the presence or absence of central nervous system invasion, the cerebrospinal fluid must be examined. Characteristically there are lymphocytic pleocytosis, high protein, and normal sugar. Morula cells of Mott are said to be nearly pathognomonic when seen. Spun sediment of spinal fluid may demonstrate organisms, but an elevated spinal fluid protein or cell count is considered evidence of brain invasion even when organisms cannot be found, if trypanosomes have been demonstrated in peripheral blood or lymph nodes. When the total protein in spinal fluid is normal, a high proportion of IgM supports the diagnosis of cerebral trypanosomiasis. Electroencephalograms, pneumoencephalograms, and angiograms reveal only nonspecific patterns, and may actually be misleading and suggest a space-occupying lesion.

Patients with trypanosomiasis often have other laboratory abnormalities that suggest but do not confirm the diagnosis. Anemia, often hemolytic, is common. The white blood cell count is usually low or normal unless there is secondary infection; there is no eosinophilia. In patients with Rhodesian disease there may be severe thrombocytopenia, often with depletion of fibrinogen and reduced complement levels. The serum albumin globulin ratio is typically reversed and the erythrocyte sedimentation rate may exceed 100 mm (Westergren).

One abnormality, which has achieved the status of near specificity for diagnosis, is the striking excess of IgM in trypanosomiasis. An IgM level 8 or more times the laboratory normal, or a level exceeding 1000 international units/ml, or an IgM-IgG ratio of ⩾3:1, have been proposed as screening tests (Whittle et al. 1977). Recent studies suggest that IgM levels are raised relatively early in over 95 per cent of patients with Gambian trypanosomiasis, but are less predictive of early Rhodesian infection. In both types, IgM may rise during treatment, and may occasionally fail to fall after successful therapy. Nevertheless, striking elevations of IgM are useful clues to diagnosis.

### TREATMENT
(Table 1)

Intravenous suramin sodium, 1 g given on days 1, 3, 7, 14, and 21, is the preferred treatment for bloodstream infection with T. brucei rhodesiense. Because the nervous system is invaded early in Rhodesian disease, suramin alone should be reserved for patients with negative spinal fluid examination who were exposed less than four weeks before illness (Buyst, 1975). Occasionally, patients may experience shock and collapse after the first intravenous dose; therefore a test dose of 100 mg should be given intravenously and the patient closely monitored for several hours before additional treatment is given. A Herxheimer's reaction (sudden high fever) may also occur. Common toxic reactions include rashes and renal damage. The urine should be examined between injections; marked proteinuria, casts, or red cells (but not mild albuminuria), indicate that suramin should be discontinued. Pentamidine isethionate is an alternate therapy for Rhodesian bloodstream trypanosomiasis and is the drug of choice for Gambian infection before central nervous system invasion (Buyst, 1975). Pentamidine is given intramuscularly for 10 daily injections of 3 mg base/kg body weight. Melarsoprol is also effective, but is avoided in patients with pre–nervous system disease because of its potential toxicity.

Once the brain is invaded, treatment usually requires arsenical compounds that cross the blood-brain barrier. Melarsoprol (Melarsenoxide/BAL; Mel B) is the drug of choice (Buyst, 1975). In critically ill patients with heavy parasitemia, it is wise to give several days of low dose suramin treatment before initiating melarsoprol. In one standard regimen, melarsoprol is administered intravenously in doses of 1.5, 2.0, and 2.2

**TABLE 1.   Drugs Used Against African Trypanosomiasis in Man***

| | | CLINICAL USE | |
| DRUG | Infection | Dose (mg/kg) | Regimen |
|---|---|---|---|
| Pentamidine isethionate | T. gambiense<br>T. rhodesiense | 3–4 (base) | 5–10 i.m. injections on consecutive or alternate days |
| Suramin sodium | T. rhodesiense<br>T. gambiense | 20 | 5 i.v. injections (in 10% solution) on days 1,3,7,14,21 |
| Tryparsamide | T. gambiense | 30–60 (max. dose is 2 g) | 12–14 weekly i.v. injections (20% solution) |
| Melarsonyl potassium | T. gambiense | 4 (max. dose is 200 mg) | 1 or more courses of 4 daily i.m. injections, separated by 7–10 days |
| Melarsoprol | T. rhodesiense<br>T. gambiense | 3.6 (max. dose is 5.5 ml of 3.6% solution in propylene glycol) | 1 or more courses of 3–4 daily i.v. injections, separated by 7–10 days |
| Melarsen sodium | T. gambiense | 20 | 10–12 i.v. injections of 10% solution every 5–7 days (course may be repeated after 1 month) |
| Nitrofural | T. rhodesiense<br>T. gambiense | 30–40 | 500 mg orally 3 times daily for 7 days (course may be repeated after 1 week) |

*Reference: Mulligan, 1970; and Buyst, 1975.

mg/kg at 48-hour intervals. One week later doses of 2.5, 3.0, and 3.6 mg/kg are administered on the same schedule, and after another week a third course of three injections, each 3.6 mg/kg, is given. Although preferred for safety, graded doses of melarsoprol may not be needed in Gambian cases. For example, in Zaire an initial dose of 3.6 mg/kg given without pretreatment is used with negligible toxicity, whereas this protocol in Burundi or Zambia has been associated with deaths in up to half of the cases.

Patients should be watched closely for serious complications of arsenic poisoning, such as encephalopathy, exfoliative dermatitis, and enteritis. The most feared complication is encephalopathy, usually heralded by headache and dizziness. Corticosteroids do not prevent arsenic encephalopathy, but may reduce the frequency of fever, exfoliative dermatitis, and enteritis. Although not well studied, corticosteroids are recommended for the immediate management of moribund patients in whom they may extend survival to permit specific therapy (Foulkes, 1975). Patients with Rhodesian disease who receive chloroquine in addition to arsenicals seem to have a better outcome; it is not clear whether this is a consequence of the antiinflammatory or antimalarial effect of chloroquine.

Treatment failures or relapses are a problem. In some areas the relapse rate is nearly 10 per cent. Relapses usually occur less than one year after treatment, but may be delayed for over two years. The majority of those relapsing after the first course of melarsoprol are cured with the second, and are not truly resistant. Patients are said to be melarsoprol-resistant only if they relapse after a second course of drug. Nitrofural, 500 mg orally three times a day for seven days, repeated after one week, is useful in cases resistant to melarsoprol. If arsenic has been well tolerated, nitrofural is combined with another course of melarsoprol in some cases. Side effects of nitrofural include polyneuropathy and hemolytic anemia. The latter occurs in patients with glucose-6-phosphate dehydrogenase deficiency, which should be excluded by the appropriate diagnostic test before nitrofural is begun.

## PROPHYLAXIS

Of the many theoretically possible ways to control trypanosomiasis, only a few are of practical value in the African environment. Tsetse fly control can be achieved on a limited geographic basis by insecticides, bush clearing, or game control, used singly or in combination. No one protocol is superior and the choices depend on local conditions. Reduction in the infected human reservoir has been used successfully to control disease transmission in many parts of West Africa. Chemoprophylaxis or case finding is seldom valuable in Rhodesian foci, where human infections are sporadic and animals the main reservoir.

For the traveler visiting endemic areas, precautions against insect bites by means of clothing, screening, and mosquito nets are advised. Chemoprophylaxis against Rhodesian strains is not recommended, but extended sojourns in areas of Gambian transmission may warrant the use of pentamidine prophylaxis. Chemoprophylaxis in any population carries a small but important risk of cryptic infection with delayed diagnosis.

### References

Barrett-Connor, E., Ugoretz, R. J., and Braude, A. I.: Disseminated intravascular coagulation in trypanosomiasis. Arch Intern Med 13:574, 1973.

Basson, W., Page, M. L., and Myburgh, D. P.: Human trypanosomiasis in Southern Africa. S Afric Med J 51:453, 1977.

Boreham, P. F.: Kinin release and the immune reaction in human trypanosomiasis caused by *Trypanosoma rhodesiense*. Trans R Soc Trop Med Hyg 64:574, 1970.

Buyst, H.: The treatment of *T. rhodesiense* sleeping sickness, with special references to its physio-pathological and epidemiological base. Ann Soc Belg Med Trop 55:95, 1975.

Davis, C. E., Robbins, R. S., Weller, R. D., and Braude, A. I. Thrombocytopenia in experimental trypanosomiasis. J Clin Investig 53:1359, 1974.

Foulkes, J. R.: An evaluation of prednisolone as a routine adjunct to the treatment of *T. rhodesiense*. J Trop Med Hyg 78:72, 1975.

Mulligan, H. W., (ed.): The African Trypanosomiases. London, George Allen and Unwin Ltd., 1970.

Poltera, A. A., Cox J. N., Owor, R.: Pancarditis affecting the conducting system and all valves in human African trypanosomiasis. Br Heart J 38:827, 1976.

Richards, W. H. G.: Pharmacologically active substances in the blood, tissues, and urine of mice infected with *Trypanosoma brucie*. Br J Pharmacol Chemother 24:124, 1965.

Whittle, H. C., Greenwood, B. M., Bidwell, D. E., Bartlett, A., and Voller, A.: IgM and antibody measurement in the diagnosis and management of gambian trypanosomiasis. Am J Trop Med Hyg 26:1129, 1977.

WHO collaborative study: Parallel evaluation of serological tests applied in African trypanosomiasis. Bull WHO 54:141, 1976.

# 164 *SPINAL EPIDURAL ABSCESS*

*Ann Sullivan Baker, M.D.*

## INTRODUCTION

Spinal epidural abscess is an uncommon disease; however, its importance stems not from its frequency but from its therapeutic implications. Effective treatment to prevent paraplegia requires early and accurate diagnosis of an often atypical and confusing group of symptoms and signs. Because the pace and evolution of the disease may be very rapid, it is important that the family practitioner, internist, and pediatrician recognize the features of the illness, make the diagnosis, and refer to the neurosurgeon for immediate treatment.

## DEFINITION

Spinal epidural infections are purulent or granulomatous collections within the spinal epidural space. They lie over or encircle the spinal cord, roots, and nerves (Baker et al., 1975; Browder and Meyer, 1927; Dus, 1960). Infection is usually localized within three to four vertebral segments, although it may extend the length of the spinal canal. Spinal epidural abscesses are acute or chronic. The acute abscess has a rapid clinical course of less than two weeks. In chronic abscesses, more than two weeks elapse between back symptoms and surgical intervention, and granulation tissue rather than pus is found in the epidural space.

## INCIDENCE

Spinal epidural abscess is less than one-twentieth as common as bacterial meningitis. Children and adults may be affected.

## ETIOLOGY

*Staphylococcus aureus* is the organism most commonly isolated from an epidural abscess and accounts for 50 per cent of cases. Streptococci, including non-Group A species, compose the second major category. *Escherichia coli* and *Pseudomonas aeruginosa* have been isolated secondary to urinary tract or abdominal infections. Rarely, anaerobic or mixed organisms from dental or upper airway infections have been isolated from spinal epidural abscesses, in contrast to their much greater frequency as the cause of brain abscess. In a few patients, no organism has been found.

## PATHOGENESIS

The most common focus for hematogenous spread to the epidural space is a skin infection, especially a furuncle. Dental and upper respiratory infections are frequent sources. Antecedent hematogenous vertebral osteomyelitis accounts for about 40 per cent of spinal epidural abscesses. A contiguous focus, such as a psoas abscess or sacral decubitus, may predispose to an epidural abscess. Congenital dermal sinuses may also be a source of infection.

In view of the frequency of transient bacteremic episodes, why do so few localize as spinal epidural abscesses? One possibility is that traumatic bleeding into the epidural space is often necessary for transmitting the infection into this sequestered site, even some time after the injury. In one series, 13 of 38 patients (30 per cent) had a history of back trauma or back surgery.

## ANATOMY

The clinical features and pathophysiology of spinal epidural abscess depend on certain key anatomic relationships. The epidural space contains fatty tissue and a rich, venous plexus (Fig. 1). Posteriorly, this space is relatively capacious, whereas anteriorly it narrows. The anterior spi-

nal artery and central arteries supply most of the spinal cord. Indeed, occlusion of the anterior spinal artery or central arteries affects the anterior four fifths of the cord.

The venous drainage of the spinal column consists of three communicating systems: (1) the internal or epidural plexus, (2) the intraosseous plexus, and (3) the external vertebral plexus. The internal network forms a meshwork around the dura, lining the adjacent bones, and connects with both the intraosseous and the external plexuses. The external plexus communicates freely with the vertebral and systemic circulations and with the intercostal, ascending lumbar, and lateral sacral veins, thus forming the well-known Batson's plexus (Batson, 1940).

## PATHOLOGY

The average abscess extends over four to five vertebral segments. The primary site of involvement is, in order of frequency: thoracic, lumbar, or cervical. The posterior thoracic or lumbar extradural space of the spinal cord is the most common location for an epidural abscess. An anterior epidural abscess is almost always secondary to vertebral osteomyelitis.

The epidural space contains either pus in acute cases or granulation tissue in chronic cases with-

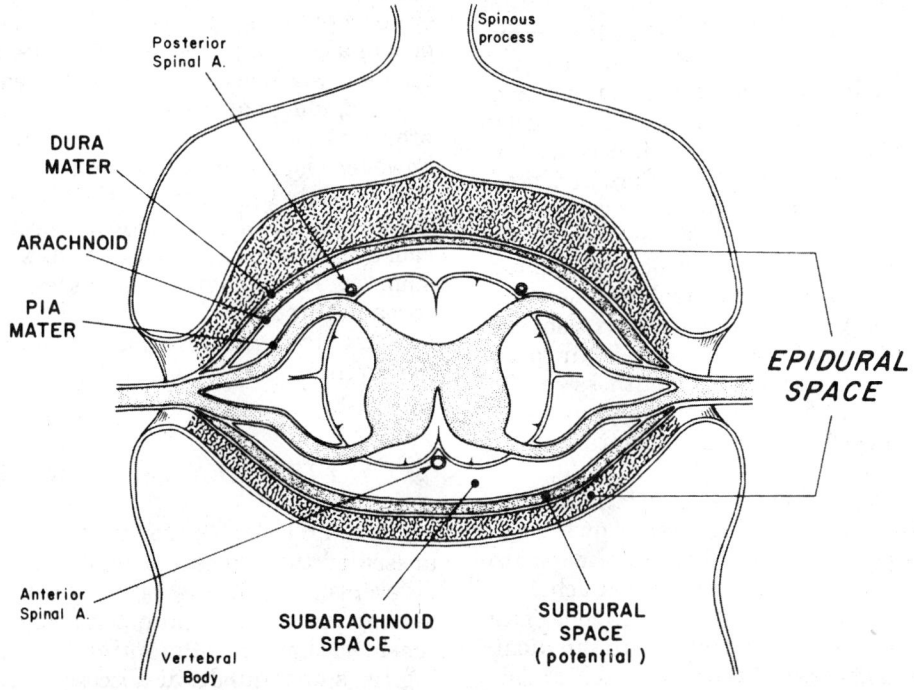

**FIGURE 1.** *Anatomic relationship of epidural space. Note the larger capacity of the posterior space compared with the anterior space and the vulnerable positions of the spinal arteries.*

out lesions in the spinal cord. In the more severe cases, examined postmortem, the spinal cord may become necrotic with early macrophage reaction in the disintegrating cord tissue, and many small arteries and veins in the subarachnoid space and spinal cord may be inflamed and thrombosed. The mechanism of the destructive changes in the spinal cord in cases of epidural abscess is not entirely clear. The lesions in the cord seem to be more extensive than can be accounted for by mechanical compression alone. Most probably, the rapidly growing infected inflammatory mass impairs the intrinsic circulation of the cord, perhaps by thrombosis. Thus, in addition to the serious effects of nerve root and cord compression from the epidural mass, there is the additional hazard of ischemic injury to the neural tissue.

## CLINICAL MANIFESTATIONS

The clinical picture of an epidural abscess was classically described by Heusner (1948) as a progression from spinal ache to root pain to weakness and finally paralysis. The spinal ache starts at the level of the affected spine. The pain is usually excruciating, often requiring large doses of narcotics. The patient may be extremely restless. Within a few days in acute cases, the patient complains of root pains radiating from the tender spinal area. Most patients appear acutely ill. Almost all have fever. The spine is tender, and, in a few patients, edema of the overlying soft tissues may occur. Reflex changes at this time are consistent with the anatomic level of the lesion, i.e., depression of the deep tendon reflexes in the legs if the abscess overlies the cauda equina, or accentuation of the deep tendon reflexes if it is over the cord. An increased concentration of protein in the spinal fluid suggests the diagnosis and warrants myelography. Untreated, the disease enters the third phase, in which motor weakness, gradual ascending numbness, and control over bladder and bowel is lost. There is a progression from root pain to weakness within an average of four to five days and, if further neglected, the illness rapidly progresses to paralysis. Paraplegia may occur within 24 hours, whereupon immediate surgical treatment is mandatory.

The course of chronic epidural infection is slower than that of acute and is spread over weeks or months. Sepsis is absent. These patients also complain of severe, excruciating spinal ache.

It is important to emphasize the extreme pain and restlessness in the patient with an acute spinal epidural abscess (Baker et al., 1975). The patients usually require large doses of narcotics. "Electric" pains or paresthesias (as described by Lhermitte) may be misinterpreted as hysterical (Liveson and Zimmer, 1972). Unfortunately, the patient with spinal epidural abscess is often labeled obstructive or malingering, and the psychiatrist may be consulted before the neurologist.

The mean peripheral white cell count is elevated in acute cases but is within normal limits in the chronic group. The cerebrospinal fluid (CSF) findings are typical of those of a parameningeal infection: the white cell count ranges from 0 to 1000 per mm³; polymorphonuclear leukocytes and lymphocytes are present in roughly equal numbers; the protein level is markedly elevated with a mean value of about 500 mg per 1000 ml; and the glucose level is normal. Those patients with accompanying bacterial meningitis will have higher CSF white cell counts and may have low cerebrospinal fluid glucose values. If the spinal puncture needle enters the abscess, a very high white cell count is found.

Radiographs of the spine may reveal osteomyelitis in a significant number of patients. If spine films, including tomography, are negative, a bone scan should be obtained. Myelograms show a partial, or most commonly, a complete block in most patients with spinal epidural abscess (Fig. 2).

## COMPLICATIONS AND SEQUELAE

Because of the rapid progression of neurologic damage, failure to make an early diagnosis of spinal epidural abscess is often disastrous. Approximately 5 per cent of patients will have residual weakness, paralysis, or death.

The epidural abscess may extend into the vertebrae and cause osteomyelitis. This progression, however, is much less common than extension from vertebral osteomyelitis to an epidural abscess. Spread of the epidural abscess may also cause retroperitoneal psoas abscess, pleural effusion, or retropharyngeal abscess. It may also spread through the vertebral system, erode through the subarachnoid space, and produce meningitis.

## DIFFERENTIAL DIAGNOSIS

The diagnosis of spinal epidural abscess will be missed if this disease is not considered in the differential diagnosis of backache in a febrile patient with local spine tenderness. The major considerations in differential diagnosis are meningitis, spinal subdural abscess, acute transverse myelopathy, problems in the vertebral or intervertebral disk space, vascular lesions, and tumors in the spinal cord.

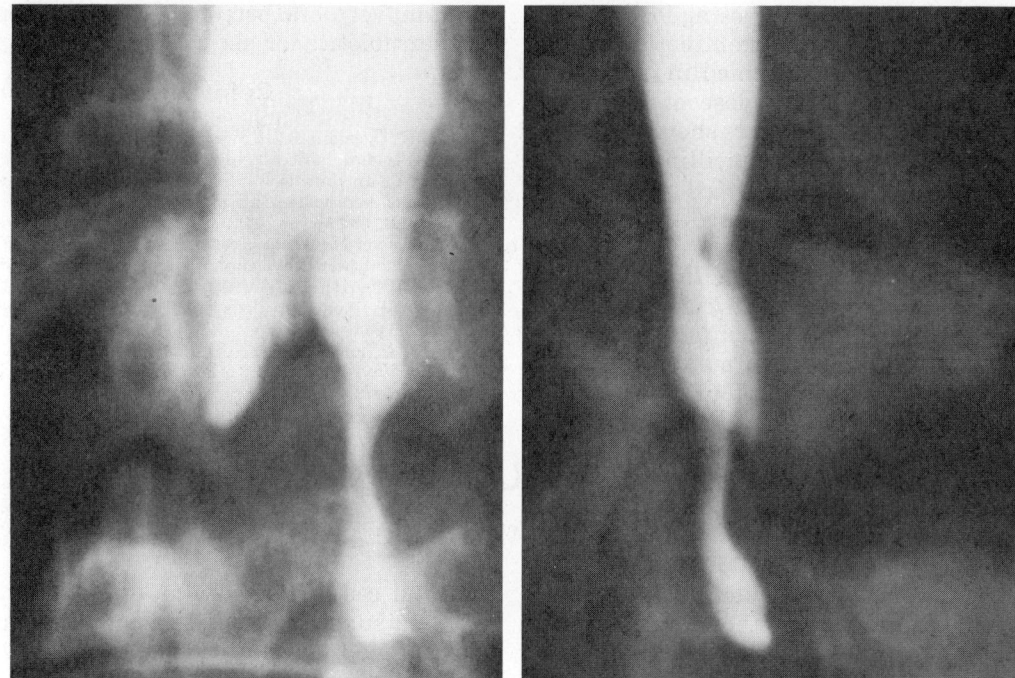

**FIGURE 2.** *Myelogram of spinal epidural abscess showing complete block.*

*Meningitis* may present with back pain, but headache is usually the major complaint. Local spine tenderness should suggest the possibility of an epidural process. *Spinal subdural abscess* is much less common but presents with signs nearly identical to those of an epidural abscess.

The onset of *acute transverse myelopathy* is usually more sudden than that of spinal epidural abscess, with paralysis occurring within 72 hours. Pain may be absent, and the myelogram is usually normal. *Infectious polyneuritis* is predominantly a motor disorder with minimal sensory disturbances. The initial symptom is usually weakness rather than back pain.

*Osteomyelitis* may start with back pain or root signs, but the cerebrospinal fluid analysis is normal. If there is associated vertebral collapse and spinal cord compression, differentiation from a spinal epidural abscess may be difficult. *Extruded disks* may produce similar symptoms, but the cerebrospinal fluid is usually clear.

Most *vascular problems* such as an epidural hematoma or interruption of the vascular supply of the cord occur with sudden paralysis, often acute pain, and no fever. *Dissecting aortic aneurysm* often presents with severe stabbing pain and may be confused with epidural abscess.

Finally, *primary spinal tumors* may present in a manner similar to that of a chronic epidural abscess. This differentiation is difficult to make without a tissue biopsy of the epidural contents.

## DIAGNOSIS AND TREATMENT

The patient with back pain, fever, and localized tenderness should have radiographs of the spine and a careful spinal puncture, with slow insertion of the needle and intermittent aspiration to ensure that epidural pus is detected. The risk of introducing infection from the epidural space is real, but is less a risk than not making the diagnosis of an epidural abscess. If involvement of the lumbar area is suspected, it is preferable to obtain the cerebrospinal fluid by lateral cervical puncture.

Signs of spinal cord or nerve root compression are an indication for myelography, preferably at the time of the spinal puncture. If a block or epidural mass is found on myelogram, laminectomy should be performed without delay, exposing the entire longitudinal extent of the abscess. If an acute abscess is found, the area is drained or packed open and subsequently closed secondarily. If the abscess is chronic and consists primarily of granulation tissue, the spinal cord should be fully decompressed and the wound closed.

When the primary abnormality is anterior, the extradural exposure should be done by removal of the pedicle or by a lateral or anterior approach. Blood cultures should be performed. The material obtained at operation should be immediately examined by Gram stain and cultured. Antibiotic treatment should be started during the operation or earlier. If there are no predisposing foci and no clues to the bacterial cause on examination of the Gram stain, a semisynthetic penicillin (nafcillin, oxacillin, or methicillin) in a dose of 1.0 g intravenously (I.V.) every two hours should be used initially. The combination of ampicillin (2.0 g I.V. every four hours) or carbenicillin (3.0 g I.V. every three hours) plus gentamicin (1 mg/kg I.V. every eight hours) is recommended in the setting of a known urinary tract focus. If penicillin allergy is present, a cephalosporin might be used in place of penicillin or semisynthetic penicillin.

Epidural abscess merits treatment with parenteral antibiotics for three to four weeks; concomitant vertebral osteomyelitis should be treated with antibiotics for six to eight weeks.

## References

Baker, A. S., Ojemann, R. G., Swartz, M. N., and Richardson, E. P., Jr.: Spinal epidural abscess. N Engl J Med 293:463, 1975.
Batson, O. V.: The function of the vertebral veins and their role in the spread of metastases. Ann Surg 112:138, 1940.
Browder, J. R., and Meyer, R.: Infection of the spinal epidural space; an aspect of vertebral osteomyelitis. Am J Surg 37:4, 1927.
Dus, B.: Spinal peripachymeningitis (epidural abscess): Report of 8 cases. J Neurosurg 17:972, 1960.
Heusner, A. P.: Nontuberculous spinal epidural infections. N Engl J Med 239:845, 1948.
Liveson, J. A., and Zimmer, A. E.: A localizing symptom in thoracic myelopathy. A variation of Lhermitte's sign. Ann Intern Med 76:769, 1972.

# 165 SUBDURAL EMPYEMA
## Ann Sullivan Baker, M.D.

Subdural empyema is a purulent collection in the potential space between the dura and the arachnoid. The term subdural abscess has been applied to this condition, but a better term is subdural empyema, which indicates suppuration in a preformed space. More than half of the cases result from extension of infection from primary foci in the paranasal sinuses, especially the frontal sinuses; chronic otitis media and mastoiditis less commonly result in subdural empyema. Subdural empyema may also occur from direct introduction of infection through operative or traumatic wounds or, rarely, by arterial hematogenous dissemination. In addition, subdural empyema is occasionally associated with bacterial meningitis with infection extending to a subdural effusion.

## INCIDENCE

Subdural empyema comprises about one-quarter of all localized intracranial bacterial infections. Mortality remains high, in the range of 20 to 40 per cent, because of errors in diagnosis, uncontrolled infection, and delayed surgical intervention.

## ETIOLOGY

The organisms vary with the initiating process (Hitchcock and Andreadis, 1964; Swartz and Karchmer, 1974). The most common organisms are streptococci, accounting for about 50 per cent of the cases. The streptococci are frequently non-group A and often anaerobic organisms that are typical of chronic rather than acute sinusitis. Gram-negative bacteria, *E. coli*, *Proteus*, and *Pseudomonas*, cause approximately 20 per cent of the total cases. *Hemophilus influenzae* has been found in subdural empyema complicating *H. influenzae* meningitis in rare cases. *Staphylococcus aureus* accounts for as much as 30 per cent of the total isolates. This is not an unexpected finding, since the common predisposing factor to subdural empyema is paranasal sinus infection (Coonrod and Davis, 1972; Kubik and Adams, 1943; Kaufman et al., 1975), in which anaerobes are important pathogens (Frederick and Braude, 1974). Anaerobic streptococci make up the largest portion of anaerobic bacteria isolated from subdural empyema, followed by Bacteroidaceae (Yoshikawa et al., 1975). Finally, unusual organisms or no organisms are found in 10 to 20 per cent of cases.

## PATHOGENESIS AND PATHOLOGY

The potential subdural space is unrestricted over and between the cerebral hemispheres but is restricted in the central basal region; hence most subdural empyemas are found either on the convexity (supratentorial region) or in the parafalx region. In cases of infection from a contiguous site, the empyema is usually located in the adjacent subdural spaces; for example, empyema following paranasal sinusitis is located primarily in the frontal subdural space. The spread in such cases occurs mainly via progressive thrombophlebitis of the mucosal veins, extending to the cerebral veins and to venous sinuses; less often, there is direct extension from bone or dura. Infection may also reach the subdural space by direct extension from osteomyelitis secondary to otogenic infection; the empyema may then be located in the adjacent temporal-parietal area.

Once the infection enters the subdural space,

pus forms rapidly and can spread widely. The extension of the infection in the subdural space depends on the primary site of origin and is influenced by gravity and anatomic boundaries. When empyema is established following otogenic infection, it usually spreads posteriorly and medially over the tentorium and toward the falx. The empyema is usually confined to the area over one cerebral hemisphere, but because purulent material may spread under the falx to the contralateral side, bilateral parafalcine collections are often encountered. If the pus is not drained, the ensuing phlebitis of the dural sinuses and cortical veins causes areas of cerebral infarction and hemorrhage. Compression of the brain by rapidly accumulating pus and the cerebral injury due to phlebitis give rise to diffuse as well as focal neurologic abnormalities.

Subdural exudate generally covers a large part of one cerebral hemisphere and ranges in volume from a few milliliters to 200 ml. The arachnoid is cloudy and thrombosis of meningeal veins may be seen. The exudate on the inner surface of the dura undergoes variable degrees of organization. There is infiltration of the underlying pia with small numbers of neutrophilic leukocytes, lymphocytes, and mononuclear cells. The thrombi in cerebral veins appear to begin on the side of the vein nearest the subdural exudate. The superficial layers of the cerebral cortex then undergo ischemic necrosis.

## CLINICAL MANIFESTATIONS

Subdural empyema is most often preceded by a flare-up of sinusitis or mastoiditis and symptoms of local pain with an increase in discharge from the nose or ear. Swelling, erythema, and local tenderness of the site overlying the primary infection may then become evident. In the early stages, pain or headache may be localized and moderate. As the illness progresses, the headache becomes generalized and severe. High fever, vomiting, and nuchal rigidity then develop. Focal or generalized seizures, hemiparesis, sensory deficits, visual field defects, and dysphasia may occur within several days. In dominant hemisphere collections, dysphasia is a frequent symptom, often appearing as a reluctance to talk and regarded by the inexperienced examiner as an expected accompaniment to the headache and systemic infection. Minimal weakness of one or more limbs progresses to complete paralysis. In some cases this is preceded by focal or generalized seizures. Papilledema may be seen. Seizures occur, owing partly to mass effect but also to the associated thrombophlebitis of cortical veins and infarction of cerebral tissue. Without treatment, progressive obtundation, coma, and death occur within 48 to 72 hours. Table 1 presents the relative frequency of symptoms and signs in 26 cases. Headache is present in every case in the early stages. The frequency of symptoms in patients with paranasal infections closely parallels that in otitic patients. Patients with pus on the convexity of the brain usually present with contralateral hemiplegia, often with focal seizures of face, arms, and legs. Sensory disturbances are less common, whereas in collections over the dominant hemisphere, aphasia is usual. The primary falcine collection begins with a lower limb monoplegia that rapidly progresses up the trunk to involve the arm but characteristically spares the face.

## DIAGNOSIS

Sinusitis, fever, and focal neurologic signs and symptoms are major diagnostic clues in the diagnosis of subdural empyema. A peripheral leuko-

**TABLE 1.** Incidence of Different Symptoms and Signs

| SYMPTOMS AND SIGNS | PARANASAL (20 CASES) AT ONSET | ESTABLISHED | OTITIC (16 CASES) AT ONSET | ESTABLISHED |
|---|---|---|---|---|
| Evidence of systemic infection | 19 | 20 (100%) | 5 | 6 (100%) |
| Paralysis (usually hemiplegia) | 13 | 20 (100%) | 4 | 6 (100%) |
| Stiff neck and Kernigism | 12 | 18 (90%) | 5 | 6 (100%) |
| Disturbed consciousness | 13 | 16 (80%) | 5 | 6 (100%) |
| Headache | 20 | 15 (75%) | 4 | 4 (66%) |
| High intracranial pressure | 8 | 15 (75%) | 2 | 3 (50%) |
| Mental changes | 10 | 12 (60%) | 3 | 4 (66%) |
| Vomiting | 10 | 10 (50%) | 4 | 4 (66%) |
| Epilepsy | 7 | 9 (45%) | 2 | 3 (50%) |
| Visual field defects | 1 | 9 (45%) | •2 | 3 (50%) |
| Sensory changes | 5 | 8 (40%) | 1 | 4 (66%) |
| Aphasia (in left hemisphere involvement) | | 100% | | 80% |

From Hitchock, E., and Andreadis, A.: J Neurol Neurosurg Psychiat 27:422, 1964.

cytosis is often present. The cerebrospinal fluid (CSF) and white blood cell formula is variable — it may contain no cells, a few polymorphonuclear and/or mononuclear cells, or, most frequently, from 50 to 1000 white blood cells; usually there is an equal number of polymorphonuclear cells and mononuclear cells. The protein concentration is increased in the CSF (a range of 75 to 300 mg/100 ml) with a normal glucose level. Gram stain of the smear and cultures of the CSF are usually negative. The combination of focal signs, cells in the CSF, and a high protein concentration indicates a parameningeal focus. In general, the early performance of a lumbar puncture is important in the evaluation of patients with possible central nervous system infection. However, if papilledema or other signs of increased intracranial pressure are present, transtentorial herniation is apt to occur following lumbar puncture. This procedure should be omitted or postponed until after a mass lesion is excluded by CAT scan.

Skull films, with sinus or mastoid films, may confirm the existence of paranasal sinus or mastoid infection. These examinations and the selective use of conventional tomograms may demonstrate and delineate bony destruction from infection. Rarely, air fluid levels may be diagnostic of a subdural or epidural process. A shift of the calcified pineal may suggest an intracranial mass effect.

Computerized axial tomography, or CAT scan, is the single most useful procedure for making the diagnosis of subdural empyema (Joubert and Stephanov, 1977; Kaufman and Leeds, 1977). Typically, a low absorption mass is identified in an extracerebral location. A thin, moderately dense margin may be visualized after the injection of intravenous contrast material. The conventional axial CAT scan frequently shows the extent of the subdural mass, although coronal scans may help to define collections at the base of the brain or about the tentorium. Coexisting brain abscess, focal cerebritis, or infarction edema is detected as well. Bony involvement may also be documented by using special settings to visualize bone. The CAT scan may be negative if collections are small and may not distinguish a sterile collection from an empyema.

The radionuclide scan can also detect subdural empyema and associated brain abscess. It is less helpful in defining the exact anatomic location of the process, that is, in distinguishing a subdural collection from meningitis or infarction, and may miss small or parafalcine collections.

Cerebral angiography reliably demonstrates extracerebral collections and may be especially helpful for bilateral or small parafalcine lesions. Demonstration of irregular contours, spasm, small vessel occlusions, or venous obstruction in association with an extracerebral mass may suggest infection as the cause. Rarely, however, is the gain significant, and angiography should be avoided when possible because of its potential morbidity in the febrile, infected, neurologically impaired patient.

**Differential Diagnosis**

Subdural empyema may present the same symptoms and signs as brain abscess. The initial stage of cerebral abscess is often milder and more insidious in onset, and the course may be more protracted. The temperature is usually normal and the neck is rarely stiff except in the case of a complicating meningitis. Although the deterioration may be more acute in some cases of subdural empyema, the fact remains that making a clinical distinction from brain abscess may be quite difficult.

The clinical resemblance between subdural empyema and thrombophlebitis of the superior longitudinal sinus is close, and reference has already been made to their possible coexistence. Favoring the diagnosis of sinus thrombophlebitis are a septic temperature, bacteremia, absence of increased intracranial pressure or stiff neck, little or no pleocytosis, and bilateral signs such as focal convulsions or paralysis occurring first on one side of the body and then on the other.

Bacterial meningitis and subdural empyema may also present in a similar fashion, that is, with depressed sensorium, fever, and nuchal rigidity. However, sinusitis, especially frontal sinusitis, is an uncommon antecedent of bacterial meningitis. In addition, meningitis in adults, unlike subdural empyema, is usually not associated with focal seizures, hemiparesis, or papilledema. These findings suggest parenchymal brain involvement. Finally, slight pleocytosis, absence of organisms, a high protein concentration, and a normal glucose level in the spinal fluid are more suggestive of subdural empyema. Tuberculous, fungal (e.g., cryptococcal), and viral meningoencephalitis may all be confused with subdural empyema. Acid-fast smears and wet preparations of the spinal fluid, cultures for *Mycobacterium tuberculosis,* viruses, and fungi, and fungal or viral antibody titers of the cerebrospinal fluid and serum are helpful in the differential diagnosis of these entities.

## COMPLICATIONS AND SEQUELAE

The mortality of subdural infections has decreased from 100 per cent to about 40 per cent since the introduction of antibiotics. A further decline in mortality has been prevented by persistent errors in diagnosis and by complications of the disease. Frank meningitis seldom accompanies subdural empyema. Administration of antibiotics to patients with subdural empyema without concomitant drainage results in a chronic illness with a course resembling that of an intraparenchymal brain abscess.

Cortical venous or major dural sinus thrombophlebitis, cerebral abscess, or infarction or herniation may all complicate subdural empyema. At least one-half of the survivors from subdural empyema will have neurologic incapacities secondary to thrombosis of surface veins, dural sinuses, and areas of cerebral infarction.

## *TREATMENT*

Subdural empyema is a life-threatening infection requiring prompt surgical drainage and intensive antimicrobial therapy. Both are crucial for a favorable outcome. Surgical management of the subdural empyema must provide for adequate drainage of all collections of purulent material. The simplest process is immediate drainage through enlarged multiple frontal burr holes. Craniotomy with contralateral placement of burr holes provides for full bilateral drainage, especially of loculated or viscous fluid, as well as for the proper exposure of parafalcine collections and cranial abscess formation. Surgical treatment of the accompanying sinusitis, frontal osteomyelitis, or mastoiditis is a secondary consideration and is usually postponed until the acute intracranial infection has subsided.

When the subdural contents are liquid, large amounts of purulent material are readily evacuated. In more chronic lesions, however, granulation tissue may be densely adherent to the underlying pia-arachnoid, making radical removal infeasible. Catheters may be left extending into each corner of the abscess cavity for drainage. At the time of surgery, purulent fluid should be obtained for a Gram-stained smear and aerobic and anaerobic cultures.

Antibiotic therapy should be instituted at the time of surgery or earlier. The initial choice of antibiotics should include penicillin, and, if recommended by the background of the case, an additional agent to cover gram-negative bacilli. Penicillin G, 20 million units/day in divided intravenous doses every four hours combined with chloramphenicol 500 to 1000 mg/kg/day in divided doses every six hours, will be effective against most of the pathogens isolated from these infections. These antibiotics are also found in good concentrations in the cerebrospinal fluid. However, when infection follows surgery or a penetrating skull injury, a penicillinase-resistant penicillin should be substituted for penicillin G. Antibiotic therapy should be refined according to the background of the case, the Gram-stained smear of the pus obtained at surgery, and the results of cultures of this material. Antibiotics that do not penetrate cerebrospinal fluid, such as cephalosporins and clindamycin, should be avoided. Although of unproven efficacy, bacitracin 500 to 2000 units/ml may be instilled into the subdural space at the time of surgery and for variable periods thereafter. Local therapy may also be beneficial when treatment requires that poorly diffusible aminoglycoside antibiotics be used. Administration of antibiotics should continue for at least three weeks after surgical drainage.

Since seizures are a frequent feature of subdural empyema, prophylactic use of anticonvulsants such as phenytoin seems reasonable. In addition, if signs of increased intracranial pressure are apparent, use of glucocorticosteroids such as dexamethasone should be considered to reduce inflammatory edema.

## References

Coonrod, J. D., and Davis, P. E.: Subdural empyema. Am J Med 53:85, 1972.

Frederick, J., and Braude, A.: Anaerobic infection of the paranasal sinuses. N Engl J Med 290:135, 1974.

Hitchcock, E., and Andreadis, A.: Subdural empyema: A review of 29 cases. J Neurol Neurosurg Psychiatr 27:422, 1964.

Joubert, M. J., and Stephanov, S.: Computerized tomography and surgical treatment in intracranial suppuration. Report of 30 consecutive unselected cases of brain abscess and subdural empyema. J Neurosurg 48:73, 1977.

Kaufman, D. M., and Leeds, N. E.: Computed tomography (CT) in the diagnosis of intracranial abscesses. Brain abscess, subdural empyema and epidural empyema. Neurology 27:1069, 1977.

Kaufman, D. M., Miller, M. H., and Steigbigel, N. H.: Subdural empyema. Analysis of seventeen recent cases and review of the literature. Medicine 54:485, 1975.

Kubik, R. S., and Adams, R. D.: Subdural empyema. Brain 66:18, 1943.

Swartz, M. N., and Karchmer, A. W.: Infections of the central nervous system. In Balows, A., et al. (eds.): Anaerobic Bacteria. Role of Disease. Springfield, Ill., Charles C Thomas, 1974.

Yoshikawa, T. T., Chow, A. W., and Guze, L. B.: Role of anaerobic bacteria in subdural empyema. Report of four cases and review of 327 cases from the English literature. Am J Med 58:99, 1975.

# 166 CEREBRAL ANGIOSTRONGYLIASIS

*Leon Rosen, M.D., Dr. P.H.*

## DEFINITION

Cerebral angiostrongyliasis results from the invasion of the human central nervous system by the rodent metastrongylid lungworm, *Angiostrongylus cantonensis* (Rosen et al., 1962).

## ETIOLOGY

Both the male and female mature adult forms of *A. cantonensis* normally live within the pulmonary arteries of rodents (species of the genus *Rattus* and some related genera). In the course of their unusual life cycle, the parasites undergo an obligatory period of development within the central nervous system of the rodent before migrating to the pulmonary arteries. In man, however, development of the parasites almost always is arrested in the central nervous system, and the nematodes usually die there.

In the complete life cycle, eggs laid by fertilized females form emboli in the terminal branches of the pulmonary arteries and hatch there, and the resultant first-stage larvae enter the bronchial system. The larvae migrate up the trachea, pass into the alimentary canal, and are excreted in the feces. The parasites then must enter a molluscan intermediate host, usually a terrestrial or amphibious snail or slug. Two further stages of development occur in the mollusc, and the parasites then reach the third or infective larval stage. Development continues when infected molluscs are eaten by a rodent of the appropriate species. After liberation from molluscan tissue by digestive juices in the alimentary tract, third-stage larvae migrate to the brain and undergo two further stages of development within the parenchyma. The young adult nematodes then migrate to the surface of the brain and enter the venous system in order to reach their final destination, the pulmonary arteries. They attain full sexual maturity after they arrive in the arteries.

## PATHOGENESIS AND PATHOLOGY

Man acquires cerebral angiostrongyliasis by accidental or intentional consumption of infected intermediate hosts (molluscs) or paratenic hosts (see below). Paratenic hosts become infected by consuming intermediate hosts. Infective larvae do not develop further in such hosts but remain viable. Although complete development of *A. cantonensis* does not occur in man, a high proportion of ingested third-stage larvae apparently do reach the human central nervous system, since disease has been observed in persons thought to have been exposed to relatively small numbers of larvae. (No multiplication of the parasite occurs in humans). The usual incubation period of the disease in man from the time of ingestion of infective larvae to the appearance of the first signs and symptoms is about two weeks (with a range of about one to four weeks).

Damage to the human host occurs as a result of the development and movement of the living parasites (for example, when they migrate to the anterior chamber of the eye), or, more commonly, as a result of a granulomatous reaction to dead or dying parasites in either the parenchyma of the central nervous system or the meninges. This inflammatory response, characterized by an abundance of eosinophilic leukocytes, gives rise to the eosinophilic pleocytosis characteristic of the disease. The degree of pathology usually is proportional to the number of parasites ingested, except in rare instances when parasites migrate to a critical area (such as the eye). Fatalities are rare, and most patients recover without sequelae. One episode of the disease does not confer immunity to subsequent exposure, and repeated episodes have been observed in individuals reexposed to infective larvae.

## CLINICAL MANIFESTATIONS, COMPLICATIONS, AND SEQUELAE

The most common clinical expression of cerebral angiostrongyliasis is a meningitis characterized by headache, nausea and vomiting, moderate stiffness of the neck and/or back, paresthesias, and low-grade or no fever. Headache commonly is severe, intractable, and bitemporal in location, and is usually the symptom that causes the patient to consult a physician. Paresthesias are of a variety of types but commonly consist of exaggerated sensitivity to touch. They usually are unilateral in distribution and are not limited to areas innervated by specific spinal segments or peripheral nerves. Unilateral facial paralysis of the lower motor neuron type occurs in about 5 per cent of patients. Other cranial nerves are affected more rarely. Fever is observed more commonly when the disease occurs in children (Char and Rosen, 1967). Living young adult parasites have occasionally been observed in the eye. Characteristically, the disease is benign and self-limited with a case-mortality ratio of well under 1 per cent. However, severe permanent sequelae (such as blindness) and death are known to occur, presumably as the result of infection with large numbers of parasites. Severe illness is characterized by somnolence or lethargy that may progress to unconsciousness. Paresthesias occasionally persist for years following mild disease.

## GEOGRAPHIC VARIATIONS IN DISEASE

Although human disease caused by *A. cantonensis* generally is similar throughout the vast geographic area (see below) in which the parasite occurs, some variations in clinical manifestations are observed. These variations are believed to reflect the number of parasites that patients have ingested. In turn, this reflects differences in the epidemiology of the disease in various geographic areas and differences in the species of, and intensity of infection in, molluscan intermediate or paratenic hosts. For example, in Taiwan, where most human infection is acquired from heavily parasitized giant African snails (*Achatina fulica*), severe disease with permanent sequelae is fairly common (Yii, 1976). On the other hand, on South Pacific islands, where the disease most commonly is acquired from lightly infected paratenic hosts, serious sequelae or deaths are rare.

## DIAGNOSIS

Cerebral angiostrongyliasis should be considered in evaluation of patients with severe headache and/or paresthesias who live in, or have recently visited, areas where *A. cantonensis* is known to occur. The range of the parasite is limited by Madagascar in the west, the Hawaiian Islands in the east, Japan in the north, and Australia in the south. Of course, *A. cantonensis* does not occur in every locality within this vast area. Since both the rodent vertebrate hosts and the molluscan intermediate hosts are commonly transported by human activity, it is probable that the geographic distribution of the parasite will continue to expand, both to new territory within the known geographic range and outside it. For example, neither rodent nor molluscan hosts of *A. cantonensis* occurred in Pacific islands before the arrival of humans. The parasite has been introduced in some of these islands (Tahiti) but not on others.

The diagnosis of cerebral angiostrongyliasis usually can be made on clinical grounds alone in association with an epidemiologic history, provided one thinks of the possibility (Rosen et al., 1967). Most, but not all, cases have a characteristic pleocytosis consisting in large part of eosinophils. It is this characteristic that led to the designation of the disease as "eosinophilic meningitis" before its cause was discovered. Most patients have cerebrospinal fluid leukocyte counts of between 100 and 2000 cells/cm in conjunction with their symptoms, and characteristically 25 to 75 per cent of the leukocytes are eosinophils. In general, persons with the highest total cell counts have the highest percentages of eosinophils. An increased number of eosinophils is observed also in the peripheral blood, but this finding is less useful because it is of lesser magnitude, is more fleeting, and is commonly observed in patients with other helmintic parasites.

Although living young adult *A. cantonensis* organisms have been recovered from the eye and cerebrospinal fluid of patients, this is a rare occurrence. Despite considerable research, there is at present no satisfactory serologic or skin test that can be used to diagnose the disease in man. Consequently, the majority of cases can be diagnosed only on the basis of clinical, epidemiologic, and cerebrospinal fluid findings.

Infections with *A. cantonensis* often are not recognized because (1) patients are not sick enough to seek medical attention, (2) a spinal tap is not done because the meningitic nature of the illness is not recognized in the absence of fever, or (3) the presence of eosinophils in the cerebrospinal fluid is not detected because of failure to use suitable staining methods.

The finding of an eosinophilic pleocytosis does not, of course, establish the diagnosis of invasion of the central nervous system by *A. cantonensis*. Such a finding does, however, strongly suggest the invasion of the central nervous system by a helmintic parasite. Other than helmintic parasites, the only known causes of a significant eosinophilic pleocytosis are the intrathecal injection of various types of foreign proteins, rabies vaccination, the insertion of rubber tubing into the central nervous system in the course of neurosurgery, and coccidioidal meningitis. Helminths other than *A. cantonensis* that invade the central nervous system of man and that can give rise to an eosinophilic pleocytosis include the cysticercus of the pork tapeworm, *Taenia solium,* and the adult forms and eggs of the lung fluke, *Paragonimus westermani.* Both *T. solium* and *P. westermani* often give rise to signs and symptoms of space-occupying lesions and convulsions when the central nervous system is involved. *Gnathostoma spinigerum,* a nematode, also has been shown to be capable of invading the human central nervous system and causing an eosinophilic pleocytosis. Although larvae of *Trichinella spiralis* are known to reach the central nervous system of humans, pleocytosis is uncommon and eosinophils have not been demonstrated. The situation with respect to *Toxocara canis* is similar to that for *T. spiralis.* The larvae of *T. canis* have been found in the human central nervous system, but an eosinophilic pleocytosis has not been described.

It should be noted that sporadic cases of eosinophilic meningitis of unknown etiology have been described from many different parts of the world. Because of their geographic distribution, it is unlikely that many of these cases were caused by *A. cantonensis.* Thus, it is probable that there are as yet unknown etiologic agents that can give rise to a clinical picture indistinguishable from that of *A. cantonensis.*

## TREATMENT

Once the diagnosis has been established, little can be done except to await recovery. Treatment is largely supportive and symptomatic. The diagnostic spinal tap often relieves headache. Aspirin and other analgesic agents are useful for fever and headache. In more severe cases, in which signs of cerebral edema may be prominent, corticosteroids or the osmotic brain-dehydrating agents such as urea or mannitol may be cautiously employed. Respiratory supportive measures, such as tracheostomy or artificial respiration, may be necessary if signs of brain stem compression appear. Recovery characteristically is slow but is usually complete.

Although thiabendazole, a broad spectrum anthelmintic, affects the development of *A. cantonensis* in rats, its use against the parasite in man has not been reported, and there is doubt as to the rationality of such use. It is suspected that most of the deleterious effects of *A. cantonensis* infection in humans are the result of reaction to dead or dying worms, and that not all parasites in a given patient die simultaneously. Consequently, if this view is correct, and if thiabendazole kills all the parasites at one time, treatment with the drug might do more harm than good.

## PROPHYLAXIS

Human consumption of raw or incompletely cooked molluscs is sometimes deliberate (e.g., the consumption of chopped *Pila* species in Thailand) and sometimes accidental (e.g., the ingestion of small slugs on carelessly washed lettuce). Paratenic hosts of *A. cantonensis* include fish, amphibians, reptiles, crustaceans, and land planarians. The consumption of raw freshwater shrimp *(Macrobrachium lar)* or food containing extracts of these animals is an important source of human infection on some Pacific islands. Terrestrial or aquatic crabs have been suspected as sources of human infection in some instances. Thus, human infection with *A. cantonensis* is determined largely by cultural factors affecting types of foods consumed and the methods of their preparation. Sporadic cases occur, however, among individuals accidentally exposed to infected molluscs in the course of work or play (for example, contamination of hands in the course of gardening).

Since most species of terrestrial molluscs are susceptible to infection with *A. cantonensis,* their relative importance depends on their abundance near human habitations, their use as food, or their tendency to frequent vegetable gardens. The importance of the various paratenic hosts depends on the frequency with which they are infected and the degree to which they are used as human food in the raw or incompletely cooked state.

Perhaps the most important measure that can be used to control *A. cantonensis* infection in man is education about the nature and source of the disease. Individual measures depend on the way humans are infected in a given area and consist of avoiding the consumption of molluscs or paratenic hosts that may contain infective larvae (both freezing and cooking are effective in destroying larvae), the careful washing of green vegetation that is consumed raw, and careful washing of hands after working in areas likely to contain molluscs. Community-wide measures consist of the control of molluscs and land planarians in vegetable gardens, and perhaps the control of rodents in such areas. Attempts to control rodents and the molluscan intermediate hosts elsewhere appear almost futile at present.

Since *A. cantonensis* is disseminated by man and has yet to reach many geographic areas that appear to be suitable for its maintenance, it obviously is desirable to avoid the introduction of molluscs or rodents from endemic areas into such parasite-free areas.

### References

Alicata, J. E., and Jindrak, K.: Angiostrongylosis in the Pacific and Southeast Asia. Springfield, Ill., Charles C Thomas, Publisher, 1970.

Char, D. F. B., and Rosen, L.: Eosinophilic meningitis among children in Hawaii. J Pediatr 70:28, 1967.

Punyagupta, S., Bunnag, T., Juttijudata, P., and Rosen, L.: Eosinophilic meningitis in Thailand. Epidemiologic studies of 484 typical cases and the etiologic role of *Angiostrongylus cantonensis*. Am J Trop Med Hyg 19:950, 1970.

Punyagupta, S., Juttijudata, P., and Bunnag, T.: Eosinophilic meningitis in Thailand. Clinical studies of 484 typical cases probably caused by *Angiostrongylus cantonensis*. Am J Trop Med Hyg 24:921, 1975.

Rosen, L., Chappell, R., Laqueur, G. L., Wallace, G. D., and Weinstein, P. P.: Eosinophilic meningoencephalitis caused by a metastrongylid lung-worm of rats. JAMA 179:620, 1962.

Rosen, L., Loison, G., Laigret, J., and Wallace, G. D.: Studies on eosinophilic meningitis. 3. Epidemiologic and clinical observations on Pacific islands and the possible etiologic role of *Angiostrongylus cantonensis*. Am J Epidemiol 85:17, 1967.

Yii, C-Y.: Clinical observations on eosinophilic meningitis and meningoencephalitis caused by *Angiostrongylus cantonensis* on Taiwan. Am J Trop Med Hyg 25:233, 1976.

Yii, C.-Y., Chen, C.-Y., Chen, E.-R., Hsieh, H.-C., Shih, C.-C., Cross, J. H., and Rosen, L.: Epidemiologic studies of eosinophilic meningitis in southern Taiwan. Am J Trop Med Hyg 24:447, 1975.

# RABIES 167

*Bosko Postic, M.D.*
*Tadeusz J. Wiktor, D.V.M.*

## DEFINITION AND ETIOLOGY

Rabies is a viral infection of the central nervous system affecting all warm-blooded animals including man. The disease is caused by rabies virus and is usually transmitted by saliva falling onto wounds inflicted by rabid animals. Overt disease, consisting of fever, excitation, convulsions, lacrimation, salivation, and dysphagia, is known as "furious rabies." The human disease is also known as hydrophobia. Another form of the disease is known as "dumb rabies." It is characterized by progressive lassitude, coma, and death. Human rabies is almost invariably fatal, except for three recently documented survivors (Hattwick et al., 1972; Porras et al., 1976).

Rabies virus belongs to a group of rhabdoviruses with a characteristic bullet-shaped form, dimensions of $75 \times 180$ nm, a ribonucleoprotein core, and a lipid envelope. Rhabdoviruses are inactivated by lipid solvents such as ether. They are described in greater detail in Chapter 4.

Rabies virus was isolated by Pasteur and co-workers in the 1880s. They discovered vaccination and introduced the widely used terms "street" and "fixed" strains. Fixed virus was produced in Pasteur's laboratory by repeated intracerebral passages of infected neural tissue in rabbits so that the incubation period became fixed at a shorter interval of five to ten days, whereas naturally circulating (street) strains produced encephalitis after a variable period of 15 to 30 days. Street strains have a wide host range and are infectious by peripheral inoculation. Transfer of infection in nature occurs by means of the virus in salivary glands. In contrast, fixed strains have diminished infectiousness when they are inoculated peripherally, and, as a rule, do not appear in the saliva of rabid animals. Fixed strains can serve for vaccine production because the original antigenicity appears to be maintained. Street strains are also antigenically stable.

## PATHOGENESIS AND PATHOLOGY

After inoculation into experimental animals, the infectious virus can persist for four to six days close to the site of injection. The infection has been shown by immunofluorescence to start in striated muscle cells close to the site of inoculation. Amputation of the limb or cutting of the nerves proximal to inoculation prevents rabies in animals. The concept of neural spread of the virus is based on this observation. Viral replication has not been demonstrated in any of the peripheral nerve structures. After mouse foot pad inoculation, the virus moves probably passively via tissue interspaces within the nerve. More recent immunofluorescent studies suggest that the earliest replication in neural cells occurs in the dorsal root ganglia. Thereafter, the virus involves the adjacent cord segment.

After this initial invasion of the central nervous system, the virus disseminates in a rapid and selective manner: It attacks the neuronal cells of the brain stem, the hippocampus, the subcortical nuclei, the limbic cortex, and the Purkinje cells in the cerebellum. In the second phase, the virus spreads from the CNS through nerves to diverse organs such as the eye, salivary glands, tongue, skin, and heart. Replication takes place in these tissues. Certain cells, such as salivary glandular epithelium, support efficiently the production of rabies virions.

The histopathology of rabies consists of (1) encephalomyelitis and (2) specific inclusions known as Negri bodies (Derakhshan, 1975).

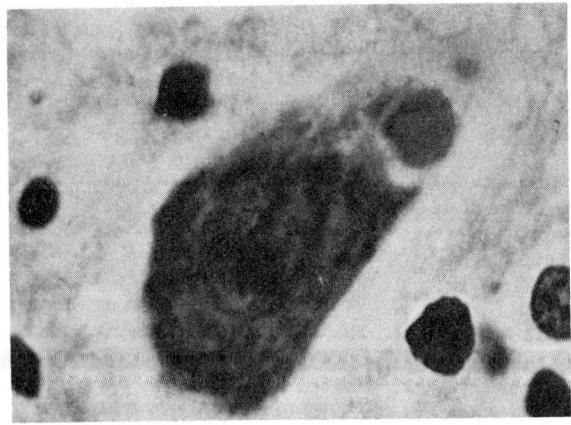

**FIGURE 1.** *Purkinje cell with intracytoplasmic eosinophilic inclusion body (hematoxylin-eosin, paraffin embedded, × 600). (From Derakhshan, I: Arch Neurol 32:75, 1975.)*

This encephalomyelitis is characterized by neuronal changes (see below) and predominantly lymphocytic infiltration, both diffuse and perivascular. Thrombosis may occur in the affected areas. Neuroglial reaction, composed mainly of astrocytes, is frequent, particularly in the substantia nigra. Oligodendroglial reaction occurs also, and has a predilection for the cord. The above changes are suggestive but not diagnostic of rabies, since other viruses cause similar changes.

Negri bodies (Fig. 1), which are specific for rabies virus encephalitis, are intracytoplasmic inclusions in neurons (Derakhshan, 1975). They are 2 to 10 $\mu$m in size and are found in the central pyramidal layer of Ammon's horn of the hippocampus, in the Purkinje cells of the cerebellum, and, less frequently, in the motor area of the cerebral cortex and medullary nuclei. Negri bodies consist of rabies virus ribonucleoprotein and are mostly acidophilic inclusions with central basophilic granules, which are demonstrable by the Seller's stain containing basic fuchsin and methylene blue. The reaction of these intracytoplasmic forms with rabies antibody, coupled to fluorescein dye or peroxidase, establishes the diagnosis of rabies histologically.

## CLINICAL MANIFESTATIONS, COMPLICATIONS, AND SEQUELAE

The usual mode of infection for man is through a bite by a rabid animal. This does not necessarily lead to infection. In 1953, Iranian workers described an accident in which a rabid wolf bit 32 persons; rabies was contracted by 60 per cent of the victims sustaining head wounds and only 30 per cent of those with peripheral bites. Unlike most infectious diseases, subclinical rabies is not recognized in humans.

Bites are not the only mode of transmission. Scratches by rabid cats have produced rabies in humans, since transfer of virus from the saliva is easily accomplished. Only one human-to-human transmission through infective saliva has been recorded. Aerosol infection of man via the respiratory route has been observed also. (Tillotson et al., 1977).

The incubation period of human rabies is long. The median is 31 to 60 days. Approximately 15 per cent of victims develop rabies after three months, and only 1.2 per cent develop disease later than 1 year after exposure.

The clinical illness in man may be divided into five stages as seen in Figure 2 (Hattwick, 1974). During the incubation period, stage 1, there are generally no symptoms, and clinical illness begins with stage 2, the prodrome, consisting of malaise, anorexia, fatigue, headache, and fever. Pain or paresthesias at or close to the site of exposure are reported in 20 to 80 per cent of cases. After a prodromal period of from two to ten days, stage 3, the phase of acute neurologic symptoms, develops. The manifestations include hyperactivity, disorientation, hallucinations, seizures, bizarre behavior, and nuchal stiffness or paralysis. The hyperactivity is usually intermittent; periods of agitation, thrashing, or other bizarre behavior last a few minutes. They occur spontaneously or may be precipitated by tactile, auditory, visual, or other stimuli. Between these periods the patient is usually cooperative and able to communicate.

Hydrophobia or the fear of water results after attempts to drink or eat produce severe, painful spasms of the pharynx and larynx and precipitate hyperactivity. Subsequently, the mere sight of water may precipitate a similar episode. Many patients experience milder hydrophobia and are willing to drink, suffering pharyngeal spasms only upon contact of water with the oral or pharyngeal mucosa. Other abnormalities include muscle fasciculations, particularly near the site of exposure, hyperventilation, hypersalivation, and focal or generalized convulsions. Paralysis generally becomes the major problem unless the patient dies abruptly. In approximately 20 per cent of patients, paralysis dominates the clinical picture ("dumb rabies"). Paralysis may be generalized, asymmetrical with maximal involvement of the bitten extremity, or ascending as in the Landry Guillain-Barré syndrome. Paralytic rabies appears frequently after exposure to some strains of rabies virus, such as those from vampire bats.

During the acute neurologic phase, the patient's mental status gradually deteriorates over

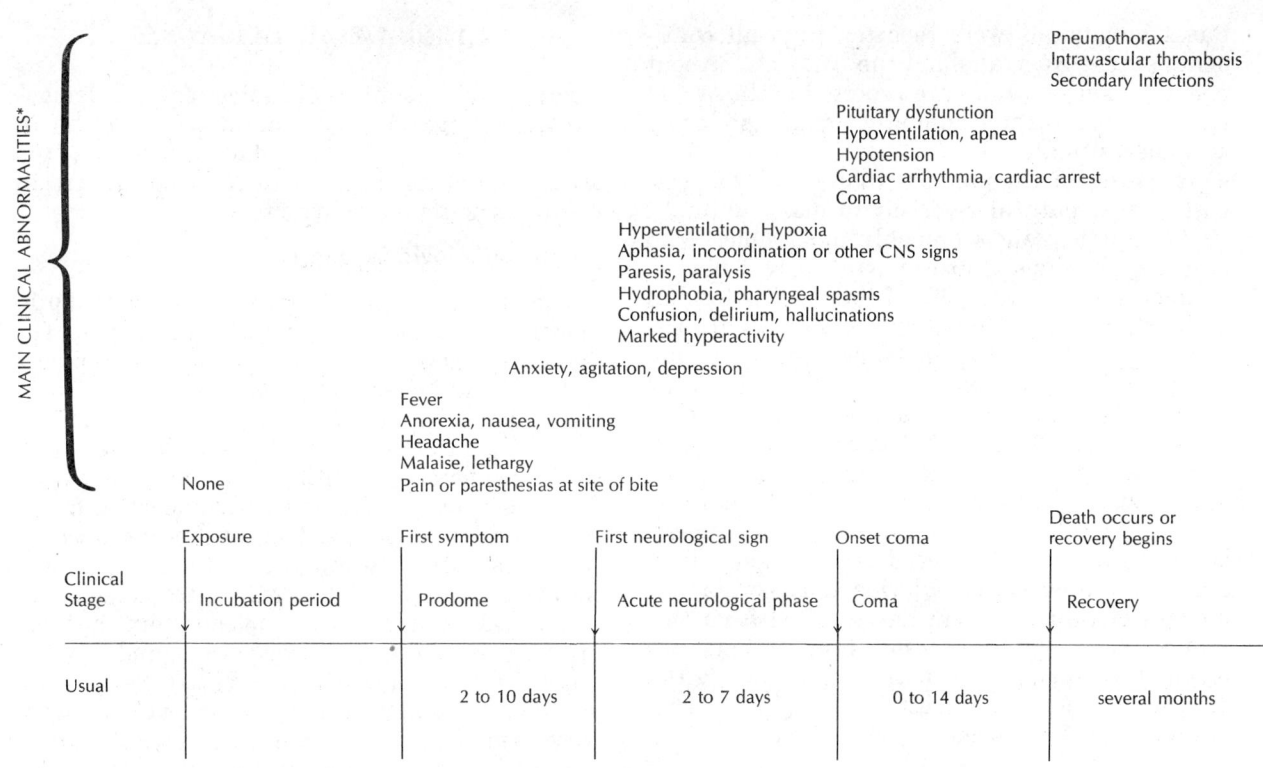

**FIGURE 2.** *The natural history of clinical rabies in man, hypothetical composite case. (From Hattwick, M.A.W.: Human Rabies, Public Health Reports, 3:229, 1974.)*

two to ten days, leading either to sudden fatal cardiac or respiratory arrest or to stage 4, the onset of coma lasting for hours or days, or rarely, months. The latter course has been seen in patients receiving modern cardiorespiratory supportive care. After a coma lasting from one to two weeks, the course has stabilized in several cases. In most, the patient died after prolonged support.

Recovery, stage 5, has been reported in three patients suffering from rabies, which was documented by exposures to rabid animals and elaborate serologic studies. In the first patient, a 6-year-old boy in the United States, and the second, a 45-year-old woman in Argentina, clinical recovery was complete or nearly complete within six months. No significant residual neurologic sequelae were observed after follow-up studies exceeding one year (Hattwick et al., 1972; Porras et al., 1972). The third patient was exposed to rabies virus aerosols and, despite previous vaccination and the presence of virus neutralizing antibody (1:32), developed rabies. He recovered partially, became ambulatory but was aphasic six months after rabies developed in April, 1977 (Tillotson et al.). In each surviving patient, the cerebrospinal fluid (CSF) contained a high level of antibody to rabies virus — approximately one third to one fourth of the serum titer. High CSF antibody is

seen in viral encephalitis but now following vaccination. In none of the survivors was rabies virus isolated.

## GEOGRAPHIC VARIATION IN DISEASE

According to the report of the World Health Organization, only the following countries were considered to be free from rabies in 1975.

**AFRICA**
Mauritius

**AMERICA**
French Guiana
Jamaica
Netherlands Antilles
Surinam
Uruguay
West Indies (St. Kitts, St. Lucia)

**ASIA**
Hong Kong
Kuwait
Singapore
United Arab Emirates

**EUROPE**
Cyprus
Denmark
Faroe Islands
Finland
Gibraltar
Iceland
Italy
Norway
Portugal
Sweden
United Kingdom

**OCEANIA**
Australia
Guam
New Zealand
Papua New Guinea

Cases in humans were reported from all continents except Australia and the Antarctic. About 700 deaths from rabies are reported to the World Health Organization annually, which is clearly an underestimate.

As stated in Chapter 64, rabies is a zoonosis with a vast natural reservoir in many animals. Global eradication is probably impossible. Wild animals, skunks and foxes particularly, emerged as important transmitters of the disease to man after 1960. In the United States, skunks are the most frequent rabid animals, accounting for approximately 50 per cent of animal cases reported in 1976. Skunks are also efficient transmitters, owing to the high content of virus in their saliva. Domestic animals, dogs, and cats have not transmitted disease in the United States since 1965; vaccination and the elimination of strays are to be credited for this reduced transmission. Raccoon rabies is enzootic in Florida and Georgia, but no case of rabies in man has resulted from this source. Approximately 1 per cent of bats are infected. Although they do not communicate the disease efficiently to terrestrial animals, several human cases have been traced to them.

## DIFFERENTIAL DIAGNOSIS

Occasionally rabies is discovered at autopsy of persons dying of an unidentified encephalitis. This usually occurs in cases with an atypical onset — lack of prodromes, lack of hydrophobia, early coma, and early paralysis. The exaggerated anxiety may be mistaken for hysteria.

On the other hand, local paresthesias at the site of the bite and hydrophobia are occasionally seen in persons who did not develop rabies. In cases of proven exposure to a rabid animal and a typical course, the differential diagnosis of rabies in man presents few problems.

Differentiation from other encephalitides may be more difficult. The enterovirus and arbovirus encephalitides commonly present diffuse alterations of the sensorium with no localizing signs and lack the characteristic waxing and waning course and hydrophobia. Cerebrospinal fluid in enteroviral and arboviral encephalitides, as well as in lymphocytic choriomeningitis, typically shows elevated leukocyte counts. In clinical rabies, CSF leukocyte counts may be normal or only slightly elevated. Herpes virus encephalitis may closely mimic clinical rabies, but brain scans often show focal herpetic lesions in contrast to the diffuse encephalitis of rabies. However, laboratory procedures may be necessary to distinguish these two infections.

## LABORATORY DIAGNOSIS

Laboratory diagnosis of rabies requires demonstration of specific inclusions (Negri bodies) in infected tissues, isolation and identification of the virus from brain tissue or saliva, and, in certain instances, special serologic tests.

### Histopathologic Diagnosis

The histopathology of rabies was discussed previously under Pathogenesis and Pathology. The diagnostic findings consist of acute encephalomyelitis and Negri bodies (Fig. 1) and immunologic identification of the inclusion content as rabies virus ribonucleoprotein. For this identification, specific rabies antibody, conjugated with a fluorescent dye, is reacted with smears of frozen sections of brain tissue. The fluorescent antibody (FA) combines with antigen in the cytoplasm of the infected cells, and under the ultraviolet microscope, rabies virus ribonucleoprotein appears bright green against a dark background.

Several procedures have recently been introduced for the diagnosis of rabies in living patients (Bryceson et al., 1975). Since FA antigen can be present in the corneal epithelium during the incubation period, the "corneal test" was introduced with varying success. A positive test indicates rabies; a negative finding, however, does not rule it out. FA staining of scrapings from the oronasal mucosa and of frozen sections of skin biopsy specimens may also be used.

### Isolation and Identification of Rabies Virus

For this purpose, young adult, weanling, or baby white mice are inoculated intracerebrally with a suspension of brain tissue. Newborn animals are most sensitive, permitting virus isolations that would otherwise be missed. Inoculated animals must be observed for sickness or death for at least four weeks. The incubation period in mice is from 9 to 18 days for street rabies virus but only 5 to 6 days for fixed strains. Rabies antigen can sometimes be detected by FA as early as the second day after inoculation in the brains of test mice. The virus must also be identified by the neutralization test. For this, antibody to rabies virus is mixed with infective brain tissue before it is inoculated into animals. In a positive test, the animals survive an otherwise lethal challenge. Neutralizing antibody in the serum or CSF of a victim can be evaluated in less than 24 hours by using the indirect FA method. In this procedure, dilutions of serum are first reacted with preparations of antigen (usually infected cells in culture); in the second step, FA against human gammaglobulin is used to detect antigen-antibody complexes that were formed during the first step of the reaction.

Antibody conjugated to peroxidase can be used instead of fluorescein, in which case preparations are examined with an ordinary light microscope.

## TREATMENT

Survival may be prolonged more than two weeks after the onset of symptoms in patients treated in intensive care units. Recovery from rabies has been reported in three patients, as described earlier. The recovery of the first patient was attributed to the anticipation and prompt treatment of hypoxemia and intracranial hypertension (through the insertion of an intraventricular catheter placed at the time of brain biopsy), as well as to the control of cardiac arrhythmia and seizures. Recovery from rabies may be obstructed by cardiac arrhythmias, cardiac arrest, pulmonary and systemic nosocomial infections, respiratory failure, and complications of neurosurgery following brain biopsy. Cardiac complications such as arrhythmia and congestive failure probably arise from the associated myocarditis or anoxia.

## PROPHYLAXIS

### Postexposure Prophylaxis

This practice dates from Pasteur and is unique in the treatment of an infectious disease. Next to vaccine injections, known as the Pasteur treatment, two more measures are equally important and should be considered in each case. These are the local treatment of the wound and the administration of rabies-immune serum, or immunoglobulin.

After a bite, local treatment of the wound should be undertaken immediately. Experimental evidence indicates that washing with soap and water is very effective. The application of 40 to 70 per cent ethyl alcohol or an antiseptic such as benzyl ammonium chloride (Zephiran) should follow. The wound should not be sutured.

The epidemiologic circumstances of the bite must be examined before initiating immunoprophylaxis. Healthy dogs and cats are quarantined for ten days. If they show no signs of rabies, no treatment is offered to bitten persons. The risks of rabies from a vaccinated domestic animal is very small. Small rodents, mice, squirrels, and rats have not transmitted rabies to man in the United States and only very rarely elsewhere. Bites by wild animals, particularly bats and skunks, are an immediate indication for treatment with all measures available.

Animal brain samples should be secured whenever feasible. The physician should not wait for laboratory confirmation of rabies by FA to initiate treatment. The laboratory results should dictate the continuation or discontinuation of the prophylactic regimen described below.

The United States Public Health Service and the World Health Organization provide postexposure guides, as shown in Table 1 (Center for Disease Control, 1976; WHO Technical Report Series, 1973). Most injuries sustained from animals suspected to be rabid call for both vaccine and serum therapy. The vaccine is given subcutaneously, frequently into the skin over the abdomen because the area is large enough for multiple injections.

Until recently, duck embryo vaccine (DEV) and nervous tissue vaccine (NTV) were used. Both contain inactivated virus. The reputation for effectiveness of NTV is based on experience in countries with a high incidence of rabies such as India. Due to the relative frequency of postvaccinal neurologic complications with NTV (0.01 to 3 per cent), DEV was preferred until 1977 (see below). It is assumed to be effective because it stimulates rabies virus-neutralizing antibodies, and rabies is rare (1:25,800) in persons so vaccinated. Local reactions occur in over half of DEV recipients, but neuroparalytic sequelae are rare (1:25,000). Multiple doses of DEV occasionally fail to stimulate antibody, which is suppressed by concurrently administered antiserum. For this reason, the full course consists of 21 daily doses of DEV vaccine, followed by boosters on the thirty-first and forty-first days whenever antiserum is used. Even with this treatment, rabies develops in individual victims.

If equine rabies anti-serum is used, the recommended dose is 40 international units per kilogram, and equal parts are instilled around the site of the bite and intramuscularly. Human rabies immunoglobulin (HRIG) is preferred because it produces fewer allergic reactions. The recommended dose is 20 international units per kilogram.

The effectiveness of serum plus vaccine treatment was established in a well-known trial in Iran in 1954 when a rabid wolf bit 18 persons. Rabies developed in three of the five victims receiving 21 injections of vaccine (NTV) alone, while only 1 of 13 persons receiving vaccine and serum succumbed to the disease.

Wiktor and Koprowski and their associates at the Wistar Institute in Philadelphia have developed a human diploid cell-derived rabies vaccine (HDCV), in which the virus was concentrated, purified, and inactivated by beta-propiolactone

## TABLE 1.
### A. LOCAL TREATMENT OF WOUNDS INVOLVING POSSIBLE EXPOSURE TO RABIES

(1) **Recommended in All Exposures**

(a) *First-aid treatment*

Since elimination of rabies virus at the site of infection by chemical or physical means is the most effective mechanism of protection, immediate washing and flushing with soap and water, detergent, or water alone is imperative (recommended procedure in all bite wounds, including those unrelated to possible exposure to rabies). Then apply either 40–70% alcohol, tincture or aqueous solutions of iodine, or 0.1% quaternary ammonium compounds.*

(b) *Treatment by or under direction of a physician*

(1) Treat as above (a) and then:
(2) apply antirabies serum by careful instillation in the depth of the wound and by infiltration around the wound;
(3) postpone suturing of wound; if suturing is necessary use antiserum locally as stated above;
(4) where indicated, institute antitetanus procedures and administer antibiotics and drugs to control infections other than rabies.

### B. SPECIFIC SYSTEMIC TREATMENT

| Nature of Exposure | Status of Biting Animal Irrespective of Previous Vaccination | | Recommended Treatment |
|---|---|---|---|
| | At Time of Exposure | During 10 Days[a] | |
| I. Contact, but no lesions; indirect contact; no contact | Rabid | — | None |
| II. Licks of the skin; scratches or abrasions; minor bites (covered areas of arms, trunk, and legs) | (a) Suspected as rabid[b] | Healthy | Start vaccine. Stop treatment if animal remains healthy for 5 days [a, c] |
| | | Rabid | Start vaccine; administer serum upon positive diagnosis and complete the course of vaccine |
| | (b) Rabid; wild animal,[d] or animal unavailable for observation | | Serum + vaccine |
| III. Licks of mucosa; major bites (multiple or on face, head, finger, or neck) | Suspect[b] or rabid domestic or wild[d] animal, or animal unavailable for observation | | Serum + vaccine. Stop treatment if animal remains healthy for 5 days[a, c] |

[a]Observation period in this chart applies only to dogs and cats.

[b]All unprovoked bites in endemic areas should be considered suspect unless proved negative by laboratory examination (brain FA).

[c]Or if its brain is found negative by FA examination.

[d]In general, exposure to rodents and rabbits seldom, if ever, requires specific antirabies treatment.

*Where soap has been used to clean wounds, all traces of it should be removed before the application of quaternary ammonium compounds because soap neutralizes the activity of such compounds.

World Health Organization Expert Committee on Rabies, Sixth Report. Geneva, 1973.

(Wiktor et al., 1964). After trials in volunteers established high immunogenicity and a low frequency of local reactions, the vaccine was used in a postexposure field trial in Iran (Wiktor et al., 1973). Forty-five persons bitten by rabid dogs and wolves were treated in 1975 by Bahmanyar and co-workers (Bahmanyar et al., 1976) with one dose of heterologous antiserum intramuscularly and only five doses of HDCV inoculated subcutaneously on days 0, 3, 7, 14, 30 with a booster on day

90. All patients survived. Judging from past experiences in similar settings, case fatalities of no less than 35 per cent could have been expected had the victims not been treated. A fatality-free therapeutic trial of this magnitude has not been previously noted with other vaccines. Thus a major breakthrough may have been achieved by HDCV in the postexposure treatment of rabies.

Experimental injection of hyperimmune serum alone after exposure usually delays the onset but does not prevent rabies. Antibodies probably neutralize the virus outside of the CNS during the early incubation period. Once the neurons are infected, antibodies are ineffective. The precise mechanism of protection produced by postexposure vaccination has not been fully defined. Both humoral and cellular immunity was induced by the inactivated rabies vaccines (Wiktor et al., 1977). In experimental animals, the HDCV induced interferon also (Wiktor et al., 1972). Thus antibody, cell immunity, and interferon may all contribute to protection.

### Pre-exposure Prophylaxis

This consists usually of four DEV or, preferably, three HDCV injections at weekly intervals, followed by a booster dose at nine weeks or later. Alternate inoculation schedules are also used. Irrespective of the type of vaccine or schedule, sera of all persons undergoing this type of immunization should be tested for neutralizing antibodies at three weeks after the booster dose. A successful pre-exposure vaccination, judged by seroconversion, allows a shorter course of one to four injections of vaccine upon exposure to a rabid animal. The titer of antibody indicating immunity has not been ascertained. The United States Center for Disease Control recommended in August, 1977, that persons working with rabies virus be surveyed annually and revaccinated if their serum antibody level should fall below 1:16.

### References

Bahmanyar, M., Fayaz, A., Nour-Salehi, S., Mohammadi, M., and Koprowski, H.: Successful protection of humans exposed to rabies infection. JAMA 236:2751, 1976.

Bryceson, A. M. D., Greenwood, B. M., Warrell, D. A., Davidson, N., Pope, H. M., Lawrie, J. H., Barnes, H. J., Bailie, W. E., and Wilcox, G. E.: Demonstration during life of rabies antigen in humans. J Infect Dis 131:71, 1975.

Center for Disease Control: Recommendations of the Public Health Service Advisory Committee on Immunization Practices: Rabies. Morbid Mortal Wkly Rep 25: Dec 31, 1976.

Derakhshan, I.: Is the Negri body specific for rabies? Arch Neurol 32:75, 1975.

Hattwick, M. A. W.: Human rabies. Public Health Rev 2:229, 1974.

Hattwick, M. A. W., Weis, T. T., Stechschulte, C. K., et al.: Recovery from rabies. A case report. Ann Intern Med 76:931, 1972.

Porras, C., Barboza, J. J., Fuenzalida, E., Adaros, H. L., Oviedo de Diaz A. M., and Furst, J.: Recovery from rabies in man. Ann Intern Med 85:44, 1976.

Tillotson, J. R., Frock, J. L., Woodruff, J. V., and Martinez, L. B.: Inhalation rabies despite effective pre-exposure vaccination. Seventeenth Interscience Conference on Antimicrobial Agents and Chemotherapy, American Society for Microbiology, Washington, D.C., 1977, Program and Abstracts, Abstract 461.

World Health Organization, Expert Committee on Rabies. Sixth Report. WHO Technical Report Series, No. 523. Geneva, World Health Organization, 1973.

Wiktor, T. J., Doherty, P. C., and Koprowski, H.: In vitro evidence of cell-mediated immunity after exposure of mice to both live and inactivated rabies virus. Proc Natl Acad Sci USA 74:334, 1977.

Wiktor, T. J., Fernandes, N. V., and Koprowski, H.: Cultivation of rabies virus in human diploid cell strain WI38. J Immunol 93:353, 1964.

Wiktor, T. J., Plotkin, S. A., and Grella, D. W.: Human cell culture rabies vaccine. Antibody response in man. JAMA 224:1170, 1973.

Wiktor, T. J., Postic, B., Ho, M., and Koprowski, H.: Role of interferon induction in the protective activity of rabies vaccines. J Infect Dis 126:408, 1972.

# HERPES SIMPLEX ENCEPHALITIS AND MENINGITIS    **168**

## Michael N. Oxman, M.D.

### DEFINITION

Symptomatic involvement of the central nervous system is a rare manifestation of herpes simplex virus (HSV) infection. It may take one of several forms depending, at least in part, upon the antigenic type of the HSV involved, the age and immunologic status of the host, and the route of infection.

Herpes simplex encephalitis is an acute necrotizing viral encephalitis that, beyond the neonatal period, is nearly always caused by HSV Type 1. It has a higher mortality rate than most other forms of viral encephalitis and appears to account for the majority of cases of sporadically occurring acute necrotizing encephalitis in the Western World. In the neonate, herpes simplex encephalitis is usually caused by HSV Type 2, which is acquired during passage through the birth canal of a mother with genital herpes. The encephalitis occurs most often as one component of a disseminated neonatal HSV infection. In the neonate, as in the adult, herpes simplex encephalitis carries a grave prognosis.

Herpes simplex meningitis is an acute aseptic meningitis that occurs mainly in young sexually active adults, frequently in association with genital herpes. It is almost always caused by HSV Type 2, which may be isolated from the spinal fluid. In contrast to herpes simplex encephalitis, herpes simplex meningitis usually follows a brief and benign course, although it may sometimes be associated with polyradiculitis and, rarely, with ascending myelitis. In some patients, the meningitis may recur in association with recurrent episodes of genital herpes.

## ETIOLOGY

Herpes simplex virus (herpesvirus hominis) is a member of the herpesvirus group (Chapter 56), which includes three other human herpesviruses: varicella-zoster virus, cytomegalovirus, and Epstein-Barr virus. All of these herpesviruses are morphologically indistinguishable and share a number of properties, including a remarkable propensity for establishing latent infections that persist for the life of the host. HSV consists of an internal core containing the viral genome, a linear molecule of double-stranded DNA with a molecular weight of 100 million. The core is enclosed within an icosahedral capsid 100 nm in diameter and is composed of 162 identical protein subunits (capsomers). This nucleocapsid is surrounded by one or two additional layers of protein and, finally, by a loose lipoprotein envelope derived from the nuclear membrane of the host cell. The complete virion is roughly spherical with a diameter of 150 to 200 nm. The envelope contains radially oriented viral glycoproteins that mediate the attachment of the virion to susceptible host cells. Only enveloped virions are fully infectious, and this accounts for the lability of HSV; infectivity is rapidly destroyed by organic solvents, detergents, proteolytic enzymes, heat, and extremes of pH. The envelope glycoproteins are antigenic and elicit neutralizing antibodies in the host. In addition to structural components of the virion, certain enzymes essential for virus replication are synthesized in infected cells — for example, a virus-specific DNA polymerase and a deoxypyrimidine kinase. These viral enzymes have proved to be important as targets for specific antiviral chemotherapy.

In contrast to the other human herpesviruses, HSV has a wide host range. HSV infection can be established in many experimental hosts, including rats, mice, hamsters, guinea pigs, rabbits nonhuman primates, and chick embryos, and in a wide variety of cell cultures established in vitro from human and animal tissues. The cytopathic effect of HSV in such cell cultures is characterized by the formation of acidophilic Cowdry Type A intranuclear inclusion bodies and multinucleated giant cells. The same cytopathology is seen in cutaneous and visceral lesions in vivo. These changes are indistinguishable from those produced by varicella zoster virus but, whereas the cytopathic effect of varicella-zoster virus in tissue culture remains focal because progeny virus remains cell associated, HSV is released into the medium by initially infected cells and rapidly spreads to infect cells throughout the culture.

There are two distinct serotypes of HSV, HSV Type 1 and HSV Type 2, which share about 50 per cent of their DNA base sequences. HSV Type 1 and HSV type 2 can be separated on the basis of antigenic, biologic, and biochemical differences (Chapter 99, Table 1), but the most obvious difference between the two types is in their clinical and epidemiologic behavior. HSV Type 1, the agent recovered from cases of acute herpetic gingivostomatitis and from most cutaneous lesions above the waist, is responsible for virtually all cases of herpes simplex encephalitis that occur in adults and in children beyond the neonatal period. HSV Type 1 has also been isolated from the spinal fluid of children, aged 6 months to 6 years, with acute benign "aseptic meningitis" (Sawanobori et al., 1974; Skoldenberg et al., 1975). HSV Type 2, the major cause of genital herpes, causes most cases of herpes simplex meningitis and more than 70 per cent of neonatal herpes simplex virus infections.

Although HSV was isolated from the brains of several patients with encephalitis early in the century, its etiologic significance was not appreciated. Because of the ubiquity of HSV and its persistence as a latent infection in most adults, it was assumed that such isolations were merely coincidental (Drachman and Adams, 1962). It was not until 1941 that Smith, Lennette, and Reames established the etiologic role of HSV in acute necrotizing encephalitis. They isolated HSV from the brain of a 4-week-old infant with encephalitis and also demonstrated Cowdry Type A intranuclear inclusions characteristic of those produced by HSV in the cerebral lesions (Smith et al., 1941). Since then a number of reports, encompassing more than 400 cases of herpes simplex encephalitis, have described the clinical, pathologic, and epidemiologic features of the disease (Haymaker et al., 1958; Drachman and Adams, 1962; Leider et al., 1965; Rawls et al., 1966; Miller et al., 1966; Olson et al., 1967; Miller and

Ross, 1968; Rappel et al., 1971; Illis and Gostling, 1972; Oxbury and MacCullum, 1973; Sarubbi et al., 1973; Whitley et al., 1977). It is now clear that most cases of sporadically occurring acute necrotizing encephalitis in the Western World are caused by HSV. Moreover, when the virus isolated from the brain in adults and children beyond the neonatal period has been typed, it has almost invariably proved to be HSV Type 1. In herpes encephalitis in the neonate, the majority of virus isolates are HSV Type 2.

The association between benign aseptic meningitis and genital herpes was first reported by Ravaut and Darré in 1904 and has been reaffirmed in a number of later studies (Craig and Nahmias, 1973). While the number of reported isolates of HSV from the spinal fluid in cases of aseptic meningitis is small, almost all of these have been HSV Type 2, and serologic studies suggest that 1 to 5 per cent of all cases of aseptic meningitis are caused by this virus (Armstrong et al., 1943; Adair et al., 1953; Stalder et al., 1973; Skoldenberg et al., 1975; Wolontis and Jeansson, 1977).

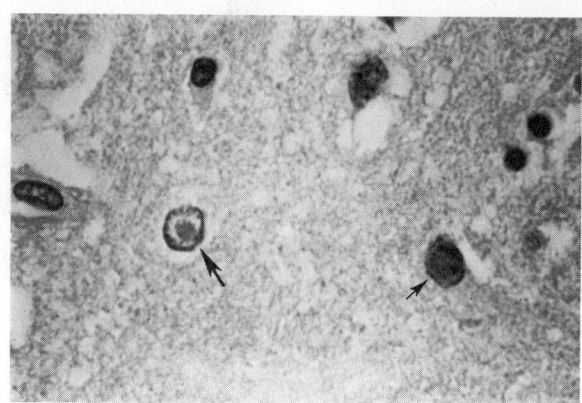

**FIGURE 1.** *Temporal lobe biopsy from a patient with herpes simplex encephalitis stained with hematoxylin and eosin. An early amphophilic Cowdry type A intranuclear inclusion body (small arrow) fills the nucleus, displacing the nucleolus to the periphery. Margination of chromatin at the nuclear membrane is already apparent. A mature eosinophilic intranuclear inclusion body (large arrow) is surrounded by a clear zone or halo. The chromatin is distributed along the nuclear membrane. (Courtesy of Dr. R. Baringer.)*

## PATHOLOGY AND PATHOGENESIS

In addition to the usual findings of viral encephalitis (that is, lymphocytic infiltration of the meninges; perivascular aggregates of lymphocytes, plasma cells, and histocytes in the cortex and subjacent white matter; and proliferation of microglia with formation of glial nodules), there are several distinctive features that serve to identify herpes simplex encephalitis (Haymaker et al., 1958; Drachman and Adams, 1962; Miller et al., 1966; Illis and Gostling, 1972).

A. Severity of the process. Lesions are not uniform in their distribution or severity, but in each case the degree of necrosis is extremely severe in the regions of greatest involvement. There are focal areas of virtually total cortical necrosis with gross softening, destruction of architecture, hemorrhage, and extensive loss of neurons and glia.

B. Topography of the lesions. Although widespread involvement is usually present at autopsy, the distribution of lesions is asymmetric, and the pathologic process is generally further advanced in one hemisphere than the other. The areas of greatest damage are in the temporal lobe, the orbital portion of the frontal lobe, and the structures forming the limbic system.

C. Inclusion bodies. Cowdry Type A intranuclear inclusion bodies are found in neurons, astrocytes, and oligodendrocytes (Fig. 1). These inclusions, the direct result of herpes simplex virus infection, are initially amphophilic and homogeneous. They fill the entire nucleus and displace the nucleolus to the periphery. The nuclear chromatin is distributed along the inner surface of the nuclear membrane. These early inclusions soon become condensed, granular, and eosinophilic, and they are then surrounded by a clear halo.

The nature and distribution of the lesions seen at autopsy are often so characteristic that the diagnosis is apparent on gross examination. In a typical case of rapidly fatal herpes simplex encephalitis (the majority of deaths occur within 2 weeks of onset) examination of the brain reveals intense hemorrhagic necrosis of the inferior and medial parts of the temporal lobe, the insula, and the orbital portion of the frontal lobe, with distinct swelling and obvious softening of the brain. The cortical surface in these areas shows engorgement of small blood vessels and petechial hemorrhages (Fig. 2). When the brain is sectioned, the cortex in the areas of major involvement is found to be congested, soft, and swollen, and there is loss of the normal demarcation between cortex and white matter. The cortex is necrotic and friable, and it contains many small hemorrhagic foci (Fig. 3), which are also present in the underlying white matter. The meninges overlying these areas of intense cortical necrosis are opaque, but they appear normal in other areas. There is often evidence of extensive cerebral edema with uncal and cerebellar tonsillar herniation. Microscopic examination reveals hyperemia and perivascular infiltration by lymphocytes,

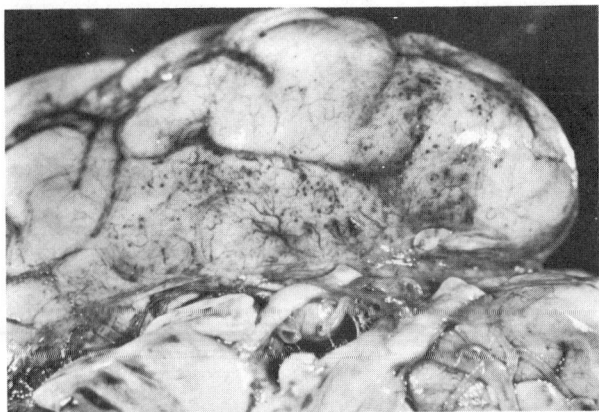

**FIGURE 2.** *Medial aspect of the temporal lobe of a patient with herpes simplex encephalitis. Note the diffuse petechial eruption and the engorgement of small blood vessels. (Courtesy of Dr. R. Baringer.)*

plasma cells, and macrophages in the meninges overlying areas of obvious cortical pathology. In the underlying brain, the necrosis is primarily cortical, but the degree of destruction varies from place to place, even within regions of maximal involvement. In some places, the entire cortex is necrotic, with disintegration of nerve cells and glia and focal hemorrhage into the destroyed tissue. In other areas, there are glial proliferation and neuronophagia. The lesions are most pronounced beneath the pia in the upper cortical laminae. Small blood vessels are engorged and show endothelial cell hypertrophy. There are perivascular collections of lymphocytes, plasma cells and large mononuclear cells, and, in areas of severe cortical necrosis, perivascular hemorrhages. Necrotic foci may progress and coalesce, giving rise to areas of cavitation. Focal necrosis,

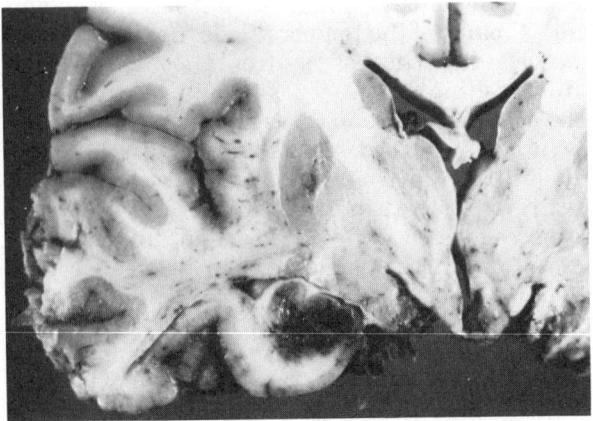

**FIGURE 3.** *The brain of a patient with fatal herpes simplex encephalitis. Coronal section through the affected temporal lobe at the level of the thalamus showing hemorrhagic necrosis involving the hippocampus and adjacent cortical tissue, and focal areas of hemorrhage in the temporal lobe cortex. Congested vessels and small hemorrhages are also visible in the subjacent white matter.*

hemorrhage, and pallor of myelin are seen in subcortical white matter in areas where the overlying cortex is severely affected, but there is no evidence of primary demyelination. Cowdry Type A intranuclear inclusion bodies (Fig. 1) are present in neurons, oligodendrocytes, and astrocytes.

Electron microscopic examination reveals viral nucleocapsids within the nuclei of infected neurons and glia. The nucleocapsids can be seen in clumps and also arrayed along the inner surface of the nuclear membrane (Fig. 4A–C). Occasionally, herpes simplex virus nucleocapsids can be seen budding through the inner lamella of the nuclear membrane in areas that are thickened by the addition of virus-specified glycoproteins (Fig. 4D). Complete enveloped virions can be seen in intercellular spaces and occasionally in the cytoplasm (Fig. 4E).

In neonatal herpes simplex encephalitis, the lesions are similar to those that are seen in the older child and adult. However, they are generally more widely and uniformly distributed, without the characteristic orbitofrontal and temporal lobe localization described above.

In addition to their importance as diagnostic criteria, these unique pathologic features of herpes simplex encephalitis reflect its pathogenesis and provide the anatomic basis for the signs and symptoms of the disease.

Clinical and pathologic evidence indicates that in herpes simplex encephalitis in children and adults infection initially involves the orbitofrontal and temporal regions of one hemisphere and only later extends to contiguous areas and to the opposite hemisphere. This localization is not explained by the selective vulnerability of a specific subset of neurons. Unlike poliovirus, which essentially infects and destroys only motor neurons, HSV is unrestricted in its capacity to infect cells within the central nervous system. In autopsy material, HSV inclusions and virions are seen in both neurons and glia over a contiguous anatomic area, as if the virus had spread from cell to cell along the base of the brain within the middle and anterior fossae (Davis and Johnson, 1979). It has been suggested that this localization may reflect the route of entry of HSV into the central nervous system. Thus, Johnson and Mims (1968) postulated that, during primary infection, HSV might infect the olfactory mucosa, enter the central nervous system via olfactory pathways, and then spread along the base of the brain. While this route of infection can lead to localized encephalitis in some animal models, it often results in meningitis with virus present in the spinal fluid. HSV is almost never recovered from the spinal fluid of children and adults with herpes simplex encephalitis. Other characteristics of herpes simplex encephalitis in humans are also inconsistent with the olfactory route of infection, at least in the majority of cases. In spite of many careful attempts at virus isolation early in the course of herpes simplex encephalitis, HSV has only rarely been recovered from the nasopharynx. Furthermore, many patients have come to autopsy with extensive orbitofrontal and temporal lobe pathology, but with little or no involvement of the olfactory bulbs.

Herpes simplex encephalitis does not always represent primary infection with HSV Type 1. In 20 to 25 per cent of patients with herpes simplex encephalitis, there is a past history of recurrent herpes labialis, an incidence no different from that in the general population. This suggests that the risk of herpes simplex encephalitis is not greatly reduced in people already infected with HSV Type 1 — that is, in people for whom herpes simplex encephalitis would represent a recurrent infection. It is now well established that during primary oropharyngeal HSV infections (which are usually asymptomatic) virus spreads centripetally to the trigeminal ganglia along branches of the trigeminal nerve and establishes latent infection in sensory neurons. Episodes of recurrent herpes labialis or of asymptomatic oropharyngeal virus shedding result when this latent HSV in the trigeminal ganglion is activated and passes centrifugally down the axon to initiate infection in the skin or oropharyngeal mucosa. Between episodes of recurrent herpes labialis, the virus remains latent in sensory neurons in the ipsilateral trigeminal ganglion. Perhaps unfortunately, sensory fibers from the trigeminal ganglia also innervate basilar structures in the middle and anterior fossae that correspond to the areas of cortex most severely involved in herpes simplex encephalitis. These considerations have led Davis and Johnson (1979) to propose that herpes simplex encephalitis results from the direct spread of HSV along nerve fibers from the trigeminal ganglion to the anterior and middle fossae. This would account for the orbitofrontal and temporal lobe localization, both in patients in whom the encephalitis is a manifestation of primary infection with HSV Type 1 and in patients with a prior history of recurrent herpes labialis, in whom encephalitis is almost certainly a recurrent infection. The recent demonstration that human superior cervical and vagus ganglia may also be latently infected with HSV Type 1 reveals another neural route by which this virus can reach the central nervous system (Warren et al., 1978).

The trigeminal route would also explain the almost exclusive role of HSV Type 1 in herpes simplex encephalitis beyond the neonatal period. HSV Type 2 is at least as neuropathic as HSV Type 1, but it is very rarely isolated from patients with primary herpes stomatitis, herpes keratitis, recurrent herpes labialis, or recurrent herpetic lesions of the facial skin. Furthermore, only HSV Type 1 has been recovered from latently infected human trigeminal ganglia. Thus, in children and adults, HSV Type 2 does not ordinarily have access to the central nervous system by the trigeminal route. We can predict that, if sustained, the recent increase in the incidence of oropharyngeal infections caused by HSV Type 2 will eventually result in an increase in the frequency with which HSV Type 2 is isolated from cases of herpes simplex encephalitis in adults.

Involvement of the central nervous system is recognized in 50 per cent or more of infants with neonatal HSV infection. In the majority, meningoencephalitis is but one component of a disseminated HSV infection in which there is extensive visceral involvement and viremic spread to the meninges and brain (Nahmias and Visintine, 1976). Pathologic changes are similar to those observed in the adult, but there is no orbitofrontal or temporal lobe localization. Lesions are widely disseminated throughout the meninges and the entire brain, and virus is readily isolated from the spinal fluid. However, 25 to 30 per cent of infants with HSV infection involving the central nervous system have no evidence of disseminated disease. Almost all such infants also have herpetic lesions of the eye, mouth, or skin. Virus is rarely isolated from the spinal fluid in infants with this localized central nervous system HSV infection, and several have had a more focal encephalitis, similar to that observed in older children and adults. Thus, although the pathogenesis of neonatal herpes simplex encephalitis usually involves the viremic spread of HSV to the central nervous system, there are some cases in which the virus may first infect the eye, mouth, or skin and then reach the brain by a neural route, perhaps via the trigeminal ganglion, as proposed in the adult.

The virus in most cases of neonatal herpes simplex encephalitis is HSV Type 2. This reflects the importance of maternal genital herpes as the source of virus in neonatal infections, and the predominance of HSV Type 2 as the cause of genital herpes. There is no detectable difference between the pathogenesis, or the nature, severity, or distribution of the pathology, in neonatal herpes simplex infections caused by HSV Type 1 and in those caused by HSV Type 2.

The risk of developing severe disease (and encephalitis) in the course of HSV infection is much greater in the neonate than in the older child or adult. In fact, beyond the neonatal period, the majority of primary HSV infections are asymptomatic. Neonatal HSV infections, on the other hand, are almost always symptomatic. The majority result in viremia and visceral dissemination, half result in central nervous system involvement, and the overall mortality is greater than 60 per cent. The factors responsible for the increased pathogenicity of HSV in the neonate have yet to be identified, but it now appears that they include a deficit in one or more components of the cellular immune response to HSV antigens, as well as the capacity of HSV to replicate in neonatal but not adult macrophages and peripheral blood leukocytes. We are even further from understanding what limits the incidence of herpes simplex encephalitis in adults, the majority of whom carry this potentially lethal virus as a lifelong tenant of their trigeminal ganglia. Reactivation of latent virus in the trigeminal ganglion with centrifugal spread to the perioral skin is certainly a common event, for at least one-quarter of the adult population is plagued by recurrent herpes labialis. The apparent rarity with which reactivated HSV spreads centrally to the meninges and brain may indicate that latency is generally established only in those neurons initially infected via axonal spread from the oral and perioral sites involved in primary infection, and that subsequent neuron-to-neuron spread within the trigeminal ganglion is uncommon.

It should be pointed out that neural and viremic spread from the ganglion are not mutually exclusive. The same immune deficit(s) that allow reactivated virus in the ganglion to replicate and spill over into the circulation may also favor spread via neural pathways.

Because of its benign course, pathologic material has not been available from cases of uncomplicated herpes simplex meningitis. The disease afflicts mainly sexually active individuals between the ages of 15 and 35 years, and approximately one-half of the documented cases have occurred in temporal association with primary herpes genitalis. Herpes simplex meningitis is almost exclusively associated with HSV Type 2. During the acute illness, HSV Type 2 can frequently be isolated from the spinal fluid and sometimes from the peripheral blood (Stalder et al., 1973; Skoldenberg et al., 1975; Hevron, 1977; Craig and Nahmias, 1973). The recovery of virus from the spinal fluid and blood has led Craig and Nahmias (1973) to propose that the route of central nervous system infection is viremic rather than neural. While this may be true in some cases, approximately one-third develop recurrent meningitis, usually accompanied by recurrent genital or perigenital herpes. These patients, as well as those in whom genital herpes is accompanied by radiculitis and ascending myelitis, suggest that activation of latent HSV Type 2 in a sacral ganglion can be followed by the direct spread of virus to the meninges and spinal cord, presumably via a neural pathway (Skoldenberg et al., 1975). This is probably the same sequence

of events that leads to the motor paralysis that occasionally accompanies herpes zoster. The isolation of HSV Type 1 from the spinal fluid in cases of acute benign aseptic meningitis in children indicates that both HSV types can cause the syndrome of benign herpes simplex meningitis.

## CLINICAL MANIFESTATIONS

### Herpes Simplex Encephalitis

The entire clinical spectrum of herpes simplex encephalitis in children and adults may not be known. It has been impossible to establish the diagnosis of herpes simplex encephalitis without demonstrating the virus or viral antigens in tissue obtained by brain biopsy or at autopsy (Johnson et al., 1968). However, brain biopsy has been reserved for patients whose clinical presentation is suggestive of the disease (that is, patients with evidence of an acute febrile encephalopathy with disordered mentation; focal cerebral signs; localization by diagnostic procedures such as electroencephalogram, brain scan, or arteriogram; and spinal fluid findings compatible with viral infection) (Whitley et al., 1977). Thus, milder, nonlocalized forms of herpes simplex encephalitis may go unrecognized. Nevertheless, analysis of recognized cases has yielded a reasonably coherent picture of the disease.

The mode of presentation, clinical manifestations, and sequelae of herpes simplex encephalitis are determined largely by the nature and distribution of the pathology — that is, acute asymmetric necrotizing encephalitis that involves primarily the orbitofrontal and temporal cortex and the limbic system. The clinical manifestations and course of the disease are quite variable, but most patients present with two recognizable groups of findings (Drachman and Adams, 1962):

1. Nonspecific changes that are seen in most forms of encephalitis. These include fever, headache, signs of meningeal irritation, nausea and vomiting, global confusion, generalized seizures, and an alteration of consciousness.
2. Changes referable to focal necrosis of the orbitofrontal and temporal cortex and the limbic system. These include anosmia, memory loss, peculiar behavior, defects of speech (especially expressive aphasia), hallucinations (particularly olfactory and gustatory hallucinations), and focal seizures.

More extensive involvement of the cerebral hemispheres is signaled by the appearance of reflex asymmetry, Babinski signs, focal (usually facial) paralysis, conjugate deviation of the eyes, ataxia, incontinence of stool and urine, hemiparesis, and coma. Cerebral edema contributes to these manifestations of herpes simplex encephalitis, and brain swelling often plays an important role in the outcome of the disease.

The most common early manifestations of herpes simplex encephalitis are fever, headache, and altered consciousness. The onset of neurologic abnormalities is often dramatic; early appearance of delirium, hemiparesis and major motor seizures, and rapid progression to coma can make the presence of a severe encephalitic process immediately obvious. In some patients, the encephalitis may progress more slowly, with expressive aphasia, paresthesias, and mental changes preceding more severe neurologic abnormalities.

Another common and important mode of presentation of herpes simplex encephalitis is one in which the most striking initial symptoms are of a "psychological" nature (Drachman and Adams, 1962; Nolan, et al., 1970; Johnson et al., 1972). There is usually a period of mild nonspecific illness lasting from one to several days and characterized by various combinations of headache, drowsiness, fever, malaise, fatigue, sore throat, rhinorrhea, photophobia, anorexia, nausea, vomiting, irritability, and abdominal pain. This is followed by the appearance of bizarre behavior characterized by disorientation, confusion, incoherent thought, memory disturbance, labile affect, and, often, sensory distortion and hallucinations. This bizarre behavior may be intermittent, alternating with periods of lethargy or sleep. The illness initially appears to be minor, and only the aberrations of behavior call attention to its serious nature. The picture is often that of an acute psychosis or delirium tremens, and many patients with herpes simplex encephalitis are admitted for psychiatric care until the appearance of localizing neurologic signs, seizures, and coma alerts their physicians to the organic nature of the disease. This is tragic, for only early diagnosis and therapy offer hope of favorably altering the grim prognosis of this disease (Whitley et al., 1977).

Fever is present initially in 80 to 90 per cent of patients and at some time during the course of the disease in almost every case. It ranges from 38 to 40.6° C (100 to 105° F) and is usually refractory to antipyretics. Headache is an early symptom in 75 per cent of patients. It is often severe and refractory to analgesics. Seizures, often focal, are also common. They occur early in 30 to 40 per cent and at some time during the course of the disease in more than 80 per cent of patients. Other localizing neurologic signs, such as cranial nerve palsies, hemiparesis, and dysphasia, occur early in the majority of patients and at some time during

the course of the disease in nearly every case. The clinical picture often suggests a space-occupying lesion in the temporoparietal area, raising the possibility of an intracranial hemorrhage or cerebral abscess. Signs of meningeal irritation are uncommon early in the course of the disease but eventually develop in more than one-half of the patients. The optic fundi often show edema and swelling of the disk, and peripapillary retinal hemorrhages. This usually reflects cerebral edema, which frequently complicates the management of patients with herpes simplex encephalitis. In some cases, however, these abnormalities are a manifestation of herpes simplex optic neuritis and retinitis, which appear to be due to contiguous spread of infection from the brain (Minckler et al., 1976; Johnson and Wisotzkey, 1977).

Although most patients with herpes simplex encephalitis present with fever, headache, alteration of consciousness, behavioral abnormalities, and localizing neurologic signs, Tucker et al. (1978) have recently described a patient with herpes simplex encephalitis whose initial illness was manifested solely as a seizure disorder. Because of the absence of fever, headache, and localizing neurologic signs until 7 days after hospital admission, the diagnosis was not made until late in the course of the disease. On rare occasions, perhaps reflecting an atypical route of entry of HSV into the central nervous system, the damage in herpes simplex encephalitis is concentrated in the brain stem. Such patients present with a brain stem encephalitis that bears little clinical resemblance to the usual case of herpes simplex encephalitis (Dayan et al., 1972).

Some cases of herpes simplex encephalitis are clearly primary infections with HSV Type 1, whereas others, occurring in patients with a history of recurrent herpes labialis and with antibody to HSV in their serum at the beginning of the illness, are almost certainly recurrent infections. Thus, it is surprising that typical herpetic lesions of the mouth, pharynx, perioral skin, or eyes are rarely present in the encephalitic patients. Furthermore, HSV is only rarely recovered from cultures of the oropharynx and has not been isolated from the blood, urine, or stool of otherwise healthy children and adults with herpes simplex encephalitis. In fact, the oropharyngeal isolation rate in patients with herpes simplex encephalitis (about 5 to 7 per cent) is no different from that in comparable patients without that disease (see Chapter 99).

The clinical course of herpes simplex encephalitis is variable, but the outlook in untreated patients is grim, with an overall mortality of 70 to 75 per cent. The illness may fluctuate in intensity during the first several days, but thereafter it generally pursues an unremitting course with progression from lethargy to coma. Coma almost always indicates severe and irreversible brain damage, for almost all comatose patients die, and the rare survivor is left with severe neurologic sequelae. The average interval from onset of symptoms to coma is 6 to 7 days, with a range of 2 days to 2 weeks. The total duration of illness is often quite short, with more than three-quarters of the deaths occurring within the first 2 weeks. The average interval from onset to death is 10 to 12 days. If recovery occurs, it usually begins during the second or third week.

Results of routine laboratory tests are normal in most patients with herpes simplex encephalitis, unless it is complicated by respiratory infection or other intercurrent illness. Some patients have a moderate leukocytosis and elevation of the erythrocyte sedimentation rate. Hyponatremia and hyposmolality are occasionally seen as a result of inappropriate secretion of antidiuretic hormone, but this can be seen in a wide variety of brain diseases.

The spinal fluid is usually abnormal from the outset, with pleocytosis and a moderately elevated protein. The spinal fluid pressure is frequently elevated, reflecting cerebral edema. However, 10 to 15 per cent of patients may have completely normal spinal fluid on the first examination and only subsequently show a rise in cell count and protein concentration. The cell count is quite variable, usually between 50 and 750 per mm$^3$, but with a range of 0 to 2500. Lymphocytes or mononuclear cells generally predominate, but there are often 10 to 25 per cent polymorphonuclear leukocytes and, especially early in the disease, most or all of the cells may be polymorphonuclear leukocytes. The protein concentration is usually elevated to between 50 and 200 mg/dl and tends to increase during the course of the disease. The glucose concentration is normal on initial examination, but may be depressed later in the disease in the presence of extensive cerebral necrosis. Erythrocytes are found in the spinal fluid initially in 40 per cent, and at some time in 70 to 80 per cent, of patients, reflecting the hemorrhagic nature of the cerebral lesions. Xanthochromia is sometimes observed. There is no clear relationship between the nature or magnitude of the spinal fluid abnormalities and the eventual outcome of the disease. HSV is almost never recovered from the spinal fluid in children and adults with herpes simplex encephalitis.

The majority of patients with proven herpes simplex encephalitis have shown temporal lobe localization on electroencephalogram, technetium brain scan, arteriogram, or computerized axial tomography, singly or in combination. The changes observed are not pathognomonic of herpes simplex encephalitis, but they do help to demonstrate the focal nature of the pathologic process and localize the area of greatest involvement for subsequent cerebral biopsy. Unfortunately, while one or more of these techniques eventually yield localizing findings in nearly every case, they often fail to do so on the first examination. The findings are nonspecific or normal in one-third of the patients during the first 5 days after the onset of neurologic signs and symptoms.

HSV infection in the newborn is usually a disseminated visceral infection with severe involvement of the liver and adrenal glands as well as many other organs (Nahmias and Visintine, 1976). The brain is affected in approximately one-half of the patients, but this may not be clinically apparent because of the severity of the disseminated visceral infection. The initial signs and symptoms of infection usually appear within the first week of life, but they may be present at birth or, rarely, appear as late as 21 days postpartum. The most common initial clinical manifestations are nonspecific, including lethargy, fever or hypothermia, vomiting, and poor feeding. Other early signs may include jaundice (with or without hepatomegaly), purpuric rash, apneic spells, respiratory distress, and cyanosis. The clinical picture resembles neonatal bacterial sepsis. Neurologic manifestations usually include generalized or focal seizures, increased intracranial pressure with a bulging fontanelle, cranial nerve palsies, opisthotonus, and flaccid or spastic paralysis. These signs and symptoms often progress to coma, decerebrate posturing, and continuous seizure activity that is difficult to control with anticonvulsants. The disease usually progresses rapidly, with death sometimes occurring within a few hours of the onset of symptoms. The mortality in untreated disseminated neonatal herpes, with or without encephalitis, is 70 to 80 per cent. The median interval from onset of symptoms to death is 7 days, and the median age at time of death is 2 weeks. In some patients with encephalitis, death results from the direct progression of neurologic symptoms. In others, the terminal events are respiratory failure or circulatory collapse with disseminated intravascular coagulation and bleeding from multiple sites. External herpetic lesions (that is, lesions of the skin, eyes, or oral cavity) are only noted at the onset of the disease in one-third of the patients. They appear at some time during the course of the disease in only about one-half of the infants with disseminated neonatal herpes.

Approximately one-third of neonates with herpes simplex encephalitis have no evidence of disseminated disease. The onset of symptoms in this group is later (average, 11 days) than in infants with disseminated disease. In one-half of these patients, the disease begins with the development of herpetic skin lesions, oropharyngeal lesions, or HSV infection of the eye, with subsequent development of signs and symptoms of encephalitis. In the remainder, the earliest manifestations of infection are lethargy, irritability, tremors, and focal or generalized seizures, but almost all of these patients also develop visible lesions of the skin, mouth, or eyes at some time during the course of the disease. These are probably the sites of initial infection from which virus then spreads to the central nervous system, perhaps by neural routes. Progression of neurologic signs and symptoms eventually leads to death in about 40 per cent of these patients, and most of the survivors are left with severe neurologic sequelae.

The spinal fluid is abnormal in both forms of neonatal herpes simplex encephalitis, but not invariably so on the first examination. There is usually a mononuclear pleocytosis with 50 to 200 cells per mm³, and the cell count rarely exceeds 400 per mm³. Polymorphonuclear leukocytes occasionally predominate, and erythrocytes are frequently present. The protein concentration is usually elevated and, in the presence of extensive cerebral necrosis, may sometimes exceed 1000 mg/dl. The glucose concentration is usually normal, but it may be depressed, and a low spinal fluid glucose concentration may sometimes reflect hypoglycemia. The spinal fluid is not discernibly different in the two forms of neonatal herpes simplex encephalitis except for the presence of virus. HSV is readily isolated from the spinal fluid of infants in whom encephalitis is associated with disseminated infection, but it is rarely recovered from the spinal fluid of infants with localized central nervous system infection. In the disseminated infection, HSV can also be isolated from lesions of the skin, from the eyes, throat, nasopharynx, blood, sputum, urine, and feces, and from multiple organs at autopsy. In infants with localized central nervous system infection, virus can be isolated from the peripheral lesions that are usually present in the skin, mouth, or eyes.

In some infants with localized central nervous system infection, electroencephalogram, brain scan, and computerized axial tomography may provide evidence of temporal lobe localization, as observed in older children and adults. This is in contrast to the diffuse bilateral involvement that characterizes the encephalitis that occurs in the course of disseminated neonatal HSV infections.

### Herpes Simplex Meningitis

Herpes simplex meningitis is an acute, generally benign, lymphocytic meningitis that occurs primarily in otherwise normal young adults, often in temporal association with genital or perigenital HSV infections (Terni et al., 1971; Craig and Nahmias, 1973; Skoldenberg et al., 1975; Hevron, 1977). It usually starts abruptly with headache, fever, photophobia, nausea and vomiting, myalgias, and nuchal rigidity. There are no seizures, focal neurologic signs, or behavioral disturbances. In most cases, the disease follows a brief, benign course, and symptoms disappear in about a week without residua. An occasional patient may develop radiculitis or ascending myelitis, with neurologic symptoms, such as dysesthesia and paresthesia, which persist for months. Approximately one-half of the documented cases of herpes simplex meningitis have occurred in the company of genital herpes, usually following the onset of the genital lesions by 5 to 10 days. Clinical and serologic data indicate that the majority of the episodes of genital herpes that are associated with herpes simplex meningitis are primary infections with HSV Type 2.

There is spinal fluid pleocytosis, with from 25 to 2500 cells per mm³. Most patients have cell counts between 100 and 500 per mm³, but one-quarter exceed 500 per mm³. Generally, 75 to 100 per cent of the cells are mononuclear, but polymorphonuclear leukocytes may predominate early in the illness. The protein is moderately elevated, to greater than 100 mg/dl in one-half of the patients, but rarely exceeding 250 mg/dl. The glucose concentration is abnormally low in about 20 per cent of samples. Virus, usually HSV Type 2, can be isolated from the spinal fluid early in the disease. Abnormalities of spinal fluid often resolve slowly, and lymphocytic pleocytosis may persist for several weeks after clinical recovery.

Recurrences of benign aseptic meningitis are reported in 25 to 30 per cent of the patients, usually in association with episodes of recurrent genital or cutaneous herpes. Such recurrences are usually milder than the initial episode.

## COMPLICATIONS AND SEQUELAE

In children and adults, herpes simplex encephalitis is entirely a disease of the central nervous system, and most of its complications and sequelae are the direct result of neuronal destruction by HSV. Complications outside the central nervous system are typical of those in any severely ill, unconscious patient with seizures. They include anoxic episodes, aspiration, pulmonary and urinary tract infections, fluid and electrolyte imbalance, cardiovascular problems, pulmonary embolus, stress ulcer, and bed sores. Inappropriate secretion of antidiuretic hormone and diabetes insipidus have also been observed.

The hemorrhagic necrosis produced by the

virus also results in cerebral edema, leading to extensive brain swelling and increased intracranial pressure. This major and almost universal complication is an important cause of death in the acute phase of the disease. By increasing the extent of cerebral necrosis, the cerebral edema also contributes to the frequency and severity of sequelae in survivors.

The development of optic neuritis and retinitis, with unequivocal evidence of HSV infection of the retina, choroid, and optic nerve, has been observed in adults with herpes simplex encephalitis (Minckler et al., 1976; Johnson and Wisotzkey, 1977). The pallor and edema of the optic disk and the retinal hemorrhages may be misinterpreted clinically as papilledema, and thus this complication may frequently be overlooked.

Reports of recurrent herpes simplex encephalitis are extremely rare and have not been documented by isolation of virus from the brain or spinal fluid. A patient with herpes simplex encephalitis may improve and be discharged from the hospital, only to return after several weeks with the recurrence of neurologic signs and symptoms. This has occurred in at least four patients with biopsy-proven herpes simplex encephalitis who have been treated with adenine arabinoside (vidarabine). Antiviral therapy of the initial episode resulted in dramatic improvement, but, after several weeks, the signs and symptoms of encephalitis returned, with progressive neurologic deterioration in spite of re-treatment with vidarabine. Repeat brain biopsy did not reveal HSV detectable by culture, electronmicroscopy, or fluorescent antibody staining. In one such patient reported (Koenig et al., 1979), the biopsy revealed extensive perivascular infiltration by plasmacytes and mononuclear cells and a pattern of cell-mediated demyelination resembling that seen in postinfectious encephalomyelitis. Thus, it appears that postinfectious encephalomeylitis, an acute, presumably autoimmune, demyelinating disease that most frequently occurs following virus infection or vaccination, may occur as a complication of herpes simplex encephalitis. However, it can be very difficult to demonstrate virus in the brain more than 2 weeks after the onset of herpes simplex encephalitis (Olson et al., 1967). Thus, the failure to detect HSV in the brain biopsies obtained during these recurrences does not rule out the possibility that the pathologic process is still directly related to the persistence of HSV or its antigens.

The case of a 9-year-old boy with recurrent episodes of organic psychosis, each of which occurred in association with an episode of recurrent herpes labialis, suggests that self-limited recurrences of herpes simplex encephalitis may occur (Shearer and Finch, 1964). This interesting possibility, which has been observed in animal models of herpes simplex encephalitis, has yet to be documented adequately in humans. The case reported is reminiscent of the association of recurrent HSV Type 2 meningitis with episodes of recurrent herpes genitalis.

The sequelae observed in patients surviving herpes simplex encephalitis reflect the severe cortical damage sustained by the temporal lobes and adjacent structures. They include memory loss, anosmia, ageusia, dysphasia, alexia and other agnosias, confusion, personality changes, hemiparesis, ataxia, autonomic nervous system dysfunction, seizures, and chorioretinitis. In some patients, memory loss, confabulation, and personality change result in a picture that closely resembles Korsakoff's psychosis.

When neonatal herpes simplex encephalitis occurs in the course of disseminated infection, the complications are primarily the result of viremia with extensive involvement of the liver, adrenal glands, lungs, and other organs and tissues throughout the body. Mortality exceeds 70 per cent, and death often results directly from virus infection and necrosis of vital organs. Severe complications include cerebral edema, status epilepticus, hypoglycemia, acidosis, pneumonitis, disseminated intravascular coagulation with hemorrhage and shock, and bacterial or fungal superinfection. More than one-half of the survivors have significant sequelae attributable to central nervous system damage. Infants with herpes simplex encephalitis without disseminated infection have a lower acute mortality, about 40 per cent. However, at least 75 per cent of the survivors have severe sequelae. The neurologic sequelae of neonatal herpes simplex encephalitis include microcephaly, multicystic encephalomalacia, porencephalic cysts, hydrocephaly, seizures, motor deficits, and varying degrees of psychomotor retardation. Ocular sequelae include corneal scarring, cataracts, chorioretinitis, and blindness. Some of these sequelae may not be recognized for months or years (Nahmias and Visintine, 1976).

In contrast to herpes simplex encephalitis, herpes simplex meningitis is usually a benign and self-limited infection free of significant complications and residua. However, an occasional patient may suffer a protracted illness with signs and symptoms of ascending myelitis or radiculitis, and 25 to 30 per cent have recurrent episodes of aseptic meningitis, often in association with recurrences of genital or cutaneous herpes. Increased intracranial pressure and papilledema have been reported in one patient with recurrent herpes meningitis, with isolation of HSV Type 2 from the spinal fluid (Stalder et al., 1973).

As with HSV infections at other sites, the

course of HSV infections of the central nervous system may be particularly severe and atypical in immunosuppressed patients, especially patients with defects in cellular immunity. Such severe and atypical infections have included fatal HSV Type 2 meningoencephalitis in renal transplant recipients (Linnemann et al., 1976); HSV Type 2 encephalitis in patients with cerebral metastases (Manz et al., 1979); and slowly progressive herpes simplex encephalitis without inflammatory changes or hemorrhagic necrosis in a patient with Hodgkin's disease (Price et al., 1973).

## GEOGRAPHIC VARIATION IN DISEASE AND EPIDEMIOLOGY

Herpes simplex viruses are worldwide in distribution without evidence of differing racial or sexual susceptibility. While many experimental animals can be infected, humans are the only known reservoir of natural infection. The principal mode of transmission is through direct contact with infected secretions, and there are no known animal vectors. HSV Type 1 is transmitted primarily by contact with oral secretions and HSV Type 2 by contact with genital secretions.

Following primary infection, these viruses establish latent infections that persist for the life of the host. Latently infected individuals serve as a stable reservoir of virus, and this explains why HSV infections are endemic in human populations everywhere, even in small, totally isolated populations in which the pool of susceptibles is too small to maintain the continuous circulation of such epidemic diseases as measles (Black, 1975). Primary and recurrent infections with both HSV types can be symptomatic or asymptomatic, and transmission can occur from either.

Age-related patterns of infection differ for HSV Type 1 and HSV Type 2. Antibodies to HSV Type 1 rise rapidly during childhood, and, by puberty, nearly all individuals in lower socioeconomic groups have been infected. Infection rates are inversely related to socioeconomic status. The incidence of infection is lower in higher socioeconomic groups, in which antibody prevalence in young adults is only 30 to 50 per cent. The major period of HSV Type 2 infection follows puberty, transmission being directly related to sexual activity.

Infection of neurons plays a crucial role in HSV latency, but symptomatic infection of the central nervous system is extremely uncommon. Herpes simplex encephalitis (beyond the neonatal period) is a rare manifestation of primary and recurrent HSV Type 1 infection. Nevertheless, it is the most common sporadic form of encephalitis in the United States, where it accounts for approximately 10 per cent of all reported cases of encephalitis of determined etiology. It also appears to be the most frequently identified form of severe sporadic encephalitis in the United Kingdom and Western Europe (Meyer et al., 1960; Olson et al., 1967; Miller and Ross, 1968; Juel-Jensen and Mac-Callum, 1972; Mandal, 1972; Center for Disease Control, 1978). The incidence almost certainly exceeds two cases per million population per year and may well be substantially higher. Herpes simplex encephalitis occurs sporadically throughout the year in all parts of the world and in patients of both sexes and all ages, reflecting the ubiquity of HSV infection. It is caused almost always by HSV Type 1. Approximately 10 per cent of the cases occur in the first year of life but, thereafter, the age-specific attack rate appears to be relatively constant. There is no seasonal variation in its occurrence, as there is with central nervous system infections caused by togaviruses and enteroviruses, and there is no temporal association with epidemic diseases such as measles, mumps, or varicella.

Neonatal herpes simplex encephalitis is a manifestation of neonatal HSV infection, which is worldwide in distribution and sporadic in occurrence. There is no discernible seasonal variation, and infection appears to be distributed about equally between males and females. The incidence of recognized neonatal HSV infections in the United States has been estimated to be about 1 in 7500 deliveries (Nahmias and Visintine, 1976) but it is probably somewhat lower, perhaps in the range of 1 in 20,000 deliveries. In the majority of cases, infection is acquired perinatally from the birth canal of a mother with genital herpes. In some cases, infection may occur in utero, as a result either of maternal viremia or of ascending infection from the cervix. Rarely, infection may be acquired postnatally from the mother, other family members, or nursery personnel with symptomatic or asymptomatic HSV infections, or by nosocomial spread from another infected infant. Most infections are caused by HSV Type 2, but there is no discernible difference in the nature or severity of the the disease caused by HSV Type 1 and HSV Type 2. Neonatal HSV infection is more common in premature infants, who comprise 40 per cent of reported cases. While this may reflect increased susceptibility to HSV, the outcome appears to be as poor in full-term infants as in premature infants. Another explanation may be a higher frequency of premature deliveries in women with severe genital herpes (Nahmias and Visintine, 1976).

Herpes simplex meningitis is also worldwide in distribution. Some cases, caused by HSV Type 1, have been reported in children. However, herpes simplex meningitis is primarily a disease of sexually active young adults, 15 to 35 years of age. In this age group, it is almost always caused by HSV Type 2. Serologic and virologic data from Sweden and the United States indicate that herpes simplex meningitis accounts for about 5 per cent of all cases of "aseptic" meningitis.

## DIAGNOSIS

Although herpes simplex encephalitis is a relatively uncommon disease, it is unique among the viral encephalitides in its susceptibility to specific antiviral therapy. It is also an extraordinarily severe disease, usually characterized by extensive and rapidly progressive cerebral necrosis. Even the most effective antiviral drug will not restore life to dead neurons, and, thus, it is not surprising that antiviral therapy has proved futile once the disease has progressed to the point at which the patient is comatose. In a recent study, 57 per cent of comatose patients died in spite of therapy with vidarabine, and all of the survivors were severely debilitated (Whitley et al., 1977). Since the mean interval from onset of symptoms to coma is only 6 to 7 days, there is an enormous premium on early diagnosis. Unfortunately, herpes simplex encephalitis is difficult to diagnose, especially early in the course of the disease, because its occurrence is sporadic and its manifestations protean. Many other pathologic processes mimic herpes simplex encephalitis.

The problem is well illustrated by the results of a recent multicenter collaborative study (Whitley et al., 1977). The clinical criteria for entry — "evidence of an acute, febrile encephalopathy with disordered mentation, focal cerebral signs, localization by diagnostic procedures (electroencephalogram, arteriogram, or brain scan, singly or in combination), and cerebrospinal-fluid findings compatible with viral infection" — were so stringent that more than one-third of the patients with herpes simplex encephalitis were already comatose when admitted to the study. Nevertheless, brain biopsy demonstrated herpes simplex encephalitis in only 56 per cent of the patients entered into the study. Most of the remaining 44 per cent proved to have some other specific diagnosis, including many requiring other forms of therapy. These included brain abscess, toxoplasmosis, tuberculosis, cryptococcal infection, leptospiral meningitis, cerebrovascular disease, metastatic tumor, toxic encephalopathy, Epstein-Barr virus infection, and more than one dozen cases of meningoencephalitis caused by RNA viruses (which are not inhibited by vidarabine). More than 10 per cent of these patients had nonviral central nervous system infections for which effective specific therapy is presently avail-

able. There is little doubt that if the clinical criteria are relaxed in order to start treatment earlier in the course of herpes simplex encephalitis, an even higher proportion of nonherpetic patients will be included. These considerations emphasize the need to establish firmly the etiology before accepting the diagnosis of herpes simplex encephalitis. Unfortunately, the only means of establishing the diagnosis of herpes simplex encephalitis is the demonstration of HSV or HSV antigens in brain tissue obtained by biopsy or at autopsy (Johnson et al., 1968; Boston Interhospital Virus Study Group, 1975; Whitley et al., 1977).

Critical to the early diagnosis of herpes simplex encephalitis is a high index of suspicion. The appearance of signs and symptoms referable to the orbitofrontal and temporal cortex and the limbic system, especially peculiar behavior, anosmia, dysphasia, memory loss, olfactory, gustatory or auditory hallucinations, and focal seizures can provide the earliest evidence of serious disease and of localization.

Routine laboratory tests are of no value in diagnosing herpes simplex encephalitis. Examination of the spinal fluid is helpful only in providing data consistent with a viral infection or in identifying bacterial, parasitic, or fungal infections. The cell count is quite variable but usually ranges from 50 to 750 per $mm^3$. Lymphocytes and mononuclear cells generally predominate but there are often 10 to 25 per cent polymorphonuclear leukocytes. The protein concentration is usually elevated, and the glucose concentration is normal on initial examination. The spinal fluid pressure is often elevated and erythrocytes are frequently present, reflecting the hemorrhagic nature of the cerebral lesions. However, 10 to 15 per cent of patients with herpes simplex encephalitis may have normal spinal fluid on the first examination, and others have a cellular response consisting predominantly of polymorphonuclear leukocytes early in the disease. The spinal fluid examination cannot rule out many alternative diagnoses, such as bacterial cerebritis, cerebral abscess, tumor, central nervous system manifestations of bacterial endocarditis, postinfectious encephalomyelitis, cerebral hemorrhage or infarction, tuberculous or fungal meningitis, or meningoencephalitis caused by other viruses.

Unfortunately, herpes simplex virus is almost never isolated from the spinal fluid in children and adults with herpes simplex encephalitis. Attempts have been made to detect HSV antigens in the spinal fluid in the hope of circumventing the need for brain biopsy to establish the diagnosis. Fluorescent antibody staining of leukocytes in spinal fluid to detect HSV antigens has not given positive results in most cases. The use of a sensitive radioimmune assay to detect an HSV-specific glycoprotein in spinal fluid is currently being evaluated (Chen et al., 1978), and preliminary results are encouraging. Other methods are also under investigation.

Serologic tests are of no value in the *early* diagnosis of herpes simplex encephalitis because of the necessity for convalescent specimens and because an increase in antibody titer, even from undetectable levels, may simply reflect the reactivation of latent HSV unrelated to the encephalitic process (Johnson et al., 1968). Furthermore, many cases of herpes simplex encephalitis represent recurrent rather than primary infection, further complicating the interpretation of serologic data. However, the presence or appearance of IgM antibody to HSV in newborns provides reliable evidence of neonatal HSV infection.

Antibodies to HSV appear in the spinal fluid of patients with herpes simplex encephalitis within 1 or 2 weeks of onset, and the presence of an altered serum/spinal fluid antibody ratio — for example, less than 20 — has been considered indicative of local antibody production (MacCallum et al., 1974; Levine et al., 1978). Unfortunately, the specificity of this test for the diagnosis of herpes simplex encephalitis is not established, and the delay in the appearance of antibody makes it unlikely that this approach will yield an early diagnosis.

The electroencephalogram is almost always abnormal and often serves to localize the area of maximum involvement. The typical pattern is one of widespread arrhythmic slow wave activity, sometimes with unilateral or regional predominance, and the appearance of periodic sharp waves or spike-and-wave complexes over one or both temporal lobes. These changes are not always present, nor are they pathognomonic of herpes simplex encephalitis. They may occur in cerebral infarcts, increased intracranial pressure, various inflammatory conditions, and encephalitis caused by other viruses. Nevertheless, they may aid in distinguishing herpes simplex encephalitis from other processes and help determine the best site for cerebral biopsy (Illis and Taylor, 1972).

Cerebral arteriography and technetium brain scan reveal a temporal lobe mass with abnormal uptake of isotope in most cases, but the changes are not specific, and they are often absent early in the course of the disease. Computerized axial tomography reveals an area of diminished attenuation in the medial portion of the temporal lobe with extension into the insular area in most patients. Mass effect and streaky enhancement on contrast administration are also seen (Davis et al., 1978; Enzmann et al., 1978; Zimmerman et al., 1980). Unfortunately, these changes are often not seen within the first 5 days of illness. Nevertheless, in most patients, computerized axial tomography has obviated the need for angiography.

While all of these studies may increase the likelihood of diagnosing herpes simplex encephalitis and help to localize the area of maximum involvement, definitive diagnosis requires cerebral biopsy. The biopsy should be performed early in order to start specific therapy as soon as possible, and tissue should be obtained from an area of obvious pathology. The medial and inferior surfaces of the temporal lobe are so regularly involved that if any doubt exists as to the site of maximum pathology, these areas should be selected. Biopsied tissue should be divided under sterile conditions into pieces for histopathologic examination, electronmicroscopy, routine bacterial and fungal cultures, and virus isolation. Care should be taken so that each sample includes cortex. In addition, impression smears should be made and fixed in chilled acetone for fluorescent antibody staining (Flewett, 1973). The tissue for histopathologic examination should be fixed in Bouin's or another acid fixative to best demonstrate intranuclear inclusions. The tissue for viral culture should be carried to the virology laboratory in ice-cold transport medium, finely minced (or dispersed with trypsin or collagenase), washed several times with tissue culture medium, and inoculated into tissue cultures of primary human embryonic kidney, diploid human lung or skin fibroblasts, or primary rabbit kidney cells. The inoculation of viable cells, rather than a clarified suspension of homogenized brain, increases the chances of isolating small amounts of virus, especially if there is antibody to HSV present in the biopsied tissue. Typical cytopathic effects are usually apparent within 48 hours, and more than 90 per cent of positive biopsies are recognized as such within 3 days of inoculation. However, tissue obtained from a minimally involved area of brain or taken more than 2 weeks after onset of disease may contain very little virus or large amounts of antibody. Under these circumstances, the appearance of cytopathic effects in tissue culture has been delayed for as long as 21 days (Johnson et al., 1972). Isolation of HSV represents the most sensitive and reliable means of establishing the diagnosis of herpes simplex encephalitis. The incidence of culture-negative biopsies in cases in which virus is subsequently isolated at autopsy is very low (in the neighborhood of 1 to 3 per cent). Fluorescent antibody staining provides a rapid means of establishing the diagnosis. Either direct or indirect fluorescent antibody staining can be used, and positive biopsies usually show diffuse, finely granular fluorescence in the cytoplasm of infected neurons and glia, often with discrete granular staining in the nucleus as well. Unfortunately, the results are positive in only 75 to 80 per cent of culture-positive biopsies. The false negatives appear to occur because the technique fails to detect HSV antigens in biopsies with a low concentration of virus (Cho and Feng, 1978). False-positive fluorescent antibody staining appears with a frequency of at least 5 per cent. It has been reported in cases of tuberculosis, cryptococcal meningitis, brain abscess, and St. Louis encephalitis. The use of HSV-specific monoclonal antibodies may improve the specificity of fluorescent antibody staining, but it is unlikely to improve its sensitivity. The identification of Cowdry Type A intranuclear inclusion bodies and the electronmicroscopic detection of herpesvirus particles (Figs. 1 and 4) are both less sensitive and less specific diagnostic techniques. Similar inclusion bodies can be produced by varicella-zoster virus, measles virus, and the human papovaviruses responsible for progressive multifocal leukoencephalopathy, and the virions of all of the herpesviruses are morphologically indistinguishable. Furthermore, at least one-third of biopsy specimens that are positive by culture and fluorescent antibody staining do not contain detectable inclusion bodies or virions. It should be emphasized that the likelihood of isolating virus from the brain in herpes simplex encephalitis is greatly reduced when tissue is obtained more than 2 weeks after the onset of symptoms (Olson et al., 1967). Although virus is almost never isolated from the lumbar spinal fluid, ventricular fluid is frequently culture-positive (Flewett, 1973). However, this may simply reflect the passage of the needle used to obtain ventricular fluid through infected brain.

The differential diagnosis of herpes simplex encephalitis encompasses most viral and many nonviral diseases of the central nervous system. It includes encephalitis produced by other viruses, particularly togaviruses and mumps virus; postinfectious encephalomyelitis; bacterial, fungal, and parasitic infections; toxic encephalopathy (for example, lead poisoning); cerebrovascular disorders; and tumors. Although other viruses are less likely to produce focal disease in the temporal lobe, the clinical distinction between herpes simplex encephalitis and other forms of viral encephalitis rests primarily on epidemiologic data and is never secure. Virus isolation and serologic data are required to establish the etiologic diagnosis. The possibility of postinfectious encephalomyelitis is raised by a history of antecedent viral illness, such as measles or varicella, or recent vaccination. Toxic encephalopathy may be suggested by a history of ingestion or exposure, and the diagnosis is sup-

ported by detection of the toxic substance in the blood, urine, or other body fluid. A thorough examination of the spinal fluid usually distinguishes fungal, parasitic, or bacterial meningitis from herpes simplex encephalitis. In these nonviral infections, the spinal fluid glucose concentration is consistently depressed. The detection of organisms on microscopic examination and culture, or of specific microbial antigens or antibodies (for example, cryptococcal antigen or antibody to *Coccidioides immitis*) by immunologic assay, often gives a rapid and definitive etiologic diagnosis. Cerebral infarction, subarachnoid hemorrhage, subdural hematoma, subdural empyema, epidural abscess, and brain tumors may also be confused with herpes simplex encephalitis. Examination of the spinal fluid is rarely helpful, but technetium brain scan, arteriography, and, especially, computerized axial tomography help to distinguish these disorders from herpes simplex encephalitis. Cerebral abscess presents a difficult differential diagnosis because fever, headache, obtundation, seizures, and other focal neurologic signs are frequent. The spinal fluid findings are not distinctive, and, while personality changes and isolated disorders of memory are more common in herpes simplex encephalitis, they may occur in brain abscess as well. The electroencephalogram and computerized axial tomography may suggest one or the other diagnosis, but none of the noninvasive diagnostic procedures is reliable enough to obviate the need for diagnostic brain biopsy. The necessity for brain biopsy to establish the diagnosis of herpes simplex encephalitis is clearly demonstrated by the fact that nearly one-half of the patients with the clinical diagnosis of herpes simplex encephalitis who have undergone brain biopsy have proved to have some other disease.

In the neonate, as in the adult, the key to the early diagnosis of herpes simplex encephalitis is a high index of suspicion (Nahmias and Visintine, 1976; Hanshaw and Dudgeon, 1978). The presence of skin lesions, oral ulcers, or keratoconjunctivitis greatly facilitates the diagnosis of neonatal HSV infection, and such lesions should be carefully sought at birth and frequently thereafter in any infant who is unwell. The skin lesions may intially be maculopapular and only later become vesicular. They are often present on the presenting part, especially the scalp. Enlarged epithelial cells and multinucleated giant cells containing acidophilic Cowdry Type A intranuclear inclusion bodies distinguish the lesions of herpes simplex from all others except varicella-zoster, which can usually be dismissed on epidemiologic grounds. These cells can be seen in Tzanck smears; material is scraped from the base of the vesicle, spread on a glass slide, fixed, and stained with

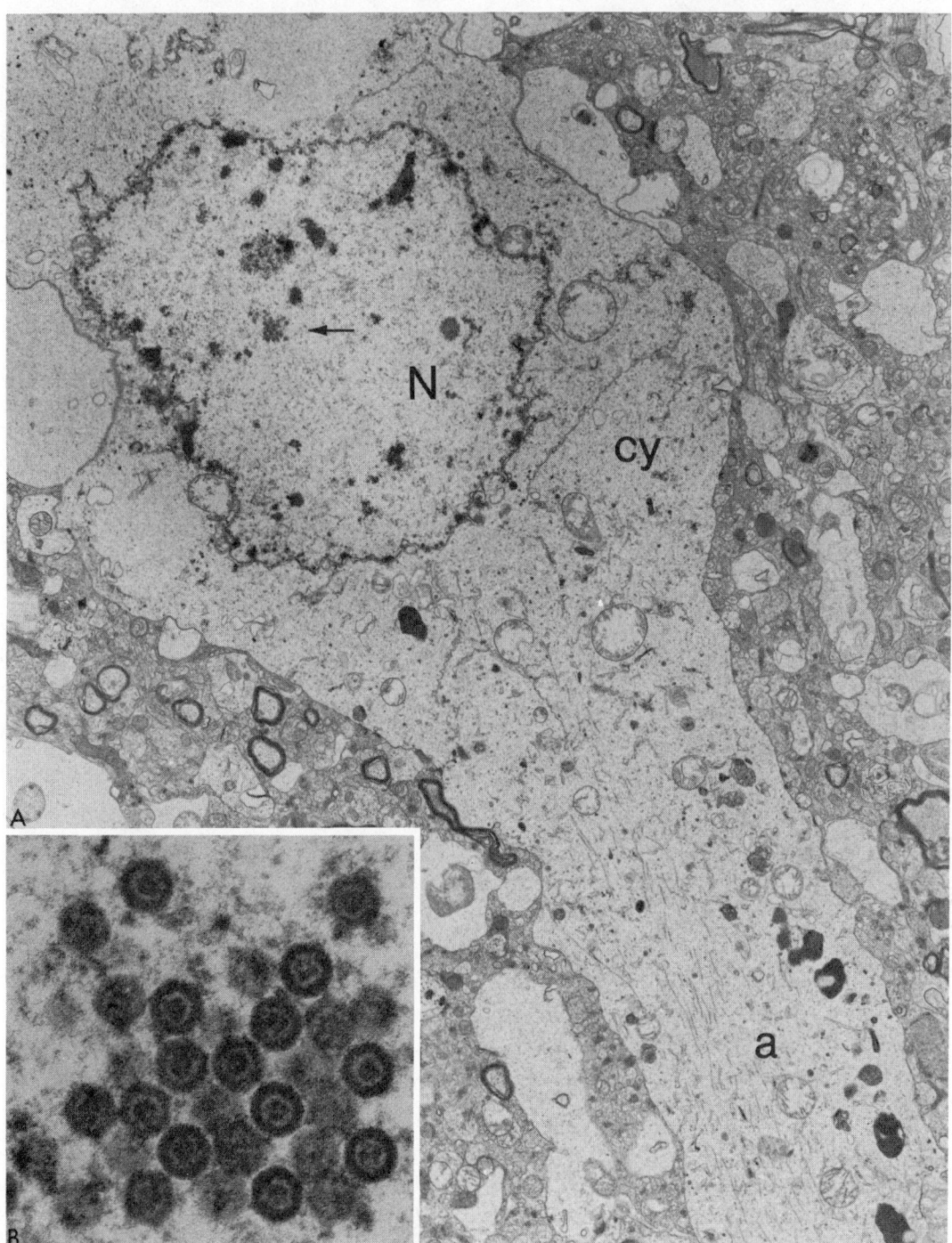

**FIGURE 4.** Herpes simplex encephalitis. *(Courtesy of Dr. H. C. Powell and Mrs. M. A. Phillips.)*
*A, Electron micrograph of a herpes simplex virus-infected neuron from the brain of a patient with herpes simplex encephalitis. The cytoplasm and axon are indicated by (cy) and (a), respectively. The nucleus (N) contains small collections of herpes simplex virus nucleocapsids (arrow). Many other herpes simplex virus nucleocapsids are adjacent to the nuclear membrane and some are in the process of budding through its inner lamella in areas thickened by the addition of herpes simplex virus-specified glycoproteins. Magnification 7200×.*
*B, The herpes simplex virus nucleocapsids indicated by the arrow in A are shown at higher magnification (90,000×) in the inset.*

*Illustration continued on following page*

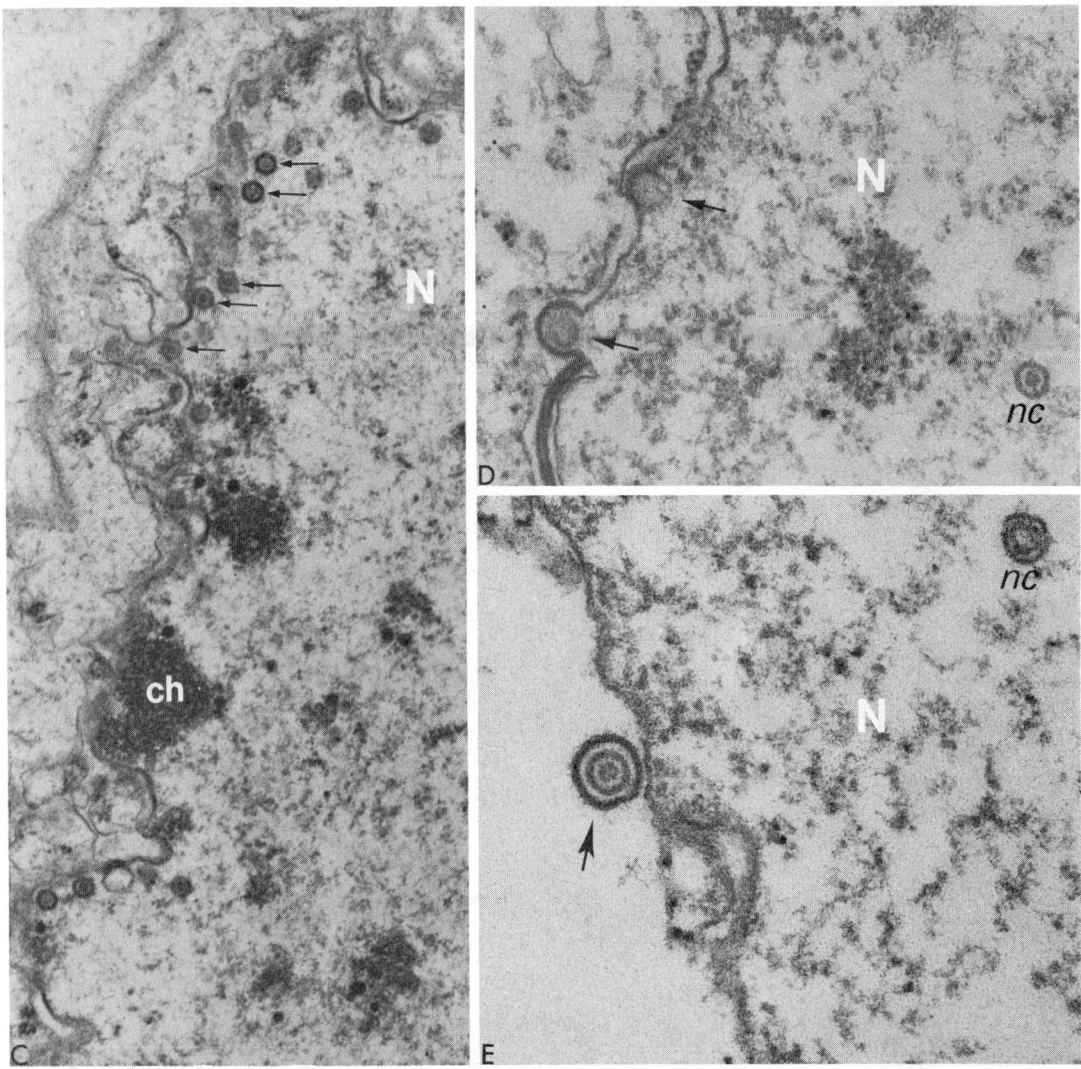

**FIGURE 4.** *Continued*

 C, *A section of the neuron in A viewed at higher magnification (30,000 ×) shows many herpes simplex virus nucleocapsids adjacent to the inner surface of the nuclear membrane (arrows). Also seen along the inner surface of the nuclear membrane are collections of condensed marginated chromatin (ch).*

 D, *Higher magnification (50,000×) showing herpes simplex virus nucleocapsids in the process of budding through the innner lamella of the nuclear membrane in areas thickened by the addition of herpes simplex virus-specified glycoprotein (arrows). Nucleocapsids within the nucleus are indicated by (nc).*

 E, *The process of budding completed, an enveloped (complete) herpes simplex virus particle (arrow) is seen in the cytoplasm adjacent to the nuclear membrane. Magnification 75,000×.*

hematoxylin-eosin, Giemsa, Papanicolaou, or Paragon multiple stain (Barr et al., 1977). A punch biopsy provides more reliable material for histopathologic examination, especially in atypical or prevesicular lesions. Tzanck smears should also be made from the base of oral ulcers and from conjunctival scrapings in infants with keratoconjunctivitis. Because more than one-half of maternal genital infections associated with neonatal herpes are clinically inapparent, cells for histopathologic examination should also be obtained from the mother's cervix, even in the absence of genital lesions. All of these materials should be carefully examined for HSV antigens by fluorescent antibody staining or with some other immunologic technique. This often gives a rapid and specific diagnosis. They may also be examined for herpes virus particles by electron microscopy. Cells scraped from all visible lesions should be immediately inoculated into tissue cultures of human embryonic kidney, diploid human fibroblast, or primary rabbit kidney cells in order to isolate the virus.

Unfortunately, visible stigmata of HSV infection are often absent at the outset of the disseminated form of neonatal herpes, and they appear at some time in only about one-half of the patients. However, virus can usually be isolated from the spinal fluid, throat, nasopharynx, sputum, blood, urine, and feces. It should be sought in any infant with the clinical picture of neonatal sepsis or meningitis in whom the bacteriologic diagnosis is not rapidly established.

The presence or appearance of IgM antibodies to HSV provides reliable evidence of neonatal infection. Unfortunately, the progression of the disease is usually so rapid that antibody is rarely present soon enough to aid in early diagnosis.

Herpes simplex meningitis is indistinguishable from the benign aseptic meningitis caused by a number of other viruses. The diagnosis should be suspected when aseptic meningitis develops in association with genital herpes. Isolation of HSV from the blood and serologic evidence of primary HSV Type 2 infection are highly suggestive, but the diagnosis is firmly established only by the isolation of HSV from the spinal fluid.

## TREATMENT

General supportive measures directed at the care of the comatose patient with seizures are extremely important. The airway must often be maintained by intubation or tracheostomy, and mechanical ventilation may be required. Frequent turning and careful skin care are essential to avoid decubitus ulcers. There must also be careful attention to the bowel, bladder, eyes, and tracheal toilet, and to the maintenance of body temperature, fluid and electrolyte balance, and blood glucose levels. Seizures may be controlled with diphenylhydantoin or phenobarbital, and diazepam may help in status epilepticus. The respiratory tract, urinary tract, skin, and intravenous sites are common loci of nosocomial infections. Such infections should be carefully sought, vigorously treated, and avoided by meticulous nursing care.

Cerebral edema with brain swelling and tentorial herniation are lethal in many cases of herpes simplex encephalitis. Large doses of corticosteroids are frequently given for this complication, but neither the effectiveness of this form of therapy nor the possibility that it may lower resistance to HSV infection has been adequately evaluated. Until they are, it is probably reasonable to use corticosteroids only when brain swelling appears to be life-threatening, and to discontinue their use as soon as possible. Osmotic diuretics, such as glycerol, may also help to control cerebral edema. An alternative approach, extensive decompressive craniotomy, has been extremely useful in selected patients (Illis and Gostling, 1972).

The discovery and development of agents capable of inhibiting the replication of HSV in tissue cultures should permit the effective specific treatment of herpes simplex encephalitis. Many of these antiviral agents are nucleoside analogs that interfere with the synthesis of HSV DNA. Unfortunately, they may also interfere with host-cell DNA synthesis and thus be toxic when administered systemically. Among the typical manifestations of such toxicity are immunosuppression and myelosuppression leading to uncontrolled bleeding and infection. Evaluation of the efficacy of antiviral agents in humans with herpes simplex encephalitis has been difficult because of the frequent failure to establish clearly the diagnosis in treated patients. The mortality in cases diagnosed clinically as herpes simplex encephalitis but negative for HSV on brain biopsy is much lower than that in untreated biopsy-proven cases, so that the inclusion of biopsy-negative patients in a treatment group results in lower mortality, regardless of the efficacy of the treatment. Variations in the stage of the disease at start of therapy, uncertainties as to the natural history of the disease in untreated patients, and difficulty in distinguishing between complications of the disease itself and complications reflecting drug toxicity have contributed to the problem. To date, three nucleoside analogs have been evaluated for the therapy of herpes simplex encephalitis in humans. In the process, we have come to the painful realization that the evaluation of therapeutic modalities can be accomplished only by means of double-blind, placebo-controlled studies in proven cases of the disease.

5-iodo-2'-deoxyuridine (idoxuridine or IDU), a thymidine analog that is effective when applied topically for the treatment of HSV keratitis, was the first antiviral drug used to treat herpes simplex encephalitis. Despite early optimism based upon case reports and uncontrolled trials, a double-blind, placebo-controlled study demonstrated lack of efficacy and unacceptable mylosuppressive toxicity (Boston Interhospital Virus Study Group, 1975). Similarly, case reports and uncontrolled trials of another pyrimidine analog, 1-B-D-arabinofuranosyl cytosine (cytosine arabinoside, cytarabine or ara-C) were thought by some to indicate efficacy until a recently completed placebo-controlled study carried out in the United Kingdom demonstrated a mortality in excess of 70 per cent in both the treated and placebo groups. Another nucleoside analog, 9-B-D arabinofuranosyl adenine (adenine arabinoside, vidarabine, or ara-A), has yielded more promising results. In a double-blind, placebo-controlled study in biopsy-proven cases of herpes simplex encephalitis, adenine arabinoside (15 mg/kg/day intravenously for 10 days) reduced the mortality, measured at 30 days, from 70 per cent to 28 per cent. The proportion of patients who survived without debilitating neurologic sequelae was increased from 20 per cent to 40 per cent. Later fatalities among patients with severe sequelae brought the mortality to 90 per cent in the placebo group and 40 per cent in the treated group at 120 days (Whitley et al., 1977). Although the number of patients in the study was small, comparable results have since been obtained in a larger group of biopsy-proven cases, all of whom were treated with this dose of adenine arabinoside. In a similar double-blind, placebo-controlled study, adenine arabinoside (15 mg/kg/day intravenously for 10 days) reduced the mortality in newborns with disseminated HSV infection and localized herpes simplex encephalitis from 74 per cent to 38 per cent. The proportion of infants who survived without significant sequelae was also increased from 11 to 29 per cent (Whitley et al., 1980).

These results are encouraging, but the mortality in treated patients is still excessive and the quality of life is poor in many survivors. Adenine arabinoside, though somewhat more active in inhibiting HSV than cellular DNA synthesis, still interferes with host-cell DNA replication and, at higher doses, produces myelosuppression and other toxic manifestations in vivo. Moreover, adenine arabinoside is relatively insoluble in aqueous solutions, and the large volume of intravenous fluid required to administer the drug frequently exacerbates cerebral edema.

Two new antiviral drugs are being evaluated in a double-blind study in parallel with adenine arabinoside, which, having already been shown to have some efficacy, can replace the placebo as a point of reference. One of these, adenine arabinoside monophosphate, a more soluble derivative of adenine arabinoside that can be administered intravenous or intramuscularly, appears to have the same mechanism of action and in vivo metabolism as the parent compound. The other, 9-(2-hydroxyethoxymethyl) guanine (acycloguanosine or acyclovir), appears to be a more selective antiviral drug. It is phosphorylated by the HSV-specified deoxypyrimidine kinase, but not by the comparable host-cell enzyme. Thus, it is taken up and converted to its active form by HSV-infected cells but not by uninfected host cells. Furthermore, acycloguanosine triphosphate, the active intracellular form of the drug, is 10 to 30 times more active in inhibiting the HSV-specified DNA polymerase than cellular DNA polymerases (Elion et al., 1977). Consequently, acycloguanosine has been a highly effective and nontoxic inhibitor of HSV in tissue culture and in animal models of herpes simplex encephalitis. Many additional compounds designed to interfere selectively with HSV-specific functions are under development and should soon be ready for testing in patients.

Interferons are natural antiviral glycoproteins produced by cells in response to virus infection. They are an important component of our natural resistance to many viruses, including HSV. When given before infection or early in infection, interferons can inhibit the replication of HSV in tissue culture and in animals without apparent toxicity. In humans, interferon has been effective against herpes simplex keratitis, and, administered perioperatively, has reduced the frequency of reactivation of latent HSV infection after surgical manipulation of the trigeminal nerve root (Pazin et al., 1979). A limited supply has prevented the evaluation of human interferon in the therapy of herpes simplex encephalitis. Recombinant DNA technology promises to increase greatly the availability of human interferon. Thus, there is a good reason to believe that interferon, alone or in combination with nucleoside analogs such as acycloguanosine, will be an effective and nontoxic treatment for herpes simplex encephalitis.

In the newborn, the early administration of human HSV immune globulin containing high levels of antibody to HSV Type 2, as well as the use of hyperthermia, needs to be evaluated, especially in combination with antiviral agents.

## PROPHYLAXIS

Herpes simplex encephalitis beyond the neonatal period is a rare complication of both primary and recurrent HSV Type 1 infections. Because we do not understand its pathogenesis and, in particular, what causes on rare occasions this otherwise temperate virus to produce a highly fatal encephalitis, we are far from developing any specific prophylactic measures. Nevertheless, it seems likely that prophylactic measures effective against primary and recurrent HSV Type 1 infections in general will also reduce the frequency of herpes simplex encephalitis. Such measures would include anything that could reduce the incidence of primary infection, interfere with the establishment of latent infections of sensory neurons, or prevent the reactivation and spread of latent virus. Because primary and recurrent HSV infections in general, and herpes simplex encephalitis in particular, are sporadic in occurrence and afflict individuals of all ages, prevention will require lifelong prophylaxis. The only practical means of achieving lifelong prophylaxis of viral infections is active immunization. However, the frequent recurrence of HSV infections and the occurrence of cases of herpes simplex encephalitis in people who already have neutralizing antibody and virus-specific cellular immunity raises doubt as to the potential efficacy of immunization. Other observations do suggest that host immunity may prevent or at least modify primary and recurrent HSV infections. The frequency and severity of recurrent herpes is markedly increased in immunosuppressed patients, particularly patients with defects in cellular immunity. Recurrent HSV infections, which occur in immune people, are generally less severe and shorter than primary infections. In animals, the passive administration of antibody to HSV can reduce the incidence and severity of the central nervous system infection that follows peripheral inoculation of virus and can also interfere with the establishment of latent infections in sensory ganglia. Similar results have been obtained by immunization with live and inactivated HSV vaccines, including vaccines that are free of all nucleic acid. This last point is important, because concerns about oncogenicity and the potential for latency and recurrence are likely to preclude the use of vaccines containing HSV DNA in otherwise normal humans. Although HSV vaccines are under active investigation, their application to patients is still years away. In any case, their effect on herpes simplex encephalitis is likely to be difficult to measure because of the rarity of the disease.

In the newborn, herpes simplex encephalitis is always a manifestation of primary infection, which is usually acquired from a mother with genital herpes. Most infections are acquired during passage through the infected birth canal or result from an ascending infection after rupture of the membranes. The risk of neonatal infection is estimated to be 50 per cent in infants delivered vaginally in the presence of active maternal genital herpes (Nahmias and Visintine, 1976). Thus, cesarean section is recommended prior to rupture of the membranes when clinically apparent genital herpes is present at term. However, more than one-half of the infants with neonatal herpes are born to mothers without clinically apparent genital herpes. Consequently, when there is a history of genital herpes in either parent, the mother's cervix and vaginal secretions should be cultured during the last month of gestation, even in the absence of symptoms of genital infection (Hanshaw and Dudgeon, 1978). Once the membranes have ruptured, there would seem to be little advantage to cesarean section, but delivery should be accomplished rapidly in order to minimize exposure of the infant to virus. Infants exposed to HSV during delivery should be isolated and closely observed for the development of peripheral lesions or signs of infection. Frequent attempts should be made to culture virus from the throat, eyes, and urine. The infant should proba-

bly be given large doses of immune serum globulin, preferably from a lot with a high titer of antibody to HSV Type 2. Although there is no evidence that passively administered antibody is protective, infants with high titers of transplacentally acquired antibody to HSV Type 2 have a more favorable outcome than infants with low antibody titers (Yeager et al., 1980). The topical application of idoxuridine or adenine arabinoside drops to the eyes, which are sometimes the portal of entry of virus, should also be considered. These recommendations are based upon limited epidemiologic data, and the assumption that the principal source of infection for the newborn is exposure to high titers of virus during passage through the birth canal (Nahmias and Visintine, 1976; Hanshaw and Dudgeon, 1978). Their efficacy is unproven.

Herpes simplex meningitis is generally a benign and self-limited infection. There is no known specific prophylaxis, except the avoidance of genital HSV infection with which it is often associated.

## References

Adair, C. V., Gauld, R. L., and Smadel, J. E.: Aseptic meningitis, a disease of diverse etiology: Clinical and etiology studies on 854 cases. Ann Intern Med 29:675, 1953.

Armstrong, C.: Herpes simplex virus recovered from the spinal fluid of a suspected case of lymphocytic choriomeningitis. Public Health Rep 58:16, 1943.

Barr, R. J., Herten, R. J., and Graham, J. H.: Rapid method for Tzanck preparations. JAMA 237:1119, 1977.

Black, F. L.: Infectious diseases in primitive societies. Science 187:515, 1975.

Boston Interhospital Virus Study Group and the NIAID Sponsored Cooperative Antiviral Clinical Study. Failure of high dose 5-iodo-2'-deoxyuridine (IDU) in the therapy of herpes simplex virus encephalitis: Evidence of unacceptable toxicity. N Engl J Med 292:599, 1975.

Center for Disease Control: Encephalitis Surveillance Annual Summary 1976, Issued December, 1978.

Chen, A. B., Ben-Porat, T., Whitley, R. J., and Kaplan, A. L.: Purification and characterization of proteins excreted by cells infected with herpes simplex virus and their use in diagnosis. Virology 91:234, 1978.

Cho, C. T., and Feng, K. K.: Sensitivity of the virus isolation and immunofluorescent staining methods in diagnosis of infections with herpes simplex virus. J Infect Dis 138:536, 1978.

Craig, C. P., and Nahmias, A. J.: Different patterns of neurologic involvement with herpes simplex virus types 1 and 2: Isolation of herpes simplex virus type 2 from the buffy coat of two adults with meningitis. J Infect Dis 127:365, 1973.

Davis, J. M., Davis, K. R., Kleinman, G. M., Kirchner, H. W., and Taveras, J. M.: Computed tomography of herpes simplex encephalitis with clinicopathological correlation. Radiology 129:409, 1978.

Davis, L. E., and Johnson, R. T.: An explanation for the localization of herpes simplex encephalitis: Ann Neurol 5:2, 1979.

Dayan, A. D., Gooddy, W., Harrison, M. J. G., and Rudge, P.: Brain stem encephalitis caused by *Herpesvirus hominis*. Br Med J 4:405, 1972.

Drachman, D. A., and Adams, R. D.: Herpes simplex and acute inclusion-body encephalitis. Arch Neurol 7:61, 1962.

Elion, G. B, Furman, P. A., Fyfe, J. A., de Miranda, P., Beauchamp, L., and Schaeffer, J. H.: Selectivity of action of an antiherpetic agent, 9-(2-hydroxyethoxymethyl) guanine. Proc Natl Acad Sci USA 74:5716, 1977.

Enzmann, D. R., Ranson, B., Norman, D., and Talberth, E.: Computed tomography of herpes simplex encephalitis. Radiology 129:419, 1978.

Flewett, T. H.: The rapid diagnosis of herpes encephalitis. Postgrad Med J 49:398, 1973.

Hanshaw, J. B., and Dudgeon, J. A.: Herpes simplex infection of the fetus and newborn. In Shaffer, A. J., and Markowitz, M. (eds.): Viral Diseases of the Fetus and Newborn, Volume 17 in series, Major Problems in Clinical Pediatrcs. Philadelphia, W. B. Saunders Co., p. 153, 1978.

Haymaker, W., Smith, M. G., van Bogaert, L., and de Chenar, C.: Pathology of viral disease in man characterized by nuclear inclusions, with emphasis on herpes simplex and subacute inclusion encephalitis. In Fields, W. S., and Blattner, R. J. (eds.): Viral Encephalitis. Springfield, Charles C Thomas, p. 95, 1958.

Hevron, J. E., Jr.: Herpes simplex virus type 2 meningitis. Obstet Gynecol 49:622, 1977.

Illis, L. S., and Gostling, J. V. T.: Herpes Simplex Encephalitis. Scientechnica Ltd., Bristol, 1972.

Illis, L. S., and Taylor, F. M.: The electroencephalogram in herpes-simplex encephalitis. Lancet 1:718, 1972.

Johnson, B. L., and Wisotzkey, H. M.: Neuroretinitis associated with herpes simplex encephalitis in an adult. Am J. Ophthalmol 83:481, 1977.

Johnson, K. P., Rosenthal, M. S., and Lerner, P. I.: Herpes simplex encephalitis. The course in five virologically proven cases. Arch Neurol 27:103, 1972.

Johnson, R. T., and Mims, C. A.: Pathogenesis of viral infections of the nervous system. N Engl J Med 278:23, 84, 1968.

Johnson, R. T., Olson, L. C., and Buescher, E. L.: Herpes simplex virus infections of the nervous system. Problems in laboratory diagnosis. Arch Neurol 18:260, 1968.

Juel-Jensen, B. E., and MacCallum, F. O.: Herpes Simplex Varicella and Zoster, Clinical Manifestations and Treatment Philadelphia, J. B. Lippincott Co., 1972.

Koenig, H., Rabinowitz, S. G., Day, E., and Miller, V.: Post-infectious encephalomyelitis after successful treatment of herpes simplex encephalitis with adenine arabinoside. N Engl J Med 300:1089, 1979.

Leider, W., Magoffin, R. L., Lennette, E. H., and Leonards, L. N. R.: Herpes-simplex-virus encephalitis. Its possible association with reactivated latent infection. N Engl J Med 273:341, 1965.

Levine, D. P., Lauter, C. B., and Lerner, M.: Simultaneous serum and CSF antibodies in herpes simplex virus encephalitis. J Am Med Assn 240:356, 1978.

Linnemann, C. C., Jr., First, M. R., Alvira, M. M., Alexander, J. W., and Schiff, G. M.: Herpesvirus hominis type 2 meningoencephalitis following renal transplantation. Am J Med 61:703, 1976.

MacCallum, F. O., Chinn, I. J., and Gostling, J. V. T.: Antibodies to herpes-simplex virus in the cerebrospinal fluid of patients with herpetic encephalitis. J Med Microbiol 7:325, 1974.

Mandal, B. K.: A survey of acute encephalitis. Publ Hlth 86:215, 1972.

Manz, H. J., Phillips, T. M., and McCullough, D. C.: Herpes simplex type 2 encephalitis concurrent with known cerebral metastases. Acta Neuropathol (Berl) 47:237, 1979.

Meyer, H. M., Jr., Johnson, R. T., Crawford, I. P., Dascomb, H. E., and Rogers, N. G.: Central nervous system syndromes of "viral" etiology: a study of 713 cases. Am J Med 29:334, 1960.

Miller, J. D., and Ross, C. A. C.: Encephalitis, a four-year survey. Lancet 1:1121, 1968.

Miller, J. K., Hesser, F., and Tompkins, V. N.: Herpes simplex encephalitis, a report of 20 cases. Ann Int Med 64:92, 1966.

Minckler, D. L., McLean, E. B., Shaw, C. M., and Hendrickson, A.: Herpesvirus hominis encephalitis and retinitis. Arch Ophthalmol 94:89, 1976.

Nahmias, A. J., and Visintine, A. M.: Herpes simplex. In Remington, J. S., and Klein, J. O. (eds.): Infectious Diseases of the Fetus and Newborn Infant, Philadelphia, W. B. Saunders Co., p. 156, 1976.

Nolan, D. C., Carruthers, M. M., and Lerner, A. M.: *Herpesvirus hominis* encephalitis in Michigan. Report of 13 cases, including six treated with idoxuridine. N Engl J Med 292:10, 1970.

Olson, L. C., Buescher, E. L., Artenstein, M. S., and Parkman, P. D.: Herpes virus infections of the human central nervous system. N Engl J Med 277:1271, 1967.

Oxbury, J. M., and MacCallum, F. O.: Herpes simplex virus encephalitis: clinical features and residual damage. Postgrad Med J 49:387, 1973.

Pazin, G. J., Armstrong, J. A., Tai Lam, M., Tarr, G. C., Jannetta, P. J., and Ho, M.: Prevention of reactivated herpes simplex infection by human leukocyte interferon after operation on the trigeminal root. N Engl J Med 301:225, 1979.

Price, R., Chernik, N. L., Horta-Barbosa, L., and Posner, J. B.: Herpes simplex encephalitis in an anergic patient. Am J Med 54:222, 1973.

Rappel, M., Dubois-Dalcq, M., Sprecher, S., Thiry, L., Lowenthal, A., Pelc, S., and Thys, J. P.: Diagnosis and treatment of herpes encephalitis, a multidisciplinary approach. J Neurol Sci 12.443, 1971.

Ravaut, P., and Darré, M.: Les réactions nerveuses au cors de herpes génitaux. Ann Dermatol Syphiligr (Paris) 5:481, 1904.

Rawls, W. E., Dyck, P. J., Klass, D. W., Greer, H. D., and Hermann, E. C., Jr.: Encephalitis associated with herpes simplex virus. Ann. Intern Med. 64:104, 1966.

Sarubbi, F. A., Jr., Sparling, P. F., and Glezen, W. P.: *Herpesvirus hominis* encephalitis, viral isolation from brain biopsy in seven patients and results of therapy. Arch Neurol 29:268, 1973.

Sawanobori, S., Onishi, S., Matsuyama, S., and Irie, H.: H.S.V-1 and acute aseptic meningitis. Lancet 1:756, 1974.

Shearer, M. L., and Finch, S. M.: Periodic organic psychosis associated with recurrent herpes simplex. N Engl J Med 271:494, 1964.

Skoldenberg, B., Jeansson, S., and Wolontis, S.: Herpes simplex virus type 2 and acute aseptic meningitis. Clinical features of cases with isolation of herpes simplex virus from cerebrospinal fluids. Scand J Infect Dis 7:227, 1975.

Smith, M. G., Lennette, E. H., and Reames, H. R.: Isolation of the virus of herpes simplex and the demonstration of intranuclear inclusions in a case of acute encephalitis. Am J Pathol 17:55, 1941.

Stalder, H., Oxman, M. N., Dawson, D. M., and Levin, M. J.: Herpes simplex meningitis: isolation of herpes simplex virus type 2 from cerebrospinal fluid. N Engl J Med 289:1296, 1973.

Terni, M., Caccialanza, P., Cassai, E., and Kieff, E.: Aseptic meningitis in association with herpes progenitalis. N Engl J Med 285:503, 1971.

Tucker, B. A., Doekel, R. C., Jr., Whitley, R. J., and Dismukes, W. E.: Herpes simplex virus encephalitis: an atypical presentation. South Med J 71:1431, 1978.

Warren, K. G., Brown, S. M., Wroblewska, Z., Gilden, D., Koprowski, H., and Subak-Sharpe, J.: Isolation of latent herpes simplex virus from the superior cervical and vagus ganglions of human beings. N Engl J Med 298:1068, 1978.

Whitley, R. J., Nahmias, A., Soong, S-J., Fleming, C. L., Galasso, G. J., and Alford, C. A.: Vidarabine therapy of neonatal herpes simplex virus infections. Pediatrics 66:495, 1980.

Whitley, R. J., Soong, S-J., Dolin, R., Galasso, G. J., Ch'ien, L. T., Alford, C. A., and the Collaborative Study Group. Adenine arabinoside therapy of biopsy-proved herpes simplex encephalitis. N Engl J Med 297:289, 1977.

Wolontis, S., and Jeansson, S.: Correlation of herpes simplex virus types 1 and 2 with clinical features of infection. J Infect Dis 135:28, 1977.

Yeager, A. S., Arvin, A. M., Urbani, L. J., and Kemp, III, J. A.: Relationship of antibody to outcome in neonatal herpes simplex infections. Infect Immun 29:532, 1980.

Zimmerman, R. D., Russell, E. J., Leeds, N. E., and Kaufman, D.: CT in the early diagnosis of herpes simplex encephalitis. Am J Radiol 134:61, 1980.

# HERPESVIRUS SIMIAE (B VIRUS) ENCEPHALITIS 169

## Joshua Fierer, M.D.

### DEFINITION

*Herpesvirus simiae* (B virus) encephalitis is a rare disease characterized by diffuse inflammation of the central nervous system consequent to infection with *H. simiae*.

### ETIOLOGY

This sporadic infection occurs in people who have had occupational exposure to monkeys or their tissues. B virus infection occurs naturally in Old World monkeys, principally *Macaca mulatta*. In the primate, *H. simiae* causes a benign, self-limited, superficial infection of the oral mucosa similar to *Herpesvirus hominis* infections in humans (Keeble et al., 1958). Structurally and antigenically, B virus is closely related to *H. hominis* (herpes simplex) (Plummer, 1964).

### PATHOGENESIS AND PATHOLOGY

Infection is acquired from infected monkeys or their tissues. Many cases, but not all, are initiated by a monkey bite, by minor trauma inflicted by a monkey, or by puncture wounds with objects that were contaminated with monkey tissue. Since an aerosol of the virus can infect experimental animals, it is possible that those patients without a history of direct trauma were infected by airborne virus (Benda and Cerva, 1969). The virus is quite neurotropic in humans. It presumably spreads along neural routes from the point of inoculation to the spinal cord and then cephalad within the central nervous system. There may also be hematogenous spread to the brain. In one patient there was circumstantial evidence that encephalitis followed reactivation of a latent infection of the trigeminal nerve (Fierer et al., 1973).

The specific pathologic changes produced by B virus are limited to regional lymph nodes and the central nervous system. Lymph nodes draining a site of inoculation may be hemorrhagic and show focal necrosis. Within the central nervous system, the pons and medulla are always involved with a lymphocytic infiltrate, glial proliferation, and edema. In some cases there is necrosis and death of neurons. Giant cells are not seen, and the microscopic appearance of the brain is not specific for B virus infection. In some patients there is a prominent myelitis of the cervical and thoracic cord that is not limited to specific tracts. Diffuse cortical encephalitis is a feature of some cases. Virus has been isolated from all affected areas of the central nervous system and from lymph nodes distal to the site of inoculation but never from blood, cerebrospinal fluid, or other organs (Davidson and Hummeler, 1960).

### CLINICAL MANIFESTATIONS

A vesicular rash may develop at the site of inoculation within two or three days of the inciting injury. This is followed by lymphangitis and regional lymphadenopathy. Within three days to five weeks fever and symptoms of central nervous system infection develop. The disease may present either as ascending myelitis with flaccid motor paralysis and bladder paresis or as a diffuse encephalitis without localizing signs. Brain stem dysfunction is often prominent, with diplopia, dysphagia, and respiratory paralysis in most patients (Davidson and Hummeler, 1960). One patient, whose illness began with a zosteriform rash in the distribution of the ophthalmic branch of the trigeminal nerve, had not been exposed to monkeys for at least ten years. The disease progressed to a diffuse encephalitis (Fierer et al., 1973).

### COMPLICATIONS AND SEQUELAE

In clinically apparent infections, death results in most cases. The few people who survive are left with residual neurologic damage of varying severity.

### GEOGRAPHIC VARIATIONS

About half the reported cases were from the United States. The rest occurred in Canada and Great Britain. This distribution probably reflects the number of individuals with occupational exposure to monkeys and their tissues.

## DIAGNOSIS

The diagnosis should be suspected in any patient who develops encephalitis or encephalomyelitis and who has had direct contact with monkeys or with monkey tissue. A definite premortem diagnosis can be established only if B virus is isolated from a skin lesion (Fierer et al., 1973). Serologic diagnosis is difficult because of extensive cross-reaction between *H. hominis* and *H. simiae* and because patients who have been immunologically primed by *H. hominis* (simplex) have increased antibody titers against that virus after infection with B virus. Antibody must be titered by virus neutralization. This should be done only in research laboratories that have facilities to protect laboratory workers from B virus infection.

## TREATMENT

There is no specific treatment. Corticosteroids and cytosine arabinoside have been used, but there is no evidence that they were beneficial.

## PROPHYLAXIS

Everyone who works with monkeys and their tissues should be aware of the potential danger of the infection and use protective clothing. Monkeys with active infections should be placed in quarantine (Perkins and Hartley, 1966). A killed virus vaccine has been developed but is not produced commercially (Hull et al., 1962). Antibody to *H. hominis* is not protective.

### References

Benda, R., and Cerva, L.: Course of air-borne infection caused by B virus (*Herpesvirus simiae*). J Hyg Epidemiol Microbiol Immunol 13:307, 1969.

Davidson, W. L., and Hummeler, K.: B virus infection in man. NY Acad Sci Ann 85:970, 1960.

Fierer, J., Bazeley, P., and Braude, A. I.: Herpes B virus encephalomyelitis presenting as ophthalmic zoster. Ann Intern Med 79:225, 1973.

Hull, R. N., Peck, F. B., Jr., Ward, T. G., and Nash, J. C.: Immunization against B virus infection. II. Further laboratory and clinical studies with an experimental vaccine. Am J Hyg 76:239, 1962.

Keeble, S. A., Christofinis, G. J., and Wood, W.: Natural virus-B infection in rhesus monkeys. J Pathol Bacteriol 76:189, 1958.

Perkins, F. T., and Hartley, E. G.: Precautions against B virus infections. Br Med J 1:899, 1966.

Plummer, G.: Serological comparison of the herpes viruses. Br J Exp Pathol 45:135, 1964.

# CENTRAL NERVOUS SYSTEM INFECTIONS CAUSED BY TOGAVIRIDAE AND RELATED AGENTS

# 170

*Monto Ho, M.D.*

## GENERAL ASPECTS OF TOGAVIRIDAE

Viral encephalitis and meningoencephalitis may be either *epidemic* (and endemic) or *sporadic* (Dickerson et al., 1952). Sporadic cases occur irrespective of time, season, and place. One example is herpes simplex encephalitis (Chapter 168), which occurs in any population at any time and place. Epidemic encephalitis occurs at particular times of the year and in particular places. The reason is that the implicated viruses are maintained in well-defined biologic reservoirs and are transmitted to man by specific biologic vectors. Togaviridae and related agents are the most important causes of epidemic encephalitis. Almost every large geographic region in the world has its own particular agent of this type. Every physician should be familiar with the arthropod-borne encephalitides peculiar to his own region.

General comments about the epidemiologic and clinical aspects of this group of viruses will be given here and will not be repeated for each agent and disease. More basic virologic material is covered in Chapter 61. There are over 350 viruses that are transmitted by arthropods or cause febrile illnesses in man and animals. In man, these range from inapparent infection to febrile diseases with or without rashes, hemorrhagic shock syndromes, and infections of the central nervous system (Theiler and Downs, 1973). The important agents causing encephalitis and infection of the central nervous system are listed in Table 1 and will be discussed here. There are subgroups of Togaviridae as well as additional virus groups such as Arenaviridae (South American hemorrhagic fevers, Lassa fever, Rift Valley fever) and Orbiviridae (Colorado tick fever), which cause infections not usually involving the central nervous system. These are discussed elsewhere. West Nile fever (flavivirus) and the *Phlebotomus* fever group usually cause febrile syndromes and belong to this category. But occasionally they involve the central nervous system. Hence, they are included in Table 1 but are not separately discussed in the text.

Many, but not all, of these agents are transmitted by arthropods, and the term arbovirus is no longer de rigueur. Nevertheless, almost all the viruses in the group that causes encephalitis and meningoencephalitis are arthropod borne. According to the new terminology, which is based on the physicochemical rather than the epidemiologic properties of these agents, most of them belong to the Togaviridae (Table 1). Some important exceptions, such as California viruses, belong to the Bunyaviridae. They are distinct from the Togaviridae because their proteins are arranged in helical symmetry. Unlike the Togaviridae, the complement fixation test is more specific for these viruses than the hemagglutination inhibition test.

## EPIDEMIOLOGY

The fact that the most important epidemic encephalitides and meningoencephalitides are transmitted by arthropods (usually mosquitoes or ticks) has profound clinical as well as public health implications. Concepts of diagnosis and prevention of these infections are largely based on the peculiar epidemiology of these viruses. For example, if a suspected case occurs during a season or in a climate or region that cannot support the presence of responsible vectors, one can safely exclude the diagnosis of this type of encephalitis. There are several basic patterns of transmission of these agents. In the most important pattern, the vector transmits the infection from the animal reservoir to man but not from man to man. The reservoirs for the viruses are usually lower vertebrates such as fowl, rodents, and pigs. Hence, these encephalitides are "zoonoses," and man is an accidental host who does not serve as a source of infection. All the major arthropod-borne encephalitides, such as eastern equine encephalomyelitis (EEE), western equine encephalomyelitis (WEE), St. Louis, Venezuelan, Japanese, California, and the tick-borne encephalitides belong to this pattern. The isolation of the patient is usually unnecessary in these diseases with the exception of Venezuelan encephalitis and Russian spring-summer encephalitis. In another pattern of transmission, the mosquito transmits the infection from man to man. This is the pattern of yellow fever and dengue, which are discussed elsewhere. Finally, some of these viruses are transmitted directly from man to man without a vector. Certain exotic hemorrhagic fevers such as Lassa fever and Marburg disease are transmitted in this pattern but no important virus causing encephalitis.

## CLINICAL MANIFESTATIONS

The patient with arthropod-borne encephalitis usually presents with signs of infection and inflammation of the central nervous system. There is fever, headache, and disturbed consciousness, ranging from lethargy to stupor and coma. Convulsions, paralysis, involuntary movements, and other localizing signs may be present. There may also be signs of meningitis.

The onset and progression of each disease varies considerably with each virus, and even with particular localities and epidemics. In general, however, the infection is of sudden onset, runs an acute or subacute course, and is strikingly different from slow virus infection of the central nervous system (see Chapter 171). No chronic infection from arthropod-borne encephalitic viruses has been described in man.

## DIAGNOSIS

Diagnosis of arthropod-borne encephalitides is not difficult during an epidemic. In isolated cases, clinical acumen and epidemiologic awareness is required. Every physician should know what is "going around." This requires communication with the local health authorities and subscription to their bulletins. In the United States, all physicians dealing with communicable diseases should subscribe to the Morbidity and Mortality Weekly Reports, available free on request from the Center for Disease Control (CDC), Atlanta, Georgia. The precise diagnosis of these infections requires laboratory proof.

## DIFFERENTIAL DIAGNOSIS

Arthropod-borne encephalitides usually have a more acute onset than herpes encephalitis. They

**TABLE 1. Togaviruses and Related Agents Causing Encephalitis**

| VIRUS FAMILY | GENUS | REPRESENTATIVE SPECIES INFECTING MAN | VECTOR | DISEASE | GEOGRAPHIC DISTRIBUTION |
|---|---|---|---|---|---|
| Togaviridae | Alphavirus | Eastern equine encephalitis (EEE) virus | Mosquito | Encephalitis | Eastern U.S., Canada, Brazil |
| | | Western equine encephalitis (WEE) virus | Mosquito | Encephalitis | Western U.S |
| | | Venezuelan equine encephalitis (VEE) virus | Mosquito | Encephalitis | Northern Latin America, Southern U.S. |
| Togaviridae | Flavivirus | St. Louis encephalitis virus | Mosquito | Encephalitis | United States |
| | | Japanese encephalitis virus | Mosquito | Encephalitis | Japan, China, Korea, Southeast Asia |
| | | Tick-borne virus group (Russian spring-summer encephalitis, Powassan encephalitis, Louping ill). Nine viruses | Tick | Encephalitis, meningoencephalitis, hemorrhagic fever | European Russia, Siberia, Central Europe; Canada, U.S. (?Powassan); United Kingdom (Louping ill) |
| | | Murray Valley encephalitis virus | Mosquito | Encephalitis | Australia, New Guinea |
| | | West Nile virus | Mosquito | Usually a febrile rash disease, occasionally meningoencephalitis | Israel, Egypt |
| Bunyaviridae | Bunyamwere | Bunyamwere and 13 other viruses | Mosquito | Fever, headache | Africa, India, South America |
| | | California group | Mosquito | Meningitis, encephalitis | United States |
| Phlebotomus fever group (ungrouped) | | Three species | Phlebotomus (sandfly) | Usually a three-day febrile illness; may be associated with aseptic meningitis | Italy, Egypt |

also appear more suddenly and have a shorter duration than encephalitides associated with tuberculosis, cryptococcosis, other fungal infections, or brain abscess. Fever is a dependable sign, and its absence is rare in arthropod-borne encephalitides. In contrast, fever may be absent in cryptococcosis, brain abscess, para- and postinfectious encephalitis, and encephalopathy due to connective tissue diseases such as disseminated lupus erythematosus.

It may not be possible to distinguish clinically between arthropod-borne encephalitis and meningoencephalitis and encephalitis due to mumps and enteroviruses. Para- and postinfectious meningoencephalitis may also be difficult to rule out. Epidemiologic and laboratory aid is essential.

In viral meningoencephalitides, the cerebrospinal fluid is usually clear and colorless. There is a moderate number of cells, usually less than 1000, over 70 per cent of which are lymphocytes. In early taps there may be a predominantly neutrophilic response. The protein concentration is only moderately elevated (<100 mg/dl) and the glucose level not at all.

## LABORATORY DIAGNOSIS

Laboratory diagnosis of diseases caused by Togaviridae and related agents is based on a serologic rise of specific antibody titer or isolation of the causative agent from the patient. The main source of viral isolation is blood. Since viremia in man lasts only a short time, the virus is frequently not isolated from the blood. But when it is, a specific diagnosis may be made. The virus is even more rarely isolated from the cerebrospinal fluid. By and large, the suckling mouse is more satisfactory and more sensitive than cell cultures for isolation of these viruses. The number of viruses involved is so large that not even well-equipped laboratories or specialized centers have the reagents and sera necessary to identify all of them. Unknown isolates should be sent to the CDC in the United States or to national public health authorities in other countries for identification or confirmation. Through these agencies, the specimen may be referred to a regional laboratory for arboviruses or to an international reference center for arboviruses designated by the World Health Organization.

The most important laboratory method in diagnosis is serologic examination. Occasionally a diagnosis is made by the height of the antibody titer, but usually it is better to demonstrate a rise of titers in paired sera because almost all togaviruses can produce infection without disease, and a large segment of the population in an endemic area may already have antibodies to a particular virus without having had disease from it. The time to collect the first serum specimen is when the diagnosis is suspected. The titer in an acute phase blood specimen is then compared with the titer of a "convalescent" specimen obtained weeks after the first one.

The main serologic tests are the complement fixation, hemagglutination inhibition, and neutralization tests. The complement fixation test is the most widely used. Antibodies that fix complement are frequently of brief duration and hence are particularly significant when they are found in acute infections. Occasionally they appear too late to be useful. The hemagglutination inhibition test in togavirology is more group-specific and less type-specific, which is the reverse of the situation in the Bunyamwere group (California viruses), influenza, and other myxoviruses. Hemagglutination-inhibiting antibodies usually appear earlier than complement-fixing and neutralizing antibodies and disappear more rapidly than neutralizing antibodies.

## TREATMENT AND CONTROL

There is no specific treatment for togavirus infections. Supportive care, however, is essential, since even patients with serious encephalitis recover. Rehabilitative care is essential for patients with residual neurologic defects.

The only widely used and well-proven human vaccine in the togavirus field is the live attenuated yellow fever vaccine, the Theiler 17-D chick embryo tissue culture strain. Formalin-inactivated mouse brain vaccine against Japanese encephalitis has been used extensively in Japan and to a lesser extent by the American armed forces. Several attenuated live vaccines are undergoing study in Japan.

There are no accepted human vaccines against the arthropod-borne encephalitides in the United States. The amount of infection and morbidity is insufficient for widespread immunization programs. Vector and reservoir control is more important, although it is by no means simply achieved.

# EASTERN EQUINE ENCEPHALOMYELITIS (EEE)

### DEFINITION

EEE is caused by an alphavirus. This frequently fatal encephalitis of children and the elderly was first described on the eastern seaboard of the United States in 1938.

### EPIDEMIOLOGY

In endemic areas more than 50 per cent of birds tested may have antibodies. This suggests a natural cycle in which birds and mosquitoes are essential links. Horses and humans are probably dead ends in the infection cycle. In most epidemics, epizootics among horses and occasionally pheasants precede human illness. Inapparent infection in man is less common in this disease than in other togavirus infections.

### PATHOLOGY

Extensive necrosis may involve large areas of the midbrain. Neuronal damage and neuronopha-

gia occur, with a predominance of neutrophils in infiltrates as an outstanding feature.

### CLINICAL MANIFESTATIONS

The severity of EEE encephalitis is notable in almost all epidemics. Cases are concentrated in the 0 to 14 and over 55 age groups.

The onset of encephalitis is abrupt in young children. In older patients there may be a longer prodromal period of malaise, headache, and nausea before drowsiness, confusion, stiff neck, or convulsions supervene. The temperature rises sharply. Nonpitting edema of the face and distal parts of the limb has frequently been described in infants during the second and third days of illness. Leukocytosis is common. CSF is under increased pressure, with 200 to 2000 cells/mm$^3$. Neutrophils may comprise over 50 per cent of the cells and may persist to the second week of illness before mononuclear cells predominate. Infants who survive the acute illness almost always have neurologic sequelae.

# WESTERN EQUINE ENCEPHALOMYELITIS (WEE)

### DEFINITION

WEE is caused by an alphavirus endemic in wildlife and in horses. Human disease was first described in 1938. It is generally less severe than EEE.

### EPIDEMIOLOGY

The WEE virus is found in wildlife in the United States, Canada, Brazil, British Guiana, and Argentina. Human disease caused by this virus has been described only in the United States, Canada, and Brazil. The virus is found in practically all sections of the United States but most frequently in the western states and western Canada. An important endemic area is the Central Valley of California. The principal vector in this area is *Culex tarsalis,* which also transmits St. Louis encephalitis.

### PATHOLOGY

Damage to the brain and spinal cord may be extensive in small children. In severe cases, the pathologic signs are similar to those of EEE.

### CLINICAL MANIFESTATIONS

The disease is more common and more severe in children. About 20 to 30 per cent of all cases occur in infants under 1 year. Fever and drowsiness are common. Convulsions occur in 90 per cent of infected infants and in 40 per cent of children between 1 and 4 years old, but rarely in adults. In all age groups remission is sudden. Even those with convulsions or in coma may recover in five to ten days. The illness ends in less severe cases in three to five days. The overall mortality is 2 to 3 per cent.

Permanent sequelae are rare in adults but are

more frequent in younger children. More than half of afflicted infants less than a month old are left with recurring convulsions or motor or behavioral disorders requiring institutionalization. Inapparent infections far outnumber clinical illness, probably in the range of 60 to 1 in young children in 1000 to 1 in adults. The spinal fluid and other laboratory findings are similar to those in St. Louis encephalitis.

# VENEZUELAN EQUINE ENCEPHALOMYELITIS (VEE)

## DEFINITION

The alphavirus that causes VEE is transmitted sporadically to man, producing a mild encephalomyelitis during epizootics afflicting horses in Venezeula, Central America, and southwestern United States.

## EPIDEMIOLOGY

The virus passes through a sylvan cycle of mosquitoes and wild rodents such as cotton rats. Many mammals and birds compose the reservoir for the virus and develop antibodies to it, but the important amplifying host for man is the horse. Viremia in horses persists for only a few days, but this is sufficient to infect mosquitoes that can then transmit the virus to man. Usually a large number of infected horses is necessary to reach an infective threshold for human disease.

## CLINICAL MANIFESTATIONS

The disease in man is not usually fatal. Children account for about half of the cases, but any age group may be affected. Usually more males than females are attacked. Clinical diagnosis is based on seizures or any three of the following features: severe drowsiness, agitation, confusion, disorientation, hallucinations, and ataxia. There may be only a short febrile illness with sudden onset of malaise, chills, fever, nausea, vomiting, headache, muscle and bone aches, and fever lasting one to four days. Convalescence with marked asthenia may last up to three weeks.

# ST. LOUIS ENCEPHALITIS (SLE)

## DEFINITION

St. Louis encephalitis is the most important epidemic encephalitis in the United States in terms of number and severity of cases. It was first recognized in 1933, when an epidemic of 1100 cases with 221 deaths occurred in the St. Louis area (Kinsella and Brown, 1934).

## EPIDEMIOLOGY

St. Louis encephalitis occurs in three distinct regions in the United States, each with distinct types of mosquito vectors. The vectors explain why this disease may occur in either rural or urban areas. In the west, principally in irrigated rural and suburban areas, the vector is the same as that for WEE, i.e., *Culex tarsalis*. In the midwestern and occasionally eastern states such as the urban area of St. Louis, Kansas City, Houston, and Dallas, the vector is the *Culex pipeinsquinquefasciatus* complex. In Florida, the vector is *Culex nigripalpus*, which is a semitropical mosquito prevalent in both rural and urban areas.

## CLINICAL MANIFESTATIONS

SLE shows a striking and unique increase of incidence with age. Children are spared, and the elderly are preferentially afflicted. The case-fatality ratio (deaths among cases) also increase with age, and most of the deaths occur among the elderly. The incubation period is 9 to 14 days.

The typical case starts abruptly with fever, headache, nuchal rigidity, nausea, vomiting, and usually somnolence, tremors, and difficulty in speaking. As a rule, the disease reaches its height within the first 24 to 48 hours of illness. Many patients show disorientation, inability to remember earlier events, slurred speech, lethargy, insomnia, and occasionally delirium, but rarely deep coma. In children, convulsions may occur. Objective findings of stiff neck and positive Kernig signs are common. The fever is highest in the first two or three days of infection and returns to normal after seven to ten days. Rarely, it persists up to a month or six weeks. Urinary frequency, dysuria, hyponatremia, and inappropriate secretion of antidiuretic hormone may occur. The white cell count varies between 12,000 and

20,000. The spinal fluid is clear and under moderate pressure. The average cell count is between 50 and 250 cells/mm³, rarely rising to 500 or 1000. In the first count one-third or even one-half of the white cells may be neutrophils. Later mononuclear cells predominate.

In mild or abortive cases the chief symptoms are fever, moderate headache, and perhaps mild systemic manifestations. Occasionally there is suspicion of a rigid neck and slight tremors. Spinal fluid reveals mononuclear cells. Symptoms of clouded consciousness, apathy, and, in some cases, night-prowling and senile dementia may follow the acute disease for weeks or months. Permanent sequelae are uncommon.

## PATHOLOGY

The basic lesions are perivascular round cell cuffing, hemorrhages, and neuronal damage. They predominate in the thalamus and substantia nigra. The cerbral cortex, cerebellum, and in particular the Purkinje cells may also be affected.

# JAPANESE ENCEPHALITIS

## DEFINITION

Japanese encephalitis is caused by a flavivirus that produces serious epidemics that affect more people in larger areas of the world than any other togavirus. The disease was distinguished from von Economo's (A) type encephalitis in 1924.

## EPIDEMIOLOGY

Like other togaviruses, Japanese encephalitis virus is maintained in extrahuman reservoirs such as wild and domestic birds that develop sustained viremia. Man is an incidental host and plays no role in its transmissions. The disease has a seasonal incidence, although in tropical regions where mosquitoes are active throughout the year, it can occur in any season. In addition to Japan, it occurs in eastern Siberia, China, Korea, Taiwan, Southeast Asia, and India. The most important vector is a rural mosquito, *Culex tritaeniorhynchus,* which prefers to bite large domestic animals but also feeds on birds and man. In Japan this virus probably overwinters in hibernating adult female mosquitoes.

## CLINICAL MANIFESTATIONS

Japanese encephalitis occurs more frequently in children than in adults. There is another peak of incidence in patients over 60 years old. In general, the disease is more severe and has a longer course, slower convalescence, higher incidence of sequelae, and higher case-fatality rate than St. Louis encephalitis. Mortality, which varies greatly from epidemic to epidemic, ranges from 10 to 40 per cent.

Encephalitis usually takes two to four days before it becomes full-blown. The presenting symptoms are headache, fever, shaking chills, nuchal rigidity, vomiting, and nausea. Several distinguishing characteristics of the encephalitis may be noted (Dickerson et al., 1952). Altered sensorium is characterized by retardation or a flattened affect. There is no anxiety or apprehension. Patients may present a mask-like facies reminiscent of Parkinsonism. The speech is thick and slow, and there are frequently coarse ocular tremors. There is an unusually severe symmetrical neurogenic paresis, which is not specifically localizing and lacks sensory abnormalities. Frequently the deep tendon reflexes are increased. The patients are extremely ill. They may be bedridden for two weeks and convalesce for four weeks. There may be long-term mental and psychiatric residual effects, with intellectual impairment, confusion, psychosis, and delusions.

The CSF is uniformly abnormal and frequently may not return to normal for seven weeks. Pleocytosis may reach 1000 cells/mm³. Blood leukocytosis is common, with a predominance of neutrophils. The erythrocyte sedimentation rate is elevated.

## PATHOLOGY

There is vascular congestion in the meninges and brain, with widespread perivascular lymphocyte infiltration and cuffing. Neuronal degeneration, neuronophagia, microglial proliferation, and petechial hemorrhages are common. The cerebral cortex and frequently the thalamus and substantia nigra are particularly involved.

## DIAGNOSIS

The specific complement fixation test is frequently unsatisfactory if only one specimen is obtained, because no titer rise may be obtained until more than five weeks after onset. Multiple hemagglutination inhibition and neutralization tests should be done to observe a diagnostic rise in titer.

# MURRAY VALLEY ENCEPHALITIS

The responsible flavivirus is antigenically related to Japanese encephalitis virus. It is enzootic in birds and mosquitoes in northern tropical Australia and New Guinea. Infection in man occurs only in these two areas. A high proportion of human infections is inapparent with an estimated ratio of inapparent to apparent infections of between 500 to 1000:1. The highest attack rate occurs in children, in whom the case-fatality rate and the incidence of serious sequelae are both higher than in older patients. Despite high infection rates, epidemics are relatively infrequent, and the population at risk is not large.

# TICK-BORNE ENCEPHALITIDES

### DEFINITION

An indefinite number of flaviviruses are transmitted by ticks and cause encephalitis. Two clinical forms are identified, a severe form occurring primarily in the Soviet Far East (Russian spring-summer encephalitis), and a milder form occurring in Central Europe (diphasic meningoencephalitis) (Henner and Hanzal, 1963).

### EPIDEMIOLOGY

Probably small wild rodents are the reservoir of these viruses, which accounts for the stationary endemicity of the disease. The larvae and nymphs of ticks grow only in field mice, whereas the adult forms feed on larger mammals. Humans are an incidental host for the virus when they are exposed to ticks in rural wooded areas. An unusual method of acquiring the infection is by consumption of raw milk from cows or sheep, which become infected by infected ticks. Of all togaviruses this one shares with the virus of VEE the distinction of creating the greatest hazard for laboratory workers. The virus may also cause infection by the respiratory route.

### CLINICAL MANIFESTATIONS

The Far Eastern or more severe form of the disease has an incubation period of 8 to 14 days. There is violent onset of headache, fever, nausea, vomiting, hyperesthesia, and photophobia. Nuchal rigidity, weakness, and drowsiness follow rapidly. At the height of illness, delirium or coma, convulsions, pareses, or paralysis may develop. Severe disease is characterized by involvement of the bulbar centers and the cervical cord. Ascending paralysis or hemiparesis may result. The more benign course is essentially that of aseptic meningitis. In the nonfatal case, fever lasts five to eight days. Convalescence may be prolonged for months. Residual paralysis typically involves the arms and shoulder girdle. The case-fatality rate is estimated to be 20 to 30 per cent, death occurring within one to seven days. Infection is more severe in children than in adults.

The Central European form is more benign and often runs a diphasic course. The first phase is a period of viremia characterized by a febrile influenza-like illness that lasts for two to seven days. The liver may be tender, and liver function tests are abnormal, but the CSF is normal. Leukopenia is characteristic. This phase is followed by an asymptomatic period of 8 to 15 days. The second phase is characterized by signs and symptoms of meningoencephalitis — that is, fever, severe headache, nuchal rigidity, nausea, and vomiting. The temperature rises rapidly to 40° C or more. There may be diplopia, blurring of vision, slowed mentation, mental confusion, and delirium. Coma is rare. Most patients recover completely. The case-fatality ranges from 0.5 to about 5 per cent depending on the locality of outbreaks. Patients have a more severe form of disease in newly endemic areas such as Austria, and are less ill in Czechoslovakia, Western U.S.S.R., and Eastern Europe. Convalescence may be prolonged, with tremors and psychic or emotional disturbances. Permanent disability is uncommon.

# POWASSAN VIRUS ENCEPHALITIS

Powassan virus was isolated in 1958 from a human case of fatal encephalitis and is distantly related to the tick-borne encephalitis virus group. Antibodies to this virus have been found in wild mammals and, very infrequently, in humans in Ontario and New York State. The evidence indicates that man was not infected by this virus in the past, but his inroads into wild habitats may cause human infections in the future.

# CALIFORNIA ENCEPHALITIS

### DEFINITION

The California virus group, now reclassified under the Bunyaviridae, was first isolated from mosquitoes in California in 1943. It was shown to cause encephalitis in man in 1952. Since then it has become the most frequently reported cause of arthropod-borne meningoencephalitis in the United States. Most patients recover.

### EPIDEMIOLOGY

The reservoir of infection is probably rodents, such as squirrels, cotton rats, and rabbits. Birds are not important in transmission of this virus. The constant and relatively immobile sylvatic reservoir may account for the constancy of infection rates in many parts of the United States. The infection is transmitted accidentally from this reservoir to man by a large variety of *Aedes* mosquitoes in rural areas. The virus is endemic in California and the Midwest, including Wisconsin and Ohio. Human infection was apparently absent before 1950.

### CLINICAL MANIFESTATIONS

This virus group causes a significant amount of inapparent infection. For example, in Kern County in the Central Valley in California, 39 per cent of rural residents were inapparently infected as demonstrated by the presence of antibodies. Encephalitis does not occur in infants but is frequent in young children. Adults may develop only meningitis.

There may be prodromal fever, headache, nausea, vomiting, and abdominal pain lasting one to four days. As in other types of encephalitides, headache, stiff neck, sensorial disturbance, and convulsions are common. The peripheral blood count is usually elevated with predominance of the neutrophils. Lymphocytosis is usually seen in the cerebrospinal fluid.

Residual neurologic defects such as recurrent seizures, depressed intellectual function, and abnormal EEG have been described. Usually the patient recovers completely, and mortality is very low.

### References

Dickerson, R. B., Newton, J. R., and Hansen, J. E.: Diagnosis and immediate prognosis of Japanese B encephalitis. Am J Med 12:277, 1952.

Hammon, W. McD., and Ho, M.: Viral encephalitis. Disease-a-Month, February, 1973.

Henner, K., and Hanzal, F.: Les encéphalites européennes à tiques. Rev Neurolog 108:697, 1963.

Kinsella, R. A., and Broun, G. O.: Clinical features of epidemic (St. Louis) encephalitis. JAMA 103:462, 1934.

Theiler, M., and Downs, W. G.: The Arthropod-Borne Viruses of Vertebrates. New Haven, Yale University Press, 1973.

# 171 SLOW INFECTIONS

### Ashley T. Haase, M.D.

### DEFINITION

Sigurdsson first introduced the term "slow infections" to capture the novel time scale of a group of chronic transmissible diseases of Icelandic sheep (Sigurdsson, 1954). The characteristics of slow infections are as follows: 1) a long preclinical phase, generally months to years, from exposure to the infectious agent to appearance of symptoms; 2) a protracted clinical course; 3) pathologic manifestations frequently confined to a single organ system, most often the central nervous system (CNS). The medical importance of slow infections became evident with the discovery by Gajdusek that degenerative diseases of man, like kuru and Creutzfeldt-Jakob disease (CJD), were transmissible diseases with incubation periods exceeding one year.

## DIVERSITY OF ETIOLOGIC AGENTS OF SLOW INFECTIONS

Diseases that fulfill Sigurdsson's criteria for slow infections are caused by viruses from most major taxonomic classes (Table 1), and by agents designated unconventional (Table 2A, because they are filterable, replicate, and transmit disease like viruses, but have other properties (Table 2B) quite unlike conventional viruses. Particularly important is the unusual resistance of these agents to commonly employed disinfectants; effective methods for inactivation are listed in

Table 2C. Slow infections frequently are called slow virus infections because they are caused by viruses or viral-like agents with one exception, Johne's disease of sheep caused by mycobacteria. However, except for the unconventional agents, the pace of viral replication is not inherently slow in animals or tissue culture. Rather, only the appearance of symptoms from cumulative pathology is slow.

## PATHOLOGY

In many slow infections the pathologic alterations are confined largely to the CNS; in immunopathologic syndromes to be described any organ system may be involved. The tissue lesions in the CNS are described as demyelinating, inflammatory, or spongiform. Unconventional agents produce a degenerative lesion giving tissue sections a spongy appearance at the light microscopic level. This is due to vacuolation primarily in neurons and neuropil. Hypertrophy and proliferation of astrocytes are also characteristic of spongiform encephalopathies. Visna and sub-

### TABLE 1. Taxonomy of Agents of Slow Infections

#### A. SLOW INFECTIONS OF MAN CAUSED BY VIRUSES

| Classification | Virus | Disease |
|---|---|---|
| *RNA Viruses* | | |
| Paramyxovirus | Measles variant | Subacute sclerosing panencephalitis (SSPE) |
| Rhabdovirus | Rabies | Rabies |
| *DNA Viruses* | | |
| Papovavirus | JC, SV40 | Progressive multifocal leukoencephalopathy (PML) |
| Parvovirus | Hepatitis A,B | Hepatitis, arteritis |

#### B. SLOW INFECTIONS OF ANIMALS CAUSED BY VIRUSES

| Classification | Virus | Disease | Host |
|---|---|---|---|
| *RNA Viruses* | | | |
| Retrovirus | Visna | Meningoencephalitis | Sheep |
| | Maedi | Pneumonitis | Sheep |
| | Progressive pneumonia (PPV) | Pneumonitis | Sheep |
| | Equine infectious anemia (EIA) | Hemolytic anemia, arteritis | Horse |
| | Gardner agent | Lower motor neuron | Feral Mouse |
| | Xenotropic C type | Hemolytic anemia, SLE-like | NZB Mouse |
| Arena Virus | Lymphocytic chorio-meningitis (LCM) | Meningitis glomerulonephritis | Mouse |
| Paramyxovirus | Canine distemper | Encephalitis | Dog |
| Togavirus | Lactate dehydrogenase (LDV) | Elevated LDH; mild nephritis | Mouse |
| Picornavirus | Theiler's agent | Demyelination | Mouse |
| *DNA Viruses* | | | |
| Parvovirus | Aleutian disease (ADV) | Arteritis, anemia, nephritis | Mink |
| Papovavirus | SV40 | Progressive multifocal leukoencephalopathy | Monkey |

**TABLE 2.   Unconventional Agents of Slow Infections**

### A. SLOW INFECTIONS CAUSED BY UNCONVENTIONAL AGENTS

| In Man | In Animals |
|---|---|
| Creutzfeldt-Jakob Disease (CJD) | Scrapie in sheep, goats |
| Kuru | Transmissible mink encephalopathy |

### B. UNUSUAL PROPERTIES OF UNCONVENTIONAL AGENTS

1. Resistance to physical, chemical treatments: Not wholly inactivated by boiling, sonication; resistant to UV irradiation, proteases, nucleases, formaldehyde, B propiolactone.
2. Genome: Small target size to UV irradiation, equivalent to molecular weight 150,000; atypical action spectrum-inactivation 237 nm greater than 254 nm.
3. Virus particles: No virus particles evident in electron micrographs of tissues with $10^8$ infectious units/g.
4. Host response: No inflammatory reaction; antigenicity questionable, as humoral or cellular immunity not demonstrable, disease unaltered in immunosuppressed animals; interferon not induced, no response to exogenously administered interferon.
5. Replication in tissue culture: Replication to low titers in explanted fragments of brain; no cytopathic effect; no interference with growth of conventional viruses.

### C. INACTIVATION OF UNCONVENTIONAL AGENTS

Autoclaving (121°C; 20 psi; 30 minutes)
Hypochlorite (Clorox NaOCl 0.5–5.0 percent) iodine disinfectants
Lipid solvents: Ether, acetone, chloroform, chloroform-butanol, 2 chlorethanol, strong detergents, 6 M urea
Carbohydrate active reagents: .01 M periodate

acute sclerosing panencephalitis (SSPE) are prototypes of inflammatory encephalitides in which lymphocytes and plasma cells infiltrate the CNS, often arrayed as cuffs around blood vessels, or collected discretely in foci (microglial nodules). Sclerosing refers to the relative firmness of the end-stage lesion vis a vis normal neural tissue. Destruction of neurons in inflammatory foci may lead secondarily to demyelination. In progressive multifocal leukoencephalopathy (PML) demyelination is primary; that is, axis cylinders are relatively preserved. Demyelination in this situation is a direct consequence of destruction of oligodendrocytes, the cells that furnish myelin sheaths in the CNS. PML is thus almost exclusively a disease of white matter (leukoencephalopathy).

## PATHOGENESIS

Persistence of virus in the face of host defense mechanisms, and the evolution of disease over a period often of years are two aspects of slow infections that require explanation and continue to inspire investigative efforts in this area.

### Mechanisms of Persistence

Mechanisms for virus persistence can be considered in a logical framework of the virus life cycle, the fate of the infected cell, and the host response to virus infection (Fig. 1). In acute infections viruses invade cells and subvert them to production of a new crop of virions. The cells often die, and virus spreads until host defenses are mobilized to limit infection. Evidently in persistent infections virus host cell interactions must be different; the destructive effects of virus growth must be mitigated in order to provide for survival of the host beyond the initial phase of infection, and host defenses must not eliminate the infecting agent. A virus may escape elimination because 1) it remains inside the cell, where humoral and cellular immunity are powerless; 2) host defense mechanisms are not evoked; and 3) defense mechanisms are ineffective. Herpetic infections, visna, and SSPE illustrate the first stratagem. Herpes virus travels to and from the nervous system in axoplasm. In visna a DNA intermediate or provirus conserves viral genetic information inside the cell, but, analogous to lysogeny, this information is not expressed. Consequently the infected cells are not detected and destroyed by immune surveillance (Haase et al., 1977). In SSPE the causative variant of measles virus remains inside the cell because the protein required for virus assembly (matrix protein) is formed aberrantly.

Unconventional agents exemplify immunologi-

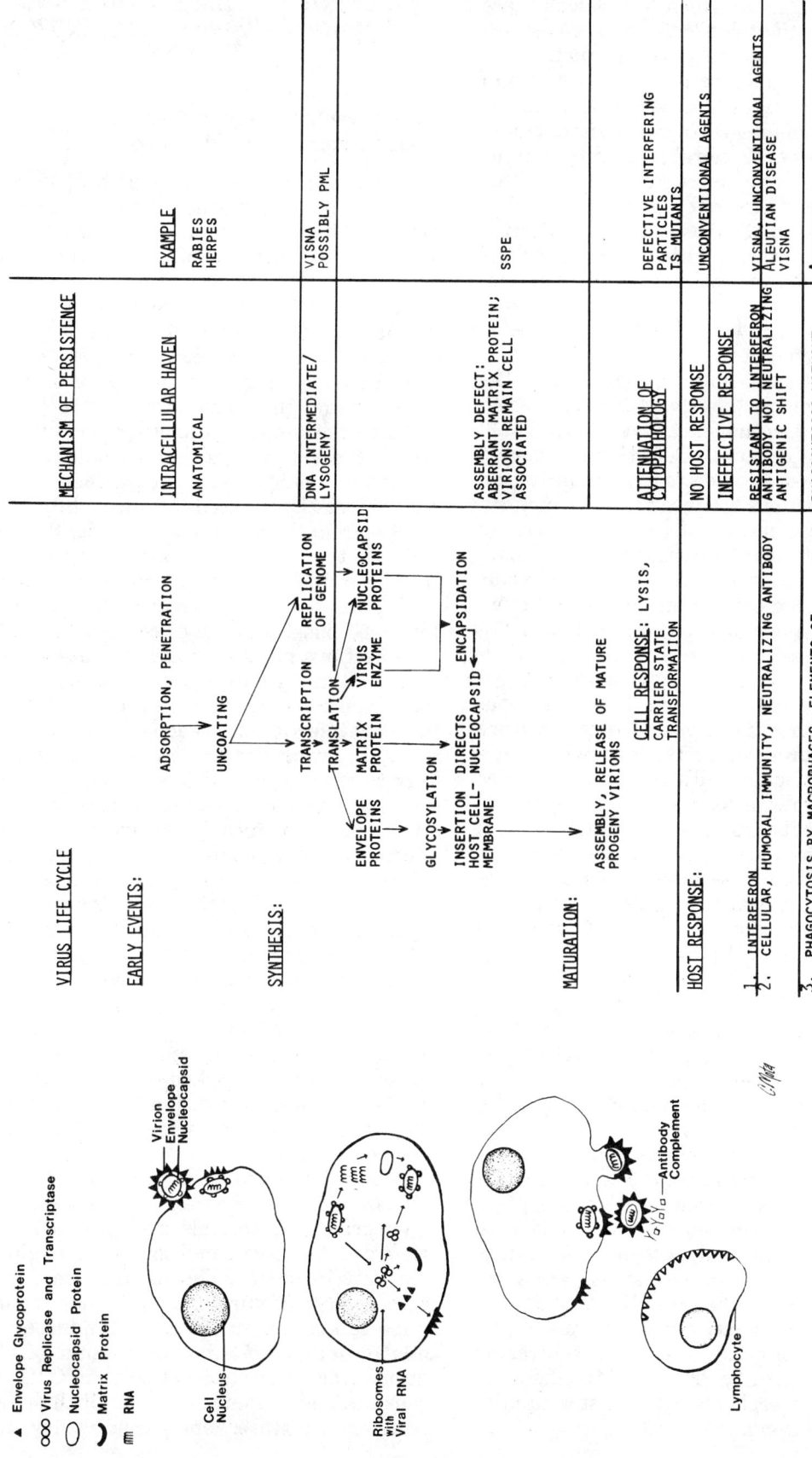

**FIGURE 1.** *Mechanisms of Virus Persistence: A generalized virus life cycle, and the attendant effects on the cell and host response, is presented schematically in the left half of the diagram; explanations proposed for persistence are tabulated in the right half.*

cally silent infections in which host defenses are not engaged. In other slow infections virus persists because the host response is ineffective. Aleutian disease is representative of a group of immune complex diseases in which antibody is produced and combines with virus without neutralizing infectivity. Humoral immunity may be ineffective too, at least temporarily, if antigenic variants arise that are not neutralized by antibody to the strain of virus-initiating infection (antigenic shift in visna). Other reasons for the failure of host defense mechanisms include phagocytosis of virus by cellular elements of the reticuloendothelial system without killing, and resistance to interferon.

Persistent infections imply moderation in the severity of viral cytopathology; otherwise susceptible cells would be consumed, or the host would succumb to acute infection. Defective interfering particles have been invoked to explain initiation of persistent infections because they diminish cytopathology. These particles have lost a portion of the genome of standard virus and can replicate only in a dual infection where standard virus supplies the missing genetic information (Huang, 1973). Such a co-infection is a competitive situation that sharply reduces the production of standard virus. Whether defective particles play a role in human infections is unknown. Their participation in the chronic infections of tissue culture cells is more securely supported by available evidence, and co-infection with defective particles prolongs some experimental infections of animals by days. Viral temperature-sensitive (ts) mutants also reduce growth of standard virions and lessen cytopathology. They arise later in persistent infections of tissue culture cells, and may play a role in the maintenance of persistent infections (Preble and Youngner, 1975).

### Slowness and Immunopathology

The tempo of viral replication, spread, and accumulation of attendant pathologic effects determine slowness. Slowness is an inherent property of the replication of unconventional agents. By contrast, the slow appearance and progress of symptoms in Aleutian disease, lymphocytic choriomeningitis, and equine infectious anemia derive from rate of expression of an immunopathologic process. In this instance virus replicates to high titer at a rate equivalent to acute infections (Porter et al., 1969), but tissue lesions occur slowly as a consequence of the formation and deposition of immune virus-antibody complexes in glomeruli and walls of blood vessels. The protracted course of infection in SSPE and PML likely reflects a complex interplay between host immunity and virus production and spread.

## CLINICAL DESCRIPTION AND DIAGNOSIS OF SLOW INFECTIONS IN MAN

### Unconventional Agents Causing Spongioform Encephalopathies

***Kuru.*** Kuru is a neurologic affliction at one time epidemic among the peoples of the Fore cultural and linguistic group inhabiting the remote mountainous regions of New Guinea. Kuru means trembling or shivering, a name derived from the most prominent symptoms, tremors of the head, trunk, and extremities. These symptoms disappear with sleep. The tremors and unsteadiness in gait are manifestations of cerebellar involvement; the symmetric cerebellar ataxia and motor dysfunction are progressively incapacitating. Flaccid paralysis, abnormalities of extraocular movements, incontinence, mental changes, and emaciation precede death, three to nine months from the onset of symptoms. Patients are afebrile, there are no inflammatory cells or increase in the protein in cerebral spinal fluid (CSF), and the pathologic changes are degenerative ones, most evident in cerebellum and pons. An infectious basis for kuru was discounted initially on these grounds, until Hadlow pointed out the remarkable similarities in the pathology of the slow infection of sheep (scrapie) and kuru in man. This stimulated renewed efforts to transmit kuru to animals, and ultimately led to the demonstration that homogenates of kuru brain would elicit a similar clinical pathologic picture in chimpanzees 13 to 18 months after inoculation.

Natural infections probably were transmitted by autoinoculation of the kuru agent into breaks in skin and mucous membranes occurring during preparation and consumption of the dead in a mourning rite. Since usually only adult women and young children of either sex were involved in this ritual, most cases of kuru occurred in these groups. The practice of cannibalism has been discontinued, with a marked decline in the overall number of cases of kuru, and the disappearance of kuru in children born since cannibalism ceased (Gajdusek, 1977).

***Creutzfeldt-Jakob Disease and other Transmissible Dementias.*** Success in transmitting kuru to experimental animals prompted a search for other degenerative conditions that might represent slow infections. The striking similarities in the pathology of kuru and CJD made the latter a prime candidate, and in 1966 Gajdusek and his collaborators reported transmission of CJD to chimpanzees. Dementias other than CJD are also transmissible in some cases that include familial Alzheimer's disease, supranuclear palsy, and sporadic presenile dementia in a variety of clinical contexts.

CJD is a rare presenile dementia of worldwide distribution most prevalent between the ages of 40 and 65. The combination of dementia, progressing noticeably from week to week, myoclonus, and an abnormal electroencephalogram, with a pattern of overall suppression on which paroxysmal bursts of high voltage slow waves are superimposed, suggest the diagnosis antemortem. Pneumoencephalogram and CT scan may disclose dilated ventricles consistent with diffuse cortical atrophy. The disease pursues a relentless downhill course with death 3 to 16 months from the onset of symptoms.

The origins and transmission of CJD are enigmatic. In about 10 per cent of cases there is a familial pattern suggesting transmission as an autosomal dominant. Clustering of disease in Jewish immigrants of Libyan origin, whose religious practices involve consumption of uncooked sheep brain, has provoked speculation that CJD may have arisen by transmission of scrapie to man. Inadvertent human transmission of CJD by corneal transplantation, and by improperly sterilized electroencephalographic electrodes has been reported.

### Conventional Agents

*Progressive Multifocal Leukoencephalopathy.* PML is a neurologic condition usually of immunologically compromised patients in which the protean symptomatology reflects the distribution of multiple foci of demyelination. Cerebral cortical involvement is most frequent with confusion, disorientation, personality change, poor memory, speech and visual disturbances, weakness, and paralysis. Dysarthria and abnormalities of sensation are common. The electroencephalogram is abnormal but not diagnostic, and, although not always useful in detecting early lesions, CT scans can be used to follow the progression of late lesions.

Eosinophilic or basophilic intranuclear inclusion bodies in enlarged oligodendroglia at the periphery of demyelinated foci first suggested viruses as the cause of PML. Subsequently, electron micrographs demonstrated viral particles with the morphologic characteristics of papovaviruses in the inclusion bodies, and the causative agent was isolated in cultures of glial cells. In most cases PML is caused by a new member of the papovavirus group, designated JC virus (Padgett et al., 1976); two reported cases of PML appear to have been caused by SV40 virus. This virus also causes a PML-like condition in macaque monkeys. Another human papovavirus, the BK agent, has been isolated from the urine of patients undergoing renal transplantation; thus far BK virus

has not been associated with disease. Serologic surveys indicate that JC and BK viruses are acquired early in life by a large proportion of populations (see Chapter 58).

Most cases of PML occur in patients with some underlying disorder that impairs host defenses. Presumably, the impaired defenses of these patients provide an opportunity for JC virus to replicate to high titer in CNS, either where it has been dormant or where it has spread, from an extraneural site or by reinfection. These explanations reconcile the ubiquitous nature of the virus with the rarity of PML (one to two cases per million in the United States).

*Subacute Sclerosing Panencephalitis (Dawson's Inclusion Body Encephalitis).* SSPE is a rare disease of children and young adults between the age of 4 and 20 years. Disease most often occurs in males from rural areas infected with measles before age 2. The initial phase is characterized by insidiously progressive deterioration of intellectual function and behavioral changes. School performance declines, and affected children are forgetful and subject to outbursts of temper. In the second phase these changes are more marked, and are associated with myoclonic movements of the head, trunk, or extremities repeated at intervals of 10 to 60 seconds. The electroencephalogram is abnormal with a pattern of periodic synchronous bursts of high voltage slow and sharp waves on a background of generalized suppression. Inflammatory lesions of the optic nerve may lead to chorioretinitis, papilledema, and pigmentary retinopathy. The terminal phase is one of profound dementia, decorticate spasticity, blindness, and hypothalamic dysfunction. Death occurs by infection or vasomotor collapse one to three years from the onset of symptoms.

Inflammatory changes in SSPE and eosinophilic intranuclear inclusion bodies pointed to a viral etiology, a suspicion heightened by finding tubular structures resembling paramyxovirus nucleocapsids in the inclusions, and by the very high titers of antibody to measles virus consistently demonstrated in the serum and CSF of these patients (Johnson et al., 1974). Later a variant of measles virus was isolated. Antigens of the measles variant can be demonstrated by immunofluorescence in cells in inflammatory foci. These foci also contain plasma cells that produce antibody to the virus; consequently the levels of IgG in CSF are elevated, and, on electrophoresis, specific bands appear (oligoclonal pattern) that can be adsorbed with viral antigens.

*Progressive Rubella Encephalitis.* Progressive motor and mental deterioration in the second decade of life has been recognized recently in patients chronically infected with rubella virus (Townsend et al., 1975). Other abnormalities include ataxia, myoclonus, elevated protein and IgG, and increased cells in the CSF. Inflammatory changes with moderate loss of neurons and cerebellar atrophy were found postmortem in addition to the calcification and deposition of basophilic granular material in the walls of blood vessels and in perivascular spaces that occur in rubella. Rubella virus was isolated in one case.

## TREATMENT AND PREVENTION

No specific therapy is available currently for slow infections. Antiviral drugs such as IuDr, Ara-A, Ara-C, and amantidine, immunopotentiation (γ-globulin, adjuvants, transfer factor), immunosuppression, and steroids have been used without success. The incidence of SSPE has declined markedly after widespread vaccination against measles. Special care must be exercised with demented patients with known or suspected spongioform encephalopathy. Corneas should not be transplanted from these patients, and the measures delineated in Table 2C should be employed to sterilize equipment, or to disinfect CSF and pathologic specimens from these patients.

## PROSPECTUS

Slow infections will continue to be the focus of major research efforts because of the possibility that far more prevalent chronic degenerative diseases of man such as multiple sclerosis (MS) may be attributed to viral infection. Higher titers and higher incidence of antibody in serum and CSF to measles virus, and epidemiologic evidence of common exposure to an environmental factor before adolescence can be cited as indirect support for a role of viruses in MS. However, direct evidence supporting a causal relationship in this and other chronic diseases has not been obtained to date.

## References

Andrewes, C. H.: The troubles of a virus. J Gen Microbiol 40:140, 1965.

Gajdusek, D. C.: Unconventional viruses and the origin and disappearance of kuru. Science 197:943, 1977.

Haase, A. T., Stowring, L., Narayan, O., Griffin, D., and Price, D.: Slow persistent infection caused by visna virus: role of host restriction. Science 195:175, 1977.

Huang, A. S.: Defective interfering viruses. Ann Rev of Microbiol 27:101, 1973.

Johnson, K. P., Byington, D. P., and Gaddis, L.: Subacute sclerosing panencephalitis. Adv in Neurol 6:77, 1974.

Padgett, B. L., Walker, D. L., ZuRhein, G. M., Hodach, A. E., and Chou, S. M.: JC papovavirus in progressive multifocal leukoencephalopathy. J. Infect Dis 133:686, 1976.

Porter, D. D., Larsen, A. T., and Porter, H. G.: The pathogenesis of aleutian disease of mink. I. *In vivo* replication and the host antibody response to viral antigen. J Exp Med 130:575, 1969.

Preble, O. T., and Youngner, J. S.: Temperature-sensitive viruses and the etiology of chronic and inapparent infections. J Infect Dis 131:467, 1975.

Sigurdsson, B.: Rida, a chronic encephalitis of sheep — with general remarks on infection which develop slowly and some of their special characteristics. British Vet J: Series of special university lectures, University of London, March, 1954.

Townsend, J. J., Baringer, J. R., Wolinsky, J. S., Malamud, N., Mednick, J. P., Panitch, H. S., Scott, R. A. T., Oshira, L. S., and Cremer, N. E.: Progressive rubella panencephalitis — late onset after congenital rubella. NEJM 292:990, 1975.

# 172  REYE'S SYNDROME

## Doris A. Trauner, M.S., M.D.

Reye's syndrome is an acute encephalopathy of childhood associated with diffuse fatty infiltration of the viscera. Before 1963 this disorder was frequently diagnosed as "acute toxic encephalopathy of unknown etiology." The full clinicopathologic syndrome was described by Reye and his co-workers in Australia in 1963, and numerous reports of this same disease from many parts of the world have since been published. The disease appears to be confined to children, with cases reported in patients 7 weeks to 22 years of age. It occurs with equal frequency in males and females. Recently, several cases have been reported in adults.

## ETIOLOGY AND PATHOGENESIS

The cause of Reye's syndrome is unknown. Numerous viruses have been associated with the prodromal illness. The most common are influenza B, A1 and A2, and varicella. Other viruses implicated in reported cases include herpes simplex, rubella, rubeola, poliovirus type I, adenovirus type III, echovirus, coxsackievirus types A, A1, B1, and B4, parainfluenza, and Epstein-Barr virus. Although a viral prodrome is present in almost all cases of Reye's syndrome, there is no evidence that the virus itself causes the encephalopathy.

There are several hypotheses regarding the cause of this disorder. Various potential toxins, including salicylates and phenothiazines, have been thought to play a possible causal role, but there is no evidence for this. However, the suggestion that a virus-toxin interaction may produce Reye's syndrome does have some foundation experimentally. Toxins such as insecticides and 4-pentenoic acid (an analogue of hypoglycin A) can produce an encephalopathy associated with fatty accumulation in the viscera of rats with viral infections. Nevertheless, no toxin or virus-toxin interaction has been identified in patients with Reye's syndrome.

Two disorders similar to Reye's syndrome are caused by exogenous toxins. Jamaican vomiting sickness is characterized by vomiting, coma, and seizures. It affects children in Jamaica and is caused by ingestion of unripe Ackee fruit, which contains the toxin hypoglycin A. Udorn encephalopathy, described from Thailand, is an acute encephalopathy of childhood that is identical to Reye's syndrome clinically and biochemically. This disorder is produced by ingestion of aflatoxin, a plant toxin present in some foods.

Patients with Reye's syndrome have elevated concentrations of serum short-chain fatty acids. These have been implicated as possible endogenous toxins. If short-chain fatty acids are injected into laboratory animals, an encephalopathy develops that has clinical and pathologic features identical to those of Reye's syndrome. Ammonia has also been considered as an endogenous toxin, but the levels of hyperammonemia seen in children with Reye's syndrome are generally lower than those required to produce coma in experimental animals. Short-chain fatty acids potentiate the effects of ammonia on the central nervous system in experimental animals, and it is possible that the presence of both toxins simultaneously may produce the encephalopathy of Reye's syndrome.

Finally, it has been suggested that some genetic factor may be involved. In a few instances Reye's syndrome has occurred in two or more family members. The presence of an inborn error of urea cycle metabolism would account for the hyperammonemia, lethargy, and coma. The activity of the mitochondrial urea cycle enzymes ornithine transcarbamylase and carbamyl phosphate synthetase have been decreased in liver biopsy specimens of patients during the acute phase of the disease. It is unlikely that this decreased activity represents an inborn metabolic error, since Reye's syndrome is not a recurrent disease and survivors exhibit no further evidence of metabolic derangements; rather, these enzyme abnormalities probably reflect mitochondrial injury during the acute illness.

## PATHOLOGY

Pathologic changes are found in liver, kidney, heart, pancreas, lungs, thymus, and brain. The liver may be enlarged and is usually yellow. Histologic examination reveals diffuse accumulation of small fatty droplets within the cytoplasm of hepatocytes (Fig. 1). There is no evidence of extensive necrosis of liver cells. Ultrastructural changes include mitochondrial swelling with distortion of cristae, dilatation of the cisternae of the rough endoplasmic reticulum, proliferation of the smooth endoplasmic reticulum, and fat droplets within the cytoplasm of hepatocytes. The glycogen content is reduced in the liver. These abnormalities disappear after the patient recovers.

The kidneys may also appear swollen and pale. Fatty infiltration is present in the proximal tubules and loops of Henle. In the heart, myocardial tissue contains fat droplets, and fibers may be swollen and vacuolated. The pancreas also contains an accumulation of fat droplets. Nonspecific intranuclear inclusions may be seen on ultrastructural examination. Histiocytes and alveolar lining cells of the lungs may also contain fat droplets.

The brain is grossly edematous and heavier, and the cortical surface is flattened. Cerebellar, tonsillar, or temporal lobe herniation may be present. The cerebral ventricles are smaller than normal. Microscopic examination of the brain reveals evidence of cellular and interstitial edema. No specific pathologic abnormalities are seen. There is no accumulation of fat. Anoxia may cause necrosis of cortical neurons, loss of cerebellar Purkinje cells, and reactive astrocytes.

## CLINICAL MANIFESTATIONS

Reye's syndrome in infants and children over 6 months of age is a biphasic illness with the features shown in Table 1. The first phase, or prodrome, is a viral illness, usually an upper respiratory infection or flu-like syndrome. This prodrome may be mild. As the child recovers from the viral illness, he begins to vomit repeatedly, and over a period of hours becomes delirious and agitated, then comatose. Generalized or focal seizures are common. Marked hyperventilation occurs with a mixed respiratory alkalosis and metabolic acidosis. Tachycardia may persist until improvement begins. Fever may be high even though no infection can be found. The liver is enlarged in the great majority of cases, even though clinical evidence of hepatic dysfunction is usually lacking.

The encephalopathy varies in severity. Several methods of staging coma in Reye's syndrome have

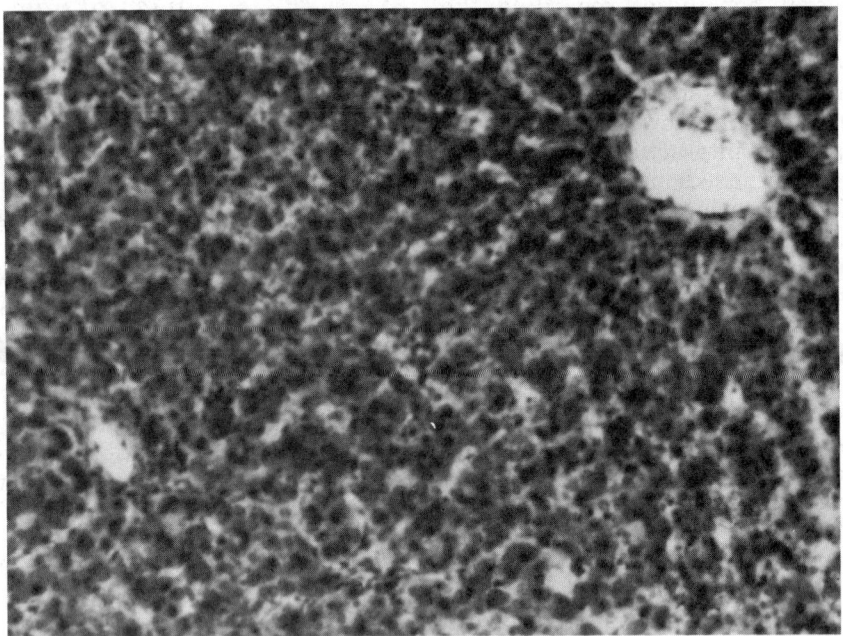

**FIGURE 1.**  *Liver biopsy from patient with Reye's syndrome; oil red O stain. Note diffuse small droplets of fat throughout specimen.*

been suggested. One commonly used set of criteria is that of Lovejoy and colleagues (1974), which consists of five stages.

Stage 1:  vomiting and lethargy.
Stage 2:  disorientation, delirium, combativeness; hyperventilation, hyperactive deep tendon reflexes, inappropriate responses to noxious stimuli.
Stage 3:  coma, hyperventilation, decorticate rigidity, preservation of pupillary reflexes.
Stage 4:  deepening coma, decerebrate rigidity, loss of oculocephalic reflexes, dilated pupils unresponsive to light, dysconjugate eye movements in response to caloric stimulation.
Stage 5:  seizures, loss of deep tendon reflexes, respiratory arrest, flaccidity.

As the coma deepens, the central nervous system dysfunction progresses in a rostral-caudal direction down the brain stem. In the final stage the brain stem stops functioning.

The clinical picture of Reye's syndrome in infants under 6 months of age differs somewhat from that in older children. Vomiting is less prominent. Respiratory abnormalities occur early and consist of marked hyperventilation and at times intermittent apnea. Seizures are common and may occur in the early encephalopathic stage. Infants tend to be limp and hypotonic with loss of primitive reflexes such as the Moro and tonic neck reflexes. The course is fulminant and the mortality and morbidity are high.

## LABORATORY ABNORMALITIES

Numerous biochemical abnormalities are present in patients with Reye's syndrome (Table 2). Abnormalities in liver function are distinctive. The prothrombin time is prolonged, and the serum glutamic oxaloacetic transaminase (SGOT), serum glutamic pyruvic transaminase (SGPT), and lactic dehydrogenase (LDH) concentrations are elevated. Yet the bilirubin concentration is typically normal. Serum creatine phosphokinase (CPK) levels are also elevated. Hyperammonemia

**TABLE 1.   Clinical Features of Reye's Syndrome**

Prodromal viral illness
Vomiting
Lethargy, delirium, coma
Hyperventilation
Seizures
Enlarged liver

**TABLE 2.   Laboratory Abnormalities in Reye's Syndrome**

Hyperammonemia
Hypoglycemia
Hypoglycorrachia
Abnormal liver function tests
Prolonged prothrombin time
Metabolic acidosis
Respiratory alkalosis
Hyperaminoacidemia
Short-chain fatty acidemia
Lactic acidemia

is present in virtually all patients early in the disease, but ammonia levels may return to normal within 24 to 48 hours.

Hypoglycemia is found in only 40 per cent of patients and is not a reliable diagnostic criterion. It is more common in children under 4 years of age. Arterial blood gas determinations may show a metabolic acidosis, respiratory alkalosis, or a mixture of both. Blood urea nitrogen is usually mildly elevated. Rarely, a significant azotemia is present, and transient anuria may occur. Although clinical evidence of pancreatitis is usually lacking, the serum amylase level may be elevated. Except for low glucose concentrations, the cerebrospinal fluid is normal.

Certain serum amino acids (alanine, glutamine, lysine, $\alpha$-amino $n$-butyrate) have been abnormally elevated. Lactic acidosis may occur. Elevated serum concentrations of the short-chain fatty acids propionate, butyrate, isobutyrate, valerate, and isovalerate have also been found in patients with Reye's syndrome.

## DIAGNOSIS

No single abnormality is pathognomonic for Reye's syndrome. Recognition of the disease is based on several criteria. The biphasic clinical course — an antecedent viral illness followed by repeated vomiting and progressing rapidly to lethargy and coma — is characteristic. This course, coupled with abnormal liver function tests, normal bilirubin levels, and a negative toxicology screen for toxins such as salicylates, leads to a diagnosis of Reye's syndrome. In doubtful or atypical cases, a biopsy of liver tissue may show diffuse accumulation of small fatty droplets.

A differential diagnosis should consider acute hepatitis, salicylate poisoning, other toxins (aflatoxin ingestion in Thailand, unripe Ackee fruit ingestion in Jamaica), encephalitis, severe hypoglycemia, and inborn errors of urea cycle metabolism.

## TREATMENT

Since the cause of Reye's syndrome is unknown, treatment is empirical. Therapy is aimed at stabilizing the patient's clinical status and correcting metabolic abnormalities.

Several procedures have been suggested to clear possible toxins from the body. Exchange blood transfusion and peritoneal dialysis have both been employed. Recent studies have found no additional benefit to the patients from these modes of therapy. A comprehensive treatment plan of intensive supportive care has been suc-cessful in many patients. This plan consists of the following steps:

1. Control respiration by nasotracheal intubation and mechanical ventilation.
2. Monitor blood pressure and central venous pressure with arterial and CVP lines.
3. Use neomycin enemas as necessary to decrease serum ammonia concentrations.
4. Administer vitamin K, 5 mg, intramuscularly or intravenously to help correct clotting abnormalities. Fresh frozen plasma can be given as well.
5. Monitor serum electrolytes, osmolality, glucose concentrations, prothrombin time, and blood urea nitrogen frequently.
6. Administer intravenous fluids consisting of 20 per cent glucose with appropriate electrolyte solutions.
7. Administer insulin, 1 unit per 5 g of glucose, every four hours intravenously. Blood glucose should be maintained at between 150 and 200 mg per 100 ml and insulin dosage altered as required to accomplish this. (Both hypertonic glucose and insulin help decrease serum accumulation of short-chain fatty acids).
8. Place the child on cooling blanket or sponge him frequently to keep temperature down to 37° C.
9. An intracranial pressure monitor should be inserted (in either the epidural or the intraventricular space) to monitor intracranial pressure continuously. Pressure should be kept below 20 mm of mercury. Control of intracranial pressure may be accomplished by the following methods:
   a. Controlled hyperventilation to a $pCO_2$ of 25 mm mercury.
   b. Intravenous mannitol ½ to 1 g per dose repeated as often as necessary. Serum osmolality should be kept below 320 to ensure continued efficacy of mannitol therapy and to decrease the incidence of complications.
   c. Paralysis of the patient with pancuronium bromide after mechanical ventilation has been instituted.

These measures should be continued until the patient begins to awaken from the coma.

## PROGNOSIS

Prognosis has become more favorable over the past several years. In Reye's original case reports (1963) there was an 80 per cent mortality. In subsequent years mortality has dropped, and with the treatment outlined above the mortality is less than 40 per cent.

Some survivors of Reye's syndrome are left

with permanent neurologic sequelae, including seizure disorders, mental retardation, and spasticity. However, many patients survive with no neurologic deficits. Since the encephalopathy is metabolic rather than structural in origin, early recognition and aggressive therapy, with particular attention to control of intracranial pressure, can result in complete recovery with return to normal function for many children with Reye's syndrome.

### EPIDEMIOLOGY

Reye's syndrome occurs sporadically and in "epidemics." The epidemic cases are geographically and temporally associated with outbreaks of influenza B infection. Sporadic cases have been reported from all parts of the world. There ap-

pears to be no clear racial or geographic predilection, although in the United States the vast majority of reported cases occur in Caucasians. With the exception of cases following influenza B infections, there is no seasonal predilection.

### References

Huttenlocher, P. R., and Trauner, D. A.: Reye's syndrome. In Vinken, P. J., and Bruyn, G. W. (eds.): Handbook of Clinical Neurology. Vol. 29. Amsterdam, North-Holland Publishing Company, 1977.
Lovejoy, F. H., Smith, A. L., Bresnan, J. J., Wood, J. N., Victor, D. J., and Adams, P. C.: Clinical staging in Reye's syndrome. Am J Dis Child 128:36, 1974.
Pollack, J. D. (ed.): Reye's Syndrome. New York, Grune & Stratton, 1975.
Reye, R. D. K., Morgan, G., and Baral, J.: Encephalopathy with fatty degeneration of the viscera. Lancet 2:749, 1963.
Trauner, D. A.: Treatment of Reye's syndrome. Ann Neurol 6:1, 1980.
Trauner, D. A., Brown, R. A., Ganz, E., and Huttenlocher, P. R.: Treatment of elevated intracranial pressure in Reye's syndrome. Ann Neurol 4:275, 1978.

# 173 POLIOMYELITIS

## Albert B. Sabin, M.D.

### DEFINITION

Poliomyelitis (infantile paralysis, acute anterior poliomyelitis, poliomyélite, Kinderlähmung, Heine-Medin disease) is a clinical-pathologic syndrome caused by enteroviruses. It is characterized by an acute febrile illness, which, in its paralytic form, presents within one or more days after onset varying degrees of usually asymmetric, flaccid paralysis of various striated muscles and sometimes also respiratory and vasomotor disturbances. The paralysis is caused by primary neuronal damage accompanied by cellular infiltration mainly in the spinal cord and medulla.

### HISTORY

Poliomyelitis is a worldwide infectious disease of human beings that probably dates back to earliest evolutionary times. The characteristic muscular atrophy and deformities resulting from paralysis of various muscles in early life has permitted identification of the disease from drawings made thousands of years ago. Poliomyelitis became a clinical entity in the 19th century after epidemics occurred in several countries. Rissler's (1888) description of the specific neuronal damage and inflammatory reaction in the central nervous

system (CNS) established poliomyelitis as a neuropathologic entity. The experimental transmission of the disease to monkeys by Landsteiner and Popper (1909) and the subsequent work of Flexner and Lewis (1909) established the viral nature of the disease. The studies of Sabin and Ward (1941a) on fatal cases of human poliomyelitis established that the human disease, in contrast to some artificial experimental models in monkeys, is predominantly an infection of the alimentary tract and of certain portions of the CNS. A collaborative effort of many investigators established that polioviruses belong to only three distinct serologic types (Committee on Typing, 1951). The work of Enders, Weller, and Robbins (1949) initiated the tissue culture era that revolutionized all further studies on poliomyelitis. Tissue cultures provided (1) simple in vitro procedures for the isolation, identification, and typing of the polioviruses as well as for determination of antibodies (Robbins et al., 1951); (2) new information on the nature and epidemiology of the disease including the fact that other viruses (Coxsackie and ECHO) can cause most cases of so-called "nonparalytic poliomyelitis" and occasionally persistent paralytic and fatal poliomyelitis; (3) the possibility of demonstrating that polioviruses of different neurovirulence exist in nature and that polioviruses with different capacities for multiplication in the nervous system, alimentary tract, and other extraneural tissues can be artificially selected in the laboratory (Sabin, 1956; 1965a); and (4) the basis for the development of both the killed (Salk) and live, attenuated, orally administered (Sabin) poliovirus vaccines. In many parts of the world, where the oral vaccine has been used on a mass scale, the paralytic disease caused by the polioviruses has almost completely disappeared (Sabin, 1965a; 1977), and the naturally occurring polioviruses have been replaced by the attenuated vaccine strains that are excreted by millions of vaccinated children and their non-immune contacts.

## ETIOLOGY

Poliomyelitis is caused by enteroviruses, a group that consists of the polioviruses, the Coxsackie A and B viruses, and the ECHO viruses. These RNA viruses have a size of 15 to 30 nm (m$\mu$), are resistant to ether, chloroform, bile, and detergents, and are stable at pH3. Some naturally occurring strains of these viruses can produce in intrathalamically inoculated monkeys paralytic disease that is associated with the characteristi-

cally located neuronal damage and inflammatory response. All naturally occurring polioviruses, ECHO viruses, Coxsackie B viruses, and some Coxsackie A viruses multiply with production of a characteristic cytopathic effect (CPE) in monkey kidney monolayer cultures (Fig. 1). Inhibition of this CPE by appropriate sera establishes their identity and serologic type. These viruses also multiply and produce CPE in various normal and malignant human cell cultures. Naturally occurring polioviruses neither multiply nor produce CPE in monolayer cultures of nonprimate tissues. Continuous serial passages in the nervous system of monkeys can select polioviruses that multiply in vitro in the nervous but not in the non-nervous tissues of human embryos (Sabin and Olitsky, 1936) and those that do not produce CPE in monkey kidney cultures (Sabin, 1954).

Although all three serotypes of poliovirus sooner or later infect almost all human beings, about 85 per cent of the persistent paralytic cases and most of the epidemics over the years have been caused by type 1 polioviruses. In the prevaccine era, the polioviruses caused only a small proportion of "abortive" or "nonparalytic" poliomyelitis and probably about 99 per cent of the

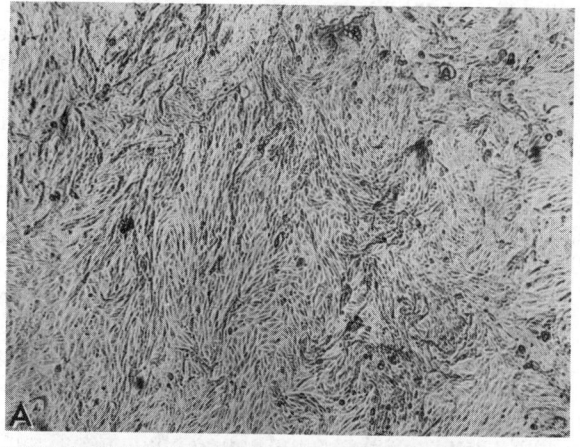

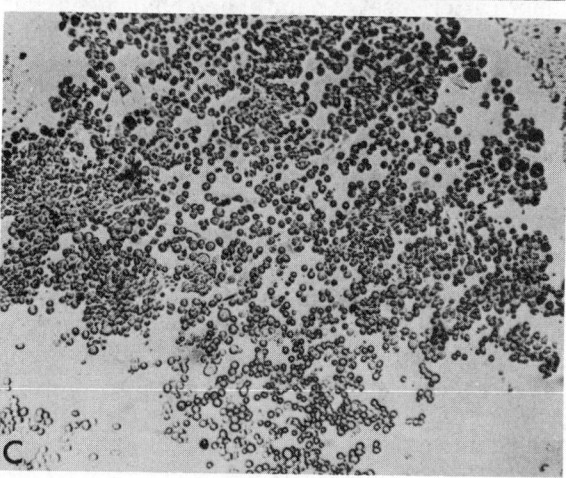

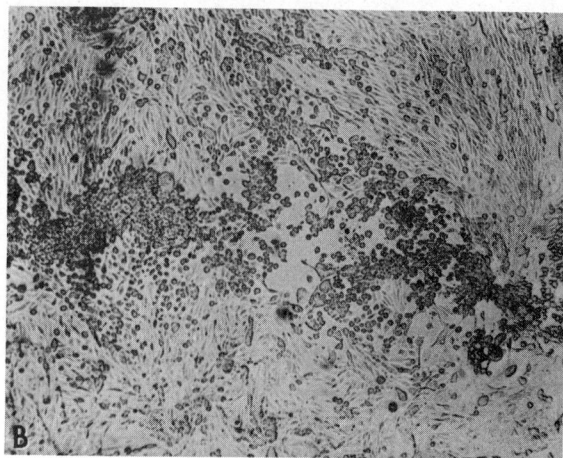

**FIGURE 1.** *Cytopathic effect (CPE) of poliovirus on monolayer grown from trypsinized monkey kidney. A, Uninfected culture; B, focal CPE; C, complete CPE.*

*persistent* paralytic cases. Paralytic poliomyelitis, occasionally severe and permanent, has been reportedly caused by Coxsackieviruses A7, A9, and B2 to B5 (Dalldorf and Melnick, 1965) and ECHO viruses types 1, 2, 4, 6, 7, 9, 11, 16, 18, and 30 (Melnick, 1965; Sabin et al., 1961 [for persistent ECHO 6 virus paralysis]). ECHO viruses types 2, 11 (Steigman, 1958; Steigman and Lipton, 1960), and 6 (Francis and Ceballos, 1959), and Coxsackievirus A7 (Grist, 1962) have been etiologically implicated in fatal cases of paralytic poliomyelitis.

Persistent lower motor neuron paralysis has recently been found to be caused by enterovirus types 70 and 71. The virus of acute hemorrhagic conjunctivitis (EV 70) has now been found in Africa, Asia, Europe, and Oceania but not yet in North or South America (Kono, 1975). With rare exceptions, the EV 70 paralytic disease occurred in 20 to 50 year old persons in association with epidemics of acute hemorrhagic conjunctivitis (Kono et al., 1977; Hung and Kong, 1979). Enterovirus 71 epidemics with persistent and also fatal lower motor neuron paralytic disease occurred in Bulgaria in 1975 (World Health Organization, 1979a) and in Hungary in 1978 (World Health Organization, 1979b). Enterovirus 71 paralytic disease occurred predominantly in very young children.

Viral studies on 497 patients with a clinical diagnosis of paralytic poliomyelitis in 1955 to 1957 incriminated polioviruses in only 57 per cent (more often in unvaccinated than in vaccinated paralytic patients), Coxsackie and ECHO viruses in 8 per cent, mumps virus in 3 per cent, herpes simplex virus in 1 per cent, mixed infections in 1 per cent, and *no evidence of viral infection in 30 per cent* (Lennette et al., 1959). In a subsequent study (Lennette et al., 1962) on 69 patients with a clinical diagnosis of poliomyelitis, 30 per cent again yielded negative results, 13 per cent had evidence of concurrent infection with Coxsackie B or ECHO viruses, 1 per cent had mumps virus, and only 52 per cent had polioviruses. Poliovirus infection was demonstrated in 75 per cent of 35 unvaccinated paralyzed patients in this group and in only 18 per cent of 17 who had received three doses of Salk vaccine, which indicated that the proportion of other causes of clinically diagnosed paralytic poliomyelitis became relatively higher as vaccination diminished the role of the polioviruses. The clinical diagnosis of paralytic poliomyelitis, even in good hospitals, is not always made on the strict criteria that would increase the probability that the disease is the result of the neuropathologic changes of poliomyelitis. Thus, Ramos-Alvarez (1967) isolated polioviruses from 91 per cent of 105 children under 2 years of age whose clinically diagnosed

paralytic poliomyelitis was associated with fever, but from none of 74 children aged 1 to 12 years when the paralytic disease was afebrile.

## PATHOLOGY

Significant virus-induced morphologic changes have been described only in the nervous system, where neuronal damage is primary and inflammatory reaction secondary. The fate of an anterior horn neuron attacked by virulent poliovirus is shown in Figure 2. The location, extent, and persistence of paralysis depend on the location and number of neurons so affected. Since any one muscle fibril is innervated by motoneurons from several levels of the spinal cord, even extensive destruction of anterior horn cells limited to one level of the spinal cord can occur in nonparalytic infections as was found in monkeys with nonparalytic poliomyelitis (Fig. 3). In experimental nonparalytic and transitory paralytic poliomyelitis in monkeys (Sabin and Ward, 1941a), one finds not only complete destruction of some neurons, resulting in neuronophagia, but also partial degenerative changes of chromatolysis and acidophilic-intranuclear inclusions from which the cells may recover (Fig. 4). The inflammatory cells in the meninges represent an overflow from the interstitial and perivascular infiltration that follows neuronal damage. The familiar spasm of the neck and back, along with other so-called signs of "meningeal irritation" actually are early manifestations of neuronal damage.

In human poliomyelitis, the extent of involvement of the spinal motoneurons observed postmortem depends on the neural pathways that first brought the virus to the CNS and on the duration of paralysis before death occurs. Figure 5A shows an essentially normal anterior horn of the lumbar cord of a patient who died within 24 hours after onset of palatal and pharyngeal paralysis. An anterior horn from the lumbar cord of a patient with bulbar poliomyelitis of somewhat longer duration shows only a few foci of neuronophagia and perivascular infiltration in the midst of a majority of intact neurons (Fig. 5B). In patients who die within a few days after onset of paralysis in the extremities the motoneurons in the lumbar cord are completely destroyed (Fig. 6). The relative distribution of neuronal lesions in the spinal cord and medulla in bulbar and spinal poliomyelitis is shown in Figure 7. Dorsal root ganglions show neuronophagia and interstitial infiltration (Fig. 8). In cynomolgus monkeys, experimentally infected by the oral route, poliovirus was demonstrated in the regional ganglia of the alimentary tract when no virus was found in the CNS (Verlinde et al., 1955).

The medulla has neuronal lesions in the nuclei of various cranial nerves, in the vestibular nuclei, and in the reticular formation. The cerebellum has neuronal lesions in the roof nuclei and vermis but not in the hemispheres. The midbrain has lesions in the periaqueductal gray matter, tectum, and tegmentum. Neuronal lesions are also present in the thalamus, hypothalamus, globus pallidus, and motor cortex, especially in area 4 of Brodmann. This localization differentiates the

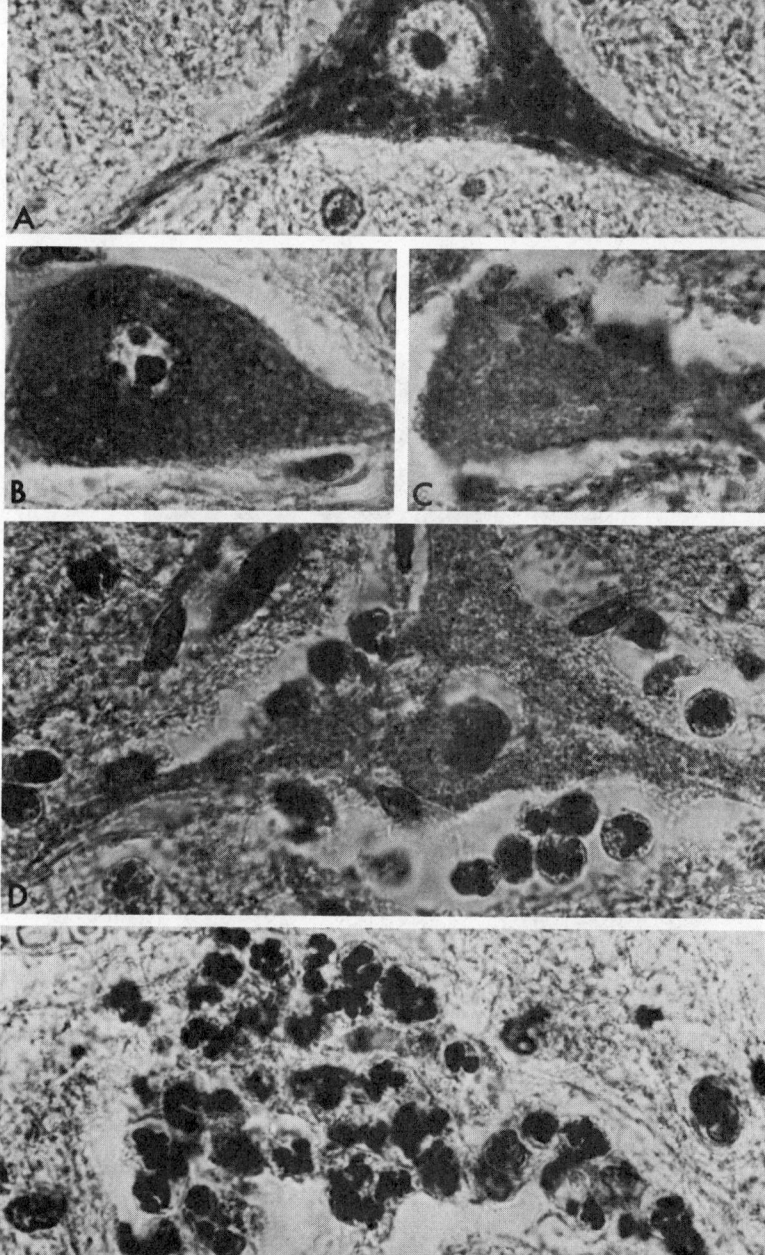

**FIGURE 2.** *Successive stages in destruction of an anterior horn cell of monkeys experimentally infected by nasal route with virulent poliovirus. A, normal appearance about three days before onset of paralysis; B, diffuse chromatolysis and three acidophilic, intranuclear inclusions grouped around the darker and larger nucleolus, found almost exclusively in monkeys sacrificed one day before onset of paralysis; C, complete acidophilic necrosis; D, polymorphonuclear leukocytes invading necrotic neuron; E, neuronophagia by polymorphonuclear leukocytes seen during the first day of paralysis. (From Sabin, A. B., and Ward, R.: J Exp Med 73:757, 1941.)*

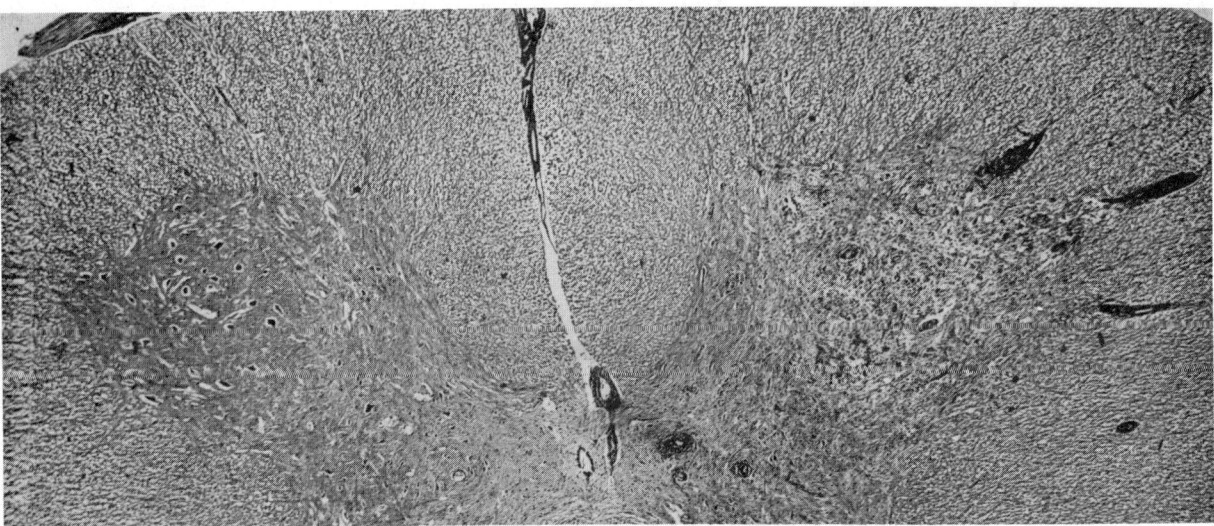

**FIGURE 3.** *Anterior horn of monkey with nonparalytic poliomyelitis. Note normal architecture on left and necrosis with inflammatory reaction and perivascular infiltration on right. (From Sabin, A. B., and Ward, R.: J Exp Med 73:757, 1941.)*

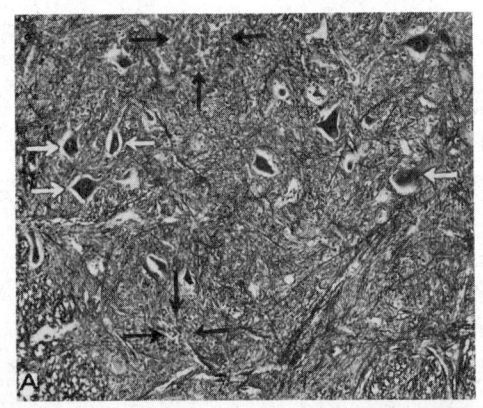

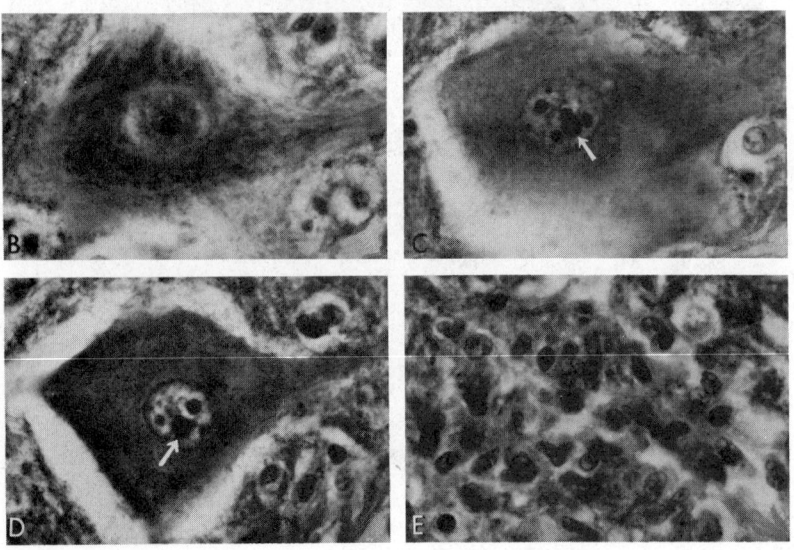

**FIGURE 4.** *A, Anterior horn in spinal cord of monkey killed two days after spontaneous recovery from paralysis of lower extremities; black arrows point to foci of glial neuronophagia shown enlarged in E and white arrows point to neurons with diffuse chromatolysis and acidophilic intranuclear inclusions shown enlarged in C and D with arrows pointing to basophilic nucleoli; B, one of only two almost normal neurons in A. (From Sabin, A. B., and Ward, R.: J Exp Med 73:757, 1941.)*

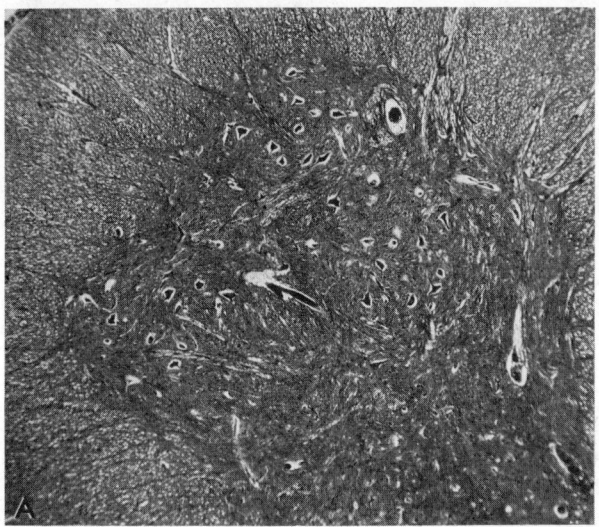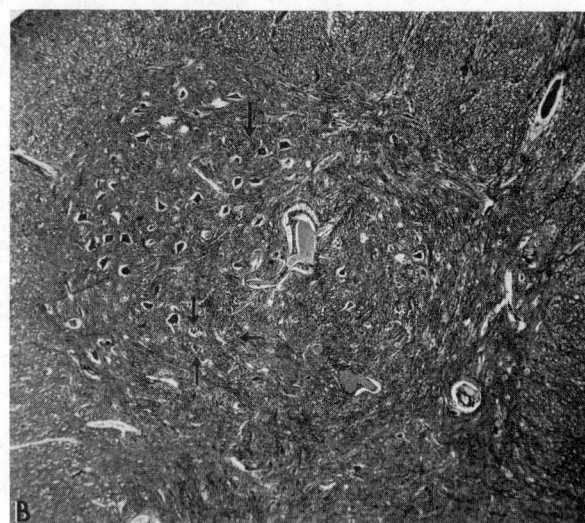

**FIGURE 5.**   A, *Essentially normal anterior horn of lumbar cord of a rapidly fatal human case of bulbar poliomyelitis. Note the large number of intact anterior horn cells and the absence of inflammatory reaction. B, Anterior horn of lumbar cord from a human case of bulbar poliomyelitis. Note foci of neuronophagia (arrows) and perivascular infiltration in the midst of many normal neurons. (From Sabin, A. B.: JAMA 120:506, 1942.)*

pathology of poliomyelitis from the more diffuse lesions seen in human encephalitis produced by a variety of different viruses.

## PATHOGENESIS

The pathogenesis of the disease in human beings is determined by (1) the extent of viral multiplication at the portal of entry in the ali-mentary tract; (2) the extent (if any) of multiplication in other extraneural tissues after the virus finds its way into the bloodstream from the lymph nodes draining the initial sites of viral multiplication; (3) the neurovirulence of the invading virus, which determines its capacity to invade the sensory neurons supplying the extraneural sites of viral multiplication and then to multiply in them sufficiently to spread to the motoneurons; and finally, (4) capacity of the virus that reaches

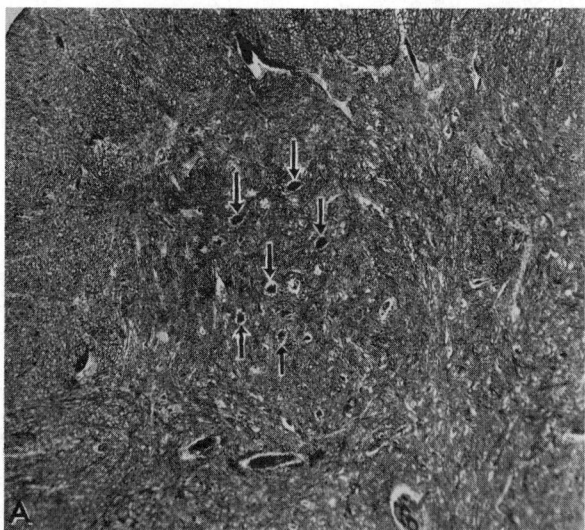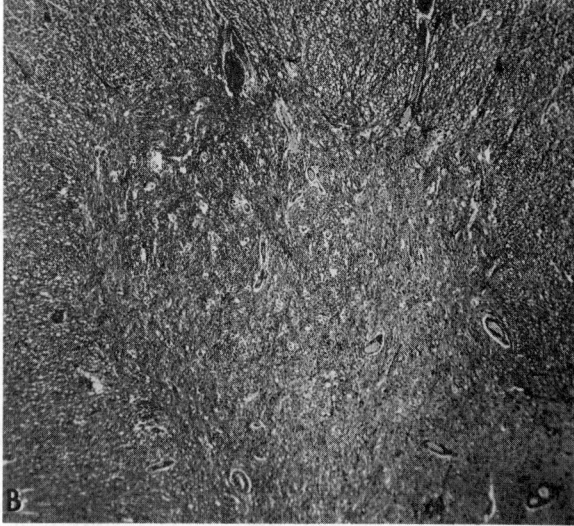

**FIGURE 6.**   A, *Anterior horn of lumbar cord from a human case of initial spinal paralysis. Note destruction of all anterior horn cells and few remaining foci of neuronophagia (arrows). B, Anterior horn of lumbar cord from a human case of initial spinal paralysis of somewhat longer duration than that in A. Note complete disappearance of all neurons. (From Sabin, A. B.: JAMA 120:506, 1942.)*

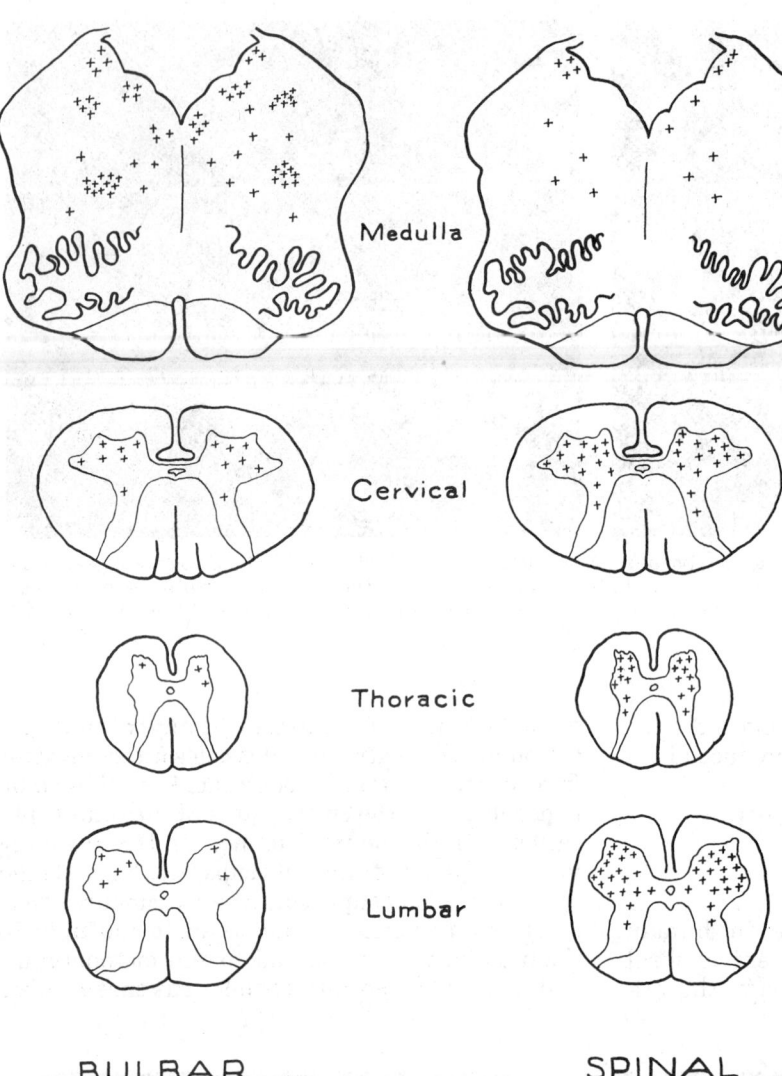

Medulla

Cervical

Thoracic

Lumbar

**FIGURE 7.** *Distribution of neuronal lesions in primary bulbar and primary spinal human poliomyelitis. (From Sabin, A. B.: JAMA 120:506, 1942.)*

BULBAR                          SPINAL

the initial motoneurons to multiply in them sufficiently to progress to and destroy the large number of motoneurons required to produce clinical paralysis.

The experimental studies on chimpanzees and cynomolgus monkeys that develop paralysis following ingestion of appropriate strains of polioviruses have been helpful in indicating potential pathogenic mechanisms but not in showing precisely what happens in man, because the relative susceptibility of the upper and lower alimentary tracts and nervous system has been found to be quantitatively different in monkeys, chimpanzees, and humans (Sabin, 1956). The source of virus spread among humans must be the feces of infected persons because virus multiplying in the oropharynx is not found in the mouth, gums, or anterior third of the tongue. Moreover, the predominant dissemination of the viruses during hot weather in countries with high standards of sanitation and hygiene in temperate climates is in accord with fecal-borne rather than with pharyngeal transmission.

Figure 9 shows a schema of the possible pathogenesis of human poliomyelitis (Sabin, 1956). The virus enters by way of the mouth on contaminated fingers or food and not by aspirated droplets. When the amount of ingested virus is less than 100,000 to one million tissue culture infective doses — and only under exceptional circumstances can it be assumed to be as much or more — it is usually swallowed without multipli-

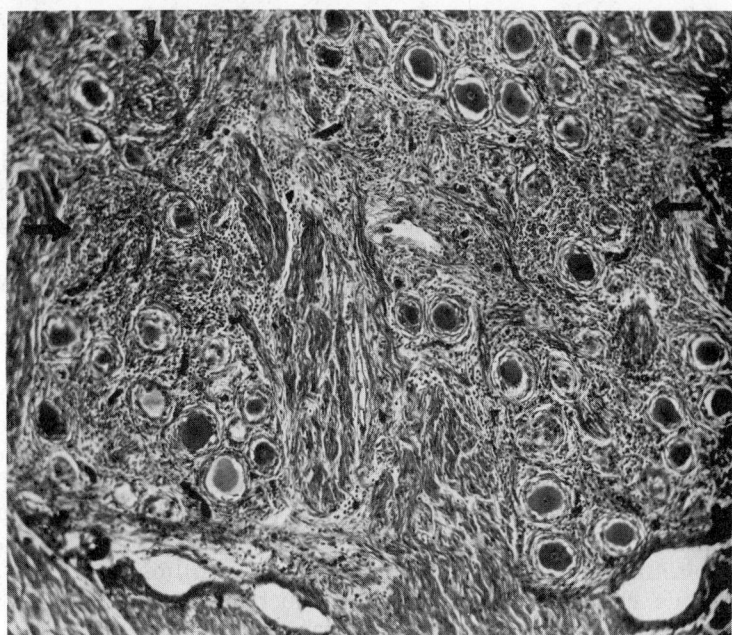

**FIGURE 8.** *Spinal dorsal root ganglion in human poliomyelitis. Note destruction of some neurons, focal neuronophagia, and interstitial cellular infiltration. (From Sabin, A. B.: JAMA 120:506, 1942.)*

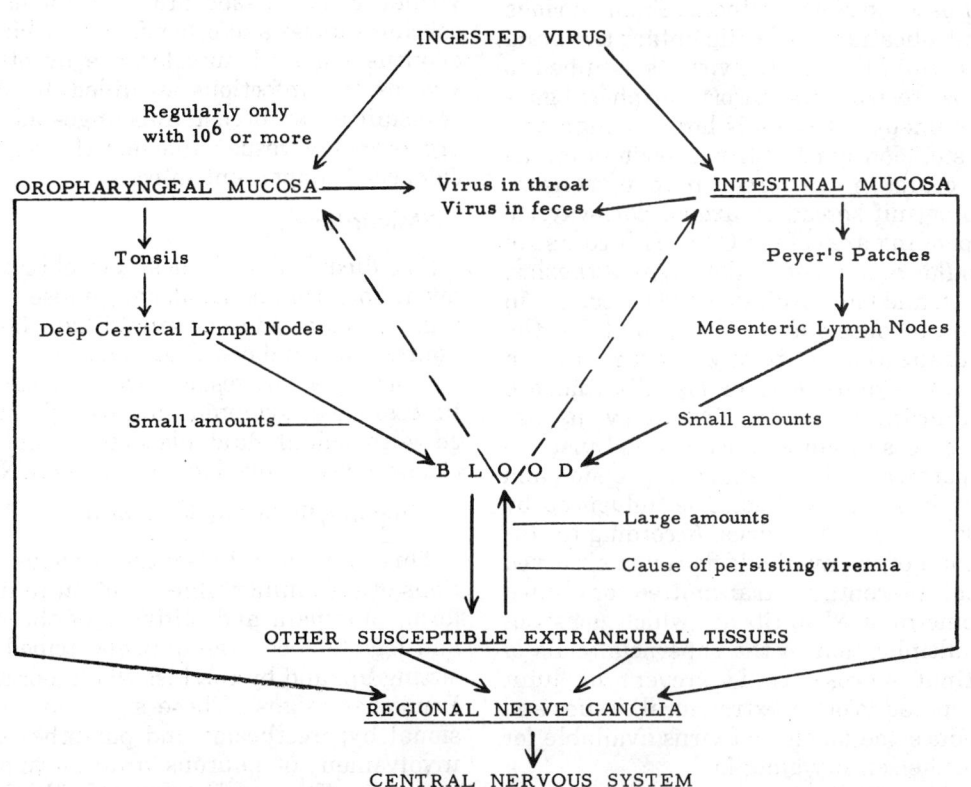

**FIGURE 9.** *Schema of possible pathogenesis of human poliomyelitis. (From Sabin, A. B.: Science 123:1151, 1956.)*

cation in the oropharynx. After passing through the stomach, the virus attaches itself to the superficial epithelium of the intestinal mucosa, and multiplication occurs within 24 hours. The virus is shed in the lumen and spreads from one superficial group of cells to another until local resistance halts further propagation, which may not happen for many weeks after initial infection and development of antibody. From the intestinal mucosa, virus is absorbed into the regional lymph nodes, from which small amounts may escape into the bloodstream before early local antibody formation. The appearance of larger amounts of virus in the bloodstream must depend on the capacity of a particular strain of virus to multiply in other extraneural tissues, because extensive multiplication of certain attenuated strains in the intestinal tract of human beings is not usually associated with detectable viremia, and intramuscular injection of as much as one million tissue culture infective doses of such a strain produces neither viremia, intestinal infection, nor antibody formation. However, with the usual paralytogenic strains, larger amounts of virus appear in the blood early after infection (Horstmann et al., 1954; Bodian and Paffenberger, 1954). Secondary spread to the oropharyngeal mucosa accounts for the high frequency of recovery of virus from the throat of patients with clinical signs of systemic illness. From various sites of multiplication in the alimentary tract and other extraneural tissues, the virus is assumed to invade the corresponding sensory peripheral ganglia. If the amount of virus is large enough and the strain sufficiently neurotropic, enough multiplication occurs in the first group of sensory neurons to permit spread by axonal pathways to the corresponding area of the CNS. This course of events would account for the hyperesthesias, paresthesias, and pain so often noted especially in adults prior to onset of paralysis, and for the different localizations of paralysis depending on the parts of the spinal cord or medulla that are invaded. After invasion of the CNS, the virus also progresses across synaptic junctions and insulated axonal pathways; the extent of progression and the number of neurons affected is influenced by the neurovirulence of the virus. According to this interpretation of the available data and observed phenomena, placentally transmitted or killed virus vaccine-induced antibody, which does not prevent multiplication in the superficial cells of the intestinal mucosa, could prevent or limit secondary spread to other extraneural tissues and thereby reduce the amount of virus available for invasion of the sensory ganglia.

According to Bodian's view of pathogenesis (1955), which is based largely on observations in chimpanzees, polioviruses multiply in the lymphatic structures and other extraneuronal tissues, invade the nervous system directly from the blood, and then spread along specific neural pathways within the nervous system. This hypothesis explains neither the prolonged multiplication of the polioviruses in the intestinal tract after the appearance of antibody nor in the presence of preexisting antibody. Moreover, if this hypothesis is correct, the effect of pre-existing antibody on primary natural infection should be all or none with regard to involvement of the nervous system, that is, complete prevention of invasion without modification of the extent of involvement when invasion is not prevented. Yet the data reported by Francis et al. (1955) indicated that the incidence of nonparalytic poliovirus infections of the CNS was not significantly affected by the killed poliovirus vaccine (Salk), and that when paralytic disease occurred in vaccinated individuals it was generally milder.

## CLINICAL MANIFESTATIONS

### Clinically Inapparent Infection

The vast majority of infections produced by polioviruses and other enteroviruses are clinically inapparent or unrecognized. Differences in virulence (i.e., tissue affinities) of naturally occurring viruses and other factors such as amount of virus ingested, interference by other enteroviruses, or infections modified by placentally transmitted or breast milk-ingested antibodies, are probably responsible for the very high incidence of inapparent infections.

### "Minor Illness"

So-called "minor illness" is characterized by fever, sore throat, headache, nausea and vomiting, anorexia, and abdominal pain lasting a few hours to a few days. Enteroviruses generally, as well as other viruses, can cause the same type of illness. These symptoms are usually not associated with spinal fluid pleocytosis and are not a consequence of involvement of the CNS.

### Nonparalytic or "Major Illness"

This illness includes the various manifestations of the "minor illness," often in more severe form, plus pain and stiffness of the neck, back, and legs (demonstrable by the tripod sign when sitting up, and by the kiss the knee, Kernig, and Brudzinski signs). These signs, as well as occasional hyperesthesias and paresthesias, indicate involvement of neurons prior to appearance of paralysis. The cerebrospinal fluid (CSF) during this period shows an increased number of leukocytes (usually between 15 and 500 cells per cubic mm with a predominance of polymorphonuclear cells early and of lymphocytes later. The protein concentration is normal or slightly elevated at first and increases later as the leukocytes disappear. Glucose level is normal. This syndrome, also called "aseptic meningitis," can be caused by many enteroviruses as well as by other viruses. Most cases of what was reported as nonparalytic poliomyelitis before the early 1950s were not caused by polioviruses.

### Paralytic Poliomyelitis

The paralytic disease, fulfilling the clinical criteria for a diagnosis of poliomyelitis, is occasionally preceded by the "minor illness" and usually by the "major illness." Excruciating muscle pain and spasm may precede or accompany onset of paralysis of the extremities. Localized hyperesthesia, fasciculation of muscle groups, loss or diminution of cremasteric and abdominal reflexes, and hyperactivity of the deep tendon reflexes may be indicators of pending paralysis. Paralysis may develop fully in one or two days or increasing weakness may be present for two or three days before the appearance of frank, flaccid paralysis associated with loss of deep tendon reflexes, which usually does not progress further after the temperature has returned to normal. The paralytic disease appears in spinal, bulbar, or bulbospinal form.

In the *spinal form* there can be asymmetric involvement of any of the muscles innervated by the motoneurons in the spinal cord — that is, legs, abdomen, back, intercostals, diaphragm, arms, shoulder girdle, or neck. Paralysis of the bladder may accompany paralysis of the legs, especially in adults and more often in males, but is usually transitory. Paralysis may remain localized in certain large muscle groups of the arms and legs but occasionally can progress to complete paralysis of both legs and arms. Paralysis of the intercostal and diaphragmatic muscles is life-threatening and causes great anxiety and restlessness in the patient. Respirations are shallow and rapid but regular, the voice is weak, cough is ineffective, and all the accessory muscles of respiration are used in the struggle to get air into the lungs.

In the *bulbar form* the muscles innervated by the cranial nerves are affected, and disturbances of respiration and circulation occur as a result of neuronal damage in the respiratory and vasomotor centers of the medulla. Weakness or paralysis of the soft palate, pharynx, and vocal cords, resulting from damage in the vagal nuclei, causes difficulty in swallowing, accumulation of pharyngeal secretions, regurgitation through the nose, nasal voice, hoarseness, and occasionally laryngeal stridor. Peripheral facial paralysis, and less often ocular palsies, pupillary disturbances, and paralysis of the tongue and masticator muscles are also seen. Involvement of the eleventh cranial motoneurons manifests itself by weakness or paralysis of the trapezius and sternocleidomastoid muscles. Involvement of the respiratory center neurons gives rise to the most serious manifestation of bulbar poliomyelitis, that is, respiratory failure resulting from irregularities in rhythm, depth, and rate. Shallow respirations with irregular periods of apnea of varying duration and Cheyne-Stokes respiration lead to acid-base imbalance, confusion, delirium, and coma. Circulatory disturbances due to involvement of the vasomotor center are indicated by a flushed, dusky facies with cherry-red lips progressing to mottled cyanosis, a pulse of 150 to 200 per minute that may be irregular and difficult to palpate, and a fluctuating blood pressure with a small pulse pressure.

The *bulbospinal form* may either begin with bulbar manifestations and descend to produce spinal manifestations, or cause ascending paralysis.

In the 90 to 95 per cent of patients who survive the most severe forms of the disease, the further course of the paralytic disease is in most instances stationary for a period of days or weeks after the temperature returns to normal. Improvement may then occur during the subsequent year or two. Atrophy of paralyzed muscles appears within less than eight weeks. When extensive paralysis occurs early in life, growth of paralyzed extremities is arrested, and severe deformities result from involvement of the back, chest, and shoulder muscles (Figs. 10 and 11).

## COMPLICATIONS

In patients with disturbances of deglutition and respiration, the airways become obstructed, and pulmonary atelectasis or pneumonia may be fatal. Long immobilization of extensively paralyzed patients may lead to decalcification of bones with high concentrations of calcium in the blood and urine and formation of kidney stones.

## GEOGRAPHIC VARIATIONS IN DISEASE

Fecal-borne microbial agents, including the polioviruses and other enteroviruses, are maximally disseminated during hot weather. Accordingly, the summer and early autumn months were the peak months for the occurrence of endemic and epidemic paralytic poliomyelitis in countries with temperate climates before the disease was controlled by vaccination. In tropical and subtropical

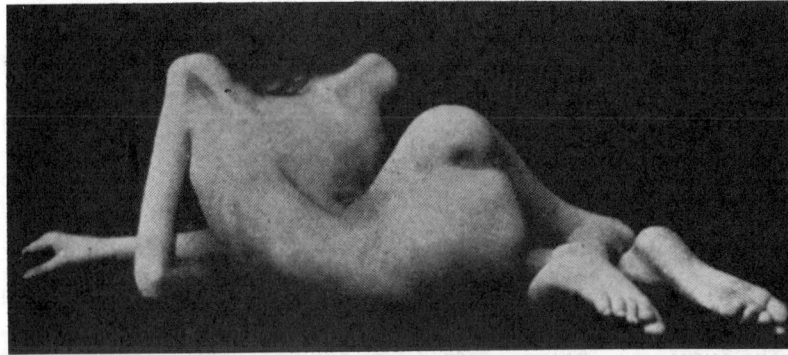

**FIGURE 10.** *Severe, untreated infantile paralysis of nine years' duration. Extensive scoliosis, contraction of both hips and both knees, double knock-knee, severe equinus of one foot, and paralysis of one arm. (From Lovett, R. W.: The Treatment of Infantile Paralysis. Philadelphia, Blakiston's Son and Company, 1916.)*

countries, dissemination of these viruses and the resulting disease occur throughout the year. In countries with poor sanitation and hygiene, which predominate in the tropical and subtropical regions of the world, dissemination of these viruses is constant and is so extensive that most children become infected very early in life. Whatever paralytic disease occurs under these conditions is truly infantile paralysis because most cases occur in children under 2 years of age. In

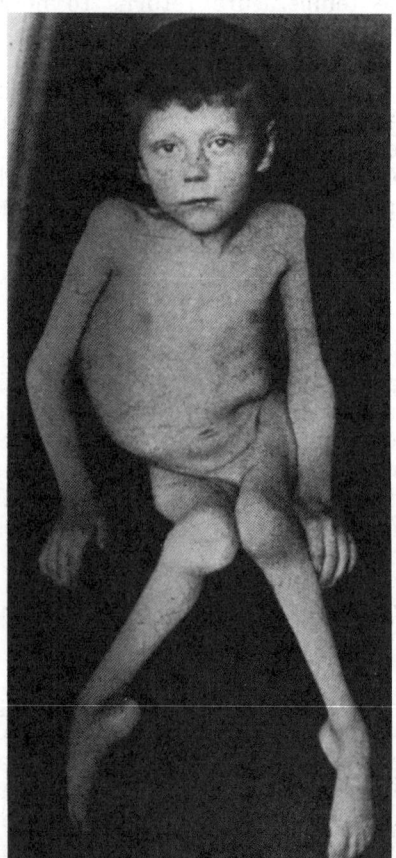

**FIGURE 11.** *Extensive paralysis and deformity in untreated infantile paralysis. (From Römer, P. H.: Epidemic Infantile Paralysis (English translation). New York, Prentice, 1913.)*

relatively small and isolated tropical and subtropical communities, paralysis was believed to be uncommon, incomplete persistent paralysis often goes unrecognized until children begin to walk, and epidemics are practically unknown. However, large epidemics have occurred in Africa and elsewhere when such population groups have left their villages and congregated in large numbers in very crowded conditions to work in large development projects. Most of the paralytic cases in these epidemics still occur in children under 2 years of age, indicating that the older children have acquired immunity from inapparent infections with viruses of lower virulence in their small communities.

Increasing numbers of older children and adults began to have paralytic poliomyelitis in countries with temperate climates when improved sanitation and hygiene, better housing with less crowding, and higher living standards for ever larger numbers of people diminished the dissemination of all enteroviruses and postponed the age at which immunity was naturally acquired. The same factors led to the accumulation of more susceptible people, which, together with increased opportunities for the spread of highly neurovirulent polioviruses provided by increasing mobility of populations, led to the emergence of large-scale summer epidemics at different times in different countries.

A study that I carried out in Brazil in 1980 showed that small epidemics, affecting children predominantly under three years, also occur with considerable frequency in tropical and subtropical areas. In Brazil, such epidemics often begin in September–December of one year and continue until March–May of the following year, lasting four to eight months instead of four to eight weeks, the usual duration of epidemics in temperate climates in the prevaccine era.

The old dogma that paralytic poliomyelitis is rare in tropical, economically underdeveloped countries until there is a marked improvement in the standard of living, sanitation, and hygiene, as reflected in decreasing infant mortality rates, has been found to be a fallacy, especially by recent surveys for residual paralysis in school-age children in Africa, Asia, and Latin America. These "lameness" surveys have shown that the number of officially reported cases is but a small and varying fraction of the actual number that can be estimated to have occurred (Sabin, 1980). Even in the absence of recognized epidemics, the estimated average annual incidence of paralytic poliomyelitis in rural and urban tropical regions has been found to be as high or higher than the average of 100 paralytic cases per annum per million total population in the USA during the five years in the pre-poliovaccine era. The lameness surveys in Ghana, Burma, and the Philippines (summarized by Sabin, 1980) and the subsequent surveys in Indonesia (World Health Organization, 1979c), Thailand (World Health Organization, 1979d), and Brazil (Sabin and Silva, 1980) yielded estimates of 123 to 589 paralytic cases for the average annual incidence per million total population in regions with limited or no vaccination programs.

## DIAGNOSIS

A clinical diagnosis of paralytic poliomyelitis is based on a history of an acute febrile illness, associated signs and symptoms of "aseptic meningitis," and appearance during the febrile period of asymmetric, flaccid, lower motor neuron type of muscle paralysis accompanied by loss of deep tendon reflexes. The paralysis usually fails to progress significantly after defervescence. Pleocytosis of the spinal fluid during the first week after onset of paralysis is essential for establishing the diagnosis of poliomyelitis, because noninflammatory lower motor neuron paralytic syndromes without pleocytosis resemble poliomyelitis but are pathologically distinct. In postmortem studies on 57 Mexican children with acute lower motor neuron paralytic disease, Ramos-Alvarez et al. (1969) found the neuropathologic changes of poliomyelitis in only 32. Among the remaining 25 without inflammatory changes in the CNS, 10 exhibited the neuropathologic changes of the Landry-Guillain-Barré syndrome and 15 presented hitherto unrecognized neuropathologic syndromes. Eight showed widespread and extensive "cytoplasmic neuronopathy" and 7 showed "nuclear neuronopathy". Although 7 of 9 patients with the Landry-Guillain-Barré syndrome showed albumino-cytologic dissociation during the first week after onset of paralysis, only 1 of the 14 patients with the other noninflammatory neuropathologic syndromes tested during the first week after onset of paralysis had a slightly elevated concentration of CSF protein. From a differential diagnosis point of view, it is noteworthy that in 23 of the 25 patients with noninflammatory paralytic syndromes, there was no fever at onset of paralysis and none exhibited nuchal or spinal rigidity. It is also noteworthy that virologic tests on the spinal cords of 17 of the patients with the noninflammatory lower motor neuron paralytic syndromes were negative, but in one of these patients (a 2-year-old child with nuclear neuronopathy who died three days after onset of paralysis), type 1 poliovirus was recovered in repeated tests from suspensions of colon, jejunum, ileum, and mesenteric lymph nodes. This important finding, as well as the presence of enteroviruses in the stools of seven other paralytic patients who showed no neuropathologic evidence of poliomyelitis, emphasizes the fact that mere isolation of a poliovirus or other enterovirus from the intestinal tract does not by itself prove an etiologic role of the virus in the paralytic condition. The statement in some textbooks (Bodian and Horstmann, 1965; Krugman et al., 1977) that the CSF may remain normal in a small proportion, or 10 per cent, of poliomyelitis cases even in the presence of severe paralysis, is not supported by acceptable evidence. The recently recognized infantile infectious botulism syndrome (Berg, 1977; Arnon et al., 1977), characterized by constipation, general weakness, paralysis of neck muscles, and dysfunction of various cranial nerves, can be confused with bulbar poliomyelitis but has no pleocytosis and usually no fever. Bell's palsy and a predominantly motor neuritis in older persons, occasionally misdiagnosed as poliomyelitis, are also without pleocytosis. A critical evaluation of the available data indicates that a diagnosis of poliomyelitis should not be made in patients without pleocytosis during the *first week* after onset of paralysis, especially when there is neither fever nor nuchal or spinal rigidity at the first appearance of paralysis.

Paralytic conditions associated with pleocytosis that occasionally are confused with paralytic poliomyelitis include transverse myelitis and postinfectious myelitis when the lesions are located predominantly in the gray matter. Encephalomyelitis caused by arboviruses, mumps, or herpesvirus have in atypical forms occasionally erroneously been diagnosed as bulbar poliomyelitis.

A valid clinical-pathologic diagnosis of poliomyelitis does not establish the etiologic diagnosis per se. However, as discussed previously under Etiology, *concurrent* infection with *naturally occurring* polioviruses (established by isolation of virus from the stools or throat and by a rising titer of antibody *shortly after onset* of paralysis) may in the prevaccine era have been responsible for about 99 per cent of all the *correctly* diagnosed cases of *persistent* poliomyelitic paralysis. Incrimination of enteroviruses in the etiology of poliomyelitic paralysis must depend not only on isolation of the virus and evidence of *concurrent* infection by antibody tests but also on the demonstration that wild polioviruses have not caused infection at the time of the clinical manifestations. In countries where paralytic poliomyelitis has become exceedingly rare following extensive use of oral poliovirus vaccine, the mere demonstration of concurrent infection with a poliovirus vaccine strain does not establish it as the etiologic agent of the paralytic condition; the mere failure to isolate other potentially neurovirulent enteroviruses from the intestinal tract shortly after onset of paralysis does not exclude the demonstrated possibility that it may have been there prior to onset of clinical illness and subsequently been replaced by poliovirus vaccine strains (Sabin, 1963; 1969; 1980).

## TREATMENT

During the acute paralytic phase of the disease, treatment should relieve pain and discomfort and deal with spinal or medullary respiratory failure or airway obstruction from aspirated fluids. If facilities are inadequate for proper home care or for prompt transfer to a hospital during an emergency, the patient should be hospitalized as soon as possible after onset of paralysis. Complete rest in a hard bed with a footboard is essential. Changes in posture are helpful for relief of discomfort and essential when the respiratory muscles are weak. Pain and muscle spasm can be relieved by judiciously applied hot packs for 20-minute periods several times a day. Aspirin and codeine relieve headache and generalized pain and discomfort. Sedatives that depress respiration should be avoided. Catheterization should be avoided for urinary retention that may respond to parasympathomimetics. Constipation and abdominal distention may be relieved by small doses of neostigmine. Voluntary movements of partly paralyzed extremities and passive movements of extensively paralyzed extremities should be started as soon as pain disappears.

Swallowing problems need special care. Mechanical suction and postural drainage should be used to prevent secretions from blocking the airway. Tracheostomy should be performed when these measures prove to be inadequate, or when paralysis of the vocal cords, ineffective cough, and laryngeal stridor result in life-threatening respiratory embarrassment — preferably before bouts of choking and cyanosis begin. Respiratory failure of medullary origin should not be treated in a tank respirator in the absence of tracheostomy or when throat secretions cannot be adequately removed. Humidified oxygen (40 to 60 per cent and in emergencies 100 per cent for brief

periods) can be given through the tracheostomy tube. A cuffed tracheostomy tube may be used for positive pressure respiration when artificial respiration is required.

Respiratory embarrassment resulting from paralysis of intercostal muscles and the diaphragm, without bulbar involvement, is best treated in a tank respirator during the acute progressive phase of paralysis as soon as the vital capacity falls to less than 50 per cent. When no tank respirator is available, Thompson's method of artificial respiration (1935) can be life-saving in patients with rapidly progressing paralysis. It consists of "lifting the pelvis of a subject in the prone position and allowing it to fall back to the floor" (Fig. 12) six to ten times per minute. This procedure, combined with the Schafer prone pressure method after the patient is lowered to the floor, produces a large respiratory exchange. When possible, weaning from the tank respirator

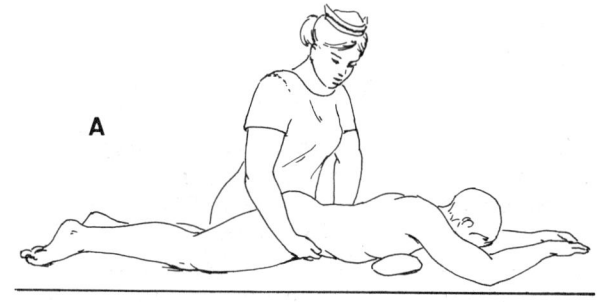

Position of patient.

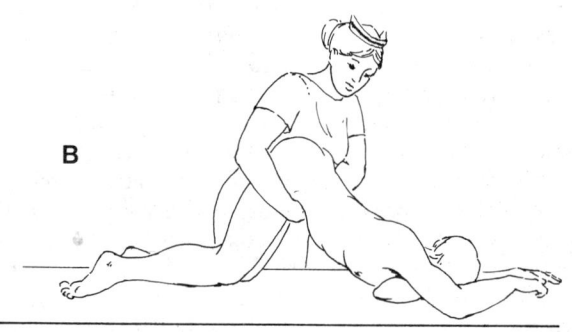

Procedure by operator.

**FIGURE 12.** *Emergency artificial respiration for spinal respiratory paralysis when tank respirator is not available. A, Patient is in prone position on a hard surface. A folded coat or small pillow is placed beneath the clavicles and upper part of chest. B, Operator, kneeling or seated on a low chair, puts one hand beneath each anterior superior spine and lifts the pelvis off the ground until the back arches and the abdomen sags down. The patient is then slowly lowered to the original position. At this point the chest may be compressed by pushing downward and forward over the lower ribs to obtain additional air exchange. (From Thompson, T. C.: JAMA 104:307, 1935.)*

should begin as soon as paralysis stops progressing. Pulmonary atelectasis, a frequent complication of respiratory failure, may require bronchoscopic aspiration. Pulmonary infection is not prevented by prophylactic antibiotics, but when it occurs it requires antibiotics for treatment.

Proper physiotherapy and orthopedic intervention, when indicated after the acute phase of paralysis is over, can help to achieve the maximum possible return of muscle function and prevent the tragic crippling deformities shown in Figures 10 and 11.

## PROPHYLAXIS

Natural infection with polioviruses, even in the absence of reinfection (Paul et al., 1951), provides lifelong immunity that is associated with neutralizing antibodies in the blood and partial or complete resistance of the intestinal tract to reinfection (Sabin, 1957; 1965a). Resistance of the intestinal tract has been found in some individuals in the absence of demonstrable neutralizing antibodies both after natural infection and after experimental infection of volunteers with attenuated strains. Placentally transmitted antibody does not confer intestinal resistance to poliovirus infection. The incomplete intestinal resistance in some persons with antibody acquired after natural infection or after ingestion of attenuated strains is characterized by brief periods of limited viral multiplication that usually are insufficient for transmission. This limited intestinal reinfection in persons with infection-acquired immunity usually induces complete resistance to subsequent infection even by very large doses. Each resistant intestinal tract represents a break of one link in the chain of transmission of polioviruses. This phenomenon provides the basis for the eradication of the naturally occurring polioviruses in large population groups, when most of the susceptible age groups are adequately immunized within a short period of time by the ingestion of poliovirus strains selected for lowest neurovirulence and maximum capacity for multiplication in the human intestinal tract.

The first practically useful vaccine was prepared by formaldehyde inactivation of polioviruses grown in monkey kidney tissue cultures (Salk et al., 1954). In adequate dosage the inactivated poliovirus vaccine (IPV) produces neutralizing antibodies that can protect against paralytic poliomyelitis caused by the polioviruses (Francis et al., 1955). The development of an acceptable live, attenuated vaccine for oral administration (OPV) depended on the acquisition of much new knowledge about the multiple properties and behavior of polioviruses in monkeys,

chimpanzees, and humans (Sabin, 1965a). The OPV in current use was ready in 1957 (Sabin, 1957) for field tests on increasingly larger numbers of persons in different parts of the world, and routine use on a mass scale began in many countries during the winter and spring of 1960. Since about 1965, OPV has come into routine use all over the world except in Sweden, Finland, and Holland.

Despite extensive reduction in the number of cases of paralytic poliomyelitis that followed the mass use of IPV, increased summer incidence and epidemics continued to occur. Because IPV has no effect on multiplication of virus in the intestinal tract, polioviruses continued to circulate in communities where IPV had been used on a large scale, and paralysis continued to occur in significant numbers among those who remained unvaccinated, or received an insufficient number of doses, or lost their vaccine-acquired immunity. Approximately 20 to 30 per cent of the paralytic cases during epidemics had received three or more doses of IPV. The antibody response to IPV is particularly poor and transitory (especially for types 1 and 3) in children and older persons who have never had natural infections with any of the three types of poliovirus. Surveys of young children who had received multiple doses of Salk vaccine in the United States and South Africa showed that about 50 per cent had no neutralizing antibodies for the important type 1 virus, and about 60 per cent had none for type 3 virus, reflecting partly a poor initial response and partly a higher loss of acquired antibody within one year. During the first five years after mass use of IPV, epidemics occurred in the United States, Canada, Australia, Finland, Hungary, Israel, Japan, and other countries. In 1959 and 1960, Finland had epidemics of a magnitude comparable to those of the prevaccine years of 1949 and 1950, despite the use of IPV on an increasingly larger scale since 1956. In 1959, four years after extensive use of IPV, the United States had 6289 reported cases of paralytic poliomyelitis, of which 5472 had residual paralysis two months after onset. In 1961, seven years after extensive use of IPV, Denmark had an epidemic of 148 paralytic cases caused by type 1 poliovirus, which on a population basis is comparable to the number of paralytic cases in the United States in 1959.

OPV has the following properties not possessed by IPV that are of special importance for a rapid elimination of the paralytic disease (Sabin, 1962):

1. Immunity can be produced quickly — within about a week — after ingestion of a single dose of any one of the three types of vaccine. Thus, when type 1 monovalent vaccine is given first,

protection is quickly obtained against the most important cause of paralytic poliomyelitis. Protection against the other two types is subsequently quickly achieved when they are given separately at a suitable interval or together in a single dose. During the winter and spring months in temperate climates when the incidence of infection by enteric viruses is low, this procedure has yielded an antibody response of 100 per cent or close to it for all three types (when low antibody titers are included) in the United States, Britain, Switzerland, Czechoslovakia, and Yugoslavia.

2. Extensive multiplication of the vaccine strains in the intestinal tract produces local resistance to reinfection that is independent of antibody in the blood.

3. Some unvaccinated persons, both children and adults, become immune by contact with young vaccinated children. During extensive community-wide programs, the incidence of such immunization has been especially high.

4. Intestinal resistance in a *large proportion of the child population,* the most important spreaders of polioviruses, leads to a break in the chain of transmission of the naturally occurring polioviruses of varying neurovirulence, which results in the elimination of the paralytic disease from the unvaccinated as well as the vaccinated persons in a community.

5. The fact that OPV begins to multiply in the intestinal tract within 24 hours after ingestion, creating the potential for immediate interference with subsequently ingested virulent polioviruses, combined with the early immunogenic effect of monovalent vaccine and the simplicity of mass administration, makes possible the rapid termination of epidemics.

The main disadvantages of OPV result from interference by enteric viruses that may be multiplying in the intestinal tract when the vaccine is ingested or when the three types of polioviruses are competing with one another after ingestion of a dose of trivalent vaccine. The types 2 and 3 vaccine strains have the advantage because they multiply more rapidly and extensively than type 1. In tropical and subtropical regions, where enteric viruses including naturally occurring polioviruses are widely disseminated throughout the year, mass administration of OPV within a period of a day or two has been shown to curtail temporarily the dissemination of the other enteric viruses as a result of a massive dissemination of the vaccine strains. Moreover, the *annual* administration of two doses of OPV, each given in a mass campaign on a single day with an interval of two months, to all children under 4 years of age, can keep a subtropical country free of paralytic poliomyelitis (Sabin, 1977; 1980). In temperate climates, where after initial mass campaigns with monovalent vaccines for all susceptible age groups, trivalent OPV is now used for routine immunization of children during the first year of life, multiple doses have proved to be as effective as the separately administered monovalent vaccines.

The rapidity with which a properly executed mass campaign with OPV can alter the incidence of paralytic poliomyelitis in a country with a large population and considerable variations in climate and social conditions is exemplified by the events in Italy with a population of 51 million during 1962 to 1966 (Fig. 13). By May 1965, the three monovalent doses and one trivalent dose had been given to 80 to 90 per cent of the children under 6 years of age in most of the northern provinces and to only about 50 to 60 per cent in most of the southern provinces. More extensive vaccination was then carried out in the southern provinces, and 80 to 90 percent of the new generations of children have continued to be vaccinated each year. According to Volpi et al. (1976), "only four cases of paralytic disease, which were not conclusively defined as poliomyelitis, were reported in 1975." In Rome in 1974 and 1975 nearly 100 per cent of all age groups had antibody for each of the three types of poliovirus (Volpi et al., 1976).

Table 1 summarizes what happened in the United States, where OPV was introduced in stages, and the mass campaigns, which covered only about 50 per cent of the total population, were followed by the routine use of trivalent vaccine for immunization of children during the first year of life (Sabin, 1978). No other country of comparable size has achieved as good a record in the complete or almost complete elimination of paralytic poliomyelitis caused by polioviruses, particularly in view of the large immigration from Mexico where paralytic polioviruses are still prevalent. The very few indigenous cases of paralytic poliomyelitis that still occur in the United States are of doubtful clinical diagnosis and are sometimes based on isolation of harmless OPV strains from the stools. Even so, it is remarkable that during the entire eight-year period of 1969 to 1976 inclusive, 18 states and the District of Columbia, with a total population of about 36 million (1970 census), did not report a single case, while the Mexican border states of California and Texas, with a combined 1970 population of a little over 31 million, reported 52 cases (6.5 per annum), some of which were probably real poliomyelitis of poliovirus etiology and some clinically or etiologically something else. This is an incredible record, since on the basis of data presented earlier under Etiology one would expect a small number of cases of persistent paralytic poliomyelitis caused by enteroviruses other than polioviruses to occur each year. Since in the 1- to

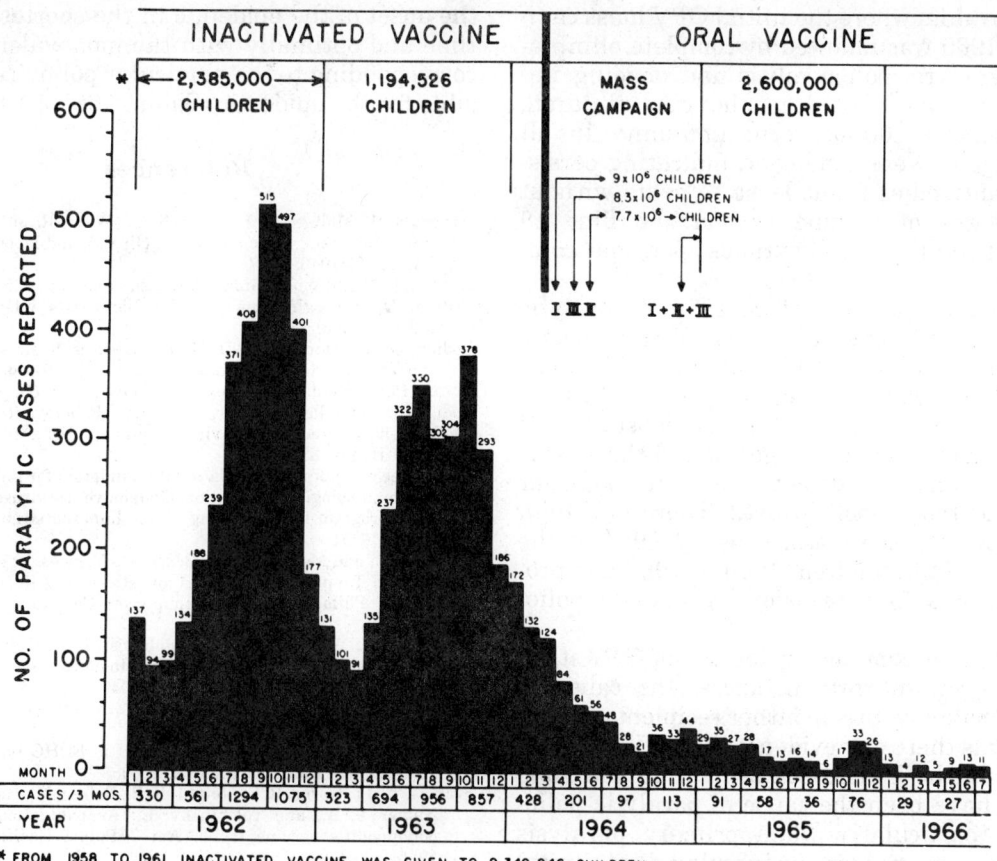

**FIGURE 13.** *Paralytic poliomyelitis in Italy from 1962–1966. (From Sabin, A. B.: Washington, D. C., PAHO Sc Pub No. 147, 1967.)*

4-year-old age group about 34 per cent of white children (82 per cent of the total population in this age group) and about 60 per cent of children of other races have had less than three doses of trivalent OPV, the extraordinary absence of paralytic poliomyelitis in the United States must be attributed partly to the ongoing documented dissemination of vaccine strains that immunize some unvaccinated persons and partly to the break in the chain of transmission of imported virulent polioviruses. A 1975 serologic survey carried out by Karzon and Wright on 341 2- to 4-year-old children in Tennessee indeed showed that close to 100 per cent had antibodies for each of the three types of poliovirus (Sabin, 1978).

A 1976 serologic survey on 3022 persons in

**TABLE 1.** Paralytic Poliomyelitis Reported in United States, 1951 to 1976

| ERA | PERIOD | TOTAL NO. FOR 5 YEARS | AVERAGE NO. PER ANNUM | APPROXIMATE NO./MILLION/ANNUM |
|---|---|---|---|---|
| No vaccine plus IPV[a], 1955 | 1951–1955 | 79,112 | 15,822 | 100 |
| IPV only | 1956–1960 | 22,291 | 4884 | 28 |
| IPV plus OPV[b] antiepidemic plus later community programs | 1961–1965 | 2,313 | 463 | 3 |
| OPV only | 1973–1976 | 24? (4 yrs) (+6 imported) | 6? | <3?/100 million |

[a]IPV, Inactivated polio vaccine (Salk).

[b]OPV, Oral polio vaccine (Sabin).

Reproduced from Sabin, A. B.: Am J Pathol 70(Supplement):136, 1978.

Czechoslovakia, where the initial OPV mass campaign in 1960 was followed by complete elimination of paralytic poliomyelitis and ongoing immunization was limited to the new children, showed almost 100 per cent immunity in all persons aged 2 years and over, indicating persistence of antibodies for at least 14 years without booster doses of vaccine beyond the first 18 months of life (Dr. V. Skovranek, personal communication).

The complete absence since 1965 of paralytic poliomyelitis and apparently also of polioviruses in Finland (population 4.7 million), which has used only IPV, cannot be explained on the basis of immunity because a 1966 serologic survey of children under 3 years of age showed that about 60 per cent had no demonstrable antibody for type 1 and type 3 polioviruses. There is a high probability that the massive use of OPV in the remainder of Europe from 1960 to 1964 has protected Finland from invasion by virulent polioviruses.

There is no acceptable evidence that OPV itself may be, even in rare instances, the cause of paralytic poliomyelitis in either recipients or contacts. Nor is there any evidence that IPV as it was prepared in the United States in 1959 and 1960 may not have been the cause of paralytic poliomyelitis (particularly when primary paralysis occasionally occurred in the inoculated extremity) (Sabin, 1963; 1969; 1977; 1978).

The strategy of initial mass vaccination of all susceptible age groups with OPV followed by ongoing vaccinations of infants concurrently with other routine immunizations has worked very well in many "developed" countries, but for a variety of reasons has been only partly effective in "developing" countries (Sabin, 1967; 1977; 1980). Mass administration of OPV *each* year to *all* children under 48 months of age, without reference to previous vaccination history, on each of two days separated by an interval of at least two months, can produce optimum results in developing countries in tropical and subtropical regions. There are valid reasons for proposing that the annual two-dose schedule should consist of 300,000 $TCID_{50}$ (50 per cent tissue culture infective doses) of only type 1 for the first dose, and of trivalent vaccine (300,000 $TCID_{50}$ of each of the three types) for the second dose (Sabin, 1977; 1980). It is difficult to set up arbitrary rules regarding the stage at which an economically developing country, with many health problems and limited health facilities, should undertake an ongoing program of vaccination against poliomyelitis. It is in such countries that OPV can be especially useful to combat epidemics but only if mass vaccination is carried out as soon as possible after the onset of the epidemic in the shortest possible time and optimally with the monovalent vaccine corresponding to the particular poliovirus responsible for the epidemic (Sabin, 1965b; 1967; 1980).

## References

Arnon, S. S., Midura, T. F., Clay, S. A., Wood, R. M., and Chin, J.: Infant botulism; epidemiological, clinical, and laboratory aspects. JAMA 237:1946, 1977.

Berg, B. O.: Syndrome of infant botulism. Pediatrics 59:321, 1977.

Bodian, D.: Emerging concept of poliomyelitis infection. Science 122:105, 1955.

Bodian, D., and Horstmann, D. M.: Polioviruses. In Horsfall, F. L., Jr., and Tamm, I. (eds.): Viral and Rickettsial Infections of Man, 4th ed. Philadelphia, J. B. Lippincott Company, 1965, p. 449.

Bodian, D., and Paffenberger, R. S., Jr.: Poliomyelitis infection in households; frequency of viremia and specific antibody response. Am J Hyg 60:83, 1954.

Committee on Typing of the National Foundation for Infantile Paralysis: Immunologic classification of poliomyelitis viruses. I. A cooperative program for the typing of one hundred strains. Am J Hyg 54:191, 1951.

Dalldorf, G., and Melnick, J. L.: Coxsackie Viruses. In Horsfall, F. L., Jr., and Tamm, I. (eds.): Viral and Rickettsial Infections of Man, 4th ed. Philadelphia, J. B. Lippincott Company, 1965, p. 492–494.

Enders, J. F., Weller, T. H., and Robbins, F. C.: Cultivation of the Lansing strain of poliomyelitis virus in cultures of various human embryonic tissues. Science 109:85, 1949.

Flexner, S., and Lewis, P. A.: The nature of the virus of epidemic poliomyelitis. JAMA 53:2095, 1909.

Francis, R. D., and Ceballos, R.: Viremia in ECHO type 6 infection. Proc Soc Exp Biol Med 101:479, 1959.

Francis, T., Jr., Korns, R. F., Voight, R. B., Boisen, M., Hemphill, F. M., Napier, J. A., and Tolchinsky, E.: An evaluation of the 1954 poliomyelitis vaccine trials. Am J Public Health 45:Suppl 5, 1955.

Grist, N. R.: Type A7 Coxsackie (type 4 poliomyelitis) virus infection in Scotland. J Hyg London 60:323, 1962.

Horstmann, D. M., McCollum, R. W., and Mascola, A. D.: Viremia in human poliomyelitis. J Exp Med 99:355, 1954.

Hung, T. P., and Kono, R.: Neurological complications of acute haemorrhagic conjunctivitis (A polio-like syndrome in adults). In Vinken, P. J., and Bruyn, G. W. (eds.): Handbook of Clinical Neurology; Neurological Manifestations of Systemic Diseases, Part I (Klawans, H. L. ed.), Amsterdam, North-Holland Publishing Company, 1979, p. 595.

Kono, R.: Apollo 11 disease or acute hemorrhagic conjunctivitis: a pandemic of a new enterovirus infection of the eyes. Am J Epidemiol 101:383, 1975.

Kono, R., Miyamura, K., Tajiri, E., Sasagawa, A., Phuapradit, P., Roongwithu, N., Vejjajiva, A., Jayavasu, C., Thongcharoen, P., Wasi, C., and Rodprasert, P.: Virological and serological studies of neurological complications of acute hemorrhagic conjunctivitis in Thailand. J. Infect Dis 135:706, 1977.

Krugman, S., Ward, R., and Katz, S. L.: Infectious Diseases in Children, 6th ed. S. Louis, C. V. Mosby Company, 1977, p. 41.

Landsteiner, K., and Popper, E.: Übertragung der Poliomyelitis acuta auf Affen. Zschr Immunitätsforsch Orig 2:377, 1909.

Lennette, E. H., Magoffin, R. L., Schmidt, N. J., and Hollister, A. C., Jr.: Viral disease of the central nervous system; influence of poliomyelitis vaccination on etiology. JAMA 171:1456, 1959.

Lennette, E., Magoffin, R. L., and Knouf, E. G.: Viral central nervous system disease: An etiologic study conducted at the Los Angeles County General Hospital. JAMA 179:687, 1962.

Melnick, J. L.: Echoviruses. In Horsfall, F. L., Jr., and Tamm, I. (eds.): Viral and Rickettsial Infections of Man, 4th ed. Philadelphia, J. B. Lippincott Company, 1965, pp. 528–529.

Paul, J. R., Riordan, J. T., and Melnick, J. L.: Antibodies to three different antigenic types of poliomyelitis virus in sera from North Alaskan eskimos. Am J Hyg 54:275, 1951.

Ramos-Alvarez, M.: Discussion. In Vaccines Against Viral and Rickettsial Diseases of Man. Pan American Health Organization Sc Pub No. 147, Washington, 1967, p. 235.

Ramos-Alvarez, M., Bessudo, L., and Sabin, A. B.: Paralytic syndromes associated with noninflammatory cytoplasmic or nuclear neuronopathy; acute paralytic disease in Mexican children, neuropatho-logically distinguishable from Landry-Guillain-Barré syndrome. JAMA 207:1481, 1969.

Rissler, J.: Zur Kenntniss der Veränderungen des Nervensystems bei Poliomyelitis anterior acuta. Nord Med Ark 20:1, 1888.

Robbins, F. C., Enders, J. F., Weller, T. H., and Florentino, G. L.: Studies on the cultivation of poliomyelitis viruses in tissue culture. V. The direct isolation and serologic identification of virus strains in tissue culture from patients with nonparalytic and paralytic poliomyelitis. Am J Hyg 54:286, 1951.

Sabin, A. B.: Pathology and pathogenesis of human poliomyelitis. JAMA 120:506, 1942.

Sabin, A. B.: Noncytopathogenic variants of poliomyelitis viruses and resistance to superinfection in tissue culture. Science 120:357, 1954.

Sabin, A. B.: Pathogenesis of poliomyelitis — reappraisal in the light of new data. Science 123:1151, 1956.

Sabin, A. B.: Properties and behavior of orally administered attenuated poliovirus vaccine. JAMA 164:1216, 1957.

Sabin, A. B.: Oral poliovirus vaccine; recent results and recommenda-tions for optimum use. Roy Soc Hlth J 82:51, 1962.

Sabin, A. B.: Is there an exceedingly small risk associated with oral poliovirus vaccine? JAMA 183:268, 1963.

Sabin, A. B.: Oral poliovirus vaccine — history of its development and prospects for eradication of poliomyelitis. JAMA 194:872, 1965a.

Sabin, A. B.: Immunization against poliomyelitis with particular reference to the tropics. Industry Trop Health 5:74, 1965b.

Sabin, A. B.: Poliomyelitis; accomplishments of live virus vaccine. In Vaccines Against Viral and Rickettsial Diseases of Man. Pan American Health Organization Sc Pub No. 147, Washington, 1967, p. 171.

Sabin, A. B.: Vaccine-associated poliomyelitis cases. Bull WHO 40:947, 1969.

Sabin, A. B.: Oral poliomyelitis vaccine: Achievements and problems in worldwide use. Bull Internat Pediatr Assn 2:6, 1977.

Sabin, A. B.: Poliomyelitis vaccination; evaluation and direction of continuing application. Am J Pathol 70(Supplement):136, 1978.

Sabin, A. B., and Olitsky, P. K.: Cultivation of poliomyelitis virus in vitro in human embryonic nervous tissue. Proc Soc Exp Biol Med 34:357, 1936.

Sabin, A. B., and Ward, R.: Nature of non-paralytic and transitory paralytic poliomyelitis in rhesus monkeys inoculated with human virus. J Exp Med 73:757, 1941a.

Sabin, A. B., and Ward, R.: The natural history of poliomyelitis. I. Distribution of virus in nervous and nonnervous tissues. J Exp Med 73:771, 1941b.

Sabin, A. B., Michaels, R. H., Spiegland, I., Pelon, W., Rhim, J. S., and Wehr, R. E.: Community-wide use of oral poliovirus vaccine; effectiveness of the Cincinnati program. Am J Dis Child 101:546, 1961.

Sabin, A. B.: Vaccination against poliomyelitis in economically under-developed countries. Bull WHO, 58:141, 1980.

Sabin, A. B., and Silva, E.: Survey for residual poliomyelitic paralysis in children of different ages in the Federal District of Brasil, Manu-script in preparation, 1980.

Salk, J. E., Krech, U., Youngner, J. S., Bennett, B. L., Lewis, L. J., and Bazeley, P. L.: Formaldehyde treatment and safety testing of experimental poliomyelitis vaccines. Am J Public Health 44:563, 1954.

Steigman, A. J.: Poliomyelitic properties of certain non-polio viruses: Enteroviruses and Heine-Medin disease. J Mt Sinai Hosp 25:391, 1958.

Steigman, A. J., and Lipton, M. M.: Fatal bulbospinal paralytic poliomyelitis due to ECHO 11 virus. JAMA 174:178, 1960.

Thompson, T. C.: A method of artificial respiration especially useful for the paralyzed patient. JAMA 104:307, 1935.

Verlinde, J. D., Kret, A., and Wyler, R.: The distribution of poliomyeli-tis virus in cynomolgus monkeys following oral administration, tonsillectomy, and intramuscular injection of diphtheria toxoid. Arch Ges Virusforsch 6:175, 1955.

Volpi, A., Ragona, G., Biondi, W., Rocchi, G., and Archetti, I.: Seroim-munity to polioviruses in an urban population of Italy. Bull W H O 54:3518, 1976.

World Health Organization: Weekly Epidemiological Record, 54:81 (16 March) 1979a.

World Health Organization: Weekly Epidemiological Record, 54:57 (23 February) 1979b.

World Health Organization: Weekly Epidemiological Record, 54:177 (9 June) 1979c.

World Health Organization: Weekly Epidemiological Record, 54:202 (29 June) 1979d.

# *ENTEROVIRAL* 174 *INFECTIONS OTHER THAN POLIOMYELITIS*

*Reisaku Kono, M.D., M.P.H.*

## *DEFINITION*

Enteroviral infections of the central nervous system other than poliomyelitis take three clini-cal forms: aseptic meningitis, encephalitis (men-ingoencephalitis), and poliolike paresis or paraly-sis. Aseptic meningitis is predominantly a syndrome of infants and children who have signs and symptoms of meningitis and a benign progno-sis. Wallgren (1925) established the concept of "aseptic meningitis" without knowledge of the viral etiology of the disease, and later Goldfield (1957) proposed the name "lymphocytic meningi-tis" for the same syndrome. When lymphocytic choriomeningitis (LCM) virus was isolated from such cases, the cause seemed to have been discov-ered, but later it became clear that LCM virus was infrequent, and other viruses were more important as etiologic agents. Accordingly, the term "viral meningitis" has been widely used to identify this disease complex, which is most often due to enteroviruses. The term "aseptic meningi-tis" applies not only to cases due to viruses but also to meningeal infections caused by *Chlamydia, Leptospira,* fungi, and some bacteria. There are also certain noninfectious causes (Krugman and Ward, 1973). Aseptic meningitis is a more suit-able clinical term than viral meningitis because the viral etiology cannot be recognized at the bedside and requires laboratory confirmation.

The encephalitis or meningoencephalitis that I refer to in this chapter is regarded as an advanced state of aseptic meningitis; meningitic inflammatory reactions spread to the central nervous system via the blood vessels but do not severely affect the parenchyma. Although encephalitic symptoms such as disturbed consciousness and convulsions occur with meningitis, they tend to be transient, and the prognosis is usually benign.

## ETIOLOGY

The enteroviruses other than poliovirus that are involved are: coxsackie virus A1 through A22 and A24; coxsackievirus B1 through B6; echovirus Types 1 through 9, 11 through 27, and 29 through 33; and enterovirus Types 68 through 71. They share some common properties with poliovirus in that the virions are ether-resistant, with cubic symmetry, and have diameters of about 20 to 30 nm and densities of 1.34 g/ml in CsCl. Their RNA genomes are single-stranded and have molecular weights of 2 to 2.8 × 10$^6$ daltons. The enteroviruses do not have as strong a neurovirulence as do poliovirus infections of primates, although the AB IV variant of coxsackievirus A7 (Voroshilova and Chumakov, 1959) and enterovirus 70 (Kono et al., 1973) display a weak but definite neurovirulence. Greater acid stability and lower buoyant density in CsCl are the main characteristics distinguishing the enteroviruses from the rhinoviruses, which are also picornaviridae but cause the common cold and are not neurotropic.

Coxsackieviruses were first distinguished from echoviruses by their pathogenicity for suckling mice, but the pathogenicity for mice was later found to vary from virus strain to strain. For example, some strains of coxsackievirus B1 through B6, A7, A9, and A16 can grow in monkey kidney cell cultures and are harmless to mice, whereas some strains of ECHOvirus 9 are pathogenic to suckling mice. Because of this variability, a subclassification of coxsackieviruses or ECHOviruses is no longer applied to new enteroviruses, and they are simply numbered as enterovirus 68, 69, 70, 71, and so forth (Melnick et al., 1974).

It is clear from the following statistical data that enteroviruses play an important role in neurologic infections. In the grand total of 23,824 viral infections of the central nervous system reported to the World Health Organization (WHO) during three years (1974 through 1976), 10,370 cases (43.5 per cent) were ascribed to enteroviruses other than poliovirus, followed in frequency by 5152 cases (21.6 per cent) of mumps virus infection (World Health Organization, 1974, 1975, 1976).

According to the aseptic meningitis surveillance summary covering the period 1969 through 1971 by the Center for Disease Control (CDC), nonpolio enteroviruses were the most prevalent cause of aseptic meningitis each year, comprising over 80 per cent of the identified etiologic agents (Center for Disease Control, 1969 to 1971 and 1971 to 1975). However, among the pathogens causing encephalitis, enteroviruses played a relatively minor role; they represented only 6.2 per cent of the total known causative agents of viral encephalitis in the CDC surveillance reports (Center for Disease Control, 1973). Table 1 summarizes the etiologic relationships among enterovirus types and clinical manifestations from past reports. Table 2 shows the reported numbers of enterovirus infections that appeared in the WHO yearly virus reports during the ten years from 1967 to 1976 (World Health Organization, 1973, 1974, 1975, and 1976). The large number of isolations of coxsackievirus A9 seems to reflect simply that coxsackievirus A9 can be easily isolated by tissue culture methods while other coxsackie A viruses require cumbersome inoculations into suckling mice; hence, fewer attempts were made to isolate other coxsackie A viruses. In spite of the small number of isolations of coxsackie A viruses, coxsackieviruses A1 and A4 have been isolated relatively frequently from patients with paralysis, although their real etiologic relationship with the disease is still uncertain.

As indicated by their generic name, enteroviruses are transient inhabitants of the human alimentary tract; hence, they are apt to be recovered from throat secretions and stools. Enteroviruses isolated from feces may or may not have an etiologic role in paralytic or other diseases that occur sporadically, since enteroviruses are often coincidentally carried in the alimentary tract of children. An isolate from nervous tissue or cerebrospinal fluid (CSF) has more etiologic significance. Although they possess the properties of enteroviruses, most strains of enterovirus 70 cannot grow in the alimentary tract but do multiply in the human conjunctiva. They are normally isolated from eye swabs but rarely from the throat or feces.

## PATHOGENESIS AND PATHOLOGY

Infections with enteroviruses show themselves through either subclinical or apparent illness, or about half of them occur in the central nervous system (World Health Organization, 1974, 1975,

**TABLE 1.    Enterovirus Types and Clinical Syndromes**

| | |
|---|---|
| Aseptic meningitis | CA 1, 2, 3, 4, 5, 6, 7, 8, 9, 10 11, 14, 16, 17, 18, 22, 24. |
| | CB 1, 2, 3, 4, 5, 6. |
| | E  1, 2, 3, 4, 5, 6, 7, 9, 11, 12, 13, 14, 15, 16, 17, 18, 19, |
| | 20, 21, 22, 23, 25, 30, 31, 32, 33. |
| | EV 71. |
| Polio-like motor paralysis | CA 1, 4, 7, 9, 10, 14. |
| | CB 1, 2, 3, 4, 5. |
| | E  1, 2, 4, 6, 7, 9, 11, 14, 16, 18, 22, 30. |
| | EV 70. |
| Encephalitis or meningoencephalitis | CA 2, 5, 6, 7, 9. |
| | CB 1, 2, 3, 4, 5. |
| | E  2, 3, 4, 6, 7, 9, 11, 14, 16, 18, 19, 33. |
| | EV 71. |

CA, coxsackievirus A Types 1, 2, etc.

CB, coxsackievirus B Types 1, 2 etc.

E, echovirus Types 1, 2 etc.

EV 70, EV 71, enterovirus Types 70 and 71.

Lines under the figure represent the types reported in outbreak.

and 1976). The primary sites of infection with enteroviruses, other than enterovirus 70, are the pharynx and intestine. In this alimentary phase, there are often no apparent signs or symptoms of infection, although sometimes there is a slight fever and a respiratory or intestinal disorder. On the other hand, the primary site of enterovirus 70 infection is the eyes, and this results in a high incidence of acute hemorrhagic conjunctivitis (AHC) (Kono and Uchida, 1977). The virus spreads from the primary site of infection to local lymph nodes, and then a transient viremia car-

**TABLE 2.    Major Enterovirus Types that Affect the Central Nervous System**

| VIRUS TYPES | TOTAL CNS DISEASE | | POLIO-LIKE PARALYSIS | |
|---|---|---|---|---|
| | No. | % | No. | % |
| Coxsackie A | | | | |
| Total | 1924 | 100.0 | 124 | 100.0 |
| CA 1 | 34 | 1.8 | 25 | 20.2 |
| CA 4 | 62 | 3.2 | 17 | 13.7 |
| CA 9 | 1515 | 78.7 | 27 | 21.7 |
| Coxsackie B | | | | |
| Total | 6286 | 100.0 | 158 | 100.0 |
| CB 1 | 346 | 5.5 | 12 | 7.5 |
| CB 2 | 1328 | 21.1 | 25 | 15.8 |
| CB 3 | 1369 | 21.8 | 40 | 25.3 |
| CB 4 | 1066 | 17.0 | 31 | 19.6 |
| CB 5 | 2106 | 33.5 | 45 | 28.5 |
| Echoviruses | | | | |
| Total | 17364 | 100.0 | 155 | 100.0 |
| E  3 | 424 | 2.4 | 7 | 4.5 |
| E  4 | 1245 | 7.2 | 5 | 3.2 |
| E  6 | 2928 | 16.9 | 19 | 12.3 |
| E  7 | 527 | 3.0 | 14 | 9.0 |
| E  9 | 3462 | 19.9 | 24 | 15.5 |
| E  11 | 1446 | 8.3 | 18 | 11.6 |
| E  14 | 413 | 2.4 | 8 | 5.1 |
| E  18 | 419 | 2.4 | 3 | 1.9 |
| E  19 | 2100 | 12.1 | 7 | 4.5 |
| E  30 | 3083 | 17.8 | 11 | 7.1 |

Compiled from WHO Yearly Virus Reports, 1967–1976.

ries it to the central organs. From these, a secondary viremia probably ensues, eventually reaching the central nervous system. It was reported that viremia was proved in five of nine blood specimens taken within five days after the onset of echovirus 4 meningitis (Ishii et al., 1968). Most enteroviruses probably infect the choroid membrane at this stage and then invade the leptomeninges and ependyma, causing aseptic meningitis. Such enteroviruses are isolated from the CSF at a high rate but have little neurovirulence. On the other hand, some strains of coxsackievirus A7 and enterovirus 70, like poliovirus, seem to have a special affinity for the motor neurons, which they destroy, causing paralysis (Horstmann and Manuelidis, 1958; Voroshilova and Chumakov, 1959; Kono et al., 1973). This neurovirulence is weaker than that of wild-type poliovirus. A diffuse meningoencephalitis may follow aseptic meningitis, but it is transitory and benign. Generally speaking, the pathogenesis and pathology of enteroviral infections of the central nervous system are not clearly understood because there have been few autopsied cases, and no suitable studies have been made in animal models.

Some host factors, like physical and/or mental strain, may precipitate the illness of the central nervous system. In the polio-like motor paralysis due to enterovirus 70, it was found that intramuscular injection of a drug seemed to provoke paralysis of the injected limb (Phuapradit et al., 1976).

## CLINICAL MANIFESTATIONS

Acute aseptic meningitis can begin abruptly with fever, headache, and signs of meningeal irritation, or it can occur diphasically with prodromal symptoms and then meningitis. The prodromal symptoms are usually fever, anorexia, malaise, and sore throat, which, after a remission for a few days, are followed by meningitis and a second temperature rise. It is likely that the alimentary phase of infection is subclinical in the former case and symptomatic in the latter.

When the central nervous system is attacked, body temperature rises, headache intensifies, and nausea and vomiting follow. During this stage, older children and adults often complain of nuchal pain, backache, or lumbago. Nuchal rigidity is often found, Kernig's and Brudzinski's signs are positive, and patellar and other deep tendon reflexes are exaggerated. However, nuchal rigidity is not so prominent as in bacterial meningitis; especially in infections of young infants, it is often absent or obscure. At the height of illness, various grades of disturbances of consciousness from somnolence to coma may appear, but convul-

sions are rather exceptional. Convulsions are considered to be the result of a diffuse meningoencephalomyelitis.

Often aseptic meningitis due to some enteroviruses (ECHOviruses 4, 6, 9, and 16 and coxsackie viruses A9 and A16) is accompanied by skin rash, and hence may be designated as meningitis exanthematica. Maculopapules, 2 to 4 mm in diameter, appear on the trunk and face most abundantly at the onset or during the second phase. The rash is sometimes scarlatina-like, vesicular, or, rarely, petechial. An enanthem may be seen on the tonsils and buccal mucosa. Meningitis is accompanied by a high incidence of rash, especially with echovirus 9 infections; in the Milwaukee epidemic of 1957, the majority of such rashes occurred in infants under 3 years old; 44 per cent were between 5 and 15 years; and 6 per cent were above 15 years (Sabin et al., 1958). I have observed skin rash in only 11 per cent of the cases of echovirus 4 meningitis in Niigata, Japan, in 1964 (Ishii et al., 1968), which suggests that the incidence of skin rash is lower in aseptic meningitis due to enteroviruses other than echovirus 9.

Aseptic meningitis due to coxsackie B viruses is often accompanied by myalgia and is called meningitis myalgica. Coxsackie B viruses tend to cause aseptic meningitis in infants and epidemic myalgia or epidemic pleurodynia in adults (see Chapter 240). If the two clinical conditions happen to manifest themselves at the same time, a coxsackie B virus etiology is suggested, although the final diagnosis cannot be made without laboratory confirmation.

One of the newer enteroviruses, enterovirus 71, was isolated from patients with the hand, foot, and mouth disease syndrome complicated by aseptic meningitis in Japan (Hagiwara et al., 1978); Sweden (Blomberg et al., 1974); and Australia (Kennett et al., 1974). Hand, foot, and mouth disease has been known to result from coxsackievurus A16 infections but has seldom led to neurologic complications. In the United States, it was reported that enterovirus 71 was isolated from the brain of a patient with encephalitis (Schmidt et al., 1974). Therefore, enterovirus 71 appears to be more neurovirulent than many other enteroviruses (Hashimoto et al., 1978).

Cerebellar and other ataxias have been observed during the course of proven infections by coxsackievirus A and B; echovirus 6 and 9 (McAllister et al., 1959); and enterovirus 71 (Ishimaru et al., 1974), but the actual etiologic relationship between ataxia and these enteroviruses remains unsolved.

Associations between Guillain-Barré syndrome and some enteroviruses have been reported but are unconfirmed (Gear, 1961 to 1962). In these cases, late examinations of CSF in patients with enteroviral meningitis may seemingly give a picture of protein increase without pleocytosis and thus lead to a misdiagnosis of Guillain-Barré syndrome. Mild paresis or paralysis may appear during the course of enterovirus infections other than poliovirus, but it occurs sporadically, and the recovery is usually complete. However, two exceptions have been recorded in the past during outbreaks of polio-like motor paralysis caused by the AB IV variant of coxsackievirus A7 (Voroshilova and Chumakov, 1959) and enterovirus 70 (Kono et al., 1977; Hung and Kono, 1979).

## COMPLICATIONS AND SEQUELAE

Enteroviral meningitis or meningoencephalitis is usually benign and resolves within two weeks. However, neonatal infections with enteroviruses, particularly with coxsackieviruses B1 through B5, require special attention (Kibrick, 1964) because they tend to be generalized diseases (encephalohepatomyocarditis) with a high fatality rate. Kibrick (1961) examined 54 newborns with disease caused by coxsackie B viruses; 45 of them had generalized infections, in which the major illness was myocarditis; one fourth of them had meningoencephalitis; and only 12 survived. The onset was abrupt and the clinical course was rapid, terminating in collapse and death within a few days. Tachycardia, tachypnea, and cyanosis were common; and cardiomegaly, hepatomegaly, and systolic murmurs were present, accompanied by electrocardiographic changes. Autopsies revealed that the patients had myocarditis (100 per cent), meningoencephalitis (76 per cent), hepatitis (43 per cent), pancreatitis (41 per cent), and adrenal cortical involvement (16 per cent). Many such illnesses are the result of infections of the mother just prior to birth (Kibrick and Benirschke, 1958), but others are transmitted by nursery personnel (Gear, 1958). Other enteroviruses are occasionally reported to cause fatal infections of newborn children, but their etiologic significance has not always been clear.

Children who experience enteroviral central nervous system diseases during their first year of life may have neurologic sequelae and lowered intelligence in later life. Sells et al. (1975) carried out a controlled follow-up study of 19 children 2½ to 8 years of age who had been hospitalized with enterovirus infection 17 to 67 months before. Three children (16 per cent) had definite neurologic impairment, 5 (26 per cent) had possible impairment, and 11 (58 per cent) were free of detectable abnormalities. Children whose illness occurred during the first year of life were found to have significantly smaller mean head circumferences, lower IQs and depressed language and speech skills. Farmer et al. (1975) reported that two of three infants who were noted to be irritable or twitching in association with coxsackie B5 meningoencephalitis in the neonatal period developed spasticity, and their intelligence was below the mean for the group six years after the onset.

Since the motor paralysis due to enterovirus 70 is a newly discovered disease and has several unique clinical features, some important clinicoepidemiologic points are described here (Kono et al., 1977; Hung and Kono, 1979). The neurologic disease usually appears two to five weeks or more after the onset of acute hemorrhagic conjunctivitis (AHC) (Fig. 1). Consequently, the relationship between conjunctivitis and the neurologic disorders is often overlooked by physicians as well as by the patients themselves. The patients sustain a systemic illness (i.e., pyrexia, general malaise, headache, nuchal pain, dizziness, and vomiting) one to three days before the onset of the neurologic symptoms. The most frequent initial symptoms are radicular pains in the muscles and limbs and aching in the lower back. Flaccid paresis or paralysis usually follows, occurring in one or more limbs, being asymmetrical and more severe in the lower limbs than in the upper, and often more proximal than distal. Tendon reflexes are abolished or diminished in the affected muscles. Cranial nerve involvement (e.g., difficulty in swallowing and facial palsy) is noted in some patients; in these cases, the interval between conjunctivitis and paralysis seems to be shorter than that found in patients with paralysis of the limbs (Fig. 1). A preponderance of male patients is usually observed. Unlike poliomyelitis, the highest incidence is found in patients who are 20 to 40 years old (Fig. 1). Pleocytosis of the CSF is found in the first three weeks from onset of neurologic symptoms, and the total protein level is raised from the second week of illness up to seven weeks or later in the CSF. Death from the disease has not been confirmed, although there was one suspicious case in Taiwan. Permanent incapacitation due to paralysis and muscular atrophy in the affected proximal muscles of the limbs is observed in roughly one fourth of the patients.

## EPIDEMIOLOGIC FEATURES AND GEOGRAPHIC VARIATION IN DISEASE

Enteroviruses have a worldwide distribution, but their spread is influenced by climatic conditions; they are prevalent in summer and early fall in the temperate zone and throughout the year in the tropics. Table 3 shows that the peak incidence

POLIO-LIKE MOTOR PARALYSIS DUE TO AHC VIRUS (ENTEROVIRUS 70)
IN DAKAR, BOMBAY, GAUHATI, BANGKOK, AND TAIPEI

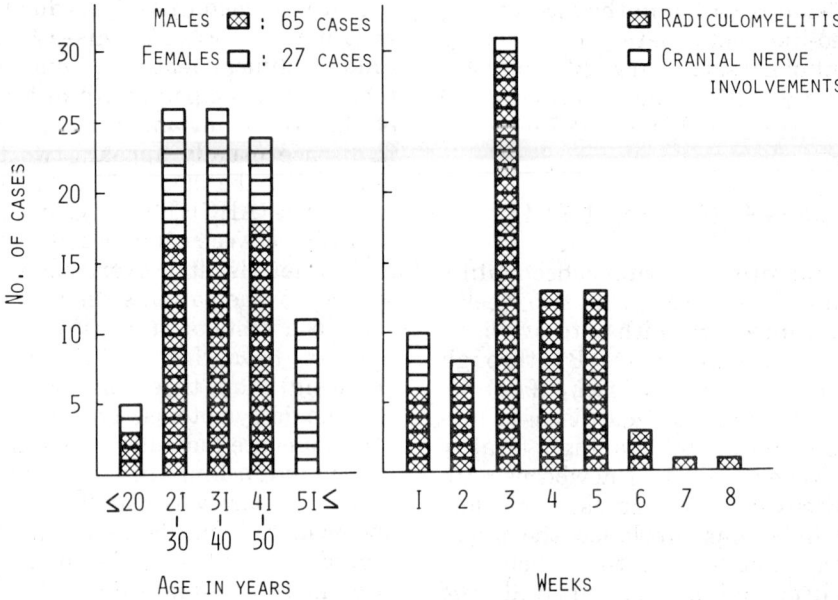

FIGURE 1.

of coxsackie A virus infection was found in July and those of coxsackie B and echo viruses occurred in August in the temperate zone of the northern hemisphere. The epidemics that occurred seemed to increase only the total number of cases, without displacing or distorting the seasonal pattern. All epidemics occurred in the season in which maximum enterovirus activity would be expected to occur in a normal, nonepidemic year.

Enterovirus infections were consistently reported more frequently in males than in females. The male to female ratio ranged from 1.33 to 1.54 in the enterovirus surveillance report, 1971 through 1975, of the Center for Disease Control (1977), but it was sometimes over 2.0.

TABLE 3. Number of Reports on Enteroviruses Other Than Poliovirus Included in the Study by Month of Collection Receipt of Specimen (1967–1973) in the Northern Hemisphere

| | VIRUS TYPE | JAN | FEB | MAR | APR | MAY | JUN | JUL | AUG | SEP | OCT | NOV | DEC | TOTAL |
|---|---|---|---|---|---|---|---|---|---|---|---|---|---|---|
| CA | No. | 81 | 53 | 72 | 74 | 229 | 529 | 700 | 559 | 365 | 333 | 236 | 108 | 3339 |
| | % | 2.4 | 1.6 | 2.2 | 2.2 | 6.9 | 15.8 | 21.0 | 16.7 | 10.9 | 10.0 | 7.1 | 3.2 | 100.0 |
| CB | No. | 128 | 113 | 152 | 187 | 417 | 807 | 1624 | 1948 | 1427 | 1054 | 512 | 247 | 8616 |
| | % | 1.5 | 1.3 | 1.8 | 2.2 | 4.8 | 9.4 | 18.8 | 22.6 | 16.6 | 12.2 | 5.9 | 2.8 | 100.0 |
| E | No. | 289 | 249 | 282 | 261 | 651 | 1210 | 2294 | 3007 | 2202 | 1899 | 840 | 374 | 13555 |
| | % | 2.1 | 1.8 | 2.1 | 1.9 | 4.8 | 8.9 | 16.9 | 22.1 | 16.2 | 14.0 | 6.1 | 2.8 | 100.0 |

CA, coxsackievirus A.

CB, coxsackievirus B.

E, echovirus.

Compiled from WHO Yearly Virus Reports, 1967–1973.

In the temperate zone, one particular type of enterovirus becomes prevalent within a particular time and space. When that occurs, the population lacks immunity against that particular enterovirus type. An epidemic of enteroviral meningitis and meningoencephalitis represents an epiphenomenon in that setting. Therefore, an enormous number of patients with summer grippe or other minor illnesses and healthy virus carriers are usually seen along with the patients with neurologic diseases during an epidemic.

In the tropical countries, several types of enteroviruses often circulate at the same time. Therefore, the local population experiences infections with many types of enteroviruses in early life. However, there is no evidence indicating that the neurologic diseases are more prevalent in the tropics than in the temperate zone.

When new types of variants of enteroviruses appear in a country, they spread from area to area. Because of a lack of immunity, all ages are affected in a pandemic fashion. For instance, enterovirus 70 appeared in West Africa in 1969 and within a few years spread to other parts of Africa, Europe, and Asia. North and South America and most parts of Oceania still remain free from AHC.

Outbreaks of polio-like motor paralysis due to the AB IV variant of coxsackievirus A7 were recorded in the 1950's in Karanganda and the U.S.S.R. (Voroshilova and Chumakov, 1959) and in the 1960's in Scotland (Grist, 1962), while paralytic outbreaks of enterovirus 70 occurred in Senegal (1970), India (1971), Thailand (1974), and China (Taiwan) (1971 through 1977) (Hung and Kono, 1979). It is likely that similar cases following AHC might have occurred but went unrecognized in other countries. At the present time, it is hard to ascribe the occurrence of the neurologic disease following AHC either to the local appearance of more neurovirulent variants or to the accumulation of such cases simply because of the enormous number of patients who had also experienced hemorrhagic conjunctivitis in their backgrounds.

### DIAGNOSIS

Recognition of the aseptic meningitis syndrome is usually not difficult. Signs of meningeal irritation should prompt laboratory examination of CSF. In enterovirus infections, the pressure of CSF increases slightly (to 200 to 300 mm of water). The CSF appears clear or somewhat cloudy but never purulent or hemorrhagic. The protein content tends to remain normal in the acute stage but increases to an abnormal level two weeks after the onset of infection. The sugar content does not decrease as it does in cryptococcal meningitis, tuberculous meningitis, and other bacterial meningitides. In contrast to the pattern of elevated protein concentration, the pleocytosis (30 to 4000 cells, average 150 cells) tends to be confined to the acute rather than to the late stage. The pleocytosis usually consists of lymphocytes, but sometimes polymorphonuclear leukocytes also appear in the early stage of illness. The pleocytosis usually returns to normal within a few weeks after the onset of meningitis.

Etiologic diagnosis can be achieved by virus isolation and/or serologic reactions. However, the materials and methods used for virus isolation differ depending on what virus is sought. For isolation of enteroviruses from patients, CSF, throat swabs, and feces are the specimens of choice, and they should be sent in a frozen state (−70°C) to the virus laboratory for inoculation into human cell cultures of fetal kidney or lung and primary monkey kidney. They should also be inoculated into suckling mice. Many types of enteroviruses are readily recovered from the CSF (echoviruses 4 and 6 and coxsackie B viruses, for example), but some types (e.g., enterovirus 70 [Kono et al., 1977] and 71 [Kennett et al., 1974]) are not. A virus isolation from CSF taken during the early stage of illness (within three to five days after the onset) renders a positive diagnosis of viral etiology. In the early stage of aseptic meningitis, the virus isolation rate from CSF was reported to be as high as 87.5 per cent and 73.0 per cent in echovirus (Ishii et al., 1968) and 18 (Wilfert et al., 1975) in meningitis, respectively. If an enterovirus has been isolated from only a throat swab or feces, a diagnosis should not be made unless serologic confirmation is possible with paired sera from the same patient, and/or epidemiologic considerations indicate that the patient has encountered the same virus type during an outbreak. Serologic confirmation is necessary because the coincidental presence of enteroviruses in the feces during an unrelated illness is frequent. Dual infections with different types of enteroviruses may also occur. Immunofluorescence can detect enterovirus antigens in cells obtained by centrifugation of CSF and makes a rapid virologic diagnosis possible (Taber et al., 1973).

Viruses other than enteroviruses must be considered. Mumps virus is one of the common causes of aseptic meningitis in infants and children; herpes simplex virus Type 2 is often a cause of meningitis of the neonate and of sexually active adults with coincidental genital herpes. Some patients with bacterial meningitis who have received inadequate antibacterial chemotherapy may mimic the clinical syndrome for aseptic meningitis, and syphilitic, leptospiral, tuberculous, cysticercal, and fungal meningitis may have to be considered in some cases. Brain abscesses may also resemble enteroviral meningitis. In cases with motor paralysis, it is of primary importance to exclude poliovirus by virus isolation and serologic methods.

## TREATMENT AND PROPHYLAXIS

There is no specific therapy for enteroviral neurologic diseases. However, the clinician often faces the problem of antimicrobial treatment of patients with encephalitis and/or meningitis, since it is usually very difficult to eliminate a bacterial etiology solely on clinical grounds during the early phases of illness. Antimicrobial treatment may be started in such cases of uncertain diagnosis and be discontinued if the CSF cultures prove to be sterile. Other treatments are symptomatic. In case of polio-like motor paralysis, physiotherapy must be given as soon as the aching of limbs and muscle pains subside and the progression of motor paralysis stops. Immunization with vaccines and prophylaxis with gamma globulin are impractical. The avoidance of possible precipitating or aggravating factors that could lead to encephalomeningitis and motor paralysis (such as intramuscular drug administration and undue physical exertion) must be emphasized to patients with enteroviral infections.

As already described, enteroviruses are present in throat secretions for about two weeks and in stools for several weeks or more. Infection spreads most often by the fecal-oral route among playmates in summer. Therefore, while it is theoretically possible to prevent infection with nonpolio enteroviruses by cutting the chain of infection, it is difficult in practice because there are many healthy virus carriers, and the environment is easily contaminated by the virus during the epidemic. Avoidance of contact with patients exhibiting acute febrile illness, especially those with a rash, is advisable for very young children. Newborns acquire infection vertically from their infected mothers or horizontally from medical personnel carrying the virus and/or contaminated utensils in the nursery. Since neonatal infections tend to be more severe, strict precautions must be taken to prevent cross-infections. Members of the institutional staffs responsible for caring for infants should be tested for carriage of enteroviruses.

Since enteroviruses are unable to withstand temperatures of over 50° C, either boiling or autoclaving or dry heat sterilization is an effective method for killing them. Sodium hypochlorite is generally used as a disinfectant for enteroviruses.

As already mentioned, enterovirus 70 is present in eye discharges for a few days after the onset of AHC. Accordingly, it is most often transmitted on the contaminated hands of patients and medical personnel or by other vehicles, particularly ophthalmologic instruments. Since it is highly communicable, contaminated utensils should not be used by healthy persons unless they are sterilized or carefully disinfected in the household. In eye clinics, AHC patients must be treated separately from non-AHC patients. The disinfection of hands of ophthalmologists and nurses and of ophthalmologic instruments is of primary importance in the prevention of institutional outbreaks.

## References

Blomberg, J., Lycke, E., Ahlfors, K., Johnsson, T., Wolontis, S., and von Zeipel, G.: New enterovirus type associated with epidemic of aseptic meningitis and/or hand, foot, and mouth disease. Lancet 2:112, 1974.

Center for Disease Control, Neurotropic Viral Diseases Surveillance: Annual encephalitis summaries. In Krugman, S., and Ward, W.: Infectious Diseases of Children and Adults. 5th ed. St. Louis, C. V. Mosby Company, 1973, p. 26.

Center for Disease Control, Neurotropic Viral Diseases Surveillance: Aseptic meningitis annual summaries 1969–1971. Atlanta, U.S. Public Health Service, Center for Disease Control, 1970, 1972, 1973.

Neurotropic Viral Diseases Surveillance: Enterovirus summary 1971–1975. Atlanta, U.S. Public Health Service, Center for Disease Control, 1977.

Farmer, K., MacArthur, B. A., and Clay, M. M.: A follow-up study of 15 cases of neonatal meningoencephalitis due to coxsackie virus B5. J Pediatr 87:568, 1975.

Gear, J. H. S.: Coxsackie virus infection in South Africa. Yale J Biol Med 34:289, 1961–1962.

Gear, J. H. S.: Coxsackievirus infections of the newborn. Progr Med Virol 1:106, 1958.

Grist, N. R.: Type A-7 coxsackie (type 4 poliomyelitis) virus infection in Scotland. J Hyg 60:323, 1962.

Goldfield, M.: Viral meningitis. Am J Med Sci 234:91, 1957.

Hagiwara, A., Tagaya, I., and Yoneyama, T.: Epidemic of hand, foot, and mouth disease associated with enterovirus 71 infection. Intervirology 9:60, 1978.

Hashimoto, A., Hagiwara, A., and Kodama, H.: Neurovirulence in Cynomolgus monkeys of enterovirus 71 isolated from a patient with hand, foot and mouth disease. Arch Virol 56:257, 1978.

Horstmann, D. M., and Manuelidis, E. E.: Russian coxsackie A-7 virus (AB IV strain) — neuropathogenicity and comparison with poliomyelitis. J Immunol 81:32, 1958.

Hung, T-P., and Kono, R.: Neurologic complications of acute hemorrhagic conjunctivitis — A polio-like syndrome in adult. In Vinken, P. J., and Bruyn, G. W. (eds.): Handbook of Clinical Neurology. Vol. 38, Amsterdam, North-Holland Publishing Company 1979, p. 595.

Ishii, K., Matsunaga, Y., Onishi, E., and Kono, R.: Epidemiological and virological studies of echovirus type 4 meningitis in Japan, 1964. Jap J Med Sci Biol 21:11, 1968.

Ishimaru, K., Ishiki, M., and Yamaoka, K.: Aseptic meningitis accompanied by hand-foot-mouth disease and ataxia. Igaku-no-ayumi 89:108, 1974 (in Japanese).

Kennett, M. L., Birch, C. J., Lewis, F. A., Yung, A. P., Locarnini, S. A., and Gust, I. D.: Enterovirus type 71 infection in Melbourne. Bull WHO 51:609, 1974.

Kibrick, S.: Viral infections of the fetus and newborn. In Perspectives in Virology, Vol. 2. Minneapolis, Burgess Publishing Company, 1961, p. 140.

Kibrick, S.: Current status of coxsackie and echo viruses in human disease. Progr Med Virol 6:27, 1964.

Kibrick, S., and Benirschke, K.: Generalized disease (severe encephalohepatomyocarditis) occurring in the newborn period due to infection with coxsackievirus group B. Pediatrics 22:857, 1958.

Kono, R., Miyamura, K., Tajiri, E., Sasagawa, A., Phuapraditt, P., Roongwithu, N., Vajjajiva, A., Jayavasu, C., Thongcharoen, C., Wasi, C., and Roodprassert, P.: Virological and serological studies of neurological complications of acute hemorrhagic conjunctivitis in Thailand. J Infect Dis 133:706, 1977.

Kono, R., and Uchida, Y.: Acute hemorrhagic conjunctivitis. Ophthalmol Dig 39:14, 1977.

Kono, R., Uchida, N., Sasagawa, A., Akao, Y., Kodama, H., Mukoyama, J., and Fujiwara, T.: Neurovirulence of acute-hemorrhagic-conjunctivitis virus in monkeys. Lancet 1:61, 1973.

Krugman, S., and Ward, W.: Infectious Diseases of Children and Adults. 5th ed. St. Louis, C. V. Mosby Company, 1973.

McAllister, R. M., Hummeler, K., and Coriell, L. L.: Acute cerebellar ataxia: Report of a case with isolation of type 9 echovirus from the cerebrospinal fluid. N Engl J Med 261:1159, 1959.

Melnick, J. L., Tagaya, I., and Von Magnus, H.: Enterovirus 69, 70 and 71. Intervirology 4:369, 1974.

Phuapradit, P., Roongwithu, U., Linsukon, P., Boongird, P., and Vejjajiva, A.: Radiculomyelitis complicating acute hemorrhagic conjunctivitis: A clinical study. J Neurol Sci 27:117, 1976.

Sabin, A. B., Krumbiegel, E. R., and Wigand, R.: Echo 9 virus disease: Virologically controlled clinical and epidemiological observations during 1957 epidemic in Milwaukee with notes on concurrent similar diseases and associated coxsackie and other echo viruses. J Dis Child 96:197, 1958.

Schmidt, N. J., Lennette, E. H., and Ho, H. H.: An apparently new enterovirus isolated from patients with disease of the central nervous system. J Infect Dis 129:304, 1974.

Sells, C. J., Carpenter, R. L., and Ray, C. G.: Sequelae of central nervous system enterovirus infections. N Engl J Med 293:1, 1975.

Taber, L. H., Mirkovic, M. R., Adam, V., Ellis, S. S., Yow, M. D., and Melnick, J. L.: Rapid diagnosis of enterovirus meningitis by immunofluorescent staining of CSF leukocytes. Intervirology 1:127, 1973.

Voroshilova, M. K., and Chumakov, M. P.: Poliomyelitis-like properties of AB IV coxsackie A-7 group of viruses. Progr Med Virol 2:106, 1959.

Wallgren, A.: Une nouvelle maladie infecteuse du system nerveux central. Acta Paediat 4:158, 1925.

Wilfert, C. M., Lauer, B. A., Cohen, M., Costenbader, M. L., and Myers, E.: An epidemic of echovirus 18 meningitis. J Infect Dis 131:75, 1975.

World Health Organization, Virus Disease Unit: WHO Yearly Virus Report. Geneva, World Health Organization, 1973 VIR/74. 18; 1974 VIR/75. 18, 1974; 1975 VIR/77. 3; and 1976 VIR/78. 1.

# *TETANUS* **175**

## *Wesley Furste, M.D., F.A.C.S.*

## *DEFINITION*

Tetanus (lockjaw) is a severe and dreaded infectious complication of wounds, caused by the toxin of *Clostridium tetani*. This disease is characterized by tonic spasms of the voluntary muscles and by a tendency to episodes of respiratory arrest.

## *ETIOLOGY*

*C. tetani* is a large, gram-positive, actively motile bacillus that in its spore-bearing form resembles a drumstick or tennis racket. Spores may develop at both ends of the bacillus, giving a dumbbell appearance. It is a strict anaerobe, and spores do not germinate in the presence of even the smallest amount of oxygen.

*C. tetani* produces two exotoxins, tetanospasmin and tetanolysin. Tetanospasmin is the neurotoxin that produces the typical muscle spasms of tetanus. This toxin is second only to *C. botulinum* toxin in potency.

The source of infection with *C. tetani* in a large number of cases of tetanus varies from accidental injuries (44.5 per cent) to surgical operations (0.7 per cent). Some of the other sources reported are otorrhea and tetanus neonatorum (Patel and Mehta, 1963).

## *PATHOGENESIS AND PATHOLOGY*

The mere presence of *C. tetani* in a wound does not necessarily mean that the patient has or will develop *tetanus*. The organisms proliferate only in the presence of an oxidation-reduction (Eh) potential far lower than that existing in normal living tissue. Thus, the Eh of living mammalian tissue is +120 millivolts, and tetanus spores do not germinate at an Eh greater than +10. Once *C. tetani* begins to grow, it produces tetanospasmin, which is transported to the central nervous system, where it becomes fixed and is responsible for the development of tetanus.

As Smith (1971) has pointed out, there have been differences of opinion concerning the site of action of tetanospasmin and the route by which it spreads, but it now seems established that the toxin spreads centrally along the nerves into the central nervous system, where it acts (Kryzhanovsky, 1975). Tetanus occurs after the intravenous injection of toxin into animals, but the route by which toxin in the blood enters the nervous system in this model is not clear. Toxin injected intramuscularly apparently spreads not only by passing in a central direction in nerves but also by absorption into the blood. After toxin accumulates in the spinal cord, a small amount is degraded to a fragment with a molecular weight of

40,000, which by itself is a potent stimulant of autonomic activity. This may explain the increased sympathetic autonomic tone often seen early in tetanus (Bizzini, 1979). Tetanus toxin also acts on the end plates, the spinal cord, and the brain, where it binds to gangliosides.

## CLINICAL MANIFESTATIONS

### Incubation Period

In a 1968 report, the U.S. Public Health Service Communicable Disease Center (now the Center for Disease Control) reported that the median incubation period for fatal cases and nonfatal cases was 7 and 8 days respectively. The range was from 1 to 54 days.

### Symptoms and Signs

Tetanus almost always appears in a general form, but occasionally it may appear as local tetanus.

Some patients have prodromal symptoms of restlessness and headaches. In others, the first symptoms are those of developing muscle rigidity, with vague discomfort in the jaws, neck, or lumbar region. In an early stage, spasm of the muscles of mastication causes trismus and difficulty with chewing, i.e., lockjaw. Sustained contraction of the facial muscles produces a distorted grin (risus sardonicus). Spasm of the pharyngeal muscles makes swallowing difficult. Stiff neck due to muscle spasm (not meningeal irritation) is another early sign. Other muscle groups become progressively involved, with tightness of the chest and rigidity of the abdominal wall, back, and limbs and the development of orthotonos, opisthotonos, or emprosthotonos (Glenn, 1946). Generalized tonic convulsions are frequent and exhausting (see Fig. 1, Chapter 5). Any sudden jar or sound (such as a hypodermic injection or the fall of an object onto the floor) excites such generalized convulsions. In association with these convulsions, there is sometimes spasm of the laryngeal and respiratory muscles, occasionally resulting in a possibly fatal acute asphyxia.

The merciless disease leaves the patient mentally clear during such episodes and throughout its course. Patients suffer great pain from the muscle spasms. As part of the sympathetic nervous system disturbances, the pulse rate is elevated, and there is profuse perspiration, labile hypertension, peripheral vasoconstriction, and cardiac arrhythmias. Fever may or may not be present as a result of the intense muscular activity. Neurologic examination discloses hyperactive tendon reflexes, often with sustained clonus. There are no sensory changes.

Local tetanus is a rare form of this disease. It is characterized by spasms and rigidity of the muscle groups near the site of injury. Symptoms may last for several weeks, disappearing finally with no sequelae. Local tetanus may progress to the generalized form, however. Local tetanus involving the head and neck is more serious because of dysphagia and laryngeal spasm.

Even when treatment is adequate, the mortality in generalized tetanus may be 50 per cent or higher (Center for Disease Control, 1974). In special centers, however, mortality is less than 10 per cent in adults (Cole and Youngman, 1969). In general, cases with the shortest incubation period are more severe and have a higher mortality than cases with incubation periods of more than 14 days. Local tetanus is mild and has a fatality rate of approximately 1 per cent.

### Laboratory Data

The diagnosis of tetanus must be based on the clinical picture, for laboratory examinations are of little assistance. The demonstration of *C. tetani* in a wound does not prove the diagnosis of tetanus; the failure to demonstrate the bacillus in a wound does not eliminate the possibility of tetanus. The cerebrospinal fluid is normal, and peripheral white blood cells may be normal or elevated.

## COMPLICATIONS AND SEQUELAE

Combinations of complications may be responsible for death. Pulmonary atelectasis may be followed by pneumonia, which seriously lessens the chances for recovery. Traumatic glossitis is seen often. Compression fractures of the vertebrae may result from the convulsive seizures. Decubital ulcers may occur. Constipation, fecal impaction, and urinary retention are often encountered. Cystitis and pyelonephritis may develop in patients requiring catheterization. Foot drop and muscle contractures may follow prolonged unconsciousness. Asphyxia from respiratory or laryngeal muscle spasm or from aspiration of secretions, vomitus, or food may be the immediate cause of death. Blood clotting problems may develop, as may fatal pulmonary emboli.

In long-term follow-up studies, irritability, sleep disturbance, fits, myoclonus, decreased libido, postural hypotension, and electroencephalographic abnormalities have been noted (Illis and Taylor, 1971).

## GEOGRAPHIC VARIATIONS IN DISEASE

The introduction of tetanus toxoid approximately four decades ago, which was followed in many parts of the world by programs of immunization of the population, contributed greatly to the control of tetanus.

In developed countries, tetanus is occurring less and less frequently (Fig. 1). In the United States, the median age of those with tetanus has been increasing steadily in the last 30 years. This corresponds with the lower percentage of elderly people with protective antitoxin titers found in serologic surveys. Urban tetanus is most often a complication of drug addiction.

In contrast, in other countries, 1,000,000 deaths (900,000 caused by neonatal tetanus) per year (according to Bytchenko of the World Health Organization) may be due to tetanus.

When tetanus does occur, however, it is the same terrifying disease regardless of the geographic area in which it occurs.

## DIAGNOSIS

Early or mild tetanus may resemble certain other conditions, but severe tetanus is likely to be confused with few other diseases.

Serum sickness may be confused with early tetanus. Tetany usually follows operations on the thyroid gland, affects the upper extremities primarily, is associated with a low blood calcium level, and is relieved by intravenous calcium.

Focal central nervous system signs and abnormalities of the cerebrospinal fluid in meningitis and encephalitis make it easy to differentiate them from tetanus. Rabies is indicated by the patient's inability to swallow as an early symptom, by drooling of saliva, and by spasms of the muscles of deglutition.

Strychnine poisoning may mimic tetanus closely, except that the muscles are relaxed between seizures in strychnine intoxication, whereas spasm tends to persist in tetanus. Cancer metastases from elsewhere in the body to the central nervous system may produce a clinical picture suggesting tetanus.

The toxicity due to phenothiazine tranquilizer drugs or to lead encephalopathy may be differentiated from tetanus by an adequately taken history and by standard screening of the blood and urine for these chemicals. Acute hysteria and acute psychoses may be quite difficult to differentiate from early or mild tetanus until the patient has been evaluated for some days.

The spasms of a localized group of voluntary muscles due to soft tissue or bone injuries may simulate local tetanus. Trismus (not due to tetanus) may occur with peritonsillar abscess, dental infections, and other local infections of the mouth and cervical regions and with dentomandibular problems.

Meningitis, hypocalcemic tetany, sepsis, or intracranial hemorrhage may be confused with neonatal tetanus.

Stiff-man syndrome, described by Moersch and Woltman in 1956, may at first be confused with subacute tetanus, but the slow progression for months or years of stiff-man syndrome eventually differentiates it from tetanus.

The failure to demonstrate a wound of entrance for *C. tetani* does not eliminate a diagnosis of tetanus, because many cases of tetanus have no demonstrable wound.

## TREATMENT

Once the diagnosis of tetanus has been established, tetanus immune globulin (human)

TETANUS — Reported Cases per 100,000 Population by Year, United States, 1950–1976

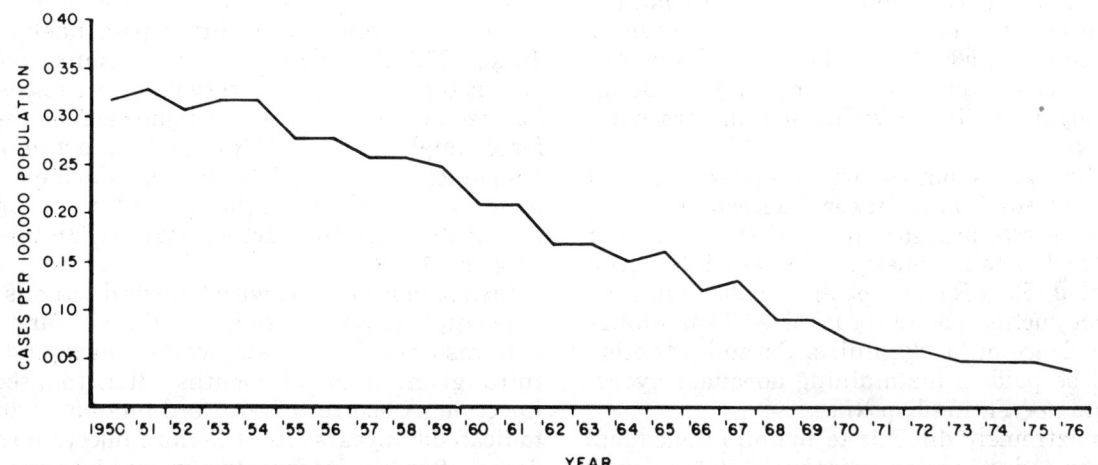

**FIGURE 1.** *Occurrence of tetanus in the United States. (From U.S. Public Health Service, Center for Disease Control: Morbid Mortal Weekly Rep 25 (no. 53), Aug. 1977.)*

(TIG[H]), 500 to 10,000 units, should be given as a deep intramuscular (I.M.) injection. Adsorbed tetanus toxoid should also be given at another site. The exact optimum dose of TIG(H) has not been established, and 500 units may be as effective as larger doses (Blake et al., 1976). Patel and his associates (1963) in Bombay, India, found no difference in mortality for doses ranging from 5000 units to 60,000 units of heterologous (equine) antitoxin and interpreted the large doses as being detrimental.

Procaine penicillin G (1.2 million units I.M. daily) should be instituted to eliminate residual tetanus bacilli in the wound. Tetracycline, 2 gm/day, can be used for patients who are allergic to penicillin. The wound itself should be carefully debrided; all foreign material and dead tissue should be removed.

The management of tetanic spasms can be difficult. Meperidine or morphine should be used to relieve the pain associated with muscle contractions, but care must be taken to avoid respiratory depression. Sedatives should be used; they also serve as muscle relaxants. Mild cases of tetanus (muscle rigidity but no generalized convulsions) can be managed with paraldehyde or thiopental. Some centers are enthusiastic about diazepam (Valium), 2 to 20 mg given intravenously every two to eight hours. Chlorpromazine, 50 to 100 mg I.M. every four to six hours, may also be used but may not control the seizures adequately. Maintaining a quiet environment and avoiding direct stimulation of the patient reduces the frequency of the seizures. If seizures cannot be controlled with sedatives, curare should be used at the lowest dose necessary to prevent seizures. Paralyzed patients are more likely to develop aspiration pneumonia and are completely dependent on mechanical ventilation.

The maintenance of an airway can be critically important. The tetanic spasms can result in asphyxia, and it may be impossible to intubate the patient due to the tetanic spasms. Therefore, tracheostomies should be done in all but the mildest cases of tetanus. A change in voice quality (hoarseness) is an indication for tracheostomy.

Cardiac arrhythmias are a major cause of death, but there is no general agreement about the methods to prevent fatal arrhythmias. Both alpha and beta adrenergic blockers have been advocated (Prys-Roberts et al., 1969). Prolonged tracheal suction should be avoided to minimize the incidence of bradycardias. Careful attention should be paid to maintaining adequate hydration and preventing hypoxia.

It is extremely difficult to maintain adequate nutrition. Adults may require up to 7000 calories daily. Only the mildest cases would be able to tolerate oral nutrition. Nasogastric tube feedings can be used, but they increase the risk of aspiration and gastrointestinal bleeding. Parenteral hyperalimentation appears to be the method of choice for providing nutrition.

Nursing care is extremely important. The tongue should be protected with a padded tongue blade. Patients should be turned frequently to prevent bed sores, to aid pulmonary toilet, and to prevent muscle contractures. Mouth care and tracheal care need to be given often.

There is no indication that either hyperbaric oxygen or corticosteroids are beneficial.

## PROPHYLAXIS

Adsorbed tetanus toxoid is the best agent to prevent tetanus (Center for Disease Control, 1977). Unfortunately, many individuals even in developed countries are not adequately immunized with tetanus toxoid (Fig. 2).

The recommended schedule for tetanus is given in Table 1. For reasons that have been outlined previously (Furste and Wheeler, 1972), the recommendations in Table 1 are based on an interval of five years for nontetanus-prone or minor wounds and of one year for tetanus-prone or major wounds. In 1978, Dull, assistant director for programs of the U.S. Public Health Service Center for Disease Control wrote about tetanus toxoid booster injections: "At times of injury when tetanus exposure is clearly felt to be possible, and the most recent Td (tetanus diphtheria toxoid) booster was more than a year earlier, an additional booster of Td is usually recommended. The next regular booster is measured from that time. Td is used instead of tetanus toxoid alone to provide continuing diphtheria protection."

The medical officers of the U.S. Armed Forces have an unequaled record of tetanus prophylaxis. Before 1972, they gave a booster dose of tetanus toxoid to all wounded or burned personnel. Since June, 1972, they have followed a similar policy, except that a five-year interval between boosters has been observed for minor injuries. As a result, for example, from 1945 to 1977, no active duty personnel of the U.S. Navy and Marine Corps have had tetanus as the result of an injury incurred while on active duty (Furste and Aguirre, 1978).

Basic immunization with adsorbed tetanus toxoid requires three injections, with the first two administered four to six weeks apart and the third given 6 to 12 months after the second injection. A booster of adsorbed tetanus toxoid is indicated ten years after the third injection or ten years after an intervening wound booster. All individuals, including pregnant women, should

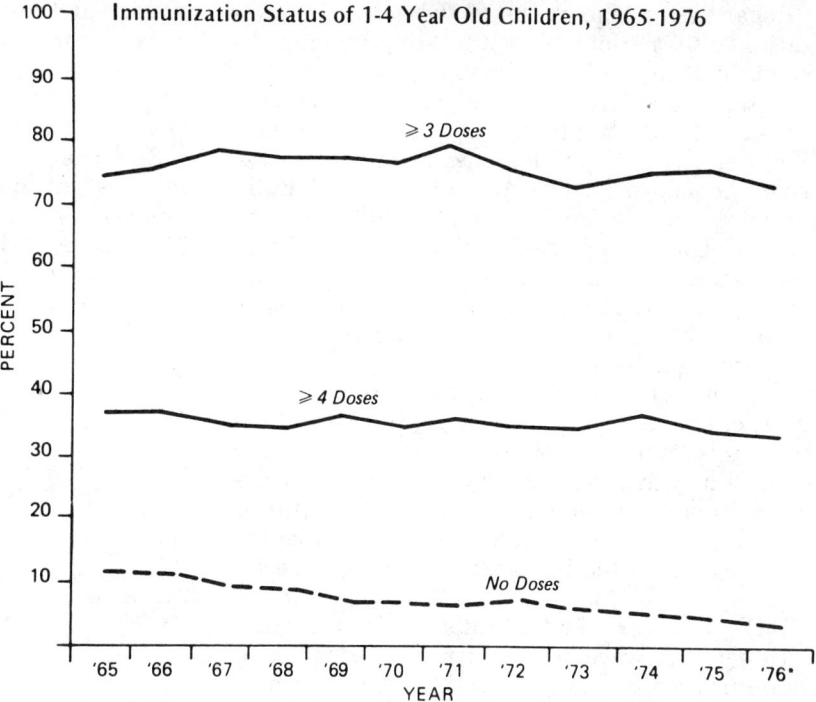

**FIGURE 2.** *Immunization status of 1- to 4-year-old children. (Figures from U.S Public Health Service, Center for Disease Control:* United States Immunization Survey: 1976. HEW Publ. No. [CDC] 78-8221. *Atlanta, Center for Disease Control, 1977, p. 9.)*

have basic immunization and booster injections when indicated. Neonatal tetanus is preventable by active immunization of the mother before or during the first six months of pregnancy. This immunization can be achieved by two intramuscular injections of adsorbed toxoid given six weeks apart. In the event that a neonate is born by a nonimmunized mother without adequate obstetric care, the infant should receive 250 to 500 units of tetanus immune globulin (human) (TIG)[H]) or 1500 I.U. of heterologous tetanus antitoxin. Active and passive immunization for the mother should also be initiated.

Each patient with a wound should receive adsorbed tetanus toxoid intramuscularly at the time of injury, either as an initial immunizing dose or as a booster for previous immunization, unless he

has received a booster or has completed his initial immunization series within the past one to ten years (Table 2). As the concentration of tetanus toxoid varies in different products, specific information on the volume of a single dose is provided on the label of the package.

**TABLE 2.　Tetanus Prophylaxis for the Injured**

1. Wound care: remove devitalized tissue and foreign bodies
2. Immunization
   A. Unimmunized patients (have not completed primary immunization)
      a. Clean minor wounds
         Give adsorbed tetanus toxoid (Td) as the initial immunizing dose and arrange for complete immunization
      b. All other wounds
         1. Give adsorbed tetanus toxoid (Td) as initial immunizing dose
         2. Give 250 to 500 units TIG(H) in a separate intramuscular injection
         3. Consider administering oral penicillin
   B. Immunized patients <10 years previously
      a. Most wounds: Adsorbed tetanus toxoid (Td) as booster unless last booster was <5 years before
      b. Severe, neglected, or old wounds (more than 24 hours old)
         Adsorbed tetanus toxoid (Td) as booster unless last booster was <1 year before
   C. Immunized patients >10 years previously
      a. Most wounds: Adsorbed tetanus toxoid as booster
      b. Severe, neglected, or old wounds (more than 24 hours old)
         1. Adsorbed tetanus toxoid booster
         2. TIG(H) 250 to 500 units in a separate intramuscular site
         3. Consider administering oral penicillin

**TABLE 1.　Tetanus Immunization Schedule**

A. Primary: Tetanus toxoid, three doses. Doses 1 and 2 administered four to six weeks apart. Third dose 6 to 12 months after second dose. Subsequent doses every ten years.
B. Pregnant women (nonimmunized): Two doses of alum-adsorbed toxoid, six weeks apart during first six months of pregnancy.
C. Incompletely immunized:
   1. If one previous dose of toxoid has been given >1 month before, give a second dose and
   2. If two previous doses of toxoid have been given, the last 6 months before, give a third dose.
   3. If three previous doses have been given, the last >5 years before, give a fourth dose.
   4. If four previous doses have been given, the last >10 years before, give a fifth dose.

Regardless of the status of the active immunization of the patient, all wounds require immediate optimal surgical care, including removal of all dead tissue and foreign bodies. Such care is essential as part of the prophylaxis against tetanus. Whether or not to provide passive immunization with homologous tetanus immune globulin (human) must be decided individually for each patient. The characteristics of the wound, conditions under which it was incurred, its treatment, its age, and the previous active immunization status of the patient must be considered.

Every wounded patient should be given a written record of the immunization provided and instructions to complete active immunization. For precise tetanus prophylaxis, an accurate and immediately available history regarding previous active immunization against tetanus is required, or rapid laboratory titration to determine the patient's serum tetanus antitoxin level is necessary.

DTP (diphtheria and tetanus toxoids combined with pertussis vaccine) is recommended for basic immunization in infants and children from 2 months through the sixth year of age, and Td (combined tetanus and diphtheria toxoid, adult type) for basic immunization of those over 6 years of age. For the latter group, Td toxoid is recommended for routine or wound boosters, but if there is any reason to suspect hypersensitivity to the diphtheria component, tetanus toxoid (T) should be substituted for Td. *A prior significant reaction to tetanus toxoid is a contraindication to another toxoid injection.*

The following precautions are recommended regarding passive immunization with heterologous tetanus antitoxin (equine).

1. Heterologous tetanus antitoxin (equine) should *not* be given except when tetanus immune globulin (human) is not available within 24 hours and only if the possibility of tetanus outweighs the danger of reaction to heterologous tetanus antitoxin.

2. Before using heterologous tetanus antitoxin, the patient should be questioned for a history of allergy and tested for sensitivity. If the patient is sensitive to heterologous antitoxin, it should not be used because the danger of anaphylaxis probably outweighs the danger of tetanus. Desensitization is not worth trying.

3. If the patient is not sensitive to heterologous tetanus antitoxin and if the decision is made to administer it for passive immunization, doses of 1500 to 3000 I.U. are given; and — for severe, neglected, or old (tetanus-prone) wounds — 3000 to 6000 I.U. are recommended.

### References

Bizzini, B.: Tetanus toxin. Microbiol Rev 43:224, 1979.
Blake, P. et al.: Serologic therapy of tetanus in the United States, 1965–1971. JAMA 235:42, 1976.
Bytchenko, B.: Personal communication, 18 June, 1978.
Cole, L., and Youngman, H.: Treatment of tetanus. Lancet 1:1017, 1969.
Communicable Disease Center, Public Health Service, U.S. Department of Health, Education, and Welfare: Tetanus surveillance. Report No. 1, February 1, 1968.
Dull, H.: Active immunization for infectious diseases. In Conn, H. (ed.): Current Therapy 1978. Philadelphia, W. B. Saunders Company, 1978, p. 86.
Furste, W., and Aguirre, A.: Preventing tetanus. Am J Nursing 78:834, 1978.
Furste, W., and Wheeler, W.: Tetanus: A team disease. Curr Prob Surg 1–62, October, 1972.
Glenn, F.: Tetanus — a preventable disease: Including an experience with civilian casualties in the battle for Manila (1945). Ann Surg 124:1030, 1946.
Illis, L. S., and Taylor, I. M.: Neurological and electroencephalographic sequelae of tetanus. Lancet 1:826, 1971.
Kryzhanovsky, G.: Tetanus: A polysystemic disease. In Comptes rendus de la Quatrième Conférence Internationale sur le Tétanos (Proceedings of the Fourth International Conference on Tetanus). Lyon (France), Lips, 1975, p. 189.
Moersch, F., and Woltman, H.: Progressive fluctuating muscular rigidity and spasm (stiff-man syndrome). Proc Staff Meet Mayo Clin 31:421, 1956.
Patel, J., and Mehta, B.: Tetanus: A study of 2007 cases. Indian J M Sci 17:791, 1963.
Patel, J., Mehta, B., Nanavati, B., Hazra, A., Rao, S., and Swaminathan, C.: Role of serum therapy in tetanus. Lancet 1:740, 1963.
Prys-Roberts, C., Corbett, J., Kerr, J., Spalding, J., and Crampton-Smith, A.: Treatment of sympathetic overactivity in tetanus. Lancet 1:542, 1969.
Smith, A.: Tetanus. In Beeson, P. B., and McDermott, W. (eds.): Cecil-Loeb Textbook of Medicine. 13th ed. Philadelphia, W. B. Saunders Company, 1971, p. 566.
U.S. Public Health Service, Center for Disease Control: Tetanus surveillance. Report No. 4. March 31, 1974.
U.S. Public Health Service, Center for Disease Control: Recommendation of the Public Health Service Advisory Committee on Immunization Practices. Morbid Mortal Weekly Rep 26:401, 1977.

# **176** *LEPROSY*

## *Robert R. Jacobson, M.D., Ph.D.*

Leprosy (Hansen's disease) is a chronic infection primarily affecting the skin, peripheral nerves, eyes, and mucous membranes. It has been known for over 2000 years and afflicts more than 12,000,000 people worldwide. The etiologic agent is a bacterium *(Mycobacterium leprae)* that has never definitely been cultured in artificial media, although it will grow in the mouse footpad (Shepard, 1960) and produce disseminated disease in the armadillo (Kirchheimer and Storrs, 1971).

There is much about the disease we do not understand, but we can manage nearly all patients satisfactorily without removing them from their normal position in society.

## PATHOGENESIS AND PATHOLOGY

There are three theories regarding transmission. The oldest holds that bacilli are shed from the skin of a patient and pass through the skin of a new host. Recently it has been argued that respiratory spread is more probable. The upper respiratory tract in a patient with active disseminated (lepromatous) disease is heavily infected, and with each cough or sneeze huge numbers of bacilli are blown out. When inhaled by a susceptible host, these bacilli presumably grow in the upper respiratory tract and disseminate therefrom via the bloodstream. The third theory suggests that insect vectors may at least occasionally transmit leprosy. Certain biting insects can take in *M. leprae* from untreated patients and transmit them to mouse footpads, where they multiply (Narayanan et al., 1977). Because no definitive studies have been done in humans, opinions vary, but the theory that transmission is respiratory seems to be favored now.

However it is transmitted, leprosy seems to be very contagious as measured by lymphocyte transformation to *M. leprae* antigens in exposed persons (Godal, 1974), yet the incidence of the disease in most areas remains very low, presumably because the overwhelming majority of people are not susceptible. Data suggest that susceptible persons have a defective cell-mediated immune (CMI) response toward *M. leprae*. Thus, when a normal person is exposed, the invading bacilli are engulfed by macrophages and destroyed, and no outward sign of infection develops. Although the macrophages in a person with the specific CMI defect ingest the bacilli, they do not fully recognize them as pathogens and allow them to multiply and disseminate to a variable degree. The source of the defective immune response to *M. leprae* is unknown. The evidence for a genetic origin is inconclusive. It is specific for *M. leprae,* since the CMI response to other pathogens is normal in patients with leprosy.

Leprologists often describe the different forms of leprosy as separate disease entities. This distinction is important clinically but tends to obscure the fact that these are different manifestations of the same disease. Since its presentation in a given patient is related to the degree of immune deficit present, any description should integrate the clinical and immunologic aspects. It is for this reason that the classification of Ridley and Jopling has gained relatively widespread

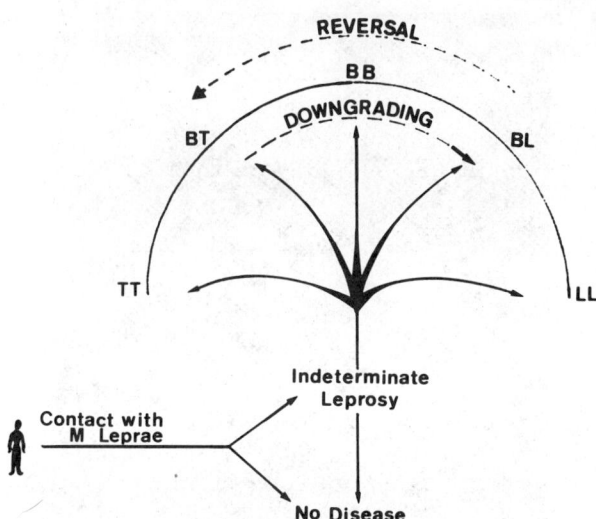

**FIGURE 1.** *The Ridley-Jopling classification of leprosy.*

acceptance (Ridley and Jopling, 1966). Figure 1 illustrates the five-part Ridley-Jopling classification. As noted, almost everyone (> 95 per cent) can apparently resist a routine exposure to this infection. The remainder develop indeterminate leprosy. Unless it heals spontaneously or is treated the disease will progress to one of the three common clinical types. Those with the greatest resistance keep the infection localized and develop tuberculoid disease (TT), while those with the least resistance develop generalized or lepromatous disease (LL). Between these two extremes is a broad zone (BT, BB, and BL), which is usually referred to as borderline (dimorphous) leprosy. The disease in a patient at either pole (TT or LL) tends to be stable, but in the broad borderline portion of the spectrum relatively wide shifts in disease type can occur. Without treatment there is a tendency for immunity to diminish with a consequent shift toward lepromatous disease. With effective chemotherapy, on the other hand, the tendency is to shift in the other direction toward tuberculoid disease with an enhanced immune response. These shifts may be accompanied by reactive episodes, referred to as downgrading (rare) or reversal reactions, respectively. Thus, although an infection may start out as BT, extensive disease may develop (downgrading), and it may be classified upon diagnosis as BB or beyond. With treatment, on the other hand, the patient's immunity and clinical course may improve (reversal), and the disease moves toward BT again. Although these immunologic shifts are seldom demonstrated histologically, they explain the course of the disease.

Biopsy sections in patients with indeterminate leprosy will usually show minimal nonspecific chronic inflammation of the upper dermis consist-

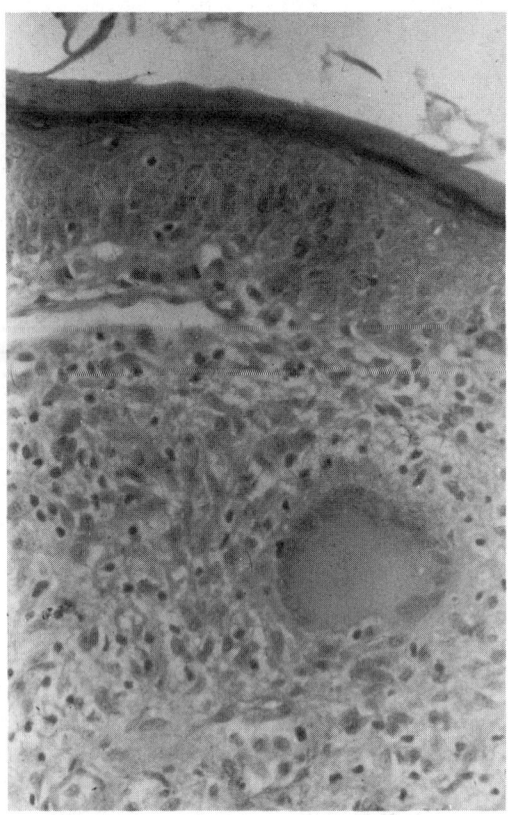

**FIGURE 2.** *Tuberculoid leprosy granuloma, consisting mainly of epithelioid cells, some lymphocytes, and a giant cell. It extends up to the epidermis.*

ing of round cells around nerves, blood vessels, and glands. These may be mistaken for a chronic nonspecific dermatitis unless leprosy is suspected and an acid-fast stain is done to demonstrate bacilli, particularly in the dermal nerves, which may have an associated infiltrate. The mycobacteria may be difficult to find because of their small numbers.

Tuberculoid leprosy is characterized by epithelioid cell granulomas containing occasional giant cells and surrounded by lymphocytes (Fig. 2). The infiltrate extends up to the epidermis and sometimes invades the basal epithelium. Nerve involvement is pathognomonic of leprosy, and in tuberculoid disease, nerve bundles are invaded and destroyed, often to the point of being unidentifiable. Bacilli are most likely to be found in the nerves but only with extreme difficulty.

The cutaneous infiltrate in lepromatous leprosy initially consists of macrophages that proliferate around dermal appendages, nerves, and blood vessels. This infiltrate gradually increases and may eventually replace much of the dermis, always, however, separated from the epidermis by a clear zone (Fig. 3). *M. leprae* organisms are found in macrophages, and their numbers steadily increase, gradually replacing the cytoplasm,

which becomes vacuolated with accumulated lipid forming foam cells. Although the infiltrate is apparent around the nerves, intraneural invasion by macrophages is seldom significant until late in advanced cases. Numerous bacilli may be seen within the nerves, however, particularly within Schwann cells. Edema and pressure from these cells filled with bacilli probably account for the gradual diminution of neural function seen in lepromatous leprosy. The gradual loss of nerve function is to be contrasted with the rapid destruction of nerves by the intense cellular infiltrates of tuberculoid leprosy and many borderline cases.

The lesions of borderline leprosy present a very mixed picture. In general, in BT leprosy the infiltrate is composed of lymphocytes, epithelioid, and giant cells as in TT disease. A clear zone may be found; however, nerves tend to be more readily identifiable, and acid-fast bacilli (AFB) are easier to find. As the disease moves toward BL, the infiltrate is composed mostly of macrophages, the clear zone becomes more prominent, bacilli steadily increase in numbers, and the infiltration of nerves becomes mostly perineural rather than intraneural. Lymphocytes are plentiful but nearly disappear as the LL end of the spectrum is reached.

## CLINICAL MANIFESTATIONS AND DIAGNOSIS

A diagnosis of leprosy should always be considered in a patient with skin lesions and sensory loss. The ideal examination would include routine laboratory studies, a G-6-PD screening test plus skin scrapings, a biopsy, examination of the eyes, a test of motor strength in the hands and feet, palpation of peripheral nerves, a sensory examination, inspection of the skin to determine the extent and type of lesions, and, in certain instances, a lepromin test.

Smears are taken by scraping the edge of small skin slits and smearing the material obtained on a microscopic slide. Since the bacillus grows best in cooler regions of the body, we routinely scrape the earlobes, elbows, and knees in addition to select lesions in newly diagnosed borderline and lepromatous patients.

A biopsy specimen should be taken entirely from within the margin of the chosen lesion. Separate sections of it are then stained for routine histopathology and AFB. The skin scrapings are also stained for AFB, and the numbers of bacilli in biopsy sections and scrapings are counted by using a semilogarithmic scale called the bacteriologic index (BI). See Figure 4. Typically, the BI on scrapings and biopsy will be 0 to 1+ in indeter-

1381

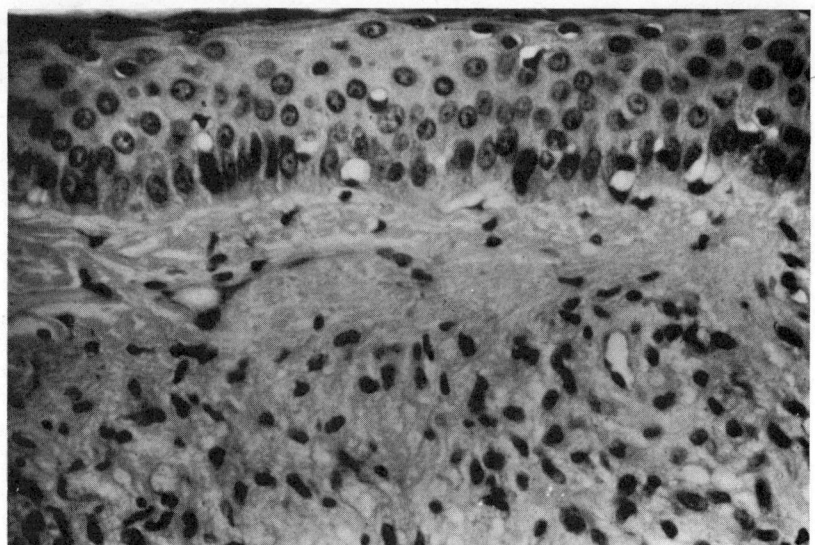

**FIGURE 3.** *Lepromatous leprosy with infiltrate consisting of macrophages, many having foamy cytoplasms. It is separated from the epidermis by a clear zone (zone of Grenz).*

minate and tuberculoid disease, 1 to 4+ in borderline disease, and 4 to 6+ in lepromatous cases. The morphologic index (MI) is also determined. This is the percentage of bacilli that appears normal in size, shape, and uniformity of staining (1 to 5 per cent in a typical newly diagnosed case). The figure is correlated to some extent with viability in that, when the MI becomes 0, the bacilli cannot be routinely grown in the mouse footpad, and the disease is no longer considered communicable.

The eyes are tested for lagophthalmus, visual acuity, circumcorneal hyperemia, tear production, corneal sensation, pupillary shape, and response to light.

Motor strength should be examined in the face, hands, and feet. The face is inspected for seventh nerve paralysis. In the hand, complete ulnar nerve paralysis will result in a partial claw-hand deformity, flattening of the hypothenar eminence and thenar web space, and wasting of the interosseous muscles. Lesser involvement will cause only weakness in the ulnar innervated muscles. The median nerve may be affected but only with or after the ulnar nerve. This combined paralysis leads to the classic complete claw-hand deformity. The radial nerve may be involved rarely, producing a wrist-drop. In the lower extremities clawtoe (posterior tibial nerve) and foot-drop (common peroneal nerve) deformities may be seen. The ulnar, median, superficial radial cutaneous, great auricular, and common peroneal nerves should be palpated for evidence of enlargement and/or tenderness.

Sensory loss will involve light touch, pain, and temperature. In general, in tuberculoid leprosy sensory loss will be confined to the lesion or lesions and in borderline disease it may be found in and around the lesions or in the lepromatous

pattern — i.e., in the distal extremities — or any combination in between. Sensory loss in the lepromatous case may advance to nearly total body anesthesia, sparing only the warmer regions such as the axillae, groin, and midline of the back. The ability to sweat is lost in insensitive areas owing to damage to autonomic fibers and destruction of sweat glands, and this often leads to severe dryness.

The lepromin test is a useful measure of immune status toward *M. leprae,* but it is not a diagnostic test. The Mitsuda-type lepromin contains $160 \times 10^6$ heat-killed *M. leprae* per ml, and 0.1 ml of this suspension is injected intradermally. A positive result consists of a tuberculin-like response (Fernandez reaction) at 48 hours and/or a nodular, occasionally ulcerated response (Mitsuda reaction) at 21 days. The test is invari-

BI

| | |
|---|---|
| 0 | NO BACILLI IN 100 OIF* |
| 1+ | 1-10 BACILLI PER 100 OIF |
| 2+ | 1-10 BACILLI PER 10 OIF |
| 3+ | 1-10 BACILLI PER OIF |
| 4+ | 10-100 BACILLI PER OIF |
| 5+ | 100-1000 BACILLI PER OIF |
| 6+ | OVER 1000 BACILLI PER OIF |

(*OIL IMMERSION FIELDS)

**FIGURE 4.** *The bacteriologic index (BI).*

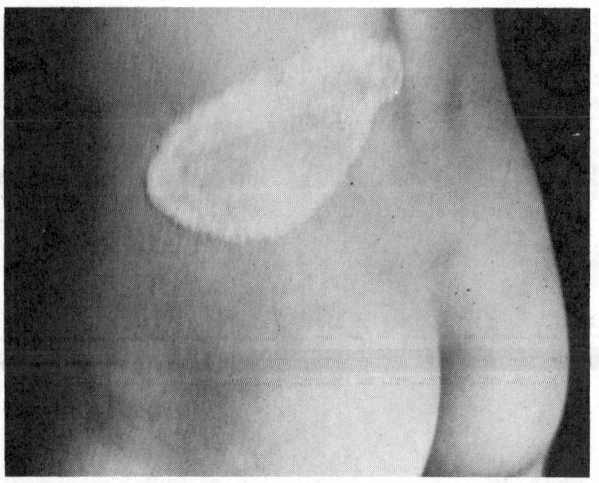

**FIGURE 5.** *Tuberculoid leprosy (TT). A large solitary lesion with a sharply demarcated raised margin and a scaly hypopigmented surface.*

ably positive in TT and BT cases, negative in BL and LL cases, and may be positive or negative in indeterminate, BB cases and the general population depending upon their ability to generate a delayed hypersensitivity response to *M. leprae.*

The skin manifestations of leprosy are remarkably varied, sometimes resembling those seen in many other skin diseases. In the section that follows the usual manifestations of the various types are described, but variations occur.

### Indeterminate Leprosy

This usually presents as a hypopigmented macule that may have slight erythema. It appears most commonly on the face, extremities, or buttocks, and more than one lesion may be present. Sensation is usually normal or only mildly dimin-

ished. The lesion appears insignificant and is most often detected during contact examinations or leprosy case-finding surveys. Diagnosis can be confirmed only by biopsy.

### Tuberculoid Leprosy

There is usually only one or at most a very few lesions with well-defined margins that vary in size from a few to 30 or more centimeters. They are hypopigmented and may be purely macular, macular with an irregularly or uniformly raised edge, or occasionally plaque-like (Fig. 5). The surface is usually scaly and sensation is absent. Only cutaneous or peripheral nerves in the area are usually enlarged and tender.

### Lepromatous Leprosy

This form of disease is usually generalized at the time of diagnosis, but occasionally patients are seen so early that only a few lesions are present. It may present in several different ways. Disseminated faint erythematous macules with vague margins may occur; if allowed to progress, they tend to increase in number, enlarge, coalesce, and become plaque-like. Second, this disease may present with generalized papular and nodular lesions (Fig. 6), and third, it may present as diffuse disease with no distinct lesions, although the skin may have a slight generalized erythema and a somewhat glossy appearance. Here as in all lepromatous cases, complete or partial loss of eyebrows and eyelashes (lateral portions) and diminished body hair may be seen. Where the infiltration becomes more pronounced, as on the face, corrugation may develop, leading to the classic leonine facies (Fig. 7). Finally, a mixed picture may occur. Another variation, referred to as the histoid variety, is most commonly

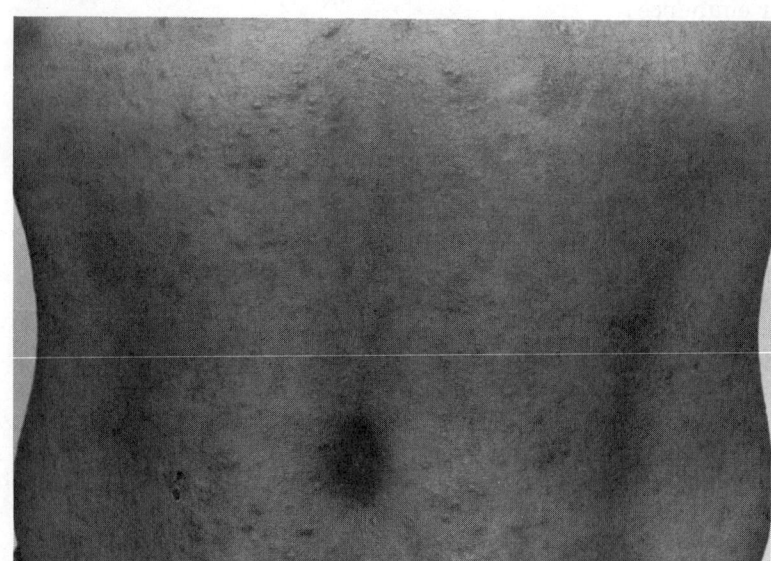

**FIGURE 6.** *Lepromatous leprosy (LL). Advanced disease with multiple papules and nodules symmetrically distributed.*

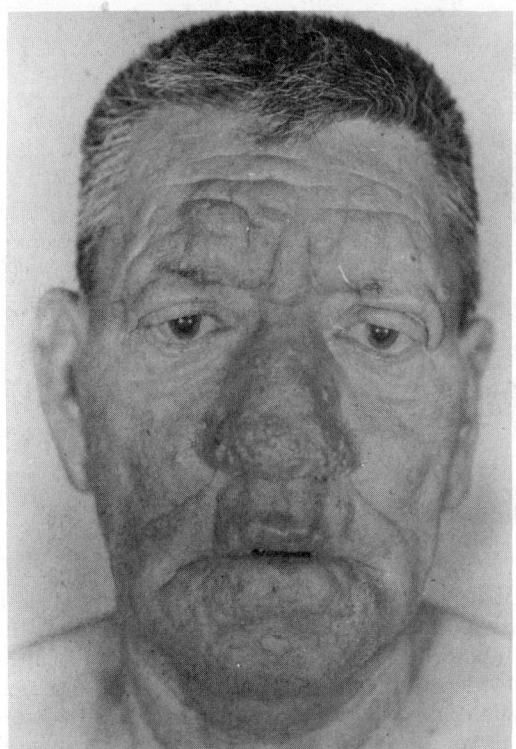

**FIGURE 7.** *Lepromatous leprosy (LL). An early leonine facies with diffuse infiltration, particularly of the nose. Note the loss of eyelashes and lateral eyebrows.*

seen in relapsed cases and presents as multiple, firm, waxy nodules. Other findings in lepromatous cases include the following:

1. There may be varying degrees of motor loss.
2. Heavy infiltration of the upper respiratory tract may cause nasal stuffiness, epistaxis, and voice changes. The nasal lesions may destroy the cartilage and bone, produce a septal perforation, and then result in collapse of the nose.
3. Small lepromatous nodules may be seen in the conjunctiva, sclera, and episclera, particularly at the corneal-scleral junction, and there may be beading of the corneal nerves. Lagophthalmos from facial nerve paralysis may cause exposure keratitis.
4. In theory, *M. leprae* organisms may be found anywhere in the body outside of the central nervous system, but only the following areas are of interest or significance clinically:
   a. A granulomatous infiltrate and multiple bacilli may be found in the liver, spleen, lymph nodes, and testes. No alteration of function is usually seen except in the testes, which may be destroyed or atrophied by the process. Gynecomastia often accompanies testicular atrophy, but a direct causal relationship has not been established.

   b. The small bones of the hands and feet occasionally contain lepromatous granulomas that may appear cystic on radiographs.
   c. *M. leprae* bacteremia is common.
5. A false-positive serologic result (VDRL) is frequently observed. The FTA will be negative, however.

### Borderline Leprosy

Borderline disease occupies most of the leprosy spectrum from localized disease with large lesions on one end to generalized disease with small lesions on the other, with all possible gradations and mixtures between. In BT disease the lesions vary in size but tend to be large. They may be macules, plaques, or annular (Fig. 8) with diminished sensation in and around many of them and sometimes small satellite lesions nearby. BB disease shows a similar picture but has more (although smaller) lesions, a higher BI, and a mixed tuberculoid-lepromatous sensory picture (Fig. 9). At the BL region, we usually find extensive disease with small lesions, a high BI, and a mostly lepromatous-type sensory loss (Fig. 10). Some borderline lesions may have indented or depressed hypopigmented centers, giving them a "punched out" appearance. Nerve involvement tends to be extensive and severe in borderline cases, and paralysis is frequent, particularly with reactive episodes. In some geographic areas, particularly India, cases are occasionally seen in which the disease in fact appears to involve only the nerves, and these are referred to as polyneuritic or pure neuritic leprosy.

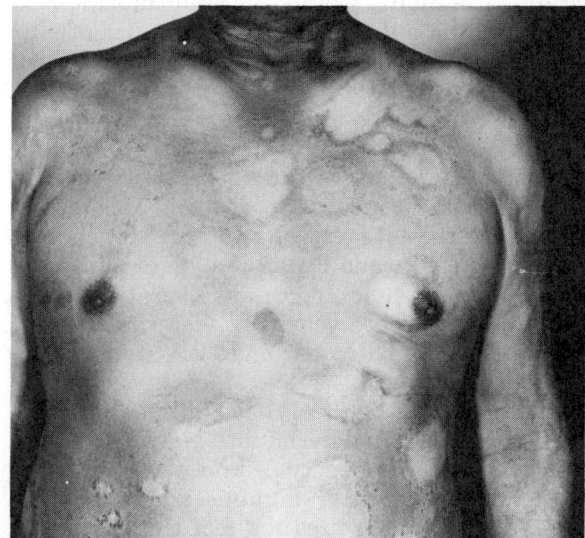

**FIGURE 8.** *Borderline tuberculoid leprosy (BT). Multiple, scaly hypopigmented lesions with sharp raised margins and a bacteriologic index of 0 to 1+.*

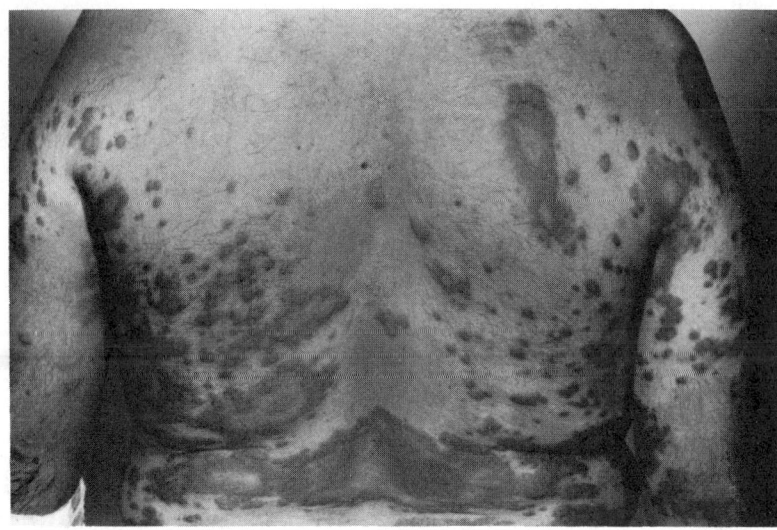

**FIGURE 9.** *Borderline leprosy (BB). The disease in this case is downgrading toward borderline lepromatous leprosy (BL), and the lesions vary from small nodules to large plaques. Note the "punched out" centers on many lesions. The bacteriologic index is 3 to 4+.*

## TREATMENT

Successful treatment requires patient education and rehabilitation as well as antibacterial therapy. The patient must understand his disease, the reasons for his treatment (to help him *and* prevent transmission of the infection), and the fact that he may temporarily feel worse (reactions) with treatment. The importance of never interrupting medications must be emphasized if the development of sulfone-resistant disease is to be minimized.

The treatment of choice is dapsone given in a dose of 50 mg daily to adult indeterminate and tuberculoid cases, and 100 mg daily to adult borderline and lepromatous cases. Response to treatment is evidenced by a fall in the MI on scrapings or biopsy to a classification of 0 in about three months and the gradual clearance of skin lesions. Therapy is continued for various periods after the patient's disease has become inactive. Inactivity is defined as at least one year of negative skin scrapings and biopsies (BI = 0) and no clinical evidence of activity. Inactivity will be attained within one to two years in tuberculoid and indeterminate cases; two to six years in borderline cases; and five to ten years in over 90 per cent of BL and LL cases. Therapy is then continued two more years in indeterminate and TT cases, five in BT cases, ten in BB cases, and for life in all BL and LL cases. Many investigators, including the author, feel that lifetime therapy is also indicated in indeterminate and BB patients who are lepromin-negative. Lifetime therapy in those with a defective immune response to *M. leprae* merely recognizes the fact that, although the BI on scrapings and biopsy may be 0, this is a relatively imprecise test and large numbers of bacilli still remain in the tissues. Some of these bacilli are viable, as has been demonstrated in studies in which persistent viable organisms have been sought (Waters et al., 1974). The failure of some lepromatous patients to attain inactive status is due to irregular intake of medication or the development of sulfone-resistant strains of *M. leprae*. Irregular or low-dose dapsone intake

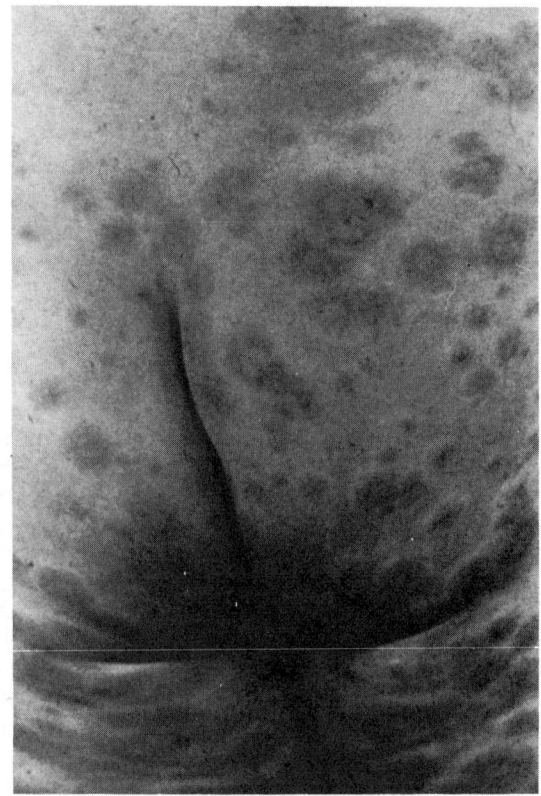

**FIGURE 10.** *Borderline lepromatous leprosy (BL). Multiple small plaques, papules, and nodules symmetrically distributed. The bacteriologic index is 4 to 5 +.*

favors development of resistant strains, which occurs step-wise after prolonged treatment (an average of 17 years in Carville's series). Drug sensitivity testing is done in mouse footpads and has demonstrated that in the United States and elsewhere primary sulfone-resistant cases may now be occurring, i.e., newly diagnosed cases in which bacilli show evidence of sulfone resistance without prior sulfone therapy. Sulfone resistance may also be demonstrated clinically by observing progression of the patient's disease in spite of a known adequate sulfone intake over a period of three to six months. Serious side effects from dapsone therapy are uncommon. Occasionally hemolytic anemias occur, particularly in G-6-PD-deficient patients, but these are usually mild and seldom require changing therapy.

Several other drugs are available for the treatment of leprosy.

1. Clofazimine (B663, Lamprene) is the treatment of choice for sulfone-resistant disease in a dose of 100 mg daily. Higher doses are anti-inflammatory and useful for the treatment of reaction. The major side effect is an uneven reddish-tan to black pigmentation of the skin that diminishes as the disease approaches negativity and clears completely if the drug is discontinued. It also is deposited in the wall of the small bowel, and doses of over 100 mg daily may produce pain and diarrhea or decreased motility with obstructive symptoms. Decreasing the dose or temporarily discontinuing the drug usually eliminates the problem.
2. Rifampin is bactericidal, but since resistance may develop within three to four years if it is given alone, it should always be used with another drug. The usual dose is 600 mg daily. A flu-like syndrome, hepatotoxicity, thrombocytopenia, and renal failure may occur as side effects, particularly if the drug is taken irregularly.
3. Ethionamide. The usual dose is 500 to 750 mg daily, and hepatotoxicity is the major side effect.
4. Prothionamide. The dose is 5 mg/kg in combination regimens.
5. Thiambutosine is given in a dose of 500 mg three times daily.
6. Thiacetazone is given in a dose of 150 mg daily.
7. Streptomycin is given in amounts of 1 g three times weekly intramuscularly. Discontinue if eighth nerve toxicity develops. Resistant strains of *M. leprae* may develop within a few years if drugs 3 to 7 are given alone. They are all, therefore, useful only in combination regimens.
8. DADDS is the diacetyl derivative of dapsone. The dose (225 mg intramuscularly every 77 days) provides extremely low blood levels of dapsone. Its use as sole therapy of multibacillary (BB, BL, and LL) disease might thus promote the development of sulfone-resistant strains, and it is therefore contraindicated. Whether it has a place as a prophylactic measure in family contacts, for the treatment of paucibacillary (indeterminate, TT, and BT) disease, or in combination regimens for multibacillary disease is under investigation.

The Fifth World Health Organization (WHO) Expert Committee on Leprosy (WHO, 1977) has recommended that combination drug therapy be given as the initial treatment for all multibacillary cases. In theory, by analogy with tuberculosis this is a sound approach and might reduce the incidence of sulfone-resistant disease or shorten the treatment period from life to a matter of years. However, there is no proof that combinations are superior to dapsone alone, nor do we know the best combinations or how long they should be given. Present recommendations call for dapsone with rifampin for at least two weeks or clofazimine for six months, followed by dapsone monotherapy.

Attempts to correct the specific CMI defect through administration of transfer factor have shown promise, but immunotherapy remains experimental (Hastings, 1977).

## COMPLICATIONS AND SEQUELAE

### Reactions

Reactions occur in about 50 per cent of leprosy patients and probably produce most of the deformities in this disease. There are basically two types:

1. *Reversal reactions* represent a delayed-type hypersensitivity response to *M. leprae* antigens. As the term implies, a change or "reversal" has apparently occurred in the individual's responsiveness to these antigens. They may occur in borderline and tuberculoid cases, usually those receiving treatment. The clinical findings are fever, neuritis, edema and erythema of pre-existing lesions (which may ulcerate), new lesions, adenopathy, and a high white blood count. Any reaction that carries a danger of a significant motor or sensory deficit or skin ulceration must be treated daily with 60 to 100 mg of prednisone or an equivalent dose of another corticosteroid. Steroids will usually control the reaction and reverse nerve damage within 24 to 48 hours if they are given early enough. Patients with a low BI (0 to 1+) may need only brief therapy, but

multibacillary patients may require months or even years of treatment. These chronic reactions should be managed by alternate day steroids to minimize side effects. As an alternative, clofazimine in a dose of 200 to 300 mg daily may control the reaction and allow the steroids to be discontinued over a period of 2 to 12 months. Care should be taken to avoid small bowel toxicity, however. Dapsone should be continued without interruption, since stopping it has no immediate effect on the reaction.

2. *Erythema nodosum leprosum* (ENL) usually occurs and is more severe in BL and LL cases under treatment but may occur in untreated patients. It seems to be the result of Arthus reactions (immune complex deposition in vessels) at multiple sites. Erythematous, often painful, nodules develop in large crops within a matter of hours. Less commonly, the lesions may be pustular, necrotic, erythema multiforme-like, or hemorrhagic. All but the mildest episodes are febrile. Neuritis, malaise, arthralgias, leukocytosis, iridocyclitis, lymphadenitis, periostitis (particularly pretibial), orchitis, and nephritis may also occur. The nephritis may be an immune complex type, and a nephrotic syndrome may occur. Stress may bring on an episode, but the precipitating cause is usually unknown. Dapsone is continued and the reaction is suppressed by thalidomide, the treatment of choice, in a dose of 100 mg four times daily. This dose usually controls the reaction within 48 hours, and it can then be tapered to a maintenance level of about 100 mg daily, which may have to be continued for years in some cases. If acute neuritis is present, corticosteroids should be used. Although very effective, their prolonged use for the treatment of ENL itself often results in serious steroid side effects even if they are given on alternate days. Thus, in fertile women in whom thalidomide is contraindicated because of its teratogenicity and in cases where thalidomide is not effective or available, clofazimine should be used as in reversal reactions. Antimonials and chloroquine are also effective in some cases, but thalidomide and clofazimine are preferred. Mild cases of ENL may require only aspirin and rest.

In Mexico and some other areas patients with diffuse lepromatous leprosy may develop a reaction called the Lucio phenomenon. Many punched-out skin ulcers develop, and patients frequently die of septic complications. High doses of corticosteroids usually control the Lucio phenomenon, but they may need to be continued for years.

### Neuritis

This complication usually occurs during reactions but may occur without other signs of reaction. The nerve is usually enlarged and tender and its function may be lost. Early high-dose corticosteroid therapy is necessary to save it. Resting it by use of a sling or splinting may also help. Surgical intervention, e.g., neurolysis or drainage of the nerve abscesses as sometimes seen in tuberculoid cases, is occasionally necessary.

### Eye Problems

Iridocyclitis is heralded by photophobia and blurring of vision. It is a medical emergency! Atropine and corticosteroids must be dropped in the eye at once to avoid permanent damage. Glaucoma may eventually occur in these cases. Lagophthalmos and decreased lacrimation are treated with a tear substitute to avoid development of an exposure keratitis.

### Injuries

Most patients have varying degrees of permanent sensory and/or motor impairment. They must be taught to use their eyes as a substitute for other sensations and to rely on protective measures such as gloves and special footwear. When injuries occur, they must be protected from trauma while healing occurs, e.g., by resting a foot with a plantar ulcer or by using a total skin-contact walking cast. Repeated trauma and infection may lead to absorption of bones in hands and feet. Proper management of these problems is essential for the success of any leprosy control program, or the patient may feel that treatment has failed and abandon it.

### Orchitis

This may accompany a reactive episode or occur independently. A short tapered course of corticosteroids will usually control the problem, but sterility may ultimately result.

### Renal Disease

Renal amyloidosis or glomerulonephritis is a complication of long-standing active leprosy or a chronic reaction. The patients usually progress to renal failure unless the underlying process is controlled.

## GEOGRAPHIC VARIATIONS IN DISEASE

Leprosy today is mostly a disease of tropical and semitropical areas and occurs mainly in the underdeveloped nations. The incidence of the disease varies markedly between countries and within a given country, and in the proportions of indeterminate, tuberculoid, borderline, and lepromatous cases. The reasons for this variation are unknown.

### CONTROL AND PROPHYLAXIS

First, the prevalence and incidence rates should be determined for each type of leprosy and case-detection surveys should be repeated at regular intervals. Outpatient treatment and close follow-up should be provided for all cases, and programs for health education should be established. Household contacts of lepromatous patients are at greatest risk, but most new cases will be detected outside the household.

The value of prophylaxis remains uncertain, and it can never be used as a substitute for active case-finding programs. Trials of BCG vaccination have shown marked variation in the degree of protection afforded. One can conclude only that BCG might be useful in areas with a high prevalence rate for tuberculoid leprosy. A specific antileprosy vaccine is under development but is many years away from regular use. Chemoprophylaxis with dapsone is plagued by administrative and medical uncertainties. For this reason, the Fifth Report by the WHO Expert Committee on Leprosy does not recommend it for large-scale control programs. Nonetheless, many workers feel that it is indicated for household contacts.

### References

Godal, T.: Growing points in leprosy research. 3. Immunological detection of sub-clinical infection in leprosy. Lepr Rev 45:22, 1974.

Hastings, R. C.: Transfer factor as a probe of the immune defect in lepromatous leprosy. Int J Lepr 45:281, 1977.

Kirchheimer, W. F., and Storrs, E. E.: Attempts to establish the armadillo (*Dasypus Novemcinctus* Linn.) as a model for the study of leprosy. I. Report of lepromatoid leprosy in an experimentally infected armadillo. Int J Lepr 39:693, 1971.

Navayanane, E. S., Kirchheimer, W. B., and Bedi, M. B. S.: Transfer of leprosy bacilli from patients to mouse footpads by *Aedes aegypti*. Lepr India 48:181, 1977.

Ridley, D. S., and Jopling, W. H.: Classification of leprosy according to immunity. A five-group system. Int J Lepr 34:255, 1966.

Shepard, C. C.: The experimental disease that follows the injection of human leprosy bacilli into footpads of mice. J Exp Med 112:445, 1960.

Waters, M. F. R., Reese, R. J. W., McDougall, A. C., and Weddell, A. G. M.: Ten years of dapsone in lepromatous leprosy: Clinical, bacteriological, and histological assessment and the finding of viable leprosy bacilli. Lepr Rev 45:288, 1974.

World Health Organization, Expert Committee on Leprosy: Fifth Report. WHO Technical Report Series No. 607. Geneva, World Health Organization, 1977.

# F VASCULAR AND HEMATOLOGIC INFECTIONS

## GRAM-NEGATIVE **177** BACTEREMIA

### William R. McCabe, M.D.

Gram-negative bacilli have assumed the paramount role in producing nosocomial infections over the past few decades. Although these organisms have become increasingly prevalent causes of hospital-acquired pulmonary, wound, and urinary tract infections, bacteremia caused by Enterobacteriaceae and Pseudomonadaceae provides the most definitive and striking example of the increasing frequency of gram-negative bacillary infections. Bacteremia caused by coliform bacilli was originally recognized shortly after the turn of the century but was considered a clinical rarity until the 1950's. Since this time, however, a progressive increase, as great as 20-fold in some hospitals, in the frequency of gram-negative bacteremia has been documented by McCabe and Jackson, 1962a; Dupont and Spink, 1969; McCabe, 1974; Young et al., 1977. The frequency of occurrence of gram-negative bacteremia currently exceeds a rate of 1 per 100 hospital admissions in many major medical centers in the United States. Estimates of the frequency of gram-negative bacteremia in the United States range from 71,000 to 300,000 episodes annually.

### DEFINITION

The term *bacteremia* indicates the presence of bacteria in the blood and, although the diagnosis may be suspected on clinical grounds, it can be confirmed only by culture of the blood. The term *septicemia* is often used interchangeably and implies the occurrence of "toxemia" and other ill-defined clinical manifestations in addition to bacteremia. Since clinical features may vary considerably depending on the duration of infection and other factors, the diagnosis of septicemia is largely dependent on subjective interpretation. Bacteremia is a more precise term that is preferable for clinical use. In some instances, bacteremia may be transient and associated with minimal clinical symptoms, but most patients with gram-negative bacteremia are acutely and severely ill.

## ETIOLOGY

Although almost all gram-negative bacteria may produce bacteremia, the term *gram-negative bacteremia* is usually reserved for bacteremias produced by members of the families Enterobacteriaceae and Pseudomonadaceae. Bacteremias caused by other gram-negative bacteria (such as meningococci, gonococci, *Brucella, Salmonella typhosa,* and *Haemophilus influenzae)* may be associated with similar clinical manifestations but are usually considered as discrete clinical entities rather than under the general term of gram-negative bacteremia.

The most frequent causative agents of gram-negative bacteremia observed in 612 patients in a Boston hospital are shown in Table 1, with *Escherichia coli* accounting for slightly more than one third of cases, and *Klebsiella pneumoniae, Pseudomonas aeruginosa,* and species of *Proteus* and *Bacteroides* following in this order. A variety of other genera of gram-negative bacilli, such as *Serratia, Acinetobacter, Providencia,* and *Flavobacter,* also are responsible for occasional instances of bacteremia, but the total number of cases caused by these less frequent species constitutes only about 10 per cent of cases of bacteremia. Mixed or polymicrobic bacteremias, in which more than one species of gram-negative

bacilli or cocci and gram-negative bacilli are isolated, occur in approximately 15 per cent of cases.

Some variation in the relative frequency of etiologic agents may occur in individual hospitals. A higher incidence of bacteremia with *Bacteroides* and other anaerobic gram-negative bacilli would be anticipated in hospitals with a large volume of abdominal and gynecologic surgery of large numbers of patients with abdominal trauma. Similarly, a higher proportion of bacteremias from *P. aeruginosa* occurs in hospitals with large numbers of patients with burns or hematologic malignancies. Outbreaks of nosocomial bacteremias caused by gentamicin-resistant *K. pneumoniae, P. aeruginosa, P. rettgerii,* and *Serratia marcescens* have also been reported in a number of hospitals.

Other factors (such as site of local infection or source of bacteremia, prior antibiotic therapy, and whether the infection is nosocomial or community-acquired) also may determine the most likely etiologic agent of bacteremia. Table 2 lists the most frequent sites of origin of gram-negative bacteremia, factors predisposing to bacteremia, and the species most often causing bacteremia originating from these sites. Generally, bacteria that comprise the major constituents of the bacterial flora of the gastrointestinal tract are the most frequent causes of bacteremia originating from the genitourinary, gastrointestinal, or female genital tract. *E. coli* is the most frequent etiologic agent in bacteremia originating from the genitourinary tract, with *Klebsiella* and *Enterobacter, Proteus,* and *Pseudomonas* being much less frequent and tending to occur only in patients with obstruction, repeated urinary infections, or protracted indwelling catheterization. Anaerobic bacilli, such as *Bacteroides,* are more frequent as the etiologic agent when the bowel or the female genital tract is the source of bacteremia.

In contrast, when bacteremia originates from unidentifiable sites, from tracheostomies or the use of ventilatory equipment, intravascular foreign bodies, or the skin, a different group of gram-negative bacilli is more prevalent. Bacteria such as *P. aeruginosa, Acinetobacter,* and *Serratia,* which are often found in dust, water, or on the human skin, become relatively more frequent.

## PATHOGENESIS AND PATHOLOGY

Gram-negative bacilli usually enter the blood from extravascular foci but also may originate from intravascular foci such as intravascular catheters, septic thrombophlebitis, or, more rarely, bacterial endarteritis, endocarditis, mycotic aneurysms, or infected vascular grafts. The latter

**TABLE 1.    Etiologic Agents in Gram-Negative Bacteria**

| ETIOLOGIC AGENT | RELATIVE FREQUENCY (PER CENT) |
|---|---|
| E. coli | 35 |
| Klebsiella-Enterobacter-Serratia sp | 27 |
| (Klebsiella, 16%; Enterobacter, 9%; | |
| Serratia, 2%) | |
| P. aeruginosa | 12 |
| Proteus sp | 11 |
| Bacteroides sp | 8 |
| Other gram-negative bacilli | 7 |
| (Acinetobacter, Alcaligenes, Hafnia, | |
| Providencia, Achromobacter, Flavobacter, etc.) | |

More than one species of gram-negative bacilli or gram-negative bacilli and gram-positive cocci are isolated from blood cultures from approximately 16 per cent of patients with gram-negative bacteremia.

types of infection usually result from localization from prior bacteremic episodes or from direct invasion of large blood vessels from areas of adjacent infection. Most often, gram-negative bacilli gain access to the blood from extravascular septic foci by passage through the lymphatics or by direct invasion of small blood vessels within a local area of infection.

Factors involved in the increasing incidence of gram-negative bacteremia are more a reflection of the population affected and changing medical practices than of the virulence of gram-negative bacilli. Several factors appear to be implicated in the continuing increase in frequency of bacteremia:

### Bacterial Characteristics

Despite the relatively limited capacity to produce invasive infection, other properties of gram-

negative bacilli make them ideal for the production of opportunistic infections. Gram-negative bacilli are ubiquitous in their distribution. Some are major components of the fecal flora, others occur as normal inhabitants of the skin, and gram-negative bacilli are also found in large numbers within the hospital environment. In addition, gram-negative bacilli are relatively resistant to moisture, drying, and some disinfectants; and some are able to persist and multiply in water. Equally important is the proclivity among gram-negative bacilli for the development of antibiotic resistance, which is much greater than that observed with gram-positive bacteria. Resistance is mediated by self-replicating, extrachromosomal genetic material termed *plasmids*. These plasmids are composed of two components: the resistance transfer factor (RTF), which is responsible for the transfer of resistance from one bac-

**TABLE 2. Factors Influencing Etiologic Agents in Bacteremia**

| SITE OF ORIGIN | PRECIPITATING EVENTS | MOST FREQUENT ETIOLOGIC AGENTS |
|---|---|---|
| Genitourinary tract | Indwelling catheters<br>Instrumentation<br>Obstruction | *E. coli*<br>*Klebsiella-*<br>    *Enterobacter-Serratia*<br>*Proteus* sp<br>*P. aeruginosa* |
| Gastrointestinal tract<br>Bowel | Obstruction<br>Perforation<br>Abscesses<br>Neoplasia<br>Diverticuli | *Bacteroides* sp<br>*E. coli*<br>*Klebsiella-*<br>    *Enterobacter-Serratia*<br>*Salmonella* |
| Biliary tract | Cholangitis<br>Obstruction (stones)<br>Surgical procedures | *E. coli*<br>*Klebsiella-*<br>    *Enterobacter-Serratia* |
| Reproductive system | Abortion<br>Instrumentation<br>Postpartum | *Bacteroides* sp<br>*E. coli* |
| Vascular system | Venous cutdowns<br>Intravenous catheters<br>Intracardiac pacemakers<br>Surgical procedures | *P. aeruginosa*<br>*Acinetobacter* sp<br>*Serratia*<br>*Erwinia*<br>*E. cloacae* |
| Skin | Leukemia<br>Agranulocytosis<br>Immunosuppressive and cancer<br>  chemotherapeutic agents | *P. aeruginosa*<br>*Acinetobacter* sp<br>*Serratia* |
| Respiratory tract | Tracheostomy<br>Mechanical ventilatory assistance | *P. aeruginosa*<br>*Klebsiella-*<br>    *Enterobacter-Serratia*<br>*Acinetobacter* sp<br>*E. coli* |
| | Aspiration | *E. coli*<br>*Bacteroides* sp<br>*Klebsiella-*<br>    *Enterobacter-Serratia* |

terium to another, is linked to resistance determinants (RD), which provide the genetic information required to enable recipient bacteria to perform the biochemical changes responsible for antibiotic resistance (Chapter 21). Transfer of RTF and RD occurs between bacteria of the same and different species. Although exposure to antibiotics per se does not induce antibiotic resistance, it does provide a selective reproductive advantage to bacteria that are resistant and enhances the development of a resistant hospital flora. For this reason, the frequency of antibiotic resistance among bacteria within a hospital tends to reflect the intensity of antibiotic usage.

## Susceptible Population

Striking changes in the characteristics of hospitalized patients have occurred over the past few decades. There has been a progressive increase in age of hospitalized patients and an increasing proportion of the hospital population is composed of patients with abnormal defense mechanisms who are most susceptible to infections with opportunistic pathogens such as gram-negative bacilli. The demonstration that the severity of the host's underlying disease is the major determinant of the outcome of gram-negative bacteremia further emphasizes the importance of the susceptible host in the pathogenesis of bacteremia (McCabe and Jackson, 1962a and b).

## Circumvention or Alteration of Host Defenses

Many procedures in hospitals, such as intravenous and bladder catheters and ventilatory assistance equipment, allow a direct means by which gram-negative bacilli may be introduced or gain access to body sites that are normally protected against bacterial ingress by host defense mechanisms. Increased likelihood of infection may result from prolonged operative procedures required by newer, more complex surgical techniques. In addition, commonly used therapeutic measures such as corticosteroids, cytotoxic agents, and irradiation therapy deleteriously affect host defense mechanisms and greatly enhance susceptibility to infection.

Thus, the modern hospital provides the optimal conditions for the occurrence of opportunistic infections (Myerowitz et al., 1971). The extensive use of antimicrobial agents results in the selection of a hospital flora composed largely of antibiotic-resistant gram-negative bacilli, while the patient population represents a concentration of patients most susceptible to infections with relatively avirulent microorganisms such as gram-negative bacilli. In addition, many therapeutic agents and procedures either deleteriously affect host defense mechanisms or provide mechanisms that circumvent normal defense mechanisms and allow access of bacteria into normally protected body sites. This combination of circumstances affords a ready explanation of the progressively increasing frequency of gram-negative bacillary infections.

The clinical features of bacteremia caused by various species of gram-negative bacteria are virtually identical regardless of the etiologic agent. In addition, intravenous administration of killed gram-negative bacteria or purified endotoxin extracted from the cell walls of gram-negative bacteria produces manifestations similar to those observed in bacteremia. This has led to the assumption that endotoxin, which is present in all gram-negative bacteria, is released during the course of infection and is the primary pathogenetic mechanism in bacteremia (Young et al., 1977). Despite the attractiveness of this concept, the actual role of endotoxin in the pathogenesis of the manifestations of gram-negative bacteremia is not clearly defined. Other studies have suggested that endotoxin per se may play a negligible role in the pathogenesis of the manifestations of certain bacteremias (McCabe, 1975).

A variety of substances (histamine, 5-hydroxytryptamine, glucocorticoids, lysosomal enzymes, epinephrine, and norepinephrine) have also been proposed as mediators of many of the clinical features observed in gram-negative bacteremia, but their actual importance in clinical infections has yet to be documented. More recent laboratory and clinical studies have indicated that concomitant activation of the coagulation, fibrinolytic, and complement systems, depicted in Figure 1, may be important in the development of the hemodynamic and hemostatic changes sometimes observed in gram-negative bacteremia. Gram-negative bacilli or their endotoxins can activate Hageman factor (Factor XII). This is followed by activation of the intrinsic clotting system and also the fibrinolytic system as a result of the conversion of plasminogen to plasmin. Concomitant activation of the coagulation and the fibrinolytic systems provides the circumstances required for the development of disseminated intravascular coagulation or consumptive coagulopathy occasionally seen in gram-negative bacteremia. The magnitude of activation of the complement system, primarily via the properdin C3-C9 pathway, has been shown to parallel the severity of bacteremia. Similarly, conversion of kallikreinogen ultimately to bradykinin, which increases vascular permeability and produces vascular dilatation, has been demonstrated to occur in gram-negative bacteremia. Thus, intravascular coagulation, fibrinolysis, and shock may result from activation of Hageman factor. These interrelated changes in the coagulation, fibrin-

Activation of Humoral Mediators by Gram-negative Bacteria

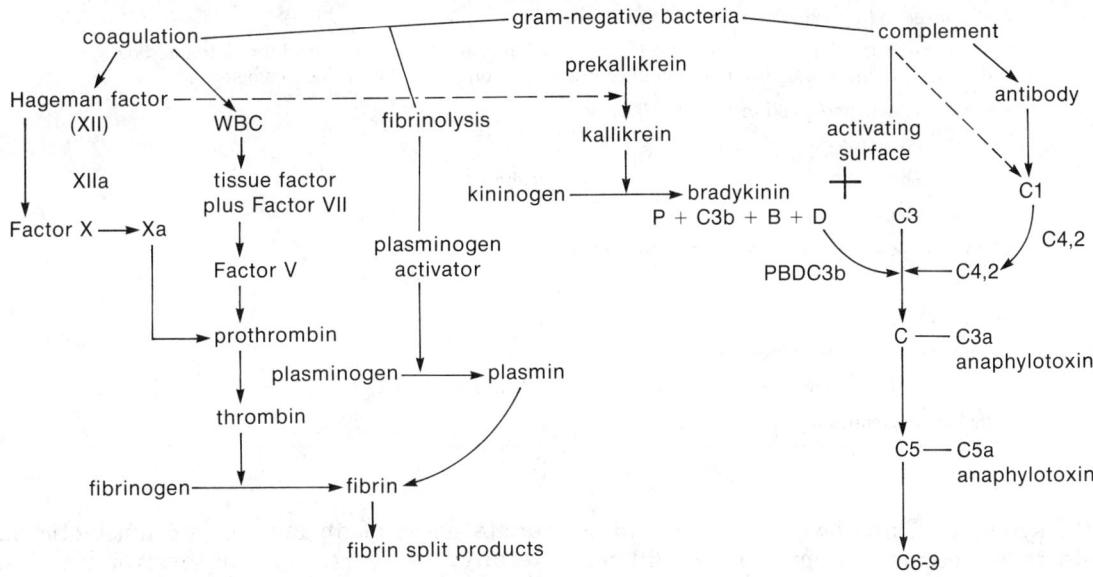

**FIGURE 1.** *In addition to its effects on the intrinsic clotting mechanism via Hageman factor, endotoxin stimulates the release of tissue factor from phagocytic leukocytes (WBC) and thereby activates the extrinsic clotting pathway. Both PMN and monocytes have been implicated as sources of procoagulant activity. In addition, macrophages are stimulated by endotoxin to release plasminogen activator. The complement system, as well as the clotting system, can also be activated as a result of gram-negative bacteremia, and there is evidence that the magnitude of activation parallels the severity of the bacteremia. Complement activation can be reproduced in vitro and in vivo by endotoxin. It appears that both the classic and the alternative complement pathways can be activated by endotoxin and by gram-negative bacteremia. Activation of complement generates the anaphylatoxins C3a and C5a, which increase vascular permeability. In additon, C3d is generated and causes the initial leukopenia that is characteristic of gram-negative bacteremia. Thus, activation of proenzymes by the bacteria or their endotoxins may cause intravascular coagulation, fibrinolysis, complement activation, and even shock.*

olytic, complement, and kinin systems as a result of contact with gram-negative bacilli or their products have been documented to occur in bacteremia and may be responsible for the pathophysiologic changes observed.

## CLINICAL MANIFESTATIONS

The diagnosis of bacteremia can be established with certainty only by isolation of the infecting organism from cultures of the blood. The rapid course and high fatality rate of bacteremia, however, often require the formulation of clinical diagnosis and initiation of treatment before the results of blood culture are known. Although there may be considerable case-to-case variation in the severity of the disease, the clinical signs of bacteremia produced by individual species of gram-negative bacilli are virtually identical. Thus, the clinical manifestations do not readily allow identification of the etiologic agent. In the typical case, shaking chills, high fever, prostration, and occasionally nausea and vomiting develop within one to two hours after manipulation, insertion, or removal of a bladder catheter or manipulation of an area of focal infection. Shock, or hypotension, usually appears within two to eight hours after the initial manifestations of

bacteremia. Regrettably, however, this typical sequence of events occurs in only 30 to 40 per cent of patients with gram-negative bacteremia, and the clinical manifestations are more subtle in the majority of patients. Table 3 lists some of the clinical manifestations that may be observed in gram-negative bacteremia. Fever is almost universal at the onset but may be minimal in uremics, the elderly, and patients receiving corticosteroids. The development of fever after genitourinary and gastrointestinal procedures, in patients with bladder or venous catheters, and in patients with leukemia or hematologic disorders, especially if associated with granulocytopenia, may be the only manifestation of bacteremia. Despite considerable variation in the magnitude of fever, higher fevers tend to occur in bacteremias caused by gram-negative bacilli than in those caused by gram-positive bacteria. Very rarely, hypothermia may be the presenting feature of bacteremia.

Hyperpnea, tachypnea, and respiratory alkalosis, in the absence of pulmonary abnormalities, may be the mode of presentation of bacteremia. Similarly, bacteremia may present as hypotension, anuria or oliguria, or acidosis without apparent cause. Clinical manifestations of bacteremia tend to be less flagrant in the elderly, and confusion, delirium or agitation, or stupor may be

**TABLE 3.   Clinical Features Suggestive of Gram-Negative Bacteremia**

| | |
|---|---|
| Chills, fever and hypotension | |
| Fever alone (particularly in patients with malignancies, hematologic, urinary tract, or gastrointestinal disorders, and following instrumentation or insertion of urinary or intravenous catheters) | |
| Hyperpnea, tachypnea, and respiratory alkalosis | |
| Oliguria and anuria | |
| Hypotension | Without |
| Thrombocytopenia | apparent |
| Change in mentation (agitation, confusion, stupor) | cause |
| Acidosis | |
| Hypothermia | |
| Evidence of urinary tract infection | |
| Evidence of pulmonary infection (associated with ventilatory assistance) | |
| Ecthyma gangrenosum | |

the initial symptom. Thrombocytopenia of mild to moderate degree occurs in approximately 60 per cent of patients and may suggest the diagnosis of bacteremia. In patients in whom bacteremia results from extension of previously localized pulmonary, genitourinary, and gastrointestinal infections, manifestations of the local infection may obscure those of bacteremia. As a result, bacteremia should always be considered a likely possibility in patients with severe pulmonary, genitourinary, and gastrointestinal infections.

Although it is generally not possible to identify the specific etiologic agent of bacteremia on the basis of clinical findings, there is one manifestation that may allow clinical identification of the specific etiologic agent. The appearance of tender, indurated, or ulcerative lesions with black, necrotic centers, ecthyma gangrenosum, or erythematous vesicles filled with cloudy fluid is almost diagnostic of bacteremia with *P. aeruginosa*, although there have been isolated reports of similar lesions in *Citrobacter* and *Aeromonas* bacteremia.

The above-described features, except for ecthyma gangrenosum, are not specific, but they should alert the physician to the possibility of bacteremia. Their occurrence should stimulate prompt collection of blood cultures and other appropriate specimens for culture and Gram stain.

## DIAGNOSIS AND TREATMENT

Optimal treatment of gram-negative bacteremia is based on (1) early recognition of bacteremia and its source; (2) identification of the etiologic agent and determination of its antimicrobial susceptibility; (3) administration of ade-

quate doses of an appropriate antibiotic parenterally; (4) correction of obstructive lesions, drainage of purulent accumulations, or removal of foreign bodies; and (5) prevention or treatment of complications.

Once the etiologic agent has been identified and its antimicrobial susceptibility determined, the treatment of bacteremia is not difficult. This is different from the usual clinical situation, however, when the physician is presented with an ill, febrile patient suspected of having bacteremia but in whom the etiologic agent and its antibiotic susceptibility are unknown. In these circumstances, two to three blood cultures should be obtained at intervals of no less than ten minutes. Appropriate specimens should also be collected from any possible site of infection, e.g., urine, sputum, purulent exudates, and intravenous catheters, for immediate Gram stain and culture. Total and differential leukocyte counts, urinalysis, and x-ray of the chest should also be included in the evaluation of patients with suspected bacteremia. Prior culture and sensitivity results that may have been obtained also may provide clues for the initiation of therapy.

Identification of the source of bacteremia can assist in estimation of the most likely etiologic agent and selection of appropriate antibiotic therapy. Those bacterial species that produce infections most often in specific organs or body sites also are the species most often found in bacteremias originating from infections at these sites. Table 2 lists the bacterial species most often isolated from blood cultures in instances of bacteremia originating from various organs. It is important to recognize that anaerobic bacteria, such as *Bacteroides* sp, are frequent causes of bacteremia originating from the gastrointestinal and female genital tracts since the antibiotic sensitivity of anaerobes varies markedly from that of aerobic gram-negative bacilli. Overall, *E. coli* is the most frequent cause of gram-negative bacteremia and is especially likely to be found in bacteremias originating from the urinary, gastrointestinal, and female reproductive systems. *Pseudomonas* is relatively more frequent in bacteremias occurring in leukemics and in patients with thermal injuries, and in infections secondary to intravascular catheters and tracheostomies.

Initial antibiotic therapy is selected on the basis of the most likely etiologic agent and its antimicrobial sensitivity pattern. Estimation of susceptibility to various antimicrobial agents should include consideration of whether the infection was hospital-acquired and a knowledge of the sensitivity patterns of bacteria indigenous to individual hospitals, since there may be considerable variation in antibiotic susceptibility patterns of gram-negative bacilli from hospital to hospital. In general, an agent is usually selected for initial therapy of suspected gram-negative bacteremia that provides the broadest spectrum of activity against the most likely causative gram-negative bacilli. Gentamicin, 1.5 mg/kg body weight every eight hours; tobramycin, 1.5 mg/kg body weight every eight hours; and amikacin, 5 mg/kg body weight every eight hours are the antimicrobials most frequently used for initial therapy of suspected gram-negative bacteremia in most centers because of the frequency of resistance to other antibiotics. After receipt of culture and antibiotic sensitivity results, it is preferable to change to a less toxic effective agent whenever possible. Clindamycin or chloramphenicol is usually administered simultaneously with one of the aminoglycosides when the concomitant presence of anaerobic gram-negative bacilli is suspected. Combined therapy with one of the above aminoglycosides and a cephalothin or carbenicillin has been proposed, but such combinations do not materially increase the spectrum of activity against aerobic gram-negative bacilli over that of the aminoglycosides, and the clinical value of synergistic effects of these agents has not been convincingly demonstrated. In addition, the use of such combinations may enhance toxicity and the likelihood of superinfection. Antibiotic treatment is continued until the patient has been afebrile for at least three to five days, and the ultimate duration is usually determined by the time required for optimal treatment of the primary infection.

Drainage of abscesses, correction of obstruction, and removal of infected intravenous or bladder catheters also constitute an important aspect of the management of bacteremia.

## COMPLICATIONS AND SEQUELAE

Shock is the most frequent and serious complication of gram-negative bacteremia. It occurs in approximately 40 per cent of such patients. Characteristically, hypotension tends to appear within six to eight hours after the first manifestations of bacteremia. Diminution in peripheral resistance, normal venous pressure, and variable alterations in cardiac output are the characteristic hemodynamic findings in shock associated with gram-negative bacteremia. Steps involved in the treatment of shock consist of (1) administration of an appropriate antimicrobial agent; (2) monitoring of central venous pressure (CVP) or wedged pulmonary capillary pressure (PWP); (3) expansion of intravascular fluid volume; (4) monitoring of arterial pressure, mental status, and urinary output; and (5) administration of vasoactive agents.

After initial evaluation has been completed and an adequate airway has been ensured, plasma volume deficits and anemia should be corrected immediately using CVP or PWP to assess the adequacy of volume replacement. Because the major functional defect in bacteremic shock is the result of diminished peripheral resistance not compensated by an adequate increase in cardiac output, attempts are made to expand plasma volume and increase cardiac output in order to provide an adequate perfusion volume. Expansion of plasma volume requires monitoring of CVP or PWP. Changes in CVP or PWP in response to volume expansion provide better indices of the adequacy of volume expansion and fluid overload than absolute values. Initially, saline, plasma, or blood is administered rapidly, then more slowly with frequent measurement of CVP or PWP until the arterial blood pressure rises. If the CVP rises to 110 to 120 mm of water and persists at this level or continues to rise, volume expansion is discontinued. Repetitive measurement of urinary output and mental status provide an assessment of perfusion of vital organs in addition to information obtained from arterial blood pressure measurements.

If blood pressure is not restored by fluid replacement, vasoactive amines should be used. Disagreement exists over the relative merits of various agents in shock. Dopamine, which has recently been used frequently in patients with bacteremic shock, should be started in a dose of 1 to 10 μg/kg/min because this amount dilates renal vessels and increases urine output. At higher doses (10 to 50 μg/kg/min), it stimulates alpha reactors so that arterial pressure rises due to peripheral vasoconstriction. Isoproterenol should be used if there is no response to dopamine and is given in a dose of 1 to 2 $\mu$g/kg/min. It stimulates myocardial contractility and heart rate and causes vasodilatation, but renal blood flow is unchanged and arrhythmias are frequent. Older patients especially must be watched closely for supraventricular tachycardias. Norepinephrine is the agent of last resort. It produces severe peripheral vasoconstriction and thrombosis that may cause irreversible ischemic injury to the extremities. Nevertheless, it may restore blood pressure when other treatment fails. Its dose is 0.05/$\mu$g/kg. The alpha adrenergic blocking agent phentolamine has also been used in dosages of 0.1 to 2 mg over a 20-minute period with reported good results. There is even more controversy over the value of corticosteroid therapy in bacteremic shock. Early controlled studies failed to demonstrate any beneficial effects of doses of steroids equivalent to 300 mg of hydrocortisone per day but, more recently, doses of 30 mg/kg of body weight of methylprednisolone were reported to be of benefit in the treatment of bacteremic shock (Schumer, 1976). Other recent studies demonstrated greater fatality rates in patients with bacteremic shock treated with large doses of steroids than in similar patients not receiving steroids (Kreger et al., 1980).

Anuria, oliguria, and retention of urea nitrogen may complicate shock. If correction of hypotension does not induce increased urine output, osmotic diuresis with 12.5 to 25 g of mannitol, given intravenously, may be attempted. Failure to obtain diuresis necessitates modification of antibiotic dosage and initiation of measures such as hemodialysis for management of renal failure.

Respiratory alkalosis often occurs early in the course of bacteremia but metabolic acidosis usually supervenes in severe shock and may require correction with bicarbonate. Pulmonary changes, termed *shock lung,* also may result from bacteremic shock and are manifested by roentgenographic evidence of diffuse opacification of the lung and severe hypoxemia, which is relatively refractory to oxygen administration.

Disseminated intravascular coagulation with thrombocytopenia, fibrinogenopenia, decreased levels of clotting Factors II, V, and VIII, and the presence of circulating fibrin split products may occur in 5 to 10 per cent of patients with bacteremia. Its occurrence is limited almost exclusively to patients with shock, and correction of the hypotension is usually associated with improvement of coagulation abnormalities. Heparin has been used in the treatment of disseminated intravascular coagulation with equivocal results.

## PREVENTION

Prevention is much more effective than treatment of gram-negative bacteremia. Care in the use of the most frequent sources of bacteremia (intravenous catheters, urinary catheters, and ventilatory equipment) can materially reduce the frequency of bacteremia. The use of these devices should be limited to instances in which they are absolutely necessary. If the use of an intravenous catheter is mandatory, it should be inserted under scrupulously sterile conditions and removed within 48 to 72 hours. Similarly, care should be exercised to ensure that bladder catheters are also inserted under sterile conditions and that closed drainage systems, which prevent contamination between the drainage tube and the collection bottle, are used. Continuous irrigation with antibiotic solutions is not of value if closed drainage systems are carefully maintained. Equipment used for ventilatory assistance and therapy should be gas-sterilized before use, and reservoir nebulizers and humidifiers removed daily and cleaned with 0.25 per cent acetic acid. Additional control measures should include insistence on strict aseptic precautions for the care of wounds, tube drainage systems, catheters, and tracheostomies, prevention of decubiti, and limitation of prophylactic antibiotics. Diligent application of techniques for infection control can materially reduce the incidence of nosocomial bacteremia and effect reductions in the costs of medical care by shortening the duration of hospitalization for many patients.

## References

DuPont, H. L., and Spink, W. W.: Infections due to gram-negative organisms. An analysis of 860 patients with bacteremia at the University of Minnesota Medical Center, 1958-1966. Medicine 48:307, 1969.

Kreger, B. E., Craven, D. E., Carling, P. C., and McCabe, W. R.: Gram-Negative Bacteremia. III Reassessment of Etiology, Epidemiology, and Ecology in 612 Patients. Am J Med 68:332, 1980.

Kreger, B. E., Craven, D. E., and McCabe, W. R.: Gram-Negative Bacteremia. IV Re-evaluation of Clinical Features and Treatment in 612 Patients. Am J Med 68:344, 1980.

McCabe, W. R.: Gram-negative bacteremia. Adv Intern Med 19:135, 1974.

McCabe, W. R.: Antibiotics and endotoxic shock. Bull NY Acad Med 51:1084, 1975.

McCabe, W. R., and Jackson, G. G.: Gram-negative bacteremia I. Etiology and ecology. Arch Intern Med 110:847, 1962a.

McCabe, W. R., and Jackson, G. G.: Gram-negative bacteremia II. Clinical, laboratory, and therapeutic observations. Arch Intern Med 110:856, 1962b.

Myerowitz, R. L., Medeiros, A. A., and O'Brien, T. F.: Recent experience with bacillemia due to gram-negative organisms. J Infect Dis 124:239, 1971.

Schumer, W.: Steroids in the treatment of clinical septic shock. Ann Surg 184:333, 1976.

Young, L. S., Martin, W. J., Meyer, R. D., Weinstein, R. J., and Anderson, E. T.: Gram-negative rod bacteremia: Microbiologic, immunologic and therepeutic considerations. Ann Intern Med 86:456, 1977.

# STAPHYLOCOCCAL 178
## BACTEREMIA

*Stephen I. Morse, M.D.*

Staphylococcal bacteremia may arise from any site of infection or colonization or after the parenteral inoculation of contaminated material (Nolan and Beaty, 1976). Coagulase-positive *Staphylococcus aureus* is far more frequently responsible for bacteremia than the coagulase-negative *S. epidermidis* and *S. saprophyticus* species. The organisms may be present in the blood transiently, intermittently, or continuously. There are two classes of staphylococcal bacteremia. In primary staphylococcal bacteremia there is no evidence of prior staphylococcal disease, whereas in secondary bacteremia there are preexisting lesions from which the bloodstream is seeded. Metastatic staphylococcal abscesses can occur in all instances of staphylococcal bacteremia, but are more frequent when endocarditis occurs.

In the 1950s and early 1960s staphylococci were the most frequent cause of hospital-acquired (nosocomial) bacteremic infections in the United States (McGowan et al., 1975). Although bacteremia caused by gram-negative organisms is now more common, staphylococcal bacteremia is still important, often difficult to treat, and kills many patients. Staphylococcal bacteremia and endocarditis is a special problem in drug addicts.

## ETIOLOGY AND PATHOGENESIS

Staphylococcal bacteremia is usually caused by *S. aureus*, which is the most pathogenic species of staphylococci and is uniquely coagulase positive. *S. epidermidis* bacteremia is an important complication of contaminated intravascular prostheses or cannulae.

Secondary bloodstream dissemination of staphylococci can occur from any extravascular primary lesion. Most often the primary site is a cutaneous abscess, cellulitis, or decubitus ulcer. Staphylococcal pneumonia and osteomyelitis are often associated with bacteremia.

Preexisting extravascular staphylococcal lesions are not found in primary bacteremia. In many patients bacteremia is a consequence of an intravascular focus, such as a contaminated catheter or prosthetic device. In others, such as drug addicts, it can be assumed that the organisms were injected parenterally. The cause of bacteremia cannot be determined in approximately one-third of all patients with staphylococcal bacteremia. It is likely that in these instances organisms are disseminated into the bloodstream from colonized areas after mild or even unrecognized trauma.

Metastatic lesions can be produced in all cases of bacteremia but are much more frequent in primary bacteremia, especially when endocarditis is present. Often, extravascular lesions of hematogenous origin are the only manifestations of episodes of transient staphylococcal bacteremia — for example, osteomyelitis. However, these metastatic lesions in turn can give rise to continuing bacteremia.

Staphylococci probably disseminate from localized abscesses into the bloodstream by invading blood vessels in the lesion and producing septic thrombi, or by traveling up the lymphatics through incompetent lymph nodes into the general circulation. Although *S. aureus* produces a number of toxins and enzymes that might promote bloodstream invasion, none of these has been shown to be of primary importance in the development of bacteremia, nor do *S. aureus* strains isolated from the blood show heightened virulence in experimental animals when compared with strains isolated from other sites.

The status of the host is of major importance in determining the occurrence of staphylococcal bacteremia. Severe staphylococcal sepsis including bacteremia does not usually occur in normal individuals. Among the factors that appear to predispose to staphylococcal bacteremia are uncontrolled diabetes mellitus, renal insufficiency requiring hemodialysis, extensive surgery, malignancies, malnutrition, corticosteroids, granulocytopenia, liver disease, and immunosuppressive drugs; all cause a decrease in local or systemic defense mechanisms, either vascular, cellular, or humoral, or a combination thereof. Therefore, the pathogenicity of staphylococcal bacteremia is as much host determined as organism determined. The same conditions that predispose to serious staphylococcal disease also favor development of other infections.

## PATHOLOGY

The pathologic findings in staphylococcal bacteremia are those of the metastatic or primary abscesses and have the same basic histopathologic findings irrespective of site. The hallmark of the abscess is the central core of liquefaction necrosis containing dead polymorphonuclear leukocytes, other cells, and bacteria, surrounded by a zone of fibrin in which viable organisms and newly recruited granulocytes are found. In *S. aureus* endocarditis, destructive lesions of the valve leaflet and valve ring are serious complications. Although abscesses may completely replace an organ, as with renal abscesses, or affect such vital sites as the brain, meninges, and myocardium, the proximate cause of death cannot always be determined in overwhelming staphylococcal sepsis.

Laboratory findings include anemia and polymorphonuclear leukocytosis with the presence of immature granulocytes ("shift to the left"). When severe infection is present the leukocyte count may be normal and neutropenia may even be seen. In these instances, however, the proportion of immature neutrophils is greatly elevated. Proteinuria and microscopic hematuria secondary to embolic phenomena and/or immune complex disease may be present.

## CLINICAL MANIFESTATIONS

The clinical manifestations of staphylococcal bacteremia are related to sepsis, primary foci, and metastatic infection (Musher and McKenzie, 1977; Nolan and Beaty, 1976; Shulman and Nahmias, 1972). *S. aureus* bacteremia from any source may be a fulminating disease beginning suddenly with high fever, chills, tachycardia, and rapidly progressive shock that kills within 24 to 48 hours. More often the disease is slower. There are no specific symptoms of staphylococcal bacteremia, as opposed to sepsis caused by other organisms, although shock is less frequent than with gram-negative bacteremia.

*S. epidermidis* bacteremia is most often primary and related to the use of contaminated intravenous catheters, cardiac valve prostheses, or shunts used to relieve hydrocephalus. Bacteremia due to *S. epidermidis* is usually less hectic, more indolent, and less dramatic in onset than *S. aureus* bacteremia.

## COMPLICATIONS AND SEQUELAE

### Endocarditis

Differentiation between staphylococcal bacteremia with and without endocarditis has an important bearing on the intensity and duration of therapy as well as on prognosis. But the differentiation is not always simple and it has now become clear that prolonged staphylococcal bacteremia does not necessarily lead to endocarditis. In general, obvious primary staphylococcal lesions are not found in patients with endocarditis, whereas they are in bacteremia without endocarditis. On the other hand, secondary embolic abscesses, splenomegaly, and hematuria are more frequent when endocarditis is present. Staphylococcal endocarditis, as in other types of bacterial endocarditis, tends to develop on previously abnormal valves, but normal valves may be infected. Endocarditis is usually recognized by changing murmurs or new murmurs and often involves the aortic valve. The tricuspid valve may be infected after intravenous injection of contaminated fluids, especially in drug addicts; murmurs may be absent in tricuspid endocarditis. A feared complication of staphylococcal endocarditis is rupture of the valve leaflet or annulus.

### Osteomyelitis

Osteomyelitis, septic arthritis, and lung abscesses are the most common secondary conditions resulting from staphylococcal bacteremia. Hematogenous osteomyelitis is a disease primarily of children under 12 years of age. The source of the hematogenous spread is not found in over half of patients, nor is bacteremia present in more than 50 per cent of patients at the time bone symptoms appear. Trauma is thought to cause transient bacteremia of *S. aureus* from the skin. For unknown reasons the organisms have a predilection for the diaphyseal ends of the femur and tibia. Usually, only one bone is involved. In adults, osteomyelitis of the vertebrae is a complication of staphylococcal bacteremia. The presenting symptom of osteomyelitis is almost always pain, and swelling of overlying soft tissue due to secondary inflammatory reaction or extension of the infection. Radiographic evidence of bone disease may not appear for two weeks or more after symptoms appear, but may be found earlier by radionuclide scanning.

### Septic Arthritis

Staphylococcal arthritis occurs both in children and in adults. In adults, infection often occurs in joints with rheumatoid arthritis or osteoarthritis. Organisms can be seen in and isolated from aspirated joint fluid.

### Pulmonary Abscesses

Multiple lung abscesses can arise hematogenously, particularly from endocarditis of the tricuspid valve. Lung abscesses may be the only evidence of right-sided endocarditis, since tricuspid lesions are often silent. The usual radiographic finding is multiple small (< 3 cm) peripheral lung densities that may cavitate and coalesce. Scanning techniques will often demonstrate lesions before they are observed on chest x-rays.

### Kidney Lesions

Septic emboli to the kidneys may cause cortical and perinephric abscesses or pyelonephritis that can be demonstrated by radiographic and scanning techniques. Proteinuria and hematuria alone suggest the noninfectious lesions of immune complex glomerulonephritis. Immune complex nephritis is a particular complication of prolonged *S. epidermidis* bacteremia.

### Cutaneous Pustules

These occur in some patients with staphylococcal bacteremia and organisms are found in the lesions. Septic emboli less commonly cause cerebral microabscesses with encephalitic symptoms.

Over 95 per cent of reported cases of pyomyositis are caused by *S. aureus*. Although blood cultures are usually sterile at the time symptoms appear they are probably hematogenous. Abscesses are usually deep within striated muscle and involvement of overlying tissues does not occur for several weeks. Uncommon in temperate zones, pyomyositis may be responsible for 1 to 2 per cent of surgical admissions to hospitals in some tropical areas ("tropical" pyomyositis) (Levin et al., 1971).

### Disseminated Intravascular Coagulation (DIC)

This occurs in staphylococcal bacteremia, but with much less frequency than in gram-negative bacteremia. Hemorrhagic skin lesions, thrombocytopenia, clotting abnormalities, and increased plasma levels of fibrinogen split products are all found (Murray et al., 1977).

## DIAGNOSIS

Bacteremia is often unsuspected and overlooked in patients who have severe underlying disorders because the basic disease may mask infection. It is mandatory, therefore, that susceptible patients be monitored carefully for superimposed infections. It is difficult to diagnose staphylococcal bacteremia on clinical grounds alone, but metastatic foci in a patient with symptoms of bacteremia may point to disseminated staphylococcal infection. However, as previously noted, staphylococcal bacteremia may occur without an overt extravascular lesion. Search for metastatic lesions must be made by radionuclide scanning, x-ray procedures, and clinical observations.

Specific diagnosis can be made only by isolation of the bacteria from the blood. Usually the organisms will grow out within 24 to 48 hours. Scrupulous attention to sterile procedures in drawing and handling the specimen is critical, particularly in the case of *S. epidermidis* bacteremia. These organisms are common in the environment and on the skin and may also be confused with environmental micrococci. Thus, the true significance of their isolation from blood cultures may be overlooked and passed off merely as contamination. Sometimes in heavy infections staphylococci can be seen within phagocytes when stained specimens of the buffy coat of peripheral blood are examined.

The species identification of *S. aureus* usually presents no problems. Although *S. aureus* may appear as gram-positive cocci in chains in liquid cultures, the characteristic clumping will be present in agar cultures. The typical colonial pigmentation, $\beta$ hemolysis, ability to grow in high concentrations of sodium chloride (e.g., 7.5 per cent), and capacity to ferment mannitol point to identification of *S. aureus,* but a positive coagulase test leaves no ambiguity and is simple to perform. The differentiation of *S. epidermidis* from other micrococci may be difficult and may require appropriate biochemical testing.

Isolation of staphylococci from primary or secondary lesions may aid diagnosis as well as prognosis, and in all instances search must be made for these foci. It should be remembered that such lesions may not be radiographically visible for several weeks after symptoms develop.

## THERAPY

There remains considerable controversy about the choice and duration of antimicrobial therapy in patients with staphylococcal bacteremia, with or without endocarditis. There are, however, certain principles that are universally accepted.

Penicillin is the most effective antistaphylococcal agent, but penicillin-resistant organisms are common; in hospitals as many as 80 per cent of *S. aureus* strains are resistant. Penicillin resistance is due to the production of the inactivating enzyme penicillinase, a $\beta$-lactamase. Therefore, initial therapy should consist of a chemically modified penicillin resistant to penicillinase. Drug sensitivities, preferably determination of both the minimal inhibitory concentration (MIC) and the minimal bactericidal concentration (MBC), should be done on the isolate. If the strain is penicillin sensitive, penicillin G can then be substituted for the semisynthetic penicillin. If the patient is known to be allergic to penicillins, a cephalosporin (cephalothin) should be used. If the patient is allergic to both penicillins and cephalosporins, vancomycin is the drug of choice. In some parts of the world virulent *S. aureus* strains have appeared that are resistant by a nonpenicillinase

**TABLE 1. Parenteral Doses of Antimicrobial Drugs in Staphylococcal Bacteremia in Adults**

A. Patients not allergic to penicillins:
  1. Initial therapy
    Oxacillin, 8–12 grams per day in divided doses every 4 hours
    *or*
    Nafcillin, 8–12 grams per day in divided doses every 4 hours
    *or*
    Methicillin, 12–16 grams per day in divided doses every 4–6 hours
  2. Definitive therapy
    a. Penicillin-sensitive staphylococcus
      Change to penicillin G, $12 \times 10^6$ units per day in divided doses every 4 hours
    b. Penicillin-resistant staphylococcus
      Continue initial therapy

B. Patients allergic to penicillin but not to cephalosporins:
  1. Initial and definitive therapy (if organism sensitive)
    Cephalothin, 12–16 grams per day given in divided doses every 4–6 hours; *or* Cefazolin 3–4 grams per day in divided doses every 6–8 hours

C. Patients allergic to both penicillin and cephalosporins *or* organisms resistant to penicillin G, semisynthetic penicillins and cephalosporins:
    Vancomycin, 2 grams per day in divided doses every 6 hours

mechanism to all penicillins and such resistance also occurs in strains of *S. epidermidis*. Some of these strains retain sensitivity to cephalothin, but usually vancomycin must be used. The combined use of the aminoglycoside gentamicin with a penicillin or cephalothin during the first two weeks of therapy has been advocated, but, although animal experiments are suggestive, there is no convincing evidence in man that combined therapy is more effective.

Table 1 presents some of the regimens employed. In the absence of antimicrobial sensitivities, penicillin G should not be used as initial therapy. Note that all agents are given parenterally in divided doses. Particular care must be used with methicillin, since it is markedly unstable in even slightly acidic solutions — for example, dextrose in water. Response to correct treatment may be slow. Even in the face of curative antibiotic doses the fever may not resolve for a week and blood cultures may remain positive for staphylococci for that period of time. This slow response should not be misinterpreted as evidence of inadequate treatment and the antibiotic regime should not be changed if adequate blood levels are obtained.

In *S. aureus* endocarditis, therapy should be continued for at least six weeks. There is, however, evidence that bacteremia uncomplicated by endocarditis will resolve with appropriate antibi-

otic therapy over a much shorter period, particularly if there is a readily identifiable and easily removed source, such as an infected catheter. It is, however, often difficult to determine clinically whether a patient does or does not have endocarditis, and reduction in the length of therapy should be done only after careful consideration. The finding that patients with endocarditis and those with severe bacteremia have high levels of teichoic acid antibodies, whereas patients with less serious disease without endocarditis generally do not, may provide a useful method for deciding on the duration of therapy (Tuazon et al., 1978).

Where a focus of infection is readily removable, such as an intravenous catheter, this should be done immediately. Similarly, the removal or replacement of more complicated intravascular devices, such as atrioventricular shunts and valve prostheses, may have to be undertaken. The same is true for foreign bodies in extravascular sites, such as bone sequestra in osteomyelitic lesions. All abscesses that are readily amenable to incision and drainage should be so treated, and in many cases surgical treatment of deep-seated lesions is necessary once antibiotic therapy has been started. Treatment failures are usually due to bacteria in a locus where antimicrobials cannot act, to inadequate serum levels of the antimicrobial agent, or to insufficient duration of drug therapy. Tests for the bactericidal capacity of the patient's serum should be done when the therapeutic response is inadequate. Although changes in staphylococcal drug sensitivity rarely, if ever, occur during therapy, cultures should be obtained. Sometimes, a mixed infection may have been unrecognized or superinfection may have taken place.

Because of the frequent occurrence in individuals with severe underlying disorders, the tendency for rapidly destructive lesions to occur and the mortality from staphylococcal bacteremia, particularly endocarditis, remain high (20 to 30 percent).

## PROPHYLAXIS

Prevention of staphylococcal disease is an exceedingly difficult problem because the organisms are present as part of the normal flora of the skin and mucous membranes, and both endogenously and exogenously derived disease can occur. Fortunately, normal individuals have a high level of resistance to serious staphylococcal disease, although minor disease, particularly of the skin, is frequent. Nevertheless, personnel with open draining lesions should be excluded from contact with highly susceptible patients and there must be scrupulous attention to sterile techniques in the operating room and in the preparation and use of intravenous devices.

## References

Hieber, J. P., Nelson, A. J., and McCracken, G. H., Jr.: Acute disseminated staphylococcal disease in childhood. Am J Dis Child 131:181, 1977.

Levin, M. J., Gardner, P., and Waldvogel, F. A.: Tropical pyomyositis. An unusual infection due to *Staphylococcus aureus*. N Engl J Med 284:196, 1971.

McGowan, J. E., Jr., Barnes, M. W., and Finland, M.: Bacteremia at Boston City Hospital: occurrence and mortality during 12 selected years (1935–1972), with special reference to hospital-acquired cases. J Infect Dis 132:316, 1975.

Murray, H. W., Tuazon, C. U., and Sheagren, J. N.: Staphylococcal septicemia and disseminated intravascular coagulation. *Staphylococcus aureus* endocarditis mimicking meningococcemia. Arch Intern Med 137:844, 1977.

Musher, D. M., and McKenzie, S. O.: Infections due to *Staphylococcus aureus*. Medicine (Balt.) 56:383, 1977.

Nolan, C. M., and Beaty, H. N.: *Staphylococcus aureus* bacteremia. Current clinical patterns. Am J Med 60:495, 1976.

Shulman, J. A., and Nahmias, A. J.: Staphylococcal infections: clinical aspects. In Cohen, J. O. (ed.): The Staphylococci. New York, John Wiley and Sons, Inc., 1972, p. 547.

Tuazon, C. U., Sheagren, J. N., Choa, M. S., Marcus, D., and Curtin, J. A.: *Staphylococcus aureus* bacteremia: relationship between formation of antibodies to teichoic acid and development of metastatic abscesses. J Infect Dis 137:57, 1978.

# *TYPHOID FEVER* 179

## *Gerald T. Keusch, M.D.*

## *DEFINITION*

Typhoid fever, which is caused by a motile, gram-negative bacillus, *Salmonella typhi*, is an acute febrile illness that was originally named for its clinical resemblance to typhus (the word typhoid means typhus-like). The names for both diseases were derived from the Greek word *typhos*, which means smoke in both a literal and a metaphoric sense, because the diseases were thought to have their origin in miasmic vapors and to cause mental clouding with high fever. Typhoid and typhus were clinically distinct, however, being designated "putrid-malignant" and "slow nervous" fevers, respectively. In fact, in all aspects of etiology, pathogenesis, and pathology, they are entirely distinct, but "typhoid" is still the accepted term for infection with *S. typhi*.

Actually, the clinical syndrome of typhoid fever can be caused by other salmonellae, including *S. enteritidis* bioserotype paratyphi A (*S. paratyphi* A), *S. enteritidis* serotype paratyphi B (*S. schottmuelleri* or *S. paratyphi* B), and on rare occasions even by *S. enteritidis* serotype typhimurium (*S. typhimurium*). Thus, some have advocated calling these various diseases "enteric fevers" because of the consistent involvement of Peyer's patches in the intestine by infecting organisms. Although this term is useful to indicate a family of infections with similar clinical manifestations, involvement of the enteric tract is not the essential feature of the disease. Rather, invasion of, and multiplication within, the mononuclear phagocytic cells in the liver, spleen, lymph nodes, and Peyer's patches by these infecting organisms is the hallmark of this syndrome.

## *ETIOLOGY*

### Microbiology

Microbiologic identification of *S. typhi* is rather simple because the biochemical reactions of this particular bacterium are different from those of all of the more than 1600 distinct salmonellae currently known. These reactions are based on the specific biochemical features of the organism and the serologic tests for identification of the envelope, somatic, and flagellar antigens. Salmonellae belong to the family Enterobacteriaceae (Chapter 31) because they all ferment glucose, reduce nitrate to nitrite, and synthesize peritrichous flagella when motile.

Biochemical features of importance in distinguishing *S. typhi* and *S. enteritidis* bioserotype paratyphi A and paratyphi B are shown in Table 1. *S. typhi*, a lactose and sucrose nonfermenting bacterium, produces a characteristic pattern that initially resembles *Shigella* more than *Salmonella*. It is anaerogenic (does not produce gas from glucose) and usually produces a trace of hydrogen sulfide ($H_2S$), which, in conjunction with motility and its inability to utilize citrate (Simmons') and to decarboxylate ornithine, is sufficient for a presumptive identification of *S. typhi*. Confirmation is easily obtained by serologic testing of agglutination patterns with commercially available antisera (Table 2).

Identification of *S. enteritidis* bioserotype paratyphi A may be confusing at first glance because, unlike nearly all other salmonellae, it does not produce $H_2S$ (10 per cent of strains produce trace amounts but only after several days in culture). Initial biochemical screening may therefore sug-

TABLE 1.   Biochemical Differences Between *S. typhi* and *S. enteritidis*

| | S. TYPHI | S. ENTERITIDIS | |
| --- | --- | --- | --- |
| | | Bioserotype paratyphi A | Serotype paratyphi B |
| Acid from glucose | + | + | + |
| Gas from glucose | − | + (trace) | + |
| H₂S production | + (trace) (5% −) | − (10% late +) | + |
| Citrate utilization | − | − (25% late +) | + |
| Lysine decarboxylase | + | − | + |
| Ornithine decarboxylase | − | + | + |

gest identification as a *Shigella, Alkalescens dispar, Citrobacter freundii* (H₂S negative variety), *Enterobacter hafnia,* or even *Yersinia enterocolitica.* Use of pooled *Salmonella* O-antigen grouping sera can quickly establish the correct genus and, in conjunction with the biochemical data and flagellar antigen typing, the species as well.

*S. enteritidis* serotype paratyphi B resembles biochemically the majority of the remaining salmonellae. Because its somatic antigens are also identical to those of *S. enteritidis* serotype typhimurium, the single most common *Salmonella* species isolated from humans, further characterization is required for specific identification. Serologic detection of flagellar antigens is essential in making this distinction.

## Serology

Salmonellae possess multiple diverse antigens. Detection of some of these antigens by agglutination with antisera is the basis for serologic classification and identification. Specific antisera are used to determine the particular kind of envelope (K), somatic (O), or flagellar (H) antigens that are present. The resulting antigenic formula is the fingerprint that helps to identify specific strains.

Envelope antigens are the most exterior of the three antigenic types; they form a capsule on the surface of the organism. In fact, colonies of *S. enteritidis* serotype paratyphi B, when left at room temperature for a few days, may form a distinctive raised moist rim composed of K polysaccharide, the so-called "slime wall." The most important K antigen, however, is the highly polymerized acidic polysaccharide, the Vi factor, found in *S. typhi, S. enteritidis* serotype paratyphi C, and in *Citrobacter.* Vi antigens cover the somatic O antigens of these bacteria and render the strains inagglutinable in anti-O serum. Vi was originally discovered in this fashion by Felix and Pitt, who also showed that Vi-positive strains of *S. typhi* were more virulent for mice (hence the designation Vi). Experimental studies in human volunteers have documented a similar role of Vi in man, although the mechanism is not clear. Vi also determines phage susceptibility but is most useful in the laboratory for rapid identification of *S. typhi* by a slide agglutination test against Vi antisera. Fresh isolates of *S. typhi* that are Vi-positive are usually poorly motile and are thus not flocculated by antiflageller antisera. Because of blocking by the Vi antigen, they are not agglutinated by anti-O sera either. However, they may be quickly identified by agglutination with anti-Vi. Boiling a suspension of these organisms in physiologic saline for 20 minutes removes the Vi (and reaction with anti-Vi) and permits agglutination with anti-O serum for confirmation of the identification of *Salmonella.*

O antigens are heat-stable oligosaccharides composed of repeating units of specific sequences of simple and amino sugars at the terminal end of

TABLE 2.   Antigenic Formulae of Certain Salmonellae

| ORGANISM | O ANTIGEN GROUP | O ANTIGENS | H ANTIGENS | K ANTIGENS |
| --- | --- | --- | --- | --- |
| *S. enteritidis* | | | | |
| bioserotype paratyphi A | A | 1, 2, 12 | a | − |
| serotype paratyphi B | B | 1, 4, 5, 12 | b:1, 2 | − |
| serotype typhimurium B | B | 1, 4, 5, 12 | i:1, 2 | − |
| bioserotype paratyphi C | C | 6, 7 | c:1, 5 | Vi |
| *S. typhi* | D | 9, 12 | d | Vi |

the lipopolysaccharide of the bacterial cell wall. Several different O antigens (designated by Arabic numerals) are usually present in each individual organism. Salmonellae with identical major O antigens are grouped together in serogroups (A, B, C, etc.), although some minor O antigens occur in more than one serogroup (Table 2). *S. typhi* is one of many organisms in group D, while *S. enteritidis* bioserotype paratyphi A is in group A, and *S. enteritidis* serotype paratyphi B is in group B. Pooled grouping antisera are commercially available for use in slide agglutination tests. A serologic distinction among the many organisms that group together in the same serogroup is made on the basis of Vi and flagellar antigens.

H antigens are flagellar proteins. In contrast to O antigens, tests for the presence of flagellar antigens are usually made in broth cultures because the organisms must be actively motile for the antigens to be detectable. Many *Salmonella* strains possess both specific and nonspecific H determinants; the latter result in significant cross-agglutination between strains. These antigens are now designated phase 1 (specific) and phase 2 (nonspecific) antigens; they are denoted by lower case Roman letters and Arabic numbers, respectively. Thus, *S. enteritidis* serotype paratyphi B expresses b antigen in phase 1 and antigens 1, 2 in phase 2 (Table 2). A fresh isolate is likely to express only one H antigen phase. In order to test for antigens of the variant phase, it is usually necessary to select colonies expressing such antigens. This is generally accomplished by the use of a phase reversal medium, a semisolid agar containing antibody to the expressed H phase. The antiserum immobolizes colonies with the homologous antigen but permits motility of organisms expressing the other phase. These organisms may then be selected for testing.

### Epidemiology

*S. typhi, S. enteritidis* bioserotype paratyphi A, and serotype paratyphi B infect only humans. Christie (1969) suggests that this evolution and adaptation to the human environment constitute an "epidemiologic rut" because every case of typhoid fever may ultimately be traced back to a human carrier. There are limited possibilities for transmission of infection. Theoretically, this situation should facilitate efforts to mount an epidemiologic attack on the organisms because the transmission routes should be easily followed.

However, this is not necessarily the case. First, while patients may excrete large numbers of viable organisms in the feces, urine, vomitus, and respiratory secretions, and although the stools of chronic carriers usually contain more than one million *S. typhi* organisms per gram, direct person-to-person transmission is rare. In addition to the human source, a vehicle is required. Second, while most infections are food-borne or water-borne, there are a multitude of secondary pathways and vehicles. For example, shellfish such as mussels, living in waters contaminated with sewage, may become highly infectious although the water itself is not. This occurs because the mussel picks up and filters out the microbial content of over 10 gallons of water per day. This marked concentration of the inoculum in the creature creates a highly infectious meal for a human. The chain of causative events in this situation involves a carrier who sheds organisms into inadequately processed sewage, which is discharged into waters inhabited by edible shellfish. It is apparently safer to swim in such polluted water than it is to eat its shellfish. Third, *S. typhi* can persist for weeks in water, ice, or even dust or dried sewage. If such organisms reach a suitable vehicle, they can multiply to an infectious dose and complete the epidemiologic life cycle by reinfecting a human subject. It is not unusual to be unable to isolate *S. typhi* from the contaminated water source when clinical cases develop, because the responsible contamination occurred two or more weeks before. Nevertheless, in the classic epidemiologic investigation of a water-borne outbreak of typhoid fever, the disease is traced backward along waterways and septic systems to the chronic carrier.

The incidence of typhoid fever will therefore be determined by the prevalence of human carriers, the adequacy of environmental sanitation, and the purity of the water supply. In industrialized nations, technical improvements in handling wastes and water have contributed to a steady decline in typhoid fever, while mass production and distribution of food, which is often poorly stored and handled, have led to an explosive increase in all other forms of salmonellosis. This is perhaps the clearest example of the limited epidemiologic potential of the Salmonellae adapted to humans and the unlimited potential of the nonadapted strains. In developing countries with poor sanitation and primitive water systems, typhoid fever remains a common endemic illness.

### Pathogenesis

Experimental studies in human volunteers infected with *S. typhi* and in mice infected with *S. enteritidis* serotype enteriditis or typhimurium ("mouse typhoid") have shed considerable light on the pathogenesis of typhoid fever. Oral administration of the virulent Quailes strain of *S. typhi* has shown that the intestine, not the pharynx, is the portal of entry. Organisms must be swallowed in order to initiate disease; gargling and expectoration of large inocula failed to cause typhoid. About 50 per cent of adult humans are infected after ingestion of $10^7$ organisms of the Quailes strain, whereas 28 per cent and 95 per cent of humans are infected by $10^5$ or $10^9$ organisms, respectively. Doses below $10^5$ do not cause disease. Limited comparisons with other Vi-positive strains have shown a similar degree of virulence. Vi-negative strains are less virulent.

Ingested organisms must traverse the stomach to reach the small bowel. Gastric acid appears to affect S. typhi less than V. cholerae, E. coli, and other salmonellae. Viable S. typhi organisms can be isolated from gastric secretions for at least 30 minutes after ingestion. Organisms reaching the proximal small intestine rapidly penetrate the mucosa and begin the process of systemic invasion and frank clinical illness. Biopsy of the proximal small intestine of humans during the incubation period of typhoid, before bacteremia occurs, shows focal inflammation and suggests that this is the site of penetration. Electron micrographs of the small bowel of animals during experimental salmonellosis have demonstrated a remarkable sequence in which the epithelial cell brush border seems to melt away in advance of the penetrating organisms but is quickly restored after invasion is complete.

In monkeys, invading S. typhi organisms are contained for a short time in the regional mesenteric nodes before spreading to the liver and spleen. In the mouse, however, transient bacteremia occurs within 20 seconds of ingestion, and bacteria reach the liver and spleen shortly thereafter. S. typhi is rapidly taken up by mononuclear phagocytes in the liver and spleen, but instead of being quickly killed by these phagocytes, the organism multiplies intracellularly. It is precisely this characteristic of S. typhi that determines the nature of the illness it produces. After this period of intracellular multiplication (corresponding to the incubation period), organisms escape into the bloodstream, cause a second bacteremia, which is now sustained, and usher in the febrile symptomatic phase of the disease. In experimental animals the duration of the symptom-free interval varies inversely with the size of the inoculum. Establishment of bacteremia seems to require a set number of viable intracellular organisms; the smaller the inoculum, the longer it takes to reach this critical mass of bacteria.

Bacteremia also leads directly to two critical events in typhoid fever — invasion of the gallbladder and the Peyer's patches of the bowel. Infection of either site leads to positive stool cultures, and invasion of the gallbladder may lead to long-term carriage of the organism. When the inflammatory response of either tissue is severe, necrosis may occur, presenting clinically as necrotizing cholecystitis or hemorrhage and/or perforation of the bowel.

The role of endotoxin in the pathogenesis of typhoid fever is unclear. Although the systemic symptoms (including chills, fever, headache, myalgia, anorexia, nausea, leukopenia, and thrombocytopenia) produced by intravenous injection of S. typhi endotoxin resemble those of the actual disease, subjects rendered unresponsive (tolerant) to these effects of S. typhi endotoxin nevertheless develop typical typhoid symptoms during experimental infection. It is possible that the intracellular location of the typhoid bacillus stimulates the release of endogenous mediators directly from leukocytes and macrophages, relegating endotoxin to an unessential role.

The histopathology of typhoid is directly related to the proliferation of large mononuclear cells. This infiltration is most pronounced in the Peyer's patches of the terminal ileum but is also prominent in the liver, spleen, and mesenteric lymph nodes. Focal hepatic necrosis and cloudy swelling of hepatic cells are responsible for abnormalities of liver function during typhoid fever.

Much of our understanding of host defenses against S. typhi has been derived from investigations of an experimental model of typhoid fever in mice produced by mouse-passaged strains of S. typhimurium or enteritidis. Although humoral antibody reduces the number of organisms in the blood of infected mice, bacterial multiplication in tissues such as the liver and spleen is unaffected. The systemic bacterial population is reduced and the infection controlled only when the intracellular bacterial activity of macrophages is activated. Circulating specific antibody appears to contribute little to the cell-mediated immune response responsible for this critical intracellular bactericidal process. Mouse typhoid, and by extrapolation human typhoid as well, has therefore been classified as a facultative intracellular infection in which the causative organism can multiply freely within nonimmune macrophages (Hornick et al., 1970). These pathogens are rapidly killed, however, by macrophages that have been activated by lymphokines from specifically sensitized T lymphocytes, which develop early in infection.

Actually, the ability of different strains of S. typhimurium to survive within normal mouse peritoneal macrophages varies considerably and constitutes a measure of the intrinsic virulence of the organism. As a consequence, the need for the development of specific cellular immunity varies as well. Furthermore, experimental studies do not completely exclude a role for humoral factors in the host defense response, in the form of either free antibody or cytophilic antibody on lymphocyte or macrophage membranes. Passive immunization of normal mice with isolated B, but not T, lymphocytes sensitized to *S. typhimurium* reduces the tissue multiplication of bacteria and enhances survival. This mechanism is probably distinct from the partial protection offered by circulating anti-Vi or O antibody in the vaccinated human, a protection that is most likely due to serum bactericidal activity during the initial transient bacteremia before the organism is sequestered inside macrophages.

## CLINICAL MANIFESTATIONS, COMPLICATIONS, AND SEQUELAE

The incubation period of typhoid fever is generally one to two weeks, but it varies inversely with the size of the inoculum, and may be as short as three days or as long as two months. Classically, clinical disease is ushered in with fever as the phase of sustained bacteremia begins. The peak temperatures typically increase in step-wise fashion over three to four days to 104 to 105° F. Nonspecific symptoms, including anorexia, malaise, lethargy, myalgia, and continuous dull frontal headache, accompany the fever. In the past, patients have been noted to have constipation rather than diarrhea, nonproductive cough with evidence of bronchitis, and a relative bradycardia for the height of the fever response. More recent observations suggest that diarrhea is in fact more commonly observed, that cough is present in only 10 to 15 per cent of patients, and that relative bradycardia is observed in fewer than 25 per cent of cases (Samantry et al., 1977; Gulati et al., 1968). Moreover, the step-wise pattern of temperature elevation is no longer common either, and sustained or intermittent fevers often occur from the outset. A small number of patients may even fail to manifest any sort of fever.

Although some patients experience spontaneous remission of illness in one week or less, high sustained fevers characteristically occur during the second and third weeks. The patient looks acutely ill and has prominent facial flushing, dry skin, dilated pupils, and an asthenic, dulled, and detached appearance. Frank prostration or, particularly in children, delirium may occur at this stage. This distinctive appearance is often referred to as "toxic," although the participation of a toxin in its genesis has not been shown. Clinical symptoms usually abate within four weeks, but may last much longer. During the second week, vague abdominal discomfort with diffuse lower quadrant tenderness and distension may be experienced. At times the examiner can readily palpate loops of bowel filled with air and fluid. The

liver and spleen are enlarged in about one third of these patients. Thus, the traditional clues to diagnosis, including the step-wise rise in fever, the relative bradycardia, and splenomegaly, may be absent. The value of splenomegaly in the diagnosis must be further discounted in regions of the world in which endemic malaria is a common cause of splenic enlargement. Rose spots, which are transient blanching rose-colored papules that often occur in the second week of fever in the periumbilical region, are not specific for typhoid fever but are very suggestive of it. Many observers feel that the presence of herpes labialis rules out the diagnosis of typhoid fever.

In a significant proportion of patients, perhaps 15 per cent of adults and 30 per cent or more of children, the onset of disease does not fit the above description. In some, the mildness of the clinical presentation is misleading, and the correct diagnosis is made only by subsequent isolation of the organism. In others, symptoms affecting the central nervous system (convulsions, meningismus, altered sensorium) or the lungs (cough, bronchitis, pneumonia), or an acute condition of the abdomen suggest focal rather than systemic disease. Isolation of *S. typhi* comes as a surprise, but this should not be the case, for a bewildering array of clinical syndromes has been reported as either the principal or an accompanying feature of typhoid. These include a number of other complications of the nervous system (encephalitis or encephalomyelitis; myelitis with spastic paraplegia; peripheral or cranial neuritis, especially involving the eighth nerve; meningitis; and Guillain-Barré syndrome), psychiatric presentations (including acute psychoses, mania, catatonia, or depression), acute myocarditis, hepatitis, necrotizing cholangitis, immune-complex nephritis, hemolytic-uremic syndrome, and osteomyelitis or septic arthritis.

Typhoid fever has been associated traditionally with two late complications: significant intestinal hemorrhage and frank perforation. These problems occur secondary to bacterial invasion of the Peyer's patches, which in turn may lead to necrosis, ulceration, and erosion of blood vessels. Although the lesions are usually restricted to the superficial mucosa, they may extend to the serosa and cause perforation, which always occurs on the antimesenteric border of the bowel. These complications occur in 2 to 3 per cent of patients, most often in the third week of illness. Many more, perhaps 20 per cent, have minor intestinal blood loss. In developing countries, an acute bowel catastrophe may be the event that brings the patient to medical attention. Typhoid perforation is clinically manifested by a sudden drop in temperature, a rise in the pulse, and rapid development of the signs of peritonitis, with pain, tenderness, rebound, and rigidity, most often in the right lower quadrant. Seventy-five per cent of perforations occur within 40 cm of the ileocecal valve and 90 per cent within 60 cm. In about one fifth of patients operated on more than 24 hours after perforation, focal abscesses will be found in the subphrenic or subhepatic spaces or in the pelvis. Perforation and massive hemorrhage are the major causes of the reported mortality rate of about 10 per cent in untreated infection.

Relapse, which is a common complication, usually occurs one to three weeks after therapy is discontinued. The signs and symptoms are similar to the first episode, but relapse is usually a milder illness that responds promptly to antimicrobials.

## GEOGRAPHIC VARIATIONS

The clinical presentation of typhoid has changed considerably throughout the world in the past three decades because of several factors related to host, agent, and environment. These changes have tended to sharpen rather than lessen the geographic variations in disease patterns. Thus, age, underlying illness, nutritional state, and R factor-mediated antimicrobial resistance of the organisms have caused differences in the severity of the disease, while water supply, environmental sanitation, and the degree of environmental contamination have contributed to differences in the prevalence of typhoid.

In industrial countries, the incidence of typhoid has steadily declined, so that most cases are now imported by young adult travelers to endemic regions (dubbed holiday typhoid in England). Complications (except for relapse) are unusual. Indeed, the sole clinical presentation can be that of fever of undetermined origin. The emergence of chloramphenicol-resistant S. typhi has led to occasional cases of severe "old-time" disease, but this is a limited phenomenon at present.

In contrast, in the developing nations intestinal perforation still occurs in as many as 10 to 20 per cent of patients hospitalized with typhoid fever. Because of the long delay before obtaining medical care, these patients are usually gravely ill when they present with high fever, profound toxemia, delirium, stupor, or even frank coma. Hypothermia and cardiovascular collapse may accompany signs of an acute abdomen. The death rate from this complication remained high in the mid-1970s, with a mortality rate of 70 to 80 per cent regardless of surgery.

In Africa and some parts of India, central nervous system and psychiatric symptoms are prominent (Scragg et al., 1969). These include acute confusional, delirious, or psychotic states; nuchal rigidity; cog-wheel extrapyramidal rigidity of extremities; incontinence; and motor seizures. Patients may occasionally be admitted to psychiatric units with a diagnosis of catatonic schizophrenia; however, the finding of fever usually leads to more appropriate medical care. Examination of the cerebrospinal fluid is invariably negative in these patients.

In these endemic regions of the world, there is a higher relative incidence of typhoid fever in children, including infants in the first two years of life, a rarity elsewhere. Although childhood typhoid in the affluent nations is typically a mild disease, it is severe in the tropics, with a high incidence of pulmonary, central nervous system, and intestinal complications (Duggan and Beyer, 1975). Because the omentum may be short or relatively immobile in this age group, extensive peritoneal soiling and early abscess formation is not uncommon. This is often worsened by delay in bringing patients to the hospital. A few specific geographic clinical associations have also been made. These are (1) a syndrome of prolonged, intermittent fever and bacteremia, persisting for as long as two years in patients with *Schistosoma mansoni* infection. It has been suggested but not proved that salmonellae infecting the gut of the worm may be the source of recurrent bacteremia, although altered blood flow due to intrahepatic fibrosis may also alter mononuclear cell function. (2) Chronic urinary tract carriage of organisms, which may be a source of sporadic or epidemic infection in patients with *Schistosoma haematobium* infection. These individuals experience intermittent bacteremia and fever. (3) Intrahepatic (as opposed to gallbladder) carriage among Chinese suffering from concomitant *Clonorchis sinensis* infection. This is associated with a spectrum of clinical manifestations ranging from asymptomatic excretion of *S. typhi* in the stool to recurrent cholangitis. In these patients, the sex ratio of carriers is close to 1:1 instead of the usual predominance of women, which is probably related to the sex distribution of cholelithiasis.

For the most part, however, geographic variations in the severity of typhoid fever and its complications appear to be related more to the adequacy of health care than to factors intrinsic to the host or microorganism.

## DIAGNOSIS

There are three methods of making the diagnosis of typhoid fever: microbiologic, serologic, and clinical. The first method is the most specific, and more than 90 per cent of untreated patients will have a positive blood culture during the first week of illness. Unfortunately, the incidence of isolations drops to 40 per cent in the face of antecedent antimicrobial therapy. However, cultures of the bone marrow are still positive 90 per cent of the time, even after a few doses of antibiotics. The yield of positive blood cultures slowly diminishes with time, but there is a concomitant rise in stool (85 per cent) and urine (25 per cent) isolates in the third and fourth weeks because of invasion of Peyer's patches and the kidneys. More recent studies (Wicks et al., 1974; Gilman et al., 1975) suggest a much lower incidence of positive stool and urine cultures, especially in the treated patient. Cultures from the center of rose spots are positive in two thirds of patients. Fecal excretion ceases by three months in 90 per cent of patients, but about 3 per cent may go on to become long-term fecal carriers (more than one year). These chronic enteric carriers may excrete *S. typhi* for life, and they are the usual source for new cases. Adults more frequently than children, and women more frequently than men, become chronic carriers, probably because of the relative incidence of gallstones in these groups.

Serologic diagnosis depends upon antibody rises to O and H antigens, detected by agglutination reactions (Widal test). Antibody to O antigens in group D develops during the first week of illness, peaks at three to four weeks, and declines after nine months to one year. A rising titer (greater than fourfold) is suggestive of acute infection but of course may be produced by any group D salmonella sharing the 9, 12 somatic antigens with *S. typhi*. Prior immunization with typhoid-paratyphoid vaccine may also result in an anamnestic antibody response of group D titers due to infection with many other salmonellae and other enteric bacteria. Additional specificity can be ascribed to the O antibody response if there is also a rise in titer of antibody to the d flagellar antigen of *S. typhi*. These antibodies rise in titer after the first week and peak in four to six weeks. However, titers remain high for years, whether stimulated by infection or vaccine, and a single determination of a high titer of flagellar antibody cannot be considered diagnostic of recent infection. The effect of vaccine may be particularly vexing, because patients often cannot remember their immunization history. It has been suggested that a distinctive and unusual H antigen be included in the vaccine to facilitate identification of vaccine-induced titers, but this has not been done. For all these reasons, a single high Widal titer or even rising titers are even less specific than most serologic tests.

Diseases that are most commonly confused with typhoid clinically include nontyphoidal salmonellosis, brucellosis, tularemia, shigellosis, tuberculosis, malaria, Rocky Mountain spotted fever, murine typhus, or even lymphoproliferative or collagen-vascular diseases. All of these diseases can present with similar high sustained fevers, splenomegaly, and, in some instances, rashes that can be confused with rose spots. Appropriate cultures will usually establish the correct diagnosis, but other laboratory tests are also useful. The white blood count is normal or reduced, but a pronounced left shift in the differential is common. The serum transaminases are often elevated without other evidence of liver disease. Anemia and occult blood in the feces are common during the third and fourth weeks of the disease, even in patients without frank perforation.

## THERAPY

Effective antimicrobial therapy has reduced the mortality rate to 1 per cent or less in recent reported series. At the same time, the incidence of relapse, which usually occurs one to three weeks after antibiotics are discontinued, has doubled to about 15 to 20 per cent. Although recrudescent illness may be severe or complicated, it is usually less severe than the original illness and responds promptly to therapy. Second and even third relapses have been reported.

Since 1948, chloramphenicol has been the chemotherapeutic standard against which the efficacy of other drugs has been measured. Typhoid fever is one of the classic infections in which in vitro sensitivity does not predict in vivo efficacy, although drugs ineffective in vitro will surely be clinically ineffective. For chloramphenicol-sensitive strains, no other agent has been found to produce a superior clinical response. Except for concern about effects on the bone marrow, chloramphenicol would be the clear-cut agent of choice. Other drugs that are nearly as effective, such as ampicillin, amoxycillin, or trimethoprim-sulfamethoxazole, are less toxic and may be chosen for the initial therapy of patients who are not severely ill. Chloramphenicol should be given orally in a dose of 60 mg/kg/day in four divided doses. Many alternate regimens have been suggested in an attempt to reduce the relapse rate, but none seem superior. One reasonable program is to continue therapy until the temperature becomes normal (usually four to eight days), then lower the oral dose to 30 mg/kg/day and treat the patient for two additional weeks. Chloramphenicol may be given intravenously in the same fashion. Because it is not absorbed well from muscle, chloramphenicol should not be given intramuscularly. Bleeding or perforation may occur during therapy, even in afebrile patients. Treatment with chloramphenicol does not prevent the carrier state.

Intravenous ampicillin (100 mg/kg/day) or oral amoxycillin (100 mg/kg/day) is also effective. Some studies suggest that amoxycillin therapy may indeed be superior to chloramphenicol in the rapidity of the response, the subsequent relapse rate, and the convalescent carrier rates (Scragg, 1976). Further experience will be required to substantiate these claims. However, both forms of ampicillin and especially amoxycillin are considerably more expensive than chloramphenicol. Ampicillin or amoxycillin is the drug of choice for chloramphenicol-resistant strains of S. typhi.

S. typhi may also be resistant to ampicillin and amoxycillin. In the typhoid outbreak in Mexico in 1972, strains resistant to these drugs and ·to chloramphenicol were recovered (Overturf et al., 1973). The recommended treatment for these organisms, as well as for patients who are unable to take penicillins or chloramphenicol because of allergy or toxicity, is trimethoprim-sulfamethoxazole, two tablets by mouth two to three times daily (Butler et al., 1977).

Hemorrhage is generally managed by conservative supportive measures, including transfusions. Occasionally, bowel resection has been employed for massive or recurrent bleeding, but this can be difficult because there are usually multiple bleeding sites in a friable bowel.

Results of surgical repair of perforations have improved with modern fluid and electrolyte replacement. Early recognition and aggressive correction of hypovolemic shock permit successful simple operative repairs, without the need for wedge excision or resection and anastomosis (Kim et al., 1975). Mortality rates should be less than 10 per cent in these circumstances, and even lower when the diagnosis is made quickly and the surgery performed rapidly.

Treatment of the chronic carrier state has always been a problem, particularly in gallbladder carriers with stones. In vitro experiments demonstrate the ease with which S. typhi can move to the interior of a gallstone and the difficulty of killing these protected organisms, even by immersing the infected stone in a very high concentration of a bactericidal antibiotic. Approximately 3 per cent of appropriately treated typhoid patients become chronic carriers. In the absence of cholelithiasis, the majority of these subjects will be cured by a course of oral ampicillin or amoxycillin, 100 mg/kg/day, plus probenecid, 30 mg/kg/day, or trimethoprim-sulfamethoxazole, 2 tablets twice daily for three months (Johnson et al., 1973). In the presence of cholelithiasis, the likelihood of cure with antimicrobials alone is much reduced, and cholecystectomy and antimicrobials may be needed. Nevertheless, an adequate course of one or both antimicrobials should be tried before a decision for surgical intervention

is made. Known chronic enteric carriers should, of course, be urged to maintain strict standards of hygiene and particularly to wash their hands thoroughly after defecation. They should not work as food handlers where there is an increased opportunity to disseminate the organism to susceptibles.

Chronic urinary carriers of S. typhi are often infected with Schistosoma haematobium or Schistosoma mansoni at the same time. The best results are obtained when the schistosomiasis is treated first, for example, with niridazole, 25 mg/kg for six days. Excellent results have been reported recently when treatment with niridazole is followed by 250 mg of amoxycillin every six hours for four weeks.

## IMMUNIZATION

Current vaccines consist of killed bacterial suspensions, prepared for subcutaneous inoculation, of either S. typhi alone (monovalent) or S. typhi in combination with S. enteritidis bioserotype paratyphi A and serotype paratyphi B (TAB). Recent studies have confirmed the original observations of Almford Wright at the turn of the century that such vaccines afford protection, at least for the S. typhi component (Warren and Hornick, 1979). Because there are virtually no data verifying the efficacy of the TAB vaccine for the nontyphi strains and the increased risk of adverse side reactions such as severe local inflammatory responses, monovalent S. typhi vaccine is the preferred vaccine. This preparation does not induce cell-mediated immunity, but stimulates the production of serum antibody to Vi, O, and H antigens. Human trials show no correlation between anti-Vi or anti-O responses and protection, but a number of studies suggest an association between anti-H antibodies and resistance. It is likely that serum antibody would assist host defenses during the initial bacteremia, before the invasion of mononuclear phagocytes, by reducing the number of organisms capable of intracellular multiplication. The mechanism of action of the antibody is unknown. Anti-H antibodies stop motility of the microorganisms, but the importance of this effect is uncertain.

Human studies have documented three key points about killed vaccines (Warren and Hornick, 1979). (1) Immunity can be overcome by increasing the bacterial inoculum. This is probably important when the route of transmission is considered because food-borne inocula may be considerably greater than water-borne inocula. (2) The method of vaccine preparation is important. Acetone-killed and preserved vaccine is more effective than the classic heat-killed, phenol-preserved vaccine. (3) Two doses are better than one; both increase the degree and duration of protection. The recommended routes and schedules for immunization are arbitrary and are based on tradition rather than data. From the field trial experiences, however, a reasonable primary schedule would include two 0.5 ml subcutaneous injections of acetone-inactivated vaccine given four weeks apart. In endemic regions, boosters should probably be given every three years. While the acetone vaccine is intended for subcutaneous (or intramuscular) inoculation, the phenol vaccine can be administered intradermally by Jet injection. However, the primary injection should be given by syringe because it is difficult to guarantee delivery of the required dose by Jet injector. The Jet method is suitable for revaccination (booster doses).

Because of new concepts of mucosal immunity, recent studies have been directed towards production of an oral vaccine in order to promote local resistance in the small intestine, the initial site of infection. There is still controversy about the efficacy of live attenuated or dead virulent oral vaccines. Live vaccines are more likely to activate mucosal and cell-mediated immune responses, but dead vaccines are safer because they preclude the possibility of reversion to virulence. The few human studies of killed oral vaccine have been disappointing. Because the critical protective antigen is undefined, these failures may represent specific faults of the vaccines rather than the general method. On the other hand, oral vaccination with a live mutant, which synthesizes incomplete O antigen because it lacks UDP-glucose-4-epimerase, is very effective (Warren and Hornick, 1979). When grown in excess exogenous galac-

tose, this mutant synthesizes complete O side chains but eventually lyses. Volunteers immunized orally with this mutant grown in excess galactose had a lower incidence of illness and duration of fecal carriage following oral challenge with virulent *S. typhi*. However, multiple doses of the vaccine were given, and the duration of the immunity was not determined.

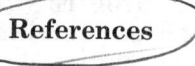

## References

Butler, T., Linh, N. N., Arnold, K., Adickman, M. D., Chau, D. M., and Muoi, M. M.: Therapy of antimicrobial resistant typhoid fever. Antimicrob Ag Chemother 11:645, 1977.

Christie, A. N.: Typhoid and paratyphoid fevers. In Infectious Diseases: Epidemiology and Clinical Practice. London, E & S Livingstone, Ltd., 1969, pp. 54–121.

Duggan, M. D., and Beyer, L.: Enteric fever in young Yoruba children. Arch Dis Childh 50:67, 1975.

Gilman, R. H., Terminel, M., Levine, M. M., Hernandez-Mendoza, P., and Hornick, R. B.: Relative efficacy of blood, urine, rectal swabs, bone marrow and Rose spot cultures for recognition of *Salmonella typhi* in typhoid fever. Lancet 1:1211, 1975.

Gulati, P. D., Saxena, S. N., Gupta, P. S., and Chuttani, H. K.: Changing pattern of typhoid fever. Am J Med 45:544, 1968.

Hornick, R. B., Greisman, S. E., Woodward, T. E., DuPont, H. L., Dawkins, A. T., and Snyder, M. J.: Typhoid fever: Pathogenesis and immunologic control. New Engl J Med 283:686, 739, 1970.

Johnson, W. D., Jr., Hook, E. W., Lindsey, E., and Kaye, D.: Treatment of chronic typhoid carriers with ampicillin. Antimicrob Ag Chemother 3:439, 1973.

Kim, J. P., Oh, S. K., and Jarrett, F.: Management of ileal perforation due to typhoid fever. Ann Surg 181:88, 1975.

Overturf, G., Martin, K. I., and Mathies, A. W., Jr.: Antibiotic resistance in typhoid fever. New Engl J Med 289:463, 1973.

Samantry, S. K., Johnson, S. C., and Chakrabarti, A. K.: Enteric fever: An analysis of 500 cases. Practitioner 218:400, 1977.

Scragg, J. N.: Further experience with amoxycillin in typhoid fever in children. Br Med J 2:1031, 1976.

Scragg, J., Rubridge, C., and Wallace, H. L.: Typhoid fever in African and Indian children in Durban. Arch Dis Childh 44:18, 1969.

Warren, J. W., and Hornick, R. B.: Immunization against typhoid fever. Annu Rev Med 30:457, 1979.

Wicks, A. C. B., Cruickshank, J. G., and Musewe, N.: Observations on the diagnosis of typhoid fever. S Afr Med J 68:1368, 1974.

# *GONOCOCCEMIA* **180**

## *J. Allen McCutchan, M.D.*

### DEFINITION

Gonococci infecting the genitalia, pharynx, or rectum may invade the blood to produce a variety of syndromes collectively called disseminated gonococcal infection (DGI). Patients with DGI usually have no symptoms of gonorrhea because DGI complicates asymptomatic infection. Arthritis-dermatitis, the most common form of DGI, is characterized by fever and chills, typical skin lesions, and arthralgias or transient arthritis. Gonococcal septic arthritis, a less common form of DGI, is a typical, culture-positive, purulent ar-

thritis with minimal systemic symptoms and negative blood cultures. Metastatic infection of the heart (endocarditis or pericarditis) or the meninges is rare. In contrast to meningococci, gonococci in the blood do not produce shock or disseminated intravascular coagulation and thus rarely kill patients.

### ETIOLOGY

*Neisseria gonorrhoeae* and gonococcal infections without gonococcemia are discussed elsewhere in this volume. Gonococci from cases of DGI are usually resistant to killing by serum, very sensitive to penicillin, nutritionally fastidious, and slow growing. These traits (DGI biotype), which help to explain some features of disseminated gonococcal infections, occur less frequently in gonococci that cause local infections.

Almost all DGI isolates resist killing by antibody and complement in normal human sera (Schoolnik et al., 1976). This resistance results from the binding of a natural IgG antibody that blocks killing by bactericidal IgM antibody (McCutchan et al., 1978). Resistant gonococci avidly bind the blocking antibody to their surfaces, but sensitive strains do not. Since many gonococci that cause only local infections also resist killing by serum but do not invade the blood, serum resistance is necessary but not sufficient for dissemination.

Gonococci that cause DGI are extremely sensitive to penicillin (minimum inhibitory concentration is less than 0.03 $\mu$g/ml) (Weisner et al., 1973). In contrast, gonococci causing local infection have become increasingly resistant (see Chapter 149). Disseminated gonococci cannot synthesize certain nutrients made by most local strains. By adding these growth factors (e.g., proline, arginine, hypoxanthine, or uracil) to nutritionally deficient media, the pattern of growth requirements (auxotype) of gonococci can be determined. Gonococci requiring either proline or the triad of arginine, hypoxanthine, and uracil (AHU), or both are isolated much more commonly from disseminated disease than from local disease. The proportion of various auxotypes varies geographically. For example, in the northwestern United States, AHU-negative strains cause about 90 per cent of recent DGI. In the southeastern United States, about 25 per cent of DGI strains are AHU-negative, and 50 per cent are proline-negative. Since the mucosal infections in patients with DGI are usually asymptomatic, it is significant that AHU-negative gonococci also cause most cases of asymptomatic urethritis (Crawford et al., 1977). Because they cause no symptoms, nutritionally dependent gonococci escape treatment and by persisting increase their chances of invading the blood. Careful examination of these traits (serum resistance, penicillin susceptibility, and auxotype) suggests that they are not genetically linked (Eisenstein et al., 1977). Each trait probably promotes dissemination independently. Identical gonococci are isolated from mucosal and disseminated sites in patients with DGI and from their contacts. Thus, it appears that only those patients initially infected with strains capable of invading the blood are at risk for DGI.

DGI strains are more difficult to grow, their colonies are smaller, and they are more sensitive to undefined, methanol-soluble toxins in agar. These properties may be related to their nutritional dependence and help to account for the difficulty encountered in growing gonococci from some patients with clinically typical DGI.

Finally, gonococci from DGI compete for iron, an essential nutrient, more successfully than other strains. In experimental infections of the chick embryo, isolates from DGI kill the embryo independently of iron, whereas local strains are rendered less virulent when iron chelators are administered (Payne et al., 1978).

## PATHOGENESIS AND PATHOLOGY

Although certain characteristics of gonococci determine their potential for dissemination, the sporadic pattern of DGI suggests that the response by the patient is more important than virulence in determining who gets DGI. If the virulence of certain strains were the key factor, epidemics of DGI would be common. Paired cases and a "microepidemic" have been reported, but infected partners of patients with DGI rarely develop infection. Two groups of patients appear to be at increased risk for gonococcemia: women during the menses and pregnancy and patients with genetic deficiency of the terminal components of complement. Alterations in levels of sex hormones may explain the increased frequency of dissemination at the menses and during pregnancy. In addition, mucin and hemoglobin, which flood the endocervix at the menses, may increase gonococcal invasiveness. When gonococci are injected into the peritoneal cavities of mice, they multiply, invade the blood, and kill the animals only if mucin and hemoglobin are added (Corbeil et al., 1978). Neisserial bacteremias recur in patients with congenital deficiency of one of the terminal components of complement (Table 1).

TABLE 1.  Association of Neisserial Bacteremias and Deficiency of the Terminal Components of Complement

| DEFICIENT C COMPONENT | TYPE OF NEISSERIAL INFECTION | | TOTAL NEISSERIAL INFECTIONS |
|---|---|---|---|
| | DGI[a] | MI[b] | |
| C6 | 2/6[c] | 5/6 | 6/6 |
| C7 | 1/11 | 4/11 | 5/11 |
| C8 | 2/8 | 1/8 | 3/8 |
| Total | 5/25 | 10/25 | 14/25 |

[a]DGI, Disseminated gonococcal infection.

[b]MI, Meningococcal infection (implies bacteremia).

[c]No. of infections/no. of complement-deficient patients at risk.

Data from Petersen et al., 1979.

Since these components (C6 through C9) mediate lysis of gonococci but not opsonization or chemotaxis, gonococci are phagocytosed but not killed in their sera. The striking association of complement deficiency with recurrent DGI emphasizes the importance of complement-mediated bacteriolysis in protection against DGI. However, since most patients with DGI have normal levels of hemolytic complement, complement deficiency explains only a minority of cases of DGI.

Susceptibility to gonococcemia, unlike that to meningococcemia, is not predictable except in these rare patients with complement deficiency. Patients with either type of neisserial bacteremia (gonococcal or meningococcal) lack complement-mediated serum bactericidal activity against their infecting strain. Patients whose serum does not kill their colonizing meningococcal strain are at high risk for meningococcemia in epidemics (Goldschneider et al., 1969). This susceptibility apparently results from inexperience with the infecting strain and can be corrected by immunization with meningococcal vaccine, which enhances bactericidal activity. Patients fail to kill DGI strains because blocking antibody protects the strains from bactericidal antibody. Since these blocking antibodies against gonococci are present in most people, almost no one can kill DGI strains. Because most carriers of gonococci do not develop DGI, something other than serum bactericidal activity must protect them from gonococcemia.

Two stages of DGI are recognized (Keiser et al., 1968). In the bacteremic (arthritis-dermatitis) stage, gonococci can be cultured from the blood and skin but not from the joints. In the septic joint stage, the blood is sterile, but gonococci are found in one or a few infected joints. Patients presenting with arthritis-dermatitis have had symptoms for an average of three days, and patients with septic joints for eight days. Not all patients with septic joints have antecedent polyarthritis or dermatitis, and some patients have features of both syndromes. It appears that bacteremia produces polyarthritis early and that septic arthritis develops only after bacteremia is over.

Joint fluid from patients with polyarthritis is sterile despite positive blood cultures. The polyarthritis resembles that seen in acute immune complex diseases (i.e., serum sickness or the prodrome of hepatitis B). Circulating immune complexes are found in the majority of DGI patients and are associated with joint disease and a history of previous gonococcal infection but not skin rash (Walker et al., 1978). A possible interpretation is that the initial polyarthritis results from immune complex disease that favors localization of circulating gonococci in joints. Since most people have natural antibodies to gonococci, the formation of immune complexes may not require an antibody response to the infection.

In gonococcal dermatitis skin biopsy shows collections of neutrophils and monocytes around small arteries in the dermis. Lysis of white cells around arterioles produces leukocytoclastic angiitis, which is often associated with allergic diseases (Seifert et al., 1974). Gonococci grow from only a minority of lesions but are frequently seen after immunofluorescent antibody staining (Barr and Danielsson, 1971). Thus, circulating gonococci seem to localize in dermal arterioles and evoke an immune cellular response.

In acute septic arthritis, the synovial membranes are invaded by an intense cellular infiltrate of polymorphonuclear leukocytes, lymphocytes, macrophages, and neutrophils. A lymphocytic perivascular infiltrate develops in the deeper synovium, and gonococci can be seen in the tissues. The synovium is destroyed and replaced by granulation tissue, and the underlying cartilage may be invaded and destroyed.

Untreated patients dying of gonococcal endocarditis in the pre-antibiotic era resembled patients with other forms of subacute endocarditis (Williams, 1938). Similar valves (aortic, mitral, pulmonary, tricuspid) were involved and similar complications (nephritis, myocarditis, splenitis, arterial emboli) were found postmortem. Most patients died of cardiac or renal failure.

A striking but unexplained feature of DGI is the inverse relationship between the degree of local inflammation and dissemination: most patients with DGI have asymptomatic local infection, and those with pelvic inflammatory disease seldom develop DGI. Thus, vigorous local inflammation may prevent dissemination. As discussed in the previous section, the nutritional fastidiousness and consequent slow growth of DGI strains may explain why they elicit little local inflammation.

## CLINICAL COURSE AND COMPLICATIONS

DGI causes clinical syndromes ranging from low-grade fever or dermatitis alone to severe metastatic infection of joints, heart, or meninges. Bacteremia is usually a complication of asymptomatic local infection, especially of the pharynx; less frequently it arises from symptomatic genital infections and rarely occurs with pelvic inflammatory disease. Dissemination occurs more frequently during the first week of the menstrual cycle or during pregnancy and perhaps most frequently after genital trauma. Most patients have an acute febrile illness with polyarthritis of the hands, knees, wrists, ankles, or feet. When poly-

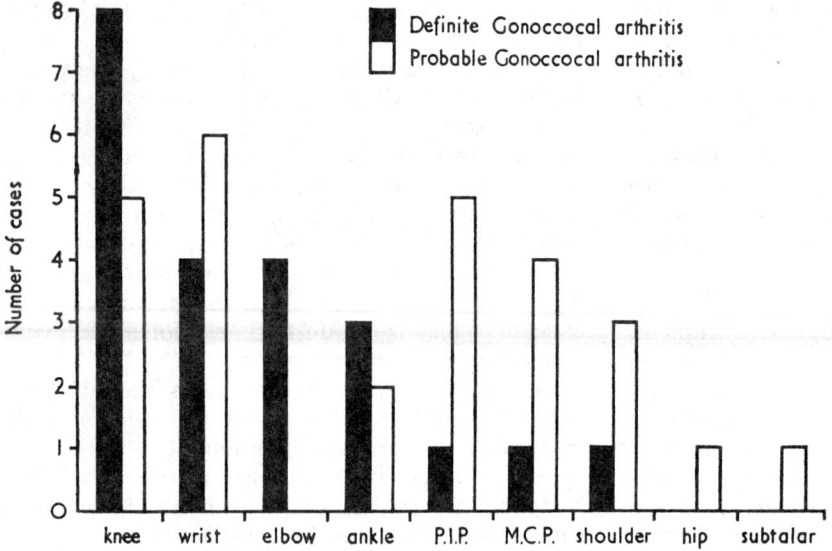

**FIGURE 1.** *Frequency of involvement of various joints in gonococcemia.*

arthritis accompanies the characteristic dermatitis in a sexually active young person, the diagnosis of disseminated gonococcal infection can be made at the bedside.

### Uncomplicated Gonococcemia (Arthritis-Dermatitis Syndrome)

The cardinal symptoms of gonococcemia are fever, chills, malaise, polyarthritis, and dermatitis. Any or all of these symptoms may be absent. In addition to arthritis and dermatitis, asymptomatic myocarditis (transient electrocardiographic changes) and hepatitis (elevated liver enzymes) can be found in about half the patients (Holmes et al., 1971). Polyarthritis occurs in about 90 per cent of patients with gonococcemia and has a migratory or additive pattern, small effusions, and less than 20,000 white cells per mm³ in sterile joint fluids (Handsfield, 1975). The knee is most commonly affected, followed by the wrists, hands, ankles, feet, elbows, and shoulders (Fig. 1). Arthralgia, often without arthritis, is usually the first symptom and is succeeded by fever, chills, malaise, and frank arthritis. Periarticular inflammation, especially tenosynovitis, is frequent. Dermatitis is present in 50 to 70 per cent of patients. Lesions start as small red papules on an erythematous base and may evolve through vesicular, pustular, hemorrhagic, and occasionally bullous or necrotic stages (Fig. 2). These skin lesions usually are tender and number between 2 and 10 per patient. They are found on the hands and feet (including the palms and soles) or near the joints but spare the head, trunk, and mucous membranes. Lesions may be in various stages of development. They evolve over one to three days, are arrested by therapy, and heal quickly (three to seven days) and completely unless they are necrotic.

### Septic Arthritis

Patients with gonococcal septic arthritis complain of severe pain in one or two joints with only minimal systemic symptoms. They often report antecedent fever, malaise, polyarthritis, or dermatitis that resolved without treatment. On average their symptoms have been present longer than those of patients with uncomplicated gonococcemia. Septic arthritis involves the same joints, especially the knees, wrists, and ankles, as gonococcal polyarthritis. Joint fluid is usually purulent with more than 20,000 leukocytes per mm³ and more than 75 per cent polymorphonuclear leukocytes. Gonococci can be grown from the joint in about half the cases and can be seen by Gram stain or fluorescent antibody staining in some of the sterile fluids. Untreated arthritis progressively destroys the joint and leads to periarticular fibrosis and adhesions between articular cartilages (Keefer and Spink, 1937). Response to treatment is slower in patients with septic arthritis than in those with polyarthritis, but residual joint dysfunction is unusual six months after treatment.

### Endocarditis

*Neisseria gonorrhoeae* was an important cause of endocarditis in the pre-antibiotic era, accounting for 20 to 25 per cent in several series (Jones, 1950; Williams, 1938), but it is rare in developed countries today. Gonococci usually infect normal cardiac valves, involve the right heart about one-third of the time, and create large vegetations that frequently embolize (Thayer, 1922). The course of untreated gonococcal endocarditis is intermediate in length and severity between the subacute disease cause by *Streptococcus viridans* and the acute disease caused by the pneumococ-

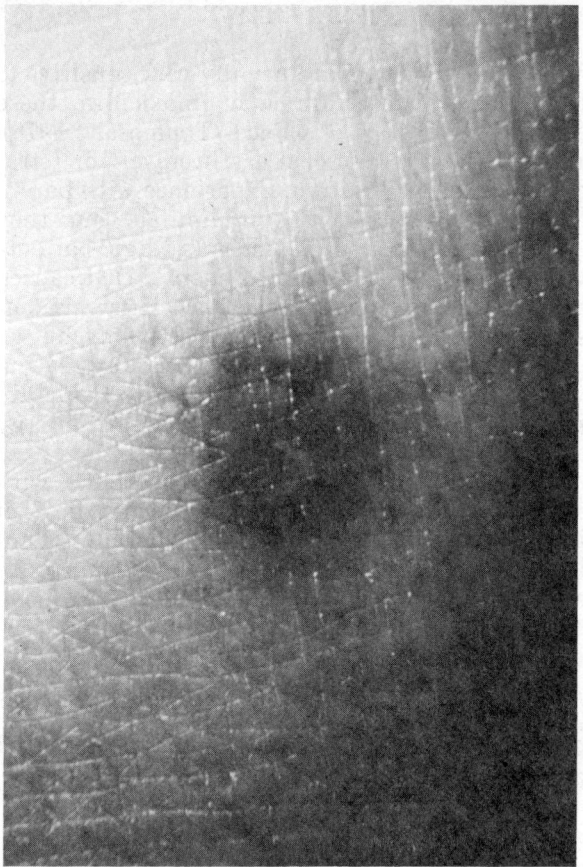

**FIGURE 2.** *Skin lesion of gonococcemia.*

cus and *Staphylococcus aureus*. Fever, chills, arthritis, skin lesions, cardiac murmurs, mild hepatitis, and markedly elevated sedimentation rates and white blood counts are characteristic. Only a new pathologic cardiac murmur or embolus differentiates clearly endocarditis from benign gonococcemia, but sustained gonococcemia, anemia, nephritis, or a very high erythrocyte sedimentation rate at presentation (>100) should suggest endocarditis. Complications include arterial emboli, myocarditis, pericarditis, nephritis with renal failure, and valvular destruction with cardiac failure. Before the antibiotic era only a few untreated patients survived. Antibiotic therapy has cured most of the recently reported cases.

### Gonococcal Meningitis

In contrast to the frequency of meningeal infection with meningococci, gonococcal meningitis is rare. Of 16 cases collected by Holmes et al. (1971), six had skin lesions, nine had arthritis, three of six had positive blood cultures, and only three of nine untreated patients died. All treated cases survived. Cerebrospinal fluids show the typical polymorphonuclear pleocytosis and low glucose levels typical of bacterial meningitis. Because

only one saccharolytic reaction differentiates meningococci from gonococci, *Neisseria* organisms isolated from cerebrospinal fluid (CSF) should not agglutinate in meningococcal capsular antiserum, should fail to grow in the absence of carbon dioxide, and should bind gonococcal fluorescent antibody before being called gonococci.

## EPIDEMIOLOGY AND GEOGRAPHIC VARIATION

Patients with DGI resemble in age and behavior the larger population of patients with gonorrhea. In the pre-antibiotic era, most cases of DGI occurred in men, probably because untreated urethritis produced prolonged infections that increased the risk of dissemination. In the early antibiotic era, when men were rapidly treated but asymptomatic women carrying gonococci remained untreated, DGI was reported predominantly in women. Now the increased recognition of asymptomatic gonorrhea in men has led to routine cultures of the urethra and pharynx in men with possible DGI. With this approach a recent prospective study found that DGI occurred in nearly equal numbers of men and women (Handsfield et al., 1976). Thus, the sex distribution and the frequency of dissemination probably depend on the number of patients carrying gonococci that can invade the blood.

The emergence in some areas of the world of the DGI biotype (auxotrophic, penicillin-sensitive, and serum-resistant gonococci) may have increased both asymptomatic disease in men and DGI in both sexes. DGI appears to have increased during the past 20 years along with uncomplicated gonorrhea. Rates of dissemination as high as 1 to 3 per cent have been calculated, but marked geographic variation occurs. In the western Pacific area, where the DGI biotype is rare (Knapp and Holmes, 1975), DGI is also rare despite high rates of gonorrhea in some populations. Penicillinase-producing *Neisseria gonorrhoeae* are found predominantly in the western Pacific, are probably not of the DGI biotype, and rarely cause DGI.

## DIAGNOSIS

DGI is diagnosed clinically from combinations of dermatitis, arthritis, symptoms of gonorrhea, or a history of recent unusual sexual exposures. Symptomatic gonorrhea occurs in only a minority of patients with DGI, but it is a helpful sign when present. Polyarthritis and typical dermatitis in a sexually active young adult is nearly diagnostic. On the west coast of the United States, where

DGI is common, gonococci cause over half the hospital admissions for acute arthritis in adults under 30 years of age. Gonococcal dermatitis is often so characteristic in location and appearance that a presumptive diagnosis can be made even in the absence of arthritis.

When gonococcemia is suspected, cultures of blood, the genitalia, pharynx, and rectum should be taken (see Chapter 149). Standard blood culture media incubated aerobically are suitable for isolation of gonococci from blood. Positive cultures are most frequently obtained from genital sites, but occasionally only the pharynx or rectum yields the gonococcus. Joint fluid, if obtained, should always be cultured and is frequently positive if many (>80,000 per mm$^3$) polymorphonuclear leukocytes are present. Immunofluorescent stains frequently detect gonococci in skin lesions and buffy coats of blood even when cultures of these sites are negative.

Gonococcemia must be distinguished from several similar diseases. Polyarthritis, dermatitis, and fever occur in Reiter's syndrome, acute rheumatic fever, meningococcemia, the prodrome of hepatitis B, and various other infections and immunologic diseases. Reiter's syndrome (arthritis, dermatitis, urethritis, and conjunctivitis) can simulate several features of gonococcemia and was unknowingly included in some early reviews of gonococcal arthritis. Outbreaks of Reiter's syndrome following epidemics of diarrhea caused by *Shigella*, *Salmonella*, or *Yersinia* are easily recognized. The endemic (or venereal) form, occurring primarily in sexually active, often promiscuous young men with the HLA-B27 histocompatibility antigen, is more easily confused with DGI. Although Reiter's disease may follow gonococcal or nongonococcal urethritis, neither gonococci nor the agents of nongonococcal urethritis are as well established antecedents of Reiter's syndrome as the agents of bacterial diarrheas. The distribution of involved joints simulates that of gonococcal arthritis, but the characteristic skin lesions of Reiter's syndrome (keratodermia blenorrhagica and balanitis circinata) differ from those of gonococcemia. In addition, Reiter's syndrome does not respond to antibiotics and often relapses. Skin lesions of acute rheumatic fever are uncommon, do not resemble gonococcal dermatitis, and progress despite antibiotics. Meningococcemia frequently produces petechiae and rarely causes lesions that are indistinguishable from gonococcal dermatitis. The prodromes of hepatitis B, serum sickness, and other immune complex diseases produce polyarthritis, but their skin lesions (petechiae, urticaria, and erythemas) are easily differentiated from gonococcal dermatitis.

## TREATMENT

Because gonococci are usually very sensitive to penicillin G, ampicillin, and amoxicillin, these are the antibiotics of choice (Thompson, 1979). Seven-day courses of oral erythromycin or tetracycline are also effective. Experience with parenteral cephem antibiotics is limited, but they should be effective in penicillin-allergic patients who are unable to take oral agents. DGI caused by penicillinase-producing gonococci is rare but should respond to cefoxitin or spectinomycin.

Table 2 lists acceptable regimens for treating various syndromes of gonococcemia. Penicillin regimens are preferred unless penicillin allergy or penicillinase-producing gonococci are involved. Although some physicians treat patients with septic arthritis for 10 to 14 days, three days of intravenous high-dose penicillin therapy (Blankenship, 1974) or seven days of oral ampicillin and amoxicillin (Handsfield et al., 1976) have been uniformly successful. Septic arthritis does not require surgical drainage (except perhaps in the hip), and intra-articular injections of antibiotics are contraindicated. Joint immobilization, repeated aspiration of purulent joint fluid, and

### TABLE 2.    Treatment of Disseminated Gonococcal Infections

**UNCOMPLICATED GONOCOCCEMIA AND SEPTIC ARTHRITIS**

**Intravenous**
1. Penicillin G, 10 million ($10^7$) units daily in four divided doses (2.5 mU) every six hours for three days; in neonates or children use 100,000 ($10^5$) u/kg/day for three to seven days
2. Cefoxitin, 8.0 g daily in four divided doses (2.0 g every six hours) for seven days
3. Cefazolin, 3.0 g daily in three divided doses (1.0 g every eight hours) for seven days

**Intramuscular**
1. Spectinomycin, 2 g intramuscularly every 12 hours for three days
2. Procaine penicillin G, 1.2 million units daily (600,000 units every 12 hours) for seven days

**Oral**
1. Ampicillin or amoxicillin, 0.5 g every six hours for seven days after either ampicillin, 3.5 g plus probenecid, 1.0 g or amoxicillin, 3.0 g
2. Tetracycline or erythromycin, 0.5 g every six hours for seven days

**GONOCOCCAL ENDOCARDITIS (INTRAVENOUS)**
1. Penicillin G, 8 million units daily intravenously (1.0 million units every three hours) for three weeks
2. Cefoxitin, 8 g daily intravenously (1.0 g every three hours) for three weeks

**GONOCOCCAL MENINGITIS (INTRAVENOUS)**
1. Penicillin G, 4 million units daily intravenously (2 g every two hours) for ten days
2. Chloramphenicol, 8 g daily intravenously (1 g every three hours) for ten days

anti-inflammatory agents may be used, but their efficacy has not been studied. Gonococcal endocarditis should be treated with three to four weeks of parenteral penicillin because experience with shorter regimens and other drugs is not available. Because of poor penetration into the CSF, high doses of penicillin G or chloramphenicol (in penicillin-allergic patients) are recommended for meningitis.

## References

Barr, J., and Danielsson, D.: Septic gonococcal dermatitis. Br Med J 1:482, 1971.

Blankenship, R. M., Holmes, R. K., and Sanford, J. P.: Treatment of disseminated gonococcal infection. N Engl J Med 290:267, 1974.

Corbeil, L. B., Wunderlich, A. C., McCutchan, J. A., and Braude, A. I.: in Brooks, G. F. (ed.): Immunobiology of Neisseria gonorrhoeae. Washington, D.C., American Society for Microbiology, 1978, p. 318.

Crawford, G., Knapp, J. S., Hale, J., and Holmes, K. K.: Asymptomatic gonorrhea in men: Caused by gonococci with unique nutritional requirements. Science 196:1352, 1977.

Eisenstein, B., Lee, T. J., and Sparling, P. F.: Penicillin sensitivity and serum resistance are independent attributes of strains of Neisseria gonorrhoeae causing disseminated gonococcal infection. Infect Immun 15:834, 1977.

Goldschneider, I., Gotschlich, E. C., and Artenstein, M. S.: Human immunity to the meningococcus. I. The role of humoral antibodies. J Exp Med 129:1307, 1969.

Handsfield, H. H.: Disseminated gonococcal infection. Clin Obstet Gynecol 18:131, 1975.

Handsfield, H. H., Weisner, P. J., and Holmes, K. K.: Treatment of the gonococcal arthritis-dermatitis syndrome. Ann Intern Med 84:661, 1976.

Holmes, K. K., Counts, G. W., and Beaty, H. N.: Disseminated gonococcal infection. Ann Intern Med 74:979, 1971.

Jones, M.: Subacute bacterial endocarditis of non-streptococcic etiology. Am Heart J 40:106, 1950.

Keefer, C. S., and Spink, W. W.: Gonococcic arthritis: Pathogenesis, mechanism of recovery and treatment. JAMA 109:1448, 1937.

Keiser, H., Ruben, F. L., Wolinsky, E., and Kushner, I.: Clinical forms of gonococcal arthritis. N Engl J Med 279:233, 1968.

Knapp, J. S., and Holmes, K. K.: Disseminated gonococcal infection caused by Neisseria gonorrhoeae with unique nutritional requirements. J Infect Dis 132:204, 1975.

McCutchan, J. A., Katzenstein, D., Norquist, D., Chikami, G., Wunderlich, A., and Braude, A. I.: Role of blocking antibody in disseminated gonococcal infection. J Immunol 121:1884, 1978.

Payne, S. M., Holmes, K. K., and Finkelstein, R. A.: Role of iron in disseminated gonococcal infections. Infect Immun 20:573, 1978.

Partain, J. O., Cathcart, E. S., and Cohen, A. S.: Arthritis associated with gonorrhea. Ann Rheum Dis 27:156, 1968.

Petersen, B. H., Lee, I. J., Synderman, R., and Brooks, G. F.: Neisseria meningitidis and Neisseria gonorrhoeae bacteremia associated with C6, C7, and C8 deficiency. Ann Intern Med 90:917, 1979.

Seifert, M. H., Warin, A. P., and Miller, A.: Articular and cutaneous manifestations of gonorrhea. Ann Rheum Dis 33:140, 1974.

Schoolnik, G. K., Buchanan, T. M., and Holmes, K. K.: Gonococci causing disseminated gonococcal infection are resistant to the bactericidal action of normal human serum. J Clin Invest 58:1163, 1976.

Thayer, W. S.: On the cardiac complications of gonorrhea. Bull Johns Hopkins Hosp 33:361, 1922.

Thompson, S. E.: Treatment of disseminated gonococcal infections. Sex Transmitted Dis 6:181, 1979.

Walker, L. C., Ahlin, T. D., Tung, K. S. K., and Williams, R. C.: Circulating immune complexes and disseminated gonorrheal infection. Ann Intern Med 88:28, 1978.

Weisner, P. J., Handsfield, H. H., and Holmes, K. K.: Low antibiotic resistance of gonococci causing disseminated infection. N Engl J Med 288:1221, 1973.

Williams, R. H.: Gonococcic endocarditis. Arch Intern Med 61:26, 1938.

# MENINGOCOCCEMIA 181

## Thomas Allan Hoffman, M.D.

### DEFINITION

Invasion of the bloodstream by *Neisseria meningitidis* causes a spectrum of disease ranging from a benign transient bacteremia to an overwhelming infection that is rapidly fatal. Meningitis commonly begins during the course of meningococcemia. Meningococcal disease occurs sporadically or as large-scale epidemics throughout the world. The incidence of meningococcal disease is highest in children from six months to one year of age and then declines. Meningococcal disease also breaks out frequently in military recruits.

### ETIOLOGY

*N. meningitidis* is a gram-negative diplococcus, commonly named the meningococcus. It grows well on solid media supplemented with blood and incubated in a moist $CO_2$-enriched atmosphere, and in liquid media used to culture blood aerobically. After 24 hours it should be subcultured onto blood agar or chocolate agar because turbidity may be difficult to recognize. Oxidase and catalase are biochemical markers for preliminary identification and sugar fermentations for final identification of the species. *N. meningitidis* ferments glucose and maltose, but not sucrose or lactose. Agglutination reactions with immune serum subdivide the species into serogroups A, B, C, X, Y, and Z, and depend upon a group-specific capsular polysaccharide antigen. The group A meningococcal polysaccharide consists mainly of acetylated mannosamine phosphate whereas the group C polysaccharide is a polymer of acetylated sialic acid (Goldschneider et al., 1969). Sialic acid is also found in the group B polysaccharide, but it is antigenically distinct from that in group C polysaccharide (Goldschneider et al., 1969). Most strains causing meningococcal disease have the polysaccharide antigen of groups A, B, or C. Group Y meningococci cause disease infrequently but more commonly than groups X and Z, which are rarely associated with disease. Meningococcal strains that lack these group-specific antigens are thought to be nonpathogenic.

The cell wall of pathogenic meningococci contains a toxic lipopolysaccharide or endotoxin. Meningococcal endotoxin appears to be chemically identical to endotoxin of enteric bacilli, but meningococcal endotoxin has greater potency for inducing the dermal Shwartzman reaction than enteric endotoxin (Davis and Arnold, 1974). Since the dermal Shwartzman reaction is the experimental equivalent of meningococcal purpura, endotoxin appears to be the cause of certain meningococcal lesions (Sotto et al., 1976).

Meningococci are susceptible to several antimicrobial agents. The activity of penicillin G against these organisms is greater than that of other penicillins or cephalothin. Minimal inhibitory concentrations of penicillin G usually range between 0.02 and 0.2 $\mu$g/ml. Chloramphenicol, erythromycin, and tetracyclines are also active against meningococci. Meningococci have appeared that are resistant to 0.01 mg of sulfadiazine per milliliter and disk sensitivity testing with sulfathiazole is reliable for determining sulfonamide susceptibility. Meningococci are not susceptible to vancomycin, polymyxin, or achievable serum levels of aminoglycoside antibiotics.

## PATHOGENESIS AND PATHOLOGY

The nasopharynx of man is the only known reservoir of meningococcal infection. Meningococci are spread from person to person by airborne droplets of infected nasopharyngeal secretions. Organisms attach to mucosal surfaces where droplets deposit. Concomitant viral respiratory infection, particularly infection by influenza viruses, appears to enhance the spread of meningococcal infection and the likelihood of nasopharyngeal carriage after exposure to meningococci. Meningococcal infection of the nasopharynx produces at most few symptoms and is usually subclinical. Asymptomatic nasopharyngeal carriage of meningococci is transient and resolves within several weeks. In a few individuals the infection invades the circulation, causing either transient bacteremia, metastatic infection that most commonly involves the meninges, or a fulminant, overwhelming systemic infection with circulatory collapse. Many of the manifestations of this fulminant form of meningococcemia can be reproduced experimentally by meningococcal endotoxin. This substance can cause hypotension,

margination of circulating leukocytes, aggregation of platelets, and disseminated intravascular clotting (Davis and Arnold, 1974; Mellins et al., 1972).

The fundamental pathologic change in meningococcemia is widespread vascular injury characterized by endothelial necrosis, intraluminal thrombosis, and perivascular hemorrhage (Sotto et al., 1976; Mellins et al., 1972; Hoffman and Edwards, 1972). Organisms in blood invade through damaged vessels in the skin and elicit a perivascular infiltration of neutrophils. Skin lesions usually contain numerous meningococci undergoing phagocytosis by neutrophils. Occlusive thrombi composed of platelets, red blood cells, and fibrin are most prominent in vessels deep in the dermis and suggest a local Shwartzman reaction (Sotto et al., 1976). Immunologic factors probably contribute to vascular injury, since the walls of damaged vessels usually contain deposits of immunoglobulins, complement, and meningococcal antigen (Sotto et al., 1976). Serous surfaces and other organs have the same vascular injury (Mellins et al., 1972), although bacteria are difficult to find in tissues other than the skin.

Patients who die of meningococcemia develop thrombosis and hemorrhage in the skin, mucous membranes, serosal surfaces, adrenal sinusoids, and renal glomeruli (Hoffman and Edwards, 1972; Wolf and Birbara, 1968). Adrenal hemorrhage is rarely extensive. Thrombosis of the glomerular capillaries may cause renal cortical necrosis, the chief characteristic of the generalized Shwartzman reaction, which can be induced experimentally by meningococcal endotoxin (Davis and Arnold, 1974). In the lung, thrombi containing numerous leukocytes are occasionally seen, and extensive intra-alveolar hemorrhage can occur. Myocarditis has been frequent in adults with fatal meningococcal infections (Hoffman and Edwards, 1972; Wolf and Birbara, 1968).

Susceptibility to meningococcal disease has been correlated with the absence of bactericidal antibody against pathogenic meningococci (Goldschneider et al., 1969). Bactericidal activity is mediated by IgG antibodies that have specificity for the meningococcal polysaccharides; however, activation of the complement system is required for expression of this activity. Asymptomatic carriage of meningococci in the nasopharynx induces a humoral antibody response and most individuals acquire immunity to meningococcal disease by age 20. Passively transferred maternal antibody provides temporary protection to infants for the first six months. Colonization with nonpathogenic meningococci seems to induce cross-reacting, protective antibodies. An episode of meningococcal disease confers group-specific immunity, but a second episode may be caused by another meningococcal serogroup. Complement deficiencies may allow repeated episodes of severe meningococcal infection.

## CLINICAL MANIFESTATIONS

The clinical pattern of meningococcemia is varied (Hoffman and Edwards, 1972; Wolf and Birbara, 1968). The mildest form is a transient bacteremic illness that begins insidiously with fever and malaise. Petechial skin lesions do not appear in this form and the symptoms resolve spontaneously within one to two days. It is learned, subsequently, that N. meningitidis was recovered from blood cultures obtained during the febrile episode.

Acute meningococcemia is more serious. After a few days of upper respiratory prodromal symptoms, the temperature rises abruptly, often after a chill. Malaise, weakness, myalgias, headache, nausea, vomiting, and arthralgias are frequent presenting symptoms. The most characteristic manifestation of meningococcemia is the skin rash, which is essential for its recognition (Wolf and Birbara, 1968). Petechiae are the most common type of skin lesion and they may be sparsely distributed over the body. Ill-defined pink macules have sometimes been noted. Maculopapular lesions also occur and are sometimes large plaque-like lesions with a central petechia. The skin lesions of meningococcemia tend to occur in crops, and on any part of the body, although the face is usually spared and involvement of the palms and soles is less common. Petechiae are occasionally present on the conjunctiva and mucous membranes. The skin rash may advance from a few ill-defined lesions to a widespread eruption within a few hours. Patients with acute meningococcemia usually present with moderate fever (average 39.5° C) and marked leukocytosis (average 19,000/mm$^3$). Signs of shock are not present. Coagulation is normal except for elevated fibrinogen (Hoffman and Edwards, 1972). Other acute phase reactants, such as the serum complement, may be elevated.

Fulminant meningococcemia is the most serious form of meningococcal disease because of the high mortality rate. This form, which is also called the Waterhouse-Friderichsen syndrome, occurs in approximately 5 to 15 per cent of the cases of meningococcal disease (Hoffman and Edwards, 1972). It begins abruptly with sudden high fever, chills, myalgias, weakness, nausea, vomiting, and headache. Apprehension, restlessness, and frequently delirium occur within the next few hours. The rash appears suddenly and is widespread, purpuric, and ecchymotic. Hemorrhages appear on the buccal mucosa and conjunctiva. Less frequently, this form presents as purpura fulminans and, rarely, no skin lesions are recognized. Typically, no signs of meningitis are present. Cyanosis, hypotension, and profound shock eventually appear. Patients with the fulminant form of meningococcemia usually present with a high fever (average of 40.6° C) and either a normal WBC count or leukopenia. The blood pressure is lowered and shock may be present. Thrombocytopenia and other changes of disseminated intravascular clotting are also present (Hoffman and Edwards, 1972). These changes include a lowered prothrombin time, an increased partial thromboplastin time, a lowered fibrinogen level, and circulating levels of fibrin split products. The cell count, glucose, and protein in the cerebrospinal fluid are usually normal even though meningococci can frequently be cultured from it. The serum complement may be lowered. Pulmonary insufficiency develops within a few hours and many patients die despite appropriate antibiotic therapy and intensive care. Patients with fatal forms of fulminant meningococcemia are not likely to survive for 24 hours after admission to the hospital.

Chronic meningococcemia is a rare form of meningococcal disease. This is an intermittent bacteremic illness that lasts for at least one week and as long as several months. The fever tends to be intermittent with afebrile periods ranging from two to ten days, during which the patient seems well. As the disease progresses the temperature rises daily and the fever may be continuous. Eventually, a skin eruption appears during the febrile episodes. The skin lesions are usually maculopapular, but may be hemorrhagic or pustular. Leukocytosis is noted during the febrile episodes but coagulation studies are usually normal.

## COMPLICATIONS AND SEQUELAE

The most frequent complication of meningococcemia is meningitis. This complication is present in approximately half the patients with meningococcal disease. Other metastatic meningococcal infections are arthritis and, rarely, pericarditis (Hoffman and Edwards, 1972; Wolf and Birbara, 1968). Although joint involvement in meningococcal disease may be that of a septic arthritis, it frequently appears as an effusion after several days of antibiotic treatment. Meningococcal infection is associated with reactivation of herpes labialis.

In fulminant meningococcemia many complications are related to the circulatory changes of overwhelming infection. Acute renal failure can necessitate dialysis. Occlusion of pulmonary vessels and pulmonary hemorrhage may produce respiratory insufficiency. Acute adrenal failure has also been described, but infrequently. Cardiac insufficiency is frequent in fatal cases of meningococcemia.

## GEOGRAPHIC VARIATIONS

Meningococcemia occurs sporadically in all inhabited areas of the world. The prevalence of meningococcal disease is highest in the spring. Meningococci have also caused massive outbreaks. Large-scale outbreaks of meningococcal disease have spread at cyclic intervals through Central African countries north of the equator. The recent outbreaks in Africa have been caused by group A meningococci. An outbreak of unusually massive proportions began in São Paulo, Brazil, during 1971. The predominant serogroup during the initial years of this epidemic was group C meningococci, but group A organisms became prevalent during the later years. The last extensive outbreak of meningococcal disease in the United States occurred during World War II when group A organisms were the prevalent serogroup. This serogroup has been subsequently replaced by group B and then by group C meningococci. Although sulfonamide-resistant meningococci were initially identified in the United States, they have subsequently been recovered in several parts of the world.

## DIAGNOSIS

Recovery of *N. meningitidis* from cultures of the blood or petechiae is the usual means for establishing the diagnosis of meningococcemia. Positive blood cultures may not be obtained until late in the course of chronic meningococcemia. Detection of group-specific meningococcal antigen in serum offers a new and rapid means of diagnosis (Hoffman and Edwards, 1972). Studies with group-specific immune sera in counterimmunoelectrophoresis have shown that serum from patients with fulminant meningococcemia contains detectable levels of the polysaccharide antigen. The concentration of antigen in serum is likely to be related to the intensity of the bacteremia and to have prognostic significance (Hoffman and Edwards, 1972).

Meningococcal disease must be differentiated from Rocky Mountain spotted fever, bacterial endocarditis, hemorrhagic fevers due to arboviruses, enteroviral infection with exanthem, thrombotic thrombocytopenic purpura, and anaphylactoid purpura. The skin lesions of disseminated gonococcemia can usually be distinguished from those of meningococcemia.

## TREATMENT

Specific antimicrobial therapy should be instituted promptly when the clinical features are suggestive of meningococcemia. The preferred drug for the treatment of meningococcal disease is penicillin G, and it should be given intravenously (Wolf and Birbara, 1968). Patients suspected of having meningococcemia should receive a high dosage of penicillin G for the initial 48 hours of therapy, since meningitis is a likely complication. Recommended initial therapy in adults with meningococcemia is one to two million units of penicillin G given by intermittent intravenous infusions every two hours; a dosage of 250,000 units/kg of body weight can be given daily in divided doses to pediatric patients. Most patients with uncomplicated meningococcemia defervesce within the first 24 hours of antibiotic therapy. Antibiotic therapy for uncomplicated meningococcemia need be given for only 4 to 5 days after defervescence occurs, and the dosage needed to complete the course of therapy in adults can be reduced to 600,000 units of procaine penicillin G given every 12 hours intramuscularly. Alternate therapy in penicillin-allergic patients is chloramphenicol hemisuccinate, which is given in a dosage of 100 mg/kg/day intravenously until defervescence occurs, and then 50 mg/kg/day orally to complete a seven- to ten-day course of therapy. The cephalosporins are contraindicated in meningococcal disease, since these agents may be inactive in cerebrospinal fluid. Sulfonamides should not be used in treatment of meningococcal disease, because some strains of meningococci are resistant to them.

Patients with fulminant meningococcemia may require supportive therapy to maintain perfusion to vital organs (Wolf and Birbara, 1968). Electrolyte-containing fluids should be administered aggressively in a critical care setting where cardiovascular monitoring is available. Rapid digitalization is indicated when evidence of cardiac insufficiency is present. A single intravenous infusion of either 30 mg of methylprednisolone per kilogram or 3 mg of dexamethazone per kilogram may be beneficial for profound hypotension that is unresponsive to other supportive measures. One additional dose can be administered four hours later if no response has occurred. A continuous infusion of dopamine or another ionotropic agent may also be needed for the management of shock. Anticoagulant therapy in fulminant meningococcemia remains controversial although it is generally accepted that heparin therapy does not improve survival in this condition.

## PROPHYLAXIS

Meningococcal disease can be prevented by vaccination with group-specific meningococcal polysaccharides and by chemoprophylaxis (Artenstein, 1975). Purified polysaccharides of group A and group C meningococci have been used to stimulate group-specific humoral bactericidal antibodies. Vaccination with these polysaccharide antigens appears to be a highly effective means of preventing disease caused by these serogroups of meningococci. A single dose of vaccine, however, does not protect younger children, especially those under two years of age. Nevertheless, use of the vaccines is indicated for the population at risk whenever an outbreak caused by group A or group C meningococci becomes evident. Vaccination with the meningococcal polysaccharides has also been used effectively in military recruit populations to control disease caused by group A and group C organisms (Artenstein, 1975). Efforts to obtain a satisfactory vaccine for group B meningococcal disease have been unsuccessful.

Household contacts of patients with meningococcal disease are an identifiable population in which the risk of acquiring illness is definable (Artenstein, 1975). The secondary attack rate is inversely proportional to age and estimated to be approximately 10 per cent in household contacts between the ages of one and four years. Meningococcal infection is postulated to be introduced commonly into families by asymptomatic adults and then spread through one or more household contacts to reach the younger family members. Person-to-person transmission can be interrupted by chemoprophylaxis, which eradicates the asymptomatic nasopharyngeal carrier state. Sulfonamides, rifampin, and minocycline are the only drugs that have been shown to eradicate meningococci from the nasopharynx. Meningococcal isolates that are susceptible to 0.01 mg of sulfadiazide per milliliter can be eradicated by a two-day course of sulfadiazine given to adults in a dosage of 2 g per day. The dosage of sulfadiazine for children from 1 to 12 years of age is 1 g per day; children under 1 year are given 500 mg per day. The rapid emergence of rifampin-resistant meningococci precludes the use of this drug in large populations; the high incidence of side effects has limited the wide acceptance of minocycline. Many experts believe that chemoprophylaxis of sulfadiazine-resistant meningococci by either of these agents is less preferable than close observation of household contacts for signs of disease (Artenstein, 1975).

### References

Artenstein, M. S.: Prophylaxis of meningococcal disease. JAMA 231:1035, 1975.

Davis, C. E., and Arnold, K.: Role of meningococcal endotoxin in meningococcal purpura. J Exp Med 140:159, 1974.

Goldschneider, I., Gotschlich, E. C., and Artenstein, M. S.: Human immunity to the meningococcus: The role of humoral antibodies. J Exp Med 129:1307, 1969.

Hoffman, T. A., and Edwards, E. A.: Group-specific polysaccharide antigen and humoral antibody response in disease due to Neisseria meningititis. J Infect Dis 126:636, 1972.

Mellins, R. B., Levine, O. R., Wigger, H. J., et al.: Experimental meningococcemia. J Appl Physiol 32:309, 1972.

Sotto, M. N., Langer, B., Hoshino-Shimizu, S., et al.: Pathogenesis of cutaneous lesions in acute meningococcemia in humans. J Infect Dis 133:506, 1976.

Wolf, R. E., and Birbara, C. A.: Meningococcal infections at an army training center. Am J Med 44:243, 1968.

# BACTEROIDES SEPTICEMIA 182

## Donald L. Bornstein, M.D.

### DEFINITION

The obligately anaerobic gram-negative bacilli of clinical importance, the *Bacteroides*, make up the major portion of the normal microflora of the intestinal tract, and are prevalent on certain areas of skin, in the oropharynx, and often in the female genital tract. Disease, surgery, or trauma involving these colonized sites is often complicated by opportunistic infection with *Bacteroides*, usually in combination with other resident anaerobic or aerobic microorganisms. Many species of the two important genera, *Bacteroides* and *Fusobacterium*, can cause suppurative infections and bacteremia, but the pre-eminent pathogen and the organism most frequently isolated from purulent sites and from the blood is *B. fragilis*. *Bacteroides* septicemia usually follows the development of a necrotizing suppurative process that has originated from and around the gastrointestinal or the female genital tract. Advanced cases may be associated with marked leukocytosis, septic thrombophlebitis, jaundice, metastatic infection, obtundation, and refractory shock. Because *B. fragilis* is generally resistant to penicillin, cephalosporins, and aminoglycosides, infection with this organism should be seriously considered when febrile illness develops or persists despite use of these agents following abdominal or pelvic surgery or in other appropriate clinical settings.

## *ETIOLOGY*

In recent years remarkable advances have been made in the isolation, cultivation, speciation, and identification of the obligately anaerobic gram-negative bacilli (Holdeman et al., 1977). The Family *Bacteroidaceae* comprises three genera: the genus *Bacteroides,* with over twenty species; the genus *Fusobacterium,* with fourteen species; and the genus *Leptotrichia,* with one species. Accurate speciation has helped to clarify the ecologic characteristics, the pathogenic potential, and the antimicrobial susceptibilities of clinical isolates of *Bacteroides* and to resolve confusion between laboratories in identifying these organisms. The specialized microbiologic methods of the anerobic research laboratories have now been simplified and adapted to the routine clinical laboratory (Sutter et al., 1975). Many large hospital bacteriology laboratories can identify *Bacteroides* isolates to the species level.

In a two-year study at the Mayo Clinic, *Bacteroides* organisms were recovered from 19 per cent of all clinical specimens that contained bacteria (Martin, 1974). Bacteremia due to *Bacteroides* has increased in incidence from 1 to 2 per cent of all positive blood cultures between 1955 and 1965 to 6 to 12 per cent in recent studies (Wilson et al., 1972; Chow and Guze, 1974). Over 60 per cent of strains of *Bacteroides* isolated from all clinical specimens and over 80 per cent of strains isolated from the blood are of the *B. fragilis* group.

The distribution of species of *Fusobacterium* and *Bacteroides* varies throughout the body, and this fact is reflected in the patterns of infection associated with the different species. In the oropharynx, fusobacteria (*F. fusiforme, F. nucleatum, F. varium*), *B. oralis, B. corrodens,* and *B. melaninogenicus* are common, while *B. fragilis* is rare. In the distal ileum and colon, in the female genital tract, and on the perineum, the *B. fragilis* group predominates, but *B. melaninogenicus* and *F. necrophorum* are also commonly present. *B. fragilis* rarely causes infections that arise above the diaphragm, although septic embolization and metastatic infection to the lungs or to the brain

can occur. Chronic sinusitis, chronic otitis media, and mastoiditis are occasionally caused by *B. fragilis.* Conversely, *Bacteroides* infection originating from an abdominal or pelvic source, a wound, or a decubitus ulcer should be considered to be due to *B. fragilis* until proved otherwise.

The distribution of *Bacteroides* organisms recovered from clinical specimens by species and site was reviewed by Martin (1974). Of 4433 clinical isolates of *Bacteroides,* 56 per cent were of the *B. fragilis* group, 25 per cent were *B. melaninogenicus,* 13 per cent were other *Bacteroides,* 4 per cent were *F. nucleatum,* and 1 per cent were other fusobacteria. *B. fragilis* was recovered from 13 per cent of 134 sputum specimens containing *Bacteroides* organisms, 65 per cent of specimens from abdominal wounds, and 87 per cent of 326 positive blood cultures for *Bacteroides.* These figures indicate the rarity of *B. fragilis* in the lung, its prevalence in abdominal sites, and its greater virulence as indicated by a disproportionate presence in the blood.

Until 1976, five subspecies were recognized within the species *B. fragilis: s.s. fragilis,* s.s. *thetaiotamicron,* ss. *distasonis,* s.s. *vulgatus,* and s.s. *ovatus.* Subsequently, each has been raised to full species rank (Cato and Johnson, 1976). Most clinical studies begun before 1977 have not distinguished among the five species, and the term *B. fragilis* used in earlier reports refers to what is now described as the *B. fragilis* group. This group shares a common habitat, many common cultural characteristics, and a common special pattern of antibiotic susceptibility. The potential virulence varies considerably, however, among these five species, from the highly pathogenic *B. fragilis* to the essentially nonpathogenic *B. ovatus.* Of the five species of the *B. fragilis* group, *B. fragilis* is the most prevalent in clinical specimens, while the other species are more prevalent in the normal bowel flora. About 70 to 80 per cent of clinical isolates described as *B. fragilis* in the recent past are truly *B. fragilis,* 10 to 20 per cent are *B. thetaiotamicron,* and 5 to 10 per cent are *B. vulgatus* or *B. distasonis* (Polk and Kasper, 1977).

## *PATHOGENESIS AND PATHOLOGY*

*Bacteroides* organisms are opportunistic pathogens without primary invasive ability, and a breach of local anatomic defenses is usually required to initiate infection. However, the intense colonization of the lower gastrointestinal tract — over $10^9$ organism per gram of stool (100 to 1000 times the number of *Escherichia coli*) — and the consequent colonization of adjacent skin surfaces and, in 50 to 70 per cent of women, of the female genital tract, pose a constant threat of infection. The oropharynx also carries a large number of other *Bacteroides* species as part of its complex microflora. Ulcerating or necrotizing inflammatory or malignant disease, trauma, or surgery involving heavily colonized skin or mucosal surfaces is the usual means of introducing *Bacteroides,* along with other indigenous flora, into normally sterile deeper tissues. Since *Bacteroides* organisms are obligate anaerobes, the presence of any necrotic tissue, foreign material, impaired blood flow, anoxia or acidosis, or aerobic bacterial growth, which reduces the redox potential (Eh) in the tissues, provides a potent stimulus for rapid bacterial growth.

Bacteremia may be initiated directly by minor injury to a colonized mucous membrane, but most important *Bacteroides* sepsis involves an established local suppurative infection. The major sources of *Bacteroides* septicemia have been the gastrointestinal tract (50 to 65 per cent of cases), the female genital tract (20 to 30 per cent), decubiti and other wounds (10 to 15 per cent), the respiratory tract (2 to 5 per cent), and the oropharynx (1 to 3 per cent).

The predisposing event involving the gastrointestinal tract has been disease (appendicitis, diverticulitis, acute pancreatitis, intestinal obstruction, vascular disease, malignancy, inflammatory bowel disease, perforated ulcer, other surgical problems), trauma (gunshot wounds), or surgery that has caused a spill of bowel contents into the peritoneum. The disease that follows depends on the magnitude of the spill, the prior health of the patient, and the subsequent medical and surgical management. A large leak can lead to frank peritonitis and gram-negative sepsis within 2 to 24 hours owing to rapidly growing facultative enteric bacilli. After the acute problem has been corrected, from 5 to 20 days after the initiating event, *Bacteroides* infection may first become apparent. An experimental animal model of the events that follow fecal contamination of the peritoneum has shown a similar biphasic illness: an early acute peritonitis and bacteremia after one to two days due to *E. coli* or *Klebsiella,* followed in all survivors by intra-abdominal abscess formation after a week or so due to *B. fragilis* (Weinstein et al., 1974).

*Bacteroides* septicemia originating in the female genital tract is usually secondary to septic abortion, to amnionitis and puerperal complications, to cesarean surgery, or to vaginal hysterectomies (Ledger et al., 1975). Less common but more serious septicemia can be seen in older women with more extensive gynecologic surgery or radiation therapy for malignant disease.

Surgical or traumatic wounds of the back, hips, buttocks, or thighs, and decubitus ulcers are often heavily soiled with fecal flora. This is an exceedingly serious problem in paraplegics and other immobile or bedridden patients. It is further intensified by diabetes mellitus, peripheral vascular disease, obesity, and fecal incontinence (Galpin et al., 1976).

Neither the lung nor the oropharynx is a common portal of entry of *Bacteroides* sepsis today. In the pre-antibiotic era, however, over 30 per cent of cases developed from the oropharynx. A severe pharyngitis with suppurative complications or Ludwig's angina was a common presentation, occasionally associated with septic thrombophlebitis of the jugular vein (Gunn, 1956). The oral *Bacteroides* organisms are highly sensitive to common antimicrobial agents, and antibiotics abort most of these infections in their early stages today. The remaining few oral and respiratory infections relate to local tissue injury and to aspiration.

When penicillins, cephalosporins, or aminoglycoside antibiotics are administered, or when oral neomycin or nonabsorbable sulfonamides are given for "preparation" of the bowel before colon surgery, significant changes occur in the microbial ecology of the bowel. These drugs suppress enterobacteria and many of the antibiotic-sensitive anaerobes and allow the more pathogenic and drug-resistant *B. fragilis* to proliferate, increasing the risk of postoperative or other opportunistic infection. The addition of erythromycin base to oral neomycin reduces the overgrowth of *B. fragilis,* and this regimen appears to be somewhat safer in regard to opportunistic infection (Nichols et al., 1973). Surgery of the bowel can be complicated by intraoperative spills, by anastomotic leaks or fistulae, and by abdominal wound infections. Surgery is often associated with antibiotic use that promotes growth of *B. fragilis.*

In 1976, Kasper and co-workers demonstrated a possible virulence factor in *B. fragilis.* Electron micrography of various species of *Bacteroides* stained with ruthenium red revealed a capsular structure on fresh isolates of *B. fragilis* that was not seen in any other species. The capsule was found to be made up of a protein-polysaccharide complex that was immunogenic. Specific capsular antibody was prepared and immunofluorescence studies demonstrated capsules on *B. fragilis* strains but on no other *Bacteroides.* Isolates of *B. thetaiotamicron, B. distasonis, B. vulgatus,* and *B. ovatus* showed no evidence of capsules by ruthenium red and no capsules by immunofluorescence (Kasper et al., 1977). More recently, an analogous specific capsular material has been demonstrated on a subspecies of *B. melaninogenicus,* ss. *asaccharolyticus.* This subspecies may soon be assigned full species status (*B. assacharolyticus*). It may be significantly more pathogenic than other isolates of *B. melaninogenicus* and may have accounted for many of the serious *B. melaninogenicus* infections (Mansheim et al., 1978). *B. thetaiotamicron, B. distasonis,* and *F. necrophorum* exhibit significant pathogenicity in some cases, and it is conceivable that some isolates of these species will eventually be shown to possess a capsule.

In addition to its association with greater virulence, possibly by an antiphagocytic effect, the capsular material of *B. fragilis* has been shown to be highly leukotactic for polymorphonuclear leukocytes. Killed *B. fragilis* or partially purified capsular material placed in the peritoneal cavity of a rat can elicit a massive accumulation of polymorphonuclear cells and abscess formation. This may explain, in part, the markedly purulent nature of the host response to *B. fragilis* infections, which has been described as being more like a pyogenic infection than a coliform infection.

Other factors that may be involved in the pathogenicity of *B. fragilis* include proteolytic and collagenolytic enzymes, heparinase, which may promote septic thrombophlebitis and interfere with anticoagulant therapy, and the presence of a toxic lipopolysaccharide. There has been controversy about whether *B. fragilis* has a typical endotoxin. An endotoxin-like material has been demonstrated that can elicit the Shwartzman reaction and can clot solutions of limulus amoebocyte lysate in relatively high concentration, but this would appear to be much less potent a toxin than most gram-negative bacteria possess. Septic shock does occur in *Bacteroides* sepsis, but it may be unrelated to any endotoxin, since it generally occurs later in the course of the illness, as seen in continuing sepsis due to gram-positive pathogens.

Beta-lactamase activity is common in *B. fragilis,* although it is not the only mechanism of penicillin or cephalosporin resistance. Recently, plasmids bearing R factors for clindamycin and for chloramphenicol have been described. Such plasmids, which may introduce a variety of other factors that enhance bacterial virulence, and their role in the pathogenesis of *Bacteroides* infections, require further careful study.

## CLINICAL PICTURE

*Bacteroides* septicemia typically appears as a prostrating and toxemic febrile illness that develops over several days in a patient hospitalized for other medical problems or recovering from recent abdominal or gynecologic surgery. A more acute onset may be seen in young women following septic abortion or puerperal complications. In contrast to gram-negative rod bacteremia, *Bacteroides* sepsis rarely originates from the urinary tract or in severely immunocompromised hosts (acute leukemics, transplant recipients). The clinical picture is usually less precipitous in onset and is more protracted than typical gram-negative bacteremia.

The majority of nonobstetrical patients are over 40 years of age, have had recent surgery or a biopsy, and have been on antibiotics or have received oral neomycin or other agents in preparation for bowel surgery. Common clinical features are a brisk peripheral leukocytosis sometimes exceeding 40,000 white blood cells per mm³, spiking fevers and repeated chills, persistence of bacteremia over several days, and, usually, some signs and symptoms of the initial infection in the abdomen, the pelvis, or an infected wound. In other patients persistent low-grade fever and malaise may be the only findings.

Jaundice (12 to 29 per cent), septic thrombophlebitis (5 to 44 per cent), septic embolization to the lungs, liver, or brain (23 to 29 per cent), and septic shock (25 to 35 per cent) can be seen in far-advanced cases and constitute a classic but uncommon syndrome of *Bacteroides* septicemia. The majority of cases will not present with these findings. The incidence of shock is similar to that seen in gram-negative bacterial sepsis, but the presentation differs, reflecting the biologic differences in the lipopolysaccharides of the *Bacteroides* and the Enterobacteriaceae.

The bacteremia and the toxemia of *Bacteroides* sepsis can persist intermittently or continuously for up to several weeks despite the use of appropriate antibiotics unless all suppurative lesions are identified and are drained effectively. Bacteremia that persists after effective drainage often indicates bacterial invasion of veins in the infected area. Septic thrombophlebitis is more common following pelvic infection or surgery. Venous cords may be palpated or clinical evidence of venous obstruction may be noted in some cases. Septic emboli to the liver and, and more often, to the lungs may be the first evidence of venous infection. Antibiotics and heparin therapy can usually correct the phlebitis, but venous ligation is still required in some cases.

Metastatic infection can develop into more extensive and life-threatening problems than the original suppurative lesion. Large or multiple liver abscesses or extensive pleuropulmonary suppuration can become the source of persistent bacteremia and further metastatic infection to the brain, to joints, to other serosal surfaces, and to the heart valves.

About 3 to 8 per cent of patients with *Bacteroides* bacteremia have only transient bacteremia — a brief fever elevation without significant toxemia. They do not have an established local infection and they recover without specific therapy. Another significant portion of cases (10 to 25 per cent) are polymicrobial; anaerobic streptococci, facultative streptococci, and enterobacteria are common associated organisms. These cases are usually associated wtih less morbidity and mortality than pure *B. fragilis* septicemia.

## COMPLICATIONS

The major hazards of *Bacteroides* septicemia are septic shock and its consequences, serious metastatic infection, septic thrombophlebitis and, rarely, bacterial endocarditis. Metastatic complications include lung, liver, spleen, myocardial and brain abscesses, empyema, meningitis, and septic arthritis. Local complications (extension, obstruction, and necrosis) at the initial site of infection can themselves be life-threatening.

The diagnosis of endocarditis due to *Bacteroides* is difficult to establish unless there is clear-cut peripheral embolization or unequivocal evidence of new valve injury, because persistent bacteremia is often due to undrained abscesses or septic thrombophlebitis. Finegold (1977) reviewed 56 case reports of *Bacteroides* endocarditis. Most cases were in older persons without predisposing valvular abnormalities; over 50 per cent of these patients died. About one half of cases were due to *B. fragilis* and originated mainly from the abdomen, pelvis, or perineum. The other cases were of dental, pharyngeal, and pulmonary origin and involved *B. melaninogenicus, B. oralis,* and fusobacteria. The validity of the diagnosis of endocarditis in many of the patients who recover on antibiotic therapy is open to question. The need for effective bactericidal therapy to cure *Bacteroides* endocarditis was underlined by Nastro and Finegold (1973), who recommend the use of intravenous metronidazole for this disease.

## DIAGNOSIS

When fever and toxemia develop or progress in a patient with puerperal or postabortal complications, gynecologic or intra-abdominal problems, chronic decubiti, or after recent abdominal or pelvic surgery, one must strongly suspect either enterobacterial or *Bacteroides* sepsis. If blood cultures are still sterile after 48 hours of incubation, *Bacteroides* septicemia is more likely, since it often takes three to seven days, and occasionally longer, for these slower growing organisms to be recognized. If the febrile illness developed or progressed despite antimicrobial therapy with a cephalosporin and an aminoglycoside, the diagnosis of *Bacteroides* sepsis is strongly supported.

Surgical wounds, decubitus ulcers, or other accessible sites that could be the source of bacteremia should be examined and swabbed for smears and anaerobic and aerobic cultures. The presence of foul-smelling exudate and of small or pleomorphic gram-negative rods on gram-stained smears should heighten suspicion. In over 70 per cent of patients, however, the seeding site is not accessible to direct culture. It must be localized by other means in order to identify the origin of the bacteremia and to render proper treatment. Thorough physical examination, including repeat rectal and pelvic examinations, plain and barium contrast x-ray films, and liver function tests, will often identify the site of a septic focus. A pocket of gas in an extra-intestinal site or in the soft tissues may indicate the source of the sepsis. Newer diagnostic techniques, nuclear scintigraphy (liver-spleen scans and gallium scans, for example), sonography, and computer-assisted axial tomography have proved to be of great value in localizing intra-abdominal and hepatic abscesses and other masses or suppurative lesions that cannot be observed by routine x-rays. They are invaluable adjuncts in finding the source of *Bacteroides* septicemia.

Diagnosis rests ultimately on recovery of the agent in blood cultures, and success here relates directly to the level of awareness of the need to obtain blood cultures and on the use of proper media and bacteriologic methods. Most *Bacteroides* organisms and fusobacteria are not very stringent anaerobes and need only moderate reduction in the redox potential (Eh) for growth. Although most *Bacteroides* strains will grow in routine blood culture media in evacuated bottles if the blood sample is injected without the introduction of air, it is generally preferable to inoculate specific anerobic blood culture media containing thioglycolate or an equivalent reducing substance in addition. Some strains of *B. melaninogenicus* require media enriched with hemin and menadione, and it is possible that some *Bacteroides* are not recoverable with commonly used bacteriologic media.

In polymicrobial bacteremia (about 10 to 25 per cent of all *Bacteroides* bacteremia) it is possible to overlook the slower growing *Bacteroides* if an enteric gram-negative rod is present. The coexisting *Bacteroides* will be detected only if the laboratory routinely subcultures all turbid blood culture bottles to two blood agar plates, one of which is cultured under anaerobic conditions. Unfortunately, this is not a routine for many laboratories. *Bacteroides* bacteremia may be recognized belatedly in such cases, after therapy aimed at the aerobic isolate has cleared this organism but allowed the *Bacteroides* to persist. Such belated recognition adds significantly to the morbidity and mortality of *Bacteroides* infection.

As a general rule, *B. fragilis,* when present in a mixed aerobic-anaerobic infection, is the most important pathogen, and the infection will not be cured without specific and effective therapy against this organism. One exception is in idiopathic lung abscess. In this condition *B. fragilis* has been isolated from over 20 per cent of cases as part of a mixed flora, but therapy with penicillin, which is normally ineffective against this organism, has been very successful. Recently, fluorescein-conjugated antisera to capsular antigens of *B. fragilis* and *B. melaninogenicus, s.s. asaccharolyticus* have become commercially available. These reagents allow rapid recognition of these pathogenic *Bacteroides* organisms in wound exudates and more rapid speciation in the laboratory, speeding diagnosis and delivery of appropriate antimicrobial therapy.

### GEOGRAPHIC CONSIDERATIONS

The extent of colonization of the bowel by the various species of *Bacteroides* and of fusobacteria does vary in different parts of the world, primarily because of dietary differences. Significant colonization with the major pathogenic species of *Bacteroides* is universal, however. The incidence of illness caused by these endogenous organisms varies in relation to the extent of obstetric infections, abdominal and pelvic surgery, and malignancy. When hospital facilities are more limited and when less extensive surgery is carried out, infection rates will appear lower. However, more fatal cases will develop in the home and will not be recognized as due to *Bacteroides.*

### TREATMENT

Because abscesses and other local suppurative lesions are the usual sources of *Bacteroides* septicemia, antimicrobial therapy must be supplemented with effective surgery in most cases. Abscesses must be drained, necrotic tissues excised, decubitus ulcers debrided, obstructed bowel or viscera relieved, and infected veins that do not respond to heparin must be ligated. Sites of metastatic infection may also require surgical drainage to terminate bacteremia. Patients who succumb to *Bacteroides* septicemia usually have collections of undrained pus at autopsy (Lawrence et al., 1977).

There are important differences in antimicrobial susceptibility among the *Bacteroides.* Most fusobacteria and many *Bacteroides* species (*B.*

*oralis, B. melaninogenicus*) are highly susceptible to penicillin G and, to a lesser extent, to the other penicillins and cephalosporins (Table 1). *B. fragilis,* however, and the related strains of the *B. fragilis* group, are intrinsically resistant to penicillins and cephalosporins, to all aminoglycosides, and to polymyxins. In 50 to 70 per cent of cases they are also resistant to tetracyclines. Fortunately, these species are susceptible to clindamycin and chloramphenicol in over 95 per cent of cases. Although both agents have been generally effective, more treatment failures have been reported with chloramphenicol, probably because this drug lacks bactericidal activity. Clindamycin, in concentrations easily achievable in the blood, is bactericidal in vitro for up to 60 per cent of isolates of *B. fragilis.* The usual doses employed in *B. fragilis* infections in adults are 450 to 600 mg of clindamycin I.V. every six hours or 0.75 to 1.0 g of chloramphenicol I.V. every six hours.

Metronidazole is an effective bactericidal drug in vitro for most obligate anaerobes and in clinical studies also. It is still on investigational status in the United States for treatment of anerobic infections. A parenteral form is under study. Metronidazole and chloramphenicol penetrate the brain tissue and cerebrospinal fluid very well, unlike clindamycin, and are useful for *B. fragilis* infections of the central nervous system. Most *Bacteroides* infections of the CNS, however, are caused by penicillin-sensitive species resident in the oropharynx. The dose of metronidazole for adults with serious *Bacteroides* infection is 750 mg every eight hours I.V. or orally.

Penicillin G (12 to 36 million units/day I.V.) is the drug of choice for serious infections due to fusobacteria and most *Bacteroides* species other than the *B. fragilis* group. In penicillin-allergic patients clindamycin or chloramphenicol is an effective alternative. Because many isolates of *B. fragilis* are inhibited in vitro by 32 $\mu$g/ml of penicillin G and because blood concentrations of this magnitude can be achieved by massive doses of penicillin (40 to 100 million units/day), some clinicians have advocated such doses for serious *B. fragilis* infection. Despite initial enthusiasm, these regimens have been unsuccessful too often and are not recommended.

Carbenicillin or ticarcillin, and the new cephalosporin, cefoxitin, have been recommended for *B. fragilis* infections. Carbenicillin inhibits 80 to 90 per cent of isolates of *B. fragilis* in vitro at 128 $\mu$g/ml. Stable blood levels of 125 to 200 $\mu$g/ml can be achieved in adults with normal renal function at a dose of 5 g I.V. every four hours. Cefoxitin, a cephamycin derivative with enhanced resistance to beta-lactamases, inhibits 70 to 75 per cent of strains of *B. fragilis* in vitro at 16 $\mu$g/ml and 85 to 90 per cent at 32 $\mu$g/ml. A dose of 2 to 3 g

### TABLE 1. Antimicrobial Susceptibility of Bacteroides and Fusobacteria[a]

| ANTIMICROBIAL AGENT | CONCENTRATION ($\mu$g/ml) | B. FRAGILIS GROUP | B. MELANINOGENICUS | BACTEROIDES SPECIES | FUSOBACTERIUM SPECIES |
|---|---|---|---|---|---|
| Penicillin G | 2 | 0 | ++-+++ | + | ++-+++ |
|  | 8 | 0-± | +++ | ++ | +++ |
| Cephalothin | 8 | 0 | ++ | + | ++-+++ |
| Gentamicin | 4 | 0 | 0-+ | 0 | 0 |
| Polymyxin | 4-8 | 0 | 0-± | 0-± | ++ |
| Tetracycline | 1-2 | ±-+ | ++ | ±-+ | +++ |
| Erythromycin | 1-2 | ± | +++ | ++ | 0-+ |
| Chloramphenicol | 8 | ++-+++ | +++ | +++ | +++ |
| Clindamycin | 4 | +++ | +++ | +++ | +++ |
| Metronidazole | 8 | +++ | +++ | ++-+++ | +++ |
| Carbenicillin | 64 | ++ | +++ | +++ | +++ |
| Cefoxitin | 16 | ++ | +++ | ++-+++ | +++ |

[a]Per cent susceptible at concentration tested: +++, over 95%; ++, over 75%; +, over 50%; ±, over 25%; 0, less than 25%.
Data from Finegold (1977), Martin (1972), and other sources.

intravenously every four hours is needed to maintain effective concentrations in the blood. Although both types of drugs appear to be effective, they are very expensive alternatives that do not appear to be superior to clindamycin in established infection. Neither drug approaches the inhibitory ratio (serum concentration/MIC) of clindamycin (Table 2).

The in vitro susceptibility patterns of the five species of the B. fragilis group are very similar. B. distasonis is somewhat more susceptible to penicillins and B. thetaiotamicron is slightly more resistant to clindamycin (Jones and Fuchs, 1976).

Recently plasmid-borne resistance to chloramphenicol and to clindamycin has been recognized, and some increase in resistance to cefoxitin has been noted (Sutter et al., 1979). Unnecessary use of these agents must be restricted, and appropriate infection control measures must be taken when plasmid-borne resistance is detected to prevent the spread of resistant B. fragilis strains. Although the prophylactic use of antibiotics active against B. fragilis in surgery must be carefully considered, early surgical use in conditions in

which an actual spill of bowel contents has occurred would appear to be clinically indicated (Thadepalli et al., 1973).

Bacteroides septicemia has a poor prognosis, despite the availability of effective antimicrobial drugs. In large collected series 25 to 45 per cent of patients have died. Important prognostic factors are age, site of infection, underlying disease, choice of antibiotic, adequacy of drainage, and promptness of recognition and treatment.

Bacteroides bacteremia arising from an obstetrical infection is a very mild illness. In 184 cases reviewed by Chow and Guze (1974) there was only one fatality (0.6 per cent), in contrast to a mortality rate of 35 to 45 per cent for nonobstetrical cases. Infection is rare in childhood, but young adults can develop serious septicemia from decubiti (in paraplegics), trauma, surgery, or appendiceal disease. Mortality is higher in the nonobstetrical group for older patients, in postsurgical cases, in bedridden patients, and in the presence of advanced diabetes, arteriosclerosis, liver or kidney disease, and malignant disease. Inadequate surgical drainage, inappropriate antibacterial therapy, and the development of septic

### TABLE 2. Inhibitory Index (I. I.) of Antimicrobial Agents Active Against B. Fragilis

| ANTIMICROBIAL AGENT | PARENTERAL DOSE | ACHIEVABLE SERUM CONCENTRATIONS[a] ($\mu$g/ml) | MIC FOR 95% OF STRAINS | I. I. (SERUM CONCENTRATION/MIC 95) |
|---|---|---|---|---|
| Clindamycin | 600 mg every six hrs | 8-10 | 3 | 3.0 |
| Chloramphenicol | 1000 mg every six hrs | 12-16 | 12 | 1.2 |
| Metronidazole | 750 mg every eight hrs | 16-24 | 8 | 2.5 |
| Carbenicillin | 5000 mg every four hrs | 125 | 128 | 1.0 |
| Cefoxitin | 2000 mg every four hrs | 30 | 32 | 0.8 |

[a]Serum concentration one hour after IV infusion or IM injection.

shock are associated with a poorer prognosis. Deferring surgery to allow an extended period of antimicrobial therapy is generally unwise; surgical drainage should be carried out as soon as the need is recognized, even if the patient appears acutely ill. When effective drainage is not possible (as in patients with multiple abdominal fistulae or severe eroding decubiti), survival rates are poor.

## PREVENTION

Neither active or passive immunization against *Bacteroides* infection is available. It is conceivable that protective anticapsular antibody can be elicited in man and that there may be a role for immunoprophylaxis in selected high-risk settings in the future.

Antimicrobial prophylaxis of postoperative infection after bowel or uterine surgery is widely practiced. If the regimen does not include an agent effective against *B. fragilis,* overgrowth of *Bacteroides* in the gut and an increased risk of *Bacteroides* infection can be anticipated. Although the inclusion of clindamycin, chloramphenicol, or cefoxitin might reduce the incidence or delay the onset of *Bacteroides* infections, the risks of prophylaxis may well outweigh any benefits. The risks of prophylaxis include: drug toxicity; hypersensitive, idiosyncratic, and other adverse reactions; microbiologic effects of altering normal flora (colonization with resistant organisms, superinfection, pseudomembranous enterocolitis); and the epidemiologic consequences (selection of R factor plasmid-bearing organisms and eventual selection of drug-resistant *B. fragilis* strains).

The best preventive measures against bacteroides sepsis are early recognition and effective treatment of localized *Bacteroides* infections.

## References

Cato, E. P., and Johnson, J. L.: Reinstatement of species rank for *Bacteroides fragilis, B. ovatus, B. distasonis, B. thetaiotamicron* and *B. vulgatus.* Int J Syst Bacteriol 26:230, 1976.

Chow, A. W., and Guze, L. B.: Bacteroidaceae bacteremia: Clinical experience with 112 patients. Medicine 53:93, 1974.

Finegold, S. M.: Anaerobic Bacteria in Human Disease. New York, Academic Press, 1977.

Finegold, S. M., Bartlett, J. G., Chow, A. W., Flora, D. J., Gorbach, S. L., Harder, E. J., and Tally, F. P.: Management of anaerobic infections. Ann Intern Med 83:375, 1975.

Galpin, J. E., Chow, A. W., Bayer, A. S., and Guze, L. B.: Sepsis associated with decubitus ulcers. Am J Med 61:346, 1976.

Gunn, A. A.: Bacteroides septicemia. J R Coll Surg Edinb 2:41, 1956.

Holdeman, L. V., Cato, E. P., and Moore, W. E. C.: Anaerobic Laboratory Manual. 4th ed. Blacksburg, Va., Virginia Poytechnic Institute and State University, 1977.

Jones, R. N., and Fuchs, P. C.: Identification and antimicrobial susceptibility of 250 *Bacteroides fragilis* subspecies tested by broth microdilution methods. Antimicrob Agents Chemother 9:719, 1976.

Kasper, D. L., Hayes, M. E., Reinap, B. G., Craft, F. O., Onderdonk, A. B., and Polk, B. F.: Isolation and identification of encapsulated strains of *Bacteroides fragilis.* J Infect Dis 136:75, 1977.

Lawrence, P. F., Tietgen, J. W., Gingrich, S., and King, T. E.: Bacteroides bacteremia. Ann Surg 186:559, 1977.

Ledger, W. J., Norman, M., Gee, C. L., and Lewis, W. P.: Bacteremia on an obstetric-gynecologic service. Am J Obstet Gynecol 121:205, 1975.

Mansheim, B. J., Solstad, C. A., and Kasper, D. L.: Identification of a subspecies-specific capsular antigen from *Bacteroides melaninogenicus,* subspecies *asaccharolyticus* by immunofluorescence and electron microscopy. J Infect Dis 136:736, 1978.

Martin, W. J.: Isolation and identification of anaerobic bacteria in the clinical laboratory. Mayo Clin Proc 49:300, 1974.

Nastro, L. J., and Finegold, S. M.: Endocarditis due to anaerobic gram-negative bacilli. Am J Med 54:82, 1973.

Nichols, R. L., Broido, P., Condon, R. E., Gorbach, S. L., and Nyhus, L. M.: Effect of pre-operative neomycin-erythromycin intestinal preparation on the incidence of infectious complications following colon surgery. Ann Surg 178:453, 1973.

Polk, B. F., and Kasper, D. L.: *Bacteroides fragilis* subspecies in clinical isolates. Ann Intern Med 86:569, 1977.

Sutter, V. L., Vargo, V. L., and Finegold, S. M.: Wadsworth Anaerobic Bacteriology Manual. 2nd ed. Los Angeles, Extension Division, University of California at Los Angeles, 1975.

Sutter, V. L., Kirby, B., and Finegold, S. M.: In-vitro activity of cefoxitin and parenterally administered cephalosporins against anaerobic bacteria. Rev Infect Dis 1:128, 1979.

Thadepalli, H., Gorbach, S. L., Broido, P. W., Norsen, J., and Nyhus, L. M.: Abdominal trauma, anaerobes and antibiotics. Surg Gynecol Obstet 137:270, 1973.

Weinstein, W. M., Onderdonk, A. B., Bartlett, J. G., and Gorbach, S. L.: Experimental intraabdominal abscesses in rats: Quantitative bacteriology of infected animals. Infect Immun 10:1250, 1974.

Wilson, W. R., Martin, W. J., Wilkowske, C. J., et al.: Anaerobic bacteremia. Mayo Clin Proc 47:639, 1972.

# 183 CLOSTRIDIAL SEPTICEMIA

## Donald L. Bornstein, M.D.

## DEFINITION

Clostridial septicemia is a rare, highly lethal illness due to heavy bacteremic seeding with pathogenic clostridia originating primarily from the uterus, colon, or biliary tract. The characteristic clinical presentation is that of high fever, extensive intravascular hemolysis due to circulating clostridial alphatoxin (lecithinase C), hypotension, and acute renal tubular necrosis. Episodes of transient clostridial bacteremia are much more common than septicemia and do not necessarily carry a serious prognosis. Clostridial myo-necrosis (gas gangrene) may give rise to transient bacteremia but is very rarely associated with septicemia and hemolysis. In rare cases, protract-ed clostridial septicemia may induce "metastatic" or "spontaneous" gas gangrene. Clostridial bac-teremia can also occur agonally or in the last hours of life, especially in patients with impaired resistance or intestinal ulceration, and may pro-duce striking postmortem changes of crepitus and gas-filled cysts in many organs.

## ETIOLOGY

Although many of the 70-odd species of *Clos-tridium* can colonize humans and cause local infections and a transient bacteremia, only a few are significant pathogens. *Clostridium perfrin-gens*, the major pathogen, causes over 90 per cent of cases of septicemia as well as the majority of cases of transient bacteremia. *C. septicum*, which may be relatively more common in patients with malignant disease, and, very rarely, *C. sordelli* or *C. novyi* account for the other cases. Clostridia are recovered from 1 to 2.5 per cent of all positive blood cultures. The large majority of isolations represent transient bacteremia; the septicemic cases are rare. In about 30 to 40 per cent of positive cultures, clostridia are mixed with other aerobes and/or anaerobes (Martin, 1974; Gorbach and Thadepalli, 1975).

A clinically apparent site of origin can be identified in less than half of the patients; an intestinal, biliary, or gynecologic origin is as-sumed for the others. Transient bacteremias due to nonpathogenic species, for example, *C. ramo-sum, C. tertium, C. difficile,* and *C. bifermentans*, arise from the same sites and from secondarily infected necrotic processes. Bacteremia with these organisms, usually benign, can produce shock or lethal illness in newborns or in severely compromised patients (Alpern and Dowell, 1971).

## PATHOGENESIS AND PATHOLOGY

The pathogenesis of clostridial septicemia in-volves colonization of a site with pathogenic clos-tridia, a local environment that promotes rapid growth of clostridia, and local factors that help to introduce organisms into the bloodstream.

Bacteremia may originate from any location that is colonized or infected with pathogenic clos-tridia.

The vast intestinal reservoirs of pathogenic and nonpathogenic clostridia are concentrated in the large intestine, but colonization of the small in-testine can occur and is favored by disordered or reverse peristalsis, antibiotic use (including some nonabsorbable drugs), and surgery, especially gastrojejunostomy or bypass jejunoileostomy.

The biliary tract is sterile in health but be-comes susceptible to colonization with enteric bacteria via portal venous blood by disease, sur-gery, or obstruction. Clostridia have been recov-ered in pure or mixed culture in 5 to 27 per cent of infected cases (Fukunaga, 1973).

The perineal area and the skin of the thighs and abdomen and, to a lesser extent, the hands, other skin areas, and the oropharynx are contam-inated with clostridia as a consequence of the heavy intestinal carriage of this organism. Clos-tridia also colonize the genital tract of 4 to 9 per cent of healthy women. Carriage increases in complicated pregnancy or after surgical interven-tion and reaches rates of 18 to 27 per cent follow-ing septic abortion.

Clostridia, like other obligate anaerobes, can proliferate in tissues only when the oxidation-reduction potential (Eh) falls or when, at any level of Eh, the pH is reduced. Rapid growth of clostridia is promoted by foreign material, lactic acid accumulation due to tissue anoxia, arterial injury or compression of vessels by edema, and above all, the presence of necrotic tissue (Oakley, 1954). While *C. perfringens* requires anaerobiosis for growth, its pathogenicity is enhanced by its ability to survive for considerable periods of time at atmospheric oxygen tensions. Even exposure to oxygen at three atmospheres pressure for several hours does not kill this hardy organism (Fredette, 1965).

Most cases of clostridial septicemia originate from the genital tract of women; a few occur after complicated term delivery, Cesarean section, gyn-ecologic surgery, or, very rarely, from infected necrotic tumors (leiomyomas or malignant le-sions), but the vast majority of cases follow sep-tic abortion. In septic abortion a foreign body (catheter, wire, slippery elm stalk) or a solution (soap, phenolics, quinine) is introduced through the cervix. In this process clostridia from the perineum or the vagina or occasionally from the foreign object itself can be introduced into the uterus, where there are usually residual necrotic fetal and placental tissues and traumatized areas of endometrium that favor the rapid heavy growth of clostridia. In addition, the pregnant uterus is a highly vascular organ and infected retained placental tissue is intimately apposed to vascular beds, a feature that is responsible for the early intense and persistent septicemia that can follow. Fortunately, only a small fraction of cases of septic abortion are followed by serious bac-teremic illness. The conditions required to permit clostridial sepsis occur in only about 0.2 to 1.5 per cent of all women hospitalized after septic abortion, which is fortunate in view of the poor salvage rate in this disease.

Dissemination of clostridia into the blood from the gastrointestinal tract is favored by ulcerative processes of the small or large intestine (bleeding peptic ulcer in a patient with a gastrojejunostomy, enteritis necroticans); intestinal obstruction; necrotic or infiltrating malignancy; abdominal catastrophe (perforation, diverticulitis, ruptured appendix, acute pancreatitis); or recent bowel surgery. Anaerobic cellulitis, decubitus ulcers, and ischiorectal abscesses have also caused septicemia. A special group at high risk for clostridial septicemia are patients with hematologic or other advanced malignant disease. Primary or metastatic disease, and cytotoxic or radiation therapy can cause intestinal ulceration that allows clostridia to enter the blood without opposition because the normal processes of resistance are damaged in these conditions. Clostridial septicemia can originate from acute cholecystitis (especially emphysematous or gangrenous cases) or surgery (operative cholangiography, common duct exploration, or cholecystectomy).

Many of the features of clostridial sepsis are due to exotoxins. Alpha toxin, the important hemolytic toxin of *C. perfringens*, is an enzyme, lecithinase C, which cleaves phosphorylcholine from lecithin to leave an insoluble diglyceride. It also acts similarly on sphingomyelin. Both lecithin and, to a lesser extent, sphingomyelin are vital structural components of the surface membranes and of mitochondrial and lysosomal membranes of mammalian cells. Although other bacteria can produce lecithinases of similar specificity, they have lower affinity or they are not released during infection in sufficient amounts to cause significant hemolysis in vivo. All the activities of alpha toxin can be neutralized by specific antitoxin or by incubation in an excess of free lecithin.

Alpha toxin has the most obvious effects on erythrocytes. It damages membrane transport mechanisms so that metabolic injury occurs that progresses to cell fragmentation, loss of volume, and formation of osmotically fragile and morphologically distinctive microspherocytes. The ensuing hemolysis releases free hemoglobin intravascularly in amounts that rapidly overload clearance by haptoglobin and the reticuloendothelial system. Injury to endothelial cells and platelets is instrumental in producing the disseminated intravascular coagulation (DIC) that is seen in the most severe cases. Alpha toxin can also damage muscle and be responsible for the severe muscle tenderness and myonecrosis seen in advanced clostridial sepsis.

The contribution of the other toxins of *C. per-*

*fringens* is not clear, although some may play an important role (see Chapters 45 and 239). Septic shock is common in clostridial sepsis and occurs within the first 12 to 24 hours of illness, a pattern that is unusual for bacteremia caused by other gram-positive organisms. This may be due to the intensity of the bacteremic seeding or may be a reflection of the toxicity of *C. perfringens* for leukocytes or other tissues. Clostridial sepsis is frequently so intense that organisms can be demonstrated on smears of the buffy coat or peripheral blood (Brooks, 1973).

The combination of massive hemolysis, sudden high fever, and hypotension causes the characteristic renal lesion of acute tubular necrosis with hemoglobinuria and subsequent oliguria or anuria. Intravenous infusion of hemoglobin solutions does not cause acute renal failure in normal man or animals, but rapid intravascular hemolysis, especially in combination with the circulatory changes of an acute febrile illness or impending shock, will produce this lesion.

At autopsy there is evidence of intravascular hemolysis such as pink discoloration of blood vessels, bronzing of the skin, icterus, hemoglobin casts in renal tubules, and erythropoiesis in the marrow. Either obvious or subtle lesions may be found at the site of origin in the uterus, gastrointestinal tract, biliary tree, or skin. Changes compatible with acute renal tubular necrosis may also be present. Welch in 1892 described masses of clostridia and gas-filled bubbles and cysts in many tissues (liver, heart, muscle, and others) and recognized that they represent the effects of continued postmortem proliferation of clostridia with accompanying gas production in the tissues. Too often these postmortem changes have been erroneously described as "gas gangrene" of the liver or of other viscera and have been misinterpreted as antemortem events. On occasion, however, patients with severely depressed resistance (advanced malignancy, acute leukemia, immunosuppression) have such overwhelming septicemia that they may develop multiple foci of metastatic gas infection during life (Boggs et al., 1958; Cabrera et al., 1965).

### CLINICAL MANIFESTATIONS

Clostridial sepsis, fever, and chills usually begin 24 to 72 hours after attempted abortion and are associated first with malaise, headache, severe myalgias, crampy or sharp abdominal pain, nausea, vomiting, and occasionally diarrhea. A foul bloody or brown vaginal discharge is noted. Within a matter of hours symptoms may increase dramatically with the development of oliguria, hypotension, and jaundice. Dark mahogany urine due to hemoglobinuria may be noticed. A characteristic bronzing of the skin can occur within several hours of the onset of hemolysis. On admission to the hospital patients are often gravely ill, jaundiced, and hypotensive. They are characteristically apprehensive, mentally alert although hypotensive, tachypneic, and often display tachycardia out of proportion to the temperature elevation. The skin may be cold and mottled and the sclerae icteric. Pelvic examination reveals red-brown, foul cervical drainage, sometimes with gas bubbles. Laceration marks around the cervix or perforation of the cervical segment may be detected. The uterus is slightly enlarged and tender, but if infection involves the myometrium or has spread to the adnexa, extreme tenderness, guarding, and an adnexal mass may be detected (Mahn and Dantuono, 1955; MacLennan, 1962).

Laboratory studies show a neutrophilic leukocytosis with leukocyte counts of 15,000 to 50,000 per $mm^3$, normal or pink to port-wine colored plasma, with plasma hemoglobin concentrations as high as 8000 mg/100 ml. Anemia is proportional to the degree of hemolysis; hematocrits may be as low as 10 per cent. The platelet count may be moderately or significantly reduced, either as an isolated finding or as part of an unfolding pattern of disseminated intravascular coagulation. Microspherocytes and deformed erythrocytes may be seen on the peripheral smear. Under observation, oliguria or anuria, increasingly refractory hypotension, and, in severe cases, hemorrhagic phenomena and bruising, as well as the laboratory stigmata of disseminated intravascular coagulation, may develop.

Clostridial septicemia arising from the biliary or gastrointestinal tract usually presents as an acute and serious febrile illness with chills and fevers but often with no other specific or localizing findings. Intravascular hemolysis is observed in 30 to 50 per cent of cases. Biliary or gastrointestinal symptoms may be the only clues to the etiology of the apparent bacteremic episode, and the underlying infections would be presumed to be due to gram-negative bacilli until blood culture results are reported.

Patients with malignant disease, especially those receiving treatment with radiation or cytotoxic agents, can rapidly develop fatal clostridial sepsis from a minor gastrointestinal focus or surgical trauma. They have fever, tachypnea, hypotension, abdominal pain or tenderness, nausea, vomiting, and coma. Crepitus may develop in the flanks or over a recent incision, and the temperature and pulse rate may become dissociated. Significant hemolysis is recognized in only 20 to 30 per cent of cases. In studies from oncologic hospitals, a striking feature was the lethality of this syndrome and the rapidity of death.

Half the deaths occur less than 12 hours after onset of symptoms, and almost all occur within 24 hours (Wynne and Armstrong, 1972). Physicians should consider clostridial sepsis in any patient with advanced malignancy who develops abdominal pain or tenderness and fever, and an effective drug for clostridia should be part of any empirical antibiotic therapy, pending the results of blood cultures.

The milder transient bacteremias, which are significantly more common than the septicemic cases, can arise in any hospitalized patient but are most common when there is a predisposing lesion or impaired resistance (cirrhosis, neutropenia, prior antibiotic therapy, immunosuppression). These illnesses have few distinctive clinical features. Blood cultures reveal either *C. perfringens* or nonpathogenic clostridia, and, with or without antibiotics, the fever usually disappears within 24 to 48 hours. Sometimes a more serious illness develops owing to progression of disease at the site of origin, but for the most part there are only serious or self-limited clostridial bacteremias with only a few cases falling between the two poles (Ramsay, 1949; Bornstein et al., 1964; Rathbun, 1968).

## COMPLICATIONS AND SEQUELAE

The major complications of clostridial sepsis are shock, massive intravascular hemolysis with hemoglobinemia and hemoglobinuria, and acute renal tubular necrosis with oliguria and renal failure. Disseminated intravascular coagulation, metastatic clostridial myonecrosis, or metastatic infection elsewhere (endocarditis, meningitis) may be encountered only rarely.

## GEOGRAPHIC VARIATIONS IN DISEASE

*C. perfringens* is present as a major component of human intestinal flora through the world. Hygienic practices vary considerably, however, and much higher carriage rates on the skin, in the oropharynx, and in the female genital tract may be expected in areas with poor sanitary facilities.

Geographic differences in rates of clostridial septicemia are probably related primarily to the level of obstetrical care and to variations in the incidence of septic abortion. With poor sanitation and home deliveries a greater incidence of puerperal clostridial infection may be anticipated. In countries where abortion is legal and freely available, cases of postabortal clostridial sepsis are rare. In countries where religious beliefs interdict rational policies on abortion or where sterile surgical facilities are not available, this preventable disease is still far too prevalent. Socioeconomic factors within a society also play a role in clostridial sepsis. In 1963, before legal abortions were freely available in the United States, postabortal septicemia accounted for 45 per cent of all puerperal mortality in New York and for 80 per cent of the puerperal mortality in black and Puerto Rican women, reflecting a greater incidence of abortion among those of poor socioeconomic status and the dangers of illegal abortion.

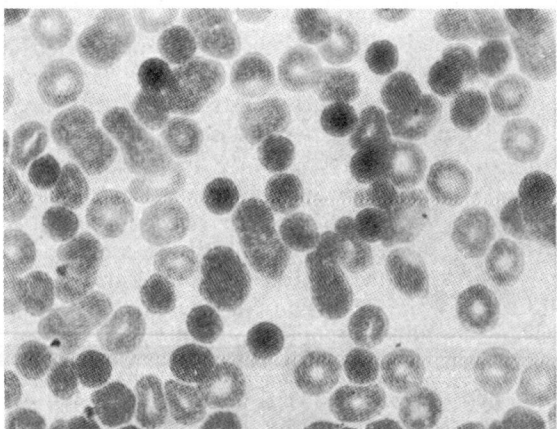

**FIGURE 1.** *Peripheral blood smear (×715) of a patient with frank hemolysis secondary to clostridial septicemia. Numerous microspherocytes are present. (From Bennett, J. M., and Healey, P. J. M.: N Engl J Med 268:1070, 1963.)*

### DIAGNOSIS

Although overt hemolysis, telltale gas shadows, or crepitus can provide clues to clostridial sepsis, they are often absent. In such a case Gram-stained smears and a high index of suspicion are required for early diagnosis.

A Wright or Gram-stained smear of peripheral blood or buffy coat may demonstrate clostridia in cases with thousands of organisms per milliliter of blood, as can be seen when there is overt hemolysis and severely impaired resistance.

Gram-stained smears of cervical drainage, of wound drainage, or of aspiration from crepitant wounds should be examined promptly. In postabortal cases the absence of plump Gram-positive rods militates against clostridial infection: their presence is supportive but may represent only vaginal carriage of *C. perfringens* or of a nonpathogenic species. A constellation of findings on Gram stains of cervical swabs that is highly associated with clostridial sepsis was described by Butler (1942): many plump Gram-positive rods with a heavy capsule (by Muir stain) associated with no more than a few ragged polymorphonuclear leukocytes (PMN's). The presence of many PMN's, active phagocytosis, or the absence of capsule augured against clostridial sepsis. If the gram-positive rods contain spores, they are not *C. perfringens*, which forms no spores in human tissues. They may represent *C. septicum* or *C. novyi*, but statistically they are more likely to represent one of the numerous nonpathogenic species.

Wright-stained blood films may show a distinctive pattern of microspherocytosis — small dense erythrocytes that have been injured by alpha toxin and are soon to lyse (Fig. 1) (Hadley and Ekroth, 1954; Bennett and Healey, 1964). Several cases had been first diagnosed when this striking abnormality was recognized in the clinical laboratory (Willis, 1969). Serial observation of serum samples for evidence of hemolysis and of urine samples for hemoglobinuria, and serial examina-

tion for new physical findings may help establish the diagnosis early. If overt hemolysis develops during observation, the diagnosis is established.

An abdominal x-ray may detect gas in the uterus, uterine wall, or free in the pelvis (Fig. 2), or gas may be found in the gallbladder or biliary tree (Fig. 3).

Cultural techniques for isolating and identifying clostridia are described in Chapter 45. Positive blood cultures will be the only evidence for clostridial bacteremia and sepsis in many cases.

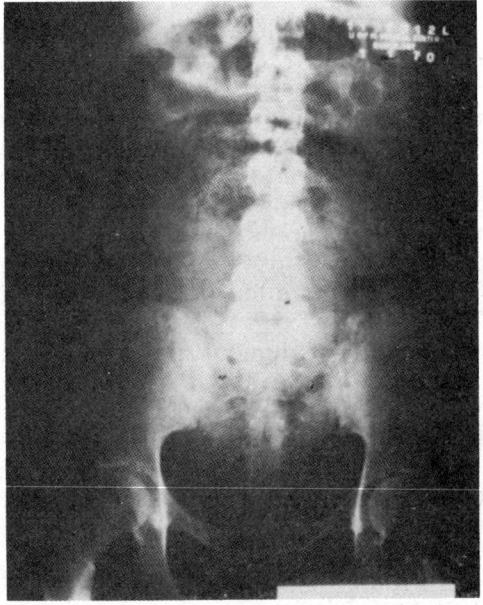

**FIGURE 2.** *Clostridial infection of the uterus. Gas bubbles can be seen in the myometrium. (From Eaton, C. J., and Peterson, E. P.: Am J Obstet Gynecol 109:1162, 1971.)*

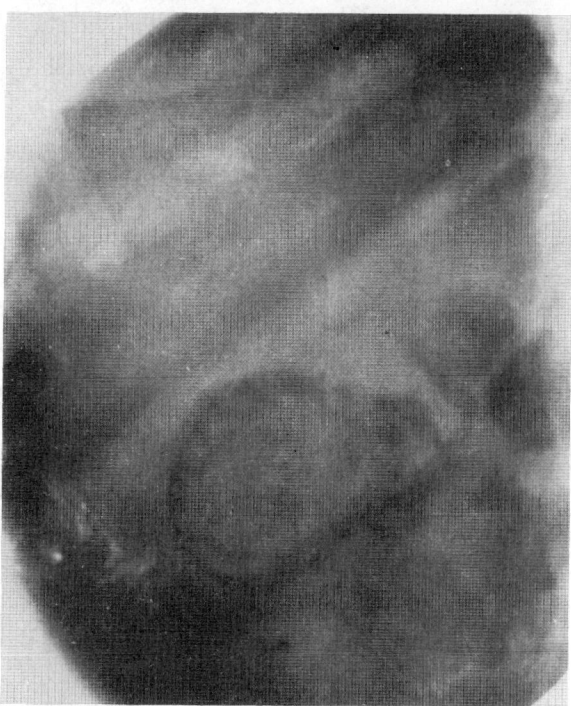

**FIGURE 3.** *Emphysematous cholecystitis. (Courtesy of Alfred Berne, M.D.)*

## TREATMENT

Clostridial septicemia carries a very poor prognosis, with a mortality of 25 to 75 per cent despite treatment. The results reflect patient delay in seeking help (especially among postabortal cases) and delays in diagnosis in the more unusual cases.

Once clostridial sepsis is suspected or proved, the treatment of choice is 3 million units penicillin G every three hours intravenously (I.V.). If the patient is allergic to penicillin, parenteral cephalosporins (cefazolin 1 g every six hours I.V.), cephalothin, cephapirin, or cephamandole 2 g every 4 hours I.V.), clindamycin (600 mg every six hours I.V.), chloramphenicol (1 g every six hours I.V.), or vancomycin (0.5 g every six hours I.V.) are effective alternatives. Aminoglycosides and polymyxins are ineffective. Tetracycline resistance is too prevalent to rely on this drug, and blood and tissue levels of erythromycin are inadequate for treatment of clostridial sepsis. Antibiotics should be begun promptly after initial cultures have been obtained in suspected cases.

Since coliforms and other enterics are even more common causes of sepsis of uterine, biliary, or intestinal origin than are clostridia, and since mixed infections can occur, an aminoglycoside, in full I.V. doses, should be added pending results of the initial cultures and adjusted for renal function. If the clinical situation suggests that *Bacteroides* may be involved, then intravenous clindamycin 600 mg every six hours, or chloramphenicol succinate 1 g every six hours should be part of the initial therapy.

Antitoxin should be used to prevent further hemolysis and tissue injury by circulating alpha toxin. Because equine antitoxin can induce serum sickness, it should be used in the absence of hemolysis only when the diagnosis of clostridial sepsis is strongly suggested. It is most effective if given before gross hemolysis has occurred. A recommended dose is 40,000 units (four vials) of monospecific anti-*C. perfringens* alpha toxin initially folowed by 20,000 to 40,000 units every six hours until hemolysis is controlled. It can be given intramuscularly or by I.V. drip; the latter may be more effective in acute hemolysis, the former may be safer. Local instillation into the uterus has been advocated but not carefully studied.

When clostridial sepsis follows septic abortion it is generally necessary to empty or to remove the uterus. There is considerable controversy about the proper surgical approach in different stages of this disease. If clostridia are demonstrated in Gram stains of cervical smears, the first decision is whether there is evidence of bacteremia. If there is no hemolysis and only moderate fever and illness, fluids and antibiotics are administered, and any retained fetal and placental tissues are removed by aspiration or by curettage. If the patient is seriously ill or if there is hemolysis, antitoxin, antibiotics, and fluids are administered and a surgical approach is chosen and carried out. If gas is found in the wall of the uterus or free in the pelvis by x-ray or sonogram, and if there is uterine or adnexal tenderness, a total abdominal hysterectomy is indicated. The decision to remove tubes and ovaries is best made after direct observation during surgery. The most controversial situation arises from the uncertainty of whether the infection has penetrated into the myometrium in a woman who is clearly ill and has hemolysis. Some would opt for curettage if such patients want to remain fertile; others would choose early hysterectomy for all patients. The best plan for these cases is uncertain but involves important personal choices for the woman as well as the physician. Hyperbaric oxygen, which is recommended by some (Perrin et al., 1970), has only limited use in serious disease and is fraught with complications (Smith et al., 1971). It does not appear to be an important alternative in frank septicemia.

If oliguria ensues, an effective means of dealing with the problems of hyperkalemia, fluid balance, and azotemia is required. Although medical management may suffice for several days, peritoneal dialysis or hemodialysis will be necessary for the more severe cases of renal tubular necrosis. If massive hemolysis and shock occur early in the illness, a protracted period of renal shutdown can be anticipated, and if facilities are available for hemodialysis, an AV shunt should be placed. Such a shunt allows, in addition, a convenient route for exchange transfusions, which have been recommended by some in the early course to remove toxic products of hemolysis and residual circulating toxins. This therapy may be lifesaving in cases of disseminated intravascular coagulation and may reduce the extent of hemoglobinuric renal injury (Rubenberg,1967; Strum, 1968).

Hypotension carries a very grave prognosis in this disease. It is best treated as other cases of septic shock (Chapter 86) by prompt correction of hypovolemia, anemia, lactic acidemia and hypoxia, by early surgical intervention to remove or drain the source of sepsis, and by appropriate antibiotic and, if indicated, antitoxin administration. Rapid and precise hemodynamic and biochemical monitoring to guide proper fluid, blood, bicarbonate, and electrolyte replacement, as well as the need for and use of pressor drugs and ventilatory support, can be lifesaving at this stage.

## PROPHYLAXIS

Clostridial sepsis is a rare disease, and specific indications for immunoprophylaxis are few. There is no effective toxoid or vaccine for active immunization in humans.

Chemoprophylaxis with parenteral penicillin does appear warranted during and after cholecystectomy or common duct exploration in elderly patients and when acute pathologic changes are encountered at surgery. Intraoperative Gram stains of bile have been urged as a guide to the choice of prophylactic antibiotics (Keighley et al., 1977).

An important general preventive measure is the removal of the need for women to seek illegal and unsterile abortions by providing birth control education and assistance and safe surgical facilities for those who require abortions. Upgrading sanitary facilities generally will reduce puerperal and post-traumatic clostridial infections.

## References

Alpern, R. J., and Dowell, V. R., Jr.: Clostridium septicum infections and malignancy. JAMA 209:385, 1969.

Alpern, R. J., and Dowell, V. R., Jr.: Non-histotoxic clostridial bacteremia. Am J Clin Pathol 55:717, 1971.

Bennett, J. M., and Healey, P. J. M.: Spherocytic hemolytic anemia and acute cholecystitis caused by Clostridium welchii. N Engl J Med 268:1070, 1963.

Boggs, D. R., Frei, E., and Thomas, L. B.: Clostridial gas gangrene and septicemia in patients with leukemia. N Engl J Med 295:1255, 1958.

Bornstein, D. L., Weinberg, A. N., Swartz, M. N., and Kunz, L. J.: Anaerobic infections: Review of current experience. Medicine 43:207, 1964.

Brooks, G. F.: Early diagnosis of bacteremia by examination of buffy coat. Arch Intern Med 132:673, 1973.

Butler, H. M.: The examination of cervical smears as a means of rapid diagnosis in severe C. welchii infection following abortion. J Pathol Bacteriol 54:39, 1942.

Cabrera, A., Tsukada, Y., and Pickren, J. W.: Clostridial gas gangrene and septicemia in malignant disease. Cancer 18:800, 1965.

Fredette, V.: Effect of hyperbaric oxygen on anaerobic bacteria and toxins. Ann NY Acad Sci 117:700, 1965.

Fukunaga, F. H.: Gallbladder bacteriology, histology, and gallstones. Arch Surg 106:169, 1973.

Gorbach, S. L., and Thadepalli, H.: Isolation of Clostridium in human infections: Evaluation of 114 cases. J Infect Dis Suppl 131:S81, 1975.

Hadley, G. G., and Ekroth, R. D.: Spherocytosis as a manifestation of postabortal C. welchii infection. Am J Obstet Gynecol 67:691, 1954.

Keighley, M. R. B., McLeish, A. R., Bishop, H. M., et al: Identification of the presence and type of biliary microflora by immediate gram stains. Surgery 81:469, 1977.

MacLennan, J. D.: The histotoxic clostridial infections of man. Bacteriol Rev 26:177, 1962.

Mahn, E., and Dantuono, L. M.: Postabortal septicotoxemia due to Clostridium welchii. Am J Obstet Gynecol 70:604, 1955.

Martin, W. J.: Isolation and identification of anaerobic bacteria in the clinical laboratory. Mayo Clin Proc 49:300, 1974.

Oakley, C. L.: Gas gangrene. Br Med Bull 10:52, 1954.

Perrin, L. E., Ostergard, D. R., and Mishell, D. R.: The use of hyperbaric oxygen in the treatment of clostridial septicemia complicating septic abortion. Am J Obstet Gynecol 106:666, 1970.

Ramsay, A. M.: The significance of Clostridium welchii in the cervical swab and blood stains in postpartum and postabortion sepsis. J Obstet Gynecol Br Commonw 56:247, 1949.

Rathbun, H. K.: Clostridial bacteremia without hemolysis. Arch Intern Med 122:496, 1968.

Rubenberg, M. L., Baker, L. R. I., McBride, J. A., Sevitt, L. H., and Brain, M. C.: Intravascular coagulation in a case of Clostridium perfringens septicemia: Treatment by exchange transfusion. Br Med J 4:271, 1967.

Smith, J. W., Southern, P. M., Jr., and Lehmann, J. D.: Bacteremia in septic abortion: Complications and treatment. Obstet Gynecol 35:704, 1970.

Smith, L. P., McLean, A. P., and Maughan, G. B.: Clostridium welchii septicotoxemia. A review and report of three cases. Am J Obstet Gynecol 110:135, 1971.

Strum, W. B., Cade, J. R., Shires, D. L., and deQuesada, A.: Postabortal septicemia due to C. welchii. Treatment with exchange transfusion. Arch Intern Med 122:73, 1968.

Welch, W. H., and Nuttall, G. H. F.: A gas-producing bacillus (Bacillus aerogenes capsulatus) capable of rapid development in the blood vessels after death. Bull Johns Hopkins Hosp 3:81, 1892.

Willis, A. T.: Clostridia of wound infection. London, Butterworths, 1969.

Wynne, J. W., and Armstrong, D.: Clostridial septicemia. Cancer 29:215, 1972.

# BRUCELLOSIS 184

## Wesley W. Spink, M.D.

### DEFINITION

Brucellosis is an infectious disease caused by bacteria in the genus *Brucella*. The disease is transmitted to humans, directly or indirectly, from the natural animal reservoirs of sheep, goats, cattle, swine, and reindeer. Acute brucellosis can simulate many other infections. Chronic brucellosis with fever, weakness, and complaints of vague origin usually has demonstrable localizing manifestations. It is unusual for chronic disease to follow acute brucellosis if properly treated.

Brucellosis has probably existed for centuries in the Mediterranean areas, causing an illness known as Mediterranean fever, Malta fever, Gibraltar fever, Neapolitan fever, Cyprus fever, and undulant fever. David Bruce first isolated brucellae from patients in Malta in 1887. Hughes described the human disease definitively in 1897. Thereafter reservoirs of the disease were traced to domestic animals (Spink, 1956).

### ETIOLOGY

Three classic species of *Brucella* cause human disease, originating from their own animal reservoirs: *Brucella melitensis* from sheep and goats, *Brucella abortus* from cattle, and *Brucella suis* from swine. Because of certain biochemical or metabolic differences, each of the species is divided into subtypes. *Br. melitensis* has three, *Br. abortus* nine, and *Br. suis* three. *Br. suis*, Subtype II, called *Brucella rangiferi tarandi*, is found in the reindeer of Alaska and Siberia and is a cause of human illness. The species *Br. canis* causes epidemic disease in dogs but has caused only a few human cases. Recognition of the species causing human illness is important epidemiologically in the control of animal reservoirs of the disease. *Br. abortus*, Strain 19, a live vaccine widely used for immunizing cattle, has caused human illness through accidental self-inoculation by veterinarians. There is no evidence that Strain 19 is transmitted from vaccinated animals to humans, either directly or indirectly.

### GEOGRAPHICAL DISTRIBUTION

The species of *Brucella* causing illness depends upon the species present in the natural reservoir of animals. Brucellosis afflicts dairy cattle in most parts of the world (Stableforth, 1959). In the United States for many years the predominant cause has been *Br. abortus*, because cattle, especially dairy herds, harbor the organisms. Range cattle in the United States and elsewhere in the world are uncommon reservoirs of brucellosis. Foci of infections due to *Br. suis* appear in workers in abattoirs where infected swine are slaughtered. *Br. melitensis* in sheep and goats is a minor problem in the United States, occurring in the southwestern part of the country. Most cases of brucellosis in the United States involve men between the ages of 20 and 50 years, principally abattoir employees, farmers, and veterinarians. Children rarely have the disease because milk is pasteurized.

In many areas, *Br. melitensis* is the predominant cause of disease because sheep and goats are infected. These areas include Mexico, Central and South America, France and southeastern Europe, countries bordering on the Mediterranean, and parts of Africa, southern Russia, Iran, and India.

Human cases originating from infected swine occur in the United States, Germany, Austria, Bulgaria, and Russia. *Br. suis* Type 4 (*rangiferi tarandus*) parasitizes reindeer in Siberia and Alaska, where it is a common, and the only, cause of human brucellosis. *Br. suis* Type 2, found in the hare and swine of Denmark and southeastern Europe, is not a cause of human disease.

There are other, less commonly distributed animal reservoirs of brucellosis that cause human disease, such as camels (*Br. melitensis*), yaks in Mongolia (*Br. abortus*), bison, elk, and moose (*Br. abortus*).

### PATHOGENESIS AND PATHOLOGY

The portals of entry for *Brucella* are minute abrasions of the skin, oropharynx, and conjunctivae. Entering the blood stream, the organisms localize preferentially in tissues having an abundance of reticuloendothelial cells such as lymph nodes, liver, spleen, and bone marrow, although the kidneys, central and peripheral nervous systems, testes, and bone are also involved (Spink, 1956). The circulating polymorphonuclear leukocytes are the first line of defense against *Brucella*, but the macrophages in the blood and tissues are the major cells that ingest and destroy the bacteria. The tissue reaction in brucellosis is primarily granulomatous. It consists of epithelioid cells, giant cells, and an infiltrate of lymphocytes and plasma cells. The lesions simulate those of sarcoidosis. Almost simultaneously with the formation of granulomas, *Brucella* disappears from the tissues.

Occasionally, however, the focal lesion becomes necrotic, and caseation appears similar to that of tuberculosis. This occurs particularly with the suppurating lesions caused by *Br. suis*, but also occasionally with *Br. melitensis* or *Br. abortus*.

Toward the second week after invasion by *Brucella*, the tissues develop hypersensitivity to *Brucella* antigens, and circulating antibodies appear. The *Brucella* hypersensitivity very likely contributes to the systemic reaction of the patient, much like the patient with tuberculosis and his reaction to tuberculin.

## CLINICAL MANIFESTATIONS

The incubation period of the disease is from one to three weeks. Brucellosis is usually an acute febrile disease with chills, sweats, headache, aches and pains, and weakness like that occurring in influenza. There are usually few or no localizing findings except lymphadenopathy and a palpable spleen and liver. With rest and supportive treatment, most patients recover within three to six months, and even earlier with tetracycline therapy. Although much has been written about a condition known as "chronic brucellosis" in which symptoms endure for years, the number of proved cases having a continued illness after 12 months is relatively small. This is particularly true of patients who have received adequate therapy. Relapses are uncommon in treated patients. Treated individuals who have illness after one year usually have a demonstrable suppurative localization, especially of the bone or joints.

## COMPLICATIONS

The most common complication involves the bones and joints. Spondylitis involving an intervertebral area of the lumbar spine, which can be associated with a sciatic distribution of severe pain, is the most frequent manifestation. The larger joints, such as the hip joint, may have localized suppuration. Brucellosis does not cause chronic polyarthritis of the smaller joints.

During the acute phase, peripheral neuritis may occur and gradually subside. Meningitis is an uncommon complication. Localization in the kidneys causes chronic pyuria, as in tuberculosis.

Orchitis, usually unilateral, mimics mumps, but sterility does not follow. Suppurative endocarditis is a rare complication, and pulmonary lesions rarely occur. Brucellosis does not cause human abortions any more frequently than other bacterial infections.

Brucellosis, like typhoid fever, does cause mental depression, especially if convalesence is prolonged. This can result in a state of chronic neurasthenia after recovery from the disease. Patients must be reassured that lingering fatigue and weakness do not imply that they have chronic brucellosis, a diagnosis that must be applied cautiously. Unless severe inflammatory complications have occurred, brucellosis does not result in sequelae.

## DIAGNOSIS

Brucellosis simulates many other febrile diseases such as infectious mononucleosis, typhoid fever, malaria, and influenza. Because the infection is an occupational disease, knowledge of exposure to potentially infected animals is a distinct aid in differential diagnosis. Likewise, the ingestion of unpasteurized milk or *fresh* milk products, such as cheese, from a questionable source is helpful. Enlarged peripheral lymph nodes and a palpable spleen are consistent with the disease.

A definitive diagnosis is dependent upon laboratory data (Alton et al., 1975). A characteristic finding in the peripheral blood is an increase in lymphocytes, which have at times a morphology like that in infectious mononucleosis. The total leukocyte count may be normal, elevated, or reduced. The erythrocyte sedimentation rate is of no aid, since it may be accelerated or normal.

The most reliable procedure for screening suspected cases of brucellosis is the tube-dilution saline agglutination test in which a reliable *Brucella* antigen is used. The test has minor limitations as far as specificity is concerned. Cross-agglutination occurs with *Vibrio cholera* and *Pasteurella tularensis* when the test is done with the sera of patients who have had these diseases or received vaccines containing these organisms. The antigen-serum mixtures should be incubated for 48 hours at 37° C and then examined. Titers of 1:100 and above are significant, although individuals who have had the disease months and years previously may have titers of 1:100 and below, and occasionally higher. "Blocking antibodies" may interfere with a clear-cut reading in the lower dilutions, where little or no agglutination may occur, and prevent complete agglutinations in the higher dilutions. When such blocking is present, centrifuging the mixtures at 3000 rpm may reveal further clumping. The presence of blocking antibody can also be detected in incubating the suspect serum with a known serum of high antibody content. Dilutions of the serum mixture are then incubated with antigen, and if blocking is present, the titer will be lower than that in the untreated serum.

Although agglutinins are rarely absent in patients with active disease, especially in those with blood cultures that reveal *Brucella* organisms, the interpretation of agglutinin titers of 1:100 or less is often difficult when the cultures remain sterile. The *Brucella* agglutinin in active disease is IgG antibody, whereas in those who have recovered from the disease it is IgM. The type of antibody present in the serum may be differentiated by adding 2-mercaptoethanol to the antigen-antibody mixtures. Under these circumstances, IgM is degraded, and no agglutination occurs.

The complement fixation, Coombs' antiglobulin, and fluorescent antibody tests add nothing to the ordinary agglutination test in routine clinical diagnosis.

Blood cultures should be made for every suspected case of brucellosis before therapy is attempted. We prefer two cultures, each performed one day apart. In the Castaneda technique, blood is introduced into rectangular bottles of 120 ml capacity. Trypticase soy broth or tryptose broth is the culture medium, and agar composed of the same basic medium is layered along one of the edges of the bottle. Ten per cent of the air is displaced with carbon dioxide. After the blood is mixed with the broth, the mixture is spread over the agar, and then the bottle is placed in the incubator at 37° C. The agar layer is examined daily for at least 21 days for evidence of bacterial colonies, which usually appear within a week. Cerebrospinal fluid, urine, and tissues minced with sterile saline solution can be cultured in the same manner.

The *Brucella* skin test is specific for the disease, and, like the tuberculin reaction, a positive test indicates past or recent exposure to the disease. Because skin reactivity may endure for years after recovery from disease, it is of little value in diagnosis. Skin testing is useful in epidemiologic studies for determining the degree of exposure to brucellosis in a population.

## TREATMENT

The physician should convey the diagnosis of brucellosis to the patient only if definitive diagnostic laboratory data support this conclusion, since popular and medical literature portray a disease leading to a life of chronic and disabling illness. Furthermore, the physician should reassure the patient that health will be restored after proper antibiotic therapy.

During the acute phase of the illness, rest is paramount. Supportive treatment should include sedation and analgesics, such as salicylates. Tetracycline should be administered orally with an initial dose of 1.0 g, followed by a second dose in four hours, and then 0.5 g four times daily for 21 days. In severe cases, 1.0 g of streptomycin daily can be given simultaneously intramuscularly for ten days. Occasional relapses may occur within one to three months for which a similar course of tetracycline should be given, with or without streptomycin. There is no advantage in giving repeated courses of therapy to any patient, particularly in those with *presumed* chronic brucellosis.

Patients with severe brucellosis accompanied by fever, marked toxicity, and anorexia can obtain marked relief from an adrenal steroid such as prednisone in an oral dose of 20 mg two to three times a day for up to five days.

*Brucella* vaccines are not recommended for "desensitization" of patients with chronic disease.

Patients who recover from brucellosis become immune to the disease. Reinfection can result in a milder febrile illness, that responds readily to tetracycline for a week or ten days, according to the foregoing schedule.

## PROPHYLAXIS

The control of human brucellosis depends upon the eradication of brucellosis in animal reservoirs. There is no suitable prophylactic vaccine for humans.

### References

Alton, G. G., Jones, L. M., and Pietz, D. E.: Laboratory Techniques in Brucellosis. 2nd ed. Geneva, World Health Organization, 1975.
Spink, W. W.: The Nature of Brucellosis. Minneapolis, University of Minnesota Press, 1956.
Stableforth, A. W.: Brucellosis. *In* Stableforth, A. W., and Galloway, I. A. (eds.): Infectious Diseases of Animals. Vol. I. Diseases Due to Bacteria. New York, Academic Press, 1959, Chapter 3.

# 185 BARTONELLOSIS

## M. Cuadra, M.D.

### DEFINITION

Bartonellosis is a human infection caused by *Bartonella bacilliformis*, a bacterium that has an affinity for vascular endothelial and red blood cells. Transmitted by certain species of *Phlebotomus*, it is confined to certain Andean valleys in Peru, Ecuador, and Colombia. The disease occurs in two stages: the first, named Oroya fever or Carrión's disease, is characterized by an acute febrile hemolytic anemia; the second stage, verruga peruana, is characterized by the appearance of hemangioma-like nodules on the skin.

### ETIOLOGY

After a short period of confusion (Strong et al., 1913), it has been firmly established that both Oroya fever and verruga peruana are caused by the same organism, *B. bacilliformis* (Noguchi, 1927a, b; Pinkerton and Weinman, 1937–38; Strong, 1945), and that the conditions represent two stages of the same disease. The experiment of Carrión, who was voluntarily inoculated with the exudate from a verruga nodule and succumbed to Oroya fever, represents one of the most solid supports for the etiologic unity of both entities. The taxonomic position of *B. bacilliformis* (Moulder, 1974) is still unsettled.

### PATHOGENESIS AND PATHOLOGY

In the stage of Oroya fever or Carrión's disease only two types of host cells are parasitized — vascular endothelial cells and red blood cells. In the stage of verruga peruana the organisms are found only in the verruga nodules; no *Bartonella* organisms can be seen in erythrocytes, although blood cultures frequently are positive. In the "verrucoma," abundant organisms are found within the cytoplasm of endothelial cells lining the vessels (angioblasts) in both human nodules (Mayer et al., 1913; Mackehenie and Weiss, 1926; Weiss, 1932; Weinman and Pinkerton, 1937; Alzamora Castro, 1945; Urteaga and Calderón, 1965) and in nodules experimentally induced in monkeys (Mayer et al., 1913; Noguchi, 1926a, b; Noguchi and Battistini, 1926; Mackehenie and Weiss, 1926; Marquez de Cunha and Muniz, 1928; Kikuth, 1931; Weinman and Pinkerton, 1937). Using the electron microscope, both intracellular (Takano, 1970) and extracellular organisms (Recavarren and Lumbreras, 1972) have been found.

This discrepancy remains to be clarified. These findings are consistent with the ability of *Bartonella* to grow intra- and extracellularly in tissue cultures (Pinkerton and Weinman, 1937).

#### Oroya Fever Stage

Neither the cycle of *B. bacilliformis* within the *Phlebotomus* nor the mechanism of penetration of the agent into or through the skin is known. Scratching of the *Phlebotomus* bite may favor penetration. From the skin (first station) the *Bartonella* organisms travel to the regional lymph nodes (second station). From there the infection enters the bloodstream and then the vascular endothelium (third station). Endothelial cells fully loaded with microorganisms have, in fact, been found by a number of authors (Strong and Tyzzer, 1915; Aldana, 1929; Pinkerton and Weinman, 1937–38; Alzamora Castro, 1940; Urteaga, 1948). The presence of *Bartonella* organisms in the blood causes symptoms (fever) if the organisms exceed a certain concentration. The time elapsing from the first station (skin) to the third one (blood) is approximately three weeks. This is the incubation period.

After infecting the endothelial cells, the parasites can involve nearly all the red blood cells of the host. It appears that when infected endothelial cells burst (Aldana, 1929, 1947), the released organisms enter the blood directly and penetrate the red blood cells. The propensity of *Bartonella* to attach to red blood cells has, in fact, been demonstrated in vitro (Cuadra, 1978). The possibility of transmission of *Bartonella* organisms from erythrocyte to erythrocyte appears to be unlikely (although intracellular organisms are viable since multiplication can be observed under the microscope in broth cultures of blood from patients with Oroya fever) because the organisms are intracellular (Cuadra and Takano, 1969) and no rupture of parasitized erythrocytes occurs within the bloodstream.

*B. bacilliformis* appears in the erythrocytes of Oroya fever patients in two discrete forms: as rods (so-called bacillary forms) and as coccoid forms. The pathogenic significance of these two forms was deduced from clinical and hematologic observations made serially on patients in different stages of Oroya fever. The clinical manifestations could be correlated with the morphologic changes of the causative organism. It was found that the bacillary form was always related, whatever its quantity, to the existence of fever; thus, at scarcely the first or second day of onset of Oroya fever, the patient has a high temperature even though there are only small numbers of intracellular rods — for example, one/1000 erythrocytes (Cuadra, 1957). During the following days, the number of the rods increases geometrically. Later, coccoid forms appear in the blood so that by the end of the second week the proportion of both forms is approximately equal. During the remission period of the fever (third week), coccoid forms increasingly predominate in number over rods. During convalescence only coccoid forms are present (see Fig. 1 in Chapter 51). If a relapse occurs as the temperature rises, bacillary forms reappear in the erythrocytes (Cuadra, 1957). From these observations it was deduced that the bacillary form and the coccoid form represent vegetative and inactive (stationary) forms respectively of *Bartonella*. The coccoid forms seem to originate from the rods by multisegmentation; rosary-like (intermediate) forms are seen frequently. A similar transformation occurs in vitro on blood agar cultures.

The anemia caused by *B. bacilliformis* is hemolytic in nature inasmuch as the lifespan of parasitized erythrocytes is notably shortened (Reynafarge and Ramos, 1961). The serum indirect bilirubin (Guzman Barrón, 1926; Hurtado et al., 1938), urobilin, and stercobilin concentrations (Urteaga, 1948), and iron stores in the spleen, liver, and lymph glands are notably increased (Strong and Tyzzer, 1915; Weiss, 1933; Urteaga, 1948). In addition, erythromyeloid hyperplasia of the bone marrow occurs (Carvallo, 1911; Hurtado et al., 1938; Urteaga, 1948), and reticulocytes in the peripheral blood are increased. *Bartonella* does not directly destroy the erythrocyte it parasitizes because intravascular hemolysis, which characteristically occurs in hemobartonellosis, never occurs in Oroya fever despite the high rate of parasitism and the significantly increased mechanical fragility of the parasitized erythrocytes (Reynafarge and Ramos, 1961). Red blood cell ghosts were found in smears of peripheral blood from Oroya fever patients and rat hemobartonellosis, slightly increased in the former and strongly in the latter (Cuadra, 1957). Neither hemagglutinins nor hemolysins are present in serum (Guzman Barrón, 1926), and the Coombs' test is negative (Reynafarge and Ramos, 1961). The finding in histologic sections of spleen, liver, and lymph nodes of large quantities of macrophages overloaded with erythrocytes (Strong, 1915; Aldana, 1929; Weiss, 1932; Urteaga, 1948) is evidence that the anemia occurs as a consequence of erythrophagocytosis (Aldana, 1929). The fact that the severity of the anemia is proportional to the degree of erythrocytic parasitism (Gonzalez Olaechea, 1932; Cuadra, 1970) indicates that only parasitized erythrocytes are phagocytized. Such selective phagocytosis implies that the macrophages can recognize parasitized erythrocytes. Since the *Bartonella* is an intracellular organism, it is not understood how this recognition occurs. It is suggested that *Bartonella* organisms release some antigen that coats the erythrocyte. The rapidity with which the anemia occurs (there is a decrease of approximately 200 to 400 thousand circulating red cells per $mm^3$ per day) is consistent with antibody-mediated phagocytosis. The anemia may also be due to an autoimmune mechanism, but there is no direct evidence for this. The anemia tends to be normocytic and normochromic during the stage of red blood cell destruction.

Hypersplenism exists in Oroya fever and may contribute to the anemia. It is evidenced by the hematologic changes that occur during the febrile period compared with those of the convalescent period. During the febrile period, in which bacillary forms of *Bartonella* are present, relative leukopenia and thrombocytopenia, and at times thrombocytopenic purpura (Ricketts, 1942) occur. When the temperature declines to normal and the convalescent period, in which only coccoid forms of *Bartonella* are present, commences, leukocytosis (at times a leukemoid reaction) and thrombocytosis occur. Large lymphocytes (40 to 60 per cent) with wide ameboid and basophilic cytoplasm are usually found. Reticulocytes also increase abruptly (10 to 30 per cent or more), and there is anisocytosis and polychromatophilia. The anemia in this stage of hematologic regeneration tends to be macrocytic and hypochromic.

The factors responsible for the functional disturbance and/or the pathologic lesions in Oroya fever are the *Bartonella* organism itself, anoxemia, and complicating salmonellosis. In pure cases of Oroya fever there is an extraordinary hyperplasia of the reticuloendothelial system in the spleen, the lymph nodes, the liver, and the bone marrow. The hyperplasia serves to increase the removal of parasitized erythrocytes and to consolidate the immunity against *Bartonella*. Zonal necrosis of the liver around the central veins of the lobules has been reported to occur in Oroya fever (Strong, 1915). Since this has been reproduced in monkeys in which neither severe anemia nor salmonellosis occurred (Noguchi, 1927), and since *Bartonella* does not invade the hepatocytes, the necrosis is probably caused by a *Bartonella* toxin circulating in blood. However, there is no significant increase of serum transaminase in typical Oroya fever. Anoxemia and *Salmonella* septicemia kill patients without producing gross pathologic lesions.

### Verruga Peruana Stage

Histologically, the verruga nodule is a dense network of blood vessels lying in a matrix or interstitium of edematous connective tissue within which lymphatic vessels, angioblasts, histiocytes, and leukocytes are associated with fibroblasts (Rocha Lima, 1913; Mackehenie, 1938; Hercelles, 1935). The relative amount of these components varies with the age and developmental stages of the nodules. Thus, according to Mackehenie (1938), early nodules are rich in histiocytes, mature ones in blood vessels and angioblasts, and old nodules in fibroblasts. The angioblasts derive from the endothelium of the vessels. They proliferate outward, forming buds of variable size (Rocha Lima, 1913). The new capillaries probably develop from the buds as a result of canalization of a lumen into which blood then flows (McCutcheon, 1948). According to the type of predominant tissue or cells, the verruga nodule may resemble a hemangioma or a fibrosarcoma. Most nodules show few leukocytes; occasionally lymphocytes or granulocytes may be present in appreciable numbers. In this latter case a secondary infection should be considered. In hematoxylin–eosin-stained sections of nodules the organisms are not visible. Sections should be fixed in Regaud's solution and stained with Giemsa's stain to demonstrate organisms (Noguchi, 1926; Pinkerton and Weinman, 1937–38). *B. bacilliformis* is doubtless present within the verruga tissue, but its precise localization, whether intracellular (Takano, 1970) or extracellular (Recavarren and Lumbreras, 1972), and the cells involved are unknown. When the nodules are full-grown, outgrowths of fibroblasts are obtained (Cuadra, 1966). The identity of the inclusion-like bodies found within cells, which presumably are densely packed *Bartonella* organisms, must be elucidated by electronmicroscopy.

## CLINICAL MANIFESTATIONS

### Oroya Fever or Carrión's Disease

The cardinal manifestations of Oroya fever (Carrión's disease) are fever, anemia, and enlargement of the spleen, lymph nodes, and liver. Fever represents the best indicator of disease activity and in most cases lasts as long as two to three weeks. It is irregular or remittent in type and considerable sweating occurs with it. Its onset may occur suddenly or be preceded by prodromal symptoms and it terminates usually by lysis. No chronic Oroya fever has been reported. The temperature reaches 39 to 40° C and is accompanied by intense toxemic manifestations (headache, malaise, pains in the bones and large joints). Anemia develops so rapidly that in a week an intense pallor of the skin and mucous membranes of the mouth and conjunctivae occurs. The

pallor is accompanied by slight jaundice. The resulting anoxemia may be reflected in clouding of consciousness, apathy, rapid pulse, and a great tendency to circulatory collapse. The enlargement of the lymph nodes (cervical, axillary, epitrochlear, inguinal) is painless and less than that in infectious mononucleosis. The spleen is less enlarged than in typhoid fever or brucellosis. The enlargement of the liver is moderate and is more marked in young people than in adults. After the fever stops, patients feel well in spite of the profound anemia, and complete recovery occurs in three to four weeks. In some patients slight edema of the face and feet; and effusion in serous cavities may occur during the first week of convalescence. This is probably due to protein deficiency (Merino, 1939). In severe forms of Oroya fever death is caused by both toxemia and anemia or by any intercurrent infection, of which salmonellosis is the most common (Cuadra, 1956).

In addition to the pattern of Oroya fever described above, in which there is a high rate of parasitism, there are cases with a very low parasitism rate throughout the course of the disease (paucibacillary form of Oroya fever) (Figs. 1 and 5). In these cases there is at most a slight anemia (Gonzalez Olaechea, 1932; Cuadra, 1970). The fever may last as long as the ordinary type or only one to three days. Between these extremes there is a range of intermediate forms.

***Complications and Sequelae.*** Approximately 40 per cent of cases of Oroya fever are complicated

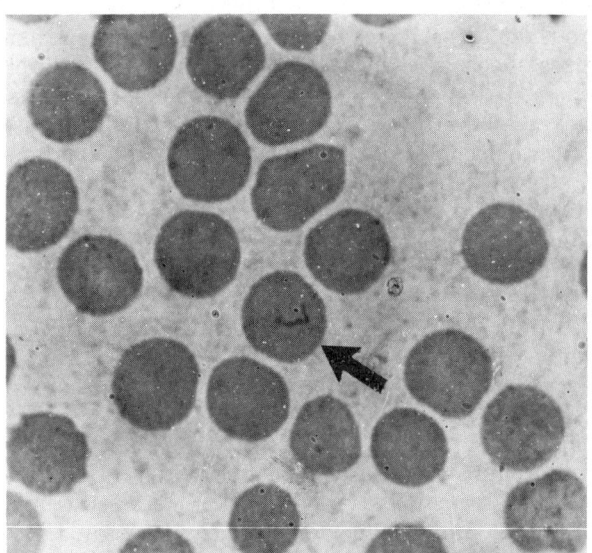

**FIGURE 1.** *Blood film of a patient suffering from a paucibacillary form of Oroya fever. A very low parasitism rate, illustrated by the photograph in which only one red blood cell (arrow) appears parasitized by a bacillary* Bartonella, *was observed throughout the course (27 days) of the disease. No antibiotics were used and the verruga peruana stage occurred 55 days after spontaneous remission of the fever.*

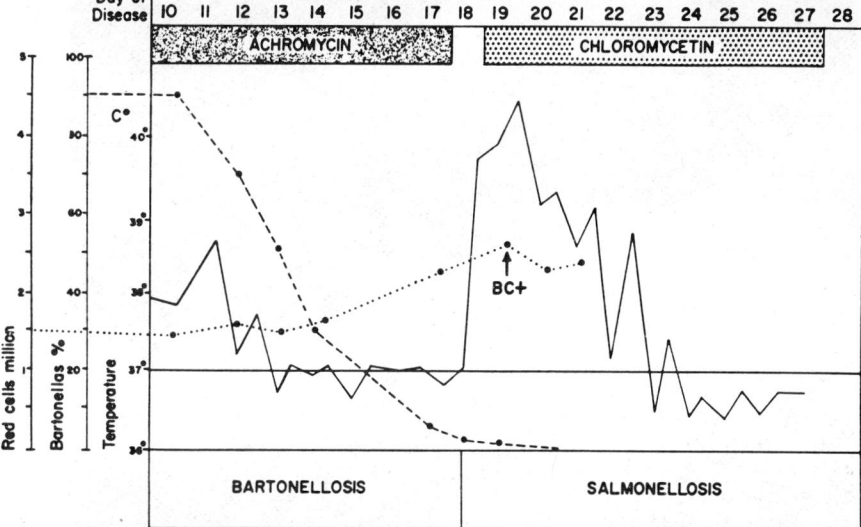

**FIGURE 2** *Salmonella bacteremia in the convalescent stage of Oroya fever (S. typhimurium). Typical response to chloramphenicol occurred with recovery of patient.*

by septicemia caused by *Salmonella* species (Tamayo, 1907; Ribeyro, 1932; Ricketts, 1948; Aldana, 1949; Cuadra, 1954; 1956), of which *S. typhimurium* is the most frequent (Colichón and Cuadra, 1954). This complication occurs during the course of Oroya fever, or, more frequently, in the period of convalescence (Fig. 2). High temperature with wide oscillations, sweating, rapid pulse, malaise, and extreme prostration are the main manifestations. Before the advent of chloramphenicol, 90 per cent of patients died within the first week (Cuadra, 1954; 1956). In contrast, the mortality of noncomplicated Oroya fever is as low as 5 per cent. The pathogenesis of the complication is not understood. Septicemia occurs in individuals who previously had solid immunity to *Salmonella*. The blockade of the macrophages of phagocytized red blood cells probably facilitates the invasion of the blood by salmonellae from the intestinal lumen or mesenteric lymph nodes. The fact that the secondary infection is not caused by agents other than *Salmonella* (e.g., *Staphylococcus, Streptococcus*) suggests that the bartonellosis selectively suppresses anti-*Salmonella* immunity.

### Verruga Peruana

One or more weeks, sometimes months, after the termination of Oroya fever, verruga peruana appear on the body as hemangiomatous nodules. The nodules may be localized in the skin (cutaneous verruga), in the subcutaneous tissue (subcutaneous verruga), in the mucous membranes (mucous verruga), or in internal organs such as muscles, bones, or viscera (Odriozola, 1898; Rebagliati, 1940). Blood capillaries, in any location,

are the only structures for which *Bartonella* shows affinity, and infection of the capillaries induces the verrucoma. The most frequent localization is apparently the skin. Perhaps because of the benignity of the disease, reports on internal verruga are scarce.

The eruption is pleomorphic (Fig. 3) as it occurs in successive episodes over a period of one to three, rarely up to six, months. It is usually preceded or accompanied by fever that varies in intensity and duration. Pains in the joints of the extremities (verrucous rheumatism), especially the knees, are very frequent and can immobilize the patient. A typical cutaneous nodule is as large as a pea, bright red in color, soft in consistency and smooth and shiny (its surface does not belong to the nodule itself but is the surface of the original skin, distended and made extremely thin by the growing nodule). A nodule is fragile and bleeds easily. On the mucous membranes nodules tend to be pedunculated. The nodules vary in size from about 1 to 2 mm in diameter (Fig. 3) up to several cm (Fig. 4). Two types are recognized: the miliary and the nodular. In the miliary type the nodules, measuring 1 to 2 mm in diameter, are distributed on the face and extremities and vary from a few to innumerable. Usually there is a heavy concentration on the legs. The eruption begins as pruritic petechiae or as small conical papules with a minute vesicle or keratinous thickening at their apex (Cuadra, 1962). The new verruga nodules emerge at the petechiae or at the base of the vesicles or the keratinous thickening and appear as red dots that grow in a few days to become a miliary lesion. The nodules may behave in one of two ways: either growth stops and they remain as miliary nodules until they degenerate

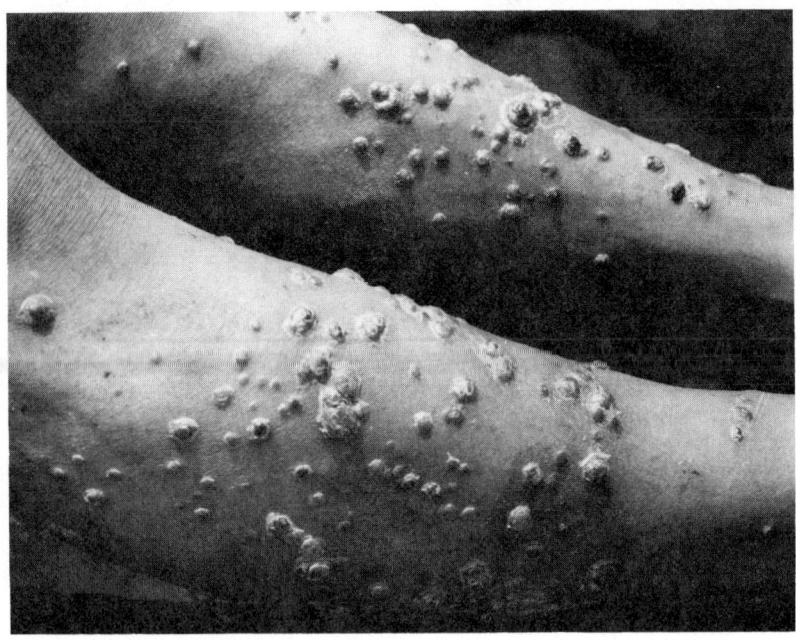

**FIGURE 3.** *Verruga peruana. The lesions vary greatly in size. The smallest, verrugas of miliary type, are early lesions. The larger, verrugas of nodular type, are old lesions. Most of the latter appear covered by keratinous thickening (corneous verruga), and a few of them are in the regressing crusted stage.*

and crust (which occurs within a few weeks), or the growth continues and produces the nodular type of eruption. The size of the nodules may vary to a large extent from pea-sized (small nodular verruga) to giant tumors (Figs. 3 and 4). Figure 4 shows one of the largest reported in the literature

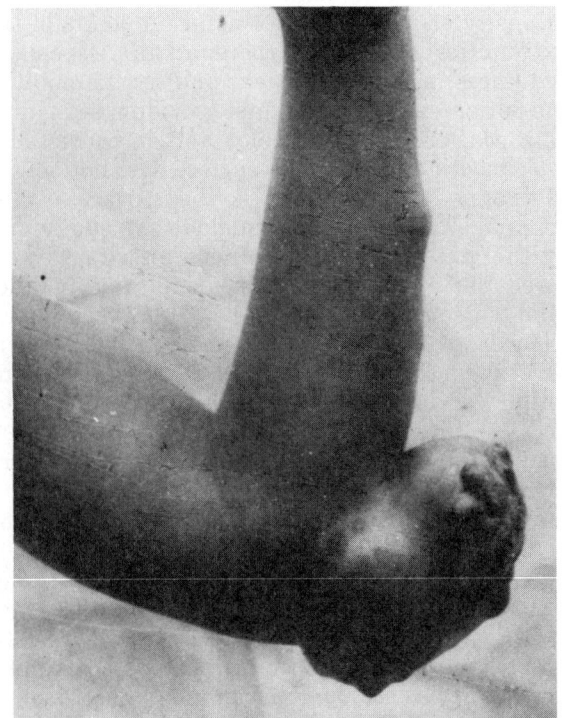

**FIGURE 4.** *Verruga peruana. A giant verrucoma. Case reported by Ricketts (1942).*

(Ricketts, 1942). Between these two extremes there is a range of middle-sized nodules; however, the small and middle-sized nodules are much more frequent than the large or giant tumors. The large verruga nodules are also called "verruga mular" because of their resemblance to certain skin tumors (probably of viral etiology) that affect mules in verrucous endemic areas. The density of the nodular eruption is in general lower than that of the miliary type; the larger the nodules the lower their density. The lifespan of the nodular type is much longer (up to six months (Odriozola, 1898) than that of the miliary type (weeks). Miliary and nodular verruga can coexist in the same individual; this fact also contributes to the pleomorphism of the eruption (Fig. 3).

Nodules localized in the subcutis tissue (subcutaneous verruga) are usually scarce and appear preferentially on the extremities. Some of these nodules are detectable only by palpation, others make a prominence above the skin or, when the growth is excessive, the skin covering them becomes distended and extremely thin.

In the internal organs (muscles, lungs, serous membranes, spleen, gastrointestinal tract, or meninges) only miliary or small nodular types have been reported. However, in the interstitium of the muscles larger nodules can be found (Odriozola, 1898).

Although verruga peruana usually occurs as a stage that follows Oroya fever, there are some important variations. (1) Eruption occuring as a primary condition — that is, cases not preceded by Oroya fever — after an incubation period of less than 40 days (Odriozola, 1898; Rebagliati,

1940). When verruga is experimentally induced in humans and monkeys, the eruption occurs mostly as a primary condition at the points of inoculation (exceptionally at a distance) after about two to three weeks of incubation. The existence of mild forms of Oroya fever (see above) and even of infection without disease suggests that "primary eruptions" are secondary to subclinical forms of Oroya fever. On the other hand, *Bartonella* inoculated by *Phlebotomus* should also be able to induce verruga nodules directly at the point of inoculation. (2) The eruption can occur precociously, that is, during the course of Oroya fever (Odriozola, 1898). (3) The usual sequence may be reversed so that the eruption precedes Oroya fever (Odriozola, 1898). (4) A second attack (relapse) of Oroya fever can follow the eruption ("retrocession") (Odriozola, 1898). (5) Some individuals can suffer periodically throughout their lives from attacks of verruga peruana (chronic verruga peruana).

Variations 2, 3, and 4, which were reported at a time when neither *Bartonella* nor secondary infections caused by *Salmonella* were known, remain to be confirmed.

**Complications and Sequelae.** Hemorrhage is the most important complication. The nodules, though appearing fragile, do not have a tendency to bleed spontaneously; bleeding is provoked by mechanical injury. Only the bleeding from nodules localized on mucous membranes (nose, larynx, trachea, bronchi, gastrointestinal tract), which are fortunately rare, may be serious. On the other hand, nodules localized on the respiratory tract, especially the larynx, may provoke serious respiratory difficulty.

Other complications, such as secondary infection or ulceration of the nodules, are infrequent.

The crusts, which are the final stage of the nodules, drop off without leaving a scar, except those that may be infected secondarily.

## GEOGRAPHIC VARIATIONS IN DISEASE

In some endemic areas of Peru, for example, Callejón de Huaylas, verruga peruana without Oroya fever occurs much more frequently than the eruption preceded by anemia. In other areas, such as the Rimac valley, the reverse is true.

## DIAGNOSIS

Fever and anemia, or fever alone, suggests Oroya fever if the patient has visited an endemic area within the preceding three weeks. Abundant *Bartonella* organisms can be found on conventional blood smears (Fig. 1 in Chapter 51). In the paucibacillary form of the disease, finding the infectious agent may be difficult. Oroya fever can be excluded in those cases only after exhaustive examinations of the blood, including thick film preparations (Figs. 1 and 5). A blood culture should be made to confirm or exclude Oroya fever and, above all, to diagnose salmonellosis.

The diagnosis of verruga peruana is suggested by the presence of the characteristic verruga nodules after residence in an endemic area. Culture and histopathology of the nodule can clarify the diagnosis in difficult cases.

## TREATMENT AND PROPHYLAXIS

Although *B. bacilliformis* is highly susceptible to many antibiotics, chloramphenicol is the antibiotic of choice because of its effectiveness against both *Bartonella* and the frequently associated *Salmonella* (Cuadra, 1956). All severely ill patients should be considered as potentially infected with *Salmonella*. Therefore, the laboratory diagnosis of bartonellosis should be established as rapidly as possible in order to initiate treatment.

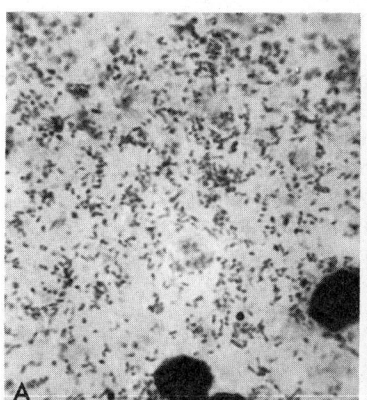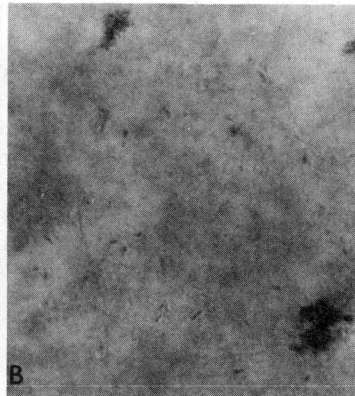

**FIGURE 5.** *Thick film preparations. A, From a patient with a high rate of parasitism involving nearly 100 per cent of red blood cells, the usual occurrence in Oroya fever. B, From a patient with a paucibacillary form of Oroya fever. Scarcely 15 organisms appear in the field.*

Chloramphenicol is administered orally to adults at an initial dose of 1 g followed by 0.5 g every six hours. In uncomplicated cases the temperature should drop abruptly within the first 24 hours (Cuadra, 1957). After the temperature is normal, treatment should be continued for five days more. In some patients a relapse may occur, usually within the first week after the termination of therapy. The relapse responds favorably to a second course of chloramphenicol (Cuadra, 1957). If there is concomitant salmonellosis, the temperature drops by lysis in three to five days. After the temperature is normal the therapy should be continued for five days more at a dose of 0.5 g every six hours. Salmonellosis occurring during the period of convalescence from Oroya fever should be treated similarly.

Blood transfusion is indicated only for patients with profound anemia. Patients who are convalescent from Oroya fever (anemia without fever) when first seen should still be treated with chloramphenicol to prevent salmonellosis and to prevent a verrucous eruption. No verruga stage occurs in patients with Oroya fever who have been treated with antibiotics. At most there is a pruriginous papulovesicular or papulokeratinous eruption, which vanishes within one to two weeks and is considered to be a frustrated form of verruga peruana (Cuadra, 1962).

The effectiveness of antibiotics against verruga peruana is doubtful, since a dramatic response has never been observed. Since *Bartonella* is a highly susceptible organism, both in patients with Oroya fever (Larrea, 1958) and in vitro (Wigand, 1952), perhaps the organisms within the verruga nodule are killed by antibiotic therapy but the tumor is still able to continue its normal evolution, or perhaps the intracellular localization of *Bartonella* within the verrucoma can protect the organism against antibiotics.

Care should be taken to avoid mechanical injury of the nodules. Hemorrhage should be stopped by compression of the bleeding nodule. Surgical extirpation, which should be as complete as possible, or cauterization may be indicated if the tumors are in a dangerous location (larynx, conjunctivae). Antibiotics are especially indicated if the nodules become secondarily infected (Biffi and Carbajal, 1904), an unusual complication. Ulcerated nodules should be protected against secondary infections. Anti-inflammatory drugs, with or without cortisone, are indicated against verrucous rheumatism.

## *PROPHYLAXIS*

All available measures should be taken to avoid being bitten by *Phlebotomus* in endemic areas either by not spending the night in such an area or by using a mosquito net, insecticide, and repellents if overnight exposure is necessary. Bartonellosis and malaria, which coexist in many areas of Peru, practically disappeared when the houses were regularly sprayed with insecticides. After spraying was discontinued both diseases returned.

Tetracycline in low doses (0.25 g every 12 hours), administered orally while in an endemic area or as a five-day treatment after leaving the area, will prevent both Oroya fever and verruga peruana. No vaccine is available.

### References

Aldana, L.: Bacteriologia de la enfermedad de Carrión. Cron Med Lima 46:237, 1929.

Aldana, L.: Estados biológicos de la *Bartonella* en la enfermedad de Carrión. Rev Sanid Polic Lima 7:391, 1947.

Aldana, L. A.: Contribución al estudio de la complicación salmonelósica en la enfermedad de Carrión. Rev Sanid Polic Lima 9:9, 1949.

Alzamora Castro, V.: Enfermedad de Carrión: Ensayo de etiopatogenia. Anal Fac Cien Med Lima 23:1, 1940.

Alzamora Castro, V.: Contribución al estudio de la bartonellosis humana o enfermedad de Carrión. Gac Med Lima 2:78, 1945.

Biffi, U., and Carbajal, G.: Sobre un caso de enfermedad de Carrión con verrucomas supurados. Cron Med Lima 21:379, 1904.

Carvallo, C.: La médula osea en la enfermedad de Carrión. Cron Med Lima 28:135, 1911.

Colichón, H., and Cuadra, M.: La salmonellosis en la verruga peruana. Rev Med Per Lima 25:30, 1954.

Cuadra, M.: La complicación salmonelósica en la bartonelosis aguda (anemia de Carrión). Rev Med Per Lima 25:3, 1954.

Cuadra, M.: Salmonellosis complication in human bartonellosis. Tex Rep Biol Med 14:97, 1956.

Cuadra, M.: Tratamiento con cloranfenicol de casos de bartoelosis aguda (enfermedad de Carrión) en periodo de inicio. Anal Fac Med Lima 40:747, 1957.

Cuadra, M.: Mecanismo de destrucción de los eritrocitos. La hemólisis intravascular. Anal Fac Med Lima 40:872, 1957.

Cuadra, M.: Erupción verrucosa frustra en pacientes tratados con antibióticos. Anal Fac Med Lima 45:302, 1962.

Cuadra, M.: Bartonellosis. Cultivo del tejido del verrucoma. Anal Fac Med Lima 40:646, 1966.

Cuadra, M., and Takano, J.: The relationship of *Bartonella bacilliformis* to the red blood cell as revealed by electron microscopy. Blood 33:708, 1969.

Cuadra, M.: Fiebre bartonellósica aguda con parasitismo escaso y anemia subclínica. Anal Progr Acad Med Lima 53:87, 1970.

Cuadra, M.: The ability of *Bartonella bacilliformis* growing in culture to attach to red blood cells. Abstract 12, International Congress of Microbiology, Munich, 1978, p. 178.

Guzman Barrón, A.: La reacción de Van den Bergh, hemoaglutininas y hemolisinas en la enfermedad de Carrión. Cron Med Lima 48:753, 1926.

Gonzalez Oechea, M.: Algunas consideraciones sobre la fiebre grave de Carrión y la infección verrucosa aguda poco anemizante. Rev Med Per Lima 46:407, 1932.

Hercelles, O.: Estudio de la *Bartonella* en los órganos y tejidos, y deducciones que de él se sacan sobre el proceso anátomoclínico de la enfermedad. Rev Med Per Lima 7:235, 1935.

Hurtado, A., Pons, J., and Merino, C.: La anemia de la enfermedad de Carrión. Anal Fac Med Lima 21:25, 1938.

Kikuth, W.: Experimentelle Untersuchungen über Oroyafieber und Verruga Peruana. Z Immunforsch 73:1, 1931.

Larrea, P.: Los antibióticos en la bartonelemia humana. Arch Per Pat Clin Lima 12:1, 1958.

Mackehenie, D., and Weiss, P.: Contribución al estudio de la verruga peruana. Gac Med Per Lima 4:51, 1926.

Mackehenie, D.: Estudio del noduloma verrucoso. Ref Med Lima 24:50, 1938.

Mayer, M., Rocha Lima, H., and Werner, H.: Untersuchungen über Verruga peruviana. Muench Med Wschr 60:739, 1913.

McCutcheon, M.: Inflamation. In Anderson, W. A. D.: Pathology. St. Louis, C. V. Mosby Company, 1948.

Marquez da Cunha, A., and Muniz, J.: Pesquisas sobre la verruga peruana. Mem Inst O Cruz 21:161, 1928.

Merino, C.: Las seroproteinas en la enfermedad de Carrión. Thesis (medicine). Lima, Faculty of Medicine of the San Marcos University, 1939.

Moulder, J. W.: The rickettsias. In Bergey's Manual of Determinative Bacteriology. 8th ed. Baltimore, The Williams & Wilkins Company, 1974, p. 882.

Noguchi, H., and Battistini, T.: Etiology of Oroya fever. I. Cultivation of *Bartonella bacilliformis*. J Exp Med 43:851, 1926a.

Noguchi, H.: Etiology of Oroya fever. III. The behavior of *Bartonella bacilliformis* in *Macacus rhesus*. J Exp Med 44:697, 1926b.

Noguchi, H.: Etiology of Oroya fever. IV. The effect of inoculation of anthropoid apes with *Bartonella bacilliformis*. J Exp Med 44:715, 1926c.

Noguchi, H.: The etiology of verruga peruana. J Exp Med 45:175, 1927a.

Noguchi, H.: Etiology of Oroya fever. VIII. Experiments on cross-immunity between Oroya fever and verruga peruana. J Exp Med 45:781, 1927b.

Noguchi, H.: Etiology of Oroya fever. VI. Pathological changes observed in animals experimentally infected with *Bartonella bacilliformis*. The distribution of the parasites in the tissues. J Exp Med 45:437, 1927c.

Odriozola, M.: La Maladie de Carrión ou la Verruga Péruvienne. Paris, 1898.

Pinkerton, H., and Weinman, D.: Carrión disease. I. Behavior of the etiological agent within cells growing or surviving in vitro. Proc Soc Exp Biol Med 37:587, 1937.

Pinkerton, H., and Weinman, D.: Carrión's disease. II. Comparative morphology of the etiological agent in Oroya fever and verruga peruana. Proc Soc Exp Biol Med 37:591, 1937–38.

Rebagliati, R. Verruga Peruana (Enfermedad de Carrión). Lima, Imprenta Torres Aguirre, 1940.

Recavarren, S., and Lumbreras, H.: Pathogenesis of the verruga of Carrión's disease. Am J Pathol 66:461, 1972.

Reynafarge, C., and Ramos, J.: The hemolytic anemia of human bartonellosis. Blood 17:562, 1961.

Ribeyro, R.: Verruga peruana y paratífico beta. Cron Med Lima 49:361, 1932.

Ricketts, G.: Contribución al estudio clínico de la enfermedad de Carrión. Thesis (medicine). Lima, 1942.

Ricketts, G.: Intercurrent infections of Carrión's disease observed in Peru. Am J Trop Med 28:437, 1948.

Rocha Lima, H.: Zur Histologie der Verruga peruviana. Verh Dtsch Pathol Ges 16:409, 1913.

Strong, R. P., Tyzzer, E. E., Brues, C. T., Sellard, A. B., and Gastiaburu, J. C.: Verruga peruviana, Oroya fever and uta, JAMA 61:1713, 1913.

Strong, R. P., and Tyzzer, E. E.: Pathology of Oroya fever. JAMA 64:965, 1915.

Strong, R. P.: Verruga peruana and Oroya fever. In Stitt's Diagnosis, Prevention and Treatment of Tropical Diseases. Philadelphia, The Blakiston Company, 1945, p. 997.

Takano, J.: Enfermedad de Carrión (Bartonellosis humana). Estudio morfológico de la fase hemática y del periodo eruptivo con el microscopio electrónico. Thesis (Medicine). Lima, Faculty of Medicine of the San Marcos University, 1970.

Tamayo, M. O.: Un ensayo de clasificación de los tifosímiles de la Verruga peruana. Cron Med Lima 14:21, 1907.

Urteaga, O.: Histopatogenia de la anemia en la Verruga peruana. Arch Per Pat Clin Lima 2:355, 1948.

Urteaga, O., and Calderón, J.: Ciclo biológico de reproducción de la *Bartonella bacilliformis* en los tejidos de pacientes de Verruga peruana o enfermedad de Carrión. Arch Per Pat Clin Lima 19:1, 1965.

Weinman, D., and Pinkerton, H.: Carrión's disease. III. Experimental production in animals. Proc Soc Exp Biol Med 37:594, 1937.

Weiss, P.: Contribución al estudio de la verruga peruana o enfermedad de Carrión. Rev Med Per Lima 4:5, 58, 1932.

Weiss, P.: Contribución al estudio de la verruga peruana. Rev Med Lat Am Buenos Aires 18:214, 1933.

Wigand, R.: Neue Untersuchungen über *Bartonella bacilliformis*. 2. Verhalten gegenüber Sulfonamide und Antibiotica in vitro. Z Tropenmed Parasitol 3:453, 1952.

# EPIDEMIC **186** (LOUSE-BORNE) TYPHUS

## R. Brezina, M.D.

### DEFINITION

Epidemic typhus is an acute infectious disease that is caused by *Rickettsia prowazekii* and transmitted from man to man by the human body louse, *Pediculus humanus corporis*. It is characterized clinically by a high fever, severe encephalitis, and a generalized macular or papular rash. The overall case fatality of untreated patients ranges from 8 to 40 per cent. Fever lasting for 14 to 18 days subsides by lysis. Antibiotic therapy shortens the duration of the disease dramatically and substantially reduces its lethality. Clinical recovery from typhus is accompanied by development of solid immunity to reinfection, but a few rickettsiae may persist in the tissues. Recrudescence of disease caused by these persisting organisms may occur decades after the primary infection (Brill-Zinsser disease).

Epidemic typhus is by far the most important rickettsiosis. In the past, outbreaks of epidemic typhus have been associated with major historical events such as wars, famines, and large migrations of populations. It still represents a serious public health problem in some countries (Tarizzo, 1978). In 1975, 10,548 cases of epidemic typhus with 146 deaths were reported to the World Health Organization. Its highest prevalence is in the developing countries of Africa (Rwanda, Burundi, Ethiopia, Uganda, Zaire) and, to a lesser extent, of Latin America (Peru, Bolivia, Ecuador, Mexico) and Asia (Afghanistan). This geographic distribution is related to the high level of louse infestation caused by low socioeconomic standards, lack of education, and climate. The high incidence of primary cases creates a reservoir of possible cases of Brill-Zinsser disease. These cases can serve as the source for future outbreaks of epidemic typhus if the population is infested with lice. Furthermore, individuals who had typhus during World War II and now live in countries without a focus of primary epidemic typhus may develop Brill-Zinsser disease.

## ETIOLOGY

*Rickettsia prowazekii* is antigenically similar to *Rickettsia typhi* and *Rickettsia canada*. Under natural conditions, it multiplies in the epithelium of the louse gut. Lice succumb to this infection within one to four weeks. *R. prowazekii* is excreted in the feces of infected lice four to five days after infection and may remain infectious, depending on the environmental temperature, for up to six months. Feces of infected lice infect human beings when driven into the skin by the process of scratching. Transmission is accomplished mainly by *Pediculus humanus corporis* (the body louse), but *Pediculus humanus capitis* (the head louse) may also be a vector. Lice can be infected experimentally via the rectum. Fleas are also susceptible to experimental infection but man is the primary reservoir of epidemic typhus. Existence of an extrahuman reservoir in domestic animals or ticks could not be confirmed experimentally (Ormsbee, 1973; Burgdorfer, 1973), but an agent indistinguishable from *R. prowazekii* has been isolated from flying squirrels (Bozeman et al., 1975).

*R. prowazekii* multiplies well in the yolk sac of chick embryos, in chick embryo cell culture, and in established lines such as mouse lymphoblasts, mouse L cells, or monkey kidney cells. The growth is restricted to the cytoplasm of the cells. The organism is unstable outside of the cells but remains viable for several years at $-70°$ C. It contains a hemolysin and toxin that kills mice within 24 hours after intravenous administration. Both the toxic and the hemolytic properties are firmly bound to viable rickettsiae.

The two major antigenic components of *R. prowazekii* are a heat-stable, soluble, group-specific antigen and a heat-labile, species-specific antigen. The group antigen, released in the aqueous phase after ether treatment, is identical to that of *R. typhi*. The species-specific antigen, which remains after thorough washing of *R. prowazekii*, distinguishes *R. prowazekii* from *R. typhi*. The common polysaccharide antigen shared with *Proteus vulgaris* strain OX 19 explains the agglutinability of the sera of acute epidemic typhus patients in the Weil-Felix reaction. Sera of patients with Brill-Zinsser disease is Weil-Felix negative. The guanine plus cytosine (G + C) content of *R. prowazekii* DNA is approximately 30 moles per cent.

The guinea pig is highly susceptible to infection and is commonly used for primary isolation. The highest titers of rickettsiae are in the brain and spleen. Mice are killed by the toxin of *R. prowazekii*. The cotton rat, *Sigmodon hispidus,* is as susceptible to infection as the chick embryo. Although mice are not susceptible to intraperitoneal infection, *R. prowazekii* can be adapted to growth in the mouse lung after serial intranasal passage.

## PATHOGENSIS AND PATHOLOGY

Infection is established by forcing infected louse feces into the skin by scratching. In rare instances, infection may be acquired by pulmonary inhalation or conjunctival absorption of airborne suspensions of the organisms. Rickettsiae may circulate in the blood well before the onset of clinical disease. During rickettsemia, organisms penetrate the endothelium of small vessels, principally those of the skin, brain, heart, and kidneys. Rickettsial growth results in cell destruction, endovasculitis, thrombosis, and hemorrhage. So-called Fraenkel's nodules consisting of accumulations of polymorphonuclear leukocytes, macrophages, and lymphoid cells are located perivascularly. In addition to the vascular lesions of the skin, necropsy reveals interstitial pneumonitis and mononuclear infiltration of the myocardium. Panencephalitis may dominate the clinical picture of epidemic typhus. Histologically, the encephalitis is also perivascular. Experimentally, the toxin of *R. prowazekii* seems to cause some of the histopathology by increasing capillary permeability, resulting in the loss of plasma and hemoconcentration. Toxic vascular damage may lead to intravascular coagulation and peripheral vascular collapse, which is the principal cause of death.

## CLINICAL MANIFESTATIONS

The incubation period of epidemic typhus ranges from 5 to 23 days, with an average of 11 days. The onset is usually abrupt with chills, fever, malaise, headache, weakness, backache, and generalized myalgia. Vomiting and vertigo occur infrequently at the onset of the disease. During the first two or three days the temperature fluctuates from normal to 39° C, and afterwards it attains a level of 39° to 40° C, where it remains until death or recovery of the patient (Fig. 1). Conjunctivitis with photophobia, orbital pain aggravated by pressure or ocular movement, and flushing of the face and the neck are common. Headache increases in severity and may be either

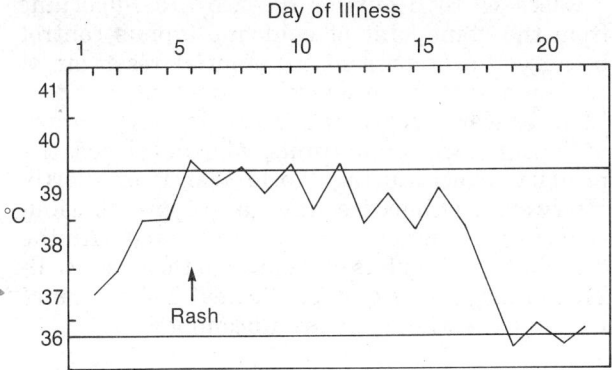

Day of Illness

**FIGURE 1.** *The temperature curve in an epidemic typhus patient untreated with antibiotics.*

generalized or most severe in the frontal region. Coughing and vomiting increase. Constipation or, less commonly, diarrhea may occur.

The appearance of a characteristic, generalized eruption, usually between the fifth and ninth days, is accompanied by progressive central nervous system (CNS) involvement. The rash, which is first apparent on the lateral chest, spreads first to the abdomen and during the next one to two days to the entire body, except the face, palms, and soles (Fig. 2). At first the skin lesions are separate macules or maculopapules about the size

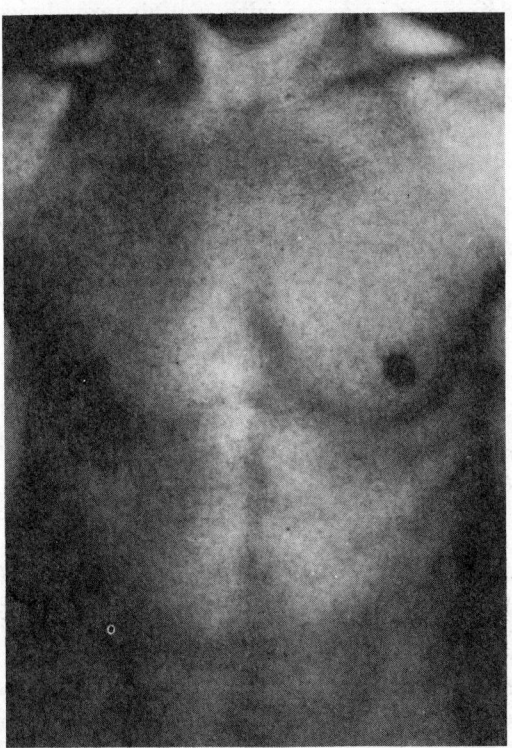

**FIGURE 2.** *The exanthem in 47 year old man on day 46 of infection with epidemic typhus (photo provided by Prof. J. A. Gaon, M.D., Medical Faculty, Sarajevo, Yugoslavia).*

of a pinhead or a lentil (2 to 4 mm in diameter) that blanch on pressure. Later on they fail to blanch, become purpuric, and form groups but do not become confluent. In some instances, there may be a transient marbled appearance of the skin before the onset of the rash. The exanthem is usually visible for 10 to 12 days, at which time it begins to change to a brown color. Desquamation occurs during convalescence.

At the end of the first week meningoencephalitis begins to dominate the clinical picture. Manifestations include psychosis, meningismus, Kernig's and Brudzinski's signs, and hyperesthesia. The second and third weeks of illness are the critical period.

Dysphagia, inability to eat and drink without assistance, and prostration develop during this stage. Stupor or coma may be interrupted by episodes of delirium and violence, which tend to subside into apathy. Catalepsy, muscle stiffness, aphasia, and hemianopsia signify diffuse brain damage. Extrapyramidal symptoms include tremor, choreiform movements, and myoclonus. Splenomegaly, cough and tachypnea, and myocarditis complete the picture of the critical period of illness. Tachycardia, hypotension, and gangrene of the toes, feet, tips of fingers, ear lobes, nose, penis, scrotum, or vulva may occur in severe cases.

Renal insufficiency manifested by albuminuria, microhematuria, and casts is common. Oliguria and azotemia are signs of fulminating, preterminal disease.

The white blood count is normal or low in the first week of illness and slightly elevated later on. The decrease in red blood cell count is accompanied by a corresponding reduction of hemoglobin. Toward the end of the first week, the serum albumin is reduced and the serum globulin increased. Increased protein and pleocytosis may be found in the spinal fluid.

In fatal cases, the terminal period is characterized by uremia, stupor, and coma. Death from epidemic typhus is caused by peripheral vascular collapse or by complications such as pneumonia. If a patient recovers, the fever generally subsides by rapid lysis in the third week of the illness. Recovery from severe encephalitis is not so rapid and the patient may be irritable or apathetic for a prolonged period. Full strength and normal mental and physical activity are regained in two or three months.

## COMPLICATIONS AND SEQUELAE

Pneumonia is one of the most important complications of epidemic typhus. Bronchopneumonia during the first week of the disease is usually of rickettsial origin. About 10 per cent of patients develop bacterial pneumonia in the third or fourth week of the disease. It may be accompanied by leukocytosis, pleuritis, and empyema. Purulent tonsillitis, otitis, parotitis, and pharyngitis are the other common bacterial complications. Thrombosis, thrombophlebitis, and gangrene are caused by the classic vascular lesions of epidemic typhus.

Serious sequelae are rare, despite extensive involvement of the central nervous system, myocardium, and kidneys during the acute stage of the disease. The most important sequelae are disturbances of the central nervous system, including deformation and enlargement of the third ventricles (Mohr et al., 1972), personality changes, impairment of mental function, epilepsy, and disorders of the cranial nerves and extrapyramidal system.

### BRILL-ZINSSER DISEASE

Brill-Zinsser disease is recrudescent epidemic typhus that appears from 4 to 50 years after the primary attack. Its clinical features are the same as those of classic epidemic typhus but with lower intensity, shorter duration, infrequent complications, and only an exceptional fatality (Fig. 3). Rickettsemia is shorter and rashes are infrequent. Although recrudescence is known to be caused by rickettsiae that persist in lymph nodes, the factors that precipitate Brill-Zinsser disease are unknown. Intercurrent diseases such as paratyphoid fever, common cold, influenza, bacillary dysentery, sunstroke, and leptospirosis preceded Brill-Zinsser disease in a recent study in East Slovakia (Mittermayer, 1978).

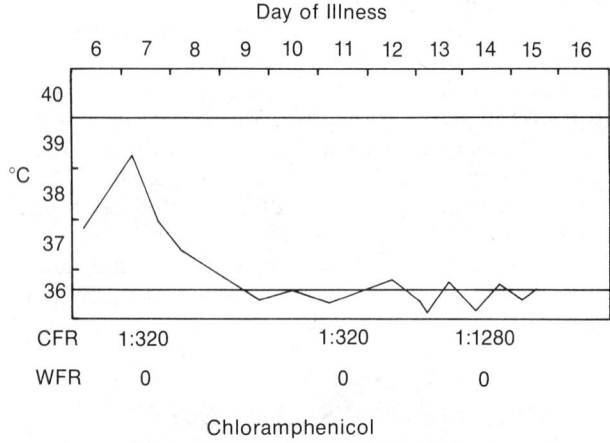

**FIGURE 3.** *The temperature curve and antibody response in a patient suffering from Brill-Zinsser disease (with permission of Prof. J. A. Gaon, M.D., Medical Faculty, Sarajevo, Yugoslavia).*

Cases of Brill-Zinsser disease are important from the standpoint of epidemic typhus control because they represent a potential reservoir of epidemic typhus in louse-infested populations. Brill-Zinsser disease can occur in any country with European immigrants who developed the primary attack during World War II or shortly afterwards. Otherwise, the geographic distribution of Brill-Zinsser disease is associated with the distribution of typhus epidemics in the past. Brill-Zinsser disease is not of public health significance in countries where lice are uncommon.

### GEOGRAPHIC VARIATIONS IN DISEASE

There are no known geographic variations in antigenic properties or virulence of wild strains of *R. prowazekii*. Variations in the severity of disease depend more on the quality of care. Because of improvement in care during World War II, the mortality dropped below 8 per cent. Under peaceful conditions, the mortality in treated sporadic cases may be less than 1 per cent.

### DIAGNOSIS

The clinical diagnosis is not difficult during epidemics or in areas with a high prevalence of epidemic typhus. It is based on the typical rash, unremitting high fever, headache, and other signs of CNS involvement. In contrast, the clinical diagnosis of Brill-Zinsser disease is difficult and depends on a careful history. The differential diagnosis of epidemic typhus includes other rickettsioses, relapsing fever, smallpox, malaria, measles, and yellow fever.

The definitive diagnosis is made in the laboratory either by isolation of *R. prowazekii* or by a rising, specific serologic test.

#### Isolation

*R. prowazekii* can be isolated during rickettsemia by inoculating a suspension of clotted blood intraperitoneally into guinea pigs or the yolk sac of the chick embryo. Several blind passages may be necessary to isolate *R. prowazekii* from the yolk sac. Guinea pigs develop a mild febrile disease after an incubation period that lasts a varying amount of time, depending on the number of rickettsiae in the inoculum. Rickettsiae can be harvested from the guinea pig brain or spleen by inoculation into yolk sacs. As early as the end of the first week after intraperitoneal inoculation, guinea pigs develop specific antibodies detectable by complement fixation (CF) or agglutination tests. The presence of rickettsiae in the patient's blood can also be demonstrated by xenodiagnosis, in which clean, hungry lice are allowed to feed on the patient. After three to four days rickettsiae are detected in the louse gut by immunofluorescence or by injection and isolation in laboratory animals.

### Serology

An increase in the titer of antibodies to *R. prowazekii* in paired, acute, and convalescent sera can be sought by several techniques. The Weil-Felix reaction for agglutinins against *Proteus vulgaris* OX 19, which starts to be positive from the fifth to eighth day, has many disadvantages: antibodies persist for a short time, there are nonspecific reactions with the sera of patients with enteric, leptospiral, and borrelial infections, it is often negative in sporadic cases of primary typhus, and it is positive in less than 20 per cent of patients with Brill-Zinsser disease. Therefore, tests using specific rickettsial antigens are recommended. The most frequently used is the CF test. It should be remembered, however, that epidemic typhus cannot be differentiated from murine (endemic) typhus with the group-specific soluble antigen but only with highly purified, species-specific *R. prowazekii* antigen. CF antibodies are detectable by the end of the first week of the disease and peak about the fourth week. Low levels of CF antibody may persist for life. Microagglutination of washed suspensions of purified rickettsiae is as sensitive as the CF test (Fiset et al., 1969). Passive hemagglutination of sheep or human O group erythrocytes sensitized with boiled, alkaline-treated rickettsiae is positive only through early convalescence and does not differentiate epidemic from murine typhus. An indirect microimmunofluorescence test (Philip et al., 1976), which determines the class of antibody made by the patient, is said to differentiate primary epidemic typhus from Brill-Zinsser disease (Ormsbee et al., 1977). Since patients with early epidemic typhus make predominantly IgM antibodies and those with Brill-Zinsser disease make IgG, differentiation by heating sera or treatment with mercaptoethanol (Ormsbee et al., 1977) is also possible.

In all these serologic tests, the possibility of cross-reactivity, not only with the typhus group rickettsiae but also with the spotted fever group (Ormsbee et al., 1977) should be taken into consideration. The specificity of serologic tests may differ in individual situations; for example, the sera of patients convalescent from epidemic typhus usually reacts with *R. canada* (see Chapter 50) in the CF and immunofluorescence tests, but only slightly or not at all in the microagglutination reaction (Urvölgyi, 1978).

## TREATMENT

Chloramphenicol and tetracycline are the only effective specific treatments for epidemic typhus. The first dose, depending on the weight of the patient, is 2 to 3 g, followed by 1 to 2 g/day, in four divided doses. Although patients become afebrile within two to three days, the antibiotic should be continued for several days after the temperature becomes normal to avoid relapses. Doxycycline, an antibiotic from the tetracycline series that persists in the blood and tissues for prolonged periods, has been effective in a single 100- to 200-mg dose (Wisseman, 1973; Huys et al., 1973). Antibiotics dramatically shorten the duration of the disease and reduce lethality practically to zero. Because they are rickettsiostatic but not rickettsiocidal, they do not affect rickettsial persistence and the possibility of recrudescent typhus.

Symptomatic therapy is aimed at relief of headache and delirium, maintenance of fluid balance, and circulatory support. Oral hygiene, skin care, and maintenance of bowel function are also important in severely ill patients.

## PROPHYLAXIS

Epidemic typhus can be prevented either by control of lice with insecticides or by active immunization of humans.

Depending on the circumstances, one or more of the following vector control techniques may be used effectively; (1) delousing of all contacts of a typhus patient; (2) delousing of small focal populations; and (3) mass delousing. Ultimately, effective louse control is dependent upon education and improvement of the standard of living in developing countries.

Resistance of lice to commonly used insecticides of the DDT, lindane, and malathion groups has been demonstrated in various areas. Resistance is usually related to the use of specific insecticides as agricultural pesticides over long periods. The use of juvenile hormones as insecticides is still in the early stages of experimental testing.

Typhus fever vaccines have been used widely and extensively, but only limited information on the effectiveness of the standard formalin-inactivated vaccine is actually available. Furthermore, commercially produced killed vaccines are not tested and standardized properly. A killed yolk-sac vaccine, used extensively during World War II, either prevented disease or greatly reduced its severity. An attenuated strain of *R. prowazekii* (Madrid E strain) has been tested experimentally by many investigators. A single dose of this live vaccine has been shown to prevent disease under epidemic conditions and to change the antibody profile of a population enough so that it could break the transmission cycle (Wisseman, 1978). The most important question at this time about the usefulness of the E strain as a vaccine is whether the attenuation is stable. Some experimental data by Soviet and Slovak investigators suggest that under appropriate selective conditions the E strain can revert to virulence. Despite this fact, live E vaccine could be administered to a population that was at very high risk of an epidemic (Wisseman, 1978).

## References

Bozeman, F. M., Masiello, S. A., Williams, M. S., and Elisberg, B. L.: Epidemic typhus rickettsiae isolated from flying squirrels. Nature (London) 255:545, 1975.

Burgdorfer, W.: Possible extrahuman reservoirs of *Rickettsia prowazekii*: Ticks. In Proceedings of the Symposium on the Control of Lice and Louse-borne Diseases. Washington, D.C., 4–6 December 1972. Washington, D. C., Pan American Health Organization, 1973, p. 109.

Fiset, P. Ormsbee, R. A., Silberman, R., Peacock, M., and Spielman, S. H.: A microagglutination technique for detection and measurement of rickettsial antibodies. Acta Virol 13:60, 1969.

Huys, J., Kayhigi, J., Freyens, P., and Vanden Berge, G.: Single-dose treatment of epidemic typhus with doxycycline. Chemotherapy 18:314, 1973.

Mittermayer, T.: Intercurrent diseases as possible provocative factors of Brill-Zinsser disease. In Kazár, J., Ormsbee, R. A., and Tarasevich, I. V. (eds.): Rickettsiae and Rickettsial Diseases, Bratislava, Veda, Publishing House of Slovak Academy of Sciences, 1978, p. 465.

Mohr, W., Weyer, F., and Asshauer, E.: Klassisches Fleckfieber. In Gsell, O., and Mohr, W. (eds.): Infektionskrankheiten. Bd. IV. Berlin, Springer-Verlag, 1972, p. 23.

Ormsbee, R. A.: The hypothesis of extrahuman reservoirs of *Rickettsia prowazekii*. In Proceedings of the Symposium on the Control of Lice and Louse-borne diseases. Washington, D.C., 4–6 December 1972. Washington, D.C., Pan American Health Organization, 1973, p. 104.

Ormsbee, R. A., Peacock, M., Philip, R., Casper, E., Plorde, J., Gabre-Kindan, T., and Wright, L.: Serologic diagnosis of epidemic typhus. Am J Epidemiol 105:261, 1977.

Philip, R. N., Casper, E. A., and Ormsbee, R. A.: Microimmunofluorescence test for the serological study of Rocky Mountain spotted fever and typhus. J Clin Microbiol 3:51, 1976.

Tarizzo, M. L.: Public health significance of rickettsial diseases. In Kazár, J., Ormsbee, R. A., and Tarasevich, I. V. (eds.); Rickettsiae and Rickettsial Diseases. Bratislava, Veda, Publishing House of Slovak Academy of Sciences, 1978, p. 539.

Urvölgyi, J.: New achievements in serological diagnosis of rickettsial diseases. In Kazár, J., Ormsbee, R. A., and Tarasevich, I. V. (eds.): Rickettsiae and Rickettsial Diseases. Bratislava, Veda, Publishing House of Slovak Academy of Sciences, 1978, p. 361.

Wisseman, C., Jr.: Concepts of typhus control and factors influencing choice of methods. In Proceedings of the Symposium on the control of lice and louse-borne diseases, Washington, D.C., 4–6 December 1972. Washington, D.C., Pan American Health Organization, 1973, p. 267.

Wisseman, C., Jr.: Prevention and control of rickettsial diseases, with emphasis on immunoprophylaxis. In Kazár, J., Ormsbee, R. A., and Tarasevich, I. V. (eds.): Rickettsiae and Rickettsial Diseases. Bratislava, Veda, Publishing House of Slovak Academy of Sciences, 1978, p. 553.

# 187  *ENDEMIC (MURINE) TYPHUS*

## R. Brezina, M.D.

### DEFINITION

Endemic flea-borne (murine) typhus is an acute febrile disease caused by *Rickettsia typhi,* which is transmitted to man by the rat flea *(Xenopsylla cheopis).* The reservoir of this zoonosis is rats and mice. Man is an accidental victim who breaks the usual rat-flea-rat cycle. Clinically, endemic typhus resembles a mild form of epidemic typhus (Chapter 186). The mortality is negligible, and late recrudescence (Brill-Zinsser disease) is unknown. Infection stimulates solid immunity not only to endemic but also to epidemic typhus.

### ETIOLOGY

*R. typhi* belongs to the typhus group (biotype) of rickettsia (see Chapter 50). This group also includes *R. prowazekii* (epidemic typhus) and *R. canada,* a recently described rickettsia that has not yet been definitely associated with human disease. *R. typhi* is very closely related to *R. prowazekii.* They share a common, thermostable, soluble antigen and another common antigen with *Proteus vulgaris* OX-19. They can be separated in complement fixation tests by antisera against a species-specific, cell-associated antigen obtained by repeated washing of the rickettsiae. They can also be differentiated by cross-challenges of vaccinated guinea pigs or by mouse-toxin neutralization tests. The guanine plus cystosine content of the DNA in *R. typhi* is approximately 30 moles per cent, similar to that of *R. prowazekii. R. typhi* is slightly more sensitive to environmental effects than *R. prowazekii,* but it can persist in flea feces for two weeks at normal humidity and room temperature, and for four months at 4° C. It grows well in the yolk sac of the chick embryo. *R. typhi* is more virulent for the guinea pig than *R. prowazekii.* In addition to fever, it causes scrotal erythema and swelling.

Adhesions develop between the testes and the tunica vaginalis so that the testes cannot be pushed up into the abdomen (Neill-Mooser reaction). The mesothelial cells of the tunica vaginalis are packed with masses of rickettsiae (Mooser's cells). White rats and mice are also highly susceptible to intraperitoneal infection and develop peritonitis with abundant rickettsiae in the peritoneal exudate. Mice die between the third and eighth days. White rats survive the infection, but *R. typhi* may persist in their brains for as long as 380 days.

The rat flea, *Xenopsylla cheopis,* is the classic vector for the transmission of the organisms from rat to rat and from rat to man. It contracts *R. typhi* by feeding on an acutely infected rat. Rickettsiae multiply in the epithelium of the gut and are shed in the feces of the flea throughout its life. Man can be infected by scratching and driving infected feces into the skin, by inhalation, by conjunctival absorption of airborne rickettsiae, or by ingestion of contaminated food. *R. typhi* multiplies in the human flea *(Pulex irritans),* the human body louse *(Pediculus humanis corporis),* and the rat louse *(Polyplax spinulosa). Xenopsylla brasiliensis* is thought to be a vector of *R. typhi* in Kenya. In the United States, infected cat flies *(Ctenocephalides felis)* have been found. In Java, *R. typhi* was isolated from a trombiculid mite, and in India from a tick *(Boophilus annulatus).*

Rats *(Rattus norvegicus* and *Rattus rattus)* are the primary reservoir of the organism. Mice can also be infected, but they are not as important a reservoir as rats.

## PATHOGENESIS AND PATHOLOGY

The pathogenesis and pathology of endemic typhus is identical to that of epidemic typhus (Chapter 186). Rickettsemia occurs during the febrile phase of infection, and rickettsiae penetrate and multiply in the endothelium of small vessels, causing vascular damage and necrosis. The pathologic findings in experimentally infected laboratory animals and in the brains of human beings at postmortem are identical to those of epidemic typhus. It is difficult to explain the mild clinical course of endemic typhus, since the pathogenesis and pathology of the diseases are so similar. Some investigators feel that the toxin of *R. prowazekii* is more potent than that of *R. typhi.*

## CLINICAL MANIFESTATIONS, COMPLICATIONS, AND SEQUELAE

The incubation period of endemic typhus varies from 4 to 15 days. The onset is sudden, but the course of the illness is more gradual than in epidemic typhus. Fever rises by steps; it may drop to normal and rise again to 40.0° C. Later in the illness, it is still remittent and varies from 38.5 to 40.0° C. In about half the cases, the rash appears first on the abdomen and spreads to the chest, back, and upper extremities. Small papules and macules are replaced later by poorly delineated roseolae. Compared with epidemic typhus, the rash is shorter in duration, skin lesions are less numerous, and petechiae are very uncommon.

Conjunctivitis may occur early in the disease. Headache and arthralgia persist throughout the course. Involvement of the central nervous system, myocardium, kidneys, and liver are less frequent and substantially less severe. The white and red blood cell counts are normal. The sedimentation rate and the concentration of serum proteins are increased.

Fever terminates by lysis after 9 to 14 days. Complications, such as thrombosis, thrombophlebitis, gangrene, azotemia, and bronchopneumonia, are infrequent. Mortality in untreated patients is about 2 per cent. Recovery is prompt without sequelae and is followed by solid immunity to *R. typhi* and cross-immunity to epidemic typhus. Clinical relapses have occurred in patients treated with a short course of antibiotics early in the disease (Wisseman et al., 1962). Spontaneous late recrudescence (Brill-Zinsser disease) has not been described.

## GEOGRAPHIC VARIATIONS

The disease occurs primarily in the tropical, subtropical, and southern temperate zones. No geographic variations are known.

## DIAGNOSIS

Endemic (murine) typhus cannot be clinically distinguished from epidemic typhus. It can also be confused with spotted fevers (Chapter 190) that occur in the same geographic areas. In endemic typhus the rash appears first on the body and spreads to the extremities; in spotted fevers the reverse is true, and the rash tends to become petechial and hemorrhagic. The incidence of the diseases in a particular area, exposure to rats, the presence of lice and the absence of the typical primary lesions of the spotted fevers may help to establish the diagnosis of endemic typhus. Viral exanthems and drug eruptions must be ruled out.

The definitive diagnosis can be made only in the laboratory by isolation of the agent or specific serologic changes. *R. typhi* can be isolated by inoculating the patient's blood into the peritoneal cavity of guinea pigs or white rats. Infected animals develop fever and scrotal swelling. Rickettsiae are easily discernible in the cells of the tunica vaginalis stained by the Giemsa, Macchiavello, or Gimenez methods. Similarly, after intraperitoneal inoculation of mice, abundant *R. typhi* can be detected in stained preparations from the peritoneal exudate. It is also possible to isolate *R. typhi* by inoculating infected blood into the chick embryo yolk sac.

Cross-reactive antibodies against *Proteus vulgaris* OX 19 (the Weil-Felix reaction) develop by the fourth day of the disease with a peak around the tenth day, but there are substantially lower antibody levels than in epidemic typhus. The complement fixation test and microagglutination reaction (Fiset et al., 1969) are the serologic methods of choice, however. The common soluble antigen shared with *R. prowazekii* makes it impossible to distinguish endemic typhus from epidemic typhus by the complement fixation test, but extensively washed rickettsial suspensions possess species-specificity in the microagglutination reaction. Endemic typhus can also be differentiated from epidemic typhus by the mouse-toxin neutralization test. As with *R. prowazekii* (Chapter 186) antibodies to *R. typhi* can be detected by the immunofluorescence test in either its macro- or micromodification (Goldwasser et al., 1959; Philip et al., 1976; Ormsbee et al., 1977). Serologic diagnosis is difficult in patients who have been vaccinated against epidemic typhus. The relative antibody titers against *R. prowazekii* and *R. typhi* may or may not be helpful. The microagglutination test against washed suspensions of *R. typhi* may be definitive if the titer rises.

## TREATMENT

Treatment of endemic (murine) typhus is the same as that of epidemic typhus. Treatment with a tetracycline should be continued for at least ten days after the onset of symptoms and for 48 hours after the patient becomes afebrile in order to prevent relapses. A single dose of 200 mg of doxycycline may also be effective against endemic typhus.

## PROPHYLAXIS

Since commensal rats and their ectoparasites are the main reservoirs and vectors of endemic typhus, prophylaxis should be directed at their elimination or control. To avoid temporary increases in human cases, rodent control measures (poisoning) should be delayed until the flea population has been reduced. The most suitable preparation for the elimination of fleas is 10 per cent DDT. Because of its residual effect, this insecticide needs to be used only once a year.

Vaccines prepared from killed *R. typhi* probably do not protect against *R. prowazekii*. Because of the mild course of endemic typhus and its rapid response to antibiotic therapy, vaccination against endemic typhus only is not necessary.

## References

Fiset, P., Ormsbee, R. A., Silberman, R., Peacock, M., and Spielman, S. H.: A microagglutination technique for detection and measurement of rickettsial antibodies. Acta Virol 13:60, 1969.

Goldwasser, R. A., Shepard, C. C., Jordan, M. E., and Fox, F. P.: The specificity of antibody response in typhus fever. Its alteration during murine typhus infection as a result of previous exposure to epidemic typhus antigen. J Immunol 83:491, 1959.

Ormsbee, R. A., Peacock, M., Philip, R., Casper, E., Plorde, J., Gabre-Kindan, T., and Wright, L.: Serologic diagnosis of epidemic typhus. Am J Epidemiol 105:261, 1977.

Philip, R. N., Casper, E. A., and Ormsbee, R. A.: Microimmunofluorescence test for the serological study of Rocky Mountain spotted fever and typhus. J Clin Microbiol 3:51, 1976.

Wisseman, C. L., Jr., Wood, W. H., Jr., Noriega, A. R., Jordan, M. E., and Rill, D. J.: Antibodies and clinical relapse of murine typhus fever following early chemotherapy. Ann Intern Med 57:743, 1962.

# 188 SCRUB TYPHUS

*Garrison Rapmund, M.D.*

## DEFINITION

Scrub typhus (Tsutsugamushi disease, mite-borne typhus, chigger-borne rickettsiosis) is characterized by a primary cutaneous lesion or eschar, fever, and rash. It is caused by *Rickettsia tsutsugamushi,* which is transmitted to man by certain larval trombiculid mites called chiggers. The disease occurs throughout Asia and the western Pacific region, reflecting the distribution of vector chiggers. Death can occur, but many infections are mild or inapparent. The immunologic heterogeneity of scrub typhus rickettsiae may explain reinfection.

## HISTORY

The disease first appeared in Western medical literature in 1879 but was known earlier in Chinese and Japanese writings. Long after 1879 the only known foci of disease were along rivers in three prefectures of northwestern Honshu Island, Japan. Disease occurred in farmers who entered low-lying grasslands to plant crops after the spring floods had subsided, hence the early name Japanese flood fever. The red larval mite called akamushi (red mite) was plentiful and was assumed to be the vector of disease (Kawamura, 1926). In 1920 Hayashi isolated from patients an organism that he called *tsutsugamushi,* meaning noxious mite, but this was probably not the disease agent (Wolbach, 1940). Nagayo and co-workers (Nagayo et al., 1930) in 1930 isolated a rickettsia-like agent from patients and called it *Rickettsia orientalis,* the name still commonly used in Japan. Ogata (Ogata, 1931) shortly thereafter isolated a similar organism from patients. He called the agent *Rickettsia tsutsugamushi,* which has become the name commonly used outside Japan.

Scrub typhus was first recognized outside Japan in Formosa by Hatori in 1915 (Blake et al., 1945) in persons who collected camphor in forests. At about the same time it was recognized in northern Sumatra by Schuffner, in Malaya by Dowden, in northern Queensland by Breinl and co-workers, and in Indochina by Lagrange (Blake et al., 1945). In the early 1920s in Malaya, Fletcher, Lesslar, and Lewthwaite (Fletcher et al., 1928) distinguished shop typhus in town dwellers from rural typhus in plantation workers. Rural typhus was similar to tsutsugamushi disease in Japan but milder. Rural typhus patients developed agglutinins to the OX-K strain of *Proteus* but not to the X-19 strain, which was agglutinated by sera from patients with shop typhus (Lewthwaite and Savoor, 1940). Rural typhus occurred in laborers and European planters who worked in terrain covered with mixed grass and low shrub vegetation, loosely referred to as scrub, hence the name scrub typhus (Fletcher et al., 1928). Scrub typhus has become the predominant name in Western literature, while in Japan it remains tsutsugamushi disease. Cross-immunity experiments in animals have proved that rural typhus in Malaya and the disease in Sumatra and Japan are caused by the same organism (Lewthwaite and Savoor, 1940).

The role of the red mite *Leptotrombidium akamushi* as a vector was established after *R. tsutsugamushi* was isolated from this mite. Its prevalence in hyperendemic foci corresponds to the incidence of disease; it transmits the disease to a monkey by feeding; its ability to infect man has been confirmed; and its principal natural host, the field vole, *Microtus montebelli,* has been shown to be infected with *R. tsutsugamushi.* The life cycle of *L. akamushi* has been established and shows that only the larval stage feeds on vertebrates. Other larval mites have been found to be vectors in other countries. *L. deliense* has been incriminated in Sumatra, Malaya, India, Indochina, and Australia (Audy, 1961). *L. fletcheri* (Vercammen-Grandjean, 1969) was the vector mite encountered in New Guinea during World War II (McCulloch, 1944), and it also transmits disease in Malaya. *L. pallida* and *L. scutellare* are prevalent in Japan in the winter, in contrast to the summer prevalence of *L. akamushi* (Tamiya, 1962). In Malaya still another vector, *L. arenicola,* has been found near sandy beaches (Upham et al., 1971). One recognized and several other proposed species are possible vectors in far eastern Siberia (Shubin et al., 1970). Thus, an array of mites, mostly of the same genus and having many characteristics in common, are vectors of scrub typhus to man, but ecologic differences such as seasonal occurrence and habitats determine the local epidemiology.

During World War II, an estimated 40,000 combatants contracted scrub typhus (Audy, 1961). Penicillin was soon found to be ineffective (Sayen et al., 1946), but in 1948 Smadel and co-workers demonstrated the value of chloramphenicol in these patients (Smadel et al., 1949). Vaccines composed of killed rickettsiae developed in Britain (Card and Walker, 1947) and the United States (Berge et al., 1949) failed to protect against all strains of the organism.

Confronted with the failure of killed vaccines and lacking a genuinely nonpathogenic strain of *R. tsutsugamushi,* Smadel and co-workers examined live rickettsiae as a vaccine, ameliorating the consequent disease with chloramphenicol (Smadel et al., 1952). From these studies in volunteers in Malaya, it was observed that immunity to challenge with the vaccine strain Karp was complete more than one year later, but challenge with a different strain, Gilliam, resulted in disease as early as four months postvaccination. Thus, the immunologic heterogeneity of rickettsial strains, documented in the laboratory (Rights et al., 1948), was confirmed in humans.

## ETIOLOGY

*Rickettsia tsutsugamushi* is a small, gram-negative microorganism that multiples intracellularly and does not grow on cell-free media. Its cell wall is composed of five layers as seen by electronmicroscopy and consists of protein, lipid, polysaccharides, and muramic and diaminopimelic acids, typical of gram-negative bacteria. The microorganism is pleomorphic but generally occurs as short rods measuring about 2.0 by 0.5 $\mu$m, visible by light microscopy. The organism is stained with basic fuchsin dyes such as those in the Giemsa and Machiavello stains. It does not possess a true capsule, but the cell is surrounded by an amorphous layer that contains soluble antigen. *R. tsutsugamushi* is immunologically heterogeneous, and classification of strains is incomplete. Nevertheless, three strains, Karp, Gilliam, and Kato, have been adopted as reference strains and have received wide use, especially in the immunofluorescence procedure for the diagnosis of human disease.

## PATHOGENESIS AND PATHOLOGY

The fundamental abnormality in scrub typhus is a disseminated focal perivasculitis with endothelial damage. Various organs develop interstitial edema, endothelial swelling in capillaries and small vessels, and infiltration of lymphocytes and large macrophages. Perivascular tissues and adventitia of vessels are widely involved, but arteritis, thrombosis, and gangrene, which are common in other rickettsial infections, are rare. The necrotizing arteritis of epidemic typhus and spotted fever is not seen in scrub typhus. Small platelet thrombi along with enlarged and hyperchromatic endothelial cells in capillaries, venules, and veins occur in the skin. Perivascular infiltration consists of lymphocytes, plasma cells, and macrophages, which need not correspond in location to the endothelial changes. Focal infiltrates are seen as an interstitial myocarditis, with myocardial fibers intact. Major coronary arteries are fully patent.

Interstitial pneumonitis and acute necrotizing bronchiolitis are seen, with only minimal changes in blood vessels, but areas of bronchopneumonia may be present. A mononuclear cell meningitis is almost always found; in half the cases of one series, meningitis occurred without brain involvement. The brain lesion consists of proliferating oligodendroglial cells and a few lymphocytes, plasma cells, and macrophages, all collected around capillaries, whose walls are disrupted and contain enlarged and hyperchromatic endothelial cells. Although these lesions are like those described by Wolbach in epidemic typhus, they are much less frequent in tsutsugamushi disease and are confined chiefly to the pons and medulla. Various authors report rickettsia-like organisms in lesions of skin vessels, heart, lung, and brain, but human tissue has not been examined by modern methods for specific identification of whole organisms or their antigens. Rickettsiae and rickettsial antigen are widely distributed in tissues of infected mice (Kundin et al., 1964).

Knowledge of pathophysiology is limited because severe disease in man has not been available for study since the advent of antibiotics. Abnormal pulmonary, myocardial, renal, and neurologic function may be caused by local reaction to the presence and multiplication of rickettsiae. The endothelial lesions presumably increase vascular permeability, but there are no published studies of peripheral vascular function similar to those for spotted fever (Moe et al., 1976), which showed increased permeability, thrombosis, and vascular occlusion before rickettsiae could be demonstrated. Schramek and co-workers report isolation of a lipopolysaccharide with endotoxin properties from *R. tsutsugamushi* (Schramek et al., 1976). Since cell wall constituents of *R. tsutsugamushi* and other rickettsiae closely resemble those of gram-negative bacteria (Perkins and Allison, 1963), and since endotoxin-like activity has been isolated from cell walls of *R. mooseri* (Wood and Wisseman, 1967), the isolation of endotoxin from *R. tsutsugamushi* would not be surprising and might provide one mechanism for the peripheral circulatory collapse seen in rapidly fatal cases. Hemorrhagic manifestations of disease described formerly were probably associated with disseminated intravascular coagulation (DIC). DIC has been well documented in one recent case (Ognibene et al., 1971). The basis for DIC is the widespread endothelial damage caused by rickettsial multiplication in endothelial cells. In the laboratory mouse, effects attributed to a rickettsial toxin have been described (Kitaoka and Tanaka, 1973). Suspensions of live rickettsiae inoculated intravenously kill mice within one hour. Very high titers of rickettsiae are required, and the relationship of this phenomenon in mice to disease in man is uncertain.

## CLINICAL MANIFESTATIONS

The incubation period is usually 8 to 10 days with extremes of 6 to 19 days. Onset is usually abrupt and is sometimes precisely timed by patients. The initial symptom is severe frontal and occipital headache followed within hours by fever to 39° C with shaking chils. Most patients also complain of general malaise, severe backache, and profuse sweating. Some have anorexia, and a few report nausea and vomiting.

Fever is remitting, rising to 40° C and higher by the fourth or fifth day. The pulse rate generally remains under 100 for a relative bradycardia during the first week of fever. In the second week, fever continues to peak near 40° C with daily remissions until it falls by lysis, around the fourteenth day. In severe cases, fever lasts for up to three weeks. Blood pressure may fall below 100 mm Hg systolic at the peak of illness but returns to normal with defervescence.

A primary lesion, or eschar, develops at the site of chigger feeding and is pathognomonic. A small papule forms within hours after the chigger has completed its painless feeding of 48 to 72 hours duration. When special attention is paid to attached chiggers (Kitaoka et al., 1974), slight burning or itching at the feeding site is sometimes recalled but is ordinarily overlooked (Kitaoka et al., 1974). The papule develops into a pustule that loses its top to become a shallow ulcer about 5 mm in diameter, surrounded by a flat red margin. The base of the ulcer usually becomes yellowish-gray, lacks exudate, and is painless by the time symptoms begin (Fig. 1). Before the end of the first week of disease, a black scab covers the ulcer (Fig. 2), which slowly regresses, leaving at most a point scar. First episodes of tsutsugamushi disease do not always have an eschar, and proven second infections usually produce no eschars, presumably because of partial immunity (Morris, 1965). As many as six (Smadel et al., 1950) eschars may appear simultaneously, and two are not unusual in persons exposed in hyperendemic areas (Kawamura, 1926). Eschars occur on every part of the body, predominating in the genital and inguinal areas, axilla, lower trunk, and neck. Eschars are frequently overlooked by patients, especially when they are located posteriorly. The portal of entry of *R. tsutsugamushi* can be so "insignificant and ephemeral" that it escapes detection on darker-skinned persons (Lewthwaite and Savoor, 1940). Furthermore, papular lesions that did not progress to ulceration have occurred at the sites of experimental intradermal inoculation into monkeys and gibbons that developed severe disease. A number of studies have shown that the skin must be thoroughly examined if all eschars are to be found and that their absence does not rule out tsutsugamushi disease. In certain series, 20 to 50 per cent of proven cases did not have eschars (Berman and Kundin, 1973; Sheehy et al., 1973; Yosano, 1953).

Lymph nodes draining the eschar are invariably enlarged and tender during the first week of disease. Generalized lymph node enlargement is also common but abates during the second week. Conjunctival hyperemia is very typical at first and about 25 per cent of cases also exhibit pharyngeal hyperemia.

Pink, maculopapular skin lesions about 0.5 cm

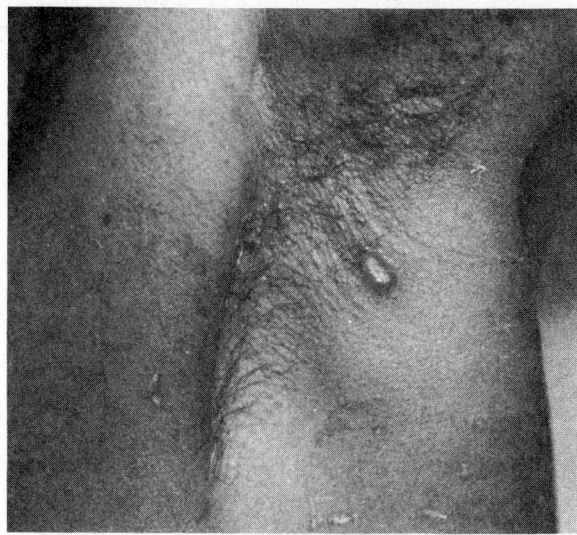

**FIGURE 1.** *Ulcerative eschar. A shallow, painless ulcer develops at the top of a papule. The ulcer has a flat, red margin.*

in diameter are present from the third to ninth day in 40 to 60 per cent of cases (Fig. 3). The rash usually begins on the face, chest, and abdomen and extends to the anterior aspects of the extremities, but it may involve all parts of the body, including the palms and soles. The buccal mucosa is occasionally involved. The rash is difficult to see in darker-skinned persons and may be present

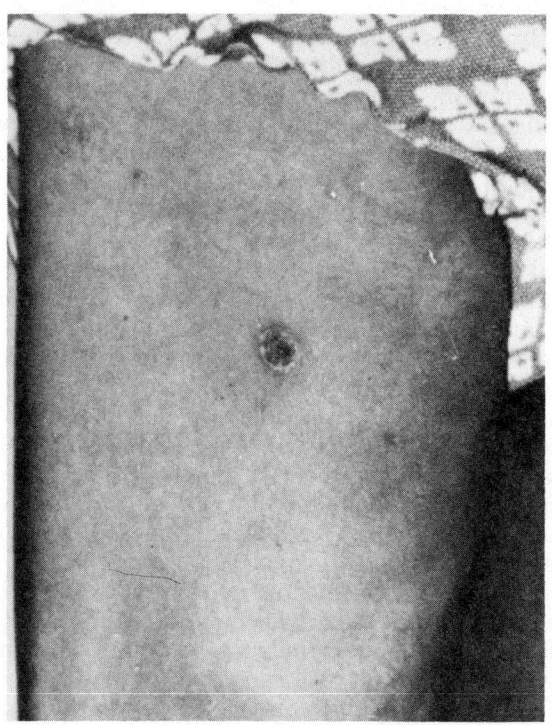

**FIGURE 2.** *Crusted eschar.*

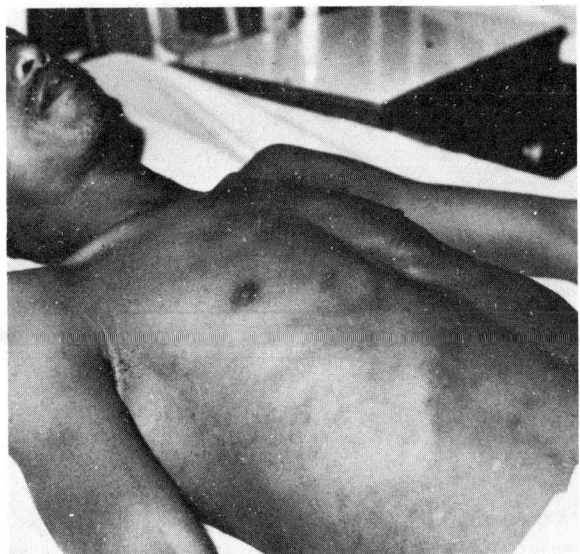

**FIGURE 3.** *Maculopapular rash is most evident here on chest and upper abdomen but may involve all parts of the body, including palms and soles.*

for only a few hours. It is not pruritic, never confluent, and almost never hemorrhagic. Purpuric lesions are described in isolated cases, but petechiae have not been reported. Subconjunctival hemorrhage and epistaxis, the principal hemorrhagic phenomena, are most common in severe disease.

Bronchitis, with moderate to severe cough, is very common. Rickettsial interstitial pneumonia is common, but physical findings are usually limited to rhonchi and occasional basilar crepitant rales. Signs of bronchopneumonia are not found. Dyspnea and cyanosis seldom occur except in fatal cases, and bacterial superinfection is rare. Although myocarditis is common at autopsy, clinical abnormalities of the heart are usually minimal. The usual findings are progressive cardiac enlargement, an apical systolic murmur, and a transient gallop rhythm, with normal central venous pressure. Electrocardiographic findings include extrasystoles, variable degrees of AV block, shifts in electrical axis, and variable T-wave changes (Ognibene et al., 1971). The spleen and liver are palpable 1 to 3 cm below the costal margins in 25 to 50 per cent of cases by the beginning of the second week.

Renal involvement is usually minor except in severely ill patients, who may develop massive albuminuria and cylindruria, oliguria, pitting peripheral edema, and, rarely, ascites.

Meningeal involvement, as evidenced by pain and tenderness in the neck muscles and some

resistance to flexion, was present in 13 per cent of one large series of patients (Sayen et al., 1946), but severe nuchal rigidity was rare. In most patients lumbar puncture revealed an elevated cerebrospinal fluid pressure, 15 cells or less with a predominance of mononuclear cells and a protein concentration of 68 to 156 mg per 100 ml. Signs of generalized cerebral involvement ranged from hyperesthesias (5 per cent) and transient mental confusion (22 per cent) to delirium (13 per cent), severe persistent restlessness (13 per cent), convulsions (6 per cent), and coma (7 per cent). Focal neurologic signs such as dysarthria, dysphagia, paraplegia, and urinary retention were less frequent. The majority of patients complained of tinnitus and deafness during the second and third weeks.

*R. tsutsugamushi* is now known to be a frequent cause of fever without rash or eschar. At one hospital in peninsular Malaysia, scrub typhus was diagnosed in 23 per cent of cases admitted for fever (Brown et al., 1976). It was also a major cause of febrile illness among American servicemen in Vietnam (Berman et al., 1973).

In the pre-antibiotic era patients usually defervesced by lysis near the end of the second week of disease. More recently, the same fever pattern has been observed in patients who were not treated because the diagnosis of scrub typhus was made only retrospectively by positive serologic tests (Berman and Kundin, 1973).

## COMPLICATIONS AND SEQUELAE

Death usually occurs between the tenth and fourteenth days of disease. Nothing in the early clinical picture points to a severe or fatal course, which usually results from progressive pneumonia and circulatory collapse, sometimes associated with an encephalitis that is manifest by delirium and coma. Convulsions, cyanosis that is resistant to oxygen therapy, and pulmonary edema are usual terminal events. In the pre-antibiotic era mortality rates in hospitalized patients ranged from less than 1 per cent (Audy, 1961) to 60 per cent (Kawamura, 1926). Elsom and co-workers (Elsom et al., 1961) found no permanent sequelae in 524 persons 11 or more years after recovery without antibiotics from severe disease contracted in the China-Burma-India region. Although rickettsiae persist for many months in lymph nodes and perhaps in other tissues after recovery, even in patients treated with antibiotics, clinical relapse some years after initial infection like that seen in epidemic typhus has never been recognized.

## GEOGRAPHIC VARIATIONS AND EPIDEMIOLOGY

In November, 1950, a nonfatal noncommunicable exanthematous febrile illness resembling tsutsugamushi disease was observed on Hachijo Island (Yosana, 1953), one of a chain of islands stretching south from Toyko Bay for several hundred miles. Unlike tsutsugamushi, it occurred in the colder months and affected many small children and women, as well as agricultural laborers. The disease prevalence matched the seasonal occurrence of the chigger *L. scutellare,* which attacks man. *R. tsutsugamushi* was isolated both from patients with so-called winter disease and from *L. scutellare* larvae. Investigation of the main Japanese islands (Tamiya, 1962) disclosed febrile disease caused by *R. tsutsugamushi* in eight widely separated prefectures, and *R. tsutsugamushi* was isolated from small mammals trapped in almost every prefecture in Japan and from several zoophilic species of chiggers not known to parasitize man. The vectors of human disease were recovered from birds, and more recent observations of *L. scutellare* in peninsular Malaysia at elevations above 5000 feet suggest that vector chiggers are dispersed over great distances by migratory birds. Widespread mild and inapparent infection with *R. tsutsugamushi* occurs in Malaysia (Brown et al., 1976; Robinson et al., 1976) just as it does in Japan.

The cardinal epidemiologic feature of scrub typhus is its highly focal nature, with outbreaks traceable to common sites of exposure. The principal determinant of epidemiology is the vector chigger, which requires a vertebrate on which to feed as a larva and a favorable microenvironment within and on the surface of the ground to complete its life cycle. Other requirements are poorly defined but are met by a variety of ecologic habitats, including: (1) grassy banks of watercourses (Audy, 1961); (2) grassland covered with kunai or lallang grass *(Imperata cylindrica)* (Audy, 1961); (3) uncultivated agricultural land that has been allowed to overgrow, or marginal land between forest and cultivated fields (Audy, 1961); (4) patches of woodland interspersed among populated rural areas (Hubert and Baker, 1963); (5) certain kinds of volcanic soil such as that found in Japan near Mt. Fuji (Asanuma et al., 1974) and offshore volcanic islands (Yosana, 1953); (6) hedgerows composed of coral rock, as in the Pescadores Islands (Cooper et al., 1964), (7) shaded areas behind sandy beaches in peninsular Malaysia (Traub, 1960; Upham et al., 1971); (8) abandoned vegetable plots and other marginal land within metropolitan areas such as Bombay (Savoor and Das, 1947); and Djakarta (Gispen et al., 1949); and (9) pockets of ecologic disturbance within the forest in which aboriginal people practice shifting slash-and-burn methods of agriculture (Cadigan et al., 1972).

In all these circumstances, the natural hosts of vector chiggers, chiefly small rodents of the genus *Rattus,* are plentiful. Larger animals (Audy, 1961), wild (Somov and Polivanov, 1972) and domestic (Kitaoka et al., 1976) fowl, and even domestic cattle (Somov et al., 1973) may also act as vector hosts. Chiggers attach to the host for several days and feed on tissue fluids rather than blood. After feeding, the larvae drop to the soil, where they develop through several additional stages into free-living adults (Traub and Wisseman, 1974). After fertilization by acquiring spermatophores deposited in the soil by males, one female adult can produce enough eggs to hatch from hundreds (Traub and Wisseman, 1974) to more than a thousand larval offspring (Neal and Barnett, 1961). The entire life cycle requires about 60 to 90 days in the laboratory but may be shorter under ideal natural conditions. Chiggers, which require a ground surface microenvironment of favorable moisture and air temperature (Gentry et al., 1963), disappear during drought, flooding, and extremes of heat and cold. Thus, in the temperate climate of Japan, scrub typhus is a seasonal disease occuring when and where the climate is favorable for a particular vector. The risk of contracting scrub typhus in the summer is greatest along certain watercourses when the temperature exceeds 20° C, which favors the prevalence of *L. akamushi.* In the winter the risk is associated with certain volcanic soil and nonriverine areas when the temperature falls to 10 to 18° C, favoring *L. scutellare* and *L. pallida* (Tamiya, 1962). In tropic and subtropic areas, the principal vector is *L. deliense.* When the tropic climate is moist throughout the year, as in Malaysia, there is little monthly fluctuation in the number of cases, whereas in tropic areas with sharp wet and dry seasons, as in India, disease is usually confined to the wet season.

Chiggers are barely visible to the naked eye as red or reddish-white spots moving across a black background such as boots. Within typical habitats, the distribution of chiggers on the ground is uneven, with collections or foci of chiggers on certain patches of ground a few meters square (Hubert and Baker, 1963). By contrast, nearby habitats of the same type can be entirely devoid of chiggers. The basis for these distribution characteristics is unknown.

The risk of disease is determined both by the distribution of vector chiggers and the presence of rickettsiae in the chigger population. It has been estimated that only one or two per cent of chiggers are infected (Kitaoka et al., 1974). Rapmund and co-workers showed, however, that all offspring of an infected adult female may be infected (Rapmund et al., 1969). Since adult chiggers are thought to have a limited range of movement, highly infectious, concentrated foci of chiggers may occur, with an attendant high risk of disease for humans exposed to them. During World War II, when military personnel moved on a broad front through terrain typical for scrub typhus vectors, disease was often limited to certain very small groups of men (Philip et al., 1946; Sayers and Hill, 1948). Highly efficient transovarial infection is a partial explanation of the very focal nature of the disease. Dohany and co-workers have recently developed an immunofluorescence procedure by which unfed chiggers collected from the ground can be speciated and examined for the presence of scrub typhus rickettsiae (Dohany et al., 1978). This provides a much needed tool for the assessment of the relative infectiousness of chigger foci. Other workers (Mirolyubova et al., 1966; Roberts et al., 1977) have shown that rickettsiae can also be identified in the tissues of larvae by immunofluorescence. The phenomenon of highly efficient transovarial transmission of rickettsiae suggests that the reservoir of *R. tsutsugamushi* in nature is the chigger itself. Infected vector chiggers transmit rickettsiae to their vertebrate hosts; surprisingly, the reverse rarely occurs. Larvae acquire rickettsiae by feeding on infected vertebrates, but for unknown reasons they rarely if ever transmit them to the next generation by transovarial passage (Traub et al., 1975; Walker et al., 1975). Thus, cyclic passage of the agent between vector and host does not appear to be a principal mechanism for maintenance of *R. tsutsugamushi* in nature.

All age groups and both sexes acquire scrub typhus. The ecologic circumstances of an area determine whether scrub typhus affects chiefly agricultural workers, individuals around the immediate environs of the home, or children and young adults who become infected on vacant land used for playing fields.

*R. tsutsugamushi* has been recovered from chiggers that are not known to feed on humans (Kitaoka et al., 1973) from tropic forest animals remote from humans (Muul et al., 1977), and from animals and chiggers in sparsely populated mountainous and subarctic terrain (Traub and Wisseman, 1974), suggesting that sylvan reservoirs of rickettsiae exist in nature. It was Audy's evolutionary view of scrub typhus that a preexisting sylvan, chigger-borne rickettsiosis has been extended and amplified by human encroachment on and alteration of primary forest, leading to creation of hyperendemic foci of vectors to which humans are exposed (Audy, 1961). A full analysis of the ecology of scrub typhus has been published by Traub and Wisseman (Traub and Wisseman, 1974). The evolutionary view is important because humans continue to alter the land, eliminating some hyperendemic foci but creating new ones elsewhere. The disease epidemiology is not static. Physicians must be alert for the appearance of new foci of scrub typhus — for example, in the vicinity of rural land settlement schemes located where forest has recently been cleared.

The current geographic distribution of scrub typhus encompasses Asia and contiguous islands of the western Pacific region, including the island continent of Australia. Known extreme limits of vector chiggers are the Maldive and Chagos Archipelagos in the Indian Ocean (Audy, 1961), the New Hebrides Islands east of New Guinea (Audy, 1961), the Tadzhik SSR in the Soviet Union adjacent to Afghanistan (Kulagin et al., 1968), and the islands of Shikotan and Kunashir in the Kuril Island chain near Japan (Somov et al., 1976). Vectors and disease have been reported from most countries on the continent of Asia, including Pakistan (Majid Khan and Gilani, 1963), India (Wanchoo et al., 1973), Burma (Win et al., 1968), Ceylon (Audy, 1961), Thailand (Trishnananda et al., 1966), and South Korea (Jackson et al., 1957), as well as Malaysia and Vietnam. Disease occurs in the Himalayan foothills, where vectors have been found in the Northeast Agency of India up to 3810 meters elevation (Varma and Mahadevan, 1973) and in Pakistan up to 2470 meters (Traub and Wisseman, 1974). Disease occurs in the Primorsk region of far eastern Siberia near the border with North Korea (Shapiro et al., 1969), in the coastal (Hsu et al., 1959; Wu et al., 1959) and southern provinces (Yu and Wu, 1959; Yu et al., 1959) of the People's Republic of China, and in Hong Kong (Webb and Hughes, 1961). In Australia, the disease occurs in the warm, moist zone of northern Queensland (Campbell and Domrow, 1974). Vectors and disease are found on Pacific islands forming a broad arc from the New Hebrides through New Guinea (Blake et al., 1945), Indonesia (Audy, 1961), the Philippines (Reisen et al., 1973) and Taiwan (Gale et al., 1974) to Japan. Vectors have not been found on Guam (Audy, 1961). In countries or regions within this broad geographic zone in which the disease has not been reported, its eventual recognition can be anticipated. There is serologic evidence of *R. tsutsugamushi* infection in rodents in eastern Iran, but human disease has not been reported there (Hamidi et al., 1974). Scrub typhus antibody and skin-test reactivity have been reported from Ruanda in central Africa (Giroud and Jadin, 1951). *R. tsutsugamushi* has not been isolated in Africa, however, Until that is accomplished, the specificity of these reactions must be questioned.

## *DIAGNOSIS*

If no eschar or rash is present, the differential diagnosis includes most etiologies contributing to fever of unknown origin syndrome, especially malaria, typhoid fever, infectious mononucleosis, leptospirosis, dengue, and other arbovirus infections. Concurrent malaria and scrub typhus are seen (Berman and Kundin, 1973). Scrub typhus must be considered in malaria patients who have persistent fever after adequate treatment, especially in southeast Asia, where such a response may be viewed as a drug-resistant falciparum infection. Ulcerative eschars in the genital area and tender regional lymph nodes may be mistaken for veneral disease (Levy, 1959).

Laboratory findings are not distinctive. Leukocyte counts may be normal. When abnormal, there is usually a leukopenia of 2000 to 4000 cells per $mm^3$ during the first week of disease with a predominance of polymorphonuclear cells and a leukocytosis of up to 25,000 cells per $ml^3$ during the second week with a predominance of small lymphocytes. Red blood cell count and hematocrit are usually normal. Total platelet count may be as low as 10,000 per $mm^3$, but its frequency and mechanism are unknown. Urinalysis may be normal at first, but in the more severe cases it usually shows moderate albuminuria, elevated specific gravity, occasional red and white blood cells, and granular casts. Nitrogen retention may occur. The serum chloride concentration is low and total protein levels are usually normal. In one series of 41 patients (Berman and Kundin, 1973), serum glutamic oxalacetic transaminase (SGOT) levels were highly variable and were not correlated with rash, severity of fever, or hepatomegaly. Hypofibrinogenemia, increased levels of circulating fibrin-split products, and general consumption of clotting factors, which are typical of disseminated intravascular coagulation (DIC), have been described in one instance (Ognibene et al., 1971).

Laboratory diagnosis is achieved by isolation of rickettsiae and by demonstration of specific antibody in convalescent serum. Intraperitoneal inoculation of white laboratory mice with whole blood or blood clot collected from untreated febrile patients should yield *R. tsutsugamushi*. Identification of rickettsiae requires at a minimum several weeks and often several months. Chloramphenicol or tetracycline rapidly eliminates rickettsemia, but mouse inoculation up to 24 hours after initiation of antibiotics occasionally yields rickettsiae. When mouse inoculation is delayed, the blood clot should be stored at or below −60° C.

Serologic diagnosis must contend with the immunologic heterogeneity of scrub typhus rickettsial strains. Bozeman and Elisberg (1963) developed an indirect immunofluorescent procedure using three strains — Karp, Gilliam, and Kato — isolated from human infections in New Guinea, Burma, and Japan, respectively. Because suspensions of whole rickettsiae are used as an antigen that is not available commercially, the test is usually performed in reference laboratories. The antigen is stable when dried on microscope slides stored frozen so that the procedure can be performed wherever fluorescent microscopy is available. Sera from some patients react with only one strain, others with two or all three. No case with a typical clinical course, or from which rickettsiae have been isolated, has been reported that failed to produce antibody against one of these strains. However, rickettsial strains that are immunologically distinct from these reference strains have been isolated from nature. The extent to which these other strains cause human disease is unknown. Shishido prepared purified complement-fixing antigens from Karp, Gilliam, and Kato strains that have been used widely in Japan (Shishido, 1962). Antibody can be detected by immunofluorescence on about the ninth day of disease, and by complement fixation on about the fourteenth day. Antibody can be detected for years by both procedures. Collection of blood specimens on filter paper for easy storage and shipment has been described by Gan and co-workers (Gan et al., 1972).

The Weil-Felix *Proteus* agglutination test has been widely used for nearly 50 years. The agglutination reaction is based on possession of common antigens by *R. tsutsugamushi* and *Proteus mirabilis* OX-K strain. Agglutinins are found as early as the ninth day of disease. Low titers of agglutinins (less than 1:100) occur in some normal individuals. Therefore, a diagnosis can be made only upon demonstration of a four-fold or greater increase in agglutinins or a high titer in a single convalescent serum specimen. However, not all scrub typhus infections stimulate these agglutinins. Indeed, in some reported case series, fewer than 25 per cent of the patients developed them. Other agents infecting man (Carley et al., 1955; Lewthwaite, 1940; Zarafonetis et al., 1946) can give rise to OX-K agglutinins. Thus, the Weil-Felix test is unreliable and with the increasing availability of other specific serologic procedures should not be relied upon.

## TREATMENT

Scrub typhus responds rapidly to antibiotics. In adults, oral tetracycline, 2.0 g per day in divided doses, clears all manifestations of disease in 36 to 48 hours. Children should be given 20 to 40 mg per kg per day in four divided doses. Chloramphenicol was the original drug of choice (Smadel et al., 1949), but it has been supplanted by tetracycline, which is less toxic and produces a faster response (Sheehy et al., 1973). Because all effective drugs are rickettsiostatic, treatment should be continued until about the fourteenth day, when the immune response is well developed. Clinical relapse with rickettsemia occurs within four to five days if treatment is stopped earlier, especially if it was begun in the first week of disease. Humoral antibody, which may be detected as early as the ninth day, does not prevent relapse. Cell-mediated immunity seems to be the principal mechanism of acquired resistance in experimentally infected mice and is assumed to play a role in humans as well (Sheehy et al., 1973). Peripheral vascular collapse should be managed as septic shock. DIC should subside quickly with antibiotic therapy. Only in instances of severe hemorrhagic diathesis should heparin therapy be necessary. Single-dose treatment of scrub typhus with 200 mg of doxycycline, a long-acting tetracycline, has been successful in Malaysia in more than 30 patients without relapse, but treatment was almost always begun on or after the seventh day of disease (Brown et al., 1978). This simplified approach must be evaluated further before it can be recommended for use earlier in disease.

## PROPHYLAXIS

No vaccine against scrub typhus is available. The immunologic heterogeneity of *R. tsutsugamushi* has proved to be an insurmountable obstacle thus far, but the limited number of immunologically distinct strains causing human disease in certain areas (Brown et al., 1976; Kitaoka et al., 1974) provides some encouragement that a vaccine may be developed eventually.

Individuals can be protected by two other means, however. Diethyltoluamide (DEET), a highly effective mite repellent suitable for skin and clothing, is sold commercially. The most effective formulation includes 50 per cent active material. Its disadvantages are that it washes off easily and has organic solvent properties that affect certain plastics used in personal and household articles. The second approach is chemoprophylaxis. Smadel first demonstrated that chloramphenicol in oral doses of 3.0 to 4.0 g every four to seven days for four weeks or longer protects persons from disease while they are taking the drug and after its discontinuance (Smadel et al., 1950). The long-acting tetracycline agent, doxycycline, would seem to be admirably suited to this purpose, but its efficacy in prophylaxis has not been examined in the field. Chemoprophylaxis should be reserved for persons who must enter known hyperendemic areas of disease for short periods.

Direct control of chiggers is also possible. The residual chlorinated hydrocarbon insecticide, dieldrin, sprayed over a hyperendemic focus of disease, eradicated vector chiggers for up to two years with one application (Traub and Dowling, 1961). Concern for the environmental impact of residual insecticides has limited the use of this highly effective chemical. In the United States, a nonresidual organophosphate, chlorpyrifos, has controlled the American chigger *Eutrombicula alfreddugesi* for four weeks with one application (Mount et al., 1978). Since this chigger is similar to scrub typhus vector chiggers, the use of chlorpyrifos should be tested against vectors in Asia. Dohany has described a systemic acaracide, dimethoate, which is effective against American chiggers. Dimethoate, an organophosphate, is placed in food for vertebrate hosts, which transfer it to chiggers during feedings (Donahy et al., 1977). Its efficacy against scrub typhus vectors is being tested. Since the mite is apparently both the vector and the reservoir of the disease, elimination of rats does not reduce the risk of disease and, in the short term, may increase it by substituting humans as the only available chigger host (Audy, 1949).

## References

Asanuma, K., Kitaoka, M., Shimizu, F., and Kano, R.: *Leptotrombidium scutellare* as a vector of scrub typhus at an endemic area of the foothills of Mt. Fuji, Japan. J Hyg Epidem Microbiol Immunol 18:172, 1974.

Audy, J. R.: Practical notes on scrub typhus in the field. J R Army Med Corps 93:273, 1949.

Audy, J. R. The ecology of scrub typhus. In May, J. M. (ed.): Studies in Disease Ecology. New York, Hafner Publishing Company, 1961.

Berge, T. O., Gauld, R. L., and Kitaoka, M.: A field trial of a vaccine prepared from Volner strain of *Rickettsia tsutsugamushi*. Am J Hyg 50:337, 1949.

Berman, S. J., and Kundin, W. D.: Scrub typhus in South Vietnam. A study of 87 cases. Ann Intern Med 79:26, 1973.

Berman, S. J., Irving, G. A., Kundin, W. D., Gunning, J., and Watten, R. H.: Epidemiology of the acute fevers of unknown origin in South Vietnam: Effect of laboratory support upon clinical diagnosis. Am J Trop Med Hyg 22:796, 1973.

Blake, F. G., Maxcy, K. F., Sadusk, J. F., Jr., Kohls, G. M., and Bell, E. J.: Studies on tsutsugamushi disease (scrub typhus, mite-borne typhus) in New Guinea and adjacent islands. Am J Hyg 41:243, 1945.

Bozeman, F. M., and Elisberg, B. L.: Serological diagnosis of scrub typhus by indirect immunofluorescence. Proc Soc Exp Biol Med 112:568, 1963.

Brown, G. W., Robinson, D. M., Huxsoll, D. L., Ng, T. S., Lim, K. J., and Sannasey, G.: Scrub typhus: A common cause of illness in indigenous populations. Trans R Soc Trop Med Hyg 70:444, 1976.

Brown, G. W., Saunders, J. P., Singh, S., Huxsoll, D. L., and Shirai, A.: Single dose doxycycline therapy for scrub typhus. Trans R Soc Trop Med Hyg 72:412, 1978.

Cadigan, F. C., Jr., Andre, R. G., Bolton, M., Gan, E., and Walker, J. S.: The effect of habitat on the prevalence of human scrub typhus in Malaysia. Trans R Soc Trop Med Hyg 66:582, 1972.

Campbell, R. W., and Domrow, R.: Rickettsioses in Australia: Isolation or *Rickettsia tsutsugamushi* and *R. australis* from naturally infected arthropods. Trans R Soc Trop Med Hyg 68:397, 1974.

Card, W. L., and Walker, J. M.: Scrub typhus vaccine: Field trial in Southeast Asia. Lancet 1:481, 1947.

Carley, J. G., Doherty, R. L., Derrick, E. M., Pope, J. M., Emanuel, M. L., and Ross, C. J.: The investigation of fever in North Queensland by mouse inoculation, with particular reference to scrub typhus. Austral Ann Med 4:91, 1955.

Cooper, W. C., Lien, J. C., Hsu, S. H., and Chen, W. F.: Scrub typhus in the Pescadores Islands: An epidemiological and clinical study. Am J Trop Med Hyg 13:833, 1964.

Dohany, A. L., Cromroy, H. L., and Cole, M. M.: Laboratory tests of dimethoate for systemic control of chiggers (Acarina: Trombiculidae), populations on rodents. J Med Ent 14:79, 1977.

Dohany, A. L., Shirai, A., Robinson, D. M., Ram, S., and Huxsoll, D. L.: Identification and antigenic typing of *Rickettsia tsutsugamushi* in naturally infected chiggers by direct immunofluorescence. Am J Trop Med Hyg 27:1261, 1978.

Elsom, K. A., Beebe, G. W., Sayen, J. J., Scheie, H. G., Cannon, G. D., and Wood, F. C.: Scrub typhus: A follow-up study. Ann Intern Med 55:784, 1961.

Fletcher, W., Lesslar, J. E., and Lewthwaite, R.: The etiology of the tsutsugamushi disease and tropical typhus in the Federated Malay States. Part I. Trans R Soc Trop Med Hyg 22:161, 1928.

Gale, J. L., Irving, G. S., Wang, H. C., Lien, J. C., Chen, W. F., and Cross, J. H.: Scrub typhus in eastern Taiwan, 1970 Am J Trop Med Hyg 23:679, 1974.

Gan, E., Cadigan, F. C., Jr., and Walker, J. S.: Filter paper collection of blood for use in a screening and diagnostic test for scrub typhus using the IFAT. Trans R Soc Trop Med Hyg 66:588, 1972.

Gentry, J. W., Cheng, S. Y., and Phang, O. W.: Preliminary observations on *Leptotrombidium (Leptotrombidium) akamushi* and *Leptotrombidium (Leptotrombidium) deliensis* in their natural habitats in Malaya. Am J Hyg 78:181, 1963.

Giroud, P., and Jadin, J.: Presence des anticorps vis-a-vis de *Rickettsia orientalis* chez les indigenes et des asiatiques vivant au Ruanda-Urindi (Congo Belge). Bull Soc Pathol Exot 44:50, 1951.

Gispen, R., Smit, A. M., and Westermann, C. D.: Epidemic scrub typhus in Batavia. Docum Neer Indon Morbis Trop 1:134, 1949.

Hamidi, A. N., Saadatezadeh, H., Tarasevich, I. V., Arata, A. A., and Farbangazad, A.: A serological study of rickettsial infections in Iranian small mammals. Bull Soc Pathol Exot 67:607, 1974.

Hsu, P. K., Su, K. C., and Chen, H. T.: Larvae of *Trombicula akamushi* var. *deliensis* as related to the epidemiology of tsutsugamushi. Acta Microbiol Sinica 1:1, 1959.

Hubert, A. A., and Baker, H. J.: The persistence of a foci of *Leptotrombidium (L.) akamushi* along a transect in Malaya. Am J Hyg 78:143, 1963.

Hubert, A. A., and Baker, H. J.: Studies on the habitats and population of *Leptotrombidium (Leptotrombidium) akamushi* and *L. (L.) deliense* in Malaya. Am J Hyg 78:131, 1963.

Jackson, E. M., Danauskas, J. X., Smadel, J. E., Cole, M., and Bozeman, F. M.: Occurrence of *Rickettsia tsutsugamushi* in Korean rodents and chiggers. Am J Hyg 66:309, 1957.

Kawai, K., Dodin, A., Wiart, J., and Capponi, M.: Étude des proprietes antigeniques de trois souches de *Rickettsia tsutsugamushi*. C R Soc Biol (Paris) 165:1857, 1971.

Kawamura, R.: Studies on tsutsugamushi disease (Japanese food fever). Bull Coll Med Univ Cincinnati 4 (Spec. nos. 1 & 2):1–229, 1926.

Kitaoka, M., and Tanaka, Y.: Rickettsial toxin and its specificity in three prototype strains, Karp, Gilliam and Kato, of *Rickettsia orientalis*. Acta Virol 17:426, 1973.

Kitaoka, M., Asanuma, K., Okubo, K., Tanegugh, H., Tsubo, M., and Hattor, K.: Seasonal occurrence of trombiculid mites species and *Leptotrombidium kawamurai* (Acarina, Trombiculidae) as a carrier of *Rickettsia orientalis* in the Nopporo area, Hokkaido, Japan. J Hyg Epidemiol Microbiol Immunol 17:478, 1973.

Kitaoka, M., Asanuma, K., and Otsuji, J.: Transmission of *Rickettsia orientalis* to man by *Leptotrombidium akamushi* at a scrub typhus endemic area in Akita Prefecture, Japan. Am J Trop Med Hyg 23:993, 1974.

Kitaoka, M., Asanuma, K., and Otsuji, J.: Experiments on chickens placed on ground endemic of classical scrub typhus in Akita Prefecture, Japan. J Hyg Epidemiol Microbiol Immunol 20:195, 1976.

Kulagin, S. M., Taresevich, I. V., Kudryashova, N. I., and Plotnikova, L. F.: The investigations of scrub typhus in the USSR. J Hyg Epidemiol Microbiol Immunol 12:257, 1968.

Kundin, W. D., Liu, C., Harmon, P., and Rodina, P.: Pathogenesis of scrub typhus infection *(Rickettsia tsutsugamushi)*, as studied by immunofluorescence. J Immunol 93:772, 1964.

Levy, B.: Scrub typhus in the differential diagnosis of venereal disease. J R Army Med Corps 105:125, 1959.

Lewthwaite, R., and Savoor, S. R.: Rickettsia diseases of Malaya. Lancet 1:255, 305, 1940.

Lewthwaite, R.: Agglutination of *Proteus* in rat-bite fever. Lancet 1:390, 1940.

McCulloch, R. N.: Notes on the habits and distribution of trombiculid mites in Queensland and New Guinea. Med J Austral 28:543, 1944.

Majid Khan, A., and Gilani, S.: Scrub typhus in Sialkot District (West Pakistan). Pakistan J Health 13:88, 1963.

Mirolyubova, L. V., Kudryashova, N. I., and Tarasevich, I. V.: The use of fluorescent serological method for determining natural infection with *Rickettsia tsutsugamushi* in trombiculid mites. Zh Mikrobiol Epidemiol Immunobiol 43:36, 1966.

Moe, J. B., Mosher, D. F., and Kenyon, R. H.: Functional and morphologic changes during experimental Rocky Mountain spotted fever in guinea pigs. Lab Invest 35:235, 1976.

Morris, J. A.: Early development in monkeys of cutaneous resistance to reinfection with *Rickettsia tsutsugamushi*. Proc Soc Exp Biol Med 119:736, 1965.

Mount, G. A., Grothaus, R. H., Reed, J. T., and Baldwin, K. F.: Area control of chigger mites with granules and concentrated sprays of chlorypyrifos. J Econ Entomol 71:27, 1978.

Muul, I., Lim, B. L., and Walker, J. S.: Scrub typhus infection in rats in four habitats in peninsular Malaysia. Trans R Soc Trop Med Hyg 71:493, 1977.

Nagayo, M., Tamiya, T., Mitamura, T., and Hagato, H.: Studies on the virus of typhus fever. Jap J Exp Med 8:319, 1930.

Neal, T. J., and Barnett, H. C.: The life cycle of the scrub typhus chigger mite. Ann Entomol Soc Am 54:196, 1961.

Ogata, N.: Aetiologie der Tsutsugamushikrankheit: *Rickettsia tsutsugamushi*. Z. Bakteriol Parasitol Infektionhr 122:249, 1931.

Ognibene, A. J., O'Leary, D. S., Czarnecki, S. W., Flannery, E. P., and Grove, R. B.: Myocarditis and disseminated intravascular coagulation in scrub typhus. Am J Med Sci 262:233, 1971.

Perkins, H. R., and Allison, A. C.: Cell-wall constituents of rickettsiae and psittacosis-lymphogranuloma organisms. J Gen Microbiol 30:469, 1963.

Philip, C. B., Woodward, T. E., and Sullivan, R. R.: Tsutsugamushi disease (scrub or mite-borne typhus) in the Philippine Islands during American reoccupation in 1944–45. Am J Trop Med 26:229, 1946.

Rapmund, G., Upham, R. W., Jr., Kundin, W. D., Manikumaran, C., and Chan, T. C.: Transovarial development of scrub typhus rickettsiae in a colony of vector mites. Trans R Soc Trop Med Hyg 63:251, 1969.

Reisen, W. K., Pollar, T. J., and Tardy, W. J.: Some epidemiological considerations of scrub typhus *(Rickettsia tsutsugamushi)* in a natural focus in the Zambales Mountains, Luzon, Republic of the Philippines. Am J Trop Med Hyg 22:503, 1973.

Rights, F. L., Smadel, J. E., and Jackson, E. B.: Studies on scrub typhus (tsutsugamushi disease). III. Heterogeneity of strains of *R. tsutsugamushi* as demonstrated by cross vaccination studies. J Exp Med 87:339, 1948.

Roberts, L. W., Muul, I., and Robinson, D. M.: Numbers of *Leptotrombidium (L.) deliense* (Acarina: Trombiculidae) and prevalence of *Rickettsia tsutsugamushi* in adjacent habitats of peninsular Malaysia. Southeast Asian J Trop Med Public Health 8:207, 1977.

Robinson, D. M., Gan, E., and Donaldson, R.: The prevalence of scrub typhus antibodies in residents of West Malaysia. Trop Geogr Med 28:303, 1976.

Savoor, S. R., and Das, M. P.: Scrub typhus (tsutsugamushi disease) in Bombay. Indian Med Gaz 82:752, 1947.

Sayen, J. J., Pond, H. S., Forrester, J. S., and Wood, F. C.: Scrub typhus in Assam and Burma. A clinical study of 616 cases. Medicine 25:155, 1946.

Sayers, M. H. P., and Hill, I. G. W.: The occurrence and identification of the typhus group of fevers in South East Asia Command. J R Army Med Corps 90:6, 1948.

Schramek, S., Brezina, R., and Tarasevich, I. V.: Isolation of a lipopolysaccharide antigen from *Rickettsia* species. Acta Virol 20:270, 1976.

Shapiro, M. I., Somov, G. P., Gopachenko, I. M., and Natsky, I. V.: Materials on epidemiology of tsutsugamushi fever in Primorsk region. Zh Mikrobiol 46:42, 1969.

Sheehy, T. W., Hazlett, D., and Turk, R. E.: Scrub typhus. A comparison of chloramphenicol and tetracycline in its treatment. Arch Intern Med 132:77, 1973.

Shishido, A.: Identification and serologic classification of the causative agent of scrub typhus in Japan. Jap J Med Sci Biol 15:308, 1962.

Shubin, F. N., Natsky, K. V., and Somov, G. P.: Concerning the vector of tsutsugamushi fever in the Far East. Zh Mikrobiol Epidemiol Immunobiol 47:112, 1970.

Smadel, J. E., Woodward, T. E., Ley, H. L., Jr., and Lewthwaite, R.: Chloramphenicol (Chloromycetin) in the treatment of tsutsugamushi disease (scrub typhus). J Clin Invest 28:1196, 1949.

Smadel, J. E., Traub, R., Frick, L. P., Diercks, F. H., and Bailey, C. A.: Chloramphenicol (Chloromycetin) in the chemoprophylaxis of scrub typhus (tsutsugamushi disease). III. Suppression of overt disease by prophylactic regimens of four-week duration. Am J Hyg 51:216, 1950.

Smadel, J. E., Ley, H. L., Jr., Diercks, F. H., Paterson, P. Y., Wisseman, C. L., Jr., and Traub, R.: Immunization against scrub typhus: Duration of immunity in volunteers following combined living vaccine and chemoprophylaxis. Am J Trop Med Hyg 1:87, 1952.

Somov, G. P., and Polivanov, V. M.: Isolation of strains of *Rickettsia tsutsugamushi* from the organs of migrant birds in the Primorie. Zh Mikrobiol Epidemiol Immunobiol 49:6, 1972.

Somov, G. P., Shubin, F. N., Kir'yanov, E. A., and Mamontova, R. M.: Serological examination of cattle as a method of detection of natural foci of tsutsugamushi fever. Zh Mikrobiol Epidemiol Immunobiol 50:63, 1973.

Somov, G. P., Shubin, F. N., Gopachenko, I. M., and Kononova, D. G.: Tsutsugamushi fever in the Kuril Islands. Zh Mikrobiol Epidemiol Immunobiol 53:69, 1976.

Tamiya, T.: Recent Advances in Studies of Tsutsugamushi Disease in Japan. Tokyo, Medical Culture, Inc., 1962.

Traub, R.: Two new species of chiggers of the genus *Leptotrombidium*. Malaysian parasites XLV. Stud Inst Med Res (Kuala Lumpur) 29:193, 1960.

Traub, R., and Dowling, M. A. C.: The duration of efficacy of the insecticide Dieldrin against the chigger vectors of scrub typhus in Malaya. J Econ Entomol 54:654, 1961.

Traub, R., and Wisseman, C. L., Jr.: The ecology of chigger-borne rickettsiosis (scrub typhus). J Med Entomol 11:237, 1974.

Traub, R., Wisseman, C. L., Jr., Jones, M. R., and O'Keefe, J. J.: The acquisition of *Rickettsia tsutsugamushi* by chiggers (trombiculid mites) during the feeding process. Ann NY Acad Sci 266:91, 1975.

Trishnananda, M., Harinasuta, C., and Vasuvat, C.: Studies on the vector of *Rickettsia tsutsugamushi* infection in Thailand. Ann Trop Med Parasitol 60:252, 1966.

Upham, R. W., Jr., Hubert, A. A., Phang, O. W., Yusof bin Mat, and Rapmund, G.: Distribution of *Leptotrobidium (Leptobrombidium) arenicola* (Acarina: Trombiculidae) on the ground in West Malaysia. J Med Entomol 8:401, 1971.

Varma, R. N., and Mahadevan, B.: The bionomics and vector potential of the scrub typhus vector *Leptotrombidium (L.) deliense* and other trombiculid populations in eastern Himalayas, India. Indian J Med Sci 27:900, 1973.

Vercammen-Grandjean, P. M.: Establissement d'us lectotype pom *Leptotrombidium (L.) akamushi* (Brumst, 1910) (Acarina: Trombiculidae). Acarologia 11:94, 1969.

Walker, J. S., Chan, T. C., Manikumaran, C., and Elisberg, B. L.: Attempts to infect and demonstrate transovarial transmission of *R. tsutsugamushi* in three species of *Leptotrombidium* mites. Ann N Y Acad Sci 266:80, 1975.

Wanchoo, S. N., Chatterjee, B. C., Rai, J., and Lamba, J. S.: Scrub typhus (an unusual outbreak in Punjab). Armed Forces Med J India 29:185, 1973.

Webb, J. S., and Hughes, D. T. D.: Scrub typhus in Hong Kong. J R Army Med Corps 107:224, 1961.

Win, K., Ohn, T., and Than, M.: Scrub typhus in Burma. Union Burma J Life Sci 1:209, 1968.

Wolbach, S. B.: Rickettsial diseases: A general survey. In Virus and Rickettsial Diseases. Cambridge, Harvard University Press, 1940.

Wood, W. H., Jr., and Wisseman, C. L., Jr.: Studies of *Rickettsia mooseri* cell walls. II. Immunologic properties. J Immunol 98:1224, 1967.

Wu, C. L., Chen, S., and Wu, K. H.: Discovery of *Trombicula akamushi* var. *deliensis* in Chekiang Province. Acta Entomolog Sinica 9:964, 1959.

Yosana, H: Studies on Shichito Fever: Winter Scrub Typhus of Izu Shichito Islands, Japan. Tokyo, Health Bureau, Tokyo Metropolitan Office, 1953.

Yu, E. S., and Wu, H. Y.: Further study on the different types of *Trombicula deliensis* and transovarian transmission of *Rickettsia orientalis*. Acta Microbiol Sinica 7:10, 1959.

Yu, E. S., Hwang, Y. L., and Liu, C. Y.: Further study on the immunology of *Rickettsia tsutsugamushi*. Acta Microbiol Sinica 7:189, 1959.

Zarafonetis, C. J. D., Ingraham, H. S., and Berry, J. F.: Weil-Felix and typhus complement fixation tests in relapsing fever, with special reference to B. *Proteus* OX-K agglutination. J Immunol 52:189, 1946.

# 189 *ROCKY MOUNTAIN SPOTTED FEVER*

*Alan L. Bisno, M.D.*

## DEFINITION

Rocky Mountain spotted fever is an acute infectious disease caused by a rickettsial agent, transmitted to man by several species of infected ticks, and characterized by fever, skin rash, myalgias, intense headache, and prostration.

## ETIOLOGY

The causative agent, *Rickettsia rickettsii*, is an obligate intracellular parasite belonging to the spotted fever group of rickettsiae. It shares a common antigen with other members of this group but may be differentiated from them serologically by means of a species-specific antigen. The organism measures approximately 1 $\mu$ by 0.2 to 0.3 $\mu$ and may be visualized under the light microscope in sections of infected tissues stained by the Gimenez, Giemsa, or Macchiavello methods. In such specimens, *R. rickettsii* often appears in pairs and surrounded by a halo, as if encapsulated.

## EPIDEMIOLOGY

The disease is limited to North and South America. It was first described during the late nineteenth century in the western United States. Its initial recognition in the mountainous areas of Montana and Idaho led to the name Rocky Mountain spotted fever. This appellation is now a misnomer, however, since, in the United States, the disease is currently much more prevalent along the Atlantic seaboard and in the southeastern states than in the Rockies. Rocky Mountain spotted fever has also been described in Canada, Mexico, Brazil, Panama, and Colombia.

Between 1906 and 1910, Howard Taylor Ricketts proved that ticks transmit the disease, described the appearance of the causative organism in human and animal tissues, and demonstrated that ticks have the capacity to transmit the rickettsiae from generation-to-generation transovarially.

Several species of ticks are known to transmit Rocky Mountain spotted fever. In the western United States, the wood tick, *Dermacentor andersoni,* is the principal vector, whereas east of the Mississippi River most cases are initiated by the bite of the American dog tick, *Dermacentor variabilis.* A third species, *Amblyomma americanum,* the Lone Star tick, is responsible for some cases in the southwestern United States. *Haemophysalis leporispalustris,* the rabbit tick, is also a natural carrier of the disease but has not been definitely implicated in spread to man. *Amblyomma cajennense* has been shown to transmit the disease in Brazil, Colombia, and Mexico. This tick, which parasitizes a number of wild and domestic animals and fowl, also avidly parasitizes man. It is a possible vector in the United States, where its range is limited to southern Texas and Florida.

Ticks become infected either transovarially or by feeding on infected animal hosts. Once infected, they can harbor the rickettsiae throughout their lifetime. Thus, the tick serves as both a vector and a reservoir of Rocky Mountain spotted

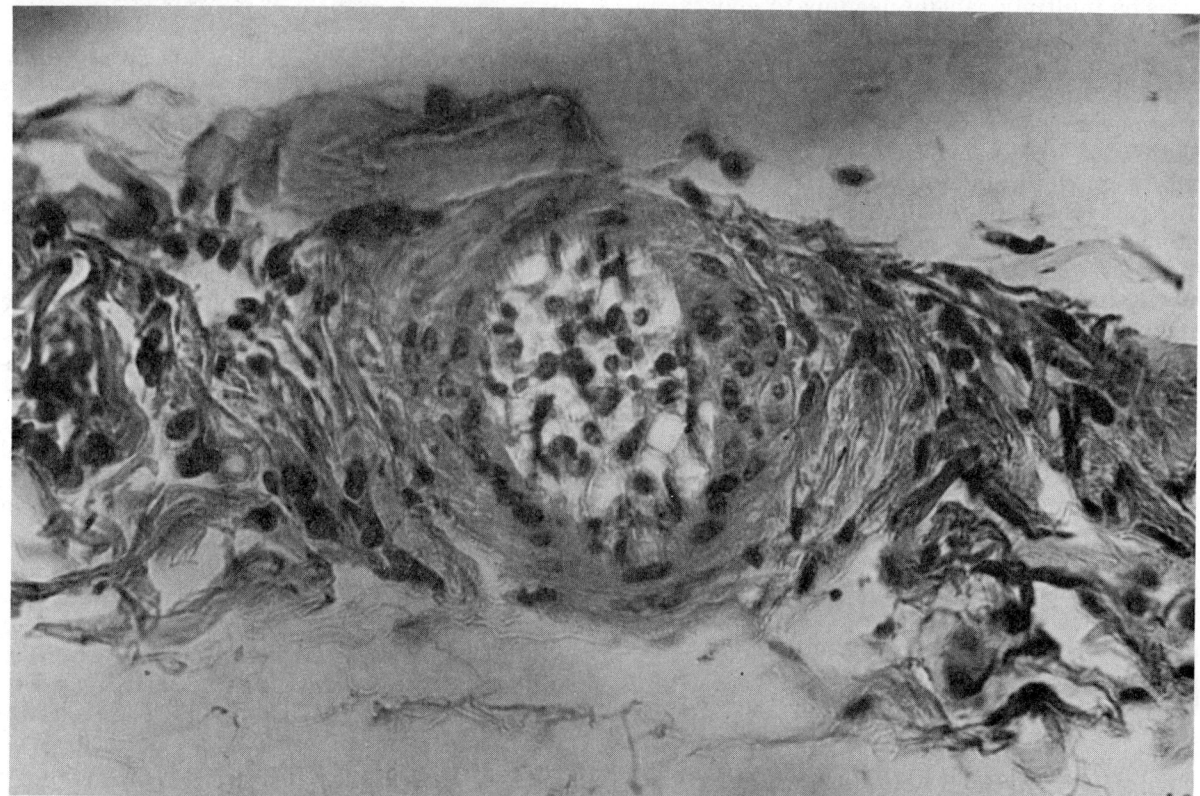

**FIGURE 1.**   *Cutaneous arteriole, demonstrating endothelial damage and mononuclear infiltration of vessel wall (hematoxylin-eosin, X400). (From Archives of Internal Medicine, Sept. 1973, 132:40. Copyright 1973, American Medical Association.)*

fever. Infection of man is an incidental event unnecessary for the persistence of *R. rickettsii* in nature. Although Rocky Mountain spotted fever is generally transmitted by tick bite, tick feces are also infectious; accidental self-inoculation, as by scratching, may cause illness. Aerosol transmission has occurred among laboratory personnel involved in rickettsial research.

Epidemiologic features of this disease are those that might be predicted from its known method of transmission. In temperate climates almost all cases occur during the warmer months of the year; approximately 60 per cent of cases occur in males and nearly 90 per cent in individuals less than 30 years of age (Hattwick et al., 1976). In the western United States most cases occur in the period April to June, the season of prevalence of *Dermacentor andersoni;* whereas in the southeastern states, cases continue throughout the summer months.

## PATHOGENESIS AND PATHOLOGY

Rocky Mountain spotted fever is characterized by rickettsial invasion of small blood vessels throughout the body. The process initially involves capillary endothelial cells, where the organisms multiply rapidly, leading to endothelial cell swelling, proliferation, and degeneration. Subsequently the lesions extend to involve veins and arterioles (Fig. 1). The pathologic process in arterioles involves the entire vascular wall, with necrosis of smooth muscle cells of the media as well as mononuclear and plasma cell infiltration of the adventitia (Fig. 2). The end result of this intense infectious vasculitis is diffuse thrombosis and microinfarction, particularly involving skin, subcutaneous tissue, and central nervous system. Necrosis of arteriolar walls leads to rupture with resultant localized areas of hemorrhage. In the brain, in addition to vascular proliferative, necrotic, and thrombotic changes, foci of cerebral astroglial proliferation (so-called "glial nodules") may be seen (Fig. 3).

The exact cause of the toxic, febrile state in Rocky Mountain spotted fever is unknown. Although products of host tissue destruction are undoubtedly involved, the rickettsial agent itself can produce both a toxin and a hemolysin, which are specifically neutralized by immune sera and which may play a role in the pathogenesis of the disease.

## CLINICAL MANIFESTATIONS

Approximately three-quarters of patients give a history of tick bite or tick exposure. The incuba-

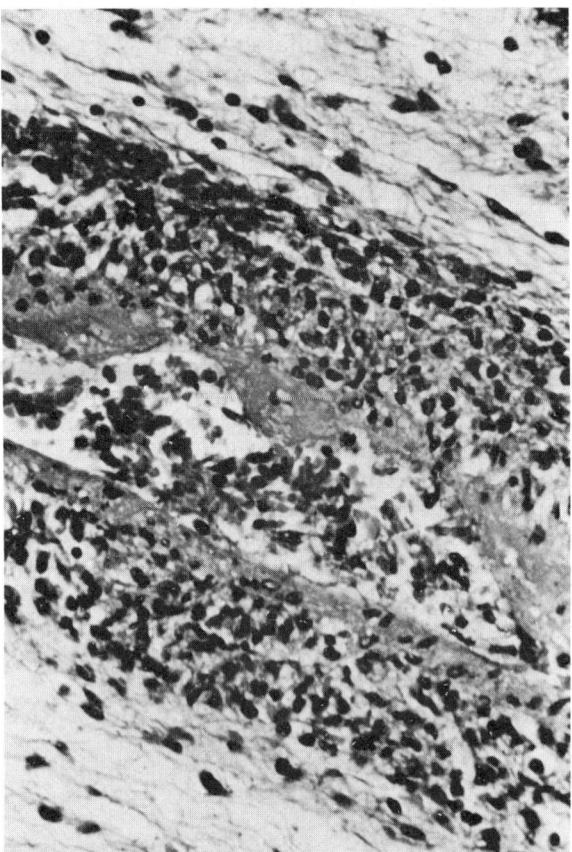

**FIGURE 2.** *Tangential section of an arteriole from seminal vesicle in a fatal case of Rocky Mountain spotted fever. The endothelium is denuded, and there is fibrin deposition along the vessel lining. Intense cellular infiltration involves all layers of the vessel (hematoxylin-eosin, X400). (Courtesy of W. Manford Gooch, M.D.)*

tion period ranges from two days to two weeks, averaging seven days. The onset is frequently abrupt, consisting of severe headache, chills, fever in excess of 102° F, generalized myalgias involving especially the back and legs, anorexia, malaise, and prostration. Additional symptoms may include nausea, vomiting, upper abdominal pain, photophobia, and arthralgias. This nondescript toxic, febrile illness resembles a number of other acute infectious processes, and specific diagnosis at this stage is extremely difficult.

The characteristic rash appears between the second and sixth day of illness (average, four days). It usually appears first as an erythematous macular eruption involving the wrists, ankles, palms, soles, and forearms (Fig. 4). The rash rapidly becomes maculopapular in character and spreads centripetally to involve the proximal extremities, trunk, and face (Fig. 5). After three to four days the lesions become petechial (Fig. 6) and, in more severe cases, may coalesce to form

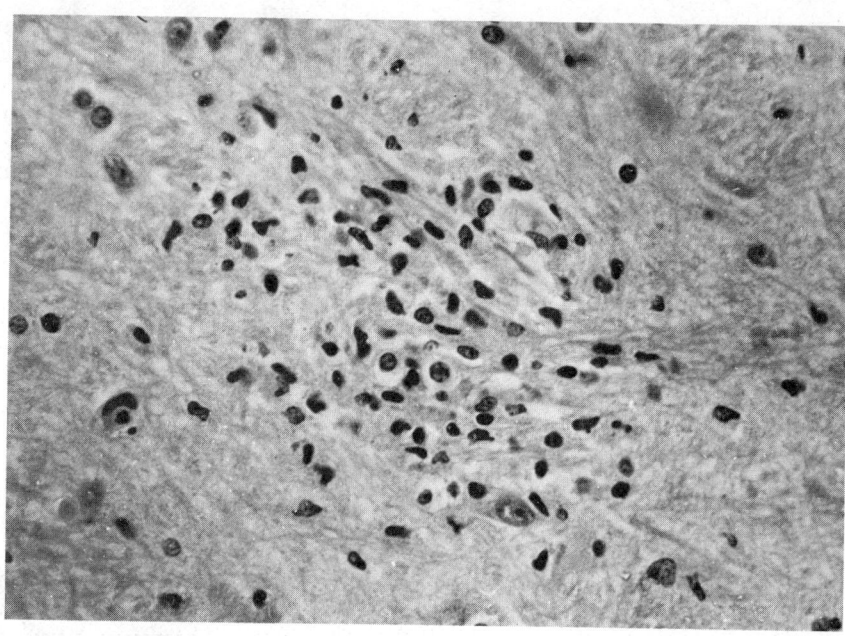

**FIGURE 3.** *Focus of cerebral astroglial proliferation ("glial nodule") in fatal case of Rocky Mountain spotted fever (hematoxylin-eosin, X400). (From Archives of Internal Medicine, Sept. 1973, 132:40. Copyright 1973, American Medical Association.)*

ecchymoses. Although the above description presents the usual features of the rash, exceptions do occur. The rash may at times begin on the trunk rather than the distal extremities. On rare occasions, the appearance of the rash may be delayed until the ninth day of illness or later, making specific diagnosis extremely difficult. Very rarely, the rash may be absent. More frequently a mild or transient rash may be overlooked, especially in black patients.

When diagnosed and treated early, the course of the disease may be relatively mild. More severe

cases, however, are characterized by profound alterations in the neurologic, hematologic, cardiovascular, and metabolic status of the patient. Neurologic abnormalities are an extremely prominent feature of the clinical illness. In addition to intense headache, these may include nuchal rigidity, delirium, stupor, coma, or grand mal seizures. Lumbar puncture may be normal or may

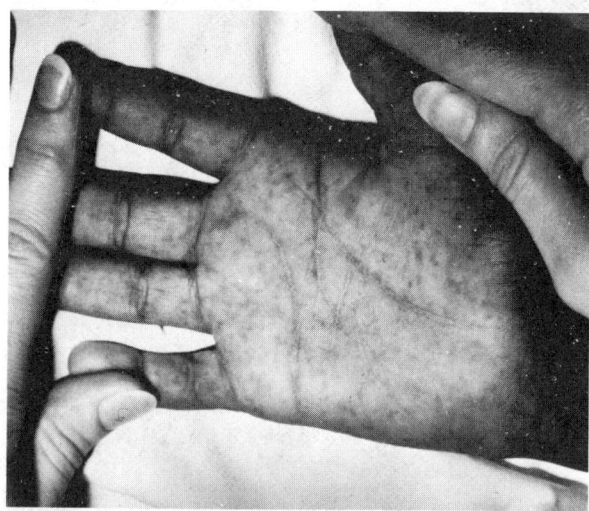

**FIGURE 4.** *Palmar rash in patient with Rocky Mountain spotted fever. (From Archives of Internal Medicine, Sept. 1973, 132:40. Copyright 1973, American Medical Association.)*

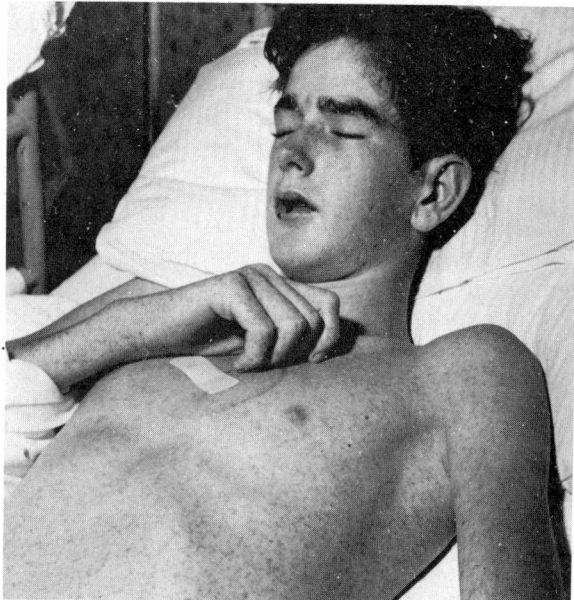

**FIGURE 5.** *Appearance of generalized rash on tenth hospital day. Bleeding about the mouth was related to mild consumptive coagulopathy. (From Archives of Internal Medicine, Sept. 1973, 132:40. Copyright 1973, American Medical Association.)*

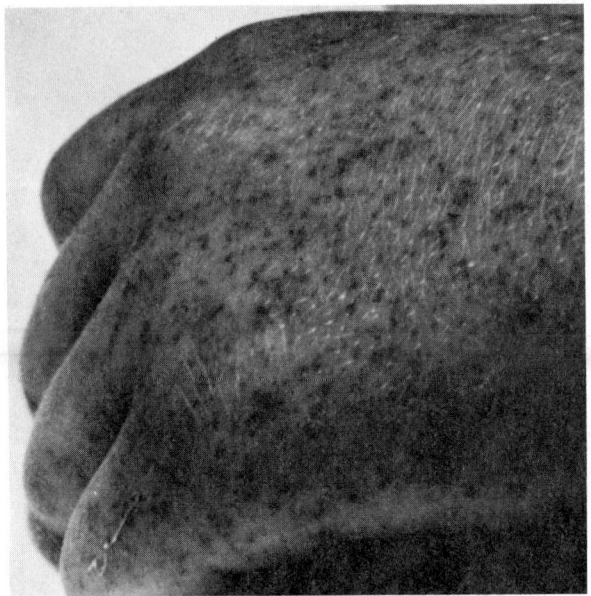

**FIGURE 6.** *Close-up view of the hand illustrates petechial nature of the rash. (From Archives of Internal Medicine, Sept. 1973, 132:40. Copyright 1973, American Medical Association.)*

show a mild pleocytosis and increase in protein concentration. Cerebrospinal fluid sugar concentration remains normal.

Approximately one-half of patients admitted to the hospital with severe forms of Rocky Mountain spotted fever exhibit thrombocytopenia. This finding is presumably due to margination of platelets at sites of vascular inflammation. In patients with fulminant infections, the diffuse intravascular coagulation that characterizes this disease gives rise to consumptive coagulopathy, manifested by hypofibrinogenemia, elevated levels of fibrin degradation products, depletion of circulating clotting factors, and severe hemorrhagic diathesis. Such a sequence of events is associated with a poor prognosis.

Another consequence of the diffuse vascular damage in Rocky Mountain spotted fever is increased capillary permeability, with the resultant loss of plasma and erythrocytes from the capillary bed into the interstitial space. Severely ill patients exhibit hypovolemia, hypoproteinemia, and edema (Fig. 7). The loss of circulating blood volume may be severe enough to lead to hypotension, oliguria, azotemia, and circulatory collapse. Marked hyponatremia is a frequent finding in seriously ill patients. Although the mechanism has not been definitively established, inappropriate secretion of antidiuretic hormone seems a likely explanation.

Although nonspecific electrocardiographic abnormalities may occur, clinically significant car-

diovascular dysfunction is more frequently secondary to circulatory collapse or to iatrogenic fluid overload during therapy. Nonproductive cough may be present, as well as localized pneumonitis. Pulmonary consolidation is uncommon. Modest hepatic as well as splenic enlargement frequently occurs, but jaundice is unusual.

## DIAGNOSIS

Since rickettsiae cannot be cultivated upon artificial media, diagnosis of Rocky Mountain spotted fever by culture of blood or tissue specimens is beyond the capability of the routine clinical laboratory. Moreover, attempts at isolation of the organism by inoculation of tissue culture, guinea pigs, or embryonated eggs may be hazardous to technical personnel in laboratories inexperienced in these procedures. Diagnostic serologic tests are available (see below), but these usually do not become positive until late in the course of the disease. Therefore, the disease must be suspected and appropriate therapy instituted on clinical grounds alone. The diagnosis of Rocky Mountain spotted fever should be strongly entertained in patients living or visiting in endemic areas who present during the warmer months of the year with an illness characterized by fever, headache, and maculopapular or petechial rash. The diagnosis is particularly likely if there is a history of tick bite or intimate exposure to ticks, but lack of such

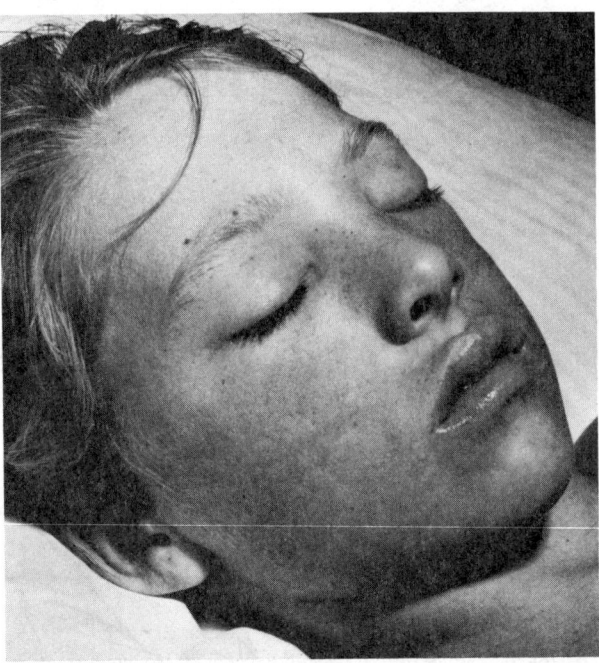

**FIGURE 7.** *Periorbital and facial edema in a child with Rocky Mountain spotted fever.*

a history by no means excludes the diagnosis. In more severely ill subjects, the presence of thrombocytopenia or hyponatremia are highly suggestive of Rocky Mountain spotted fever. Total and differential leukocyte counts are variable but are usually within normal limits. Anemia is frequently present.

The differential diagnosis is a broad one, involving a variety of febrile rash illnesses. In the early rash stage, the disease is frequently misdiagnosed as measles, although measles does not usually occur during the summer. The petechial rash and neurologic abnormalities may lead to the diagnosis of meningococcal meningitis. Time lost during consequent administration of penicillin or its congeners, which are ineffective against *R. rickettsii*, may have disastrous results. Additional diseases to be differentiated include other rickettsioses (murine typhus and, to a lesser extent, rickettsialpox), infectious mononucleosis, typhoid fever, and the various viral exanthemata.

Two types of serologic tests are generally available. The Weil-Felix agglutination reaction depends upon a fortuitous cross-antigenicity between rickettsiae and certain strains of *Proteus*, namely OX-2 and OX-19. *Proteus* OX-K agglutinins are of no value in diagnosis of Rocky Mountain spotted fever. The complement-fixation test is performed with purified rickettsial antigens. In either agglutination or complement-fixation tests a four-fold or greater rise of serum antibody titers between acute and convalescent phases of illness is diagnostic. If only a single convalescent serum sample is available, Weil-Felix titers of 1:320 or greater and complement-fixation titers of 1:16 or greater, when accompanied by a compatible clinical picture, confirm the diagnosis. Other serologic tests, such as the microagglutination or immunofluorescent antibody procedures, are still largely investigational. Regardless of the test used, serum antibody titers do not ordinarily achieve diagnostic levels until the second or third week of illness (Table 1).

Recently, investigators have demonstrated rickettsiae by immunofluorescence technique in biopsies of skin lesions taken from two patients on days four and eight of their illnesses (Woodward et al., 1976). In other studies, peripheral blood monocytes from monkeys experimentally infected with *R. rickettsii* have been maintained in in vitro tissue cultures on glass coverslips. In such preparations it has been possible to visualize rickettsiae within monocytes within three to five days after specimen collection. Both the skin biopsy and monocyte culture techniques are promising new approaches to earlier laboratory diagnosis of Rocky Mountain spotted fever.

**TABLE 1. Time of Development of Elevated Weil-Felix and Complement Fixation (CF) Titers***

| TEST | DAYS AFTER ONSET OF SYMPTOMS | | | |
|---|---|---|---|---|
| | 1–7 | 8–14 | 15–21 | >22 |
| OX-2 | 1/9 (11%)† | 11/33 (33%) | 5/10 (50%) | 5/6 (83%) |
| OX-19 | 0/14 (0%) | 16/40 (40%) | 11/15 (73%) | 4/5 (80%) |
| OX-K | 0/10 (0%) | 0/19 (0%) | 0/9 (0%) | 0/1 (0%) |
| CF | 1/4 (25%) | 7/17 (41%) | 3/4 (75%) | 8/8 (100%) |

*Weil-Felix titers of 1:320 or greater and complement fixation titers of 1:16 or greater were considered elevated.

†No. positive/No. tested (per cent positive).

Reproduced from Torres et al. (1973) with permission.

## TREATMENT

Specific antimicrobial therapy is the cornerstone of management of the patient with Rocky Mountain spotted fever. It has cut the case-fatality ratio from 20 per cent to the current figure of approximately 5 per cent. Both tetracycline and chloramphenicol are effective, and there is no convincing evidence of superiority of either drug over the other in treatment of this disorder.

Because of the potentially serious hematologic side effects of chloramphenicol therapy, tetracycline is preferred in the usual case. Before the antibiotic era, para-aminobenzoic was used with good results, but this drug is no longer employed. Penicillin, cephalosporins, or aminoglycosides (streptomycin, kanamycin, gentamicin) are of no value. Sulfonamides may actually have a deleterious effect and should be avoided.

Insofar as is known, the various tetracycline preparations are essentially equivalent in treatment, although adequate data are lacking for some of the newer preparations. Tetracycline may be administered in a total dosage of 25 to 40 mg/kg body weight per day, given in equally divided doses every six hours by mouth. (Some authorities also favor an initial loading dose of 25 mg/kg.) Since the majority of patients with Rocky Mountain spotted fever are children, the hazard of dental problems in tetracycline-treated subjects in the first decade of life must be kept in mind. The risk associated with a single course of therapy, however, is small and must be balanced against the risk of serious side effects from the alternative drug, chloramphenicol. Tetracycline is relatively contraindicated in patients with compromised renal function. If administered, it should be used in decreased dosage. Tetracyclines have been associated with severe and even fatal hepatotoxic reactions. Significant toxicity has usually been associated with high dose intravenous therapy in patients with severe pyogenic infections. Most, but not all, instances have occurred in women in the last trimester of pregnancy. Thus, intravenous tetracycline should not be administered in doses greater than 2 g per day to adults (proportionately less in children) and should probably not be used at all in women late in pregnancy (to prevent both hepatotoxicity in the mother and abnormal tooth development in the fetus). In patients requiring intravenous therapy, the choice of tetracycline vs chloramphenicol must be individualized, taking into account the patient's clinical status and the potential adverse effects of each drug.

Chloramphenicol should be administered in a total dosage of 50 mg/kg of body weight per day, divided into four equal doses to be given every six hours. The drug is well absorbed from the gastrointestinal tract but may be given by the intravenous route if necessary. Chloramphenicol is inactivated primarily by liver enzymes and should be given in decreased dosage to patients with hepatic insufficiency. The principal side effects are dose related, reversible marrow depression and very rare instances of non–dose related, usually irreversible aplastic anemia.

If treatment is initiated early in the course of the disease, the patient usually becomes afebrile in three or four days. Relapses are uncommon unless treatment is begun within the first one to two days of illness.

Supportive care is particularly critical in severely ill patients. Loss of fluid, electrolytes, and protein from the intravascular space may lead to hypotension, circulatory collapse, oliguria, and azotemia. Therefore, monitoring of central venous pressure and replacement of volume are crucial features of management. Fluid therapy should include judicious replacement of electrolytes but also may require colloid-containing solutions such as plasma or albumin. When anemia is severe, whole blood transfusions may be required. Care must be taken, however, to avoid fluid overload and precipitation of pulmonary edema in these patients, some of whom may, in addition, have myocardial and renal compromise. In patients with hyponatremia without evidence of significant volume depletion, the diagnosis of inappropriate secretion of antidiuretic hormone should be entertained, since therapy of this entity requires fluid restriction. In the occasional patient who exhibits the full-blown syndrome of disseminated intravascular coagulation, prompt heparin therapy is indicated. Subjects with

impaired levels of consciousness require meticulous nursing care to prevent decubitus ulcers or aspiration. A high protein diet is ordinarily indicated in patients able to eat.

Adrenal corticosteroids decrease the toxicity and fever of Rocky Mountain spotted fever. In view of the many problems associated with their use, these agents should ordinarily be avoided. If prescribed at all, they should be given in pharmacologic doses only to the most severely ill patients and their use limited to a few days.

## PREVENTION

The most effective measures involve prevention of tick exposure by avoiding tick-infested areas and by keeping household pets tick-free. Wearing protective clothing (long-sleeved garments, trousers tucked into lace-up boots) is often impractical in hot weather when risk is the greatest. Impregnation of clothing with tick repellent may be a useful measure when risk of tick-exposure is high.

As a rule, infected ticks are unable to transmit the disease unless attached for a period of a few hours. Therefore, one of the most practical and effective measures is careful examination of all exposed persons at least twice daily. Care should be taken to avoid crushing attached ticks while removing them and to avoid scratching the area of the bite, since infective tick juices or feces may be inoculated. After removal of the tick, the area of attachment should be washed with soap and water or treated with a disinfectant. There is no evidence that antibiotic treatment of infected individuals during the incubation period will prevent the development of the disease.

A Rocky Mountain spotted fever vaccine is available, but it is incompletely effective. The vaccine is recommended only for certain high-risk groups, such as laboratory personnel working with *R. rickettsii* or persons whose occupation necessitates continuous exposure in endemic areas. The vaccine should not be given to persons hypersensitive to eggs. A new vaccine, consisting of formalin-killed rickettsiae derived from chick embryo tissue culture, appears in animal studies to be more effective than the commercial vaccine currently available. The tissue-culture–derived vaccine has not yet been extensively tested in man.

## References

Hattwick, M. A. W., O'Brien, R. J., and Hanson, B. F.: Rocky Mountain spotted fever: epidemiology of an increasing problem. Ann Intern Med 84:732, 1976.

Torres, J., Humphreys, E., and Bisno, A. L.: Rocky Mountain spotted fever in the mid-South. Arch Intern Med 132:340, 1973.

Woodward, T. E., Pedersen, C. E., Jr., Oster, C. N., Bagley, L. R., Romberger, J., and Snyder, M. J.: Prompt confirmation of Rocky Mountain spotted fever: identification of rickettsiae in skin tissues. J Infect Dis 134:297, 1976.

# OTHER RICKETTSIAL SPOTTED FEVERS  **190**

R. Brezina, M.D.

# FIÈVRE BOUTONNEUSE

Fièvre boutonneuse (South African tick bite fever, Kenya tick typhus, Indian tick typhus) is a mild or moderately severe, acute febrile disease caused by *Rickettsia conorii*. It is characterized by a primary lesion (tâche noire) at the site of tick attachment, a maculopapular exanthem, headache, photophobia, arthralgia, and diffuse myalgia. Fièvre boutonneuse is widely distributed along the Mediterranean and the Black and Caspian Sea littorals (Spain, France, Italy, Greece, Rumania, Bulgaria, Turkey, Israel, U.S.S.R., Morocco, Algeria, Libya, and Egypt). Kenya tick typhus and South African tick bite fever, which occurs in the bush areas of West, Central, and East Africa and in all parts of the Union of South Africa (Gear, 1954), and Indian tick typhus are apparently variants of the same disease. Rickettsial strains identical to *R. conorii* have also been isolated in Pakistan, Thailand, and Malaysia.

## *ETIOLOGY*

Rickettsiae of the spotted fever group are divided into several antigenic subgroups (see Chapter 50). *R. parkeri*, which causes disease only in guinea pigs, and *R. conorii* make up subgroup B of the spotted fever group (Lackman et al., 1965). They cross-react in toxin-neutralization tests in mice and in complement fixation tests with the soluble, group-specific antigen. They can be distinguished by complement fixation tests performed with the cell-associated antigen derived from repeated washing of *R. conorii*. This CF test against mouse antibodies differentiates *R. conorii* from all other rickettsiae of the spotted fever group. *R. conorii* can also be separated from *R. rickettsii* (Rocky Mountain spotted fever) and *R. sibirica* (North Asian tick typhus) by toxin-neutralization tests in mice.

Except for lower virulence for the guinea pig, the morphologic and biologic properties of *R. conorii* are similar to those of *R. rickettsii* (Chapter 50). *R. conorii* causes fever and scrotal swelling in guinea pigs but not scrotal necrosis and death. Intravenous injections of mice with heavy suspensions of viable *R. conorii* cause acute toxic deaths. Strains of *R. conorii* collected in the Mediterranean region, Kenya, South Africa, and India are antigenically indistinguishable. *R. conorii* grows relatively well in the chick embryo yolk sac. Rickettsiae are found in both the cytoplasm and the nucleus of infected cells. *R. conorii* elicits cross-reactive antibody to *Proteus* OX-2 and OX-19 antigens. The guanine plus cytosine (G + C) content of the DNA in *R. conorii* is approximately 32.5 moles per cent.

The most important vector and arthropod host of *R. conorii* in the Mediterranean, Caspian, and Black Sea regions and in parts of the Indian subcontinent is the dog tick, *Rhipicephalus sanguineus*. In Europe, other species of the genera *Ixodes* and *Dermacentor* can probably be vectors. In Africa, *R. conorii* has been isolated from *Haemaphysalis leachii*, *Rhipicephalus sanguineus*, *Amblyomma hebraeum*, *Rhipicephalus appendiculatus*, *Rhipicephalus everts*, *Hyalomma aegypticum*, and *Rhipicephalus simus*. *H. leachii* and *R. simus* are the most important vectors. All stages of *H. leachii*, a dog tick, are infective. Transovarial transmission provides a permanent reservoir of *R. conorii*. In Malaysia, *R. conorii* was isolated from *Ixodes granulatus* and *Haemaphysalis* species. *R. conorii* has been isolated from rats and mice in South Africa, Kenya, and Malaysia (Marchette, 1965), where they may be important reservoirs. The reservoir animals of Indian tick typhus are unknown.

## *PATHOGENESIS AND PATHOLOGY*

Because fatal human cases of fièvre boutonneuse are unknown, the pathologic changes have been studied in experimentally infected guinea pigs. Rickettsemia occurs during the early febrile period, after the rickettsiae invade the body through the tick bite. Secondary invasion of the endothelium of capillaries, arterioles, and venules leads to thrombosis and formation of perivascular nodules. There is less necrosis of these small vessels than in Rocky Mountain spotted fever.

## CLINICAL MANIFESTATIONS

The incubation period of fièvre boutonneuse varies from three to six days. The onset is usually abrupt with chills and fever to 39 to 40° C, conjunctivitis, myalgia, and arthralgia. Disturbances of the sensorium may occur in more severe cases. The rash, which usually appears between the second and fifth days of fever, consists of pink, lentil-sized maculopapules (Fig. 1). The rash is noted first on the extremities and rapidly spreads to the trunk, scalp, face, palms, and soles. Exanthems were present in 100 per cent of 73 cases reported from Sicily (Romano, 1977). Fever, often remittent, continues for approximately 10 to 20 days, the rash for 5 to 10 days. The primary lesion (tâche noire, Fig. 2), which ranges from the size of a pinhead to that of a lentil, ulcerates and forms a brown to black eschar. It is usually accompanied by regional lymphadenopathy. Splenomegaly, hepatomegaly, transitory proteinuria- and hematuria, and signs of meningeal irritation may occur. Bradycardia and hypotension are unusual.

## COMPLICATIONS AND SEQUELAE

Complications are extremely rare. In the group of 73 patients with fièvre boutonneuse reported from Sicily, complications included microhematuria and albuminuria, bronchopneumonia and bronchitis, myocarditis, hypotension, and meningismus (Ferrarini et al., 1977).

There are no permanent sequelae. Insomnia and irritability may occur during convalescence. Recovery is accompanied by the development of solid immunity.

## GEOGRAPHIC VARIATIONS

Fièvre boutonneuse, African tick bite fever, Kenya tick typhus, and Indian tick typhus are thought to represent geographic variations of one disease caused by the same agent. The rickettsiae isolated from patients with each of these diseases are morphologically and antigenically indistinguishable from type strains of *R. conorii*. The vectors and the virulence of *R. conorii* (see etiology) strains may differ depending on the geographic areas from which they were collected. Strains of *R. conorii* with extremely low virulence have been isolated in Malaysia (Marchette, 1965).

## DIAGNOSIS

A primary eschar and typical exanthem and contact with tick-infected dogs in an endemic area strongly suggest the diagnosis. Other exanthematous diseases, including rickettsial infections, are difficult to exclude clinically, especially when the primary lesion is absent in abortive cases of fièvre boutonneuse.

The guinea pig is the animal of choice for primary isolation. A few days after intraperitoneal inoculation of infected blood, guinea pigs develop fever and scrotal swelling without necrosis. *R. conorii* can also be isolated by inoculation of blood, infected guinea pig tissue, or tick suspensions into the chick embryo yolk sac.

Serologic diagnosis is based on the examination of sera by complement fixation tests against the soluble group-specific antigen or, more specifically, against the highly purified species-specific cell-associated antigens. The species-specific antigen differentiates *R. conorii* from all other rick-

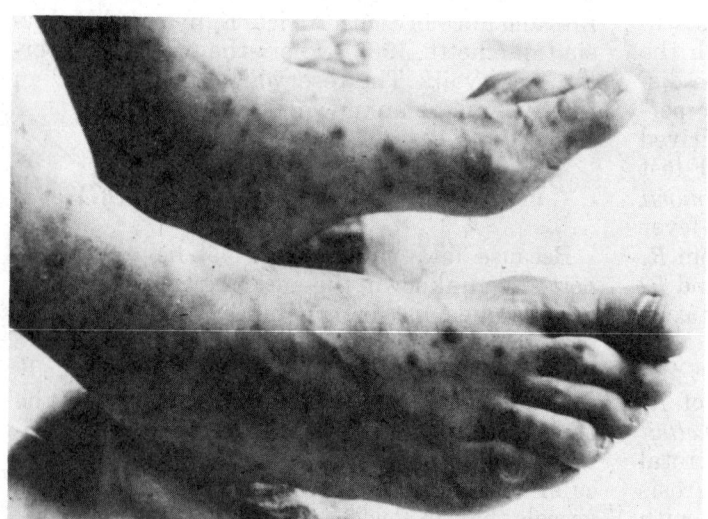

**FIGURE 1.** *The maculopapular rash on the lower extremities of a patient with fièvre boutonneuse (photo kindly provided by Prof. V. Scaffidi, M.D., University of Palermo, Italy).*

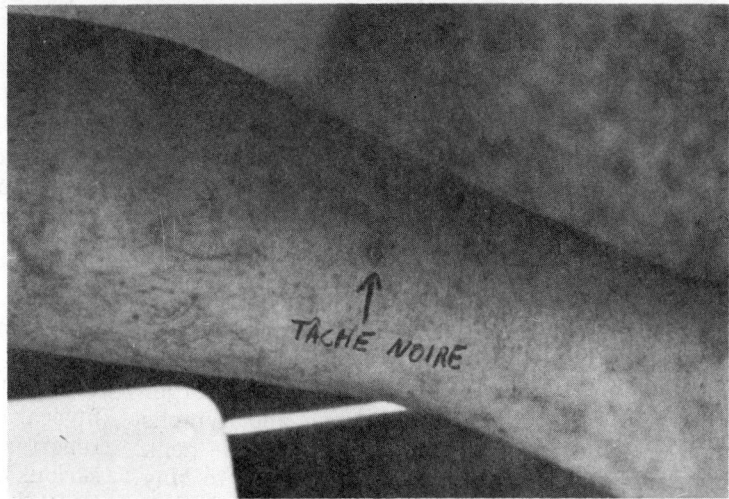

**FIGURE 2.** *The primary lesion (tâche noire) in a patient with fièvre boutonneuse (photo kindly supplied by Prof. O. Restivo, M.D., Department of Infectious Diseases, Caltanissetta, Italy).*

ettsial species of the spotted fever group. So does the microimmunofluorescence test (Philip et al., 1976), which makes it possible to establish the exact diagnosis as early as the fourth to eighth day of the disease by examination of skin lesions as described for Rocky Mountain spotted fever (Woodward et al., 1976). The Weil-Felix reactions do not distinguish fièvre boutonneuse from most other rickettsial infections.

### TREATMENT

As with other rickettsioses, chloramphenicol and the tetracyclines are the drugs of choice. Patients generally become afebrile within two to three days of the institution of 2 g per day of either antibiotic. Treatment should be continued four to seven days after the temperature returns to normal.

### PROPHYLAXIS

Fièvre boutonneuse is usually a sporadic disease of low incidence and low mortality. Under these circumstances, the only practical control measures are tick repellents and removal of ticks before attachment. Detachment or any handling of infected ticks should be done carefully to avoid contamination of the skin and environment with highly infectious tick juices.

# ASIAN TICK-BORNE TYPHUS

Asian tick-borne typhus is an acute febrile infection, caused by *Rickettsia sibirica*. It is characterized by the sudden onset of headache, myalgias, a maculopapular (or, less frequently, a petechial) exanthem, chills, and fever. The fever is usually remittent and lasts from 6 to 17 days, depending on the severity of the disease. It occurs not only in Siberia, the Far East, Central Asia, Armenia, Azerbaijan, Mongolia, and Pakistan, but also in the European part of the U.S.S.R., especially in the Tula region and the Bashkir A.S.S.R.

### ETIOLOGY

*R. sibirica* and *R. rickettsii* (Rocky Mountain spotted fever) belong to subgroup A of the spotted fever group (Lackman et al., 1965). The close antigenic relationship of these two species was first proved by mouse toxin-neutralization tests with immune guinea pig sera (Bell and Stoenner, 1960). This test, used in combination with a complement fixation system using washed *R. sibirica* and immune guinea pig sera or soluble antigen and immune mouse sera, differentiates *R. sibirica* from other species of the spotted fever group. The morphologic and biologic properties of *R. sibirica*, including its occurrence both in the cytoplasm and the nucleus of infected cells, are similar to those of the other species of the spotted fever group. The experimentally infected guinea pig develops fever, splenomegaly, and scrotal swelling. *R. sibirica* grows comparatively well in the chick embryo yolk sac and kills most embryos within four to five days. It proliferates in guinea pig kidney and chick embryo cell cultures, as well as in various established cell lines.

*R. sibirica* has been isolated from many species of ixodid ticks *(Dermacentor silvarum, D. marginatus, D. pictus, D. nuttali, Haemaphysalis concinna, H. japonica, H. punctuata, Hyalomma marginatum, Ixodes persulcatus)*, from several species of gamasid ticks, and from chiggers *(Trombicula autumnalis* and *Trombicula zachvatkini)*. It multiplies in the salivary glands, testes, and ovaries. Except for *H. concinna*, transstadial and transovarial transmission occurs in all tick vectors. Therefore, ticks are not only vectors but also the primary reservoir. Adult ticks parasitize larger wild and domestic animals; larvae and nymphs feed on small wild animals and birds. The peak incidence of human cases occurs in April to May and corresponds to the highest activity of adult ticks. Many domestic and wild animals that are hosts of ticks have been shown to harbor *R. sibirica* and have been implicated as possible reservoirs (Tarasevich et al., 1977).

## PATHOGENESIS AND PATHOLOGY

Following the tick bite, rickettsemia occurs and an eschar (tâche noire) develops at the site. It resembles a cigarette burn or a black button-like lesion with a central dark necrotic area and a surrounding reddish areola. This local lesion is accompanied by regional lymphadenitis and is probably the primary site of rickettsial propagation, as Woodward et al. (1976) demonstrated in Rocky Mountain spotted fever.

The pathologic lesions in fatal cases resemble those of Rocky Mountain spotted fever and other rickettsioses. Damage to the endothelium of capillaries, small arteries, and veins leads to thrombosis and formation of reactive perivascular nodules.

## CLINICAL MANIFESTATIONS

The incubation period of about five to seven days is followed by sudden fever, headache, myalgia, and conjunctivitis. The fever may reach 40° C or more and may persist for seven to ten days. It is usually remittent and ends by lysis. Soviet authors distinguish subclinical, mild, and severe forms of the disease. In addition to the primary lesion and fever, the most distinct clinical sign is a pink to red maculopapular eruption, which infrequently becomes petechial or hemorrhagic. It appears on about the third to fourth febrile day on the extremities and rapidly spreads over the entire body, including the scalp, face, palms, and soles. The exanthem persists during the febrile period.

There are no characteristic changes in the white blood cell count. The sedimentation rate is slightly elevated. Splenomegaly and hepatomegaly may occur with little disturbance of function. Involvement of the central nervous system or the cardiovascular system is unusual.

## COMPLICATIONS AND SEQUELAE

Complications are uncommon, but pneumonia, myocarditis, nephritis, and meningitis have been reported. Convalescence may be prolonged, but no serious or permanent sequelae occur. In contrast to Rocky Mountain spotted fever, relapses have not been observed. Recovery from the disease is accompanied by development of solid immunity to reinfection with *R. sibirica* and to infections caused by other rickettsiae of the spotted fever group.

## GEOGRAPHIC AND VARIATIONS OF THE DISEASE

There are no reliable data on differences in the clinical picture and severity of this disease.

## DIAGNOSIS

The clinical diagnosis is based on the presence of the primary lesion, regional lymphadenitis, fever, and the maculopapular rash in a patient exposed to ticks in an endemic area. Other rickettsial infections and viral exanthems must be excluded, especially if there is no primary eschar.

The definitive diagnosis can be established only in the laboratory. Intraperitoneal inoculation of infected blood into male guinea pigs causes fever and scrotal swelling with a serofibrinous exudate in the tunica vaginalis. Surviving guinea pigs develop specific antibody that can be demonstrated by the CF test with washed *R. sibirica* antigen.

By the end of the first week, the Weil-Felix reaction is positive with *Proteus* OX-2 and later with *Proteus* OX-19 antigen. During the first ten days of the disease, the sera of about 10 per cent of patients react with *Proteus* OX-K antigen. Complement-fixing antibody is detectable by the tenth day. To distinguish Asian tick-borne typhus from other spotted fevers, highly purified washed corpuscular antigen must be used in the complement fixation or microagglutination tests. Microimmunofluorescence will also distinguish these organisms (Philip et al., 1976).

## TREATMENT

Chloramphenicol and the tetracyclines are equally effective. Patients generally become afebrile after two to three days of treatment with 2 g per day of either antibiotic.

## PROPHYLAXIS

Control measures are aimed at avoiding tick bites by using repellents, by wearing clothing that interferes with attachment, and by prompt removal of attached ticks. Vaccines of purified killed suspensions of *R. sibirica* and ether-treated *R. sibirica* have been used. Kekcheeva (1963) recommended a so-called chemovaccine of the live *R. sibirica* suspension attenuated by the addition of tetracycline.

# QUEENSLAND TICK TYPHUS

Queensland tick typhus is an acute febrile exanthematous disease caused by *Rickettsia australis*. It was first recognized at Atherton in North Queensland (Andrew et al., 1946; Brody, 1946), and its etiology was established by demonstration of rickettsiae in smears from the peritoneal fluid of mice inoculated with blood from the infected patient (Andrew et al., 1946). The primary lesion or eschar is a common feature of the disease, whether it occurs in North or South Queensland.

## ETIOLOGY

*R. australis* and *R. akari* (see Chapter 191) belong to subgroup C of the spotted fever rickettsiae (Lackman et al., 1965). *R. australis* shares the common soluble antigen of this group. It can be differentiated from the others by complement fixation with washed corpuscular antigens, by cross-challenge of immunized guinea pigs, and by toxin-neutralization tests in mice (Bell and Stoenner, 1950; Bozeman et al., 1960). It can be best distinguished from *R. akari* by complement fixation tests with immune mouse sera. The morphologic and biologic properties of *R. australis* are similar to those of the other spotted fever rickettsiae, except that acute mouse toxicity has not been demonstrated. Although guinea pigs and adult mice are susceptible to intraperitoneal inoculation with *R. australis*, the best results are achieved with weaned or newborn mice.

The Australian ticks *Ixodes holocyclus* and *Ixodes tasmani* are the major vectors of *R. australis* (Campbell and Domrow, 1978). Epidemiologic evidence implicates these ticks as reservoirs as well. Specific complement-fixing antibodies and evidence of active infection have been found in several species of marsupials and wild rodents, including bandicoots, opossums, kangaroos, and mice (Cock and Campbell, 1965, cited by Campbell and Domrow, 1978).

## PATHOGENESIS AND PATHOLOGY

The pathogenesis and pathology of Queensland tick typhus are similar to those of the other species of the spotted fever group of rickettsiae.

## CLINICAL MANIFESTATIONS

The incubation period varies from seven to ten days after the tick bite. A primary eschar is common but is not always easily found. Regional lymph nodes are enlarged and tender. The disease is not fatal and is characterized by a mild course with headache, malaise, and a maculopapular rash on the face, scalp, trunk, palms, and soles. Complications and sequelae are infrequent.

## DIAGNOSIS

A primary lesion, rash, and fever in an individual exposed to ticks in the endemic area provide strong clinical evidence of the diagnosis. Scrub typhus (Chapter 188) is the only other exanthematous rickettsial infection that occurs in Australia. Furthermore, the macular rash of scrub typhus begins on the trunk and spreads later to the upper and lower extremities. The reverse is usually true in Queensland tick typhus.

The laboratory diagnosis is established by the isolation of *R. australis* from suckling or weaned mice and guinea pigs injected intraperitoneally with the blood of the patient. *R. australis* does not cause acute toxicity in the mouse.

The Weil-Felix reactions are positive with *Proteus* OX-19 and OX-2 antigens. The complement fixation reaction is positive and the soluble antigens of the spotted fever group and specifically when washed suspensions of *R. australis* are used as the antigen. It can also be differentiated by cross-challenge of immune guinea pigs and by toxin-neutralization tests in mice.

## TREATMENT

Tetracycline or chloramphenicol is effective in the doses used for the other diseases of the spotted fever group of rickettsiae.

## PROPHYLAXIS

The control measures are aimed at preventing tick bites. No effective vaccine is available.

### References

Andrew, R., Bonnin, J. M., and Williams, S.: Tick typhus in North Queensland. Med J Aust 2:253, 1946.

Bell, E. J., and Stoenner, H. G.: Immunologic relationships among the spotted fever group of rickettsias determined by toxin neutralization test in mice with convalescent animal serum. J Immunol 84:171, 1960.

Bozeman, F. L., Humphries, J. W., Campbell, J. M., and O'Hara, P. L.: Laboratory studies of the spotted fever group of rickettsiae. In Symposium on the Spotted Fever Group of Rickettsiae. Med Sci Pub No. 7, Walter Reed Army Institute of Research. Washington, D.C., U. S. Government Printing Office, 1960, pp. 7-11.

Brody, J.: A case of tick typhus in North Queensland. Med J Aust 1:511, 1946.

Campbell, R. W., and Domrow, R.: Rickettsioses in Australia: Ecology of Rickettsia tsutsugamushi and Rickettsia australis. In Kazár, J. Ormsbee, R. A., and Tarasevich, I. V. (eds.): Rickettsiae and Rickettsial Diseases. Bratislava, Veda, Publishing House of Slovak Academy of Sciences, 1978, p. 505.

Ferrarini, E., Distefano, G. and Barca, S.: Esperienze cliniche su una casistica di rickettsiosi dermotifose. Minerva med Siciliana 68:2369, 1977.

Gear, J.: The rickettsial diseases of Southern Africa. A review of recent studies. J Clin Sci 5:158, 1954.

Kekcheeva, N. (1963) cited in Zdrodovskij, P. F., and Golinevich, H. M.: La rickettsiose à tiques d'Asie. Bull WHO 35:105, 1966.

Lackman, D. B., Bell, J. E., Stoenner, H. G., and Pickens, E. G.: The Rocky Mountain spotted fever group of Rickettsias. Hlth Lab Sci 2:135, 1965.

Marchette, N. J.: Rickettsioses — tick typhus, Q fever, urban typhus in Malaya. J Med Entomol 2(4):339, 1965.

Philip, R. N., Casper, E. A., and Ormsbee, R. A.: Microimmunofluorescence test for the serological study of Rocky Mountain spotted fever and typhus. J Clin Microbiol 3:51, 1976.

Romano, A.: Osservazioni su 73 casi di febbre bottonosa verificatisi nella Provincia di Trapani nel decenio 1966–1975. Minerva med Siciliana 68:2365, 1977.

Tarasevich, I. V., Panfilova, S. S., and Fetisova, N. F.: Ecological geography of rickettsioses of tick spotted fever group (in Russian). In A. D. Lebedev (ed.): Medicinskaja geografia, Vol. 8. Moskva, Viniti, 1977, pp. 7-103.

Woodward, T. E., Pedersen, C. F., Oster, C. N., Bagley, L. R., Romberger, J., and Snyder, M. J.: Prompt confirmation of Rocky Mountain spotted fever: Identification of rickettsiae in skin tissues. J Infect Dis 134:297, 1976.

# 191 RICKETTSIALPOX

## Garrison Rapmund, M.D.

## DEFINITION AND ETIOLOGY

Rickettsialpox is a febrile disease distinguishable by the presence of a primary cutaneous lesion, or eschar, and a papulovesicular eruption. The disease is caused by *Rickettsia akari*, a member of the spotted fever group of rickettsiae and is transmitted to man by the bite of a bloodsucking mite, *Allodermanyssus sanguineus*, an ectoparasite of the house mouse (Huebner et al., 1946; Huebner, Jellison, and Pomerantz, 1946). The disease was first described by Greenberg (1947) in 1946 in New York City and shortly thereafter in the Soviet Union by Drobinskii (1962). The incidence has declined sharply in the last 15 years, but a recent case report (Wong et al., 1979) proves that the disease has not disappeared. More likely, rickettsialpox is being overlooked by physicians, which is unfortunate because the disease can be severe, although nonfatal, and specific therapy is available.

## CLINICAL MANIFESTATIONS

After an incubation period of 10 to 24 days, patients have sudden onset of fever, chills, headache, and malaise. A rash follows, usually within one to four days, consisting of red maculopapules 2 to 10 mm in size and ranging in number from a few scattered lesions to a diffuse rash over most of the body, including the mucous membranes. Involvement of the palms and soles is rare. Two to three days later vesicles form at the apices of the papules, and then crust and fall off, leaving pigmented areas but no scars. The rash persists for three to eight days and is not pruritic. Patients are not infectious for others. The fever is remittent with peaks ranging from 38.5° to 40.5°C, falling to normal after about seven days. Headache is usually frontal and can be severe. The primary cutaneous lesion can be located anywhere, developing at the site of the mite feeding. By the time a rash develops, the lesion is either ulcerated or crusted with a black top. Patients are unaware of the mite feeding and usually overlook the developing lesion as well. In up to 10 per cent of patients the primary lesion is not evident. The disease abates spontaneously in 10 to 14 days, without sequelae. Occasionally the clinical course of disease can be so mild that patients remain ambulatory. A leukopenia of 2500 to 5000 cells per cubic millimeter is seen in the acute phase, lymphocytes predominating, sometimes with large vacuolated mononuclear cells also present. Heterophil antibody is absent.

## GEOGRAPHIC VARIATIONS IN DISEASE

Rickettsialpox is an urban domiciliary disease. In the first recognized epidemic in New York City in 1946 (Greenberg et al., 1947), the disease affected middle income families living in multistoried apartment blocks. American cases were contracted infrequently in single family dwellings or at work. Disease was always associated with places having large house-mouse populations and heavy infestations of the rodent mite *A. sanguineus*. The circumstance favoring mouse proliferation was incomplete incineration of garbage in basement incinerators, which also provided warmth needed for mite proliferation. In the years after 1946 several hundred cases were reported annually in New York City and isolated outbreaks occurred in other northeastern American cities. In 1949 Drobinskii (1962) described a "vesicular rickettsiosis" in urban populations in the Donetz Basin of the Ukraine that closely resembled the disease in America. Subsequently the disease agent, called by Russian workers *Dermacentroxenus murinus* (Zdrodovskii et al., 1960), was shown to be serologically identical to *R. akari* isolated in New York City. Rickettsialpox was reported clinically in the 1950s from equatorial Africa (Central African Republic) by LeGac and coworkers (1953) and from southern Africa by Gear (1954). By 1963 disease incidence was reported to be much reduced, ascribed to improved rodent control (Lackman, 1963). Now the disease seems to have disappeared. Case reports have disappeared from the medical literature, and in New York City no cases have been reported in recent years.

But has the disease really disappeared? Evidence suggests that *R. akari* exists in nature apart from man. The rickettsia has been isolated from a single specimen of wild-caught reed vole in Korea (Jackson et al., 1957). The rickettsia is passed transovarially in *A. sanguineus* mites; so this mite as well as its rodent host may serve as a natural reservoir. *A. sanguineus* has been recovered in diverse locations around the world since its first description in Egypt in 1914. Finally, the ubiquitous tropical rat mite, *Liponyssus bacoti*, is capable experimentally of transmitting *R. akari* to mice by feeding and of passing *R. akari* transovarially to its progeny but it is not an efficient vector (Philip and Hughes, 1948). However, a thorough investigation of the natural ecology of *R. akari* has not been undertaken. Physicians should consider rickettsialpox in any patient with a vesicular eruption.

## DIAGNOSIS

The clinical differential diagnosis must take into account varicella, typhoid fever, infectious mononucleosis, other spotted fever rickettsial infections such as fièvre boutonneuse, murine typhus, and, at least formerly, mild smallpox. A specific laboratory diagnosis is possible by isolation of *R. akari* from acute phase blood inoculated into laboratory mice or guinea pigs and from the fourteenth day on by detection of complement-fixing antibody in convalescent serum (Rose, 1949). The specific antigen used in complement fixation is derived from washed *R. akari* organisms. Convalescent serum contains antibody that reacts with spotted fever group CF antigen but does not contain agglutinins to *Proteus* OX-19, OX-2, or OX-K strains at significant dilutions of serum (>1:100). Since *Proteus* agglutinins to strains OX-19 and/or OX-2 are usually present at these serum dilutions in other spotted fever infections, their absence serves to differentiate rickettsialpox from other members of the spotted fever group of diseases, especially when a vesicular eruption is absent.

## TREATMENT

Rose (1949) reported that chlortetracycline, administered in 1 g doses every six hours, produced rapid clinical response in 24 hours. Tetracycline, 250 mg every six hours, should be equally effective although its use has not been described.

### References

Drobinskii, I.R.: Gamazov'y rikketsioz. Klinika I diagnostika. Kishinev: Akademiya Naul Moldarskoi SSR, 1962.

Gear, J.: The rickettsial diseases in Southern Africa. A review of recent studies. South African J Clin Sci 5:158, 1954.

Greenberg, J., Pelliteri, O.J., and Jellison, W.L.: Rickettsialpox — a newly recognized rickettsial disease. III. Epidemiology. Am J Pub Hlth 37:860, 1947.

Huebner, R. J., Jellison, W. L., and Pomerantz, C.: Rickettsialpox — a newly recognized rickettsial disease. IV. Isolation of a rickettsia apparently identical with the causative agent of rickettsialpox from *Allodermanyssus sanguineus*, a rodent mite. Public Health Rep 61:1677, 1946.

Huebner, R.J., Stamps, P., and Armstrong, C.: Rickettsialpox — a newly recognized rickettsial disease. I. Isolation of the etiological agent. Public Health Rep 61:1605, 1946.

Jackson, E.B., Danauskas, J.X., Coale, M.C., and Smadel, J.E.: Recovery of *Rickettsia akari* from the Korean vole *Microtus fortis pelliceus*. Am J Hyg 66:301, 1957.

Lackman, D.B.: A review of information on rickettsialpox in the United States. Clin Ped 2:296, 1963.

Le Gac, P.: Research on rickettsial pox in Oubangui-Chari. West African Med J 2(n.s.):42, 1953.

Philip, C.B., and Hughes, L.E.: The tropical rat mite *Liponyssus bacoti* as an experimental vector of rickettsialpox. Am J Trop Med 28:697, 1948.

Rose, H.M.: The clinical manifestations and laboratory diagnosis of rickettsialpox. Ann Int Med 31:871, 1949.

Wong, B., Singer, C., Armstrong, D., and Millian, S.J.: Rickettsialpox. Case report and epidemiologic review. JAMA 242:1998, 1979.

Zdrodovskii, P.F., and Golinevich, H.M.: The rickettsial diseases. New York, Pergamon Press, 1960, p. 340.

# 192  *TRENCH FEVER*

## *Garrison Rapmund, M.D.*

### *DEFINITION AND ETIOLOGY*

Trench fever is a louse-borne febrile disease that is indistinguishable clinically from many other infections. It was first widely recognized during World War I in Europe when epidemics occurred in military personnel engaged in trench warfare. In Europe the disease is also called Wolhynian fever after a district in Poland where epidemic disease occurred. The causative agent, *Rochalimaea quintana,* originally considered a *Rickettsia,* is distinguished from rickettsiae by its ability to grow extracellularly on bacteriologic media and in the lumen of the louse gut. One form of the disease consists of recurrent febrile episodes with intervening afebrile periods of roughly five days, hence the specific name quintana. The disease has many other patterns including a single three- to four-day fever, continuous fever for several months, and relapsing fever at irregular intervals for many months (Byam, 1919; Strong, 1918).

### *CLINICAL MANIFESTATIONS*

Like epidemic typhus, the disease is transmitted to man through infected louse feces. Patients inoculate themselves by scratching skin contaminated with louse feces. The incubation period is 9 to 25 days. At onset, patients experience severe headache, usually postorbital, profuse sweating, pain in the lower back that extends to both legs by the second or third day, neck pain simulating meningitis, and fever of 38.5 to 40° C. Mild sore throat occurs without catarrhal rhinitis or bronchitis. Muscle and bone pain, especially in the tibiae, is very typical. Abdominal pain simulating appendicitis occurs. A macular rash of discrete spots 1 centimeter or less in diameter occurs on the anterior chest and abdomen, rarely elsewhere, on the second and third days and lasts at the most for several days. The most striking physical finding is an enlarged spleen, which is often found on the first day and persists throughout the clinical course. A mild leukocytosis may accompany the acute phase (Hurst, 1942; Mohr, 1956; Zdrodovskii and Golinevich, 1960).

The disease always remits completely without specific therapy. Occasionally convalescence is protracted, and *Rochalimaea* organisms may circulate in the blood for many months in asymptomatic convalescent patients (Vinson et al., 1969). Relapse after a year or more of good health has also been described (Mohr and Weyer, 1964).

### *GEOGRAPHIC VARIATIONS*

The distribution of the disease has never been accurately established. Specific antibody has been found in persons in Europe (Weyer et al., 1962), and in Tunisia, Burundi, Ethiopia, Mexico, and Bolivia (Meyers and Wisseman, 1973; Vinson, 1973), but broad-scale seroepidemiologic studies have not been undertaken. The only known reservoir of *Rochalimaea* is man. This agent does not pass transovarially in the louse, *Pediculus humanis* (Weyer, 1962), which parasitizes only man. There is evidence that movement of infected persons can introduce the disease to new areas, as in Greece and Iraq in World War I (Hurst, 1942). Infected human lice have been found in Mexico City (Varela, 1969) but no naturally occurring disease has been reported in the western hemisphere. Recently, Weiss and co-workers (1978) identified as a strain of *R. quintana* a microorganism isolated by Baker (1946) in 1943 from voles *(Microtus pennsylvanicus)* captured in Grosse Isle, Quebec, Canada. Grosse Isle was a quarantine station in the St. Lawrence River where in 1847 thousands of immigrants died of epidemic typhus and were buried. As Weiss and his colleagues point out, thorough study of voles and other small rodents elsewhere has failed to recover this agent. This finding probably represents an unusual isolated extension of *R. quintana* from man to voles rather than extension of disease from voles to man.

### *DIAGNOSIS*

Until recently the diagnosis could be confirmed only by allowing rickettsia-free lice to feed on patients and identifying the organism growing extracellularly in the louse intestinal lumen (xenodiagnosis). Now the organism can be cultured on specially prepared blood agar (Varela et al., 1969), and specific antibody can be detected by a variety of serologic procedures including complement fixation (Weyer et al., 1962), passive hemagglutination (Cooper et al., 1976), and enzyme immunoassay (Hollingdale et al., 1978). Antibodies appear within several weeks of the onset of disease and persist in some cases for years. Studies of volunteers during World War I show that persons are susceptible to reinfection and disease within three to six months of the initial attack, but an assessment of immunity to trench fever by current methods has not been reported (Byam, 1919; Strong, 1918). Trench fever may be particularly difficult to distinguish clinically from malaria, influenza, and relapsing fever caused by *Borrelia recurrentis*.

## TREATMENT AND PROPHYLAXIS

Rapid clinical response to treatment with tetracycline and chloramphenicol has been reported (Mohr and Weyer, 1964). The disease can be controlled by measures that curtail louse infestation and decontaminate lousy clothing. Dry louse feces remain infectious for many months.

Although it has not been reported in recent years, cases of trench fever surely must continue to occur in louse-infested populations. Recent advances in laboratory diagnosis should improve the chances of recognizing endemic disease.

### References

Baker, J. A.: A rickettsial infection in Canadian voles. J Exp Med 84:37, 1946.

Byam, W.: Trench Fever. London, Oxford University Press, 1919.

Cooper, M. D., Hollingdale, M. R., Vinson, J. W., and Costa, J.: A passive hemagglutination test for the diagnosis of trench fever. J Infect Dis 134:605, 1976.

Hollingdale, M. R., Herrmann, J. E., and Vinson, J. W.: Enzyme immunoassay of antibody to *Rochalimaea quintana:* Diagnosis of trench fever and serologic cross-reactions among other rickettsiae. J Infect Dis 137:578, 1978.

Hurst, A.: Trench fever. Br Med J 2:318, 1942.

Meyers, W. F., and Wisseman, C. L., Jr.: Louse-borne diseases worldwide: Trench fever. Serologic studies of trench fever employing a microagglutination procedure. In Proceedings of the International Symposium on the Control of Lice and Louse-borne Diseases. Publication No. 263. Washington, D.C. Pan American Health Organization, 1973, pp. 79–81.

Mohr, W.: Das Wolhynische Fieber. Med Wochenschr 10:220, 1956.

Mohr, W., and Weyer, F.: Spätrückfälle bei wolhynischem Fieber. Dtsch Med Wochenschr 89:244, 1964.

Strong, R. P. (ed.): Trench Fever. Report of Commission Medical Research Committee, American Red Cross. London, Oxford University Press, 1918.

Varela, G.: Nuevas rickettsias encontradas en la Republica Mexicana, fiebre Q y fiebre de las trincheras. Ga Med Mexico 85:275, 1955.

Varela, G., Vinson, J. W., and Molina-Pasquel, C.: Trench fever. II. Propagation of *Rickettsia quintana* on cell-free medium from the blood of two patients. Am J Trop Med Hyg 18:708, 1969.

Vinson, J. W., Varela, G., and Molina-Pasquel, C.: Trench fever. III. Induction of clinical disease in volunteers inoculated with *Rickettsia quintana* propagated on blood agar. Am J Trop Med Hyg 18:713, 1969.

Vinson, J. W.: Louse-borne diseases worldwide: Trench fever. Geographic distribution of trench fever. Proceedings of the International Symposium on the Control of Lice and Louse-borne Diseases. Publication No. 263. Washington, D.C., Pan American Health Organization, 1973, pp. 76–78.

Weiss, E., Dasch, G. A., Woodman, D. R., and Williams, J. C.: Vole agent identified as a strain of the trench fever rickettsia, *Rochalimaea quintana*. Infect Immun 19:1013, 1978.

Weyer, F.: Experimente zur Frage der transovariellen Übertragung von Rickettsien. Z Tropenmed Parasitol 13:409, 1962.

Weyer, F., Vinson, J. W., Mannweiler, E., and Mohr, W.: Serologische Untersuchungen bei wolhynischem Fieber. Z Tropenmed Parasitol 23:187, 1962.

Zdrodovskii, P. F., and Golinevich, H. M.: The Rickettsial Diseases. London, Pergamon Press, 1960, pp. 431–440.

# CHRONIC Q FEVER 193

## Walter P. G. Turck, M.D., F.R.C.P.

### DEFINITION

Chronic Q fever is a chronic disease caused by persistent infection with *Coxiella burnetii* and characterized by prolonged illness, continuous or recurrent fever, and the development of sinister complications within the cardiovascular system. In the majority of cases it is associated with a chronic hepatitis and thrombocytopenia. In contrast to the negligible mortality of acute disease (see Chapter 110) even in the absence of antibiotic therapy, untreated chronic Q fever with cardiovascular complications is invariably fatal. Although in most reports endocarditis is the dominant feature, the term chronic Q fever is preferred to Q fever endocarditis to encompass the whole spectrum of disease — from the simple prolonged fever extending over weeks and months in which there is minor hepatic involvement, to the insidious but grossly destructive endocarditis accompanied by granulomatous hepatitis or even cirrhosis.

### ETIOLOGY

The disease is caused by *C. burnetii*, a species of bacteria belonging to the family Rickettsiaceae. *C. burnetii* is named after H. R. Cox, who was a codiscoverer of the agent of Q fever in the United States after its discovery in Australia, and F. M. Burnet, the Australian who first isolated the organism. It is a short rod that grows only intracellularly in vacuoles outside the nucleus. In contrast to other rickettsiae, *C. burnetii* is resistant to drying and relatively high temperatures. It can be cultured in chick embryos and cell cultures and readily infects guinea pigs, rabbits, hamsters, and mice.

## PATHOGENESIS AND PATHOLOGY

The ability of *C. burnetii* to cause persistent and latent infection, a serologic milieu that allows the organism to become embedded within and directly destroy heart valves, and the development of immune-complex phenomena seem to be the main factors contributing to the pathogenesis of chronic Q fever.

*C. burnetii* may persist in various hosts as latent or overt and protracted infection. In the experimentally infected guinea pig the organism may be found in kidney tissue for as long as 526 days after infection, and it can be isolated from the placenta of animals infected up to 92 days before conception. In the pregnant guinea pig *C. burnetii* exists in the spleen throughout gestation, but in the placenta only in early and late pregnancy. Experimentally, both in domestic ruminants and in humans, it has been shown that the infective agent, after causing an initial mild or inapparent infection, remains latent until parturition, when large numbers may be found in placentae and birth fluids, in feces and urine, and later in milk. In naturally acquired human infection the urine may remain infective for four months. *C. burnetii* may be recovered from the placentae of women two to three years after their initial Q fever infection, and also in subsequent pregnancies. The rickettsemia of acute Q fever usually lasts no more than 15 days, but rare instances of rickettsemia persisting for more than 12 months have been recorded (Robson and Shimmin, 1959).

Although high titers of complement-fixing antibodies to phase I and phase II antigens of *C. burnetii* may be found in chronic Q fever, the role of these antibodies in its pathogenesis is not entirely clear. Phase II complement-fixing antibody develops relatively early but persists in some patients for more than ten years after the initial infection, suggesting persistence of rickettsiae. Phase I complement-fixing antibody, which is also a neutralizing antibody, develops late in acute Q fever, if at all, but when it does appear it correlates with prolonged incapacity in the older patient and a complicated illness.

Marmion (1959) has suggested that absence of phase I antibody in the early stages may allow seeding of *C. burnetii* throughout the body. Later, after phase I antibody has appeared, *C. burnetii* may be limited to an intracellular location where it cannot be reached by antibody. Antibody may thereby contribute to latency. However, the duration of the latent state is possibly related to the physiologic and metabolic state of the cell rather than to the level of antibody of the host. Experimentally, reactivation of latent infection has been provoked by x-rays and multiple cortisone injections (Sidwell et al., 1964). The factors that cause the rickettsiae to reappear in large numbers in the placenta at parturition are unknown.

The impression gained from accounts of the clinical picture is that chronic Q fever arises most readily when acute Q fever is superimposed upon another disease such as chronic rheumatic valvulitis or alcoholic liver disease. However, apart from the frequent demonstration of evidence of pre-existing heart disease, it has not been possible to substantiate this theory pathologically. Although in some cases the underlying cardiac lesion does not appear to play a significant role clinically, such patients who have come to autopsy, or whose heart valves have been replaced, have invariably shown evidence of Q fever endocarditis. Accompanying lesions such as hepatitis or glomerulonephritis may contribute materially to the disability of the patient even to the extent of overshadowing any due to endocarditis.

Q fever endocarditis affects the aortic valve more frequently than the mitral valve. In some patients, both valves may be affected. The aortic valve lesion may be superimposed upon chronic rheumatic valvulitis, but congenital bicuspid aortic valves are commonly found, and in rare instances subaortic stenosis and syphilitic aortitis have been the underlying lesions. In a large number of cases the macroscopic picture has been that of a florid and destructive endocarditis. Large vegetations, either firm and granular or friable and fungating, are found arising from the valve cusps. The cusps are frequently ulcerated or perforated and a ruptured sinus of Valsalva may be present. False aneurysms of the aortic wall may develop behind the aortic valve cusps, and may extend into the intraventricular septum and ventricular wall. The valve cusps are often fused and may be heavily calcified. On occasion the picture is less dramatic, with tiny vegetations similar to those found on the cusps of an affected valve in acute exacerbation of rheumatic valvular disease. Fibrosis and adhesions may extend from the mitral valve to the tips of the papillary muscles.

Microscopically, the vegetations are composed of fibrinoid material embedded in and fused with the collagen of the valve and overlaid with thrombus. There is an infiltrate of large mononuclear cells and neutrophils. At the bases of the infected cusps there may be ingrowth of large reticulum cells, and swelling and proliferation of endothelial cells lining the valve leaflets may be present. Microcolonies of rickettsiae with tinctorial characteristics of *C. burnetii* may be found within degenerating infected cells in the center of the vegetations or scattered extracellularly owing to breakdown of the cells.

A similarly destructive picture may be seen in the tissues around a valve prosthesis or in a homograft valve when chronic Q fever develops as a complication of open heart surgery.

Cardiovascular involvement is not restricted to heart valves. Coronary, carotid, and renal arteritis and abdominal aortitis have been described. Vasculitis may also involve the venous system, causing thrombophlebitis, deep venous thrombosis, and pulmonary embolism and infarction. Q fever infection in a large ventricular aneurysm has been described (Willey et al., 1979).

Myocarditis is not uncommon. Microscopically, numerous small foci of necrotic and swollen muscle fibers are distributed throughout the myocardium, resembling lesions seen in acute rickettsial fevers such as typhus. Evidence of ischemic heart disease has been found at autopsy in some instances, but this has been either accompanied by more florid structural damage in or around the valve or associated with coronary arteritis. Pericardial effusions may occur, but pathologic evidence of chronic pericarditis is rare.

Multiple large emboli frequently lodge in the iliac arteries as saddle emboli or in the popliteal arteries where mycotic aneurysms may develop. Splenic, renal, femoral, radial, and cerebral emboli are regular features of the disease.

Hepatic involvement almost invariably accompanies Q fever endocarditis. From liver biopsy and postmortem studies there is clear evidence that the histologic changes in Q fever hepatitis (see Chapter 110) can persist and progress, although they are variable and nonspecific (Turck et al., 1976). The most consistent feature of the chronic lesion is an infiltration of the portal tracts with lymphocytes and occasional plasma cells. In a few cases patchy parenchymal necrosis, parenchymal granulomata, and prominence of sinusoidal Küpffer cells may be seen. Periportal or diffuse fatty change is not uncommon. These appearances may persist for more than a year and may progress to portal tract fibrosis and cirrhosis. Although rickettsiae have never been seen in histologic sections of liver in chronic Q fever, isolation of the organism from hepatic tissue has sometimes been achieved.

In the kidneys of patients with endocarditis, renal infarcts secondary to embolization or arteritis are common. Hematuria occurs infrequently, but proteinuria is invariably present and may be heavy. A diffuse glomerulonephritis, similar to that found in the secondary immunologic disease that may accompany subacute bacterial endocarditis, has been seen in some patients at autopsy. Renal biopsy specimens show either hypercellularity of the glomeruli, capsular adhesions and diffuse mesangial thickening, or glomerulosclerosis. In such cases electron microscopy may show granular deposits on glomerular basement membranes and fusion of the foot processes of the epithelial cells, and immunofluorescence studies show granular distribution of immunoglobulins and C3 in the glomeruli. Serum complement is reduced (Dathan and Heyworth, 1975).

Acute tubular necrosis occurred in one fatal case, and rickettsia-like organisms were noted in the tubular epithelium in another case with mild membranous glomerulonephritis.

Although *C. burnetii* has been frequently isolated from splenic tissue, the morphology of the spleen is unremarkable, apart from occasional splenic infarction and microscopic evidence of hypertrophy and hyperplasia of the endothelial cells of the sinuses. No *Coxiella* organism has ever been found in lymph nodes, in contrast to observations in persistent infections with rickettsiae of epidemic typhus, Rocky Mountain spotted fever, and scrub typhus.

Examination of the lungs occasionally reveals peripheral infarction, interstitial pneumonitis, or pleural effusions.

In most cases there is elevation of the IgG and IgM. In some instances the elevation of IgM is the dominant feature, but in other cases normal or low levels of IgM have been recorded. The variability of IgM levels probably reflects a nonspecific immunopathologic reaction rather than a response to continuous intravascular antigenic stimulation by *C. burnetii* (Kazár et al., 1977). Even when IgM is elevated the most specific Q fever antibodies may be found in the IgG fraction.

Thrombocytopenia is common, but the cause is not clear. Marrow examination shows no reduction in numbers of megakaryocytes nor abnormal megakaryocyte morphology. The combination of thrombocytopenia, persistent liver disease, glomerulonephritis with deposition of immunoglobulins and complement on glomerular basement membranes, and a coupled rise of IgG and IgM with reduction of complement in the serum strongly suggests that immune complex formation and deposition occurs.

*C. burnetii* may be isolated by guinea pig inoculation from blood or unfixed tissue from heart valve, spleen, kidney, or embolus. Infectivity titrations of organ suspensions may indicate the primary focus.

## CLINICAL FEATURES

The onset is insidious. Persistent or recurrent fever is often the only symptom, although it may be accompanied by sweats and rigors. Its commencement may date from an illness strongly suggestive of acute Q fever, but an asymptomatic interval of weeks, months, or even years may be recognized. A few patients with endocarditis remain afebrile but present with angina and progressive dyspnea. There may be a history of previous medical treatment for rheumatic or congenital heart disease, previous valve surgery, alcoholic liver disease, diabetes, pneumoconiosis, lymphoma, or other conditions associated with impaired immune mechanisms.

On physical examination those patients without endocarditis have few signs apart from hepatomegaly, splenomegaly, and, occasionally, a petechial rash.

Patients with endocarditis have signs of the underlying cardiac disease, which may include finger clubbing, splenomegaly, murmurs, embolic phenomena, and anemia. In such cases hepatomegaly and petechial rashes are particularly common, but jaundice and ascites are infrequent.

Patients whose illness is complicated by hepatitis, myocarditis, or pericarditis may have signs and symptoms of the complication in addition to the persistent fever.

Occasionally, patients present with signs of chronic active hepatitis without any clinical evidence of active infective endocarditis. Episodes of deep venous thrombosis and pulmonary embolism may occur at any time in the illness.

Very rarely chronic Q fever may be silent and cryptic, detected only on incidental serologic testing (Willey et al., 1979).

## COMPLICATIONS AND SEQUELAE

Arterial embolism is common, particularly in the cerebral and popliteal arteries, but all major arteries may be affected. Arteritis may involve coronary arteries with myocardial ischemia and infarction, or carotid and cerebral arteries with secondary cerebral ischemia or hemorrhage.

Pulmonary embolism, occasionally massive and fatal, may follow deep venous thrombosis.

Progression from hepatitis to cirrhosis associated with the development of ascites and fatal hepatic failure has been recorded.

Hematuria occurs less frequently than in subacute bacterial endocarditis. Rarely, there may be heavy proteinuria, or even a frank nephrotic syndrome due to an immune complex glomerulonephritis that may terminate in renal failure (Dathan and Heyworth, 1975). Neuropsychiatric complications are rare, but two patients displayed fatalistic personality change and paranoid psychosis respectively.

Without treatment, Q fever endocarditis is invariably fatal. Death may be due to pulmonary embolism or to intractable cardiac failure arising from progressive destruction of the affected valve or from an associated chronic myocarditis.

## GEOGRAPHIC VARIATIONS IN DISEASE

Chronic Q fever under the age of 30 is exceedingly rare. The male preponderance may be extreme. In Australia, Q fever endocarditis appears to be exclusively a disease of males.

Despite the worldwide prevalence of Q fever, the geographic distribution of chronic Q fever appears to be far more restricted. Over half the cases reported have occurred in the British Isles, and another quarter in Australia. A few cases have occurred in France, Switzerland, Spain, Portugal, Greece, Yugoslavia, and South Africa, but, interestingly, no reports have emerged from Italy, where so much Q fever occurred during World War II. In the United States, where persistent fever and protracted illness have been well recognized, cases of Q fever endocarditis have been reported very infrequently. No cases have been reported from Canada, South America, East Africa, Russia, the Indian subcontinent, or Far East Asia.

Since only just over 100 cases have been recorded, failure to recognize chronic Q fever probably accounts for this geographic imbalance. Experience in the British Isles and Australia in recent years indicates that increasing awareness of the disease has been accompanied by an apparent increase in incidence (Turck et al., 1976; Wilson et al., 1976).

## DIAGNOSIS

The diagnosis should be considered whenever a patient with clinical evidence of infective endocarditis presents with hepatomegaly, biochemical evidence of liver involvement, thrombocytopenia, and negative bacterial blood cultures. Endocarditis due to fungal or exotic bacterial infection may have to be excluded. The diagnosis of chronic Q fever should also be suspected in any patient with fever of unknown origin, persistent hepatitis, myocarditis, or pericarditis, particularly when parent increase in incidence (Turck et al., 1976; epidemiologic background, as outlined in Chapter 110.

Confirmation of the diagnosis is obtained serologically by means of the complement fixation test using phase I and phase II antigens of *C. burnetii*. In view of the chronicity of the infection a single estimation usually suffices, the height of the antibody titer being more important than a rising titer. Both phase I and phase II antibody are elevated, the latter usually being slightly higher than the former. In patients with clinical evidence of endocarditis, a titer of complement-fixing antibody to phase I greater than 1:200 is strongly suggestive of chronic Q fever. Titers of phase I antibody greater than 1:200 in patients without clinical evidence of endocarditis indicate probable cryptic infection. When phase I antibody is detected in patients with valvular heart disease but at titers below this figure, the diagnosis should not be rejected, even if the abnormal heart valve is considered to be free of infective endocarditis, since such results may represent chronic Q fever in evolution. In those circumstances attempts should be made to isolate the organism from the blood by guinea pig inoculation. If signs or symptoms in such patients are mild or absent, repeat testing for phase I antibody should be performed after an interval of one month. Titers that do not fall confirm chronic infection. Since high titers of complement-fixing antibody frequently exist in Q fever endocarditis, prozone phenomena may cause the unwary to record false negative results. Positive sera are often anticomplementary, probably because of circulating immune complexes.

Guinea pig inoculation of embolus or valve tissue obtained at operation may establish the diagnosis where it was unsuspected previously.

## *TREATMENT*

Tetracycline is the mainstay of antibiotic therapy in chronic Q fever, but recent clinical reports suggest that in Q fever endocarditis, lincomycin, 2 g per day, in combination with tetracycline, 1 g per day, may be even more effective in eradicating the infection. Co-trimoxazole has been used with encouraging results, but experience with this drug combination is limited. Rifampicin, which is more potent than tetracycline in vitro, may also prove effective (Kimbrough et al., 1979). In view of the indolent and destructive nature of the disease, even those patients with low titers of antibody to phase I complement-fixing antigen who may have chronic Q fever in evolution should receive the full antibiotic regimen. Antibiotic therapy should be maintained for at least 12 months and withdrawn only in the presence of clinical, biochemical, and serologic evidence suggesting quiescence of the disease.

Valve replacement should be reserved for those patients requiring it for hemodynamic reasons. Antibiotic therapy should be continued post-operatively for at least one year. Continued careful monitoring of patients after antibiotic withdrawal is mandatory.

## *PROPHYLAXIS*

Acute Q fever should be suspected and treated adequately. In all elderly patients and in patients with underlying disease who have illness characterized by prolonged fever, pneumonitis, or hepatitis, it is particularly vital that tetracycline not be discontinued prematurely.

Patients with valvular heart disease should be advised not to pursue occupations where the risk of Q fever is high, nor to spend their vacations in areas where Q fever is endemic, nor to drink raw milk. If a satisfactory vaccine becomes available, such patients should be immunized, bearing in mind that live vaccines are not suitable for this purpose.

Experimental evidence suggests that it is important to be alert to the possibility of reactivation of latent disease by x-ray or corticosteroid therapy in patients who are known to have had Q fever.

### References

Dathan, J. R. E., and Heyworth, M. F.: Glomerulonephritis associated with *Coxiella burnetii* endocarditis. Br Med J 1:376, 1975.

Kazár, J., Schramek, Š., and Brezina, R.: Analysis of serum immunoglobulins in a patient with chronic Q fever and endocarditis. Bratisl Lek Listy 67:109, 1977.

Kimbrough, R. C., Ormsby, R. A., Peacock, M., Rogers, W. R., Bennetts, R W., Roof, J., Krause, A., and Gardner C.: Q fever endocarditis in the United States. Ann Intern Med 91:400, 1979.

Marmion, B. P.: Latency and rickettsial infections. Proc 6th International Congress of Tropical Medicine and Malaria, Lisbon, Sept, 1958. 5:711, 1959.

Robson, A. O., and Shimmin, C. D. G. L.: Chronic Q fever. I. Clinical aspects of a patient with endocarditis. Br Med J 2:980, 1959.

Sidwell, R. W., Thorpe, B. D., and Gebhardt, L. P.: Studies of latent Q fever infections. II. Effects of multiple cortisone injections. Am J Hyg 79:320, 1964.

Turck, W. P. G., Howitt, G., Turnberg, L. A., Fox, H., Longson, M., Matthews, M. B., and Das Gupta, R.: Chronic Q fever. Q J Med 45:193, 1976.

Willey, R. F., Matthews, M. B., Peutherer, J. F., and Marmion, B. P.: Chronic cryptic Q fever infection of the heart. Lancet 2:270, 1979.

Wilson, H. G., Neilson, G. H., Galea, E. G., Stafford, G., and O'Brien, M. F.: Q fever endocarditis in Queensland. Circulation 53:680, 1976.

# 194 *MALARIA*

## *David Francis Clyde, M.D., Ph.D.*

### *DEFINITION*

Malaria is a disease characterized by fever, anemia, and splenomegaly, and is often attended by dangerous complications. It results from infection of hepatic parenchymal cells and erythrocytes by sporozoa of the genus *Plasmodium*. Four species may infect humans: *Plasmodium falciparum* produces malignant tertian, subtertian, or falciparum malaria; *Plasmodium vivax* produces benign tertian or vivax malaria; *Plasmodium ovale* produces benign tertian or ovale malaria; *Plasmodium malariae* produces benign quartan or malariae malaria.

These parasites are carried by female *Anopheles* mosquitoes. Their development in the mosquito is sexual (sporogony), and in the human asexual (schizogony) (see Chapter 78). A few cases of malaria occur through congenital transmission, blood transfusion, or shared syringes in drug users.

### *ETIOLOGY, DISTRIBUTION, AND GEOGRAPHIC VARIATIONS*

Because malaria transmission is dependent on the presence of *Anopheles* mosquitoes, it occurs primarily in rural areas. The degree of endemicity is determined by several factors, the principal ones being: (1) *the reservoir* — the prevalence of infection in the community; (2) *the vector* — the abundance of *Anopheles* mosquitoes and their species suitability as hosts for the parasite; and (3) *the victim* — the presence of a susceptible human population.

Malaria is distributed mainly between latitudes 45° north and 40° south (Fig. 1). The most common type, caused by *P. vivax*, occurs also in temperate regions, whereas *P. falciparum* is largely confined to the tropics. *P. malariae* is considerably rarer and has a focal distribution. *P. ovale*, rather than *P. vivax*, is the benign relapsing type of malaria in West Africa, but it is found less frequently in other parts of Africa and is rare elsewhere. It has this distribution because *P. vivax* (but not *P. ovale*) requires Duffy blood group receptors on erythrocytes in order to penetrate the erythrocyte membrane, and these receptors are lacking in many Africans, particularly West Africans (Miller et al., 1976).

In the cooler parts of endemic areas, vivax malaria is first to appear each spring, while *P. falciparum* and *P. malariae* infections appear later in the summer. In tropical countries, all species of *Plasmodium* may occur in the humid lowlands, particularly at the peak periods of *Anopheles* mosquito breeding at the beginning and end of the rainy season. In the highlands *P. falciparum* disappears, although *P. vivax* may persist at altitudes higher than 2500 meters. In the individual untreated patient, falciparum infections (when not fatal) persist for up to one year, vivax up to five years, and malariae much longer.

The distribution and prevalence of the different kinds of malaria are modified by various human genetic traits. Glucose-6-phosphate dehydrogenase, essential to parasite metabolism, may be deficient in the erythrocytes of certain people, and these erythrocytes are from 2 to 80 times as resistant to invasion by *P. falciparum* as are normal erythrocytes. Various hemoglobinopathies, particularly the presence of Hbs, also result in premature death of intra-erythrocytic *P. falciparum*. The geographic distribution of people having these traits — in Africa, the eastern Mediterranean, and parts of Asia, and their descendants elsewhere — is such that it has been assumed that possession of the trait confers a selective advantage against malaria.

This advantage permits patients to survive and enhances their ability to develop immunity to malaria. At the same time, they remain infective to the mosquito and thus maintain transmission. People who are relatively asymptomatic because of enhanced partial immunity or in the intervals between paroxysms, are usually ambulatory, remain at their rural homes, and thus constitute reservoirs of infection to the mosquito. The stage of the parasite infective to the mosquito, the circulating gametocyte, appears early in the vivax or malariae attack, but does not appear for some 10 days after the first falciparum paroxysm and even then is not immediately infective — an important epidemiologic factor.

### *PATHOGENESIS AND PATHOLOGY*

The exoerythrocytic stage of the malaria parasite in the liver is not pathogenic nor does a local inflammatory reaction occur. Pathology is associated with the erythrocytic phase, in which large

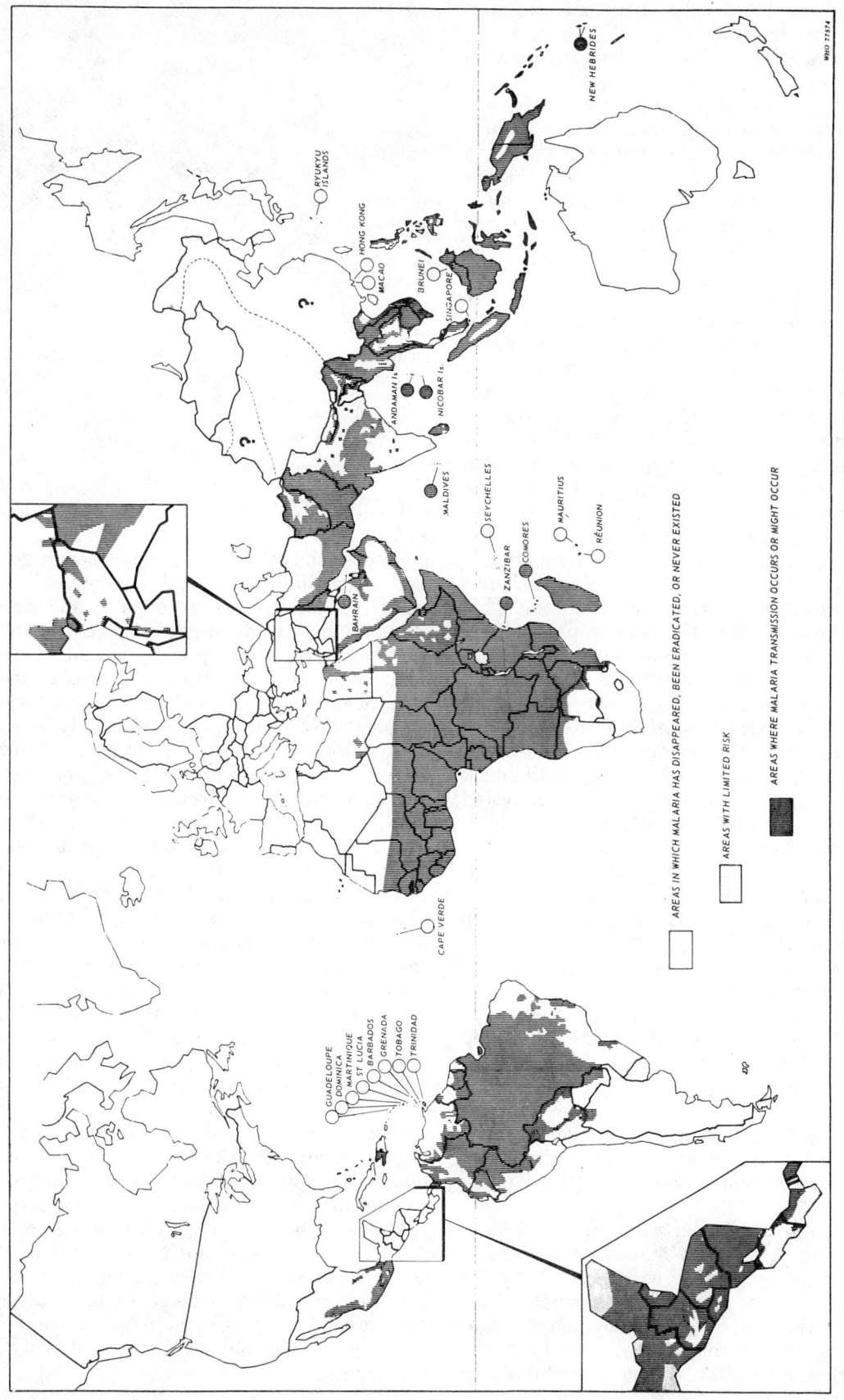

**FIGURE 1.** *Distribution of malaria in 1976. (Courtesy of the World Health Organization.)*

numbers of red blood cells, both infected and uninfected, are destroyed.

In vivax/ovale and malariae infections destruction of erythrocytes is limited, in the former to a maximum of 2 per cent because reticulocytes are preferentially invaded, and in malariae because only older erythrocytes are invaded and each schizogonic cycle is lengthy. In contrast, the hemolysis in falciparum infections, which involve erythrocytes of all ages, may be so extensive that hemoglobinuria results.

Many erythrocytes are sequestered by the reticuloendothelial system, particularly in the spleen, where parasitized cells are either phagocytosed by macrophages or hemolyzed. Destruction of circulating and sequestered erythrocytes, parasitized as well as unparasitized, quickly produces a severe anemia. This is accompanied by thrombocytopenia. The principal site of platelet destruction is the spleen. Infected erythrocytes and free merozoites are also phagocytosed in the circulation; monocytes, which show an absolute increase in numbers, play a major role, despite an overall leukopenia. Monocytes, polymorphonuclear leukocytes, and visceral reticuloendothelial cells remove hemozoin from the circulation. This malarial pigment colors the organs, particularly the spleen, liver, and brain, slate-gray or black.

The spleen may be enlarged and slate-colored, weighing 1000 grams or more after protracted infections. The reticuloendothelial elements are markedly hyperplastic, and the cells contain malarial pigment in brown blocks or small black masses. In acute malaria the spleen is congested and soft with a distended capsule, and is susceptible to spontaneous or traumatic rupture. Thrombosis and areas of infarction occur in the arterioles, while the pulp may be hemorrhagic. The follicles are reduced in size and rarely contain phagocytosed pigment. In chronic malaria, fibrosis of trabeculae is a prominent feature, and the organ becomes hard and shrunken.

The liver may be enlarged and discolored owing to black pigmentation of the endothelial and Küpffer cells. Hepatic parenchymal cells do not take up this malarial pigment but, as with the spleen pulp, may contain dark yellow hemosiderin and show vacuolization and cloudy swelling. Small necrotic foci may occur in the portal areas and in the central zones of the liver lobules.

The brain may be similarly discolored. Particularly in severe falciparum malaria, the cerebral capillaries are engorged with, and may be plugged by, masses of parasitized erythrocytes (Fig. 2). Areas of necrosis ringed by hemorrhages develop around the thrombosed vessels in the subcortical white matter, the pons, medulla, and

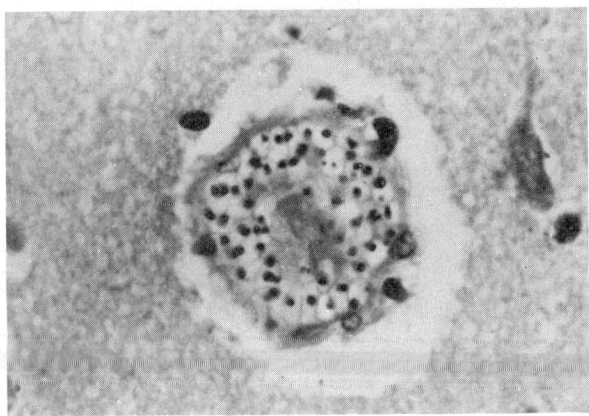

**FIGURE 2.** *Blood vessel in brain largely blocked by parasitized erythrocytes adherent to endothelium and to each other. A granule of pigment marks each parasitized red cell. (Courtesy of G. W. Hunter, III. In Hunter, G. W., et al.: Tropical Medicine. 5th ed. Philadelphia, W. B. Saunders Company, 1976.)*

cerebellum, but not in the gray matter (Young, 1976).

Because the basic pathologic process is generalized and includes anemia, disseminated intravascular coagulation, tissue anoxia, and necrosis, other organs are damaged, particularly in falciparum infections. Symptoms resembling those of acute toxic, focal, or interstitial myocarditis and pneumonitis may occur. In chronic malariae infections of African children especially, a nephrotic syndrome with excretion of large amounts of albumin and massive edema has been observed. Severe falciparum infections may produce glomerulonephritis with nitrogen retention and uremia. This is characteristically associated with the hemoglobinuria of blackwater fever. Gastrointestinal lesions may simulate appendicitis. In the placentas of infected women, erythrocytes in the intervillous spaces (maternal portions) but not in the chorionic villi (fetal portion) are parasitized. Congenital malaria may be transmitted to the fetus by a nonimmune infected woman. Although this is a rare event in regions where mothers have acquired a considerable degree of immunity, the birth weight of such infected babies is often subnormal.

Biochemical abnormalities are prominent during the acute attack. Plasma proteins are reduced, the albumin-globulin ratio is reversed, and the serum potassium and euglobulin levels are increased. Cholesterol, lecithin, and glucose concentrations increase during the febrile paroxysms. Disturbance of the glycogenetic function of the liver results in a decrease in levulose and galactose tolerance. Bilirubin appears in the plasma in quantities that parallel the intensity of the infection.

*Acquired immunity* greatly modifies these pathologic processes. Malaria infections produce partial immunity that is primarily strain-specific but to a lesser extent species-specific. Cross-immunity between species is absent; an attack of falciparum malaria, for example, does not decrease the severity of a vivax infection. This partial immunity develops during acute or chronic malaria, while erythrocytic parasitemia persists. It confers tolerance to the present infection as well as to new infections by the same strain, so that clinical phenomena cease in the face of persistent detectable parasitemia. Agglutinins, precipitins, complement-fixing, and fluorescent antibodies appear. Soon after parasites become patent, immunoglobulins M, A, and G increase in parallel with the rising parasite density. After the parasitemia peaks, IgM and IgA levels decline; but IgG remains elevated for a long time. Long-persisting IgG fluorescent antibodies are a valuable epidemiologic indication of past infection. Peaked elevations of IgM indicate infection within the past three months.

Transplacental passage of IgG from a malarious mother provides the neonate with protection that diminishes in strength over about 12 weeks. The breast milk of infected women also contains protective IgG and is doubly protective because it is also deficient in para-aminobenzoic acid, which is essential to plasmodial metabolism.

The antigens stimulating production of the IgG-related antibodies are complex and are not only species-specific but, for the erythrocytic cycle, largely stage-specific. In humans, inoculation by irradiated biting mosquitoes of live falciparum and vivax sporozoites has resulted in "sporozoite neutralizing antibody" that provides solid immunity against further sporozoite inocula of each species for up to six months (Clyde et al., 1973). Furthermore, "merozoite inhibitory" and "gametocyte-sterilizing" antibodies have been demonstrated in animal models. No practical vaccine against human malaria is available, however.

## CLINICAL MANIFESTATIONS

The clinical triad characteristic of malaria consists of periodic fever, splenomegaly, and anemia. The periodicity of the fever is related to maturation of erythrocytic schizonts and their synchronous release into the plasma as the red cells are ruptured (Fig. 3). Parasite pigment in the circulation is thought to cause leukocytes to release endogenous pyrogen into the serum, which, together with prostaglandins, stimulates hypotha-

lamic temperature sensors. Splenomegaly and to a lesser extent hepatomegaly reflect the great increase in reticuloendothelial cells, which are phagocytic for merozoites, pigment, erythrocyte remnants, whole parasitized erythrocytes, and sometimes unparasitized erythrocytes. Anemia results from the cyclical destruction of parasitized erythrocytes and concomitant lysis of large numbers of uninfected erythrocytes. Consequently, it is normocytic and normochromic.

The *intrinsic incubation period* (the interval between the infecting bite and elevation of temperature to 37.8° C) in falciparum malaria is 11 to 14 days, in vivax 11 to 15 days, in ovale 14 to 26 days, and in malariae 21 to 28 days. It is usually a day or two longer than the appearance of parasites in the erythrocytes, which indicates the end of the *prepatent period*. In the temperate climates of northern Europe and Asia, vivax infections may incubate for nine months or longer, and ovale malaria has been known to behave similarly. Before the onset of the first paroxysm of fever, prodromal symptoms of malaise, headache, anorexia, and a slightly elevated temperature may occur.

Thereafter, clinical malaria may develop into one of two types. The more serious, produced by *P. falciparum*, may be fatal, owing to (1) the capacity of this parasite to enter both reticulocytes and mature erythrocytes, develop rapidly, and thus build up high levels of parasitemia, and (2) the tendency of infected erythrocytes to agglutinate and adhere to vascular endothelium, plugging capillaries and producing thrombosis with local anoxia and ischemia in many organs, most dangerously the brain.

*Falciparum malaria* may develop insidiously, with various nonspecific symptoms including gradually increasing pyrexia, headache, and gastrointestinal disturbances. Or it may have an abrupt onset of the paroxysmal type popularly associated with malaria — initial sensations of chilliness, often with marked shivering, followed by a prolonged hot stage, terminating in sweating and a fall in temperature with temporary relief of the symptoms of intense throbbing headache, nausea, and vomiting. When it occurs, the periodicity of fever is around 36 hours, but the fever can continue for 24 hours or more without relief of symptoms. The spleen becomes palpable and painful. Prostration is a marked feature of the acute attack in a nonimmune patient. Mental confusion warns of the extremely dangerous complication of cerebral malaria that may develop rapidly.

Vivax, ovale, and malariae infections, although less life-threatening, are also accompanied by marked symptoms. The fever at first may be

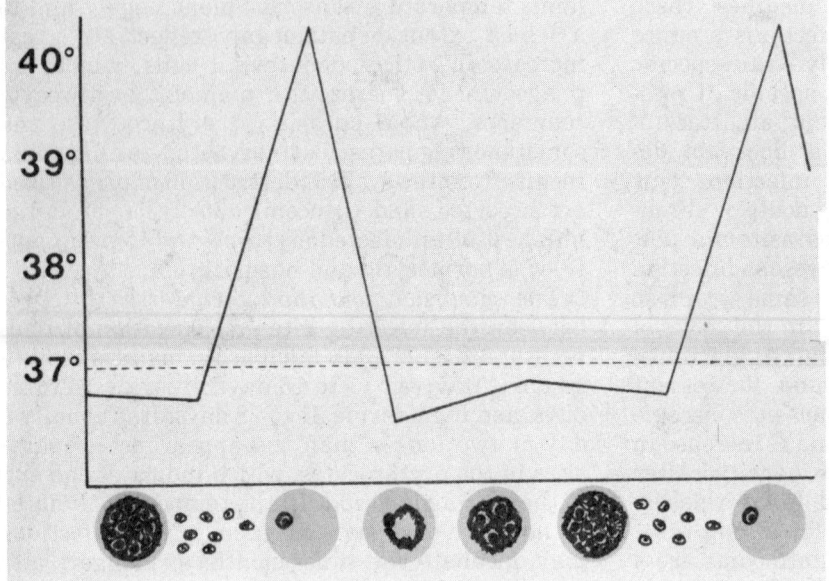

**FIGURE 3.** *Relationship between periodicity of fever and rupture of malaria parasites from erythrocytes.*

sustained or irregular in periodicity owing to the presence of two or more groups of parasites maturing on alternate days. Soon, however, one group begins to dominate and the characteristic periodicity of fever is established. In vivax and ovale infections the intervals are 40 to 50 hours, and in malariae they are 72 hours. The onset is more abrupt in vivax than in ovale and malariae, which tend to run a milder course. The paroxysm commences with a rigor, during which the temperature rises rapidly to peaks as high as 41° C, although the patient feels chilly or cold. Nausea and vomiting are prominent, and the pulse is rapid and weak. Within an hour a sensation of heat develops, accompanied by severe headache and continual nausea and vomiting. The skin is dry. This stage is followed by profuse sweating lasting two to three hours, during which the temperature and pulse rate subside. The paroxysm usually lasts 10 to 12 hours and is accompanied by a moderate leukocytosis, but in the relatively asymptomatic intervals between paroxysms leukopenia with monocytosis prevails.

The primary untreated attack of *P. malariae* terminates spontaneously in three weeks to six months. Thereafter, latent infections with a few circulating parasites may persist and set up recrudescent attacks for as long as 40 years. Such latent infection is also sufficient to establish the disease in another person receiving that blood by transfusion.

The primary attack of falciparum malaria in a nonimmune patient is short and severe. If untreated and not fatal, it subsides within three weeks. Recrudescences of latent blood stages may occur for a year.

*Mixed infections*, usually consisting of *P. falciparum* and *P. vivax*, may occur. *P. falciparum* initiates the clinical symptoms. Only when it has run its course do the vivax symptoms become manifest. Similarly, *P. vivax* predominates over *P. malariae* in mixed infections.

## COMPLICATIONS AND SEQUELAE

Complications of malaria attacks may be life-threatening. Unless the attack is cured quickly, anemia is an increasingly severe problem, and dehydration and disturbances of alkali reserve and electrolyte balance develop. The acutely enlarged spleen may rupture spontaneously or by trauma in vivax infections. Nephrosis with marked albuminuria may occur in chronic malariae infections.

Falciparum infections are much more liable than the others to produce serious complications. Although plugging of capillaries by infected erythrocytes occurs throughout the body, one organ system is usually most affected. When this is the brain, *cerebral malaria* develops, either gradually with increasing headache, confusion, and psychotic manifestations lapsing into delirium and coma, or suddenly with abrupt rise in temperature sustained at high levels, convulsive seizures (particularly in children), and coma. Cerebral edema develops, and the cerebrospinal fluid pressure may increase. The condition can be fatal within a few hours.

Other complications of falciparum infections include the following. (1) *Bilious remittent fever*, in which the liver is the main organ affected, is characterized by continuous vomiting (sometimes of coffee-ground vomitus from gastric hemorrhage), epigastric and liver tenderness, and marked jaundice. (2) *Algid malaria*, in which the adrenal gland fails and the gastrointestinal tract is extensively involved, leads to shock, prostration, syncope, and circulatory collapse. The temperature may not be elevated. Diarrhea, sometimes bloody, is often present. (3) *Acute renal failure* due to tubular necrosis is characterized clinically by prolonged oliguria leading to anuria. (4) *Blackwater fever*, with hemoglobinuria due to massive sudden hemolysis is believed to be triggered by hypersensitivity to drugs including quinine. (5) *Pneumonic malaria*, a rare complication, is accompanied by pulmonary edema.

*Recurrent attacks* generally follow inadequate treatment. The untreated primary attack of vivax malaria may persist for two months; toward the end of that time the paroxysms diminish and then cease, but in at least 50 per cent of the cases relapses develop from latent exoerythrocytic stages in the liver within a few weeks to a year or more later. Untreated relapses may continue for as long as five years at a steadily decreasing intensity. The untreated primary ovale attack tends to subside spontaneously within three weeks; relapses occur infrequently and then rarely persist longer than one year.

### DIAGNOSIS

The diagnosis of malaria depends on identification of parasites in blood smears. Morphology and species differentiation are described in Chapter 78. The thick blood film, in which a dried drop of defibrinated blood is dehemoglobinized before staining with Giemsa stain buffered to pH 7.0 to 7.2, is superior to the usual methyl alcohol-fixed thin film because low densities of parasitemia may be detected. A minimum of 100 oil immersion fields should be examined in the thin film. Leukocytes containing malarial pigment may be seen. Leukopenia and monocytosis are usual. In the rare cases in which parasitemia is not detected in thick films taken morning and afternoon for three consecutive days but clinical indications persist, sternal puncture and examination of the stained marrow smear may reveal the parasites.

Immunodiagnosis has limited clinical usefulness but positive indirect hemagglutination (IHA) and indirect fluorescent antibody (IFA) tests are valuable for epidemiologic surveys and, with the complement fixation test, for screening potential blood donors. Wassermann and Kahn reactions are often positive in malaria.

Malaria must be differentiated from other systemic infectious diseases, particularly typhoid fever, brucellosis, miliary tuberculosis, diverti-

culitis, and abscesses of the liver, kidney, or pelvis. Tropical diseases such as visceral leishmaniasis, extra intestinal amebiasis, and relapsing fever may resemble malaria. In temperate zone countries, a patient who is comatose from cerebral malaria poses a particularly difficult and critical diagnostic problem if no history of recent tropical sojourn is available. Because cerebral malaria may be so quickly fatal, it must be considered in any unconscious or semiconscious patient who has an undiagnosed fever, and appropriate blood microscopy undertaken without delay.

### TREATMENT

The specific chemotherapy of malaria is directed at (1) prompt abatement of the acute clinical attack and its complications by rapid elimination of asexual erythrocytic parasites (using blood schizontocidal drugs), (2) prevention of relapses of vivax or ovale malaria by destruction of their latent exoerythrocytic stages in the liver (using tissue schizontocidal drugs), (3) prevention of the initial attack by suppression of parasites entering the blood from the liver (using suppressive prophylactic drugs) or by destroying them when they first enter the body (using casual prophylactic drugs — still largely theoretical), and (4) prevention of transmission of malaria via the mosquito by interference with gametogony (gametocytocidal and sporontocidal drugs).

#### Abatement of the Attack

Blood schizontocidal drugs used in the treatment of the acute attack of malaria include the 4-aminoquinolines chloroquine, hydroxychloroquine, amodiaquine, and quinine. Except for falciparum malaria originating in areas of known resistance to the 4-aminoquinolines, chloroquine is the drug of choice. Symptoms are generally relieved within 24 hours, and parasites are cleared from the blood by about 60 hours, although *P. malariae* may persist for several days. Infections produced by strains of *P. falciparum* sensitive to these drugs will be cured, but gametocytes of this species are not damaged, although those of the other species will disappear rapidly.

*Dosage.* The initial dose of chloroquine per kilogram of body weight is 10 mg of the base (equivalent to 17 mg of chloroquine sulfate or diphosphate). This is followed by three doses of 5 mg (base) per kg, at 6, 24, and 48 hours after the initial dose. Hydroxychloroquine sulfate may be used similarly. Alternatively, amodiaquine 10 mg (base) per kg (equivalent to 13 mg of amodiaquine dihydrochloride) may be used on the first day, then 7 mg (base) per kg daily on the second and third days.

In severe illness with vomiting, parenteral treatment may be necessary. Chloroquine hydrochloride may be given intramuscularly in doses of 5 mg (base) per kg, injected every six hours until treatment by mouth is resumed. Alternatively, and particularly if cerebral malarial threatens, quinine dihydrochloride may be given intravenously in a dose of 10 mg/kg in normal saline diluted to 1 mg/ml, administered very slowly at a flow rate of 1 mg per minute. This should be repeated every 9 hours (in adults) or 12 hours (in children) until oral treatment is feasible. Because of the hazard of circulatory collapse from rapid or excessive intravenous administration of quinine, pulse and blood pressure must be monitored frequently. Parenteral treatment should not be continued longer than two days: if parasitemia does not diminish, the parasites are drug resistant (see below).

Complications of malaria occur most commonly in falciparum infections. In the treatment of cerebral malaria, quinine given intravenously as described above may be lifesaving. To alleviate cerebral and pulmonary edema, and in massive hemolysis with hemoglobinuria (blackwater fever), dexamethasone 4 to 6 mg may be used every four to six hours. In patients with renal failure, fluid management is necessary, drug dosage, particularly of quinine, should be reduced, and peritoneal or hemodialysis may be necessary if the plasma urea concentration nears 200 mg per 100 ml. On the other hand, acute dehydration requires fluid replacement. Symptoms such as convulsions, shock, and hyperpyrexia should be managed according to general principles. Anemia should be treated with iron or, if severe, by blood transfusion.

Pregnancy is not a contraindication to administration of these antimalarials, since malaria itself constitutes a much greater hazard.

The side effects of treatment may be difficult to distinguish from the symptoms of the disease. Vomiting is sometimes brought on by the intensely bitter taste of the 4-aminoquinolines and quinine. Children are given coated tablets or syrup preparations, and a tasteless base preparation of amodiaquine is available. Side effects of the 4-aminoquinolines include headache and pruritus, and more rarely an eruption resembling lichen planus, depigmentation of the hair, discoloration of the nails, visual disturbances, and (after higher doses of chloroquine than are used in malaria) retinal damage. Quinine produces cinchonism, early signs of which have been used as an indication of effective dosage and include giddiness, tinnitus, and transitory deafness. Permanent

deafness, amblyopia, and blindness have occurred in patients who were overdosed or had an idiosyncratic reaction to quinine. When quinine is given intravenously too rapidly, circulatory collapse and death may occur owing to cardiac depression and vasodilatation. Patients with renal failure should receive no more than half the usual doses.

Resistance to 4-aminoquinolines is apparent when appropriate treatment does not reduce parasitemia and relieve symptoms in 24 hours. Falciparum malaria in much of South America and Panama and in Southeast Asia from New Guinea and the Philippines west to Assam is resistant to these drugs. Oral treatment with quinine sulfate must be instituted immediately in the following regimen:

| | |
|---|---|
| Adults: | 650 mg every 8 hours |
| 6 to 12 years: | 325 mg every 8 hours |
| 3 to 6 years: | 160 mg every 6 hours |
| 1 to 3 years: | 80 mg every 4 hours |
| Less than 1 year: | 80 mg every 6 hours |

This treatment should continue for 14 days. While some strains of *P. falciparum* may be eliminated by shorter courses, others may recrudesce after the full 14 days of treatment. Additional drugs must then be given with the quinine. One combination consists of sulfadiazine 500 mg every six hours for five days (adult dosage) with pyrimethamine 25 mg every 12 hours for three days (folinic acid 10 mg/kg is also given daily to counteract hematologic toxicity of pyrimethamine).

Alternative methods for treating drug-resistant falciparum malaria include the above quinine schedule for 3 rather than 14 days with a full dose of a tetracycline for seven days; or, when quinine is not used, a combination of trimethoprim with a long-acting sulfonamide for three days; or a single dose of sulfadoxine 1 g with pyrimethamine 50 mg. A newly developed 4-quinolinemethanol compound, mefloquine, has proved effective in adults when given in a 1.5 g single dose.

Consideration must be given to the potentially dangerous side effects of long-acting sulfonamides, particularly the development of erythema multiforme, and to the question of inducing bacterial resistance by indiscriminate use of drugs such as the sulfonamides, trimethoprim, and tetracycline.

Severe or complicated cases are treated by intravenous administration of quinine as described above.

Malaria in partially immune patients may be treated with lower doses of schizontocides.

### Prevention of Vivax and Ovale Relapses

Destruction of the latent exoerythrocytic stages of *P. vivax* and *P. ovale* in the liver is achieved by administering 8-aminoquinoline drug primaquine. Patients treated for acute attacks of vivax or ovale malaria with blood schizontocides should also receive primaquine diphosphate 0.45 mg/kg body weight (containing 0.25 mg/kg of base primaquine) each day for 14 consecutive days; for adults, this amounts to 15 mg (base) daily. The course of primaquine may commence concurrently with the blood schizontocide but, if vomiting is a problem, it can be delayed for two or three days until the patient is stabilized. In pregnancy, use of primaquine should be delayed until after the first trimester. Some strains of *P. vivax*, notably the Chesson of New Guinea (now being found more widely in Southeast Asia), may require twice the daily dosage.

*Side effects of treatment* consist of hemolytic reactions to primaquine in individuals whose erythrocytes are deficient in glucose-6-phosphate dehydrogenase (G-6-PD). These reactions tend to be severe in some Mediterranean Caucasians and Southeast Asians and milder in some Africans. Acute intravascular hemolysis occurring in these individuals is self-limited because only the older erythrocytes are affected. Because the larger dosage regimen used in Chesson-type vivax malaria may bring on hemolytic reactions, G-6-PD–deficient patients infected with this type should be given no more than the 0.25 mg (base) per kg course, to be repeated should relapse take place later. Alternatively, primaquine may be given once a week for eight weeks, in the amount of 0.75 mg (base) per kg each dose. The drug should be discontinued in patients developing hemolytic anemia or methemoglobinemia manifested by marked cyanosis.

### Prevention by Suppression of Parasitemia

Chemoprophylaxis of malaria is effective only if a drug to which the local parasites are susceptible is taken regularly.

Chloroquine is the most widely used suppressive drug, and is taken by mouth once each week in the amount of 5 mg (base) per kg body weight, which, for an adult, is 300 mg base. Amodiaquine or hydroxychloroquine may be used in the equivalent dosage. All may be taken in suitably divided doses at shorter intervals (e.g., daily) or, in the case of partially immune patients, at intervals of two weeks without increasing the quantity. People who visit malarious areas should continue the treatment for six weeks after the last possible exposure. During or following visits to areas of high vivax transmission, primaquine may be taken in addition to the 4-aminoquinolines.

Pyrimethamine, in a once-weekly dosage of 25 mg (for those aged 10 years or more), 12.5 mg (ages 4 to 10), or 6.25 mg (children under 4 years), or *proguanil* in a daily dosage of 100 mg for adults (proportional for children) may be used alone, but resistance by *P. falciparum* may develop rapidly, requiring either the addition of chloroquine to the regimen or a change to that drug.

Resistance to 4-aminoquinolines, notably chloroquine, by *P. falciparum* in Southeast Asia and South America is often accompanied by resistance to pyrimethamine and proguanil. Because these multi-drug-resistant parasites may be suppressed by sulfones and sulfonamides, which are ineffective against *P. vivax* and *P. malariae*, and because pyrimethamine, proguanil, and the 4-aminoquinolines remain effective against *P. vivax* and *P. malariae*, combinations of drugs are used for prophylaxis in these regions. These combinations include chloroquine (weekly or daily) with dapsone 25 mg (daily; adult doses listed), proguanil 100 mg with dapsone 25 mg (daily), chloroquine with sulfadoxine 500 mg (weekly), chloroquine with primaquine 45 mg (base) (weekly), or, most commonly, pyrimethamine 25 mg with sulfadoxine 500 mg (weekly). The last combination has not been approved for use in the United States. Dapsone has produced agranulocytosis.

### Prevention of Transmission

For epidemiologic purposes, the nonpathogenic circulating gametocytes of *P. falciparum* may be destroyed or their development in the mosquito inhibited by primaquine or (provided the parasites are not resistant) by proguanil or pyrimethamine. Gametocytes of the other species are eliminated during routine treatment of the acute attack by chloroquine, quinine, and so forth. Primaquine as a single dose in the amount of 0.75 mg (base; adult dose listed) is the most effective gametocytocide and sporontocide.

## *PROPHYLAXIS*

Attainment of the goal of worldwide malaria eradication through destruction of *Anopheles* mosquitoes by spraying houses with residually acting insecticides has proved more elusive than was expected when the World Health Organization sponsored the campaign in 1956. Although nearly 40 per cent of people at risk have been freed of the threat of malaria, a resurgence of the disease is again threatening the health and economic well-being of entire populations in South and Central America, Southeast Asia, the Indian subcontinent, and equatorial Africa. The disease is also being imported increasingly to countries in the temperate zones. One factor has been the development of resistance to insecticides by mosquitoes. More significant factors include adverse international economic trends and the expense of unexpectedly protracted eradication campaigns. Strengthening of these campaigns by mass chemoprophylaxis has been partly counteracted by the spread since 1960 of parasites resistant to chloroquine.

In these circumstances, control of malaria must revert to a variety of measures directed against the vector and the parasite, including mosquito source reduction by water management; larvicidal, and biologic control methods; continuation on a selective basis of the attack on adult mosquitoes by use of residually acting insecticides and space sprays; separation of people from the night-feeding mosquitoes by use of house screening and bed nets; and reduction of the parasite reservoir in humans by use of chemoprophylaxis and sporontocidal drugs (Russell et al., 1963).

### References

Clyde, D. F., Most, H., McCarthy, V. C., and Vanderberg, J. P.: Immunization of man against sporozoite-induced falciparum malaria. Am J Med Sci 266:169, 1973.

Miller, L. H.: Mason, S. J., Clyde, D. F., and McGinniss, M. H.: The resistance factor to *Plasmodium vivax* in blacks. N Engl J Med 295:302, 1976.

Russell, P. F., West, L. S., Manwell, R. D., and Macdonald, G.: Practical Malariology. 2nd ed. London, Oxford University Press, 1963.

Young, M. D.: Malaria. In Hunter, G. W., Swartzwelder, J. C., and Clyde, D. F. (eds.): Tropical Medicine. 5th ed. Philadelphia, W. B. Saunders Company, 1976.

# 195 *BABESIOSIS*

## Michael G. Groves, D.V.M., Ph.D.
## Charles E. Davis, M.D.

### DEFINITION

Babesiosis is a tick-borne protozoan disease that affects primarily wild and domestic animals. It is a major veterinary medical problem in many areas of the world, but until recently human disease was considered a medical curiosity limited exclusively to splenectomized individuals. Within the last decade, however, interest in human babesiosis has been stimulated by several case reports in people uncompromised by splenectomy and by the isolation of *Babesia* from the blood of asymptomatic individuals. Most of the recognized infections of intact individuals have occurred near Nantucket Island, a wooded, tick-infested, recreation area off the northeastern shore of the United States.

### ETIOLOGY

*Babesia* organisms are small, malaria-like protozoan parasites of red blood cells (RBC). Although they are classified in the same subphylum (Sporozoa) as plasmodia, they are placed in a different class (Piroplasmea) because they are small, nonpigmented, and pyriform (see Chapter 16). For many years, *Babesia* were called *Piroplasma* because of their shape, and the disease is still sometimes referred to as piroplasmosis.

Since Babes first observed *Babesia* in the red blood cells (RBC) of Romanian cattle in 1888, more than 70 species have been identified. Table 1 summarizes the host and geographic distribution of some of the more common *Babesia* species. For many years, the various species were thought to be quite host-specific. Although most *Babesia* species do display at least a limited host preference, a few, like *B. divergens,* which infects cattle, rodents, and splenectomized primates, cause infections across both species and generic boundaries.

*Babesia* organisms do not necessarily retain their typical morphology in aberrant hosts. Nevertheless, the species of the host and the intraerythrocytic morphology of the parasite are the principal taxonomic criteria by which the organisms are identified. Understandably, the definitive identification of the *Babesia* species that occasionally spill over from animal transmission cycles to infect man may be difficult. However, three species have been identified with some degree of certainty: *B. bovis* and *B. divergens,* which normally infect cattle, and *B. microti,* which usually infects rodents. The bovine *Babesia* species *(B. divergens* and *bovis)* have caused most of the infections of splenectomized human beings, while *B. microti* is responsible for all known infections of intact individuals.

The principal vectors of *Babesia* are several

TABLE 1. Principal *Babesia* of Domestic and
Wild Animals

| PARASITE | USUAL HOST | DISTRIBUTION |
|---|---|---|
| B. bigemina | Cattle | Europe, Africa, Australia, South America |
| B. bovis | Cattle | Europe, Africa, Asia, East Indies |
| B. divergens | Cattle | Northern Europe, United Kingdom |
| B. ovis | Sheep and goats | Southern Europe, Middle East, U.S.S.R., Southeast Asia, Africa |
| B. motasi | Sheep and goats | Same as B. ovis |
| B. equi | Horse | Tropical and subtropical areas of the world |
| B. caballi | Horse | Same as B. equi |
| B. trautmani | Swine | Southern Europe, U.S.S.R., Central and South Africa |
| B. canis | Dog | Tropical and subtropical areas of the world |
| B. microti | Rodents | North America and Europe |

species of hard ticks in the family *Ixodidae*. The principle vector on Nantucket Island in the United States is *Ixodes dammini*, which was probably imported in the 1930s when a large number of wild deer were shipped from Michigan to Nantucket to replenish hunting stock (Spielman, 1976; Spielman et al., 1979). In 1893, Smith and Kilborne proved the tick transmission of *B. bigemina* in cattle and thereby created a unique historic niche for *Babesia* as the first pathogenic protozoan proven to be transmitted to mammals by an arthropod. Within the tick, *Babesia* organisms proceed through a developmental cycle that results in a generalized infection. The infection is carried over from one stage in the tick life cycle to another; that is, from larva to nymph to adult (transstadial transmission). *Babesia* organisms can also pass from an infected female to her offspring, which produces infective larvae that have never taken a blood meal (transovarial transmission).

*Ixodes* are three-host ticks; that is, the larva, nymph, and adult seek a new host (of the same or different species) for a blood meal. *I. dammini* feeds primarily on the white-footed deer mouse (larvae and nymphs) and deer (adults), but all three stages feed on, and can infect, man with *Babesia microti* (Dammin, 1978). Thus, a history of a bite by a mature tick may not be obtained. It is easy to overlook a bite by the very small larval form. Other *Ixodes* ticks transmit the other *Babesia* spp. The role of dog ticks and *Dermacentor* spp in the transmission of *Babesia* is controversial.

The detailed life cycle of *Babesia* organisms has not been completely worked out. In contrast to plasmodia, the development of *Babesia* organisms in the mammalian host occurs exclusively within the RBC. After invading the RBC, new tropho-

zoites are apparently formed by budding (Rudzinska and Trager, 1977). Budding produces pairs and tetrads, but the organisms remain as ring and oval forms. They do not develop into schizonts. Instead, these new parasites are released into the bloodstream when the infected RBC lyses, and they infect other RBC's.

Ring forms are occasionally seen extracellularly, especially in very heavy infections. *Babesia* organisms are not pigmented because they completely metabolize hemoglobin. This absence of the brownish, hemoglobin-derived pigment (hemozoin) is an important differential point between *Babesia* and *Plasmodium falciparum*. When stained by the Giemsa technique, the cytoplasm of *Babesia* is blue, but it contains a compact mass of red chromatin. Only a small percentage of the erythrocytic forms survive after ingestion by ticks. This has given rise to speculation that some intraerythrocytic developmental change occurs in a small number of the parasites to make them infectious for the tick. Various babesial forms observed in the gut contents of ticks are thought to be sexual stages that presumably unite to form the zygote. The zygote, then, undergoes a succession of multiple fission divisions in the gut cells of the tick. The numerous vermicules that are formed by these divisions invade other tissues and multiply. When the ovary is involved, the infection is transmitted to the guts of developing larval offspring. A final division in the salivary gland or in lymph cells produces infective *Babesia* organisms that closely resemble the trophozoites found in the mammalian host.

## PATHOGENESIS AND PATHOLOGY

The pathophysiology of *babesiosis* has been studied primarily in animals and has been found to vary greatly depending on the host and the species or strain of parasite. The disease is often quite mild. The one consistent finding throughout all infections is the invasion and destruction of RBC's by the parasites. The ability of at least some *Babesia* organisms to penetrate erythrocytes depends on the alternative complement pathway as well as on C3 and C5 (Chapman and Ward, 1977). Complement components may promote penetration of the RBC by damaging its membrane or by promoting adherence of *Babesia* to the RBC by acting as its receptor. In any event, hypocomplementemia and transient glomerulonephritis occur in experimental babesiosis (Annable and Ward, 1974).

Electron microscopy of RBC penetration by *B. microti* (Rudzinska, et al., 1976) showed that the merozoite first touches its anterior end to the RBC and then quickly becomes attached to it. The RBC membrane invaginates and forms a vacuole that disappears as the red cell membrane disintegrates. Thus, when the process is complete, the *Babesia* organism lies free in the cytoplasm separated from the RBC only by the babesial membrane.

Lysis of erythrocytes is responsible for many of the most severe manifestations of babesiosis. Hemolytic anemia, bilirubinemia, hemoglobinemia, hemoglobinuria, and renal failure with hemoglobinuriac nephrosis occur in fatal cases. For unknown reasons, erythrocytes seem to lyse after *Babesia* multiply by budding.

Wright and Mahoney (1974) ascribe the early dramatic findings of hypotension, vascular congestion, and anoxia that occur in bovine babesiosis to the release of kallikreins. The role of pharmacologic mediators in human disease is unknown.

Splenomegaly is a uniform finding in babesiosis of animals and occurs in many human infections. The spleen may be two to five times its normal size with soft, dark red pulp and prominent lymphoid follicles. In some infections, large numbers of parasitized RBC's line the walls of the capillaries and small blood vessels. These "sticky cells" cause sludging of the blood and capillary occlusion that can result in ischemia and necrosis of the affected organ. The brain is frequently affected in animal babesiosis. In the liver, stasis of blood in hepatic sinusoids leads to swelling, cellular degeneration, and necrosis, especially around the central veins. The enlarged liver and other organs are bile-stained. Erythrophagocytosis in the spleen and liver is common. Proliferation of hematopoietic tissue in the bone marrow, spleen, and liver is extensive.

After recovery from the initial illness, animals continue to carry the parasite at low levels for months and even years. *B. microti* parasitemias have been documented in people for up to 18 weeks following recovery from acute disease (Western et al., 1970). The persistence of the parasites may be explained by antigenic variation. Like the African trypanosomes (Chapter 196), *Babesia* may be capable of eluding the immune response by altering their surface antigens (Mahoney, 1977). These chronic infections appear to be important in maintaining the humoral and cellular defense mechanisms, however. If the parasitemia is eliminated, either spontaneously or by successful chemotherapy, the host becomes susceptible to reinfection.

Splenic function is extremely important in the maintenance of resistance to babesiosis. Many *Babesia* species do not infect secondary hosts unless they have been splenectomized. Further-more, the spleen restricts the degree of parasitemia and therefore the severity of the disease. Of the 20 cases of acute human babesiosis summarized in Table 2, only splenectomized individuals died. Removal of the spleen from chronically infected animals increases the parasitemia and may precipitate a fatal infection. Cellular immunity is probably also an important factor in restricting parasitemia. Hamsters given antilymphocyte serum before infection with *B. microti* develop dramatic fulminating disease (Wolf, 1974).

## CLINICAL MANIFESTATIONS

The severity and the clinical manifestations of acute human babesiosis depend upon the presence of a spleen (Table 2). Five of the six reported *Babesia* infections of splenectomized people were fulminating, and four ended fatally within a week. Fever, chills, anemia, vomiting, hemoglobinuria, and jaundice are the most common findings. Renal failure, hypotension, and coma may occur in fatal cases. One of the two nonfatal infections was mild like those of intact individuals (Scholten et al., 1968). Interestingly, a probable seventh case of babesiosis in a splenectomized subject was diagnosed serologically two years after the original illness (Grunwaldt, 1977). The individual lived in the area of the United States where infections with *B. microti* are endemic, had a history of a tick bite two weeks before the symptoms started, and recovered spontaneously.

To date, only *B. microti* has caused overt disease in persons with spleens, and these infections have been restricted to the northeastern United States. The disease is typically nonfatal, with a gradual onset and a protracted recovery. Clinically, it is characterized principally by fever, fatigue, myalgia, and anemia. Splenomegaly, nausea, chills, and sweating are seen less commonly. The severe manifestations of hemoglobinemia do not occur.

The laboratory manifestations in splenectomized and intact individuals vary chiefly in the magnitude of their response. The major changes are secondary to hemolysis and abnormal liver function. Anemia, decreased hemoglobin concentration, elevated erythrocyte sedimentation rate, reticulocytosis, and elevated serum glutamic oxaloacetic transaminase and lactic dehydrogenase are consistent findings. Proteinuria, elevated bilirubin, and a modest leukopenia may also occur. Splenectomized individuals may develop azotemia, thrombocytopenia, and hypocomplementemia.

A third form, inapparent or subclinical babesiosis, may be the most common form of the disease.

TABLE 2. Summary of the First 20 Human Cases of Acute Babesiosis

| LOCATION | ORGANISM | NORMAL HOST | NUMBER OF CASES | AGE OF PATIENT | SPLEEN | DEATH | YEAR OF REPORT | AUTHOR(S) |
|---|---|---|---|---|---|---|---|---|
| Yugoslavia | B. bovis | Cattle | 1 | 33 | No | Yes | 1957 | Skrabalo |
| California, U.S.A. | Unknown | — | 1 | 46 | No | No | 1968 | Scholten et al. |
| Ireland | B. divergens | Cattle | 1 | 47 | No | Yes | 1968 | Fitzpatrick et al. |
| Yugoslavia | B. divergens | Cattle | 1 | 27 | No | Yes | 1971 | Skrabalo |
| France | Unknown | — | 2 | 61 & 53 | No | No | 1976–79 | Bazin et al.; Healy |
| Georgia, U.S.S.R. | (B. divergens?) | (Cattle?) | 1 | 49 | No | Yes | 1978 | Rabinovich et al. |
| Nantucket Island, Massachusetts, U.S.A. | B. microti | Rodents | 8 | 48–73 | Yes | No | 1970–77 | [a] |
| Long Island, New York, U.S.A. | B. microti | Rodents | 1 | 57 | Yes | No | 1977 | Parry et al. |
| Shelter Island, New York, U.S.A. | B. microti | Rodents | 2 | 54, 59 | Yes | No | 1977 | Grunwaldt |
| | (B. microti?) | (Rodents?) | 1 | 64 | No | No | 1977 | Grunwaldt |
| Martha's Vineyard, Massachusetts, U.S.A. | B. microti | Rodents | 1 | | Yes | No | 1978 | Miller et al. |

[a]Ruebush et al., 1977; Anderson et al., 1974; Western et al., 1970; and Scharfman and Taft, 1977.

Thirty-eight of 101 people in an enzootic area of animal babesiosis in rural Mexico reacted positively to an indirect hemagglutination test, and *Babesia*, probably of rodent origin, was isolated in splenectomized hamsters from three asymptomatic carriers (Osorno et al., 1976). In the same study, 29 individuals living in Mexico City were all negative for antibody. In a similar survey on Nantucket Island, the *B. microti* endemic area of the United States, 10 of 133 sera from asymptomatic individuals with a recent history of fever or tick bite were positive by a fluorescent antibody test (Ruebush et al., 1977). This survey also found evidence of undiagnosed infections in unselected patients undergoing routine diagnostic tests. Eleven of 577 specimens were seropositive for *Babesia*. *B. microti* was isolated in splenectomized hamsters from the blood of one seropositive patient nine weeks after discharge from the hospital, and rare *Babesia* organisms were seen in thin blood smears of another seropositive individual. An additional asymptomatic case of babesiosis was discovered in Georgia (United States) on routine blood smear (Healy et al., 1976). This person gave no history of tick bite or fever. The species of *Babesia* was not identified.

## COMPLICATIONS AND SEQUELAE

The development of a chronic low-level parasitemia following acute disease has been discussed above (see section on *Pathogenesis and Pathology*). No long-term side effects have been attributed to these parasitemias in either animals or man, although patients frequently complain of fatigue for four to eight weeks following the disappearance of parasites from routine blood smears. Until more information is available, patients who have recovered from babesiosis must

be considered carriers and should not be used as blood donors. If splenectomy of a possible *Babesia* carrier is required, the patient should be closely observed, and peripheral blood smears should be carefully monitored for signs of an acute exacerbation.

## GEOGRAPHIC VARIATIONS IN DISEASE

*Babesia* species, like their tick vectors, are distributed throughout most of the tropical and temperate areas of the world (Table 1). Animal babesiosis, however, is more prevalent in tropical and subtropical zones due to the longer tick seasons. Paradoxically, acute human babesiosis has only been diagnosed in temperate, nonmalarious areas. Clinical disease may be suppressed in malarious areas either by antimalarial antibody that cross-reacts with *Babesia* (Chisholm et al., 1978) or by prophylactic antimalarial drugs, an unlikely possibility because antimalarial compounds are not very effective against *Babesia*. It seems more likely that babesiosis is overlooked in these areas because it is misdiagnosed as malaria. This diagnostic error is common even in temperate climates. Because the disease is self-limited in normal individuals, any treatment may appear to be effective. Fatal babesiosis in splenectomized persons could certainly mimic fulminating drug-resistant malaria, since the resistance of these individuals to *Plasmodium* would also be severely compromised.

By far the largest concentration of reported human babesiosis cases has occurred in a small area of the northeastern United States. All affected persons were 48 years of age or older, possessed a spleen, and contracted the infection on one of four coastal islands (Table 2). The age distribution of acute infections is interesting. It seems unlikely that older individuals were exposed more frequently to the vectors or that they all had some form of splenic dysfunction. Babesiosis in young animals is often asymptomatic, and at least two of the asymptomatic patients on Nantucket Island (Ruebush, 1978) were less than 23 years old. The reason for this age-related susceptibility to disease may provide important information about the pathogenesis of babesiosis.

The causative agent in the northeastern United States has been identified as *B. microti*. Because this parasite is widely distributed throughout North America and Europe but seems to produce disease only in this location, it has been suggested that a more virulent strain of the organism has emerged on these islands. A number of other factors (such as an abundant *B. microti* reservoir in the form of the white-footed mouse; a vector tick, *Ixodes dammini*, which feeds both on mouse and man; and an intimate tick–man contact on islands that are popular summer vacation areas) have certainly contributed to the establishment of this endemic focus of disease.

## DIAGNOSIS

The diagnosis of acute disease depends upon the demonstration of *Babesia* in peripheral blood smears stained with either Wright's or Giemsa's stain. The parasites may be pyriform, round, ameboid, rod- or ring-shaped (Fig. 1), and are frequently mistaken for *Plasmodium*. Pairs and tetrads ("maltese-cross" forms) are common. *Babesia* organisms differ from plasmodia in that they do not produce hemozoin pigment in the RBC and do not develop into schizonts or gametocytes.

The diagnosis of chronic babesiosis is more difficult because parasites are scarce in the peripheral blood. Serodiagnosis by the indirect fluorescent antibody, complement fixation, capillary tube agglutination, or indirect hemagglutination tests is sensitive and reliable in malaria-free areas. The immunofluorescent test is especially useful. Infected individuals develop very high titers that drop to 1:64 or less within 8 to 12 months (Chisholm et al., 1978). Thus, a titer greater than 1:64 usually indicates active or recent infection. However, because many *Babesia* antigens cross-react with those of *Plasmodium* (Chisholm et al., 1978), serology is of limited value in areas endemic for malaria. The presence of parasites in chronic infections is usually detectable only by subinoculating large quantities of blood into a susceptible animal (usually splenectomized). Asymptomatic infections of animals

have been detected by administering corticosteroids and monitoring blood smears for an exacerbation of the parasitemia.

## TREATMENT

Although the antimalarial drug chloroquine has been the most common chemotherapeutic agent used in the treatment of human babesiosis, clinical and laboratory findings do not support its use. Patients treated with the drug fail to eliminate their parasitemias, and the drug is ineffective against experimental *B. microti* and *B. rodhaini* infections in rodents (Miller et al., 1978). The aromatic diamidines pentamidine isethionate and diminazene aceturate (Berenil) may be more useful. Both drugs are effective in the treatment of animal babesiosis and have been used in humans for the treatment of other parasitic diseases. However, they were only partially successful against experimental *B. microti* infections of hamsters (Miller et al., 1978). One patient with human *B. microti* infection has been treated with an unstated dose of diminazene and cleared his parasitemia but developed Guillain-Barré syndrome (Ruebush, 1978). Since diminazene can cause central nervous system toxicity in dogs, it is possible that this complication was caused by the drug. On the other hand, many patients with African trypanosomiasis have been treated with I.M. (intramuscular) diminazene, 5 mg/kg for three doses on alternate days, without serious side effects (Temu, 1975).

Pentamidine has not been used in human babesiosis but has been successful against *Pneumocystis* infections (Chapter 124) and African trypanosomiasis with minimal toxicity in a dose of 2 to 3 mg/kg I.M. daily for ten days. The combination of trimethoprim and sulfamethoxazole (Septra, Clotrimoxazole) has also been used successfully against *Pneumocystis* and also has antimalarial activity. Since it is virtually free of serious toxicity during short-term treatment, it should probably be tried against nonfulminating babesiosis.

Until more information is available, it is probably prudent to give only symptomatic treatment to intact individuals with babesiosis since all have recovered. Patients who are asplenic or otherwise compromised and develop fulminating disease should probably be treated with one of the diamidines. These drugs should be used with caution, however, because of their intrinsic toxicity and because some animals treated with these drugs for experimental babesiosis died despite an impressive reduction in their parasitemia (Miller et al., 1978).

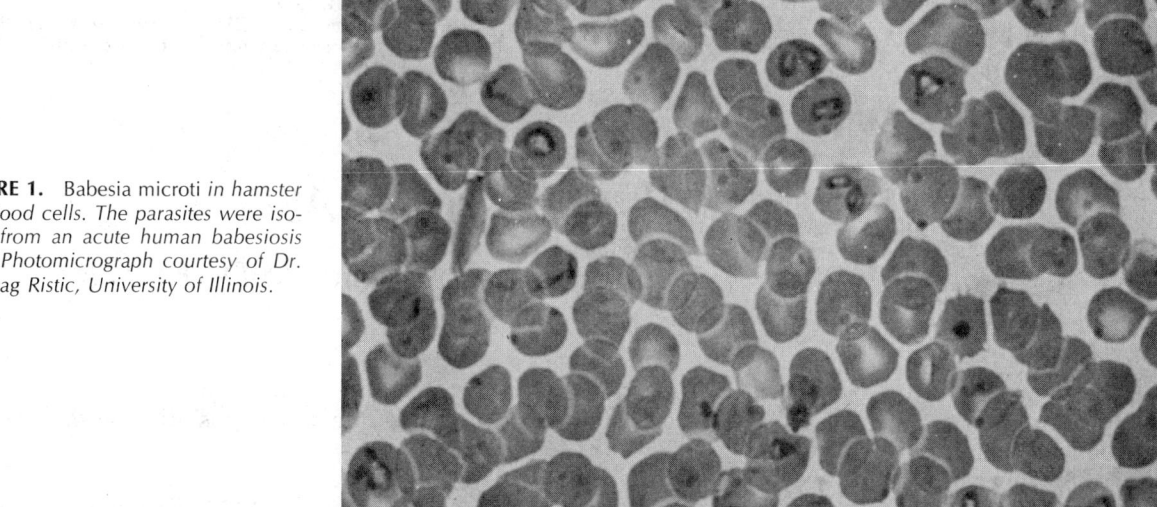

**FIGURE 1.** Babesia microti *in hamster red blood cells. The parasites were isolated from an acute human babesiosis case. Photomicrograph courtesy of Dr. Miodrag Ristic, University of Illinois.*

## *PROPHYLAXIS*

Prevention of human babesiosis would depend on: (1) reduction of ticks below disease maintenance levels, (2) removal of susceptible reservoir animals, or (3) isolation of humans from vector ticks. The institution of any of these measures is impractical because of the rare incidence of this disease and our limited knowledge of the control of wildlife babesiosis.

## References

Annable, C. R., and Ward, P. A.: Immunopathology of the renal complications of babesiosis. J Immunol 112:1, 1974.

Babés, V.: Sur l'hémoglobinurie bactérienne du boeuf. C R Acad Sci (Paris) 107:692, 1888.

Bazin, C., Lamy, C., Piette, M., Gorenflot, A., Duhamel, C., and Valla, A.: Un nouveau cas de babesiose humaine. Nouv Presse Med 5:799, 1976.

Chapman, E., and Ward, P. A.: *Babesia rodhaini*: Requirement of complement for penetration of human erythrocytes. Science 196:67, 1977.

Chisholm, E. S., Ruebush, T. K. II, Sulzer, A. J., and Healy, G. R.: *Babesia microti* infection in man: Evaluation of an indirect immunofluorescent antibody test. Am J Trop Med Hyg 27:14, 1978.

Dammin, G. J.: Babesiosis *In* Weinstein, L., and Fields B. N. (eds.): Seminars in Infectious Disease. Vol. 1. New York, Stratton Intercontinental, 1978, pp. 169-199.

Fitzpatrick J. E. P., Kennedy, C. C., McGeown, M. G., Oreopoulos, D. G., Robertson, J. H., and Soyannwo, M. A. O.: Human case of piroplasmosis (babesiosis). Nature 217:861, 1968.

Grunwaldt, E: Babesiosis on Shelter Island. NY State J Med 77:1320, 1977.

Healy, G. R.: Babesia infections in man. Hosp Pract 14:107, 1979.

Healy, G. R., Walzer, P. D., and Sulzer, A. J.: A case of asymptomatic babesiosis in Georgia. Am J Trop Med Hyg 25:376, 1976.

Mahoney, D. F.: Babesiosis of domestic animals. In Kreier, J. P. (ed.): Parasitic Protozoa. Vol IV. New York, Academic Press, 1977, pp. 1-52.

Miller, L. H., Neva, F. A., and Gill, F.: Failure of chloroquine in human babesiosis *(Babesia microti)*. Case report and chemotherapeutic trials in hamsters. Ann Intern Med 88:200, 1978.

Osorno, M., Vega, C., Ristic, M., Roble, C., and Ibarra, S.: Isolation of *Babesia sp.* from asymptomatic human beings. Vet Parasitol 2:111, 1976.

Parry, M. F., Fox, M., Burka, S. A., and Richar, W. J.: *Babesia microti* infection in man. JAMA 238, 1282, 1977.

Rabinovich, S. A., Voronina, C. K., Stepanova, N. I., Maruashvily, T. L., Bakradza, M. S., Odisharia, M. S., and Gvasalia, M. J.: The first detection of human babesiosis in the U.S.S.R. Int Congress of Parasitology 4:43, 1978 (Abstr.).

Ruebush, T. K. II: Human babesiosis in the United States. Ann Intern Med 88:263, 1978.

Ruebush, T. K. II, Cassady, P. B., Marsh, H. J., Lisker, S. A., Voorhees, D. B., Mahoney, E. B., and Healy, G. R.: Human babesiosis on Nantucket Island. Clinical features. Ann Intern Med 86:6, 1977.

Ruebush, T. K. II, Juranek, D. D., Chisholm, E. S., Snow, P. C., Healy, G. R., and Sulzer, A. J.: Human babesiosis on Shelter Island. Evidence for self-limited and subclinical infections. N Engl J Med 297:825, 1977.

Rudzinska, M. A., and Trager, W.: Formation of merozoites in intraerythrocytic *Babesia microti*: An ultrastructural study. Can J Zool 55:928, 1977.

Rudzinska, M. A., Trager, W., Lewengrub, S. J., and Gubert, E.: An electron microscopic study of *Babesia microti* invading erythrocytes. Cell Tissue Res 169:323, 1976.

Scharfman, W. B., and Taft, E. G.: Nantucket Fever. An additional case of babesiosis. JAMA 238:1281, 1977.

Scholten, R. G., Braff, E. H., Healey, G., and Gleason, N.: A case of babesiosis in man in the United States. Am J Trop Med Hyg 17:810, 1968.

Skrabalo, Z.: Babesiosis. In Marcial-Rojas, R. A. (ed.): Pathology of Protozoal and Helminthic Diseases. Baltimore, The Williams & Wilkins Company, 1971.

Skrabalo, Z., and Deanovic, Z.: Piroplasmosis in man. Report on a case. Doc Med Geogr Trop 9:11, 1957.

Smith, T., and Kilbourne, F. L.: Investigation into the nature, causation, and prevention of Texas or south cattle fever. Washington D.C., U.S. Department of Agriculture Bur Anim Ind Bull 1:1, 1893.

Spielman, A.: Human babesiosis on Nantucket Island: Transmission by nymphal *Ixodes* ticks. Am J Trop Med 25:784, 1976.

Spielman, A., Carlton, C. M., Piesman, J., and Carlton, M. D.: Human babesiosis on Nantucket Island, U.S.A. Description of the vector *Ixodes dammini*, N. sp. *(Acarina Ixodidea)*. J Med Entomol 15:218, 1979.

Temu, S. E.: Summary of cases of human early trypanosomiasis treated with Berenil at E.A.T.R.O. Trans R Soc Trop Med Hyg 69:277, 1975.

Western, K. A., Benson, G. D., Gleason, N. N., Healy, G. R., and Schultz, M. G.: Babesiosis in a Massachusetts resident. N Engl J Med 282:854, 1970.

Wolf, R. E.: Effects of antilymphocyte serum and splenectomy on resistance to *Babesia microti* infection in hamsters. Clin Immunol Immunopathol 2:381, 1974.

Wright, I. G., and Mahoney, D. F.: The activation of plasma kallikrein in acute *Babesia argentina* infections of splenectomized calves. Z Parasitenkd 43:271, 1974.

# 196    TRYPANOSOMIASIS

## W. H. R. Lumsden, D.Sc., M.D., F.R.C.P.E., F.R.S.E.

Trypanosomiasis of man is surpassed only by malaria as an infection that inhibits the development of tropical lands. There are two distinct forms of trypanosomiasis, American trypanosomiasis or Chagas' disease and African trypanosomiasis or sleeping sickness. Both are transmitted by blood-sucking insects, infect other vertebrates in addition to man, and occur mainly in rural environments. But they differ in the mechanisms of their transmission and are caused by different species of trypanosomes. *Trypanosoma cruzi*, the agent that causes Chagas' disease, belongs to the section Stercoraria of *Trypanosoma*. Stercoraria are transmitted, as the name indicates, via the feces of blood-sucking insects. *Trypanosoma brucei*, the agent of African sleeping sickness, belongs to the section Salivaria, which are transmitted via the bite or saliva of the vector (Hoare, 1972). Because their geographic distributions differ and because of linguistic barriers between investigators, the two diseases have been studied independently and will be described separately in this chapter. Nevertheless, there are many general similarities between their clinical course, pathology, and epidemiology, and instructive comparisons may be drawn.

## AMERICAN TRYPANOSOMIASIS — CHAGAS' DISEASE

### Definition and Geographic Distribution

Chagas' disease is caused by infection with *Trypanosoma (Schizotrypanum) cruzi*, which is transmitted by blood-sucking bugs (Hemiptera). The disease occurs in Central America, Panama, Guatemala, and Costa Rica, and in all the states of South America as far south as central Argentina. It has been estimated that 30 million people are at risk of infection and 7 million infected. There are probably more cases of cardiac disease in the world due to Chagas' disease than to any other cause.

### Etiology and Transmission

*Trypanosoma cruzi* exists in two morphologic forms in the vertebrate (Fig. 1). Amastigotes are rounded, nonmotile, aflagellate forms, about 3 $\mu$m in diameter that multiply by binary fission inside the cells of many different tissues of the body but particularly in muscle cells. Amastigotes multiply until nearly all the cytoplasm of the cell is consumed, resulting in a mass of amastigotes surrounded by the remains of the cell membrane. This structure is called a pseudocyst. When the pseudocyst ruptures, the amastigotes transform into trypomastigotes — motile forms about 15 to 20 $\mu$m long with a flagellum and undulating membrane. These nonmultiplying forms serve two purposes: to disseminate the infection from cell to cell and to initiate infection in the vector. The insects are nocturnally active blood-sucking bugs of the family Reduviidae, subfamily Triatominae (*Triatoma, Rhodnius*, and *Panstrongylus* spp, Chapter 18). In the midgut of these bugs the ingested trypomastigotes transform into epimastigotes — motile, multiplying forms with a flagellum and a short undulating membrane. These proliferate in the lumen of the midgut and eventually invade the hindgut. In the rectum trypomastigotes are formed again; these are the infective forms. The bugs defecate when they feed, and trypomastigotes in the feces enter the body of a new vertebrate through the bite, skin abrasions, or the intact mucous membranes.

In addition to man, a wide variety of wild and domestic animals can be infected with *T. cruzi*–like organisms. These animals may be important reservoirs of infection. *T. cruzi* has been isolated from wild mammals and triatomes in the southern and southwestern United States. It is assumed that human disease is virtually nonexis-

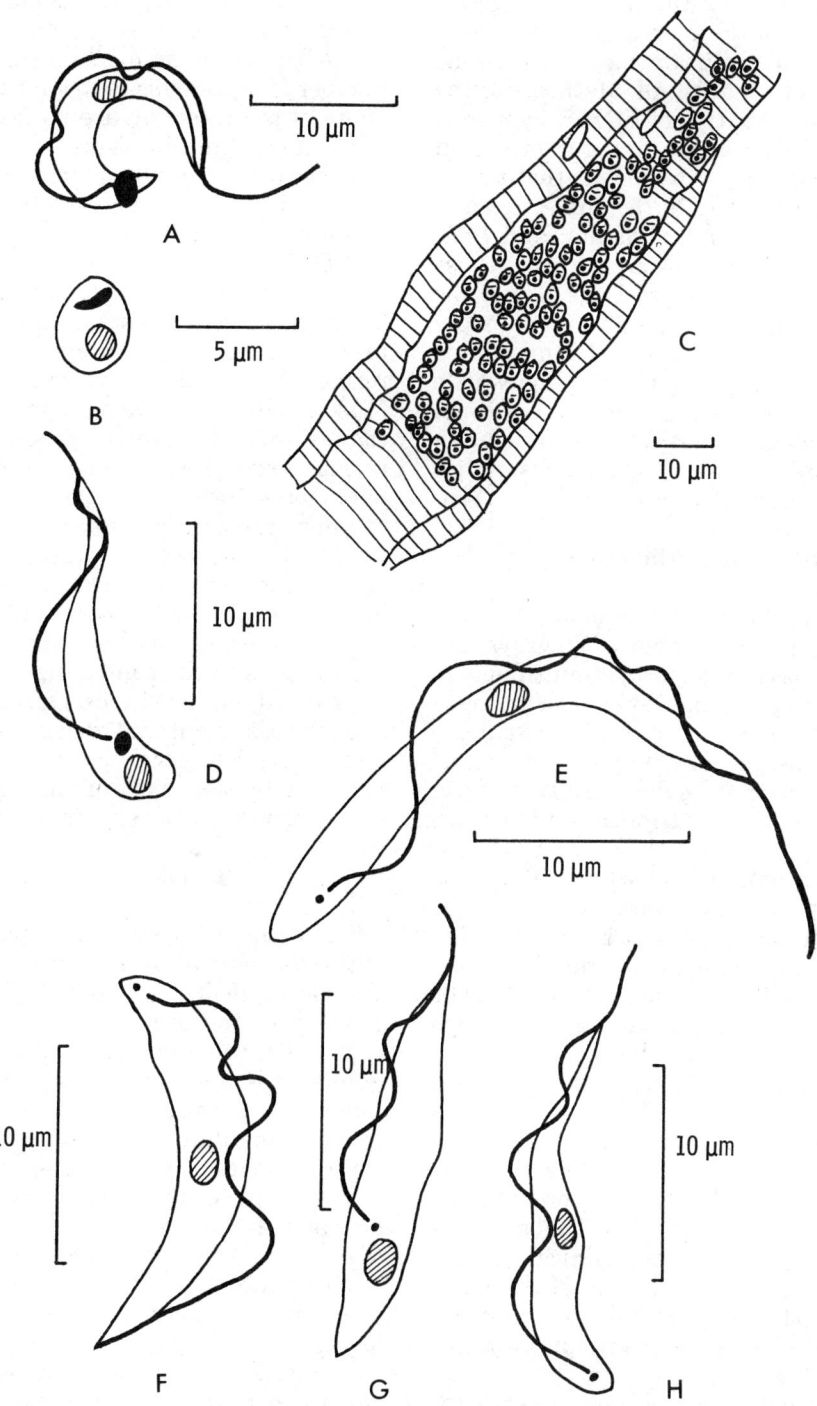

**FIGURE 1.** Trypanosoma cruzi: A, *Trypomastigote from mammalian blood;* B, *amastigote from mammalian cell;* C, *pseudocyst packed with amastigotes in mammalian muscle;* D, *epimastigotes from midgut of bug vector.* Trypanosoma brucei: E, *Long slender form from mammalian blood;* F, *short stumpy form from mammalian blood;* G, *epimastigote form from salivary gland of* Glossina; H, *metacyclic trypomastigote from salivary gland of* Glossina.

tent in these areas because man does not live in close association with either the vector or these mammalian reservoirs. It is difficult to judge the magnitude of the threat of the nonhuman reservoirs because many of these organisms may well be transmitted exclusively among wild animals and not impinge upon man at all. Methods for the infraspecific characterization of *T. cruzi* by means of isoenzyme patterns are now giving information on this point. In one case it was clear that the *T. cruzi* organisms circulating in the domestic environment in man, cats, dogs, rodents, and *Panstrongylus megistus* were different from those found in sylvatic mammals and bugs. Thus, the most common epidemiologic picture is probably transmission to man in the house by domiciliated bugs sheltered in crevices of mud-and-wattle walls or palm-leaf roofs, with only an occasional introduction of trypanosomes from sylvatic environments. Transmission by blood transfusion has also become an important hazard.

## Pathology and Pathogenesis

At the site of inoculation (chagoma), *T. cruzi* multiplies mainly in macrophages. When systemic dissemination occurs, *T. cruzi* multiplies in cells of many different tissues. There is a predilection for nerve cells and muscle cells, particularly of the heart and the gut. The pathological effects of the acute stage seem to be due mainly to direct damage to these cells by multiplication of the organisms.

Later in the chronic phase, when circulating and intracellular organisms are very few, the mechanisms of pathology are more controversial. In addition to direct damage to muscle tissue, destruction of the autonomic nerve-ganglion cells that control function seems to be important. One school of thought holds that the onset of symptoms is determined by the proportion of these cells that is damaged during the acute stage and the rate of further loss of cells naturally by senescence (Köberle, 1968). The other school represents the damage as a continuing, progressive, immunologically mediated process. This mechanism has received support from clinical studies that show widespread inflammation of the heart in the absence of parasites and from experimental studies that show similar lesions in mice injected with extracts of *T. cruzi*.

In its reproductive stages, *T. cruzi* evades the immune response by living within the cytoplasm of the cells of the host. In this location the amastigotes provoke little host reaction. The immunologic response to the breakdown products of the parasitized cells may be greater than that to the organisms themselves. However, there is a humoral response to the circulating trypomastigotes. This antibody is the basis of the complement fixation test. There is no evidence of the antigenic variability that is characteristic of the African trypanosomes.

The immunologic mechanisms that reduce the number of organisms to low levels after the acute phase of the infection are poorly understood, but cell-mediated mechanisms are likely to be operative because immune macrophages can kill *T. cruzi* and delayed hypersensitivity skin reactions to soluble antigens of *T. cruzi* become positive (WHO, 1974).

A severe inflammatory reaction characterized by lymphangitis, edema, and infiltration of polymorphonuclears, lymphocytes, and monocytes is responsible for the appearance of the chagoma. Muscle cells that have become packed with amastigotes are called pseudocysts. These rupture and release toxic products and the developing trypomastigotes, provoking the early inflammatory response consisting primarily of neutrophils, followed by lymphocytes, plasma cells, and histiocytes. In chronic disease, these lesions become granulomatous with pseudotubercles and giant cells in affected muscles. Adjacent cells degenerate. Lesions in the central nervous system (CNS) consist of lymphocytic perivascular cuffing, focal endarteritis, neuronal degeneration, and leptomeningitis. The focal nature of the vascular and neuroglial lesions may produce glial nodules scattered throughout the brain.

## Clinical Manifestations

Three stages of Chagas' disease can be recognized: the primary lesion, the acute stage, and the chronic stage. The primary lesion marks the site of entry of the organism into the body and appears after an incubation period of one to two weeks. It is not invariably present. When infection occurs through a skin abrasion, the primary lesion is an inflamed swelling of the skin, some 10 cm in diameter, called a chagoma. If the portal of entry is the conjunctiva, a common route, the primary lesion is a unilateral, bipalpebral edema of the conjunctiva (Romaña's sign).

When the acute stage of the disease is recognized, it follows the appearance of the primary lesion by 7 to 14 days and lasts some 30 days. It is characterized by pyrexia, headache, facial and generalized edema, and signs of heart damage. The acute stage occurs mostly in children and is believed to cause a mortality of about 5 per cent. Meningoencephalitis or heart failure is the usual cause of death. The acute stage is usually not recognized, however. When it does occur, it often resolves with little or no immediate damage.

After this stage, the infection becomes latent, and the individual may remain healthy and asymptomatic for the rest of his life.

The infection is probably rarely eliminated, however, and an unknown proportion of cases enters the so-called chronic phase. This stage is characterized by disturbances of the function of the hollow organs, particularly the heart, esophagus, and colon. The cardiac changes include myocardial insufficiency, cardiomegaly, disturbances of atrioventricular conduction, and the Adams-Stokes syndrome. Disturbances of peristalsis in the esophagus and colon lead to distention of these organs (megaesophagus and megacolon). Food may accumulate in the lower esophagus, and the patient may be able to transfer it to the stomach only by a jolt, such as that produced by jumping off a chair to the floor. Huge quantities of feces may accumulate in the colon. Megacolon and megaesophagus occur because of invasion and destruction of cells of the autonomic ganglia.

Sudden death on exertion is a common terminal event in chronic Chagas' disease. Many macabre anecdotes illustrate the frequency of this type of death. One of the most impressive is that football teams from affected communities may carry a large number of reserves to replace the losses occasioned by the rigor of the game! The late effects of Chagas' disease appear mainly in the third to fifth decades of life. They are of great social significance because they tend to occur when the family responsibilities of the subject are at their most demanding.

## Diagnosis

A distinction should be made between protozoologic and serologic diagnosis because each gives fundamentally different information. Protozoologic diagnosis, which depends on the actual demonstration of the organism, proves that the patient is still infected. It has two implications: the pathologic process is continuing and the patient is still a source of infection to vector insects. Serologic positivity is evidence only of past infection with either *T. cruzi* or some other antigenically similar agent. False positive and negative results are not infrequent.

### Protozoologic Diagnosis

This procedure is usually straightforward during the acute phase of the disease. The organisms are multiplying actively and amastigotes are plentiful in tissue cells. Consequently, trypomastigotes are also plentiful in the peripheral blood. Trypomastigotes can be detected in the peripheral blood by examination of thin or thick films stained with Romanowsky stain. Later, however, organisms become very scarce and can be demonstrated only by the use of multiplicative methods. *T. cruzi* is comparatively easy to cultivate on simple blood-agar slants and these may be used. However, the most sensitive method is generally believed to be xenodiagnosis, the process of allowing laboratory-bred, uninfected bugs to feed on the patient and examining the gut of these bugs subsequently for the presence of *T. cruzi* epimastigotes or trypomastigotes. The method, although sensitive, has obvious shortcomings: it is distasteful to patients, it is slow (since bugs may not show infection for as long as 90 days), and it is dangerous to the personnel who perform it.

*Trypanosoma (Herpetosoma) rangeli*, a nonpathogenic organism that occurs in man in Guatemala and El Salvador in Central America and in Colombia, Venezuela, and Chile in South America, is readily distinguished from *T. cruzi* in the peripheral blood. It is much longer — up to 36 $\mu$m long — and its kinetoplast is much smaller than that of *T. cruzi*. It also is transmitted by triatomid bugs.

### Serologic Diagnosis

Complement fixation, introduced in the 1930's, demonstrated the wide distribution and high prevalence of antibodies to *T. cruzi* in South America and established it as an important cause of disease. It is still the most widely used test, although there have been problems with variability of the antigen that is derived from *T. cruzi* cultures (Lumsden, 1973; WHO, 1974). Some of the more modern tests for recognition of humoral antibody, such as immunofluorescence (IF) and enzyme-linked immunosorbent assay (ELISA), are coming into use (PAHO, 1975).

## Geographic Variations

Because the disease is chronic and occurs mainly in rural communities that are often largely illiterate and deficient in health records, it is difficult to document the anecdotal geographic variations in the disease. However, the acute stage of the disease is more frequently recognized in western Argentina than elsewhere and the "mega" conditions occur most commonly in southern Brazil.

## Treatment

The disease arouses a fear out of proportion to the chance of infection because it is widely accepted in South America that there is no really effective chemotherapy against it. The most active drug available so far is a nitrofurazone compound, nifurtimox (Bayer 2502 or Lampit) (Lumsden, 1972). It appears to be effective against circulating trypomastigotes but less so against the intracellular amastigotes.

An experimental imidazole (R07-1051, *N*-benzyl-2-nitro-1-imidazolacetamide) may be useful against circulating and intracellular *T. cruzi* (Lugones et al., 1974). There is good evidence that it may cure acute Chagas' disease and a possibility that it may also be effective against chronic disease.

### Prophylaxis and Control

Control measures are limited to those that reduce contact between the vectors and man. Measures to improve housing and to use materials that do not provide shelter for the bugs are obvious but are often precluded economically. The disease is one of poverty-stricken rural communities. When housing cannot be improved, spraying with the insecticide benzene hexachloride (BHC) is widely used.

## AFRICAN TRYPANOSOMIASIS — SLEEPING SICKNESS

### Definition and Geographic Distribution

Sleeping sickness is caused by infection with *Trypanosoma (Trypanozoon) brucei*, which is transmitted by blood-sucking tsetse flies (Muscidae: *Glossina*). The disease occurs widely in sub-Saharan Africa from Senegal in the west to Ethiopia in the east and as far south as Zambia and Rhodesia. It is not coextensive with the distribution of the vector tsetse flies. Instead, it occurs focally within that distribution, depending on the habits and customs of the people and the ecologic characteristics of the local flies and wild animals (Ford, 1971).

### Etiology and Transmission

*T. brucei* exists in the vertebrate in only one morphologic form, the trypomastigote (Fig. 1). The trypomastigote is pleomorphic, however, and may occur as "long slender," 23 to 30 $\mu$m in length with a long flagellum, or "short stumpy" forms, 17 to 22 $\mu$m in length. The short stumpy forms have no, or only a very short, free flagellum. The long slender trypomastigote is the reproductive form in the vertebrate. The function of the short stumpy form is more controversial, but it is generally believed that it has altered respiratory metabolism that permits it to survive

in the gut of *Glossina* and infect this vector insect.

*T. brucei* is divided into three subspecies only because of differences in host range and in the characteristics of the diseases they cause (Mulligan, 1970). All are identical morphologically. *T.b. brucei* is by definition noninfectious for man but infects a wide variety of domestic and wild artiodactyls, including cattle, waterbuck, bushbuck, and buffalo. The other two species infect man as well as lower animals. *T.b. gambiense* causes a slowly developing disease (Gambian disease) with an incubation period that may last many months and a course that may permit the patient to survive for many years. *T.b. rhodesiense* is also infectious for man, but it is associated with a rapidly progressive disease (Rhodesian disease) that has a short incubation period and usually kills the patient within a few months. These are the classic courses of the two diseases, but evidence is accumulating that there may be a significant number of subclinical cases.

All three subspecies of *T. brucei* are transmitted by the bite of tsetse flies (*Glossina* spp), which typically inhabit woodland or forest. Short stumpy trypomastigotes from the circulation of an infected patient are ingested in the blood meal of the fly and multiply first as trypomastigotes in the midgut of the fly. Later, infection extends to the salivary glands and after about 15 days, metacyclic, mammal-infective forms develop (Mulligan, 1970). These are trypomastigotes clothed in a glycoprotein outer coat, which equips them for survival in the mammalian host. These forms are injected into a mammal during the next blood meal of the fly. It was formerly thought that the entire development of the trypanosome in the fly took place in the lumina of the gut and in the salivary glands, but recent evidence indicates that organisms may alternatively pass through the intestinal wall and the hemocoele to reach the salivary glands.

The patterns of transmission and maintenance of *T.b. rhodesiense* and *T.b. gambiense* differ. In the rapidly progressive Rhodesian disease, infected humans cannot provide a continuous source of infection in nature because they are soon removed from the scene by treatment, hospitalization, or death. Thus, this type of disease is a true zoonosis; humans are infected by flies that acquired their infection from wild animals. Intrahuman cycles of transmission are unimportant. A preponderance of males are infected because it is mainly men who go hunting, fishing, or honey-gathering (or, as tourists, go game-watching) and expose themselves to attack by flies that usually feed only on wild animals.

In the more slowly progressive Gambian disease, humans are available to provide long-term sources of infection for flies, and purely intrahuman cycles of transmission are more frequent. Thus, in the classic epidemiology of West African sleeping sickness a small population of flies is concentrated in a riverine forest by the prevailing aridity of the surrounding terrain and feeds repetitively on the people coming to the river bed to collect water. Women and children are infected most often because they visit the river bed more frequently.

## Pathology and Pathogenesis

*T. brucei* differs from *T. cruzi* in the behavior it adopts to evade the immune response of the host. Instead of sheltering themselves within cells, the organisms alter their external antigens about every five or six days. Thus, the infection consists of a series of waves of parasitemia, each one differing antigenically from those that preceded it and from those that will follow. This antigenic change occurs in the "outer coat," a glycoprotein layer outside the plasmalemma that is the true boundary of the cell. The mechanism of the change is probably by selection of the minor component of the population by antibody against the major component. The antigens of *T. brucei* can, therefore, be divided into two classes: the variable antigens contributed by this outer coat and the stable antigens — internal run-of-the-mill cell constituents such as enzymes and structural proteins.

The multiplicity and rapid succession of variable antigens bombards the immune response like a succession of infections by different organisms and induces a profuse production of IgM antibody, the antibody that is stimulated by new particulate antigens. The towering IgM levels produced both in serum and in cerebrospinal fluid (CSF) are characteristic of trypanosomiasis, are exploited for diagnostic purposes, and may be responsible for many of the manifestations of the disease. This profuse production of antibody causes hyperplasia of the reticuloendothelial system, particularly the lymph nodes and the spleen. The small lymphocytes in the germinal centers are replaced by macrophages and plasma cells. The patient eventually becomes immunosuppressed, and the lymph nodes become atrophic and fibrotic.

The high levels of IgM and antigen-antibody complexes are thought to cause many of the pathologic manifestations of trypanosomiasis. The markedly elevated erythrocyte sedimentation rate is caused by the high immunoglobulin levels. Antigen-antibody complexes are thought by some investigators to contribute directly to the pathology of trypanosomiasis by immune injury to the blood vessels and by stimulating the production of "kinins" and other mediators, which are elevated during trypanosomiasis (Boreham, 1968). Glomerulonephritis occurs during the course of trypanosomiasis and has been taken as evidence of the importance of immune complex disease.

Immune complexes and mediators have also been blamed for the destruction of red blood cells and platelets that often occurs during the course of trypanosomiasis. There is also evidence, however, that parasite metabolites or even protein toxins may be responsible for destruction of these formed elements of the blood (Davis et al., 1974; Tizard et al., 1978). Immunosuppression precedes the late atrophy of the germinal centers and may also be caused by massive antigenic stimulation and immune complexes.

Cardiac dilatation and hypertrophy is usually caused by myocarditis but may also be associated with valvulitis, pancarditis, pericarditis, or lesions of the conduction system. Interstitial hemorrhage and interstitial and perivascular mononuclear infiltration are characteristic.

The most attention, however, has been devoted to the late-stage changes in the CNS, which include diffuse meningoencephalitis, swelling of the brain, and dura-arachnoid adhesions. The membranes are "felted" on to the surface of the brain and there is infiltration by lymphocytes. The infiltration of lymphoid cells into the brain via the Virchow-Robin space surrounding the blood vessels is particularly striking. This layer of perivascular cuffing around the vessels is sometimes 20 to 30 cells thick and separates them from the brain substance. Morula or Mott cells, lymphoid cells containing a large mulberry-like eosinophilic mass, are found in these "cuffs," in the brain substance, and in the lymph nodes. These are thought to be IgM-secretory plasma cells that have failed to externalize their secretion. They are very characteristic although not pathognomonic of sleeping sickness.

The immediate cause of the cerebral damage in sleeping sickness is still uncertain, but it seems likely that the neural damage is mediated by immunologic reactions that take place around the blood vessels and invade the brain substance.

## Clinical Manifestations

As in Chagas' disease, three stages can be recognized: the primary lesion, the early stage, and the late stage. The primary lesion, called the trypanosome chancre, develops at the site of the infected tsetse bite after a period of two to three weeks. It is an indurated, inflamed area about 10 cm in diameter that resolves in a week or two to an area of shiny desquamation. It seems to be more frequent in the rapidly progressive Rhodesian disease than in the Gambian disease. Local multiplication of trypanosomes in the chancre is followed in the early stage by dissemination of the organisms, which multiply as trypomastigotes in the blood and interstitial fluids of most tissues. This early stage is characterized by fever, debilitation, anemia, and cardiac signs, including tachycardia and right bundle branch block. The fever tends to be intermittent, with weekly peaks that correspond to the waves of parasitemia. Each of these waves is different antigenically from those that precede or succeed it. By this phenomenon of antigenic variation, the trypanosome avoids the effects of humoral antibody.

During this early stage, the organism is multiplying not only in the blood but also in the tissue fluids, particularly in the lymphatics. The distribution of lymphadenopathy varies but is particularly prominent in the nodes of the posterior cervical triangle. This finding, called Winterbottom's sign, was well known to the 18th-century slavers and used by them to exclude individuals with sleeping sickness from their shipments. Localized edema of the face and other tissues is common. Caucasians may develop a fugitive, erythematous circinate rash, mainly on the trunk and shoulders. Disseminated intravascular coagulation (Barrett-Connor et al., 1973) or thrombocytopenia (Robins-Browne et al., 1975) may occur during this stage.

There is no clear distinction or period of latency between this early stage and the late stage of the disease. Although there is often invasion of the CNS very early in the disease, the late stage can be defined clinically by the onset of symptoms of interference with mental function, headache, irritability, insomnia, and changes in mood. These progress to the more obvious signs of tremors of the hands, muscle fasciculations (particularly of the tongue), muscular rigidity, indistinct speech, difficulty in walking, and, finally, somnolence gradually deepening to coma and loss of sphincter control. Death is usually due to bronchopneumonia or other intercurrent infections.

The foregoing is a short summary of the main characteristics of a very variable and protean disease. Both types, Gambian and Rhodesian, are fundamentally similar and differ primarily in the speed of their progression. In Gambian disease the onset may be mild and unnoticed, so that the first signs are those of mental damage and somnolence. The typical duration of disease is about three years to death. In Rhodesian disease, the onset is almost invariably acute, but it may be followed by a relatively asymptomatic and afebrile period until the disease resumes its progress

and leads to death six to nine months after onset. In general, the disease is more acute in Europeans than in Africans, but its manifestations are quite variable in both groups.

## Diagnosis

### Protozoologic Diagnosis

The problems of establishing the diagnosis of *T. brucei* infections are similar to those of *T. cruzi* infections. The recognition of organisms in the early stage is simple because the concentrations in the blood are high. They are readily recognized in wet blood films or in thin or thick blood films or in aspirates of chancres or lymph nodes stained with Romanowsky stains. In the later stages of the disease, organisms are scanty, so concentrative or multiplicative methods must be used. For blood, double centrifugation, that is, a first centrifugation just sufficient to deposit the erythrocytes followed by a second centrifugation of the supernatant and examination of the pellet, is often successful. There are other more sensitive methods of concentration. Blood samples taken in microhematocrit tubes are centrifuged and examined microscopically, preferably directly in the tube. The trypanosomes are concentrated in the plasma immediately above the buffy layer. Anion-exchange/centrifugation or anion-exchange/filtration methods are probably the most sensitive. The blood is diluted with buffers of suitable osmolarity and pH and passed through anion-exchange columns. Blood cells are adsorbed to the anion exchanger; trypanosomes pass through unimpeded and can be found in the eluate on direct microscopic examination or after centrifugation or filtration. The filter membrane may be fixed and stained before examination. Examination of the CSF is also important. Increases in the cell count about 5 cells/mm$^3$, a protein content above 40 mg/100 ml, or the presence of trypanosomes indicates that the infection has entered the late stage and changes the choice of antitrypanosomal drugs.

As a multiplicative method, blood, lymph node aspirate, or CSF should be inoculated into laboratory rodents. This is effective for Rhodesian infections but less so for Gambian, which typically produces only very low parasitemias that may be difficult to recognize. Other more susceptible hosts for *T.b. gambiense* are inconvenient and expensive.

### Serologic Diagnosis

The antigenic variability of *T. brucei* has impeded the development of serologic diagnostic tests, but CF, immunofluorescent, and ELISA tests for antibody to stable antigens are becoming available (Lumsden, 1972). The simple, nonspecific estimation of serum IgM by radial immunodiffusion is also useful. High concentrations in the serum of an individual exposed to an endemic area should stimulate an intensive search for trypanosomes and trypanosomal antibody.

## Geographic Variations

The more slowly progressive Gambian disease is characteristic of the western and northern part of the distribution from Senegal on the African west coast through west and central Africa as far as the Sudan and Uganda. The rapidly progressive Rhodesian disease is characteristic of eastern Africa from Ethiopia and eastern Uganda south to Zambia and Rhodesia. These distinctions, however, are not hard and fast; for example, virulent infections have been reported from eastern Nigeria and mild infections from Malawi.

## Treatment

In contrast to the situation in Chagas' disease, effective curative and prophylactic chemotherapy is available for African trypanosomiasis. Successful treatment depends, however, on early recognition of the disease and the use of drugs appropriate for the stage of infection. The important distinction is between the early stage of the disease, when CNS invasion is absent or minimal, and the late-stage disease, when CNS involvement is well established. Successful treatment of late disease depends on the use of drugs that cross the blood-brain barrier. Patients with CNS symptoms, abnormal cerebrospinal fluid, or trypanosomes in the spinal fluid should be treated as late disease. Because the nervous system is invaded early in Rhodesian trypanosomiasis, patients who have been infected longer than four weeks should be treated as if they had late disease.

Intravenous suramin sodium, 1 g on days 1, 3, 7, and 14, is the treatment of choice for early infections. A test dose of 100 mg should be given and the patient carefully monitored for a few hours before the remainder of the first dose is given because some patients experience shock and collapse after intravenous suramin. Common toxic reactions include rashes and renal damage. Suramin should be discontinued if proteinuria or marked changes in the urine sediment occur. Pentamidine is a good alternative for early disease in a daily dose of 3 mg base per kg intramuscularly for ten days. When CNS invasion is established or suspected, melarsoprol must be used, often after a preliminary course of suramin, which clears the parasitemia and improves the general condition of the patient so that he can withstand the toxic effects of melarsoprol (Melarsen-oxide/BAL; Mel B). Melarsoprol should be administered cautiously intravenously at 48-hour intervals. In one recommended schedule, 1.5, 2.0, and 2.2 mg/kg are given the first week; one week later 2.5, 3.0 and 3.6 mg/kg are administered, and after another week a final course of three injections of 3.6 mg/kg is given. Patients should be watched closely for signs of arsenic poisoning such as encephalopathy, exfoliative dermatitis, or enteritis.

## Control and Prevention

Prevention of infection with Rhodesian trypanosomes is primarily a matter of personal protection against tsetse bites; no general attack against the tsetse is feasible because of the huge areas of country involved. Prevention of Gambian disease can be accomplished by measures against the vector including clearing of the forest and the use of insecticides because the infested forest areas are usually circumscribed. Prophylactic chemotherapy with pentamidine has also been widely employed against *T.b. gambiense*, but the success of this method is dependent on well-organized survey teams and regular surveillance of the infected areas. The usual prophylactic dose of pentamidine isethionate is 250 mg intramuscularly every six months. It is better, however, to permit the short-incubation, acute Rhodesian disease to declare itself and treat the patient early. The problem with chemoprophylactic campaigns is the possibility of suppression of the disease so that it is only recognized in the late stages, when radical cure is more difficult to accomplish.

## References

Barrett-Connor, E., Ugoretz, R. J., and Braude, A. I.: Disseminated intravascular coagulation in trypanosomiasis. Arch Intern Med 131:574, 1973.

Boreham, P. F. L.: Immune reactions and kinin formation in chronic trypanosomiasis. Br J Pharmacol Chemother 32:493, 1968.

Davis, C. E., Robbins, R. S., Weller, R. D., and Braude, A. I.: Thrombocytopenia in experimental trypanosomiasis. J Clin Invest 53:1359, 1974.

Ford, J.: The Role of the Trypanosomes in African Ecology. Oxford, Clarendon Press, 1971.

Hoare, C. A.: The Trypanosomes of Mammals. Oxford, Blackwell Scientific Publications, 1972.

Köberle, F.: Chagas' disease and Chagas' syndrome: The pathology of American trypanosomiasis. In Dawes, B. (ed.): Advances in Parasitology. Vol. 6. London, Academic Press, 1968.

Lugones, H., Rabinovich, B., Cerisola, J. A., Ledesma, O., and Barclay, C.: Preliminary results of the anti-*T. cruzi* activity of RO7-1051 in man. In Proceedings of the Third International Congress of Parasitology 3:1297, 1974.

Lumsden, W. H. R.: Trypanosomiasis. Br Med Bull 28:34, 1972.

Lumsden, W. H. R.: Demonstration of antibodies to protozoa. In Weir, D. M. (ed.): Handbook of Experimental Immunology. 2nd ed. Oxford, Blackwell Scientific Publications, 1973.

Mulligan, H. W. (ed.): The African Trypanosomiases. London, George Allen and Unwin, 1970.

Pan American Health Organization: New Approaches in American Trypanosomiasis. Washington, D.C., Pan American Health Organization, 1975.

Robins-Browne, R. M., Schneider, J., and Metz, J.: Thrombocytopenia in trypanosomiasis. Am J Trop Med Hyg 24:226, 1975.

Tizard, I., Nielson, K. H., Seed, J. R., and Hall, J. E.: Biologically active products from African trypanosomes. Microbiol Rev 42:661, 1978.

World Health Organization: Immunology of Chagas' disease. Bull WHO 50:459, 1974.

# 197 BANCROFTIAN AND MALAYAN FILARIASIS

Abraham I. Braude, M.D., Ph.D.

## DEFINITION

Bancroftian and Malayan filariasis are infections that are transmitted by mosquitoes and located in the lymphatics, in which adult worms can cause inflammation or obstruction and release microfilariae that enter the peripheral blood at night. Bancroftian filariasis occurs throughout the tropics and subtropics, including Central Africa, North Africa along the Mediterranean, Southeast Asia, the Philippines, Indonesia, China, Korea, Japan, Polynesia, the West Indies, Venezuela, Brazil, and Colombia. Malayan filariasis is much less extensive, but foci are found in India and Southeast Asia, including Burma, Malaysia, Vietnam, Borneo, and Indonesia. Manson proved that mosquitoes suck the filarial larvae from the blood of patients and thus demonstrated for the first time that arthropods can be a vector of a parasitic infection.

## ETIOLOGY

Bancroftian filariasis is caused by *Wuchereria bancrofti*. The adults are white, thread-like worms with tapering ends. The males can measure 1.5 inches and the females twice as long. The two exist intertwined in human lymphatic vessels and lymph nodes, in which they mate, and the female gives birth to minute eel-like embryos, the microfilariae. These remain coiled within the egg shell when first developed but later elongate and retain the shell as a thin delicate sheath. The microfilaria is a diminutive worm with graceful sweeping curves and a pointed tail. In blood smears, the sheathed larva measures 245 to 295 microns. It has rudimentary organs, no alimentary canal, and numerous nuclei except in the rear end of the tail. This absence of terminal nuclei is used to differentiate it from *Brugia malayi*, whose tail is swollen at the tip with two nuclei. The larvae of bancroftian filariasis were proved to be the cause of this disease by the Brazilian physician, Wucherer, who found them in the urine of patients with chyluria and whose name has become identified with the parasite. Further development of *W. bancrofti* takes place in the mosquito after the larvae are ingested with a blood meal obtained by biting an infected person at night during the periodic entry of microfilariae into the circulation. The larva loses its sheath in the stomach of the mosquito, leaves the alimentary canal, and migrates to the breast muscles, in which it changes its shape and structure within ten days to become infective for man. In maturing to the infectious third stage, the microfilaria grows to 1.5 to 2.0 mm and becomes filiform. Then, it goes to the head of the mosquito and down into the proboscis. When the mosquito bites a warm, moist skin, the larvae creep out and penetrate through the mosquito bite. The infectious larvae then migrate to lymph nodes and lymph vessels, in which they mature, sexually mate, and produce embryos in about one year after the bite.

The adult worms do not multiply in people, nor do the larvae multiply in mosquitoes, so that the extent and severity of human infection depend on the total number of bites each person receives from an infected vector. In addition, the filariae are not highly infective for human beings because many larvae fail to penetrate the skin after a mosquito bite or cannot reach the lymphatics if they do penetrate. Others are injured by the immune response in the lymphatics, so that microfilariae never enter the blood for further transmission. This situation was common in American troops in the South Pacific in World War II, when soldiers frequently had inguinal lymphadenitis and lymphangitis of the spermatic cord but rarely had microfilariae in the blood. Because of these obstacles to infection, an enormous number of bites is required to maintain the disease in a community; perhaps as many as 15,000 infective bites per person are needed to ensure transmission (Hairston and DeMerllon, 1968).

The filaria belonging to the genus *B. malayi* are smaller than *W. bancrofti*. Male adult forms of *B. malayi* measure only 0.5 to 1.0 and the females 1.5 to 2.2 inches in length. The sheathed larvae are also smaller than those of *W. bancrofti*; the microfilariae of *B. malayi* have a length of only 175 to 230 microns. The life cycles of the two species of filaria are the same, but the mosquito vectors are somewhat different. The important vectors of bancroftian filariasis are *Culex, Anopheles* and *Aedes* mosquitoes, whereas Malayan filariasis is transmitted primarily by members of the genera *Mansonia* and *Anopheles*. Both forms of filariasis exhibit nocturnal periodicity, a condition in which the number of microfilariae in the peripheral blood increases at night and decreases during the day. As a result, both forms of disease are transmitted by mosquitoes that bite at night when there are more than 15 microfilariae per drop of blood, the minimum number that can infect mosquitoes. An exception to this periodicity in bancroftian filariasis is seen under two circumstances: (1) If the infected person changes his sleeping habits and stays awake at night, the microfilariae increase in the peripheral blood during the day. This change in periodicity occurs about a week after daytime sleeping begins. (2) In the Polynesian islands (Samoa, Fiji, Tonga, and Cook islands) the microfilariae are found in the blood at all times but increase after noon and decrease after sunset. This is known as the subperiodic form of filariasis, and the filaria involved is regarded by some (Manson-Bahr and Muggleton, 1952) as a separate variety or species, to be designated *Wuchereria pacifica*. Most authorities feel this distinction is not justified because, under close scrutiny, the two forms appear to be identical, except that the adult worms in most periodic cases are slightly longer.

## PATHOGENESIS AND PATHOLOGY

The adult worms cause lymphatic inflammation and obstruction in the scrotum, spermatic cords, epididymis, testis, arms, legs, abdomen, and retroperitoneal area. Lymphangitis and lymphadenitis are thought to be allergic reactions to worm secretions or antigens liberated from dead filariae periodically so that the attacks of chills and fever are recurrent. Obstruction probably results from the lymphangitis and secondary fibrosis rather than from simple mechanical blockade by the worm. Lymph varices are among the early signs of lymphatic obstruction, and if they rupture, lymph (chyle) is released into the peritoneum, kidney, bladder, scrotum, or bowel. Chyluria and chylous ascites are manifestations of this phenomenon. Obstruction of the smaller sub-cutaneous lymphatic vessels produces lymphedema of the scrotum, vulva, legs, arms, and breast. As lymphedema gives way to subcutaneous fibrosis and hyperkeratosis, the skin takes on the character of elephant hide and becomes thick, hard, and dry from loss of sweat glands.

In contrast to the adult worms, microfilariae contribute little to the pathology of the disease. In fact, there is a negative correlation between lymphatic obstruction and positive blood smears for microfilariae. There may be 20,000 microfilariae per milliliter of blood from people with no symptoms, and negative blood smears in patients with elephantiasis. This is probably because the adults have died before lymphatic injury becomes severe enought to produce clinical disturbances. A positive correlation exists, however, between clinical severity and the development of rapid infection with many worms. Thus, foreigners residing in endemic areas seldom show symptoms for 10 to 15 years, whereas American troops in the South Pacific developed lymphangitis, lymphadenitis, and swelling of the genitalia or arms in about nine months (Huntington et al., 1944). The difference can probably be explained by the speed and intensity of infection. Europeans and Americans living in the tropics under peacetime conditions can protect themselves well enough from night-biting mosquitoes to avoid heavy infections. The troops in the South Pacific, on the other hand, were heavily exposed to the day-biting mosquitoes *(Aëdes scutellaris polynesiensis)* near native villages, and received bites from more infected mosquitoes in a few weeks than foreigners residing in other endemic regions would get in years. Individual variation in sensitization to worm antigens probably explains why, among persons with equal exposure to infection, some develop lymphangitis and lymphedema, and some do not. Biopsies showing acute lymphangitis with no adult worms in sight are consistent with the idea that inflammatory lesions are the result of allergy to worm antigens carried along the lymph channels rather than a nonspecific reaction to the intact worm.

The tissue reaction in lymph nodes and lymph vessels is an infiltration of histiocytes, lymphocytes, and eosinophils, along with hyperplasia of the lymphatic endothelium. The lymphatic wall becomes thickened and edematous so that its lumen narrows and dilatation occurs beyond it. Within the dilatations of the lymph vessels and nodes lie the tightly coiled adult worms. Later, small granulomas appear in the lymph nodes. When the active inflammation is replaced by fibrosis, sclerotic lymph channels become permanently obstructed. The granulomatous tissues are eventually absorbed, and the scar sometimes calcifies around dead worms. The obstructed lymph channels develop varices; in some areas, they become obliterated, fibrous strands.

The location of elephantiasis depends on which lymph nodes are obstructed. Obstruction of the para-aortic nodes blocks drainage of lymph from the tunica vaginalis, epididymis, and spermatic cord so that hydrocele develops (Jordan, 1955) without edema of the scrotal skin, which drains into the superficial inguinal glands. In patients with elephantiasis of the leg, the obstruction is in the inguinal or iliac group of nodes.

## CLINICAL MANIFESTATIONS

After an incubation period of about one year, the acute stage begins with frequent attacks of fever to 104° F, lymphangitis, and lymphadenitis. The lymphangitis usually occurs on the legs, hands, and scrotum, where it produces tenderness and red streaks or cord-like swellings that extend peripherally from the infected swollen lymph nodes in the groin, axilla, or epitrochlear region. In the early attacks, the pain and swelling of the scrotum, spermatic cord, testis, or limb may be only mild and transient, but later the lymphedema becomes more marked and persistent. Abdominal lymphangitis may produce a clinical picture suggesting an acute abdomen if there is pain, or unexplained fever if painless. The fever and chills last for several days and then stop suddenly with profuse sweating. The clinical picture during acute attacks varies with the population and their location. In American troops exposed to the nonperiodic strain of *W. bancrofti* in the South Pacific islands, for example, the attacks of lymphangitis were often accompanied by headache, backache, fatigue, nausea, and mental depression, but fever was unusual. Lymphangitis of the spermatic cord and orchitis were the most common clinical signs in these soldiers.

After a couple of years of recurring attacks, permanent edema sets in and most often causes swelling of the legs, scrotum, and penis. Lymphatic obstruction causes subcutaneous lymph varices. These soft, lobular, elastic structures develop in the groin or axilla. Numerous varices also develop within the scrotum and on its surface, a condition known as "lymph scrotum." It has a characteristic velvety feel and produces a steady ooze from the skin after surface blebs rupture. If the thoracic duct is obstructed, the urinary lymphatics may rupture into the bladder and produce chyluria. The chyluria tends to be transient, lasting usually for only a few days at a time but sometimes for months. The incidence of chyluria varies considerably from one geographic zone to another. Rupture of lymphatics in the peritoneal or pleural spaces can produce chylous ascites or chylothorax.

Hydrocele is probably the most common sign of long-standing bancroftian filariasis. The significance of this finding as a sign of filariasis tends to be ignored in areas of low endemicity and exaggerated in highly endemic areas. It may affect as many as 40 per cent of the male population (Nelson, 1979).

Filariasis caused by *Brugia malayi* usually produces a more acute clinical picture than bancroftian filariasis. Elephantiasis of the limbs is common, but the genitalia and bladder are usually spared.

## COMPLICATIONS AND SEQUELAE

Although patients with filariasis have a morbid fear of developing elephantiasis, especially of the genitalia, this complication occurs in only a small percentage of cases. Elephantiasis most often affects the legs but can occur in any part of the body, including the arms, breast, scrotum, and vulva (Fig. 1). The mistaken belief that elephantiasis is an inevitable consequence of bancroftian filariasis has caused much unnecessary mental anguish and neurotic problems, which can thus be serious sequelae of the disease.

Elephantiasis is further complicated by attacks of inflammation in the swollen part. These may be due to filariasis itself or to secondary bacterial infection.

Elephantiasis appears to be a function of high rates of microfilarial infection. In areas with microfilarial rates over 10 per cent, elephantiasis is one of the most common complications. In areas with lower rates, hydrocele and chyluria predominate (Edeson, 1972).

## GEOGRAPHIC VARIATIONS IN DISEASE

Chyluria has been the most important and frequent clinical manifestation of bancroftian filariasis in the temperate zone countries such as Japan. In 111 cases of filariasis reported in 1961 from Ehime, Japan, 103 (92.8 per cent) had chyluria, but only four had hydrocele, and another four had elephantiasis. Among 3407 cases of filariasis in Sri Lanka, on the other hand, only two had chyluria and 2983 (87.5 per cent) had elephantiasis (Sasa, 1976).

Another interesting symptom reported from Sri Lanka is chest pain. Among students at the University of Ceylon, this was the second most common symptom (after headache) in early bancroftian filariasis. The pain was usually precordial, retrosternal, or infraclavicular and worse at night. It was also recurrent and severe enough to suggest a myocardial infarction (Wijetunge, 1967).

The periodicity of *W. bancrofti* infection also follows geographic patterns. The periodic form, in which the microfilariae enter the blood at night, occurs in the tropics throughout the world, whereas the nonperiodic diurnal form occurs in Polynesia. *B. malayi*, which is limited to Asia, produces a somewhat different clinical picture than *W. bancrofti*. Infections by *B. malayi* tend to have a shorter incubation period, to involve the upper limbs more frequently, and to be free of genital or urinary disease.

In Puerto Rico, serial observations over 40 years show a tendency toward a declining incidence of microfilaremia and the emergence of a persistent subclinical form of bancroftian filariasis. In a study of intrascrotal organs in 330 autopsies, 23.9 per cent had filarial worms, and hydroceles were found in 59.5 per cent of those with filariasis. In about 90 per cent the worm was dead and encased in a scar that was sometimes calcified (Galindo et al., 1962). This unexpectedly high incidence of filarial infection in an asymptomatic population suggests that a decline in overt clinical manifestations in certain parts of the world does not necessarily mean a disappearance of the disease.

In Malaya, there is evidence that Brugian filariasis can cause the syndrome of tropical pulmonary eosinophilia. The distribution of tropical eosinophilia in Malaya tends to follow the pattern of filariasis, and the filarial skin and complement fixation tests are strongly positive in tropical eosinophilia (Janssens, 1974). Diethylcarbamazine, which is effective in filariasis, also cures tropical eosinophilia. Tropical eosinophilia is usually a subacute or chronic illness of young men aged 20 to 30 and produces nocturnal asth-

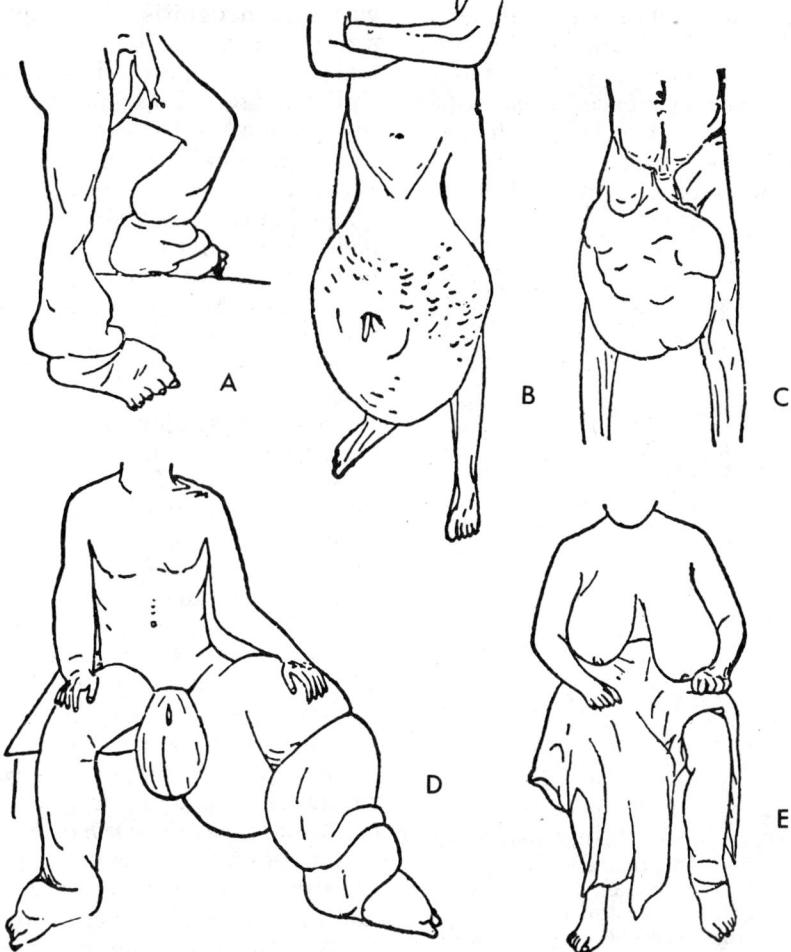

**FIGURE 1.** *Extreme cases of elephantiasis sketched by A. C. Chandler from photographs. A, Legs and feet. B, Scrotum. C, Varicele of inguinal lymph node. D, Scrotum and legs. E, Breasts. (Chandler, A. C.: Introduction to Parasitology. New York, John Wiley and Sons, 1955.)*

matic attacks, fever, and eosinophilia ranging from 20 to 90 per cent with total leukocyte counts as high as 50,000. This syndrome is also seen in patients with Bancroftian filariasis. Microfilaremia does not occur in tropical eosinophilia, but microfilariae are found in pulmonary granulomas. It is likely that animal as well as human species of *Wuchereria* and *Brugia* filariae cause the disease, and the tendency to involve the lung may represent a genetic susceptibility in certain people, such as Asiatic Indians, who display by far the highest incidence of the disease.

## DIAGNOSIS

Biopsy is contraindicated because it can worsen lymphatic obstruction. Short of biopsy, demonstration of microfilariae in the blood is the most specific test for diagnosis of either bancroftian or malayan filariasis, but they can be found only in the intermediate stages of the disease. They do not usually circulate in the blood for the first two or three years of infection and disappear in older infections when the adult organisms die and leave behind lymphatic pathology, the "tombstones of their obstructive existence." If parasitemia is heavy, the microfilariae can be demonstrated easily in Giemsa-stained smears of blood taken between 10 P.M. and 2 A.M. In a wet prepa-

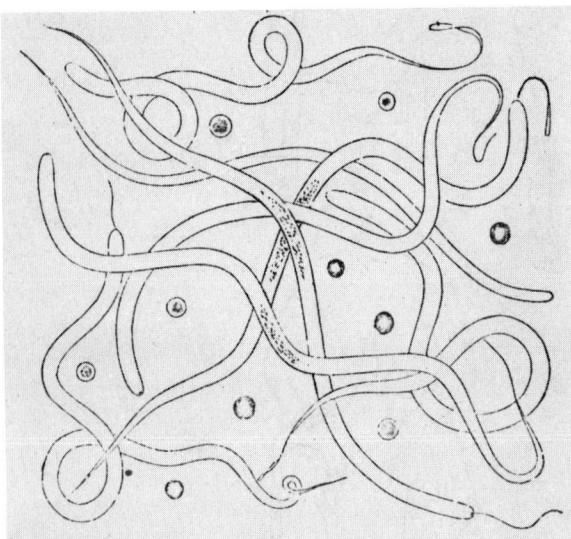

**FIGURE 2.** *Living microfilariae observed by T. R. Lewis (1872) in a drop of blood from the finger of a European woman suffering from chyluria. A few red blood corpuscles have been introduced to show the relative size of the microfilariae. This was the first description of microfilariae in the blood. (From a woodcut made by T. R. Lewis to show a composite picture of several fields. Eighth Annual Report of the Public Health Commissioner with the Government of India. Calcutta Office of Superintendent of Gov. Prints, 1872, p. 243.)*

ration of the blood under a coverslip, the microfilaria is seen in constant motion, coiling and uncoiling itself increasingly and lashing the blood corpuscles in all directions (Lewis, 1872) (Fig. 2). If parasitemia is light, the blood should be passed through a membrane filter with a 5 $\mu$m pore, so that the microfilariae (but not the blood cells) are collected on the membrane, where they can be stained. In the Pacific areas where the nonperiodic strains prevail, blood should be examined in the early afternoon. The nocturnal forms of microfilariae can be driven from lung capillaries into the circulation in the daytime by giving 100 mg of diethylcarbamazine orally and making smears one hour later. This technique is risky, however, for patients who may have onchocerciasis and loa loa infections because it may cause severe allergic reaction when the worms are killed (Nelson, 1979; WHO report, 1974).

In the early stages before blood smears are positive, the clinical signs are usually typical enough to make the diagnosis. In an endemic area, recurrent attacks of "elephantoid" fever with lymphadenitis and lymphangitis of a limb, scrotum, or spermatic cord are almost enough to make the diagnosis. The attack starts with a chill; the fever comes down in three to five days; the lymphatics are swollen and tender; and the overlying skin is inflamed. The diagnosis is more difficult if there is only recurrent fever without lymphangitis. When abscesses form in the lymph node or lymphatic vessels, the diagnosis can be made by finding remnants of dead filarial worms in the pus. Microfilariae can be found in fluid from hydroceles that result from rupture of a lymph vessel. They are also seen in chylous urine.

Recurrent streptococcal lymphangitis (relapsing erysipelas) is important in differential diagnosis. The titer of antistreptolysin O is characteristically elevated, and a trial with penicillin abruptly terminates the fever and prevents future attacks of streptococcal lymphangitis. Unfortunately, streptococci are difficult to isolate from the bullae that are characteristic of this condition, and cultures of biopsies of the deep lymphatics may be needed to find the organism. In sporotrichosis, there is thickening of the lymphatics, but there is no fever and no local erythema or pain. Although the fungus cannot be seen in smears of the pus, the diagnosis is easily made by culture of *Sporothrix schenckii*.

Hereditary lymphedema (Milroy's disease) can be difficult to distinguish from filariasis. The familial history and the involvement of both legs are helpful since elephantiasis tends to be unilateral. Lymphangiography is useful in the early stages of filarial elephantiasis when the lymphatic vessels are dilated and tortuous because the lymphatics are hypoplastic in Milroy's disease. In advanced elephantiasis, the lymphatics atrophy, and lymphangiography loses its differential value.

The occurrence of nonfilarial elephantiasis must be kept in mind in the highlands of East Africa where there is no filariasis because the altitude is too great for mosquitoes to live. People cultivating the red clays of Africa develop non-filarial elephantiasis of the legs secondary to the absorption of aluminosilicate and silicon from the soil through the skin of the feet. Irritation of the different lymphatics by particles of these substances causes fibrosis and obstructive lymphopathy (Price and Henderson, 1979).

Many patients with filariasis have eosinophilia, but this sign is too nonspecific to be of much help in diagnosis. There are no serologic tests of value because it has not been possible to obtain enough antigen of *W. bancrofti*. The reason for this problem is that there is no susceptible laboratory animal in which to propagate the worm.

## TREATMENT

Both bancroftian and Malayan filariasis can be cured with diethylcarbamazine (Hetrazan), which kills both adult worms and microfilariae. Treatment is usually started with a small oral dose of 0.25 mg/kg and then gradually increased to 6 mg/kg per day. A total dose of 72 mg/kg is then given in divided doses at daily or weekly intervals as best tolerated (WHO Report, 1974). Schedules vary from 6 mg/kg once daily to 3 mg/kg three times daily. The schedule is less important than the total dose in achieving a high cure rate. Febrile reactions occur after the first dose and are especially severe in infections by *B. malayi*, which is much more susceptible to diethylcarbamazine. In addition to fever, patients complain of headache, nausea, and painful swellings of the lymph nodes and lymph vessels early in the course of treatment. In some patients, filarial abscess may occur along the lymphatics during treatment as a result of an allergic reaction to the dead worm. If care is taken to start treatment with small doses and to increase them slowly, severe symptoms can be avoided. These allergic reactions result from the release of antigens upon disintegration of killed microfilariae or adult worms. The reactions respond to Phenergan in doses of 10 mg. Phenergan is also useful with aspirin in controlling attacks of filarial lymphangitis in patients who are not under treatment with diethylcarbamazine. After diethylcarbamazine therapy, the microfilariae disappear from the blood in a period ranging from several days to a few weeks, but relapses can occur. For this rea-

son, blood smears should be reexamined, and another course of treatment should be given if microfilariae are still present.

Although radical cure of infection with chemotherapy can eliminate the febrile attacks, the acute lymphangitis, and early lymphedema, it does little to improve the stigmata of chronic filariasis such as elephantiasis, chronic hydrocele, chyluria, or draining sinuses. Instead, it is necessary to resort to nonspecific treatment for these problems. Hydroceles and scrotal elephantiasis can be corrected by surgery, but precautions must be taken to protect the spermatic cord and testes during the operation. Excisional treatment of elephantiasis of the limbs, on the other hand, is often unsatisfactory, and this condition should be treated conservatively with pressure bandages and elevation of the swollen part during bed rest. The swelling in elephantiasis of the leg, for example, diminishes considerably in a week if the foot of the bed is raised as much as possible. If an elastic stocking is applied before the patient leaves the bed, recurrent swelling and discomfort is minimized. The patient can then be mobilized and even undertake useful work. Prednisone, in doses of 40 mg per day, helps to soften the tissues and reduce the swelling if it is given for a few weeks before the elastic bandage is applied.

Chyluria should be treated with diethylcarbamazine to eliminate the obstructing worms. In chyluric patients, such treatment does not produce the side effects otherwise found in treating filariasis. It is difficult to evaluate chemotherapy, however, because chyluria undergoes frequent remissions and exacerbations. Since eating fat provokes chyluria, fatty foods are restricted. Some success has been achieved by repeated injection of 25 per cent sodium iodide or 3 per cent silver nitrate into the renal pelvis through retrograde catheters. A cure rate of 51.5 per cent has been reported in Japan with this treatment (Sasa, 1976). In very severe cases, chyluria has been radically cured by surgical removal of collateral lymph vessels that empty into the renal pelvis.

## PROPHYLAXIS

Mass chemotherapy has been used against the parasite, and insecticides against the mosquitoes, but each approach has met with difficulties. When diethylcarbamazine is used for treatment of whole populations in endemic areas, it meets resistance because of the febrile reactions in carriers of filariasis. Yet it is worth pursuing despite the missed doses from febrile reactions and the problems in getting the drug to many people because microfilariasis rates can be reduced greatly by mass treatment and then retreatment of positive carriers (Edeson, 1972). The microfilariasis rates were reduced in this way from 26.0 per cent to 0.7 per cent in Malaysia, and an 82 per cent cure rate was obtained in the Ryuka islands by giving one course of treatment to known microfilaria carriers.

Prevention of filariasis through mosquito control has met two serious obstacles. One of these is the resistance acquired by *Culex fatigans* to insecticides. This mosquito is the chief vector of bancroftian filariasis in many parts of the world and is almost impossible to control because population growth has overwhelmed the attempts in large cities to provide sanitation and disposal of waste waters. The problem with Malayan filariasis is even worse because the subperiodic (diurnal) type in Malaya and Indonesia has a reservoir in monkeys and is transmitted in the forests by mosquitoes that bite rubber plantation workers in the daytime (Nelson, 1979).

### References

Chandler, A. C.: Introduction to Parasitology. New York, John Wiley and Sons, 1955, p. 469.

Edeson, J.: Filariasis. Br Med Bull 28:60, 1972.

Galindo, L., von Lichtenberg, F., and Boldizon, C.: Bancroftian filariasis in Puerto Rico: Infection pattern and tissue lesions. Am J Trop Med Hyg 11:739, 1962.

Hairston, N., and DeMerllon, B.: On the inefficiency of transmission of *Wuchereria bancrofti* from mosquito to human host. Bull WHO 38:935, 1968.

Huntington, R., Fogel, R., Eichold, A., and Dickson, J.: Filariasis among American troops in a South Pacific Island. Yale J Biol Med 16:529, 1944.

Janssens, P.: Filariasis. In Woodruff, A. W. (ed): Medicine in the Tropics. Edinburgh, Churchill Livingstone, 1974, p. 244.

Jordan, R.: Notes on elephantiasis and hydrocoele due to *Wuchereria bancrofti*. J Trop Med Hyg 58:113, 1955.

Lewis, T. R.: On a *Haematozoan* inhabiting human blood, its relation to chyluria and other diseases. Eighth annual report of the Public Health Commissioner with the Government of India. Calcutta Office of Superintendent of Government Prints, 1872, p. 243.

Manson-Bahr, P., and Muggleton, W.: Further research on filariasis in Fiji. Trans R Soc Trop Med Hyg 46:301, 1952.

Nelson, G.: Current concepts in parasitology: Filariasis. N Engl J Med 300:1136, 1979.

Price, E., and Henderson, W.: Silica and silicates in femoral lymph nodes of bare-footed people in Ethiopia with special reference to elephantiasis of the lower limbs. Trans R Soc Trop Med Hyg 73:640, 1979.

Sasa, M.: Human filariasis. Baltimore, University Park Press, 1976.

Wijetunge, H.: Clinical manifestations of early Bancroftian filariasis. A study of 212 cases of microfilariaemia. J Trop Med Hyg 70:90, 1967.

World Health Organization Expert Committee on Filariasis: Third report. WHO Tech Rep Ser 542:1, 1974.

# 198 *FUNGEMIA*

## *John E. Edwards, Jr., M.D.*

### DEFINITION

Fungemia denotes fungi in the circulating venous or arterial blood.

### ETIOLOGY

*Candida* is by far the most frequent fungus isolated from the blood. Candidemia has become a major problem in centers in which critically ill patients are managed. The emergence of this problem over the past three decades is a result of new therapeutic modalities; candidemia and candidiasis are, for the most part, iatrogenic conditions.

Although *Candida albicans* is the most frequent species of *Candida* found in blood and was once thought to be the only pathogenic species of the genus *Candida*, it is now clear that several *Candida* species can cause disseminated candidiasis. These species include *C. tropicalis, C. pseudotropicalis, C. guilliermondii, C. stellatoidea, C. krusei,* and *C. parapsilosis.* A blood isolate of any of these species has the same significance as isolation of *C. albicans.*

Second in frequency to *Candida* species in isolation from human sources are organisms of the genus *Torula.* This yeast has low pathogenicity but can produce extensive disease in immunocompromised patients. The clinical setting for *Torula* infection is similar to that for *Candida*; the predisposing factors are practically identical for both organisms. Thus, catheter-associated *Torula* fungemia, like catheter-associated candidemia, resolves without disseminated disease.

*Cryptococcus, Histoplasma, Rhodotorula, Geotrichium,* and *Trichosporon* are only rarely recovered from blood (Sheehy et al., 1976; Winston et al., 1977). In unusual instances of fungal endocarditis, *Aspergillus, Paecilomyces, Homodendrum,* and *Curvularie* also have been recovered from blood (Hartford, 1974). Despite the fact that aspergillosis is the second most common cause of disseminated mycosis in the compromised host, and widespread hematogenous seeding undoubtedly occurs, aspergilli are almost never cultured from blood. Since aspergilli are common laboratory contaminants, it is difficult to know whether a positive blood culture actually represents an *Aspergillus* fungemia. In one series, 20 per cent of patients with cryptococcal meningitis had positive blood cultures (Butler et al., 1964). *Rhodotorula* organisms have been recovered from blood occasionally, but in four cases of *Rhodotorula* fungemia, no disseminated fungal disease was present (Louria et al., 1967). One case of *Rhodotorula* septicemia has been associated with the picture of endotoxic shock. Patients with histoplasmosis may have positive blood cultures and the organism may be seen in peripheral smears.

## PATHOLOGY AND PATHOGENESIS

*Candida* and *Torula* fungemia occur more frequently in the following clinical settings: (1) intravenous hyperalimentation, (2) intravenous polyethylene catheters, (3) immunosuppressive drug therapy, (4) postoperative complications, (5) cancer, and (6) multiple antibiotic therapy. Burn patients, heroin addicts, and patients receiving prosthetic cardiac valves are at special risk for developing candidemia and/or endocarditis.

Disseminated candidiasis and candidemia probably originate from the gastrointestinal tract. Two important observations substantiate that hypothesis. (1) An investigator drank a suspension of *C. albicans* and became candidemic and candiduric afterward. This heroic experiment is almost irrefutable evidence that the gastrointestinal route can be a source for dissemination (Krause et al., 1969). (2) H. H. Stone (Stone et al., 1974) injected suspensions of *Candida* into various levels of canine and primate gastrointestinal tracts and found that the yeasts crossed the gastrointestinal tract and entered the bloodstream. To determine whether the yeasts gained entrance into the blood from colonized wounds, he injected *Candida* into canine muscles, fat, and granulating pouches and found no subsequent candidemia. In patients who have been treated with multiple antibiotics, candida probably overgrow the gastrointestinal tract because the resident bacteria are suppressed. This risk is compounded after abdominal surgery because the gastrointestinal trauma may facilitate entry of organisms through injured mucosa or open vessels. The pathogenesis of candidemia after hyperalimentation is not fully understood. Since high glucose concentrations promote the growth of yeasts, it is theoretically possible for hyperglycemia to foster growth of organisms that enter the bloodstream from the gastrointestinal tract or skin. Another possibility is that the foreign body (hyperalimentation catheter) may provide a site for the localization and multiplication of circulating yeasts that come from the gastrointestinal tract. Catheters acquire vegetations that are evidence of prolific growth after localization on the catheter.

## CLINICAL MANIFESTATIONS

If contamination is excluded, growth of fungi in blood cultures can represent fungemia with or without underlying disseminated mycosis of various organs. Clinical recognition of the complications that result from the fungemia are of utmost importance, not only for diagnosing the fungemia but also for determining its significance. Unfortunately, with the exception of blood cultures, there are practically no laboratory tools to assist in detection of fungemia.

There are several peripheral manifestations that suggest candidemia. Candidal endophthalmitis is one of the more easily recognizable. The lesions begin in the chorioretina, extend into the vitreous, and are covered by an overlying vitreous haze (Fig. 1). The chorioretinal-vitreal reaction has the appearance of a cottonball, off-white in color. Both experimental and clinical evidence suggest that when candidal eye lesions are present, there is a high likelihood that other organs are involved as well (Edwards et al., 1974). Although the evidence is incomplete, it appears that many patients with candidemia have ocular lesions. Therefore, patients must have thorough serial ocular examinations, preferably with an indirect ophthalmoscope. By far the most common species cultured from *Candida* endophthalmitis has been *C. albicans*. Experimental evidence suggests that other species may have less predilection for the eye. Because of the frequency, importance, and significance of these lesions, any patient who is predisposed to candidemia should have a thorough baseline ocular examination and regular evaluations for hematogenous *Candida* endophthalmitis.

Macronodular skin lesions are another peripheral sign of candidemia and disseminated candidiasis (Bodey and Luna, 1974). The lesions are 0.5 to 1.0 cm in diameter and pink to red in color. Either single or multiple lesions may occur (see Chapter 211). Occasionally they have a hemorrhagic base. *Candida* organisms have been found more often in biopsy sections than by culture of the lesion. Finding the lesion and demonstrating the causative organism may not increase the frequency of diagnosis of disseminated candidiasis but may reduce the time required, because blood cultures may become positive only after several days (often after the patient has died).

Hematogenous *Candida* osteomyelitis and arthritis may also be clues to candidemia and underlying disseminated candidiasis. Candida osteomyelitis may affect the spine (intervertebral disks and adjacent vertebrae), wrist, femur, neck, costochondral junction, scapula, and proximal humerus. Diagnosis is made by biopsy (usually percutaneous); blood cultures are generally nega-

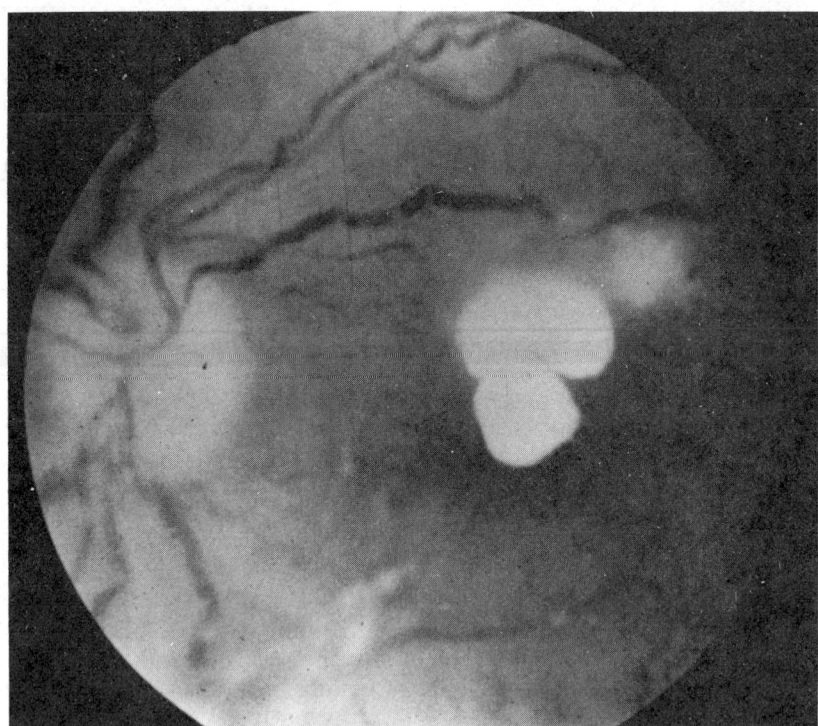

**FIGURE 1.** *Typical, relatively advanced Candida chorioretinitis involving the macula. (From Fishman, L. S., Griffin, J. R., Sapico, F. L., et al.: Hematogenous Candida endophthalmitis — a complication of candidemia. N Engl J Med 286:675, 1972.)*

tive. *Candida* arthritis usually follows direct hematogenous infection but can also develop after extension from an adjacent area of hematogenous osteomyelitis or from direct inoculation into the joint.

In addition to these "peripheral manifestations," visceral infection should be sought in the patient who is predisposed to candidemia and disseminated candidiasis. Frank myocarditis, which occurs in about half of the patients with disseminated candidiasis, may cause chest pains, congestive heart failure, or cardiac arrhythmias. Diffuse candidal brain involvement may first produce obtundation, and later focal neurologic findings or frank meningitis. Hematogenous pyelonephritis occurs, renal function may fail rapidly, and *Candida* may be found in the urine. The shock syndrome that has been described might be related to the endotoxin-like substance in its cell wall.

The clinical manifestations of *Torula* septicemia are less well defined than those of *Candida* septicemia, primarily because the experience has been much smaller. A review of 10 cases (Pankey and Dalaviso, 1973) indicated that rapid elevation of temperatures was characteristic. In this series, hypotension was not seen; in other series, an endotoxic shock-like picture has been described (Valdivieso et al., 1976). Since this organism is distributed to multiple organs during he-

matogenous infection one would expect the focal manifestations observed in candidemia, but there are only a few reports of such findings. Several comprehensive reviews of *Torula* septicemia fail to mention involvement of the eye, skin, bone, or joint. Instead, *Torula* produces disseminated disease in the lung and kidney and in the mucosa of the gastrointestinal and genitourinary tracts, uterus, and fallopian tubes.

A review of 26 patients with progressive disseminated histoplasmosis revealed that in 54 per cent of the patients, the organism was recovered from blood (Smith and Utz, 1972). Indirect evidence suggests that many, if not all, cases of primary pulmonary histoplasmosis disseminate hematogenously. Culture of both blood and bone marrow may assist in the diagnosis of disseminated histoplasmosis.

Clinically detectable *Aspergillus* fungemia is so rare that it is impossible to derive a meaningful account of the clinical manifestations of the fungemic period.

Rarely, cryptococci may be recovered from blood. In one series of 19 patients with different forms of cryptococcosis (ranging from isolated pulmonary infection to meningitis and disseminated disease), blood culture was positive in three patients (Lewis and Rabinovich, 1972). Again, data are too limited to construct a representative clinical picture for cryptococcal septicemia.

## DIAGNOSIS

Reviews of blastomycosis, sporotrichosis, mucormycosis, and coccidioidomycosis fail to demonstrate the occurrence of positive blood cultures. Widespread organ involvement and subcutaneous nodules (which are consistent with hematogenous spread rather than direct inoculation) suggest that these fungi disseminate hematogenously.

The diagnosis of fungemia is made by blood culture. Venting the routine blood culture bottles improves the rate of recovery of candida. The time required to detect growth of candida may be reduced by placing an aliquot of blood directly onto agar or into the Castaneda bottle, which contains a layer of agar on the side. Blood cultures for fungi should be held for at least 21 days to allow the slower growing organisms to become visible. A lysis of polymorphonuclear leukocytes may facilitate recovery of intracellular *Candida*. Experiments in dogs suggest that right atrial or arterial cultures may give a higher yield than peripheral venous cultures. Gas-liquid chromatography of the serum for mannose is being evaluated in *Candida* septicemia for rapid diagnosis. Radioimmunoassay techniques for the detection of *Candida* and *Aspergillus* antigen in serum are also under study.

In addition to culturing blood for fungi, a peripheral smear may help identify fungemia due to *Candida, Geotrichia,* and *Histoplasma.* Figure 2 shows candida in peripheral blood.

High or rising precipitin titers for *Candida* antigens in selected patients may help confirm the presence of disseminated candidiasis. However, the incidence of false-negative titers is high, especially in the terminally ill or severely immunocompromised patient, so that the value of the test is limited. Kozinn et al. (1976) have reviewed the value of *Candida* precipitins.

Because of the low rate of positive blood cultures, the diagnosis of a fungemia is often made only after complications of the disseminated form of the disease become evident.

## TREATMENT AND PROPHYLAXIS

The treatment for fungemias other than those caused by *Candida* and *Torula* is described in each chapter for the specific disseminated mycosis, because the fungemia is a manifestation of the disseminated infection.

In some patients with *Candida* and *Torula* septicemia, removal of the catheter is followed by clearance of *Candida* or *Torula* organisms from the blood, with no identifiable sequelae. However, in the severely immunocompromised patient (Young et al., 1974) or the complicated postsurgical patient, it is dangerous to assume that a catheter-associated fungemia is "benign" until proven otherwise. Some patients in whom the fungemia clears after removal of the catheter may have disseminated disease despite negative follow-up blood cultures. With any patient who has candidemia, whether or not it is associated with an indwelling polyethylene catheter, a thorough examination should be performed to detect both peripheral and deep organ involvement, and serial blood cultures should be obtained. If the

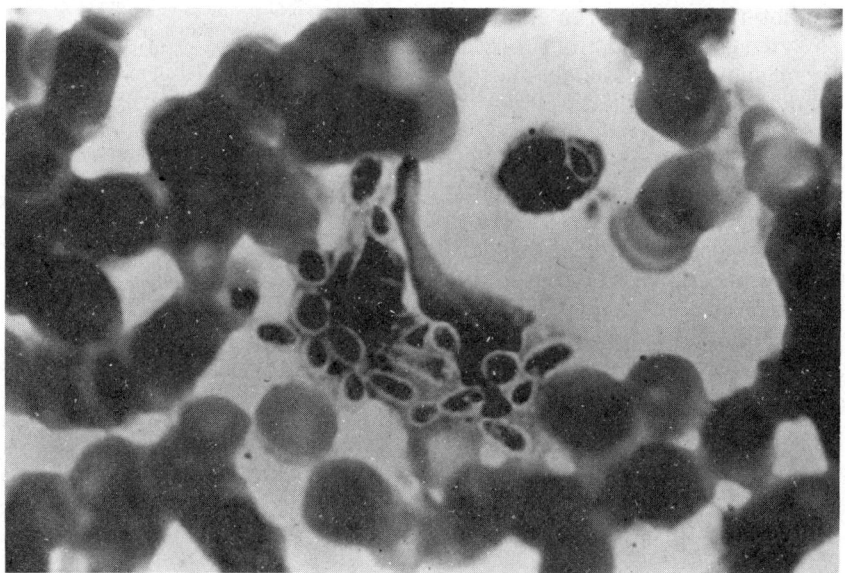

**FIGURE 2.**   Candida *in a peripheral blood smear. (Courtesy of Dr. Jack S. Remington.)*

**TABLE 1. Management of Candidemia Associated with Intravenous Catheters**

**AXIOM:** Vast majority of patients with catheter-associated candidemia have disseminated candidiasis.

**PLAN:**
1. Remove catheter.
2. If patient has inexplicable worsening course: Treat
3. If patient has stable course:
   a. Eliminate predisposing factors
   b. Complete evaluation:
      (1) Physical examination: eyes, blood smear, skin, bone, muscle, auscultation, neurologic
      Other studies: EKG, EMG, spinal tap (if indicated), muscle biopsy (if clinical myositis is present)
      (2) Serologic tests: Candida precipitins
      (3) Repeat blood cultures

If result is positive, treat; if negative, continue observation with extreme caution.

titers of *Candida* precipitins exceed 1:8 by counterimmunoelectrophoresis or if they are rising, dissemination rather than benign candidemia is more likely. However, since some patients, especially those who are terminally ill, may not be able to mount an antibody response during dissemination, a negative titer is of limited value. If the patient's course is inexplicably worsening, antifungal therapy should be initiated while a decision regarding the significance of the fungemia is made. An algorithm for the management of candidemia is diagrammed in Table 1.

Once the decision to treat has been made, several options are available. Because most *Candida* strains are highly susceptible to amphotericin B, this drug is the mainstay of therapy for candidemia and disseminated candidiasis. If the patient is deteriorating rapidly, the addition of 5-fluorocytosine (5-FC) to the regimen may help to achieve therapeutic antifungal levels sooner than the use of amphotericin B alone. In addition, the two drugs are synergistic for many *Candida* strains. The organism should be tested for susceptibility to 5-FC and to the synergistic action of 5-FC with amphotericin B. Many isolates of *Candida* are completely resistant to 5-FC on initial isolation, and others become resistant during therapy. The length of therapy and the total amount of medication necessary to treat disseminated candidiasis are unknown. A reasonable approach is to treat the patient wiht 0.5 mg/kg amphotericin B intravenously daily. A dose of 1.0 g 5-fluorocytosine every three hours can be added

if the organism is susceptible or if the course is fulminant. One or both drugs can be given until substantial clinical improvement is evident and then withheld as the patient is watched cautiously for recurrent signs of infection.

Minimizing the use of broad spectrum antibiotics, hyperalimentation catheters and fluids, steroids, and antineoplastic therapy will reduce the incidence of candidemia and perhaps *Torula* septicemia. Prophylactic oral nystatin may be useful in burn patients and postsurgical patients. However, its usefulness in the severely immunocompromised patient is not clear. Flushing intravenous lines with small quantities of amphotericin B has been attempted, but the value of that technique has not been established.

## References

Bodey, G. P., and Luna, M.: Skin lesions associated with disseminated candidiasis. JAMA 229:1466, 1974.

Butler, W. T., Alling, D. W., Spickard, A., and Utz, J. P.: Diagnostic and prognostic value of clinical and laboratory findings in cryptococcal meningitis. N Engl J Med 270:59, 1964.

Edwards, J. E., Jr., Foos, R. Y., Montgomerie, J. Z., Shaw, V., and Guze, L. B.: Ocular manifestations of *Candida* septicemia: Review of seventy-six cases of hematogenous *Candida* endophthalmitis. Medicine 53:47, 1974.

Fishman, L. S., Griffin, J. R., Sapico, F. L. et al: Hematogenous *Candida* endophthalmitis — a complication of candidemia. N Engl J Med 286:675, 1972.

Harford, C. G.: Postoperative fungal endocarditis. Fungemia, embolism, and therapy. Arch Intern Med 134:116, 1974.

Kozinn, P. J., Galen, R. S., Taschdjian, C. L., Goldberg, P. L., Protzman, W., and Kozinn, M. A.: The precipitin test in systemic candidiasis. JAMA 235:628, 1976.

Krause, W., Matheis, H., and Wulf, K.: Fungemia and funguria after oral administration of *Candida albicans*. Lancet 1:598, 1969.

Lewis, J. L., and Rabinovich, S.: The wide spectrum of cryptococcal infections. Am J Med 53:315, 1972.

Louria, D. B., Blevins, A., Armstrong, D., Burdich, R., and Lieberman, P.: Fungemia caused by "nonpathogenic" yeasts. Arch Intern Med 119:247, 1967.

Pankey, G. A., and Dalaviso, J. R.: Fungemia caused by *Torulopsis glabrata*. Medicine 52:395, 1973.

Sheehy, T. W., Honeycutt, B. K., and Spencer, J. T.: *Geotrichum* septicemia. JAMA 235:1035, 1976.

Smith, J. W., and Utz, J. P.: Progressive disseminated histoplasmosis. A prospective study of 26 patients. Ann Intern Med 76:557, 1972.

Stone, H. H., Kolb, L. D., Currie, C. A., Geheber, C. E., and Cuzzell, J. Z.: Candida sepsis: Pathogenesis and principles of treatment. Ann Surg 179:697, 1974.

Valdivieso, M., Luna, M., Bodey, G. P., Rodriguez, V., and Groschel, D.: Fungemia due to *Torulopsis glabrata* in the compromised host. Cancer 38:1750, 1976.

Winston, D. J., Balsley, G. E., Rhodes, J., and Linne, S. R.: Disseminated *Trichosporon capitatum* infection in an immunosuppressed host. Arch Intern Med 137:1192, 1977.

Young, R. C., Bennett, J. E., Geelhoed, G. W., and Levine, A. S.: Fungemia with compromised host resistance. Ann Intern Med 80:605, 1974.

# INFECTIVE 199
# ENDOCARDITIS AND
# OTHER INTRAVASCULAR
# INFECTIONS

*Lawrence R. Freedman, M.D.*

Intravascular infection is established when circulating microorganisms colonize platelet-fibrin vegetations covering altered vascular endothelium. Intravascular infection within the heart is referred to as infective endocarditis (IE). These infections occur in all parts of the world and affect approximately 60 per 1,000,000 persons per year.

There are few examples in medicine in which simple and inexpensive diagnostic methods are sufficient to indicate the presence of a lethal disease that can be cured with antibiotics. Nevertheless, despite the technical simplicity of diagnosis, many patients die or suffer the consequences of serious arterial embolization or heart valve damage because of a long delay in establishing the diagnosis or because the diagnosis is not thought of at all. Part of the reason for this delay is that the clinical picture is nonspecific and does not conform to the "classic textbook description" derived from observation of patients with long-established disease in the preantibiotic era.

Prevention of IE with antibiotics is theoretically possible in about 25 per cent of persons in whom the infection develops. However, patients at risk are often unaware of the need for antibiotic prophylaxis in the face of procedures known to induce bacteremia, and physicians and dentists often do not prescribe prophylactic measures despite having facts available that should have warranted their doing so.

So it is that merely having the information and the means available to prevent, diagnose, and treat potentially fatal illness does not ensure that the disease will be prevented, diagnosed, or treated correctly. In addition, several dramatic technical advances in medicine (chronic hemodialysis, cardiac surgery) have created a new population of patients who are at special risk for developing IE. It is no wonder that there is considerable interest in intravascular infections in the clinic and in the laboratory.

## DEFINITION

Infective endocarditis is a microbial infection of a platelet-fibrin vegetation located on the endo-thelial surface of the heart. Similar infections occur less frequently within the vascular system outside the heart: mycotic aneurysms, infections of aortic prosthetic grafts, infections of patent ductus arteriosus and coarctation of the aorta, and septic thrombophlebitis. The principles of pathogenesis, prevention, and treatment are similar for all of these infections.

It has been customary in the past to divide patients with infective endocarditis into categories of acute (malignant) and subacute (lente) endocarditis. The differences of clinical course and infecting microorganism (subacute, predominantly alpha-hemolytic streptococci; acute, staphylococci, pneumococci, gonococci), although statistically valid, overlap sufficiently to argue against continuing the distinction. The lethal complications of infection, aortic valve perforation or cerebral embolization, are frequent and may occur with any type of infection. It is therefore incumbent upon the physician to establish the diagnosis and begin treatment as soon as possible. The decision to begin treatment in the absence of definite proof of the diagnosis is not an easy one and will, of course, be influenced by the clinical state of the patient. However, the idea that a prolonged evolution in the past argues for a relatively benign evolution in the future is a dangerous premise on which to establish a therapeutic decision.

## PATHOGENESIS

The development of any intravascular infection depends upon the presence of a lesion of the vascular endothelium susceptible to infection, and the arrival at that lesion of sufficient organisms capable of establishing infection. Experimental studies have shown that the endothelial injury susceptible to infection may be so small as to escape detection. When endothelial damage was produced in rabbits by the mere placement of a plastic catheter within the heart chambers, the intravenous inoculation of only $10^3$ streptococci (viridans group) or staphylococci (*aureus* species) was sufficient to produce infection in 25 per cent of animals. (Larger inocula produce infection regularly under these circumstances.) Vegetations in the rabbit are more susceptible to infection with *Staphylococcus aureus* than with streptococci, and still less susceptible to infection with *Escherichia coli*. Although it is not clear how many factors influence the ability of bacteria to colonize such vegetations, one of them seems to be increased stickiness of those gram-positive cocci that produce dextran. Infections in the left side of the heart in rabbits achieve higher microbial populations than infections in the right heart and have a more severe "clinical" course; right heart infections are rarely fatal and often have an evolution leading to spontaneous sterilization (without antibiotics). In rabbits infection is much more difficult to establish in the vena cava or aorta than in the left heart (Freedman and Valone, 1979).

All of these experimental phenomena have their counterparts in human disease. In man, vegetations (or areas of endothelial damage) susceptible to becoming infected are found in the following conditions: rheumatic heart (valvular) disease, congenital heart disease (except for atrial septal defect, which rarely becomes infected), mitral valve prolapse (a forme fruste of Marfan's syndrome?), Marfan's syndrome, idiopathic hypertrophic subaortic stenosis, patent ductus arteriosus, coarctation of the aorta, peripheral arteriovenous fistulas (either on the fistula or in the heart), indwelling intravenous or intra-arterial plastic catheters or intracardiac pacemakers, prosthetic valve surgery, placement of prosthetic aortic grafts, and myocardial infarction.

Sterile valvular vegetations are frequent at autopsy in patients with cancer and in patients who had disseminated intravascular coagulation during life. These vegetations probably result from generalized hypercoagulability or valve damage by circulating immune complexes. In addition, unknown mechanisms induce susceptibility of heart valves to infection by chronic hemodialysis and intravenous drug usage.

It is often difficult to identify the source of bacteremia that initiates the infection because the number of bacteria required to induce infection may be too small to detect, since the first symptoms of IE may be too vague and insidious to pinpoint the onset of infection, and because there are so many causes of bacteremia that it is difficult to be certain of the relation between a particular bacteremia-producing event and the onset of infection.

Bacteremia often occurs after any procedure that breaks the normal mucosal or epithelial barrier. Bacteremia can occur after almost any dental treatment. It is more frequent with gingival disease and results from procedures as nontraumatic as tooth-brushing, gingival irrigation, nasotracheal suctioning, and chewing hard candy.

In the gastrointestinal tract, bacteremia is provoked by liver biopsy, gastroscopy, sigmoidoscopy, and barium enema. In the genitourinary tract, bacteremia has been documented during normal delivery, cesarian section, normal menstruation, and uterine dilatation and curettage. Urinary tract instrumentation and prostatectomy produce bacteremia. The risk is higher with established urinary tract infections. Virtually any procedure that involves cannulation of veins, arteries, or the heart can give rise to bacteremia. Particularly dangerous is total parenteral nutrition, from which 27 per cent of patients developed bacteremia in one series. Bacteremia can also arise from any local infection, especially if manipulated or incised, and from any severe infection in patients with impaired defense mechanisms. In many patients with infective endocarditis, no source of bacteremia is apparent.

Infective endocarditis is thought to develop frequently on normal heart valves. In the laboratory, normal endocardium is resistant to infection. It is often not possible, however, to rule out tiny underlying endocardial lesions; even at autopsy, the reason for the development of an impressive vegetation may not be apparent. Nevertheless, there is general agreement (and considerable clinical and experimental evidence to support the view) that infective endocarditis begins when circulating microorganisms colonize sterile vegetations covering a damaged endothelium.

The platelet-fibrin vegetation, once colonized by bacteria, grows quickly by the further deposition of platelets and fibrin, thus rapidly isolating the bacteria from the few polymorphonuclear leukocytes that might arrive from the vessels in the heart valve or from the circulation. *This "protection" of bacteria from phagocytic cells* is one of the most important features of the infection and creates, in fact, an infection in a *zone of localized agranulocytosis*. This phenomenon explains why cure of these infections requires prolonged administration of bactericidal antibiotics. Intensive antibiotic therapy may also be needed for the old bacterial colonies, at the base of infected vegetations that metabolize at a much slower rate than those on the surface. Thus, even bactericidal antibiotics that depend for their activity on active bacterial cell-wall synthesis are less effective in sterilizing these deep colonies than in sterilizing rapidly growing bacteria (Durack and Beeson, 1978).

At first, the vegetation remains fairly constant in size because of a balance between growth, resorption, and fragmentation. New surface growth of the vegetation is due to the continued deposition of circulating bacteria. Growth of the vegetation due to its continual reseeding is compensated for by resorption at its base or fragmentation and embolization. One of the hallmarks of these infections is *constant bacteremia* with little variation in the number of circulating bacteria over long periods of time.

There are four mechanisms by which these infections affect the patient:

1. *Constant bacteremia* produces fever, loss of appetite, anemia, splenomegaly, and metastatic infection.

2. *Local invasion* can produce disturbances of cardiac conduction, myocardial infarction, valve ring abscesses and pericarditis, mycotic aneurysm of the sinus of Valsalva, and valve perforation.

3. *Peripheral embolization* of fragments of infected vegetation are responsible for mycotic aneurysm formation and septic infarction of any organ. Most commonly, these emboli involve the brain, spleen, kidneys, bone, and myocardium. Abscesses in these organs may be a source of reinfection of the vegetation and consequent treatment failure. Emboli from mycotic vegetations are larger than in bacterial endocarditis and occlude major vessels.

4. *Circulating immune complexes* are another distinctive feature of infective endocarditis. Aside from patients with salmonellosis, brucellosis, leprosy, and quartan malaria, it is unusual to find viable bacteria in the bloodstream simultaneously with their specific antibody, yet this is the rule in infective endocarditis. The simultaneous presence of antigen (bacteria) and antibody leads to the formation of circulating immune complexes. In other infections the presence of antibody and the availability of polymorphonuclear leukocytes effectively block the shedding of bacteria into the blood. In infective endocarditis this mechanism is ineffective. Gram-negative bacteria, which are destroyed by antibody and complement without requiring leukocytes, can consequently establish persistent intravascular infection only rarely.

Circulating immune complexes probably cause petechiae, Osler and Janeway lesions, arthritis, and, most important, glomerulonephritis. Immune complexes may be detected as cryoprecipitates and stimulate antibody formation against globulins (rheumatoid factor).

## EPIDEMIOLOGY AND BACTERIOLOGY

The frequency of infective endocarditis and the types of bacteria isolated depend on the population under study. For example, in Western Europe and North America, streptococci (excluding group A) and staphylococci account for about 90 per cent of the infecting microorganisms. In Nigeria, on the other hand, streptococci are rarely recovered from patients with infective endocarditis.

In narcotic addicts with endocarditis, infections with certain organisms tend to cluster in different cities in the United States. *Staphylococcus aureus* is prevalent in some areas, enterococci in others, and *Pseudomonas aeruginosa* in others. The explanation for this is not clear, since specific microorganisms are not found in the drugs or equipment used for injections in specific geographic locations. In addicts with *S. aureus* infections, skin and mucous membranes were often colonized with the infecting bacteria, thus suggesting that they spread to the heart from the carrier sites.

Although streptococci and staphylococci are the most common causes, almost any bacteria can infect a susceptible intravascular site including, rarely, tubercle bacilli, meningococci, *Brucella* spp., and rickettsiae. *Candida albicans* and *Aspergillus* spp. have produced such infections but viruses and cell-wall–defective bacteria have not been proved to cause infective endocarditis in man. *Candida* endocarditis occurs mainly in drug addicts and recipients of prosthetic heart valves. *Candida albicans* and *Candida parapsilosis* are the main species of *Candida* involved in endocarditis and also always require underlying valve injury to cause infection of the heart. For this reason, nearly all cases of *Candida* endocarditis in addicts affect the mitral or aortic valves, in contrast to staphylococci, which often attack the right side of the heart.

Extracardiac intravascular infections are frequently caused by bacteriologic contamination during surgery or accidental trauma. *Salmonella* spp. are among the most common bacteria recovered from spontaneous infections of abdominal aortic aneurysms. The explanation for this peculiar predilection is not known, since *Salmonella* very rarely cause infective endocarditis.

Recovery of more than one bacterial species from the blood of patients with infective endocarditis, although unusual, is being reported with increasing frequency. The antibiotic sensitivities of bacteria recovered in these "double infections" may differ considerably, thus complicating the choice of antibiotics and the evaluation of bactericidal drug activity in the serum.

## PROPHYLAXIS

Although it would appear to be a simple matter to prevent infective endocarditis, the problem is complex (Everett and Hirschmann, 1977; Kaplan et al., 1977; Sipes et al., 1977; Sternon, 1975). If one starts with those patients given a diagnosis of endocarditis, about 50 per cent are unaware of any cardiac abnormality or predisposing condition, and about 50 per cent (probably more) have no evident source of bacteremia. Thus, with our present understanding of the disease, it would be possible to prevent only about 25 per cent of identified cases.

Many patients in apparent good health have "innocuous" heart murmurs — should they be protected? In a recent study of "normal" young women, between 6 and 28 per cent were considered to have mitral valve prolapse, regarded by some authorities as the underlying lesion in one-third of patients with infective endocarditis and mitral valve insufficiency.

Another problem is to decide against which organisms to direct antibiotic prophylaxis. For example, it is customary to cover high risk of infection by staphylococci after open heart surgery with prophylactic penicillins that are resistant to $\beta$-lactamase. The only studies of the efficacy of this prophylaxis found no difference between treated and nontreated patients except for infections in the treated group that were resistant to the antibiotics administered.

Finally, there is no evidence in man that prophylactic antibiotics work, even for reasonably well-defined procedures involving dental manipulations. The low frequency of infection and the ethical impossibility of withholding antibiotics from susceptible patients prevent investigation of the problem.

Nevertheless, despite these difficulties and unknown factors, there is general agreement that prophylactic antibiotics should be given to patients subjected to procedures described below. The patients are those with a history of infective endocarditis, valvular heart disease, prosthetic valves or aortic grafts, coarctation of the aorta, patent ductus arteriosus, and, perhaps, prolapse of the mitral valve.

It is astonishing how often patients with known heart disease are not aware of the risk of developing infective endocarditis and of the recommendations for prophylactic antibiotics. It is equally astonishing how infrequently dentists ask their patients about a history of heart disease. Some patients who have developed endocarditis of prosthetic heart valves after dental extraction believed that their heart surgery eliminated the risk of endocarditis. This problem was not discussed by their physicians and they were not told, at least for a while, that the risk of endocarditis is probably greater than before operation and that the risk will always remain.

The following procedures increase the risk of endocarditis:

1. *Oropharyngeal procedures,* such as dental extraction, dental prophylaxis, oral surgery, and rigid-tube bronchoscopy. The frequency of bacteremia varies after these procedures, but it is generally detected in 30 to 80 per cent of patients. The bacteria recovered from the blood are those resident in the mouth, especially various streptococci.

2. *Urologic procedures,* such as instrumentation or catheterization of the urethra and prostatectomy. The frequency of bacteremia varies between about 10 and 80 per cent of patients, the higher rates being seen with established urinary infections. The urinary tract is considered to be the portal of entry in about 50 per cent of patients with group D streptococcus endocarditis.

3. *Gastrointestinal procedures,* such as sigmoidoscopy, upper GI tract endoscopy, barium enema, colonoscopy, and liver biopsy. About 10 per cent of patients undergoing these examinations develop bacteremia. The bacteria in the blood may be any of those in the normal bowel flora. After barium enema and sigmoidoscopy, blood cultures often reveal enterococci.

4. *Gynecologic procedures,* such as normal pregnancy, uterine dilation and curettage, and cesarian section. The frequency of bacteremia in these patients is reported to be low. Nevertheless, obstetric and gynecologic procedures are believed to be the source of group D streptococcal endocarditis in about 20 per cent of patients. The problem of defining the indications for antibiotic prophylaxis is well illustrated by considering the procedure of insertion of an intra-uterine device. Although no bacteremia was detected in one group of 84 patients, in others with infective endocarditis it is highly probable that insertion of an IUD was the source of infection.

The choice of antibiotics will depend on the probability that certain bacteria will cause bacteremia after a given procedure. The dose of antibiotics has not been established by studies in man. There are two clues that past recommendations are inadequate. One such clue is the failure of prophylaxis in a number of patients and another is the failure of recommended doses for man to prevent infective endocarditis in rabbits. The problem is complicated, and the recommendations of the American Heart Association for antibiotic prophylaxis in the prevention of infective endocarditis have recently been revised (Table 1).

The basic prophylaxis for dental procedures and surgery of the upper respiratory tract is either penicillin or penicillin plus streptomycin. Parenteral antibiotics are preferred. Regimen A or B is recommended for patients with congenital, rheumatic, or other acquired heart disease. Regimen C is recommended in these instances for patients allergic to penicillin. Regimen B is recommended for patients with prosthetic heart valves, and for these patients Regimen D in the case of allergy to penicillin. These recommendations are intended to prevent infection with non–group A streptococci. For instrumentation and surgery of the genitourinary or gastrointestinal tract, at which time enterococcus bacteremia might be provoked, the recommendation is to administer penicillin plus gentamicin or streptomycin, or ampicillin plus gentamicin or streptomycin. For patients allergic to penicillin, vancomycin plus streptomycin is recommended.

## CLINICAL FINDINGS

Infective endocarditis may produce symptoms related to any organ, with or without fever, and with or without evidence of heart disease. Symptoms range from vague complaints of poor health to those of an acute illness of the central nervous system. Many patients are referred to the hospital for possible intestinal cancer, or arthritis, or back pain. The nonspecific symptoms in these patients are the reason why the interval between the onset of symptoms and diagnosis is usually several weeks and often many months.

The clinical findings are related to bacteremia (fever, weight loss, anemia, splenomegaly), local invasion of the infection (valve perforation, congestive heart failure, cardiac arrhythmias), peripheral emboli (symptoms of embolization, infarction, abscess formation, any mycotic aneurysm), and circulating immune complexes (skin lesions, arthritis, glomerulonephritis) (Kaye, 1976; Sternon, 1975; Weinstein and Schlesinger, 1974).

Patients usually have fever and a heart murmur, but other signs of infective endocarditis may be absent. Fever may be slight or absent in 5 to 15 per cent of patients. Similarly, there may be no heart murmur (about 15 per cent of patients). But absence of both fever and heart murmur is exceedingly rare. A changing quality of systolic

**TABLE 1.   Prophylaxis of Infective Endocarditis***
(Risk of infection with non–group A streptococci from the upper respiratory tract)

| DRUG | TIME OF ADMINISTRATION | PREPARATION† | DOSE |
|---|---|---|---|
| A. Penicillin (parenteral-oral) | Before procedure 30 min to 1 hr | ACPG + PPG | 1,000,000 units I.M. 600,000 units I.M. |
| | After procedure every 6 hr for 8 doses | PV | 500 mg orally |
| OR: Penicillin (oral) | Before procedure 30 min to 1 hr | PV | 2.0 g orally |
| | After procedure every 6 hr for 8 doses | PV | 500 mg orally |
| B. Penicillin + Streptomycin | Before procedure 30 min to 1 hr | ACPG + PPG + streptomycin | 1,000,000 units I.M. 600,000 units I.M. 1.0 g I.M. |
| | After procedure every 6 hr for 8 doses | PV | 500 mg orally |
| C. Patients Allergic to Penicillin (parenteral-oral) | During procedure over 30 min to 1 hr | vancomycin | 1.0 g I.V. (start 30 min to 1 hr before procedure) |
| | After procedure every 6 hr for 8 doses | erythromycin | 500 mg orally |
| D. Patients Allergic to Penicillin (oral) | 1½–2 hr before procedure | erythromycin | 1.0 g orally |
| | After procedure every 6 hr for 8 doses | erythromycin | 500 mg orally |

*For details concerning these recommendations and for children's dosages, see Kaplan, E. L., et al.: A. H. A. Committee Report: Prevention of bacterial endocarditis. Circulation 56:139A, 1977.

†ACPG — aqueous crystalline penicillin G; PV — penicillin V (phenoxymethyl penicillin); PPG — procaine penicillin G.

heart murmurs is unusual and to be expected only in exceptional cases. Even when present this finding is often difficult to interpret.

The murmur of aortic insufficiency is easily recognized, and may be an ominous prognostic sign. Clubbing of the fingers, Osler's nodes, retinal "Roth spots," and Janeway lesions (Table 2) are unusual today. Migrating polyarthritis and osteomyelitis are seen occasionally.

The laboratory findings are seldom helpful (except for blood cultures). There may be an anemia without reticulocytosis, an elevated titer of rheumatoid factor, decreased levels of complement, circulating immune complexes, and cryoglobulinemia. There may be laboratory findings associated with infarctions or abscess in any organ and, of course, the findings in the blood (azotemia) and urine (hematuria, red cell casts, proteinuria) typical of glomerulonephritis. In addition, patients may develop the clinical syndrome of disseminated intravascular coagulation.

### DIAGNOSIS

*The diagnosis of infective endocarditis depends on the culturing of bacteria from the blood.* It is necessary to obtain cultures aerobically and anaerobically. *Bacteria may be cultured from the blood in this infection in the absence of fever.* Since there is insignificant filtration of bacteria in the peripheral circulation, there is no advantage in obtaining cultures from arterial blood — venous blood is satisfactory. Occasionally, special culture techniques are necessary to cultivate fungi or mycobacteria and microorganisms with peculiar nutritional requirements. In infections due to *Coxiella burnetti* (Q fever), serologic evidence of infection is essential for diagnosis.

Because of the constancy of the bacteremia in infective endocarditis, three to five blood culture pairs (aerobic and anaerobic) are sufficient to establish the diagnosis in about 90 per cent of patients who will ever have a positive blood culture. Occasionally, it takes several days, and rarely, weeks, for the microorganisms to be detectable in blood cultures.

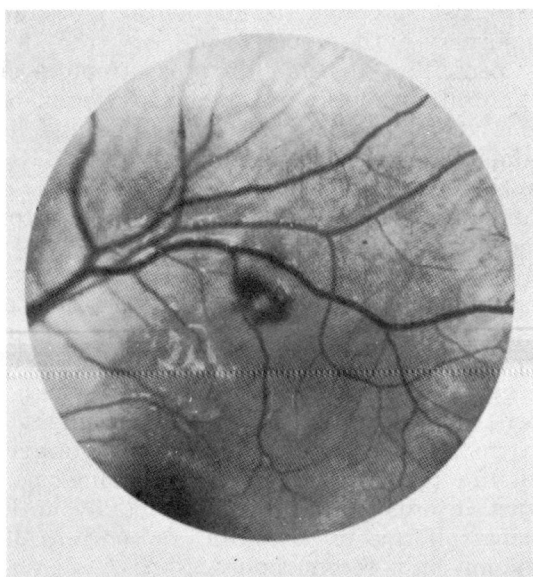

**FIGURE 1.** *Roth spot (hemorrhage with white center) in a patient with subacute bacterial endocarditis. (From Cogan: Ophthalmic Manifestations of Systemic Vascular Disease, W. B. Saunders Co., 1974.)*

A certain number of patients have infective endocarditis detected at autopsy in whom it was not possible to culture microorganisms from the blood during life. This may be due to several phenomena:

1. Prior administration of antibiotics. The administration of even small quantities of antibiotics may suppress bacterial growth (without sterilization of the lesion) in the vegetation for prolonged periods of time. We have recently followed a patient whose daily blood cultures were sterile for 12 days after the administration of a few doxycycline tablets. Blood cultures became consistently positive from the thirteenth day onward. The practice of treating febrile illnesses with antibiotics without undertaking bacteriologic studies to establish the nature of the infection is generally to be condemned.

2. Infection with peculiar microorganisms whose

### TABLE 2.  Comparison of Small Focal Lesions
### Characteristic of Endocarditis

| LESION | LOCATION | |
|---|---|---|
| Osler node | Pads of fingers and toes, thenar or hypothenar eminence, soles | Raised, *tender*, discolored (bluish, pink, or red), pea sized. Last several hours to several days |
| Janeway lesion | Palms or soles | Small area of erythema or hemorrhage, sometimes raised but *never* painful |
| Roth's spots (Fig. 1) | Retina | Round hemorrhage with white center near disk |

growth needs are not satisfied by "routine" culture media. Examples are tubercle bacilli, *Coxiella burnetti*, and vitamin $B_6$-dependent streptococci.

3. The biology of the infection. Infections on the right side of the heart are occasionally accompanied by negative blood cultures. Blood cultures in patients with infections of the abdominal aorta are negative about 50 per cent of the time. Experiments in rabbits show that the density of bacterial populations in these locations is lower than in vegetations in the left side of the heart. This could explain the negative blood cultures in these clinical circumstances.

4. Rarely, infective endocarditis is seen at autopsy for which none of the above explanations for negative blood cultures is applicable.

*Echocardiography* may provide evidence of vegetations on heart valves. Vegetations do not necessarily indicate infection, since nonbacterial thrombotic endocarditis, found frequently in patients with cancer, may produce a clinical picture very similar to that of infective endocarditis, but with negative blood cultures. A negative echocardiogram does not rule out vegetations.

*Heart antibodies* occur with infective endocarditis, but it is not yet clear how useful these will be in diagnosis.

*Radioactive scanning* of the heart after administration of technetium-99-labeled pyrophosphate or after injection of radioactive-labeled antibodies to the infecting organism has been useful in the laboratory, but has not yet been applied to human infections.

## DIFFERENTIAL DIAGNOSIS

Infective endocarditis may mimic a wide variety of disorders and may be superimposed on underlying unrelated disease. The clinical features of infective endocarditis may not be distinguishable from those of nonbacterial thrombotic endocarditis (often seen in patients with cancer), atrial myxoma, or endothelial tumors. The presence of circulating immune complexes, cryoglobulinemia, rheumatoid factor, hypocomplementemia, and arteritis in skin biopsy has led to the mistaken diagnosis of collagen-vascular disease and treatment of patients with endocarditis with adrenocortical steroids.

Any febrile patient with clinical evidence of glomerulonephritis should be suspected of having endocarditis. In the aged the diagnosis may be exceptionally difficult, and some authors have gone so far as to recommend culturing the blood of any elderly person who doesn't feel well.

A difficult problem arises in the interpretation of positive blood cultures without other signs of infective endocarditis. In these instances it is necessary to try to determine the source of the bacteremia. Even when a peripheral source for bacteremia is evident, it is possible that the peripheral infection is secondary to endocarditis.

## TREATMENT

The principles of antibiotic treatment in infective endocarditis are determined by two important features of the pathologic lesion: (1) the ineffective participation of polymorphonuclear leukocytes and (2) the decreased metabolic activity of bacteria located at the base of infected vegetations.

The vegetation of infective endocarditis can be considered a zone of "localized agranulocytosis," so that bactericidal antibiotics are needed to sterilize the lesions. Treatment of infective endocarditis with bacteriostatic antibiotics may suppress clinical signs and symptoms, but signs of infection invariably reappear when antibiotics are discontinued. In view of the lowered metabolic activity of bacteria buried in vegetations and in view of the dependence of penicillin upon bacterial cell-wall synthesis, it is not surprising that even bactericidal antibiotics must be administered for prolonged periods of time.

Benzyl penicillin is the mainstay of treatment for streptococcal endocarditis and a $\beta$-lactamase–resistant penicillin for staphylococcal endocarditis. Drugs for the treatment of less common infections are selected according to in vitro antibiotic sensitivities.

It is not a simple matter to know when to start antibiotic treatment if the causative organism has not been isolated from the blood. If the clinical diagnosis is clear, therapy can be started immediately after obtaining three to five blood cultures. If the patient has already received antibiotics and the clinical diagnosis is uncertain, it may be advisable to wait up to several weeks in an effort to identify the causative microorganism. These are decisions that require judgment; the risk of blind treatment without an established diagnosis or sensitivities of the organism must be weighed against the risk of sudden cerebral embolism or valve perforation.

It is relatively easy to judge response to treatment when there is prompt disappearance of fever, reduction in size of the spleen, cessation of new skin petechiae, and increase in general well-being. On the other hand, low-grade fever (often due to drug hypersensitivity) commonly persists throughout treatment. It is important, therefore, to examine indirect indices of the effectiveness of treatment: reticulocyte response in anemic patients, decrease in titer of rheumatoid factor, and decrease in circulating immune complexes. Unfortunately, none of these changes is conclusive evidence of response, nor is absence of change a conclusive argument for lack of response. As a rough guide to effective antibiotic treatment it is common practice to adjust antibiotics so as to achieve a peak bactericidal effect in vitro with a dilution of serum of at least 1/4 to 1/8. This is easily achieved with infections with streptococci of the viridans type, and bacteriologic cure is the rule. Experimental studies have substantiated this relation in viridans streptococcal infections. In staphylococcal infections, however, it is frequently impossible to achieve in vitro evidence of satisfactory bactericidal levels in the serum and yet such patients may also be cured bacteriologically. Despite experimental evidence suggesting the usefulness of serum bactericidal levels as a guide to proper therapy, conclusive proof is lacking that this relation holds in man.

Some infections do not respond to antibiotics despite in vitro effectiveness as measured by sensitivity testing. For example, the treatment of endocarditis due to *Candida* and other fungi is unsatisfactory, and infections on prosthetic valves are usually impossible to sterilize without removal of the valve (Duma, 1977). It may be necessary to observe patients for several years after the treatment of fungal endocarditis to be certain that the infection has been eradicated. *Candida* endocarditis should be treated postoperatively with 8.0 g 5-fluorocytosine orally, daily, and 40 mg amphotericin B every other day. The 5-fluorocytosine should be continued for six weeks and the amphotericin B for a total dose of 1200 mg.

In contrast to the uncertainty regarding the effectiveness of antibiotics in the prophylaxis of infective endocarditis, there is no question regarding their effectiveness in treatment of the established infection. Choice of antibiotic depends, obviously, on the bacteria or fungi recovered from the bloodstream. The relapse rate in this disease can be related inversely to the duration of treatment with effective antibiotics.

Many reports appear in the literature on the successful use of antibiotics for short periods of time in small numbers of patients. These reports are useful in indicating which antibiotics can work, but they do not tell us how regularly they work. For example, the relapse rate after a two-week penicillin-streptomycin treatment of penicillin-sensitive ($< 0.1$ $\mu$g/ml-MIC) viridans streptococcus infections is between 6 and 10 per cent. After four weeks of treatment no relapses are reported. Clearly, two weeks of this treatment program can work, but four weeks works better. The life-threatening consequences of this infection are such that antibiotics should be administered so as to reduce to a minimum (zero, if possible) the rate of relapse. Antibiotics should be administered parenterally. There are reports of the successful use of oral antibiotics in patients

with infective endocarditis, but the uncertainties of intestinal absorption of large quantities of antibiotics would seem to introduce a dangerous element of uncertainty in the treatment of a lethal disease. If long-term intravenous or intramuscular therapy cannot be pursued, oral treatment can be substituted, with frequent monitoring of serum bactericidal activity.

A major cause of death in infective endocarditis is congestive heart failure due to aortic valve perforation. We do not know whether treatment that sterilizes a valve more rapidly is more likely to prevent dangerous local complications. Nevertheless, it is logical to assume that the most rapid sterilization of valves is one of the goals of therapy. For this reason, treatment programs have been adjusted recently to take into consideration experimental data in rabbit endocarditis that show that for penicillin-sensitive streptococcal and staphylococcal infections, the addition to a penicillin of an aminoglycoside that is synergistic in vitro significantly speeds the sterilization of the valve.

Although there is no conclusive evidence that this occurs in man, the following recommendations take into consideration data derived from experimental studies.

*Penicillin-sensitive viridans streptococci (MIC $< 0.1$ $\mu$g/ml)*: penicillin, 10 to 20 million units I.V.; or 1.6 million units (procaine penicillin) I.M. every six hours for four weeks, plus streptomycin, 0.5 I.M. every 12 hours for two weeks.

*Other streptococci (MIC $\geq 0.1$ $\mu$g/ml + enterococci)*: penicillin, 20 million units I.V. for six weeks, plus streptomycin, 1.0 g I.M. every 12 hours (or 0.5 g every six hours) for two weeks, then 0.5 g I.M. every 12 hours (or 0.25 g every six hours) for four weeks.

In the case of vestibular or auditory impairment, streptomycin may be discontinued after four weeks for the treatment of penicillin-resistant streptococci. Cephalosporins should not be used for the treatment of penicillin-resistant streptococci, since clinical results have been unsatisfactory.

*Staphylococci sensitive to penicillin (MIC $< 0.1$ $\mu$g/ml)*: as for penicillin-sensitive streptococci, but with administration of 20 million units of penicillin and continuing treatment for six weeks.

*Other staphylococci (penicillinase producers)*: methicillin, oxacillin, or nafcillin 2 g every four hours I.V. for six weeks plus gentamicin, 3 to 5 mg/kg I.M. daily in three divided doses every eight hours for two weeks.

There is disagreement whether aminoglycosides are necessary for penicillin-sensitive streptococcal or staphylococcal infection and many authorities do not recommend their use. In the case of penicillin allergy, it is possible to substitute vancomycin, 0.5 g I.V. every six hours. Some authors believe cephalothin or cefazolin should be given to patients with penicillin allergy because they feel these cephalosporins are as effective in staphylococcal endocarditis as $\beta$-lactamase–resistant semisynthetic penicillins. It is difficult to evaluate the relative effectiveness of different antibiotics in staphylococcal endocarditis, since comparative clinical studies have not been done. In addition, many patients with staphylococcal endocarditis reported in the literature had right heart infection due to intravenous narcotic usage; the likelihood is that infections in the right heart are easier to sterilize than those in the left heart. It may thus not be possible to translate the results of treatment of right heart infections to infections of the left heart.

In circumstances where streptomycin or gentamicin is recommended, it is reasonable to substitute tobramycin or amikacin according to in vitro sensitivity tests. Antibiotic dosages should be adjusted to avoid toxic blood levels and still obtain peak serum bactericidal concentrations of 1/8.

The treatment of endocarditis due to other microorganisms is determined by the antibiotic sensitivities demonstrated in vitro. As a general rule, it is desirable to associate an aminoglycoside with a penicillin (or cephalosporin). In *Pseudomonas* endocarditis, carbenicillin is given in a dose of 2.5 g I.V. every two hours with gentamicin, 100 mg I.V. every six hours. When antibiotic treatment must be initiated in the absence of a bacteriologic diagnosis, the regimen chosen is that for treatment of either enterococcal or penicillin-resistant staphylococcal infection.

*Anticoagulants* have no place in the treatment of infective endocarditis. On the other hand, there is no contraindication to their use for other reasons in patients receiving proper antibiotic treatment for infective endocarditis. Patients with prosthetic heart valves receiving long-term anticoagulant treatment may experience difficulties in the regulation of their anticoagulants as an initial sign of the presence of infective endocarditis. It is generally felt that the risk of discontinuing anticoagulants in these patients exceeds that of continuing them during antibiotic treatment.

Whereas in the pre-antibiotic era virtually all patients died of infection, today it is exceptional not to be able to sterilize intravascular vegetations. Mortality, on the other hand, remains between 0 to 5 per cent and 30 to 40 per cent depending on the patient population under study. Factors of obvious importance to the outcome of treatment include age, associated disease, alcoholism, drug addiction, severity and nature of underlying heart disease, and embolic complications. Although there is variation from one series to another, valve perforation (and resulting congestive heart failure) and neurologic complications are among the most serious.

Valve perforation with resultant congestive heart failure is usually an indication for surgical replacement of the damaged valve with a prosthesis. This complication may occur as late as one week after the institution of antibiotic therapy and has been noted in about 25 per cent of patients with streptococcal endocarditis. Surgery is lifesaving in such patients, and is successful even when carried out within hours of starting antibiotic therapy. It is desirable, however, to delay surgery as long as possible in order to achieve maximal antibiotic effectiveness before exposing the prosthetic valve to possible infection.

In patients with prosthetic heart valves who develop infective endocarditis, it is usually but not always necessary to replace the valve in order to eliminate the infection. Antibiotics without surgery are often successful in patients who acquire endocarditis many months or years after insertion of a prosthetic valve, and whose infection is caused by a drug-sensitive organism. Mortality is considerable when such infections require surgery. In some patients, osteomyelitis or splenic abscess may serve as a source of reinfection of heart valves after antibiotic therapy is completed.

In rare patients with severe renal insufficiency due to immune complex glomerulonephritis renal function does not improve despite sterilization of the intravascular infection. Immune complexes have been found to persist in the circulation of these patients, an indication for their removal by plasmapheresis.

If the patient cannot withstand heart surgery, he can be treated effectively with continuous suppressive drug therapy given orally or even intramuscularly. Dicloxacillin, for example, can be given in doses of 1.0 g three times daily for suppression of staphylococcal bacteremia in patients with inoperable endocarditis.

## References

Duma, R. J.: Infections of Prosthetic Heart Valves and Vascular Grafts. Baltimore, University Park Press, 1977.

Durack, D. T., and Beeson, P. B.: Pathogenesis of Infective Endocarditis. In Rahimtoola, S. H. (ed.): Infective Endocarditis. New York, Grune and Stratton, 1978.

Everett, E. D., and Hirschmann, J. V.: Transient bacteremia and endocarditis prophylaxis — a review. Medicine 56:61, 1977.

Freedman, L. R., and Valone, J.: Experimental infective endocarditis. Prog Cardiovasc Dis 22:169, 1979.

Kaplan, E. L., Anthony, B. F., Bisno, A., Durack, D., Houser, H., Millard, H. D., Sanford, J., Shulman, S. T., Stillerman, M., Taranta, A., and Wenger, N.: A.H.A. Committee Report: Prevention of bacterial endocarditis. Circulation 56:139A, 1977.

Kaye, D.: Infective Endocarditis. Baltimore, University Park Press, 1976.

Sipes, J. M., Thompson, R. L., and Hook, E. W.: Prophylaxis of infective endocarditis: A reevaluation. Ann Rev Med 28:371, 1977.

Sternon, J.: Les endocardites bactériennes de l'adulte. Clinique, anatomie pathologique, thérapeutique et prophylaxie. Paris, Masson et Cie, 1975.

Weinstein, L., and Schlesinger, J. M.: Pathoanatomic, pathophysiologic and clinical correlations in endocarditis. N Engl J Med 291:832, 1974.

# 200 *MYOCARDITIS AND PERICARDITIS*

*A. Martin Lerner, M.D.*

Infections and inflammation within the myocardium, endocardium, or pericardium are always a potential threat to life that may develop during systemic infections or as a primary focus of infection. The major infectious causes of myopericardial dysfunction in the United States are enteroviruses, certain pyogenic bacteria, *Mycobacterium tuberculosis,* and a few fungi.

## *ETIOLOGIC AGENTS*

### Enterovirus

Enteroviruses, pyogenic bacteria, *Mycobacterium tuberculosis,* and fungi *(Candida, Aspergillus)* are the most important infectious causes of myopericarditis, but the heart and pericardium may also be involved in many systemic infections (Table 1) (Fowler and Monitsas, 1973). Available data, however, indicate that enteroviruses are the dominant cause of so-called "idiopathic" myopericarditis. Because of difficulties inherent in diagnosing enteroviral infections, the incidence of enteroviral infections is probably greatly underestimated. Over a 6-year period, Grist and Bell at the Regional Virus Laboratory (Ruchill Hospital, Glasgow, Scotland) examined sera from 385 patients with suspected heart disease (Grist and Bell, 1974). On the basis of their studies of type-specific neutralizing antibodies, they suggested that coxsackieviruses belonging to Group B accounted for at least half of the cases of acute myocarditis and an additional one-third of the cases of acute nonbacterial pericarditis. These cases occurred throughout the year, but fewest cases were found in the first quarter, and most in the second and third quarters of the year. This incidence corresponds to the seasonal distribution of enterovirus infections. Serologic results inferred that (compared with coxsackieviruses) influenza viruses, adenoviruses, *Chlamydia,* Q fever, and *Mycoplasma pneumoniae* contributed few cases.

In order to sharpen the criteria for the diagnosis of enteroviral myopericarditis, we have proposed the following scheme for evaluating diagnostic criteria (Lerner et al., 1975).

1. High Order Associations (H).

   A. Virus is isolated from the myocardium, endocardium, or pericardial fluid; or
   B. Type-specific virus is localized in the myocardium, endocardium, or pericardium at sites of pathologic change by methods of immunofluorescence or peroxidase-labeled antibody. These studies may be possible only at autopsy. Specimens must be properly taken and stored ($-50°$), but cannot be placed in formalin.

   H-order associations are strengthened if virus isolated from the myocardium produces similar heart disease in an experimental model (for example, mouse).

2. *Moderate-Order Associations (M):* (moderate probability of a true positive diagnosis).

   A. Virus is isolated from pharynx or feces, and a fourfold rise in type-specific neutralizing, hemagglutinating-inhibiting, or complement-fixing antibodies is demonstrated; or
   B. Virus is isolated from pharynx or feces, and a concomitant titer in serum of 1/32 or greater of type-specific immunoglobulin M (IgM) (mercaptoethanol-sensitive) neutralizing or hemagglutinating-inhibiting antibodies is demonstrated.

   The evidence used to establish a moderate-order association (M) can attain a higher order of probability (H) if significant numbers of appropriate controls do not show the findings of 2A or 2B.

3. Low-Order Associations (L).

   A. Virus is isolated from pharynx or feces; or
   B. A fourfold rise in type-specific neutralizing, hemagglutinating-inhibiting, or complement-fixing antibodies is demonstrated; or
   C. A single serum shows a titer of 1/32 or greater of type-specific IgM (mercaptoethanol-sensitive) neutralizing or hemagglutinating-inhibiting antibodies.

   A low-order association (L) can attain a higher (moderate) order of probability if significant numbers of appropriate controls do not

**TABLE 1.   Infectious Causes of Myopericarditis**

| | |
|---|---|
| **VIRUSES**<br>Adenoviruses<br>Cytomegalovirus<br>Enteroviruses (coxsackieviruses, Groups A and B, echoviruses, polioviruses)<br>Epstein-Barr virus<br>Hepatitis A virus<br>Herpes simplex viruses, Type 1 and Type 2<br>Influenza viruses A and B<br>Lymphocytic choriomeningitis virus<br>Mumps virus<br>Rubella virus<br>Vaccinia virus<br>Varicella-zoster virus | **FUNGI**<br>*Actinomyces israelii*<br>*Aspergillus* sp.<br>*Blastomyces dermatitidis*<br>*Candida* sp.<br>*Coccidioides immitis*<br>*Cryptococcus neoformans*<br>*Histoplasma capsulatum*<br>*Nocardia asteroides*<br>*Sporothrix schenckii* |
| **PYOGENIC BACTERIA**<br>*Corynebacterium diphtheriae*<br>*Neisseria gonorrhoeae*<br>*Neisseria meningitidis*<br>*Pasteurella (Francisella) tularensis*<br>*Pseudomonas pseudomallei*<br>*Staphylococcus aureus*<br>*Streptococcus pneumoniae*<br>*Streptococcus pyogenes*<br>Various aerobic gram-negative bacilli<br>*Bacteroides* and *Peptostreptococci* | **PARASITES**<br>*Echinococcus granulosus*<br>*Entamoeba histolytica*<br>*Plasmodium* sp.<br>*Schistosoma* sp.<br>*Toxoplasma gondii*<br>*Treponema pallidum*<br>*Trichinella spiralis*<br>*Trypanosoma cruzi* |
| **MYCOBACTERIA**<br>*Mycobacterium chelonei*<br>*Mycobacterium tuberculosis* | **RICKETTSIA**<br>*Rickettsia burnetii*<br>*Rickettsia mooseri*<br>*Rickettsia rickettsii*<br><br>**OTHER**<br>*Chlamydia psittaci*<br>*Mycoplasma pneumoniae* |

show the findings of 3A, 3B, or 3C. For instance, a CF titer $>1/32$ is more suggestive of a recent infection if $<5$ per cent age-matched controls have titers $\geq 1/32$.

Only high-order associations can be accepted as firm evidence for a viral infection as the etiology of myopericarditis.

High-order associations with acute myocardiopathies have been established in man for coxsackieviruses Group A, Types 4 and 16; coxsackieviruses Group B, Types 1, 2, 3, 4, 5, and 6; and echoviruses, Types 9, 11, and 22 (Table 2). Lower degrees of evidence are available for coxsackieviruses Group A, Types 1, 2, 5, 8, and 9; and echoviruses, Types 1, 4, 6, 7, 14, 16, 19, 25, and 30. Therefore, we conclude that coxsackieviruses belonging to Group B (Types 1 through 6) are established causes of virus myocardiopathy. There are also data implicating certain coxsackieviruses belonging to Group A and some echoviruses (Table 2). Coxsackieviruses may cause 23 per cent of acute virus myocardiopathies (Bell and Grist, 1968). No estimate of the proportion of cases due to echoviruses is available (Bell and Grist, 1970).

A characteristic postvaccinial myopericarditis has been observed 10 to 14 days after primary smallpox vaccination. Severe local reactions have occurred, but generalized vaccinia is not accompanied by heart disease. When congestive heart failure ensues, it responds dramatically to corti-costeroids, digoxin, and diuretics without sequelae (Matthews and Griffith, 1974).

### Bacteria

Significant changes in the incidence of several bacterial pathogens in purulent pericarditis were shown in an 86-year review of autopsy experience with 200 patients at the Johns Hopkins Medical institutions by Klacsmann, Bulkley, and Hutchins (Klacsmann et al., 1977). They studied 145 patients with purulent pericarditis at Johns Hopkins from 1889 through 1943 (Group 1) and compared them with 56 patients admitted since 1943 (Group 2). The median age of patients in Group 1 was 22 years, but it was 49 years in the later period. Whereas 80 per cent of the cases formerly were caused by aerobic, gram-positive cocci *(Streptococcus pneumoniae, Staphylococcus aureus, Streptococcus pyogenes),* these organisms accounted for 44 per cent of the cases since 1943. On the other hand, gram-negative bacilli *(E. coli, Proteus* sp., and *Pseudomonas aeruginosa, Salmonella* sp., *Shigella* sp., *Neisseria meningitidis)* were 39 per cent in Group 2, but only 5 per cent in Group 1. This remarkable increase in the occurrence of gram-negative bacilli in Group 2 was due to more infections with *E. coli, Proteus,* and *Pseudomonas.*

### Mycobacteria

The number and percentage of cases of tuber-

**TABLE 2. Coxsackieviruses or Echoviruses Associated with Acute Phase of Virus Myocardiopathy**

| ENTEROVIRUS | ORDER OF ASSOCIATION* |
|---|---|
| Coxsackieviruses A | |
| Types 1 | L, M |
| 2 | L, M |
| 4 | H |
| 5 | L, M |
| 8 | L, M |
| 9 | L, M |
| 16 | H |
| Coxsackieviruses B | |
| Types 1 | H |
| through 6 | |
| Echoviruses | |
| Types 1 | L, M |
| 4 | L, M |
| 6 | L, M |
| 7 | L, M |
| 9 | H |
| 11 | H |
| 14 | L, M |
| 16 | L, M |
| 19 | L, M |
| 22 | H |
| 25 | L, M |
| 30 | L, M |

*L = low; M = moderate; H = high.

culous pericarditis varies with the prevalence of tuberculosis in the region. There are rare postoperative infections of the pericardium and mediastinum due to rapid growing mycobacteria—for example, *M. chelonei.*

### Fungi

*Candida* and *Aspergillus* pericarditis occur in immunocompromised patients receiving cancer chemotherapy (Franklin et al., 1976). *Histoplasma capsulatum* uncommonly causes pericarditis either as an isolated infection or as part of disseminated disease.

## PATHOGENESIS AND PATHOLOGY

The anatomy of the pericardium has an influence on both the pathogenesis of infection and the physiologic consequences of infection. The parietal pericardium separates the heart and proximal segments of the main vessels (aorta, pulmonary artery and veins, superior and inferior vena cava) from surrounding mediastinal tissues. A central tendon fuses the diaphragm with the pericardium. Laterally, *the parietal pericardium* is separated by pleura from the external surface of the lungs. On each side, a phrenic nerve passes vertically between the membranes of pleura and pericardium. The *visceral pericardium* is continuous with interstitial tissues of the myocardium. The

pericardial sac normally contains 15 to 20 ml of clear fluid (Hipona and Paredes, 1976).

A fine capillary endomyocardial lymphatic system arises in the endocardium and interstitial areas of the myocardium and condenses into collecting channels subjacent to myocardial fibers. Lymphatic channels coalesce to form tertiary lymphatic vessels, or lymphatic trunks, which again join at the epicardium in a septal lymphatic system. The subepicardial tissues, therefore, have a diffuse lymphatic network.

Lymph flows from endocardial and interstitial myocardium to epicardial lymphatics, and, finally, to tracheobronchial lymph nodes in the mediastinal collecting system. The parietal pericardium has no lymphatics (Kline, 1969; Miller, 1970; Cohen, 1976; Drinker and Field, 1931).

### Pathologic Physiology of Pericardial Effusion

Blockade of lymphatics in the mediastinum *plus* epicardium causes pericardial effusion. Impedance of venous drainage from the heart at the coronary sinus facilitates formation of pericardial effusion. Isolated mediastinal lymphatic obstruction causes pleural effusion but not pericardial effusion.

### Pathologic Anatomy

*Virus Pericarditis.* Usually, both pericardium and myocardium are simultaneously affected (myopericarditis). Clinically, there may be predominantly myocarditis or pericarditis. The acute process may be benign with a mixed inflammatory response limited to interstitial areas of the heart and indistinguishable from acute rheumatic fever with carditis (Fig. 1). In benign myopericarditis, muscle-cell necrosis is minimal and recovery is anatomically and physiologically complete. An intervening ventricular arrhythmia can lead to death, but this is unusual. Virulent infections have varying degrees of interstitial myocarditis and myocardial cellular necrosis (Fig. 2). Lesions heal with permanent scar and sometimes with myocardial calcification. Virus-induced myocardial necrosis is indistinguishable from that of myocardial infarction secondary to coronary atherosclerosis and thrombosis (Woods et al., 1975). Of course, in virus myocarditis, coronary arteries and veins are patent, and vasculitis is absent. Coronary atherosclerosis does not prevent, however, supervening virus myocarditis.

The special tropism of enteroviruses for the human heart is virus-specific and age-specific. These viruses attach as the result of specific interaction between outer capsid viral protein and enterovirus receptors on cell membranes. The subunit structure of the outer protein capsid (capsomeres) determines species, tissue, and age specificities

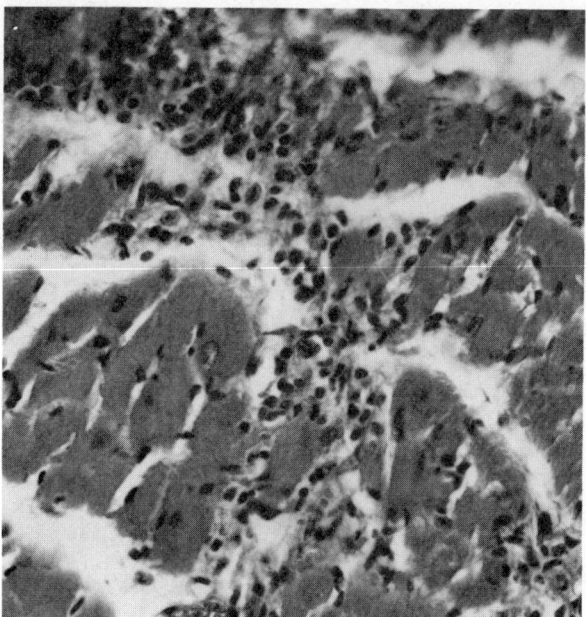

**FIGURE 1.** *Benign coxsackievirus A9 myocarditis (acute infectious phase of myocardiopathy). With this virus strain, complete healing occurs without sequela; there is no late noninfectious phase. Myocarditis was induced by coxsackievirus A9, strain 711, in 8-month-old Swiss mice by intraperitoneal inoculation of $10^5 TCD_{50}$. An area of moderate focal inflammation was seen after 9 days. (Reprinted from Progress in Medical Virology, by permission.)*

for infection, as well as antigenicity. Enterovirus receptors on cell membranes are present in limited number ($1$ to $10 \times 10^4$ per cell). Coxsackievirus B all share the same receptor, but this is distinct from the poliovirus receptor. Adenoviruses Types 2 and 5 also share the coxsackievirus B receptor (Lonberg-Holm et al., 1976).

Infections with enteroviruses are common. By adult life, most people in the United States have neutralizing antibodies to many of the viruses. Contagium spreads from person to person by the fecal-oral route. (Transplacental spread of coxsackievirus and echoviruses also occurs). Spread to the heart is presumably hematogenous and occurs at about 5 per cent of all symptomatic coxsackievirus infections.

Once myopericarditis is established, it may be a progressive infection leading to death (especially in newborns), or it may be self-limited, or relapsing. There is both clinical and experimental evidence to suggest that the inflammatory reaction is due to an immunopathologic process (Wilson et al., 1969). During the early stages of the infection in the mouse model of myopericarditis, viruses are shed from the cell surface through vacuoles that fuse with the plasma membrane. Virus is discharged from infected cells as they lyse. Later in the process, myonecrosis results

from the activity of cytotoxic T-lymphocytes; B-lymphocytes and macrophages do not play an important role (Lerner, 1969; Wong et al., 1977).

There is evidence that stress, such as forced swimming, enhances viral virulence, especially with coxsackievirus B3. The myocardium transforms into a wholly necrotic, inflamed, calcified mass (Fig. 3). This is accompanied by increased replication of the virus (Fig. 4). (Gatmaitan et al., 1970). The mechanism of this reaction to stress is unknown, but interferon production is delayed. Exercise is also a potent immunosuppressive agent (Reyes and Lerner, 1976). Adrenal corticoids also exacerbate infection, and stress may act through that mechanism. Additional adverse influences on experimental myocarditis include genetic susceptibility of mice, pregnancy, male sex, and undernutrition (Grodums, 1972). Whether these factors contribute to human infection is not known.

*Pyogenic Pericarditis.* Acute purulent pericarditis induces a thickened (8 to 12 mm) pericardium usually containing 500 to 2000 ml of viscid fibrinous or frankly yellow purulent exudate and granulation tissue under varying degrees of tension. The left lower lung may be adhering to the thoracic wall. Pericardium is often adherent to myocardium and covered with "cottage-cheese–like" material. On the other hand, there may be a fibrinous granulomatous pericarditis and no free fluid (Liedtke et al., 1976; Cameron, 1975; Das and Ray, 1976).

*Bacteria.* Most adult patients developing pyogenic pericarditis today have chronic underlying conditions or diseases (for example, recent thoracic surgery, chronic renal failure, carcinoma, myocardial infarctions, diabetes mellitus, myeloproliferative disorders, or sickle cell anemia) (Liedtke et al., 1976). In contrast to the preantibiotic era, primary infectious diseases in patients without underlying diseases account for only 22 per cent of the cases of purulent pericarditis since 1943 at the Johns Hopkins Medical Institutions. Pneumonia, meningitis, otitis media, subacute bacterial endocarditis, skin infections, and endometritis are primary infections that can spread to the pericardium. Extension of infection from the lung to the pericardium is now less common (20 per cent of cases versus 64 per cent before 1943), but perforating injury to the chest wall (for example, surgery, trauma) as a cause of pericarditis increased to 24 per cent from 4 per cent. Rupture of myocardial abscess, embolization from acute endocarditis, and extension from a subdiaphragmatic suppurative lesion are other routes of infection. Some patients with meningococcemia develop pericarditis 4 to 16 days after treatment begins. The exudate is sterile, and symptoms respond to anti-inflammatory drugs. This condition

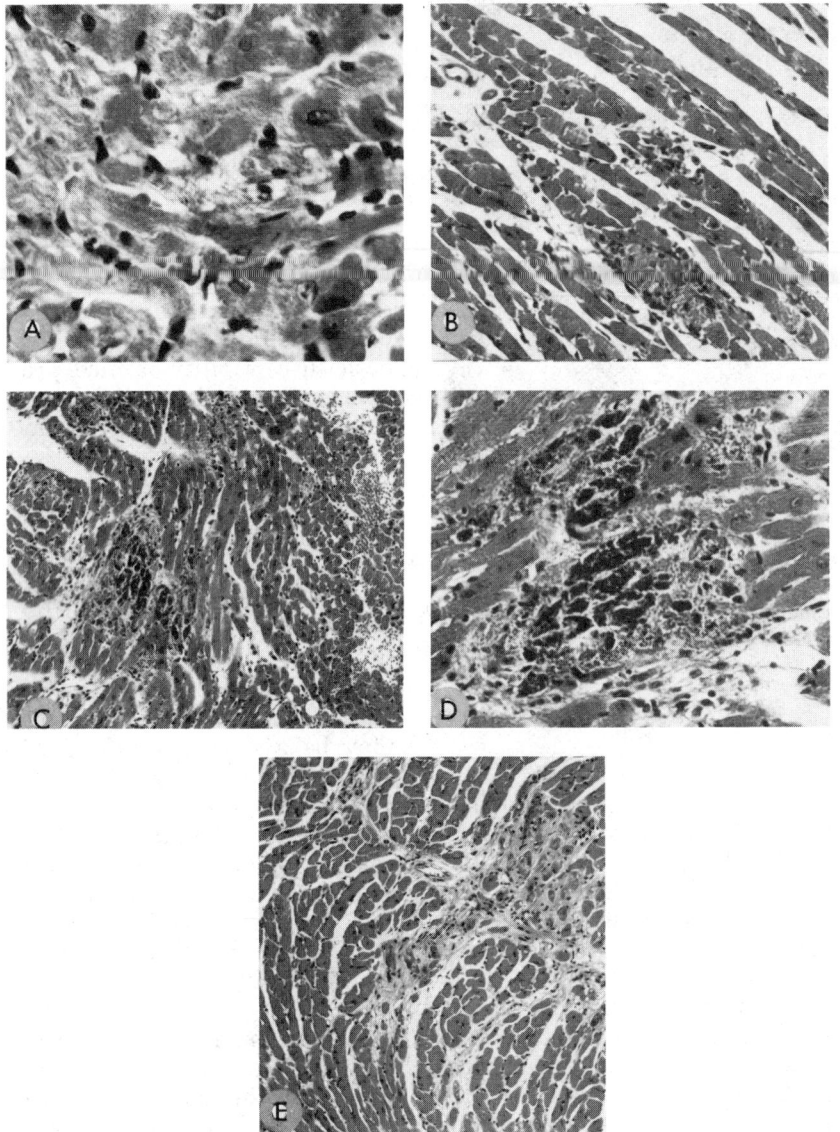

**FIGURE 2.** *Pathologic changes in coxsackievirus B-3 myocarditis are shown. All sections were stained with hematoxylin and eosin. (Reprinted from* The American Journal of Pathology, *by permission.)*

*A, Isolated eosinophilic changes in muscle fibers in myocardium of an 18-day-old weanling mouse on day 3 of infection. Pathologic areas have darkened homogeneous staining along mid-left margin and right upper corner of section (× 415).*

*B, Sixth day of infection in a 22-day-old mouse. A pale, necrotic myocardial fiber is infiltrated and surrounded by mononuclear cells. An adjacent fiber is undergoing advanced eosinophilic changes (× 415).*

*C, Ninth day of infection in a 26-day-old mouse. There is fine and coarse mineralization of necrotic myocardial fibers. Clusters of pale necrotic fibers with mononuclear cells are also present (× 90).*

*D, Higher magnification of same area as in Figure 2C (× 225).*

*E, Day 126 of infection in a 141-day-old mouse. A fibrotic scar is shown containing residual myocardial fibers. Some of the latter show early mineralization (× 90).*

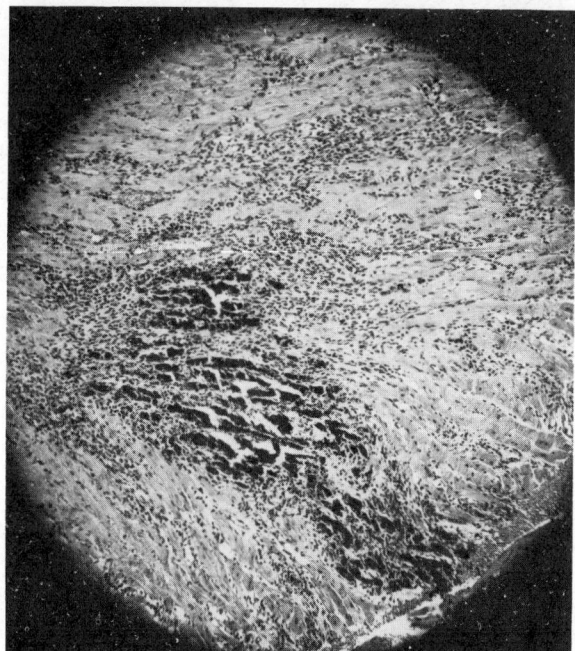

**FIGURE 3.** *Effect of swimming on pathologic findings in acute coxsackievirus B3 myocardiopathy. The extensively involved myocardium of a 27-day-old mouse on the thirteenth day after infection is shown (HE × 90). (Reprinted from Progress in Medical Virology, by permission.)*

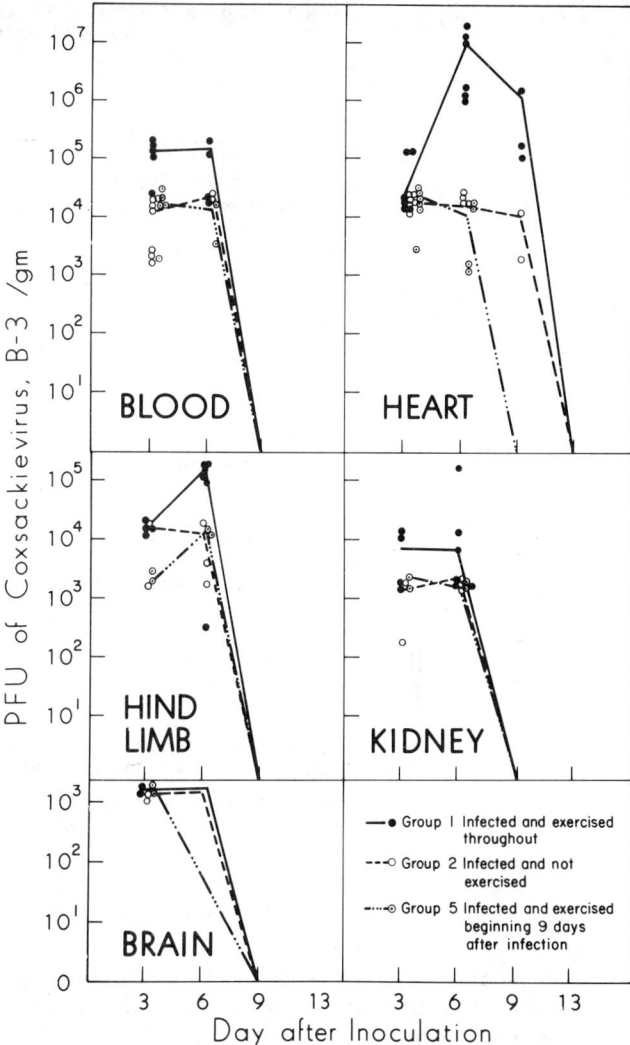

**FIGURE 4.** *Effect of swimming on multiplication of coxsackievirus B3 in several tissues. (Reprinted from Progress in Medical Virology, by permission.)*

is believed to represent a hypersensitivity response to bacterial antigens (Morse et al., 1971).

*Fungus Myopericarditis.* These systemic infections often complicate cancer chemotherapy. The heart as well as the kidneys, gastrointestinal tract, lungs, brain, liver, and thyroid are often simultaneously affected. Opportunistic *Candida* and *Aspergillus* species are the most frequent. Myocardial abscesses are uniformly present. Palpable 3 to 15 mm white-yellow nodules with or without hyperemic borders distribute themselves randomly through both ventricles. Fibrinous pericarditis may also occur.

If histologic secretions are stained with periodic acid-Schiff or silver-methenamine stains, microcolonies of fungi can be seen in the pericardial and myocardial abscesses. Depending upon the patient's underlying disease, the inflammatory response varies from none to marked acute suppuration. Microcolonies may also infiltrate between myocardial fibers. Myocardial fibers can show coagulative necrosis. Coronary vessels occasionally are invaded by pseudohyphae *(Aspergillus),* but valves remain free (Franklin et al., 1976).

## CLINICAL MANIFESTATIONS
(Table 3)

Irrespective of the infectious agent, the symptoms and signs are similar, except that, in bacterial myopericarditis, they are generally more dramatic than in viral. In cases ascribed by Sainani, Dekate, and Rao to coxsackieviruses B, Types 2, 3, 4, or 5; dyspnea (16 of 19 patients); pain in the chest (15 of 19 patients); and malaise and fever (12 of 19 patients) were common, but cough, myalgia, arthralgia, preceding upper respiratory infections, nausea, vomiting, or diarrhea occurred in only a minority (Sainani et al., 1975).

**TABLE 3.** Clinical Findings in Pyogenic Pericarditis and Coxsackievirus
B Myopericarditis

| | PYOGENIC*† (PER CENT) | COXSACKIE- VIRUS B* (PER CENT) |
|---|---|---|
| SYMPTOMS/SIGNS | | |
| Acutely ill (toxic, fever, dyspnea) | 100*† | 58 |
| Raised jugular venous pulse | 100 | 21 |
| Enlarged cardiac dullness | 100 | 74 |
| Adynamic pericardium | 100 | 11 |
| Muffled heart sounds | 94 | 11 |
| Hepatomegaly | 94 | 21 |
| Paradoxic pulse | 88 | 11 |
| Cardiac tamponade | 88 | 0 |
| Pleural effusion | 56 | 5 |
| Pericardial friction rub | 38 | 26 |
| Ascites | 31 | 0 |
| Pitting edema | 25 | 5 |
| Apical systolic murmur | 10 | 68 |
| | | |
| LABORATORY | | |
| Polymorphonuclear leukocytosis | 100 | 74 |
| Enlarged cardiac silhouette | 100 | 74 |
| Abnormal EKG (low voltage; ↓ST, ↑ST segments) | 100 | 100 |
| Arrhythmia | rare | common |
| Pericardiocentesis with isolation of bacterium or virus from fluid | 100* | rare |
| Pericardial fluid | exudate | usually exudate |

*Estimates of occurrence of symptoms/signs are made from the following references: Klacsmann et al., 1977, and Sainani et al., 1975.

†Isolation of etiologic organism is routine prior to therapy. This is possible in only about 40% of cases of tuberculous pericarditis.

All patients with pyogenic pericarditis have toxic signs and become acutely ill with anorexia, fever, chills, and chest pain. Physical findings also help differentiate pyogenic pericarditis from virus myopericarditis. Raised jugular venous pulsations (16 of 16 patients); adynamic pericardiums with impalpable apical pulses (16 of 16 patients); muffled heart sounds (15 of 16 patients); hepatomegaly (15 of 16 patients); paradoxic pulses (14 of 16 patients); and cardiac tamponade (14 of 16 patients) are the striking physical findings of pyogenic pericarditis (Klacsmann et al., 1977). Pleural effusions (9 of 16 patients), ascites (5 of 16 patients), and pitting edema (4 of 16 patients) are also more common in purulent pericarditis. None of these signs are common in coxsackievirus, Group B myopericarditis.

Pericardial friction rubs are heard to the left of the midsternal border while the patient is sitting up, leaning forward, and not breathing. The rubs are accentuated during inspiration or expiration and may be mono-, di- or tri-phasic, corresponding to atrial or ventricular systole or early ventricular diastole. At phonocardiogram, systolic murmurs or clicks may be detected. Pericardial or pleuropericardial friction rubs are often also palpable (Spodick, 1971).

The heart may not be enlarged in patients with cardiac disability that results from virus cardiomyopathies. Further, there may be no pericardial rubs, no arrhythmia, no congestive heart failure, questionable ischemic myocardial pain, and no congestive heart failure. However, systolic time intervals may be prolonged, indicating myocardial dysfunction. The latter tests, along with usual observations (clinical findings, EKG, chest x-ray, phonocardiogram, echocardiogram), should be used to follow convalescent patients (Weissler, 1974). Cardiac catheterization is needed to confirm pulmonary embolization or restrictive/constrictive cardiomyopathies before decisions are made to perform pericardial drainage or decortication.

## DIAGNOSIS

### Microbiologic Diagnosis

In human enterovirus infections, virus often multiplies in the heart when the same virus is no longer recoverable from pharynx or feces, the initial sites of infection. When acute myocardiopathy is discovered, antibody titers may already have risen. On the other hand, if a chronic myocardiopathy has been induced, replicating virus may not even be present in the heart at the time of clinical presentation. The etiologic diagnosis of a virus myocardiopathy is difficult.

Criteria for the diagnosis of enterovirus myopericarditis have been outlined (see *Etiologic Agents*). Rhesus-kidney tube cultures and intraperitoneal inoculations of suckling mice are best for isolation of enteroviruses from throat or rectal swabs, blood, or pericardial fluid. Enteroviruses are rarely recovered from pericardial fluid. Pyogenic pericarditis is proved by isolation of the causative bacteria at pericardiocentesis or from blood cultures. Tubercle bacilli are isolated from pericardial fluid in about 40 per cent of cases. Gram, acid-fast, and methenamine silver stains of pericardial exudates must be examined.

### Serologic Diagnosis

Within 3 days after onset of a virus myocardiopathy, IgM neutralizing antibodies are often found in sera, but, when bloods are taken several weeks later, fourfold rises in titers are often not demonstrable. IgM antibodies normally disappear from sera about 39 days later. Considerable cross-reacting IgM neutralizing antibody occurs among the coxsackievirus B serotypes. Schmidt, Magoffin, and Lenette demonstrated IgM antibody to Group B coxsackieviruses in 27 per cent of 148 patients with pericarditis, 25 per cent of 92 patients with myocarditis, and 8 per cent of 259 controls taken from age- and place-matched patients with pneumonia (Schmidt et al., 1973). The data were not diagnostic in the individual patient. These are M-order associations.

Chances for demonstrating significant increases in neutralizing antibodies to enteroviruses are greatly reduced if the titer in the acute-phase serum is 1/32 or greater. Neutralizing-antibody responses are highly type-specific in primary or initial infections with any of the five immunotypes of Group B coxsackievirus. However, in subsequent infections heterotypic responses occur with increasing frequency, and presumably arise from a booster effect of the current infecting virus on the level of antibodies to other enteroviruses with which the individual has previously been infected. Titers of heterotypic antibody frequently exceed those of homotypic antibody. Neutralizing antibodies to Group B coxsackievirus, Types 1 through 5, are frequently found at titers of 1/64 to 1/512 in patients without other evidence of current coxsackievirus infections. The prevalence of neutralizing antibody at these high residual titers precludes diagnosis on the basis of elevated neutralizing antibody in the absence of a fourfold or greater increase in titer. The finding of IgM antibodies is a reliable indicator of recent infection but does not preclude heterotypic reactions that may be of greater magnitude. However, even in initial infections with coxsackievirus, complement-fixing antibodies are invariably 7S immunoglobulins. Antibodies to heart muscle, γ globulins bound to the myocardium, decreases in serum complement, and biologic false-positive serologic tests for syphilis have occasionally been found in patients with idiopathic myocardiopathies.

### Other Laboratory Findings

Electrocardiograms in purulent and coxsackievirus B myopericarditis show low voltage and ST segment elevation and/or depression. On the other hand, left ventricular hypertrophy, systolic murmurs, and arrhythmias (sinus bradycardia, atrial fibrillation, complete heart block, and low voltage) are more frequent in the virus myopericarditis. Leukocytosis, an enlarged cardiac silhouette, and an elevated erythrocyte sedimentation rate are frequent in both acute pyogenic and virus pericarditis.

*Radiography.* (Echocardiogram, Isotopic Scan, Angiocardiogram, Pericardiocentesis with Contrast Material).

A sonolucent space on echocardiograph (ultrasound) separating the ventricular wall motions from nonmoving pericardial echo indicates pericardial effusion. Echocardiograms validate the presence of significant pericardial effusion, but a negative examination does not exclude significant effusion. In fact, a pericardiocentesis has relieved severe cardiac tamponade after an echocardiogram failed to reveal a diagnostic sonolucent space.

Intravenous radioisotope (technetium-99 bound to serum albumin or technetium-99 per technetate) outlines the intracardiac blood pool, and this is compared with the cardiac silhouette at chest x-ray. At angiocardiography, the distance between the endocardial surface of a cardiac chamber and its adjacent pericardial/pleural lung surface is determined.

At pericardiocentesis, contrast material may be injected directly into the pericardial sac.

### Pericardiocentesis

Pericardiocentesis has the risk of hemopericardium and cardiac tamponade. This procedure is most safe when done by a cardiothoracic surgeon in the operating room with electrocardiographic monitoring, and with advice and inoculations for culture/stains of pericardial fluids by physicians with special competence in infectious diseases.

## COMPLICATIONS

The possible courses that enteroviral myopericarditis infection may take are diagramed in Fig-

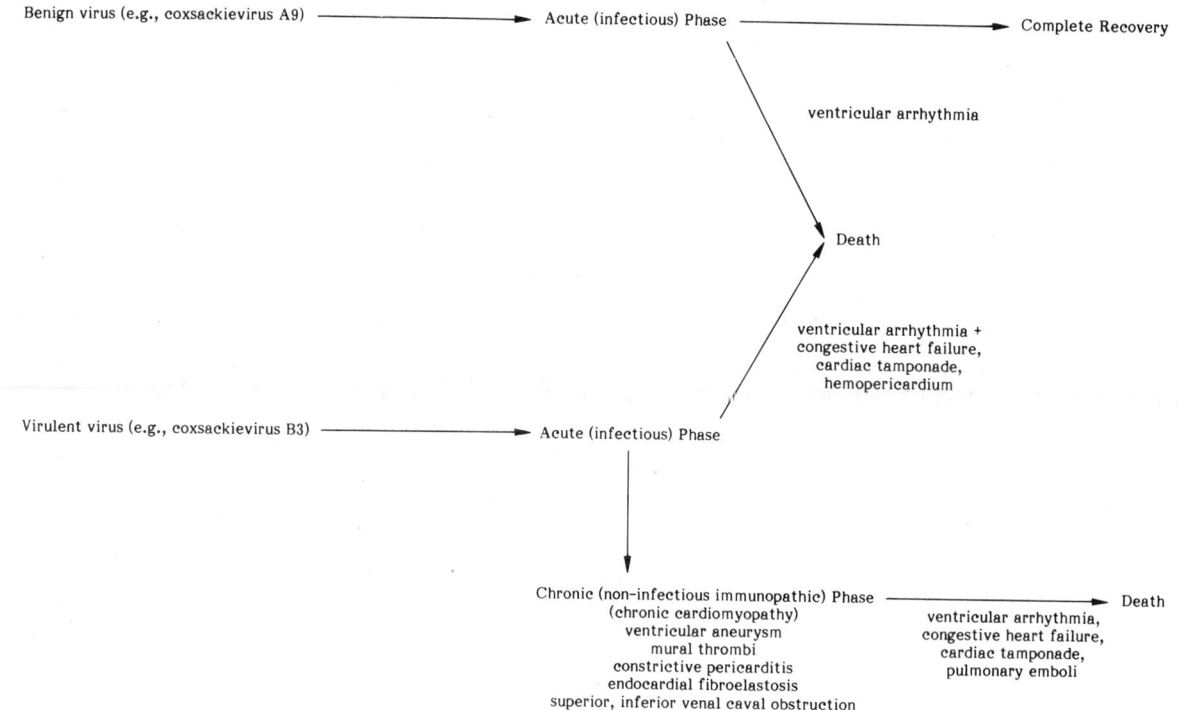

**FIGURE 5.** *Possible courses of coxsackievirus murine myocardiopathy.*

ure 5. This scheme is based on clinical observations and data obtained from experimental murine infections. The histologic lesion produced in mice as the result of coxsackievirus B3 infections is shown in Figure 2. This produces permanent myocardial injury (Wilson et al., 1969) that may progress to a cardiomyopathy. The mild, focal infection produced by coxsackievirus 49 (Fig. 1) does not progress to congestive failure.

Roberts and Ferrans described idiopathic cardiomyopathies as (1) dilated and (2) hypertrophic (Roberts and Ferrans, 1975). In hypertrophic cases, the ventricular septum is often thicker than the free ventricular wall. There is indirect (low-order) serologic evidence that both forms may result from enteroviral infection. Some cases of myocarditis may affect the subendocardium (for example, mumps), resulting in endocardial fibroelastosis (St. Geme, Jr., et al., 1966).

The prognosis in purulent bacterial pericarditis is good if the specific etiologic diagnosis is made early and proper therapy instituted. At follow-up several months after treatment ended, only 3 of 16 patients had died, and those that recovered had no residua (Klacsmann et al., 1977).

Tuberculous pericarditis can progress to fibrosis and calcification. This process causes constrictive pericarditis, which ultimately results in myocardial failure.

## TREATMENT

### Purulent Pericarditis

Purulent pericarditis is a medical and surgical emergency because of the tendency for cardiac tamponade and shock to develop rapidly. Pericardial drainage by pericardiostomy is rarely sufficient (Das and Ray, 1976). Decortication is usually necessary in order to drain adequately the otherwise closed space and to prevent the development of adhesive pericarditis and later constriction. Antibacterial therapy for 4 to 6 weeks (Table 4) is necessary. Local instillation of antibiotics into the pericardial sac is not indicated.

### Tuberculous Pericarditis

This complication of tuberculosis is treated with the same antituberculous agents that are used to treat pulmonary infection. However, adrenal corticosteroids are also indicated and should be given promptly. They promote the reabsorption of the effusion and reduce the risk of constrictive pericarditis (Rooney et al., 1970). If the diagnosis is not made until constrictive pericarditis has already developed, then surgical excision of the fibrotic pericardium is required. Pericardiectomy may actually precipitate left ventricular failure in patients who have had longstanding pericardial constriction.

**TABLE 4.  Treatment of Enterovirus Myopericarditis and Purulent  Pericarditis**

| ETIOLOGIC AGENT(S) | TREATMENT | |
| | Medical | Surgical |
| --- | --- | --- |
| Enterovirus myopericarditis | Acute phase (first 14 days of disease). Avoid: corticosteroids, anti-coagulants, exercise, alcohol. Use: digitalis, diuretics, anti-arrhythmic agents.* Chronic phase (after 14 days of disease). Corticosteroids (see text); otherwise as for acute phase | Pericardiocentesis† Pericardiocentesis† or pericardiectomy† |
| **Purulent Pericarditis** Gram-positive cocci *Staphylococcus aureus* *Streptococcus pneumoniae* *Streptococcus pyogenes* | Penicillin G: 30,000,000 u/day, I.V. (for 4 to 6 weeks) or Methicillin, 1.5 g I.V., q 4 h (for 4 to 6 weeks) with resistant staphylococci | Tube drainage†/ decortication†/ pericardiectomy† |
| Gram-negative bacilli *Esch. coli, Proteus, Enterobacter, Pseudomonas* | Two appropriate antibiotics: carbenicillin, 20 to 30 g/day, I.V. (for 4 to 6 weeks) gentamicin, 3 to 5 mg/kg/day, I.V. in 3 divided doses‡ (for at least 2 weeks) amikacin, 15 mg/kg/day, I.V. in 2 divided doses (for at least 2 weeks). cephalothin, 1.5 g q 4 h I.V. (for 4 to 6 weeks) ampicillin, 1.5 g q 4 h, I.V. (for 4 to 6 weeks) | Tube drainage†/ decortication†/ pericardiectomy† |
| Hemophilus influenza b | ampicillin, 400 mg/kg/day chloramphenicol, 100 mg/kg/day | |
| Fungi *(Aspergillus, Candida)* | Amphotericin B, 20 to 45 mg/kg/day I.V. (for 10 weeks) | Tube drainage†/ decortication†/ pericardiectomy† |
| *Mycobacterium tuberculosis* | Corticosteroids (see text) plus two of the following: isoniazid, 300 mg/day (for 2 years) ethambutol, 15 to 25 mg/kg/day (for 2 years) rifampin, 600 mg/day (for 2 years) | Tube drainage†/ decortication†/ pericardiectomy† |

*Use for congestive heart failure or arrhythmia.

†Use for cardiac tamponade/or constrictive pericarditis.

‡Watch for oto- or nephrotoxicity especially after second week of treatment.

### Enterovirus Pericarditis

No specific therapy is available. Once the diagnosis is suspected, patients are treated exactly as are patients with myocardial necrosis due to coronary atheromatous disease. Those without evidence of muscle necrosis should rest for about 30 days; others with destruction of muscle should rest for 3 months or more. Arrhythmias, congestive failure, angina-like pain, and cardiomegaly are all poor prognostic signs. Alcohol, strenuous exercise, and reserpine should be avoided during convalescence.

Adrenal corticosteroids are avoided during the acute infectious phase (about the first 14 days), but, if the disease lasts longer, patients should receive adrenal steroids. After an initial dose of 20 mg prednisone four times a day, the amount is decreased by 25 per cent weekly until the lowest effective dose is reached. At times, patients with congestive heart failure that is refractory to digitalis and diuretics respond dramatically to prednisone.

### Fungus Pericarditis

Intravenous amphotericin B is given for 4 to 6 weeks in *Candida* or *Aspergillus* myocarditis (Table 4).

## Parasitic Pericarditis

American trypanosomiasis (Chagas' disease), trichinosis, toxoplasmosis, amebiasis, and echinococcosis are systemic parasitic diseases sometimes producing myopericarditis (Turner, 1975). Treatment is that of the systemic disease. Echinococcal cysts of the heart must be carefully removed surgically to avoid anaphylaxis and allergic phenomena resulting from dissemination of cysts to other organs, or their rupture into the pericardial cavity (Heyat et al., 1971).

## References

Bell, E. J., and Grist, N. R.: Coxsackievirus infections in patients with acute cardiac disease and chest pain. Scott Med J 13:47, 1968.

Bell, E. J., and Grist, N. R.: Echoviruses, carditis, and acute pleurodynia. Lancet 1:326, 1970.

Cameron, E. W. J.: Surgical management of staphylococcal pericarditis. Thorax 30:678, 1975.

Cohen, J. L.: Neoplastic pericarditis. In Spodick, D. (ed): Pericardial Diseases. Philadelphia, F. A. Davis Co., 1976, p. 257.

Das, P. B., and Ray, D.: Surgical management of pyogenic pericarditis. International Surgery 61:483, 1976.

Drinker, C. K., and Field, M. E.: Absorption from pericardial cavity. J Exp Med 53:143, 1931.

Fowler, N. O., and Monitsas, G. T.: Infectious pericarditis. Prog Cardiovasc Dis 16:323, 1973.

Franklin, W. G., Simon, A. B., and Sodeman, T. M.: Candida myocarditis without valvulitis. Am J Cardiol 38:924, 1976.

Gatmaitan, B. G., Chason, J. L., and Lerner, A. M.: Augmentation of the virulence of murine coxsackievirus B-3 myocardiopathy by exercise. J Exp Med 131:1121, 1970.

Grist, N. R., and Bell, E. J.: A six-year study of coxsackievirus B infections in heart disease. J Hyg 73:165, 1974.

Grodums, E. I.: The effect of reserpine upon experimental coxsackievirus B-3 infection in mice. Can J Microbiol 18:577, 1972.

Heyat, J., Mokhtari, H., Hajaliloo, J., and Shakibi, J. G.: Surgical treatment of echinococcal cyst of the heart. Report of a case and review of the world literature. J Thorac Cardiovasc Surg 61:755, 1971.

Hipona, F. A., and Paredes, S.: The radiology of pericardial disease. In Spodick, D. (ed): Pericardial Diseases. Philadelphia, F. A. Davis Co., 1976, p. 91.

Klacsmann, P. G., Bulkley, B. H., and Hutchins, G. M.: The changed spectrum of purulent pericarditis. An 86-year autopsy experience in 200 patients. Am J Med 63:666, 1977.

Kline, I. K.: Lymphatic pathways in the heart. Arch Path 88:638, 1969.

Lerner, A. M.: Coxsackievirus myocardiopathy. J Infect Dis 120:496, 1969.

Lerner, A. M., Wilson, F. M., and Reyes, M. P.: Enteroviruses and the heart (with special emphasis on the probable role of coxsackieviruses, group B types 1-5). II. Observations in humans. Mod Concepts Cardiovasc Dis 44:11, 1975.

Liedtke, A. J., DeJoseph, R. L., and Zelis, R.: Echocardiographic observations in inflammatory pericarditis. Ann Intern Med 84:573, 1976.

Lonberg-Holm, K., Crowell, R. L., and Philipson, L.: Unrelated animal viruses share receptors. Nature 259:679, 1976.

Matthews, A. W., and Griffiths, I. D.: Postvaccinial pericarditis and myocarditis. Br Heart J 36:1043, 1974.

Miller, A. J.: Some observations concerning pericardial effusions and their relationship to the venous and lymphatic circulation of the heart. Lymphology 3:76, 1970.

Morse, J. R., Onetsky, M. T., and Hudson, J. A.: Pericarditis as a complication of meningococcal meningitis. Ann Intern Med 74:212, 1971.

Reyes, M. P. and Lerner, A. M.: Interferon and neutralizing antibody in sera of exercised mice with coxsackie B-3 myocarditis. Proc Soc Exp Biol Med 151:333, 1976.

Roberts, W. C., and Ferrans, V. J.: Pathologic anatomy of the cardiomyopathies. Idiopathic dilated and hypertrophic types, infiltrative types, and endomyocardial disease with and without eosinophilia. Human Path 6:287, 1975.

Rooney, J. J., Crocco, J. A., and Lyons, H. A.: Tuberculous pericarditis. Ann Intern Med 72:73, 1970.

Sainani, G. S., Dekate, M. P., and Rao, C. P.: Heart disease caused by coxsackievirus B infection. Br Heart J 37:819, 1975.

Schmidt, N. J., Magoffin, R. L., and Lennette, E. H.: Association of group B coxsackieviruses with cases of pericarditis, myocarditis, or pleurodynia by demonstration of immunoglobulin M antibody. Infect Immun 8:341, 1973.

Spodick, D. H.: Acoustic phenomena in pericardial disease. Am Heart J 81:114, 1971.

St Geme, Jr., J. W., Noren, G. R., and Adams, Jr., P.: Proposed embryopathic relation between mumps virus and primary endocardial fibroelastosis. N Engl J Med 275:339, 1966.

Turner, J. A.: Parasitic causes of pericarditis. West J Med 122:307, 1975.

Weissler, A. M.: Noninvasive cardiology. Clinical cardiology monographs. New York, Grune & Stratton, 1974.

Wilson, F. M., Miranda, Q. R., Chason, J. L., and Lerner, A. M.: Residual pathologic changes following murine coxsackie A and B myocarditis. Am J Path 55:253, 1969.

Wong, C. Y., Woodruff, J. J., and Woodruff, J. F.: Generation of cytotoxic T lymphocytes during coxsackievirus B-3 infection. II. Characterization of effector cells and demonstration of cytotoxicity against viral-infected myofibers. J Immunol 118:1165, 1977.

Wood, J. D., Nimmo, M. J., and Mackay-Scollay, E. M.: Acute transmural myocardial infarction associated with active coxsackievirus B infection. Am Heart J 89:283, 1975.

# 201 KAWASAKI SYNDROME (THE MUCOCUTANEOUS LYMPH NODE SYNDROME)

## Marian E. Melish, M.D.

## DEFINITION

Kawasaki syndrome or the mucocutaneous lymph node syndrome (MCLS, MLNS) is an acute, febrile, exanthematous childhood illness of unknown etiology. It was first recognized in Japan by Dr. Tomisaku Kawasaki in 1967 (Kawasaki, 1967; Kawasaki et al., 1974). Since its first description, more than 25,000 cases have been reported to the national research committee from all over Japan.

The disease was recognized independently in Hawaii by Melish, Hicks, and Larson, who encountered 12 cases between 1971 and 1974 (Melish et al., 1974, 1976, 1979). Without knowledge of the Japanese experience, these American workers independently identified the same diagnostic criteria. Since 1974, Kawasaki syndrome has been recognized worldwide in children of all racial and ethnic groups, but the highest prevalence has been reported among Japanese children in Japan and Hawaii (Melish et al., 1979).

## ETIOLOGY

The etiology of Kawasaki syndrome is unknown. No bacterial or viral agent has been isolated consistently; reports of a rickettsial etiology have not been confirmed. Nevertheless, Kawasaki syndrome is suspected to have a microbial component because the sudden onset of a febrile, largely self-limited, exanthematous disease strongly resembles an infectious disease. A pronounced tendency for time-space clusters of cases also favors an infectious etiology.

## CLINICAL MANIFESTATIONS, COMPLICATIONS, AND SEQUELAE

At present, the diagnosis of Kawasaki syndrome is based on strict adherence to clinical criteria and exclusion of other clinically similar diseases. The principal diagnostic criteria are listed in Table 1. To fit the diagnosis of Kawasaki syndrome, the patient should meet five of the six criteria. In practice, most patients have all of the first five criteria, whereas the sixth, lymphadenopathy, is seen in 70 per cent of cases or less.

The clinical course of the illness is best described as triphasic with an acute febrile phase, a subacute phase, and a convalescent phase. Fever is generally the first sign of illness and is followed within one to three days by discrete vascular injection of bulbar conjunctivae, changes in the mouth, hands, and feet, an erythematous rash, and lymphadenopathy. The most distinctive features of the syndrome are moderate, often painful, swelling and firm induration of the hands and feet. The skin is so tightly stretched and shiny that it resembles acute scleroderma with fusiform swelling of the fingers. The palms and soles take on a diffuse, deep red-purple color during the acute stage. The erythematous rash is diffuse and may be morbilliform, urticarial, polymorphous, or scarlatiniform, but not vesicular, bullous, or petechial. The associated features of aseptic meningitis, diarrhea, and hepatic dysfunction may occur during the acute phase. Children are moderately to severely ill, extremely irritable, and anorectic throughout this acute period.

After a mean of 11 days (range 6 to more than 25) the fever, rash, and lymphadenopathy subside, and the subacute phase begins. This stage is characterized by persistent anorexia, irritability, thrombocytosis, and desquamation of the palms and soles. When arthritis, arthralgias, and myocardial dysfunction occur, they are seen during this phase, which lasts from approximately the eleventh to the twenty-fifth day after the onset of fever. The convalescent phase lasts from the time all signs of illness have disappeared until the sedimentation rate has returned to normal, usually six to eight weeks after onset.

The associated features of Kawasaki syndrome (Table 2) attest to the multisystem involvement of the disease. Pyuria/urethritis is seen in over two thirds of cases during the acute phase. Aseptic meningitis associated with irritability, lethargy, meningismus, or semicoma complicates the course of about one fourth of patients during the acute stage. The cerebrospinal fluid (CSF) contains 25 to 100 white cells that are predominantly lymphocytes; the glucose and protein levels are normal. About one fourth of patients have diarrhea and abdominal pain. Liver involvement occurs in approximately 10 per cent and consists primarily of obstructive jaundice with mild ele-

---

**TABLE 1. Principal Diagnostic Criteria**

1. Fever, persisting for greater than 5 days (mean 11 days), usually > 39° C
2. Conjunctival injection without purulent exudate or corneal involvement
3. Changes in the mouth consisting of:
   (a) Erythema, fissuring, and crusting of the lips
   (b) Diffuse oropharyngeal erythema
   (c) "Strawberry" tongue
4. Changes in the peripheral extremities consisting of:
   (a) Induration and swelling of hands and feet during acute febrile stage
   (b) Erythema of palms and soles during acute febrile stage
   (c) Desquamation of finger and toetips approximately two weeks after onset of fever progressing to extensive peeling of palms and soles
   (d) Transverse grooves across fingernails two to three months after onset
5. Erythematous rash of morbilliform, multiforme, urticarial, or scarlatiniform character
6. Enlarged lymph node mass measuring greater than 1.5 cm in diameter, usually unilateral in the cervical region.

TABLE 2.    Associated Features in Order of Frequency

Pyuria and urethritis
Arthralgia and arthritis
Aseptic meningitis
Diarrhea
Abdominal pain
Obstructive jaundice
Hydrops of gallbladder
Myocardopathy
Pericardial effusion
Acute mitral insufficiency
Myocardial infarction

vations of the liver enzymes. Both American and Japanese patients have developed acute gallbladder hydrops late in the acute period. This complication is manifested by a right upper quadrant abdominal mass, which resolves spontaneously in two to three weeks. It can be monitored by repeated ultrasound examinations. Arthralgia and arthritis, mainly of the large weight-bearing joints such as the knee, hip, and ankle, may complicate the subacute phase of the illness, but they are also self-limited and rarely persist longer than two weeks. During the subacute and convalescent phases of the illness, approximately one fifth of patients have clinical cardiac abnormalities including myocardiopathy with congestive heart failure, pericardial effusion, acute mitral insufficiency, and acute myocardial infarction. Kawasaki originally described the illness as "benign febrile mucocutaneous lymph node syndrome" (Kawasaki, 1967). It was soon recognized, however, that a small proportion of patients, approximately 2 per cent, died suddenly during the subacute or early convalescent phase. Coronary artery disease with aneurysm formation and thrombosis is the main cause of death.

Laboratory abnormalities in Kawasaki syndrome are generally nonspecific and nondiagnostic. The white blood cell count is greater than 20,000 with a left shift in more than half the patients during the acute febrile phase. The sedimentation rate and C-reactive protein level are uniformly elevated in the acute stage and gradually subside to normal six to ten weeks after the onset of fever. All patients develop thrombocytosis. Unlike the white blood count, the platelet count is normal during the acute stage but rises after the tenth day to levels of 600,000 to 1.8 million by the fifteenth to twenty-fifth day of illness. The period of the elevated platelet count is the period of greatest risk of coronary thrombosis.

Immunoglobulins IgG, IgA, and IgM are normal. IgE may be modestly to moderately elevated in the subacute phase compared with the convalescent values (Kusakawa and Heiner, 1976). The SGOT and SGPT levels may also be modestly elevated. The SGOT, creatine phosphokinase and lactic dehydrogenase may be elevated in patients with myocarditis or myocardial infarction.

## PATHOGENESIS AND PATHOLOGY

The pathologic changes of Kawasaki syndrome are better understood than the etiology. The cardinal pathologic feature is multisystem arteritis of the medium-sized muscular arteries. In fatal cases the most profound changes occur in the coronary arteries, with scattered and variable involvement of other blood vessels. The cardiac pathology varies with the stage of illness. The main changes in the few patients who have died during the first ten days of illness were pancarditis and acute perivasculitis of the coronary arteries and aorta. An inflammatory infiltrate was also noted in the AV conduction system of these patients. The coronary arteries were patent.

The most typical pathologic changes are seen in the hearts of children who die from day 15 to day 50, the period during which more than 70 per cent of deaths occur. These patients have severe panvasculitis of the coronary arteries with coronary aneurysms. The immediate cause of death is either coronary thrombosis or rupture of the coronary aneurysm. Massive myocardial infarction may occur. Pericarditis, myocarditis, and endocarditis are less pronounced than in the early deaths, and some fatal cases have had a variable degree of extracardiac vasculitis (Fujiwara and Hamashima, 1978). The extraparenchymal portion of the musculoelastic arteries such as the mesenteric, adrenal, splenic, renal, and genital arteries is most frequently involved. Extracoronary aneurysms are rare but do occur, especially in the axillary and mesenteric arteries.

The pathologic features of fatal Kawasaki syndrome are indistinguishable from those of what had been known as infantile periarteritis nodosa (IPN) (Landing and Larson, 1976). IPN was a rare pathologic entity diagnosed only at autopsy. The clinical course of these patients was similar to that of patients with Kawasaki syndrome. Therefore, the Kawasaki syndrome appears to be the clinical expression of an illness that, in its most severe form (the 2 per cent who die), has the pathologic features of IPN. It is likely that similar but less severe vascular changes are present in the vessels of all children with the disease. Although the names are confusingly similar, IPN differs considerably from adult or classic periarteritis not only in the ages affected but also in the vessels involved (Landing and Larson, 1976).

Late deaths that occur from more than 50 days to years after the clinical illness are characterized by coronary scarring, aneurysms with recanalization, and old myocardial infarction with fibrosis. Active inflammation of vessels is not a feature of the late deaths, but the cardiac and vascular pathologic changes appear to be caused by the vasculitis of the acute episode.

## EPIDEMIOLOGY AND GEOGRAPHIC VARIATIONS IN DISEASE

Kawasaki syndrome is overwhelmingly a disease of young children. In Japan and in our series in Hawaii, the incidence peaks at 1 year of age with almost equal numbers affected in the first and second years of life. Eighty per cent of patients are less than 4 years of age, and the age-specific incidence declines steadily to age 8. Very few cases occur after 10 years of age. In Japan and Honolulu, there is a male predominance of over 1.5:1 (Kawasaki et al., 1974; Melish et al., 1976; Landing and Larson, 1976). The epidemiology has been most carefully studied in Japan, where the MCLS research committee of the Ministry of Health and Welfare has conducted four nationwide surveys involving more than 10,000 patients. There were no clear geographic or urban-rural differences in the incidence of the disease in children aged 0 to 4 years. There has been a steady increase in the reported yearly incidence since the survey began. There were no dramatic seasonal differences, although a few more cases occurred in the summer. Nearly all cases were sporadic with no evidence of secondary cases in the school, home, or neighborhood. In a small case-control study, affected children showed few important differences from neighborhood controls except that they were more likely to have had pharyngitis, eczema, urticaria, or allergic rhinitis at some time before the development of Kawasaki syndrome. Diet, general health, and environment were unremarkable and equivalent to that of controls (Yanigawa et al., 1975).

Since its first description in the English language, Kawasaki syndrome has been reported worldwide among children of all racial groups. Outside of Japan, the largest collection of cases has been reported from Hawaii. Clusters of cases have been encountered in the continental United States; scattered cases have been reported from other areas of the world. Among 90 cases in Hawaii, children of Japanese ancestry were markedly overrepresented compared with their proportion of the population; Caucasian children were markedly underrepresented. Chinese, Polynesian, and Filipino children and children of mixed race appeared to have an intermediate incidence (Melish et al., 1979).

Because this disease appears to be most prevalent in Japan and among Japanese children in Hawaii, a unique genetic susceptibility is suspected. HLA typing of cases compared with controls has been studied with conflicting results. No single HLA antigen has been common to all cases. A report from Japan showing a modest excess in frequency of HLA antigen BW 22 subtype $J_2$ differs from the negative findings of three other studies.

## DIAGNOSIS

The diagnosis of Kawasaki syndrome is entirely a clinical one based on firm adherence to the clinical criteria and exclusion of other possible causes. For example, leptospirosis and infection with streptococci and other bacteria should be ruled out by cultures and serologies. As a minimum, patients should meet five of the six principal diagnostic criteria (Table 1). The clinical course should also be typical. If hand and foot desquamation and thrombocytosis do not occur within 12 to 20 days after the onset of fever, the diagnosis of Kawasaki syndrome should be seriously questioned.

## TREATMENT

Effective therapy for Kawasaki syndrome awaits discovery of its etiology and pathogenesis. The present treatment is supportive and consists of a careful program of repeated clinical and laboratory evaluations designed to detect and manage arthritis and serious cardiac and vascular abnormalities.

Because inflammatory vasculitis is the major pathologic change, anti-inflammatory agents have been investigated as supportive therapy. For example, aspirin is an attractive therapeutic agent because it is anti-inflammatory and inhibits platelet aggregation. We have found that aspirin administered in standard anti-inflammatory doses of 80 to 100 mg/kg/day shortens the mean duration of fever compared with untreated controls. Approximately two thirds of patients become afebrile within two days of starting aspirin therapy; the remaining third remains febrile for several days (Melish et al., 1979). Salicylate levels can be monitored 48 hours after starting therapy. The therapeutic anti-inflammatory level is 1.5 to 2.5 mg/dl. Once fever has been controlled, aspirin dose should be reduced to 10–20 mg/kg/day and continued for the additional six to eight weeks that the sedimentation rate remains elevated.

Corticosteroids have been used in the United States and Japan. A recent controlled study demonstrated that corticosteroids are contraindicated because they increased the frequency of aneurysms in patients studied by routine aortography approximately four weeks after the onset of disease. Aneurysms developed in 11 per cent of patients who received aspirin, 20 per cent of those on no anti-inflammatory therapy, and 65 per cent of those on corticosteroids (Kato et al., 1979). Corticosteroids may also increase the platelet count without decreasing platelet adhesiveness. For these reasons, corticosteroids are specifically contraindicated in Kawasaki syndrome.

Hospitalization is desirable during the acute febrile stage to facilitate diagnostic testing, but patients can be managed as outpatients if they are seen frequently. Blood, urine, throat, and stool cultures must be obtained to exclude a treatable bacterial disease. Streptococcal infection should also be excluded by serial antistreptococcal antibody titers. If available, leptospiral cultures and serology should be obtained. Chest radiograph and EKG should be performed to monitor cardiac function. Careful follow-up with repeated physical examinations is mandatory to detect arthritis and cardiac disease, which usually appear after the acute symptoms have cleared.

If cardiac decompensation occurs, the patient should be hospitalized for anticoagulation and digitalization. Angiography should not be performed on every child with Kawasaki syndrome but may be helpful in the minority with overt cardiac disease. Biplanar echocardiography may be a useful noninvasive method of detecting and evaluating aneurysms at the origin of the coronary arteries (Yoshida et al., 1979).

## PROGNOSIS

In Japan approximately 2 per cent of children with Kawasaki syndrome die in the subacute or early convalescent phase. Ten to 20 per cent develop coronary aneurysms detectable by routine angiography. Resolution of angiographic abnormalities over a 1 year follow-up period has been noted in a third of those with aneurysms (Kato et al., 1975). Kawasaki syndrome is self-limited in the overwhelming majority of patients. If cardiac damage is not detected by careful follow-up through the convalescent period, it is not likely to pose major clinical problems in the next three to five years. However, because some degree of coronary vasculitis may be present in all patients, long-term follow-up studies of complicated and uncomplicated cases are needed to determine whether they may be susceptible to premature coronary atherosclerosis.

## References

Fujiwara, H., and Hamashima, Y.: Pathology of the heart in Kawasaki disease. Pediatrics 61:100, 1978.

Kato, H., Koike, S., and Yokoyama, T.: Kawasaki disease: Effect of treatment on coronary artery involvement. Pediatrics 63:175, 1979.

Kato, H., Koike, S., Yamamoto, M., Ito, Y., and Yano, E.: Coronary aneurysms in infants and young children with acute febrile mucocutaneous lymph node syndrome. J Pediatr 86:892, 1975.

Kawasaki, T.: Acute febrile mucocutaneous syndrome with lymphoid involvement with specific desquamation of the fingers and toes. Jap J Allergy 16:178, 1967.

Kawasaki, T., Kosaki, F., Okawa, S., Shigematsu, I., and Yanagawa, H.: A new infantile febrile mucocutaneous lymph node syndrome (MLNS) prevailing in Japan. Pediatrics 54(3):271, 1974.

Kusakawa, S., and Heiner, D.: Elevated levels of immunoglobulin E in the acute febrile mucocutaneous lymph node syndrome. Pediat Res 10:108, 1976.

Landing, B. H., and Larson, E. J.: Are infantile periarteritis nodosa with coronary artery involvement and fatal mucocutaneous lymph node syndrome the same? Comparison of 20 patients from North America with patients from Hawaii and Japan. Pediatrics 59:651, 1976.

Melish, M. E., Hicks, R. M., and Dean, A. G.: Kawasaki syndrome in Hawaii (abstract). Pediat Res 13:451, 1979.

Melish, M. E., Hicks, R. M., and Larson, E. J.: Mucocutaneous lymph node syndrome in the United States (abstract). Pediat Res 8:427, 1974.

Melish, M. E., Hicks, R. M., and Larson, E. J.: Mucocutaneous lymph node syndrome in the United States. Am J Dis Child 130:599, 1976.

Yanigawa, H., Shigematsu, I., and Kawasaki, T.: Epidemiological aspects of so-called "Kawasaki disease": Presented to the 15th SEAMO-Tropical Medicine Seminar. Bangkok, Thailand, November 24–28, 1975.

Yoshida, H., Funabashi, T., Nakaya, S., and Taniguchi, N.: Mucocutaneous lymph node syndrome: A cross-sectional echocardiographic diagnosis of coronary aneurysms. Am J Dis Child 133:1244, 1979.

# 202 DENGUE AND OTHER HEMORRHAGIC FEVERS

Abraham I. Braude, M.D., Ph.D.
Amorn Leelarasamee, M.D.

## DEFINITION

The hemorrhagic fevers are a collection of diverse epidemic virus infections transmitted by arthropod bites or contact with rodents. They are severe, life-threatening illnesses with fever, thrombocytopenia, hemorrhages, shock, and neurologic disturbances.

## ETIOLOGY

The viruses known to cause the hemorrhagic fever syndrome are shown in Table 1. They belong mainly to the families Togaviridae and Arenaviridae. The viruses causing dengue, Kyasanur forest disease, Omsk hemorrhagic fever, and yellow fever belong to the genus *Flavivirus* in the togavirus family; and Junin, Lassa, Muchupo, and Pichinde viruses are arenaviruses. The virus of Crimean hemorrhagic fevers is listed with the family Bunyaviridae but only tentatively, because it is morphologically similar but antigenically dissimilar to the bunyaviruses.

Marburg and Ebola viruses have striking similarities in size, shape, and ultrastructure that they share with no other viruses. For this reason, they are considered the first representatives of a new group. Their superficial similarity to rabies virus does not warrant their classification as a rhabdovirus. The togaviruses are described in Chapter 61, the arenaviruses in Chapter 62, the bunyaviruses in Chapter 8, and Marburg-Ebola viruses in Chapter 66.

The viruses spread by arthropods are also placed in a category known as the *Arbovirus group*. This grouping, based on transmission, is considered useful, even though nearly all members are characterized well enough by modern methods to be classified according to the taxonomic scheme in Chapter 8. Two groups of arthropods are responsible for transmission. The mosquito *Aedes aegypti* is the main vector of dengue, yellow fever, and chikungunya fever, although other species of *Aedes* have been shown occasionally to carry dengue and yellow fever viruses. Because *A. aegypti* is a domestic mosquito, it spreads disease in urban areas. The cycles for transmission of dengue and chikungunya viruses appear to involve only human beings and mosquitoes. Yellow fever virus, on the other hand, is transmitted from monkey to monkey, from monkey to person, and from person to person.

## PATHOGENESIS AND PATHOLOGY

Not every patient infected with the hemorrhagic fever viruses develops the hemorrhagic fever syndrome. On the contrary, benign febrile illnesses may be the only clinical evidence of infection, and the reason why other patients develop increased vascular permeability and come down with lethal hemorrhages and shock is largely a mystery. This question has been studied most extensively in dengue, a disease in which a child with an apparently benign fever may suddenly develop severe abdominal pain, intestinal bleeding, and shock. There appear to be three factors in the pathogenesis of dengue hemorrhagic shock. One of these is the existence of four serotypes of dengue virus. The second is the presence on these four serotypes of cross-reacting antigenic determinants that give no lasting protection against heterologous serotypes. The third is a previous dengue infection. Infection with the first serotype sensitizes the child to produce a secondary type of immune response to infection with the

second serotype, so that IgG is generated. This IgG is believed to bind but not neutralize the heterologous serotype of dengue virus. There is evidence that such ineffectual neutralization by bound antibody not only enhances the growth of virus but also produces damage by immune complexes composed of IgG and viral antigen (Sobel et al., 1975; Theofilopoulos et al., 1976). Growth enhancement would occur when virus antibody complexes are attached to human monocytes by their Fc receptors so that entry into the cell is facilitated. Damage from immune complexes has been attributed to complement activation (Russel, 1971). During the shock stage of dengue infections, blood levels of complement components Clq, C3, C4, C5–C8, and C3 proactivator were depressed (Bokish et al., 1973), and there were low levels of blood-clotting Factor XII (Hageman factor) and activation of intravascular clotting. From these data, a hypothesis has been formulated that proposes that massive viral synthesis produces excess viral antigen for complexing with IgG, that the complexes activate complement to provide C3A and C5A, and that these complement-cleavage products increase capillary permeability by their anaphylatoxin activity (i.e., release of histamine and other mediators from mast cells). The immune complexes can also produce intravascular coagulation.

The malignant form of dengue has appeared mainly since the end of World War II and can be traced to an increased movement of people between rural and urban areas so that the chance for exposure to a new serotype is increased. There is no reason to believe that reinfection is important in the pathogenesis of the other hemorrhagic fevers, however, because the syndromes have been seen in accidental laboratory infections acquired thousands of miles from endemic areas. Although it is possible that immune complexes could develop in the nondengue hemorrhagic fevers as a result of antibody formation during their incubation and prodromal periods, there is no evidence in them of such complexes.

Biopsies of nonfatal, uncomplicated cases and autopsies both show findings consistent with a vascular injury in dengue. In skin biopsies in volunteers with benign illnesses, there were endothelial swelling, perivascular edema, and infiltration of mononuclear cells in or around small blood vessels (Sabin, 1952). The outstanding findings in fatal cases were edema, petechial hemorrhages in all tissues including the heart, some blood in the intestines and stomach, and fluid in the serous cavities. In other words, the most common finding was that resulting from diffuse, general capillary oozing of fluid and cells (Hammon et al., 1960).

Experimental infection of guinea pigs with Junin virus produces a disease that resembles human Argentine hemorrhagic fever (AHF). In

**TABLE 1. Viral Classification of Hemorrhagic Fevers**

| VIRUS (FAMILY:GENUS) | | DISEASE | VECTOR |
|---|---|---|---|
| *Togaviridae:* | *Flavivirus* | Dengue | *Aedes aegypti* (and other mosquitoes) |
| | | Kyasanur forest disease | *Haemaphysalis* (ticks) |
| | | Omsk hemorrhagic fever | *Dermacentor* (ticks) |
| | | Yellow fever | *Aedes aegypti* |
| *Togaviridae:* | *Alphavirus* | Chikungunya fever | *Aedes aegypti* |
| *Bunyaviridae:* | Possible member | | |
| | Crimean hemorrhagic fever-Congo virus | Crimean hemorrhagic fever | *Hyalomma marginatum* (ticks) |
| *Arenaviridae:* | *Arenavirus* | | |
| | Junin virus | Argentine hemorrhagic fever | *Calomys*[a] *laucha* |
| | Lassa virus | Lassa fever | *Mastomys natalensis* |
| | Machupo virus | Bolivian hemorrhagic fever | *Calomys callosus* |
| *Marburg-Ebola* group: | | | |
| | Marburg virus | Marburg virus disease | Unknown |
| | Ebola virus | Ebola virus disease | Unknown |

[a]The species *Calomys* comprises wild mice and *Mastomys* house rats.

this model, both clotting and complement systems are activated at the same time, with complement activation occurring through the classic pathway as would occur with immune complexes. Complement activation occurs in human cases of AHF also, with total serum-complement activity reduced to 68 per cent of control values in severe or moderate cases during the early acute stage. Complement-fixing antibodies, however, do not appear until 12 to 17 days, when clinical recovery begins. Moreover, the profile of change in the complement components is not that of complement activation by immune complexes, and there has been no binding of C3 or immunoglobulins in glomeruli or other vessels in fatal cases. In addition, there has been no histologic evidence that disseminated intravascular coagulation (DIC) contributes to the lesions (deBracco et al., 1978). For these reasons, it is believed that neither immune complexes or DIC are involved in the pathogenesis of human AHF.

The autopsy findings in other forms of viral hemorrhagic fever disclose little that would help in determining the pathogenesis of bleeding. Lassa fever resembles dengue hemorrhagic fever in its tendency for severe edema as well as hemorrhage to be present throughout all tissues. The occurrence of severe edema with the bleeding indicates that increased capillary permeability

from diffuse vascular injury is the basic disturbance, and that it results from infection of the capillary endothelium, from the action of pharmacologic mediators such as histamine, or from both. In other hemorrhagic fevers, edema is less prominent or absent so that focal vascular injury and coagulation disturbances are the likely defects. In human infections due to Marburg, Ebola, Junin, Lassa, and yellow fever viruses, there are hepatic lesions that might help to explain the hemorrhagic disorder. In yellow fever, for example, the prothrombin time is characteristically prolonged, indicating a disturbance in hepatic synthesis of prothrombin and the other clotting factors measured by the prothrombin screening test. In general, however, the pathogenesis of bleeding in the viral hemorrhagic fevers needs further study.

## CLINICAL MANIFESTATIONS, DIAGNOSIS, AND TREATMENT

Separate chapters are devoted to yellow fever (Chapter 143), Lassa fever (Chapter 204), Marburg virus disease (Chapter 252), and Ebola virus disease (Chapter 253). This discussion takes up mainly the other viral hemorrhagic fevers listed in Table 1.

# DENGUE

Dengue may start as an explosive urban epidemic in the rainy season and affect large numbers of people. It may also attack tourists or other travelers who visit endemic areas. Epidemics of dengue were known in the Caribbean countries

and United States of America in the early 19th century, shifted westward to Texas between 1885 and 1920, and back to the southeastern United States between 1920 and 1950. Each of the American epidemics was preceded by an Asian outbreak, and both probably spread from Africa, the original home of *Aedes aegypti*, through slave traffic (Ehrenkranz et al., 1971). In recent years, an outbreak of dengue Type 4 infection began in French Polynesia (Tahiti and Moorea) in early 1979 after never before appearing outside Southeast Asia. A few years earlier, a dengue epidemic due to Types 1, 2, and 3 broke out in the Caribbean and represented the first time that Type 1 virus had been isolated in the Western Hemisphere.

After an incubation period of five to eight days, the nonfatal, uncomplicated form of dengue starts abruptly with severe generalized aches, excruciating muscle pains, severe headache, pain behind the eyes, and fever to 104°F. Fever lasts three to six days. After two to three days the fever may rapidly subside but reappears again at a lower peak than the first. The two separated peaks give the fever curve an appearance of a saddleback. A transient punctate rash may appear on the knees and elbows early in the illness, and a morbilliform or scarlatiniform rash develops between the third and fifth days on the trunk. From there, it spreads to the face and extremities and may desquamate. Generalized lymphadenopathy is usually present, and leukopenia is prominent. During convalescence, the patient is often exhausted for weeks.

*Hemorrhagic dengue* is almost exclusively Asiatic now, although many cases of dengue, shown serologically to be due to Type 1 virus, were hemorrhagic in epidemics that broke out in Durban in 1927 and Athens in 1928 (Theiler et al., 1960). Dengue viruses were first isolated in 1956 from hemorrhagic fever patients by Hammon in Manila. The patients were children between the ages of 6 months and 16 years (median 5 to 9 years) who had extensive petechiae, ecchymoses, nose bleeds, melena, and shock. Thrombocytopenia as low as 10,000 and a prolonged bleeding time were the most prominent laboratory abnormalities (Hammon, 1973). The severe myalgias of classic dengue were usually not present. Hemorrhages started on the third and fourth days of fever (Fig. 1) when leukopenia was replaced by leukocytosis in about one third of patients. Part of the leukocytosis may have resulted from hemoconcentration. Fluid loss from the vessels into the tissues raised the hematocrit over 50 per cent during shock. The fatality rate in the Manila outbreak was 10 per cent and has been 4 to 12 per cent in other epidemics. Dengue viruses belonging to Types 2, 3, and 4 were isolated from the specimens of blood and serum, and from mosquitoes.

Subsequent epidemics of hemorrhagic fever have occurred repeatedly in Bangkok and also in Singapore, South Vietnam, and Calcutta. In each of these, as well as in rare sporadic cases recently described in Curaçao and Jamaica, the clinical pattern has been substantially the same as that described by Hammon (van Der Sar, 1979; Fraser et al., 1978). The World Health Organization has formulated a classification of dengue hemorrhagic fever into four clinical grades of severity (WHO, 1975):

Grade I: Fever, constitutional symptoms, and positive tourniquet test.

Grade II: Grade I plus spontaneous bleeding into skin, gums, gastrointestinal tract, and elsewhere.

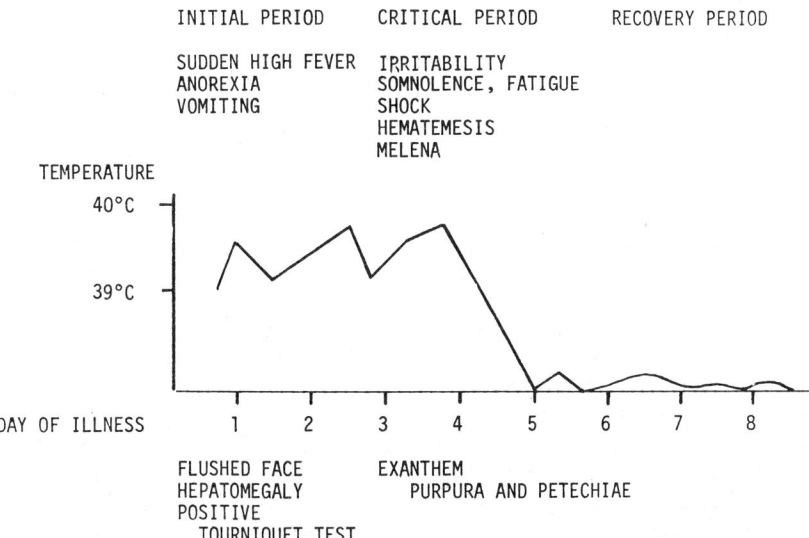

**FIGURE 1.** *Febrile response and clinical course in dengue hemorrhagic fever. (Courtesy Prasert Thongcharoen, M.D.)*

Grade III: Grade II plus circulatory failure and
agitation.

Grade IV: Profound shock; blood pressure unobtainable.

In all stages, there is thrombocytopenia and hemoconcentration. Grades III and IV are also called the *dengue shock syndrome.*

## DIAGNOSIS

Hemorrhagic fever is easy to recognize during an outbreak of dengue in Bangkok and other known epidemic areas of Asia. In the rare child who comes down with the illness when visiting an endemic area, the diagnosis can be confirmed by measuring hemagglutination-inhibition (HI) and complement-fixation (CF) antibodies to dengue Subtypes 1, 2, 3, and 4. The HI antibodies rise early in the illness, and recent dengue infection is indicated by a rise in HI titer of at least four-fold. In first infections, there is usually a type-specific rise to one virus with lower rises to other types. In second or third infections, a secondary type of response occurs, which shows an increase of antibody reacting broadly to all dengue serotypes and to other flaviviruses but to higher titer (>1:640) against one of the dengue types. Virus isolation can be made by inoculation of .015 ml of serum intracerebrally in 1- to 4-day-old Swiss mice or baby hamsters. Monolayer cell cultures are inoculated with 0.1 ml and observed for cytopathogenic changes. A variety of cell lines are used, including chick embryo, hamster kidney, Vero, HeLa, BHK-21, and others. Presumed isolates can be sent to WHO regional reference centers for identification.

The disease closely resembles fulminant meningococcal purpura, and the distinction may not be possible until the blood culture is positive for the meningococcus one or two days after it is drawn.

## TREATMENT

Treatment depends on the stage of the disease (Fig. 1). Patients who are beginning to show signs of hypovolemia, such as orthostatic hypotension but no bleeding, are given intravenously 5 per cent dextrose in normal saline until these signs are corrected and the hematocrit stabilized. It is imperative to avoid aspirin for relief of fever or headache because of the drug's adverse effect on bleeding. The relatives of the patient should be alerted to the possible need for blood donation.

If there is hemorrhage, a falling hematocrit, shock, and thrombocytopenia, the patient should receive whole blood and platelet transfusions. An aluminum hydroxide antacid suspension is taken orally for gastric bleeding. Additional fluids are given intravenously in the form of 5 per cent dextrose in saline, and, if this does not correct hypotension, the patient should receive plasma or plasma expanders other than dextran. Dextran carries the risk of causing platelet dysfunction and further bleeding. Adrenal steroids, norepinephrine, epinephrine, dopamine, or other sympathicoamines appear to be contraindicated.

## PROPHYLAXIS

The prevention of dengue depends on control of *A. aegypti.* This has been accomplished in urban areas in which yellow fever was prevalent in the western hemisphere and has also provided freedom from dengue when epidemics of dengue swept through neighboring Caribbean islands. In contrast to yellow fever, for which an effective vaccine is available, vaccination against dengue carries the theoretical risk of sensitizing the person so that hemorrhagic fever would be more likely to occur (Ehrenkranz et al., 1971). Although attenuated experimental live vaccines appear to give protection, the need for vaccines against all four types and the risk of sensitization have probably discouraged the development of a vaccine.

# CHIKUNGUNYA FEVER

Chikungunya fever resembles dengue in its transmission by *A. aegypti,* its benign clinical syndrome, its ability to cause hemorrhagic fever, and its prominence in Southeast Asia and Africa.

Like dengue, the usual picture of chikungunya fever is "break-bone fever." After an incubation period of 3 to 12 days, there is a sudden onset of high fever with severe muscle and joint pains that are so severe that the patient literally folds up and becomes immobile. The fever may go away

any time during the first week and reappear one to three days later at a lower level. This febrile relapse is accompanied in three fourths of cases by a maculopapular pruritic rash on the trunk and limbs. In addition to these dengue-like features, there is a leukopenia of 4000 to 5000. In contrast to dengue, retroorbital pain does not occur, and headache is mild. The main sequelae are crippling joint pains that may return periodically over the next four months.

Much more rarely, chikungunya virus can cause hemorrhagic fever. An outbreak of chikungunya hemorrhagic fever occurred along with dengue hemorrhagic fever in Bangkok in 1962. Nearly 90 per cent of those involved in these epidemics were children under 10 years old. They had a fever up to 104° F, vomiting, abdominal pain, and a positive tourniquet test. Purpura occurred in three fourths of the patients. The overall mortality in the combined epidemic was about 10 per cent, but there is evidence that chikun-gunya hemorrhagic fever was milder (Dasane-yavaja et al., 1963). Chikungunya hemorrhagic fever has also occurred in Calcutta, Madras, and Vellore, India, but not in Africa. Thus, Asiatic children appear to be uniquely susceptible to hemorrhagic fever by chikungunya as well as dengue viruses. These outbreaks have been distinguished from dengue hemorrhagic fever by isolation in suckling mice of chikungunya virus from the blood of patients during the first five days of illness.

# KYASANUR FOREST DISEASE

Kyasanur forest disease (KFD) was discovered in 1957 following the death of wild monkeys and human beings in Mysore State in India (Work, 1958). It is transmitted by several species of hard ticks belonging to the genus *Haemaphysalis,* and the reservoir consists of small rodents such as voles and forest rats. Rhesus and Langur monkeys are also infected but, like man, are not part of the natural chain.

The illness occurs about four to eight days after exposure to ticks in the forest and has a sudden onset of headache, fever, severe prostration, severe pains in the lower back and extremities, and insomnia. The fever has a biphasic course like that described in dengue and chikungunya fever. The phases are separated by an afebrile period of 10 to 20 days, with the second fever lasting 2 to 10 days. During the second phase, there may be evidence of meningoencephalitis, such as severe headache, vertigo, tremors, and mental changes (Webb and Rao, 1961).

There is no skin eruption, but after three or four days, there is bleeding from the gums as well as epistaxis, hemoptysis, hematemesis, and melena. Death results from blood loss, intrapulmonary hemorrhage, and shock in the second week. Bronchopneumonia is also present in some cases. The mortality among virologically proven cases in the 1957 outbreak in India was about 5 per cent.

The chief laboratory findings are a severe leukopenia of 2000 or less and thrombocytopenia. In those cases with signs of meningoencephalitis, the cerebrospinal fluid may have an increase in protein and mononuclear cells, ranging from 5 to 70 per $mm^3$. Autopsies have shown massive hemorrhage into the gastrointestinal tract, hemorrhage into the lungs, pneumonia, and occasional focal areas of necrosis in the liver. Erythrophagocytosis is prominent in the spleen and liver. No encephalitis has been found.

Patients are treated with enough fluids to restore hydration, blood pressure, and urinary output; and plasma is given to those who do not respond to normal intravenous saline. Those who recover may have prolonged muscle weakness, but there are no permanent sequelae.

Virologic diagnosis is made by isolation of KFD virus from serum during the long period of viremia. The virus multiplies readily in suckling or 3-week-old mice after intracerebral, subcutaneous, or intraperitoneal inoculation. It will also multiply in various tissue culture cell lines, where it may produce no cytopathogenic effect but can be recognized by the hemadsorption phenomenon. The virus is easily identified by complement fixation or neutralization with specific antiserum. Serologic diagnosis is made by complement fixation or hemagglutination-inhibition tests with blood samples taken during the acute and convalescent stages of the disease.

There is no vaccine for the disease, and prophylaxis depends entirely on preventing tick bites. To some extent, this can be done by applying repellents, such as dimethyl phthalate, and by wearing protective clothing. Persons in endemic forest areas should make a careful search for ticks and remove them from the skin.

# OMSK HEMORRHAGIC FEVER

This infection resembles Kyasanur forest disease very closely in its clinical manifestations (Gajdusek, 1953). Both are due to togaviruses belonging to *Flavivirus* group B and are transmitted by ticks. Omsk hemorrhagic fever occurs in Omsk and Novosibirsk in western Siberia, and possibly Bukovina in northern Romania. It has its reservoir in water voles and the Asiatic ground squirrels (or susliks). Human infections occur from bites of the tick *Dermacentor* or after contact with muskrats killed by fur trappers. The muskrats, which are not part of the primary cycle, are infected by bites from ticks infected with the virus acquired from voles or susliks. Treatment of Omsk hemorrhagic fever is the same as that of other hemorrhagic fevers. The mortality is less than 3 per cent and the incidence of the disease has dropped since the epidemics in 1945 through 1948. A formalin-inactivated mouse brain vaccine is reported to be effective in lowering the incidence of disease. Prophylaxis involves mainly protective gloves in handling carcasses of muskrats.

# CRIMEAN HEMORRHAGIC FEVER

## *ETIOLOGY*

Infection of human beings with the virus of Crimean hemorrhagic fever (CHF) occurs during spring and summer from the bites of infected ticks in Central Asia and the Crimea. This hemorrhagic fever virus is antigenically identical to a virus, designated Congo virus, which was isolated from cattle, goats, febrile patients, and *Hyalomma* ticks in equatorial Africa and Pakistan. Even though hemorrhagic fever due to this virus has not been described in equatorial Africa, the agent of the disease is now referred to as Crimean-Congo hemorrhagic fever virus (or CHF-Congo virus).

## *CLINICAL MANIFESTATIONS*

About four to eight days after a tick bite, patients become acutely ill with fever to 104° F, diffuse myalgia, flushing of the face and neck, conjunctival infection, and severe hemorrhages. As in the other hemorrhagic fevers, bleeding begins on about the fourth day with petechiae, ecchymoses, melena, and hematemesis. There are also nosebleeds and bleeding from the gums. The liver is enlarged in half the patients, and the spleen in a few. The mortality rate in man reaches 50 per cent from hemorrhage, shock, and neurologic complications. As many as 20 per cent of patients have evidence of meningoencephalitis with stiff neck, mental changes, and coma. During the prolonged convalescence, there may be postinfectious neuritis.

## *DIAGNOSIS*

The clinical pattern of hemorrhagic fever with neurologic disease is easily recognized as that of the CHF syndrome in Central Asia. If it should occur in Africa, however, it would need to be distinguished from other African hemorrhagic fevers by virus isolation. CHF-Congo virus can be isolated from blood by inoculation of serum into newborn mice. Other laboratory findings are severe leukopenia to 1000 per mm³, severe thrombocytopenia, proteinuria, and hematuria.

The epidemiologic history is also helpful in diagnosis because the disease is spread by ticks in regions where cattle are raised. Milkmaids are infected by the ticks on teats of dairy cows, and cowhands by ticks in the cowpastures. Thus, in contrast to dengue, CHF is a rural disease.

## *TREATMENT*

Blood transfusion is needed to combat the blood loss and shock. Platelet transfusions, avoidance of aspirin, and use of plasma or plasma expanders other than dextran are important measures for preventing more severe bleeding.

## *PROPHYLAXIS*

There is no vaccine. The most practical method for preventing the disease has been education of milkers and cowhands in the risks of tick infestation, so that they can take steps to avoid these vectors. Since the infection can also spread to hospital personnel, strict isolation is required to protect those involved in the care of the patient.

# ARGENTINE HEMORRHAGIC FEVER

## *ETIOLOGY*

Argentine hemorrhagic fever, caused by Junin virus (Chapter 62), is an epidemic disease primarily of young rural men working in the rich agricultural region of Argentina known as the humid pampa. Epidemics involving 300 to 1000 cases occur every year.

The disease is transmitted in the urine of rodents of the genus *Calomys* that develop immune tolerance to Junin virus so that they have steady viremia. The immune tolerance is explained by acquisition of infection within the first week after birth and the failure of an antibody response to develop against the virus. A chronic infection of the salivary glands and kidney results in constant excretion in saliva and urine. Other weanling rodents can develop neutralizing antibody that terminates the viremia but not the kidney infection, so that infected urine persists. When corn is harvested in the pampa, the harvest workers are exposed to the infected urine of *Calomys* rodents and come down with hemorrhagic fever.

## CLINICAL MANIFESTATIONS

After an incubation period of 8 to 14 days, the patients become ill with malaise, fever, hemorrhages, leukopenia, and thrombocytopenia. The onset of the symptoms is relatively gradual and slow when compared with the abrupt onset of other hemorrhagic fevers (Arribalzaga, 1955). Patients complain of headache, generalized myalgia, nausea, and vomiting. The face is flushed, the conjunctivae inflamed, and the eyelids swollen. An enanthem occurs in the mouth and eyes, and a light exanthem also develops. Neither the spleen nor liver are enlarged, and the chest x-ray is negative. About 50 per cent of patients are troubled with loss of equilibrium. There may also be tremors of the tongue and limbs. Most patients develop hypotension and signs of hemoconcentration before shock becomes definite. Hemorrhages begin on the fifth day when the gums bleed and petechiae appear on the axillae and chest. In severe cases, there are widespread hemorrhages from mucous membranes, epistaxis, hematemesis, hematuria, and melena. Death occurs from hemorrhage, shock, secondary bacterial infection, and renal failure. Those who recover become afebrile in about eight days and improve quickly after a profuse diuresis. Some patients relapse four to six weeks after the onset of symptoms, with fever and cerebellar signs that subside within a few days.

## DIAGNOSIS

Junin virus is recovered from the blood during the first week by inoculation of guinea pigs or newborn mice. Guinea pigs die in about two weeks from a hemorrhagic disease resembling human AHF. The hemorrhages occur on the skin, intestine, adrenals, and mesenteric lymph nodes. The antibody response is generally too slow to help in diagnosis of the acute illness, but complement fixation and neutralization tests on serial samples of serum make a retrospective diagnosis. The virus must be handled in specialized laboratories, because fatal infections have occurred in laboratory workers.

Other laboratory findings are severe leukopenia (lasting about a week), severe thrombocytopenia, azotemia, pronounced proteinuria, and a fall in serum albumin.

## TREATMENT

Patients must be monitored closely for the first signs of hypotension and hemoconcentration so that intravenous saline or plasma can be started before frank shock appears. The treatment outlined for dengue hemorrhagic fever also applies for AHF. The observation that recovery occurs when antibody appears in the blood suggests that convalescent serum may have a place in treatment or even prophylaxis (deBracco et al., 1978). This idea was examined in a double-blind study in which patients received intravenously 500 ml of either convalescent plasma with antibodies against Junin virus or normal plasma obtained from donors without a history of AHF (Maiztegui et al., 1979). The mortality fell from 16.5 per cent in 97 patients given nonimmune plasma to 1.1 per cent in 91 who were given convalescent immune plasma (P<0.01). Ten patients treated with immune plasma developed late neurologic complications, which were generally benign and self-limiting. The association between treatment with immune plasma and a late neurologic relapse suggests either that the neurologic disease has an immunologic mechanism or that immune plasma prevented death in those who had infection of the central nervous system but could not prevent late neurologic complications. No other form of treatment has proved so effective as immune plasma in reducing the mortality of AHF.

The mortality is about 10 to 15 per cent. Those who recover have no sequelae, although convalescence may be long.

# BOLIVIAN HEMORRHAGIC FEVER

Both the etiologic agent, the epidemiology, and the clinical features of Bolivian hemorrhagic fe-

ver (BHF) are closely related to those of Argentine hemorrhagic fever (AHF). Machupo virus is antigenically and morphologically similar to Junin virus and is transmitted to man from *Calomys callosus* by the same processes.

The disease first came to serious attention between 1959 and 1962 when it occurred near San Joaquin, Bolivia. It produced a similar clinical picture to that of AHF: fever to 104° F, severe myalgias, intention tremors of the hands and tongue, melena, hematemesis, petechiae of the skin and pharynx, hypotension, leukopenia, and proteinuria. Death usually occurred after seven to ten days from severe hypotension and shock. There were 050 cases and 115 deaths in a population of 2500. (This attack rate and severity was so great that people fled their homes in terror.)

The epidemic was finally terminated by eradication of *Calomys* from the vicinity of San Joaquin. The high population of *Calomys* had been attributed to attrition in the population of cats from fatal poisoning with DDT that had been heavily sprayed for malaria control. The situation is similar to that in West Africa, where Lassa fever broke out when control of the house rat enabled *Calomys* to infest human dwellings.

In recent years the disease has been found to spread among people by direct contact. In an outbreak in 1971 of 20 cases in Cochabamba, Bolivia, all patients had been exposed to a 20 year old nursing student who later died of the disease (Mercado et al., 1971).

# HEMORRHAGIC FEVER WITH RENAL SYNDROME (HFRS) (KOREAN HEMORRHAGIC FEVER)

Korean hemorrhagic fever (KHF) is the name given to an epidemic form of hemorrhagic fever with renal involvement. This disease first generated interest when it broke out among United Nations troops in 1951, but similar diseases had been reported in Manchuria in 1942, the Soviet Union in 1950, Scandinavia in 1951, Eastern Europe in 1962, and Japan in 1964. In Korea the disease was acquired by farmers and soldiers stationed in rural areas from the excreta of a wild rodent, *Apodemus agrarius coreae*. The disease has remained endemic near the demilitarized zone between North and South Korea. The related hemorrhagic fever in Scandinavia and Finland, known as nephropathia epidemica, is transmitted by the bank vole *Clethrionomys glareolus*.

## *ETIOLOGY*

Earlier studies by Japanese and Russian investigators indicated that the causative agent was viral because the disease could be transmitted to volunteers by injecting blood or urine from febrile patients, and the agent was filterable (Brummer-Korvenkontio et al., 1980). In 1978, Lee propagated the agent serially in adult *A. agrarius* and demonstrated specific immunofluorescent reactions when lung tissues of the rodents reacted with sera from patients convalescing from Korean hemorrhagic fever. The agent could not be cultivated in continuous cell cultures of African green monkey kidney, dog embryo, porcine kidney, human embryo lung (W1–38), mink kidney, or Chinese hamster lung; nor in primary cell cultures prepared from rhesus monkey kidney, duck and chicken embryo, rat liver, and human embryonic liver. No infections could be established in suckling white mice, weaned mice, hamsters, guinea pigs, rats, or rabbits. Antisera to Lassa, Machupo, Marburg, and Ebola viruses gave no fluorescence when reacted with infected *A. agrarius* lung tissues, but raised titers of antibody to the agent of KHF were found by the fluorescent antibody method in Finnish patients with nephropathia epidemica (NE) (Lee and Lee, 1979). Thus, the agents of KHF and NE appear to be closely related if not the same.

## *PATHOGENESIS AND PATHOLOGY*

In addition to shock, acute renal failure and pulmonary edema kill the patient. In early deaths, retroperitoneal edema is marked but not in deaths that occur later. There are hemorrhages from distended small vessels in the right atrium, anterior pituitary, adrenal medulla, and especially the renal medulla, where intense vascular congestion separates the tubules that undergo focal necrosis, resembling that seen in lower nephron nephrosis (Lukes, 1954). The necrosis may be limited to the tubules or involve the pyramids. The shock is oligemic and secondary to the loss of plasma into the tissues. There is a reduced cardiac output and increased peripheral resistance.

## CLINICAL MANIFESTATIONS

The disease occurs in three phases: invasion, toxic, and convalescent (Powell, 1953). The invasion stage starts suddenly, and the symptoms are those of any acute febrile illness. After an incubation period of 10 to 30 days, the illness begins with chilliness or chills, high fever reaching 104 to 106° F by the third day, severe myalgias, and frontal headaches. Photophobia and pain on moving the eyes are especially prominent and last into the second stage. Some patients complain of sore throat, dry cough, or diarrhea, but these are mild and transient. The main physical findings are a flush of the face and neck, giving a characteristic "sunburned" appearance, a relative bradycardia, generalized lymph node enlargement with no tenderness, normal heart and lungs, negative neurologic examination, and only occasional splenomegaly. The temperature falls rapidly to subnormal levels on the third to sixth day, along with a drop of blood pressure to near shock levels.

The toxic stage starts about the fourth day with defervescence. Thus, the disappearance of fever is not a hopeful sign as it is in most infections because it indicates the start of a more severe illness. The patients feel worse and develop a sense of desperation; prostration increases, and extreme restlessness develops. Hematemesis, hemoptysis, and melena begin, abdominal pain increases, and thirst becomes intense but cannot be satisfied because of intense vomiting. Renal failure with oliguria or anuria sets in between the fourth and ninth days. Disorientation, delirium, coma, and convulsive seizures develop in the severest cases. The systolic blood pressure drops to 80 mm Hg, and shock may become irreversible. Ocular hemorrhages vary from conjunctival petechiae to the typical "red eyes" of severe episcleral bleeding. Severe petechiae also occur in the soft palate, pharynx, axillae, chest, scapulas, and arms. Almost all patients have some evidence of uremia. Periorbital, severe conjunctival, facial, and pulmonary edema are features of the uremic phase. The heart is usually normal, but a few deaths have occurred from myocardial failure and ventricular fibrillation. Abdominal tenderness is usually severe and raises the question of an acute surgical problem.

The convalescent stage starts about ten days to two weeks after onset of illness. The symptoms usually disappear suddenly. Immediately after the oliguria subsides, marked polyuria begins with daily urine outputs of 4 to 10 liters and marked thirst. This diuretic phase may last as long as two to three months.

## LABORATORY DIAGNOSIS

Heavy proteinuria begins about the fourth day of illness when oliguria occurs. During the polyuric phase the specific gravity of the urine is below 1.010 and remains low for up to three months. Creatinine levels of 5 to 6 mg per 100 ml are common during the uremic phase. A polymorphonuclear leukocytosis of 20,000 to 40,000 is uniformly present in the toxic stage and can reach 100,000 in patients with a myeloid type of leukemoid reaction. Atypical lymphocytes are also common, reaching 5 to 25 per cent. Thrombocytopenia is present between the fourth and tenth days, falling to 20,000 or less, but the prothrombin time and other clotting factors are normal. The hematocrit depends on the balance between the loss of blood and water into the circulation. Loss of plasma can raise the hematocrit to 70 per cent in shock.

Specific diagnosis is made by demonstrating rising antibody titers to the KHF agent in lung tissues of *Apodemus agrarius jejudoici* by the indirect fluorescent antibody techniques of Lee et al. (1978). A rise in titer in serial samples must be obtained because antibodies from a past infection can still be present ten years later.

## TREATMENT

Fluids must be kept at the minimum requirements needed to replace what is lost in the urine, feces, vomitus, sweat, and evaporation during fever. This can be determined by measuring output and weighing the patient. If the overpowering thirst is allowed to determine water intake, the patient becomes overloaded with fluid and suffers pulmonary edema. When vomiting is severe, 10 per cent glucose in water should be given intravenously in minimal quantities and saline should be avoided. Mild hypotension is treated by placing the patient in the Trendelenburg position and bandaging the extremities. When the hematocrit reaches high levels (55 to 60 per cent) in more advanced shock, the patient should receive plasma or salt-free human albumin. Pressors such as 1-norepinephrine are ineffective. The treatment of severe renal failure is probably best accomplished by early and frequent dialysis. Either peritoneal or extracorporeal hemodialysis may be used. Frequent dialysis cuts down on the need for strict water restriction, makes fluid balance easier to manage, and helps avoid serious problems with hyperkalemia and other electrolyte disturbances. If dialysis cannot be done, the hyperkalemia should be treated with intravenous glucose and insulin and calcium chloride to protect against the cardiotoxic effects of potassium. Enemas of potassium-binding resins (such as Kayexelate, a sodium cycle resin), given two to four times daily, can prevent dangerous levels of potassium, but rectal impaction is a risk when these are given to severely dehydrated patients. Sodium bicarbonate may be needed to keep the plasma bicarbonate above 15 mEq per liter.

During the diuretic phase of convalescence, fluid intake must be carefully maintained to prevent dehydration and shock. For this reason, the patient should be kept in the hospital until the urine is concentrated to 1.020.

The mortality depends on the quality of the care. In early reports, before the pathophysiology and treatment were understood, one third of the patients died in some outbreaks, and the overall death rate was 15 per cent. Troops in Korea receiving better treatment had a mortality of about 6 per cent, and no deaths have occurred in specialized centers for treating hemorrhagic fever.

The main sequela is persistent disturbance in renal tubular function, which occurs in only a few patients. This may last for many years without causing serious disability.

### References

Arribalzaga, R.: Una nueva enfermedad epidémica a german desconocido: Hipertermia nefrotóxica, leukopenica y enantemática. Dia Méd 27:1204, 1955.

Bokish, V., Franklin, H., Russel, P., Dixon, F., and Müller-Eberhard, H.: The potential pathogenic role of complement in dengue hemorrhagic shock syndrome. J Immunol 102:412, 1973.

Brummer-Korvenkontio, M., Vaheri, A., Hori, T., H. von Bonsdorff, C., Vuorimies, J., Manni, T., Penttinen, K., Oker-Blom, N., and Lëhdevirta, J.: Nephropathia epidemica: Detection of antigen in bank voles and serologic diagnosis of human infection. J Infect Dis 141:131, 1980.

Dasaneyavaja, A., Robin, Y., and Yenbutia, D.: Laboratory observations related to prognosis in Thai hemorrhagic fever. J Trop Med Hyg 66:35, 1963.

deBracco, M., Rimoldi, M., Cossio, P., Rabinovich, A., Maiztegui, J., Carballal, G., and Arana, R.: Argentine hemorrhagic fever. N Engl J Med 299:216, 1978.

Ehrenkranz, N. J., Ventura, A., Cuadrado, R., Pond, W., and Porter, J.: Pandemic dengue in Caribbean countries and the southern United States—past, present, and potential problems. N Engl J Med 285:1460, 1971.

Fraser, H., Wilson, W., Thomas, E., and Sissons, J.: Dengue shock syndrome in Jamaica. Br Med J 1:893, 1978.

Gajdusek, D.: Acute infectious hemorrhagic fevers and mycotoxicoses in the Union of Soviet Socialist Republics. Medical Science Publications no. 2. Washington, Army Medical Service Graduate School, 1953, pp. 19–35.

Hammon, W.: Dengue hemorrhagic fever. Do we know its cause? Am J Trop Med Hyg 22:82, 1973.

Hammon, W., Rudnick, A., Sather, G., Rogers, K., and Morse, L.: New hemorrhagic fevers of children in the Philippines and Thailand. Trans. Assoc Am Physicians 73:140, 1960.

Lee, H., and Lee, P.: Etiological relation between Korean haemorrhagic fever and nephropathia epidemica. Lancet 1:186:1979.

Lee, H., Lee, P., and Johnson, K.: Isolation of the etiologic agent of Korean hemorrhagic fever. J Infect Dis 137:298, 1978.

Lukes, R.: The pathology of 39 fatal cases of epidemic hemorrhagic fever. Am J Med 16:639, 1954.

Maiztegui, J., Fernandez, N., and Damilano, A.: Efficacy of immune plasma in treatment of Argentine haemorrhagic fever and association between treatment and a late neurological syndrome. Lancet 2:1216, 1979.

Mercado, R., Valverde, L., Webb, P., Peters, C., and Johnson, K.: Hemorrhagic fever. Bolivia Morbid Mortal Weekly Rep May 1, 1971, p. 162.

Powell, G.: Clinical manifestations of epidemic hemorrhagic fever. JAMA 151:1261, 1953.

Russel, P.: Immunopathologic mechanism in the dengue shock syndrome. In Amos, B. (ed.): Progress in Immunology. New York, Academic Press, 1971, pp. 831–838.

Sabin, A.: Research on dengue during World War II. Am J Trop Med Hyg 1:30, 1952.

Sobel, A., Bodusch, V., and Müller-Eberhard, H.: C1q deviation test for the detection of immune complexes, aggregates of IgG, and bacterial products in human sera. J Exp Med 142:139, 1975.

Theiler, M., Casals, J., and Moutousses, C.: Etiology of the 1927–1928 epidemic of dengue in Greece. Proc Soc Exp Biol Med 103:244, 1960.

Theofilopoulos, A., Wilson, C., and Dixon, F.: The Raji cell radioimmune assay for detecting immune complexes in human sera. J Clin Invest 57:169, 1976.

van Der Sar, A.: An outbreak of dengue hemorrhagic fever in Curaçao. Trop Geogr Med 25:119, 1979.

Webb, H., and Rao, R. L.: Kyasanur forest disease: A general clinical study in which some cases with neurological complications were observed. Trans R Soc Trop Med Hyg 55:284, 1961.

Work, T.: Russian spring–summer virus in India. Kyasanur forest disease. Progr Med Virol 1:248, 1958.

World Health Organization: Technical guides for diagnosis, treatment, surveillance, prevention and control of Dengue hemorrhagic fever. Geneva, 1975.

# 203 *INFECTIOUS MONONUCLEOSIS*

*David A. Stevens, M.D.*

### DEFINITION

Infectious mononucleosis has fascinated physicians for many reasons. It is perhaps most intriguing as a self-limited lymphoproliferative disorder, a "leukemia that turns itself off." Seroepidemiologic studies provide convincing evidence that a primary infection with the Epstein-Barr virus is its cause (Evans et al., 1968). Thus, only individuals who are negative for antibody to Epstein-Barr virus develop infectious mononucleosis, and after they do, antibody to the virus can be demonstrated.

### ETIOLOGY

The Epstein-Barr virus is a human herpesvirus, with an affinity for lymphocytes (Diehl et al.,

1968; Henle et al., 1968). It is shed from the throat during infectious mononucleosis. Like the three other human herpesviruses, after the primary infection a prolonged latent period ensues. The virus can later reactivate from its dormant focus and shed from the throat of seropositive normal individuals. This residence in the pharynx presumably explains the long epidemiologic association of infectious mononucleosis with oral contact, the so-called "kissing disease."

Epstein-Barr virus is the most common cause of human infection. For example, we found that 97 per cent of healthy adult blood donors are seropositive, indicating previous infection. This has been shown by a variety of serologic techniques with population groups from all over the world, including remote tribesmen.

The virus is also under scrutiny because of a proposed etiologic association with two human cancers: Burkitt's lymphoma, a disease endemic to parts of Africa and New Guinea, and nasopharyngeal carcinoma, a disease endemic to persons of Southern Chinese and North African ancestry (Epstein et al., 1965). Cases of both diseases also occur worldwide. This association is made because of the high antibody titers against the virus in these cancer patients (and the presence of antibodies to Epstein-Barr viral antigens that are unusual in seropositive healthy individuals), the presence of the viral genome in the nucleic acid of the tumors, and a capacity of the virus to induce lymphoproliferation in human cells in vitro and in primates in vivo. If the virus causes these cancers, its association with both benign and malignant diseases suggests that cofactors are important in the cancers.

## EPIDEMIOLOGY

Perhaps only one third of infections with Epstein-Barr virus result in typical symptoms of infectious mononucleosis. In college students this incidence is approximately 50 per cent. About one third of patients with infections in the college age group are asymptomatic, and the remainder (about 20 per cent) present with various illnesses (predominantly upper respiratory) that do not resemble infectious mononucleosis. The asymptomatic infections and the other nondescript illnesses may produce heterophilic antibody (described below).

The incidence of infectious mononucleosis in the United States is estimated to be 45 per 100,000 persons per year. Its striking affinity for the high school and college age population is illustrated by the incidence in the 15- to 19-year age group of 343 per 100,000 persons per year. The reported lower incidence in developing countries may reflect inattention to this relatively benign disease and/or infection in early childhood because of differing hygienic practices. This is discussed further in the next section.

The incubation period, derived inferentially from epidemiologic studies (largely among military cadets) is 6 to 60 days (Hoagland, 1967).

## PATHOGENESIS

Lymphoproliferation is prominent. About 5 per cent of circulating leukocytes are actively synthesizing DNA, approximately the same percentage as that found in acute leukemia and chronic granulocytic leukemia. This proliferation lasts three to four months.

The target cell of the Epstein-Barr virus is the B lymphocyte. This cell is the only lymphocyte with receptors for the virus. The viral infection presumably results in an antigenic alteration in these cells that then induces a defensive response in the T-lymphocyte population. This response of the T lymphocytes is presumed to bring the infection under control.

If this infected B cell is transplanted beyond the control mechanisms of the patient, it has neoplastic properties. Thus, when blood from a patient with infectious mononucleosis is transplanted to a hamster, a disseminated tumor will result, and all the tumor cells will have B-lymphocyte markers.

The number of B lymphocytes increases in the first week of illness, and the T lymphocytes peak one to two weeks later. Most of the atypical lymphocytes are T cells, and there is some variation at different times in the illness. With all this activity involving both T and B lymphocytes, it is not surprising that cell-mediated immunity is depressed. For example, tuberculin-positive patients become tuberculin-negative during infectious mononucleosis. Depression in both T- and B-lymphocyte function can be defined by the use of selective mitogens. Recent studies in our laboratory provide support for the role of cellular immunity in terminating the disease, because there is a close temporal relationship between the onset of cellular reactivity and Epstein-Barr virus antigens and disappearance of symptoms.

The lymph nodes enlarge as a result of infiltration by atypical lymphocytes and their hyperplasia in the follicles. The architecture of the nodes is not usually disturbed, unless the atypical cells flood the medullary portion and produce a picture that stimulates the infiltrative pattern of leukemia. Other lymphoid tissues such as the tonsils also enlarge as a consequence of infiltration and proliferation by atypical lymphocytes. The spleen increases two to three times in size and becomes hyperemic and soft. The atypical cells may also infiltrate the trabeculae and capsule so that the organ is easily ruptured. In the liver, the atypical cells may infiltrate the portal areas, sinusoids, and areas of scattered parenchymal necrosis, producing a picture very similar to that caused by hepatitis A or B virus.

## CLINICAL MANIFESTATIONS

After the incubation period two cardinal findings, pharyngitis and cervical adenitis, appear. Sore throat is the most common symptom and is found in 80 to 85 per cent of cases. Pharyngitis is found on examination in over 90 per cent of patients and the absence of pharyngitis should make one question the diagnosis of infectious mononucleosis. Pharyngitis is almost always associated with adenopathy, particularly the cervical lymph glands. Nontender enlargement of axillary, inguinal, and mediastinal glands may also occur. The incidence of adenopathy is greater than 90 per cent. Pharyngitis without adenitis is a characteristic of those diseases that mimic infectious mononucleosis and are discussed under Differential Diagnosis.

The other common findings are splenomegaly in one fourth to three fourths of cases, and hepatomegaly in one sixth to one half. Many liver enzymes are elevated, but the most sensitive biochemical test is that for lactic dehydrogenase, which is abnormal in more than 90 per cent of cases, and is increased disproportionately in relation to the other tests of liver function. Jaundice occurs in 5 to 10 per cent of patients. Fever (present in over 95 per cent of cases and lasting one to three weeks) and lethargy are also common and prominent. Headache is common, and nausea, chills, sweats, cough, and myalgias may also occur. Rhinitis, sputum production, pleurisy, arthralgias, and diarrhea suggest other infections.

There are other clinical and laboratory findings that receive less attention and may even be misleading. Petechiae on the palate are found in one fourth to one half of patients, and periorbital edema occurs in one third. The blood uric acid level is elevated in one fifth of cases. One third will have cold agglutinins in the serum (and one fourth of these will show hemolysis by sensitive assays). If ampicillin is given to a patient with infectious mononucleosis, a morbiliform rash is almost universal. The mechanism of this association is unknown.

In uncomplicated illness these clinical findings all resolve by the fourth week.

## DIAGNOSIS

In the diagnostic laboratory, the hallmarks of the disease are the atypical lymphocyte and the heterophilic antibody.

The atypical lymphocyte takes several forms, and one of the most common is virtually indistinguishable from the blast cell that is produced by stimulating lymphocytes with antigen or mitogen in vitro. The nucleus may be oval or irregular, contain nucleoli, and have a foamy cytoplasm. These cells generally appear in the peripheral blood on the second to twelfth day of illness, persist for two to eight weeks, and amount to at least 20 per cent of the total leukocytes at the peak of the fever when total mononuclear cells form over 50 per cent of all leukocytes.

The heterophilic antibody is an IgM antibody (Wollheim and Williams, 1966). Opinions on significant titers range from 1:56 to 1:224. The titer should decrease less than one eighth after absorption with guinea pig cells (Forssman antigen), and at least one eighth after absorption with beef cells. There is good evidence that any titer over 1:80 is diagnostic, so that absorption steps are unnecessary at that level. Any titer of 1:8 to 1:10 that persists after guinea pig absorption is probably diagnostic as well, and is not due to other conditions in which heterophilic antibody is found (notably hepatitis and serum sickness).

The heterophilic antibody appears in the first two weeks of illness (after the atypical lymphocytes appear), reaches a peak titer in the second or third week, and may persist up to eight months (Davidsohn, 1962). This antibody may reappear up to two years afterward and may cause confusion over possible "second attacks" of infectious mononucleosis. The heterophilic antibody may rise in titer or turn positive in this interval in response to various intercurrent illnesses and does not represent recurrence of infectious mononucleosis. The picture is clear when the antibody reappears with a typical clinical syndrome such as mumps, especially when mumps virus is isolated. It may be confusing, however, when the intercurrent illness resembles infectious mononucleosis. We have investigated several such reputed "second attacks" with antibody studies of Epstein-Barr virus and found no evidence that second attacks of infectious mononucleosis could occur.

Agglutination of sheep erythrocytes is the traditional method for demonstrating the heterophilic antibody as in the Paul-Bunnell test (Paul and Bunnell, 1932). However, antibodies also lyse ox erythrocytes in infectious mononucleosis, and the test for these is the most sensitive for heterophilic antibody with the fewest false positives. Because this test is more difficult technically, it is generally unavailable. Since the use of horse erythrocytes can detect low titers of agglutinating antibody, commercial kits utilizing this antibody in slide tests have been prepared. If the Paul-Bunnell test is negative in patients with the clinical signs of infectious mononucleosis, the horse cell test should be applied.

Absorption with beef cells removes all antisheep and antihorse cell antibodies because the beef cell apparently contains all the heterophilic antigens. These properties form the basis for the differential absorption test described above. In addition, the sheep cell receptor for the heterophilic antibody in infectious mononucleosis is sensitive to papain, a feature distinguishing it from the receptors for heterophilic antibodies that appear in other diseases.

After primary Epstein-Barr virus infection, a symptomatic illness with the classic features of infectious mononucleosis is more common in those over 15 years of age. Moreover, when the infection resembles infectious mononucleosis the heterophilic test is more often positive in patients over 15 years old (seven eighths of those over 15 versus two thirds of those under 15). The confusing illnesses that resemble infectious mononucleosis but produce negative test results for antibody to Epstein-Barr virus and negative sheep cell agglutinins are most common in those under 15 years of age. The reason for the age-dependent differences in manifestations of Epstein-Barr virus infection is not understood.

Other antibodies are formed in infectious mononucleosis, and the concentrations of the major serum immunoglobulins are increased, especially IgM. The other antibodies include rheumatoid factor, a macroglobulin with specificity against the fetal erythrocyte i antigen, cryoglobulins, lymphocytotoxic antibodies of broad specificity, antibodies against Newcastle disease virus (which has nothing to do with the etiology of the disease), and antibodies against smooth muscle. Less commonly, low titers of antinuclear antibodies are found, and VDRL tests are false positive.

### The Antiviral Response

Antibodies directed against the capsid of Epstein-Barr virus can be detected by immunofluorescence soon after onset of infection. In some cases, when sera had been collected for other purposes, capsid antibody appeared during the incubation period. These antibodies persist for life without change in titer.

Antibodies also appear against antigens that form early in the viral replicative cycle and are termed early antigen. Two types of antibody against early antigen have been described—those producing restricted (R) patterns of immunofluorescence and those producing diffuse patterns (D). Antibodies against early antigen are rare in normal adults, occurring in less than 1 of 8, and when present they are usually of the R specificity.

About 60 per cent of infectious mononucleosis patients have D type antibody against early antigen that disappears a few months after onset of infection.

Antibodies to a nuclear, nucleic-acid–associated antigen, referred to as EBNA (Epstein-Barr nuclear antigen), first appear two months or more after infection. These are usually assayed by an indirect immunofluorescence technique employing antibodies directed against complement, which is fixed in the nuclear antigen-antibody reaction. A traditional complement fixation antibody test has been devised with cellular extract, which appears to detect the same or a very closely related antigen.

As with other infections, IgM antibodies are a feature of the primary infection but can give cross-reactions with IgM antibody produced after cytomegalovirus infection. We have shown that IgA antibodies to Epstein-Barr viral capsid are also transiently present in the serum in infectious mononucleosis and absent from healthy adults. This antibody is found in the sera of patients with nasopharyngeal carcinoma.

These antibodies are potentially useful in diagnosis. Demonstration of antibodies to viral capsid antigen at a level greater than 1:320 or, more significantly, a fourfold increase in titer or higher during an acute illness, supports the diagnosis of primary EBV infection. Likewise, antibodies to early antigen or, even better, a fourfold change in titer over an acute illness, supports this diagnosis, as does the presence of IgM or IgA antiviral antibodies. These antibodies only rarely represent a reactivated infection. The antibody to EBNA may help differentiate primary EBV infection from those diseases that resemble infectious mononucleosis. If the infection is a primary one, antibodies to EBNA should be absent, since these appear after the acute stage. People who have been infected with EBV at some time in the past should have antibodies to both viral capsid antigens and EBNA.

Some of these tests will not be available in routine laboratories, nor are they necessary in most cases of infectious mononucleosis. However, there are problems in differential diagnosis between infectious mononucleosis and other infectious diseases, and sometimes between infectious mononucleosis and malignant lymphoproliferative diseases such as leukemia and lymphoma, that will warrant the performance of such serologic studies in a specialized laboratory.

Several studies have shown no relation between the heterophilic and EBV antigens or antibodies. Therefore, the mechanism for the production of heterophilic antibodies (and the other antibodies lacking Epstein-Barr specificity) in infectious mononucleosis is still a mystery.

## DIFFERENTIAL DIAGNOSIS

The sore throat of infectious mononucleosis must be distinguished from streptococcal sore throat, diphtheria, Vincent's angina, primary herpes simplex pharyngitis and tonsillitis, adenovirus pharyngitis, and herpangina. In none of these diseases does the patient develop the characteristic blood picture of infectious mononucleosis, and some are rapidly distinguished by smear or culture and by the characteristic appearance of the throat. The typical vesicular lesions of herpes simplex and herpangina are described elsewhere in this text. Herpes simplex virus can be isolated in 24 to 48 hours and the herpetic giant epithelial cells demonstrated from the base of the lesion in Tzanck preparations in a few minutes. Herpangina is a disease of children below the age of 7, whereas mononucleosis occurs mainly in high school and college age persons.

The blood picture must be differentiated from that of several diseases resembling infectious mononucleosis.

### Post-Transfusion Mononucleosis

This is probably the disease most frequently resembling infectious mononucleosis. Post-transfusion mononucleosis occurs with an estimated frequency of 3 to 67 per cent following blood transfusion. The incidence rises with the amount of blood perfused, the freshness of the blood, and the length of perfusion times during the massive transfusions of cardiopulmonary bypass, the most common setting for this disease. The clinical picture is similar to that of infectious mononucleosis except that pharyngitis is rare and adenopathy is uncommon. The absence of laboratory features of infectious mononucleosis described above (with the exception of atypical mononuclear cells in the peripheral blood) is thus helpful. Several studies (using serologic tests and virus isolation) have suggested that cytomegalovirus is the cause of most cases of post-transfusion mononucleosis, although one case caused by Epstein-Barr virus has been reported. In some of the cytomegalovirus-related cases, the blood donors were found to be excreting cytomegalovirus. Since in most studies there are a few cases not associated with either cytomegalovirus or Epstein-Barr virus, there is yet another agent or agents that can cause this syndrome.

### Cytomegalovirus Mononucleosis

Cytomegalovirus can cause a disease similar to infectious mononucleosis in the absence of transfusions. Some studies have implicated cytomegalovirus as etiologic in half the cases of heterophilic-negative infectious mononucleosis. The peripheral blood picture in cytomegalovirus mononucleosis strikingly resembles that of infectious mononucleosis, as most patients have more than 50 per cent mononuclear cells in their peripheral blood, and more than 50 per cent of these are atypical. The age range of patients is similar to that in infectious mononucleosis, and except for the heterophilic antibody, many of the aberrant antibodies seen in infectious mononucleosis are also found in cytomegalovirus mononucleosis. Differentiation from infectious mononucleosis can be made by the fact that sore throat is rare and adenopathy, hepatomegaly, and splenomegaly occur in only a small minority of patients with cytomegalovirus mononucleosis. Prominent features are myalgia, headache, cough, hepatitis, and a fever that lasts two to five weeks. These patients may develop bronchopneumonia, polyneuritis, myocarditis, or pericarditis, although these are occasionally seen in infectious mononucleosis as well. The presence of antibody to cytomegalovirus does not appear to protect against cytomegalovirus mononucleosis. The antibody rise in this illness is frequently delayed beyond that usually noted in acute viral infections, and this point may be helpful in planning the collection of paired serum specimens for diagnostic purposes.

### Acute Infectious Lymphocytosis

This term has unfortunately been applied to Paul-Bunnell–negative infectious mononucleosis, but it should be reserved for a distinct syndrome of unknown cause in children. Epidemics have been reported in institutions. Hepatomegaly, splenomegaly, and adenopathy are absent, as is heterophilic antibody. The leukocyte count is elevated above $20,000/mm^3$, and in some series the lowest count recorded was $38,000/mm^3$. Although the increase is due to lymphocytes, they are all typical in appearance. Eosinophilia is frequently seen. Diarrhea is sometimes part of the syndrome, and in some institutional outbreaks the lymphocytosis was found in children who were asymptomatic and even afebrile. Aseptic meningitis, respiratory symptoms, and rashes are more common in this disorder than in infectious mononucleosis. The percentage of lymphocytes in the marrow is increased, unlike the situation in infectious mononucleosis, in which the marrow is normal.

### Toxoplasmosis

This may produce an illness like infectious mononucleosis when acquired in the postnatal period. Adenopathy and a relative lymphocytosis are common, whereas other clinical features of infectious mononucleosis are much less frequent. A maculopapular rash, pneumonitis, myocarditis, and encephalitis are rare complications of this disease, and are seldom seen in infectious mononucleosis. Serologic tests are helpful in differentiation.

### Other Etiologies

*Listeria monocytogenes* or parainfluenza virus rarely causes syndromes resembling infectious mononucleosis, and some drugs can result in atypical lymphocytes. The most common of these are phenytoin and para-aminosalicyclic acid.

### Angioimmunoblastic Lymphadenopathy

This nonmalignant but progressive lymphoproliferative disease resembles infectious mononucleosis in that it causes adenopathy, fever, and other systemic symptoms, and sometimes hepatosplenomegaly and gammaglobulin abnormalities. However, the patients are usually over 50 years old, and the pathologic changes in the lymph nodes are distinctive.

Differential diagnosis from malignant lymphoproliferation has been mentioned. The histopathology of a lymph node obtained by biopsy in infectious mononucleosis may closely resemble that of lymphoma, with mixed lymphoid proliferation and follicular hyperplasia, effacement of the node architecture, infiltration of the sinuses and capsule, and even the presence of Reed-Sternberg cells.

## COMPLICATIONS

Neurologic involvement is one of the most common complications. In neurologically normal patients with infectious mononucleosis 25 to 30 per cent will have an abnormal electroencephalogram. Clinically apparent involvement is estimated to occur in 1 to 7 per cent of patients, particularly males. The most common symptoms are headache and meningismus. Neurologic involvement usually occurs in the first three weeks after other symptoms of infectious mononucleosis, but may precede them by as much as 18 days. The most common manifestations are encephalitis, aseptic meningitis, or Guillain-Barré syndrome, although a variety of other neurologic syndromes have been described. These manifestations appear to respond to adrenal steroids. The mortality from neurologic involvement is estimated to be 4 to 11 per cent, but some of these estimates are from the older literature and include some patients with Guillain-Barré syndrome who would probably be saved with present treatment.

Splenic rupture is responsible for one fourth to one third of the deaths due to infectious mononucleosis and may occur weeks after the acute illness.

Airway obstruction may occur suddenly. Warning signs are dysphagia, drooling, muffled voice, and dyspnea. Steroids may be helpful in reducing airway edema.

Other reported complications include pneumonitis, hematuria, thrombocytopenia, purpura, disseminated intravascular coagulation, neutropenia, agranulocytosis, malabsorption, stomatitis, pancreatitis, orchitis, nephritis, the nephrotic syndrome, bacterial superinfection, Reye's syndrome, and involvement of the abdominal nodes mimicking appendicitis. Various ocular and electrocardiographic abnormalities have been described. Lethargy, which is characteristic in the acute phase, may persist in some patients for months after resolution of all other clinical and laboratory abnormalities.

A few instances of fatal infection in male siblings because of progressive lymphoproliferation and multisystemic involvement have been recorded and are presumably due to undefined selective congenital immunodeficiencies.

## TREATMENT

There is no specific treatment. Bed rest and, in severe cases, prednisone have been prescribed for symptomatic relief. It is given for one week starting with a dose of 40 to 60 mg and reducing it by 5 mg daily. There is no evidence that either treatment has a beneficial effect on the uncomplicated disease. However, neurologic involvement, airway edema, thrombocytopenia, and hemolysis apparently respond to adrenal steroids. Vigorous sports should be avoided in patients with splenomegaly to lessen the risk of splenic rupture.

### References

Davidsohn, E., and Lee, C.: The laboratory in diagnosis of infectious mononucleosis (with additional notes on epidemiology, etiology, and pathogenesis). Med Clin N Am 46:225, 1962.

Diehl, V., Henle, G., Henle, W., and Kohn, G.: Demonstration of a herpes group virus in cultures of peripheral leukocytes from patients with infectious mononucleosis. J Virol 2:663, 1968.

Epstein, M., Barr, Y., and Achong, B.: Studies with Burkitt's lymphoma. Wistar Symp Monogr 4:69, 1965.

Evans, A., Niederman, J., and McCollum, R.: Seroepidemiological studies of infectious mononucleosis with EB virus. N Engl J Med 279:1121, 1968.

Henle, G., Henle, W., and Diehl, V.: Relation of Burkitt's tumor-associated herpes-type virus to infectious mononucleosis. Proc Natl Acad Sci USA 59:94, 1968.

Hoagland, R. J.: Infectious Mononucleosis. New York, Grune & Stratton, 1967.

Paul, J., and Bunnell, W.: The presence of heterophile antibodies in infectious mononucleosis. Am J Med Sci 183:90, 1932.

Wollheim, F., and Williams, R.: Studies on the macroglobulins of human serum. 1. Polyclonal immunglobulin class M (IgM) increase in infectious mononucleosis. N Engl J Med 274:61, 1966.

# 204 *LASSA FEVER*

## *Abraham I. Braude, M.D., Ph.D.*

### *DEFINITION*

Lassa fever is a severe infection caused by an arenavirus. The disease is named for Lassa, a lonely herdsmen's village in the northern Nigerian Sudan where the first outbreak was recognized in 1969. The virus is spread to man from its reservoir, a multimammate rat, and from one person to another in households and hospitals. The outstanding symptoms are fever, prostration, severe pharyngitis, vomiting, abdominal pain, and dyspnea. Serous effusions, facial edema, generalized hemorrhages, and fatal shock occur later. The mortality rate is between 30 and 50 per cent.

### *ETIOLOGY*

The Lassa fever virus is one of four arenaviruses pathogenic for man; the others cause lymphocytic choriomeningitis, Argentine hemorrhagic fever, and Bolivian hemorrhagic fever. The term arenavirus is taken from the Latin word *arenosus*, which means sandy and refers to the characteristic granules seen by electron microscopy in infected cells (Rowe et al., 1970). Like other arenaviruses, Lassa virus is released from infected cells by budding and has an envelope formed from the plasma membrane. Its nucleic acid is single-stranded RNA (Chapter 62).

The apparent recent emergence of the disease suggests the possibility that Lassa virus is a virulent mutant of lymphocytic choriomeningitis virus or some nonpathogenic arenavirus.

### *PATHOGENESIS AND PATHOLOGY*

Man is infected through contact with *Mastomys natalensis,* a multimammate rat widespread in Africa. Lassa virus was recovered from tissues of *Mastomys* captured in houses occupied by Lassa fever patients during the 1972 epidemic in Sierra Leone. Ironically, the more vicious *Rattus rattus* seems to protect communities from Lassa fever by competing for food and space and thus driving away *Mastomys* and its Lassa virus. The rodents have easy access to the open African dwellings to which they are attracted by grains and food that are stored without protection. *Mastomys* sheds virus in the urine for long periods of time and spreads the infection to human beings by crawling over the beams and rafters of huts or houses and urinating on the sleeping inhabitants, their personal articles, and their food. The portal of entry is thus surmised to be inhalation of virus, direct contact with infected urine, or eating contaminated food. The prominence of sore throat and abdominal pain early in the illness would fit with a gastrointestinal or inhalational route of infection. Spread from patient to medical personnel takes place after direct contact, exposure to respiratory droplets, and accidental cuts from needles or scalpels. Airborne dissemination is the best way to explain infections in hospital visitors or patients who had no direct contact with hospitalized cases of Lassa fever and who developed prominent respiratory symptoms. Infection in households is probably transmitted by eating contaminated food or drinking infected water. Lassa virus has been recovered from the throat two to three weeks after symptoms began, and from the urine four to five weeks thereafter. Viremia is heavy enough to explain the spread of infection by sharp instruments. There are records of infection that occurred after sticking a finger with a needle being used for intravenous injection of fluid. One death from Lassa fever was the result of a cut received while performing an autopsy. Thus Lassa virus differs from other arenaviruses in the ease with which it spreads from person to person.

Whether the portal of entry is the throat, gastrointestinal tract, or lung, a persistent viremia develops that carries the Lassa virus to all organs, apparently damaging capillaries everywhere so that water and blood is lost into the tissues, producing edema and hemorrhages. Thrombocytopenia and other coagulation disturbances contribute to these hemorrhages, which have been noted in the skin, intestine, myocardium, and kidney. A distinctive lesion has been found throughout the liver where the virus has been seen by electron microscopy. Individual hepatocytes, or groups of hepatocytes, undergo eosinophilic necrosis with no accompanying inflammatory exudate, inclusions, or fatty changes. Unusual lesions also occur in the spleen where the malpighian bodies have been found depleted of lymphocytes and surrounded by an eosinophilic zone of coagulation necrosis. Focal pneumonitis has also been present (Edington and White, 1972; Frame et al., 1970).

## CLINICAL MANIFESTATIONS

Symptoms usually start gradually after an incubation period of 7 to 17 days. An exact incubation period was calculated in the case of a pathologist who cut her finger on January 25, 1970 with a scalpel while freeing the ribs of a dead patient with Lassa fever in Jos, Nigeria. Ten days later, on February 3, the pathologist had a severe chill, felt severe muscle pains, and became very tired. The next day her temperature was over 102° F, and her throat became so sore she could hardly swallow. On February 11 she complained of greatly increased malaise, her skin became flushed, and petechiae began to appear. Her course thereafter was steadily downhill. Blood oozed from anywhere an injection had been made, oliguria set in, and she became hypothermic to 94.6°. Her white count, which had been low, suddenly jumped to over 37,000, a puzzling feature noted in other Lassa cases. She went into shock and her respirations became labored, but she remained conscious until her death on February 18, 15 days after the illness began (Fuller, 1974).

The features of this case are typical of the severe form of Lassa fever with its fatality rate of 41 per cent in Africans to 64 per cent in whites (Frame et al., 1970; Monath, 1975). In milder cases the mortality rate is only 8 per cent (Monath et al., 1974). In most patients the onset is more insidious than that described in the pathologist, possibly because she gave herself a massive inoculum of Lassa virus from a fatal case. The symptoms of chills, fever, and muscle aches are regularly seen at the beginning, but they are usually not bad enough to see a doctor until four to nine days after they start. Sometimes there is improvement on the second and third days before the progressive illness sets in. Sore throat is usually present after the third day and may become so severe that swallowing is impossible. In about half the patients, pains are also noticed in the head, chest, and abdomen. Headache is mild but persistent and either frontal or generalized. The abdominal pain may be localized over the liver, or diffuse and colicky, with frequent loose stools. Chest pain tends to occur along the costal margins or under the sternum and is made worse by a frequent nonproductive cough (Monath, 1974).

The severe sore throat is accompanied by an exudative pharyngitis and tonsillitis. The yellowish or white exudate may coalesce to form a pseudomembrane. Aphthous ulcers with a yellow center and bright red rim may occur singly or in clusters on the back of the throat, buccal mucosa, and palate. The cervical and submaxillary lymph nodes are enlarged and often tender. Axillary lymphadenopathy is also present.

Signs of capillary leakage, such as facial edema, pleural effusion, and ecchymoses occur in the more severe cases. The pleural effusion, which is a clear serous fluid, is accompanied by dyspnea. Rales are more common than edema or serous effusions, last only a few days, and are not accompanied by signs of heart failure. It is also of interest that the edema does not tend to be dependent. The blood pressure is low (systolic under 90 mm Hg) during the acute stage, but shock occurs only in fatal cases.

## COMPLICATIONS AND SEQUELAE

Abortion and hearing loss are the only two complications of Lassa fever. Women with severe Lassa fever often abort within four days of admission (Fabiyi, 1975), and others may deliver a dead fetus during convalescence. The death rate from Lassa fever in pregnant women is twice that in nonpregnant women (Monath, 1975).

About half the patients have symptoms referable to the eighth nerve, and a few continue to have trouble hearing after recovery from the acute illness. Ataxia may also be a problem in convalescence (Fuller, 1974).

## GEOGRAPHIC VARIATIONS IN DISEASE

There are no clinical differences in the Lassa fever syndrome seen in Nigeria, Sierra Leone, and Liberia, the three epidemic areas of the disease.

## DIAGNOSIS

The disease should be suspected in anyone living in, or coming from, Nigeria, Sierra Leone, or Liberia and who becomes ill with fever, prostration, severe ulcerative pharyngitis, cervical adenopathy, rales, cough, and abdominal pain. Leukopenia and proteinuria are also useful diagnostic points, and a history of employment in a hospital in these epidemic regions is important. The pharyngitis is perhaps the distinctive feature of the illness because no other tropical infection is characterized by this combination of a severe sore throat with severe febrile prostration. It resembles infectious mononucleosis, but mononucleosis is seldom seen in the tropics. Streptococcal sore throat and diphtheria would be important diagnostic considerations if there were no facilities for bacteriologic diagnosis, but otherwise the distinction is easy to make. Dengue hemorrhagic fever and yellow fever are tropical diseases with severe prostration and bleeding, but the rash of dengue and the jaundice of yellow fever are not seen in Lassa fever.

The specific diagnosis of Lassa fever can be made by serologic tests and virus isolation. Lassa virus can be rapidly isolated from the throat, blood, and urine in Vero cells and other tissue culture cell lines, and by mouse inoculation. Such isolation should be attempted, however, only in laboratories equipped with iron-clad safety precautions against laboratory infection with this lethal virus (such as the Maximum Security Laboratory at the Center for Disease Control [CDC]). Lassa virus can be isolated from the blood, throat, and urine for at least two weeks and rarely more than three. Hence, quarantine for three weeks is probably long enough.

Serologic diagnosis is made by complement fixation, neutralization, and indirect immunofluorescence. Complement-fixing antibody does not appear until two weeks after onset of infection, and antigenic differences in strains from different outbreaks have been noted that could give negative results in proven infections if a nonreacting strain is used for complement fixation. Thus, sera from Lassa fever patients in Nigeria did not fix complement in the presence of strains from Liberia and Sierra Leone (Monath, 1975). Such antigenic differences have not been encountered with the indirect immunofluorescence test. For this reason, and also because it has been positive with sera as early as seven days after onset of infection, it is probably the diagnostic test of choice in Lassa fever. The test must also be done in high-security laboratories because live virus is used to prepare the antigenic substrates to which the human sera are applied. The reaction between human serum and Lassa virus is detected on slides with fluorescein isothiocyanate-conjugated antihuman immunoglobulin.

### TREATMENT

Transfusions of immune plasma have been given to Lassa fever patients who recovered, but their number is too small to draw conclusions about the value of such immunotherapy. One patient died after such treatment, possibly because renal failure was precipitated by the plasma (White, 1972). Otherwise, treatment is supportive and should be directed at relieving the sore throat, removing pleural fluid when such effusions compromise breathing, treating the bleeding disorder with transfusions of platelets, and replacing blood lost by hemorrhage. Dialysis may be of value for patients with renal failure. Ribavarin, an antiviral drug used successfully against Lassa virus infections in monkeys, may help in treating patients with Lassa fever (Jahrling et al., 1980).

### PREVENTION

Current epidemiologic information would suggest that prevention of Lassa fever will require rodent control, isolation of patients, and personal precautions by hospital personnel or laboratory workers who must deal with infected excreta, blood specimens, or tissues. *Mastomys natalensis* are the rodents that must be controlled, since the virus has been found in no other animal reservoir. Unfortunately the crowded living conditions, poor sanitation, open houses, and unprotected food storage that encourage this rodent in epidemic areas are too widespread and too difficult to change. A more realistic approach is to prevent spread in the hospital where the source of nosocomial outbreaks is a patient admitted with an unexplained fever. A high index of suspicion should prevail in West Africa in epidemic areas so that the index case can be spotted and isolated. Surgeons, nurses, pathologists, and laboratory technicians are among those at greatest risk and should be most alert to the danger of infection from cases of unexplained fever with sore throat who might have the Lassa syndrome. Although food and water are vehicles for transmission, the danger of this route of transmission from the index cases is minimized in African hospitals by the practice of feeding patients with food brought by their relatives. Isolation of index cases should be carried out in a way that would not allow airborne dissemination. In addition, linens, bedpans, and other utensils must be carefully handled and sterilized because the virus is shed in excreta for at least two weeks.

Travelers who arrive from West Africa with pharyngitis and fever should be hospitalized in strict isolation. Throat swabs and urine and blood samples should be collected for shipment to a diagnostic center by a physician wearing a mask and protective clothing. High-risk contacts known to have had intimate contact, including face-to-face conversation, should be identified and kept under close surveillance if the diagnosis is confirmed. It should be kept in mind that Lassa fever is not highly communicable outside the home or hospital. At least five patients have traveled aboard commercial airplanes, but no secondary cases have been found among airline passengers (Editorial note, 1978).

### References

Edington, G., and White, H.: The pathology of Lassa fever. Trans R Soc Trop Med Hyg 19:670, 1970.

Fabiyi, A.: In discussion of paper by Monath, T., 1975.

Frame, J., Baldwin, J., Gocke, D., and Troup, J.: Lassa fever, a new virus disease of man from West Africa. I. Clinical description and pathological findings. Am J Trop Med Hyg 19:670, 1970.

Fuller, J. G.: Fever! The Hunt for a New Killer Virus. New York, Ballantine Books, 1974, pp. 183–205.

Jahrling, P., Hesse, R., Eddy, G., Johnson, K., Callis, R., and Stephen, E.: Lassa virus infections of rhesus monkeys: pathogenesis and treatment with ribavarin. J Infect Dis 141:580, 1980.

Monath, T. P.: Lassa fever: Review of epidemiology and epizootiology. WHO Bull 52:577, 1975.

Monath, T., Maher, M., Casals, J., Kissling, R., and Cacciapuoti, A.: Lassa fever in the Eastern Province of Sierra Leone, 1970–1972. II. Clinical observation and virologic studies on selected hospital cases. Am J Trop Med Hyg 23:1140, 1974.

Rowe, W., Murphy, F., Bergold, G., Lasak, J., Hotchin, J., Johnson, K., Lehman-Grube, F., Mims, C., Traub, E., and Webb, P.: Arenaviruses: Proposed name for a newly defined virus group. J Virol 5:651, 1970.

U.S. Public Health Service, Center for Disease Control: Editorial note: Suspected Lassa fever—Washington, D.C. Morbid Mortal Weekly Rep May 26, 1978, p. 182.

White, H.: Clinical findings in 23 cases of Lassa fever hospitalized in Jos, Nigeria. Trans R Soc Trop Med Hyg 66:390, 1972.

# G DERMAL INFECTIONS, EXANTHEMS, AND INFESTATIONS

## *IMPETIGO* **205**

*Marian E. Melish, M.D.*

### DEFINITION AND ETIOLOGY

There are two clinically and bacteriologically distinct superficial skin infections that are commonly called "impetigo." These two basic forms are: (1) the thick crusted variety that is primarily of streptococcal origin, and (2) the bullous form that is caused exclusively by coagulase-positive staphylococci. Either or both may be referred to as impetigo. In the United States, however, the term impetigo generally refers to the thick crusted variety and "bullous impetigo" to the staphylococcal form.

Bacterial culture of typical crusted impetigo lesions generally yields either group A β-hemolytic streptococci or a mixed flora of group A streptococci and coagulase-positive staphylococci. Several lines of evidence indicate that the streptococcus is the primary etiologic agent and the staphylococcus merely a secondary invader or "fellow traveler."

1. Streptococci are frequently isolated in pure culture from typical thick crusted lesions, whereas staphylococci are almost never encountered alone.

2. Sequential cultures of typical lesions show the same strain of streptococci as permanent residents, whereas staphylococci of varying types are only intermittently present.

3. Early lesions are often purely streptococcal; later cultures yield mixed flora. An increasing yield of staphylococci as the lesion ages suggests that staphylococci are secondary invaders.

4. Treatment of patients with antibiotics active against streptococci, but not staphylococci, gives as good a cure rate as treatment directed against both organisms (Dajani et al., 1972; Dillon, 1970).

A number of different M types (see Chapter 24) are associated with impetigo, particularly those of higher numbers; for example, M-33, M-49 (Red Lake), and M-52 to M-61. Many strains cannot be typed by antibody to known M types and are iden-

tified by antisera to their T antigens (Chapter 24).

Only strains of *Staphylococcus aureus* that produce epidermolytic toxin (see Chapter 5) cause bullous impetigo. Pustular folliculitis (Chapter 205) is the superficial dermatitis commonly caused by nontoxigenic strains of staphylococci.

### IMPETIGO (STREPTOCOCCAL PYODERMA)

#### Pathogenesis and Pathology

Direct inoculation of group A hemolytic streptococci into superficial abrasions or compromised areas of skin is the usual route of infection. The most common skin conditions predisposing to impetigo are insect bites, maceration (by sweat or rhinorrhea), atopic dermatitis, and eczema. Biopsy of lesions is not needed for diagnosis and is rarely indicated. The typical pathology is restricted to the epidermis and is characterized by subcorneal inflammatory infiltrate containing bacteria, polymorphonuclear leukocytes, and scattered areas of liquefactive degeneration. There may be a perivascular cellular infiltrate within the dermis.

#### Clinical Manifestations

This thick crusted superficial skin infection is exceedingly common, especially in children. It is sufficiently distinctive to be diagnosed and treated on clinical grounds alone (Fig. 1). The typical lesion begins as an erythematous papule or an erythematous zone surrounding an abrasion or insect bite. Small vesicles may appear transiently, but these are rarely appreciated because the lesion rapidly evolves to the crusted form. The usual lesion varies in size from a few millimeters to 1 to 2 cm and consists of a central crusted plaque surrounded by a discrete erythematous margin. The crust is thick, raised, and of an amber or dirty honey color. Lesions are generally not

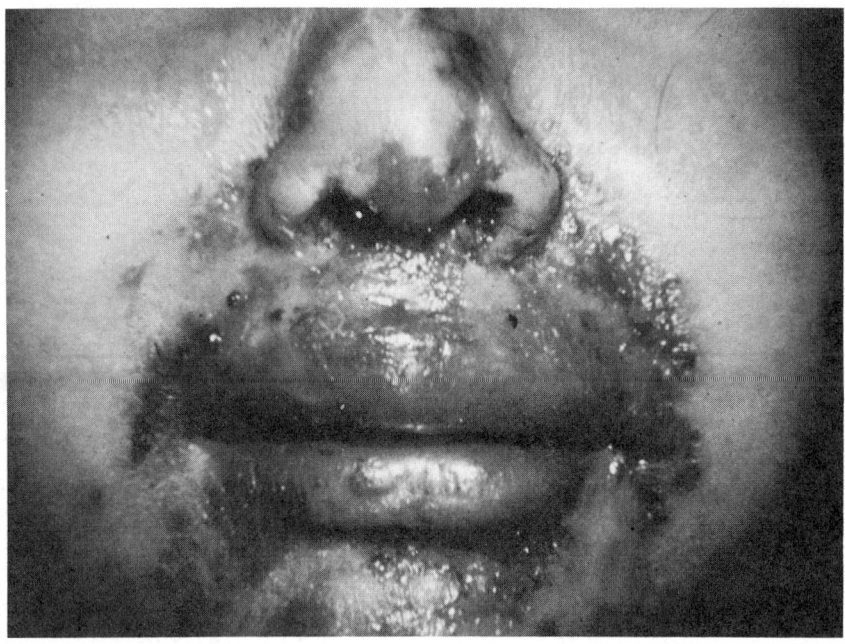

**FIGURE 1.** *Common impetigo. Extensive thick crusted lesions are present around the nose and mouth of this preschool child. The lesion is a dark yellow-brown crust composed of dried cloudy serous exudate. This lesion is predominantly streptococcal.*

purulent; when the crust is removed, a cloudy amber fluid issues from the moist erythematous base. With time, lesions may become extensive and coalescent, particularly on the scalp. Systemic signs are unusual even in patients with extensive impetigo; the appearance of fever and pain generally heralds development of a significant cellulitis. For this reason, there is frequent delay in seeking medical attention; several series in children in the United States demonstrated a two to three week period of lesions before patient presentation. This delay is even more likely in tropical areas or medically underserved regions where sores are frequently considered a normal attribute of childhood. Lesions are only moderately tender to touch. Exposed areas such as the face and extremities are most often involved. Regional adenitis is common.

### Complications and Sequelae

Impetigo is usually indolent and may remain stable for considerable periods. Many lesions heal spontaneously, particularly in people with good personal hygiene, but the infection may spread from the dermis and cause deeper suppurative disease, including cellulitis, lymphadenitis, and bacteremia. Neglected lesions may also form chronic ulcers with erosion through the dermis.

The most important complication of streptococcal impetigo, however, is acute poststreptococcal glomerulonephritis. The pathogenesis of this complication is similar to that described for experimental immune-complex disease with glomerular deposition of IgG, complement, and fibrin.

### Geographic Variations in Disease

Climate dramatically affects the prevalence of impetigo. It occurs during warm humid seasons in temperate areas but year around in tropical areas. It is strikingly less common in arid climates. Warm humid weather apparently enhances the establishment of impetigo by providing maximum opportunities for inoculation sites (insect bites and abrasions on uncovered limbs) and for bacterial multiplication.

Impetigo is generally endemic but may spread in epidemic fashion among people who are in close contact such as families, schools, military camps, and athletic teams.

### Diagnosis and Treatment

The diagnosis of impetigo can usually be made clinically. Cultures of the lesions are not necessary unless the presentation is atypical or the response to therapy is poor. Serum antibodies to the enzymes of group A streptococci are most often measured as an aid to establishing the diagnosis of poststreptococcal glomerulonephritis. The antibody response to streptolysin O after impetigo is often poor, but antibodies are uniformly produced to hyaluronidase and DNAse B.

Multiple studies have demonstrated the superiority of systemic antibiotic therapy over local measures such as scrubbing, soaking, or topical antibiotics. One dose of intramuscular benzathine penicillin (600,000 units for patients weighing less than 60 pounds, 1.2 million units for patients weighing more than 60 pounds) or a 10-day course of oral penicillin, erythromycin, or lincomycin has been demonstrated to be equivalent in efficacy and superior to local therapy. Systemic antibiotic therapy is important for all but the most trivial lesions to prevent deeper suppurative disease and bacteremia. Antibiotic therapy will not prevent the complication of acute poststreptococcal nephritis, at least in part because so much antigenic exposure has already occurred during the delay between first appearance of the lesion and therapy (Anthony et al., 1967; Dillon, 1968).

### Prophylaxis

Prevention of impetigo depends on maintenance of good general hygiene, bathing of insect bites and abrasions, and recognition of early lesions. Scrubbing and application of antibiotic ointment to incipient lesions will prevent development of extensive disease.

## BULLOUS IMPETIGO

### Pathogenesis and Pathology

Staphylococci from the focus of infection within the epidermis produce epidermolytic toxin that acts locally to separate the granular cells of the superficial epidermis and form the characteristic thin-roofed bullae. Histologic examination of the bullae demonstrates a cleavage plane high in the epidermis at the granular cell layer just below the stratum corneum (Fig. 2). Staphylococci and polymorphonuclear leukocytes are seen within the bullae. Epidermolytic toxin can be demonstrated within bullae fluid. Biopsy is diagnostic but is rarely needed unless extensive lesions suggest another diagnosis.

### Clinical Manifestations, Complications, and Sequelae

Bullous impetigo presents a completely different clinical picture from the thick crusted appearance of the streptococcal disease. It can be recognized by the presence of superficial thin-walled, flaccid bullae ranging in size from 0.5 to 3 cm in diameter that erupt on otherwise normal-appearing skin (Fig. 3). There is only a small ring of erythema surrounding the bullae. They may be grouped or coalescent. The fluid within the bulla is generally thin and varies in appearance from slightly cloudy to frankly purulent. Bullae rupture easily and spontaneously, revealing a moist, circular erythematous plaque (Fig. 4). Soon after rupture a thin, varnish-like crust forms over the surface of this plaque. Bullous impetigo is usually localized to a few lesions or a few areas of the body; however, widely disseminated disease may result when the skin has been macerated or

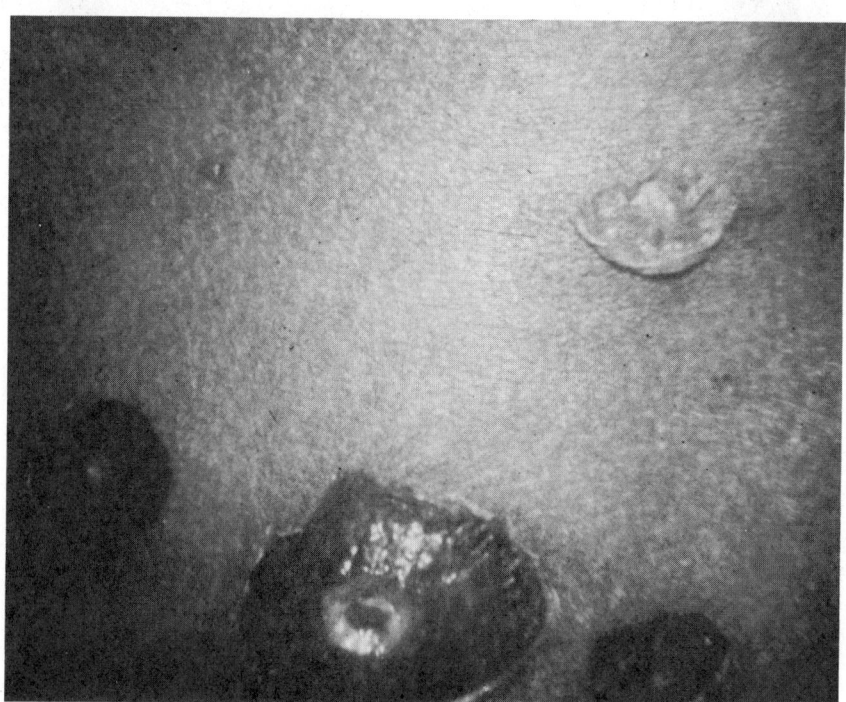

**FIGURE 2.** *Bulla in bullous impetigo. The lesion is composed of a cavity containing leukocytes, organisms, and epidermolytic toxin. The cleavage plane is located at the granular cell layer.*

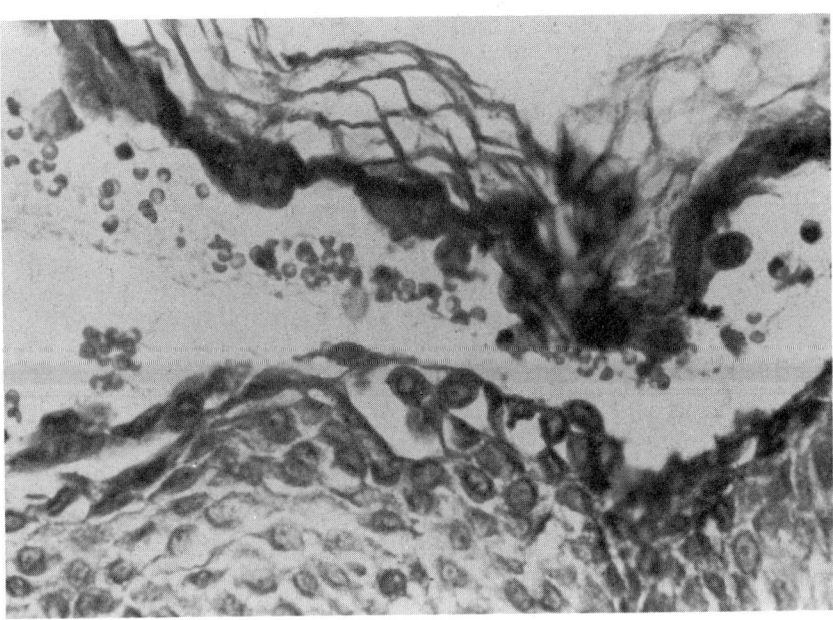

**FIGURE 3.** *Bullous impetigo. In contrast to common impetigo, bullous impetigo is composed of superficial bullae that rupture spontaneously, revealing a moist surface that may dry to a thin collodion-like veneer.*

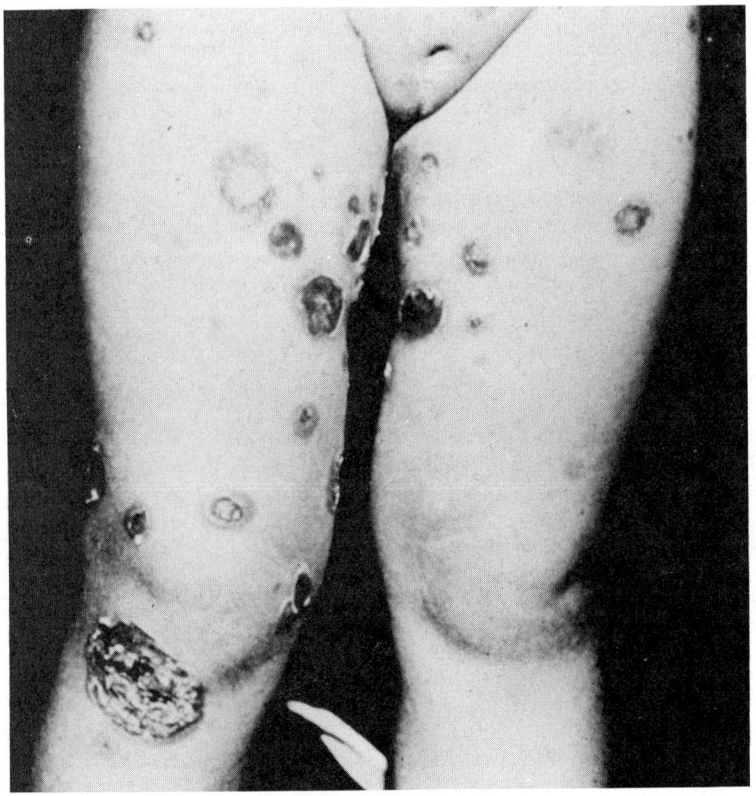

**FIGURE 4.** *Bullous impetigo.*

soaked. Coagulase-positive staphylococci that produce the epidermolytic toxin are recovered from the bullae.

If neglected or untreated, bullous impetigo may progress to involve large areas of skin. Disseminated staphylococcal septicemia may also occur. Although antitoxin to epidermolytic toxin develops after an episode of bullous impetigo, the disease can develop and progress despite serum antibody (Melish et al., 1978).

### Diagnosis

Bullous impetigo occurs both in endemic and epidemic patterns. In neonates, the disease has been seen frequently in association with common nursery epidemics of staphylococcal disease. Among older children and adults, disease is generally sporadic and relatively uncommon compared to streptococcal impetigo. The lesions of bullous impetigo are generally correctly identified when present in small groups in a single area. Single lesions may be mistaken for thermal burns. Extensive, coalescent lesions are likely to be confused with generalized bullous dermatoses such as dermatitis herpetiformis pemphigus and bullous erythema multiforme (Stevens-Johnson syndrome). A firm diagnosis can be made by aspirating intact bullae and demonstrating staphylococci and polymorphonuclear leukocytes within the fluid. Skin biopsy is definitive and occasion-ally necessary (Dillon, 1968; Melish and Glasgow, 1978).

### Treatment

Systemic antistaphylococcal antibiotics, usually given by the oral route, eradicate the infection. Infections may progress rapidly if untreated, particularly in neonates and individuals with pre-existing skin disease. Staphylococci that produce epidermolytic toxin are overwhelmingly penicillin-resistant, at least in North America and Europe, and should be treated either with β-lactamase-resistant penicillins, cephalosporins, erythromycin, or lincomycin.

### References

Anthony, F. B., Perlman, L. V., and Wannamaker, L. W.: Skin infections and acute nephritis in American Indian children. Pediatrics 39:263, 1967.

Dajani, A. S., Ferrieri, P., and Wannamaker, L. W.: Natural history of impetigo. II. Etiologic agents and bacterial interactions. J Clin Invest 51:2863, 1972.

Dillon, H. C.: Impetigo contagiosa: Suppurative and non-suppurative complications. Am J Dis Child 115:530, 1968.

Dillon, H. C.: The treatment of streptococcal skin infections. J Pediatr 76:676, 1970.

Melish, M. E., and Glasgow, L. A.: The staphylococcal scalded skin syndrome: The expanded clinical syndrome. J Pediatr 78:958, 1971.

Melish, M. E., Stuckey, M., and Sprouse, S.: Development of antibody to staphylococcal epidermolytic toxin (ET). Clin Res 26:188A, 1978.

# PYOGENIC SKIN INFECTIONS
# 206

### Marian E. Melish, M.D.

Most of the infections considered in this chapter are more extensive and involve deeper tissue planes than superficial impetigo.

Only bacterial skin infections that elicit a pyogenic response and are not usually a manifestation of a specific systemic disease are included. Thus, cutaneous anthrax, erysipeloid, actinomycotic mycetoma, and swimming pool granuloma (*Mycobacterium marinum*) are not considered.

Although *Staphylococcus aureus* and group A β-hemolytic streptococci are the most common causes of pyogenic skin infections, a rich array of other bacteria may be involved in certain environmental and clinical situations. These clinical settings and the clinical manifestations are sometimes specific enough to permit the institution of appropriate treatment while awaiting the results of smears and cultures.

## FOLLICULITIS, FURUNCULOSIS, AND CARBUNCLES

### DEFINITION

This group of infections is characterized by a common origin in hair follicles, the formation of abscesses with central purulence, and a common etiology that is nearly always coagulase-positive staphylococci (*S. aureus*). The lesions differ in extent. *Folliculitis* is limited to small abscesses involving single hair follicles with only a small amount of surrounding tissue reaction. *Furuncles* develop in hair follicles but become larger and deeper inflammatory nodules surrounded by a large zone of intense tissue reaction. *Carbuncles*, which are composed of several interconnecting furuncles or abscesses, are much wider and deeper.

## ETIOLOGY

Coagulase-positive staphylococci cause the overwhelming majority of these infections. Rarely, other organisms may cause the same lesions in the immunocompromised host or in persons who have experienced unusual environmental exposure. For example, *Pseudomonas aeruginosa* can cause folliculitis associated with the use of heavily contaminated hot tubs or whirlpools. These lesions occur only on the areas of the body that have been immersed and resolve spontaneously if use of the tubs is discontinued.

## PATHOGENESIS AND PATHOLOGY

Lesions are limited to hair-bearing areas and are most common in the axillae, perineum, extremities, neck, and around the breast. They appear to arise de novo without preexisting foci. Poor personal hygiene, occlusion and maceration of the skin, and warm, moist, tropical climates appear to be powerful predisposing factors to the development of these lesions. Nevertheless, trouble may occur in persons with meticulous hygiene. Environmental exposure to virulent staphylococci has also been the source of widespread outbreaks of folliculitis and furunculosis in infants residing in normal newborn nurseries. In addition to infants, adolescents, young adults, and diabetics are more susceptible to these infections. Experimentally, folliculitis can be induced regularly in laboratory animals and in man when coagulase-positive staphylococci are applied to mildly traumatized or occluded skin. Infection cannot be induced in normal, unmanipulated skin, even with extremely large inocula. In either experimental or natural infections, a thick-walled abscess eventually becomes established in the hair follicle. Lesions have a purulent necrotic center that may rupture spontaneously. Although most are well contained by the surrounding inflammatory reaction, infection may spread to adjacent tissues and cause a diffuse cellulitis or metastasize to distant sites hematogenously.

## DIAGNOSIS AND MANAGEMENT

The diagnosis can be made by inspection (Fig. 1) and confirmed by Gram stain. If the lesions or

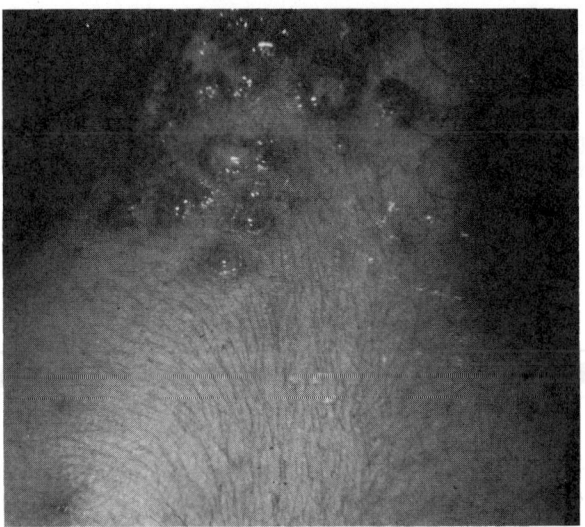

**FIGURE 1.** *Superficial staphylococcal furunculosis. All stages in the development of superficial staphylococcal skin abscesses are depicted here from early folliculitis to multiple nodular furuncles to a small carbuncle made up of interconnecting furuncles.*

history are atypical or if organisms other than *Staphylococcus aureus* are seen in the Gram stain, cultures must be obtained.

Early lesions may be treated with warm soaks to encourage spontaneous drainage. Larger, localized lesions must be incised and drained. Patients with an extensive carbuncle or a furuncle associated with cellulitis may also require an oral antistaphylococcal antibiotic, such as dicloxacillin or cephalexin (0.5 g four times a day for seven to ten days). Penicillinase-negative *S. aureus* should be treated with 1.0 g of penicillin V four times a day. Patients must be cautioned that draining lesions are a hazard to others and should not be allowed to work as food handlers or have contact with hospitalized patients. After adequate drainage, the erythema and edema subside, but a dense scar frequently follows all but the most trivial lesions.

## COMPLICATIONS AND SEQUELAE

Local or metastatic spread of infection, the most serious complication, can usually be avoided by prompt drainage. If the patient is already febrile and systemically ill when first evaluated, blood and the lesion should be cultured and metastatic foci should be sought in the heart, bones, joints, brain, and muscles.

## PROPHYLAXIS

Certain patients are predisposed to recurrent disease. These individuals should have careful physical examinations, with particular attention to underlying disease, nutritional status, personal hygiene, and any potential breaks in the skin barrier. Chronic dermatoses such as eczema, icthyosis, or seborrhea may be predisposing factors and should be treated. A meticulous regimen of personal hygiene and antibiotic ointment for use on all minor wounds and early lesions should be prescribed. No other regimens are of proven value. Staphylococcal vaccines have been widely used but have never been adequately evaluated.

# WOUND INFECTIONS

When the protective barrier of the skin is breached by traumatic or surgical invasion, infection may be introduced and develop in the skin and adjacent tissues. The ubiquitous, coagulase-positive staphylococcus and group A streptococcus are most often responsible for wound infections. However, a variety of other organisms may be introduced under specific environmental conditions. These organisms require specific consideration.

## HUMAN BITE WOUND INFECTIONS

Human bites frequently result in rapidly progressive destructive infections of soft tissues, tendons, joints, and bones. The hand is commonly infected after tooth lacerations to the fist or full mouth bites to the hand or fingers. Signs of infection develop rapidly within 24 hours of injury. Bite wound infections are nearly always polymicrobial. Normal mouth flora, particularly anaerobic streptococci, oral spirochetes, staphylococci, aerobic streptococci, and mouth aerobes, are involved. The pus is malodorous because of the presence of anaerobic bacteria. Bite wounds should be carefully inspected and irrigated, and devitalized tissue should be debrided. The wounds should not be sutured primarily, because adequate drainage is very important. Penicillinase-resistant penicillins or cephalosporins directed at staphylococci and mouth bacteria may be given even before signs of infection appear, because the fully developed infection is so destructive.

Patients who present with an established infection after a human bite frequently require radical débridement, deep wound culture, and high-dose systemic antibiotics directed at the organisms isolated from the deep wound culture (Shields et al., 1975).

## ANIMAL BITES

Animal bites (also see Chapter 241) are less likely to become infected than human bites. *Pasteurella multocida,* a short gram-negative rod that is sensitive to penicillin, is particularly likely to infect dog, cat, and rat bites. Other organisms, most prominently streptococci and staphylococci but also *Seminus* and *S. multiformis* (Chapter 241), also infect animal bites. The principles of preventive management include careful inspection, débridement, and copious irrigation of the wound. Primary suturing increases the likelihood of infection. If the wound is closed, penicillin $\overline{V}$ (500 mg four times a day) should be given to prevent infection with *Pasteurella multocida,* and the wound should be inspected daily. Infection may develop despite careful early management. Characteristically, there is rapid progression to cellulitis and/or abscess formation with severe local pain and edema. Lymphadenopathy and systemic signs of illness are frequent. In the case of rat and cat bites, tenosynovitis and osteomyelitis may also occur because the sharp teeth can penetrate and inoculate tendons, joint spaces, and the periosteum.

## SOIL-CONTAMINATED WOUNDS

When wounds are contaminated with soil, a wide variety of organisms may be inoculated and cause infections. Prominent pathogens for this group of wound infections are the gram-negative enteric bacilli and the gas-forming anaerobic clostridia that are responsible for gas gangrene and tetanus. Preventive practices are very important in handling dirty wounds. The wound must be completely explored for foreign material, debrided adequately, and irrigated. Primary closure should be avoided. Clostridial cellulitis and myonecrosis (gas gangrene) can be prevented only by making the local environment unsatisfactory for the growth of clostridia. This requires removal of foreign material and devitalized tissue and provision for oxygen to enter the wound.

An established wound infection should be surgically inspected for its full extent and any foreign material removed. Bullae, tissue crepitation, and/or gas in tissue on x-ray suggests clostridial infection. Deep wound culture and Gram stain should be made. If the Gram stain shows gram positive rods, and there is clinical evidence of clostridial cellulitis, extensive surgical débridement with multiple incisions into the involved tissue must be made. Large intravenous doses of penicillin (200,000 units/kg) should be given. Necrotic muscle containing gram-positive rods and gas in the tissue establish the diagnosis of gas gangrene and constitute a medical emergency. Amputation or extensive débridement and hyperbaric oxygen treatment should be instituted immediately (see Chapter 238).

Wound infections that are not obviously clostridial should be managed in a similar way. Deep wound culture and Gram stain should be taken at the time of débridement. A penicillinase-resistant penicillin plus an aminoglycoside should be given for all significant infections, pending the results of cultures and sensitivities. If the primary Gram stain suggests the presence of *Bacteroides,* clindamycin can be substituted for the semisynthetic penicillin until the cultures are completed.

## WATER-CONTAMINATED WOUNDS

Organisms found in stagnant fresh water, particularly *Aeromonas hydrophila,* pseudomonads, and coliforms, may infect wounds that are sustained in fresh water. *Aeromonas* causes a particularly rapid progressive necrotizing infection. Wounds sustained in salt water may be contaminated with *Vibrio parahemolyticus* and other noncholera vibrios. Deep culture, adequate surgical exploration and exposure, and careful follow-up are especially important measures in the management of traumatic wounds sustained under unusual circumstances because unusual bacteria may be encountered.

## SURGICAL WOUNDS

Surgical wound infections are caused primarily by coagulase-positive staphylococci and group A streptococci. Occasionally, the anaerobic and aerobic enteric flora infect abdominal incisions after surgery for peritonitis or gross fecal contamination.

The condition of the wound plays a major role in its resistance to infection. The presence of a hematoma, necrotic tissue, diminished blood flow, and foreign bodies all decrease innate local resistance. The type of suture material is also impor-

tant; braided silk sutures are more likely to form a nidus of infection than monofilament nylon or wire.

The nature of the infecting organism dictates the clinical manifestations. Group A $\beta$-hemolytic streptococci, which cause surgical infections far less commonly than coagulase–positive staphylococci, present the most immediate and serious problem. Within one to two days after the operation, the patient may develop high fever, leukocytosis, tachycardia, and even vascular collapse. Erysipelas may develop around the wound. Often, however, the wound appears normal, but large numbers of gram-positive cocci are seen in the deep wound aspirate. Because streptococcal postoperative wound infections may cause fulminant disease, a high degree of suspicion, careful wound evaluation, and deep cultures are essential measures in the management of patients who develop fever soon after surgery. Penicillin at a dose of 200,000 units/kg/day should be started intravenously. If the Gram stain shows gram-positive cocci that are not clearly differentiated from staphylococci, methicillin, or oxacillin should be used instead of penicillin at doses of 200 mg/kg/day.

Staphylococci and enteric bacilli usually cause a less dramatic illness. Early signs of infection are insidious and begin four to six days after surgery with wound tenderness, low-grade fever, and mild systemic signs, such as lethargy and anorexia. The wound may look normal, but careful inspection and removal of sutures may reveal evidence of infection deep within the wound. Gram stain of the exudate distinguishes between staphylococci and enterics, which are the usual causes of this common, more indolent presentation. The wound should be opened to allow drainage and to determine the extent of involvement. Antibiotics are given to prevent dissemination of the infection but are less important than adequate surgical drainage. Staphylococcal infections should be treated with an antistaphylococcal penicillin. Gram-negative infections of abdominal wounds, particularly when the drainage is foul-smelling, are likely to be caused by *Bacteroides fragilis.* In this case, therapy with chloramphenicol, clindamycin, or metronidazole is required. An aminoglycoside is currently preferred for aerobic enteric flora.

# ERYSIPELAS

Erysipelas is a specific form of superficial cellulitis that involves the dermis and uppermost subcutaneous tissue. It is caused exclusively by

group A $\beta$–hemolytic streptococci that pack and obstruct the superficial lymphatics beneath the involved skin. Erysipelas has a characteristic appearance consisting of a rapidly enlarging, deeply erythematous plaque with a sharply demarcated, raised border. The involved area is indurated, tender, and may have a "peau d'orange" appearance (Fig. 2). Large tension bullae may develop within the erythematous zone because the lymphatics are obstructed by streptococci.

Group A streptococci may be recovered either from the advancing margin or from the central primary wound, if present, but a punch biopsy from the center of the erysipeloid lesion is the most reliable way to obtain the organism for Gram stain and culture. The portal of entry may be a surgical wound or an excoriated insect bite but is most frequently inapparent. Erysipelas may occur on any area of the body; we have seen it most frequently as a circumferential, rapidly progressive lesion on the extremities, but it is also common on the face or in association with surgical wounds.

Patients with erysipelas are frequently febrile and toxic. Because of the characteristic rapid progression we initiate therapy with 600,000 units of procaine penicillin twice daily for the first 24

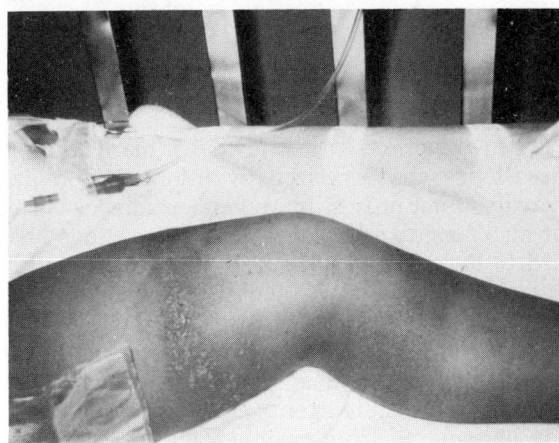

**FIGURE 2.**  *Erysipelas. This form of superficial streptococcal cellulitis presents with a sharply demarcated, slightly elevated, tender erythroderma, here forming a band around the thigh and calf of a child. Small bullae are seen at the uppermost extent of the lesions.*

to 48 hours followed by 500 mg of penicillin V four times each day for ten days.

# CELLULITIS

Cellulitis refers to infections that involve primarily the subcutaneous tissues with some secondary involvement of the dermis. Clinically, cellulitis is manifest as an area of edema, erythema, warmth, and tenderness. Because the area of involvement is primarily in the subcutaneous tissue, the lateral margins of the infection appear indistinct, and the edema and erythema merge into the surrounding area.

A wide variety of organisms may cause cellulitis, particularly after trauma or in immunocompromised hosts, but group A streptococci and *Staphylococcus aureus* are by far the most common organisms. In children under 5 years, *Haemophilus influenzae* Type b is a frequent cause of cellulitis, especially on the face.

Staphylococcal and streptococcal cellulitis may have identical clinical appearances. Both are associated with cutaneous trauma and tend to be more frequent on the extremities. Aspiration of both the central and lateral margins of the cellulitis or a punch biopsy of the central area should be done in all cases in an attempt to recover an agent for culture. Blood cultures may also be positive. Therapy should be started before the culture results are known and should include an antistaphylococcal agent, unless Gram stain of the aspiration or punch biopsy clearly shows strep-

tococci. Streptococcal cellulitis should be treated with penicillin by the same routes and doses listed above for erysipelas. Cefazolin (1.0 g I.M. four times daily for two days) followed by cephalexin (500 mg orally four times daily for ten days) is good treatment for staphylococci and satisfactory for streptococci until the culture results are known. Gram-negative bacilli and fungi may also cause cellulitis in the immunocompromised host. For these patients, maximal efforts should be made to obtain an etiologic agent, including the use of skin biopsy. Empiric therapy for cellulitis in the immunocompromised host should include coverage for *Pseudomonas aeruginosa* gram-negative enterics, staphylococci, and streptococci by using an aminoglycoside such as gentamicin at 3 to 5 mg/kg/day plus an antistaphylococcal penicillin or cephalosporin in the doses given above.

As an adjunct to antibiotics, warm compresses may be applied to promote suppuration and drainage. If frank abscesses occur within the lesion, surgical drainage is indicated.

The prognosis of cellulitis in the normal host is excellent after antibiotics are begun. Cellulitis may disseminate hematogenously or to contiguous underlying foci, such as bone, joint, or muscle. Careful follow-up should be planned to search for evidence of local or distant spread.

# NECROTIZING CELLULITIS AND NECROTIZING FASCIITIS

These infections are known by many names, but all are characterized by inflammation and necrosis of not only skin and subcutaneous tissue but also fascia and muscle. Terms that have been used to describe infections in this group include "necrotizing fasciitis," "acute hemolytic streptococcal gangrene," "synergistic necrotizing cellulitis," "progressive synergistic gangrene," and "gangrenous erysipelas." An array of individual agents and multiple agents acting synergistically may be isolated from patients who present with similar clinical manifestations. Synergistic infection is not essential in the pathogenesis; single agents may be equally destructive.

## CLINICAL MANIFESTATIONS

Patients first present with severe or extensive cellulitis that frequently contains a dusky area in the center indicative of poor perfusion (Fig. 3). Induration is extensive and may extend beyond the area of erythema. The local and systemic disease usually progresses despite antibiotics. Blebs and areas of frank necrosis become apparent within the involved area, and systemic signs of illness, fever, and debilitation progress. Patients may develop edema, hypoproteinemia, and proteinuria. Hypocalcemia secondary to deposition of calcium in necrotic tissues is frequent.

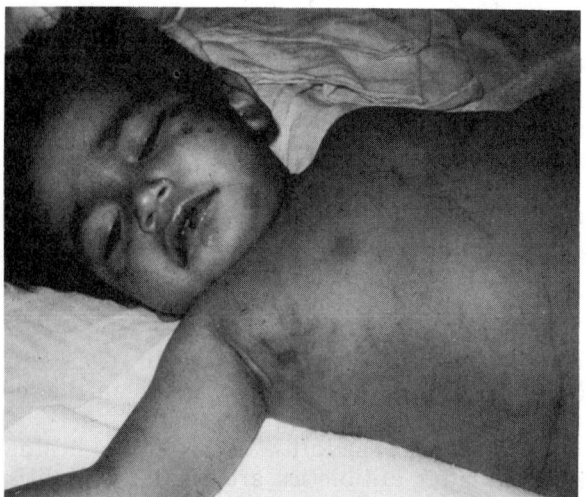

**FIGURE 3.** Necrotizing fasciitis. The cutaneous signs of extensive necrotizing fasciitis in this child were small central necrotic areas within a large area of erythema and induration (outlined in pencil on the child's chest). At surgery, he was found to have necrosis of the fascia of the latissimus dorsi muscles posteriorly and the pectoralis major muscles anteriorly.

## DIAGNOSIS

Necrotizing fasciitis/cellulitis should be suspected if the cellulitis is extensive, contains necrotic areas, or fails to respond promptly to appropriate antibiotic therapy. Specific microbiologic diagnosis is made by culture of blood and Gram stain and culture of wound aspirate, or by punch biopsy. Anaerobic cultures are essential.

Determination of the tissue plane involved by incision and exploration is more important than the microbiologic diagnosis. The involved tissue should be incised down to the fascia, and a probe introduced laterally from the incision. If the fascia or subcutaneous tissue is necrotic, the probe moves easily through the tissue. Thin, malodorous fluid frequently oozes from the incision. This fluid and necrotic tissue should be stained and cultured.

## THERAPY

After the presence of necrotic fascia or muscle is confirmed, extensive surgical débridement is the sine qua non of effective therapy. All necrotic tissue extending to the margins of healthy bleeding tissue must be debrided. If initial débridement is limited, it needs to be repeated. To delay or limit surgery results in "a bigger wound in a sicker patient" (Rea and Wyrick, 1973; Stone and Martin, 1972).

Intensive antibiotic therapy and meticulous supportive care are essential adjuncts to surgery. Anaerobic and aerobic streptococci, coagulase-positive staphylococci, and gram-negative bacilli are the bacteria that are most frequently encountered. If staphylococci are seen on Gram stain, a penicillinase-resistant penicillin such as methicillin should be given intravenously in doses of 200 mg/kg/day. If both gram-positive and gram-negative organisms are seen, an aminoglycoside such as gentamicin should be added at 3 to 5 mg/kg/day until the culture results are known. If the gram-negative bacilli in the smear are small and encapsulated, or if the necrotizing fasciitis/cellulitis follows abdominal surgery, antibiotics must be selected that cover *Bacteroides fragilis*. Unlike other anaerobes, *B. fragilis* is resistant to penicillin and must be treated with chloramphenicol, clindamycin or metronidozole

## PROGNOSIS

Extensive necrotizing cellulitis is a serious illness. Patients may die if not treated promptly and intensively. Supportive care must include fluid therapy, correction of hypocalcemia, and adequate nutrition. Convalescence is prolonged. Skin grafting and physical therapy may be required because of extensive surgical débridement.

# TROPICAL PYOMYOSITIS

## DEFINITION AND ETIOLOGY

Tropical pyomyositis is an acute staphylococcal infection of skeletal muscle that occurs spontaneously in the absence of other known foci of infection. Myositis secondary to hematogenous spread from a distant focus or to local spread from a contiguous site of infection in the bone or overlying soft tissue is excluded from this definition. Patients with tropical pyomyositis rarely develop septicemia, and hematogenous spread to other organs is distinctly unusual. Isolated, staphylococcal pyomyositis may account for as many as 4 per cent of hospital admissions in the tropics (Levin et al., 1971; Horn and Master, 1968), but it is very rare in temperate climates.

## PATHOGENESIS AND CLINICAL MANIFESTATIONS

The pathogenesis of tropical pyomyositis is unknown. Attempts to explain its high prevalence in the tropics have been unsuccessful. There is no convincing evidence that any tropical disease or parasite is responsible either for damaging the affected muscle or seeding it with staphylococci. A history of recent trauma can be elicited from about 20 per cent of patients, and it seems likely that at least some of the cases develop from seeding of a traumatized muscle during a transient, asymptomatic bacteremia.

The muscles of the leg and trunk are most commonly affected. The typical patient presents with fever, leukocytosis, and a history of a few days of localized muscle pain and tenderness. A firm swelling may be present over the affected muscle, but local heat and erythema are absent until the infection breaks through the muscle into the overlying tissue. One or more muscles may be affected.

## DIAGNOSIS AND TREATMENT

The diagnosis of tropical myositis is established by cultivating S. aureus from aspiration or surgical drainage of an infected muscle in a patient with negative blood cultures and no other detectable focus of infection. If blood cultures are positive, the patient should be carefully evaluated for the presence of endocarditis or other foci of infection in the bone or joints. Streptococcus pneumoniae and group A streptococci have been isolated from rare cases of isolated pyomyositis.

The cornerstone of treatment is surgical drainage of all muscle abscesses. A penicillinase-resistant penicillin should be administered intravenously in doses of 100 to 200 mg/kg/day until the cultures and sensitivities are completed. Penicillinase-negative S. aureus and the rare isolates of streptococci should be treated with similar doses of I.V. penicillin G. If the patient becomes afebrile promptly, and there is no evidence of endocarditis or osteomyelitis, antibiotics can be discontinued after the abscess has resolved.

### References

Horn, C. V., and Master, S.: Pyomyositis tropicans in Uganda. E Afr Med J 35:463, 1968.

Levin, M. J., Gardner, P., and Waldvogel, F. A.: "Tropical" pyomyositis: An unusual infection due to Staphylococcus aureus. N Engl J Med 284:196, 1971.

Rea, W. J., and Wyrick, J. J.: Necrotizing fasciitis. Ann Surg 172:957, 1973.

Shields, C., Patzakis, M. S., Myers, M. H., and Harvey, J. P., Jr.: Hand infections secondary to human bites. J Trauma 15:235, 1975.

Stone, H. H., and Martin, J. D.: Synergistic necrotizing cellulitis. Ann Surg 175:702, 1972.

# THE STAPHYLOCOCCAL SCALDED SKIN SYNDROME    207

Marian E. Melish, M.D.

## DEFINITION AND ETIOLOGY

Staphylococcus aureus is associated with a spectrum of dermatologic diseases that range from localized bullae to diffuse exfoliative disease with systemic toxemia. These conditions are caused by an epidermolytic toxin that is produced only by S. aureus. In the localized form of the disease, called bullous impetigo, the toxin is produced in a focus of infected skin, remains at that site, and produces localized bullae. By contrast, in the other two forms of the scalded skin syndrome, the toxin is produced at a site that may be distant from the skin, is disseminated hematogenously, and produces widespread skin disease at sites distant from the focus of infection. The two generalized forms of the scalded skin syndrome are associated with systemic toxemia and present clinically as either an acute generalized exfoliative disease or an acute nonstreptococcal scarlatiniform eruption.

These toxin-mediated diseases have been called a bewildering variety of names. The diffuse exfoliative form of the disease has been known as Ritter's disease and pemphigus neonatorum when it occurs in neonates and as Lyell's disease and toxic epidermal necrolysis when it occurs in children and adults. We prefer to refer to the entire spectrum of dermatologic diseases caused by the epidermolytic toxin as the staphylococcal scalded skin syndrome (SSSS) and to the clinical varieties as the diffuse exfoliative form of SSSS, the scarlatiniform variety of SSSS, and bullous impetigo. SSSS may be a cumbersome term, but it is encompassing, descriptive, and etiologic rather than eponymic.

## PATHOGENESIS AND PATHOLOGY

The skin changes are caused by a soluble protein exotoxin, epidermolytic toxin, that is elaborated in vitro and in vivo by *S. aureus*, primarily but not exclusively those belonging to phage group II. Epidermolytic toxin can be detected in the blood during the early stages of the exfoliative diseases (Melish et al., 1972). At least two separate antigenic forms of the toxin, referred to as epidermolytic toxins A and B, have been isolated in the United States and in Japan (Kondo et al., 1925). Both have molecular weights of about 25,500, but they differ in other physical properties. Toxin A is sometimes called the stable toxin because it is resistant to boiling. Toxin B is referred to as labile toxin because it is inactivated at 60° F. Toxin A is chromosomally determined, but toxin B may be extrachromosomally mediated because it can be eliminated by DNA intercalating agents (Warren et al., 1974). Between 70 and 90 per cent of toxin–positive *S. aureus* produce A, up to 30 per cent produce A and B, but only 15 per cent produce toxin B only (Melish et al., 1979).

The toxin causes the separation of granular cells within the epidermis (Fig. 1). Intact cells lose their attachments to each other, and a cleavage plane develops just below the stratum corneum. There is no inflammatory response. Antitoxic antibody develops after infection and appears to be protective against the hematogenous dissemination of toxin that is responsible for the generalized manifestations of the scalded skin syndrome. Antitoxic antibody does not prevent local production and action of the toxin. Bullous impetigo and secondary infections of other skin lesions such as bullous varicella may occur and progress despite the presence of antitoxic antibody.

The generalized forms of the scalded skin syndrome occur almost exclusively in children less than 5 years old. There are only twelve reports of

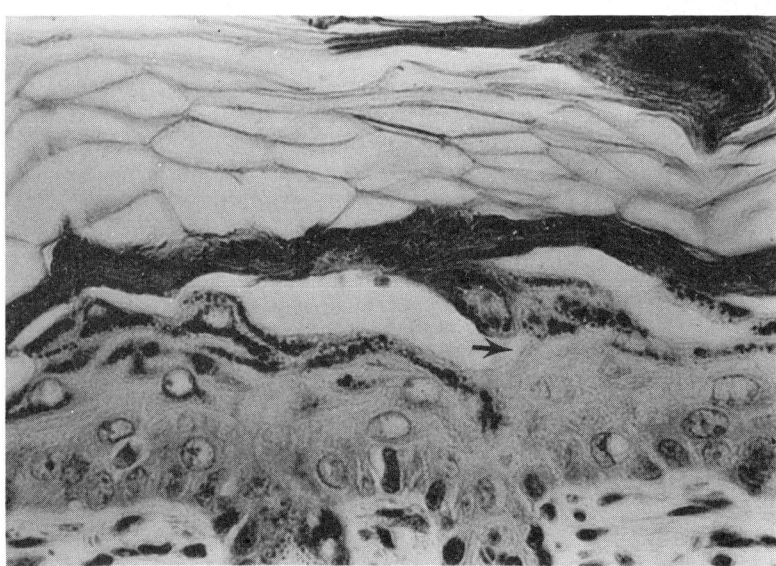

**FIGURE 1.**  *Site of action of epidermolytic toxin. In this early lesion, a cleavage plane is developing at the granular cell layer high in the epidermis.*

staphylococcal toxic epidermal necrolysis in adults, and all have been immunocompromised or have had renal failure. This age-related susceptibility to generalized disease has been explained by a survey of antibody prevalence in people of different ages. In the United States, more than three-quarters of the population over 10 years of age but only one-quarter of children less than 2 years old have antibody to epidermolytic toxin A. Antitoxic antibody develops early in life, probably from minor, inapparent infections with toxin-producing staphylococci (Melish et al., 1979). Although bullous impetigo occurs in the presence of antibody to epidermolytic toxin, immunity even to the diffuse forms of the disease is unusual because humoral immunity to other staphylococcal extracellular products or toxins does not prevent staphylococcal infections.

## CLINICAL MANIFESTATIONS

### Bullous Impetigo

The lesion is a superficial, localized bulla arising on areas of apparently normal skin (also see Chapter 204). The bullae are flaccid and contain clear, pale to dark yellow fluid. They usually appear on moist or opposing surfaces of the skin, such as the diaper area, the neck, and the axilla, and are easily denuded by slight trauma. The lesions are superficial and heal without scarring or systemic illness. Nikolsky's sign, in which the outer layer of the skin is easily rubbed off by slight friction, is not present, and there is no exfoliation beyond the local lesion.

Bullous varicella is a variant of localized SSSS that usually occurs two to five days after the onset of the skin lesions of chickenpox. Variable numbers of the varicella lesions become secondarily infected with staphylococci. Small crops of bullae may develop around each secondarily infected vesicle. After the bullae become denuded, the clinical appearance of denuded skin surrounding crusted varicella lesions is very characteristic.

### Diffuse Exfoliative Disease

This illness generally begins with the sudden appearance of a diffuse scarlatiniform erythroderma. This rash is tender to the touch and has a rough sandpaper-like texture. In the early stages, it is indistinguishable from the rash of streptococcal scarlet fever except for its tenderness. Within one to three days, generalized bullae appear in the skin, the Nikolsky sign becomes positive, and the epidermis separates and peels off in large sheets, revealing a moist, red surface beneath (Figs. 2 and 3). Areas of exfoliation generally involve most of the body surface but are occasionally limited to smaller areas. Bullae in

this disease are quite transient, and diffuse erythroderma with large areas of exfoliation may be all that is seen when the patient presents. Cultures of aspirates from intact bullae are generally sterile, but a focus of staphylococcal infection is found at a distant site. This focus is often trivial, such as conjunctivitis or throat colonization, but serious infections like bacteremia, omphalitis, osteomyelitis, endocarditis, or major wound infections also occur. The patient is usually febrile, irritable, and in pain. Small infants may develop serious problems with dehydration and temperature regulation secondary to evaporative losses. Within 24 hours, the exposed exfoliative areas dry with a thin, shiny, varnish-like crust. Cracks and fissures develop spontaneously in the skin surrounding the eyes and mouth. Secondary desquamation of large, thick flakes of skin follows during the next five to seven days. Within 14 days from the onset, the skin has healed without scarring.

### Staphylococcal Scarlatiniform Eruption

Children with this form of the staphylococcal scalded skin syndrome develop a generalized erythroderma that is usually associated with fever. The skin has a roughened sandpaper-like texture with increased erythema in skin creases similar to the rose-red, transverse Pastia's lines in the skin over the fold of the elbow in patients with scarlet fever. The appearance of the skin in these early stages can be indistinguishable from streptococcal scarlet fever. There are important clinical differences, however. In the staphylococcal disease, the skin is tender to the touch, and there is no palatal enanthem or strawberry tongue. The resolution of the rash differs markedly from that of streptococcal scarlet fever as well. Within two to four days of the onset, cracks and fissures develop about the eyes and mouth. Thick flakes appear and the entire skin surface undergoes desquamation within ten days of onset. This pattern of desquamation differs from the fine, branny flaking that begins on the fingers ten days or longer after the onset of streptococcal scarlet fever.

The staphylococcal scarlatiniform eruption and diffuse exfoliative SSSS are identical during the initial stage of generalized erythroderma and the final stage of secondary desquamation, but the intermediate stages of bullae formation and generalized exfoliation do not occur in the scarlatiniform disease.

## DIAGNOSIS

The clinical presentation of diffuse exfoliative disease or toxic epidermal necrolysis may be iden-

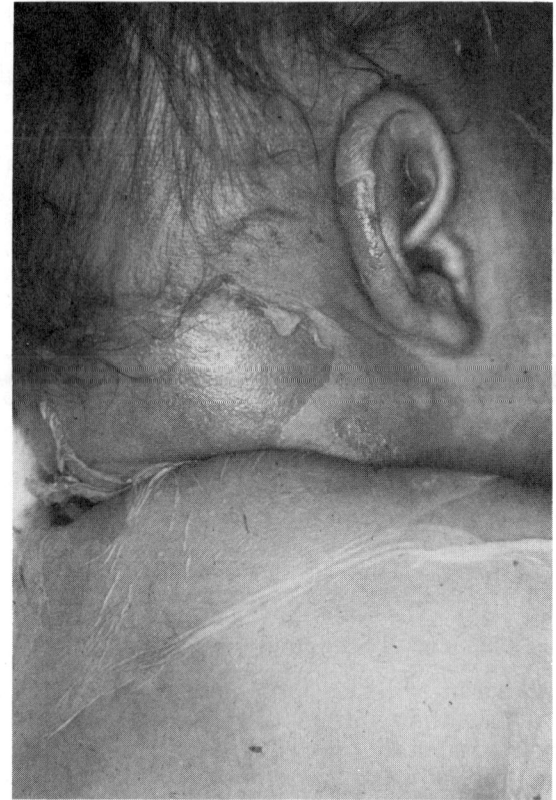 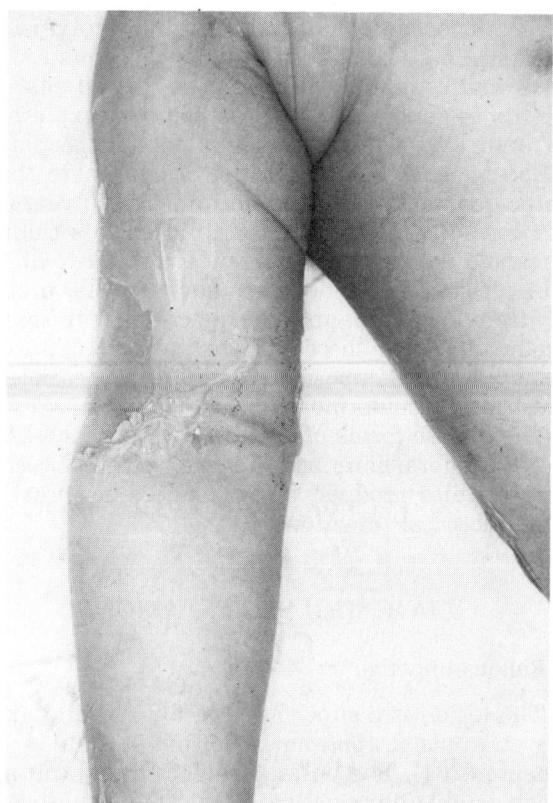

**FIGURES 2 and 3.** *Generalized staphylococcal scalded skin syndrome (toxic epidermal necrolysis). Extensive superficial skin separation is seen in this child who had generalized tender erythroderma with increased erythema in skin creases, transient flaccid bullae, and extensive denudation of skin, revealing a moist, red surface that rapidly dried. In this child, staphylococcal epidermolytic toxin was disseminated from a focus of infection in the eye. (Photographed by Mitsuo Tottori, M.D.)*

tical whether it is caused by staphylococcal epidermolytic toxin or is of the idiopathic variety. The idiopathic type of toxic epidermal necrolysis has been associated with hypersensitivity reactions to drugs, viral infections, and graft-versus-host reaction. It is far more rare than the staphylococcal disease and usually occurs in adults. Despite the clinical similarity, the idiopathic variety has a completely different histologic appearance. In the idiopathic variety, the inflammatory response is intense, the epidermis is necrotic, and a cleavage plane develops either at the level of the dermal-epidermal junction or within the upper dermis. In the staphylococcal variety, the cleavage plane develops just below the cornified layer, and there is no inflammatory reaction within the epidermis (Fig. 1). A simple punch skin biopsy can make this differentiation. Even simpler, one can obtain a frozen section of bulla roof or freshly exfoliative skin (Fig. 4). If only cornified cells with one epidermal cell layer are seen, the process is toxin-mediated. The full epidermis is present in the idiopathic variety. Many clinicians are satisfied with a diagnosis in

children of staphylococcal toxic epidermal necrolysis based upon the typical clinical appearance plus identification of a focus of staphylococcal infection. If the clinical appearance and biopsy suggest staphylococcal disease, a search must be made for the infective focus. Blood, wounds, eye exudates, and the throat should be cultured. Osteomyelitis, septic arthritis, or other occult foci should be sought if the source of infection is not obvious. Because the skin disease is toxin-mediated, its severity is not necessarily related to the severity of the infection; the focus is often trivial, and purulent conjunctivitis is the most common infection in our experience. The importance of making the correct etiologic diagnosis is to ensure effective therapy. An antistaphylococcal antibiotic aimed at eradicating the focus of staphylococcal infection is indicated for staphylococcal disease. Corticosteroids are contraindicated because they have no beneficial effect on toxin-mediated skin changes and may enhance the infection. On the other hand, the idiopathic variety is primarily an inflammatory condition, and corticosteroids are indicated.

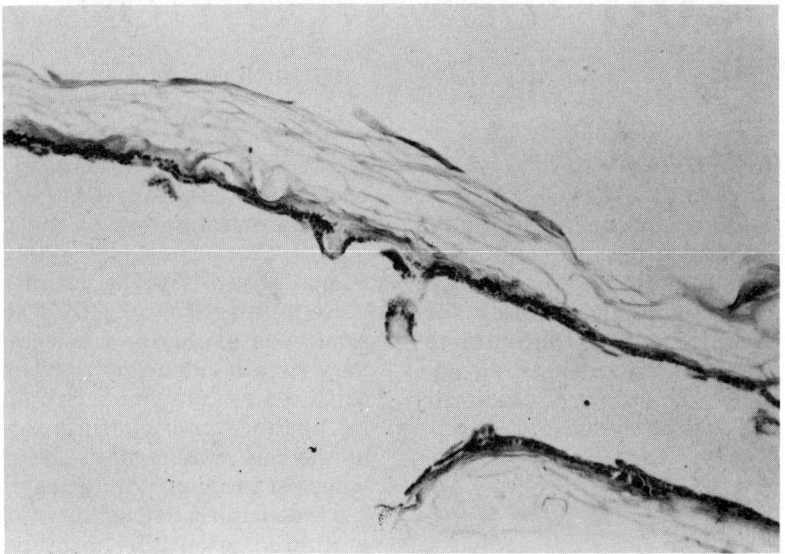

**FIGURE 4.** *Rapid diagnosis of SSSS. Firm diagnosis of SSSS can be made by skin biopsy or by examination of an excised bulla roof, as seen here. Only the stratum corneum and uppermost granular cell layer are present, indicating SSSS. A deeper cleavage plane is seen in idiopathic toxic epidermal necrolysis, Stevens-Johnson syndrome, and other bullous exfoliative diseases.*

## TREATMENT

In severe cases with considerable loss of skin surface, we prefer to hospitalize patients and administer intravenous antistaphylococcal antibiotics, usually methicillin at 200,000 mg per kg per day or another penicillinase-resistant penicillin in high doses. Almost all phage group II *S. aureus* produce penicillinase. Weight, urine output, and temperature are closely monitored. Small children may be dehydrated or hypothermic because of the evaporation of fluid from denuded skin. The patient is nursed on clean linen and handled as little as possible. We do not apply topical therapy or dressings of any kind. Once the focus of infection has been identified, therapy should be continued as indicated for the basic condition. If the infection is minor, intravenous therapy is discontinued in three to five days when the skin begins to heal, and oral therapy is given for a total treatment course of 10 days. Staphylococcal scarlatiniform rash may be treated at home with oral antistaphylococcal therapy, providing that the focus of infection is minor. When the skin disease is limited, the nature of the underlying infection should dictate the route, duration, and intensity of therapy. Bullous impetigo and bullous vari-

cella should also be treated with oral antistaphylococcal drugs. Local therapy should be avoided because of the dangers of skin maceration and sensitization to topical antimicrobials.

The prognosis for recovery from the skin disease is excellent once the underlying infection is controlled. The skin heals without scarring within 14 days of the institution of antibiotic therapy. The mortality is low (5 per cent even in infants) provided that prompt therapy and proper supportive care are given during the acute phase. Mortality from the idiopathic disease in adults is much higher and may be over 50 per cent.

## References

Kondo, I., Sakurai, S., and Sarai, Y.: Two serotypes of exfoliation (epidermolytic toxin) and their distribution in staphylococcal strains isolated from patients with scalded skin syndrome. J Clin Microbiol 1:397, 1975.

Melish, M. E., Glasgow, L. A., and Turner, M. D.: The staphylococcal scalded skin syndrome: Isolation of a new exfoliative toxin. J Infect Dis 1255:129, 1972.

Melish, M. E., Sprouse, S., and Stuckey, M.: Development of antibody to staphylococcal epidermolytic toxin (abst.). Clin Res 78:188A, 1979.

Warren, R., Rogolsky, M., Wiley, B. B., and Glasgow, L. A.: Effect of ethidium bromide on elimination of exfoliative toxin and bacteriocin production in *Staphylococcus aureus*. J Bacteriol 118:980, 1974.

# 208 *DERMATOPHYTOSIS*

*Richard B. Stoughton, M.D.*

## DEFINITION

The dermatophytoses are the superficial fungus infections of the skin. The fungi are confined to the dead stratum corneum, hair, and nails. These organisms are nourished by keratin and can survive only in the keratin structures. Dermatophytosis is classified broadly into tinea versicolor, tinea nigra, tinea capitis, tinea cruris, tinea corporis, tinea pedis, and onychomycosis.

## ETIOLOGY

Sabouraud (1910) discovered the relationship between certain skin fungi and specific diseases. Emmons (1934) classified these pathogenic fungi into three main genera: *Trichophyton, Microsporum,* and *Epidermophyton.* Each of the many species in these genera may produce clinical variations. At least 35 species have been identified in superficial skin infections (Ajello, 1968).

## PATHOGENESIS AND PATHOLOGY

The organisms of dermatophytosis live in balance with the functional changes in the stratum corneum, hair, and nails. These constantly growing structures shed at the surface (stratum corneum), at the ends (nails), or at the base (hair). The infection can maintain itself only if the fungi invade at a rate equal to the rate of sloughing (stratum corneum), or the rate of extension (nail), or the rate of growing out (hair). Thus, there is a dynamic, perpetual battle between the invading force of the organism and the counterflow of the biologic river in which it has to survive. There are factors in serum and in live epidermal cells that make it impossible for the dermatophytic fungus to survive. Thus, when the organism invades beyond the stratum corneum into the nucleated epidermis the host factors rapidly destroy the invading organism. Again we see the precarious balance that the organism must maintain if it is to survive. If it invades too fast it will provoke a lethal response; if it invades too slowly it will be ejected.

The first contact of the organism with its host is in the top layer of the stratum corneum. This lipid film contains a variety of chemical agents derived from sweat, sebaceous glands, and the keratinization process. Sebaceous glands contribute triglycerides that are hydrolyzed by surface bacteria to fatty acids. Many of these fatty acids are potent inhibitors of the growth of dermatophytes. These endogenous antibiotics limit the invasion of much of the cutaneous surface by dermatophytes. The soles of the feet do not have sebaceous glands and this may account for the very high incidence of dermatophyte infection of this area as compared with elsewhere. It is rare, for instance, to see a fungus infection of the sole of the foot extend onto the dorsum of the foot, where sebaceous glands are present.

Tinea capitis caused by *Microsporum audouini* is limited essentially to prepuberty. The disease is cured spontaneously at puberty and practically never starts in adults. The enormous increase of sebaceous glands at puberty probably explains spontaneous regression of *M. audouini* tinea capitis at puberty and its absence in adults. During the 1940s *M. audouini* tinea capitis was epidemic but has been relatively uncommon since. The episodic nature of tinea capitis epidemics is unexplained.

The immunologic state is important in determining the type of infection. In subjects infected for the first time with *Trichophyton rubrum* mild erythema and scaling develop slowly and gradually spread peripherally. As delayed skin tests to the trichophyton antigen become reactive, the clinical course becomes more intense and rapid. Some patients who cannot develop delayed hypersensitivity to the organism usually have enhanced immediate-type hypersensitivity and tend to be atopic. In them, tinea pedis is chronic, scaling, and noninflammatory. Recent studies (Ray et al., 1976) have implicated the complement system and chemotaxis in the resistance to *Candida albicans* infections. Typical pustules can be created in newborn mice by applying *C. albicans* to the skin under occlusion. Polymorphonuclear leukocytes densely infiltrate the epidermis (pustule) and *C. albicans* is walled off in the epidermis with *no* invasion of the lower layers of the skin. In mice deficient in the fifth component of complement (C5) this experiment evoked a minimal response of polys (lack of the chemotactic agent C5α) and *C. albicans* invades the deep skin and subcutaneous tissues. *C. albicans* infections (moniliasis) are common in diabetes mellitus, a disease with defective chemotaxis.

These examples of the biologic complexities involved in host-parasite relationships of dermatophytic infections illustrate that it is hardly a static process taking place in a dead layer.

Dermatophytes live only in the stratum corneum, hair, or nails, where their hyphae or spores can be identified with special stains — for example, periodic acid-Schiff.

Lymphocyte invasion of the corium, particularly in the upper layer, is evidence of an active immunologic response to dermatophytes. Along with this early invasion of lymphocytes there is a breakdown of the cytoplasm of the nucleated epidermal cells and a subsequent widening of spaces between the cells. This epidermal response, known as spongiosis, is also seen in a variety of eczematous diseases. The organisms rarely penetrate beneath the epidermis but may invade deeply into the horny matrix of the hair or nail. When the immune response is inactive, many dermatophytes may be seen in the stratum corneum with very little, if any, inflammation in the corium.

## CLINICAL MANIFESTATIONS

### Tinea Pedis (Athlete's Foot, Ringworm of the Feet)

This is probably the most common fungus infection in man. The organism can be isolated from 25 to 40 per cent of the feet of normal adults whether symptomatic or not. The most common form of tinea pedis is manifested by redness, scaling, and occasional vesiculation on the soles of the feet and particularly in the toe webs, usually between the fourth and fifth toes. There is some question whether the toe web type of tinea pedis is complicated by bacterial infection, but the lesions on the soles are caused primarily by the dermatophyte. *Trichophyton mentagrophytes* is the most common cause of tinea pedis but *Trichophyton rubrum* is also frequently involved. *Epidermophyton floccosum* is not usually found in this infection. These three organisms account for over 95 per cent of fungus infections of the soles of the feet.

Minimal scaling is found in many subjects but seldom bothers anyone enough to send him to the doctor. Those who consult the physician usually do so because of intense pruritus or very noticeable scaling or vesiculation. This disease occurs in acute episodes building up to its maximum severity in seven to sixteen days and then spontaneously subsiding over the next two to three weeks. It is common in individuals wearing unventilated shoes in moist and warm climates. In societies where shoes are rarely used, this type of acute tinea pedis is rarely seen. The more acute vesicular type of tinea pedis most often occurs in patients with a positive delayed skin test to trichophyton antigen. Those having a negative delayed test to *Trichophyton* but a positive immediate test for hypersensitivity usually show a chronic scaling, erythematous type of tinea pedis,

frequently caused by *T. rubrum*. This latter type of tinea pedis is difficult to eradicate and seldom undergoes spontaneous remission.

The clinical picture is highly suggestive of a fungus infection but proof resides in demonstrating hyphae in the stratum corneum. This can be done by treating scales from the lesion by the potassium hydroxide technique, which is the most reliable for distinguishing the presence of the dermatophytic infection (see below). Culturing the lesion will give positive results in only about 50 per cent of active clinical infections. Cultural identification of the exact organism is not necessary for the diagnosis of tinea pedis.

### Tinea Manus (Ringworm of the Hands)

In contrast to tinea pedis, tinea manus is relatively rare. The usual cause is *T. rubrum* and the infection is almost always associated with the chronic dry scaling type of *T. rubrum* tinea pedis.

In general, chronic scaling of the hands is not a fungus infection and is more likely an eczematous reaction of contact dermatitis, neurodermatitis, or atopic dermatitis.

### Tinea Cruris (Jock Itch)

This occurs mainly in the inguinal areas, where there is increased moisture and warmth, and is more common in males than females. There is a sharp strongly erythematous, scaling border. The area behind the advancing margin has less erythema but as many scales as the margin. The inflammatory margin is the most characteristic feature of this disease. The three organisms most often associated with this type of fungus infection are: *E. floccosum, T. rubrum,* and *T. mentagrophytes.*

### Tinea Corporis (Tinea Carcinata, Tinea Glabrosa)

Superficial fungus infections of areas other than the hands, feet, groin, and scalp express themselves in different ways. These infections are much more common in hot, humid climates than in the cool northern latitudes. The lesions are usually circinate, have an active spreading erythematous inflammatory border, and heal behind the advancing border. The term "ringworm" is probably derived from this lesion. They frequently regress without treatment. In patients with underlying disease such as diabetes or lymphoma these lesions may become enormous and spread over most of the body.

The classic annular lesion of tinea circinata may be caused by a variety of dermatophytes, but most commonly in the United States by *Microsporum audouini, Microsporum canis,* and *T. mentagrophytes.*

Occasionally no clearing occurs behind the advancing border and a large plaque of eczematous vesicular lesions develops. This more inflammatory type of ringworm can be caused by an endothrix, *Trichophyton* or *M. canis*. In severe inflammatory ringworm, known as kerion, there are large vesicles, extensive edema, and pustulation. Kerion is self-curing because the intense inflammatory response sterilizes the lesion. Self-sterilization also makes it difficult to demonstrate the offending organism.

Majocchi's granuloma is a variant of this more inflammatory ringworm that involves hair follicles, particularly in the lower extremities and usually is caused by deep infection of the skin with *T. rubrum*. It is best treated with griseofulvin.

### Tinea Capitis (Ringworm of the Scalp)

Inflammation of the scalp can be induced by many species of dermatophytes belonging to the genera *Microsporum* and *Trichophyton*. The type of infection can be mild or severe, depending upon the organism.

The most common type of tinea capitis in the United States is caused by *Microsporum audouini*. It causes epidemics and during the 1940s was severe in the United States, but occurs only sporadically now in children and practically never in adults. The infection is easily transmitted from one child to another and is difficult to control during epidemic periods. Broken hairs are the first obvious sign of the disease, and are responsible for partial alopecia of the scalp. Scaling and mild erythema around the broken hairs in tinea capitis usually help to distinguish it from alopecia areata, trichotillomania, and other causes of hair loss.

### Onychomycosis

Fungus infections of the toenails are very common. They are more likely to occur in men than in women and are unusual before puberty. Other cutaneous disease may give nail changes that can resemble those produced by fungus infections of the nail. Probably less than half of distorting afflictions of the nail are caused by fungi; the most common are *T. rubrum* and *T. mentagrophytes*. *Epidermophyton* and *Microsporum* rarely cause nail infections. In Asia, *T. violaceum* has been reported as a fairly common agent in fingernail infections.

It is interesting to note that onychomycosis is not common in societies where it is not customary to use footwear. Shoes may account for the much higher incidence of fungus infections of toenails as compared to the fingernails.

Onychomycosis ordinarily is not a severe disease but one of cosmetic importance. Men usually ignore a fungus infection of the toenails and are not disturbed if told to learn to live with their disease. Women are distressed by infection of the toenails, particularly if they wear open toed shoes. Both men and women are upset by fungus infection of the fingernails and are frequently desperate to have the fingernails cleared by therapy. Onychomycosis of the fingernails is most often caused by *T. rubrum*. It is rare to have a *T. rubrum* infection of the hand or fingernail and not have it on the feet and toenails. The big toenail seems to be the most often infected by a fungus, but all other nails can be so involved. Usually one or two nails of the foot are involved and the other nails are spared. Secondary bacterial infection is a rare complication of severe onychomycosis. The nail may become severely disfigured and impinge upon footwear so that it has to be cut down or filed.

### Tinea Versicolor

This superficial fungus infection of the skin is relatively easy to diagnose. It is characterized by discolored, slightly hyperpigmented spots or plaques on the chest and back. These lesions have a slight scale and gentle trauma with the fingernail will expose a branny-type scaling within the lesion. The disease is most common in young adults but may occur at practically any age. It is much more common in hot humid areas than in dry cold areas. Its tendency to recur after treatment probably results from widespread presence of the organism. Infection is a matter of individual susceptibility because this disease is usually not contracted even after intimate contact.

### Tinea Nigra

As the name implies, the disease is characterized by black discolorations of the skin, resembling stains of silver nitrate. They usually occur on the palms or sides of the fingers. The disease is more common in South America than in the United States. The organism causing this disease is *Cladosporium wernecki*.

## COMPLICATIONS AND SEQUELAE

By far the majority of dermatophyte infections are mild, self-limited, and completely reversible with little or no permanent change in the invaded tissue. The repair process causes no permanent damage.

Severe tinea capitis, tinea barbae, or trichophyton granuloma are rare causes of scarring. Some organisms are more likely to cause permanent damage and severe inflammation may destroy or scar the skin, even when the infection is caused by an organism such as *T. rubrum*, which is usually benign.

Secondary infection with pathogenic bacteria is unusual but when it occurs is generally caused by *Staphylococcus aureus* or certain types of Group A streptococci. Secondary streptococcal skin infection can rarely lead to acute glomeronephritis.

## GEOGRAPHIC VARIATIONS

There are many differences in the incidence of the various clinical types of dermatophyte infection in different parts of the world. The incidence of the type of organism causing a given clinical type of infection also will vary.

In India, tinea pedis occurs less frequently than in the United States, where it is the commonest dermatophyte infection, probably because occlusive shoes are worn by the vast majority in the United States. *Epidermophyton* is a relatively rare cause of dermatophytosis in India but common in the United States. The same is true for *T. mentagrophytes,* a common cause of tinea pedis in the United States.

Tinea capitis seems to be caused by different organisms in different parts of the world. *T. tonsurans* is a common offender in Mexico and *T. violaceum* is common in India.

Tinea versicolor is a common problem in tropical areas and relatively rare in cold, dry climates.

## DIAGNOSIS

The clinical features described above are most helpful in the diagnosis of fungus infections. To substantiate the clinical impression two laboratory methods are very useful.

The first is called the KOH preparation, which refers to the 10 per cent potassium hydroxide solution that is used to digest the scales that are put onto a glass slide under a cover slip. After heating over a mild flame just to the point of boiling, the slide is examined under $40 \times$ magnification with subdued lighting. The hyphae of the fungus show up as clearly outlined, branched filaments, which are easily distinguished from the cell outlines of the skin cells. It is best to learn this technique from one with experience before attempting it by yourself.

The other laboratory method is to culture the skin scales on Sabouraud's medium. Dermatophytes take 7 to 14 days to grow at room temperature. Usually, the organism can be classified by its gross and microscopic characteristics but this requires considerable experience. Often a KOH preparation will be positive and the culture negative.

The diagnosis of tinea pedis should be made cautiously from clinical features alone because it can mimic other diseases. Dyshidrosis, a variant of atopic eczema and neurodermatitis, can give a similar clinical picture. Dyshidrosis is usually bilateral and tina pedis is not. Dyshidrosis tends to be more intensely pruritic and is frequently associated with lesions of neurodermatitis or atopic dermatitis elsewhere on the body. The lesions of dyshidrosis will rarely reveal the presence of hyphae in the lesions. Contact dermatitis can mimic dermatophytosis of the feet. The most common cause of contact dermatitis of the feet is allergy to something in the shoes. Patch tests to elements in the shoes will show such allergy. Occasionally psoriasis can mimic tinea pedis but lesions of psoriasis elsewhere on the skin and nails distinguish it from a fungus infection.

The organism in tinea cruris or corporis is best identified by scraping horny material from the inflamed, advancing margin, and making a KOH preparation. The hyphae can then be demonstrated under the microscope. Again, the KOH preparation is more reliable than culture for demonstrating the organism.

In tinea capitis the fungi can easily be seen in the hair on KOH preparations. Greenish fluorescence of the hair under black light is characteristic of tinea capitis due to *Microsporum,* including *M. canis, M. ferrugineum,* and *M. distortum.* The other types of tinea capitis do not fluoresce. Cultures are helpful in distinguishing these organisms.

Onychomycosis is diagnosed by KOH preparation or culture. It is best to scrape away superficial debris and use the scales beneath for examination. Many nonpathogenic fungi are saprophytic on human toenails and rarely cause disruption of the nail. Nail distortion can occur with many other dermatoses such as psoriasis, eczema, and lichen planus so it is important not to ascribe the nail disease to a saprophyte that is cultured.

In tinea versicolor the hyphae and spores are sometimes called "spaghetti and meatballs." The stratum corneum is invaded by thick masses of these hyphae and spores and they are easy to see on the KOH preparation. They are difficult to culture and standard culture media are of no value in identification of the organism.

In tinea nigra a KOH preparation will disclose the dark green segmented hyphae and the organism is fairly easy to culture on standard media. This disease is occasionally misdiagnosed as junctional nevus or melanoma and unnecessary surgery is performed.

## TREATMENT

The only systemic drug for dermatophyte infections is griseofulvin. It is particularly useful in resistant cases of tinea pedis, tinea manus, onychomycosis, and tinea cruris, and is the only treatment for tinea capitis. Griseofulvin should be used with considerable discretion, however, because tinea pedis, tinea manus, onychomycosis, and tinea cruris tend to recur soon after discontinuing the drug even though it takes up to 12 to 18 months to clear onychomycosis and up to two to three months to clear tinea pedis or tinea manus. Tinea capitis responds rapidly and completely.

The standard dosage is 500 mg/day of micronized griseofulvin. The crystals of griseofulvin are ground to a very small size (micronized) to facilitate absorption through the gastrointestinal tract. Griseofulvin sometimes causes headaches but very few other complaints. Although it can cause porphyria and liver tumors in animals it has been relatively safe in patients for the past 15 years.

Most dermatophytic infections are treated first with topical formulations of fungistatic or fungicidal agents. One of the oldest is precipitated sulfur 2 to 5 per cent in a cream or ointment. Many agents introduced in the past ten years have a wider spectrum of activity against yeasts and bacteria. Because some tinea infections are complicated by bacterial secondary infection and some tinea infections are mimicked by bacterial and yeast infections, these newer agents are usually preferred. Miconazole and clotrimazole are the most widely used examples of these broad spectrum agents. Tolnaftate is also widely used but its spectrum is confined to dermatophytes and it is inactive against most yeasts and bacteria.

These antifungal drugs are supplied in 1 per cent concentration in liquid or cream vehicles. Generally, the liquid preparations are more active and better tolerated by the patient. They are applied as a thin layer twice a day to the affected area. Occasionally allergic reactions occur with either miconazole or clotrimazole and medication must be stopped. The period of treatment varies greatly. In tinea corporis or tinea cruris the lesions usually respond well in two weeks or less. In tinea pedis or tinea manus treatment is often prolonged indefinitely and usually without a cure.

Tinea pedis or tinea manus is treated topically with a potent antifungal agent such as tolnaftate, miconazole, or clotrimazole. All are available in lotions and creams. The main problem in tinea pedis is that the very thick, horny layer on the bottoms of the feet prevents penetration of the antifungal drugs to the depths of the stratum corneum where the fungus may reside. Most patients improve with topical therapy but the infection is likely to reappear from external reinfection. The answer may be in a combination of topical therapy and oral griseofulvin. The most difficult type of tinea pedis to treat is chronic, scaling nonvesicular lesions over large areas of both soles. Topical antifungal agents offer little in this disease. During oral griseofulvin therapy the majority of these infections subside but the disease recurs soon after griseofulvin is stopped.

The usual course of tinea cruris infection is for spontaneous flares, which frequently subside on their own without treatment but do respond rapidly to topical tolnaftate, miconazole, or clotrimazole. In about 10 per cent of the subjects the infection is fairly persistent and resistant, and although topical agents are of some benefit they do not eradicate the disease. Only rarely is it necessary to give oral griseofulvin to treat this problem. The same agents that work topically for tinea pedis (see above) are effective in the management of tinea cruris.

Some forms of tinea capitis tend to be more inflammatory than those caused by *M. audouini* and on rare occasions may give rise to large boggy draining lesions of the kerion type. Although usually self-healing the severe inflammatory types of tinea capitis are treated with griseofulvin.

Closely related to tinea capitis is tinea barbae. This is an inflammation of the beard area and is usually caused by a zoophilic fungus. This can also be easily controlled with oral griseofulvin.

Topical antifungal agents are of little, if any, value in the management of onychomycosis because they do not penetrate deeply enough to reach the fungus in the nail bed and nail plate. More than 50 per cent of toenail infections subside after oral griseofulvin. The faster growing fingernails respond in six months, whereas the toenails need to be treated for one year. When griseofulvin is stopped the nail infection almost invariably returns. Since griseofulvin cannot be taken indefinitely it is not used as widely as in the past. Topical antifungal agents may help prevent reinfection of the fingernails after griseofulvin therapy. Removal of the nail is generally ineffective because the new nail becomes reinfected even when prophylactic topical antifungal agents are used. The patient should be advised that there is no satisfactory treatment for onychomycosis.

Tinea versicolor responds readily to precipitated sulfur or selenium sulfide. Tolnaftate, miconazole, and clotrimazole also seem to be effective. If topical treatment is applied only once a day in a very thin layer, the fungi will not be recognizable after two to three weeks. If treatment is stopped then the disease will frequently recur, but application of one of these fungicides once or twice a week will prevent recurrence. Discoloration will remain sometimes five to six months after the disease process and the responsible fungi have been cleared from the area.

## PROPHYLAXIS

Since almost all attempts to clear the environment of dermatophytes have met with failure, we must assume that exposure of the population to dermatophytes is inevitable. Nevertheless, tinea pedis would be a relatively rare disease if the population did not wear shoes. In most societies this is an impractical suggestion, but the individual who suffers from resistant severe tinea pedis may get considerable relief by wearing open shoes or sandals. There is little gain in forbidding people with scaly feet from entering locker rooms or swimming pool areas. About 25 per cent of people without scaly feet carry dermatophytes on their feet and about 50 per cent of subjects with scaly feet do not have tinea pedis. In any event, it is the inborn host resistance that determines susceptibility rather than the size or frequency of the inoculum.

Occasionally an infected pet (cat or dog) will pass on tinea corporis to a group of children. In this case, elimination of the infection of the pet will prevent spread of the disease. The same situation holds for infection of farmers by animal carriers.

Eliminating local moisture can help tinea cruris. Loose underclothes, drying powders, and air conditioned rooms are helpful but usually not curative or fully effective in prophylaxis.

Epidemic tinea capitis (*M. audouini*) depends on spread by direct or intermediate contacts. Yet extreme measures of isolation and protection of children during the USA epidemic in the 1940s seemed to be of little help in containing the spread of this disease.

Topical antifungal drugs seem to prevent recurrent dermatophytosis in patients who are easily reinfected, especially with stubborn infections due to tinea pedis, onychomycosis, or tinea cruris that had required treatment with oral griseofulvin.

### References

Ajello, L.: A taxonomic review of the dermatophytes and related species. Sabouraudia 6:147, 1968.
Conant, N.F., Smith, D.T., Baker R.D., et al.: Manual of Clinical Mycology. 3rd ed. Philadelphia, W. B. Saunders Company, 1971.
Emmons, E.W.: Dermatophytes. Natural grouping based on the form of the spores and accessory organs. Arch Derm Syph 30:337, 1934.
Hildick-Smith, G., Blank, H., and Sarkany, I.: Fungus Diseases and Their Treatment. Boston, Little, Brown & Company, 1964.
Ray, T.L., Baker, D., and Weupper, K.: Experimental cutaneous candidiasis. Role of stratum corneum. J Invest Dermatol 66:278, 1976.
Sabourand, R.: Les Teignes. Paris, Masson et Cie, 1910.

# *SPOROTRICHOSIS* **209**

## *Abraham I. Braude, M.D., Ph.D.*

### DEFINITION

Sporotrichosis is a chronic infection due to the soil fungus *Sporothrix schenckii*. In most cases suppurating nodules form along the lymphatics of the skin and subcutaneous tissues. Hematogenous dissemination is rare, but pulmonary infection occurs occasionally from inhaled fungi.

### ETIOLOGY

The fungus *S. schenckii* is dimorphic on Sabouraud's agar. At room temperature its growth is mycelial, but in the tissues it takes the form of tiny cigar-shaped, gram-positive yeast cells. These yeast cells are seen abundantly in lesions of the testicle and other experimental lesions but are rarely found in infected lesions of patients. The yeast stage can develop in culture if the organism is incubated under $CO_2$ at 37° C on blood agar containing cystine.

### PATHOGENESIS AND PATHOLOGY

The fungus lives as a saprophyte on vegetation and penetrates the hands or feet when the skin is broken. Many cases have followed injury by thorns or wood splinters. Sporotrichosis is primarily an occupational disease in people working with plants. Sphagnum moss is an important source of infection.

From 7 to 40 weeks after penetrating the skin the fungus produces at the incubation site a reddish-purple necrotic nodule, the sporotrichotic chancre. This lesion has marked hyperkeratosis and intradermal microabscesses that rupture into the dermis. The most distinctive feature is a suppurative granuloma that contains polymorphonuclears in the center of a zone of histiocytes and giant cells. The entire lesion is surrounded by lymphocytes and plasma cells (Lurie, 1963). Occasionally the lesion at the inoculation site remains confined to the skin or epidermis without lymphatic involvement and has been called fixed cutaneous sporotrichosis. In the vast majority of cases the fungus spreads from the chancre up the extremities and evokes nodular lesions along the thickened lymphatics. It seems that tolerance for higher temperatures is essential for lymphatic spread beyond the cooler superficial tissues at the inoculation site. Thus, conidia of strains isolated from fixed cutaneous lesions without lymphangitis cannot grow at 37° C even though they multiply at 35° C. Conidia from isolates recovered from lymphangitic or disseminated infections multiply at both 35° and 37° C. Microscopically, the nodules along the lymphatics are also granulomas with abscesses in their center. Sometimes asteroid bodies can be found scattered irregularly in the pus (Splendore, 1980). These bodies are spherical structures measuring 5 to 10 $\mu$ in diameter and resemble spores. When stained by the periodic acid-Schiff method, the wall seems to have a double contour. This round structure is surrounded by eosinophilic material arranged in the form of a star. Similar radial formation of eosinophilic material has been found around schistosome ova (Hoeppli, 1932), microfilaria, and *Entomophthora coronata,* the cause of African nasal phycomycosis. Known as the Splendore-Hoeppli phenomenon, it is thought to result from an antigen-antibody reaction.

Primary infections of the extremities almost never become disseminated through the bloodstream. In the rare case of disseminated infection the portal of entry is thought to be the gastrointestinal tract, and lesions predominate in the skin, bones, muscles, and joints. Occasionally the liver, testicles, eye, and lung may also be involved. Sporotrichosis of the central nervous system is the most unusual form of disseminated infection and produces a granulomatous basilar meningitis. The rarity of any form of disseminated infection can be appreciated from the fact that in South Africa, where 3300 cases of sporotrichosis had been seen by 1963, only five were disseminated (Lurie, 1963). More recently, sporotrichosis has shown a tendency to be an opportunistic infection that disseminates in compromised patients with such disorders as Hodgkin's disease, multiple myeloma, leukemia, diabetes, nephrosis, and especially alcoholism (Lynch et al., 1970). The disseminated lesions have the same granulomatous appearance as those described in primary lymphocutaneous infection. In some disseminated lesions abundant yeast forms have been visible.

## CLINICAL MANIFESTATIONS

### Primary Cutaneous Sporotrichosis

The primary lesion is usually found on the hands or fingers but can appear on any exposed part of the body, including the face. It starts as a small red papule and progresses to a pustular nodule of firm, rubbery consistency. An ulcer forms on the pustule, exudes pus on pressure, and is frequently surrounded by tiny papules. Later the lesion may be covered by a hard scab. In about 20 per cent of cases, there is no extension of disease along the lymphatics. This is especially likely to be the case in endemic areas where repeated exposure to the fungus is thought to sensitize or immunize the patient so that infection is confined to the area of inoculation. In these infections, known as the fixed cutaneous form, the lesions may also be verrucous, papillomatous, acneiform, or nonulcerative papules.

In most patients, however, the infection begins to spread along the lymphatics in about a week after the primary lesion appears. A chain of hard, red discrete lumps extends up the arm or leg to the axilla or groin, and the intervening lymphatics become red and thickened. The epitrochlear lymph node frequently enlarges, but the axillary or inguinal glands usually do not. The disproportion between symptoms and findings is striking; there is no pain, fever, or other constitutional symptoms. Older nodules may rupture to produce fistulas or ulcers, but these remain relatively indolent.

### Disseminated Sporotrichosis

There are two forms of disseminated infection. In one, the patient has multiple, scattered, dusky red skin nodules. These may begin anywhere, with one nodule and then multiple nodules appearing on the trunk, face, scalp, arms, and legs. Most of these patients also have lesions in the bones or joints and may complain of migratory arthritis, with joint swellings and effusion. A few patients develop metastatic deep-seated abscesses of the muscles, including the trapezius, biceps, gastrocnemius, and triceps (Lurie, 1963). Lymphangitis is not a characteristic feature of disseminated disease, but lymphadenopathy is found in some cases. Meningitis and brain infection are exceedingly unusual. Metastatic lung nodules and mucosal lesions are also rare. Sporotrichosis of mucous membranes may occur in the nasopharynx, mouth, or larynx and may produce ulcers, soft scars, and suppurating nodules with regional lymphadenopathy. Sporotrichosis of bone in these patients usually causes local swelling over the area of bone destruction. Warmth and tenderness may also be present. Sinuses drain from the bone through the skin, and adjacent joints become infected by contiguous spread. The bones of the arms, legs, wrists, ankles, hands, and feet are most often infected. In contrast to the classic lymphocutaneous infection, this form of disseminated sporotrichosis may be accompanied by mild fever (<39° C), anorexia, and weight loss.

The other form of disseminated sporotrichosis has only one metastatic focus that involves primarily a joint but sometimes the eye, genitourinary tract, or bone. Because any one of these occurs with no contiguous skin lesion and without direct trauma into the infected site, each is presumed to be infected by hematogenous spread.

### Primary Pulmonary Sporotrichosis

In primary pulmonary sporotrichosis the patient usually has slight respiratory symptoms, if any, until the disease becomes well advanced. A number of cases have been identified when routine x-ray examinations disclosed an upper lobe infiltrate or cavity. These infiltrates resemble those of tuberculosis (Fig. 1), and patients are often given antituberculous drugs even though tubercle bacilli are never seen or cultured. When symptoms occur, a mild or moderate cough is noted at first, and a small amount of sputum may be produced. Chest pain, fever, chills, night sweats, and hemoptysis are not the rule when the disease is first recognized, and there are no skin nodules or other signs of disseminated infection. Later, however, fever, hemoptysis (Fig. 1), and respiratory insufficiency may become prominent.

### Traumatic Synovitis

Penetrating injury of a joint or tendon sheath may cause synovitis. It has been suggested that these infections tend to occur in alcoholics because the fungus can penetrate deeper than in the ordinary patient, whose coordination and sensitivity to pain are not affected during gardening. Traumatic synovitis tends to involve the wrist, which becomes swollen, painful, and red (Kedes et al., 1964; DeHaven et al., 1972; Marrocco et al., 1975). The diagnosis is usually missed and the patient treated unsuccessfully with antituberculous drugs and synovectomy. A diagnosis of chronic granulomatous synovitis is made from the infected synovium, but no etiology can be found by the pathologist because the fungus cannot be seen microscopically, and routine cultures for bacteria are negative. Cases are on record in which multiple surgical procedures were done over a period of seven years without a correct diagnosis.

### Ocular Sporotrichosis

The fungus has a predilection for the conjunctiva and eyelids but may infect any part of the eye, either exogenously or endogenously (Francois, 1972). It is a special hazard to laboratory workers who handle the fungus. Primary sporotrichosis of the eyelid starts as a hard inflammatory nodule that involves the overlying skin and underlying conjunctiva. Primary sporotrichosis of the conjunctiva produces small, hard, yellow nodules, usually on the inner surface of the lids but also on the bulbar conjunctiva. Both conjunctival and palpebral nodules become abscesses that discharge pus and are accompanied by enlarged preauricular lymph nodes. The cornea is resistant to spread of infection from the conjunctiva, and sportrichotic ulcers are rare. In-

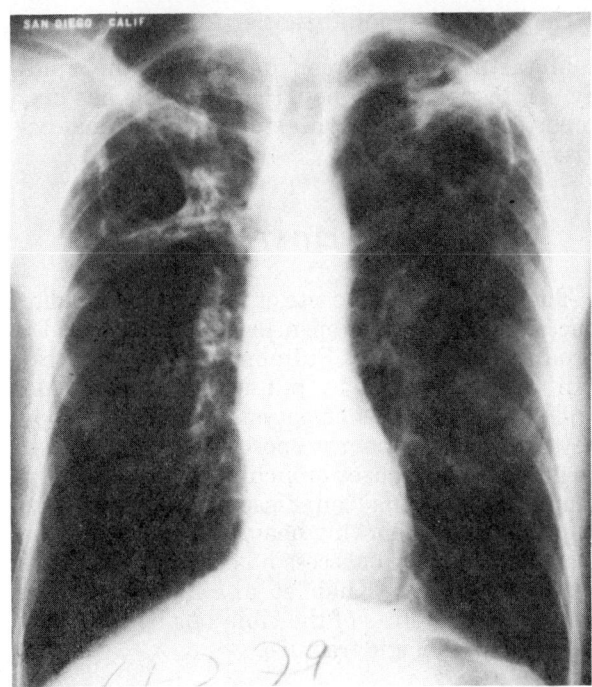

**FIGURE 1.** *Pulmonary sporotrichosis with bilateral apical cavities resembling tuberculosis. Patient was treated unsuccessfully for tuberculosis despite negative smears and cultures of sputa for mycobacteria. Diagnosis of sporotrichosis was made by repeated culture of* Sporothrix schenckii *from sputum. Chief clinical problem had been ten years of marked hemoptysis that did not abate with treatment of sporotrichosis and required therapeutic embolization of the bleeding vessel.*

traocular sporotrichosis is relatively common and may be caused by traumatic inoculation or metastatic spread during hematogenous dissemination. Several cases of intraocular sporotrichosis have followed cataract surgery. The first lesion is usually a nodular iritis.

### Central Nervous System Sporotrichosis

Both meningitis and brain abscess have occurred but are exceedingly rare. One of the reported infections started two years after a myelogram was done for a herniated intervertebral disk and was probably a form of inoculation sporotrichosis. The patient complained of occipital headache and dizziness for a year (Shoemaker et al., 1957). He also lost weight, became confused, and deteriorated neurologically until his death. Another case occurred in a 58-year-old farmer who also suffered from confusion, weakness, ataxia, weight loss, and impaired vestibular function (Klein et al., 1966). He responded to treatment with amphotericin B. In a third case no neurologic symptoms were noted during the course of disseminated sporotrichosis, but suppurative granulomas were scattered throughout the cerebral cortex at postmortem examination (Collins, 1947).

## Genitourinary Sporotrichosis

Metastatic lesions can develop in the epididymis, testis, and kidney. Pyonephrosis has been reported in a patient with stones in the renal pelvis.

## COMPLICATIONS

These depend on the site of infection. Secondary bacterial infection of open lesions may spread to produce septicemia. Pulmonary sporotrichosis can be complicated by pulmonary insufficiency and severe chronic hemoptysis. If hilar adenopathy occurs in pulmonary sporotrichosis, it may be so great that it causes bronchial obstruction. Pulmonary infections can disseminate hematogenously or by swallowing heavily infected sputum; a case of perirectal abscess has been attributed to swallowed fungi (Khan et al., 1975). Sporotrichotic osteomyelitis of the tibia has been complicated by pathologic fracture.

## GEOGRAPHIC VARIATIONS IN DISEASE

The common denominator of sporotrichosis throughout the world is occupational exposure during agricultural work and gardening. In certain areas, however, special forms of exposure have been noted. For example, in a huge epidemic in South Africa, nearly 3000 cases occurred in gold miners who were infected by exposure of skin abrasions to *S. schenckii* growing as a saprophyte on timbers supporting the mine. In the United States, several epidemics of cutaneous sporotrichosis have been traced to sphagnum moss contaminated with the fungus (Powell et al., 1978). In Mexico, where sporotrichosis is the most common fungus infection, the pattern of disease varies with age, sex, and occupation. Thus, women get lesions on their fingers from weaving baskets of grass, children on the face from scratches of branches, and men on the fingers and wrists from collecting grasses or on the legs from thorns (Rippon, 1974). Steady exposure to spores in endemic areas of Mexico is thought to produce immunity and sensitization to antigens of *S. schenckii* so that infections remain localized to the inoculation site and take on the character of verrucous, acneiform, plaque-like, papular, or crusted weeping lesions that behave more like allergic reactions than infections. Patients in endemic areas develop strong intradermal allergic reactions to sporotrichin, an antigen of *S. schenckii*.

The nutritional status of the population is probably another important factor in determining the incidence and severity of sporotrichosis. The declining frequency in France has been attributed to improved nutrition, whereas the high frequency in the poor areas of Latin America can be correlated there with poor diets. Nutritional disturbances would also account for the increased prevalence of sporotrichosis in alcoholics, and its tendency to become disseminated in patients with an underlying illness. Thus sporotrichosis appears to be an opportunistic infection, and its geographic or clinical pattern can be explained to some extent on this premise.

## DIAGNOSIS

### Lymphocutaneous Sporotrichosis

The fungus cannot be seen upon microscopic examination of biopsied material or pus in most cases. Cultural isolation is always successful, however, if pus is taken from an unbroken nodule or ulcer and inoculated into Sabouraud's agar at room temperature. The growth at first has the soft creamy character of bacterial colonies and later develops a wrinkled dark-brown appearance without the cotton-like filament of most molds. Microscopically, typical clusters of pear-shaped spores are found at the tips of tiny conidiophores arising from the tangled mass of delicate branched mycelia. If the mold or pus is inoculated intraperitoneally into mice or rats, numerous yeast forms will be seen in lesions of the peritoneal cavity or testicle, where they take the form of gram-positive, cigar-shaped rods within polymorphonuclear leukocytes.

Recovery of the organism is so reliable that sporotrichosis can be recognized in a week or two and thus differentiated from other chronic infections of the subcutaneous tissues such as tularemia, blastomycosis, coccidioidomycosis, syphilis, and mycobacterial infections. The lymphangitic ("sporotrichoid") forms of *Mycobacterium marinum* and *Mycobacterium kansasii* infections cannot be distinguished from sporotrichosis clinically, but skin injuries in an aquarium or swimming pool point to *M. marinum*.

### Disseminated Cutaneous Sporotrichosis

In contrast to the lymphocutaneous type, subcutaneous nodules are scattered all over the body, and no primary lesion is found. As the scattered nodules grow, they soften and form a central depression with hard peripheries. Although they may run their course without ulcerating, when perforation does occur, the indolent ulcers are indistinguishable from those in the localized form of the disease. Pus aspirated from the unbroken disseminated nodules may have numerous cigar-shaped, gram-positive yeast forms of *S. schenckii*, so that this less typical clinical variety of sporotrichosis can be more easily identified in the laboratory. The combination of bone or joint lesions with such skin lesions should always suggest the possibility of sporotrichosis, especially in alcoholics or immunosuppressed patients.

### Extracutaneous Sporotrichosis

Sporotrichosis of joints is difficult to differentiate from rheumatoid arthritis, because both diseases may be multiarticular, chronic, and relapsing; the joint fluids both have high neutrophil counts; the chronic inflammatory response in synovial biopsies looks the same in both diseases; the fungus is not usually seen in the tissues in sporotrichosis; and in both diseases subcutaneous nodules may occur. In addition, rheumatoid arthritis and articular sporotrichosis respond somewhat to rest, heat, salicylates, and intra-articular steroids. The diagnosis of sporotrichosis can be suspected if a synovial fistula to the skin develops and if the small joints of the foot are affected. Culture of the synovial biopsy will always be positive.

In osseous sporotrichosis the lesion is osteolytic, and x-ray examination shows destruction of bone without reactive osteoblastic change (Gladstone and Littman, 1971). About two thirds of patients have distant skin lesions from which the fungus can be cultured, if not seen in direct examination. Nearly 80 per cent have signs of joint involvement, and over 40 per cent have draining sinuses from which positive cultures can be made.

In pulmonary or meningeal sporotrichosis differential diagnosis centers first around tuberculosis. In pulmonary sporotrichosis the fungus grows heavily from the sputum, and sputum culture on Sabouraud's medium is imperative in any patient with upper-lobe cavities whose sputum has no acid-fast bacilli in smears. This test will also help exclude histoplasmosis, which can be endemic in the same regions as sporotrichosis and is another important cause of upper-lung cavitation with negative acid-fast smears in the sputum.

Limited experience in the rare cases of meningeal sporotrichosis indicates that *S. schenckii* can also be readily grown from the spinal fluid. In addition to clinical signs of a chronic basilar meningitis, meningeal sporotrichosis produces cerebrospinal fluid changes like those of tuberculosis—i.e., low sugar levels, moderate lymphocytosis, and elevated protein levels.

### TREATMENT

The common lymphangitic form of sporotrichosis is almost invariably and dramatically cured by saturated potassium iodide. This should be given orally in starting doses of 10 drops three times daily after meals and gradually increased to the point of maximum tolerance. Treatment should be continued for a month after lesions disappear. Additional local therapy may be required for cutaneous ulcers, which should be painted with tincture of iodine. It may also be necessary to excise epidermal lesions, because these may not subside with oral iodides. Systemic sporotrichosis is resistant to iodides but often responds well to intravenous treatment with amphotericin B, given in a total dose of 1.5 to 2.0 g over a period of six to eight weeks. There is some evidence that intravenous miconazole may be of value in patients who do not respond to amphotericin B because of drug resistance, clinical resistance, or drug intolerance (Rohwedder and Archer, 1976). Miconazole is given in a dose of 800 to 1000 mg three times daily through a central venous catheter to avoid phlebitis. The chief side effects of miconazole are itching and water retention due to inappropriate secretion of antidiuretic hormone. Antipruritic drugs and water restriction can control these problems.

Heat treatment has been advocated for skin lesions in patients who cannot tolerate iodides or amphotericin B. An attempt is made to kill the fungus in the lesions by raising the temperature of the infected area above 39° C for an hour or more four times daily. This can be done with hot packs or an electric heating pad.

### PROPHYLAXIS

Sporotrichosis can be prevented when epidemic sources are identified. For example, in a recent epidemic traced to sphagnum moss, the incriminated moss was buried in order to control the outbreak (Powell et al., 1978). Other lots of sphagnum moss are stored indoors, the storage buildings are scrubbed monthly with a disinfectant, and the moss is cultured regularly for *S. schenckii*. The massive epidemic in South African gold mines was controlled by disinfecting the timber where *S. schenckii* was growing as a saprophyte. Laboratory infections can be prevented by reasonable precautions among technicians, who should be made aware of the risk of autoinoculation, especially of the eyelids. For the most part, however, the simple precautions needed to prevent infection in agriculture workers are difficult to enforce because they cannot afford the clothing needed to protect their hands, legs, and feet.

### References

Collins, W.: Disseminated ulcerating sporotrichosis with widespread visceral involvement: Report of a case. Arch Derm Syph (Chicago) 56:523, 1947.

DeHaven, K., Wilde, A., and O'Duffy, J.: Sporotrichosis arthritis and tenosynovitis. J Bone Joint Surg 54A:874, 1972.

Francois, J.: Sporotrichosis. In Francois, J.: Oculomycoses. Springfield, Ill., Charles C Thomas, 1972, p. 375.

Gladstone, J., and Littman, M.: Osseous sporotrichosis. Am J Med 51:121, 1971.

Hoeppli, R.: Histologic observation in experimental schistosomiasis Japonica. Chinese Med J 43:1179, 1932.

Kedes, L., Siemienski, J., and Braude, A.: The syndrome of the alcoholic rose garden. Sporotrichosis of the radial tendon sheath. Ann Intern Med 61:1139, 1964.

Khan, F., Guarneri, J., and Sierra, M.: Primary pulmonary sporotrichosis complicated by perirectal abscess. Am Rev Resp Dis 112:119, 1975.

Klein, R., Ivens, M., Seabury, S., and Dascomb, H.: Meningitis due to Sporotrichum schenckii. Arch Intern Med 118:145, 1966.

Lurie, H.: Histopathology of sporotrichosis. Arch Pathol 75:421, 1963.

Lynch, P., Voorhees, I., and Harrell, E.: Systemic sporotrichosis. Ann Intern Med 73:23, 1970.

Marrocco, G., Tihen, W., Goodnough, C., and Johnson, R.: Granulomatous synovitis and osteitis caused by Sporothrix schenckii. Am J Clin Pathol 64:345, 1975.

Powell, K., Taylor, A., Phillips, B., Blakey, D., Campbell, G., Kaufman, L., and Kaplan, W.: Cutaneous sporotrichosis in forestry workers. JAMA 240:232, 1978.

Rippon, J.: Sporotrichosis. In Medical Mycology. Philadelphia, W. B. Saunders Company, 1974, p. 250.

Rohwedder, J., and Archer, G.: Pulmonary sporotrichosis: Treatment with miconazole. Am Rev Resp Dis 114:403, 1976.

Shoemaker, E., Bennett, H., Fields, W., Whitcomb, F., and Halpert, B.: Leptomeningitis due to Sporotrichum schenckii. Arch Pathol 64:222, 1957.

Splendore, A.: Sobre acultura d'uma nova especie de cogumello pathogenico. Rev Soc Sci S Paulo 3:62, 1908.

# 210 CHROMOBLASTOMYCOSIS

## Alberto Thomaz Londero, M.D.

### DEFINITION

Chromoblastomycosis is a chronic indolent granulomatous infection, usually confined to the skin, caused by several dematiaceous fungi, which develop in the tissue as round, dark-brown bodies and multiply by equatorial splitting.

### ETIOLOGY

Five closely related dematiaceous fungi are the etiologic agents of chromoblastomycosis. They are: *Acrotheca aquaspersa, Cladosporium carrionii, Fonsecaea pedrosoi, Fonsecaea compactum,* and *Phialophora verrucosa.*

### EPIDEMIOLOGY

The mycosis primarily affects rural adults, usually between 30 and 50 years of age. The infection is rare in children, even in highly endemic areas, and is more frequent among males than females. All races seem to be susceptible to the infection, and its prevalence is closely related to the social and economic habits of the people.

### CLINICAL MANIFESTATIONS

In chromoblastomycosis, cutaneous lesions are nearly always unilateral and situated on an exposed part of the body. They occur on the lower limbs, upper limbs, face, and trunk, in that order of frequency.

Bopp (1959) classified the lesions in two types: (1) nodular or tumoral and (2) smooth or vegetating plaque-like lesions. The plaque-like lesions may be subdivided into tuberculoid, syphiloid, psoriasiform, and mycetoma-like subtypes. The noncharacteristic early lesions are still another type.

The noncharacteristic early lesions have been described as either a pink scaly papule, a nodule that ulcerates, a subcutaneous abscess, a ringworm-like lesion, a superficial ulceration with a slightly verrucoid basis, or an erythematous violaceous pustule. A nodule or a papule has been reported to be the starting lesion in experimental inoculations in man.

Nodular or tumoral lesions are characteristic of the mycosis, but usually they are seen in the distal part of the lower limbs. At first a hemispheric, soft or fibrous, glistening pink to violaceous, small nodule is seen. After months or perhaps years, other nodules appear in adjacent areas or ascend irregularly along the limbs, covering large areas (Fig. 1). As the lesions progress the nodules became raised, up to 1 or 2 cm above the skin, sometimes pedunculated. Their surface may be smooth or verrucoid. These crops of nodules are hard and dry, but, when pressed, a caseous or purulent secretion emerges. Some nodules may ulcerate, and from the ulceration many tumoral lobulated masses arise, resembling the florets of the cauliflower. At the proximal part of the limb these nodular overgrowths usually are isolated and moderately elevated from the skin, presenting a violaceous surface that is sometimes covered by dirty, grayish crusts.

Plaque-like lesions are seen almost exclusively on the upper limbs, face, and trunk. These lesions result from the eccentric progress of the small initial infiltrated area. After months or perhaps years, they became round or oval lesions, elevated

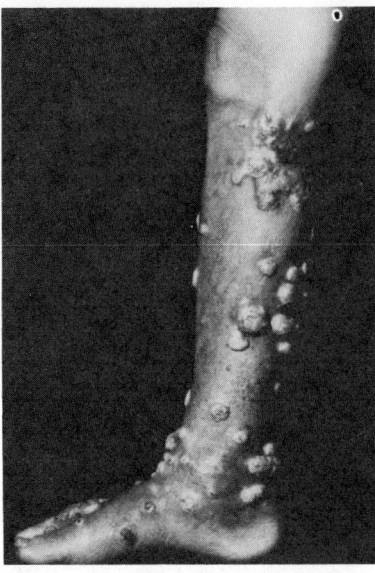

**FIGURE 1.** *Nodular or tumoral form of chromoblastomycosis. (Courtesy of Dr. C. Bopp, Brazil.)*

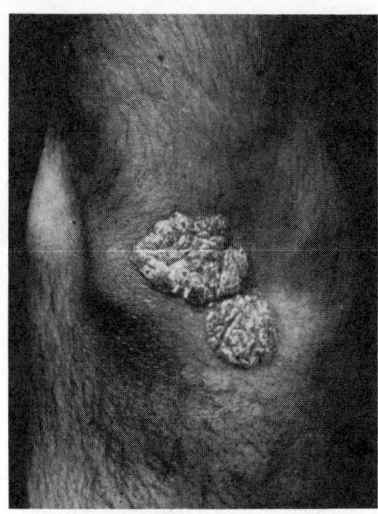

**FIGURE 2.** *Psoriasiform subtype of the plaque-like form of chromoblastomycosis.*

up to 1 to 5 mm above the skin, measuring 5 to 10 cm in diameter, sometimes greater. These lesions are formed or packed papillomatous vegetations, either denuded and pink colored or covered by horny, grayish crusts. Pus or caseous material may be obtained by pressing, and when the crusts are picked up the surface bleeds easily. Sometimes the plaque-like lesions extend over a large area of the body. In those cases the surface becomes smooth and glistening, pink or violaceous, and covered by grayish crusts.

The plaque can heal spontaneously in the center or on a segment of the border of the lesion. If the remaining lesion is semilunar, elevated, and heavily infiltrated, it is considered to be of the tuberculoid subtype. If the atrophic cicatricial area is bordered by an infiltrated and ulcerated serpiginous or arciform lesion that progresses centrifugally, it is called the syphiloid subtype. On the other hand, if the area has some slightly infiltrated plaques, whose surface is a conglomerate of closed minute papillae covered by micaceous adherent scales, it is called the psoriasiform subtype (Fig. 2). The mycetomatoid subtype is a heavily infiltrated plaque with scattered mammillated elevations containing apertures at their apex, through which pus may drain.

Primary lesions on the mucous membranes of the nose, eye, larynx, and vulva are rare. Disseminated hematogenous lesions of the skin or internal organs, especially the brain, are also unusual. Lymphatic spread may cause lymphangitis and regional lymphadenopathy.

## COMPLICATIONS AND SEQUELAE

The most frequent complication is elephantiasis of the extremities. It is caused by lymphatic blockade from extensive fibrosis in the deeper tissues. Another complication is secondary bacterial infection producing ulcerations that are sometimes extensive. Scars take the form of smooth, atrophic areas of glistening skin and result from spontaneous partial healing of the lesions, or from treatment.

## DIAGNOSIS

Diagnosis of chromoblastomycosis can only be established by demonstrating the infective agent in the lesion.

### Clinical Diagnosis

Chromoblastomycosis may be suspected in advanced cases, especially in patients presenting the tumoral form. The early lesions must be differentiated from bacterial infections and the initial lesions of the other subcutaneous mycosis. The circumscribed tumoral, plaque-like, and mixed types of the mycosis must be differentiated from similar lesions seen in other mycoses (e.g., lobomycosis, sporotrichosis, blastomycosis, tropical mossy foot, yaws, syphilis, tuberculosis, lupus erythematosus, lupus vulgaris, leishmaniasis, and psoriasis.

### Laboratory Diagnosis

Mycologic diagnosis is very simple and inexpensive. A little drop of pus or caseous material, obtained by squeezing the lesions or puncturing a

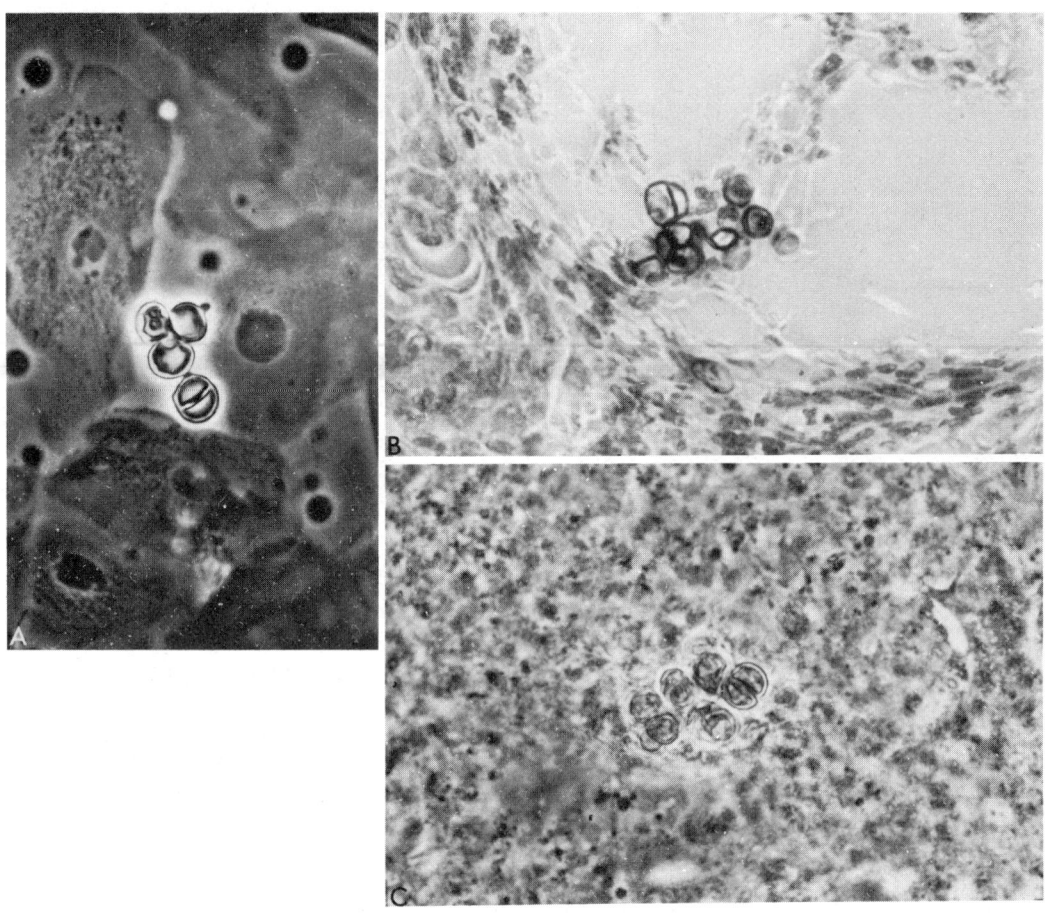

**FIGURE 3.**   *Pigmented fungus cells in pus from lesions (left) and in tissue (right) (250 ×).*

small abscess, should be placed on a slide with 10 per cent potassium hydroxide and examined under a coverglass. Crusts should be removed and mounted in the same way. All the agents of chromoblastomycosis present identical forms in tissue or pus. They appear as single or clustered round, dark-brown, thick-walled bodies, 8 to 12 μm in diameter, some of them dividing by splitting (Fig. 3). In the epithelial crusts the fungal elements are seen occasionally as brown septate-branching hyphae, 2 to 5 μm in width, germinating from sclerotic bodies. The diagnosis may also be made by histologic examination and culture of biopsied tissue.

Cultures of crusts, pus, exudate, and biopsied tissue should be placed on Mycosel or Sabouraud's dextrose agar, in tubes or plates, and incubated at 25 to 30° C (see Chapter 76).

## PATHOGENESIS AND PATHOLOGY

The agents of chromoblastomycosis are soil-inhabiting fungi, but they have been isolated more frequently from wood than from soil itself (Gezuele et al., 1972). *F. pedrosoi* and *P. verrucosa* have been recovered from rotting wood, wood pulp, and plant debris. *C. carrionii* has been isolated from fence posts in Australia, and Salonen and Ruokola (1969) recovered *P. verrucosa* from the wooden furniture and floor of rustic saunas in Finland.

The fungus enters the skin through an abrasion or trauma caused by decaying wood. Inadequate nutrition, immunologic deficiency, and poor general health seem to play a role in allowing the infection to evolve.

The lesions appear at the site of the trauma and remain circumscribed for some time. After months, the lesions spread slowly to adjacent areas through the superficial lymphatics, extending after many years over large areas of the body. Some lesions may heal and form scars. Metastatic lesions, located some distance from uninvolved areas, may be caused by autoinoculation and either by lymphatic or, more rarely, by hematogenous spread. There is no known transmission from person to person.

The chromoblastomycotic lesions, usually confined to the skin, are sharply limited. Histologic section under low-power microscopic observation shows hyperkeratosis, pseudoepitheliomatous hyperplasia, papillomatosis, and microabscesses. A granulomatous infiltrate of the upper and lower dermis is also seen. The pleomorphic infiltrate, composed of lymphocytes, plasma cells, some eosinophils, and multinulceated giant cells, of either the Langhans or the foreign-body type, surrounds the tuberculoid granulomata and the microabscesses. Dermal tuberculoid granulomas are formed by clusters of epithelioid cells. Microabscesses consist of masses of polymorphonuclear leukocytes surrounded by histiocytes or epidermal cells. Usually there is slight fibrosis. Fungal elements may be seen within granuloma, the microabscess, and giant cells. They are described under *Diagnosis*.

Secondary bacterial invasion, with or without ulceration, may obscure the histologic picture of chronic inflammation by evoking a pyogenic reaction.

## GEOGRAPHIC VARIATIONS IN THE DISEASE

With the exception of the frigid polar regions, chromoblastomycosis has been reported from every continent in the world, but its geographic distribution is not uniform. In the New World almost all cases have been reported in a belt limited by 30° N and 30° S. In this zone there are highly endemic circumscribed areas, such as Costa Rica and the Dominican Republic. In Europe most cases have been seen in countries above 45° N, with the greatest number appearing in Finland. In Africa the endemic zone is below the equator, with a highly endemic area in the Malagasy Republic. In Asia, with the exception of Japan, the mycosis has not been frequently reported. In Australasia almost all cases have been reported in Australia.

Throughout the world, *F. pedrosoi* is the agent most commonly isolated from chromoblastomycosis. It prevails in humid areas with more than 2000 mm annual rainfall. *C. carrionii*, the agent isolated next most frequently, infects patients in regions with less than 600 mm annual rainfall (Mexico, Venezuela, South Africa, Malagasy Republic, and Australia). *P. verrucosa*, less frequently found as an agent of chromoblastomycosis, generally occurs in patients living in the temperate regions of the New World, and sporadically in patients from Africa and Asia. *F. compac-*

*tum* has been isolated sporadically from patients in the New World, Europe, and Asia. *A. aquaspersa* is an occasional cause of the infection in Mexico, Costa Rica, and Brazil.

## TREATMENT

In the early small lesions the most suitable treatment is local heat administered as a water bath or infrared rays (Conti-Diaz et al., 1969). Heat treatment can be combined with perilesional infiltration of amphotericin B. The drug is infiltrated weekly for three months in a concentration of 40 mg/5 ml of 2 per cent procaine solution (Costello et al., 1959).

Patients with nonextensive lesions, especially those caused by *C. carrionii*, can be treated with 5-fluorocytosine in a dose of 100 mg/kg body weight daily, in three daily doses for 8 to 12 weeks. Treatment may be stopped three weeks after the first negative culture (Boreilli, 1972). An alternative is thiabendazole in a dose of 25 mg/kg body weight daily, for 6 to 22 months (Bayles, 1971).

Advanced cases may be treated with a combination of 50 mg amphotericin B intravenously three times a week and 5-fluorocytosine, at a level of 50 mg/kg body weight, three times a day for three months (Bopp, 1976).

## PROPHYLAXIS

The exposed parts of the body, especially the distal parts of the limbs, must be covered during work in the fields or with wood.

## References

Bayles, M. A. H.: Chromomycosis. Treatment with thiabendazole. Arch Derm 104:476, 1971.

Bopp, C.: Cromoblastomicose. Contribuição ao estudo de alguns de seus aspectos. Thesis. Porto Alegre, Livraria Globo, 1959.

Bopp, C.: Cura da cromoblastomicose por novo método de tratamento. Med Cut ILA 13:285, 1976.

Borelli, D.: *Acrotheca aquaspersa* nova species agente de cromomicosis. Acta Cient Venez 23:193, 1972.

Conti-Diaz, I. A., Vignale, R. A., and Pereira, M. E. P.: Cromoblastomicosis tratada con termoterapia local. Med Cut ILA 3: 383, 1969.

Costello, M. J., DeFeo, C. P., Jr., and Littman, M. L.: Chromoblastomycosis treated with local infiltration of amphotericin B solution. Arch Derm 79:184, 1959.

Gezuele, E., Mackinnon, J. E., and Conti-Diaz, I. A.: The frequent isolation of *Phialophora verrucosa* and *Phialophora pedrosoi* from natural sources. Sabouraudia 10:266, 1972.

Ridey, M. F.: The saprophytic occurrence of fungi causing chromoblastomycosis. *In:* Recent Advances in Botany. Univ. Toronto Press, Toronto, 1961, p. 312.

Salonen, A. and Ruokola, A. L.: Mycoflora of the Finish "sauna." Mycopathologia 38:327, 1969.

# 211 MONILIASIS OF THE SKIN

## J. E. Edwards, Jr., M.D.

Although chronic mucocutaneous candidiasis is not the most common form of *Candida* cutaneous infection, it will be considered in detail in this chapter because of its importance in elucidating immunologic mechanisms operative against *Candida*.

## CHRONIC MUCOCUTANEOUS CANDIDIASIS

### Definition

This term applies to a heterogeneous group of stubborn *Candida* infections of the skin, mucous membranes, hair, and nails that persist and recur in spite of therapy. These infections occur in patients with specific immunologic abnormalities.

### Etiology

Thymus-derived lymphocytes (T cells) are abnormal (see section on Pathogenesis and Pathology) in most patients with chronic mucocutaneous candidiasis, but the cause of the T-cell disorder is not known. In some forms, genetic factors are obvious from familial trends. Several mechanisms, all speculative, have been considered responsible for failure of cellular immunity: (1) failure of antigen recognition by the T-cell, (2) failure of T-cell mediator production (macrophage inhibition factor [MIF]), (3) abnormality in the inflammatory cell itself (defective monocyte chemotaxis), (4) inhibition of T-cell function by a population of suppressor cells, (5) abnormal thymic function, and (6) immune tolerance for a specific antigen shared by *Candida* organisms.

### Pathogenesis and Pathology

T-cell dysfunction is evident from the following observations (Stiehm, 1977): in approximately half of patients there is cutaneous anergy to *Candida* antigen, in 80 per cent there is diminished synthesis of lymphocyte MIF (in vitro) after stimulation with *Candida* antigen, and in approximately one-third of patients lymphocyte transformation by *Candida* antigen is depressed. Various combinations of these T-cell abnormalities exist. Some patients, whose lymphocytes undergo transformation, do not synthesize MIF, but virtually all patients with negative transformation lack MIF production. Diminished MIF production is closely correlated with cutaneous anergy. However, the number of T cells, the lymphocyte proliferative responses to phytohemagglutinins, and the allogenic cells are usually normal. The quantity of B lymphocytes and serum immunoglobulins is also normal.

Certain patients with chronic mucocutaneous candidiasis have had additional immunologic abnormalities, such as cutaneous anergy to other delayed hypersensitivity skin-test antigens (e.g., streptokinase-streptodornase, tetanus toxoid, and mumps). Their lymphocyte transformation to PHA and other mitogens and their monocyte chemotaxis may be defective. In addition, anti-*Candida* antibody may be absent from salivary IgA immunoglobulins. Various degrees of thymic aplasia are also observed.

Generally, the earlier the onset of chronic mucocutaneous candidiasis, the more severe the immune abnormalities. Some patients with early onset disease and severe immune abnormalities have had negative skin tests to all common antigens, including *Candida,* and cannot be sensitized to dinitrochlorobenzene. An additional group, with even more severe defects, has had evidence of thymus dysfunction as demonstrated by reduced numbers of circulating T cells and reduced proliferation responses to phytohemagglutinins.

In the resultant infection of the mucous membranes, skin, and nails, chronic inflammation with plasma cells and lymphocytes is associated with hyperkeratosis and parakeratosis in the epidermis. Deep involvement into the dermis is rare. Giant cells and fungi may be seen in the epidermis. Candidal granuloma, the most severe cutaneous form, is characterized by pronounced papillomatosis, hyperkeratosis, and dense infiltrate in the dermis of lymphoid cells, neutrophils, plasma cells, and multinucleated giant cells. The infiltrate may extend to the subcutis. Organisms have been found only in the stratum corneum.

### Clinical Manifestations

Most forms of chronic mucocutaneous candidiasis begin in infancy or within the first two decades. Rarely, the onset may be after age 30. The more severe immunologic abnormalities are usually present in infections of early onset. Thrush is usually the first sign of the disease, followed by nail infection and then by cutaneous moniliasis.

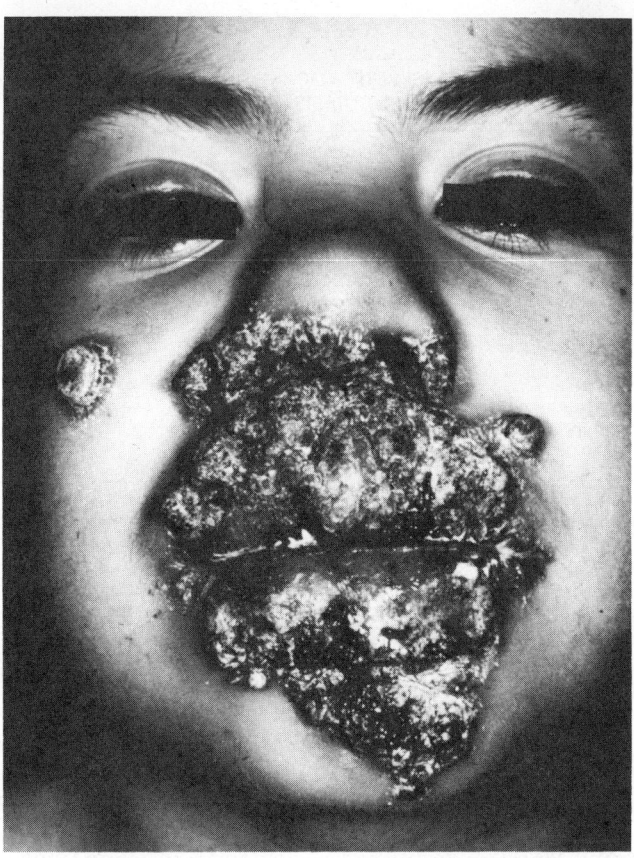

**FIGURE 1.**　*Severe disfiguration from Candida granuloma involving the perioral area. (Courtesy of Dr. Victor New-comer.)*

The spectrum of severity ranges from chronic involvement of a single nail to disfigurement by the worst form of infection, candidal granuloma (Fig. 1).

Endocrine disorders are associated with chronic mucocutaneous candidiasis in half the patients. These are hypoparathyroidism, Addison's disease, hypothyroidism, and diabetes. Pernicious anemia, ovarian insufficiency, chronic active hepatitis, hepatic cirrhosis, alopecia, depigmentation, cheilosis, blepharitis, keratoconjunctivitis, corneal ulcers, iron deficiency anemia, chronic pulmonary disease, malabsorption, hemolytic anemia, and thymoma have also accompanied this disease.

Stiehm has proposed the working classification of these disorders outlined in Table 1. In addition, this form of candidiasis has been described in patients with thymic dysplasia and agammaglobulinemia (Swiss type agammaglobulinemia), and thymic dysplasia without agammaglobulinemia (Nezelof-Allibone syndrome).

### Complications and Sequelae

If cutaneous involvement and the immunodeficiencies are severe enough, the condition may

be fatal, usually as a result of disseminated bacterial infection. Surprisingly, disseminated candidiasis has been a rare complication of chronic mucocutaneous candidiasis. Squamous carcinoma of the mouth and esophageal carcinoma may develop at the site of chronic candidal inflammation. Inflammation may cause loss of hair and nail, and scarring. In addition to direct complications of candidal infection, these patients may develop thymomas and sequelae related to their endocrine disorders.

### Geographical Variations

There are no known geographical variations.

### Diagnosis

Diagnosis of chronic mucocutaneous candidiasis is based on finding refractory candidal infections and the characteristic immunologic abnormalities, genetic background, and endocrinopathies. Proof of chronic candidiasis is established by biopsy and by demonstration of the typical histopathologic signs. Classification of the disease type requires skin testing with the appropriate antigens, evaluation of in vitro lymphocyte

TABLE 1.

| | SEVERITY OF CANDIDIASIS | ENDOCRINOPATHY | INHERI-TANCE |
|---|---|---|---|
| I. Early onset chronic mucocutaneous candidiasis | Moderate to severe | Common | Sporadic |
| Subtype candidal granuloma | Severe | Common | Sporadic |
| II. Late onset CMC | Mild | Rare | Sporadic |
| III. Familial CMC | Mild to moderate | Rare | Autosomal recessive |
| IV. Juvenile familial polyendocrinopathy with candidiasis (candida-endocrinopathy syndrome) | Mild to moderate | Always | Autosomal recessive |

From Stiehm, E. R.: Chronic mucocutaneous candidiasis. Clinical perspectives, pp. 96–99. In Edwards, J. E., Jr. (moderator): Severe candida infections. Clinical perspective, immune defense mechanisms, and current concepts of therapy. Ann Intern Med 89:91–106, 1978.

function, and assessment of immunoglobulin status. The endocrinopathy must also be identified.

### Treatment and Prophylaxis

Efforts to correct immune deficiencies with transfer factor, levamisole (a synthetic anthelmintic agent capable of T-cell activation), and thymus extracts (thymosin fraction 5 or fetal thymus) are still experimental and their effects are doubtful. Amphotericin B has been the mainstay of treatment. It is given in a dose of 0.5 mg/kg intravenously every other day for two to four weeks, depending on the clinical response. 5–Fluorocytosine (5–FC) in a dose of 100 mg/kg can be given alone or in conjunction with amphotericin B. 5–FC is taken in divided doses every six hours orally and should be continued as long as clinical improvement occurs. Both drugs are repeated as tolerated for relapses. Topical preparations of these and other antifungal drugs may also be of value. Amphotericin B is applied in 2 per cent concentration as a lotion and 5–FC as a 1 per cent solution. Miconazole nitrate ointment (2 per cent) or Mycostatin ointment can be applied twice daily to the skin lesions in place of amphotericin B or 5–FC.

## OTHER CUTANEOUS CANDIDAL INFECTIONS

### Candida Intertrigo

This common disease affects any skin surfaces that are close enough to provide a warm moist environment. The crural folds, interdigital areas of hands and feet, submammary area, submaxil-lary area, gluteal folds, and ear folds are examples. The first lesions are vesicopustules that enlarge, rupture, macerate the skin, and produce fissures. The lesions have a scalloped border rimmed by a white necrotic epidermis with the appearance of overhanging scales. The base of the lesion is erythematous, and satellite flaccid vesicopustules or white colloid macules often appear on adjacent skin. These may coalesce and extend the area of involvement. Although *Candida* may be cultured from an intertriginous area of inflammation, one should not conclude that *Candida* is the cause without proof by biopsy of cutaneous invasion by *Candida* organisms. Even without biopsy, however, a presumptive diagnosis is enough to undertake a therapeutic trial.

In addition to intertrigo, candidiasis of the skin may take on a miliary appearance from the erythematous macules or vesicopustules resembling miliaria rubra or a drug eruption.

### Candidal Paronychia

This is an inflammatory reaction around the nail attributed to candidal infection. The exact role *Candida* play in this reaction is not clear, however, since many skin bacteria, in addition to *Candida*, are usually cultured from the infected area. The importance of *Candida* as the primary pathogen has been challenged.

Because frequent immersion of the hands in water is highly correlated with this condition, there is a high incidence of it in dishwashers and laundry workers. Young children may develop a candidal paronychia as a complication of thumb-sucking. Diabetics have a higher incidence of paronychia than do those who are not diabetics.

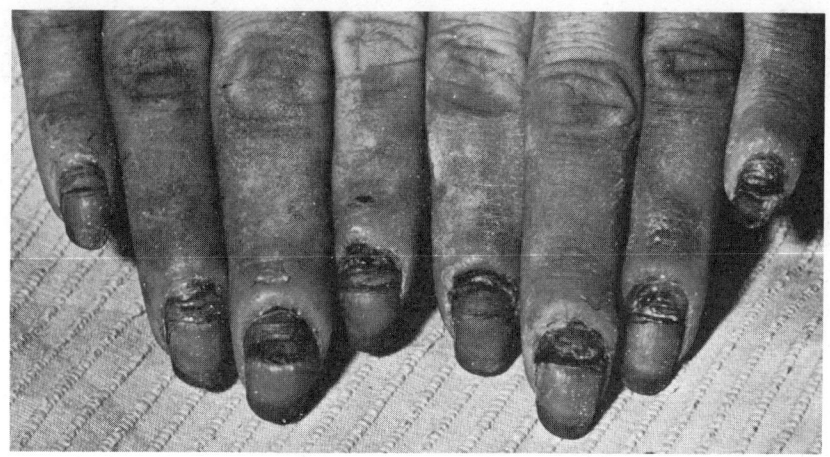

**FIGURE 2.**  Candida *paronychia. (Courtesy of Dr. Victor Newcomer.)*

The clinical appearance of a paronychia is that of a relatively well localized periungual inflammation that becomes warm, glistening, and tense. It may extend under the nail and gradually destroy the nail plate so that the nail develops secondary thickening, ridging, and discoloration (Fig. 2). Pain varies from severe to mild or may even be absent. The histologic changes include acanthosis and parakeratosis in the presence of chronic inflammatory infiltration. Candidal hyphae are seen penetrating the stratum corneum. The specific diagnosis is made by Gram stain, potassium hydroxide preparation, or culture showing predominantly *Candida* organisms. Major complications are loss of the nail and/or cellulitis of the finger.

### Cutaneous Genital Candidiasis

This condition is a direct extension of candidal vaginitis. In addition to the vulvar skin, the urethral orifice and urethral mucosa may be involved. As the infection progresses, the vulva becomes very red and the skin erodes. The process may spread onto the perineum and contiguous areas (Fig. 3).

Genital candidiasis in men is thought to be a venereal infection acquired from the infected vagina. The process begins on the penis as vesicles that evolve into painful, itchy, burning patches resembling thrush. It can spread to the thighs, gluteal folds, buttocks, and scrotum.

### Perianal Candidiasis

*Candida* may be one of the numerous microorganisms associated with pruritus ani, either alone or in combination. *Candida* has been implicated as the predominant cause in some cases, resulting in erythema that progresses to maceration and generally intense pruritus, especially at night (Fig. 4). It can spread to the anal canal and cause frank proctitis.

### Generalized Cutaneous Candidiasis

This is an unusual form of cutaneous candidiasis seen primarily in infants. It causes a widespread eruption that is particularly severe in the genitocrural folds, anal region, axillae, hands,

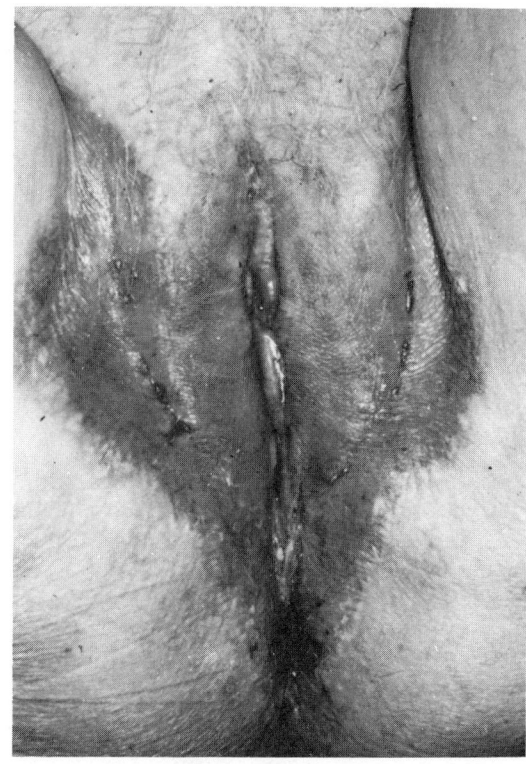

**FIGURE 3.**  *Severe vulvar and intercrural Candida intertrigo. (Courtesy of Dr. Victor Newcomer.)*

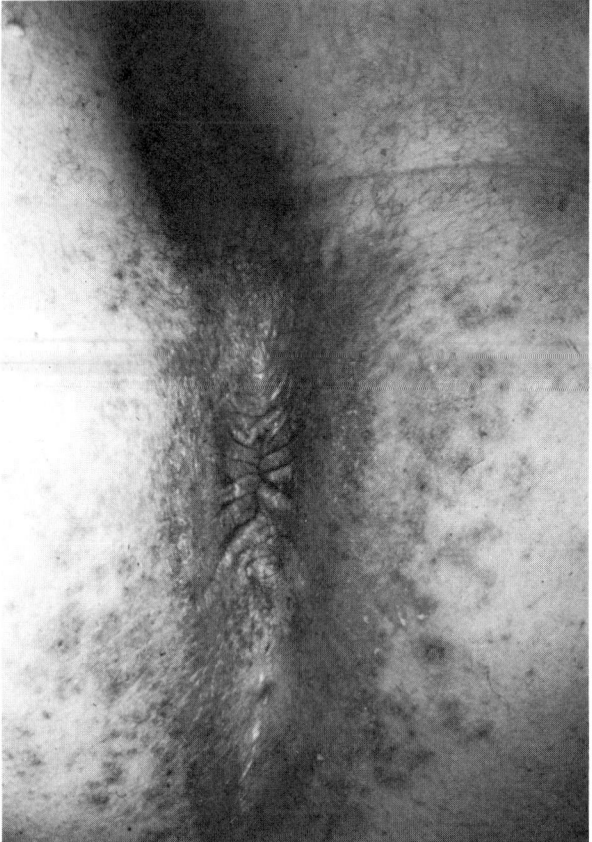

**FIGURE 4.** *Perianal candidiasis. (Courtesy of Dr. Victor Newcomer.)*

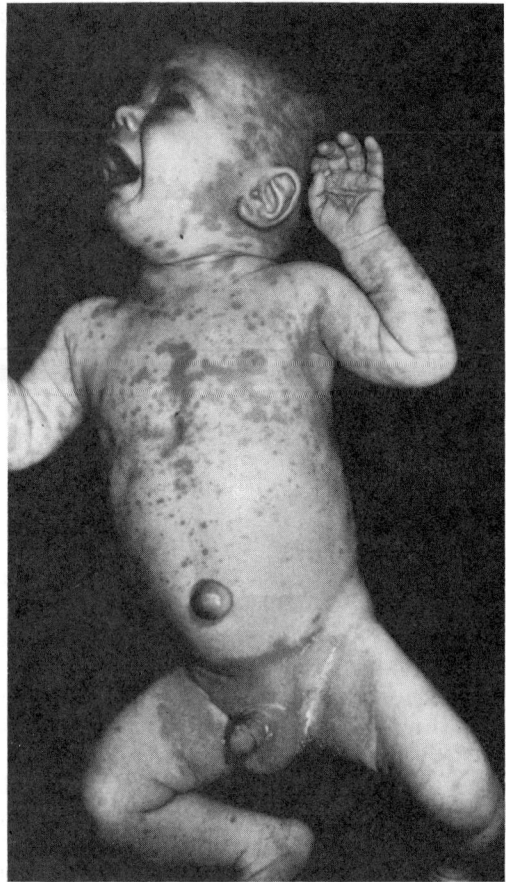

**FIGURE 5.** *Generalized cutaneous candidiasis that began in the diaper distribution in this patient. (Courtesy of Dr. Victor Newcomer.)*

and feet. The process begins as vesicles or vesicopustules that rupture and leave a denuded surface. Eventually it spreads peripherally, and large confluent areas develop (Fig. 5). Paronychia occurs and the mucocutaneous area may be involved. This condition may simulate acrodermatitis enteropathica, seborrheic dermatitis, psoriasis, contact dermatitis, and pityriasis rubra pilaris.

### Macronodular Cutaneous Lesions of Disseminated Candidiasis

These are lesions of disseminated candidiasis in which multiple blood cultures are positive (Bodey and Luna, 1974). They are pink to red lesions 0.5 to 1.0 cm in diameter and occur either as single lesions or scattered over the entire body (Fig. 6). Occasionally, they have a hemorrhagic base. Organisms have been demonstrated most frequently on histologic sections of punch biopsy.

### Candidal Diaper Rash

*Candida* is a very common cause of diaper rash in infants. The initial perianal localization sug-

gests that the gastrointestinal tract is the site of origin. Spread to the diaper area occurs rapidly and is facilitated by cutaneous maceration from wet diapers. Scaly macules and vesicles characterize the rash, which is very uncomfortable because of itching and burning (Fig. 7). Diagnosis is made by scraping the involved area (simple swabbing is inadequate) and demonstrating the organisms on potassium hydroxide preparation or culture.

### Additional Forms of Cutaneous Candidiasis

Candida may cause onychomycosis with extensive nail plate involvement, but this is usually associated with paronychia. Erosia interdigitalis blastomycetica is a term applied to a form of candidal infection that occurs between the fingers (Fig. 8) or between the toes and extends onto the sides of the digits. It causes a red base, maceration, and pain. Candidal folliculitis may also occur (Fig. 9).

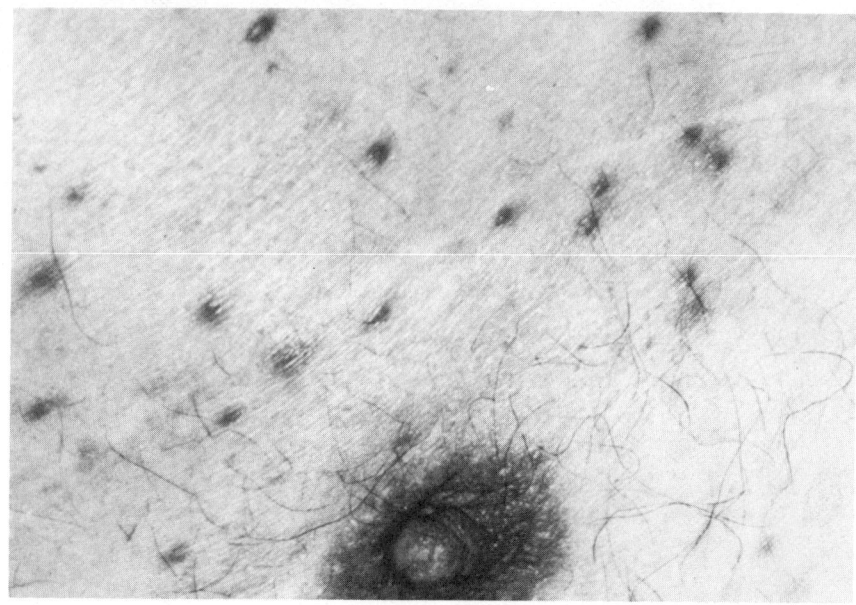

**FIGURE 6.** *Typical macronodular lesions of disseminated candidiasis. (Courtesy of Dr. Gerald P. Bodey.)*

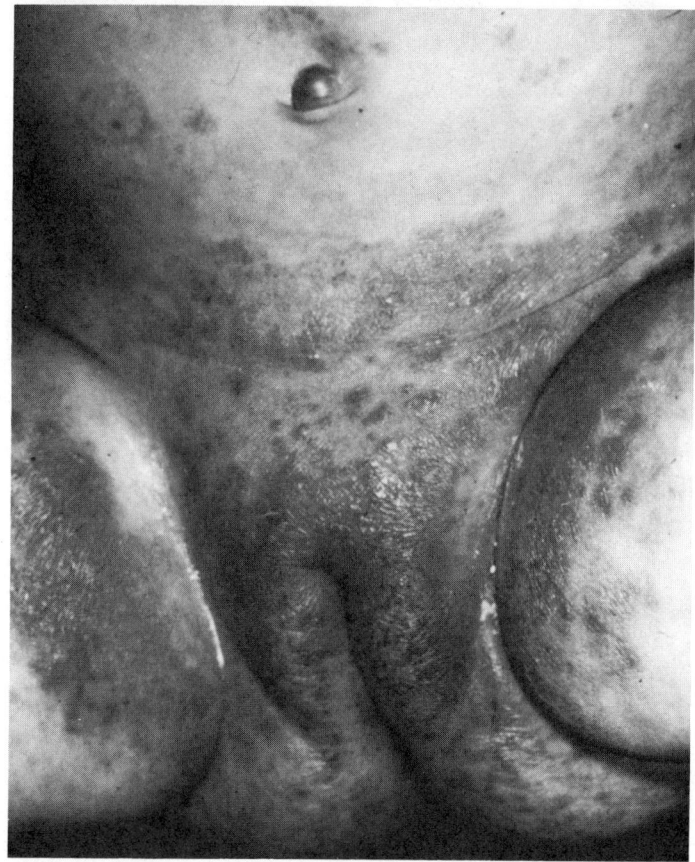

**FIGURE 7.** *Typical* Candida *diaper rash. (Course of Dr. Victor Newcomer.)*

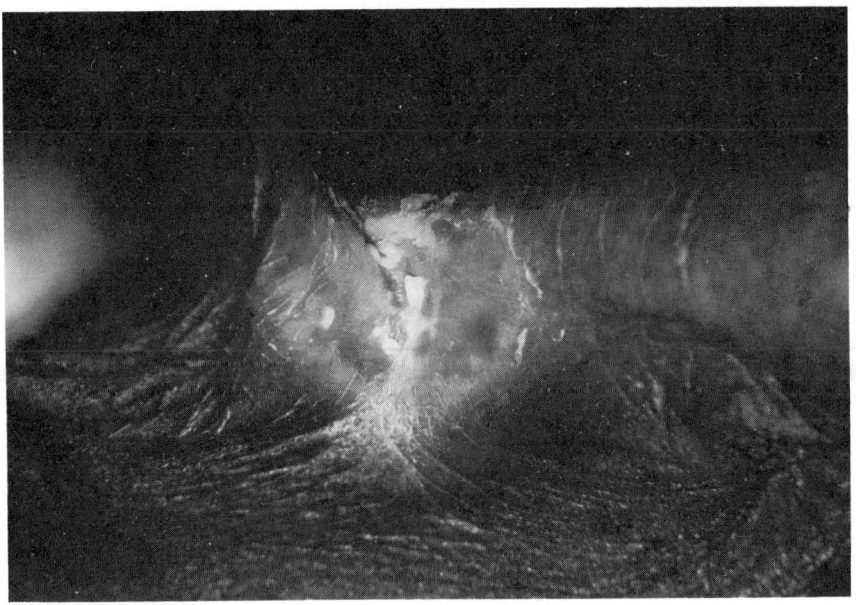

**FIGURE 8.** *Erosio interdigitalis blastomycetica. (Courtesy of Dr. Arnold Gurevitch.)*

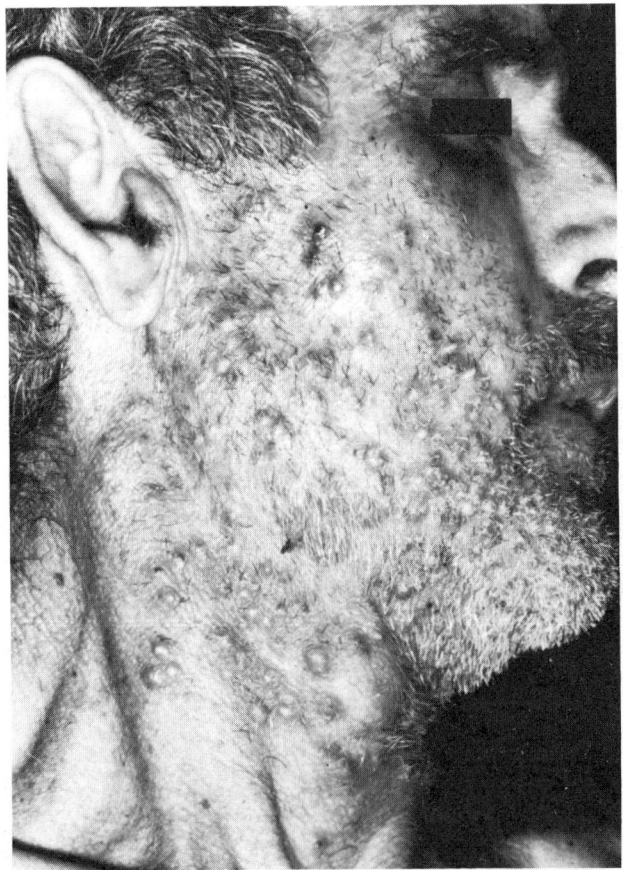

**FIGURE 9.** *Severe* Candida *folliculitis. (Courtesy of Dr. Victor Newcomer.)*

## TREATMENT AND PROPHYLAXIS

Successful treatment of all forms of mucocutaneous candidiasis requires the elimination of local irritation and moisture. The hands must be spared excessive immersion in dish water, thumb-sucking must stop, moist skin should be dried, and diapers should be changed more frequently. Powders or creams can reduce skin moisture, especially in intertriginous areas. Vaginal, oral, or gastrointestinal candidiasis must be treated if it is the source of cutaneous disease (such as vulvar disease).

Chronic mucocutaneous candidiasis and cutaneous candidiasis not associated with T-cell defects are usually treated with either nystatin or amphotericin B topical preparations. Amphotericin B 3 per cent in vanishing cream base or 100,000 units of nystatin in the same base can be used with equal efficacy. On the other hand, calamine lotion is relatively ineffective by comparison (Stritzler, 1966). For candidal paronychia, either the 3 per cent amphotericin B or resorcin (3 per cent in 70 per cent isopropyl alcohol) lotions can be followed by application of a cream containing 3 per cent iodochlorhydroxyquin. Candidal diaper rash has been treated successfully with nystatin powder or cream in combination with a corticosteroid such as Mycolog cream (Squibb). Other successful compounds include amphotericin cream or lotion, Castellani paint, 1 per cent gentian violet applied once daily, or chlordantoin lotion (Sporostecin [Ortho]). The agents used for diaper rash are generally successful for pruritus ani as well.

Two newer antifungal agents—miconazole and clotrimazole—are currently undergoing trial for their efficacy in controlling mucocutaneous candidiasis (Cullen, 1977; Keczkes et al., 1975). Initial studies with both compounds are encouraging; however, further evaluation of their advantages over existing agents is necessary.

Finally, correction of iron deficiency has been associated with rapid improvement of clinical manifestations in some patients with chronic mucocutaneous candidiasis. It has been postulated that iron deficiency contributes to an immune deficiency against *Candida* (Higgs and Wells, 1972).

### References

Bodey, G. P., and Luna, M:.: Skin lesions associated with disseminated candidiasis. JAMA 229:1466, 1974.

Cullen, S. I.: Cutaneous candidiasis: Treatment with miconazole nitrate. Cutis 19:126, 1977.

Higgs, J. M., and Wells, R. S.: Mucocutaneous candidiasis. Br J Dermatol 86, Supplement 8:88, 1972.

Keczkes, K., Leighton, I., and Good, C. S.: Topical treatment of dermatophytoses and candidoses. Practitioner 214:412, 1975.

Kozinn, P. J., and Taschdgian, C. L.: Candidiasis (unit 17–18). In Dennis, D. J., Dobson, R. L., and McGuire, J. (eds): Clinical Dermatology. Hagerstown, Harper and Row, 1977.

Stiehm, E. R.: Chronic mucocutaneous candidiasis. Clinical aspects, pp. 96–99. In Edwards, J. E., Jr. (moderator): Severe candida infections: Clinical perspectives, immune defense mechanisms, and current concepts in therapy. Ann Intern Med 89:91–106, 1978.

Stritzler, C.: Cutaneous candidiasis treated with topical amphotericin B. Arch Dermatol 93:101, 1966.

# *LOBOMYCOSIS* **212**

### José Lisbôa Miranda, M.D.

Lobomycosis (keloidal blastomycosis, Jorge Lôbo's disease, Lobo's mycosis) is an autonomous, chronic fungus infection that produces lesions only in the skin. Its etiologic agent has probably not yet been cultured. The disease has been found in humans living in the torrid zone of the Americas and in dolphins from the waters of the Florida and Surinam coasts.

The epidemiology and pathogenesis of the disease are still unclear, since it is difficult to reproduce experimentally in animals. Immunologic studies have been inconclusive, and there is no effective treatment for this infection. Diagnosis can be easily made because its clinical and histopathologic features are characteristic and the parasites are very abundant in the lesion.

## DEFINITION

Lobomycosis is a chronic skin infection characterized chiefly by slow-growing, keloid-like tumors caused by a fungus that abounds in the tissues as round, thick-walled cells and excites a massive proliferation of histiocytes and giant cells in the dermis.

## ETIOLOGY

The causative agent of lobomycosis has not yet been cultured, and whatever fungi that have been isolated and reported should be considered as contaminants. Several names were proposed for the fungus, but it is best to call it *Loboa loboi*. Using this name discourages the use of names based on cultures of contaminants. Also, with our present knowledge there is no reason for classifying the fungus in the genus *Paracoccidioides*.

## HISTORY

The disease was first described in a preliminary report in 1930 by Jorge Lobo, who published further studies of the case in 1931 and 1933. The patient had keloidal skin lesions without any lymphatic or visceral involvement. Lobo gave an accurate account of the main histopathologic features of the disease and of the morphology of the parasite as seen in tissues. He could not reproduce the infection in guinea pigs, rats, or Rhesus monkeys but claimed to have obtained cultures of the fungus on Sabouraud's glucose agar. Intradermal and complement fixation tests for *Paracoccidioides brasiliensis* were negative in his patient, and he concluded from all those findings that he had found a new clinical form of blastomycosis caused by a new fungus species.

The cultures first obtained by Lobo were probably contaminants, since a fungus like the one originally described has never again been isolated from other patients with the disease. Furthermore, the original strain appears to have been lost and a colony of *P. brasiliensis* mislabeled with its name (Carneiro, 1952; Da Fonseca Filho, 1955).

## EPIDEMIOLOGY

Lobomycosis has a limited geographic distribution. All human cases of the disease have lived in tropical forest areas of South and Central America, chiefly the Amazon basin. Most patients have been reported from Brazil, but the infection has been found also in French Guiana, Surinam, Venezuela, Colombia, Panama, and Costa Rica.

The disease is not as rare as first thought, and increasing numbers of reports have appeared during the last 15 years. There are published references to 101 patients (Miranda, 1972), but many other cases are unreported and it is now considered a relatively frequent fungus infection in Amazon State (Brazil).

This mycosis does not appear to have a racial preference. The majority of the cases reported were in mulattos because they predominate in the area where the disease occurs. However, it has been found also in Brazilian Indians (Baruzzi et al., 1967), in 13 Negroes from Surinam (Wiersema and Niemel, 1965), and in a white Portuguese male living in Amazon State, Brazil (Lacaz et al., 1955).

Most patients are adult males who have worked on rubber plantations or in other agricultural occupations. The infection has been found in females very rarely.

It is difficult to determine the age at the time of acquisition of the disease because most patients seek medical care many years, even decades, after the first lesions are apparent. The age at diagnosis varies between 20 and 83 years old.

The lesions are found commonly on exposed skin, particularly ear lobes and legs (Fig. 1*A, B, E*). Many patients state that the lesions appeared at sites of previous injuries, including snake and insect bites. There are no data suggesting that this mycosis is contagious from person to person.

Natural infection of animals was not known until recently. A first reported case of lobomycosis in a bottle-nosed dolphin *(Tursiops truncatus)* on the west coast of Florida in 1971 (Migaki et al., 1971) was followed by findings in another infected dolphin *(Sotalia guianensis)* in the estuary of the Surinam river (De Vries and Laarman, 1973), in one on the east coast of Florida, and still another captured in the Gulf of Mexico (Caldwell et al., 1975).

The ecology of the parasite is unknown. The fact that the fungus cannot be grown from tissue obtained from humans or naturally infected dolphins and that most attempts to reproduce the disease experimentally in animals have not been successful suggest the existence of an obligatory natural host of the parasite. However, there is no proof to substantiate this theory.

## CLINICAL MANIFESTATIONS

Lobomycosis is a chronic disease of the skin without systemic involvement. Cases are known in which the infection has persisted for several decades without impairment of the general health of the patient.

The characteristic feature of the lesion is a very slow-growing keloid-like tumor surrounded by apparently normal skin (Fig. 1*C*). In addition to this typical clinical aspect, one can sometimes see papules, verrucoid, nodular lesions, or infiltrated plaques.

The isolated keloid-like lesion is freely movable and usually has a smooth, shiny surface with telangiectases. Old lesions may become scaly or verrucous and occasionally ulcerate or become pedunculated. Large lobulated tumors may be produced by confluence of several growing nodules (Fig. 1*E*). The lesions may remain confined to one area, growing in diameter or showing new nodules in the surrounding skin, or they may be scattered to several different regions of the body.

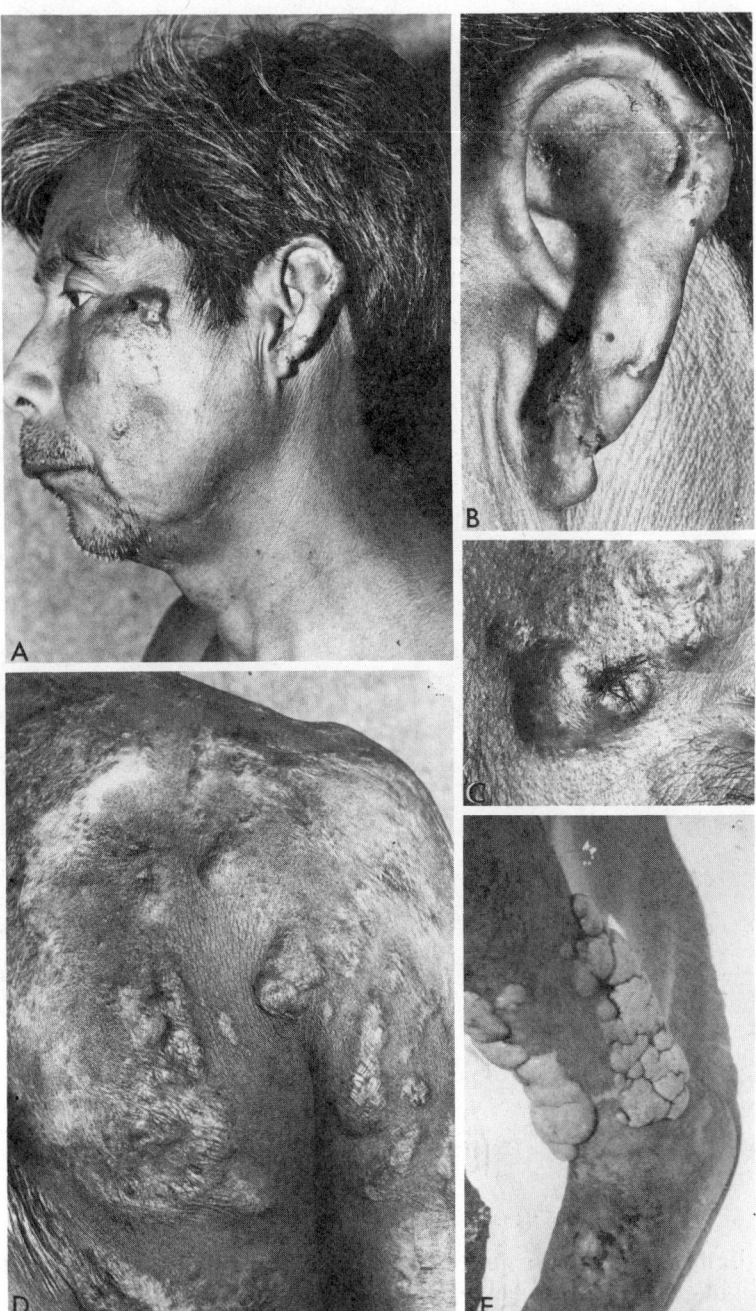

**FIGURE 1.** *Lobomycosis. A, Cutaneous lesions on zygomatic area and ear. B, Close-up of the ear showing nodular lesions on helix and ear lobe. Note traumatic erosion on ear lobe. C, Close-up of zygomatic arch showing keloid-like lesions surrounded by apparently normal skin. The stitches were done to repair the biopsy area. D, Keloid-like tumors, infiltrated plaques, hypertrophic scarring and wrinkled atrophic skin are shown in a Brazilian Indian. E, Lobulated tumors resulting from confluence of growing nodules.*

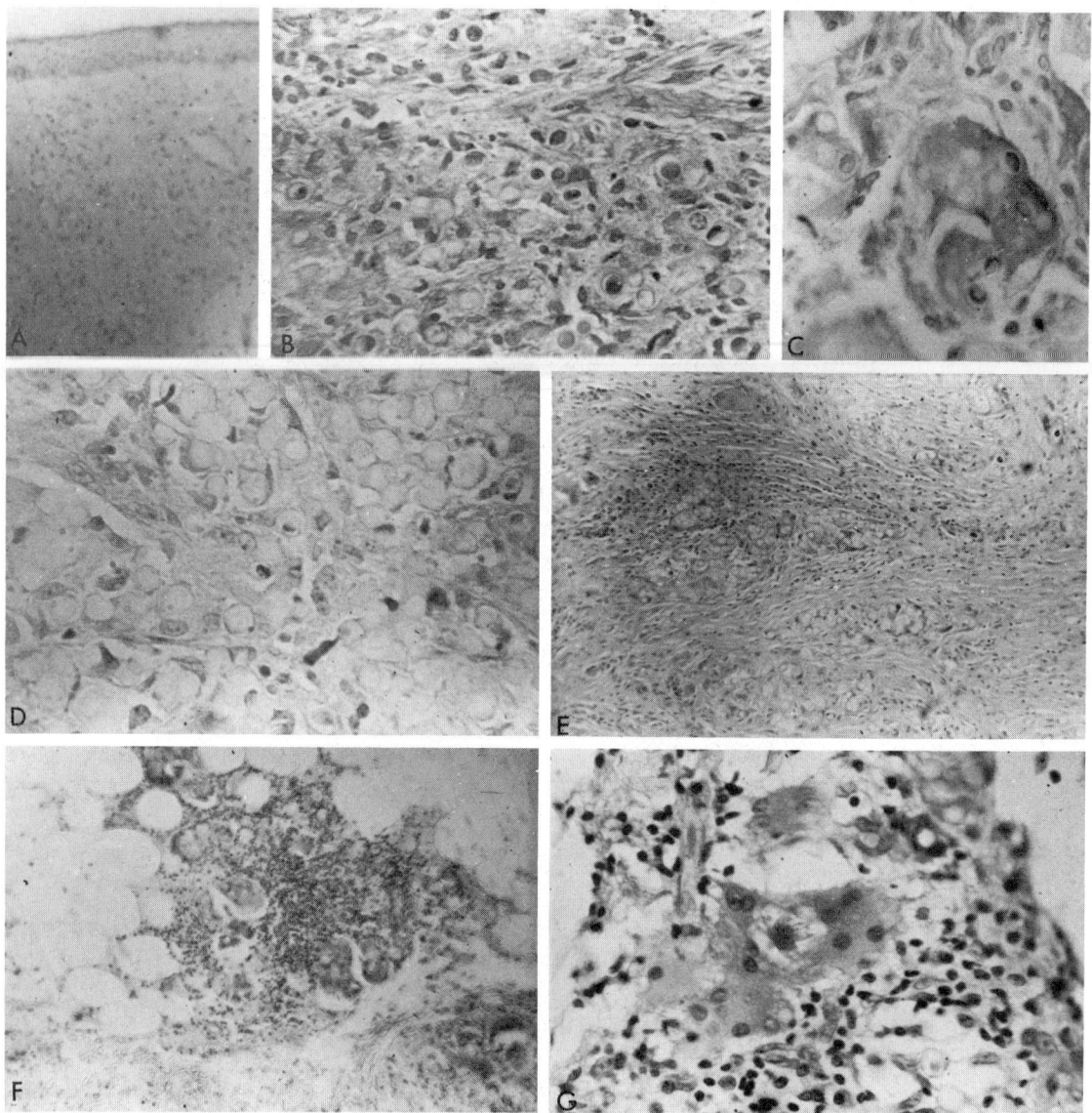

**FIGURE 2.** *Lobomycosis. A, Stretched epidermis with disappearance of rete pegs. Subpapillary dermis with narrow band of normal connective tissue (H & E, × 120). B, Proliferation of histiocytes and numerous parasites (PAS, × 480). C, Giant cells filled with parasites (PAS, × 480). D, Abundant fungi seen as empty cells, giving a sieve-like appearance (H & E, × 480). E, Collagen fibers dividing the lesion into lobules (H & E, × 120). F, Lesion penetrating the hypodermis. Fat cells are seen (PAS, × 120). G, Asteroid body in a giant cell (PAS, × 480).*

Symptoms are negligible, and only a few patients complain of slight pruritus. As a rule regional lymph nodes are not involved, but occasionally they become enlarged.

A somewhat different clinical appearance is seen in infected Brazilian Indians (Fig. 1D). They present, besides the characteristic keloid-like tumors, papules and infiltrated plaques like those seen in tuberculoid leprosy. In its classic form the lesions of lobomycosis have no tendency to heal spontaneously, but in the Brazilian Indians one can see hypertrophic scarring and wrinkled atrophic skin following a natural involution of the nodules.

## PATHOLOGY AND PATHOGENESIS

The histopathologic picture is characteristic and diagnostic. The lesions are located in the dermis, but the epidermis shows some changes.

The epidermis frequently is atrophic and may be stretched, with disappearance of the rete pegs

(Fig. 2A) owing to pressure from the diffuse dermal lesion. When ulceration occurs, the borders show acanthosis or pseudoepitheliomatous hyperplasia. In old scaly lesions there is hyperkeratosis and focal parakeratosis.

The whole dermis is obliterated by a massive infiltrate consisting mainly of histiocytes and giant cells (Fig. 2B, C). The parasites abound in the affected area, and because many organisms seem to be empty cells, the skin sections have a sieve-like appearance (Fig. 2D). A narrow band of normal connective tissue is frequently present in the subpapillary dermis (Fig. 2A), but sometimes the lesions reach the epidermis and even destroy its basal layer. In the same way, the dermal infiltrate may occasionally extend downward into the upper hypodermis (Fig. 2F). Giant cells are more numerous in the center of the lesions, while at the borders the histiocytes predominate in such a way as to give an appearance of cultured cells (Fialho, 1938). The histiocytes are large with foamy cytoplasm and eccentric nuclei. The giant cells vary in size and disposition of nuclei and contain many parasites (Fig. 2C) and sometimes asteroid bodies (Fig. 2G). Small foci of lymphocytes and plasma cells may be found at the periphery of the histiocytic proliferation. Collagen fibers are seen dividing the entire lesion into lobules. In old lesions there is an increase of these collagen fibers (Fig. 2E). There is no necrosis in the affected tissues.

A striking feature in the tissue sections of lobomycosis is the great abundance of parasites (Fig. 3A). They are seen in long chains (Fig. 3A), in rosettes (Fig. 3D), or isolated (Fig. 3A). The author (Miranda, 1972a) found the maximum diameter to be $15.2\mu$, the minimum $6.0\mu$, and the average $9.6\mu$. Organisms of apparently small diameter may be only segments of cells (Wiersema and Niemel, 1965). The relative uniformity in size of the yeasts distinguishes them from the yeast cells of *P. brasiliensis.* Many of the organisms appear as empty cells; some are deformed; some have a homogeneous cytoplasmic mass that may be shrunk at the center of the cell, while in others the cytoplasm is seen as irregular masses or dust-like material. The wall of the fungus is $1\mu$ in thickness, and the parasite has no capsule. Both wall and cytoplasm are PAS-positive. In PAS- or silver-stained specimens some cells show the walls with radiating spines (Figs. 3H and 4B). Scanning electron microscopy (Abreu and Miranda, 1972; Miranda, 1972b) seems to corroborate the impression that the radiations are part of the parasite's wall and not a host-tissue reaction. Those observations revealed a thick three-layer wall whose outermost layer was made of irregular overlapping scales (Fig. 4C, D).

The fungus apparently reproduces by single, double, and rarely by three or more gemmations (Fig. 3C). Cryptosporulation with numerous small buds around the mother cell, such as that observed in *P. brasiliensis,* is not seen in lobomycosis. Buds have a tendency to remain permanently attached to the cell from which they originate, which explains the long chains of parasites. Because the parasites may have multiple buddings, those chains sometimes are branched (Fig. 3B). It is estimated that 90 per cent of the organisms found in the lesions are strung together (Wiersema and Niemel, 1965). The walls of the parasites continue from one cell to another as short, narrow, bridge-like structures. This connection may be severed by pressure and a bud scar shows at the site of the fracture (Fig. 3G).

Following the several stages of budding, the yeast-like cell first appears pear-shaped (Fig. 3E), then exhibits a finger-like projection with a nodular end (Fig. 3F) that widens to a knob-like aspect (Fig. 3E), finally growing up to form a new cell. At the beginning, the cytoplasm of both cells is continuous (Fig. 4A), but later communication is interrupted.

The pathogenesis of lobomycosis is still unclear. The infection probably follows direct implantation of the fungus into the skin. This is in accordance with the belief of many patients that the first lesions appeared at the site of a previous injury. It also explains why most sufferers show the disease on exposed skin areas. The occurrence of lesions at scattered regions of the body might suggest hematogenous spread of the organism, but autoinoculation is more likely to be the cause. This latter possibility would also explain the appearance of new satellite nodules around the original one.

Some authors (Leite, 1954; Teixeira, 1962; Wiersema and Niemel, 1965) have tried to reconstruct the pathogenesis of the infection from the pathologic findings. They postulate that the large size of the parasites, their rigid wall, and their disposition to chains of cells do not permit hematogenous or lymphatic dissemination. The proliferating histiocytes and giant cells of the host and the causative agent of the disease do not seem to harm each other. There is no sign in the lesions of digested parasites or tissue necrosis. The fungi are apparently not killed.

Most attempts to infect animals by inoculation of material from humans have failed. The few successful attempts did not clarify our understanding of the disease. Material from dolphins' lesions has not been infectious for laboratory animals. A few successful experimental infections were obtained with difficulty using hamsters (Guimarães, 1964; Sampaio and Dias, 1970; Wiersema and Niemel, 1965), rats (Azulay et al., 1970), and tortoises (Sampaio et al., 1971).

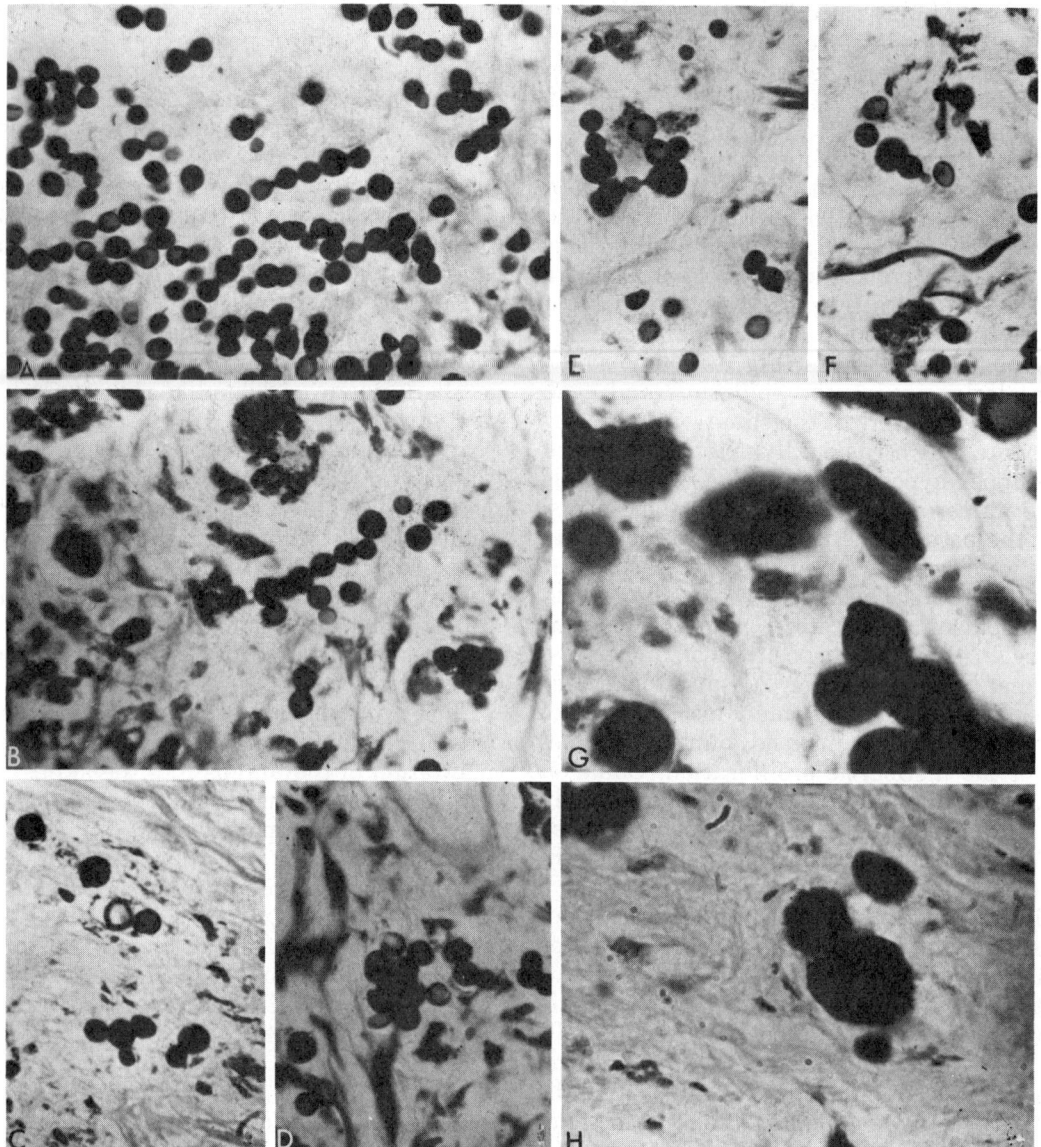

**FIGURE 3.** *Lobomycosis. A, Abundance of parasites with little variation in size. Fungi are isolated or arranged in chains. Narrow tubes connect the cells (methenamine silver, × 480). B, Branched chain of parasites (methenamine silver, × 480). C, Cell showing three buds (Grocott, × 480). D, Fungi arranged in rosette (methenamine silver, × 480). E, First stage of budding: pear-shaped cell at lower right quadrant. At center is a further stage of reproduction: the knob-like aspect of the bud (methenamine silver, × 480). F, Early stage of budding: finger-like projection with nodular ending (methenamine silver, × 480). G, Bud scar where connecting tube was severed (methenamine silver, × 1200). H, Parasite's wall with radiating spines (Grocott, × 1200).*

## DIAGNOSIS

Clinical diagnosis is based on the finding of slow-growing nodules resembling keloids on agricultural workers who live or have lived in the torrid zone of the Americas. Brazilian Indians with the disease present with infiltrated plaques, hypertrophic scars, and atrophic wrinkled lesions, as well as the typical keloids. True keloids, leprosy, and xanthomatoses should be considered in the differential diagnosis. Old verrucous lobomycosis lesions may resemble chromomycosis, tuberculosis verrucosa cutis, or chronic pyogenic infection.

The diagnosis is confirmed by direct histopathologic examination. For the direct examination, the material obtained through scarification of a lesion or from a biopsied nodule is digested in 10 per cent potassium hydroxide. The parasites appear as numerous yeast-like cells with thick re-

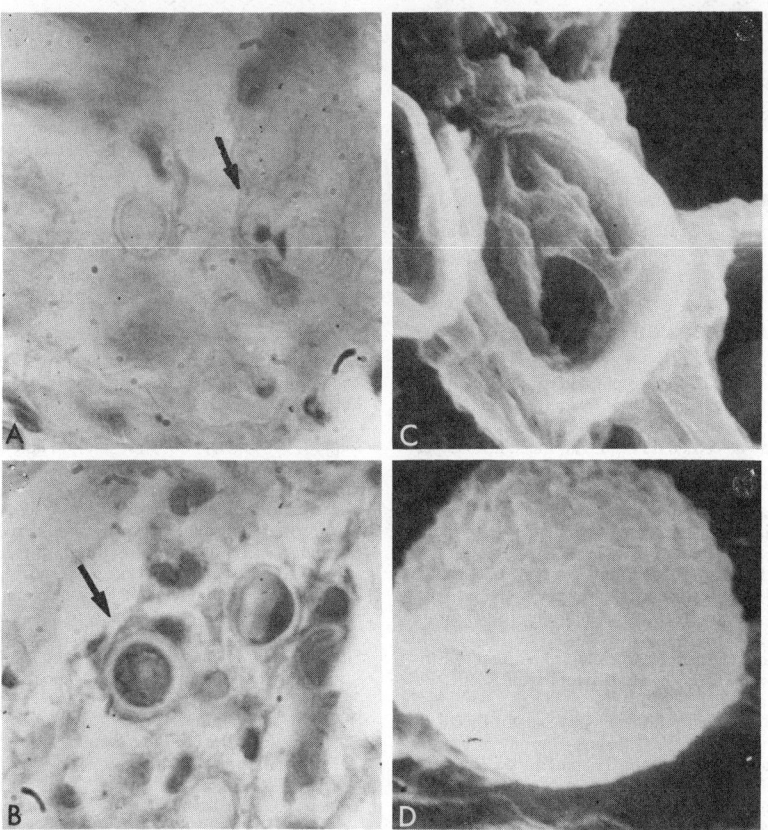

**FIGURE 4.** *Lobomycosis. A, The arrow points to budding cell showing continuity of its cytoplasm with that of the mother cell (PAS, × 1200). B, Fungus wall with radiating spines (PAS, × 1200). C, Thick three-layered wall of the parasite (scanning electron microscopy, × 5000). D, Parasite's wall with irregular overlapping scales (scanning electron microscopy, × 5000).*

fractile walls. Often they are arranged in chains, but isolated cells are also frequently seen. Most organisms show single or double budding, rarely three or more gemmulations. Each cell is attached to the next by a short and narrow tubular structure. The fungi have little variation in size, averaging 9 to 10μ in diameter. The histopathologic picture is typical, showing a dense dermal infiltrate with intense proliferation of histiocytes, the presence of giant cells, and a great abundance of parasites. The fungus does not have cryptosporulation (numerous small buds) like *P. brasiliensis,* their buds are not connected to the mother cell by a broad base as in *Blastomyces dermatitidis,* and the organism does not show a capsule like *Cryptococcus neoformans.* Transmission electron microscopy demonstrates the parasite to be multinucleated (Furtado et al., 1967).

The fungus cannot be cultivated in vitro. Serology and skin tests do not contribute to the diagnosis of the disease. Complement fixation test with the polysaccharide antigen of *P. brasiliensis* and paracoccidioidin skin test are negative or weakly positive (Lacaz et al., 1955; Fonseca and Lacaz, 1971). Immunofluorescence studies (Silva et al., 1968) showed that *Loboa loboi* is more closely related antigenically to some strains of *P. brasiliensis* than to others. It also has antigens in common with the yeast forms of *Histoplasma capsulatum, B. dermatitidis, Candida albicans,* and the mycelial form of *Coccidioides immitis.* However, labeled serum globulins from three patients with lobomycosis did not stain cells of *L. loboi* from tissues and yeast-like cells of *P. brasiliensis.*

## COMPLICATIONS, SEQUELAE, AND PROGNOSIS

The only frequent complications observed are traumatic ulceration and secondary bacterial infection of ulcerated lesions. Lesions may increase in size until they cover extensive areas and produce incapacitating deformities.

The prognosis is good as far as general health is concerned, but the lesions persist without self-healing.

## TREATMENT AND PROPHYLAXIS

There is no specific treatment for the disease. Wide surgical excision of the lesion is the only effective procedure, although recurrences are frequent.

No prophylaxis can be advised since the ecology of the fungus and the pathogenesis of infection are still unknown.

### References

Abreu, W. M., and Miranda, J. L.: Microscopia electrônica scanning: Agente da micose de Jorge Lobo. An Bras Dermat 47:115, 1972.

Azulay, R. D., Carneiro, J. A., and Andrade, L. C.: Blastomicose de Jorge Lôbo. Contribuiçao ao estudo da etiologia, inoculação experimental, immunologia e patologia da doença. An Bras Derm Sif 45:47, 1970.

Baruzzi, R. G., D'Andretta, C., Jr, Carvalhal, S., Ramos, O. L., and Pontes, P. L.: Ocorrência de blastomicose queloideana entre índios Caiabí. Rev Inst Med Trop S Paulo 9:135, 1967.

Caldwell, D. K., Caldwell, M. C., Woodard, J. C., Ajello, L., Kaplan, W., and McClure, H. M.: Lobomycosis as a disease of the Atlantic bottle-nosed dolphin (Tursiops truncatus Montagu, 1821). Am J Trop Med Hyg 24:105, 1975.

Carneiro, L. S.: Contribuiçao ao Estudo Microbiológico do Agente Etiológico da Doença de Jorge Lôbo. Thesis, University of Recife. Recife, Imprensa Industrial, 1952.

Da Fonseca Filho, O.: Deep skin and pulmonary mycosis in Brazil. In Sternberg, T. H., and Newcomer, V. D. (eds.): Therapy of Fungus Diseases. An International Symposium. Boston, Little Brown & Company, 1955, p. 56.

De Vries, G. A., and Laarman, J. J.: A case of Lobo's disease in the dolphin Sotalia guianensis. Aquatic Mammals 1:26, 1973.

Fialho, A.: Blastomicose do tipo 'Jorge Lôbo.' Hospital (Rio de J) 14:903, 1938.

Fonseca, O. J. M., and Lacaz, C. S.: Estudo das culturas isoladas de blastomicose queilodiforme (doença Jorge Lobo). Denominação ao seu agente etiológico. Rev Inst Med Trop S Paulo 13:225, 1971.

Furtado, J. S., Brito, T., and Freymuller, E.: Structure and reproduction of Paracoccidioides loboi. Mycologia 59:286, 1967.

Guimarães, F. N.: Inoculações em hamsters da blastomicose sulamericana (doençã de Lutz), da blastomicose queloidiforme (doença de Lôbo), e da blastomicose dos índios do Tapajós-Xingú. Hospital (Rio de J) 66:581, 1964.

Lacaz, C. S., Sterman, L., Monteiro, E. V. L., and Pinto, D. O.: Blastomicose queloideana. Comentários sobre novo caso. Rev Hosp Clín Fac Med S Paulo 10:254, 1955.

Leite, J. M.: Doença de Jorge Lôbo. (Contribuiçao ao seu Estudo Anátomo-patológico). Thesis, University of Recife. Revista da Veterinaria, 1954.

Lôbo, J.: Nova espécie de blastomicose. Brasil Méd 44:1327, 1930.

Lôbo, J.: Um caso de blastomicose produzido por uma espécie nova, encontrada em Recife. Rev Med Pernambuco 1:763, 1931.

Lôbo, J.: Contribuiçao ao estudo das blastomicoses. An Bras Derm Sif 8:43, 1933.

Migaki, G., Valerio, M. G., Irvine, B., and Garner, F. M.: Lobo's disease in an Atlantic bottle-nosed dolphin. J Am Vet Med Assoc 159:578, 1971.

Miranda, J. L.: Lôbo's mycosis. In Marshall, J. (ed.): Essays on Tropical Dermatology. Vol. 2. Amsterdam, Excerpta Medica, 1972a, p. 356.

Miranda, J. L.: Lobomicose (blastomicose queilodiforme, micose de Jorge Lobo, morbus Jorge Lobo). An Bras Dermat 47:273, 1972b.

Sampaio, M. M., and Dias, L. B.: Experimental infection of Jorge Lobo's disease in the cheek pouch of the golden hamster (Mesocricetus auratus). Rev Inst Med Trop S Paulo 12:115, 1970.

Sampaio, M. M., Dias, L. B., and Scaff, L.: Bizarre forms of the etiologic agent in experimental Jorge Lobo's disease in tortoises. Rev Inst Med Trop S Paulo 13:191, 1971.

Silva, M. E., Kaplan, W., and Miranda, J. L.: Antigenic relationship between Paracoccidioides loboi and other pathogenic fungi determined by immunofluorescence. Mycopathologia (Den Haag) 36:97, 1968.

Teixeira, G. A.: Doença de Jorge Lôbo. Aspectos microscópicos. Hospital (Rio de J) 62:813, 1962.

Wiersema, J. P., and Niemel, P. L. A.: Lôbo's disease in Surinam patients. Trop Geogr Med 17:89, 1965.

# 213 MYCOBACTERIAL INFECTIONS OF THE SKIN

Wayne M. Meyers, M.D., Ph.D.

In 1882 Robert Koch identified *Mycobacterium tuberculosis* as the cause of tuberculosis. Thus, by priority this bacillus became the "typical" mycobacterium. Other mycobacteria, however, were soon observed that differed from *M. tuberculosis*, and these became known as "atypical" mycobacteria. In 1954 Timpe and Runyon first classified atypical mycobacteria into four groups on the basis of their growth characteristics. This system, known as the Runyon Classification (Table 1) has undergone so many modifications that it has been more or less abandoned in favor of a new system that recognizes ten species or species complexes of mycobacteria pathogenic for man: *M. leprae, M. tuberculosis* complex, *M. ulcerans, M. marinum, M. kansasii, M. szulgai, M. simiae, M. avium-scrofulaceum-intracellulare* complex, *M. xenopi*, and *M. fortuitum* complex. All of these mycobacteria except *M. simiae* and *M. xenopi* are known to cause diseases of the skin. *M. leprae*, the cause of leprosy, is discussed in Chapter 175.

**TABLE 1. Classification of the Atypical Mycobacteria That Cause Lesions of Skin in Man (Runyon System)**

| GROUP | PIGMENT PRODUCTION IN CULTURE | GROWTH RATE | SPECIES IDENTIFIED |
|-------|-------------------------------|-------------|--------------------|
| I | Photochromogens[a] | Slow | M. kansasii<br>M. marinum |
| II | Scotochromogens[b] | Slow | M. scrofulaceum<br>M. szulgai |
| III | Nonphotochromgens[c] | Slow | M. avium<br>M. intracellulare<br>(Battey) |
| IV | Variable | Rapid | M. fortuitum<br>M. chelonei |

[a]Pigment produced only on exposure to light.

[b]Pigment produced in dark or light.

[c]Nonpigmented.

Note: M. ulcerans has not been classified in the Runyon system.

# M. TUBERCULOSIS INFECTION

## DEFINITION AND ETIOLOGY

M. tuberculosis is the predominant cause of cutaneous tuberculosis, but M. bovis, sometimes called M. tuberculosis (var. bovis), also infects the skin. Cutaneous tuberculosis is classified as follows:

1. *Primary inoculation tuberculosis.* Infection starts in the skin.

2. *Reinfection tuberculosis.* The skin becomes infected in a patient sensitized by co-existing or previous tuberculosis.

3. *Tuberculids.* Some authorities believe that tuberculids are local hyperergic reactions to mycobacteria or their antigens that are spread hematogenously to the skin from foci of active tuberculosis. Others, however, consider tuberculids a misnomer for a phenomenon that is unrelated to tuberculosis. The skepticism about tuberculids as an entity may be explained in part by their rarity in countries with relatively little active tuberculosis (Iden et al. 1978). The various forms of tuberculids are: erythema induratum, lichen scrofulosorum, papulonecrotic tuberculid, and lupus miliaris disseminatus faciei. Tuberculids will not be discussed in this chapter.

## EPIDEMIOLOGY

With the marked reduction of pulmonary tuberculosis in many countries, cutaneous tuberculosis has become rare. Tuberculosis of the skin is more common in colder humid climates and is uncommon in tropical Africa, even though pulmonary tuberculosis is highly prevalent there. For example, in Kenya, Verhagen et al. (1968) found only 14 patients with cutaneous tuberculosis among 3168 patients with skin disease.

## PATHOGENESIS AND PATHOLOGY

### Primary Tuberculosis

*Primary Inoculation Tuberculosis.* In patients who have not been sensitized to M. tuberculosis, the inoculation of tubercle bacilli into the skin produces a local lesion and enlargement of regional lymph nodes. This is *primary inoculation tuberculosis* and is analogous to the Ghon complex. Within two weeks after inoculation into the skin there is an infiltration of polymorphonuclear leukocytes, necrosis, and ulceration. In approximately six weeks this acute reaction is replaced by epithelioid cells and giant cells. Tubercles may develop in the later stages, but caseation is not a constant feature. Acid-fast bacilli are abundant in early lesions but gradually decrease and become rare as granulomas develop.

*Generalized Miliary Tuberculosis of the Skin.* In anergic patients with fulminating tuberculosis of other organs there may be hematogenous spread to the skin. In the dermis there is a perivascular infiltration of polymorphonuclear leukocytes and lymphocytes. Acid-fast bacilli are easily demonstrated in vessels and surrounding tissues. Tuberculoid granulomas develop in older lesions.

### Reinfection Tuberculosis

Patients who are sensitized to M. tuberculosis, either by previous infection or by co-existing tuberculosis, usually develop local delayed-type hy-

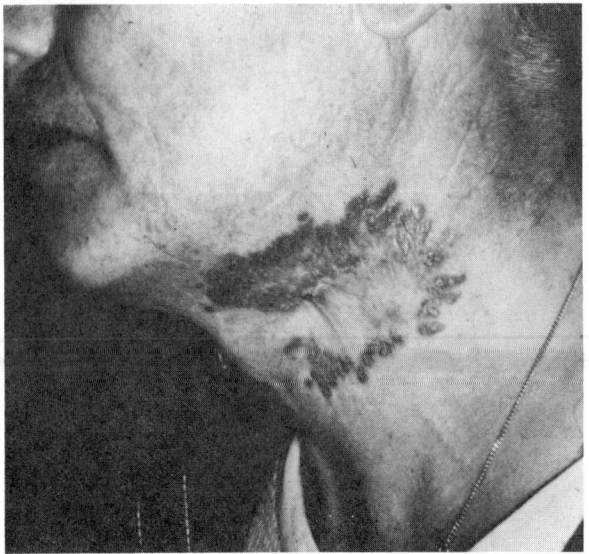

**FIGURE 1.** *Lupus vulgaris. Lesion began in the central scarred area and in 40 to 50 years enlarged to its present size. AFIP 75-15588. (Photograph by Dr. B. Rasaiah).*

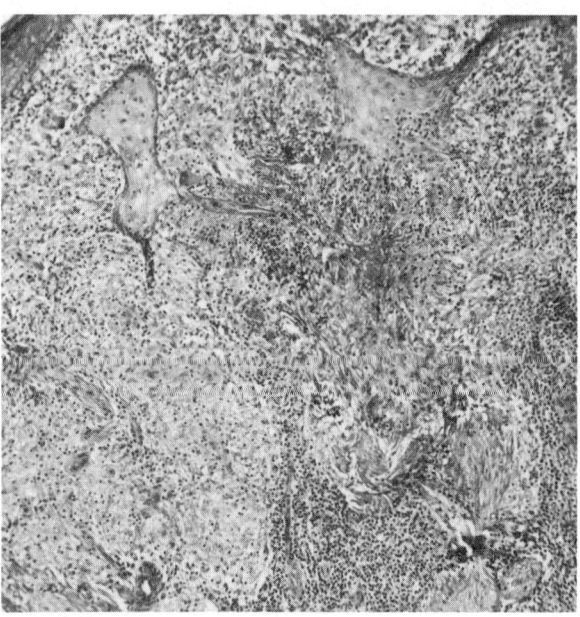

**FIGURE 2.** *Lupus vulgaris. In the dermis, there is an admixture of lymphocytes, epithelioid cells, giant cells, and plasma cells without caseation necrosis. × 40, AFIP 57-9803.*

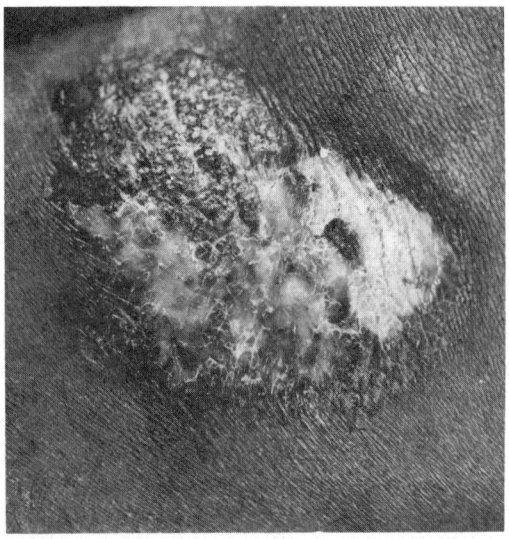

**FIGURE 3.** *Tuberculosis verrucosa cutis on leg. The surface of the lesion is hyperkeratotic and verrucose. AFIP 53-1664.*

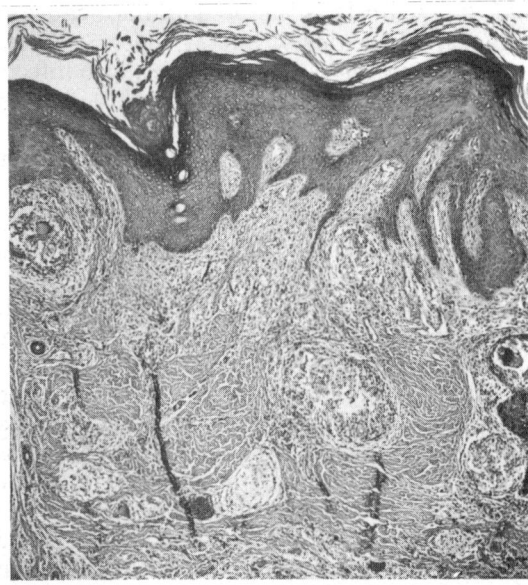

**FIGURE 4.** *Tuberculosis verrucosa cutis showing hyperkeratosis and acanthosis. There are several granulomas in the dermis. × 40, AFIP 58-4939.*

persensitivity reactions when reinfected by *M. tuberculosis*. Histopathologic changes in the common variants of these lesions are as follows:

*Lupus Vulgaris.* In the dermis there are admixtures of epithelioid cells, giant cells, lymphocytes, and plasma cells (Fig. 2). There often are tuberculoid granulomas with only slight necrosis or none. Acid-fast bacilli are rare. Squamous cell carcinomas may develop at the borders of the lesion.

*Tuberculosis Verrucosa Cutis.* In the upper dermis there are marked hyperkeratosis and parakeratosis with abscesses containing polymorphonuclear leukocytes (Fig. 4). Pseudoepitheliomatous hyperplasia may be marked. There may be tuberculoid granulomas with slight to moderate necrosis. Acid-fast bacilli are uncommon but are more numerous than in lupus vulgaris.

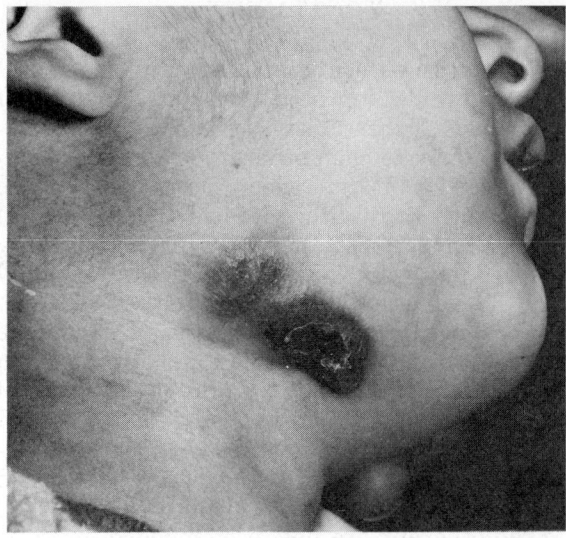

**FIGURE 5.** *Scrofuloderma in a child. There is cervical lymphadenitis with a communicating sinus tract and ulcer. AFIP 53-11701.*

*Scrofuloderma.* A tract of necrosis extends through the dermis and ulcerates the epidermis (Fig. 6). Tuberculoid granulomas with caseation necrosis often surround the ulcer and sinus tract. Acid-fast bacilli are usually readily demonstrable.

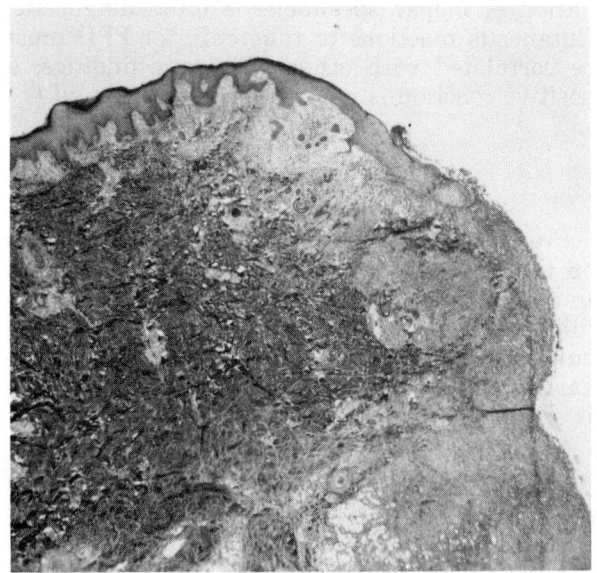

**FIGURE 6.** *Scrofuloderma, showing edge of sinus tract (right) with granulomas and necrosis in surrounding tissues. This ulcer and sinus was in the chest wall of a patient in Zaire who died of pulmonary tuberculosis. The sinus communicated with the diseased lung. × 18, AFIP 78-729.*

*Tuberculosis Cutis Orificialis.* The mucous membrane is ulcerated with acute inflammatory cells in the ulcer base and a mixture of acute and chronic inflammation beneath the base. In long-standing lesions there may be tuberculoid granulomas with caseation. Acid-fast bacilli are abundant.

## CLINICAL MANIFESTATIONS

### Primary Tuberculosis

*Primary Inoculation Tuberculosis.* Approximately 0.15 per cent of all primary tuberculosis occurs in the skin. Infants and those whose occupations bring them in contact with tuberculosis are at risk, for example, "prosector's paronychia" in those who perform autopsies (Goette et al., 1978). Lesions appear as papules or crusted ulcers about two weeks after infection. These ulcers, or "tuberculous chancres," gradually enlarge to up to 5 cm in diameter. Often, about one month after infection, there is regional painful lymphadenopathy. Most infections subside after several months without therapy. Miliary dissemination from the skin is rare. A serious form of primary tuberculosis has been reported in subjects who have undergone circumcision by circumcisers with active tuberculosis.

*Generalized Miliary Tuberculosis of the Skin.* This rare complication of tuberculosis is usually seen in infants. There are widely disseminated small erythematous macules, papules, or vesicles in the skin. Prognosis is poor.

### Reinfection Tuberculosis

*Lupus Vulgaris.* Lupus vulgaris is the most common form of cutaneous tuberculosis and is more frequent in women. Peak incidences occur at ages 20 years and 50 years. Horwitz (1960) studied 3902 patients with lupus vulgaris in Denmark and found that one-third of them eventually developed pulmonary tuberculosis, one-third had pulmonary tuberculosis before the onset of lupus vulgaris, and one-third had onset of pulmonary tuberculosis and lupus vulgaris simultaneously. Three-quarters of all patients with lupus vulgaris had tuberculosis of other organs.

Lupus vulgaris involves the head and neck most commonly but may occur anywhere, and usually there is a single lesion (Fig. 1). There is an early small red papule that gradually expands peripherally. As the lesion enlarges foci of healing and active growth occur with atrophic or hypertrophic scarring and ulceration. This process, if not treated, may continue for decades and cover large areas of the skin. Loss of function of vital structures (e.g., eyelids) and disfigurement are serious sequelae. Skin cancers, usually squamous cell carcinomas, are not uncommon in long-standing lesions.

*Tuberculosis Verrucosa Cutis.* Tuberculosis verrucosa cutis is a disease of adults. Lesions are most frequent on exposed parts of the body (e.g., hands). Individuals exposed to patients or cadavers with tuberculosis are at risk. "Prosector's" and "anatomist's" wart are synonyms for lesions in those who perform autopsies. Lesions begin as papules, become hyperkeratotic, and resemble verrucae vulgaris. These "warts" gradually expand peripherally to form verrucose, reddish-brown, irregular patches (Fig. 3). Regional lymphadenopathy is usually absent. The course is protracted, often for years, but there may be spontaneous healing.

*Scrofuloderma (Tuberculosis Colliquativa Cutis).* Scrofuloderma is an extension of tuberculosis into the skin from underlying structures such as lymph nodes, bone, or lung. A subcutaneous swelling progresses into cold abscesses, multiple ulcers, and sinus tracts. Lesions on the neck are common, especially in children, and develop from mycobacterial cervical lymphadenitis (Fig. 5). Lincoln and Gilbert (1972), in 340 patients throughout the world with culturally proven nontuberculous mycobacterial cervical lymphadenitis found that 208 were caused by scotochromogens, 108 were caused by organisms in the *M. avium-intracellulare* complex, 21 were in Runyon group I (probably *M. kansasii*), and three were rapid growers. *M. scrofulaceum* is the most frequently identified scotochromogen. *M. bovis* is a well-known cause of scrofuloderma. The course is protracted but eventually heals with residual keloidal scars.

*Tuberculosis Cutis Orificialis.* Tuberculosis cutis orificialis arises by autoinoculation of mucous membranes from internal tuberculosis and is rare where there are effective tuberculosis control programs. There are shallow crusted ulcers in or around the mouth, anus, or vulva. Although the lesions regress with effective chemotherapy, involvement of orifices often portends a poor prognosis.

## TREATMENT

All patients with cutaneous tuberculosis should be studied to determine if there are other foci of tuberculosis. Tuberculosis of the skin usually responds rapidly to chemotherapy. The drugs commonly used for internal tuberculosis are effective. Combined therapy with isoniazid (300 mg orally) and streptomycin (1 to 2 g daily IM) is commonly employed, but isoniazid alone is effective in many cases. The duration of chemotherapy is variable. Some believe that isoniazid therapy should be continued for up to three years and streptomycin for two months. Rifampicin (daily oral doses of 600 mg), ethambutol (15 to 25 mg/kg daily), and 0.5 gr. cycloserine may be used in patients infected with mycobacteria that are resistant to isoniazid or streptomycin. Calciferol (vitamin $D_2$) and radiotherapy are not recommended.

Small lesions of lupus vulgaris and tuberculosis verrucosa cutis may be excised if there is no fever or evidence of spread to lymph nodes. Surgery for scrofuloderma lessens morbidity. Tuberculostatic drug therapy should precede surgical intervention for cutaneous tuberculosis.

## DIAGNOSIS

Identification of mycobacteria requires cultivation. In primary tuberculosis acid-fast organisms may be seen in Ziehl-Neelsen-stained smears or by fluorescent microscopy of auramine-rhodamine-stained smears. Histopathologic evaluation of biopsy specimens is often diagnostic. Cutaneous reactions to tuberculin or PPD must be correlated with other diagnostic findings; a positive reaction is never diagnostic by itself.

## PROPHYLAXIS

Prevention of cutaneous tuberculosis depends on the effective control of systemic tuberculosis in man. Some cases of cervical adenitis and scrofuloderma can be prevented by control of tuberculosis in cattle and pasteurization of milk. The early treatment of all patients with tuberculosis is essential.

# MYCOBACTERIUM ULCERANS INFECTION (BURULI ULCER)

## DEFINITION AND ETIOLOGY

*M. ulcerans* is a slow-growing organism that infects the skin and subcutaneous tissues of man, giving rise to indolent ulcers with undermined edges. *M. ulcerans* grows optimally on routine mycobacterial media at 32° C and elaborates a cytotoxin (Hockmeyer et al., 1978) that causes necrosis of skin and subcutaneous tissue. Growth in culture is usually inhibited at temperatures above 35° C, but a rare strain will grow at 37° C. Large undermined ulcers, almost certainly caused by *M. ulcerans,* were first described by Cook in Uganda in 1897 (Connor and Lunn, 1966), but *M. ulcerans* was not identified until 1948 in Australia (MacCallum et al., 1948).

## EPIDEMIOLOGY

All major endemic foci are located in swampy terrain of tropical or subtropical countries. The largest known foci are in Uganda (Barker, 1972) and Zaire (Meyers et al. 1974a). The source of *M. ulcerans* in nature is unknown. Infection probably begins when *M. ulcerans* is introduced into the skin by minor trauma or by hypodermic needle (Meyers et al. 1974c), presumably from the contaminated surface of the skin. Spread from patient to patient is rare. Persons of all age groups are infected, but the highest frequency of infection occurs in the second and third decades.

## PATHOGENESIS AND PATHOLOGY

*M. ulcerans* organisms elaborate a toxin that causes necrosis of the dermis, panniculus, and deep fascia (Krieg et al., 1974) (Figs. 10 and 11).

Early lesions are closed, but the necrosis spreads to the overlying dermis and epidermis, and in two to three months produces an ulcer with undermined borders and a necrotic base. Microscopically, there is contiguous coagulation necrosis of the deep dermis and panniculus with destruction of all tissue including nerves, appendages, and vessels. There is interstitial edema without conspicuous inflammatory cells. Extracellular clumps and masses of acid-fast bacilli are found in the necrotic areas, especially in the ulcer bed (Figs. 11 and 12). Necrosis may spread to the deep fascia and muscle, and rarely to bone. In the healing phase there is a granulomatous response and eventual scarring.

## CLINICAL MANIFESTATIONS

The first sign is a firm, painless, nontender, movable nodule 1 to 2 cm in diameter in the subcutaneous tissue. Within one to two months the nodule becomes fluctuant, spreads peripherally, and, ulcerates. The border of the ulcer is undermined up to 15 cm or more, and the adjacent skin is edematous (Fig. 7). Even with large ulcers, there is usually no regional lymphadenopathy or systemic symptoms. Ulcers may remain small and heal within a few months without treatment, or spread rapidly, undermining the skin of large areas, even an entire leg, thigh, or arm. Occasionally, important structures such as an eye are lost (Fig. 8). Lesions tend to heal spontaneously in months or years, but without therapy contrac-

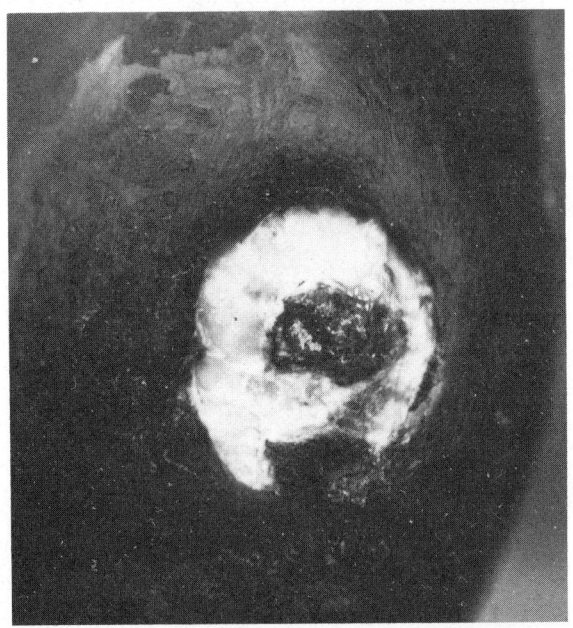

**FIGURE 7.** Mycobacterium ulcerans *infection in the deltoid area of a Zairian boy. Lesion developed at the site of a hypodermic injection. The border of the ulcer was undermined and there is a necrotic slough in the base. AFIP 76-11034-5.*

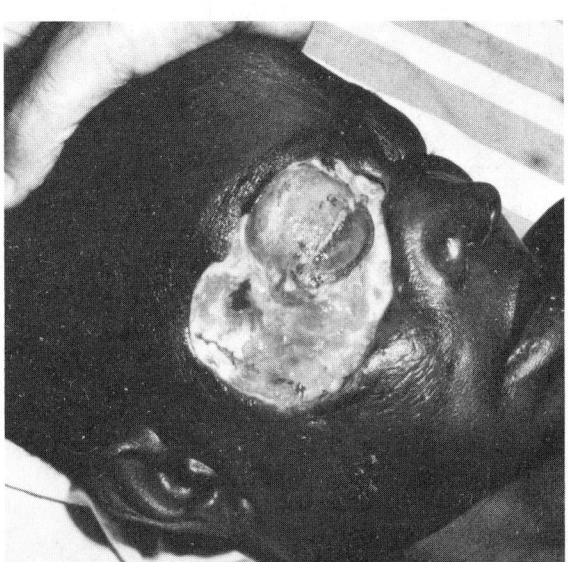

**FIGURE 8.** Mycobacterium ulcerans *infection in a Zairian woman. The eye was lost because of damage to the eyelids. AFIP 76-11034-6.*

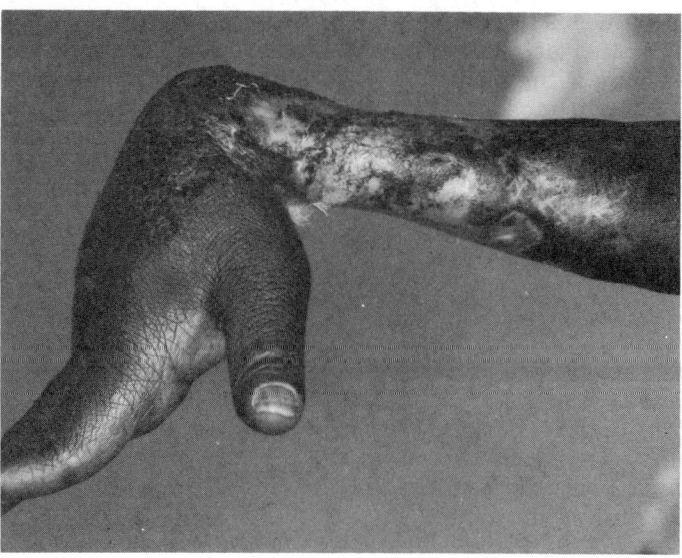

**FIGURE 9.**   Mycobacterium ulcerans *infection of forearm and wrist. Lesion is healed but the scar has caused a contraction deformity with subluxation at the wrist. AFIP 65-2982-1. (Photographed by Dr. D. H. Connor).*

tion deformities and lymphedema may result (Fig. 9).

### TREATMENT

Early pre-ulcerative nodules are excised and closed primarily. Ulcers are widely excised and skin is grafted. Continuous heating at 40° C (e.g.,

by a heated water jacket) will promote healing without wide excision, but this must be used cautiously when vital structures are threatened (Meyers et al., 1974b). Amputation of limbs is rarely necessary and should be done only as a last resort. Rifampicin promotes healing of pre-ulcerative nodules or small ulcers but has not been adequately evaluated. Other antimicrobial agents are ineffective. Physical therapy must be insti-

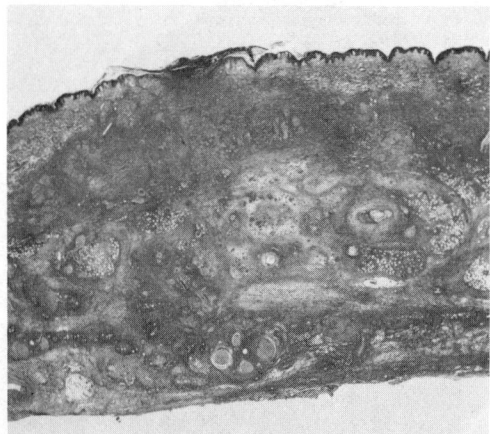

**FIGURE 10.**   Mycobacterium ulcerans *infection, preulcerative lesion. This section, through the center of the lesion, shows massive coagulation necrosis in the lower dermis and subcutaneous tissue. × 4, AFIP 65-1411.*

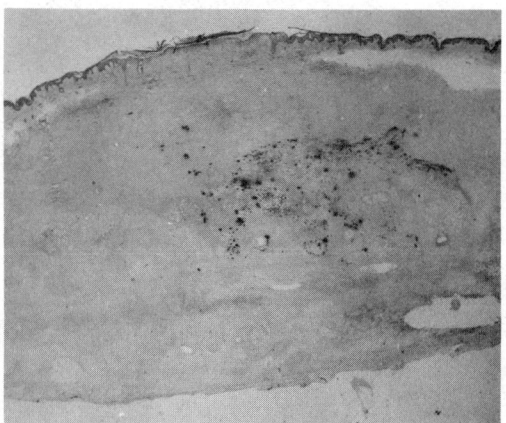

**FIGURE 11.**   Mycobacterium ulcerans *infection. This is a parallel section of the lesion in Figure 10 stained by the Ziehl-Neelsen method. There are many clumps of acid-fast bacilli in the necrotic area. × 4, AFIP 65-1413.*

tuted early when there is danger of contraction deformities.

### DIAGNOSIS

Smears from the necrotic base of ulcers, stained by the Ziehl-Neelsen technique, often reveal clumps of acid-fast bacilli. Biopsy specimens of the necrotic base and undermined periphery of the ulcer usually reveal necrosis of the dermis and subcutaneous tissue and acid-fast bacilli and establish the diagnosis. Culture of *M. ulcerans* from exudates or biopsy specimens is successful in 50 to 75 per cent of active lesions, but visible growth often requires six to eight weeks. Skin tests are of no diagnostic value.

### PROPHYLAXIS

There is no effective prophylaxis, but vaccination with BCG may give short-lived protection (Uganda Buruli group, 1969).

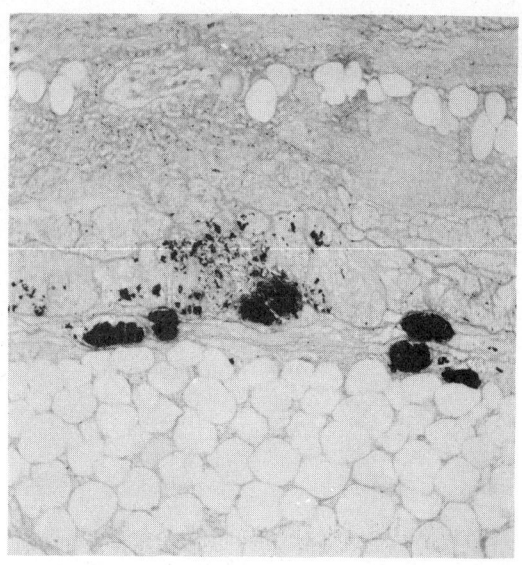

**FIGURE 12.** Mycobacterium ulcerans *infection showing large numbers of acid-fast bacilli in the subcutaneous area of the edge of an ulcer. The surrounding tissue is nonviable and there are many "ghosts" of fat cells. Ziehl-Neelsen stain.* × 80, AFIP 65-5851.

# MYCOBACTERIUM MARINUM INFECTION

### DEFINITION AND ETIOLOGY

Aronson (1926) first identified *M. marinum* in marine fish in an aquarium in Philadelphia. Linell and Norden (1954) isolated this mycobacterium from patients who developed granulomas of the skin after swimming in a pool in Sweden; hence infections by *M. marinum* are commonly called "swimming pool granulomas." *M. marinum* grows within two weeks at 30 to 32° C on mycobacterial media, but growth is inhibited at 37° C. *M. balnei* is a synonym for *M. marinum*.

### EPIDEMIOLOGY

*M. marinum* infections have been reported from Australia, Belgium, England, Germany, Israel, Japan, Sweden, and the United States (including Hawaii), and the organism is presumed to be ubiquitous. Most patients have been in contaminated swimming pools. Philpott et al. (1963), for example, described 290 patients who had been in a single swimming pool in Colorado. Occasionally a hobbyist who keeps tropical fish, or people who work or swim in bayous, rivers, or coastal or brackish water are infected (Miller and Toon,

1973; Zeligman, 1972). Sometimes the patient has not been exposed to any known source of *M. marinum*. The organism is introduced into the skin at sites of trauma, and there is no evidence of man-to-man transmission. In nature, water-dwelling animals can become infected from water contaminated with *M. marinum* and in turn shed *M. marinum* into the water. The "water flea," Daphnia, can serve as a host. Because of cross-reactivity with other mycobacterial antigens, epidemiologic studies based on skin testing are not valid.

### PATHOGENESIS AND PATHOLOGY

Incubation periods are often difficult to establish in natural infections, but usually last from one to six weeks. A laboratory infection is reported that became clinically apparent ten days after an accident, and *M. marinum* was cultured at 15 days (Chappler et al., 1977). The low temperature growth requirement limits infections to the skin, usually to the focus of inoculation. The disease, however, may spread along the lymphatics and may resemble sporotrichosis (Dickey, 1968). Spread may be enhanced by local infiltration with corticosteroids (Aaronson and Park,

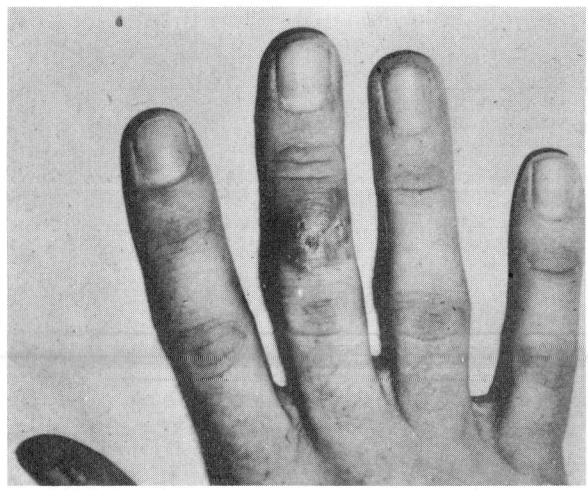

**FIGURE 13.** Mycobacterium marinum *infection, "swimming pool granulomas," on dorsum of middle finger. There is a small draining ulcer in the center of the nodule. AFIP 75-12395.*

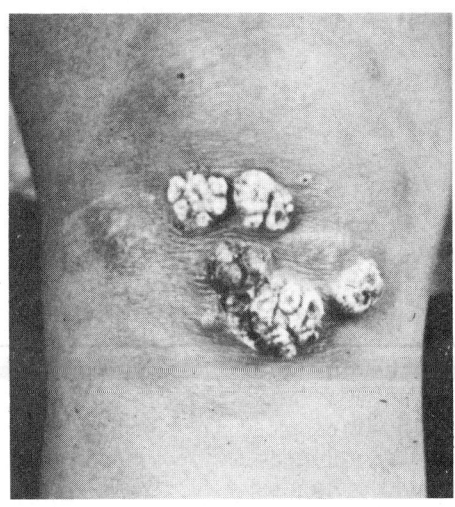

**FIGURE 14.** Mycobacterium marinum *infection, "swimming pool granuloma," on knee showing verrucose nature of this lesion that had persisted for 6 years. AFIP 75-12396.*

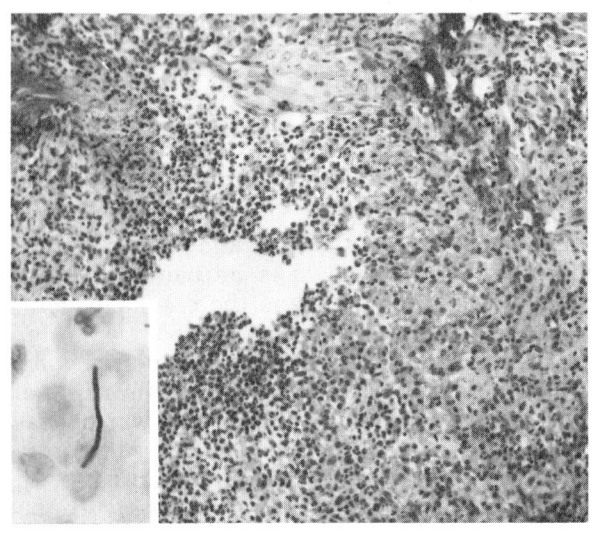

**FIGURE 15.** Mycobacterium marinum *infection, "swimming pool granulomas," showing a mixed inflammatory reaction in dermis. × 100, AFIP 73-3053. Inset: A single M. marinum in area of inflammation. Ziehl-Neelsen, × 1190, AFIP 73-3054. These sections are from the lesions shown in Figure 13.*

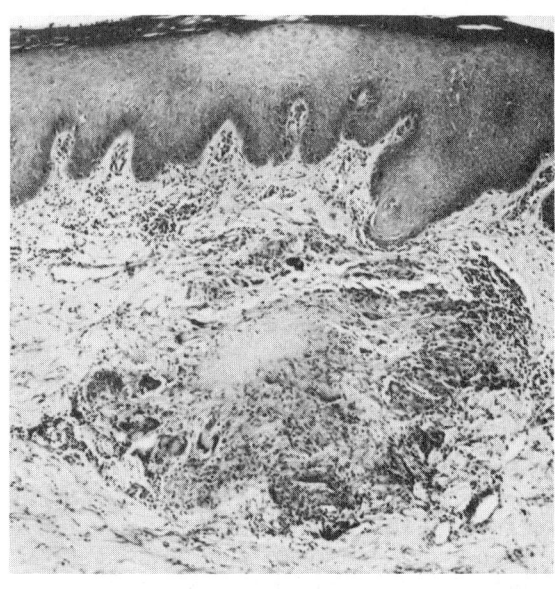

**FIGURE 16.** Mycobacterium marinum *infection, "swimming pool granulomas," showing granuloma with necrosis in dermis. × 40, AFIP 69-9675.*

1974). In early lesions a mixture of lymphocytes, histiocytes, and polymorphonuclear leukocytes infiltrates the dermis (Fig. 15). In older lesions there are tuberculoid granulomas that may show caseation necrosis (Fig. 16). Acid-fast rods with crossbands that are wider and longer than *M. tuberculosis,* although scarce, are often seen in the granulomas. In immunosuppressed patients *M. marinum* may mimic undermined lesions caused by *M. ulcerans.*

## CLINICAL MANIFESTATIONS

The earliest sign is usually a mildly tender erythema at the inoculation site. This erythema develops into a papule that gradually enlarges into an erythematous or violaceous nodule that occasionally ulcerates and discharges pus (Fig. 13). Older lesions may become verrucose (Fig. 14). Because bony prominences are prone to trauma, the hands, elbows, and knees are sites of predilection (Philpott et al., 1963), and the bursae of the elbows and knees are sometimes invaded. Sporotrichoid *M. marinum* infections are uncommon. Spontaneous cure is the rule, usually requiring three months to three years for complete resolution, but infections have persisted 4 to 17 years.

## TREATMENT

Most lesions are self-healing. Because of the protracted course of the disease, many patients demand therapy. The following drugs have been used orally with some success; tetracycline, 1 to 2 g daily (Kim, 1974; Izumi et al., 1977); minocycline, 100 mg twice daily, and trimethoprim, 60 mg, plus sulfamethoxazole, 800 mg, twice daily. Antituberculosis drugs, including streptomycin, isoniazid, and ethambutol, have been tried with varying success. When possible, surgical excision or curettage and electrodesiccation have been recommended as the treatments of choice.

## DIAGNOSIS

Diagnosis requires cultivation of *M. marinum* from the lesion because histopathologic changes are not specific. Positive skin tests, even with antigens prepared from *M. marinum,* are not diagnostic owing to strong cross-reactions with other mycobacteria (Judson and Feldman, 1974).

## PROPHYLAXIS

Adequate maintenance of swimming pools (Philpott et al., 1963) interrupts epidemics; however, sporadic cases cannot be prevented except by avoiding potentially contaminated sources such as home aquariums.

# MYCOBACTERIUM KANSASII INFECTION

## DEFINITION AND ETIOLOGY

Typical *M. kansasii* strains grow at 37° C and are photochromogens, but there are nonchromogenic and scotochromogenic strains that are otherwise identical. *M. kansasii* commonly infects the lungs, but only approximately ten patients with skin lesions have been reported. *M. kansasii* infections protect against *M. tuberculosis* infections in the guinea pig and hence are more closely related to *M. tuberculosis* than any other mycobacterium except BCG (Palmer and Long, 1966). Consequently, cross-reactions to skin-test antigens of *M. kansasii* and *M. tuberculosis* are common.

## EPIDEMIOLOGY

In nature, *M. kansasii* is found most frequently in tap water but occasionally also in cows and swine. *M. kansasii* infections are worldwide in distribution, and in the United States occur most frequently in the Midwest and Southwest. Among 1185 consecutive patients admitted to a Denver, Colorado, hospital during the period 1960 to 1964, 4.2 per cent had atypical mycobacteriosis, and 60 per cent of these were infected by *M. kansasii* (Fischer et al., 1968). Pulmonary infections are acquired by inhalation and are probably transmissible. The mode of primary infections of the skin is not known but may be by inoculation.

## PATHOGENESIS AND PATHOLOGY

The length of the incubation period of primary cutaneous lesions is not known. One infection occurred approximately one year after a local injury. Histopathologic changes in pulmonary and systemic lesions are similar to those caused by *M. tuberculosis* (i.e., granulomas with caseation). Acid-fast bacilli are few and difficult to find in smears and tissue sections.

Lesions of the skin that have spread from primary infections elsewhere have often been seen in immunosuppressed patients. These lesions show a variable acute and chronic inflammatory response that is sometimes pyogenic. Acid-fast organisms may be numerous. No systemic spread has been reported from primary lesions of the skin.

## CLINICAL MANIFESTATIONS

Primary lesions of the skin may present as single nodules or as sporotrichoid spread. Some nodular lesions are preceded by erythematous tender swellings. In patients with sporotrichoid spread the lesions appear on the hand and extend to the forearm but do not involve the lymph nodes. Chronic infections may last as long as 22 years. Four patients with disseminated *M. kansasii* have been reported; they had erythema induratum, abscesses, cellulitis, and ulcers of the skin (Fraser et al., 1975; Hirsh and Saffold, 1976).

### TREATMENT

Treatment with antibiotics or by chemotherapy should be based on sensitivity studies on cultured organisms. Primary lesions have healed after four months of combined therapy with isoniazid, para-aminosalicylic acid, and streptomycin. One immunosuppressed patient with disseminated

disease responded to specific transfer factor (Hirsh and Saffold, 1976).

### DIAGNOSIS

Diagnosis requires the cultivation of *M. kansasii* from biopsy specimens or exudates. Skin reactions to mycobacterial antigens are not specific.

### PROPHYLAXIS

No prophylactic measures are known.

# INFECTIONS CAUSED BY THE "RAPID-GROWING" MYCOBACTERIA

### DEFINITION AND ETIOLOGY

This group of organisms grows within five days (usually in 48 hours) on routine laboratory media at 32 to 37° C. Nomenclature of the "rapid-growers" is imprecise: Some employ the term "*M. fortuitum* complex" for all members of this group, whereas others (e.g., Inman et al., 1969) separate *M. fortuitum* from *M. chelonei* because of their antigenic and biochemical differences. Stanford et al. (1972) concluded that *M. abscessus, M. runyonii,* and *M. borstelense* are synonymous with *M. chelonei.*

### EPIDEMIOLOGY

These ubiquitous organisms are common saprophytes in soil and water. *M. fortuitum* and *M. chelonei* have been reported from nearly all continents. Cruz (1938) first identified *M. fortuitum* as the cause of an injection abscess in the arm of a patient in Brazil. Penetrating wounds of the skin, including surgical wounds and hypodermic injections, may introduce the organism (Hand and Sanford, 1970). In local epidemics of "injection abscesses" the injected medication may be contaminated (Inman et al., 1969). Although these organisms may cause disease in amphibians, rodents, and other animals, there are no epidemiologic data linking disease in man to these sources.

### PATHOGENESIS AND PATHOLOGY

The incubation period is ordinarily two to seven months. The early histopathologic changes have not been described. The earliest lesion presented

for medical examination is a fluctuant abscess that may form one or more sinuses that discharge pus. In closed lesions the predominant feature is liquefactive necrosis with an intense polymorphonuclear leukocytic infiltrate into the dermis and subcutaneous tissue. In chronic lesions there is fibrosis of the abscess wall or sinus tract. Epithelioid cell granulomas with suppuration and caseation have been described (Moore and Fredrichs, 1953). Acid-fast bacilli are present but are often scarce in tissue sections. Most lesions of the skin and subcutaneous tissue remain localized. There may be regional lymphadenopathy. Systemic spread is rare, but immunosuppression may cause multiple skin lesions and dissemination (Graybill et al., 1974). Pulmonary infections are common, but there is no evidence that pulmonary disease has arisen from skin infections.

### CLINICAL MANIFESTATIONS

Mild local inflammation develops within a few days at the site of an injection or injury. These changes are minor and the physician often does not see the patient until there is a subcutaneous nodule, fluctuation, or ulceration. Lesions are painless and are frequently on the buttocks and deltoid areas (usual sites of injections), and range from 1 cm in diameter to those that cover the entire buttock (Fig. 17). Larger lesions may have multiple sinuses. Regional lymph nodes may be enlarged and tender. Healing requires several months to over two years.

### TREATMENT

Incision and drainage is adequate therapy for most abscesses. Repeated incisions may be nec-

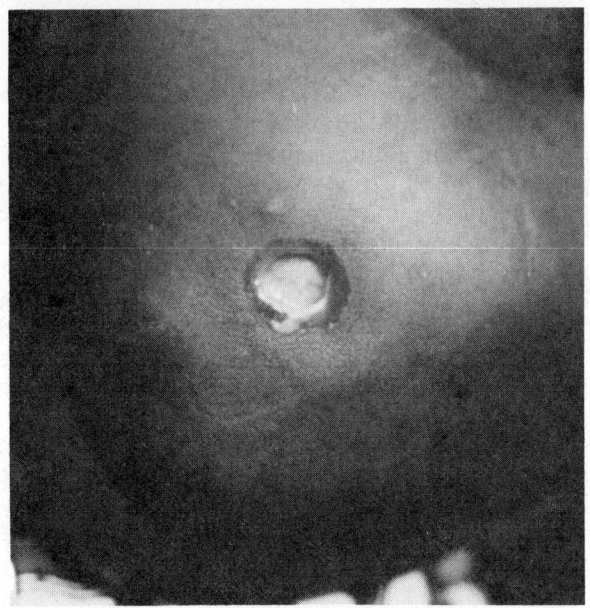

**FIGURE 17.** *Injection ulcer caused by* M. fortuitum *in buttock of Zairian infant. Infant had received a hypodermic injection at this site approximately 2 months previously. AFIP 78-3306.*

out recurrence. *M. fortuitum* and *M. chelonei* are frequently resistant to antibiotics and chemotherapy. Nevertheless, sensitivity tests should be performed, and if the organism proves to be sensitive, specific therapy should be given. Drug therapy, like incision and drainage, requires prolonged treatment.

### DIAGNOSIS

There may be a history of trauma, but the incubation period is long and many patients forget they have had injections or an injury. Diagnosis depends on identifying the mycobacteria in exudates or biopsy specimens. In closed lesions exudate may be obtained by needle aspiration. If acid-fast stains are not routinely done on exudates, the diagnosis may be missed, and the bacteria misidentified as "diphtheroids" on Gram stains. Because the organisms grow rapidly on simple media, the diagnosis can be made within a few days.

### PROPHYLAXIS

Infections acquired by hypodermic injections are preventable by ensuring sterility and practicing antisepsis of the skin (Vandepitte et al., 1969). Many infections acquired in hospitals and clinics could be prevented by asepsis in wound care.

essary to maintain drainage. If practicable, sinuses may be excised. On the mistaken clinical diagnosis of a pre-ulcerative *M. ulcerans* infection, the author excised an abscess on the deltoid area that was caused by *M. chelonei*. The skin was closed primarily and the wound healed with-

# MISCELLANEOUS AND UNCOMMON MYCOBACTERIAL INFECTIONS OF THE SKIN, SCOTOCHROMOGENIC MYCOBACTERIA AND THE M. AVIUM-SCROFULACEUM-INTRACELLULARE COMPLEX

This is a composite of mycobacteria. Their nomenclature and interrelationships, involving both Runyon groups II and III organisms, present problems in identification. The most common pathogenic scotochromogen is *M. scrofulaceum (M. marianum)*, found in soil and water and sometimes cultured as a contaminant in secretions and tissues from humans. Primary *M. scrofulaceum* infections of the skin are rarely if ever

reported with positive identification of the etiologic agent. *M. scrofulaceum* is a common cause of cervical lymphadenitis and scrofuloderma in children (Lincoln and Gilbert, 1972). One patient on corticosteroid therapy developed multiple cutaneous nodules, cellulitis, and ulcers caused by the scotochromogen *M. szulgai* (Sybert et al., 1977).

Organisms of the *M. avium-intracellulare* com-

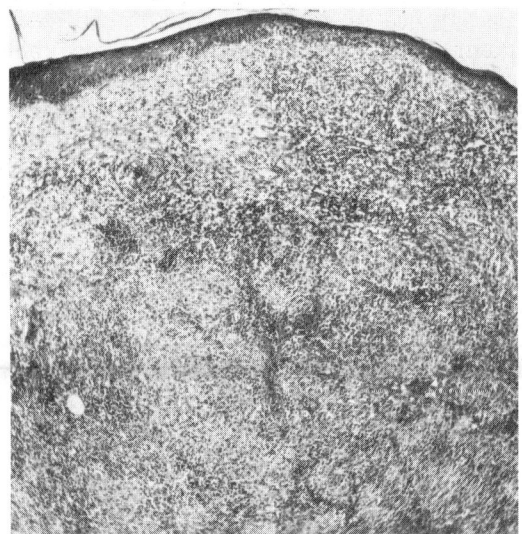

**FIGURE 18.** *Dermal granulomas caused by unidentified mycobacteria in a nodule on the wrist of an 84 year old woman from Minnesota (USA). The dermis is replaced by an infiltration of histiocytes, lymphocytes, and polymorphonuclear leucocytes. × 56, AFIP 74-894.*

### Skin Lesions Caused by Unidentified Mycobacteria

A group of 29 patients in the period 1957 to 1971 from north central United States and Canada developed indurated erythematous papules, primarily of the extremities, and regional lymphadenitis (Feldman and Hershfield, 1974). The lesions ulcerated and were found to contain numerous intracellular and extracellular acid-fast bacilli in exudates and histopathologic sections. The organisms could not be cultured (Figs. 18 and 19). The mycobacterium causing these infections has not been identified, but it was not *M. leprae* as originally suspected. Several cutaneous mycobacterial infections reminiscent of these have occurred in immunosuppressed patients and have been studied at the Armed Forces Institute of Pathology. The acid-fast bacilli in these lesions have not been identified (Figs. 20 and 21).

### Complications of Vaccination with the Bacillus of Calmette-Guerin (BCG)

Occasionally, vaccination with BCG (a viable attenuated strain of *M. bovis*), which is given to prevent tuberculosis or to treat cancer, results in progressive disease. Local lupus vulgaris-like lesions with or without regional lymphadenopathy may develop. Immunosuppressed patients can develop fatal systemic infections (Aungst, 1975). Most progressive infections by BCG respond to isoniazid therapy.

lex rarely cause primary skin lesions. An ulcer of the foot caused by a "Runyon group III" organism occurred in a patient who claimed to have had a minor abrasion at the site about one month before the lesion appeared (Schmidt et al., 1972). This patient responded to combined isoniazid, cycloserine, and streptomycin therapy.

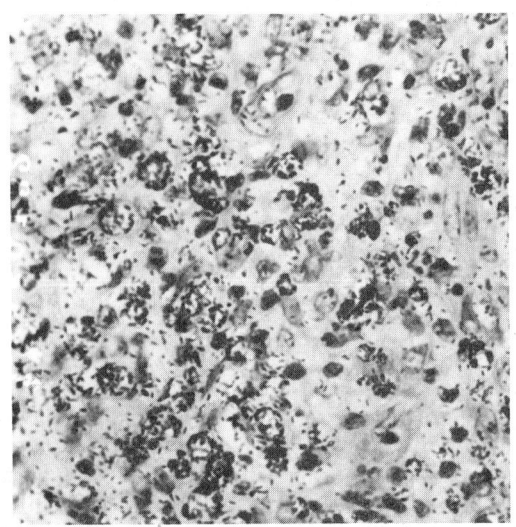

**FIGURE 19.** *Higher magnification of lesion of Figure 18 showing masses of acid-fast bacilli in infiltration. This area is undergoing necrosis. × 485, AFIP 74-896.*

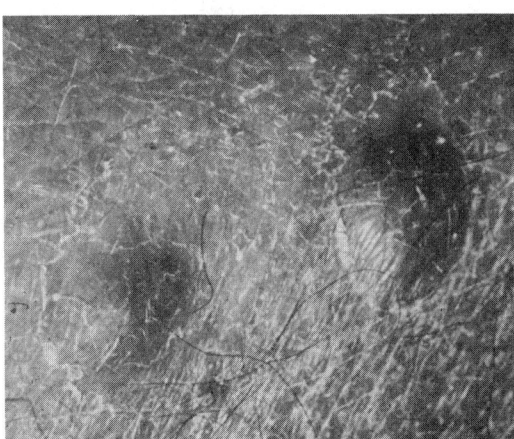

**FIGURE 20.** *Two of many similar nodules in the skin of a 51 year old man under immunosuppressive therapy following an organ transplant. Nodules were caused by an unidentified mycobacterium. AFIP 75-12220-1.*

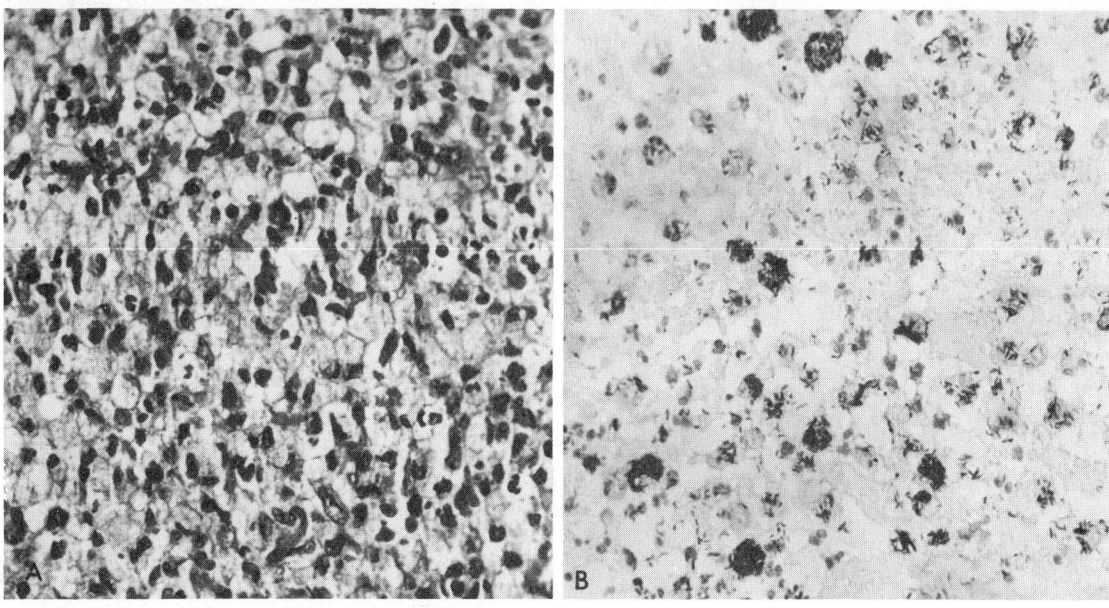

**FIGURE 21.** A, *Histiocytic infiltration of dermis in lesion shown in Figure 20. × 440, AFIP 74-889. B, Parallel section stained by Ziehl-Neelsen method and showing clumps of acid-fast bacilli in histiocytes. × 440, AFIP 74-890.*

# References

Aaronson, C. M., and Park, C. H.: Sporotrichoid infection due to *Mycobacterium marinum:* Lesion exacerbated by corticosteroid infiltration. South Med J 67:117, 1974.

Aronson, J. D.: Spontaneous tuberculosis in salt water fish. J Infect Dis 39:315, 1926.

Aungst, C. W., Sokal, J. E., and Jager, B. V.: Complications of BCG vaccination in neoplastic diseases. Ann Intern Med 82:666, 1975.

Bailey, R. K., Wyles, S., Dingley, M., Hesse, F., and Kent, G. W.: The isolation of high catalase *Mycobacterium kansasii* from tap water. Notes. Am Rev Resp Dis 101:430, 1970.

Barker, D. J. P.: Epidemiology of *Mycobacterium ulcerans* infection. Trans R Soc Trop Med Hyg 67:43, 1973.

Chappler, R. R., Hoke, A. W., and Borchardt, K. A.: Primary inoculation with *Mycobacterium marinum*. Letter. Arch Dermatol *113*:380, 1977.

Connor, D. H., and Lunn, F.: Buruli ulceration. A clinicopathologic study of 38 Ugandans with *Mycobacterium ulcerans* ulceration. Arch Pathol 81:183, 1966.

Cruz, J. C.: *Mycobacterium fortuitum*, um novo bacilo acido-resistente patogenico para o homem. Acta Med Rio de Janeiro 1:297, 1938.

Dickey, R. F.: Sporotrichoid mycobacteriosis caused by *M. marinum (balnei)*. Arch Dermatol 98:385, 1968.

Feldman, R. A., and Hershfield, E.: Mycobacterial skin infections by an unidentified species: A report of 29 patients. Ann Intern Med 80:445, 1974.

Fischer, D. A., Lester, W., and Schaefer, W. B.: Infections with atypical mycobacteria. Five years' experience at the National Jewish Hospital. Am Rev Resp Dis 98:29, 1968.

Fraser, D. W., Buxton, A. E., Naji, A., Barker, C. F., Rudnick, M., and Weinstein, A. J.: Disseminated *Mycobacterium kansasii* infection presenting as cellulitis in a recipient of a renal homograft. Am Rev Resp Dis 112:125, 1975.

Goette, D. K., Jacobson, K. W., and Doty, R. D.: Primary inoculation tuberculosis of the skin. Prosector's paronychia. Arch Dermatol 114:567, 1978.

Graybill, J. R., Silva, J., Fraser, D. W., Lordon, R., and Rogers, E.: Disseminated mycobacteriosis due to *Mycobacterium abscessus* in two recipients of renal homografts. Am Rev Resp Dis 109:4, 1974.

Hand, W. L., and Sanford, J. P.: *Mycobacterium fortuitum*—a human pathogen. Ann Intern Med 73:971, 1970.

Heineman, H. S., Spitzer, S., and Pianphongsant, T.: Fish tank granuloma. A hobby hazard. Arch Intern Med *130*:121, 1972.

Hirsh, F. S., and Saffold, O. E.: *Mycobacterium kansasii* infection with dermatologic manifestations. Arch Dermatol 112:706, 1976.

Hockmeyer, W. T., Krieg, R. E., Reich, M., and Johnson, R. D.: Further characterization of *Mycobacterium ulcerans* toxin. Infect Immun 21:124, 1978.

Horwitz, O.: Lupus vulgaris cutis in Denmark 1895–1954: Its relation to the epidemiology of other forms of tuberculosis. Epidemiology and course of the tuberculous infection based on 3902 cases from the Finsen Institute, Copenhagen. Acta Tuberc Scand (Suppl) 49:1, 1960.

Iden, D. L., Rogers, R. S., and Schroeter, A. L.: Papulonecrotic tuberculid secondary to *Mycobacterium bovis*. Arch Dermatol 114:564, 1978.

Inman, P. M., Beck, A., Brown, A. E., and Stanford, J. L.: Outbreak of injection abscesses due to *Mycobacterium abscessus*. Arch Dermatol 100:141, 1969.

Izumi, A. K., Hanke, W., and Higaki, M.: *Mycobacterium marinum* infections treated with tetracycline. Arch Dermatol 113:1067, 1977.

Judson, F. N., and Feldman, R. A.: Mycobacterial skin tests in humans 12 years after infection with *Mycobacterium marinum*. Am Rev Resp Dis 109:544, 1974.

Kim, R.: Tetracycline therapy for atypical mycobacterial granuloma. Letter. Arch Dermatol 110:299, 1974.

Koch, R.: Die Aetiologie der Tuberkulose. Berl Klin Wochnschr 19:221, 1882.

Krieg, R. E., Hockmeyer, W. T., and Connor, D. H.: Toxin of *Mycobacterium ulcerans*. Production and effects on guinea pig skin. Arch Dermatol 110:783, 1974.

Lincoln, E. M., and Gilbert, L. A.: Disease in children due to mycobacteria other than *Mycobacterium tuberculosis*. Am Rev Resp Dis 105:683, 1972.

Linell, F., and Norden, A.: *Mycobacterium balnei*. A new acid-fast bacillus occurring in swimming pools and capable of producing skin lesions in humans. Acta Tuberc Scand (Suppl) 33:1, 1954.

MacCallum, P., Tolhurst, J. C., Buckle, G., and Sissons, H. A.: A new mycobacterial infection in man. J Pathol Bacteriol 60:93, 1948.

Meyers, W. M., Connor, D. H., McCullough, B., Bourland, J., Morris, R., and Proos, L.: Distribution of *Mycobacterium ulcerans* infections in Zaire, including the report of new foci. Ann Soc Belg Med Trop 54:147, 1974a.

Meyers, W. M., Shelly, W. M., and Connor, D. H.: Heat treatment of *Mycobacterium ulcerans* infections without surgical excision. Am J Trop Med Hyg 23:924, 1974b.

Meyers, W. M., Shelly, W. M., Connor, D. H., and Meyers, E. K.: Human *Mycobacterium ulcerans* infection developing at sites of trauma to skin. Am J Trop Med Hyg 23:919, 1974c.

Miller, W. C., and Toon, R.: *Mycobacterium marinum* in gulf fishermen. Arch Environ Health 27:8, 1973.

Moore, M., and Frerichs, J. B.: An unusual acid-fast infection of the knee with subcutaneous, abscess-like lesions of the gluteal region. Report of a case with a study of the organism, *Mycobacterium abscessus* n. sp. J Invest Dermatol 20:133, 1953.

Palmer, C. E., and Long, M. W.: Effects of infection with atypical mycobacteria on BCG vaccination and tuberculosis. Am Rev Resp Dis 94:553, 1966.

Philpott, J. A., Woodburne, A. R., Philpott, O. S., Schaefer, W. B., and Mollohan, C. S.: Swimming pool granuloma. A study of 290 cases. Arch Dermatol 88:158, 1963.

Schmidt, J. D., Yeager, H., Jr., Smieth, E. B., and Raleigh, J. W.: Cutaneous infection due to a Runyon Group III atypical mycobacterium. Am Rev Resp Dis 106:469, 1972.

Stanford, J. L., Pattyn, S. R., Portaels, F., and Gunthorpe, W. J.: Studies on *Mycobacterium chelonei*. J Med Microbiol 5:177, 1972.

Sybert, A., Tsou, E., and Garagusi, V. R.: Cutaneous infection due to *Mycobacterium szulgai*. Am Rev Resp Dis 115:695, 1977.

Timpe, A., and Runyon, E. H.: Relationship of "atypical" acid-fast bacilli to human disease: Preliminary report. J Lab Clin Med 44:202, 1954.

Uganda Buruli Group: B.C.G. vaccination against *Mycobacterium ulcerans* infection (Buruli ulcer). First results of a trial in Uganda. Lancet 1:111, 1969.

Vandepitte, J., Desmyter, J., and Gatti, F.: Mycobacteria, skins, needles. Lancet 2:691, 1969.

Verhagen, A. R., Koten, J. W., Chaddah, V. K., and Patel, R. I.: Skin diseases in Kenya. A clinical and histopathological study of 3168 patients. Arch Dermatol 98:577, 1968.

Zeligman, I.: *Mycobacterium marinum* granuloma. A disease acquired in the tributaries of Chesapeake Bay. Arch Dermatol 106:26, 1972.

# 214 *SYPHILIS OF THE SKIN*

## *Daniel M. Musher, M.D.*

## *DEFINITION*

Syphilis of the skin results from infection by *Treponema pallidum* during sexual encounters or from hematogenous spread thereafter. The first skin lesion is called a chancre and is limited to the area of inoculation. The disseminated lesions may involve any part of the skin and assume multiple forms. The properties of *T. pallidum* are described in Chapter 49.

## *CLINICAL MANIFESTATIONS AND PATHOLOGY*

Syphilitic chancres are skin lesions that result from intimate, usually sexual, contact and therefore most frequently appear in the genital, perineal, or anal area as well as in and around the mouth; however, any part of the body may be affected. After about three weeks of incubation, one or more papules appear at the site of inoculation. Papules ulcerate within a few days and produce a chancre. The typical syphilitic chancre is 0.5 to 2 cm in diameter, with firm, raised margins and a slight exudate over the central, ulcerated area (Fig. 1). Although chancres are usually round, they may follow tissue lines and become elongated, as seen in lesions around the prepuce or vulvae. Untreated chancres resolve spontaneously after three to six weeks. Although solitary lesions were once thought to be characteristic, multiple lesions frequently occur.

Histologic examination of the papule reveals a relatively acellular center rich in mucopolysaccharides and a periphery infiltrated by polymorphonuclear leukocytes, lymphocytes, and macrophages. As the chancre evolves, the center becomes necrotic, and plasma cells and macro-phages come to predominate at the periphery. Endothelial proliferation and perivascular infiltration by lymphocytes and plasma cells are characteristic of a well-developed lesion.

Disseminated (secondary) syphilis appears three to eight weeks after the appearance of the chancre, presumably as a result of hematogenous dissemination of *T. pallidum* from the primary lesion. Occasionally, disseminated lesions appear before the chancre has resolved completely. At first, there is an evanescent macular rash, which is usually overlooked by the patient, especially if the patient is dark-skinned. A few days later a widespread, symmetric, papular eruption is noted (Fig. 2). The papules are discrete and usually 0.5 to 2 cm in size; they may be smooth, scaly, follicular, or, rarely, pustular, although a papulosquamous appearance is most common. The eruption is red, dusky, or reddish brown. The entire trunk and the extremities, including the palms and soles, are usually involved; lesions on the palms and soles are usually macular and reddish brown, although they may be hyperkeratotic or pustular. Hypo- or hyperpigmentation may be seen. Annular lesions are common in blacks and occur especially on the face (Fig. 3). Mucous membrane lesions in secondary syphilis are small, ulcerated areas with grayish borders that resemble aphthous ulcers but are painless. Condylomas (condyloma lata) are large, flat, whitish, vegetative, and plaque-like confluent lesions that occur in warm, moist areas, especially in the perineal area. Although classically described as a manifestation of disseminated syphilis, condylomas may be seen late in primary infection; in either case they result from local spread of treponemes either from chancres or from disseminated skin lesions. In cases of "malignant" syphilis, disseminated lesions all resemble primary chancres in

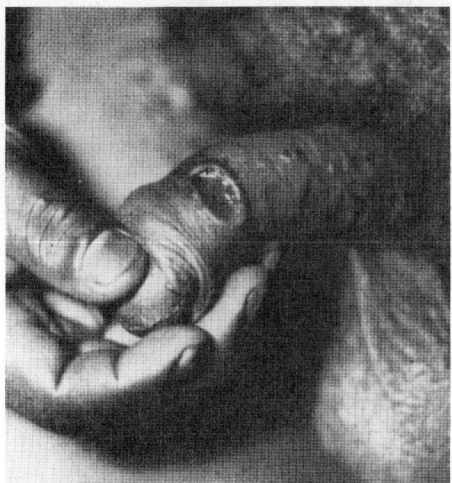

**FIGURE 1.** *Chancre of shaft of penis. (From Howles, J. K.: A Synopsis of Clinical Syphilis. St. Louis, C. V. Mosby Company, 1943.)*

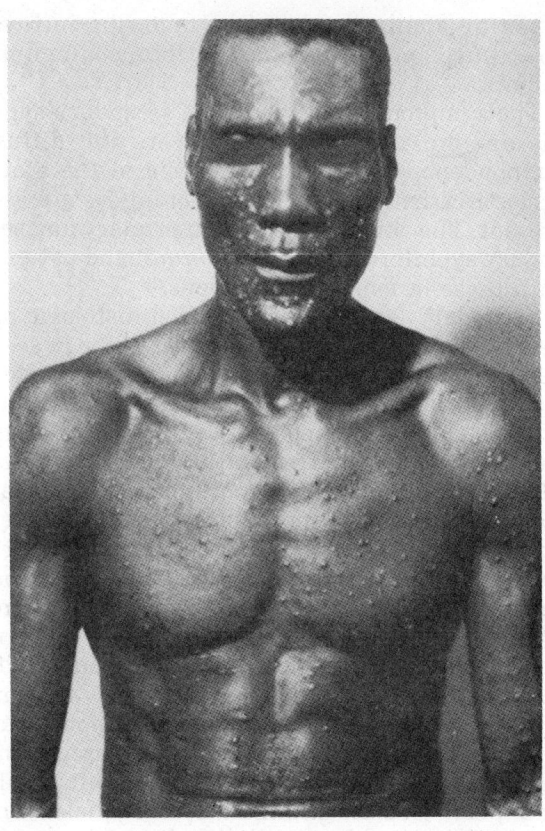

**FIGURE 2.** *Papules of secondary syphilis on trunk, arms, face and forehead. (From Howles, J. K.: A Synopsis of Clinical Syphilis. St. Louis, C. V. Mosby Company, 1943.)*

**FIGURE 3.** *Annular syphilis of secondary syphilis with hyperpigmentation in centers of lesions. (From Howles, J. K.: A Synopsis of Clinical Syphilis. St. Louis, C. V. Mosby Company, 1943.)*

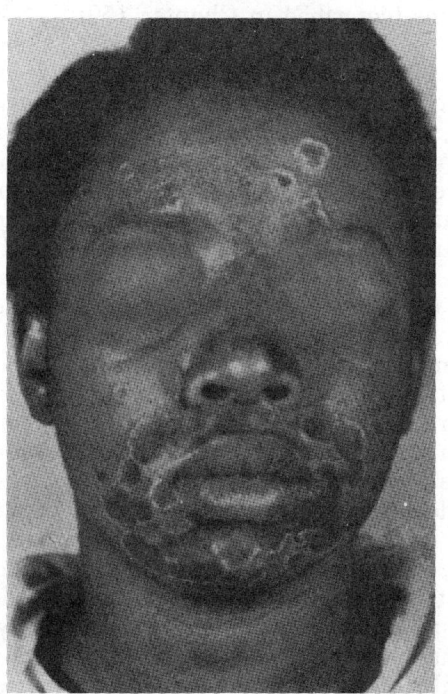

a picture similar to that seen following intravenous infection of *T. pallidum* into nonimmune rabbits.

The symptoms and findings of secondary syphilis are malaise, low-grade fever, and diffuse lymphadenopathy; patchy alopecia of the scalp, periostitis, iritis, and aseptic meningitis are also present. The skin lesions of both primary and secondary syphilis contain *T. pallidum,* and patients with these lesions are contagious.

Secondary lesions have a varied histologic appearance. Inflammatory cells are regularly seen, but the nature of the inflammation varies considerably from case to case. In lesions with the "classic" histologic appearance, plasma cells are the prominent cell. Frequently, however, the infiltrate contains a mixture of lymphocytes, macrophages, and polymorphonuclear leukocytes, and any of these cells may predominate. In a recent study, microabscesses were seen in 20 per cent of secondary lesions. In some cases, macrophages predominate and produce a picture suggestive of histiocytosis. True granulomas with giant cells may also be seen, especially in more chronic lesions, but caseation does not occur. Opinions differ on the frequency of vascular dilation, enlargement of vascular endothelial cells, and perivascular inflammation. Follicles and sweat glands are frequently involved and may be the focal point of histologic abnormalities.

As pointed out in Chapter 150, secondary syphilis is followed by an asymptomatic state called latent syphilis. Late syphilis follows after months or years of latency. Benign late (tertiary) syphilis most commonly involves the skin alone, although other manifestations (described in Chapter 150) such as periostitis, perichondritis, or gummas of other organs may also be present. The pathogenesis of these lesions is obscure. Treponemes are usually not found, and it is believed that an immunologic reaction is responsible. Although there appears to be no relation between the location of primary or disseminated lesions and the location of gummas, tertiary involvement tends to occur in areas that are frequently traumatized. Tertiary skin lesions usually occur singly, although a few asymmetric areas may be involved simultaneously. They most commonly affect the face, neck, and extremities. Indurated, nodular lesions that describe an arc or an irregular full circle are characteristic. Peripheral hyperpigmentation is seen, and there is often central scarring. These lesions may be indolent or aggressive; frequently tissue destruction occurs, producing small nodular ulcers or large, confluent ulcerated areas (Fig. 4). If untreated, these may persist for several years. Late syphilitic lesions are characterized by prominent vascular changes with endothelial proliferation and infiltration by plasma cells, lym-

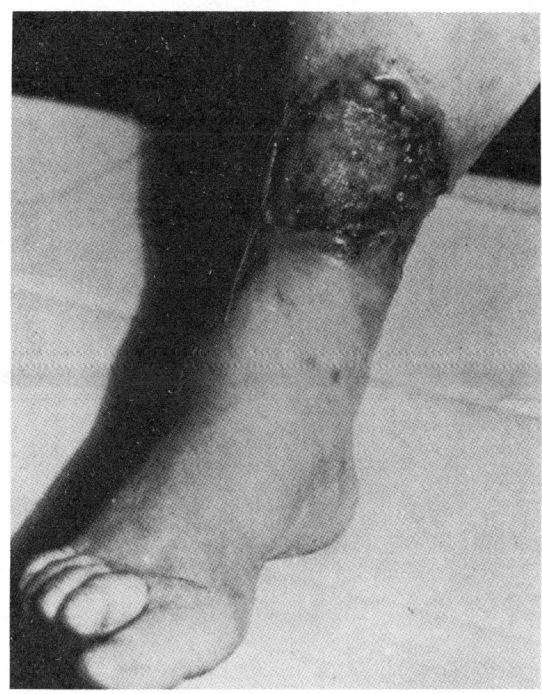

**FIGURE 4.**   *Gumma. (From Howles, J. K.: A Synopsis of Clinical Syphilis. St. Louis, C. V. Mosby Company, 1943.)*

phocytes, histiocytes, and fibroblasts. There are granulomas with epithelioid and giant cells and frequent central necrosis.

## DIAGNOSIS

Syphilitic chancres of the genital area may be confused with herpetic lesions, soft chancre (chancroid), traumatic sores (especially if secondarily infected), fixed drug eruptions, erosions due to Reiter's or Behcet's syndrome, and, rarely, carcinoma or granuloma inguinale. Chancres of the mouth or tongue may resemble aphthous ulcers and similar lesions due to syndromes such as Behçet's. The lack of pain and the general appearance may also suggest carcinoma. Disseminated (secondary) syphilis must be differentiated from other causes of diffuse, symmetric rashes such as acute exanthems, pityriasis rosea, psoriasis, erythema multiforme, allergic reactions, or other dermatitides. The association of diffuse lymphadenopathy and splenomegaly may also raise the possibility of infectious mononucleosis or lymphoma. Late (tertiary) lesions of the skin need to be differentiated from other chronic infections such as tuberculosis, blastomycosis, or leprosy. They may simulate the lesions of discoid lupus erythematosus, especially when they occur on the face. Sarcoidosis, basal cell carcinoma, or cutaneous involvement by lymphoma may cause confusion. Ulcers from stasis or factitious causes must also be differentiated.

The finding of treponemes on dark-field examination of exudate from chancres or from secondary lesions is relatively sensitive and highly specific in establishing the diagnosis of syphilis. Saprophytic spirochetes, which may be found normally in the mouth, may be mistaken for *T. pallidum,* but they usually can be distinguished by their size, coiling, and motility. As mentioned above, treponemes are not found in gummatous lesions. VDRL antibodies are present in 75 per cent of patients with chancres when first seen for the infection, and the VDRL reaction is positive in high titer in virtually all patients with disseminated and late dermatologic disease. The diagnosis of disseminated syphilis of the skin is usually made by physical examination and confirmed by the VDRL reaction, since it may be difficult to obtain an adequate specimen for dark-field examination. The fluorescent treponemal antibody absorption (FTA-ABS) test is positive in 90 per cent of patients when they seek medical attention for a chancre. This test is positive in all those with secondary or tertiary skin disease and is most useful in evaluating skin lesions resembling those of syphilis but caused by a disease like systemic lupus erythematosus, which produces a false-positive VDRL. The *treponema pallidum* agglutinating test is easier to perform than, and gives results comparable to, the FTA-ABS, which it is replacing in many laboratories.

## TREATMENT

Primary and secondary syphilis are both treated with one injection of 2.4 million units of benzathine penicillin. Patients who are allergic to this drug may receive erythromycin or tetracycline orally in a dose of 500 mg four times daily for 15 days. Treponemes have been eradicated from chancres within a few hours of the first antibiotic dose. Late syphilis is treated with 2.4 million units of benzathine penicillin each week for three weeks. Patients who are allergic to penicillin should be given 500 mg of tetracycline or erythromycin by mouth four times daily for 30 days. Skin lesions in both early and late forms resolve promptly once proper treatment has been initiated.

### References

Abell, E., Marks, R., and Jones, E. W.: Secondary syphilis: A clinico-pathological review. Br J Dermatol 93:53, 1975.

Chapel, T. A.: The variability of syphilitic chancre. Sex Transm Dis 5:68, 1978.

Jeerapaet, P., and Ackerman, B. A.: Histologic patterns of secondary syphilis. Arch Dermatol 107:373, 1973.

Olansky, S.: Late benign syphilis (gumma). In Youmans, J. B.(ed.): Syphilis and other venereal diseases. Med Clin North Am 48 (3):653, 1964.

Olansky, S., and Norins, L. C.: Venereal diseases: Syphilis and other treponematosis. In Fitzpatrick, T. B. et al.(eds.): Dermatology in General Medicine. New York, McGraw Hill Book Company, 1971, pp. 1955–1989.

Pariser, R. J., and Mehr, K. A.: Pustules in secondary syphilis. Sex Transm Dis 5:115, 1978.

# *YAWS, PINTA, AND BEJEL* **215**
## *Peter M. Moodie, M.D., B.S., D.T.M. & H.*

### DEFINITIONS

Yaws, pinta, and bejel are endemic nonvenereal treponemal infections of humans (treponematoses). They share many clinical, pathologic, and immunologic features with venereal syphilis, and the causative treponemes are morphologically identical to each other and to *Treponema pallidum* (Chapter 49).

The endemic treponematoses are characterized by a superficial primary lesion at the site of inoculation and secondary, blood-borne, satellite lesions that are usually superficial. Destructive granulomas of skin, subcutaneous tissues, bones, and joints are tertiary manifestations of yaws and bejel, and pigmented tertiary skin changes of pinta.

Yaws, pinta, and bejel constitute a clinical and pathologic spectrum of diseases in which bejel most resembles venereal syphilis, pinta least resembles venereal syphilis, and yaws occupies an intermediate position. Differentiation of the treponematoses, including venereal syphilis (Chapter 214), is based on clinical, epidemiologic, and geographic considerations and may be difficult in the individual case.

*Yaws* (frambesia, pian, buba, bouba, parangi) is a disease of the humid tropics throughout the world. *Pinta* (carate, mal del pinto, tian, lota, azul) is confined to parts of Latin America and the Caribbean. *Bejel* (or endemic syphilis) occurs in cooler, drier climates in all regions of the world except the Americas, under a variety of local names—for example, bejel or balash in the Mid-

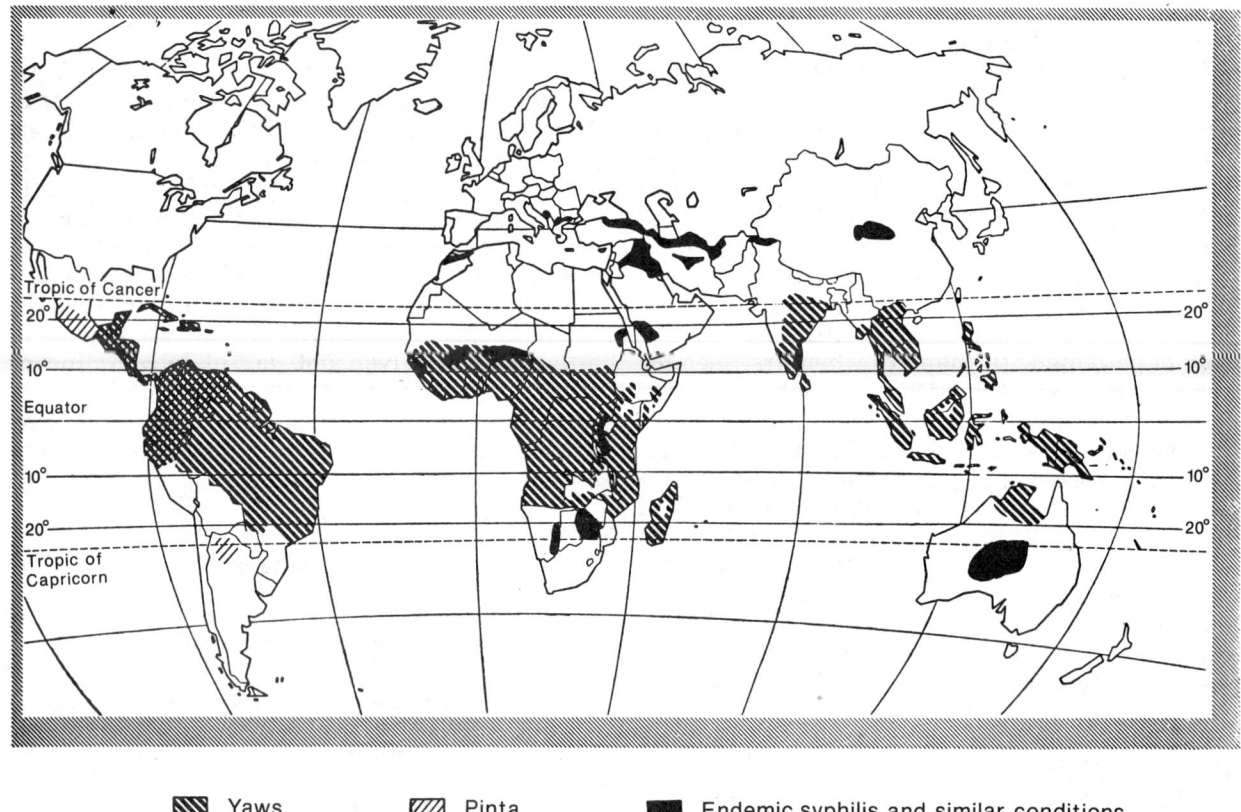

NN Yaws          ///// Pinta          ■ Endemic syphilis and similar conditions

**FIGURE 1.** *Geographical distribution of the endemic treponematoses about 1950, at the beginning of the WHO-supported mass eradication campaign. (Modified from World Health Organization: International Work in Endemic Treponematoses and Venereal Infections 1948–1963. Geneva, World Health Organization, 1965.)*

dle East, dichuchwa in Botswana, irkintja in Central Australia, njovera in Rhodesia, siti in Gambia, and skerlievo in Bosnia.

Once widespread throughout the rural tropics and subtropics (Fig. 1), the endemic treponematoses were greatly reduced in incidence or eradicated locally by mass treatment campaigns with penicillin. However, they still occur in remote rural communities with poor hygiene, and their sequelae may be encountered in areas where the endemic infection has been eradicated.

## ETIOLOGY

The treponemes cannot be cultured on artificial media or otherwise distinguished from each other in the laboratory but have been given the following specific names: *Treponema pertenue* (yaws), *Treponema carateum* (pinta), and *Treponema pallidum* (bejel, endemic syphilis). Sometimes the agent of bejel is referred to as *T. pallidum II* or *T. pallidum endemicum* to distinguish it from *T. pallidum* of venereal syphilis.

There is a continuing controversy about the origins and interrelationships of the treponematoses. Hackett (1963) believes that they have all evolved from pinta over about 15,000 years into distinct treponemal species with relatively fixed disease-producing characteristics. Hudson (1958) holds that they all derived from a yaws-like disease in Africa about 100,000 years ago and that the organisms are no more than intraspecific strains of *T. pallidum*. Willcox (1974) considers the evolution of treponemal diseases to be continuing through the natural selection of strains suited to local conditions and modes of transmission. Turner and Hollander (1957) have demonstrated characteristic, but not particularly consistent, differences in the lesions produced by inoculating and passing the treponemes of syphilis, yaws, and bejel in laboratory hamsters and rabbits. Pinta treponemes did not produce lesions and could not be passed in these animals, but Kuhn et al. (1968) have produced typical pinta lesions in inoculated chimpanzees.

The reservoir of yaws, pinta, and bejel is humans. Yaws may have an additional animal reservoir of unknown significance in human disease, in West African cynocephalic baboons (Hardy, 1976). In endemic areas, the incidence of yaws is highest in children, who therefore form the main reservoir. The main reservoir of pinta is older children and young adults.

## PATHOGENESIS AND PATHOLOGY

### Source

The sources of the infectious agents of yaws, pinta, and bejel are cases with active primary or secondary lesions, which are usually on the skin in yaws and pinta and in the mouth or on the lips in bejel.

Because treponemes are fragile and are very easily killed by drying, they are short-lived in the external environment. They survive best in serum or living cellular material, and the diseases are usually acquired by direct contact of the abraded or minimally injured epithelium with an exudative lesion. Pinta lesions are not normally exudative but are characteristically pruritic. Scratching the lesions causes oozing of infectious serum.

### Indirect Transmission

Indirect transmission of bejel may occur through shared eating and drinking utensils, toothpicks, and tobacco pipes, as well as by kissing or biting. Biting insects may play a part in the mechanical transmission of pinta, and sucking flies in the transmission of yaws and bejel. The fingers of children may also transfer infection. Child-to-mother transmission of yaws and bejel is not uncommon. Indirect skin-to-skin spread by way of floors, furniture, clothing, bedding, or the ground underfoot is unlikely unless the time interval between contamination and inoculation is very brief.

Venereal transmission is rare because of the rarity of genital lesions in adults. Congenital transmission does not occur.

### Susceptibility and Immunity

Susceptibility is general. More than 80 per cent of adults in highly endemic areas may show serologic evidence of past infection. Susceptibility is altered by acquired immunity, but in a variable and unpredictable manner. Cross-immunity occurs between each of the endemic treponematoses (particularly yaws and bejel) and between the endemic treponematoses and venereal syphilis but is not complete and may be overcome by a large inoculum of treponemes. Immunity to homologous strains of treponemes is stronger and develops more rapidly but is also incomplete.

### Incubation Period

In most cases the time from inoculation to the appearance of the primary lesion varies from a few weeks to a few months. The results of animal studies suggest that the incubation period is directly related to the size of the infecting dose, which may be as small as a single organism.

### Pathology of Primary Infection

As in venereal syphilis, the basic pathologic processes in the endemic treponematoses may be grouped into three characteristic but often overlapping stages. The primary stage includes the relatively slow development of an inflammatory reaction at the inoculation site. During this stage, organisms multiply in the primary lesion, spread to the regional lymph nodes and the blood, and are disseminated throughout the body. Histopathologically, early edema of the corium is followed by infiltration with lymphocytes, plasma cells, and polymorphonuclear leukocytes associated with micro-abscesses. Unless it is secondarily infected, the primary lesion heals slowly with minimal scarring.

### Pathology of Secondary Lesions

Yaws and bejel, but not pinta, may pass through a latent phase before the appearance of secondary lesions. The usual sites of secondary lesions are the skin in pinta, the skin and subperiosteum in yaws, and the skin, subperiosteum, and mucous membranes in bejel. The secondary lesions usually contain numerous treponemes but show a greater and more accelerated tissue reaction than primary lesions. They develop and heal faster than the primary lesions in yaws and bejel and induce pronounced hyperplasia (of epithelium or periosteum) and marked perivascular, round-cell cuffing. Allergic reactions of the syphilide ("ide") type may also occur, particularly in bejel and yaws. These lesions contain very few treponemes and are probably not infectious.

### Pathology of the Tertiary Stage

Tertiary lesions are usually grossly destructive (gummas of skin, subcutaneous tissues, or bone in yaws and bejel) or grossly hyperplastic (hyperkeratosis or hyperostosis in yaws and bejel; hyperkeratosis and hyperpigmentation in pinta). Bone lesions commonly show a mixture of hyperplastic and destructive processes. Superficial gummas commonly ulcerate. The histopathology features necrosis, epithelioid and giant-cell aggregation, capillary obstruction, and fibrous tissue scarring. Surface scars are usually depigmented.

The histopathologic aspects of the three stages may be viewed as the result of three grades of immunologic response to treponemes: (1) slowly developing cell-mediated immunity and relatively ineffective humoral immunity in the primary stage; (2) fairly effective cell-mediated and humoral immunity in the secondary stage; and (3) a late, cell-mediated local hypersensitivity reaction to a few surviving treponemes in the tertiary stage.

## CLINICAL MANIFESTATIONS

The following descriptions emphasize the typical clinical features of the various stages of the endemic treponematoses. Atypical lesions are common in the individual case, and the stages may overlap. Very few clinical manifestations are unique to a particular treponemal disease, including venereal syphilis. With the probable exception of Bosnian endemic syphilis (now eradicated), the endemic treponematoses do not attack the central nervous system, the eye, the cardiovascular system, or the abdominal viscera (Turner, 1959).

### Primary Infection

The primary papilloma of yaws ("mother yaw") usually occurs on the lower leg, face, or arm in children and may also occur on the breast or hip of nonimmune women nursing infected children. The lesion begins as a papule, without prodromal or general symptoms, and evolves slowly and rel-

atively painlessly into a raised pseudogranulomatous lesion as large as 8 cm in diameter. It appears to be bursting through the skin, and oozes serum or becomes covered with a thin, tough scab. Untreated, it may take 6 to 12 months to heal and usually leaves a faint, slightly pitted circular scar. It is usually accompanied by moderate, nontender regional lymphadenopathy.

The primary oral lesion of bejel is seldom noticed. On the lips, nipple, or elsewhere on the skin it is similar to an extragenital chancre of venereal syphilis.

The primary lesion of pinta is an itchy red papule, usually on the exposed skin of the dorsum of the foot or hand. It occurs rarely on the trunk. It spreads slowly and becomes more raised and scaly but never ulcerates unless it is scratched or injured. Regional lymph nodes may enlarge. The primary lesion usually persists for years, overlapping with the secondary manifestations and eventually becoming indistinguishable from them.

### Secondary Manifestations

In yaws, multiple secondary lesions may appear either before the primary lesion heals or up to several years later. Their appearance is accompanied by fever, malaise, bone and joint pains, and headache. The skin lesions vary in appearance from large, oozing or crusted papillomas that resemble the typical primary lesion (Fig. 2) to small, scattered or diffuse papular lesions like syphilides. Hyperplastic subperiosteal changes

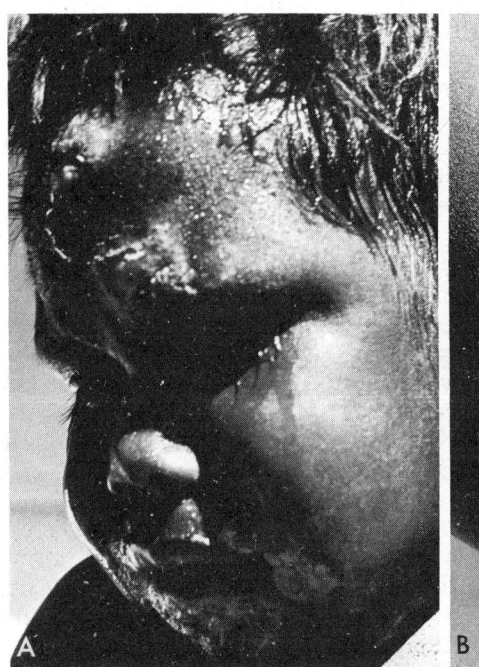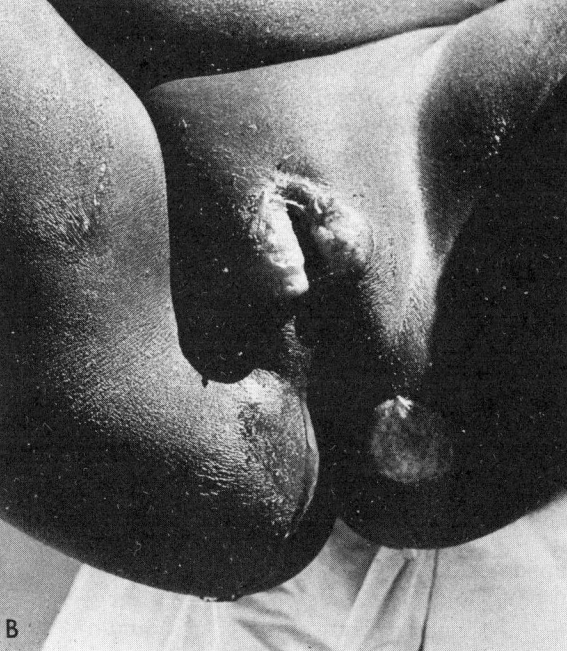

**FIGURE 2.** A and B, Secondary yaws: papillomas of face, genitalia, and buttocks.

with or without small foci of rarefaction may be visible in x-rays, particularly of the anterior cortex of the tibia, the ulna, and the small bones of the hands and feet. Scaly or papillomatous lesions of the soles and palms are not uncommon. General lymphadenopathy is common. The lesions heal in a few months, usually without permanent structural change or scarring.

In pinta, pruritic, erythematous macules or papules erupt 5 to 12 months after the first appearance of the primary lesion. They are usually widespread and are accompanied by generalized lymphadenopathy. The lesions persist without intervening latency, but they often appear in crops that later coalesce into irregular patterns. Plantar and palmar hyperkeratoses have been reported only in Cuban pinta. Pigmentation in various colors appears as the lesions enter the tertiary stage.

In bejel, secondary manifestations include macular and papular rashes (syphilides), condylomatous papillomas in the skin folds, "split papules" at the corners of the mouth, oral mucous patches, laryngitis and pharyngitis, periostitis, and generalized lymphadenopathy. Scaly lesions of the palms and soles may also appear. Relapses, especially of the "-ide" lesions, may alternate with periods of latency over several years. Bone pain is common in some populations.

### Tertiary Manifestations

Tertiary yaws and bejel cause nodular or ulcerative necrosis (gummas of skin and subcutaneous tissue); gummas and subperiosteal thickening of the long bones, and plantar hyperkeratosis (Fig. 3). Nasopalatal destructive lesions (gangosa), de-

struction of joints (particularly the interphalangeal joints in yaws), and mobile soft tissue nodules near the joints (juxta-articular nodes) occur in both diseases, but are more common in yaws. Healed ulcerative lesions leave thin depigmented scars (Hackett, 1957; Hackett and Loewenthal, 1960).

Tertiary pinta lesions are generally limited to dyspigmented patches (gray, black, bluish, purplish, red, coppery), which may heal spontaneously or become depigmented (leukodermic) in the center before they heal as atrophic white patches. Aortitis has been reported in some cases of Cuban pinta.

The progress of untreated treponemal diseases through the three stages is not inevitable. Primary lesions may be so insignificant that they are never noticed, and spontaneous cure during one of the periods of latency before the onset of tertiary manifestations is the rule rather than the exception in yaws and bejel.

## COMPLICATIONS AND SEQUELAE

Complications and sequelae are uncommon in the primary and secondary stages. Joint effusions may occur in yaws and bejel. Respiratory obstruction and dysphagia have been reported in bejel due to extensive laryngeal or pharyngeal involvement during the secondary stage (Hudson, 1958). Plantar hyperkeratosis or papillomas in secondary yaws and bejel may become ulcerated and make walking painful and difficult. The minor subperiosteal changes in secondary yaws and bejel and the very rare massive periostitis of the nasal processes of the maxillae (goundou) are mainly of cosmetic importance.

Functional handicaps may follow secondarily infected skin lesions that ulcerate and cause deep scarring and contractures. Polydactylitis in childhood yaws may be temporarily disabling.

Destructive tertiary lesions of bone and subcutaneous and submucous tissues in yaws and bejel are responsible for nearly all the serious permanent sequelae in the endemic treponematoses. Spontaneous fractures may occur and heal imperfectly. Gross bony deformities, particularly of the tibia and ulna; destruction or partial resorption of the phalanges, metacarpals, metatarsals, and tarsal bones (Fig. 4); palatal perforation; pharyngeal stenosis; and scar-tissue contractures of joints, tendons, and fascia may be severely disabling. Gangosa, a massive and grossly mutilating gummatous destruction of the nose, mouth, nasal septum, palate, and pharynx is a late complication of yaws and occasionally of bejel (Fig. 5).

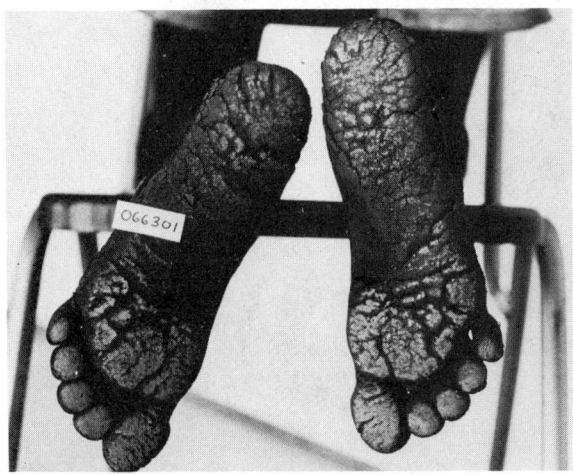

**FIGURE 3.**  *Tertiary yaws: plantar hyperkeratosis.*

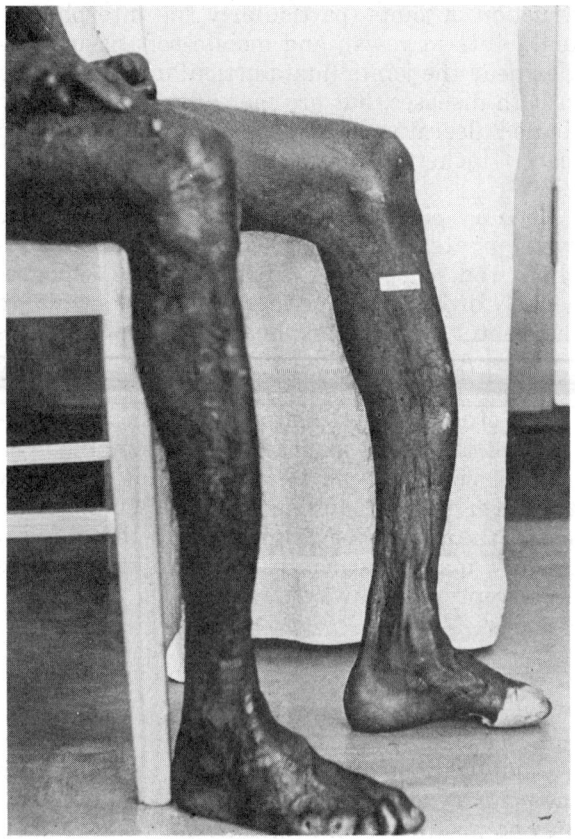

**FIGURE 4.** *Tertiary yaws: tibial osteitis and bowing; contractures and partial resorption of phalanges.*

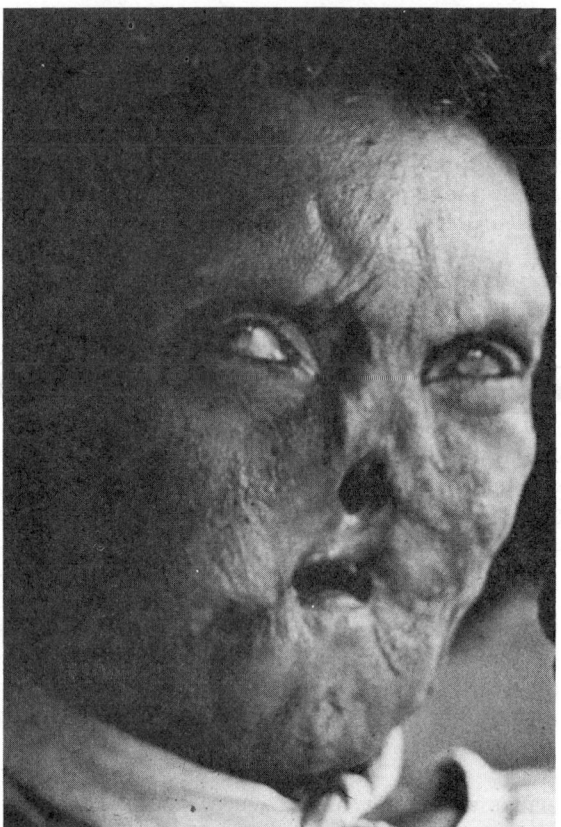

**FIGURE 5.** *Tertiary yaws: facial scarring following gangosa.*

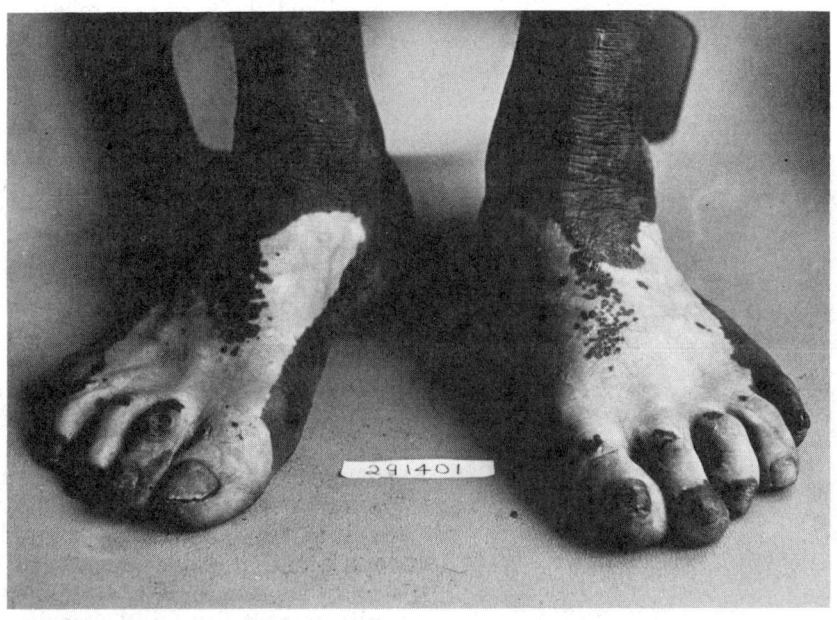

**FIGURE 6.** *Tertiary yaws: symmetrical depigmentation of feet.*

The sequelae of pinta are patches of permanently depigmented, atrophic areas of skin. Similar sequelae may occur in yaws and bejel (Fig. 6).

## GEOGRAPHIC VARIATIONS

Variations in the clinical features of the endemic treponematoses appear to be related more to climate, clothing, behavior, and life style than to geography or race in the usual sense. These factors may act to select strains, but they certainly also influence the age of onset and the site and type of primary (and possibly secondary and tertiary) lesions. Because all treponemes are highly sensitive to penicillin, the tetracyclines, erythromycin, chloramphenicol, and other antibiotics, local variations in the extent and frequency of general exposure to these antibiotics (for any kind of infection) is another potent factor that influences the pattern of clinical treponemal disease. The "incidental" cure of many treponemal infections at an early stage in their evolution decreases the rate of transmission as well as the incidence of late disease and complications. There is no evidence anywhere in the world of development of resistance by treponemes to antibiotics.

The geographic variation of greatest significance is the restriction of pinta to the Americas, where today it is a disease of remote jungle Amerindian communities in Mexico, Venezuela, Colombia, Peru, and Ecuador, and probably in parts of Argentina, Chile, Dominican Republic and Haiti (Willcox, 1976).

## DIAGNOSIS

The firm diagnosis of one of the nonvenereal treponematoses depends on establishing two or more of the following: (1) a history of exposure to the disease; (2) appropriate clinical or radiologic findings; (3) the presence of typical treponemes; and (4) treponemal seroreactivity. The diagnosis is most difficult to establish in patients with early primary lesions, atypical secondary lesions, and latent disease discovered by routine serologic screening.

In all suspected cases, a history of contact with other cases or residence in an endemic area should be pursued. In possible secondary, latent, and tertiary disease, a history of earlier lesions should be sought and a search made for a primary scar and minor abnormalities of bone and skin. In adult latent or tertiary disease, evidence of neurologic and cardiovascular syphilis should be specifically excluded before making the diagnosis of endemic treponematosis.

An essential step in early primary infection is darkfield microscopy of fresh exudate or a saline suspension of material swabbed or scraped from the lesion. This can confirm the presence of treponemes before serologic tests become positive, but it is also important in later primary and secondary stages. If darkfield microscopy is unsuccessful, immunofluorescent staining of scrapings or biopsy material may confirm the presence of treponemes. Treponemes are rarely found in "–ide" lesions, but may be found in lymph node aspirates in the secondary stage.

All the serologic tests for venereal syphilis become positive after three to four weeks in yaws and bejel, and during the secondary rash in pinta. Nonspecific reactions such as the Cardiolipin Wassermann reaction (CWR), Venereal Disease Research Laboratory (VDRL) test, rapid plasma reagin (RPR) test, and the Reiter protein complement fixation (RPCF) test may be converted to false positivity by other tropical diseases, and should be confirmed by treponeme-specific tests such as the fluorescent treponemal antibody-absorption (FTA-ABS) test, the *Treponema pallidum* hemagglutination (TPHA) test, or the *Treponema pallidum* immobilization (TPI) test. Quantitative versions of the serologic tests are helpful in evaluating current or recent disease activity and the evidence for spontaneous or therapeutic cure.

Venereal syphilis is generally increasing in incidence in areas where endemic treponematosis has been reduced, and the two diseases may coexist in the same community. In these areas, a specific diagnosis of one or the other may be often impossible without a detailed and accurate history.

## TREATMENT

Penicillin is the antibiotic of choice unless it is contraindicated by allergy. Primary and secondary stages of yaws and bejel and all stages of pinta respond rapidly and completely to a single intramuscular injection of long-acting penicillin. The recommended adult dose is 1.2 mega units of procaine penicillin G in oil with 2 per cent aluminum monostearate (PAM), or 1.2 mega units of benzathine penicillin. Infected children and adult household contacts should receive 0.6 mega units, and child contacts 0.3 mega units. Standard four- to five-day courses of tetracycline or erythromycin may be substituted.

Late latent and tertiary yaws and bejel should be treated in the same way as late venereal syphilis; for example, PAM or benzathine penicillin 0.6 mega units twice weekly or daily for 15 to 20 doses.

Local treatment of early lesions is usually unnecessary. Reconstructive surgery may be indicated in late tertiary yaws and bejel with deformities.

## PROPHYLAXIS

Individual prophylaxis depends entirely on attention to personal hygiene and appropriate precautions when in contact with early cases. Community prophylaxis is important and depends on general improvement of living conditions, case finding, and treatment of cases and contacts (particularly household contacts). Early latent cases of yaws and bejel may exceed clinical cases by ratios of 5:1 or more. For this reason, community protection cannot be achieved by clinical case finding alone.

Public health authorities should be notified of cases diagnosed in hospitals and clinics even in areas where it is not a statutory requirement.

## References

Hackett, C. J.: An International Nomenclature of Yaws Lesions. Monograph Series No. 36. Geneva, World Health Organization, 1957.
Hackett, C. J.: On the origin of the human treponematoses. Bull WHO 29:7, 1963.
Hackett, C. J., and Loewenthal, L. J. A.: Differential Diagnosis of Yaws. Monograph Series No. 45. Geneva, World Health Organization, 1960.
Hardy, P. H.: Pathogenic treponemes. In Johnson, R. C. (ed.): The Biology of the Parasitic Spirochetes. New York, Academic Press, 1976, p. 107.
Hudson, E. H.: Non-Venereal Syphilis: A Sociological and Medical Study of Bejel. London, E. & S. Livingstone Ltd., 1958.
Kuhn, U. S. G., Varela, G., Chandler, F. W., and Bsuna, C. G.: Experimental pinta in the chimpanzee. JAMA 206:829, 1968.
Turner, L. H.: Notes on the Treponematoses with an Illustrated Account of Yaws. Bulletin No. 9, Institute for Medical Research, Federation of Malaya. Kuala Lumpur, Government Press, 1959.
Turner, T. B., and Hollander, D. H.: The Biology of the Treponematoses. Monograph Series No. 35. Geneva, World Health Organization, 1957.
Willcox, R. R.: Changing patterns of treponemal disease. Br J Vener Dis 50:169, 1974.
Willcox, R. R.: The epidemiology of the spirochetoses: A worldwide view. In Johnson, R. C. (ed.): The Biology of the Parasitic Spirochetes. New York, Academic Press, 1976, p. 133.

# 216 LOAIASIS

## B. A. Southgate, M.B., B.S., F.F.C.M.

### DEFINITION

Loaiasis is the state of infection with the filarial nematode *Loa loa*. This infection is confined to the equatorial rain forest regions of West and Central Africa, particularly cleared areas on the edge of natural forests where trees such as rubber have been planted. One exception is the focus situated in moist savanna in the southwest of Sudan.

The principal countries affected by loaiasis are Zaire, Cameroon, Angola, Gabon, Congo (Brazzaville), Central African Empire, Chad, and Sudan. Autochthonous cases have been reported from Equatorial Guinea, Sierra Leone, Guinea, Ghana, Benin, Ruanda, Burundi, and Senegal, but infection in these countries is very rare and some reports require confirmation. In East Africa the infection is rare, but cases have been reported from Uganda, Ethiopia, Zambia, and Malawi.

### ETIOLOGY

The causative agent of loaiasis, *L. loa* is transmitted to man by the bites of large tabanid flies of the genus *Chrysops*. The most important species involved are *C. silacea* and *C. dimidiata,* but all species of *Chrysops* can transmit *L. loa. C.*

*zahrai* and *C. distinctipennis* may be locally important vectors, and *C. langi, C. centurionis,* and *C. longicornis* are subjects of current research as possible vectors.

*L. loa* is closely related to a number of other sibling species of the same genus that infect nonhuman primates, particularly baboons, mandrills, vervet monkeys, and gorillas in endemic regions. Although occasional cases of human infection are acquired from other primates, it seems certain that human loaiasis is primarily an anthroponosis, and the problems of an animal reservoir of infection can be ignored in considering etiology and control.

### PATHOGENESIS AND PATHOLOGY

All three phases of the life cycle of *L. loa* that occur in the human body can be involved in the pathogenesis of loaiasis. The most serious and sometimes fatal pathologic lesions occur as a result of either the human immune response to the parasite or specific drug treatment of the infection.

A characteristic wheal frequently appears at the site of an infected *Chrysops* bite if infective third-stage larvae from the vector reach the subcutaneous tissues. This wheal is particularly pronounced in previously infected subjects and may progress to a small induration lasting for several days in heavily infected individuals. The lesion, which results from both immediate and delayed hypersensitivity, indicates the presence of circulating IgE or reaginic antibody and a well-developed, cell-mediated immune response to the infective larvae of *L. loa*.

The most common and widely studied lesions of loaiasis are associated with subcutaneous and transocular migrations of the sexually mature adult worms. These give rise to transient episodes of local tissue inflammation and edema. The swellings usually range in size from 2 to 20 cm in diameter, but occasionally involve a whole limb, most often the arm. The exact pathogenesis of these tissue reactions is still uncertain. Some workers hold that they are a response to mechanical damage of the tissues by the rapid (at least 1 cm/minute) movement of the large adult worms. Others postulate that they result from the immunologic lysis of large numbers of microfilariae shortly after they are produced by the migrating adult female. Histologic sections usually contain adult worms, surrounded by an edematous reaction containing polymorphonuclear neutrophils and eosinophils, plasma cells, and macrophages. Sometimes a dead adult worm will be seen. In these cases, the reaction tends to be lymphocytic, producing a granuloma and later a fibrous nodule.

The third main element in the pathogenesis of loaiasis is the interaction between the embryo worms or microfilariae and either circulating antimicrofilarial IgG antibodies or the specific therapeutic drug diethylcarbamazine citrate. The two most important organs in which these reactions occur are the kidneys and the brain.

Renal damage can be demonstrated by the presence of proteinuria, microfilariae in the urine, and occasionally the nephrotic syndrome. Proteinuria is often provoked or made worse by administration of diethylcarbamazine. Two theories have been proposed to explain the glomerular lesions: penetration of and mechanical damage by circulating microfilariae, and precipitation of antigen-antibody complexes on the glomerular endothelium.

A more severe and sometimes fatal aspect of loaiasis is the production of meningoencephalitis by the administration (often unsupervised self-administration) of diethylcarbamazine to patients with high-density microfilaremia. The syndrome does occur rarely without drug therapy, probably due to specific immune responses. Diethylcarbamazine causes massive invasion of the cerebrospinal fluid by microfilariae when it is administered to heavily infected persons. Cerebral hypoxia and coma result from capillary obstruction by masses of moribund or dead microfilariae. Two distinct pathologic features are seen in fatal cases: an acute and diffuse edema of the brain with many occluded capillaries, and localized, partially necrotic granulomas containing much microfilarial debris. These chronic granulomas appear to be long-standing reactions around dying microfilariae, and their presence in the brain may determine whether diethylcarbamazine administration will precipitate an episode of acute meningoencephalitis. Some workers have attributed the cerebral lesions in loaiasis to a Jarisch-Herxheimer type reaction caused by the liberation of enormous quantities of specific neurotropic somatic toxins from microfilariae by diethylcarbamazine. The histologic evidence, however, indicates that such a mechanism could only be secondary in importance to cerebral hypoxia and edema resulting from capillary blockade. A frequent complication of meningoencephalitis in loaiasis is retinal hemorrhage and retinal exudates. Although the exact mechanism is obscure, it is probably associated with raised intracranial venous pressure. Retinal lesions occur most often in individuals with pre-existing retinopathy of another cause.

A report from Nigeria implicates *L. loa* as the etiologic agent of a form of endomyocardial fibrosis associated with eosinophilia, fever, skin irritation, and transient localized subcutaneous swellings, particularly of the face. This report clearly needs further investigation.

## CLINICAL MANIFESTATIONS

The hypersensitivity reactions associated with the entry of infective *L. loa* larvae into the body after *Chrysops* bites can cause intense itching and irritation. The scratching of infected material into this painful site may be an important cause of secondary pyoderma in areas of high *Chrysops* density and loaiasis transmission.

Between 6 and 12 months after entry into the body, worms attain sexual maturity and start their migrations through the connective tissues. The pathologic reactions to these migrations, which are mainly subcutaneous, give rise to the most common clinical effect of loaiasis, the so-called Calabar swelling. This is a firm area of edema, usually painless but sometimes showing signs of acute inflammation and becoming hot, tender, and painful. The swellings are often accompanied by pruritus and fever and, if they occur near a joint, can cause limitation of movement. Calabar swellings are most frequent on the hands and arms, but patients complain most vigorously when they occur on the face, particularly the bridge of the nose. They can, however, occur on any part of the body. Swelling is usually transient, lasting a few days or rarely a few weeks, and has often been graphically described as a "hen's egg" or "wasp sting" swelling. Less commonly, worm migrations produce fugitive swelling of a complete limb, usually the arm.

Transocular migration of adult worms is a common phenomenon, and the worms are easily seen migrating across the conjunctiva. Their presence can cause painful conjunctivitis and lacrimation.

At any stage of loaiasis, subcutaneous or deep abscesses may occur, usually in areas of inflammation surrounding a dead adult worm.

Proteinuria is common in loaiasis, and a fully developed nephrotic syndrome occurs occasionally. Both may be precipitated or exacerbated by diethylcarbamazine therapy.

Meningoencephalitis appears as a severe and progressive headache leading rapidly to coma. It is most common in heavily infected adults and is usually provoked by diethylcarbamazine treatment. However, it must be stressed that a history of drug treatment may be impossible to obtain, since the drug is widely sold by retail stores in endemic areas. Furthermore, self-medication may have a totally different objective from the treatment of loaiasis, for diethylcarbamazine frequently causes the visible expulsion of some intestinal roundworms in feces, and patients or their relatives may not connect the taking of a "worm" medicine with questions about self-treatment for Calabar swellings or pruritus. Retinal hemorrhage is always a grave prognostic sign in cerebral loaiasis. Even after recovery, there is usually complete or partial blindness.

## COMPLICATIONS AND SEQUELAE

The main complications and sequelae of long-standing loaiasis are lichenification of the skin in areas where multiple Calabar swellings have occurred. Abscesses, meningoencephalitis, and renal complications have been described above.

## GEOGRAPHIC VARIATIONS IN DISEASE

The only geographic variations recorded in the clinical picture of loaiasis relate to the local intensities of transmission, and hence to the numbers of live adult worms and microfilariae in the body at any given time. The frequency of clinical manifestations, their severity, and the frequency of complications are directly correlated with worm burdens. No evidence has yet been presented of geographic strain variation in the pathogenicity of L. loa.

## DIAGNOSIS

The typical history of loaiasis is diagnostic, given the fugitive swellings with or without pain and fever, and the occasional dramatic migration of an adult worm across the eye. Worms in the conjunctiva or under the skin can be easily removed surgically under local anesthesia and identified by a parasitologist.

A definitive diagnosis of loaiasis can be made only by recovery and identification of the adult worms or the typical sheathed microfilariae in peripheral blood. However, it must be remembered that many patients with loaiasis are amicrofilaremic, either because they have unisexual infections or because a very light infection with both sexes has not permitted mating. Further, a vigorous immune response appears to render a few heavily infected persons amicrofilaremic. Conversely, many persons with microfilaremia may have no signs or symptoms of clinical loaiasis.

Since the microfilariae of L. loa are diurnally periodic, blood samples for examination should be taken as close as possible to 12 noon. Microfilariae must be counted as well as identified in blood samples of known volume in order to plan treatment schedules for the individual patient and to assess the effectiveness of control measures in community surveys. Depending on the desired degree of sensitivity, blood sample sizes are usually 20 $mm^3$, 100 $mm^3$, 1 ml, or 10 ml. The first two sample volumes are usually obtained by stylet puncture of skin to produce capillary blood from the finger, thumb, heel, or earlobe. Volumes of 1 ml or 10 ml require venipuncture. Three main methods for processing the blood are available: smearing, fixing, and staining on a glass microscope slide; hemolysis and counting in a counting-chamber; or concentration and filtration through a Millipore or Nuclepore membrane. Details of the techniques can be found in textbooks of medical helminthology such as Muller (1975).

Hypereosinophilia of 60 to 90 per cent (20,000 to 50,000 per $mm^3$) is common in loaiasis and is useful as confirmatory evidence in diagnosis. Serodiagnosis and skin testing are the subjects of intensive research but for the present are too nonspecific to be of value to the practitioner.

## TREATMENT

The drug of choice in the treatment of loaiasis is diethylcarbamazine. In different dosages, it is effective against all the life-cycle stages of L. loa that occur in humans—adult worms, microfilariae, and infective larvae. Diethylcarbamazine has no effect on L. loa in vitro. In vivo, it is an extremely effective microfilaricide in small doses, apparently inducing an opsonin-like effect which sensitizes microfilariae to destruction by phagocytes, primarily the Kupffer cells in the liver. In larger doses it kills adult worms more slowly, apparently by inducing them to migrate to the dermis, where they are killed by a mechanism akin to that of a foreign body reaction.

Dosage schedules in loaiasis should be planned according to circulating microfilarial densities. Dosages refer to oral administration of diethylcarbamazine citrate, and are planned to bring about radical cure in adults.

1. For amicrofilaremic patients:

    Day 1, 50 mg in one dose
    Day 2, 100 mg in one dose
    Day 3, 200 mg in divided doses every 12 hours
    Day 4, 400 mg in divided doses every 12 hours
    Day 5 to day 26, 600 mg in divided doses three times daily

2. For microfilaremic patients with less than 30 microfilariae per $mm^3$ blood:

    Day 1, 6.25 mg ⎫
    Day 2, 12.5 mg ⎪
    Day 3, 25 mg ⎬ in one dose each day
    Day 4, 50 mg ⎪
    Day 5, 100 mg ⎭
    Day 6, 200 mg in divided doses every 12 hours
    Day 7, 400 mg in divided doses every 12 hours
    Day 8 to day 29, 600 mg in divided doses three times daily

3. For microfilaremic patients with more than 30 microfilariae per $mm^3$ blood:

    As in (2) above, with the addition of oral prednisone 20 mg daily for the first seven days of treatment.

The adult doses given above are regarded as suitable for a 70-kg patient; doses for children should be reduced accordingly on a dose-for-weight basis. All treated patients should be given a follow-up blood examination after six months, and further therapy should be given if necessary.

Individual inflammatory lesions of loaiasis should be treated by the application of cold compresses and antihistamine creams to the affected area to relieve itching and pain. Visible adult worms in the eye or the skin should be removed under local anesthesia by passing a curved bayonet-edged surgical needle under them and gently extracting them by traction through a small incision, controlled by a mounted needle.

### *PROPHYLAXIS*

Personal prophylaxis against *L. loa* can be achieved by taking 200 mg of diethylcarbamazine citrate twice daily for three consecutive days once a month. Less specific measures are the use of insect repellents such as dimethylphthalate when in areas where *Chrysops* is present, and the careful screening of houses against insects.

Community prophylaxis by environmental and insecticidal control of *Chrysops* breeding sites has been tried, but measures have not been developed that are practical and cheap.

### References

Fain, A.: Les problemes actuels de la loase. Bull WHO 56:155, 1978.
Muller, R.: Worms and Disease. London, William Heinemann Medical Books Ltd., 1975, p. 142.
Sasa, M.: Human Filariasis. Baltimore, University Park Press, 1976, p. 122.

# *DRACUNCULIASIS* **217**

## D. W. Belcher, M.D.

### DEFINITION

Dracunculiasis is an acquired infection of subcutaneous and connective tissues caused by a large nematode, *Dracunculus medinensis*. Because of its unique clinical presentation—a long, string-like worm protruding from a shallow skin ulcer—it has been recognized since ancient times. Local names like guinea worm (Africa) and Medina worm (Middle East and Nile valley) reflect its endemic distribution. In these areas and in India and in Pakistan it is a major health problem because it incapacitates many farmers (Belcher et al., 1975).

## ETIOLOGY AND LIFE CYCLE

Man becomes infected when he drinks unfiltered water containing *Cyclops* infected with *D. medinensis* larvae. After the *Cyclops* are digested by gastric secretions, larvae are freed and penetrate the intestinal wall. In about six weeks they migrate to subcutaneous tissues, where they mature into worms. Males die after fertilizing the female, a few months after entering the human host. Males are absorbed or encysted in experimental animals, while the fertilized female burrows deeper into connective tissue until its uterus becomes distended with an estimated three million embryos. About eight months after entering the human host, the gravid female worm begins to migrate back to subcutaneous tissue, usually in the legs. Ten to 14 months after infection, the female emerges through the skin to release larvae into the water. The stage is now set for a new cycle. Larvae are released into water through the prolapsed uterus over a two- to four-week period before the worm dies. Repeated contact with water produces vigorous contraction of the uterus which expels the embryos.

*D. medinensis* is an obligate parasite that alternates between man, the definitive host, and its intermediate arthropod host. In 1870 Fedchenko discovered that a freshwater crustacean, *Cyclops* (water flea), contained *D. medinensis* larvae. He suggested that infected *Cyclops* were the source of guinea worm disease. His report is the first that showed that an arthropod could serve as the intermediate host for an agent of human disease. Since *Dracunculus* larvae possess no boring apparatus, only large predatory *Cyclops* strains that can ingest larvae become infected. These include *C. leukarti* (West Africa, Middle East, India) and *C. hyalinus* (West Africa, India). Endemic areas are sharply demarcated tropical locations because disease transmission is dependent upon an appropriate *Cyclops* species and a water temperature above 19° C. Warm water is necessary for larvae to complete their two- to three-week development period inside the *Cyclops* host.

Since *Cyclops* organisms propagate best in stagnant surface water, communities that are dependent on ponds, cisterns (Iran), and step-down wells (India) for drinking water have the greatest risk of infection. Water becomes contaminated when patients with guinea worm infections wade in to obtain water or bathe their ulcers to relieve pain.

*D. medinensis* is the only member of the Dracunculidae family that is known to infect man. A related nematode, *D. insignis,* infects North American mammals such as the raccoon and fox, but not man. Although *D. medinensis* infections of dogs, cats, monkeys, and several domesticated animals are known, no definite reservoir host has been demonstrated.

## EPIDEMIOLOGY AND GEOGRAPHIC VARIATIONS

The actual number of cases per year is unknown because official statistics grossly underestimate the extent of the problem. Dracunculiasis is not a notifiable disease in endemic areas. Because most patients are from rural areas, they are likely to have poor access to clinics and to prefer traditional treatment methods. Thirty years ago, an estimated 48 million persons were infected annually in areas with long dry seasons and ponds, cisterns, or step-down wells as water sources.

West Africa, Ethiopia, the Nile valley, Saudi Arabia, Iran and the Middle East, and Pakistan and India are endemic areas because water supplies are poor, an appropriate *Cyclops* species is present, and the water temperature is above 19° C. (Fig. 1). Previous foci in the West Indies and northeastern South America are no longer active because of improved economic conditions and better water supplies (Reddy et al., 1969).

Peak attack rates occur in adult males aged 16 to 44 years, probably because of their heavy seasonal farming activities and increased consumption of contaminated water. Females are infected as often as males in communities that use a common source of water. Infants and toddlers are rarely infected because they are breast-fed.

The source of water in tropical areas varies with the season. During a rainy season lasting two or three months, ponds fill and overflow as small streams. Villagers collect roof water in barrels and water pots. As the dry season progresses, these sources are expended and shallow surface ponds are used. Near the end of the dry season, the volume of pond water becomes low, so that the density of *Cyclops* is increased. Experimental evidence shows that infected *Cyclops* organisms lie near the bottom, where low pond volume may increase the likelihood of their being scooped up with drinking water (Muller, 1970a). Seasonal rains interrupt the transmission of dracunculiasis because the increased water volume and turbidity reduce the density of *Cyclops*. In areas where wells and cisterns are used, *Cyclops* tend to persist in larger numbers and transmission periods are longer.

Agricultural activities in the tropics have clear seasonal patterns. Land-clearing and planting are done at the end of the dry season, just before the rains. This peak farming period coincides with the major transmission period of dracunculiasis. When the patent worm emerges about one

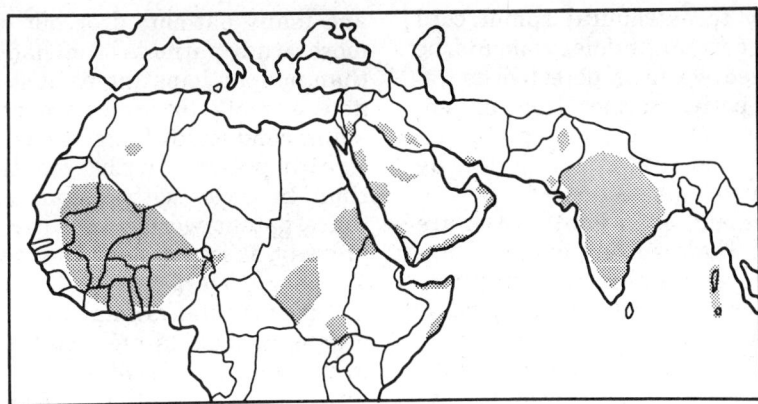

**FIGURE 1.** *Geographic distribution of dracunculiasis.*

year later, ulcers located on the feet or ankles and secondary bacterial infections can incapacitate the farmer at this critical time. In southern Ghana three out of four adult farmers are affected in some villages. The impact of this painful and disabling illness on communities where it recurs year after year is difficult to measure. Adults lying around with guinea worm ulcers and swollen legs explain the ill-kept and listless atmosphere of some of these villages (Kale, 1977a).

Some people who use larvae-contaminated water do not develop dracunculiasis, but little is known about factors that influence individual host resistance. The effect of gastric acidity on the infectivity of ingested larvae is controversial. However, gastric emptying time is clearly an important factor. Experimental animals that have rapid passage of infected cyclops through the stomach are more readily infected (Muller, 1970b). This observation suggests that gastric contents interfere with the infectivity of larvae. The fact that previously infected adults acquire fewer patent worms suggests that acquired immunity limits infection.

## PATHOGENESIS AND CLINICAL MANIFESTATIONS

The infected patient is asymptomatic for about one year, the prepatency period. Shortly before emerging, the female worm migrates to a subcutaneous location where she lies in a fibrous tunnel. Localized skin changes develop over the anterior end, apparently caused by the premature release of larvae into subcutaneous tissue. Localized swelling, accompanied by intense burning or itching, is followed within a few days by the formation of a blister made up of granulation tissue, fibrin, and a sterile yellow fluid containing eosinophils and larvae. Within a week the blister ruptures, leaving a shallow, 1- to 2-cm erosion. In its center is a tiny hole through which a portion of the uterus may protrude. Such ulcerations are not disabling unless they are numerous, located near a joint, or secondarily infected (Price and Child, 1971).

The vast majority of patients have one to three patent worms. Only 10 per cent develop four or more lesions. One third of skin lesions are on the foot and ankle and one half are on the leg. The rest occur on the trunk and arms and, rarely, on the head and neck. One to three days before the appearance of skin lesions, about one third of patients develop prodromal symptoms including fever, generalized urticaria, dizziness, vomiting, diarrhea, and occasionally dyspnea.

A small number of gravid females do not reach the surface of the skin and produce deep, sterile abscesses causing swollen extremities. Cryptic infection by nonemergent worms is often confused with bacterial pyomyositis of the extremities (Davey, 1971). Clinical differentiation between these two conditions is usually possible because pyomyositis is characterized by fever, induration with marked tenderness, and occasionally scaling of the overlying skin. In contrast, the abscesses of dracunculiasis are much less tender, and patients are generally afebrile. There is often an associated eosinophilia attributed to release of larvae into tissue. Other parasitic skin conditions caused by nonhuman hookworm or the Tumbu fly can be differentiated because they are smaller in size and occur in a wider range of anatomic locations.

## COMPLICATIONS AND SEQUELAE

Nonemergent female worms sometimes invade other organs. Infrequent extracutaneous manifestations of dracunculiasis include genitourinary symptoms, retroplacental bleeding, pericarditis, pulmonary scarring, ophthalmic disease, and paraplegia secondary to extradural spinal cord involvement. The underlying etiology should be suspected if a calcified worm is detected on radiography or if the patient comes from an endemic area. More commonly, the unexpected diagnosis is established at surgery or by examination of the histologic sections.

Periarticular tissue and even joint spaces are invaded occasionally. The resulting pain and immobility cause knee and ankle contractures, which leave patients crippled and unable to work. Bony ankylosis is rare.

Prolonged incapacitation may occur secondary to cellulitis and abscess formation. Ulcers involving the lower extremity are frequently secondarily infected because patients continue to farm, make unsuccessful attempts to extract a worm, or apply local herb poultices. Colonization with *Streptococcus, Staphylococcus,* or coliforms produces a local cellulitis or a spreading infection along the subcutaneous worm track. These may be the "fiery serpents" described by Moses during the exodus through the Sinai peninsula in Numbers 21. Other complications include bacterial abscesses, septic arthritis, and large, persistent ulcerations. These painful conditions prevent normal activity for months. Numerous cases of fatal tetanus originating in guinea worm ulcerations have been reported from West Africa.

## DIAGNOSIS

In endemic areas dracunculiasis can be diagnosed on clinical grounds. The diagnosis is usually obvious when the slender, string-like uterus protrudes from the ulcer or if the long serpentine configuration of the subcutaneous worm can be seen or palpated. Microscopic examination of ulcer fluid to identify larvae is rarely used. Fluorescent antibody tests are positive six months or more before the worm emerges, but this technique is feasible only in a research setting. Eosinophilia of about 15 per cent may be helpful in diagnosis. Nonemergent, calcified worms in atypical locations are occasionally an incidental finding on radiographs.

## TREATMENT

Four drugs are currently used to treat dracunculiasis. Niridazole was the first agent tested, but the high prevalence of side effects has shifted the interest of clinicians to metronidazole (Kulkarni and Nagalotimath, 1975), thiabendazole, and mebendazole (Kale, 1977). Published results of trials are difficult to interpret because different criteria of efficacy are used, control groups are infrequent,

and many patients drop out of studies. Furthermore, study patients often had lighter worm loads than nonparticipating patients, so that they were able to walk to clinics where the research was being conducted. Drug treatment was less effective in patients with recently emerged worms than in those with lesions of longer duration. Since patent worms only live two to four weeks anyway, it is not clear that the drugs are useful (Belcher, 1975).

Experimental animal work suggests that niridazole, metronidazole, and thiabendazole provide symptomatic relief and make patent worms easier to extract (Muller, 1970b). These effects are apparently related to a nonspecific anti-inflammatory action (Muller, 1971b). No direct toxicity or interference with guinea worm metabolism has been demonstrated (Muller, 1971a).

None of these drugs affect either the latent larvae or the pre-emergent worm. For weeks after a completed drug course, viable adult worms continue to emerge in patients with heavy infections. Diethylcarbamazine, which is used in filariasis, destroys latent *Dracunculus* larvae but has no effect on the adults. It is not recommended for mass chemotherapy in latent asymptomatic cases.

Since drug treatment reduces pain and swelling within a few days, treatment of individual patients with currently available drugs (Table 1) should be considered. Cost may preclude widespread application in developing countries. Repeated courses are necessary for symptomatic relief as new worms emerge.

Because well-designed comparative drug trials are unavailable, the drug of choice is unclear; however, the shorter course required for thiabendazole should promote better compliance by patients with instructions. After chemotherapy, some physicians use local anesthesia and make multiple incisions along the worm track to remove the entire female.

In isolated areas, the use of traditional therapy will continue. The protruding worm is tied to a piece of wood and a few centimeters are extracted each day for two to three weeks. Frequent moistening of the ulcer facilitates removal, because water produces uterine contraction, expulsion of

**TABLE 1.   Drugs Used in Treatment of Dracunculiasis**

| Drug | Schedule | Duration |
|------|----------|----------|
| Thiabendazole | 25 mg/kg twice a day | 2 days |
| Metronidazole[a] | 500 mg three times a day | 7 days |
| Mebendazole | 400 mg twice a day | 7 days |
| Niridazole | 25 mg/kg in divided doses | 7 days |

[a]25 mg/kg in children (maximum 500 mg/day); generally not used in pregnant women.

larvae, and reduced worm resistance to traction. Patients are advised to elevate the affected limb, cleanse the wound, and apply clean dressings. Secondary bacterial complications are treated with antibiotics.

## PROPHYLAXIS AND CONTROL

There appears to be little likelihood for some years that piped water or bore wells can be afforded in most rural communities where dracunculiasis is prevalent, although this is the most direct approach to interrupting transmission. Since the epidemiology and seasonality of dracunculiasis are well understood, several methods of achieve control can be considered.

Because man is the definitive host, eradication of the infection in patients would be one means of controlling dracunculiasis. Unfortunately, drugs that will suppress latent human infection are not yet available. Even if effective anthelmintics were available, residents in endemic areas generally have poor access to regular medical services. Furthermore, patients have depended on traditional treatment for years. There may be a long time lag before modern clinical care is sought, particularly when patients are too ill to walk.

Another approach is to educate residents of endemic areas to avoid water sources contaminated by patients suffering from dracunculiasis, but there are numerous obstacles to successful education programs. Residents often have supernatural explanations for the appearance of dracunculiasis in some individuals or communities while others are spared. The long incubation period of about one year also makes it difficult to explain the transmission cycle to local inhabitants in an effort to modify their behavior. The construction of walls that prevent wading in water reservoirs and platforms that are combined with a device to lower a utensil into the pond have proved useful in helping to end the transmission cycle.

Control methods can also be directed at the intermediate host. Because cyclops are macroscopic crustaceans, they can be removed from water by filtering through a cloth. Thirsty farmers working in fields some distance from a village rarely take time to filter nearby pond water. Boiling is also effective, but few households will regularly boil all their drinking water if wood and other fuels are scarce.

Biologic and chemical approaches have been used to suppress *Cyclops* populations during the transmission season. Large year-round ponds might be successfully stocked with *Cyclops*-consuming fish, but transient seasonal rural ponds are best managed by periodic application of chemical compounds (Muller, 1971b). Several compounds have been field tested. In Iran widespread chlorination of cisterns has met with marked success (Sahba et al., 1973). In India, however, the taste of chlorinated water was poorly accepted. DDT is also effective but affects other life forms and is not recommended in water used for drinking purposes.

Abate (tetramethyl thiophenylene-phosphorothioate), an organophosphorus insecticide originally developed for control of mosquitoes, is one of the more successful anti-*Cyclops* chemicals (Lyons, 1973). Abate in a sand granule form at one part per million suppresses *Cyclops* for six weeks. In areas where ponds are associated with short transmission periods, Abate could be applied near the end of the dry season in two courses at a four-week interval. Repeated cycles of Abate would be required to suppress *Cyclops* effectively in areas where water sources are associated with longer transmission periods. Zirame (zinc dimethyldithiocarbamate), a molluscicide, has also been used successfully in village ponds at 3 to 10 ppm. To achieve interruption of dracunculiasis transmission for several consecutive years in communities located at some distance from government facilities, local community participation and support are essential.

## References

Belcher, D. W., Wurapa, F. K., Ward, W. B., and Lourie, I. M.: Guinea worm in southern Ghana: Its epidemiology and impact on agricultural productivity. Am J Trop Med Hyg 24:243, 1975.

Belcher, D. W., Wurapa, F. K., and Ward, W. B.: Failure of thiabendazole and metronidazole in the treatment and suppression of guinea worm disease. Am J Trop Med Hyg 24:444, 1975.

Davey, W. W.: Guinea worm disease versus pyomyositis. In Companion to Surgery in Africa. Edinburgh, E. & S. Livingstone, 1971, p. 100.

Kale, O. O.: The clinico-epidemiologic profile of guinea worm in the Ibaden district of Nigeria. Am J Trop Med Hyg 26:208, 1977a.

Kale, O. O.: Clinical evaluation of drugs for dracontiasis. Tropical Doctor 7:15, 1977b.

Kulkarni, D. R., and Nagalotimath, S. J.: Guinea worms and metronidazole. Trans R Soc Trop Med Hyg 69:169, 1975.

Lyons, G. R.: The control of guinea worm with Abate: A trial in a village in northern Ghana. Bull WHO 49:215, 1973.

Muller, R.: Laboratory experiments in the control of cyclops transmitting guinea worm. Bull WHO 42:563, 1970a.

Muller, R.: Pathology and chemotherapy of dracunculiasis infection in rhesus monkeys. Trans R Soc Trop Med Hyg 64:24, 1970b.

Muller, R.: The possible mode of action of some chemotherapeutic agents in guinea worm disease. Trans R Soc Trop Med Hyg 63:843, 1971a.

Muller, R.: Dracunculus and dracunculiasis. In Dawes, B. (ed.): Advances in Parasitology. New York, Academic Press, 1971b, pp. 73–151.

Price, D. L., and Child, P. L.: Dracontiasis (dracunculiasis, dracunculosis, medina worm, guinea worm). In Marcial-Rojas, R. A. (ed.): Pathology of Protozoal and Helminthic Diseases with Clinical Correlation. Baltimore, The Williams & Wilkins Company, 1971, pp. 852–863.

Reddy, C. R. R. M., Narasaiah, I. L., and Parvathi, G.: Epidemiological studies on guinea worm infection. Bull WHO 40:521, 1969.

Sahba, G. H., Afraa, F., Fardin, A., and Ardalan, A.: Studies in dracontiasis in Iran. Am J Trop Med Hyg 22:343, 1973.

# 218 *CUTANEOUS ONCHOCERCIASIS*

*Horacio Figueroa Marroquin*

*Cutaneous onchocerciasis* is the term applied to certain dermal changes in man caused by an infestation with *Onchocerca volvulus*.

The first recorded observation of the skin lesions produced by *O. volvulus* dates back to 1875, when O'Neill discovered microfilariae in patients with craw-craw, a condition identified with filaric scabies. In 1893 Leuckart reported filariae in tumors excised from natives of Ghana by German missionaries. He named the parasite *Filaria volvulus*. In 1910 Raillet and Henry classified it in the genus *Onchocerca* as *Onchocerca volvulus*.

For many years the parasite was regarded as a curiosity that could infect man with no untoward effects. Robles in Guatemala discovered, after excising many nodules, that infestation with *O. volvulus* resulted in blindness (Robles, 1919). This news was received with skepticism, and it was not until 17 years later in 1932 that Hissette observed ocular lesions in the Belgian Congo similar to those found by Robles and Pacheco Luna in Guatemala.

## ETIOLOGY

The etiologic agent of onchocerciasis is *Onchocerca volvulus*, a nematode of the superfamily Filarioidea, genus *Onchocerca*, species *volvulus*. It is transmitted from man to man by several species of Simuliidae. The main vectors are *S. damnosum* in Africa, *S. ochraceum* in Mexico and Guatemala, and *S. metallicum* in Venezuela. These insects are known as buffalo gnats or black flies.

## PATHOGENESIS AND PATHOLOGY

Adult parasites live in nodules or onchocercomas. The nodules are either superficial or deeply embedded in the tissues. The parasites also live free in the tissues with no inflammatory reaction. In Africa most of the nodules are located from the waist down, whereas those in the Americas usually appear from the waist up.

Two regions are observed in sections of nodules (Fig. 1)—a central region or stroma where the thread-like adult worms are found, and a peripheral section formed by fibrous tissue. The female liberates her embryos around the nodule, from which site they migrate to the skin and eyes (Figueroa, 1972).

Although several theories have been advanced to explain the symptoms produced by *O. volvulus*, most authorities favor the idea of an allergic reaction to substances liberated by the disintegration of microfilariae.

There are no specific pathologic findings. The most frequent are hyperkeratosis, acanthosis, papillomatosis, and perivascular inflammation.

## CLINICAL MANIFESTATIONS

Regardless of geographic location, nodules, eye lesions, and dermatitis are uniformly present. This triad is found in Africa, Mexico, Central America, and South America, but with some geographic differences. There are striking differences between African and American onchocerciasis. Lymphatic symptoms, elephantiasis, and hanging groin are never seen in Mexico and Guatemala, whereas "erysipela de la costa" (coast erysipelas) and "mal morado" (purple disease) are never observed in Africa.

### Skin Lesions

The findings usually include pruritus, erythema, papules, scab-like eruptions, pigmentation, depigmentation, and lichenification, all intermingled in the different lesions. The types of lesions vary according to the geographic location.

## GEOGRAPHIC VARIATIONS

### Yemen and Asia

The typical form of onchocercal dermatitis found in Yemen is "sowda" (Fig. 2). The name is taken from its main characteristic, a black pigmentation of the skin (*sowda* is Arabic for black). It is usually observed in one or both of the lower limbs. Intense pruritus, papules, thickening and roughness of the skin, and hypertrophy of the inguinal glands are present (Anderson and Fuglsang, 1900). It is very unusual to find micro-

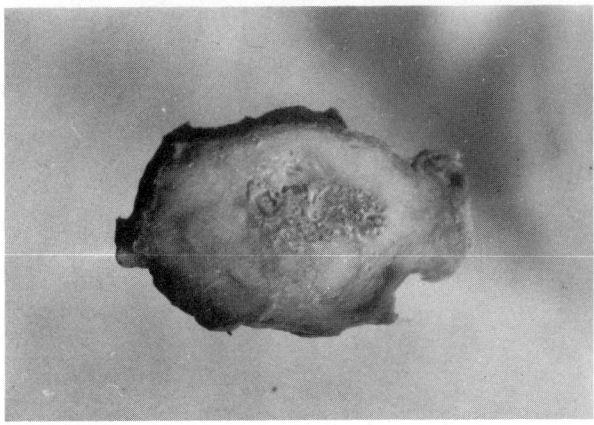

**FIGURE 1.** *Section of a nodule showing the two main portions: the central part, or stroma, and the peripheral fibrous capsule.*

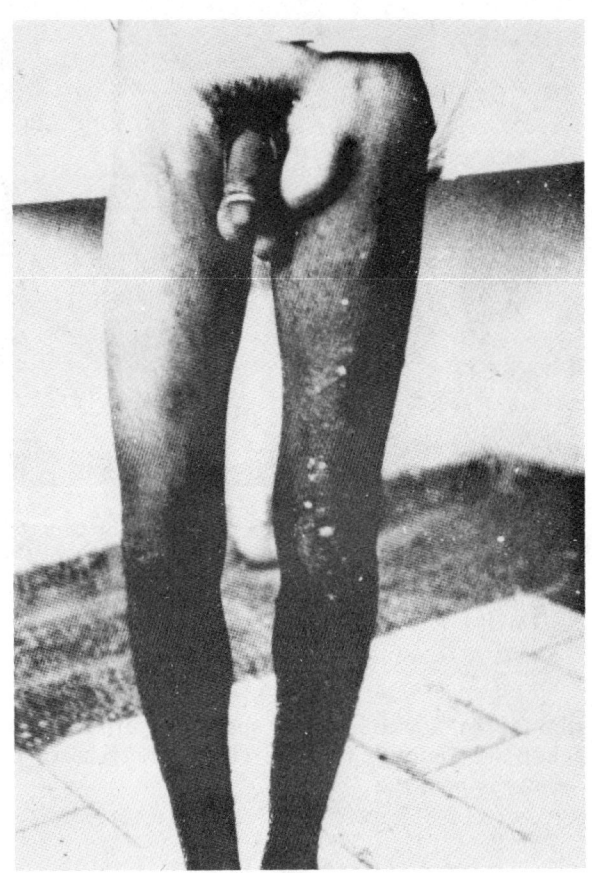

**FIGURE 2.** *A typical case of sowda from Yemen. (From Buck, A. A.: Onchocerciasis. Geneva, World Health Organization [monograph], 1974.)*

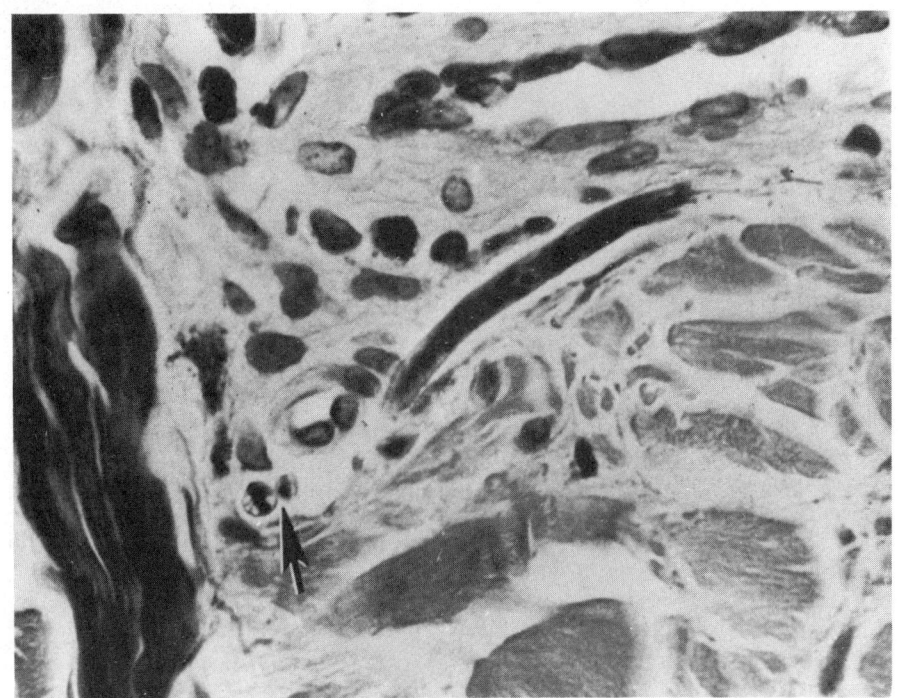

**FIGURE 3.** *Microfilaria in the mid-dermis in a case of sowda (Giemsa stain). (From Buck, A. A.: Onchocerciasis. Geneva, World Health Organization [monograph], 1974.)*

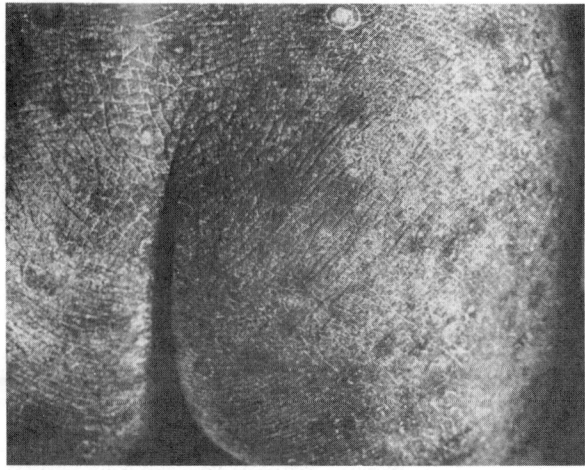

**FIGURE 4.** *Pigmentation of the skin in an early case of onchocercal dermatitis. Round and small spots of pigmentation. (From Connor, D. H.: Pathology of onchocerciasis and main geographic characteristics of the disease. Geneva, World Health Organization, Pub. No. 298, 1974.)*

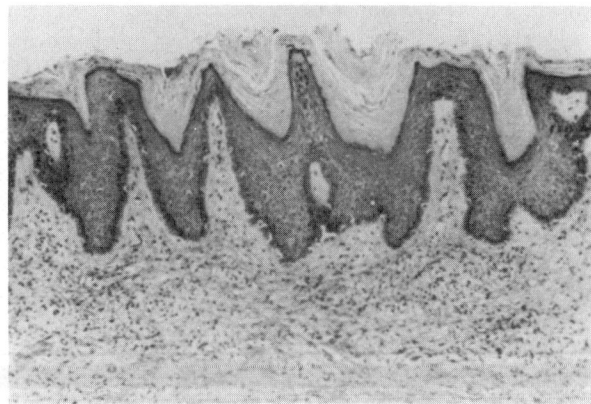

**FIGURE 5.** *Slight acanthosis, elongation of the rete ridges, pigmentation of the basal layer and inflammatory cell infiltrates (hematoxylin-eosin). (From Connor, D. H.: Pathology of onchocerciasis and main geographic characteristics of the disease. Geneva, World Health Organization, Pub. No. 298, 1974.)*

filariae in a skin biopsy specimen unless it is taken deep enough (Fig. 3). The Mazzotti test (see below) is positive.

### Africa

Pruritus is one of the main symptoms but is not unique to the African disease. It can be mild or acute, localized or generalized, continuous or intermittent, and it sometimes disappears spontaneously.

Round pigmented spots (Fig. 4) result from hyperkeratosis, increased pigmentation of the basal epidermis, and perivascular inflammation (Fig. 5). Depigmentation also occurs and resembles vitiligo. Discolored bands alternating with normally pigmented skin give the appearance of what is known as leopard skin (Buck, 1974). It usually appears on the shins (Fig. 6). In long-standing cases, the skin resembles that of various animals (Reber and Hoeppli, 1964). With lizard skin, pigmentation increases and the skin becomes scaly and geometrically squared like the skin of an alligator (Fig. 7). Histologically, there is hyperkeratosis, separation of the corneous stratum, perivascular infiltration, and atrophy of the epidermis (Fig. 8). When the lesions are very old, atrophy of the papillary body, which histologically looks like the skin of an old man, ensues. Because of its shiny and scaly appearance it is known as xeroderma ichthyosiformes, or fish skin (Fig. 9). When the skin atrophies completely it loses its elasticity and resembles crushed tissue or crushed paper. There are fewer dermal papillae and almost complete disappearance of elastic fibers (Fig. 10) but no hyperkeratosis.

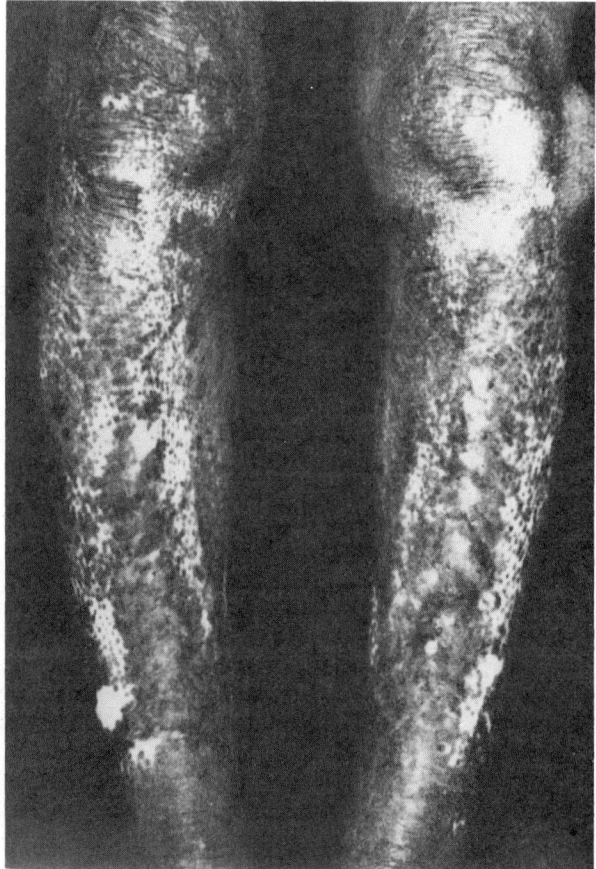

**FIGURE 6.** *A case of "leopard skin." Depigmentation is more common at the shins. (From Buck, A. A.: Onchocerciasis. Geneva, World Health Organization [monograph], 1974.)*

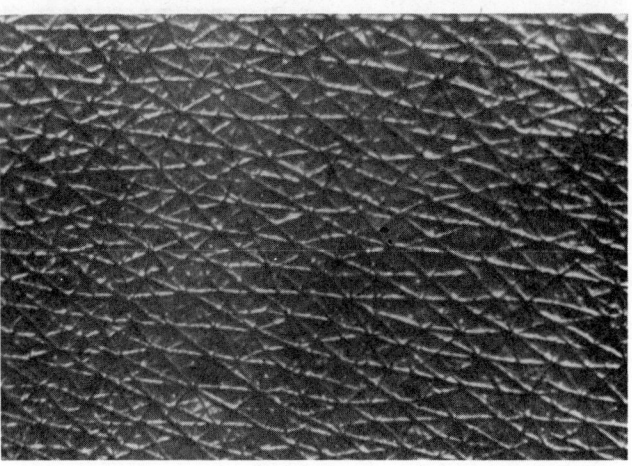

**FIGURE 7.** *"Lizard skin." Increased pigmentation. Skin alterations in onchocercal dermatitis. (From Reber, W. W., and Hoeppli, R.: The relationship between macroscopic skin alterations, histological changes and microfilaria in one hundred Liberians with onchocercal dermatitis. Z Tropenmed Parasitol 15 (2), July 1964.)*

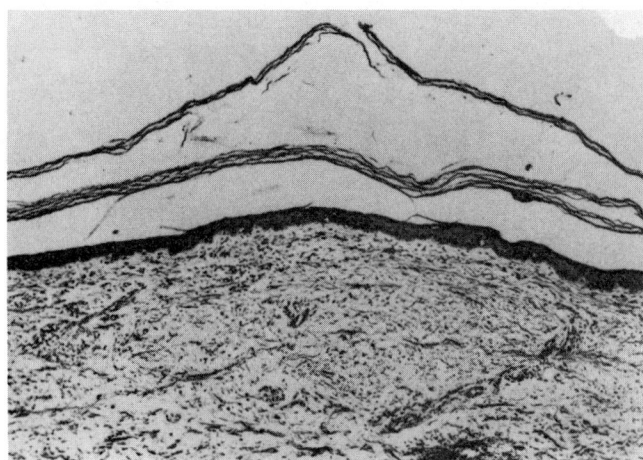

**FIGURE 8.** *"Lizard skin." Separation of the keratin, atrophy of the epidermis, and chronic inflammation of the dermis. (From Connor, D. H.: Pathology of onchocerciasis and main geographic characteristics of the disease. Geneva, World Health Organization, Pub. No. 298, 1974.)*

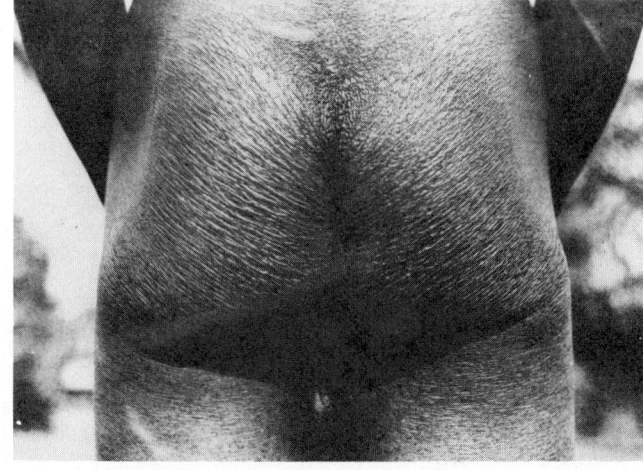

**FIGURE 9.** *A case of xeroderma ichthyosiformes, fish skin. (From Watson, M.: L'onchocercose africaine humaine, 1950.)*

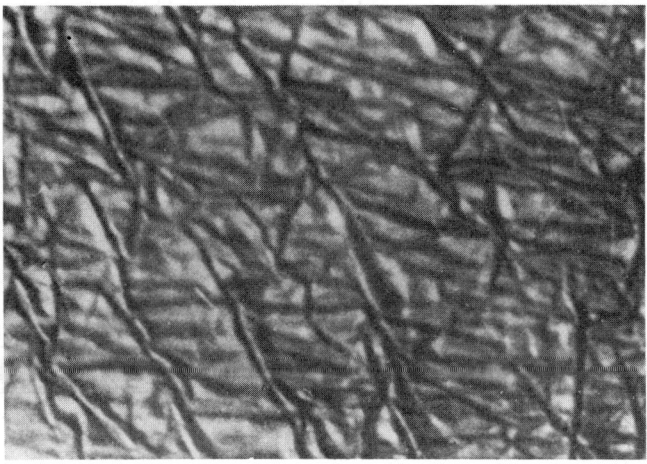

**FIGURE 10.** *Crushed tissue or crushed paper appearance of xeroderma ichthyosiformes. The skin is thin and pale and loses its elasticity and luster. (From Reber, W. W., and Hoeppli, R.: The relationship between macroscopic skin alterations, histological changes and microfilaria in one hundred Liberians with onchocercal dematitis. Z Tropenmed Parasitol 15(2), July 1964.)*

In African onchocerciasis lymphatic obstruction causes "hanging groin" (Fig. 11). The skin atrophies, becomes flaccid, and hangs like a bag containing lymph nodes (Buck, 1974) (Fig. 12).

### Central America and Mexico

Onchocerciasis in Mexico and Guatemala is known as Robles disease. The most typical form is erysipela de la costa (coast erysipelas), so-called for its resemblance to streptococcal erysipelas. First the skin becomes tense, smooth, and shiny, and acquires a red pigmentation. Then it becomes edematous, and when the face is affected, the lips, nose, ears, and eyelids become swollen and in-

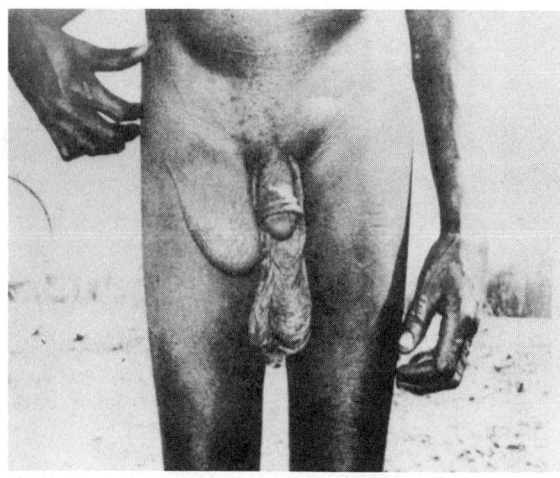

**FIGURE 11.** *Unilateral hanging groin. The inguinal glands are enlarged. (From Buck, A. A.: Onchocerciasis. Geneva, World Health Organization [monograph], 1974.)*

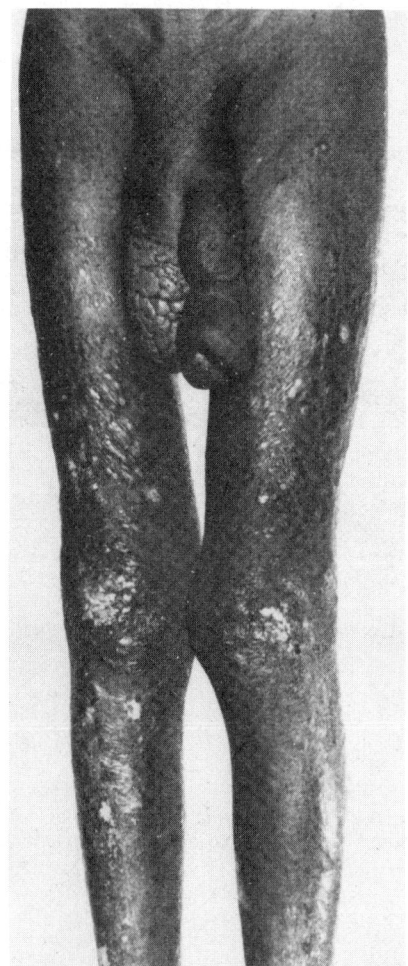

**FIGURE 12.** *Elephantoid changes of the penis, the scrotum, and the thighs. (From Buck, A. A.: Onchocerciasis. Geneva, World Health Organization [monograph], 1974.)*

tensely pruritic (Fig. 13). In chronic disease the skin loses elasticity, atrophies, becomes wrinkled, and causes a leonine face (Fig. 14).

Sometimes the color of erysipelas is replaced by a blue cast to the skin, called mal morado in Mexico (Salazar Mallen, 1962).

In Mexico and Guatemala almost all the skin manifestations are seen, but with differences. Hyperpigmentation, especially of the face and chest, occurs but not very intensely. Depigmentation is also present, not as leopard skin but rather as small or medium sized spots (Fig. 15). Onchocercotic scabies is frequent and is accompanied by pruritus, itching lesions, and papules that sometimes resemble craw-craw (Fig. 16).

One type of onchocercotic dermatitis that appears commonly on the ears, chest, and arms resembles the keratinization observed in vitamin A deficiency. The skin becomes dry, and pin-point papules appear as a result of obstruction of the pilosebaceous ducts (Fig. 17).

Lichenification is also common in the form of thick folds on the anterior surface of the arm (Fig. 18); the skin becomes very thick and dry.

Pseudosowda is a new kind of dermatitis that resembles sowda in that it is also black; however, it lacks some of the characteristics of true sowda (Fig. 19).

All the skin lesions mentioned are almost always bilateral. Biopsy specimens taken from the lesions are usually positive for microfilariae.

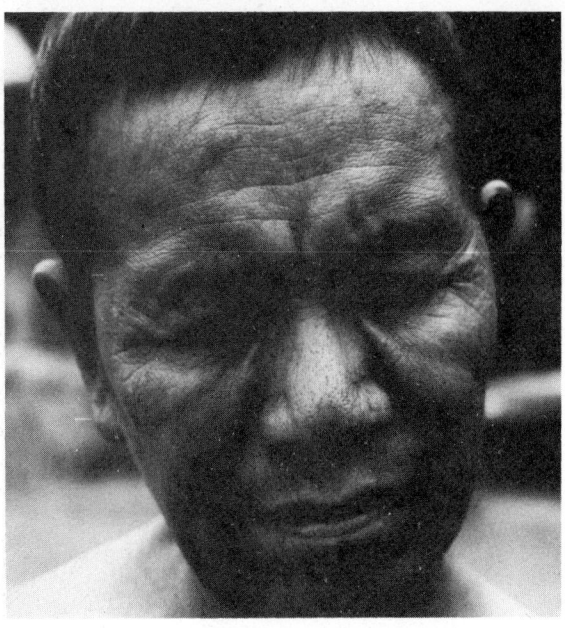

**FIGURE 14.** *"Leonine facies" in a case of severe, chronic onchocercal dermatitis.*

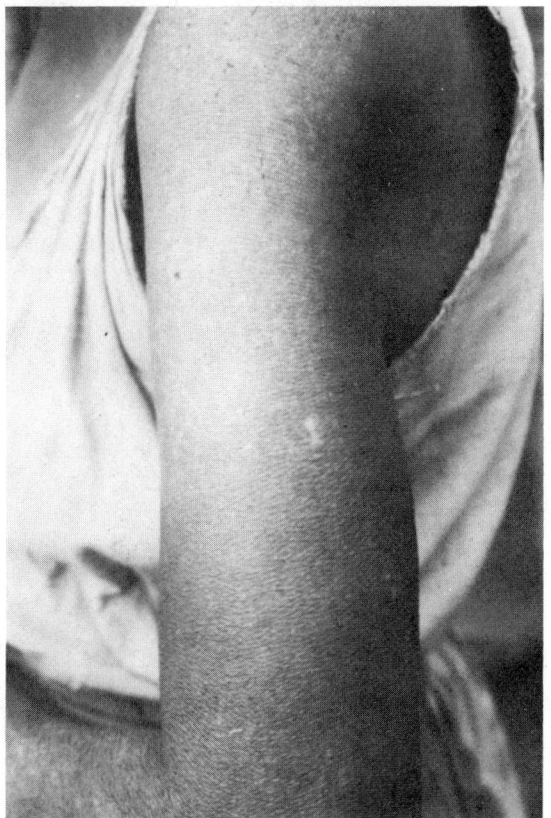

**FIGURE 15.** *Pinpoint depigmentation of the skin in a case of onchocercal dermatitis.*

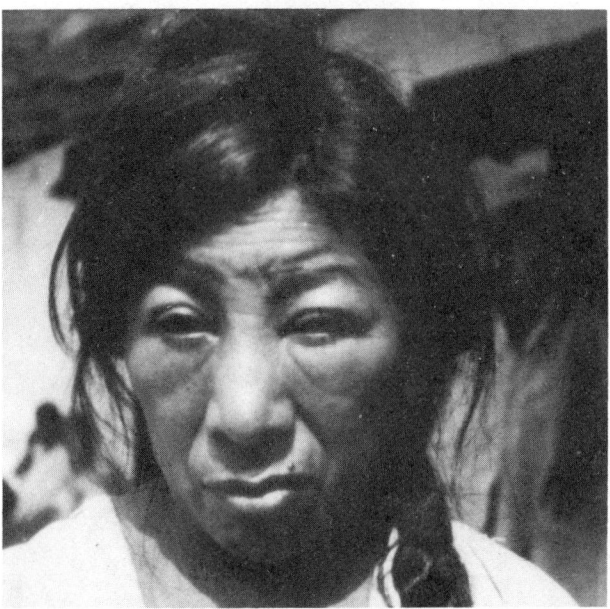

**FIGURE 13.** *Erisipela de la costa.*

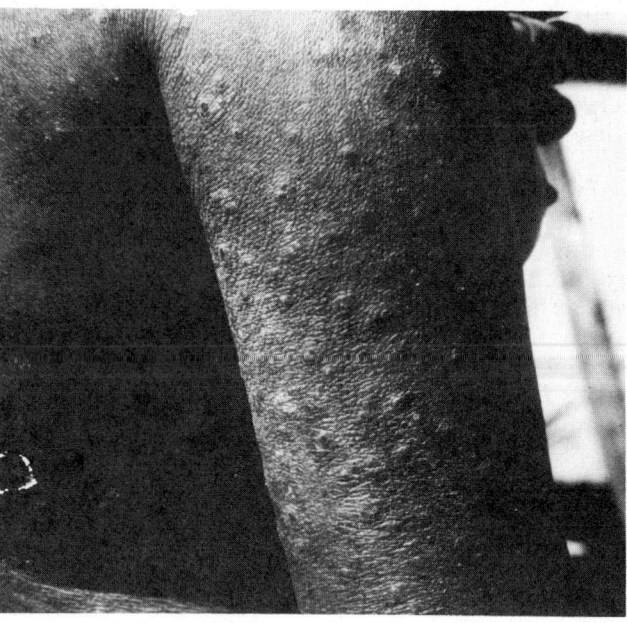

**FIGURE 16.** *Scabies-like onchocercal dermatitis in a very old and severe case.*

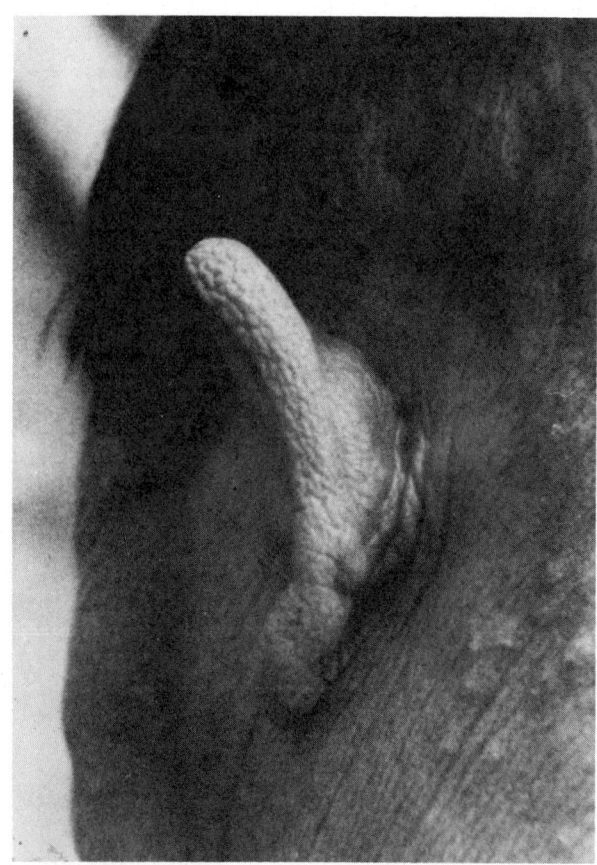

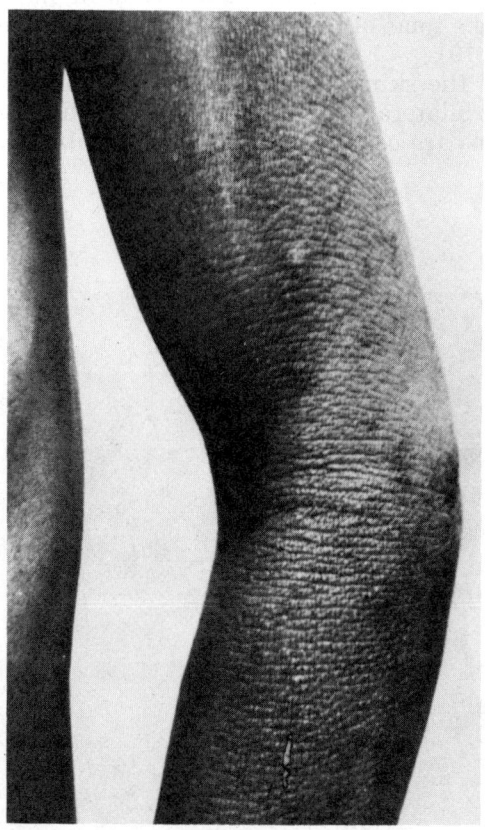

**FIGURE 17.** *Pinpoint papules caused by plugging of the pilose-baceous follicles. The ear is frequently enlarged and displaced from its normal position.*

**FIGURE 18.** *Lichenification in a severe case of onchocercal dermatitis. Transverse and prominent folds of the skin appear.*

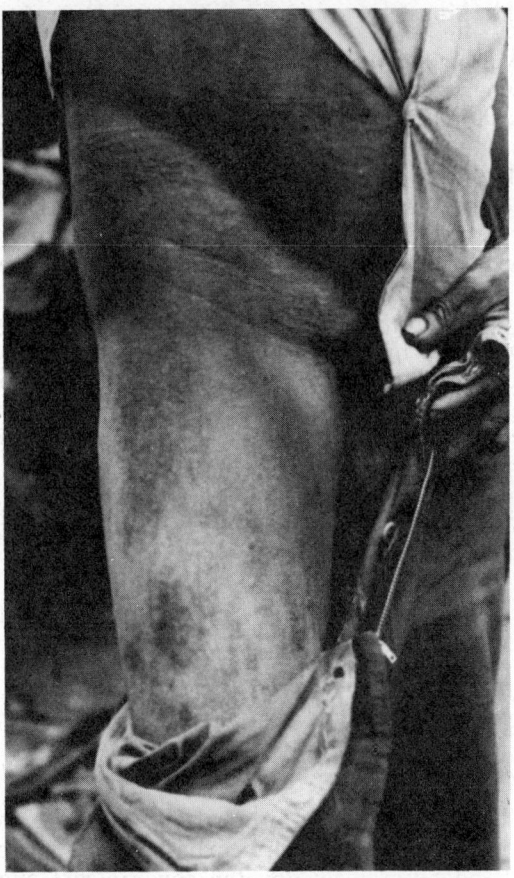

**FIGURE 19.** *A case of pseudo sowda. The inguinal nodes are somewhat enlarged. The black coloration of the skin is also seen in the thorax and arms.*

### South America

South American onchocerciasis is found in Venezuela, Colombia, Ecuador, and Brazil. The skin lesions there resemble those observed in Africa more than those found in Mexico and Guatemala. Pruritus and scabies-like onchodermatitis as well as atrophy and hypertrophy of the skin occur. More acute manifestations have been found in a geographic focus of onchocerciasis recently discovered by Rassi and his colleagues (1977) in the Amazonian Federal Territory. As in Africa, there are conditions that closely resemble hanging groin (Fig. 20). Skin depigmentation appears as white small spots covering the entire body, in some cases giving the patient a mottled appearance (Fig. 21). Xeroderma ichthyosiformes or fish skin (Fig. 22) and acute atrophy of the skin also have been observed (Fig. 23). Erythematous dermatitis, like that in erysipela de la costa, is present (Fig. 24).

### DIAGNOSIS

Diagnosis is easy when the triad of nodules, eye lesions, and skin changes is found. However, there are persons with the disease in whom none of these signs are observed. In such cases, microfilariae can sometimes be found in the anterior chamber of the eye.

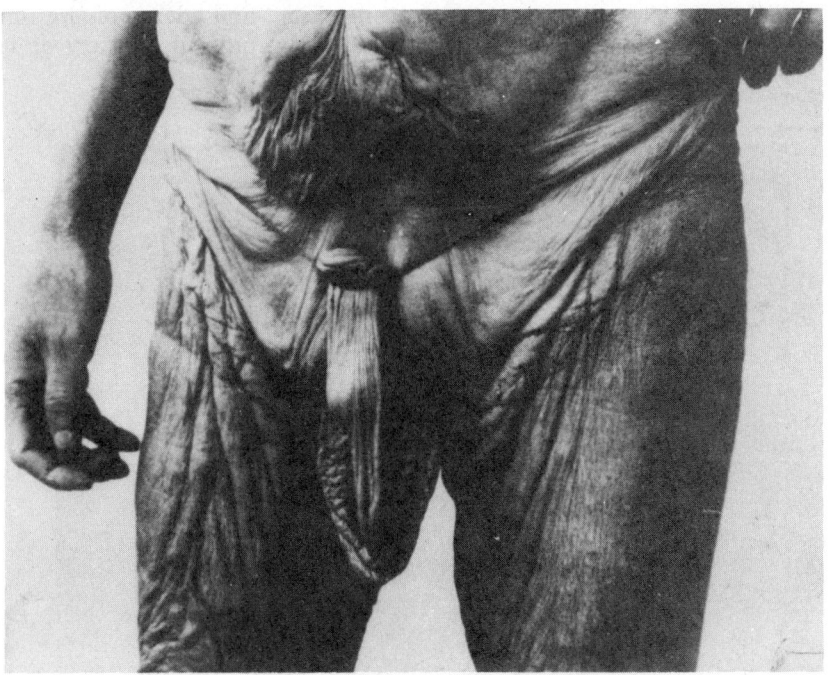

**FIGURE 20.** *Hanging groin and atrophy of the skin. (From Rassi, E., et al.: Discovery of a new onchocerciasis focus in Venezuela. Bull Pan Am Health Organ 11 (1): 41, 1977.)*

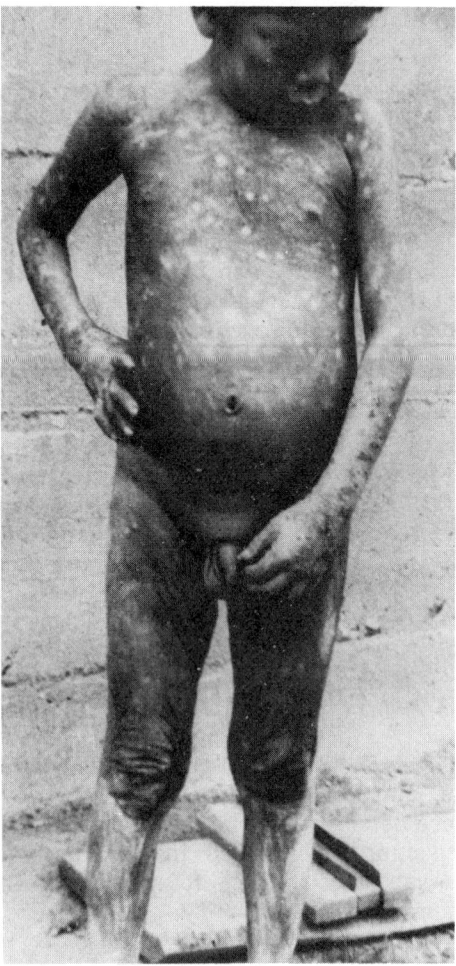

**FIGURE 21.** *Generalized depigmentation. Small white spots covering almost the entire body (mottled depigmentation). (From Rassi, E., et al.: Discovery of a new onchocerciasis focus in Venezuela. Bull Pan Am Health Organ 11 (1): 41, 1977.)*

## Skin Biopsy

A skin site is selected where experience in a given geographic region has demonstrated that microfilariae are more likely to be found. The suprascapular or deltoid region, iliac crest, and malleolus (Yemen) are common sites. A skin fold is pinched to avoid bleeding and snipped with a razor blade. The excised skin snip is placed in a drop of water or saline on a microscope slide, and 30 minutes later the microfilariae are counted under the microscope. For maximum accuracy a biopsy may be taken from three of the sites mentioned. Another procedure is to raise a thin portion of the skin with a needle and cut it at the base with a razor blade, or use a corneal scleral punch of 2.3 to 3 mm bite.

In countries where there are other microfilariae (*Dipetalonema streptocerca* in Africa and *Mansonella ozzardi* in the Americas) besides *O. volvulus* that may be infecting the skin, it is necessary to differentiate them. The length and location of the cephalic and caudal nuclei are different in stained preparations.

When no microfilariae show up in the biopsy it is necessary to resort to the Mazzotti test.

## Mazzotti Test

The test consists of an oral dose of one or two 50 mg tablets of diethylcarbamazine. Patients with onchocerciasis develop severe local symptoms in 30 minutes to a few hours after ingesting the drug. The symptoms include localized or generalized pruritus and papular erythema, eye congestion, and edema of the limbs or face. Less frequently, painful axillary or inguinal adenop-

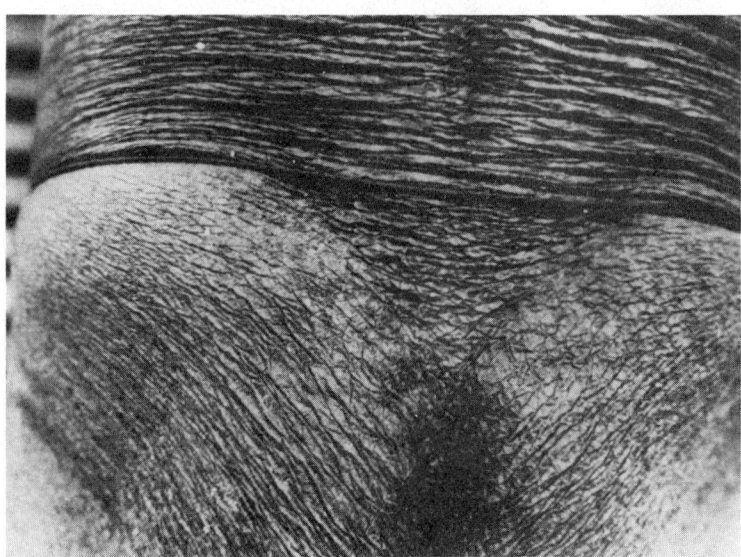

**FIGURE 22.** *Fish skin (xeroderma ichthyosiformes). There is atrophy of the skin. (From Rassi, E., et al.: Discovery of a new onchocerciasis focus in Venezuela. Bull Pan Am Health Organ 11(1):41, 1977.)*

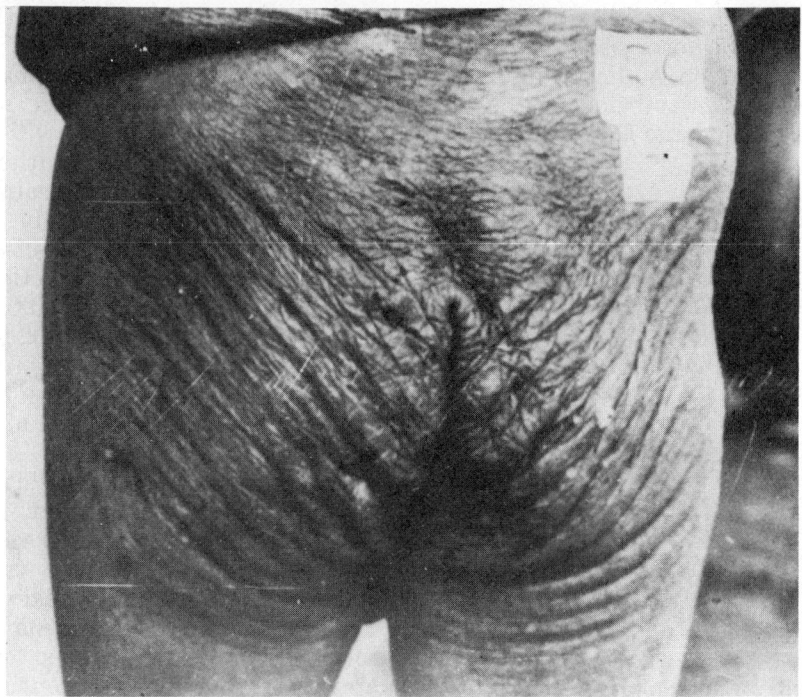

**FIGURE 23.** *Complete atrophy of the skin. (From Rassi, E., et al.: Discovery of a new onchocerciasis focus in Venezuela. Bull Pan Am Health Organ 11(1):41, 1977.)*

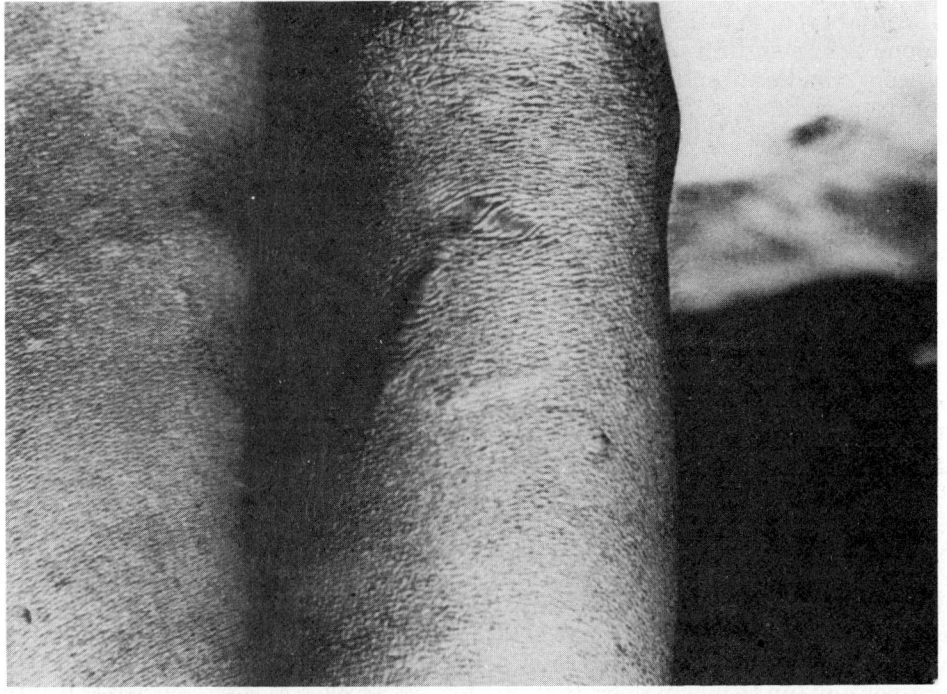

**FIGURE 24.** *Lichenification, thickening of the skin, and "erisipela de la costa" appearance.*

athy, fever, and headache are observed. In infected patients who have never been exposed to the drug, a positive reaction is almost universal; if the drug has been taken previously, the test may be negative (Figueroa and Garcia, 1972).

## PROGNOSIS

In patients with chronic and massive infestations, prognosis is not good because the disease can lead to complete blindness. Widespread dissemination of microfilariae may cause several systemic reactions.

## TREATMENT

Treatment can be surgical or chemotherapeutic, and must be individualized according to the severity of the lesions and general state of the patient. Treatment must be initiated before lesions become irreversible.

### Surgical Treatment: Nodulectomy

This is the most common treatment in Americans, and it has decreased the incidence of ocular and cutaneous invasion. All palpable nodules are anesthetized with 2 per cent Novocain with epinephrine. The overlying skin is dissected until the nodule can be identified by its white color or by palpation. With dissecting forceps and curved scissors the lips of the incision are widened in order to isolate and excise the nodule. A finger is inserted into the cavity to ensure that the entire nodule has been removed, and then the incision is closed with one or two sutures. All this should be done with aseptic and antiseptic precautions.

If there are deep nodules or free filariae the treatment is only palliative; if not, recovery is excellent.

### Chemotherapy

The drugs in common use are diethylcarbamazine, which kills microfilariae, and suramin (Germanine, Antripol, Moranil), which kills adult parasites and microfilariae.

*Diethylcarbamazine.* Reaction to this drug, which can be violent, calls for caution in undernourished or heavily infested patients. After two or three days the reaction subsides and the patient can continue taking the drug without any problem. To minimize the reaction, Antistin (100 mg) or Betamethazone (1 mg three times a day) may be administered during the first three or four days of treatment.

Diethylcarbamazine can be given in several dosages. An average dose is from 6 to 10 mg/kg of body weight per day (up to 600 mg per day), in three divided doses at meal times. Other schedules give 2 mg/kg body weight, three times daily for two to three weeks (Mazzotti, 1962) or 100 mg twice daily for 15 days.

Treatment of acute infections starts with lower doses that are gradually increased. Periodic treatment is palliative and not without risk.

*Suramin.* This is a synthetic drug derived from urea. A 10 per cent solution of the white powder is given intravenously. In patients weighing 60 kg or more, the usual dose is 1 g weekly for six or seven weeks. In patients weighing less than 60 kg, the first dose is 0.01 g/kg, and the six remaining doses are each 0.02 g/kg (Rivas, 1965). Treatment is stopped if significant proteinuria develops. Before starting treatment, the patient can be challenged with 0.1 g of the drug to determine sensitivity.

The drug kills adult parasites and microfilariae. It can cause serious toxic reaction to the patient, including edema and renal injury, and is contraindicated in patients with kidney disease. It can also cause severe exfoliative dermatitis, urticaria, and hyperkeratosis in the palms and soles. It is not recommended for mass treatment, and its use has been discontinued after several deaths in trials carried out in Africa and Guatemala (Aguilar et al., 1955). But in Venezuela, where it is still being used, 2432 cases were reported treated in 1974 with no deaths.

## References

Aguilar, G., Barrera, M., et al.: Proyecto piloto de una campaña de tratamiento médico de la oncocercosis, basado en la adminístración de suramina sódica (U.S.P. XIII). Bol Of Sanit Panama, 38(2), Feb. 1955.

Anderson, J., and Fuglsang, H.: Clinical aspects of onchocerciases in Uganda and Yemen Arab Republic compared with rain forest and savanna focus in Cameroon. World Health Organization–ONCHO Series No. 102. Mimeographed.

Buck, A. A.: Onchocerciasis. Symptomatology, Pathology, Diagnosis. Geneva, World Health Organization [monograph], 1974.

Castro, F.: Histological findings in some onchocercal dermatitis. Unpublished data. Pathol Laboratory, General Hospital, Guatemala.

Figueroa Marroquin, H.: Enfermedad de Robles. ¿Como salen las microfilarias del oncocercoma? Rev Invest Salud Publica 32:9, 1972.

Figueroa Marroquin, H., and Garcia, G. C.: Especificidad de la reacción de Mazzotti en el diagnóstico de la enfermedad de Robles. Rev Semana Médica Centroamérica Panamá 29(240), January 12, 1972.

Hissette, J.: Mémoire sur l'onchocerca volvulus "Leuckart," et ses manifestations oculaires au Congo Belge. Ann Soc Belge Med Trop 12(4), Dec. 1932.

Mazzotti, L.: Tratamiento de la oncocercosis. Rev Salud Publica Mexico. Epoca 5. 4(6), Nov.-Dec. 1962.

O'Neill, J.: On the presence of a filaria in craw craw. Lancet, Feb. 20, 1875.

Rassi, E., et al.: Discovery of a new onchocerciasis focus in Venezuela. Bull Pan Am Health Organ 11(1):41, 1977.

Reber, W. W., and Hoeppli, R.: The relationship between macroscopic skin alterations, histological changes and microfilaria in one hundred Liberians with onchocercal dermatitis. Z Tropenmed Parasitol 15(2), July 1964.

Rendon, A., Tito, B.: La "oncocercosis," enfermedad desconocida aparece en el país. Diaro "Universal," Section 2, Ecuador, August 30, 1980.

Rivas, A., et al.: La oncocercosis en Venezuela. Acta Med Venezol (Suppl 1), Dec. 1965.

Robles, R.: Onchocercose humaine au Guatemala produisant la cécité et "l'erysipele du littoral" (erisipela de la costa). Bull Soc Pathol Exot Paris 7, July 1919.

Salazar Mallen, M.: Los síntomas cutáneos de la oncocercosis. Rev Salud Publica Mexico, Epoca 5,. 4(6), Nov.-Dec., 1962.

# CUTANEOUS LARVA MIGRANS (CREEPING ERUPTION)

## 219

### Charles E. Davis, M.D.

## DEFINITION

Cutaneous larva migrans and creeping eruption are synonyms for the prolonged migration of dog and cat hookworm larvae in the skin of man. Because they have penetrated the skin of an "abnormal" host, these parasites cannot complete their life cycle. Instead, they wander for weeks or months in the epidermis and leave a pruritic, elevated, erythematous trail along the path of their migration. By contrast, reactions at the site of skin penetration by *Necator americanus, Ancylostoma duodenale* (human hookworms), and *Strongyloides stercoralis* are only a macule or papule without migration and are called "ground itch."

## ETIOLOGY

By far the most common cause of cutaneous larva migrans is *Ancylostoma braziliense,* the hookworm of dogs and cats (Beaver, 1956). In 1926, Kirby-Smith et al. identified larval nematodes in skin biopsies of people in Florida with creeping eruption. Experiments on human volunteers by these investigators (White and Dove, 1928 and 1929) with third-stage infective filariform larvae of *A. braziliense* reproduced the disease that was seen in thousands of people in the southeastern United States. Many similar trials (Dove, 1932; Maplestone, 1933) with *A. caninum,* the dog hookworm, established that it could also cause creeping eruption but usually penetrated the skin less readily and migrated for less than 2 weeks. Other experiments and observations (Fulleborn, 1926a; Mayhew, 1947) established that *Uncinaria stenocephala,* the European dog hookworm, and the cattle hookworm *(Bunostomum phlebotomum)* could occasionally cause cutaneous larva migrans that was also of shorter duration than typical creeping eruption caused by *A. braziliense.*

Experiments with *Ancylostoma duodenale, Necator americanus,* and *Strongyloides stercoralis* (Beaver, 1945; Fulleborn, 1930; Fulleborn, 1926) indicated that these natural parasites of people cause creeping eruption rarely and only in sensitized individuals, either during or recently after intestinal infection.

The development and life cycle of the hookworms of dogs and cats is the same as the human hookworm (see Nemathelminthes, Chapter 79). After ova are passed in the feces, rhabditiform larvae hatch within 24 hours under ideal conditions in moist, sandy soil in subtropical or tropical zones. After feeding on bacteria and organic debris, the larvae molt twice, grow, and become slender, nonfeeding, infectious filariform larvae. These larvae stand upright on pieces of dirt or other organic material and wait for a warm-blooded host. They penetrate the skin on contact and reach the circulation of the normal host by migration to capillary beds. They remain localized in the skin of "abnormal" hosts and die after a few weeks to months.

*A. braziliense,* the usual cause of typical cutaneous larva migrans, is distributed most heavily in the southeastern and southern United States, the coastal regions of Mexico, Central America, and the tropical and subtropical coastal areas of South America and Africa. It also occurs in India, Southeast Asia, the Philippines, Taiwan, and Hong Kong. Because moist and warm sandy soil, loam, or humus favors development of the larvae, typical high risk areas include swimming beaches, sand piles, and crawl spaces under houses where dogs and cats defecate.

## PATHOGENESIS AND PATHOLOGY

Penetration of the skin appears to be mechanical but is probably aided by collagenases. The adherence of caked earth or sand to the skin probably also adds purchase to the slender, filariform larvae that usually penetrate through a hair follicle. A small papule or macule may develop at the site of invasion. After 2 to 3 days, the larvae begin to migrate in the stratum germinativum with the corium as a floor and the stratum granulosum as a roof (Fig. 1). Local infiltration of eosinophilic and lymphocytic leukocytes and the movements of the larvae cause intense pruritis. Secondary bacterial infection from inoculation of bacteria by scratching may induce surrounding cellulitis and polymorphonuclear infiltration. It

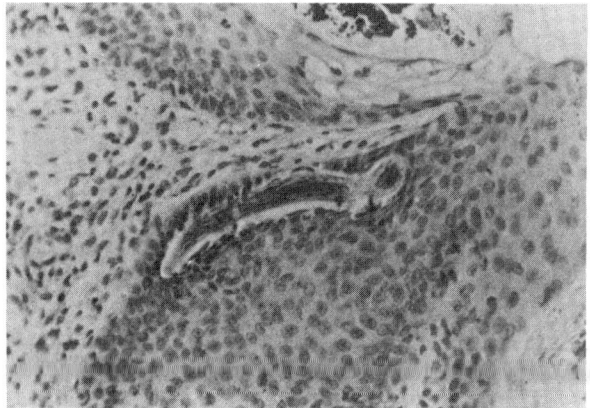

**FIGURE 1.** *Longitudinal section of a larva of Ancylostoma sp. in the lower layers of the epidermis around a hair follicle in the skin of the back. (From Meyers, Wayne M., and Neafie, Ronald C.: Creeping eruption. In Binford, C. H., and Connor, D.H. (eds.): Pathology of Tropical and Extraordinary Diseases, Vol. 2. Washington, D.C., Armed Forces Institute of Pathology, 1976.)*

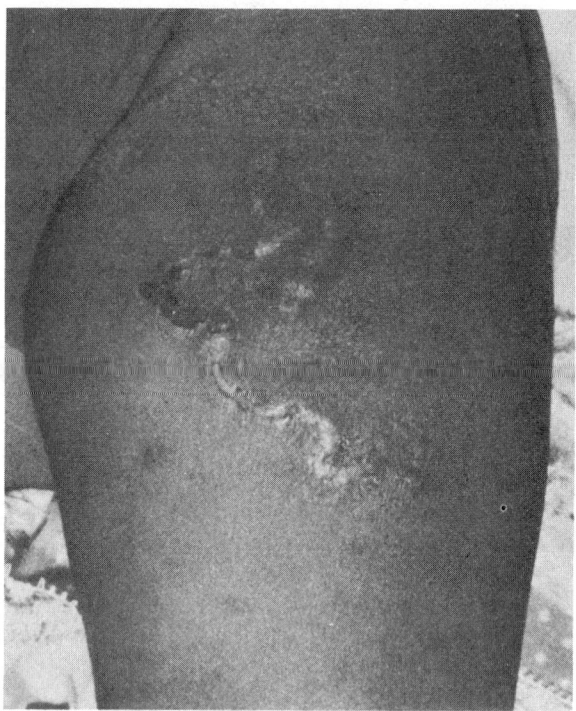

**FIGURE 2.** *Creeping eruption on the thigh of an 11-month-old child. The most recent portion of the tract is on the upper left. (From Meyers, Wayne M., and Neafie, Ronald C.: Creeping eruption. In Binford, C. H., and Connor, D. H. (eds.): Pathology of Tropical and Extraordinary Diseases, Vol. 2. Washington, D.C., Armed Forces Institute, 1976.)*

is likely that penetration into the capillary beds of the dermis of the usual host is aided by enzymes that are ineffective against the dermal structures of the human being in whom the migration seems aimless and serpentine.

Since human hookworms and *S. stercoralis* cause creeping eruption primarily in sensitized individuals, it would seem that they are temporarily confined to the skin of these individuals by immune reactions.

There have been scattered reports of human intestinal infections with adult *A. braziliense*. Many of these probably represent infections with distinct but closely related species. It is possible, however, that *A. braziliense* may rarely complete its life cycle in the human being because transient pulmonary infiltrations, eosinophilia, and cough (Loeffler's syndrome) have been reported in conjunction with cutaneous larva migrans (Wright and Gold, 1946). The mere demonstration of hookworm ova in the stools of patients with cutaneous larva migrans must be interpreted with caution, however, because the ova of many hookworms are identical.

## CLINICAL MANIFESTATIONS

Lesions may be single or multiple and occur most often on the hands, feet, and buttocks of sunbathers and on the hands, shoulders, and torso of plumbers, pipefitters, and others who work under buildings and crawlspaces of houses where dogs and cats defecate. A sensation of tingling or itching at the time of penetration may be recalled by the patient. A pruritic, red papule forms within a few hours to a day after penetration. Migration

begins 2 to 3 days later and causes a conspicuous, elevated, serpiginous, erythematous, intensely pruritic tunnel that marks the trail of the migrating larva. The larva, which may migrate at a rate of 1 to 2 cm per day, lies just in advance of the conspicuous portion of its trail. The unoccupied portion of the burrow dries and becomes crusted within a few days, but the larva of *A. braziliensis* continues its migration for up to 1 year, circling on its own trail and producing a serpentine design (Fig. 2). The path is so serpentine that the larva usually lies only a few centimeters from the site of penetration even after months of migration. The local pruritis is enough to bring on prominent insomnia and anorexia.

Symptoms from the migration of *A. caninum, Unicinaria stenocaphala,* and *Bunostomum phlebotomum* (see *Etiology*) are indistinguishable, but the worm usually dies and the symptoms disappear within 2 weeks instead of several months. The human hookworms and *S. stercoralis* usually cause only "ground itch," a localized pruritic macule or papule at the site of penetration, but they occasionally migrate in the skin of sensitized victims for a few days or weeks. *S. stercoralis* also causes a rare form of creeping eruption called *larva currens* that is unique in two of its clinical characteristics (Fulleborn, 1926; Caplan, 1949). First, the migration is perianal because it occurs by autoinoculation of filariform larvae that mature at the anus. Second, the migration is incredibly rapid. Instead of the rate of 1 to 2 cm per day that is characteristic of *A. braziliense* larvae, the perianal migration of *S. stercoralis* may advance at a rate of 10 cm in the first 2.5 hours. Obvious migration does not continue after 1 or 2 days; fleeting burrows at distant sites and urticarial wheals replace the typical picture of larva migrans and underscore the hypersensitive nature of this syndrome.

Cutaneous larva migrans causes only a low-grade eosinophilia and no other laboratory abnormalities.

## COMPLICATIONS AND SEQUELAE

Secondary infections from autoinoculation of bacteria by scratching are common and are usually manifest by cellulitis. In the rare instances of Loeffler's syndrome, there are cough, transient pulmonary infiltrates, and eosinophilia to 50 per cent.

## GEOGRAPHIC VARIATIONS IN DISEASE

There are no known geographic variations in cutaneous larva migrans, but *A. caninum* occurs as far north as New York City (Dormand and Van Ostrand, 1958) and Montreal (Choquette and Gelinas, 1950) in the Western Hemisphere. Since its northern distribution probably exceeds that of *A. braziliense,* it is likely that cutaneous larva migrans in temperate and northern climates is milder and of shorter duration than that in subtropical and tropical climates.

## DIAGNOSIS

The diagnosis of cutaneous larva migrans can almost always be made clinically. The patient should recall exposure of the affected part of the body to the earth and often remembers a tingling or itching sensation that occurred within a few hours of exposure. Even without a typical history, the characteristics of the lesions are pathognomonic. Only lesions caused by *Gnathostoma spinigerum* and bot flies are easily confused with cutaneous larva migrans caused by hookworm larvae.

*G. spinigerum*, a natural parasite of the intestine of dogs, cats, and other carnivores, requires two waterborne intermediate hosts (microscopic crustaceans and either a fish, frog, or snake). Man becomes infected by eating the incompletely cooked flesh of the fish, frog, or snake. The larvae migrate and cause visceral larval migrans in man that may involve the lungs, meninges, and eyes. The cutaneous form may be indistinguishable clinically from creeping eruption caused by hookworm larvae except that it commonly causes nodules and abscesses that do not occur in creeping eruption. Gnathostomiosis is restricted to Israel, the Indian subcontinent, Southeast Asia, and the Far East.

Larvae of the bot flies of horses *(Gasterophilus* spp.) and cattle *(Hypoderma* spp.) may also migrate superficially and be indistinguishable from true creeping eruption, but they frequently migrate into deeper tissue temporarily, leaving gaps in their trail. This condition should be considered in patients with creeping eruption who also have heavy exposure to livestock.

All larvae that migrate in the skin lie just in advance of their burrow and may be removed, examined, and identified by a skin biopsy of this area. This procedure is seldom necessary, however, because *A. braziliense* and the larvae of other hookworms cause the vast majority of creeping eruption.

## TREATMENT

The traditional treatment is freezing the area around the leading edge of the tunnel with ethyl chloride spray or carbon dioxide snow. Because this treatment does not always provide permanent relief and is impractical if there are multiple lesions, treatment with local and oral anthelmintics is becoming more popular. Thiabendazole, 25 mg per kg orally twice daily for 2 days, has been used most commonly. A suspension of thiabendazole (500 mg per 5 ml) may be applied to the leading area in addition to, or instead of, oral therapy. Oral mebendazole at 1 to 2 mg per kg may be equally effective, and an ointment made up of mebendazole tablets and tetracaine ointment (for the pruritis) was recently reported to cure four patients with typical creeping eruption (Winter and Fripp, 1978).

## PROPHYLAXIS

Dogs and cats should be prohibited from public beaches, and people should avoid contact with beaches on which these animals are permitted. Sandboxes in which children play should be covered to protect them from dogs and cats. Workmen who come into contact with the soil under buildings and crawl spaces under houses should wear protective clothing. Finally, dogs and cats should be dewormed periodically.

## References

Beaver, P.: Immunity to *Necator americanus* infection. J Parasitol 31 (Suppl.):18, 1945.

Beaver, Paul C.: Parasitological Reviews. Larva migrans. Exp Parasitol V:587, 1956.

Caplan, J. P.: Creeping eruption and intestinal strongyloidiasis. Br Med J 1:396, 1949.

Choquette, L. P. E., Gelinas, L. de G.: The incidence of intestinal nematodes and protozoa in dogs of the Montreal area. Can J Comp Med 24:33, 1950.

Dormand, D. W., and Van Ostrand, J. R.: A survey of *Toxocara caris* and *Toxocara cati* in the New York City area. NY State J Med 58 (Part 2): 2793, 1958.

Dove, W.: Further studies on *Ancylostoma braziliense* and the etiology of creeping eruption. Am J Hyg 15:664, 1932.

Fulleborn, F.: Hautquaddeln und "Autoinfection" bis Strongyloid estragern. Arch. Schiffs- U. Tropen-Hyg 30:721, 1926.

Fulleborn, F.: Experimental erzeugte "Creeping eruption." Dermatol Wochschr 83:1474, 1926.

Fulleborn, F.: Über die durch die larvae von *Ancylostoma caninum* verursachten Hauterscheinungen. Giorn Clin Med Festschr f Prof Gabbi Part 1:37, 1930.

Kirby-Smith, J., Dove, W., and White, G.: Creeping eruption. Arch Dermatol Syphilol 13:137, 1926.

Maplestone, P. A.: Creeping eruption caused by hookworm larvae. Indian Med Gaz 68:251, 1933.

Mayhew, R. L.: Creeping eruption caused by the larvae of the cattle hookworm *Bunostomum phelobotomum*. Proc Soc Exp Biol Med 66:12, 1947.

White, G., and Dove, W.: The causation of creeping eruption. JAMA 90:1701, 1928.

White, G., and Dove, W.: A dermatitis caused by larvae of *Ancylostoma caninum*. Arch Dermatol Syphilol 20:191, 1929.

Winter, P. A. D., and Fripp, P. J.: Treatment of cutaneous larva migrans (Sandworm disease). S Afr Med J 52:556, 1978.

Wright, D. O., and Gold, E. M.: Löffler's syndrome associated with creeping eruption. Arch Intern Med 78:303, 1946.

# 220 *CUTANEOUS AMEBIASIS*

## *Francisco Biagi, M.D.*

## *DEFINITION*

Cutaneous amebiasis is an ulcer of the skin that sometimes extends to the contiguous mucous membranes. It can occur as a complication of intestinal or hepatic amebiasis or as a primary infection with exogenous trophozoites of *Entamoeba histolytica*. It is sporadically seen in geographic areas where amebiasis is severe and common. Cutaneous amebiasis should always be included in the differential diagnosis of skin lesions in endemic areas because it is often fatal if untreated but is easy to diagnose and responds promptly to treatment.

The etiology and epidemiology of amebiasis are discussed in Chapter 130 (Amebic Dysentery).

## *PATHOGENESIS AND CLINICAL MANIFESTATIONS*

The source of the trophozoites of *E. histolytica* and their pathway to the skin determine the location of amebic skin lesions.

1. When the skin is invaded by trophozoites from fistulae or surgery on intestinal amebiasis, the lesions are located on the perineum or the anterior abdominal wall (Fig. 1).

2. Trophozoites from spontaneous or surgical drainage of a liver abscess are located on the skin over the abdominal wall or the base of the right hemithorax. These lesions sometimes communicate with the lungs.

3. Trophozoites may be directly implanted from the exterior:

   a. Genital lesions may develop in infants with acute intestinal amebiasis because infected feces are held in contact with the skin by diapers (Fig. 2). This type of cutaneous amebiasis is more common in girls.

   b. Penile lesions may occur after rectal intercourse (Fig. 3).

   c. Rarely, cutaneous amebiasis may occur on the nose or face (Fig. 4) after implantation of trophozoites by contaminated fingers or hands. These lesions may occur in patients with no other evidence of amebiasis.

The basic pathologic process is lysis of the tissues with formation of ulcers. The inflammatory response is minimal. *E. histolytica* produces several enzymes that may be capable of degrading skin.

The ulcers are painful, bleed easily, and grow rapidly. The edges are well-defined, thick, and dark red. Small early lesions resemble cutaneous leishmaniasis. These ulcers may become very large and destroy the skin, mucous membranes, and subcutaneous tissues. Muscles are usually not invaded. The process may destroy the external genitalia. If untreated, the lesions may spread from the perineum, abdomen, thorax, or face, and become so large that the patient dies (Fig. 5).

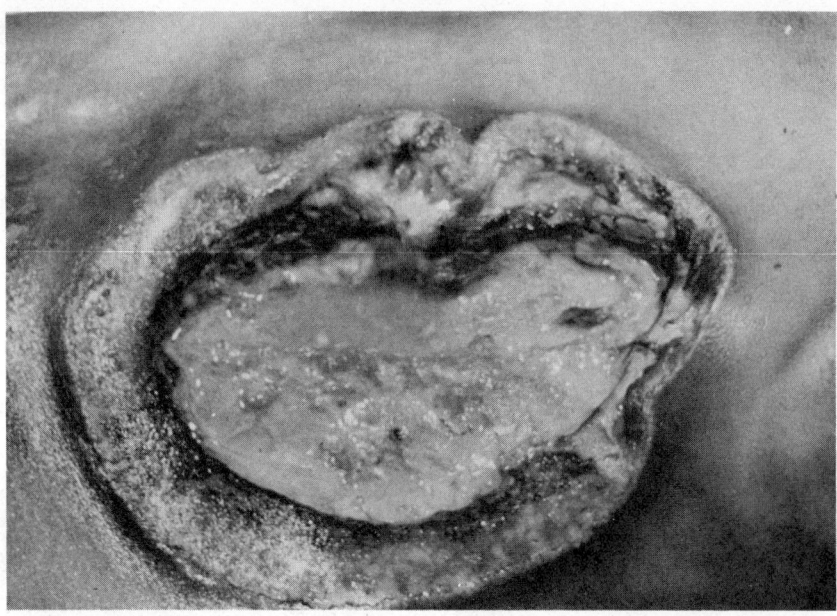

**FIGURE 1.** *Cutaneous amebiasis of the abdomen after surgery for unsuspected amebic appendicitis.*

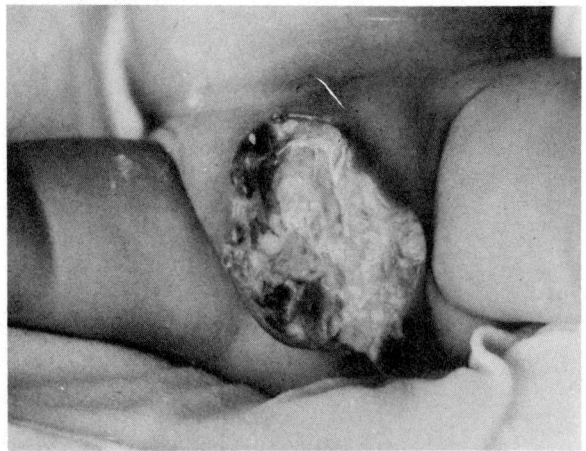

**FIGURE 2.** *Infant with acute intestinal amebiasis and genital amebiasis secondary to reinvasion of trophozoites.*

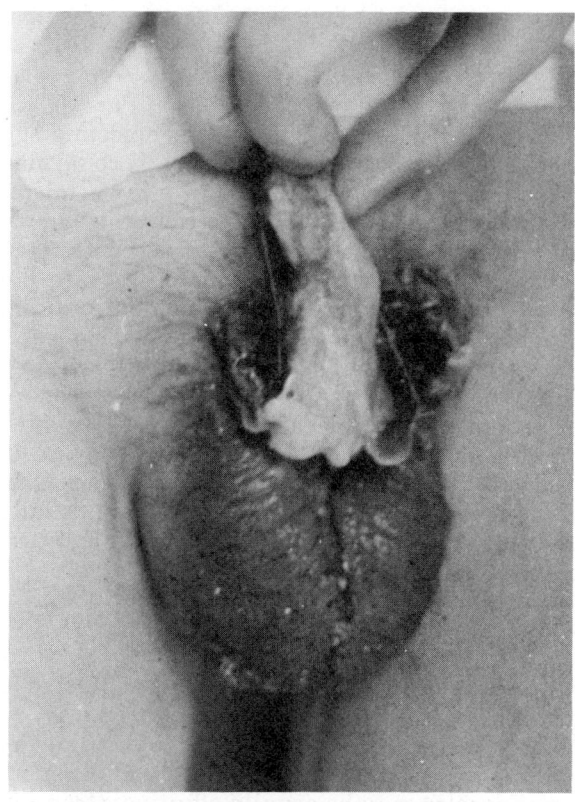

**FIGURE 3.** *Cutaneous amebiasis of the penis.*

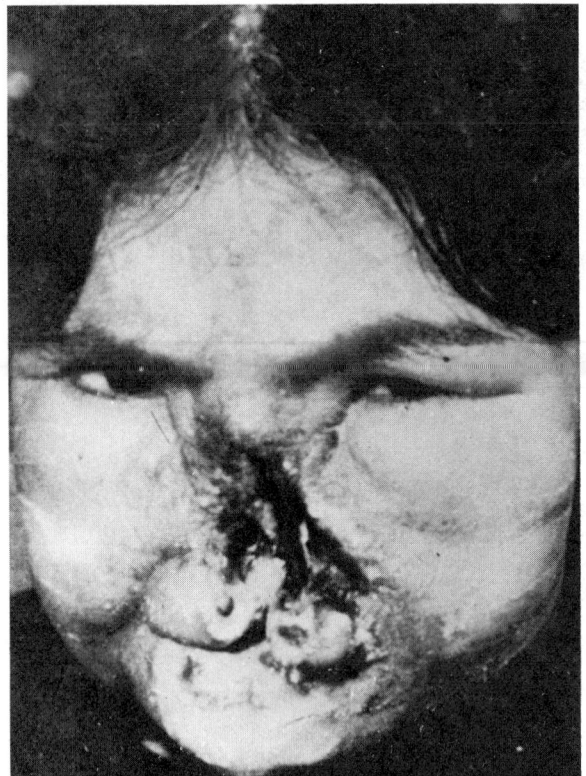

**FIGURE 4.**  *Cutaneous amebiasis of the face.*

good healing with little fibrosis. This prompt, complete healing may occur because of the minimal inflammatory reaction provoked by amebae. Reconstructive surgery is usually not necessary. If the lesions have grown too large (more than 20 cm in diameter), however, the patient usually dies in spite of appropriate therapy.

## PROPHYLAXIS

In addition to general measures to control or avoid amebiasis (Chapter 130), a few specific principles for prevention of cutaneous amebiasis

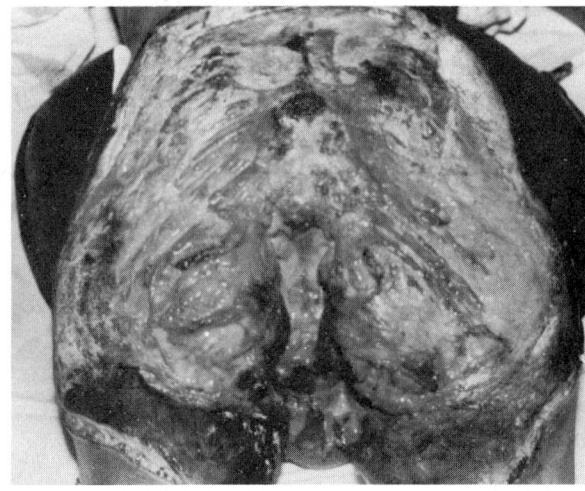

**FIGURE 5.**  *Fatal cutaneous amebiasis of the perineal and gluteal regions.*

## DIAGNOSIS

The history, clinical findings, and epidemiology should suggest the diagnosis, which is confirmed by demonstrating trophozoites in a fresh microscopic preparation of a scraping from the edge of the ulcer. The smears can be stained with iron-hematoxylin to bring out details of the internal structure and permit more precise identification. Trophozoites can also be shown on histologic sections of skin biopsies stained with iron-hematoxylin or hematoxylin and eosin, but this procedure takes longer. The amebae may also be cultivated in one of the standard egg and rice flour media (Chapter 78) from a scraping or biopsy of the edge of the ulcer. Serologies for amebiasis are usually positive.

## TREATMENT

Emetine or dehydroemetine is very effective (1 mg/kg of body weight daily for ten days) (Fig. 6). Nimorazole is also very effective (20 to 40 mg/kg of body weight daily for ten days), and other nitroimidazoles may be equally effective. Granulation of the skin is rapid and clean and produces

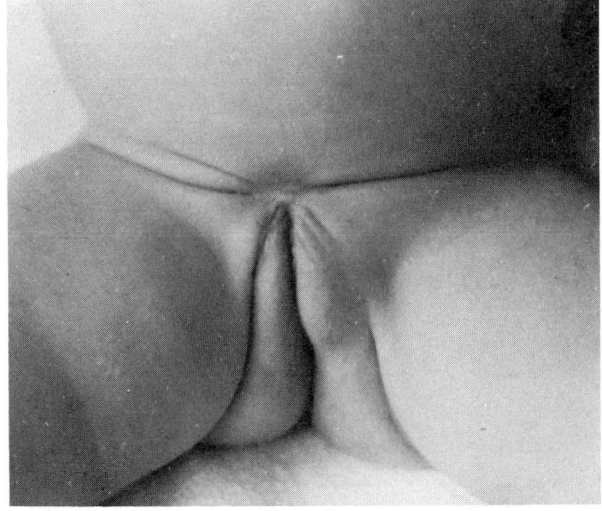

**FIGURE 6.**  *Healed cutaneous amebiasis after emetine. (Same case as Fig. 2)*

can be listed: (1) Amebiasis should be treated early, preferably during the carrier state; (2) infants with diarrhea should be cleaned and changed frequently; and (3) surgery of amebic bowel lesions or liver abscesses should be done carefully with minimal tissue contamination. If appendicitis is shown to be amebic by histopa-thology, fecal examination, or serology, anti-amebic therapy should be started promptly.

### References

Biagi, F.: Amibiasis cutánea. Prensa Med Mex 30 (5–6): 155, 1965.
Meleney, F. L., and Meleney, H. E.: Gangrene of the buttock, perineum and scrotum due to *Entamoeba histolytica*. Arch Surg 30:980, 1953.

# CUTANEOUS AND MUCOCUTANEOUS LEISHMANIASIS (ORIENTAL SORE, ESPUNDIA)

# 221

### Anthony D. M. Bryceson

## DEFINITION

Cutaneous leishmaniasis is an infection with one of the cutaneous species of parasites of the genus *Leishmania* (see Table 1). It is usually a zoonosis transmitted by phlebotomine sandflies between wild or peridomestic animals, especially rodents or carnivores. Man is infected when he interrupts the natural cycle. Human infection is characterized by one or several chronic sores that usually heal spontaneously. In parts of South and Central America, severe mutilating metastatic lesions of the mouth and nose are seen.

## ETIOLOGY AND EPIDEMIOLOGY

The morphology and biology of *Leishmania* are described in Chapter 78 (Hommel, 1978).

In the Old World the innumerable names of this disease (Delhi or Baghdad boil, Biskra button, Aleppo evil, bouton de Crete, little sister) testify to its scope and familiarity throughout the Mediterranean basin, the Near and Middle East, and parts of India. Four epidemiologic situations are recognized.

"Rural" leishmaniasis throughout these areas is caused by *L. tropica major*. The disease is a zoonosis among the desert gerbils *(Rhomobomys opimus)* and is transmitted to man by *Phlebotomus papatasi*. When village settlements are close to gerbil colonies, 100 per cent of the population may become infected, usually in early childhood. Travelers, hunters, and soldiers also get the dis-ease. In "urban" leishmaniasis, the parasite *L. tropica minor* is adapted to dogs and to man, either of which can act as a reservoir. *P. sergenti* is the main vector. This disease was formerly the scourge of Middle Eastern cities. Every adult inhabitant bore the scars, and few visitors were spared.

In Africa two distinct zoonoses exist. In West Africa the situation is "rural." Human cases are uncommon and sporadic. The vector and reservoir are not definitely established, but rodents and dogs are probably involved. In Ethiopia and Kenya the disease is caused by *L. aethiopica* and is confined to the highlands, where the reservoir is the rock hyrax *(Procavia)*. The vector, *P. longipes,* bites villagers at night in their houses. A few isolated cases of cutaneous leishmaniasis have been reported in Central and Southern Africa. Their epidemiology is unknown.

In the New World, cutaneous leishmaniasis is endemic in Central and South America as far south as the Parana Estuary in the east and the Peruvian Andes in the west. In this extensive and varied terrain many different zoonoses exist, each associated with its own reservoirs and vector and a particular pattern of human disease (Lainson and Shaw, 1978). Two main groups of parasites are distinguished, those of *L. mexicana* and of *L. brasiliensis. L. mexicana,* which grows easily in NNN medium and in the hamster, is responsible for most of the cutaneous leishmaniasis in Central America and a little in Brazil. Rates of infection among forest rodents may be as high as 20 per cent, but the vector is not attracted to man,

**TABLE 1.   Epidemiology of Cutaneous Leishmaniasis**

| OLD WORLD | | | | |
|---|---|---|---|---|
| **Parasite** | **Vector to Man** | **Reservoir** | **Geography** | **Human Disease** |
| *L. tropica minor* (*L. t. tropica*) | *Phlebotomus sergenti* | Man, dog | Middle East, Mediterranean | "Urban" sores and leishmaniasis recidiva |
| *L. tropica major* | *Phlebotomus papatasi* and others | Rodents, especially *Rhomobomys* | Middle East, India, China, Mediterranean, ? West Africa | "Rural" sores |
| *L. aethiopica* | *Phlebotomus longipes* | Rock hyrax | Ethiopian and Kenyan highlands | Simple sores and diffuse cutaneous leishmaniasis |
| NEW WORLD | | | | |
| *L. mexicana mexicana* | *Lutzomyia olmeca* | Numerous forest rodents | Yucatan, Belize, Guatemala | "Chicle ulcer," "bay sore" in forest workers; diffuse cutaneous leishmaniasis |
| *L. mexicana amazonensis* | *Lutzomyia flaviscutella* | Numerous rodents (marsupials, fox) | Amazonian Brazil, Trinidad; ? = *L. pifanoi,* Venezuela | Rare, single skin lesions; diffuse cutaneous leishmaniasis |
| *L. brasiliensis brasiliensis* | *Psychodopygus wellcomei, Lutzomyia* spp | Several forest rodents | All Amazon forests, especially Brazil | Single or few large, persistent, destructive skin ulcers. Oronasal metastases common: espundia |
| *L. brasiliensis guyanensis* | *Lutzomyia umbratilis* | Unknown | Guyanas, Surinam, into Brazil and Venezuela | "Forest yaws," "pian-bois," ? oronasal metastases |
| *L. brasiliensis panamensis* | *Lutzomyia trapidoi, Psychodopygus panamensis,* and others | Rodents, sloths, primates | Panama, Costa Rica, Colombia | Skin ulcers, ? oronasal metastases |
| *L. peruviana* | *Lutzomyia verrucarum,* ? *Lutzomyia peruensis* | Dogs | Peru, west slopes of Andes to 3000 meters, Argentinian highlands | "Uta;" single or few skin lesions healing in one year |

so human infection is rare except in Mexican chicle collectors who are exposed to intense contact with infective sandflies at the time of maximum transmission. *L. brasiliensis,* which grows poorly in NNN medium and in the hamster and has a distinctive phase of development in the hind gut of the sandfly, is responsible for most of the disease in South America, including mucocutaneous leishmaniasis. All the vectors of *L. brasiliensis* are highly anthropophilic and will bite man viciously by night or day, so that the rate of infection among those who enter the forest is high. In Panama the natural sloth-sandfly cycle takes place in the treetops rather than on the forest floor, but the vector rests on the lower parts of tree trunks, from which it is attracted to man.

Cutaneous leishmaniasis presents a formidable obstacle to the development of the Central and South American forests. This is particularly true in Brazil, where new settlers and workers in the forest, such as those employed on the trans-Amazonian highway, become infected and run the risk of developing mutilating oronasal metastatic lesions.

In the Peruvian Andes and Argentinian highlands the parasite *L. peruviana* has adapted to the high, dry climate and sparse vegetation. The dog is the reservoir, and transmission is domiciliary.

Epidemiologic data are summarized in the table.

## PATHOGENESIS

The patterns of disease in man are partly determined by the parasite and partly by man's response to the parasite (Bryceson, 1975; Ridley, 1979). Dermatotropic species of *Leishmania* are sensitive to temperatures above 35° C and will grow only on the exposed, cooler areas of skin. Some species are more immunogenic and allergenic than others. *Leishmania* organisms may eventually destroy the macrophages in which they multiply but do not otherwise damage their host directly. Resistance to *Leishmania* depends on the development of specific cell-mediated immunity. The capacity of individuals to mount such a response varies, and consequently cutaneous leishmaniasis presents a spectrum of disease similar to that seen in leprosy. At one end of the spectrum is diffuse cutaneous leishmaniasis, characterized by an abundance of parasites, absence of lymphocytes in lesions, dermal insensitivity to injection of leishmanin (a suspension of promastigotes), and poor prognosis. At the other end are the self-healing sores, characterized by relatively scanty parasites, marked lymphocytic infiltration, and leishmanin sensitivity. Accompanying cell-mediated immunity is delayed hypersensitivity to numerous parasite antigens, which seems to cause the destructive pathology of leishmanial ulcers, which in turn seems to be an essential step toward healing, unlike the situation in leprosy. In the chronic conditions of mucocutaneous leishmaniasis and leishmaniasis recidiva the normal balance between immunity and hypersensitivity has been lost, so that healing is prevented.

## PATHOLOGY

At the site of inoculation there is a massive infiltration of monocytes and histiocytes, which take up the parasites and support their growth. The lesion then becomes surrounded by or mixed with lymphocytes and a few plasma cells. Macrophages develop into epithelioid cells, and parasites diminish. Later, tubercles composed of loosely packed cells may develop. The overlying dermis ulcerates. The epidermis shows hyperkeratosis, acanthosis, pseudo-epitheliomatous hyperplasia, intraepidermal necrosis, and ulceration. Healing is accompanied by fibrosis.

In diffuse cutaneous leishmaniasis, cell-mediated immunity fails to develop, and the disease spreads to other parts of the skin (Convit et al., 1972). Histologic study shows masses of heavily parasitized macrophages with little or no lymphocytic infiltration or epidermal change.

In leishmaniasis recidiva, failure to heal is associated with extreme chronicity, a tuberculoid histology with epithelioid giant cells but no caseation, and scanty or undetectable parasites.

Metastatic lesions of *L. brasiliensis* arise in the mucosa of the nose and mouth and show at first a typical leishmanial granuloma with numerous parasites. The parasites later become scanty, and can be seen also in cells in cartilage, which is rapidly invaded and destroyed. There is vasculitis with edema, necrosis, and fibrosis.

## CLINICAL MANIFESTATIONS

The earliest lesion is a small erythematous papule, appearing two to eight weeks after the sandfly bite. It may itch slightly. The prototype is the "urban" sore, caused by *L. tropica minor,* which grows slowly into a nodule 1 to 2 cm across, and after a period of weeks or months forms a central crust overlying a shallow ulcer with an elevated margin (Fig. 1). The edge of the lesion is characteristically studded with small satellite papules. The sore usually remains in this state for a few more months and then heals gradually, leaving a depressed, mottled scar. The whole pro-

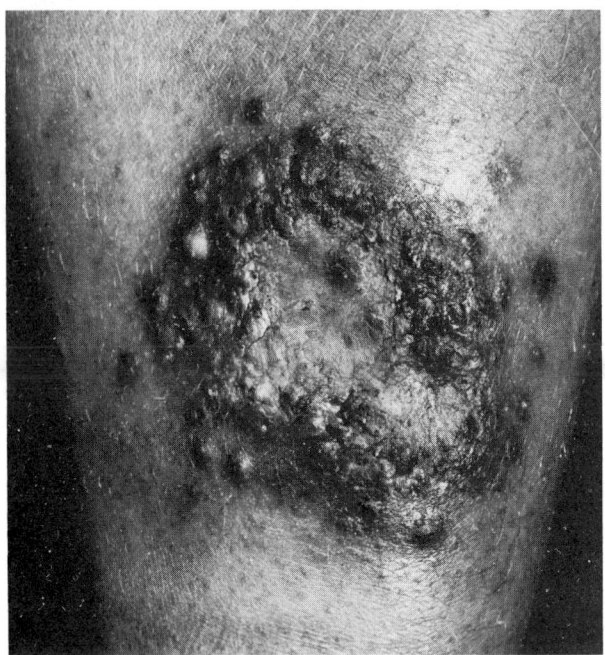

**FIGURE 1.** *Oriental sore from the Middle East, showing the classic appearance of cutaneous leishmaniasis caused by L. tropica: elevated lesion with central crusting, satellite papules, and little peripheral inflammation. (Courtesy of St. John's Hospital for Diseases of the Skin, London.)*

cess takes from three months to two years. The most common site is the face, followed by the arms and legs. Soles, palms, axillae, and scalp are usually spared. There may be one or several sores.

## COMPLICATIONS AND SEQUELAE

Healing is usually followed by lifelong immunity. Second infections are seen in only about 2 in 1000 cases of oriental sore, usually in older patients or in those taking corticosteroid drugs. Immunity is usually species-specific, but *L. tropica major* protects against *L. tropica minor.* About 1 per cent of patients with urban sores develop leishmaniasis recidiva (lupoid leishmaniasis). In this condition the ulcer fails to heal completely. It either spreads peripherally from the central scar or heals and recrudesces at the edge of the scar. The lesion lasts for many years and resembles cutaneous tuberculosis. This complication is less common with *L. tropica major* and *L. aethiopica* and is not seen in the New World.

Diffuse cutaneous leishmaniasis develops in the rare patient without cellular immunity. This complication is associated with only two species of parasite (see next section).

## GEOGRAPHIC VARIATIONS

The diverse epidemiology of cutaneous leishmaniasis is associated with many different clinical patterns. Some of these patterns are distinct, while others are themselves a spectrum of disease that merges into other patterns.

There are many variants of the typical pattern of the Old World oriental sore. "Rural" sores, caused by *L. tropica major,* are commonly multiple, rapid in evolution, more florid, and produce more scarring. West African sores, usually found on the limbs, are often multiple and extremely crusty. Ethiopian lesions are solitary, facial, milder, and slower in evolution, often lasting several years before healing with little or no ulceration. Primary lesions affecting the mucocutaneous border of the nose are common and are extremely chronic and disfiguring.

Ethiopia and Kenya are the only Old World countries where diffuse cutaneous leishmaniasis is found. It is a rare condition, occurring in perhaps 1 in 100,000 cases of leishmaniasis. The primary nodule does not ulcerate. After a period of months or years it spreads locally, and the disease is disseminated to other parts of the skin, notably the face and the extensor surfaces of the limbs. These infiltrative and nodular lesions may resemble lepromatous leprosy (Fig. 2) and do not heal spontaneously. The viscera are not involved, and the patient feels well.

In the New World, many sores conform to the Old World prototype, especially "uta" due to *L. peruviensis* and the majority of lesions due to *L. m. mexicana,* the "chicle ulcer" or "bay sore" (Fig. 3) of forest workers in Yucatan and ·Central America that is commonly seen on the face and heals in less than six months. *L. m. mexicana* lesions are, however, especially common on the pinna, where they may last for many years, slowly destroying the cartilage (Fig. 4).

Primary lesions of *L. b. brasiliensis* are often frankly and deeply ulcerative. They occur most commonly on the limbs, are often multiple, and heal spontaneously. American Indians commonly develop transient mild infections, so that by the age of 40 almost all are sensitive to leishmanin. They rarely develop mucocutaneous lesions. Lesions due to *L. b. guyanensis,* known as "forest yaws" or "pian bois," and *L. b. panamensis* have a tendency to produce nodular or cord-like lesions in the draining lymphatic vessels.

### American Mucocutaneous Leishmaniasis

Primary lesions of *L. b. brasiliensis* are followed after a period ranging from a few days to 25 years by metastatic lesions of the nose or mouth, most commonly on the mucocutaneous borders, but sometimes on the palate or larynx

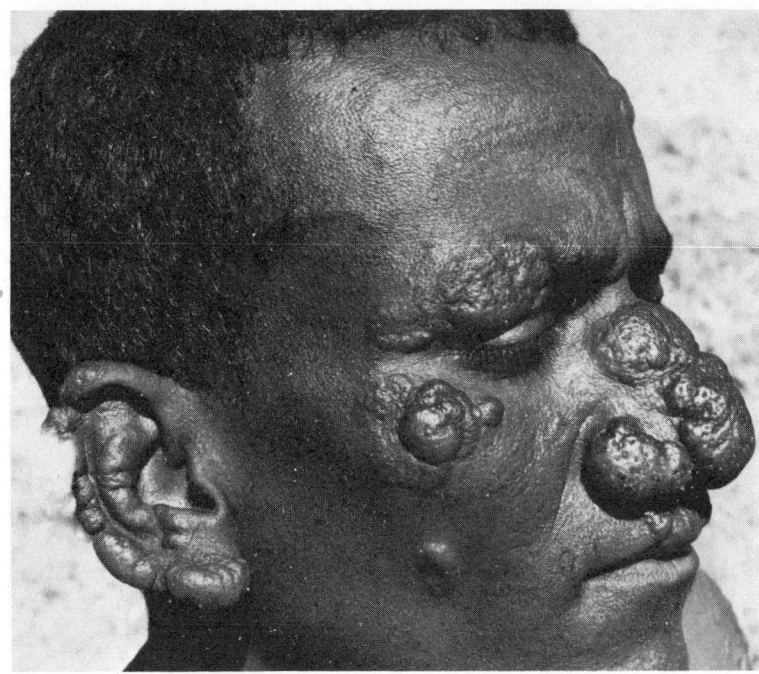

**FIGURE 2.** *Diffuse cutaneous leishmaniasis caused by* L. aethiopica *in an Ethiopian. Note the resemblance with post-kala-azar dermal leishmaniasis and lepromatous leprosy. (Courtesy of Dr. A. Bryceson and Trans. R Soc Trop Med Hyg.)*

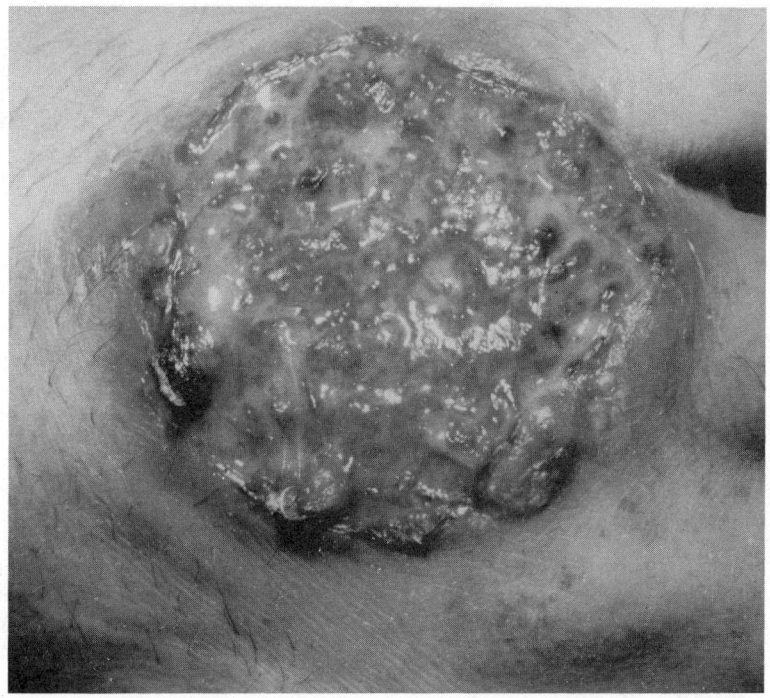

**FIGURE 3.** *Ulcer on back of hand caused by* L. mexicana mexicana *in Belise. (Courtesy of Dr. A. Bryceson.)*

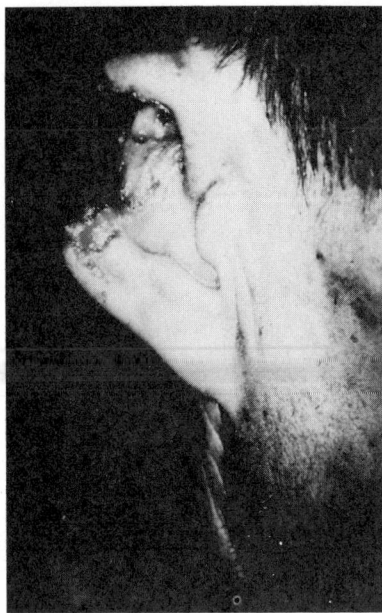

**FIGURE 4.** *Chronic destructive lesion caused by* L. mexicana mexicana *on the pinna of a Mexican chiclero. (Courtesy Dr. J. E. Ash.)*

yp formation, and then ulceration and perforation of the septum. Alternatively, large protruding granulomas of the nose and lips develop (Fig. 5). The lesion heals slowly, if at all, after many years. Scarring may constrict the nose or mouth, producing gross deformity and making eating difficult. Secondary sepsis is common and increases the patient's debility. The prevalence of this complication, sometimes called espundia (Portuguese for sponge), varies from 2 per cent in Panama, where few cases of the disease are due to *L. b. brasiliensis,* to 80 per cent in Paraguay, where most cases of the disease are due to this agent. The complication is usually prevented by adequate chemotherapy of the primary lesion.

Diffuse cutaneous leishmaniasis has been described in Venezuela, northern Brazil, Mexico, and Texas. Its clinical features are the same as in Ethiopia.

## DIAGNOSIS

Leishmaniasis must be suspected as the cause of any chronic nodule or ulcer in a person who lives in or has recently visited an endemic area. Typical sores can be diagnosed on sight. Diagnosis is confirmed by finding parasites in stained slit-skin smears taken from a nonulcerated part of the lesion (Fig. 6). The slit must reach the dermis; the smears must contain tissue juice, not

and rarely on the conjunctiva or external genitalia (Marsden and Nonata, 1975). Nasal obstruction is the most common early symptom. These lesions may arise many years after the primary lesion has healed. At first there is crusting or pol-

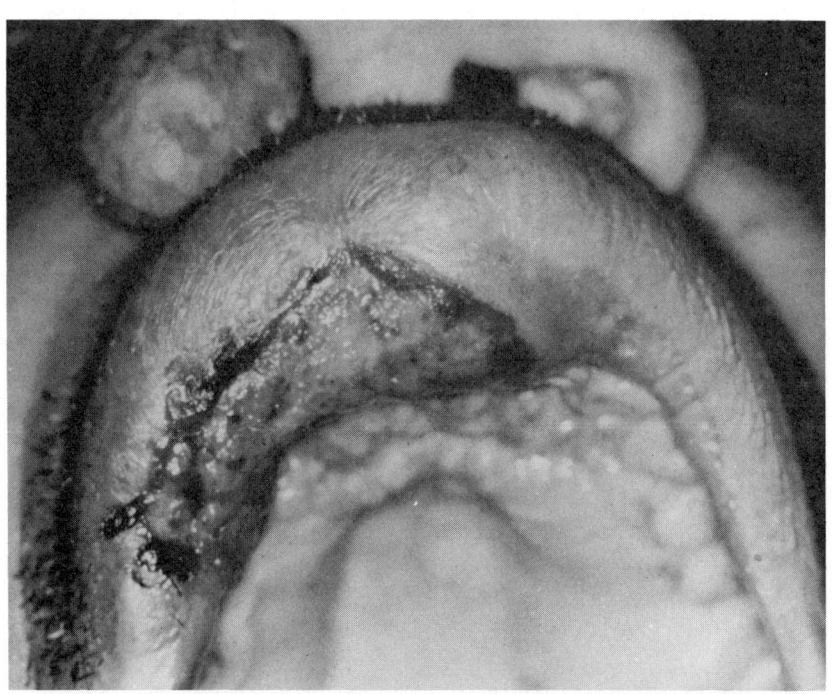

**FIGURE 5.** *Mucocutaneous leishmaniasis caused by* L. braziliensis. *There is granulomatous infiltration of the palate, ulceration of the lip, and a polypoid lesion in the right nostril. (Courtesy of Professor A. Pons.)*

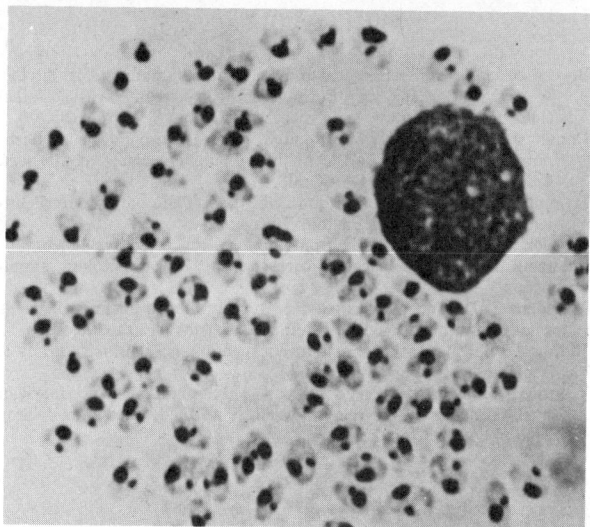

**FIGURE 6.** *Macrophage containing numerous amastigotes of* Leishmania *in a smear from the tail of* Oryzomys capito, *a rodent reservoir of* L. mexicana. *A similar appearance is seen in slit skin smears from human cutaneous lesions or marrow aspiration smears in visceral leishmaniasis. (Courtesy of Dr. R. Lainson, Dr. J. Shaw, and Trans R Soc Trop Med Hyg.)*

blood or pus. If this technique is unsuccessful, the crust should be removed, the ulcer cleaned of all debris, and smears made of tissue scraped from the base of the ulcer. These methods are simpler and more likely to show parasites than biopsy. In healing lesions of leishmaniasis recidiva and in mucocutaneous lesions, parasites are scanty, and culture of tissue juice or biopsy tissue may be necessary (Chapter 140).

### Leishmanin (Montenegro) Test

Leishmanin is a suspension of $10^6$ promastigotes in 1 ml of 0.5 per cent phenolsaline. The test is performed by injecting 0.1 ml of leishmanin intradermally into the volar surface of the forearm. A palpable nodule, 5 mm or more in diameter after 48 to 72 hours, is considered positive. The test is an index of delayed hypersensitivity but not necessarily of immunity to *Leishmania*. It is not species-specific. It is used to map out the extent of past infection in a community and may help in the diagnosis of individual patients.

The leishmanin test becomes positive as the lesion ulcerates and is of diagnostic value in patients who do not live in endemic areas; it also may help to distinguish lupoid leishmaniasis from cutaneous tuberculosis, late syphilis, blastomycosis, histoplasmosis, and other fungal granulomas that may be histologically similar.

Antibodies may be detected by indirect immunofluorescence in over 90 per cent of patients with American mucocutaneous leishmaniasis, and in a smaller proportion of patients with simple sores from the New World (Walton et al., 1972). Serologic tests have not generally been found helpful in the diagnosis of cutaneous leishmaniasis in the Old World.

## TREATMENT

Treatment is unsatisfactory. In most parts of the world lesions heal spontaneously, and the systemic use of toxic drugs is seldom justified. Any patient with a lesion that could be due to *L. brasiliensis* should be thoroughly treated with systemic pentavalent antimony as described in Chapter 140.

### Local Treatment

Success has been claimed for local infiltration with 2 per cent berberine sulfate, 15 per cent mepacrine, or 0.3 to 0.8 ml sodium stibogluconate. The local application of heat, whereby the lesion is held at 40 to 43° C for several hours daily, is usually successful.

Leishmaniasis recidiva heals poorly and may require intralesional injections of corticosteroids combined with a course of antimony, or curettage and skin grafting.

### Systemic Treatment

Most cases respond to a course of pentavalent antimony, which is usually not toxic and should be given until the lesion is nearly healed (see Chapter 140). *L. brasiliensis* lesions are treated until they are well healed. Failure to respond is usually due to inadequate dosage or duration of treatment. *L. mexicana* lesions are said to respond to a single (painful) repository injection of cycloguanil pamoate, 5 mg/kg body weight. This drug is otherwise ineffective. Established American mucocutaneous lesions often fail to respond to antimony or relapse after its use. Amphotericin B is then the drug of choice (see Chapter 140). 5-Fluorocytosine has also been used successfully in a dose of 5 g daily for 10 days. Diffuse cutaneous leishmaniasis responds initially to antimony in South America but is resistant in Ethiopia. Amphotericin B- or pentamidine may then be tried, but frequent relapses are the rule.

## PROPHYLAXIS

Detailed epidemiologic knowledge has permitted attacks on the reservoir of this disease in Central Asia and in Middle Eastern cities, where demolition of mud buildings and antimalarial spraying have reduced the number of sandflies. Immunization with live, virulent organisms is practiced on a mass scale in Russia and in the Middle East.

Prevention in South America is difficult. Intensity of transmission in the forest and lack of detailed epidemiologic information make mass prophylaxis a hopeless approach at the moment. People who are obliged to enter the forest should try to apply insect repellents every few hours and sleep under a fine mesh netting, even though these procedures are uncomfortable and inconvenient, and wear long sleeved shirts and trousers.

## References

Bryceson, A. D. M.: Mechanisms of disease in leishmaniasis. In Taylor, A., and Muller, R. (eds.): Pathogenic Processes in Parasitic Infections. Oxford, Blackwell Scientific Publications, 1975, p. 85.

Convit, J., Pinardi, M. E., and Rondon, A. J.: Diffuse cutaneous leishmaniasis: A disease due to an immunological defect of the host. Trans Soc Trop Med Hyg 66:603, 1972.

Hommel, M.: The genus *Leishmania*: biology of the parasite and clinical aspects. Bull Inst Pasteur 76:5, 1978.

Lainson, R., and Shaw, J. J.: Epidemiology and ecology of leishmaniasis in Latin America. Nature (Lond) 273:(parasitology suppl) 595, 1978.

Marsden, P. D., and Nonata, R. R.: Mucocutaneous leishmaniasis: A review of clinical aspects. Rev Soc Bras Med Trop 9:309, 1975.

Ridley, D. S.: The pathogenesis of cutaneous leishmaniasis. Trans R Soc Trop Med Hyg 73:150, 1979.

Walton, B. C., Brooks, W. H., and Aronja, I.: Serodiagnosis of American leishmaniasis by indirect fluorescent antibody test. Am J Trop Med Hyg 21:296, 1972.

# 222 VARICELLA

## Michael N. Oxman, M.D.

Varicella (chickenpox) and herpes zoster (shingles, zoster) are distinct clinical entities caused by a single member of the herpesvirus group, *Herpesvirus varicellae* (varicella-zoster virus, VZV). The differences between these two diseases are due to differences in the host and in the circumstances of infection rather than to differences in the etiologic agent.

Varicella, an acute, highly contagious exanthematous disease that occurs most often in childhood, is the result of primary infection of a susceptible individual. It is characterized by a short or absent prodromal period and a generalized pruritic rash consisting of successive crops of lesions that progress rapidly from macules and papules to vesicles, pustules, and crusts. In normal children systemic symptoms are usually mild, and serious complications are extremely rare. In adults and in immunologically compromised individuals of any age, varicella is more likely to be associated with an extensive eruption, high fever, severe constitutional symptoms, pneumonia, and other life-threatening complications.

## ETIOLOGY

Heberden (1767) is credited with first differentiating varicella from smallpox, but more than a century later such authorities as Osler (1892) deemed it necessary to emphasize that the two diseases were indeed etiologically distinct. Steiner in 1875 transmitted the disease to volunteers by the inoculation of vesicle fluid from patients with varicella. Tyzzer described the histopathology of the skin lesions of varicella in 1906 and called attention to the characteristic multinucleated giant cells and intranuclear inclusion bodies. However, it was not until 1952 that Weller and Stoddard succeeded in isolating and propagating the virus from varicella vesicle fluid in vitro.

*Herpesvirus varicellae* is a member of the herpesvirus group. Other members pathogenic for humans include the herpes simplex viruses (see Chapter 56), the cytomegaloviruses, and the Epstein-Barr virus of infectious mononucleosis. All of these herpesviruses are morphologically indistinguishable and share a number of properties, including a remarkable propensity for establishing latent infections that may persist for the life of the host. Varicella-zoster virus (VZV) consists of an icosahedral capsid 100 nm in diameter that encloses the viral genome, a linear molecule of double-stranded DNA with a molecular weight of about 100 million daltons. The capsid is composed of 162 protein subunits (capsomers), which resemble elongated hexagonal or pentagonal prisms with an axial hole (Fig. 1B). The nucleocapsid is surrounded by one or two additional layers of protein and, finally, by a loose lipoprotein envelope derived from the nuclear membrane of the host cell and containing radially oriented viral glycoproteins on its surface (Fig. 1A). The complete virion is roughly spherical with a diameter of 150 to 200 nm (Almeida et al., 1962). Only enveloped virions are infectious, and this accounts for the lability of VZV; infectivity is rapidly destroyed

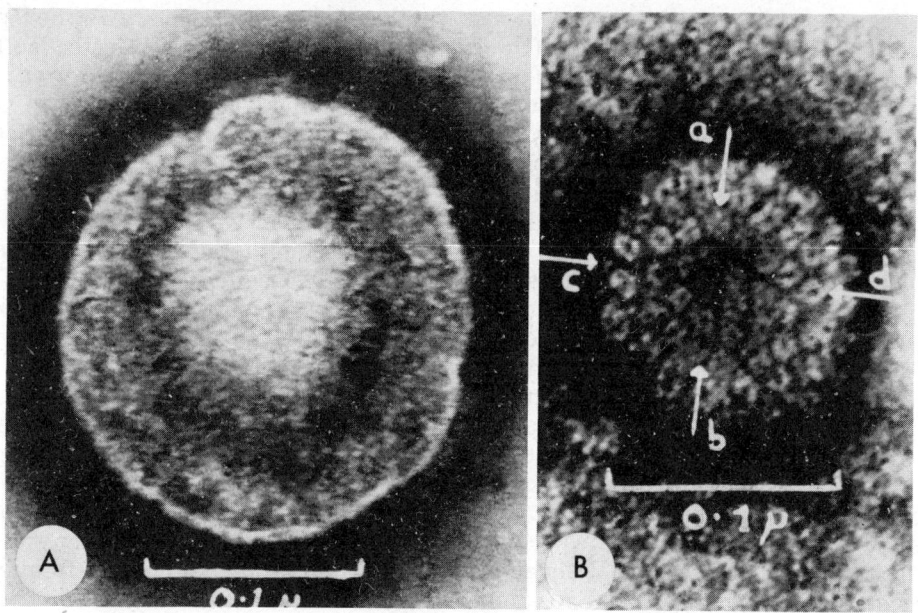

**FIGURE 1.** *Varicella-zoster virus stained with phosphotungstic acid. A, Intact particle showing envelope with radially oriented glycoproteins on its surface. B, Rupture of the envelope reveals the nucleocapsid within. (From Almeida, J. D., Howatson, A. F., and Williams, M. G.: Virology 16:353, 1962.)*

by organic solvents, detergents, proteolytic enzymes, heat, and extremes of pH. In addition to structural components of the virion, certain enzymes essential for virus replication are synthesized in infected cells, e.g., a virus-specific DNA polymerase and a virus-specific deoxypyrimidine kinase. These are of potential importance as targets for specific antiviral chemotherapy (Richman and Oxman, 1978).

There is only one VZV serotype. A number of antigens are present in the virion and are produced in infected cells, but these are identical in viruses isolated from patients with varicella and herpes zoster throughout the world (Weller, 1976; Taylor-Robinson and Caunt, 1972; Weller et al., 1958). However, some VZV antigens cross-react with antigens of other members of the herpesvirus group, and this limits the usefulness of certain serologic tests (Weller, 1976; Taylor-Robinson and Caunt, 1972; Weller, 1979).

None of the common laboratory animals are susceptible to infection by VZV, but the virus can be isolated and propagated in vitro in monolayer cultures of a variety of human (and certain simian) cells (Weller, 1976; Taylor-Robinson and Caunt, 1972; Weller, 1979). The cytopathic effect in such cell cultures is characterized by the formation of acidophilic intranuclear inclusion bodies and multinucleated giant cells similar to those seen in the cutaneous lesions of the disease. These changes are indistinguishable from those pro-

duced by herpes simplex virus, but whereas herpes simplex virus is released into the medium by initially infected cells and rapidly spreads to infect the remaining cells in the culture, the cytopathic effect of VZV remains focal. This is because infectious VZV remains cell-associated and is not released into the medium; by the initially infected cells; infection proceeds from cell to cell only by direct contact, and the initial foci of infection gradually enlarge. Serial passage of VZV in tissue culture requires the transfer of infected cells.

## PATHOGENESIS AND PATHOLOGY

Our concept of the pathogenesis of varicella is based primarily on circumstantial evidence and analogy with experimental models of other exanthematous diseases. The virus probably enters through the mucosa of the upper respiratory tract and oropharynx. Initial multiplication here results in dissemination of small amounts of virus by way of the blood and lymphatics (the primary viremia). This virus is removed by the reticuloendothelial system, which is probably the major site of virus replication during the remainder of the incubation period. The incubating infection is partially contained by nonspecific defenses (e.g., interferon) and developing immune responses. In most individuals, virus replication eventually overwhelms these defenses so that about two weeks after infection a much larger viremia (the secondary viremia) occurs (Feldman and Epp, 1979). This causes fever and malaise and disseminates virus throughout the body, especially to the skin and mucous membranes, where foci of infection are initiated by the infection of capillary endothelial cells (Tyzzer, 1906; Bruusgaard, 1932; Cheatham et al., 1956; Johnson, 1940; Eisenbud, 1952). The appearance of lesions in successive crops probably reflects a cyclic viremia that, in the normal host, is terminated by specific humoral and cellular immunity after about three days. These host responses also limit the progression of focal lesions in the skin and other organs.

Serum antibody to VZV is an important factor in immunity to exogenous reinfection. People with detectable serum antibody to VZV do not become ill after exogenous exposure, whereas those devoid of serum antibody to VZV develop varicella (Gershon and Krugman, 1975; Zaia and Oxman, 1977). Moreover, passive immunization can prevent varicella in susceptible individuals exposed to exogenous VZV (Ross, 1962; Brunell et al., 1969; Gershon et al., 1974). However, there is no apparent correlation between the endogenous antibody response and the severity of varicella (Feldman et al., 1975; Gold, 1966; Brunell et al., 1975); cellular immune responses and perhaps interferon are more important than humoral immunity in limiting the extent and duration of VZV infection (Feldman et al., 1975; Rand et al., 1977; Armstrong et al., 1970; Stevens et al., 1975; Gershon and Steinberg, 1979).

Pneumonia and other complications of varicella reflect a failure to limit virus replication and dissemination. Their frequency in newborns and in patients with congenital, acquired, or iatrogenic immunodeficiencies is almost certainly due, in large part, to depressed cellular immunity. The reason for the greater severity of varicella in normal adults than in children, however, is unknown.

The characteristic changes in infected cells, which can be observed in tissue culture as well as in vivo, are "ballooning degeneration" with the formation of intranuclear inclusion bodies and multinucleated giant cells (Taylor-Robinson and Caunt, 1972). Individual infected cells become greatly enlarged with pale vacuolated cytoplasm. The nuclei exhibit margination of chromatin and contain inclusion bodies. Early in the course of the infection, the inclusion bodies may be homogeneous and moderately basophilic, and they often fill the nucleus. However, they rapidly evolve into sharply demarcated acidophilic inclusion bodies that are separated from the deeply basophilic ring of marginated chromatin at the nuclear membrane by a clear zone or halo. Mul-

tinucleated giant cells are formed primarily by the fusion of adjacent infected cells (Johnson, 1940). Neither multinucleated giant cells nor intranuclear inclusions are found in the vesicular lesions caused by poxviruses (smallpox, vaccinia) or enteroviruses (echoviruses, coxsackieviruses).

The initial event in the formation of the cutaneous lesions of varicella is probably infection of capillary endothelial cells in the papillary dermis, with subsequent spread of virus to epithelial cells in the epidermis, hair follicles, and sebaceous glands (Tyzzer, 1906; Bruusgaard, 1932; Lipschutz, 1921; Taylor-Robinson and Caunt, 1972; Cheatham et al., 1956; Olding-Stenkvist and Grandien, 1976). In early papular lesions, the epithelium is slightly elevated owing to swelling of the infected epithelial cells and to edema and vascular congestion of the underlying dermis. In the superficial dermis, capillary endothelial cells are swollen, and their nuclei frequently contain intranuclear inclusions. Similar inclusions may be seen in the nuclei of fibroblasts in the surrounding connective tissue, which is edematous and infiltrated sparsely by mononuclear cells. Superficial lymphatics are dilated, and cells lining these structures are also swollen and may contain intranuclear inclusions. In the epidermis, the cells initially involved are those of the germinal layer and the deeper portion of the stratum spinosum. These cells show ballooning degeneration with loss of intercellular bridges, and they soon become separated by intercellular edema (acantholysis). A few small multinucleated giant cells, containing three to eight nuclei, can usually be seen at the base and periphery of these early epithelial lesions. The papular lesions rapidly evolve into intraepidermal vesicles as a result of infection and degeneration of more epithelial cells and the influx of edema fluid, which elevates the uninvolved stratum corneum to form a delicate clear vesicle (Fig. 2A). At this stage, the vesicle fluid contains fibrin, degenerating and "ballooned" epithelial cells, and abundant cell-free infectious varicella-zoster virus. Multinucleated giant cells with eosinophilic intranuclear inclusions are readily found in the walls and base of the vesicle (Fig. 2B). Polymorphonuclear leukocytes and a smaller number of macrophages then invade from the underlying dermis, and the vesicle fluid becomes cloudy. The fluid is subsequently absorbed, with the formation of a flat adherent crust which is eventually detached by the regrowth of subjacent epithelial cells. The lesion can evolve from papule to early crusting in 8 to 12 hours. Lesions of uncomplicated varicella usually heal without scarring. Lesions in mucous membranes develop in the same way, but the thin roof of the vesicle breaks down quickly, producing a shallow ulcer that heals rapidly.

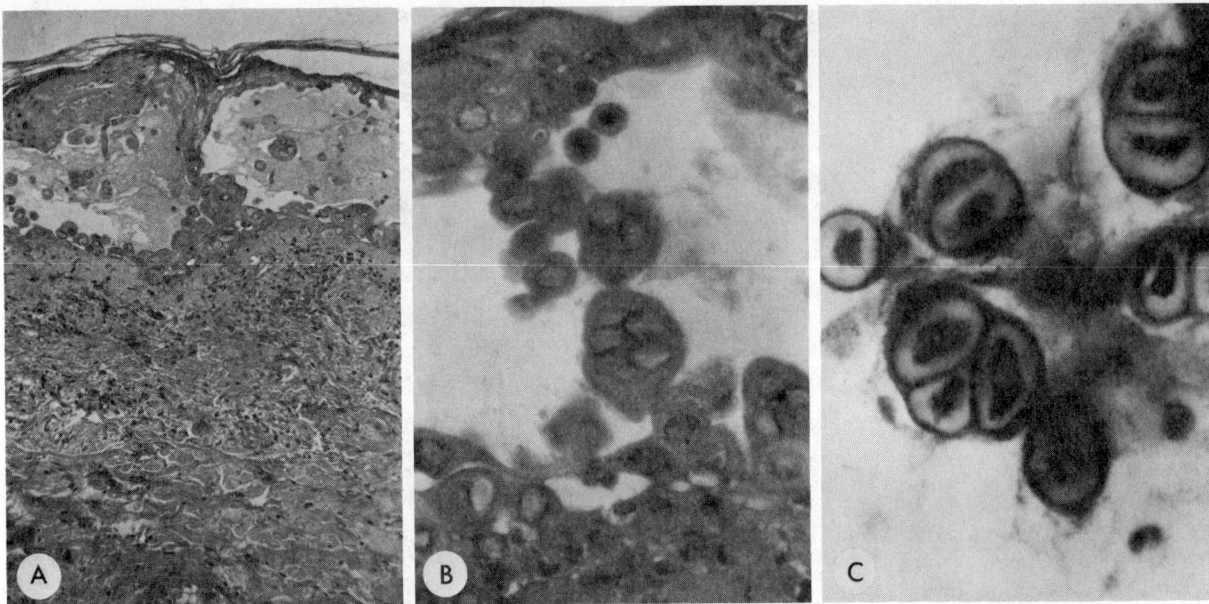

**FIGURE 2.** *Varicella, early vesicle. A, Intraepidermal vesicle. Infected epithelial cells show acantholysis, "ballooning degeneration," intranuclear inclusions, and multinucleated giant cell formation. Underlying dermis shows edema and mononuclear cell infiltration (hematoxylin-eosin stain × 200). (Courtesy of Dr. R. J. Barr.) B, Multinucleated giant cells in the walls and base of the vesicle (hematoxylin-eosin stain × 800). (Courtesy of Dr. R. J. Barr.) C, Tzanck smear from the base of the vesicle, showing multinucleated giant cells with intranuclear inclusion bodies (hematoxylin-eosin stain. × 2000).*

In fatal varicella, focal lesions have been found in the mucous membranes of the respiratory, gastrointestinal, and genitourinary tracts, in the serosa of the pleural and peritoneal cavities, and in the parenchyma of virtually every organ, the lungs being the most frequent site of severe involvement (Taylor-Robinson and Caunt, 1972; Krugman et al., 1977; Cheatham et al., 1956; Christie, 1974; Johnson, 1940; Eisenbud, 1952). There is widespread vascular damage, with characteristic acidophilic intranuclear inclusions in the endothelial cells lining small blood vessels and lymphatics; capillaries within individual lesions are often destroyed, with thrombosis and hemorrhage. In varicella pneumonia, the pleura are studded with hemorrhagic nodules, and the lungs show widely disseminated interstitial pneumonia with numerous foci of hemorrhagic necrosis. Alveoli are filled with red cells, fibrin, inclusion-bearing mononuclear cells, and occasional multinucleated giant cells. Typical acidophilic inclusions are also seen within hyperplastic alveolar septal cells, swollen capillary endothelial cells, fibroblasts, and bronchiolar and tracheobronchial epithelial cells. Similar areas of vascular damage and focal necrosis are found in the liver, spleen, and other organs.

When meningoencephalitis occurs as an isolated complication of varicella, the pathologic changes resemble those seen in measles, mumps, and other "postinfectious" encephalitides; there is perivascular demyelination and round-cell infiltration, suggesting an allergic encephalitis. However, direct invasion by VZV may also be involved, especially in cases of meningoencephalitis that occur during disseminated visceral infection (McCormick et al., 1969; Takashima and Becker, 1979).

## CLINICAL MANIFESTATIONS

### Prodrome

In young children prodromal symptoms are infrequent and the illness usually begins, after an incubation period of 14 or 15 days, with the rash. The rash may be accompanied by low-grade fever and malaise. In older children and adults the rash is often preceded by two to three days of fever, chills, malaise, headache, anorexia, severe backache, and, in some patients, sore throat and dry cough. A fleeting scarlatiniform rash may occur occasionally just before or coincident with the vesicular eruption.

### Rash

The most striking feature of the lesions of varicella is their rapid progression from macules to

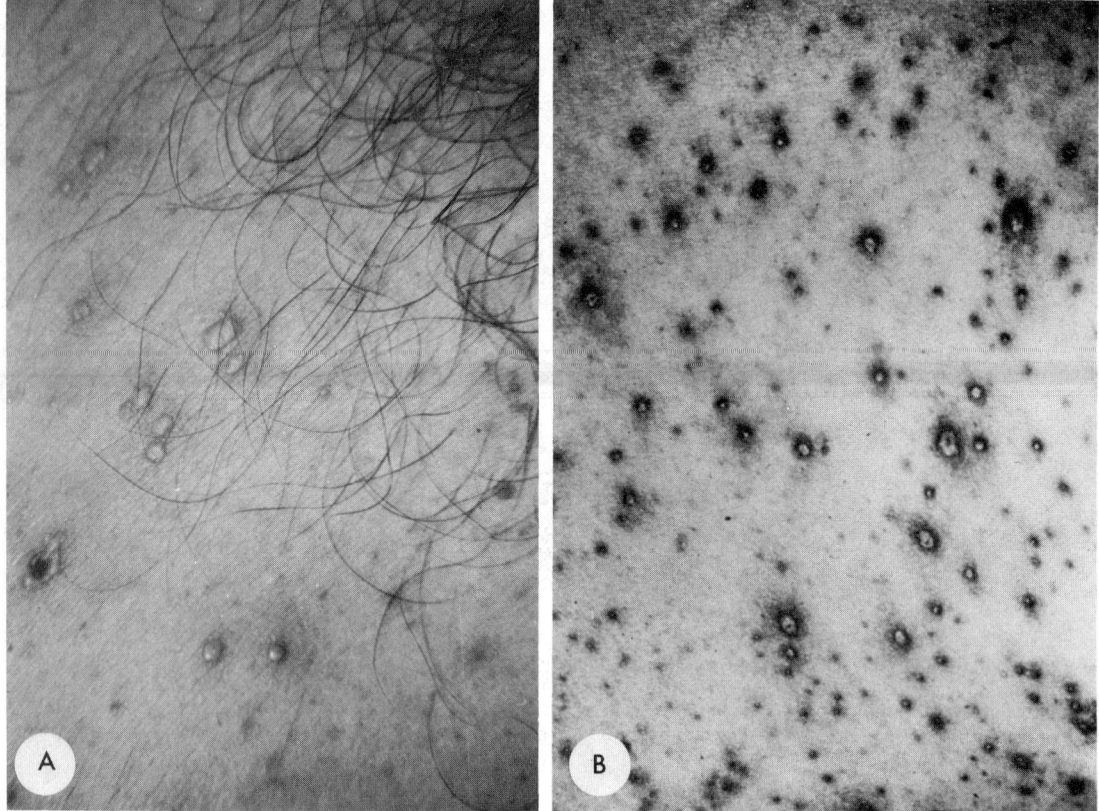

**FIGURE 3.**   *Varicella. A, Superficial, thin-walled, elliptical vesicles with their long axis parallel to the skin folds. B, Lesions in all stages of evolution.*

papules to vesicles to pustules to crusts. The entire transition may take only 8 to 12 hours. The typical superficial, thin-walled vesicle of varicella looks like a drop of water lying on the skin. It is usually 2 to 3 mm in diameter and elliptical; its long axis is parallel to the folds of the skin (Fig. 3A) and it is surrounded by an irregular area of erythema, which gives the lesions the appearance of a "dewdrop on a rose petal" (Wesselhoeft, 1944). The vesicle fluid soon becomes cloudy and the lesion begins to dry. Drying begins in the center, first producing an umbilicated appearance and then a crust. Crusts fall off in one to three weeks, depending on the depth of the skin involvement, leaving shallow pink depressions that gradually disappear. Scarring is rare in uncomplicated varicella.

Vesicles also develop in the mouth, occurring most commonly over the palate. Mucosal vesicles rupture so rapidly that the vesicular stage may be missed. They are usually shallow ulcers, 2 to 3 mm in diameter. Vesicles may also appear on other mucous membranes, including those of the pharynx, larynx, trachea, gastrointestinal tract, and vagina, as well as on the conjunctivae.

The lesions of varicella appear in successive crops on the trunk, scalp, face, and extremities. The distribution is central, with lesions concen-

trated on the trunk and proximal parts of the extremities. A few lesions are not uncommon on the palms and soles. The rash tends to be more profuse in hollows and protected parts of the body than on prominent and exposed parts. Thus it is denser in the hollow of the small of the back and the furrow between the shoulder blades than on the scapulae and buttocks, and more profuse on the medial than on the lateral aspects of the limbs. Vesicles often appear earlier and in larger numbers in areas of inflammation, such as diaper rash, sunburn, or eczema.

A distinctive feature of varicella is the simultaneous presence in any one area of the skin of lesions in all stages of evolution (Fig. 3B). This is due to the rapid development of individual lesions and the appearance of successive crops involving the same anatomic areas. In the typical case, three crops of lesions appear over a three-day period, but there are wide variations, ranging from a single crop of a few scattered lesions to a series of five or more crops developing over a period of one week with innumerable lesions over the entire body. In general, the mildest cases are seen most frequently in infants, and the most severe in adults. Inapparent infections occur but are rare (Ross, 1962).

Fever usually persists as long as new lesions

continue to appear, and its height is generally proportional to the severity of the rash. In typical cases it rarely exceeds 102° F; it may be absent in mild cases and rise to 105° F in severe cases with extensive rash. Prolonged fever or recurrence of fever after defervescence may accompany secondary bacterial infection or other complications. Headache, malaise, myalgia, and anorexia accompany the fever and are more severe in older children and adults. However, the most distressing symptom is usually pruritus, which is present throughout the vesicular stage.

## COMPLICATIONS AND SEQUELAE

In the normal child varicella is a benign disease rarely attended by serious complications. The most frequent complication is staphylococcal or streptococcal infection of skin lesions, which may produce impetigo, furuncles, cellulitis, and, occasionally, erysipelas. These local infections often lead to scarring and, very rarely, to septicemia with metastatic infection of other organs (Bullowa and Wishik, 1935; Krugman et al., 1977). Bullous lesions may be produced when vesicles are infected with staphylococci that elaborate exfoliative toxin (Melish, 1973). Secondary bacterial pneumonia is rare, occurs mainly in children under seven years old, and responds to antibiotics (Bullowa and Wishik, 1935; Weinstein and Meade, 1956). In contrast to the normal host, bacterial superinfection is frequent and life-threatening in leukopenic patients, especially children with leukemia.

Other complications account for the increased morbidity and mortality of varicella in adults, in newborns, and in immunocompromised patients of any age (Krugman et al., 1977; Weinstein and Meade, 1956; Juel-Jensen and MacCallum, 1972; Gold and Nankervis, 1973; Triebwasser et al., 1967; Cheatham et al., 1956; Feldman et al., 1975; Haggerty and Eley, 1956; Gershon et al., 1972).

Varicella is generally more severe in adults. Fever and constitutional symptoms are more prominent and prolonged. The rash is more profuse and complications more frequent. Primary varicella pneumonia is the major complication of adult varicella. It is rarely observed in normal children; adults account for more than 90 per cent of reported cases (Bullowa and Wishik, 1935; Krugman et al., 1977; Weinstein and Meade, 1956; Triebwasser et al., 1967).

The incidence of primary varicella pneumonia depends on the population of patients studied and the diagnostic criteria employed. Roentgenographic evidence of pneumonia was found in 16 per cent of healthy male military recruits with varicella, but clinical signs of pneumonia were present in only 4 per cent (Weber and Pellecchia, 1965). The incidence and severity are substantially higher in older patients and in the subset of adults with varicella admitted to hospitals (Weinstein and Meade, 1956; Triebwasser et al., 1967). Pneumonia generally appears one to six days after onset of rash, and the degree of pulmonary involvement correlates best with the severity of the cutaneous eruption. Some patients are asymptomatic, but others develop cough, dyspnea, tachypnea, high fever, pleuritic chest pain, cyanosis, and hemoptysis. The severity of the symptoms is usually out of proportion to the physical findings in the chest, but the roentgenogram typically reveals diffuse nodular densities throughout both lung fields, often peribronchial in distribution, with a tendency to concentrate in the perihilar regions and at the bases. Roentgenographic abnormalities disappear more slowly than do the symptoms of pneumonia, and occasionally the pulmonary lesions calcify and persist for years (Krugman et al., 1977; Gold and Nankervis, 1973; Triebwasser et al., 1967; Mackay and Cairney, 1960). The mortality in adults with varicella pneumonia has been estimated to be between 10 and 30 per cent, but it is probably closer to 10 per cent if immunocompromised patients are excluded (Krugman et al., 1977; Triebwasser et al., 1967; Young, 1976). It is clear from postmortem examination of fatal cases that the pneumonia is only one manifestation of widespread hematogenous dissemination, with evidence of varicella infection in virtually every organ examined (Triebwasser et al., 1967).

When an infant acquires VZV infection in utero but is born before the transplacental passage of sufficient maternal antibody to modify the infection during its incubation period (i.e., when the rash of varicella occurs in the mother less than five days before or within two days after delivery or, begins in an infant between five and ten days of age), the result is severe disseminated varicella (Meyers, 1974; Krugman et al., 1977; Gold and Nankervis, 1973; Young, 1976). This fact implies that immature prenatal and neonatal defenses cannot restrain VZV replication and dissemination. Varicella early in pregnancy has, on rare occasions, been associated with a characteristic syndrome of congenital malformations, which include cicatricial skin scarring in a dermatomal distribution and hypoplastic limbs (Krugman et al., 1977; Young, 1976; Williamson, 1975).

The morbidity and mortality of varicella are markedly increased in immunocompromised patients, including patients with leukemia and other malignancies who are receiving corticosteroids, chemotherapeutic agents, or radiotherapy at the time of infection; patients receiving corticosteroids for such diseases as nephrotic syndrome and rheumatic fever; and patients with congenital immunologic deficiencies (Cheatham et al., 1956; Feldman et al., 1975; Haggerty and Eley, 1956; Gershon et al., 1972; Scheinman and Stamler, 1969; Lux et al., 1970; Hattori et al., 1976). These patients have extensive involvement of the lungs, liver, central nervous system, and other organs, almost certainly as a result of prolonged high-level viremia (Feldman and Epp, 1979; Myers, 1979). In one series, 19 of 60 children with leukemia who were receiving therapy at the time of infection had visceral dissemination, and four died (Feldman et al., 1975). There was varicella pneumonia in all four fatal cases and fulminant encephalitis in two. Varicella hepatitis was also frequently present but was not fatal in the absence of pneumonia. Disseminated varicella occurred more frequently in children with absolute lymphopenia (less than 500 lymphocytes per cubic millimeter). Immunosuppressed and corticosteroid-treated patients may also develop hemorrhagic complications of varicella that range in severity from mild febrile purpura to severe and often fatal purpura fulminans and malignant varicella with purpura (Juel-Jensen and MacCallum, 1972; Christie, 1974; Charkes, 1961; Marcy and Kibrick, 1977). The etiology of these hemorrhagic complications is complex and probably not the same in every case. In some, thrombocytopenia may be associated with the underlying disease, its therapy, and the direct effect of VZV infection on the bone marrow. (Espinoza and Kuhn, 1974). In others, particularly malignant varicella and purpura fulminans (Juel-Jensen and MacCallum, 1972; Marcy and Kibrick, 1977), the primary factor may be infection of vascular endothelial cells so that endothelial damage initiates disseminated intravascular coagulation and thrombotic purpura.

Central nervous system complications occur in approximately one case of varicella per 1000. The most common manifestation is acute cerebellar ataxia, which ordinarily begins a few days after the onset of rash and is usually benign. (Underwood, 1935; Johnson and Milbourne, 1970). Meningoencephalomyelitis, transverse myelitis, peripheral neuritis, and Reye's syndrome (acute encephalopathy with fatty degeneration of the viscera) are less common. The pathogenesis of these complications is not well understood. (Takashima and Becker, 1979). Direct virus infection of the central nervous system is involved in some cases (McCormick et al., 1969), whereas others may be associated with an allergic response to altered neural tissues or with circulating immune complexes. VZV is not found in the brain or liver in Reye's syndrome.

Other rare complications of varicella are myo-carditis, hepatitis, nephritis, orchitis, appendicitis, pancreatitis, arthritis, keratitis, and iritis. The pathogenesis of these complications has not been delineated, but direct parenchymal infection and vasculitis induced by endothelial VZV infection are responsible in at least some instances.

## GEOGRAPHIC VARIATIONS IN DISEASE AND EPIDEMIOLOGY

Varicella is worldwide in distribution, and there is no evidence of differing racial or sexual susceptibility. Humans are the only known reservoir of infection, and arthropod vectors play no known role in transmission. Varicella is endemic in metropolitan communities in temperate climates, with a regularly recurring prevalence in winter and spring and periodic epidemics when susceptibles accumulate. In urban areas of the United States, 90 per cent of cases occur in children under 10 and fewer than 5 per cent in individuals over 15 years old (Gordon, 1962; Weller, 1976). In tropical and less developed regions, infection is delayed, and varicella is seen more often in adults. In a survey of parturient women in New York City, only 4.5 per cent of those born in the United States lacked antibody to VZV, whereas 16 per cent of those from Latin America were seronegative (Gershon et al., 1976).

Despite the lability of the virus, varicella is highly contagious. Attack rates of 87 per cent among susceptible siblings in households and nearly 70 per cent among susceptible patients on hospital wards have been reported (Gordon, 1962; Ross, 1962). Most cases of varicella are clinically apparent, although the exanthem may be so sparse and transient that it is unnoticed. A typical patient is probably infectious for one to two days (rarely, three to four days) before the exanthem appears, and for four or five days thereafter—i.e., until the last crop of vesicles has crusted (Evans, 1940). The immunocompromised patient, who may experience successive crops of lesions for one week or more, is infectious for a longer period. The average incubation period of varicella is 14 or 15 days, with a range of 10 to 23 days (Gordon, 1962; Ross, 1962). Varicella is thought to be acquired and transmitted mainly via the respiratory tract by airborne droplets (Leclair et al., 1980), but also by direct contact and, less frequently, by indirect contact. Unlike smallpox, varicella crusts are not infectious, and the duration of infectivity of droplets containing the labile VZV must be relatively limited. The mechanism by which VZV is shed is unclear. Viremia occurs during the prodromal stage, when varicella can be transmitted to the fetus in utero and by blood transfusion from a donor incubating the infection. Lesions are not confined to the skin, but occur also in the respiratory, genitourinary, and gastrointestinal tracts. Though infectiousness is thought to depend largely upon virus shed from the upper respiratory tract, VZV has only rarely been isolated from pharyngeal secretions, whereas it can regularly be recovered from vesicular fluid (Weller, 1976).

An attack of varicella confers lasting immunity. The rare second attacks that have been reported are probably examples of cutaneous dissemination in patients with herpes zoster.

## DIAGNOSIS

Varicella can usually be recognized by the character and evolution of the rash, particularly after exposure within the preceding two to three weeks (Wesselhoeft, 1944; Krugman et al., 1977; Christie, 1974). Characteristic diagnostic features include (1) a papulovesicular eruption accompanied by fever and mild constitutional symptoms; (2) crops of lesions with a predominantly central distribution including the scalp; (3) rapid evolution from macules to papules to delicate thin-walled vesicles and, finally, to crusts; (4) the presence of lesions in all stages of development in any one anatomic area throughout the acute disease; and (5) lesions in the oral mucous membranes. Severe varicella, especially in immunosuppressed patients, may resemble smallpox or generalized vaccinia. Conversely, mild variola, especially when modified by vaccination, may be indistinguishable from varicella. Generalized vaccinia, especially in patients with immunologic defects or eczema, may also be confused with varicella. Since the distinction between varicella and these poxvirus infections cannot be made with certainty on clinical grounds, prompt laboratory diagnosis is mandatory. However, the eradication of smallpox and the consequent cessation of smallpox vaccination should eliminate this diagnostic problem.

Disseminated herpes simplex may occasionally resemble varicella, especially in immunosuppressed individuals or patients with eczema. However, the distribution of lesions is rarely typical of varicella, and there may be an obvious concentration of lesions at the site of the primary or recurrent infection (e.g., the mouth or external genitalia).

Other diseases that may be confused with varicella include impetigo, the vesicular exanthems of coxsackievirus and echovirus infections, rickettsialpox, insect bites, papular urticaria, scabies, contact dermatitis, dermatitis herpetiformis,

drug eruptions, secondary syphilis, and erythema multiforme. The character, distribution, and evolution of the lesions, together with a careful epidemiologic history, usually differentiate these diseases from varicella (Krugman et al., 1977). When any doubt exists, the clinical impression should receive laboratory confirmation.

Multinucleated giant cells and epithelial cells containing acidophilic intranuclear inclusion bodies distinguish the cutaneous lesions produced by VZV from all others except herpes simplex (Fig. 2). These cells can be demonstrated in Tzanck smears; material is scraped from the base of an early vesicle and stained with hematoxylin-eosin, Giemsa, Papanicolaou, or Paragon multiple stain (Blank et al., 1951; Barr et al., 1977) (Fig. 2C). Every physician should use this simple procedure for the evaluation of any patient with a vesicular eruption. Punch biopsies provide more reliable material for histologic examination and also facilitate diagnosis in the prevesicular stage. Sputum from patients with varicella pneumonia may contain desquamated respiratory epithelial cells with acidophilic intranuclear inclusions, but such cells are also found in patients with measles pneumonia. The identification of herpesvirus particles in vesicle fluid or biopsy material by electronmicroscopy provides another rapid and reliable diagnostic technique. However, neither electronmicroscopy nor Tzanck smears can distinguish VZV from herpes simplex virus infections.

In addition to the isolation of VZV from fresh vesicle fluid inoculated into suitable tissue cultures, VZV infection can be diagnosed in 12 to 24 hours by identifying VZV antigens in vesicle fluid or extracts of crusts by gel-precipitation techniques using antiserum to VZV (Uduman et al., 1972). Direct fluorescent antibody staining of cellular material from fresh vesicles or prevesicular lesions is another rapid and specific method of diagnosis, and it can identify individual infected cells and structures (Esiri and Tomlinson, 1972; Aoyama et al., 1974; Weller, 1979; Olding-Stenkvist and Grandien, 1976). These techniques can also document VZV infection of specific tissues.

Serologic tests allow a retrospective diagnosis by comparing acute and convalescent sera, and can be used to identify susceptible candidates for isolation or prophylaxis. The complement fixation (CF) test has two disadvantages (Weller, 1976; Schmidt, 1980): (1) a rise in CF titer to VZV or herpes simplex virus is not diagnostic if antibody to both viruses increases, because infection by either virus can induce a heterologous anamnestic response, and (2) CF antibody drops within months after varicella infection and may reach undetectable levels. Thus, many adults who are immune to varicella may be CF antibody-negative. An indirect fluorescent antibody test has problems of specificity similar to those of the CF test (Schmidt, 1980). The VZV neutralization test, which is both sensitive and specific, is available only in the research laboratory, but several additional serologic tests that are sensitive and specific have recently been described. These include: (1) an immunofluorescence assay for antibody to VZV-induced membrane antigen (VZMA) (Gershon and Krugman, 1975; Zaia and Oxman, 1977; Williams et al., 1974), which can distinguish between VZV immune and susceptible adults; (2) an immune adherence hemagglutination test, which is slightly less sensitive than the VZMA test but which may prove more practical (Kalter et al., 1977); and (3) a rapid $^{125}$I-staphylococcal protein A radioimmunoassay, which is more sensitive than the VZMA test and easier to perform than the immune adherence hemagglutination test (Richman et al., 1981).

## TREATMENT

There is no specific therapy for varicella. Cool compresses or calamine lotion locally and antihistamines orally may help control itching. Fingernails should be kept short and clean to minimize secondary skin infections from scratching. Bacterial infections of local lesions are treated with warm soaks; systemic antimicrobial drugs are indicated for bacterial cellulitis, sepsis, or pneumonia.

Treatment of varicella encephalitis and varicella pneumonia is supportive and symptomatic (Krugman et al., 1977; Marcy and Kibrick, 1977). There is little evidence that corticosteroids are effective in either disease, and they are not recommended. Antibiotics are useless in varicella pneumonia unless there is bacterial superinfection.

Inhibitors of VZV administered early in varicella may reduce the incidence and severity of complications, especially in immunosuppressed patients. VZV-immune serum globulin (VZIG) (Brunell et al., 1969; Gershon et al., 1974), adenine arabinoside (Ara-A) (Johnson et al., 1975; Whitley et al., 1976), and human interferon (Merigan et al., 1978) have such therapeutic potential but are still undergoing controlled clinical trials. Newer and more specific inhibitors of VZV replication, such as acycloguanosine (Elion et al., 1977), are even more promising and are also being evaluated clinically. Systemic cytosine arabinoside (Ara-C) or iododeoxyuridine (IUdR) should *not* be used in patients with varicella or its complications because they are too toxic and harmful and are likely to affect adversely the outcome of the disease, especially in immunosuppressed patients (Richman and Oxman, 1978).

## PROPHYLAXIS

Varicella is almost always a benign disease in normal children. Since infection results in lifelong immunity, its acquisition in childhood eliminates the problem of varicella in the adult. Consequently, no preventive measures are recommended for a normal child who has been exposed to varicella.

On the other hand, varicella is potentially fatal in susceptible patients undergoing immunosuppressive therapy, patients with an immunosuppressive malignancy such as Hodgkin's disease, susceptible newborn infants, and even normal adults. Thus it is desirable to prevent or modify varicella in these high-risk individuals. Potential approaches include passive immunization, active immunization, chemoprophylaxis, and prevention of exposure.

Passive immunization with large doses (0.6 to 1.2 ml/kg) of standard human immune serum globulin (ISG) administered within three days of exposure attenuates but does not prevent varicella in normal children (Ross, 1962). The capacity of ISG to modify varicella in immunosuppressed patients is uncertain (Geiser et al., 1975). Passive immunization with VZIG (which contains a high titer of antibody to VZV) prevents varicella in susceptible normal children when administered within three days of exposure (Brunell et al., 1969) and modifies the disease in immunosuppressed children (Gershon et al., 1974). One third of the immunosuppressed recipients develop subclinical infection, and the disease is mild in most of the others. Similarly, zoster immune plasma (ZIP) obtained from otherwise healthy individuals during convalescence from varicella or herpes zoster will modify or prevent varicella in susceptible high-risk children when it is administered within five days of exposure (Geiser et al., 1975; Balfour et al., 1977). The incubation period is prolonged in those VZIG and ZIP recipients who develop clinical disease. In contrast to the favorable outcome in passively immunized children is the 32 per cent mortality reported in a group of 106 leukemic children with unmodified varicella (Hattori et al., 1976).

The scarcity of VZIG and the difficulty of rapidly determining susceptibility to VZV has limited the use of VZIG to high-risk children without a history of varicella. VZIG is not marketed commercially but may be obtained for patients who meet the criteria for its use from the American

Red Cross Blood Services—Northeast Region through 13 regional blood centers in the United States (Center for Disease Control, 1981). The following is a list of the criteria for VZIG use:

1. One of the following underlying illnesses or conditions

    A. Leukemia or lymphoma
    B. Congenital or acquired immunodeficiency
    C. Under immunosuppressive treatment
    D. Newly born of a mother who had onset of varicella less than 5 days before delivery or within 48 hours after delivery

2. One of the following types of exposure to varicella or zoster patient

    A. Household contact
    B. Playmate contact (more than one hour play indoors)
    C. Hospital contact (in same two- to four-bed room or adjacent beds in a large ward)
    D. Newborn contact (newborn whose mother developed varicella within five days before delivery or within 48 hours after delivery)

3. Negative or unknown prior history of varicella

4. Age of less than 15 years
    *or*
    15 years or older and either

    A. VZV antibody-negative or
    B. Highly likely on epidemiologic grounds to have never experienced VZV infection

5. Time elapsed after exposure is such that VZIG can be administered within 96 hours of exposure.

New serologic tests for rapid identification of susceptible individuals (Gershon and Krugman, 1975; Zaia and Oxman, 1977; Williams et al., 1974; Kalter et al., 1977; Richman et al., 1981) and a new technique for preparing VZIG from outdated bank blood with high titer antibody to VZV (Zaia et al., 1978) will greatly increase the availability and application of VZIG. Since exposure to VZV may go unrecognized, many immunosuppressed patients who would otherwise develop varicella without prophylactic VZIG might benefit from maintenance prophylaxis with VZIG on a monthly or bimonthly schedule. Postexposure VZIG prophylaxis might also be considered for susceptible adults, especially pregnant women.

An experimental live VZV vaccine (Hattori et al., 1976; Izawa et al., 1977; Gershon, 1980) is immunogenic, but questions of safety, degree of attenuation, and capacity to induce latent infec-

tion are likely to preclude its use in normal children (Brunell, 1977).

Chemoprophylaxis has not been developed for VZV. Exposure of susceptible patients to VZV warrants reduction in the dosage of corticosteroids to physiologic levels and elimination or reduction of immunosuppressive drugs until the varicella has resolved or until it is clear that they have escaped infection. Such patients should receive VZIG immediately after exposure.

No attempts need to be made to prevent exposure of susceptible normal children; patients with varicella need only be kept at home until all vesicles have crusted (Weller, 1976; Krugman et al., 1977). On the other hand, rigid isolation should be enforced to prevent infection of susceptible immunosuppressed patients and newborn infants. Contact with patients with varicella and herpes zoster, and with persons who may be incubating varicella, must be avoided (Weller, 1976; Krugman et al., 1977; Marcy and Kibrick, 1977; Leclair et al., 1980). If such exposure occurs or is suspected, VZIG prophylaxis is warranted.

## References

Almeida, J. D., Howatson, A. F., and Williams, M. G.: Morphology of varicella (chickenpox) virus. Virology 16:353, 1962.

Aoyama, Y., Kurata, T., Kurata, K., Hondo, R., and Ogiwara, H.: Demonstration of viral antigens in herpes simplex and varicella-zoster infection. Recent Adv RES Res 14:90, 1974.

Armstrong, R. W., Gurwith, M. J., Waddell, D., and Merigan, T. C.: Cutaneous interferon production in patients with Hodgkin's disease and other cancers infected with varicella or vaccinia. N Engl J Med 283:1182, 1970.

Balfour, H. H., Jr., Groth, K. E., McCullough, J., Kallis, J. M., Marker, S. C., Nesbit, M. E., Simmons, R. L., and Najarian, J. S.: Prevention or modification of varicella using zoster immune plasma. Am J Dis Child 131:693, 1977.

Barr, R. J., Herten, R. J., and Graham, J. H.: Rapid method for tzanck preparations. JAMA 237:1119, 1977.

Bastian, F. O., Rabson, A. S., Yee, C. L., and Tralka, T. S.: Herpesvirus varicellae: Isolated from human dorsal root ganglia. Arch Pathol 97:331, 1974.

Blank, H., Burgoon, C. F., Baldridge, G. D., McCarthy, P. L., and Urbach, F.: Cytologic smears in diagnosis of herpes simplex, herpes zoster, and varicella. JAMA 146:1410, 1951.

Brunell, P. A.: Protection against varicella. Pediatrics 59:1, 1977.

Brunell, P. A., Gershon, A. A., Uduman, S. A., and Steinberg, S.: Varicella-zoster immunoglobulins during varicella, latency, and zoster. J Infect Dis 132:49, 1975.

Brunell, P. A., Ross, A., Miller, L. H., and Kuo, B.: Prevention of varicella by zoster immune globulin. N Engl J Med 280:1191, 1969.

Bruusgaard, E.: The mutual relation between zoster and varicella. Br J Dermatol 44:1, 1932.

Bullowa, J. G. M., and Wishik, S. M.: Complications of varicella. I. Their occurrence among 2,534 patients. Am J Dis Child 49:923, 1935.

Center for Disease Control: Varicella-Zoster Immune Globulin—United States. Morbid Mortal Wkly Rep 30:15, January 23, 1981.

Charkes, N. D.: Purpuric chickenpox: Report of a case, review of the literature, and classification by clinical features. Ann Intern Med 54:745, 1961.

Cheatham, W. J., Weller, T. H., Dolan, T. F., and Dower, J. C.: Varicella: Report of two fatal cases with necropsy, virus isolation, and serologic studies. Am J Pathol 32:1015, 1956.

Christie, A. B.: Chickenpox; herpes zoster. In Infectious Diseases: Epidemiology and Clinical Practice. 2nd ed. Edinburgh, Churchill Livingstone, 1974, pp. 259–277, 278–290.

Eisenbud, M.: Chickenpox with visceral involvement. Am J Med 12:740, 1952.

Elion, G. B., Furman, P. A., Fyfe, J. A., de Miranda, P., Beauchamp, L., and Schaeffer, H. J.; Selectivity of action of an antiherpetic agent, 9-(2-hydroxyethoxymethyl) guanine. Proc Natl Acad Sci USA 74:5716, 1977.

Esiri, M. M., and Tomlinson, A. H.: Herpes zoster: Demonstration of virus in trigeminal nerve and ganglion by immunofluorescence and electron microscopy. J Neurol Sci 15:35, 1972.

Espinoza, C., and Kuhn, C.; Viral infection of megakaryocytes in varicella with purpura. Am J Clin Pathol 61:203, 1974.

Evans, P.: An epidemic of chickenpox. Lancet 2:339, 1940.

Feldman, S., and Epp, E.; Detection of viremia during incubation of varicella. J Pediatr 94:746, 1979.

Feldman, S., Hughes, W. T., and Daniel, C. B.: Varicella in children with cancer: Seventy-seven cases. Pediatrics 56:388, 1975.

Geiser, C. F., Bishop, Y., Myers, M., Jaffe, N., and Yankee, R.: Prophylaxis of varicella in children with neoplastic disease: Comparative results with zoster immune plasma and gamma globulin. Cancer 35:1027, 1975.

Gershon, A. A.: Live attenuated varicella-zoster vaccine. Rev Infect Dis 2:393, 1980.

Gershon, A. A., Brunell, P. A., Doyle, E. F., and Clapps, A. A.: Steroid therapy and varicella. J Pediatr 81:1034, 1972.

Gershon, A. A., and Krugman, S.: Seroepidemiologic survey of varicella: Value of specific fluorescent antibody test. Pediatrics 56:1005, 1975.

Gershon, A. A., Raker, R., Steinberg, S., Topf-Olstein, B., and Drusin, L. M.: Antibody to varicella-zoster virus in parturient women and their offspring during the first year of life. Pediatrics 58:692, 1976.

Gershon, A. A., and Steinberg, S. P.: Cellular and humoral immune responses to varicella-zoster virus in immunocompromised patients during and after varicella-zoster infections. Infect Immun 25:170, 1979.

Gershon, A. A., Steinberg, S., and Brunell, P. A.: Zoster immune globulin, a further assessment. N Engl J Med 290:243, 1974.

Goffinet, D. R., Glatstein, E. J., and Merigan, T. C.: Herpes zoster-varicella infections and lymphoma. Ann Intern Med 76:235, 1972.

Gold, E.: Serologic and virus-isolation studies of patients with varicella or herpes-zoster infection. N Engl J Med 274:181, 1966.

Gold, E., and Nankervis, G. A.: Varicella-zoster viruses. In Kaplan, A. S. (ed.): The Herpesviruses. New York, Academic Press, 1973, pp. 327–351.

Gordon, J. E.: Chickenpox: An epidemiological review. Am J Med Sci 244:362, 1962.

Haggerty, R. J., and Eley, R. C.: Varicella and cortisone. Pediatrics 18:160, 1956.

Hattori, A., Ihara, T., Iwasa, T., Kamiya, H., Sakurai, M., Izawa, T., and Takahashi, M.: Use of live varicella vaccine in children with acute leukaemia or other malignancies. Lancet 2:210, 1976.

Izawa, T., Ihara, T., Hattori, A., Iwasa, T., Kamiya, H., Sakurai, M., and Takahashi, M.: Application of a live varicella vaccine in children with acute leukemia or other malignant diseases. Pediatrics 60:805, 1977.

Johnson, H. N.: Visceral lesions associated with varicella. Arch Pathol 30:292, 1940.

Johnson, M. T., Luby, J. P., Buchanan, R. A., and Mikulec, D.: Treatment of varicella-zoster virus infections with adenine arabinoside. J Infect Dis 131:225, 1975.

Johnson, R., and Milbourne, P. E.: Central nervous system manifestations of chickenpox. Canad Med Ass J 102:831, 1970.

Juel-Jensen, B. E., and MacCallum, F. O.: Herpes Simplex Varicella and Zoster. Philadelphia, J. B. Lippincott Company, 1972.

Kalter, Z. G., Steinberg, S., and Gershon, A. A.: Immune adherence hemagglutination: Further observations on demonstration of antibody to varicella-zoster virus. J Infect Dis 135:1010, 1977.

Krugman, S., Ward, R., and Katz, S. L.: Varicella-zoster infections. In Infectious Diseases of Children. 6th ed. St. Louis, C. V. Mosby Company, 1977, pp. 451–471.

Leclair, J. M., Zaia, J. A., Levin, M. J., Congdon, R. G., and Goldmann, D. A.: Airborne transmission of chickenpox in a hospital. N Engl J Med 302:450, 1980.

Lipschutz, B.: Untersuchungen über die Ätiologie der Krankheiten der Herpesgruppe (Herpes zoster, Herpes genitalis, Herpes febrilis). Arch Dermatol 136:428, 1921.

Luby, J. P., Ramirez-Ronda, C., Rinner, S., Hull, A., and Vergne-Marini, P.: A longitudinal study of varicella-zoster virus infections in renal transplant recipients. J Infect Dis 135:659, 1977.

Lux, S. E., Johnston, R. B., Jr., August, C. S., Say, B., Penchaszadeh, V. B., Rosen, F. S., and McKusick, V. A.: Chronic neutropenia and abnormal cellular immunity in cartilage-hair hypoplasia. N Engl J Med 282:231, 1970.

Mackay, J. B., and Cairney, P.: Pulmonary calcification following varicella. N Z Med J 59:453, 1960.

Marcy, S. M., and Kibrick, S.: Varicella and herpes zoster. In Hoeprich, P. D. (ed.): Infectious Diseases. 2nd ed. Hagerstown, Md., Harper & Row, Inc., 1977, pp. 744–758.

McCormick, W. F., Rodnitzky, R. L., Schochet, S. S., Jr., and McKee, A. P.: Varicella-zoster encephalomyelitis. Arch Neurol 21:559, 1969.

Melish, M. E.: Bullous varicella: Its association with the staphylococcal scalded skin syndrome. J Pediatr 83:1019, 1973.

Merigan, T. C., Rand, K. H., Pollard, R. B., Abdallah, P. S., Jordan, G. W., and Fried, R. P.: Human leukocyte interferon for the treatment of herpes zoster in patients with cancer. N Engl J Med 298:981, 1978.

Meyers, J. D.: Congenital varicella in term infants: risk reconsidered. J Infect Dis 129:215, 1974.

Meyers, M. G.; Viremia caused by varicella-zoster virus; association with malignant progressive varicella. J Infect Dis 140:229, 1979.

Olding-Stenkvist, E., and Grandien, M.: Early diagnosis of virus-caused vesicular rashes by immunofluorescence on skin biopsies. Scand J Infect Dis 8:27, 1976.

Osler, W.: The Principles and Practice of Medicine. New York, D. Appleton and Company, 1892, p. 65.

Rand, K. H., Rasmussen, L. E., Pollard, R. B., Arvin, A., and Merigan, T. C.: Cellular immunity and herpesvirus infections in cardiac-transplant patients. N Engl J Med 296:1372, 1977.

Reboul, F., Donaldson, S. S., and Kaplan, H. S.: Herpes zoster and varicella infections in children with Hodgkin's disease. Cancer 41:95, 1978.

Richman, D. D., Cleveland, P. H., Oxman, M. N., and Zaia, J. A.: A rapid $^{125}$-I-staphylococcal protein A radioimmunoassay for antibody to varicella-zoster virus. J Infect Dis. 1981, in press.

Richman, D. D., and Oxman, M. N.: Antiviral agents. In Weinstein, L., and Fields, B. N. (eds.): Seminars in Infectious Diseases. Vol. 1. New York, Stratton Intercontinental Medical Book Corp., 1978, pp. 200–255.

Rifkind, D.: The activation of varicella-zoster virus infections by immunosuppressive therapy. J Lab Clin Med 68:463, 1966.

Ross, A. H.: Modification of chicken pox in family contacts by administration of gamma globulin. N Engl J Med 267:369, 1962.

Scheinman, J. I., and Stamler, F. W.: Cyclophosphamide and fatal varicella. J Pediatr 74:117, 1969.

Schimpff, S., Serpick, A., Stoler, B., Rumack, B., Mellin, H., Joseph, J. M., and Block, J.: Varicella-zoster infection in patients with cancer. Ann Intern Med 76:241, 1972.

Schmidt, N. J.: Varicella-zoster virus. In Lennette, E. H., Balows, A., Hausler, W. J., Jr., and Truant, J. P. (eds.): Manual of Clinical Microbiology, Third Edition. Washington, American Society for Microbiology, 1980, pp. 798–806.

Sokal, J. E., and Firat, D.: Varicella-zoster infection in Hodgkin's disease. Am J Med 39:452, 1965.

Steiner: Zur Inokulation der Varicellen. Wien Med Wochenschr 25:306, 1875.

Stevens, D. A., Ferrington, R. A., Jordan, G. W., and Merigan, T. C.: Cellular events in zoster vesicles: Relation to clinical course and immune parameters. J Infect Dis 131:509, 1975.

Stevens, J. G.: Latent herpes simplex virus and the nervous system. Curr Top Microbiol Immunol 70:31, 1975.

Takashima, S., and Becker, L. E.: Neuropathology of fatal varicella. Arch Pathol Lab Med 103:209, 1979.

Taylor-Robinson, D., and Caunt, A. E.: Varicella Virus. Vienna, Springer-Verlag, 1972.

Triebwasser, J. H., Harris, R. E., Bryant, R. E., and Rhoades, E. R.: Varicella pneumonia in adults. Medicine 46:409, 1967.

Tyzzer, E. E.: The histology of the skin lesions in varicella. Philipp J Sci 1:349, 1906.

Uduman, S. A., Gershon, A. A., and Brunell, P. A.: Rapid diagnosis of varicella-zoster infections by agar-gel diffusion. J Infect Dis 126:193, 1972.

Underwood, E. A.: The neurological complications of varicella; a clinical and epidemiological study. Brit J Children's Dis 32:83, 1935.

Weber, D. M., and Pellecchia, J. A.: Varicella pneumonia: Study of prevalence in adult men. JAMA 192:527, 1965.

Weinstein, L., and Meade, R. H.: Respiratory manifestations of chicken pox. Arch Intern Med 98:91, 1956.

Weller, T. H.: Varicella-herpes zoster virus. In Evans, A. S. (ed.): Viral Infections of Humans, Epidemiology and Control. New York, Plenum Medical Book Company, 1976, pp. 457–480.

Weller, T. H.: Varicella and Herpes Zoster. In Lennette, E. H., and Schmidt, N. J. (eds): Diagnostic Procedures for Viral, Rickettsial and Chlamydial Infections, Fifth Edition. Washington, American Public Health Association, 1979, pp. 375–398.

Weller, T. H., and Stoddard, M. B.: Intranuclear inclusion bodies in cultures of human tissue inoculated with varicella vesicle fluid. J Immunol 68:311, 1952.

Weller, T. H., and Witton, H. M.: The etiologic agents of varicella and herpes zoster: Serologic studies with the viruses as propagated *in vitro* J Exp Med 108:869, 1958.

Weller, T. H., Witton, H. M., and Bell, E. J.: The etiologic agents of varicella and herpes zoster: Isolation, propagation, and cultural characteristics *in vitro*. J Exp Med 108:843, 1958.

Wesselhoeft, C.: The differential diagnosis of chicken pox and smallpox. N Engl J Med 230:15, 1944. •

Whitley, R. J., Ch'ien, L. T., Dolin, R., Galasso, G. J., and Alford, C. A., Jr.: Adenine arabinoside therapy of herpes zoster in the immunosuppressed. N Engl J Med 294:1193, 1976.

Williams, V., Gerson, A., and Brunell, P. A.: Serologic response to varicella-zoster membrane antigens measured by indirect immunofluorescence. J Infect Dis 130:669, 1974.

Williamson, A. P.: The varicella-zoster virus in the etiology of severe congenital defects. Clin Pediatr 14:553, 1975.

Young, N. A.: Chickenpox, measles and mumps. In Remington, J. S., and Klein, J. O. (eds.): Infectious Diseases of the Fetus and Newborn Infant. Philadelphia, W. B. Saunders Company, 1976, pp. 521–586.

Zaia, J. A., Levin, M. J., Wright, G. G., and Grady, G. F.: A practical method for preparation of varicella-zoster immune globulin. J Infect Dis 137:601, 1978.

Zaia, J. A., and Oxman, M. N.: Antibody to varicella-zoster virus-induced membrane antigen: Immunofluorescence assay using monodisperse glutaraldehyde-fixed target cells. J Infect Dis 136:519, 1977.

# *HERPES ZOSTER* **223**

## Michael N. Oxman, M.D.

Herpes zoster (shingles, zoster) is a localized disease that occurs most frequently in elderly people and is characterized by unilateral radicular pain and a vesicular eruption that is limited to the dermatome innervated by a single spinal or cranial sensory ganglion. It is caused by varicella-zoster virus (VZV), the same virus that causes varicella. In contrast to varicella, which follows primary exogenous VZV infection, herpes zoster appears to represent activation of an endogenous infection that has persisted in latent form after an earlier attack of varicella.

### ETIOLOGY

The relationship of herpes zoster to varicella was first noted by von Bokay in 1888, who observed that susceptible children acquired varicella after contact with individuals with herpes zoster (Weller, 1976; Bruusgaard, 1932). Lipschutz (1921) noted that the skin lesions of herpes zoster were histologically identical to those of varicella.

Kundratitz (1922) and Bruusgaard (1932) inoculated children with zoster vesicle fluid and demonstrated that the same agent caused both diseases. Some developed varicella-like lesions at the site of inoculation; others developed, in addition, generalized varicella. Uninoculated children in contact with affected recipients developed typical varicella after a normal incubation period and transmitted the disease to other contacts. Children who had previously had varicella developed no disease when inoculated with zoster vesicle fluid or when exposed to children who had developed varicella after such inoculation. Vesicles from the site of inoculation and in the generalized exanthem were histologically identical

with those of ordinary varicella and herpes zoster. In early studies, antigens from vesicles and crusts of varicella and herpes zoster were shown to react equally well in complement fixation tests with convalescent sera from patients with either disease (Taylor-Robinson and Caunt, 1972). Final proof of their common cause was provided when Weller and his colleagues found that the viruses recovered from patients with varicella and herpes zoster were identical (Weller, 1976). The properties of the virus are described in the previous chapter on varicella (Chapter 222).

### PATHOGENESIS AND PATHOLOGY

The neurologic implications of the segmental distribution of the lesions of herpes zoster were recognized as long ago as 1831 by Richard Bright, and the inflammatory changes in the corresponding sensory ganglion and spinal nerve were first described by von Barensprung in 1862. The definitive work is that of Head and Campbell (1900), who correlated postmortem examinations of 21 persons with herpes zoster with the clinical observations on 450 individuals with the disease. They described acute lymphocytic inflammation, focal hemorrhage, and neuronal destruction in sensory ganglia, the degeneration of sensory nerve fibers linking the affected neurons peripherally to the involved skin and centrally to the spinal cord and brain, and the later fibrosis of severely involved ganglia and nerves. They were also able to map the area of skin (dermatome) innervated by each of the sensory ganglia. Their findings have been repeatedly confirmed by a number of subsequent studies (Stern, 1937; Denny-Brown et al., 1944; Muller and Winkelmann, 1969; Esiri and Tomlinson, 1972; Bastian et al., 1974; Aoyama et al., 1974), some of which employed newer techniques such as electronmicroscopy and fluorescent antibody staining to demonstrate virus and viral antigen within neurons and satellite cells in the sensory ganglia, and within peripheral sensory nerves early in the disease. Together, these observations indicate that in herpes zoster, active infection of sensory neurons precedes involvement of the skin.

Although the histopathology of the skin lesions of herpes zoster and varicella is the same, herpes zoster is accompanied by acute inflammation of the corresponding sensory nerve and ganglion. The ganglion shows intense lymphocytic infiltration, necrosis of nerve cells and fibers, endothelial proliferation and lymphocytic cuffing of small vessels, focal hemorrhage, and inflammation of the ganglion sheath (Head and Campbell, 1900; Denny-Brown et al., 1944). Satellite cells and neurons contain characteristic acidophilic intranuclear inclusions, virus particles visible by electronmicroscopy, and VZV antigens demonstrable by immunofluorescence (Esiri and Tomlinson, 1972; Ghatak and Zimmerman, 1973; Bastian et al., 1974; Aoyama et al., 1974; Juel-Jensen and MacCallum, 1972). Some neuronal degeneration and lymphocytic infiltration is also generally present in adjacent ganglia on the same side. The peripheral nerve shows diffuse lymphocytic infiltration and focal hemorrhage, with axonal degeneration and demyelination of sensory fibers; virus particles and VZV antigens are present in Schwann and perineural cells. These inflammatory and degenerative changes can be traced distally to branches innervating the affected skin. The inflammatory reaction in the ganglion also extends proximally to the posterior nerve root and into adjacent segments of the cord or brain stem. This segmental myelitis is predominantly unilateral and involves the posterior horns more than the anterior ones. There is degeneration of nerve fibers in the posterior columns and inflammatory changes in the gray matter of the posterior and anterior horns, with perivenous lymphocytic infiltration, scattered neuronal necrosis and neuronophagia. These changes may extend two or more segments from the one corresponding to the cutaneous eruption. A mild lymphocytic leptomeningitis is generally present and is most intense over the involved segments and nerve roots. Marked inflammation and degeneration of the anterior nerve root within the meninges and in the portion contiguous to the involved sensory ganglia can produce a true motor radiculitis (Denny-Brown et al., 1944) and, when extensive, results in fibrosis of the ganglion and nerve (Head and Campbell, 1900). These observations, as well as the isolation of VZV from the sensory gan-

glion, cerebrospinal fluid, and central nervous system tissue (Aoyama et al., 1974; Bastian et al., 1974; Shibuta et al., 1974; Hogan and Krigman, 1973; McCormick et al., 1969; Gold and Robbins, 1958; Feldman et al., 1973), indicate that the pathologic changes in herpes zoster are the direct result of VZV infection.

Lesions in the skin, lungs, and other organs in fatal cases of disseminated herpes zoster are identical with those observed in fatal cases of varicella (Merselis et al., 1964).

The pathologic findings in zoster meningoencephalitis (or encephalomyelitis) vary from focal mononuclear cell infiltration in the leptomeninges (Juel-Jensen and MacCallum, 1972; Norris et al., 1970) to acute necrotizing encephalitis with perivenous encephalomalacia, myelin and axonal degeneration, macrophage infiltration, and typical intranuclear inclusions and virus particles in glial cells (McCormick et al., 1969). Virus has been isolated from the brain in at least two such fatal cases (McCormick et al., 1966) and from the cerebrospinal fluid in a patient with meningoencephalitis who recovered (Feldman et al., 1973).

The contralateral hemiplegia that sometimes develops in patients with ophthalmic zoster appears to be caused by segmental granulomatous angiitis (Laws, 1960; Gilbert, 1974; Dolin et al., 1978; Linnemann and Alvira, 1980). The angiitis is probably due to VZV infection of the vessel wall, which results from the contiguous spread of virus from the involved ganglion and cranial nerves.

The pathogenesis of herpes zoster is not fully understood, but clinical, epidemiologic, and pathologic data, as well as analogy with recurrent herpes simplex virus infections (Stevens, 1975; Chapter 99), support the following model (Hope-Simpson, 1965). During varicella, VZV passes from skin and mucosal lesions into the contiguous endings of sensory nerves and travels centripetally up the sensory fibers to the sensory ganglia. In the ganglia, a latent infection is established in sensory neurons, and the virus then persists silently and harmlessly; it is no longer infectious and does not multiply, but it retains the capacity to revert to full infectiousness. Herpes zoster occurs with the highest frequency in dermatomes in which the rash of varicella achieves the greatest density (Hope-Simpson, 1975; Stern, 1937), and this is probably because, during varicella, larger amounts of virus are transmitted to the corresponding ganglia, and latent infections are established in more sensory neurons. If reactivation occurs at random, zoster should occur most frequently in areas of skin innervated by ganglia with the most latently infected neurons.

Although the latent virus in the ganglia re-

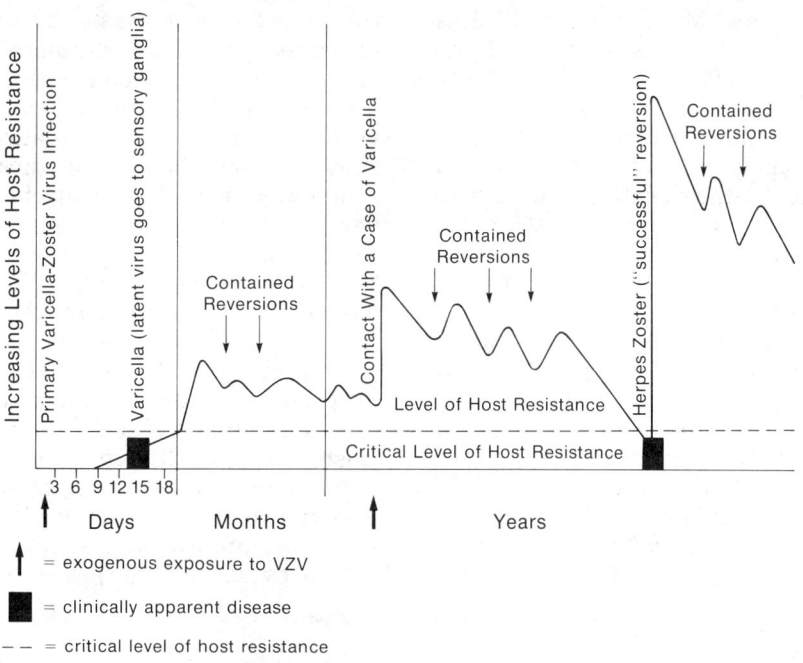

**FIGURE 1.**  *Pathogenesis of herpes zoster. (Modified from Hope-Simpson, R.E.: Proc R Soc Med 58:9, 1965.)*

tains its potential for full infectivity, reversions are sporadic and infrequent. The mechanisms involved in the reactivation of latent VZV are unclear, but a number of conditions have been associated with the occurrence and localization of herpes zoster. These include immunosuppression in Hodgkin's disease and other malignancies; administration of immunosuppressive drugs and corticosteroids; irradiation of the spinal column; tumor involvement of the cord, dorsal root ganglion, or adjacent structures; local trauma; surgical manipulation of the spine; heavy-metal poisoning or therapy; and frontal sinusitis, as a precipitant of ophthalmic zoster (Head and Campbell, 1900; Shanbrom et al., 1960; Hope-Simpson, 1965; Juel-Jensen and MacCallum, 1972; Marcy and Kibrick, 1977; Schimpff et al., 1972; Feldman et al., 1973; Reboul et al., 1978).

Even when latent virus does revert, usually nothing perceptible happens. The minute dose of infectious virus that results is immediately neutralized by circulating antibody or destroyed by cellular immune responses before it can infect other cells and multiply enough to cause perceptible damage. The small quantity of viral antigen released into the bloodstream during such "contained reversions" stimulates host immune responses, raising the level of host resistance (Fig. 1). A similar boost in the level of host resistance may follow contact with a patient with varicella (Fig. 1). When host resistance falls to the point at which reactivated virus can no longer be contained, reversion is "successful." Virus mul-

tiplies and spreads within the ganglion, causing neuronal necrosis and intense inflammation, and this is usually accompanied by severe neuralgia. Infectious VZV then spreads antidromically down the sensory nerve, causing intense neuritis, and is released around the nerve endings, where it produces the characteristic cluster of zoster vesicles. The frequent occurrence of neuralgia several days before the rash appears and the presence of degenerative changes in cutaneous nerve fibrils on the first day of the eruption (Muller and Winkelmann, 1969) provide additional evidence that infection in the sensory ganglion precedes involvement of the skin. Spread of the ganglionic infection proximally along the posterior nerve root results in local leptomeningitis, spinal fluid pleocytosis, and myelitis. Infection of motor neurons in the anterior horn and inflammation of the anterior nerve root occasionally cause local palsies, and extension of infection within the central nervous system may cause meningoencephalitis, a rare complication of herpes zoster (Dolin et al., 1978).

During each successful reversion, hematogenous dissemination of virus from the ganglion often produces aberrant vesicles in uncomplicated herpes zoster (Oberg and Svedmyr, 1969) and stimulates an anamnestic immune response that terminates or may even prevent the cutaneous lesions. Sometimes this results in radicular pain without eruption (zoster sine herpete), but with a coincident rise in antibody to VZV. The occurrence of this syndrome has now been well documented (Juel-Jensen and MacCallum, 1972; Easton, 1970; Luby et al., 1977), as have completely asymptomatic rises in antibody to VZV that presumably reflect "contained reversions" (Luby et al., 1977). If the anamnestic response is delayed or deficient, as it appears to be in many immunosuppressed patients, the duration and severity of the local infection are increased, and the hematogenous dissemination of VZV is more prolonged and extensive (Feldman et al., 1977; Mazur et al., 1979).

Hope-Simpson considered the level of antibody to be the critical determinant of the host's capacity to contain VZV reversions (Hope-Simpson, 1965). However, it now appears that cellular immunity is more important in resistance to recurrent VZV infections (Miller and Brunell, 1970; Schimpff et al., 1972; Feldman et al., 1973; Rand et al., 1977; Arvin et al., 1980; Meyers et al., 1980).

## CLINICAL MANIFESTATIONS

### Prodrome

The first symptom of herpes zoster is usually pain and paresthesia in the involved dermatome. This generally precedes the eruption by several days and varies from superficial itching, tingling, or burning to severe, deep pain. It may be constant or intermittent, and it is often accompanied by tenderness and hyperesthesia of the skin in the involved dermatome. The pre-eruptive pain of herpes zoster may simulate pleurisy, myocardial infarction, duodenal ulcer, cholecystitis, biliary or renal colic, appendicitis, prolapsed intervertebral disk, or early glaucoma, and it may thus lead to serious misdiagnosis. Constitutional symptoms, including headache, malaise, and fever, occur in about 5 per cent of patients, mostly in children, and may precede the rash by one or two days (Burgoon et al., 1957; Rogers and Tindall, 1972; Juel-Jensen and MacCallum, 1972).

A few patients experience acute segmental neuralgia without ever developing a cutaneous eruption, a syndrome called zoster sine herpete (Juel-Jensen and MacCallum, 1972; Lewis, 1958; Easton, 1970). Although zoster sine herpete may explain some cases of trigeminal neuralgia and perhaps an occasional case of facial (Bell's) palsy, most patients with this syndrome do not have serologic evidence of herpes zoster.

### Rash

The most distinctive feature of herpes zoster is the localization of the rash, which is nearly always unilateral, does not cross the midline, and is usually limited to the area of skin innervated by a single sensory ganglion (Fig. 2). Individual sensory ganglia are not attacked at random; herpes zoster occurs with greatest frequency in those areas in which the rash of varicella is most abundant (Hope-Simpson, 1965; Stern, 1937). The areas supplied by the trigeminal nerve, particularly the ophthalmic division, and the trunk from

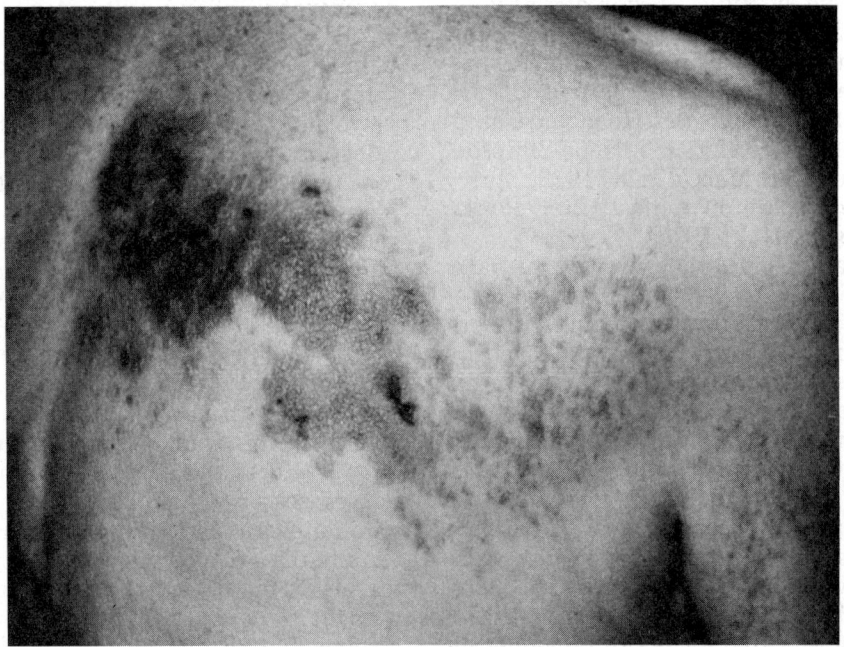

**FIGURE 2.**    *Herpes zoster in the right second thoracic dermatome involving primarily skin innervated by the posterior primary division and by the posterior branch of the lateral cutaneous nerve (Courtesy Dr. D. A. Lopez).*

T3 to L2 are most frequently affected; the thoracic region alone accounts for two thirds of reported cases, and lesions rarely occur below the elbows or knees (Head and Campbell, 1900; Hope-Simpson, 1965; Burgoon et al., 1957; Juel-Jensen and MacCallum, 1972). Regional lymphadenopathy occurs in the majority of cases, and the spinal fluid frequently shows a mild pleocytosis, predominantly lymphocytic, and an elevated protein content. Although individual lesions of herpes zoster and varicella are usually indistinguishable, those of herpes zoster tend to evolve more slowly and often consist of closely grouped vesicles on an erythematous base rather than the discrete, randomly distributed vesicles of varicella. The lesions begin as erythematous maculopapules that often first appear where superficial branches of the affected sensory nerve are given off—e.g., the posterior primary division and the lateral and anterior branches of the anterior primary division of the spinal nerves (Head and Campbell, 1900; Stern, 1937). Vesicles form within 12 to 24 hours and evolve into pustules by the third day. These dry up and crust in seven to ten days. Crusts generally persist for two to three weeks. In normal individuals, new lesions continue to appear for one to four days (occasionally for as long as seven days), and virus may be recovered from lesions for as long as a week after the appearance of the rash. The severity and duration of the rash are greatest in older individuals and least in children (Burgoon et al., 1957; de Moragas and Kierland, 1957; Brown, 1976; Juel-Jensen and MacCallum, 1972). Segmental pain, a prominent feature of herpes zoster in older individuals, generally remits as the crusts fall off. Pain is seldom a significant symptom of herpes zoster in children.

From 10 to 15 per cent of reported cases of herpes zoster involve the ophthalmic division of the trigeminal nerve. The rash of ophthalmic zoster may extend from the level of the eye to the vertex of the skull, but it does not cross the midline of the forehead. When only the supratrochlear and supraorbital branches are involved, the eye is usually spared. Involvement of the nasociliary branch, as evidenced by a herpetic rash on the tip and side of the nose (Fig. 3), occurs in about one third of patients and is usually accompanied by conjunctivitis and occasionally by keratitis, scleritis, iridocyclitis, extraocular muscle palsies, ptosis, and mydriasis. Thus, when ophthalmic zoster involves the side of the nose, careful attention must be given to the condition of the eye. VZV is not, however, as pathogenic for the eye as herpes simplex virus.

Herpes zoster affecting the second and third divisions of the trigeminal nerve and other cranial nerves is uncommon, but when it occurs, it

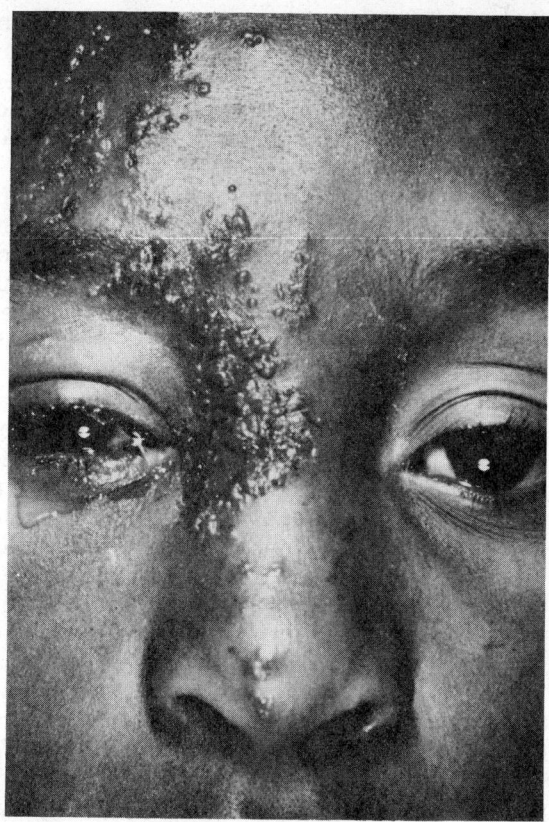

**FIGURE 3.** *Herpes zoster of the ophthalmic division of the fifth cranial nerve. Involvement of the nasociliary branch results in lesions on the tip and side of the nose and unilateral conjunctivitis. (Courtesy of Dr. D. A. Lopez.)*

may produce symptoms and lesions in the mouth, ears, pharynx, or larynx (Denny-Brown et al., 1944; Eisenberg, 1978; Clark, 1979; Christie, 1974). The so-called Ramsay Hunt syndrome, which consists of facial palsy in combination with herpes zoster of the external ear or tympanic membrane, with or without tinnitus, vertigo, and deafness, results from involvement of the facial and auditory nerves (Denny-Brown et al., 1944).

### Complications

Postherpetic neuralgia (pain persisting after all crusts have fallen off) is uncommon in patients under 40 years of age, but occurs in more than one third of patients 60 years old or older, especially those with ophthalmic zoster (Burgoon et al., 1957; de Moragas and Kierland, 1957; Juel-Jensen and MacCallum, 1972). Anesthesia in the involved dermatome is another common sequela that is particularly troublesome when it occurs in the area innervated by the ophthalmic nerve (Juel-Jensen and MacCallum, 1972). Postherpetic neuralgia is refractory to treatment but usually remits spontaneously in one to six months.

When the rash is particularly severe, there may be superficial gangrene with delayed healing and subsequent scarring. As in varicella, secondary bacterial infection may also delay healing and cause scarring. Severe or unrecognized ophthalmic zoster may cause corneal or conjunctival ulcers and scarring. Rarely, secondary bacterial infection may result in panophthalmitis.

Most other complications of herpes zoster appear to be associated with spread of virus from the involved ganglion, either via the bloodstream or by direct neural extension. When patients with herpes zoster are carefully examined, 17 to 35 per cent are found to have at least a few vesicles in areas remote from the involved dermatome; this is due presumably to hematogenous dissemination of virus from the affected ganglion, nerve, or skin (Oberg and Svedmyr, 1969; Juel-Jensen and MacCallum, 1972). The disseminated lesions usually appear within a week of onset of the segmental eruption and, if few in number, are easily overlooked. More extensive dissemination, producing a varicella-like eruption (generalized herpes zoster), occurs in 2 to 10 per cent of unselected patients with localized zoster, most of whom have immunologic defects due to underlying malignancy (particularly lymphomas) or immunosuppressive therapy (Burgoon et al., 1957; de Moragas and Kierland, 1957; Oberg and Svedmyr, 1969; Rogers and Tindall, 1972; Merselis et al., 1964).

On rare occasions, most often in children, infection disseminates widely from a small, painless area of zoster (Rogers and Tindall, 1972), so that the zoster is unnoticed and the disseminated eruption is mistaken for varicella. This probably explains the occasional reports of second attacks of varicella.

Motor paralysis occurs in 1 to 5 per cent of patients with herpes zoster owing to spread of infection from the sensory ganglion to adjacent parts of the nervous system (Head and Campbell, 1900; Denny-Brown et al., 1944; Juel-Jensen and MacCallum, 1972; Christie, 1974; Grant and Rowe, 1961; Thomas and Howard, 1972). Paralysis usually begins within two weeks of onset of the rash and almost always involves muscle groups with innervation that is contiguous with that of the affected dermatome; oculomotor and facial palsies are seen with cephalic zoster, unilateral diaphragmatic paralysis with homolateral cervical zoster, paralysis of the trunk and limbs with zoster involving corresponding dermatomes, and dysfunction of the bladder and anus with sacral zoster (Head and Campbell, 1900; Kendall, 1957; Brostoff, 1966; Juel-Jensen and Mac-Callum, 1972; Christie, 1974; Thomas and Howard, 1972; Izumi and Edwards, 1973; Jellinek and Tulloch, 1976). Rare cases in which the involved myotome and dermatome are widely separated may represent the result of more extensive mye-

litis (Christie, 1974; Thomas and Howard, 1972). Total or functional recovery occurs in most cases.

Although a lymphocytic pleocytosis, with or without an increase in protein in the cerebrospinal fluid, is a regular feature of uncomplicated herpes zoster, the incidence of acute symptomatic meningoencephalitis is exceedingly low. When this rare complication does occur, its clinical manifestations are similar to those of varicella meningoencephalitis; there is a relatively high frequency of ataxia and other cerebellar signs, and a low mortality (Appelbaum et al., 1962). Most cases probably represent VZV infection, with virus reaching the central nervous system by direct extension from the involved sensory ganglia or by the hematogenous route during disseminated herpes zoster (McCormick et al., 1969; Gold and Robbins, 1958). Guillain-Barré syndrome may also follow herpes zoster.

### Herpes Zoster in the Immunosuppressed Host

Certain types of malignancy, especially Hodgkin's disease and lymphocytic leukemia, and the administration of immunosuppressive therapy (e.g., radiation, antimetabolites, antilymphocyte serum, and corticosteroids) to patients with malignancies and nonmalignant diseases (Schimpff et al., 1972; Goffinet et al., 1972; Feldman et al., 1973; Reboul et al., 1978) markedly increase the incidence and severity of herpes zoster. In fact, serious complications of herpes zoster occur almost exclusively in such immunosuppressed patients. From 20 to 50 per cent of patients with Hodgkin's disease develop herpes zoster, with the highest incidence in patients with far advanced disease and those receiving radiation and combination chemotherapy (Schimpff et al., 1972; Goffinet et al., 1972; Feldman et al., 1973; Rand et al., 1977; Reboul et al., 1978; Atkinson et al., 1980). The severity of the disease is also increased; necrosis of skin and scarring are relatively common, as is postherpetic neuralgia; and the incidence of cutaneous dissemination is 25 to 50 per cent. Approximately 10 per cent of patients with disseminated cutaneous lesions develop widespread, frequently fatal visceral involvement, particularly of the lungs, liver, and brain (McCormick et al., 1969; Merselis et al., 1964). The incidence of herpes zoster is also markedly increased in immunosuppressed kidney, heart, and bone marrow transplant recipients (Luby et al., 1977; Rifkin, 1966; Rand et al., 1977; Atkinson et al., 1980).

The cellular rather than the humoral response to VZV appears to determine the response of these patients to herpes zoster (Miller and Brunell, 1970; Feldman et al., 1973; Rand et al., 1977; Gold, 1966; Brunell et al., 1975; Armstrong et al.,

1970; Stevens et al., 1975; Arvin et al., 1980; Meyers et al., 1980). Lymphocyte blastogenesis and interferon production after exposure to VZV antigens, both of which are indicators of cellular immunity, appear to correlate well with resistance to VZV replication and dissemination.

## EPIDEMIOLOGY

Herpes zoster occurs sporadically throughout the year without seasonal prevalence and affects both sexes and all races with equal frequency. As expected with a disease that reflects the reactivation of latent endogenous infection, the occurrence of herpes zoster is independent of the prevalence of varicella, and there is no convincing evidence that zoster can be acquired by contact with persons with varicella or with zoster (Hope-Simpson, 1965; Seiler, 1949; Burgoon et al., 1957). Rather, the incidence of herpes zoster is determined by factors that influence the host-parasite relationship. One of these is age. The rate of occurrence is in the range of 3 to 5 per 1000 persons per year, and although the disease may be seen in any age group, including children, more than two thirds of reported cases occur in individuals over 50 years of age, and less than 10 per cent of cases occur in persons under the age of 20 years (Gordon, 1962; Hope-Simpson, 1965; Seiler, 1949; Burgoon et al., 1957; de Moragas and Kierland, 1957; Oberg and Svedmyr, 1969; Miller and Brunell, 1970; Rogers and Tindall, 1972). Hope-Simpson's tabulation of data from 192 cases occurring over a 16-year period in a population of 3500 individuals showed that the annual incidence per 1000 rises from 0.74 in children under 10 years of age to a plateau of approximately 2.5 between ages 20 and 50, and thereafter increases to reach a level of over 10 in octogenarians. The incidence of zoster among those who have already had an attack appears to be at least as high as that of first attacks in individuals of comparable age. Second attacks comprise approximately 4 per cent of reported series, and third attacks are not unheard of. Hope-Simpson estimated that if a cohort of 1000 people were to live to be 85 years old, half would have had an attack of zoster and ten would have two attacks. However, multiple episodes of zoster-like disease, especially in the same anatomic location, are far more likely to be recurrent zosteriform herpes simplex virus infections. The incidence of herpes zoster in immunosuppressed patients is increased by 20- to 100-fold, and the severity of the disease is also increased. The increased incidence and severity of herpes zoster in older individuals, as well as in individuals of any age who are immunosuppressed, is correlated with a deficient cell-mediated immune response to VZV antigens (Miller, 1980; Rand et al., 1977; Arvin et al., 1980; Meyers et al., 1980).

Patients with herpes zoster are infectious. Virus can be isolated from vesicles in uncomplicated herpes zoster for up to seven days after the appearance of the rash and for much longer periods in immunocompromised individuals. However, herpes zoster is less contagious than varicella; the infection rate in susceptible household contacts appears to be only about one third that of varicella (Gordon, 1962; Bruusgaard, 1932; Hope-Simpson, 1965; Seiler, 1949).

## DIAGNOSIS

In the pre-eruptive stage, herpes zoster is easily confused with other causes of pain such as pleurisy, myocardial infarction, cholecystitis, appendicitis, renal colic, or collapsed intervertebral disk. When the eruption appears, the diagnosis is almost always obvious.

Zosteriform herpes simplex eruptions are often impossible to distinguish from herpes zoster on clinical grounds or by the complement fixation test. Multiple recurrences at the same site are common in herpes simplex but exceedingly rare in herpes zoster. Virus isolation or the identification of VZV (or herpes simplex virus) antigens in material obtained from the lesions is the only reliable means of differential diagnosis (see Chapters 99 and 222 for details).

Contact dermatitis, burns, vaccinia autoinoculation, and localized bacterial skin infections may resemble herpes zoster, but a careful history and examination of the lesions (including a Tzanck smear with the identification of multinucleated giant cells and intranuclear inclusion bodies) eliminates any confusion.

## TREATMENT

The neuralgia of herpes zoster can often be relieved by analgesics; narcotics carry a risk of addiction if pain persists. Cool compresses and calamine lotion may reduce the discomfort and hasten the drying of vesicular lesions. A bland ointment or olive oil dressing may help soften and separate the crusts.

Topical application of 5 to 40 per cent iododeoxyuridine (IUdR) in 100 per cent dimethylsulfoxide (DMSO), beginning early in the course of uncomplicated herpes zoster, shortens the vesicular phase and accelerates healing, and may also reduce the duration of pain (Juel-Jensen and MacCallum, 1972; Wildenhoff et al., 1979). However, these effects are small, and this preparation of IUdR is not licensed for use in the United States. The cost and undefined long-term toxicity of such high concentrations of drug and solvent may deter its use elsewhere.

Local corticosteroids have no place in the therapy of VZV infections. However, the results of two small controlled trials suggest that the oral administration of 48 mg of triamcinolone or 40 mg of prednisolone per day, beginning during the early eruptive phase of the disease, may reduce the duration of postherpetic neuralgia in otherwise healthy patients over 60 years of age (Eaglstein, 1970; Keczkes and Basheer, 1980). The possibility that such large doses of corticosteroid may induce VZV dissemination warrants a larger controlled trial to confirm these results. Corticosteroids are contraindicated in immunosuppressed patients, because danger of disseminated infection is increased.

Inhibitors of VZV replication have been used in attempts to control the multiplication and dissemination of VZV in immunosuppressed patients with herpes zoster. Cytosine arabinoside (Ara-C) and IUdR are contraindicated because they are ineffective and toxic (Richman and Oxman, 1978). In nontoxic doses, intravenous adenine arabinoside (Ara-A) accelerates the clearance of virus from vesicles, shortens the period of new vesicle formation, and reduces the duration and intensity of pain in immunosuppressed patients (Whitley et al., 1976). Its effect on late complications has not been evaluated. Also being evaluated is a more soluble (and thus more easily administered) monophosphate derivative of ara-A. More encouraging still is the advent of a new generation of antiviral drugs specifically designed to take advantage of the presence of VZV-specific enzymes. The first of these, 9-(2-hydroxyethoxymethyl) guanine (acycloguanosine or acyclovir), is phosphorylated by the VZV-specified deoxypyrimidine kinase but not by the comparable host-cell enzyme (Elion et al., 1977). Thus, it is taken up and converted to its active form by VZV-infected cells but not by uninfected host cells. In addition, the active intracellular form of the drug, acyclovir triphosphate, inhibits the VZV-specified DNA polymerase to a greater extent than host-cell DNA polymerases. Consequently, acyclovir is a highly effective and nontoxic inhibitor of VZV in tissue culture. It is now being evaluated in immunosuppressed patients with herpes zoster. Interferon also appears to be effective. When administered to immunosuppressed patients with early localized herpes zoster, large parenteral doses of human interferon significantly reduce progression of disease within the primary dermatome, cutaneous dissemination, visceral complications, and postherpetic neuralgia (Merigan et al., 1978).

In general, the clinical course of herpes zoster appears to be unrelated to the serologic response to VZV. Nevertheless, the increased severity and widespread dissemination observed in some immunosuppressed patients with a deficient or delayed humoral response (Schimpff et al., 1972; Rifkind, 1966; Mazur et al., 1979) and the safety of VZIG led Stevens and Merigan (1980) to conduct a double-blind controlled therapeutic trial of VZIG in immunosuppressed patients with herpes zoster. Despite a much higher titer of antibody to VZV, the VZIG did not appear superior to the normal serum globulin control in preventing dissemination or diminishing postherpetic pain.

Suspected infection of the eye by VZV needs prompt treatment by an ophthalmologist. Mydriatics are used to prevent synechiae. Corticosteroids are sometimes recommended if uveitis is present. Topical antiviral drugs (IUdR, Ara-A) are of unproven efficacy in ophthalmic zoster, but they should probably be employed whenever corticosteroids are used.

## PROPHYLAXIS

Reactivation of latent VZV and the development of herpes zoster is limited by immune mechanisms, especially cellular immunity. The increased severity of herpes zoster in some patients with a deficient humoral response to VZV (Schimpff et al., 1972; Rifkind, 1966; Mazur et al., 1979) and the capacity of antiviral antibody to prevent reactivation of latent herpes simplex virus in an animal model (Stevens, 1975) suggest, however, that prophylactic VZIG might suppress herpes zoster in immunosuppressed patients. A clinical trial of VZIG prophylaxis in immunosuppressed patients is now underway to examine this possibility.

## References

Aoyama, Y., Kurata, T., Kurata, K., Hondo, R., and Ogiwara, H.: Demonstration of viral antigens in herpes simplex and varicella-zoster infection. Recent Adv RES Res 14:90, 1974.

Appelbaum, E., Kreps, S. I., and Sunshine, A.: Herpes zoster encephalitis. Am J Med 32:25, 1962.

Armstrong, R. W., Gurwith, M. J., Waddell, D., and Merigan, T. C.: Cutaneous interferon production in patients with Hodgkin's disease and other cancers infected with varicella or vaccinia. N Engl J Med 283:1182, 1970.

Arvin, A. M., Pollard, R. B., Rasmussen, L. E., and Merigan, T. C.: Cellular and humoral immunity in the pathogenesis of recurrent herpes viral infections in patients with lymphoma. J Clin Invest 65:869, 1980

Atkinson, K., Meyers, J. D., Storb, R., Prentice, R. L., and Thomas, E. D.: Varicella-zoster virus infection after marrow transplantation for aplastic anemia or leukemia. Transplantation 29:47, 1980.

Barr, R. J., Herten, R. J., and Graham, J. H.: Rapid method for Tzanck preparations. JAMA 237:1119, 1977.

Bastian, F. O., Rabson, A. S., Yee, C. L., and Tralka, T. S.: Herpesvirus varicellae: Isolated from human dorsal root ganglia. Arch Pathol 97:331, 1974.

Brostoff, J.: Diaphragmatic paralysis after herpes zoster. Br Med J 2:1571, 1966.

Brown, G. R.: Herpes Zoster: Correlation of age, sex, distribution, neuralgia, and associated disorders. South Med J 69:576, 1976.

Brunell, P. A., Gershon, A. A., Uduman, S. A., and Steinberg, S.: Varicella-zoster immunoglobulins during varicella, latency, and zoster. J Infect Dis 132:49, 1975.

Bruusgaard, E.: The mutual relation between zoster and varicella. Br J Dermatol 44:1, 1932.

Burgoon, C. F., Burgoon, J. S., and Baldridge, G. D.: The natural history of herpes zoster. JAMA 164:265, 1957.

Christie, A. B.: Chickenpox: herpes zoster. In Infectious Diseases, Epidemiology and Clinical Practice, 2nd ed. Edinburgh, Churchill Livingstone, 1974, pp. 278–290, 1974.

Clark, J.: Herpes zoster of right glossopharyngeal nerve. Lancet 1:38, 1979.

de Moragas, J. M., and Kierland, R. R.: The outcome of patients with herpes zoster. Arch Dermatol 75:193, 1957.

Denny-Brown, D., Adams, R. D., and Fitzgerald, P. J.: Pathologic features of herpes zoster: A note on "geniculate herpes." Arch Neurol Psychiat 51:216, 1944.

Dolin, R., Reichman, R. C., Mazur, M. H., and Whitley, R. J.: Herpes zoster–varicella infections in immunosuppressed patients. Ann Intern Med 89:375, 1978.

Eaglstein, W. H., Katz, R., and Brown, J. A.: The effects of early corticosteroid therapy on the skin eruption and pain of herpes zoster. JAMA 211:1681, 1970.

Easton, H. G.: Zoster sine herpete causing trigeminal neuralgia. Lancet 2:1065, 1970.

Eisenberg, E.: Intraoral isolated herpes zoster. Oral Surg 45:214, 1978.

Esiri, M. M., and Tomlinson, A. H.: Herpes zoster: Demonstration of virus in trigeminal nerve and ganglion by immunofluorescence and electron microscopy. J Neurol Sci 15:35, 1972.

Feldman, S., Chaudary, S., Ossi, M., and Epp, E.: A viremic phase for herpes zoster in children with cancer. Pediatrics 91:597, 1977.

Feldman, S., Hughes, W. T., and Kim, H. Y.: Herpes zoster in children with cancer. Am J Dis Child 126:178, 1973.

Gershon, A. A., Steinberg, S., and Brunell, P. A.: Zoster immune globulin, a further assessment. N Engl J Med 290:243, 1974.

Ghatak, N. R., and Zimmerman, H. M.: Spinal ganglion in herpes zoster. Arch Pathol 95:411, 1973.

Gilbert, G. J.: Herpes zoster ophthalmicus and delayed contralateral hemiparesis. JAMA 229:302, 1974.

Goffinet, D. R., Glatstein, E. J., and Merigan, T. C.: Herpes zoster-varicella infections and lymphoma. Ann Intern Med 76:235, 1972.

Gold, E.: Serologic and virus-isolation studies of patients with varicella or herpes-zoster infection. N Engl J Med 274:181, 1966.

Gold, E., and Robbins, F. C.: Isolation of herpes zoster virus from spinal fluid of a patient. Virology 6:293, 1958.

Gordon, J. E.: Chickenpox: An epidemiological review. Am J Med Sci 244:362, 1962.

Grant, B. D., and Rowe, C. R.: Motor paralysis of the extremities in herpes zoster. J Bone Joint Surg 43A:885, 1961.

Head, H., and Campbell, A. W.: The pathology of herpes zoster and its bearing on sensory localisation. Brain 23:353, 1900.

Hogan, E. L., and Krigman, M. R.: Herpes zoster myelitis. Arch Neurol 29:309, 1973.

Hope-Simpson, R. E.: The nature of herpes zoster: A long-term study and a new hypothesis. Proc R Soc Med 58:9, 1965.

Izumi, A. K., and Edwards, J.: Herpes zoster and neurogenic bladder dysfunction. JAMA 224:1748, 1973.

Jellinek, E. H., and Tulloch, W. S.: Herpes zoster with dysfunction of bladder and anus. Lancet 2:1219, 1976.

Juel-Jensen, B. E., and MacCallum, F. O.: Herpes Simplex Varicella and Zoster. Philadelphia, J. B. Lippincott Company, 1972.

Keczkes, K., and Basheer, A. M.: Do corticosteroids prevent post-herpetic neuralgia? Br J Dermatol, 102:551. 1980.

Kendall, D.: Motor complications of herpes zoster. Br Med J 1:616, 1957.

Laws, H. W.: Herpes zoster ophthalmicus complicated by contralateral hemiplegia. Arch Ophthalmol 63:273, 1960.

Lewis, G. W.: Zoster Sine Herpete. Br Med J 2:418, 1958.

Linnemann, C. C., and Alvira, M. M.: Pathogenesis of varicella-zoster angitis in the CNS. Arch Neurol 37:239, 1980.

Lipschutz, B.: Untersuchungen über die Ätiologie der Krankheiten der Herpesgruppe (Herpes zoster, Herpes genitalis, Herpes febrilis). Arch Dermatol 136:428, 1921.

Luby, J. P., Ramirez-Ronda, C., Rinner, S., Hull, A., and Vergne-Marini, P.: A longitudinal study of varicella-zoster virus infections in renal transplant recipients. J Infect Dis 135:659, 1977.

McCormick, W. F., Rodnitzky, R. L., Schochet, S. S., Jr., and McKee, A. P.: Varicella-zoster encephalomyelitis. Arch Neurol 21:559, 1969.

Mazur, M. H., Whitley, R. J., and Dolin, R.: Serum antibody levels as risk factors in the dissemination of herpes zoster. Arch Intern Med 139:1341, 1979.

Merigan, T. C., Rand, K. H., Pollard, R. B., Abdallah, P. S., Jordan, G. W., and Fried, R. P.: Human leukocyte interferon for the treatment of herpes zoster in patients with cancer. N Engl J Med 298:981, 1978.

Merselis, J. G., Jr., Kaye, D., and Hook, E. W.: Disseminated herpes zoster. Arch Intern Med 113:679, 1964.

Meyers, J. D., Flournoy, N., and Thomas, E. D.: Cell-mediated immunity to varicella-zoster virus after allogeneic marrow transplant. J Infect Dis 141:479, 1980.

Miller, A. E.: Selective decline in cellular immune response to varicella-zoster in the elderly. Neur 30:582, 1980.

Miller, L. H., and Brunell, P. A.: Zoster, reinfection or activation of latent virus? Am J Med 49:480, 1970.

Muller, S. A., and Winkelmann, R. K.: Cutaneous nerve changes in zoster. J Invest Derm 52:71, 1969.

Norris, F. H., Jr., Leonards, R., Calanchini, P. R., and Calder, C. D.: Herpes-zoster meningoencephalitis. J Infect Dis 122:335, 1970.

Oberg, G., and Svedmyr, A.: Varicelliform eruptions in herpes zoster—some clinical and serological observations. Scand J Infect Dis 1:47, 1969.

Rand, K. H., Rasmussen, L. E., Pollard, R. B., Arvin, A., and Merigan, T. C.: Cellular immunity and herpesvirus infections in cardiac-transplant patients. N Engl J Med 296:1372, 1977.

Reboul, F., Donaldson, S. S., and Kaplan, H. S.: Herpes zoster and varicella infections in children with Hodgkin's disease. Cancer 41:95, 1978.

Richman, D. D., and Oxman, M. N.: Antiviral agents. In Weinstein, L., and Fields, B. N. (eds.): Seminars in Infectious Diseases. Vol. 1. New York, Stratton Intercontinental Medical Book Corp., 1978, pp. 200–255.

Rifkind, D.: The activation of varicella-zoster virus infections by immunosuppressive therapy. J Lab Clin Med 68:463, 1966.

Rogers, R. S., and Tindall, J. P.: Herpes zoster in children. Arch Dermatol 106:204, 1972.

Schimpff, S., Serpick, A., Stoler, B., Rumack, B., Mellin, H., Joseph, J. M., and Block, J.: Varicella-zoster infection in patients with cancer. Ann Intern Med 76:241, 1972.

Seiler, H. E.: A study of herpes zoster particularly in its relationship to chickenpox. J Hyg 47:253, 1949.

Shanbrom, E., Miller, S., and Haar, H.: Herpes zoster in hematologic neoplasias: Some unusual manifestations. Ann Intern Med 53:523, 1960.

Shibuta, H., Ishikawa, T., Hondo, R., Aoyama, Y., Kurata, K., and Matumoto, M.: Varicella virus isolation from spinal ganglion. Archiv fur die gesamte Virusforschung 45:382, 1974.

Stern, E. S.: The mechanism of herpes zoster and its relation to chicken-pox. Br J Dermatol 49:263, 1937.

Stevens, D. A., Ferrington, R. A., Jordan, G. W., and Merigan, T. C.: Cellular events in zoster vesicles: Relation to clinical course and immune parameters. J Infect Dis 131:509, 1975.

Stevens, D. A., and Merigan, T. C.: Zoster immune globulin prophylaxis of disseminated zoster in compromised hosts. Arch Intern Med 140:52, 1980.

Stevens, J. G.: Latent herpes simplex virus and the nervous system. Curr Top Microbiol Immunol 70:31, 1975.

Taylor-Robinson, D., and Caunt, A. E.: Varicella Virus. Vienna, Springer-Verlag, 1972.

Thomas, J. E., and Howard, F. M., Jr.: Segmental zoster paresis—a disease profile. Neurology 22:459, 1972.

Weller, T. H.: Varicella-herpes zoster virus. In Evans, A. S. (ed.): Viral Infections of Humans: Epidemiology and Control. New York, Plenum Medical Book Company, 1976, pp. 457–480.

Whitley, R. J., Ch'ien, L. T., Dolin, R., Galasso, G. J., and Alford, C. A., Jr.: Adenine arabinoside therapy of herpes zoster in the immunosuppressed. N Engl J Med 294:1193, 1976.

Wildenhoff, K. E., Ispen, J., Esmann, V., Ingemann-Jensen, J., and Poulsen, J. H.: Treatment of herpes zoster with idoxuridine ointment, including a multivariate analysis of symptoms and signs. Scand J Infect Dis 11:1, 1979.

Zaia, J. A., and Oxman, M. N.: Antibody to varicella-zoster virus-induced membrane antigen: Immunofluorescence assay using monodisperse glutaraldehyde-fixed target cells. J Infect Dis 136:519, 1977.

# 224 *SMALLPOX, VACCINIA AND COWPOX*

*A. Ramachandra Rao, M.B., B.S., B.S.Sc.*

# SMALLPOX

## DEFINITION

Smallpox is an infection caused by *Poxvirus variolae*. It is characterized by high fever, severe constitutional symptoms and a characteristic rash two to three days later. The rash evolves through different stages, finally producing scabs, which separate and leave scars.

## ETIOLOGY

### Agent of Infection

The infectious agent is a filterable virus, *Poxvirus variolae*. It is one of the large viruses, measuring about $300 \times 200$ m$\mu$. It was described by Bruist as spherical bodies seen in material collected from the lesions of smallpox. Later, they were studied in greater detail by Paschen, and these bodies are currently known as the elementary bodies or Paschen-Bruist bodies. By suitable staining, these can be demonstrated easily under the ordinary microscope in smears made of scrapings from the base of lesions in the papulovesicular stage of the rash.

There are mainly two strains of variola virus: variola major, which produces the classic Asiatic smallpox, and variola minor, which produces the milder variety, called alastrim. These two viruses breed true, and each confers immunity against the other. Recently, another strain has been isolated, variola intermedius or variola tanzania, which was reported to be prevalent in some parts of Africa and Indonesia.

The host range of smallpox is very limited. Besides man, the monkey is the only animal that develops clinical disease similar to that in man when infected. However, the disease in monkeys is invariably mild and nonfatal.

Variola virus can be grown on the chorioallantoic membrane of the developing chick embryo. It produces small dome-shaped grayish-white pock-like lesions on the membrane within 48 to 72 hours after the inoculation of the infectious material. Variola virus can also be grown on several tissue culture lines. The two strains, v. major and v. minor, can be differentiated by their behavior on the chorioallantoic membrane (Nizamuddin and Dumbell, 1961), and the third strain lies between the two.

The antigenic structure of variola virus is rather complex. It seems to consist of V antigen, which is bound to the elementary bodies, and soluble LS antigens. Besides these, it has precipitating, hemagglutinating, and complement-fixing antigens, which are all employed in the serologic studies. It is claimed that variola and vaccinia share a common protein antigen, which is responsible for resistance to infection with smallpox.

Variola virus is one of the most stable viruses. It resists drying and freezing. It is highly stable for several years in a freeze-dried state, and is relatively resistant to the commonly used chemical disinfectants. It is sensitive to ultraviolet rays and gamma radiation. Even tropical sun destroys the virus in a matter of a few hours.

### Transmission of Infection

*Sources of Infection.* Theoretically speaking, there are three types of sources: inanimate, non-human animate, and human. There were historic records of smallpox outbreaks occurring during the 19th century, in which inanimate sources such as cotton and used clothes were incriminated. But it is doubtful whether human sources were carefully investigated and excluded then. In recent times, when the methods of epidemiologic surveillance have been well developed, an outbreak has rarely been traced to inanimate sources. Similarly, there is no evidence so far, either epidemiologic or otherwise, to show that any nonhuman animate sources play any role in the transmission of smallpox. No animal reservoirs or insect vectors have been described so far.

The only known source, therefore, is man. A man suffering from smallpox is the most common source, if not the only one. Though a patient suffering from smallpox is potentially infectious from the first day of the disease until the last scab separates off, there is enough evidence (Rao et al., 1968a) to show that maximum transmission occurs only during the first two weeks. Although scabs contain plenty of viable virus, it is doubtful whether they play much role in the transmission of the disease since the virus in the scab is not in the free state that would allow it to be inhaled easily.

Some claims have been made (Rao, 1972) about the occurrence of subclinical (inapparent) infections in smallpox. These are more of academic than epidemiologic interest. So far there has been no report of any outbreak of smallpox, anywhere in the world, with subclinical infection as the source.

*Transfer of Infection.* Although variola virus is voided through several portals of exit from a smallpox patient, air-sampling studies (Meikeljohn et al., 1961; Downie et al., 1965) and epidemiologic studies (Rao et al., 1968a) clearly suggest that the infectious agent is transferred mainly through nasopharyngeal droplets of the patient in the early stages of the disease. Smallpox is therefore a contact disease and not an airborne disease, as was once thought. Very rarely, infection is transmitted by virus carried over long distances by air.

The infected droplets are inhaled, with the nasopharynx as the portal of entry. Occasionally, one may see a case of variola inoculata, with virus entering through a break in the skin. The placenta is not a barrier to the virus. However, the incidence of congenital smallpox is not as high as one would expect (Rao, 1972), probably because of the high fetal death rate in the pregnant woman with smallpox.

*Factors Influencing the Transmission Pattern.* Recent studies on the epidemiology of smallpox (Rao et al., 1968a) indicate that there are several factors that determine the pattern of transmission. The transmission rate is greater from cases of ordinary and flat varieties than hemorrhagic and modified, greater from the unvaccinated than the vaccinated, and greater from children than adults. Thus, unvaccinated children suffering from ordinary and flat varieties of smallpox are responsible for greater transmission of the disease in the family or community.

As far as the host is concerned, the most important determinant is the immunity status of the contact who is exposed to the patient. For all age groups, even on close familial exposure, only 3 per cent of vaccinated contacts develop the disease compared with nearly 40 per cent of the unvaccinated contacts.

Among the environmental factors, low socioeconomic status and overcrowding enhance the possibility of transmission of infection. Meteorologic factors per se do not seem to influence directly the transmission pattern, although a definite seasonal variation in the prevalence of the disease has been universally observed.

## PATHOGENESIS AND PATHOLOGY

Most of our knowledge about the fate of variola virus after entry into the nasopharynx of man was gained from the experimental evidence gathered so far with the allied vaccinia virus in animals. It is now clear that the virus, after entering through the nasopharynx of the susceptible host, initially multiplies in the cells of the bronchioles and alveoli of the lungs. There, it produces minimal lesions and quickly passes through the regional lymph nodes into the blood, producing primary viremia. From the blood, it immediately disappears into the cells of the reticuloendothelial system, where it multiplies throughout the incubation period. At the end of this period, it enters the blood again as a severe "virus shower," producing secondary viremia, which corresponds to the pre-eruptive stage of the disease. In about 24 to 48 hours, the virus leaves the blood to settle in the skin and mucous membranes, producing the typical lesions of the disease. So far, attempts to isolate the virus either from the blood or from nasopharyngeal secretions during the incubation period have not been successful. However, it has been isolated from the blood during the pre-eruptive stage, when the secondary viremia occurs.

The first changes in the skin occur in the capillaries of the dermis. Perivascular infiltration occurs with swelling of the lining endothelium. Then the malpighian cells of the epidermis become edematous due to proliferation of cells as well as to intercellular edema. The epithelial layer is thickened, and cell walls break down, resulting in the formation of multilocular vesicles. During the pustular stage, however, these septa break down. Finally, when scabs are formed, new epithelium grows under the scabs. The crusts separate, leaving scars.

On the mucous membranes, lesions break down easily and quickly because there is no horny layer. In the viscera, there is cloudy swelling with mononuclear cell infiltration and focal hemorrhages.

## CLINICAL MANIFESTATIONS

### Variola Major

*Clinical Classification.* Smallpox presents in several clinical forms. Because the clinical features, the course, and even the prognosis vary from one form to another, great importance is attached to the clinical classification of the disease. Curshmann (1875) classified the disease into hemorrhagic and nonhemorrhagic forms, and subdivided the former into purpura variolosa and variola pustulosa hemorrhagica and the latter into confluent, semiconfluent, discrete, and mod-

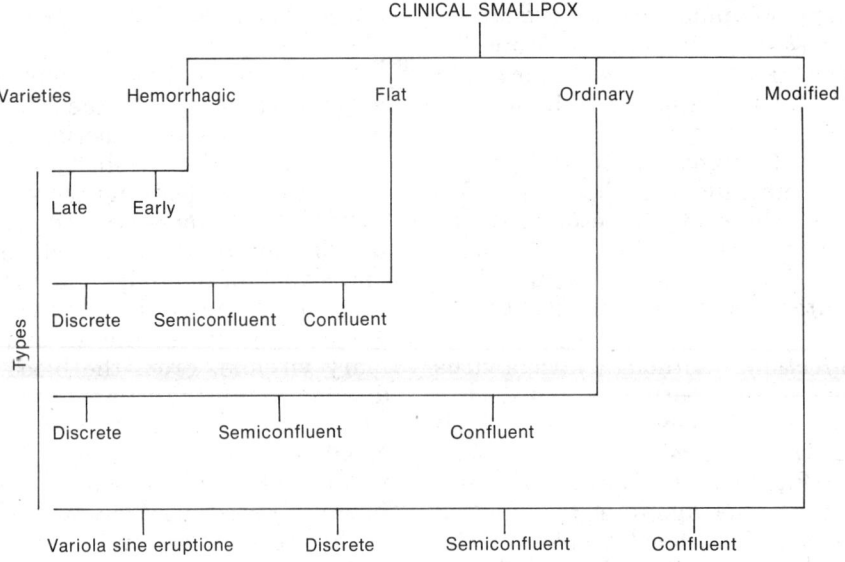

**FIGURE 1.** *Classification scheme of clinical smallpox (Rao's).*

ified. This classification was based mainly on the density of rash, and some of the names are misleading. Dixon (1962), on the other hand, avoided the use of the name hemorrhagic and classified smallpox into nine clinical types: fulminating, malignant confluent, malignant semiconfluent, benign confluent, benign semiconfluent, discrete, mild, abortive, and variola sine eruptionae. Rao (1972), from his vast clinical experience of having treated nearly 30,000 cases of variola major, theorized that hemorrhagic smallpox is a clinical entity different from the nonhemorrhagic form, and that the nature and evolution of the rash, rather than the density alone, are the criteria for classification of a case. Accordingly, he classified smallpox into four main clinical varieties: hemorrhagic, flat, ordinary, and modified. For detailed description, however, he further subdivided these four varieties into twelve types (Fig. 1 and Table 1).

*Clinical Features.* Each stage of the disease has its own characteristics. A careful consideration of these is very essential for a proper understanding of the course and even for assessing the prognosis. There is no clear-cut demarcation between stages, but for descriptive purposes, smallpox can be divided into three stages.

*Incubation Stage.* This period is usually not considered as a clinical stage of the disease, since no clinical manifestations are visible. However, when the virus is actively multiplying in the reticuloendothelial system during this period, it has to be considered as a part of the disease process. To determine the exact duration of this period is very difficult. It is impossible to know the actual time of entry of the virus into the host, and similarly, the actual time of appearance of the first clinical manifestation is also difficult to elicit. From available data regarding single and brief exposures in various outbreaks of smallpox, it has been found that the incubation period of smallpox is about 12 to 14 days and may range from 7 to 21 days.

*Pre-eruptive Stage.* Smallpox can occur without a rash but not without fever and other constitutional symptoms preceding the rash. This

**TABLE 1.** Frequency of Occurrence of Different Clinical Varieties of Smallpox with Reference to Vaccinal Status

| VACCINAL STATUS | | CLINICAL VARIETIES | | | | |
|---|---|---|---|---|---|---|
| | | Hemorrhage | Flat | Ordinary | Modified | Total |
| Vaccinated | Cases | 115 | 45 | 2377 | 861 | 3378 |
| | Frequency[a] | 3.4 | 1.3 | 70.0 | 25.3 | 100.0 |
| Unvaccinated | Cases | 85 | 236 | 3147 | 76 | 3544 |
| | Frequency | 2.4 | 6.7 | 88.8 | 2.1 | 100.0 |

[a]Represents percentage of total cases in that group.

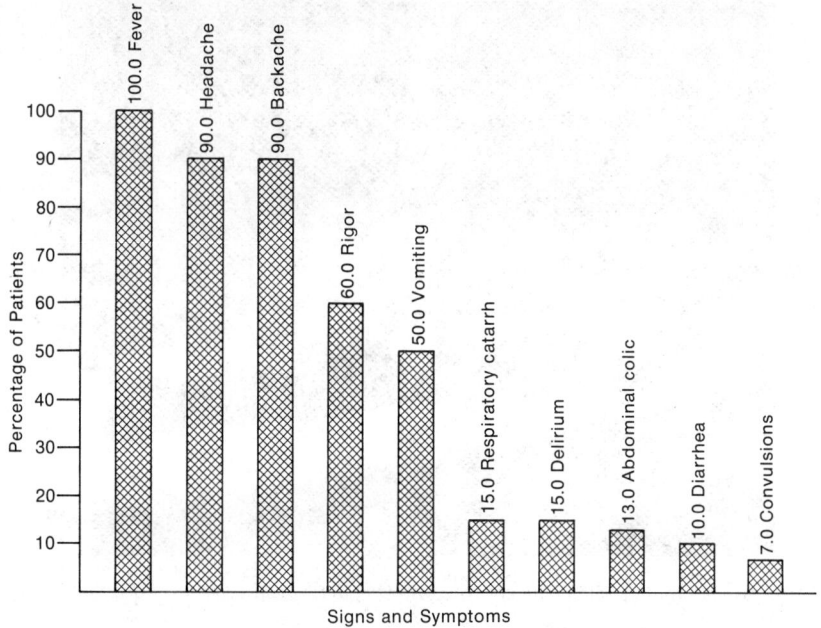

**FIGURE 2.** *Frequency of occurrence of signs and symptoms in the pre-eruptive stage of smallpox.*

pre-eruptive syndrome is so characteristic of smallpox that its occurrence is a "must" for diagnosis. This stage is characterized by a sudden onset of fever with or without rigor and is accompanied by severe constitutional symptoms (Fig. 2). The fever may be of varying degree, temperature ranging from 102° F to 105° F. Various types of rash have been described during this stage but have rarely been found in endemic areas, because cases are almost never seen by doctors during this stage. When such rashes are present, they are confined to an area between the loins and groins (bathing-trunk type) and are transient, disappearing in the wake of the specific rash. The duration of this stage is about two to three days but may be prolonged in some severe types.

*Eruptive Stage.* The characteristics of the lesions, their evolution, and their distribution vary with different varieties and types. Hence, it is necessary to describe this stage separately in each of the clinical types.

### ORDINARY VARIETY

*Order of Appearance of the Rash.* The lesions appear on the mucous membranes first (enanthem). The buccal mucous membrane, tongue, palate, and pharynx are involved usually. The rash appears as minute reddish spots about 24 to 48 hours before the appearance of the rash on the skin (exanthem). The enanthem is not present in all cases. The exanthem usually starts on the forehead with angry-looking flea-bite-like mac-

ules, which rapidly appear on the whole face, proximal portions of the extremities, trunk, and lastly, on the distal portions of the extremities. The whole process usually does not take more than 24 to 36 hours, after which no more fresh lesions appear.

*Evolution of the Rash.* Lesions on the mucous membranes rapidly evolve into papules and vesicles and break down by about the sixth to eighth day of fever. Lesions on the skin are slower to evolve. The macules are raised over the skin, becoming papules in about 24 to 48 hours. An opalescent fluid collects within them, making them vesicles in another 48 hours. By about the tenth day, the fluid becomes opaque, giving them the appearance of pustules. Actually, these so-called pustules do not contain pus but only tissue debris. Between the tenth and fourteenth day, these pustules mature and increase in size. After this, resolution starts, with flattening of the lesions, slow absorption of the fluid, and thickening of the central portion of the lesion. By about the twentieth day, the central portion hardens, forming a scab, which separates in another ten days to leave a depigmented scar. The whole period of this evolution may vary from case to case, depending upon several factors such as the immunity status of the patient and the severity of the disease.

*Distribution of the Rash.* The rash of smallpox has a characteristic distribution. It is relatively more dense on the peripheral parts of the body than on the central region (centrifugal distribution) (Fig. 3). On the trunk it is more dense on

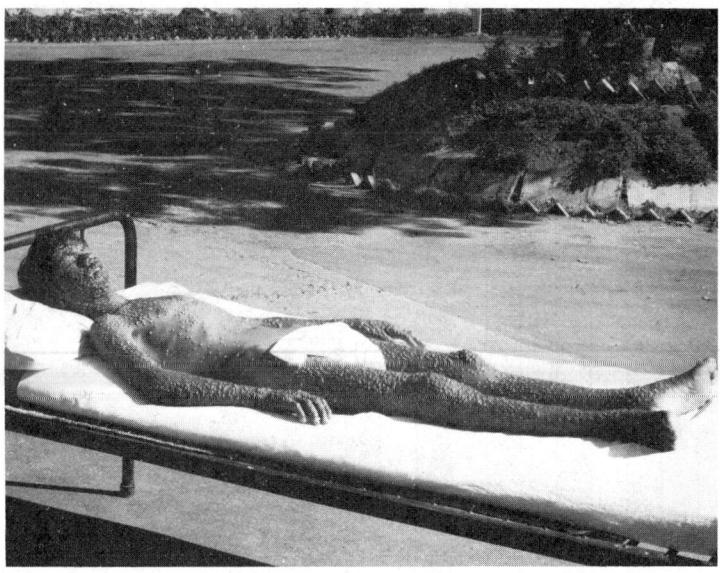

**FIGURE 3.** *A case of ordinary semiconfluent type, showing the typical centrifugal distribution of the rash.*

the back (Fig. 4) than on the front (Fig. 5); on the front, it is more dense on the chest than on the abdomen; and on the abdomen, it is more dense on the upper half than on the lower (Gaspirini's sign) (Fig. 6). On the extremities, it is more dense on the distal portions, extensor aspects, and convexities than on the proximal portions, flexor aspects, and concavities, respectively. The rash is relatively more profuse on the folds of the axillae than on the apex. On the face, it is more dense on the upper half. Invariably, lesions are found on the palms and soles.

*Individual Characteristics of the Lesions.* The lesions are fairly deep-set in the skin and feel shotty. They are circular in pattern. During the vesicular and pustular stages, they appear multilocular with fibrinous strands separating the vesicular cavity into several compartments. Due to retraction of these strands and due to loss of fluid tension, a dimple with a black spot is often formed on the apex of the lesion, a process known as umbilication (Fig. 7). This may disappear as the pustule matures. At a given time, and at a particular site of the body, all the lesions are found to be more or less in the same stage of evolution (absence of pleomorphism). This is because, unlike chickenpox, the rash occurs only in one crop.

*Constitutional Symptoms.* The fever of the pre-eruptive stage comes down appreciably as the rash appears and continues to be low, between

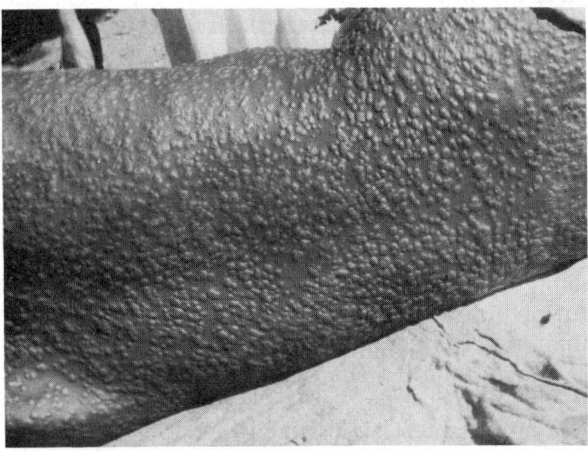

**FIGURE 4.** *Dense rash of smallpox on the back of the patient.*

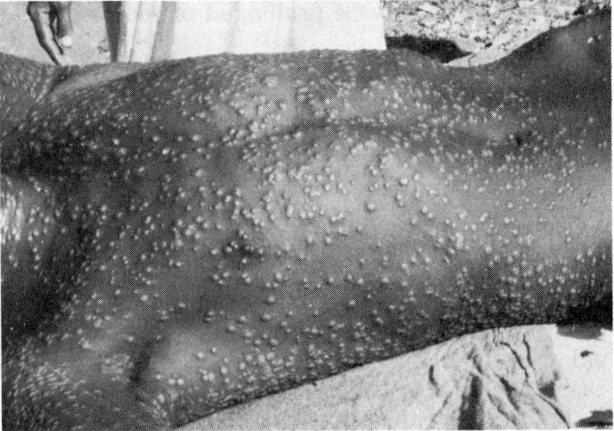

**FIGURE 5.** *Relatively less dense rash on the front in the same patient shown in Figure 4.*

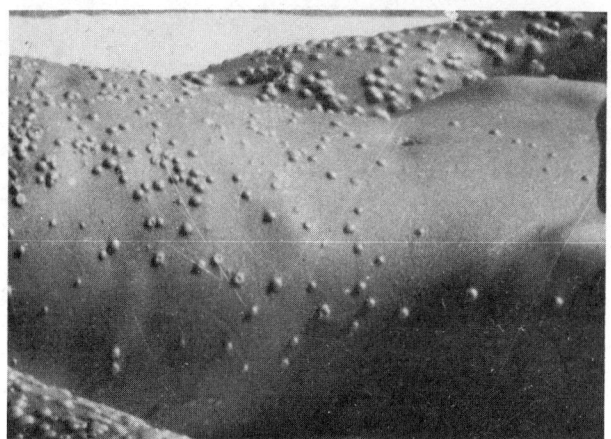

**FIGURE 6.** *Typical Gaspirini's sign.*

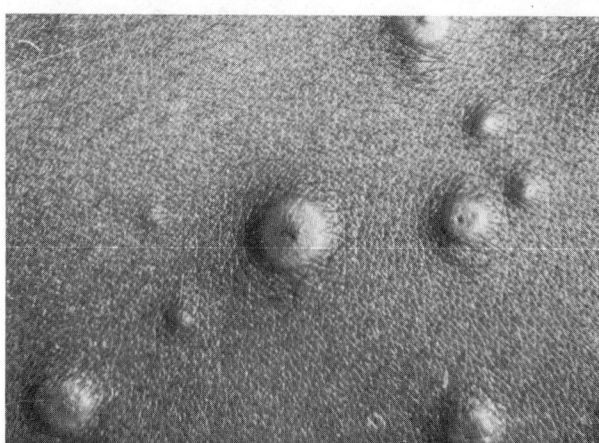

**FIGURE 7.** *Deep-set lesions of smallpox with typical umbilication.*

100° and 102° F, until about the eighth day, after which it rises again, remaining high until the scabbing starts. After scabbing is completed, the temperature comes down to normal by lysis in almost all uncomplicated cases. It may remain high in unvaccinated patients and in those with complications even after scabbing is over.

About 70 per cent of all cases in vaccinated patients and about 90 per cent of unvaccinated patients belong to this variety. Depending upon the density of the rash, this variety is divided into three types: ordinary confluent, ordinary semi-confluent, and ordinary discrete (Fig. 8). The ordinary confluent is far more common in the unvaccinated, and the ordinary discrete type is more prevalent in the vaccinated.

### HEMORRHAGIC VARIETY

In this highly fatal variety of smallpox, hemorrhages occur in the skin and/or mucous membranes. The pre-eruptive stage is considerably prolonged and is associated with very severe constitutional symptoms. This variety is far more common in adults and women, especially if pregnant. It is as prevalent in the vaccinated as in the unvaccinated. These observations suggest that it is not a lack of immunity alone that is responsible for this highly fatal variety. If lack of immunity were responsible, this variety should have been very common in young unvaccinated children, which is not the case. One school of thought believes that it is caused by a different strain of virus, but epidemiologic evidence (Rao et al., 1968a) does not support this view. Blood coagulation studies (Roberts et al, 1966; McKenzie et al., 1966) showed coagulation abnormalities in the hemorrhagic variety that were absent in the nonhemorrhagic variety. In experimental variola

in monkeys (Rao et al., 1968b), hemorrhagic smallpox could be produced by cortisone administration before variolation. Variola infection in pregnant women, pregnant monkeys, and cortisone-treated monkeys behaved in an almost identical manner. It is therefore possible that some hormonal disturbances, especially of corticosteroids, may be one of the factors that determine the occurrence of this fatal variety of smallpox. This variety is of two types.

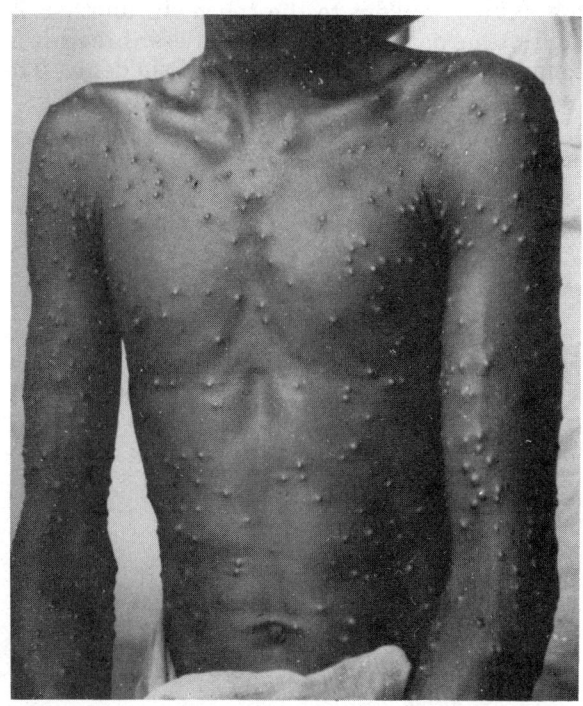

**FIGURE 8.** *A case of ordinary discrete type.*

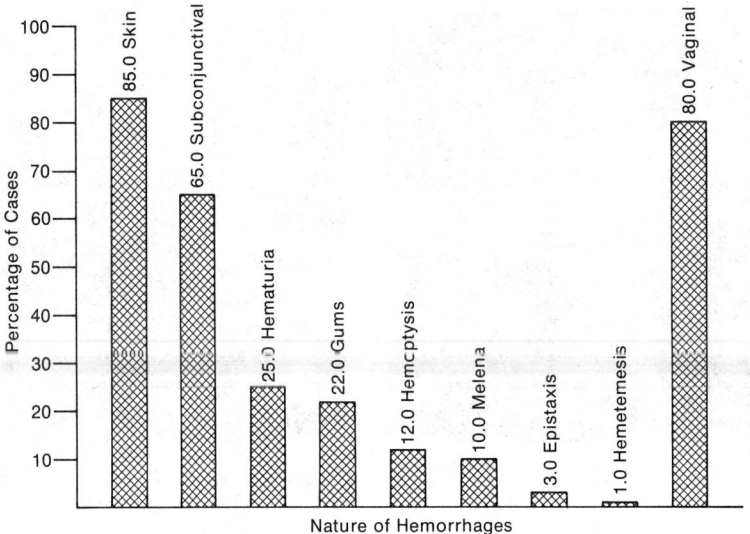

**FIGURE 9.** *Frequency of occurrence of hemorrhages in early hemorrhagic type.*

*Early Hemorrhagic Type.* In these cases, hemorrhages appear before onset of the rash, and patients may even die before the rash is seen. There is a sudden onset of fever with rigor, a splitting headache, excruciating backache, and vomiting. The patient is highly toxic, pale, and has an anxious look. On the third or fourth day, the whole body has a generalized flush with fine petechiae. Simultaneously, bleeding occurs through different mucous membranes (Fig. 9). By about the fifth day, the skin color changes to purple, and the skin is velvety to the touch. In another 24 hours, the patient becomes restless, breathless, complains of chest pain, and dies suddenly. The patient is conscious until the end and knows of his impending death.

Ninety per cent of the cases are adults above the age of 14 years, and 70 per cent are women. Sixteen per cent of smallpox cases among pregnant women belong to this variety as against only 0.9 per cent of nonpregnant women and 0.8 per cent of men in the same age group (15 to 44 years). This type is equally common in both vaccinated and unvaccinated patients.

*Late Hemorrhagic Types.* In this type, the hemorrhages occur after the appearance of the rash. As in the early type, the pre-eruptive stage is prolonged and is associated with very severe consti-

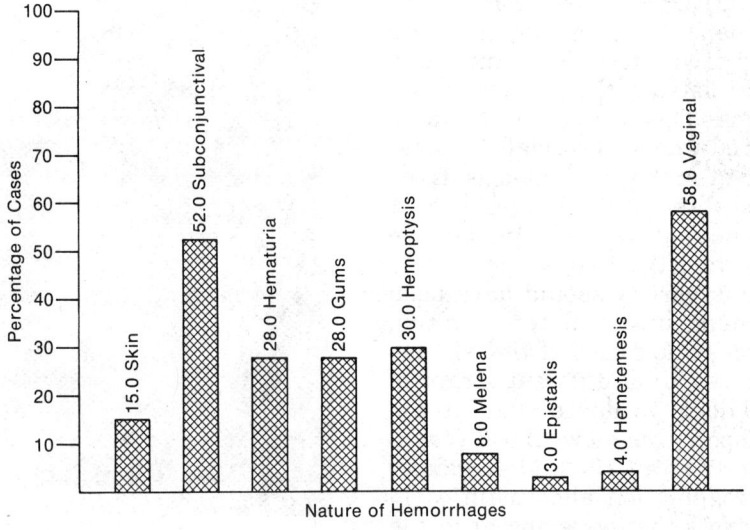

**FIGURE 10.** *Frequency of occurrence of hemorrhages in late hemorrhagic type.*

tutional symptoms. As in the ordinary variety, the rash appears, and the lesions evolve through macules, papules, and vesicles. In many cases, hemorrhages occur into bases of the lesions as well as into various mucous membranes (Fig. 10). The lesions appear flat and dark and do not evolve further. These patients may survive until about the eighth day of fever. They are highly toxic and have high fever throughout the course. There may be a few survivors and their convalescence is very prolonged. Survival is greater in those in whom hemorrhages have not occurred into the lesions.

Eighty per cent of these cases are adults. There is not much sex difference in frequency of occurrence of this type, except that pregnant women are more susceptible. It is equally prevalent in the vaccinated and the unvaccinated.

### FLAT VARIETY

In this variety also, the pre-eruptive stage may be prolonged and is associated with fairly severe constitutional symptoms, which may continue even after the appearance of the rash. The enanthem, which is frequently seen in this variety, is very severe. As in the ordinary variety, the exanthem occurs, and the lesions evolve through macules and papules. In the early vesicular stage, instead of projecting on the skin, the lesions flatten with hemorrhages occurring into their bases, and appear buried in the skin. This variety differs from the late hemorrhagic type by the absence of hemorrhages into the mucous membranes. There is very little fluid in the lesions. They are not multilocular, do not present any umbilication, and are invariably surrounded by an erythematous areola. The patient is febrile throughout the course and is highly toxic. On or about the tenth day, patients invariably develop respiratory complications like viral pneumonitis and usually die. In survivors, scabbing starts and ends early. The scabs, which are very minute, separate off easily, leaving superficial scars.

Nearly 75 per cent of cases of this variety are children under the age of 14 years. Eighty per cent of total cases are among the unvaccinated. Depending upon the density of the rash, this variety is subdivided into three types: flat confluent, flat semiconfluent, and flat discrete. Of the three, the flat confluent type is the most severe and is common in the unvaccinated. Unlike the hemorrhagic variety, the vaccinated always fare better in the flat variety.

### MODIFIED VARIETY

There is considerable modification in the characteristics of the lesions, their evolution and distribution, and even in the constitutional symptoms in these cases. The extreme modification occurs in the type called variola sine eruptionae, in which patients present no rash on the skin. Though most cases of the modified variety have very few lesions, the number of lesions or the density of rash is not the criterion for classification in this variety.

The pre-eruptive stage lasts two to three days and usually has milder constitutional symptoms. The temperature comes down to normal as soon as the rash appears on the skin and does not rise again. An enanthem is very rare in this variety. The skin lesions evolve through macules, papules, and vesicles very rapidly. Without going through the pustular stage, the rash scabs off and is completed by the tenth day of fever or earlier. The distribution of the rash may not conform to the classic pattern. The lesions are superficial and neither multilocular nor umbilicated. The scabs are superficial and separate early, leaving faint scars, which may not persist for more than five years.

Nearly 90 per cent of cases of this variety occur in the vaccinated. Depending on the density of rash, this variety is subdivided into four types: modified confluent, modified semiconfluent, modified discrete, and variola sine eruptionae. Modified discrete alone accounts for nearly 99 per cent of all cases of this variety; the other types are very rare. Variola sine eruptionae is very difficult to diagnose clinically. The patients have the usual pre-eruptive syndrome, but it is not followed by any rash on the skin. Some may have an enanthem. A history of close exposure to a case of smallpox, with fever and characteristic constitutional symptoms even in the absence of rash, should suggest the possibility of variola sine eruptionae. Virus can sometimes be isolated from the blood during the febrile stage.

*Prognosis.* Prognosis in smallpox depends mainly on the clinical type and the vaccination status of the patient. Since immunity after vaccination is not permanent, the time lag between the last successful vaccination and the onset of the present attack also influences prognosis. Table 2 shows the case-fatality rates of different clinical varieties and types of smallpox with reference to vaccination status. In general, chances of survival among the vaccinated are greater in all types except the hemorrhagic, which is fatal regardless of the vaccination status. Contacts of smallpox cases who are vaccinated for the first time during the incubation period also seem to have better chances of survival than those who are never vaccinated. In pregnancy, prognosis is uniformly bad in all varieties except modified.

### Variola Minor (Alastrim)

This is a milder form of smallpox, predominantly confined to certain parts of the world such

TABLE 2.   Case-Fatality Rates in Smallpox with Reference to Clinical
Varieties and Vaccinal Status

| | CLINICAL VARIETIES | | | | | | | | | |
|---|---|---|---|---|---|---|---|---|---|---|
| | Hemorrhagic | | Flat | | Ordinary | | Modified | | Total | |
| VACCINAL STATUS | Cases | CFR[a] | Cases | CFR | Cases | CFR | Cases | CFR | Cases | CFR |
| Unvaccinated | 22 | 100.0 | 120 | 22.1 | 1296 | 36.2 | 15 | 0.0 | 1453 | 42.7 |
| Unsuccessfully vaccinated | 59 | 96.6 | 88 | 96.6 | 1425 | 27.2 | 16 | 0.0 | 1589 | 33.3 |
| Primarily vaccinated during incubation period | 4 | 100.0 | 28 | 96.4 | 426 | 20.6 | 44 | 0.0 | 502 | 23.6 |
| With primary vaccination scars only | 111 | 94.0 | 45 | 66.7 | 2302 | 3.3 | 808 | 0.0 | 3266 | 6.5 |
| With primary and revaccination scars | 4 | 100.0 | nil | nil | 75 | 0.0 | 53 | 0.0 | 182 | 3.0 |

[a]CFR, Case-fatality rate.

as Africa and South America. The incubation period is a little longer than that of variola major. The constitutional symptoms of the pre-eruptive stage are generally mild, and the evolution of the rash is rapid. Although it may be difficult to differentiate these cases from those of the modified variety of variola major, they breed true. Thus, variola minor can produce only variola minor in even unvaccinated contacts, whereas a modified case of variola major can produce a hemorrhagic or flat variety in the unvaccinated. The average case-fatality rates for alastrim are not more than 0.5 per cent. Hemorrhagic cases are reported to be very rare with variola minor.

## COMPLICATIONS AND SEQUELAE

### Complications

Complications in smallpox may involve any system or organ; the most common is the respiratory system. Almost all cases in unvaccinated children and most in unvaccinated adults, except those cases belonging to the modified variety, develop a respiratory complication, ranging from simple bronchitis to the usually fatal viral pneu-

monitis. Even among the vaccinated, bacterial pneumonias are common in the severe types. Hemorrhagic and flat cases are usually associated with terminal pulmonary edema.

Gastrointestinal complications are comparatively rare in smallpox. Diarrhea may occur in a few patients during the second week of the illness. Very severe mucous colitis is a frequent complication in flat confluent cases as a result of extensive involvement of the mucous membrane of the descending colon.

Encephalitis occurs in about 1 in 500 cases of smallpox. It is more common in adults and is associated with the milder types. On or about the fifth day of fever, the patient becomes drowsy and in the next few days becomes semicomatose or even comatose. Signs of meningeal irritation are rare. The cerebrospinal fluid is usually sterile but is under increased pressure and may contain more cells than normal. These cases recover slowly in about two or three weeks with some temporary disability like dysarthria and an ataxic gait. Even from these disabilities, they recover in about two or three months.

About 2 per cent develop arthritis, which is far more common in unvaccinated children (80 per cent) and is mostly associated with the ordinary

TABLE 3.   Case-Fatality Rates in Smallpox Among Men and Pregnant
and Nonpregnant Women (Age Group 15–44 Years)

| | PREGNANT WOMEN (377)[a] | | | NONPREGNANT WOMEN (1228)[a] | | | MEN (1720)[a] | | |
|---|---|---|---|---|---|---|---|---|---|
| CLINICAL VARIETIES | Vacci-nated | Unvac-cinated | Total | Vacci-nated | Unvac-cinated | Total | Vacci-nated | Unvac-cinated | Total |
| All varieties | 27.2 | 61.1 | 36.6 | 3.6 | 34.7 | 9.6 | 4.1 | 30.2 | 7.8 |
| Nonhemorrhagic varieties | 8.7 | 46.3 | 14.5 | 1.9 | 31.4 | 7.5 | 1.9 | 25.2 | 5.2 |

[a]Number of cases of smallpox treated.

variety of cases (94 per cent). The elbow (86 per cent) is the most common joint involved. In about 6 per cent of cases, multiple joints are involved. This complication normally occurs during the fourth week of illness. It starts with a sudden rise in temperature and tenderness around the affected joint in an otherwise normally convalescing child. Within 48 hours, the joint becomes swollen, and there is marked limitation of movements. The fever soon disappears, but the arthritis progresses and in untreated cases ends in ankylosis. The joint disease acts like suppurative arthritis, but the constitutional symptoms are absent. The fluid from the joint is turbid but invariably sterile.

The eye is affected in about 2 per cent of all cases of smallpox. Complications include conjunctivitis, keratitis, and especially corneal ulcer, which by itself accounts for nearly 70 per cent of all ocular complications. These occur in both the vaccinated and the unvaccinated, in all age groups, and in the mild as well as the severe varieties. Even cases of the modified variety develop eye complications. The virus can be isolated from the tears of the affected eye (Kempe et al., 1969). Luckily, corneal ulcer is rarely bilateral. In about 35 to 40 per cent of cases of corneal ulcer and keratitis, blindness may result in the affected eye.

Other complications are otitis media, temporary deafness, suppurative parotitis, orchitis, bed sores, multiple abscesses, peripheral neuritis, and alopecia.

### Sequelae

Disfiguration is one of the permanent sequelae of smallpox. Permanent pitted scars are notably observed on the face. The depth of the scars seems to depend upon the depth of the lesions during the acute phase of the disease. Recent studies indicate that nearly 30 per cent of survivors of smallpox may not have any visible scars five years after the attack. The scars seem to persist more in cases of the ordinary variety than in others; more in males than in females; more in children than in adults; and more in the unvaccinated than in the vaccinated. Treatment in any form during the acute stage does not seem to alter or minimize the scarring.

## GEOGRAPHIC VARIATIONS IN DISEASE

Smallpox in its classic form (variola major) was prevalent all over the world during the 19th century and early part of this century. Later, several countries controlled the disease. However, some countries in Africa, Southeast Asia, and South America continued to be endemic until recently. Variola major was replaced by the less virulent alastrim in Africa and South America, but Southeast Asia, especially India and Pakistan, had only the classic variety, variola major. It is not known why this change to alastrim has occurred in other countries but not in India and Pakistan. In any case, for purposes of global eradication, both forms were tackled, and the whole world is now smallpox-free.

## DIAGNOSIS

### Introduction

Now that the whole world is declared smallpox-free, paradoxically, a correct diagnosis of smallpox becomes of vital importance. Any case misdiagnosed as smallpox anywhere in the world will create a grave international emergency. On the other hand, if a real case of smallpox should be missed and given another diagnosis, it could flare up into a big outbreak, especially now that vaccination is disappearing and immunity is waning. Since such a tragedy would undo the excellent work that has been done all over the world during the last decade, there is still a need for physicians to be well acquainted with the diagnosis of smallpox. Further, every clinically diagnosed case of smallpox should be confirmed by epidemiologic and laboratory findings. Every suspected case should also be subjected to the same methods. A good coordination between the clinician, epidemiologist, and virologist is essential for correct diagnosis of smallpox.

### Differential Diagnosis

Diagnosis during the pre-eruptive stage is almost impossible, since several communicable diseases (such as influenza, dengue, and scarlet fever) have similar signs and symptoms. However, when there is a definite history of contact with a proven case of smallpox, smallpox should be suspected even in the pre-eruptive stage if the typical signs and symptoms of the pre-eruptive syndrome are present.

After the appearance of rash, several exanthematous fevers caused by viruses, rickettsiae, bacteria, and spirochetes have to be kept in mind, especially chickenpox, measles, dengue, typhus fevers, enteric fevers, scarlet fever, and secondary syphilis. In addition, some skin diseases and drug or allergic rashes also may simulate smallpox. A few of the important conditions that resemble smallpox merit detailed consideration.

*Chickenpox.* Of all the exanthematous fevers, this is the disease that causes maximum confusion with smallpox. The important characteristics of chickenpox that differ from smallpox are the absence of a typical pre-eruptive syndrome, the superficial nature of the lesions, and the pleomorphism of the rash. These clinch the diagnosis.

*Dengue.* In about 20 per cent of cases of dengue, there is a papular rash similar to that of smallpox. The joint pains of the pre-eruptive stage and the saddleback-type of temperature are characteristic of dengue. Further, the rash in dengue does not evolve beyond the papular stage, is transient, and disappears in one or two days without leaving any mark.

*Measles.* Rarely, measles causes confusion. The characteristic catarrhal symptoms of the pre-eruptive stage of measles are invariably absent in smallpox. Further, the rash of measles does not evolve beyond the papular stage, and it is discolored and desquamates and does not scab like smallpox.

*Generalized Vaccinia.* This occurs in a few children after primary vaccination. The rash appears on or about the tenth day after vaccination. The confusion arises only when this rash appears in contacts of smallpox who have been vaccinated during the incubation period. When there is a history of exposure to smallpox, such cases have to be isolated as though they are smallpox until proven otherwise by the laboratory.

*Secondary Syphilis.* Some cases of secondary syphilis give a typical history of a pre-eruptive syndrome similar to that of smallpox. The important differentiating feature is that the papules of syphilis are hard, while those of smallpox are early vesicles. If a syringe needle is passed horizontally through the papule, the papule does not split in syphilis but splits easily in smallpox. This simple "needle test" has been very useful in differential diagnosis. Further, there is no evolution of rash in syphilis. It scales off, leaving no scars.

### Clinical Diagnosis

*History.* For clinical diagnosis of smallpox eliciting a history is as important as the clinical examination. There are three types of history to be elicited.

HISTORY OF SUSCEPTIBILITY. At the outset, the clinician has to ascertain whether or not the patient with rash is suceptible to smallpox. For instance, a person who has evidence of a successful vaccination (visible scars of vaccination) reported to have been done within three to four years before the present attack and a person who has evidence of a previous attack of smallpox (pitting on the face) within about 10 to 15 years before the present attack can normally be considered as not susceptible to smallpox. In such cases, one has to think twice before making a diagnosis of smallpox. One also has to bear in mind that such persons also may get smallpox under exceptional cir-

cumstances, but such circumstances are very rare.

HISTORY OF EXPOSURE. Careful inquiry should be made about the movements of the patient during a period of three to four weeks before the onset of rash and whether during that period he has come in contact with a patient with a similar rash, either among the immediate family members, relatives, friends, neighbors, travelers, shoppers, schoolmates, and fellow workers or at a funeral of someone who died from an eruptive fever. It is very difficult to elicit this history, especially from the illiterate, unless leading questions are put. Experience in a recent intensive antismallpox drive in endemic areas has shown that in several outbreaks, the source of infection could not be found.

HISTORY OF ONSET. As stated earlier, the onset of the disease in smallpox has some special characteristics. Every effort should be made to elicit a correct and detailed history of onset. This would help more in diagnosis than the clinical findings.

*Clinical Examination.* No diagnosis should be made by examining the patient in an artificial light. The patient should be thoroughly examined by exposing his body as much as decency permits. The stage of the rash has to be decided first. One should then determine whether the stage of rash is consistent with the history of duration of fever as furnished by the patient. For example, if the patient has a papular or papulovesicular rash, and if fever is present for six days, then the diagnosis is more in favor of smallpox. On the other hand, with such a history in a case of chickenpox, one would find scabs, pustules, vesicles, papules, and even macules simultaneously. Further, the important diagnostic triad (history of typical pre-eruptive syndrome, deep-set lesions in the skin, and absence of pleomorphism) must not be forgotten. These are a "must" for diagnosis of smallpox.

*Laboratory Diagnosis.* Diagnosis must be confirmed in all cases by the laboratory. Specimens should be collected and dispatched to the nearest virus laboratory, in the shortest time possible and in the prescribed manner for sending pathologic specimens. Special kits with instructions for collection and dispatch of specimens are supplied by the World Health Organization. Details regarding the different laboratory methods employed for diagnosis of smallpox are described in greater detail elsewhere in this book. The one that establishes the diagnosis is isolation of the virus either on the chorioallantoic membrane of the developing chick embryo or in tissue culture. This, however, takes nearly 48 to 72 hours to give a final report. When there is an electron microscope, diagnosis can be made in about two hours. A provisional diagnosis is made by demonstration of elementary bodies in the smears taken from the bases of the lesions and especially by detection of the antigen in the vesicular fluid by precipitation in gel, but neither test can differentiate smallpox from vaccinia. In the early stages of smallpox, scrapings from the base of the lesions are smeared on clean glass slides for all the tests. In the vesiculopustular stages, the fluid should be collected and sent for examination. During the scabbing stage, the scabs are the best material. In completely recovered cases, for which no scabs are available, serum can be collected and sent for antibody determinations. Positive serologic findings have to be considered along with the clinical and epidemiologic findings before a final opinion can be given.

When smallpox is suspected, all preventive measures must be taken immediately, without waiting for laboratory reports. Such a case should be considered to be smallpox until proved otherwise.

## TREATMENT

In the absence of any specific antiviral drugs, treatment of smallpox is mostly symptomatic and is directed toward alleviation of suffering and prevention of complications.

Several antiviral drugs have been tried in treatment of smallpox. These include 4-bromo 3-methyl, isothiazole 5-carboxaldehyde thiosemicarbazone (Rao et al., 1965; Ramachandra Rao et al., 1966a); N-methyl isatin beta thiosemicarbazone (Rao et al., 1969b); and CG662, a urea derivative of diphenylsulfone (Rao et al., 1969b). None proved effective, and some of these were toxic to the patients.

Smallpox patients do not usually need antiviral drugs. Hemorrhagic cases invariably die from bleeding and no antiviral drug could save them. They need sedatives and hypnotics. Cases of the modified variety do not need any treatment. Cases belonging to the other two varieties can be treated with any antibiotic with the hope of preventing bacterial complications. Although experience has shown that this approach may help, in the absence of any controlled studies, no one can confirm the utility of these drugs. No external application of any kind helps either in altering the course of the disease or the process of evolution of the lesions.

Use of corticosteroids in the treatment of smallpox is a controversial subject. There are some physicians who claim that steroids hasten the recovery and even reduce the fatality rates. But these opinions are based on uncontrolled studies and hence are not reliable. On the other hand, in experimental variola in monkeys, administration of cortisone has produced very severe varieties of

smallpox associated with high mortality (Rao et al., 1968b). Use of steroids in any form in the treatment of smallpox is to be discouraged.

Good nursing is by far the most important measure in the management of smallpox. Kind words, pleasing bedside manners, assurance, and moral support from the attending physicians and nurses do far more in helping smallpox patients to recover than any drugs. Nursing of these cases is very difficult and requires great patience and skill. Special attention has to be paid to oral hygiene and to care of the eyes, bowels, and bladder.

During the early stages of the disease in severe types, there may be dehydration due to loss of fluids into the lesions and also to the low intake of fluids by the patient because of difficulty in swallowing. Intravenous transfusions may have to be administered. The patients should be encouraged to take plenty of fluids. During the convalescence, patients should be given highly nutritious food in adequate quantities to hasten recovery and reduce the period of convalescence.

### Treatment of Complications

*Respiratory.* Respiratory complications can be treated with any antibiotics. If they are of viral origin, this treatment may not help, but bacterial complications may respond favorably in some cases, especially in the vaccinated.

*Neurologic.* Encephalitis cases do not need any special drugs. Recovery is the rule, unless they die of the severity of the attack itself. These cases do need special nursing, such as nasal feeding, bladder catheters, and treatment or prevention of bedsores.

*Osteoarticular.* Early detection of this complication is very important if one wants to prevent permanent disability. Any sudden rise in temperature in a normally convalescing patient should arouse suspicion of arthritis. Immobilization of the joint and administration of phenylbutazone with steroids in adequate doses have been found to be very useful in the management of these cases. At this stage of the disease, there seems to be no harm in administration of steroids.

*Ophthalmic.* Bathing the eyes daily with normal saline and application of any broad-spectrum antibiotic ophthalmic ointment may prevent bacterial infection of viral lesions. Steroids in any form should be scrupulously avoided in the eyes.

## PROPHYLAXIS

### Immunization

*Active Immunization.* No discovery made in recent years has saved so many millions of lives from dreaded diseases as "smallpox vaccination."

Thanks to Edward Jenner, this disease is already becoming a disease of the past. Prior to Jenner's discovery, variolation (inoculation of variola virus into the skin) was in vogue in several countries and was being practiced until recently in some parts of Africa, Afghanistan, and Nepal. Variolation is always associated with a great risk of inducing smallpox itself in the variolee instead of protecting him from it.

Smallpox vaccination is the introduction of vaccinia virus into the basal layers of the skin. Being antigenically similar, vaccinia confers immunity against variola infection. In the manufacture of smallpox vaccine, vaccinia virus propagated on the skin of certain animals like sheep and calves is used, and this vaccine is known as dermal vaccine. Vaccine containing the virus propagated on the chorioallantoic membrane of the developing chick embryo is called avian vaccine. This is also used in some countries. Until recently, glycerolated liquid vaccine was being used for vaccination. After the introduction of the global smallpox eradication program, the liquid vaccine was replaced all over the world by freeze-dried vaccine. This has the advantage of being stable even in hot tropical climates.

When there was still a risk of exposure to smallpox, there were no contraindications to smallpox vaccination, except that vaccination was better avoided or postponed in those who were suffering from any acute diseases or chronic debilitating diseases; eczema and other chronic skin diseases; diseases affecting the reticuloendothelial (RES) system; and malignant diseases. It was also avoided in those who were under treatment with cytotoxic drugs, steroids, or radiation, and in pregnant women. The right age for vaccination was either within the first month of life or between one and two years. Neonatal vaccination has the fewest complications. The technique of vaccination is to give multiple punctures with a bifurcated needle with 5 to 15 strokes per insertion.

Now that the world is free from smallpox, the need for smallpox vaccination is very limited. Other pox diseases are contracted from animals, and it is quite likely that human beings will be exposed more and more to these diseases, which can be prevented by smallpox vaccination. Hence, one has to consider whether there is any need for smallpox vaccination on a limited scale to prevent these diseases.

*Passive Immunization.* After exposure to smallpox, vaccination administered during the incubation period did not offer protection, unless it was given very early during the incubation period. Injection of hyperimmune antivaccinia gamma globulin along with smallpox vaccination has been found (Kempe et al., 1961) to reduce the attack rate considerably.

### Chemoprophylaxis

Certain drugs have been tried in prophylaxis of smallpox. They have been given only to exposed contacts along with vaccination. The drugs used were 4-bromo 3-methyl, isothiazole 5-carboxaldehyde thiosemicarbazone (Ramachandra Rao et al., 1966); *N*-methyl isatin beta thiosemicarbazone (Bauer et al., 1963; Rao et al., 1969a); and CG662 (Rao et al., 1969a). None was found to be effective enough to warrant use on a mass scale in the global eradication program.

# VACCINIA

Vaccinia is not a disease that occurs in nature either in man or animals. It is induced either artificially or accidentally.

## VACCINIA VIRUS

Vaccinia virus belongs to the *Poxvirus* group of viruses. It is only a laboratory virus and is not found in nature. Originally, it was used by Jenner, and the present virus was derived from his original virus. What actually was the origin of the original virus is still not definitely known. Some believe that it was derived from variola, and others feel that it was a derivative of cowpox virus. In its morphology, it is similar to the variola virus, but it has a far wider host range. Antigenically, the two viruses are almost identical.

Vaccinia can be grown on the chorioallantoic membrane of the developing chick embryo, on which it produces pock-like lesions similar to those of variola, except that they are larger in size and flat. There are several strains of vaccinia virus, but for vaccination purposes, only the dermal strain is used.

## COURSE OF VACCINIA

Artificially, man has been deliberately inoculated with vaccinia virus to induce immunity against the allied virus, variola. In a previously unvaccinated person or a completely nonimmune person, vaccination produced a typical reaction that is called a jennerian take or primary reaction. The incubation period is about three to four days. On about the fourth day of vaccination, a papule appears at the site of vaccination, which evolves through vesicle and pustule by about the ninth day. The pustule matures and reaches maximum size by about the twelfth day. Usually, there are some constitutional symptoms like fever, headache, and regional lymphadenitis. Slowly these abate, the lesion shrinks, and a scab appears by about the twentieth day, after which the scab falls off, leaving a permanent scar. The whole course may be modified or accelerated in partially immune persons. Accordingly, the reactions of vaccination have been classified as follows.

### Primary Reaction

This occurs in nonimmune persons, and the course of this reaction is as described above.

### Major Reaction

This occurs in partially immune individuals. On examination after one week, a vesicular or pustular lesion or an area of definite induration or congestion surrounding a central lesion, which may be a scab or ulcer, is manifest.

### Equivocal Reaction

All reactions other than the two above are equivocal. These reactions may occur in immune individuals; they may also follow insertion of inactivated vaccine or vaccination with a poor technique.

The first two reactions are considered successful. People with equivocal reaction would have to be vaccinated again with a fresh potent vaccine and with a good technique to ensure adequate protection.

## COMPLICATIONS OF VACCINATION

Normally, complications after vaccination are rare, but occasionally they were found, especially in nonendemic areas of smallpox. These may be local or general.

### Local

Some strains of vaccinia virus have produced very aggressive skin reactions. Even with less aggressive strains, very severe local reactions have occurred, which were usually the result of secondary bacterial infection of the vaccinia lesion and due to bad aftercare of the vaccination site. Similarly, local infection with clostridia may result in tetanus or gas gangrene.

### General

*Autovaccinia.* If vaccinia virus was transferred from the original site of vaccination to other areas by scratching, the virus could multiply in all such areas and produce the same type of vaccinial reaction. This is called autovaccinia. It caused no problem if the lesions were not infected with other nonviral microbes. Similarly, accidental inoculation of the eye has resulted in vaccinial conjunctivitis.

*Exanthematous Reactions.* Several types of rashes appeared on the skin after vaccination but had nothing to do with vaccinia virus. They were probably allergic reactions.

*Generalized Vaccinia.* This was occasionally seen in children after primary vaccination. The transient viremia following primary vaccination resulted in localization of the virus in the skin of some children and produced a generalized rash. This was similar to the rash of smallpox. The lesions evolved in the same manner as those of smallpox, but were fewer in number and not distributed like smallpox. Rarely, these cases were fatal.

*Eczema Vaccinatum.* This is a rare complication. It occurs as a result of accidental implantation of vaccinia virus in an eczematous area of the skin. It is considered in some parts of the world to be one of the serious complications of vaccination. This complication has occurred even in the eczematous contacts of vaccinees.

*Progressive Vaccinia (Fig. 11).* Though infrequent, this is considered to be one of the most fatal complications of vaccination. It was reported more frequently among persons who had some defective immunologic mechanism such as congenital agammaglobulinemia or diseases of the reticuloendothelial system; or in those who were under treatment with steroids, cytotoxic drugs, and radiation. This was a highly fatal complication, and the children were saved only if this complication was anticipated and vaccination was done under cover of antivaccinia gamma globulin.

*Postvaccinial Encephalitis.* This also was a serious complication after vaccination. This occurred mostly after primary vaccination. The frequency of this complication varied very widely from country to country, and it is not clear whether this was due to some ethnic differences in the people, climatic factors, or the criteria employed by the physicians in its diagnosis. It was very rare after revaccination. At one time it was thought that this complication occurred if the primary vaccination was done late in life, around 5 years. But now there is enough evidence that it was more common in children vaccinated during the first year of life, and several countries switched to the age group 1 to 2 years for primary vaccination. It was very rare after neonatal vaccination.

The common fatal complications, namely, progressive vaccinia, eczema vaccinatum, and post-

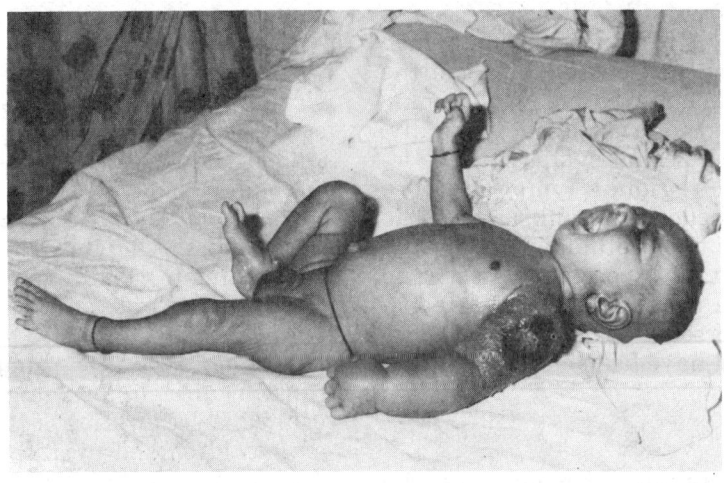

**FIGURE 11.** *A fatal case of progressive vaccinia (vaccinia gangrenosa)*

vaccinial encephalitis, have been very rare after neonatal vaccination, and that is the reason that

the WHO once recommended neonatal vaccination in all endemic areas of smallpox.

# COWPOX

This is mainly a disease of cattle, caused by *Poxvirus bovis*. Man becomes infected accidentally. It is mostly an occupational disease of farm hands and dairy workers. The lesion in the cow occurs on the udder and teats, and the worker may become infected while milking the infected animal if he has a break in the skin on his fingers. The primary lesion, a vesicle, appears usually on the fingers. It may be associated with local edema, lymphangitis, and regional lymphadeni-

tis. There may or may not be any fever. Rarely, generalized rash appears, and recovery is the rule. Diagnosis is easy and can be confirmed by inoculating the suspected material onto the chorioallantoic membrane of the developing chick embryo. On the chorioallantoic membrane, it produces lesions similar to those of vaccinia or variola, but unlike them, the cowpox virus produces hemorrhagic ulcerating pocks. There is cross-immunity among these three viruses.

## References

Bauer, D. J., St. Vincent. L., Kempe, C. H., and Downie, A. W.: Prophylactic treatment of smallpox contacts with *N*-methyl isatin beta thiosemicarbazone. Lancet 2:494, 1963.

Curshmann, H. In Ziemssen: Cyclopedia of the Practice of Medicine. Vol. 2. London, Samson Low, Martson Low, Searle, 1875. (Cited by Dixon, C. W.: 1962).

Dixon, C. W.: Smallpox. London, J. & A. Churchill Limited, 1962.

Downie, A. W., Meiklejohn, G., St. Vincent, L., Rao, A. R., Sundarababu, B. V., and Kempe, C. H.: The recovery of smallpox virus from patients and their environment in a smallpox hospital. Bull WHO 33:615, 1965.

Kempe, C. H., Dekking, F., St. Vincent, L., Rao, A. R., and Downie, A. W.: Conjunctivitis and subclinical infection in smallpox. J Hyg (Camb) 67:631, 1969.

Kempe, C. H., Bowles, C., Meiklejohn, G., Berge, T. O., St. Vincent, L., Sundarababu, B. V., Govindarajan, S., Ratnakannan, N. R., Downie, A. W., and Murray, V. R.: The use of vaccinia hyperimmune gammaglobulin in the prophylaxis of smallpox. Bull WHO 25:41, 1961.

McKenzie, P. J., Githens, J. H., Harwood, M. E., Roberts, J. R., Rao, A. R., and Kempe, C. H.: Hemorrhagic smallpox—Specific bleeding and coagulation studies. Bull WHO 33:773, 1966.

Meiklejohn, G., Kempe, C. H., Downie, A. W., Berge, T. O., St. Vincent, L., and Rao, A. R.: Air sampling to recover variola virus in the environment of a smallpox hospital. Bull WHO 25:63, 1961.

Nizamuddin, M., and Dumbell, K. R.: A simple laboratory test to distinguish the virus of smallpox from Alastrim. Lancet 1:68, 1961.

Ramachandra Rao, A., McFedzean, J. A., and Kamalakshi, S.: An iso-

thiazole thiosemicarbazone in the treatment of variola major in man. Lancet 1:1072, 1966a.

Ramachandra Rao, A., McKendric, G. D. W., Velayudhan, L., and Kamalakshi, S.: Assessment of an isothiazole thiosemicarbazone in the prophylaxis of contacts of Variola major. Lancet 1:1072, 1966b.

Rao, A. R.: Smallpox. Bombay, Kothari Book Depot, 1972.

Rao, A. R., Jacobs, E. S., Kamalakshi, S., Appaswasmy, M. S., and Bradbury: Epidemiological studies of smallpox—A study of intrafamilial transmission in a series of 254 infected families. Ind J Med Res 56:1826, 1968a.

Rao, A. R., Jacobs, E. S., Kamalakshi, S., et al.: Chemoprophylaxis and chemotherapy in variola major. Part 1. An assessment of CG662 and Marboran in prophylaxis of contacts of variola major. Ind J Med Res 57:477, 1969a.

Rao, A. R., Jacobs, E. S., Kamalakshi, S., et al.: Chemoprophylaxis and chemotherapy in variola major. Part 2. Therapeutic assessment of CG662 and Marboran in treatment of variola major in man. Ind J Med Res 57:484, 1969b.

Rao, A. R., McFedzean, J. A., and Squires, S.: The laboratory and clinical assessment of an isothiazole thiosemicarbazone (M&B 7714) against poxviruses. Ann NY Acad Sci 130:118, 1965.

Rao, A. R., Savithri Sukumar, M., Kamalakshi, S., Paramasivam, T. V., Parasuram, A. R., and Shantha, M.: Experimental Variola in monkeys. Part 1. Studies on the disease-enhancing property of cortisone in smallpox. Ind J Med Res 56:1855, 1968b.

Roberts, J. F., Coffee, G., Creel, S. M., Gall, A., Githens, J. H., Rao, A. R., Sundarababu, B. V., and Kempe, C. H. Hemorrhagic smallpox. 1. Preliminary hematologic studies. Bull WHO 35:607, 1965.

World Health Organization: Report of WHO Expert Committee on Smallpox Eradication. Technical Report Series No. 493. Geneva, World Health Organization, 1972.

*Gilbert M. Schiff, M.D.*

## DEFINITION

Measles (rubeola) is a highly contagious viral disease of childhood that is recognized by a typical prodrome of fever, conjunctivitis, coryza, cough, and enanthem followed by a generalized maculopapular eruption. Complications are common, and some are of a serious nature. Measles has occurred in all countries since antiquity. Because the measles virus has been cultivated in tissue culture, it has been possible to develop reliable diagnostic laboratory tests and effective vaccines. Widespread use of the vaccines has altered the familiar epidemiologic patterns of the disease and has reduced the incidence.

## ETIOLOGY

The measles virus is a member of the paramyxovirus group and is closely related to canine distemper and rinderpest viruses. On examination by the electronmicroscope, the virus appears as a circular structure 1200 to 1500 Å in diameter with an outer lipoprotein envelope 100 to 200 Å in width and containing short spikelike projections. The envelope surrounds an inner core of elongated nucleocapsid consisting of spirally arranged protein units dispersed around an RNA nucleic acid. The envelope contains hemagglutination and complement-fixation antigens, and the nucleocapsid contains a complement-fixation antigen. The virus is stable at lower temperatures but relatively unstable at room and body temperature.

Measles virus requires the entire virion to produce infection. Infection produces two types of giant cells in the body. One type consists of large, multinucleated lymphoid giant cells, which are present in lymphoid tissues and occasionally contain inclusion bodies. The second type is the syncytial epithelial giant cell found in the upper and lower respiratory tract. These cells may contain 40 or more nuclei and inclusion bodies in the nucleus and cytoplasm. These cells may be readily found in nasal secretions.

Infection with measles virus results in the development of neutralizing, hemagglutination-inhibition, and complement-fixation antibodies. The neutralizing and hemagglutination-inhibition antibodies generally parallel each other and first appear within a few days after onset of the rash. They reach peak titers two to four weeks later and persist for many years (probably for life). The complement-fixation antibodies appear and peak somewhat later, and disappear after 6 to 12 months or more. The primary antibody response to measles infection is characterized by the production of both IgM and IgG immunoglobulins, with disappearance of IgM after 21 days.

Measles infection stimulates the development of cellular immunity. Patients incapable of responding with humoral immunity have nonetheless been protected against subsequent measles virus challenge.

## PATHOGENESIS AND PATHOLOGY

Measles virus enters the body via the upper respiratory tract (or possibly by the conjunctival sac), multiplies locally, and soon spreads to the regional lymphoid tissues. Following a primary viremia, the virus disseminates and multiplies throughout the reticuloendothelial system. A secondary viremia then takes place and seeds the respiratory tract and conjunctival sac. Ultimately the virus localizes in the skin and/or other organs. Replication of the virus in leukocytes aids in dissemination.

The lesions of measles are generalized throughout the body, and multinucleated giant cells are found widely in hypoplastic lymphoid organs. The epithelial cells of the upper respiratory tract and bronchi may lose their cilia and their ability to secrete mucus and contain intranuclear and cytoplasmic inclusions. Koplik's spots are inflamed, submucosal glands, in which the endothelium of the inflamed vessels proliferates and becomes necrotic. The cutaneous lesions are caused by a serous perivascular exudate into the epidermis and by vacuolization and necrosis of the epithelial cells, which eventually form vesicles. Both Koplik's spots and skin lesions have foci of syncytial giant cells. The lesions in measles encephalitis are described under Complications.

## CLINICAL MANIFESTATIONS

Measles is a seven- to ten-day illness. Following an incubation period of 8 to 12 days, there are two to four days of prodromal symptoms and then an eruptive phase. The prodromal period begins with malaise and fever, followed within 24 hours by a copious coryza, a dry brassy cough, and conjunctivitis. These symptoms become progressively more severe until the sixth day, when there is rapid improvement. The temperature varies from 101 to 105° F during the early rash stage, and falls rather quickly to normal about the third day of the rash. The conjunctivitis is frequently associated with photophobia. The cough may persist in a mild form for one or two weeks. Small bluish-white spots on a red areolar base (Koplik's spots) appear in the buccal mucosa opposite the molars two days before the onset of the rash. They rapidly spread over the entire oral mucous membrane during the next few days. Examination of the blood during the prodromal period shows a leukopenia.

The eruption begins behind the ears and on the forehead, and then spreads onto the face and neck within 24 hours. Soon afterward, the eruption spreads to the chest and downward over the trunk and extremities; the soles and palms are spared. The rash is initially maculopapular, light pink, and discrete. Later, it becomes deeper red and may remain discrete or coalesce. By the fifth day, the color has become brownish, and the lesions eventually become desquamative. At the height of the illness, usually two days after the appearance of the rash, the child appears miserable. He is covered with a maculopapular rash, has a high fever, malaise, copious nasal discharge, a distressful cough, swollen and inflamed eyes, photophobia, and Koplik's spots on the buccal mucosa. However, there is usually a relatively uneventful, short convalescence.

Modified measles occurs in infants who have residual maternal antibody and in children who have been given immune globulin early in the incubation period. The incubation period is prolonged, the prodromal symptoms diminished or absent, Koplik's spots few in number or absent, and the eruption mild and discrete. Hemorrhagic measles is a rare severe form featuring a sudden rise in temperature to 105 to 106° F; convulsions, delirium, stupor, and coma; and marked respiratory distress. There is hemorrhage into the cutaneous lesions and mucous membranes. The outcome is usually fatal.

"Atypical measles" is a newer syndrome that occurs in children who have previously been immunized with inactivated (and in some cases live, attenuated) measles vaccine (Fulginiti et al., 1967). There is high fever, interstitial pneumonitis, edema of the extremities, myalgia, and prostration. An atypical rash occurs that may be urticarial, vesicular, petechial, or maculopapular. The rash tends to be located primarily on the extremities and appears on the palms and soles. Atypical measles frequently resembles the exanthem of Rocky Mountain spotted fever.

## COMPLICATIONS

Complications of measles are common. They can be caused by the virus, secondary bacterial invasion, or both. Sudden appearance of leukocytosis is indicative of a bacterial complication. The most common complication is otitis media. This is generally caused by secondary invasion by beta-hemolytic streptococci, pneumococci, or *Haemophilus influenzae*. Bacterial invasion of the lower respiratory tract causes the next most frequent complication. There may be bronchiolitis (in infants), bronchopneumonia, or lobar pneumonia. The bacteria involved are beta-hemolytic streptococci, pneumococci, or staphylococci. Giant cell pneumonias occur in patients with immunologic deficiencies. The pulmonary complications account for over 90 per cent of measles-related deaths.

Upper respiratory tract complications include laryngotracheitis or obstructive laryngitis. These are caused by extension of the usual respiratory tract inflammation found in measles and may result in a need for tracheostomy.

Acute encephalitis occurs in approximately 0.1 per cent of measles cases. The encephalitis varies in severity from mild to fulminant. Usually it appears suddenly during the eruptive stage, but can precede the rash. The fever returns, and there may be headache, confusion, convulsions, and coma, as a result of cerebral edema, hemorrhages, cellular infiltration, and perivascular demyelination. Paresis of the limbs or bladder indicates myelitis. The cerebrospinal fluid is characterized by a pleocytosis in which lymphocytes are predominant, protein level is elevated, and glucose concentration is normal. Although measles virus has been recovered from the brain tissue of patients, some feel that the encephalitis is caused by activation of a second latent virus or by an allergic phenomenon. The mortality rate is 15 per cent; 25 per cent have significant residual neurologic deficiences, and 60 per cent recover fully.

An uncommon complication is the development of subacute sclerosing panencephalitis (SSPE) (Detels et al., 1973). This is a progressive deteriorating neurologic disease with a fatal outcome. Pathologically, there is perivascular lymphocytic and plasma cell infiltration, astrocyte hypertrophy, neuroglial proliferation, and demyelination in the brain. Measles-like virus has been recovered from the brain tissue of patients with SSPE. These patients also exhibit very high titers of measles antibody in the cerebrospinal fluid and serum. The disease begins insidiously several months to years (average five years) after the child has had clinical measles. There are also documented cases in which the child's only *known* experience with measles virus was the receipt of attenuated measles vaccine. However, in none of these vaccine-associated cases were studies done before vaccination to rule out previous subclinical measles. Subtle disturbances in mental and emotional activity occur at the onset. The child's memory may begin to fail, and his performance may decline at school. Nightmares, crying spells, and involuntary movements or "spasms" become prominent. Coordination becomes poor, seizures develop, and ataxia appears. The electroencephalogram exhibits a characteristic suppression-burst pattern. There may be temporary remissions, but a general downhill course ensues, ending in death 6 to 12 months later.

There are several theories concerning the pathogenic mechanisms involved. Most believe that the measles virus becomes latent in the brain, and some unknown mechanism later reactivates the latent virus. Such a triggering event may involve a second virus (McDonald, 1977). Others advocate the concept of a hypersensitivity mechanism, pointing out the simultaneous presence of virus and high levels of specific antibody (Termeislen, 1973).

There has been much consternation that the inoculation of an attenuated measles virus vaccine might create a favorable circumstance for the development of the chronic carrier state of the virus in the brain with a predisposition to subsequent SSPE. This fear is apparently unfounded. The widespread use of further attenuated measles vaccines to prevent active measles could conceivably decrease or eliminate cases of SSPE.

## GEOGRAPHIC CONSIDERATIONS

Measles is found all over the world. In most areas it is endemic with epidemics occurring every six to seven years. In island populations, however, the epidemiology is much different in that the disease is not endemic, and explosive outbreaks occur when the virus is reintroduced (Panum, 1940). The epidemiology of measles is changing in countries practicing widespread immunization of the young. In these countries, outbreaks of measles are occurring in older adolescents and young adults rather than in elementary school-age children (Werner et al., 1977).

The severity of measles varies around the world. It is more severe in children in underdeveloped countries and in island populations, where more adults become ill.

## DIAGNOSIS

In cases of typical measles, the clinical diagnosis is reliable. The observation of Koplik's spots strengthens the diagnosis. The difficulty comes in cases of modified or atypical measles. In such circumstances laboratory diagnosis is required for confirmation. Laboratory diagnosis may be accomplished by isolation of the measles virus in tissue culture systems or through documentation

of a significant (four-fold or greater) rise in antibody titer in acute and convalescent blood specimens. A serologic diagnosis is preferred because of the relative difficulty in growing the virus from clinical specimens. Nasopharyngeal secretions taken during the acute period of the illness are the best source for isolation of the virus. Measles virus grows in human and simian renal cells and in human amnion cells. A typical cytopathic effect is found in cell cultures featuring the formation of syncytia or multinucleated giant cells, with intranuclear and intracytoplasmic inclusion bodies. The hemagglutination-inhibition antibody test is the most practical serologic test.

The diseases most likely to be confused with measles are rubella, scarlet fever, erythema infectiosum, exanthem subitum, Rocky Mountain spotted fever, enteroviral infections, and drug eruptions. Laboratory tests are available for the diagnosis of rubella, scarlet fever, Rocky Mountain spotted fever, and enteroviral infections.

In rubella the prodromal period is unremarkable. The rash is discrete, spreads quickly, and disappears by 72 hours without desquamation. Posterior auricular and/or occipital adenopathy is quite prominent. In adults, there may be joint symptoms that mimic rheumatoid arthritis.

In scarlet fever, the rash occurs within 12 hours of the prodromal period of high fever, vomiting, and sore throat. The rash is an erythematous, punctiform eruption that blanches on pressure. It first appears on the flexural surfaces of the extremities and rapidly becomes generalized. A characteristic circumoral pallor is present. The characteristic "strawberry tongue" and a membranous tonsillitis help in making the diagnosis. Group A hemolytic streptococci are cultured from the nasopharynx, and there is usually a rise in the titer of antistreptolysin O.

Erythema infectiosum (fifth disease) has a characteristic rash without any prodromal symptoms. There is first a "slapped cheek" appearance. Then a secondary generalized discrete maculopapular rash that may be pruritic and remains for five days or more appears; it resembles a "chicken-wire" effect as it fades. Finally, there is a variable period lasting for weeks in which the eruption recurs after stimulation of the skin with sunlight or hot baths. Lymphadenopathy and low-grade fever may be present but are frequently absent. The disease tends to occur in explosive classroom epidemics. Occasionally adults become involved and may develop transient arthralgia or arthritis. Although it is believed to be of viral etiology, no specific viral agent has been recovered from patients with erythema infectiosum.

Exanthem subitum is a disease of young infants characterized by several days of high fever, irritability, and a discrete maculopapular rash of

48 hours. The fever abates dramatically when the eruption occurs. No etiologic agent has been discovered.

Rocky Mountain spotted fever (RMSF) is frequently confused with typical measles but is most likely to be mistaken for atypical measles. In RMSF, there is a three- to four-day prodrome of fever, chills, headache, and malaise followed by a maculopapular and petechial eruption with a centrifugal distribution including the palms and soles. A history of tick bite or discovery of a tick on the child's body suggests the diagnosis. The scalp should be searched as a likely place for ticks. Laboratory tests include recovery of rickettsial organisms from the ticks, the Weil-Felix agglutination test, and complement fixation antibody assay. A Giemsa stain of skin biopsy may disclose coccobacilli in the endothelial cells.

Many of the enteroviruses can cause a rubella-like rash. Frequently, there are other signs of enteroviral infection such as aseptic meningitis, pleurodynia and herpangina. These infections tend to occur in the summer in the northern hemisphere and can be identified by recovery of the viruses from stools, spinal fluid, or throat cultures and by specific serologic tests.

Occasionally a drug eruption will mimic the rash of measles. Differential diagnosis is based on lack of prodromal symptoms and a history of drug administration.

## TREATMENT

There is no specific treatment for measles. Symptomatic treatment and supportive therapy include bed rest, hydration, eye washes, dim lighting, antipyretics, and non-narcotic cough medications. Antibiotics are indicated when secondary bacterial invasion occurs. Routine prophylactic antibiotics are to be discouraged except in high-risk children with chronic illnesses such as heart disease, cystic fibrosis, tuberculosis, and immunopathologic deficiencies. Adrenal corticosteroids have not been of proven benefit in the treatment of measles encephalitis.

Antiviral agents have been empirically given to patients with SSPE. Amantadine, 5–iodo–2–deoxyuridine, and cytosine arabinoside have failed to alter the downhill course significantly. However, a newer antiviral agent, Isoprinosine, has given some favorable indications of effectiveness in early noncontrolled trials.

## PREVENTION

It is desirable to prevent or modify measles infection in children under 5 years of age, in chronically ill patients, and in patients who are immunosuppressed. Immune human globulin serum (gamma globulin) in a dose of 0.25 ml/kg body weight administered within 48 hours of exposure will prevent measles infection. Measles may be modified by a dose of 0.05 ml/kg body weight of immunoglobulin given within six days of exposure. The advantage of modifying measles infection is that not only will a milder disease occur, but natural immunity will develop. However, in order to ensure the development of immunity, patients given immune globulin should be immunized no sooner than six weeks after the administration of immune globulin or after 15 months of age unless there is a contraindication for the vaccine.

Highly effective, safe vaccines are available for measles (Proceedings 1962; Rauh and Schmidt, 1965). In the 1960s both inactivated and attenuated live measles vaccines were developed. The inactivated vaccines required a series of primary inoculations, and it soon became evident that subsequent boosters would be required to maintain vaccine-induced immunity. Because the attenuated live vaccine had a high rate of side effects when given alone, measles immune globulin was recommended for simultaneous administration. In 1965, further attenuated live measles vaccines were developed that were associated with an acceptable rate of side effects and produced long-standing immunity after one subcutaneous inoculation.

Measles vaccines have dramatically lowered the incidence of measles since their introduction (Krugman, 1977). A resurgence of measles in the United States in 1970 to 1971 (cases occurring among previously immunized children) was attributed to improper use of the vaccines (Linneman et al., 1972). Vaccination may fail in patients under 1 year of age when maternal antibody may still be present, when too much measles immune globulin is used, or if vaccine is stored improperly. The resurgence of measles cases brought up the consideration of routine "booster" immunization. It appears unnecessary at this time, but a final decision awaits the results of continued surveillance of vaccinees.

Further attenuated vaccine is recommended for routine use at 15 months of age. Recent studies have indicated that there were significantly more vaccine failures in children who were vaccinated under 15 months of age, probably because of the presence of maternal antibody (Yeager et al., 1977). The measles vaccine may be given alone or in combination with other viral vaccines. Revaccination is recommended in children who previously received inactivated measles vaccine, or who received measles immune globulin to prevent measles. Exposed adults may be vaccinated if they have no history of measles. Contraindications to vaccination include (1) children with altered immune status due to underlying disease and/or therapy, and (2) pregnancy.

## References

Detels, R., Brody, J. A., McNew, J., and Edgar, A. H.: Further epidemiological studies of subacute sclerosing panencephalitis. Lancet 2:11, 1973.

Fulginiti, V. A., Eller, J. J., Downie, A. W., and Kempe, C. H.: Altered reactivity to measles virus. JAMA 202:1075, 1967.

Krugman, S.: Present status of measles and rubella immunization in the United States: A medical progress report. J Pediatr 90:1, 1977.

Linneman, C. C., Jr., Rotte, T. C., Schiff, G. M., and Youtsey, J. L.: A seroepidemiologic study of a measles epidemic in a highly immunized population. Am J Epidemiol 95:238, 1972.

McDonald, R.: SSPE (subacute sclerosing panencephalitis) Clin Pediatr 16:124, 1977.

Panum, P. L.: Observations Made During the Epidemic of Measles on the Faroe Islands in the Year 1846. Berkeley, Delta Omega Society, 1940.

Proceedings of the International Conference on Measles Immunization. Am J Dis Child 103:211, 1962.

Rauh, L. W., and Schmidt, R.: Measles immunization with killed virus vaccine. Am J Dis Child 109:232, 1965.

Termeislen, V.: SSPE and measles virus: Current state of our knowledge. Neuropädiatric 4:347, 1973.

Werner, L. B., Corwin, R. M., Nieburg, P. F., and Feldman, H. A.: A measles outbreak among adolescents. J Pediatr 90:17, 1977.

Yeager, A. S., Davis, J. H., Ross, L. A., and Harvey, B.: Measles immunization: Successes and failures. JAMA 237:347, 1977.

# *RUBELLA* **226**

## *Gilbert M. Schiff, M.D.*

### DEFINITION

Rubella is a childhood disease highlighted by a three-day generalized maculopapular rash, posterior auricular and/or occipital lymphadenopathy, and low-grade fever. The disease is endemic throughout the world and occurs in periodic epidemics. Rubella is not considered as contagious as measles or chickenpox, requiring relatively close exposure for transmission. Adults with rubella tend to develop arthralgia or arthritis.

The disease has serious implications when it occurs in a pregnant woman. The rubella virus can create an intrauterine infection and cause fetal death, spontaneous abortion, or a variety of congenital anomalies. For this reason, it is desirable to prevent rubella.

The isolation of the etiologic agent in 1962 in tissue culture was followed by the development of diagnostic laboratory tests and live, attenuated vaccines (Parkman et al., 1962; Weller and Neva, 1962; Schiff and Sever, 1966). A severe, widespread epidemic in 1964–65 provided many cases of acquired and congenital rubella for study, and the availability of the newly developed diagnostic tools permitted great advancement in our knowledge of the disease. Widespread application of rubella vaccines has reduced the incidence of rubella (and congenital rubella), changed its epidemiology, and provides a basis for effective control.

### ETIOLOGIC AGENT

The rubella virus is an RNA virus classified in the togavirus group. The 60 nm viral particles are made up of a 150s nucleocapsid with single-stranded RNA and a surrounding lipid-containing envelope. Three proteins have been detected: two glycoproteins and a capsid protein. The virus hemagglutinates at low temperatures only.

The virus is stable for years at $-70°$ C, for short periods at $-20°$ C, and thermolabile at room and body temperature. It can be inactivated by radiation, chemicals (chloroform, formalin, or beta-propriolactone), and low pH ($<6.5$) or high pH ($>8.1$).

Rubella virus can be grown in many tissue culture cell lines. In some cell lines ($RK_{13}$, SIRC) there is a direct cytopathic effect, while in others (primary African green kidney, Vero) the virus is detected only by interference with a superinfecting enterovirus. Some workers feel that the interference method is the most sensitive for recovering rubella virus from clinical specimens.

Subhuman primates and rodents have successfully been given experimental rubella infections. These animals do not develop clinical signs of illness. Intrauterine infection has been reported in rabbits, mice, and ferrets. Specific antisera can best be made in African green monkeys and ferrets.

Rubella infection generates neutralizing, hemagglutination-inhibition, and complement-fixation antibodies. Neutralizing and hemagglutination-inhibition antibodies parallel each other and are a reliable index of immunity. These antibodies first appear at the time of clinical symptoms and reach a peak two to four weeks later. They remain for long periods of time, if not for life. Complement-fixation antibodies develop a week or two after the onset of symptoms, peak two to four weeks later, and disappear six months to two years later.

There are conflicting reports on the effect of rubella infection on cell-mediated immunity.

## CLINICAL MANIFESTATIONS

Subclinical infection with rubella virus occurs at least as often as clinical infection. The incubation period varies from 12 to 21 days. There is little prodromal symptomatology. Illness begins with the appearance of posterior auricular, occipital, and/or cervical lymphadenopathy that is usually nontender. Within a day or two a maculopapular rash begins on the face and rapidly spreads downward over the rest of the body, sparing the palms and soles. The discrete rash turns into an erythematous blush and disappears without desquamation by the third to fourth day. The rash is usually nonpruritic. A low-grade fever may accompany the eruptive period. Lymphadenopathy may persist for a week or so. Some children have a mild to moderate sore throat. Early in the illness there may be a leukopenia, but later the white cell count is within normal limits or may be slightly elevated.

In adults constitutional symptoms are usually more severe and adenopathy less so. Adults frequently (25 per cent) develop arthralgia and/or arthritis. The joint manifestations usually appear when the rash is disappearing but may occur earlier, or may occur without the rash. The arthritis resembles acute rheumatoid arthritis and may persist for weeks. Joint involvement is 10 to 25 times more common in women than men, and occurs in about 1 per cent of children.

The virus may be found in the nasopharynx for a week to ten days before the onset of rubella and for up to two weeks afterward. The peak period of viral shedding in the nasopharynx occurs during the eruptive phase. Viremia and viruria have been detected from six days after exposure to virus until soon after the appearance of the rash (Schiff et al., 1969).

## COMPLICATIONS

Except for arthralgia and arthritis, complications from rubella are very uncommon. There have been reports of thrombocytopenic purpura and encephalitis with coma, post-encephalitic sequelae, and death.

Recently, a fatal degenerative neurologic disease very similar to subacute sclerosing panencephalitis (SSPE) has been found in several patients with congenital rubella (Weil, 1975). The patients were all in their second decade. They presented with signs like those in SSPE, and had very high rubella antibody titers in cerebrospinal fluid and serum. Rubella-like virus has been recovered from the brain tissue of one of these patients. There were thousands of patients born with congenital rubella in 1964–65 who are now in their second decade of life, but an epidemic of rubella-associated SSPE has not materialized.

## GEOGRAPHIC VARIATIONS

Rubella is distributed worldwide and is endemic in most locations. Epidemics occur every seven to ten years. Island populations may be spared outbreaks for longer periods but often experience explosive epidemics that affect those born since the previous outbreak.

Although there appears to be only one serologic type of rubella virus, there is some evidence that the virus varies in its teratogenic potential in different locations (Cockburn, 1969). Thus, in Japan, the incidence of teratogenic effect of the virus is much less than it is elsewhere.

## DIAGNOSIS

There are many viral infections that can produce a symptom complex similar to that of rubella. These infections are caused by viruses that do not appear to have teratogenic potential. Also, rubella may produce an atypical clinical picture or be subclinical. *A clinical diagnosis of rubella is unreliable and requires laboratory confirmation.* This is especially true when a pregnant woman is in some way involved. There are two reliable methods of making a laboratory diagnosis of rubella: (1) isolation of the virus, and (2) serologic test. Virus may be recovered from the nasopharynx for up to two weeks after appearance of the rash. The isolation of the virus requires tissue culture systems and may take a week to ten days. The most sensitive method for isolation of the virus is the enteroviral interference technique. A more practical method of laboratory diagnosis is the demonstration of a fourfold or greater rise in hemagglutination-inhibition antibody in paired specimens taken at the time of clinical illness and two to three weeks later. When the first specimen is collected a week or two after onset of symptoms, the complement-fixation antibody test may be used.

Blood counts and urinalysis are not useful in the diagnosis of acute rubella.

For the determination of immune status to rubella, the hemagglutination-inhibition antibody assay is most practical. This antibody is a good index of immunity and persists after natural infection. The complement-fixation antibody disappears within a year or two after natural infection and is therefore not a valuable assay for the determination of immune status.

## CONGENITAL RUBELLA

Although rubella had been recognized as a entity for many years previously, it was in 1941 that Gregg first noted the teratogenic potential of the disease (Gregg, 1942). Since that time much information has been compiled concerning the extent, pathogenesis, pathology, clinical manifestations, diagnosis, and economic impact of congenital rubella. Intrauterine infection with rubella virus often results in a child with one or more birth abnormalities, although the infection may be entirely subclinical. In the newborn with congenital rubella infection, there is active multiplication of the rubella virus in the nasopharynx, urine, cerebrospinal fluid, and many internal organs. Circulating antibody is present at the same time. Virus shedding continues for months to years, whereas the antibody level persists for years and then may disappear. During the first few weeks of life the antibody is both IgM and IgG; later only IgG persists.

The viremia that occurs in the mother leads to infection of the fetal tissues. The infection may be restricted to the placenta, or it may progress to widespread involvement of many fetal tissues. The viral infection in the fetus causes degenerative and inflammatory reactions with intravascular thrombosis. Fewer parenchymal cells are found in infected organs. The timing of the initial fetal infection determines the type of teratogenic effects that result. A chronic infection occurs that may produce continuous damage throughout gestation and in the neonatal and early life of the infant.

The occurrence of fetal infection during the first trimester of pregnancy appears to be most critical. The generally accepted rates for subsequent anomalies are 50 per cent, 20 per cent, and 4 per cent if maternal rubella occurs in the first, second, or third month of pregnancy, respectively. Subclinical maternal infection can produce anomalies. The incidence of stillbirths and spontaneous abortion caused by maternal infection may be as high as 75 per cent.

The clinical manifestations of congenital rubella are varied. Some may be life-threatening, some may result in handicaps that require institutional care, and some are only temporary. The major abnormalities are cardiac lesions such as patent ductus arteriosus, pulmonary and aortic stenosis, coarctation of the aorta, and atrial and/ or ventricular septal defects; ocular lesions such as unilateral or bilateral cataracts, glaucoma, and chorioretinitis; deafness, unilateral or bilateral, partial, or complete; microcephaly; mental retardation, and generalized growth retardation. There may be acute, self-limited lesions such as thrombocytopenic purpura, anemia, hepatitis, interstitial pneumonitis, myocarditis, encephalitis, and radiolucencies of the long bones.

The laboratory diagnosis of congenital rubella is easily made by isolation of the virus from the nasopharynx and/or documentation of elevated IgM antibodies in the first few weeks of life. The newborn with congenital rubella is literally pouring out virus in the nasopharynx. Physicians should be aware that many, if not most, congenital rubella cases may be subclinical, and laboratory diagnosis becomes essential. The differential diagnosis includes cytomegalovirus disease, toxoplasmosis, and syphilis. Laboratory tests are available for each of these entities.

Many of the abnormalities are amenable to surgical correction and medical therapy. Early intervention in hearing and speech deficiencies is crucial if proper social adjustments are to be made. Amantadine, an antiviral drug, has been shown to be effective against rubella virus in vitro (Maassab and Cockran, 1964) but was disappointing in a few cases of congenital rubella in children. At best, amantadine temporarily decreased viral shedding.

## TREATMENT

Since there is no specific treatment for rubella, it is fortunate that the disease is seldom severe enough to require even supportive treatment. The arthralgia/arthritis is treated with analgesics. Corticosteroids are not indicated.

Encephalitis requires supportive therapy; corticosteroids have been administered, but their effectiveness has not been determined. Patients with thrombocytopenic purpura often require corticosteroids and platelet transfusions.

Amantadine has not been used in clinical cases of acquired rubella.

## PREVENTION

Administration of immune globulin has been reported to prevent or modify rubella infection. However, the value of immune globulin for the exposed pregnant woman is controversial. The controversy is the result of several variables that can confuse the interpretation of clinical trials if they are not well controlled: immune status of the recipient, accurate diagnosis of rubella infection, variation in dose of immune globulin, variation in rubella antibody titer of immune globulin, and variation in the time of administration of immune globulin in relation to time of exposure. The important goal in administering immune globulin to a susceptible pregnant woman is prevention of viremia. Experimental human challenge studies have shown that viremia is first detected on day 6 after intranasal administration of rubella virus. In practice it is difficult to pinpoint the time of exposure. It must be taken into consideration that a person with clinical symptoms of rubella has been contagious for a week or so before the onset of symptoms. A series of human experimental rubella challenge studies indicated that a specifically prepared, high titered (2048) immune globulin prevented clinical symptoms and signs and viremia when rubella virus was given 24 hours later, but viremia occurred when commercially available immune globulin (titer 64–256) was used (Schiff, 1969).

The hazard of administering immune globulin to the exposed susceptible pregnant woman is that it might convert a clinical disease into a subclinical infection without preventing the viremia. Therefore, it is imperative, if immune globulin is administered, that pre-administration and follow-up antibody titers be assayed to determine if subclinical infection has occurred. This would be important if termination of pregnancy were to be considered for rubella infection. Certainly, in cases in which termination of pregnancy are not permissible under any circumstances, immune globulin should be administered to the exposed woman as the one positive measure that might be helpful. Twenty ml of immune globulin is the recommended dose.

Several effective, safe, live attenuated rubella vaccines have been developed (Buynak et al., 1969; Musser and Hilrabeck, 1969; Huggelen et al., 1969). These vaccines are over 95 per cent effective in stimulating the development of antibody to protective levels. The vaccines cause few side effects in children, and are not transmitted to susceptible contacts. The duration of vaccine-induced immunity can be determined only by continuous monitoring of vaccinees, but studies to date reveal persistence of immunity in over 90 per cent for at least seven to nine years (Schiff et al., 1974).

In adult women, the vaccines are equally effective but produce a higher incidence of side effects, including parethesias and/or temporary joint manifestations, which may mimic rheumatoid arthritis. The vaccines should not be given to women who are pregnant or become pregnant within two months of vaccination on the theoretical grounds that the vaccines may be teratogenic. It has been proved that vaccine strain viruses can cross the placenta, but there has been no proof that they are indeed teratogenic. The vaccines can be given to women of childbearing age if the following recommendations are heeded:

(1) the woman has been tested and shown to lack rubella hemagglutination (HI) antibody, (2) pregnancy has been ruled out, (3) the woman will not get pregnant for eight weeks after vaccination, and (4) postvaccination blood test is performed to confirm the development of antibody.

In the United States, rubella vaccination is part of the well-baby routine care. The vaccine may be given singly or in combination with other vaccines at 15 months of age or older. The goal is to create a "herd immunity" and thus indirectly protect pregnant women. After almost ten years of administering rubella vaccines to well babies and pre-pubertal children, there has been a dramatic reduction in cases of acquired and congenital rubella, but outbreaks of cases have occurred among nonvaccinated teenagers and young adults (Krugman, 1977). Thus an effective herd immunity has not been achieved. The danger of rubella vaccination at an early age is that lifelong immunity from natural disease in childhood may be prevented, and that vaccine-induced immunity will wane in the childbearing age.

In England, the rubella vaccination program provides for vaccination of girls at puberty. The overall effect of this program has not been determined.

An effective rubella control program should not rely on vaccination alone. Equally important are identification of susceptible women of childbearing age by antibody testing so that careful vaccination or intelligent management may be instituted if exposure occurs during pregnancy, and use of laboratory tests to diagnose the infection properly.

# References

Buynak, E. B., Larson, V. M., McAleer, W. Y., Mascoli, C. C., and Hilleman, M. R.: Preparation and testing of duck embryo cell culture rubella vaccine. Am J Dis Child 118:347, 1969.

Cockburn, W. C.: World aspects of the epidemiology of rubella. Am J Dis Child 118:112, 1969.

Gregg, N. M.: Congenital cataract following German measles in the mother. Trans Ophthalmol Soc Aust 3:35, 1942.

Huggelen, C., Sigel, M. M., Zygraich, N., Peetermans, B. S., Colinet, G., Leyton, R., Raupp, W. G., Pinto, C. A., Garg, S. G., Boyle, J. J., and Haff, R. F.: Safety testing of rubella virus vaccine (Cendehill strain): Preparation in primary rabbit kidney cells. Am J Dis Child 118:362, 1969.

Krugman, S.: Present status of measles and rubella immunization in the United States: A medical progress report. J Pediat 90:1, 1977.

Maassab, H. F., and Cockran, K. W.: Rubella virus. Inhibition in vitro by amantadine hydrochloride. Lancet 287:1443, 1964.

Musser, S. J., and Hilrabeck, L. Y.: Production of rubella virus vaccine: live, attenuated in canine renal cell cultures. Am J Dis Child 118:362, 1969.

Parkman, P. O., Buercher, E. L., and Artenitein, M. S.: Recovery of rubella virus from army recruits. Proc Soc Exp Biol Med 111:225, 1962.

Schiff, G. M.: Titered lots of immune globulin (IG): Efficacy in the prevention of rubella. Am J Dis Child 118:322, 1969.

Schiff, G. M., Donath, R., and Rotte, T.: Experimental rubella clinical and laboratory features of infection. Am J Dis Child 118:269, 1969.

Schiff, G. M., Rauh, J. R., Linnemann, C. C., Jr., Shea, F., Rotte, T. C., and Trimble, S.: Rubella vaccinees in a public school system. A 4½ year follow-up. Am J Dis Child 128:180, 1974.

Schiff, G. M., and Sever, J. F.: Rubella. Recent laboratory and clinical advances. Progr Med Virol 8:30, 1966.
Weil, M. F., Itabashi, H. H., Cremer, N. E., Oshiro, L. S., Lennette, E. H., and Carnay, F.: Chronic progressive panencephalitis due to rubella virus simulating subacute sclerosing panencephalitis. N Engl J Med 292:994, 1975.
Weller, T. H., and Neva, F. A.: Propagation in tissue culture of cytopathic agents from patients with rubella-like illness. Proc Soc Exp Biol Med 111:215, 1962.

# *WARTS* 227

## Seppo Pyrhönen, M.D.

### ETIOLOGY

Human warts are induced by human papilloma viruses (HPV), a subgroup of the papovavirides (see Chapter 58). They are stable, cubical, icosahedral viruses with a diameter of 52 to 55 nm; occasionally tubular forms are observed. The viral capsid is composed of 72 capsomer units. The genome of HPV is a covalently closed, circular, double-stranded DNA with a molecular weight of about $5 \times 10^6$. Five main subtypes (HPV-1 to 5) of HPV DNA have been found in different warts (Coggin and zur Hausen, 1978), and additional microheterogeneity of genomes within the viruses of a single wart has been demonstrated (Favre et al., 1977). The structural proteins of the various subtypes also differ. Different protein patterns and serologic groups corresponding to genetic subtypes have been demonstrated. The total number of different proteins varies between the groups, but the exact numbers are still unknown. In many respects the human papilloma viruses so far identified are still far from being fully characterized, and additional subtypes are likely to be found.

### PATHOGENESIS

Warts are generally regarded as a simple hyperplasia rather than a true neoplasm. In the normal epidermis, cell division is limited to the basal layer of cells. In warts mitotic figures are seen in cells of higher layers. Proliferation of keratinocytes and elongation of rete pegs accompany the development of protruding papilloma topped by extensive hyperkeratosis.

Warts are transmitted either by autoinoculations from one site of the body to another or from one person to another, both directly by contact with wart tissue and indirectly by contact with contaminated objects. The incubation period after experimental inoculation averages about four months but varies from a few weeks up to two years (Rowson and Mahy, 1967). Microtrauma and pressure probably aid in skin penetration by the virus. Accordingly, the most common sites for lesions are the palmar and plantar areas. Hyperhidrosis and certain hormonal states (puberty, pregnancy) may predispose the patient to infection. After infection, latent virus may become manifest during immunosuppression or immunodeficiency.

The number of viral particles in wart tissue seems to be highly variable. Viruses are abundant in plantar warts, particularly within a year after their appearance (Shirodaria and Matthews, 1975). By contrast, genital warts rarely contain detectable virus. Virus particles cannot be found in the proliferating cells of the wart; they first appear within the nucleoli of the cells in the stratum spinosum. In the stratum granulosum, nucleoli disappear and may be replaced by virus particles. Virus aggregates can be seen in the stratum corneum. Thus, virus maturation seems to be linked to cell differentiation.

It has been suggested that warts are made up of proliferating epidermal cells that arise from a single clone of infected cells (Murray et al., 1971). Another possible mechanism of origin is infection and subsequent transformation of adjacent cells into wart tumor cells. This type of multicellular origin has been suggested for genital warts (Friedman and Fialkow, 1976).

Warts are self-limiting tumors. Their natural lifespan varies from a few months to decades but averages about two years. Cell-mediated immunity (Morison, 1974; Ivanyi and Morison, 1976) and specific antibodies, particularly of the IgG class (Pyrhönen and Johansson, 1975), probably limit growth, produce spontaneous resolution, and prevent reinfection.

### PATHOLOGY

Warts are local accumulations of hyperplastic epithelial cells. The basement membrane remains intact and the basal cells appear normal. Hyperplasia (acanthosis) occurs in the stratum spinosum. The keratinization pattern differs from normal skin. Parakeratosis in cells of the stratum corneum and thickening (hyperkeratosis) of this layer and the underlying stratum granulosum are characteristic. Certain features predominate in warts on different skin sites. Hyperkeratosis is marked in plantar and common warts. Plane warts show acanthosis but little papillomatosis or hyperkeratosis. Acanthosis and papillomatosis without hyperkeratosis are the typical histopathologic forms of warts on thin skin and genital warts of the vagina and cervix. Two types of intranuclear inclusions occur in warts. Eosinophilic and basophilic inclusions first appear in the nuclei of cells in the stratum spinosum and increase in size in the overlying, more superficial layers. The basophilic inclusions are viral in origin. The eosinophilic inclusions are caused by abnormal keratinization of wart tissue.

Histopathologic findings during spontaneous regression of plane and common warts differ. In plane warts, a dense mononuclear cell infiltration of the upper dermis and epidermis occurs first and is replaced by spongiosis and necrotic eosinophilic cells (Tagami et al., 1977). During regression of common warts, there is no infiltration of mononuclear cells. Instead, blood vessels are occluded with thrombi (Matthews and Shirodaria, 1973). The epidermis retains the typical structure of common warts.

## CLINICAL MANIFESTATIONS

Skin warts are the most common disease caused by HPV. The appearance of warts varies remarkably depending on the site and the duration of the tumor. The *common wart* (verruca vulgaris), a round papillomatous tumor with a horny surface, is most often located on the dorsal aspects of the hands and fingers. Larger and older lesions develop a verrucous surface with clefts. These warts are usually 1 to 10 mm in size, but they may form lesions 2 cm or more in diameter. Warts located on areas of soft skin like the eyelids, face, neck, and nasolabial area have slender finger-like projections, 2 to 10 mm long on a narrow base, and are called *filiform warts*. Flat and smooth warts, *plane warts* or verruca plana, are found primarily on the face and dorsal aspects of the hands but also occur on the extensor surfaces of the arms and legs. They are flat-topped, round, slightly raised, 2- to 6-mm lesions with a granular surface. Plantar, palmar, and subungual warts do not project but lie deep in the epidermis. The most typical of these are the so-called *plantar warts,* which may be of several different types: a single wart, multiple warts containing small satellite warts around a central primary lesion, or a mosaic wart, which is a thick coalescence of smaller warts with extensive involvement of the sole of the foot. Warts may cover a large area of the skin, particularly on the head and neck re-

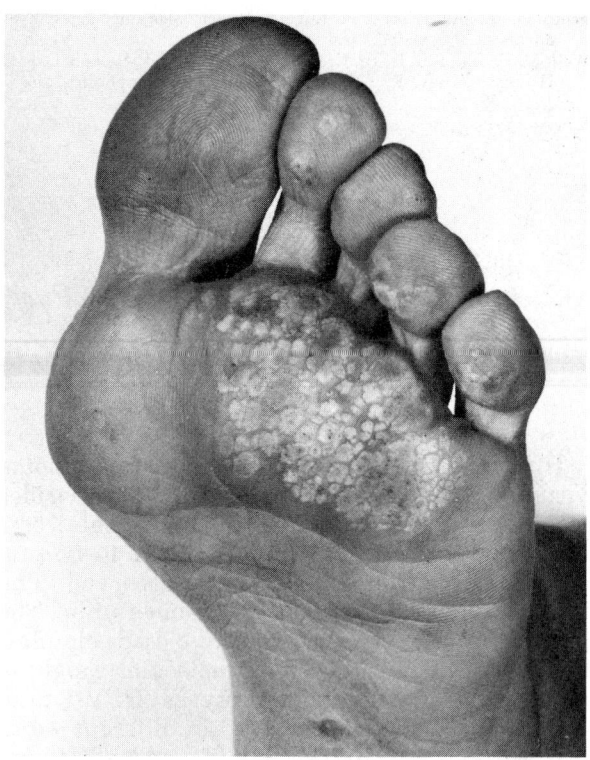

**FIGURE 1.** *Typical mosaic type of plantar wart with extensive involvement of the sole.*

gion. This disease is called *epidermodysplasia verruciformis.*

Another group of HPV tumors is *genital* or *venereal warts* (condyloma acuminata). Transmission is mainly venereal (Oriel, 1971). In males the lesions are usually located on the glans penis and prepuce but also occur in the urethra and occasionally in the bladder and ureters. In females the lesions are most frequent on the external genitals and perianal area but also occur frequently in the vagina and on the cervix. The warts often have a cauliflower-like appearance, but the virus may affect the cervical and vaginal epithelium without producing typical papillary condylomatous lesions (Purola and Savia, 1977).

Papillomatous tumors sometimes occur in the larynx. At least some of these *laryngeal papillomas* are induced by HPV, particularly in children. Infection may be acquired from vaginal condylomata during delivery (Cook, 1973).

Different clinical types of warts are preferentially associated with some types of HPVs. Typical plantar warts have been associated with HPV-1, multiple common warts mainly with HPV-2, and multiple flat warts with HPV-3. Subtypes 3 and 5 have been found in epidermodysplastic lesions (Orth et al., 1978), and at least some condylomas are caused by HPV-4.

## COMPLICATIONS AND SEQUELAE

The vast majority of warts are benign tumors; malignant transformation is rare. A simple cutaneous wart almost never becomes malignant, but the lesions in about 20 per cent of patients with epidermodysplasia verruciformis undergo malignant changes (zur Hausen, 1977). These tumors can spread to other tissues and even produce destruction of the underlying bone. Malignant conversion seems to depend on the virus type, HPV-5 being associated with malignant forms, while HPV-3 is found in benign lesions.

Malignant transformations of condylomata have also been reported (zur Hausen, 1977), and the distinction between verrucous carcinoma and benign condyloma may be difficult. Exceptional extension of growth may lead to a giant condyloma called Buschke-Loewenstein's tumor. Clinically, these appear to be malignant, but the tumor is usually found to be benign histologically. Women with typical genital condylomata frequently have premalignant dysplasia of the vaginal and cervical epithelium (Purola and Savia, 1977; zur Hausen, 1977). This dysplasia may develop into cervical carcinoma.

Juvenile laryngeal papillomas may also sometimes be transformed into malignant tumors, particularly if the papillomas were treated by x-rays.

After appropriate therapy or spontaneous recovery, cutaneous warts usually leave no detectable sequelae. Plantar warts may cause painful scars that interfere with normal walking for a long time. Periungual warts may scar the nail matrix and cause permanent deformity. Plane warts can cause spotty hyperpigmentation, especially in dark-skinned people. Certain warts, especially in soft and moist skin, may develop into large masses with secondary bacterial infection and ulceration.

## GEOGRAPHIC VARIATIONS IN DISEASE

Warts are common diseases with a worldwide distribution. The highest incidence is during childhood and adolescence. Most people have had some kind of wart by the age of 20. The incidence is probably similar throughout Europe and the United States, but warts are much less common in most tropical regions (Rook et al., 1972).

## DIAGNOSIS

There is usually no doubt about the clinical diagnosis of viral warts. However, a few other lesions can simulate these common warts. Simple calluses and corns, especially on the sole of the foot, are probably confused most often with warts. The correct diagnosis can be verified by removing the thick covering of horny cells. In warts, the infected central area has a white surface in which the capillary loops are seen as bleeding points or as thrombosed black dots. In contrast, calluses have a smooth, normal epidermis under the horny layer. Molluscum contagiosum (Chapter 228) may also mimic warts. The surface of these small, pearly tumors is smooth except for a central umbilicus from which infected cell debris can be extruded. Seborrheic warts and squamous cell papillomas or keratoacanthomas can also simulate viral warts but are seen mainly in older people. The discrete horny papules of punctate keratoderma that develop during childhood or early adult life can sometimes mimic plantar warts. The differential diagnosis also includes intradermal foreign bodies (glass and splinters, for example), neurofibroma, and painful scars. The definitive diagnosis can be established by histologic examination of tissue. This is most important in cases of venereal warts, when malignancy must be excluded. Gynecologic condylomata also can be identified by vaginal and cervical cytologic examinations (Purola and Savia, 1977).

## TREATMENT AND PROPHYLAXIS

Therapy that might lead to permanent scarring or other sequelae should be avoided because most warts will involute spontaneously within two years. Warts that are painful, subject to trauma and infection, or cosmetically objectionable should be treated. Sometimes treatment is indicated to prevent further dissemination. The type of therapy should be determined by the type and location of the wart and the response to treatment. The treatment may include destructive therapy such as electrocoagulation, curettage, cryotherapy, or superficial radiotherapy, but less destructive treatment should be favored, especially for plantar warts, to avoid scarring. Daily application of one of the following agents often leads to the resolution of plantar as well as other types of warts: 10 to 20 per cent glutaraldehyde solution, 15 to 20 per cent lactic and salicylic acid in flexible collodion, or 20 to 40 per cent salicylic acid ointment or plaster. The combination of one of these agents with curettage often gives good results. Cantharidin, 0.7 per cent solution in acetonecollodion 1:1, is especially effective against common warts, particularly in the periungual area. Genital warts are usually treated by a weekly application of 20 per cent podophyllin in tincture of benzoin or in alcohol. The surrounding normal skin should be covered with a protective ointment. Podophyllin should never be used for pregnant women. The therapy of recurrent warts has included application of topical antiviral agents like iododeoxyuridine (IDU), topical anti-tumor agents such as 5-fluorouracil and bleomycin, and immunotherapy with dinitrochloroben-zēne (DNCB), smallpox vaccination, or autogenous wart vaccines. Some of these agents may be help-ful but their efficacy is unproved.

Because of the lack of a vaccine and the ubiq-uitous nature of HPV, there is no effective pro-phylaxis for common warts. Genital warts can be prevented by avoiding infected sexual contacts. Avoiding common bathing and swimming pools may prevent some exposure to HPV, but other sources of infection are widespread throughout the environment.

### References

Cook, T. A.: Maternal condyloma linked to lesions in babies. JAMA 224:1475, 1973.

Coggin, J. R., Jr., and zur Hausen, H.: Workshop on papillomaviruses and cancer. Cancer Res. 39:545, 1979.

Favre, M., Orth, G., Croissant, O., and Yaniv, M.: Human papilloma virus DNA: Physical mapping of the cleavage sites of *Bacillus amyloliquefaciens* (BamI) and *Haemophilus parainfluenzae* (HpaII) endonucleases and evidence for partial heterogeneity. J Virol 21:1210, 1977.

Friedman, J. M., and Fialkow, P. J.: Viral "tumorigenesis" in man: Cell markers in condylomata acuminata. Int J Cancer 17:57, 1976.

Ivanyi, L., and Morison, W. L.: In vitro lymphocyte stimulation by wart antigen in man. Br J Dermatol 94:523, 1976.

Matthews, R. S., and Shirodaria, P. V.: Study of regressing warts by immunofluorescence. Lancet 1:689, 1973.

Morison, W. L.: In vitro assay of cell-mediated immunity to human wart antigen. Br J Dermatol 90:531, 1974.

Murray, R. F., Hobbs, J., and Payne, B.: Possible clonal origin of com-mon warts (verruca vulgaris). Nature 232:51, 1971.

Oriel, J. D.: Natural history of genital warts. Br J Vener Dis 47:1, 1971.

Orth, G., Jablonska, S., Favre, M., Croissant, O., Jarzabek-Chorzelska, M., and Rzesa, G.: Characterization of two types of human papil-lomaviruses in lesions of epidermodysplasia verruciformis. Proc Natl Acad Sci USA 75:1537, 1978.

Purola, E., and Savia, E.: Cytology of gynecologic condyloma acumi-natum. Acta Cytol 21:26, 1977.

Pyrhönen, S., and Johansson, E.: Regression of warts. An immunolog-ical study. Lancet 1:592, 1975.

Rook, A., Wilkinson, D. S., and Ebling, F. J. G.: Textbook of Derma-tology. Vol. I, 2nd ed. Oxford, Blackwell Scientific Publications, 1972, p. 550.

Rowson, K. E. K., and Mahy, B. W. J.: Human papova (wart) virus. Bact Rev 31:110, 1967.

Shirodaria, P. V., and Matthews, R. S.: An immunofluorescence study of warts. Clin Exp Immunol 21:329, 1975.

Tagami, H., Takigawa, M., Ogino, A., Imamura, S., and Ofugi, S.: Spontaneous regression of plane warts after inflammation. Arch Dermatol 113:1209, 1977.

zur Hausen, H.: Human papillomaviruses and their possible role in squamous cell carcinomas. Curr Top Microbiol Immunol 78:1, 1977.

# 228  *HAND-FOOT-MOUTH DISEASE*

*David I. Minkoff, M.D.,*
*and James D. Connor, M.D.*

### DEFINITION

Hand-foot-mouth disease is a mild exanthe-matous infection of children due to coxsackievi-ruses A. Its name comes from a characteristic ve-sicular eruption of the hands, feet, and mouth and must not be confused with foot and mouth disease of cattle.

### ETIOLOGY

Since the isolation of coxsackieviruses in 1947 by Dalldorf and Sickles (1948) and subsequent recognition of two distinct biologic groups, A and B, recurring clinical patterns of disease caused by specific coxsackievirus serotypes have been rec-ognized. One such epidemic was investigated by Robinson, Doane, and Rhoades in 1957. It was linked with coxsackievirus A16 and was charac-terized by vesiculo-ulcerative lesions of the oro-pharynx and exanthems on the hands and feet. Alsop subsequently reported an epidemic in Bir-mingham, England, in 1960 and gave the name hand-foot-mouth disease to the syndrome he ob-served. Many epidemics have been reported since then with similar clinical characteristics and demonstration of coxsackievirus A16 as the etio-logic agent of hand-foot-mouth syndrome. Clini-cal cases associated with coxsackieviruses A5 and A10 have also been described.

### PATHOLOGY

The characteristic histologic change is a subep-idermal vesicle with a mixed inflammatory exu-date of lymphocytes, monocytes, and polymorpho-nuclear leukocytes. The overlying dermis shows extensive acantholysis with reticular degeneration. Intracytoplasmic inclusions have been seen. There are no multinucleated giant cells on Tzanck preparations from active vesicles.

## CLINICAL MANIFESTATIONS

The illness is typically mild without obvious prodromal signs and seldom lasts over a week. In one outbreak, the disease was so mild that only 2 per cent of the patients had fever. However, the same virus may cause aseptic meningitis, paralysis, a life-threatening systemic disease resembling measles, myocarditis, and death.

The incubation period is usually three to five days. Mild fever, sore mouth, and refusal to eat are the most common presenting symptoms (Richardson and Leibovitz, 1965). The oral lesions begin as small red macules and then form vesicles on an erythematous base in the pharynx, soft palate, buccal mucosa, gingivae, and tongue. The vesicles are 1 to 3 mm in diameter but may coalesce to form bullae. Some vesicles may ulcerate while others absorb without breaking the mucous membrane. Those that break down form shallow ulcers 1 to 2 cm across in the oropharynx, with yellowish gray bases and hyperemic margins. These are often so painful that children refuse to eat. The exanthem is maculopapular and often evolves to vesicles containing clear watery fluid. The vesicles measure 0.5 to 1 cm in diameter and have a narrow rim of erythema around the base of the lesion. They usually appear on the back of the hands and the lateral margins of the feet; less often they are found on the palms, soles, and between the fingers and toes. The number varies from as few as 2 or 3 to 30 to 40. They are nonpruritic, rarely painful, and usually absorbed in three to four days without scarring. The buttocks are sometimes involved, and scattered single vesicles may appear over the proximal extremities, penis, ear lobes, and face. During the acute illness there may also be malaise, anorexia, abdominal pain, diarrhea, cough, coryza, chest pain, and headache.

The disease is most common in preschool children from birth to age 4. There is no sex predilection. The incidence of infection is difficult to determine because disease in most cases is too mild to warrant the patient seeing a doctor. In epidemics, the high attack rate of the virus can be demonstrated because clinical illness develops in more than half of the contacts in affected households. In epidemics, up to 44 per cent of asymptomatic contacts without a past history of hand-foot-mouth disease have evidence of infection as demonstrated by stool culture and/or neutralizing antibody titer rises.

## DIAGNOSIS

The diagnosis is usually made when vesicular ulcerative stomatitis occurs along with exanthems of the hands and feet during a mild febrile illness. The leukocyte count ranges from 3750 to 16,200, occasionally with an atypical lymphocytosis. If coxsackievirus A16 is cultured or neutralizing antibody rises fourfold or more, the diagnosis is established. Inoculation of stool (not a rectal swab) into tissue culture and suckling mice produces a viral isolation rate of 75 to 80 per cent in most series. Twenty-five to 50 per cent of throat swabs and vesicle fluid cultures from patients are found to contain coxsackievirus.

It is not uncommon to find that a high neutralizing antibody titer is already present in "acute phase" serum two to seven days after onset of symptoms, and that the antibody titer may not rise in convalescent serum.

The differential diagnosis must first take into account the possibility of herpes simplex stomatitis because the distribution of these vesicular lesions may be similar to those of hand-foot-mouth infection. Herpes infection can be distinguished by the fact that it often involves the perioral structures and may be accompanied by high fever and cervical and submandibular lymphadenopathy, all of which are unusual with hand-foot-mouth disease. Herpangina, caused by another coxsackie A virus, most frequently involves the anterior fauces, tonsillar pillars, soft palate, and uvula, and is not commonly associated with lingual, buccal mucosal, or gingival lesions. Erythema multiforme may involve the mouth and skin, but typical target or iris lesions are the rule, and its association with other underlying viral infections and drug ingestions is well known. Aphthous stomatitis does not present with fever or systemic signs or symptoms and is localized to the anterior mouth alone. It is not known to be caused by a specific viral agent and has a tendency to recur in certain individuals, occasionally after trigger stimuli.

## GEOGRAPHIC VARIATIONS

Although first reported in Canada, outbreaks have occurred in areas of the world as widely separated as South Africa (Gear, 1962), Australia, Japan (Togaya and Tachibana, 1975), and the United States (Adler et al., 1970). The Japanese outbreaks have been the most extensive, involving thousands of cases.

## TREATMENT

There is no specific drug therapy.

## References

Adler, J. L., Mostow, S. R., Mellin, H., et al.: Epidemiologic investigation of Hand-Foot-Mouth disease. Am J Dis Child 120:309, 1970.

Dalldorf, G., and Sickles, G.: An unidentified, filterable agent isolated from the feces of children with paralysis. Science 108:61, 1948.

Gear, J.: Coxsackie virus infections in Southern Africa. Yale J Biol Med 34:289, 1962.

Richardson, H. B., and Leibovitz, A.: "Hand-Foot-Mouth disease" in children. J Pediatr 67:6, 1965.

Robinson, C. R., Doane, F. W., and Rhoades, A. J.: Report of an outbreak of febrile illness with pharyngeal lesions and exanthem: Toronto, summer, 1957. Isolation of group A Coxsackie virus. Can Med Assoc J: 79(8):1958.

Togaya, I., and Tachibana, K.: Epidemic of hand, foot, and mouth disease in Japan 1972–1973: Difference in epidemiologic and virologic features from the previous one. Jpn J Med Sci Biol 28:231, 1975.

# 229 *MOLLUSCUM CONTAGIOSUM*

*Roy Postlethwaite, B.Sc., M.D.*

## DEFINITION

Molluscum contagiosum is a benign epidermal tumor of characteristic appearance. It occurs only in human beings and is caused by a poxvirus (Postlethwaite, 1970).

## ETIOLOGY

An unclassified member of the pox group, molluscum contagiosum virus (Fig. 1) is distinct from the parapoxviruses and resembles vaccinia virus in size ($300 \times 240$ nm) and shape and in its linear, duplex DNA genome with a molecular weight of $118 \times 10^6$ (Parr et al., 1977). It differs from vaccinia in some structural details (Peters and Küper, 1970), in G + C (guanine plus cytosine) content and base sequence of its DNA, and in some properties of its DNA-dependent RNA polymerase (Shand et al., 1976). Virion DNA from different patients shows genetic and structural heterogeneity. Homologous sera react weakly with viral antigen in complement fixation, precipitation, immunofluorescence, and neutralization tests. There is no cross-reactivity with vaccinia, cowpox, mousepox, rabbitpox, or fowlpox antigens. Molluscum virus fails to reactivate other poxviruses and has not consistently been grown in serial passage outside man. An etiologic relationship to similar rare lesions in chimpanzees and red kangaroos has not been established.

## PATHOGENESIS AND PATHOLOGY

An ordered array of proliferating epidermal cells extends as pear-shaped lobules into the dermis (Lever and Schaumburg-Lever, 1975), compressing papillae but not breaching the basement membrane (Fig. 2). The surrounding epidermis is undermined and stretched over the projecting tumor, and a central pore appears over the degenerating apical portions, which are rich in molluscum inclusion bodies. Virus growth is confined to the epidermis (Epstein and Fukuyama, 1973; Vreeswijk et al., 1976) and is associated with extensive development of gap junctions and increased turnover of basal cells. The phagosomes of these basal cells contain virions but do not fuse with lysosomes (Vreeswijk et al., 1977). Released viral cores cluster alongside the Golgi apparatus, centrioles, and spindle fibers of cells in early mitosis where second-stage uncoating may occur. Nuclear DNA synthesis declines as the viral DNA begins to replicate in the cytoplasm of the infected prickle cell layer and tiny eosinophilic inclusions appear. Granular masses of viroplasm are pinched off in developing membranes to form immature and then mature virions. The inclusions become basophilic and packed with progeny virions as infected cells migrate synchronously to the surface. Inclusions of up to 30 $\mu$m in diameter displace the nuclear remnant and occupy virtually the entire cell (Fig. 3). As glassy molluscum bodies, they reach the horny layer within a week and are shed by 9 to 15 days. The precise relationship of infection to cell division, whether virus is transmitted between cells, and the mechanisms of initiation and maintenance of infection remain to be elucidated.

Molluscum virus does not grow reproducibly in cell cultures. Even without propagation, however, it is cytotoxic and induces interference, interferon, and a transient "transformed" phenotype (Barbanti-Brodano et al., 1974) in cell cultures. Along with the lack of reactivating capacity, these properties are consistent with the behavior of a mutant, defective, or partially inactivated virus, which achieves partial genome expression but is unable to synthesize uncoating protein except in human skin in situ (La Placa et al., 1967;

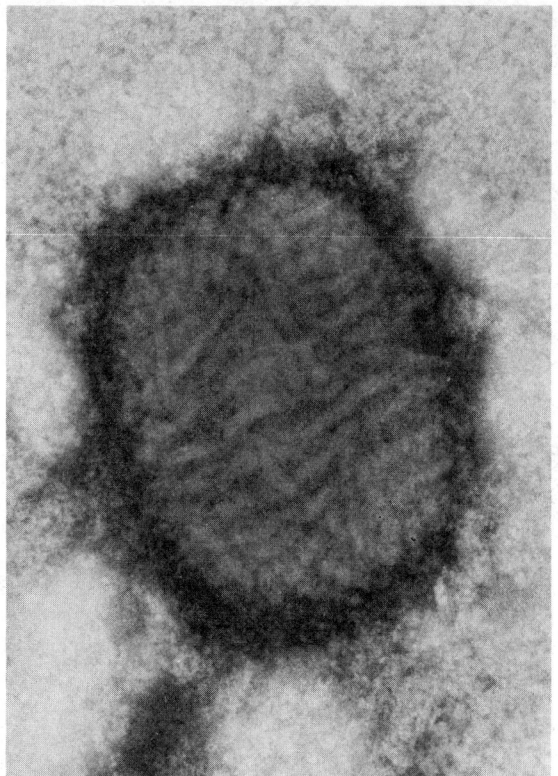

**FIGURE 1.** *Molluscum contagiosum virion negatively stained with ammonium molybdate. × 210,000. (Courtesy Dr. D. W. Gregory.)*

McFadden et al., 1979). In cell cultures, indeed, ingested virions are either destroyed in phagolysosomes like heated vaccinia virus or, after first-stage uncoating, remain as cytoplasmic cores that fail to become fully uncoated (Prose et al., 1969). Anecdotal reports suggest that some viral properties are relatively heat-labile, and in vitro growth has been reported at 30° C but not at 37° C. Another report of virus growth in cell cultures suggested a novel mechanism of DNA replication (Francis and Bradford, 1976) because of the surprising failure of base analogues and of rifampicin and methisazone to inhibit viral replication. Confirmation and extension of these findings are awaited.

Although viral antigen is present in all lesions, the cellular response is usually slight and antibody may not be detectable. However, inflammatory reactions, cellular infiltration around regressing lesions, tuberculin-type responses after experimental inoculation, and the predominance of IgG antibody in most patients (Shirodaria and Matthews, 1977), sometimes only after treatment, all suggest that specific sensitization occurs when viral antigens reach subepidermal tissues. The relationship of these responses to immunity, regression, recurrence, and the age distribution of the disease is unknown.

## CLINICAL MANIFESTATIONS

The incubation period of experimental infection ranges from 14 days to 6 months. Up to 20 or

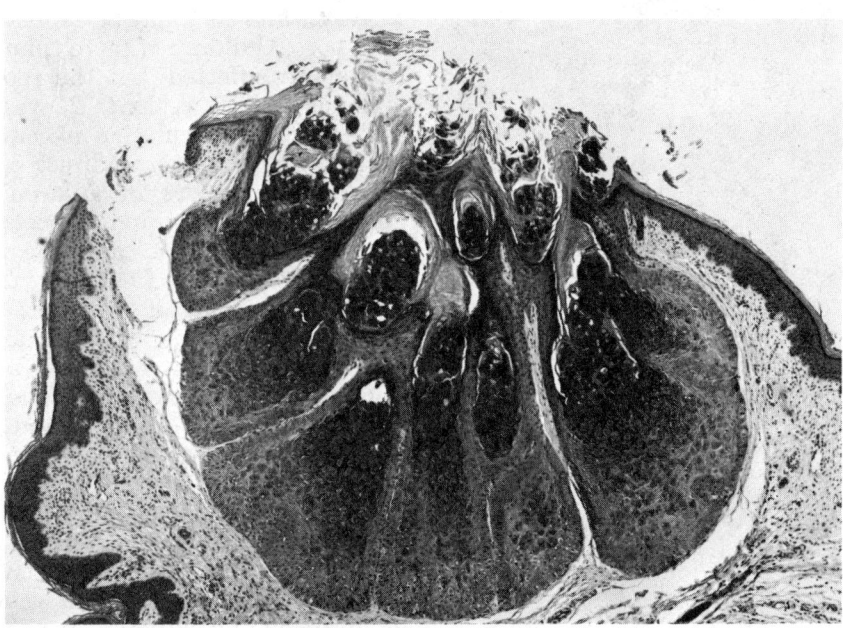

**FIGURE 2.** *Molluscum contagiosum. Section through entire lesion. Hematoxylin and eosin stain. × 37. (Courtesy Dr. S. W. B. Ewen.)*

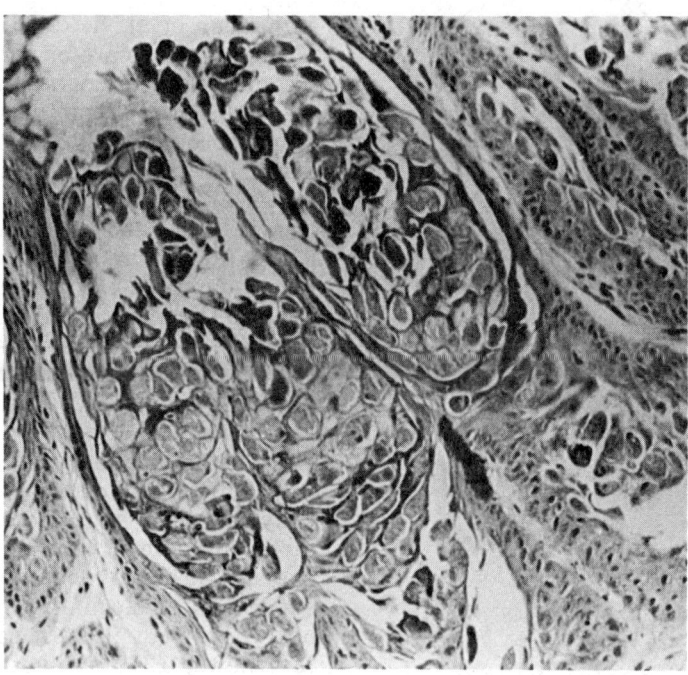

**FIGURE 3.** *Molluscum contagiosum. Section through apical part of lesion showing molluscum bodies. Phloxine-tartrazine stain. ×160. (From Postlethwaite, R; Watt, J. A.; Hawley, T. G.; Simpson, I., and Adam, H. Features of molluscum contagiosum in the northeast of Scotland and in Fijian village settlements. Journal of Hygiene, Cambridge 65:281, 1967.)*

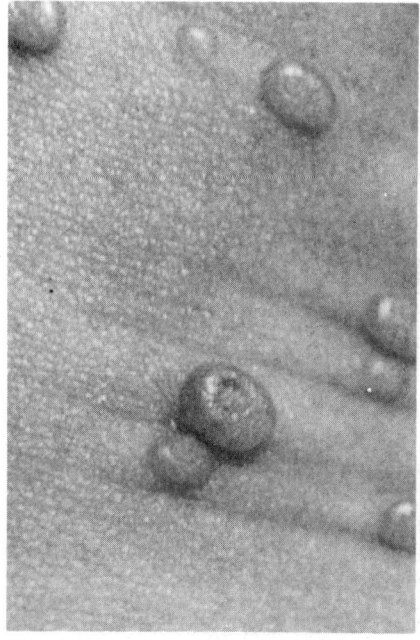

**FIGURE 4.** *Molluscum contagiosum lesions. ×2½. (Courtesy Dr. R. F. Menzies.)*

more discrete pearly papules about 2 to 7 mm in diameter appear singly or in groups on the face, neck, trunk (Fig. 4), and limbs. They are rare on the palms, soles, and mucous membranes. A cheesy white core may be expressed from the central pore. Children of more than 1 year are most commonly affected, but the reported age range extends from 6 weeks to 72 years. Lesions may itch and autoinoculation is common. Outbreaks suggesting direct or indirect contagion are recorded in wrestlers, in children's homes, and in association with swimming pools and beauty parlors. However, most cases are sporadic, experimental infection is frequently unsuccessful, and the precise mode of transmission is unknown. Venereal infections, with genital lesions and an appropriate contact history, are recognized with increasing frequency in young adults (Lynch, 1972; Wilkin, 1977). Both indigenous and imported infections have been reported. A specific diagnosis in the sexual partner is more usually inferred than proved. Lesions regress spontaneously or after trauma or bacterial infection; new ones appear intermittently during a total course of six months to four years. The presence of antibody and skin hypersensitivity in patients without lesions may imply inapparent, unrecognized, or unreported infection.

## COMPLICATIONS AND SEQUELAE

Minor bleeding after trauma, secondary bacterial infection, and perilesional depigmentation may occur. Conjunctivitis may complicate eyelid lesions. An eczematous reaction occurs in 10 per cent of patients after a month or more and may represent a nonspecific or an immunologic response to the extension of products of the lesions into the dermis. The claim that treatment of preexisting eczema with topical steroids predisposes to molluscum contagiosum is disputed. Subjects treated with immunosuppressive drugs (Rosenberg and Yusk, 1970), and those with atopic dermatitis or lymphoid malignancy sometimes develop several hundred lesions within a few days. This phenomenon also occurs rarely in apparently normal patients. Extensive chronic infection in a patient with atopic dermatitis was attributed to impaired cellular immunity (Pauly et al., 1978). New lesions may appear two months or more after apparent cure.

## GEOGRAPHICAL VARIATIONS IN DISEASE

Regional variations in prevalence and age distribution (Rook et al., 1972) of this worldwide condition reflect local patterns of hygiene, living conditions, social customs, and possibly climate. A prevalence of 0.1 per cent in dermatology outpatients in Scotland contrasts with 4.5 per cent of an entire population and 22 per cent of children under 10 in villages in Fiji and New Guinea (Sturt et al., 1971), respectively. Household spread is rare in Aberdeen, Scotland, but common in Fiji. The peak age incidence is 10 to 12 years in Aberdeen, predominantly in boys attending public swimming baths; 2 to 3 years in the Pacific Islands, with both sexes equally affected; and 1 to 4 years in the Congo. Infrequent infection among adults in countries with widespread infection in early childhood may reflect persisting specific immunity, which, combined with the long incubation period, may also contribute to the low prevalence during the first year of life.

## DIAGNOSIS

Diagnostic difficulties (Molluscum contagiosum, 1968) arise with giant, isolated, miliary, and confluent lesions, and those in unusual locations such as the soles of the feet and the glans penis. Secondarily infected lesions simulate furuncles or folliculitis, and eyelid lesions may resemble chalazions or sebaceous cysts. Some mistaken diagnoses include (Mehregan, 1961) epithelioma, basal cell carcinoma, keratoacanthoma, and verruca vulgaris. The presence of multiple lesions or freezing with ethyl chloride to accentuate the central dimple may help establish the diagnosis.

Molluscum bodies are readily recognized by microscopic examination of expressed core material, either unstained or stained by the Giemsa or Papanicolaou techniques. Virions may be detected by Morosow's stain or by electron microscopy (Fig. 1). Biopsies may be examined histologically (Fig. 2) or by immunofluorescence and electronmicroscopy for viral antigen and viral particles, respectively. Molluscum virus cannot be directly isolated from lesions in standard tissue culture lines, but three different types have been recognized by restriction endonuclease analysis of viral DNA (Parr et al., 1977). Antibodies may be demonstrated by gel diffusion and immunofluorescence techniques.

## TREATMENT

Since lesions resolve spontaneously, treatment should not cause scarring. Removal of the central core with a needle or curette, puncture with a toothpick dipped in Liquor iodi fortis, and freezing with liquid nitrogen or dry ice are all advocated but can be painful. Treatment with 0.9 per cent cantharidin in equal parts of acetone and flexible collodion, or twice daily application of 0.05 per cent tretinoin (vitamin A acid) cream (Papa and Berger, 1976), is effective and painless. Twice weekly applications of trichloroacetic acid or 20 per cent podophyllin in 95 per cent ethanol must be continued for several weeks. Methisazone, an antiviral agent for other poxviruses, is not effective. Successful treatment relieves associated dermatitis or conjunctivitis. Follow-up examinations for four months are necessary to treat previously undetected lesions.

## PROPHYLAXIS

There is no specific prophylaxis. General measures include successful treatment of patients and their exclusion from, for instance, communal swimming pools until cured. The general principles of epidemiology and hygiene should be applied to common source outbreaks. Patients with genital lesions should be examined for other sexually transmitted diseases and followed up by contact-tracing and health education. Similarly, patients with other sexually transmitted infections should be examined for coexistent molluscum contagiosum.

## References

Barbanti-Brodano, G., Mannini-Palenzona, A., Varoli, O., Portolani, M., and La Placa, M.: Abortive infection and transformation of human embryonic fibroblasts by molluscum contagiosum virus. J Gen Virol 24:237, 1974.

Epstein, W. L., and Fukuyama, K.: Maturation of molluscum contagiosum virus (MCV) in vivo: Quantitative electron microscopic autoradiography. J Invest Dermatol 60:73, 1973.

Francis, R. D., and Bradford, H. B., Jr.: Some biological and physical properties of molluscum contagiosum virus propagated in cell culture. J Virol 19:382, 1976.

La Placa, M., Portolani, M., Mannini-Palenzona, A., Barbanti-Brodano, G., and Bernardini, A.: Further studies on the mechanism of the cytopathic changes produced by the molluscum contagiosum virus into human amnion cell cultures. G Microbiol 15:205, 1967.

Lever, W. F., and Schaumburg-Lever, G.: Histopathology of the Skin. 5th ed. Philadelphia and Toronto, J. B. Lippincott Company, 1975.

Lynch, P. J.: Molluscum contagiosum venereum. Clin Obst Gynecol 15:966, 1972.

McFadden, G., Pace, W. E., Purres, J., and Dales, S.: Biogenesis of poxviruses: transitory expression of molluscum contagiosum early functions. Virology 94:297, 1979.

Mehregan, A. H.: Molluscum contagiosum—a clinicopathologic study. Arch Dermatol 84:123, 1961.

Molluscum contagiosum. Br Med J 1:459, 1968.

Papa, C. M., and Berger, R. S.: Venereal herpes-like molluscum contagiosum: Treatment with tretinoin. Cutis 18:537, 1976.

Parr, R. P., Burnett, J. W., and Garon, C. F.: Structural characterization of the molluscum contagiosum virus genome. Virology 81:247, 1977.

Pauly, C. R., Artis, W. M., and Jones, H. E.: Atopic dermatitis, impaired cellular immunity, and molluscum contagiosum. Arch Dermatol 114:391, 1978.

Peters, D., and Küper, H.: The nucleoid structure of molluscum contagiosum virus during maturation. Arch Ges Virusforsch 31:137, 1970.

Postlethwaite, R.: Molluscum contagiosum—a review. Arch Environ Health 21:432, 1970.

Prose, P. H., Friedman-Kien, A. E., and Vilček, J.: Molluscum contagiosum virus in adult human skin cultures: An electron microscopic study. Am J Pathol 55:349, 1969.

Rook, A., Wilkinson, D. S., and Ebling, F. J. G. (eds.): Textbook of Dermatology. 2nd ed. Oxford, Blackwell Scientific Publications, 1972.

Rosenberg, E. W., and Yusk, J. W.: Molluscum contagiosum. Eruption following treatment with prednisone and methotrexate. Arch Dermatol 101:439, 1970.

Shand, J. H., Gibson, P., Gregory, D. W., Cooper, R. J., Keir, H. M., and Postlethwaite, R.: Molluscum contagiosum—a defective poxvirus? J Gen Virol 33:281, 1976.

Shirodaria, P. V., and Matthews, R. S.: Observations on the antibody responses in molluscum contagiosum. Br J Dermatol 96:29, 1977.

Sturt, R. J., Muller, K. H., and Francis, G. D.: Molluscum contagiosum in villages of the West Sepik district of New Guinea. Med J Aust 2:751, 1971.

Vreeswijk, J., Leene, W., and Kalsbeek, G. L.: Early interactions of the virus molluscum contagiosum with its host cell. Virus-induced alterations in the basal and suprabasal layers of the epidermis. J Ultrastruct Res 54:37, 1976.

Vreeswijk, J., Leene, W., and Kalsbeek, G. L.: Early host cell-molluscum contagiosum virus interactions. II. Viral interactions with the basal epidermal cells. J Invest Dermatol 69:249, 1977.

Wilkin, J. K.: Molluscum contagiosum venereum in a women's outpatient clinic: A venereally transmitted disease. Am J Obstet Gynecol 128:531, 1977.

# 230 *MYIASIS*

## *Alexander W. Pierce, Jr., M.D.*

## *DEFINITIONS*

The order Diptera includes all insects with only one pair of functional wings—flies, gnats, and mosquitoes. Diptera undergo complete metamorphosis and transform from ovum to larva to pupa to the adult insect (imago). Parasitic disease of man and other vertebrates caused by larvae of Diptera (maggots) is termed myiasis.

The typical larva is a cylindrical, headless, legless, segmented, white or gray maggot. The length ranges from 2 to 30 millimeters. The anterior end may be prominently tapered. Larvae respire through two posterior respiratory spiracles that are frequently mistaken for eyes. The morphology of different species and, on occasion, developmental stages of the same species may vary markedly.

A newly hatched larva is termed the first instar. After a period of feeding and growth, the larva molts and discloses a second instar. The number of repetitions of this process varies with the species, but there are usually three developmental stages or instars. The skin of the final instar does not shed but hardens into a dark, protective shell that encloses a nonfeeding semiquiescent pupa. Pupation of all the Diptera that produce myiasis occurs in the soil. Weeks to months later, varying both with the species and the climatic conditions, an adult fly emerges from the pupal case. Most adult females are oviparous, but a few give birth to live larvae.

Obligate parasites feed and develop in nature only in living tissue. They may be host-specific. Incidental parasitism is the invasion of an unusual host by an obligate parasite. The symptoms of the incidental host may differ from those of the usual host because the parasite may fail to complete normal growth and development or may behave in an unusual manner. Facultative parasites feed and develop in dead and decaying organic matter under most circumstances but occasionally infect a living organism. A temporary parasite lives free of its host during part of its existence.

Accidental parasitism refers to infection resulting from the unknowing transfer of an infectious parasite from a previous location. Accidental myiasis is usually the result of the ingestion of food on which oviposition has occurred.

## ETIOLOGY

Dipterous species that cause human myiasis may be divided into four groups: (1) obligate myiasis-producing Diptera for which man is a favored host, (2) obligate myiasis-producing Diptera for which man is an incidental host, (3) facultative myiasis-producing Diptera, and (4) accidental myiasis-producing Diptera. Diptera that cause facultative and accidental myiasis are traditionally differentiated, although many species are classified in both groups.

The Diptera listed in Table 1 are obligate parasites for which man may be the host.

The primary screwworm (*Cochliomyia hominivorax*), the Old World screwworm (*Chrysomyia bezziana*), and the larvae of *Wohlfahrtia magnifica* are the most virulent dipterous larvae. The human botfly (*Dermatobia hominis*) and the tumbu fly (*Cordylobia anthropophaga*) account for the majority of human disease caused by Dipterous larvae that are obligatory parasites. Attacks by the Congo floor maggot (*Auchmeromyia luteola*) are not considered true myiasis by many authorities. Man is, however, the only known host for this temporary parasite.

Obligate parasites that may incidentally infect man are listed in Table 2.

Larvae of the *Gasterophilus* spp are gastrointestinal parasites of horses. Cattle and deer are the usual hosts for larvae of the *Hypoderma* species. Larvae of the sheep botfly, *Oestrus ovis*, infect the nasal passages and paranasal sinuses of sheep and goats. *Rhinoestrus purpureus* larvae cause similar infections of horses. *Wohlfahrtia opaca* and *W. vigil* are probably a single species. *W. opaca vigil* larvae usually infect mink and fox pups. The antelope is the primary host for larvae of *C. rodhaini*. Larvae of *Cuterebra* sp infect rodents and lagomorphs.

More than 150 dipterous species have been implicated in facultative myiasis of man. Among the most common are the larvae of *Phormia* spp, *Phoenicia* spp, *Sarcophaga* spp, *Calliphora* sp, and the common house fly, *Musca domestica*. Rarely, deliberate inoculation of a necrotic wound with larvae of a facultative dipterous species has been used to facilitate wound débridement.

Over 50 dipterous species have been reported to cause accidental human gastrointestinal myiasis. The most frequently reported species are the cheese skipper (*Piophila casei*), the rat-tailed maggot (*Eristalis tenax*), and *M. domestica*.

Specific identification of dipterous larvae requires entomologic expertise. Differentiation of the obligate parasites *C. hominivorax* and *C. bezziana* from their respective facultative counterparts, *C. macelleria* and *C. megacephala*, has been particularly difficult. Species identification of the first larval instar is not always possible.

## PATHOGENESIS AND PATHOLOGY

Screwworm flies oviposit up to several hundred eggs next to minor integumentary lesions such as

**TABLE 1.  Human Obligatory Myiasis**

| GEOGRAPHIC DISTRIBUTION | GENUS/SPECIES | ANATOMIC LOCALIZATION |
|---|---|---|
| North America and South America | *Cochliomyia hominivorax* (primary screwworm) | Aural, ophthalmic, genitourinary, nasopharyngeal, integumentary |
| Africa, Asia and Indonesia | *Chrysomyia bezziana* (Old World screwworm) | Aural, ophthalmic, genitourinary, nasopharyngeal, integumentary |
| Asia, Africa and Europe | *Wohlfahrtia magnifica* | Aural, ophthalmic, genitourinary, nasopharyngeal, integumentary |
| Central America and South America | *Dermatobia hominis* (human botfly) | Integumentary |
| Africa | *Cordylobia anthropophaga* (tumbu fly) | Integumentary |
| Africa | *Auchmeromyia luteola* (Congo floor maggot) | Bloodsucking |

**TABLE 2.  Human Incidental Myiasis**

| GEOGRAPHIC DISTRIBUTION | GENUS/SPECIES | ANATOMIC LOCALIZATION |
|---|---|---|
| Worldwide | Gasterophilus nasalis | Integumentary |
| | Gasterophilus intestinalis | Integumentary |
| | Gasterophilus hemorrhoidalis | Integumentary |
| Africa | Cordylobia rodhaini | Integumentary |
| North America | Wohlfahrtia opaca | Integumentary |
| | Wohlfahrtia vigil | |
| Europe, Asia and North America | Hypoderma lineatum | Integumentary, ophthalmic |
| | Hypoderma bovis | |
| Europe | Hypoderma diana | Integumentary, ophthalmic |
| North America | Cuterebra buccata | Integumentary, nasopharyngeal |
| Europe, Asia, Africa, and Australia | Oestrus ovis | Ophthalmic, nasopharyngeal |
| Europe, Asia, and Africa | Rhinoestrus purpureus | Ophthalmic, nasopharyngeal |

scratches, insect bites, or abrasions. The ova are glued to adjacent intact skin. Upon hatching, the first instar of the primary screwworm (*C. hominivorax*) enters the break in the integument and actively invades, digests, and liquefies normal tissue. The first larval instar of the Old World screwworm (*C. bezziana*) remains superficial, but the second instar is invasive. The growth rate of these biophagous larvae is remarkable. The primary screwworm increases in size 15-fold in eight days. It is believed that previously infected wounds attract gravid females of the species for further oviposition.

*Wohlfahrtia magnifica* is larviparous. Larviposition of the 100 to 200 first larval instars is adjacent to minor integumentary lesions of a mammalian host. The first instar is invasive and biophagous.

The human botfly (*D. hominis*) oviposits 15 to 25 ova on the ventral surface of a captured, but unharmed, insect vector, usually a mosquito. The egg hatches in 5 to 15 days, and the first larval instar abandons the chorion while the vector is in contact with a mammalian host. The larva does not penetrate intact skin but may penetrate even minimal lesions such as the bite of the mosquito vector. Once established in the subcutaneous tissue, the larvae do not migrate but live singly in furuncular lesions. Their lifespan averages five to ten weeks but may last up to three months.

The tumbu fly (*C. anthropophaga*) oviposits several hundred ova in the soil, usually in sand contaminated by urine or feces. Oviposition occurs only in shaded places. Larvae hatch in one to three days and remain viable awaiting a host for one to two weeks. When the soil is disturbed, the larvae extend themselves upward from the soil and wave actively, seeking a host. After attachment, the larva penetrates intact skin. These maggots also dwell singly in subcutaneous furuncular lesions. The usual three instars are passed in eight to ten days, whereupon the larva leaves the wound and returns to the soil for pupation.

Gravid *A. luteola* flies oviposit on dry soil or sand in shaded areas, usually in the crevices of huts. The larvae, the Congo floor maggots, live in crevices and emerge at night to attach to a human host by means of powerful mouth hooks. The maggot sucks blood for 15 to 20 minutes, then detaches and returns to its hiding place, returning to the host the following evening. Sleep disturbances with heavy infestations are the sole symptoms caused by this sanguinivorous, temporary parasite. Moreover, it is not known to be the vector for any other infectious agent.

Dipterous species whose larvae fail to grow and develop as incidental parasites in man include *Gasterophilus* spp, *O. ovis*, *R. purpureus*, and probably the *Cuterebra* species. *Gasterophilus* species, *O. ovis*, and *R. purpureus* larvae fail to develop beyond the first instar in man. *Hypoderma* spp may achieve normal larval development in humans, but the extended subcutaneous wandering of the parasite is not comparable to the highly directed migration that occurs in the preferred bovine host. Human infection by *W. opaca vigil*, *C. rodhaini*, and the *Cuterebra* sp is rare.

Oviposition on a living host by Diptera species that are facultative parasites is generally on diseased, frequently necrotic, exposed, and neglected tissues. Similarly, a fetid discharge from a body orifice, such as the ear, urethra, or vagina, or the external accumulation of body excrement perianally in a neglected and debilitated elderly individual may invite oviposition by facultative Diptera species.

## CLINICAL MANIFESTATIONS

Symptoms and signs of myiasis are related to the infected organ or tissue. Classifications of myiasis based on organ system involvement are more useful clinically than those based on the identity of the infecting parasite. The most commonly involved organ is the skin. Integumentary myiasis may be either furuncular or a creeping eruption.

Furuncular myiasis is characterized by one or more erythematous nodules, each with one or more ulcers (Fig. 1). Visualization of single or multiple motile larvae is diagnostic and easily achieved by careful inspection. There is usually a serous or purulent discharge from the ulcer. The discharge may be stained with blood or larval feces. A single large furuncle with several ulcers and containing numerous larvae is characteristic of infections by the screwworms or larvae of *W. magnifica.* Infection by tumbu fly larvae is manifested by multiple furuncles, each with a single maggot. One to three furuncles of long duration, each with a single maggot, are characteristic of *D. hominis* infection. *Wohlfahrtia opaca vigil* in-

fections usually present with 5 to 15 pustulofuruncular lesions of 1 to 5 mm on the neck, upper trunk, or arms of an infant. Each furuncle contains one to four larvae.

In man, infection by larvae of *Gasterophilus* spp produces a creeping eruption. The lesions are visible, palpable, serpiginous, intradermal tracts. The larva is found distal to the more prominent end of the tract. The lesion will be single and pruritic. By contrast, the lesions of cutaneous larva migrans due to the dog and cat hookworm, *Ancylostoma braziliense,* are multiple and on skin surfaces that have been in contact with the soil.

Larvae of *Hypoderma* spp produce furuncular myiasis in cattle and deer after extensive migration through tissue. The furuncles in cattle are known as warbles. In man, the maggot migrates in the subcutaneous tissue over extensive distances, frequently disappearing and re-emerging at a distant site. The general direction of the larval migration is cephalad. The subcutaneous tracts are not sharply demarcated. They may be tender at the site of the most recent migration and become increasingly tender and inflamed as furuncles form. Several furuncles at several sites may form and resolve before the definitive surface furuncle with ulcer formation develops. The definitive warble is usually on the shoulder, neck, or head and may be associated with diffuse edema.

Nasopharyngeal myiasis may be fatal. Infection usually occurs in debilitated patients with antecedent nasopharyngeal disease. The screwworms and the larvae of *W. magnifica* pro-

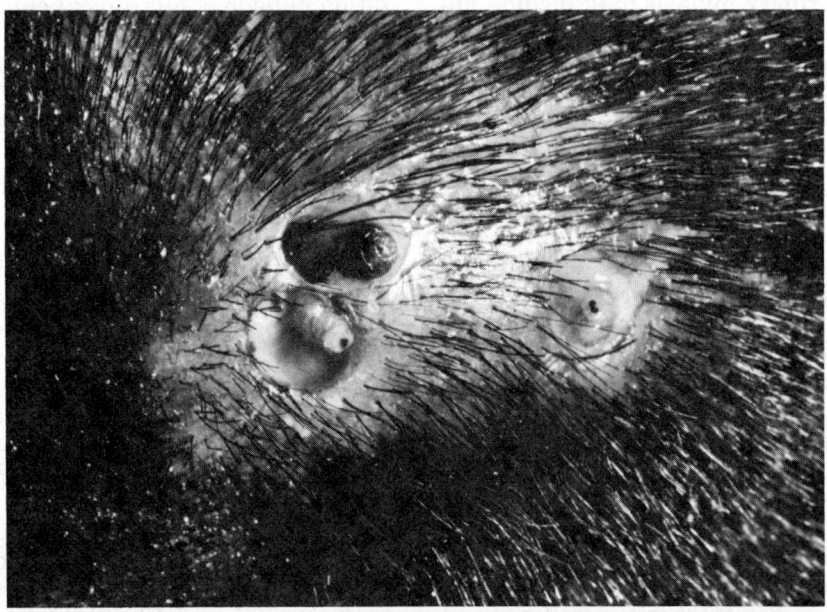

**FIGURE 1.** *Furuncular myiasis of the scalp. The parasite is* Cochliomyia hominivorax.

duce extensive tissue destruction that may in-volve the paranasal sinuses. The palate or nasal septum may be perforated. There may be exten-sion into the eye or through the calvarium into the central nervous system. Manifestations in-clude a malodorous, serosanguineous, or purulent nasal discharge, nasal obstruction, pain, and the sensation of "something moving." Less destruc-tive nasopharyngeal lesions are produced by the incidental parasites *O. ovis* and *R. purpureus*.

These same maggots, *O. ovis* (the sheep botfly) and *R. purpureus* (the equine head maggot), may be found in ophthalmomyiasis. External ophthalmic involvement with conjunctivitis is usual, but the first larval instar has been found in both the anterior and posterior chambers of the eye in association with uveitis. *Cuterebra* species may also be found in either the anterior or pos-terior chamber and may produce multiple linear and arcuate subretinal tracts. These tracts are believed to be diagnostic by virtue of their extent, size, and circuity even in the absence of a visible larva. Rarely, the larva of *Hypoderma* spp mi-grates into the orbit and produces extensive ocu-lar damage.

Aural myiasis usually occurs in the presence of pre-existing diseases of the external ear. *Phoen-icia* species have been recovered from the exter-nal ear, however, in the absence of known ante-cedent pathology. Pain and noise are the major manifestations of myiasis of the external auditory canal. The larva of *Hypoderma* spp may produce extensive middle ear damage in the course of its wandering. The screwworms and *W. magnifica* may invade the middle ear directly or extend into the middle ear from the paranasal sinuses.

Symptoms of urinary myiasis may include ab-dominal pain, dysuria, frequency, urgency, gross hematuria, priapism, and spontaneous ejacula-tion. The ejaculate may contain larvae. Urethral obstruction may occur. There is usually anteced-ent urogenital disease. It is hypothesized that oviposition occurs at the urethral meatus, and the first larval instar migrates into the posterior ur-ethra or bladder. The larvae are usually faculta-tive parasites, and these infections generally re-mit spontaneously when the maggots are passed.

Larvae of facultative Diptera organisms may be found in excrement, leading to confusion about their origin. Oviposition in excrement after its passage is far more common than infection of the gastrointestinal tract. Most ova deposited in food do not survive passage through the gastrointes-tinal tract. Classification of this benign infesta-tion as myiasis is controversial. It has therefore been called pseudomyiasis. Symptoms attributed to enteric myiasis include malaise, pallor, abdom-inal pain, diarrhea, hematochezia, vomiting, and anorexia.

## COMPLICATIONS AND SEQUELAE

Most infections by dipterous larvae result in uncomplicated cutaneous myiasis. "Ver du Cayor," furuncular myiasis due to tumbu fly lar-vae, may leave persistent, pigmented scars. *Hy-poderma* species may invade the spinal canal with resulting paresis. Inflammation, edema, and suppuration may be manifestations of the larval infection and do not necessarily require antimi-crobial therapy. Rarely, isolated granulomatous lesions of viscera have been attributed to dipter-ous larvae. A larva of *Gasterophilus* sp has been found in a pulmonary coin lesion, and a *Hypo-derma* sp has been demonstrated in a hepatic granuloma.

## GEOGRAPHIC VARIATIONS

Although myiasis due to certain dipterous lar-vae is endemic to specific geographic regions, and case clusters of human myiasis may be seen in association with epizootics in domestic animals, human myiasis is usually seen as isolated cases. The geographic distribution of the Diptera species for which myiasis is obligatory is shown in Tables 1 and 2. Case importation has been repeatedly documented, however. Instances of infection by both *D. hominis* and *C. anthropophaga* have been documented on the North American continent. Climatic conditions have a major influence on pu-pation, and many species such as the primary screwworm will not maintain sustained coloni-zation outside a subtropical climate.

## DIAGNOSIS

Diagnosis requires the demonstration of dipter-ous larvae in tissue or wounds. Preservation of maggots for entomologic identification is impor-tant and can be achieved by placing specimens in a solution of 70 to 80 per cent alcohol. If an an-tiseptic has been applied to the wound, the spec-imens should be rinsed in saline before suspen-sion in alcohol. Figure 2 illustrates some of the maggots that are common causes of human myi-asis. Saprophytic species may be reared on blood agar plates at 30° C, but obligate dipterous larvae require specialized rearing techniques. In the United States, an entomologic identification ser-vice is provided by the Department of Agricul-ture, Animal and Plant Health Inspection Ser-vice, Post Office Box 969, Mission, Texas 78572.

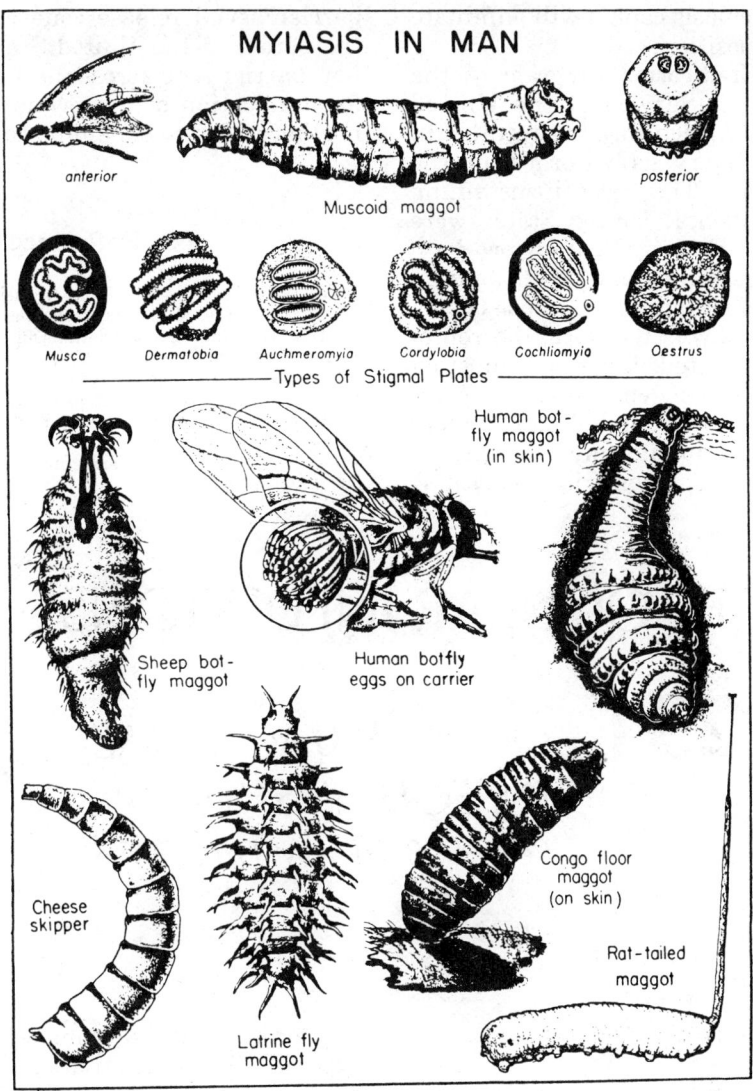

**FIGURE 2.** *Agents of human myiasis. (From Newson, H. D.: Order Diptera. In Hunter, G. W., Swartzwelder, J. C., and Clyder, D. F. (eds.): Tropical Medicine. 5th Ed. Philadelphia, W. B. Saunders Company, 1976.)*

### TREATMENT

Removal of the maggots is curative. This is usually easily accomplished by saline irrigation and extraction with forceps. Large furuncles with multiple larvae produced by obligate parasites such as the screwworms or larvae of *W. magnifica* may require surgical enlargement of an ulcer under local anesthesia to achieve complete removal of all the maggots. The local application of oils, paraffin, chloroform, or ether to interfere with larval respiration will produce increased larval activity and migration to the surface. Extensive surgical débridement may be required for nasopharyngeal myiasis. Antimicrobial therapy should be employed for culturally documented secondary bacterial infections.

### PROPHYLAXIS

Good personal and environmental hygiene is the most effective prophylaxis. These measures include appropriate disposal of human and animal excreta and screening of homes and public buildings. Endemic or epidemic outbreaks may require spraying with chlorinated hydrocarbons to control the adult fly and veterinary care for domestic animals. Prompt, appropriate therapy for pyoderma or pediculosis capitis will eliminate potential sites of oviposition.

The Screwworm Eradication Program of the Agricultural Research Service of the United States Department of Agriculture has resulted in eradication of the primary screwworm from the southern United States. The last self-sustaining colonies in the continental United States were eliminated by 1966. This eradication program consists of aerial release of irradiated pupae from which infertile male flies emerge. Because the female *C. hominivorax* mates but once, the reproductive cycle is interrupted. Livestock infection by *C. hominivorax* is still endemic along the Mexican border, however, and when hot and dry conditions favor pupation, human myiasis may be seen in association with epidemics in livestock. A barrier aerial release zone is maintained along the border of the United States with Mexico. A new barrier zone across the Tehuantepec isthmus for eradication of the primary screwworm from northern Mexico should be completed by 1982.

### References

James, M. T.: The Flies That Cause Myiasis in Man. U.S. Department of Agriculture, Miscellaneous Publication No. 631. Washington, D.C., U.S. Government Printing Office, 1947.

James, M. T., and Harwood, R. T.: Herms's Medical Entomology. 6th ed. London, The Macmillan Company, 1969.

Newsom, H. D.: Order Diptera. In Hunter, Swartzwelder, and Clyde (eds.): Tropical Medicine. 5th ed. Philadelphia, W. B. Saunders Company, 1976.

Zumpt, F.: Myiasis in Man and Animals of the Old World. London, Butterworth, 1965.

# H. OCULAR INFECTIONS

# 231 *OCULAR BACTERIAL INFECTIONS*

*Perry S. Binder, M.D., F.A.C.S.*

## INTRODUCTION

The hallmark of an ocular infection is a red eye. The location of the erythema usually occurs near the infected structure. For instance, the eyelid margins are red in cases of blepharitis; the conjunctiva are injected in bacterial and viral conjunctivitis; and the deep blood vessels adjacent to the cornea and sclera are dilated (ciliary flush) in cases of iritis. Erythema of all ocular structures suggests a severe infection of the entire globe and orbit, such as panophthalmitis (abscess of the globe). The presence of edema, in addition to erythema, suggests severe or advanced infection or inflammation. The presence of an ocular discharge is not normal, and its character indicates the type of disease that caused it. For example, the discharge is watery in allergies, serosanguinous in severe viral conjunctivitis, and purulent in bacterial infections.

The first symptoms of an ocular infection are a mild sensation of a foreign body and tearing and sensitivity to sunlight. More advanced infection causes pain and decreased vision. The sensation of a foreign body is common in patients with any type of mild conjunctivitis, and any source of irritation to the fifth nerve reflexly stimulates the lacrimal gland and causes tearing.

Sensitivity to light is usually produced by a corneal abnormality, or an intraocular inflammation or infection that affects the pigmented tissues of the eye. Decreased vision is a very serious sign of advanced infection and is usually associated with an opacity in the path of light from the cornea to the retina, such as a corneal abscess or severe intraocular inflammation that clouds the vitreous.

A careful history is important in the evaluation of a patient with a red eye. Factors that predispose to infection include recent or previous trauma, previous infections, contacts with family members or friends who have acute red eyes, diabetes mellitus, malnutrition, and diseases or drugs that diminish cell-mediated immunity. The use of ocular medications and their frequency of administration must be determined because they can produce toxic and/or allergic changes. Unlabeled bottles with red tops contain medications that dilate the pupil; green-topped bottles contain medications that constrict the pupil. Milky white drops are usually glucocorticoids, and clear drops in clear bottles are usually anesthetics.

The examination of the patient with a red eye must be done carefully in order to avoid contaminating the physician's hands and instruments. Because ocular viral infections are highly contagious, it is important to clean carefully any instruments that may have come in contact with an infected eye before examining another patient. It is best not to touch a patient who you suspect has viral conjunctivitis.

The routine administration of antibiotics, topical glucocorticoids, or topical anesthetics to every patient with a red eye is inappropriate because this treatment does not help the patient and may make his condition worse. For example, steroids aggravate a herpes simplex infection of the cornea, and anesthetics, which are toxic to the cornea, can produce severe sloughing of the entire epithelium, subsequent scarring, and neovascularization. The administration of antibiotics before obtaining cultures of a corneal abscess may hinder later efforts to determine the cause of infection by temporarily suppressing growth.

Most patients with *redness,* a *sudden* change in *vision,* or ocular *pain* (RSVP) should be examined immediately and referred to an ophthalmologist (an M.D.) for evaluation. Referral to an optometrist (a doctor of optometry, who is not an M.D.), who is untrained in the diagnosis and therapy of ocular disease, only delays accurate diagnosis and appropriate therapy.

# ORBITAL CELLULITIS

## ETIOLOGY AND PATHOGENESIS

Orbital cellulitis is an acute inflammation of the orbital tissues that may threaten the patient's vision or even his life if it is not diagnosed and treated immediately. It may be produced by spread of an infection from either nearby structures or distant foci. In children, ethmoiditis is a common focus of spread to the orbit. In adults, infections of the other sinuses are equally common foci. Sinus infections spread to the orbit by causing thrombophlebitis of the communicating veins between the orbit and sinuses.

*Haemophilus influenzae* is the most common cause of orbital cellulitis in children less than 5 years of age. *Staphylococcus aureus,* group A streptococci, and pneumococci are the predominant organisms in adults and also occur in children. When the infection spreads from chronic sinusitis, anaerobic bacteria may be prominent (Frederick and Braude, 1974). Almost any microorganism may be introduced by penetrating trauma or during surgery.

## CLINICAL MANIFESTATIONS

The clinical presentation depends upon the location of the infection in the orbit. The infected area displaces the globe in the opposite direction (proptosis). For instance, a superior abscess produces a downward displacement of the globe.

The patient may or may not be systemically ill. There is usually orbital pain and eyelid erythema with edema of the upper lid (Fig. 1). The eye usually protrudes (proptosis), and the lids are usually swollen shut with a discharge that may or may not be purulent. Early in the disease, the cornea and conjunctiva are uninvolved. As the proptosis progresses, however, the cornea can become exposed, ulcerated and perforated, which may lead to panophthalmitis. If the apex of the orbit is affected, the optic nerve and cranial nerves III through VI may be infected. This complication

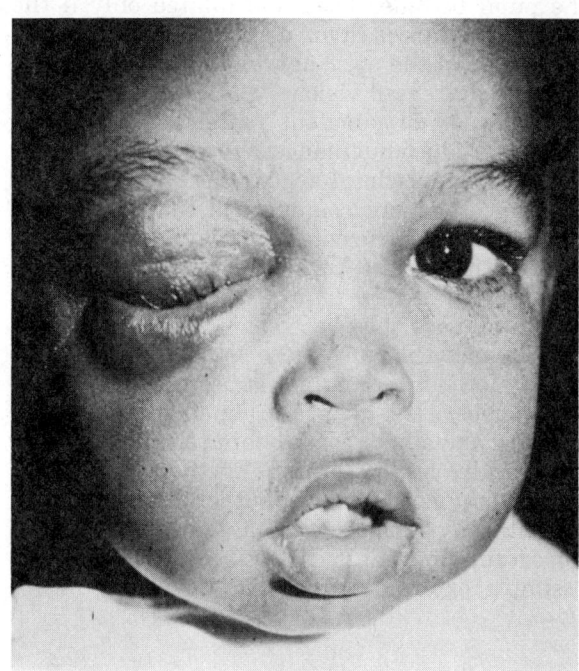

**FIGURE 1.** Haemophilus influenzae *orbital cellulitis in a 2-year-old. The eyelid edema is sharply demarcated by the orbital septum in the upper and lower eyelids.*

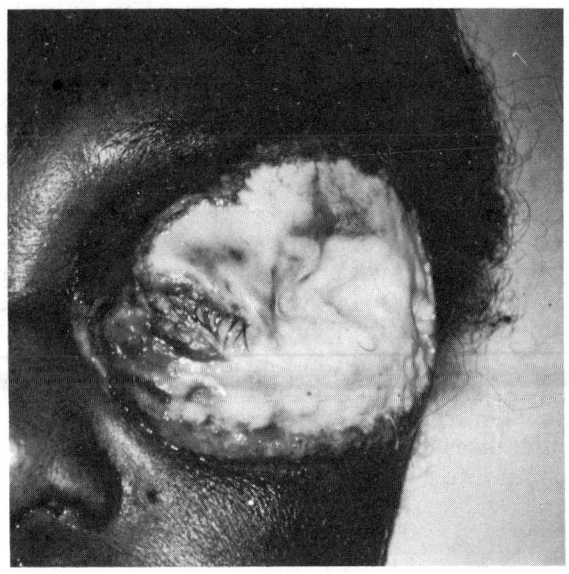

**FIGURE 2.** Pseudomonas *orbital abscesses in a diabetic following a minor injury to the skin of the left upper eyelid.*

causes optic neuritis with decreased vision and an afferent pupillary defect with decreased extraocular muscle movements (progressive ophthalmoplegia). The extraocular muscle movements become restricted slowly, but with advanced disease, there are no extraocular muscle movements. The pupil becomes fixed and dilated only if the cavernous sinus is involved. Compression and/or infiltration of the optic nerve produces optic neuritis and decreased vision.

The pocket of purulent material may either point or produce fluctuance. When the pus is confined to the episcleral space, there is less eyelid swelling and more conjunctival involvement at the site of the extraocular muscle insertions near the junction of the cornea and sclera (limbus). This causes severe pain when the patient attempts to move the eye.

Some bacteria cause these signs and symptoms over a slower time course. Tuberculous or syphilitic periostitis and granulomas may produce swelling and a hard mass behind the globe either unilaterally or bilaterally. Erythema and pain may or may not be prominent, and most of these patients may be thought to have an orbital tumor. Opportunistic organisms can infect the orbit from a simple external lesion and slowly produce a large external orbital mass before they produce the typical signs and symptoms of acute orbital cellulitis (Fig. 2).

## DIAGNOSIS AND THERAPY

It is easy to make a diagnosis when a patient presents with a rapid onset of lid and orbital swelling with erythema of the eyelid, proptosis of the globe, pain in the eye and orbit, and decreased vision. The presence of a pointing abscess or a fluctuant mass in a systemically ill patient is further evidence of orbital infection. The extent of the infection is determined by examining the retina and by measuring the patient's visual acuity, pupillary reaction, corneal sensation, and extraocular muscle movements. Sinus x-rays may confirm disease of an adjacent sinus, and ultrasound can be used to define the extent of the abscess within the orbit.

Blood cultures are usually positive in children with orbital cellulitis caused by *H. influenzae,* but are frequently negative in children and adults when staphylococci, streptococci, pneumococci, or anaerobes have spread from the paranasal sinuses. Since there is usually no external drainage from the orbital infection, and it is usually undesirable to aspirate the orbital abscess, therapy is often directed at the most likely organism. If there is clinical or radiologic evidence of sinusitis, sinus aspiration usually yields the responsible organism. In the absence of definitive bacteriology, children less than 5 years of age are usually treated with I.V. ampicillin at 200 mg per kg per day or chloramphenicol (50 mg per kg per day). A specific antistaphylococcal antibiotic may be added to this regimen. Since *Staphylococcus aureus* is the most common cause of orbital cellulitis in older children and adults, they are usually treated with a penicillinase-resistant penicillin at 200 mg per kg per day. This treatment is also adequate for pneumococci and group A streptococci.

Surgical decompression of the orbit is necessary only in cases of optic nerve compression and/or progressive exposure of the cornea. Topical hotpacks and daily evaluation of the visual acuity and extraocular muscle movements are important adjuncts to the systemic antibiotics. With appropriate therapy, the signs and symptoms abate rapidly, and the patients are left without sequelae (Gombos, 1973; Trevor-Roper, 1974).

# INFECTION OF THE EYELIDS AND OCULAR ADNEXAE (LACRIMAL GLAND, LACRIMAL DUCTS AND LACRIMAL SAC)

## *DEFINITION AND CLINICAL MANIFESTATIONS*

Infection of the eyelids and adnexae produces redness and swelling of the involved structure(s) and ultimate compromise of the particular function (for example, interference with tearing when the tear ducts or lacrimal sac is occluded). Chronic infection produces permanent changes in the structures and may cause permanent loss of function.

The sty, or hordeolum, is an acute staphylococcal abscess of the oil-secreting glands of the eyelids. It may occur on the inner lid (internal hordeolum) when the meibomian glands are involved and on the outer surface of the lid (external hordeolum—Fig. 3) when the glands of Zeiss and Moll are infected. The patient develops acute localized swelling of the lid with pain and erythema. In time, the abscess may point through the skin of the lid. The conjunctiva and remainder of the eye are usually uninvolved. Extension of the infection into the entire eyelid produces a lid abscess (Fig. 4).

A chalazion is a sterile granulomatous inflammation of the meibomian glands. It may or may not follow a hordeolum, but many patients with chalazia have a history of previous episodes of acute inflammation. The lesion develops slowly, and patients may only notice a "lump" in their eyelids. Chalazia seldom subside spontaneously. If chalazia become large enough to induce abnormal curvatures in the cornea, they can cause visual symptoms.

Chronic low-grade infection of the oil-secreting glands by *Staphylococcus aureus* and/or *Staphylococcus epidermidis* (blepharitis) is another common disease of the eyelid. This infection produces a vascularized and erythematous lid margin with scale formation, loss of lashes, production of white lashes, misdirection of lashes, and deposits around the base of the eyelashes (collarettes—Fig. 5). Staphylococcal exotoxins erode the superficial corneal epithelium, and the bacteria metabolize the oil to nonesterified free fatty acids, which destabilize the tear film and add to the disruption of the corneal epithelium. These patients may develop a punctate pattern of erosions on the inferior cornea, ulceration of the cornea at the junction of the cornea and sclera (limbus), or other acute inflammatory lesions of the cornea with neovascularization (phlyctenulosis) (Smolin and Okumoto, 1977).

The corneal debris seen at the base of the lashes may also consist of greasy scales from coexistent seborrheic dermatitis. The conjunctiva is often mildly injected. Staphylococcal blepharitis is common in patients with atopic dermatitis and in the immunologically suppressed. A previous history of hordeola and chalazia is common. The destruction of the tear film produces a dry, gritty feeling, and the patients may sometimes complain of a foreign body in the eye. Scarring of the eyelids may cause the lashes to rub on the cornea

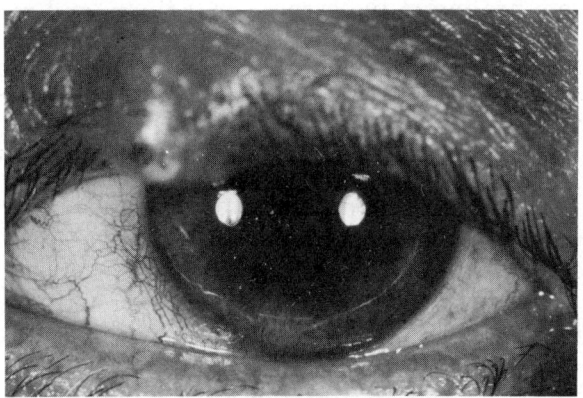

**FIGURE 3.** *Typical external hordeolum.*

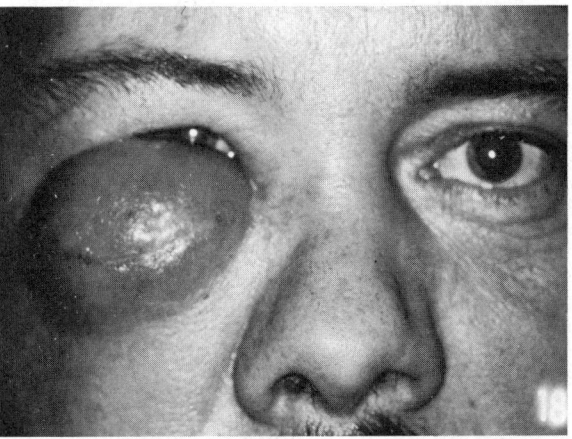

**FIGURE 4.** *Pneumococcal eyelid abscess following repair of a blow-out fracture. The infection is limited by the orbital septum. The old incision was reopened, and a drain was placed in the wound after removal of 15 ml of pus.*

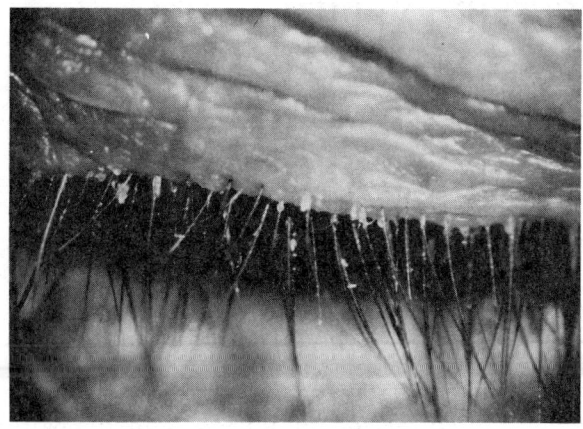

**FIGURE 5.** *Chronic staphyloccal eyelid infection with collarettes at the base of the lashes.*

and produce corneal scarring. These patients may complain of photophobia from the abnormalities in their corneal epithelium. Other common presenting complaints include burning, itching, and red eyelid margins. Chronic, untreated blepharitis may cause inferior corneal scarring and loss of vision. When the area of erythema is fixed in the corners of the eye and spares the central lids (angular blepharitis), either staphylococci or *Moraxella* may be responsible for the infection.

Infection of the lacrimal ducts (canaliculitis) usually produces a unilateral red eye. There is localized redness and swelling in the area in which the duct opens into the eyelid (punctum), and granular material can usually be expressed from the duct. If the infection is untreated, purulent conjunctivitis may result. Fungi or *Actinomyces* usually cause this infection. Other bacteria rarely cause canaliculitis.

Dacryoadenitis is a rare unilateral infection of the lacrimal gland that occurs in children as a

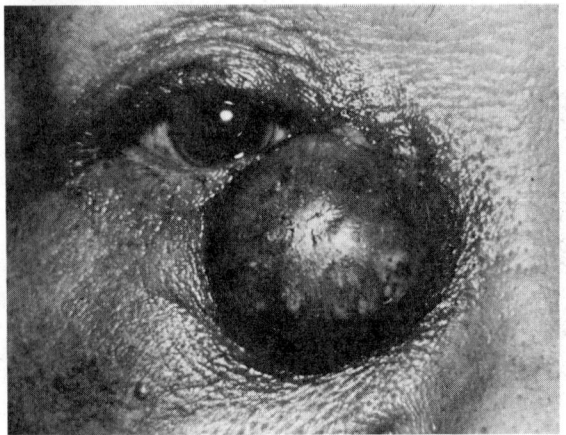

**FIGURE 6.** *This was the third recurrence of this chronic pneumococcal dacryocystitis. Note the nasal location in comparison with the eyelid abscess in Figure 4.*

complication of mumps, measles, or influenza and in adults as a complication of gonococcal bacteremia. Other purulent infections of the lacrimal gland may follow penetrating injuries to the eyelid. Patients develop pain, swelling, and redness in the upper outer quadrant of the orbit in which the lacrimal gland is located.

When the duct from the lacrimal sac becomes occluded, usually near its opening into the nose, stagnation in the sac promotes infection. Most cases are unilateral. Patients complain of tearing (from lacrimal duct obstruction), redness, swelling, and tenderness over the area of the tear sac that is adjacent to the nose below the junction of the upper and lower lids (Fig. 6).

Pressure over the sac usually expresses purulent material from the ducts. The most common offending organisms are *Staphylococcus aureus, Streptococcus pneumonia,* or *Haemophilus influenza,* although almost any organism may infect the sac. In severe cases, the abscess may point through the skin or a fistula may develop. In contrast to canaliculitis, concomitant unilateral conjunctivitis is uncommon.

## DIAGNOSIS AND TREATMENT

All of these infections of the eyelid and ocular adnexae are treated as localized abscesses. The infected area is drained by massage or surgery; heat is applied; and topical or systemic antibiotics are given.

Topical heat and instillation of antibiotic drops (10 per cent sulfacetamide or 0.5 per cent chloromycetin) for a minimum of six times a day is recommended for acute hordeolum. If the lesion points, incision and drainage promote rapid healing. Chalazia do not respond to this treatment, and excision is recommended for cosmetic purposes.

Treatment of staphylococcal blepharitis is designed to decrease the number of organisms, promote healing of the corneal epithelium, and restabilize the tear film. Patients are instructed to "scrub" the eyelid margins at the base of the lashes daily with a cotton-tipped applicator moistened in dilute baby shampoo. This treatment promotes drainage from the stagnant oil glands and cleans the lid margin. Topical antibiotic drops (10 per cent sulfacetamide or tetracycline) should be instilled at a minimum of six to eight times per day initially, and antibiotic ointments (erythromycin, bacitracin, or tetracycline) should be applied to the base of the lashes four times a day with a cotton-tipped applicator. Artificial tears should be applied frequently to smooth out the tear film.

In severe, recurrent cases, oral tetracycline

(250 mg four times daily) may be added to the treatment schedule, but the major cause of treatment failure is noncompliance with or incorrect use of the eyelid scrubs.

Cultures of hordeola and blepharitis are usually not necessary because the diagnosis is obvious, and they are always caused by *S. aureus*. If a culture is taken, a broth-moistened, cotton-tipped applicator should be rubbed gently to and fro across the base of the lashes after the lids have been compressed between two applicators to express material from the meibomian glands.

Infection of the lacrimal ducts is controlled by removal of the organism by expression, irrigation of the ducts with an antibiotic (gantrisin), application of topical heat, and frequent instillation of topical antibiotics (sulfacetamide or chloromycetin). If *Actinomyces* is isolated, tetracycline (500 mg orally every eight hours until two weeks after clinical cure) may be necessary but does not replace irrigation to keep the canaliculi patent.

Infections of the lacrimal sac (dacryocystitis) cannot be cured until the obstruction in the nasal lacrimal duct is relieved. If the duct fails to open by repeated digital pressure on the lacrimal sac, the nasal lacrimal system should be probed. Infection of the sac is treated with topical and systemic antibiotics chosen on the basis of cultures and sensitivities, irrigation with antibiotics, and hot packs. Pointing lesions should be incised and drained. If the nasal lacrimal duct cannot be unobstructed, a new opening into the nose is produced surgically (dacryocystorhinostomy). The site of obstruction in chronic recurrent cases can be determined clinically by staining the tear film with fluorescein or radiographically by injecting radiopaque dyes into the lacrimal duct system (dacryocystography). Applying a radioactive tracer to the tear film and following its path is another technique that has been used to locate obstruction.

Purulent dacryoadenitis is treated with heat and topical and systemic antibiotics chosen according to the cultures of the red eye or penetrating wound. Diagnostic biopsy of the chronically infected, swollen lacrimal gland is seldom necessary.

# CONJUNCTIVITIS

## *ETIOLOGY*

The normal conjunctival flora consists of *S. epidermidis*, *S. aureus*, diphtheroids, some gram-negative rods, a few other aerobic organisms (Locatcher-Khorazo and Seegal, 1972), and two major anaerobes (*Propionibacterium acnes* and *Peptostreptococcus* species) (Perkins et al., 1975). The conjunctival sac is difficult to sterilize because of easy contamination from the eyelid margins. Positive cultures can be obtained from 80 to 95 per cent of normal eyes when a cotton swab moistened in a broth medium is rubbed gently back and forth across the conjunctival sac without contamination from the eyelid margins. Fungi can be cultured from 2 to 22 per cent of normal patients, and viruses from 1 per cent of conjunctival cultures (Table 1).

Most ophthalmologists have regarded "conjunctivitis" as a mild, self-limited disease and until recently have felt that the etiology of conjunctivitis could be established by clinical signs and symptoms supported by Gram and Giemsa smears of the conjunctiva and cultures of the conjunctival sac. Unfortunately, the same aerobic organisms are found in cultures of the normal and infected conjunctival sac. There is no increase in aerobic bacteria during bacterial conjunctivitis (Leibowitz et al., 1976). However, there is some

**TABLE 1.  Normal Conjunctival Flora**

| AEROBIC BACTERIA | ANAEROBIC BACTERIA |
|---|---|
| *Staphylococcus epidermidis* | *Propionibacterium acnes* |
| *Staphylococcus aureus* | *Peptostreptococcus* species |
| *Corynebacterium* species | *Lactobacillus* species |
| *Micrococcus* species | *Clostridium* species |
| *Streptococcus* species | *Eubacterium* species |
| Gram-negative rods | |
| *Streptococcus pneumonia* | **FUNGI** |
| *Bacillus* species | *Candida* species |
| | *Aspergillus* species |
| **VIRUSES** | *Rhodotorula* species |
| Adenoviruses | |

new evidence that anaerobic organisms may play a role in the etiology of conjunctivitis (Perkins et al., 1975).

## *CLINICAL MANIFESTATIONS AND DIAGNOSIS*

A patient with conjunctivitis has a red eye. Conjunctivitis is an extremely common disease and may present unilaterally or bilaterally. The patient may awaken with matter on the lid margins, and the lids may be "stuck together." The conjunctiva is injected in all areas but is usually not as severely injected adjacent to the junction between the cornea and sclera (limbus). The conjunctiva on the surface of the eyelids (palpebral conjunctiva) and on the surface of the eyeball (bulbar conjunctiva) is usually affected. The application of one drop of $2\frac{1}{2}$ per cent phenylephrine usually clears this injection temporarily, whereas a red eye caused by glaucoma or iritis is unaffected by this agent.

Tearing is a nonspecific response to inflammation and is not diagnostic. The discharge in conjunctivitis ranges from minimal and serous to profuse and purulent. This profuse, purulent discharge is diagnostic only in neisserian infections (*Neisseria gonorrhoeae* or *Neisseria meningitidis*), where it is extremely thick and appears to pour out between the eyelids (Fig. 7). Purulent conjunctivitis in a newborn child can be caused by *Neisseria,* almost any other bacterium, chemicals such as silver nitrate, and *Chlamydia* (inclusion blenorrhea). A purulent discharge in a newborn should be considered to be gonorrhea until proved otherwise because this organism can produce blindness in a very short time. In most cases of bacterial conjunctivitis, however, the discharge can be of any type. It may also vary in severity and change in quality during the course of the disease from serous to purulent.

The presence of conjunctival membranes (not mucus), which can be removed and peeled off the conjunctival surface, suggests a diagnosis of diphtheria. Immediate therapy is indicated because this organism can penetrate the intact epithelium and produce blindness within hours (Chandler and Milam, 1978).

A palpable preauricular node is most commonly found in viral infections but occasionally occurs in bacterial disease. Its presence during purulent

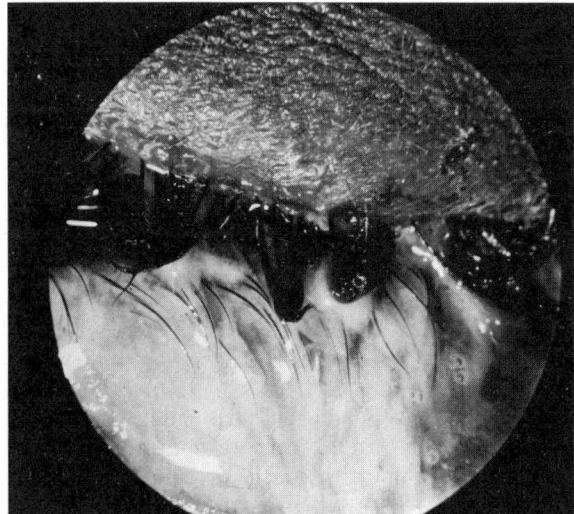

**FIGURE 7.** *Purulent gonococcal conjunctivitis. The pus is so profuse that it will return within minutes of irrigation.*

conjunctivitis suggests severe infections such as tularemia, glanders, and granulomatous diseases. Most cases of bacterial conjunctivitis do not cause systemic symptoms or affect the peripheral white count.

Patients complain of mild discomfort or a feeling of "something in the eye." They are usually comfortable, and few are sensitive to the sunlight or a flashlight. The visual acuity and intraocular pressures are normal. Patients complain of itching and burning, but ocular itching is more commonly associated with allergy. The presence of blood beneath the conjunctiva is rare in bacterial conjunctivitis. It is more commonly associated with severe viral conjunctivitis, especially adenovirus infection. The bacterial causes of subconjunctival hemorrhage are the pneumococcus, *Haemophilus,* or Koch-Weeks bacillus. Eyelid disease such as blepharitis or disease of the lacrimal ducts can produce a concomitant conjunctivitis and should be sought in patients with unilateral conjunctivitis.

The diagnosis of a bacterial conjunctivitis can be made clinically in the presence of the appropriate signs and symptoms (Table 2). A Giemsa smear of the conjunctival sac shows a predominance of polymorphonuclear leukocytes in only about 50 per cent of patients with a clinical diagnosis of bacterial conjunctivitis (Leibowitz et al., 1976a). Gram stains are even less rewarding; bacteria are found in smears from only about 12 per cent of patients with a clinical diagnosis of bacterial conjunctivitis (Leibowitz et al., 1976a).

Cultures of the conjunctiva in injected eyes also have a poor yield; only about 30 per cent of patients with clinical bacterial conjunctivitis harbor pathogenic organisms, and more than 50 per cent of patients with a clinical diagnosis of viral conjunctivitis harbor the same organisms (Leibowitz et al., 1976a). These results, coupled with the expense of the diagnostic tests, have discouraged their use in the routine diagnosis of conjunctivitis. The poor correlation between the clinical and laboratory diagnoses of bacterial (and viral) conjunctivitis should make us less dogmatic about the clinical manifestations that we have considered to be specific for a given type of conjunctivitis.

**TABLE 2.   Signs and Symptoms of Bacterial Conjunctivitis**

| SIGNS | SYMPTOMS |
| --- | --- |
| Preauricular node | Burning |
| Purulent discharge | Itching |
| Matted eyelashes | Pain |
| Conjunctival injection | Foreign body sensation |
| Eyelid disease | Photophobia |
| Subconjunctival hemorrhage | Tearing |

## THERAPY

The time-honored treatment of conjunctivitis has been the instillation of topical antibiotic drops four times a day. The reason this regimen was chosen is not clear because there is good evidence that this frequency of medication does nothing to the normal conjunctival flora (Binder et al., 1975; Binder and Worthen, 1976; Leibowitz et al., 1976b). In fact, it is almost impossible to sterilize the conjunctival sac under ideal conditions, and the normal flora return after topical therapy is discontinued.

While it is clear that this regimen of antibiotic drops decreases the signs and symptoms of conjunctivitis when compared with placebo artificial tears, it is not clear why topical steroids or a steroid in combination with an antibiotic are even better at decreasing the signs and symptoms of conjunctivitis (Leibowitz et al., 1976b). In spite of these findings, steroids should never be used in the routine treatment of "conjunctivitis" because they predispose patients to cataracts and glaucoma and potentiate infections of the cornea with herpes simplex virus.

The recommended treatment of conjunctivitis (bacterial or viral) is the application of topical antibiotic drops at least six times a day because four times per day has no effect on the conjunctival flora (Binder et al., 1975; Binder and Worthen, 1976). The application of a hot pack over the closed eyelids after the use of eye drops makes the patient more comfortable but usually does not affect the course of the disease. An antibiotic that is not allergenic or toxic is the best choice, and most ophthalmologists recommend chloramphenicol or sulfacetamide as the drug of first choice. Neomycin-containing drops are highly allergenic, and like other aminoglycosides such as gentamicin are toxic to the epithelium of the cornea when used frequently.

The drops are continued for about 48 hours after signs and symptoms are gone. If a patient has not improved after 48 hours and has been using the drops appropriately, it is possible there is an underlying problem such as infection of the lacrimal system, the eyelid, or the cornea. Alternatively, the original diagnosis of conjunctivitis may have been incorrect, and the patient may have iritis or glaucoma. The most likely cause of conjunctivitis persisting beyond 48 hours of proper therapy is an adenovirus infection that may last two to three weeks. In case of doubt, it is best to refer the patient to an ophthalmologist.

Gonococcal conjunctivitis must be treated immediately. All patients should be hospitalized, and the purulent drainage cultured on Thayer-Martin media or chocolate agar. Topical penicillin G drops, prepared by diluting the parenteral preparation to 10,000 units per ml, should be instilled hourly. Hourly 30 per cent sulfacetamide may be substituted. Systemic penicillin (50,000 U per kg per day I.V. in two doses), topical atropine, and very frequent irrigation of the eyes are also mandatory.

# BACTERIAL CORNEAL ULCERS

## ETIOLOGY

The normal eye has very effective defenses against infection. The eyelids and lashes prevent foreign debris from striking the eye. The lashes wash the tears across the cornea and cleanse the eyes. Tears also contain secretory immunoglobulins and lysozymes that help prevent infection. The corneal epithelium and the underlying strong band of collagenous tissue (Bowman's layer) act as strong barriers to infection and injury by foreign bodies. The eye becomes susceptible to infection only when these defense mechanisms are altered.

Most bacterial ulcers occur after trauma to the cornea disrupts the epithelium. A mild injury such as a fingernail scratch or a glancing blow from a tree branch or a moderately severe injury such as a foreign body can disrupt the epithelium of the cornea, which permits bacterial colonization. In most instances of mild trauma, the eye heals without complications, but this type of mild trauma may proceed to frank abscess formation in a few cases.

In the presence of predisposing factors such as concomitant eyelid infection (blepharitis or dacryocystitis), decreased corneal sensation due to a fifth nerve lesion (neurotrophic keratitis), or decreased tear film (keratoconjunctivitis sicca), even very mild trauma can produce ulceration.

Contaminated ocular solutions, contaminated makeup (Wilson and Ahern, 1977), or contaminated soft or hard contact lenses also promote the progression of an ulcerative process (Krachmer and Purcell, 1978). Topical anesthetics or steroids severely increase the risk of infection and should not be prescribed. Only those organisms capable of epithelial colonization and penetration can produce spontaneous infections (*Neisseria gonorrhoeae, Corynebacterium diphtheria,* and Koch-Weeks bacillus).

## PATHOGENESIS, CLINICAL MANIFESTATIONS, AND DIAGNOSIS

Once the organisms penetrate the corneal stroma, they can proliferate freely. They may spread either into superficial areas or into the deep stroma. In the past, ophthalmologists attempted to identify the infecting organism by the morphology of the corneal abscess and the location of the abscess. It is true that some bacteria such as the pneumococcus and *Pseudomonas* produce fairly typical ulcerations, but the accepted and superior practice is to scrape and culture the abscesses in order to obtain a definitive diagnosis. Too much emphasis has been placed on the clinical morphology of the abscess.

All corneal ulcer cases must be cultured, and most should be admitted to the hospital. Neurotrophic keratitis, herpes simplex keratitis, and corneal transplant rejections can present with findings similar to bacterial corneal abscesses. It is very important to make the correct diagnosis because these diseases require different therapy.

Injury to the cornea causes the sensation of a foreign body because the corneal nerves are exposed. An interruption of the normally smooth optical surface also produces a dispersion of light rays with the production of glare and photosensitivity. Any infection in the cornea is usually associated with pain and internal ocular inflammation (iritis). An inflamed iris and ciliary body produce severe pain when they are moved, as occurs when light is shined into the eye. Increased opacity in the corneal stroma also decreases vision. In summary, patients with corneal ulcers experience pain, the sensation of a foreign body, photophobia, and decreased vision.

The hallmark of bacterial corneal ulceration is pus. The stroma, which is normally crystal clear, becomes opaque and the surface irregular. An overlying epithelial defect is almost always present. The underlying stroma becomes soft and mushy and is often discolored to a white, yellow, or brown color (Fig. 8). The stromal abscess may be single or interconnected with other smaller abscesses. The ulcer is usually located near the center of the cornea. A similar abscess in the periphery of the cornea is usually associated with a specific organism such as *Staphylococcus aureus, Haemophilus aegypticus,* or *Moraxella lacunata,* but cultures and scrapings must always be performed.

Bacterial ulceration produces pus on the surface of the cornea, the conjunctiva, and the lid

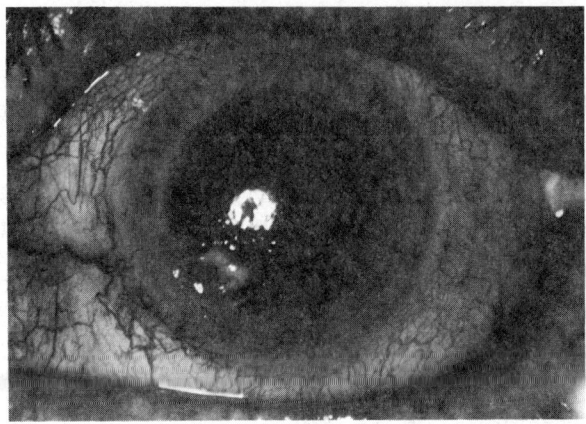

**FIGURE 8.** Staphylococcus aureus *corneal ulcer in a 65-year-old man with rheumatoid arthritis and mild dry eyes. The patient had been treated with topical steroids for two months before the infection.*

margins, which causes matted eyelashes (Fig. 9). As the corneal abscess enlarges, the cornea swells and becomes opaque in areas adjacent to the ulcerative process, and folds are produced in the back layer of the cornea (Descemet's membrane) that appear as white lines.

Increased ocular inflammation produces pus in the anterior chamber (hypopyon), which appears as a yellow to white layer in the inferior part of the anterior chamber (Fig. 10). This severe intraocular inflammation causes constriction of the pupil (miosis), which fails to dilate even in a dark room. With advanced infection, the lens may become opaque (cataract), the entire eye may become infected, or the cornea may perforate. The conjunctiva is always severely injected and is usually edematous. The lids are red and may be swollen. All of these signs depend on the duration of the infection, the pathogenicity of the orga-

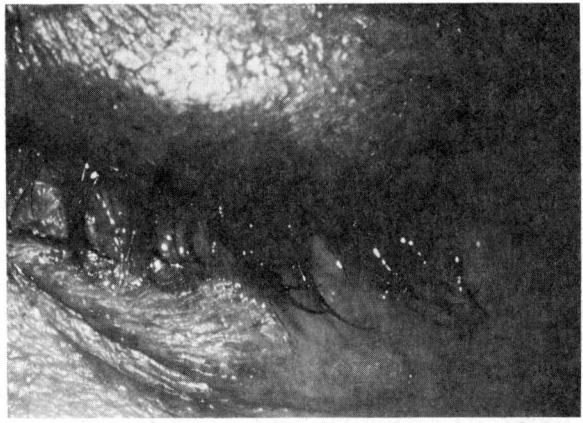

**FIGURE 9.** *Matted eyelashes in a case of a bacterial corneal ulceration.*

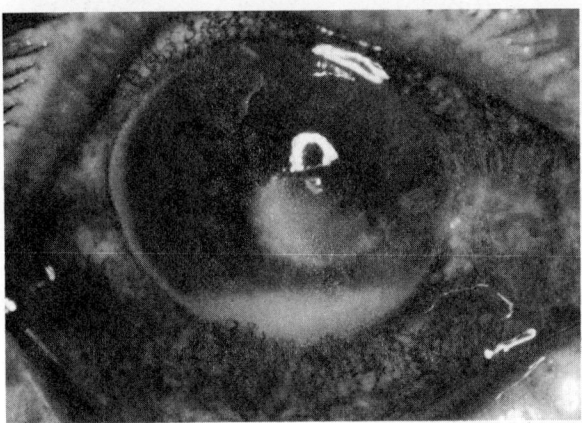

**FIGURE 10.** *This* Moraxella lacunata *ulcer occurred one week after a "scratch" to the eye of a 45-year-old chronic alcoholic.*

nism, previous antibiotic therapy, and predisposing factors such as topical steroid therapy.

A history of a foreign body injury with the associated signs and symptoms described above is usually indicative of bacterial ulceration, but patients with viral corneal ulceration, neurotrophic keratitis, or recent corneal transplantation may have similar clinical findings. In order to establish a specific diagnosis, all corneal ulcers must be carefully examined and cultured.

Because very few organisms can be obtained by scraping the cornea, it is important to make smears for Gram, Giemsa, potassium hydroxide, and acid-fast stains and to plate the cultures directly from the spatula that is used to scrape the cornea (Jones, 1980). Because this procedure is technically difficult and because the area of tissue to be scraped is small, the procedure is usually performed under magnification with a slit-lamp microscope by an ophthalmologist. Diagnostic paracentesis of the anterior chamber is necessary only in severely advanced cases with deep stromal abscesses.

The most common bacteria cultured from bacterial corneal ulcers are *S. pneumonia, S. aureus, Pseudomonas,* and *Moraxella,* but almost every bacterium has been isolated from corneal ulcerations. More and more so-called nonpathogens have been isolated as opportunists from eyes of patients with decreased cell-mediated immunity or after treatment with corticosteroids.

### TREATMENT

Bacterial corneal ulcers may be treated topically with frequent instillation of antibiotic drops and systemic or periocular injections of antibiotics. The antibiotic is selected on the basis of the Gram stain and modified according to the results of the cultures. When no organisms are seen in the Gram stain, one must assume that the ulcer is caused by a penicillin-resistant staphylococcus or *Pseudomonas aeruginosa* until proved otherwise (Jones, 1980). This decision is based on the fact that more than 50 per cent of *S. aureus* isolated from corneal ulcers produce penicillinase and that *Pseudomonas* ulcers are so virulent that they can perforate a cornea in one day if not treated promptly and appropriately.

The topical treatment of choice for Pseudomonas is 0.3 per cent gentamicin drops. *Staphylococcus aureus* infections may be treated with chloramphenicol (1.0 g orally every six hours) or with 200 mg per kg per day I.V. of a penicillinase-resistant penicillin. *Pseudomonas aeruginosa* ulcers can be treated with 2.5 g of carbenicillin I.V. every two hours. The dose and circumstances under which subtenon's gentamicin is given are described below.

Topical antibiotic drops should be applied hourly around the clock until the signs and symptoms abate and should be continued a minimum of six times a day for at least seven to ten days after the corneal ulcer completely resolves. If therapy is discontinued prematurely, especially for *Pseudomonas* ulcers, the keratitis may relapse or become exacerbate. In cases of superficial ulceration, topical therapy may be all that is necessary. In very severe cases of ulceration, it may be necessary to use a continuous antibiotic irrigation system in which a special plastic contact lens is attached to an intravenous infusion bottle containing antibiotics.

Periocular injections of antibiotics are also used in modern therapy. These injections are made underneath the conjunctiva or under the deep fibrofatty capsule that surrounds the globe (Tenon's capsule). Most ophthalmologists prefer a sub-

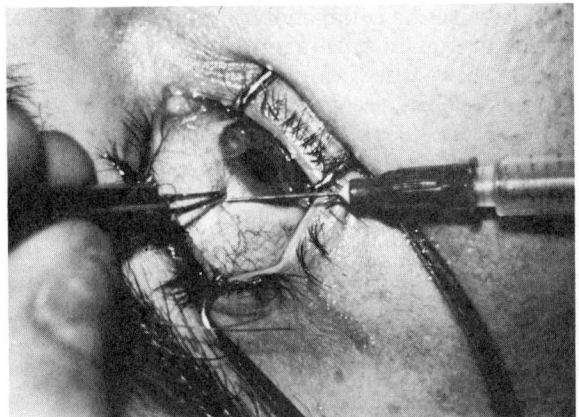

**FIGURE 11.** *Example of a subconjunctival injection of antibiotics with a 25-gauge needle and topical cocaine anesthesia. About 1½ ml of antibiotic can be injected at one time.*

tenon's injection with a 25-gauge needle (Fig. 11) under topical anesthesia, although there is some evidence that higher aqueous levels of antibiotics may be obtained by subconjunctival injection (Patterson, 1973). It is clear that periocular injection provides higher levels of antibiotics in the ocular tissue and fluid than those obtained with intravenous or intramuscular injection (Baum, 1977). Recommended dosages of subconjunctival and subtenon's injections have been published and are presently in use (Jones, 1980; Baum, 1977). Gentamicin (60 mg by subtenon's injection or 20 mg by subconjunctival injection) is effective treatment for staphylococcal and *Pseudomonas* corneal ulcers.

The periocular injection is repeated daily until the signs of infection decrease. The frequency of repeated injections is limited primarily by discomfort to the patient and by the condition of the periocular tissues. Since this mode of therapy produces measurable blood levels of antibiotics, renal function should be evaluated during repeated therapy with nephrotoxic drugs.

Intravenous and intramuscular routes of therapy were in vogue until periocular injections were used. Systemic therapy provides acceptable ocular fluid levels of antibiotics in inflamed eyes but not as high as those obtained with periocular injection (Baum, 1977). Intraocular injections are not performed in the routine treatment of most bacterial corneal ulcers, but may be the therapy of choice for endophthalmitis (Peyman, 1977).

In addition to antibiotic therapy, patients with corneal ulcers are treated with medications that dilate the pupil and paralyze the ciliary body. These parasympatholytic (cycloplegic) agents such as atropine (red-topped bottles) help to decrease the discomfort of ciliary spasm caused by iritis and help prevent glaucoma secondary to fibrin adhesion of the iris and lens. In some cases of *Pseudomonas* ulceration, it may be necessary to neutralize the collagenolytic enzymes produced by this organism with agents such as 0.01 M disodium ethylenediaminotetraacetate (EDTA). Steroids are not recommended in the early treatment of corneal ulcers. Studies have shown that steroids aggravate existing cases of corneal ulcers and cause exacerbations or relapses of *Pseudomonas* keratitis (Burns, 1969).

The following parameters should be specifically measured in patients with bacterial corneal ulcers before beginning antibacterial therapy and daily during the entire course of treatment: best obtainable visual acuity, size of corneal abscess, size of corneal epithelial defect, height of a hypopyon, and pupillary diameter. Measurements are made with a light beam ruler on the slit-lamp

microscope. All of the findings decrease as the infection improves except the pupil size, which becomes larger (assuming the patient is being treated with daily cycloplegic agents). The medications are tapered as the signs and symptoms improve. Any underlying disease or abnormality is treated concurrently. Medications are continued for several days after the abscess has resolved.

Some patients recover good visual acuity, but most are left with a corneal opacity which may interfere with vision. When the opacity is severe, a corneal transplant (Fig. 12) and a cataract extraction are required. Any underlying disease process or predisposing factor should be eliminated and the patient instructed to return if inflammation recurs after treatment is discontinued.

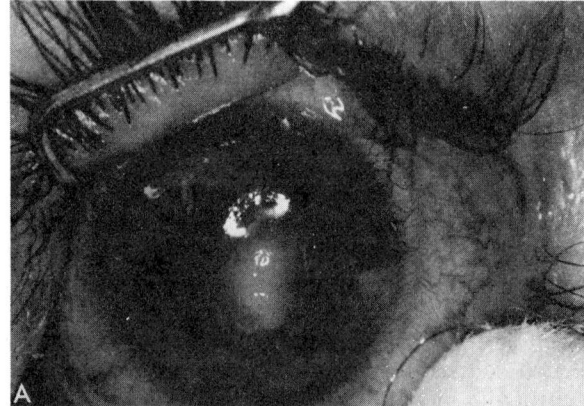
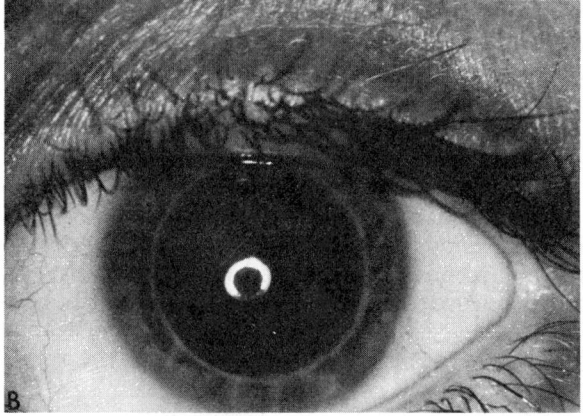

**FIGURE 12.** A, *Six-year-old boy with an allergic conjunctivitis which was treated with steroids. He developed a Staphylococcus aureus infection and required general anesthesia for a subconjunctival injection of antibiotics (11/18/76). B, This patient underwent a corneal transplant in December, 1976, because of corneal scarring and finger counting vision. His vision with glasses after surgery is 20/30 (5/2/80).*

## References

Baum, J. L.: Antibiotic administration in the treatment of bacterial endophthalmitis. I. Periocular injections. Surv Ophthalmol 21:332, 1977.

Binder, P. S., Abel, R. A., Jr., and Kaufman, H. E.: The effect of chronic administration of a topical antibiotic on the conjunctival flora. Ann Ophthalmol 7:1429, 1975.

Binder, P. S., and Worthen, D. M.: A continuous-wear hydrophilic lens. Prophylactic topical antibiotics. Arch Ophthalmol 94:2109, 1976.

Burns, R. P.: *Pseudomonas aeruginosa* keratitis: Mixed infections of the eye. Am J Ophthalmol 67:257, 1969.

Chandler, J. W., and Milam, D. F.: Diphtheria corneal ulcers. Arch Ophthalmol 96:53, 1978.

Frederick, J., and Braude, A. I.: Anaerobic infections of the paranasal sinuses. N Engl J Med 290:1177, 1974.

Gombos, G. M.: Handbook of Ophthalmologic Emergencies. Medical Examination Publishing Company, Inc., 1973, p. 55.

Jones, D. B.: Strategy for the initial management of suspected microbial keratitis. In Symposium on Medical and Surgical Diseases of the Cornea. C. V. Mosby Co. St. Louis, Mo. 1980, p. 86.

Krachmer, J. H., and Purcell, J. J., Jr.: Bacterial corneal ulcers in cosmetic soft contact lens wearers. Arch Ophthalmol 96:57, 1978.

Leibowitz, H. M., Pratt, M. V., Flagstad, I. J., Berrospi, A. R., and Kundsin, R.: Human conjunctivitis. I. Diagnostic evaluation. Arch Ophthalmol 94:1747, 1976a.

Leibowitz, H. M., Pratt, M. V., Flagstad, I. J., Berrospi, A. R., and Kundsin, R.: Human conjunctivitis. II. Treatment. Arch Ophthalmol 94:1752, 1976b.

Locatcher-Khorazo, D., and Seegal, B. C.: The bacterial flora of the healthy eye. In Microbiology of the Eye. St. Louis, C. V. Mosby Company, 1972, p. 13.

Patterson, C. A.: Intraocular penetration of C$^{14}$-labelled penicillin after subtenons or subconjunctival injection. Ann Ophthalmol 5:17, 1973.

Perkins, R. E., Kundsin, R. B., Pratt, M. V., Abrahamsen, I., and Leibowitz, H. M.: Bacteriology of normal and infected conjunctiva. J Clin Microbiol 1:147, 1975.

Peyman, G. A.: Antibiotic administration in the treatment of bacterial endophthalmitis. II. Intravitreal injections. Surv Ophthalmol 21:331, 1977.

Smolin, G., and Okumoto, M.: Staphylococcal blepharitis. Arch Ophthalmol 95:812, 1977.

Trevor-Roper, P. D.: Diseases of the Orbit. Int Ophthalmol Clin 14:323, 1974.

Wilson, L. A., and Ahern, D. G.: Pseudomonas-induced corneal ulcers associated with contaminated eye mascaras. Am J Ophthalmol 84:112, 1977.

# *VIRAL* **232**
# *KERATOCONJUNCTIVITIS*

*Herbert E. Kaufman, M.D.*

## *HERPES SIMPLEX*

In the United States and Europe, herpes simplex infection is the most common corneal infection and the most important ocular virus disease from the point of view of morbidity and mortality. Its importance stems not only from the frequency of initial attacks, but from its likelihood of recurrences with progressive scarring and morbidity, and also from the fact that this is one of the few virus diseases that may be successfully treated with chemotherapeutic agents.

### Clinical Manifestations

#### Primary Herpes Simplex

Primary herpes simplex most commonly occurs between the ages of six months and five years (Duke-Elder, 1965). In its classic form it involves not only the eyes, but also areas of skin, most commonly the face. In children with eczema, the primary infection with herpes simplex can be an acute disseminated infection with a generalized rash as well as necrotic lesions of the liver and other organs, and encephalitis (Kaposi's varicelliform eruption). The mortality in this type of infection may be as high as 50 per cent. Most commonly, primary herpes simplex is associated with blisters over the face and lips, sometimes lesions elsewhere on the body. With this there may be an acute keratoconjunctivitis, and sometimes an involvement of the cornea, with preauricular lymphadenopathy and fever. The very severe form of the disease is rare, and by the age of 15 years up to 90 per cent of people may have antibodies indicating previous infection by herpes simplex, but most of these have had no clinical manifestations of disease. It is clear, therefore, that the most common type of ocular infection with herpes simplex is the so-called recurrent, or secondary, herpes simplex which develops in the presence of circulating antibodies even though there may be no history of previous infection.

### Dendritic Keratitis

As virus infection begins in the cornea, small punctate epithelial spots or tiny vacuoles may appear in the corneal epithelium. As the disease progresses, these rapidly coalesce to form the familiar, branching dendritic figure (Fig. 1). Although corneal sensation may be lost early in infection with herpes simplex, in our experience this has not been an invariable sign of herpes simplex infection.

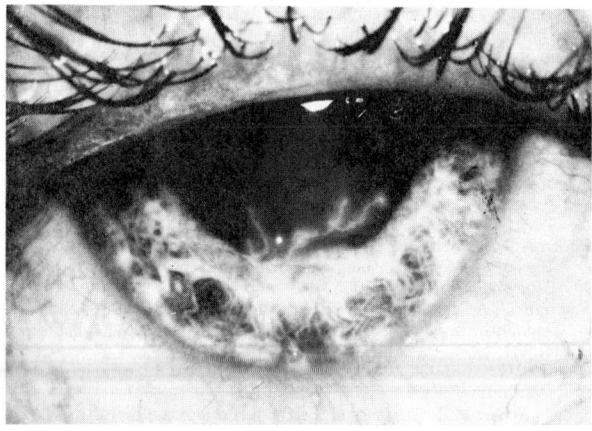

**FIGURE 1.** *Typical dendritic lesion caused by herpes simplex infection of the superficial cornea. Stained with fluorescein.*

The symptomatology of herpetic infection varies widely in patients of different age groups. In older adults this disease tends to be relatively asymptomatic, in that the eye is not red and pain is not severe. In children and even in young adults, this is not the case. In children, herpes simplex is one of the most common causes of the red, sore, painful eye. In a young child, a red eye with pain and photophobia and the absence of obvious conjunctivitis should suggest herpes simplex infection until proven otherwise. Especially in infants and young children, the morphology of the corneal infection loses its dendritic character and large areas of the cornea appear to be involved by ulceration and vascularization in a process whose etiology frequently is not apparent until virus cultures are done. The reason for this apparent pleomorphism may be that infants come to an ophthalmologist only later in the course of the disease. Pleomorphism is a common clinical finding.

In the early dendritic ulcer, and in the dendritic ulcer with some stromal involvement beneath it, multiplying virus is generally present in the cornea. When virus cultures are done on such patients, most are positive, and virus multiplication appears responsible for the tissue damage. If corticosteroids are used inadvertently on dendritic ulcers, the ulcers usually extend and invade the stroma and the cornea may perforate. The typical adult with epithelial herpes simplex complains only of a foreign body sensation, and may have little redness and reaction around the eye. The physician should be especially alert to the patient who complains of a foreign body sensation of the cornea without a clear history of having been struck in the eye by a foreign body. The patient, for example, who awakens with a foreign body sensation would be most likely to have some primary corneal disease rather than a true foreign body injury, since any epithelial damage is felt as a foreign body injury.

### Stromal Herpes

The original epithelial defect, if left untreated, may progress to a much larger map-like lesion, and may invade the stroma. The involvement of the corneal stroma seems to take three clinically different forms which are treated differently:

1. Stromal ulceration may occur with direct invasion of the stroma and is facilitated by the inadvertent administration of corticosteroids.

2. In the absence of ulceration, however, virus may also directly invade the stroma causing a cheesy white infiltrate with iritis that is difficult to treat.

3. A third type of stromal involvement probably does not represent direct viral invasion, but may represent a true hypersensitivity reaction. This hypersensitivity disease can be mimicked by injecting sensitized animals with dead herpes antigen, and is seen in infected animals who have previously been sensitized to the virus. It consists primarily of a round patch of corneal edema (disciform edema) and, like many types of hypersensitivity reaction, responds rapidly to very small doses of topical corticosteroid (Fig. 2).

Stromal herpes may also be accompanied by severe iritis, which may persist for long periods of time and usually is amenable to corticosteroid treatment with coverage by an antiviral agent. Herpetic retinitis has been seen in a few neonatal cases of disseminated herpes but is rare.

### Recurrent Herpes Simplex

In the eye, recurrent herpes simplex causes much greater morbidity than on the lips and else-

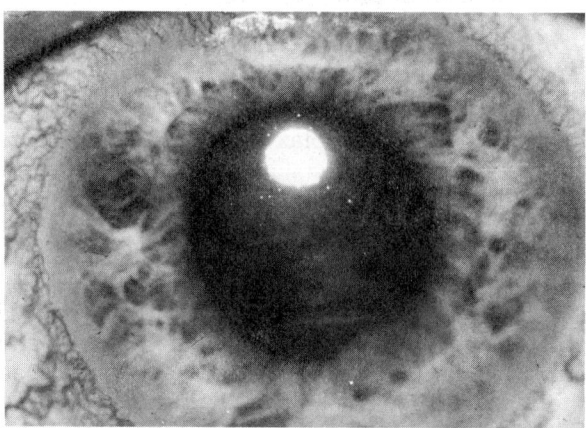

**FIGURE 2.** *Patch of corneal edema with folds in Descemet's membrane caused by hypersensitivity to herpes virus.*

where. The progressive scarring of the cornea makes it one of our most serious clinical problems. The chance for recurrence after a first attack of herpes is almost 25 per cent within two years. After two or more attacks the chances are approximately 43 per cent of a recurrence within two years.

Patients with recurrent herpes, as well as some who remain asymptomatic, intermittently excrete virus in the tears and in the saliva for months or even years. There is some possibility that herpes simplex virus also may remain latent in the trigeminal ganglion, but the relationship of this to recurrent ocular disease is unclear.

The mechanisms by which recurrences occur are uncertain, but most patients with recurrent herpes have high stable levels of neutralizing antibody in their blood before their recurrences. Similarly, no definite correlation with local IgA secretory antibody has been found, although we have found that such antibody to herpes virus is produced in the eye.

### Therapy of Herpes Simplex

Two basic groups of herpes simplex virus are known to infect man, Type I and Type II. Type I is generally responsible for recurrent disease of the eye, lips, and face, whereas Type II is associated primarily with genital infections, has a reservoir in the male genitourinary tract, and may occasionally cause keratitis in infants. Most therapeutic studies have been done with Type I virus, which seems slightly more susceptible to chemotherapy than Type II.

IDU (iodo-deoxyuridine) has been proved by several controlled studies to be effective in the treatment of corneal herpes. It is used either as drops or as ointment, and has been valuable over the years for the control of epithelial disease in which multiplying virus plays a prominent part. On hypersensitivity-like disciform edema of the cornea it has no apparent effect, since multiplying virus is of little importance. Corticosteroids can reactivate local herpes and make local herpes infection worse, and clinical studies indicate that the addition of IDU to corticosteroids greatly increases the safety of this drug. Even with antivirals, however, corticosteroids should be used carefully and in minimal quantities.

In some recurrent ulcers, the problem is not direct reinvasion by herpes virus giving a new dendritic lesion, but rather an erosion of the epithelium. In these erosions, the epithelium does not attach well to its basement membrane because of previous basement membrane damage, and is peeled off by the motion of the lids. This recurrent-erosion type of ulcer is not caused by multiplying virus, does not have the irregular dendritic projections of its margins, and must be recognized and treated by patching and other techniques that favor epithelial healing rather than by frequent administration of antiviral compounds that do not help in the absence of multiplying virus.

IDU, although valuable over the years, is not an ideal antiviral drug. It is relatively insoluble, causes some cases of allergies, produces resistant virus in tissue culture and rarely in man, and has been shown in our laboratory to be teratogenic in rabbits, although no such problem has been seen in other species. Newer, superior drugs have been developed. The primary among these is trifluorothymidine, which is far more effective than IDU or adenine arabinoside for topical administration. For deep keratitis and herpes iritis intravenous adenine arabinoside with high systemic antiviral activity but very low toxicity has been shown to be effective.

The prevention of recurrent herpes also may be possible through the use of interferon. Interferon inducers such as Poly I:C and tilorone were studied extensively and found to be very effective in rabbits and other rodents. In monkeys and man, however, these interferon inducers seem to have only a minimal effect that disappears rapidly. This would suggest that they will not be clinically useful. Human interferon, on the other hand, effectively prevents herpes infection in monkeys, even when given as drops as seldom as twice a day. Studies are in progress in humans to determine whether recurrent herpes is preventable.

## ADENOVIRUS INFECTION

Infection due to adenovirus is fairly common in the United States and can be more serious than many physicians realize. Many syndromes are presently associated with adenovirus infection. For example, types 1, 2, and 5 can cause a febrile disease in young children, and this can be accompanied by gastrointestinal symptoms. Types 3, 4, and 7 cause pharyngoconjunctival fever or an acute respiratory disease. Types 2, 3, 4, 5, 6, 7, 8, and 9, as well as others, can be associated with a simple conjunctivitis. Most of the epidemic keratoconjunctivitis, however, appears due to type 8, although cases caused by types 3, 7, 19, and 22 have also been reported. In spite of the large number of types, all of these agents, except the avian adenoviruses, share a specific complement-fixing antigen and produce generally similar cytopathogenic changes in tissue culture.

### Ocular Manifestations of Adenovirus Infection

A simple, mild follicular conjunctivitis is associated with many types of adenovirus infection.

Often, this is unilateral, and associated with pharyngitis, lymphadenopathy (usually either preauricular or submaxillary), and severe gastrointestinal symptoms, coryza, or even meningismus. Similarly, conjunctivitis due to adenovirus is sometimes acquired through swimming pool contacts, without either apparent systemic manifestations or enlargement of the preauricular or submaxillary nodes. In most cases the conjunctivitis is mild, but in epidemic keratoconjunctivitis it can be severe and disabling (Duke-Elder, 1965; and Kaufman, 1964).

Epidemic keratoconjunctivitis (EKC) is most commonly caused by adenovirus type 8, and is rarely associated with systemic symptoms of fever, nausea, vomiting, and adenopathy. The conjunctivitis is sometimes mild, but may be so severe as to cause petechiae and bleeding into the conjunctiva and even pseudomembrane formation. EKC tends to be bilateral, although unilateral cases sometimes occur. It is common for one eye to be more severely involved than the other. During the acute phase of adenovirus infection, symptoms may be severe. Pain, redness of the eye, and severe photophobia often are present and, on some occasions, the symptoms are so severe that patients are too uncomfortable to read; some even require hospitalization. The keratitis of this disease usually begins within two weeks after the onset of symptoms of conjunctivitis but may be more delayed. In the initial phases it is common to see subepithelial corneal infiltrates that are small, round translucent infiltrates varying widely in their distribution and number (Fig. 3). During the initial formation of the subepithelial infiltrates, tiny pits in the epithelium, which stain with fluorescein, sometimes occur over the infiltrates. The *acute* phase of EKC usually lasts from four to six weeks. After this time, however, although symptoms of conjunctivitis and epithe-

lial pits may disappear, the subepithelial infiltrates may persist for years.

The presently available antiviral agents have not been shown to be effective in adenovirus infection, but, occasionally, if the disease is severe and there is significant iritis, corticosteroids may give some symptomatic benefit. In addition, corticosteroids seem to temporarily make the subepithelial infiltrates smaller and may be of limited use when these infiltrates are central and reduce vision.

*The most important fact about EKC is that it is frequently spread by the general physician or ophthalmologist through unwashed hands or unsterile tonometers.*

## VACCINIA

Vaccinia keratitis is uncommon, but can be devastating. In many ways, although not recurrent, the acute infection is similar to herpes simplex keratitis, and may even produce dendritic lesions. Its morphology can be similar to that of herpes simplex, and the problems of treating it are similar. Very frequently, a vaccinated patient will present with vesicles on the upper lid and some swelling of the lid which may be severe and diffuse. In such patients it is always important to ask about a history of previous vaccination both of the patient and of members of the family.

Although many patients with lid lesions who do not have definite corneal involvement will remain free of direct ocular involvement, IDU and the other agents active against ocular DNA viruses are also effective against vaccinia. Many physicians prefers to instill IDU into the eye several times a day to minimize the likelihood of corneal infection. Immune globulin and other forms of treatment have not been found to be effective in the treatment of ocular vaccinia.

## VARICELLA-ZOSTER

Primary infection of the eye in patients with chickenpox can occur with lid lesions, a red elevated "pock" on the conjunctiva, or direct infection of the cornea with scarring of the corneal stroma. This is relatively uncommon, however.

Involvement of the first division of the fifth nerve, however, is much more likely to involve the eye, since the cornea is innervated by the nasociliary branch of the first division of the trigeminal nerve. This branch innervates both the eye and the tip of the nose and when the tip of the nose is involved with herpetic vesicles, eye involvement is relatively common and should be suspected (Fig. 4).

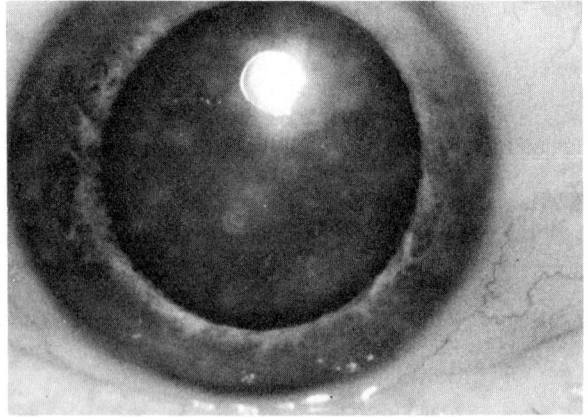

**FIGURE 3.** *Subepithelial infiltrates of the cornea caused by adenovirus.*

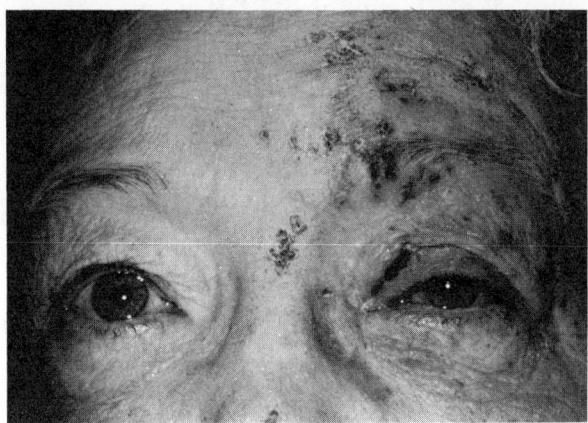

**FIGURE 4.** *Herpes zoster involvement of face and nose.*

The eye is involved as a severe iridocyclitis that lasts for months or even years. In zoster the cornea may be denervated and the eye dry. It is common to see serious corneal disease. It may be treated with cycloplegics and mydriatics to dilate the pupil and prevent the formation of iris adhesions; corticosteroid therapy may be necessary. In addition to the iritis, primary involvement of the cornea may cause corneal ulcers (dendritic ulcers) and, less commonly dense white corneal scarring. In addition, optic neuritis, ophthalmoplegia, and pupillary paralysis have all been observed after herpes zoster, and ocular motor paralyses should be recognized as a rare but definite part of this syndrome.

The treatment of ophthalmic zoster with specific antivirals is in its infancy, but systemic ad-

enine arabinoside may prove to be useful. In England, high concentrations of IDU in dimethyl-sulfoxide are used topically on the skin with apparent good success.

### OTHER VIRUSES

Virtually all the exanthems can produce a mild conjunctivitis and even keratitis with punctate stippling of the cornea. The condition in which this is most common is measles, where the keratitis and mild iritis may make it desirable to reduce the light level for the patient for the purposes of comfort. In North America and Europe, severe corneal disease from these infections is rare and the ocular irritation is generally transient, but in parts of Africa, measles can produce severe corneal scarring and blindness.

On occasions, systemic infection with a variety of viruses can also produce an iritis and a disturbance of the pigment epithelium of the eye as well as optic neuritis. Although the frequency and importance of viral uveitis is uncertain, viruses may be an important cause of nonspecific iridocyclitis. Placoid pigmentery epitheliopathy, a transient depigmenting choroiditis that does not cause permanent visual loss, occurs after viral upper respiratory infections.

### References

Duke-Elder, S.: System of Ophthalmology. Vol. 8, p. 310. St. Louis, C. V. Mosby Co., 1965.
Kaufman, H. E.: Viral diseases. Int Ophthalmol Clin, 4:267, 1964.

# OCULAR FUNGAL, PARASITIC, CHLAMYDIAL, AND RICKETTSIAL INFECTIONS

## 233

*Perry S. Binder, M.D., F.A.C.S.*

## OCULAR FUNGAL INFECTIONS

### ORBITAL FUNGAL INFECTIONS

#### Etiology

The most common causes of orbital fungal infections are the *Phycomycetes (Mucor* and *Rhi-*

*zopus)*, but almost any fungus can cause either primary or secondary infections of the orbit. These infections can be secondary to trauma (with or without retained foreign material), to immune suppression, and, most commonly, to spread from infected paranasal sinuses. There are also a few reports of spontaneous orbital infections in normal people without apparent antecedent sinus involvement (Schwartz et al., 1977).

### Clinical Manifestations

Most cases of cerebrorhinoorbital phycomycosis (CROP) occur in diabetics. Diabetics in good control may suddenly develop facial pain, sinusitis, and/or rhinitis, and become obtunded within hours. Alternatively, a diabetic who has just recovered from ketoacidosis may suddenly develop the same rapid progression of symptoms. Infected wounds or spontaneous infections of the skin about the orbit can also spread into the orbit. In addition to diabetes, acidosis in infancy, leukemia, and lymphomas also predispose patients to CROP.

The early orbital manifestations of CROP are similar to bacterial infections of the orbit and include a lid droop (ptosis), injection and edema of the lids and conjunctiva (chemosis), and proptosis. As the infection progresses, the lids become more involved and may become gangrenous. Because the *Phycomycetes* have a predilection for invasion of blood vessels, ischemic necrosis and infarction of all structures in the orbit and nose may occur. The extent of involvement can be more easily outlined when the necrotic areas are cleaned with hydrogen peroxide.

Involvement of the cranial nerves as they enter the orbital apex may produce extraocular muscle palsies, convulsions, hemiplegia, hemianesthesia, and death. This infection causes bilateral disease rarely and only after one side is severely affected. The patients are febrile, systemically ill, and have a peripheral leukocytosis.

### Diagnosis and Treatment

A diabetic who develops facial pain, sinusitis, and rhinitis with neurologic signs and symptoms fits easily into the diagnosis of CROP. Roentgenograms of the sinuses are usually abnormal and may show an air-fluid level. Portions of the palate and nose may be ischemic or necrotic. The best way to make the diagnosis is by examination of wet mounts, smears, histologic sections, and cultures of biopsies from the orbit, sinuses, or skin. Histologic examination of biopsy specimens demonstrates the organisms (nonseptate hyphae in the case of *Phycomycetes*), vascular thrombosis, coagulative necrosis, and gangrene.

Treatment includes the surgical removal of foreign bodies and necrotic tissue, control of the underlying disease process, and systemic antifungal therapy. Amphotericin B (0.7 to 1.0 mg/kg/day I.V.) is the treatment of choice for the phycomycoses. Sensitive *Candida* and other yeasts may be treated with 150 mg/kg/day of 5-fluorocytosine, which is well absorbed orally, in combination with a lower, nontoxic dose of amphotericin to suppress the emergence of 5-fc-resistant mutants (see Chapter 155). CROP causes a severe illness in immunosuppressed patients and has a mortality rate as high as 68 per cent (Schwartz et al., 1977).

## FUNGAL INFECTIONS OF THE EYELIDS AND OCULAR ADNEXA

Fungal infections of the eyelids are rare. They usually cause rashes, ulcers, granulomas, nodules, or verrucous lesions on the lid margin and surrounding skin. The diagnosis is made by scraping the lesion onto a glass slide, treating the scrapings on the slide with potassium hydroxide to eliminate the keratin, and examining the slide microscopically for mycelial elements. Another portion of the scrapings may be cultured for fungi. Treatment is by topical application of antifungal agents. The subject of fungal eyelid infections has been well reviewed recently (Ostler et al., 1978).

Fungal infection of the lacrimal system is much more common and is usually associated with a stone in the lacrimal sac (dacryolith) or an obstructed lacrimal drainage system (canaliculitis). *Candida albicans* is the most common organism associated with dacryoliths, but many other fungi and bacteria may be involved (Wolter, 1977). Canaliculitis is usually caused by bacteria. Actinomyces is the most common, but fusobacteria have also been reported (Weinberg et al., 1977).

Patients complain of unilateral tearing, conjunctivitis, or discharge. The eyelid or skin overlying the nasal lacrimal sac or canalicular system may be injected (Fig. 1), and solid lesions may be outlined when radiopaque dyes are injected into the canalicular system. In canaliculitis, firm con-

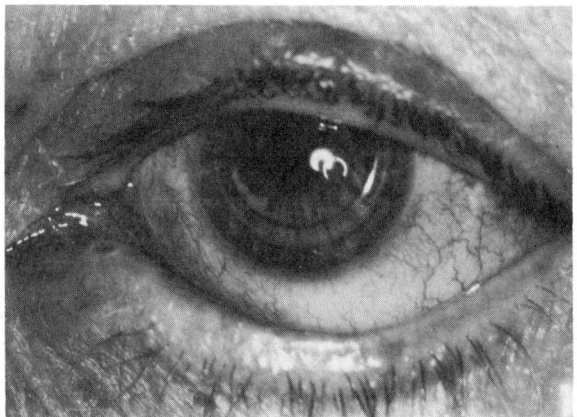

**FIGURE 1.** *Actinomyces canaliculitis. The punctum is swollen and the adjacent eyelid and conjunctiva are infected. (Eye infections with this branching, filamentous bacterium have traditionally been included with fungal eye infections.)*

cretions can be seen at the opening of the puncta. The dacryolith or canalicular obstruction should be removed and cultured and the canalicular system irrigated with penicillin diluted to 10,000 units per ml. Topical sulfacetamide drops should be used for treatment of *Actinomyces* and *Fusobacterium* canaliculitis. After removal of dacryoliths, *C. albicans* and other fungi should be treated with topical antifungal agents as described for fungal infections of the cornea.

## CONJUNCTIVAL FUNGAL INFECTION

### Etiology

Some fungi are normal inhabitants of the conjunctival sac and may be cultured from 2 to 20 per cent of normal eyes. After treatment of nonspecific inflammation with topical antibiotics or corticosteroids, fungi may be cultured from a much higher percentage. Most are nonpathogens and rarely produce ocular disease except in the immunodeficient or after severe ocular trauma.

### Diagnosis and Clinical Manifestations

Most fungal infections of the conjunctiva occur in a setting of chronic conjunctivitis that has not responded to antibiotic therapy, but in the early stages they can resemble almost any "conjunctivitis." Fungi can produce deep purulent lesions with ulcerating nodules, granulomatous lesions surrounding ulcers, pseudomembranes, or large polypoid growths. Follicular conjunctivitis with a palpable preauricular node is a rare manifestation of fungal infection. Skin lesions are usually present. Fungal infections should be considered in all cases of chronic conjunctivitis with or without concomitant skin disease that have not responded to standard therapy and in any conjunctivitis in a compromised host. The clinical manifestations of the most common causes of fungal conjunctivitis are listed in Table 1. The organisms may be identified by examination of conjunctival scrapings with potassium hydroxide, by

biopsy of the conjunctiva, and by cultures of the scrapings and biopsies on standard fungal media.

### Treatment

Predisposing factors, such as infection of the lacrimal system and chronic antibiotic and/or corticosteroid therapy, must be eliminated or discontinued. Eyelid lesions may be treated with the standard topical antifungal agents that are used to treat skin disease. Topical diluted amphotericin B, natamycin (pimaricin), or miconazole may also be used in the same doses used for fungal infections of the cornea. Surgical excision of large conjunctival lesions with cautery may accelerate healing. Systemic amphotericin B or oral 5–fluorocytosine may be useful in specific cases. Scarring usually follows resolution of the lesions and may cause the eye lashes to rub on the cornea (trichiasis).

## FUNGAL CORNEAL INFECTIONS

### Etiology

The normal cornea is rarely infected by fungi, but damage to the normal protective mechanisms permits fungal invasion. Patients who are predisposed to fungal corneal ulceration include those who have received topical corticosteroid therapy, immunosuppressed patients, and those with antecedent or concurrent bacterial ulceration or herpes simplex keratitis.

### Clinical Manifestations

Most patients have a history of antecedent ocular trauma, especially trauma due to plant material or to accidents that occur during outdoor activity. Many have received topical antibiotics or steroids before the diagnosis of fungal keratitis is made, but a significant proportion have not had antecedent trauma or therapy (Forster and Rebell, 1975a).

The patient complains of pain, photophobia, tearing, and decreased vision. The conjunctiva is

**TABLE 1.    Clinical Manifestations of Fungal Conjunctivitis[a]**

| | |
|---|---|
| *Sporothrix schenckii* | Ulcerating nodules, purulent discharge, lymphadenopathy |
| *Blastomyces* | Ulcer surrounded by granuloma, lymphadenopathy |
| *Coccidioides immitis* | Nodules, peripheral corneal vascularization |
| *Rhinosporidiosis* | Unilateral pink polypoid growths resembling granulomas; pus may be expressed from center of growth |
| *Candida albicans* | Pseudomembranous conjunctivitis |
| *Ringworm fungi* | Diffuse conjunctivitis |

[a]After Ostler, H. B., et al.: J Cont Ed Ophthalmol, Feb., 1978, p. 3.

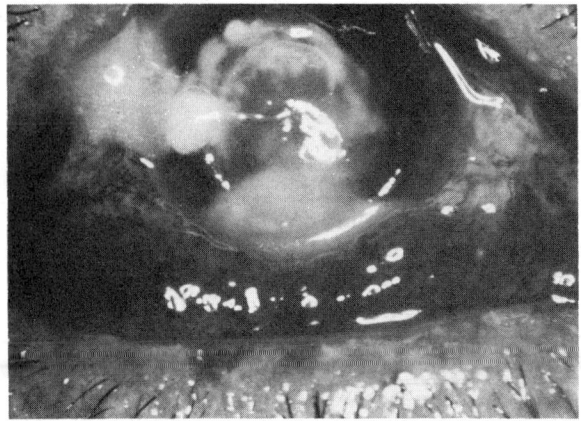

**FIGURE 2.** Aspergillus *ulcer after foreign body injury. Large clumps of leukocytes are adherent to the posterior corneal surface (plaques) above the ulcer. A fluffy hypopyon can be seen below.*

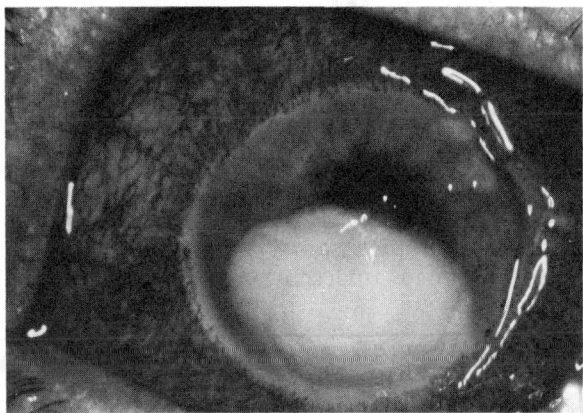

**FIGURE 3.** Candida *ulcer in a chronic diabetic. Only a small corneal abscess can be seen because of the very large hypopyon filling most of the anterior chamber.*

injected, and the eyelids are swollen. The corneal abscess may be accompanied by a hypopyon (Fig. 2). Mycelial fungi (molds) tend to produce a gray-white elevated lesion with a stromal abscess whose edges are "feathery." Satellite lesions are common. Lesions that are caused by yeasts are more yellow-white and tend to be single and focal. They resemble bacterial ulcers (Fig. 3). Occasionally, white blood cells adhere to the posterior surface of the stromal lesion in solid plaques (Fig. 2). An accurate clinical diagnosis cannot be made on the basis of the morphology of the lesion alone. The differential diagnosis includes chronic herpes simplex stromal keratitis and bacterial stromal abscess.

### Diagnosis

A fungal ulcer should be suspected in any patient who presents with a stromal corneal abscess and a history of foreign body trauma from plant material, a history of a chronic corneal ulcer that has not responded to standard therapy, or a history of antecedent treatment with corticosteroids. Fungal ulcers are also common in the immunosuppressed or after strokes that cause chronic corneal exposure.

The lesion is cultured in the same fashion as bacterial ulcers (Chapter 231) with a platinum spatula under microscopic control. Glass slides are prepared for a potassium hydroxide mount, Gram stain, Giemsa stain, acid-fast stain, and special stains for fungi such as the Gridley, periodic acid-Schiff (PAS), or Gomorri methenamine silver (GMS) stain. These stains supplement each other and increase the percentage of positive diagnoses (Polack, 1973). The scrapings are also directly streaked onto media appropriate for bacterial and fungal culture (Forster and Rebell, 1975a). If the index of suspicion is high and no organisms are seen on the slides, a biopsy of the edge of the lesion may reveal the fungi. It is rarely necessary to perform an anterior chamber paracentesis. The organisms most frequently cultured from keratomycoses are listed in Table 2.

### Treatment

The necrotic cornea is usually removed at the time of diagnostic scraping. The lesions are then treated with topical antifungal agents. The topical application of one of the polyene antibiotics such as amphotericin B or natamycin (pimaricin) either directly to the ulcer (amphotericin B or natamycin) or subconjunctivally (amphotericin B) is standard therapy. Topical and oral therapy

**TABLE 2.   Causes of Keratomycosis**

| COMMON | RARE |
| --- | --- |
| Fusarium | Tetraploa |
| Cephalosporium | Curvularia |
| Candida | Phialophora |
| Aspergillus | Nocardia[a] |
| Penicillium | |

[a]This filamentous, branching bacterium is included because the disease is similar to that caused by fungi.

**TABLE 3.   Medical Therapy for Keratomycosis**

| | |
|---|---|
| *Amphotericin B* | |
| Topical | 0.01 to 2.5 mg/ml, every two to three hours |
| Subconjunctival | 0.15 to 2.0 mg as necessary |
| *Natamycin* | 50 mg/ml topically every one to two hours |
| *5-Fluorocytosine* | |
| Topical | 10 to 15 mg/ml, every one to two hours |
| Oral | 50 to 150 mg/kg/day in four divided doses |

with 5-fluorocytosine is effective against *Candida, Cryptococcus,* and some strains of *Aspergillus* and *Penicillium* (Table 3). Newer agents with a broader antifungal spectrum that are less toxic to the eye include clotrimazole and miconazole. Amphotericin B or natamycin should be used until the responsible organism is identified (Table 3). Concomitant cycloplegics and antibiotics should also be given.

If the infection fails to respond to medical therapy, it is necessary to excise the superficial cornea and cover the infected cornea with conjunctiva (conjunctival flap). After the eye heals, a corneal transplant should be done. An emergency corneal transplant is only necessary for acute perforations in order to halt the disease process (Forster and Rebell, 1975b). Fungal ulcers rarely progress to endophthalmitis.

## INTRAOCULAR FUNGAL INFECTIONS

### Etiology

Fungi can be introduced into the interior of the eye through a corneal ulceration, by intraocular trauma with retained intraocular plant material, cataract surgery, or from metastatic spread (Fig. 4). The infection usually presents as a fulminant endophthalmitis. It should be treated with topical, subconjunctival, systemic, and intravitreal antifungal agents and by surgical removal of the foreign body and infected vitreous (vitrectomy) (Snip and Michaels, 1976). Rarely, the fungal infection presents as retinal and vitreal inflammation (Fig. 5) instead of a fulminating infection. The diagnosis and management of fungal endophthalmitis is discussed in Chapter 234.

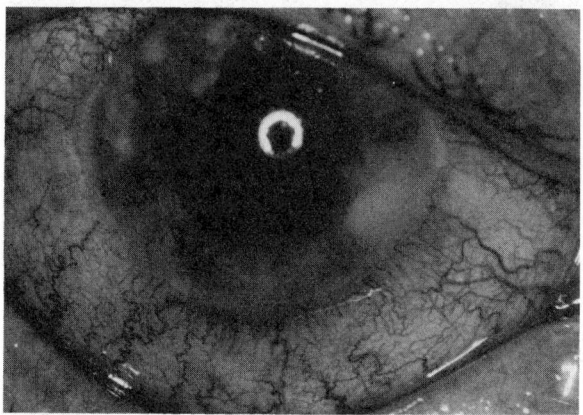

**FIGURE 4.**   *Large, elevated, white nodules scattered over the surface of the iris in a patient with disseminated coccidioidomycosis.*

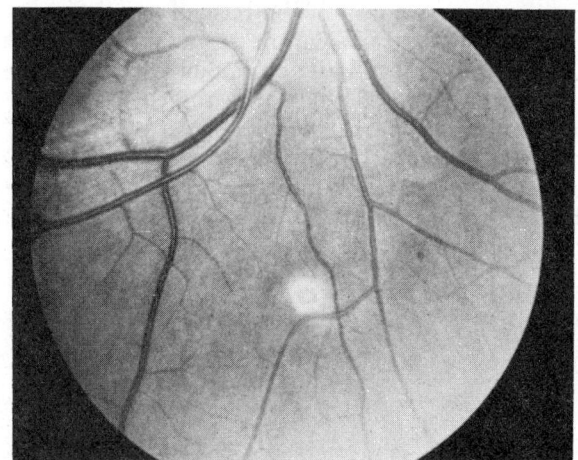

**FIGURE 5.**   *Isolated, focal, yellow-white retinal abscess in a patient with disseminated coccidioidomycosis.*

# OCULAR PARASITIC INFECTIONS

## ORBITAL PARASITIC INFECTIONS

Parasitic orbital infections are rare. Trichinosis, cysticercosis, echinococcosis, and onchocerciasis produce granulomatous infections and mild irritation until the organisms die, when they produce a severe inflammatory reaction. Trichina cysts within the extraocular muscles cause pain on eye movement, extraocular muscle paralysis, and edema of the conjunctiva and eyelids that re-

**TABLE 4.   Causes of Parasitic Infections of the Eyelids**[a]

| | |
|---|---|
| *Pediculus humanis* | *Demodex folliculorum* |
| Leishmaniasis | *Enterobius vermicularis* |
| Loa-loa | *Ascaris lumbricoides* |
| *Ancylostoma duodenale* | *Necator americanus* |
| *Trichinella spiralis* | Schistosoma |
| Flukes | Sparganum |
| Echinococcus | Cysticercus |

[a]After Ostler, H. B., et al.: J Cont Ed Ophthalmol, Feb., 1978, p. 3.

semble Chagas' disease (Romaña's sign). All of these organisms tend to invade the globe more frequently than the orbit.

## PARASITIC INFECTIONS OF THE EYELIDS AND OCULAR ADNEXA

The two most common parasites that affect the eyelids are lice (Fig. 6) and mites. The specific organisms include *Pediculus humanis* var. *capitis,* the head louse; *Pediculus humanis* var. *corporis,* the body louse; *Phthirus pubis,* the crab louse; and *Demodex folliculorum,* the common mite of hair follicles and sebaceous glands (Table 4).

*Phthirus pubis* produces complaints similar to those of staphylococcal blepharitis. High magnification examination of the base of the eyelashes may reveal the transparent organism (Fig. 7) or the nits. The nits should be removed and the eyelid margins treated by smothering the organisms with ointment and directly killing them with 0.25 per cent physostigmine (eserine ointment) or careful application of 1 per cent gamma benzene hexachloride (Kwell). The pubic area should also be treated with Kwell.

*Demodex folliculorum* is a common contaminant of the hair follicle (Coston, 1967). Slit-lamp examination of the base of the eyelashes reveals a fine or waxy brownish debris. If the lashes are pulled out and examined microscopically, the mite may be seen attached to the base. Itching is the main symptom. *Demodex* may also carry staphylococci into the hair follicle. The treatment is to maintain good eyelid hygiene and to kill the mites by applying camphor, acetone, or ether to

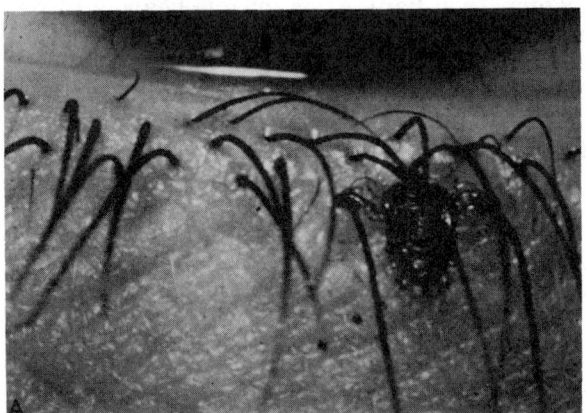

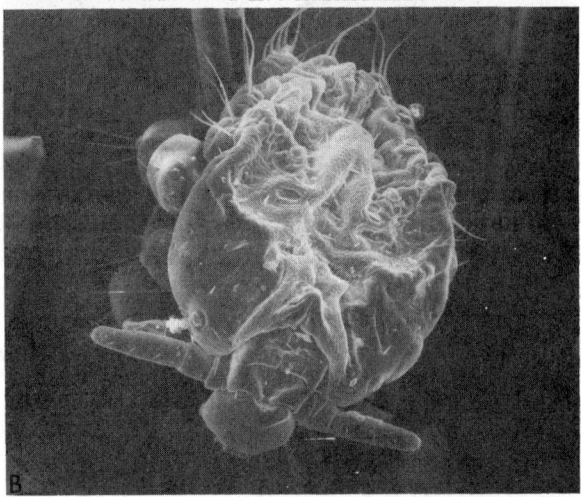

**FIGURE 7.**   A, Phthirus pubis *on eyelid margin. The patient complained of itching and redness. B, Scanning electron micrograph of* Pediculus humanis *removed from the base of an eyelash. (× 128).*

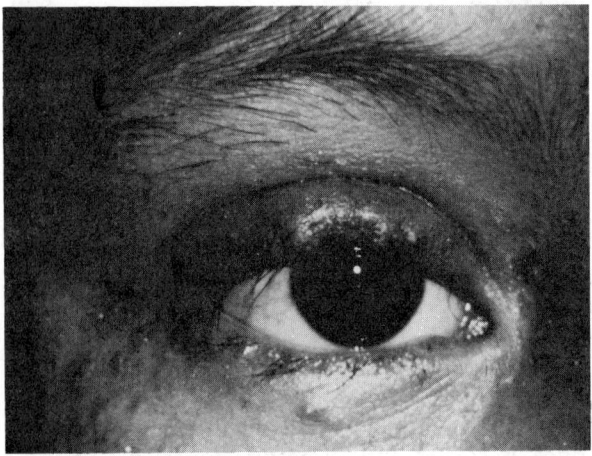

**FIGURE 6.**   Tinea capitis *infection of the eyelid. Note loss of lashes above, scarred and irregular lid margin, and depigmentation.*

the lid margin with a cotton-tipped applicator (using care to avoid the cornea) or by topical application of 10 per cent sulfacetamide ointment (Ostler et al., 1978).

Other parasites that infect the eyelids produce chronic lid infections that may present as nodules, depigmented areas (Fig. 6), hyperkeratosis, edema, loss of lashes, or erythema (Table 4). After the organisms are removed and identified microscopically, the affected area is treated topically as described above.

## CONJUNCTIVAL PARASITIC INFECTIONS

Parasitic conjunctival disease is very rare in the United States but common in areas where the parasites listed in Table 4 and 5 are endemic. The ease of jet travel, however, has increased the number of patients with parasitic conjunctivitis in nonendemic areas. Therefore, the possibility of a parasitic infection should be considered in any patient who presents with conjunctivitis following a trip into an endemic area. Unfortunately, the manifestations of some parasitic infections occur months to years after exposure (Duke-Elder, 1965).

### Clinical Manifestations and Diagnosis

Tearing, photophobia, itching, erythema, chemosis, and mass lesions of the conjunctiva are common to all parasitic infections of the conjunctivae. Concomitant disease of the eyelids and periorbital skin is frequent. A history of recent exposure to an endemic area is helpful. The organism may be directly visualized in the conjunctiva or in a biopsy of a conjunctival mass. Eosinophils are prominent in Giemsa smears of conjunctival scrapings. Corneal lesions may be present. Many patients also have symptoms and signs of systemic infection with the parasite. Some of the clinical presentations are listed in Table 5.

### Treatment

If an organism is either visible or thought to be alive and near the surface of the eye, the topical application of 4 to 10 per cent cocaine paralyzes the organism (Hennessy et al., 1977) so that it can be removed with a blunt forceps. Topical physostigmine ointment (eserine) can also be used for this purpose and to smother the organism. Deep burrowing or encysted parasites must be excised surgically. Patients are also treated systemically with the appropriate antiparasitic drug. The eye is carefully monitored for the acute ocular inflammation that occurs when the organisms die, and topical corticosteroids and cycloplegic agents such as atropine are given to control this inflammatory response. The number of eosinophils in serial conjunctival Giemsa smears decreases as the disease is controlled.

## PARASITIC CORNEAL INFECTIONS

Corneal infections usually spread from the conjunctivae. The etiology cannot be established by the type and appearance of the corneal lesions alone (Table 5). The organism can only rarely be visualized in the corneal stroma. The diagnosis

TABLE 5.  Clinical Manifestations of Conjunctival and Corneal Parasitic Infection[a]

**PROTOZOA**
| | |
|---|---|
| Leishmaniasis | Ulcerating granuloma, gelatinous avascular nodules, peripheral corneal vascularization, corneal abscess |

**NEMATHELMINTHES**
| | |
|---|---|
| Loa loa | Visible movement under conjunctiva, irregular symptoms |
| Onchocerciasis | Chronic conjunctivitis, diffuse edema and erythema, conjunctival pigmentation, conjunctival nodules, peripheral corneal vascularization, fluffy (temporary) or discrete superficial (permanent) corneal opacities |

**PLATYHELMINTHES**
| | |
|---|---|
| Schistosomiasis | Conjunctival tumors |
| Echinococcosis | Conjunctival cyst |
| Cysticercosis | Conjunctival cyst |

**ARTHROPODS**
| | |
|---|---|
| Ocular myiasis | Irregular foreign body sensation, maggot visible in conjunctiva, marginal corneal ulcers, subconjunctival mass |

[a]After Ostler, H. B., et al.: J Cont Ed Ophthalmol, Feb., 1978.

frequently must be established by obtaining the organism from the cornea or from other organs. Treatment is directed toward decreasing the corneal inflammation and eliminating the organism systemically.

## INTRAOCULAR PARASITIC INFECTIONS

### Etiology

Most intraocular parasitic infections are produced by organisms that enter the globe hematogenously or directly from adjacent orbital or conjunctival infections. Living parasites usually do not cause intraocular inflammation but may produce cataracts, lens dislocation, vitreous hemorrhage, or retinal detachment. When the organism dies, it elicits severe inflammation that usually destroys the eye in spite of appropriate therapy.

### Clinical Manifestations and Diagnosis

Patients often have no ocular complaints when only the posterior segment is involved. The first symptoms may be severe and may include inflammation, bleeding, cataracts, retinal scars, and/or detachment. If the symptoms suggest infection of the anterior part of the eye, the vitreous and retina should be examined (Table 6).

A history of exposure to an endemic area or the ingestion of uncooked meat adds further to the suspicion of a parasitic infection. The visual acuity is usually unaffected by early infection. Even if only minimal inflammation can be detected, examination may reveal floating cysts in the vitreous, tracks under the retina (Gass and Louis, 1976), or chorioretinal scars; or the organism may be seen (rarely) with an ophthalmoscope or at the slit lamp (Fig. 8) (Fitzgerald and Ruben, 1974). The parasites tend to avoid the light and make visualization by the ophthalmoscope difficult.

When isolated intraocular parasitic infections occur, the specific complement fixation tests and stool examinations for ova and parasites are negative.

### Treatment

The parasite must be removed alive without disturbing the intraocular structures. This type of operation is technically difficult but must be attempted because dead parasites produce such severe inflammation that blindness may result (Hutton et al., 1976). Successful treatment without surgery has been reported but is rare (Fitzgerald and Ruben, 1974). Cycloplegics and periocular corticosteroids are essential adjuncts to surgery.

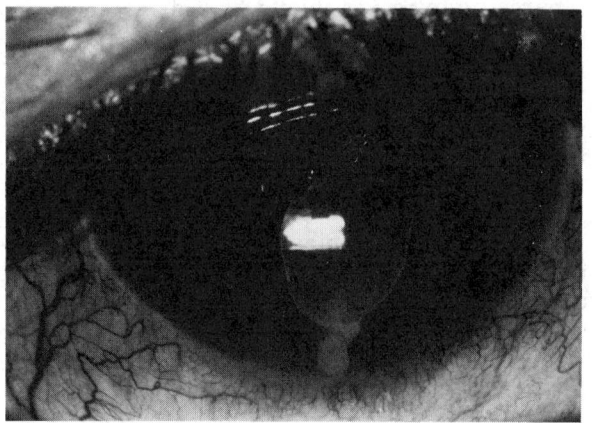

**FIGURE 8.**  *Free-floating cyst (Cysticercus) in anterior chamber.*

**TABLE 6.  Characteristics of Intraocular Parasitic Infection**[a]

| | |
|---|---|
| **PROTOZOA** | |
| Leishmaniasis | Endophthalmitis following corneal perforation |
| **NEMATHELMINTHES** | |
| Loa loa | Free floating in vitreous |
| Onchocerciasis | Choroiditis, iritis, "retinal degeneration" with pigment dispersion |
| **PLATYHELMINTHES** | |
| Echinococcosis | Vitreous cysts |
| Cysticercosis | Chorioretinal scars, vitreous cysts |
| Coenurosis | Vitreous cysts |
| **ARTHROPODS** | |
| Oculomyiasis | Subretinal scars ("tracks"), endophthalmitis |

[a]After Ostler, H. B., et al.: J Cont Ed Ophthalmol, Feb., 1978.

# CHLAMYDIAL AND RICKETTSIAL INFECTIONS

## CHLAMYDIAL AND RICKETTSIAL INFECTIONS OF THE EYELIDS AND OCULAR ADNEXA

These infections are extremely rare and are always associated with active conjunctivitis (Ostler et al., 1978). Rickettsiae and Chlamydiae are sensitive to tetracycline, and the eyelid and conjunctival lesions clear simultaneously during topical and systemic therapy.

## CONJUNCTIVAL CHLAMYDIAL DISEASES

### Trachoma

*Etiology.* *Chlamydia* is divided into two species or groups, *C. psittaci* and *C. trachomatis*. *C. psittaci* causes ornithosis or psittacosis. Trachoma, inclusion conjunctivitis, and lymphogranuloma venereum (LGV) are caused by *C. trachomatis*. Unlike those of *C. psittaci*, the intracellular inclusion bodies of this species stain with iodine. All *Chlamydial* organisms show a common lipopolysaccharide group antigen, but they can be separated by other type-specific cell-wall antigens. The subgroup of *C. trachomatis* that causes trachoma and inclusion conjunctivitis (TRIC agents) can be divided into nine antigenic types (A through I) by microimmunofluorescence. Types A, B, and C cause trachoma in hyperendemic areas (Afro-Oriental), where poor social conditions and poor hygiene favor eye-to-eye transmission. Inclusion conjunctivitis (occidental

trachoma or paratrachoma), which is caused by Types D through I, is spread from the genital areas to the eyes. The agents of lymphogranuloma venereum can be divided into three separate antigenic types. The types of *C. psittaci* do not cross-react with those of *C. trachomatis*.

The history of trachoma and the discovery of its etiology are nicely outlined by Duke-Elder (Duke-Elder, 1965b).

*Diagnosis.* Trachoma is the major cause of preventable blindness in the world. The organism infects the conjunctiva and produces hypertrophy of the lymphoid follicles underneath the upper eyelid and nonspecific inflammation of the remaining conjunctiva. When untreated, this process causes scarring of the conjunctiva (Fig. 9), dry eyes, and inturning of the scarred upper eyelid margin (entropion), so that the lashes continuously rub the cornea (trichiasis). Corneal infection and scarring (Fig. 10) eventually result in blindness.

Certain characteristic lesions (Table 7) strongly suggest the diagnosis. An ingrowth of blood vessels from the superior junction of the cornea and sclera (limbus) into the clear corneal stroma (corneal pannus) and an overlying disturbance of the corneal epithelium (punctate keratitis) are particularly characteristic of trachoma (Table 7). The diagnosis is established by the clinical presentation and the demonstration of the organism in smears or cultures. Blunt scrapings of the superficial conjunctiva under topical anesthesia with a platinum spatula should be stained by the Giemsa technique and examined microscopically. If intracytoplasmic inclusion bodies are found, a

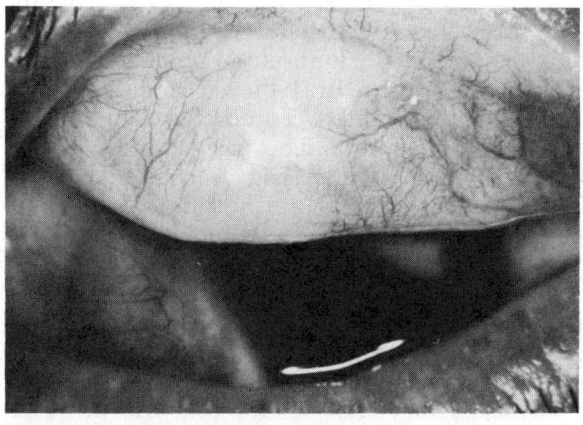

**FIGURE 9.** *Severe conjunctival scarring on the everted upper eyelid in a patient with end-stage trachoma.*

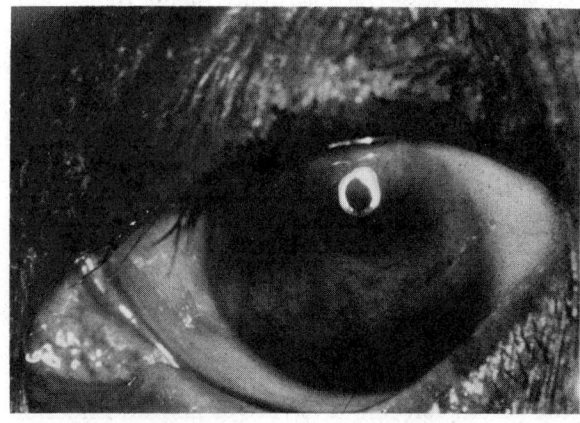

**FIGURE 10.** *Diffuse corneal scarring of the superior and central cornea in a patient with advanced trachoma*

**TABLE 7.  Clinical Findings in Trachoma**

| | |
|---|---|
| Eyelids: | Papillae, follicles, scarring, trichiasis |
| Limbus: | Follicles, Herbert's pits, scars |
| Cornea: | Pannus, keratitis, scars |

definitive diagnosis can be made. Iodine stains or special fluorescent antibody stains may also be used. Unfortunately, it is difficult to find inclusions in scrapings. The types of white blood cells in the scrapings help to stage the disease. Polymorphonuclear leukocytes and lymphocytes are prominent in acute disease, whereas monocytes and lymphoblasts are predominant in the chronic stage. The conjunctival scrapings may be cultured in Hela cells, where they cause typical iodine-positive, intracytoplasmic inclusions. Serologic tests for group-specific antibody or type-specific antibody and tests of cell-mediated immunity, such as migration-inhibition factor (MIF) to type-specific antigens, may be helpful.

*Treatment.* Hyperendemic trachoma is difficult to treat because of continuous reexposure. Treatment must include improvement of hand and facial hygiene to prevent reinfection by eye-to-eye and hand-to-eye contact. The treatment of choice is topical and systemic tetracycline. Tetracycline ointment should be applied twice a day for 60 days or on an intermittent schedule of five days each month for six months. Oral tetracycline (1 gram each day for three to six weeks), vibramycin (3 to 5 mg/kg initially, followed by 2 to 5 mg/kg for three to six weeks), or sulfonamides (2 to 4 gm per day for three to six weeks are effective systemic therapy. Most patients respond within 12 to 17 weeks after starting therapy (Dawson, 1973; Yoneda et al., 1975). All members of the same social group should be treated to eliminate repeated transmission of the infection. The anatomic ocular complications must be treated to prevent or arrest corneal scarring. Surgical correction of the lids, the use of artificial tears, and corneal transplantation may all be necessary.

## Paratrachoma (Endemic, Occidental Paratrachoma)

*Etiology.* Paratrachoma is a sexually transmitted infection caused by *Chlamydia trachomatis* of Types D through I. It is transmitted by genital secretions either to the genital area or to the eyes. The clinical presentation depends on the age of the contact and the portal of entry. Neonates develop inclusion blennorrhea (TRIC ophthalmia neonatorum), and adults develop either inclusion conjunctivitis or genital infection (TRIC urethritis, cervicitis, proctitis).

*Inclusion Blennorrhea (TRIC Ophthalmia Neonatorum).* Newborns are exposed to *Chla-*

*mydia* during passage through the infected birth canal. After 5 to 12 days, the infant develops a severe mucopurulent discharge from one or both eyes, with swelling and redness of the lids and diffuse conjunctival injection. Unlike the adult with inclusion conjunctivitis whose conjunctiva reacts by producing lymphoid follicles, the newborn does not produce follicles until 3 months of age. Giemsa stains of the conjunctival scrapings reveal diagnostic intracellular inclusions in 50 to 90 per cent of the cases (Yoneda et al., 1975), a much higher yield than in adults with inclusion conjunctivitis. Conjunctival cultures of the infant and cervical cultures of the mother are also usually positive.

The infants are treated with topical tetracycline or sulfa ointment at least six times per day for five to six weeks, and both parents are treated for chronic inclusion conjunctivitis. The ocular complications are usually mild and include minimal conjunctival scarring and some neovascularization of the superior cornea, but a rare patient may develop considerable scarring (Markham et al., 1977).

*Adult Inclusion Conjunctivitis (Oculogenital Inclusion Conjunctivitis).* *C. trachomatis* causes asymptomatic, nonspecific urethritis in men and chronic cervicitis with or without vaginal discharge in women. The infection is transferred to the eye by the hands or by direct transfer from the genitals to the eye. The incubation period varies from 4 to 12 days (Dawson, 1973). The disease presents in sexually active adults, usually 18 to 30 years of age, as acute (or chronic) unilateral or bilateral conjunctivitis with a palpable preauricular node, conjunctival lymphoid follicles, and mild mucopurulent discharge. Fever and respiratory symptoms are absent. Lymphoid follicles are most prominent in the lower conjunctiva but can spread to the entire conjunctiva. Conjunctival infection is moderate. The patient complains of tearing, a mild foreign body sensation, and lid fullness. The corneal epithelium becomes involved in the second week. Sequelae include scarring, opacities, and, rarely, iritis.

The patients are treated with systemic tetracycline or sulfa in the same doses prescribed for trachoma but only for three weeks. Topical ointments may also be used if the response to therapy is unsatisfactory. All sexual consorts must be treated to prevent reinfection. If untreated, the disease becomes chronic and produces corneal scarring.

## CONJUNCTIVAL RICKETTSIAL INFECTIONS

Rickettsiae may infect the eye as part of the generalized rickettsial illness. They have a predilection for vascular endothelium and may produce angiitis with necrosis and thrombosis of conjunctival and intraocular vessels. Rickettsial conjunctivitis is characterized by subconjunctival hemorrhage, erythema, and edema. The organisms may be cultured from conjunctival scrapings. Topical and systemic tetracycline or chloramphenicol is the treatment of choice.

## INTRAOCULAR RICKETTSIAL INFECTIONS

The manifestations of intraocular rickettsial infections include venous engorgement, retinal edema, papilledema, cytoid bodies, retinal hemorrhages, arteriolar branch occlusions, and severe inflammation (Smith and Burton, 1977). Although these findings are not diagnostic, they suggest rickettsial infection in a patient with an acute febrile exanthematous illness. Systemic tetracycline, as given for the generalized illness, is the only treatment necessary.

### References

Coston, T.: *Demodex folliculorum* blepharitis. Trans Am Ophthalmol Soc 65:361, 1967.

Dawson, C.: Therapy of diseases caused by *Chlamydia* organisms. Int Ophthalmol Clin 13:93, 1973.

Duke-Elder, S.: System of Ophthalmology. VIII. Diseases of the Outer Eye. Part I. Parasitic Infections of the Conjunctiva. London, Henry Kimpton, 1965a, p. 398.

Duke-Elder, S.: System of Ophthalmology. VIII. Diseases of the Outer Eye. Part I. Trachoma. London, Henry Kimpton, 1965b, p. 258.

Fitzgerald, C. R., and Ruben, M. L.: Intraocular parasite destroyed by photocoagulation. Arch Ophthalmol 91:162, 1974.

Forster, R. K., and Rebell, G.: The diagnosis and management of keratomycoses. I. Cause and diagnosis. Arch Ophthalmol 93:975, 1975a.

Forster, R. K., and Rebell, G.: The diagnosis and management of keratomycoses. II. Medical and surgical management. Arch Ophthalmol 93:1134, 1975b.

Gass, J. D. M., and Louis, R. A.: Subretinal tracts in ophthalmomyiasis. Arch Ophthalmol 94:1500, 1976.

Hennessy, D. J., Sherrill, J. W., and Binder, P. S.: External ophthalmomyiasis caused by *Estrus ovis.* Am J Ophthalmol 84:802, 1977.

Hutton, W. L., Vaiser, A., and Snyder, W. B.: Pars plana vitrectomy for removal of intravitreous *Cysticercus.* Am J Ophthalmol 81:571, 1976.

Markham, R. H. C., Richmond, S. J., Walshaw, N. W. D., and Easty, D. L.: Severe persistent inclusion conjunctivitis in a young child. Am J Ophthalmol 83:414, 1977.

Ostler, H. B., Thygeson, P., and Okumoto, M.: Infectious diseases of the eye. J Cont Ed Ophthalmol, Feb 1978, p. 3.

Polack, F. M.: Diagnosis and treatment of keratomycosis. Int Ophthalmol Clin 13:75, 1973.

Schwartz, J. N., Donnelly, E. H., and Klintworth, G. K.: Ocular and orbital phycomycosis. Surv Ophthalmol 22:3, 1977.

Smith, T. W., and Burton, T. C.: The retinal manifestations of Rocky Mountain spotted fever. Am J Ophthalmol 84:259, 1977.

Snip, R. C., and Michaels, R. G.: Pars plana vitrectomy in the management of indigenous *Candida* endophthalmitis. Am J Ophthalmol 82:699, 1976.

Weinberg, R. J., Sartoris, M. J., Buerger, G. F., Jr., and Novak, J. F.: *Fusobacterium* in presumed Actinomyces canaliculitis. Am J Ophthalmol 84:371, 1977.

Wolter, J. R.: *Pityrosporum* species associated with dacryoliths in obstructive dacryocystitis. Am J Ophthalmol 84:806, 1977.

Yoneda, C., Dawson, C. R., Daghfous, T., Hoshiwara, I., Jones, P., Messadi, M., and Schachter, J.: Cytology as a guide to the presence of chlamydial inclusions in Giemsa-stained conjunctival smears in severe endemic trachoma. Br J Ophthalmol 59:116, 1975.

# ENDOPHTHALMITIS **234**

## Burt R. Meyers, M.D.

### DEFINITION

Endophthalmitis is an inflammation of the interior of the eye that may involve the vitreous body and/or the anterior chamber. The inflammatory process may spread to the uvea or the retina. If all the tunics are involved, the process is called panophthalmitis. Endophthalmitis may be caused by infection, blood, retained lens material, trauma, and neoplasm. It may be classified according to the anatomic location of the inflammation (anterior or posterior), the type of infectious agent (bacterial or fungal), or the route of entry of the infectious agent (endogenous or exogenous). Infection acquired during trauma, ophthalmic surgery, or by direct extension from adjacent tissues is called exogenous. Endophthalmitis acquired by hematogenous, lymphatic, or neural pathways is classified as endogenous.

Bacteria and fungi, including strains of questionable pathogenicity for other tissues, are the most common causes of endophthalmitis. Parasites and viruses cause occasional infections of the globe, but rickettsial and chlamydial infections are extremely uncommon.

### ETIOLOGY AND PATHOGENESIS

#### Exogenous Endophthalmitis

The bacteria and fungi that make up the normal flora of the conjunctivae are the most common causes of endophthalmitis acquired at the time of trauma or surgery. Infants usually acquire an aerobic flora similar to the aerobic vaginal flora of the mother. *Staphylococcus epidermidis*, streptococci, *Escherichia coli*, and *Staphylococcus aureus* have been isolated at birth and persist through the fifth day even after topical penicillin or silver nitrate therapy. Cultures of more than 10,000 healthy conjunctivae have shown that *S. epidermidis* is the most common isolate, followed by *S. aureus* and diphtheroids. Other gram-positive bacteria and Enterobacteriaceae are isolated less frequently (Locatcher-Khorazo and Gutierrez, 1972). This pattern of normal flora is independent of age, season, and sex. There is no significant geographic variation in the conjunctival flora. The cultural results from many different countries are strikingly similar (Locatcher-Khorazo and Seegal, 1972). Obligate anaerobes are rarely isolated from normal conjunctivae. In the United States, fungi have been recovered much less frequently than bacteria from healthy eyes; 1.5 per cent of the age group from 10 with 18 years were positive compared with 4.4 per cent of adults (Locatcher-Khorazo and Seegal, 1972). Comparative reports of the incidence of fungi recovered from healthy eyes range from 2.5 per cent in the U.S.S.R. (Ovsepian and Osipian, 1965) to 52 per cent in Spain (Vasquez de Parga and Pereira, 1965). Over 80 species of fungi belonging to 50 genera have been isolated from the conjunctivae, but *Aspergillus* species are by far the most common. The bacterial flora of the eyelid margins and the conjunctival sac are the same, but fungi are more common on the lid margin. Urban dwellers have a lower incidence of fungal isolates than those in rural settings. The instillation of topical steroids and antibiotics, a warm, moist climate, an agricultural environment, and advanced age increase the number of fungal isolates from the conjunctivae. The local microbial flora is probably prevented from causing infections by local protective mechanisms such as lid closure, mechanical washing by the tears, and the lysozyme and IgA in the tears.

Endophthalmitis following surgery or trauma is usually caused by the introduction into the interior of the eye of one of these members of the normal conjunctival flora. The commonest cause of endophthalmitis after surgery, most often a cataract extraction, is staphylococci. Gram-negative bacteria including Enterobacteriaceae and *Pseudomonas* spp have become more prominent since the advent of preoperative topical antibiotics. The most common causes of fungal endophthalmitis after surgery or trauma are *Candida* spp, *Aspergillus* spp, *Fusarium*, *Penicillium*, *Cephalosporium*, *Alternaria*, and *Allescheria boydii (Monosporium apiospermum)*. Abrasions and ulcers from contact lenses have also been the portal of entry for fungal endophthalmitis.

The interior of the eye can also be infected by direct extension of orbital cellulitis or sinusitis, but the globe is remarkably resistant to invasion unless the natural defenses are breached by surgery or trauma. *S. aureus* is the most common microbe that extends into the globe from the orbit or sinuses, but the Phycomycetes (*Rhizopus* and *Mucor*) and *Aspergillus* have a predilection to invade local blood vessels and can also extend through facial planes into the globe.

### Endogenous Ophthalmitis

Endogenous endophthalmitis usually occurs from seeding of the globe during hematogenous infection. When the infection is localized, the vessels of the choroid and ciliary body are often involved. The first intraocular focus is often in the choroid and retina, with direct extension into the vitreous body. The retina may become necrotic, especially with fungal infections. *Candida* spreads through the intraocular tissues, whereas Phycomycetes invade the vascular supply and cause thrombosis of the retinal artery. Abscesses of the vitreous body and choroid and uveitis are frequent complications. Granulomatous chorioretinitis also occurs. Endogenous endophthalmitis can be caused by *Aspergillus*, *Cryptococcus neoformans*, *Blastomyces dermatitidis*, and *Sporothrix schenckii*, but *Candida* spp (usually *C. albicans*) are the most common causes of endogenous fungal endophthalmitis (Meyers et al., 1973). Metastatic endophthalmitis from bacteremia due to *S. aureus*, pneumococci, meningococci, *Streptococcus pyogenes*, *E. coli*, *Klebsiella*, and *Pseudomonas* spp has also been reported. Endophthalmitis may follow puerperal sepsis, pneumococcal pneumonia, endocarditis, and meningitis.

Endophthalmitis complicates 0.3 to 6 per cent of cases of meningococcemia. The tubercle bacillus and *Treponema pallidum* may also involve the globe secondary to hematogenous spread. *T. pallidum* has been found in the anterior chamber many years after the initial diagnosis of primary syphilis.

The prominence of *Candida* as a cause of endophthalmitis parallels the increasing incidence of candidemia. The rising number of patients with underlying malignancies, main-line drug addiction, intravenous or intra-arterial catheters, indwelling urinary catheters, and parenteral hyperalimentation increases the incidence of candidemia and secondary endophthalmitis. Periocular devices such as encircling bands placed around the eye at the time of surgery for retinal detachment can become contaminated and cause orbital and intraocular infection. Disseminated aspergillosis is a significant cause of endophthalmitis and death in leukemia patients. Unfortunately, the diagnosis is frequently made at necropsy.

*Toxocara* and *Toxoplasma* are the most common causes of parasitic intraocular infections. *Toxoplasma* usually causes posterior uveitis and is discussed in Chapters 235 and 248. Intraocular infection with *Toxocara* is discussed in Chapter 250, and viral ocular infections are discussed in Chapter 232.

## CLINICAL MANIFESTATIONS

Endophthalmitis may present as an acute fulminating infection or as a more prolonged, subacute disease. In a patient who has either bacteremia or fungemia the development of eye symptoms of even the mildest degree should alert one to the possibility of ophthalmic infection. Complaints of eye irritation, pain, photophobia, blurred vision, or loss of vision are most common. Redness, hyperemia, and edema of the conjunctiva are early findings. Chemosis of the lids and proptosis follow.

Ophthalmic examination may reveal decreased vision with scotomas. Yellow-white opaque lesions may be seen on the retina and appear to be growing into the vitreous (Fig. 1). The iris may be involved and on slit-lamp examination a flare and cells are noted in the anterior chamber. The vitreous body may also appear hazy. In fungal endophthalmitis the retinal lesions may be fluffy with indistinct borders and look like cotton-wool spots.

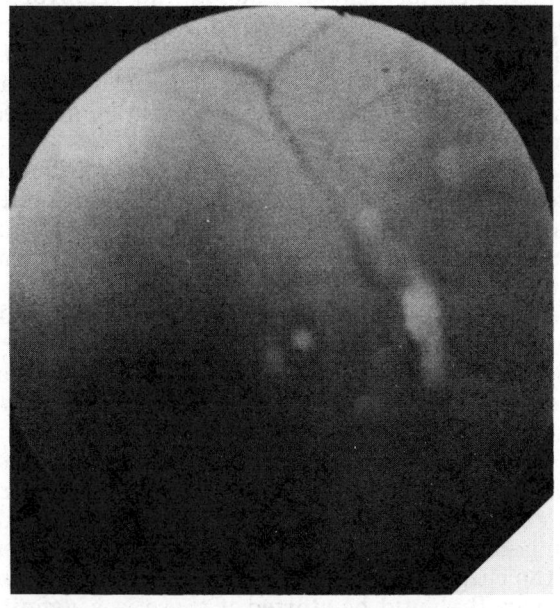

**FIGURE 1.**

If the disease is secondary to local extension from the nasal sinuses there are usually complaints of facial pain and headache; tenderness over the maxillary or frontal sinus will usually be elicited. Radiographs of the sinuses may reveal distortion of the normal architecture, bony erosion, and fluid.

Patients are usually febrile with a leukocytosis and a left shift. Endophthalmitis may be the first manifestation of meningococcemia or occur concomitantly with bacterial pneumonia. In this event blood cultures should be performed before therapy is initiated.

The subacute form of this disease may occur 6 to 12 weeks after trauma, eye surgery, or fungemia. Endophthalmitis secondary to intravenous drug abuse usually has a subacute presentation. These patients may have no history of chills or fever and present with only minor eye complaints of blurring, redness, or irritation. An eye complaint in an addict warrants a thorough ophthalmoscopic examination.

In subacute endophthalmitis blood cultures are usually negative, and the peripheral white count is normal. Aspiration of the vitreous body for smear and culture may establish the etiology. Paracentesis of the anterior chamber is positive less frequently. The presence of either white blood cells or bacteria in the Gram stain of aspirated fluid suggests a suppurative infection. Fluids should be cultured for fungi and aerobically and anaerobically for bacteria. Serologic determinations for *Candida* precipitins and agglutinins have not been of value. The hemagglutination test for *Toxocara* may be reactive, but cross-reactions with gastrointestinal nematode infections have limited its usefulness.

Noninfectious endophthalmitis secondary to metastatic bronchogenic carcinoma, melanoma, and primary reticulum cell sarcoma causes similar symptoms and signs. Behçet's syndrome usually involves the uvea but can cause endophthalmitis. Asteroid hyalitis (inflammation of the vitreous body with star-shaped inclusions) may produce endogenous opacities, but these are of no clinical importance. Endophthalmitis phakoanaphylactica, a sterile, postoperative inflammatory process, must be considered after cataract surgery. Phacolytic glaucoma, a condition in which lens protein leaks through the intact lens capsule, may cause severe sterile inflammation and glaucoma.

## GEOGRAPHIC VARIATIONS

Postoperative bacterial and fungal endophthalmitis and endogenous *Candida* endophthalmitis associated with hospitalization, radical surgery for neoplasms, and indwelling lines are diseases of medical progress and occur more frequently in industrialized countries. *Toxocara* and *Toxoplasma* eye infections have been reported most frequently from the United States but depend on exposure to cats *(Toxocara cati* and *Toxoplasma)* or dogs *(Toxocara canis)* and probably occur worldwide. Except for *Candida, Aspergillus,* and *Cryptococcus,* the fungi that cause endogenous endophthalmitis are restricted in their distribution. *Coccidioides* occurs in the arid southwest region of the United States, Mexico, and Argentina; *Blastomyces dermatitidis* (North American blastomycosis) in the southeastern United States, Canada, and Africa; and *Histoplasma capsulatum* primarily in the Mississippi and Ohio river valleys of the United States but also in Central and South America. The bacteria that cause endophthalmitis and the fungi that cause exogenous endophthalmitis are ubiquitous. As noted in the *Etiology and Pathogenesis* section, the conjunctivae of people from rural environments and moist, warm climates are more frequently colonized with fungi, but there is no clear-cut evidence that exogenous fungal endophthalmitis is more common in these populations.

## TREATMENT AND SEQUELAE

Bacterial infections of the globe are usually very destructive. Early therapy is mandatory in order to avoid enucleation and save vision (Peyman and Sanders, 1975). Since the etiology of most cases is not known when therapy is started, it is necessary to give broad-spectrum antibiotic coverage for both gram-positive and gram-negative bacteria. For example, the antibiotic regimen must cover beta-lactamase–producing *S. aureus* and *Pseudomonas aeruginosa* since these are common causes of this condition. Furthermore, the route of administration and the pharmacology of the antibiotics must be carefully considered because most antibiotics do not penetrate into the eye very well. It is believed that antibiotics diffuse from the blood into the aqueous and that inflammation increases diffusion. Lipophilic compounds like chloramphenicol achieve higher intraocular levels than the penicillins, cephalosporins, or aminoglycosides. Protein-binding decreases penetration, so antibiotics like methicillin, cephaloridine, and gentamicin with a relatively high percentage of free drug should be selected. Therapeutic concentrations of trimethoprim-sulfamethoxazole have been detected in the anterior chamber, but the levels in the vitreous are unknown. Many antibiotics reach reasonable levels in the aqueous after systemic administration, but penetration into the vitreous is usually very poor. These observations and the

high frequency of treatment failures have prompted the use of periocular injections to increase antibiotic penetration into the globe. Based on these considerations, therapy should be started with cephaloridine or methicillin 2 g I.V. every four hours. The drug should be given as a pulse because the high serum levels diffuse into the eye against a gradient more effectively. Gentamicin sulfate should also be given parenterally in a dose of 5 mg/kg daily in three divided doses. Topical and periocular administration (by an ophthalmologist) of gentamicin is also recommended. Some authorities believe that intraocular antibiotics should be administered; however, complications are increased with this procedure, the benefits are not certain, and it is considered an experimental procedure. When blood or intraocular culture reports are available and antibiotic sensitivities known, more specific therapy should be given. Therapeutic efficacy is not increased by multiple drugs, and continued use of combinations may increase toxicity and superinfection. The optimal duration of therapy is unknown, but parenteral antibiotics should probably be given for four to six weeks.

Inflammation can destroy vision and cause cataracts, retinal detachment, and glaucoma. Topical and periocular administration of corticosteroids reduce inflammation of the retina and choroid in an animal model, and clinical studies have suggested that their use with antibiotics has been of value in preserving vision. Intravitreal administration of corticosteroids is also considered an experimental procedure.

Coexisting infections such as meningitis, pneumonia, or endocarditis must be treated effectively. Débridement of wounds and removal of foreign bodies, indwelling lines, and urinary catheters is necessary to prevent further hematologic seeding. If contiguous structures such as the sinuses are involved, they should be drained immediately.

Studies of the comparative efficacy of different treatment regimens are not available, since only case reports have been presented in the literature. When antimicrobial therapy fails, enucleation or evisceration is necessary. Data derived from clinical studies of postoperative endophthalmitis revealed that 66 per cent of patients were blinded by inflammatory destruction or enucleation. Additional patients were left with almost useless vision.

Subacute endophthalmitis is more difficult to diagnose. If blood cultures are negative and there is either a history or a strong suspicion of prior fungemia, the vitreous should be aspirated. Even if the cultures are negative, therapy with amphotericin B should be started if there is a definite history of previous candidemia.

Data on the intraocular penetration of antifungal drugs are also scanty (Leopold, 1973). Amphotericin B penetrates into the inflamed rabbit eye, but the intraocular levels of this compound and of 5-fluorocytosine in man have been measured only rarely. 5-Fluorocytosine has been used to treat only a few patients with endophthalmitis, and its efficacy is unknown. Data are also unavailable on miconazole, a newer antifungal agent.

Amphotericin B is the drug of choice for proven or suspected fungal endophthalmitis. A total of 1 to 2 g should be given intravenously over a four- to six-week period, although regression of lesions has been observed with less. The earliest response to therapy is decreased inflammation and clearing of the vitreous haze; regression of vitreous inflammation may take longer. Visual acuity will improve if the patient is responding to antifungal therapy.

The combination of 5-fluorocytosine (150 mg/kg/day) with nontoxic doses of amphotericin B (0.3 to 0.4 mg/kg/day) to prevent 5-fluorocytosine resistance has been used successfully in a few cases of postsurgical candidal endophthalmitis (Jones, 1978), but this regimen should probably not be used routinely until more information on the intraocular concentrations of 5-fluorocytosine is available.

Débridement, surgical drainage, and removal of all intraocular and intravascular devices should prevent further hematologic seeding. Periocular corticosteroids are recommended by some clinicians. Intraorbital injections of corticosteroids and amphotericin B have been attempted, but the efficacy and safety of these agents by this route are unclear.

Tuberculosis of the eye, a rare condition, usually presents as choroiditis with whitish tubercles on the retinal surface, but tuberculous endophthalmitis has also been reported. Standard systemic antituberculous therapy should be administered and other sites of infection thoroughly sought.

Intraocular syphilis is treated with 15 daily intramuscular injections of 600,000 units of procaine penicillin.

## PROPHYLAXIS

Preoperative antibiotics have been recommended to prevent postoperative endophthalmitis. Most studies compare different drug regimens, and comparative data without antibiotics are unavailable. Improvement of surgical techniques may have lowered the rate of infection. Postoperative infections often occur in spurts, which suggests that the source of these infections may be contaminated instruments or eye solutions. Elective surgery should never be performed in the presence of eye, lid, or adjacent infections of the face. Trauma to the eye should be attended to at once by an ophthalmologist. The incidence of candidemia can be lowered by avoiding the use of unnecessary antibiotics, and by removal or frequent replacement of intravascular lines and Foley catheters. The eyes of candidemic patients should be examined even in the absence of symptoms. If lesions are seen or suspected, antifungal therapy should be instituted promptly after appropriate cultures are obtained.

## References

Jones, D. B.: Therapy of postsurgical fungal endophthalmitis. Ophthalmology 85:357, 1978.

Leopold, I. H. (ed.): Symposium on Ocular Therapy. Vol. 6. St. Louis, C. V. Mosby Company, 1973.

Locatcher-Khorazo, D., and Gutierrez, E.: Unpublished data quoted in Locatcher-Khorazo, D., and Seegal, B. C.: Microbiology of the Eye. St. Louis, C. V. Mosby Company, 1972, p. 15.

Locatcher-Khorazo, D., and Seegal, B. C.: Microbiology of the Eye. St. Louis, C. V. Mosby Company, 1972.

Meyers, B. R., Lieberman, T. W., and Ferry, A. P.: Candida endophthalmitis complicating candidemia. Ann Intern Med 79:647, 1973.

Ovsepian, T. L., and Osipian, L. L.: Mycologic flora of the conjunctival sac. Zh Eksp Klin Med 5:78, 1965.

Peyman, G. A., and Sanders, D. R.: Advances in Uveal Surgery, Vitreous Surgery and the Treatment of Endophthalmitis. New York, Appleton Century Crofts-Prentice Hall, 1975.

Vasquez de Parga, A. S., and Pereiro, M.: Flora micotica de la conjunctiva. Arch Soc Oftal Hisp Am 25:168, 1965.

# 235 *OCULAR INFLAMMATORY DISEASE—IRITIS, CYCLITIS, CHOROIDITIS ("UVEITIS")*

*Perry S. Binder, M.D., F.A.C.S.*

## DEFINITION

The pigmented tissues of the eye are the iris, ciliary body, and choroid. These structures, which are collectively known as the uvea, respond to infection, trauma, and other stimuli by becoming inflamed. When the front of the eye (anterior uvea) is inflamed, the process may be described as iritis, cyclitis, or iridocyclitis. Inflammatory processes may also be restricted to the choroid (choroiditis) or involve all of the pigmented ocular tissues (panuveitis). Uveitis is a general word that means inflammation of the pigmented tissues of the eye, regardless of the cause. Uveal inflammation may spread to any other ocular structure. As a result, endophthalmitis (infection of the interior of the eye) and panophthalmitis (infection of the interior of the eye plus all the tunics) are potential complications of uveitis.

## CLASSIFICATION

Uveitis may be classified according to the pathologic process produced by the inflammation, the location of the inflammation (for example, anterior or posterior uveitis) or the agents that cause the inflammation. The system outlined in Table 1, which was modified from Hogan and Zimmerman (1962), classifies uveitis according to the type of inflammation and lists the major known causes of each kind of uveal response.

## SUPPURATIVE UVEITIS

### Exogenous Suppurative Uveitis

Acute suppurative inflammation of the uvea usually follows eye infection or trauma with or without the introduction of foreign bodies. Bacteria, fungi, chemicals, and organic materials may elicit massive polymorphonuclear responses. This type of inflammation may involve other ocular structures initially and be more prominent in the uvea only because of its great vascularity.

## NONSUPPURATIVE UVEITIS

This is the most common type of "uveitis." It is usually divided into nongranulomatous and granulomatous varieties.

### Nongranulomatous Variety

*Exogenous* nongranulomatous uveitis is produced by trauma (either external or surgical) to any of the ocular tissues or follows systemic immune processes such as serum sickness or rejections of corneal transplants.

*Endogenous* nongranulomatous uveitis is the most common type of uveitis. It can be caused by several viruses (including herpes simplex and herpes zoster), idiopathic ocular inflammations (such as Behçet's disease), systemic diseases (such as ankylosing spondylitis), or systemic allergic reactions to penicillin and other drugs.

### Granulomatous Variety

*Exogenous* granulomatous uveitis is caused only by sympathetic ophthalmia in which severe ocular inflammation develops in a previously healthy eye after penetrating injury to the *opposite* eye.

*Endogenous* granulomatous uveitis may occur during the course of infections with several bacteria, viruses, fungi and parasites. It is a complication of tuberculosis and syphilis, almost certainly a complication of visceral larva migrans *(Toxocara)*, and probably of histoplasmosis. No etiology has been found for certain other diseases, such as Vogt-Koyanagi-Harada disease, a diffuse disease of the uvea, auditory apparatus, and skin.

## UNCLASSIFIED

The causes of uveitis listed in Table 1 will probably change as our knowledge of the various diseases increases. Some causes of uveitis may also cause more than one type of tissue response, but I have chosen to keep the table simple in order to provide an overview. The pathologic features of each category have been documented by Hogan

**TABLE 1.  Classification of Uveitis**

I. Suppurative Uveitis
  A. Exogenous suppurative uveitis
    1. Secondary to ocular or orbital infection
    2. Secondary to ocular trauma
II. Nonsuppurative Uveitis
  A. Nongranulomatous uveitis
    1. Exogenous nongranulomatous uveitis
      a. Secondary to trauma or surgery
      b. Serum sickness
      c. Corneal graft rejection
    2. Endogenous nongranulomatous uveitis
      a. Allergies and hypersensitivities
      b. Behçet's disease
      c. Fuch's heterochromic iridocyclitis
      d. Juvenile rheumatoid arthritis
      e. Viral diseases—herpes simplex, herpes zoster, measles, mumps, influenza, whooping cough
      f. Ankylosing spondylitis
      g. Reiter's syndrome
      h. Cyclitis (pars planitis)
      i. Lens-induced uveitis
      j. Glaucomatocyclitic crisis
      k. Unknown causes
  B. Granulomatous uveitis
    1. Exogenous granulomatous uveitis
      a. Sympathetic ophthalmia
      b. Phacoanaphylactic endophthalmitis
    2. Endogenous granulomatous uveitis
      a. Bacterial—tuberculosis, leprosy, syphilis, brucellosis, leptospirosis, rickettsial
      b. Mycotic—histoplasmosis, coccidioidomycosis, cryptococcosis, blastomycosis, actinomycosis, candidiasis
      c. Parasitic—cysticercosis, *Toxocara canis*, onchocerciasis, toxoplasmosis
      d. Viral—cytomegalovirus infection
      e. Nontraumatic, noninfectious—sarcoidosis, rheumatoid arthritis, juvenile xanthogranuloma, histiocytosis X, Vogt-Koyanagi-Harada syndrome, Chediak-Higashi syndrome, Eales's disease

and Zimmerman (1962), and an excellent historic review of uveitis, as well as an in-depth review of individual entities, can be found in Duke-Elder and Perkins (1966).

The anatomic classifications of uveitis either may be general (anterior, posterior, or diffuse) or may refer to the specific tissues and the agent, e.g., keratoiritis of herpes simplex, sclerokeratitis in rheumatoid disorders, and toxoplasma chorioretinitis. Vogt-Koyanagi-Harada disease causes uveal meningitis. All types of uveitis may be acute or chronic and mild to severe. All have a great tendency to recur.

## PATHOLOGY, CLINICAL MANIFESTATIONS AND COMPLICATIONS

The signs and symptoms of uveitis (Table 2) vary depending upon the type of inflammation, the tissues of the eye that are involved, the temporal course of the disease (acute vs. chronic), the state of health of the patient, and the previous use of systemic or ocular medications.

Inflammation of the iris causes photophobia, pain, tearing, and decreased vision. The blood vessels next to the junction of the cornea and the sclera are engorged (ciliary flush). With increased inflammation, vascular dilatation and increased permeability of the small blood vessels in the iris permit the exudation of protein and cells into the anterior chamber. Early in the disease process, there is only a slight increase in the turbidity of the aqueous. In severe, late disease, large quantities of fibrin form sheets over the surface of the iris, lens, and posterior cornea; and the aqueous can become almost gel-like in consistency (plastic iritis).

The early cellular exudation consists primarily of polymorphonuclear leukocytes that look like small, motile, white specks in the aqueous. Later in the disease process, chronic inflammatory cells appear and may ingest and carry iris pigment to the back of the cornea or to the lens surface. The cells may deposit on the posterior surface of the

**TABLE 2.  Signs and Symptoms of Uveitis**

| SIGNS | SYMPTOMS |
|---|---|
| Ciliary flush | Pain |
| Conjunctival chemosis | Tearing |
| Band keratopathy | Decreased vision |
| Keratic precipitates | Photophobia |
| Hypopyon | |
| Small, irregular pupil | |
| Lens-iris adhesions (synechiae) | |
| Iris nodules | |
| Posterior subcapsular cataract | |
| Low intraocular pressure | |
| Cloudy aqueous/vitreous | |
| Choroidal lesions | |
| Necrotoxic retinitis | |

cornea in "agglutinated" clumps (keratic precip-itates, KP's—Fig. 1) or on the surfaces of the iris or lens. If large numbers of these cells are present, they may form a layered mass (hypopyon) in the bottom of the anterior chamber (Fig. 2). The fibrin and cellular debris can "glue" the iris to the lens (posterior synechia), (Fig. 3) or to the peripheral edge of the cornea (peripheral anterior synechia). Severe inflammation may cause bleeding into the anterior chamber (hemorrhagic iritis).

The character and distribution of the cells and the changes in the iris seen through the slit-lamp biomicroscope help to classify the type of iritis. In nongranulomatous uveitis, there are small, fine keratic precipitates composed of lymphocytes and plasma cells (Fig. 1). The inflammatory reaction in the iris is not severe. The stroma of the iris changes only slightly. Nodules do not form on its surface, and formation of synechiae is minimal. On the other hand, granulomatous uveitis causes a cellular reaction in the iris that is severe enough to produce thickening, loss of surface pat-

tern, nodules, synechiae between the lens and iris, and greasy, large, white cellular precipitates of epithelioid cells and lymphocytes on the posterior surface of the cornea (mutton-fat KP's).

Inflammation of the iris causes a small pupil (miosis) that is slowly reactive to light. Synechiae make the pupil irregular (Fig. 4). If the process is severe, the pupil does not move under any circumstances. Chronic inflammation can cause atrophy of the iris, which may make it lighter or darker than the fellow eye (heterochromia irides).

When the ciliary body is involved (cyclitis), all the signs and symptoms worsen. There is a greater tendency for the conjunctiva to swell (chemosis), and the intraocular pressure becomes low due to decreased function of the ciliary body. Isolated involvement of the ciliary body is uncommon. Chronic cyclitis causes only slight inflammation in the anterior chamber and few symptoms. It is more common for the ciliary body to be associated with inflammation of the iris in anterior uveitis and with the choroid in posterior uveitis.

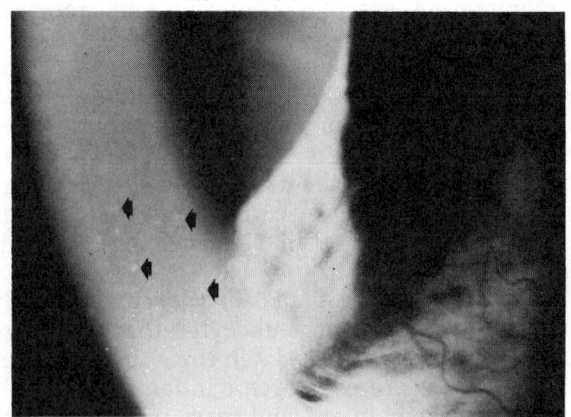

**FIGURE 1.**  *Slit-lamp photograph of inferior cornea with many clumps of cells on its posterior surface (arrows).*

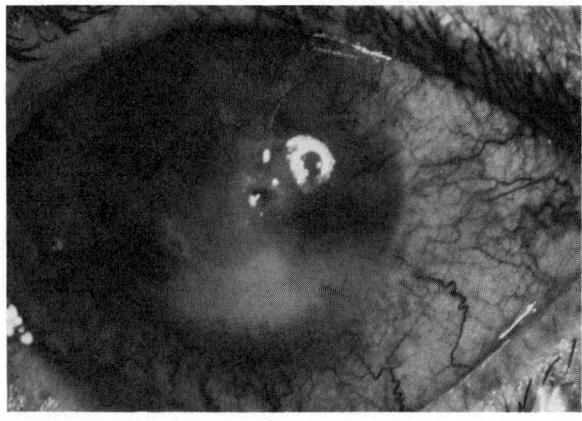

**FIGURE 2.**  *Anterior chamber with white blood cells filling the bottom one third of the chamber (hypopyon) in a patient with severe iritis after blunt trauma.*

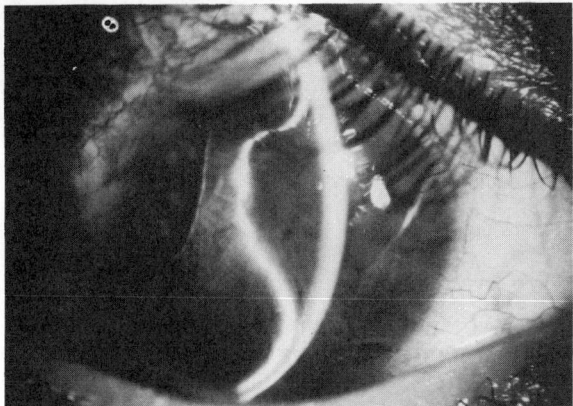

**FIGURE 3.** Slit-lamp photo demonstrating a pupil that has become adherent to the lens (posterior synechia) in a patient with Reiter's syndrome and iritis.

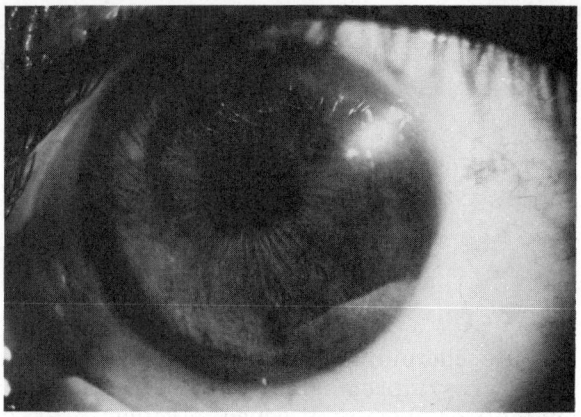

**FIGURE 4.** Irregular pupil due to partial adhesion of the iris to the lens surface.

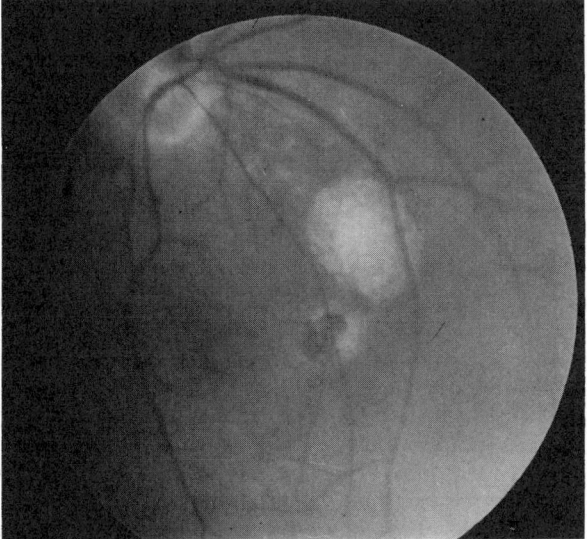

**FIGURE 5.** Two choroidal scars. The smaller lesion appears somewhat more advanced with some overlying hyperplasia of pigment cells.

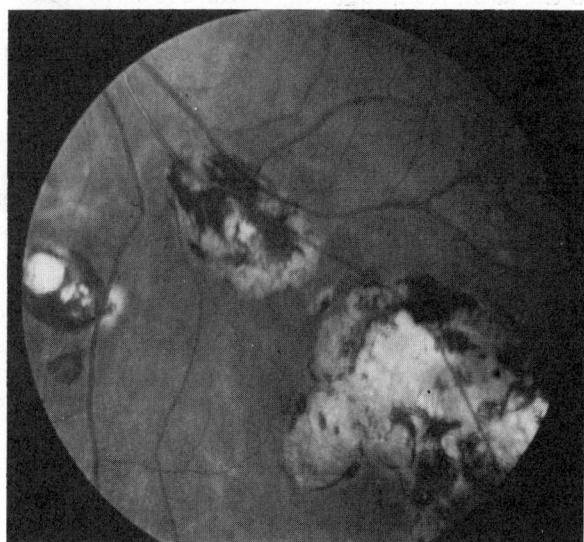

**FIGURE 6.** Multiple inactive chorioretinal scars with central depigmented areas and peripheral pigment hyperplasia. These lesions are nonspecific.

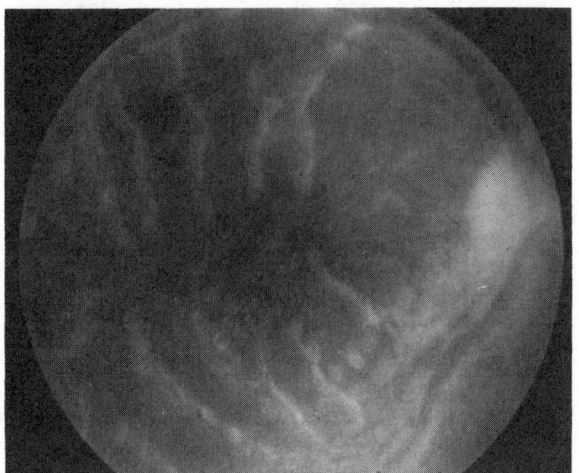

**FIGURE 7.** Diffuse retinitis in a patient with sarcoidosis. There is diffuse retinal edema, and the retinal vessels are "sheathed" with inflammatory cells. Fluid collected in the macula had reduced the vision to 20/200.

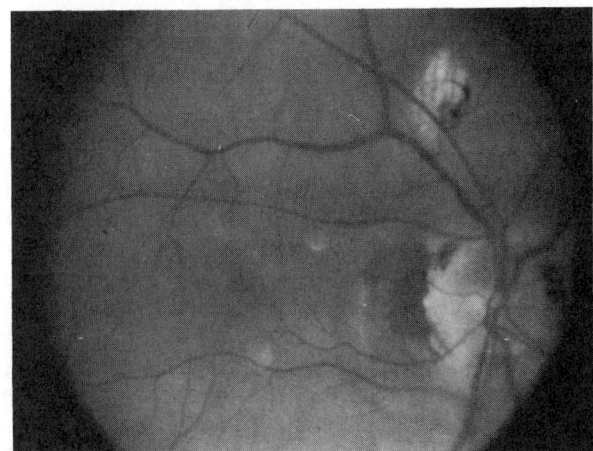

**FIGURE 8.** Retinal hemorrhage adjacent to the optic nerve head in a patient with presumed ocular histoplasmosis. Note the choroidal scar above the optic nerve.

**TABLE 3.  Complications of Uveitis**

| | |
|---|---|
| Iris depigmentation and atrophy (heterochromia) | Calcium deposits on cornea |
| | Glaucoma (many types) |
| Posterior subcapsular cataract | Corneal scarring |
| Retinal detachment | Phthisis bulbi |
| Vitreous opacification | Scleritis |
| Macular edema | Low pressure (hypotony) |
| Retinal hemorrhage | |

Acute choroiditis does not produce external signs or symptoms, and must be diagnosed ophthalmoscopically. It causes a yellow, gray, or white ill-defined lesion behind the retina. It has an overlying haze that looks like the headlight of a car as seen through fog, because it is covered by exudative fluid and cells (Fig. 5). In a later, more chronic stage, the inflamed area becomes more sharply demarcated, and the lesion changes in color due to atrophy of the choroid and scar formation (white) or proliferation of pigment cells at the edge of the scar (black) (Fig. 6).

Severe inflammation of the vitreous causes changes that are similar to those in the aqueous and suggests concomitant inflammation of the ciliary body. In the rare instances when the cellular exudation extends from the inflamed ciliary body and choroid into the uninvolved anterior segment, patients develop visual complaints only if the macula, retina (Fig. 7), vitreous, or optic nerve is involved.

Continued inflammation finally affects all layers of the globe and produces the complications listed in Table 3. Some of these changes, such as cataracts, macular edema, glaucoma, and retinal hemorrhages (Fig. 8) may occur early. The rest are late complications.

## HISTORY AND LABORATORY EVALUATION

An accurate history is probably the most important tool for establishing the correct diagnosis of uveitis. It tells us what physical findings to look for and what laboratory test(s) to order. An outline of a uveitis questionnaire is shown in Table 4. The items in parentheses are the major causes or associations of each historic item.

Many of the ocular findings in patients with uveitis can only be identified with the slit-lamp biomicroscope or ophthalmoscope (Table 2). After the history and physical examination are completed, the clinician should list in order of likelihood the types of uveitis the patient might have and order the appropriate laboratory test(s) to confirm the diagnosis (Table 5).

## TREATMENT OF UVEITIS

The major objective in the treatment of uveitis is to prevent loss of vision. If the cause is established, the disease or infection producing the inflammation should be treated promptly and appropriately. Surgical procedures may be necessary for diagnosis or to eliminate the cause of inflammation. Finally, efforts should be made to decrease the intraocular inflammation and prevent the ocular complications.

Corticosteroids are the main group of drugs that are used to treat noninfectious ocular inflammation, but other anti-inflammatory agents are sometimes necessary. Although corticosteroids are very effective, they produce many adverse systemic and ocular side effects, such as cataracts; glaucoma; poor wound healing after cataract and corneal surgery; and potentiation of fungal, bacterial, and viral infections, especially herpes simplex keratitis. These effects are so common that their *indiscriminate* use to treat a red or irritated eye must be condemned.

Corticosteroids may be used topically as eye drops or ointments applied as frequently as every hour or as infrequently as every week. As little as 0.005 per cent dexamethasone once daily has successfully suppressed corneal transplant rejections, and as frequent as hourly 1 per cent prednisolone acetate drops have been required to suppress severe anterior ocular inflammation.

Periocular steroids are necessary to treat many patients with posterior uveitis and an occasional patient with anterior inflammation that is unresponsive to topical therapy. Most ophthalmologists prefer to inject soluble, short-acting steroids underneath the fibro-fatty capsule that surrounds the globe (Tenon's capsule). Long-acting steroids should not be used unless the anti-inflammatory effect of the short-acting compounds is too transient (Schlaegel, 1970).

If topical and periocular steroids do not control the ocular inflammation, systemic steroids must be used. The risks of systemic complications from steroids must be balanced against the possibility of visual loss in these occasional patients (Schlaegel, 1975).

The pupil should be dilated in almost all pa-

**TABLE 4.   Uveitis Questionnaire**

**PAST HISTORY AND PRESENT ILLNESS**

*Acute onset with pain, redness, photophobia* (herpes simplex, Beh[4]cet's disease, recurrent toxoplasmosis, ankylosing spondylitis, Vogt-Koyanagi-Harada syndrome)

*Insidious onset with white eyes and decreased vision* (cyclitis, juvenile rheumatoid arthritis, heterochromic iritis, posterior uveitis)

*Unusual skin lumps* (juvenile xanthogranuloma, sarcoidosis)

*Change in eye color* (Fuch's heterochromic iridocyclitis)

*History of glaucoma* (glaucomatocyclitic crisis)

*Urinary tract disease* (Reiter's syndrome)

*Mental retardation, hydrocephalus* (toxoplasmosis)

*Ulcers of mouth and genital tract* (Behçet's disease)

*Recent acute febrile respiratory illness* (acute iritis and papillitis)

*Previous ocular infection* (herpes simplex)

*Change of skin and hair color* (Vogt-Koyanagi-Harada syndrome, herpes zoster, Behçet's disease, Chediak-Higashi syndrome)

*Cough and weight loss* (tuberculosis)

*Raw meat ingestion* (toxoplasmosis, trichinosis, cysticercosis)

*PICA (Toxocara)*

*Abnormal gestation* (rubella, cytomegalovirus)

*Decreased hearing or tinnitus* (Vogt-Koyanagi-Harada syndrome)

*Ocular trauma or previous cataract surgery* (sympathetic ophthalmia, lens-associated inflammations)

*History of drug abuse or hyperalimentation (Candida)*

*History of arthritis* (juvenile rheumatoid arthritis, Reiter's syndrome)

*History of venereal disease* (gonorrhea, syphilis)

*Diarrhea or blood in stool* (ulcerative colitis, bacillary dysentery)

**FAMILY HISTORY**

Recent travel (parasites)

Family members with tuberculosis

Exposure to endemic areas of coccidioidomycosis, histoplasmosis; pets *(Toxocara)*

**ALLERGY**

Pollens, food and drug allergies (rare acute iritis)

Recent injections (serum sickness)

**OCCUPATION**

Farmer (brucellosis)

Hunter (tularemia)

**MEDICATIONS**

Systemic steroids, immunosuppressive agents (cytomegalovirus)

---

tients with ocular inflammation in order to prevent the fibrin that is deposited in the anterior chamber from forming adhesions between the iris and lens, iris and cornea, or iris and filtering angle (peripheral anterior synechia). Strong cycloplegic agents such as atropine also have some anti-inflammatory effect. The prevention of synechiae also reduces the frequency of the complications of glaucoma and pupil distortion.

Patients who do not respond to corticosteroids or who develop ocular or systemic complications of steroids may require different therapy. Systemic anti-inflammatory therapy with indomethacin or aspirin occasionally helps resolve inflammation that has been unresponsive to steroids (Hanna, 1970). Severe, progressive, chronic uveitis that is unresponsive to steroids alone may respond to the addition of azathioprine or chlorambucil (Andrasch et al., 1978; Foster, 1980). The inflamed peripheral retina in chronic cyclitis (pars planitis) may respond to freezing (cryotherapy) (Aaberg et al., 1973).

More recently, there have been attempts to boost cell-mediated immunity by BCG vaccinations or systemic transfer factor. Other newer therapeutic modalities that have been used in the treatment of various ocular inflammations include the intraocular injection of steroids, antibiotics, and antifungal agents and the surgical removal of diseased tissues, such as the vitreous (mechanical vitrectomy) or the lens (phakoemulsification). The new antiviral agents (adenine arabinoside and trifluorthymidine) have been used successfully to treat epithelial herpes simplex, and adenine arabinoside has been effective against active intraocular and intraretinal herpes simplex infection. Topical interferon is currently being investigated in the treatment of patients with recurrent herpes simplex heratitis. As our knowledge of the etiology and pathogenesis of uveitis increases, the category of unknown causes of uveitis will decrease, additional forms of treatment will be developed, and fewer patients will suffer loss of vision.

**TABLE 5.   Laboratory Evaluation of Uveitis**

**GENERAL TESTS**
Complete blood count (systemic infection)
Differential blood count for eosinophils (*Toxocara*)
Sedimentation rate (ankylosing spondylitis)
Calcium (sarcoidosis)
Serum lysozyme (any granulomatous disease)
**MICROBIOLOGY**
Blood cultures (*Candida*)
Stool examinations (ova and parasites)
Cultures of biopsies and ocular paracenteses for bacteria, mycobacteria, fungi, and
    viruses
**SERUM IMMUNOLOGIC TESTS**
Microhemagglutination assay–Treponema (MHA-TP)
Bentonite flocculation and indirect hemagglutination for cysticercosis and echino-
    coccosis
Specific complement fixation tests for viral diseases
Toxoplasma dye test or fluorescent-antibody test
Anti-lens antibodies (lens-induced uveitis)
HLA B27 (ankylosing spondylitis, Reiter's disease, juvenile rheumatoid arthritis)
HLA B5 (Behçet's disease)
VDRL, FTA-ABS (syphilis)
Antinuclear antibody (juvenile rheumatoid arthritis, chronic iridocyclitis)
**SKIN TESTS**
Blastomycosis, tuberculosis, coccidioidomycosis, histoplasmosis
Anergy to *Candida, Trichophyton,* and mumps (sarcoidosis)
Dinitrochlorobenzene to establish normal delayed hypersensitivity reaction
Intradermal saline injection—pustule formation (Behçet's disease)
Casoni test (Echinococcosis)
**SPECIFIC TESTS FOR CELL-MEDIATED IMMUNITY AGAINST SUSPECTED
AGENTS**
Lymphocyte transformation studies
Migration-inhibition factor
**URINALYSIS (REITER'S)**
**X-RAYS**
Sacroiliac views (ankylosing spondylitis)
Chest (tuberculosis, sarcoidosis, coccidioidomycosis, histoplasmosis)
Skull (histiocytosis, toxoplasmosis)
Skeletal (sarcoidosis)
Orbit and ocular (foreign body)
**SURGICAL BIOPSIES**
Conjunctiva and lacrimal gland (sarcoidosis)
**SKIN AND PERIOCULAR NODULES**
Leprosy, sarcoidosis, Wegener's granulomatosis, juvenile xanthogranuloma, fungal
    granulomas
**AQUEOUS OR VITREOUS PARACENTESIS**
Eosinophils (*Toxocara*), bacteria, fungi (endophthalmitis), macrophages (phacolytic
    glaucoma), immunoglobulin levels (intraocular infection), tumor cells (reticulum
    cell sarcoma)

## References

Aaberg, T. M., Cesarz, T. J., and Flickinger, R. R.: Treatment of pe-
    ripheral uveoretinitis by cryotherapy. Am J Ophthalmol 75:085,
    1973.
Andrasch, R. H., Pirofsky, B., and Burns, R. P.: Immunosuppressive
    therapy for severe chronic uveitis. Arch Ophthalmol 96:247, 1978.
Duke-Elder, S., and Perkins, E. S.: System of Ophthalmology. Vol. IX.
    Diseases of the Uveal Tract. London, Henry Kimpton, 1966, p. 39.
Foster, C. S.: Immunosuppressive therapy for external ocular inflam-
    matory disease. Ophthalmology 87:140, 1980.
Hanna, C.: Non-steroid anti-inflammatory agents: Past and present.

In Kaufman, H. E. (ed.): Ocular Anti-Inflammatory Therapy.
    Springfield, Ill., Charles C Thomas, 1970, p. 139.
Hogan, M. J., and Zimmerman, L. E.: Ophthalmic Pathology. 2nd ed.
    Philadelphia, W. B. Saunders Company, 1962, p. 373.
Schlaegel, T. F., Jr.: Depot corticosteroids by the cul-de-sac route. In
    Kaufman, H. E. (ed.): Ocular Anti-Inflammatory Therapy. Spring-
    field, Ill., Charles C Thomas, 1970, p. 117.
Schlaegel, T. F., Jr.: Diagnosis and management of minimal recur-
    rences of macular histoplasmosis. Int Ophthalmol Clin 15:167,
    1975.
Schlaegel, T. F.: Diseases of the Uvea. In Duane, T. D. (ed.): Clinical
    Ophthalmology. Vol. 4. Hagerstown, Md., Harper and Row, 1976,
    Chapters 31–67.

# I. MUSCULOSKELETAL INFECTIONS

## BACTERIAL ARTHRITIS 236

Patrick J. Kelly, M.D.
Robert H. Fitzgerald, Jr., M.D.

### DEFINITION

This entity is also known as infectious arthritis, septic arthritis, suppurative arthritis, and pyoarthrosis. Granulomatous infections such as those caused by *Mycobacterium, Brucella,* and fungi are discussed in other chapters.

### ETIOLOGY

#### Adults

*Staphylococcus aureus* causes three fourths of all joint infections (Kelly, 1977). Beta-hemolytic streptococci (nearly all group A), *Streptococcus pneumoniae,* and *Neisseria gonorrhoeae* are the only other bacteria that cause a sizable number of infections. All gram-negative bacilli together account for 10 to 20 per cent of infections. Bacterial arthritis due to obligate anaerobic bacteria is infrequent (Ziment et al., 1969). Many different anaerobic organisms, often in mixed culture, have been isolated from joints. Most mixed anaerobic infections are due to the contiguous spread of infection from adjacent soft tissue infections. *Haemophilus influenzae* arthritis is rare in adults (Krauss et al., 1974).

#### Children

The principal organisms isolated from infected joints in children are *S. aureus* and *H. influenzae* type B. They occur with approximately equal frequency in children between 6 months and 5 years of age. In older children, *S. aureus* predominates. Group A hemolytic streptococci and the pneumococci are isolated less frequently. Gram-negative bacilli such as *Pseudomonas aeruginosa* are much less common causes of arthritis except as complications of direct puncture wounds of metatarsophalangeal joints.

Nearly all cases of bacterial arthritis are due to hematogenous spread of bacteria to the joint.

The bacteria evoke hyperemia and edema of the synovial membrane, which becomes infiltrated with leukocytes. Small vessels may rupture and cause microscopic hemorrhages. Fluid accumulates in the joint space and probably interferes with normal nutrition of the cartilage. The most devastating aspect of bacterial arthritis is the inflammatory damage to articular cartilage. The leukocytes in the joint release lysosomal enzymes that can digest cartilage and seem to destroy tissue. Since bacterial antigens, especially endotoxin, are themselves chemotactic, inflammation may persist after viable bacteria are killed (Braude et al., 1963; Curtiss and Klein, 1963; Dingle, 1973). The proteolytic enzymes produced by bacteria may also help destroy the joint. Inflammation can denude the joint of cartilage, but it rarely leads to spontaneous ankylosis in the adult. If the articular plate is penetrated by the infection, frank osteomyelitis can result. Pannus may form if the infection is not promptly controlled.

#### Predisposing Conditions

The principal predisposing factor is infection outside the joint. However, bacterial arthritis can occur following a bacteremia without any other apparent focus of infection. The knee, hip, and shoulder are most often affected. There is often no explanation for localization of infection in a particular joint, but previously damaged joints, especially those with rheumatoid arthritis, seem particularly vulnerable. (Hypocomplementemia may also increase the susceptibility of rheumatoid joints [Hunder and McDuffie, 1973]). Bacterial arthritis is also associated with diseases and treatment in which immune mechanisms are impaired, such as malignancy, diabetes mellitus, and sickle cell anemia. Patients with sickle cell anemia are especially prone to *Salmonella* infections, probably because of decreased splenic function as well as iron overload. High local concentrations of injected corticosteroids may also predispose to joint infection and may account for the increase in the incidence of shoulder joint infections that has been observed in the last ten years (Chartier et al., 1959; Kelly, 1977). Heroin addicts are peculiarly disposed to infections of axial skeletal joints with *P. aeruginosa* and *Serratia marcescens*. There is no explanation for the unusual distribution of these infections or for their unusual etiology (Kido et al., 1973).

Patients who develop gonococcal arthritis may be predisposed to disseminated infection by a deficiency of serum bactericidal activity (McCutchan et al., 1978). The strains that cause disseminated infections are often auxotrophs and differ from strains of *N. gonorrhoeae* that are limited to mucosal surfaces (see Chapter 179). Patients with congenital absence of one of the terminal complement components (C6 through C8) are uniquely predisposed to disseminated neisserial infections (Lee et al., 1978).

Infections of prosthetic arthroplasties are initiated either at the time of surgery or any time afterward by the hematogenous route. Operative sepsis, when due to organisms of low virulence, may not become apparent for several weeks. The prosthetic joint apparently remains susceptible to hematogenous infection indefinitely. These late infections often originate from urinary tract infections. Residual synovium, the pseudocapsule, or the bone in which the prosthesis is anchored may be infected (Wilson et al., 1975).

## CLINICAL MANIFESTATIONS

### Adults

The infection usually starts abruptly with fever, pain, and swelling of the affected joints. Rarely, multiple joints may be affected simultaneously. Gonococcal arthritis is often preceded by migrating polyarthritis. Gonococcal infections involve small joints more commonly than do staphylococcal infections. The infected joint is characteristically warm, painful, tender, and swollen with joint fluid. Movement of the joint, either active or passive, produces pain. Occasionally, these signs of joint infection are less dramatic so that the diagnosis is delayed. Infected rheumatoid joints are often mistaken for an exacerbation of the rheumatoid process. Other noninfectious conditions, such as gout and Reiter's syndrome, may mimic infection. Patients with gonococcal arthritis may or may not have clinical evidence of genital infection or pharyngitis. Many patients have characteristic skin lesions (Ackerman et al., 1965), especially when multiple joints are involved.

The most direct avenue to diagnosis of bacterial arthritis is aspiration of joint fluid. Infected fluids are usually yellow, turbid, and have a friable mucin clot. The white blood cell count is 10,000 to 100,000 and most of the cells are granulocytes. The protein content is elevated and the glucose concentration is almost always less than half the serum value. Gram stains are often positive except in gonococcal infections. A specific etiologic diagnosis is made by culturing the joint fluid. Blood cultures should also be obtained because in many cases *Neisseria meningitidis* and *N. gonorrhoeae* cannot be recovered from joint fluid cultures but can be grown from blood cultures. All joint fluids should be cultured on chocolate agar for *Neisseria* and *H. influenzae*.

Most patients with septic arthritis have leukocytosis and elevated erythrocyte sedimentation rates, an exception being patients with acute gonococcal infections. X-rays show only enlargement of the joint space and soft tissue swelling due to edema of periarticular structures. After several weeks of infection, rarefaction of subchondral bone develops along with narrowing of the joint space because of destruction of the articular cartilage.

Infections of prosthetic joints may cause characteristic signs and symptoms of inflammation, especially those infections that begin in the immediate postoperative period. There is usually drainage (sometimes bloody), which contains the responsible bacteria; blood cultures may also be positive. Delayed infections often occur without producing any signs of inflammation, and pain is the only symptom. Radiographic evidence of a loose prosthesis and an elevated erythrocyte sedimentation rate may be the only clues preoperatively that there is an infection. The diagnosis is made by surgical exploration, biopsy, and culture (Fitzgerald et al., 1977).

### Children

Bacterial arthritis in children presents with more characteristic symptoms and signs than does acute hematogenous osteomyelitis. Bacterial arthritis must be distinguished from rheumatic fever and rheumatoid arthritis. The most difficult distinction to make is that between benign, self-limited, sterile inflammation of the hip and bacterial arthritis of the hip. In bacterial infections, the patient is younger, the temperature and erythrocyte sedimentation rate are elevated, polyarticular involvement is more likely, and cell counts of joint fluid are higher. In the final analysis, only a positive culture or isolation of the organism from a focus in another system or from the blood may give the final answer (Molteni, 1978).

## DIFFERENTIAL DIAGNOSIS

Suppurative bacterial arthritis must be distinguished from arthritis caused by mycobacteria, *Brucella* organisms, syphilis, *Streptobacillus moniliformis, Salmonella* organisms, fungi, and viruses. Arthritis can be caused by any of the 3 species of *Brucella* and usually has an acute onset with purulent joint fluid. Like pyogenic arthritis, *Brucella* arthritis attacks the large joints, especially the hips, ankles, and sacroiliac joints and cannot be distinguished on clinical grounds from acute pyogenic arthritis. *Brucella* organisms can be cultured from the joint fluid and blood, and serum agglutinins usually reach a titer of 1:320 or more. Mycobacterial (usually *M. tuberculosis* but sometimes *M. kansasii* or *M. intracellulare*) arthritis is milder than pyogenic arthritis and may last for months or years without recognition. It is often confused with rheumatoid arthritis. Only about 50 per cent of patients with skeletal tuberculosis have active concomitant pulmonary tuberculosis, and there is often a history of antecedent local trauma to the affected joint, or of steroid injections. The mild clinical manifestations are attributed to the fact that the joint inflammation from caseating granulomas is milder than that with acute suppuration. Next to the spine, tuberculous arthritis attacks chiefly the hips or knees. The warm, swollen soft tissues around these joints have a peculiar doughy consistency and are not usually red. A surprising feature is the cell count of the joint fluid: there are usually over 10,000 cells/mm$^3$ and the majority are often polymorphonuclears. Acid-fast smears are positive in only 30 per cent but cultures of the fluid or synovial biopsy tissue yield the tubercle bacillus in over 80 per cent of cases. Biopsies of the synovium show granulomas in over 90 per cent.

Septic arthritis due to *Salmonella, E. coli,* and other enteric bacilli is an acute pyogenic infection but occurs mainly in sickle cell disease, systemic lupus erythematosus, chronic rheumatoid arthritis, and other debilitating diseases. These infections tend to be monoarticular and usually in the knee. Arthritis due to *E. coli* is often accompanied by *E. coli* cystitis or pyelonephritis. Because of the underlying problems, these gram-negative bacillus infections show a poor response to treatment. *Pseudomonas aeruginosa* has become the most important nonenteric gram-negative bacillus causing arthritis. It is especially prominent as a cause of monoarticular infection in heroin addicts, in whom it has a predilection for the sternoclavicular and sacroiliac joints.

Three other bacterial infections must also be kept in mind in the differential diagnosis of septic arthritis. *Streptobacillus moniliformis,* the cause of rat bite fever, produces a very painful migratory polyarthritis in 50 per cent of cases, and tends to involve large joints. Syphilis produces migratory polyarthralgia due to periostitis in the secondary stage, Clutton's joints in older children (8 to 16 years), and Charcot joints in tabes dorsalis. The painless bilateral hydroarthrosis of Clutton's joints, and the noninflammatory neuropathic joint of Charcot's disease are easy to distinguish from acute bacterial arthritis. The third bacterial infection to be considered is septic bursitis. This is a disease of the olecranon (80 per cent) and prepatellar bursae, and is sometimes confused with infection of the elbow or knee joints themselves. It is not, however, associated with septic arthritis and is recognized by the characteristic swelling of the bursa, by a history of trauma or sustained pressure, and by examination of bursa fluid, which is purulent and usually infected with staphylococci.

Bacterial arthritis must also be differentiated from acute viral arthritis due to rubella, mumps, hepatitis B, and certain togaviruses. Before its eradication, smallpox was also a cause of infectious arthritis. Most of these tend to be polyarticular and can cause severe pain. Rubella arthritis is a common problem in adolescents and adults. It usually starts when the rash is fading and it involves both large and small joints. Because of its migratory polyarticular nature, it tends to resemble rheumatic fever or rheumatoid arthritis more than septic arthritis. Although massive effusions can occur in large joints, much more commonly fusiform swellings develop in the fingers. All manifestations usually go away in 5 to 10 days. Mumps arthritis is also polyarticular and migrates to large and small joints, but is rare. Varicella is another rare cause of arthritis; it can produce pain and a monoarticular effusion in the knee without erythema. The synovial fluid has a few thousand lymphocytes. The polyarthritis of hepatitis B virus infection occurs in the preicteric stage, is usually a symmetric disease of distal joints, but may affect large joints as well. Patients with hepatitis may seem to have various forms of acute arthritis, only to have the diagnosis clarified when jaundice appears. The two togaviruses that cause prominent joint symptoms are both alphaviruses: Chikungunya fever virus and Ross River virus. Chikungunya fever is a disease of Southeast Asia and Africa in which joint pain is so severe that the patient literally folds up from the immobilizing discomfort. The crippling joint pains may return periodically over the next four months. The occurrence of a maculopapular rash and the leukopenia help differentiate this disease from pyogenic infections. In addition, joint swelling and redness is not common. Ross River virus also causes an illness with febrile rash and is endemic in Australia, but has recently caused a large outbreak in Fiji, where a number of American tourists became infected. The disease in Australia, known as epidemic polyarthritis is characterized by mild joint pains and is transmitted by bites of *Aedes vigilax* and *Culex annulirostris*.

Any of the deep fungus infections can produce arthritis by extension from adjacent areas of osteomyelitis. This form of secondary fungal arthritis is most common in mycetomas, and easily recognized by the characteristic antecedent infection of the bone and soft tissues (Chapter 238). Occasionally, however, the agents of mycetoma, such as *Petriellidium boydii,* can be inoculated directly into the joint and cause primary arthritis, especially of the knee. Coccidioidomycosis and sporotrichosis are much more important causes of fungal arthritis and need to be distinguished from bacterial arthritis. Primary pulmonary coccidioidomycosis can be accompanied by a transient arthritis in which the joints are painful, tender, swollen, and red. The fungus is not present in the joint and the arthritis disappears. In about 33 per cent of cases of chronic dissemination, *Coccidioides immitis* invades the joints, usually the ankle, but the knee, elbow, wrist, shoulder, and hand are also infected in the order of frequency listed, and often more than one at a time. The infection starts as an acute arthritis with swelling and redness but later causes a chronic monoarticular arthritis. This may occur without evidence of coccidioidomycosis elsewhere, usually involves the knee, and no adjacent bone involvement is seen on x-ray examination. *Coccidioides immitis* is readily cultured from joint fluid, synovial biopsy tissue, or drainage from articular sinuses. In sporotrichosis, arthritis can be secondary either to hematogenous dissemination or trauma. The hematogenous form of arthritis can be one of several sites of disseminated infection with migratory joint swellings and effusions, or it may be the only metastatic focus. Traumatic synovitis results from penetrating injury of a joint or tendon sheath and tends to occur in alcoholic gardeners because the fungus can penetrate deeper when pain is blunted by inebriation. It tends to involve the wrist, which becomes swollen, painful and tender. Unless the synovium is biopsied and cultured with *Sporothrix* in mind, the diagnosis is usually missed and the patient mistakenly treated for tuberculosis after granulomas are seen in the joint tissue. *Candida* arthritis can also be hematogenous or traumatic. Hematogenous infection sometimes spreads to two or more joints and affects the knee, hip, and elbow in that order of frequency. Traumatic candidal arthritis is a complication of steroid injec-

tion. In contrast to other fungal infections, the arthritis is not granulomatous, and causes a polymorphonuclear exudate in acute infections. The yeast is seen and grown with ease in the joint fluid.

## COMPLICATIONS AND SEQUELAE

### Adults

Although bacterial arthritis is not a common disease, death attributable to this disorder has occurred in as many as 15 per cent of proven cases (Kelly, 1977). Spread to bone and ligaments around the joint can lead to a markedly unstable joint and necessitate external support or a surgical arthrodesis after infection is controlled. In adults, spontaneous bony ankylosis is not common. Because of loss of bone or poor positioning during the healing period, flexion contractures, inequality of limb length, and a painful joint may result. Persistent drainage may occur, especially if there is secondary osteomyelitis.

### Children

Delay in diagnosis and therefore delay in treatment are the most important factors adversely affecting prognosis. One study of 49 patients indicated that 31 per cent were functionally impaired as the result of their infections (Howard et al., 1976). Bacterial arthritis of the hip may have serious sequelae such as discrepancies in limb length, persistent pain, and limitation of hip motion. These complications may require arthrodesis of the hip, epiphysiodesis to correct leg length, or an osteotomy to correct deformity. The hip and shoulder joints are especially prone to late sequelae because the ends of the bone are within the joint space. With accumulation of pus, increased pressure compromises the blood supply, and necrosis of the femoral or humeral head can occur. The destruction of joints seems to be equally likely with *S. aureus* and *H. influenzae* infections.

## GEOGRAPHIC VARIATIONS

Geographic variation in the occurrence of bacterial arthritis is not striking if granulomatous infections are excluded. Large series with late follow-up are now available from North America (Morrey et al., 1975; Howard et al., 1976; Newman, 1976; Nade, 1977), Australia, and England, and no major differences in pattern are evident.

## *TREATMENT*

### Adults

It is necessary to identify the specific microorganism responsible for the infection and determine its susceptibility to antibacterials. If the diagnosis is established early, antibacterial treatment alone may cure the patient. Most antibiotics are transported into the synovial fluid, and concentrations are approximately equal to serum levels (Nelson, 1971; Parker and Schmid, 1971; Marsh et al., 1974). There is no reason to inject antibiotics directly into the joint space. Pneumococci and beta-hemolytic streptococci should be treated with penicillin G. There are no convincing data to guide one in deciding how long the patient with *S. aureus* arthritis should receive antibiotics. However, it appears to us that a month of parenteral antibacterials is a helpful, albeit an arbitrary guide. Uncomplicated gonococcal arthritis can be cured with seven to ten days of either oral ampicillin, 2 g/day, or tetracycline, 2 g/day. More acutely ill patients should be treated with intravenous penicillin G in a dose of 10 million units/day for three days or until improvement occurs. Treatment is then continued with ampicillin for a total of ten days' combined therapy.

There is controversy regarding removal of infected joint fluid. Experiments in animal models support a hypothesis that infected joint fluid interferes with metabolism of cartilage (Curtiss and Klein, 1965) and that its removal diminishes this damage (Daniel et al., 1975). On this basis surgeons favor removal of infected joint fluid. Easily accessible joints such as the knee, ankle, and shoulder can be aspirated by needle and syringe. If the fluid thickens or if the joint is one that is not easily aspirated—for example, the hip or sacroiliac joint—it may be necessary to open the joint and remove infected material by suction-irrigation. However, some cautionary notes must be made: (1) Addition of antibacterials to the irrigant may not only be unnecessary but can be harmful because potentially toxic antibacterials can be absorbed by synovial tissues and the antibacterial may be damaging to articular cartilage. (2) Suction-irrigation may allow entry of secondary invaders and cause superinfection, especially if kept in place beyond three to four days. Some authorities believe that periodic distention of the joint prevents adhesions.

Open drainage has been advocated recently (Ballard et al., 1975), as it was after World War I (Willems, 1919). Establishing open drainage may be necessary if purulent material tends to loculate in the recesses of the joint. This method may be useful in post-traumatic joint infections, which represent a different category of patients from those with hematogenous septic arthritis.

In the adult, the following brief outline suggests the management of bacterial arthritis when the diagnosis and institution of treatment have been delayed and one is faced with a surgical as well as a medical problem.

1. Débridement and arthrodesis are recommended for the knee, ankle, elbow, wrist, and subtalar joints. Compression by means of the Hoffman apparatus is useful.

2. For the hip, joint resection should be done, followed by skeletal traction and gradual ambulation with an ischial weight-bearing brace for three months.

3. For the glenohumeral, sternoclavicular, and acromioclavicular joints, débridement of the joint and immobilization in a sling are recommended. The treatment of infected prosthetic joints is often difficult. Most acute infections should be treated by removal of the prosthesis, surgical débridement, and four weeks of parenteral antibiotics, chosen according to the in vitro susceptibility of the pathogen. In some cases, if the components are not loose and there is no x-ray evidence of osteomyelitis, it may be possible to suppress the infection without removing the prosthesis. Once the infection has been brought under control, these patients should receive oral antibiotics indefinitely. Some patients with infections due to bacteria of low virulence, for example, *Staphylococcus epidermidis,* can be treated by removal of the prosthesis, débridement, and antibiotics with reinsertion of a new prosthesis in six months (Wilson, 1978).

### Children

It appears that bacterial arthritis of the hip in the child is best treated by immediate open surgical drainage. This statement may be controversial, but long-term follow-up studies suggest that the majority of bad results from bacterial arthritis occur after hip infections. In one series, 50 per cent of the late results were unsatisfactory. In the other joints that are more accessible to needle aspiration, daily needle aspiration may be adequate; if not, open drainage is preferable to no drainage. Management of late sequelae are discussed above.

In summary, early diagnosis, identification of the causative organism, and proper choice of antibacterial agent, plus removal of infected joint material, are the essential steps in the treatment of infections of the joint. Early diagnosis is all too often not established, and when first seen, some patients have irreparably injured joints. Once invasion of bone has occurred and ligamentous structures have been damaged, it seems likely that stability, mobility, and freedom from pain will have been lost.

## References

Ackerman, A. B., Miller, R. C., and Shapiro, L.: Gonococcemia and its cutaneous manifestations. Arch Dermatol 91:227, 1965.

Ballard, A., Burkhalter, W. E., Mayfield, G. W., Dehne, E., and Brown, P. W.: The functional treatment of pyogenic arthritis of the adult knee. J Bone Joint Surg [Am]57:1119, 1975.

Braude, A. I., Jones, J. L., and Douglas, H.: The behavior of *Escherichia coli* endotoxin (somatic antigen) during infectious arthritis. J Immunol 90:297, 1963.

Chartier, Y., Martin, W. J., and Kelly, P. J.: Bacterial arthritis: Experiences in the treatment of 77 patients. Ann Intern Med 50:1462, 1959.

Curtiss, P. H., Jr., and Klein, L.: Destruction of articular cartilage in septic arthritis. I. In vitro studies. J Bone Joint Surg [Am] 45:797, 1963.

Curtiss, P. H., Jr., and Klein, L.: Destruction of articular cartilage in septic arthritis. II. In vivo studies. J Bone Joint Surg [Am] 47:1595, 1965.

Daniel, D., Akeson, W., and Amiel, D.: The effect of joint lavage in preventing cartilage destruction in an experimentally produced *Staphylococcus aureus* joint infection (abstract). J Bone Joint Surg [Am]57:583, 1975.

Dingle, J. T.: The role of lysosomal enzymes in skeletal tissues. J Bone Joint Surg [Br] 55:87, 1973.

Fitzgerald, R. H., Nolan, D. R., Ilstrup, D. M., Van Scoy, R. E, Washington, J. A. II, and Coventry, M. B.: Deep wound sepsis following total hip arthroplasty. J Bone Joint Surg 59:847, 1977.

Howard, J. B., Highgenboten, C. L., and Nelson, J. D.: Residual effects of septic arthritis in infancy and childhood. JAMA 236:932, 1976.

Hunder, G. G., and McDuffie, F. C.: Hypocomplementemia in rheumatoid arthritis. Am J Med 54:461, 1973.

Kelly, P. J.: Infections of bones and joints in adult patients. Instructional Course Lectures 26:3, 1977.

Kido, D., Bryan, D., and Halpern, M.: Hematogenous osteomyelitis in drug addicts. Am J Roentgenol Rad Ther Nucl Med 118:356, 1973.

Krauss, D. S., Aronson, M. D., Gump, D. W., and Newcombe, D. S.: *Hemophilus influenzae* septic arthritis: A mimicker of gonococcal arthritis. Arthritis Rheum 17:267, 1974.

Lee, T. J., Utsinger, P. D., Snyderman, R., Yount, W. J., and Sparling, P. F.: Familial deficiency of the seventh component of complement associated with recurrent bacteremic infections due to *Neisseria*. J Infect Dis 138:359, 1978.

Marsh, D. C., Jr., Matthew, E. B., and Persellin, R. H.: Transport of gentamicin into synovial fluid. JAMA 228:607, 1974.

McCutchan, J. A., Katzenstein, D., Norquist, D., Chikami, G., Wunderlich, A., and Braude, A. I.: Role of blocking antibody in disseminated gonococcal infection. J Immunol 121:1884, 1978.

Molteni, R. A.: The differential diagnosis of benign and septic joint disease in children: Clinical, radiologic, laboratory, and joint fluid analysis, based on 37 children with septic arthritis and 97 with benign aseptic arthritis. Clin Pediatr 17:19, 1978.

Morrey, B. F., Bianco, A. J., Jr., and Rhodes, K. H.: Septic arthritis in children. Orthoped Clin North Am 6:923, 1975.

Nade, S.: Choice of antibiotics in management of acute osteomyelitis and acute septic arthritis in children. Arch Dis Child 52:679, 1977.

Nelson, J. D.: Antibiotic concentrations in septic joint effusions. N Engl J Med 284:349, 1971.

Newman, J. H.: Review of septic arthritis throughout the antibiotic era. Ann Rheum Dis 35:198, 1976.

Parker, R. H., and Schmid, F. R.: Antibacterial activity of synovial fluid during therapy of septic arthritis. Arthritis Rheum 14:96, 1971.

Willems, C.: Treatment of purulent arthritis by wide arthrotomy followed by immediate active mobilization. Surg Gynecol Obstet 28:546, 1919.

Wilson, M. R., Fitzgerald, R. H., Jr., and Coventry, M. B.; Reconstruction (delayed) by total hip arthroplasty after resection arthroplasty for infection. Proc Sci Meet Hip Soc 6:149, 1978.

Wilson, P. D. Jr., Salvati, E. A., and Blumenfeld, E. L.: The problem of infection in total prosthetic arthroplasty of the hip. Surg Clin North Am 55:1431, 1975.

Ziment, I., Davis, A., and Finegold, S. M.: Joint infection by anaerobic bacteria: A case report and review of the literature. Arthritis Rheum 12:627, 1969.

# 237 *BACTERIAL OSTEOMYELITIS*

*Robert H. Fitzgerald, Jr., M.D.*
*Patrick J. Kelly, M.D.*

## DEFINITION

Although osteomyelitis refers to an inflammation of the marrow (myelitis) of bone *(osteo)*, the term is generally understood to signify an infection of either the cortical or the medullary portion of a bone. Pyogenic or bacterial osteomyelitis can be subdivided into hematogenous and secondary forms of osteomyelitis; the latter includes osteomyelitis from a contiguous focus of infection and post-traumatic and postoperative osteomyelitis. The selection of treatment requires further subdivision into acute and chronic stages according to the clinical signs and symptoms and the pathologic changes.

## PATHOGENESIS AND PATHOLOGY

The exact pathophysiologic changes in hematogenous osteomyelitis are incompletely understood. Although the initial pathologic changes may occur in various anatomic locations, the relatively high frequency of involvement of the metaphyses suggests that this site is vulnerable to infection. The vascular anatomy of the metaphysis (end arteries, capillary loops, and venous sinusoids) creates the necessary environment for the propagation of infective emboli (Trueta, 1959). Hobo (1921) demonstrated that the afferent capillary has no phagocytes and that in the efferent venous sinusoid, phagocytosis by leukocytes and endothelial cells is ineffective.

The infective embolus probably enters through the nutrient artery and lodges in the metaphyseal end artery–venous sinusoid. The local nidus of sepsis creates arterial occlusion. Both the host's humoral and cellular responses and the toxins released by the invading bacteria combine to produce tissue necrosis. The resulting debris, exudate, and acidosis increase the local pressure, which further compromises the circulation and promotes more necrosis. When defense mechanisms fail to eradicate the bacteria, an abscess (Brodie's abscess) surrounded by a fibrous membrane and a wall of dense bone may occur (Fig. 1). The infection may then become quiescent only to undergo recrudescence. Frequently, the bacteria are destroyed, and serous fluid or fibrous tissue fills the cavity. More frequently, the necrosis and increased pressure spread the infection through the paths of least resistance: the haversian and Volkmann canals and the intramedullary space. As the process continues, the pus forms a subperiosteal abscess and deprives the cortex of its periosteal blood supply. If the endosteal blood supply is occluded simultaneously, the entire cortex can become necrotic and sequestrated (Fig. 2). New periosteal bone is formed, and this creates an involucrum about the necrotic bone (the sequestrum). A reactive synovitis frequently occurs in adjacent joints. Healing with resolution of the infection may occur at any stage,

by natural recovery or through the influence of antimicrobial agents.

Hematogenous osteomyelitis in adults is uncommon and usually affects the axial skeleton of patients in the fifth and sixth decades of life. An underlying debilitating condition such as diabetes mellitus is frequently noted. Most commonly, the thoracolumbar segments of the spinal column

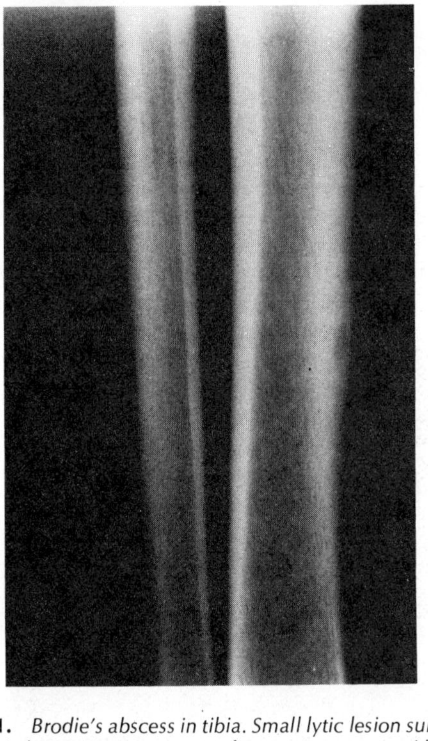

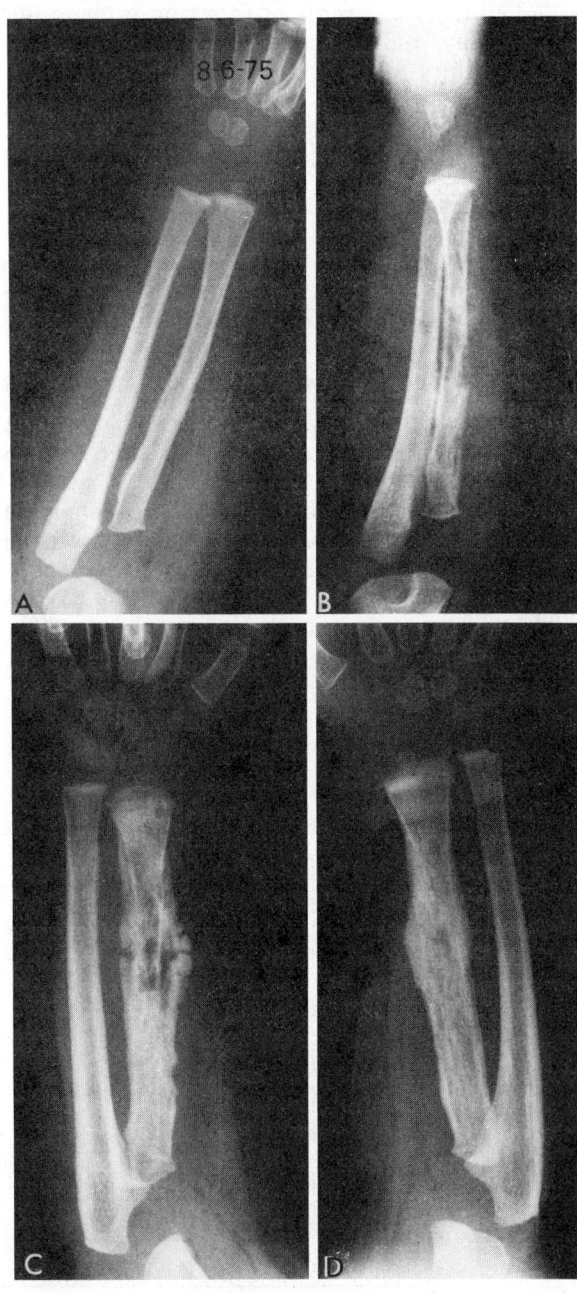

**FIGURE 2.** *Acute osteomyelitis of radius and ulna in a child. A, Soft tissue changes can be seen within the first week after onset of symptoms. B, Lytic destruction of osseous architecture is seen in the third week. C, Elevation of periosteum with new periosteal bone formation has resulted in sequestration of entire radius. D, Healing of osteomyelitic process is well demonstrated.*

**FIGURE 1.** *Brodie's abscess in tibia. Small lytic lesion surrounded by sclerotic bone. Note attempt to form a sinus tract, with erosion of sclerotic bone.*

are involved. An antecedent infection of the pelvic organs or instrumentation of the urogenital tract is frequently associated with vertebral osteomyelitis and is considered to create a bacteremia, with retrograde seeding of the vertebral body through the interconnecting plexus of valveless veins, as described by Batson (1957). Arterial seeding through posterior spinal arteries into the nutrient artery is also believed to occur, and this is undoubtedly the route of infection in drug addicts (Wiley and Trueta, 1959). The vertebrae have capillary arcades and venous sinusoids adjacent to the vertebral end plate, reminiscent of the metaphysis of a long bone in a growing child. The intervertebral disk space becomes involved only after the end plate has been destroyed by the infection.

## ETIOLOGY

### Hematogenous Causes

*Staphylococcus aureus* causes 80 to 90 per cent of hematogenous bone infections in children (Morrey and Peterson, 1975). Group A beta hemolytic streptococci are seen most frequently in children under 3 years. Gram-negative bacteria, other than *Haemophilus influenza,* are encoun-

tered very infrequently in children, except for those with sickle cell anemia who are susceptible to infection with *Salmonella enteritidis.*

Adults with acute vertebral osteomyelitis are also most often infected with *S. aureus.* Enteric gram-negative bacilli such as *Escherichia coli* also cause vertebral osteomyelitis, especially when the infection originates in the urinary tract. In drug addicts *Pseudomonas aeruginosa, Serratia marcescens,* or *S. aureus* often causes osteomyelitis.

### Contiguous Focus

Bone infections that originate from contiguous soft tissue infections can have various bacterial etiologies and may even be due to mixtures of bacteria from multiple genera. *S. aureus* is the most common etiology, but various gram-negative bacteria can cause osteomyelitis in this clinical setting (Fierer et al., 1979). Identification of the etiologic agent can be difficult in these cases because many have received an antibiotic for their soft tissue infection, which prevents the growth of the primary pathogen but allows the superficial overgrowth of antibiotic-resistant, colonizing bacteria in the wound. A specific syndrome of osteomyelitis due to *P. aeruginosa* has been recognized in patients who sustain a puncture wound of the foot.

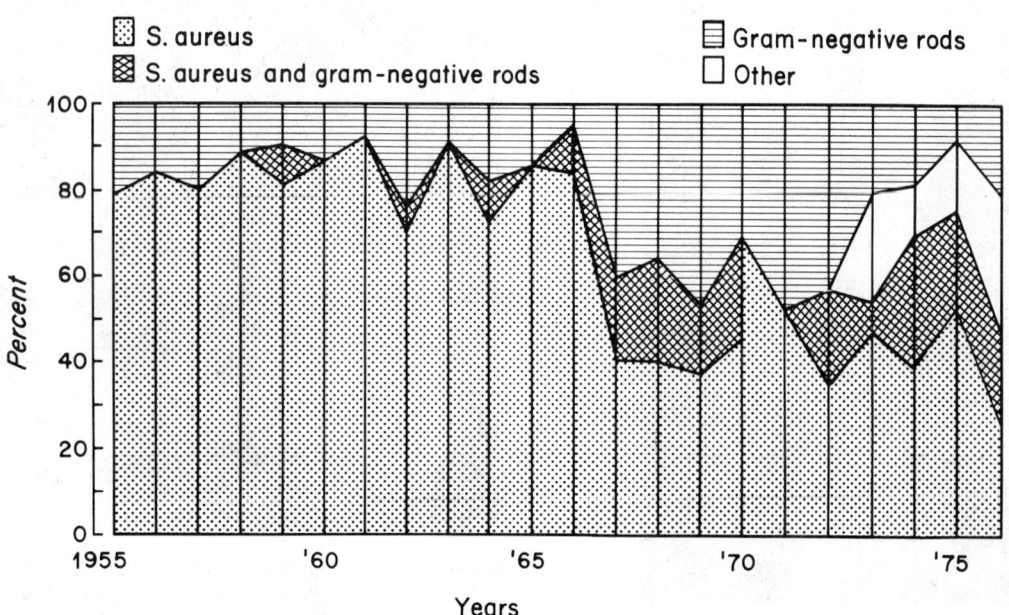

**FIGURE 3.** *Isolates recovered from tissue cultures obtained at debridement in patients with chronic osteomyelitis.*

## Post-traumatic and Postoperative Causes

Whereas *S. aureus* is the cause of hematogenous osteomyelitis in the vast majority of patients, contamination of traumatic wounds with soil and water results in infections due to a diverse group of microorganisms. Gram-negative bacilli have been isolated in more than half the patients, and even fungi are occasionally isolated in post-traumatic osteomyelitis. When anaerobic bacteria are isolated, it is usually as part of a mixed culture containing facultative anaerobes.

The microbiologic findings in chronic hematogenous osteomyelitis are different from those in post-traumatic and postoperative osteomyelitis. Gram-positive bacteria, especially *S. aureus,* are isolated in patients with postoperative and chronic hematogenous osteomyelitis. Gram-negative bacilli predominate in post-traumatic osteomyelitis. The increasing frequency of post-traumatic osteomyelitis is reflected in our overall experience with the microbiologic findings in chronic osteomyelitis (Fig. 3). *S. aureus,* formerly the causal organism in 80 per cent of patients with chronic osteomyelitis, is still most frequently isolated, but gram-negative bacilli and anaerobes are cultured with increasing frequency.

## CLINICAL MANIFESTATIONS

### Hematogenous

Acute hematogenous osteomyelitis is primarily a disease of children between the ages of 3 and 15 years. The abrupt onset of pain of increasing severity, frequently after minor trauma, and fever are the cardinal symptoms. Irritability, lethargy, and dehydration are usually present as well. The principal signs are tenderness, erythema, and swelling. The joints of the involved extremity are held in flexion, and the enveloping muscles are in spasm. Unless done gently, passive motion in the adjacent joints is resisted. Fluctuation is not found until the abscess cavity has ruptured through the periosteum. Pseudoparalysis is frequent. Leukocytosis, with counts as high as 30,000/mm³, and a shift to the left usually occur. An elevated erythrocyte sedimentation rate is characteristic. Although roentgenographic examination in the acute phase demonstrates a normal osseous pattern, careful inspection frequently identifies alteration of the soft tissues. A localized destructive process surrounded by a zone of decalcification in the metaphysis is observed 10 to 14 days after the onset of the disease (Fig. 4). Subsequently, the periosteal shadow at the same level is elevated, and periosteal calcifi-

cation may occur. In the untreated patient, the periosteum may be elevated in a circumferential fashion, creating an involucrum of the entire bone. Eventually, the trabeculae of the metaphysis are eroded, giving a moth-eaten appearance (Fig. 4*B*).

Before definitive roentgenographic changes of the osseous structure are seen, a technetium–99 scan frequently demonstrates the area of involvement. The earliest detectable change may be a decrease in uptake of the isotope in the metaphysis. Increased uptake occurs a few days later. Because the isotope is normally concentrated in the metaphysis, it may be difficult to distinguish changes due to infection, and a normal scan does not exclude the diagnosis within the first five days of infection.

Hematogenous osteomyelitis has a predilection for the metaphyseal region of a long tubular bone. The distal femoral and the proximal and distal tibial metaphyses are the most frequent sites of involvement. Infection of the proximal femoral metaphysis is intracapsular and frequently is associated with septic arthritis of the hip. The humerus, fibula, radius, and ulna are involved less frequently. The pelvis is infected but only uncommonly. In the child with spinal involvement, the arterial blood supply to the disk space results in

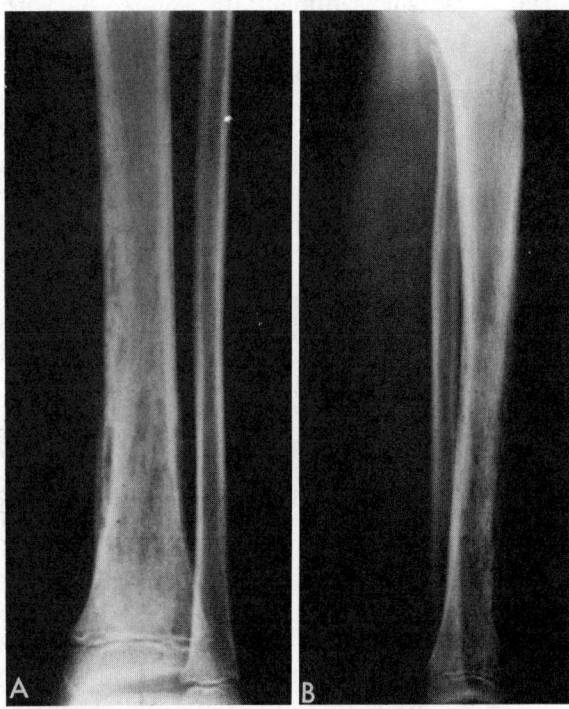

**FIGURE 4.**   *Anteroposterior (A) and lateral (B) views. Patient with osteomyelitis of distal tibial metaphysis. Periosteal elevation and localized lytic destruction with surrounding zone of decalcification are well illustrated.*

disk space infections rather than vertebral osteomyelitis, as seen in the adult.

A subacute form of the disease is occasionally encountered in a child who has received inadequate antimicrobial therapy. This illness has few systemic symptoms and a persistence of regional physical findings. Although the leukocyte count may have returned to normal as the result of incomplete therapy, the erythrocyte sedimentation rate remains elevated. Roentgenographic changes usually are seen.

Although the patient with acute vertebral hematogenous osteomyelitis may have severe back pain and systemic signs of acute sepsis, the clinical signs and symptoms are frequently insidious, with little systemic reaction. Localized pain to the area of involvement is the most characteristic symptom. There is usually severe paraspinal spasm and splinting to prevent spinal motion. Palpation and percussion over the afflicted area precipitate exquisite pain.

There is frequently a normal or slightly elevated leukocyte count. Elevation of the erythrocyte sedimentation rate is the most frequent abnormal laboratory finding. During acute systemic disease, the causal organism may be identified with cultures of blood and tissue obtained by needle biopsy of the vertebral body. In the subacute and chronic phases of the disease, the causal organism is difficult to isolate. As with other types of acute osteomyelitis, roentgenographic findings are normal for the first 10 to 14 days. The earliest changes include narrowing of the disk space and demineralization of the end plate. Erosion of the vertebral body and end plate follows (Fig. 5). Loss of vertebral height frequently occurs. During the early phase, a technetium-99 scan can be helpful in identifying the level involved.

Blood cultures are positive in approximately two thirds of patients with acute osteomyelitis. In the remaining third, the diagnosis is made by aspiration of a contiguous abscess or needle biopsy of the subperiosteal space or metaphysis. If needle aspiration yields only sterile blood, it may be necessary to repeat the procedure if the patient has not responded to empiric therapy. Open biopsy of the affected vertebrae may be necessary to establish the diagnosis in adults.

## Osteomyelitis from a Contiguous Focus of Infection

Osteomyelitis secondary to exogenous contamination or spread from a contiguous focus of infection that has been incompletely treated is being seen with increasing frequency (Fitzgerald et al., 1975). This form of osteomyelitis usually occurs after a puncture wound to the foot but also after an inadequately treated soft tissue abscess or septic arthritis. The patients usually have re-

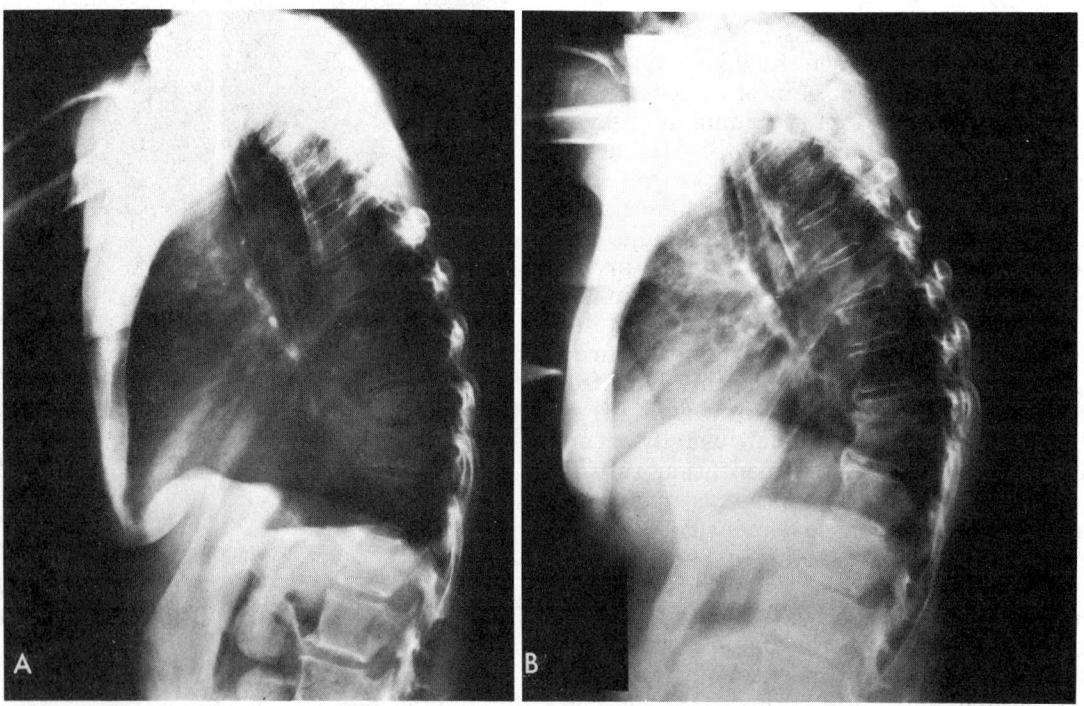

**FIGURE 5.** *Vertebral osteomyelitis. Periapical abscess with hematogenous seeding of the T9 and T10 vertebrae. A, Erosion of end plates, with collapse of disk space. B, Spontaneous fusion is occurring.*

ceived incomplete antimicrobial therapy, which changed their clinical picture. They are frequently afebrile but have a limp or a painful extremity with regional muscular spasm. The sedimentation rate is usually elevated.

Because most of these patients are seen late during the course of the infection, characteristic roentgenographic changes are present. Surgical débridement is invariably necessary in their treatment. A retained foreign body is common after puncture wounds. When a foreign body is not encountered, the central focus involves a cartilaginous surface (articular, epiphyseal, apophyseal, or some combination of these).

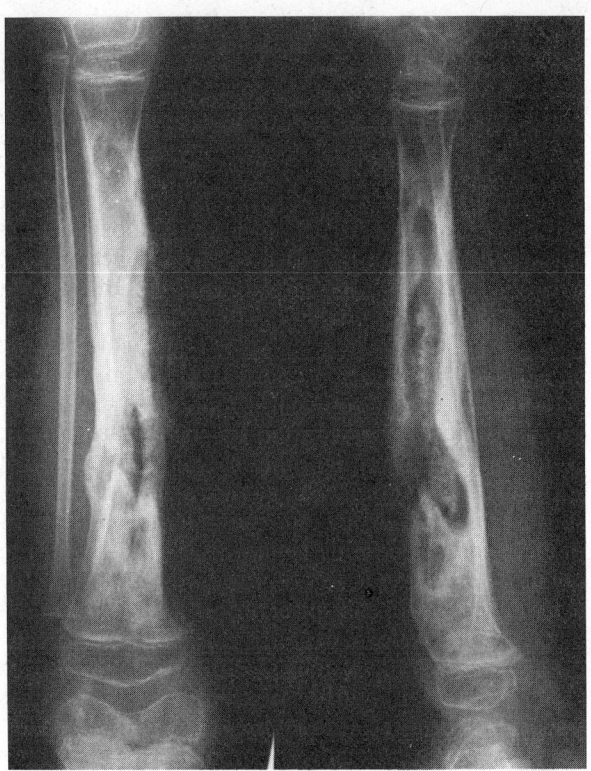

**FIGURE 6.** *Chronic osteomyelitis of tibia, with sequestrum in intramedullary canal.*

## Post-traumatic and Postoperative Osteomyelitis

The neurovascular and other soft tissue injuries associated with fractures and dislocations of the musculoskeletal system increase the risk of infection in patients with severe traumatic injuries. The areas of involvement reflect the high incidence of traumatic injuries to the tibia and femur and, to a lesser extent, the bones of the upper extremity. Concomitant nonunion of fractures in as many as one third of the patients with post-traumatic osteomyelitis was noted by Fitzgerald and Kelly (in press).

With the improved diagnostic techniques and therapeutic modalities in the treatment of acute hematogenous osteomyelitis, the incidence of chronic hematogenous osteomyelitis has decreased and should continue to do so. The most common sites of involvement (the femur, tibia, and humerus) reflect the high incidence of osteomyelitis in these sites in children. The femur and tibia constitute almost 80 per cent of the long bones involved. Disease of the soft tissues about the involved bone can vary considerably. Contracted scar with little healthy tissue is noted in patients who have had repeated surgery or chronic drainage.

Laboratory tests are rarely of value in patients with chronic osteomyelitis. Roentgenographic examination of the involved extremity demonstrates deformity with a mixture of lucent and sclerotic changes. Although sequestrum may be noted on routine roentgenograms, tomography may be needed to visualize the sclerotic changes (Fig. 6).

Although comparisons are difficult, the prognosis in patients with either post-traumatic or postoperative osteomyelitis is similar to that in patients with chronic hematogenous osteomyelitis. Successful eradication of the infection is most frequent in the upper extremity, followed by the femur and tibia. Infection recurs more often in patients with a concomitant nonunion than in those with a united but infected fracture. Gram-negative bacilli are often isolated in pure or mixed culture in recurrent infections.

The incidence of osteomyelitis and postoperative wound infection after musculoskeletal surgery is unknown. The incidence of postoperative wound sepsis has been reported to vary from 1.0 to 7.4 per cent (Howard, 1964; Patzakis et al., 1974). However, most major institutions have reported an incidence of deep wound infection of 1 to 2 per cent after musculoskeletal surgery (Fitzgerald, 1979), the infection rate varying with the type of surgery. Elective procedures without the implantation of foreign bodies and procedures performed on children have a low infection rate (0.5 per cent) (Patzakis et al., 1974). In surgery after fractures and dislocations, especially with an open injury, the infection rate is usually 1 to 2 per cent. Procedures for implantation of a foreign body, especially the newer ones involving implantation of a total joint arthroplasty, have an infection rate of approximately 1 per cent (Fitzgerald et al., 1977).

Osteomyelitis frequently develops from infections after surgery that involves a foreign body: a plate, screws, a rod, or a total joint arthroplasty (Burri, 1975). Most infections are due to gram-positive bacteria acquired in the operating rooms. In recent years, anaerobic isolates have been identified in almost 25 per cent of such infections (Fitzgerald et al., 1977).

The prognosis is poor when sepsis occurs after the implantation of the foreign body. In general, the infection does not respond to treatment until the foreign body is removed. When infection occurs after open reduction and internal fixation of an acute fracture, débridement of the wound is done, leaving the foreign bodies in situ until first-stage osseous healing occurs. Then the internal fixation device is removed, and cast immobilization is used until the fracture is healed. When an infection develops after an open fracture or fracture-dislocation, gram-negative bacilli predominate.

## TREATMENT OF OSTEOMYELITIS

### Acute Hematogenous Osteomyelitis

This is often a life threatening disease in children because of the associated staphylococcal bacteremia. Early treatment with antibiotics often obviates the need for surgery (Morrey and Peterson, 1975). If bony destruction is present on the initial radiograph or if there is soft tissue fluctuance indicating abscess formation, surgical débridement is necessary to prevent bone necrosis. Blood cultures should be obtained and abscesses aspirated before starting antibiotics. Since most infections are caused by *S. aureus* organisms that produce penicillinase, therapy should be started with a penicillinase-resistant beta lactam antibiotic. If a penicillin-sensitive strain of *S. aureus* is isolated, penicillin G is the treatment of choice (Table 1). Parenteral therapy should be continued for three to four weeks (Waldvogel, 1970). However, cooperative patients may be treated with parenteral therapy until they are afebrile for three days and then oral drugs for a total of four weeks of therapy (Bryson et al., 1979). The high doses of dicloxacillin and cephalexin used in these studies are rarely tolerated by children, and comparable studies of oral therapy have not been done in adults.

Treatment of vertebral osteomyelitis in adults varies with the clinical condition of the patient. Immobilization of the spinal column relieves pain and promotes new bone formation, fusion of the involved disk space, and healing of the infection (Fig. 5). Antibiotics are administered intravenously until the patient is afebrile and has no systemic symptoms. Oral therapy can be continued for a total of four weeks if the pathogen is susceptible to orally absorbed antibiotics.

**TABLE 1.    Antibiotics Used in the Treatment of Osteomyelitis**

| ORGANISM | AGE | ANTIBIOTICS |
|---|---|---|
| *S. aureus* (beta-lactamase producing) | Adult | Oxacillin 3 every six hours or cefazolin 1 g every six hours |
| | Child | Oxacillin 200 mg/kg/day or cefazolin 60 mg/kg/day |
| *S. aureus* (beta-lactamase negative) | Adult | Penicillin G 2 mega units every four hours or cefazolin 1 g every six hours |
| | Child | Penicillin G 0.5 mega units/kg or cefazolin 60 mg/kg/day |
| *H. influenzae* and | Child | Ampicillin 100 mg/kg or chloramphenicol 100 mg/kg |
| *S. enteritidis* | Adult | Ampicillin 2 g every six hours or co-trimoxazole 2 tabs twice daily |
| *P. aeruginosa* | Adult | Carbenicillin 3 g every two hours plus gentamicin 1.5 mg/kg every eight hours |

In chronic hematogenous and post-traumatic osteomyelitis, it is essential to excise infected granulation tissue, including the dead and infected bone. Saucerization of the infected cavities of bone by unroofing procedures is frequently necessary. Once all the infected and dead tissues have been excised, the dead space can be eradicated at a subsequent operation. When the femur or humerus is involved, there is frequently sufficient healthy soft tissue to permit delayed primary or secondary closure over an irrigation-suction system. A myocutaneous flap or a muscle pedicle and split-thickness skin graft can be used to obliterate the dead space when the tibia, ulna, or radius is involved (Ger, 1977). Alternatively, the wound can be packed open, and, when a healthy granulating bed has been achieved, a split-thickness skin graft can be applied. Papineau (1973) has had good results with the application of cancellous bone grafts in the cavity with secondary split-thickness skin graft. In the distal forearm and hand, abdominal and thoracic pedicle flaps have been used with success.

When osteomyelitis is associated with a nonunion of a fracture, control of the infection has first priority. In the past, the nonunion has been treated with a bone graft or internal fixation only after eradication of the infection and healing of soft tissue have occurred. However, with the advent of rigid external fixation devices, the fracture can be rigidly stabilized while the infection is being treated. Frequently, union occurs, thus obviating the need for subsequent internal fixation and bone grafting (Fig. 7).

Results of susceptibility studies are considered in the selection of specific antimicrobial therapy in the adult with chronic osteomyelitis. The polymicrobic nature of post-traumatic osteomyelitis frequently necessitates the administration of more than one antibiotic. Parenteral therapy of four weeks in duration is essential if successful eradication is to be achieved (Dich et al., 1975). If secondary bacterial invasion occurs with the isolation of nosocomial organisms from the irrigation-suction tubes or wound drainage, they should be treated with specific antimicrobial therapy. When the causal organism(s) is susceptible to an oral agent, the oral agent should be administered for 8 to 12 weeks following completion of parenteral therapy.

The recovery of a mixed flora consisting of gram-negative and gram-positive isolates from specimens of deep tissue can be difficult to evaluate. If necessary, multiple antimicrobial agents should be administered in order to treat all of the isolates. When anaerobic isolates are recovered from tissue cultures, specific antimicrobial therapy for the anaerobic isolate is necessary. If un-

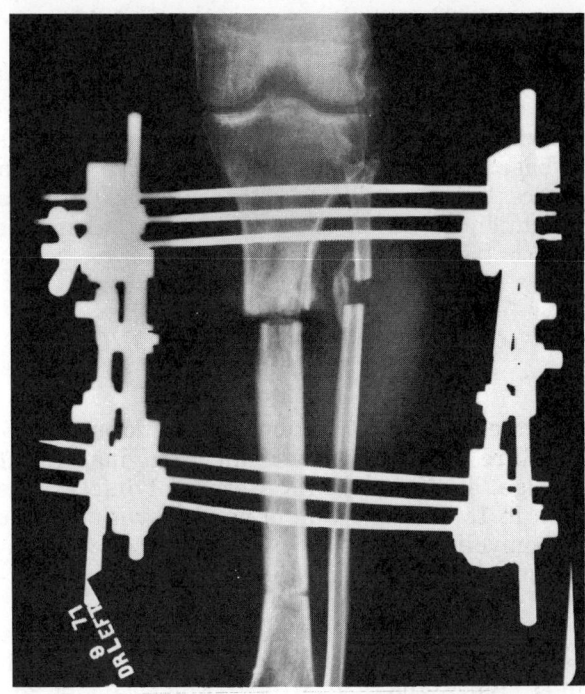

**FIGURE 7.** *Post-traumatic osteomyelitis after a compound fracture of tibia and fibula with extensive soft tissue loss. The osteomyelitis of ununited tibial fracture was treated with sequestrectomy and saucerization. An external fixation device (Vidal modification of the Hoffman apparatus) was applied after saucerization and sequestrectomy. A muscle pedicle graft was subsequently placed in soft tissue defect. Tibial union occurred over the ensuing six months.*

treated, anaerobes are often isolated from the bone when recurrent infection develops.

When second-stage surgical débridements are performed, additional specimens should be analyzed to ensure that the bacteria remain susceptible to the antibiotic drug used. Frequently, a gram-negative bacillus that is initially susceptible to the antimicrobial administered develops resistance, necessitating change of the treatment.

Irrigation-suction tubes are valuable in the management of the dead space that remains after saucerization of an osteomyelitic cavity (Kelly et al., 1970). In the past, such irrigation systems were empirically used for three weeks. Contamination of an irrigation-suction system with secondary gram-negative bacillary organisms is common after the reversal of the system if clotting or leakage occurs. Reversal of the system can lead to nosocomial colonization of the wound. Irrigation-suction tubes continue to be used in the management of osteomyelitis, but specimens of ingress and egress tubes for culture should be obtained every third day. The irrigation-suction system should be discontinued after five days, or after the first negative culture is obtained. The irrigation-suction tubes are rarely needed beyond ten days.

Creation of healthy tissue, both osseous and soft, with a good blood supply is the fundamental principle on which the treatment of osteomyelitis is based. Failure to remove inadequate fixation devices or to provide adequate stabilization of a nonunion by either internal or external means can contribute to recurrent infection.

## COMPLICATIONS OF CHRONIC OSTEOMYELITIS

Three major complications of chronic osteomyelitis are seen: recurrent infection, malignant change, and amyloidosis. Recurrent infection is seen in 15 to 20 per cent of patients with chronic osteomyelitis and is usually associated with inadequate antimicrobial therapy, inadequate surgical treatment, or both.

Malignant change in association with chronic osteomyelitis can be carcinomatous or sarcomatous (Baitz and Kyle, 1964; Fitzgerald et al., 1976). Either tumor can occur as a consequence of post-traumatic or hematogenous osteomyelitis. Both types of malignant change probably result from a long-standing reparative process: either hyperplastic reparative epithelium or stimulated reticuloendothelial elements become neoplastic. Squamous cell carcinoma occurs in 0.2 to 1.7 per cent of patients with osteomyelitis (Sedlin and Fleming, 1963). The incidence in patients with wounds that drain for 20 to 30 years appears to be higher. Fitzgerald et al. (1976) reported that 19 of the 23 patients with squamous cell carcinoma complicating chronic osteomyelitis had post-traumatic osteomyelitis. All of the patients had long-standing osteomyelitis, the duration ranging from 18 to 72 years (mean, 42 years).

The clinical features of squamous carcinoma include a draining sinus that spontaneously develops a foul odor, increased pain, and increased drainage that is often bloody. An enlarging mass or a pathologic fracture may occur. Males predominate in a ratio of 10 to 1. Because osteomyelitis is tolerated for a longer duration in the lower extremity than in the upper, the femur and tibia are the most frequent sites of involvement.

Routine laboratory evaluations, including those of the sedimentation rate and leukocyte count, are of limited diagnostic value. A routine roentgenogram of the chest should be performed to evaluate the possibility of pulmonary metastasis. Osseous roentgenograms usually demonstrate lytic and sclerotic changes indistinguishable from chronic osteomyelitis (Fig. 8). However, a severely destructive lesion clearly different from the usual osteomyelitic process can be seen in some cases (Fig. 9).

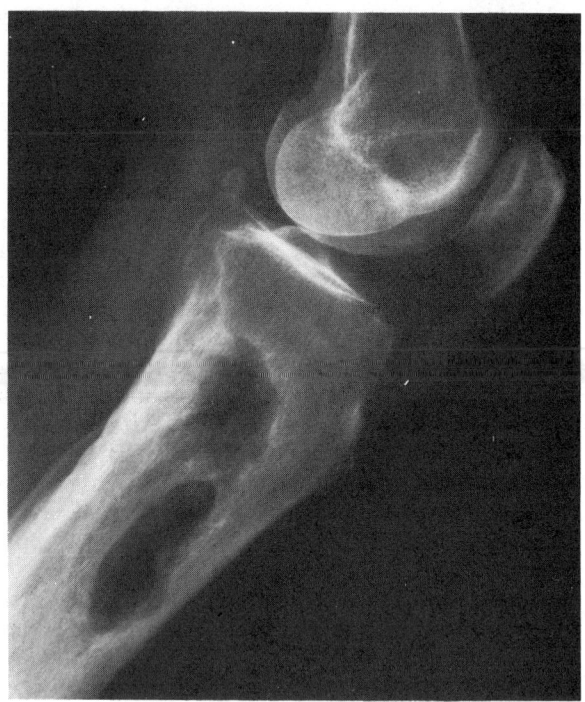

**FIGURE 8.** *Squamous cell carcinoma in chronic osteomyelitis of tibia. Findings are indistinguishable from those of chronic osteomyelitis without carcinomatous change.*

Histologically, low-grade (Broders' classification), malignant-appearing squamous epithelium invading bone is seen. With ablative surgery (which is the treatment of choice), the prognosis for patients with carcinomatous degeneration is good. Only 2 of 21 patients who received aggressive surgical treatment reported by Fitzgerald et al. (1976) had metastatic disease and died secondary to the malignancy. Regional lymphadenopathy is usually inflammatory. Regional lymphadenectomy need not be performed unless lymphadenopathy persists longer than three months after ablative surgery.

Sarcomatous change in chronic osteomyelitis is much less common (Baitz and Kyle, 1964). Approximately 20 acceptable examples have been documented in the literature. Liposarcoma, myeloma, reticulum cell sarcoma, polymorphic sarcoma, myxofibrosarcoma, synovial sarcoma, and unclassified sarcomas have been reported. Pathologic fracture or a growing mass is the most common variety. Biopsy makes the histologic diagnosis. The prognosis for patients with sarcomatous degeneration is similar to that of patients with sarcomas without osteomyelitis.

The association of amyloidosis with long-standing osteomyelitis and tuberculosis was recognized years ago. Modern drug therapy has significantly limited this complication of osteomyelitis (Dahlin, 1949; Sherman, 1949; Cohen, 1967). Secondary amyloidosis is seen with equal frequency in

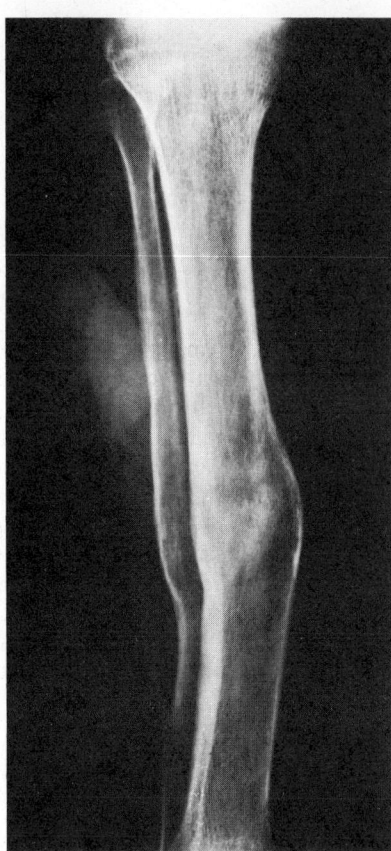

**FIGURE 9.** *Squamous cell carcinoma in chronic osteomyelitis of tibia. Large soft tissue defect located posteriorly with a fungating soft tissue mass is demonstrated. It is highly suggestive of malignant change.*

patients with chronic hematogenous and post-traumatic osteomyelitis. In general, chronic or recurring osteomyelitis will have been present for 20 years or more before amyloidosis becomes evident. Most patients in whom secondary amyloidosis develops secondary to chronic osteomyelitis have infection of bones of the lower extremity.

Hepatosplenomegaly, a common finding in primary amyloidosis, is noted infrequently. Occasionally, peripheral edema of the involved extremity is seen. Laboratory evaluation of renal function is helpful in identifying the patient who has secondary amyloidosis. The serum creatinine and blood urea nitrogen levels are elevated. Proteinuria is seen on routine urinalysis. Renal biopsies are necessary to confirm the diagnosis. Hypertension is present in a minority of the patients with secondary amyloidosis. Improvement can be achieved by eradication of the infection. Hopefully, the improved prognosis for patients with

osteomyelitis will make this complication of historic interest.

## References

Baitz, T., and Kyle, R. A.: Solitary myeloma in chronic osteomyelitis: Report of case. Arch Intern Med 113:872, 1964.

Batson, O. V.: The vertebral vein system. Am J Roentgenol 78:195, 1957.

Bryson, Y. J., Connor, J. D., LeClerc, M., and Giammona, S. T.: High-dose oral dicloxacillin treatment of acute staphylococcal osteomyelitis in children. J Pediatr 94:673, 1979.

Burri, C.: Post-traumatic Osteomyelitis. Bern, Hans Huber Medical Publishers, 1975.

Cohen, A. S.: Amyloidosis. N Engl J Med 277:522; 574; 628, 1967.

Dahlin, D. C.: Secondary amyloidosis. Ann Intern Med 31:105, 1949.

Dich, V. Q., Nelson, J. D., and Haltalin, K. C.: Osteomyelitis in infants and children: A review of 163 cases. Am J Dis Child 129:1273, 1975.

Fierer, J., Daniel, D., and Davis, C.: The fetid foot: Lower extremity infections in patients with diabetes mellitus. Rev Infect Dis 1:210, 1979.

Fitzgerald, R. H., Jr.: Laboratory diagnosis of postoperative sepsis of the musculoskeletal system. Orthop Clin North Am 10:361, 1979.

Fitzgerald, R. H., Jr., Brewer, N. S., and Dahlin, D. C.: Squamous-cell carcinoma complicating chronic osteomyelitis. J Bone Joint Surg [Am] 58:1146, 1976.

Fitzgerald, R. H., Jr., and Kelly, P. J.: Recurrent sepsis, malignant change, and sarcoidosis following post-traumatic osteomyelitis. In Hierholzer, G., and Lob, G. (eds.): Posttraumatic Osteomyelitis. New York, Springer Verlag, 1980.

Fitzgerald, R. H., Jr., Landells, D. G., and Cowan, J. D. E.: Osteomyelitis in children: Comparison of hematogenous and secondary osteomyelitis. Can Med Assoc J 112:166, 1975.

Fitzgerald, R. H., Jr., Nolan, D. R., Ilstrup, D. M., Van Scoy, R. E., Washington, J. A., II, and Coventry, M. B.: Deep wound sepsis following total hip arthroplasty. J Bone Joint Surg [Am] 59:847, 1977.

Ger, R.: Muscle transposition for treatment and prevention of chronic post-traumatic osteomyelitis of the tibia. J Bone Joint Surg [Am] 59:784, 1977.

Hobo, T.: Zur Pathogenese der akuten haematogenen Osteomyelitis, mit Berücksichtigung der Vitalfärbungslehre. Acta Sch Med Univ Imp Kioto 4:1, 1921.

Howard, J. M. (Chairman): Postoperative wound infections: The influence of ultraviolet irradiation of the operating room and of various other factors. Ann Surg 160 Suppl:1, 1964.

Kelly, P. J., Martin, W. J., and Coventry, M. B.: Chronic osteomyelitis. II. Treatment with closed irrigation and suction. JAMA 213:1843, 1970.

Morrey, B. F., and Peterson, H. A.: Hematogenous pyogenic osteomyelitis in children. Orthoped Clin North Am 6:935, 1975.

Papineau, L.-J.: L'excision-greffe avec fermeture retardée délibérée dans l'ostéomyélite chronique. Nouv Presse Med 2:2753, 1973.

Patzakis, M. J., Harvey, J. P., Jr., and Ivler, D.: The role of antibiotics in the management of open fractures. J Bone Joint Surg [Am] 56:532, 1974.

Sedlin, E. D., and Fleming, J. L.: Epidermoid carcinoma arising in chronic osteomyelitic foci. J Bone Joint Surg [Am] 45:827, 1963.

Sherman, M. S.: Acute and chronic osteomyelitis. Surg Clin North Am 29:117, 1949.

Trueta, J.: The three types of acute haematogenous osteomyelitis: A clinical and vascular study. J Bone Joint Surg [Br] 41:671, 1959.

Waldvogel, F. A., Medoff, G., and Swartz, M. N.: Osteomyelitis: A review of clinical features, therapeutic considerations, and unusual aspects. N Engl J Med 282:198; 260; 316, 1970.

West, W. F., Kelly, P. J., and Martin, W. J.: Chronic osteomyelitis. I. Fractures affecting the results of treatment in 186 patients. JAMA 213:1837, 1970.

Wiley, A. M., and Trueta, J.: The vascular anatomy of the spine and its relationship to pyogenic vertebral osteomyelitis. J Bone Joint Surg [Br] 41:796, 1959.

# 238 MYCETOMA

Taralakshmi V. Venugopal, M.D.
Pankajalakshmi V. Venugopal, M.D.

## DEFINITION

Mycetoma is a chronic, suppurative, granulomatous disease of the subcutaneous tissues and bones. It is characterized by localized swellings with multiple sinuses discharging granules or grains that are the microcolonies of the causal agents.

## ETIOLOGY

The etiologic agents of this clinical entity range from bacteria (actinomycotic mycetoma) to fungi (eumycotic or maduromycotic mycetoma). They exist free in nature as soil saprophytes or plant pathogens and enter the tissues through abrasion or implantation.

Actinomycotic mycetoma is caused by aerobic species of the actinomycetes group, belonging to the genera *Nocardia, Streptomyces,* and *Actinomadura* (Table 1). Eumycotic mycetoma is associated with a variety of fungi (Table 2), the most common being *Madurella mycetomii, Petriellidium boydii,* and *Acremonium* species *(Cephalosporium* species).

## PATHOGENESIS AND PATHOLOGY

Mycetoma generally affects those parts of the body surface that come into contact with the soil. The agents from the soil are introduced into the tissues through traumatic or imperceptible abrasions of the skin. After a period of quiescence, during which the organisms possibly adapt themselves to the host environment, an acute suppurative inflammation results. The enzymes of the pus facilitate the burrowing and spreading of the infection in the soft tissues and bones. This leads to the formation of sinuses communicating with the skin surface through which the granules or microcolonies of the organism are discharged.

The size, shape, color, and texture of the granules vary with the infecting agent. Actinomycotic mycetomas have granules composed of filamentous mycelium of bacterial width and without any chlamydospores. In eumycotic mycetoma, the granules consist of broad septate hyphae with well-defined walls and chlamydospores.

The histologic appearance of the granules in tissue sections is characteristic for most of the species of organisms (Figs. 1 through 7). The initial response of the host tissue to all agents of mycetoma is an acute suppurative reaction. This pyogenic reaction persists in actinomycotic mycetoma, whereas the true fungi evoke a foreign body response with the formation of granuloma with epithelioid hyperplasia and multinucleated giant cells (Fig. 8).

## CLINICAL MANIFESTATIONS

The exact duration of the incubation period of mycetoma is not known, and it may vary from a few days to several months. The disease may develop at any age, but the maximal incidence occurs in the 21 to 40 age group. Men are affected five times as often as women. The most common location of the infection is on the foot, although no site is exempt from mycetoma.

The condition often begins as a small, painless subcutaneous nodule at the site of previous injury, which then softens, forming a sinus that discharges pus. Gradually, multiple nodules develop, ulcerate, and drain through sinus tracts (Figs. 9 and 10). The tracts may remain open for months, or heal only to open again in other areas (Fig. 11). The discharge may be serosanguineous, seropurulent, or purulent, and often contains the characteristic granules (Fig. 12), which can be white, yellow, cream, pink, red, brown, or black, depending on the etiologic agent. As the disease progresses, the surrounding tissue becomes swollen and deformed by fibrous tissue reaction and multiple sinus formation (Figs. 13 and 14 A, B). Pain is not a serious complaint when only the soft tissues are invaded. However, the condition can be very painful if there is involvement of bone or secondary bacterial infection. Often the disease exists for a number of years before the patient seeks medical advice. The general health is not affected, although the disease may incapacitate the patient.

*Text continued on page 1770.*

**TABLE 1    Common Causal Agents of Actinomycotic Mycetoma**

| AGENT | GRAIN Color | GRAIN Approximate Diameter (mm) | GEOGRAPHIC DISTRIBUTION | RAINFALL (mm/year) |
|---|---|---|---|---|
| Actinomycetes: | | | | |
| *Nocardia asteroides* | White | 0.5 | Ubiquitous | 1000–2000 |
| *Nocardia brasiliensis* | White | 0.2 | Mexico, South America, Africa, India | 500–1500 |
| *Nocardia caviae* | White | 0.5 | Ubiquitous | — |
| *Actinomadura madurae* | White to yellow | 2 | Africa, India, North and South America, Europe | 250–500 |
| *Actinomadura pelletierii* | Red to pink | 1 | Africa, India, North and South America | 500–800 |
| *Streptomyces somaliensis* | White to yellow | 1 | Africa, North and South America, Arabia, Israel, India | 50–250 |

**TABLE 2.    Common Causal Agents of Eumycotic Mycetoma**

| AGENT | GRAIN Color | GRAIN Approximate Diameter (mm) | GEOGRAPHIC DISTRIBUTION | RAINFALL (mm/year) |
|---|---|---|---|---|
| Fungi | | | | |
| *Madurella mycetomii* | Black to brown | 1 | Africa, India, Indonesia, North and South America, Europe | 250–500 |
| *Madurella grisea* | Black to brown | 1 | North and South America, Africa, India | — |
| *Leptosphaeria senegalensis* | Black | 1 | Senegal, Chad, Mauritania, India | 250–500 |
| *Pyrenochaeta romeroi* | Black | 1 | Mexico, South America, Africa | — |
| *Phialophora jeanselmei* | Brown to black | 1 | North America, Martinique, Congo, Europe | — |
| *Petriellidium boydii* | White to pale yellow | 1 | North and South America, Europe, Africa, India | 1000–2000 |
| *Acremonium* species (*Cephalosporium* species) | White to yellow or black | 1 | North and South America, Africa, Europe, India, Japan, Thailand, Malaysia | — |
| *Neotestudina rosatti* | Yellow | 1 | Somali, Senegal | — |

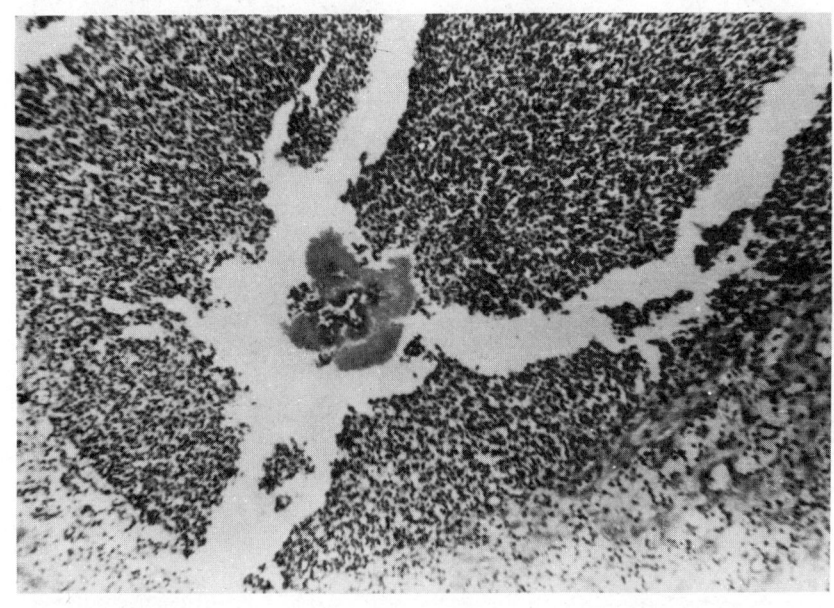

**FIGURE 1.**    *Small granule of* N. asteroides *surrounded by inflammatory cells. Hematoxylin and eosin stain. (×100)*

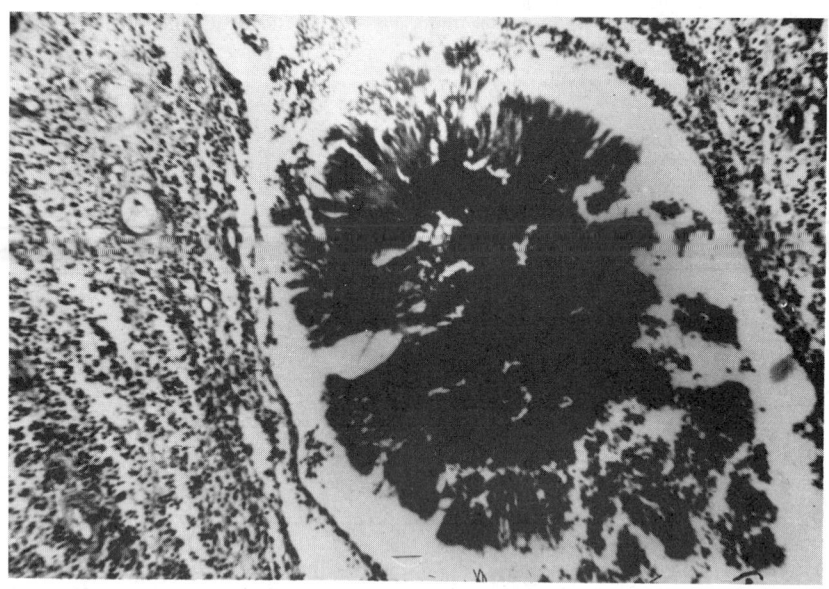

**FIGURE 2.**   *Large granule of* A. madurae *in subcutaneous tissue with characteristic fringe at the periphery. Hematoxylin and eosin stain. (×100)*

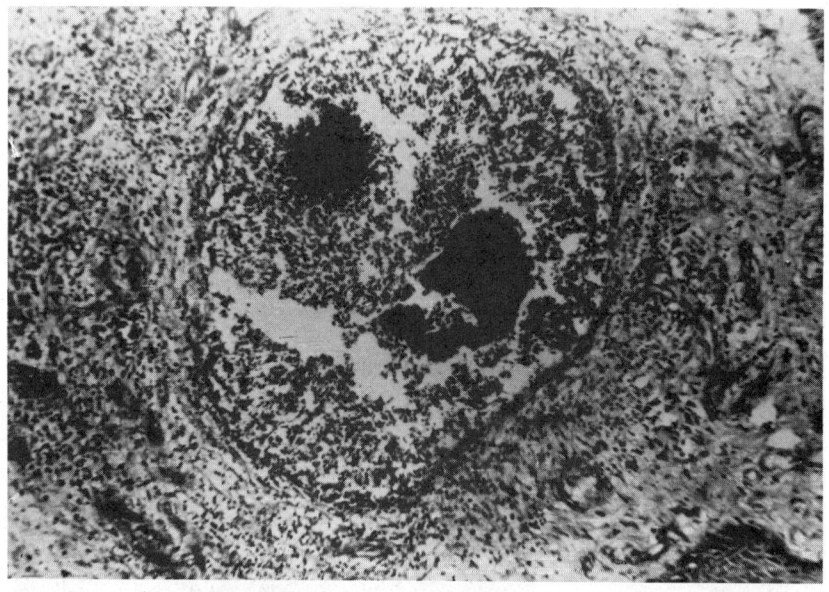

**FIGURE 3.**   *Granules of* A. pelletierii *with densely staining homogeneous matrix. Hematoxylin and eosin stain. (×100)*

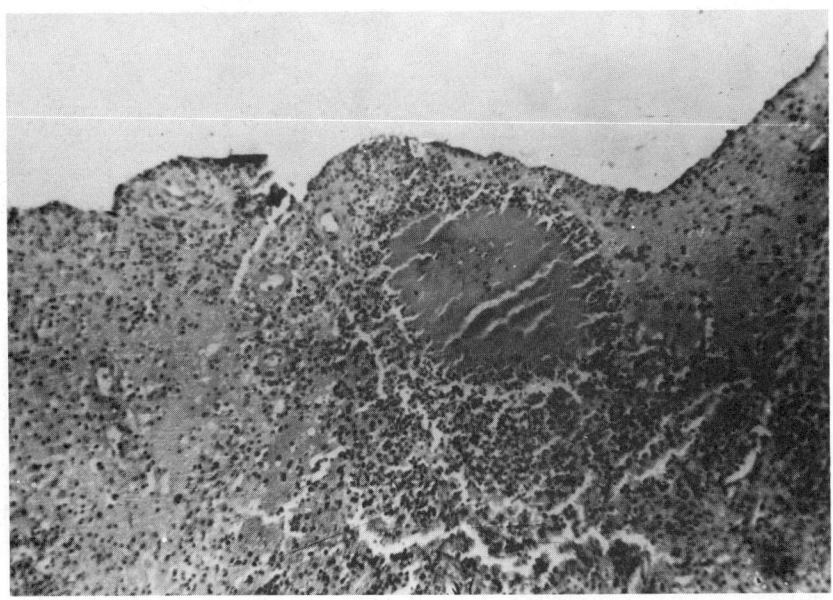

**FIGURE 4.** *Weakly stained amorphous granule of* S. somaliensis. *Hematoxylin and eosin stain.* (×100)

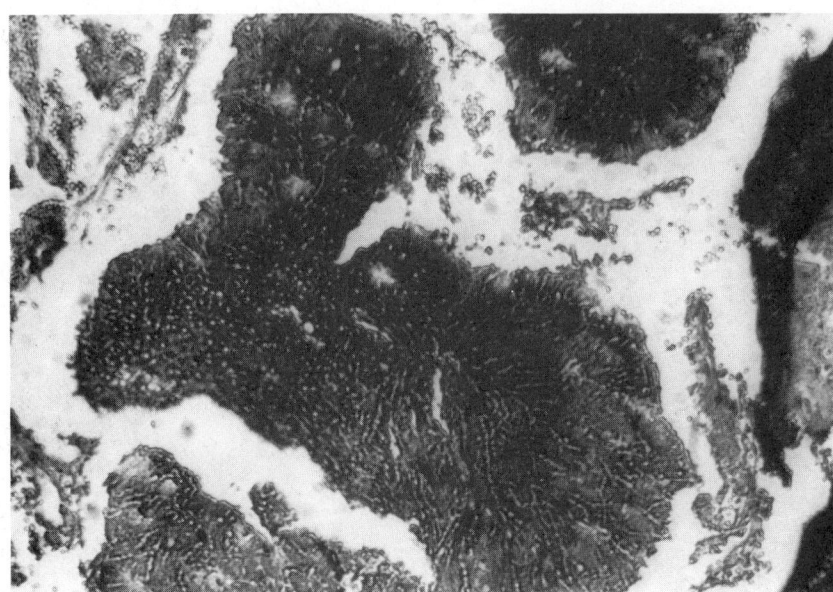

**FIGURE 5.** *Granules of* M. mycetomii *with hyphae embedded in interstitial cement. Hematoxylin and eosin stain.* (×100)

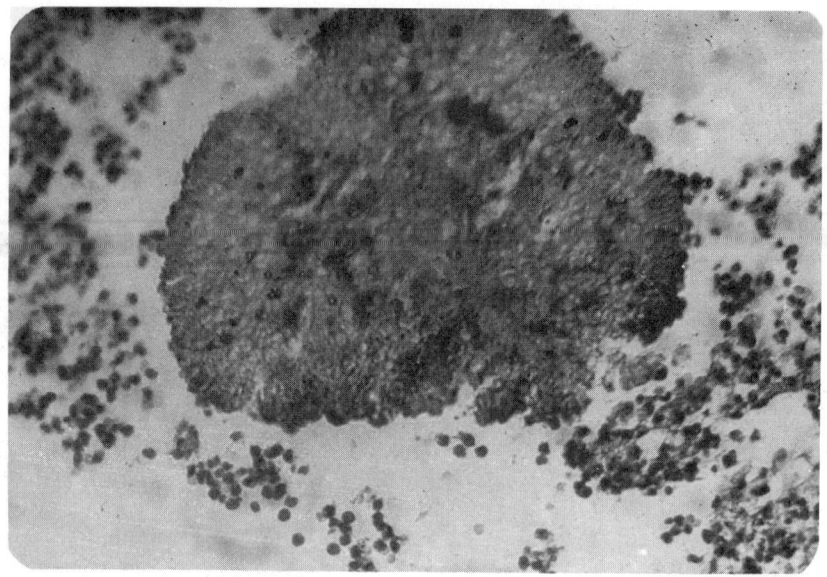

**FIGURE 6.** *Light colored granule of* A. boydii *in tissue. Hematoxylin and eosin stain. (×450)*

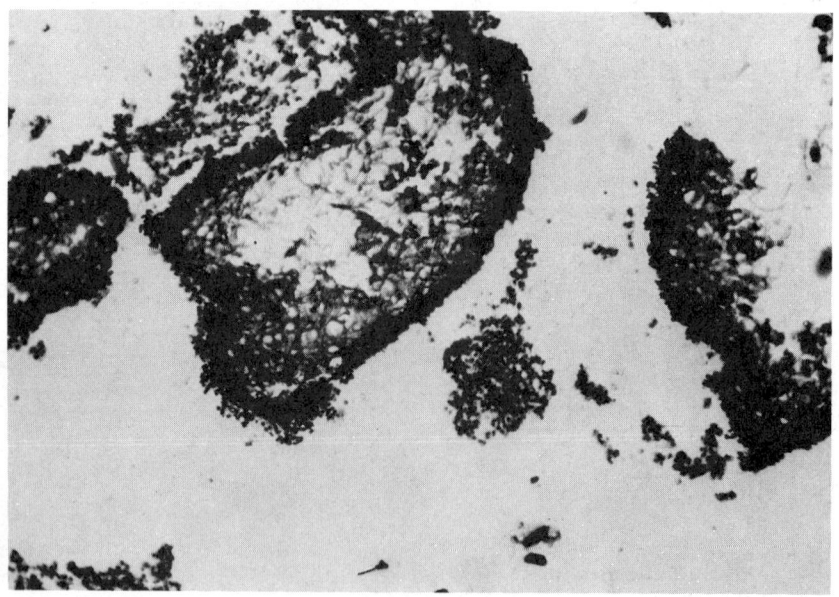

**FIGURE 7.** *Granules of* L. senegalensis *with large vesicles. Hematoxylin and eosin stain. (×100)*

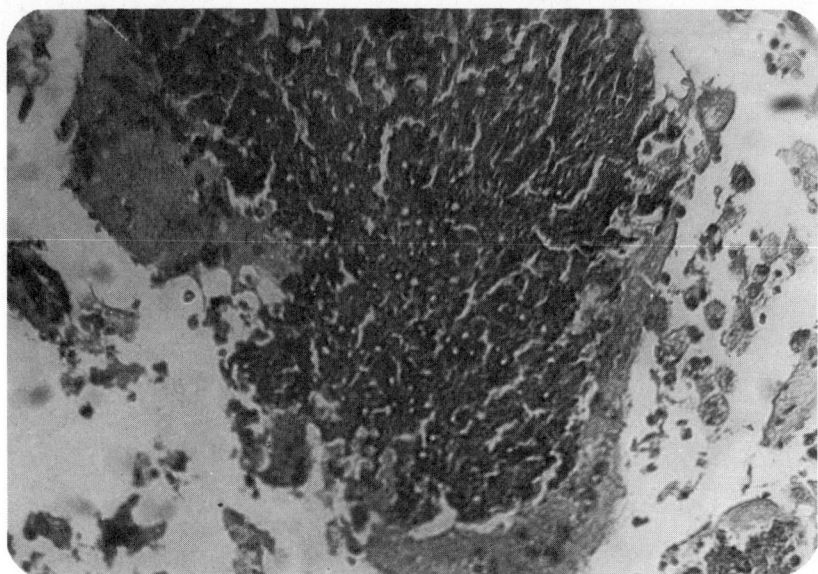

**FIGURE 8.** *Large giant cells surrounding the granule of* M. mycetomii. *Hematoxylin and eosin stain. (×100)*

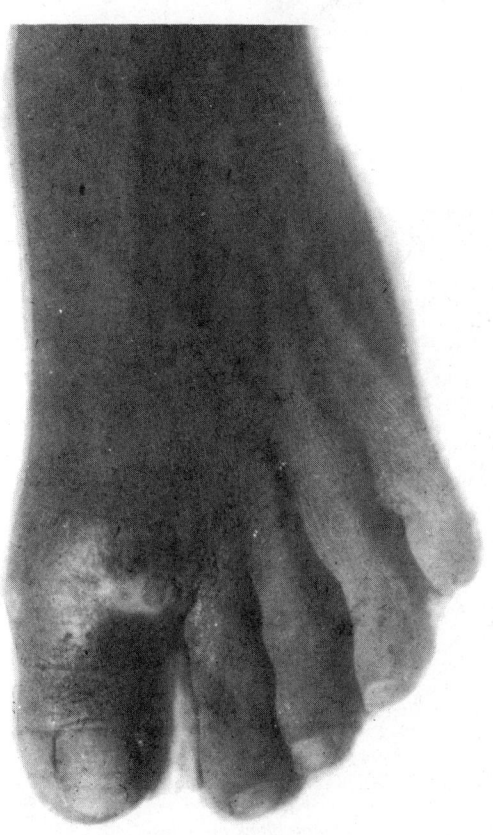

**FIGURE 9.** *Mycetoma caused by* M. mycetomii *with nodules at the base of the great toe.*

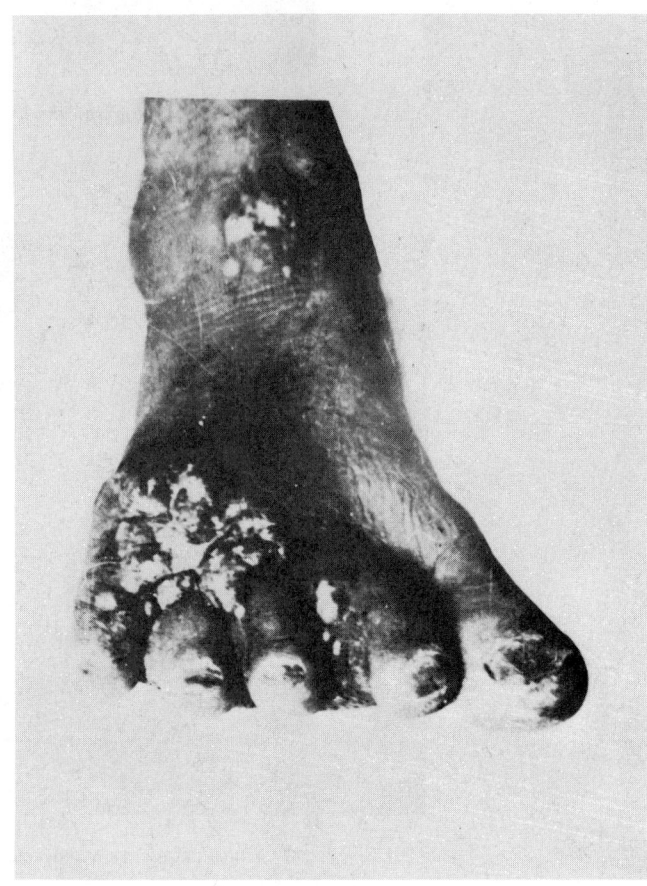

**FIGURE 10.** *Mycetoma of the foot caused by* A. pelletierii.

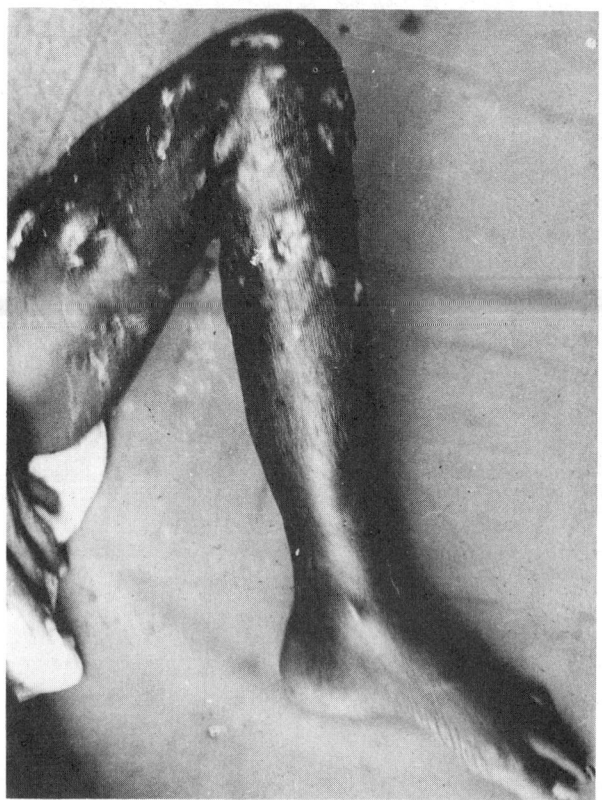

**FIGURE 11.** *Mycetoma of the thigh and leg caused by* N. brasiliensis.

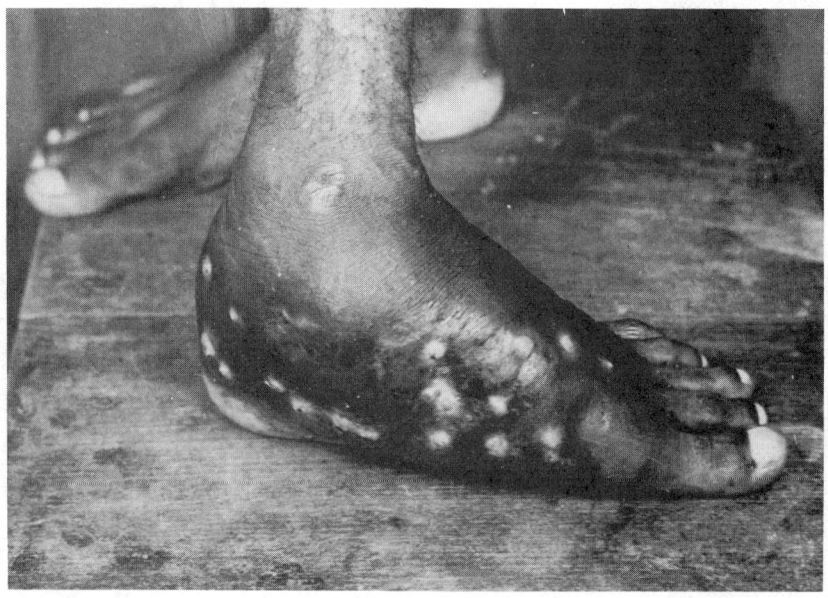

**FIGURE 12.** *Mycetoma caused by* M. mycetomii *with sinuses discharging black granules.*

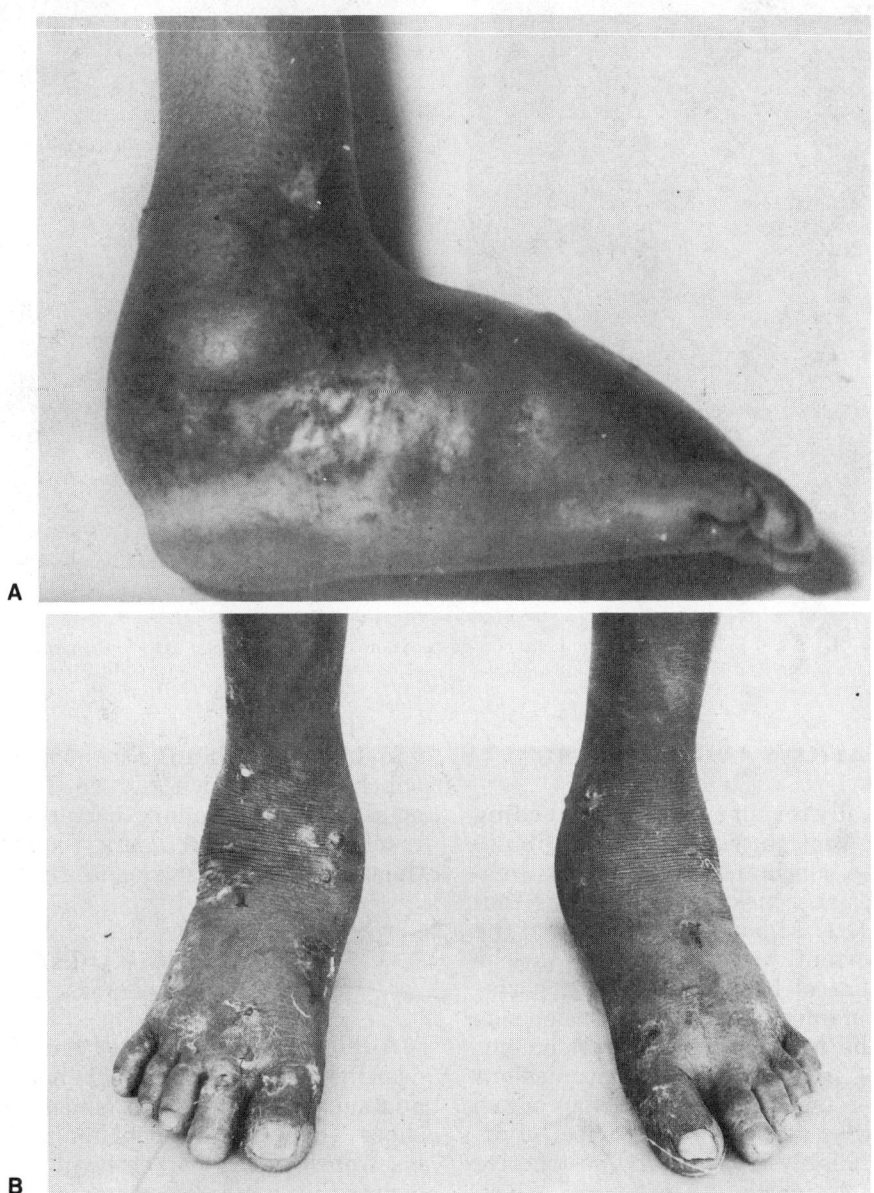

**FIGURE 13.** A and B, *Mycetoma of the foot caused by* A. madurae.

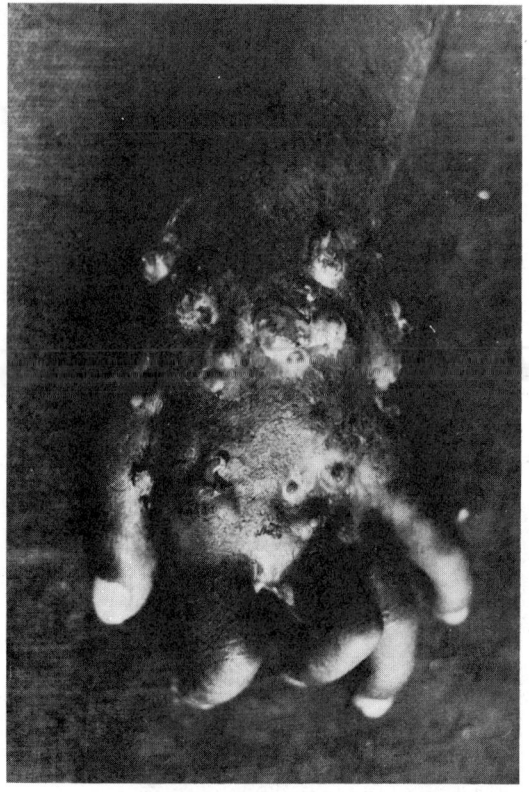

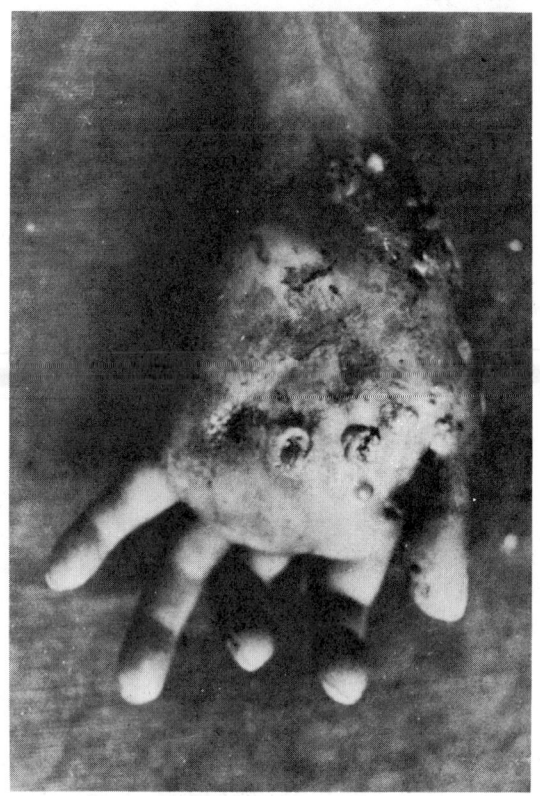

A                                                                                            B

**FIGURE 14.**   A and B, Mycetoma of the hand caused by M. mycetomii. A, Dorsal aspect. B, Palmar aspect.

## COMPLICATIONS AND SEQUELAE

Mycetoma usually remains localized, extending slowly by direct contiguity along fascial planes and invading the subcutaneous tissue, fat, ligaments, muscles, and bones but sparing the tendons until very late. Although penetration of the bone is an important feature of mycetoma, the degree and extent of bone involvement varies with the species of infecting agent. It also depends on the site of the lesion, stage of development, and intensity of infection. The osseous lesions (periostitis and round cavities of various sizes) may evolve slowly, as with localized foci of *M. mycetomii* or be highly invasive and destructive lesions, as with *Actinomadura pelletierii* (Cockshott, 1968).

Destruction of the ligaments and articular surfaces results in ankylosis of the affected joints.

When the infection occurs in the head, neck, chest, or buttocks region, visceral invasion by contiguity is not rare. Hematogenous spread is very rare, whereas lymphatic spread of mycetoma agents to regional lymph nodes with consequent enlargement have been reported (Koshi et al., 1972; Symmers, 1978). This is most commonly found in *Nocardia* and *Streptomyces* infections in which encapsulation is rare (Hassan and Mahgoub, 1972). Secondary bacterial infection may result in large open ulcers. Extensive fibrosis in the tissue may cause elephantiasis.

## GEOGRAPHIC VARIATIONS IN DISEASE

Although mycetoma has been reported from all over the world, it is more commonly seen in tropic and subtropic regions in which few people wear shoes. The species responsible for mycetoma varies from country to country, and the etiologic agents that are common in one region are rarely reported from others (Tables 1 and 2).

Climate exerts some influence on the prevalence of the disease and distribution of the causative agents. *M. mycetomii* and *Streptomyces somaliensis* are found in dry arid regions with sandy soils and thorny vegetation, where the rainfall ranges from 50 to 500 mm per year (Vanbreuseghem, 1967). Mycetoma caused by *M. mycetomii* is common in Africa, but the organism has been found in several regions of the world. In

Sudan 70 per cent of all recorded cases are caused by *M. mycetomii* (Mahgoub, 1968), and this is the major cause of black grain mycetoma in India, which is responsible for most of the cases encountered in the dry arid regions of the North (Mohapatra and Bhargava, 1967; Andleigh, 1957; Harbans Singh, 1976).

*S. somaliensis* has been reported mainly from Africa, including Sudan, Somalia, Senegal, Ethiopia, Nigeria, Republic of South Africa, and Tanzania, and in the western hemisphere from Brazil and Mexico. In Sudan it accounts for 20 per cent of mycetoma cases (Mahgoub, 1968). Three to 10 per cent of mycetomas in India are due to *S. somaliensis*, which is more common in the southern region of the country (Grueber and Kumar, 1970).

*A. pelletierii* infection is especially prevalent in relatively humid areas that have a rainfall of 500 to 800 mm or more per year (Rey, 1961). This agent has been reported mainly from African and Latin American countries. The infection is not seen in northern India, and most of the cases reported from the southern region were from Tamilnadu (Venugopal et al., 1978).

*Nocardia* is more commonly seen in wet forest countries, and small grain mycetoma due to *Nocardia brasiliensis* is prevalent in Mexico, Central and South America, and Africa. *Nocardia* species, once considered rare in Asia, were found to be present in a considerable percentage of cases in India (Venugopal et al., 1977).

*Leptosphaeria senegalensis* infection, which is native to Africa (seen in Senegal and Chad only), has also been encountered in a significant number of cases from southern India (Klokke et al., 1968; Reddy et al., 1972).

*Actinomadura madurae* as a causative agent of mycetoma has mainly been reported from North and South America, Africa, and Asia. It is the predominant pathogen in India, along with *M. mycetomii*.

Only a few sporadic cases of mycetoma have been recorded in Europe, Canada, and the United States, and in the last two areas, *Petriellidium boydii* is the most common agent.

Although certain agents of mycetoma show some geographic and ecologic prevalence, most of them have been found all over the world, and it is quite probable that they are ubiquitous, awaiting the proper circumstances for expression.

The factors that determine the susceptibility of humans to mycetoma are unknown. Wounds, personal hygiene, nutrition, general health of the patient, and virulence of the causative agent may all play a role. Sensitization of the body by repeated infections may be a prerequisite to the development of mycetoma in a given individual (Mahgoub and Murray, 1973).

## DIAGNOSIS

### Clinical Diagnosis

A fully developed mycetoma can be easily diagnosed on sight by the presence of the pathognomonic triad of swelling, formation of sinuses, and grains in the discharge. Diagnosis may be very difficult in the early stages, especially when the lesion is located at an unusual site.

### Radiologic Diagnosis

The radiologic manifestations of mycetoma are late sequelae and are of no help in the early diagnosis of the disease. However, certain radiologic features help to distinguish different types of mycetoma to some extent. In eumycotic mycetoma the lesion takes the form of single or multiple, punched-out lytic areas with well-defined walls and little sign of bone reaction, owing to localized masses of grains that gradually replace the osseous tissue and marrow with absence of sequestration (Fig. 15). In actinomycotic mycetoma, both osteolytic and osteosclerotic changes are present at the same time (Fig. 16). The affected bone thickens as fresh lamellae are deposited beneath the active periosteum (Mahgoub, 1968). The size and number of cavities in the bone

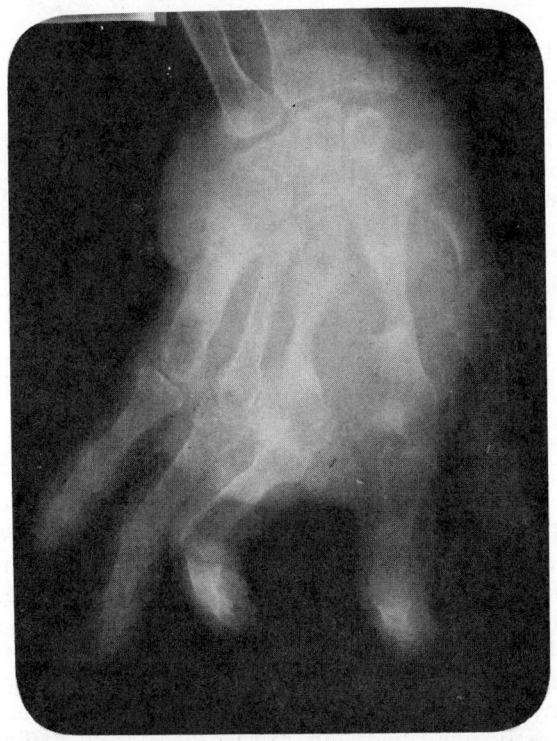

**FIGURE 15.** *Mycetoma. X-ray of foot showing osteolytic lesions due to* M. mycetomii.

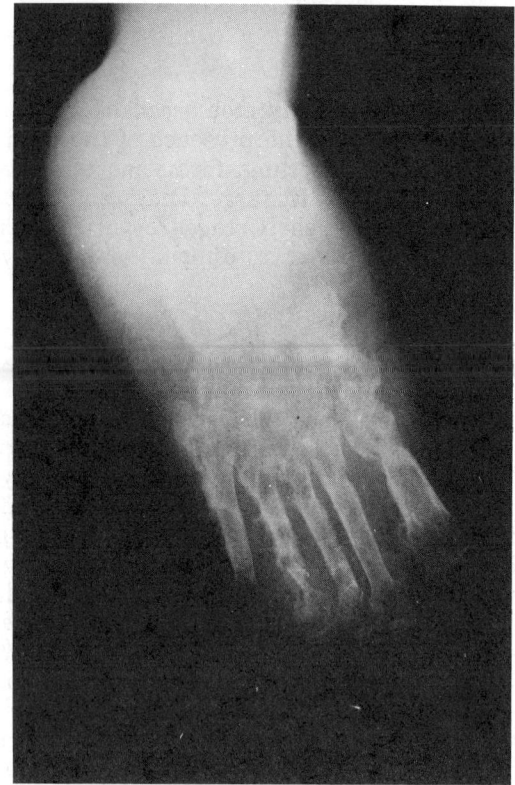

**FIGURE 16.** *Mycetoma. X-ray of foot showing osteosclerotic and osteolytic lesions due to* A. madurae.

may give a clue to the identity of the causal agent (Destombes et al., 1958; Delahaye et al., 1962). A few large single cavities generally suggest *M. mycetomii* infection; large multiple cavities with limited destruction suggest *A. madurae*; and a large number of small cavities with extensive fuzzy destruction of bones are probably caused by *A. pelletierii* or *S. somaliensis*. Extensive bone destruction without cavities is generally suggestive of *N. asteroides* (Desai et al., 1970).

## *LABORATORY DIAGNOSIS*

### Direct Examination

The pus, serosanguineous fluid that either drains from or is aspirated from unopened lesions, scraping of sinuses, or biopsy material, should be examined for the presence of granules. The gross and microscopic morphologic characteristics of the granules help in differentiating actinomycotic mycetoma from eumycotic mycetoma and botryomycosis. The causative agent can often be at least partly identified, but precise species identification depends on culture.

The granules should be washed in sterile saline and examined microscopically in a drop of 10 per cent potassium hydroxide. Actinomycotic granules are further stained by Gram's and Kinyoun's acid-fast methods after crushing. The dimensions of the filaments in the granule and the color, shape, size, texture, internal morphology, and staining properties are important in the identification of the causative agent. The actinomycotic granules consist of tangled masses of delicate branching gram-positive filaments, 0.5 to 1 $\mu$ in diameter, which may break up into bacillary and coccoid forms. *Nocardia* species are partially acid-fast, whereas *Actinomadura* and *Streptomyces* organisms are not. Eumycotic granules contain wide septate hyphae with hyphal swellings and chlamydospores.

### Culture

A deep biopsy is ideal for culture, as it is free from any external contamination. Granules from open lesions should be washed repeatedly with sterile saline. The material is cultured on Sabouraud's dextrose agar slants with and without chloramphenicol (0.05 mg/ml) and is incubated at both 26° C and 37° C. The organisms isolated in pure form are further studied for cultural, morphologic, physiologic, and biochemical properties, and species identification is made accordingly. The characteristics of the common agents are given in Tables 3 and 4.

### Histopathology

Histologic sections of the biopsy material stained by hematoxylin and eosin are examined for the presence of characteristic granules within the abscess cavities. If no granule is seen, deeper sections should be examined. Mere histologic examination of the biopsy material not only establishes the diagnosis of the disease but also allows specific identification of the causal agent in 94 per cent of mycetomas (Klokke et al., 1968). However, histologic examination has its limitations, and it should always be supplemented by culture for final identification.

Sections of actinomycotic mycetoma are further stained by Brown and Brenn's modification of Gram's and Kinyoun's acid-fast methods, and eumycotic mycetomas are stained by Bauer chromic acid Schiff and Gomori Grocott's methenamine silver stains. A detailed morphologic study of the organism in the granule should be made for establishing the identity of different species.

### Immunologic Diagnosis

Although precipitins, agglutinins, and complement-fixing antibodies have been demonstrated in the patient's serum, immunologic diagnosis of mycetoma is of only academic value because no

**TABLE 3. Histological and Cultural Characteristics of Common Causal Agents of Actinomycotic Mycetoma**

| ORGANISM | HISTOLOGY (H & E STAIN) | CULTURE Macroscopic | Microscopic |
|---|---|---|---|
| N. asteroides | Small; round, oval or vermiform; homogeneous loose clumps of filaments; partially stained by hematoxylin. | Fast-growing, glabrous, chalky, folded or wrinkled, white to orange pink; no enzymatic activity | Delicate branched filaments fragmenting into bacillary and coccoid forms; gram-positive, partially acid-fast |
| N. brasiliensis | Same as above | Fast-growing, small, heaped, wrinkled or folded, yellow to orange; enzymatically active | Same as above |
| N. caviae | Same as above | Resembles N. asteroides; differentiated by special tests | Same as above |
| A. madurae | Large; round or lobulated; center eosinophilic, amorphous; dense basophilic mantle peripherally surrounded by an eosinophilic fringe; clubs | Slow-growing, glabrous or waxy, wrinkled and folded, white to cream color colonies; adherent to the medium; enzymatically active | Delicate branched nonfragmenting filaments and arthrospores; gram-positive, not acid-fast |
| A. pelletierii | Small; round or irregular with denticulate edge: homogeneous matrix staining deeply with hematoxylin; no clubs | Very slow growing; small, glabrous, waxy, wrinkled or irregularly folded, pink to coral red colonies | Delicate branched nonfragmenting filaments; gram-positive, not acid-fast |
| S. somaliensis | Variable size; round or oval with smooth borders; center amorphous and lightly stained; no clubs | Fast-growing, glabrous, folded or wrinkled, cream to brown in color | Delicate branched nonfragmenting filaments and arthrospores; gram-positive, not acid-fast |

standard antigen was available until recently. However, this method is gaining importance as a highly useful diagnostic procedure, especially in the very early stages of the disease, during which the granules are not found.

Demonstration of precipitins by immunodiffusion test has been useful in identifying the causal agents of mycetoma (Mahgoub, 1964; Murray and Mahgoub, 1968). Counterimmunoelectrophoresis has been found to be more sensitive than immunodiffusion for the diagnosis of early cases of mycetoma (Gumaa and Mahgoub, 1975).

Skin tests are of some value in actinomycotic mycetoma, but eumycotic mycetoma patients fail to react (Murray and Moghraby, 1964).

### TREATMENT

Ideal specific therapy depends upon the identification of the causative agent and determination of its drug sensitivity. Unlike eumycotic mycetoma, actinomycotic mycetoma responds to chemotherapy. Treatment should be continued for several months after clinical cure to prevent a relapse. Surgical procedures such as exploration and drainage of sinus tracts, débridement of diseased tissue, and removal of bone cysts assist greatly in healing. Favorable responses have been reported with drug therapy alone in actinomycotic mycetoma even when there are extensive long-standing lesions involving the bone and lymphatics (Mahgoub, 1976).

The treatment of choice for nocardial mycetoma is sulfonamide or its derivatives. The commonest drug used is sulfadiazine, and the dose varies from 3 to 8 g per day. Long-acting sulfonamides such as sulfadimethoxine and sulfamethoxypyridazine have been reported to be useful (Vipulyasekha and Vathanabhuti, 1960).

In mycetomas caused by A. madurae, A. pelletierii, and S. somaliensis, streptomycin has been used most successfully. Clinical improvement is noticed with an initial dose of 3 g daily for three weeks, decreasing to 2 g and then 1 g daily for similar intervals (Abbot, 1956; Lynch, 1964). Other broad spectrum antibiotics, either singly or in combination, have been used with some success.

Dapsone (diaminodiphenylsulfone) has a beneficial effect on N. brasiliensis mycetoma (González Ochoa et al., 1952). It has been reported to be effective in a case of black grain mycetoma due to Madurella grisea (Neuhauser, 1955). In vitro studies have shown that the drug causes inhibition of growth of M. grisea, A. madurae, S. somaliensis, and N. brasiliensis (Mackinnon et al., 1958). A preliminary course of broad spectrum antibiotics combined with a prolonged course of dapsone in a dosage of 100 mg twice daily, together with immobilization of the affected part, has been found effective in the treatment of mycetomas caused by fungi as well as actinomycetes (Cockshott, 1957; Cockshott and Rankin, 1960).

Recently, a combination of sulfamethoxazole and trimethoprim has given encouraging results

**TABLE 4.  Histologic and Cultural Characteristics of Causal Agents of Eumycotic Mycetoma**

| ORGANISM | HISTOLOGY (H & E STAIN) | CULTURE Macroscopic | CULTURE Microscopic |
|---|---|---|---|
| *M. mycetomii* | Large, dark brown, lobulated; compact type with even distribution of brownish cement intersected by a network of hyphae; vesicular type with peripheral localization of brown cement around hyaline hyphae and chlamydospores; brown pigment particles in hyphal cells | Slow-growing, cottony to membranous, flat or folded, white, yellowish brown or brown with diffusible pigment; growth better at 37° C | Branched septate hyphae with chains of chlamydospores; black sclerotia; rare phialides and conidia |
| *M. grisea* | Small, oval or lobed; hollow center with loose hyaline hyphae; dark colored periphery with dense network of hyphae and chlamydospores embedded in brown cement; brown granules of intracellular pigment absent | Slow-growing, leathery, folded, black colonies with gray mycelium; red diffusible pigment | Fine septate hyphae and larger moniliform hyphae with chains of chlamydospores; sterile pycnidia. |
| *L. senegalensis* | Small, irregular, tubular or hollow; central core of hyaline hyphae; periphery dense with black hyphae and large vesicular cells imbedded in black cement | Fast-growing, gray-brown colony with black reverse, rare diffusible rose pigment | Dark brown or black perithecia; septate ascospores |
| *P. romeroi* | Small, tubular, central network of hyphae with thick band of chlamydospores in the periphery; dark swollen cells in the outer edge surrounded by an eosinophilic zone | Rapid-growing, dark gray, floccose; white periphery; black pigment in reverse | Brownish black pycnidia; elliptical conidia |
| *P. jeanselmei* | Small, vermiform, crescent-shaped; hollow center; hyphae and chlamydospores brown; cement absent. | Slow-growing, leathery, black and moist; later velvety, reverse black | Toruloid yeast cells; moniliform cells; long unbranched phialides |
| *P. bovdii* | Large; round or lobulated; broad septate hyaline hyphae with numerous, swollen hyphal cells (<20 $\mu$) | Rapid-growing, white, cottony, or fluffy; later grayish white, reverse gray to black | Hyaline hyphae, ovoid to pyriform conidia borne singly or in groups; dark brown perithecia; evanescent asci and ascospores |
| *Acremonium* spp (*Cephalosporium* spp) | Small, irregular; hyaline hyphae with numerous swollen cells (>12 $\mu$) surrounded by an eosinophilic zone | Slow-growing, white, glabrous colony; later downy, diffusible violet | Hyaline hyphae; curved septate conidia in mucoid clusters at the tips of conidiophores |
| *N. rosatii* | Small, polyhedral; center basophilic with vesicles and few hyphae; periphery with narrow septate hyphae imbedded in cement | Slow-growing, dark, flat or wrinkled colonies with light gray aerial mycelia; reverse dark brown | Black perithecia; kidney-shaped ascospores |

in the treatment of actinomycotic mycetoma (Mahgoub, 1972). Clinical cure was obtained in 70 per cent of the treated patients between the second and seventh months (González Ochoa, 1975).

Until recently, there had been no specific therapy for eumycotic mycetoma, and the prognosis was poor. Complete surgical excision of the early lesions may prevent spread. Griseofulvin and penicillin, when combined with surgery, have been reported to be effective by reducing the post-surgical recurrence rate (Mahgoub, 1976). Am-putation is necessary for advanced cases. Miconazole and ketoconazole have given favorable results in mycetomas due to *P. boydii*.

## PROPHYLAXIS

Prevention is not possible at present, but the disease is likely to disappear with better standards of living. Since trauma, often inflicted by a thorn, is generally found to be the basis of mycetoma, shoes would be a practical control measure.

# References

Abbott, P.: Mycetoma in the Sudan. Trans R Soc Trop Med Hyg 50:11, 1956.

Andleigh, H. S.: Etiology of maduromycosis in India. Mycopathol Mycol Appl 8:138, 1957.

Cockshott, W. P.: The therapy of mycetoma. W Afr Med J 6:101, 1957.

Cockshott, W. P.: Radiological patterns of the deep mycoses. In Wolstenholme, G. E. W., and Porter, R. (eds.): Systemic Mycoses. London, J. & A. Churchill Ltd., 1968, p. 113.

Cockshott, W. P., and Rankin, A. M.: Medical treatment of mycetoma. Lancet 2:1112, 1960.

Delahaye, R. P., Destombes, P., and Moutounet, J.: Les aspects radiologiques des mycétomes. Ann Radiol (Paris) 5:817, 1962.

Desai, S. C., Pardanani, D. S., Sreedevi, N., and Mehta, R. S.: Studies on mycetoma. Indian J Surg 32:427, 1970.

Destombes, P., Andre, M., Segretain, G., Mariat, F., Camain, R., and Nazimoff, O.: Contribution a l'étude des mycétomes en Afrique francaise. Bull Soc Pathol Exot 51:815, 1958.

González Ochoa, A.: Tropical deep fungous infections—mycetoma. In Orlando Canizares (ed.): Clinical Tropical Dermatology. Oxford, Blackwell Scientific Publications, 1975, p. 24.

González Ochoa, A., Shiels, J., and Vázquez, P.: Acción de la 4:4'-diamino-difenil-sulfona frente a Nocardia brasiliensis. Gac Med Mexico 82:345, 1952.

Grueber, H. L. E., and Kumar, T. M.: Mycetoma caused by Streptomyces somaliensis in North India. Sabouraudia 8:108, 1970.

Gumaa, S. A., and Mahgoub, E. S.: Counterimmunoelectrophoresis in the diagnosis of mycetoma and its sensitivity as compared to immunodiffusion. Sabouraudia 13:309, 1975.

Hassan, E. A. M., and Mahgoub, E. S.: Lymph node involvement in mycetoma. Trans R Soc Trop Med Hyg 66:165, 1972.

Klokke, A. H., Swamidasan, S., Anguli, R., and Verghese, A.: The causal agents of mycetoma in South India. Trans R Soc Trop Med Hyg 62:509, 1968.

Koshi, G., Victor, N., and Chacko, J.: Causal agents in mycetoma of the foot in Southern India. Sabouraudia 10:14, 1972.

Lynch, J. B.: Mycetoma in the Sudan. Ann R Coll Surg Engl 35:319, 1964.

Mackinnon, J. E., Artagaveytia-Allende, R. C., and Gracia-Zorron, N.: The inhibitory effect of chemotherapeutic agents on the growth of the causal organisms of exogenous mycetomas and nocardiosis. Trans R Soc Trop Med Hyg 52:78, 1958.

Mahgoub, E. S.: The value of gel diffusions in the diagnosis of mycetoma. Trans R Soc Trop Med Hyg 58:560, 1964.

Mahgoub, E. S.: Clinical aspects. In Wolstenholme, G. E. W., and Porter, R. (eds.): Systemic Mycoses. London, J. & A. Churchill Ltd. 1968, p. 125.

Mahgoub, E. S.: Treatment of actinomycetoma with sulfamethoxazole plus trimethoprim. Am J Trop Med Hyg 21:332, 1972.

Mahgoub, E. S.: Medical management of mycetoma. Bull WHO 54:303, 1976.

Mahgoub, E. S., and Murray, I. G.: Mycetoma. London, William Heinemann Medical Books Ltd., 1973.

Mohapatra, L. N., and Bhargava, S.: Mycetoma. Indian J Ortho 1:172, 1967.

Murray, I. G., and Mahgoub, E. S.: Further studies on the diagnosis of mycetoma by double diffusion in agar. Sabouraudia 6:106, 1968.

Murray, I. G., and Moghraby, I. M. E.: The value of skin tests in distinguishing between maduromycetoma and actinomycetoma. Trans R Soc Trop Med Hyg 58:557, 1964.

Neuhauser, I.: Black grain maduromycosis caused by Madurella grisea. Arch Derm 72:550, 1955.

Reddy, C. R. R. M., Sundareshwar, B., Pattabhi Rama Rao, A., and Reddy, S. S.: Mycetoma: Histopathological diagnosis of causal agents in 50 cases. Indian J Med Sci 26:733, 1972.

Rey, M.: Les mycetomes dans ouest africain. Paris, R. Foulon et Cie, 1961.

Singh, H.: Black grain perianal mycetoma. Indian J Surg 38:530, 1976.

Symmers, W. St. C.: The lymphoreticular system—lymphadenitis caused by actinomycetes and true fungi. In Symmers, W. St. C. (ed.): Systemic Pathology. Edinburgh, Churchill Livingstone, 1978, p. 616.

Vanbreuseghem, R.: Early diagnosis, treatment and epidemiology of mycetoma, Rev Med Vet Mycol 6:49, 1967.

Venugopal, T. V., Venugopal, P. V., Paramasivan, C. N., Shetty, B. M. V., and Subramanian, S.: Mycetomas in Madras. Sabouraudia 15:17, 1977.

Venugopal, T. V., Venugopal, P. V., Kamalakannan, R., Annamalai, R., Shetty, B. M. V., Subramanian, S., and Shanmugasundaram, T. K.: Mycetomas caused by Streptomyces pelletierii in Madras, India. Arch Derm 114:204, 1978.

Vipulyasekha, S., and Vathanabhuti, S.: Treatment of nocardial mycetoma with sulphamethoxypyridazine. Br J Derm 72:188, 1960.

# CLOSTRIDIAL MYONECROSIS

# 239

## Donald L. Bornstein, M.D.

## DEFINITION

Clostridial myonecrosis (gas gangrene) is a rapidly progressive, highly toxemic, and life-threatening illness caused by the invasion of previously healthy skeletal muscle by pathogenic clostridia. Most cases occur following serious injuries or surgical procedures. Although the organisms often contaminate traumatic or surgical wounds, myonecrosis is very rare because its development requires special conditions in the injured tissue. The involved muscle and the overlying soft tissues undergo necrosis and autolysis with little inflammatory cell reaction (myonecrosis). Severe toxemia with tachycardia, hypotension, and mental changes accompanies this process.

## ETIOLOGY

Over 70 species of Clostridium can be isolated from man and his environment, but only six seem able to induce myonecrosis: C. perfringens (C. welchii), C. septicum, C. novyi (C. oedematiens), C. sordelli (C. bifermentans), and, very rarely, C. histolyticum and C. fallax. Of these, C. perfringens, Type A, is by far the most important pathogen, accounting for 90 to 95 per cent of cases of myonecrosis. C. septicum and C. novyi, Type A, cause the balance of cases of civilian gas gangrene. More than one pathogenic species of clostridia may be isolated from a wound.

C. perfringens is prominent among the normal bowel microflora in man and may be 10 to 100 times more prevalent than *Escherichia coli* in fecal specimens. Clostridia can be found on the skin, especially over the buttocks, thighs, and perineum, and less frequently in the vagina and in the diseased biliary tract. Our environment is heavily contaminated with clostridia, which can be found on clothing, in the air of operating rooms, in water, on food, in dust, and in soil. The ability of clostridia to form spores allows them to persist in the environment under adverse conditions.

## PATHOGENESIS AND PATHOLOGY

The virulence of pathogenic clostridia is a consequence of their potent exotoxins and their ability to grow rapidly under favorable growth conditions. There is apparently no difference in the virulence of strains of *C. perfringens* that are isolated from cases of gas gangrene and strains that are commensals. Isolates from normal bowel flora and from fatal cases of myonecrosis are not distinguishable in toxin production or in animal virulence tests. Rather, myonecrosis occurs because damaged tissue presents this common enteric organism with an unusual opportunity to proliferate and thereby brings out the full latent toxigenic and invasive characteristics of the species.

Pathogenic clostridia are obligate anaerobes and cannot proliferate unless the oxidation-reduction or redox potential (Eh) of their microenvironment is reduced well below the +120 mv potential of well-oxygenated human tissues. They are not killed in atmospheric concentrations of oxygen but they will not multiply in such conditions. Lacerated, crushed, or dead tissues have redox potentials of as low as −150 to −250 mv and provide excellent growth conditions.

With impaired blood flow in tissue, anaerobic glycolysis occurs, lactic acid accumulates, and pH falls. A fall in pH creates new opportunities for clostridia to grow. *C. perfringens,* which could not grow at redox potentials above +60 mv at pH 7.4, was able to grow at an Eh of +160 mv when the pH was reduced to 6.4 (Oakley, 1954).

Like other anaerobic infections, many infections with *C. perfringens* are endogenous. Exogenous infection is more likely only in cases of major trauma in which gross contamination with soil, water, or foreign material has occurred.

Wounds at highest risk for developing gas gangrene are those produced by high velocity missiles, severe compound fractures, and badly contaminated crush injuries. In all of these, muscle is lacerated, circulation and local perfusion is badly compromised, clothing, dirt, and foreign material are buried deep within a wound, and pH and Eh fall. Clostridia from the skin, clothing, or external sources are often introduced along with other bacteria. The longer this dangerous situation persists before effective surgical care is initiated, the greater the risk of gas gangrene (Langley and Winkelstein, 1945).

The major toxin of *C. perfringens* is the alpha toxin, a lecithinase C, which has lethal, hemolytic, and necrotizing activities. This toxin can cause massive hemolysis by its action on the cell membranes of erythrocytes, as in clostridial septicemia (Chap. 183) or after intravenous administration to experimental animals. When injected intramuscularly, however, hemolysis is not significant, perhaps because the toxin is fixed at the injection site where it damages tissue and increases vascular permeability. Alpha toxin is believed to initiate the injury to myofibril membranes that triggers the invasion of previously normal muscle.

The severe toxemia observed in gas gangrene, however, is not due to alpha toxin itself, because alpha toxin is not usually detected in the circulation, gross hemolysis is not seen, and specific antitoxin does not reduce the toxemia. Excision of all affected muscle or, in some cases, hyperbaric oxygen therapy can reverse the toxemia. Products of clostridia-infected muscle, as yet uncharacterized, appear to be responsible for toxemia.

The role of the other toxins in the genesis of clostridial myonecrosis is obscure, except for their potent leukocidal activity, which eliminates phagocytosis and facilitates invasion by the organism. The major toxin of *C. novyi* is also a lecithinase C, but the major toxin of *C. septicum,* which produces an equally severe myonecrosis, has no lecithinase activity.

The important pathologic change in myonecrosis is a progressive destruction of muscle. The process disrupts the sarcolemma and fragments the muscle fibers, but the myofibrils are preserved. There is gas and edema between the muscle fibers, some loss of reticulin and collagen, and karyolysis. There is no vascular congestion, no marked fibrin deposition, and no neutrophilic exudate (Robb-Smith, 1945) (Fig. 1). Electronmicrographs suggest a primary attack on the lecithin in the cell membranes of muscle where small membrane gaps can be observed (Strunk et al., 1967).

With the exception of uterine infections (Chap. 183), serious clostridial wound infection is confined to skeletal muscle. Necrosis of the overlying connective tissue and skin in clostridial infection is a secondary phenomenon. There is no evidence that clostridia can cause a primary destructive or invasive infection of skin or soft tissues, a fundamental distinction that has been obscured in some recent reviews.

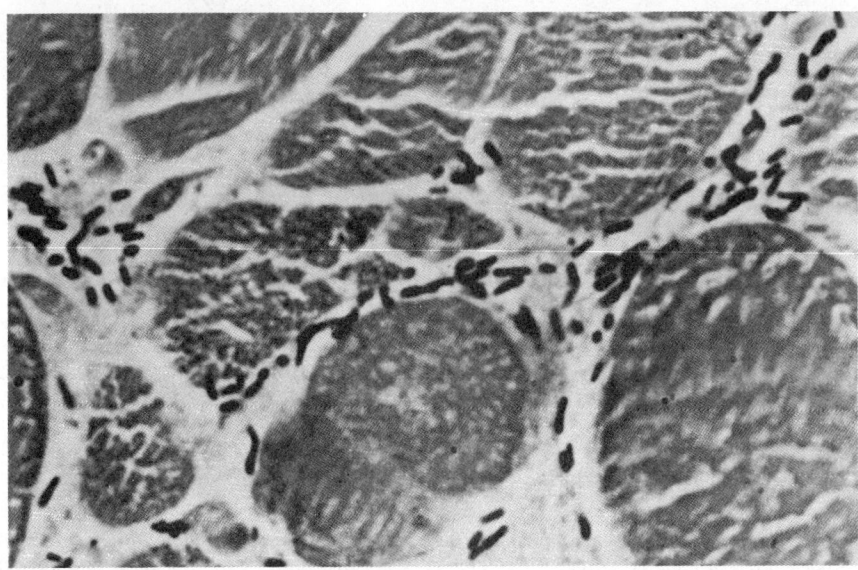

**FIGURE 1.** *Pathologic changes in muscle in clostridial myonecrosis (×400). Necrotic muscle fibers are separated by gas and edema fluid. Many clostridia are present with minimal inflammatory response. (From Boyd, N. A., Walter, P. D., and Thomson, R. O.: J. Med Microbiol 5:459, 1972.)*

Localized infections with clostridia can occur almost anywhere if organisms are introduced into a normally sterile area such as the pleural space, peritoneum, subarachnoid space, a joint, the brain, the eye, or the gallbladder. Although local tissue injury, edema, gas formation, and purulence or abscess formation may ensue, and although bacteremia may on rare occasions develop from such a site, these are rarely progressive, toxemic, or life-threatening infections, and they respond to antibiotic therapy and simple drainage procedures (Bornstein et al., 1964).

## CLINICAL MANIFESTATIONS

Sixty to 70 per cent of civilian gas gangrene follows trauma, usually a major injury that breaks the skin, crushes tissue, introduces dirt and foreign materials, compromises the vascular supply, and in most cases badly fractures one or more long bones. The thigh and/or hip are involved in most cases. Motorcycle or other traffic accidents, falls, crushing by industrial or farm machinery, gunshot wounds, and penetrating injuries are the most common precipitating events. The common features in these cases are ill-advised, early internal fixation of contaminated open fractures, primary wound closure, inadequate débridement, unrelieved tension in fascial compartments, or application of tight casts (Fig. 2).

Twenty to 30 per cent of cases follow clean surgical procedures. Biliary surgery with common duct exploration (Fig. 3), bowel surgery, orthopedic procedures on the hip or femur, amputation, or attempted vascular repair for arterial insufficiency of the leg are the most common offenders.

The remaining 10 to 15 per cent of cases occur after intramuscular injections, minor trauma or superficial lesions in patients with impaired circulation, and in immunosuppressed patients. There are also cases of "spontaneous" and "metastatic" gas gangrene. Intragluteal injection of epinephrine is the most common cause of post-injection gas gangrene. Epinephrine should never be injected in the buttocks because it constricts blood flow and can introduce clostridial spores into ischemic tissue. Ischemic or neuropathic ulcers and decubitus ulcers have served as other points of entry. Neutropenia, immunosuppression, advanced Hodgkin's disease, and acute leukemia all predispose to clostridial myonecrosis. Minor trauma such as an infiltrated intravenous infusion or an infected venipuncture site can usher in atypical, rapidly advancing, and usually fatal myonecrosis. "Spontaneous" or "idiopathic" gas gangrene involves a previously uninjured site. Occult bowel leakage (diverticulitis, necrotic malignancy, fistulae) that drains down along the iliopsoas sheath can sometimes initiate myonecrosis in the upper thigh or buttock. Other muscle groups have been seeded by heavy clostridial bacteremia originating from a carcinoma or an ulcerated lesion of the bowel. *C. septicum* has been involved in many of the reported cases. Very rarely in advanced myonecrosis a metastatic

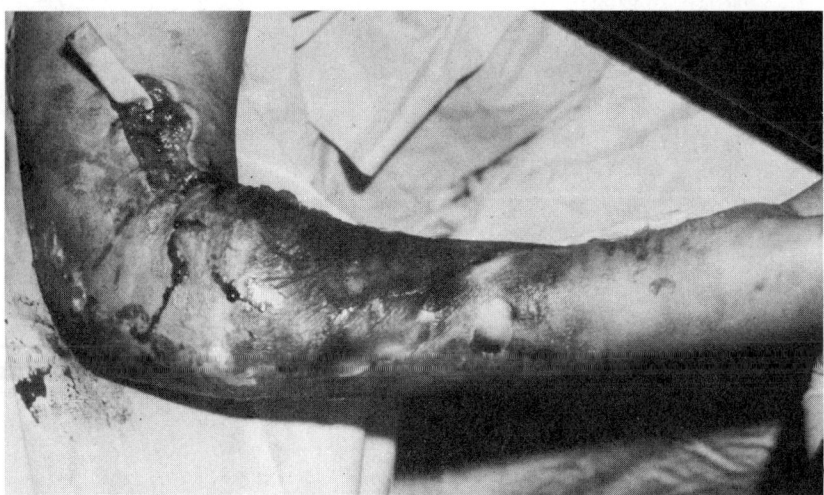

**FIGURE 2.** *Gas gangrene of the forearm following an open fracture of the proximal ulna resulting from a fall. When the cast was opened because of severe pain, discoloration, serous discharge, bleb formation, and frank necrosis of the skin were apparent. Amputation above the elbow was required.*

patch of disease will develop at a new and distant site presumably because of blood-borne spread.

The first symptom of myonecrosis in most cases is the development of heaviness or pain in the affected area beginning 6 to 120 hours (usually 24 to 48 hours) after injury. The pain is unrelenting and increases in degree and in extent. The painful area is not red and inflamed but appears cool, pale, and swollen, often with tense, white, shiny skin. Crepitus is not prominent because it is obscured by the increasing edema, which is most severe in infections caused by *C. novyi*. The

area becomes swollen and tense, and a dark, thin, serous fluid drains from existing wounds. A blotchy bronze or brown discoloration and thin-walled blebs filled with dark fluid containing clostridia but few white cells develop in the affected skin. These changes progress to patches of frank necrosis in the initial sites of involvement, while pain, edema, and discoloration advance to involve new areas.

With the onset of pain and edema, a marked systemic reaction appears, with myalgias, tachycardia, sweating, and restlessness that are dis-

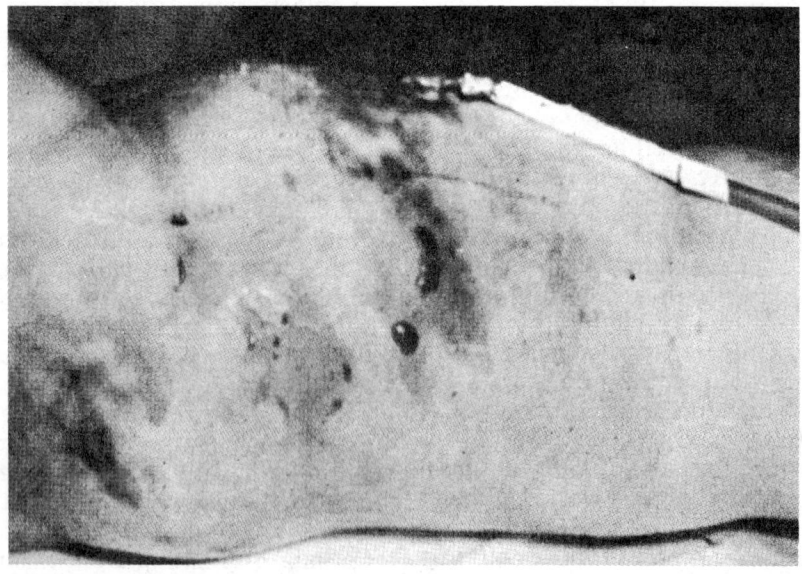

**FIGURE 3.** *Gas gangrene of the abdominal wall following gallbladder surgery. The patient survived after extensive resection of necrotic muscle and soft tissue. (From Bornstein, D. L., et al.: Medicine 43:207, 1964. Courtesy of The Williams & Wilkins Company.)*

proportionate to the local changes and to the low-grade fever. Within several hours a rapidly advancing toxemic state with prostration, hypotension, and either agitation or signs of obtundation appears. Most patients are febrile, some with rigors and high fever; a few are hypothermic. Without prompt and effective therapy, refractory septic shock, circulatory failure, central nervous system depression, and death soon follow (MacLennan, 1962; Altemeier and Fullen, 1971).

## COMPLICATIONS AND SEQUELAE

The major complication in survivors of myonecrosis is loss of a limb by amputation or weakness caused by extensive removal of necrotic muscle. Defects in the abdominal wall from myonecrosis may be of such magnitude that extensive and prolonged plastic surgery may be needed before the patient can resume a normal life (Phillips et al., 1974).

## GEOGRAPHIC VARIATIONS

Although the content of clostridia in soils varies geographically, the major reservoir of pathogenic clostridia is the human intestinal tract, which does not. The most important geographic factor in the incidence of myonecrosis is the level of hygiene and the availability of medical facilities at which effective primary surgical care of contaminated open fractures, crush injuries, and penetrating wounds can be carried out. Local customs such as the use of contaminated soil or other natural materials as poultices for traumatic wounds may introduce infection.

## DIAGNOSIS

Early recognition and prompt therapy are vital to minimize tissue destruction and death. Definitive diagnosis in early cases can be made only by surgical examination of muscle in the affected area. Persistent pain in a high-risk surgical or traumatic wound should always be evaluated. Casts should be split, sutured wounds opened, and dressings taken down to evaluate the state of the wound and to obtain smears and cultures.

If local edema or early skin discoloration is found, or if the patient appears unduly toxemic, confused, or hypotensive, prompt muscle exploration is required. The finding of clostridia on Gram-stained smears of wound exudate with only a few neutrophils supports the diagnosis of gas gangrene. Once gas gangrene is considered, exploration should not be deferred. A two-hour delay may cost a patient a limb that could otherwise have been saved. First priority for operating room use must be granted for this emergency (Altemeier and Fullen, 1971). Crepitus in a wound in the absence of local pain or systemic signs also requires limited surgical exploration of the underlying muscle, but is a lesser emergency.

The first changes in involved muscle are pallor, edema, loss of tone, and poor contractility when pinched. With further involvement an unhealthy brick red color appears that progresses to a brown or gray "cooked meat" appearance. The excised muscle does not bleed freely and soon becomes necrotic with green-black discoloration, liquefaction, and gas bubbles. The extent of myonecrosis must be determined surgically because it is often greater than the skin changes might indicate.

Gram-stained smears from the gangrenous muscle reveal plump gram-positive rods (with some discoloration and no spores in *C. perfringens*) and very few leukocytes. The rare cases of anaerobic streptococcal myositis, which can mimic early stages of clostridial myonecrosis, are clearly distinguished by large numbers of streptococci and heavy neutrophilic infiltration (Chap. 240). Wound and blood cultures are obtained to confirm the diagnosis, to speciate the clostridia, to determine the extent of other bacterial contamination, and to rule out any associated bacteremia. *C. perfringens* bacteremia can be detected in 5 to 10 per cent of patients with advanced myonecrosis. The bacteremia is rarely heavy and is only occasionally associated with significant in vivo hemolysis caused by circulating alpha toxin, although significant anemia and some degree of hyperbilirubinemia are commonly seen in myonecrosis due to other causes.

If muscle is not involved, surgical examination can identify and help correct other infections, such as necrotizing fasciitis or crepitant or noncrepitant cellulitis. In civilian practice, many crepitant infections are not caused by clostridia but rather by facultatively anaerobic gram-negative bacilli, or nonclostridial obligate anaerobes. Gram stains will give clues to the etiologic agents and will guide the initial antimicrobial therapy. Culture of *C. perfringens* from a wound does not make the diagnosis of myonecrosis because it may represent simple contamination, anaerobic cellulitis (a gas infection that spreads along superficial fascial plains without muscle involvement and that is treated by limited débridement), or a localized ("Welch") abscess (Wilson, 1960).

X-ray films can sometimes differentiate the feathery or fern-like pattern of gas within muscle bundles that generally signifies myonecrosis from the linear patterns or rounded or irregular pockets of gas in subcutaneous tissues due to other crepitant processes (Fig. 4). Because these x-ray findings may be late in developing, surgical exploration should not be delayed in their absence.

There are no other specific tests for the early detection of myonecrosis. Leukocytosis, anemia, elevated transaminase, and slight hyperbilirubinemia are common. An increase in the blood of myoglobin and muscle enzymes (creatine phosphokinase, aldolase, LDH isozymes) is not helpful because they are also elevated by the trauma or surgery that preceded the development of myonecrosis. Laboratory studies of fluid and electrolyte balance, renal function, hepatic function, and the blood picture are required for proper management of this disease and its complications.

Without muscle examination it may not be possible to distinguish between clostridial myonecrosis and a variety of other crepitant or necrotizing infections of the skin and soft tissues. Necrotizing fasciitis—a mixed infection with hemolytic streptococci, staphylococci, or gram-negative bacilli—and synergistic necrotizing cellulitis due to aerobic gram-negative rods plus peptostreptococci or *Bacteroides* are likely to be the most confusing because they cause local pain, discoloration and necrosis of the skin, and marked systemic reactions (Ledingham and Tehrani, 1975). Necrotizing fasciitis of the perineum is frequently misdiagnosed as gas gangrene (Finegold, 1977).

## TREATMENT

Complete excision of diseased muscle has been the only effective treatment for gas gangrene in the past. It has been repeatedly observed that when affected muscle was overlooked or could not be removed, the disease progressed despite antibiotics or antitoxin.

Myonecrosis in an extremity may involve only a few muscle bundles if it is detected at an early stage. If these are excised a functional limb can be salvaged. When surgery is delayed, the necrosis may be so extensive that there is no alternative to amputation. Postoperative gas gangrene of the abdominal wall generally requires extensive resection.

The toxemia clears fairly soon after surgery, and most patients who were not comatose, in refractory shock, or in extremis before surgery go on to recover. The surgical wound is left open under sterile dressings for periodic inspection of muscle at the resected margins.

The overall recovery rate in patients who receive competent surgical care is about 75 to 85 per cent (Altemeier and Fullen, 1971; Langley and Winkelstein, 1945). Prognosis is worse in postoperative cases and in patients with advanced age, underlying illness, abdominal wall involvement, and especially, immunocompro-

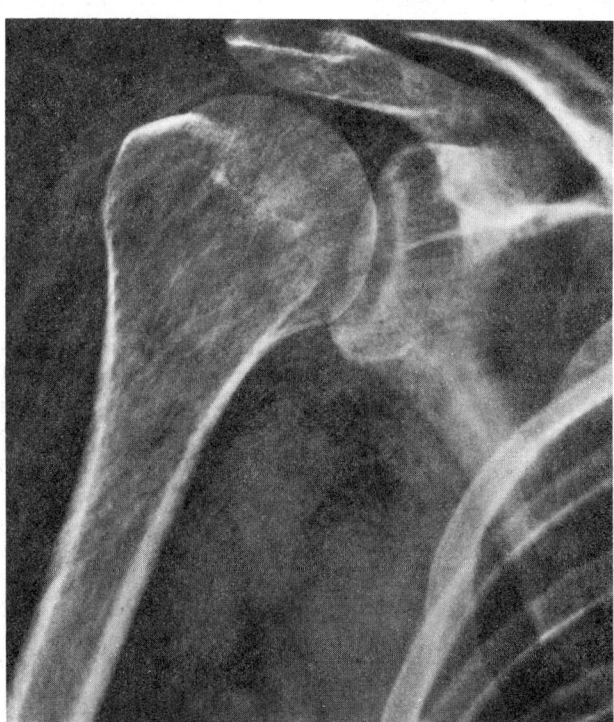

**FIGURE 4.** *Regular linear pattern of gas within muscle bundles in "spontaneous" clostridial myonecrosis of the shoulder in a young man with advanced Hodgkin's disease.*

mised status. Even better recovery rates (85 to 95 per cent) are seen when disease is limited to the extremities.

Surgery must be supplemented with prompt fluid replacement to correct hypovolemia, which can progress rapidly to refractory hypotension in these critically ill patients. Fluid balance, urine output, central venous pressure, cardiac status, and renal function must be monitored.

Aqueous penicillin is recommended in doses of 16 to 24 million units/day. Cephalosporins (cefazolin, 1 gm I.V. every six hours), clindamycin (600 mg I.V. every six hours), or chloramphenicol (1.0 gm I.V. every four to six hours) can be given to patients who are allergic to penicillin. Although antibiotics cannot penetrate the heavily infected necrotic tissues, they help prevent invasion of healthy muscle and can treat bacteremia. An aminoglycoside is needed if Gram stains reveal heavy gram-negative rod contamination and if the clinical course raises concern about associated gram-negative bacteremia. Smears of clostridial exudates must be interpreted cautiously, however, because some clostridia do not retain the Gram stain and appear as gram-negative rods.

Extensive military experience with polyvalent clostridial antitoxin has shown a high incidence of unpleasant and occasionally dangerous serum sickness reactions without clear-cut therapeutic effect in myonecrosis. Despite intravenous infusion and local infiltration of large amounts of antitoxin, the spread of infection was not prevented and the toxemia was not reversed. Antitoxin is no longer generally recommended for therapy, although some clinicians still favor its use (Altemeier and Fullen, 1971). Antitoxin should be given to patients with associated clostridial septicemia and significant hemolysis.

In some patients the disease is too extensive for resection. This group includes some whose disease has spread extensively despite initial surgery (amputation), some in whom diagnosis or transport was delayed, and a few whose disease progressed very rapidly. In 1961 the use of hyperbaric oxygen (HBO) was reported as a dramatic development for these hopeless cases. The first report in English reviewed two cases with myonecrosis (Brummelkamp et al., 1961). By 1963 a series of 25 cases had been reported, and in 1972 the results of 130 cases treated by HBO therapy in Amsterdam were tabulated (Roding et al., 1972).

The objective of HBO therapy is to raise the Eh of tissues by oxygen saturation to a level at which pathogenic clostridia cannot continue the process of myonecrosis. The inspired partial pressure of oxygen is over 2000 mm Hg, arterial $pO_2$ reaches 1700 Hg, venous $pO_2$ values are about 100 mm Hg, and tissue $pO_2$ values of 200 to 300 mm Hg

have been recorded. Proponents of HBO therapy claim that the hyperoxia reduces toxemia dramatically and terminates the disease process. Experimental studies indicate that C. perfringens is inhibited but not killed by oxygen at 3 ATA, and that alpha toxin is not destroyed. One study suggests that the release of alpha toxin is inhibited by HBO (Gottlieb, 1971). Experimental studies in animals have not shown therapeutic effects comparable to the reported clinical experience. There are complications of hyperbaric oxygen therapy related to oxygen toxicity and to hazards of decompression: nausea, vomiting, dizziness, convulsions, tympanic membrane injury, abdominal distention, aeroembolism, and pulmonary complications.

Unfortunately, despite two decades of experience, five international congresses, major expenditures for construction and staffing of hyperbaric facilities, and a clinical experience of over 800 cases of "gas gangrene," the exact role of HBO therapy in the management of myonecrosis is still very unclear because it rests on uncontrolled studies and because muscle was not examined in many treated cases. It seems that HBO can arrest disease in some cases, but it is uncertain if it is safe to rely on this therapy instead of surgery in all cases. To resolve this question a large, well-planned and well-monitored collaborative study involving several centers over several years will be required, since myonecrosis is such a rare disease. Since HBO facilities are limited in number and distribution, the questions raised in HBO therapy are academic for much of the world. For the present, prompt surgical excision appears to be the surest therapy for proven myonecrosis.

### PROPHYLAXIS

Active immunization is not employed because gas gangrene is so rare (0.5 to 1 case per million per year) and because the incubation period after injury is so short. Toxoids of alpha toxin can be prepared, but the many antigenic subtypes of C. perfringens, Type A, limit the development of an effective antibacterial vaccine.

Many cases of gas gangrene have developed despite passive immunization of both military personnel and civilians with polyvalent horse antitoxin shortly after injury. Antitoxin is no longer stocked by the United States military services for prevention (or treatment) of gas gangrene.

Antibiotic prophylaxis is widely practiced for contaminated traumatic injuries. If given early and in large doses, penicillin may offer some degree of protection (Owen-Smith and Matheson, 1968). However, if a wound is not adequately débrided, myonecrosis can develop despite any amount of antibiotic.

Penicillin prophylaxis is strongly recommended to prevent postoperative gas gangrene after mid-thigh amputations for vascular disease and after orthopedic surgery of the hip or femur, both "clean" surgical procedures that carry a special risk (Parker, 1969). The operative site should be prepared with a 30-minute povidone-iodine scrub that can kill the clostridial spores that are so commonly found on the thighs and buttocks. Antimicrobial prophylaxis is also recommended for biliary tract surgery when there is emphysematous cholecystitis, when common duct exploration is planned, or when intraoperative Gram stains of bile reveal clostridia. It is less likely that significant anticlostridial protection would be afforded by antibiotics in "contaminated" surgery such as large bowel resection.

Prevention of gas gangrene rests on proper initial surgical care of contaminated traumatic wounds. The wound must be thoroughly cleaned, all foreign material must be removed, dead tissues must be débrided, tissue spaces must be obliterated, compression within fascial compartments must be relieved, arterial injuries should be repaired, primary closure must be avoided, open reduction with prosthetic implantation should be delayed, any casts that are applied should be bivalved, and hypovolemia or shock must be treated promptly. If these principles are followed, over two thirds of cases of clostridial myonecrosis can be prevented.

## References

Altemeier, W. A., and Fullen, W. D.: Prevention and treatment of gas gangrene. JAMA 217:806, 1971.

Bornstein, D. L., Weinberg, A. N., Swartz, M. N., and Kunz, L. J.: Anaerobic infections. Review of current experience. Medicine 43:207, 1964.

Brummelkamp, W. H., Hogendijk, J. L., and Boerema, I.: Treatment of anaerobic infections (clostridial myositis) by drenching the tissues with oxygen under high atmospheric pressure. Surgery 49:299, 1961.

Finegold, S. M.: Anaerobic Bacteria in Human Disease. New York, Academic Press, 1977, pp. 386–432.

Gottlieb, S. F.: Effect of hyperbaric oxygen on microorganisms. Ann Rev Microbiol 25:111, 1971.

Langley, F. H., and Winkelstein, L. B.: Gas gangrene. A study of 96 cases treated in an evacuation hospital. JAMA 128.783, 1945.

Ledingham, I. M., and Tehrani, M. A.: Diagnosis, clinical course and treatment of acute dermal gangrene. Br J Surg 62:364, 1975.

MacLennan, J. D.: The histotoxic clostridial infections of man. Bacteriol Rev 26:177, 1962.

Oakley, C. L.: Gas gangrene. Br Med Bull 10:52, 1954.

Parker, M. T.: Post-operative clostridial infections in Britain. Br Med J 3:671, 1969.

Phillips, J., Heimbach, D. M., and Jones, R. C.: Clostridial myonecrosis of the abdominal wall. Management after extensive resection. Am J Surg 128:436, 1974.

Owen-Smith, M. S., and Matheson, J. M.: Successful prophylaxis of gas gangrene of the high velocity missile wound in sheep. Br J Surg 55:36, 1968.

Robb-Smith, A. H. T.: Tissue changes induced by Clostridium welchii Type A filtrates. Lancet 2:362, 1945.

Roding, B., Groenveld, P. H. A., and Boerema, I.: Ten years of experience in the treatment of gas gangrene with hyperbaric oxygen. Surg Gynec Obstet 134:579, 1972.

Strunk, S. W., Smith, C. W., and Blumberg, J. M.: Ultrastructural studies on the lesion produced in skeletal muscle fibers by crude Type A C. perfringens toxin and its purified alpha fraction. Am J Pathol 50:89, 1967.

Wilson, T. S.: The significance of Clostridium welchii infections and their relationship to gas gangrene. Can J Surg 4:35, 1960.

# 240 *NONCLOSTRIDIAL ANAEROBIC CELLULITIS*

## H. Harlan Stone, M.D.

With the exception of various types of clostridial sepsis and possibly rare instances of isolated peptostreptococcal gangrene, essentially all anaerobic soft tissue infections are caused by the synergistic action of a mixed bacterial flora, containing several species of aerobic and anaerobic bacteria. Clinical manifestations vary considerably but are primarily determined by the tissue planes involved and the general resistance to infection of the patient. Indeed, specific pathogen combinations appear to be only of secondary importance in establishing the clinical presentation as well as the eventual outcome.

As a general rule, the course of the infection is one of progressive tissue destruction, eventually leading to a fatal septicemia caused by the aerobic component, with or without an associated anaerobic bacteremia. Although specific parenteral antibiotic therapy may offer temporary control of the local process and the bacteremia, excision of all necrotic tissue and appropriate management of the resultant open contaminated wound are the absolute requisites for survival of the patient.

## *ETIOLOGY*

The usual method for classification of infection on the basis of specific etiologic agent or agents is not practical in the case of nonclostridial anaerobic sepsis because the infectious process is almost always due to a *microbial synergism* between different aerobic and anaerobic bacteria (Giuliano et al., 1977). At times, there may be only one aerobic and one anaerobic species, thereby creating a dual symbiosis, as in Meleney's cellulitis (aerobic *Staphylococcus aureus)* and anaerobic *Peptostreptococcus* (Meleney, 1931). Polymicrobial synergistic infections, however, are far more common and are caused by one or more aerobic gram-negative rods *(Escherichia coli, Klebsiella pneumoniae, Enterobacter aerogenes)* in combination with many different species of anaerobic bacteria, including peptostreptococci, *Bacteroides fragilis, Bacteroides melaninogenicus, Bacteroides corrodens,* and fusobacteria.

## PATHOGENESIS

The basic problem is the introduction of a mixture of aerobic and anaerobic bacteria into compromised tissues. The infected tissues often display poor vitality secondary to a generalized illness like diabetes or to local trauma from surgery or accidental causes. The site of infection is often near the rectum, from which the polymicrobial fecal flora can initiate infection.

In a polymicrobial flora, if there are both aerobic and anaerobic bacteria, potentiation of virulence for each component is possible. Aerobic organisms appear to reduce significantly the local redox potential by taking up most if not all of the available tissue oxygen, thereby providing an environment more conducive to anaerobic growth. The greater the quantity of oxygen extracted from tissues infected by aerobic species, the greater the number and the more fastidious the anaerobes that can be supported in a mixed flora. The aerobic gram-negative enteric bacilli are especially well adapted to serve in this capacity because they are facultative organisms that thrive even after tissue oxygen is depleted. In addition, gram-negative bacilli can produce a lethal bacteremia.

Anaerobic organisms bring catabolic enzymes to the bacterial symbiosis. It would seem that gangrene results from the direct action of these exotoxins on host cells or thrombotic occlusion of vessels by these toxins. Since tissue barriers are easily breached and immunoglobulins are probably destroyed by anaerobic proteolysis, it is not surprising that bacteremia is exceedingly common whenever anaerobic organisms participate in an infection.

## CLINICAL MANIFESTATIONS

### General Features

Anaerobic soft tissue infections characteristically produce a fetid odor. As a general rule, there is spiking fever to 39° or 40° C; leukocytosis exceeds 15,000 mm³ with a significant shift to immature polymorphonuclear forms; and the patient appears exceedingly toxic and may be irrational as well. The jaundice of a septic hemolytic anemia may also be present.

Previously documented or heretofore unsuspected diabetes mellitus often complicates the clinical picture by progressing to overt ketoacidosis. Since renal failure may also pre-exist, development or worsening of antecedent uremia is common. Extremes of nutrition are often noted, with patients being either extremely obese or obviously malnourished. Infants, preschool children, and the elderly are the usual victims of these infections.

### Specific Features

#### Meleney's Cellulitis

The first report of an aerobic-anaerobic symbiosis in clinical infection was made by Meleney in 1924. In this instance, a dual synergism was established between the aerobic *S. aureus* and an anaerobic *Streptococcus,* now classified as *Peptostreptococcus.* The infection is usually a postoperative complication in a compromised patient.

The initial lesion is either an unimpressive area of cellulitis or a small area of cutaneous gangrene. Over a period of several days, the extent of tissue necrosis enlarges, the more centrally located eschar sloughs, and an ever-expanding ulcer results. Despite relatively healthy appearing granulations in the wound base and at its margin, the lesion steadily progresses.

The infection responds to intravenous oxacillin in a dose of 1.0 g every four hours. Patients allergic to penicillin can be given 600 mg clindamycin every four hours I.V. Wound excision and closure by a delayed split skin graft are usually necessary also.

#### Polymicrobial Synergistic Gangrene

Most infections caused by a polymicrobial symbiosis of bacteria with strikingly different oxygen requirements harbor one or more facultatively aerobic enteric gram-negative rods, a multitude of various anaerobic species, and often the enterococcus. The enteric bacteria may be *E. coli, K. pneumoniae, E. aerogenes,* and *Proteus mirabilis,* and the anaerobes often consist of *B. fragilis, B. melaninogenicus, Fusobacterium nucleatum, F. necrophorum,* and various peptostreptococci.

The major determinant of which type of septic process develops is not the inoculum but the resistance of the patient. Diabetes mellitus, renal failure, advanced liver disease, malnutrition, obesity, malignancy, and immunosuppressive therapy are critical factors that promote synergistic gangrene.

The incubation period varies between three and seven days. It is longer than the incubation period for infectious gangrene due to aerobic *Streptococci* or *Clostridia* alone but generally more rapid in onset and progression than necrosis caused by individual aerobic gram-negative rods, fungi, or the dual symbiosis of Meleney's cellulitis. Only the odor of gas gangrene is more offensive. Often the discharging exudate has the appearance of feces, so much so that a bowel fistula must be ruled out.

Several terms have been used to label these infections. Specific tissue planes along which the process spreads and the region of body involved have been the more popular determinants in classification.

1. Polymicrobial gangrene primarily confined to the skin, subcutaneous fat, and Scarpa's fascia is called *synergistic necrotizing fasciitis* (Defore et al., 1977). Seldom is there deeper penetration unless a surgical or traumatic wound has already bridged the external oblique fascia, as in cases involving the abdominal wall.

2. The same symbiotic infectious gangrene involving those tissues below the deep enveloping fascia is referred to as *synergistic necrotizing cellulitis* (Stone and Martin, 1972). Because there has been no dissection into the superficial subcutaneous fat, the skin overlying the process seldom reflects what is beneath. All soft tissues within the same fascial compartment appear to be equally necrotic, with only vessel and nerve conduit remaining intact. The first observable lesion may be a small skin ulcer that drains a thin brown fluid with a fecal odor and is surrounded by dermal necrosis and sometimes accompanied by crepitation due to gas in the tissues. Fever and toxemia are prominent.

Not only the contained muscle but also all fascial confining walls must be excised. Amputation, even as radical as hip disarticulation and hemipelvectomy, may be required. On occasion, both synergistic necrotizing fasciitis and cellulitis may be present.

3. In *Fornier's cellulitis* there is necrosis of the scrotum, penis, and perineum (Benjamin, 1979; Lee and Oh, 1979). Usually the testicles have been spared.

Most cases of synergistic gangrene are initiated by contamination of adjacent tissues by large bowel contents. A perianal source is common. Trauma or operative perforation of the colon produces synergistic gangrene almost as frequently as does perianal contamination. Similar bacteria may be introduced into a traumatic wound from sources outside the intestinal tract.

## DIAGNOSIS

In Meleney's cellulitis the peptostreptococci are best recovered from the advancing edge of the ulcer even though *S. aureus* can be grown from any part of the lesion.

A fetid odor is diagnostic of anaerobic infection in polymicrobial synergistic gangrene. Further insight into the etiology is obtained when bacteria seen in Gram stain of the exudate do not grow in aerobic culture the next day. In fact, peptostreptococci can be identified in smears of fetid drainage if streptococci seen in the Gram stain have not grown aerobically in 48 hours. By then, however, a laboratory with ordinary anaerobic competence can recover peptostreptococci in simple commercial anaerobic jars. *Bacteroides* sp and fusobacteria may be more difficult to isolate and identify.

Clinically, synergistic gangrene must be differentiated from anaerobic streptococcal myonecrosis and clostridial myonecrosis. The last two syndromes, in contrast to synergistic gangrene, are primarily infections of muscles. The purulent drainage from the wound of streptococcal myonecrosis also distinguishes it from synergistic infection, and there is no mixed infection on smear.

## TREATMENT

The basic principles of treatment are centered about total excision of all necrotic tissue, maintenance of an open wound with almost daily dressing changes and repeated débridement when necessary, and eventual closure of the surface defect by split-thickness skin graft in cases with a sizable gap, or by delayed primary closure or spontaneous wound contracture if only a small separation persists. Survival can be correlated almost uniformly with the specific anatomic planes involved and thus the potential for all gangrenous tissue to be excised.

Antibiotics are given to control the often attendant bacteremia and to increase local tissue resistance against reinfection when fresh tissues are exposed to inoculation at the time of surgical débridement. Since exudate smears are not always reliable and since definitive culture data are seldom available for several days, wound appearance is the main determinant by which antibiotics should be selected. In addition, more than one antimicrobial agent may be required, because a polymicrobial flora is often present in the blood as well as within the wound. Systemic antibiotics should be continued until wound closure has been obtained.

The aerobic gram-negative bacilli are treated with tobramycin or gentamicin in a dose of 100 mg every eight hours I.V. along with carbenicillin 2.0 g I.V. every two hours. For the anaerobic component of the synergism, clindamycin 600 mg every six hours I.V., or metronidazole 200 mg every four hours orally should be selected. Chloramphenicol may be extremely useful because it is often effective against enteric gram-negative bacilli and most anaerobic bacteria, and if the patient can take oral medication, it can give as high levels by that route as intravenously.

Topical agents are likewise useful, providing higher concentrations on the wound surface and within the discharging exudate than could be achieved by a parenteral route alone. Local bacterial populations and thus total quantity of necrotizing toxin are thereby reduced.

Antimicrobial agents used for direct application to the wound surface should not freely bind to tissue proteins. Various aminoglycosides, cephaloridine, and mafenide are generally recommended.

## PROGNOSIS

Approximately one half of the deaths occur within the first week of therapy from uncontrolled infection. Inability or failure to excise all infected tissue, ineffective antibiotic therapy, and significant impairment in the mechanism of host resistance appear to be the more responsible factors. Although late deaths are sometimes due to recurrent sepsis, the major complications of diabetes mellitus, renal disease, and surgical management of massive tissue defects are the most common reasons for the delayed fatalities.

The overall mortality rate is 40 per cent, being greatest in cases of polymicrobial synergistic gangrene in the elderly compromised patient.

### References

Benjamin, B. I.: Fornier's gangrene. Br J Urol 51:312, 1979.
Defore, W. W., Jr., Mattox, K. L., Dang, M. H., Crawford, R., and Jordan, G. L.: Necrotizing fasciitis; a persistent surgical problem. Journal of the American College of Emergency Physicians 6:62, 1977.
Giuliano, A., Lewis, F., Jr., Hadley, K., and Blaisdell, F. W.: Bacteriology of necrotizing fasciitis. Am J Surg 134:52, 1977.
Lee, C., and Oh, C.: Necrotizing fasciitis of the genitalia. Urology 13:604, 1979.
Meleney, F. L.: Bacterial synergism in disease processes with a confirmation of the synergistic bacterial etiology of a certain type of progressive gangrene of the abdominal wall. Ann Surg 94:961, 1931.
Meleney, F. L.: Hemolytic *Streptococcus* gangrene. Arch Surg 9:317, 1924.
Stone, H. H., and Martin, J. D., Jr.; Synergistic necrotizing cellulitis. Ann Surg 175:702, 1972.

# PLEURODYNIA 241

## Melvin I. Marks, M.D.

### DEFINITION

Pleurodynia is an acute viral infection characterized by the sudden onset of pleuritic chest pain, fever, headache, and generalized malaise. Synonyms for this syndrome include Bornholm disease, devil's grip, and epidemic myalgia. Although the infection usually involves the striated intercostal muscles, abdominal pain may be prominent, and other organ systems can be involved.

### ETIOLOGY

The most common cause of pleurodynia is an infection due to coxsackievirus B. All six types of the B group viruses have been cultured from patients with this syndrome, and infection with multiple types have been documented as well. Coxsackievirus A, echovirus, and herpes simplex virus infections have also been associated with this syndrome infrequently. Coxsackieviruses A4 and A6 and echovirus Type 8 are recently reported examples.

### PATHOGENESIS AND PATHOLOGY

The pathogenesis of this disease is inferred from clinical experience and experimental animal infections. The viruses gain entry via the human gastrointestinal tract. A viremia follows with seeding of virus to the striated intercostal muscles. In some patients the testicles, myocardium, pericardium, and the brain or meninges may also be infected. Although it is stated that the pleura is not involved in this infection, patients with pleural effusion have been described.

IgM is the first class of antibody to increase, and later the IgG level is elevated (Schmidt et al., 1973). These immunoglobulins stop viral replication and terminate the infection. T lymphocytes are stimulated by the viral antigen and appear to contribute to the severity of local inflammation (Woodruff and Woodruff, 1974).

Deaths from pleurodynia have not been recorded, and pathologic studies of human tissues are not available. Coxsackievirus B causes intense myositis in suckling mice and hamsters. Histopathologic examination of striated muscle lesions reveals necrosis with nuclear pyknosis, loss of cross-striations, fragmentation, and hyaline degeneration.

### CLINICAL MANIFESTATIONS

Approximately one fourth of the patients with pleurodynia have prodromal headache, malaise, anorexia, and diffuse myalgia. This prodrome usually lasts two to three days but may last for as long as ten days. The incubation period is approximately two to five days. The most common clinical feature of pleurodynia is sudden, sharp, paroxysmal pain over the lower ribs or sternum (Sylvest, 1934; Bain et al., 1961). The chest pain is accentuated by deep breathing, coughing, and movement and may radiate to the shoulders, neck, and scapula. A local area of hyperesthesia is sometimes present over the affected part of the chest. Abdominal pain also occurs frequently and may be the only manifestation, particularly in younger patients. The severe knife-like pleuritic pain has been called the "devil's grip" by some patients. A painful episode may last several seconds to a few minutes, and the patient is remarkably symptom-free between such attacks. The pain has been severe enough to simulate coronary occlusion, rib fracture, cholecystitis, or pulmonary embolization.

The fever can occasionally be diphasic, as in other enteroviral infections. Nonproductive cough, nausea, vomiting, diarrhea, and shaking chills have also been described in pleurodynia.

Despite the severe symptoms in some patients, most young patients have a mild illness, and coxsackievirus infections may be asymptomatic in one half to two thirds of individuals.

Children and young adults seem to be most commonly affected with pleurodynia, although the age range is great. There is no sex predilection. Coxsackievirus B infections have been documented in some young infants with only fever, paroxysmal crying, tachycardia, and features suggestive of intussusception in others (Dery et al., 1974).

The physical examination of patients with pleurodynia is often unrewarding. Tachycardia may accompany the fever and is occasionally disproportionately severe. A pleural friction rub has been noted in as many as one fourth of patients with pleurodynia; pleural effusion may also be present. Localized tenderness may be present over the area of pleurodynia. Sore throat sometimes occurs and may occasionally be due to exudative pharyngotonsillitis.

The course of pleurodynia is usually benign and lasts three to five days, but symptoms may persist for several months and may cause serious morbidity. Deaths have not been reported.

### COMPLICATIONS AND SEQUELAE

The disease runs an uncomplicated course in most patients. Pleurodynia is one manifestation of systemic coxsackievirus infections and may therefore have other features of coxsackievirus disease, such as meningoencephalitis, myocarditis, pericarditis, pleuritis, hepatitis, or bronchitis. As many as 10 per cent of men may have orchitis, and 30 per cent of these will suffer relapses of testicular pain and swelling one to six months later.

### GEOGRAPHIC VARIATIONS IN DISEASE

Pleurodynia is a worldwide disease of the summer and autumn months. Its incidence parallels that of coxsackievirus infections. The disease is usually sporadic in the community. Nevertheless, epidemic outbreaks have been described in several communities in the warmer months. The name Bornholm disease refers to an outbreak of pleurodynia on the Danish island of Bornholm in 1930 (Sylvest, 1934). Person-to-person contact is probably the most critical factor in communicability. Coxsackieviruses have also been isolated from sewage, shellfish, and flies.

### DIAGNOSIS

The sudden onset of sharp pain, its intermittent character, location, and the absence of other causes usually make the diagnosis easy. The season and the prevalence of similar illness in family members or in the community are also clues. Pre-eruptive herpes zoster is differentiated by the more consistent pain, and costochondritis is differentiated by swelling of the costochondral junction. Although the abdominal pain may be severe, the physical examination of the abdomen is usually negative. If a pleural effusion is present, pneumonia, malignancy, tuberculosis, pulmonary infarct, and other causes of this condition must be excluded.

Laboratory studies are usually normal in pleurodynia. These include chest radiograph, electrocardiogram, and urinalysis. The white blood cell count is usually between 3000 and 8000 cells/mm$^3$, and polymorphonuclear leukocytes often predominate. Creatine phosphokinase may sometimes be elevated as evidence of injury to striated muscle.

Coxsackievirus B and the other viruses causing pleurodynia can be isolated from the throat and/or feces of these patients. Although the recovery rate of viruses is highest in the first week, they may be present in the stools for two to three weeks and sometimes for months. Coxsackie B viruses can be isolated in human diploid fibroblast cell lines as well as in human epithelial and rhesus monkey kidney tissues. Most of the other viruses causing this syndrome can also be cultured in these cell lines; however, certain coxsackieviruses A (Types 9 and 16) require inoculation of suckling mice or other more specialized techniques for cultivation and identification. Coxsackieviruses are serotyped by neutralization, which also serves to characterize the humoral antibody response. Antibody responses to infection are limited to the infecting virus, but occasionally heterotypic booster responses are noted. Multiple infections with several serotypes have also been documented. The virus may be isolated from the cerebrospinal fluid or pericardium in aseptic meningitis or pericarditis.

## TREATMENT AND PROPHYLAXIS

Although experimental studies have indicated some activity for thiourea derivatives and other chemical agents against coxsackieviruses in vitro and in vivo, the application of these chemicals to the prevention or therapy of human disease has not yet been reported. Analgesics can control pain. Although non-narcotic analgesics may be tried first, codeine and even meperidine (Demerol) may be necessary. Narcotics should be avoided in patients with serious underlying lung disease, because depression of respiration and cough may be harmful. Indomethacin may be a useful alternative in these situations.

Prevention of pleurodynia is not possible. However, malnourished individuals, newborns, and immunocompromised hosts should avoid direct contact with patients with pleurodynia or other coxsackievirus infections.

### References

Bain, H. W., McLean, D. M., and Walker, S. J.: Epidemic pleurodynia (Bornholm disease) due to coxsackie B-5 virus. Pediatrics 27:889, 1961.

Dery, P., Marks, M. I., and Shapera, R.: Clinical manifestations of coxsackievirus infections in children. Am J Dis Child 128:464, 1974.

Schmidt, N., Magoffin, R., and Lennette, E.: Association of group B coxsackieviruses with cases of pericarditis, myocarditis, or pleurodynia by demonstration of immunoglobulin M antibody. Infect Immun 8:341, 1973.

Sylvest, E.: Epidemic myalgia: Bornholm Disease. Copenhagen, Levin and Munksgaard, 1934.

Woodruff, J., and Woodruff, J.: Involvement of T lymphocytes in the pathogenesis of coxsackievirus B, heart disease. J Immunol 113:1726, 1974.

# J. INFECTIONS ACQUIRED FROM ANIMALS

## BITES: P. MULTOCIDA, S. MONILIFORMIS, AND S. MINOR

## 242

### J. L. Ryan, Ph.D., M.D.

Animal bites are responsible for approximately 1.2 per cent of the surgical problems handled in hospital emergency rooms in the United States. These bites are due primarily to the more than 100 million canine and feline pets in the United States. Other countries also have significant dog and cat populations, and the problem of domestic animal bites and infections resulting from these bites is therefore international in scope. Studies in the United States and Great Britain indicate that nearly three-fourths of the animal-related injuries are dog bites; cat bites and scratches account for the majority of the remainder. Most of these bites cause no infections, but many patients have developed cellulitis and lymphangitis. About 5 per cent of dog bites and 29 per cent of cat bites that are severe enough to require medical attention have infectious complications (Kizer, 1979). More invasive infections have also occurred following these bites. The annual incidence of animal bites in the United States has been estimated at 3.5 million; it represents a major medical problem in the United States and very likely in all countries that maintain large pet populations.

## P. MULTOCIDA INFECTION

Animal bite wounds are infected by various aerobic and anaerobic bacteria (Goldstein et al., 1978). The pathogen most often isolated has been *Pasteurella multocida*. This organism is recovered from 50 per cent of infected dog bites and 80 per cent of infected cat bites and scratches (Kizer, 1979; Francis et al., 1975). *P. multocida* is a gram-negative, coccobacillary organism that resides in the oropharynx and gingiva of many animals including dogs, cats, rats, rabbits, opossum, bear, lions, and others (Saphir and Carter, 1977; Owen et al., 1968). Careful studies have demonstrated that at least 50 per cent of dogs and 70 per cent of cats harbor this organism (Saphir and Carter, 1977; Owen et al., 1968; Bailie et al., 1978). In veterinary medicine, *P. multocida* is well known for the infections it causes among birds. Outbreaks of hemorrhagic septicemia due to *P. multocida* have also been reported in horses, cattle, sheep, reindeer, swine, cats, ducks, chickens, rabbits, and mice (Tindall and Harrison, 1972). Similarly, *P. multocida* has been reported to cause a broad spectrum of disease in man (Henderson, 1963). Exposure to animals may result in asymptomatic oropharyngeal carriage of *P. multocida* by man (Jones and Small, 1973).

The ability of *P. multocida* to be pathogenic in man depends on both bacterial and host properties. The bacteria usually have a hyaluronic acid capsule, and at least four antigenic types have been defined. There are also eleven different O antigens. These outer membrane components may increase the pathogenicity of the organism by preventing opsonization and phagocytosis. In animal models of infection, *P. multocida* can multiply rapidly in extracellular spaces and body cavities before phagocytosis begins (Collins, 1977). Host factors are equally important in determining the pathogenic potential of *P. multocida*. Defects in humoral immunity appear to predispose patients to invasive disease. Innate or acquired deficiencies of immunoglobulin or complement may result in inadequate opsonization and less efficient chemotaxis and phagocytosis. Chronic liver disease and chronic pulmonary disease are frequently associated with severe *P. multocida* infection. Defects in cellular immunity do not appear to predispose to infection with *P. multocida*.

*P. multocida* causes three types of clinical disease in man. The first is local soft tissue infection that may become complicated by tenosynovitis or osteomyelitis (Francis et al., 1975; Tindall and Harrison, 1972; Henderson, 1963). This is most frequently a complication of cat bites and scratches or dog bites. Patients with rheumatoid arthritis appear to be predisposed to joint infections with *P. multocida* following injuries from cats (Spagnuolo, 1978). Soft tissue injuries are characterized by their rapid onset, frequent abscess formation, and slow resolution despite specific antimicrobial therapy.

The second clinical syndrome of *P. multocida* infection is local disease of the respiratory tract. It most often occurs in patients with chronic lung disease and may be associated with defects in local humoral immune mechanisms. This syndrome is not directly related to animal bites (Hubbert and Rosen, 1970) and is usually correlated instead with domestic animal association. Bronchiectasis has been the most common predisposing illness, and the disease occurs after aspiration of secretions. It may cause pneumonia, pleural effusions, or abscesses (Beyt et al., 1979).

The third clinical syndrome is disseminated *P. multocida* infection. It frequently involves the gastrointestinal tract and may spread to many other tissues including the meninges. This syndrome has occurred most often in patients with chronic liver disease. In Laennec's cirrhosis and ascites, the syndromes of spontaneous bacterial peritonitis (SBP) and sepsis due to *P. multocida* have been reported following animal bites or scratches (Bearn et al., 1955; Palutke et al., 1973; Normann et al., 1971; Gerding et al., 1976). Since there may be a latent period between the exposure and the clinical presentation, a history of animal bite should always be sought when patients with cirrhosis and ascites present with febrile illness. SBP is felt to be of hematogenous origin, and metastatic infections in multiple other sites including the appendix, joints, and cardiovascular system have occurred (Henderson, 1963; Jones and Small, 1973).

Local infections with *P. multocida* are treated with antimicrobial drugs in addition to débridement and drainage. Penicillin is the drug of choice, given as procaine penicillin 600,000 units intramuscularly twice daily. Ampicillin in an oral dose of 500 mg four times daily or tetracycline in the same oral dosage is also effective. Treatment must be continued for two to four weeks because the organism tends to produce chronic and deep tissue involvement. The median MBC for *P. multocida* is 0.78 $\mu$g/ml of penicillin G and 3.12 $\mu$g/ml of tetracycline (Stevens et al., 1979). Therapeutic failures have been recorded with both oxacillin and erythromycin. Antimicrobial sensitivity testing is necessary because some penicillin-resistant strains have been found. Bacteremia is treated with 2,000,000 units of benzylpenicillin intravenously every six hours and meningitis with the same dose every three hours. Patients allergic to penicillin should be given 1.0 gm chloramphenicol succinate every four hours intravenously for *P. multocida* meningitis.

Antibiotic prophylaxis for *P. multocida* infection does not appear to be warranted in dog bite victims, but controlled trials have not been carried out (Callaham, 1978). Since the rate of infection after cat bites and scratches is much higher, prophylactic therapy should be beneficial, but again, no controlled trials have been reported.

## RAT-BITE FEVER

Infections due to *Streptobacillus moniliformis* and *Spirillum minor* are usually caused by the bite of a rat, and the disease resulting from these infections has been called rat-bite fever. Both organisms are present as normal flora in the oropharynx of many rodents. The clinical syndrome of rat-bite fever caused by each of these organisms overlaps, and it may be difficult to determine the specific etiology of the disease without cultural or serologic information. Rat-bite fever has been known since ancient times in India and has been recognized by the medical community since the early nineteenth century (Roughgarden, 1965).

### Streptobacillary Fever

*Streptobacillus moniliformis* is a pleomorphic, gram-negative rod that is a facultative anaerobe and is well known for its ability to convert spontaneously to L-form variants in culture. It grows best in medium supplemented with serum but has frequently been recovered from standard blood culture media. Typical puff-ball colonies are seen in liquid medium. The organism was studied in some detail after the 1926 outbreak of a febrile disease associated with raw milk consumption in Haverhill, Massachusetts. It was recovered from blood in over half of those in whom blood culture was attempted. It is of interest that cow's milk is a poor medium for growth of *S. moniliformis*, and

aside from the epidemiologic association with milk consumption in the affected population, the only direct evidence of milk contamination was the presence of antibody to *S. moniliformis* in one cow from the implicated dairy (Parker and Hudson, 1926). The epidemic was abruptly terminated by initiation of pasteurization. It has become common terminology to refer to *S. moniliformis*-caused disease that is not attributable to a rat bite as Haverhill fever (Lambe, 1974).

The incubation time of streptobacillary fever is generally less than ten days and often as short as two days. Most patients have no evidence of infection at the site of the rat bite when the disease becomes clinically apparent. Fever to 40° C (104° F) is common, and many patients have a morbilliform or petechial rash. It is most prominent on the extremities, including the palms and soles, and becomes evident early in the course of the disease. Polyarthritis is a prominent finding in streptobacillary rat-bite fever. It occurs in 50 per cent of infected patients and is often the major complaint. Large joints are most frequently affected and are painful and tender. Joint effusions are occasionally present. In untreated cases the arthritis may persist for months to years. Mortality is very low in uncomplicated cases, but severe complications including endocarditis, pneumonia, metastatic abscess, and anemia have been reported (Roughgarden, 1965; Tabor and Feigen, 1979). Endocarditis of a previously diseased valve has been the most frequent fatal complication of *S. moniliformis* infection, but most reported cases occurred before the modern antibiotic era. The prognosis appears to be much better with antibiotics (McCormack et al., 1967; Hamburger and Knowles, 1953).

In streptobacillary fever there is a mild leukocytosis and a low incidence (15 to 25 per cent) of false-positive serologic tests for syphilis. The therapy of choice is 600,000 units of penicillin per day for at least seven days. Increased doses should be used if a prompt response is not obtained. In complicated cases, such as endocarditis, doses of 10 to 15 million units per day of penicillin have been recommended for four weeks. Streptomycin, tetracycline, and chloramphenicol represent alternate modes of therapy that should be considered when penicillin allergy exists or when a resistant organism is encountered (Stokes et al., 1951).

Streptobacillary fever may occur after a bite from laboratory or pet rats as well as wild rats (Cole et al., 1969). Cases have been reported secondary to bites from other mammals and there are many cases for which there is no history of an animal bite. It may be confused with other diseases, particularly of rickettsial origin, in the ab-

TABLE 1.  Differential Features of Streptobacillary Fever and Sodoku

|  | STREPTOBACILLARY FEVER | SODOKU |
|---|---|---|
| Isolation of organism | Culture in serum-supplemented medium | Requires animal inoculation |
| Incubation period | Usually less than ten days | Frequently more than ten days |
| Local inflammation | Rare | Frequent |
| Regional lymphadenopathy | Rare | Frequent |
| Arthritis | Frequent | Rare |
| Rash | Frequent, morbilliform, petechial | Frequent, macular, red-brown |
| False-positive serologic test for syphilis | Less than 25 % | At least 50 % |
| Leukocytosis | Mild | Often absent |
| Specific serology | Helpful | Unavailable |
| Complications | Uncommon, severe | Very rare |

sence of cultural or serologic information (Portnoy et al., 1979). Most often, however, it is confused with sodoku.

### Sodoku

Sodoku, or spirillary fever, is rat-bite fever secondary to infection with *Spirillum minor*. *S. minor* has not been reproducibly cultured in artificial medium. The organism is a gram-negative spiral rod, relatively short at 2 to 5 $\mu$m and containing two to six spirals. It is actively motile. When the diagnosis of spirillary fever is under consideration, the organism should be sought in blood smears and tissue exudates. Animal inoculation is usually necessary to confirm the diagnosis. One ml of blood should be administered intraperitoneally to mice or guinea pigs and the animal blood examined for characteristic organisms one to three weeks later.

Infection with *S. minor* occurs most commonly after rat bites, but as with streptobacillary fever, there are reports of sodoku secondary to the bites of other rodents and animals that eat rodents (Roughgarden, 1965). The incubation period is generally longer than ten days and frequently there is persisting evidence of inflammation at the site of the bite. Regional lymphadenopathy is relatively common but frank arthritis is rare. Table 1 illustrates criteria that may be helpful in the differentiation of spirillary fever from streptobacillary fever. Most patients with sodoku manifest a macular red-brown rash that spreads from the initial lesion. If untreated, the signs and symptoms abate, but relapse occurs with new onset of fever, increased local inflammation, and more severe rash. Complications of the disease are rare, but endocarditis has been reported. Uncomplicated disease had a relatively low mortality in the pre-antibiotic era and mortality with appropriate treatment has been negligible. Penicillin is so effective that it is necessary to give procaine penicillin in a dose of 600,000 units intramuscularly twice a day for only one day. Streptomycin and tetracycline are alternative modes of therapy. Sodoku remains a rare disease in the United States; most cases have been reported from Japan.

### References

Bailie, W. E., Stowe, E. C., and Schmitt, A. M.: Aerobic bacterial flora of oral and nasal fluids of canines with special reference to bacteria associated with bites. J Clin Microbiol 7:223, 1978.

Bearn, A. G., Jacobs, K., and McCarty, M.: *Pasteurella multocida* septicemia in man. Am J Med 18:167, 1955.

Beyt, B. E., Sondag, J., Roosevelt, T. S., and Bruce, R.: Human pulmonary pasteurellosis. JAMA 242:1647, 1979.

Callaham, M. L.: Treatment of common dog bites; infection risk factors. Journal of the American College of Emergency Physicians 7:83, 1978.

Cole, J. S., Stoll, R. W., and Bulger, R. J.: Rat-bite fever. Am Intern Med 71:979, 1969.

Collins, F. M.: Mechanisms of acquired resistance to *Pasteurella multocida* infection: A review. Cornell Vet 67:103, 1977.

Francis, D. P., Holmes, M. A., and Brandon, G.: *Pasteurella multocida*: Infections after domestic animal bites and scratches. JAMA 233:42, 1975.

Gerding, D. N., Khan, M. Y., Ewing, J. E., and Hall, W. H.: *Pasteurella multocida* peritonitis in hepatic cirrhosis with ascites. Gastroenterology 70:413, 1976.

Goldstein, E. J. C., Citron, D. M., Wield, B., Blachman, U., Sutter, V. L., Miller, T. A., and Finegold, S. M.: Bacteriology of human and animal bite wounds. J Clin Microbiol 8:667, 1978.

Hamburger, M., and Knowles, H. C.: *Streptobacillus moniliformis* infection complicated by acute bacterial endocarditis. Arch Intern Med 92:216, 1953.

Henderson, A.: *Pasteurella multocida* infection in man; a review of the literature. Antonie van Leeuwenhoek 29:359, 1963.

Hubbert, W. T., and Rosen, M. A.: *Pasteurella multocida* infection in man unrelated to animal bite. Am J Pub Health 60:1109, 1970.

Jones, F. L., and Small, C. E.: Infections in man due to *Pasteurella multocida*; importance of human carrier. Penn Med 76:41, 1973.

Kizer, K. W.: Epidemiologic and clinical aspects of animal bite injuries. Journal of the American College of Emergency Physicians 8:134, 1979.

Lambe, D. W.: Haverhill fever and rat-bite fever. Am J Clin Pathol 62:444, 1974.

McCormack, R. C., Kaye, D., and Hooke, E. W.: Endocarditis due to *Streptobacillus moniliformis*. JAMA 200:77, 1967.

Normann, B., Nilehn, B., Rays, J., and Karlberg, B.: A fatal human case of *Pasteurella multocida* septicemia after cat bite. Scand J Infect Dis 3:251, 1971.

Owen, C. R., Buker, E. O., Bell, J. F., and Jellison, W. L.: *Pasteurella multocida* in animal mouths. Rocky Mtn Med J 65:45, 1968.

Palutke, W. A., Boyd, C. B., and Carter, G. R.: *Pasteurella multocida* septicemia in a patient with cirrhosis. Am J Med Sci 266:305, 1973.

Parker, F., and Hudson, N. P.: The etiology of Haverhill fever (erythema arthriticum epidemicum). Am J Pathol 2:357, 1926.

Portnoy, B. L., Satterwhite, T. K., and Dyckman, J. D.: Rat-bite fever misdiagnosed as Rocky Mountain spotted fever. South Med J 72:607, 1979.

Roughgarden, J. W.: Antimicrobial therapy of rat bite fever. Arch Intern Med 116:39, 1965.

Saphir, D. A., and Carter, G. R.: Gingival flora of the dog with special reference to bacteria associated with bites. J Clin Microbiol 3:344, 1977.

Spagnuolo, P. J.: *Pasteurella multocida* infectious arthritis. Am J Med Sci 275:359, 1978.

Stevens, D. L., Higbee, J. W., Oberhofer, T. R., and Everett, E. D.: Antibiotic susceptibilities of human isolates of *Pasteurella multocida*. Antimicrob Agents Chemother 16:322, 1979.

Stokes, J. F., Gray, I. R., and Stokes, E. J.: *Actinomyces muris* endocarditis treated with chloramphenicol. Br Heart J 13:247, 1951.

Taber, L. H., and Feigen, R. D.: Spirochetal infections. Pediat Clin N Am 26:377, 1979.

Tindall, J. P., and Harrison, C. M.: *Pasteurella multocida* infections following animal injuries, especially cat bites. Arch Dermatol 105:412, 1972.

# *TULAREMIA* **243**

## Joseph H. Bates, M.D.

### DEFINITION

Tularemia is an infectious disease of endemic nature caused by the bacterium *Francisella tularensis*. Although the disease is primarily found in rodents, many cases occur in man and in various kinds of wild life. The first description of a case in man was by Martin, an opthalmic surgeon, in 1907 (Simpson, 1928). The causative organism was reported in 1911 by McCoy and Chapin who described a "plague-like disease among ground squirrels" in Tulare County, California, and called the organism *Bacterium tularense*. The human disease was called "deer fly fever" in Utah and "rabbit fever" elsewhere. Edward Francis in 1921 recognized the unity of the disease in rodents and man, and gave it the descriptive name tularemia (Francis, 1921). Ohara described an acute febrile disease in Japan transmitted by rabbits in 1925, and working with Francis showed that it was tularemia. In 1928, when Suvorov described tularemia in Astrakhan, the USSR was the scene of several outbreaks.

### ETIOLOGY

Although first called *B. tularense,* the organism was soon placed in the genus *Pasteurella* because of similarities with *Pasteurella pestis*. In 1947 a new genus, *Francisella,* was established, since the organism did not belong in any of the genera in which it had been placed previously. (British investigators maintain that the organism belongs to the Brucella group.) *F. tularensis* is a minute, gram-negative, pleomorphic rod that may appear coccoid. It will not grow on ordinary media but will grow on blood-dextrose-cystine agar and other enriched media containing cystine. The disease is endemic on four continents and it appears that variation in the organisms does occur. Tularemia organisms occurring in North America are usually more virulent than the Asian and European varieties, although the less virulent forms are also found in North America. There may be other differences among the varieties, including biochemical reactions, habitat, and mode of transmission.

### PATHOGENESIS AND PATHOLOGY

Mechanisms for human infection with *F. tularensis* are highly variable. The earliest descriptions associated with the disease with skinning and dressing of wild rabbits and with bites by the deer fly, *Chrysops discalis* commonly found on horses. Careful investigative studies later showed that the common wood tick, *Dermacentor andersoni* harbored tularemia organisms, and presently 11 different species in North America are known to be naturally infected (Hopla, 1974). Transovarian transmission of *F. tularensis* in ticks was long thought to occur and the tick was suspected as being the natural reservoir for the organism, but recent work has shown that this is not true. A more likely natural reservoir is a multiple-host system of disease involving various highly susceptible rabbits, hares, and ticks. The tick is infected after taking a blood meal from an infected animal. The bacteria multiply in the tick, penetrate the gut, and spread to the salivary glands. There they can be injected into the next host along with the saliva or they may persist in the tick gut and be transmitted by tick fecal matter at the time of the blood meal. Naturally infected ticks in the USSR include *Dermacentor sictus* and *Dermacentor marginatus,* in Europe *Ixodes ricinusand,* and in Japan *Haemayshysalis flavis* and *Ixodes japonensia.*

Many vertebrates may become infected and over 100 different species of wild animals, 25 species of birds, and several species of fish and amphibians have been found naturally infected. Cricetine rodents and hares are extremely susceptible; rabbits, squirrels, and beavers are moderately susceptible; and carnivora and domestic animals show low susceptibility. In the USSR the vole, muskrat, mouse, and hamster are the most frequent sources of human infection. In Europe and in Japan it is primarily hares and field mice. In North America, hares, rabbits, voles, muskrats, and sheep are primarily involved in the northern regions, and in the southern areas rabbits and ticks are most important. Minor vectors include fleas, mosquitoes (ten different species), tabanid flies, and mites.

Tularemia may also be acquired by ingestion of infected meat and contaminated water, and by inhalation. The first report of water-borne tularemia and the first major outbreak from water were recognized in the USSR, where infected voles had contaminated the water. The organism has been isolated from thoroughly cooked meat and has been shown to be capable of penetrating the intact epidermis of humans.

Man-to-man transmission of tularemia has not been proved but the organism can be cultured from the sputum, pharynx, and gastric washings of patients who have tularemic pneumonia. Almost all nonimmune laboratory investigators who study tularemia acquire the disease, and respiratory exposure is suspected as the most likely mode of infection. Immunized human volunteers exposed to aerosol challenge developed chest roentgenographic abnormalities, fever, and malaise after three to five days. An outbreak of an influenza-like illness in northern Sweden was shown to have been airborne tularemia resulting from the inhalation of dust from dried vole fecal material deposited in haystacks (Dahlstrand, 1971).

Asymptomatic infection has been shown to occur in endemic areas where exposure to ticks and infected animals is common. Sequential serologic surveys among Indians and Eskimos in Alaska and animal trappers in Montana indicate that serologic and skin test conversion occurs in the absence of recognized disease. The absence of clinical illness after infection may be explained by one factor or a combination of factors: infection with a strain of markedly decreased virulence, a route of infection that favors the development of asymp-

tomatic infection, and infection in a resistant host.

The most common site for the organism to invade humans is the skin, where an ulcer with surrounding inflammation develops in approximately half of all cases. The ulcer extends deeply and shows coagulation necrosis resembling caseation. About the margins there are polymorphonuclear leukocytes and epithelioid cells. The bacteria in the ulcer and in all other lesions are difficult to demonstrate with routine staining methods. When fluorescent antibody-staining methods are used the organisms are readily identified and are usually located intracellularly in monocytes, macrophages, and polymorphonuclear leukocytes. Extracellular organisms are uncommon except in necrotic areas, where they are abundant.

Lymph node involvement is characteristically confined to the regional nodes draining the involved ulcer, but may become generalized with associated hepatic and splenic enlargement. The lesions closely resemble tuberculosis with caseation necrosis, Langhans giant cells, epithelioid cells, and mononuclear cells predominating. At other times an acute necrotizing process leading to marked suppuration may evolve. Similar lesions may be found in the spleen and liver.

The lung is involved either by inhalation of organisms or by hematogenous dissemination. In experimental animals after inhalation of organisms in aerosol form, the earliest lesions are noted in the alveolar ducts and alveoli where polymorphonuclear cells collect in increased number (Baskerville, 1976). This development is followed by capillary congestion, bronchial inflammation, and necrosis of bronchial epithelium. Within 72 hours marked arteritis of medium and large vessels occurs. These later changes are similar to those described among fatal human cases. Experimental respiratory tularemia in the monkey shows that the primary sites of infection are the respiratory bronchioles and alveolar ducts, where the organisms are rapidly phagocytized by alveolar macrophages. In man the most frequently found pulmonary lesions at autopsy are areas of focal necrosis beneath the pleura, which may coalesce to produce consolidation of an entire lobe or lung. Abscesses of varying sizes up to 10 centimeters in diameter may occur, and pleural involvement varying from slight thickening to extensive effusion also develops in many nonfatal cases.

Many other organs and tissues including the bone marrow, pharynx, esophagus, stomach, ileum, appendix, colon, adrenals, pericardium, kidney, meninges, and brain have been involved with the necrotic lesion of tularemia. In each the lesion is primarily a necrotizing granuloma.

## CLINICAL MANIFESTATIONS

In North America tularemia shows a remarkable seasonal variation with two peaks during the year. An early spring and summer peak occurs in areas where tularemia is tick-borne, as in the south-central states. Hand contact with blood or tissue of infected animals, especially rabbits, is the most common source of infection in other regions of the United States, and this form peaks between November and February. Several clinical types are recognized and most cases can be placed into one of four categories: ulceroglandular, oculoglandular, glandular, and typhoidal (Dienst, 1963). Less common presentations include primary respiratory disease, meningitis, and a gastrointestinal form with severe diarrhea. The incubation period may not be possible to determine, since a specific vector contact cannot be recalled in many cases. In those cases with a reliable vector history the incubation period ranges between a few fours to two weeks, with an average period of five days. The clinical type does not alter the incubation period.

The clinical picture is extremely variable owing to the several portals of entry and the great fluctuations in degree of morbidity. The disease may present as a prolonged disorder with low-grade fever and adenopathy, suggesting a lymphoma. The most frequent complaints are chills and fever followed by headache, backache, generalized muscle aches, malaise, and weakness. Delirium, stupor, or marked restlessness are frequent among patients with acute toxemia. These patients are usually free of any demonstrable central nervous system infection and the cause for these symptoms has never been explained. Upon specific treatment the central nervous system symptoms clear rapidly. Hepatic and splenic enlargement occurs in a few cases. Jaundice is uncommon and seen only in the severely ill patient. Cutaneous manifestations are usually limited to the ulcer and enlarged regional lymph nodes, but in exceptional cases macular, papular, vesicular, and pustular eruptions are a major feature. A petechial rash over the trunk and proximal portion of the extremities can be seen and typical erythema nodosum has been described as a rare manifestation.

### Ulceroglandular Tularemia

Ulceroglandular tularemia is the most common type and occurs in from 50 to 80 per cent of all cases. The primary lesion is a papule at the point of inoculation, usually on the finger or hand if acquired by direct animal contact, but on almost any site if vector borne. The papule rapidly becomes painful and swollen and suppurates in the center, leaving an ulcer 3 to 5 mm in diameter. Some ulcers may be as large as 2 cm in diameter. Tenderness and pain in the regional lymph nodes begins about 24 hours later and becomes severe. If left untreated or misdiagnosed and improperly treated the overlying skin becomes thinned and the nodes drain spontaneously in about one-half of the cases. In a few patients lymphangitic nodules (simulating sporotrichosis) are found along the course of the lymphatics draining the inoculation site. Most ulceroglandular cases do not present with the overwhelming toxic infection seen with other forms.

### Glandular Tularemia

Glandular tularemia shows no visible primary lesion even upon careful scrutiny. In all other respects, the disease process simulates the ulceroglandular type. The glandular form accounts for 10 to 15 per cent of all cases, and the most common site of involvement is the axillary node group. These are the least toxic of all tularemic patients and usually present with fever and localized adenopathy. The involved nodes may be very tender and show marked erythema of the overlying skin.

### Oculoglandular Tularemia

This form accounts for only 3 to 5 per cent of all cases. The primary site of entry is the conjunctival sac. Unilateral involvement is usual with associated enlargement of the cervical and preauricular lymph nodes. Photophobia, excessive lacrimation, and decreased visual acuity are common. The conjunctiva is very reddened and there may be small ulcerations. Membrane formation and corneal ulceration are rare. Late sequelae are seldom seen.

### Typhoidal Tularemia

Typhoidal tularemia is the most serious form of the disease and has the highest mortality. There is no primary lesion and no regional lymphadenopathy. Fever, malaise, aching, mental confusion, and extreme toxicity are the primary features. Most cases occurring in laboratory workers are typhoidal. The frequency of this form varies from 10 to 30 per cent. The patients are acutely ill with dehydration, vomiting, and meningismus. Diarrhea is a frequent complication. Pleuropulmonary involvement is most frequent in this form and may complicate 40 per cent of cases. In untreated patients, the mortality rate is approximately 30 per cent.

### Uncommon Forms

Oropharyngeal tularemia, primarily found in the pediatric group, presents as exudative pharyngitis (Tyson, 1976). Pustular lesions on the tonsils with membrane formation, cervical lymph node involvement, high fever, and marked difficulty in swallowing is the usual presentation. The process may progress to tracheal obstruction and death. Infection is probably introduced by ingestion of food or water contaminated with *F. tularensis* or by hand contact with the mouth after handling an infected animal.

Gastrointestinal tularemia is more commonly encountered in Europe and the USSR than in North America or Asia. These patients develop acute, watery diarrhea with fever and cramping abdominal pain. Bloody diarrhea or acute hemorrhage with minimal diarrhea secondary to superficial ulcerations in the colon is rare.

## COMPLICATIONS AND SEQUELAE

Most observers agree that pleuropulmonary tularemia usually results from hematogenous dissemination of local infection elsewhere in the body (Miller, 1969), but primary respiratory tract infection can also occur. It is a necrotizing process that heals with fibrosis and calcification. Residual pleural thickening is common. The chest roentgenographic features are variable and may be confused with tuberculosis, mycotic infection, acute bacterial pneumonia, lymphoma, and carcinoma of the lung. Almost any roentgenographic pattern may appear and tularemia must be considered in all cases of diagnostically perplexing pneumonia in those regions where tularemia occurs. Roentgenographic appearances described include lobar consolidation with or without hilar adenopathy, pleural effusion, bronchopleural fistula and empyema, upper lobe interstitial infiltration, and massive mediastinal adenopathy without lung involvement.

Pneumonia complicates 10 to 30 per cent of cases of tularemia. The most common pulmonary complaints are cough, pleuritic pain, dyspnea, and sputum production. Hemoptysis is rare. A few patients have no respiratory complaints and the pulmonic process is discovered only by roentgenogram.

Pericardial involvement with effusion is usually associated with pneumonia. Cardiac tamponade or constrictive pericarditis may develop, requiring pericardectomy.

Tularemic meningitis and encephalitis are rare complications. The symptoms are headache, stiff neck, and delirium. The cerebrospinal fluid usually shows less than 1000 cells per cubic millimeter with lymphocytes predominating. The protein content is elevated above 100 and the sugar is less than 30 mg/ml. Bloody spinal fluid may be seen. Most reported patients with this complication have succumbed, in part due to a delayed or missed diagnosis.

## GEOGRAPHIC VARIATIONS IN DISEASE

The disease in North America is more variable in severity than in Europe or Asia; North American patients may show extreme toxicity or the disease may be mild. Asymptomatic infections occur as evidenced by conversion of serial serologic tests. In Europe and Asia, most illness is mild. In regions where ticks are abundant or where rabbit contact is frequent, ulceroglandular and glandular tularemia are common. In the USSR and eastern European countries water contamination with *F. tularensis* is more common, resulting in water-borne outbreaks in man presenting with gastrointestinal complaints.

## DIAGNOSIS

The most important step in making the diagnosis of tularemia is to include it in the differential diagnosis. The initial symptoms simulate those of influenza; after the disease is well advanced with ulceration and adenopathy, streptococcus infection may be considered. When there is nodular lymphangitis sporotrichosis is mimicked. The uncommon cases that present as generalized lymphadenopathy and fever may suggest lymphoma or infectious mononucleosis. The typhoidal form is similar to typhoid fever, and if pneumonia is present any of a number of acute and chronic bacterial pneumonias must be included as diagnostic possibilities. Sera from patients with tularemia may contain antibodies that cross-agglutinate with *Brucella abortus* and *Brucella melitensis,* but the highest titer is almost always against *F. tularensis.* Upon examination of enlarged lymph nodes the pathologist may suggest a histopathologic diagnosis of tuberculosis or cat-scratch fever.

Once the clinical diagnosis has been raised it is relatively easy to confirm or exclude it. The best method is the serum agglutination test. An agglutination titer of 1:80 or above is highly suspicious. It is always desirable to show a four-fold or greater rise in titer from the acute to the convalescent serum taken ten days to two weeks later. Antibodies first appear about the second week, but in some cases the appearance of anti-bodies is very much delayed and they may not be detectable for up to 30 days or more. The patients with the greatest toxicity are more likely to show a delayed antibody response. The agglutination titer can reach very high levels of up to 1:40,000 and greater although the usual peak titer is in the range of 1:1024. Positive agglutination tests may persist for life, but most patients show a low level of 1:80 or below within three years after recovery.

A tularemia skin test has been used primarily as an investigative tool. It is an intradermal test read 48 hours after application and is a measure of delayed hypersensitivity. It is positive in more than 90 per cent of cases during the first week of illness even when the agglutination test remains negative.

The organism can be cultured readily from infected tissues such as the skin ulcer, suppurative lymph nodes, and sputum from those with pulmonic involvement; however, it is not routinely isolated in clinical laboratories because laboratory workers who are not specifically immunized are at high risk of acquiring the disease and the special media containing cystine required for the growth of the organism are not utilized. The guinea pig and rabbit can be inoculated with pus, sputum, or infected tissue; the animal will die within one to two weeks and at autopsy focal necrosis of the liver and spleen is evident. Specific staining of infected tissues from inoculated animals or from human tissue by fluorescent antibody techniques will show intracellular organisms within macrophages and polymorphonuclear leukocytes and extracellular organisms in areas where necrosis is marked.

The white blood cell count may range from low normal to marked leukocytosis. The differential count is usually normal and there may be a mild anemia. The sedimentation rate is increased.

## TREATMENT

Streptomycin is the drug of choice for treatment of tularemia. The bacteriostatic concentration for most strains of F. tularensis is less than 0.4 $\mu$g/ml. The dose for adults is generally 1 to 2 g daily with a treatment period of 10 to 14 days. The clinical response is dramatic except in the most advanced cases. If the patient is gravely ill with advanced pneumonia or meningitis at the time chemotherapy is begun death may not be averted. Frequently streptomycin must be begun on the basis of only a clinical suspicion when serologic proof is lacking. The physician should have no reservation about streptomycin chemotherapy in this situation, since early treatment dramatically reduces the incidence of serious complications and death.

Chloramphenicol and tetracycline are also somewhat effective. Relapse after treatment with these drugs may be as high as 30 per cent, but retreatment with the same drug is usually effective. Laboratory reports indicate that gentamicin is bactericidal for the organism in vitro, and limited clinical experience indicates that this drug may be as effective as streptomycin.

General supportive measures are important in the very ill patient. Most deaths occur from extensive pneumonia producing the "adult respiratory distress syndrome." The use of corticosteroids in these patients has been limited, but there are no data to indicate that these medications are effective.

Mortality rates before specific chemotherapy ranged from 7 to 31 per cent; since the advent of streptomycin the mortality rate has been less than 6 per cent.

## PROPHYLAXIS

Defense against tularemia involves resistance to facultative intracellular infection. Although serum agglutination antibodies appear after naturally acquired infection as well as in vaccinated subjects, this antibody confers no significant protection in animal challenge experiments. Strong immunity follows natural infection or immunization with a live attenuated strain of F. tularensis (Burke, 1977). The immunity is cell mediated and long lasting. A phenol-killed vaccine has been tried but the protection that results is very incomplete.

### References

Baskerville, A., and Hambleton, P.: Pathogenesis and pathology of respiratory tularemia in the rabbit. Br J Exp Pathol 57:339, 1976.

Burke, S. D.: Immunization against tularemia: Analysis of the effectiveness of liver Francisella tularensis vaccine in prevention of laboratory acquired tularemia. J Infect Dis 135:55, 1977.

Dahlstrand, S., Ringertz, O., and Zetterberg, B.: Airbone tularemia in Sweden. Scand J Infect Dis 3:7, 1971.

Dienst, F. T., Jr., Tularemia: A perusal of three hundred thirty-nine cases. J Louisiana Med Soc 115:114, 1963.

Francis, E., The occurrence of tularemia in nature as a disease of man. Pub Health Dep 36:1731, 1921.

Hopla, C. E.: The ecology of tularemia. Adv Vet Sci Comp Med 18:25, 1974.

Miller, R. P., and Bates, J. H.: Pleuropulmonary tularemia, a review of 29 patients. Am Rev Resp Dis 99:31, 1969.

Simpson, W. M.: Tularemia (Francis' disease). Clinical and pathological study of 48 non-fatal cases and one rapidly fatal case, with autopsy occurring in Dayton, Ohio. Ann Int Med 1:1007, 1928.

Tyson, H. K.: Tularemia: An unappreciated cause of exudative pharyngitis. Pediatrics 58:864, 1976.

# 244 *PLAGUE*

*Alexander L. Kisch, M.D.*

## DEFINITION

Plague is a severe acute or chronic enzootic or epizootic bacterial infection produced by *Yersinia pestis.* It is acquired in endemic areas throughout the world (Fig. 1). Over 200 species of wild rodents (e.g., marmots, squirrels, field mice, prairie dogs, and gerbils), commensal rodents (e.g., *Rattus rattus, R. norvegicus, Mus musculus),* lagomorphs (e.g., rabbits and hares), and certain other mammalian species (e.g., dogs, cats, coyotes, and guinea pigs) are susceptible (Pollitzer, 1954; Rust et al., 1971). Rodents, which are relatively resistant to *Y. pestis,* are the reservoir in which the pathogen is maintained between epidemics of plague. Asymptomatic or, more often, life-threatening infection is sporadically and incidentally transmitted to humans from this natural animal reservoir through the bite of infected fleas (e.g., *Xenopsylla cheopis*) or, rarely, of other ectoparasites (e.g., lice and ticks). Plague may also be acquired by direct contact with living or dead infected animals or with contaminated rodent burrow soil. Human populations in geographic areas adjoining enzootic regions are at particular risk of epidemic plague during periods when sanitation is disrupted or when rodents are not controlled and there is transmission of *Y. pestis* from sylvatic to urban rat populations. The great historic plague epidemics of mankind have usually occurred when plague-infected rat fleas, deprived of their normal hosts by massive rat epizootics and die-offs, have sought and infected human beings instead. With the development of modern high-speed transportation, introduction of unrecognized cases of human or rodent plague into nonendemic areas via air travel and container freighting is an ever-present hazard. Bacteremic pulmonary seeding during the bubonic or septicemic forms of the disease may produce secondary plague pneumonia. Explosive epidemics of highly fatal primary pneumonic plague can then result from human-to-human ("demic") respiratory transmission of *Y. pestis* via droplet aerosols (Fig. 2). There has been an increase in reported cases of plague in the last decade (Table 1).

## ETIOLOGY

The causative bacterium of plague, recently reclassified in the genus *Yersinia,* belongs to the family Enterobacteriaceae. Credit for its isolation in Hong Kong during the plague pandemic of 1894 is shared by the French bacteriologist A. E. J. Yersin and the Japanese bacteriologist S. Kitasato (Bibel and Chen, 1976). *Y. pestis* is a gram-negative, nonmotile, aerobic and facultatively anaerobic, nonhemolytic, pleomorphic coccobacillus 1 to 2 $\mu$m in length whose bipolar staining results in a characteristic "safety-pin" appearance. This appearance is more easily recognized in smears of clinical specimens than of cultured organisms by use of Wayson's or Giemsa stain (Sonnenwirth, 1974) (see chapter 37.)

## PATHOGENESIS AND PATHOLOGY

Although human plague may be acquired by inhalation or by mucous membrane inoculation, the most common route of infection is by the bite of a flea infected by a blood meal from an infected rodent. *Y. pestis* proliferates in the flea gut, where organisms lacking envelope antigen (Fraction I) replicate and block the proventriculus. Organisms regurgitated by such "blocked fleas" are then inoculated intradermally into human beings when fleas refeed. In some highly immune people, a pustule may develop at the bite but is more often absent. Usually, in less resistant people, the injected organisms spread via lymphatic channels to the regional lymph nodes. These become enlarged due to inflammation, edema, thrombosis, and hemorrhagic necrosis, forming the buboes characteristic of the disease. Bacilli replicating at these sites extracellularly and surviving intracellularly in mononuclear phagocytes (Janssen and Surgalla, 1969) become resistant to phagocytosis. Early bacteremic dissemination establishes suppurative foci throughout the body in the distant lymph nodes, skin, lungs, spleen, liver, and central nervous system. Concentrations of more than 100 *Y. pestis* organisms per ml of blood are common and are associated with a poor prognosis (Butler et al., 1976).

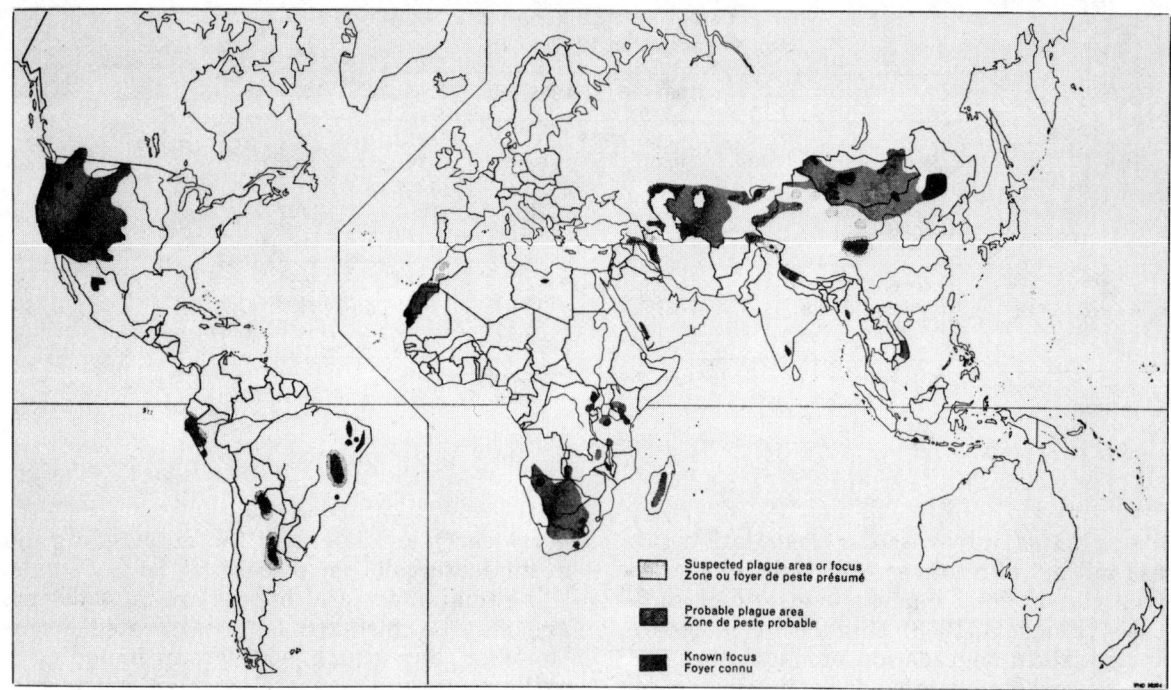

**FIGURE 1.** *Known and probable foci and areas of plague, 1969. (Reprinted with permission of World Health Organization from WHO Expert Committee on Plague, Fourth Report, WHO Technical Report Series No. 447. Geneva, World Health Organization, 1970.)*

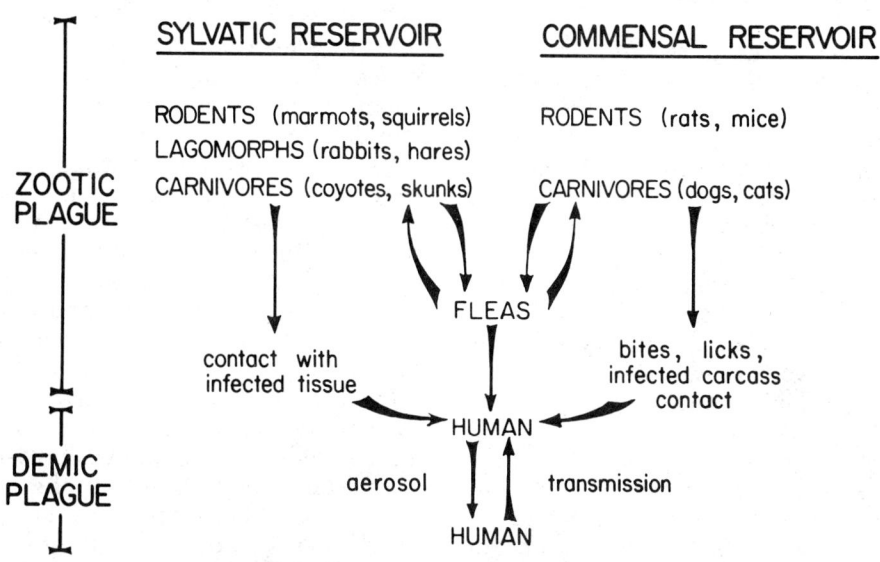

**FIGURE 2.** *Epidemiologic features of plague.*

**TABLE 1.** Human Cases of Plague Reported to the World Health
Organization 1961 to 1976[a]

|  | 1961–64 | 1965–68 | 1969–72 | 1973–76 |
|---|---|---|---|---|
| Africa | 734 | 233 | 322 | 454 |
| Asia[b] | 2038 | 7500 | 13591 | 4004[c] |
| Europe | 0 | 0 | 0 | 0 |
| South America | 1847 | 2138 | 1242 | 1127 |
| United States | 4 | 11 | 21 | 46 |
| Total world cases | 4623 | 9882 | 15173 | 5631[c] |
| Total world deaths | 615 | 539 | 625 | 394 |
| % Mortality | 13.3 | 5.45 | 4.12 | 6.99 |

[a]Modified after Reed et al., 1970 and World Health Organization, 1977.
[b]Does not include mainland China, which is not a participating member of the World Health
Organization.
[c]Based on incomplete reporting of cases from Viet Nam (1975–76) and Burma (1976).

Disseminated intravascular coagulation produces capillary fibrin thrombi in renal glomeruli, adrenal glands, skin, lungs, and elsewhere in fatal cases (Finegold, 1968). Circulating endotoxin, fibrinogen-fibrin degradation products, thrombocytopenia, and consumption of clotting factors are characteristically identifiable even in nonfatal cases. The term "black death," long identified with plague (Nohl, 1961), may well have referred to the diffuse hemorrhagic, necrotic changes in the skin plus the marked hypoxia and cyanosis that result from pneumonia. Patients may succumb so rapidly to overwhelming plague septicemia and toxemia that pathologic lesions characteristic of plague may not have time to develop.

## CLINICAL MANIFESTATIONS

Fever begins two to ten days after exposure, often without accompanying chills. There is usually tachycardia, headache, generalized aching, prostration, severe malaise, and conjunctivitis. Abdominal pain, nausea, vomiting, and diarrhea may also be present. Bubonic plague, the most common clinical form of the disease, begins with localized pain and tenderness in lymph nodes (e.g., inguinal, axillary) accompanying the systemic symptoms, and may precede the appearance of palpable and visible adenitis by a day or longer. When relatively mild, self-limited, and benign, the early adenitis has been designated "pestis minor." Usually, however, the affected lymph nodes become grossly enlarged, exquisitely painful, and so excruciatingly tender that the patient shrinks to avoid the examiner's touch or refuses to permit palpation. Motion of the affected area is avoided, and patients with a groin bubo typically flex the corresponding thigh in their attempt to immobilize the lesion and lessen the pain. This extreme tenderness of the buboes appears early and is one of the outstanding diagnostic features of the disease.

Inguinal or femoral buboes are most common, and may be mistaken for incarcerated herniae. However, any lymph node group including the axillary, cervical, supraclavicular, epitrochlear, and even mediastinal nodes (Fig. 3) may be affected. Involvement of deep iliac nodes may cause a clinical picture impossible to differentiate from acute appendicitis. Buboes at multiple sites are not unusual. The rare tonsillar form of plague is a subtype of the bubonic form and results from bacteremic seeding or from primary localization in pharyngeal lymphoid tissue of bacilli inoculated onto mucous membranes. It has occurred after crushing infected fleas and lice between the teeth.

Fully developed buboes vary in length from 1 to 10 cm, are usually oval or round in shape, and may be formed by the fusion of two or more lymph nodes. With development and progression of periadenitis, the fully developed bubo becomes fixed and doughy or boggy in consistency. The overlying skin may become reddened, edematous, sometimes hemorrhagic, and rarely ulcerated. Bubo suppuration with fluctuance is common, and resolution after institution of specific antibiotic therapy may be slow. Spontaneous drainage is not common in treated cases, and surgical incision and drainage of pus may occasionally become necessary.

In the relatively uncommon primary septicemic form of plague, no obvious focus of lymphadenitis may be evident The clinical presentation is one of fulminant septic shock or of secondary plague pneumonia. Whereas plague pneumonia produces cough, rales, rhonchi, and signs of pulmonary consolidation on physical examination, it may sometimes be detected only by x-ray. Secondary plague pneumonia occurs in less than 5 per cent of cases of bubonic plague.

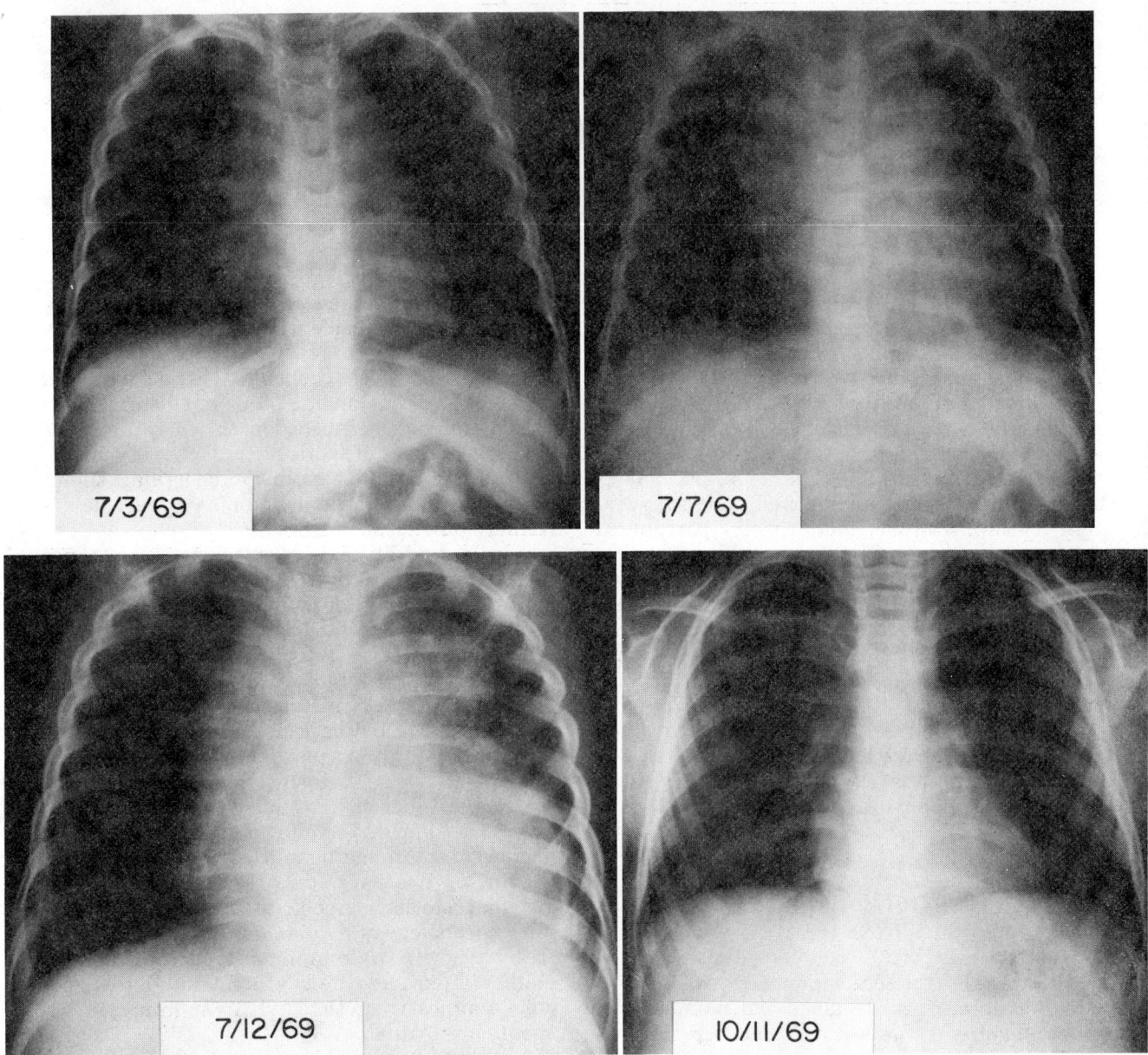

**FIGURE 3.** *Serial chest roentgenograms taken during the course of bubonic plague in a 3-year-old boy who also exhibited plague meningitis after initial therapy with penicillin. Hilar lymphadenopathy and pulmonary infiltration present on the fourth hospital day (upper left) progressed after four (upper right) and nine (lower left) days, and were associated with clinical evidence of myocarditis. Film three months later (lower right) has reverted to normal appearance. (From Reed, W. P., et al.: Medicine 49:465, 1970. © 1970 The Williams & Wilkins Co., Baltimore.)*

Primary plague pneumonia is even less common, but it is a fulminating, highly contagious illness, virtually always fatal if untreated. It causes fever, severe systemic toxicity, and rapidly progressive symptoms and signs of respiratory insufficiency. Large amounts of bloody, frothy sputum teeming with *Y. pestis* organisms beginning 12 to 24 hours after onset of fever characterize this form of the disease. Plague meningitis may develop from bacteremic seeding of meninges. It

has usually occurred in patients, often children, initially treated with penicillin, ampicillin, or other suboptimal antibiotic therapies, and it is observed with increased frequency in patients with axillary buboes.

Pericarditis and myocarditis occasionally occur, and signs of congestive heart failure may develop during the acute phase of illness or during convalescence.

Asymptomatic and self-limited pharyngeal carriage of *Y. pestis* in over 10 per cent of healthy contacts of plague cases, as well as in a similar proportion of bubonic plague patients themselves, has been recorded. However, multiple cases of disease within households more likely reflect environmental acquisition than person-to-person respiratory transmission.

## COMPLICATIONS AND SEQUELAE

Disseminated intravascular coagulation, bacteremic or endotoxemic shock, and secondary plague pneumonia are the principal early complications of untreated or partially treated plague. The late complications, in some instances attributable to delayed or suboptimal antimicrobial therapy, include *Y. pestis* meningitis, metastatic abscess formation, delayed bubo suppuration, cardiac failure, and, rarely, peripheral symmetrical gangrene.

The case-fatality rate of untreated bubonic plague is between 50 and 80 per cent, while that of the septicemic and meningitic forms of the disease is even higher; untreated plague pneumonia is an almost invariably and rapidly fatal complication.

With early diagnosis and institution of antibiotics, survival from bubonic plague approaches 100 per cent and has even been recorded in the primary pneumonic form of the disease.

## GEOGRAPHIC VARIATION IN DISEASE

Differences in the seasonal incidence of bubonic plague outbreaks exist among endemic areas in different parts of the world. The differences appear to be chiefly determined by climatic conditions that may alter the availability and efficiency of insect vectors; plague epidemics are most likely to occur when temperature and humidity are high. Epizootic plague outbreaks in urban rat populations produce die-offs that characteristically result in clustered cases of bubonic plague in the contiguous human settlement. Secondary pneumonic plague cases may then give rise to endemic outbreaks of primary pneumonic plague. In contrast, persistent infection of wild rodents in sylvatic or rural settings results in sporadic cases of plague in individuals and domestic animals who enter this ecologic setting for occupational or recreational reasons. Variations in the clinical features of plague attributable to specific antigenic components of *Y. pestis* or to geography-related strain variation have not been described.

## DIAGNOSIS

Bubonic plague must be differentiated from adenitis caused by such other infectious agents as *Staphylococcus aureus, Streptococcus pyogenes, Franciscella tularensis, Pasteurella multocida,* and *Chlamydia trachomatis;* from the etiologic agent of cat-scratch disease; and from a wide variety of other febrile illnesses (Reed et al., 1970). The diagnosis deserves serious consideration in any acutely ill, febrile patient who has tender inguinal or axillary adenopathy and gives a history of possible recent residential, occupational, or recreational exposure to plague-infected rodent fleas or animal carcasses. It should also be considered when cases of pneumonia occur in clusters. Even with a high index of suspicion, the early diagnosis of sporadic cases of septicemic plague, of bubonic plague with occult (e.g., intra-abdominal) adenitis, or of primary pneumonic plague may be extremely difficult or impossible.

Needle aspiration of suspicious lymph nodes (with utmost caution to avoid aerosols when expelling aspirated fluids from syringes) should be performed routinely and usually yields diagnostic material. An 18- or 19-gauge needle on a 10- to 20-ml syringe containing 1 ml of sterile, nonbacteriostatic saline is inserted aseptically into the bubo and aspirated back and forth until a small amount of bloody or purulent fluid is obtained. Smears of lymph fluid, peripheral blood buffy coats, and other body fluids (e.g., sputum, tracheal secretion, and cerebrospinal fluid) should be fixed in absolute methanol to kill the organisms; Giemsa or Wayson's stain then usually reveals the characteristic bipolar staining and "safety-pin" morphology of *Y. pestis* far better than Gram stain (Fig. 4). Immunofluorescent staining of methanol-fixed smears is a rapid and highly specific diagnostic method when appropriate reagents are available.

Aspirated body fluids may be cultured on ordinary bacteriologic media, and two or more blood cultures should be obtained. The organism grows well but slowly on solid media, forming convex grayish colonies that are 1 to 3 mm in diameter after 48 hours. Prior antimicrobial therapy may significantly delay or prevent recovery of *Y. pestis* in cultures. Except for the demonstration of diagnostic antibody titers in acute and convalescent sera by the sensitive and specific passive hemagglutination technique of Chen and Meyer (1966), other laboratory methods are of no specific diagnostic value; leukocytosis, laboratory parameters typical of disseminated intravascular coagulation, and SGOT level elevation are commonly present. Roentgenologic evidence of pulmonary infection should be sought. *Because of the high mortality and the risk of pneumonic transmission when treatment of plague is delayed, specific pre-*

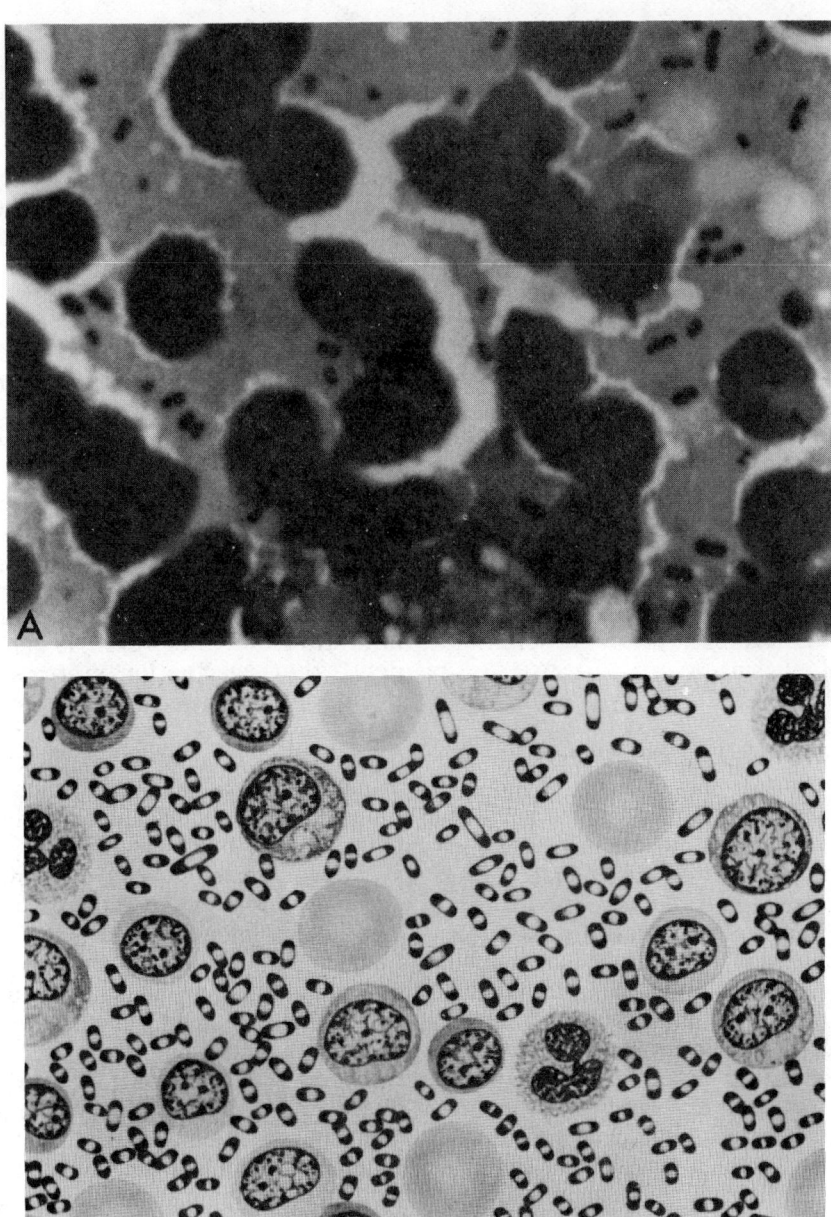

**FIGURE 4.** Yersinia pestis. A, *Gram-stained smear of bubo aspirate reveals many gram-negative bacilli exhibiting characteristic bipolar staining appearance and polymorphonuclear leukocytic exudate. Magnification 960×. (Courtesy of John Ulrich, Ph.D., University of New Mexico, Albuquerque, N.M.) B, Drawing of bubo aspirate shows "safety-pin" appearance of Y. pestis organisms with Wayson's stain. (From Muir, R.: Bacteriological Atlas. 2nd ed. Edinburgh, E. and S. Livingstone, 1937.)*

*sumptive antimicrobial therapy should be urgently instituted on clinical and epidemiologic grounds without awaiting bacteriologic confirmation.*

## TREATMENT

Supportive therapy may be needed for hypoxia, hypovolemia, circulatory insufficiency, disseminated intravascular coagulation, and pain. Strep-

tomycin, 30 mg/kg/day should be given intramuscularly in divided doses every 6 to 12 hours for 7 to 10 days, together with tetracycline 0.5 every 6 hours orally, or, if necessary, intravenously. The combination of antibiotics is justified by the intracellular location of *Y. pestis* and by the possibility of rapid development of high level resistance to streptomycin alone. Tetracycline therapy is continued for two weeks. *Y. pestis* may still be cultured from bubo contents after several days of antibiotic administration. Either tetracycline or a sulfonamide has been effective alone in mild to moderately severe cases but is not recommended. Intravenous chloramphenicol (50 to 75 mg/kg/day in six-hourly divided doses) should be substituted for tetracycline in pregnant patients and for treatment of plague meningitis because it readily penetrates the cerebrospinal fluid. Despite the apparent in vitro susceptibility of Y. pestis to penicillin and ampicillin, these antibiotics are ineffective in vivo and *have no place in the therapy of plague;* Y. pestis meningitis has frequently been observed as a complication of such treatment. Prolonged fever and an increased incidence of complications have been noted in patients treated with peroral trimethoprim-sulfamethoxazole (Butler et al., 1976). Although gentamicin has cured a few cases of plague septicemia, streptomycin is the antibiotic of choice because the accrued evidence of its efficacy is unequivocal.

Incision and drainage of buboes for diagnostic purposes is not warranted, but may become necessary when fluctuant buboes persist despite adequate antimicrobial therapy.

## PROPHYLAXIS

Plague is a quarantinable disease. As soon as the diagnosis is suspected, local and national health agencies must be notified so that epidemiologic investigations may be expedited to define the source of infection and public health measures may be instituted, including rodent and vector control to prevent wider dissemination. Strict hospital isolation of patients suspected of having plague is desirable because cough, sputum production, and auscultatory signs frequently appear late in both primary and secondary plague pneumonia. Strict isolation should be continued until specific antimicrobial treatment has been in effect for 72 hours. The risk of household or nosocomial transmission of Y. pestis infection to contacts of patients who have bubonic plague but no pneumonia is minimal, and well-controlled studies of the efficacy of antibiotic prophylaxis of pneumonic spread are not available. Therefore, administration of prophylaxis or "abortive treatment" with oral tetracycline (30 mg/kg) or sulfadiazine (60 mg/kg) daily in six hourly divided doses for ten days should be strictly limited to those believed to have had close and significant exposure to infected respiratory or other secretions. All other case contacts should be placed under surveillance, and their temperatures measured twice daily for ten days. Case contacts who develop fever or other clinical findings compatible with the diagnosis of plague should be hospitalized promptly for confirmation of the diagnosis and for antimicrobial therapy.

All specimens from suspected plague cases should be handled with gloves and transported with extreme caution; attendants as well as laboratory personnel should be alerted to the possible diagnosis. Nosocomially acquired Y. pestis infections have occurred only rarely.

In geographic areas in which sylvatic plague is endemic, hunters should avoid direct hand contact with the carcasses of rodents or wild carnivores that are potentially plague-infected or flea-bearing.

Immunization with formalin-killed plague vaccines stimulates production of antibodies. These are detectable by the passive hemagglutination test and afford limited protection against illness and death after Y. pestis infection is acquired naturally or in the laboratory. The killed vaccines are preferred to live, attenuated vaccines because they appear to produce greater immunity with fewer and milder local reactions. However, the protection afforded by such vaccines is incomplete and transient, and there is no convincing evidence that vaccination protects against human pneumonic plague. Primary immunization for adults consists of intramuscular injection of two 0.5-ml doses of vaccine four or more weeks apart and a further dose of 0.2 ml one to three months later. Thereafter, booster injections of 0.2 ml intramuscularly are required at six-month intervals for maintenance of immunity. Vaccination against plague is not required by any country as a condition for entry and is not routinely recommended for individuals living in or traveling to plague-endemic areas unless exposure to plague-infected rodents is specifically anticipated. Laboratory and field personnel engaged in Y. pestis-related research should maintain vaccine-induced immunity. A history of plague immunization should under no circumstances eliminate plague from a differential diagnosis when it would otherwise be considered.

## References

Bibel, D. J., and Chen, T. H.: Diagnosis of plague: An analysis of the Yersin-Kitasato controversy. Bacteriol Rev 40:633, 1976.

Butler, T., Levin, J., Linh, N. N., Chan, D. M., Adickman, M., and Arnold, K.: *Yersinia pestis* infection in Viet Nam. II Quantitative blood cultures and detection of endotoxin in the cerebrospinal fluid of patients with meningitis. J Infect Dis 133:493, 1976.

Chen, T. H., and Meyer, K. F.: An evaluation of *Pasteurella pestis* Fraction-1-specific antibody for the confirmation of plague infections. Bull WHO 34:911, 1966.

Finegold, M. J.: Pathogenesis of plague. Am J Med 45:549, 1968.

Janssen, W. A., and Surgalla, M. J.: Plague bacillus: Survival within host phagocytes. Science 163:950, 1969.

Nohl, J.: The Black Death. A Chronicle of the Plague. London, Unwin Books, 1961.

Pollitzer, R.: Plague. World Health Organization Monograph No. 22, Geneva, World Health Organization, 1954.

Reed, W. P., Palmer, D. L., Williams, R. C., Jr., and Kisch, A. L.: Bubonic plague in the southwestern United States. Medicine 49:465, 1970.

Rust, J. H., Jr., Cavanaugh, D. C., O'Shita R., and Marshall, J. D., Jr.: The role of domestic animals in the epidemiology of plague. II. Antibody to *Yersinia pestis* in sera of dogs and cats. J Infect Dis 124:527, 1971.

Sonnenwirth, A. C.: Yersinia. In Lennette, E. H., Spalding, E. H., and Truant, J. P. (eds.): Manual of Clinical Microbiology. Washington, D.C., American Society for Microbiology, 1974, p. 222.

World Health Organization Expert Committee on Plague: Fourth Report. World Health Organization Technical Report Series No. 447. Geneva, World Health Organization, 1970.

World Health Organization Weekly Epidemiologic Record 52:229, 1977.

# ERYSIPELOID  **245**

## Chantal Freland, Ph.D.
## Doctor in Bio-Chemistry

## DEFINITION AND HISTORY

Erysipeloid is a skin infection of man that is acquired by handling infected animal tissues. It is caused by *Erysipelothrix rhusiopathiae,* which also infects many wild and domestic animals. Infections of hogs (swine erysipelas) and poultry cause major economic losses to the agricultural industry. Infection of humans is called erysipeloid because the disease resembls streptococcal erysipelas. Arthritis of the joints underlying erysipeloid lesions is common in humans and is a major manifestation of swine erysipelas. Systemic infection is rare in man, but septicemia and endocarditis have been reported.

In 1873, Fox and Baker described a skin infection of the hands and fingers of butchers and named it erythema serpens. In 1882, Pasteur and Thuillier first isolated *Erysipelothrix* from a diseased pig. Two years later, Rosenbach isolated *E. rhusiopathiae* from erysipeloid lesions of man and proved the existence of a link between the human cutaneous complaint erythema serpens and swine erysipelas. Rosenbach named the human disease erysipeloid, but it was often called the "Rouget" of Rosenbach. In 1912, Gunther described the first cases of septicemia with endocarditis caused by *E. rhusiopathiae.*

When the general medical population became aware of the epidemiology of erysipeloid, case reports proliferated (Gilchrist, 1904) until it was realized that erysipeloid was a common occupational disease that was usually self-limited. Since that time, the more unusual manifestations of *Erysipelothrix* infection have been emphasized, and about 40 cases of septicemia or endocarditis have been reported.

## ETIOLOGY AND EPIDEMIOLOGY

*E. rhusiopathiae* is a gram-positive bacillus that may be either short and coccobacillary or filamentous. It is nonencapsulated, nonsporulating, and nonmotile regardless of the temperature. Its growth is stimulated by carbon dioxide, reduced oxygen tension, and the addition of blood, serum, or ascitic fluid. Under these conditions, the colonies appear in 24 hours at 37° C as pinpoint, round, regular, smooth colonies that are either transparent or slightly tinged with blue. Rough colonies occasionally occur and are larger and irregular (see Chapter 27).

*Erysipelothrix* resembles *Listeria,* lactobacilli, and corynebacteria most closely but can be differentiated from these organisms and most other gram-positive bacteria by its production of $H_2S$. It is also readily differentiated from *Listeria* because it is nonhemolytic and nonmotile. About 20 serotypes of *Erysipelothrix* can be distinguished by bacterial agglutination. These serotypes, which are designated by arabic numerals, are used infrequently because they are not linked to virulence nor to colonization of certain animals.

*E. rhusiopathiae* is distributed widely in the animal kingdom, where it may behave as either a saprophyte or a pathogen. It has been isolated from the following groups of animals: (1) mammals (swine, sheep, horse, cow, kangaroo, roebuck, mink, wild boar, dolphin, cat, rabbit, rat, and mouse); (2) fish (perch, pike, sardine, and many others); (3) crustaceans (crab, lobster, and shellfish); and (4) domestic and wild birds (turkey, duck, chicken, sparrow, and blackbird).

Some strains of *Erysipelothrix* are not virulent and colonize only animals, but most are capable of causing disease under appropriate conditions. The susceptibility of animals varies with age, intercurrent disease (enteropathies and parasitic diseases), the season (May to August), and the degree of environmental contamination.

The manifestations of *Erysipelothrix* infection vary from animal to animal. Because of its economic importance, swine erysipelas has been described most thoroughly. Four clinical types of disease occur in swine: (1) acute septicemia that is often fatal within three to five days; (2)

"diamond-back" or "diamond-skin" disease in which red to purple, rhomboid-shaped skin lesions occur on the back; (3) chronic mitral endocarditis; and (4) arthritis, which may either occur independently or complicate any of the other types of infection (Gledhill, 1948).

*Erysipelothrix* occurs throughout the world but is most prevalent in temperate climates. It is especially common in Germany, France (swine), North America (turkey, fish), South America, and Australia (sheep).

Humans do not contract the disease spontaneously. They acquire *Erysipelothrix* only from infected animals, their by-products (meat, bones, fish scales, and crustacean shells), and perhaps from plants or soil that have been contaminated by animals. Human-to-human transmission does not occur. Humans are almost always infected through abraded skin, but this route has not been proved in all septicemic cases.

The survival of *Erysipelothrix* in the external environment depends on the temperature and pH. It is sensitive to heat but resistant to cold. The most favorable range of pH is between 5.8 and 8.6. It develops as well in sea water as in fresh water.

Domestic animals can be infected by the ingestion of contaminated food, but this route of infection remains very questionable in man.

These observations stress the zoonotic nature of this disease which affects primarily farmers, ranchers, butchers, abbatoir workers, veterinarians, and fishermen. Middle-aged men are most commonly affected (Klauder, 1938).

Finally, attention should be drawn to the marked predominance of human disease in autumn, which follows the peak incidence of animal disease during May to August.

## PATHOGENESIS AND PATHOLOGY

Erysipeloid is characterized by marked inflammation and edema of the skin. The epidermis is edematous, infiltrated with polymorphonuclear leukocytes, and necrotic. The corium is infiltrated with lymphocytes, mast cells, and polymorphonuclears. The bacilli are located throughout the infected skin but are concentrated deep in the corium around the capillaries.

The virulence of *Erysipelothrix* is usually tested in laboratory mice. Most strains kill mice, but there are marked variations in the median lethal dose. The virulence factors have not been determined but are associated with rapid growth rates and with the production of neuraminidase (Krasemann and Muller, 1975). A glycoprotein extracted from the cell wall of *Erysipelothrix*

causes dermal necrosis and high fevers in rabbits (Leimbeck et al., 1975).

Intravenous inoculation of live organisms, dead organisms, and even a cell-free, crude extract of culture filtrates causes polyarthritis in swine, dogs, and rabbits (White et al., 1971). This cell-free extract, which contains murein and many different proteins, binds rapidly to the synovium and persists for many months. It causes cytopathic effects in synovial cell cultures after a single brief exposure (White et al., 1976). Because of clinical and histologic similarities, experimental *Erysipelothrix* arthritis has been used as a model for rheumatoid arthritis.

## CLINICAL MANIFESTATIONS, COMPLICATIONS, AND SEQUELAE

### Erysipeloid (Rosenbach's "Rouget")

This common, localized, cutaneous form is by far the most frequent. The lesion follows accidental inoculation along the back of the hand or the thumb. Clinical manifestations begin within the next 12 to 48 hours around the vestige of the initial injury and consist of a pruritic, purplish-red patch that is slightly indurated and bordered by a clear-cut, slightly raised margin. The lesion gradually spreads over the hand, evolving centrifugally while the center recovers (Erlich, 1946).

Sensations of pressure, itching, and burning are common. Arthralgia of the neighboring small joints occurs occasionally. Lymphangitis and satellite lymphadenopathy occur in about 10 per cent of cases and may be more common in cases of ichthyologic origin. Fever and other signs of systemic involvement are rare. Recovery occurs in two or three weeks, often spontaneously.

In rare cases, localized erysipeloid may spread and cause diffuse generalized skin lesions that are identical to the initial lesion. This rare complication is accompanied by generalized lymphadenopathy and fever.

There is no immunity to erysipeloid; it recurs readily.

### Septicemic Form

Only about 40 cases of this serious disease have been reported (Freland, 1977). If the septicemia was preceded by clinically apparent erysipeloid, there is a latent phase and even apparent recovery before the onset of symptoms. Most cases of septicemia have a preceding history of contact and an erysipeloid lesion. When there is no history of erysipeloid, the earliest symptoms are a low-grade fever, weakness, and malaise. In either case, the fever soon becomes more severe and is accompanied by rigors, generalized myalgia, anorexia, and weight loss. Purpura, splenomegaly, and arthralgia may occur (Coste, 1954).

Endocarditis develops in 75 per cent of septicemic cases. Half of the cases of endocarditis occur on previously normal valves. The aortic valve is commonly affected (Freland, 1977). The symptoms and complications of *Erysipelothrix* endocarditis are not unique. Cerebral (Silberstein, 1965), renal, and pulmonary complications have been described (Proctor, 1965; Russel and Lamb, 1940; and Freland, 1977).

## GEOGRAPHIC VARIATIONS IN DISEASE

Most cases of erysipeloid and *Erysipelothrix* endocarditis have been reported from Western Europe, the United States, and other agriculturally developed countries in the temperate zone. The prevalence of infection is directly related to the number of people in close contact with animal reservoirs. There is no apparent geographic variation in the manifestations or severity of infection.

## DIAGNOSIS

An individual with a history of contact with an animal reservoir or their by-products (meat, bones, crab shells) and an erysipelas-like lesion on the hand is likely to have erysipeloid. Streptococcal erysipelas commonly affects the face and causes bright red lesions that are markedly indurated and spread rapidly. There are usually multiple bullae on the skin. Joints are not affected. Erysipeloid, by contrast, affects the hands, evolves more slowly, causes purplish-red lesions, and frequently causes arthritis of neighboring joints. Bullae are less dramatic and may be absent. Most other causes of dermatitis either differ in appearance or are not localized to the hands.

The definitive diagnosis is made by culture of a skin biopsy. Any coccobacillary, coryneform, or filamentous gram-positive bacillus isolated from such a lesion must be tested for the microbiologic characteristics of *Erysipelothrix*. It can be quickly differentiated from all similar bacteria by the production of $H_2S$. Its other differential characteristics are given under Etiology and in Chapter 27, Table I.

The diagnosis of septicemia is made by blood culture. It is especially important that *Erysipelothrix* in blood cultures is not misidentified as contaminating coryneform bacteria. The diagnosis of endocarditis in patients with *Erysipelothrix* endocarditis is primarily clinical (see Chapter 199). Immune complex glomerulonephritis, rheu-

matoid factor, and depression of serum complement levels strongly suggest the diagnosis of endocarditis. The aortic valve is most commonly affected. The vegetations are large and bulky and may be ulcerated.

## TREATMENT AND PROPHYLAXIS

Although erysipeloid usually heals spontaneously in a few weeks, recovery is hastened, and complications prevented, by treatment with penicillin. The organism is exquisitely sensitive to penicillin, and infections can usually be cured by injection of 1.2 million units of benzathine penicillin. Oral penicillins (250 mg four times a day for seven days) or daily injections of 600,000 units of procaine penicillin are also effective. One g per day in four divided doses for five to seven days of erythromycin or tetracycline is effective alternate therapy for penicillin-allergic individuals.

Endocarditis has been successfully treated with 10 to 12 million units of penicillin per day for four to five weeks along with streptomycin 1 g per day for ten days.

*Erysipelothrix* infections can be controlled by care in the handling of reservoir animals and their by-products. Gloves and protective aprons are helpful. Control of reservoirs in herds of domestic animals can be achieved by vaccination (see Chapter 27) and by improving techniques of animal husbandry and meat inspection. Except for personal protection, these measures will have little effect on erysipeloid contracted from fish and crustaceans.

## References

Coste, F., Domart, A., and Antoine, B.: Manifestations articulaires au cours d'une septicémie à *Erysipelothrix rhusiopathiae*. Rev Rhun 21:47, 1954.

Erlich, J. C.: *Erysipelothrix rhusiopathiae* infection in man. Arch Intern Med 78:565, 1946.

Freland, C.: Les infections à *Erysipelothrix rhusiopathiae*. Revue générale à propos de 31 cas de septicémies avec endocardite relevé dans la littérature. Path Biol 25:345, 1977.

Gilchrist, T. C.: Erysipeloid with a record of 329 cases, of which 32 were caused by crab bites or lesions produced by crabs. J Cutan Dis 22:507, 1904.

Gledhill, A. W.: Swine erysipelas infection *(E. rhusiopathiae)* in man and animals. Proc Roy Soc Med 41:330, 1948.

Klauder, J. V.: Erysipeloid as an occupational disease. JAMA 111:1345, 1938.

Krasemann, C., and Muller, H. E.: The virulence of *Erysipelothrix rhusiopathiae* strains and their virulence production. Zentrabl Bakteriol (Orig A) 231(1–3):206, 1975.

Leimbeck, R., Bohm, K. H., Ehard, H., and Schulz, L.-C.: Studies on the toxic components of *Erysipelothrix rhusiopathiae:* Detailed characterization of an extracted endotoxin. Zentrabl Bakterio (Orig A) 232(2–3):266, 1975.

Procter, W. I.: Subacute bacterial endocarditis due to *E. rhusiopathiae*. Report of a case and review of the literature. Am J Med 38:820 1965.

Russel, W. O., and Lamb, M. E.: Erysipelothrix endocarditis, a complication of erysipeloid. Report of a case with necropsy. JAMA 114:1045, 1940.

Silberstein, E. B.: Erysipelothrix endocarditis. Report of a case with cerebral manifestations. JAMA 191:862, 1965.

White, T. G., Mirikitani, F. K., and Hargrove, P.: The effects of bacterial extract on synovial cells in tissue culture. In Vitro 12:702, 1976.

White, T. G., Puls, J. L., and Mirikitani, F. K.: Rabbit arthritis induced by cell-free extracts of *Erysipelothrix*. Infect Immun 3:715, 1971.

# 246 *ANTHRAX*

*Werner Dutz, M.D.*

## DEFINITION

Anthrax ($\alpha\nu\vartheta\rho\alpha\xi$: charcoal, carbuncle; synonyms: malignant pustule, malignant edema, splenic fever, woolsorters disease, charbon, Milzbrand) is a disease caused by *Bacillus anthracis* or its spores, ingested from infected pastures by herbivorous animals or indirectly derived from infected carcasses by carnivorous animals. Man is infected by contaminated products, such as skins, bone, horsehair, bristles, bone meal, or wool.

## HISTORY

Anthrax has been known since antiquity and was described in the *Iliad,* and in the collection of Hippocratic texts by Pliny and Galen. The epidemiology is hinted at in the Bible: ". . . and it shall become fine dust over the land of Egypt and become boils breaking out in sores in man and beast throughout the land of Egypt." (Exodus 9:9.)

The study of anthrax led to the development of modern bacteriology, serology, and immunology. Microorganisms were first seen in 1863 by Davaine, who proved their infectivity. Robert Koch isolated the bacillus in pure culture in the vitreous of cow's eyes in 1876 and established Koch's postulates. Pasteur clarified the pathogenicity and performed the first successful vaccination of sheep with attenuated bacilli (Vallery-Radot, 1960).

## GEOGRAPHIC VARIATION AND INCIDENCE

The massive plague-like spread of anthrax over the southern part of Europe in the 18th and 19th centuries has been stemmed by mandatory vaccination. Anthrax persists in the arid and semiarid regions of the Middle East, in Africa, Asia, and South America. Wild living animals are often affected. A proper worldwide estimate of disease frequency in animals and man cannot be made. Anthrax is underreported owing to lack of inter-est, lack of facilities, and sometimes deliberately to prevent economic problems with wool or hide exports (Brachman and Fekety, 1958).

Anthrax epidemics in livestock occur more frequently during draught, when closed-cropped grazing and digging for roots lead to closer contact with spores. Animals feed then on thorny plants that they normally shun. The resulting injuries of the jaws form a portal of entry. Malnutrition reduces host resistance. In time of need livestock owners are forced to slaughter animals at the first signs of infection. Farmers, shepherds, butchers, and women spinning wool with hand spindles, carpet weavers, and wool merchants are most frequently infected. Bathhouse epidemics occur in the Middle East, where epilation of the skin is practiced and the body is rubbed down with rough wool that is occasionally contaminated with anthrax spores. Epidemics of inhalation anthrax in woolsorters have been described by Eppinger in Western countries at the turn of the century. Osler noticed that the danger of infection from wool is inversely proportionate to its greasiness. Most infections in the textile industry occur in the carding departments, where the washed and degreased wool is fluffed up. Pulmonary anthrax epidemics occur more frequently in well-ventilated factories, where spores remain longer suspended in the air. Detection of industrial dust contamination is best achieved by the infection of detergent-pretreated, defatted dust material into mice and microscopic examination with fluorescent antianthrax globulin (Brachman and Fekety, 1958). Sporadic infections with infected bristles of shaving brushes, contaminated bone meal fertilizer, or from leather products are continuously reported from all countries of the world (Federation Proceedings, 1967; Dutz and Kohout, 1971).

## BACTERIOLOGY AND PATHOPHYSIOLOGY

*B. anthracis* is a large ($2.5 \times 10 \mu$) rod-shaped spore-forming gram-positive organism that cannot be differentiated by morphologic criteria or on the usual culture media from the nonpathogenic *B. cereus*. *B. anthracis* lies singly or in pairs in tissue. The characterisic "box car" or "bamboo rod" long chains appear on agar cultures. Stab cultures in gelatin produce the classic inverted fir tree pattern.

Sporulation occurs after the death of the host. The dormant spores are extremely resistant to chemicals, heat, and environmental changes. Pastures once contaminated remain so indefinitely. The transformation of a dormant spore into a vegetative one can be observed under the phase microscope. Dormant spores are refractile, whereas germinated ones are dark and nonrefractile. The growth of the vegetative cell occurs after the germinated spore has been phagocytosed by a macrophage (Federation Proceedings, 1967).

The virulence of *B. anthracis* is proved by animal inoculation. The polysaccharides in the bacillary capsule determine the virulence of the strain. Host phagocytes form a vesicular membrane around avirulent and hypovirulent bacilli, whereas no membrane formation can be detected around virulent ones. The virulence of given strains of *B. anthracis* varies greatly and depends, among other things, on the number of animal passages before sporulation. Growth above or below temperature optimum or on poor nutritional media reduces virulence.

The pathogenicity of a given strain also depends on toxin production (see Chapter 28). The toxins are generated in the bacillary cytoplasm and their release is proportional to the $CO_2$ tension of the medium. Anthrax toxins lead to a detachment of cytoplasmic processes of endothelial cells, subsequent increased vascular permeability, platelet thrombi, stasis, and thrombosis. There is extensive edema and hemorrhage due to capillary wall dissolution and venous obstruction. Injection of pure anthrax toxin into the spinal fluid leads to centrally induced systemic anoxic changes, marked disorganization of the electroencephalogram pattern, and cerebral death.

The phagocytosis of *B. anthracis* depends on host nutrition. Lysin deficiency leads to phagocytic paralysis (Gray, 1963). Meat-fed rats are resistant to a dosage of bacilli that kills grain-fed littermates (Dutz and Kohout, 1971). Herbivorous animals are therefore more susceptible to infection than carnivores. Most of our own patients with anthrax ate meat very rarely and suffered from relative protein malnutrition. Lysine deficiency after a pure plant-protein diet may explain the particular susceptibility of village populations during times of draught and starvation (Dutz and Kohout, 1971; Gray, 1963).

Experimental infection with a standard toxic strain leads to an orderly progressive physiologic alteration of predictable pattern. All animal strains cause leukocytosis, low plasma pH, hyponatremia, hypocalcemia, and respiratory alkalosis superimposed on metabolic acidosis. Glycogen depletion of the liver, hypoxia, and respiratory failure occur preterminally. Hyperphosphatemia, hyperchloremia, and hyperpotassemia depend on the degree of hemolysis (Federation Proceedings, 1967).

Death in Rhesus monkeys is dosage related. Toxemia and death occur 20 hours after the injection of $10^{10}$ spores and two hours after $10^{11}$ spores, if a bacillus of standard virulence and toxicity is used. Lymph nodes may clear up to $10^8$ spores from the circulation. Bacillary clearance occurs in some species, predominantly in the spleen. Horses, sheep, and guinea pigs develop splenomegaly and often die after splenic rupture (Federation Proceedings, 1967). Splenomegaly, however, is not a feature of human anthrax (Dutz and Kohout, 1971).

The clinical appearance of the disease in any given species depends on the route of infection, the number, virulence, and toxin content of the infective strain and the host resistance, which is mostly related to the nutritional state.

## PATHOLOGY

The different forms of human anthrax are schematically presented in Figure 1. Cutaneous infection is by far the most frequent and occurs in two forms:

1. A necrotic sore with little accompanying swelling and tissue reaction. The anthrax bacilli are contained early by macrophages. There is little neutrophilic infiltration. The lesion is characterized by vascular thrombosis, interstitial hemorrhage, and tissue necrosis. No putrefaction occurs unless there is superinfection. (The classic terminology of anthrax pustule or carbuncle is definitely wrong; there is no liquefaction necrosis or pus formation.) The necrotic eschar heals without scarring (Fig. 2).

2. *Malignant edema:* This infection with toxic strains of *B. anthracis* starts with blisters similar to a second degree burn or erysipelas. The blister breaks down rapidly and a necrotic eschar develops surrounded by massive edema, which may distort the face beyond recognition, extend from a primary sore on the eyelid to encompass half the thorax or spread over an entire extremity. The edema in one of our cases with an eschar at the nape of the neck extended to the abdomen and distended the subcutaneous tissue over the sternum to a thickness of 10 cm. The erythrocytes ooze freely out of the vessels and may impart a bluish to black discoloration to the swelling (Fig. 3).

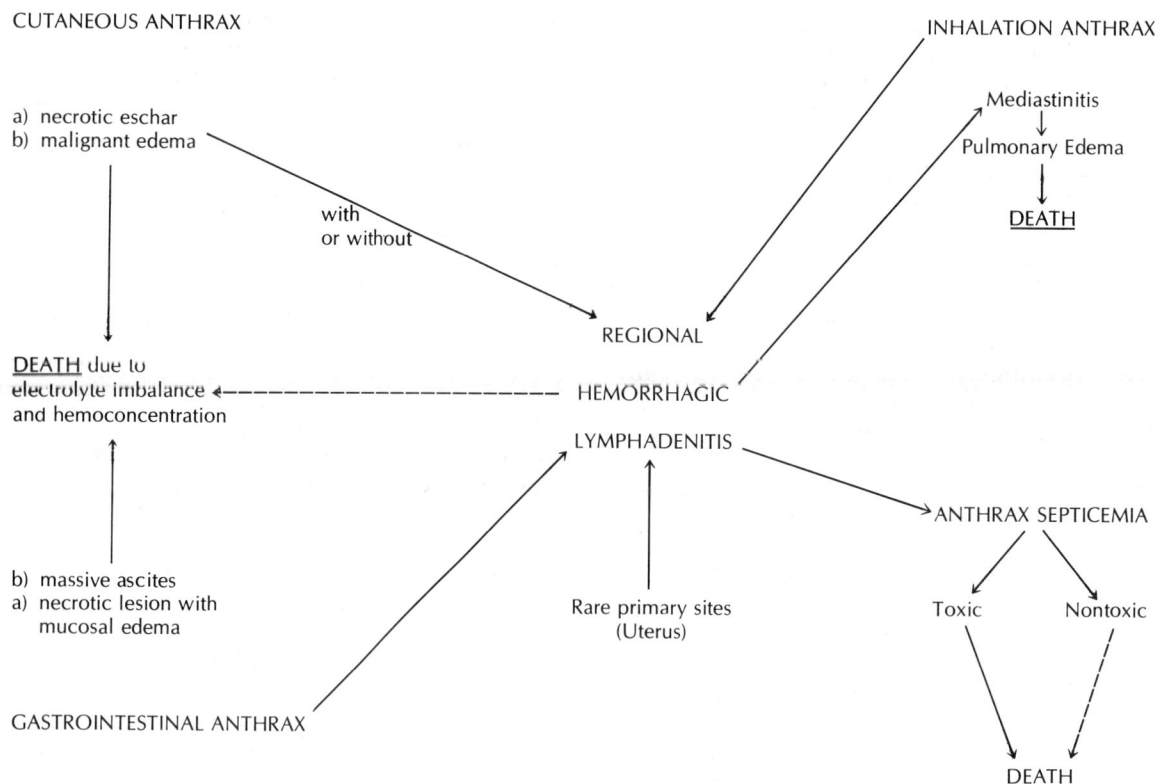

**FIGURE 1.** *Interrelationship of hemorrhagic lymphadenitis to anthrax forms.*

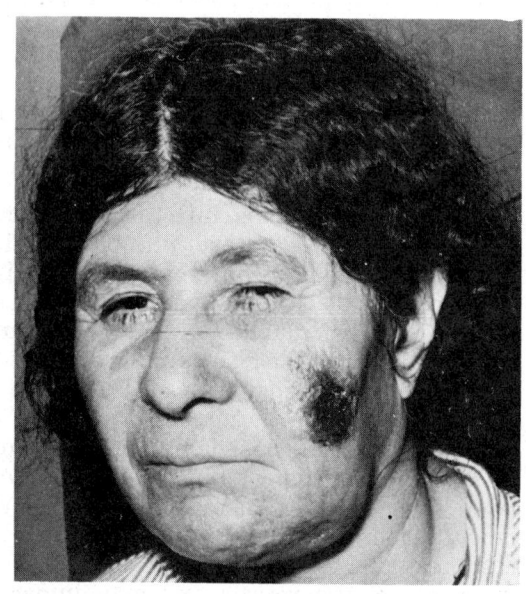

**FIGURE 2.** *Necrotic eschar of anthrax.*

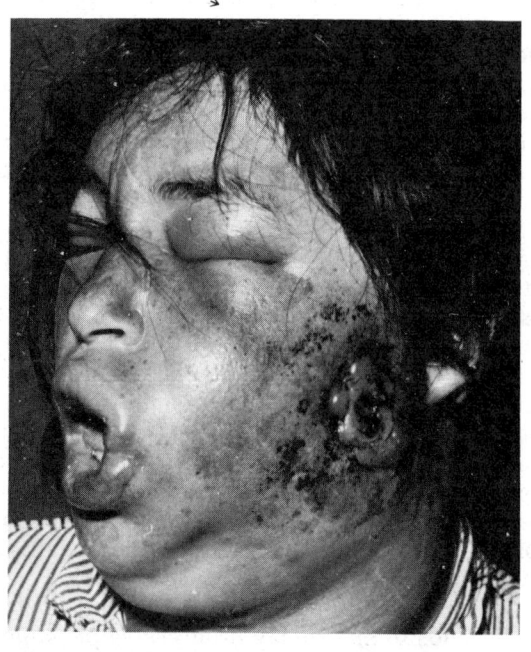

**FIGURE 3.** *Malignant edema of face. Acute lesion with cutaneous blisters and early eschar formation.*

Spread of bacilli along the lymphatics leads to anthrax lymphadenitis. The phagocytes of the marginal and intermediate sinusoids engulf and kill most of the bacilli. The sinusoids dilate with hemorrhage, the lymph node structure disintegrates and all lymphatics become blocked in overwhelming infections. Such lymph nodes are swollen, soft, and dark red to blue black. Septicemic dissemination follows the hemorrhagic lymphadenitis (Fig. 4).

Splenic enlargement in man occurs rarely. We found a splenic enlargement of 400 g in only one of 25 deaths from all different forms of anthrax. Bacilli can be found in the Kupffer cells and leukocytosis in the hepatic sinusoids.

Gastrointestinal anthrax develops after ingestion of massively contaminated material in the stomach, or more frequently, the terminal ileum and ileocecal region. There are single or multiple necrotic ulcers up to 5 cm in size, surrounded by massive mucosal edema, which may obstruct the bowel. Fluid may be lost into the abdominal cavity so rapidly and massively that fatal dehydration occurs. The bowel loops in other patients are filled with many liters of fluid. The regional lymph nodes are swollen and hemorrhagic and the entire mesentery may be dark red. Death is usually due to fluid and electrolyte loss.

Inhalation anthrax is characterized by pulmonary edema. Ross showed that the inhaled spores are taken up by the alveolar pneumocytes and transported to the regional lymph nodes (Dutz and Kohout, 1971). Germination occurs during the transport. The result is a massive hilar lymphadenopathy with mediastinal edema and hemorrhage, followed by secondary pulmonary edema and hydrothorax. There are no necrotic lesions in the lung or bronchi, since the spores are diffusely scattered throughout the entire lung and are secondarily concentrated in the hilar lymph nodes. Studies in textile factories showed that up to 1300 spores may be inhaled in particles of 5 $\mu$ over a five-hour period without infection (Brachman and Fekety, 1958). If anthrax bronchopneumonia follows anthrax septicemia it takes the form of hemorrhagic bronchopneumonia.

Anthrax infections by other routes are rare. Anthrax of the endometrium has followed attempted or completed abortion and puerperal fever has occurred after delivery in contaminated stables.

One complication of anthrax septicemia is hemorrhagic meningitis. The cerebrospinal fluid is hemorrhagic, vessels are disrupted and/or thrombosed. The brain substance or the ganglion cells are undisturbed at autopsy because death occurs rapidly after the onset of toxic anthrax meningitis.

### CLINICAL PATTERN

Skin lesions occur after abrasions or prolonged contact with infected material. Lesions of the lip are frequent in weavers and spinners who wet the thread in their mouths, infections of the bearded skin occur after shaving, lesions of the eyelids are frequent in hot arid countries, where the material is rubbed into the skin with the back of the hand (Amidi et al., 1977). Butchers have infections of fingers and forearm; the nape of the neck and back is frequently infected in porters of hides. Lesions of the intertriginous areas between the legs, at the beltline, and in the region of the collar are not infrequent.

The first symptom in cutaneous anthrax is itching at the site of inoculation after two to three hours, followed by a small papule that rapidly becomes vesicular. A dark brown eschar is formed within 36 hours. The necrotic eschar separates within a few days without leaving a scar. This form of the disease has little morbidity, causes no general symptoms, and is rarely seen by physi-

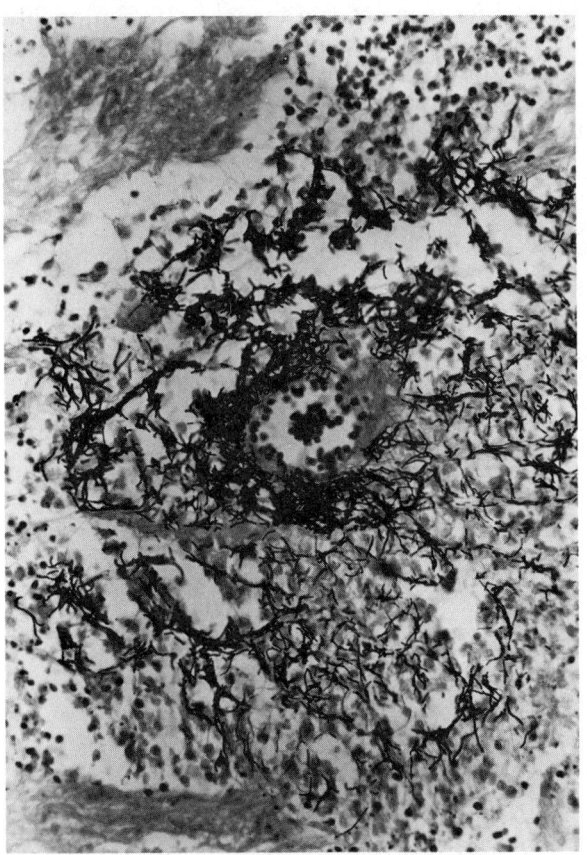

**FIGURE 4.** *Brown and Bren stain. Magnification 800×. Anthrax bacilli in dilated lymphatics. Note periarteriolar clustering.*

cians. Malignant edema is at the other end of the spectrum of cutaneous anthrax. The lesion starts as one or more small vesicles that may resemble burn blisters. Necrosis follows within one or two days and is surrounded by slightly raised small blisters with a hemorrhagic rim. Subcutaneous edema may distort the features, grotesquely close both eyes, and prevent breathing through the nostrils or eating and drinking with the enlarged lips. All possible transition forms between the two types of cutaneous anthrax may occur.

Leukocytosis with up to 20,000 WBC, 80 per cent neutrophils, and a shift to the left is the earliest systemic manifestation. Moderate fever of 38 to 39° C may accompany severe forms of cutaneous anthrax. Electrolyte disturbances and hemoconcentration are proportionate to the extent of the edema. Renal failure with papillary necrosis and shock precede death by septicemia. The patient is often free of anxiety and his mental state remains clear despite his critical condition.

Gastrointestinal anthrax probably occurs more frequently than stated. Most cases are recognized after death. Clinical diagnosis is extremely difficult. We observed one case at laparotomy for bowel obstruction of unknown etiology, who recovered uneventfully after penicillin therapy. Undoubtedly many mild cases escape detection. Symptoms of gastrointestinal anthrax are rapidly developing and refilling ascites, cholera-like diarrhea, moderate to severe fever with chills relatively late in the illness as a sign of septicemia,

leukocytosis, and hemoconcentration. Radiographs show signs of intestinal obstruction. Fluid loss from the bowel may reach 12 liters within 24 hours. Hematemesis in gastric anthrax and moderate melena in ileocecal anthrax may occur (Dutz and Kohout, 1971; Nalin et al., 1977).

The initial symptoms of inhalation anthrax are nonspecific. The patient may be afebrile, complain of increasing shortness of breath and grippe-like symptoms, and show leukocytosis. Occasionally there is nonproductive cough. The patient dies after five to seven days in shock with tachypnea, tachycardia, and cyanosis. Fulminating cases with an onset of chills and high fever, rapidly developing dyspnea, and vascular collapse leading to death within 24 to 48 hours are also described. The massive hilar adenopathy and mediastinal hemorrhage is evident in chest x-rays as a widening of the hilus, followed by a massive widening of the mediastinum with clear and sharp borders (Vassal, 1975). The absence of pain associated with other forms of rapidly developing mediastinitis, the marked leukocytosis, and the history or possibility of professional exposure should raise the suspicion of anthrax infection (Fig. 5).

Patients with anthrax septicemia should be examined for signs of meningeal irritation, mental changes, delirium, and unconsciousness, which are sequentially associated with anthrax meningitis. The spinal fluid is frankly bloody and bacilli may be seen on direct smears or cultured from it.

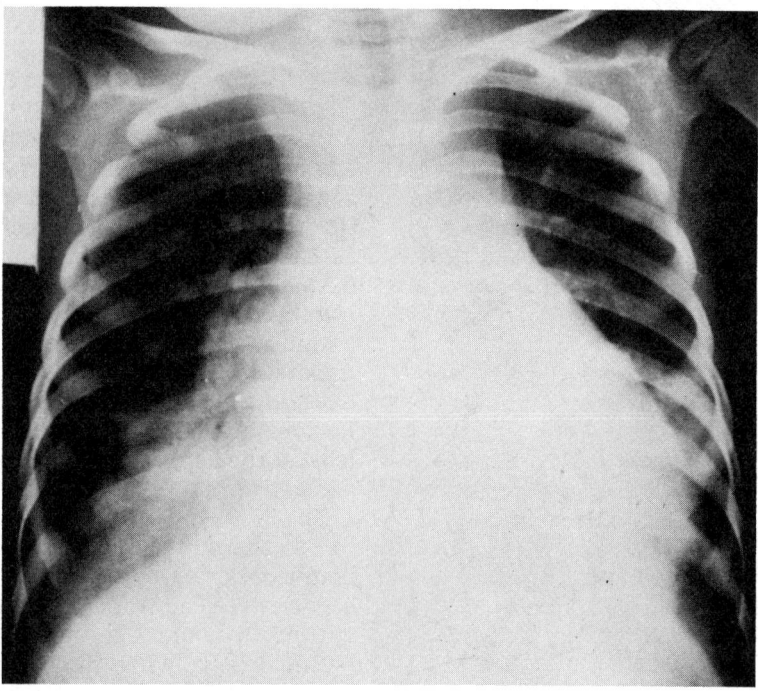

**FIGURE 5.** *Chest x-ray. Marked mediastinal widening in inhalation anthrax.*

## DIAGNOSIS

The clinical appearance of the eschar and the malignant edema of cutaneous anthrax are characteristic and easy to recognize in endemic areas. It is sometimes difficult to obtain viable bacilli from the eschar or the edematous skin. Perforation of the epidemic with a thin dental root canal needle helps to obtain material from the deeper layers and permits easy inoculation of media as well as the preparation of smears. The finding of single or double gram-positive bacilli in conjunction with the clinical lesion are sufficient evidence for diagnosis. Inhalation anthrax and gastrointestinal anthrax are more difficult to diagnose without invasive methods. Treatment should be started on suspicion alone. Recovery of bacilli from the blood stream in septicemia usually comes too late for clinical purposes. The indirect microhemagglutination test of Buchanan is very specific. A rising titer confirms the identity of the infection after it has run its course.

## THERAPY

*B. anthracis* is sensitive to sulfonamides, penicillin, and the broad spectrum antibiotics. Early diagnosis and treatment before the onset of septicemia are essential. Penicillin is the drug of choice, but good results are obtained with any of the following dosage schedules for cutaneous anthrax (Federation Proceedings, 1967; Gold, 1966): Sulfadiazine, initial 3 g, then 1 g every four hours; phenoxymethyl penicillin, 500 mg orally four times daily for seven days; aqueous procaine penicillin, 600,000 units intramuscularly twice daily for five days; tetracycline 0.5 g every four hours and erythromycin 0.2 g every four hours. The tetracyclines and erythromycin are the preferred therapy (Gold, 1955). Higher dosages are used if indicated either by antibiotic sensitivity tests or by the clinical status of the patient, particularly in malignant edema and internal anthrax. Nalin et al. (1977) used 6 g per day chloramphenicol for five days followed by 4 g per day for 18 days until marrow depression occurred, to cure a case of intestinal anthrax. All drugs prevent further dissemination and systemic invasion of the organisms. They have little effect on the established local lesion, which passes through its usual cycle more or less unchanged. Penicillin leads, in our own experience, to a sterilization of the local lesion within 24 hours. Occasionally a febrile reaction and a temporary increase in the edema lasting from several hours to two days occur after treatment is started. Penicillin in doses up to 20 million units per day intravenously has been spectacularly successful in some cases of an-

thrax septicemia and intestinal, pulmonary, and meningeal anthrax with bacteria of low toxicity. It has little effect in well-established toxic septicemic anthrax, where the sudden release of toxins may accelerate death.

Careful monitoring of electrolytes and proper fluid replacement are absolutely essential in the therapy of malignant edema and intestinal and septicemic anthrax. Fluid and electrolyte requirements may approach those in cholera (see Chapter 127, Dutz and Kohout, 1971; Nalin, 1977). Fluid replacement is particularly important shortly after the institution of antibiotic therapy and the subsequent toxin release. Toxemia leads to adrenal exhaustion and supportive therapy with 100 to 200 mg Solu-Cortef intravenously daily followed by decreasing oral dosage has been recommended (Yeganeh-Doust et al., 1968).

Serum therapy, has been superseded by antibiotics and sulfonamides. Topical treatment with antibiotics is useless. Excision and surgical tampering with lesions of the skin should be avoided.

## PROPHYLAXIS

Vaccination of professionally exposed persons is recommended wherever raw materials from countries with endemic anthrax are used. Veterinarians, leather workers, brushmakers, and vendors of bone meal fertilizer should also be protected. The case of a secretary who succumbed to inhalation anthrax although she had never entered the factory and worked in a neighboring office building suggests that all employees should be vaccinated. An absorbed anthrax vaccine according to USPHS standard regulation 73 is commercially available. Three subcutaneous injections of 0.5 cc at two-week intervals followed by boosters after 6, 12, and 18 months, and thereafter once yearly are recommended for complete protection.

The ultimate eradication of anthrax depends largely on vaccination of herds of domesticated animals. Burying of the infected carcasses in deep pits with subsequent covering with lime has been recommended. Too many pastures throughout the world, however, are infected to render this a practical method. Mass vaccination of humans is cumbersome and therefore only indicated in particularly endangered individuals.

### References

Amidi, S., Dutz, W., Kohout, E., and Ronaghy, H. A.: Anthrax in Iran. Z Tropenmed Parasitol 24:250, 1977.

Brachman, P. S., and Fekety, F. R.: Industrial anthrax. Ann NY Acad Sci 70:575, 1958.

Dutz, W., and Kohout, E.: Anthrax. Pathol Annu 6:209, 1971.

Gold, H.: Anthrax: A report of 117 cases. AMA Arch Int Med 96:387, 1955.
Gray, I.: Lysine deficiency and host resistance to anthrax. J Exp Med 117:497, 1963.
Nalin, D. R., et al.: Survival of patient with intestinal anthrax. Am J Med 62:130, 1977.
Proceedings of the conference on progress in the understanding of anthrax. Fed Proc 26:1483, 1967.

Vallery-Radot, R.: The life of Pasteur. N.Y., Dover Publ., Inc., 1960.
Vessal, K., et al.: Radiological changes in inhalation anthrax. Clin Radiol 26:471, 1975.
Yeganeh-Doust, J., et al.: Corticosteroids in treatment of malignant edema of chest wall and neck (anthrax). Dis Chest 53:773, 1968.

# 247 GLANDERS (FARCY)

*Charles E. Davis, M.D.*

## DEFINITION AND HISTORY

Glanders is an infection of horses, mules, and donkeys caused by *Pseudomonas mallei,* the glanders bacillus. Although the natural disease occurs almost exclusively in equines, many other animals and man have occasionally contracted glanders from infected solipeds. Glanders presents in one of three forms: acute fatal septicemia; chronic glanders of the lung and other organs; and farcy, which is the name given to chronic glanders of the skin, subcutaneous tissue, and lymphatics.

Glanders is now primarily of historic interest. It was eliminated from the United States, Canada, and western Europe by 1939. The last known human case in the United States was reported in 1938 (Herold and Erikson, 1938). In fact, *P. mallei* rarely infected man even when it was a common, worldwide disease of horses. In 1906, Robins could find only 156 reported cases in the world literature. The effects of World War I on sanitation and on equine contact in cavalry units temporarily increased the number of cases in the western world, but all industrialized countries had passed effective control acts by 1920 that legislated the destruction of infected equines. This legislation and the replacement of cavalry by motorized vehicles has eliminated glanders from the world except for a few foci in Asia, Africa, and the Middle East.

Despite the fact that it was never common, glanders is one of the oldest diseases known. Hippocrates and Aristotle both described glanders, and Aristotle actually named the disease "malleus," which is derived from the Greek word meaning malignant or epidemic. *P. mallei* was isolated in pure culture and proved to be the etiologic agent of glanders in 1882 by Loeffler and Schutz in Germany and by Bouchard, Charrin, and Capitan in France.

## ETIOLOGY

*P. mallei* was originally named *Bacillus mallei* by Zopf in 1885. Since that time, it has been temporarily placed in various ill-defined genera of bacteria including *Pfeifferella, Actinobacillus, Loefferella, Acinetobacter,* and *Malleomyces.* The species name has always been mallei. Because it is a nonfermentative, oxidase-positive, gram-negative bacterium, *P. mallei* seemed most closely related to the pseudomonads but did not fit the definition exactly because of its nonmotility. It was finally placed in the *Pseudomonas* genus in the eighth edition of Bergey's manual (Doudoroff and Palleroni, 1974) because of its many similarities to *P. pseudomallei* (Wetmore and Gochenour, 1956; Redfearn et al., 1966), the cause of meliodosis (a glanders-like disease of man). Among its many similarities to *P. pseudomallei* and the other pseudomonads are its oxidative attack on glucose, reduction of nitrate to nitrite, and its guanine plus cytosine content of $69 \pm 1.0$ per cent (Mandel, 1966). An additional significant relationship between *P. mallei* and *P. pseudomallei* is that several temperate phages isolated from *P. pseudomallei* can lyse strains of *P. mallei* but not other pseudomonads (Smith and Cherry, 1957). Finally, it was shown that *P. mallei* and *P. pseudomallei* accumulate poly-B-hydroxybutyrate as a cellular reserve material (Miller et al., 1948; Levine and Wolochow, 1960), a common characteristic among the nonfluorescent aerobic pseudomonads (Forsyth et al., 1958).

*P. mallei* is easily differentiated from *P. pseudomallei* and the other pseudomonads because it is nonmotile, requires 48 hours to form well-developed colonies, and grows best on media supplemented with 4 per cent glycerol. In addition to these major biologic differences, it can also be differentiated from *P. pseudomallei* on the basis of several other biochemical tests (see Table 7, Chapter 33).

P. mallei and P. pseudomallei also cross-react extensively in serologic reactions. They cross-react almost completely in agglutination (Cravitz and Miller, 1950) and fluorescent antibody (Moody et al., 1956) reactions with serum prepared against whole live or formalin-killed bacteria and also share at least one heat-stable antigen (Fournier, 1967) that is probably located in the lipopolysaccharide. Because the two organisms were so similar but P. pseudomallei contained two other heat-stable antigens and was flagellated, Fournier (1967) hypothesized that P. mallei evolved from the free-living P. pseudomallei when the glanders bacillus adapted to a strict parasitic existence in equines.

## PATHOGENESIS AND PATHOLOGY

The virulence of individual strains of P. mallei for susceptible laboratory animals varies greatly, but the reasons for this variability are not known. Furthermore, certain animals (cattle and rats) are almost completely resistant to both natural and experimental glanders. Among the equines, horses are the best adapted animal. Chronic infections are common in horses, whereas mules and donkeys usually die of acute disease within 10 to 30 days. Man seems to be fairly resistant to glanders and may develop either acute or chronic disease.

Man acquires glanders by contact with infected nasal secretions of equines. The organism usually enters the body through an abrasion or scratch, but primary nasal infection also occurs (Mendelson, 1950). The possibility of aerosol transmission is strongly reinforced by the frequency of laboratory-acquired disease. With the possible exceptions of Brucella, the plague bacillus, and Pasteurella tularensis, no bacterium is as dangerous to work with in the laboratory as P. mallei. Several members of one laboratory became ill a few days after a centrifuge tube was broken (Jennings, 1963). In another laboratory specifically designed to work with P. mallei, 50 per cent of the laboratory personnel became ill within one year (Howe and Miller, 1947). Human to human transmission is also well documented.

The classic lesion of glanders is a tuberculoid nodule. In the acute pulmonary form of the disease, diffuse necrotizing pneumonia may accompany multiple abscess-like pulmonary nodules. The acute nodule is 1 to 4 mm in size and dark red because of hemorrhage. As it ages, it becomes gray, firm, and organized. Calcification may occur in old pulmonary nodules (M'Fadyean, 1900; Frothingham, 1901).

Nodules occur most commonly in the lungs, mucous membranes of the nose, lymphatics, and skin. The spleen, liver, testes, and bones are less commonly affected. Instead of organizing and healing, nodules may ulcerate and discharge a thick, sticky, purulent, highly infectious exudate into the bronchus or from the skin or the nose (the characteristic nasal discharge of glanders).

The center of acute nodules is thick pus composed of polymorphonuclear leukocytes. In older nodules, the necrotic center is surrounded by epitheliod and giant cells. The entire nodule is surrounded by fibrous tissue.

In farcy, the nodules occur in the skin or subcutaneous tissue and frequently break down and ulcerate. The lymphatics that drain these superficial nodules become firm and stand out as hard cords, the so-called "farcy-pipes." The local lymph nodes, which become firm and enlarge, are referred to as "farcy buds." Farcy can occur in human beings but is much more common in horses.

Very little work has been done on the virulence factors of P. mallei. It synthesizes an antigenically complete lipopolysaccharide that presumably contributes to the manifestations of acute, fatal septicemia. Neither capsules nor exotoxins have been described. Mallein, a product obtained by autoclaving, filtering, and concentrating tenfold a 10- to 14-day culture of P. mallei, induces delayed hypersensitivity reactions in the skin of people and animals with glanders. Early investigators were struck with the similarities between glanders and tuberculosis because the growth of P. mallei was enhanced by glycerol; mallein induced delayed hypersensitivity reactions in infected animals; and glanders produced pulmonary nodules that were tuberculoid in nature. While the diseases are only slightly similar and the organisms very dissimilar, these characteristics of glanders suggest that some of its pathologic manifestations are characteristic of a facultative intracellular parasite.

## CLINICAL MANIFESTATIONS

Untreated glanders in man has been described as an intensely painful, loathsome disease from which few recover (Jennings, 1963). It may be acute or chronic and may be localized primarily either in the respiratory organs or in the skin or subcutaneous tissue. The manifestations are partly determined by the route of infection and, as alluded to in Pathogenesis and Pathology, may vary with the virulence of the strain of P. mallei. One to five days after accidental inoculation of the skin, the patient develops a nodule with surrounding lymphangitis. As this type of infection progresses, typical "farcy pipes" and "farcy buds" form. If the mucous membranes are involved, mucopurulent drainage from the nose, eye, or lips is soon replaced by extensive, disfiguring granulomatous lesions that may ulcerate and drain tenacious pus.

The septicemic form of the disease may occur either primarily or secondary to localized disease. It is characterized by early onset of anorexia, malaise, fever, nausea, and myalgia. Erysipeloid lesions on the face and limbs develop and are quickly followed by a generalized pustular eruption. Ulcerations of the nasal septum cause a mucopurulent, blood-streaked discharge. Bronchopneumonia or nodular, necrotizing pneumonia occurs very commonly and may cause severe cough and pleuritic pain. Cervical lymphadenopathy, splenomegaly, and jaundice are common. The skin pustules finally become suppurative and metastatic lesions in the muscles, bones, spleen, and liver often precede fatal collapse, which usually occurs within two weeks in untreated patients. A slight leukocytosis and left shift are usual, but leukopenia also occurs.

Chronic disease most commonly involves the skin and musculoskeletal system (83 per cent), the lymphatics (50 per cent), and the nose (50 per cent) (Robins, 1906). Patients who recover from septicemia after developing chronic disease and patients with chronic glanders may develop septicemia at any time during the course of the disease (Mendelson, 1950).

## COMPLICATIONS AND SEQUELAE

Most patients with untreated, acute septicemia die. The chief complication of chronic glanders is the development of disfiguring lesions of the skin, subcutaneous tissue, and face. The lesions of the nose and lips, which resemble those of cutaneous leishmaniasis and other granulomatous diseases of the mucous membranes, are not only disfiguring but also interfere with breathing, eating, and swallowing. Patients may also live for many years with the nodules of metastatic glanders in the musculoskeletal system or viscera before they finally succumb to a fatal episode of septicemia.

## GEOGRAPHIC VARIATIONS IN DISEASE

When glanders was a worldwide disease, there were no known geographic variations in its manifestations or course. Individual variation in the virulence of strains and the variable susceptibility of mammalian species seemed to be independent of geographic location. The only known foci of infection in the 1980s are in remote, underdeveloped areas of Asia, Africa, and the Middle East.

## DIAGNOSIS

Microscopic examination of pus from skin or subcutaneous nodules, nasal drainage, or sputum shows polymorphonuclear leukocytes and small gram-negative bacilli that tend to stain irregularly in the Gram and methylene blue stains. The microscopic appearance of *P. mallei* is not distinctive. It cannot be differentiated from *P. pseudomallei* or most other common gram-negative bacilli. The specimen should be inoculated onto nutrient agar, glycerol agar, blood agar, or all three media. If the source of the specimen is likely to be contaminated, it should be inoculated onto agar containing a 1 to 200,000 dilution of crystal violet to suppress gram-positive organisms. Gram-negative colonies that develop after 24 to 48 hours should be worked up as possible *P. mallei*. The fastest way to differentiate *P. mallei* from *P. pseudomallei* is by examination of a hanging-drop preparation of a culture grown at room temperature. *P. mallei* is nonmotile. Its other characteristics are given in the text and tables in Chapter 33. Either primary material or the isolated, suspected bacterium should also be inoculated intraperitoneally into male guinea pigs. Moderate or large doses produce localized peritonitis that involves the scrotum. The testicles become enlarged and finally form a caseous mass that breaks through the scrotum (Straus' reaction). This reaction is specific for *P. mallei* and *P. pseudomallei*. Organisms can also be identified as either *P. mallei* or *P. pseudomallei* by immunofluorescence with fluoresceinated antiserum against formalinized *P. mallei* or *P. pseudomallei*.

A high percentage of infected people and equines have developed a firm, indurated nodule about 24 to 48 hours after intradermal inoculation of 0.1 ml of commercial mallein at a dilution of 1 to 10,000. False positives are uncommon. Mallein may induce an antibody response and should not be injected until serologic studies are completed.

The complement fixation and bacterial agglutination tests are valuable diagnostic techniques (Cravitz and Miller, 1950). The agglutination test is more sensitive than the complement fixation test (CF), but the CF is more specific. Normal people often have agglutination titers of 1:20 to 1:160, and patients with meliodosis may have high titers. Glanders almost always causes agglutination titers of greater than 1:320. A complement fixation titer of 1:20 or greater is specific for glanders. Patients with meliodosis do not develop CF antibodies to *P. mallei*.

Acute glanders could be confused with any acute bacterial septicemia, especially typhoid, brucellosis, and meliodosis. The blood count may not be high enough to exclude typhoid fever or brucellosis, which usually cause white counts of less than 10,000 per mm³, and acute meliodosis may closely resemble glanders. Chronic glanders may be confused with sporotrichosis and other mycotic infections of the skin and subcutaneous tissue, with other granulomatous infections of the nose and mouth, and with pulmonary tuberculosis. A history of exposure to equines in an endemic area and proper bacteriologic and serologic techniques should quickly establish the correct diagnosis.

## TREATMENT

*P. mallei* is resistant to penicillin but sensitive to sulfonamides, streptomycin, the tetracyclines, and chloramphenicol. The natural disease in man and experimental glanders in laboratory rodents responds to treatment with sulfonamides (Howe and Miller, 1947; Cravitz and Miller, 1950; Miller et al., 1948). The optimal dose and duration of therapy is unknown. The results of treatment of experimental glanders with streptomycin and tetracycline are contradictory.

## PROPHYLAXIS

Glanders has been virtually eliminated from the developed world by procedures like those laid down in the British Glanders or Farcy Order of 1907 and similar legislation in the United States and Canada at the same time. According to these laws, every animal with clinical evidence of glanders or a positive mallein test was considered a diseased animal and slaughtered. The carcasses were burned, the area disinfected and all equine contacts tested with mallein. Reactors were destroyed. These procedures were effective because of the relatively limited host range of the natural disease.

## References

Cravitz, L., and Miller, W. R.: Immunologic studies with *Malleomyces mallei* and *Malleomyces pseudomallei*. J Infect Dis 86:46, 1950.

Doudoroff, M., and Palleroni, N. J.: Pseudomonadaceae. In Bergey's Manual of Determinative Bacteriology. 8th ed. Baltimore, The Williams & Wilkins Company, 1974, p. 217.

Forsyth, W. G. C., Hayward, A. C., and Roberts, J. B.: Occurrence of poly-B-hydroxybutyric acid in aerobic gram-negative bacteria. Nature (London) 182:800, 1958.

Fournier, J.: The thermostable antigens of *Pseudomonas pseudomallei* and of *Malleomyces mallei* and their communities. Ann Inst Pasteur 112:93, 1967.

Frothingham, L.: The diagnosis of glanders by the Straus method. J Med Res 6:331, 1901.

Herold, A. A., and Erikson, C. G.: Human glanders—case report. South Med J 1022, 1938.

Howe, C., and Miller, W. R.: Human glanders: Report of 6 cases. Ann Intern Med 26:93, 1947.

Jennings, W. E.: Glanders. In Hull, T. G. (ed.): Diseases Transmitted from Animals to Man. 5th ed. Springfield, Ill., Charles C Thomas, 1963, p. 264.

Levine, H. B., and Wolochow, H.: Occurrence of poly-B-hydroxybutyrate in *Pseudomonas pseudomallei*. J. Bacteriol 79:805, 1960.

Mandel, M.: Deoxyribonucleic acid base composition in the genus *Pseudomonas*. J Gen Microbiol 43:273, 1966.

M'Fadyean, J.: The curability of glanders. J Comp Pathol Ther 13:55, 1900.

Mendelson, R. W.: Glanders. U.S. Armed Forces Med 1:781, 1950.

Miller, W. R., Pannel, L., Cravitz, L., Tanner, W. A., and Ingalls, M. S.: Studies on certain biological characteristics of *Malleomyces pseudomallei* I. Morphology, cultivation, viability, and isolation from contaminated specimens. J Bacteriol 55:115, 1948.

Miller, W. R., Pannel, L., and Ingalls, M. S.: Experimental chemotherapy in glanders and meliodosis. Am J Hyg 47:205, 1948.

Moody, M. D., Golman, M., and Thomason, B. M.: Staining bacterial smears with fluorescent antibody. J Bacteriol 72:357, 1956.

Redfearn, M. S., Palleroni, N. J., and Stanier, R. Y.: A comparative study of *Pseudomonas pseudomallei* and *Bacillus mallei*. J Gen Microbiol 43:293, 1966.

Robins, G. D.: Chronic glanders in man. Studies from the Royal Victoria Hospital, Montreal 2, No. 1, 1906.

Smith, P. B., and Cherry, W. B.: Identification of malleomyces by specific bacteriophages. J Bacteriol 74:668, 1957.

Wetmore, P. W., and Gochenour, W. S.: Comparative studies of the genus *Malleomyces* and selected *Pseudomonas* species. I. Morphological and cultural characteristics. J Bacteriol 72:79, 1956.

# 248 TOXOPLASMOSIS

Jack S. Remington, M.D.
Rima McLeod, M.D.*

## DEFINITION

In the past, the term toxoplasmosis has been used imprecisely to refer to both infection and disease due to *Toxoplasma gondii*. The distinction between infection and disease caused by this organism is important clinically and epidemiologically. *Toxoplasma* infection refers to the presence of the protozoan in individuals with or without clinical manifestations. Toxoplasmosis refers to the disease caused by the organism. *Toxoplasma* infection is usually asymptomatic in older children and adults; but when signs and symptoms are present, they are usually of short duration (acute) and self-limited. Chronic *Toxoplasma* infection describes persistence of the organism in the cyst form without clinical manifestations. The term chronic toxoplasmosis is best reserved to describe the disease in which active *Toxoplasma* infection is the proven cause of persistent or recrudescent clinical manifestations (e.g., encephalitis in infants; myocarditis, chorioretinitis, or lymphadenopathy). Throughout the world, *Toxoplasma* infection occurs with significantly greater frequency than toxoplasmosis.

## ETIOLOGY

### Classification of the Organism

*T. gondii* is an obligate intracellular protozoan. It has an enteroepithelial and extraintestinal cycle in members of the cat family and only an extraintestinal cycle in all other mammalian and avian hosts. The organism is classified among the Sporozoa and exists in three forms: trophozoite, cyst, and oocyst (Fig. 1).

*Trophozoites (Tachyzoites).* The trophozoite (Fig. 1A and B) is crescent or oval, with one end pointed and the other rounded. It measures approximately 3 by 7 $\mu$m. It stains well with either Wright's stain or Giemsa stain. The nucleus is centrally located, and there are no flagella, cilia,

*Recipient of a fellowship award from the Giannini Foundation.

This work was supported by Public Health Service grant A104717 from the National Institute of Allergy and Infectious Diseases.

or pseudopods. Trophozoites are found in tissues during the acute stage of infection and invade all mammalian cells except non-nucleated erythrocytes. Multiplication is by endodyogeny (i.e., two *Toxoplasma* organisms form within each parent cell). Division continues until the host cell ruptures or a tissue cyst forms. Desiccation, freezing and thawing, and gastric secretions kill trophozoites.

Trophozoites can be propagated in the laboratory in the peritoneum of mice, in tissue culture, or in eggs. Antigens of trophozoites are used in complement fixation and hemagglutination tests for diagnosis of *Toxoplasma* infection, and whole trophozoites are used in the Sabin-Feldman dye test, agglutination test, and fluorescent antibody method.

*Cysts.* The tissue cyst (Fig. 1C) develops within host cells and may contain thousands of organisms. Cysts range in size from 10 to 100 $\mu$m and stain well with periodic acid–Schiff (PAS) stain. The cyst wall also stains with silver. Because cysts may be present in tissues ingested by carnivorous animals or humans, they are important in transmission. It seems likely that they are also the source of recrudescent disseminated infection in the immunosuppressed individual and in older children and adults who develop chorioretinitis. Cysts are demonstrable as early as the eighth day of infection in animals and may remain viable in multiple tissues throughout the life of the host. Skeletal and heart muscle and brain are the most common sites of chronic (latent) infection in humans, although cysts may exist in virtually every organ. Peptic or tryptic digestive fluids disrupt the cyst wall, thereby liberating viable *T. gondii,* which can survive several hours of exposure to these digestive enzymes. Freezing ($-20°$ C) and thawing, heating to $60°$ C, or desiccation destroys tissue cysts.

*Oocysts.* The oocyst (Fig. 1E to H) is oval and measures 10 to 12 $\mu$m in diameter. Only members of the cat family have been reported to excrete oocysts (Fig. 2), and cats have systemic infection with *T. gondii* as well. After a cat eats food containing cysts or contaminated with oocysts, *T. gondii* are released into the lumen of the stomach or small intestine. After invasion of the epithelial cells of the small intestine (Fig. 1D) (Dubey et al., 1972), the organism undergoes an asexual cycle

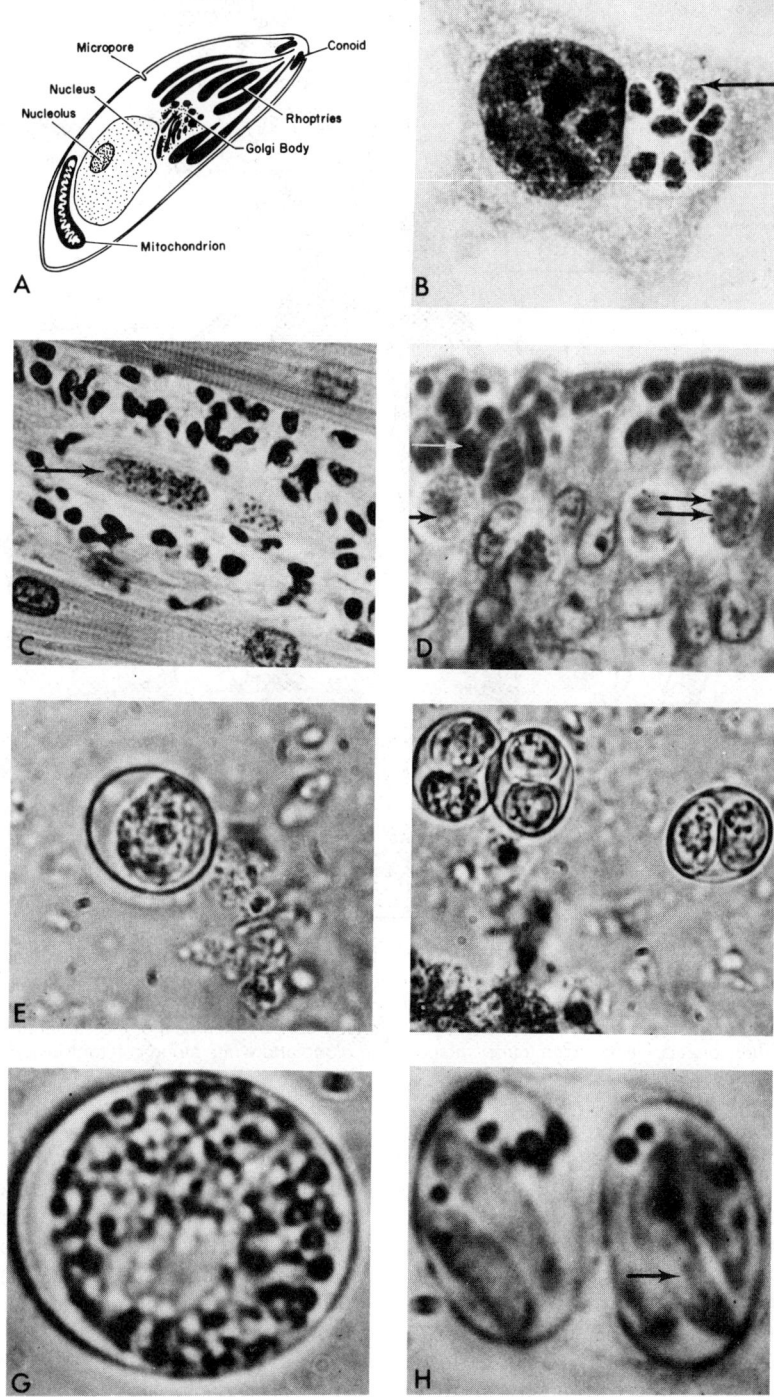

**FIGURE 1.** *The forms of Toxoplasma. A, Trophozoite, schematic representation. (Courtesy of W. M. Hutchinson, Glasgow.) B, Trophozoites (arrow) in vacuole in the cytoplasm of cell cultured in vitro. C, Tissue cyst (arrow) in human myocardium. Note that cyst conforms to shape of muscle fiber. In brain, cysts are spherical. D, Schizonts (white arrow). Male (double arrow) and female (black arrow) gametocytes in the cat ileum. (From Dubey, J., and Frenkel, J. K.: J Protozool 19:155, 1972.) E, Unsporulated oocyst. F, Sporulated oocyst. G, Unsporulated oocyst (higher magnification). H, Unsporulated oocyst (higher magnification) in which two sporozoites (arrow) are visible. (From Dubey, J., Miller, N., and Frenkel, J.: J Exp Med 132:636, 1970.)*

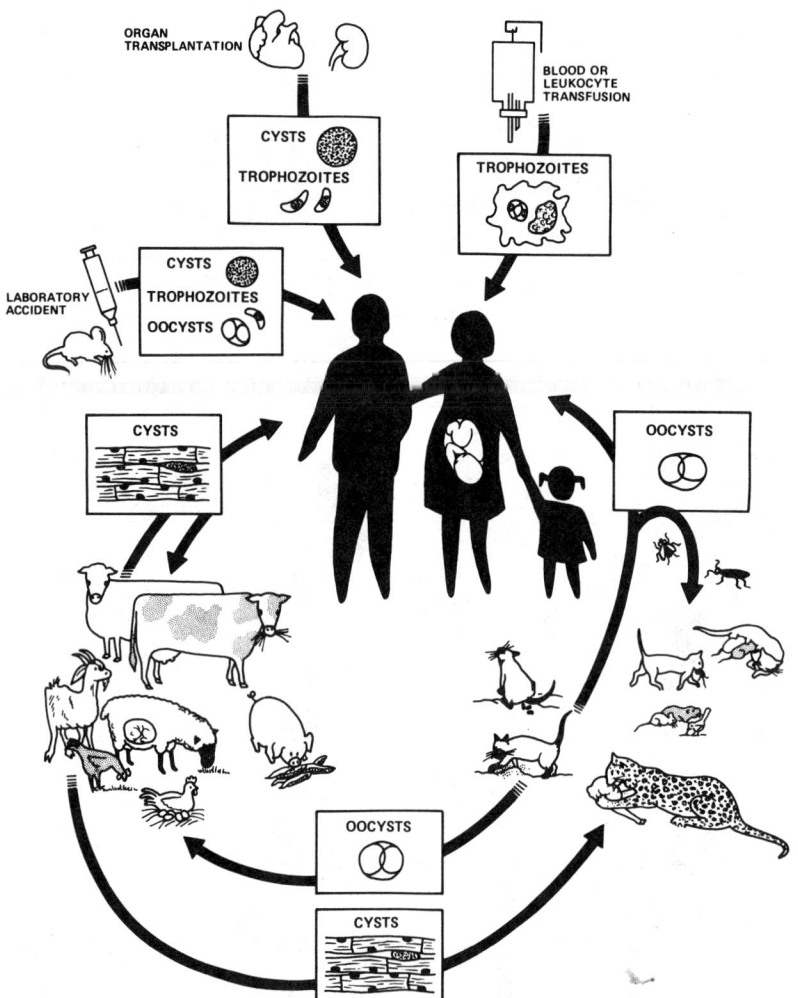

**FIGURE 2.**  *Life cycle and modes of transmission of* Toxoplasma gondii. *Infection in man and other animals occurs primarily after ingestion of either the cyst or the oocyst. Released organisms invade the intestinal epithelium, spread to tissues (either hematogenously or via lymphatics), and form cysts. When man or other animals (including the cat) eat infected tissues (from any animal) or mature oocysts (excreted only by members of the cat family), the life cycle is completed. Laboratory accidents, organ transplantation, and blood and white blood cell transfusion also have been implicated in transmission of the organism.*

(schizogony) and then a sexual cycle (gametogony), resulting in development of the noninfectious, unsporulated oocyst (Fig. 1E and G). The time by which a cat begins to excrete oocysts ranges from 3 to 24 days after the infection and depends on the form of the organism with which the cat has become infected. This excretion continues for 7 to 20 days, and as many as 10 million oocysts may be shed in the feces in a single day. Renewed oocyst excretion has been reported to occur when a cat becomes reinfected with *Toxoplasma* organisms or is acutely infected with *Isospora*. Maturation (sporulation) (Fig. 1F and H), which is required for the oocyst to become infectious, occurs only after the oocysts have been excreted. Sporulation occurs in 2 to 3 days at 24° C, in 5 to 8 days at 15° C, and in 14 to 21 days at

11° C. Oocysts do not sporulate below 4° C or above 37° C. Under favorable conditions (e.g., warm, moist soil), oocysts remain infectious for several months to over a year. Dry heat (over 66° C) or boiling water renders oocysts noninfectious. Ingestion of oocysts has been shown to cause infection.

## Life Cycle and Modes of Transmission of *T. gondii*

*T. gondii* is ubiquitous and can infect herbivorous, omnivorous, and carnivorous animals, including all orders of mammals, some birds, and some reptiles. Most commonly, *T. gondii* infects man or other animals when organisms are released from ingested cysts or oocysts. The trophozoites invade the intestinal epithelium and spread hematogenously or via lymphatics to tissues, where they form cysts. When man or other animals (including the cat) eat infected tissues (from any animal) or mature oocysts (excreted only by members of the cat family), the life cycle is completed. Members of the family Felidae, including both domestic and feral cats, appear to be the definitive hosts in this life cycle because they are the only animals that are known to shed oocysts. Oocysts have been found in the feces of approximately 1 per cent of cats in diverse areas of the world (including Costa Rica, Germany, Japan, and the United States).

The major routes of acquisition of *Toxoplasma* organisms are ingestion and transplacental transmission. Less common modes of transmission are through blood transfusion, leukocyte transfusion, organ transplantation, and laboratory accident (Fig. 2). Reinfection from an exogenous source has not been recognized as a cause of clinical illness.

*Ingestion.* *T. gondii* is acquired principally by eating food containing cysts or contaminated with oocysts. In most areas of the world, approximately 10 per cent of lamb and 25 per cent of pork contain cysts; the prevalence of cysts in beef is not known. Ingestion of oocysts can result from direct contact with any material contaminated by infected cat feces. Flies, cockroaches, and probably other insects can transport oocysts to food.

*Transplacental Transmission.* *Toxoplasma* organisms may be transmitted transplacentally to the fetus in utero or at vaginal delivery. This transmission can occur only if infection is acquired by the mother during pregnancy. Infection acquired by the mother during pregnancy most often results in birth of an uninfected infant but may also result in spontaneous abortion, stillbirth, or birth of a premature or full-term infected infant. Approximately one third of infants born to mothers who acquire infection during pregnancy are infected. In infants born to mothers infected during the first trimester, congenital infection is least common (approximately 17 per cent) but disease is most severe; in infants born to mothers infected during the third trimester, congenital infection is most common (approximately 65 per cent) but is usually asymptomatic. *Toxoplasma* infection that is acquired by the mother during pregnancy is symptomatic in only about 10 to 20 per cent of cases; but whether or not the infection is symptomatic, the fetus is still at risk.

The following are guidelines for ascertaining the risk to the fetus of a woman who has been infected before the pregnancy in question. A woman who acquired *Toxoplasma* infection at any time before gestation will not deliver an infected infant. A woman who had acute *Toxo-* *plasma* infection during one pregnancy, whether or not she delivered an infected infant, will not give birth to a child infected with *T. gondii* in a subsequent pregnancy. Although investigators have presented data to the contrary, their studies lacked appropriate controls and the data have not been confirmed. If there is a risk to the fetus in these settings, it must be exceedingly low. *Toxoplasma* has, however, been isolated on rare occasions from abortuses of women with chronic (latent) infection. The frequency of *Toxoplasma* infection as a cause of abortion is unknown and is the subject of considerable controversy.

*Transmission by Blood or Leukocyte Transfusion.* Parasitemia has been reported to persist in otherwise normal persons for up to one year after acquisition of infection, and *Toxoplasma* organisms have been recovered from leukocytes of individuals without recognized clinical evidence of *Toxoplasma* infection. Particularly noteworthy is the high incidence of isolation of the organism from the blood of patients who have chronic myelogenous leukemia and high antibody titers to *Toxoplasma*. The organism can survive for up to 50 days in whole citrated blood stored at 4° C. This poses a particular threat to immunodeficient patients who require multiple blood transfusions.

## PATHOGENESIS AND PATHOLOGY

### Pathogenesis

After they are released from cysts or oocysts, the organisms enter cells of the gastrointestinal tract, where they multiply, disrupt cells, and then infect contiguous cells. Extracellular organisms or organisms within leukocytes may be transported via the lymphatic system and bloodstream to where they can invade every organ and tissue. Proliferating trophozoites usually produce necrotic foci of invaded cells. These foci are surrounded by an intense cellular reaction. The outcome of the acute process depends primarily on the immune response of the host. Both humoral and cell-mediated immunity are important. In some apparently normal people and especially in immunodeficient patients, the acute infection may progress and cause potentially lethal lesions, such as acute necrotizing encephalitis, pneumonitis, or myocarditis. With development of the normal immune response, trophozoites disappear from the tissues.

A unique aspect of the infection is that organisms persist as cysts in multiple organs for the lifespan of the host. The tissue cysts, which are characteristic of chronic infection, provoke little or no inflammatory response. Either rupture of cysts or persistence of viable trophozoites within monocytes and macrophages may be the source of the recurrent parasitemias that occur in some asymptomatic individuals with chronic infection. Cysts are the likely source of organisms that cause recrudescent disease in immunocompromised patients or chorioretinitis in older children and adults with congenital toxoplasmosis.

## Pathology

The meager information on the pathologic changes of toxoplasmosis in immunologically normal people is derived largely from lymph node biopsy, because most of these infections are asymptomatic and self-limited. There is limited information concerning changes in other organs. Pathology has been defined most clearly in congenitally infected infants and in immunosuppressed individuals with disseminated infection.

There are considerable variations in the degree of organ and tissue involvement in infants with congenital infection. In some instances, autopsy reveals only central nervous system (CNS) and eye involvement, whereas in other instances there is wide dissemination of lesions and organisms. The central nervous system is never spared. In extraneural organs, whose tissues can regenerate, residual lesions may be so slight that they are easily overlooked. In the central nervous system and eye, on the other hand, the inability of nerve cells to regenerate leads to more severe, permanent damage.

The pathologic changes described below are the same in adults and congenitally infected infants unless otherwise specified.

*Lymph Node.* In older children and adults, the histopathologic changes in toxoplasmic lymphadenitis are distinctive (Fig. 3). The characteristic lesion is a reactive follicular hyperplasia with irregular clusters of epithelioid histiocytes that encroach upon and blur the margins of germinal centers. There is also an associated focal distension of sinuses with monocytoid cells. Giant cells are absent, and *T. gondii* can be demonstrated only rarely.

*Eye.* The earliest changes in the eye are single or multiple foci of necrosis. The infiltrate consists largely of lymphocytes, plasma cells, and mononuclear phagocytes. Intra- and extracellular trophozoites and numerous cysts may be found in the retinal lesions. It has been suggested that the retinitis originates from cyst rupture. Granulomatous inflammation of the choroid is secondary to the necrotizing retinitis. Iridocyclitis, glaucoma, and cataracts may occur as complications of the chorioretinitis.

*Central Nervous System (CNS).* In acute infection, there is a focal or diffuse meningoencephalitis with necrosis and microglial nodules. Multinucleated giant cells are not a characteristic feature. Perivascular mononuclear inflammation is frequent and is contiguous to areas of necrosis. Occasionally there is necrosis of vessel walls. Areas of necrosis may mimic mass lesions, and intra- and extracellular trophozoites are usually found at the periphery of areas of necrosis. Cysts in the brain may occur during acute infection or reflect infection of long duration (Fig. 4). The extent and location of CNS involvement, as well as the size of lesions, vary considerably. The lesions in the CNS in adults and congenitally infected infants are similar. Periaqueductal or periventricular vasculitis with necrosis is a unique aspect of severe congenital infection. Necrotic tissue sloughs into the ventricles, obstructing the aqueduct of Sylvius or the foramen of Monro and causing internal hydrocephalus. Calcification of necrotic areas is especially prominent in congenital infection but may also occur in infected older children or adults.

*Lung.* Pulmonary infection may cause clinically significant interstitial pneumonitis in congenitally infected infants and in immunocompromised patients, and uncommonly in individuals without apparent underlying disease. In each of these settings, there are thickened and edematous alveolar septa that, along with peribronchial areas, may be infiltrated with mononuclear cells, occasional plasma cells, and rare eosinophils. The walls of small blood vessels may also be infiltrated with lymphocytes and mononuclear cells, and *Toxoplasma* organisms may be present in endothelial cells. Both trophozoites and cysts have been seen within alveolar lining cells. Necrosis within granulomatous foci is prominent in some patients with disseminated toxoplasmosis and malignancy but is rarely seen in infants or in patients without malignancy. In many cases, there is some bronchopneumonia, often caused by superimposed infection with other organisms.

*Heart.* Myocarditis is found in congenital infection, in infection of immunocompromised individuals, and rarely in severe acute infection of apparently normal individuals. Cysts and large aggregates of trophozoites occur within muscle fibers (Fig. 1C). Single organisms are found adjacent to and within areas of necrotic tissue. Foci of inflammatory cells (lymphocytes, plasma cells, mononuclear cells, and occasional eosinophils) are associated with hyaline necrosis and fragmentation of myocardial cells, usually without organisms. Hemorrhagic pericarditis has also been reported in some patients with toxoplasmosis.

*Kidney.* In congenital toxoplasmosis and disseminated infection in older children and adults, the pathologic changes in the kidney resemble those in other organs (i.e., necrosis and the presence of cysts, trophozoites, and inflammatory

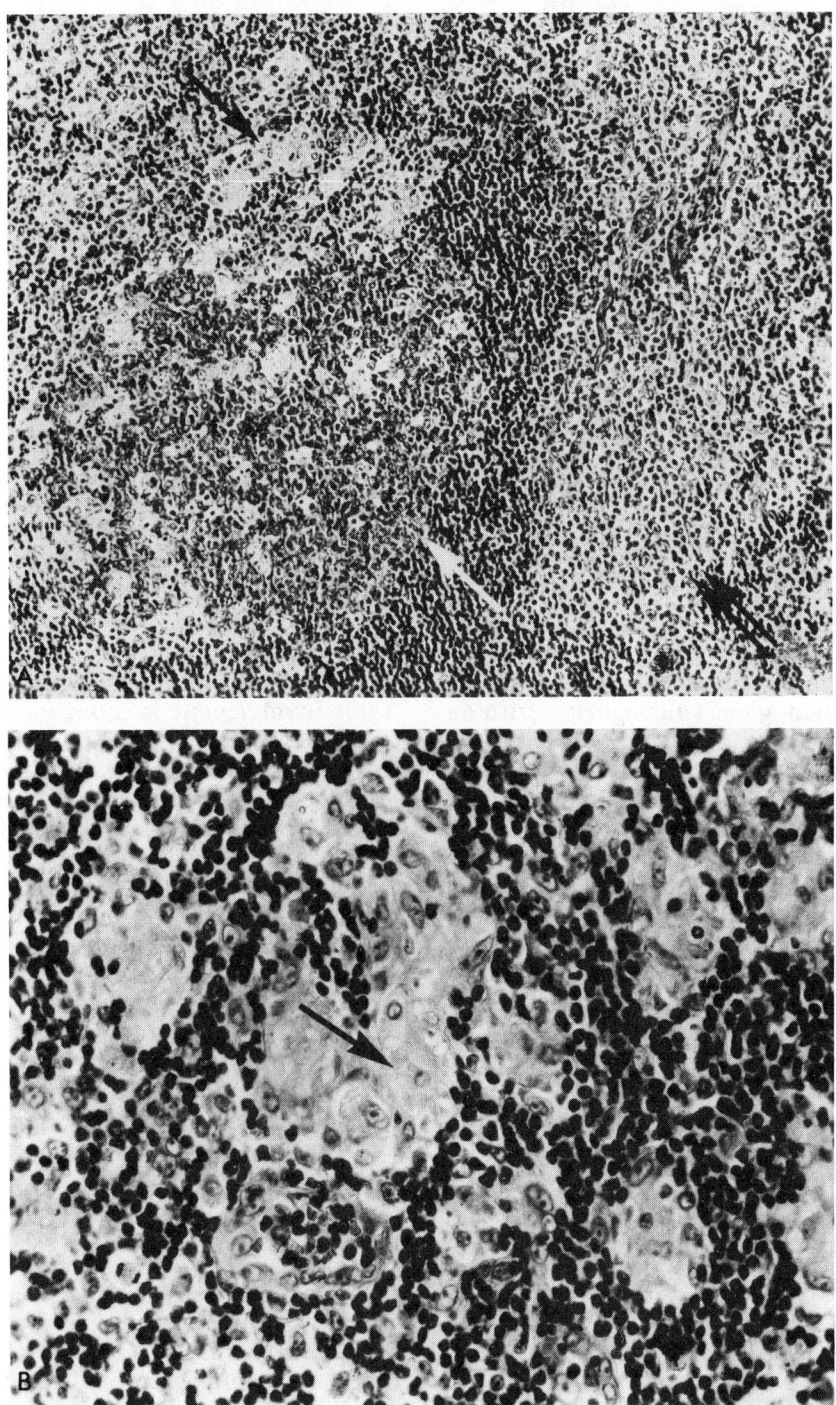

**FIGURE 3.** *Characteristic lymph node pathology in lymphadenitis due to Toxoplasma. A, Epithelioid cells (black arrow) encroach upon and blur margins of germinal center (white arrow), and there is focal distension of subcapsular and trabecular sinuses by "monocytoid" cells (double black arrows). B, Irregular clusters of epithelioid cells (arrow) scattered throughout paracortical lymphoid stroma. (From Dorfman, R. F., and Remington, J. S.: N Engl J Med 289:878, 1973.)*

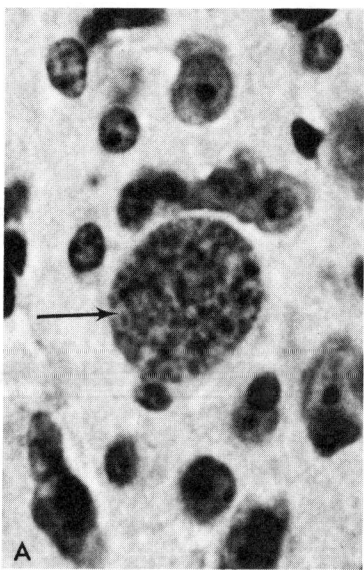
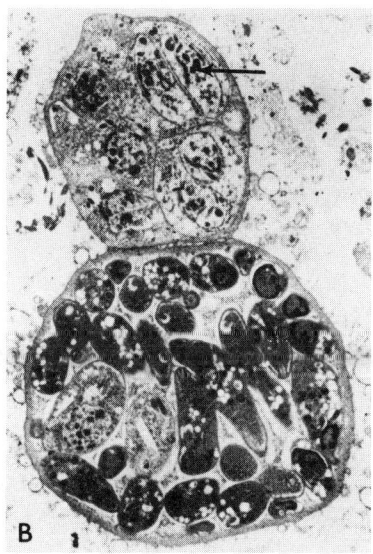

**FIGURE 4.** *Infection of central nervous system with Toxoplasma. A, Cyst (arrow) in brain is seen in acute infection as early as eight days, or in chronic (latent) infection. B, Electronmicrograph of central nervous system Toxoplasma infection. The diagnosis may be established by electronmicroscopic identification of organisms (arrow) when light microscopic examination is not definitive. (From Ghatak, N. R., Poon, T. P., and Zimmerman, H. M.: Arch Pathol 89:337, 1970.)*

cells). Necrosis may occur in both glomeruli and tubules. In addition, glomerulonephritis with deposits of IgM, fibrinogen, and *Toxoplasma* antigen and antibody has been reported.

*Other Sites.* *Toxoplasma* organisms and foci of necrosis have been found in the adrenal cortex, testes, and ovaries of infected infants; and organisms, usually without inflammation, have been found in the pituitary. Cysts or trophozoites with or without inflammation have been reported in multiple organs including liver, spleen, bone marrow, thyroid, pancreas, adipose tissue, and skin in infected infants and adults. Pancreatic involvement has been a prominent finding in infection in immunocompromised patients. Involvement of skeletal muscles varies from parasitized fibers without pathologic changes to focal areas of infiltration or widespread myositis with necrosis.

*Immunoglobulin Abnormalities.* Monoclonal gammopathy of the IgG class has been described in infants with congenital toxoplasmosis. IgM levels may be elevated in newborns with congenital toxoplasmosis.

## CLINICAL MANIFESTATIONS

### Lymphadenopathy and Other Manifestations

The most commonly recognized clinical manifestation of acute acquired toxoplasmosis is lymphadenopathy. The cervical nodes (either a single posterior cervical node or multiple nodes) are involved most frequently, and discovery of their involvement is often incidental. Asymptomatic lymphadenopathy may mimic lymphoma. Involvement of a pectoral node may be mistaken for carcinoma of the breast in females. Suboccipital, supraclavicular, axillary, and inguinal nodes are also involved frequently. It is important to recognize that the mediastinal, mesenteric, and retroperitoneal nodes may also be involved. With infection of the mesenteric or retroperitoneal nodes, there may be abdominal pain and fever to 40° C. Involved lymph nodes are usually discrete and vary in firmness; they may be tender but do not suppurate. Fever, malaise, myalgias, headache, sore throat, maculopapular rash (which spares the palms and soles), hepatosplenomegaly, and reactive (atypical) lymphocytes may be present. The lymphadenopathic form of toxoplasmosis is self-limited, but lymphadenopathy and/or malaise may persist or recur for months.

Rarely, someone who seems to be normal immunologically may develop any of the following, alone or in combination: myocarditis, pericarditis, polymyositis, hepatitis, pneumonitis, encephalitis, or meningoencephalitis. None of the signs or symptoms from involvement of these organs are specific for infection with *T. gondii.* Some of these patients have died.

### Ocular Involvement

*Toxoplasma* has been estimated to cause approximately 35 per cent of cases of chorioretinitis in the United States and Central and Western Europe. In the older child and adult, ocular disease is most frequently a consequence of congenital *Toxoplasma* infection, but chorioretinitis has been estimated to occur in approximately 1 per cent of patients with acute acquired *Toxoplasma* infection.

Active chorioretinitis may produce blurred vision, scotomas, pain, photophobia, or epiphora (O'Connor, 1974). Central vision may be impaired or lost if the macula is involved. Strabismus may be an early sign of chorioretinitis in children. Associated systemic signs of infection are uncommon. Since ocular involvement may cause the only clinical sign of infection in newborns, newborn infants require ophthalmologic examination to exclude toxoplasmosis. As inflammation subsides, vision improves, but often only incompletely. Episodic flares of chorioretinitis are common and destroy retinal tissue. These multiple recurrences may result in glaucoma.

On ophthalmoscopic examination the acute lesions appear as yellowish white, cotton-like patches that have elevated, indistinct margins surrounded by a zone of hyperemia. The inflammatory exudate in the vitreous may obscure the fundus. Older lesions are atrophic, whitish gray plaques with distinct borders and black spots of choroidal pigment. The lesions may be single or, more commonly, multiple and are usually located near the posterior pole of the retina, although they may be peripheral. Lesions of varying age may be seen simultaneously (Fig. 5). Less commonly, a panuveitis and papillitis with optic atrophy may occur. Isolated anterior uveitis due to toxoplasmosis has never been proved.

### Special Considerations

*Toxoplasmosis in the Immunocompromised Patient.* All forms of toxoplasmosis that occur in normal individuals also occur in immunocompromised individuals (Ruskin and Remington, 1976). Acute toxoplasmosis in the immunocompromised patient may be due to reactivation of latent infection or to acquisition of infection from exogenous sources, including organ transplants and blood or leukocyte transfusions. Immunosuppressed patients with the greatest predilection for life-threatening toxoplasmosis are those receiving immunosuppressive therapy for lymphoproliferative disorders (especially Hodgkin's disease), for hematologic malignancy, or for prevention of organ graft rejection. In immunosuppressed patients the infection is often fulmi-

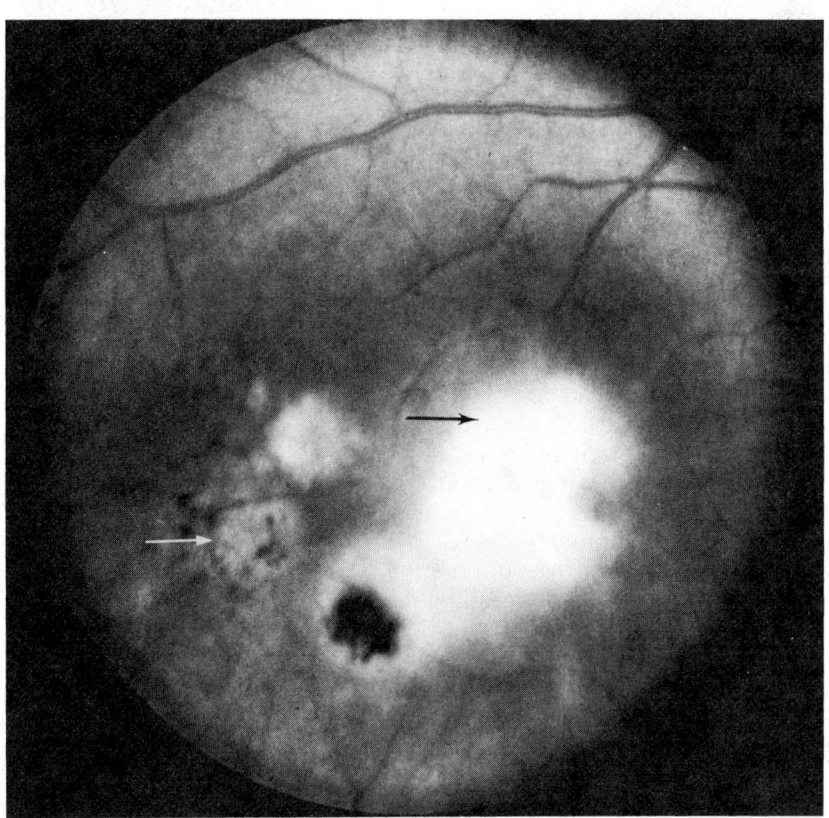

**FIGURE 5.** *Chorioretinitis due to* Toxoplasma. *The characteristic lesion is a focal necrotizing retinitis with cotton-like patches in the fundus. Note that the acute lesions (black arrow) have indistinct borders and appear soft and white, while older lesions (white arrow) are whitish-gray, sharply outlined, and spotted by accumulations of choroidal pigment. (From O'Connor, G. R.: Ocular toxoplasmosis. In Locatcher-Khorazo, D., and Seegal, B. C. (eds.): Microbiology of the Eye. St. Louis, The C. V. Mosby Company, 1972, p. 199.)*

nant and rapidly fatal. Since effective therapy is available, it is incumbent on clinicians to be aware of the clinical presentation in this type of patient.

The most characteristic clinical manifestations of toxoplasmosis in immunocompromised patients result from brain involvement, which is present in over 50 per cent of documented cases. The symptoms and signs are manifestations of diffuse encephalopathy, meningoencephalitis, or cerebral mass lesions and include changes in mental status, headache, seizures, and focal neurologic deficits. The diagnosis of brain involvement can be made by finding trophozoites in a biopsy specimen or in material aspirated from mass lesions that resemble a brain abscess on computerized axial tomography scan. The cerebrospinal fluid typically shows a mononuclear pleocytosis, a moderate elevation in protein concentration, and a normal glucose level. In any immunosuppressed patient with symptoms or signs of brain involvement, the diagnosis of toxoplasmosis must be excluded. Other manifestations of the disease in immunocompromised patients may be nonspecific or reflect inflammation and necrosis of the organs involved, particularly the heart and lungs.

*Toxoplasmosis and Toxoplasma Infection in the Pregnant Woman.* Toxoplasma infection acquired in pregnancy causes symptoms in only about 10 to 20 per cent of mothers; but the fetus is at risk whether symptoms are present or not. Guidelines regarding toxoplasmosis and *Toxoplasma* infection in the pregnant woman have been offered earlier under the heading Transplacental Transmission.

*Congenital Toxoplasmosis.* Most infected newborns are asymptomatic at birth. Some asymptomatic infants may never suffer untoward sequelae of the infection; others will develop chorioretinitis, strabismus, blindness, epilepsy, or psychomotor or mental retardation at any time (weeks, months, or even years later). Those with clinically apparent infection at birth may have all or any combination of the following: a mild nonspecific illness, fever, hypothermia, vomiting, diarrhea, jaundice, rash (most commonly petechiae due to thrombocytopenia), hydrocephalus, microcephaly, cerebral calcifications, microphthalmia, strabismus, cataracts, glaucoma, chorioretinitis, optic atrophy, deafness, lymphadenopathy, pneumonitis, myocarditis, hepatosplenomegaly, convulsions, psychomotor retardation, other CNS signs, anemia, abnormal bleeding, thrombocytopenia, eosinophilia, monocytosis, and abnormal cerebrospinal fluid with xanthochromia, mononuclear pleocytosis, and high protein (grams per cent). *Toxoplasma* does not cause fetal malformations.

## COMPLICATIONS AND SEQUELAE

The lymphadenopathic form of acquired toxoplasmosis is usually self-limited but may persist or recur for months in the presence or absence of constitutional symptoms.

Mental retardation, epilepsy, spasticity, palsies, and severe impairment of vision are common when clinical signs of infection are present at birth. Deafness also may occur. Microcephaly has been reported in approximately 13 per cent and hydrocephalus in approximately 28 per cent of infants with signs or symptoms of toxoplasmosis involving the CNS. These serious sequelae are a threat to all congenitally infected infants whether or not they are symptomatic in the newborn period.

Ocular toxoplasmosis is characterized by frequent relapses. It may result in glaucoma or loss of vision and ultimately may necessitate enucleation.

Acute infection is extremely serious in immunodeficient patients. Although mortality is high, the actual death rate is unknown.

## GEOGRAPHIC VARIATIONS IN DISEASE AND INFECTION

There are considerable geographic variations in prevalence of infection with *Toxoplasma* (Fig. 6). In all areas surveyed, the prevalence of positive serologic reactions increases with age. Generally, there is less human infection in cold regions, in hot and arid areas, and at high elevations. Exceptions do exist: Eskimos, once thought to be free of this infection, have been found to have prevalence rates of 13 to 46 per cent, whereas some isolated tropical communities have little or no *Toxoplasma* infection. It is interesting that these tropical communities do not have known exposure to domestic or feral cats. However, there are also populations who are infected with *T. gondii* and who have no known exposure to cats. The variations in prevalence and incidence of infection from area to area cannot be explained.

The actual incidence of congenital toxoplasmosis is unknown. Approximations per 1000 live births are as follows: Vienna, 6 to 7; Paris, 3; New York City, 1.3; and Mexico City, 2.

## DIAGNOSIS

The diagnosis of acute infection with *Toxoplasma* is made by isolation of *T. gondii* from blood or body fluids. It is also made by demonstration of trophozoites in sections or prepara-

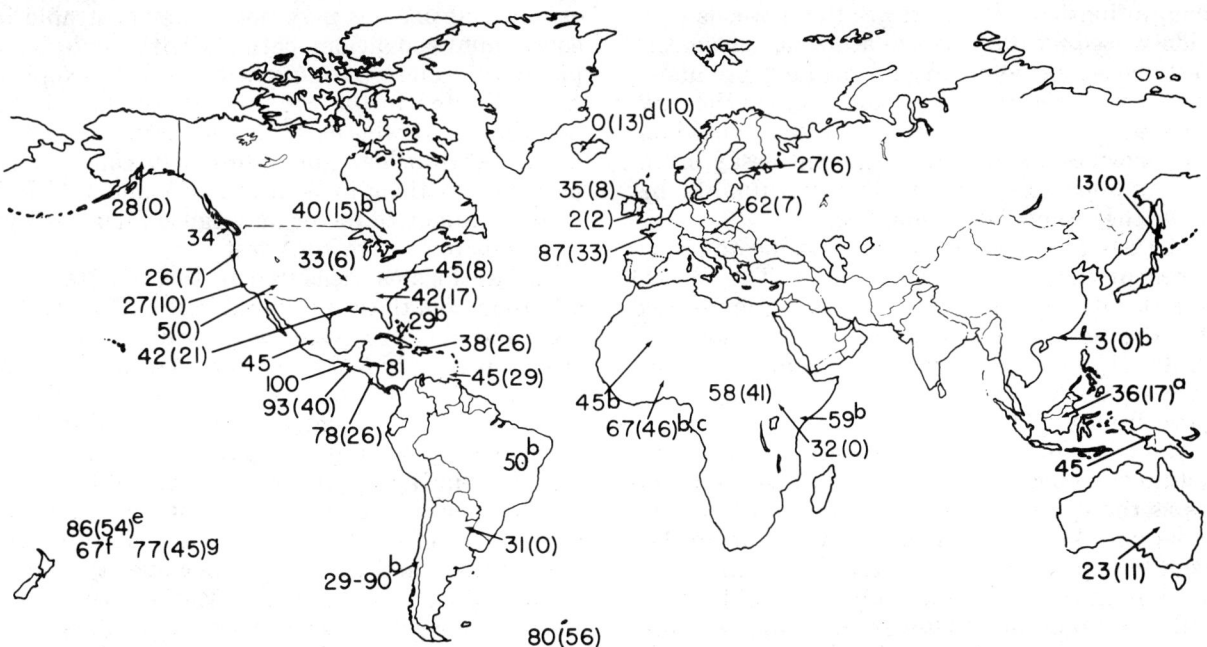

**FIGURE 6.** *Prevalence of antibodies against* Toxoplasma gondii *in individuals in selected locales. Unless otherwise specified, figures outside parentheses equal per cent of positive adults of approximately 30 to 40 years of age; figures inside parentheses equal per cent of positive children less than 10 years of age. a, IHA antibodies, others were IFA or dye test; b, adults with either age range not clearly specified or wider age range than approximately 30 to 40 years of age; c, "juveniles"; d, although 14 individuals between 30 and 39 years of age had no* Toxoplasma *antibody, 29 per cent of 14 individuals 40 to 49 years of age did have* Toxoplasma *antibody; e, Society Island; f, American Samoa; g, Tahiti.*

tions of tissues and body fluids; of cysts in the placenta or tissues of a fetus or newborn; and of characteristic lymph node histology. Serologic tests are also useful for diagnosis.

### Isolation Procedures

The organism can be isolated by inoculation of body fluids, leukocytes, or tissue specimens into the peritoneal cavity of mice or into tissue cultures. Body fluids should be processed and inoculated immediately; tissues and blood may be stored at 4° C overnight. Freezing or treating specimens with formalin kills the organism.

Mice should be examined for *Toxoplasma* organisms in their peritoneal fluid at six to ten days after inoculation, or earlier if they die. Mice surviving for six weeks should be tested for *Toxoplasma* antibody in their serum. If antibody is present, definitive diagnosis is made by visualization of *Toxoplasma* cysts in the mouse brain. If no cysts are seen in mice with *Toxoplasma* antibody, portions of brain, liver, and spleen from the mice should be inoculated into other mice.

Isolation of *T. gondii* from body fluids reflects acute infection, as does isolation from the blood in most patients. Persistent parasitemia in asymptomatic people with latent infection appears to be rare, except perhaps in chronic my-

elogenous leukemia. Isolation from tissues (e.g., skeletal muscle, lung, brain, or eye) obtained by biopsy or at autopsy may reflect the presence of tissue cysts and thus is not proof of acute infection.

### Histologic Diagnosis

Demonstration of trophozoites in tissue sections or smears (e.g., brain biopsy, bone marrow aspirate) or in body fluids (e.g., cerebrospinal fluid, amniotic fluid) establishes the diagnosis of acute toxoplasmosis. Although it is difficult to see the trophozoite with ordinary stains, immunofluorescent antibody techniques have been successful. Demonstration of the tissue cyst is diagnostic of infection with *Toxoplasma* but does not differentiate between acute and chronic infection. Numerous cysts in any organ usually indicate recent acute infection. The presence of cysts in the placenta or tissues of the newborn infant establishes the diagnosis of congenital infection. The characteristic histologic criteria are sufficient to establish the diagnosis of toxoplasmic lymphadenitis (Fig. 3) (Dorfman and Remington, 1973).

### Serologic Tests

The Sabin-Feldman dye test, indirect fluorescent antibody (IFA) tests, and the indirect hemagglutination (IHA) test are the methods most widely used for diagnosis of acute toxoplasmosis. Tests for antigenemia are particularly promising (although experimental) for diagnosis in the newborn and in the immunocompromised individual. The enzyme-linked immunosorbent assay or radioimmunoassay are potentially valuable because they allow for automation.

The dye test is sensitive and specific and measures primarily IgG antibodies. The World Health Organization (WHO) has recommended that dye test titers be expressed in International Units (IU/ml). An international standard reference serum for this purpose is available on request from WHO.

The IFA test is the most widely available procedure and appears to measure the same antibodies as the dye test. In both tests, the titers tend to be parallel. Dye test and IFA test antibodies usually appear one to two weeks after infection, reach high titers (≥1:1000) in six to eight weeks, and then gradually decline over months to years; low titers (1:4 to 1:64) commonly persist for life (Fig. 7). The antibody titer does not correlate with severity of illness.

The IgM-fluorescent antibody (IgM-IFA) test has special value for the diagnosis of acute infection with *T. gondii* because IgM antibodies appear faster (as early as five days after infection) and disappear sooner than IgG antibodies. In most cases, IgM-IFA test antibodies rise rapidly (to levels of 1:80 to ≥1:1000) and fall to low titers (1:10 or 1:20) or disappear within a few weeks or months (Fig. 7). In some patients, they remain positive at low titers for as long as several years. IgM antibodies in the neonate represent synthesis in utero by the infected fetus because IgM does not normally pass the placental barrier. IgM *Tox-*

*oplasma* antibodies may not be demonstrable in some immunodeficient patients with acute toxoplasmosis, most patients with active toxoplasmosis limited to the eye, and approximately 25 per cent of newborns with congenital toxoplasmosis. Antinuclear antibodies may cause false-positive reactions in both the IFA and IgM-IFA tests; rheumatoid factor may cause false-positive reactions in the IgM-IFA test.

The antibodies measured in the IHA test are different from those measured in the IFA and dye tests and may persist for years. Since IHA titers rise later than IFA or dye test titers, the IHA test may be helpful when these titers have stabilized. Because IHA test antibody may be absent in proven congenital infections, it should not be tested for in the diagnosis of congenital toxoplasmosis. There is a great need for proper standardization of methodology for this and all other serologic tests, and particularly for quality control of commercial kits that are often used by laboratories inexperienced in performing these serologic tests.

The complement fixation (CF) test also measures antibodies that may appear several weeks later than those measured in the IFA and dye tests and that may persist for years. A single positive CF test does not indicate acute infection, nor does a negative CF test exclude toxoplasmosis. A significant rise in CF titer (i.e., two serial dilutions performed in parallel on sera obtained several weeks apart) establishes recent infection.

Guidelines for interpretation of test results are presented in Table 1.

The level of *Toxoplasma* antibody in cerebrospinal fluid or aqueous humor may be used to demonstrate local production of antibody in active ocular or CNS toxoplasmosis. Local antibody

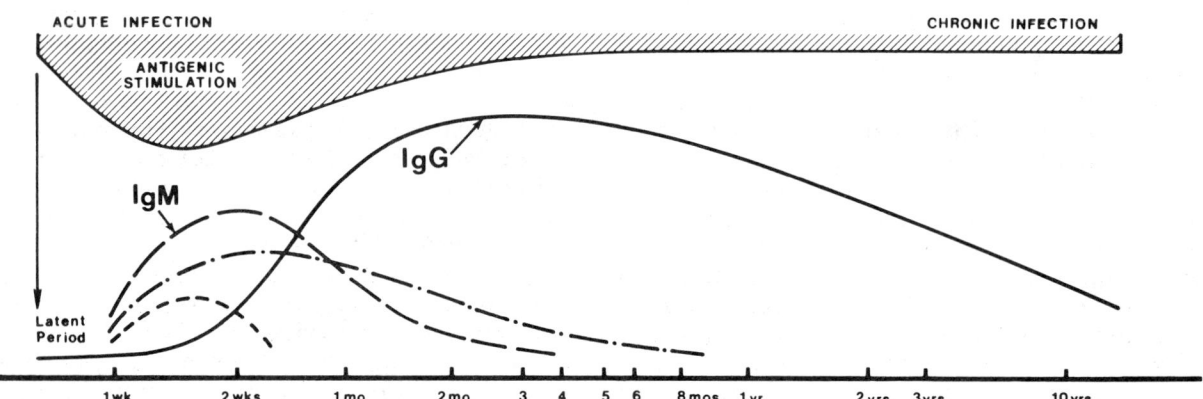

**FIGURE 7.** *Antibody response in Toxoplasma infection in humans. IgM antibodies (— —), detectable by the IgM-IFA test, reach their maximum titer within the first few weeks after infection and may decline within a few weeks (– –) or persist for months (—•—). IgG antibodies (——), detectable by either the Sabin-Feldman dye test or the conventional IFA test, reach their maximum titer within two months, maintain a plateau for months or years, and then decline, but usually persist at a low titer for life. (Data from Desmonts, G.: Feuillets de Biologie 16:61, 1975.)*

**TABLE 1.** Guidelines[a] for Interpretation of Commonly Employed Serologic Tests for Diagnosis of Toxoplasmosis

| TEST (ABBREVIATION) | POSITIVE TITER | TITER IN ACUTE INFECTION | TITER IN CHRONIC (LATENT) INFECTION | DURATION OF ELEVATION OF TITER | SPECIAL CONSIDERATIONS |
|---|---|---|---|---|---|
| Sabin-Feldman dye test | 1:4 undiluted[b] | ≥1:1000 | 1:4 to 1:2000 | years | (1) There are no known cross reactions or false-positives in man. (2) The World Health Organization has recommended that titers be expressed in IU/ml. |
| Indirect fluorescent antibody (IFA) test | 1:10[c] | ≥1:1000 | 1:8 to 1:2000 | years | (1) The same recommendation for expression of test results in IU/ml applies. (2) Antibody measured is the same as that measured in the dye test. (3) Antinuclear antibodies may cause false-positive results. |
| Indirect fluorescent antibody test for IgM *Toxoplasma* antibodies (IgM-IFA) | 1:2 infants[c] 1:10 adults[c] | ≥1:80 | negative to 1:20 | weeks to months; occasionally years | (1) Either antinuclear antibodies or rheumatoid factor (IgM) may cause false-positive results. Rheumatoid factor may be absorbed from serum with heat-aggregated IgG. |
| Indirect hemagglutination (IHA) test | 1:16[c] | ≥1:1000 | 1:16 to 1:256 | years | (1) Not useful for diagnosis of congenital toxoplasmosis. (2) Antibodies by IHA rise later than antibodies measured by dye test and IFA. This test may be especially useful when a rising IHA titer can be demonstrated. |
| Complement fixation (CF) test | 1:4[c] | varies among laboratories | negative to 1:8 | years | (1) Antigen preparations used for this test have not been standardized. (2) See (2) under IHA. |

[a]These guidelines are useful in the interpretation of test results, but exceptions to these generalizations may occur.
[b]In some cases of eye disease, the dye test may be positive only in undiluted serum.
[c]These values are representative, but normal values for each laboratory may differ significantly.

production is assessed by application of the following equation:

$$C = \frac{\text{antibody titer in body fluid}}{\text{antibody titer in serum}}$$
$$\times \frac{\text{concentration of gamma globulin in serum}}{\text{concentration of gamma globulin in body fluid}}$$

A significant correlation coefficient [c] is ≥8 and reflects local antibody production due to active infection of the CNS or eye. If the dye test serum titer is ≥1000, it is usually not possible to demonstrate significant local antibody production by application of this formula. This formula has been applied by using dye test titers and IgM-IFA test titers.

*Acute Acquired Toxoplasma Infection in the Immunocompetent Person.* In settings in which acute acquired *Toxoplasma* infection is suspected in the immunocompetent person, a negative dye test or IFA test virtually excludes the diagnosis. The diagnosis of recent acute acquired infection

is confirmed if there is a seroconversion from a negative to a positive titer (in the absence of transfer of antibody by transfusion), or if there is a serial two-tube rise in titer when sera drawn at three-week intervals are run in parallel. Although suggestive of active infection, one high titer in any test is not diagnostic.

The following guidelines are helpful in interpretation of test results, but exceptions may occur. A dye test or IFA test titer of 1:1000 or greater in the presence of a high IgM-IFA test titer (1:80 or greater) is probably diagnostic of recent acute infection in the presence or absence of symptoms. In immunologically normal people with positive titers in the dye test or IFA test, the absence of IgM-IFA test antibodies almost always excludes the diagnosis of acute infection.

*Ocular Toxoplasmosis.* The diagnosis of ocular toxoplasmosis in older children and adults is difficult because the titer of antibody in the serum does not necessarily correlate with presence of active lesions in the fundus. Indeed, low serologic test titers (1:4 to 1:64) are usual in patients with active toxoplasmic chorioretinitis. For practical purposes, toxoplasmic chorioretinitis is probably excluded if serologic tests are negative when performed on undiluted serum. If retinal lesions are characteristic and serologic tests are positive, the diagnosis can be made with a high degree of confidence. If the retinal lesion is atypical and the serologic test is positive, the diagnosis of toxoplasmosis is only presumptive; a high prevalence of antibodies in the normal population precludes the assumption of a causal relationship in this situation.

*Active Infection in the Immunocompromised Individual.* The available diagnostic techniques, including the IgM-IFA test, are at times insufficient for detection of active infection in immunocompromised patients because antibody response may be abnormal. Serologic tests should be performed to screen for *Toxoplasma* infection in immunocompromised individuals to identify those patients who are at risk for primary infection or reactivation of latent infection (see also the section Prophylaxis).

*Toxoplasmosis and Toxoplasma Infection in the Pregnant Woman.* Any woman who is considering becoming pregnant should have a *Toxoplasma* serologic test performed to determine whether she has *Toxoplasma* infection before pregnancy. (See Transplacental Transmission for a complete discussion of risks to the fetus in relation to *Toxoplasma* infection acquired by the mother before pregnancy versus during pregnancy.)

In the absence of a routine screening program in which *Toxoplasma* serologic tests are performed each month in the pregnant woman, an IgM-IFA test should be performed if any other serologic test is positive at any titer. If the IgM-IFA test is unavailable, the serologic test should be repeated in three weeks in order to determine if the titer is stable or rising. If the IgM-IFA test is negative and an IFA or dye test titer is stable and less than 1:1000 (300 IU), no further evaluation is necessary. Because titers in the dye test or IFA test usually stabilize at high levels ($\geq$1:1000) six to eight weeks or longer after acquisition of infection, if the dye test or IFA test titer is $\geq$1:1000 (300 IU) and stable (regardless of titer in the IgM-IFA test), the infection was acquired at least four weeks earlier and probably more than eight weeks before the serum was obtained. Thus, for practical purposes, if the dye test or IFA test titer is $\geq$1:1000 and stable when measured in the first two months of pregnancy, the fetus is not at risk.

Whereas titers in the dye test or IFA test may have stabilized and peaked by eight weeks after onset of infection, titers in the complement fixation or indirect hemagglutination test may continue to rise for four to six months or longer after acquisition of infection. Therefore, rises in the last two tests may not be helpful in defining when the infection occurred relative to the time of conception.

A common problem is the interpretation of serologic test results in an asymptomatic woman who is tested for *Toxoplasma* antibody late in the first trimester or in the second trimester of pregnancy. Her IFA or dye test titer is found to be in the range of 1:2000, her IgM-IFA test titer is negative, and no significant rise in titer in any test is demonstrable. It is impossible to determine whether her infection occurred before, at, or after conception in this situation.

*Congenital Toxoplasmosis.* Guidelines for interpreting serologic test results in a mother just delivered of an infant suspected of having congenital toxoplasmosis are given in Table 2. These interpretations of serologic test results are not absolutes but can be used until sufficient data upon which to base a definitive advisory statement become available.

Diagnosis of acute toxoplasmosis in the neonate is based on finding either persistent or rising titers in the dye test or IFA test, or a positive IgM-IFA test (at any titer) in the absence of a placental leak. Since rheumatoid factor may be present in a newborn with congenital infection, it is important to exclude the presence of this antibody in an infant with a positive IgM-IFA test. If a placental leak of maternal blood has occurred, the IgM-IFA test titer in the neonate will fall significantly within a week, since the half-life of IgM is approximately three to five days. Passively transferred maternal antibodies may require six to twelve months or longer, depending on the original titer, to disappear from the infant's serum. Synthesis of *Toxoplasma* antibody by the infected infant is usually demonstrable by the third month of life if the infant is not treated, but it may be delayed until the sixth or ninth month if the infant is treated. Thus, at the time the infant begins to synthesize antibody, infection may be documented serologically even when IgM antibodies are not demonstrable. This may be accomplished by computation of the specific "antibody load," i.e., the ratio of specific serum antibody titer to the level of serum IgG in mother and infant. For example, in an uninfected infant with only maternal antibody, there is no change in antibody load because, as the titer of antibody decreases in the infant's serum, total IgG decreases in a similar manner. During the second and third months, the amount of IgG synthesized by the infant increases. Because this newly synthesized IgG does not contain *Toxoplasma* antibodies, the antibody load decreases and will continue to decrease as IgG synthesis in the child

**TABLE 2. Guidelines for Interpretation of Antibody Test. Results in a Mother Just Delivered of a Child Suspected of Having Congenital Toxoplasmosis**

| CONGENITAL INFECTION IN CHILD | SEROLOGIC TEST RESULTS IN MOTHER | |
| --- | --- | --- |
| | Dye Test[a] | IgM Fluorescent Antibody Test |
| Most often present | 300 to 3000 IU/ml (1:1200 to 1:12,000) | Positive |
| Often present | 1000 to 3000 IU/ml (1:4000 to 1:12,000)[b] | Negative |
| Seldom present | 300 to 1000 IU/ml (1:1200 to 1:4000)[b] | Negative |
| Possible[c] | < 300 IU/ml | Positive |
| Excluded | < 300 IU/ml | Negative |

[a]Figures in parentheses indicate approximate titers expressed as reciprocal of serum dilution, which correspond to the titers expressed in international units.
[b]There is no information concerning interpretation of high dye test titers in a mother just delivered of a child suspected of having congenital toxoplasmosis in regions in which a significant number of infected mothers have high dye test titers (e.g., Central America).
[c]Usually present if maternal dye test is rising after delivery; usually absent if maternal dye test is not rising.

Adapted from Remington and Desmonts, 1976.

progresses. In congenitally infected infants, the production of antibody may vary considerably from one case to another. Early and delayed antibody production can be demonstrated by increases in antibody load.

## THERAPY

### Therapy in Specific Clinical Settings

The need for and duration of therapy are determined by the clinical severity of the illness and by the individual who is infected.

Most immunologically normal patients with the lymphadenopathic form of acute toxoplasmosis do not require specific treatment. Indication for treatment in these cases is the presence of severe and persistent symptoms. Evidence of damage to vital organs is also an indication for therapy in the apparently normal individual. Infections acquired in laboratory accidents or via transfusions may be more severe than naturally acquired infections and probably should be treated.

Patients with active chorioretinitis should be treated with specific drug therapy. Corticosteroids are usually added to the regimen when there is potential for serious visual impairment secondary to macular or optic nerve involvement.

Toxoplasmosis should be treated in a patient whose resistance to infection is compromised by an underlying disease or by therapy (e.g., corticosteroids or cytotoxic drugs). Either serologic evidence of acute infection in an immunocompromised patient, whether or not signs and symptoms of infection are present, or the demonstration of trophozoites in tissue, regardless of serologic test titers, is an indication for therapy. In 80 per cent of immunocompromised patients in whom the diagnosis was established antemortem, improvement occurred when specific therapy was administered. The major problem lies in making the diagnosis early enough to institute treatment.

If a pregnant woman who acquires infection at any time during pregnancy is treated, the chance of congenital infection in her infant is decreased but not eliminated. In one series, the incidence of infection was decreased from 17 per cent to 5 per cent, and in another series it was decreased from 60 per cent to 23 per cent. The drugs effective in the only two reported studies were spiramycin in the study from France and pyrimethamine plus sulfonamide in the study from Germany. Because of the potential teratogenicity of pyrimethamine, sulfadiazine (which is highly effective in animal models when used alone) should be used alone if treatment is to be given in the first trimester of pregnancy. Spiramycin (not available in the United States) has also been used safely for treatment during the first trimester of pregnancy. Because of the high probability of severe damage when infection occurs early in fetal life, therapeutic abortion has been recommended by some authorities. Because the risk of transmission of the infection to the fetus is low (approximately 15 per cent) in the first trimester and because the incidence of congenital toxoplasmosis can be reduced significantly by interpartum therapy, other authorities recommend treatment rather than abortion, reasoning that this would result in saving a significant number of healthy fetuses. The decision about mode of therapy ultimately must be made with the well-informed pregnant patient who is aware of the risks discussed above. There are no carefully controlled studies to support the contention that a pregnant woman who has *Toxoplasma* antibody and a history of habitual abortion will benefit from treatment.

Both symptomatic and asymptomatic infants with congenital toxoplasmosis should be treated in an effort to prevent further destruction of vital organs. Guidelines for treatment of congenitally infected infants in whom the diagnosis is strongly suspected are outlined in Table 3. The guidelines are those of Dr. Jacques Couvreur, who has treated over 100 cases of congenital toxoplasmosis using this regimen.

### Therapeutic Agents

***Pyrimethamine Plus Sulfadiazine or Trisulfapyrimidines.*** Pyrimethamine and sulfadiazine act synergistically against *Toxoplasma* in vivo with a combined activity that is eight times the amount expected if their effects were merely additive. There are no reports of controlled clinical trials in which adult humans with severe symptomatic toxoplasmosis were treated with this combination; nevertheless, clinical experience confirms their efficacy. There is evidence that treatment of an acutely infected pregnant woman may prevent infection of her fetus (see above under Therapy in Specific Clinical Settings). The simultaneous use of both drugs is indicated except during the first trimester of pregnancy. Comparative tests have shown that sulfapyrazine, sulfamethazine, and sulfamerazine are about as effective as sulfadiazine. All the other sulfonamides tested (sulfathiazole, sulfapyridine, sulfadimetine, and sulfisoxazole) are much less effective.

***Pyrimethamine.*** In adults, a loading dose of 100 to 200 mg pyrimethamine should be given orally in two divided doses on the first day of treatment. In young children, a loading dose of 2 mg/kg body weight should be given for the first two to three days of treatment. Infants are given 1 mg/kg body weight as a loading dose. A maintenance dose for all ages is 1 mg/kg body weight (with a maximum of 25 mg) in one dose. Administration of the maintenance dose at three- to four-day intervals has been suggested in view of the drug's half-life of four to five days. Since there are no data concerning absorption of the drug in

---

**TABLE 3.   Guidelines for Therapy of Congenital Toxoplasmosis***

**DRUGS**

1. *Pyrimethamine + sulfadiazine or trisulfapyrimidines:* 21-day course.
   a. Pyrimethamine: 1 mg/kg by the oral route every two to three or even four days (since the half-life of pyrimethamine is four to five days).
   b. Sulfadiazine: 50 to 100 mg/kg/day by the oral route in two daily divided doses.
2. *Spiramycin*[a]: 30- to 45-day course. 100mg/kg/day by the oral route in two daily divided doses.
3. *Corticosteroids* (prednisone or methylprednisolone): 1 to 2 mg/kg/day by the oral route in two divided doses. Continued until the inflammatory process (e.g., high cerebrospinal fluid protein, chorioretinitis) has subsided; dosage then to be tapered progressively to nil.
4. *Folinic acid:* 5 mg twice weekly during pyrimethamine treatment.

**INDICATIONS**

1. *Overt congenital toxoplasmosis:* Pyrimethamine + sulfadiazine + folinic acid: 21 days. During the first year of life, the child is given three to four courses of pyrimethamine + sulfadiazine, separated with spiramycin courses of 30 to 45 days.[a] No treatment is usually given after 12 months of age.
2. *Overt congenital toxoplasmosis with evidence of inflammatory process* (chorioretinitis, high cerebrospinal fluid protein content, generalized infection, jaundice): As in (1) above + corticosteroid treatment.
3. *Subclinical congenital toxoplasmosis:* As in (1) above.
4. *Healthy newborn in whom serologic testing has not provided definitive results but maternal infection was acquired during pregnancy:* One course of pyrimethamine + sulfadiazine for 21 days, followed by spiramycin. Then wait for laboratory evidence for diagnosis.

---

[a]If spiramycin is not available, we recommend continued use of the pyrimethamine-sulfonamide combination for the total period of therapy.

*Courtesy of Dr. Jacques Couvreur, Laboratoire de Sérologie Néonatale et de Recherche sur la Toxoplasmose, Institut de Puériculture, Paris.

Adapted from Remington and Desmonts, 1976.

the patient who is very ill, daily administration is recommended in this situation. Daily therapy is recommended for the active infection in the eye. Pyrimethamine is available only in tablet form. For infants, this may be crushed and administered with food or fluid.

Pyrimethamine is a folic acid antagonist and therefore produces a dose-related, reversible, and usually gradual depression of the bone marrow. Thrombocytopenia, leukopenia, and anemia may occur. All patients treated with pyrimethamine should have platelet and peripheral blood cell counts twice weekly.

Folinic acid (calcium leucovorin) should be administered in conjunction with pyrimethamine therapy to prevent suppression of the bone marrow. The optimal frequency for administration of folinic acid is unknown. An oral dose of 5 to 10 mg is recommended daily in older children and adults, or 5 mg twice weekly in infants. Bakers' yeast (three to four cakes daily) may be used if folinic acid is not available to prevent toxicity due to pyrimethamine. Unlike folic acid, neither folinic acid nor Bakers' yeast inhibits the action of pyrimethamine on *T. gondii*.

*Sulfadiazine or Trisulfapyrimidines.* Sulfadiazine or trisulfapyrimidine is administered in the following doses. In older children and adults, the loading dose is 50 to 75 mg/kg body weight; thereafter, a daily dose of 75 to 100 mg/kg body weight is administered in four divided doses at intervals of approximately six hours. In infants, the loading dose is 50 to 100 mg/kg body weight; thereafter, a total daily dose of 100 to 150 mg/kg body weight is administered in two or four divided doses every six hours. Tablet and liquid oral forms and intravenous forms are available.

The potential toxic effects of sulfonamides (e.g., crystalluria, hematuria, and rash) must be carefully monitored.

*Other Drugs.* Trimethoprim alone or in combination with a sulfonamide has not been proved effective in humans, but the activity of this combination in vitro and in vivo in animal models warrants carefully controlled clinical trials. This combination is significantly less active than is the combination of pyrimethamine with sulfadiazine.

### Duration of Therapy

The optimal duration of specific therapy of toxoplasmosis is unknown. Patients who appear to be immunologically normal but have severe and persistent symptoms or damage to vital organs (e.g., chorioretinitis, myocarditis) require specific therapy for at least four to six weeks, or possibly longer.

In the immunocompromised patient, therapy should continue for at least four to six weeks *beyond* complete resolution of all signs and symptoms of active disease. Careful follow-up of these patients is imperative because relapse may occur, requiring prompt reinstitution of therapy. Although therapy may be effective against *T. gondii* trophozoites and may induce a beneficial response clinically, it does not eradicate the cyst form from the CNS and perhaps from other tissues.

Desmonts and Couvreur treated the acutely infected pregnant woman with 2 to 3 grams spiramycin daily, administered orally in four divided doses. This regimen was administered intermittently from the time of diagnosis until term. A three-week course of treatment was alternated with a two-week interval without treatment. Another treatment regimen was used by Kraubig et al. in Germany. It consisted of a course of sulfonamide and pyrimethamine followed by one to two courses of sulfonamide administered alone or in combination with pyrimethamine. Each course of therapy was given for approximately two weeks. The courses of treatment were alternated with three- to four-week intervals without treatment. Pyrimethamine was not given in the first trimester of pregnancy.

Infants with congenital toxoplasmosis should be treated as outlined in Table 3.

### PROPHYLAXIS

Measures for prophylaxis against *Toxoplasma* involve intervention in the cycle of transmission. Prevention of infection by *T. gondii* is most important in immunodeficient patients and seronegative pregnant women.

Meat should be heated to 60° C to kill cysts. Freezing to −20° C will kill cysts in meat, but freezers available commercially in most areas of the world do not reach or maintain this temperature reliably. Hands should be washed after touching uncooked meat. Fruits and vegetables may be contaminated with oocysts and should be washed. Contact with cat feces should be avoided.

Although there are no definitive data to allow a firm recommendation regarding the use of whole blood or leukocyte transfusions or organ transplants when donors are seropositive for *Toxoplasma* antibodies, the following are our recommendations: Blood or blood products donated by people with *Toxoplasma* antibody should not be used in immunosuppressed recipients, and organs of those with *Toxoplasma* antibody should not be given to seronegative recipients.

A nontoxic drug that eliminates the organism in the tissue cyst form as well as in the trophozoite form is needed to prevent the devastating complications of recrudescent infection in immunocompromised patients.

For prevention of transmission of *Toxoplasma* to the fetus, see Therapy in Specific Clinical Settings.

There is no effective vaccine to prevent infection with *Toxoplasma*. Because maternal immunity appears to prevent congenital transmission of *T. gondii*, development of a vaccine for use in nonimmune women of childbearing age should be explored. Vaccines that prevent oocyst development in household cats could interrupt the life cycle of *T. gondii*.

### References

Desmonts, G.: Serodiagnostic de la toxoplasmose. Intérêt et limites des différentes méthodes. Leur application au diagnostic de la toxoplasmose acquise. Feuillets de Biologie 6:61, 1975.

Dorfman, R. F., and Remington, J. S.: Value of lymph node biopsy in the diagnosis of acute acquired toxoplasmosis. N Engl J Med 289:878, 1973.

Dubey, J. P., Miller, N. L., and Frenkel, J. K.: Characterization of the new fecal form of *Toxoplasma gondii*. J Parasitol 56:447, 1970.

Dubey, J. P., Swan, G. V., and Frenkel, J. K.: A simplified method for isolation of *Toxoplasma gondii* from the feces of cats. J Parasitol 58:1005, 1972.

Feldman, H. A.: Toxoplasmosis. N Engl J Med 279:1370 and 1431, 1968.

Ghatak, N. R., Poon, T. P., and Zimmerman, H. M.: Toxoplasmosis of the central nervous system in the adult: A light and electron microscopic study of three cases. Arch Pathol 89:337, 1970.

O'Connor, G. R.: Ocular toxoplasmosis. In Locatcher-Khorazo, D., and Seegal, B. C. (eds.): Microbiology of the Eye. St. Louis, The C. V. Mosby Company, 1972, p. 199.

O'Connor, G. R.: Manifestations and management of ocular toxoplasmosis. Bull NY Acad Med 50:192, 1974.

Remington, J. S., and Desmonts, G.: Toxoplasmosis. In Remington, J. S., and Klein, J. O. (eds.): Infectious Diseases of the Fetus and Newborn Infant. Philadelphia, W. B. Saunders Company, 1976, p. 191.

Ruskin, J., and Remington, J. S.: Toxoplasmosis in the compromised host. Ann Intern Med 84:193, 1976.

Siim, J. C.: Acquired toxoplasmosis. JAMA 147:1641, 1951.

# 249 *TRICHINELLOSIS*

## *Z. S. Pawlowski, M.D.*

### DEFINITION

Trichinellosis is a zoonotic infection caused by *Trichinella spiralis*. Symptomatic infections have an acute allergic phase and a protracted phase with muscle inflammation and degeneration, metabolic disorders, and restoration of damaged muscle tissue. Trichinellosis may be fatal when it is not diagnosed and treated properly (Gould, 1970).

### ETIOLOGY

Man may ingest infectious larvae of *T. spiralis* in the incompletely cooked muscle tissue of many domestic or wild animals. The most common source of trichinellosis is infected pork; less common sources (Fig. 1) include the meat of wild animals—e.g., polar bear (Alaska, Siberia); wild boar (Europe, Hawaii); brown or black bear (Canada); bush pig or warthog (Africa) and the domesticated dog (Alaska, Indonesia) and horse (Italy) (Pawlowski, 1980).

Within three days after they are ingested, larvae become adult worms and penetrate into the mucosa of the small intestine. As early as the fifth day after infection, the first newborn *T. spiralis* larvae are produced by fertilized female worms (Fig. 2) (Gould et al., 1963). After migration through lymphatics and blood vessels, the larvae invade the fibers of striated muscles. A few may reach the myocardium or internal organs, but they encyst only in skeletal muscle. Encapsulation of coiled larvae takes a minimum of 17 days after they enter the muscle fibers. One female worm produces about 1500 larvae. In intensive infections more than 1000 larvae may be present per g of human deltoid muscle. Encysted larvae are gradually destroyed by the host and become calcified after six to eight years.

The life cycle is identical in man, hog, rat, and other infected animals. Traditionally, hogs have acquired trichinellosis from uncooked garbage containing infected porkscraps. Rats can also be infected by uncooked garbage and serve as another source of infection for domestic or wild hogs. With the exceptions of Australasia, the Pacific islands other than Hawaii, China, and Japan, trichinellosis is endemic throughout the temperate regions of the world wherever pork is eaten. Cooking garbage before it is fed to hogs, meat inspection, and public education have greatly reduced the prevalence of trichinellosis in Europe and the United States (Fig. 3) (Zimmerman et al., 1973).

### PATHOGENESIS AND PATHOLOGY

Adult worms provoke a mononuclear cellular infiltration of the small intestinal mucosa. Intes-

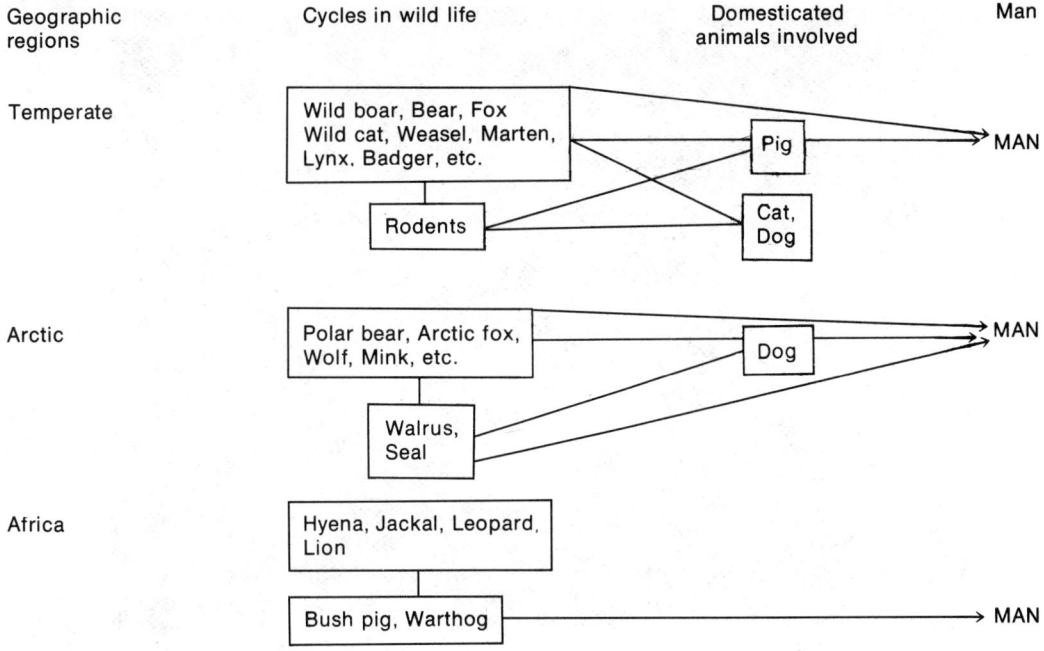

| Geographic regions | Cycles in wild life | Domesticated animals involved | Man |
|---|---|---|---|

**Temperate**

Wild boar, Bear, Fox Wild cat, Weasel, Marten, Lynx, Badger, etc.

Rodents

Pig

Cat, Dog

→ MAN

**Arctic**

Polar bear, Arctic fox, Wolf, Mink, etc.

Walrus, Seal

Dog

→ MAN

**Africa**

Hyena, Jackal, Leopard, Lion

Bush pig, Warthog

→ MAN

**FIGURE 1.** *Transmission of trichinellosis to man in different geographic regions.*

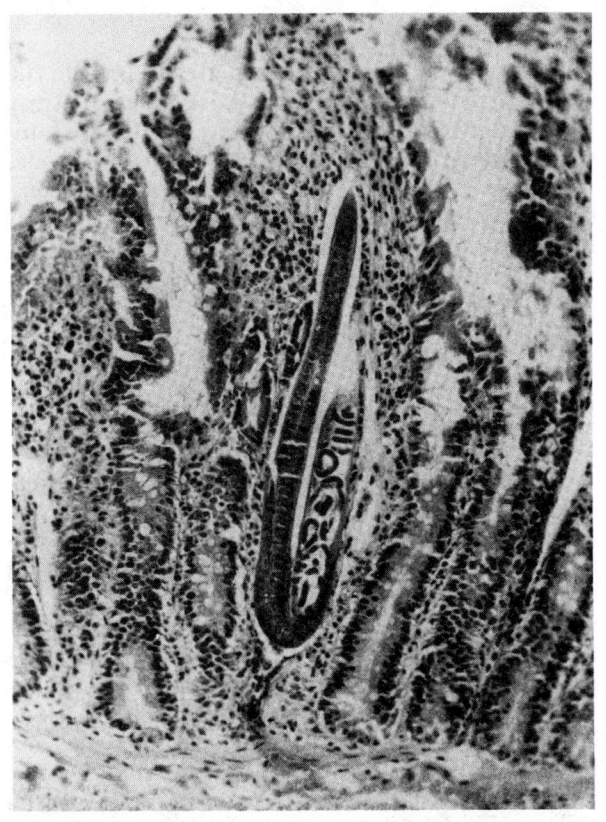

**FIGURE 2.** *Gravid adult female* Trichina *embedded in a villus of the small intestine. Note second generation filariform larvae within the uterus in the right portion of the segment. × 120 (From Gould, S. E., Hinerman, E. L., Batsakis, J. G., and Beamer, P. R.: Am J Clin Pathol 40:197, 1963.)*

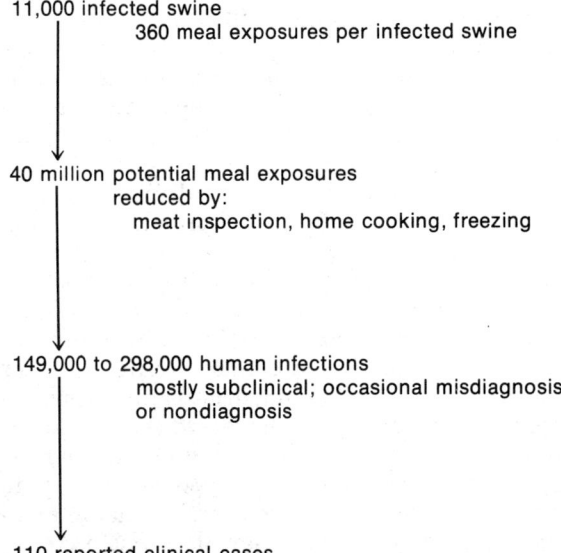

11,000 infected swine
    360 meal exposures per infected swine

40 million potential meal exposures
    reduced by:
        meat inspection, home cooking, freezing

149,000 to 298,000 human infections
    mostly subclinical; occasional misdiagnosis
    or nondiagnosis

110 reported clinical cases

**FIGURE 3.** *Estimate of transmission rate of trichinellosis in the United States (Zimmerman et al., 1973).*

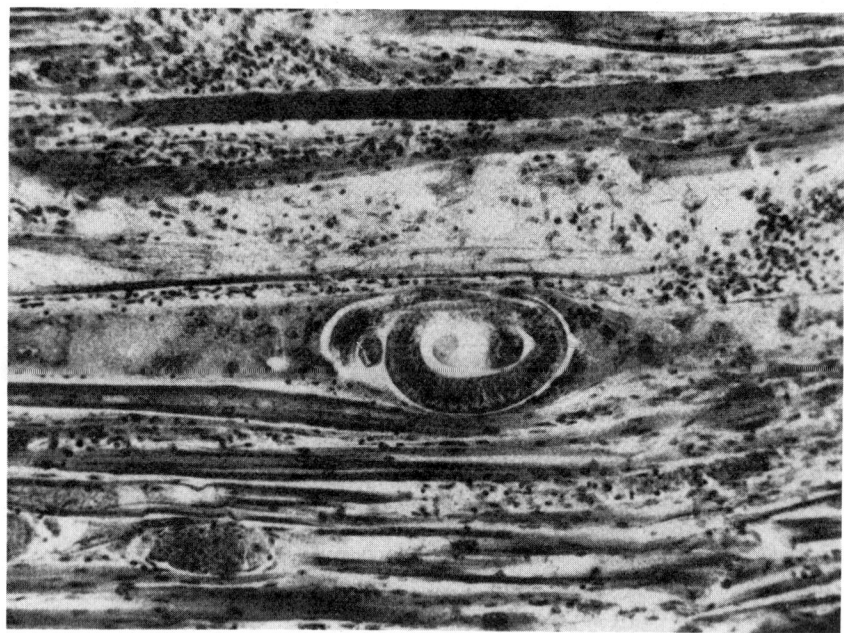

**FIGURE 4.** *Encysted* Trichina *larva in human skeletal muscle fiber four weeks after infection. The fiber has under-gone basophilic transformation, and the muscle nuclei seem to be increased in number. The cyst wall has not yet formed. Note the degeneration of adjacent fibers and infiltration of histiocytes and leukocytes including eosinophils. × 125 (From Gould, S. E., Hinerman, E. L., Batsakis, J. G., and Beamer, P. R.: Am J Clin Pathol 40:197, 1963.)*

tinal infection rarely causes abdominal symptoms but plays an important role in stimulating immunologic processes. In an immune host, the life-span of adult worms is much shorter, and females produce fewer larvae. When *T. spiralis* larvae invade the muscle, they disturb the local ultrastructure and the metabolic process of adjacent muscle fibers, resulting in basophilic transformation (Fig. 4). A myositis follows, characterized by muscle fiber damage, cellular infiltration, fibrous tissue production, and finally destruction of muscle fibers and encapsulation of larvae. In the months and years that follow, the encapsulated larvae gradually die, provoking an intense granulomatous reaction or foreign body cellular response that ends in a fibrotic scar or calcification. This process may be responsible for prolonged muscular symptoms.

In early trichinellosis the most severe symptoms are caused by hypersensitivity and inflammatory reactions. Small vessel vasculitis is manifested by hemorrhagic conjunctivitis, splinter hemorrhages under the fingernails and periorbital edema. Fever and malaise are thought to be due to absorption of toxic products of the larvae and to the development of hypersensitivity to these substances. Larvae may induce acute myocarditis, although encystment does not occur in the myocardium.

In the later stages of severe trichinellosis, metabolic disorders characterized by hypoalbumine-

mia and hypopotassemia secondary to muscle tissue damage may dominate the clinical picture. Muscle contractures and atrophy may follow untreated severe trichinellosis.

At any stage of trichinellosis, unexpected complications may occur owing to hypersensitivity or migration of *T. spiralis* larvae into tissues other than muscle.

## CLINICAL MANIFESTATIONS

Trichinellosis is frequently asymptomatic (Fig. 3) when the intensity of infection is less than 1 larva per g of deltoid muscle tissue. On the other hand, the frequency and severity of allergic reactions may be out of proportion to the size of the inoculum. The incubation period is between 5 and 46 days, but in intensive infections it may be shorter (5 to 10 days). During the incubation period, abdominal pain, diarrhea, and nausea may occur but are uncommon (12 per cent). The disease usually begins with allergic manifestations characterized by fever, malaise, myalgia, periorbital edema, and eosinophilia. Fever is usually over 38° C and may be remittent for one to three weeks. Malaise is often severe and persists longer than fever. Myalgia, which is particularly severe in the ocular, brachial, and crural muscles, may continue for months. Some muscles are painful when examined or used. Periorbital edema is present in 86 per cent of patients and is often complicated by subconjunctival and subungual hemorrhages; all these signs disappear within one to two weeks.

Eosinophilia, which is usually greater than 20 per cent and may be greater than 50 per cent, frequently persists for several months and is often the only sign of trichinellosis. In very serious cases, the number of eosinophils may be low. The blood leukocyte count is usually greater than 10,000/mm$^3$. The first chemical evidence of a muscle disorder is elevation of the serum creatine phosphokinase (CPK) and the serum transaminase levels that may be observed by the second week of the disease. By the third week, hypoalbuminemia may occur with concentrations of as low as 2.5 gm/100 ml. Despite hypergammaglobulinemia, the total serum protein level may be quite low. Severe hypoalbuminemia causes hydrostatic edema, mainly of the back and lower extremities. Hypopotassemia usually accompanies hypoalbuminemia and may cause cardiac disorders in the later stages of trichinellosis. Recovery from these metabolic disorders may take as long as two to four months in patients with untreated severe disease. Muscle atrophy and contractures may also occur.

The course of trichinellosis may be asymptomatic with mild eosinophilia only; abortive with myalgia only; mild with moderate fever and typical symptoms that disappear within three weeks; moderate with high fever and metabolic disorders; or severe with high fever, severe metabolic disorders and cardiac, pulmonary, or cerebral complications. Severe disease may be fatal.

## COMPLICATIONS AND SEQUELAE

Hypersensitivity reactions, intense cardiac involvement, and adrenal cortical insufficiency are responsible for the early deaths in fulminating trichinellosis. Deaths that occur between the third and fifth weeks of disease are usually due to cardiac, pulmonary, or cerebral complications.

In early trichinellosis, myocardial inflammation causes decreased cardiac contractability and conduction disorders. Later in the disease, hypoalbuminemia and hypopotassemia further impair cardiac function. Pneumonitis, bronchitis, and Loeffler's syndrome are unusual complications of early trichinellosis, but secondary bacterial pneumonia is common after the third week of severe disease. Meningitis, encephalopathy, and focal neurologic impairment are rare complications that occur only during the larval migratory phase of severe trichinellosis.

Recovery can be slow. Myalgia, inflammation around encapsulated larvae, and impaired elec-tromyography may last for years after the infection. The symptoms and signs of muscular involvement during severe untreated trichinellosis usually disappear within one to three years without permanent sequelae. Contractures and atrophy are very rare. Permanent impairment of the eye, central nervous system, heart, or lung can be caused by ectopic localization of larvae.

## GEOGRAPHIC VARIATIONS

In the last two decades, two new strains of *T. spiralis* have been found: *T. spiralis nativa* in the Arctic and *T. spiralis nelsoni* in Africa south of the Sahara. Both strains are less infective for man than classic *T. spiralis,* but the Arctic strain seems to be more immunogenic, more pathogenic, and less sensitive to corticosteroid therapy. The African strain seems to be much less pathogenic and less infective. A new species, *T. pseudospiralis,* has been found in wild animals in Asia but not in man. These larvae were less coiled and unencapsulated.

The different range of hosts available within the geographic distribution of *T. spiralis* causes geographic differences in the transmission and epidemiology of trichinellosis (Fig. 1). Infections of wild animals serve an important role as a reservoir and source of infection whenever man joins the natural cycle by eating the raw or undercooked meat of wild animals.

## DIAGNOSIS

Fever, malaise, and myalgia are common in many infectious diseases, but the clinical signs of periorbital edema, conjunctival hemorrhages, and marked eosinophilia are more specific for trichinellosis. A group of people, such as a family or a party of hunters, who all ingest the same suspicious food and who present these signs and symptoms can be given the clinical diagnosis of trichinellosis. Food intoxication and acute gastroenteritis must be considered when gastrointestinal symptoms are present.

In the allergic phase of the disease, trichinellosis must be differentiated from typhoid, septicemia, and influenza on the one hand, and serum sickness, drug allergy, and collagen vascular diseases on the other. Trichinellosis is sometimes first diagnosed by an ophthalmologist when eye signs are prominent.

Elevated serum transaminase and creatine phosphokinase levels are helpful in establishing the diagnosis. The intradermal skin test, which is read within 15 minutes and reflects immediate hypersensitivity, becomes positive three weeks after infection. If positive, it is helpful, but many false-negative reactions are reported. The most useful specific serologic tests for trichinellosis are bentonite flocculation (the bentonite is treated with an extract of muscle larvae) and counter-immunoelectrophoresis of the patient's serum against larval extracts. These tests also become positive three weeks after infection. The indirect fluorescent antibody test becomes positive earlier but is less widely available.

Definitive diagnosis is made by finding larvae in muscle biopsies or by finding adult worms in the gastrointestinal mucosa at autopsy if early death occurs. The deltoid, biceps, and gastrocnemius muscles yield the highest number of positive biopsies. Part of the biopsy section should be compressed between glass slides for direct microscopic examination (Fig. 5), part should be digested before examination (Fig. 6), and part should be fixed and sectioned for staining (Fig. 4).

## TREATMENT

Ethanol may help prevent infection if it is drunk concurrently or a few hours after ingestion of infected meat. Gastric lavage also has some prophylactic value. Saline purgatives and anthelmintics (piperazine or thiabendazole both at daily dose of 50 mg/kg for five days) may be able to prevent the disease if taken a few days after ingestion of infected meat. Piperazine, tetramisole, pyrantel, or mebendazole should be taken at any stage of the disease to eliminate adult *T. spiralis* (Campbell and Blair, 1974).

In severe allergic trichinellosis, high doses of corticosteroids and circulatory support may save the lives of heavily infected patients. Smaller doses of corticosteroids readily alleviate the symptoms and signs of mild disease. In light or abortive cases, only antipyretics and analgesics are needed. When metabolic disorders dominate, replacement therapy with albumin and potassium may be necessary. Prompt institution of treatment and intensive rehabilitative care accelerate recovery from severe disease.

## PROPHYLAXIS

The individual can protect himself from trichinellosis by cooking all meat thoroughly, especially pork, wild boar, or bear meat. Cooking until meat changes from pink to gray (65° C) provides a good margin of safety. Public health control measures include surveillance of the wildlife population and introduction of preventive measures such as cooking garbage and offal fed to pigs, rodent control, meat inspection, deep-freezing carcasses or canned meat products for at least 36 hours at −30° C, and sanitary education of pig-breeders, hunters, butchers, and consumers.

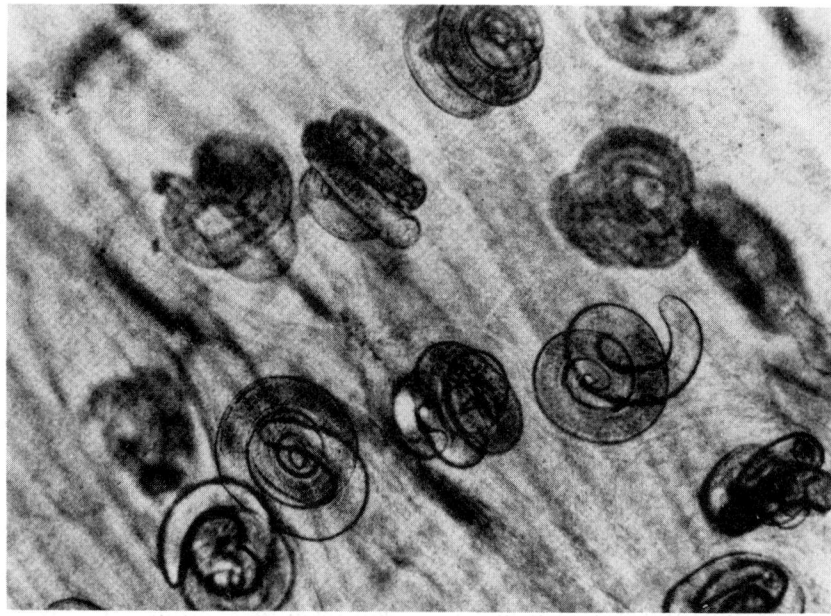

**FIGURE 5.**   *Encysted larvae in compressed, unstained skeletal muscle seen by stereoscopic microscopy (× 75). The cyst walls are transparent. (From Gould, S. E., Hinerman, E. L., Batsakis, J. G., and Beamer, P. R.: Am J Clin Pathol 40:197, 1963.)*

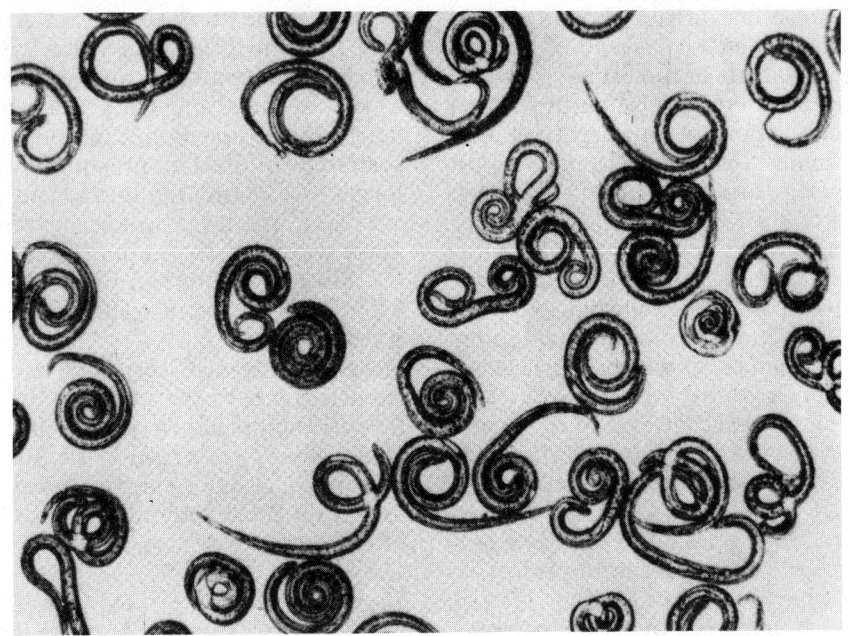

**FIGURE 6.** *Larvae freed from cysts by digestion of ground muscle at 37° C in 1 per cent HCl and 1 per cent pepsin. The tightly coiled forms are motile. Elongated or partially uncoiled larvae are dead or dying. × 40 (From Gould, S. E., Hinerman, E. L., Batsakis, J. G., and Beamer, P. R.: Am J Clin Pathol 40:197, 1963.)*

### References

Campbell, W. C., and Blair, L. S.: Chemotherapy of *Trichinella spiralis* infections: A review. Exp Parasitol 35:304, 1974.

Gould, S. E. (ed.): Trichinosis in Man and Animals. Springfield, Ill., Charles C Thomas, 1970.

Gould, S. E., Hinerman, E. L., Batsakis, J. G., and Beamer, P. R.: Diagnostic patterns: *Trichinella spiralis.* Am J Clin Pathol 40:197, 1963.

Kim, C. W. (ed.): Proceedings of the Third International Conference on Trichinellosis. New York, Intext Educational Publishers, 1974.

Kim, C. W. and Pawlowski, Z. (eds.): Proceedings of the Fourth International Conference on Trichinellosis. Warsaw, 1978.

Pawlowski, Z. S.: Control of Trichinellosis. In Proceedings of the Fifth International Conference on Trichinellosis. Noordwijk aan Zee, 1980.

Zimmermann, W. J., Steele, J. H., and Kagan, I. G.: Trichiniasis in the U.S. population, 1966–1970. Prevalence and epidemiologic factors. Health Services Rep 88:606, 1973.

# VISCERAL LARVA MIGRANS 250

## Carolyn Coker Huntley, M.D.

### DEFINITION

Visceral larva migrans (VLM) is a clinical syndrome characterized by eosinophilia and evidence of visceral involvement caused by the larval migratory phase of roundworms indigenous to lower animal species. A similar disease may also occur during the larval migratory phases of *Ascaris lumbricoides, Ancylostoma duodenale, Necator americanus,* and *Strongyloides stercoralis,* roundworms whose definitive host is man.

### ETIOLOGY

*Toxocara canis,* the common roundworm of dogs, has most often been incriminated as the cause of VLM, and the syndrome has become synonymous with *T. canis* infection in the minds of many physicians. Other animal roundworms can, however, cause an illness indistinguishable from *T. canis* infection. These helminths include *Toxocara cati; Ascaris suum,* the pig roundworm; *Capillaria hepatica,* a rat liver parasite requiring another rat or cat as the intermediate host; and *Dirofilaria immitis,* the dog heart worm that is considered to be the most common cause of tropical eosinophilia in the western hemisphere. The role of *T. cati* in VLM is unknown because of the difficulty of distinguishing this parasite from *T. canis* in tissue sections. *Toxascaris leonina* has been suspected as the cause of VLM in northern Canada (Unruh et al., 1973) because of the prevalence of this parasite and the absence of *T. canis* in the dog population of this area.

*T. canis* is an almost universal infection of puppies owing to transplacental passage of larvae. Ova are found in the stools of the pup by 3 weeks of age. After a period of embryonation in the soil at appropriate conditions of temperature and moisture, ova become infective and may remain viable for years. Dogs are most heavily infected between the ages of 3 weeks and 6 months, after which the worms are often discharged spontaneously. Human beings become infected by ingesting infective ova in soil. The ova are very sticky and cling to the hair of animals and fomites so that transmission can occur without direct contact with contaminated soil.

*A. suum,* the common roundworm of pigs, may infect farmers who are exposed to infected pigs (Phills et al., 1972). The mode of infection is the same as that for *T. canis.*

*C. hepatica,* a rat liver parasite, requires a second host (a rat or cat) before becoming infective for man. The intermediate host eats the infected rat and, without acquiring the infection, excretes noninfective ova in the feces. These ova mature in the soil and become infectious for man. The rarity of this infection in man is difficult to understand considering the high prevalence of *C. hepatica* infection in rats.

## PATHOGENESIS AND PATHOLOGY

After embryonated ova are ingested, second-stage larvae of *T. canis* are released from the ova in the small bowel. The second stage larvae penetrate the bowel and migrate via the lymphatics and venules to the portal system (Sprent, 1958). *T. canis* larvae do not mature past the second stage in man and therefore remain small. Their average length is 320 $\mu$m and their maximum diameter 14 to 20 $\mu$m. In primary infections the larvae migrate from the portal system to the lung and from there throughout the body, including the spinal cord and brain. Studies of experimental toxocariasis in mice, which are good models of human disease, show that migration of larvae through the liver of immune mice is slowed and that most larvae remain in the liver. Very large livers are found in children who have been repeatedly infected with *T. canis.*

The microscopic pathology varies with the location of the parasite. Eosinophilic granulomas predominate in the lungs and liver, but intact larvae may be difficult to find in biopsy specimens. The larvae may escape from the granuloma and be found some distance from the site of the original inflammatory reaction. There is little tissue reaction in the central nervous system except for hemorrhagic tracts along the path of larval migration.

The second-stage larvae of *A. suum* also migrate to the liver and lung, where they elicit marked eosinophilic and granulomatous reactions. In the lung they mature to third- and fourth-stage larvae and do not migrate into the systemic circulation, presumably because of their larger size. Although larvae can be found in sputum and are swallowed, they rarely mature to adult worms in the human gastrointestinal tract.

Unlike the other helminths that cause VLM, *C. hepatica* develops into the adult form in the liver (Cochrane et al., 1957). After penetration of the bowel, larvae of *C. hepatica* migrate directly to the liver, where they mature, mate, and produce large numbers of ova. In autopsied cases the liver is massively enlarged with an intense inflammatory reaction consisting of many eosinophils and giant cells surrounding both the adult worms and the ova.

## CLINICAL MANIFESTATIONS

The clinical picture of *T. canis* infection depends on the size of the infecting dose. Massive infections that cause the visceral larva migrans syndrome are acquired most commonly by small children between the ages of 1 to 4 years who eat dirt. Boys have VLM more often than girls in a ratio of 2:1. Minor infections are probably much more common than we realize and can occur at any age in individuals who have contact with infected soil and have hand-to-mouth habits such as smoking or nail biting. Minor infections are of no clinical importance unless one of the *T. canis* larvae migrates to the eye (Fig. 1). It is also possible that one or more larvae that migrate to the brain may set up an epileptic focus and lead to idiopathic epilepsy (Glickman et al., 1979). Eye involvement is seen in children older than 4 years and occasionally in adults. There are three basic types of eye lesions: (1) central granulomas, (2) peripheral granulomas, which may be accompanied by elevated retinal folds extending to the disk, and (3) diffuse endophthalmitis with retinal detachment (Wilkinson and Welch, 1971). The patient may present with a blind eye or the lesion may be seen on routine ophthalmoscopic examination. It is not known whether the larva migrates to the eye at the time of initial infection or whether it migrates to the eye from another organ, months or years after the primary infection. It is known that larvae may remain alive in nonhuman primate hosts for many years following a single infection, but the disease is usually benign and self-limited.

Typical VLM caused by massive infection with *T. canis* is most often characterized by fever, pulmonary symptoms, including cough and/or

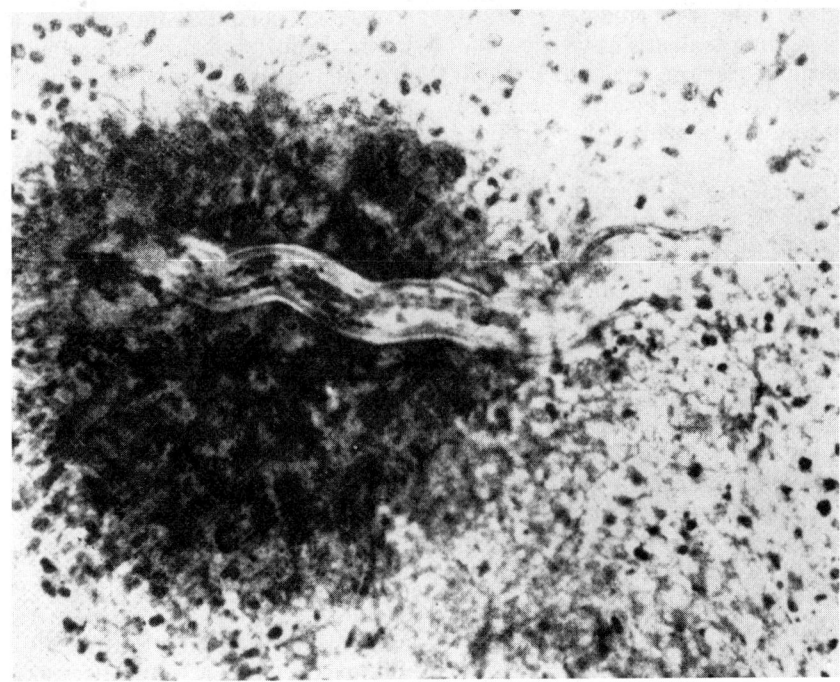

**FIGURE 1.**   *Ocular VLM. Nematode larva in eosinophilic abscess of vitreous membrane × 400. (From Wilder, Helenor C.: Trans Am Acad Ophthalmol Otolaryngol 55:99, 1950.)*

wheezing, rales, and hepatomegaly (Huntley et al., 1965). A history of pica is usually elicited, and other conditions associated with pica, such as lead poisoning or hydrocarbon ingestion, may coexist. Less common symptoms and signs include abdominal pain, vomiting, papular skin lesions, lymphadenopathy, and muscle pain. Central nervous system symptoms occur in 15 to 20 per cent of the patients and include seizures (Huntley et al., 1965), ataxia, coma, hemiparesis (Anderson et al., 1975), and Guillain-Barré syndrome (Phillips et al., 1969). Fatalities have occurred as a result of myocarditis (Becroft, 1964), a bronchiolitis-like syndrome, and encephalitis (Mikhael et al., 1974).

The marked eosinophilia usually associated with this disease (Beaver et al., 1952) may be discovered accidentally or in association with fever, cough, and wheezing. There is no absolute eosinophil count above which the disease should be considered, since the daily count varies widely in known cases, but spectacularly high counts can be seen with a leukocytosis of above 100,000 and 80 to 90 per cent eosinophils. Liver function tests, even in patients with massive hepatomegaly, are only slightly or transiently abnormal. Serum immunoglobulin concentrations are abnormal in most cases. IgE is markedly elevated (Huntley, 1976). IgG and IgM are moderately elevated, but IgA is usually normal. The immunoelectrophoretic pattern is one of a polyclonal hypergammop-

athy. Antibodies to group A and B human erythrocytes are often of the IgG type, and titers of such antibodies may be extremely high (Huntley et al., 1969). It has been suggested that *T. canis* infection of pregnant women in tropical countries may contribute to the increased incidence of ABO hemolytic disease of newborns in these areas (Huntley et al., 1976). Antibodies to human IgG as determined by the latex agglutination test (rheumatoid factors) are present in half of the cases (Huntley et al., 1966). Antinuclear antibodies are not present, but serum precipitins to proteins of cow's milk are present in 20 per cent of the patients, usually those with iron deficiency anemia. Chest radiographs may be normal, or the lungs may be hyperinflated with or without fluffy infiltrates.

## COMPLICATIONS AND SEQUELAE

Ocular *T. canis* infection may be asymptomatic or may lead to a blind eye as the result of retinal detachment. Unnecessary enucleation has been carried out in some cases because of the similarity of this lesion to retinoblastoma. Eye lesions may occur during the acute phase of the disease or as a late complication.

As a generalized *T. canis* infection, VLM is rarely fatal and is usually self-limited. Theoretically, recurrent infections could cause liver failure, but this has not been reported. Persistent myoclonic seizures leading to death have occurred in at least one patient. Serum antibodies to *T. canis* have been reported to be encountered more frequently in children with seizures than in normal children.

Massive *A. suum* infection can lead to respiratory failure, and *C. hepatica* infection to liver failure.

## GEOGRAPHIC VARIATIONS IN DISEASE

VLM is a worldwide disease that occurs primarily in tropical and temperate areas. Twenty-four per cent of 800 soil samples from public places in Britain contained viable ova of *T. canis* (Seah et al., 1975). Infections have been reported from all parts of the United States, Canada, Australia, and Great Britain, but the disease is more prevalent in tropical countries where hygienic conditions are poor and dogs are numerous.

## DIAGNOSIS

VLM should be considered in a young child with leukocytosis and hypereosinophilia who has a dog and eats dirt. The diagnosis is confirmed if larvae of *T. canis* are identified in a liver biopsy. If the child lives on a farm and is exposed to pigs, the syndrome may be caused by *A. suum* rather than *T. canis*. Since pica may lead to more than one type of parasitic infection, these patients should be examined for other intestinal helminths. *Strongyloides stercoralis* may cause massive eosinophilia and visceral involvement in the elderly and the immunosuppressed and should be considered in these patients, especially if gastrointestinal symptoms are prominent. If routine stool examination is negative for *Strongyloides*, larvae may be seen by direct examination of liquid stools following catharsis. Flotation techniques are ineffective.

Serologic diagnosis has been hampered because of the lack of a specific antigen that does not cross-react either with other helminth antigens, human A and B blood group substances, or Forssman antigen. Larval antigens or whole larvae of *T. canis* have been utilized in immunoprecipitation, tanned cell hemagglutination, enzyme-linked immunosorbent assays (ELISA), and fluorescent antibody techniques (Cypess et al., 1977; Glickman et al., 1978). Secretory-excretory antigens also offer promise for the development of a reliable test (Savigny and Tizard, 1977). A macromolecular antigen recently extracted in our laboratory from adult *A. suum* worms precipi-

tates the serum from rabbits infected with *T. canis*. It does not precipitate the serum of rabbits infected with *A. suum* nor cross-react with Forssman antigen or A and B blood group substances. Preparing this antigen, which may be identical with an important *T. canis* larval antigen, does not require working with the infective stage of the worm and shows promise for use with ELISA or radioimmunoassay techniques. The most commonly used test in the United States at present is the ELISA against *T. canis* larval antigen. Its reliability is difficult to prove in humans because the diagnosis is usually made clinically without a liver biopsy.

## TREATMENT

There is no proof that any treatment is effective against *T. canis* infections of humans. Diethylcarbamazine (Hetrazan) decreases the numbers of larvae recovered from the carcasses of infected mice (Dafalla, 1972; Pike, 1960). Thiabendazole did not decrease the numbers of larvae in similar experiments (Dafalla, 1972). If intestinal infection with *A. lumbricoides* is present in association with *T. canis* in humans, adult *Ascaris* should be eliminated from the gastrointestinal tract by an appropriate antihelmintic agent before the use of diethylcarbamazine. Diethylcarbamazine causes adult *Ascaris* worms to migrate, which can result in bowel perforation or obstruction of the intestine or common bile duct. Ocular infections with *T. canis* should be treated with antihelmintic agents cautiously and only in association with steroids. Steroids may be helpful in the treatment of *T. canis* endophthalmitis without other drugs. Severe respiratory symptoms, wheezing, and dyspnea must be treated like any other type of asthma. Iron deficiency should be treated when present, and pica must be strictly prevented.

## PROPHYLAXIS

It is not generally appreciated that *T. canis* infection is an increasing problem in the world today because of the burgeoning population of dogs, which are usually infected during the early months of life. The ova are very resistant to destruction, and families sometimes have to move to a new home if dirt-eating by children cannot be prevented. Proper disposal of canine feces combined with frequent worming of dogs during the first 6 months of life would reduce the prevalence of infected soil (Seah et al., 1975). As long as infected animals are allowed to roam free and contaminate the soil in areas frequented by children, the incidence of VLM and serious ocular infections with *T. canis* will continue to increase.

## References

Anderson, D. C., Greenwood, R., Fishman, M., and Kagan, I. G.: Acute infantile hemiplegia with cerebrospinal fluid eosinophilic pleocytosis: An unusual case of visceral larva migrans. J Pediatr 86:247, 1975.

Beaver, P. C., Snyder, C. H., Carrera, G. M., Dent, J. H., and Lafferty, J. W.: Chronic eosinophilia due to visceral larva migrans; report of 3 cases. Pediatrics 9:7, 1952.

Becroft, D. M.: Infection by the dog roundworm *Toxocara canis* and fatal myocarditis. N Z Med J 63:729, 1964.

Cochrane, J. C., Sagorin, L., and Wilcocks, M. G.: *Capillaria hepatica* infection in man. S Afr Med J 31:751, 1957.

Cypess, R. H., Karol, M. H., Zidian, J. L., Glickman, L. T., and Gitlin, D.: Larva-specific antibodies in patients with visceral larva migrans. J Infect Dis 135(4):633, 1977.

Dafalla, A. A.: A study of the effect of diethylcarbamazine and thiabendazole on experimental *Toxocara canis* infection in mice. Am J Trop Med Hyg 75:158, 1972.

de Savigny, D. H., and Tizard, I. R.: Toxocaral larva migrans: The use of larval secretory antigens in hemagglutination and soluble antigen fluorescent antibody tests. Trans R Soc Trop Med Hyg 71(6):581, 1977.

Glickman, L., Schantz, P., Domeroske, R., and Cypess, R.H. : Evaluation of serodiagnostic tests for visceral larva migrans. Am J Trop Med Hyg 27(3):492, 1978.

Glickman, L. T., Cypess, R. H., Crumrine, P. K., and Gitlin, D. A.: Toxocara infection and epilepsy in children. J Pediatr 94:75, 1979.

Hogarth-Scott, R. S.: Visceral larva migrans—an immunofluorescent examination of rabbit and human sera for antibodies to the ES antigens of the second stage larvae of *Toxocara canis, Toxocara cati* and *Toxascaris leonina* (Nematoda). Immunology 10:217, 1966.

Huntley, C. C.: Of worms and asthma, or Tullis revisited. N Eng J Med 294:1295, 1976.

Huntley, C. C., Costas, M. C., and Lyerly, A.: Visceral larva migrans syndrome: Clinical characteristics and immunologic studies in 51 patients. Pediatrics 36:523, 1965.

Huntley, C. C., Costas, M. C., Williams, R. C., Lyerly, A. D., and Watson, R. G.: Anti-gamma-globulin factors in visceral larva migrans. JAMA 197:552, 1966.

Huntley, C. C., Lyerly, A., and Patterson, M. V.: Isohemagglutinins in parasitic infections. JAMA 208:1145, 1969.

Huntley, C. C., et al.: ABO hemolytic disease in Puerto Rico and North Carolina. Pediatrics 57:875, 1976.

Mikhael, N. Z., Montpetit, V. J. A., Orizaga, M., Rowsell, H. C., and Richard, M. T.: *Toxocara canis* infestation with encephalitis. Can J Neurol Sci 1:114, 1974.

Phillips, J. A., McLean, W. T., and Huntley, C. C.: Letter: Co-existing Guillain-Barré and visceral larva migrans syndromes. Pediatrics 44:142, 1969.

Phills, J. A., Harrold, A. J., Whiteman, G. V., and Perelmutter, L.: Pulmonary infiltrates, asthma and eosinophilia due to *Ascaris suum* infestation in man. N Engl J Med 286:965, 1972.

Pike, E. H.: Effect of diethylcarbamazine, oxophenarsine hydrochloride and piperazine citrate on *Toxocara canis* larvae in mice. Exp Parasitol 9:223, 1960.

Seah, S. K., Hucal, G., and Law, C.: Dogs and intestinal parasites: A public health problem. Can Med Assoc J 112:1191, 1975.

Sprent, J. F. A.: Observations on the development of *Toxocara canis*. Parasitology 48:184, 1958.

Unruh, D. H. A., King, J. E., Eaton, R. D. P., and Allen, J. R.: Parasites of dogs from Indian settlements in Northwestern Canada: A survey of wide public health implications. Can J Comp Med 27:25, 1973.

Wilder, H. C.: Nematode endophthalmitis. Trans Am Acad Ophthalmol Otolaryngol 55:99, 1950.

Wilkinson, C. P., and Welch, R. B.: Intraocular *Toxocara*. Am J Ophthalmol 71:921, 1971.

# *LEPTOSPIROSIS* 251

## George A. Edwards, B.A., M.D.

### DEFINITION

Leptospirosis is a spirochetal disease of animals and man caused by pathogenic members of the genus *Leptospira*. Several leptospiral serotypes have been associated with presumably distinct diseases or syndromes, e.g., *L. icterohaemorrhagiae* with "Weil's disease," *L. canicola* with "canicola fever," *L. pomona* with "swineherd's disease," and *L. grippotyphosa* with "swamp fever" or "mud fever," but use of such terms as synonyms for leptospiral infections is confusing and inaccurate, as it has become evident that no clinical syndrome is exclusively attributable to a specific serotype and that no serotype invariably causes the same pattern of illness. In the interest of accuracy and clarity, the generic term leptospirosis should be used, regardless of the infecting serotype. The disease is worldwide in distribution and ranks among the most important of the zoonoses.

### ETIOLOGY

Landouzy, in 1883, and Weil, in 1886, published clinical accounts of patients with a form of infectious jaundice that appeared to differ from the usual catarrhal jaundice with which they were familiar. The syndrome was later given Weil's name, and cases were reported from various localities in Europe and the Orient. However, the etiologic agent remained unknown until 1915, when Inada and his co-workers isolated a spirochete from the blood of a patient with Weil's syndrome. Noguichi subsequently assigned the organism to a new genus, the *Leptospira,* and named it *Leptospira icterohaemorrhagiae*.

Taxonomy of the leptospires has been troublesome from the beginning and is still evolving. On the basis of recent recommendations of the World Health Organization, the genus is now considered monospecific and is designated as *Leptospira interrogans* (Pan American Health Organization,

1976). Within the one species there are some 130 serotypes (serovars) that fall into 16 serogroups on the basis of common antigenic components. The biology of these remarkable pathogens is discussed in Chapter 42.

## EPIDEMIOLOGY

All pathogenic leptospires are harbored by animal hosts and are communicated either directly or indirectly via water and soil (Alston and Broom, 1958). The infectiousness of animals results primarily from the emission of leptospires in urine, rarely from the illness itself, although man can acquire the disease through contact with tissues of infected animals as well as through direct or indirect contact with urine. Organisms that are shed in urine can survive in neutral or slightly alkaline water or moist soil for weeks if the temperature exceeds 22° C. In warm seasons, fresh water in ponds, slow-moving streams, drains, canals, and mud may remain infectious for prolonged intervals following contamination.

The leptospires are essentially parasites of mammals, of which the rodents and a few domestic animals play a dominant role in the transmission of infection to man. Rats and mice are the pre-eminent rodent hosts. Because their association with man is worldwide and ranges from chance contact in the course of recreational and vocational activities to shared housing, it is not surprising that leptospirosis knows no geographic limits. Domestic animals, particularly dogs, pigs, and cows, are the major sources of human infection in the developing countries. Leptospirosis can occur in humans of all ages, at all seasons, and in both sexes, but is primarily a disease of young adults, of warm weather (summer and autumn), and of men (Johnson, 1976). It is a threat to pet owners, certain occupational groups, and those fond of outdoor sports. Hunters, fishermen, and swimmers are at risk because surface waters in rural areas are likely to be contaminated by animal carriers. Among occupational groups most vulnerable to infection are workers in the fish and poultry industries, veterinarians, miners, sewer workers, those engaged in animal husbandry, abattoir workers, and hand laborers in grain, rice, vegetable, and sugar cane fields.

## PATHOGENESIS AND PATHOLOGY

The intraperitoneal inoculation of guinea pigs with leptospires is followed by rapid invasion of the bloodstream and, after 24 hours, by the presence of organisms in virtually all organs and tissues (Green and Arean, 1964). As the disease progresses, the organisms spread unchecked through the tissues and can be recovered from the cerebrospinal fluid, brain, and anterior chamber of the eye in the absence of visible irritation or hemorrhage. This observation led Green and Arean (1964) to conclude that leptospires penetrate tissues mechanically and are not necessarily carried into tissues by hemorrhage. Their conclusion is supported by the clinical observation in human disease that leptospires regularly invade the subarachnoid space and anterior chamber of the eye without inciting significant inflammation. The type of tissue injury caused by virulent leptospires has not been fully clarified, but it appears to be toxic in nature. The hemolysins produced by pathogenic leptospires in vitro and probably in vivo account for intravascular hemolysis, while hemorrhage appears to result from damage to endothelial cells by a cytotoxin. Leptospiral virulence appears to depend on toxin production.

Death due to anicteric leptospirosis is exceedingly rare; hence, knowledge of morbid anatomy in leptospirosis has been gained principally from the study of fatal cases of Weil's disease (Arean, 1962). At autopsy, the only gross changes of note are bile staining of tissues and extensive ecchymoses or petechiae in striated muscle, kidneys, adrenals, liver, stomach, spleen, and lungs, with less extensive bleeding elsewhere. The most prominent alterations in the kidney occur in the tubular epithelium, where damage ranges from cloudy swelling to complete necrosis and desquamation. Tubules may be dilated and the lumina of medullary tubules may contain cellular casts, blood, bile-stained hyaline casts, and other debris. Interstitial edema, scattered hemorrhages, and areas of mononuclear cell infiltration are characteristic. In patients with acute renal failure, the pathologic findings are those of nonspecific acute tubular necrosis. Histologic examination of the liver discloses dissociation of liver cords with separation of hepatocytes, focal areas of necrosis around central veins, an increase in the number of binucleated liver cells, slight to moderate infiltration by neutrophils and round cells, and inspissation of bile in canaliculi. Overall, the pathologic changes in the liver are nonspecific and unimpressive and show little correlation with the degree of functional impairment. Leptospires are rarely demonstrable in hepatic tissues, and acute yellow atrophy is a very uncommon finding.

In skeletal muscle, there is focal loss of cross-striations, vacuolation, and hyalinization early in the disease, and necrosis in the later stages. Leptospiral antigens can be demonstrated in areas of muscle degeneration. Hemorrhagic pneumonitis in localized or confluent patches is found in patients with pulmonary symptoms. Hemorrhages are the only characteristic lesions in other organs.

## CLINICAL CHARACTERISTICS

### General Features

The manifestations and severity of leptospiral infection can vary greatly. A physician who knows the protean features of leptospirosis and understands its natural course seldom fails to appreciate the possibility of that diagnosis when confronted with a victim of the disease. Approximately 10 to 15 per cent of patients present with the distinctive features of Weil's disease—e.g., jaundice, hemorrhage, and renal damage—and virtually all deaths due to leptospirosis occur in this group of patients. Fortunately, the majority of patients experience an acute, benign, anicteric, self-limited illness (Edwards and Domm, 1960).

### Incubation Period

The incubation period averages 10 days, with a usual range of 7 to 13 days. However, isolated opportunities for exposure such as laboratory or water accidents indicate an extreme range of 2 to 26 days.

### Phases of Illness

Leptospirosis is a biphasic illness, a fact that can best be appreciated from observations of anicteric patients (Edwards, 1959). The initial "septicemic" or "leptospiremic" phase is characterized by the clinical manifestations of an acute systemic infection and by the presence of leptospires in the blood and cerebrospinal fluid. Defervescence and symptomatic improvement occur after four to seven days of acute illness, coincident with the disappearance of leptospires from the blood and spinal fluid. Following an asymptomatic interval of 24 to 72 hours, the second, or "immune," phase is ushered in by the reappearance of fever and often by a recurrence or intensification of headache. This phase of illness is characterized clinically and from the laboratory standpoint by manifestations related to the development of immunity and by the appearance of circulating IgM antibodies. Leptospires cannot be recovered from blood or cerebrospinal fluid after the first week but make their appearance in the urine around the middle of the second week. The variable severity, manifestations, and morbidity of the second phase are in sharp contrast to the monotonous clinical picture of the first phase. Many patients experience no symptoms in the second phase; others remain symptomatic for only one to three days; and a few have extended morbidity.

### Manifestations

*First Phase.* Typically, the illness begins with the abrupt onset of headache, chills, fever, severe muscle aching, anorexia, nausea, vomiting, and prostration. Headache is frontal (sometimes bitemporal or occipital) and is intense, unremitting, rarely throbbing, and tends to persist several days. Repeatedly, patients with headache and nuchal rigidity have been found to have normal cerebrospinal fluid when lumbar puncture has been performed in anticipation of finding evidence of meningitis. Muscular discomfort is usually maximal in the calf and lumbar areas; fever is universal and usually spiking in character; chills may recur over a period of three to five days; anorexia, nausea, and vomiting are quite common; and constipation is the rule, although a few patients have diarrhea. A significant number of patients complain of abdominal pain, which is probably caused by involvement of muscles of the abdominal wall rather than by inflammation of the gastrointestinal tract. Cough, dyspnea, and chest pain have been prominent symptoms in some reported series but not in others. Nevertheless, involvement of the respiratory system is an important feature of the first phase. Hemoptysis is infrequent.

Patients examined early in the course of illness are febrile, dehydrated, and lethargic, and may be confused or delirious. Relative bradycardia and normal or low blood pressure are the rule. Muscle tenderness may be marked in the presence of severe myalgia, and nuchal rigidity is often present. The most characteristic and valuable physical sign is suffusion of the conjunctivae, found in 80 to 85 per cent of cases. The eyes have a bright pink appearance similar to that resulting from exposure when swimming in fresh water. Photophobia and burning are common complaints, but purulent exudate and chemosis are rarely found. Infrequent findings include splenomegaly, hepatomegaly, lymphadenopathy, rash (macular, maculopapular, blotchy, urticarial, or even hemorrhagic), and rales or signs of pulmonary consolidation. Death is unusual in the first week of illness, even among patients with Weil's disease. The nonspecific manifestations of this phase suggest such diagnoses as bacterial pneumonia, typhus, tularemia, acute bronchitis, and viral infection.

### Second Phase

MENINGITIS. Aseptic meningitis is the principal manifestation of the immune phase of illness. Approximately 50 per cent of all patients exhibit signs and symptoms, but fewer than half of these have the full-blown picture of meningitis, with excruciating headache, stiffness of the neck, and vomiting. Some of these latter patients are prostrated for a week or longer and may require narcotic analgesics for symptomatic relief. Patients with severe headache may experience considerable relief from lumbar puncture. Around 30 to 35 per cent of patients have pleocytosis despite the absence of symptoms and signs of meningitis, while the remaining 15 to 20 per cent have normal spinal fluid throughout the course of the illness.

Neither the development nor the severity of meningitis can be correlated with the severity of other manifestations of leptospirosis. It is not unusual for a patient who has had an insignificant first-phase illness to seek medical attention only following the onset of severe symptoms due to meningitis. Hence, the concept of "pure" leptospiral meningitis has arisen. Fortunately, a careful history usually brings to light an account of the antecedent febrile illness.

In meningitis, the leukocytes in the cerebrospinal fluid range from fewer than 10 to over 1000 per mm$^3$. Although neutrophils may predominate initially, the percentage of lymphocytes rises thereafter, and lymphocytosis of the spinal fluid may persist six to eight weeks after the patient becomes asymptomatic. Protein values are elevated to the range of 80 to 120 mg per mm$^3$ early in the course of meningitis but then decline. Glucose values are usually normal but fall occasionally. Xanthochromic spinal fluid may be found in jaundiced patients.

OTHER NERVOUS SYSTEM LESIONS. A variety of lesions of the nervous system may develop in the immune phase. Fortunately, these are uncommon, but they may be devastating. They include encephalitis, myelitis, radiculitis, the Guillain-Barré syndrome, and peripheral nerve lesions. The optic, oculomotor, facial, glossopharyngeal, auditory, and spinal nerves may be affected. These lesions resemble those that occur as sequelae of certain infections, vaccinations, and hypersensitivity to antibiotic agents and antisera and are thought to have the same pathogenesis.

UVEITIS. Some authors have reported uveal tract involvement in a high percentage of their patients, but others have found it infrequently, apparently because it is easily overlooked. There have been reports of the isolation of viable leptospires from the aqueous humor of patients with lesions of the uveal tract, but it is not certain that uveitis is always due to persistence of organisms in the anterior chamber. It is of interest that no evidence of preceding leptospiral infection was found in large numbers of patients with unexplained uveitis. In contrast to other manifestations of leptospirosis, uveitis first becomes evident during convalescence or after a latent period of several weeks or months. The prognosis for cure is excellent, but visual impairment may be permanent.

## Special Features

### Weil's Disease

The term Weil's disease is a convenient designation for severe leptospirosis characterized by icterus, azotemia, hemorrhage, anemia, vascular collapse, and disturbances in consciousness. In contrast to benign anicteric leptospirosis, Weil's disease is a dramatic, life-threatening illness. It cannot be equated with illness due to *L. icterohaemorrhagiae* infection, as every pathogenic serotype has the potential for causing such a syndrome. Although fairly insignificant from a numerical standpoint, this variant of leptospirosis far overshadows the anicteric form with respect to morbidity and mortality. As might be anticipated, incomplete syndromes in which one or more of the major manifestations are absent have improved prognoses.

A basic pattern of illness is common to all variants of leptospirosis, and the onset and first phase of Weil's disease, before jaundice appears, are indistinguishable from those of anicteric leptospirosis. The distinctive manifestations of the syndrome (jaundice, hemorrhage and renal damage) first become evident around the third to fifth day of illness and reach their peak in the second week. Nevertheless, a biphasic temperature curve is usually discernible, and leptospires disappear from blood and cerebrospinal fluid around the seventh day. However, fever in the immune phase tends to be more prominent than in anicteric disease and may persist for two to three weeks.

The clinical picture may be dominated by hepatic, renal, or hemorrhagic manifestations, but death usually results from renal failure or hemorrhage rather than from hepatic failure. Fortunately, as methods of management of dehydration, shock, and acute renal failure have improved, the mortality rate of Weil's disease in developed countries has declined in recent years from 25 to 40 per cent to 5 per cent or less.

### Hepatic Damage

Hepatic enlargement and tenderness are the rule in the presence of jaundice but are rarely found in its absence. Serum bilirubin levels usually remain below 20 mg per 100 ml, with the conjugated fraction predominating, but extreme hyperbilirubinemia has been recorded in some cases, usually in those with the triad of acute renal failure, hemolytic anemia, and severe liver involvement. There is evidence that bilirubin excretion is blocked at the subcellular level. Prothrombin production is usually normal, but if it is impaired, the deficiency can be corrected with vitamin K or one of its precursors.

It is fortunate that essential hepatocellular functions are less severely compromised than the extent of jaundice might imply and that complete resolution of hepatic damage is the rule in surviving patients.

### Renal Damage

Renal dysfunction is common in leptospirosis. Proteinuria, transient oliguria, microscopic hematuria, and modest elevations of blood urea nitrogen are detected in 70 per cent of patients in the first phase, but with rare exceptions, major renal damage is limited to patients with Weil's disease. Renal injury is aggravated by shock, extreme hyperbilirubinemia, and possibly hemoglobinemia in severely ill patients. Renal failure was once the primary cause of death, but this is no longer necessarily true, as the incidence of acute tubular necrosis can be reduced by vigorous attention to fluid and blood replacement in the first phase of illness, and survival can be enhanced by use of modern methods of managing acute renal failure, including dialysis if necessary.

### Cardiac Involvement

Electrocardiographic changes in the form of T-wave abnormalities and minor disturbances of conduction are relatively common in leptospirosis, but clinically significant cardiac manifestations are infrequent. Premature ventricular contractions, atrial flutter, ventricular tachycardia, and paroxysmal atrial fibrillation have been described, and patients with evidence of myocardial damage, e.g., dilatation, ventricular gallop rhythm, or frank congestive heart failure, have been reported.

### Anemia

Anemia is a common feature of Weil's disease but rarely occurs in the absence of jaundice. It is multifactorial in origin (i.e., due to hemolysis, hemorrhage, and azotemia) and may be severe.

### Laboratory Features

#### Peripheral Blood

White blood cell counts vary from low to slightly elevated in anicteric leptospirosis, but jaundiced patients have significant leukocytosis, usually in the range of 15,000 to 30,000 per $mm^3$, although extreme degrees of leukocytosis may occur. Neutrophilia is so characteristic of the first stage of illness that its absence virtually negates the diagnosis of leptospirosis. Anemia is not a feature of anicteric leptospirosis but may be severe in Weil's disease. Thrombocytopenia is rarely clinically significant.

### Blood Chemistry

Jaundice occurs in approximately 15 per cent of cases. Bilirubin levels remain below 20 mg per 100 ml in two-thirds of these, but in the remaining cases may reach 40 to 60 mg per 100 ml. Transaminase and alkaline phosphatase levels are usually elevated in jaundiced patients, although rarely more than threefold. In anicteric patients, the values tend to be normal or nearly so. Anicteric patients tend to maintain normal serum urea nitrogen levels, but as many as 25 per cent have elevations in the range of 20 to 60 mg per 100 ml, sometimes in the presence of normal urine. Patients with Weil's disease often have azotemia, and serum urea nitrogen values greater than 100 mg per 100 ml are characteristic in patients with acute tubular necrosis.

### Urine

Urinalysis often discloses proteinuria, casts, and red and white blood cells early in the disease. However, the urine clears rapidly except in patients who sustain acute tubular necrosis.

## PROPHYLAXIS

Leptospiral vaccines for human use were first developed more than 50 years ago, but several important problems remain to be solved. Killed vaccines have received the most attention, but live vaccines composed of virulent strains cultured in special media are being tested. Although the general use of vaccines cannot be justified because of the sporadic nature of leptospirosis, their use for the protection of workers in certain high-risk occupations is probably worthwhile. Unfortunately, the killed vaccines afford minimal protection against heterologous serotypes, and vaccines must be custom manufactured by using the specific serotype to which exposure is anticipated.

Until safe, potent polyvalent vaccines are developed, other approaches to the control of leptospirosis should be used. Educational campaigns are needed to alert outdoor recreationalists, pet owners, and certain occupational groups to the hazards of the disease. The danger of swimming or wading in surface waters to which domestic or wild animals have access should be publicized. Pet owners, veterinarians, and livestock workers should be encouraged to protect themselves from contact with the urine or tissues of sick animals by wearing rubber gloves and aprons, and laborers in sugar cane and rice fields, abattoirs, and pig farms should be provided with protective clothing, including shoes. The incidence of infection due to *L. icterohaemorrhagiae* in urban areas can be reduced by water purification, sewage and waste disposal systems, and vigorous rodent control programs.

## COMPLICATIONS AND SEQUELAE

There are few sequelae of leptospiral infections. The liver and kidneys recover full function in patients who survive Weil's disease, except for a few patients left with permanent impairment of renal concentration. Leptospiral uveitis usually resolves completely, although there have been reported instances of blindness and cataract formation. Meningitis clears without residuals, but recovery from the "postinfectious" lesions of the nervous system is prolonged and may be incomplete.

As a statistical possibility, chronic systemic leptospirosis can be ignored. Only one such case has been documented, that of a patient who was probably immunodeficient. Although leptospires may persist in the anterior chamber of the eye and in the renal tubules for many months, little or no damage is caused by their presence in the kidneys, and surprisingly little reaction results from their presence in the eye other than an indolent uveitis.

## GEOGRAPHIC VARIATIONS

Published accounts of leptospirosis seem to indicate that the disease is much more severe in some geographic areas than others. Reports from Latin America and the Caribbean islands depict leptospirosis as a serious hepatonephritic syndrome, yet public health authorities believe large numbers of anicteric cases go unrecognized. On the other hand, in developed countries where clinicians are aware of the anicteric form of the disease, patients with Weil's disease constitute a minority of all cases of leptospirosis. Thus, it is probable that the reported geographic variations in severity of leptospirosis are more apparent than real and can be attributed to differences in awareness of the full clinical spectrum of the disease.

It is reasonable to expect the experience of the United States in regard to leptospirosis to be recapitulated in Latin America and other developing countries in the next few decades. Between 1905 and 1974 the percentage of cases of leptospirosis due to *L. icterohaemorrhagiae* fell from 90 per cent before 1946 to 40 per cent between 1949 and 1961 and to 20 per cent between 1965 and 1974. Prior to 1948, a total of 299 cases were

reported, the vast majority of the patients were jaundiced, and the mortality rate was approximately 25 per cent. In contrast, of the 791 cases reported between 1965 and 1974, less than 15 per cent of the patients were icteric, and of these less than 5 per cent died.

## DIAGNOSIS

The laboratory diagnosis of leptospirosis depends on isolation of the organisms by bacteriologic methods or serologic tests. Dark-field microscopy, once widely used for identification of the spirochetes in body fluids, is no longer considered reliable. The blood or cerebrospinal fluid should be cultured in the first week of illness and the urine after the middle of the second week. Leptospiruria is usually limited to two to four weeks but sometimes persists for months. Since only a minority of patients exhibit leptospiruria, failure to recover the organisms from urine does not exclude the diagnosis. A special semisolid medium such as Fletcher's, Korthof's, or Stuart's is required for culture. Inoculation of guinea pigs or hamsters is preferred to culture if specimens are contaminated.

Leptospiral antibodies appear in the blood around the end of the first week and usually reach their peak titer in the third or fourth week. There are a number of satisfactory serologic tests in use, but the microscopic agglutination-lysis test is regarded as most specific and is often used in confirming results of other tests. Blood for serologic tests should be collected in both the acute and convalescent phases of illness. A rise in titer of fourfold or greater is considered diagnostic, but if only a single specimen is available, a titer in the range of 1:1600 provides strong presumptive evidence of leptospirosis. Unfortunately, definitive identification of the infecting serotype by serologic test is impossible because of extensive cross-agglutination, nor is there a reliable diagnostic serologic test in the first week of illness.

## TREATMENT

Leptospires have in vivo sensitivity to a wide variety of antimicrobial drugs including the penicillins, tetracyclines, chloramphenicol, and erythromycin. Antibiotic therapy seems to be beneficial if it is initiated within the first four days of illness (Kocen, 1962). Therapy begun after the fifth day cannot be expected to alter the course of illness, and the use of antimicrobials in the treatment of jaundice or meningitis has no rationale. Soluble penicillin in a daily dose of 2.4 million units and tetracycline in a dose of 2 g daily are the most widely used regimens, with penicillin being preferred by most authorities. Headache should be relieved, volume depletion corrected, and blood replaced in Weil's disease.

## References

Alston, J. M., and Broom, J. C.: Leptospirosis in Man and Animals. Edinburgh and London, E. & S. Livingstone Ltd., 1958.
Arean, V. M.: The pathologic anatomy and pathogenesis of fatal human leptospirosis (Weil's disease). Am J Pathol 40:393, 1962.

Edwards, G. A.: Clinical characteristics of leptospirosis. Am J Med 27:4, 1959.
Edwards, G. A., and Domm, B. M.: Human leptospirosis. Medicine 39:117, 1960.
VIII Inter-American Meeting on Foot-and-Mouth Disease and Zoonose Control. Pan American Health Organization: Scientific Publication No. 316. Washington, D.C., World Health Organization, 1976.
Green, J. H., and Arean, V. M.: Virulence and distribution of *Leptospira icterohaemorrhagiae* in experimental guinea pig infections. Am J Vet Res 25:264, 1964.
Johnson, R. C.: The Biology of Parasitic Spirochetes. New York, Academic Press, 1976.
Kocen, R. S.: Leptospirosis: A comparison of symptomatic and penicillin therapy. Br Med J 1:1181, 1962.

# MARBURG VIRUS DISEASE 252

## R. Siegert, M.D.

### DEFINITION

Marburg virus disease is a hemorrhagic fever with a high mortality rate which first appeared in Germany and Yugoslavia in 1967. It is named after the city where most of the cases occurred, and where the etiology of the disease was elucidated. The agent, which has not yet been classified, is a coated RNA virus of unusual shape and length. The primary source of infection in 1967 was monkeys imported from Africa, and at first the disease was also referred to as green or vervet monkey disease. A minor outbreak occurred in 1975 in South Africa. So far, only 34 cases have been observed.

### ETIOLOGY

The clinical symptoms, pathologic and anatomic findings, epidemiology, and fruitless microbiologic and serologic diagnosis all indicated a hitherto unknown disease (Siegert et al., 1968). From material obtained from patients, Marburg virus was first grown in guinea pigs and in monkey kidney cell cultures. Cytoplasmic antigen inclusions were demonstrated in organs of guinea pigs and dead patients, and also in infected cell cultures, using immunofluorescence-labeled antisera from guinea pigs and patients. Finally, a virus was revealed by electron microscopy in the serum and tissues of patients and likewise in infected animals, thus meeting the Henle-Koch postulates for an infectious agent (Siegert et al., 1967).

### PATHOGENESIS AND PATHOLOGY

Incubation periods for primary infections via monkey blood and organs lasted three to seven days, and five to nine days for secondary infections via human contacts. The most severe symptoms and all fatalities were observed only in primary infections. The main reason for these pathogenic differences is probably that the virus loses its virulence when passaged in humans. However, differences may also be the result of varying infective doses, since the virus concentrations found in monkeys and their excretions were higher than those found in patients (Siegert, 1978).

All the cases examined revealed viremia, marked by high fever and lasting an average of 14 days. Marburg virus was carried hematogenously to all organs. Virus propagation leads to diffuse necrosis, and to functional disturbances in various parenchymatous organs. Fatalities occurred only during the acute stage of the disease.

The persistence of the virus in the liver, testes, and eye in the presence of circulating antibodies was of particular pathogenetic interest. It was verified in three patients by isolating the virus in a liver sample, in semen samples, and in ocular fluid two to three months after inception of the disease. Virus persistence was also suggested by the relapsing hepatitis observed in five cases at intervals of 4 to 73 days after fever had disappeared.

Repeated examinations of all the patients have yielded no signs of late organ damage, so that the prognosis is favorable once the patient has survived the acute stage of the disease. In spite of extensive necrosis, the liver structure can be expected to regenerate.

Frequent testicular and ovarian damage, together with the fact that the disease was transmitted in one case via semen, raised the question whether germinal transmission of Marburg virus to offspring is possible. However, no evidence of this has been found in animal experiments.

The pathologic changes resulting from Marburg virus disease were closely studied in five patients who died between the eighth and sixteenth days. Since death occurred at the climax of the disease or at the beginning of the convalescent phase, nothing is known about possible early changes.

Macroscopic findings were noncharacteristic and yielded little information. The important findings in microscopic examination of various tissues were limited to the liver, kidney, and lung. The most striking of these were hemorrhages and parenchymal necroses, which occurred without any appreciable inflammatory reactions (Gedigk et al., 1968).

Necrosis in the liver was severe. The individual and group necroses in the liver cells were scattered irregularly over all the zones of the lobes and were characterized by changes in the cytoplasm—partly homogeneous, partly lumpy—and by positive PAS reactions and increased eosin staining. Cytoplasmic degeneration, with nucleolysis and formation of structures resembling Councilman bodies, was noted. Maximal alteration was observed in the second week, after which the cells degenerated rapidly and were resorbed. The defects were replaced by hepatogenic formations, and therefore liver structure can be expected to return to normal. Hepatitis caused by Marburg virus differs in regard to combination, distribution pattern, and development of lesions from classic forms of hepatitis, namely, yellow fever, leptospirosis, and other hemorrhagic fevers.

There were also hemorrhages and necroses in the testes, ovaries, pancreas, and kidneys; in each case, they indicated a severe tubular insufficiency. In addition, follicular necroses and perifollicular hemorrhages were found in the pulpa of the spleen and in the medulla of the lymph nodes, which showed a striking paucity of cells and dense deposits of eosinophilic, PAS-positive material. Later, plasma-cellular monocytoid infiltrations were also found. In the lungs, edema was seen, with an accumulation of alveolar macrophages in fluid-filled alveoli.

Most of the fatalities had a glial nodular encephalitis distributed throughout the brain (Jacob, 1971). The process resembled that of other forms of encephalitis, especially louse-borne typhus and infections with arboviruses.

## CLINICAL MANIFESTATIONS

All 34 patients were adults aged 18 to 64 years. They were closely observed clinically and showed uniform symptoms (Martini et al., 1968; Stille and Böhle, 1971; Gear et al., 1975). Marburg virus disease began suddenly, with brief and noncharacteristic prodromes: marked malaise, tor-por, and pain in the head, limbs, and muscles. Within a few hours, body temperature rose to more than 39° C.

The fever, accompanied by relative bradycardia, reached its climax on the third and fourth days, continued between 38° and 40° C up to the second week, and then gradually declined. Some of the patients had a second attack of fever around the twelfth to fourteenth day. Altogether, fever lasted from 12 to 22 days.

Gastrointestinal disturbances were present from the beginning. At first, marked nausea and occasionally uncontrolled vomiting were observed. Later, there was profuse watery diarrhea, which led to extreme dehydration in certain patients.

The most reliable symptom was a maculopapular, nonpruritic rash, which appeared in every patient between the fifth and eighth day, almost always beginning on the face and then spreading to the trunk and extremities. It consisted of livid red pinhead-sized papillae, which then developed into an extensive exanthem. In the more serious cases, the exanthem on the face and trunk merged into a dark red, diffuse erythema. Some of the patients also developed scrotal or labial dermatitis. Petechial skin hemorrhages occurred less frequently. The exanthem disappeared within a few days. After the sixteenth day, all the patients showed a fine exfoliative desquamation, especially on the soles and palms.

Simultaneously, most of the patients developed a dark red enanthem on the hard and soft palates, sometimes with glassy vesicles. In addition, there was noticeable conjunctivitis, with photophobia and increased secretion.

Between the third and sixth day, many of the patients showed a swelling of the lymph nodes in the neck, throat, and axillae. These were pea- to bean-sized, soft, and slightly sensitive to pressure. The spleen was not palpable.

From the fourth day on, half of the patients showed a hemorrhagic diathesis, with spontaneous bleeding from the nose and gums, hematuria, and hemorrhages in the gastrointestinal tract. Younger female patients also had genital hemorrhages. In the severe cases, large hematomas developed at injection sites, and bleeding from the punctures was hard to arrest.

Almost all of the parenchymatous organs were affected. The most obvious alteration was in the liver, which was seriously damaged in all cases. Some livers showed an extreme increase in the serum transaminase level, although neither icterus nor hepatic coma ensued. Electrocardiographic changes indicated myocarditis. When the disease reached its crisis, there were frequent disturbances in heart rhythm and signs of insufficiency. A drop in blood pressure was observed only in the terminal stage. In severe cases there was considerable kidney damage, with proteinuria, oliguria, and anuria, as well as microhematuria and retention of urinous substances.

In many of the patients, certain symptoms, including marked restlessness, depressive and sullen behavior, myoclonia, tremor, hyperesthesia, and paresthesia, indicated that the central nervous system was also affected. Some patients became confused, lost consciousness, and died in cerebral coma; two of them were convulsive. One woman developed a severe psychosis, and another a postinfectious myelitis with flaccid paralysis of both legs. The cell count and protein content of the cerebrospinal fluid remained within the normal range in the cases examined.

The laboratory findings revealed characteristic changes. A marked increase in serum glutamic oxaloacetic transaminase (SGOT) and serum glutamic pyruvic transaminase (SGPT) was noted in virtually all the patients during the second week. The SGOT values were always higher than the SGPT levels, in extreme cases attaining values of more than 5000 units/ml.

Bilirubin values were slightly increased, if at all, only during the terminal stages of the disease. Creatinine and urea levels increased only in cases of anuria. Hypokalemia appeared in connection with vomiting and diarrhea. The total serum protein concentration occasionally decreased to less than 5 per cent. In a few patients, elevated serum amylase levels were noted.

The hematologic changes consisted of marked leukopenia, with cell counts sometimes as low as 1000/mm³. Excessive leukocytosis was observed only in patients with pulmonary complications. The blood sedimentation rate was rarely abnormal.

The hemopoietic system in all the patients was affected during the first few days. This was shown mainly by a critical decline in platelets, which sometimes dropped to as low as 10,000/mm³. Some investigators regard the hematologic picture seen in patients with Marburg disease as characteristic of disseminated intravascular coagulopathy, which is found in various exanthematous viral and arboviral diseases and produces prolonged prothrombin times and increased fibrinogen degradation products.

## COMPLICATIONS AND SEQUELAE

Various complications appeared at the crisis of the disease: bronchopneumonia, edema in the lower leg, unilateral orchitis with painful swelling of the scrotum. There was one case each of pericarditis, psychosis, and postinfectious myelitis and uveitis. Shock and anuria may complicate the terminal picture.

Twenty-three per cent of patients died from cardiac and circulatory failure, complete anuria, and cerebral coma.

The prognosis was favorable for all patients who survived the acute phase, even though convalescence was slow. During late convalescence, certain patients suffered a single relapse of hepatitis, with raised transaminase levels and slight fever. Recovery from liver damage, as ascertained by biopsy, was complete in all cases.

Sequelae also appeared: extensive alopecia, sharp pain in the liver region, and inability to tolerate alcohol. These sequelae persisted for some time. Some patients developed unilateral testicular atrophy, with oligospermia, loss of libido, and impotence, although the ketosteroids remained normal. Neurovegetative disturbances such as hyperhidrosis and fatigability lasted for many years.

## DIAGNOSIS

Both of the recorded outbreaks of Marburg virus disease had a connection with Africa, where the disease probably originated. Therefore, differential diagnostic considerations can be limited mainly to African febrile hemorrhagic diseases.

Protozoal diseases (malaria, trypanosomiasis) can be ruled out by negative blood smears, and bacterial diseases (leptospirosis, shigellosis, typhoid fever, plague) can be eliminated by negative blood or stool cultures as well as by the failure of suspected cases to respond clinically to high doses of broad spectrum antibiotics. Other important possibilities include certain virus diseases (chikungunya and Rift Valley fever, dengue, smallpox, hepatitis). The most important differential diagnosis is that between Lassa and yellow fever and Marburg and Ebola virus disease (Wulff and Conrad, 1977).

The earliest symptom of Lassa fever is a severe sore throat, usually with exudative or ulcerative pharyngitis, which makes it difficult or impossible for the patient to swallow. This severe pharyngitis is generally lacking in Marburg virus disease and yellow fever. Maculopapular rash is a prominent feature of Marburg virus disease but is never seen in yellow fever and only rarely in Lassa fever. Jaundice is common in yellow fever but does not occur in the other diseases. The immediate medical problem in Lassa fever is hypotension and shock, whereas in Marburg virus disease shock appears to be a terminal event resulting from blood loss and/or overwhelming bacterial superinfection.

## *TREATMENT AND PROPHYLAXIS*

Therapy is symptomatic. Antibiotics, singly or combined, had no effect on the viral process. However, their early use is recommended in order to prevent secondary bacterial infections. Convalescent plasma was used in some cases, but its effect is uncertain. The patient must be promptly treated for any complications that may arise; for instance, if the platelet level falls, platelets or fresh blood must be transfused. If disseminated intravascular coagulation sets in, intravenous heparin may be effective. Adequate replacement of fluid and electrolytes was especially important in patients with vomiting and diarrhea. Cardiac and circulatory drugs were necessary in most cases. Hypoproteinemia was treated with up to 30 g of human albumin daily. Corticosteroids had no effect. Therapy with human interferon on a trial basis is advisable.

Prevention and control measures in Marburg and Frankfurt consisted of destroying all monkeys and cell cultures they had yielded. All animal housing and laboratories were thoroughly disinfected. There were no further primary infections after these steps had been taken (Hennessen et al., 1968).

The patients were kept completely isolated in quarantine wards, as with cases of smallpox, and were attended by volunteer physicians and nurses. The medical personnel all wore completely protective clothing in order to prevent contact, especially with blood from the patients. The patients were not released until two weeks after complete recovery. The men with orchitis were advised to be sexually continent as a precautionary measure. That this measure was justified is shown by the later seminal infection of a woman by her husband.

All primary and secondary contact persons were kept under observation and were given daily medical examinations. The general public and all medical personnel were kept informed, which proved to be psychologically effective.

The World Health Organization formulated recommendations for the capture, transportation, export and import, buying and selling, quarantine, and veterinary inspection of monkeys. In addition, national regulations were issued for protective measures in monkey and cell experiments.

Preclusion of Marburg virus from all live virus vaccines produced from monkey kidney cells was of particular importance. The 1967 outbreak led to worldwide efforts to find a suitable replacement for monkey kidney cells in vaccine production. As a result, they are no longer used.

Experience so far indicates that Marburg virus disease is very rare. Still, as long as the natural reservoir and means of transmission of the agent are not known, there are no means of primary prevention. No vaccine is available for endangered laboratory personnel.

## References

Gear, J. S. S., Cassel, G. A., Gear, A. J., Trappler, B., Clausen, L., Meyers, A. M., Kew, M. C., Bothwell, T. H., Sher, R., Miller, G. B., Schneider, J., Koornhof, H. J., Gomperts, E. D., Isaäcson, M., and Gear, J. H. S.: Outbreak of Marburg virus disease in Johannesburg. Br Med J 1:489, 1975.

Gedigk, P., Bechtelsheimer, H., and Korb, G.: Die pathologische Anatomie der "Marburg-Virus"-Krankheit (sog. "Marburger Affenkrankheit"). Dtsch Med Wochenschr 93:590, 1968.

Hennessen, W., Bonin, O., and Mauler, R.: Zur Epidemiologie der Erkrankung von Menschen durch Affen. Dtsch Med Wochenschr 93:582, 1968.

Jacob, H.: The neuropathology of the Marburg disease in man. In Martini, G. A., and Siegert, R. (eds.): Marburg Virus Disease. Berlin, Springer-Verlag, 1971, p. 54.

Martini, G. A., Knauff, H. G., Schmidt, H. A., Mayer, G., and Baltzer, G.: Über eine bisher unbekannte, von Affen eingeschleppte Infektionskrankheit: Marburg-Virus-Krankheit. Dtsch Med Wochenschr 93:559, 1968.

Siegert, R.: Marburgvirus-Krankheit. In Röhrer, H. (ed.): Handbuch der Virusinfektionen bei Tieren. Vol. 6. Jena, Gustav Fischer Verlag, 1978, p. 579.

Siegert, R., Shu, H. L., and Slenczka, W.: Isolierung und Identifizierung des "Marburg-Virus." Dtsch Med Wochenschr 93:604, 1968.

Siegert, R., Shu, H. L., Slenczka, W., Peters, D., and Müller, G.: Zur Ätiologie einer unbekannten, von Affen ausgegangenen menschlichen Infektionskrankheit. Dtsch Med Wochenschr 92:2341, 1967.

Stille, W., and Böhle, E.: Clinical course and prognosis of Marburg virus ("green monkey") disease. In Martini, G. A., and Siegert, R. (eds.): Marburg Virus Disease. Berlin, Springer-Verlag, 1971, p. 10.

Wulff, H., and Conrad, I. L.: Marburg virus disease. In Kurstak, E., and Kurstak, C. (eds.): Comparative Diagnosis of Viral Diseases. Vol. 2. Human and Related Viruses, Part B. New York, Academic Press, 1977, p. 3.

# EBOLA VIRUS DISEASE 253

*R. Siegert, M.D.*

## DEFINITION

Ebola virus disease is a hemorrhagic fever with a high mortality rate. Clinically, it is extremely similar to Marburg virus disease, and central Africa is the natural habitat of both. However, the agent, which is named after a river in Zaire, shares no antigen with Marburg virus, despite their extensive morphologic similarity. Neither the natural hosts of Ebola virus nor its habitat and transmission are known. In 1976 there was an epidemic in southern Sudan and northern Zaire, and several hundred cases were observed. Another outbreak occurred in 1979 in the Yambio-Nzara district of southern Sudan, where the first cases were identified in 1976 (World Health Organization, 1979).

## ETIOLOGY

Isolation and identification of the agent were made by means of investigations similar to those that clarified the etiology of Marburg virus disease (Bowen et al., 1977; Johnson et al., 1977; Pattyn et al., 1977). Although Ebola virus is an independent agent antigenically, it is very closely related to Marburg virus in structure and pathogenic properties.

## PATHOGENESIS AND PATHOLOGY

Since detailed pathologic and anatomic information is lacking, it has not yet been possible to analyze the pathogenic mechanism. The incubation period is given as 4 to 16 days, with an average of 7 days. Subsequently, viremia always develops, and the virus appears in all organs. Persistence must also be expected, since the virus was isolated in the semen of one patient on the thirty-ninth and the sixty-first day after the onset of the disease. The infection conveys immunity of an undetermined duration.

No representative description of pathologic changes is yet available. So far, histologic examinations have been restricted to liver specimens from three virologically verified patients from Zaire. These specimens showed fatty degenerations and necroses distributed in a focal pattern. Inflammatory reactions were remarkably slight. Eosinophilic inclusion bodies of varying size were found in the cytoplasm of the hepatocytes. These bodies, together with the presence of structures resembling Councilman bodies, made tentative histologic diagnosis possible.

## CLINICAL MANIFESTATIONS

The disease begins suddenly, with fever, gastrointestinal symptoms, and pain in the limbs as prodromes (Brès, 1977; Emond et al., 1977). On the third day, diarrhea, pharyngitis, and a dry cough usually set in, and on the fifth day the characteristic symptoms appear: hepatitis without jaundice, morbilliform exanthems, and, in severe cases, hemorrhagic diathesis with spontaneous bleeding. In pregnant patients there are massive metrorrhagias and miscarriages. Torpor, tremor, and convulsions indicate that the central nervous system is affected. Alopecia and loss of weight are frequent accompanying symptoms. Mortality is reported as ranging from 30 to 89 per cent with death occurring between the fourth and tenth day. Convalescence is slow. Nothing is known about possible complications or sequelae, nor are any clinicochemical findings available.

## DIAGNOSIS

The principles of differential diagnosis of Marburg virus disease also apply to Ebola virus disease.

## TREATMENT AND PROPHYLAXIS

Therapy is symptomatic. A laboratory worker with a relatively light case received more than 80 million units of human interferon and about 800 ml of immune plasma. This serotherapy led to an immediate decrease of the virus titer in the blood, but it is not clear which therapy was responsible for recovery (Emond et al., 1977).

Prevention and control measures were limited mainly to ascertaining and quarantining those with the disease as well as primary contacts (Brès, 1977). In addition, attending physicians and nurses wore protective clothing, and disinfection measures were taken. The above-mentioned laboratory worker was isolated in a low-pressure plastic tent. Vaccines are not yet available. The World Health Organization has drawn up detailed recommendations for procedures in any future outbreaks. The most recent outbreak in southern Sudan (1979) began with hospital spread, which amplified transmission into the community.

### References

Bowen, E. T. W., Lloyd, G., Harris, W. J., Platt, G. S., Baskerville, A., and Vella, E. E.: Viral haemorrhagic fever in southern Sudan and northern Zaire. Lancet 1:571, 1977.

Brès, P.: WHO report of the informal consultation on the Marburg virus-like disease outbreaks in the Sudan and Zaire in 1976, held at the London School of Hygiene and Tropical Medicine, 4 and 5 January 1977. Geneva, World Health Organization, 1977.

Emond, R. T. D., Evans, B., Bowen, E. T. W., and Lloyd, G.: A case of Ebola virus infection. Br Med J 2:541, 1977.

Johnson, K. M., Lange, J. V., Webb, P. A., and Murphy, F. A.: Isolation and partial characterisation of a new virus causing acute haemorrhagic fever in Zaire. Lancet 1:569, 1977.

Pattyn, S., Groen, G. van der, Jacob, W., Piot, P., and Courteille, G.: Isolation of Marburg-like virus from a case of haemorrhagic fever in Zaire. Lancet 1:573, 1977.

World Health Organization: Viral haemorrhagic fever surveillance. Weekly Epidem. Rec. 54:319, 1979.

# 254  *CAT SCRATCH DISEASE*

### *Warren J. Warwick, M.D.*

## *DEFINITION*

Cat scratch disease (cat scratch fever, cat scratch syndrome, cat claw fever, benign inoculation lymphoreticulosis, nonbacterial regional lymphadenitis, cat adenitis) is an acute, benign, self-limited disease of the regional lymph nodes. The most specific feature is subacute regional lymphadenitis, almost always preceded by a granulomatous skin reaction at the site of a skin injury, which is usually a scratch by a cat. This skin lesion is important in establishing the diagnosis because no lymphangitis develops between the skin lesion and the enlarged lymph nodes. The enlarged lymph nodes become necrotic and are filled with pus in one third of reported cases. Fever, mild and of short duration, is the only common constitutional symptom.

## *ETIOLOGY*

The unknown causative agent is presumed to be a virus or chlamydia. The several reports of isolation of an agent from cases of cat scratch disease have not been confirmed by other laboratories.

## *EPIDEMIOLOGY*

### Subjects

Although cat scratch disease can occur at any age, children and young adults are most often affected. Cat scratch disease affects both sexes equally and all races. Excluding obvious bacterial infections, it is the most common cause of localized lymphadenopathy during the middle years (Carithers et al., 1969).

### Seasonal Variation

Cat scratch disease that is severe enough to be diagnosed and reported has a strong seasonal variation. In the temperate zone of Europe and North America three fourths of cases have been observed to occur between September and February (Warwick, 1967). However, factors influencing transmission of cat scratch disease may operate differently in other climates and environments. In the subtropical climate of Florida, three fourths of cases have been seen in the last six months of the year (Carithers et al., 1969) and in temperate-zone Japan most cases have been reported in summer and autumn (Miupa et al., 1975). In tropical areas the seasonal variation may be different or nonexistent.

### Cat Scratches and Cat Contact

The significance of cat contact, which was reported early by Daniels and MacMurray (1954) and Debré and Job (1954) to occur in nine tenths of cases, may be incidental, for 90 per cent of children in the United States have similar exposure to cats. Nevertheless, the hallmark of this disease historically (Carithers, 1970) and clinically (Warwick, 1967) has been a preceding cat scratch. Since many of the cases of cat scratch disease that occur without a preceding cat scratch follow a puncture of the skin, the focus for epidemiologic studies should be on the type of injury rather than on the cat. Although the name cat scratch disease appropriately recognizes that over half the cases follow a cat scratch, many early workers preferred the name benign inoculation lymphoreticulosis, thereby emphasizing the mode of injury rather than the usual inoculating agent.

### Epidemics

Although familial outbreaks of cat scratch disease occur, infectivity is low, fewer than one fifth of exposed family members acquiring symptomatic disease. Most family outbreaks are associated with a kitten in the household. Epidemics of cat scratch disease occur during the months of greatest likelihood of sporadic occurrence (Warwick, 1967).

## CLINICAL MANIFESTATIONS

Cat scratch disease usually begins with an isolated lesion at the site of a cat scratch occurring a week or so earlier. Two or three weeks after the first lesion the patient notices a slightly painful swollen lymph node and has slight malaise for a few days with a low fever, reduced appetite, and an occasional ache. His white blood count is slightly elevated, and there is slight eosinophilia. The constitutional symptoms and the local discomfort regress rapidly. The lymphadenopathy disappears in another three to four weeks. The patient's symptoms have been so mild that he has not come to his doctor for consultation.

### Primary Lesion

Despite early reports that primary lesions were present in only half the cases, careful research has shown that the primary lesion can be found in 95 per cent of cat scratch disease patients (Carithers et al., 1969). Since the primary lesion usually begins one to two weeks after the inoculating skin injury and lasts a variable period of one to four weeks, it is probably a constant phenomenon that is missed when it is looked for late in the course of cat scratch disease. It may begin as early as three days after the cat scratch or as late as a month, and rarely lasts several months. It does not itch. The primary lesion is usually a single papule but may consist of multiple papules along a cat scratch. The early papule is red, 2 to 5 mm in diameter, and there is no associated lymphangitis. Later, the papule may be reddish purple, scaly, vesicular, or pustular. All primary lesions are sterile. The pathologic sign is granuloma formation that resembles the pathologic process of the lymph nodes. Primary lesions heal without a scar.

Failure to find a primary lesion should alert the clinician to consider another diagnosis.

### Regional Lymphadenopathy

Every patient with cat scratch disease has lymphadenopathy. The adenopathy may affect only one node in mild cases but may involve all or most of the lymph nodes in several sequential regional chains in severe cases. Although adenopathy is occasionally painless, a local tenderness usually calls attention to the node enlargement. When the enlargement is rapid, acute tenderness may be present.

The enlargement of the lymph nodes follows the appearance of the primary lesion—in over half of cases it develops between one and two weeks and in two thirds of cases by three weeks after the inoculating cat scratch. Rarely, the lymphadenopathy may not appear for seven to ten weeks. In such cases a primary lesion may be hard to find or even absent.

Once started, the nodal pathology progresses toward suppuration. In mild cases this occurs infrequently, perhaps 10 per cent of the time. In more severe cases with substantial lymph node enlargement, suppuration may occur in half the cases.

Lymph node regression varies directly with severity of illness: in 10 per cent regression occurs by two weeks, in 25 per cent by four weeks, in 50 per cent by six weeks, in 75 per cent by nine weeks, and in 95 per cent by six months after onset of the enlargement.

The site of lymph node involvement parallels the sites of frequency of cat scratches: epitrochlear and axillary nodes in two thirds of cases, cervical and submandibular in one fourth, preauricular (Parinaud's ocular glandular syndrome) in one tenth, and inguinal and femoral nodes in one tenth. Nevertheless, lymph nodes in almost every location in the body, including the mediastinum and the mesentery, may be involved.

Lymphadenopathy in an unusual location, when accompanied by an inoculating skin injury, a primary lesion, and absence of lymphangitis, should alert the physician to a suspicion of cat scratch disease. On the other hand, the diagnosis of cat scratch disease should not be made in the absence of lymphadenopathy.

### Parinaud's Oculoglandular Syndrome

Parinaud's syndrome has been found in 2 to 18 per cent of cat scratch disease patients. Cat scratch disease is probably the only cause of this unusual syndrome. Inoculation appears to be in the conjunctiva, where one or more atypical primary lesions—gray, yellow, or reddish necrotic nodular or granulomatous lesions—develop in the retrotarsal area. When such lesions are associated with a preauricular lymph node enlargement, with or without cervical node involvement or constitutional symptoms, a clinical diagnosis of cat scratch disease may be made. The conjunctival lesion heals in one to three weeks without injury to the eye.

### Systemic Symptoms

Although over two thirds of diagnosed patients are only mildly ill, constitutional symptoms can be important. In patients with milder lymphadenopathy fever may be associated in one third of cases, whereas in more severe illness fever may be present in three fourths of cases. Fever is usually low, 38° C, but rarely it may exceed 39° C. Generalized or local aching, malaise, anorexia, nausea, and abdominal pain are seen more often in older patients and in patients with extensive lymph node involvement.

## COMPLICATIONS

Table 1 contains a test of many of the reported atypical manifestations associated with cat scratch disease. These are rare, sometimes only

**TABLE 1.  Atypical Signs of Cat Scratch Disease**

Parinaud's oculoglandular syndrome

Lymphadenopathy

    Bilateral
    Generalized
    Mesenteric hilar

Skin reactions

    Erythema annulare
    Erythema multiforme
    Papular vesicular rash
    Maculopapular rash
    Thrombocytopenic purpura
    Erythema nodosum
    Nonthrombocytopenic purpura

Miscellaneous

    Pneumonia
    Pharyngitis
    Osteolytic granuloma
    Subacute iriditis
    Nonspecific nongonococcal urethritis
    Lymphedema
    Herpes zoster
    Thyroiditis
    Anicteric hepatitis
    Submaxillary and parotid localization
    Encephalitis
    Hepatomegaly
    Splenomegaly
    Optic neuritis

one observation, but they demonstrate the many variations of symptomatology that can make diagnosis difficult. Encephalitis is the most important symptom and has been reported in over 30 patients.

The association of encephalitis (Lyon, 1971; Warwick, 1967) with cat scratch disease is hard to establish in a given case. The afflicted patients have abrupt onset of convulsions and coma. The clinical impression of encephalitis is supported by findings of mild pleocytosis. The patients regain consciousness within two to ten days and recover completely. About one third have transient neurologic problems lasting a few months to a year. Although not proved beyond a doubt, deaths have been seen in suspected cases of encephalitis attributed to cat scratch disease.

## DIAGNOSIS

Since the etiologic agent is unknown, the diagnosis of cat scratch disease requires matching symptoms to a syndrome: (1) There must be regional lymphadenopathy; (2) there must be no other cause for the lymphadenopathy; (3) a primary lesion is present; (4) a cat scratch or other puncture wound precedes the other symptoms; (5) the disease shows a benign course with spontaneous recovery.

When these five criteria are satisfied a presumptive diagnosis of cat scratch disease may be made. When atypical features are present or when the syndrome is incomplete, the diagnosis can usually be confirmed by finding: (6) typical histopathology on biopsy of the primary lesion or the affected lymph node; (7) a positive Hanger-Rose skin test.

### Biopsy

The pathology of the skin lesion and of the skin test is one of dermal necrosis within a zone of acellular necrobiosis, which is in turn inside a zone of epithelial cells and giant cells surrounded by a thin layer of small lymphocytes (Johnson and Helwig, 1969; Czarnetzki et al., 1975).

The lymph node changes of early lymphoid hyperplasia, later granuloma, and finally microabscess formation are separately characteristic but not diagnostic of cat scratch disease. When all three histologic phases are present in the same lymph node, however, the trio is distinctive (Campbell, 1977). When Campbell's observations of the simultaneous presence of lymphoid hyperplasia, granulomas, and microabscess in the same lymph node are found, the diagnosis of cat scratch disease may be made on as firm or firmer ground than the finding of a positive Hanger-Rose skin test.

## Hanger-Rose Skin Test

The development of a skin test antigen by Hanger and Rose (Carithers, 1970) made it possible for clinicians to assign a common cause to many benign lymphadenopathies. The Hanger-Rose antigen is prepared from pus from proven cases of cat scratch disease. The pus is tested to prove that it is sterile by conventional aerobic, anaerobic, and viral cultures and animal inoculations. The pus is diluted, usually in a ratio of 1 part pus to 4 or 5 parts sterile distilled water. It is then heated to inactivate any undetectable agent, checked again for sterility, and tested on known cases to prove potency and on normals to prove specificity. One tenth of the Hanger-Rose antigen is injected intradermally, and the reaction is read at 48 hours. Induration of 5 mm or more or erythema of 10 mm or more is regarded as a positive test.

Antigens vary in both sensitivity and specificity. Not all antigens give positive skin tests in all proven cases of cat scratch disease. In fact, only 90 per cent of proven cases react positively to potent skin test antigens, and a variable proportion of healthy normal subjects have positive skin tests. The frequency of positive skin tests in healthy normals varies from 4 per cent in nonendemic areas to 10 per cent in endemic areas. Almost one fifth of family contacts and one fourth of veterinary workers have positive skin tests.

The relatively high background of positive tests and the substantial number of false-negative tests indicate that the Hanger-Rose skin test is not to be substituted for clinical judgment or pathologic studies. The Hanger-Rose skin test has been and is a valuable aid in diagnosis, but with 5 to 10 per cent false-positive and false-negative results, it cannot be used as the sole arbiter of a diagnosis. The scientific foundation for the Hanger-Rose skin test awaits identification of the causative agent.

Despite 35 years of use with no untoward reactions reported, questions of the safety of the Hanger-Rose antigen continue to be raised—especially concerning viral hepatitis, a slow virus, or an incomplete virus. Autoclaving at 4.5 kg, 100° C for 10 minutes (Kalter et al., 1977), heating at 56° C for 12 hours (Carithers, 1977), or sterilizing with gamma radiation (Bradstreet and Gidherd, 1977) has been recommended to make the antigen safe.

Since there is no antigen available commercially, persons studying cat scratch disease continue to make their own antigen. In view of the problems of specificity, sensitivity, and safety, new workers in the field of cat scratch disease are advised to collaborate with workers still active in cat scratch disease research in preparation of new Hanger-Rose antigen from pus from suppurative lymph nodes.

The Hanger-Rose skin test has been accepted as evidence of a delayed type hypersensitivity response to the cat scratch disease antigen. Therefore, the observations by Schulkind and Ayoub (1974) that cat scratch disease patients show no in vitro lymphocyte transformation when exposed to cat scratch disease antigen when the Hanger-Rose skin test is positive was unexpected. Cat scratch disease patients also showed lymphocyte transformation, unresponsiveness to *C. albicans* and PHA. These in vitro types of unresponsiveness were of shorter duration than similar changes seen in sarcoid, cancer, or protein-caloric malnutrition, being closer to the transient state produced by acute viral infections.

The pathology of the Hanger-Rose skin test has been studied recently by Czarnetzki and co-workers (1975). They found that 15 patients with cat scratch disease, 3 of 12 patients with sarcoidosis, 1 of 12 with tuberculosis, and none of 12 controls showed a common pathology—a granulomatous reaction with epithelioid cells, plasma cells, lymphocytes, and giant cell areas of necrobiosis.

These two studies suggest a possible etiologic link between cat scratch disease and sarcoidosis.

## Laboratory Studies

No laboratory test is helpful in establishing the diagnosis of cat scratch disease. Laboratory tests are, however, of great aid in establishing that a patient with lymphadenopathy does not have another disease. The exclusion of other causes of lymphadenopathy is a major step in arriving at a diagnosis. Hematologic studies show no neutropenia, rare leukocytosis, and occasional eosinophilia; the occasionally elevated sedimentation rate is related to fever.

Cultures for bacteria, fungi, mycobacteria, and viruses are sterile. Agglutination tests for syphilis, *Brucella*, tularemia, and melitensis are negative, as are the heterophil tests. Skin tests for mycobacteria and fungi are negative. Although low titers against chlamydial antigens develop in many patients who have suppurative lymph nodes, these titers are not helpful in diagnosis.

## Differential Clinical Diagnosis

The lymphadenopathy of cat scratch disease, especially when suppuration occurs, may be misdiagnosed as a purulent bacterial lymphadenopathy. When cat scratch disease is the cause, antibiotic treatment will not alter the course of the illness, and when the diagnosis is missed, prolonged antibiotic therapy only exposes the patient to the expense and hazards of over-treatment.

On the other hand, when the lymph node enlargement is solid and of long duration, the question of lymphoma may arise. Since the pathology of cat scratch disease may not be specific, confusion with lymphoma or Hodgkin's disease can lead to serious errors in treatment.

## TREATMENT

Supportive symptomatic treatment is indicated. Antibiotics do not change the course of the disease, nor does cortisone. Suppurative nodes should be aspirated. Incision and drainage are contraindicated because draining sinuses frequently result. Excision of the affected nodes may be indicated when a draining sinus is present, when the symptoms are atypical, when constitutional symptoms are severe (i.e., encephalitis), when diagnosis is urgent, or when malignancy is suspected.

## References

Bradstreet, C. M., and Digherd, N. W.: Cat-scratch fever skin-test antigen (letter). Lancet 1:913, 1977.
Campbell, J. A.: Cat-scratch disease. Pathol Annu 12:277, 1977.
Carithers, H. A.: Cat-scratch disease; notes on its history. Am J Dis Child 119:200, 1970.
Carithers, H. A.: Cat-scratch skin test antigen; purification by heating. Pediatrics 60:928, 1977.
Carithers, H. A., Carithers, C. M., and Edwards, R. O., Jr.: Cat-scratch disease: Its natural history. JAMA 207:312, 1969.
Czarnetzki, B. M., Pomeranz, J. R., Khandekar, P. K., Wolinsky, E., and Belcher, P. W.: Cat-scratch disease skin test. Studies of specificity and histopathologic features. Arch Dermatol 111:736, 1975.
Daniels, W. B., and MacMurray, F. G.: Cat-scratch disease; report of 160 cases. JAMA 154:1247, 1954.
Debré, R., and Job, J. C.: La maladie des griffes de chat. Acta Paediat Suppl Upps 43:1, 1954.
Johnson, W. T., and Helwig, E. B.: Cat-scratch disease. Histopathologic changes in the skin. Arch Dermatol 100:148, 1969.
Kalter, S. S., Rodriguez, A. P., and Heberling, R. L.: Cat-scratch disease skin-test antigen preparation (letter). Lancet 2:606, 1977.
Lyon, L. W.: Neurologic manifestations of cat-scratch disease. Report of a case and review of the literature. Arch Neurol 25:23, 1971.
Margileth, A. M.: Cat-scratch disease: Nonbacterial regional lymphadenitis. The story of 145 patients and a review of the literature. Pediatrics 42:803, 1968.
Miupa, T., Topinuki, I. W., and Tanahashi, Y.: Cat-scratch disease. J Exp Med 117:373, 1975.
Schulkind, M. L., and Ayoub, E. M.: Cell-mediated immunity in cat-scratch disease. J Pediatr 85:199, 1974.
Warwick, W. J.: The cat-scratch syndrome, many diseases or one disease. Prog Med Virol 9:256, 1967.

# 255 COLORADO TICK FEVER

## Alan G. Barbour, M.D.
## Spotswood L. Spruance, M.D.

## DEFINITION

Colorado tick fever is a viral disease characterized by a biphasic course and leukopenia. It is transmitted by ticks in the Rocky Mountain area and the Pacific slope of the United States and Canada.

## ETIOLOGY AND EPIDEMIOLOGY

At the end of the 19th century, physicians in the newly settled Rocky Mountain region of the United States recognized a mild, tick-borne disease that was distinct from Rocky Mountain spotted fever. In 1944, Florio reported the successful transmission of Colorado tick fever to human volunteers and to hamsters by the injection of serum from patients with the disease. Florio later noted that the agent would pass through bacterial filters, and the causative organism was subsequently shown to be a double-stranded RNA virus. Colorado tick fever virus is presently classified in the genus *Orbivirus* of the family Reoviridae. Human virus isolates have been of one major serotype. An unclassified tick-borne virus, the Eyach virus, isolated in the Federal Republic of Germany, has partial antigenic cross-reactivity with the Colorado tick fever virus.

Colorado tick fever is acquired from the bite of infected ticks. The disease occurs almost exclusively in the area of distribution of the wood tick, *Dermacentor andersoni* (Fig. 1). Infection of travelers and vacationers may lead to the appearance of the disease outside of western North America. The virus has been recovered from other ticks in the endemic area, but *D. andersoni* is the only tick known to transmit the disease to man (Eklund et al., 1955).

*D. andersoni*, a hard-body tick, resides at 1200 to 3300 meters altitude in regions of brushy and evergreen vegetation, such as sagebrush and juniper. It is scarce in heavy timber or open grassland. Female ticks lay their eggs under dead vegetation. The six-legged larvae that emerge find a small mammal such as a ground squirrel, feed for a few days, and drop off to molt into nymphs. The eight-legged nymphs hibernate unfed and seek

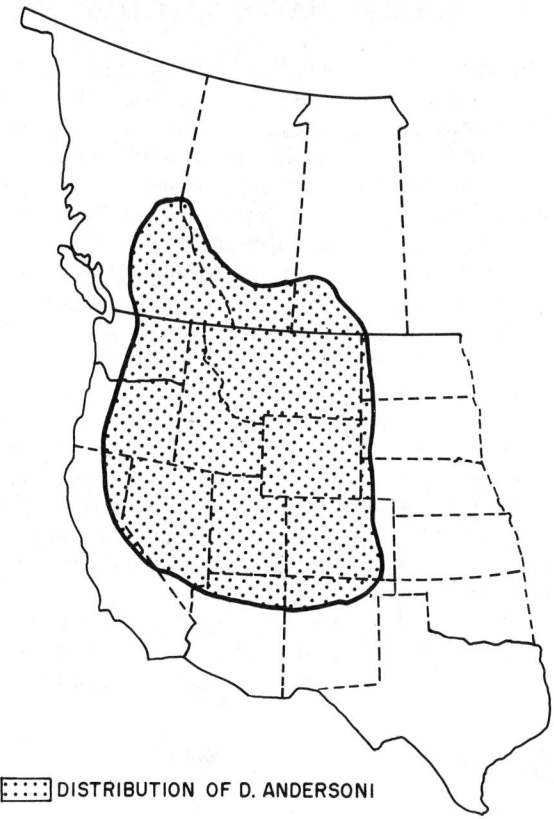

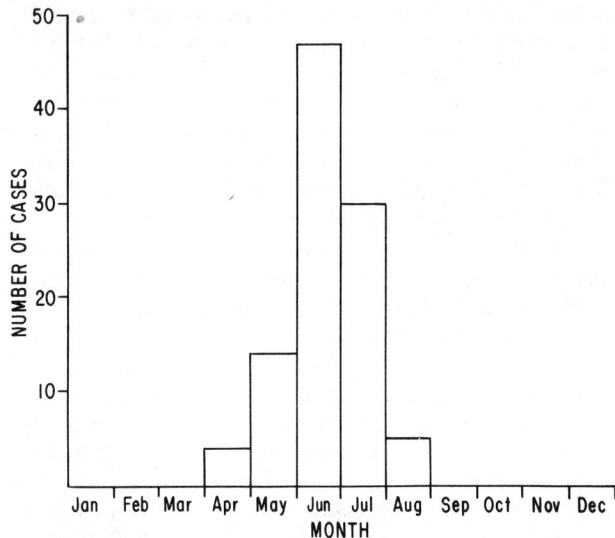

**FIGURE 2.** *Month of onset of 100 cases of Colorado tick fever in Utah.*

**FIGURE 1.** *Distribution of* Dermacentor andersoni *in the western United States and Canada. (Adapted from Eklund, C. M., Kohls, G. M., and Brennan, J. M.: JAMA 157:335, 1955.)*

another small mammal in the spring. After feeding for four to nine days, the nymphs fall off and molt into adults. The adults seek larger mammal hosts, including deer and man. Female ticks attach and feed for 6 to 13 days, drop off to lay eggs, and die. The male may feed for only a few hours before seeking an attached female to mate. A cycle of inapparent infections between the immature stages of the tick and small mammals maintains the virus in the endemic area. The virus overwinters in nymphal ticks and may also persist in hibernating animals. Transovarial passage of the virus by the tick has not been demonstrated.

Man acquires infected adult ticks by contact with grass stalks and low shrubs while hiking, camping, or engaging in other outdoor activities. Although most patients with Colorado tick fever report possible exposure to ticks, only one half have been aware of a tick bite or attachment. The high proportion of Colorado tick fever patients who are adult males reflects their more frequent exposure to the vector. As many as 15 per cent of individuals in high-risk occupations, such as forest rangers, may possess neutralizing antibody against the virus.

Colorado tick fever occurs in the late spring and summer (Fig. 2), the seasons when adult *D. andersoni* ticks are most active. The peak incidence of human cases occurs during April and May at lower altitudes and during June and July at higher elevations. Rarely, cases may occur at atypical times of the year in recipients of infected blood or in laboratory workers who are accidentally inoculated.

## PATHOGENESIS AND PATHOLOGY

Viremia is a regular occurrence in Colorado tick fever. The virus can be recovered from the plasma for approximately one week and from the erythrocyte fraction of blood for up to 120 days after onset of the disease. The duration of viremia corresponds with the lifespan of red cells. Its intra-erythrocytic location protects the virus from neutralizing antibody. Because the mature erythrocyte lacks functional ribosomes that are essential to viral replication, it is likely that infection of red cells begins in hematopoietic cells. Virions and evidence of viral replication have been seen by electronmicroscopy within erythrocyte precursors in the bone marrow of infected patients.

Leukopenia with the nadir at the beginning of the second febrile episode is characteristic of Colorado tick fever. Neutrophils and lymphocytes are both decreased in number. Because lymphocytes appear to recover more quickly, neutropenia is observed more commonly. There is an increase in the proportion of immature neutrophils in the peripheral blood, and examination of the bone marrow reveals a maturation arrest in the neutrophil series. The white cell count may remain depressed for up to seven days after clinical recovery. The pathogenesis of the leukopenia is unknown, but it may be caused by infection of stem cells in the bone marrow. Alternatively, because Colorado tick fever virus is an interferon inducer, high systemic or local hematopoietic tissue levels of interferon may depress the white cell count.

Thrombocytopenia, disseminated intravascular coagulation, and hemorrhage occur rarely. Focal necrosis and swelling of the capillary epithelium were seen on postmortem examination of one patient. Meningitis and encephalitis occur rarely and are probably the result of infection rather than immunologic injury. The virus has been recovered from the cerebrospinal fluid of one patient with encephalitis and from the CSF of experimentally infected volunteers without neurologic symptoms. There were intracytoplasmic inclusion bodies in the Purkinje cells and neurons of the midbrain in one fatal case. In mice, there is an apparent predilection of the virus for brain as well as for heart muscle, spleen, lymphoid tissue, and bone marrow.

## CLINICAL MANIFESTATIONS

The incubation period is usually three to five days, but it may be as long as ten days. There are no prodromal manifestations. The onset is sudden, and symptoms are commonly maximal within hours. Patients often report chilliness without true rigors. The triad of fever, headache, and myalgia, notably of the back and legs, is usual. Retro-orbital pain and pain elicited by ocular movements are other common complaints. Respiratory symptoms are very rare. Abdominal pain and vomiting occur occasionally.

The course of Colorado tick fever is distinctive (Fig. 3). A majority of patients experience a biphasic fever in which a two- to three-day febrile period is followed by a remission of one or two days before the onset of another two- to three-day febrile period ("saddle-back" fever). The remaining patients have a single febrile episode or, more rarely, three bouts of fever.

Physical findings are meager. A mild, transient rash occurs in approximately 5 to 10 per cent of patients; it may be macular, maculopapular, or

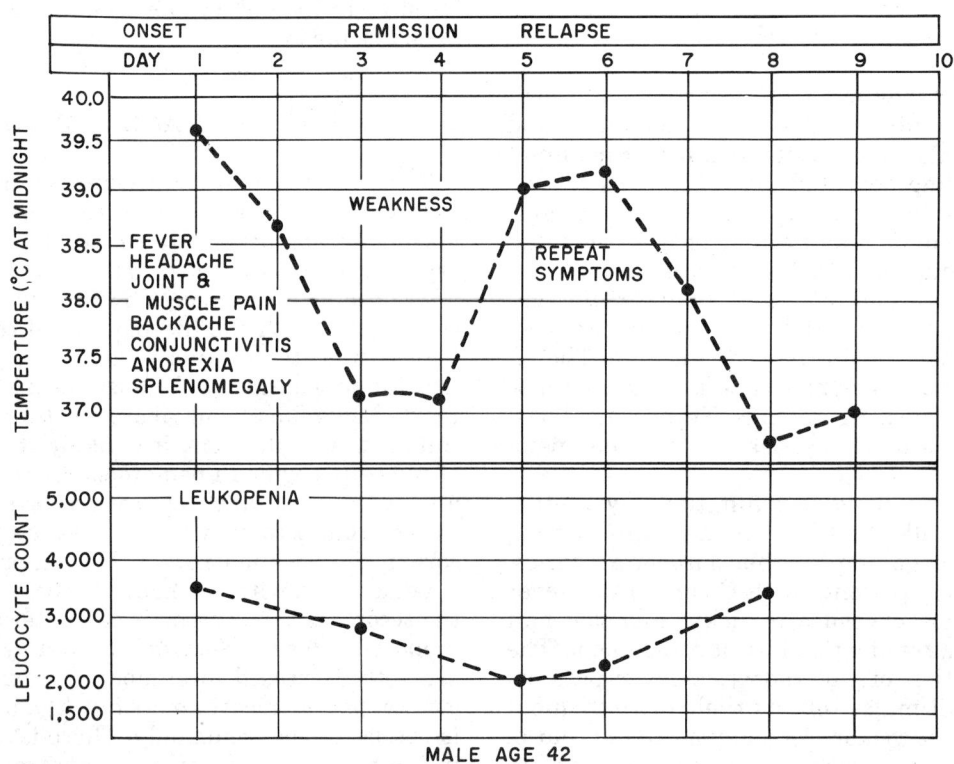

**FIGURE 3.** *Temperature curve, clinical findings, and leukocyte count during the course of Colorado tick fever. (Adapted from Johnson, E. S., Napoli V. M., and White, W. C.: Am J Clin Pathol 34:118, 1960.)*

petechial. Tachycardia, a flushed face, injection of the conjunctiva and pharynx, and a palpable spleen are other findings that may be observed. There is usually no unusual local reaction at the site of the tick bite.

## COMPLICATIONS AND SEQUELAE

Complications of Colorado tick fever are rare and usually occur only in children. Encephalitis, meningitis, meningoencephalitis, and a hemorrhagic state resembling the hemorrhagic syndrome of dengue have occurred. Adults have developed pericarditis and myocarditis.

Many patients, especially those over 30 years of age, experience a prolonged convalescence with complaints of malaise and weakness. There is no apparent association between the length of convalescence and the duration of viremia. Immunity is usually life-long, but there is one documented case of reinfection (Goodpasture et al., 1978).

In laboratory animals, Colorado tick fever virus crosses the placenta and is teratogenic. Of the six known cases of Colorado tick fever in pregnant women, one woman aborted, four delivered normal infants, and one delivered an infant with multiple congenital abnormalities.

## DIAGNOSIS

Usually the biphasic course and the leukopenia should suggest Colorado tick fever, particularly if there is a history of tick exposure. Dengue is the closest clinical analog of Colorado tick fever but can be distinguished by the mutually exclusive epidemiologic features of the two diseases. Dengue is transmitted by *Aedes* mosquitoes in tropic and subtropic regions. Influenza may have a similar abrupt onset and may also be accompanied by leukopenia but usually causes prominent respiratory complaints such as sore throat, cough, and chest pain. In areas that are endemic for Colorado tick fever, the disease is commonly confused with Rocky Mountain spotted fever (Spruance and Bailey, 1973). This rickettsial disease, although tick-borne, is at present seldom documented in the Rocky Mountain area. Rocky Mountain spotted fever can be distinguished by the progressive rash that appears two to four days after onset, a tendency to cause leukocytosis, and a more severe, unremitting course. Tick-borne relapsing fever, caused by *Borrelia* species and transmitted by soft-body ticks of the genus *Ornithodoros,* can closely mimic Colorado tick fever. In relapsing fever, the leukocyte count is usually within normal limits, and the spirochete can be seen in blood smears obtained from the patient during a febrile episode or from rats inoculated with the patient's blood. The *Proteus* OX-K agglutination may be reactive in relapsing fever, and the *Proteus* OX-2 and/or OX-19 serologic reactions are positive in Rocky Mountain spotted fever. Specific complement fixation tests are also available for relapsing fever and Rocky Mountain spotted fever. Tularemia may be tick-borne but is usually accompanied by an ulcer at the tick bite and by lymphadenopathy. The agglutination test for tularemia is positive after 10 to 14 days.

Leukopenia, as noted above, is very common during Colorado tick fever. Leukocyte counts of between 2000 and 3000 per $mm^3$ are common. The lowest values occur during the beginning of the second febrile period. The white cell count may be normal during the initial stages of the illness. On blood smear, "toxic" neutrophils and atypical lymphocytes may be seen.

The diagnosis is confirmed by isolating the virus from blood, by identifying the agent in red cells by fluorescent antibody staining, or by serology. Because the viremia is cell-associated and because neutralizing antibody may be present in the plasma, a blood clot or erythrocytes washed free of plasma is the appropriate specimen for virus isolation and fluorescent antibody studies (Emmons, 1979). Red cells are homogenized and injected intraperitoneally or intracerebrally into suckling mice for virus isolation. The injection is usually lethal for mice, but serial passage may be necessary for isolation. The identification is verified by neutralization tests in mice. The direct fluorescent antibody stain of a peripheral blood clot is positive in virtually all human cases six days or more after onset and for up to several weeks thereafter (Emmons and Lennette, 1966). False-negative tests may occur during the first few days of the disease. A fourfold rise in neutralizing antibodies, complement-fixing antibodies, or antibodies in the indirect immunofluorescence assay is diagnostic. The presence of complement-fixing antibodies in a single convalescent specimen in association with the typical clinical syndrome is strong evidence for the disease. Diagnostic tests for Colorado tick fever are available only from a few state or regional reference laboratories in the endemic area.

## TREATMENT

Treatment is symptomatic. Analgesics and antipyretics such as salicylates are usually adequate for control of headache and myalgia. When a patient with tick exposure is seriously ill, one should consider other tick-borne diseases such as Rocky Mountain spotted fever, relapsing fever, and tularemia.

## *PREVENTION*

The cornerstone of prevention is avoidance of tick bites. Individuals who are outdoors in the endemic area during spring and summer should inspect their clothing, hair, and skin periodically with special attention to the hairline and axillae. If an attached tick is discovered, it can be removed by gentle backward traction. Trying to "unscrew" the tick will often only break off the body and leave the mouth parts embedded. A physician removing a tick from a patient should insert the tip of a needle under the head of the tick before applying traction with forceps. Application of an organic solvent such as alcohol or nail polish remover to the tick may aid detachment. A lighted match or other flame should not be used.

An experimental vaccine has been prepared from inactivated virus. Immunized volunteers developed high titers of neutralizing antibody. Possible utilization of a vaccine would appear to be justifiable only for laboratory personnel and outdoor workers at high risk of exposure in the restricted ecologic niche of *D. andersoni*.

The Colorado tick fever patient is not contagious and need not be isolated at home or in the hospital. However, the patient's blood products should be considered potentially hazardous and should not be used for transfusion for at least six months after recovery.

### References

Eklund, C. M., Kohls, G. M., and Brennan, J. M.: Distribution of Colorado tick fever and virus carrying ticks. JAMA 157:335, 1955.
Emmons, R. W.: Colorado tick fever. In Beran, G. (ed.): CRC Handbook of Zoonoses. Section B: Viral Zoonoses. Cleveland, CRC Press, Inc., 1981.
Emmons, R. W., and Lennette, E. H.: Immunofluorescent staining in the laboratory diagnosis of Colorado tick fever. J Lab Clin Med 68:923, 1966.
Florio, L., Steward, M. O., and Mugrage, E. R.: The experimental transmission of Colorado tick fever. J Exp Med 80:165, 1944.
Goodpasture, H. C., Poland, J. D., Francy, D. B., Bowen, G. S., and Horn, K. A.: Colorado tick fever: Clinical, epidemiologic, and laboratory aspects of 228 cases in Colorado in 1973–1974. Ann Intern Med 88:303, 1978.
Spruance, S. L., and Bailey, A.: Colorado tick fever: A review of 115 laboratory confirmed cases. Arch Intern Med 131:288, 1973.

# K.   ILLNESSES SIMULATING INFECTIONS

# 256 *FACTITIOUS AND DELUSIONAL ILLNESSES SIMULATING INFECTIONS*

## J. Allen McCutchan, M.D.

### *INTRODUCTION*

Certain illnesses simulate infections but are self-inflicted or delusional. In order to deceive their physicians, psychologically disturbed patients may injure themselves by causing factitious infections. These patients sometimes present additional signs or symptoms of other hereditary, metabolic, immunologic, or traumatic conditions (Aduan et al., 1979; Petersdorf and Bennett, 1957; Rumans and Vosti, 1978). Because of the multiple and sometimes exotic agents and syndromes of infection, the possibility of deception is often overlooked until extensive diagnostic evaluations have been repeated several times.

Factitious illnesses seen at two major medical centers in the United States have been recently reviewed (Aduan et al., 1979; Rumans and Vosti, 1978). The cases collected in these series suggest that these diseases are uncommon but not rare. For example, factitious fever accounted for 32 of 342 (9 per cent) cases referred to the National Institutes of Health for evaluation of prolonged, unexplained fever. The first part of this chapter describes the clinical syndromes, psychopathology, diagnosis, and management of these difficult and confounding patients. The second part deals with delusional illnesses that simulate infection.

### *DEFINITIONS*

*Factitious illness* is the simulation or production of illnesses with the intent of deception. In *simulated disease,* data or symptoms are falsified to mimic illness when none exists (for example, heating a thermometer to simulate fever). *Self-inflicted disease* is unacknowledged self-injury that produces real illness. Although illnesses (for example, lung cancer) may result from chronic self-injury (smoking), the intent is not to injure or defraud, and activity is not concealed. In contrast to those who intentionally deceive their physicians, patients with delusional illnesses believe they have a disease when none exists. Thus, *delusional disease* is obsessive belief in a non-existent illness (for example, delusions of parasitosis) after reassurance by a physician. Rarely, parents cause simulated disease in their children, medical personnel falsify clinical data about patients, and groups of patients may share delusions (epidemic hysteria).

Several conditions related to factitious illness require definition and differentiation. *Malingering* refers to fraudulent illness practiced for some clear gain (Asher, 1959). Because the gain may be socially acceptable (for example, escape from prison camps in wartime), malingerers are not necessarily psychologically disturbed or sociopathic. Physicians can usually recognize malingering easily because the motive (for example, transfer from jail to the hospital) is obvious. *Munchausen's syndrome* refers to a distinct subgroup of chronic fraudulent illnesses in which wandering, homeless men repeatedly simulate dramatic acute illnesses (Cramer et al., 1971).

## PATHOGENESIS

Factitious illnesses occur in patients who have both the motivation and skills to simulate or produce illness. The motivation is not well understood, and the degree of psychological disturbance varies widely. Psychiatric diagnoses in these patients range from malingering to schizophrenia, but many patients lack easily recognizable psychological disturbances. Malingerers achieve secondary gains from their illness, which most physicians recognize in obviously sociopathic persons. When apparently well-adjusted people use self-inflicted illness to avoid responsibility, gain attention, or manipulate others, malingering is not so obvious. Patients with chronic factitious illness include several groups with moderately severe psychological disturbances often described as "borderline personalities" (Asher, 1959). Munchausen's syndrome describes a group of male wanderers who present in dramatic fashion to hospital emergency rooms with elaborate false medical histories and assumed identities. They often submit to extensive, invasive, and potentially dangerous diagnostic and therapeutic procedures and then abruptly leave against medical advice. Their motivation and psychopathology are not understood. More common, but less easily recognized, are young, usually female, medical and paramedical personnel. These patients have a variety of psychiatric syndromes ranging from neuroses, conversion reactions, borderline personalities, and transient psychoses. Many of them appear to have an underlying personality disorder characterized by hostility, dependency, hysteria, and self-destruction. Because psychopathology in these patients is not necessarily obvious, their physicians often fail to consider the possibility of fraudulent illness and to deny it when consultants suggest it. Further self-destructive behavior in the form of suicide is unusual but must be borne in mind.

Medical and paramedical workers are heavily represented among patients with factitious illnesses for several reasons. They have the necessary skills, knowledge, and access to equipment. They may have selected a medical career because of the need to form dependent relationships with physicians. Moreover, their hostility and dependency toward physicians may have developed because of their relative occupational status or individual relationships with physicians. Other persons with the equipment and skills necessary for self-infection are intravenous drug users and insulin-dependent diabetics.

## CLINICAL SYNDROMES

Factitious illnesses can be classified by the methods of deception, the diseases they mimic, or the psychopathology of the patients. The following classification divides these illnesses by clinical syndrome.

### Factitious Fever

#### Simulated Fever

Falsification of temperatures to mimic prolonged unexplained fever is the most widely recognized factitious infectious disease. By definition, real fever and its symptoms are absent, but some of these patients deliberately prolong a real febrile illness. Objective evidence of a real disease early in its course often dissuades the physician from considering the diagnosis of factitious prolongation of the fever.

The two major techniques for falsifying fever are warming the thermometer or substituting thermometers with preset recordings. Various sources of heat (water, light bulbs, cigarette lighters, and hair dryers) have been used. Patients may also submit fraudulent temperature records taken at home or in other hospitals. The major clues to the diagnosis are lack of objective signs of disease, bizarre temperature patterns, other factitious symptoms, and manipulative behavior during temperature recording. When these patients are examined immediately after a high temperature is recorded, they have neither the tachycardia, skin warmth, and flushing of high fever, nor the cool, wet skin found after recent defervescence. Temperature readings more than 41.1° C and rapid, nonphysiologic changes in fever should arouse suspicion. Carefully monitored temperature recordings show no fever. This syndrome occurs most commonly in paramedical personnel whose knowledge of hospital routine makes it easy for them to deceive the nursing staff. Other factitious diseases may coexist with fever but usually do not.

The illustrative cases outlined below were reported by Rumans and Vosti (1978). The first patient's age, sex, occupation, history of emotional problems, and methods of deception are typical of factitious fever in paramedical personnel. The second case illustrates the problem of factitious prolongation of fever after a real febrile illness in a school-age adolescent.

## Case 1

A 28-year-old registered nurse was admitted after a 10-day course of pain in the right lower abdominal quadrant. Her intrauterine contraceptive (Dalkon shield) was removed without improvement. Admission temperature was 37.0° C with a pulse of 70. Pelvic exam revealed only minimal tenderness; complete blood count was normal; cultures of blood, urine, and cervix were negative; and radiologic examination of colon and intravenous pyelogram were normal. Laparoscopy and cystoscopy discovered no disease. On oral cephalosporin therapy, she had repeatedly elevated temperatures as high as 40° C without accompanying tachycardia. The nursing staff was instructed to measure the temperature very carefully with a nurse in attendance at the bedside. Despite these instructions, the patient was able repeatedly to manipulate those responsible for obtaining an accurate record of her temperature; that is, she would leave the bed to go to the bathroom with the thermometer in place or she would wear electric hair curlers while her temperature was taken. Frequent measurements gave the following pattern of temperature: 10:15 A.M., 38.6° C; 10:45 A.M., 36.6° C; 11:15 A.M., 37.2° C; 12 Noon, 39.5° C; 12:30 P.M., 37.3° C. Corresponding pulse rates were 80 to 94/minute. No antipyretics were given.

The patient was confronted with these findings by her private gynecologist. She denied any attempted manipulation of the thermometer. A significant past history for emotional problems was obtained, including a history of child abuse. In addition, she had recently experienced a stormy breakup with a boyfriend of long standing and described marked distress with her job. She was discharged with no antibiotics and subsequently returned to work. There has been no recurrence of fever or abdominal pain.

## Case 2

A 16-year-old woman student had persistent fever for 6 months following acute right otitis media with drainage. Ampicillin for 2 months failed to affect the fevers (38.5 to 39.0° C), and the patient stayed home from school. After stopping ampicillin, her fevers increased to between 39 and 40° C, but diaphoresis, chills, weight loss, and drainage were absent. The patient attended school but went to bed promptly on arriving home. Admission temperature was 39.0° C with pulse of 70/minute. The right ear canal was red, but the tympanic membrane was normal. CBC was normal, sedimentation rate was 27 mm/minute. Radiographic exam of mastoids and chest, blood cultures, and bone marrow exam were normal. When rectal temperature measurements were carefully monitored because of the lack of tachycardia with fever, she remained afebrile.

### Self-Inflicted Fever

Fever, without local signs of infection, may result from skillful intravenous injection of sterile pyrogens, cultures of bacteria, other contaminated material (such as sputum, urine, or feces), or allergens such as foreign proteins. Blood cultures may document the presence of bacteremia. Repeated isolation of the same organism may simulate endocarditis. Polymicrobial bacteremia might suggest an occult biliary tract, gastrointestinal, or genitourinary infection. Ingestion or intravenous injection of allergens is a less common method of producing fever and may simulate febrile rheumatologic, metabolic, or infectious diseases. Since the fever is real, these patients have the usual signs and symptoms of fever and defervescence.

The cases below were reported by Aduan and his colleagues at the National Institutes of Health in Bethesda (Aduan et al., 1979). The patient described in Case 3 produced polymicrobial bacteremia probably by intravenous injection of feces. In Case 4, a patient with access to pure cultures of bacteria injected herself subcutaneously many times. In the hospital, she produced *Staphylococcus aureus* and *Pseudomonas* bacteremia with hypotension probably by deep subcutaneous or intravenous self-injection.

## Case 3

A 25-year-old, white licensed practical nurse was admitted with fever and abdominal pain for 10 months. Nine years before admission, the patient had suffered right lower quadrant pain and had undergone an exploratory laparotomy with removal of a right ovarian cyst and a normal appendix. One year before admission, because of recurrent abdominal pain, she underwent a second exploratory laparotomy with a right oophorectomy and removal of a left ovarian cyst. Ten months before admission, she developed fever and abdominal pain. Initial urine and blood cultures grew *Klebsiella* species. Subsequent blood cultures grew *Clostridia* species, *E. coli*, anaerobic diphtheroids, and another species of *Klebsiella*. Because a pelvic abscess was suspected, the patient underwent her third exploratory laparotomy, which revealed only splenomegaly. Seven months before admission, she was evaluated at a major hospital center. Blood cultures were again positive for multiple different organisms. *E. coli*, two *Bacillus* species, *Pseudomonas maltophilia*, and *Klebsiella* sp. Celiac angiography suggested a splenic abscess, and the patient underwent her fourth exploratory laparotomy. Again, only splenomegaly was found. Four months before admission, she again developed abdominal pain, fever, and shock. Repeat celiac angiography was negative, but subsequent abdominal radiographic contrast studies suggested a pancreatic cyst. Because of continued episodes of pain, she required three additional hospitalizations and large doses of narcotic analgesics. Factitious fever had been considered by this patient's referring physician but was not proved.

At admission, her temperature was 37.2° C rectally. Physical examination revealed numerous areas of induration on her buttocks and anterior thighs bilaterally from intramuscular injections of analgesics. A grade 2/6 systolic murmur was heard. Multiple well-healed surgical scars were noted on the abdomen. Leukocyte count was 4000/mm with a normal differential count; erythrocyte sedimentation rate was 70 mm/hour. Other laboratory serologic tests were negative. The patient complained of severe abdominal pain and had multiple temperature spikes up to 40° C rectally. Two days after admission, she had an episode of polymicrobial bacteremia with blood cultures growing *Klebsiella*, *E. coli*, *Proteus morgani*, and Group D streptococcus. Subsequent blood cultures were negative. Extensive diagnostic evaluation failed to reveal a septic focus. Because of the high index of suspicion of factitious fever or self-induced bacteremia, the patient's room was searched. Several syringes, needles, and an open bottle of local anesthetic (lidocaine) were found.

A psychiatric consultant made a diagnosis of borderline personality disorder. The patient denied self-injection or possession of needles and syringes and never admitted to inducing either her fevers or infections. She was referred for inpatient psychiatric care at another institution.

During the next 3 months, she had an unsuccessful trial of psychotherapy. Hypnosis, with posthypnotic suggestion, was used unsuccessfully to treat her persistent abdominal pain (conversion reaction). She made four suicide attempts during this period and underwent 14 electroconvulsive treatments. Some progress was made by using behavior modification. The final psychiatric diagnosis was (1) hysterical personality, severe, with depressive neurosis, or (2) borderline state with hysterical features.

## Case 4

A 28-year-old, white laboratory technologist had a 5-year history of fever and recurrent skin lesions. She claimed to have a lifelong history of skin lesions attributed to "staphylococcal infections." At age 15, she had an apparent episode of acute rheumatic fever manifested by arthritis and a heart murmur. Over the next 6 years, she received penicillin prophylaxis. Her heart murmur was subsequently not heard. Five years before admission, she developed the first of many episodes of fever, chills, and erythematous skin lesions on the extremities. Blood cultures were negative, a heart murmur was again heard, however, and a presumptive diagnosis of subacute bacterial endocarditis was made. The patient was treated for 4 weeks with antibiotics. Her fever and skin lesions recurred when the antibiotics were withdrawn, and the patient was treated for an additional 6 weeks with antibiotics for a presumed relapse of endocarditis.

Intermittent fever and erythematous skin lesions continued, and the patient was referred to a major hospital center for evaluation of a possible immune deficiency. No clear-cut abnormalities were found. During that hospitalization, the patient had two subcutaneous abscesses that required incision and drainage.

At admission, she was afebrile (37° C rectally). Physical examination revealed well-healed sites of prior incision and drainage procedures on the left lower extremity and upper extremities. She had no acute or chronic skin lesions. A grade 1/6 systolic murmur was heard. Routine evaluations were unrevealing, with the exception of an elevated antistreptolysin-O titer of 500 Todd units.

The patient had no fever or skin lesions during a 10-day hospitalization and was discharged, only to return 6 days later with a 2-day history of fever to 38.3° C. At readmission, the patient noted the spontaneous development of a tender posterior calf lesion associated with fever of 38.9° C to 39.4° C. She had a temperature of 38.2° C rectally. A 1-cm, raised, erythematous lesion with 8 cm of surrounding induration was present on the left posterior calf. There appeared to be a pinpoint-sized break in the skin at the center of the lesion. Leukocyte count was 16,000/mm with a left shift; erythrocyte sedimentation rate was 102 mm/hour. Blood cultures obtained at admission were negative. The patient was treated with heat and elevation of the extremity and intravenous antibiotics.

Because the skin lesion appeared to have been self-induced, psychiatric consultation was obtained. A diagnosis was made of borderline personality disorder with self-destructive behavior. The patient was confronted with the suspicion that her fever and skin lesions were self-induced, and she vehemently denied these charges. The next day she developed fever and hypotension. Physical examination was unrevealing. Leukocyte count was 27,000/mm with a left shift. Blood cultures subsequently grew S. aureus and Pseudomonas dimenuta. She was treated with intravenous fluids and antibiotics and made an uneventful recovery.

A second psychiatric consultation was obtained. The patient eventually admitted that she had been inducing the recurrent episodes of fever and skin lesions over the past 2 years. In fact, she further admitted to having falsified or induced episodes of "fever" since age 12. She stated that she had obtained pure cultures of streptococcus from the hospital laboratory in which she worked. Upon returning home, she would inject the culture material into the deep subcutaneous tissues with a needle and syringe. She did not, however, admit any responsibility for the episode of sepsis noted above. The patient was referred for outpatient psychotherapy.

## Self-Inflicted Local Infections

### Skin and Subcutaneous Tissues

Infections of the skin or subcutaneous tissues are simulated or actually produced by injections, excoriation, or repeated wounding with heat, chemicals, or instruments. *Dermatitis artefacta* was recognized and described early in this century (Sneddon and Sneddon, 1975). Either infectious or noninfectious skin diseases are simulated, and inadvertent superinfections are not unusual. *Subcutaneous abscesses* may be mistaken for erythema nodosum, Weber-Christian's

disease, immune deficiency, recurrent furunculosis, or thrombophlebitis. Cellulitis combined with subcutaneous injection of air may simulate gas gangrene.

### Case 5

A right-handed, 20-year-old man was transferred from jail to University Hospital in San Diego for left knee arthritis and fever. He reported progressive pain in the knee since "bumping" it on a bed in jail. On examination, he had needle tracks consistent with a history of heroin addiction and numerous, amateur tatoos in the form of swasticas. Temperature was 102° F, WBC was 10,400, and sedimentation rate was 8. There was minimal swelling of the medial left knee centered on three small puncture wounds. Aspiration of the joint was unsuccessful and 5 cc of sterile fluid was washed into the joint and cultured. This fluid grew scant amounts of nonpathogenic *Neisseria, Gaffkya,* diphtheroids, *Streptococcus viridans,* and *Hemophilus parahemolyticus.* On high-dose intravenous penicillin for possible gonococcal arthritis, swelling and erythema progressed, and an x-ray showed gas under the patella. On the third hospital day, frank pus was aspirated during arthrocentesis, and the knee was surgically explored. A necrotizing fasciitis of the capsular fascia was drained of foul-smelling pus containing gram-negative rods, gram-positive cocci, and polymorphonuclear leukocytes. Cultures of necrotic tissue grew heavy, β-hemolytic streptococci (not Groups A, B, D, E, or F), moderate *Streptococcus viridans,* and scant penicillin-sensitive *Bacteroides.* Exploration revealed no necrosis or obvious infection of the knee joint, and sterile effusion was aspirated from the joint. The patient was treated with high-dose penicillin, chloramphenicol, and multiple drainage procedures. He was discharged on the twenty-fourth day with a healing wound. Mild joint dysfunction remained 3 years later. The patient was questioned several times by his physicians but denied injecting anything into his leg.

This patient's infection with mixed anaerobic and aerobic mouth flora was almost certainly the result of injecting his saliva into the periarticular and subcutaneous tissues of his knee. When this flora is inoculated into tissues (for example, with human bites), it typically produces the necrotizing, gas-producing, subcutaneous, and fascial infection seen in this patient. The diagnosis of self-injection is supported by his sociopathic personality, the secondary gain afforded by hospitalization, his familiarity with needles, and his history of self-injection as evidenced by tatooing.

### Septic Arthritis

The following patient illustrates that septic arthritis may be produced by injection of body fluids into the joint space rather than near the joint as in the previous example.

### Case 6

A 32-year-old, insulin-dependent, diabetic woman with multiple complications was admitted to University Hospital in San Diego for 3 days of fever to 103° F, chills, and left leg swelling. Four months before admission, an "insect bite" had resulted in a large abscess over the lateral left leg that grew only *S. aureus* and responded to surgical drainage and cephalosporins. The wound healed well, leaving only a small, shallow ulcer in the wound scar over the knee laterally. On admission, she appeared chronically ill with fever of 100.5° F and multiple signs of her diabetic complications, including retinopathy, cataracts, peripheral neuropathy, and generalized weakness. Her skin had multiple 1 to 3 cm ulcers on arms, legs, face, and chest. The back was spared. The lesions were excoriated but not infected, and they resembled lesions seen during an earlier admission. There was brawny pitting edema of both legs, which was greater on the left. The left leg was slightly warm and tender, and Homans' sign was present. Laboratory studies revealed leukocytosis of 12,700, mild azotemia (creatinine = 1.9), and hyperglycemia (glucose = 437). Culture of urine grew 20,000 *Candida parapsilosis,* and the left leg ulcer was sterile. On the second hospital day, a left-knee effusion developed and was aspirated of grossly purulent fluid containing 198,000 leukocytes that were 98 per cent neutrophils. Gram stain revealed budding yeast and large gram-positive rods. *Candida parapsilosis* and *Lactobacillus* were grown in moderate amounts from repeated aspirates. Her arthritis ultimately required surgical drainage of the knee joint and subcutaneous tissues. The patient responded slowly to cefazolin, gentamicin, 5-fluorocytosine, a local instillation of amphotericin B. Cultures at 17 days were sterile.

Because the excoriated skin lesions and the unusual microbiology of the arthritis suggested self-injection, she was asked if she had injected the knee. She admitted to exploring the overlying wound on multiple occasions with her insulin needle "to help it drain," but not to injecting anything.

Psychiatric evaluation revealed a history of attempted suicide, depression over recent death of a diabetic roommate, and the long-held expectation that she would "die in my twenties" from diabetes. In addition, she related "riding with Hell's Angels" and working as a prostitute in the past, but said she was no longer sexually active because of fecal incontinence.

This young woman with a history of self-destructive behavior and advanced diabetes had two organisms *(Candida* and *Lactobacillus)* only rarely found in infected joints. Because the overlying ulcer was sterile and did not communicate with the joint, she appears to have injected urine or vaginal flora into the joint. Simultaneous hematogenous seeding of the joint with these organisms is unlikely. Her familiarity, as a diabetic, with needles and urine collections probably provided her the means for further self-destructive behavior.

### DIAGNOSIS

Factitious diseases are often difficult to recognize because the patient may not appear overtly disturbed, and the illness may seem plausible. Physicians justifiably fear overlooking rare or unfamiliar diseases when an illness is atypical. Recurrent bacterial infections may suggest one of the rare genetic defects of cellular or humoral immunity. Abnormal numbers or functions of leukocytes, antibody production, or complement components do predispose to recurrent bacterial infections. Before undertaking an exhaustive search for such defects, however, consideration should be given to fraudulent disease. In addition to fear of missing a diagnosis, many physicians have difficulty believing that a patient is intentionally deceiving them. Recognition of fraudulent diseases requires both a knowledge of fraudulent syndromes and a willingness to entertain the diagnosis. Systematic attempts to find objective evidence of fraud can confirm the diagnosis and save the patient from unnecessary and dangerous diagnostic tests and therapy.

Atypical clinical or microbiologic features are the most important clue to fraudulent infectious diseases. Knowledge of the pathogenesis of most infections is enough to alert well-informed physicians that many fraudulent diseases "don't make sense." For instance, polymicrobial bacteremia in patients without compromised immunity or an identifiable site of infection suggests intravenous injection of bacteria. This suspicion is strengthened by the isolation of organisms that make up the flora found in feces, saliva, vaginal secretions, or on the skin. Fever without changes in other vital signs, rapid defervescence without diaphoresis, temperature of 41.1° C or higher, or prolonged fevers without objective signs of inflammation should suggest simulated fever.

Age, sex, occupation, and psychiatric history are helpful in diagnosis. Young, female medical and paramedical workers (for example, nurses and laboratory technicians) or students are the most frequently represented groups. Self-injection requires experience with and access to needles and syringes. Medical and paramedical personnel, laboratory workers, diabetics, and intravenous drug abusers are the groups with such experience. Atypical illness in these groups should arouse suspicion of self-inoculation. In persons with a knowledge of microbiology and access to pure cultures, self-injection may lead to repeated isolation of the same organism from blood or from recurrent subcutaneous abscesses.

Motivation in the form of secondary gain is an important clue. Adolescent students who have been legitimately ill may prolong convalescence to avoid returning to school or home. Prisoners may use factitious or self-inflicted illness to escape the dangers or tedium of jail, or addicts may seek opiates. In many patients, however, the motivation is not so clear.

A number of techniques are useful to detect stimulated fevers. The most effective is immediate measurement of fever at several sites with a responsible observer continuously present. Assessment of other vital signs, skin warmth and moisture, and measurement of the temperature of freshly voided urine can also help. Checking the serial number of glass thermometers makes substitution of preheated ones more difficult.

Major corroborative evidence of self-injection can be found by searching the patient's room for the apparatus used (syringe and needle, bacterial cultures). Additional clues are needle marks over veins or sites of infection and the resolution of chronic infections when they are rendered inaccessible by casting the affected limb.

The diagnosis of fraudulent disease is made by careful exclusion of other explanations for the patient's illness and enough positive evidence that the means is clear. It is often hard to understand the patient's motivation, and most patients are unwilling to admit to fraud even if confronted with the evidence.

When the diagnosis cannot be made with certainty, physicians may wish to explore the patient's social and psychiatric history for psychopathology. The value of this approach to diagnosis and therapy has not been determined. Techniques such as Amytal interviews, projective psychometric testing, hypnosis, or analytic psychotherapy have not been systematically applied to these patients, and aggressve attempts to explore the patient's psychopathology may be contraindicated.

## MANAGEMENT

Most physicians experienced with this problem agree on the basic principles of management when the diagnosis of fraudulent illness is made. The first step is to ask for psychiatric help to evaluate the patient's psychopathology with emphasis on their potential for self-destruction. Next, the physicians, nurses, and others involved in the patient's care should be told the diagnosis and plan of management. Since these patients may arouse strong emotional reactions in those caring for them, an opportunity to deal with these feelings away from the patient is thereby provided. The need to maintain a nonjudgmental, supportive attitude should be emphasized to the staff. Next, the patient is confronted with the evidence for fraudulent illness in a sympathetic, but realistic, manner. Those involved must be prepared for anger and hostility as a result of confrontation and not attack the patient's defenses in reaction. The possibility of flight (almost invariable in Munchausen's syndrome) or even suicide should be recognized. By expressing concern for the patient's medical and emotional problems, the physician may be able to redefine the illness and direct therapy at the underlying psychopathology. Practical and emotional support, limitation of self-destructive behavior, and exploration of the social pressures on the patient are the immediate goals. Strengthening and preserving the patient's fragile defenses is the ultimate goal.

Self-inflicted illness requiring further medical therapy can be treated on a medical ward. When outpatient therapy is arranged and the immediate consequences of confrontation have passed, patients may be discharged. The medical consequences of self-inflicted disease can be serious and even life-threatening. Careful medical management of infections and, when possible, measures to prevent further manipulation are mandatory. In doing so, the physician communicates his continuing support for the patient and emphasizes the importance of stopping the injurious behavior.

After the diagnosis of factitious infection is made, it is important to entertain alternative diagnoses. Obviously a correct diagnosis of factitious disease does not protect the patient from developing "real" complications or unrelated naturally occurring illnesses. The consequences of incorrect diagnosis or inadequate treatment of self-inflicted diseases are potentially severe. Jokes about the high mortality of malingering and hysteria abound.

# DELUSIONAL ILLNESSES

## *DELUSIONAL INFESTATIONS (DELUSIONS OF PARASITOSIS)*

Delirious or psychotic patients may suffer hallucinations or delusions of infestation that are dramatic and easily recognized. In contrast, other patients with delusions of infestation by worms or insects ("parasitosis") are otherwise not obviously psychotic. They cling tenaciously to their delusion despite reassurance and can sometimes involve others in their delusion. They present their physicians with evidence of the infestations in the form of household or bodily detritus (vegetable material from their stools, bits of skin, nasal mucus, thread, and so on). When the nonparasitic nature of this material is demonstrated, they often collect more and may refer themselves to specialists in parasitology or infectious diseases or to entomologists. Most patients localize the infestation to the skin or hair, but the mouth, nose, subcutaneous tissues, bowel, or internal organs may be involved. In some cases, insects are described as biting, rather than infesting the patient. Another variation is that parasites are feared obsessively, but delusions are absent. Excoriation and artifactual dermatitis may result from scratching or attempts to remove the "parasites" with instruments, heat, or caustics. Real arthropod infestations may precede and trigger the delusional one. Real cutaneous or systemic diseases (especially if pruritic) may be misinterpreted by the patient as caused by parasites. Medications (for example, monoamine oxidase inhibitors) or psychostimulants (for example, amphetamines, cocaine, or methylphenidate) may cause delusions of parasitosis. In addition, a variety of social or psychological stresses may be linked to the delusion. An illustrative example of social stress leading to similar delusions in three housewives was observed by Wilson in Los Angeles during the Second World War (Wilson, 1952). Each had unwillingly yielded to social pressure by allowing soldiers or defense workers to share their homes during the wartime housing shortage. They became convinced that the unwanted houseguests had brought insects into their homes and that these insects were attacking them.

The psychiatric diagnosis underlying delusions of parasitosis and the degree of psychopathology are controversial. "Monosymptomatic hypochondriacal psychosis" describes the major elements of the syndrome. These anxious patients suffer a persistent, unshakable delusion, but reject psychiatric diagnoses or therapy, retain their underlying personality, continue to function socially, and rarely become severely depressed or overtly schizophrenic. Diagnosis of delusory infestation is made when the patient repeatedly rejects alternative explanations for the "parasites" or for his symptoms. Obviously, examination of the patient for real infestations or other diseases must precede attempts at reassurance. Scabies is notoriously deceptive and should be excluded if itching and unusual skin lesions are present, regardless of how bizarre the patient's explanations for these findings may seem.

Treatment for delusions of infestation have been frustrating to both physicians and psychiatrists. The recognition that these patients refuse referral and do not benefit from psychotherapy has led some physicians to attempt supportive, informal psychotherapy bolstered by antipsychotic agents (Gould and Gragg, 1976). Pimoxide, a diphenyl butylpiperidine antipsychotic agent, may have specific value for them (Munro, 1978).

## *DELUSIONAL EPIDEMICS (EPIDEMIC HYSTERIA)*

Rapidly developing epidemics usually result from exposures of groups to toxins or microorganisms. Contagious spread of delusional or hysterical symptoms within groups can simulate infections or intoxications. A number of such outbreaks of subjective symptoms within closed groups are best explained as mass hysteria (Sirois, 1974). Typically, young women in institutions (for example, schools or hospitals) rapidly develop similar, dramatic, subjective symptoms (for example, fainting, hyperventilation, or weakness). In one case, fainting, headache, nausea, and weakness spread rapidly within an American high school marching band after a moderate heat stress (Levine, 1977).

These epidemics may have several patterns. Sudden, explosive outbreaks spread within minutes and may be preceded by a few cases during slower, prodromal stages. A small outbreak may be followed in hours or days by a second, more prominent wave. Cumulative epidemics may build over several weeks, usually within closed institutional settings. The inciting event may be a real or hysterical illness within a group predisposed to hysteria by anxiety. The role of anxiety is illustrated by outbreaks of symptoms simulating poliomyelitis (benign myalgic encephalomyelitis or Icelandic disease) in nurses during epidemics of poliomyelitis (McEvedy and Beard, 1970).

The diagnosis should be considered when dramatic, subjective symptoms spread within a group under stress. Various combinations of weakness, headache, hyperventilation, myalgias, fainting, abnormal movements, tremor, globus, pain, nausea, and vomiting have been reported. Objective signs of disease such as fever or diarrhea are absent. Careful clinical and epidemio logic investigations eliminate the possibility of infection or intoxication.

Management of epidemic hysteria is dispersion of the group, isolation of affected individuals, and careful search for objective signs of illness. Confrontation or exhortation has not been effective and may aggravate the outbreak.

## References

Aduan, R. P., Fauci, A. S., Dale, D. C., Herzberg, J. H., and Wolff, S. M.: Factitious fever and self-induced infection. Ann Intern Med 90:230, 1979.

Asher, R.: Malingering. Trans Med Soc Lond 75:145, 1959.

Cramer, B., Gershberg, M. R., and Stern, M.: Munchausen Syndrome. Arch Gen Psychiatry 24:573, 1971.

Gould, W. M., and Gragg, T. M.: Delusions of parasitosis. Arch Dermatol 112:1745, 1976.

Levine, R. J.: Epidemic faintness and syncope in a school marching band. JAMA 238:2373, 1977.

McEvedy, C. P., and Beard, A. W.: Concept of benign myalgic encephalomyelitis. Br Med J 1:11, 1970.

Munro, A.: Two cases of delusions of worm infestation. Am J Psychiatry 135:2, 1978.

Petersdorf, R. G., and Bennett, I. L.: Factitious fever. Ann Intern Med 46:1039, 1957.

Rumans, L. W., and Vosti, K. L.: Factitious and fraudulent fever. Am J Med 65:745, 1978.

Sirois, F.: Epidemic hysteria. Acta Psychiatrica Scandinavia Supplementum 252, 1974.

Sneddon, I., and Sneddon, J.: Self-inflicted injury: a follow-up study of 43 patients. Br Med J 3:527, 1975.

Wilson, J. W.: Delusions of parasitosis (Acarophobia). Arch Dermatol Syphilis 66:577, 1952.

# INDEX

Note: Page numbers in *italics* indicate illustrations;
page numbers followed by t indicate tables.